Contributors

Chapter 13: Liver (Non-neoplastic diseases)

Kenneth W. Barwick, M.D.
Chief of Anatomic Pathology
Baptist Medical Center
Jacksonville, Florida

Chapter 17: Kidney (Non-neoplastic diseases)

Nelson G. Ordóñez, M.D.
Professor of Pathology
The University of Texas M.D. Anderson Cancer Center
Houston, Texas

Chapter 23: Bone Marrow

Richard D. Brunning, M.D.
Professor of Laboratory Medicine and Pathology
Head, Hematopathology Laboratory
University of Minnesota Medical School
Minneapolis, Minnesota

**Chapter 28: Neuromuscular System
(Peripheral nerves; Skeletal muscle)**

Juan M. Bilbao, M.D.
Associate Professor of Neuropathology
University of Toronto Faculty of Medicine;
Associate Pathologist
St. Michael's Hospital
Toronto, Ontario, Canada

Lee Cyn Ang, MBBS, FRCPC, FRCPath
Associate Professor of Pathology
University of Toronto Faculty of Medicine
Toronto, Ontario, Canada;
Staff Neuropathologist
Department of Pathology
Sunnybrook Health Science Centre
North York, Ontario, Canada

**Chapter 28: Neuromuscular System
(Central nervous system)**

Marc K. Rosenblum, M.D.
Chief, Neuropathology and Autopsy Service
Memorial Sloan-Kettering Cancer Center;
Associate Professor of Pathology
Cornell University Medical College
New York, New York

Chapter 29: Pituitary Gland

Juan M. Bilbao, M.D.
Associate Professor of Neuropathology
University of Toronto Faculty of Medicine;
Associate Pathologist
St. Michael's Hospital
Toronto, Ontario, Canada

Ackerman's

SURGICAL PATHOLOGY

JUAN ROSAI, M.D.

Chairman, Department of Pathology
James Ewing Alumni Chair in Pathology
Memorial Sloan-Kettering Cancer Center;
Professor of Pathology
Cornell University Medical College
New York, New York

EIGHTH EDITION
with 3295 illustrations, 898 in color

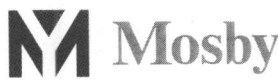 Mosby

St. Louis Baltimore Boston Carlsbad Chicago Naples New York Philadelphia Portland
London Madrid Mexico City Singapore Sydney Tokyo Toronto Wiesbaden

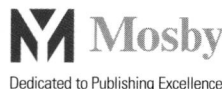

Dedicated to Publishing Excellence

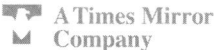 A Times Mirror
Company

Publisher: Anne S. Patterson
Senior Managing Editor: Lynne Gery
Project Manager: Carol Sullivan Weis
Senior Production Editor: Pat Joiner
Design Manager: Sheilah Barrett
Manufacturing Manager: Theresa Fuchs

EIGHTH EDITION (two volumes)
Copyright © 1996 by Mosby–Year Book, Inc.

Previous editions copyrighted 1953, 1959, 1964, 1968, 1974, 1981, 1989

Printed in the United States of America
Composition by Accu-color/Beaumont Book Division, Inc.
Printing/binding by Von Hoffmann Press, Inc.

Mosby–Year Book, Inc.
11830 Westline Industrial Drive
St. Louis, Missouri 63146

Library of Congress Cataloging in Publication Data
Rosai, Juan. 1940–
　　Ackerman's surgical pathology.—8th ed./Juan Rosai.
　　　　p. cm.
　　7th ed. cataloged under Ackerman.
　　Includes bibliographical references and index.
　　ISBN 0-8016-7004-7
　　1. Pathology, Surgical. I. Ackerman, Lauren Vedder, 1905–.
Surgical pathology. II. Title
　　[DNLM: 1. Pathology, Surgical. WO 142 R788a 1995]
RD57.A2 1995
617' .07—dc20
DNLM/DLC
for Library of Congress　　　　　　　　　　　　95-36167
　　　　　　　　　　　　　　　　　　　　　　　　CIP

95 96 97 98 99 / 9 8 7 6 5 4 3 2 1

Ackerman's

SURGICAL PATHOLOGY

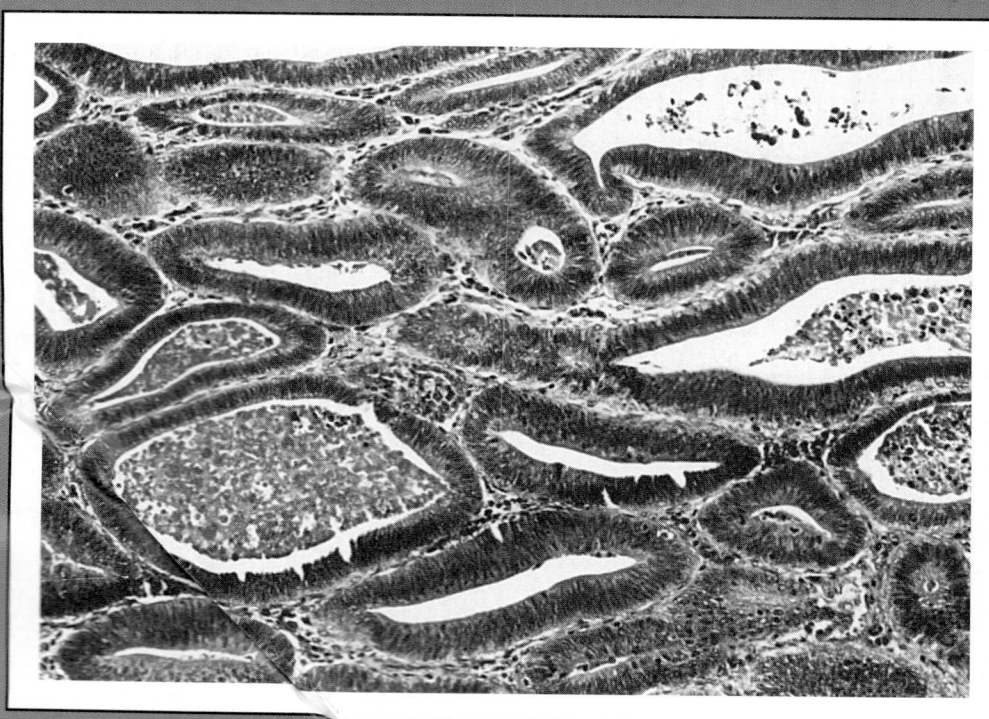

Endometrial-type carcinoma of prostate. Microscopic appearance is reminiscent of that of the usual type of endometrial adenocarcinoma. This tumor is of large duct prostatic origin.

To my wife, Maria Luisa Carcangiu

To my teachers,
Eduardo F. Lascano (1908-1990)
Lauren V. Ackerman (1905-1993)

Preface to eighth edition

There have been several significant developments in surgical pathology during the seven years that have elapsed since the previous edition of this book was published. The diagnostic applications of immunohistochemical techniques have continued to expand at a brisk rate as the result of a seemingly endless proliferation of newly discovered markers. The explosive development of molecular techniques during the past decade and their almost miraculous suitability to the study of routinely processed human tissue has already had a profound impact in the field, and every indicator tells us that this is only the beginning. Less dramatically but just as powerfully, internal and external regulatory forces are exerting an increasing influence over the practice of the specialty.

An attempt has been made to incorporate in this new edition the most important material related to these issues. Several other changes have been made. The clinicopathologically oriented format introduced in the previous edition for selected neoplasms has been adopted for virtually all major tumor types. This includes a greatly enlarged section on special techniques, in which recent findings derived from immunohistochemistry, cytogenetics, and molecular pathology are described, particularly when purported to be of diagnostic or prognostic significance. Consequently, the listing of prognostically significant parameters has been considerably lengthened. Various recommendations and guidelines concerning the practice of surgical pathology produced by several organizations (in particular by the burgeoning Association of Directors of Anatomic and Surgical Pathology) have been incorporated in the form of appendixes. A brief section on normal anatomy and histology as it pertains to the pathologic aspects of the corresponding sites has been added to virtually all chapters.

All of the electron micrographs that have been added to this edition are generously provided by Dr. Robert A. Erlandson, Director of the Diagnostic Electron Microscopy Laboratory at Memorial Sloan-Kettering Cancer Center. Nearly all of the other new illustrations have been reproduced in color, whether incorporated in the text or displayed in the form of multipictorial plates.

As in previous editions, most of the book has been written by one individual, in the hope that whatever may be missing as a result has been compensated for by what somebody, in another context, has referred to as "the ultimate simplicity of one voice speaking." Along those lines, a constant attempt has been made to preserve as much as possible the pragmatic flavor given to this work by its begetter, Dr. Lauren V. Ackerman. Thus and despite its predictable deficiencies, this edition should be viewed as a tribute to the vision, energy, and dedication of that towering figure of American surgical pathology, who died in 1993 at the age of 88 years.

The coherence goal notwithstanding, it was apparent that there exist highly specialized areas that could not have been covered adequately without the contribution of experts. I was fortunate to have the collaboration of Dr. Kenneth W. Barwick, Baptist Medical Center, Jacksonville, Florida, for the section on medical diseases of the liver; Dr. Juan M. Bilbao, St. Michael's Hospital, Toronto, for the sections on peripheral nerves and skeletal muscle (with the latter in collaboration with Dr. Lee C. Ang) and the chapter on the pituitary gland; Dr. Richard D. Brunning, University of Minnesota, for the chapter on bone marrow; Dr. Nelson G. Ordóñez, M.D. Anderson Hospital, Houston, for the section on medical diseases of the kidney; and Dr. Marc K. Rosenblum, of my own department, for the completely rewritten section on the central nervous system.

Some of the contributions to the text and illustrations made by Drs. José Costa, John S. Morrow, Hector A. Rodriguez-Martinez, Richard K. Sibley, Morton E. Smith, and Robert A. Vickers in years past remain in the present edition. There are many other colleagues who have shared their material with me in one form or another over the course of the years and who may recognize that material in the photographs of this book; it would be too difficult to acknowledge them individually, but I wish here to thank them all for their trust and courtesy.

The contribution of my wife, Maria Luisa Carcangiu, to this edition was even greater than for the previous one. She made countless suggestions during the preparation; critically reviewed the entire manuscript at the draft, galley proof, and page proof stages; selected and organized the bibliographic material; personally chose most of the material for the new illustrations; and—last but not least—prodded me mercilessly during my moments of prostration. Thanking her for her labor of love—which included spending a whole sabbatical year at Memorial on the project—would be almost inappropriate. As before—more so than before—this book is hers as much as mine.

Finally, I want to express my appreciation to Rita Freed and Cindy Behrman for transcribing and improving the innumerable revisions that this manuscript has undergone in the course of the past three years.

Juan Rosai, M.D.
New York, New York

Preface to first edition

This book can be only an introduction to the vast field of surgical pathology: the pathology of the living. It does not pretend to replace in any way the textbooks to general pathology, its purpose being merely to supplement them, assuming that the reader has a background in or access to those texts. The contents are not as complete as they might be because emphasis has been placed on the common rather than the rare lesions and are, to a great extent, based on the author's personal experiences.

This book has been written for the medical student as well as for those physicians who are daily intimately concerned with surgical pathology. This must of necessity include not only the surgeon and the pathologist, but also those physicians in other fields who are affected by its decisions, such as the radiologist and the internist. Gross pathology has been stressed throughout with an attempt to correlate the gross findings with the clinical observations. The many illustrations have been selected as typical of the various surgical conditions, although in a few instances the author has been unable to resist showing some of the more interesting rare lesions he has encountered. Concluding each chapter there is a bibliography listing those references which are not only relatively recent and readily available, but also those which will lead the reader to a more detailed knowledge of the subject.

Dr. Zola K. Cooper, Assistant Professor of Pathology and Surgical Pathology, has written one of the sections on Skin, and Dr. David E. Smith, Assistant Professor of Pathology and Surgical Pathology, has written the chapter on Central Nervous System. Both of these members of the Department are particularly well qualified for their respective roles because of their background and present responsibilities in these fields. Their efforts on my behalf are most gratefully acknowledged.

Many members of the Surgical Staff at Barnes Hospital have given much help both knowingly and unwittingly. I am particularly grateful to Dr. Charles L. Eckert, Associate Pro-

fessor of Surgery, for letting me bother him rather constantly with my questions and for giving freely of his experience. Dr. Richard Johnson, who succeeded me as Pathologist at the Ellis Fischel State Cancer Hospital, agreeably made available all the material there, and Dr. Franz Leidler, Pathologist at the Veterans Hospital, has been most cooperative.

Thanks must be given to Dr. H.R. McCarroll, Assistant Professor of Orthopedics, for constructively criticizing the chapter on Bone and Joint, and to Dr. C.A. Waldron for helping me with the chapters related to the Oral Cavity. Among other faculty friends and colleagues who were especially helpful, I would like to mention Dr. Carl E. Lischer, Dr. Eugene M. Bricker, Dr. Heinz Haffner, Dr. Thomas H. Burford, Dr. Carl A. Moyer, Dr. Evarts A. Graham, Dr. Robert Elman, Dr. Edward H. Reinhard, Dr. J. Albert Key, Dr. Glover H. Copher, Dr. Margaret G. Smith, and Dr. Robert A. Moore.

Mr. Cramer K. Lewis, of our Department of Illustration, has been very patient with my demands, and his efforts and skill have been invaluable. Miss Marion Murphy, in charge of our Medical Library, and her associates gave untiringly of their time.

Because of recent advances in anesthesia, antibiotics, and pre- and postoperative care, modern surgery permits the radical excision of portions or all of various organs. There is a need today for contemplative surgeons, men with a rich background in the fundamental sciences, whether chemistry, physiology, or pathology. The modern surgeon should not ask himself, "Can I get away with this operation?" but rather, "What does the future hold for this patient?" It is hoped that this book may contribute in some small fashion toward the acquisition of this attitude.

Lauren V. Ackerman, M.D.
St. Louis, Missouri

Contents

APPENDIXES

PLATES

Ackerman's

SURGICAL PATHOLOGY

19 Female reproductive system

Vulva
Vagina
Uterus-cervix
Uterus-corpus
Fallopian tube
Ovary
Placenta

Vulva

NORMAL ANATOMY

The vulva is composed of the following anatomic portions: mons pubis, clitoris, labia minora, labia majora, vulvar vestibule and vestibulovaginal bulbs, urethral meatus, hymen, Bartholin's and Skene's glands and ducts, and vaginal introitus.[1,4]

The labia majora are lined by keratinized skin containing all three cutaneous adnexae: hair follicles, sebaceous glands, apocrine gland, and sweat (eccrine) glands.[3] The labia minora are covered by nonkeratinized stratified squamous epithelium in their vestibular surfaces but have a thin keratin layer laterally. Skin adnexae are usually absent, but in some individuals one may encounter both sweat and sebaceous glands.

The Bartholin's gland is the major vestibular gland and has a tubuloalveolar structure. It is made up of acini composed of mucus-secreting columnar cells and a duct lined by transitional epithelium.[2] Minor vestibular glands are of simple tubular type and are lined with a mucus-secreting columnar epithelium that merges with the stratified squamous epithelium of the vestibule.

Skene's or periurethral glands are analogous to the male prostate gland; they are lined by a pseudostratified mucus-secreting columnar epithelium that merges with the transitional-type epithelium of the ducts, which in turn joins with the stratified squamous epithelium of the vestibule.

The hymen is lined by nonkeratinized stratified squamous epithelium on both surfaces.

The clitoris contains erectile tissue similar to that in the corpora cavernosa of the penis.

Most of the vulvar lymphatics drain to the superficial inguinal nodes, but those in the clitoris empty directly into the deep chain.

CONGENITAL ABNORMALITIES

Ectopic mammary tissue can occur in the vulvar region, along the primitive milk line that extends in the embryo from the axilla to the groin.[12] This tissue is subject to many of the physiologic and pathologic changes that occur in the normally situated breast. These include swelling and secretion of milk during pregnancy,[12] cysts,[12a] fibroadenoma,[5,7] phylloides tumor,[11] and carcinoma.[6,9,10,12a] The latter has been reported in association with bilateral breast carcinoma.[8] In addition, it is likely that ectopic mammary tissue is the source of the common benign vulvar tumor known as papillary hydradenoma (see p. 1329).

SO-CALLED CHRONIC VULVAR DYSTROPHIES

There exists a group of vulvar diseases that are pathogenetically unrelated but that have several features in com-

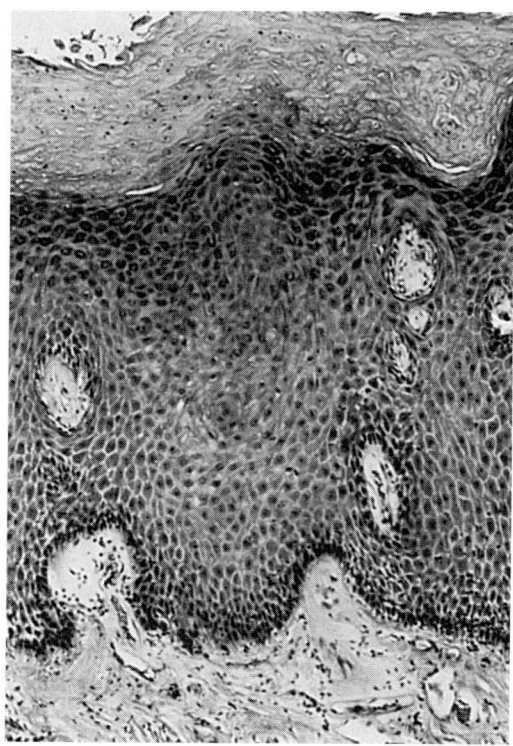

Fig. 19-1 Keratosis and chronic inflammation. Note especially acanthosis and lack of dermal homogenization in contrast to pattern of lichen sclerosus et atrophicus.

mon at the clinical level. They usually present as irregular patchy areas of thickened skin, often accompanied by severe pruritus. The color is usually white, in which case the clinically descriptive term *leukoplakia* has been traditionally used. In other instances, the lesions are red or a mixture of both colors. They are easily traumatized and excoriated. In some of these lesions the vulvar soft tissues are atrophied and shrunken, in which case the term *kraurosis* has been employed.

In the presence of a lesion with some of these clinical features, it is essential to reach a specific diagnosis, and this often necessitates the performance of a biopsy.[15] Multiple biopsies are necessary if the lesion is large or varies in appearance from place to place. The differential diagnosis includes the following categories:

1 Specific dermatoses such as psoriasis, lichen planus, or lichen simplex chronicus (see Chapter 4).
2 Squamous intraepithelial lesions (see p. 1323).
3 So-called chronic vulvar dystrophy. In turn, this highly questionable term[17] encompasses two diseases, which, although sometimes coexisting, should be regarded as separate: lichen sclerosus and squamous cell hyperplasia.

Lichen sclerosus (et atrophicus) of the vulva may occur in any age group, including children.[14] In the latter group, the vulvar region represents the most common location, and there is a high incidence of spontaneous involution at the time of puberty.[16] The microscopic features are similar to those seen in this disorder when it occurs elsewhere in the skin (see Chapter 4). The often-repeated statement that

lichen sclerosus of the adult vulva is a precancerous condition has not been substantiated in the better documented series of this disorder. Thus squamous cell carcinoma developed in only one of 92 patients in one series[13] and in twelve (4%) of 290 patients followed for a mean period of 12.5 years in another.[19]

Squamous cell hyperplasia (keratosis) is characterized microscopically by acanthosis, prominent stratum granulosum, and hyperkeratosis, often associated with mild dermal chronic inflammatory infiltrate (Figs. 19-1 and 19-2). Atypia is absent.

Occasionally, the features of lichen sclerosus and squamous cell hyperplasia are seen to coexist, in which case the term *mixed vulvar dystrophy* has been used.[18] Furthermore, the changes of vulvar intraepithelial neoplasia (VIN) are sometimes superimposed on them. Failure to appreciate the existence of these various combinations is probably responsible for the widely different figures given regarding the precancerous connotations of these various entities.[18]

INFLAMMATORY DISEASES

Syphilis in women often manifests itself initially in the vulvar region. The fully developed syphilitic chancre is composed microscopically of plasma cells, lymphocytes, and histiocytes and is covered by a zone of ulceration infiltrated by neutrophils and necrotic debris. The microscopic appearance is not entirely specific, but the combination of numerous plasma cells and endarteritis should alert to the diagnosis. Sometimes, the possibility of syphilis is first suggested on the basis of the microscopic examination of an enlarged inguinal lymph node if this node shows a combination of capsular and pericapsular fibrosis, follicular hyperplasia, plasma cell infiltration, and endarteritis. The latter, which represents the most useful clue to the diagnosis, is particularly well seen in or outside the nodal capsule (see Chapter 21).

Granuloma inguinale is a chronic infection caused by *Calymmatobacterium granulomatis,* a gram-negative, nonmotile, encapsulated bacillus. It begins as a soft elevated granulomatous area that enlarges very slowly by peripheral extension and ulcerates (see Fig. 11-158, *A*). Microscopically, there is a dense dermal inflammatory infiltrate composed of histiocytes and plasma cells, with a scattering of small abscesses.[26] The diagnosis rests on demonstration of Donovan bodies, which are seen as small round encapsulated bodies inside the cytoplasm of the histiocytes. They can be seen in H&E sections but are best demonstrated with the Giemsa or Warthin-Starry stain (see Fig. 11-181, *B*). Pronounced pseudoepitheliomatous hyperplasia that may accompany chronic lesions should be distinguished from the very rare squamous cell carcinoma that may arise in such areas.[20] The disease can spread to the retroperitoneum and simulate a soft tissue neoplasm.[21]

Lymphogranuloma venereum is a venereal disease produced by *Chlamydia* organisms corresponding to serotypes L1, L2, and L3. It mainly affects lymph vessels and lymphoid tissue. The initial small ulcer at a site of venereal contact is often unnoticed. The first clinical manifestation is swelling of inguinal lymph nodes caused by stellate abscesses surrounded by pale epithelioid cells[23] (see Fig. 21-

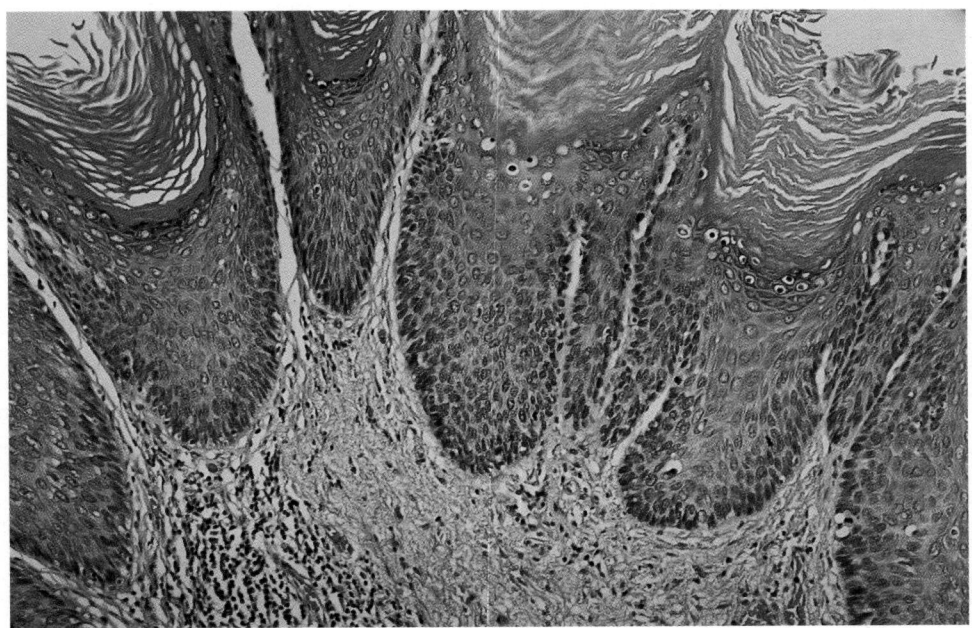

Fig. 19-2 Marked squamous cell metaplasia (keratosis) of vulva associated with papillomatosis and chronic inflammation of the underlying stroma. There is no significant atypia.

19). There is extensive scarring as the disease progresses, often leading to fistulas and strictures of the urethra, vagina, and rectum. The diagnosis can be confirmed by intradermal skin test (Frei test), complement fixation test, or immunofluorescence.[22] Serum immunoglobulin levels are usually markedly elevated. Rainey[27] reported eleven cases of squamous cell carcinoma or adenocarcinoma engrafted on lymphogranulomatous strictures. Most of the tumors were located in the anorectal area.

Crohn's disease involving the vulva has been reported on several occasions.[24,25,28a] In some cases, the vulvar lesions are associated with perineal disease and fistula formation, but in others they are separated from the anal lesions by normal tissue. Grossly, erythematous areas appear that later ulcerate (Fig. 19-3). Microscopically, noncaseating granulomas may be found. The process reported as *vulvitis granulomatosa* is probably related to Crohn's disase in that some of the patients have subsequently developed either intestinal Crohn's disease or cheilitis granulomatosa.[22a]

Necrotizing fasciitis of the vulva may be seen in diabetic women and is associated with a high mortality rate; wide excision of the diseased tissue is the treatment of choice.[28]

Vulvar vestibulitis is a recently described disorder characterized microscopically by a chronic inflammatory infiltrate predominantly involving the mucosal lamina propria and the periglandular/periductal connective tissue of the vestibular region.[25a]

HUMAN PAPILLOMA VIRUS AND VULVAR PATHOLOGY

There are several vulvar diseases in which a causative role for human papilloma virus (HPV) has been suggested. They are condyloma (acuminatum and flat), vulvar intraepithelial neoplasia (VIN), invasive squamous cell carcinoma (includ-

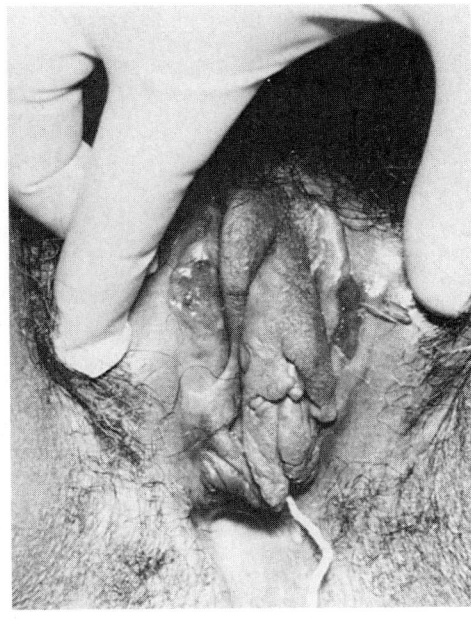

Fig. 19-3 Crohn's disease of vulva. There are edema, hyperemia, and areas of ulceration. Microscopically, granulomas were identified. Patient had extensive intestinal and anal lesions of Crohn's disease.

ing those of the urethra, see later section),[28b] and verrucous carcinoma.[29,31,36,40] All types of association (synchronous and metachronous) have been described among these conditions, supporting a common pathogenetic mechanism.[37] The etiologic role of HPV in the development of condyloma is

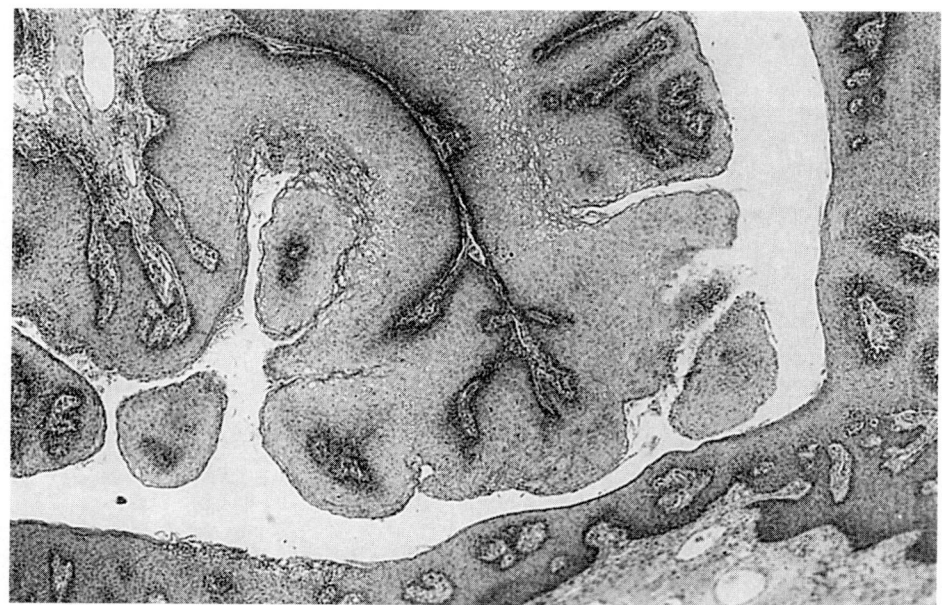

Fig. 19-4 Condyloma acuminatum with complicated papillary arrangement of well-differentiated squamous cells with intact basement membrane.

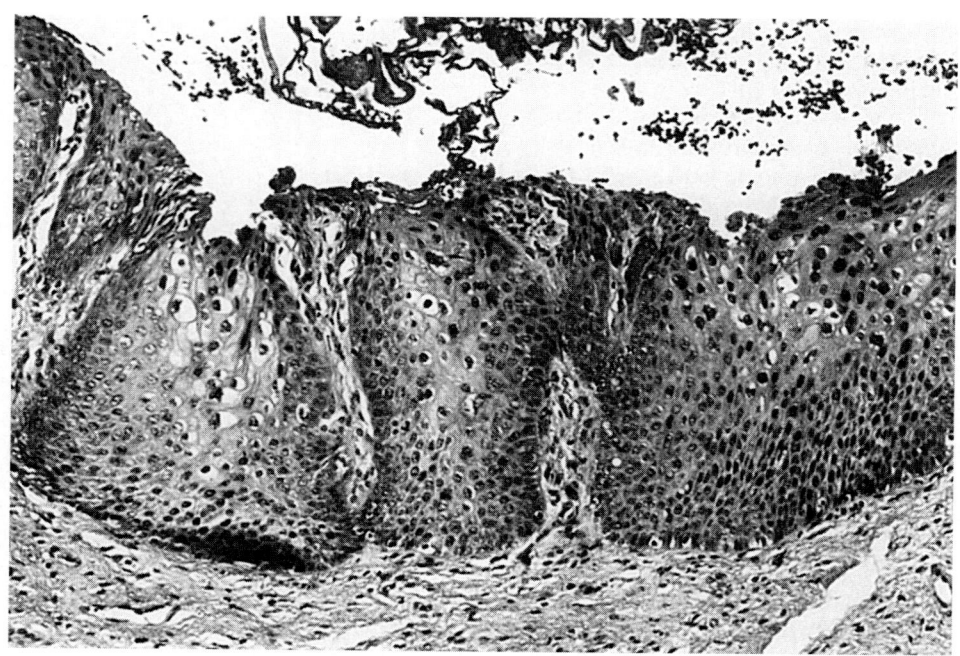

Fig. 19-5 Flat condyloma of vulva. Viral effect is seen in the form of cytoplasmic swelling and pallor, nuclear pleomorphism, and presence of occasional multinucleated malpighian cells. Maturation pattern is somewhat disturbed but still preserved.

proved; its common presence in the other diseases has been shown by a variety of means.[34,35]

In the case of HPV 16, the oncogenic activity has been found to be related to the encoding of two transferring proteins, E6 and E7. The E7 protein binds to the retinoblastoma tumor suppressor gene product pR6, whereas the E6 protein forms complexes with the cellular p53 protein.[43]

Whether the various pathologic manifestations depend on the type of HPV involved, the response elicited by the host, or the addition of other factors remains to be determined.

From a practical standpoint, it is important to classify these conditions separately in view of their widely different natural history and treatment.

CONDYLOMA

Vulvar *condyloma* is a venereal disease caused by HPV, usually type 6.[32] The better known form is *condyloma acuminatum,* which is characterized grossly by one or several soft elevated masses of variable but usually small size. Microscopically there is a complicated papillary arrangement of well-differentiated undulating squamous epithelium supported by delicate, well-vascularized connective tissue stalks containing mononuclear inflammatory cells (mainly CD4$^+$ and CD8$^+$ cells)[38] (Fig. 19-4).

The other form of condyloma, which is actually much more common, is the *flat condyloma* (not to be confused with the *condyloma latum* of syphilis). The cytologic features are similar in both forms. Koilocytosis of the malpighian epithelium (see p. 1358) and lymphocytic infiltration of the stroma are regular features (Fig. 19-5). A typical condyloma shows minimal basal or parabasal cell atypia, orderly maturation, and a smooth transition to koilocytotic intermediate and superficial cells; mitoses may be numerous but are all typical.[30,39] In contrast, the lesions of VIN exhibit abnormal mitoses and nuclear pleomorphism, enlargement, and hyperchromasia in the basal and parabasal cell layers (see later section). The DNA content of condylomas is diploid and polyploid (including tetraploidy and octaploidy), in contrast to the aneuploid pattern seen in most cases of VIN.[41]

Sometimes one sees verrucopapillary vulvar lesions in children or adults that lack the cytologic markers of condyloma; these are often referred to as *squamous papillomas* and usually contain genital HPV types by PCR.[37a] Conversely, there may be multinucleated atypia of the epithelial cells associated with reactive conditions in the absence of HPV infection.[37b]

The traditional therapy for condyloma consisted of podophyllin application. Microscopically, this results in epidermal pallor, necrosis of keratinocytes, and marked increase in mitosis; these changes wane after 72 hours and are essentially gone by 1 week.[42] The treatment of choice of these lesions at present is with carbon dioxide laser.[33]

SQUAMOUS INTRAEPITHELIAL LESIONS

The spectrum of abnormalities seen in atypical proliferative lesions of the vulvar skin and generically designated as vulvar intraepithelial neoplasia (VIN) is wider than that exhibited by equivalent lesions in the vagina (VAIN) or cervix (CIN).[53a] Traditionally, they have been segregated into specific types on the basis of clinical and pathologic features.[49,58]

The type of VIN classically known as *Bowen's disease* or *carcinoma in situ* presents as a slightly elevated, plaque-like lesion with a red velvety appearance (Fig. 19-6).[44,45] It is usually centered in the labia majora, and it may extend to the perineum and anus. Microscopically, there is hyperkeratosis and parakeratosis, acanthosis, and a variable number of multinucleated dyskeratotic cells and abnormal mitoses involving the entire thickness of the epidermis (Fig. 19-7).

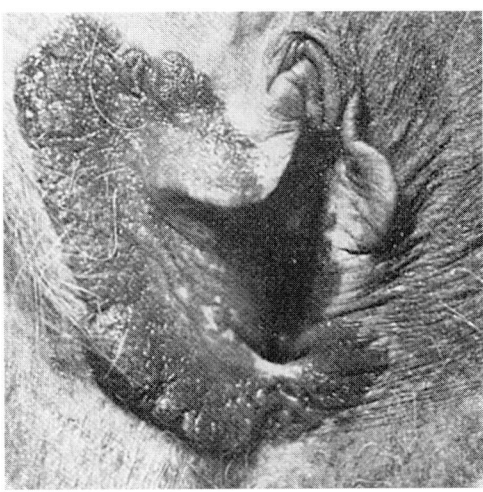

Fig. 19-6 Carcinoma in situ involving wide area of vulva as elevated plaque. (From Gonin R: Maladie de Bowen-Erythroplasie des muqueuses. Dermatologica **92**:74-79, 1946.)

The acrotrichium (intraepidermal portion of the hair follicle) is often involved, whereas the acrosyringium (intraepidermal portion of the sweat gland) is usually spared.[57,59] The large majority of these lesions show an aneuploid DNA pattern. Only a few will stain for HPV in immunohistochemical preparations,[48] but hybridization studies have shown a strong association with HPV-16.[52,55] If left untreated, invasive carcinoma will develop in about 10% of the cases. The therapy depends on the age of the patient and the size, configuration, and distribution of the lesions. Small localized lesions may be treated by wide local excision or skinning vulvectomy.[50] A relationship has been found between the recurrence rate and presence of tumor at the surgical margins in the initial specimen.[51]

The type of VIN designated as *bowenoid papulosis* presents as multiple, often pigmented, papules in or near the vulva of young patients. Clinically, they resemble verrucae, small condylomas, or nevi, but microscopically they show a degree of cytologic atypia approaching that of Bowen's disease.[54] The distinction is largely made on clinical grounds, but some microscopic differences have been described, the most important being that in bowenoid keratosis the dysplastic cells are present in a background of relatively orderly epithelial maturation and that the acrotrichium is usually spared.[57,60] Spontaneous regression has been observed, and response to conservative therapy is the rule, even if recurrences are common.[46]

The similarities in morphologic appearance, ploidy pattern and p53 expression between Bowen's disease and bowenoid papulosis, their occasional coexistence,[47] and the fact that both are statistically associated with HPV[61] suggest an etiologic and pathogenetic link between the two. This has led to the proposal to group them under the term bowenoid dysplasia[60] and incorporate them into the VIN concept while still acknowledging the important differences they exhibit in age of appearance and risk of development of invasive carcinoma.[53] According to this proposal, such lesions could be diagnosed as VIN, Bowen's disease type and VIN, bowenoid papulosis type, respectively. Another proposed morphologic approach is to divide VIN into two types: warty or bowenoid (which includes both Bowen's disease and bowenoid papulosis) and basaloid or undifferentiated. The latter type, which resembles CIN III, shows a lesser degree of association with HPV than the warty type.[56] Yet another scheme is to divide VIN into classic type (which includes Bowen's disease, bowenoid papulosis, warty VIN, carcinoma in situ, and basaloid VIN) and a "variant" or differentiated type. The latter, which is characterized by maturation, variable degrees of hyperplasia, keratinization and parabasal atypia, is less likely to contain HPV nucleic acids than the classic form.[53a]

INVASIVE SQUAMOUS CELL CARCINOMA
General features

Squamous cell carcinoma accounts for approximately 95% of the malignant tumors of this organ. The mean age at presentation is between 60 and 74 years. Risk factors include number of lifetime sexual partners, cigarette smoking, immunodeficiency, and genital granulomatous disease.[66,70,72] Vulvar carcinoma is frequently associated with malignant tumors elsewhere in the lower genital tract, notably the uterine cervix.[90] This has led to the hypothesis that the epithelium of the entire lower genital tract (cervix, vagina, vulva, and perianal area) reacts as a single tissue field to certain carcinogenic stimuli.[97,104]

On the basis of epidemiologic and virologic studies, it has been suggested that there are two types of vulvar carcinoma: the most common occurring in older women and not related to HPV and the other occurring in younger women and related to HPV (see p. 1321).[62,65,94,105]

Morphologic features

Invasive squamous cell carcinoma of the vulva arises most commonly on the labia majora but may be found on the labia minora or in the region of the clitoris[72a,75,96] (Figs. 19-8 and 19-9). Microscopically, most cases have a well-differentiated appearance, although those located in the clitoris tend to be more anaplastic (Fig. 19-10). VIN is often present at the margins.[109]

Some high-grade squamous cell carcinomas show focal areas of glandular differentiation, analogous to those sometimes seen in squamous cell carcinomas of other organs.[95] The suggestion that these tumors are analogous to the adenoid squamous cell carcinomas of sun-damaged skin[106] is not warranted because they differ greatly from them in microscopic appearance, histogenesis, and natural history.

Spread and metastases

Regional lymph node metastases occur in about 20% of the cases.[78] Tumors of the labia spread first to inguinal lymph nodes, whereas those located in the clitoris may metastasize directly into the deep nodes. It should be noted that ulceration and inflammation in vulvar carcinoma often lead to reactive enlargement of inguinal lymph nodes, which may be confused clinically with metastatic disease.

Therapy

The usual treatment of invasive carcinoma is radical vulvectomy with bilateral radical inguinal lymph node dissection.[71,77,80] Iliac lymphadenectomy and pelvic exenteration are reserved for advanced cases.[86] Early cases can be treated with a more conservative approach in the form of wide local excision[81]; it has been shown that leaving a 1-cm tumor-free surgical margin results in a high rate of local

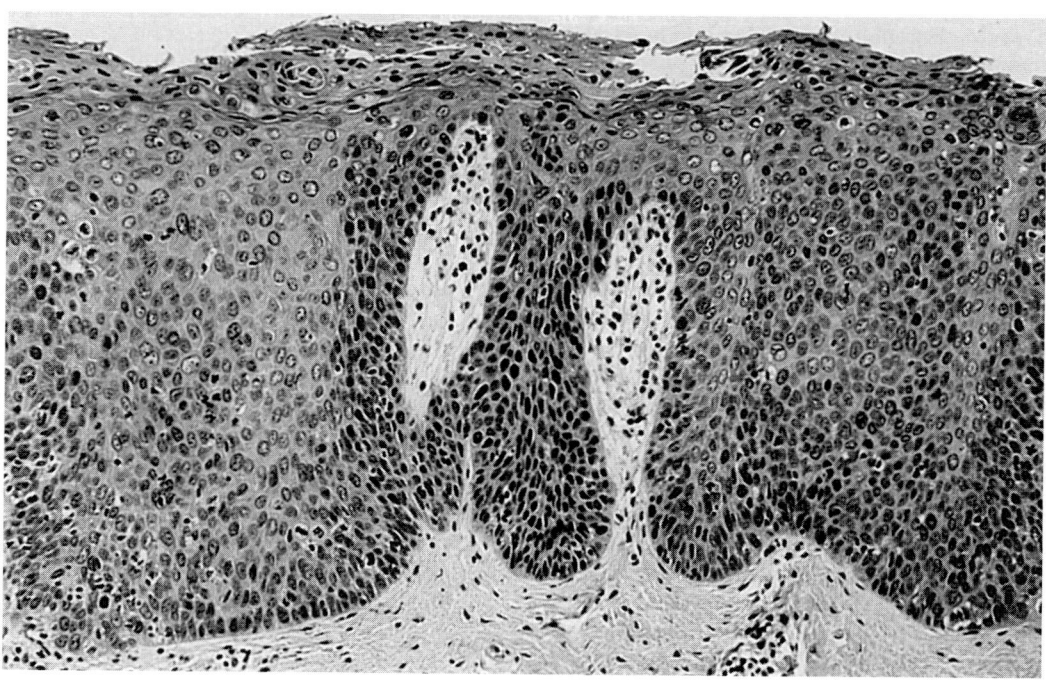

Fig.19-7 Squamous cell carcinoma in situ. There is disorganization of all layers with prominent variation in size and shape of cells, but basement membrane is intact.

control.[82] Alternative methods include radiation therapy alone and the combination of wide local excision and radiation therapy.[101]

Prognosis

The overall 5-year survival rate in patients treated for vulvar squamous cell carcinoma has been in the 50% to 75% range in most large series.[74,84,101]

The most important prognostic factors are included in the staging system (Table 19-1) and are represented by tumor diameter, depth of invasion, and lymph node status.* The latter is by far the most significant parameter. In cases with involved nodes, the presence of extracapsular spread and large size of the metastatic focus are poor prognostic indicators.[83,99] Infiltrative margins and vascular invasion in the primary tumor correlate with the incidence of nodal metastases.[64,102] A well-differentiated cytologic appearance and the presence of hyperkeratotic dysplastic skin at the edge of the cancer have been associated with a significantly better prognosis in some series.[79,87] DNA ploidy status does not seem to be an independent prognostic determinator.[63]

Microinvasive carcinoma

The term *microinvasive carcinoma* has been applied to vulvar carcinomas in which the depth of penetration is less than 5 mm (Fig. 19-11). Some authors have suggested that inguinal lymphadenectomy be foregone in these patients because of the low incidence of lymph node metastases.[107] However, enough exceptions have been reported to cast serious doubts on the wisdom of this recommendation[73,98] and on the very use and definition of the term.[68,69,76,103,108] Perhaps the only invasive carcinomas for which a conservative surgery is indicated are those that are both well differentiated and very superficial (3 mm or less).

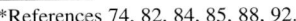

*References 74, 82, 84, 85, 88, 92.

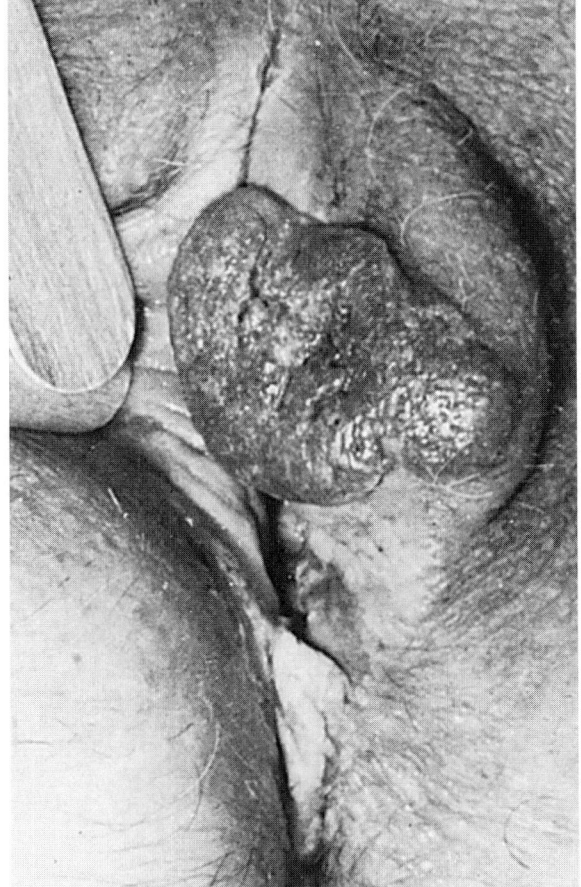

Fig. 19-8 Large ulcerating carcinoma of vulva associated with leukoplakia. (Courtesy Dr. R. Johnson, Columbia, MO.)

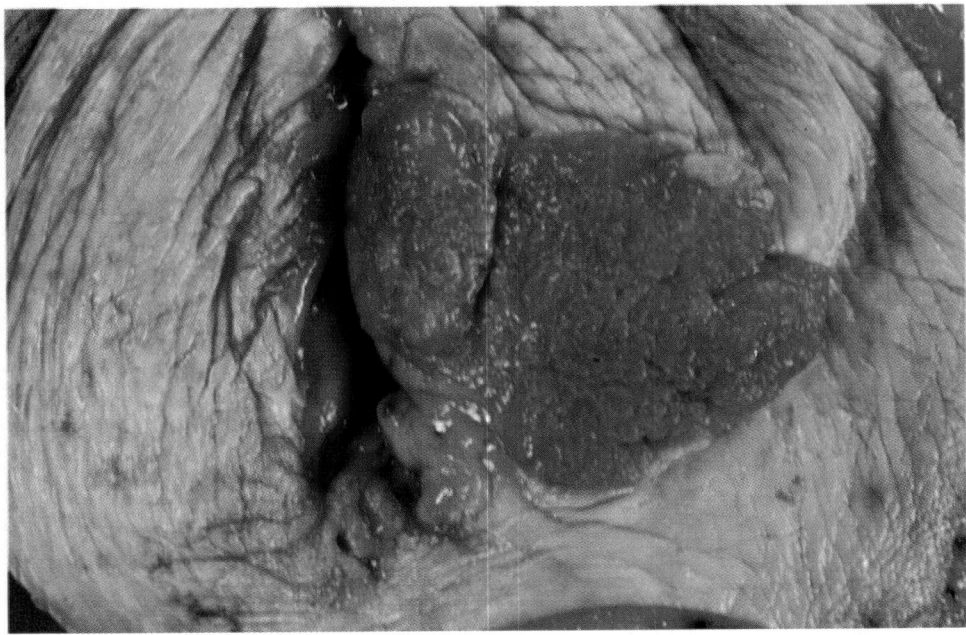

Fig. 19-9 Squamous cell carcinoma of the vulva involving clitoris and labia.

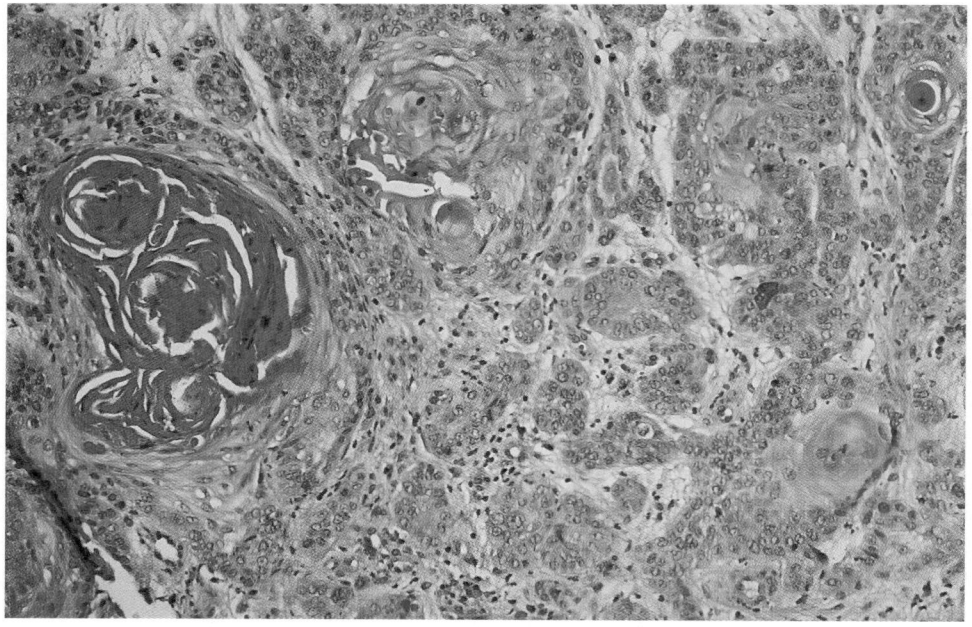

Fig. 19-10 Well-differentiated squamous cell carcinoma of vulva.

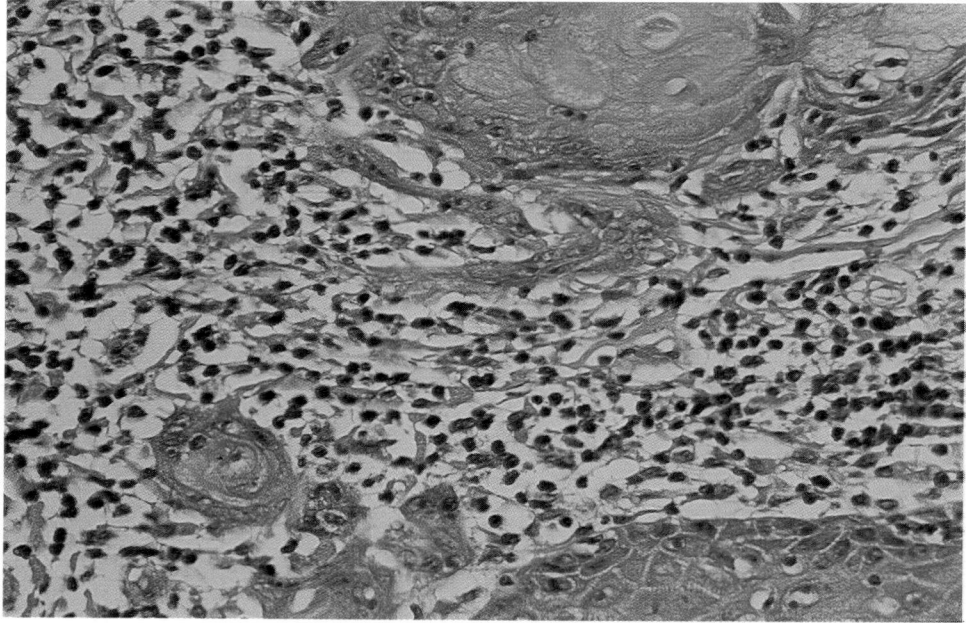

Fig. 19-11 Microinvasive carcinoma of vulva. Small clusters of malignant epithelium are seen detaching from the in situ component and invading a heavily inflamed stroma.

Other microscopic types

Verrucous carcinoma is a special type of squamous cell carcinoma of the vulva, similar to its more common counterpart in the upper aerodigestive tract. It may grow to huge dimensions, has a typical exophytic appearance, and infiltrates locally (Fig. 19-12). Metastases are practically nonexistent,[89,91] and therefore inguinal lymphadenectomy is not necessary.

The differential diagnosis of verrucous carcinoma includes condyloma acuminatum and conventional squamous cell carcinoma. It is distinguished from the former by its generally larger size and the presence of club-shaped fingers of epithelium invading the underlying stroma in a well-circumscribed ("pushing") fashion.[100] The distinction from squamous cell carcinoma rests entirely on two criteria, which often go together: the presence of cytologic atypia and/or a clearly infiltrative pattern of growth. The occurrence of either of these features removes the lesion from the verrucous carcinoma category and puts it into the squamous cell category. Immunohistochemically, staining for keratin is more uniform and homogeneous in verrucous carcinoma than in squamous cell carcinoma.[67] Tumors having the overall appearance of verrucous carcinoma but exhibiting focal squamous cell features as previously defined are designated by some as *hybrid carcinomas.*

Warty carcinoma should not be used as a synonym for verrucous carcinoma, despite the fact that the gross appearance of the latter has sometimes been described as "warty." The term warty carcinoma, if used at all, should be reserved for the squamous cell carcinomas in which the tumor cells display marked pleomorphism, enlargement, atypia, and multinucleation. These features are often associated with koilocytotic atypia in the adjacent epithelium. HPV DNA is often detected in these tumors.[93]

Lymphoepithelioma-like carcinoma has been described in the vulvar region, but the single reported case was negative for EBV.[134a]

PAGET'S DISEASE

Paget's disease is a malignant glandular tumor of the vulva that could be viewed either as a sweat gland carcinoma arising primarily from the intraepidermal portion of the glands (acrosyringium) or as a carcinoma of multipotential cells located along the epidermal basal layer that differentiate along glandular (sweat gland) lines.[127] Clinically, it presents as a crusting, elevated scaling erythematous rash in the labia majora, labia minora, and/or perineal skin (Fig. 19-13). Microscopically, the epidermis contains large pale tumor cells that form solid nests, glandular spaces, or a continuous layer along the epidermal basement membrane and also in pilosebaceous structures and sweat ducts. A cleft often develops between the row of malignant cells and the overlying keratinocytes, resulting in a low-power appearance sometimes reminiscent of an acantholytic suprabasal bulla. Paget's disease can also be misinterpreted as malignant melanoma. It should be noted that the presence of melanin granules in some tumor cells *does not* rule out the diagnosis of Paget's disease. Histochemically, some or all of the tumor cells contain acidic mucus, as evidenced by their positivity for Mayer's mucicarmine and aldehyde fuchsin

Table 19-1 FIGO staging for carcinoma of the vulva

Stage 0	
T1S	Carcinoma in situ; intraepithelial carcinoma.
Stage I	
T1 N0 M0	Tumor confined to the vulva and/or perineum— 2 cm or less in greatest dimension, nodes are negative.
Stage II	
T2 N0 M0	Tumor confined to the vulva and/or perineum— more than 2 cm in greatest dimension, nodes are negative.
Stage III	
T3 N0 M0	Tumor of any size with
T3 N1 M0	1) Adjacent spread to the lower urethra and/or the vagina, or the anus, and/or
T1 N1 M0	2) Unilateral regional lymph node metastasis.
T2 N1 M0	
Stage IVA	
T1 N2 M0	Tumor invades any of the following:
T2 N2 M0	Upper urethra, bladder mucosa, rectal mucosa, pelvic bone, and/or bilateral regional node metastasis
T3 N2 M0	
T4 any N M0	
Stage IVB	
Any T	Any distant metastasis including
Any N, M1	pelvic lymph nodes

Rules for Clinical Staging
The rules for staging are similar to those for carcinoma of the cervix

TNM Classification of Carcinoma of the Vulva (FIGO)

T	*Primary tumor*
Tis	Preinvasive carcinoma (carcinoma in situ)
T1	Tumor confined to the vulva and/or perineum— ≤2 cm in greatest dimension
T2	Tumor confined to the vulva and/or perineum— >2 cm in greatest dimension
T3	Tumor of any size with adjacent spread to the urethra and/or vagina and/or to the anus
T4	Tumor of any size infiltrating the bladder mucosa and/or the rectal mucosa, including the upper part of the urethral mucosa and/or fixed to the bone
N	*Regional lymph nodes*
N0	No lymph node metastasis
N1	Unilateral regional lymph node metastasis
N2	Bilateral regional lymph node metastasis
M	*Distant metastasis*
M0	No clinical metastasis
M1	Distant metastasis (including pelvic lymph node metastasis)

From SGO handbook. Staging of gynecologic malignancies. Chicago, 1994, Society of Gynecologic Oncologists.
See also Appendix G.

stains.[118] Immunohistochemically, they are reactive for low-molecular-weight keratin, EMA, CEA, and B72.3[125,126,130,131] (Fig. 19-14). In the majority of the cases, they also stain for

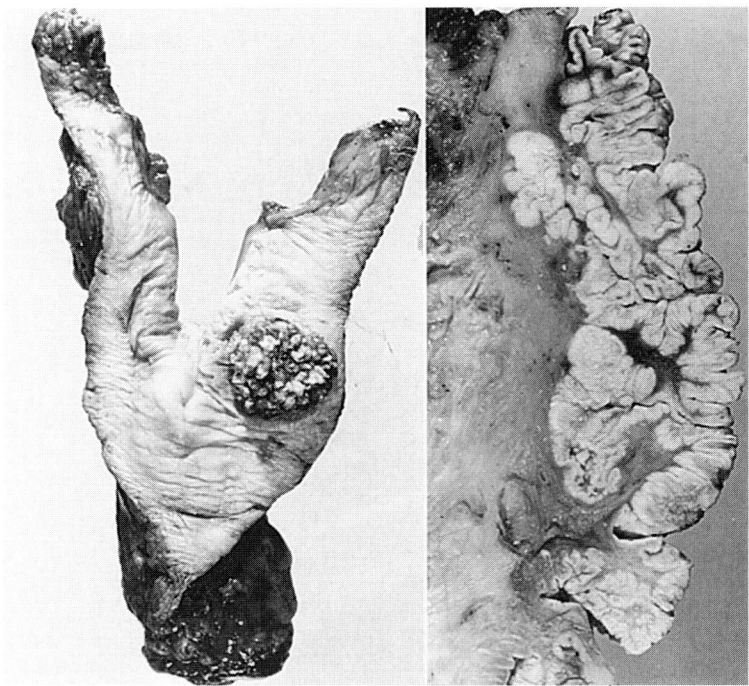

Fig. 19-12 Outer aspect and cut surface appearance of verrucous carcinoma of vulva. Tumor forms large exophytic mass, which invades the underlying stroma in a pushing fashion. (Courtesy Dr. J. Costa, Lausanne, Switzerland.)

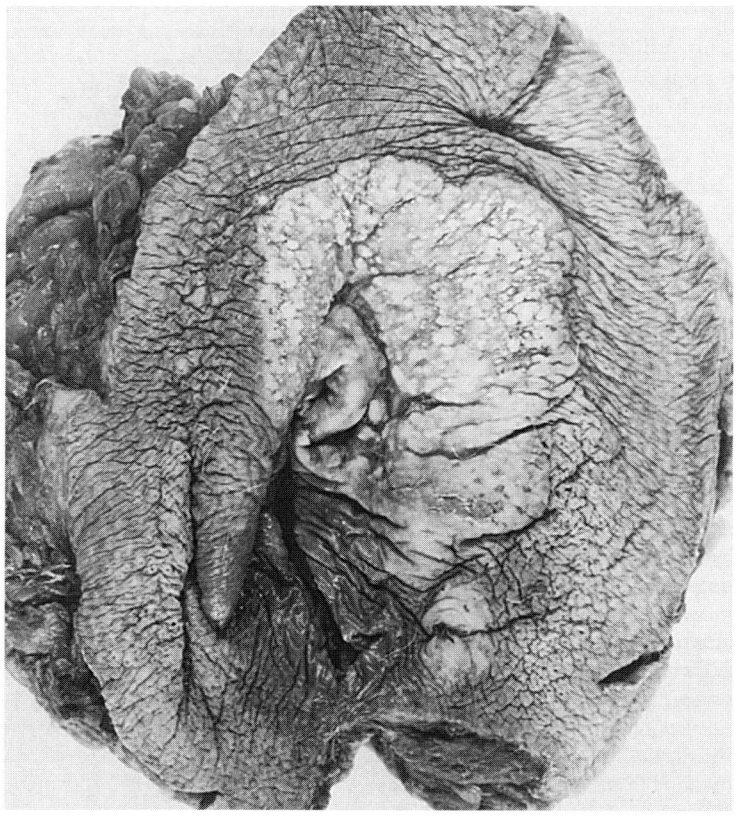

Fig. 19-13 Paget's disease of vulva in 87-year-old woman. Disease involves labia majora and labia minora. Note clinical similarity to leukoplakia. (From Fenn ME, Morley GW, Abell MR: Paget's disease of vulva. Obstet Gynecol **38:**660-670, 1971.)

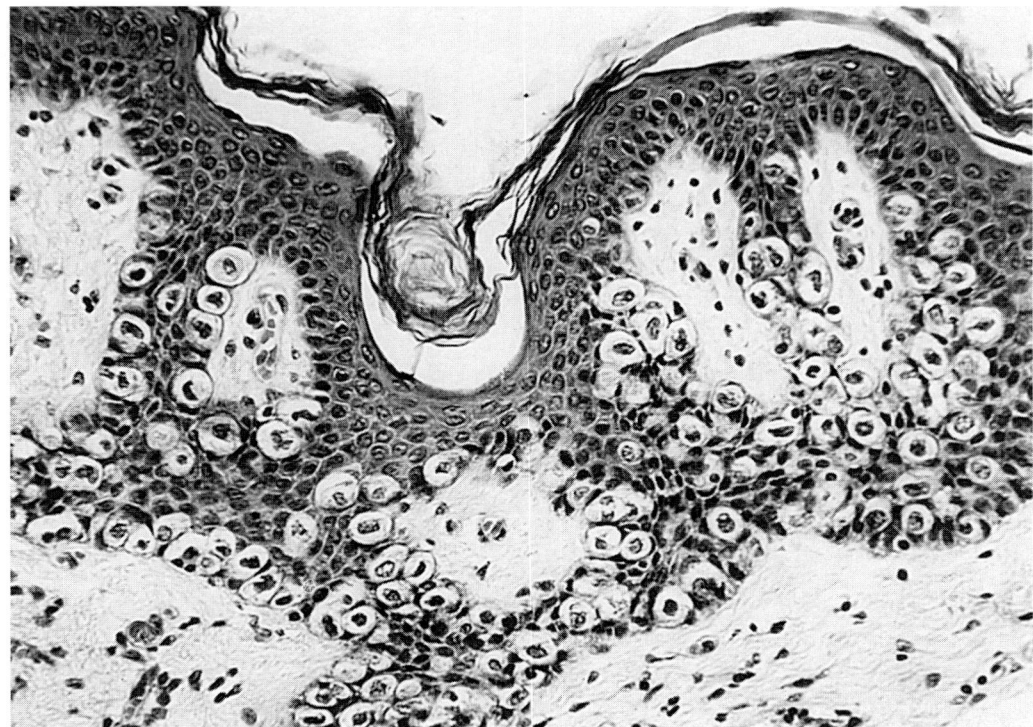

Fig. 19-14 Paget's disease of vulva in 60-year-old woman. Paget cell are large, clear, and concentrated in the basal portion of the epithelium.

GCDFP-15, a marker of apocrine differentiation. S-100 protein stain is positive in about one third of the cases, but HMB-45 is negative.[114,128] The ultrastructural features are indicative of glandular rather than keratinocytic or melanocytic differentiation.[129] Overexpression of c-erbB-2 oncoprotein and of the *ras* oncogene product p21 has been found in about half the cases.[121,124]

Paget's disease of the vulva differs in several respects from Paget's disease of the breast. The latter is nearly always associated with an underlying carcinoma that may be intraductal or invasive, and the intraepidermal malignant cells are more often than not mucin-negative. In contrast, the majority of the cases of vulvar Paget's disease are not associated with an invasive underlying carcinoma and are usually (although not always) positive for mucin stains, as previously indicated.[110,119,120] The incidence of underlying invasive carcinoma in vulvar Paget's disease ranges from zero to 30% depending on the series.[112,113,122] Occasionally, Paget's disease is seen in association with VIN, in keeping with its presumed origin from multipotential epidermal basal cells.[117]

If no invasive component is found in the resected specimen, the prognosis is good. Metastases do not occur under these circumstances, although local recurrence may supervene, sometimes in the form of invasive carcinoma.[116] Therefore excision should include a margin of normal skin and the subcutaneous tissue to incorporate all sweat glands. Unfortunately, the microscopic extent of the disease is often greater than that suspected from clinical examination, and this should be taken into account at the time of surgery.[115] Frozen sections are useful to determine the status of the margins.[111] The disease may also recur in the vulvar split-thickness skin graft.[123]

OTHER EPITHELIAL TUMORS

Hidradenoma papilliferum is a benign vulvar tumor that usually presents as a small, well-circumscribed nodule covered by normal skin. Occasionally, it ulcerates through the skin and clinically may simulate carcinoma.[133] Microscopically, it has a complex papillary glandular pattern, with stratification and some degree of pleomorphism; a myoepithelial layer is usually apparent (Fig. 19-15). Traditionally, this tumor has been regarded as of sweat gland derivation. However, its remarkable morphologic and immunohistochemical similarity with intraductal papilloma of breast and nipple adenoma suggests an origin from ectopic mammary tissue (see p. 1319). All acceptable examples of this tumor have behaved in a benign fashion.[141,148] However, a case of intraductal carcinoma of mammary-type apocrine epithelium has been reported arising from this tumor.[143]

Benign lesions of skin adnexal type occur in the vulva. These include *syringoma, chondroid syringoma* (benign mixed tumor),[135,146] *benign pilar tumor,*[134] *warty dyskeratoma,*[139] and *keratoacanthoma.*[145]

Basal cell carcinoma of the vulva usually presents as nodular masses in the labia majora of elderly patients; it may grow very large and ulcerate.[138] Its microscopic appearance and behavior are the same as those of basal cell carcinomas elsewhere in the skin; solid, keratotic, and adenoid types have been described. The differential diagnosis

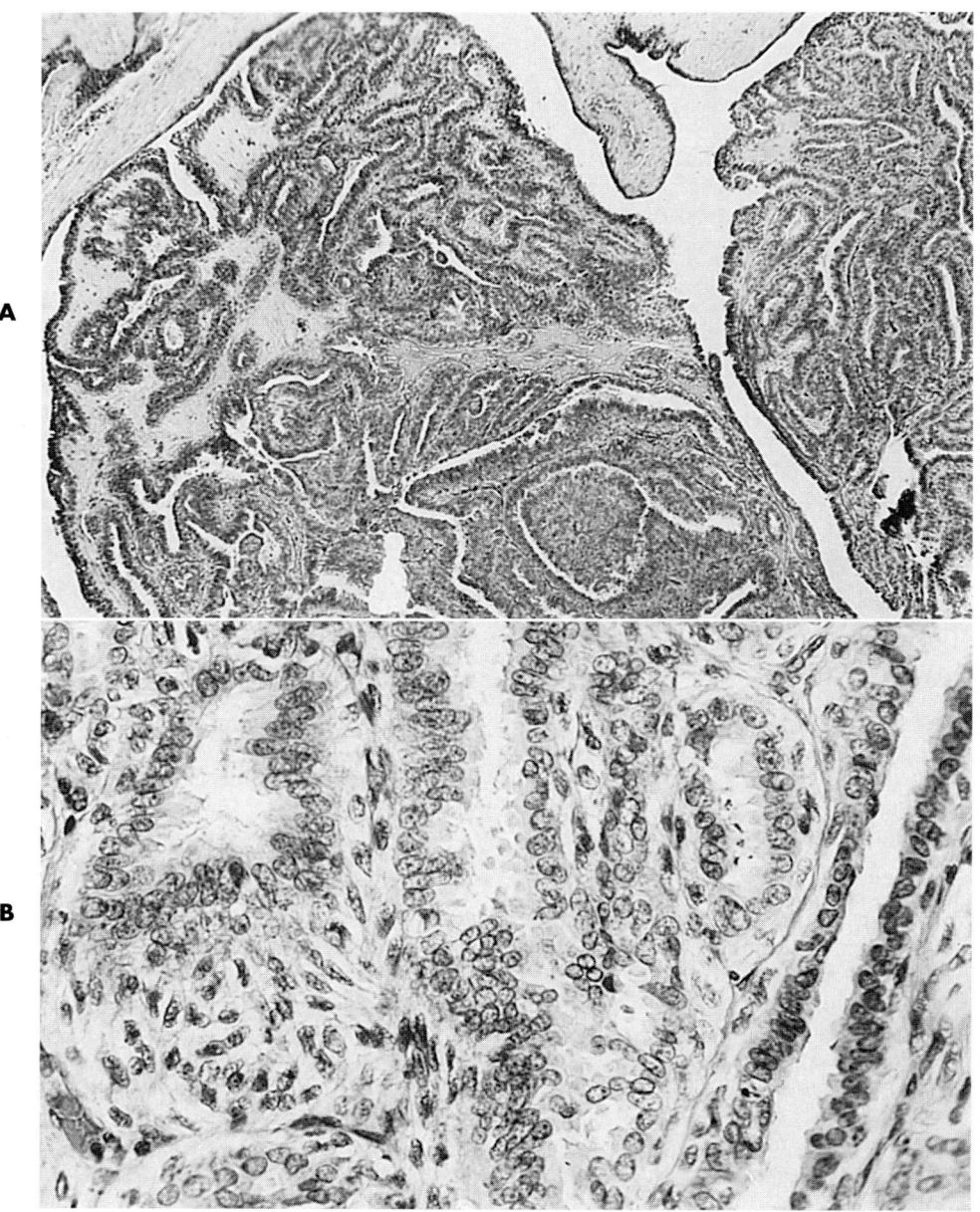

Fig. 19-15 Typical hidradenoma papilliferum of vulva. Note apparent encapsulation and papillary pattern. **B,** Same specimen shown in **A** at higher magnification. Double layer of cells and characteristic cellular pattern can be seen.

includes basaloid carcinoma (see later section) and the basaloid changes sometimes seen as a component of Bowen's disease and invasive squamous cell carcinoma. It should be remembered that, as elsewhere in the skin, basal cell carcinoma may exhibit abrupt squamous differentiation of possible pilar type, a change that does not affect the natural history of the lesion; such tumors should not be referred to as basosquamous carcinomas.

The incidence of nodal metastases in vulvar basal cell carcinoma is extremely low and is largely restricted to the deeply invasive lesions.[144]

Basaloid (squamous cell) carcinoma has an appearance analogous to its counterpart in the upper aerodigestive tract. Peripheral palisading is prominent; in some cases there is a well-developed adenoid cystic–like appearance. These features suggest an early differentiation toward glandular structures.[132,142]

Merkel cell carcinoma has been reported in the vulva, sometimes in association with Bowen's disease.[136,137] Its behavior has been very aggressive.[140]

Sweat gland carcinoma of the vulva, exclusive of Paget's disease, is exceptional; it may present with a variety of mor-

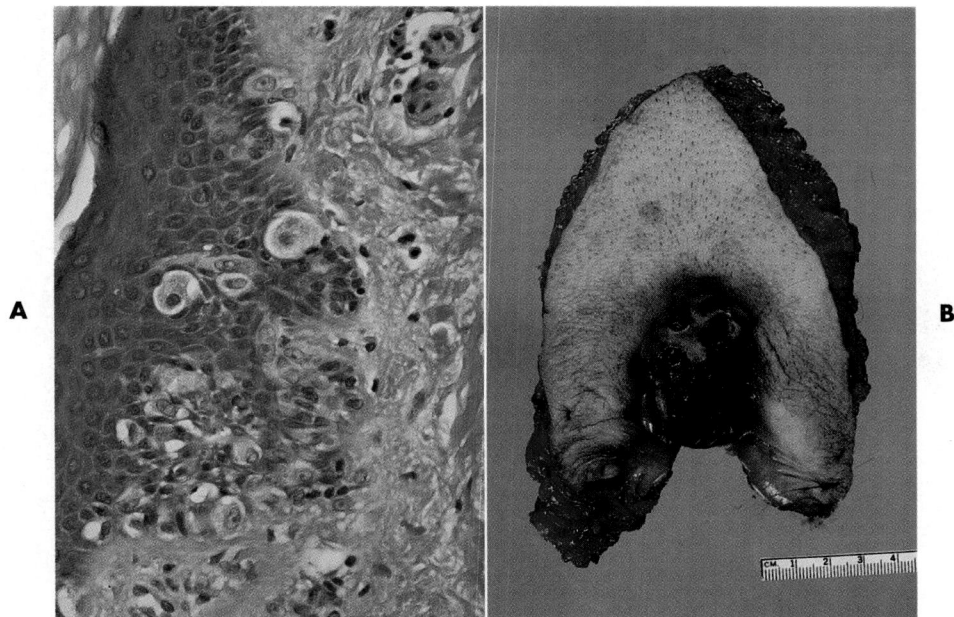

Fig. 19-16 Melanoma of vulva. **A,** This portion of the tumor is primarily intraepidermal and appears in the form of large pagetoid cells. **B,** Gross appearance of advanced malignant melanoma of vulva. The tumor is large, polypoid, and deeply pigmented.

phologic patterns and should be distinguished from metastatic adenocarcinoma.[147] A case has been described showing mucinous and neuroendocrine features.[144a]

MELANOCYTIC TUMORS

Melanocytic nevi occur in the vulva, particularly in the labia majora. Those seen in adults are nearly always of intradermal or compound type. Sometimes, a prominent junctional component is seen in nevi of younger women, in which the enlarged junctional nests vary in size, shape, and position, and may lead to an overdiagnosis of malignant melanoma.[151,158] The term *genital nevus* is sometimes employed for this microscopically troublesome lesion.

Malignant melanoma is the second most common malignant tumor of the vulva, but it is much less frequent than squamous cell carcinoma.[153] The large majority of the patients are older than 50 years at the time of diagnosis, a fact of great importance in the differential diagnosis with genital nevus.[157] The microscopic appearance is similar to that of malignant melanoma of the skin (see Chapter 4) (Fig. 19-16, *A*). Most lesions are advanced (Clark's level III or IV) at the time of diagnosis[159] (Fig. 19-16, *B*). The usual treatment is radical vulvectomy with bilateral inguinal lymph node dissection, but small lesions with depths of ≥1.75 mm may be treated with wide local excision.[152,155] The overall 5-year survival rate is about 35%.[150] Lymph node status, level or thickness of the primary tumor, and ulceration are the most important prognostic parameters.[149,154,156,160] There is some suggestion that the DNA ploidy pattern may also provide prognostic information.[159a]

OTHER TUMORS AND TUMORLIKE CONDITIONS

Fibroepithelial polyp is a superficially located benign lesion composed of a loose myxoid stroma covered by normal squamous epithelium. Bizarre, stellate, frequently multinucleated stromal cells may be present[161,169,187] (Fig. 19-17). As in other sites where this lesion may occur, desmin immunoreactivity may be present.[185]

Aggressive angiomyxoma is a soft tissue neoplasm that usually arises within the perineum. It often presents as a vulvar mass and clinically simulates a Bartholin gland cyst.[164,195] Most patients are in the second or third decade of life, but cases have also been reported in children.[205] A similar tumor occurs in males in the scrotal region.[176a]

Grossly, the appearance is gelatinous and ill-defined. Microscopically, a hypocellular myxomatous stroma devoid of atypicality or mitotic activity is seen intermingling with sizable vessels having dilated lumina and occasional hyaline thickening of the adventitia (Fig. 19-18). This tumor is distinguished from the more common and innocuous fibroepithelial polyp already described because of its larger size, deeper location, and lack of bizarre stromal cells. The ultrastructural and immunohistochemical features are those of primitive mesenchymal cells focally exhibiting myofibroblastic ("myoid") traits.[194] A case analyzed cytogenetically showed a chromosomal translocation involving the region 12q14-15.[178a]

Recurrence into the ischiorectal and retroperitoneal spaces is common, probably because of the difficulties encountered in achieving a complete surgical excision.[191]

Angiomyofibroblastoma has been described as a benign vulvar tumor characterized by alternating hypercellular and hypocellular areas admixed with small blood vessels. Spindle and plump stromal cells aggregate around the vessels (Fig. 18-19). These cells are immunoreactive for vimentin and desmin but not for actin or keratin. This tumor is said to differ from aggressive angiomyxoma by virtue of its circumscribed borders, higher cellularity, abundance of blood ves-

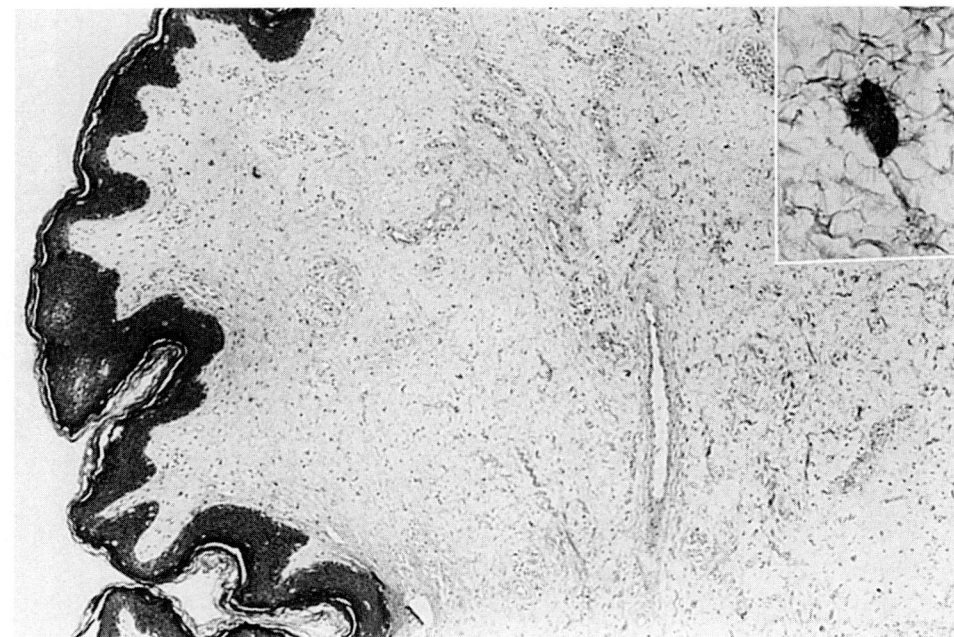

Fig. 19-17 Benign vulvar polyp composed of myxoid stroma. **Inset** shows one of stromal multinucleated cells often found in this lesion.

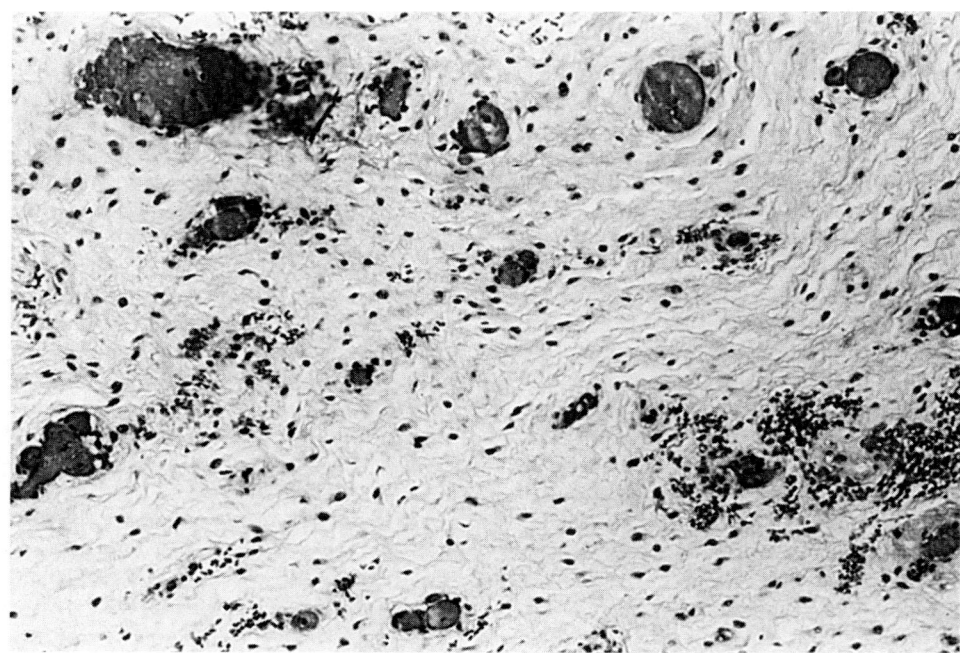

Fig. 19-18 Aggressive angiomyxoma of vulvar region. Large dilated blood vessels are irregularly distributed in hypocellular myxoid mass. Numerous foci of fresh hemorrhage are present around vessels.

sels, plump stromal cells, minimal stromal mucin, and rarity of red blood cell extravasation.[170,174] However, enough common features and transitions occur between it and aggressive angiomyxoma to suggest that they are closely related entities.[194]

Other primary tumors and tumorlike conditions that have been seen to occur in the vulva are *endometriosis, leiomyoma* (including a myxoid variety that can simulate aggressive angiomyxoma),[185a] *leiomyosarcoma* (including the epithelioid and myxoid varieties),[186,197] *hemangioma,*[203] *angiokeratoma,*[184] *epithelioid hemangioendothelioma,*[196] *angiosarcoma,*[186a] *glomus tumor,*[194a] benign and malignant *granular cell tumors* (some with accompanying pseudoepitheliomatous hyperplasia),[190,206] *schwannoma,*[176] *neurofibroma(tosis),*[172,175] *malignant peripheral nerve sheath*

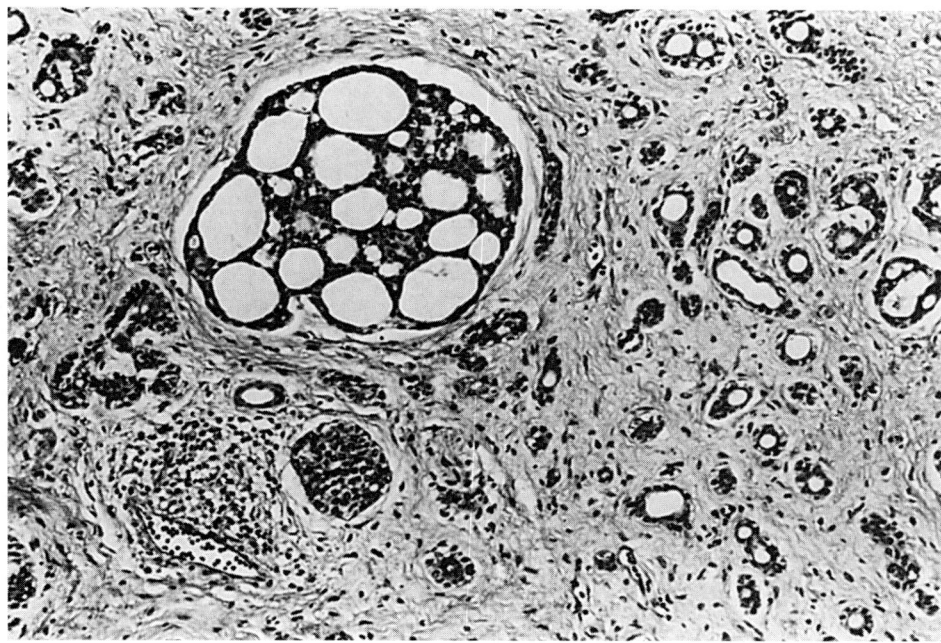

Fig. 19-19 Bartholin's gland carcinoma of adenoid cystic type. Widely invasive tumor shows focally prominent cribriform features.

tumor,[199,201] *sclerosing lipogranuloma,*[179] *yolk sac tumor,*[168] *rhabdomyosarcoma,*[173,174] *benign lymphoid hyperplasia,*[180] *malignant lymphoma,*[177] *verruciform xanthoma,*[192] *glomus tumor,*[178] *Langerhans' cell granulomatosis (histiocytosis X),*[162,188,200] *nodular fasciitis,*[171] *postoperative spindle-cell nodule,*[181a] *malignant fibrous histiocytoma,*[198] *dermatofibrosarcoma protuberans,*[163,165] *paraganglioma,*[166] *alveolar soft part sarcoma,*[193] and *epithelioid sarcoma.*[202]

The latter tumor is of importance because of its relatively high frequency at this site and the fact that it tends to run a more aggressive course here than in its usual location in the distal extremities. This may be at least partially result from the fact that this tumor, when located in the vulva, often exhibits rhabdoid features, known to be associated with an aggressive course.[204] As a matter of fact, it may be difficult to decide whether to designate a given vulvar tumor as an epithelioid sarcoma or as a malignant rhabdoid tumor.[182,189] In this regard, it may be pertinent to note that most authors favor the interpretation that the latter represents a phenotype that can be exhibited by a variety of neoplasms, including epithelioid sarcoma, malignant melanoma, and undifferentiated carcinoma (see Chapter 25).[181]

Metastases to the vulva usually originate from the cervix (almost 50%), endometrium, kidney, or gastrointestinal tract.[167] Most are expressions of generalized disease.[183]

LESIONS OF BARTHOLIN GLANDS AND RELATED STRUCTURES

Cysts and abscesses of Bartholin's glands are the result of chronic bacterial inflammation, especially from gonorrhea.[225] The lining of the cyst, which is usually of transitional or squamous type, can be destroyed partially or totally by the inflammatory infiltrate. The nature of the cyst can be estab-lished by the presence of residual mucinous glands in the fibrotic and inflamed connective tissue that forms the cyst wall. The secretion product is a nonsulfated sialomucin.[221] Sometimes, extravasation of this mucus into the stroma may induce changes similar to those seen in "mucocele" of the oral cavity.[214] The cyst may be treated by excision or marsupialization.[207] Occasionally, the inflammatory infiltrate is found to have the features of *malakoplakia.*[220]

Mucous cysts of the *vulvar vestibule* are usually solitary and lined by mucin-producing columnar cells.[215]

Benign tumors of this area include adenoma of minor vestibular glands (which may well represent focal hyperplastic changes secondary to trauma and inflammation),[208] mucinous cystadenoma,[209] and papilloma.[212]

Carcinomas of Bartholin's gland may take the form of squamous cell carcinoma (the most common), adenocarcinoma, transitional cell carcinoma, small cell carcinoma, and adenoid cystic carcinoma[210,211,213,216-219,222-224] (Figs. 19-19 and 19-20). Lymph node metastases are common. HPV is often found in the squamous cell type.[213]

LESIONS OF THE FEMALE URETHRA

Urethral caruncle has the appearance of a small raspberry protruding from the meatus; it bleeds easily and may become infected. It occurs only in the female urethra and is not a true neoplasm but rather a reactive polypoid lesion. Microscopically, chronic inflammatory cells, dilated vessels, and hyperplastic epithelium are seen in varying proportions. Mistaken diagnoses of malignancy can result from overinterpretation of islands of reactive epithelium or scattered bizarre stromal or lymphoid cells. There is a tendency for these lesions to recur following excision, probably because of persistence of the original inciting factors.[242]

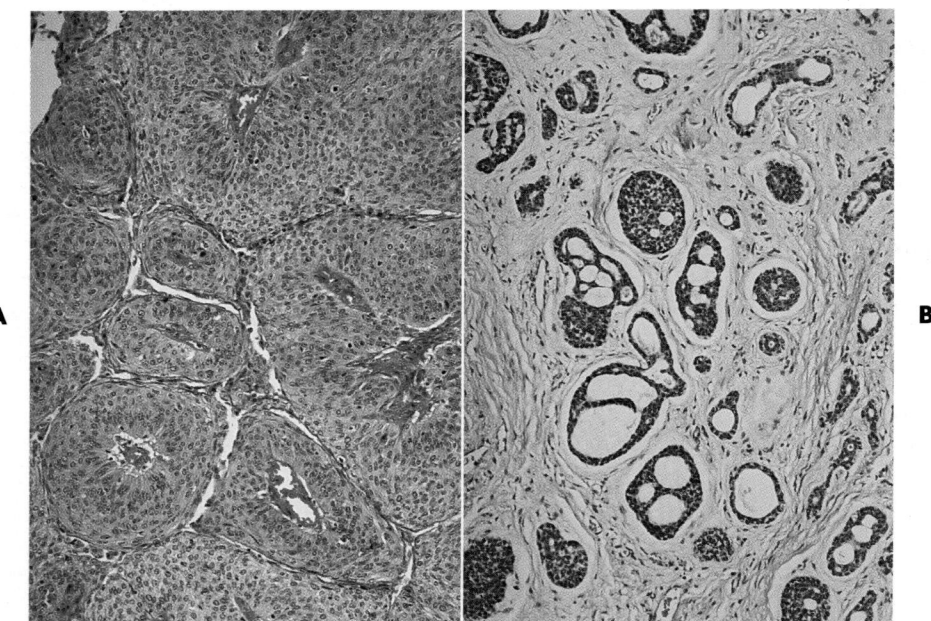

Fig. 19-20 Bartholin's gland carcinoma **A,** This tumor has an appearance reminiscent of transitional cell carcinoma of the urinary tract. **B,** This neoplasm has the appearance of an adenoid cystic carcinoma.

So-called *nephrogenic (mesonephric) adenoma* is a metaplastic change resulting from inflammation rather than a true neoplasm. It is microscopically similar to the more common lesions located in the bladder neck.[230,241] Similarly, an occurrence in the urethra of mucinous epithelium of *colonic* type can also be explained on a metaplastic basis, although a congenital origin is also possible.[233]

Prolapse of the urethral mucosa can occur in childhood and clinically simulate a vulvovaginal neoplasm.[227]

Urethral carcinoma occurs in elderly patients and presents with bleeding or dysuria.[226,234] The majority of the cases arise from the meatus, at the junction of the transitional and squamous epithelium.[236] In a series of thirty-five cases, nineteen were anterior (vulvourethral), four were posterior (vesicourethral), and twelve involved the entire urethra.[244]

Microscopically, most urethral carcinomas are of squamous cell type.[239] Other types include transitional cell carcinoma, columnar/mucinous adenocarcinoma,[238] and clear cell (mesonephroid) adenocarcinoma.[247] Interestingly, nearly half of the carcinomas reported as arising in urethral diverticula have been adenocarcinomas of either conventional or clear cell type.[228,229] HPV has been detected by PCR techniques in a high proportion of urethral carcinomas.[246]

The prognosis of urethral carcinoma is relatively poor, except when the disease is limited to the anterior portion of the urethra.[237] In one large series, the 5-, 10-, and 15-year actuarial survival rates were 41%, 31%, and 22%, respectively.[231] The usual treatment is radiation therapy,[231,243,245] but depending on their size and location they can also be treated by surgery alone or surgery plus irradiation.[232,240]

Malignant melanoma of the urethra is a highly aggressive neoplasm that is treated by total urethrectomy with bilateral inguinal lymph node dissection.[235]

Malignant lymphoma can exceptionally present as a urethral tumor.[240a]

Metastatic tumors in the urethra usually originate in other portions of the female genital tract, particularly endometrium.[239]

REFERENCES
NORMAL ANATOMY

1 McLean JM: Anatomy and physiology of the vulvar area. In Ridley CM, ed: The vulva. New York, 1988, Churchill Livingstone.

2 Rorat E, Ferenczy A, Richart RM: Human Bartholin gland, duct, and duct cyst. Arch Pathol **99:**367-374, 1975.

3 van der Putte SC: Anogenital "sweat" glands. Histology and pathology of a gland that may mimic mammary glands. Am J Dermatopathol **13:**557-567, 1991.

4 Wilkinson EJ, Hardt NS: Vulva. In Sternberg SS, ed: Histology for pathologists. New York, 1992, Raven Press.

CONGENITAL ABNORMALITIES

5 Burger RA, Marcuse PM: Fibroadenoma of the vulva. Am J Clin Pathol **24:**965-968, 1954.

6 Di Bonito L, Patriarca S, Falconieri G: Aggressive "breast-like" adenocarcinoma of vulva. Pathol Res Pract **188:**211-214, 1992.

7 Foushee J, Smith H, Pruitt AB Jr: Vulvar fibroadenoma from aberrant breast tissue. Report of two cases. Obstet Gynecol **29:**819-823, 1967.

8 Guerry RL, Pratt-Thomas HR: Carcinoma of supernumerary breast of vulva with bilateral mammary cancer. Cancer **38:**2570-2574, 1976.

9 Rose PG, Roman LD, Reale FR, Tak WK, Hunter RE: Primary adenocarcinoma of the breast arising in the vulva. Obstet Gynecol **76:**537-539, 1990.

10 Simon KE, Dutcher JP, Runowicz CD, Wiernik PH: Adenocarcinoma arising in vulvar breast tissue. Cancer **62:**2234-2238, 1988.

11 Tbakhi A, Cowan DF, Kumar D, Kyle D: Recurring phylloides tumor in aberrant breast tissue of the vulva. Am J Surg Pathol **17:**946-950, 1993.

12 Tow SH, Shanmugaratnam K: Supernumerary mammary gland in the vulva. Br Med J **5314:**1234-1236, 1962.

12a van der Putte SC: Mammary-like glands of the vulva and their disorders. Int J Gynecol Pathol **13:**150-160, 1994.

SO-CALLED CHRONIC VULVAR DYSTROPHIES

13 Hart WR, Norris JH, Helwig EB: Relation of lichen sclerosus et atrophicus of the vulva to development of carcinoma. Obstet Gynecol **45**:369-377, 1975.

14 Janovski NA, Ames S: Lichen sclerosus et atrophicus of the vulva. A poorly understood disease entity. Obstet Gynecol **22**:697-708, 1963.

15 Kiryu H, Ackerman AB: A critique of current classification of vulvar diseases. Am J Dermatopathol **12**:377-392, 1990.

16 Lascano EF, Montes LF, Mazzini MA: Lichen sclerosus et atrophicus in childhood. Report of 6 cases. Obstet Gynecol **24**:872-877, 1964.

17 Lawrence WD: Non-neoplastic epithelial disorders of the vulva (vulvar dystrophies). Historical and current perspectives. Pathol Annu **28** (Pt 2):23-51, 1993.

18 Rodke G, Friedrich EG Jr, Wilkinson EJ: Malignant potential of mixed vulvar dystrophy (lichen sclerosus associated with squamous cell hyperplasia). J Reprod Med **33**:545-550, 1988.

19 Wallace HJ: Lichen sclerosus et atrophicus. Trans St. John's Hosp Dermatol Soc **57**:9-30, 1971.

INFLAMMATORY DISEASES

20 Alexander LJ, Shields TL: Squamous cell carcinoma of the vulva secondary to granuloma inguinale. Arch Dermatol **67**:395-402, 1953.

21 Barnes R, Masood S, Lammert N, Young RH: Extragenital granuloma inguinale mimicking a soft-tissue neoplasm. A case report and review of the literature. Hum Pathol **21**:559-561, 1990.

22 Douglas CPL: Lymphogranuloma venereum and granuloma inguinale of the vulva. J Obstet Gynaecol Br Commonw **69**:871-880, 1962.

22a Guerrieri C, Ohlsson E, Rydén G, Westermark P: Vulvitis granulomatosia. A cryptogenic chronic inflammatory hypertrophy of vulvar labia related to cheilitis granulomatosa and Crohn's disease. Int J Gynecol Pathol **14**:352-359, 1995.

23 Koteen H: Lymphogranuloma venereum. Medicine (Baltimore) **24**:1-69, 1945.

24 Kremer M, Nussenson E, Steinfeld M, Zuckerman P: Crohn's disease of the vulva. Am J Gasteroenterol **79**:376-378, 1984.

25 Lavery HA, Pinkerton JHM, Sloan J: Crohn's disease of the vulva. Two further cases. Br J Dermatol **113**:359-363, 1985.

25a Prayson RA, Stoler MH, Hart WR: Vulvar vestibulitis. A histiopathologic study of 36 cases, including human papillomavirus in situ hybridization analysis. Am J Surg Pathol **19**:154-160, 1995.

26 Pund ER, Greenblatt RB: Specific histology of granuloma inguinale. Arch Pathol **23**:224-229, 1937.

27 Rainey R: The association of lymphogranuloma inguinale and cancer. Surgery **35**:221-235, 1954.

28 Roberts DB: Necrotizing fasciitis of the vulva. Am J Obstet Gynecol **157**:568-571, 1987.

28a Vettraino IM, Merritt DF: Crohn's disease of the vulva. Am J Dermatopathol **17**:410-413, 1995.

HUMAN PAPILLOMA VIRUS AND VULVAR PATHOLOGY; CONDYLOMA

28b Ashfaq R, Vuitch F: Human papilloma virus and carcinomas of the female urethra. J Urol Pathol **2**:195-202, 1994.

29 Crum CP, Burkett BJ: Papillomavirus and vulvovaginal neoplasia. J Reprod Med **34**:566-571, 1989.

30 Crum CP, Fu YS, Levine RU, Richart RM, Townsend DE, Fenoglio CM: Intraepithelial squamous lesions of the vulva. Biologic and histologic criteria for the distinction of condylomas from vulvar intraepithelial neoplasia. Am J Obstet Gynecol **144**:77-83, 1982.

31 Della Torre G, Donghi R, Longoni A, Pilotti S, Pasquini G, De Palo G, Pierotti MA, Rilke F, Della Porta G: HPV DNA in intraepithelial neoplasia and carcinoma of the vulva and penis. Diagn Mol Pathol **1**:25-30, 1992.

32 Di Bonito L, Falconieri G, Bonifacio-Gori D: Multicentric papillomavirus infection of the female genital tract. A study of morphologic pattern, possible risk factors and viral prevalence. Pathol Res Pract **189**:1023-1029, 1993.

33 Ferenczy A: Laser treatment of patients with condylomata and squamous carcinoma precursors of the lower female genital tract. CA **37**:334-347, 1987.

34 Gross G, Hagedorn M, Ikenberg H, Rufli T, Dahlet C, Grosshans E, Gissmann L: Bowenoid papulosis. Presence of human papillomavirus (HPV) structural antigens and of HPV 16-related DNA sequences. Arch Dermatol **121**:858-863, 1985.

35 Gupta J, Pilotti S, Rilke F, Shah K: Association of human papillomavirus type 16 with neoplastic lesions of the vulva and other genital sites by in situ hybridization. Am J Pathol **127**:206-215, 1987.

36 Ikenberg H, Gissmann L, Gross G, Grussendorf-Conen E-I, zur Hausen H: Human papillomavirus type 16-related DNA in genital Bowen's disease and in bowenoid papulosis. Int J Cancer **32**:563-565, 1983.

37 Kovi J, Tillman RL, Lee SM: Malignant transformation of condyloma acuminatum. A light microscopic and ultrastructural study. Am J Clin Pathol **61**:702-710, 1974.

37a McLachlin CM, Kozakewich H, Craighill M, O'Connell B, Crum CP: Histologic correlates of vulvar human papillomavirus infection in children and young adults. Am J Surg Pathol **18**:728-735, 1994.

37b McLachlin CM, Mutter GL, Crum CP: Multinucleated atypia of the vulva. Report of a distinct entity not associated with human papillomavirus. Am J Surg Pathol **18**:1233-1239, 1994.

38 McMillan A, Bishop PE, Fletcher S: An immunohistological study of condylomata acuminata. Histopathology **17**:45-52, 1990.

39 Nuovo GJ, O'Connell M, Blanco JS, Levine RU, Silverstein SJ: Correlation of histology and human papillomavirus DNA detection in condyloma acuminatum and condyloma-like vulvar lesions. Am J Surg Pathol **13**:700-706, 1989.

40 Sawchuk WS: Vulvar manifestations of human papillomavirus infection. Dermatol Clin **10**:405-414, 1992.

41 Shevchuk MM, Richart RM: DNA content of condyloma acuminatum. Cancer **49**:489-492, 1982.

42 Wade TR, Ackerman AB: The effects of resin of podophyllin on condyloma acuminatum. Am J Dermatopathol **6**:109-122, 1984.

43 Werness BA, Levine AJ, Howley PM: Association of human papillomavirus types 16 and 18 E6 proteins with p53. Science **248**:76-79, 1990.

SQUAMOUS INTRAEPITHELIAL LESIONS

44 Abell MR, Gosling JRG: Intraepithelial and infiltrating carcinoma of the vulva. Bowen's type. Cancer **14**:318-329, 1961.

45 Barclay DL, Collins CG: Intraepithelial cancer of the vulva. Am J Obstet Gynecol **86**:95-106, 1963.

46 Berger BW, Hori Y: Multicentric Bowen's disease of the genitalia. Spontaneous regression of lesions. Arch Dermatol **114**:1698-1699, 1978.

47 Bergeron C, Neghashfar Z, Canaan C, Shah K, Fu Y, Ferenczy A: Human papillomavirus type 16 in intraepithelial neoplasia (bowenoid papulosis) and coexistent invasive carcinoma of the vulva. Int J Gynecol Pathol **6**:1-11, 1987.

48 Crum CP, Braun LA, Shah KV, Fu Y-S, Levine RU, Fenoglio CM, Richart RM, Townsend DE: Vulvar intraepithelial neoplasia. Correlation of nuclear DNA content and the presence of a human papilloma virus (HPV) structural antigen. Cancer **49**:468-471, 1982.

49 Crum CP, Liskow A, Petras P, Keng WC, Frick HC II: Vulvar intraepithelial neoplasia (severe atypia and carcinoma in situ). A clinicopathologic analysis of 41 cases. Cancer **54**:1429-1434, 1984.

50 Forney JP, Morrow CP, Townsend DE, DiSaia PJ: Management of carcinoma in situ of the vulva. Am J Obstet Gynecol **127**:801-806, 1977.

51 Friedrich EG Jr, Wilkinson EJ, Fu YS: Carcinoma in situ of the vulva. A continuing challenge. Am J Obstet Gynecol **136**:830-843, 1980.

52 Gupta J, Pilotti S, Rilke F, Shah K: Association of human papillomavirus type 16 with neoplastic lesions of the vulva and other genital sites by in situ hybridization. Am J Pathol **127**:206-215, 1987.

53 Husseinzadeh N, Newman NJ, Wesseler TA: Vulvar intraepithelial neoplasia. A clinicopathological study of carcinoma in situ of the vulva. Gynecol Oncol **33**:157-163, 1989.

53a Kaefner HK, Tate JE, McLachlin CM, Crum CP: Vulvar intraepithelial neoplasia. Morphological phenotype, papillomavirus DNA, and coexisting invasive carcinoma. Hum Pathol **26**:147-154, 1995.

54 Kimura A: Condylomata acuminata with pigmented papular lesions. Dermatologica **160**:390-397, 1980.

55 Macnab JCM, Walkinshaw SA, Cordiner JW, Clements JB: Human papillomavirus in clinically and histologically normal tissue of patients with genital cancer. N Engl J Med **315**:1052-1058, 1986.

56 Park JS, Jones RW, McLean MR, Currie JL, Woodruff JD, Shah DV, Kurman RJ: Possible etiologic heterogeneity of vulvar intraepithelial neoplasia. A correlation of pathologic characteristics with human papillomavirus detection by in situ hybridization and polymerase chain reaction. Cancer **67**:1599-1607, 1991.

57 Patterson JW, Kao GF, Graham JH, Helwig EB: Bowenoid papulosis. A clinicopathologic study with ultrastructural observations. Cancer **57**:823-836, 1986.

58 Prat J: Pathology of vulvar intraepithelial lesions and early invasive carcinoma. Hum Pathol **22**:877-883, 1991.

59 Shatz P, Bergeron C, Wilkinson EJ, Arseneau J, Ferenczy A: Vulvar intraepithelial neoplasia and skin appendage involvement. Obstet Gynecol **74**:769-774, 1989.

60 Ulbright TM, Stehman FB, Roth LM, Ehrlich CE, Ransburg RC: Bowenoid dysplasia of the vulva. Cancer **50**:2910-2919, 1982.

61 Walts AE, Koeffler HP, Said JW: Localization of p53 protein and human papillomavirus in anogenital squamous lesions. Immunohistochemical and in situ hybridization studies in benign, dysplastic, and malignant epithelia. Hum Pathol **24**:1238-1242, 1993.

INVASIVE SQUAMOUS CELL CARCINOMA

62 Andersen WA, Franquemont DW, Williams J, Taylor PT, Crum CP: Vulvar squamous cell carcinoma and papillomaviruses. Two separate entities? Am J Obstet Gynecol 165:329-335, 1991.

63 Ballouk F, Ambros RA, Malfetano JH, Ross JS: Evaluation of prognostic indicators in squamous carcinoma of the vulva including nuclear DNA content. Mod Pathol 6:371-375, 1993.

64 Binder SW, Huang I, Fu YS, Hacker NF, Berek JS: Risk factors for the development of lymph node metastasis in vulvar squamous cell carcinoma. Gynecol Oncol 37:9-16, 1990.

65 Bloss JD, Liao SY, Wilczynski SP, Macri C, Walker J, Peake M, Berman ML: Clinical and histologic features of vulvar carcinomas analyzed for human papillomavirus status. Evidence that squamous cell carcinoma of the vulva has more than one etiology. Hum Pathol 22:711-718, 1991.

66 Brinton LA, Nasca PC, Mallin K, Baptiste MS, Wilbanks GD, Richart RM: Case-control study of cancer of the vulva. Obstet Gynecol 75:859-866, 1990.

67 Brisigotti M, Moreno A, Murcia C, Matias-Guiu X, Prat J: Verrucous carcinoma of the vulva. A clinicopathologic and immunohistochemical study of five cases. Int J Gynecol Pathol 8:1-7, 1989.

68 Buckley CH, Butler EB, Fox H: Vulvar intraepithelial neoplasia and microinvasive carcinoma of the vulva. J Clin Pathol 37:1201-1211, 1984.

69 Buscerna J, Woodruff JD, Parmley TH, Genadry R: Carcinoma in situ of the vulva. Obstet Gynecol 55:225-230, 1980.

70 Carter J, Carlson J, Fowler J, Hartenbach E, Adcock L, Carson L, Twiggs LB: Invasive vulvar tumors in young women. A disease of the immunosuppressed? Gynecol Oncol 51:307-310, 1993.

71 Collins CG, Lee FYL, Roman-Lopez JJ: Invasive carcinoma of the vulva with lymph node metastasis. Am J Obstet Gynecol 109:446-452, 1971.

72 Crum CP: Carcinoma of the vulva. Epidemiology and pathogenesis. Obstet Gynecol 79:448-454, 1992.

72a Czernobilsky B, Gat A, Evron R, Dgani R, Ben-Hur H, Lifschitz-Mercer B: Carcinoma of the clitoris. A histologic study with cytokeratin profile. Int J Gynecol Pathol 14:274-278, 1995.

73 Dipaola GR, Gomez-Rueda N, Arrighi L: Relevance of microinvasion of carcinoma of the vulva. Obstet Gynecol 45:647-649, 1975.

74 Donaldson ES, Powell DE, Hanson MB, van Nagell JR: Prognostic parameters in invasive vulvar cancer. Gynecol Oncol 11:184-190, 1981.

75 Dvoretsky PM, Bonfiglio TA: The pathology of vulvar squamous cell carcinoma and verrucous carcinoma. Pathol Annu 21(Pt 2):23-45, 1986.

76 Dvoretsky PM, Bonfiglio TA, Helmkamp BF, Ramsey G, Chuang C, Beecham JB: The pathology of superficially invasive, thin vulvar squamous cell carcinoma. Int J Gynecol Pathol 3:331-342, 1984.

77 Edsmyr F: Carcinoma of the vulva. An analysis of 560 patients with histologically verified squamous cell carcinoma. Acta Radiol (Diagn) (Stockh) 217(Suppl):1-135, 1962.

78 Figge DC, Tamimi HK, Greer BE: Lymphatic spread in carcinoma of the vulva. Am J Obstet Gynecol 152:387-394, 1985.

79 Gosling JRG, Abell MR, Prolette BM, Loughrin TD: Infiltrative squamous cell (epidermoid) carcinoma of vulva. Cancer 14:330-343, 1961.

80 Green TH Jr, Ulfelder H, Meigs JV: Epidermoid carcinoma of the vulva. An analysis of 238 cases. Part I. Etiology and diagnosis. Part II. Therapy and end results. Am J Obstet Gynecol 75:834-864, 1958.

81 Hacker NF, Van der Velden J: Conservative management of early vulvar cancer. Cancer 71:1673-1677, 1993.

82 Heaps JM, Fu YS, Montz FJ, Hacker NF, Berek JS: Surgical-pathologic variables predictive of local recurrence in squamous cell carcinoma of the vulva. Gynecol Oncol 38:309-314, 1990.

83 Homesley HD: Lymph node findings and outcome in squamous cell carcinoma of the vulva (editorial). Cancer 74:2399-2402, 1994.

84 Homesley HD, Bundy BN, Sedlis A, Yordan E, Berek JS, Jahsan A, Mortel R: Assessment of current International Federation of Gynecology and Obstetrics staging of vulvar carcinoma relative to prognostic factors for survival (a Gynecologic Oncology Group study). Am J Obstet Gynecol 164:997-1003, 1991.

85 Homesley HD, Bundy BN, Sedlis A, Yordan E, Berek JS, Jahsan A, Mortel R: Prognostic factors for groin node metastasis in squamous cell carcinoma of the vulva (a Gynecologic Oncology Group study). Gynecol Oncol 49:279-283, 1993.

86 Hopkins MP, Morley GW: Pelvic exenteration for the treatment of vulvar cancer. Cancer 70:2835-2838, 1992.

87 Husseinzadeh N, Wesseler T, Schneider D, Schellhas H, Nahhas W: Prognostic factors and the significance of cytologic grading in invasive squamous cell carcinoma of the vulva. A clinicopathologic study. Gynecol Oncol 36:192-199, 1990.

88 Husseinzadeh N, Zaino R, Nahhas WA, Mortel R: The significance of histologic findings in predicting nodal metastases in invasive squamous cell carcinoma of the vulva. Gynecol Oncol 16:105-111, 1983.

89 Japaze H, Van Dinh T, Woodruff JD: Verrucous carcinoma of the vulva. Study of 24 cases. Obstet Gynecol 60:462-466, 1982.

90 Jimerson GK, Merrill JA: Multicentric squamous malignancy involving both cervix and vulva. Cancer 26:150-153, 1970.

91 Kraus FT, Perez-Mesa C: Verrucous carcinoma. Clinical and pathologic study of 105 cases involving oral cavity, larynx and genitalia. Cancer 19:26-38, 1966.

92 Kunschner A, Kanbour AI, David B: Early vulvar carcinoma. Am J Obstet Gynecol 132:599-606, 1978.

93 Kurman RJ, Toki T, Schiffman MH: Basaloid and warty carcinomas of the vulva. Distinctive types of squamous cell carcinoma frequently associated with human papillomaviruses. Am J Surg Pathol 17:133-145, 1993.

94 Kurman RJ, Trimble CL, Shah KV: Human papillomavirus and the pathogenesis of vulvar carcinoma. Curr Opin Obstet Gynecol 4:582-585, 1992.

95 Lasser A, Cornog JL, Morris JM: Adenoid squamous cell carcinoma of the vulva. Cancer 33:224-227, 1974.

96 Macafee CHG: Some aspects of vulvar cancer. J Obstet Gynaecol Br Commonw 69:177-195, 1962.

97 Mitchell MF, Prasad CJ, Silva EG, Rutledge FN, McArthur MC, Crum CP: Second genital primary squamous neoplasms in vulvar carcinoma. Viral and histopathologic correlates. Obstet Gynecol 81:13-18, 1993.

98 Nakao CY, Nolan JF, DiSaia PJ, Futoran R: Microinvasive epidermoid carcinoma of the vulva with an unexpected natural history. Am J Obstet Gynecol 120:1122-1123, 1974.

99 Paladini D, Cross P, Lopes A, Monaghan JM: Prognostic significance of lymph node variables in squamous cell carcinoma of the vulva. Cancer 74:2491-2496, 1994.

100 Partridge EE, Murad T, Shingleton HM, Austin JM, Hatch KD: Verrucous lesions of the female genitalia. I. Giant condylomata. Am J Obstet Gynecol 137:412-418, 1980.

101 Perez CA, Grigsby PW, Galakatos A, Swanson R, Camel HM, Kao MS, Lockett MA: Radiation therapy in management of carcinoma of the vulva with emphasis on conservation therapy. Cancer 71:3707-3716, 1993.

102 Ross MJ, Ehrmann RL: Histologic prognosticators in stage I squamous cell carcinoma of the vulva. Obstet Gynecol 70:774-784, 1987.

103 Sedlis A, Homesley H, Bundy BN, Marshall R, Yordan E, Hacker N, Lee JH, Whitney C: Positive groin lymph nodes in superficial squamous cell vulvar cancer. A gynecologic oncology group study. Am J Obstet Gynecol 156:1159-1164, 1987.

104 Sherman KJ, Daling JR, Chu J, McKnight B, Weiss NS: Multiple primary tumours in women with vulvar neoplasms. A case-control study. Br J Cancer 57:423-427, 1988.

105 Toki T, Kurman RJ, Park JS, Kessis T, Daniel RW, Shah KV: Probable non-papillomavirus etiology of squamous cell carcinoma of the vulva in older women. A clinicopathologic study using in situ hybridization and polymerase chain reaction. Int J Gynecol Pathol 10:107-125, 1991.

106 Underwood JW, Adcock LL, Okagaki T: Adenosquamous carcinoma of skin appendages (adenoid squamous cell carcinoma, pseudoglandular squamous cell carcinoma, adenoacanthoma of sweat gland of Lever) of the vulva. A clinical and ultrastructural study. Cancer 42:1851-1858, 1978.

107 Wharton JT, Gallager S, Rutledge FN: Microinvasive carcinoma of the vulva. Am J Obstet Gynecol 118:159-162, 1974.

108 Wilkinson EJ, Rico MJ, Pierson KK: Microinvasive carcinoma of the vulva. Int J Gynecol Pathol 1:29-39, 1982.

109 Zaino RJ, Husseinzadeh N, Nahhas W, Mortel R: Epithelial alterations in proximity to invasive squamous carcinoma of the vulva. Int J Gynecol Pathol 1:173-184, 1982.

PAGET'S DISEASE

110 Alguacil-Garcia A, O'Connor R: Mucin-negative biopsy in extra-mammary Paget's disease. A diagnostic problem. Histopathology 15:429-431, 1989.

111 Bergen S, Di Saia PJ, Liao SY, Berman ML: Conservative management of extra-mammary Paget's disease of the vulva. Gynecol Oncol 33:151-156, 1989.

112 Curtin JP, Rubin SC, Jones WB, Hoskins WJ, Lewis JL Jr: Paget's disease of the vulva. Gynecol Oncol 39:374-377, 1990.

113 Fenn ME, Morley GW, Abell MR: Paget's disease of vulva. Obstet Gynecol 38:660-670. 1971.

114 Guarner J, Cohen C, De Rose PB: Histogenesis of extramammary and mammary Paget cells. An immunohistochemical study. Am J Dermatopathol 11:313-318, 1989.

115 Gunn RA, Gallager HS: Vulvar Paget's disease. A topographic study. Cancer 46:590-594, 1980.

116 Hart WR, Millman JB: Progression of intraepithelial Paget's disease of the vulva to invasive carcinoma. Cancer 40:2333-2337, 1977.

117 Hawley IC, Husain F, Pryse-Davies J: Extramammary Paget's disease of the vulva with dermal invasion and vulval intra-epithelial neoplasia. Histopathology 18:374-376, 1991.

118 Helm KF, Goellner JR, Peters MS: Immunohistochemical stains in extramammary Paget's disease. Am J Dermatopathol **14**:402-407, 1992.

119 Helwig EB, Graham JH: Anogenital (extramammary) Paget's disease. A clinicopathological study. Cancer **16**:387-403, 1963.

120 Jones RE Jr, Austin C, Ackerman AB: Extramammary Paget's disease. A critical reexamination. Am J Dermatopathol **1**:101-132, 1979.

121 Keatings L, Sinclair J, Wright C, Corbett IP, Watchorn C, Hennessy C, Angus B, Lennard T, Horne CH: c-*erb*B-2 oncoprotein expression in mammary and extramammary Paget's disease. An immunohistochemical study. Histopathology **17**:243-247, 1990.

122 Lee SC, Roth LM, Ehrlich C, Hall JA: Extramammary Paget's disease of the vulva. A clinicopathologic study of 13 cases. Cancer **39**:2540-2549, 1977.

123 Misas JE, Larson JE, Podczaski E, Manetta A, Mortel R: Recurrent Paget disease of the vulva in a split-thickness graft. Obstet Gynecol **76**:543-544, 1990.

124 Mori O, Hachisuka H, Nakano S, Sasai Y, Shiku H: Expression of *ras* p21 in mammary and extramammary Paget's disease. Arch Pathol Lab Med **114**:858-861, 1990.

125 Nadji M, Morales AR, Girtanner RE, Ziegels-Weissman J, Penneys NS: Paget's disease of the skin. A unifying concept of histogenesis. Cancer **50**:2203-2206, 1982.

126 Olson DJ, Fujimura M, Swanson P, Okagaki T: Immunohistochemical features of Paget's disease of the vulva with and without adenocarcinoma. Int J Gynecol Pathol **10**:285-295, 1991.

127 Paget GE, Rowley A, Woodcock AS: Paget's disease of the vulva. J Pathol Bacteriol **67**:256-258, 1954.

128 Reed W, Oppedal BR, Eeg Larsen T: Immunohistology is valuable in distinguishing between Paget's disease, Bowen's disease and superficial spreading malignant melanoma. Histopathology **16**:583-588, 1990.

129 Roth LM, Lee SC, Ehrlich CE: Paget's disease of the vulva. A histogenetic study of five cases including ultrastructural observations and review of the literature. Am J Surg Pathol **1**:193-206, 1977.

130 Urabe A, Matsukuma A, Shimizu N, Nishimura M, Wada H, Hori Y: Extramammary Paget's disease. Comparative histopathologic studies of intraductal carcinoma of the breast and apocrine adenocarcinoma. J Cutan Pathol **17**:257-265, 1990.

131 Watanabe S, Ohnishi T, Takahashi H, Ishibashi Y: A comparative study of cytokeratin expression in Paget cells located at various sites. Cancer **72**:3323-3330, 1993.

OTHER EPITHELIAL TUMORS

132 Abell MR: Adenocystic (pseudoadenomatous) basal cell carcinoma of vestibular glands of vulva. Am J Obstet Gynecol **86**:470-482, 1963.

133 Anderson NP: Hidradenoma of the vulva. Arch Dermatol **62**:873-891, 1950.

134 Avinoach I, Zirkin HJ, Glezerman M: Proliferating trichilemmal tumor of the vulva. Case report and review of the literature. Int J Gynecol Pathol **8**:163-168, 1989.

134a Axelsen SM, Stamp IM: Lymphoepithelioma-like carcinoma of the vulvar region. Histopathology **27**:281-283, 1995

135 Carneiro SJC, Gardner HL, Knox JM: Syringoma. Three cases with vulvar involvement. Obstet Gynecol **39**:95-99, 1972.

136 Chen KTK: Merkel's cell (neuroendocrine) carcinoma of the vulva. Cancer **73**:2186-2191, 1994.

137 Copeland LJ, Cleary K, Sneige N, Edwards CL: Neuroendocrine (Merkel cell) carcinoma of the vulva. A case report and review of the literature. Gynecol Oncol **22**:367-378, 1985.

138 Cruz-Jimenez PR, Abell MR: Cutaneous basal cell carcinoma of vulva. Cancer **36**:1860-1868, 1975.

139 Duray PH, Merino MJ, Axiotis C: Warty dyskeratoma of the vulva. Int J Gynecol Pathol **2**:286-293, 1983.

140 Loret de Mola JR, Hudock PA, Steinetz C, Jacobs G, Macfee M, Abdul-Karim FW: Merkel cell carcinoma of the vulva. Gynecol Oncol **51**:272-276, 1993.

141 Meeker JH, Neubecker RD, Helwig EF: Hidradenoma papilliferum. Am J Clin Pathol **37**:182-195, 1962.

142 Merino MJ, LiVolsi VA, Schwartz PE, Rudnicki J: Adenoid basal cell carcinoma of the vulva. Int J Gynecol Pathol **1**:299-306, 1982.

143 Pelosi G, Martignoni G, Bonetti F: Intraductal carcinoma of mammary-type apocrine epithelium arising within a papillary hydradenoma of the vulva. Report of a case and review of the literature. Arch Pathol Lab Med **115**:1249-1254, 1991.

144 Perrone T, Twiggs LB, Adcock LL, Dehner LP: Vulvar basal cell carcinoma. An infrequently metastasizing neoplasm. Int J Gynecol Pathol **6**:152-165, 1987.

144a Rahilly MA, Beattie GJ, Lessells AM: Mucinous eccrine carcinoma of the vulva with neuroendocrine differentiation. Histopathology **27**:82-86, 1995.

145 Rhatigan RM, Nuss RC: Keratoacanthoma of the vulva. Gynecol Oncol **21**:118-123, 1985.

146 Rorat E, Wallach RC: Mixed tumors of the vulva. Clinical outcome and pathology. Int J Gynecol Pathol **3**:323-328. 1984.

147 Wick MR, Goellner JR, Wolfe JT III, Su WPD: Vulvar sweat gland carcinomas. Arch Pathol Lab Med **109**:43-47, 1985.

148 Woodworth H Jr, Dockerty MB, Wilson RB, Pratt JH: Papillary hidradenoma of the vulva. A clinicopathologic study of 69 cases. Am J Obstet Gynecol **110**:501-508, 1971.

MELANOCYTIC TUMORS

149 Benda JA, Platz CE, Anderson B: Malignant melanoma of the vulva. A clinical-pathologic review of 16 cases. Int J Gynecol Pathol **5**:202-216, 1986.

150 Bradgate MG, Rollason TP, McConkey CC, Powell J: Malignant melanoma of the vulva. A clinicopathological study of 50 women. Br J Obstet Gynaecol **97**:124-133, 1990.

151 Christensen WN, Friedman KJ, Woodruff JD, Hood AF: Histologic characteristics of vulvar nevocellular nevi. J Cutan Pathol **14**:87-91, 1987.

152 Das Gupta T, D'Urso J: Melanoma of female genitalia. Surg Gynecol Obstet **119**:1074-1078, 1964.

153 Jaramillo BA, Ganjei P, Averette HE, Sevin B-U, Lovecchio JL: Malignant melanoma of the vulva. Obstet Gynecol **66**:398-401, 1985.

154 Johnson TL, Kumar NB, White CD, Morley GW: Prognostic features of vulvar melanoma. A clinicopathologic analysis. Int J Gynecol Pathol **5**:110-118, 1986.

155 Look KY, Roth LM, Sutton GP: Vulvar melanoma reconsidered. Cancer **72**:143-146, 1993.

156 Podratz KC, Symmonds RE, Taylor WF, Williams TJ: Carcinoma of the vulva. Analysis of treatment and survival. Obstet Gynecol **61**:63-74, 1983.

157 Ragnarsson-Olding B, Johansson H, Rutqvist LE, Ringborg U: Malignant melanoma of the vulva and vagina. Trends in incidence, age distribution, and long-term survival among 245 consecutive cases in Sweden 1960-1984. Cancer **71**:1893-1897, 1993.

158 Rock B: Pigmented lesions of the vulva. Dermatol Clin **10**:361-370, 1992.

159 Ronan SG, Eng AM, Briele HA, Walker MJ, Das Gupta TK: Malignant melanoma of the female genitalia. J Am Acad Dermatol **22**:428-435, 1990.

159a Scheistroen M, Trope C, Koern J, Pettersen EO, Abeler VM, Kristensen GB: Malignant melanoma of the vulva. Evaluation of prognostic factors with emphasis on DNA ploidy in 75 patients. Cancer **75**:72-80, 1995.

160 Tasseron EW, van der Esch EP, Hart AA, Brutel de la Riviere G, Aartsen EJ: A clinicopathological study of 30 melanomas of the vulva. Gynecol Oncol **46**:170-175, 1992.

OTHER TUMORS AND TUMORLIKE CONDITIONS

161 Abdul-Karim FW, Cohen RE: Atypical stromal cells of lower female genital tract. Histopathology **17**:249-253, 1990.

162 Axiotis CA, Merino MJ, Duray PH: Langerhans cell histiocytosis of the female genital tract. Cancer **67**:1650-1660, 1991.

163 Barnhill DR, Boling R, Nobles W, Crooks L, Burke T: Vulvar dermatofibrosarcoma protuberans. Gynecol Oncol **30**:149-152, 1988.

164 Bégin LR, Clement PB, Kirk ME, Jothy S, McCaughey WTE, Ferenczy A: Aggressive angiomyxoma of pelvic soft parts. A clinicopathologic study of nine cases. Hum Pathol **16**:621-628, 1985.

165 Bock JE, Andreasson B, Thorn A, Holck S: Dermatofibrosarcoma protuberans of the vulva. Gynecol Oncol **20**:129-135, 1985.

166 Colgan TJ, Dardick I, O'Connell G: Paraganglioma of the vulva. Int J Gynecol Pathol **10**:203-208, 1991.

167 Dehner LP: Metastatic and secondary tumors of the vulva. Obstet Gynecol **42**:47-57, 1973.

168 Dudley AG, Young RH, Lawrence WD, Scully RE: Endodermal sinus tumor of the vulva in an infant. Obstet Gynecol **61**:76S-78S, 1983.

169 Elliott GB, Elliott JDA: Superficial stromal reactions of lower genital tract. Arch Pathol **95**:100-101, 1973.

170 Fletcher CD, Tsang WY, Fisher C, Lee KC, Chan JK: Angiomyofibroblastoma of the vulva. A benign neoplasm distinct from aggressive angiomyxoma. Am J Surg Pathol **16**:373-382, 1992.

171 Gaffney EF, Majmudar B, Bryan JA: Nodular fasciitis (pseudosarcomatous fasciitis) of the vulva. Int J Gynecol Pathol **1**:307-312, 1982.

172 Gersell DJ, Fulling KH: Localized neurofibromatosis of the female genitourinary tract. Am J Surg Pathol **13**:873-878, 1989.

173 Hays DM, Raney RB Jr, Lawrence W Jr, Gehan EA, Soule EH, Tefft M, Maurer HM: Rhabdomyosarcoma of the female urogenital tract. J Pediatr Surg **16**:828-834, 1981.

174 Hays DM, Shimada H, Raney RB Jr, Tefft M, Newton W, Crist WM, Lawrence W Jr, Ragab A, Beltangady M, Maurer HM: Clinical staging and treatment results in rhabdomyosarcoma of the female genital tract among children and adolescents. Cancer **61**:1893-1903, 1988.

174a Hisaoka M, Kouho H, Aoki T, Daimaru Y, Hashimoto H: Angiomyofibroblastoma of the vulva. A clinicopathologic study of seven cases. Pathol Int **45:**487-492, 1995.

175 Hood AF, Lumadue J: Benign vulvar tumors. Dermatol Clin **10:**371-385, 1992.

176 Huang HJ, Yamabe T, Tagawa H: A solitary neurilemmoma of the clitoris. Gynecol Oncol **15:**103-110, 1983.

176a Iezzoni JC, Fechner RE, Wong LS, Rosai J: Aggressive angiomyxoma in males. A report of four cases. Am J Clin Pathol **104:**391-396, 1995.

177 Kaplan MA, Jacobson JO, Ferry JA, Harris NL: T-cell lymphoma of the vulva in a renal allograft recipient with associated hemophagocytosis. Am J Surg Pathol **17:**842-849, 1993.

178 Katz VL, Askin FB, Bosch BD: Glomus tumor of the vulva. A case report. Obstet Gynecol **67:**43S-45S, 1986.

178a Kazmierczak B, Wanschura S, Meyer-Bolte K, Caselitz J, Meister P, Bartnitzke S, Van de Ven W, Bullerdiek J: Cytogenetic and molecular analysis of an aggressive angiomyxoma. Am J Pathol **147:**580-585, 1995.

179 Kempson RL, Sherman AI: Sclerosing lipogranuloma of the vulva. Report of a case. Obstet Gynecol **101:**854-856, 1968.

180 Kernen JA, Morgan ML: Benign lymphoid hamartoma of the vulva. Report of a case. Obstet Gynecol **35:**290-292, 1970.

181 Kudo E, Hirose T, Fujii Y, Hasegawa T, Ino H, Hizawa K: Undifferentiated carcinoma of the vulva mimicking epithelioid sarcoma. Am J Surg Pathol **15:**990-1001, 1991.

181a Manson CM, Hirsch PJ, Coyne JD: Post-operative spindle cell nodule of the vulva. Histopathology **26:**571-574, 1995.

182 Matias C, Nunes JF, Vicente LF, Almeida MO: Primary malignant rhabdoid tumour of the vulva. Histopathology **17:**576-578, 1990.

183 Mazur MT, Hsueh S, Gersell DJ: Metastases to the female genital tract. Analysis of 325 cases. Cancer **53:**1978-1984, 1984.

184 McNeely TB: Angiokeratoma of the clitoris. Arch Pathol Lab Med **116:**880-881, 1992.

185 Mucitelli DR, Charles EZ, Kraus FT: Vulvovaginal polyps. Histologic appearance, ultrastructure, immunocytochemical characteristics, and clinicopathologic correlations. Int J Gynecol Pathol **9:**20-40, 1990.

185a Nemoto T, Shinoda M, Komatsuzaki K, Hara T, Kojima M, Ogihara T: Myxoid leiomyoma of the vulva mimicking aggressive angiomyxoma. Pathol Int **44:**454-459, 1994.

186 Newman PL, Fletcher CD: Smooth muscle tumours of the external genitalia. Clinicopathological analysis of a series. Histopathology **18:**523-529, 1991.

186a Nirenberg A, Ostor AG, Slavin J, Riley CB, Rome RM: Primary vulvar sarcomas. Int J Gynecol Pathol **14:**55-62,1995.

187 Ostor AG, Fortune DW, Riley CB: Fibroepithelial polyps with atypical stromal cells (pseudosarcoma botryoides) of vulva and vagina. A report of 13 cases. Int J Gynecol Pathol **7:**351-360, 1988.

188 Otis CN, Fischer RA, Johnson N, Kelleher JF, Powell JL: Histiocytosis X of the vulva. A case report and review of the literature. Obstet Gynecol **75:**555-558, 1990.

189 Perrone T, Swanson PE, Twiggs L, Ulbright TM, Dehner LP: Malignant rhabdoid tumor of the vulva. Is distinction from epithelioid sarcoma possible? A pathologic and immunohistochemical study. Am J Surg Pathol **13:**848-858, 1989.

190 Robertson AJ, McIntosh W, Lamont P, Guthrie W: Malignant granular cell tumour (myoblastoma) of the vulva. Report of a case and review of the literature. Histopathology **5:**69-79, 1981.

191 Rotmensch EJ, Kasznica J, Hamid MA: Immunohistochemical analysis of hormone receptors and proliferating cell nuclear antigen in aggressive angiomyxoma of the vulva. Int J Gynaecol Obstet **41:**171-179, 1993.

192 Santa Cruz J, Martin SA: Verruciform xanthoma of the vulva. Am J Clin Pathol **71:**224-228, 1979.

193 Shen J-T, D'Ablaing G, Morro CP: Alveolar soft part sarcoma of the vulva. Report of first case and review of literature. Gynecol Oncol **13:**120-128, 1982.

194 Skalova A, Michal M, Husek K, Zamecnik M, Leivo I: Aggressive angiomyxoma of the pelvioperineal region. Immunohistological and ultrastructural study of seven cases. Am J Dermatopathol **15:**446-451, 1993.

194a Sonobe H, Ro JY, Ramos M, Diaz I, Mackay B, Ordóñez NG, Ayala AG: Glomus tumor of the female external genitalia. A report of two cases. Int J Gynecol Pathol **13:**359-364, 1994.

195 Steeper TA, Rosai J: Aggressive angiomyxoma of the female pelvis and perineum. Report of nine cases of a distinctive type of gynecologic soft tissue neoplasm. Am J Surg Pathol **7:**463-475, 1983.

196 Strayer SA, Yum MN, Sutton GP: Epithelioid hemangioendothelioma of the clitoris. A case report with immunohistochemical and ultrastructural findings. Int J Gynecol Pathol **11:**234-239, 1992.

197 Tavassoli FA, Norris HJ: Smooth muscle tumors of the vulva. Obstet Gynecol **53:**213-217, 1979.

198 Taylor RN, Bottles K, Miller TR, Braga CA: Malignant fibrous histiocytoma of the vulva. Obstet Gynecol **66:**145-148, 1985.

199 Terada KY, Schmidt RW, Roberts JA: Malignant schwannoma of the vulva. A case report. J Reprod Med **33:**969-972, 1988.

200 Thomas R, Barnhill D, Bibro M, Hoskins W, Hambidge W: Histiocytosis-X in gynecology. A case presentation and review of the literature. Obstet Gynecol **67:**46S-49S, 1986.

201 Thomas WJ, Bevan HE, Hooper DG, Downey EJ: Malignant schwannoma of the clitoris in a 1-year-old child. Cancer **63:**2216-2219, 1989.

202 Ulbright TM, Brokaw SA, Stehman FB, Roth LM: Epithelioid sarcoma of the vulva. Evidence suggesting a more aggressive behavior than extra-genital epithelioid sarcoma. Cancer **52:**1462-1469, 1983.

203 Weinshel LR: Benign tumors of vulva. Am J Surg **71:**210-215, 1946.

204 Weissmann D, Amenta PS, Kantor GR: Vulvar epithelioid sarcoma metastatic to the scalp. A case report and review of the literature. Am J Dermatopathol **12:**462-468, 1990.

205 White J, Chan YF: Aggressive angiomyxoma of the vulva in an 11-year-old girl. Pediatr Pathol **14:**27-37, 1994.

206 Wolber RA, Talerman A, Wilkinson EJ, Clement PB: Vulvar granular cell tumors with pseudocarcinomatous hyperplasia. A comparative analysis with well-differentiated squamous carcinoma. Int J Gynecol Pathol **10:**59-66, 1991.

LESIONS OF BARTHOLIN GLANDS AND RELATED STRUCTURES

207 Andersen G, Christensen S, Detlefsen GU, Kern-Hansen P: Treatment of Bartholin's abscess. Marsupialization versus incision, curettage and suture under antibiotic cover. A randomized trial with a 6-months follow-up. Acta Obstet Gynecol Scand **71:**59-62, 1992.

208 Axe S, Parmley T, Woodruff JD, Hlopak B: Adenomas in minor vestibular glands. Obstet Gynecol **68:**16-18, 1986.

209 Chapman GW Jr, Hassan N, Page D, Mostoufi-Zadeh M, Leyman D: Mucinous cystadenoma of Bartholin's gland. A case report. J Reprod Med **32:**939-941, 1987.

210 Copeland LJ, Sneige N, Gershenson DM, McGuffee VB, Abdul-Karim F, Rutledge FN: Bartholin gland carcinoma. Obstet Gynecol **67:**794-801, 1986.

211 Copeland LJ, Sneige N, Gershenson DM, Saul PB, Stringer CA, Seski JC: Adenoid cystic carcinoma of Bartholin gland. Obstet Gynecol **67:**115-120, 1986.

212 Enghardt MH, Valente PT, Day DH: Papilloma of Bartholin's gland duct cyst. First report of a case. Int J Gynecol Pathol **12:**86-92, 1993.

213 Felix JC, Cote RJ, Kramer EE, Saigo P, Goldman GH: Carcinomas of Bartholin's gland. Histogenesis and the etiological role of human papillomavirus. Am J Pathol **142:**925-933, 1993.

214 Freedman SR, Goldman RL: Mucocele-like changes in Bartholin's glands. Hum Pathol **9:**111-114, 1978.

215 Friedrich EG Jr, Wilkinson EJ: Mucous cysts of the vulvar vestibule. Obstet Gynecol **42:**407-414, 1973.

216 Jones MA, Mann EW, Caldwell CL, Tarraza HM, Dickersin GR, Young RH: Small cell neuroendocrine carcinoma of Bartholin's gland. Am J Clin Pathol **94:**439-442, 1990.

217 Leuchter RS, Hacker NF, Voet RL, Berek JS, Townsend DE, Lagasse LD: Primary carcinoma of the Bartholin gland. A report of 14 cases and review of the literature. Obstet Gynecol **60:**361-368, 1982.

218 Milchgrub S, Wiley EL, Vuitch F, Albores-Saavedra J: The tubular variant of adenoid cystic carcinoma of the Bartholin's gland. Am J Clin Pathol **101:**204-208, 1994.

219 Mossler JA, Woodard BH, Addison A, McArty KS: Adenocarcinoma of Bartholin's gland. Arch Pathol Lab Med **104:**523-526, 1980.

220 Paquin ML, Davis JR, Weiner S: Malacoplakia of Bartholin's gland. Arch Pathol Lab Med **110:**757-758, 1986.

221 Rorat E, Ferenczy A, Richart RM: Human Bartholin gland, duct and duct cyst. Histochemical and ultrastructural study. Arch Pathol **99:**367-374, 1975.

222 Rosenberg P, Simonsen E, Risberg B: Adenoid cystic carcinoma of Bartholin's gland. A report of five new cases treated with surgery and radiotherapy. Gynecol Oncol **34:**145-147, 1989.

223 Scinicariello F, Rady P, Hannigan E, Dinh TV, Tyring SK: Human papillomavirus type 16 found in primary transitional cell carcinoma of the Bartholin's gland and in a lymph node metastasis. Gynecol Oncol **47:**263-266, 1992.

224 Wheelock JB, Goplerud DR, Dunn LJ, Oates JF III: Primary carcinoma of the Bartholin gland. A report of ten cases. Obstet Gynecol **63:**820-824, 1984.

225 Wilkinson EJ: Pathology of the vulva and vagina. In Wilkerson EJ, ed: Contemporary issues in surgical pathology, vol 9. New York, 1986, Churchill-Livingstone.

LESIONS OF THE FEMALE URETHRA

226 Benson RC, Tunca JC, Buchler DA, Uehling DT: Primary carcinoma of the female urethra. Gynecol Oncol **14:**313-318, 1982.

227 Capraro VJ, Bayonet-Rivera NP, Magoss I: Vulvar tumor in children due to pro-lapse of urethral mucosa. Am J Obstet Gynecol **108:**572-575, 1970.

228 Clayton M, Siami P, Guinan P: Urethral diverticular carcinoma. Cancer **70:**665-670, 1992.

229 Evans KJ, McCarthy MP, Sands JP: Adenocarcinoma of a female urethral diver-ticulum. Case report and review of the literature. J Urol **126:**124-126, 1981.

230 Furusato M, Takaki K, Joh K, Suzuki M, Chiba S, Nakata Y, Kakimoto S, Aizawa S, Ishikawa E: Nephrogenic adenoma in female urethra. Acta Pathol Jpn **33:**1009-1015, 1983.

231 Garden AS, Zagars GK, Delclos L: Primary carcinoma of the female urethra. Results of radiation therapy. Cancer **71:**3102-3108, 1993.

232 Grigsby PW, Corn BW: Localized urethral tumors in women. Indications for conservative versus exenterative therapies. J Urol **147:**1516-1520, 1992.

233 Jarvi OH, Marin S, de Boer WGRM: Further studies of intestinal heterotopia in urethral caruncle. Acta Pathol Microbiol Immunol Scand (A) **92:**469-474, 1984.

234 Johnson DE, O'Connell JR: Primary carcinoma of female urethra. Urology **21:**42-44, 1983.

235 Kim CJ, Pak K, Hamaguchi A, Ishida A, Arai Y, Konishi T, Okada Y, Tomoyoshi T: Primary malignant melanoma of the female urethra. Cancer **71:**448-451, 1993.

236 Marshall FC, Uson AC, Melicow MM: Neoplasms and caruncles of the female urethra. Surg Gynecol Obstet **110:**723-733, 1960.

237 Mayer R, Fowler JE Jr, Clayton M: Localized urethral cancer in women. Cancer **60:**1548-1551, 1987.

238 Meis JM, Ayala AG, Johnson DE: Adenocarcinoma of the urethra in women. A clinicopathologic study. Cancer **60:**1038-1052, 1987.

239 Mostofi FK, David CJ Jr, Sesterhenn IA: Carcinoma of the male and female ure-thra. Urol Clin North Am **19:**347-358, 1992.

240 Narayan P, Konety B: Surgical treatment of female urethral carcinoma. Urol Clin North Am **19:**373-382, 1992.

240a Ohsawa M, Mishima K, Suzuki A, Hagino K, Doi J, Aozasa K: Malignant lym-phoma of the urethra. Report of a case with detection of Epstein-Barr virus genome in the tumor cells. Histopathology **24:**525-529, 1994.

241 Odze R, Begin LR: Tubular adenomatous metaplasia (nephrogenic adenoma) of the female urethra. Int J Gynecol Pathol **8:**374-380, 1989.

242 Palmer JK, Emmett JL, McDonald JR: Urethral caruncle. Surg Gynecol Obstet **87:**611-620, 1948.

243 Prempee T, Amornmarn R, Patanaphan V: Radiation therapy in primary carci-noma of the female urethra. Part II. An update on results. Cancer **54:**729-733, 1984.

244 Rogers RE, Burns B: Carcinoma of the female urethra. Obstet Gynecol **33:**54-57, 1969.

245 Wegnaupt K, Gerstner GJ, Kucera H: Radiation therapy for primary carcinoma of the female urethra. A survey over 25 years. Gynecol Oncol **17:**58-63, 1984.

246 Wiener JS, Walther PJ: A high association of oncogenic human papillomaviruses with carcinomas of the female urethra. Polymerase chain reaction-based analysis of multiple histological types. J Urol **151:**49-53, 1994.

247 Young RH, Scully RE: Clear cell adenocarcinoma of the bladder and urethra. A re-port of three cases and review of the literature. Am J Surg Pathol **9:**816-826, 1985.

Vagina

NORMAL ANATOMY

The vagina is a tubular structure derived from the paired müllerian ducts that extend from the vestibule of the vulva to the uterus.[4] It is composed of three main layers: mucosa, muscularis, and adventitia. The mucosa is composed of stratified squamous epithelium resting on loose connective tissue stroma. The squamous epithelium can be divided, as in the exocervix, into three main zones: basal, intermediate, and superficial.[2] This epithelium is responsive to steroid hormones, its appearance depending on the age of the patient and the time of the menstrual cycle.[3]

The subepithelial stroma or lamina propria contains elastic fibers and a rich venous and lymphatic network. Polygonal to stellate stromal cells—some multinucleated—may be present.

The wolffian (mesonephric) duct in the vagina is represented by the Gartner's duct, which runs deeply along the lateral vaginal walls. Microscopically, one usually sees a small single duct, sometimes surrounded by a cluster of small glands, all of them lined by a simple cuboidal epithelium. The presence of inspissated eosinophilic secretion in the lumen is a characteristic feature of these remnants.

The lymphatic drainage of the vagina is rather complex. The vessels in the upper anterior wall join those of the cervix and terminate in the medial chain of the external iliac nodes (interiliac nodes). Those in the posterior vagina drain into deep pelvic, rectal, and aortic nodes. Some of those of the lower vagina (including the hymenal portion) go to the interiliac nodes; others traverse the paravesical spaces and drain into the inferior gluteal nodes. Finally, the vessels that anastomose with those from the vulva drain to the femoral nodes.[1,2]

ADENOSIS AND RELATED LESIONS

Adenosis of the vagina was originally described as a partial or complete conversion of the vaginal mucosa from squamous to endocervical-type glandular epithelium,[17] but the concept has been expanded to embrace the presence of any müllerian-type glandular epithelium in the vagina. Sandberg[16] found occult vaginal adenosis in nine (41%) of twenty-two vaginas from postpubertal patients obtained at autopsy but in none of thirteen prepubertal patients. Kurman and Scully[10] obtained similar results, suggesting that vaginal adenosis can arise on a congenital basis but that steroid hormones may play a stimulatory role in their development. Excess mucous discharge is the most common complaint in the symptomatic cases. Grossly, adenosis appears as red granular spots or patches that do not stain with Lugol's solution. Microscopically, there are mucin-producing glandular cells similar to those seen in the endocervix, sometimes admixed with a lesser number of cells of tubal or endometrial type[7] (Fig. 19-21).

Depending on the relative amounts of these components, a *mucinous (endocervical)* and a *tuboendometrial* form of vaginal adenosis have been described. Exceptionally, intestinal metaplasia is also encountered.[11] The glandular cells may be in the lamina propria or may line the surface of the vagina (Fig. 19-21). As a result, they may be identified in cytologic smears, which represent a useful means for the detection of this disorder.[15] Accompanying chronic inflammation and squamous metaplasia (mature, immature, or atypical) are very frequent. The latter, which is poor in cytoplasmic glycogen, can obliterate the glandular lumen and appear as a peg continuous with the surface, a feature that may cause confusion with vaginal intraepithelial neoplasia (VAIN) or even squamous cell carcinoma.[13] One should be aware, however, that lesions with the features of VAIN can superimpose themselves on foci of adenosis; the identifying features are the same as those described for similar lesions in the chapter on the uterine cervix.

Sometimes the squamous metaplasia is so extensive that the only evidence of a pre-existing adenosis is found in the form of rare intercellular pools or intracellular droplets of mucin, as shown by mucicarmine stain. It has been suggested that, as these women grow older, vaginal adenosis regresses by the process of squamous metaplasia.[14]

Microglandular hyperplasia can develop within lesions of vaginal adenosis following the use of oral contraceptives; it is important not to confuse this benign lesion with clear cell adenocarcinoma.[15]

A definite relationship between vaginal adenosis and exposure in utero to diethylstilbestrol (DES) has been documented. The reported incidence of adenosis in the exposed population has varied from 35% to more than 90% in the different series.[5] Sonek et al.[18] have shown that the incidence of vaginal adenosis and related colposcopic abnormalities is close to 100% if the drug was begun during or before the eighth week of pregnancy and only 6% if it was begun during the fifteenth week or later. The microscopic features of adenosis in women exposed in utero to DES are identical to those seen in women before the DES era.[12]

Transverse ridges and other structural anomalies are also related to DES administration.[8,9] They are found in the upper vagina or cervix in about one fourth of the exposed population and have been described as cockscomb cervix, rims, collars, hoods, and pseudopolyps. Microscopically, the ridge is composed of a core of fibrous tissue lined by mucinous epithelium, metaplastic squamous epithelium, or, rarely, tubal or endometrial epithelium. Although both vaginal

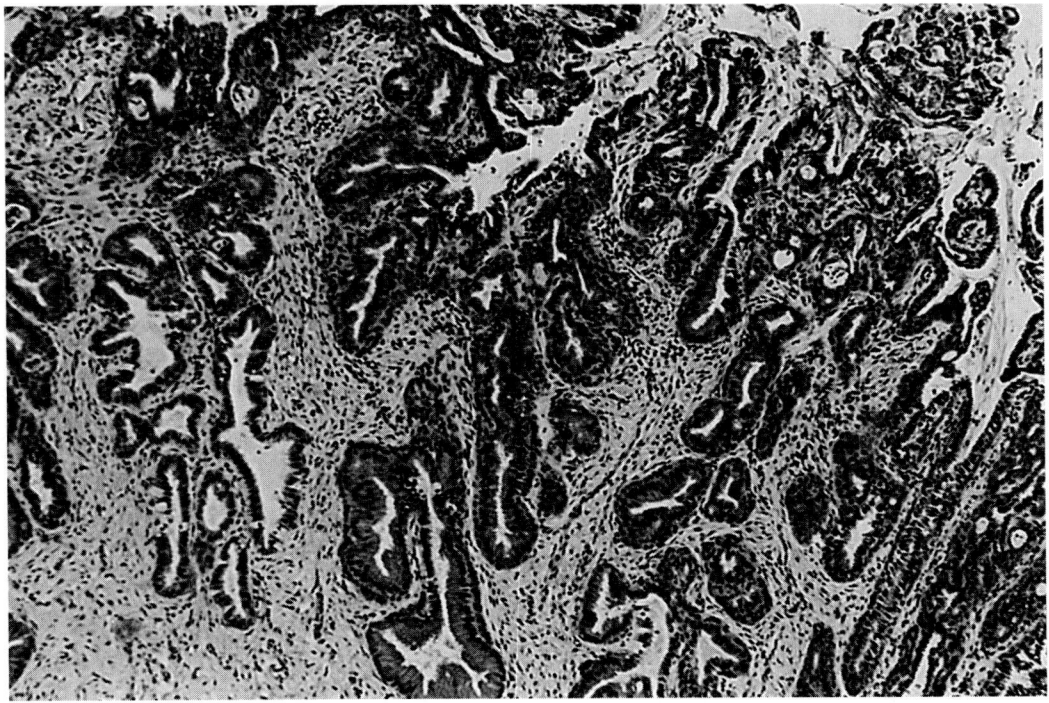

Fig. 19-21 Persistent vaginal adenosis in 27-year-old woman who had had a partial vaginectomy 7 years previously for same condition. (Slide contributed by Dr. C. Kaplan, Stony Brook, NY.)

adenosis and clear cell carcinoma are related to DES exposure (see p. 1345), it seems that the potential for the development of carcinoma from adenosis is exceedingly small.

DES-related lesions featuring immature squamous metaplasia, atypical metaplasia, and VAIN I usually revert to normal following biopsy or therapy; lesions in the VAIN II or III categories (usually characterized by an aneuploid DNA pattern by microspectrophotometry) tend to persist and recur after biopsy or therapy.[6]

OTHER NON-NEOPLASTIC LESIONS

The adult vagina is impervious to most bacterial infections. However, the overgrowth of facultative and anaerobic bacterial flora may result in a condition known as *bacterial vaginosis.* Microscopically, the most important finding is the presence of squamous cells covered with coccobacilli ("clue cells").[25] Indolent infections caused by *Trichomonas vaginalis* and *Candida albicans* are relatively common, especially during pregnancy.[27] *Lymphogranuloma venereum* can involve the vagina during the late stage of the disease and result in stricture. *Xanthogranulomatous reactions*[28] and *malakoplakia*[20] may occur as a result of unusual bacterial infections and lead to pseudotumor formation or strictures (Fig. 19-22). The use of *tampons* can result in gross vaginal ulcers.[21]

Occasionally, following vaginal hysterectomy, the **tubal fimbria** may become entrapped in the healing vaginal apex, a finding that must not be confused with a neoplastic process.[19] The clinical presentation is that of "granulation tissue" at the vaginal apex, usually appearing within 6 months following a hysterectomy.[26]

Endometriosis of the vagina is rare.[23] Its most common occurrence is in episiotomy scars.

Cysts of the vagina can be of several different types.[22] The most common is the *epithelial inclusion cyst,* lined by squamous epithelium and sometimes resulting from surgery or trauma. Another common type is characterized by a simple lining of mucin-secreting, tall columnar, nonciliated epithelium of endocervical type, sometimes associated with focal squamous metaplasia; this has been designated *müllerian cyst* and can be found anywhere in the vagina. *Mesonephric (Gartner's duct) cyst* is rare; it is located in the anterolateral or lateral vaginal wall and is lined by low cuboidal epithelial cells, sometimes ciliated, that do not secrete mucin. Other rare cystic lesions of the vagina include *urothelial cysts* (located in the suburethral portion and probably arising from paraurethral glands and Skene's ducts), *emphysematous vaginitis,*[22,24] and the already mentioned *endometriosis.*

BENIGN TUMORS

Intramural papilloma having a branching configuration and a lining of a single layer of cuboidal cells has been rarely described in children. It may present in the surface as polyps or intramurally. It is sometimes referred to as *mesonephric papilloma,* but ultrastructural studies suggest that the lesion is instead of müllerian derivation.[44]

Squamous papilloma may be seen in the adult vagina but less commonly than in the cervix. Many of the cases are probably of viral (HPV) etiology.

Tubulovillous adenoma of the vagina morphologically similar to its colorectal counterpart has been described.[35]

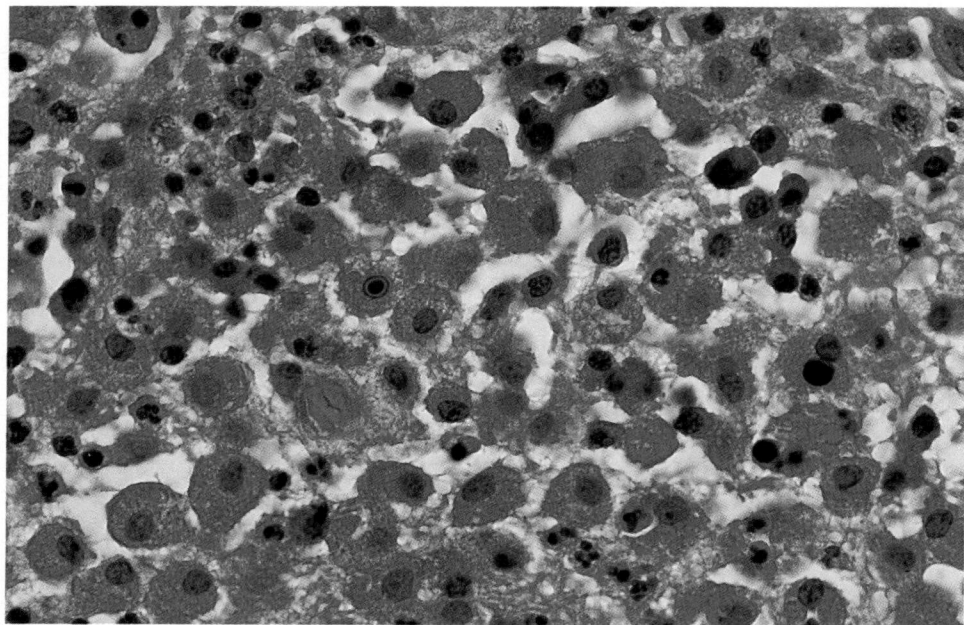

Fig. 19-22 Malakoplakia of vagina. This PAS stains shows numerous histiocytes containing particulate material in their cytoplasm.

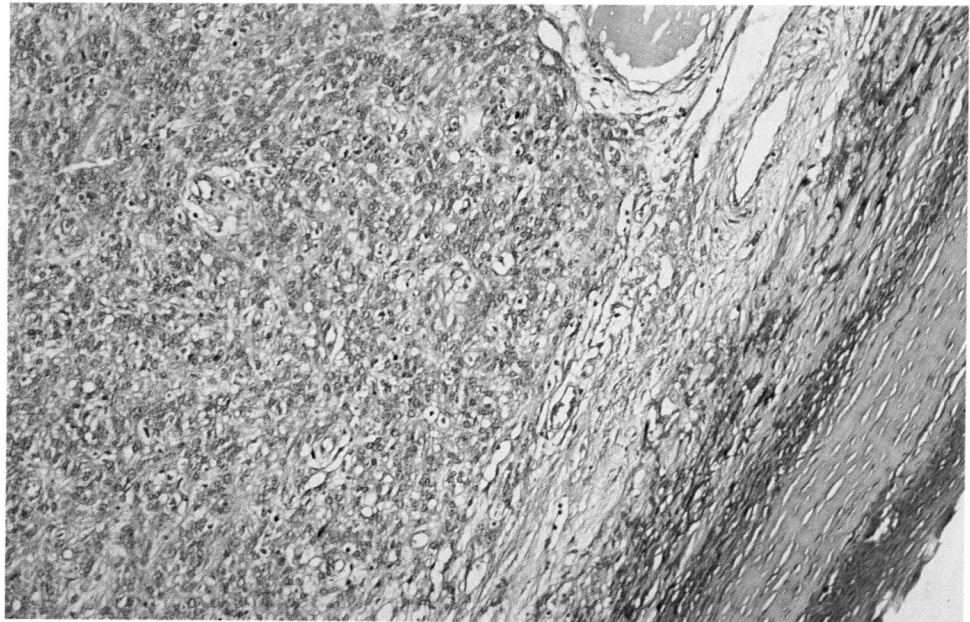

Fig. 19-23 Benign mixed tumor of vagina. The neoplasm, which is growing beneath an intact epithelium, simulates a mesenchymal neoplasm because of the solid configuration and the spindle shape of the tumor cells.

Benign mixed tumor is usually located in or near the hymenal ring. It is composed of small stromal-type spindle cells intermixed with mature squamous cells and glands lined by mucinous epithelium[39] (Fig. 19-23). Ultrastructural and immunohistochemical studies have conclusively proved its epithelial nature,[30] and the renaming of this tumor as spindle-cell epithelioma has been proposed.[30] The lesion is benign, but it may recur locally.[30,45]

Leiomyoma is the most common benign mesenchymal tumor of the vagina.[42] The patients are adults, and any region of the vagina can be affected.

Rhabdomyoma presents as a polypoid mass.[31] All of the reported cases have occurred in adult patients, an important differential point with botryoid rhabdomyosarcoma. Microscopically, the lesion consists of interweaving and haphazardly oriented bundles of spindle- to strap-shaped cells, some

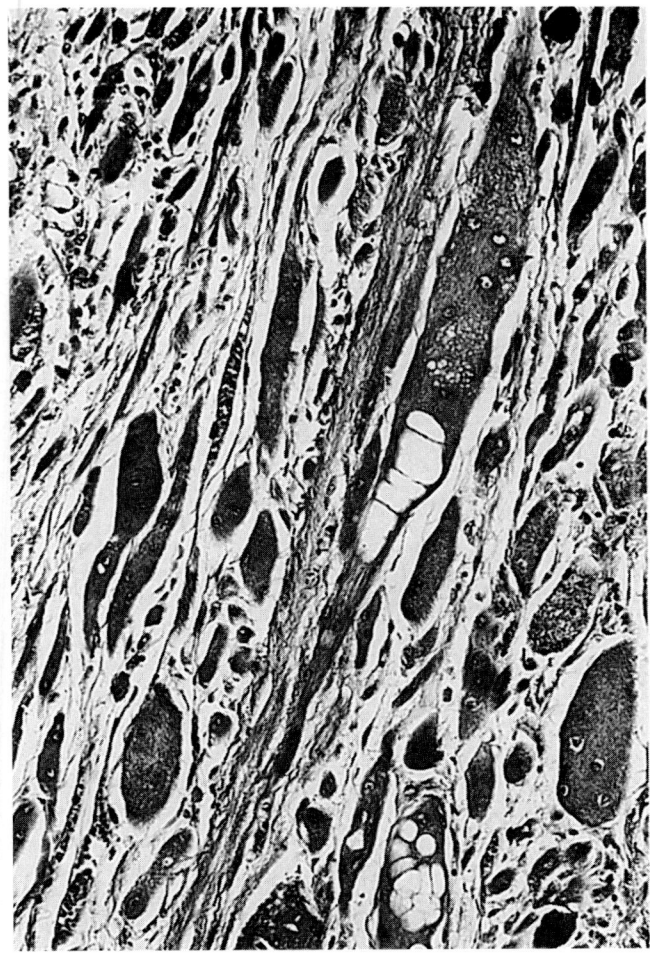

Fig. 19-24 Rhabdomyoma of vagina. Huge strap cells with cytoplasmic vacuolization are present. Cross striations were identified in several of them.

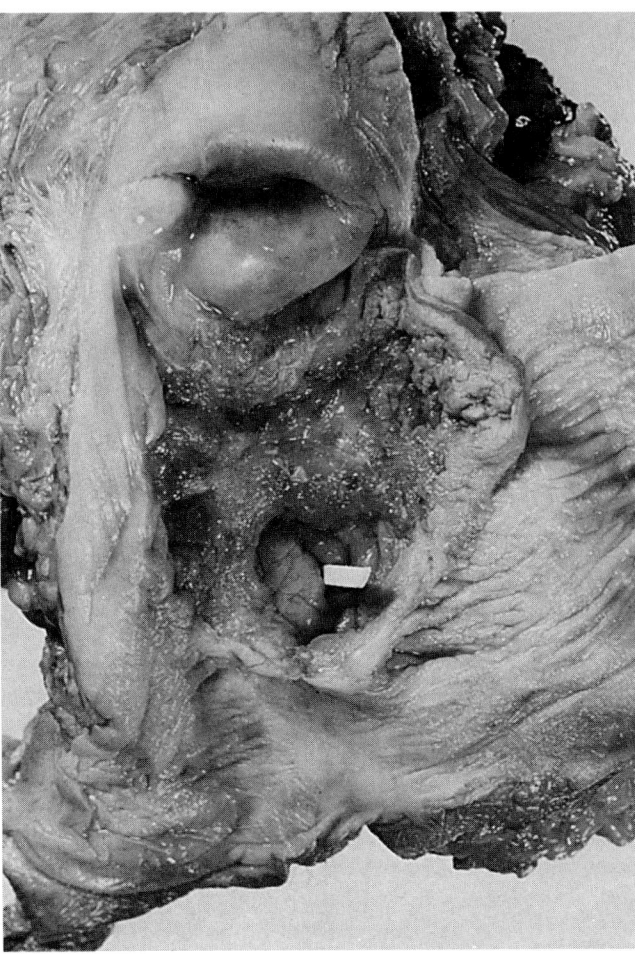

Fig. 19-25 Ulcerating carcinoma of vagina that had infiltrated recto vaginal septum. It was removed by pelvic exenteration.

with cross striations[37] (Fig. 19-24, *A*). Mitoses are scanty or absent, and there is no concentration of neoplastic cells beneath the epithelium.

Aggressive angiomyxoma can present as a protruding intravaginal mass and extend through the paravaginal soft tissue.[41] This entity is more fully described on p. 1331.

Other reported benign vaginal tumors are *hemangioma, hemangiopericytoma,*[38] *glomus tumor,*[40] *benign "triton" tumor,*[29] *angiomyolipoma,*[33] *schwannoma,*[34] *neurofibroma,*[36] *blue nevus,*[43] *Brenner's tumor,*[32] and *female adnexal tumor of probable wolffian origin.*[33a]

MALIGNANT TUMORS
Squamous cell carcinoma

Primary carcinoma of the vagina is much less common than carcinoma of the vulva or cervix.[49,61] It is largely a disease of the elderly (Fig. 19-25). HPV has been incriminated as a possible causative agent, as it has been for microscopically similar tumors of cervix and vulva.[57,60,62]

Since most carcinomas involving the vagina represent direct extension from cervical carcinomas, only vaginal tumors that spare the uterine cervix are regarded as primary. Those involving both areas are classified as cervical carcinomas with vaginal extension, regardless of the relative proportion of involvement.

Up to 20% of the patients successfully treated for CIN or invasive squamous cell carcinoma of the cervix will have abnormal cytologic smears, and some will develop a similar tumor in the vagina at a later date.[63] This event seems to be more common in those patients who were treated by irradiation alone than in those who had only surgery; the average interval is 5 or 6 years.[52,63] Therefore patients who had cervical carcinoma should have follow-up examinations for the rest of their lives, with special attention to the possibility of a vaginal recurrence or a new primary vaginal carcinoma. The area for biopsy may be detected by colposcopy, Schiller's test, or multiple smears taken from all sectors of the vagina.[58] Vaginal carcinoma can also develop following hysterectomy for benign disease; therefore regular PAP tests are still indicated after this operation.[48]

Most primary vaginal carcinomas are grossly nodular or ulcerative.[81] The upper third and the anterior or lateral walls are the most common sites of origin.[76] A few cases have been described as arising in surgically constructed neovaginas.[74]

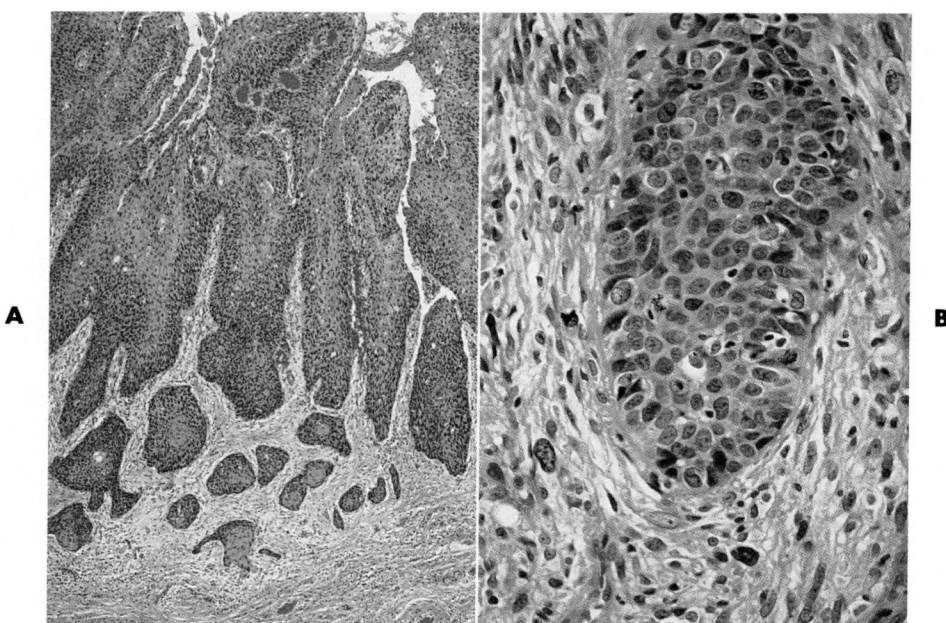

Fig. 19-26 A, Well-differentiated squamous cell carcinoma of vagina invading the superficial stroma. **B,** Spindle-cell (sarcomatoid) carcinoma of vagina. Elongated cells with a sarcoma-like appearance surround a well-defined nest having a clear-cut epithelial appearance.

Table 19-2 FIGO staging for carcinoma of the vagina

Stage 0	Carcinoma in situ, intraepithelial carcinoma.
Stage I	The carcinoma is limited to the vaginal wall.
Stage II	The carcinoma has involved the subvaginal tissue but has not extended on to the pelvic wall.
Stage III	The carcinoma has extended on to the pelvic wall.
Stage IV	The carcinoma has extended beyond the true pelvis or has clinically involved the mucosa of the bladder or rectum. Bullous edema as such does not permit a case to be allotted to Stage IV.
Stage IVA	Spread to adjacent organs and/or direct extension beyond the true pelvis.
Stage IVB	Spread to distant organs.

From SGO handbook. Staging of gynecologic malignancies. Chicago, 1994, Society of Gynecologic Oncologists.
See also Appendix G.

Microscopically, about 95% of the vaginal carcinomas are conventional squamous cell carcinomas of varying degrees of differentiation, their morphologic appearance duplicating that of their more common cervical counterparts (Fig. 19-26, *A*).

Vaginal carcinoma is usually treated by a combination of external and intracavitary radiation[59,73,78]; local excision can be employed for small tumors[66] and radical surgery for selected cases located in the upper vaginal third or posterior wall.[53,55,56] The overall 5-year survival rate is between 40% and 50%.[56,70,75] The prognosis is closely related to the stage of the disease (Table 19-2)[66,68] and is similar whether the patient has a previously treated cervical carcinoma or not.[67] Most recurrences occur within 1 year of therapy and carry an ominous prognosis. Upper lesions tend to recur locally, whereas lower lesions are more commonly associated with pelvic sidewall and distal recurrence.[80]

The existence of *microinvasive (superficially invasive) carcinoma* as a distinct clinical entity in the vagina has been proposed, but the concept faces the same theoretic and practical difficulties for a precise definition as in the vulva (see p. 1325).[69] Some of the reported cases have followed treatment for cervical carcinoma.[54]

Squamous intraepithelial lesions

Atypical squamous epithelial lesions of the vagina have been designated as *vaginal intraepithelial neoplasia* (VAIN), borrowing the terminology from the analogous lesions in the cervix (CIN).[77] It should be noted that the vaginal lesions usually arise from native squamous epithelium, in contrast to most cervical cases, which originate from *metaplastic* squamous epithelium. VAIN is multifocal in about one half of the cases and very frequently associated with concomitant, subsequent, or prior (in situ or invasive) neoplasms of the lower genital tract.[46,50,58] The upper third of the vagina is the most common site, in which case the vaginal and cervical lesions may be confluent.[64] The type of treatment depends largely on the extent of the disease and may consist of local excision, partial or total vaginectomy, CO_2 laser therapy, or administration of topical 5-fluorouracil.[47,50,51]

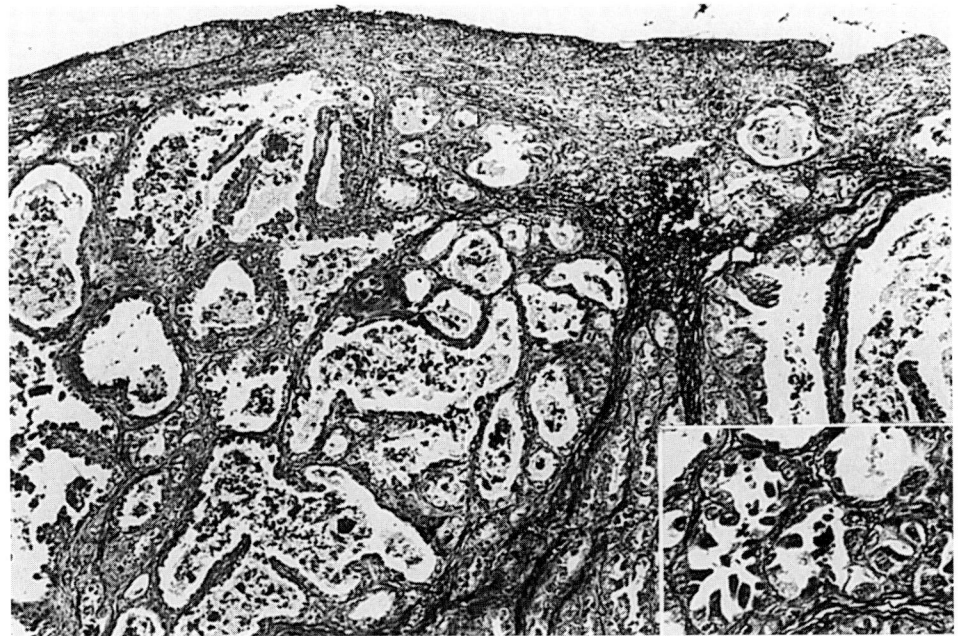

Fig. 19-27 Clear cell (mesonephroid) carcinoma of vagina in patient who was exposed to diethyl-stilbestrol during intrauterine life. **Inset** shows typical appearance of tumor cells, which protrude into lumen of glands.

Other microscopic types

Verrucous carcinoma is an extremely well-differentiated variant of squamous cell carcinoma. Like its vulvar and cervical counterparts, it invades locally but is practically never associated with lymph node metastases. The local spread can be quite extensive and reach the rectum and coccyx.[71] It should be distinguished from condyloma acuminatum, which may rarely involve the vagina; the criteria are the same as those described in the section on the vulva. HPV has been demonstrated in some cases of vaginal verrucous carcinoma.[65]

Spindle-cell (sarcomatoid) carcinoma has an appearance analogous to that more often seen in tumors of the upper aerodigestive tract; it should not be confused with a mixed müllerian tumor[72,79] (Fig. 19-26, *B*).

Other types that have been rarely described in the vagina include **transitional cell carcinoma**[47a] and **lymphoepithe-lioma-like carcinoma.**[53a]

Clear cell (adeno)carcinoma

This tumor type is also known as mesonephroid (adeno)carcinoma, both terms being preferable to the older designation, *mesonephric carcinoma.*[89,98] It characteristically occurs in the anterior or lateral wall of the upper vagina or in the uterine cervix of children, adolescents, and young adults. The average age at the time of diagnosis is 17 years. It is extremely rare before the age of 12 and after the age of 30 years. In two thirds of the patients, there is a history of prenatal exposure to DES and related nonsteroid estrogens.[90,93,100] However, the risk of carcinoma in the exposed population is low; it has been estimated to be 1 in 1000.[86,93] It has been found to be higher for those patients whose mothers began therapy before the twelfth week of pregnancy.[87]

Steroid estrogens do not seem to be associated with this complication. Most patients present with vaginal bleeding or discharge, but 16% of those studied by Herbst et al.[88] were asymptomatic. There is a very common association with vaginal adenosis, cervical ectropion, and occasional coexistence of transverse vaginal or cervical ridges. These features strongly suggest the existence of a DES-related disturbance in the development of the lower müllerian tract. Grossly, the larger tumors may involve most of the vagina. The majority are polypoid and nodular; others are flat or ulcerated, with an indurated or granular surface.[96] Most of the tumors are only superficially invasive at the time of diagnosis.

Microscopically, there are tubules and cysts lined by clear cells alternating with more solid areas and papillary formations[94] (Fig. 19-27). Mitotic figures are variable but usually scanty. The tumor cells have an abundant clear cytoplasm because of the presence of glycogen and sometimes fat. Intracytoplasmic mucin is either absent or scanty. Hobnail-shaped cells frequently are seen protruding into the glandular lumen. These cells can be detected by cytologic examination,[99] but about one fourth of patients will have a negative vaginal smear. The microscopic differential diagnosis needs to be made primarily with microglandular hyperplasia, which can occur in areas of vaginal adenosis, and the Arias-Stella reaction related to pregnancy or progestational agents. It is of interest that whereas the lesions of vaginal adenosis are usually strongly positive for mucin stain, this is almost never the case for the cells of clear cell adenocarci-

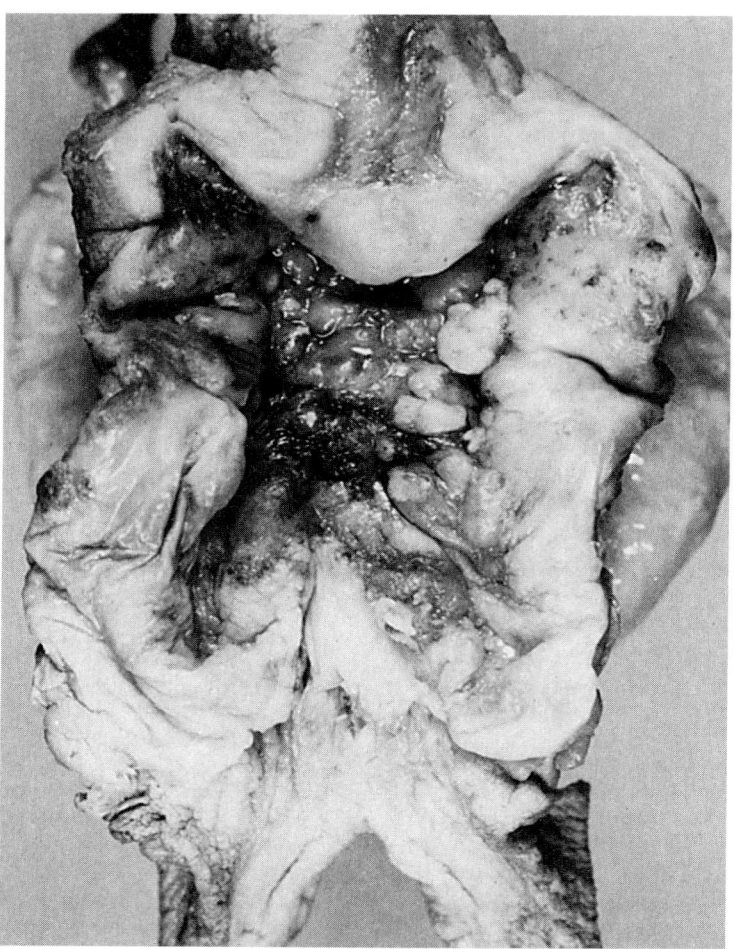

Fig. 19-28 Primary mucus-secreting adenocarcinoma of vagina in 45-year-old patient. Vaginal adenosis was identified in nontumoral vagina.

noma. The explanation given is that this tumor tends to arise from the tuboendometrial rather than the mucinous form of adenosis; support for this interpretation comes from a study showing tuboendometrial epithelium in 95% of clear cell adenocarcinomas (usually in greater concentrations at the margin of the tumor) and the presence of atypical changes in 80% of them.[97]

Ultrastructurally, the appearance of clear cell carcinoma is very similar regardless of the architecture or cytologic features as seen by light microscopy and is comparable to the clear cell carcinomas of the endometrium and ovary seen in older women.[82]

The prognosis is relatively good. Small, asymptomatic tumors usually are cured by surgery. Tumors that are large, that are close to the resection margins, or that have penetrated more than 3 mm into the wall tend to recur locally.[95] Metastases occur to pelvic lymph nodes (and sometimes those in the supraclavicular region) and lungs. In the series of Herbst et al.,[88] 24% of the patients developed persistent or recurrent disease, and 16% have died. The recur–rences can occur very late after the treatment of the primary tumor.[92]

Other adenocarcinoma types

Mucinous adenocarcinoma of vagina has been described in middle-aged and elderly patients. Its microscopic features are indistinguishable from those of its more common endocervical counterpart (Fig. 19-28). In a few cases, the appearance is reminiscent of enteric epithelium.[83,101]

Mesonephric (wolffian) adenocarcinoma is an exceptionally rare tumor located paravaginally, along the course of the wolffian-derived ducts of Gartner.[91]

Endometrioid adenocarcinoma is thought to arise on the basis of vaginal endometriosis.[85] This is also the presumed origin for most cases of adenocarcinomas located in the retrovaginal septum and having no mucosal involvement of either the vagina or rectum; this supposition is based on the fact that endometriosis is sometimes detected together with or preceding the carcinoma,[84] and because of the well-known predilection of this condition for the retrovaginal septum.[102]

Neuroendocrine carcinoma

Small cell carcinoma can occur in the vagina, either in a pure form or associated with squamous or glandular elements.[103,105,106] One case has been reported in a back-

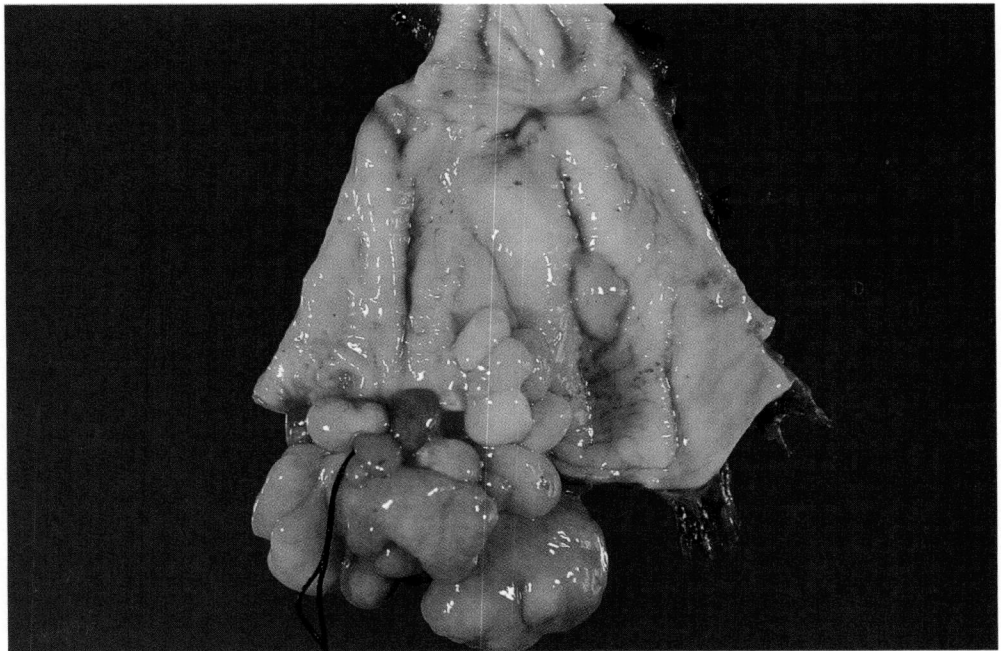

Fig. 19-29 Typical botryoid rhabdomyosarcoma of vagina. The grape-like configuration of this lesion is characteristic.

ground of atypical adenosis.[107] A high proportion of these tumors will show electron microscopic and immunohistochemical evidence of endocrine differentiation.[104,108,109] Most cases have been treated by a combination of radiation therapy and chemotherapy.[105]

Other malignant tumors

Botryoid rhabdomyosarcoma (sarcoma botryoides) is a rare polypoid invasive tumor that usually arises from the anterior vaginal wall[121] (Fig. 19-29). Approximately 90% of the cases occur in girls under 5 years of age, with close to two thirds appearing during the first 2 years. Grossly, it presents as a conglomerate of soft polypoid masses resembling a bunch of grapes—hence its name.

Microscopically, a myxoid stroma is seen containing undifferentiated round or spindle cells (Fig. 19-30). Some of these cells contain a bright eosinophilic granular cytoplasm suggestive of rhabdomyoblastic differentiation. Their racquet- or strap-shaped form mimics that of the cells seen during normal muscle embryogenesis. Cross striations may or may not be present. An important diagnostic feature is the crowding of the tumor cells around blood vessels and, most important, beneath the squamous epithelium. The latter results in a distinctive subepithelial dense zone (the "cambium layer" of Nicholson). Invasion of the overlying epithelium can be seen. Foci of neoplastic cartilage may be found; these tend to occur in older patients and/or in tumors located higher in the vagina or cervix; they are said to be associated with a better prognosis. Botryoid tumors probably represent a variation in the growth pattern of embryonal rhabdomyosarcoma, as a result of their location immediately beneath an expansile epithelial lining. They cause death more often by direct extension than by distant metastases.

Of the fifteen autopsied cases reviewed by Hilgers et al.,[123] the tumor was confined to the pelvis in about half.

The treatment of this tumor, traditionally consisting of radical surgery,[122,138] is now primarily based on chemotherapy, which can be combined with radiation therapy and/or surgery depending on the circumstances.[120]

Yolk sac tumor (endodermal sinus tumor) typically affects infants under 2 years of age and is more commonly located in either the posterior wall or the fornices.[117,142] Clinically, it stimulates botryoid rhabdomyosarcoma. Microscopically, the most important differential diagnosis is with clear cell (adeno)carcinoma, a tumor with which it has been confused in the past. Immunohistochemically, reactivity for alpha-fetoprotein favors yolk sac tumor, and reactivity for Leu-M1 favors clear cell carcinoma.[143] In early series, most patients with vaginal yolk sac carcinoma had died with generalized metastases,[130] but the combination of surgical excision and multidrug chemotherapy (sometimes with the addition of radiation therapy) has resulted in several long-term cures.[125,138]

Malignant melanoma can occur as a primary vaginal tumor in elderly patients.[116,131,136] It presents as a soft polypoid mass, blue or black, frequently ulcerated (Fig. 19-31). Most cases are located in the lower one third and in the anterolateral aspect.[110] Microscopically, the appearance is the same as that of the cutaneous melanomas, although they tend to show greater anaplasia and pleomorphism. An intraepithelial component of lentiginous appearance ("junctional activity") should be looked for to substantiate a local origin, although this feature can be destroyed by the tumor ulceration. The prognosis is extremely poor.[119,127] The melanocytes that have been identified in 3% of normal vaginas[129] most likely represent the cell of origin of this neoplasm,

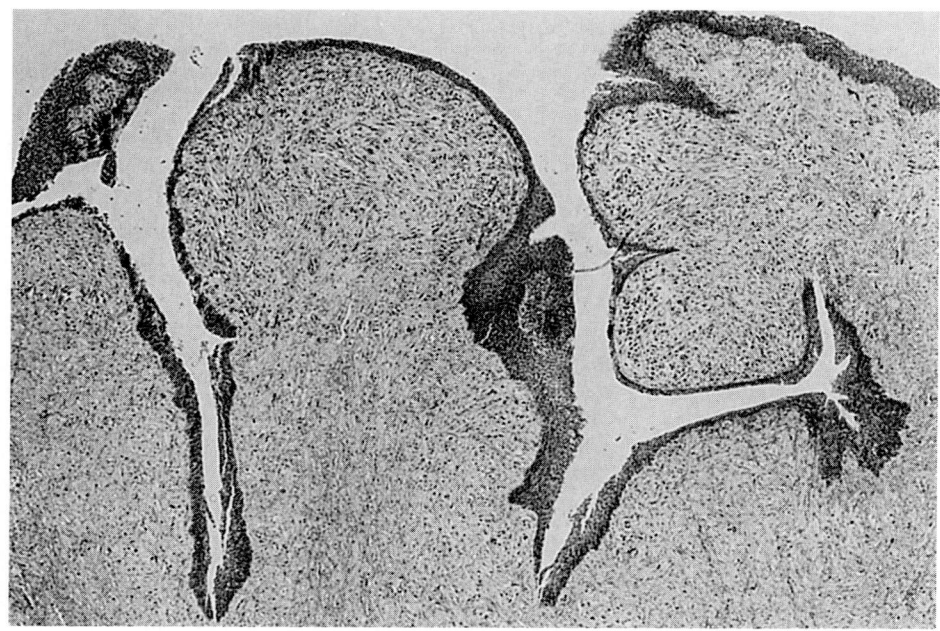

Fig. 19-30 Botryoid rhabdomyosarcoma of vagina with polypoid configuation and intact overlying epithelium. (Slide contributed by Dr. H. Ulfelder, Boston.)

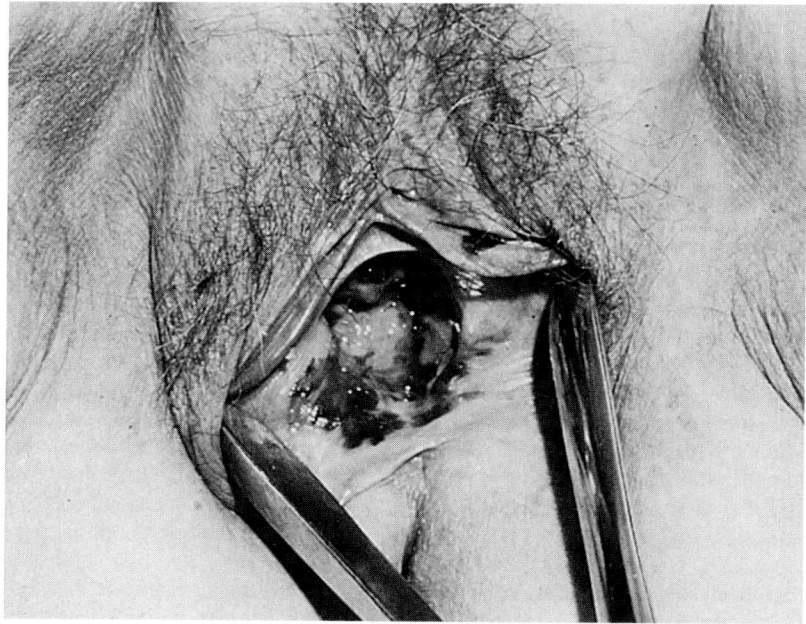

Fig. 19-31 Malignant melanoma of vagina. (From Norris HJ, Taylor HB: Melanomas of the vagina. Am J Clin Pathol **46:**420-426, 1966.)

sometimes through a preceding stage of melanosis or atypical melanocytic hyperplasia.[111,124]

Malignant lymphoma can affect the vagina secondarily or sometimes as the only site of involvement; nearly all cases are of non-Hodgkin's type.[115,118,133] Vaginal involve-

ment can also occur in acute granulocytic leukemia (granulocytic sarcoma).[118]

Malignant mixed tumor of the vagina (not to be confused with the neoplasm discussed on p. 1342) is characterized microscopically by a biphasic pattern of glands and spindle

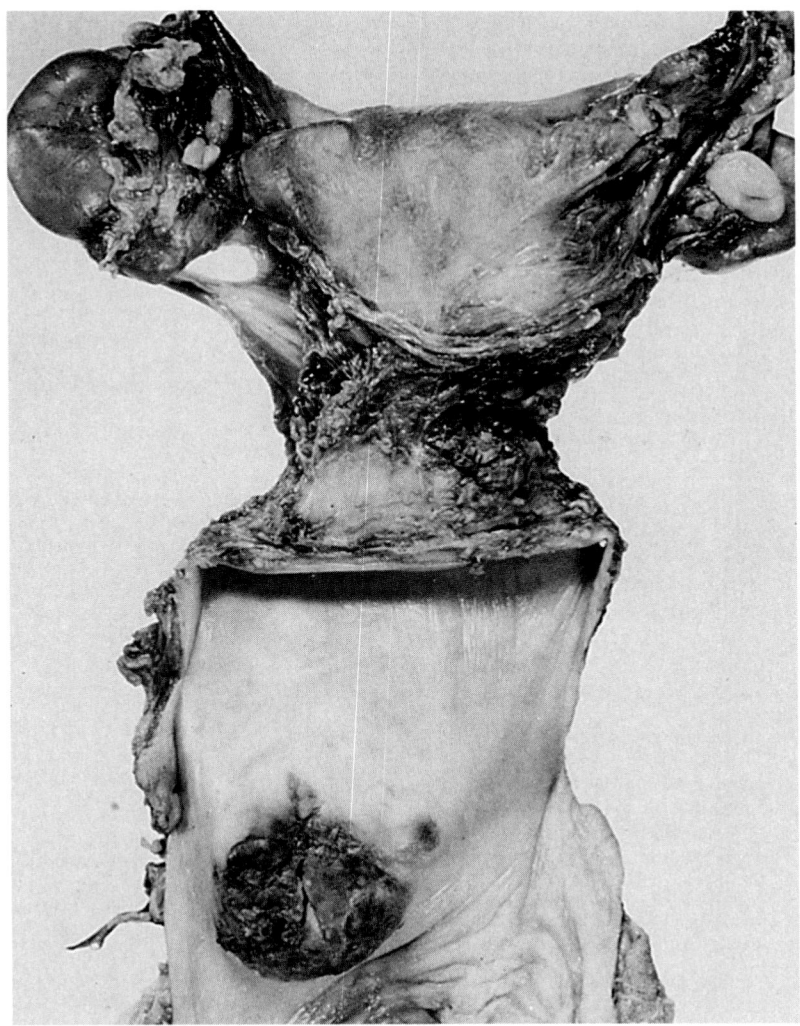

Fig. 19-32 Ulcerating large leiomyosarcoma of vagina occurring in 62-year-old woman.

cells. Its superficial resemblance to synovial sarcoma has led some observers to erroneously propose a mesenchymal origin for this neoplasm.[132] Some of the cases have been located in the upper lateral portion, and the possibility that they may arise from Gartner's ducts or related mesonephric rests has been suggested.[139]

Leiomyosarcoma can attain a large size and ulcerate (Fig. 19-32). The majority of the cases manifest their malignancy only through local recurrence. The criteria used by Tavassoli and Norris[141] were the presence of moderate to marked atypism and five or more mitotic figures per ten high-power fields. Poorly differentiated tumors are associated with a high mortality rate.[137]

Other primary malignant tumors that have been reported in the vagina are *mixed müllerian tumor,*[134] *stromal sarcoma* of endometrial type,[134] *malignant peripheral nerve sheath tumor,*[134] *angiosarcoma*[135] (sometimes arising as a complication of radiation therapy[113]), and *alveolar soft part sarcoma.*[112,114,128a]

Metastatic carcinoma to the vagina arises most commonly in the uterine cervix and endometrium, followed by the ovary, large bowel, and kidney.[126,128,140] Some cases represent direct extension, and others are distant metastases. The metastases from endometrial adenocarcinoma are often submucosal and located in the upper third of the organ. The routine practice of preoperative radiation therapy for uterine adenocarcinomas associated with uterine enlargement has reduced their frequency.

TUMORLIKE LESIONS

Fibroepithelial polyps may be seen in adult women (especially during pregnancy) or in neonates.[151] They are probably not true neoplasms but rather manifestations of hormone-induced localized hyperplasia of the loose subepithelial connective tissue zone[145]; others may represent the end stage of granulation tissue.[147] Microscopically, they are formed of a central fibrovascular core and a covering of normal-appearing squamous epithelium. Sometimes the stroma is markedly edematous[145]; in other instances it is hypercellular and/or contains scattered highly atypical stromal cells of stellate shape[144,146,149,152] (Fig. 19-17). These stromal cells are immunoreactive for vimentin, desmin, and steroid receptors but usually not for actin.[148,150] The clinical appearance, nuclear atypia, and desmin immunoreactivity may lead to a mistaken diagnosis of botryoid rhabdomyosarcoma.[151] The slow pace of growth at the clinical level and the fact that a cambium layer, epithelial invasion, and cross striations are absent are among the distinguishing features.

Postoperative spindle-cell nodule is a pseudosarcomatous vaginal lesion that occurs a few weeks following hysterectomy or some other surgical procedure in the region and presents as a small friable reddish mass in the vaginal vault.[153,154] Microscopically, it shows ulceration, granulation tissue, and a very hypercellular spindle-cell proliferation characterized by a fascicular pattern of growth, many mitotic figures, and numerous extravasated red blood cells, resulting in a Kaposi's sarcoma–like appearance.[153] It may be confused with sarcoma, particularly leiomyosarcoma. Immunohistochemically, there may be reactivity for low-molecular-weight keratin. Clues to its recognition are the distinctly fascicular pattern, the Kaposi's sarcoma–like areas, the absence of pleomorphism, the fact that the mitoses—although abundant—are all typical, and, most important, the history of a recent operation in the area.

REFERENCES

NORMAL ANATOMY

1 Hafez ESE, Evans TN, eds: The human vagina. New York, 1978, North-Holland.
2 Krantz KE: The gross and microscopic anatomy of the human vagina. Ann NY Acad Sci 83:89-104, 1959.
3 Robboy SJ, Prade M, Cunha G: Vagina. In Sternberg SS, ed: Histology for pathologists. New York, 1992, Raven Press Ltd.
4 Ulfelder H, Robboy SJ: The embryological development of the human vagina. Am J Obstet Gynecol 126:769-776, 1976.

ADENOSIS AND RELATED LESIONS

5 Antonioli DA, Burke L: Vaginal adenosis. Analysis of 325 biopsy specimens from 100 patients. Am J Clin Pathol 64:625-638, 1975.
6 Fu YS, Reagan JW, Richart RM, Townsend DE: Nuclear DNA and histologic studies of genital lesions in diethylstilbestrol-exposed progeny. I. Intraepithelial squamous abnormalities. Am J Clin Pathol 72:503-520, 1979.
7 Hart WR, Townsend DE, Aldrich JO, Henderson BE, Roy M, Benton B: Histopathologic spectrum of vaginal adenosis and related changes in stilbestrol-exposed females. Cancer 37:763-775, 1976.
8 Herbst AL, Poskanzer DC, Robboy SJ, Friedlander L, Scully RE: Prenatal exposure to stilbestrol. A prospective comparison of exposed female offspring with unexposed controls. N Engl J Med 292:334-339, 1975.
9 Jefferies JA, Robboy SJ, O'Brien PC, Bergstralh EJ, Labarthe DR, Barnes AB, Noller KL, Hatab PA, Kaufman RH, Townsend DE: Structural anomalies of the cervix and vagina in women enrolled in the Diethylstilbestrol Adenosis (DESAD) Project. Am J Obstet Gynecol 148:59-66, 1984.
10 Kurman RJ, Scully RE: The incidence and histogenesis of vaginal adenosis. An autopsy study. Hum Pathol 5:265-276, 1974.
11 Merchant WJ, Gale J: Intestinal metaplasia in stilboestrol-induced vaginal adenosis. Histopathology 23:373-376, 1993.
12 Robboy SJ, Hill EC, Sandberg EC, Czernobilsky B: Vaginal adenosis in women born prior to the diethylstilbestrol era. Hum Pathol 17:488-492, 1986.
13 Robboy SJ, Scully RE, Welch WR, Herbst AL: Intrauterine diethylstilbestrol exposure and its consequences. Pathologic characteristics of vaginal adenosis, clear cell adenocarcinoma, and related lesions. Arch Pathol Lab Med 101:1-5, 1977.
14 Robboy SJ, Szyfelbein WM, Goellner JR, Kaufman RH, Taft PD, Richard RM, Gaffey TA, Prat J, Virata R, Hatab PA, McGorray SP, Noller KL, Townsend D, Lobarthe D, Barnes AB: Dysplasia and cytologic findings in 4589 young women enrolled in Diethylstilbestrol Adenosis (DESAD) Project. Am J Obstet Gynecol 140:579-586, 1981.
15 Robboy SJ, Welch WR: Microglandular hyperplasia in vaginal adenosis associated with oral contraceptives and prenatal diethylstilbestrol exposure. Obstet Gynecol 49:430-434, 1977.
16 Sandberg EC: The incidence of distribution of occult vaginal adenosis. Trans Pac Coast Obstet Gynecol Soc 35:36-48, 1967.
17 Siders DB, Parrott MH, Abell MR: Gland cell prosoplasia (adenosis) of vagina. Am J Obstet Gynecol 91:190-203, 1965.
18 Sonek M, Bibbo M, Wied GL: Colposcopic findings in offspring of DES-treated mothers as related to onset of therapy. J Reprod Med 16:65-71, 1976.

OTHER NON-NEOPLASTIC LESIONS

19 Bilodeau B: Intravaginal prolapse of the fallopian tube following vaginal hysterectomy. Am J Obstet Gynecol 143:970-971, 1982.
20 Chalvardjan A, Picard L, Shaw R, Davey R, Cairns JD: Malacoplakia of the female genital tract. Am J Obstet Gynecol 138:391-394, 1980.
21 Danielson RW: Vaginal ulcers caused by tampons. Am J Obstet Gynecol 146:547-548, 1983.
22 Deppisch LM: Cysts of the vagina. Classification and clinical correlations. Obstet Gynecol 45:632-637, 1975.
23 Gardner HL: Cervical and vaginal endometriosis. Clin Obstet Gynecol 9:358-372, 1966.
24 Kramer K, Tobón H: Vaginitis emphysematosa. Arch Pathol Lab Med 111:746-749, 1987.
25 Robboy SJ, Welch WR: Selected topics in the pathology of the vagina. Hum Pathol 22:868-878, 1991.
26 Silverberg SG, Frable WJ: Prolapse of fallopian tube into vaginal vault after hysterectomy. Histopathology, cytopathology, and differential diagnosis. Arch Pathol 97:100-103, 1974.
27 Sobel JD: Vaginal infections in adult women. Med Clin North Am 74:1573-1602, 1990.
28 Strate SM, Taylor WE, Forney JP, Silva FG: Xanthogranulomatous pseudotumor of the vagina. Evidence of a local response to an unusual bacterium (mucoid *Escherichia coli*). Am J Clin Pathol 79:637-643, 1983.

BENIGN TUMORS

29 Azzopardi JG, Eusebi V, Tison V, Betts CM: Neurofibroma with rhabdomyomatous differentiation. Benign "triton" tumour of the vagina. Histopathology 7:561-572, 1983.
30 Branton PA, Tavassoli FA: Spindle cell epithelioma, the so-called mixed tumor of the vagina. A clinicopathologic, immunohistochemical, and ultrastructural analysis of 28 cases. Am J Surg Pathol 17:509-515, 1993.
31 Chabrel CM, Beilby JOW: Vaginal rhabdomyoma. Histopathology 4:645-651, 1980.
32 Chen KTK: Brenner tumor of the vagina. Diagn Gynecol Obstet 3:255-258, 1981.
33 Chen KT: Angiomyolipoma of the vagina. Gynecol Oncol 37:302-304, 1990.
33a Daya D, Murphy J, Simon G: Paravaginal female adnexal tumor of probable wolffian origin. Am J Clin Pathol 101:275-278, 1994.
34 Ellison DW, Mac Kenzie IZ, McGee JO: Cellular schwannoma of the vagina. Gynecol Oncol 46:119-121, 1992.
35 Fox H, Wells M, Harris M, McWilliam LJ, Anderson GS: Enteric tumours of the lower female genital tract. A report of three cases. Histopathology 12:167-176, 1988.
36 Gersell DJ, Fulling KH: Localized neurofibromatosis of the female genitourinary tract. Am J Surg Pathol 13:873-878, 1989.
37 Gold JH, Bossen EH: Benign vaginal rhabdomyoma. A light and electron microscopic study. Cancer 37:2283-2294, 1976.
38 Hiura M, Nogawa T, Nagai N, Yorishima M, Fujiwara A: Vaginal hemangiopericytoma. A light microscopic and ultrastructural study. Gynecol Oncol 21:376-384, 1985.
39 Sirota RL, Dickersin GR, Scully RE: Mixed tumors of the vagina. Am J Surg Pathol 5:413-422, 1981.
40 Spitzer M, Molho L, Seltzer VL, Lipper S: Vaginal glomus tumor. Case presentation and ultrastructural findings. Obstet Gynecol 66:86S-88S, 1985.
41 Steeper TA, Rosai J: Aggressive angiomyxoma of the female pelvis and perineum. Report of nine cases of a distinctive type of gynecologic soft tissue neoplasm. Am J Surg Pathol 7:463-475, 1983.
42 Tavassoli FA, Norris HJ: Smooth muscle tumors of the vagina. Obstet Gynecol 53:689-693, 1979.
43 Tobon H, Murphy AI: Benign blue nevus of the vagina. Cancer 40:3174-3176, 1977.
44 Ulbright TM, Alexander RW, Kraus FT: Intramural papilloma of the vagina. Evidence of müllerian histogenesis. Cancer 48:2260-2266, 1981.
45 Wright RG, Buntine DW, Forbes KL: Recurrent benign mixed tumor of the vagina. Gynecol Oncol 40:84-86, 1991.

MALIGNANT TUMORS
Squamous cell carcinoma; squamous intraepithelial lesions; other microscopic types

46 Aho M, Vesterinen E, Meyer B, Purola E, Paavonen J: Natural history of vaginal intraepithelial neoplasia. Cancer 68:195-197, 1991.
47 Audet-Lapointe P, Body G, Vauclair R, Drouin P, Ayoub J: Vaginal intraepithelial neoplasia. Gynecol Oncol 36:232-239, 1990.

47a Bass PS, Birch B, Smart C, Theaker JM, Wells M: Low-grade transitional cell carcinoma of the vagina. An unusual cause of vaginal bleeding. Histopathology **24**:581-583, 1994.

48 Bell J, Sevin B-U, Averette H, Nadji M: Vaginal cancer after hysterectomy for benign disease. Value of cytologic screening. Obstet Gynecol **64**:699-702, 1984.

49 Benedet JL: Vaginal malignancy. Curr Opin Obstet Gynecol **3**:73-77, 1991.

50 Benedet JL, Sanders BH: Carcinoma in situ of the vagina. Am J Obstet Gynecol **148**:695-700, 1984.

51 Caglar H, Hertzog RW, Hreshchyshyn MM: Topical 5-fluorouracil treatment of vaginal intraepithelial neoplasia. Obstet Gynecol **58**:580-583, 1981.

52 Choo YC, Anderson DG: Neoplasms of the vagina following cervical carcinoma. Gynecol Oncol **14**:125-132, 1982.

53 Davis KP, Stanhope CR, Garton GR, Atkinson EJ, O'Brien PC: Invasive vaginal carcinoma. Analysis of early-stage disease. Gynecol Oncol **42**:131-136, 1991.

53a Dietl J, Horny HP, Kaiserling E: Lymphoepithelioma-like carcinoma of the vagina. A case report with special reference to the immunophenotype of the tumor cells and tumor-infiltrating lymphoreticular cells. Int J Gynecol Pathol **13**:186-189, 1994.

54 Eddy GL, Singh KP, Gansler TS: Superficially invasive carcinoma of the vagina following treatment for cervical cancer. A report of six cases. Gynecol Oncol **36**:376-379, 1990.

55 Gray LA, Christopherson WM: In situ and early invasive carcinoma of the vagina. Obstet Gynecol **34**:226-230, 1969.

56 Houghton CRS, Iversen T: Squamous cell carcinoma of the vagina. A clinical study of the location of the tumor. Gynecol Oncol **13**:365-372, 1982.

57 Ikenberg H, Runge M, Goppinger A, Pfeiderer A: Human papillomavirus DNA in invasive carcinoma of the vagina. Obstet Gynecol **76**:432-438, 1990.

58 Kanbour AI, Klionsky B, Murphy AI: Carcinoma of the vagina following cervical cancer. Cancer **34**:1838-1841, 1974.

59 Kucera H, Vavra N: Radiation management of primary carcinoma of the vagina. Clinical and histopathological variables associated with survival. Gynecol Oncol **40**:12-16, 1991.

60 Macnab JCM, Walkinshaw SA, Cordiner JW, Clements JB: Human papillomavirus in clinically and histologically normal tissue of patients with genital cancer. N Engl J Med **315**:1052-1058, 1986.

61 Manetta A, Gutrecht EL, Berman ML, Di Saia PJ: Primary invasive carcinoma of the vagina. Obstet Gynecol **76**:639-642, 1990.

62 Merino MJ: Vaginal cancer. The role of infectious and environmental factors. Am J Obstet Gynecol **165**:1255-1262, 1991.

63 Murad TM, Durant JR, Maddox WA, Dowling EA: The pathologic behavior of primary vaginal carcinoma and its relationship to cervical cancer. Cancer **35**:787-794, 1975.

64 Nwabineli NJ, Monaghan JM: Vaginal epithelial abnormalities in patients with CIN. Clinical and pathological features and management. Br J Obstet Gynaecol **98**:25-29, 1991.

65 Okagaki T, Clark BA, Zachow KR, Twiggs LB, Ostrow RS, Pass F, Faras AJ: Presence of human papillomavirus in verrucous carcinoma (Ackerman) of the vagina. Immunocytochemical, ultrastructural, and DNA hybridization studies. Arch Pathol Lab Med **108**:567-570, 1984.

66 Perez CA, Arneson AN, Dehner LP, Galakatos A: Radiation therapy in carcinoma of the vagina. Obstet Gynecol **44**:862-872, 1974.

67 Perez CA, Arneson AN, Galakatos A, Samanth HK: Malignant tumors of the vagina. Cancer **31**:36-44, 1973.

68 Peters WA III, Kumar NB, Morley GW: Carcinoma of the vagina. Factors influencing treatment outcome. Cancer **55**:892-897, 1985.

69 Peters WA III, Kumar NB, Morley GW: Microinvasive carcinoma of the vagina. A distinct clinical entity? Am J Obstet Gynecol **153**:505-507, 1985.

70 Prempree T, Viravathana T, Slawson RG, Wizenberg MJ, Cuccia CA: Radiation management of primary carcinoma of the vagina. Cancer **40**:109-118, 1977.

71 Ramzy I, Smout MS, Collins JA: Verrucous carcinoma of the vagina. Am J Clin Pathol **65**:644-653, 1976.

72 Raptis S, Haber G, Ferenczy A: Vaginal squamous cell carcinoma with sarcomatoid spindle cell features. Gynecol Oncol **49**:100-106, 1993.

73 Reddy S, Lee MS, Graham JE, Yordan EL, Phillips R, Saxena VS, Hendrickson FR, Wilbanks GD: Radiation therapy in primary carcinoma of the vagina. Gynecol Oncol **26**:19-24, 1987.

74 Rotmensch J, Rosenshein N, Dillon M, Murphy A, Woodruff JD: Carcinoma arising in the neovagina. Case report and review of the literature. Obstet Gynecol **61**:534-538, 1983.

75 Rubin SC, Young J, Mikuta JJ: Squamous carcinoma of the vagina. Treatment complications and long-term follow-up. Gynecol Oncol **20**:346-353, 1985.

76 Rutledge F: Cancer of the vagina. Am J Obstet Gynecol **97**:635-655, 1967.

77 Sherman ME, Paull G: Vaginal intraepithelial neoplasia. Reproducibility of pathologic diagnosis and correlation of smears and biopsies. Acta Cytol **37**:699-704, 1993.

78 Spirtos NM, Doshi BP, Kapp DS, Teng N: Radiation therapy for primary squamous cell carcinoma of the vagina. Stanford University experience. Gynecol Oncol **35**:20-26, 1989.

79 Steeper TA, Piscioli F, Rosai J: Squamous cell carcinoma with sarcoma-like stroma of the female genital tract. Clinicopathologic study of four cases. Cancer **52**:890-898, 1983.

80 Tarraza MH Jr, Muntz H, Decain M, Granai OC, Fuller A Jr: Patterns of recurrence of primary carcinoma of the vagina. Eur J Gynaecol Oncol **12**:89-92, 1991.

81 Whelton J, Kottmeier HL: Primary carcinoma of the vagina. A study of a Radium-hemmet series of 145 cases. Acta Obstet Gynecol Scand **41**:22-40, 1962.

Clear cell (adeno)carcinoma; other adenocarcinoma types

82 Dickersin GR, Welch WR, Erlandson R, Robboy SJ: Ultrastructure of 16 cases of clear cell adenocarcinoma of the vagina and cervix in young women. Cancer **45**:1615-1624, 1980.

83 Fox A, Wells M, Harris M, McWilliam LJ, Anderson GS: Enteric tumours of the lower female genital tract. A report of three cases. Histopathology **12**:167-176, 1988.

84 Granai CO, Walters MD, Safaii H, Jelen I, Madoc-Jones H, Moukhtar M: Malignant transformation of vaginal endometriosis. Obstet Gynecol **64**:592-595, 1984.

85 Haskel S, Chen SS, Spiegel G: Vaginal endometrioid adenocarcinoma arising in vaginal endometriosis. A case report and literature review. Gynecol Oncol **34**:232-236, 1989.

86 Herbst AL, Anderson D: Clear cell adenocarcinoma of the vagina and cervix secondary to intrauterine exposure to diethylstilbestrol. Semin Surg Oncol **6**:343-346, 1990.

87 Herbst AL, Anderson S, Hubby MM, Haenszel WM, Kaufmann RH, Noller KL: Risk factors for the development of diethylstilbestrol-associated clear cell adenocarcinoma. A case-control study. Am J Obstet Gynecol **154**:814-822, 1986.

88 Herbst AL, Robboy SJ, Scully RE, Poskanzer DC: Clear-cell adenocarcinoma of the vagina and cervix in girls. Analysis of 170 registry cases. Am J Obstet Gynecol **119**:713-724, 1974.

89 Herbst AL, Scully RE: Adenocarcinoma of the vagina in adolescence. A report of 7 cases including 6 clear-cell carcinomas (so-called mesonephromas). Cancer **25**:745-757, 1970.

90 Herbst AL, Ulfelder H, Poskanzer DC: Adenocarcinoma of the vagina. Association of maternal stilbestrol therapy with tumor appearance in young women. N Engl J Med **284**:878-881, 1971.

91 Hinchey WW, Silva EG, Guarda LA, Ordonez NG, Wharton JT: Paravaginal Wolffian duct (mesonephros) adenocarcinoma. A light and electron microscopic study. Am J Clin Pathol **80**:539-544, 1983.

92 Jones WB, Tan LK, Lewis JL Jr: Late recurrence of clear cell adenocarcinoma of the vagina and cervix. A report of three cases. Gynecol Oncol **51**:266-271, 1993.

93 Melnick S, Cole P, Anderson D, Herbst A: Rates and risks of diethylstilbestrol-related clear-cell adenocarcinoma of the vagina and cervix. An update. N Engl J Med **316**:514-516, 1987.

94 Nordqvist SRB, Fidler WJ Jr, Woodruff JM, Lewis JL: Clear cell adenocarcinoma of the cervix and vagina. A clinicopathologic study of 21 cases with and without a history of maternal ingestion of estrogens. Cancer **37**:858-871, 1976.

95 Robboy SJ, Herbst AL, Scully RE: Clear-cell adenocarcinoma of the vagina and cervix in young females. Analysis of 37 tumors that persisted or recurred after primary therapy. Cancer **34**:606-614, 1974.

96 Robboy SJ, Scully RE, Welch WR, Herbst AL: Intrauterine diethylstilbestrol exposure and its consequences. Pathologic characteristics of vaginal adenosis, clear cell adenocarcinoma, and related lesions. Arch Pathol Lab Med **101**:1-5, 1977.

97 Robboy SJ, Young RH, Welch WR, Truslow GV, Prat J, Herbst AL, Scully RE: Atypical vaginal adenosis and cervical ectropion. Association with clear cell adenocarcinoma in diethylstilbestrol-exposed offspring. Cancer **54**:869-875, 1984.

98 Silverberg SG, DeGiorgi LS: Clear cell carcinoma of the vagina. Cancer **29**:262-272, 1972.

99 Taft PD, Robboy SJ, Herbst AL, Scully RE: Cytology of clear-cell adenocarcinoma of the genital tract in young females. Report of 95 cases from the registry. Acta Cytol (Baltimore) **18**:279-290, 1974.

100 Welch WR, Prat J, Robboy SJ, Herbst AL: Pathology of prenatal diethylstilbestrol exposure. Pathol Annu **13**(Pt 1):201-216, 1978.

101 Yaghsezian H, Palazzo JP, Finkel GC, Carlson JA Jr, Talerman A: Primary vaginal adenocarcinoma of the intestinal type associated with adenosis. Gynecol Oncol **45**:62-65, 1992.

102 Young EE, Gamble CH: Primary adenocarcinoma of the rectovaginal septum arising from endometriosis. Report of a case. Cancer **24**:597-601, 1969.

Neuroendocrine carcinoma

103 Chafe W: Neuroepithelial small cell carcinoma of the vagina. Cancer **64:**1948-1951, 1989.

104 Fukushima M, Twiggs LB, Okagaki T: Mixed intestinal adenocarcinoma. Argentaffin carcinoma of the vagina. Gynecol Oncol 23:387-394, 1986.

105 Hopkins MP, Kumar NB, Lichter AS, Peters WA, Morley GW: Small cell carcinoma of the vagina with neuroendocrine features. A report of three cases. J Reprod Med **34:**486-491, 1989.

106 Miliauskas JR, Leong AS: Small cell (neuroendocrine) carcinoma of the vagina. Histopathology 21:371-374, 1992.

107 Prasad CJ, Ray JA, Kessler S: Primary small cell carcinoma of the vagina arising in a background of atypical adenosis. Cancer 70:2484-2487, 1992.

108 Rusthoven JJ, Daya D: Small-cell carcinoma of the vagina. A clinicopathologic study. Arch Pathol Lab Med **114:**728-731, 1990.

109 Ulich TR, Liao S-Y, Layfield L, Romansky S, Cheng L, Lewin KJ: Endocrine and tumor differentiation markers in poorly differentiated small-cell carcinoids of the cervix and vagina. Arch Pathol Lab Med 110:1054-1057, 1986.

Other malignant tumors

110 Borazjani G, Prem KA, Okagaki T, Twiggs LB, Adcock LL: Primary malignant melanoma of the vagina. A clinicopathological analysis of 10 cases. Gynecol Oncol **37:**264-267, 1990.

111 Bottles K, Lacey CG, Miller TR: Atypical melanocytic hyperplasia of the vagina. Gynecol Oncol 19:226-230, 1984.

112 Carinelli SG, Giudici MN, Brioschi D, Cefis F: Alveolar soft part sarcoma of the vagina. Tumori **76:**77-80, 1990.

113 Chan WW, Sen Gupta SK: Postirradiation angiosarcoma of the vaginal vault. Arch Pathol Lab Med **115:**527-528, 1991.

114 Chapman GW, Genda J, Williams T: Alveolar soft-part sarcoma of the vagina. Gynecol Oncol **18:**125-129, 1984.

115 Chorlton I, Karnei RF Jr, Norris HJ: Primary malignant reticuloendothelial disease involving the vagina, cervix, and corpus uteri. Obstet Gynecol **44:**735-748, 1974.

116 Chung AF, Casey MJ, Flannery JT, Woodruff JM, Lewis JL Jr: Malignant melanoma of the vagina. Report of 19 cases. Obstet Gynecol **55:**720-727, 1980.

117 Copeland LJ, Sneige N, Ordonex NG, Hancock KC, Gershenson DM, Saul PB, Kavanagh JJ: Endodermal sinus tumor of the vagina and cervix. Cancer **55:**2558-2565, 1985.

118 Harris NL, Scully RE: Malignant lymphoma and granulocytic sarcoma of the uterus and vagina. A clinicopathologic analysis of 27 cases. Cancer **53:**2530-2545, 1984.

119 Hasumi K, Sakamoto G, Sugano H, Kasuga T, Masubuchi K: Primary malignant melanoma of the vagina. Study of four autopsy cases with ultrastructural findings. Cancer **42:**2675-2686, 1978.

120 Hays DM, Shimada H, Raney RB Jr, Tefft M, Newton W, Crist WM, Lawrence W Jr, Ragab A, Beltangady M, Maurer HM: Clinical staging and treatment results in rhabdomyosarcoma of the female genital tract among children and adolescents. Cancer **61:**1893-1903, 1988.

121 Hays DM, Shimada H, Raney RB Jr, Tefft M, Newton W, Crist WM, Lawrence W Jr, Ragab A, Maurer HM: Sarcomas of the vagina and uterus. The Intergroup Rhabdomyosarcoma Study. J Pediatr Surg **20:**718-724, 1985.

122 Hilgers RD: Pelvic exenteration for vaginal embryonal rhabdomyosarcoma. A review. Obstet Gynecol **45:**175-180, 1975.

123 Hilgers R, Malkasian GD Jr, Soule EH: Embryonal rhabdomyosarcoma (botryoid type) of the vagina. A clinicopathologic review. Am J Obstet Gynecol **107:**484-502, 1970.

124 Kerley SW, Blute ML, Keeney GL: Multifocal malignant melanoma arising in vesicovaginal melanosis. Arch Pathol Lab Med **115:**950-952, 1991.

125 Kohorn EI, McIntosh S, Lytton B, Knowlton AH, Merino M: Endodermal sinus tumor of the infant vagina. Gynecol Oncol 20:196-203, 1985.

126 Mazur MT, Hsueh S, Gersell DJ: Metastases to the female genital tract. Analysis of 325 cases. Cancer **53:**1978-1984, 1984.

127 Morrow CP, DiSaia PJ: Malignant melanoma of the female genitalia. A clinical analysis. Obstet Gynecol Surv **31:**233-271, 1976.

128 Nerdrum TA: Vaginal metastasis of hypernephroma. Report of three cases. Acta Obstet Gynecol Scand 45:515-524, 1966.

128a Nielsen GP, Oliva E, Young RH, Rosenberg AE, Dickersin GR, Scully RE: Alveolar soft-part sarcoma of the female genital tract. A report of nine cases and review of the literature. Int J Gynecol Pathol 14:283-292, 1995.

129 Nigogosyan G, De La Pava S, Pickren JW: Melanoblasts in the vaginal mucosa. Origin for primary malignant melanoma. Cancer 17:912-913, 1964.

130 Norris HJ, Bagley GP, Taylor HB: Carcinoma of the infant vagina. A distinctive tumor. Arch Pathol **90:**473-479, 1970.

131 Norris HJ, Taylor HB: Melanomas of the vagina. Am J Clin Pathol **46:**420-426, 1966.

132 Okagaki T, Ishida T, Hilgers RD: A malignant tumor of the vagina resembling synovial sarcoma. A light and electron microscopic study. Cancer 37:2306-2320, 1976.

133 Perren T, Farrant M, McCarthy K, Harper P, Wiltshaw E: Lymphomas of the cervix and upper vagina. A report of five cases and a review of the literature. Gynecol Oncol **44:**87-95, 1992.

134 Peters WA III, Kumar NB, Anderson WA, Morley GW: Primary sarcoma of the adult vagina. A clinicopathologic study. Obstet Gynecol **63:**699-704, 1985.

135 Prempree T, Tang C-K, Hatef A, Forster S: Angiosarcoma of the vagina. A clinicopathologic report. A reappraisal of the radiation treatment of angiosarcomas of the female genital tract. Cancer **51:**618-622, 1983.

136 Ragnarsson-Olding B, Johansson H, Rutqvist LE, Ringborg U: Malignant melanoma of the vulva and vagina. Trends in incidence, age distribution, and long-term survival among 245 consecutive cases in Sweden 1960-1984. Cancer **71:**1893-1897, 1993.

137 Rastogi BL, Bergman B, Angervall L: Primary leiomyosarcoma of the vagina. A study of five cases. Gynecol Oncol **18:**77-86, 1984.

138 Rutledge F, Sullivan MP: Sarcoma botryoides. Ann NY Acad Sci **142:**694-708, 1967.

139 Shevchuk MM, Fenoglio CM, Lattes R, Frick HC II, Richart RM: Malignant mixed tumor of the vagina probably arising in mesonephric rests. Cancer 42:214-233, 1978.

140 Stander RW: Vaginal metastases following treatment of endometrial carcinoma. Am J Obstet Gynecol **71:**776-779, 1956.

141 Tavassoli FA, Norris HJ: Smooth muscle tumors of the vagina. Obstet Gynecol **53:**689-693, 1979.

142 Young RH, Scully RE: Endodermal sinus tumor of the vagina. A report of nine cases and review of the literature. Gynecol Oncol **18:**380-392, 1984.

143 Zirker TA, Silva EG, Morris M, Ordonez NG: Immunohistochemical differentiation of clear-cell carcinoma of the female genital tract and endodermal sinus tumor with the use of alpha-fetoprotein and Leu-M1. Am J Clin Pathol **91:**511-514, 1989.

TUMORLIKE LESIONS

144 Abdul-Karim FW, Cohen RE: Atypical stromal cells of lower female genital tract. Histopathology 17:249-253, 1990.

145 al-Nafussi AI, Rebello G, Hughes D, Blessing K: Benign vaginal polyp. A histological, histochemical and immunohistochemical study of 20 polyps with comparison to normal vaginal subepithelial layer. Histopathology 20:145-150, 1992.

146 Chirayil SJ, Tobon H: Polyps of the vagina. A clinico-pathologic study of 18 cases. Cancer 47:2904-2907, 1981.

147 Halvorsen TB, Johannesen E: Fibroepithelial polyps of the vagina. Are they old granulation tissue polyps? J Clin Pathol 45:235-240, 1992.

148 Hartmann CA, Sperling M, Stein H: So-called fibroepithelial polyps of the vagina exhibiting an unusual but uniform antigen profile characterized by expression of desmin and steroid hormone receptors but no muscle-specific actin or macrophage markers. Am J Clin Pathol 93:604-608, 1990.

149 Miettinen M, Wahlstrom T, Vesterinen E, Saksela E: Vaginal polyps with pseudosarcomatous features. A clinicopathologic study of seven cases. Cancer **51:**1148-1151, 1983.

150 Mucitelli DR, Charles EZ, Kraus FT: Vulvovaginal polyps. Histologic appearance, ultrastructure, immunocytochemical characteristics, and clinicopathologic correlations. Int J Gynecol Pathol 9:20-40, 1990.

151 Norris HJ, Taylor HB: Polyps of the vagina. Cancer 19:227-232, 1966.

152 Ostor AG, Fortune DW, Riley CB: Fibroepithelial polyps with atypical stromal cells (pseudosarcoma botryoides) of vulva and vagina. A report of 13 cases. Int J Gynecol Pathol 7:351-360, 1988.

153 Proppe KH, Scully RE, Rosai J: Postoperative spindle cell nodules of genitourinary tract resembling sarcomas. A report of eight cases. Am J Surg Pathol 8:101-108, 1984.

154 Young RH, Clement PB: Pseudoneoplastic lesions of the lower female genital tract. Pathol Annu 24(Pt 2):189-226, 1989.

Uterus—cervix

NORMAL ANATOMY

The cervix is the lower portion of the uterus, which connects this organ to the vagina through the endocervical canal. It is divided into a portion that protrudes into the vagina (*portio vaginalis*) and one that lies above the vaginal vault (*supravaginal portion*). The outer surface of the portio vaginalis is known as the exocervix or ectocervix, and the portion related to the endocervical canal corresponds to the endocervix. The opening of the endocervical canal onto the exocervix is known as the *external os*, whereas the grossly indistinct upper limit of the endocervical canal is designated the *internal os*.

Most of the exocervix is covered by nonkeratinizing squamous epithelium that in child-bearing age is composed of three layers: basal cell, midzone (stratum spongiosum), and superficial. The portion of the midzone immediately above the basal layer is referred to as the suprabasal layer. The morphologic appearance of the various layers varies with age; in the postmenopausal period the cells are atrophic and exhibit a high nucleocytoplasmic ratio. These changes should not be misinterpreted as evidence of CIN.

Histochemically, the cells above the basal layer show variable amounts of glycogen, readily appreciated in sections with a PAS stain and clinically by the application of the iodine (Lugol or Schiller's) test. Immunohistochemically, the cells of the basal layer are positive for low-molecular-weight keratin and tissue polypeptide antigen (TPA) but not for high-molecular-weight (epidermal type) keratin or for involucrin.[4,5,10-12] The latter two markers become positive in the cells above the basal layer. Basal cells are also immunoreactive for estrogen receptors.[6]

The glandular mucosa of the endocervix is formed by a layer of columnar mucus-secreting cells, the histochemical reactivity for the mucin depending on the time of the menstrual cycle.[3] These cells rest on a normally inconspicuous layer of subcolumnar "reserve" cells, which are also positive for TPA.[4] These "reserve" cells (in particular, those located at or near the squamocolumnar junction) are primarily involved in the processes of squamous metaplasia, CIN, and carcinoma. The glandular epithelium is immunoreactive for estrogen receptors.[6] In addition to lining the surface, it invaginates into the stroma to produce elongated clefts (usually less than 5 mm deep but sometimes as deep as 1 cm or more), usually referred to as endocervical glands.

The area where the squamous and glandular epithelia meet is known as the squamocolumnar junction (Fig. 19-33). It should be noted that this junction is not located in the anatomic external os but rather in the adjacent exocervix, a fact that renders it easily accessible to the colposcope. The portion of endocervical mucosa covering the exocervix is sometimes referred to as *ectropion* and, inaccurately, as *erosion*. This is a very unstable region, in which replacement of one epithelium for another repeatedly occurs, a process that Robert Meyer allegorically referred to as "the fight of the epithelia." Today, this area is more prosaically known as the *transformation zone*.

Scattered endocrine cells are found both in the normal endocervix and exocervix,[1,2] and melanocytes have been occasionally detected along the exocervical basal layer.[7]

The stroma of the cervix is mainly made up of fibrous tissue admixed with elastic fibers and scattered smooth muscle fibers.

Mesonephric rests are remnants of the wolffian ducts that are found surrounded by the endocervical stroma in about a third of women. They are composed of tubules lined by a single row of cuboidal cells; they typically contain an inspissated deeply eosinophilic secretion in the lumen.

Ectopic and/or *metaplastic tissues* sometimes found in the cervix include cutaneous adnexae (sebaceous glands and hair follicles)[8] and mature cartilage islands.[9] The latter should not be confused with a mixed müllerian tumor or a botryoid rhabdomyosarcoma.

SQUAMOUS AND OTHER METAPLASIAS

Various types of metaplastic changes of the cervical epithelium occur, their appearance being related to the type of mucosa affected. Squamous metaplasia, by far the most common (to the point that some regard it as a normal finding) is centered on the transformation zone; transitional metaplasia involves the exocervical squamous epithelium; and tubal, tuboendometrial, and intestinal metaplasia affect the glandular epithelium of the endocervix.

The term **squamous metaplasia** is used to designate the focal or extensive replacement of the mucus-secreting glandular epithelium by stratified squamous epithelium, which, in its late stage, is morphologically indistinguishable from the epithelium normally lining the exocervical portion. The

1353

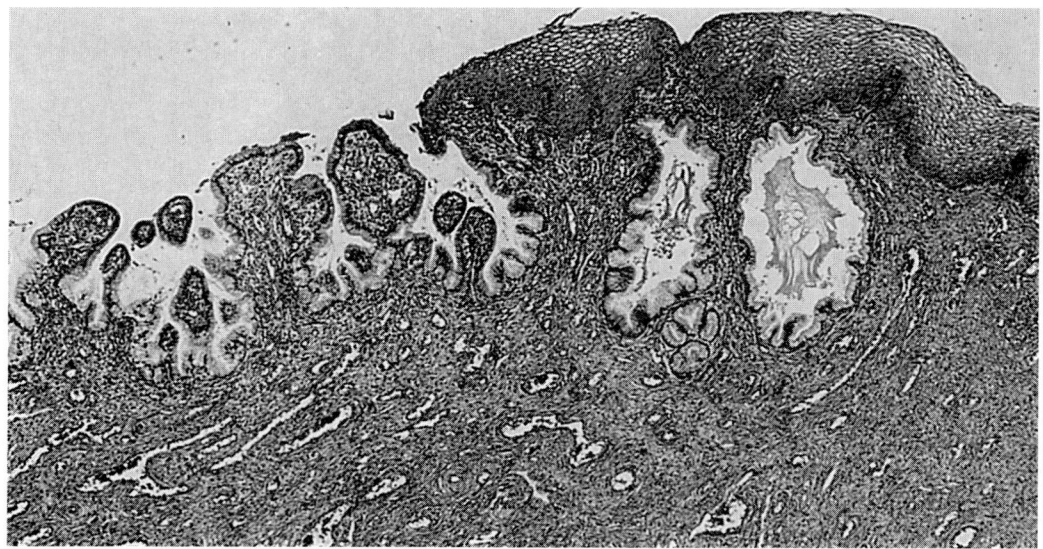

Fig. 19-33 Squamocolumnar junction of uterine cervix. It is in this area that most dysplasias and carcinomas in situ arise.

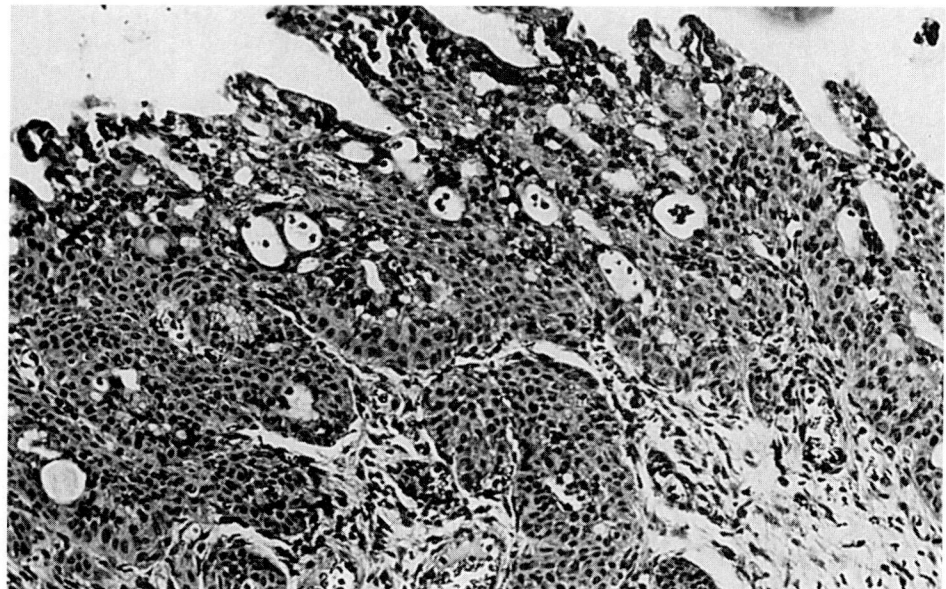

Fig. 19-34 Extensive squamous metaplasia of cervix. Individual cells are uniform, and there is considerable inflammation.

pathogenesis of this process, also known as *prosoplasia,* has been a subject of a heated controversy over the years. It is now generally agreed that it most commonly arises on the basis of proliferation and metaplasia of reserve cells. It is possible that in other instances it results from direct ingrowth into the endocervical mucosa of mature native squamous epithelium from the exocervix, possibly as a healing mechanism of a true cervical erosion.[18] Strictly speaking, the latter is not a metaplastic process but rather one of "squamous epithelization." However, it is common usage to employ the term squamous metaplasia regardless of the presumed mechanism for the change.

Some degree of squamous metaplasia is present in almost every uterine cervix during the child-bearing years. Most commonly, the process involves only the superficial epithelium and is recognized by the presence of squamous epithelium overlying endocervical glands. In other instances, it affects the glandular component as well, resulting in a complex microscopic appearance that can be confused with invasive carcinoma by the inexperienced (Fig. 19-34).

Ultrastructural and immunohistochemical markers of squamous epithelium appear *pari passu* with the morphologic changes.[16,20] Variations within this theme, probably representing various stages within a continuum, have been described as *reserve cell hyperplasia* and as *immature, intermediate,* and *mature squamous metaplasia.*[14] A further nuance is *atypical immature metaplasia,* a lesion combining the features of immature metaplasia with some degree of cytologic atypia.[14]

Although most cervical carcinomas arise in areas of the cervix that sometime in the past had been involved by squamous metaplasia, the latter process has no premalignant connotations per se. Actually, it is so common and insignificant that, unless quite extensive and/or involving the glandular component, we tend to ignore it altogether in our pathology reports.

A somewhat different appearance is seen often in the cervix of prolapsed uteri. The clinical appearance is usually referred to as "leukoplakic." Microscopically, the process involves mainly the exocervical portion and is characterized by the appearance of granular and horny layers in the epithelium. This process, which is also unrelated to carcinoma, is best designated as **hyperkeratosis.**

Transitional metaplasia is seen in the exocervix of older women and it is often associated with atrophy. It morphologically resembles transitional (urothelial) epithelium, and it involves the entire thickness of the mucosa. The nuclei are oval and devoid of atypical features. Their long axes, which are arranged perpendicularly to the surface, often exhibit longitudinal grooves. The term transitional metaplasia is probably a misnomer, inasmuch as the condition probably represents instead basal cell hyperplasia.

Tubal metaplasia is diagnosed when a specimen from the endocervix (usually from the upper portion) is found to contain all three cell types found in the normal fallopian tube (i.e., ciliated, secretory, and intercalated).[19,21] In many instances, the appearance of the metaplastic epithelium combines features of tubal and endometrial mucosa, in which case the term *tuboendometrial (tuboendometrioid) metaplasia* is employed.[13,19a,22] Diagnostic difficulties may result from the fact that these glands may be deeply seated, irregularly shaped, cystically dilated, and/or accompanied by a hypercellular, edematous, or myxoid stroma.[19b] Staining for Ki-67 and M1B1 is of some help in the differential diagnosis from in situ and invasive endocervical adenocarcinoma.[19a] Tubal metaplasia is often found after conization, and it has therefore been suggested that it represents aberrant differentiation following injury.[17] This condition can be identified in cytologic preparations.[15]

Intestinal metaplasia is a much rarer condition, which may be accompanied by extravasation of mucin into the stroma.[23]

INFLAMMATORY LESIONS

Chronic cervicitis is an extremely common condition in adult females, at least at the microscopic level. It affects preferentially the squamocolumnar junction and endocervix, and it may be accompanied by hyperemia, edema, fibrosis, and metaplastic changes in the epithelium. The etiology is variable.[34] In most cases the disease is asymptomatic, but it

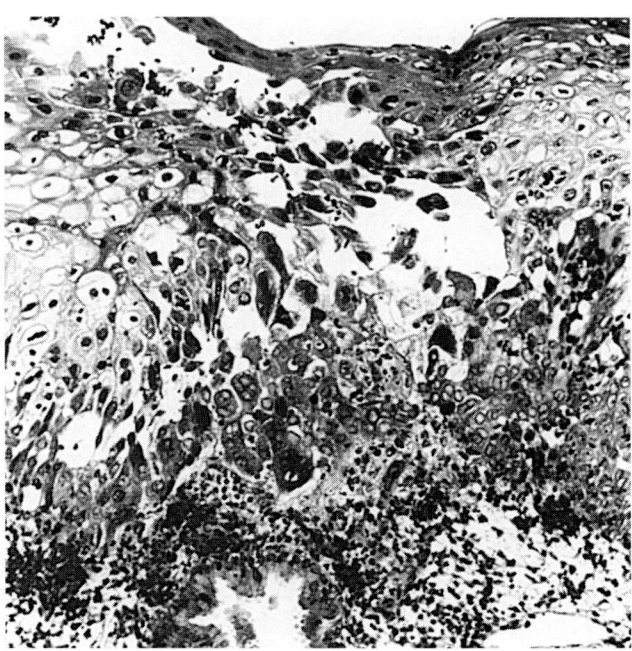

Fig. 19-35 Herpes simplex infection of cervix.

is of importance because it may lead to endometritis, salpingitis, and "pelvic inflammatory disease" through ascending intraluminal spread, chorioamnionitis and other complications during pregnancy, and it may also play a role in the initiation or promotion of cervical neoplasia.

Herpes simplex infection of the cervix is now recognized as a relatively common occurrence. The microscopic appearance at the time of biopsy is usually that of an intense nonspecific inflammation with ulceration. Only rarely are diagnostic multinucleated squamous cells with intra-nuclear inclusions encountered[33] (Fig. 19-35). The diagnosis can be confirmed by immunocytochemical demonstration of the viral antigen.[24,31a]

Chlamydia trachomatis infection is now recognized as the most common venereal disease in the Western world. The microscopic appearance in the cervix is that of a chronic nonspecific inflammation, with reactive epithelial atypia and sometimes prominent formation of lymphoid follicles.[30,36] The organisms are not visible in routine histologic slides and only with difficulty in cytologic preparations, but they can be detected by immunocytochemical techniques.[36] Culture isolation is regarded as the standard for diagnosis of active infection. Chlamydial cervicitis can be associated with CIN, but there is no evidence of a causal relationship.[32]

Syphilis can affect the cervix, usually in the form of a primary chancre.[35]

Amebiasis may produce a polypoid and ulcerated mass in the cervix clinically simulating carcinoma, and it may also engraft itself upon a pre-existing cervical carcinoma.

Actinomycosis of the cervix occurs, but it needs to be distinguished from the more common pseudoactinomycotic radiate granules that may form around microorganisms or biologically inert substances.[27]

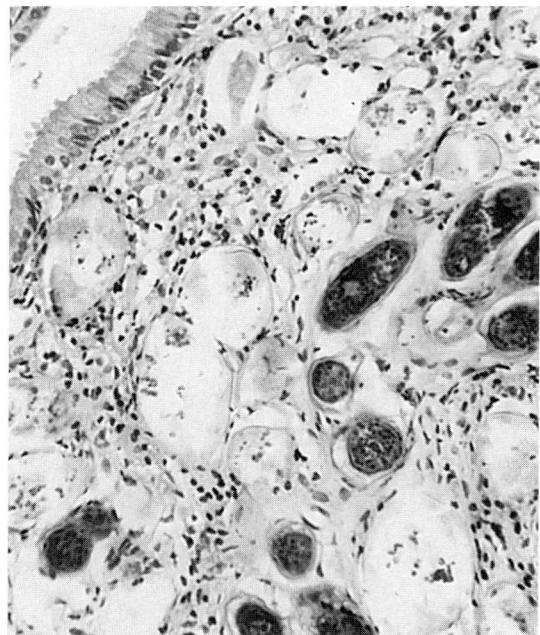

Fig. 19-36 Bilharziasis (schistosomiasis) presenting as cervical polyp in African woman. (Courtesy Dr. A. Schmamann, Johannesburg, South Africa.)

Bilharziasis (schistosomiasis), common in Africa and Central America, can involve any portion of the female genitalia tract, including the cervix[26] (Fig. 19-36).

Malakoplakia rarely occurs in the cervix, sometimes in association with disease in the uterine corpus, pelvis, or kidney.[28]

Ceroid granuloma of the type more commonly seen in the gallbladder has been exceptionally found to involve the cervix.[25]

Localized arteritis of the cervix has been described, accompanied by inflammation and ulceration, and apparently restricted to this anatomic site.[29,31]

NON-NEOPLASTIC GLANDULAR LESIONS

Endocervical polyps are not true neoplasms but probably are the result of chronic inflammatory changes ("chronic polypoid cervicitis"). They are usually small but may reach several centimeters in diameter. Microscopically, dilated endocervical glands are seen in an edematous, inflamed, and fibrotic stroma. The surface epithelium usually shows squamous metaplasia. CIN can develop from these polyps but not more so than in the cervix as a whole; Hertig[42] found only five cases he diagnosed as carcinoma in situ in 1600 polyps. Occasionally, the configuration of these polyps is that of a branching papillary structure, in which case the term *papillary endocervicitis* is employed.[55]

Nabothian cysts are thought to develop from blockage of the endocervical glands secondarily to inflammation and associated changes; they appear grossly as cystic spaces filled with mucoid material and microscopically as cystically dilated glands lined by a flattened epithelium, sometimes

focally absent. Occasionally they extend deeply into the cervical wall, a phenomenon that should not be mistaken for malignancy.[38]

Tunnel clusters, as described by Fluhmann, are the result of localized proliferation of endocervical glands (clefts), with side channels growing out from them. This is often accompanied by dilatation resulting from the accumulation of inspissated, deeply eosinophilic secretion in the lumen.[49]

Microglandular hyperplasia of the endocervical epithelium occurs in women using oral contraceptive drugs and, less frequently, during pregnancy.[47,54] It may also be seen in the absence of these conditions and even in postmenopausal patients.[37] As a matter of fact, the very relationship between microglandular hyperplasia and oral contraception or other hormonal perturbations has been questioned.[41a] Microscopically, the typical case is characterized by a complex proliferation of small glands lined by flat epithelial cells with little or no atypia (Fig. 19-37, *A*). Accompanying squamous metaplasia is frequent, resulting in a complex microscopic picture that may be confused with carcinoma. Additional features that may lead to overdiagnosis include areas of solid proliferation, pseudoinfiltrative pattern, signet ring cells, focal atypia, and occasional mitotic figures.[56] The intervening stroma invariably shows chronic inflammation. Immunocytochemical reactivity for CEA is nil, a useful feature in the differential diagnosis with endocervical adenocarcinoma.[53]

Arias-Stella reaction, as seen during pregnancy, can involve the endocervical glands. The nuclear abnormalities are similar to those seen more commonly in the endometrial mucosa and should not be confused with malignancy.[39,48]

Diffuse laminar endocervical glandular hyperplasia is a non-neoplastic condition characterized by a proliferation of medium-sized, evenly spaced, well-differentiated glands within the inner third of the cervical wall, sharply separated from the underlying stroma, and often accompanied by chronic inflammation[46]; it should not be confused with adenoma malignum, from which it is distinguishable because of the fact that stromal infiltration, desmoplastic stromal response, and cytologic atypia are absent.

Mesonephric duct vestiges can undergo cystic dilatation[52] or be affected by florid and even atypical hyperplastic changes[43,45,49a,51,56] (Plate XIII-A). This hyperplasia may have a lobular, diffuse, or ductal pattern.[41] Rare malignant tumors arising from these structures also occur (see p. 1375).[40] Mesonephric remnants are also rarely involved by in situ squamous cell carcinoma of the cervix.[48a] It is doubtful whether the rare benign polypoid lesion found in the cervix and vagina of young children and described as *mesonephric papilloma* is related to these remnants.[44,50] Microscopically, it is a superficially located lesion composed of delicate connective tissue stalks covered by a layer of cuboidal cells and is probably of müllerian derivation.

NON-NEOPLASTIC STROMAL LESIONS

Multinucleated stromal giant cells can be present beneath the cervical epithelium and be mistaken for a malignancy. They are often accompanied by edema and may result in a vaguely polypoid-appearing lesion.[59,62] These cells are of a reactive fibroblastic/myofibroblastic nature

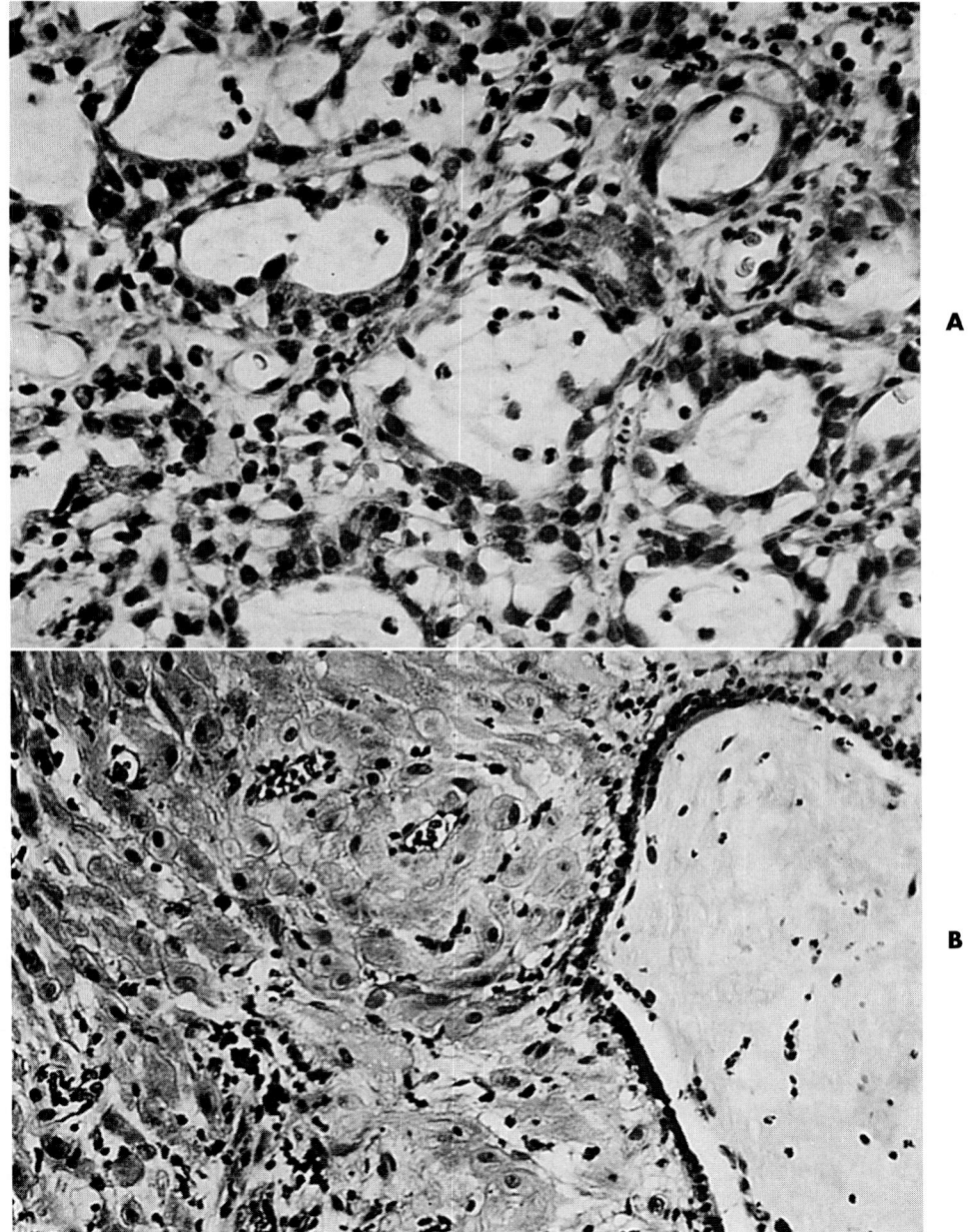

Fig. 19-37 A, Microglandular hyperplasia of endocervical epithelium. This benign change associated with use of cyclic artificial progestogens may be mistaken for cancer. **B,** Decidual reaction in cervix. Note large decidual cells growing diffusely through cervix. Clinically, patient was thought to have early carcinoma of cervix.

and analogous to those seen in other sites covered by mucosal membranes, such as the vulva, vagina, anus, oral cavity, and nasal cavity.[57,64]

Decidual reaction in the cervix during pregnancy usually presents as multiple, small, yellowish or red elevations of the cervical mucosa. They are soft and friable and bleed easily with trauma. Rarely, they develop into fungating masses difficult to distinguish grossly from carcinoma.[58,60] Microscopically, the decidual cells are characterized by abundant

pale granular cytoplasm and bland nuclei (Fig. 19-37, *B*). Immunostains for keratin are negative.

Placental-site nodule appears as a well-defined hyalinized lesion located immediately beneath the mucosa; it is composed of intermediate trophoblast exhibiting cytoplasmic vacuolization.[65,67] Some nuclear atypia may be present. This lesion can be confused with carcinoma and with neoplastic cartilage. Immunohistochemically, the trophoblastic cells are reactive for keratin (another factor that may lead to a mistaken diagnosis of malignancy) but also for human placental lactogen.

Endometriosis of the cervix presents as blue or reddish nodules and may result in abnormal uterine bleeding. Both endometrial glands and stroma are needed to establish the diagnosis. However, the proportion of the two components may vary greatly from case to case. On occasion, the process is composed almost exclusively of endometrial stroma and may be confused with a neoplasm.[61]

Necrobiotic granulomas resembling tuberculosis or rheumatoid nodules have been seen following cervical surgery.[63] They are probably histologically and pathogenetically analogous to those described postoperatively in the prostate (see Chapter 18).

Florid mesenchymal reactions can develop from the cervical stroma as a result of various surgical interventions and lead to confusion with sarcoma.[66] Some of these have a nodular fasciitis–like appearance and may be looked upon as the genitourinary equivalent of this soft tissue lesion.

HUMAN PAPILLOMA VIRUS (HPV) AND CERVICAL PATHOLOGY

HPV has been linked to various types of cervical diseases, ranging from the relatively innocuous condyloma acuminatum (see p. 1359) to the sometimes fatal invasive squamous cell carcinoma.[80,90,103] HPV comprises a family of DNA viruses, of which more than 60 types have been characterized. It can be detected by electron microscopy (as intranuclear crystalline and occasionally filamentous inclusions), but its specific identification depends on immunohistochemical or molecular virologic analysis with in situ or Southern blot hybridization.[74,82,87,91,97] The latter test is currently regarded as the "gold standard" for the detection of HPV. Of the many HPV types known, those most often encountered are HPV-6 and HPV-11, and less commonly HPV-16.[94]

HPV infection of the cervix is transmitted venereally and it has a predilection for the metaplastic squamous epithelium. It may remain dormant for long periods or become productive, with release of infectious virus in the terminally differentiated squamous epithelium.

The morphologic hallmark of HPV infection of the cervical squamous epithelium is *koilocytosis,* also known as *koilocytotic atypia,* a change that is said to be related to expression of the viral E4 protein and the disruption that this causes in the cytoplasmic keratin matrix.[100] The koilocyte is a superficial or intermediate mature squamous cell characterized by a sharply outlined perinuclear vacuolation, dense and irregular staining peripheral cytoplasm, and an enlarged nucleus with an undulating (raisin- or prune-like) nuclear membrane and a rope-like chromatin pattern. Binucleation and multinucleation can occur.[101] It is important that these nuclear changes—which may be accompanied by either a diploid or polyploid nuclear DNA distribution[109]—be present somewhere in the lesion for the diagnosis of koilocytosis (and, by inference, HPV infection) to be made, or else other forms of cytoplasmic clearing (notably those related to glycogen accumulation) will be mistakenly included in this category.[95,110] This is particularly the case for the condition known as postmenopausal squamous atypia, in which perinuclear halos can be very prominent.[87a] This is not to imply that HPV infection does not occur in the absence of koilocytosis, because it certainly does. Sometimes, the only abnormality seen in HPV-infected cells is nuclear enlargement, and occasionally there are no detectable changes at all.[75,98,115]

The most interesting and difficult problem that these HPV-induced cervical lesions pose is in relation to the differential diagnosis, coexistence, and possible causation of CIN and invasive carcinoma.[68,69,77,114] It seems obvious, in retrospect, that many cases diagnosed in the past as mild or moderate dysplasia (CIN I and II) would now be reported as HPV-induced koilocytotic atypia.[72] It has also become apparent that HPV-associated lesions are often seen together with (or preceding those of) CIN or, sometimes, invasive cervical carcinoma.[96,99,108] Actually, the high frequency of this association on a worldwide basis,[72a] the topographic continuity between the two processes,[105] and the respective age distributions of the affected populations[78] all suggest an underlying dependence and perhaps a continuum between the two.[86a,106] This concordance is not apparent between cervical carcinoma and other infections of the cervix.[73] The association between HPV and cervical neoplasia is particularly strong for squamous cell tumors, but it has also been documented for both in situ and invasive adenocarcinoma[76,83,84,92,112] and for adenosquamous carcinoma.[89] The HPV proteins E6 and E7 are thought to play an important role in this process by their interaction with the p53 protein and the Rb-susceptibility gene product, respectively.[74a,100]

Following the realization that koilocytotic atypia equals HPV infection, an attitude took hold in some quarters that the presence of this change in a cervical biopsy was indicative of a benign process. This is not necessarily the case. These biopsies should be evaluated according to the standard criteria applied to CIN. The added presence of the HPV-associated component should be mentioned in the diagnosis but should not modify the diagnostic or clinical approach toward them.[88]

The features in a cervical biopsy exhibiting the signs of HPV-infection that indicate the additional presence of CIN are the presence of atypia along the basal layers, a disorderly pattern of maturation, and abnormal mitotic figures.[113] A definite association exists between high-degree atypia (CIN III), an aneuploid DNA pattern, p53 overexpression, and the presence of HPV type 16.[79,85,86,108a] Along similar lines, the presence of the HPV-16 genome has been documented in most invasive cervical carcinomas and in histologically normal neighboring epithelium.[93] In one study, HPV-18 was found to be associated with low-grade intraepithelial lesions but not high-grade invasive lesions.[93a] In another, HIV-16 and HPV-18 were found to be associated with higher densities of Ki-67–positive cells than others, such as HPV-6 and HPV-11.[67b] Whether typing of the viral strain could be of use for prognostic or therapeutic purposes remains to be determined.[70,81,107,111] It is of interest that the probability of finding direct evidence of HPV infection in cervical squamous intraepithelial lesions decreases proportionally to the degree of atypia, reaching low levels in CIN III.[71,104] These findings have been explained by postulating that an intact squamous epithelium is needed for virus replication.

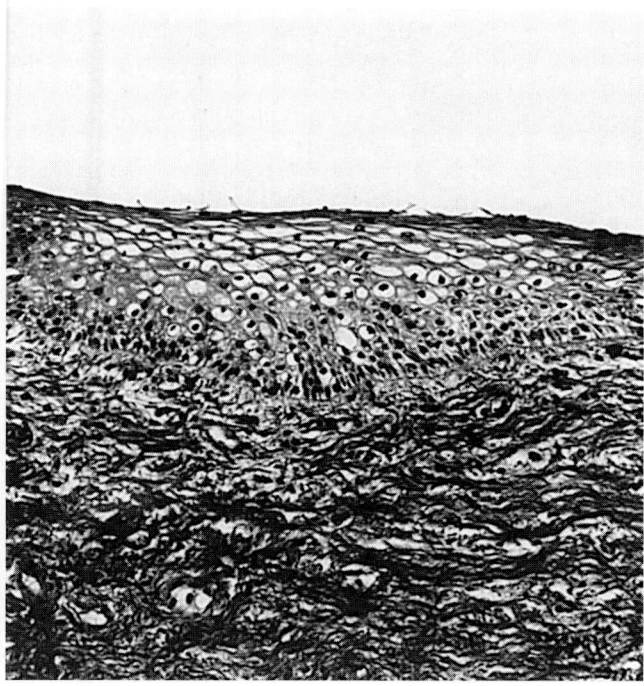

Fig. 19-38 Minimal condylomatous changes of cervix.

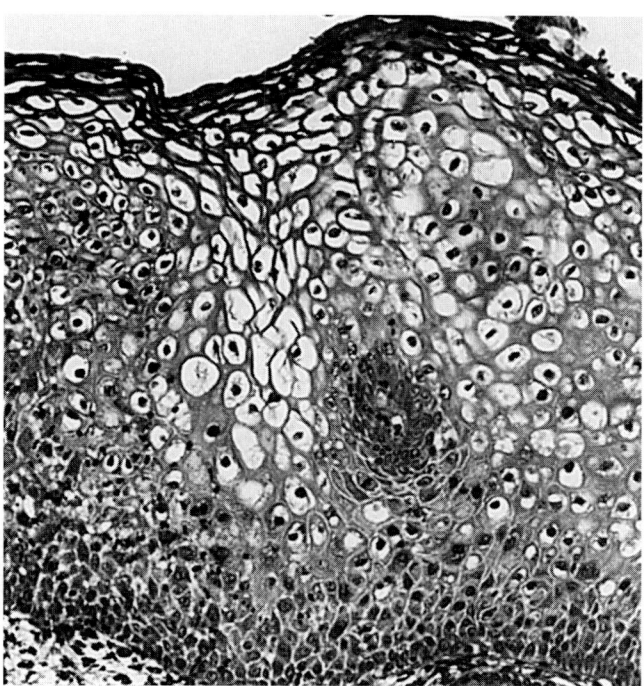

Fig. 19-39 Moderate condylomatous changes of cervix.

Benign squamous neoplasms

Condyloma acuminatum is a grossly polypoid lesion characterized microscopically by papillomatosis, acanthosis, koilocytosis, and a variable degree of inflammatory infiltration of the stroma. An undulating appearance of the epithelium is a characteristic feature on low-power examination. A mild degree of atypia in the squamous component is common and needs not be mentioned; if more severe, it should be evaluated and graded as for the flat squamous intraepithelial lesions (i.e., condyloma with CIN II or III).

Condyloma acuminatum is an HPV-induced lesion (see p. 1358); HPV-6 and HPV-11 are found in 70% to 90% of the cases, but occasionally other types—such as HPV-16—are encountered. When the latter is the case, high-grade cytologic atypia is often found.

Other morphologic manifestations of HPV infection of the cervix (which are actually much more common than condyloma acuminatum) include lesions variously described as flat, spiked, and inverted condyloma and warty atypia.[112] Many HPV infections are clinically inapparent. Microscopically, these clinically different lesions share the following features: relatively normal basal cell layer, expanded or hyperplastic parabasal cell layer, orderly maturation, mitotic activity (but few or no abnormal mitoses), and koilocytosis (Figs. 19-38 and 19-39).

Squamous papilloma is a polypoid lesion composed of a fibrovascular stalk covered by mature squamous epithelium. It has also been designated as fibroepithelial papilloma, fibroepithelioma, and ectocervical polyp. Microscopically, the lack of an arborizing pattern and—most important—the absence of koilocytotic changes distinguish this lesion from condyloma acuminatum. The nature of this process is not clear; in at least some instances, squamous papilloma probably represents condyloma in which the recognizable morphologic changes of HPV infection have subsided. The differential diagnosis also includes the papillary form of CIN (in which case the atypical changes present in the epithelium of the polypoid lesion are also seen in the adjacent flat epithelium),[102] verrucous carcinoma (see p. 1368), and well-differentiated squamous cell carcinoma (see p. 1365).

Inverted transitional cell papilloma, similar to its more common bladder counterpart, has been recently described in the cervix.[67a]

TUMORS
Cervical intraepithelial neoplasia (CIN)

The terminology of cervical intraepithelial lesions composed of squamous epithelium and thought to represent the precursors of invasive carcinoma has evolved over the years and continues changing today. The concept is of great practical and historical importance, since it represents the main model on which the theory of the existence of morphologically identifiable precursor lesions of cancer has been built (a general model that, one should add, has recently found strong support from molecular studies). The basic premises are the following:

1. Nearly all invasive cervical carcinomas are preceded by a stage in which the abnormal cells are confined to the epithelium (intraepithelial stage).[134]
2. These intraepithelial lesions share many of the cytologic features of the invasive stage, mainly manifested by enlargement, irregularities, and hyperchromasia of the nuclei; increase in mitotic activity; and alteration of the maturation pattern. There is also a diminution or absence of cytoplasmic glycogen, this being the reason

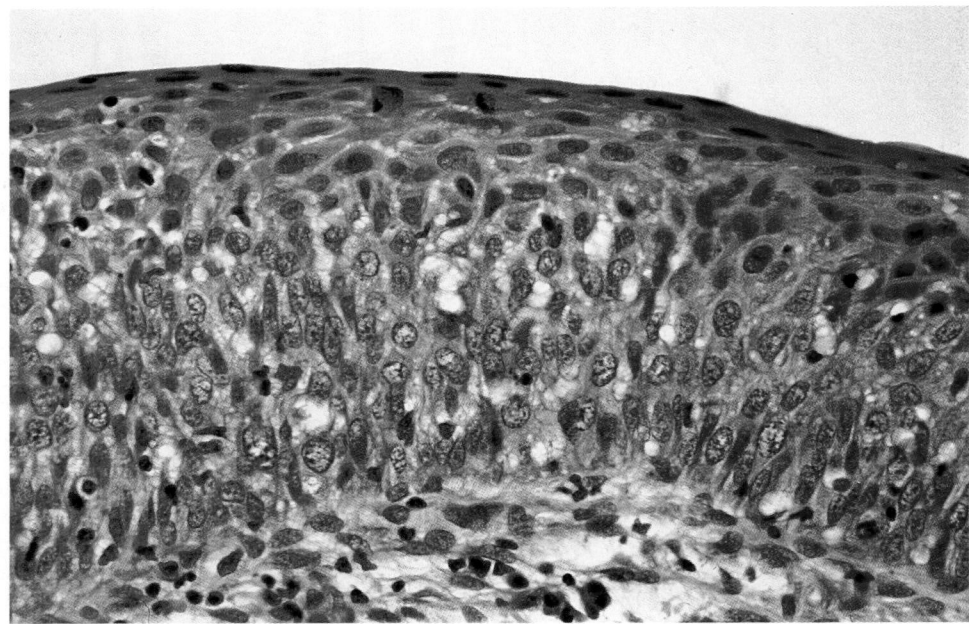

Fig. 19-40 Moderate dysplasia of uterine cervix (CIN II). There is proliferation and atypia in the lower two thirds, but some surface maturation is still apparent.

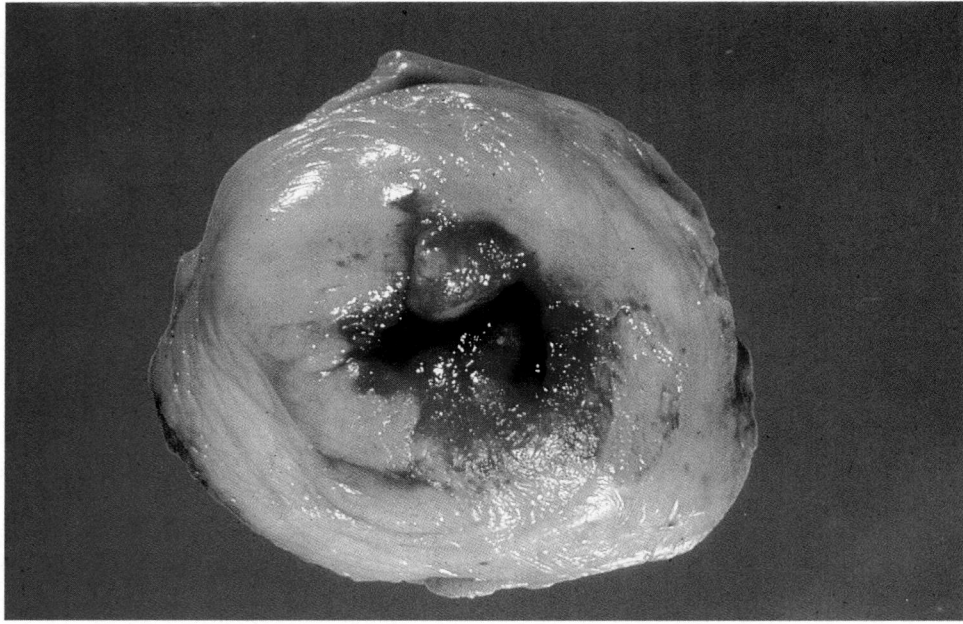

Fig. 19-41 Gross appearance of carcinoma in situ (CIN III) extensively involving the uterine cervix. (Courtesy Dr. Hector Rodriguez-Martinez, Mexico City.)

for the decrease or lack of staining in the iodine (Lugol or Schiller's) test.

3 A continuous range of morphologic abnormalities exists among these lesions, thus providing a rough indication of the likelihood with which they would evolve into invasive carcinoma if left untreated.[150] These morphologic abnormalities correlate with cyto-genetic, DNA ploidy, cell proliferation, and molecular changes. For instance, autoradiographic studies have shown a continuum in the proportion of cells in DNA synthesis, their number paralleling the degree of atypia.[161] Low-grade lesions usually have a euploid or polyploid pattern, whereas high-grade lesions are generally aneuploid.[119,152,157] A similar relationship has been found among morphologic aberrations and prolif-erating cell nuclear antigen,[145,164] nucleolar organizer

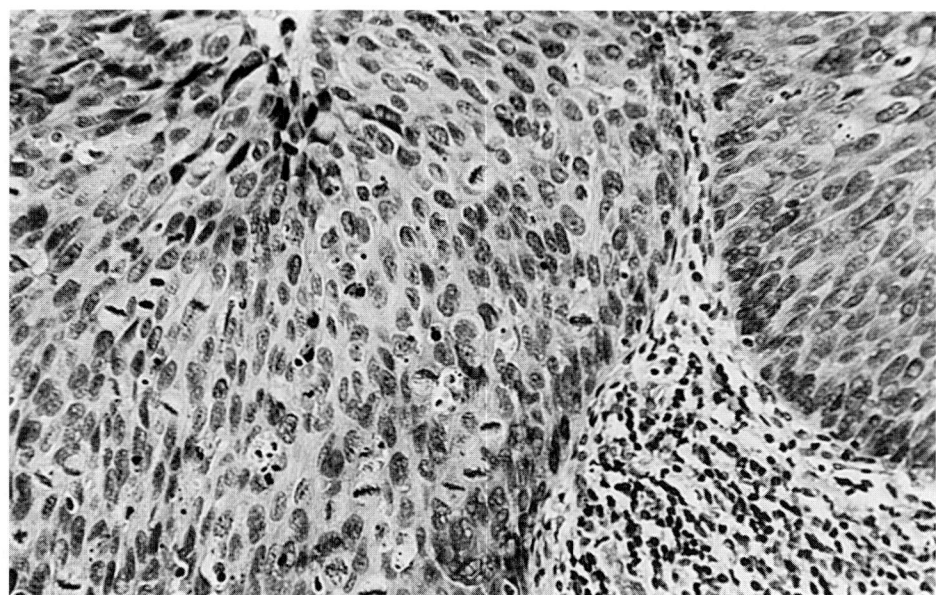

Fig. 19-42 Squamous cell carcinoma in situ. Complete disorganization throughout all layers with numerous normal and typical mitotic figures is demonstrated.

region,[137a,169] and aberrant expression of various keratins,[165,166] p53 protein,[115a,154] and *ras* oncogene.[162] The available evidence suggests the existence of a sequence of events that in some cases leads to progression to a full-blown invasive malignancy but that in others stops at a given stage or regresses altogether. The often held assumption that the most severe forms will *inevitably* lead to invasive carcinoma is unproved and unprovable.[138,147] The milder forms are particularly unstable.[126,159] In one study, follow-up evaluation after conservative therapy showed regression in 62% of the cases, persistence in 22%, and progression to a more severe lesion in 16%.[148] The more severe lesions regress less frequently and may persist for long periods. Petersen[153] studied the course of 127 untreated patients with such severe lesions. Invasive carcinoma had developed in 11% at the end of 3 years, in 22% at the end of 5 years, and in 33% at the end of 9 years.

4 In the large majority of cases, the process involves not the native squamous epithelium of the exocervix but rather areas of squamous metaplasia located at the transformation zone and in its endocervical side.[132] It practically always involves the surface epithelium, as well as the glandular elements, but by definition shows no stromal invasion. It often ends abruptly, and its extent is highly variable. Occasionally it seems to consist of only a minute focus removable by a simple biopsy; more commonly, it involves large areas of the cervix. Extension up the endocervical canal is particularly common,[130] but it may also grow along the portio and upper vagina[125,155,168] or extend into mesonephric remnants.[163a] In exceptional instances, it has been seen to extend into the vagina to the introitus or into the endometrial cavity and even the fallopian tubes.[135,163]

Sometimes, the intraepithelial change as seen in a cervical biopsy represents only the peripheral manifestation of a more proximally located invasive carcinoma that is diagnosed only by endocervical curettage.

5 The microscopic criteria for the diagnosis of these lesions should be the same regardless of the circumstances. This is true if they are found in the pregnant woman; such changes do not routinely regress postpartum, despite early statements to the contrary. It is also true if they are found following treatment of invasive squamous cell carcinoma with radiation therapy, a change found in approximately one quarter of the patients and sometimes referred to as *postirradiation dysplasia.* The available evidence suggests that this is not merely a reaction of a previously normal epithelium to the radiation but rather the expression of a basically abnormal mucosa. Indeed, postirradiation dysplasia appearing within 3 years after treatment is associated with poor prognosis.[172]

All of the previously listed basic tenets have been accepted, the current controversy centering on the number of recognizable steps within that range (2, 3, or 4) and the best way to name them.

The classic approach, unchallenged for half a century, has been that of designating these lesions as either dysplasia or carcinoma in situ. The term *dysplasia* was used when the atypical cytologic features mentioned were accompanied by a partial retention of the normal maturation pattern and a preservation of the organization of the basal layer[121,128] (Fig. 19-40). By contrast, the term *carcinoma in situ* was employed when there was no differentiation at any level (despite some occasional flattening of the surface cells) and the basal cell was disorganized[137,140,156] (Figs. 19-41 to 19-43). Dysplasia was further subdivided into mild, moderate,

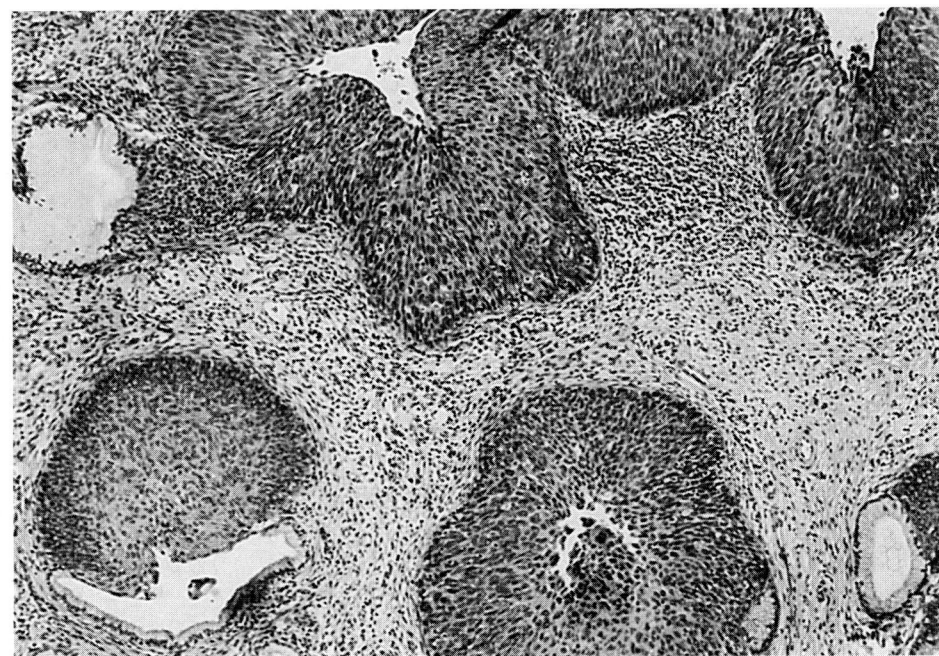

Fig. 19-43 Squamous cell carcinoma in situ. Lesion has extended into glands and partially or completely replaced them. This is not evidence of invasion.

and severe, depending on the severity of the changes. Carcinoma in situ was further subdivided by some authors into parabasal cell (51%), keratinizing cell (37%), pleomorphic cell (3%), and small cell (1.5%) types.[170]

Most of the seminal studies documenting the relationship between these changes and the development of invasive carcinoma have been done using this terminology, which, however, came under attack on the grounds that it implies a significant biologic difference between dysplasia and carcinoma in situ that probably does not exist and also because it may lead to a radically different approach to therapy (i.e., follow-up with cytologic studies in the case of dysplasia as opposed to surgical therapy for carcinoma in situ), which does not seem justified. That the difference between severe dysplasia and carcinoma in situ is based on rather subtle and subjective criteria, and that these criteria vary according to the individual pathologist and institution has been repeatedly proved.[129,131,133]

In the hope of eliminating these problems, the alternative term *cervical intraepithelial neoplasia* (CIN) was proposed, with a subdivision into three grades: CIN I as the equivalent of mild dysplasia, CIN II of moderate dysplasia, and CIN III of severe dysplasia and carcinoma in situ.[157] When it seemed as if this terminology was finally on its way to replacing that of dysplasia/carcinoma in situ,[120,122,167] a new one was proposed, referred to as the Bethesda classification.[149] In this scheme, which was designed for cervical cytologic specimens (see p. 1377) but which some would like to see applied also to histologic samples, the preferred generic term is *squamous intraepithelial lesion* (SIL), with a subdivision into low and high grades. The low-grade lesion corresponds to CIN I (as well as some HPV-induced lesions that do not

qualify as CIN; see p. 1358), whereas the high-grade lesion corresponds to CIN II and III.

One of the rationales for this new approach is the problem represented by the difficulty often encountered in distinguishing CIN I from HPV-related flat condylomatous changes and the overdiagnosis of CIN that can occur as a result.[116] A suggested way to deal with this problem within the context of the CIN terminology is to designate those doubtful cases as either "borderline CIN"[127] or "CIN with HPV-related changes."[158] Whichever scheme is ultimately chosen, one hopes that it will be applied to both cytologic and histologic specimens.

At a practical level, and regardless of the terminology used, these lesions can be safely treated by conization, electrodiathermy, cryosurgery, laser, or the recently introduced loop electrosurgical excision, all of them done under colposcopic guidance, assuming that a proper cytologic follow-up can be assured.* In most series, conization has resulted in control of even the most severe forms in over 90% of the patients.[136,141] In making the final decision regarding the timing and type of therapy for this group of lesions, the microscopic diagnosis is only one of the factors to be considered, albeit a very important one. The extension of the lesion, age of the patient, parity, and the desire to have more children all have to be considered. Both the surface and the possible depth of involvement have to be taken into account. Anderson and Hartley[117] calculated that destruction of tissue to a depth of 2.92 mm would eradicate all involved glands in 95% of the patients, whereas destruction to a depth of 3.8 mm would eradicate 99.7%. Whether all patients with low-grade CIN require therapy remains a contentious issue.[160]

---

*References 123, 139, 142, 144, 146, 171.

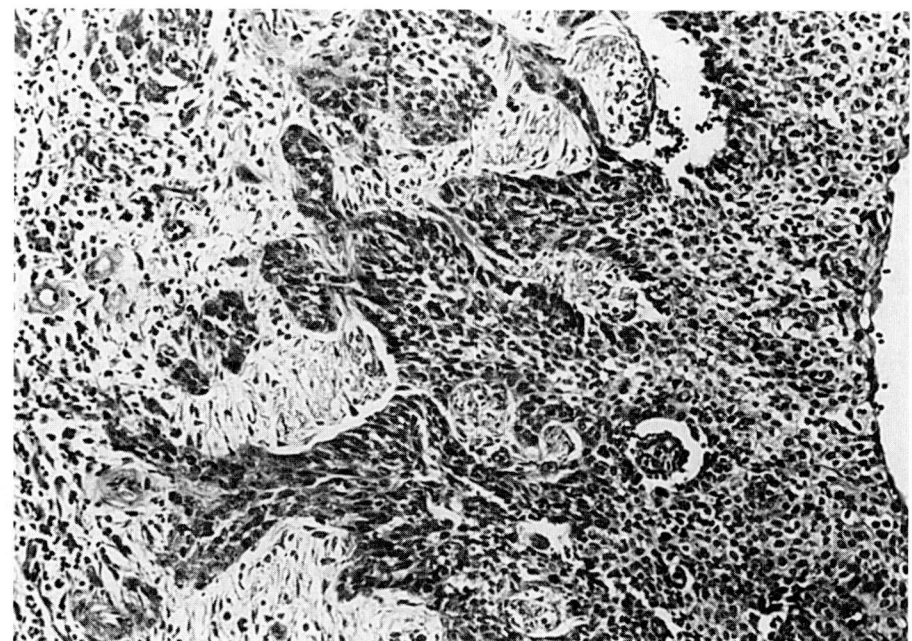

Fig. 19-44 Microinvasive carcinoma of cervix. In situ malignant changes are seen together with foci of beginning stromal invasion.

The pathologic report of a cervical biopsy specimen containing this group of lesions should include the degree of abnormality according to the agreed terminology for that institution, the presence or absence of endocervical gland involvement, and the presence or absence of HPV-related or any other associated changes. The report on a conization specimen should also include the status of the surgical margins, of which the endocervical one is the most important. Positive margins and involved glands are independent predictors of residual or recurrent disease.[124,151]

Once the pathologist has made the diagnosis of CIN in a cervical biopsy, it is the responsibility of the gynecologist to determine the presence or absence of invasive carcinoma, especially in the case of the high-grade lesions. Cold knife cervical sampling and the proper sectioning of tissue should establish whether or not invasive carcinoma exists. If the latter is found, conventional methods of therapy may be instituted. Whenever the therapy is conservative, long-term follow-up (longer than 5 years) with periodic cytologic examination is imperative. In one series, patients with continuing abnormal cytology after initial treatment of CIN III (carcinoma in situ) were found to be twenty-five times more likely to develop invasive carcinomas than women with normal follow-up cytology.[143]

In addition to HPV-related koilocytotic atypia, the differential diagnosis of CIN includes florid squamous metaplasia and transitional metaplasia (see p. 1355). It should also be mentioned that the iodine test, used to delineate the extent of cervical disease prior to conization, can induce shrinkage, cytoplasmic eosinophilia and vacuolization, and pyknosis in the epithelial cells (particularly when they are abnormal).[118]

Microinvasive squamous cell carcinoma

Invasive squamous cell carcinomas in which the depth of stromal invasion is minimal (5 mm or less) have been segregated from the others and designated as "microinvasive carcinoma," "superficially invasive carcinoma," or "carcinoma with early stromal invasion"[178,189-191] (Fig. 19-44). This corresponds rather closely to stage IA carcinoma in the FIGO system, defined as a lesion with a maximum depth of invasion of 5 mm and a maximum horizontal spread of 7 mm.[175,196]

Regardless of the terminology used, there is justification for the separation since the natural history of the lesion is quite different from that of the ordinary invasive carcinoma and more akin to that of high-grade CIN/carcinoma in situ.[174,184,192] Accordingly, the treatment can be generally conservative, although it needs to be individualized.[175,176,179,189a,198a] Ng and Reagan[191] diagnosed as microinvasive carcinomas sixty-six (8.4%) of the cervical squamous cell carcinomas they reviewed. The area of microinvasion originated practically always from a focus of CIN. The majority of the tumors were located in the anterior lip of the cervix. They emphasized the common occurrence of pleomorphism, cellular differentiation, presence of conspicuous nucleoli, and individual cell keratinization. Since these features are rarely seen together in CIN, their presence in an apparently intraepidermal cervical lesion should stimulate the search for areas of incipient invasion.[181] Another feature that should raise the suspicion of beginning stromal invasion is the presence of a desmoplastic stroma rich in acid mucosubstances and characterized by metachromatic staining properties.[182] In the area of invasion, there is a breach of the basement membrane, a feature traditionally

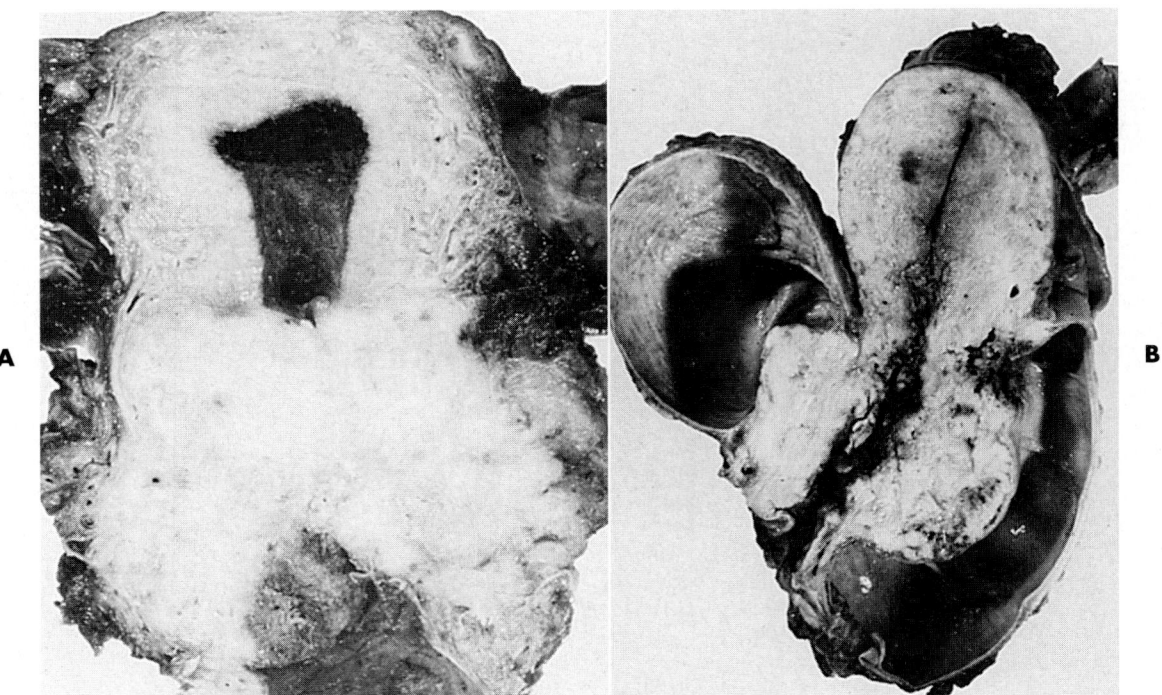

Fig. 19-45 Advanced squamous cell carcinoma of uterine cervix. **A,** Tumor replaces whole circumference of cervix and invades both parametria. **B,** Extensive neoplasm has invaded vagina, urinary bladder, and anterior rectal wall. (Courtesy Dr. H. Rodriguez-Martinez, Mexico City.)

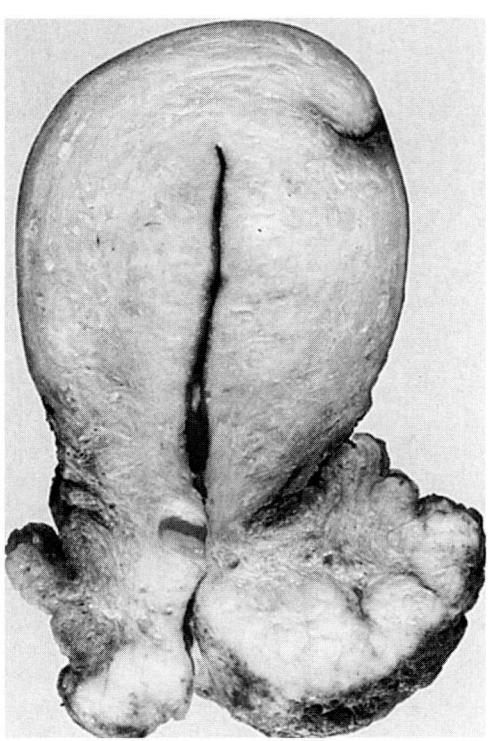

Fig. 19-46 Gross appearance of predominantly exophytic squamous cell carcinoma of cervix.

evaluated with reticulin stains and now also with immuno-stains for basement membrane components such as type IV collagen, laminin, or fibronectin.[185,193,198]

A comprehensive review of the literature by Benson and I Norris[173] revealed that the overall risk for lymph node metastasis in microinvasive carcinoma is around 1%. This excellent prognosis also applies to the subset of tumors showing lymphatic invasion and/or confluent pattern of stromal growth, as long as their depth of invasion does not exceed 5 mm.[180,186,187,194,195] A further refinement and possible modification of the definition of microinvasive carcinoma was introduced by Hasumi et al.[183] These authors found that one (0.9%) of 106 patients with invasion up to 3 mm had lymph node metastases, whereas four (13.19%) of twenty-nine patients with invasion of 3.1 to 5 mm had nodal metastases; on the basis of these findings, they recommend conservative surgery (as for CIN) for the first group and aggressive therapy (as for invasive carcinoma) for the second. This article and others have led to an ongoing controversy about the exact definition of the term, most authors now favoring a 3-mm cutoff point.[177,183,197,199] Recent evidence suggests that tumor volume may be the most reliable criterion for the definition of microinvasive carcinoma and the prediction of likelihood of nodal metastases.[173a]

Invasive squamous cell carcinoma

General features

Invasive squamous cell carcinoma of the cervix is still the most common malignant tumor of the female genital tract in

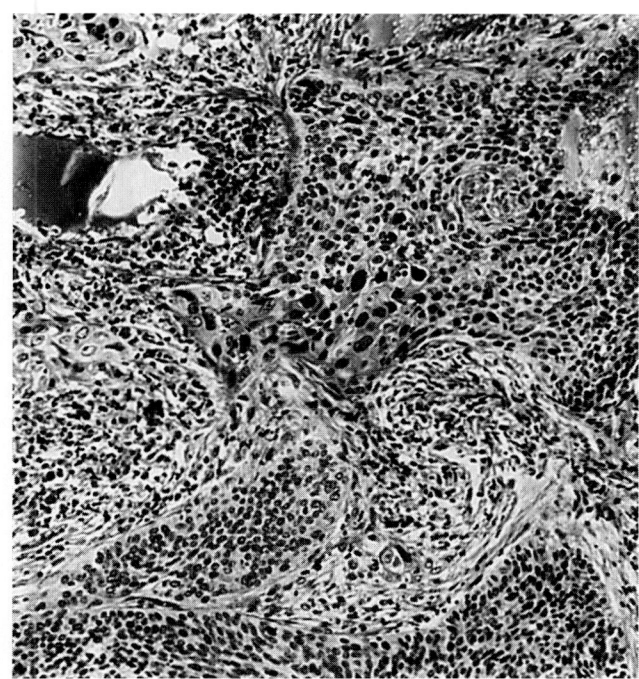

Fig. 19-47 Large cell keratinizing carcinoma of cervix.

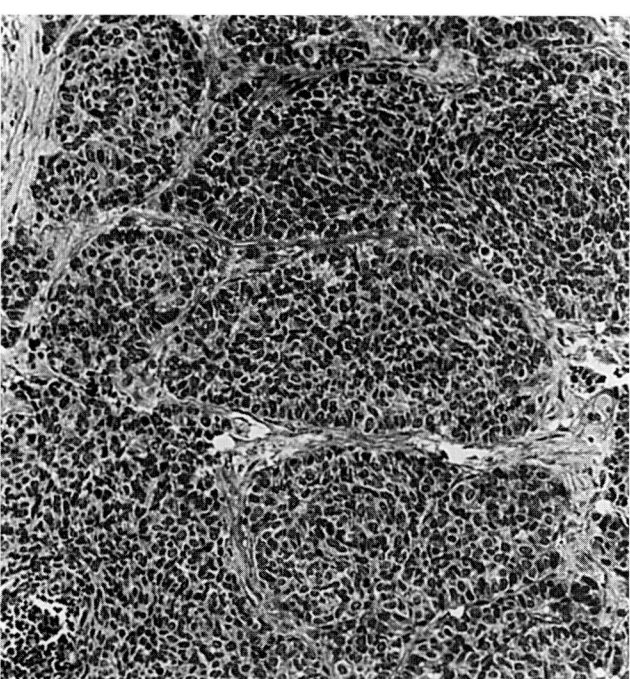

Fig. 19-48 Small cell carcinoma of cervix.

most countries and the most frequent neoplasm among women in many of them.[207] In the United States, the incidence rate has decreased during the last several decades both among blacks and whites, presumably as a result of the widespread use of cervical cytologic screening programs, which have counteracted increases anticipated from changes in risk factor prevalence.[201,208] The tumor appears most often in the older age groups but also occurs, with increased *relative* frequency, in young white females.[203] Evidence exists supporting the association of early marriage, multiparity, and low economic level with a high incidence of cervical carcinoma.[200,204] The single most important factor is probably age at first intercourse.[202,204] This tumor has a low incidence in Jewish women and is practically nonexistent in nuns.

The relationship between invasive cervical carcinoma and viruses is a complex and controversial topic. Herpes virus II and Epstein-Barr virus, although statistically associated with tumor development, do not seem to be causally related to it.[209,212] HTLV-1 and HIV viruses, when present, adversely affect the prognosis of patients with cervical carcinoma and may be associated with a rapidly progressive clinical course, but there is no conclusive evidence for a direct oncogenic effect for them.[205,206,210-212] The virus most closely implicated in the etiology of cervical carcinoma is HPV; this was discussed on p. 1358.

The possible relationship of oral contraceptives and other hormones (including diethylstilbestrol exposure in utero) to cervical carcinoma remains controversial.[208]

Morphologic features

Grossly, cervical carcinoma may be polypoid or deeply infiltrative (Figs. 19-45 and 19-46). The bulky carcinomas that grow out of the cervix are less likely to invade surrounding structures than are the infiltrating ones.

Some tumors are either clinically inapparent or simply missed by the examiner and are first discovered on pathologic examination of a uterus removed for a benign condition.[219] Still others develop in the cervical stump left from a supracervical hysterectomy, an operation that (for this very reason) is performed only exceptionally at present.[221]

Microscopically, three major categories of cervical squamous cell carcinoma exist, although admixtures and intermediate forms abound: large cell nonkeratinizing (Fig. 19-47), keratinizing, and small cell[214,216,222] (Fig. 19-48). The latter should be distinguished from small cell neuroendocrine carcinoma, a tumor morphologically similar to small cell carcinoma of the lung and exhibiting features of neuroendocrine differentiation; electron microscopy and immunohistochemistry may be necessary for this purpose (see p. 1375).

Some squamous cell carcinomas are accompanied by acantholysis, which may result in a pseudoglandular pattern.[213] Amyloid deposition in the stroma has been documented in some other cases.[213,218,223] On occasion, cervical squamous cell carcinoma is found to be associated with intense infiltration by mature eosinophils, with or without accompanying peripheral blood eosinophilia; production of eosinotactic and eosinopoietic substances by the tumor cells has been suggested as the pathogenetic mechanism.[215,220]

Mucicarmine stains will demonstrate the presence of scattered droplets of cytoplasmic mucin in a minority of cases having the morphologic features of squamous cell carcinoma in routinely stained sections, a finding analogous to that sometimes encountered in carcinomas of the lung and other sites. These tumors have been variously referred to as

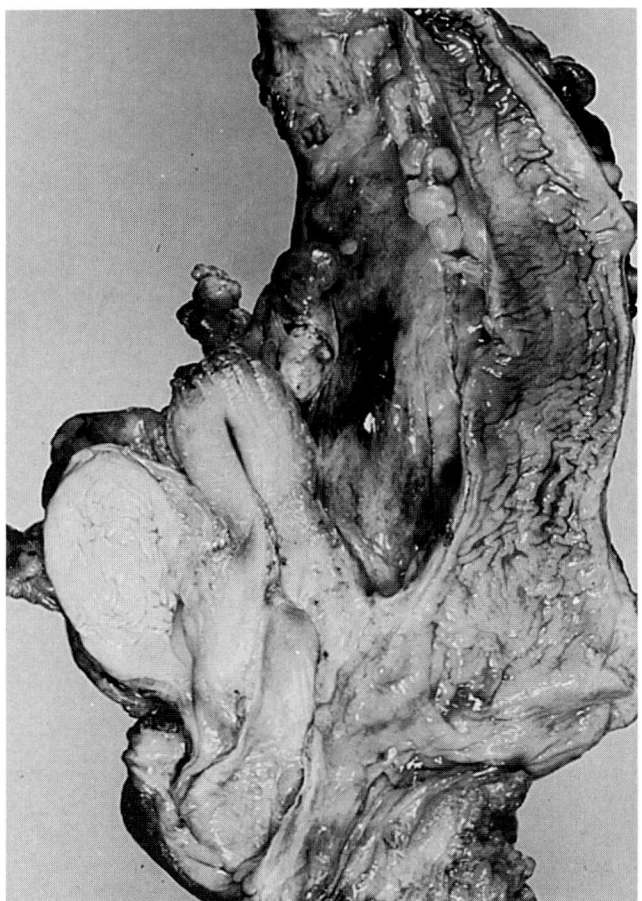

Fig. 19-49 Specimen from pelvic exenteration that has been sectioned so that intimate relation between bladder, cervix, vagina, and large bowel can be seen. There was persistent carcinoma in cervix with invasion of right parametrium. There were no involved lymph nodes of thirty examined.

mucoepidermoid carcinoma (a misleading term), adenosquamous carcinoma (less objectionable but not ideal), and squamous (cell) carcinoma with mucin secretion.[217] Whatever term one may wish to employ, it is important to regard this tumor as a morphologic variation on the theme of squamous cell carcinoma rather than adenocarcinoma (see p. 1368).

Immunohistochemical and other special techniques

Immunohistochemically, squamous cell carcinomas of the cervix express keratins (nearly 100% of the cases), CEA (90%),[224] and blood group antigens.[230] The range of keratins found in the tumor varies somewhat depending on the subtype, but it is very wide.[229] There may also be reactivity for cathepsin B (although not as frequently as in adenocarcinoma)[227] and for parathyroid hormone–related gene (although these tumors rarely give rise to hypercalcemia).[224a]

Immunoreactivity for progesterone receptor has been found in the majority of the cases.[226]

In contrast to the situation in many other human malignancies, the p53 gene is rarely mutated in cervical squamous cell carcinoma; this is also true for the biologically related MDM2 gene.[225]

Aneuploidy has been the rule in DNA studies of cervical squamous cell carcinoma, but there is often considerable heterogeneity within the same lesion.[228]

Spread and metastases

Cervical carcinoma spreads characteristically by direct extension to the vagina, corpus (endometrium or myometral wall), parametrium, lower urinary tract, and uterosacral ligaments.[235]

Lymph node metastases are also common. The pattern of involvement generally proceeds in a sequential fashion. The first station is represented by the paracervical, hypogastric, obturator, and external iliac groups and the second by the sacral, common iliac, aortic, and inguinal groups.[232] The incidence of nodal involvement is directly related to the stage of the disease. Hematogenous metastases were rare in older series, but with better control of the local lesion, they have increased in frequency.[235] Lungs (9%) and bones (4%) are the most common sites.[231,233,234] Ovarian metastases are less common than in endometrial adenocarcinoma, but they do occur.[236]

Treatment

Invasive carcinomas of the cervix can be treated by surgery, irradiation, or a combination of both modalities.[245,250] The choice depends on the extent of the tumor, the general condition of the patient, and the expertise available at the institution where the patient is treated. Early lesions can be treated just as effectively with hysterectomy or intracavitary radium[239,240]; for stage IIa lesions, irradiation alone and a combination of irradiation and surgery have yielded equivalent results in randomized studies.[248] If an occult invasive cervical carcinoma is found in a specimen from a simple hysterectomy done for another reason, additional therapy is indicated, usually in the form of a radical re-operation.[243]

Lack of prompt response (within 1 to 3 months) to radiation therapy is a predictor of likely recurrence and an indicator that adjuvant chemotherapy should be considered.[241] The latter has also been tried to increase the number of operable patients as well as a postoperative measure, with some encouraging preliminary results.[242]

In cases of postirradiation relapse of cervical carcinoma, pelvic exenteration should be seriously considered because a considerable number of the patients will have the persistent tumor confined to the pelvis.[246] This operation removes all pelvic viscera and lateral pelvic lymph node–bearing tissue (Figs. 19-49 and 2-8). At laparotomy, the surgeon should examine the upper abdomen carefully, particularly the periaortic area, for evidence of spread outside the pelvis. Any suspicious lymph nodes or liver nodules should be submitted to the pathologist for frozen section before the operative procedure is begun. Gross appraisal of enlarged extrapelvic nodes is unreliable, whereas frozen section examination is a highly accurate procedure.[237] The study of the surgical specimen should include a careful examination

Table 19-3 FIGO staging for carcinoma of the cervix uteri

Stage 0	Carcinoma in situ, intraepithelial carcinoma.
Stage I	The carcinoma is strictly confined ot the cervix (extension to the corpus should be disregarded).
Stage IA	Preclinical carcinomas of the cervix, that is those diagnosed only by microscopy.
Stage IA-1	Minimal microscopically evident stromal invasion.
Stage IA-2	Lesions detected microscopically that can be measured. The upper limit of the measurement should not show a depth of invasion of more than 5mm taken from the base of the epithelium, either surface or glandular, from which it originates, and a second dimension, the horizontal spread, must not exceed 7mm. Larger lesions should be classified as Stage IB.
Stage IB	Lesions of greater dimensions that Stage IA-2, whether seen clinically or not. Pre-formed space involvement should not alter the staging but should be specifically recorded so as to determine whether it should affect treatment decisions in the future.
Stage II	The carcinoma extends beyond the cervix but has not extended to the pelvic wall. The carcinoma involves the vagina but not as far as the lower third.
Stage IIA	No obvious parametrial involvement
Stage IIB	Obvious parametrial involvement
Stage III	The carcinoma has extended to the pelvic wall. On rectal examination, there is no cancer-free space between the tumor and the pelvic wall. The tumor involves the lower third of the vagina. All cases with a hydronephrosis or nonfunctioning kidney are included unless they are known to be due to other causes.
Stage IIIA	No extension to the pelvic wall.
Stage IIIB	Extension to the pelvic wall and/or hydronephrosis or nonfunctioning kidney.
Stage IV	The carcinoma has extended beyond the true pelvis or has clinically involved the mucosa of the bladder or rectum. A bullous edema as such does not permit a case to be allotted to Stage IV.
Stage IVA	Spread of the growth to adjacent organs.
Stage IVB	Spread to distant organs.

Notes about the staging

Stage IA carcinoma should include minimal microscopically evident stromal invasion as well as small cancerous tumors of measurable size. Stage IA should be divided into those lesions with minute foci of invasion visible only microscopically as Stage IA-1 and macroscopically measurable microcarcinomas as stage IA-2, in order to gain further knowledge of the clinical behavior of these lesions. The term "1B occult" should be omitted.

The diagnosis of both Stage IA-1 and IA-2 cases should be based on microscopic examination of removed tissue, preferably a cone, which must include the entire lesion. The lower limit of stage IA-2 should be measured macroscopically (even if dots need to be placed on the slide prior to measurement), and the upper limit of Stage IA-2 is given by the measurement of the two largest dimensions in any given section. The depth of invasion should not be more than 5mm taken from the base of the epithelium, either surface or glandular, from which it originates. The second dimension, the horizontal spread, must not exceed 7mm. Vascular space involvement, either venous or lymphatic, should not alter the staging but should be specifically recorded, as it may affect treatment decisions in the future.
Lesions of greater size should be classified as Stage IB.

From SGO handbook. Staging of gynecologic malignancies. Chicago, 1994, Society of Gynecologic Oncologists.
See also Appendix G.

of the lymph nodes, the lateral edges of the resection, and the local extent of the tumor. Microscopically, the nodes, vessels, and adjacent organs should be examined for evidence of tumor. The finding of greater prognostic relevance in the pathologic evaluation of pelvic exenteration specimens is the presence or absence of lymph node metastases.[249]

Other indications for pelvic exenteration are locally invasive carcinoma of the rectum, severe pelvic irradiation necrosis, and recurrent carcinoma of the endometrium. The 5-year survival rate for patients undergoing this formidable procedure for postirradiation persistence of carcinoma of the cervix is notably high considering the circumstances; it was approximately 25% in early series[238,244] and has now reached the remarkable figure of 73% at one institution.[247]

Prognosis

The prognosis of cervical carcinoma is related to the following parameters:

1 *Clinical stage* (Table 19-3).[251] As for most other human malignancies, this is the most important prognostic determinator.
2 *Nodal status.* This is another crucial predictor, which is incorporated into the staging scheme.[259,266]
3 *Size* of the largest involved node[261] and *number* of positive nodes.[262]
4 *Tumor size,* as determined by measurement of the tumor greatest diameter[264,269] or by volumetric techniques.[254]
5 *Depth of invasion.*[260,271]
6 *Endometrial extension.* The presence of this feature decreases the survival rate by a factor of 10% to 20%.[268]
7 Microscopic evidence of *parametrial involvement.*[263]
8 *Blood vessel invasion.*[253,278]
9 *Microscopic grade.* Whether the degree of tumor differentiation as evaluated in routinely stained sections correlates with survival independently from staging remains a controversial issue.[273,274] If a correlation

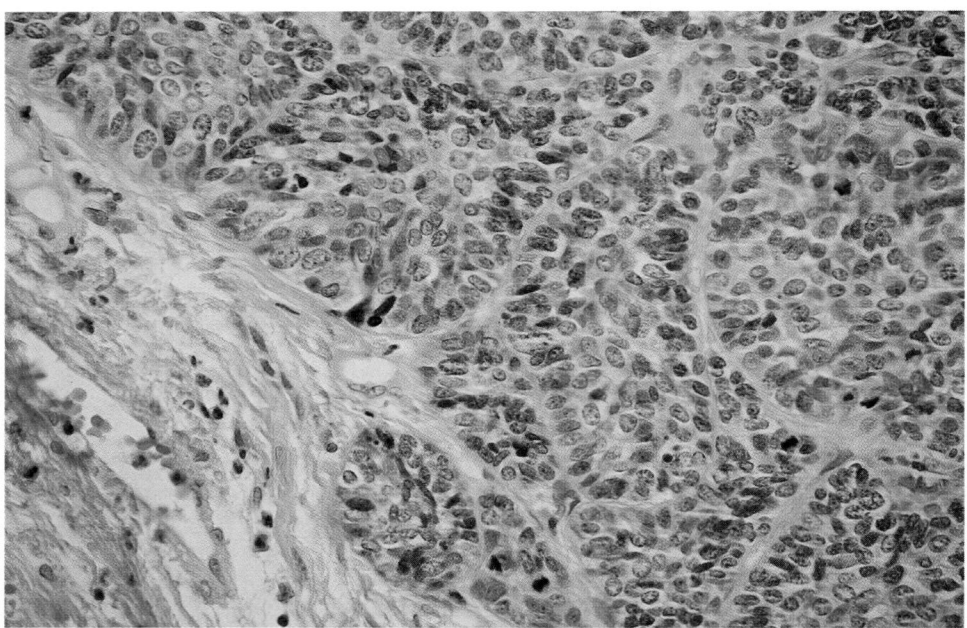

Fig. 19-50 Basaloid (squamous cell) carcinoma of uterine cervix. The tumor grows in the form of well-defined nests showing peripheral palisading.

exists, it must be minimal indeed, whether one uses the Reagan-Ng or the Broders' method of grading.[275,278]

10 *Microscopic type.* A similar comment applies to this parameter, which is roughly related to microscopic grade. Some authors have found a better prognosis with the large cell nonkeratinizing type and a worse prognosis with the small cell type,[277] but others have found no correlation between microscopic classification and prognosis.[255,256]

11 *Tumor-associated tissue eosinophilia.* It has been claimed that a markedly eosinophilic infiltrate in the carcinoma is associated with a statistically improved survival.[252] This is in accord with results obtained in other locations concerning this morphologic finding.

12 *Keratin profile* as evaluated immunohistochemically. No predictive value seems to be attached to this parameter.[276a]

13 *Cell proliferation index.* High S-phase rates as determined by flow cytometry are correlated to both a poorly differentiated histologic appearance and decreased short-term survival.[276]

14 *Lack of detection of HPV DNA,*[270] stromal infiltration by S-100 protein–positive *Langerhans' cells,*[265] and expression of c-*erb*B-2,[257,267] *ras* oncogene,[272] and Tn antigen (a precursor of MN blood group antigen)[258] have all been found to relate to an unfavorable outcome. It remains to be determined how many of these parameters will prove to have independent prognostic value.

15 *Angiogenesis.* No evidence has been found between the density of microvessels and prognosis in cervical squamous cell carcinoma.[271a]

Other microscopic types

Verrucous carcinoma is a highly differentiated variant of squamous cell carcinoma with a polypoid pattern of growth,

an extremely well-differentiated cytologic appearance, and a capacity for local invasion but not for metastatic spread. Some cases have been found to extend into the endometrial cavity.[286] Verrucous carcinoma should be distinguished both from condyloma acuminatum and from ordinary squamous cell carcinoma with a prominent papillary pattern of growth.[284] The general gross and microscopic features of this tumor have been described in Chapter 4.

Spindle-cell carcinoma (sarcomatoid carcinoma, squamous cell carcinoma with sarcoma-like stroma) is morphologically analogous to the homonymous tumor in the upper aerodigestive tract; it should be distinguished from mixed müllerian tumor (see p. 1379).[285]

Basaloid (squamous cell) carcinoma is characterized by prominent peripheral palisading, an infiltrative growth pattern, and minimal stromal reaction[279,280] (Fig. 19-50). The behavior of this tumor is aggressive, as is also the case with the homonymous neoplasm in the upper aerodigestive tract.

Lymphoepithelioma-like carcinoma resembles its more common counterpart in the upper respiratory tract by virtue of the large size of the tumor cells, vesicular nuclei with prominent nucleoli, syncytial appearance, and heavy lymphocytic infiltration.[281,283,287] This tumor type shows considerable overlap with the *circumscribed* type of cervical carcinoma described by Japanese authors (Fig. 19-51).[282]

Transitional cell carcinoma having an appearance similar to the homonymous tumor located in the bladder or ovary can occur in the cervix; it should be distinguished from other papillary lesions of the cervix and from inverted transitional cell papilloma.[278a]

Adenocarcinoma

Primary adenocarcinomas make up 5% to 15% of all carcinomas of the cervix. This percentage is higher in Jewish women,[323] and it has been suggested that its relative incidence is on the rise for the general population, particularly

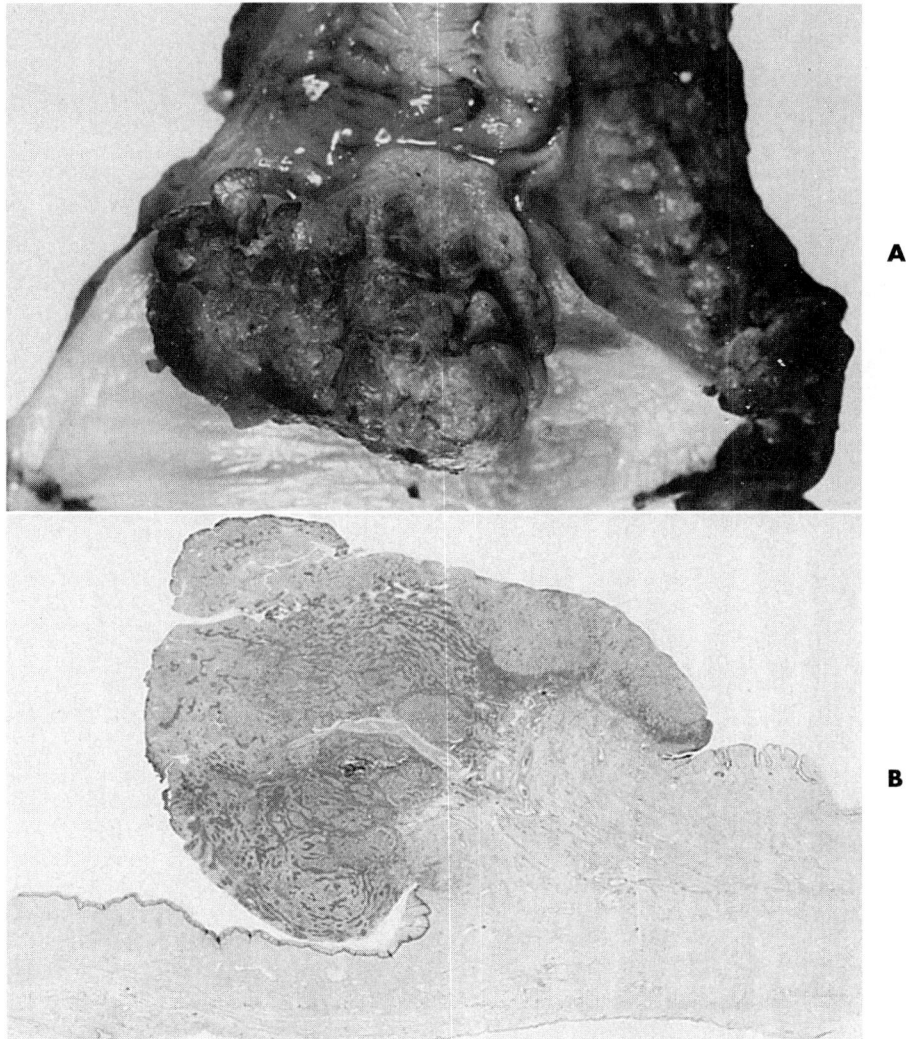

Fig. 19-51 Gross specimen **(A)** and whole-mount section **(B)** of circumscribed carcinoma of cervix. Tumor is polypoid, has pushing margins, and is associated with dense inflammatory infiltrate.

in young women.[360,367,369,380,390] An association has been found between the long-term use of oral contraceptives and the development of endocervical neoplasia in young patients,[313,389] but this has been contested by others.[336]

The tumor presents no distinguishing gross characteristics. Microscopically, the most common pattern is that of a well-differentiated glandular pattern with mucin secretion, some of which can leak into the stroma[346,363,381,395] (Fig. 19-52). Cervical adenocarcinoma can be poorly differentiated, can be papillary and can have psammoma bodies (thus resembling ovarian papillary serous carcinoma),[315,373,379] or can have an endometrioid appearance.[372] Some of the latter are extremely well differentiated,[301a,396] and a few have coexistent or subsequent endometrioid carcinoma in the ovary.[341] An association between ordinary endocervical adenocarcinoma and ovarian mucinous adenocarcinoma (and occasionally even tubal adenocarcinoma) has also been recorded.[333,354]

Histochemically, Alcian blue and mucicarmine-positive material is found intracellularly in nearly all cases.[381] The staining pattern is different from that of normal endocervical glands but similar to that of in situ adenocarcinoma.[321a] CEA and 1C5 are also consistently present immunohistochemically.[297,299,349] These features are of some value in the differential diagnosis with endometrial adenocarcinoma with endocervical involvement,[294] since mucin and CEA tend to be present only focally and superficially (apically and luminally) in the latter.[297,383] Keratin is consistently expressed, whereas vimentin is not.[302] Markers common to gastric, intestinal, and pancreatobiliary epithelial cells (such as M1 and cathepsin E) are commonly present.[383a] Cervical adenocarcinomas have also been shown to contain argyrophilic cells[352] and a variety of peptide hormones[387] and also to express hormone receptors[314,357] and the enzyme amylase.[322] Basement membrane, as investigated immunohistochemically with type IV collagen or

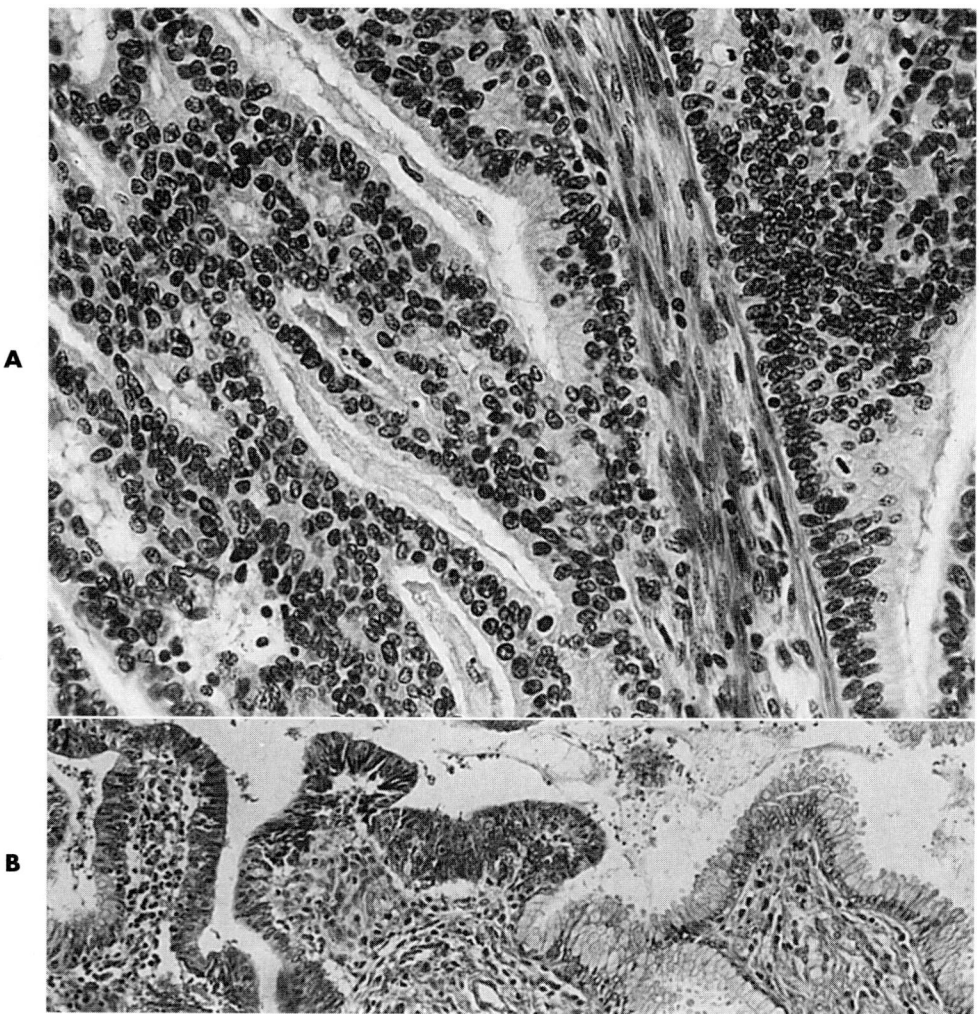

Fig. 19-52 Adenocarcinoma of cervix. Tumor shown in **A** is well differentiated and mucin producing. Tumor shown in **B** involves only portion of endocervical gland shown.

laminin, may be present around the tumor cell even in the invasive tumors, but usually in a discontinuous fashion.[386,393]

The prognosis in cervical adenocarcinoma depends on the clinical stage, amount of tumor (as determined by tumor volume), microscopic grade, and nodal status.* In most series, the overall prognosis has been less favorable than for the squamous cell counterpart.[330,347,361] There is not much difference among the various histologic subtypes, although the endometrioid variety is said to behave slightly better.[376] The presence of nodal metastases is an ominous prognostic sign.[292] Increased serum levels of CA125 and overexpression of c-erbB-2 and nm23-H1 proteins have also been found to represent poor prognostic factors.[304,343,356a]

The preferred therapies are radiation alone or a combination of radiation and surgery.[305,321,329] The incidence of residual tumor in the hysterectomy specimens after intracavitary treatment is much higher than for squamous cell carcinoma.[344]

---

*References 290, 306, 330, 342, 345, 358.

In situ and microinvasive adenocarcinoma

In situ[318,328,336,362,368] and microinvasive[384] stages of cervical adenocarcinoma exist. Instances of glandular dysplasia have also been described,[334,335] with the ensuing proposal to group the dysplastic and the in situ adenocarcinomatous lesions under the term "cervical intraepithelial glandular neoplasia."[317,392] Some of the in situ lesions have been shown to precede the development of invasive adenocarcinoma, just as squamous carcinoma in situ (CIN III) precedes invasive carcinoma of the same type.[293] The mucus secreted by the in situ malignant glands may be similar to those of the normal endocervical mucosa or may resemble the pattern of intestinal goblet cells.[317] Most lesions are positive for CEA, less than half for keratin, and one tenth for secretory component, those figures being lower than for the invasive tumors.[332] It should be mentioned in this context that almost half of the invasive cervical adenocarcinomas and about 75% of their in situ counterparts have an associated CIN of the conventional squamous type of the overlying epithe-

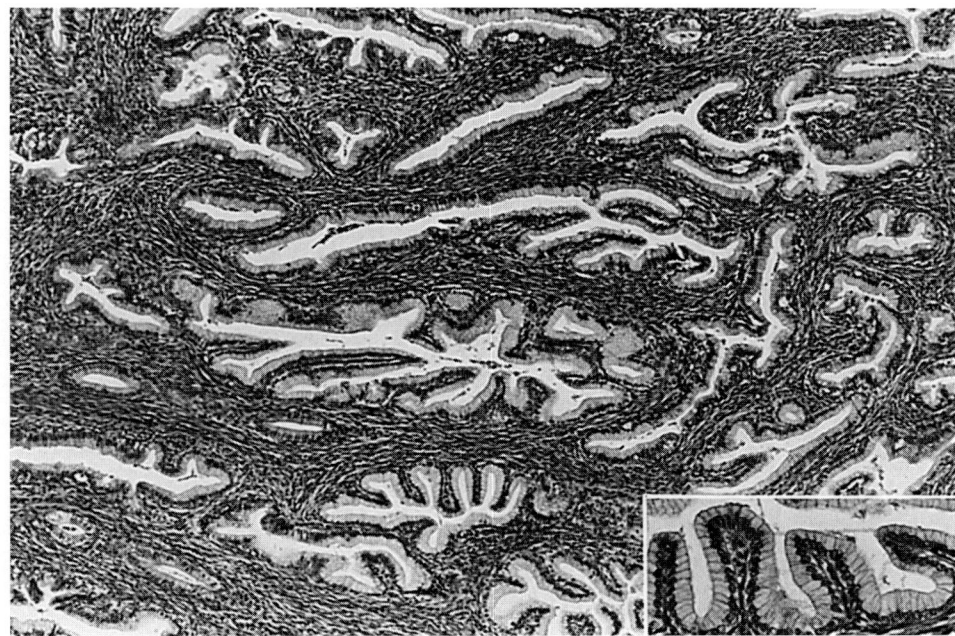

Fig. 19-53 Well-differentiated adenocarcinoma of cervix (so-called adenoma malignum). **Inset** shows remarkably well-differentiated appearance of tumor cells.

lium.[298,355,391] Conization is the treatment of choice for in situ adenocarcinoma of the cervix.[289]

Morphologic variants of cervical adenocarcinoma

Adenoma malignum (minimal deviation adenocarcinoma) is a type of cervical adenocarcinoma so well-differentiated structurally and cytologically that it can be diagnosed only as malignant because of the presence of distorted glands with irregular outlines deeply positioned in the cervix and the fact that a portion of the infiltrating tumor is associated with a stromal response[316,338,340,365] (Fig. 19-53). About half of the cases have small foci with a less well-differentiated appearance. Vascular and perineurial invasion may be present. A minor component of argyrophilic cell can be detected in most of the cases.[316] The fact that these tumors, like the more obvious adenocarcinomas, are CEA positive is of importance in the differential diagnosis with benign lesions such as microglandular hyperplasia.[359,382] Parenthetically, there is no convincing evidence that adenoma malignum and conventional cervical adenocarcinoma are causally related to microglandular hyperplasia.[336] The differential diagnosis also includes the condition known as *florid deep glands,* in which atypia, architectural disarray, and desmoplastic stromal reaction are lacking.[302a]

Adenoma malignum constitutes about 1% of all endocervical adenocarcinomas. Some cases are associated with the Peutz-Jeghers syndrome.[316,397] The prognosis is poor.

Villoglandular (papillary) adenocarcinoma presents as an exophytic polypoid lesion with papillae lined by endocervical, endometrial, or intestinal-type epithelium showing mild atypia. The appearance of the superficial portion is similar to that of colorectal villous adenoma. Most cases are associ-

ated with adenocarcinoma in situ and/or CIN.[337] The prognosis is excellent.[394]

Adenosquamous (mixed) carcinoma combines the patterns of adenocarcinoma with a well-defined squamous component[295] (Figs. 19-54 and 19-55). This tumor type seems to be particularly common during pregnancy.[319] It is likely that the cell of origin of adenosquamous carcinomas and most adenocarcinomas of the cervix is the same as for the ordinary squamous cell carcinoma (i.e., the subcolumnar reserve cell).[296,348,371]

Adenocarcinoma as previously defined should be distinguished from squamous cell carcinoma without glandular formations but with histochemically demonstrable intracellular mucin (see p. 1365).[385]

Adenosquamous carcinomas have been shown in some series to have a worse overall prognosis than pure squamous cell carcinoma or adenocarcinoma. This is probably due to the fact that most of them are poorly differentiated tumors,[311] as supported by the greater proportion of high ploidy stem cells found in these lesions when subjected to DNA analysis.[310] However, when compared grade by grade and stage by stage with adenocarcinomas and squamous cell carcinomas, no prognostic differences are found.[301,326]

Auersperg et al.[291] have shown that most cervical carcinomas that appear undifferentiated at the light microscopic level still exhibit traits of squamous and/or glandular differentiation at the ultrastructural level.

Glassy cell carcinoma has been described as a distinct type of poorly differentiated adenosquamous carcinoma.[320] It occurs in a younger age group (mean age, 41 years) than other cervical neoplasms and often has been associated with pregnancy. The tumor cells have a moderate amount of cyto-

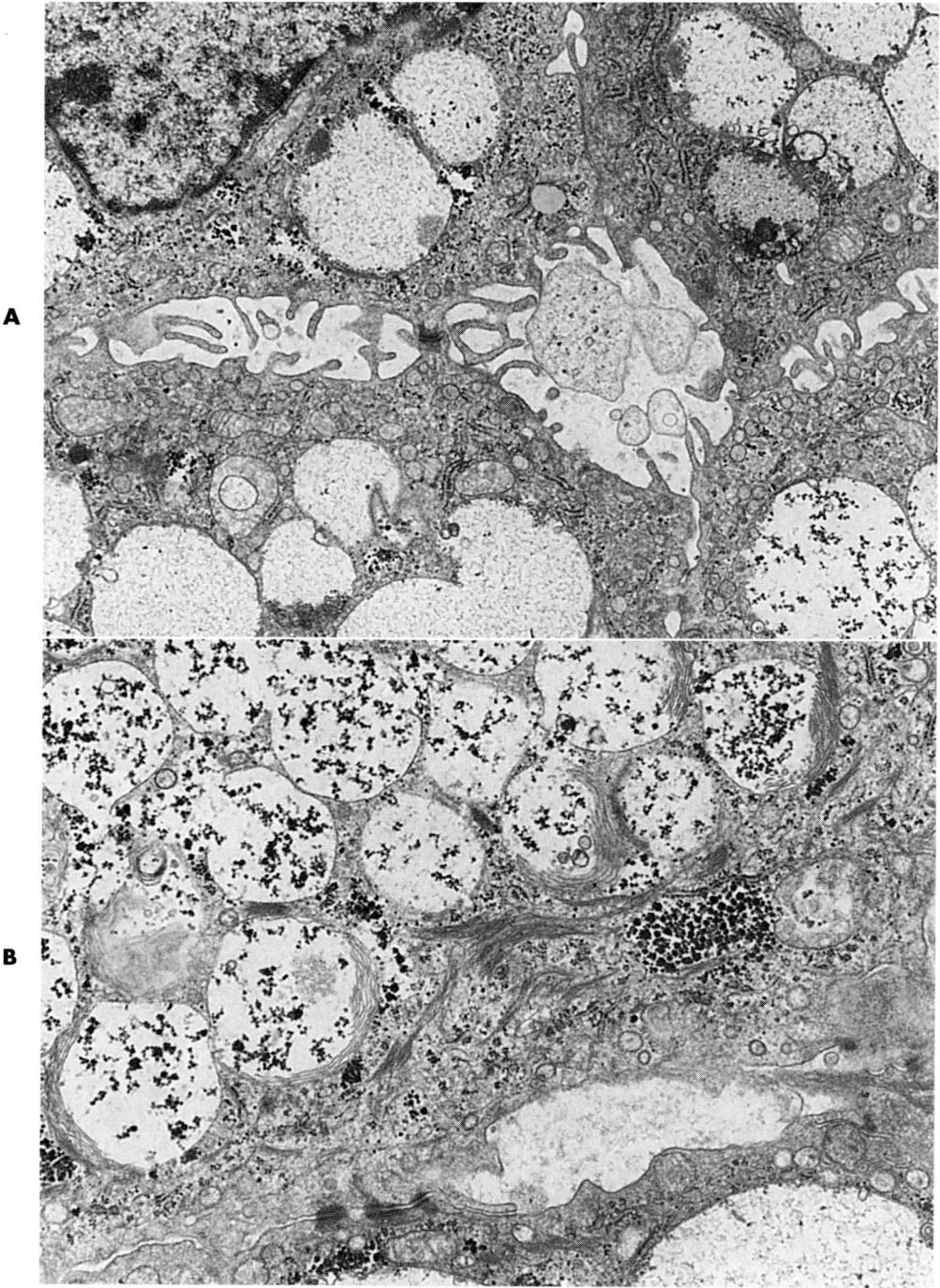

Fig. 19-54 Ultrastructural appearance of adenosquamous carcinoma of cervix. **A,** Large mucous secretory vacuoles, true lumen formation, and scattered glycogen may be noted in tumor cells. **B,** Note tonofiliments in addition to secretory products.

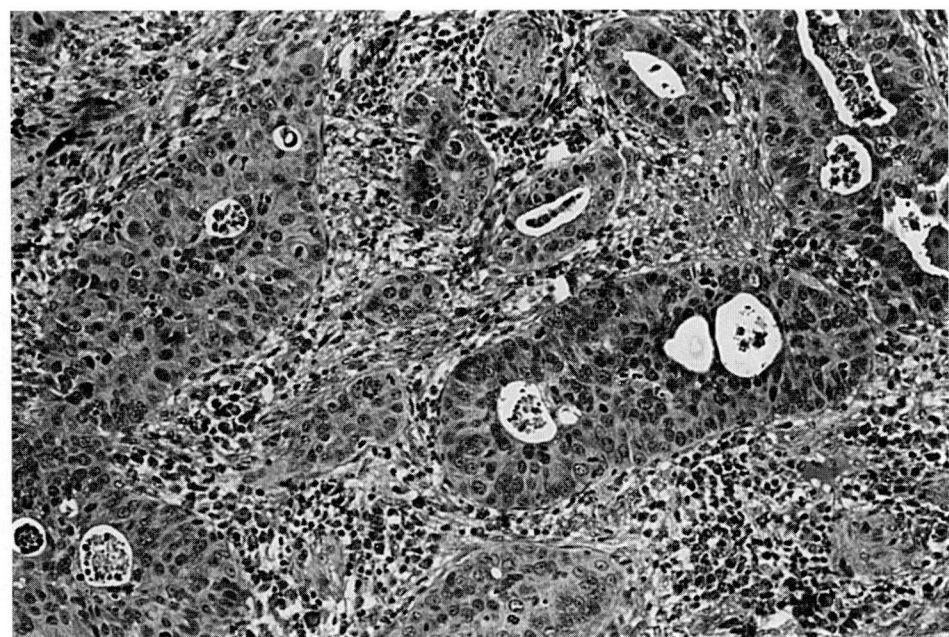

Fig. 19-55 Adenosquamous carcinoma of cervix. Glandular formations blend with foci of squamous differentiation.

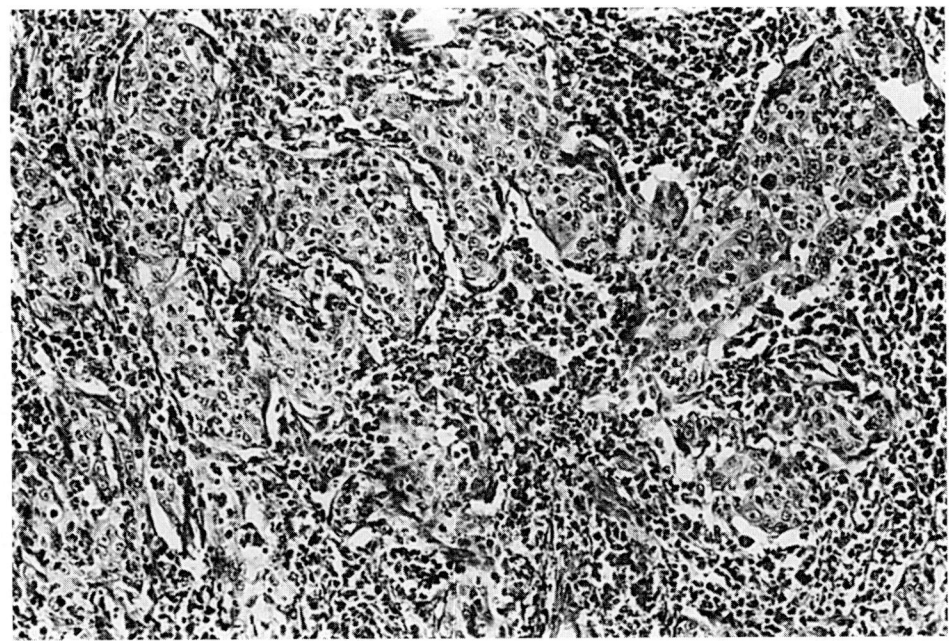

Fig. 19-56 So-called glassy cell carcinoma of cervix. Solid nests of tumor cells with glassy acidophilic cytoplasm are surrounded by very heavy infiltrate rich in eosinophils.

plasm with a ground-glass or finely granular appearance, a prominent eosinophilic and PAS-positive cell wall, and large nuclei with prominent nucleoli. Mitoses are numerous. A prominent inflammatory infiltrate often rich in eosinophils is regularly seen in the adjacent stroma, and this may be accompanied by peripheral blood eosinophilia (Fig. 19-56).

In pure cases of glassy cell carcinoma, glandular or squamous differentiation is absent, although it can be consistently detected by ultrastructural examination.[388] Other cases show an admixture with mucin-producing adenocarcinoma and/or clear-cut squamous foci, raising the question whether it is justified to regard glassy cell carcinoma as a

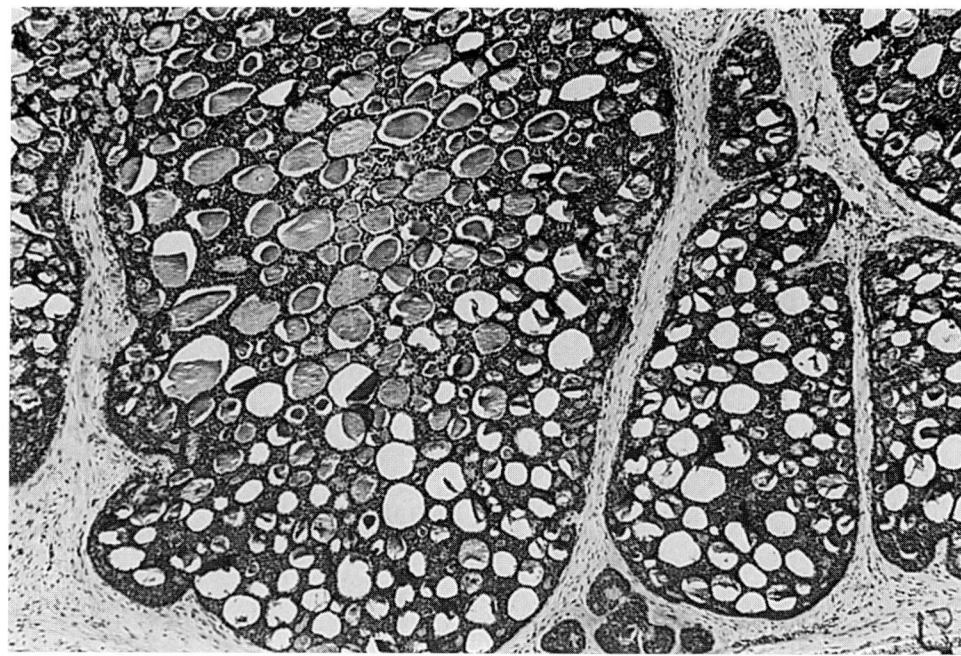

Fig. 19-57 Adenoid cystic carcinoma of uterine cervix. Appearance is similar to that of homonymous salivary gland tumor. (Slide contributed by Dr. G. Finkel, Port Jefferson, NY.)

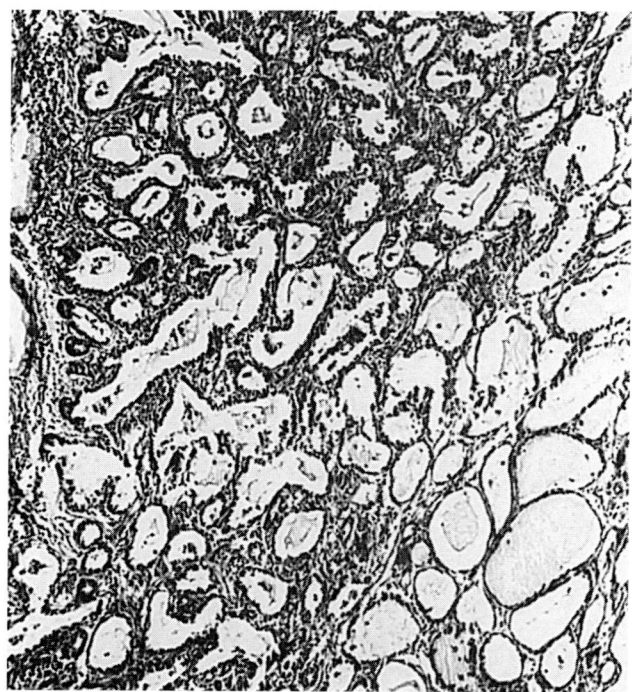

Fig. 19-58 Clear cell (mesonephroid) carcinoma of cervix. Glands have a branching configuration, and some are cystically dilated.

distinct entity.[300,356] The prognosis is poor, a fact probably related to its poorly differentiated nature.[353,366]

Adenoid cystic carcinoma is a specific variant of cervical adenocarcinoma that tends to occur in elderly multigravid black women[312] and that is associated with a particularly poor prognosis.[309,331] The morphologic appearance is similar to that of the homonymous tumors of salivary glands (Fig. 19-57). Like the former, it may be cribriform (the most common pattern) or grow in a predominantly solid fashion.[288] It needs to be distinguished from the already mentioned basaloid carcinoma, also known as adenoid basal carcinoma[308] (see p. 1368).

Clear cell carcinoma (formerly called *mesonephric carcinoma*) of the cervix is of müllerian rather than of mesonephric origin. The presence of in situ changes in the area of the squamocolumnar junction in some of the cases[375] and the electron microscopic features[303] seem to provide conclusive evidence for this interpretation. Glands lined by large cells with abundant clear cytoplasm are characteristic[307] (Fig. 19-58). "Hobnail" cells are common, as well as intraglandular papillary projections. Grossly, the tumor is usually exophytic. This is the most common form of cervical carcinoma in young females, although it occurs in all age groups.[324,364] The prognosis is relatively good. In the thirteen cases studied by Hart and Norris,[327] the actuarial survival rate was 55% at 5 years and 40% at 10 years. The relationship with intrauterine diethylstilbestrol exposure and other features of this tumor are the same as for the analogous vaginal neoplasms.[325,370,378] It is also evident, however, that morphologically identical cases occur in the absence of exposure to this hormone, particularly in older women.[339]

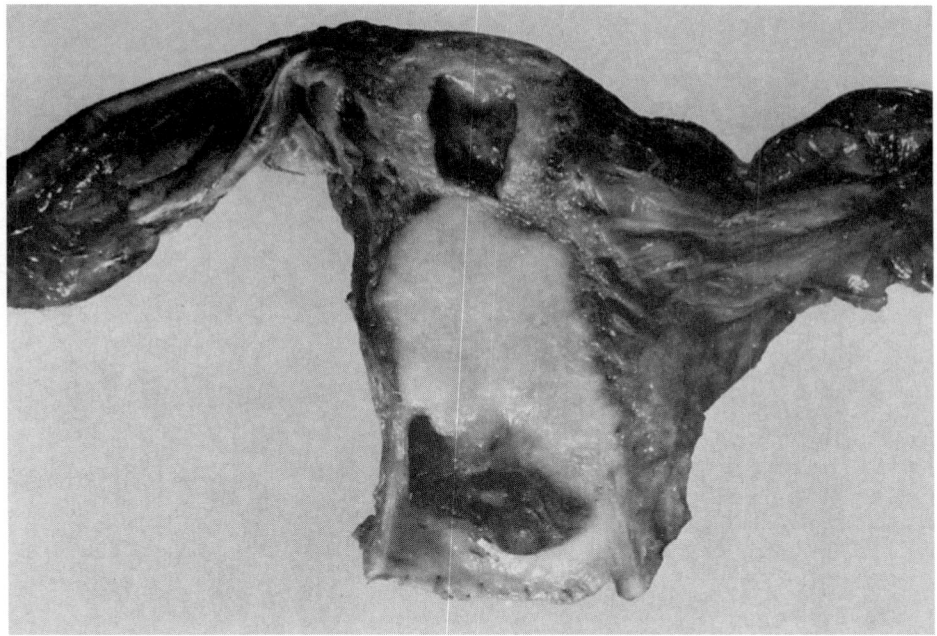

Fig. 19-59 Neuroendocrine carcinoma of uterine cervix. Large neoplasm has completely replaced cervix and is extending into parametrium. (Courtesy Dr. J. Albores-Saavedra and Dr. H. Rodriguez-Martinez, Mexico City.)

Mesonephric (adeno)carcinoma is a very rare tumor. Most of the cases that have been reported as such in the past probably represent müllerian-type adenocarcinomas or yolk sac tumors. True mesonephric carcinomas are often found adjacent to mesonephric hyperplasia (sometimes florid and atypical) and may exhibit a variety of patterns, such as ductal (resembling endometrioid adenocarcinoma), small tubular, retiform, solid, sex-cord–like, and spindle[296a,350,374] (Plate XIII-B).

An exceptionally rare adenocarcinoma of *small intestinal (enteric) type* containing numerous Paneth's cells has been described.[351,377]

Neuroendocrine carcinoma

A small number of cervical carcinomas exhibit various degrees of neuroendocrine differentiation, as detected by conventional morphologic, ultrastructural, histochemical, and/or immunohistochemical criteria.[401,422] These tumors have been variously called *carcinoid tumor, apudoma, argyrophil cell carcinoma, (extrapulmonary) small cell carcinoma, (neuro)endocrine carcinoma,* and *carcinoma with (neuro)endocrine differentiation,* the choice in terminology depending on the degree of differentiation of the tumor, the extent of endocrine features present, and the observer's bias[399,407,411,417] (Fig. 19-59). The age distribution is the same as for squamous cell carcinoma. They also show a similar association with HPV.[398,416] The carcinoid syndrome is invariably absent, but some cases have been seen in association with Cushing's syndrome.[410] In contrast to squamous cell carcinoma, CIN changes in the adjacent epithelium are

extremely rare.[400,416] A possible precursor lesion in the form of endocrine cell hyperplasia of the cervix has been identified.[402]

The better differentiated members of this group have an organoid arrangement, with trabecular, insular, glandular, and spindle patterns of growth (Fig. 19-60). Most cases are pure, but others are combined with squamous cell carcinoma[415] or adenocarcinoma.[406,413,414] Some of these combined tumors have been referred to as amphicrine carcinomas.[405]

Argyrophilic (but not argentaffin) granules can be demonstrated in some of the cases. Amyloid may be deposited in the stroma. Ultrastructurally, a variable number of dense core secretory granules are found in all but the most undifferentiated types. Immunohistochemically, positivity may be found for neuron-specific enolase,[408] chromogranin (but only in the better differentiated examples), serotonin, other generic neuroendocrine markers,[418,419] and a variety of peptide hormones.[420] They also commonly express keratin (befitting their epithelial nature) and CEA.[420]

In contrast to the classic carcinoid tumors of the appendix, small bowel, or lung, the large majority of these cervical neoplasms are histologically and clinically aggressive. Mitoses and areas of necrosis are common, and the prognosis is generally poor.[423] In this regard, they resemble the "atypical carcinoid tumors" and even the small cell carcinomas of the lung.[398] A definite relationship exists between degree of microscopic differentiation and clinical behavior, the outcome being particularly bleak for the small cell carcinomas.[399,403,409,412,421] Current evidence supports the concept that, as in the lung, small cell carcinomas of the

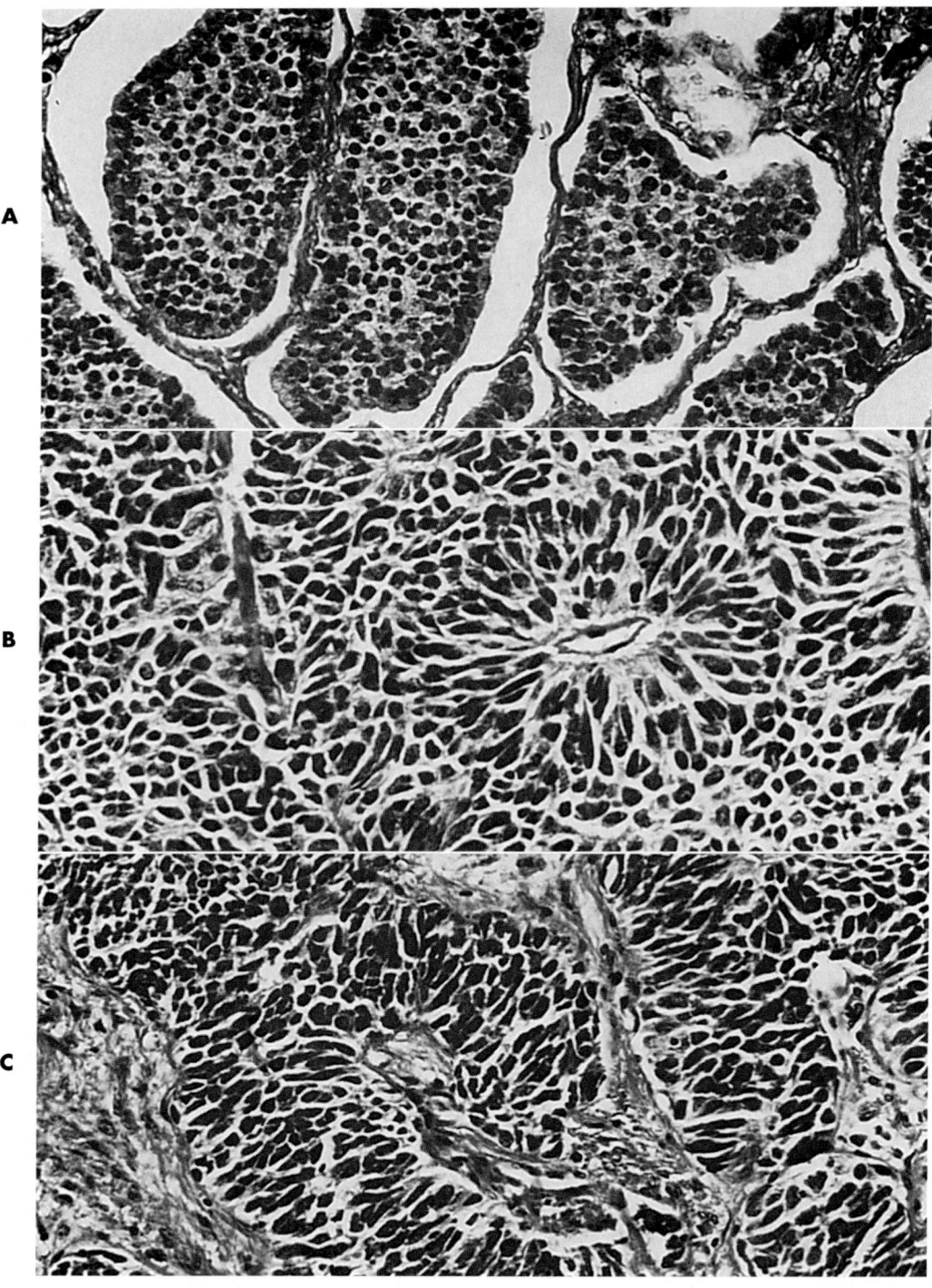

Fig. 19-60 Different morphologic patterns exhibited by neuroendocrine carcinoma of cervix. **A,** So-called insular or classic pattern, with solid nests of small cells exhibiting peripheral palisading and retraction from stroma. **B,** Perivascular arrangement of tumor cells. **C,** Thick trabeculae with serpiginous pattern of growth. (Courtesy Dr. J. Albores-Saavedra and Dr. H. Rodriguez-Martinez, Mexico City.)

cervix show heterogeneity in their morphologic and functional properties; some will show evidence of endocrine differentiation, and some will not.[404]

Cytology

The broadest and most successful application of clinical cytology has been in the diagnosis of invasive carcinoma of the uterine cervix and precursor lesions through the technique popularized by George Papanicolaou at Cornell University and universally known as the Pap test.[442] Today, it is widely used both as a screening test in asymptomatic populations and in the follow-up of patients with cervical carcinomas treated by either conservative surgery or irradiation.[440,444]

Mass cytologic screening has shifted the presentation of cervical carcinoma from the clinical to the preclinical stage.[434,435] This is an established fact, the statement that the incidence of cervical carcinoma was already declining prior to the introduction of this diagnostic method notwithstanding. Incidentally, the accuracy of this statement has been disputed.[425,432] Following mass screening, there has been a reduction of 38% to 57% in the overall incidence of invasive carcinoma and a reduction of 67% in the incidence of clinically evident carcinoma (stages Ib to IV).[426,427,429,433,451] Whereas in the prescreening era invasive carcinoma contributed approximately 80% of all diagnosed cases, at the present time it makes up only 16% to 35% of the cases, the remaining being carcinomas in the intraepithelial stage.[428,432] This has resulted in an increased cure rate for the screened population and in an increase in the survival times for the patients with invasive carcinoma.[430,432,433,448] For instance, Christopherson and Scott[428] reported a 70% decrease in the mortality from carcinoma of the uterine cervix between 1970/1971 and 1955/1956 in women younger than 60 years of age.

The diagnostic accuracy of cervical cytology is high. In a series reviewed by Patten,[447] it was 96% for CIN and 94% for invasive carcinoma. Wied et al.[458] reported practically identical findings.

However, in the evaluation of some remarkably high figures, one cannot escape the suspicion that they might have been influenced by the fact that the same person diagnosed the cytology specimen and the cervical biopsy. To avoid subconscious bias, it is better for these two functions to be performed by two different individuals.[441] Seybolt[452] demonstrated this fact by distributing twenty-five problem cases to eight authorities in cytopathology and requesting them to interpret the cytology slides independently of the histology. There was no universal agreement in any case, and in some instances the disagreements were quite disparate. The conclusion from this survey was that it is not always possible to determine the exact histologic change in the cervix on the basis of the cytology smear. However, a more important demonstration was that if a cervical abnormality was present, this was detected by cytologic examination in the large majority of the cases.

Careful attention to technical factors is essential to achieve good results. The smear should be promptly fixed and carefully stained. Air-dried smears are grossly inadequate in this regard. Even if squamous cells can be rehydrated, they never exhibit the fine structural details of wet-fixed material; glandular cells are even more distorted. It is also highly desirable that the specimen be secured by a trained individual. Self-made samples, obtained with a pipette, are not nearly so satisfactory. Invasive carcinoma is detected at almost the same rate as with the material obtained by the physician, but the accuracy for is considerably lower. Furthermore, the percentage of unsatisfactory specimens approaches 20%.[429,439] It is also important for the detection of early carcinoma that an endocervical sample be examined in addition to the ordinary specimen from the exocervix and vaginal pool; this can be obtained by the use of a special brush.[437]

Special techniques are also applicable to cytology smears, including immunohistochemistry, in situ hybridization, and DNA cytometry.[431]

The terminology used in cervicovaginal cytology has evolved in the course of years, sometimes adapting names from the histopathology lexicon but more often devising some of its own. Papanicolaou's original system had five "classes" of increasing atypia. Although this nomenclature fulfilled a very important role in the establishment of the technique, it was eventually abandoned because of the vagueness of the information provided. A "class III" smear, for instance, could represent anything from a CIN II (moderate dysplasia) to an invasive carcinoma. Therefore it was progressively replaced in the 1960s by the nomenclature then in vogue among histopathologists (i.e., negative, benign atypia, dysplasia [mild, moderate, or severe] carcinoma in situ, and invasive carcinoma)[441,452,453] (Figs. 19-61 to 19-64). During the 1970s, many institutions switched to the CIN system for both cytologic and histologic specimens (see p. 1362). In 1988, a proposal was made at a meeting in Bethesda to classify squamous intraepithelial lesions (SIL) in the following categories: (1) atypical squamous cells of undetermined significance, (2) low-grade SIL, (3) high-grade SIL, and (4) squamous cell carcinoma.[445,446,455-457] In this scheme, low-grade SIL corresponds to HPV-associated cellular changes, mild dysplasia, and CIN I, whereas high-grade SIL corresponds to moderate and severe dysplasia, carcinoma in situ, and CIN II and III. The rationale for grouping HPV-related changes (koilocytosis) and CIN I within the low-grade SIL group is based on the many similarities that exist between the lesions, which makes their separation difficult. A similar reasoning lies behind the decision to combine CIN II and III lesions in the category of high-grade SIL. The term "atypical squamous cells of undetermined significance" was proposed at the same meeting for cases in which the findings do not fulfill the criteria for either benign reactive change or SIL; as such, it has a more restricted meaning than the more traditional terms "atypia" and "inflammatory atypia."[445] The system has been criticized on the basis that it may lead to overtreatment of many individuals whose smears are placed into the low-grade SIL category.[436]

The great success of the Pap test has led to overexpectations on the part of clinicians and the public at large and the unreasonable demand that every case of carcinoma be detected with it. One should not forget that it is and will remain a *screening* test and that—as such—it will inevitably be associated with a "false-negative rate."[449] The reasons

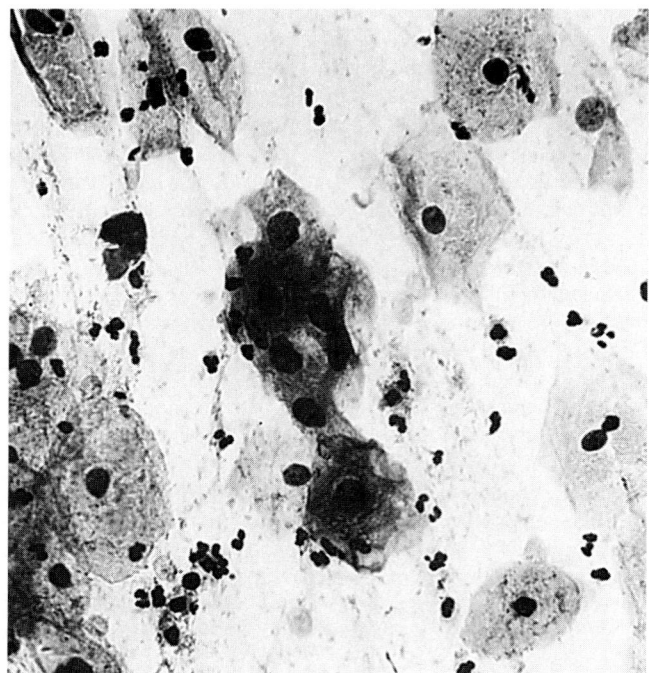

Fig. 19-61 Condylomatous changes mainly manifested in form of perinuclear clear haloes.

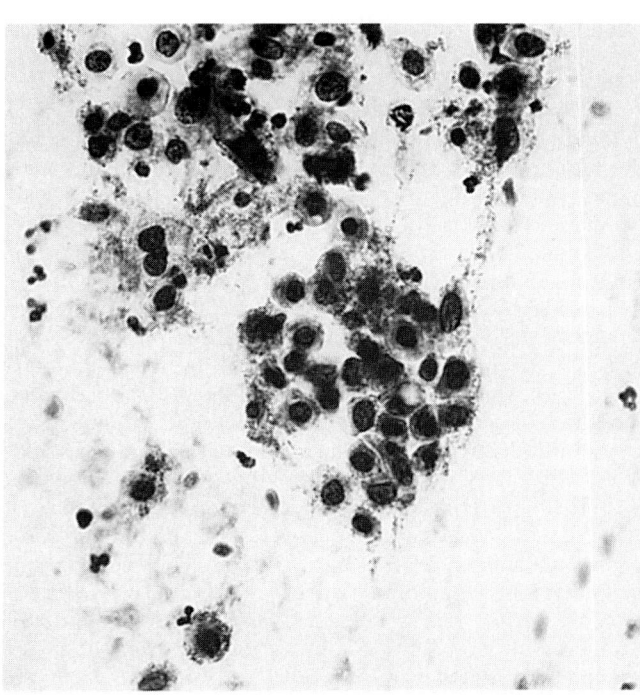

Fig. 19-62 Severe dysplasia. Nuclei are hyperchromatic, and amount of cytoplasm is scanty.

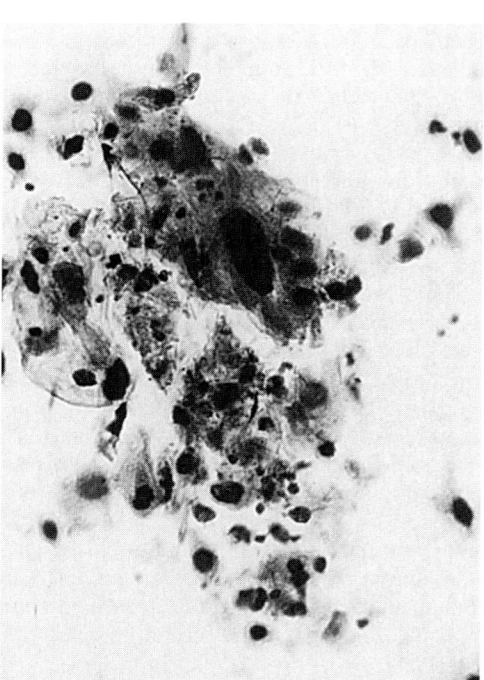

Fig. 19-63 Invasive squamous cell carcinoma. One of tumor cells has particularly large and deeply staining nucleus. Cytoplasm is relatively abundant.

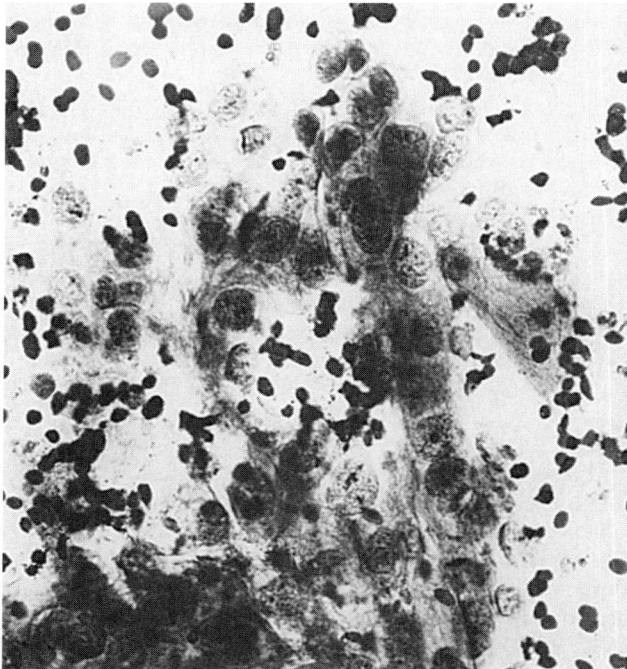

Fig. 19-64 Cervical adenocarcinoma. Nuclei are vesicular and contain prominent nucleoli.

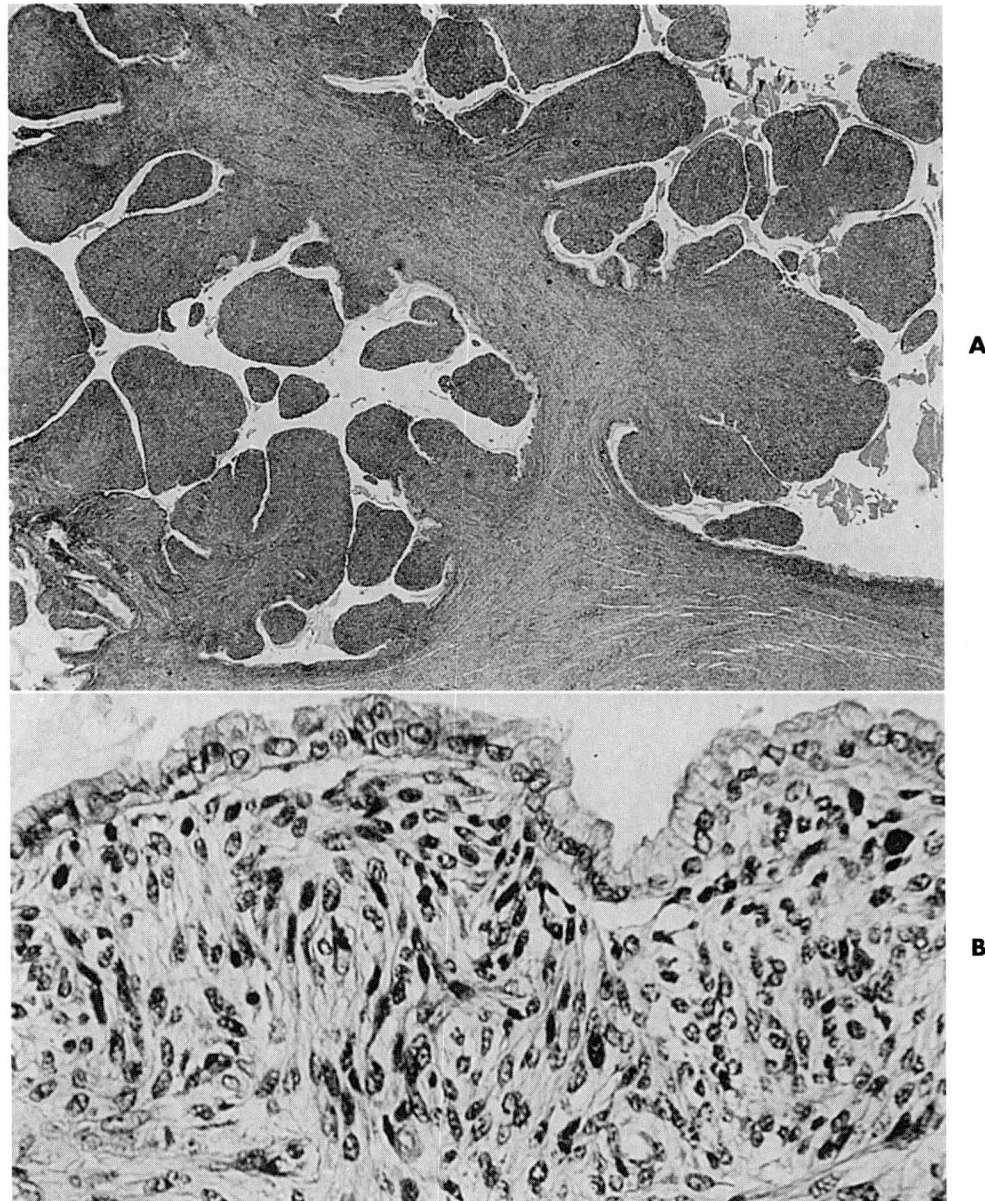

Fig. 19-65 A, Papillary adenofibroma of uterine cervix of adult. Stout ramifying connective tissue core is covered by endocervical epithelium. **B,** High power of same lesion shown in **A.**

include inadequacy of the sample, insufficient time devoted to screening, human fatigue, and (much more rarely) inadequate interpretation by the screener and/or pathologist.[443,450,454] In a recent study, rescreening of 25% of cervical smears yielded an "error-screening rate" of 5%,[454] but the total false-negative rate is probably much higher.

At present, several automated screening devices that analyze either conventionally or monolayered prepared cervical smears are being evaluated in an attempt to reduce the manual screening workload of cytology laboratories and, hopefully, contribute to a diminution of the false-negative rate.[424,438,459]

OTHER TUMORS AND TUMORLIKE CONDITIONS

Carcinomas of one type or another comprise about 99% of all primary cervical malignancies. The remaining 1% is made up of a variety of neoplasms.[468,504] ***Botryoid rhabdomyosarcoma*** presents in children and adolescents as a myxoid polypoid mass covered by attenuated epithelium.[470,473,490] The appearance is generally similar to that of the homonymous vaginal tumor. However, some of the cervical cases occurring in older patients have been seen to contain cartilage and to be associated with a better prognosis.[475] ***Mixed müllerian tumors*** also present as poly-

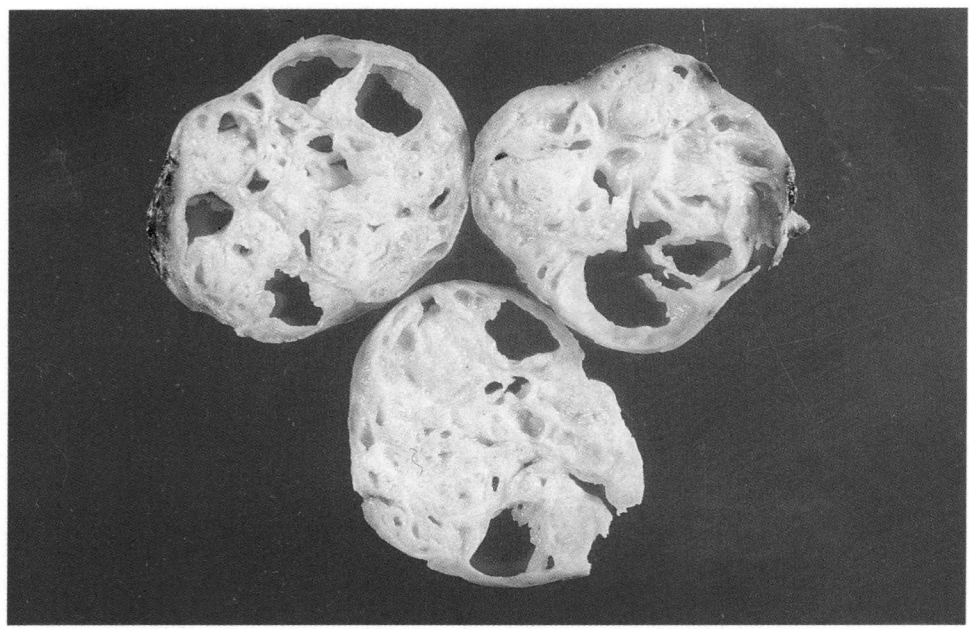

Fig. 19-66 Gross appearance of müllerian adenosarcoma of cervix. This tumor was extremely well differentiated and could qualify as an adenofibroma. (Courtesy Dr. Juan José Segura, San José, Costa Rica.)

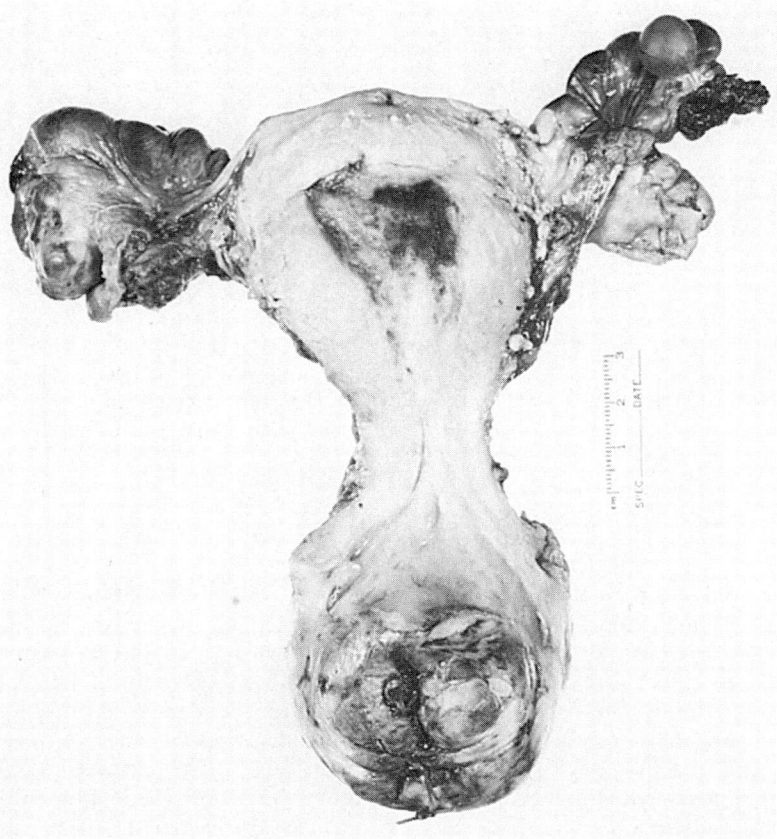

Fig. 19-67 Large cervical leiomyoma complicated by ulceration, hemorrhage, and necrosis.

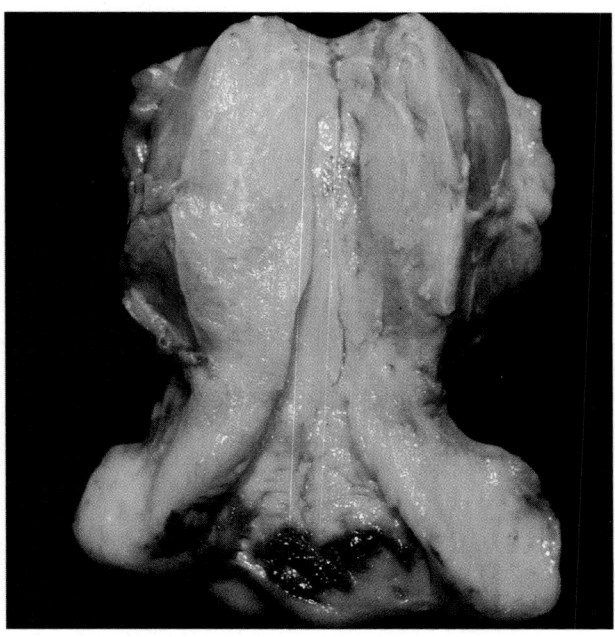

Fig. 19-68 Gross appearance of blue nevus of cervix. (Courtesy Dr. Luis Spitale, Córdoba, Argentina.)

poid masses but occur in older patients; they look like their more common counterpart in the uterine corpus. The type with homologous stroma, also known as carcinosarcoma,[463] needs to be distinguished from spindle cell carcinoma (squamous cell carcinoma with sarcoma-like stroma) (see p. 1368).[499] *Müllerian adenosarcoma*[486a,502] and *stromal sarcoma* of endometrial type also occur in the cervix, the former sometimes in association with ovarian sex-cord differentiation[484]; this includes the better differentiated and presumably benign variant of this tumor originally described as *papillary adenofibroma*[462,506] (Figs. 19-65 and 19-66). *Smooth muscle tumors,* both benign and malignant, also occur in the cervix (Fig. 19-67); the diagnostic criteria are the same as for those in the uterine corpus, but the ratio may be slightly different (comparatively more leiomyosarcomas are found in the cervix).[480]

Other rare primary cervical tumors and tumorlike conditions include *teratoma,*[482,486b] *glial polyp (glioma),* and *ganglioneuroma*[491]; *yolk sac (endodermal sinus) tumor* (closely simulating the clinical appearance of botryoid rhabdomyosarcoma)[474]; *extrarenal Wilms' tumor*[467]; *traumatic (amputation) neuroma*[466]; *neurofibroma*[481]; *pigmented schwannoma*[500]; *pigmented neuroectodermal tumor*[498]; *melanosis* (sometimes developing after cryotherapy for CIN)[477,485]; *blue nevus*[493,501] (Fig. 19-68); *cellular blue nevus; malignant melanoma*[487]; *choriocarcinoma*[488]; *benign mesenchymoma*[503]; *hemangioma; angiosarcoma*[472]; *osteosarcoma*[469]; and *alveolar soft sarcoma.*[461,479,492a,496]

Malignant lymphomas of the cervix present with vaginal bleeding and a subepithelial mass without obvious ulceration; most are diffuse large cell lymphomas and many are accompanied by extensive fibrosis.* An important differen-

tial diagnosis is with lymphoma-like lesions resulting from focally florid lymphoid proliferation associated with chronic cervicitis or as an expression of infectious mononucleosis[505]; these are identified by the polymorphic nature of the infiltrate (including mature plasma cells, small lymphocytes, and neutrophils), surface ulceration, minimal or no sclerosis, and evidence of polyclonality by immunoperoxidase staining. *Granulocytic sarcoma (chloroma),*[460,497] *Hodgkin's disease,*[495] *inflammatory pseudotumor,*[464] and *sinus histiocytosis with massive lymphadenopathy (Rosai-Dorfman's disease)*[492] can also present initially as a cervical mass.

Metastatic carcinomas to the cervix can originate from genital or extragenital organs; the most common sites are the ovary, large bowel, stomach, breast, and kidney.[486,489] Some of them simulate clinically and pathologically the appearance of primary cervical carcinoma. Knowledge of the clinical findings may make this mistake avoidable.

REFERENCES
NORMAL ANATOMY

1 Fetissof F, Dubois MP, Heitz PU, Lansac J, Arbeille-Brassart B, Jobard P: Endocrine cells in the female genital tract. Int J Gynecol Pathol **5**:75-87, 1986.

2 Fetissof F, Serres G, Arbeille B, de Muret A, Sam-Giao M, Lansac J: Argyrophilic cells and ectocervical epithelium. Int J Gynecol Pathol **10**:177-190, 1991.

3 Gilks CB, Reid PE, Clement PB, Owen DA: Histochemical changes in cervical mucus-secreting epithelium during the normal menstrual cycle. Fertil Steril **5**:286-291, 1989.

4 Loning T, Kuhler C, Caselitz J, Stegner HE: Keratin and tissue polypeptide antigen profiles of the cervical mucosa. Int J Gynecol Pathol **2**:105-112, 1983.

5 Malecha MJ, Miettinen M: Patterns of keratin subsets in normal and abnormal uterine cervical tissues. An immunohistochemical study. Int J Gynecol Pathol **11**:24-29, 1992.

6 Nonogaki H, Fujii S, Konishi I, Nanbu Y, Ozaki S, Ishikawa Y, Mori T: Estrogen receptor localization in normal and neoplastic epithelium of the uterine cervix. Cancer **66**:2620-2627, 1990.

*References 465, 471, 476, 478, 483, 494.

7 Osamura RY, Watanabe K, Oh M: Melanin-containing cells in the uterine cervix. Histochemical and electron-microscopic studies of two cases. Am J Clin Pathol **74:**239-242, 1980.

8 Robledo M, Vazquez J, Contreras-Mejuto F, Lopez-Garcia G: Sebaceous glands and hair follicles in the cervix uteri. Histopathology **21:**278-279, 1992.

9 Roth E, Taylor HB: Heterotopic cartilage in the uterus. Obstet Gynecol **27:**838-844, 1966.

10 Smedts F, Ramaekers F, Troyanovsky S, Pruszczynski M, Robben H, Lane B, Leigh I, Plantema F, Vooijs P: Basal-cell keratins in cervical reserve cells and a comparison to their expression in cervical intraepithelial neoplasia. Am J Pathol **140:**601-612, 1992.

11 Warhol MJ, Antonioli DA, Pinkus GS, Burke L, Rice RH: Immunoperoxidase staining for involucrin. A potential diagnostic aid in cervicovaginal pathology. Hum Pathol **13:**1095-1099, 1982.

12 Whittaker JR, Samy AM, Sunter JP, Sinha DP, Monaghan JM: Cytokeratin expression in cervical epithelium. An immunohistological study of normal, wart virus-infected and neoplastic tissue. Histopathology **14:**151-160, 1989.

SQUAMOUS AND OTHER METAPLASIAS

13 al-Nafussi A, Rahilly M: The prevalence of tubo-endometrial metaplasia and adenomatoid proliferation. Histopathology **22:**177-179, 1993.

14 Crum CP, Egawa K, Fu YS, Lancaster WD, Barron B, Levine RU, Fenoglio CM, Richart RM: Atypical immature metaplasia (AIM). A subset of human papilloma virus infection of the cervix. Cancer **51:**2214-2219, 1983.

15 Ducatman BS, Wang HH, Jonasson JG, Hogan CL, Antonioli DA: Tubal metaplasia. A cytologic study with comparison to other neoplastic and non-neoplastic conditions of the endocervix. Diagn Cytopathol **9:**95-103, 1993.

16 Feldman D, Romney SL, Edgcomb J, Valentine T: Ultrastructure of normal, metaplastic, and abnormal human uterine cervix. Use of montages to study the topographical relationship of epithelial cells. Am J Obstet Gynecol **150:**573-688, 1984.

17 Ismail SM: Cone biopsy causes cervical endometriosis and tubo-endometrioid metaplasia. Histopathology **18:**107-114, 1991.

18 Johnson LD, Easterday CL, Gore H, Hertig AT: Histogenesis of carcinoma in situ of the uterine cervix. A preliminary report of the origin of carcinoma in situ in subcylindrical cell anaplasia. Cancer **17:**213-229, 1964.

19 Jonasson JG, Wang HH, Antonioli DA, Ducatman BS: Tubal metaplasia of the uterine cervix. A prevalence study in patients with gynecologic pathologic findings. Int J Gynecol Pathol **11:**89-95, 1992.

19a McCluggage WG, Maxwell P, McBride HA, Hamilton PW, Bharucha H: Monoclonal antibodies Ki-67 and M1B1 in the distinction of tuboendometrial metaplasia from endocervical adenocarcinoma and adenocarcinoma in situ in formalin-fixed material. Int J Gynecol Pathol **14:**209-216, 1995.

19b Oliva E, Clement PB, Young RH: Tubal and tubo-endometrioid metaplasia of the uterine cervix. Unemphasized features that may cause problems in differential diagnosis—A report of 25 cases. Am J Clin Pathol **103:**618-623, 1995.

20 Puts JJG, Moesker O, Kenemans P, Vooijs GP, Ramaekers FCS: Expression of cytokeratins in early neoplastic epithelial lesions of the uterine cervix. Int J Gynecol Pathol **4:**300-313, 1985.

21 Suh KS, Silverberg SG: Tubal metaplasia of the uterine cervix. Int J Gynecol Pathol **9:**122-128, 1990.

22 Yeh IT, Bronner M, Li Volsi VA: Endometrial metaplasia of the uterine endocervix. Arch Pathol Lab Med **117:**734-735, 1993.

23 Young RH, Clement PB: Pseudoneoplastic glandular lesions of the uterine cervix. Semin Diagn Pathol **8:**234-249, 1991.

INFLAMMATORY LESIONS

24 Adams RL, Springall DR, Levene MM: The immunocytochemical detection of herpes simplex virus in cervical smears. A valuable technique for routine use. J Pathol **143:**241-247, 1984.

25 al Nafussi AI, Hughes D, Rebello G: Ceroid granuloma of the uterine cervix. Histopathology **21:**282-284, 1992.

26 Berry A: A cytopathological and histopathological study of bilharziasis of the female genital tract. J Pathol Bacteriol **91:**325-338, 1966.

27 Bhagavan BS, Ruffier J, Shinn B: Pseudoactinomycotic radiate granules in the lower female genital tract. Relationship to the Splendore-Hoeppli phenomenon. Hum Pathol **13:**898-904, 1982.

28 Chen KTK, Hendricks EJ: Malakoplakia of the female genital tract. Obstet Gynecol **65:**84S-87S, 1985.

29 Crow J, McWhinney N: Isolated arteritis of the cervix uteri. Br J Obstet Gynaecol **86:**393-398, 1979.

30 Kiviat NB, Paavonen JA, Wolner-Hanssen P, Critchlow CW, Stamm WE, Douglas J, Eschenbach DA, Corey LA, Holmes KK: Histopathology of endocervical infection caused by *Chlamydia trachomatis,* herpes simplex virus, *Trichomonas vaginalis,* and *Neisseria gonorrhoeae.* Hum Pathol **21:**831-837, 1990.

31 Marrogi AJ, Gersell DJ, Kraus FT: Localized asymptomatic giant cell arteritis of the female genital tract. Int J Gynecol Pathol **10:**51-58, 1991.

31a Marsella RC, Buckner SB, Bratthauer GL, O'Connor DM, O'Leary TJ: Identification of genital herpes simplex virus infection by immunoperoxidase staining. Appl Immunohistochem **3:**184-189, 1995.

32 Mitao M, Reumann W, Winkler B, Richart RM, Fujiwara A, Crum CP: Chlamydial cervicitis and cervical intraepithelial neoplasia. An immunohistochemical analysis. Gynecol Oncol **19:**90-97, 1984.

33 Naib ZM, Nahmias AJ, Josey WE: Cytology and histopathology of cervical herpes simplex infection. Cancer **19:**1026-1031, 1966.

34 Paavonen J, Critchlow CW, DeRouen T, Stevens CE, Kiviat N, Brunham RC, Staam WE, Kuo CC, Hyde KE, Corey L, Eschenbach DA, Holmes KK: Etiology of cervical inflammation. Am J Obstet Gynecol **154:**556-564, 1986.

35 Tchertkoff V, Ober WB: Primary chancre of cervix uteri. NY State J Med **66:**1921-1924, 1966.

36 Winkler B, Crum CP: Chlamydia trachomatis infection of the female genital tract. Pathogenetic and clinicopathologic correlations. Pathol Annu **22**(Pt 1):193-223, 1987.

NON-NEOPLASTIC GLANDULAR LESIONS

37 Chumas JC, Nelson B, Mann WJ, Chalas E, Kaplan CG: Microglandular hyperplasia of the uterine cervix. Obstet Gynecol **66:**406-409, 1985.

38 Clement PB, Young RH: Deep nabothian cysts of the uterine cervix. A possible source of confusion with minimal-deviation adenocarcinoma (adenoma malignum). Int J Gynecol Pathol **8:**340-348, 1989.

39 Cove H: The Arias-Stella reaction occurring in the endocervix in pregnancy. Recognition and comparison with an adenocarcinoma of the cervix. Am J Surg Pathol **3:**567-568, 1979.

40 Ferenczy A, Braun L, Shah KV: Human papillomavirus (HPV) in condylomatous lesions of cervix. A comparative ultrastructural and immunohistochemical study. Am J Surg Pathol **5:**661-670, 1981.

41 Ferry JA, Scully RE: Mesonephric remnants, hyperplasia, and neoplasia in the uterine cervix. A study of 49 cases. Am J Surg Pathol **14:**1100-1111, 1990.

41a Greeley C, Schroeder S, Silverberg SG: Microglandular hyperplasia of the cervix. A true "pill" lesion? Int J Gynecol Pathol **14:**50-54, 1995.

42 Hertig A: Proceedings of Eighteenth Seminar of the American Society of Clinical Pathologists, October 1952, Chicago, Ill.

43 Inai K, Arihiro K, Tokuoka S, Katsube Y, Fujiwara A: Mesonephric duct hyperplasia of the uterus. Report of two cases and three other cases of mesonephric duct remnant with findings of mucin histochemistry and lectin binding immunohistochemistry. Acta Pathol Jpn **39:**457-464, 1989.

44 Janovski NA, Kasdon EJ: Benign mesonephric papillary and polypoid tumors of the cervix in childhood. J Pediatr **63:**211-216, 1963.

45 Jones MA, Andrews J, Tarraza HM: Mesonephric remnant hyperplasia of the cervix. A clinicopathologic analysis of 14 cases. Gynecol Oncol **49:**41-47, 1993.

46 Jones MA, Young RH, Scully RE: Diffuse laminar endocervical glandular hyperplasia. A benign lesion often confused with adenoma malignum (minimal deviation adenocarcinoma). Am J Surg Pathol **15:**1123-1129, 1991.

47 Kyriakos M, Kempson RL, Konikov NF: A clinical and pathologic study of endocervical lesions associated with oral contraceptives. Cancer **22:**99-110, 1968.

48 Rhatigan RM: Endocervical gland atypia secondary to Arias-Stella change. Arch Pathol Lab Med **116:**943-946, 1992.

48a Samaratunga H, Beresford A, Davison A: Squamous cell carcinoma in situ involving mesonephric remnants. A potential diagnostic pitfall. Am J Surg Pathol **18:**1265-1269, 1994.

49 Segal GH, Hart WR: Cystic endocervical tunnel clusters. A clinicopathologic study of 29 cases of so-called adenomatous hyperplasia. Am J Surg Pathol **14:**895-903, 1990.

49a Seidman JD, Tavassoli FA: Mesonephric hyperplasia of the uterine cervix. A clinicopathologic study of 51 cases. Int J Gynecol Pathol **14:**293-299, 1995.

50 Selzer I, Nelson HM: Benign papilloma (polypoid tumor) of the cervix uteri in children. Report of 2 cases. Am J Obstet Gynecol **84:**165-169, 1962.

51 Shah KH, Kurman RJ, Scully RE, Norris HS: Atypical hyperplasia of mesonephric remnants in the cervix (abstract). Lab Invest **42:**149, 1980.

52 Sherrick JC, Vega JG: Congenital intramural cysts of uterus. Obstet Gynecol **19:**486-493, 1962.

53 Speers WC, Picaso LG, Silverberg SG: Immunohistochemical localization of carcinoembryonic antigen in microglandular hyperplasia and adenocarcinoma of the endocervix. Am J Clin Pathol **79:**105-107, 1983.

54 Taylor HB, Irey NS, Norris HJ: Atypical endocervical hyperplasia in women taking oral contraceptives. JAMA **202:**637-639, 1967.

55 Young RH, Clement PB: Pseudoneoplastic glandular lesions of the uterine cervix. Semin Diagn Pathol **8:**234-249, 1991.

56 Young RH, Scully RE: Atypical forms of microglandular hyperplasia of the cervix simulating carcinoma. A report of five cases and review of the literature. Am J Surg Pathol **13:**50-56, 1989.

NON-NEOPLASTIC STROMAL LESIONS

57 Abdul-Karim FW, Cohen RE: Atypical stromal cells of lower female genital tract. Histopathology **17:**249-253, 1990.

58 Bausch RG, Kaump DH, Alles RW: Observations on the decidual reaction of the cervix during pregnancy. Am J Obstet Gynecol **58:**777-783, 1949.

59 Clement PB: Multinucleated stromal giant cells of the uterine cervix. Arch Pathol Lab Med **109:**200-202, 1985.

60 Clement PB, Young RH, Scully RE: Nontrophoblastic pathology of the female genital tract and peritoneum associated with pregnancy. Semin Diagn Pathol **6:**372-406, 1989.

61 Clement PB, Young RH, Scully RE: Stromal endometriosis of the uterine cervix. A variant of endometriosis that may simulate a sarcoma. Am J Surg Pathol **14:**449-455, 1990.

62 Elliott GB, Elliott JDA: Superficial stromal reactions of lower genital tract. Arch Pathol **95:**100-101, 1973.

63 Evans CS, Goldman RL, Klein HZ, Kohout ND: Necrobiotic granulomas of the uterine cervix. A probable postoperative reaction. Am J Surg Pathol **8:**841-844, 1984.

64 Hariri J, Ingemanssen JL: Multinucleated stromal giant cells of the uterine cervix. Int J Gynecol Pathol **12:**228-234, 1993.

65 Huettner PC, Gersell DJ: Placental site nodule. A clinicopathologic study of 38 cases. Int J Gynecol Pathol **13:**191-198, 1994.

66 Kay S, Schneider V: Reactive spindle cell nodule of the endocervix simulating uterine sarcoma. Int J Gynecol Pathol **4:**255-257, 1985.

67 Young RH, Kurman RJ, Scully RE: Placental site nodules and plaques. A clinicopathologic analysis of 20 cases. Am J Surg Pathol **14:**1001-1009, 1990.

HUMAN PAPILLOMA VIRUS (HPV) AND CERVICAL PATHOLOGY; BENIGN SQUAMOUS NEOPLASMS

67a Albores-Saavedra J, Young RH: Transitional cell neoplasms (carcinomas and inverted papillomas) of the uterine cervix. A report of four cases. Am J Surg Pathol **19:**1138-1145, 1995.

67b Al-Saleh W, Delvenne P, Greimers R, Fridman V, Doyen J, Boniver J: Assessment of Ki-67 antigen immunostaining in squamous intraepithelial lesions of the uterine cervix. Correlation with the histologic grade and human papillomavirus type. Am J Clin Pathol **104:**154-160, 1995.

68 Ambros RA, Kurman RJ: Current concepts in the relationship of human papillomavirus infection to the pathogenesis and classification of precancerous squamous lesions of the uterine cervix. Semin Diagn Pathol **7:**158-172, 1990.

69 Arends MJ, Wyllie AH, Bird CC: Papillomaviruses and human cancer. Hum Pathol **21:**686-698, 1990.

70 Barnes W, Delgado G, Kurman RJ, Petrilli ES, Smith DM, Ahmed S, Lorincz AT, Temple GF, Jenson AB, Lancaster WD: Possible prognostic significance of human papillomavirus type in cervical cancer. Gynecol Oncol **29:**267-273, 1988.

71 Bergeron C, Barrasso R, Beaudenon S, Flamant P, Croissant O, Orth G: Human papillomaviruses associated with cervical intraepithelial neoplasia. Great diversity and distinct distribution in low- and high-grade lesions. Am J Surg Pathol **16:**641-649, 1992.

72 Binder MA, Cates GW, Emson HE, Valnicek SJ, MacLachlan TB, Schmidt EW, Popkin DR, Ferenczy A: The changing concepts of condyloma. A retrospective study of colposcopically directed cervical biopsies. Am J Obstet Gynecol **151:**213-219, 1985.

72a Bosch FX, Manos MM, Muñoz N, Sherman M, Jansen AM, Peto J, Schiffman MH, Moreno V, Kurman R, Shah KV, International Biological Study on Cervical Cancer (IBSCC) Study Group: Prevalence of human papillomavirus in cervical cancer. A worldwide perspective. J Natl Cancer Inst **87:**796-802, 1995.

73 Boyle CA, Lowell DM, Kelsey JL, Li Volsi VA, Boyle KE: Cervical intraepithelial neoplasia among women with papillomavirus infection compared to women with *Trichomonas* infection. Cancer **64:**168-172, 1989.

74 Chapman WB, Lorincz AT, Willett GD, Wright VC, Kurman RJ: Evaluation of two commercially available in situ hybridization kits for detection of human papillomavirus DNA in cervical biopsies. Comparison to Southern blot hybridization. Mod Pathol **6:**73-79, 1993.

74a Chen JJ, Reid CE, Band V, Androphy EJ: Interaction of papillomavirus E6 oncoproteins with a putative calcium-binding protein. Science **269:**529-531, 1995.

75 Colgan TJ, Percy ME, Suri M, Shier RM, Andrews DF, Lickrish GM: Human papillomavirus infection of morphologically normal cervical epithelium adjacent to squamous dysplasia and invasive carcinoma. Hum Pathol **20:**316-319, 1989.

76 Cooper K, Herrington CS, Lo ES, Evans MF, McGee JO: Integration of human papillomavirus types 16 and 18 in cervical adenocarcinoma. J Clin Pathol **45:**382-384, 1992.

77 Crum C: Genital papillomaviruses and related neoplasms. Causation, diagnosis and classification (Bethesda). Mod Pathol **7:**138-145, 1994.

78 Crum CP, Egawa K, Barron B, Fenoglio CM, Levine RU, Richart RM: Human papilloma virus infection (condyloma) of the cervix and cervical intraepithelial neoplasia. A histopathologic and statistical analysis. Gynecol Oncol **15:**88-94, 1983.

79 Crum CP, Ikenberg H, Richart RM, Gissman L: Human papilloma virus type 16 and early cervical neoplasia. N Engl J Med **310:**880-883, 1984.

80 Crum CP, Roche JK: Molecular pathology of the lower female genital tract. The papillomavirus model. Am J Surg Pathol **14**(Suppl 1):26-33, 1990.

81 Cuzick J, Terry G, Ho L, Hollingworth T, Anderson M: Human papillomavirus type 16 in cervical smears as predictor of high-grade cervical intraepithelial neoplasia. Lancet **339:**959-960, 1992.

82 Delvenne P, Fontaine M, Delvenne C, Nikkels A, Boniver J: Detection of human papillomaviruses in paraffin-embedded biopsies of cervical intraepithelial lesions. Analysis by immunohistochemistry, in situ hybridization, and the polymerase chain reaction. Mod Pathol **7:**113-119, 1994.

83 Duggan MA, Benoit JL, McGregor SE, Inoue M, Nation JG, Stuart GCE: Adenocarcinoma in situ of the endocervix. Human papillomavirus determination by dot blot hybridization and polymerase chain reaction amplification. Int J Gynecol Pathol **13:**143-149, 1994.

84 Farnsworth A, Laverty C, Stoler MH: Human papillomavirus messenger RNA expression in adenocarcinoma in situ of the uterine cervix. Int J Gynecol Pathol **8:**321-330, 1989.

85 Franquemont DW, Ward BE, Andersen WA, Crum CP: Prediction of "high-risk" cervical papillomavirus infection by biopsy morphology. Am J Clin Pathol **92:**577-582, 1989.

86 Genest DR, Stein L, Cibas E, Sheets E, Zitz JC, Crum CP: A binary (Bethesda) system for classifying cervical cancer precursors. Criteria, reproducibility, and viral correlates. Hum Pathol **24:**730-736, 1993.

86a Ho GYF, Burk RD, Klein S, Kadish AS, Chang CJ, Palan P, Basu J, Tachezy R, Lewis R, Romney S: Persistent cervical dysplasia. J Natl Cancer Inst **87:**1365-1371, 1995.

87 Johnson TL, Kim W, Plieth DA, Sarkar FH: Detection of HPV 16/18 DNA in cervical adenocarcinoma using polymerase chain reaction (PCR) methodology. Mod Pathol **5:**35-40, 1992.

87a Jovanovic AS, McLachlin CM, Shen L, Welch WR, Crum CP: Postmenopausal squamous atypia. A spectrum including "pseudo-koilocytosis." Mod Pathol **8:**408-412, 1995.

88 Kaufman R, Koss LG, Kurman RJ, Meisels A, Okagaki T, Patten SF, Reid R, Richart RM, Wied GL: Statement of caution in the interpretation of papilloma virus–associated lesions of the epithelium of uterine cervix. Am J Obstet Gynecol **146:**125, 1983.

89 Kenny MB, Unger ER, Chenggis ML, Costa MJ: In situ hybridization for human papillomavirus DNA in uterine adenosquamous carcinoma with glassy cell features ("glassy cell carcinoma"). Am J Clin Pathol **98:**180-187, 1992.

90 Koss LG: Cytologic and histologic manifestations of human papillomavirus infection of the female genital tract and their clinical significance. Cancer **60:**1942-1950, 1987.

91 Kurman RJ, Sanz LE, Jenson AB, Perry S, Lancaster WD: Papillomavirus infection of the cervix. I. Correlation of histology with viral structural antigens and DNA sequences. Int J Gynecol Pathol **1:**17-28, 1982.

92 Leminen A, Paavonen J, Vesterinen E, Wahlstrom T, Rantala I, Lehtinen M: Human papillomavirus types 16 and 18 in adenocarcinoma of the uterine cervix. Am J Clin Pathol **95:**647-652, 1991.

93 Macnab JCM, Walkinshaw SA, Cordiner JW, Clements JB: Human papilloma virus in clinically and histologically normal tissue of patients with genital cancer. N Engl J Med **315:**1052-1058, 1986.

93a McLachlin CM, Tate JE, Zitz JC, Sheets EE, Crum CP: Human papillomavirus type 18 and intraepithelial lesions of the cervix. Am J Pathol **144:**141-147, 1994.

94 Mitao M, Nagai N, Levine RU, Silverstein SJ, Crum CP: Human papilloma-virus type 16 infection. A morphological spectrum with evidence for late gene expression. Int J Gynecol Pathol **5:**287-296, 1987.

95 Mittal KR, Chan W, Demopoulos RI: Sensitivity and specificity of various morphological features of cervical condylomas. An in situ hybridization study. Arch Pathol Lab Med 114:1038-1041, 1990.

96 Mittal KR, Miller HK, Lowell DM: Koilocytosis preceding squamous cell carcinoma in situ of uterine cervix. Am J Clin Pathol 87:243-245, 1987.

97 Nagai N, Nuovo G, Freidman D, Crum CP: Detection of papillomavirus nucleic acids in genital precancers with the in situ hybridization technique. Int J Gynecol Pathol 6:366-379, 1987.

98 Nuovo GJ: Human papillomavirus DNA in genital tract lesions histologically negative for condylomata. Analysis by in situ, Southern blot hybridization and the polymerase chain reaction. Am J Surg Pathol 14:643-651, 1990.

99 Nyeem R, Wilkinson EJ, Grover LJ: Condylomata acuminata of the cervix. Histopathology and association with cervical neoplasia. Int J Gynecol Pathol 1:246-257, 1982.

100 Paquette RL, Lee YY, Wilczynski SP, Karmakar A, Kizaki M, Miller CW, Koeffler HP: Mutations of p53 and human papillomavirus infection in cervical carcinoma. Cancer 72:1272-1280, 1993.

101 Prasad CJ, Sheets E, Selig AM, McArthur MC, Crum CP: The binucleate squamous cell. Histologic spectrum and relationship to low-grade squamous intraepithelial lesions. Mod Pathol 6:313-317, 1993.

102 Qizilbash AH: Papillary squamous tumors of the uterine cervix. A clinical and pathologic study of 21 cases. Am J Clin Pathol 61:508-520, 1974.

103 Richart RM: Causes and management of cervical intraepithelial neoplasia. Cancer 60:1951-1959, 1987.

104 Richart RM, Nuovo GJ: Human papillomavirus DNA in situ hybridization may be used for the quality control of genital tract biopsies. Obstet Gynecol 75:223-226, 1990.

105 Saito K, Saito A, Fu YS, Smotkin D, Gupta J, Shah K: Topographic study of cervical condyloma and intraepithelial neoplasia. Cancer 59:2064-2070, 1987.

106 Schiffman MH, Bauer HM, Hoover RN, Glass AG, Cadeli DM, Rush BB, Scott DR, Sherman ME, Kurman RJ, Wacholder S, et al.: Epidemiologic evidence showing that human papillomavirus infection causes most cervical intraepithelial neoplasia. J Natl Cancer Inst 85:958-964, 1993.

107 Sedlacek TV, Sedlacek AE, Neff DK, Rando RF: The clinical role of human papilloma virus typing. Gynecol Oncol 42:222-226, 1991.

108 Syrjanen KJ: Human papillomavirus (HPV) infections of the female genital tract and their associations with intraepithelial neoplasia and squamous cell carcinoma. Pathol Annu 21(Pt 1):53-89, 1986.

108a ter Harmsel B, van Belkum A, Quint W, Pronk A, Kuijpers J, Ramaekers F, Tandon A, Smedts F: p53 and human papilloma virus type 16 in cervical intraepithelial neoplasia and carcinoma. Int J Gynecol Pathol 14:125-133, 1995.

109 Vallejos H, Delmistro AD, Kleinhaus S, Braunstein JD, Halwer M, Koss LG: Characterization of human papilloma virus types in condylomata acuminata in children by in situ hybridization. Lab Invest 56:611-615, 1987.

110 Ward BE, Burkett B, Petersen C, Nuckols ML, Brennan C, Birch LM, Crum CP: Cytologic correlates of cervical papillomavirus infection. Int J Gynecol Pathol 9:297-305, 1990.

111 Weaver MG, Abdul-Karim FW, Dale G, Sorensen K, Huang YT: Outcome in mild and moderate cervical dysplasias related to the presence of specific human papillomavirus types. Mod Pathol 3:679-683, 1990.

112 Willett GD, Kurman RJ, Reid R, Greenberg M, Jenson AB, Lorincz AT: Correlation of the histologic appearance of intraepithelial neoplasia of the cervix with human papillomavirus types. Emphasis on low grade lesions including so-called flat condyloma. Int J Gynecol Pathol 8:18-25, 1989.

113 Winkler B, Crum CP, Fujii T, Ferenczy A, Boon M, Braun L, Lancaster WD, Richart RM: Koilocytotic lesions of the cervix. The relationship of mitotic abnormalities to the presence of papillomavirus antigens and nuclear DNA content. Cancer 53:1081-1087, 1984.

114 Wright TC Jr, Richart RM: Role of human papillomavirus in the pathogenesis of genital tract warts and cancer. Gynecol Oncol 37:151-164, 1990.

115 Yang GC, Demopoulos RI, Chan W, Mittal KR: Superficial nuclear enlargement without koilocytosis as an expression of human papillomavirus infection of the uterine cervix: an in situ hybridization study. Int J Gynecol Pathol 1:283-287, 1992.

TUMORS
Cervical intraepithelial neoplasia (CIN)

115a Akasofu M, Oda Y: Immunohistochemical detection of p53 in cervical epithelial lesions with or without infection of human papillomavirus types 16 and 18. Virchows Arch 425:593-602, 1995.

116 Al-Nafussi AI, Colquhoun MK: Mild cervical intraepithelial neoplasia (CIN 1). A histological overdiagnosis. Histopathology 17:557-561, 1990.

117 Anderson MC, Hartley RB: Cervical crypt involvement by intraepithelial neoplasia. Obstet Gynecol 55:546-550, 1980.

118 Benda JA, Lamoreaux J, Johnson SR: Artifact associated with the use of strong iodine solution (Lugol's) in cone biopsies. Am J Surg Pathol 11:367-374, 1987.

119 Bibbo M, Dytch HE, Alenghat E, Bartels PH, Wied GL: DNA ploidy profiles as prognostic indicators in CIN lesions. Am J Clin Pathol 92:261-265, 1989.

120 Buckley CH, Butler EB, Fox H: Cervical intraepithelial neoplasia. J Clin Pathol 35:1-13, 1982.

121 Christopherson WM: Dysplasia, carcinoma in situ, and microinvasive carcinoma of the uterine cervix. Hum Pathol 8:489-501, 1977.

122 Christopherson WM, Gray LA Sr: Dysplasia and preclinical carcinoma of the uterine cervix. Diagnosis and management. Semin Oncol 9:265-279, 1982.

123 Coppleson M, Pixley E, Reid B: Colposcopy. A scientific and practical approach to the cervix in health and disease. Springfield, IL, 1971, Charles C Thomas, Publisher.

124 Demopoulos RI, Horowitz LF, Vamvakas EC: Endocervical gland involvement by cervical intraepithelial neoplasia grade III. Predictive value for residual and/or recurrent disease. Cancer 68:1932-1936, 1991.

125 Foote FW Jr, Stewart FW: The anatomical distribution of intraepithelial epidermoid carcinomas of the cervix. Cancer 1:431-440, 1948.

126 Fox CH: Biologic behavior of dysplasia and carcinoma in situ. Am J Obstet Gynecol 99:960-974, 1967.

127 Fox H, Buckley CH: Current problems in the pathology of intra-epithelial lesions of the uterine cervix. Histopathology 17:1-6, 1990.

128 Fu YS, Reagan JW, Richart RM: Definition of precursors. Gynecol Oncol 12:S220-S231, 1981.

129 Govan ADT, Haines RM, Langley FA, Taylor CW, Woodcock AS: Changes in the epithelium of the cervix uteri. J Obstet Gynaecol Br Commonw 73:883-896, 1966.

130 Gusberg SB, Moore DB: The clinical pattern of intraepithelial carcinoma of the cervix and its pathologic background. Obstet Gynecol 2:1-14, 1953.

131 Holmquist ND, McMahan CA, Williams OD: Variability in classification of carcinoma in situ of the uterine cervix. Arch Pathol 84:334-345, 1967.

132 Howard L, Erickson CC, Stoddard LD: A study of the incidence and histogenesis of endocervical metaplasia and intraepithelial carcinoma. Cancer 4:1210-1223, 1951.

133 Ismail SM, Colclough AB, Dinnen JS, Eakins D, Evans DM, Gradwell E, O'Sullivan JP, Summerell JM, Newcombe R: Reporting cervical intra-epithelial neoplasia (CIN). Intra- and interpathologist variation and factors associated with disagreement. Histopathology 16:371-376, 1990.

134 Johnson LD, Nickerson RJ, Easterday CL, Stuart RS, Hertig AT: Epidemiologic evidence for the spectrum of change from dysplasia through carcinoma in situ to invasive cancer. Cancer 22:901-914, 1968.

135 Kanbour AI, Stock RJ: Squamous cell carcinoma in situ of the endometrium and fallopian tube as superficial extension of invasive cervical carcinoma. Cancer 42:570-580, 1978.

136 Killackey MA, Jones WB, Lewis JL: Diagnostic conization of the cervix. Review of 460 consecutive cases. Obstet Gynecol 67:766-770, 1986.

137 Klavins JV: Intra-epithelial carcinoma with differentiated surface cells and dysplasia. Definition and separation of these lesions. Acta Cytol (Baltimore) 7:351-356, 1963.

137a Kobayashi I, Matsuo K, Ishibashi Y, Kanda S, Sakai H: The proliferative activity in dysplasia and carcinoma in situ of the uterine cervix analyzed by proliferating cell nuclear antigen immunostaining and silver-binding argyrophilic nucleolar organizer region staining. Hum Pathol 25:198-202, 1994.

138 Kolstad P, Klein V: Long-term follow-up of 1121 cases of carcinoma in situ. Obstet Gynecol 48:125-129, 1976.

139 Kolstad P, Stafl A: Atlas of colposcopy. Baltimore, 1972, University Park Press.

140 Kraus FT: Gynecologic pathology. St. Louis, 1967, The C.V. Mosby Co., p. 174.

141 Kreiger JS, McCormack LJ: Graded treatment for in situ carcinoma of the uterine cervix. Am J Obstet Gynecol 101:171-182, 1968.

142 Matseoane S, Williams SB, Navarro C, Hedriana H, Mushayandebvu T: Diagnostic value of conization of the uterine cervix in the management of cervical neoplasia: a review of 756 consecutive patients. Gynecol Oncol 47:287-291, 1992.

143 McIndoe WA, McLean MR, Jones RW, Mullins PR: The invasive potential of carcinoma in situ of the cervix. Obstet Gynecol 64:451-458, 1984.

144 McIndoe GA, Robson MS, Tidy JA, Mason WP, Anderson MC: Laser excision rather than vaporization. The treatment of choice for cervical intraepithelial neoplasia. Obstet Gynecol 74:165-168, 1989.

145 Mittal KR, Demopoulos RI, Goswami S: Proliferating cell nuclear antigen (cyclin) expression in normal and abnormal cervical squamous epithelia. Am J Surg Pathol 17:117-122, 1993.

146 Montz FJ, Holschneider CH, Thompson LD: Large-loop excision of the transformation zone. Effect on the pathologic interpretation of resection margins. Obstet Gynecol 81:976-982, 1993.

147 Murphy WM, Coleman SA: The long-term course of carcinoma in situ of the uterine cervix. Cancer **38**:957-963, 1976.

148 Nasiell K, Roger V, Nasiell M: Behavior of mild cervical dysplasia during long-term follow-up. Obstet Gynecol **67**:665-669, 1986.

149 National Cancer Institute Workshop: The 1988 Bethesda System for reporting cervical/vaginal cytologic diagnoses. JAMA **262**:931-932, 1988.

150 Ostor AG: Natural history of cervical intraepithelial neoplasia. A critical review. Int J Gynecol Pathol **12**:186-192, 1993.

151 Paterson-Brown S, Chappatte OA, Clark SK, Wright A, Maxwell P, Taub NA, Raju KS: The significance of cone biopsy resection margins. Gynecol Oncol **46**:182-185, 1992.

152 Perticarari S, Presani G, Michelutti A, Facca MC, Alberico S, Mandruzzato GP: Flow cytometric analysis of DNA content in cervical lesions. Pathol Res Pract **185**:686-688, 1989.

153 Petersen O: Spontaneous course of cervical precancerous conditions. Am J Obstet Gynecol **72**:1063-1071, 1956.

154 Pollanen R, Soini Y, Vahakangas K, Paakko P, Lehto VP: Aberrant p53 protein expression in cervical intra-epithelial neoplasia. Histopathology **23**:471-474, 1993.

155 Przybora LA, Plutowa A: Histological topography of carcinoma in situ of the cervix uteri. Cancer **12**:263-277, 1959.

156 Reagan JW, Seidemann IL, Saracusa Y: Cellular morphology of carcinoma in situ and dysplasia or atypical hyperplasia of the uterine cervix. Cancer **6**:224-235, 1953.

157 Richart RM: Cervical intraepithelial neoplasia. Pathol Annu **8**:301-328, 1973.

158 Richart RM: A modified terminology for cervical intraepithelial neoplasia. Obstet Gynecol **75**:131-133, 1990.

159 Richart RM, Barron BA: A follow-up study of patients with cervical dysplasia. Am J Obstet Gynecol **105**:386-393, 1969.

160 Richart RM, Wright TC Jr: Controversies in the management of low-grade cervical intraepithelial neoplasia. Cancer **71**:1413-1421, 1993.

161 Rubio CA, Lagerlöf B: Autoradiographic studies of dysplasia and carcinoma in situ in cervical cones. Acta Pathol Microbiol Scand (A) **82**:411-418, 1974.

162 Sagae S, Kudo R, Kuzumaki N, Hisada T, Mugikura Y, Nihei T, Takeda T, Hashimoto M: Ras oncogene expression and progression in intraepithelial neoplasia of the uterine cervix. Cancer **66**:295-301, 1990.

163 Salm R: Superficial intra-uterine spread of intra-epithelial cervical carcinoma. J Pathol **97**:719-723, 1969.

163a Samaratunga H, Beresford A, Davison A: Squamous cell carcinoma in situ involving mesonephric remnants. A potential diagnostic pitfall. Am J Surg Pathol **18**:1265-1269, 1994.

164 Shurbaji MS, Brooks SK, Thurmond TS: Proliferating cell nuclear antigen immunoreactivity in cervical intraepithelial neoplasia and benign cervical epithelium. Am J Clin Pathol **100**:22-26, 1993.

165 Smedts F, Ramaekers F, Leube RE, Keijser K, Link M, Vooijs P: Expression of keratins 1, 6, 15, 16, and 20 in normal cervical epithelium, squamous metaplasia, cervical intraepithelial neoplasia, and cervical carcinoma. Am J Pathol **142**:403-412, 1993.

166 Smedts F, Ramaekers F, Robben H, Pruszczynski M, van Muijen G, Lane B, Leigh I, Vooijs P: Changing patterns of keratin expression during progression of cervical intraepithelial neoplasia. Am J Pathol **136**:657-668, 1990.

167 Suprun HZ, Schwartz J, Spira H: Cervical intraepithelial neoplasia and associated condylomatous lesions. A preliminary report on 4,764 women from northern Israel. Acta Cytol (Baltimore) **29**:334-340, 1985.

168 Takeuchi A, McKay DB: The area of the cervix involved by carcinoma in situ and anaplasia (atypical hyperplasia). Obstet Gynecol **15**:134-145, 1960.

169 Thickett KM, Griffin NR, Griffiths AP, Wells M: A study of nucleolar organizer regions in cervical intraepithelial neoplasia and human papillomavirus infection. Int J Gynecol Pathol **8**:331-339, 1989.

170 Tweeddale DN, Roddick JW: Histologic types of squamous-cell carcinoma in situ of the cervix. Obstet Gynecol **33**:35-40, 1969.

171 Walton LA, Edelman DA, Fowler WC Jr, Photropulos GJ: Cryosurgery for the treatment of cervical intraepithelial neoplasm during the reproductive years. Obstet Gynecol **55**:353-357, 1980.

172 Wentz WB, Reagan JW: Clinical significance of postirradiation dysplasia of the uterine cervix. Am J Obstet Gynecol **106**:812-817, 1970.

Microinvasive squamous cell carcinoma

173 Benson WL, Norris HJ: A critical review of the frequency of lymph node metastasis and death from microinvasive carcinoma of the cervix. Obstet Gynecol **49**:632-638, 1977.

173a Burke TW: Factors affecting recurrence and survival in stage I carcinoma of the uterine cervix. Oncology (Huntingt) **6**:111-119, 1992.

174 Brudenell M, Cox BS, Taylor CW: The management of dysplasia, carcinoma in situ and microcarcinoma of the cervix. J Obstet Gynaecol Br Commonw **80**:673-679, 1973.

175 Burghardt E, Girardi F, Lahousen M, Pickel H, Tamussino K: Microinvasive carcinoma of the uterine cervix (International Federation of Gynecology and Obstetrics Stage IA). Cancer **67**:1037-1045, 1991.

176 Christopherson WM, Gray LA, Parker JE: Microinvasive carcinoma of the uterine cervix. A long-term follow-up study of eighty cases. Cancer **38**:629-632. 1976.

177 Clement PB, Scully RE: Carcinoma of the cervix. Histologic types. Semin Oncol **9**:251-264, 1982.

178 Copeland LJ, Silva EG, Gershenson DM, Morris M, Young DC, Wharton JT: Superficially invasive squamous cell carcinoma of the cervix. Gynecol Oncol **45**:307-312, 1992.

179 Creasman WT, Fetter BF, Clarke-Pearson DL, Kaufmann L, Parker RT: Management of stage IA carcinoma of cervix. Am J Obstet Gynecol **153**:164-172, 1985.

180 Fennell RH: Review. Microinvasive carcinoma of the uterine cervix. Obstet Gynecol Surv **33**:406-411, 1978.

181 Genadry R, Olson J, Parmley T, Woodruff JD: The morphology of the earliest invasive cell in low genital tract epidermoid neoplasia. Obstet Gynecol **51**:718-722, 1978.

182 Hartveit F, Sandstad E: Stromal metachromasia. A marker for areas of infiltrating tumour growth? Histopathology **6**:423-428, 1982.

183 Hasumi K, Sakamoto A, Sugano H: Microinvasive carcinoma of the uterine cervix. Cancer **45**:928-931. 1980.

184 Jones WB, Mercer GO, Lewis JL Jr, Rubin SC, Hoskins WJ: Early invasive carcinoma of the cervix. Gynecol Oncol **51**:26-32, 1993.

185 Kudo R, Sato T, Mizuuchi H: Ultrastructural and immunohistochemical study of infiltration in microinvasive carcinoma of the uterine cervix. Gynecol Oncol **36**:23-29, 1990.

186 Langley FA, Crompton AC: Epithelial abnormalities of the cervix uteri. New York, 1973, Springer-Verlag, New York, Inc.

187 Lehman MH Jr, Benson WL, Kurman RJ, Park RC: Microinvasive carcinoma of the cervix. Obstet Gynecol **48**:571-578, 1976.

188 Leung K-M, Chan W-Y, Hui P-K: Invasive squamous cell carcinoma and cervical intraepithelial neoplasia III of uterine cervix. Morphologic differences other than stromal invasion. Am J Clin Pathol **101**:508-513, 1994.

189 Margulis RR, Ely CW Jr, Ladd JE: Diagnosis and management of stage IA (microinvasive) carcinoma of cervix. Obstet Gynecol **29**:529-538, 1967.

189a Morris M, Mitchell MF, Silva EG, Copeland LJ, Gershenson DM: Cervical conization as definitive therapy for early invasive squamous carcinoma of the cervix. Gynecol Oncol **51**:193-196, 1993.

190 Mussey E, Soule EH, Welch JS: Microinvasive carcinoma of the cervix. Am J Obstet Gynecol **104**:738-744, 1969.

191 Ng ABP, Reagan JW: Microinvasive carcinoma of the uterine cervix. Am J Clin Pathol **52**:511-529, 1969.

192 Ostor AG: Studies on 200 cases of early squamous cell carcinoma of the cervix. Int J Gynecol Pathol **12**:193-207, 1993.

193 Richards CJ, Furness PN: Basement membrane continuity in benign, premalignant and malignant epithelial conditions of the uterine cervix. Histopathology **16**:47-52, 1990.

194 Roche WD, Norris HJ: Microinvasive carcinoma of the cervix. The significance of lymphatic invasion and confluent patterns of stromal growth. Cancer **36**:180-186, 1975.

195 Rubio CA, Söderberg G, Einhorn N: Histological and follow-up studies in cases of micro-invasive carcinoma of the uterine cervix. Acta Pathol Microbiol Scand (A) **82**:397-410, 1974.

196 Sevin BU, Nadji M, Averette HE, Hilsenbeck S, Smith D, Lampe B: Microinvasive carcinoma of the cervix. Cancer **70**:2121-2128, 1992.

197 Simon NL, Gore H, Shingleton HM, Soong S-J, Orr JW, Hatch KD: Study of superficially invasive carcinoma of the cervix. Obstet Gynecol **68**:19-24, 1986.

198 Stewart CJ, McNicol AM: Distribution of type IV collagen immunoreactivity to assess questionable early stromal invasion. J Clin Pathol **45**:9-15, 1992.

198a Ueki M, Okamoto Y, Misaki O, Seiki Y, Kitsuki K, Ueda M, Sugimoto O: Conservative therapy for microinvasive carcinoma of the uterine cervix. Gynecol Oncol **53**:109-113, 1994.

199 van Nagell JR, Greenwell N, Powell DF, Donaldson ES, Hanson MB, Gay EC: Microinvasive carcinoma of the cervix. Am J Obstet Gynecol **145**:981-991, 1983.

Invasive squamous cell carcinoma
General features

200 Devesa SS: Descriptive epidemiology of cancer of the uterine cervix. Obstet Gynecol **63**:605-612, 1984.

201 Devesa SS, Young JL Jr, Brinton LA, Fraumeni JF Jr: Recent trends in cervix uteri cancer. Cancer **64:**2184-2190, 1989.

202 Herrero R, Brinton LA, Reeves WC, Brenes MM, Tenorio F, de Britton RC, Gaitan E, Garcia M, Rawls WE: Sexual behavior, venereal diseases, hygiene practices, and invasive cervical cancer in a high-risk population. Cancer **65:**380-386, 1990.

203 Larsen NS: Invasive cervical cancer rising in young white females. J Natl Cancer Inst **86:**6-7, 1994.

204 La Vecchia C, Franceschi S, Decarli A, Fasoli M, Gentile A, Parazzini F, Regallo M: Sexual factors, venereal diseases, and the risk of intraepithelial and invasive cervical neoplasia. Cancer **58:**935-941, 1986.

205 Maiman M, Fruchter RG, Serur E, Remy JC, Feuer G, Boyce J: Human immunodeficiency virus infection and cervical neoplasia. Gynecol Oncol **38:**377-382, 1990.

206 Miyazaki K, Yamaguchi K, Tohya T, Ohba T, Takatsuki K, Okamura H: Human T-cell leukemia virus type I infection as an oncogenic and prognostic risk factor in cervical and vaginal carcinoma. Obstet Gynecol **77:**107-110, 1991.

207 Nair BS, Pillai R: Oncogenesis of squamous carcinoma of the uterine cervix. Int J Gynecol Pathol **11:**47-57, 1992.

208 Piver MS: Invasive cervical cancer in the 1990s. Semin Surg Oncol **6:**359-363, 1990.

209 Rapp F, Jenkins FJ: Genital cancer and viruses. Gynecol Oncol **12:**S25-S41, 1981.

210 Rellihan MA, Dooley DP, Burke TW, Berkland ME, Longfield RN: Rapidly progressing cervical cancer in a patient with human immunodeficiency virus infection. Gynecol Oncol **36:**435-438, 1990.

211 Schwartz LB, Carcangiu ML, Bradham L, Schwartz PE: Rapidly progressive squamous cell carcinoma of the cervix coexisting with human immunodeficiency virus infection: clinical opinion. Gynecol Oncol **41:**255-258, 1991.

212 Wong KY, Collins RJ, Srivastava G, Pittaluga S, Cheung AN, Wong LC: Epstein Barr virus in carcinoma of the cervix. Int J Gynecol Pathol **12:**224-227, 1993.

Morphologic features

213 Aho HJ, Talve L, Maenpaa J: Acantholytic squamous cell carcinoma of the uterine cervix with amyloid deposition. Int J Gynecol Pathol **11:**150-155, 1992.

214 Benda JA: Pathology of cervical carcinoma and its prognostic implications. Semin Oncol **21:**3-11, 1994.

215 Bostrom SG, Hart WR: Carcinomas of the cervix with intense stromal eosinophilia. Cancer **47:**2887-2893, 1981.

216 Clement PB, Scully RE: Carcinoma of the cervix. Histologic types. Semin Oncol **9:**251-264, 1982.

217 Colgan TJ, Auger M, McLaughlin JR: Histopathologic classification of cervical carcinomas and recognition of mucin-secreting squamous carcinomas. Int J Gynecol Pathol **12:**64-69, 1993.

218 Gondo T, Ishihara T, Kawano H, Uchino F, Takahashi M, Iwata T, Matsumoto N, Yokota T: Localized amyloidosis in squamous cell carcinoma of uterine cervix. Electron microscopic features of nodular and star-like amyloid deposits. Virchows Arch [A] **422:**225-231, 1993.

219 Heller PB, Barnhill Dr, Mayer AR, Fontaine TP, Hoskins WJ, Park RC: Cervical carcinoma found incidentally in a uterus removed for benign indications. Obstet Gynecol **67:**187-190, 1986.

220 Kapp DS, LiVolsi VA: Intense eosinophilic stromal infiltration in carcinoma of the uterine cervix. A clinicopathologic study of 14 cases. Gynecol Oncol **16:**19-30, 1983.

221 Miller BE, Copeland LJ, Hamberger AD, Gershenson DM, Saul PB, Herson J, Rutledge FN: Carcinoma of the cervical stump. Gynecol Oncol **18:**100-108, 1984.

222 Ng ABP, Atkin NB: Histological cell type and DNA value in the prognosis of squamous cell cancer of uterine cervix. Br J Cancer **28:**322-331, 1973.

223 Tsang WY, Chan JK: Amyloid-producing squamous cell carcinoma of the uterine cervix. Arch Pathol Lab Med **117:**199-201, 1993.

Immunohistochemical and other special techniques

224 Bychkov V, Rothman M, Bardawil WA: Immunocytochemical localization of carcinoembryonic antigen (CEA), alpha-fetoprotein (AFP), and human chorionic gonadotropin (HCG) in cervical neoplasia. Am J Clin Pathol **79:**414-420, 1983.

224a Dunne FP, Rollason T, Ratcliff WA, Marshall T, Heath DA: Parathyroid hormone–related protein gene expression in invasive cervical tumors. Cancer **74:**83-89, 1994.

225 Kessis TD, Slebos RJ, Han SM, Shah K, Bosch XF, Munoz N, Hedrick L, Cho KR: p53 gene mutations and MDM2 amplification are uncommon in primary carcinomas of the uterine cervix. Am J Pathol **143:**1398-1405, 1993.

226 Konishi I, Fujii S, Nonogaki H, Nanbu Y, Iwai T, Mori T: Immunohistochemical analysis of estrogen receptors, progesterone receptors, Ki-67 antigen, and human papillomavirus DNA in normal and neoplastic epithelium of the uterine cervix. Cancer **68:**1340-1350, 1991.

227 Mitchell KM, Hale RJ, Buckley CH, Fox H, Smith D: Cathepsin-D expression in cervical carcinoma and its prognostic significance. Virchows Arch [A] **422:**357-360, 1993.

228 Nguyen HN, Sevin BU, Averette HE, Ramos R, Ganjei P, Perras J: Evidence of tumor heterogeneity in cervical cancers and lymph node metastases as determined by flow cytometry. Cancer **71:**2543-2550, 1993.

229 Smedts F, Ramaekers F, Link M, Lauerova L, Troyanovsky S, Schijf C, Voojis GP: Detection of keratin subtypes in routinely processed cervical tissue. Implications for tumour classification and the study of cervix cancer aetiology. Virchows Arch **425:**145-155, 1994.

230 To ACW, Soong S-J, Shingleton HM, Gore H, Wilkerson JA, Hatch KD, Phillips D, Dollar JR: Immunohistochemistry of the blood group A, B, H isoantigens and Oxford Ca antigen as prognostic markers for stage IB squamous cell carcinoma of the cervix. Cancer **58:**2435-2439, 1986.

Spread and metastases

231 Barmeir E, Langer O, Levy JI, Nissenbaum M, DeMoor NG, Blumenthal NJ: Unusual skeletal metastases in carcinoma of the cervix. Gynecol Oncol **20:**307-316, 1985.

232 Henriksen E: The lymphatic spread of carcinoma of the cervix and the body of the uterus. Am J Obstet Gynecol **58:**924-942, 1949.

233 Ratanatharathorn V, Powers WE, Steverson N, Han I, Ahmad K, Grimm J: Bone metastasis from cervical cancer. Cancer **73:**2372-2379, 1994.

234 Tellis CJ, Beechler CR: Pulmonary metastasis of carcinoma of the cervix. A retrospective study. Cancer **49:**1705-1709, 1982.

235 Uqmakli A, Bonney WA Jr, Palladino A: The nonlymphatic metastases of carcinoma of the uterine cervix. A prospective analysis based on laparotomy. Cancer **41:**1027-1033, 1978.

236 Young RH, Gersell DJ, Roth LM, Scully RE: Ovarian metastases from cervical carcinomas other than pure adenocarcinomas. A report of 12 cases. Cancer **71:**407-418, 1993.

Treatment

237 Bjornsson BL, Nelson BE, Reale FR, Rose PG: Accuracy of frozen section for lymph node metastasis in patients undergoing radical hysterectomy for carcinoma of the cervix. Gynecol Oncol **51:**50-53, 1993.

238 Bricker EM, Butcher HR Jr, Lawler WH Jr, McAfee CA: Surgical treatment of advanced and recurrent cancer of the pelvic viscera. An evaluation of ten years' experience. Ann Surg **152:**388-402, 1960.

239 Hamberger AD, Fletcher GH, Wharton JT: Results of treatment of early stage I carcinoma of the uterine cervix with intracavitary radium alone. Cancer **41:**980-985, 1978.

240 Hopkins MP, Morley GW: Radical hysterectomy versus radiation therapy for stage IB squamous cell cancer of the cervix. Cancer **68:**272-277, 1991.

241 Jacobs AJ, Faris C, Perez CA, Kao MS, Galakatos A, Camel HM: Short-term persistence of carcinoma of the uterine cervix after radiation. An indicator of long-term prognosis. Cancer **57:**944-950, 1986.

242 Jones WB: New approaches to high-risk cervical cancer. Advanced cervical cancer. Cancer **71:**1451-1459, 1993.

243 Kinney WK, Egorshin EV, Ballard DJ, Podratz KC: Long-term survival and sequelae after surgical management of invasive cervical carcinoma diagnosed at the time of simple hysterectomy. Gynecol Oncol **44:**24-27, 1992.

244 Kiselow M, Butcher HR, Bricker EM: Results of the radical surgical treatment of advanced pelvic cancer. Ann Surg **166:**428-437, 1967.

245 Morgan LS, Nelson JH: Surgical treatment of early cervical cancer. Semin Oncol **9:**312-330, 1982.

246 Morley GW: Pelvic exenterative therapy and the treatment of recurrent carcinoma of the cervix. Semin Oncol **9:**331-340, 1982.

247 Morley GW, Hopkins MP, Lindenauer SM, Roberts JA: Pelvic exenteration, University of Michigan. 100 patients at 5 years. Obstet Gynecol **74:**934-943, 1989.

248 Perez CA, Camel HM, Kao MS, Hederman MA: Randomized study of preoperative radiation and surgery or irradiation alone in the treatment of stage IB and IIA carcinoma of the uterine cervix. Final report. Gynecol Oncol **27:**129-140, 1987.

249 Perez-Mesa C, Spjut HJ: Persistent postirradiation carcinoma of cervix uteri. A pathologic study of 83 pelvic exenteration specimens. Arch Pathol **75:**462-474, 1963.

250 Thar TL, Million RR, Daly JW: Radiation treatment of carcinoma of the cervix. Semin Oncol **9:**299-311, 1982.

Prognosis

251 Baltzer J, Lohe KJ: What's new in prognosis of uterine cancer? Pathol Res Pract **178:**635-641, 1984.

252 Bethwaite PB, Holloway LJ, Yeong ML, Thornton A: Effect of tumour associated tissue eosinophilia on survival of women with stage IB carcinoma of the uterine cervix. J Clin Pathol **46:**1016-1020, 1993.

253 Boyce JG, Fruchter RG, Nicastri AD, DeRegt RH, Ambiavagar PC, Reinis M, Macasaet M, Rotman M: Vascular invasion in stage I carcinoma of the cervix. Cancer **53:**1175-1180, 1984.

254 Burghardt E, Baltzer J, Tulusan AH, Haas J: Results of surgical treatment of 1028 cervical cancers studied with volumetry. Cancer **70:**648-655, 1992.

255 Goellner JR: Carcinoma of the cervix. Clinicopathologic correlation of 196 cases. Am J Clin Pathol **66:**775-785, 1976.

256 Gunderson LL, Weems WS, Hebertson RM, Plenk HP: Correlation of histopathology with clinical results following radiation therapy for carcinoma of the cervix. Am J Roentgenol Radium Ther Nucl Med **120:**74-87, 1974.

257 Hale RJ, Buckley CH, Fox H, Williams J: Prognostic value of c-*erb*B-2 expression in uterine cervical carcinoma. J Clin Pathol **45:**594-596, 1992.

258 Hirao T, Sakamoto Y, Kamada M, Hamada S, Aono T: Tn antigen, a marker of potential for metastasis of uterine cervix cancer cells. Cancer **72:**154-159, 1993.

259 Hopkins MP, Morley GW: Prognostic factors in advanced stage squamous cell cancer of the cervix. Cancer **72:**2389-2393, 1993.

260 Inoue T: Prognostic significance of the depth of invasion relating to nodal metastases, parametrial extension, and cell types. A study of 628 cases with stage IB, IIA, and IIB cervical carcinoma. Cancer **54:**3035-3042, 1984.

261 Inoue T, Chihara T, Morita K: The prognostic significance of the size of the largest nodes in metastatic carcinoma from the uterine cervix. Gynecol Oncol **19:**187-193, 1984.

262 Inoue T, Morita K: The prognostic significance of number of positive nodes in cervical carcinoma stages IB, IIA, and IIB. Cancer **65:**1923-1927, 1990.

263 Inoue T, Okumura M: Prognostic significance of parametrial extension in patients with cervical carcinoma stages IB, IIA, and IIB. A study of 628 cases treated by radical hysterectomy and lymphadenectomy with or without postoperative irradiation. Cancer **54:**1714-1719, 1984.

264 Kamura T, Tsukamoto N, Tsuruchi N, Saito T, Matsuyama T, Akazawa K, Nakano H: Multivariate analysis of the histopathologic prognostic factors of cervical cancer in patients undergoing radical hysterectomy. Cancer **69:**181-186, 1992.

265 Nakano T, Oka K, Takahashi T, Morita S, Arai T: Roles of Langerhans' cells and T-lymphocytes infiltrating cancer tissues in patients treated by radiation therapy for cervical cancer. Cancer **70:**2839-2844, 1992.

266 Noguchi H, Shiozawa I, Sakai Y, Yamazaki T, Fukuta T: Pelvic lymph node metastasis of uterine cervical cancer. Gynecol Oncol **27:**150-158, 1987.

267 Oka K, Nakano T, Arai T: c-*erb*B-2 Oncoprotein expression is associated withpoor prognosis in squamous cell carcinoma of the cervix. Cancer **73:**664-671, 1994.

268 Perez CA, Camel HM, Askin F, Breaux S: Endometrial extension of carcinoma of the uterine cervix. A prognostic factor that may modify staging. Cancer **48:**170-180, 1981.

269 Perez CA, Grigsby PW, Nene SM, Camel HM, Galakatos A, Kao MS, Lockett MA: Effect of tumor size on the prognosis of carcinoma of the uterine cervix treated with irradiation alone. Cancer **69:**2796-2806, 1992.

270 Riou G, Favre M, Jeannel D, Bourhis J, Le Doussal V, Orth G: Association between poor prognosis in early-stage invasive cervical carcinomas and non-detection of HPV DNA. Lancet **335:**1171-1174, 1990.

271 Robert ME, Fu YS: Squamous cell carcinoma of the uterine cervix—a review with emphasis on prognostic factors and unusual variants. Semin Diagn Pathol **7:**173-189, 1990.

271a Rutgers JL, Mattox TF, Vargas MP: Angiogenesis in uterine cervical squamous cell carcinoma. Int J Gynecol Pathol **14:**114-118, 1995.

272 Sagae S, Kuzumaki N, Hisada T, Mugikura Y, Kudo R, Hashimoto M: *ras* Oncogene expression and prognosis of invasive squamous cell carcinomas of the uterine cervix. Cancer **63:**1577-1582, 1989.

273 Smiley LM, Burke TW, Silva EG, Morris M, Gershenson DM, Wharton JT: Prognostic factors in stage IB squamous cervical cancer patients with low risk for recurrence. Obstet Gynecol **77:**271-275, 1991.

274 Stendahl U, Eklund G, Willen R: Prognosis of invasive squamous cell carcinoma of the uterine cervix. A comparative study of the predictive values of clinical staging IB-III and a histopathologic malignancy grading system. Int J Gynecol Pathol **2:**42-54, 1983.

275 Stock RJ, Zaino R, Bundy BN, Askin FB, Woodward J, Fetter B, Paulson JA, DiSaia PJ, Stehman FB: Evaluation and comparison of histopathologic grading systems of epithelial carcinoma of the uterine cervix; Gynecologic Oncology Group studies. Int J Gynecol Pathol **13:**99-108, 1994.

276 Strang P: Cytogenetic and cytometric analyses in squamous cell carcinoma of the uterine cervix. Int J Gynecol Pathol **8:**54-63, 1989.

276a van Bommel PF, Kenemans P, Helmerhorst TJ, Gallee MP, Ivanyi D: Expression of cytokeratin 10, 13, and involucrin as prognostic factors in low stage squamous cell carcinoma. Cancer **74:**2314-2320, 1994.

277 Wentz WB, Lewis GC Jr: Correlation of histologic morphology and survival in cervical cancer following radiation therapy. Obstet Gynecol **26:**228-232, 1965.

278 Zaino RJ, Ward S, Delgado G, Bundy B, Gore H, Fetter G, Ganjei P, Frauenhoffer E: Histopathologic predictors of the behavior of surgically treated stage IB squamous cell carcinoma of the cervix. A Gynecologic Oncology Group study. Cancer **69:**1750-1758, 1992.

Other microscopic types

278a Albores-Saavedra J, Young RH: Transitional cell neoplasms (carcinomas and inverted papillomas) of the uterine cervix. A report of four cases. Am J Surg Pathol (in press).

279 Daroca PJ Jr, Dhorandhar HN: Basaloid carcinoma of uterine cervix. Am J Surg Pathol **4:**235-239, 1980.

280 Dinh TV, Woodruff JD: Adenoid cystic and adenoid basal carcinomas of the cervix. Obstet Gynecol **65:**705-709, 1985.

281 Halpin TF, Hunter RE, Cohen MB: Lymphoepithelioma of the uterine cervix. Gynecol Oncol **34:**101-105, 1989.

282 Hasumi K, Sugano H, Sakamoto G, Masubuchi K, Kubo H: Circumscribed carcinoma of the uterine cervix, with marked lymphocytic infiltration. Cancer **39:**2503-2507, 1977.

283 Mills SE, Austin MB, Randall ME: Lymphoepithelioma-like carcinoma of the uterine cervix. A distinctive, undifferentiated carcinoma with inflammatory stroma. Am J Surg Pathol **9:**883-889, 1985.

284 Randall ME, Andersen WA, Mills SE, Kim JAC: Papillary squamous cell carcinoma of the uterine cervix. A clinicopathologic study of nine cases. Int J Gynecol Pathol **5:**1-10, 1986.

285 Steeper TA, Piscioli F, Rosai J: Squamous cell carcinoma with sarcoma-like stroma of the female genital tract. Cancer **52:**890-898, 1983.

286 Tiltman AJ, Atad J: Verrucous carcinoma of the cervix with endometrial involvement. Int J Gynecol Pathol **1:**221-226, 1982.

287 Weinberg E, Hoisington S, Eastman AY, Rice DK, Malfetano J, Ross JS: Uterine cervical lymphoepithelial-like carcinoma. Absence of Epstein-Barr virus genomes. Am J Clin Pathol **99:**195-199, 1993.

Adenocarcinoma

288 Albores-Saavedra J, Manivel C, Mora A, Vuitch F, Milchgrub S, Gould E: The solid variant of adenoid cystic carcinoma of the cervix. Int J Gynecol Pathol **11:**2-10, 1992.

289 Andersen ES, Arffmann E: Adenocarcinoma in situ of the uterine cervix. A clinico-pathologic study of 36 cases. Gynecol Oncol **35:**1-7, 1989.

290 Angel C, Du Beshter B, Lin JY: Clinical presentation and management of stage I cervical adenocarcinoma. A 25 year experience. Gynecol Oncol **44:**71-78, 1992.

291 Auersperg N, Erber H, Worth A: Histologic variation among poorly differentiated invasive carcinomas of the human uterine cervix. J Natl Cancer Inst **51:**1461-1477, 1973.

292 Berek JS, Hacker NF, Fu Y-S, Sokale JR, Leuchter RC, Lagasse LD: Adenocarcinoma of the uterine cervix. Histologic variables associated with lymph node metastasis and survival. Obstet Gynecol **65:**46-52, 1985.

293 Boon ME, Baak JPA, Kurver PJH, Overdiep SH, Verdonk GW: Adenocarcinoma in situ of the cervix. An underdiagnosed lesion. Cancer **48:**768-773, 1981.

294 Caron C, Tetu B, Laberge P, Bellemare G, Raymond PE: Endocervical involvement by endometrial carcinoma on fractional curettage. A clinicopathological study of 37 cases. Mod Pathol **4:**644-647, 1991.

295 Choo YC, Naylor B: Coexistent squamous cell carcinoma and adenocarcinoma of the uterine cervix. Gynecol Oncol **17:**168-174, 1984.

296 Christopherson WM, Nealon N, Gray LA Sr: Noninvasive precursor lesions of adenocarcinoma and mixed adenosquamous carcinoma of the cervix uteri. Cancer **44:**975-983, 1979.

296a Clement PB, Young RH, Keh P, Östör AG, Scully RE: Malignant mesonephric neoplasms of the uterine cervix. A report of eight cases, including four with a malignant spindle cell component. Am J Surg Pathol **19:**1158-1171, 1995.

297 Cohen C, Shulman G, Budgeon LR: Endocervical and endometrial adenocarcinoma. An immunoperoxidase and histochemical study. Am J Surg Pathol **6:**151-157, 1982.

298 Colgan TJ, Lickrish GM: The topography and invasive potential of cervical adenocarcinoma in situ, with and without associated dysplasia. Gynecol Oncol **36:**246-249, 1990.

299 Cooper P, Russell G, Wilson B: Adenocarcinoma of the endocervix. A histochemical study. Histopathology **11:**1321-1330, 1987.

300 Costa MJ, Kenny MB, Hewan-Lowe K, Judd R: Glassy cell features in adenosquamous carcinoma of the uterine cervix. Histologic, ultrastructural, immunohistochemical, and clinical findings. Am J Clin Pathol **96:**520-528, 1991.

301 Costa MJ, Kenny MB, Judd R: Adenocarcinoma and adenosquamous carcinoma of the uterine cervix. Histologic and immunohistochemical features with clinical correlation. Int J Surg Pathol **1:**181-190, 1994.

301a Costa MJ, McIlnay KR, Trelford J: Cervical carcinoma with glandular differentiation. Histological evaluation predicts disease recurrence in clinical Stage I or II patients. Hum Pathol **26**:829-837, 1995.

302 Dabbs DJ, Geisinger KR, Norris HT: Intermediate filaments in endometrial and endocervical carcinomas. The diagnostic utility of vimentin patterns. Am J Surg Pathol **10**:568-576, 1986.

302a Daya D, Young RH: Florid deep glands of the uterine cervix. Another mimic of adenoma malignum. Am J Clin Pathol (in press).

303 Dickersin GR, Welch WR, Erlandson R, Robboy SJ: Ultrastructure of 16 cases of clear cell adenocarcinoma of the vagina and cervix in young women. Cancer **45**:1615-1624, 1980.

304 Duk JM, De Bruijn HW, Groenier KH, Fleuren GJ, Aalders JG: Adenocarcinoma of the uterine cervix. Prognostic significance of pretreatment serum CA 125, squamous cell carcinoma antigen, and carcinoembryonic antigen levels in relation to clinical and histopathologic tumor characteristics. Cancer **65**:1830-1837, 1990.

305 Eifel PJ, Burke TW, Delclos L, Wharton JT, Oswald MJ: Early stage I adenocarcinoma of the uterine cervix. Treatment results in patients with tumors less than or equal to 4 cm in diameter. Gynecol Oncol **41**:199-205, 1991.

306 Eifel PJ, Morris M, Oswald MJ, Wharton JT, Delclos L: Adenocarcinoma of the uterine cervix. Prognosis and patterns of failure in 367 cases. Cancer **65**:2507-2514, 1990.

307 Fawcett KJ, Dockerty MB, Hunt AB: Mesonephric carcinoma of the cervix uteri. Clinical and pathologic study. Am J Obstet Gynecol **95**:1068-1079, 1966.

308 Ferry JA, Scully RE: "Adenoid cystic" carcinoma and adenoid basal carcinoma of the uterine cervix. A study of 28 cases. Am J Surg Pathol **12**:134-144, 1988.

309 Fowler WC Jr, Miles PA, Surwit EA, Edelman DA, Walton LA, Photopulos GJ: Adenoid cystic carcinoma of the cervix. Obstet Gynecol **52**:337-342, 1978.

310 Fu YS, Reagan JW, Fu AS, Janiga KE: Adenocarcinoma and mixed carcinoma of the uterine cervix. II. Prognostic value of nuclear DNA analysis. Cancer **49**:2571-2577, 1982.

311 Fu YS, Reagan JW, Hsiu JG, Storaasli JP, Wentz WB: Adenocarcinoma and mixed carcinoma of the uterine cervix. Cancer **49**:2560-2570, 1982.

312 Gallager HS, Simpson CB, Ayala AG: Adenoid cystic carcinoma of the uterine cervix. Report of 4 cases. Cancer **27**:1398-1402, 1971.

313 Gallup DG, Abell MR: Invasive adenocarcinoma of the uterine cervix. Obstet Gynecol **49**:596-603, 1977.

314 Ghandour FA, Attanoos R, Nahar K, Gee JW, Bigrigg A, Ismail SM: Immunocytochemical localization of oestrogen and progesterone receptors in primary adenocarcinoma of the cervix. Histopathology **24**:49-56, 1994.

315 Gilks CB, Clement PB: Papillary serous adenocarcinoma of the uterine cervix. A report of three cases. Mod Pathol **5**:426-431, 1992.

316 Gilks CB, Young RH, Aguirre P, De Lellis RA, Scully RE: Adenoma malignum (minimal deviation adenocarcinoma) of the uterine cervix. A clinicopathological and immunohistochemical analysis of 26 cases. Am J Surg Pathol **13**:717-729, 1989.

317 Gloor E, Hurlimann J: Cervical intraepithelial glandular neoplasia (adenocarcinoma in situ and glandular dysplasia). A correlative study of 23 cases with histologic grading, histochemical analysis of mucins, and immunohistochemical determination of the affinity for four lectins. Cancer **58**:1272-1280, 1986.

318 Gloor E, Ruzicka J: Morphology of adenocarcinoma in situ of the uterine cervix. A study of 14 cases. Cancer **49**:294-302, 1982.

319 Glücksmann A: Relationships between hormonal changes in pregnancy and the development of "mixed carcinoma" of the uterine cervix. Cancer **10**:831-837, 1957.

320 Glücksmann A, Cherry CP: Incidence, histology, and response to radiation of mixed carcinomas (adenocanthomas) of the uterine cervix. Cancer **9**:971-979, 1956.

321 Greer BE, Figge DC, Tamimi HK, Cain JM: Stage IB adenocarcinoma of the cervix treated by radical hysterectomy and pelvic lymph node dissection. Am J Obstet Gynecol **160**:1509-1513, 1989.

321a Griffin NR, Wells M: Characterisation of complex carbohydrates in cervical glandular intraepithelial neoplasia and invasive adenocarcinoma. Int J Gynecol Pathol **13**:319-329, 1994.

322 Griffin NR, Wells M, Fox H: Modulation of the antigenicity of amylase in cervical glandular atypia, adenocarcinoma in situ and invasive adenocarcinoma. Histopathology **15**:267-279, 1989.

323 Gusberg SB, Corscaden JA: The pathology and treatment of adenocarcinoma of the cervix. Cancer **4**:1066-1072, 1951.

324 Hameed K: Clear-cell carcinoma of the uterine cervix. Am J Obstet Gynecol **101**:954-958, 1968.

325 Hanselaar AG, Van Leusen ND, De Wilde PC, Vooijs GP: Clear cell adenocarcinoma of the vagina and cervix. A report of the Central Netherlands Registry with emphasis on early detection and prognosis. Cancer **67**:1971-1978, 1991.

326 Harrison TA, Sevin BU, Koechli O, Nguyen HN, Averette HE, Penalver M, Donato DM, Nadji M: Adenosquamous carcinoma of the cervix. Prognosis in early stage disease treated by radical hysterectomy. Gynecol Oncol **50**:310-315, 1993.

327 Hart WR, Norris HJ: Mesonephric adenocarcinomas of the cervix. Cancer **29**:106-113, 1972.

328 Helper TK, Dockerty MB, Randall LM: Primary adenocarcinoma of the cervix. Am J Obstet Gynecol **63**:800-808, 1952.

329 Hopkins MP, Schmidt RW, Roberts JA, Morley GW: The prognosis and treatment of stage I adenocarcinoma of the cervix. Obstet Gynecol **72**:915-921, 1988.

330 Hopkins MP, Sutton P, Roberts JA: Prognostic features and treatment of endocervical adenocarcinoma of the cervix. Gynecol Oncol **27**:69-75, 1987.

331 Hoskins WJ, Averette HE, Ng ABP, Yon JL: Adenoid cystic carcinoma of the cervix uteri. Report of six cases and review of literature. Gynecol Oncol **7**:371-384, 1979.

332 Hurlimann J, Gloor E: Adenocarcinoma in situ and invasive adenocarcinoma of the uterine cervix. An immunohistologic study with antibodies specific for several epithelial markers. Cancer **54**:103-109, 1984.

333 Jackson-York GL, Ramzy I: Synchronous papillary mucinous adenocarcinoma of the endocervix and fallopian tubes. Int J Gynecol Pathol **11**:63-67, 1992.

334 Jaworski RC: Endocervical glandular dysplasia, adenocarcinoma in situ, and early invasive (microinvasive) adenocarcinoma of the uterine cervix. Semin Diagn Pathol **7**:190-204, 1990.

335 Jaworski RC, Pacey NF, Greenberg ML, Osborn RA: The histologic diagnosis of adenocarcinoma in situ and related lesions of the cervix uteri. Adenocarcinoma in situ. Cancer **61**:1171-1181, 1988.

336 Jones MW, Silverberg SG: Cervical adenocarcinoma in young women. Possible relationship to microglandular hyperplasia and use of oral contraceptives. Obstet Gynecol **73**:984-989, 1989.

337 Jones MW, Silverberg SG, Kurman RJ: Well-differentiated villoglandular adenocarcinoma of the uterine cervix. A clinicopathological study of 24 cases. Int J Gynecol Pathol **12**:1-7, 1993.

338 Kaku T, Enjoji M: Extremely well-differentiated adenocarcinoma ("adenoma malignum") of the cervix. Int J Gynecol Pathol **2**:28-41, 1983.

339 Kaminski PF, Maier RC: Clear cell adenocarcinoma of the cervix unrelated to diethylstilbestrol exposure. Obstet Gynecol **62**:720-727, 1983.

340 Kaminski PF, Norris HJ: Minimal deviation carcinoma (adenoma malignum) of the cervix. Int J Gynecol Pathol **2**:141-152, 1983.

341 Kaminski PF, Norris HJ: Coexistence of ovarian neoplasms and endocervical adenocarcinoma. Obstet Gynecol **64**:553-556, 1984.

342 Kaspar HG, Dinh TV, Doherty MG, Hannigan EV, Kumar D: Clinical implications of tumor volume measurement in stage I adenocarcinoma of the cervix. Obstet Gynecol **81**:296-300, 1993.

343 Kihana T, Tsuda H, Teshima S, Nomoto K, Tsugane S, Sonoda T, Matsuura S, Hirohashi S: Prognostic significance of the overexpression of c-*erb*B-2 protein in adenocarcinoma of the uterine cervix. Cancer **73**:148-153, 1994.

344 Kjorstad KE, Bond B: Stage IB adenocarcinoma of the cervix. Metastatic potential and patterns of dissemination. Am J Obstet Gynecol **150**:297-299, 1984.

345 Kleine W, Rau K, Schwoeorer D, Pfleiderer A: Prognosis of the adenocarcinoma of the cervix uteri: a comparative study. Gynecol Oncol **35**:145-149, 1989.

346 Konishi I, Fujii S, Nanbu Y, Nonogaki H, Mori T: Mucin leakage into the cervical stroma may increase lymph node metastasis in mucin-producing cervical adenocarcinomas. Cancer **65**:229-237, 1990.

347 Korhonen MO: Adenocarcinoma of the uterine cervix. Prognosis and prognostic significance of histology. Cancer **53**:1760-1763, 1984.

348 Kudo R, Sagae S, Hayakawa O, Ito E, Horimoto E, Hashimoto M: Morphology of adenocarcinoma in situ and microinvasive adenocarcinoma of the uterine cervix. A cytologic and ultrastructural study. Acta Cytol **35**:109-116, 1991.

349 Kudo R, Sasano H, Koizumi M, Orenstein JM, Silverberg SG: Immunohistochemical comparison of new monoclonal antibody 1C5 and carcinoembryonic antigen in the differential diagnosis of adenocarcinoma of the uterine cervix. Int J Gynecol Pathol **9**:325-336, 1990.

350 Lang G, Dallenbach-Hellweg G: The histogenetic origin of cervical mesonephric hyperplasia and mesonephric adenocarcinoma of the uterine cervix studied with immunohistochemical methods. Int J Gynecol Pathol **9**:145-157, 1990.

351 Lee KR, Trainer TD: Adenocarcinoma of the uterine cervix of small intestinal type containing numerous Paneth cells. Arch Pathol Lab Med **114**:731-733, 1990.

352 Lee SJ, Rollason TP: Argyrophilic cells in cervical intraepithelial glandular neoplasia. Int J Gynecol Pathol **13**:131-132, 1994.

353 Littman P, Clement PB, Henriksen B, Wang CC, Robboy SJ, Taft PD, Ulfelder H, Scully RE: Glassy cell carcinoma of the cervix. Cancer **37**:2238-2246, 1976.

354 LiVolsi VA, Merino MJ, Schwartz PE: Coexistent endocervical adenocarcinoma and mucinous adenocarcinoma of ovary. A clinicopathologic study of four cases. Int J Gynecol Pathol 1:391-402, 1983.

355 Maier RC, Norris HJ: Coexistence of cervical intraepithelial neoplasia with primary adenocarcinoma of the endocervix. Obstet Gynecol 56:361-364, 1980.

356 Maier RC, Norris HJ: Glassy cell carcinoma of the cervix. Obstet Gynecol 60:219-224, 1982.

356a Mandai M, Konishi I, Koshiyama M, Komatsu T, Yamamoto S, Nanbu K, Mori T, Fukumoto M: Altered expression of nm23-H1 and c-erbB-2 proteins have prognostic significance in adenocarcinoma but not in squamous cell carcinoma of the uterine cervix. Cancer 75:2523-2529, 1995.

357 Masood S, Rhatigan RM, Wilkinson EW, Barwick KW, Wilson WJ: Expression and prognostic significance of estrogen and progesterone receptors in adenocarcinoma of the uterine cervix. An immunocytochemical study. Cancer 72:511-518, 1993.

358 Matthews CM, Burke TW, Tornos C, Eifel PJ, Atkinson EN, Stringer CA, Morris M, Silva EG: Stage I cervical adenocarcinoma. Prognostic evaluation of surgically treated patients. Gynecol Oncol 49:19-23, 1993.

359 Michael H, Grawe L, Kraus FT: Minimal deviation endocervical adenocarcinoma. Clinical and histologic features, immunohistochemical staining for carcino-embryonic antigen, and differentiation from confusing benign lesions. Int J Gynecol Pathol 3:261-276, 1984.

360 Miller BE, Flax SD, Arheart K, Photopulos G: The presentation of adenocarcinoma of the uterine cervix. Cancer 72:1281-1285, 1993.

361 Moberg PJ, Einhorn N, Silfversward C, Soderberg G: Adenocarcinoma of the uterine cervix. Cancer 57:407-410, 1986.

362 Muntz HG, Bell DA, Lage JM, Goff BA, Feldman S, Rice LW: Adenocarcinoma in situ of the uterine cervix. Obstet Gynecol 80:935-939, 1992.

363 Nguyen GK, Daya D: Cervical adenocarcinoma and related lesions. Cytodiagnostic criteria and pitfalls. Pathol Annu 28(Pt 2):53-75, 1993.

364 Nordqvist SRB, Fidler WJ Jr, Woodruff JM, Lewis JL Jr: Clear cell adenocarcinoma of the cervix and vagina. A clinicopathologic study of 21 cases with and without a history of maternal ingestion of estrogens. Cancer 37:858-871, 1976.

365 Norris HJ, McCauley KM: Unusual forms of adenocarcinoma of the cervix. An update. Pathol Annu 28(Pt 1):73-95, 1993.

366 Pak HY, Yokota SB, Paladugu RR, Agliozzo CM: Glassy cell carcinoma of the cervix. Cytologic and clinicopathologic analysis. Cancer 52:307-312, 1983.

367 Parazzini F, La Vecchia C: Epidemiology of adenocarcinoma of the cervix. Gynecol Oncol 39:40-46, 1990.

368 Qizilbash AH: In-situ and microinvasive adenocarcinoma of the uterine cervix. A clinical cytologic and histologic study of 14 cases. Am J Clin Pathol 64:155-170, 1975.

369 Reagan JW: Cellular pathology and uterine cancer. Ward Burdick Award Address. Am J Clin Pathol 62:150-164, 1974.

370 Robboy SJ, Herbst AL, Scully RE: Vaginal and cervical abnormalities related to prenatal exposure to diethylstilbestrol (DES). In Blaustein A, ed: Pathology of female genital tract. New York, 1977, Springer-Verlag, New York, Inc., pp. 87-101.

371 Rollason TP, Cullimore J, Bradgate MG: A suggested columnar cell morphological equivalent of squamous carcinoma in situ with early stromal invasion. Int J Gynecol Pathol 8:230-236, 1989.

372 Rombaut RP, Charles D, Murphy A: Adenocarcinoma of the cervix. A clinico pathologic study of 47 cases. Cancer 19:891-900, 1966.

373 Rose PG, Reale FR: Serous papillary carcinoma of the cervix. Gynecol Oncol 50:361-364, 1993.

374 Rosen Y, Dolan TE: Carcinoma of the cervix with cylindromatous features believed to arise in mesonephric duct. Cancer 36:1739-1747, 1975.

375 Roth LM, Hornback NB: Clear-cell adenocarcinoma of the cervix in young women. Cancer 34:1761-1768, 1974.

376 Saigo PE, Cain JM, Kim WS, Gaynor JJ, Johnson K, Lewis JL: Prognostic factors in adenocarcinoma of the uterine cervix. Cancer 57:1584-1593, 1986.

377 Savargaonkar PR, Hale RJ, Pope R, Fox H, Buckley CH: Enteric differentiation in cervical adenocarcinomas and its prognostic significance. Histopathology 23:275-277, 1993.

378 Scully RE, Robboy SJ, Welch WR: Pathology and pathogenesis of diethylstilbestrol-related disorders of the female genital tract. In Herbst AL, ed: Intrauterine exposure to diethylstilbestrol in the human. Chicago, IL, 1978, American College of Obstetricians and Gynecologists, pp. 8-22.

379 Shintaku M, Ueda H: Serous papillary adenocarcinoma of the uterine cervix. Histopathology 22:506-507, 1993.

380 Shorrock K, Johnson J, Johnson IR: Epidemiological changes in cervical carcinoma with particular reference to mucin-secreting subtypes. Histopathology 17:53-57, 1990.

381 Sorvari TE: A histochemical study of epithelial mucosubstances in endometrial and cervical adenocarcinomas. With reference to normal endometrium and cervical mucosa. Acta Pathol Microbiol Scand 207(Suppl):1-85, 1969.

382 Steeper TA, Wick MR: Minimal deviation adenocarcinoma of the uterine cervix ("adenoma malignum"). An immunohistochemical comparison with microglandular endocervical hyperplasia and conventional endocervical adenocarcinoma. Cancer 58:1131-1138, 1986.

383 Tamimi HK, Gown AM, Kim-Deobald J, Figge DC, Greer BE, Cain JM: The utility of immunocytochemistry in invasive adenocarcinoma of the cervix. Am J Obstet Gynecol 166:1655-1661, 1992.

383a Tenti P, Romagnoli S, Silini E, Zappatore R, Giunta P, Stella G, Carnevali L: Cervical adenocarcinomas express markers common to gastric, intestinal, and pancreatobiliary epithelial cells. Pathol Res Pract 190:342-349, 1994.

384 Teshima S, Shimosato Y, Kishi K, Kasamatsu T, Ohmi K, Uei Y: Early stage adenocarcinoma of the uterine cervix. Histopathologic analysis with consideration of histogenesis. Cancer 56:167-172, 1985.

385 Thelmo WL, Nicastri AD, Fruchter R, Spring H, Di Maio T, Boyce J: Mucoepidermoid carcinoma of uterine cervix stage IB. Long-term follow-up, histochemical and immunohistochemical study. Int J Gynecol Pathol 9:316-324, 1990.

386 Toki N, Kaku T, Tsukamoto N, Matsumura M, Saito T, Kamura T, Matsuyama T, Nakano H: Distribution of basement membrane antigens in the uterine cervical adenocarcinoma. An immunohistochemical study. Gynecol Oncol 38:17-21, 1990.

387 Ueda G, Yamasaki M, Inoue M, Tanaka Y, Hiramatsu K, Inoue Y, Abe Y: Immunohistochemical demonstration of peptide hormones in cervical adenocarcinomas with argyrophil cells. Int J Gynecol Pathol 2:373-379, 1984.

388 Ulbright TM, Gersell DJ: Glassy cell carcinoma of the uterine cervix. A light and electron microscopic study of five cases. Cancer 51:2255-2263, 1983.

389 Valente PT, Hanjani P: Endocervical neoplasia in long-term users of oral contraceptives. Clinical and pathologic observations. Obstet Gynecol 67:695-704, 1986.

390 Vesterinen E, Forss M, Nieminen U: Increase of cervical adenocarcinoma. A report of 520 cases of cervical carcinoma including 112 tumors with glandular elements. Gynecol Oncol 33:49-53, 1990.

391 Weisbrot IM, Stabinsky C, Davis AM: Adenocarcinoma in situ of the uterine cervix. Cancer 29:225-233, 1972.

392 Wells M, Brown LJR: Glandular lesions of the uterine cervix. The present state of our knowledge. Histopathology 10:777-792, 1986.

393 Yavner DL, Dwyer IM, Hancock WW, Ehrmann RL: Basement membrane of cervical adenocarcinoma. An immunoperoxidase study of laminin and type IV collagen. Obstet Gynecol 76:1014-1019, 1990.

394 Young RH, Scully RE: Villoglandular papillary adenocarcinoma of the uterine cervix. A clinicopathologic analysis of 13 cases. Cancer 63:1773-1779, 1989.

395 Young RH, Scully RE: Invasive adenocarcinoma and related tumors of the uterine cervix. Semin Diagn Pathol 7:205-227, 1990.

396 Young RH, Scully RE: Minimal-deviation endometrioid adenocarcinoma of the uterine cervix. A report of five cases of distinctive neoplasm that may be misinterpreted as benign. Am J Surg Pathol 17:660-665, 1993.

397 Young RH, Welch WR, Dickersin GR, Scully RE: Ovarian sex-cord tumor with annular tubules. Cancer 50:1384-1402, 1982.

Neuroendocrine carcinoma

398 Abeler VM, Holm R, Nesland JM, Kjorstad KE: Small cell carcinoma of the cervix. A clinicopathologic study of 26 patients. Cancer 73:672-677, 1994.

399 Albores-Saavedra J, Larraza O, Poucell S, Rodriguez-Martinez HA: Carcinoid of the uterine cervix. Additional observations on a new tumor entity. Cancer 38:2328-2342, 1976.

400 Ambros RA, Park JS, Shah KV, Kurman RJ: Evaluation of histologic, morphometric, and immunohistochemical criteria in the differential diagnosis of small cell carcinomas of the cervix with particular reference to human papillomavirus types 16 and 18. Mod Pathol 4:586-593, 1991.

401 Barrett RJ II, Davos I, Leuchter RS, LaGasse LD: Neuroendocrine features in poorly differentiated and undifferentiated carcinomas of the cervix. Cancer 60:2325-2330, 1987.

402 Chan JK, Tsui WM, Tung SY, Ching RC: Endocrine cell hyperplasia of the uterine cervix. A precursor of neuroendocrine carcinoma of the cervix? Am J Clin Pathol 92:825-830, 1989.

403 Gersell DJ, Mazoujian G, Mutch DG, Rudloff MA: Small-cell undifferentiated carcinoma of the cervix. A clinicopathologic, ultrastructural, and immunocytochemical study of 15 cases. Am J Surg Pathol 12:684-698, 1988.

404 Groben P, Reddick R, Askin F: The pathologic spectrum of small cell carcinoma of the cervix. Int J Gynecol Pathol 4:42-57, 1985.

405 Hammar SP, Insalaco SJ, Lee RB, Bockus DE, Remington FL, Yu A: Amphicrine carcinoma of the uterine cervix. Am J Clin Pathol 97:516-522, 1992.

406 Husain AN, Gattuso P, Abraham K, Castelli MJ: Synchronous adenocarcinoma and carcinoid of the uterine cervix. Immunohistochemical study of a case and review of literature. Gynecol Oncol 33:125-128, 1990.

407 Ibrahim NBN, Briggs JC, Corbishley CM: Extrapulmonary oat cell carcinoma. Cancer 54:1645-1661, 1984.

408 Inoue M, Ueda G, Nakajima T: Immunohistochemical demonstration of neuron-specific enolase in gynecologic malignant tumors. Cancer 55:1686-1690, 1985.

409 Johannessen JV, Capella C, Solcia E, Davy M, Sobrinho-Simôes M: Endocrine cell carcinoma of the uterine cervix. Diagn Gynecol Obstet 2:127-134, 1980.

410 Jones HW III, Plymate S, Gluck FB, Miles PA, Greene JF Jr. Small cell non-keratinizing carcinoma of the cervix associated with ACTH production. Cancer 38:1629-1635, 1976.

411 Mackay B, Osborne BM, Wharton JT: Small cell tumor of cervix with neuroepithelial features. Cancer 43:1138-1145, 1979.

412 Miller B, Dockter M, el Torky M, Photopulos G: Small cel carcinoma of the cervix: a clinical and flow-cytometric study. Gynecol Oncol 42:27-33, 1991.

413 Mullins JD, Hilliard GD: Cervical carcinoid ("argyrophil cell" carcinoma) associated with an endocervical adenocarcinoma. A light and ultrastructural study. Cancer 47:785-790, 1981.

414 Silva EG, Kott MM, Ordonez NG: Endocrine carcinoma intermediate cell type of the uterine cervix. Cancer 54:1705-1713, 1984.

415 Stahl R, Demopoulos RI, Bigelow B: Carcinoid tumor within a squamous cell carcinoma of the cervix. Gynecol Oncol 11:387-392, 1981.

416 Stoler MH, Mills SE, Gersell DJ, Walker AN: Small-cell neuroendocrine carcinoma of the cervix. A human papillomavirus type 18-associated cancer. Am J Surg Pathol 15:28-32, 1991.

417 Tateishi R, Wada A, Hayakawa K, Hongo J, Ishii S, Terakawa N: Argyrophil cell carcinomas (apudomas) of the uterine cervix. Light and electron microscopic observations of 5 cases. Virchows Arch [A] 366:257-274, 1975.

418 Ueda G, Shimizu C, Shimizu H, Saito J, Tanaka Y, Inoue M, Tanizawa O: An immunohistochemical study of small-cell and poorly differentiated carcinomas of the cervix using neuroendocrine markers. Gynecol Oncol 34:164-169, 1989.

419 Ueda G, Yamasaki M, Inoue M, Tanaka Y, Inoue Y, Abe Y, Tanizawa O: Immunohistochemical demonstration of HNK-1-defined antigen in gynecologic tumors with argyrophilia. Int J Gynecol Pathol 5:143-150, 1986.

420 Ulich TR, Liao S-Y, Layfield L, Romansky S, Cheng L, Lewin KJ: Endocrine and tumor differentiation markers in poorly differentiated small cell carcinoids of the cervix and vagina. Arch Pathol Lab Med 110:1054-1057, 1986.

421 van Nagell JR Jr, Donaldson ES, Wood EG, Maruyama Y, Utley J: Small cell cancer of the uterine cervix. Cancer 40:2243-2249, 1977.

422 Walker AN, Mills SE, Taylor PT: Cervical neuroendocrine carcinoma. A clinical and light microscopic study of 14 cases. Int J Gynecol Pathol 7:64-74, 1988.

423 Yamasaki M, Tateishi R, Hongo J, Ozaki Y, Inoue M, Ueda G: Argyrophil small cell carcinomas of the uterine cervix. Int J Gynecol Pathol 3:146-152, 1984.

Cytology

424 Bartoo GT, Lee JS, Bartels PH, Kiviat NB, Nelson AC: Automated prescreening of conventionally prepared cervical smears: a feasibility study. Lab Invest 66:116-122, 1992.

425 Boyes DA: The British Columbia screening program. Obstet Gynecol Surv 24:1005-1011, 1969.

426 Bryans FE, Boyes DA, Fidler HK: The influence of a cytological screening program upon the incidence of invasive squamous cell carcinoma of the cervix in British Columbia. Am J Obstet Gynecol 88:898-906, 1964.

427 Christopherson WM, Mendez WM, Ahuja EM, Lundin FE, Barker JE: Cervix cancer control in Louisville, Kentucky. Cancer 26:29-38, 1970.

428 Christopherson WM, Scott MA: Trends in mortality from uterine cancer in relation to mass screening. Acta Cytol (Baltimore) 21:5-9, 1977.

429 Coleman SA, Rube IF, Kashgarian M, Erickson CC: An appraisal of the irrigation cytology method for uterine cancer detection. Acta Cytol (Baltimore) 14:502-506, 1970.

430 Cramer DW: The role of cervical cytology in the declining morbidity and mortality of cervical cancer. Cancer 34:2018-2027, 1974.

431 Davey DD, Gallion H, Jennings CD: DNA cytometry in postirradiation cervical-vaginal smears. Hum Pathol 23:1027-1031, 1992.

432 Dickinson L, Mussey ME, Kurland LT: Evaluation of the effectiveness of cytologic screening for cervical cancer. II. Survival parameters before and after inception of screening. Mayo Clin Proc 47:545-549, 1972.

433 Dickinson L, Mussey ME, Soule EH, Kurland LT: Evaluation of the effectiveness of cytologic screening for cervical cancer. I. Incidence and mortality trends in relation to screening. Mayo Clin Proc 47:534-544, 1972.

434 Erickson CC, Everett BE Jr, Graves LM, Kaiser RF, Malmgren RA, Rube I, Schreier PC, Cutler SJ, Sprunt DH. Population screening for uterine cancer by vaginal cytology. JAMA 162:167-173, 1956.

435 Fidler HK, Boyes DA, Worth AJ: Cervical cancer detection in British Columbia. J Obstet Gynaecol Br Commonw 75:392-404, 1968.

436 Herbst AL: The Bethesda System for cervical/vaginal cytologic diagnoses. A note of caution (editorial). Obstet Gynecol 76:449-450, 1990.

437 Hoffman MS, Sterghos S Jr, Gordy LW, Gunasekaran S, Cavanagh D:Evaluation of the cervical canal with the endocervical brush. Obstet Gynecol 82:573-577, 1993.

438 James LP, Knapp D: New cervical cytology preparation device shows improved sensitivity to abnormal findings over the conventional Papanicolaou smear. Acta Cytol 36:579, 1992.

439 Klinken L, Koch F, Albrechtsen R: Comparison of pipette and smear methods in population screenings for carcinoma of the uterine cervix. Dan Med Bull 19:138-140, 1972.

440 Kohn G: The postradiation vaginal smear. Its usefulness as a routine procedure. Acta Obstet Gynecol Scand 33:264-282, 1953.

441 Konikov NF, Kempson RL, Piskie V: Cytohistologic correlation of dysplasia, carcinoma-in-situ, and invasive carcinoma of the uterine cervix. Am J Clin Pathol 51:463-469, 1969.

442 Koss LG: Diagnostic cytology and its histopathologic bases, ed. 3. Philadelphia, 1979, JB Lippincott Co.

443 Koss LG: The Papanicolaou test for cervical cancer detection. A triumph and a tragedy. JAMA 261:737-743, 1989.

444 Koss LG: Cervical (Pap) smear. New directions. Cancer 71:1406-1412, 1993.

445 Kurman RJ, Malkasian GD Jr, Sedlis A, Solomon D: From Papanicolaou to Bethesda. The rationale for a new cervical cytologic classification. Obstet Gynecol 77:779-782, 1991.

446 Luff RD: The Bethesda System for reporting cervical/vaginal cytologic diagnoses. Report of the 1991 Bethesda workshop. The Bethesda System Editorial Committee. Hum Pathol 23:719-721, 1992.

447 Patten SF: Diagnostic cytology of the uterine cervix. Baltimore, 1969, Williams & Williams.

448 Petersen O: Spontaneous course of cervical precancerous conditions. Am J Obstet Gynecol 72:1063-1071, 1956.

449 Ramzy I, Mody DR: Gynecologic cytology. Practical considerations and limitations. Clin Lab Med 11:271-192, 1991.

450 Robertson JH, Woodend B: Negative cytology preceding cervical cancer: causes and prevention. J Clin Pathol 46:700-702, 1993.

451 Ruch RM, Blake C, Abou A, Lado M, Ruch WA Jr: The changing incidence of cervical carcinoma. Am J Obstet Gynecol 89:727-731, 1964.

452 Seybolt JF: Thoughts on the "numbers game." Acta Cytol (Baltimore) 12:271-273, 1968.

453 Seybolt JF, Johnson WD: Cervical cytodiagnostic problems. A survey. Am J Obstet Gynecol 109:1089-1103, 1971.

454 Sherman ME, Kelly D: High-grade squamous intraepithelial lesions and invasive carcinoma following the report of three negative Papanicolaou smears. Screening failures or rapid progression? Mod Pathol 5:337-342, 1992.

455 Sherman ME, Schiffman MH, Erozan YS, Wacholder S, Kurman RJ: The Bethesda System. A proposal for reporting abnormal cervical smears based on the reproducibility of cytopathologic diagnoses. Arch Pathol Lab Med 116:1155-1158, 1992.

456 Solomon D: The Bethesda Sytem for reporting cervical/vaginal cytologic diagnosis. An overview. Int J Gynecol Pathol 10:323-325, 1991.

457 The Bethesda System for Reporting Cervical/Vaginal Cytologic Diagnoses. Acta Cytol 37:115-124, 1993.

458 Wied GL, Legorreta G, Mohr D, Rauzy A: Cytology of invasive cervical carcinoma and carcinoma in situ. Ann NY Acad Sci 97:759-766, 1962.

459 Wilbur DH, Cibas ES, Merritt S, et al: ThinPrep™ Processor. Clinical trials demonstrate an increased detection rate of abnormal cervical cytologic specimens. Am J Clin Pathol 10:209-214, 1994.

OTHER TUMORS AND TUMORLIKE CONDITIONS

460 Abeler V, Kjorstad KE, Langholm R, Marton PF: Granulocytic sarcoma (chloroma) of the uterine cervix. Report of two cases. Int J Gynecol Pathol 2:88-92, 1983.

461 Abeler V, Nesland JM: Alveolar soft-part sarcoma in the uterine cervix. Arch Pathol Lab Med 113:1179-1183, 1989.

462 Abell MR: Papillary adenofibroma of the uterine cervix. Am J Obstet Gynecol 110:991-993, 1971.

463 Abell MR, Ramirez JA: Sarcomas and carcinosarcomas of the uterine cervix. Cancer **31**:1176-1192, 1973.

464 Abenoza P, Shek Y, Perrone T: Inflammatory pseudotumor of the cervix. Int J Gynecol Pathol **13**:80-86, 1994.

465 Aozasa K, Saeki K, Ohsawa M, Horiuchi K, Mishima K, Tsujimoto M: Malignant lymphoma of the uterus. Report of seven cases with immunohistochemical study. Cancer **72**:1959-1964, 1993.

466 Barua R: Post-cone biopsy traumatic neuroma of the uterine cervix. Arch Pathol Lab Med **113**:945-947, 1989.

467 Bell DA, Shimm DS, Gang DL: Wilms' tumor of the endocervix. Arch Pathol Lab Med **109**:371-373, 1985.

468 Benitez E, Rodriguez HA, Rodriguez-Cuevas H, Chavez GB: Adenoid cystic sarcoma of the uterine cervix. Report of a case and review of 4 cases. Obstet Gynecol **33**:757-762, 1969.

469 Bloch T, Roth LM, Stehman FB, Hull MT, Schwenk GR Jr: Osteosarcoma of the uterine cervix associated with hyperplastic and atypical mesonephric rests. Cancer **62**:1594-1600, 1988.

470 Brand E, Berek JS, Nieberg RK, Hacker NF: Rhabdomyosarcoma of the uterine cervix. Sarcoma botryoides. Cancer **60**:1552-1560, 1987.

471 Chorlton I, Karnei RF Jr, Norris HJ: Primary malignant reticuloendothelial disease involving the vagina, cervix, and corpus uteri. Obstet Gynecol **44**:735-748, 1974.

472 Clement PB: Miscellaneous primary tumors and metastatic tumors of the uterine cervix. Semin Diagn Pathol **7**:228-248, 1990.

473 Copeland LJ, Gershenson DM, Saul PB, Sneige N, Stringer CA, Edwards CL: Sarcoma botryoides of the female genital tract. Obstet Gynecol **66**:262-266, 1985.

474 Copeland LJ, Sneige N, Ordonez NG, Hancock KC, Gershenson DM, Saul PB, Kavanagh JJ: Endodermal sinus tumor of the vagina and cervix. Cancer **55**:2558-2565, 1985.

475 Daya DA, Scully RE: Sarcoma botryoides of the uterine cervix in young women: a clinicopathological study of 13 cases. Gynecol Oncol **29**:290-304, 1988.

476 Delgado G, Smith JP, Declos G, Gallagher S: Reticulum cell sarcoma of the cervix. Am J Obstet Gynecol **126**:691-694, 1976.

477 Deppisch LM: Cervical melanosis. Obstet Gynecol **62**:525-526, 1983.

478 Ferry JA, Young RH: Malignant lymphoma, pseudolymphoma, and hematopoietic disorders of the female genital tract. Pathol Annu **26**(Pt 1):227-263, 1991.

479 Foschini MP, Eusebi V, Tison V: Alveolar soft part sarcoma of the cervix uteri. A case report. Pathol Res Pract **184**:354-358, 1989.

480 Fraga M, Prieto O, Garcia-Caballero T, Beiras A, Forteza J: Myxoid leiomyosarcoma of the uterine cervix. Histopathology **25**:381-383, 1994.

481 Gersell DJ, Fulling KH: Localized neurofibromatosis of the female genitourinary tract. Am J Surg Pathol **13**:873-878, 1989.

482 Hanai J, Tsuji M: Uterine teratoma with lymphoid hyperplasia. Acta Pathol Jpn **31**:153-159, 1981.

483 Harris NL, Scully RE: Malignant lymphoma and granulocytic sarcoma of the uterus and vagina. A clinicopathologic analysis of 27 cases. Cancer **53**:2530-2545, 1984.

484 Hirschfield L, Kahn LB, Chen S, Winkler B, Rosenberg S: Müllerian adenosarcoma with ovarian sex cord-like differentiation. Cancer **57**:1197-1200, 1986.

485 Hytiroglou P, Domingo J: Development of melanosis of uterine cervix after cryotherapy for epithelial dysplasia. A case report and brief review of the literature on pigmented lesions of the cervix. Am J Clin Pathol **93**:802-805, 1990.

486 Imachi M, Tsukamoto N, Amagase H, Shigematsu T, Amada S, Nakano H: Metastatic adenocarcinoma to the uterine cervix from gastric cancer. A clinicopathologic analysis of 16 cases. Cancer **71**:3472-3477, 1993.

486a Jones MW, Lefkowitz M: Adenosarcoma of the uterine cervix. A clinicopathological study of 12 cases. Int J Gynecol Pathol **14**:223-229, 1995.

486b Khoor A, Fleming MV, Purcell CA, Seidman JD, Ashton AH, Weaver DL: Mature teratoma of the uterine cervix with pulmonary differentiation. Arch Pathol Lab Med **119**:848-850, 1995.

487 Kristiansen SB, Anderson R, Cohen DM: Primary malignant melanoma of the cervix and review of the literature. Gynecol Oncol **47**:398-403, 1992.

488 Lee JD, Chang TC, Lai YM, Hsueh S, Soong YK: Choriocarcinoma of the cervix. Acta Obstet Gynecol Scand **71**:479-481, 1992.

489 Lemoine NR, Hall PA: Epithelial tumors metastatic to the uterine cervix. A study of 33 cases and review of the literature. Cancer **57**:2002-2005, 1986.

490 Loughlin KR, Retik AB, Weinstein HJ, Colodny AH, Shamberger RC, Delorey M, Tarbell N, Cassady JR, Hendren WH: Genitourinary rhabdomyosarcoma in children. Cancer **63**:1600-1606, 1989.

491 Luevano-Flores E, Sotelo J, Tena-Suck M: Glial polyp (glioma) of the uterine cervix. Report of a case with demonstration of glial fibrillary acidic protein. Gynecol Oncol **21**:385-390, 1985.

492 Murray J, Fox H: Rosai-Dorfman disease of the uterine cervix. Int J Gynecol Pathol **10**:209-213, 1991.

492a Nielsen GP, Oliva E, Young RH, Rosenberg AE, Dickersin GR, Scully RE: Alveolar soft-part sarcoma of the female genital tract. A report of nine cases and review of the literature. Int J Gynecol Pathol **14**:283-292, 1995.

493 Patel DS, Bhagavan BS: Blue nevus of the uterine cervix. Hum Pathol **16**:79-86, 1985.

494 Perren T, Farrant M, McCarthy K, Harper P, Wiltshaw E: Lymphomas of the cervix and upper vagina: a report of five cases and a review of the literature. Gynecol Oncol **44**:87-95, 1992.

495 Retikas DG: Hodgkin's sarcoma of the cervix. Report of a case. Am J Obstet Gynecol **80**:1104-1107, 1960.

496 Sahin AA, Silva EG, Ordonez NG: Alveolar soft part sarcoma of the uterine cervix. Mod Pathol **2**:676-680, 1989.

497 Seo IS, Hull MT, Pak HY: Granulocytic sarcoma of the cervix as a primary manifestation. Case without overt leukemic features for 26 months. Cancer **40**:3030-3037, 1977.

498 Sobel N, Carcangiu ML: Primary pigmented neuroectodermal tumor of the uterine cervix. Int J Surg Pathol **2**:31-36, 1994.

499 Steeper TA, Piscioli F, Rosai J: Squamous cell carcinoma with sarcoma-like stroma of the female genital tract. Cancer **52**:890-898, 1983.

500 Terzakis JA, Opher E, Melamed J, Santagada E, Sloan D: Pigmented melanocytic schwannoma of the uterine cervix. Ultrastruct Pathol **14**:357-366, 1990.

501 Uehara T, Izumo T, Kishi K, Takayama S, Kasuga T: Stromal melanocytic foci ("blue nevus") in step sections of the uterine cervix. Acta Pathol Jpn **41**:751-756, 1991.

502 Vellios F: Papillary adenofibroma-adenosarcoma. The uterine cystosarcoma phyllodes. In Fenoglio CM, Wolff M, eds: Progress in surgical pathology, vol. 1. New York, 1980, Masson Publishing USA, Inc., pp. 205-219.

503 Volpe R, Canzonieri V, Gloghini A, Carbone A: "Lipoleiomyoma with metaplastic cartilage" (benign mesenchymoma) of the uterine cervix. Pathol Res Pract **188**:799-801, 1992.

504 Walker AN, Mills SE: Unusual variants of uterine cervical carcinoma. Pathol Annu **22**(Pt 1):277-310, 1987.

505 Young RH, Harris NL, Scully RE: Lymphoma-like lesions of the lower female genital tract. A report of 16 cases. Int J Gynecol Pathol **4**:289-299, 1985.

506 Zaloudek CJ, Norris HJ: Adenofibroma and adenosarcoma of the uterus. Cancer **48**:354-366, 1981.

Uterus—corpus

NORMAL ANATOMY

The adult nulliparous uterus is a hollow, pear-shaped organ that weighs 40 to 80 g and measures 7 to 8 cm along its longest axis. It is divided into the *cervix* (discussed in the preceding section of this chapter) and the *corpus*. The portion of the corpus cephalad to a line connecting the insertion of the fallopian tubes is the *fundus*. The two lateral regions of the fundus associated with the intramural portion of the fallopian tubes are referred to as the *cornua*. The portion of the corpus that connects with the cervix is called the *isthmus* or *lower uterine segment*.

The uterine cavity has a triangular shape and a length of approximately 6 cm. It is lined by the endometrial mucosa, which constitutes the inner layer (myometrium) of the organ. It is surrounded by a thick muscular layer and a serosal covering, the latter extending to the point of peritoneal reflection (which is lower in the posterior than the anterior aspect).

The uterine lymph vessels drain to a rich network of lymph nodes, the main groups being parametrial and paracervical; internal (hypogastric), external and common iliac; periaortic; and inguinal.

The endometrial mucosa is made up of glands and stroma. It is divided into a deeply seated *basal* layer and a superficial *functional* layer. The basal layer is the equivalent of the reserve cell layer of other epithelia and is responsible for the regeneration of the endometrium following menstruation. It is made up of weakly proliferative glands and spindled stroma. The functional layer has been subdivided into two strata, the *compactum* (toward the surface) and the *spongiosum* (close to the basalis). The stroma is mainly composed of endometrial stromal cells (whose appearance changes considerably during the menstrual cycle, see later section) and vessels (of which the spiral arterioles are the most distinctive). Other components include the stromal granulocyte (thought to be either a subpopulation of T lymphocytes or of macrophages) and inconstant stromal foamy cells (lipid-containing cells of disputed histogenesis).

During child-bearing age, the normal endometrium undergoes a series of sequential changes in the course of the ovulatory cycle that prepare it to receive the ovum. If the ovum is not fertilized, the proliferative endometrium is cast off by menstruation, and the cycle repeats itself. A normal endometrial cycle is associated with changes in both endometrial glands and stroma that allow the pathologist to diagnose microscopically the phase of the menstrual cycle.[11] In a classic article, Noyes et al.[14] set forth specific criteria by which an accurate dating of the endometrium was made possible (Figs. 19-69 and 19-70 and box).

MICROSCOPIC FEATURES FOR DATING ENDOMETRIUM

Proliferative phase

Early (fourth-seventh day)—thin regenerating surface epithelium; straight, short, narrow glands; compact stroma, with some mitotic activity and large nuclei

Mid (eighth-tenth day)—columnar surface epithelium; longer, curving glands; variable amount of stromal edema; numerous mitoses in naked nuclei of stroma

Late (eleventh-fourteenth day)—undulant surface; tortuous glands showing active growth and pseudostratification; moderately dense, actively growing stroma

Secretory phase

36-48 hours after ovulation—no microscopic changes apparent

Sixteenth day—subnuclear vacuolation of epithelium appears

Seventeenth day—orderly row of nuclei with homogeneous cytoplasm above them and large vacuoles below

Eighteenth day—vacuoles decrease in size; nuclei approach base of cell

Nineteenth day—few vacuoles; appearance of intraluminal secretion

Twentieth day—peak of acidophilic intraluminal secretion

Twenty-first day—tissue edema appears rather abruptly

Twenty-second day—edema reaches its peak

Twenty-third day—spiral arterioles become prominent

Twenty-fourth day—collections of predecidual cells appear around arterioles

Twenty-fifth day—predecidua appears under surface epithelium

Twenty-sixth day—predecidua appears as solid sheet of well-developed cells; polynuclear cell infiltration appears

Twenty-seventh day—polynuclear infiltration becomes prominent; areas of focal necrosis and hemorrhage begin to appear

Twenty-eighth day—necrosis and hemorrhage prominent

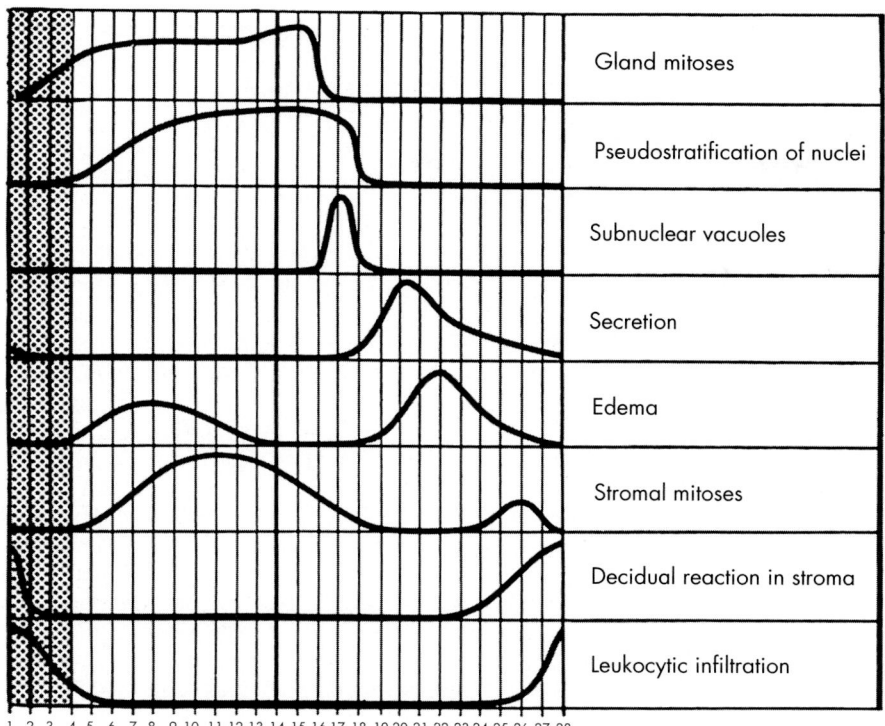

The chart shows the following rows (labeled on the right):

- Gland mitoses
- Pseudostratification of nuclei
- Subnuclear vacuoles
- Secretion
- Edema
- Stromal mitoses
- Decidual reaction in stroma
- Leukocytic infiltration

1 2 3 4 5 6 7 8 9 10 11 12 13 14 15 16 17 18 19 20 21 22 23 24 25 26 27 28

Fig. 19-69 Cyclic changes in endometrium. Approximate relationship of useful microscopic changes. (After Latour; from Noyes RW, Hertig AT, Rock J: Dating the endometrial biopsy. Fertil Steril **1**:3-25, 1950.)

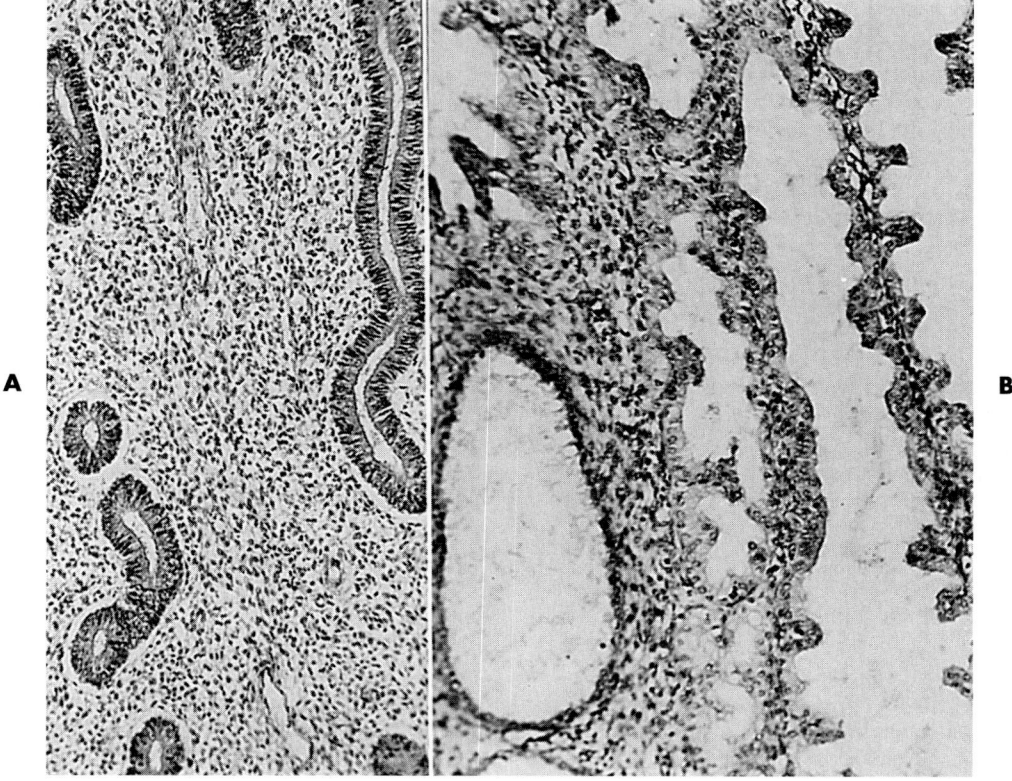

A   B

Fig. 19-70 Sequential endometrial changes during normal menstrual cycle. **A,** Late proliferative endometrium. Note straight elongated glands and lack of vascularity. **B,** Late secretory endometrium. Note sawtooth epithelium and intraluminal secretion, edematous stroma, and congested blood vessels.

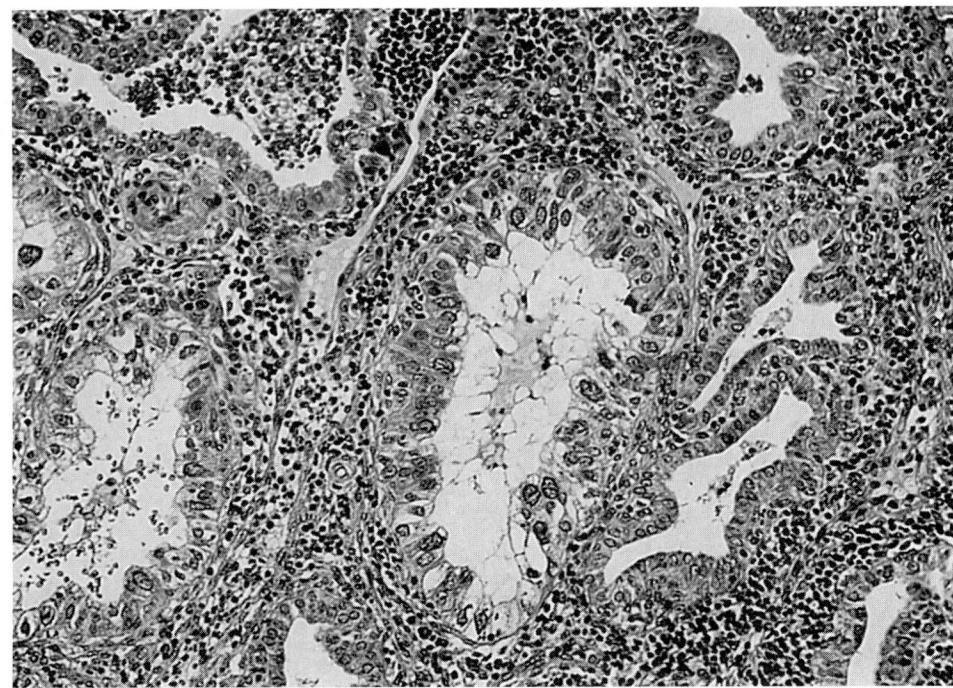

Fig. 19-71 Gestational hyperplasia and Arias-Stella reaction of endometrium occurring in early pregnancy. Nuclear atypia is characteristic of this normal anatomic variation. (From Kraus FT: Gynecologic pathology. St. Louis, 1967, Mosby.)

In general, the changes are quite uniform throughout the functional endometrium.[12] When this is not the case, the dating should be based on the most advanced area rather than on the average morphologic picture.[13] The surface epithelium is less responsive to the hormonal influences than the glandular epithelium. Radioautographic studies have shown that cell proliferation is highest on the eighth to tenth day in the upper third of the functional layer and that it decreases to nearly zero levels by the nineteenth day.[8] For subnuclear vacuolation to be regarded as evidence of ovulation, it should be present in at least 50% of the functional glands present in the section. A markedly compact stroma may simulate predecidua. One of the earlier signs of the menstrual phase (and also of pathologic crumbling of the stroma) is the presence of nuclear dust at the base of the glandular epithelium.[7] Neutrophils, which are seen in large numbers in areas of tissue degradation (beginning on day 26) are very rare during the other days of the cycle; they should be distinguished from the already mentioned stromal granulocytes, which do not stain for chloroacetate esterase.[15]

The nuclear crowding, squamoid appearance, and focal cytoplasmic acidophilia seen in late menstrual and postcurettage specimens should not be confused with a malignant process. The possibility of overdiagnosis is even greater in the rare instances in which the menstrual endometrium is seen within the lumen of blood vessels.[4] It should be noted that endometrial tissue can also be found in myometrial vessels independently from menstruation.[16]

The basal layer of the endometrium is not subject to the influence of progesterone. Therefore if biopsies are taken in the premenstrual phase for evidence of secretory activity (ovulation) and contain only the basal layer, a proper evaluation cannot be made. Similarly, the mucosa of the lower uterine segment responds only sluggishly to the hormonal stimulations and should be disregarded for dating purposes.[8] This mucosa gradually merges with that of the endocervix; the hybrid endometrial-endocervical appearance of both glands and stroma allows its recognition in D&C specimens.

Biopsies to determine anovulatory cycles are most informative when performed about 2 days before the expected onset of menstruation.

The reappearance of glandular secretion and stromal edema once predecidual reaction is established—leading to the simultaneous presence of these three features in an endometrial specimen—is evidence that a fertilized ovum has implanted; this pattern is referred to as *gestational hyperplasia.*[9] An exaggerated expression of this phenomenon is the *Arias-Stella reaction,* in which secretory or proliferative changes in the endometrial glands are accompanied by prominent nuclear changes, manifested by hyperchromasia and marked enlargement (Figs. 19-71 and 19-222). Normal and abnormal mitoses may also be present.[2a] These changes are almost always focal and may also occur in the cervix, endocervical polyps, adenomyosis, and endometriosis.[1,2] They are more often seen in postabortion curettings (present in 20% to 70% of the cases and persisting for weeks), but they are also seen in normal orthotopic or ectopic pregnancies, hydatidiform mole, choriocarcinoma, and (very rarely) following the administration of exogenous hormones.[3,6,9a] In hydatidiform mole and choriocarcinoma, the nuclei of the endometrial cells may attain gigantic sizes. The most important differential diagnosis is with so-called in situ and clear cell types of endometrial adenocarcinoma.

Another interesting pregnancy-related endometrial alteration (often associated with the Arias-Stella reaction) is the focal appearance of optically clear nuclei in the glandular cells, simulating viral inclusions; these are due to the replacement of normal chromatin by a fine filamentous network that is immunoreactive for biotin.[10,16a,17]

Exceptionally, decidual reaction is seen in the postmenopausal endometrium in the absence of an exogenous or endogenous source of progesterone excess.[5]

CURETTAGE AND BIOPSY

Tissue from the endometrial cavity taken for diagnostic purposes has been traditionally obtained by *dilatation* of the cervical canal and *curettage* of the endometrial cavity (D&C). As a sampling technique, it is unsurpassed. If it is properly performed, very few endometrial lesions (perhaps only those located deep in a cornu) should escape detection. It has been regarded for a long time as the method of choice for the detection and typing of lesions presumed to be localized, such as polyps and carcinoma.[23] Information about endocervical extension of an endometrial neoplasm can be obtained by performing a *fractional curettage* (i.e., a separate sampling from the endometrial and endocervical cavities during the same procedure). The endocervical specimen should be obtained first so as to minimize contamination from the endometrium. However, even when this precaution is taken, small isolated tumor fragments may be found in endocervical specimens in cases without actual infiltration of the cervix. Therefore it is our policy to report the presence of endocervical extension of a tumor *only* if cancer and normal endocervical glands are seen *in the same fragment.* Otherwise, we simply record the presence of carcinoma in the material submitted from the endocervix and let the clinician decide whether this is significant on the basis of the findings at the time of curettage.

Regeneration of the endometrium proceeds very rapidly after curettage. Complete restoration occurs in 2 or 3 days in most instances.[24] Exceptionally, intrauterine adhesions develop, resulting in amenorrhea and other menstrual abnormalities. This condition, known as *Asherman's syndrome,* is seen most often after postpartum or postabortal curettages and is thought to be the result of a subclinical uterine infection.[19,20]

Endometrial biopsy is a safe alternative to D&C for the evaluation of infertile or dysmenorrheic patients.[18,21] At present, this procedure (as carried out with various suction devices) has become the choice method for the initial approach to patients with suspected endometrial hyperplasia or carcinoma.[19a] Kahler et al.,[22] in their study of 160 patients, demonstrated that when the endometrial biopsy was performed successfully (137 patients), the tissue obtained was truly representative of the endometrium in all but six, as proved by subsequent D&C or hysterectomy. Furthermore, no endometrial carcinoma was missed when sufficient tissue was obtained.

EFFECTS OF HORMONE ADMINISTRATION
Estrogen therapy

Exogenous administration of estrogen preparations exposes the endometrium to a potent stimulus.[47] Endometrial hyperplasia is present in 15% to 30% of post-menopausal women receiving estrogen therapy alone, with some of the cases having an atypical pattern.[46] Furthermore, several case-control population studies have linked the exogenous administration of estrogens to the subsequent appearance of endometrial adenocarcinoma.[25,32] The risk is said to be four to eight times greater in this population.[43,48] The addition of progestin to the medication protects the endometrium and reduces the incidence of hyperplasia and carcinoma.[44]

Fortunately, the large majority of these tumors are well differentiated and superficial and are associated with an excellent prognosis compared with those occurring in postmenopausal women unexposed to exogenous estrogens.[42]

Progestational agents

Owing to the widespread use of progestational agents for therapeutic and contraceptive purposes, a new endometrial morphology has emerged.[29,36] The pathologist should be thoroughly familiar with the variety of changes that the "pill" may induce in the endometrium in order not to confuse them with pathologic conditions. The effect of these agents is exerted on the glands and stroma and differs more according to the regimen used than to the actual drug employed.[35,38] In the *combined program,* pills of the same mixture, representing a combination of progestogen and estrogen, are taken on consecutive days. They can be administered *continuously* for therapeutic purposes or *cyclically* (for 20 to 21 days with 7-day to 8-day intervals) for contraception or therapy.[29] In the *sequential program,* no longer used, predominantly estrogenic pills were taken for 14 to 16 days followed by progestin-dominant pills for 5 or 6 days. The changes to be described are those to be expected in a previously normal endometrium.

In the **continuous combined program,** the glands are small, straight, and inactive, with no mitoses or secretion. The stroma is very prominent and edematous, is infiltrated by some neutrophils, and shows striking pseudodecidual changes[26] (Fig. 19-72). The latter, which may appear as fragments of frankly necrotic decidua, are distinguished from the decidua of pregnancy by the completely atrophic glandular pattern. The stromal reaction may be so florid as to simulate a sarcoma.[30] Foci of endometriosis respond in a similar manner. This must be kept in mind whenever lesions of any pelvic organ are being evaluated microscopically, especially by frozen section (Fig.19-73).

In the **cyclic combined program,** the glands show little or no evidence of proliferation. There is a short, poorly developed stage of secretory activity, reaching a peak about the fourteenth or fifteenth day, followed by regression of the glands.[37] Pseudodecidual changes appear in the stroma about the twentieth day of the cycle (fifteenth day of treatment). Development of spiral arterioles is inhibited. After prolonged therapy, glandular secretion and stromal pseudodecidual changes become inconspicuous or recede altogether. The stroma acquires an atrophic, fibroblast-like appearance and may form characteristic small polypoid projections covered by atrophic surface epithelium[27] (Fig. 19-74). On very rare occasions, focal glandular changes of the Arias-Stella type may appear in patients taking contraceptive pills. In most cases, discontinuation of the hormones

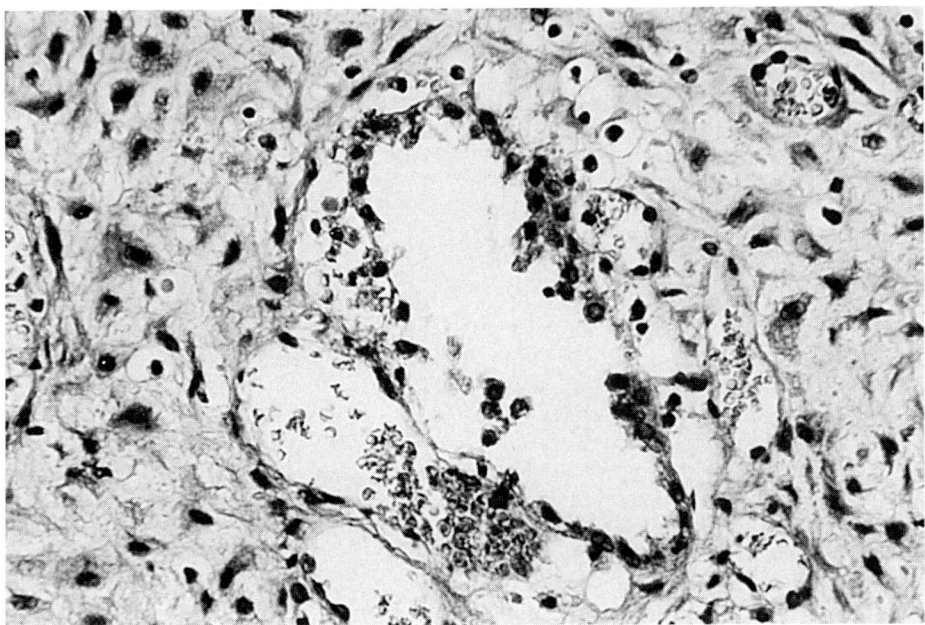

Fig. 19-72 Marked deciduoid reactin of endometrium following combined contraceptive program. Glandular epithelium is inactive and stromal vessels are markedly dilated.

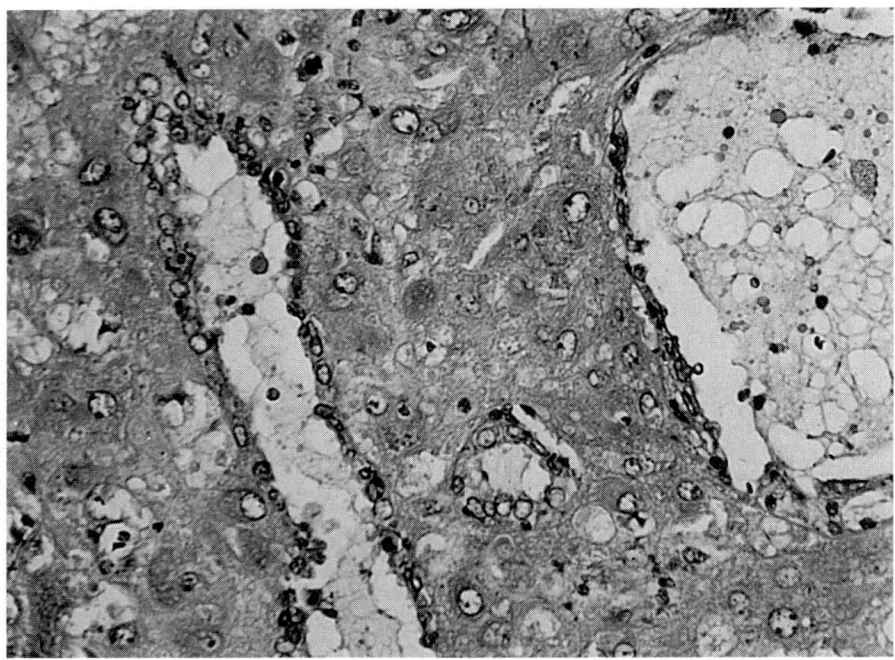

Fig. 19-73 Biopsy of endometriosis of rectosigmoid area in patient who had been receiving Enovid. Note marked deciduoid proliferation.

results in a restoration of a normal endometrial pattern in a matter of weeks.[31]

The *sequential program* more nearly parallels the normal cycle and results in a somewhat similar endometrial morphology.[34] The glands show signs of proliferation, followed by tortuosity and the appearance of well-developed secretory changes. The stroma shows inconspicuous pseudodecidual changes. Thus the endometrial morphology on the twenty-sixth day of a cycle induced by sequential therapy (the day after treatment is completed) is roughly analogous to that of the eighteenth or nineteenth day of a normal menstrual cycle. Regressive changes and crumbling of

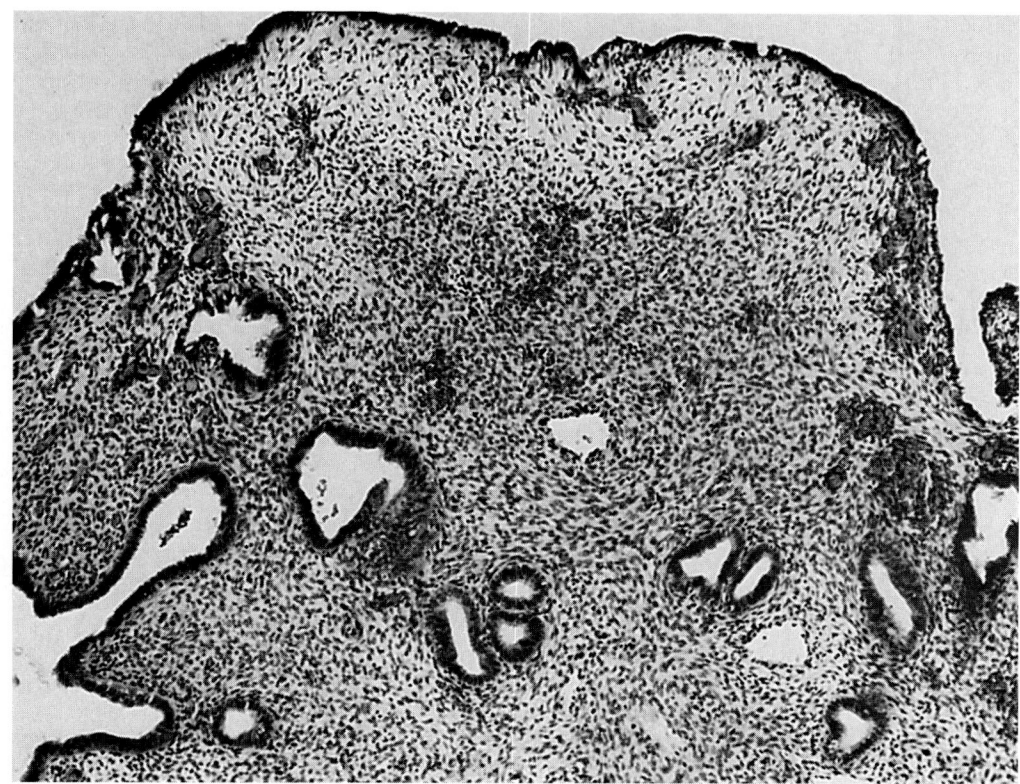

Fig. 19-74 Typical polypoid appearance of endometrium in patient taking oral contraceptives.

stroma, resulting in withdrawal bleeding, occur soon there-after.

The sequential program was discontinued in the United States and Canada in 1976 because of several reports suggesting that it promoted the development of endometrial adenocarcinoma.[28,40,41] This complication is probably not the direct result of the hormones being administered sequentially but rather a result of the difference in net estrogenic effect with the combined preparations. Most of these tumors have been well differentiated and are very superficial, and the prognosis generally has been good.

There are other complications resulting from the prolonged use of contraceptive pills, regardless of the program used. Early studies in England and in the United States have shown an increased incidence of thrombophlebitis and pulmonary embolism.[39,45] Morphologically, the vascular changes are widely distributed and involve arteries and veins. They include thrombi and intimal thickening with endothelial proliferation.[33] With present regimens, the incidence of these complications has decreased substantially.

ENDOMETRITIS

Acute endometritis is seen usually in association with abortion, the postpartum state, or instrumentation. Gonococcal endometritis is rarely seen by the pathologist because of its very transient nature. It should be remembered that neutrophils are normally present in the endometrium in days 26, 27, and 28.[77]

Chronic endometritis, characterized by an infiltrate of lymphocytes and plasma cells, may follow pregnancy or abortion, be the result of an IUD, or be accompanied by mucopurulent cervicitis and/or pelvic inflammatory disease (PID).[60,76,79] If the diagnosis is suspected clinically, cultures should be taken. The most common symptoms are vaginal bleeding and pelvic pain.[79] It should be emphasized that lymphoid follicles, with or without germinal centers, are a normal occurrence in the functional layers of the endometrial mucosa and therefore should not be considered as evidence of chronic endometritis. Actually, some authors believe that they are more common in normal than in abnormal endometria.[82] Therefore identification of plasma cells constitutes the most important criterion for the diagnosis of chronic endometritis, whether by conventional criteria or—as suggested by some—by immunostaining the sections for immunoglobulins[57] (Figs. 19-75 and 19-76).

The possibility of inflammation should be suspected—and plasma cells searched for—whenever there is an absence of a normal cyclic pattern, a focal mononuclear infiltrate, inflammatory cells in the glandular lumina, dense stroma, a stellate stromal pattern of proliferation, or foci of necrosis or calcification. Glandular alterations commonly accompany the inflammatory reaction, to the point that endometrial dating becomes impossible. The presence of neutrophils in the endometrial surface is a good predictor of PID, especially if combined with plasma cells in the endometrial stroma.[70]

Intrauterine devices inserted for the purpose of contraception result in many biologic changes.[56,68,84] In one series, only 29% of symptomatic patients and 40% of asymptomatic patients with a polyethylene IUD had a normal

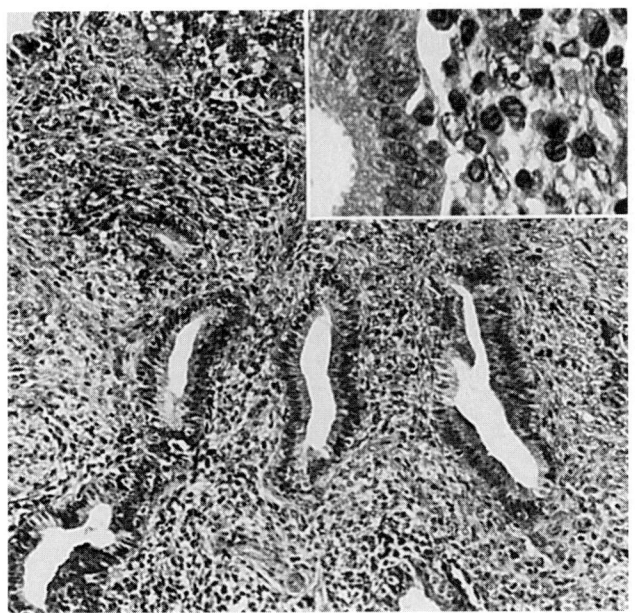

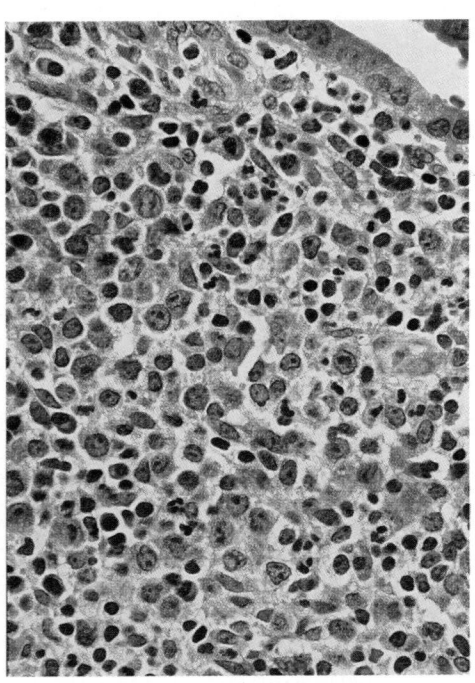

Fig. 19-75 Chronic endometritis. Endometrial glands are abnormally shaped and irregularly distributed. Inflammatory and fibroblastic reaction is seen in stroma. **Inset** shows several plasma cells in endometrial stroma.

Fig. 19-76 Chronic endometritis with a large number of plasma cells and immunoblasts.

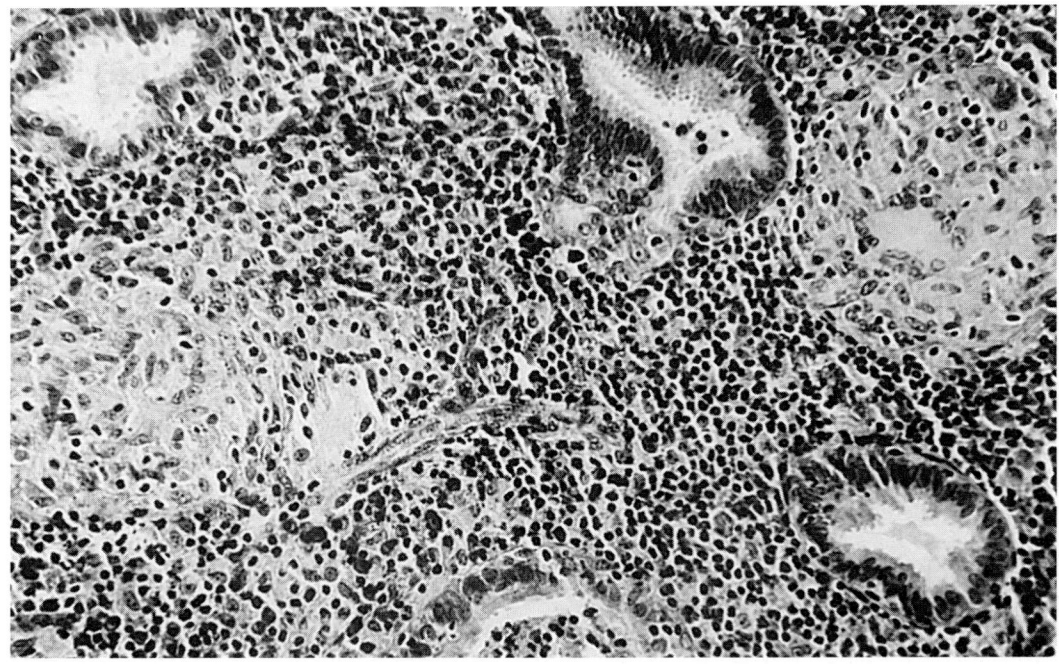

Fig. 19-77 Endometrial tuberculosis with characteristic tubercles, associated chronic inflammation, and irregularly shaped glands.

endometrial appearance on biopsy.[74] The most common change is focal or extensive chronic endometritis, which may be accompanied by necrosis and squamous metaplasia.[78,81] On occasion, the inflammation spreads through the fallopian tubes to produce PID and sometimes tubo-ovarian abscesses.[85,87] One of the agents involved in the inflammatory process is *Actinomyces;* in one series, the infection rate in IUD users was 12.6%.[51,54,69,73] The organisms can be detected in microscopic sections or in cytology preparations,[63] but care should be exercised in distinguishing them from pseudoactinomycotic radiate granules; the latter lack central branching filaments and diphtheroid forms.[52]

Pyometra refers to the accumulation of pus within the endometrial cavity. It is the consequence of the combined effect of obstruction and infection. Whiteley and Hamlett[88] reviewed thirty-five cases in postmenopausal patients. Only five were secondary to carcinoma; the remaining thirty were the result of benign cervical stricture originating from senile atresia, surgery, or cauterization.

Hematometra is the accumulation of blood within the endometrial cavity, usually as a result of cervical occlusion. This may lead to the disappearance of the endometrial mucosa and its replacement by sheets of lipid-containing histiocytic cells, a process known as *histiocytic* or *xanthogranulomatous endometritis*[53]*;* this is not to be confused with the more common histiocytic reaction seen in the stroma of endometrial adenocarcinomas, whether spontaneously or following irradiation.[80]

Sometimes the histiocytes are found to contain a yellowish-brown cytoplasmic pigment, in which case the term *ceroid-containing histiocytic granuloma* has been used.[83]

Endometrial tuberculosis is rare in the United States but still common in other parts of the world.[67] Menstrual disturbances are common. The microscopic diagnosis is based on the demonstration of acid-fast bacilli in tubercles or culture. The presence of plasma cells and leukocytes probably results from secondary infection.[62] Tubercles may be missed unless multiple levels of curettings are examined (Fig. 19-77). Since the granulomas tend to concentrate in the superficial functional layers of the endometrium, it is recommended that the biopsy be taken during the late secretory phase.

Chlamydial infection is now recognized as a major sexually transmitted disease; cases associated with endometritis have been identified through the immunohistochemical demonstration of chlamydial antigens in endometrial epithelial cells.[75,89] These cases are associated with severe acute and/or chronic inflammation.

Viral infection of the endometrium is probably more common than generally suspected. Cytomegalovirus endometritis and diffuse papillomatosis (condyloma) have both been documented[58,86]; the former can have a granulomatous quality.[61]

Coccidioidomycosis of the uterus has been reported in the United States in a few cases as a localized infection; it probably results from a clinically inapparent and completely resolved primary lung infection.[55,64]

Malakoplakia of the endometrium has been reported, one of the cases being recurrent and another associated with endometrial adenocarcinoma.[72]

Sarcoidosis of the uterus occurs, but it remains a diagnosis of exclusion.[65] In contrast to tuberculosis, the granulomatous reaction usually spreads to the myometrium.[59] Granulomatous endometritis can also follow hysteroscopic resection of the endometrium.[49]

Giant cell arteritis may involve the uterus and other female genital organs of elderly women, either as an isolated finding or as part of generalized giant cell arteritis.[50] Exceptionally, *periarteritis nodosa* will be first diagnosed because of its involvement of the female genital tract.[71]

The myometrium is usually spared in most types of endometritis (sarcoidosis excluded) unless the inflammation is very severe.

Follicular myometritis has been described as a component of inflammatory pelvic disease.[66]

METAPLASIA

The endometrial glands and stroma are subject to a variety of metaplastic changes, many of them hormonally induced. They are often accompanied by hyperplastic changes in the endometrial glands but can occur independently from them and therefore need to be evaluated separately. They should not be regarded by themselves as evidence for the existence of a malignant tumor. At the same time, it should be realized that endometrial metaplasias, like endometrial hyperplasias, tend to be associated with endometrial adenocarcinoma and that they are more common in populations at high risk for the development of endometrial carcinoma (such as those in the United States) than in low-risk populations (such as those in Japan).[102] These metaplasias include:

1 *Squamous metaplasia.* This can be encountered in normal or hyperplastic endometrium, sometimes in association with leiomyoma or uterine polyps.[94,98] Frank keratinization is very rare (ichthyosis uteri). A more common finding is the presence of nonkeratinizing squamoid cells occurring either diffusely (adenoacanthosis)[95] or in the form of berry-like aggregates (morules)[97] (Fig.19-78). Most are seen in premenopausal women, in those receiving exogenous hormones, or in association with polycystic ovarian disease.[93,102a] This change is distinguished from well-differentiated endometrial adenocarcinoma with squamous metaplasia ("adenoacanthoma") because of the benign appearance of the glandular elements.[100]

2 *Ciliated cell (tubal) metaplasia.* Scattered ciliated cells are normally present in the endometrial mucosa; when markedly increased in number, the appearance thus resembles that of a fallopian tube, and the term listed above is used.[106] Ciliated cell metaplasia may be seen in an otherwise normal organ but occurs more commonly in the setting of endometrial hyperplasia.

3 *Papillary metaplasia* (syncytial papillary hyperplasia, papillary syncytial change). This alteration is characterized by the presence of syncytial to papillary aggregates of eosinophilic cells along the surface epithelium. It is often seen in association with prolonged estrogen stimulation.[103] It has been variously regarded as a metaplastic change, a hyperplastic change, and a retro-

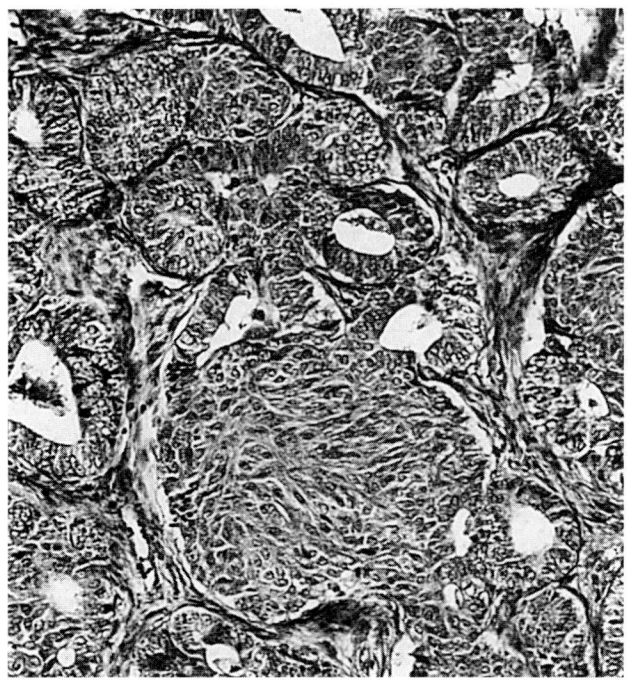

Fig. 19-78 Squamous metaplasia of endometrium (morules).

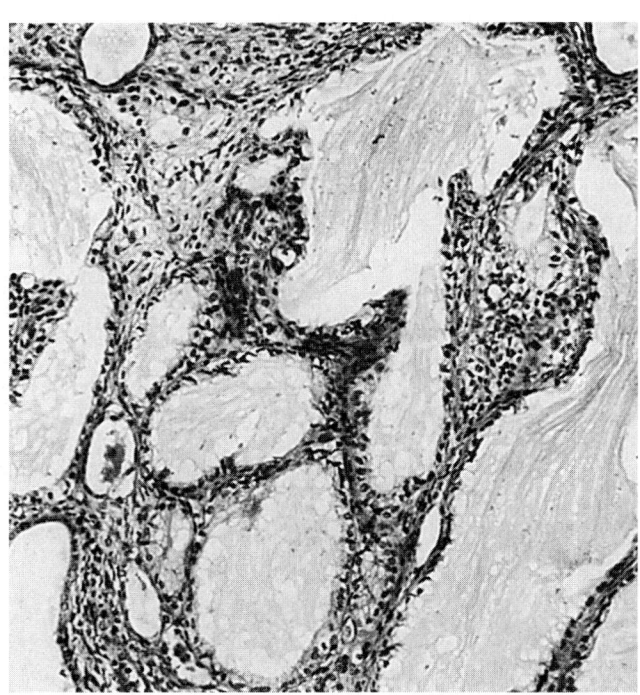

Fig. 19-79 Mucinous metaplasia of endometrium.

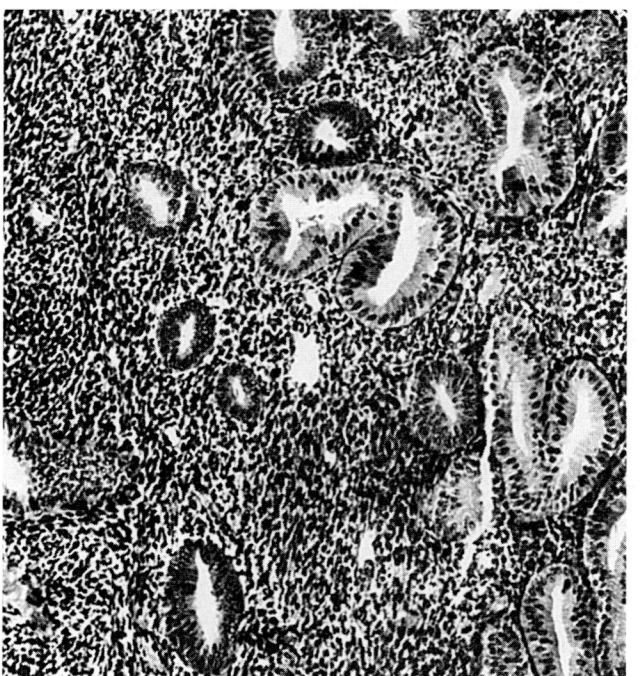

Fig. 19-80 Eosinophilic metaplasia of endometrium.

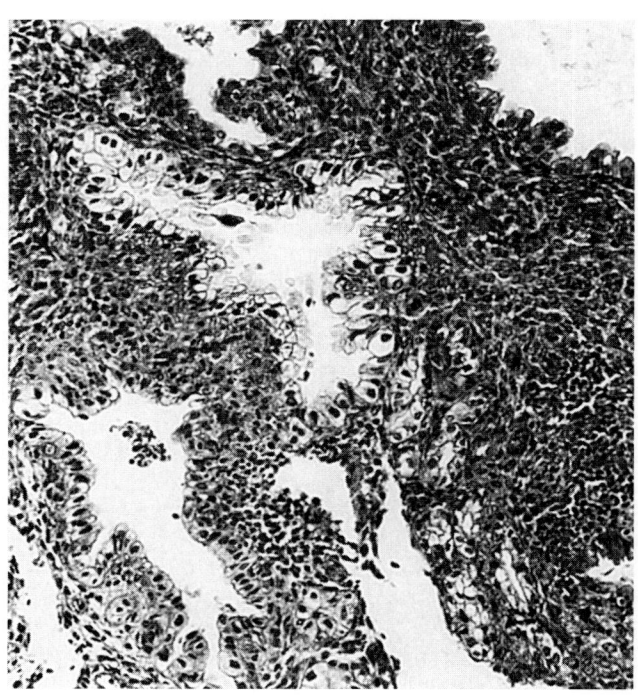

Fig. 19-81 Clear cell metaplasia of endometrium.

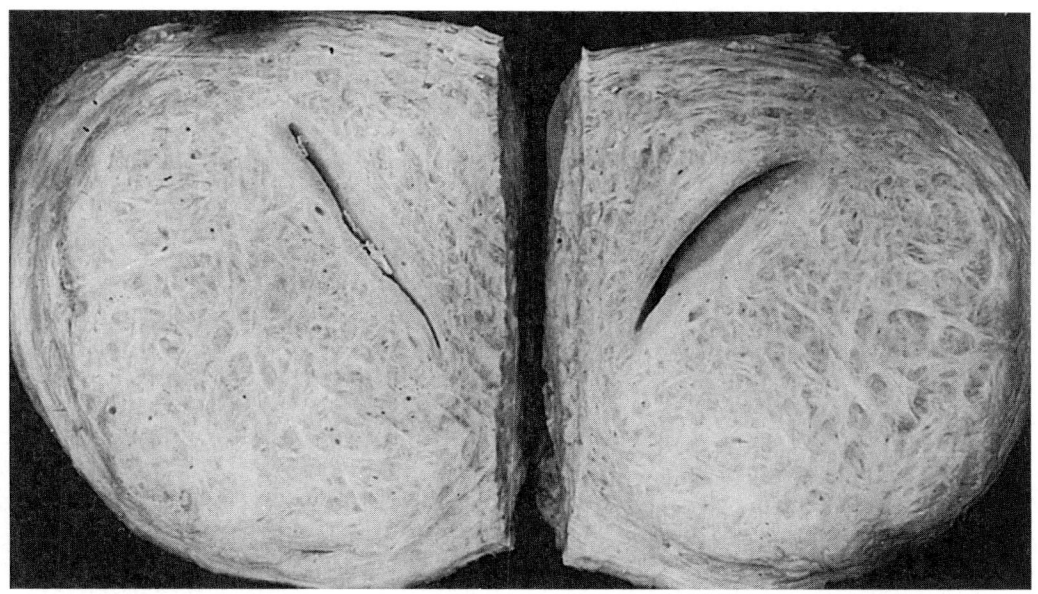

Fig. 19-82 Typical gross appearance of uterine adenomyosis. Ill-defined whorled proliferation of myometrial muscle results in thickening of wall. Circumscription of leiomyoma is lacking. (Courtesy Dr. E.F. Lascano, Buenos Aires.)

gressive alteration associated with acute endometrial breakdown.[99,109]

4 *Mucinous metaplasia.* In this condition, the endometrial mucosa reverts to a pattern morphologically, histochemically, and ultrastructurally similar to that of the endocervical mucosa[96,105] (Fig. 19-79).

5 *Eosinophilic (oxyphilic) metaplasia.* This is another estrogen-induced lesion, characterized by strong acidophilia of the cytoplasm[90] (Fig. 19-80). It is distinguished from atypical endometrial hyperplasia by the absence of atypical nuclear features.[100,101]

6 *Hobnail and clear cell (mesonephric or mesonephroid) metaplasia.* In these closely related metaplastic changes, the epithelium is clear, with tall cells having apically located nuclei (Fig. 19-81). The differential diagnosis is with clear cell (mesonephroid) adenocarcinoma).[101]

7 *Intestinal metaplasia.* In this exceptionally rare form, the endometrium resembles intestinal mucosa.[108]

8 *Stromal metaplasia.* These include the formation within the endometrial stroma of islands of smooth muscle,[92] cartilage,[104] and bone.[91] It should be noted that in some instances the presence of cartilage or bone is the result of retained fetal parts.[107]

ADENOMYOSIS AND ENDOMETRIOSIS

Adenomyosis refers to the presence of islands of endometrial glands and stroma within the myometrium, whereas *endometriosis* is the term employed for the occurrence of endometrial tissue outside the uterus. These two disorders are usually regarded as closely related, but their microscopic appearance—and probably their pathogenesis—is somewhat different. Furthermore, they often occur independently of each other. In most cases, adenomyosis is made up of the nonfunctional (basal) layer of the endometrium, is sometimes connected with the mucosa, and has been viewed by some as representing a complex endometrial diverticulosis. Endometriosis, on the other hand, is composed of the functional layers of the endometrium, and as such, it goes through proliferative, secretory, and menstrual changes similar to those of its orthotopic counterpart. However, studies using conventional morphologic techniques and cell proliferation markers have shown that the endometriotic lesions are consistently more proliferative than the normally located endometrium, both during the menstrual cycle and in postmenopause.[112,122]

Many pathogenetic theories have been proposed over the years for endometriosis: origin from congenital müllerian or wolffian rests, implantation of endometrium (spontaneous or induced by hysterosalpingography), lymphatic or hematogenous spread, and serosal metaplasia.[120,130] Different pathogenetic mechanisms may be operative depending on the nature and location of the lesion but a metaplastic change of the secondary müllerian system represented by the pelvic mesothelium is probably the most common and important mechanism.[125a]

Both endometriosis and adenomyosis may result in pelvic pain, characteristically associated with the menstrual period. Between 30% and 40% of women with endometriosis are infertile, but the exact mechanism remains obscure. Exceptionally, adenomyosis may lead to rupture at the time of pregnancy.

Adenomyosis results grossly in an enlarged and globular uterus because of the myometrial hypertrophy that regularly accompanies it.[116,123] The diagnosis may be suspected on cut section in the presence of depressed small cystic lesions in obvious but ill-defined bulging zones of muscle hypertrophy (Fig. 19-82). In elderly women, the uterus may appear atrophic despite extensive adenomyosis. Leiomyomas in uteri with adenomyosis may themselves be involved by the process.

Microscopically, the diagnosis of adenomyosis depends on the criteria used by the pathologist, some of which are

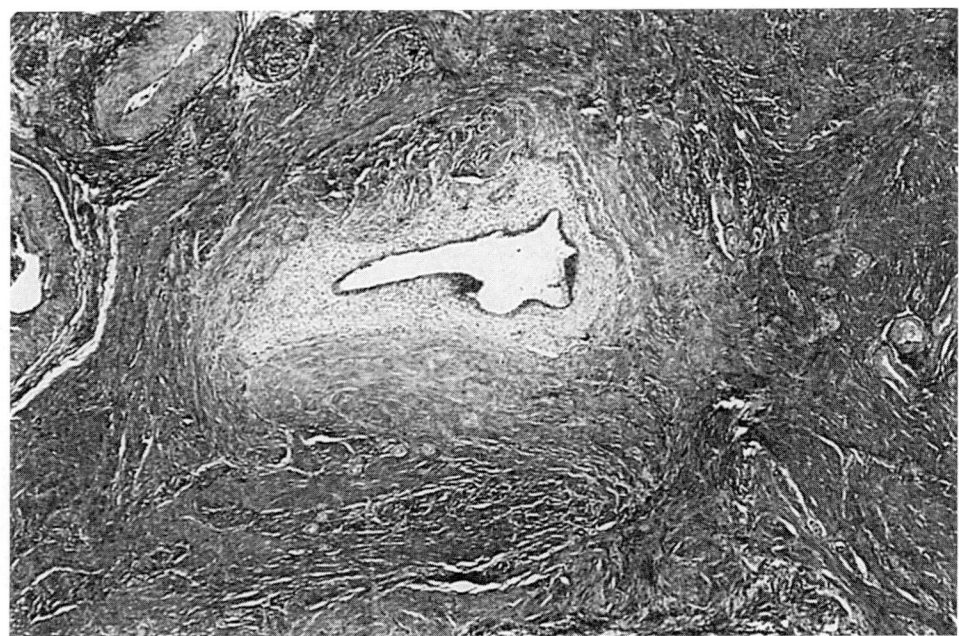

Fig. 19-83 Uterine adenomyosis. Islands of endometrial glands surrounded by endometrial stroma are seen deeply embedded in myometrium.

very liberal indeed. The interphase between endometrium and myometrium is normally an irregular one, without interposition of a submucosal layer; invaginations of the endometrial basal layer into the superficial portions of the myometrium should be regarded as a normal finding. By convention, the diagnosis of adenomyosis should be reserved for those cases in which endometrial glands and stroma are seen in the myometrium at a distance of at least one low-power field from the endometrial-myometrial junction (Fig. 19-83).

Microscopically, the endometrium of adenomyosis usually has a proliferative appearance, consistent with its basal layer derivation. When the normally located endometrium is in the secretory phase, this is true only in one quarter of the foci of adenomyosis.[124] These foci can be involved by any of the diseases affecting the orthotopic endometrium, including hyperplasia and adenocarcinoma.[132] It is important to recognize this phenomenon, lest a case of in situ or superficial endometrial adenocarcinoma associated with similar changes in the foci of adenomyosis be misinterpreted as a deeply invasive malignancy.[118] Some small islands of adenomyosis are made up predominantly of endometrial stroma (*stromal adenomyosis* or *adenomyosis with sparse glands*); however, any sizable intramyometrial focus composed entirely of endometrial stroma is likely to represent an endometrial stromal sarcoma.[117a]

Endometriosis is thought to occur in 1% to 7% of women in the United States.[111,126] It can be located in the cervix, vagina, vulva, rectovaginal septum, ovary, fallopian tube, uterine ligaments, appendix, small and large bowel, bladder and ureters, pelvic peritoneum, hernia sacs, lymph nodes, kidney, and skin and even within skeletal muscles, peripheral nerves, pleura, lung, and nasal cavity.[120] Spontaneous cutaneous endometriosis is limited to the umbilicus and

inguinal area.[129] In other locations, such as the lower abdominal wall, it practically always arises in surgical scars (particularly those from cesarean sections).[131]

Grossly, endometriosis appears as bluish cystic nodules, often surrounded by fibrosis (Plate XIII-C). Exceptionally, it may present as multiple polypoid masses grossly simulating a neoplastic process *(polypoid endometriosis or endometriotic polyposis).*[125]

Microscopically, endometrial glands and stroma are seen, often embedded in a dense fibrous mass exhibiting signs of fresh and old hemorrhage.[115] Rarely, endometriotic foci undergo prominent mucinous metaplasia, a change that can result in a mistaken diagnosis of well-differentiated mucinous adenocarcinomas. Such change has been interpreted as a metaplasia toward endocervical-type epithelium and designated as *endocervicosis.*[115] In other instances, it may exhibit prominent myxoid change and simulate pseudomyxoma peritonei.[115a]

Although well-documented cases of endometriosis of lymph nodes exist, most cases so designated are made up of glands lined by ciliated or nonciliated cuboidal epithelium unaccompanied by stroma, limited to the capsule or cortical area of the node[117]; as such, they are more reminiscent of fallopian tube than endometrial epithelium and are better designated as endosalpingiosis. They have been found in about 14% of nodes in females but practically never in males.[121]

Endometriosis may be associated with perineurial invasion.[128] It may also undergo malignant transformation.[119] The most common form is endometrioid adenocarcinoma,[113,125] but clear cell carcinoma, endometrial stromal sarcoma, and mixed müllerian tumor have also been reported.[110,114] The described benign glandular inclusions in pelvic nodes can give rise to borderline and malignant serous tumors.[127]

The treatment of endometriosis may be hormonal or surgical depending on the circumstances.[122a]

DYSFUNCTIONAL UTERINE BLEEDING AND HYPERPLASIA

Normal menstruation is defined as the bleeding from secretory endometrium—associated with an ovulatory cycle—not exceeding a length of 5 days. Any bleeding not fulfilling these criteria is referred to as an ***abnormal uterine bleeding.*** Some of these are the result of an identifiable lesion, such as endometriosis, submucous myoma, endometrial polyp, or cancer, particularly in the postmenopausal patient. In most series, approximately 5% to 15% of the cases of postmenopausal bleeding are due to endometrial carcinoma and a similar proportion to endometrial polyps.[163,171] The only finding on D&C in over half of postmenopausal bleeders is an atrophic endometrium[141]; vascular degenerative changes in the uterine blood vessels have been suggested as a possible etiology in these cases.[166]

Bleeding not associated with an organic cause in women of child-bearing age belongs to the large and somewhat nebulous category known as ***dysfunctional uterine bleeding.*** Examination of specimens obtained on D&C or endometrial biopsy is a continuous source of frustration for the pathologist. Sometimes, provided with minimal clinical information or material taken at an inappropriate moment of the menstrual cycle, one is unable to recognize any abnormality. At the most, changes can be detected that only confirm what the gynecologist already knows—i.e., that the patient has an abnormal bleeding. These include the presence of fibrin clumps in the endometrial stroma (a finding not usually present in the normal menstrual endometrium)[172] or the appearance of fragmented pieces with dense stromal cellularity (a process known as *stromal crumbling*).

On the other hand, if a thorough clinical study is available, examination of a correctly timed biopsy can be quite informative.[142-144] Cases of dysfunctional uterine bleeding can be divided in two large categories: those associated with ovulation and the more numerous ones in which ovulation has not occurred. A hybrid group in which ovulatory and anovulatory cycles alternate is frequently seen in premenopausal patients.

In the ovulatory group, bleeding may occur because of an *inadequate proliferative phase.* This is recognized by a disparity between the endometrial pattern observed and that expected from the time of the cycle (i.e., an endometrium chronologically in the fourteenth day with a morphologic appearance suggestive of the fourth to seventh day) or by the fact that the morphologic signs of proliferation (such as pseudostratification of nuclei or mitotic activity) are inconspicuous.

Bleeding resulting from an *inadequate secretory phase* (underdeveloped secretory endometrium, luteal phase inadequacy) is recognized by analogous criteria. Traditionally, it has been recommended that the curetting or biopsy should be obtained on the twelfth postovulatory day or 2 days prior to the expected menstruation. However, recent studies suggest that an earlier biopsy taken on the seventh or eighth postovulatory day may be more informative.[139,167] According to Noyes,[170] biopsies should be taken of at least two

menstrual cycles, and both the basal temperature shift and the onset of succeeding menses should be used as points of reference to time the length of the secretory phase. The "date" obtained from the endometrial biopsy should be more than 2 days retarded before the diagnosis of underdeveloped secretory endometrium is entertained. Hormone administration often corrects this defect.[150,167]

Another type of defect seen in the ovulatory group of bleeders is known as *irregular shedding of the endometrium.* The term refers to a regularly recurring menorrhagia in which the bleeding phase of the cycle requires 7 days or more for completion, without subsequent prolongation of the cycle.[164] This is due to a lag in the shedding of the secretory endometrium, which is normally completed by the fourth day of menstruation.[165] The tissue should be obtained 5 or more days after the onset of menstrual bleeding, the diagnosis depending on the detection of retained secretory endometrium in addition to fragmented menstrual and/or early proliferative endometrium. It has been estimated that 10% to 17% of cases of functional bleeding belong to this category.[177]

The term *membranous dysmenorrhea* is given to a rare condition characterized by the painful passage of an endometrial cast of the uterus during the first few days of menstruation. This cast has the microscopic appearance of decidua. The disease is thought to result from a hyperprogestational response and may be induced by the administration of high doses of progesterone.[153]

An *anovulatory cycle* can be recognized, at its earliest stage, by finding a proliferative endometrium at a time of the cycle when a secretory pattern would be expected. Most commonly, the prolonged unremitting estrogen stimulation results in ***endometrial hyperplasia.*** All grades of this phenomenon occur, ranging from one distinguished only with difficulty from a normal exuberant proliferative endometrium (so-called *disordered proliferative endometrium*) to an atypical one that approaches the appearance of adenocarcinoma. Accordingly, we grade our cases of endometrial hyperplasia as *mild* (simple), *moderate* (adenomatous), or *severe* (atypical) (Fig. 19-84). We disregard for this purpose the presence or absence of cystic changes, since they are only a secondary feature of the process and can be found in the absence of hyperplasia. There is, however, a rough inverse relationship between the presence and prominence of the cystic changes and the degree of glandular hyperplasia. In most cases of "cystic hyperplasia," the degree of glandular proliferation is mild to moderate. Another approach is to divide the hyperplasias into *simple* and *complex* on the basis of their architecture, and subdivide each of these into *typical* and *atypical* on the basis of their cytology. A comparison of some of the proposed classifications of endometrial hyperplasia is presented in the box.

Endometrial hyperplasia is most commonly seen during the perimenopausal period. However, it can also be encountered in younger patients, even adolescent ones.[161] Some of these develop as the result of estrogenic stimulation in the Stein-Leventhal syndrome and in estrogen-secreting ovarian neoplasms.

The distinction between an extreme case of hyperplasia and a well-differentiated adenocarcinoma is very difficult,

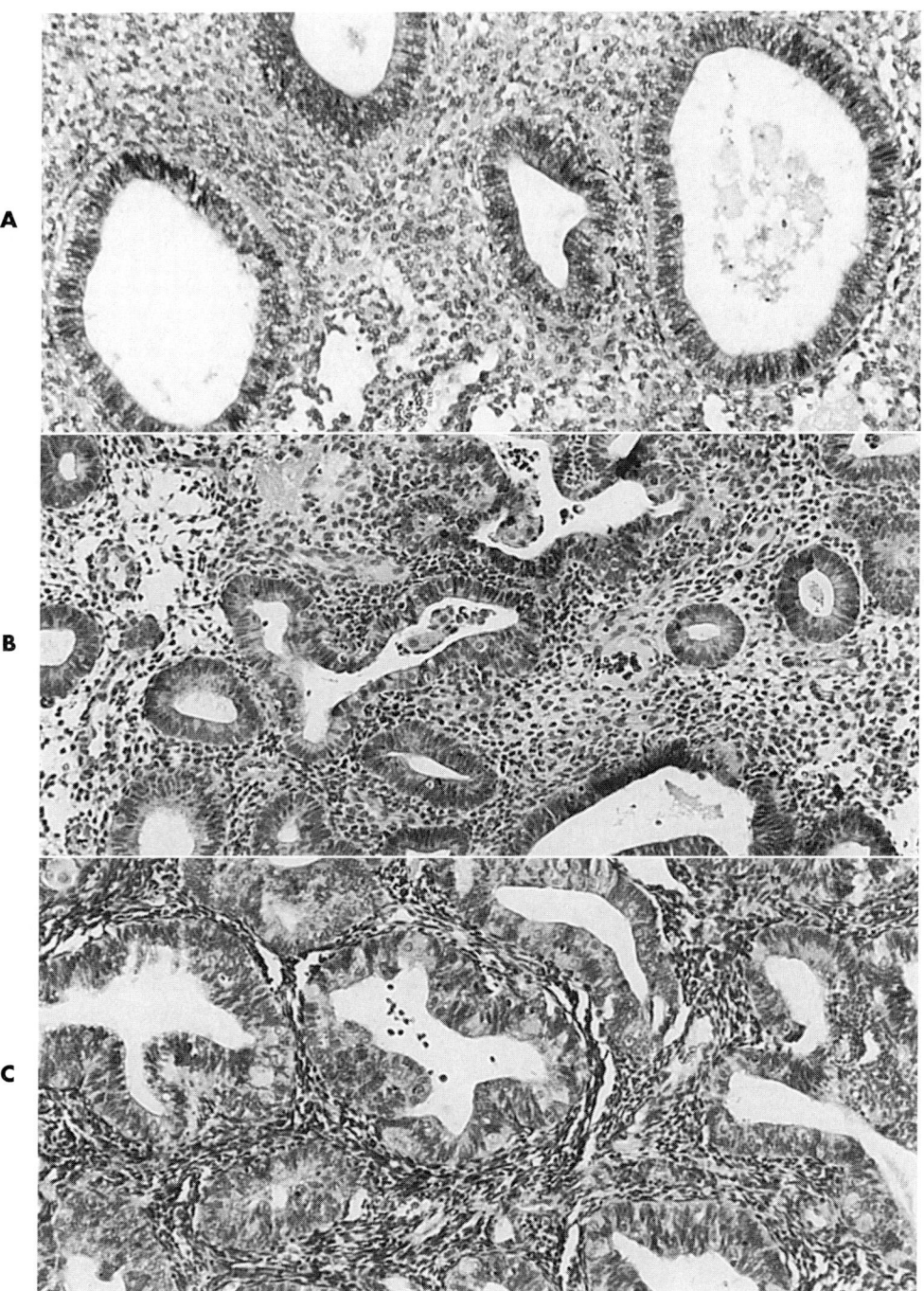

Fig. 19-84 Microscopic appearance of endometrial hyperplasia of mild degree **(A)**, moderate degree **(B)**, and severe degree **(C)**. With increasing severity of disease, cystic changes in glands and amount of stroma diminish, whereas epithelial proliferation becomes more intense.

largely because of the fact that endometrial hyperplasia and carcinoma represent different points in a disease continuum at the morphologic, ultrastructural, biochemical, immunocytochemical, and cytodynamic levels.[146,147,151,155,178] Microscopic features favoring carcinoma include marked pleomorphism with loss of polarity, complex ramification of disorderly arranged glands, extensive papillary formations, confluent glandular pattern with a solid or cribriform appearance, and desmoplastic stroma (Table 19-4).[156,159,169,176] Fox and Buckley[148] have remarked on the importance of true intraglandular cellular bridges devoid of stromal support and the presence of neutrophils and nuclear debris within glandular lamina. It should be noted that the most superficial portions of the tumor may show microglandular patterns simulating microglandular hyperplasia and other metaplastic patterns.[157a] Whether quantitative morphology (particularly nuclear morphometry), immunohistochemistry (with the MSN-1 antibody), flow cytometry, PCR for nonrandom X chromosome inactivation, or other techniques will assist or replace conventional morphology in this difficult problem remains to be seen.[134-136,145,167a,168,174]

Gore and Hertig[152] have designated an endometrial pattern characterized by endometrial glands composed of large cells with abundant eosinophilic cytoplasm as *carcinoma in situ* (Fig. 19-85). Since the assumption that this change inevitably progresses to invasive adenocarcinoma has never been proved and since this alteration has, on occasion, been reversed by hormone manipulations,[179] this and similar patterns[133,179] are now regarded by most as morphologic variants of hyperplastic/metaplastic processes.[169,181]

In some instances, metaplastic changes of various types (squamous, ciliated, clear cell, and others) are seen superimposed on a picture of endometrial hyperplasia. As already stated (see p. 1405), it is important for them to be evaluated separately and for the hyperplasia to be graded independently from them. An endometrium does not necessarily become hyperplastic because it contains a metaplastic change; similarly, a hyperplastic endometrium does not become necessarily malignant because it is accompanied by focal metaplasia of squamous or some other type. Another lesion that is sometimes confused with hyperplasia is adenomatous polyp, a lesion recognized by its dense fibrotic stroma and thick-walled vessels[184] (see p. 1407).

The relationship between hyperplasia and carcinoma has been a hotly debated subject.* On the basis of the considerable collective experience that has accumulated on the subject, the following statements can be safely made:

1 Most cases of endometrial carcinoma are preceded by a stage of hyperplasia. This is especially true in the younger woman and/or in cases of well-differentiated endometrioid adenocarcinoma, in which this sequence approaches 100%. In the classic series of Hertig and Sommers,[157] *all* patients with endometrial adenocarcinoma who had adequate material from curettage examined 15 years or less before the development of adenocarcinoma had an abnormal endometrial pattern.

2 Overall, relatively few patients with hyperplasia will subsequently develop cancer. Therefore the mere presence of hyperplasia is not a basis for hysterectomy.

3 The more severe the hyperplasia, the more likely it is to be followed by carcinoma. This is particularly true in regard to the *cytologic* changes, even if these assume even greater significance when coupled with *architectural* changes.[158] This correlation has been demonstrated both using conventional morphologic evaluation and with morphometric techniques.[136]

In the case of mild hyperplasia (often accompanied by cystic changes) the risk is very small. Thus in a series of 544 premenopausal women followed for periods ranging up to 24 years, less than 0.4% developed carcinoma.[162] Conversely, the incidence of carcinoma in women with *severe* (adenomatous or atypical) *hyperplasia* has been in the

*References 138, 160, 173, 175, 176, 182.

COMPARISON OF SOME PROPOSED CLASSIFICATIONS OF ENDOMETRIAL HYPERPLASIA

Campbell and Barter (1961)[138]
Benign hyperplasia
Atypical hyperplasia, type I
Atypical hyperplasia, type II
Atypical hyperplasia, type III
Beutler, Dockerty, and Randall (1963)[137a]
Cystic proliferation
Glandular hyperplasia
Glandular hyperplasia with atypical epithelial proliferation
Gusberg and Kaplan (1963)[154]
Mild adenomatous hyperplasia
Moderate adenomatous hyperplasia
Marked adenomatous hyperplasia
Gore and Hertig (1966)[152]
Cystic hyperplasia
Adenomatous hyperplasia
Anaplasia
Carcinoma in situ
Vellios (1972)[182]
Cystic hyperplasia
Adenomatous hyperplasia
Atypical hyperplasia
Tavassoli and Kraus (1978)[181]
Cystic hyperplasia
Adenomatous hyperplasia
Atypical hyperplasia
Hendrickson and Kempson (1980)[155]
Hyperplasia
  Without atypia
  With mild atypia
  With moderate atypia
  With severe atypia
Kurman and Norris (1986)[160]
Hyperplasia
  Simple
  Complex
Atypical hyperplasia
  Simple
  Complex

neighborhood of 15%.[140,154] Tavassoli and Kraus[181] analyzed the pathologic findings in forty-eight hysterectomy specimens resected usually within 1 to 6 months after a diagnosis of atypical endometrial hyperplasia (including so-called adenocarcinoma in situ) had been made in a curettage specimen. Lesions interpreted as well-differentiated adenocarcinomas were found in twelve instances (25%). In only one case was there myometrial extension, and this measured only 2 mm. Persistent hyperplasia was found in most of the other cases. The authors concluded that, although atypical endometrial hyperplasia poses a threat of carcinoma, this can be easily eliminated by either medical (progestogen therapy) or surgical (hysterectomy) means. The great efficacy of hormonal therapy in controlling most cases of endometrial hyperplasia and in avoiding hysterectomy in surgically high-risk postmenopausal patients has been demonstrated repeatedly.[149,180]

The term *atypical secretory hyperplasia* has been applied to a pattern of architectural abnormalities and cellular atypia within a secretory endometrium, with the atypical glands resembling those seen in the sixteenth to the seventeenth day of the normal cycle.[137,183] This change should be distinguished from the Arias-Stella reaction. The natural history of this condition is not well known. Judging from our experience, it would seem that a conservative therapeutic approach is justified.

Table 19-4 Differential microscopic criteria between endometrial hyperplasia and adenocarcinoma

Microscopic criteria	Adenomatous hyperplasia	Atypical hyperplasia	Adenocarcinoma
Nuclei			
Profiles	Smooth and oval	Irregular	Irregular
Size	Uniform	Large, variable	Large, variable
Nucleoli	Small, round	Large, irregular	Large, irregular, spiculated
Mitoses	Numerous in stroma and glands	Numerous	Variable
Cytoplasm	Abundant, amphophilic	Sometimes scant; may be very abundant, with dense eosinophilia	Scant, pale, amphophilic
Glands			
Lining epithelium	Tall columnar, single layered	Stratification, loss of polarity	Loss of polarity
Profiles	Dilated, irregular, with out-pouching and infoldings	Irregular, with intraglandular tufting *but no bridging*	Irregular, with cribriform pattern and intraglandular bridging
Size	Variable	Variable	Variable
Stroma	Usually abundant, cellular	Scant, with crowding	Scant

Adapted from Tavassoli F, Kraus FT: Endometrial lesions in uteri resected for atypical endometrial hyperplasia. Am J Clin Pathol **70**:770-779, 1978.

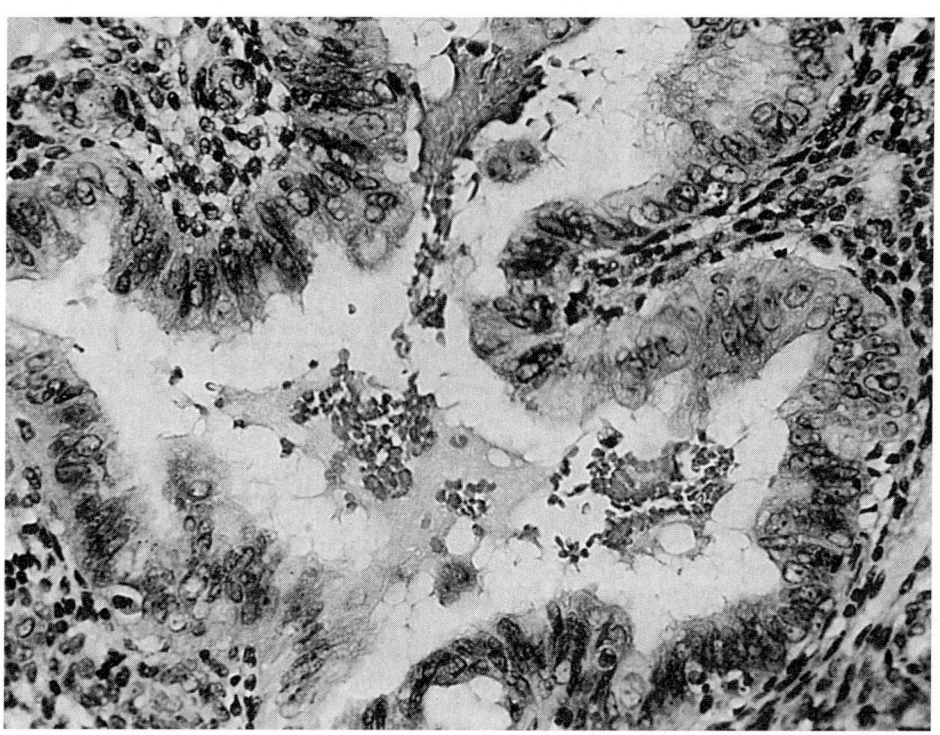

Fig. 19-85 Endometrial hyperplasia of type sometimes designated as carcinoma in situ of endometrium. Cells are large with abundant clear eosinophilic cytoplasm and some disorientation. These changes were focal in nature in the curettage specimen. No invasive carcinoma was found in hysterectomy specimen. Patient was well 13 years later.

TUMORS
Endometrial polyps

The large majority of endometrial polyps are not true neoplasms but probably represent circumscribed foci of hyperplasia (Fig. 19-86). The glands usually show some degree of cystic change. They may be lined by an active pseudostratified epithelium containing mitotic figures or, in the postmenopausal patient, by a flat, inactive epithelium (Fig. 19-87).

The glands and stroma of the polyp are unresponsive to progesterone stimulation and retain their integrity throughout the menstrual cycle. In material obtained from D&C, where usually only fragments of the polyp are obtained, the distinction with endometrial hyperplasia is made by examining the stroma. In the latter condition, the stromal cells are active, with large vesicular nuclei and occasional mitotic figures, whereas the stroma of a polyp is composed of spindle (fibroblast-like) cells, contains abundant extracellular connective tissue, and has large blood vessels with thick walls. Not infrequently, both conditions coexist, pointing to a common pathogenesis. Exceptionally, endometrial polyps are found to contain atypical stromal cells.[185b]

Endometrial polyps have been reported in women taking tamoxifen for breast carcinoma; some of these have exhibited stromal decidualization.[185a]

Rarely, polyps composed of functional endometrium are encountered. The diagnosis is made on the gross features of the lesion rather than on the microscopic pattern of glands and stroma and is therefore difficult or even impossible to make on a D&C specimen.

Endometrial polyps having smooth muscle fibers (not connected with blood vessel walls) in addition to the customary glands and stroma are designated as ***adenomyomatous polyps*** (polypoid adenomyomas).[188] They have a char-

acteristic hard consistency and a grayish color (Fig. 19-88). An important variant on the theme is the ***atypical polypoid adenomyoma***.[187,190] These tend to occur in premenopausal women (average age, 40 years) and present with abnormal uterine bleeding. Some are associated with Turner's syndrome.[185] Microscopically, they are identified by the fact that the glands occurring between the endometrial stroma

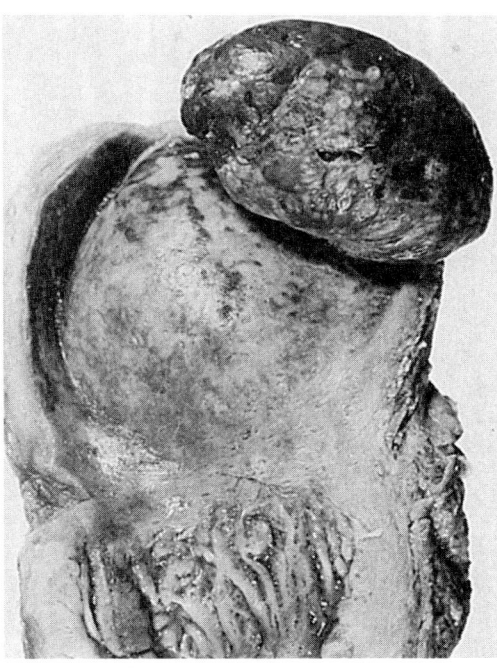

Fig. 19-86 Large benign endometrial polyp distending endometral cavity.

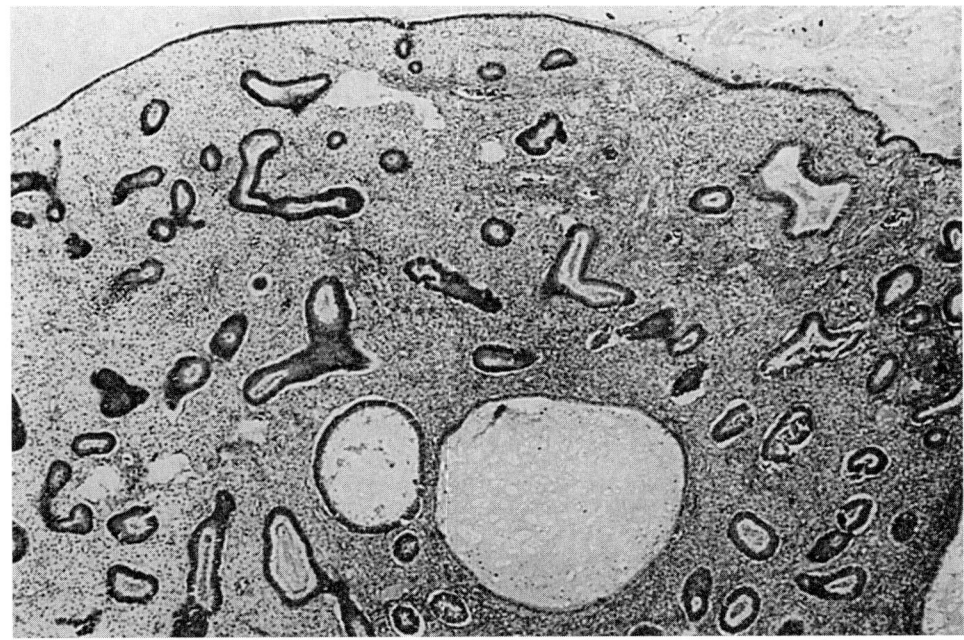

Fig. 19-87 Endometrial polyp of usual type. Glands are cystically dilated and somewhat hyperplasic. Stroma is of fibroblastic type and contains numerous blood vessels. Surface epithelium is attenuated.

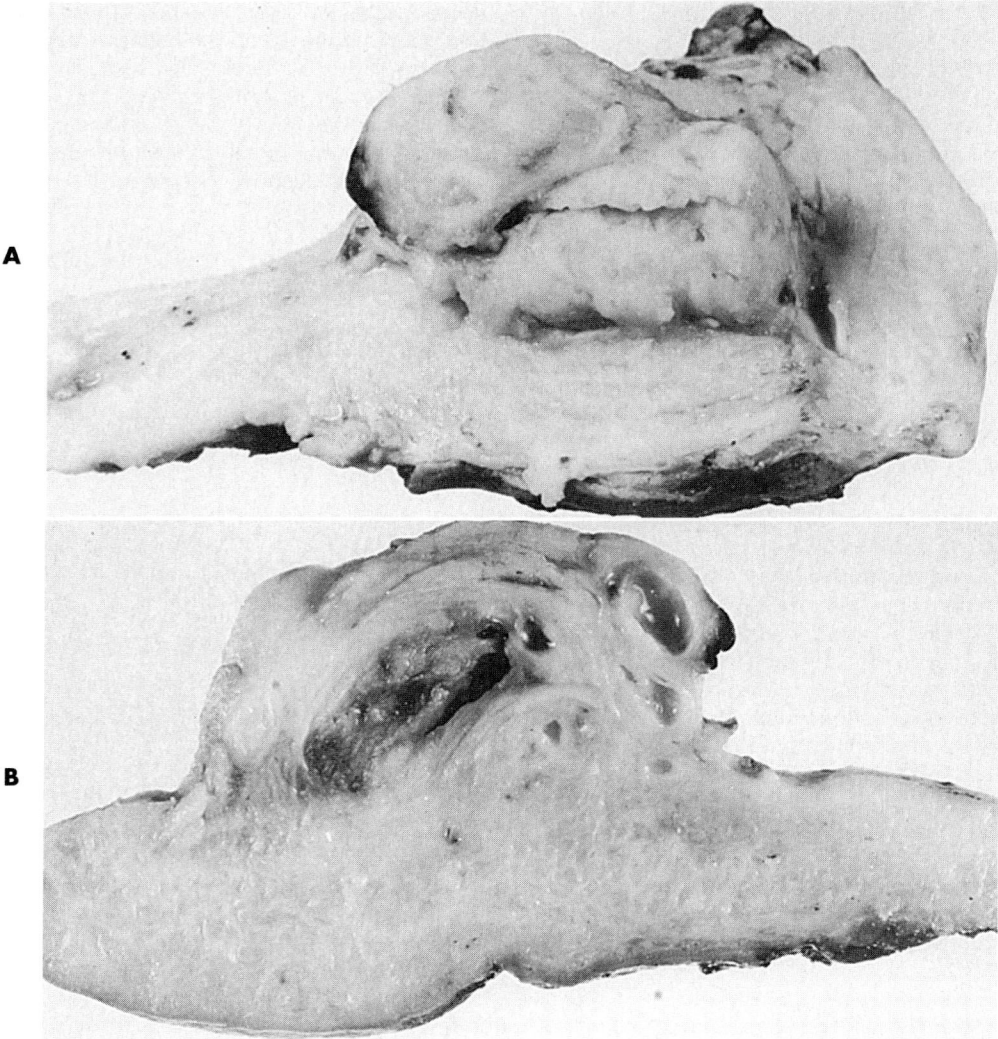

Fig. 19-88 External appearance **(A)** and cross section **(B)** of endometrial polyp of adenomyomatous type.

and smooth muscle exhibit varying degrees of hyperplasia and atypia, sometimes approaching the appearance of carcinoma in situ (Fig. 19-89). The danger is to misdiagnose them as adenocarcinomas with myometrial invasion. The behavior is generally benign, but cases have been seen with local recurrences, carcinomatous transformation,[186a,189] and coexistent endometrial or ovarian endometrioid carcinoma.[186,187a]

Endometrial carcinoma

General and clinical features

Carcinoma of the endometrium is the most common gynecologic malignancy in the United States, and its incidence is rising.[202,207,208] It typically occurs in elderly patients; approximately 80% are postmenopausal at the time of diagnosis. It has been suggested that endometrial carcinoma can be divided in two distinct types on the basis of their pathogenesis: one—by far the more common—occurring as a result of excess estrogenic stimulation and developing against a background of endometrial hyperplasia[197,198] and the other developing de novo.[191,193,206a] Patients at high risk for the first category include the obese, diabetic, hypertensive, infertile; those with failure of ovulation (including the Stein-Leventhal syndrome) and dysfunctional bleeding; long-standing estrogen users; those with severe degrees of endometrial hyperplasia, and—to a much lesser degree—those with functioning granulosa cell tumors and thecomas.[196,203,205]

In the majority of patients with Stein-Leventhal syndrome, the endometrial pathology is that of hyperplasia and, as such, it will regress with medical therapy.[199] However, a few well-documented cases of carcinoma have been reported; these have almost always been of a well-differentiated nature, and myometrial invasion, if present at all, has been minimal. Fechner and Kaufman[194] pointed out

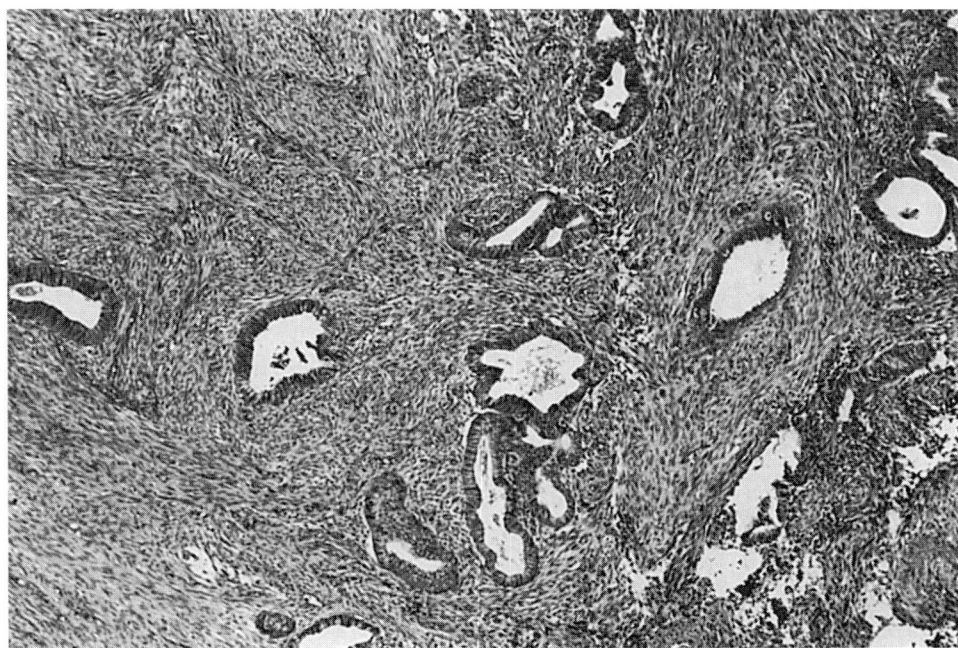

Fig. 19-89 Atypical polypoid adenomyoma. Stroma is composed of very cellular smooth muscle. Glands, which are irregularly distributed, show pseudostratification of nuclei and other atypical cytologic features. This lesion should not be confused with invasive endometrial adenocarcinoma.

that the lesion may be reversible when treated by curettage followed by therapy directed toward reestablishment of ovulation and have urged a conservative approach to these patients. In support of this policy, they emphasized the fact that not a single case of well-differentiated adenocarcinoma in a patient with Stein-Leventhal syndrome has been proved to metastasize, recur locally, or cause death. The situation is quite similar regarding the relationship between endometrial pathology and functioning ovarian tumors (see p. 1512).

Gonadal dysgenesis (Turner's syndrome) can also be associated with endometrial adenocarcinoma, usually of the well-differentiated type. McCarty et al.[201] found thirteen reported cases; eleven patients had received replacement estrogen therapy, usually in high doses and for prolonged periods. It is not clear whether this association represents a complication of long-term estrogen exposure or a rare expression of the Turner phenotype. Interestingly, almost two thirds of the carcinomas exhibited squamous differentiation.[192]

Some cases of endometrial carcinoma have been seen years after pelvic irradiation for some other condition, but whether these are spontaneous or radiation-induced is not clear.[204]

Recently several reports have appeared suggesting that patients who receive tamoxifen as long-term treatment for breast carcinoma may be at an increased risk for the development of endometrial adenocarcinoma[192a,195]; of particular concern is the fact that in two series a significant number of these cases have been high-grade tumors associated with a poor prognosis.[200,206]

Pathologic features

Grossly, carcinoma of the endometrium may form broad-based polypoid masses or infiltrate diffusely into the myometrium (Fig. 19-90). In general, extensive myometrial invasion is accompanied by clinically detectable uterine enlargement. However, notable exceptions occur; sometimes deep myometrial extension is accompanied by a normal-sized uterus. At times, the tumor begins in a cornu and is missed by D&C.

Microscopically, about 80% of endometrial malignant epithelial tumors are conventional adenocarcinomas, which are usually divided into well (grade I, 50%), moderately (grade II, 35%), and poorly differentiated (grade III, 15%) tumors (Figs. 19-91 and 19-92). The FIGO grading system is primarily based on the growth pattern (relative proportion of glandular and solid areas) but it also makes provisions for nuclear atypia.[222a]

The better differentiated tumors closely recapitulate the light and electron microscopic features of the non-neoplastic endometrium,[211,215] hence the term "endometrioid" that is used for them. Their architectural and cytologic features have been described on p. 1403. Over a quarter of the carcinomas have papillary (villoglandular) foci, either on the surface or in the invasive areas.[209,210] These tumors should be sharply separated from the much more aggressive papillary serous carcinomas (see p. 1413).

The stroma of endometrial adenocarcinoma usually has a desmoplastic quality. It may contain collections of foamy cells, probably the result of tumor necrosis and a good marker for the presence of carcinoma.[217] However, these

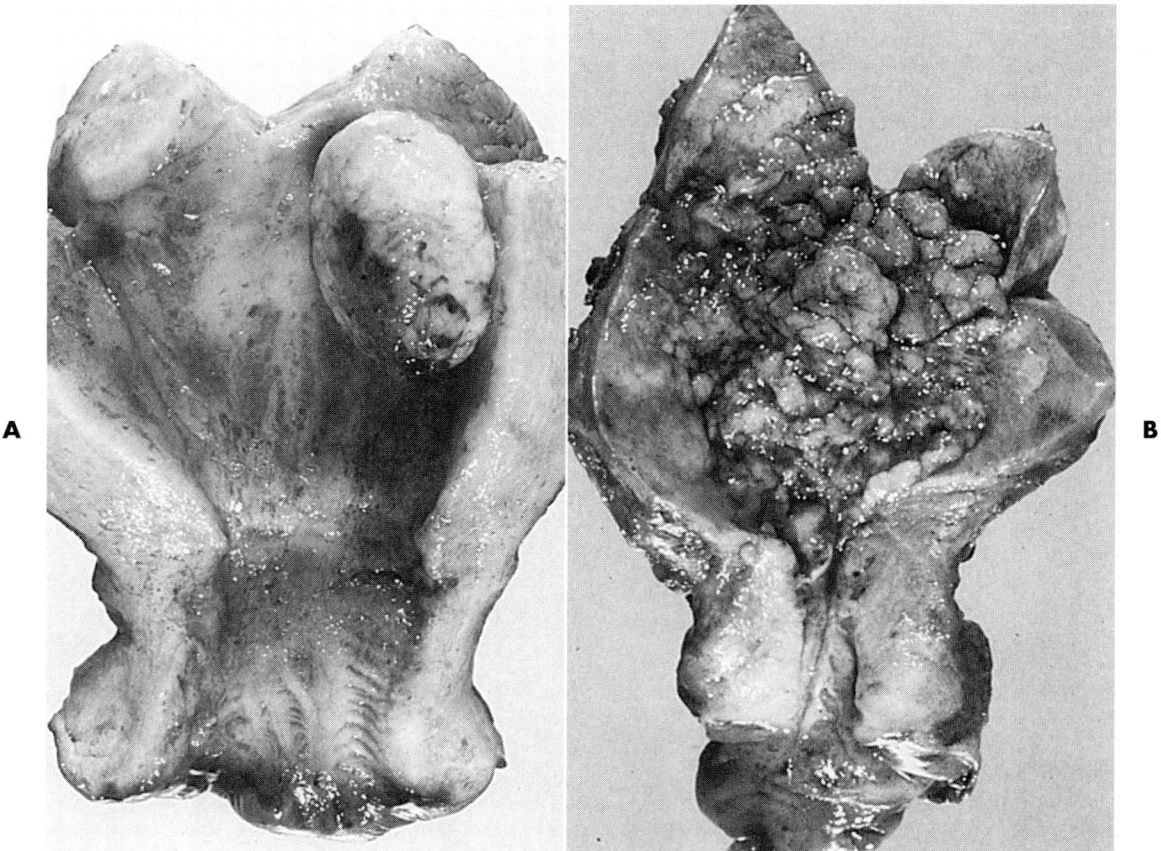

Fig. 19-90 Two gross appearance of endometrial adenocarcinoma. Lesion shown in **A** has a distinctly polypoid appearance and relatively smooth outer surface, whereas lesion shown in **B** involves most of endometrial cavity and has irregular cerebroid configuration. (Courtesy Dr. J. Costa, Lausanne, Switzerland.)

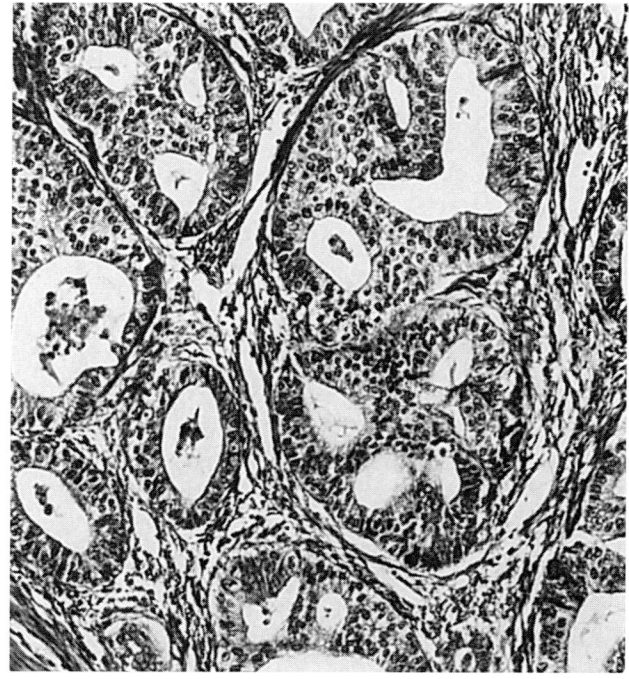

Fig. 19-91 Well-differentiated adenocarcinoma of so-called endometrioid type.

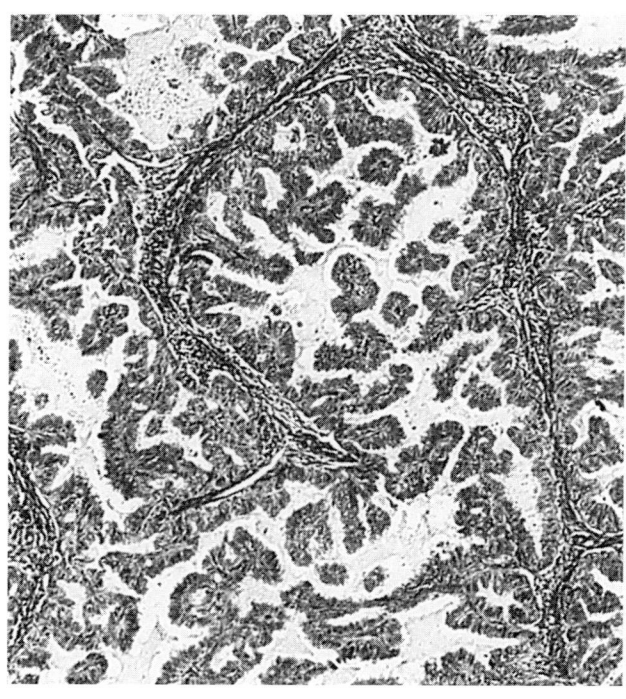

Fig. 19-92 Adenocarcinoma with papillary pattern of growth.

cells can also be seen in hyperplasia and, exceptionally, in otherwise normal endometria. They are said to form from endometrial stroma rather than histiocytes.[213] They are fat positive and mucin negative, in contrast to the mucin-positive macrophages sometimes seen in the stroma of benign endometrial polyps.[222]

The non-neoplastic endometrium of a uterus harboring an adenocarcinoma is often hyperplastic, is sometimes atrophic, and only exceptionally exhibits a normal proliferative or secretory pattern; when it does, the assumption has been made that the carcinoma has arisen in a "progesterone-refractory" mucosal area.[221]

The frequency and extent of myometrial invasion by carcinoma are directly related to the microscopic grade of the tumor.[220a] Care should be exercised to distinguish true myometrial extension by carcinoma from expansion of the endometrial-myometrial junction and from atypical or malignant changes involving pre-existent foci of adenomyosis[218]; the latter condition is recognized by the presence of endometrial stroma around the intramyometrial proliferating glandular foci.[216] Extension of the endometrial carcinoma into the cervix occurs in over 10% of the cases, usually by direct invasion,[214,220] but sometimes by implantation following D&C.[212] This may be grossly evident or become apparent only on microscopic examination; it may involve the surface only, the fibrous stroma, or both.[219,220] The presence and type of cervical extension—which influences the staging of the tumor—is best detected by fractional curettage; care should be exercised in distinguishing bona fide cervical extension from isolated tumor fragments, or else a high false positive rate will occur.[219]

Variants and other microscopic types

Numerous morphologic forms of endometrial adenocarcinoma have been described. Some, such as adenoacanthoma, adenosquamous carcinoma, secretory carcinoma, and ciliated carcinoma, are thought to represent variants of ordinary ("endometrioid") adenocarcinoma. Others, notably papillary serous carcinoma, clear cell carcinoma, and mucinous adenocarcinoma, are regarded as being of nonendometrioid type, although any of them can be seen coexisting with endometrioid adenocarcinoma.

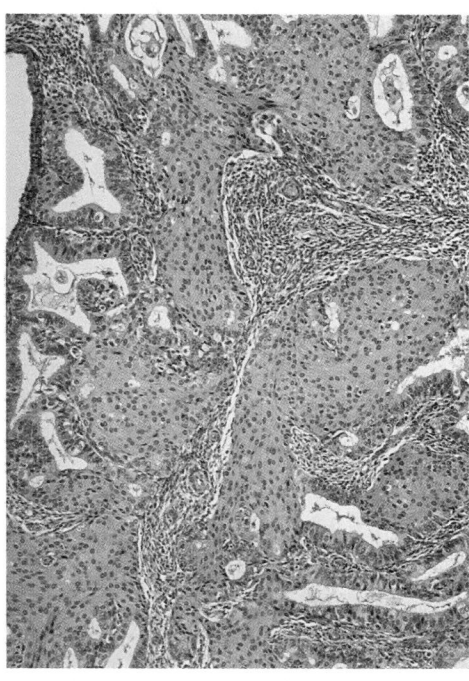

Fig. 19-93 Well-differentiated adenocarcinoma with squamous metaplasia (so-called adenoacanthoma).

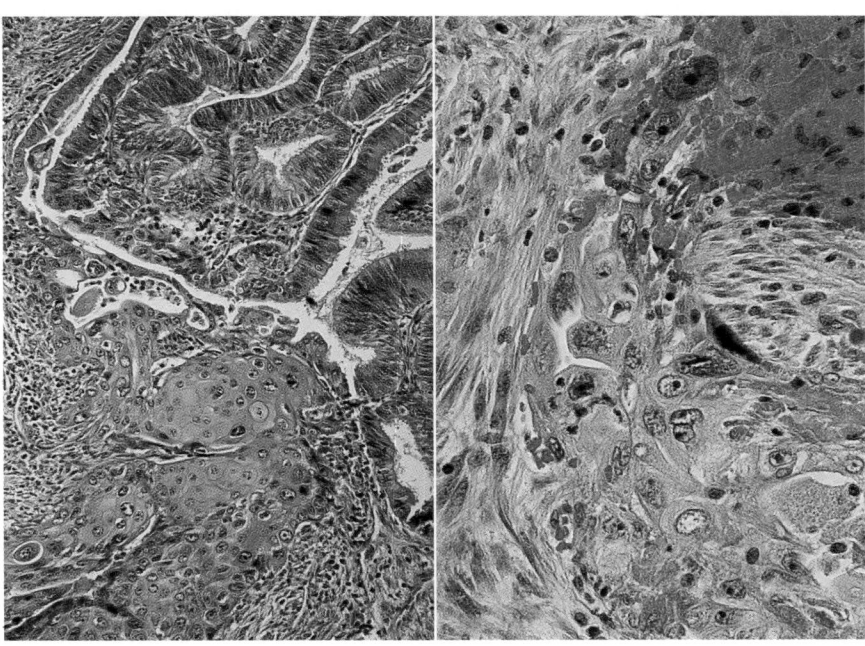

Fig. 19-94 Endometrial adenocarcinoma with squamous metaplasia. In contrast to the case shown in Fig. 19-93, the squamous component has markedly atypical cytologic features.

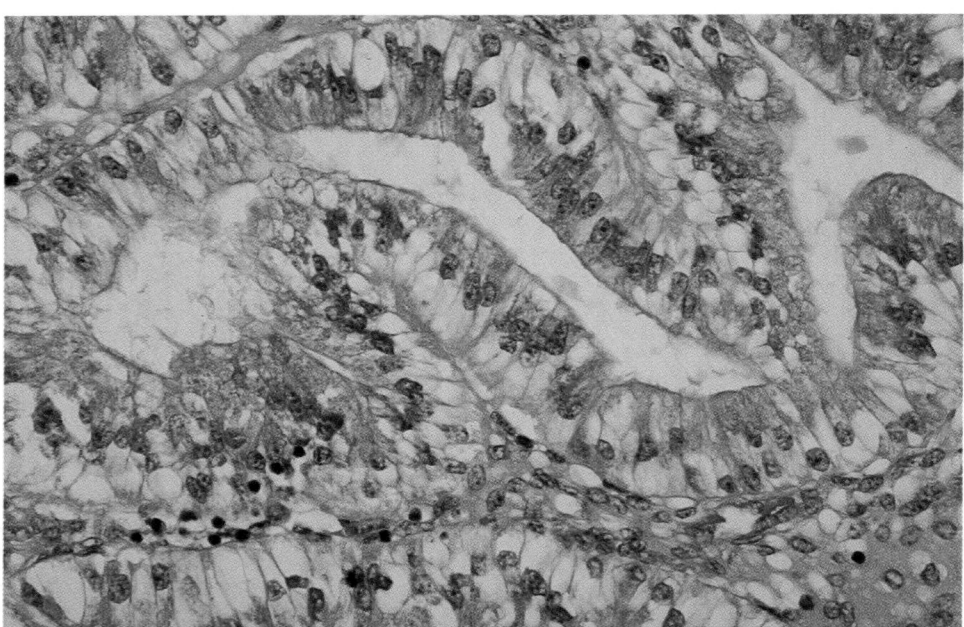

Fig. 19-95 Secretory carcinoma of endometrium. This well-differentiated lesion is composed of cells with abundant clear to finely granular cytoplasm. This tumor type should not be equated with clear cell carcinoma.

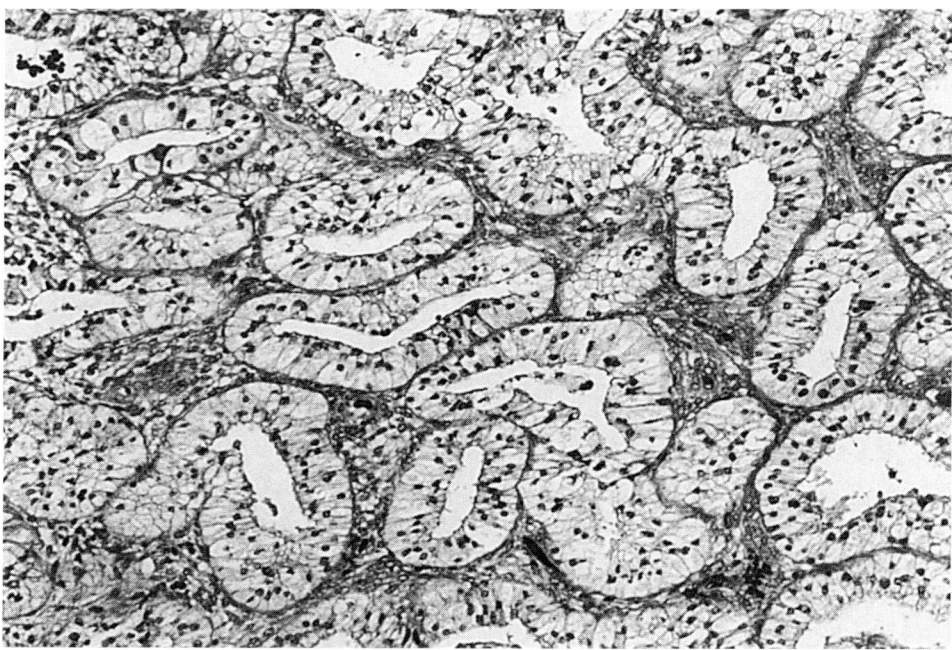

Fig. 19-96 So-called secretory carcinoma of endometrium. Lesion is very well differentiated and composed of cells with abundant cytoplasm, which is clear and finely granular. This tumor should not be equated with mesonephroid carcinoma.

Adenoacanthoma is the term traditionally given to the endometrioid adenocarcinoma containing similarly well-differentiated (benign-appearing) squamous elements derived from metaplasia of the tumor glands (Fig. 19-93). Its natural history closely parallels that of the ordinary adenocarcinoma of similar degree of differentiation.[271]

Adenosquamous (mixed) carcinoma refers to the endometrioid carcinoma containing malignant-appearing squamous elements[248] (Fig. 19-94). In some series the incidence of this tumor type has been notably high—up to 30% of all uterine carcinoma and on the rise[248,249]—but this was not our experience or that of others.[226,235] Patients with

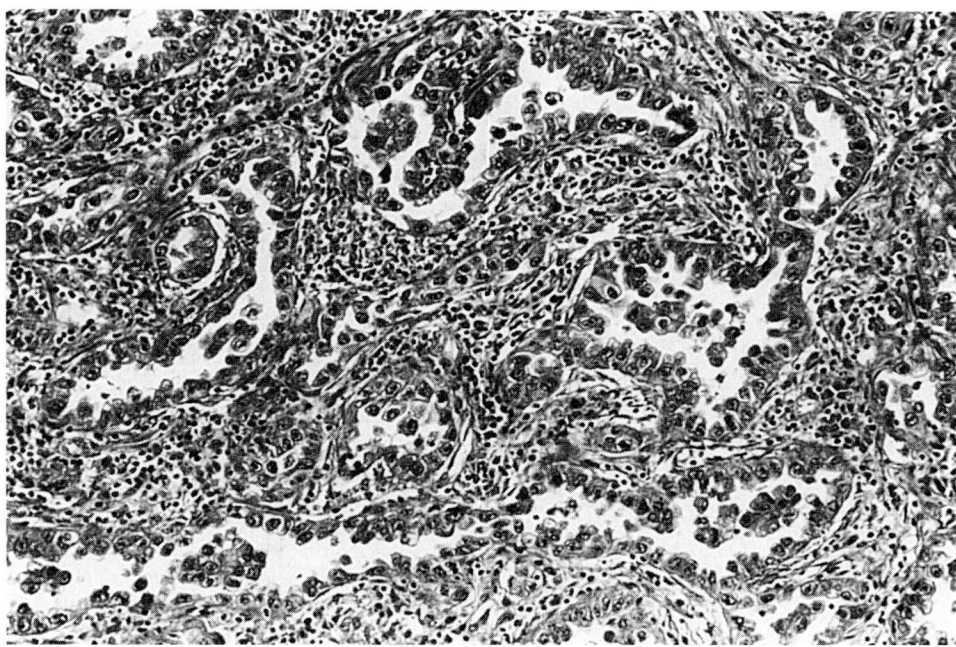

Fig. 19-97 Papillary serous carcinoma of endometrium invading myometrium. Tubular and papillary formations are present. Cytologic appearance is reminiscent of clear cell (mesonephroid) carcinoma.

adenosquamous carcinoma are said to have a worse prognosis than those with adenocarcinoma or adenoacanthoma. However, several studies have shown that, stage by stage and grade by grade, there are no prognostic differences between pure adenocarcinoma, adenoacanthoma, and adenosquamous carcinoma.[257,270] Thus it would appear that the bad reputation that the latter tumors have is the result of the fact that most of them are basically high-grade adenocarcinomas, whereas the reverse is true for the adenoacanthomas. In other words, once an endometrial adenocarcinoma is clinically staged and microscopically graded into well-differentiated, intermediate, and poorly differentiated categories, the presence and appearance of a focal squamous component would seem immaterial.[270] Morphologic studies have suggested—and immunocytochemical studies have supported—the notion that adenoacanthoma and adenosquamous carcinoma represent a spectrum of squamous metaplasia in a single tumor type rather than two independent entities.[266]

Glassy cell carcinoma is a special type of adenosquamous carcinoma that has occasionally been reported in the endometrium; its appearance is similar to that of its more common cervical counterpart.[231,234]

Secretory carcinoma is characterized by neoplastic glands having subnuclear vacuolization resembling that of a normal 17-day secretory endometrium and accompanied by a late secretory pattern in the adjacent noninvolved endometrium[264] (Figs. 19-95 and 19-96). This tumor is not believed to be a specific type of endometrial carcinoma but rather the expression of a pattern that may be present diffusely or focally in a well-differentiated carcinoma, usually as a result of progesterone stimulation.[245] It should be distinguished from the clear cell carcinoma described later.[230]

Ciliated carcinoma is an extremely rare variant of endometrial adenocarcinoma that is composed predominantly of ciliated cells[236]; it needs to be distinguished from the much more common ciliated cell metaplasia (see p. 1399).

Mucinous adenocarcinoma is a tumor subtype characterized by abundant mucin secretion.[247] It is distinguished from mucinous metaplasia by virtue of its architectural and cytologic atypia. It should be noted that scattered foci of mucin positivity are often found in ordinary endometrial adenocarcinoma and that they are not necessarily an indication of endocervical origin.[258,263] The distinction between endometrial mucinous adenocarcinoma and primary endocervical adenocarcinoma cannot be made on the basis of morphologic or histochemical features but rather depends on differential biopsy and fractional curettage.[254] Parenthetically, some of the histochemical features of the mucin produced by these tumors suggest the existence of enteric differentiation.[246b]

On occasion, endometrial adenocarcinomas of mucinous or mixed mucinous-endometrioid type exhibit a conspicuous microglandular pattern associated with eosinophilic mucinous intraluminal secretion and prominent acute inflammation, the overall picture simulating the appearance of endocervical microglandular hyperplasia.[269]

Papillary serous carcinoma (formerly also known as tubal carcinoma) is a highly aggressive form of endometrial adenocarcinoma closely resembling ovarian papillary serous carcinoma[233a,237,242,246] (Plate XIII-D). It is characterized by a complex papillary pattern of growth, a high degree of cytologic atypia (pleomorphism, hyperchromasia, giant nucleoli), numerous mitoses, extensive necrosis, psammoma bodies (30% of the cases), and prominent myometrial invasion (Fig. 19-97). It should be distinguished from the

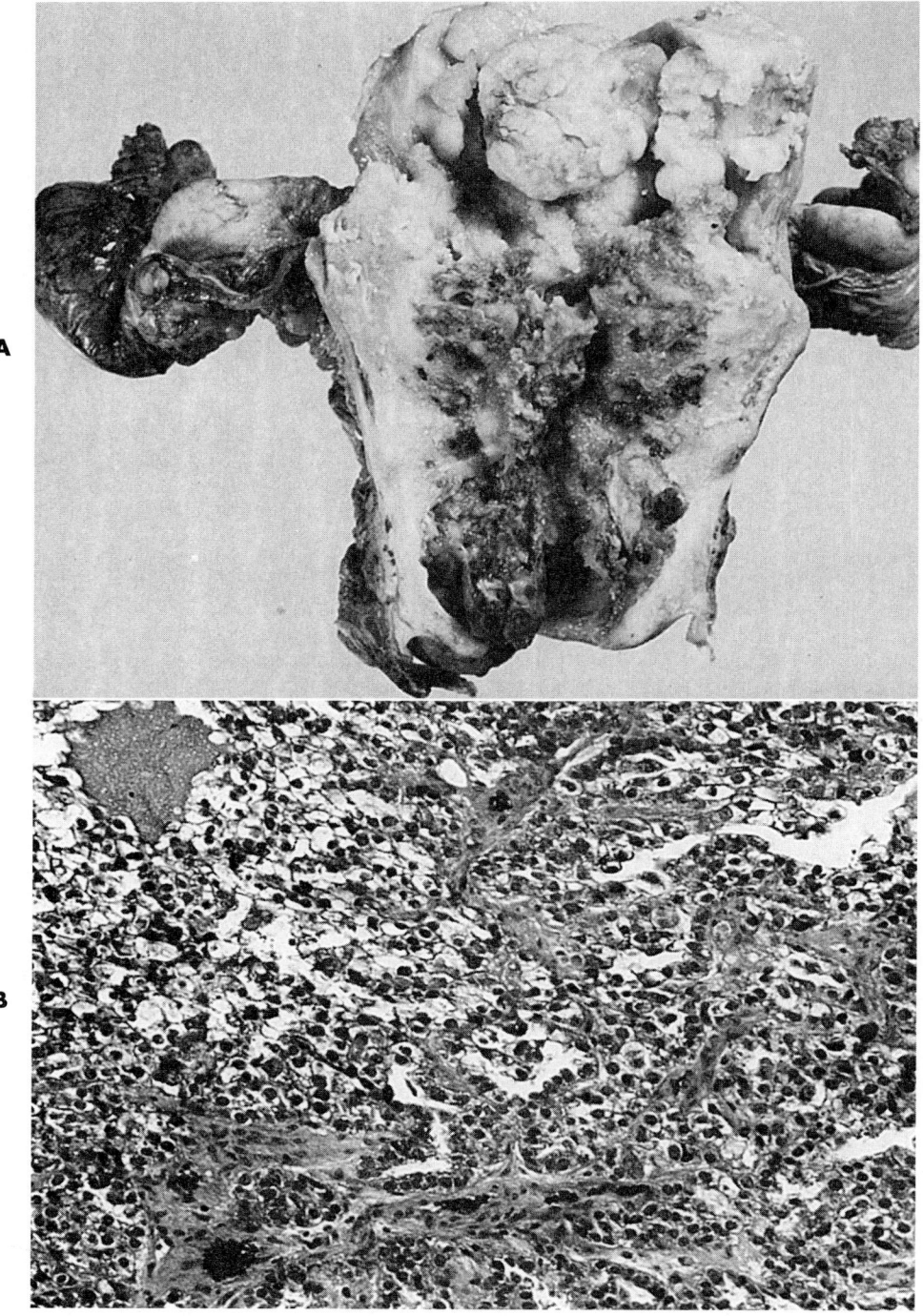

Fig. 19-98 Endometrial adenocarcinoma of clear cell (mesonephroid) type occurring in 71-year-old woman. **A,** Large polypoid masses fill endometrial cavity. Extension into myometrium and endocervix is evident. **B,** Microscopic appearance of clear cell (mesonephroid) carcinoma. Tumor grows in glandular and solid formations. Tumor cells have clear cytoplasm and their nuclei are markedly hyperchromatic.

already mentioned (and much more common) endometrial adenocarcinoma with a villoglandular pattern of growth, with which it shares several architectural features[232] (see p. 1409). A key aspect in this regard is the consistently high-grade nature of its cytologic features, which are also apparent on Pap smears.[244]

Uterine papillary serous carcinoma can coexist with endometrioid adenocarcinoma, be confined to an endometrial polyp, or be entirely intramucosal.[229,259,260] It can also occur in association with serous ovarian carcinoma,[229] and it may follow radiation therapy for carcinoma of the cervix.[250]

Clear cell carcinoma is composed of large clear cells with distinct cellular margins containing greater or lesser amounts of glycogen[245] (Fig. 19-98). Papillary formations and "hobnail" cells found in this variant of adenocarcinoma resemble those seen in the ovarian, cervical, and vaginal tumors formerly called "mesonephric carcinomas." However, their presence in superficial endometrial carcinomas, as a focal change in ordinary adenocarcinomas, and, exceptionally, even in benign endometrial polyps[245] and otherwise normal endometria[233] is evidence against a relationship with mesonephric remnants. The ultrastructural features of this tumor are also supportive of a müllerian rather than a mesonephric derivation.[253,255] Most patients are post menopausal, and there seems to be no relationship to intrauterine diethylstilbestrol exposure, as there is for somewhat similar tumors occurring in the vagina and cervix.

Although earlier articles emphasized the similarities that clear cell carcinoma bears with ordinary ("endometrioid") adenocarcinoma,[245,261] recent series suggest instead that it is more closely related to papillary serous carcinoma, both in terms of morphology and natural history.[228,246a]

Small cell carcinoma usually presents grossly as bulky (sometimes polypoid), ill-defined, and invasive. Microscopically, its appearance is similar to that of its more common cervical counterpart. It may be associated with areas of ordinary adenocarcinoma or be seen as a component of mixed müllerian tumor.[239,251] Immunohistochemically, there is often reactivity for NSE but rarely for chromogranin. Dense-core secretory granules can be detected ultrastructurally. The behavior is very aggressive.[265] As in the lung, cervix, and other sites, tumors with similar high-grade neuroendocrine features but composed of cells of intermediate or large size exist.[224] In this context, it should be noted that a minor population of endocrine cells—as detected with argyrophilic stains—is present in 25% to 50% of otherwise typical endometrial adenocarcinomas.[227,262] Some of these cells have been found to contain chromogranin, NSE, serotonin, somatostatin, ACTH, and indolamines.[225,240]

Squamous cell carcinoma occurring in the endometrium in a pure form is extremely rare.[223,241] Some cases have developed in elderly patients with pyometra, presumably on the basis of a pre-existing endometrial squamous metaplasia.[238] Others have occurred in association with mucinous glands of presumably heterotopic cervical origin.[267] One reported case was associated with *spindle-cell (sarcomatoid)* changes.[268] Another was of the *verrucous type*.[256]

Giant cell carcinoma is a rare pleomorphic form of high-grade endometrial adenocarcinoma featuring poorly cohesive sheets and nests of bizarre multinucleated giant cells.[243]

Endometrial carcinoma with trophoblastic differentiation should be distinguished from the tumor just mentioned

and from gestational choriocarcinoma.[243a] The multinucleated syncytiotrophoblast-like cells present in the tumor are strongly immunoreactive for hCG.[252]

Oxyphilic cell carcinoma is a recently described variant of endometrioid carcinoma characterized by a predominant or exclusive component of large eosinophilic (oxyphilic) cells.[252a]

Endometrioid carcinoma with *sertoliform (sex cord–like) differentiation* similar to that more commonly seen in ovarian endometrioid tumors has been reported.[264a]

Cytology

Unfortunately, the success of mass screening in reducing invasive cervical carcinoma has not had the same effect on endometrial carcinoma.[274] The routine Pap smear is not adequate for the detection of this tumor,[273] the positive rate being only 50%.[273] With cervical scrapings, this rate is 60%, and with vaginal pool material it reaches 75%.[283,285] The presence of normal endometrial cells in a cervical cytologic specimen should raise the possibility of endometrial hyperplasia or carcinoma and is an indication for histologic examination of the endometrium.[280] Several cytologic methods have been employed to increase the positive rate, such as endometrial aspiration, tampon smear, endometrial lavage, endometrial brushing, the jet wash technique, and suction curettage.[272,275-279] Of these, the latter is preferred by many because of its high degree of accuracy and patient acceptance.[276] However, the widespread applicability of any of these methods to mass screening still remains problematic.[281,282,284]

Immunohistochemical and other special techniques

Immunohistochemically, endometrial adenocarcinomas are positive for keratin (especially keratins 7, 8, 18, and 19),[296,297] vimentin (65% of the cases),[289] CEA (although less so than cervical carcinomas and generally limited to areas of squamous metaplasia),[303] CA125,[299] IgA and secretory component,[302] *Ulex europaeus,* agglutinin I, and amylase (12% of the cases).[304] Co-expression of keratin and vimentin is common.[300] Some tumor cells have also been found to contain GFAP.[297]

Estrogen and progesterone receptors, as detected by biochemical analysis or immunocytochemistry, are present in most cases of endometrial adenocarcinoma.[286,290,291,295,298] Endometrioid carcinoma shows the highest degree of positivity for both receptors, followed by adenosquamous carcinoma, papillary serous carcinoma, and clear cell carcinoma. The presence of hormone receptors correlates with FIGO stage, FIGO grade, and nuclear grade. The degrees of estrogen and progesterone receptor positivity are often similar.[288]

Overexpression of p53 (presumably as a result of mutation) is found in less than half of the cases; it is more likely to be present in high-grade endometrioid and papillary serous carcinoma than in other tumors.[287,293,299a] An inverse correlation has been detected between p53 overexpression and steroid hormone receptor status.[294]

Mutations of c-Ki-*ras* gene are frequent in adenocarcinomas showing infiltrative features and a desmoplastic stromal response.[302a]

DNA aneuploidy is present in approximately one quarter of the cases; positive tumors tend to be of advanced surgical stage and higher microscopic grade, associated with deeper

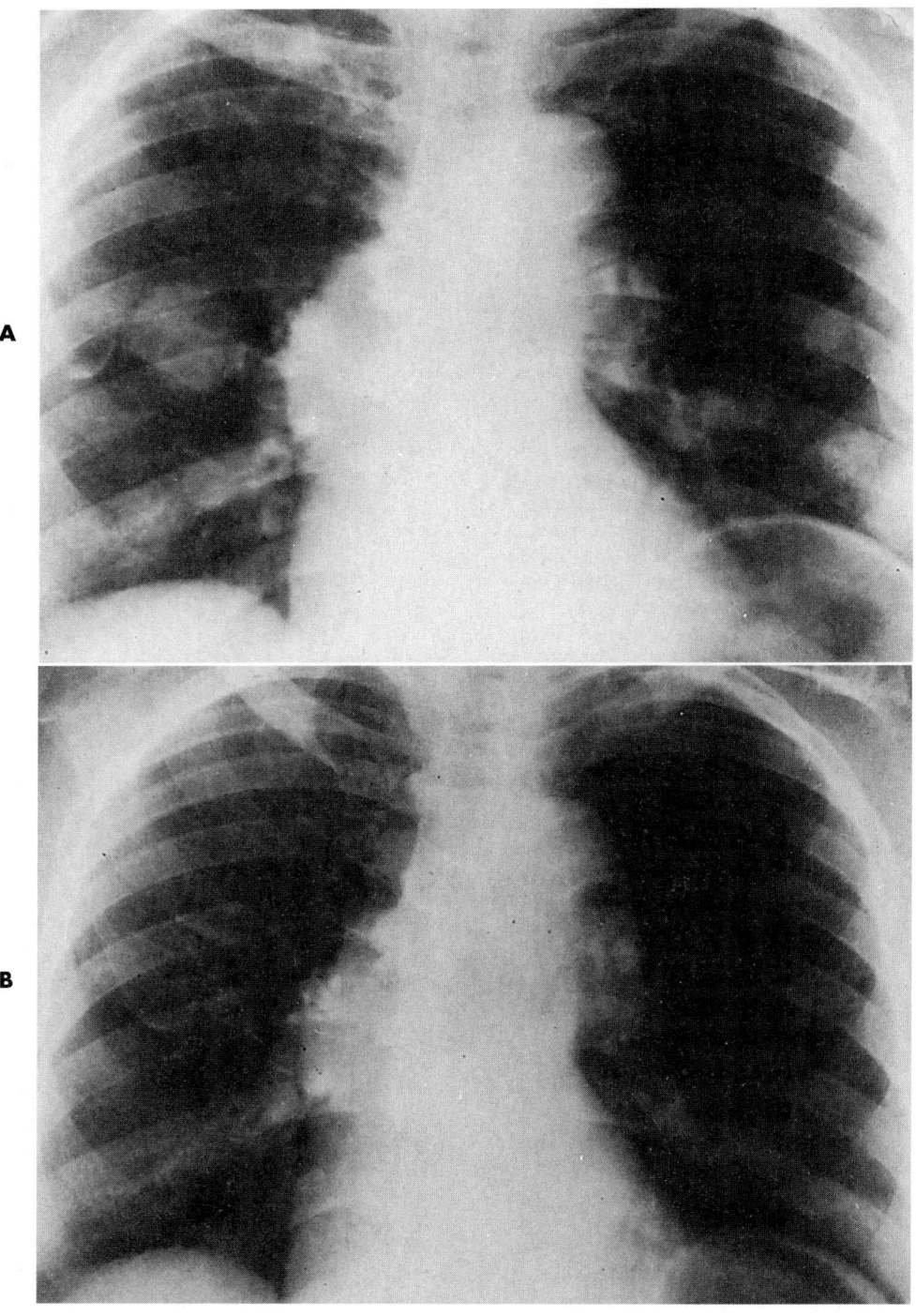

Fig. 19-99 A,Pulmonary metastases from endometrial carcinoma in 74-year-old woman. **B,** Following progesterone therapy, metastases completely disappeared. Patient also was given full course of radiotherapy to pelvis. She remained in remission for several months.

myometrial invasion, and accompanied by lymph node metastases. Multivariate analysis studies suggest that DNA ploidy may be an independent prognostic factor.[292] As expected, aneuploidy is the rule in papillary serous carcinoma.[301]

Spread and metastases

The most common sites of extrauterine spread in endometrial adenocarcinoma are the pelvic and para-aortic lymph nodes and the ovaries. Nodal metastases occur in about 5% to 25% of clinically stage I tumors and are more likely to occur in invasive high-grade tumors (even if such tumors are superficial), in large sized and/or deeply invasive tumors regardless of grade, in tumors with cervical extension, and in tumors with vascular invasion.[305,307,310]

About 8% of endometrial carcinomas are accompanied by a simultaneous ovarian carcinoma. When they are of similar microscopic types—which is usually the case—it becomes difficult to decide whether there are two independent tumors or whether one of the sites represents a metastasis. Features favoring a metastatic nature for the ovarian tumor include the following: smaller size, bilateral involvement, multinodular pattern of growth, presence of associated surface implants, and prominent lymphatic or vascular invasion within the ovarian stroma. Immunohistochemical and DNA flow cytometric studies may be of some value for the distinction between metastatic and independent tumors, but at present the decision rests largely on conventional clinicopathologic criteria such as those listed previously.[309]

The most common sites of recurrence of endometrial carcinoma are the vaginal vault and pelvis. Papillary serous carcinoma characteristically spreads throughout the abdominal cavity in a fashion similar to that of ovarian serous carcinoma. Metastases of this tumor in the bladder can simulate a primary neoplasm of this organ.[311]

Distant metastases of endometrial carcinoma are more common in the lung, liver, bone, central nervous system, and skin. The latter tend to occur in the head and neck region, particularly the scalp.

On occasion, the keratin present in endometrial carcinoma with squamous metaplasia desquamates into the uterine cavity and from there travels via the fallopian tube to produce implants in the peritoneal surface, leading to the formation of foreign body granulomas.[306] This finding should not be regarded as evidence of metastatic disease in the absence of viable neoplastic cells. Follow-up data on these patients suggest that these keratin granulomas have no prognostic significance and that they should be distinguished from viable tumor implants.[308]

Therapy

The usual treatment of endometrial carcinoma is total abdominal hysterectomy with bilateral salpingo-oophorectomy, sometimes accompanied by removal of the pelvic and periaortic lymph nodes. Radiation therapy, which until recently was administered routinely in conjunction with surgery (either preoperatively or postoperatively), is no longer favored. Tumor sterilization by radiation, as determined by histopathologic study of the hysterectomy specimen, was often obtained for tumors limited to the endometrium but only rarely for tumors invading the myometrium.[315] Progestational agents, although not curative, can induce striking temporary regressions in the primary tumor as well as in the metastases. Well-differentiated lesions are more likely to respond (Figs. 19-99 and 19-100); this is in keeping with the fact that, as already indicated, an association exists between microscopic degree of differentiation and presence of estrogen and progesterone receptors.

The treatment of papillary serous carcinoma following operation (which should include a staging laparotomy) remains controversial; some centers advocate whole abdominal radiation therapy, whereas other recommend multidrug chemotherapy.[313,314]

Tumor relapse may appear in the form of local recrudescence (50%), distant metastases (28%), or both (21%); the median interval is between 1 and 2 years.[312] Local recurrences can be treated successfully with aggressive radiation therapy.[314a]

Prognosis

Factors of prognostic importance in endometrial adenocarcinoma are the following:

1 *Clinical stage,* as defined by the FIGO system[319,320,336] (Table 19-5).
2 Level of *infiltration* of the myometrial wall.[323,326,328,330]
3 *Microscopic grade* of differentiation, as defined by the FIGO system.[328,337,339,342a] As already stated, this is primarily based on architectural rather than nuclear features, except for the papillary serous and clear cell types.[344] A relationship exists between microscopic grade and level of invasion (well-differentiated tumors being more superficial), but there is correlation between grade and survival within a given stage.[335]
4 *Cervical extension.* This is associated with a somewhat worse prognosis, regardless of the nature or extent of the change.[325,333]
5 *Estrogen dependence.* As a group, tumors associated with—and probably resulting from—chronic estrogenic stimulation have a better prognosis than the others. This includes most tumors in young patients (<40 years) and those associated with the Stein-Leventhal syndrome, functioning ovarian tumors, and exogenous estrogen administration.[318,332,338] Along the same lines, adenocarcinomas associated with hyperplasia in the residual endometrium have a better prognosis than those lacking this feature.[318]
6 *Microscopic type.* Among the various morphologic variants, the papillary serous type and clear cell types are the most aggressive, with a definite tendency for upper abdominal spread for the former. Adenosquamous carcinomas are also highly malignant, but this is probably only a reflection of the fact that they are poorly differentiated tumors. Conversely, the excellent prognosis associated with grade I endometrioid adenocarcinoma, adenoacanthoma, and secretory carcinoma probably relates to their well-differentiated nature.[323,341,343]
7 *Lymph vessel invasion.* Tumor permeation of lymph vessels is a poor prognostic sign.[327]
8 *Blood vessel invasion.* The presence of blood vessel invasion is an important prognostic factor in stage I

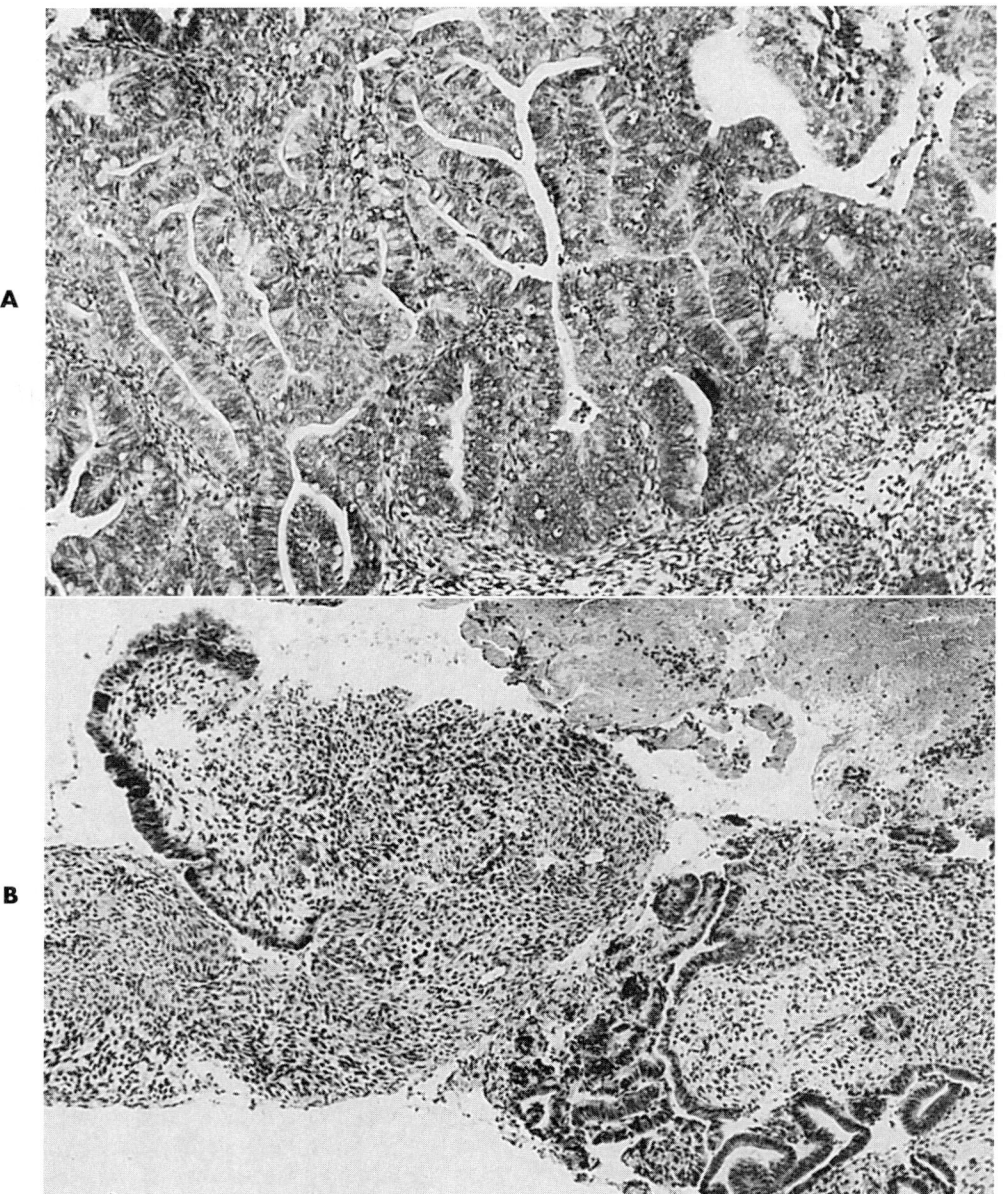

Fig. 19-100 A, Well-differentiated adenocarcinoma of endometrium invading stroma. Patient was treated for 3 weeks with progestogens and curettage was repeated twice. **B,** Repeat curettage. Endometrium shows progestogen effect without evidence of carcinoma. Patient was well 7 years after last curettage and has been pregnant twice. (From Kempson RL, Pokorny GE: Adenocarcinoma of the endometrium in women aged forty and younger. Cancer **21:**650-662, 1968.)

adenocarcinoma; this feature has often been found to be associated with perivascular lymphocytic infiltration.[316]

9 *Hormone receptor status.* Multivariate analyses have shown that the estrogen receptor status (whether measured biochemically or immunohistochemically) is a significant predictor of survival.[322,324]

10 *p53 overexpression.* This parameter has been found to be associated with tumor type, grade, and stage.[317a,337b,338a]

11 *HER-2/*neu *expression.* Intense overexpression of this oncogene is said to be associated with a poor overall survival.[329]

12 *Epidermal growth factor receptor.* Expression of this marker is said to correlate with microscopic grade and a shorter survival rate.[337a]

13 *DNA ploidy.* Aneuploid tumors are associated with high microscopic grade, high clinical stage, and poor prognosis; it has been claimed that tumor aneuploidy has independent prognostic value.[317,321,331,334]

Table 19-5 FIGO staging for carcinoma of the corpus uteri

Stage IA	Grade 1,2,3
	Tumor limited to endometrium.
Stage IB	Grade 1,2,3
	Invasion to less than óne-half the myometrium.
Stage IC	Grade 1,2,3
	Invasion to more than one-half the myometrium.
Stage IIA	Grade 1,2,3
	Endocervical glandular involvement only.
Stage IIB	Grade 1,2,3
	Cervical stromal invasion.
Stage IIIA	Grade 1,2,3
	Tumor invades serosa and/or adnexa, and/or positive peritoneal cytology.
Stage IIIB	Grade 1,2,3
	Vaginal metastases.
Stage IIIC	Grade 1,2,3
	Metastases to pelvic and/or paraaortic ymph nodes.
Stage IVA	Grade 1,2,3
	Tumor invasion of bladder and/or bowel mucosa.
Stage IVB	Distant metastases including intraabdominal and/or inguinal lymph nodes.

Histopathology—degree of differentiation:

Cases of carcinoma of the corpus should be classified (or graded) according to the degree of histologic differentiation, as follows:

Grade 1 = 5% or less of a nonsquamous or nonmorular solid growth pattern
Grade 2 = 6-50% of a nonsquamous or nonmorular solid growth pattern
Grade 3 = more than 50% of a nonsquamous or nonmorular solid growth pattern

Notes on pathological grading:

1) Notable nuclear atypia, inappropriate for the architectural grade, raises the grade of a Grade 1 or Grade 2 tumor by 1.
2) In serous adenocarcinomas, clear-cell adenocarcinomas, and squamous cell carcinomas, nuclear grading takes precedence.
3) Adenocarcinomas with squamous differentiation are graded according to the nuclear grade of the glandular component.

Rules related to staging:

1) Because corpus cancer is now staged surgically, procedures previously used for determination of stages are no longer applicable, such as the findings from fractional D&C to differentiate between Stage I and Stage II.
2) It is appreciated that there may be a small number of patients with corpus cancer who will be treated primarily with radiation therapy. If that is the case, the clinical staging adopted by FIGO in 1971 still would apply, but designation of that staging system would be noted.
3) Ideally, width of the myometrium should be measured along with the width of tumor invasion.

From SGO handbook. Staging of gynecologic malignancies. Chicago, 1994, Society of Gynecologic Oncologists.
See also Appendix G.

14 *Cell proliferation.* The degree of tumor cell proliferation, as determined by S-phase fraction, was found in one series to be a strong predictor of outcome.[340] High mitotic rate has also been found to be a sign of aggressiveness in stage I grade I adenocarcinomas.[342]

Endometrial stromal tumors

Tumors composed of endometrial stroma tend to occur in middle-aged women (average age, 45 years) and often present with vaginal bleeding.[358] They have been divided according to the type of margin into (1) a benign category (stromal nodule) having pushing margins and (2) a malignant category characterized by infiltrating margins.[369] The latter can be further subdivided on the basis of the mitotic count into a low-grade (endolymphatic stromal myosis) variety and a high-grade (stromal sarcoma) variety.

Features common to the benign type and both malignant types include a soft, yellow-to-orange, gross appearance and a microscopic pattern featuring uniform small cells closely resembling those of the endometrial stroma, individually enveloped by reticulin fibers, which characteristically encircle small vessels that resemble spiral arterioles (Fig. 19-101). Other features include foci of hyalinization, scattered foamy cells, and aggregates of epithelium-like formations (to be discussed in more detail later). The similarity of the tumor cells to normal endometrial stromal cells is also evident ultrastructurally and functionally[346,354]; these cells contain estrogen and progesterone receptors, and the tumors respond to administration of progestins.[371,376,377] Their immunohistochemical profile is variable. Reactivity for vimentin is the rule, positivity for actin and desmin is common, reactivity for keratin is focal and inconstant, and negativity for S-100 protein is universal.[353,357,360]

The prominent vascularization that is typical of these tumors may result in a mistaken diagnosis of hemangiopericytoma, particularly in metastatic sites.[373] Diagnostic confusion can also arise with malignant lymphoma, undifferentiated carcinoma, and pseudosarcomatous changes in the endometrial stroma.

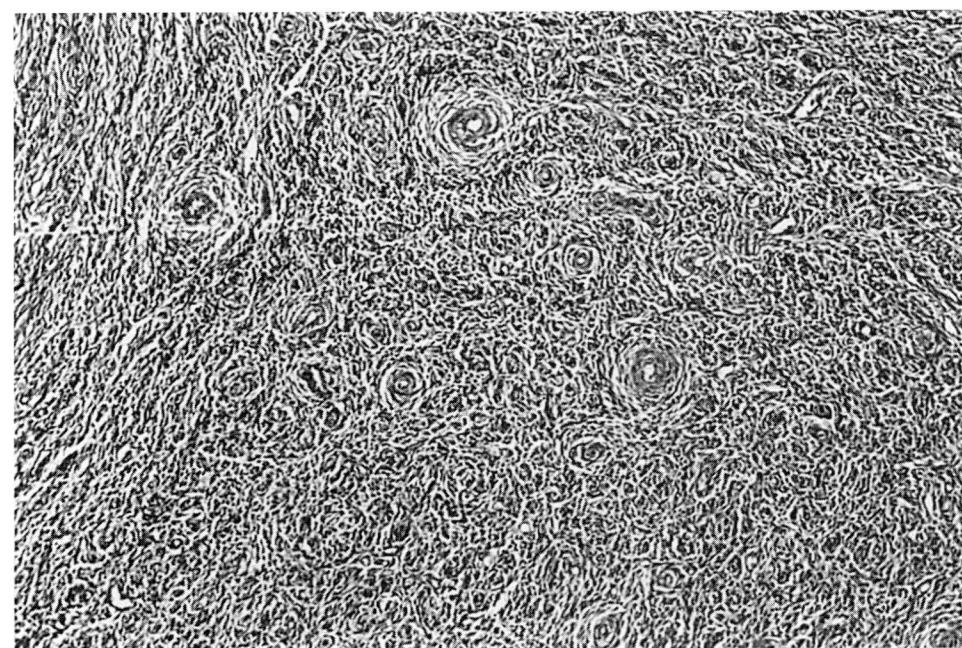

Fig. 19-101 Low-grade endometrial stromal sarcoma. Concentric arrangement of small uniform tumor cells around vessels of spiral arteriole type is characteristic of this tumor type.

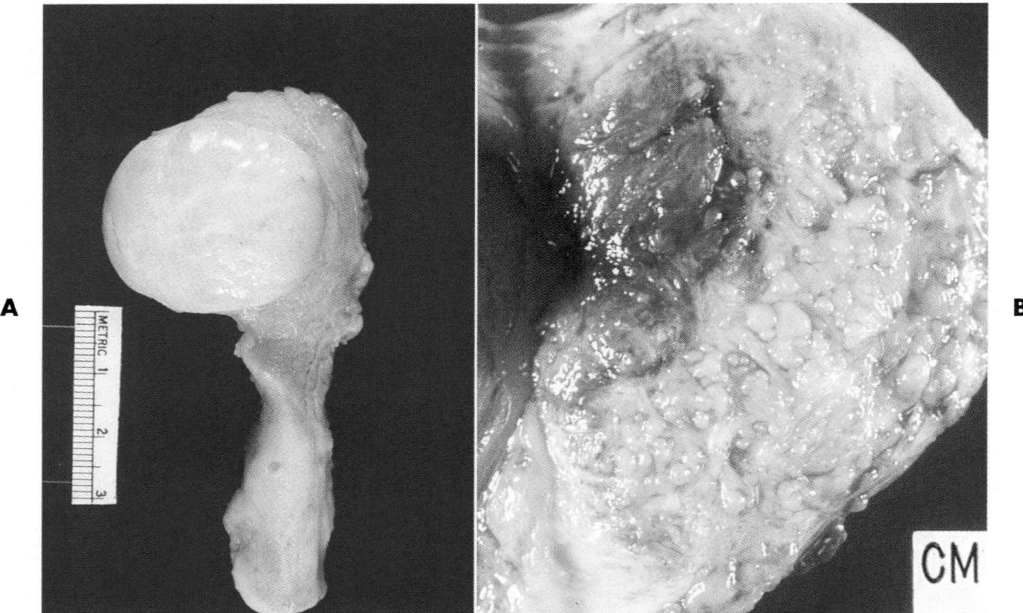

Fig. 19-102 A, Endometrial stromal nodule. The lesion is characteristically well circumscribed, and it has a yellow color. **B,** Low-grade endometrial stromal sarcoma showing diffuse permeation of the myometrium in the form of small nodules bulging on the cut surface.

Stromal nodules appear grossly as solitary sharply circumscribed masses (Fig. 19-102, *A*). They do not invade veins, lymphatics, or the myometrium. The prognosis is excellent; recurrence did not occur in any of the sixty cases studied by Tavassoli and Norris,[375] even when some irregularities in the margin, high mitotic counts, or glandular foci were present.

Low-grade stromal sarcomas, traditionally designated *endolymphatic stromal myosis,* infiltrate the myometrium and have a particular tendency to permeate lymph vessels (Fig. 19-102, *B*). The latter feature sometimes can be detected grossly by the presence of yellowish, ropy, or ball-like masses filling dilated channels. They may also present as polypoid masses (Plate XIII-E). The local invasion may

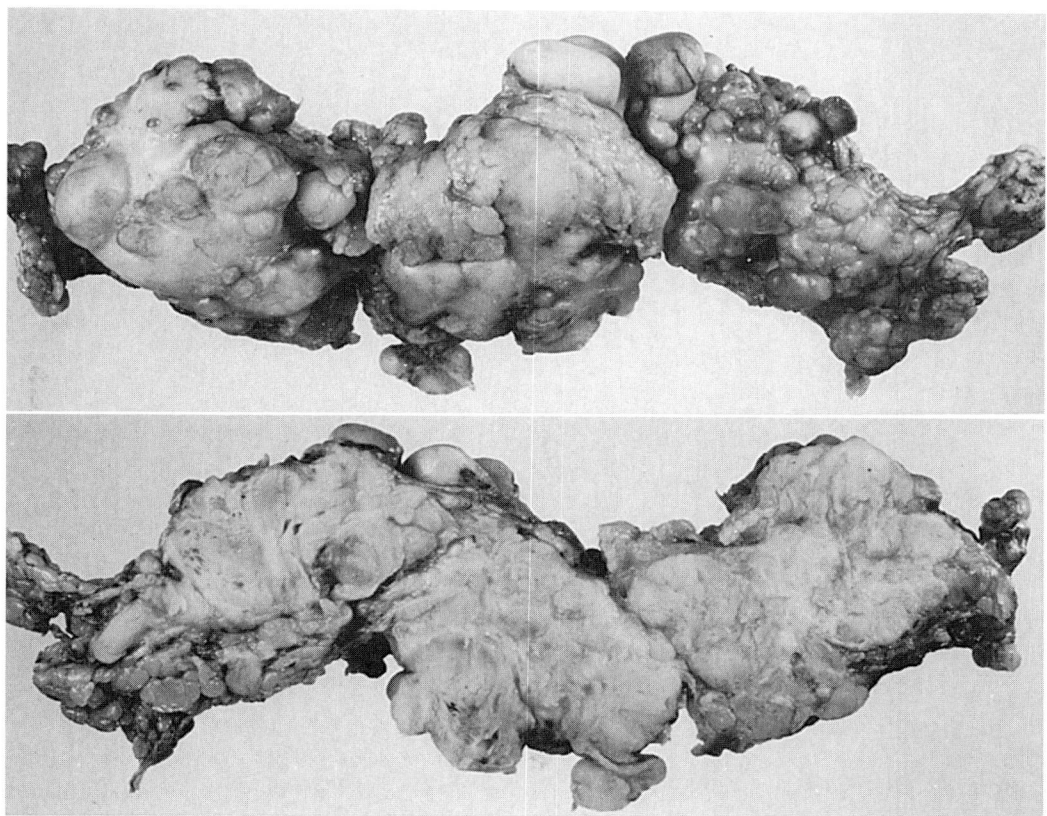

Fig. 19-103 External view and cross section of peritoneal implant of low-grade endometrial stromal sarcoma (so-called endolymphatic stromal myosis). Primary tumor had been removed 2 years previously from 53-year-old partient.

extend into the broad ligament, tubes, and ovaries (Fig. 19-103). Microscopically, the tumors should contain fewer than ten mitoses per ten high-power fields in the most active areas in order to qualify for this category. Their natural history is characterized by slow clinical progression, repeated local recurrences (in the pelvis, ovary, other intra-abdominal sites, and anterior abdominal wall), and a relatively favorable prognosis. Of the twenty patients reported by Norris and Taylor,[369] only one died of the tumor, but 31% had persistent or recurrent tumor at the time of last follow-up. Others have reported late pulmonary metastases, sometimes simulating microscopically the appearance of hemangiopericytoma or of so-called benign mesenchymal cystic hamartoma.[345]

High-grade stromal sarcomas show the same propensity for local and vascular invasion as the low-grade variety. They are distinguished from the latter only by virtue of their high mitotic count (ten or more mitoses per ten high-power fields). Grossly, they are often a diffuse growth involving the entire endometrial surface (Fig. 19-104). Patients with high-grade sarcoma have a poorer prognosis, with a tendency for recurrence in the pelvis and metastases to distant sites, particularly the lung. Of the fifteen patients reviewed by Norris and Taylor,[369] four were free of disease, seven had died, and another four were living with tumor. Although this and other early articles showed an excellent correlation

between mitotic activity and outcome,[364] this has not been nearly as apparent in larger, more recent series.[349]

Size of the tumor and extrauterine extension are important prognostic features. Stromal neoplasms less than 4 cm in diameter practically never recur, and tumors confined to the uterus at the time of the initial surgery very rarely do so, regardless of the variety to which they belong. DNA ploidy analysis is also thought to have prognostic significance.[347,355,362]

Some high-grade endometrial stromal sarcomas have a marked degree of nuclear pleomorphism and atypicality and lack a distinctive vascular pattern; these ***poorly differentiated endometrial sarcomas*** behave in a very aggressive fashion.[352,356,358,379]

A minor smooth muscle component may be seen in endometrial stromal tumors, a not surprising finding in view of the close histogenetic relationship of the two cell types. When this component is sizable (one third or more of the tumor mass), the neoplasm is referred to as ***combined smooth muscle–stromal tumor or (nodular) stromomyoma;*** no cases of malignant behavior have been reported in these combined tumors so far.[370,375] A variation on the theme is represented by the exceptional case exhibiting both smooth and skeletal muscle differentiation[367]; it is important not to confuse this lesion with a malignant mixed müllerian tumor.[367]

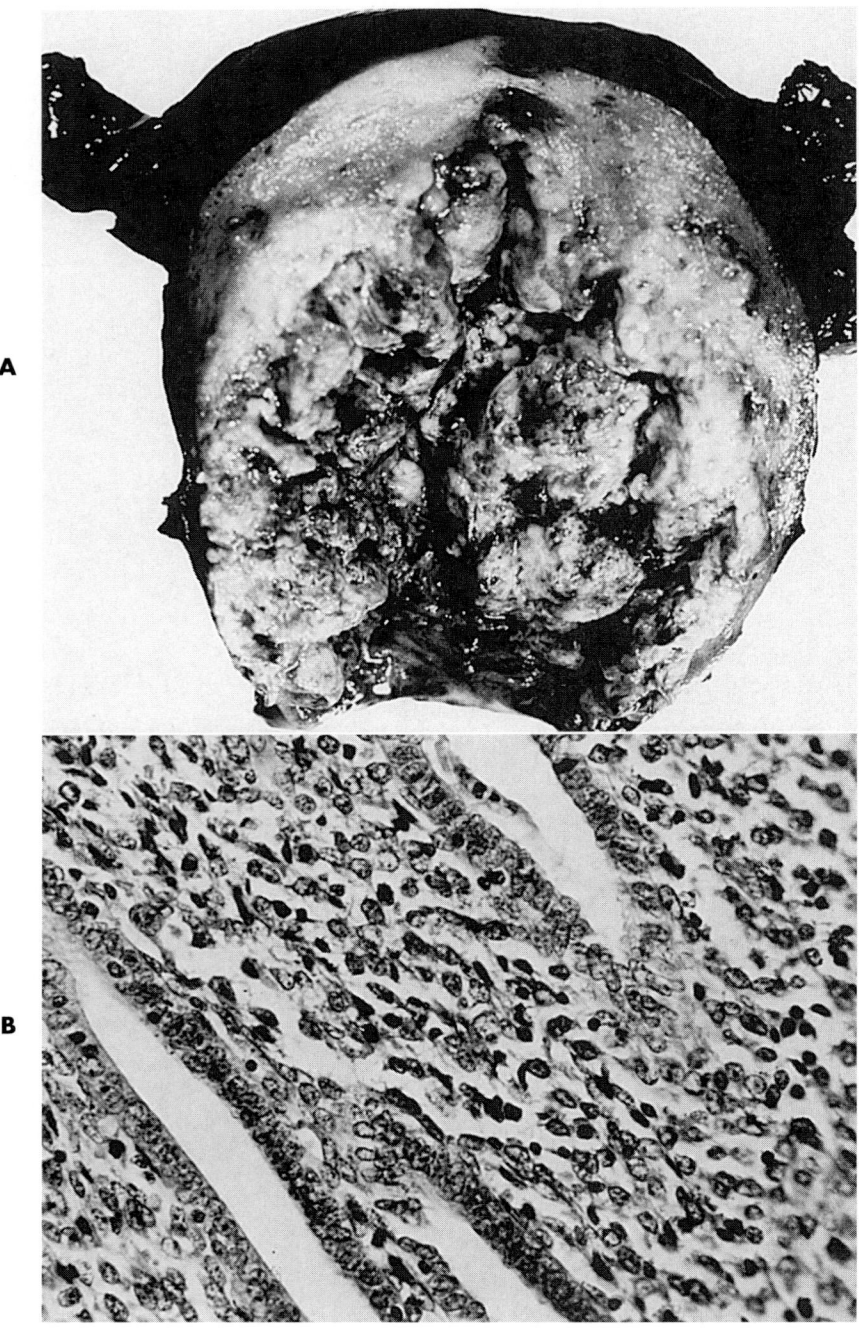

Fig. 19-104 **A,** High-grade endometrial stromal sarcoma replacing entire endometrial cavity. **B,** Same lesion shown in **A**. Note uniform cells, vesicular nuclei, and fine nucleoli. Mitotic figures, not seen here, were numerous in other areas of neoplasm. Patient died with pelvic recurrence and distant metastases 4 months after surgery.

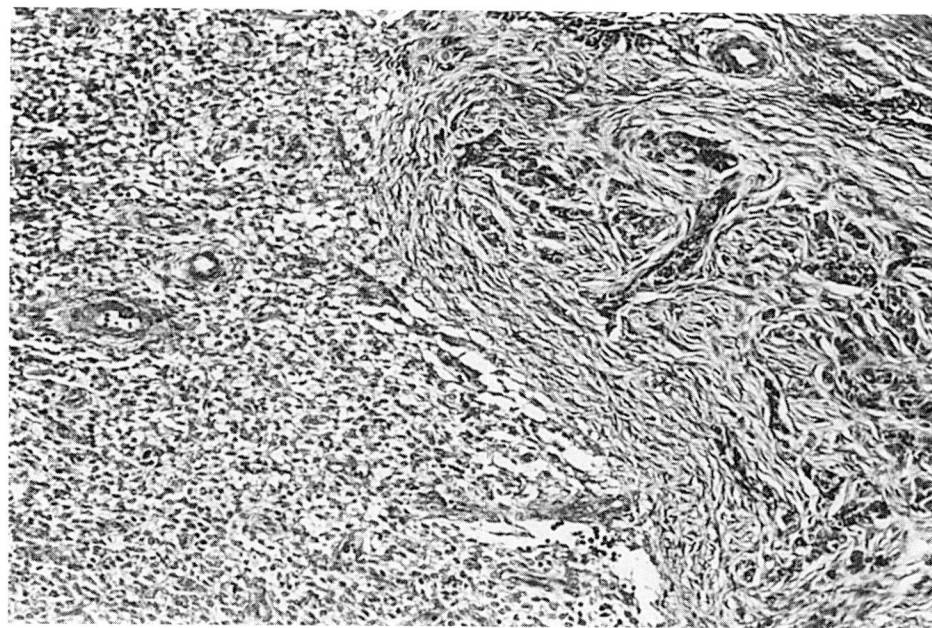

Fig. 19-105 Endometrial stromal tumor containing formations resembling sex-cord structures. There is sharp separation between the two components.

The previously mentioned epithelium-like formations may appear in endometrial stromal tumors in the form of solid masses, glandular structures, or anastomosing cords. The nature of these formations is not clear. Clement and Scully[350] have likened them to those of ovarian sex-cord neoplasms (particularly granulosa cell tumors) and have referred to the tumors containing them as *uterine tumors resembling ovarian sex-cord tumors* (Fig. 19-105). Others have suggested a smooth muscle derivation, based on ultrastructural and immunohistochemical findings.[366,374] Uterine tumors in which these structures predominate have invariably behaved in a benign fashion.[350] The uterine neoplasm known as *plexiform tumor* or *tumorlet* and variously claimed to be of endometrial stromal,[365] myofibroblastic,[359] and smooth muscle derivation[361,363] is a closely related variation, and it is therefore not surprising that similar histogenetic arguments have been raised (Plate XIII-F). The ultrastructural[361] and immunohistochemical evidence (actin and desmin positivity[348,365]) clearly points toward a smooth muscle nature. This lesion is always an incidental finding, it usually measures less than 1 cm, and its behavior is always benign.

A different type of epithelium-like formation than can be seen in endometrial stromal tumor is represented by endometrioid glandular foci having a benign, atypical, or carcinomatous appearance.[351]

Tumors with the appearance of endometrial stromal neoplasms may be found in the cervix,[368] ovary (see p. 1522), pelvis, and retroperitoneum.[378] Some of these are seen in association with endometriosis, from which presumably they have arisen.[372]

Malignant mixed müllerian tumor (mixed mesodermal tumor)

Malignant mixed müllerian tumors are rare uterine neoplasms that are seen practically always in postmenopausal patients, although exceptions occur.[383] They present with uterine bleeding and enlargement. The usual location is the uterine body, particularly the posterior wall in the region of the fundus.[380,398,400] Grossly, they present as large, soft, polypoid growths involving the endometrium and myometrium, sometimes protruding from the cervix (Fig. 19-106). Foci of necrosis and hemorrhage are common.

Microscopically, the characteristic feature is the *admixture of carcinomatous and sarcoma-like elements,* resulting in a characteristic biphasic appearance. The carcinomatous component is usually of glandular type, whether endometrioid, clear cell, or papillary serous.[403] As a rule, it is of poorly differentiated appearance and high-grade nature; therefore a careful search for stromal elements should be carried out whenever such patterns are found in an endometrial D&C, particularly if accompanied by extensive necrosis and hemorrhage. Squamous cell, undifferentiated, and primitive neurectodermal patterns may also be seen.[391] The appearance of the sarcomatous component is the basis for the time-honored division of these neoplasms into a homologous and a heterologous variety. In the former, the malignant stroma is formed by either round cells resembling those of the endometrial stroma or by spindle cells resembling leiomyosarcoma or fibrosarcoma. In the latter, specific heterologous mesenchymal elements (such as skeletal muscle, cartilage, bone, or fat) also are present (Fig. 19-107). Identification of cross striations, or of skeletal muscle markers by immunocytochemistry,[397] is required to document the presence of a rhabdomyosarcomatous component (Figs. 19-108 to 19-110). The distinction between these two varieties may require the study of numerous sections and therefore may not be possible on material obtained by curettage. Actually, the malignant stroma may be so inconspicuous in such a specimen as to be missed altogether, the lesion being misdiagnosed as an ordinary adenocarcinoma. This is particularly the case for the peritoneal metastases, in which the stromal component is often scanty or altogether absent. Since the epithelial elements can form papillae and be accompanied by psammoma bodies, a confusion with metastatic papillary serous cystadenocarcinoma from the ovary may occur. Parenthetically, cases have been reported of coexistent uterine malignant mixed müllerian tumor and ovarian serous adenocarcinoma.[394a] Exceptionally, a rhabdoid component is present.[396a]

The very fact that it is the epithelial component of the tumor that shows the most capability for invasion and metastases suggests that these tumors should be primarily regarded as carcinomas rather than sarcomas, employing a reasoning analogous to that currently accepted for carcinomas with sarcoma-like stroma of the upper aerodigestive tract and other sites.[381,403,405a] Immunohistochemical and ultrastructural studies support this view: Keratin is always detectable in the epithelial areas, but is also present in the sarcomatous component in over half of the cases[390]; by electron microscopy, hybrid epithelial/stromal cells coexist with those having purely epithelial or stromal features.[384,396] An additional supportive finding is the concordant pattern of p53 staining in the carcinomatous and sarcomatous areas, which would be difficult to explain if these tumors were biclonal.[381a,395]

Malignant mixed müllerian tumors are easily distinguished from teratomas by their occurrence in an older age group and by the absence of skin appendages, glia, thyroid, and other tissue; it should be noted, however, that they may exceptionally contain neuroectodermal elements.[391] They should also be clearly separated from botryoid rhabdomyosarcoma (sarcoma botryoides). The latter term should be reserved for the tumor of childhood or adolescence arising from the cervix or vagina and lacking a carcinomatous component.

Mixed müllerian tumors are highly aggressive neoplasms, more so than even the higher grades and the more unfavorable variants of endometrial carcinoma.[389] Extension into the pelvis, lymphatic and vascular permeation, and distant lymph-borne and blood-borne metastases are common. If the tumor has extended to the serosa of the uterus or beyond at the time of surgery, the prognosis is hopeless.[392] The only patients with some chance of cure are those in whom the tumor is restricted to the inner half of the myometrium

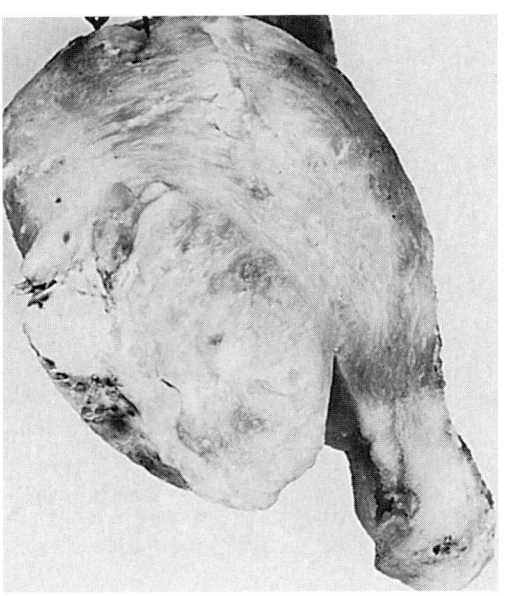

Fig. 19-106 Polypoid malignant mixed müllerian tumor of uterus. Metastases in peritoneal cavity appeared 1 year following surgery.

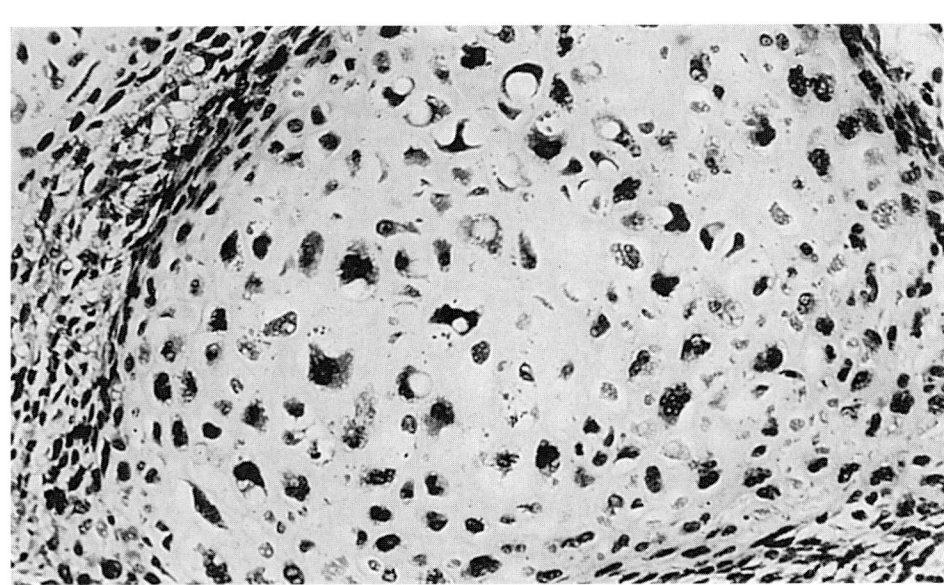

Fig. 19-107 Area of cartilaginous differentiation in malignant mixed müllerian tumor shown in Fig. 19-106.

at the time of surgery. This determination implies a thorough sampling of the hysterectomy specimen by the pathologist.

In many series, tumors having only homologous stromal elements (called "carcinosarcomas" by Norris and Taylor[400]) have been found to have a slightly better prognosis than those with heterologous elements, a fact that may justify their separation.[393,398,400,402] It should be pointed out, however, that the difference between the two is small, in some series absent altogether, and far outweighed by the stage of the disease.[382,388,405] Total abdominal hysterectomy with bilateral salpingo-oophorectomy and pelvic lymphadenectomy is the treatment of choice. The response to radiation therapy and chemotherapy has been generally poor, although some encouraging reports have appeared.[394] The most common sites of recurrent disease are lung and abdominal cavity.[404]

Norris and Taylor[399] made the disturbing observation that 30% of the patients with heterologous malignant mixed müllerian tumors and 13% of those with homologous tumors that they studied had a history of previous irradiation to the pelvic area, usually given for some benign disorder. The median interval between irradiation and the time of diagnosis of the tumor was 16.4 years both in their series and in that of Doss et al.[386] Postirradiation uterine sarcomas tend to occur in a younger age group and spread earlier to the pelvis than comparable tumors not related to irradiation.[387,406]

Mixed müllerian tumors and other sarcomas of the endometrial stroma have also been seen in association with

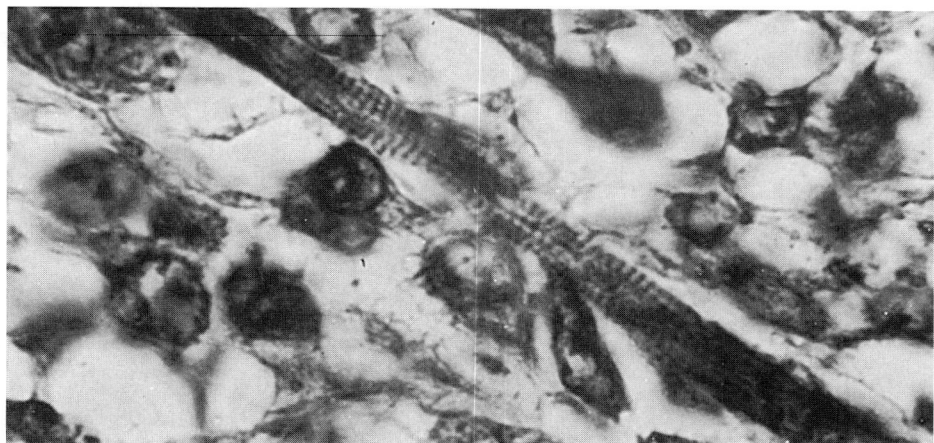

Fig. 19-108 Striated muscle cells in malignant mixed müllerian tumor.

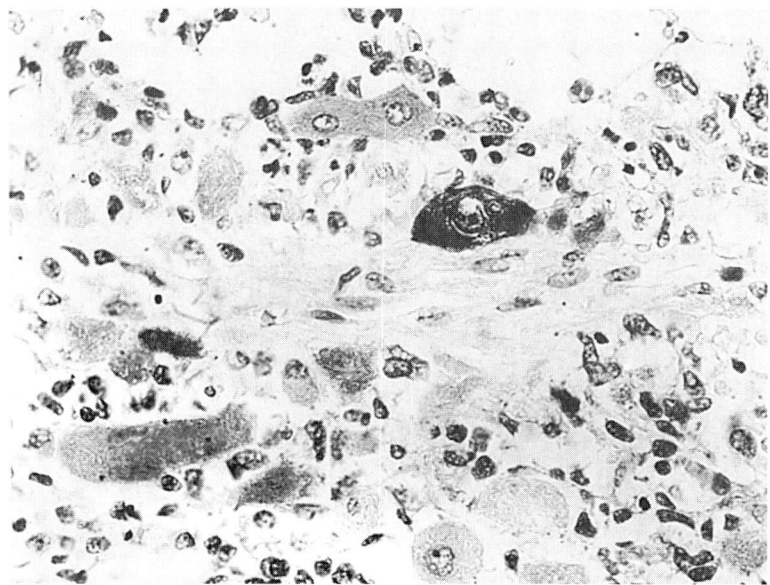

Fig. 19-109 Rhabdomyosarcomatous component in mixed müllerian tumor demonstrated by myoglobin stain with immunoperoxidase technique.

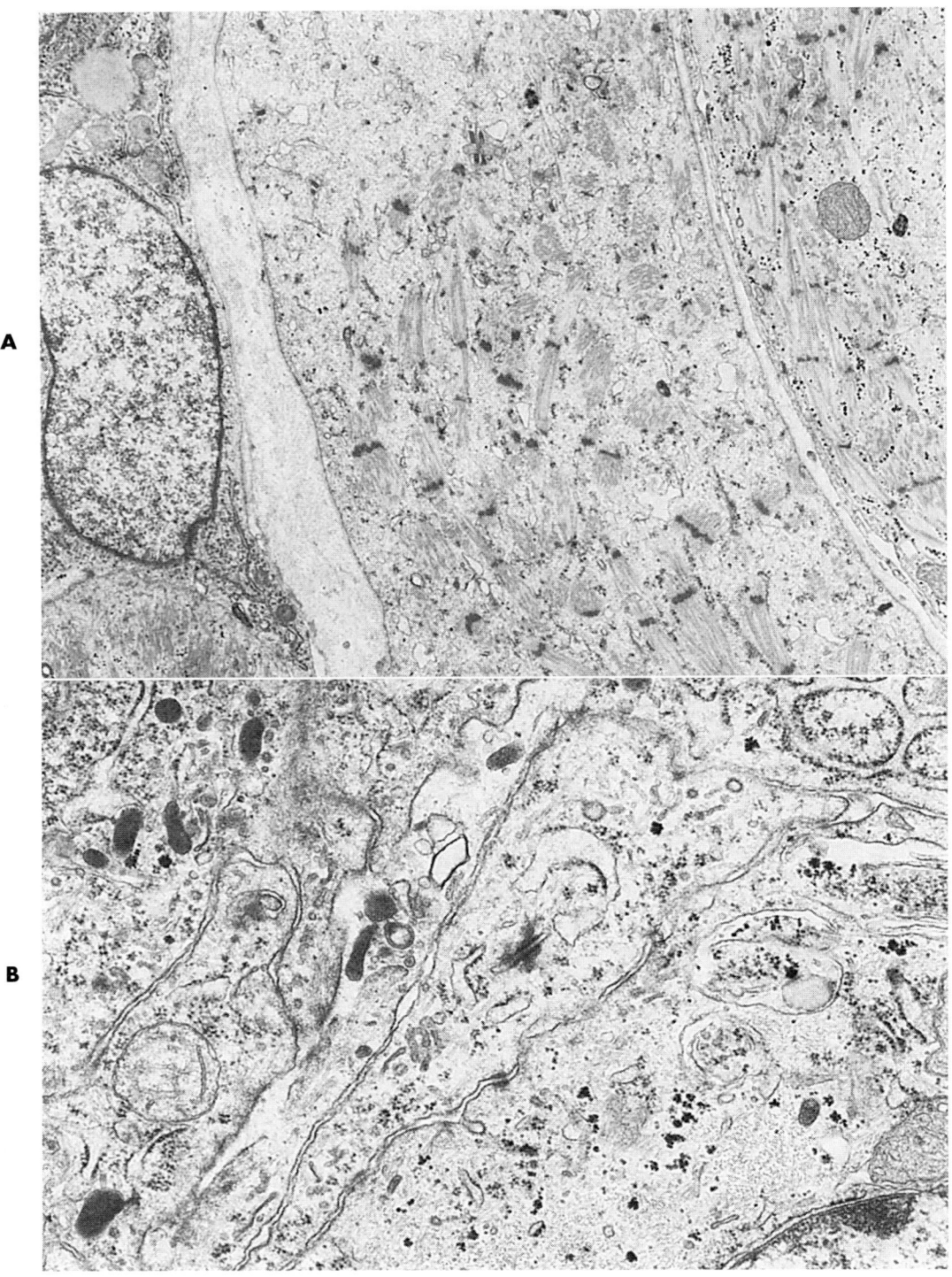

Fig. 19-110 Mixed müllerian tumor of uterine cervix with area of rhabdomyosarcomatous differentiation. A, Note Z-band formation. B, Area showing epithelial differentiation; paranuclear microfilaments
similar to those of endometrial carcinoma are present.

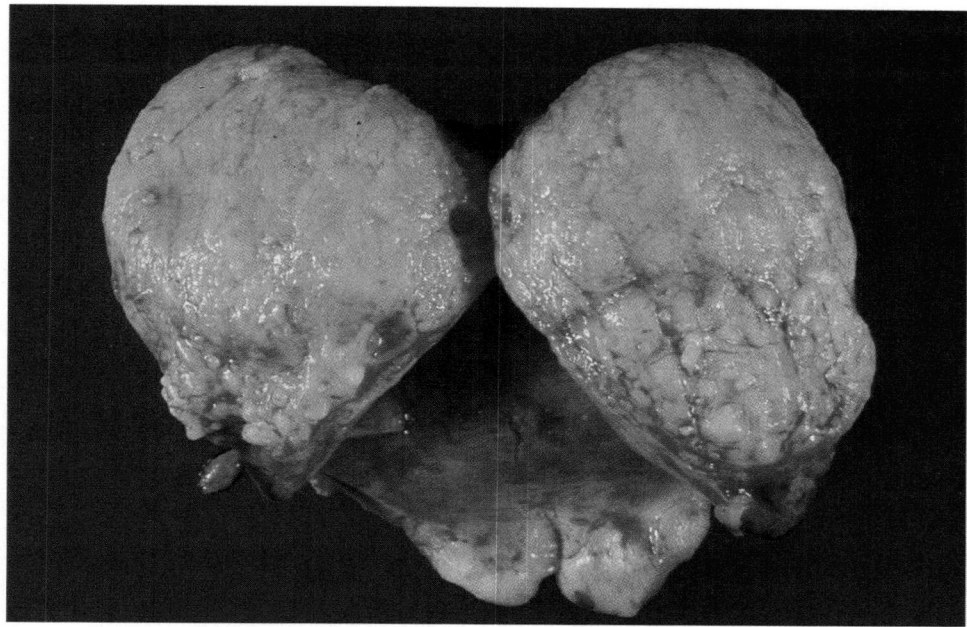

Fig. 19-111 Müllerian adenosarcoma. The tumor shows a lesser degree of necrosis and hemorrhage than the usual malignant mixed müllerian tumor.

chronic estrogenic stimulation (ovarian thecoma, polycystic ovarian disease, and prolonged estrogen therapy).[401]

These tumors can arise in extrauterine locations, the most common sites being ovary and pelvic structures.[392] Their morphologic and immunohistochemical features are similar to those of their uterine counterparts.[385]

Müllerian adenosarcoma and related tumors

Müllerian adenosarcoma is a distinctive type of uterine tumor, generally regarded as a low-grade variant of mixed müllerian tumor.[409,412,414,418] Like the latter, it usually presents in elderly individuals as a bulky polypoid growth filling the endometrial cavity, less commonly as an intramural nodule (Fig. 19-111). Microscopically, it is also composed of an admixture of epithelial and stromal elements. Its distinguishing feature is the fact that the epithelial (glandular) component appears benign, giving to the lesion a striking similarity to phylloides tumor of the breast (Fig. 19-112). The stromal elements usually resemble endometrial stroma by light and electron microscopic examination.[415,419] As a rule, they do not appear as bizarre and undifferentiated as in the classic mixed müllerian tumor, although multinucleated giant cells and heterologous elements occur in about 20% of the cases. The latter are usually of skeletal muscle type, but peculiar components such as angiosarcoma have also been observed.[407,421] Extensive areas of stromal fibrosis may result in a deceptively benign appearance.[412]

We prefer to view müllerian adenosarcomas not as a type of mixed müllerian tumor but rather as a variant of endometrial stromal sarcoma having the capacity to induce the formation and/or proliferation of glands. Support for this interpretation comes from the fact that sex-cord–like differentiation (a well-known feature of endometrial stromal sarcomas) has been occasionally found in them.[411,417] Additional support is provided by the cases in which a typical adenosarcoma is overgrown by a pure sarcoma having a higher grade and exhibiting a higher mitotic rate than the sarcomatous component of the associated adenosarcoma. This development is analogous to that well known to occur in phylloides tumor of the breast, a fact that strengthens the analogy between the two models. These *müllerian adenosarcomas with sarcomatous overgrowth* behave in an aggressive fashion and are often associated with postoperative recurrence or metastases and a fatal outcome.[408,418]

Uterine adenofibroma and the related conditions papillary adenofibroma, papillary cystadenofibroma, lipoadenofibroma, adenomyomatosis[416,417a,420,424,426-428] are regarded as the benign counterparts of müllerian adenosarcoma, but the dividing line between the two groups is not sharp (Fig. 19-113). As a matter of fact, tumors with the characteristic features of uterine adenofibroma have occasionally been found to invade myometrium and pelvic veins.[413] The problems in separating them are analogous to those encountered in trying to separate benign from malignant phylloides tumors of the breast. Criteria found to be useful in separating müllerian adenosarcomas from müllerian adenofibromas include two or more stromal mitoses per ten high-power fields, marked stromal cellularity, and significant stromal cell atypia.[409] Cases have been reported of papillary adenofibroma involved by adenocarcinoma.[422]

Like mixed müllerian tumors and endometrial stromal sarcomas, müllerian adenosarcomas can be seen outside the uterine corpus. Cases have been described in the cervix, ovary, round and broad ligaments, and pelvic wall.[410,425]

A tumor purported to be the morphologic counterpart of müllerian adenosarcoma—i.e., composed of malignant epithelium and benign stroma—has been reported under terms such as *müllerian carcinofibroma* or *carcinomesenchymoma*.[423] The analogy is ingenious but probably unwarrented.

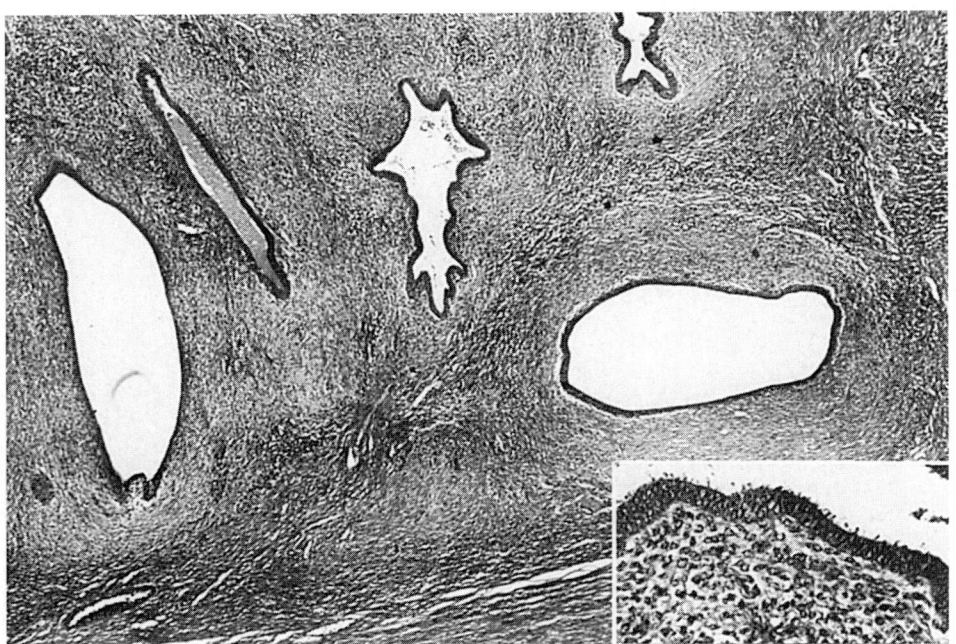

Fig. 19-112 Müllerian adenosarcoma. Glands have proliferative but benign appearance. They are surrounded by extremely cellular stroma, better seen in **inset.**

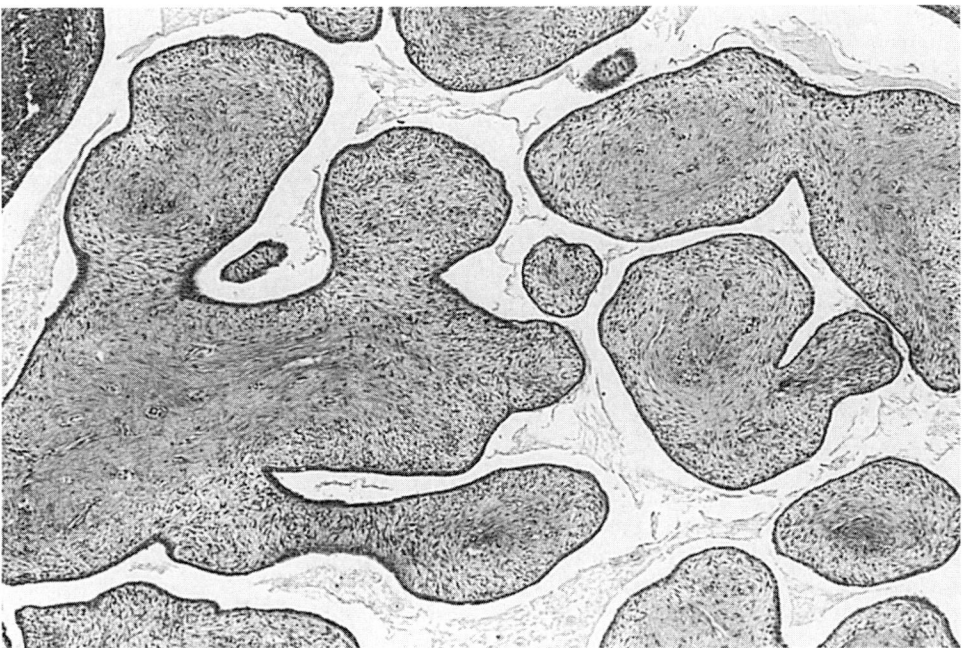

Fig. 19-113 Uterine adenofibroma. Low-power appearance is very reminiscent of phylloides tumor of breast. Stromal component is cellular but microscopically benign.

Leiomyoma

Leiomyomas of the uterus are extremely common neoplasms. The overall incidence is between 4% and 11%, but it rises to nearly 40% in women over the age of 50 years. Clinically apparent lesions are less common in parous than nulliparous women and premenopausal than postmenopausal women.[456] They are much more common in black women, in whom they have a tendency to be very numerous (Fig. 19-114).

Many of these tumors are small and go undetected; a systematic and meticulous study of 100 consecutive hysterectomy specimens revealed leiomyomas in 77 of them, 84% of the tumors being multicentric.[434]

These tumors occur subserosally, intramurally, or submucosally (Figs. 19-114 to 19-117) and produce symptoms referable to their size and location. They may become large enough to block the ureters, interfere with pregnancy, or cause inflammatory complications. In rare instances, uterine leiomyomas have been associated with polycythemia, which regressed after the tumor was excised.[451]

Submucosal tumors often result in secondary endometrial changes that range from gland distortion to atrophy and ulceration. They may fill the endometrial cavity and emerge from the cervical canal as polypoid growths ("myoma nascens") (Fig. 19-118). Under these circumstances, their surface is usually ulcerated and infected, the gross appearance thus simulating that of a malignant neoplasm.

It is difficult to make a diagnosis of leiomyoma when only a few small fragments of smooth muscle are present in a curettage specimen. Unless these fragments show an obvious increase in cellularity or definite hyaline changes, one is unable in most instances to decide whether they originated in a submucosal leiomyoma or whether they represent normal superficial myometrium curetted out by a vigorous operator.

Grossly, the cut surface of a typical leiomyoma has a raw silk appearance. Microscopically, the tumor is formed by interlacing bundles of smooth muscle cells separated by a greater or lesser amount of well-vascularized connective tissue. Ultrastructurally, the features are those of smooth muscle cells with varying degrees of differentiation.[444] The stroma may contain a scattering of lymphocytes. Mast cells

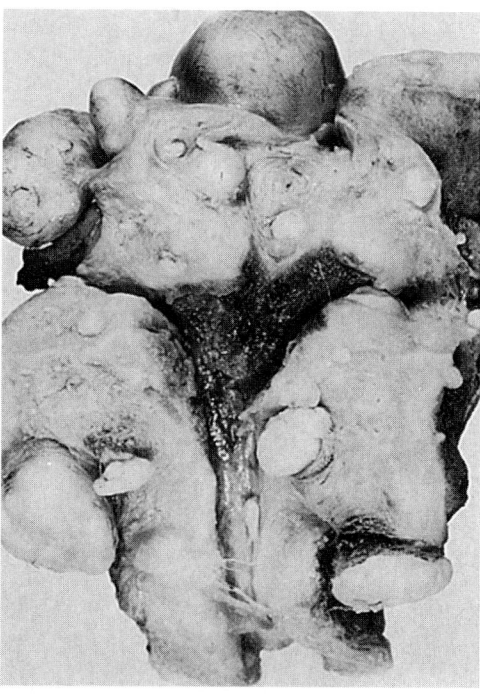

Fig. 19-114 Innumerable leiomyomas of uterus.

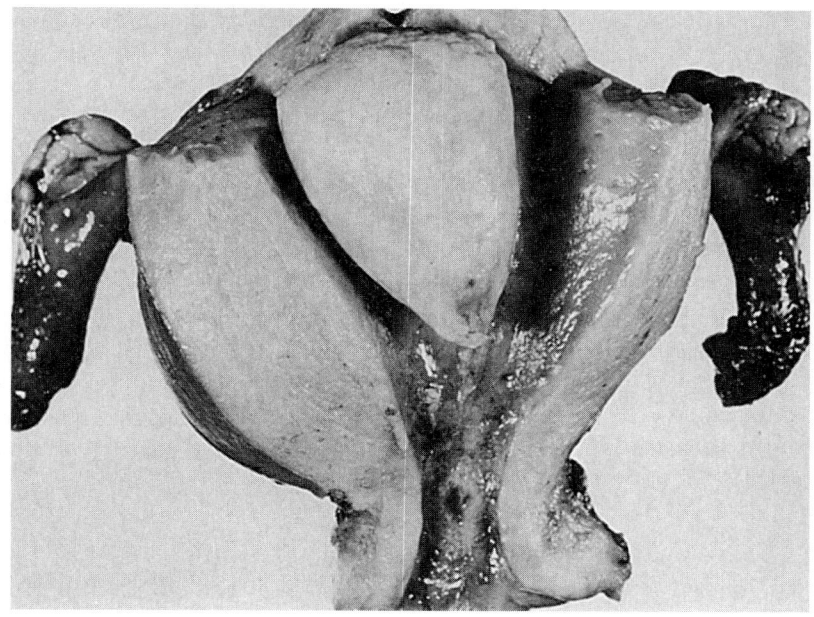

Fig. 19-115 Single leiomyoma growing within endometrial cavity and causing prominent signs and symptoms because of its location.

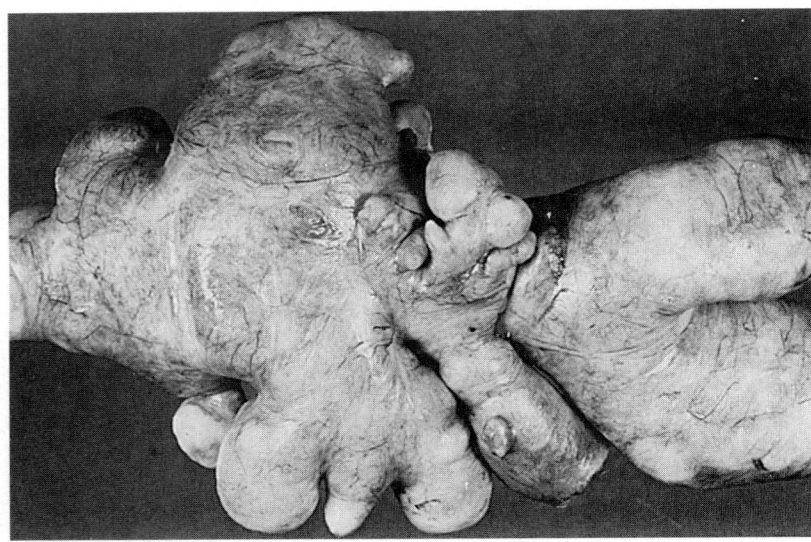

Fig. 19-116 Huge leiomyoma weighing over 1500 g growing mainly within peritoneal cavity.

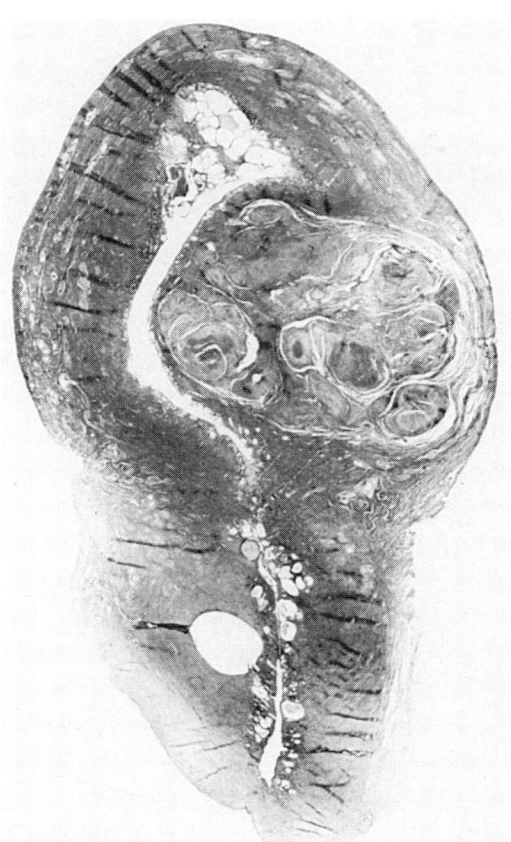

Fig. 19-117 Whole-mount section of hysterectomy specimen showing large leiomyoma in intramural and submucous location. Endometrium shows cystic atrophy. (Courtesy Dr. C. Perez-Mesa, Columbia, MO.)

are often conspicuous in contrast with leiomyomas of other sites.[445a,446a]

Cytogenetic alterations are common in uterine leiomyomas. The most consistent are rearrangements of 6p, del(7q), +12, and +(12:14).[441,452]

The treatment of uterine leiomyomas (including that of most of the many variants listed later) varies depending on the size and number of lesions, the age of the patient, and her desire to have children. Most asymptomatic leiomyomas need not be excised. Malignant transformation, if it happens at all, is such a rare event in these tumors that for practical purposes it can be disregarded. Symptomatic neoplasms can be treated by hysterectomy or, in the case of patients who desire to become pregnant, by myomectomy.[430] Medical therapy includes administration of gonadotropin-releasing hormone analogues, such as leuprolide acetate depot. This may result in a decrease in the size of the leiomyoma—probably as a result of ischemic injury and cellular atrophy—but it does not result in significant pleomorphism or increased mitotic activity.[433,437,439]

Leiomyoma variants

Many variations of the basic theme previously described exist. Most of these are the result of secondary changes and are detectable in approximately 65% of the cases. These include hyaline degeneration (63%), mucoid or myxomatous degeneration (19%), calcification (8%), cystic changes (4%), and fatty metamorphosis (3%). There is no relation between symptomatology and the presence of these changes.[457]

Red degeneration (present in 3% of the cases) can result in abdominal pain, vomiting, and fever. This change is characterized by extensive coagulative necrosis and is often associated with pregnancy or the use of contraceptive drugs (Fig. 19-119).

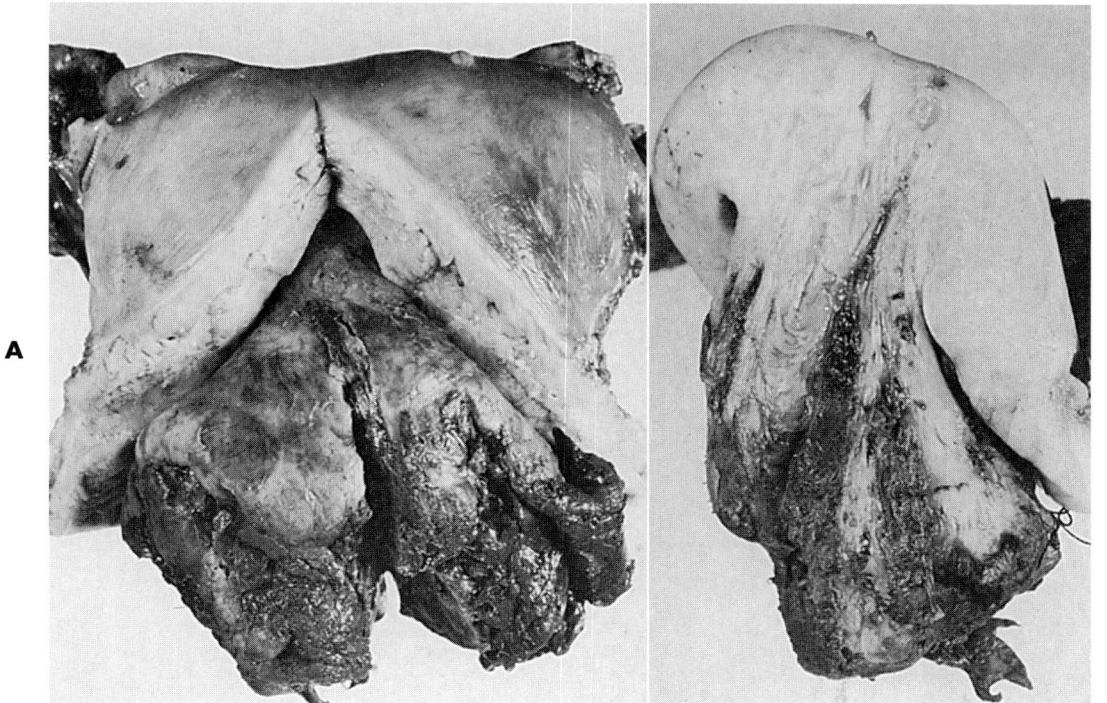

Fig. 19-118 A, Large submucosal leiomyoma presenting as polypoid mass in cervical canal and upper vagina. Note necrotic ulcerated surface. **B,** Gross section shows that tumor is implanted in fundus and has, in deep portion, typical appearance of leiomyoma.

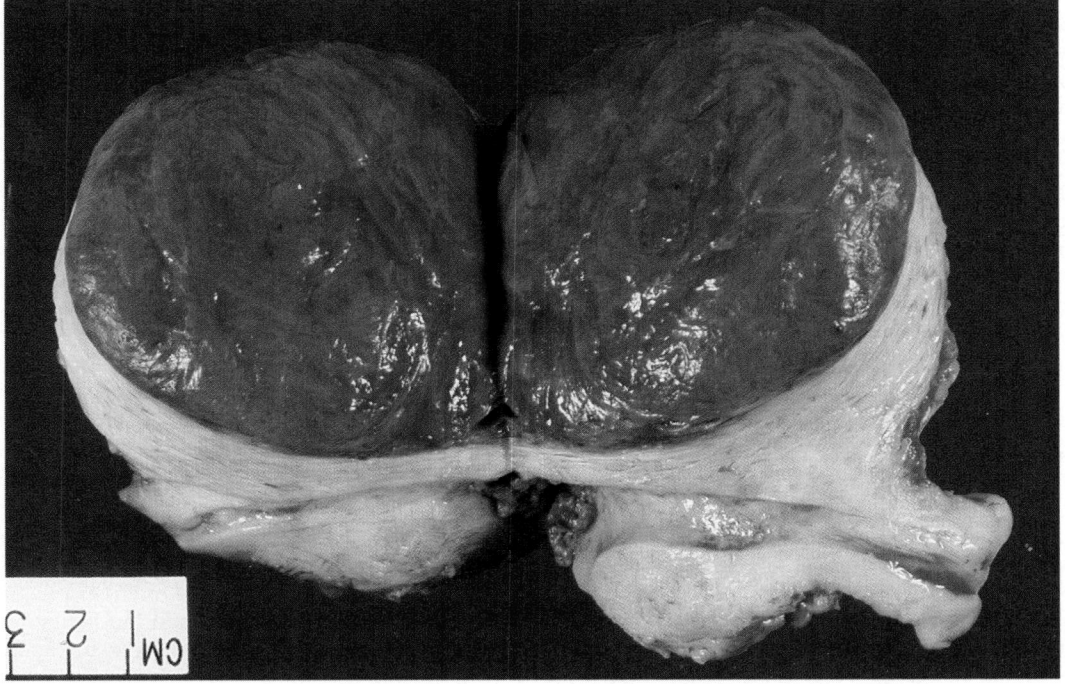

Fig. 19-119 This leiomyoma has undergone massive red degeneration.

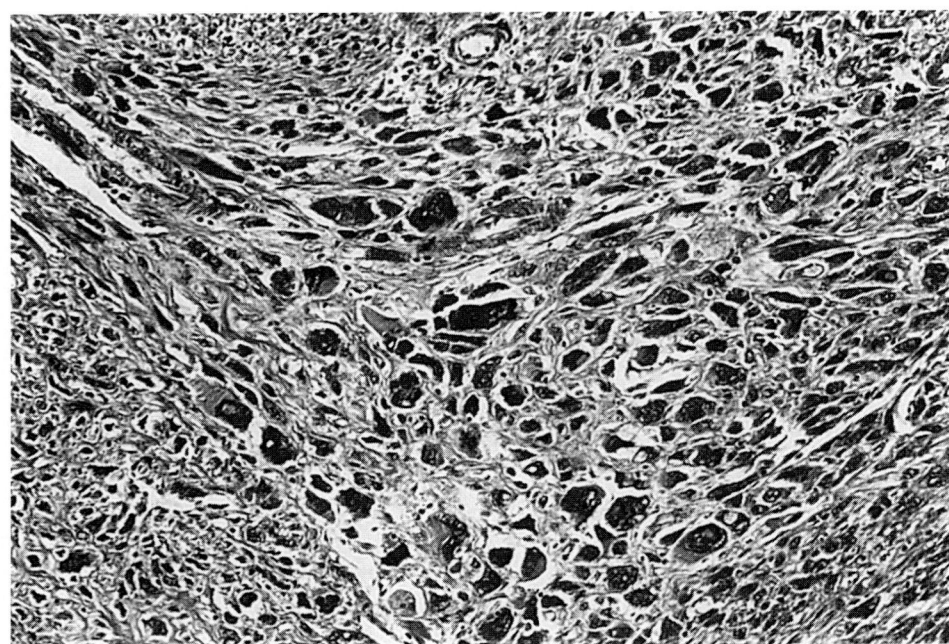

Fig. 19-120 So-called symplasmic leiomyoma. Huge hyperchromatic nuclei are present in many of tumor cells, but mitotic activity is nil. This lesion is benign and should not be overdiagnosed as leiomyosarcoma.

Apoplectic leiomyoma is pathogenetically related to red degeneration. It is seen in patients taking birth-control pills and is characterized by stellate zones of recent hemorrhage within nodules of hypercellular smooth muscle, with few or no mitotic figures.[450]

Hydropic degeneration is characterized by the accumulation of edema fluid, often associated with collagen deposition. The appearance may simulate intravenous leiomyomatosis or myxoid leiomyosarcoma.[432]

Leiomyoma with lymphoid infiltration may simulate a malignant lymphoma because of the massiveness of the inflammatory component, which is made up of small lymphocytes, immunoblasts, and plasma cells. Germinal centers may be present. The surrounding myometrium is relatively unaffected.[436,438]

Cellular leiomyoma is a term reserved for those tumors having increased cellularity but neither atypical features nor an excessive number of mitotic figures. Their natural history seems to be the same as for the ordinary leiomyoma. The differential diagnosis includes leiomyosarcoma and endometrial stromal neoplasms.[455a]

Atypical, bizarre, symplasmic or pleomorphic leiomyoma contains bizarre tumor cells with variation in size and shape, hyperchromatic nuclei, and multinucleated forms but no increased mitotic activity (Fig. 19-120). Rarely, the entire tumor is composed of such cells. It may occur spontaneously but is often seen in patients taking progestin compounds.[435,459]

Mitotically active leiomyoma refers to tumors having from five to fifteen mitotic figures per ten high-power fields but lacking cytologic atypia.[455,460] They are discussed in more detail on p. 1435.

Leiomyolipoma contains an admixture of smooth muscle and mature adipose tissue.[443,458,460a] It is believed that this tumor and the even rarer *lipoma* result from adipose metaplasia in leiomyomas.[458]

Palisaded leiomyoma is characterized by a degree of nuclear palisading such as to simulate a neurilemoma.

Benign leiomyoblastoma (clear cell or epithelioid leiomyoma) is partially or totally composed of rounded or polygonal cells, its appearance being similar to that of its more common counterpart in the gastrointestinal tract (Fig. 19-121). Mixtures of epithelioid, clear cell, and plexiform patterns occur frequently enough to suggest that they represent variants of a single entity.[442,445] A transition to typical smooth muscle is sometimes observed. Ultrastructural studies have also provided support for the smooth muscle derivation of this peculiar neoplasm, as well as for several other myometrial tumors of unusual appearance.[448,449]

Parasitic leiomyoma is the term given to the uterine leiomyoma that has become separate from the uterus and has acquired vascular connections with the omentum, pelvic wall, or other intra-abdominal sites, such as the cecal wall.

Leiomyoma with skeletal muscle differentiation has been reported in a single instance.[447]

Diffuse leiomyomatosis is the term given to involvement of almost the entire myometrium by innumerable, ill-defined leiomyomas, many of microscopic size.[431,449a] This extremely rare condition should be distinguished from the nebulous *primary myometrial hypertrophy* or *myometrial hyperplasia,* defined as a uterus weighing over 120 g in the absence of any myometrial lesion.[434a,446]

Intravenous leiomyomatosis is an extremely rare condition characterized by the growth of mature smooth muscle

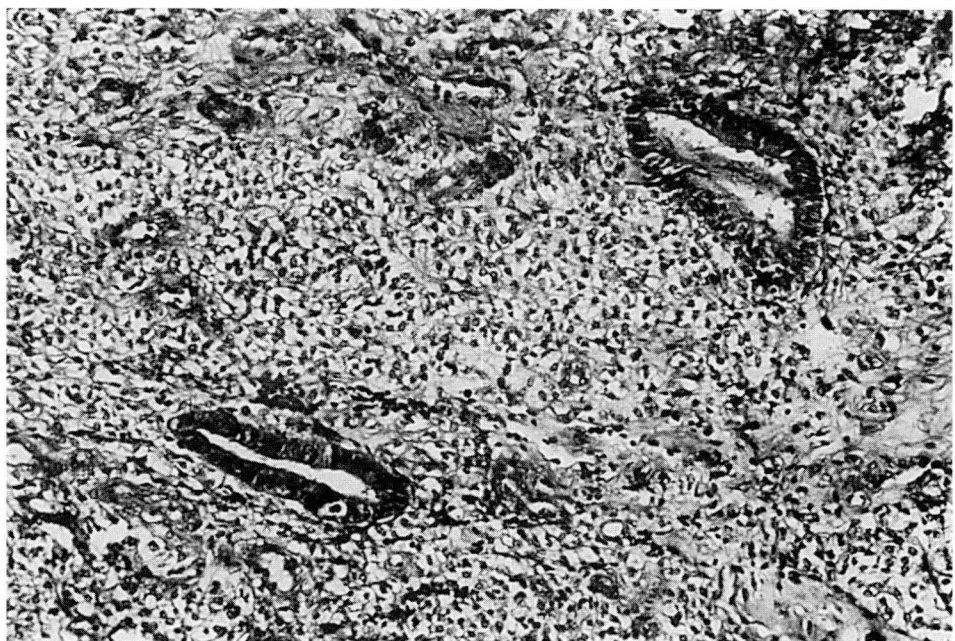

Fig. 19-121 Leiomyoblastoma showing diffuse infiltration of endometrial stroma and entrapment of endometrial glands. Tumor cells have clear cytoplasm and well-defined cell membranes. Immunocytochemistry for desmin was strongly positive. It is rare for leimyoblastoma to infiltrate endometrium diffusely in this fashion.

inside the lumen of uterine and pelvic veins[440,454] (Fig. 19-122). It is often associated with typical uterine leiomyomas, and it may arise from them.[453] The clinical and gross features are similar to those of the form of endometrial sarcoma traditionally known as endolymphatic stromal myosis, except for the fact that grossly apparent involvement of veins is more prominent. The distinction is microscopic— intravenous leiomyomatosis is composed of elongated smooth muscle cells, whereas the former condition is made up of round or oval endometrial stromal cells. The two processes may well be histogenetically related in view of the occurrence of occasional hybrids (combined muscle-stromal tumors) and the close kinship between the endometrial stroma and the myometrial smooth muscle. Mitotic figures are rare or absent. The vessel permeation often extends to vessels in the broad ligament and in uterine and iliac veins; from there, it can proceed along the vena cava and even reach the right atrium.[430a] However, distant metastases are exceptionally rare, and the long-term prognosis is excellent.[449b] Cases have been described in which the microscopic appearance of the intravenous masses was that of leiomyolipomas.[429]

Leiomyosarcoma

Leiomyosarcomas occur in an older average age group than leiomyomas (median age, 54 years). The time-honored assumption that most leiomyosarcomas arise from preexisting leiomyomas is probably incorrect. The fact that in one large series 67% of the leiomyosarcomas were solitary militates against this possibility.[482] Some leiomyosarcomas are grossly similar to ordinary leiomyomas, but the majority are soft or fleshy, with necrotic or hemorrhagic areas and signs of invasiveness[466] (Fig. 19-123).

Microscopically, they are hypercellular tumors composed of oval to spindle cells with the morphologic, ultrastructural, and immunohistochemical features of smooth muscle cells; actin and myosin are consistently present in their cytoplasm[475] (Fig. 19-124).

An important microscopic criterion in the distinction between uterine leiomyomas and leiomyosarcomas is the number of mitotic figures. Tumors with fewer than five mitoses per ten high-power fields ($\times 675$) in the most active areas behave practically always as benign tumors, even in the presence of atypical cells, hyperchromatic nuclei, and multinucleated forms. Conversely, most tumors with ten or more mitoses per ten high-power fields behave as malignant neoplasms, even if atypia is minimal (but see the exceptions in the subsequent discussion). The behavior of tumors with five to nine mitoses per ten high-power fields is less predictable, but a certain number will metastasize.[472] Fortunately, only a small minority of uterine smooth muscle tumors belong to this gray zone. They are designated as *smooth muscle tumors of undetermined, intermediate, or borderline category.* The acronym *STUMP* (smooth muscle tumor of unknown or undetermined malignant potential) has been used in some circles as an alternative term.

Mitotic count in uterine smooth muscle tumors has been criticized because of its apparent lack of standardization and reproducibility.[480] There is little question that it can be influenced by a variety of factors, such as the thickness of the slide, microscope magnification, tumor sampling, and observer's criteria for mitoses.[468] Apparently, the interval

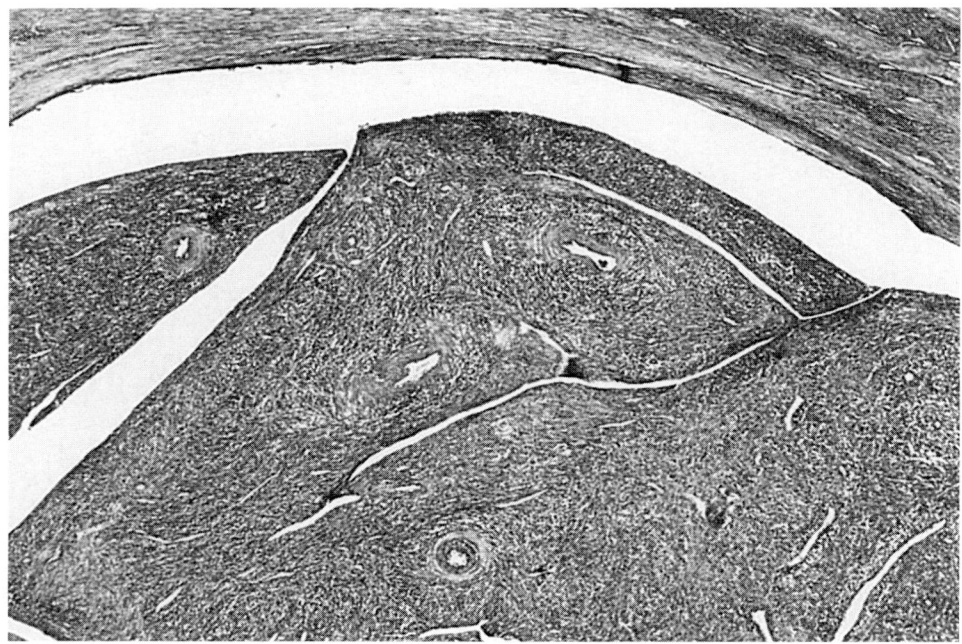

Fig. 19-122 Intravenous leiomyomatosis. Large vein located in subserosal region of uterus is filled by polypoid mass composed of smooth muscle mass. Thick-walled blood vessels are prominent within this mass.

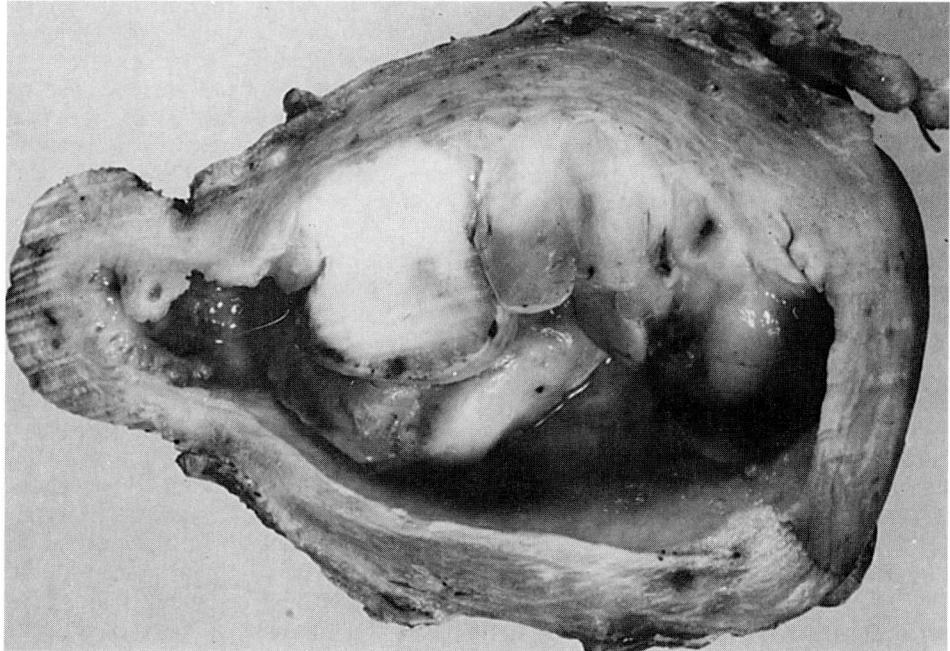

Fig. 19-123 Large polypoid leiomyosarcoma in 69-year-old woman. Patient died 2 years later with metastatic disease.

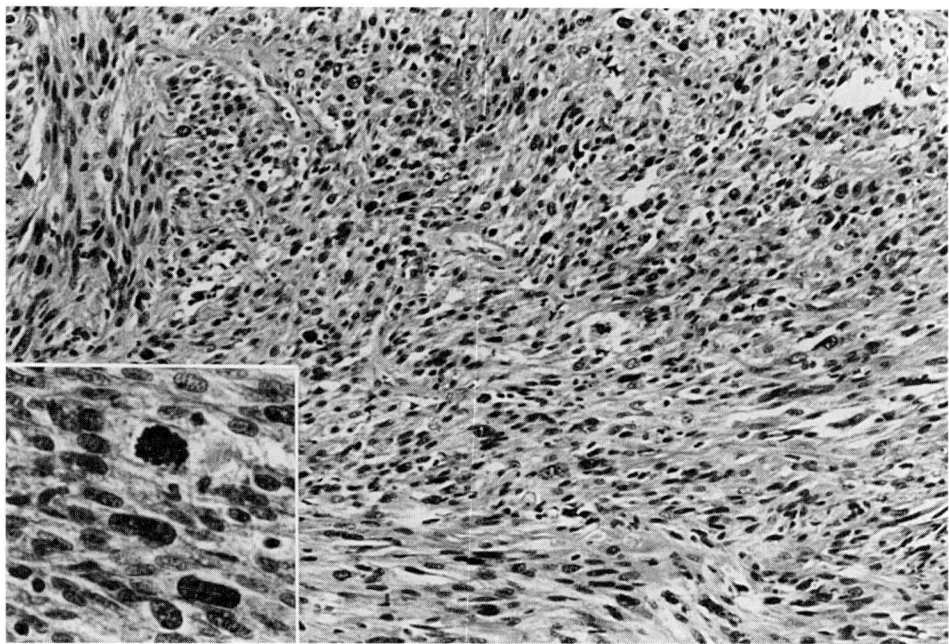

Fig. 19-124 Uterine leiomyosarcoma. This highly cellular tumor shows nuclear atypically and high mitotic activity. **Inset** shows abnormal mitotic figure and several deeply hyperchromatic nuclei.

between excision and fixation is not important.[470] A common mistake is to misinterpret small pyknotic nuclei from smooth muscle cells, mast cells, or lymphocytes as mitoses. A good practice is to scan the sections for a very active area, do the counting in ten consecutive fields in that area, and repeat the procedure a minimum of four times. An ample number of blocks should be taken in borderline tumors. Kempson[469] recommends at least ten sections or one section for each centimeter of diameter, whichever is greater. The section should have a thickness as close as possible to 5 µm. "High-power magnification" is meant to imply a 10× eyepiece and a 40× objective. Only unquestionable mitotic figures should be counted as such. If these conditions are scrupulously observed, mitotic counting will remain as an important microscopic criterion for the distinction between leiomyoma and leiomyosarcoma, at least in the uterus.[469,471b] In most cases, however, high mitotic activity is accompanied by one or more of the following features: hypercellularity, tumor cell necrosis, extensive myxoid stroma, giant cell formation, pleomorphism, and hyperchromasia.[471]

The trend in recent times has been to move from exclusive reliance on mitotic count to an approach that incorporates additional histopathologic characteristics such as cytologic atypia and coagulative tumor cell necrosis. For instance, we and others have seen cases of uterine smooth muscle tumors (most of them in young patients) that were *grossly and microscopically* typical of leiomyomas; yet focally they had a mitotic count ranging from five to fifteen per ten high-power fields. Under these circumstances, we have elected not to designate these tumors as leiomyosarcomas but rather as *mitotically active leiomyomas* (see p. 1432). An exception of an opposite sort to the foregoing statements regarding mitotic counts is the *metastasizing leiomyoma*, in which an apparently benign uterine smooth muscle tumor (with little or no mitotic activity) is accompanied by nodules in the lungs or regional lymph nodes having the same histologic appearance.[461,481,483] Inadequate sampling may account for some of the discrepancies; also, the possibility of the pulmonary tumors representing independent neoplasms should be considered for some of the cases.[465]

Bell et al.[463] have analyzed 213 cases of "problematic" smooth muscle tumors with this combined morphologic approach, have emphasized the importance of coagulative necrosis, and have divided the tumors into five categories as listed in the box on p. 1436.

Occasional leiomyosarcomas have an epithelioid or clear cell appearance and are referred to as ***malignant leiomyoblastomas*** or ***clear cell (epithelioid) leiomyosarcomas.*** Again, it would seem that mitotic counting is the best means to distinguish them from their more common benign counterpart; other helpful features are their large size, infiltrating margins, absence of hyalinization, and presence of necrosis.[464,474] The epithelioid component of these tumors may simulate metastatic carcinoma.[479]

Myxoid leiomyosarcomas represent a rare but important variant of leiomyosarcoma of uterus and broad ligament.[473] Grossly, they have a gelatinous appearance and an apparently well-circumscribed border. Microscopically, they are invasive and highly myxomatous; focally, bundles of typical smooth muscle cells alternate with nondescript mesenchymal cells (Fig. 19-125). For this variant of leiomyosarcoma, the metastatic mitotic count rule does not apply; they tend to recur and metastasize whether mitoses are scanty[473] or numerous.[477]

Exceptionally, leiomyosarcomas are seen to contain a large population of osteoclast-like giant cells[467,476]; the

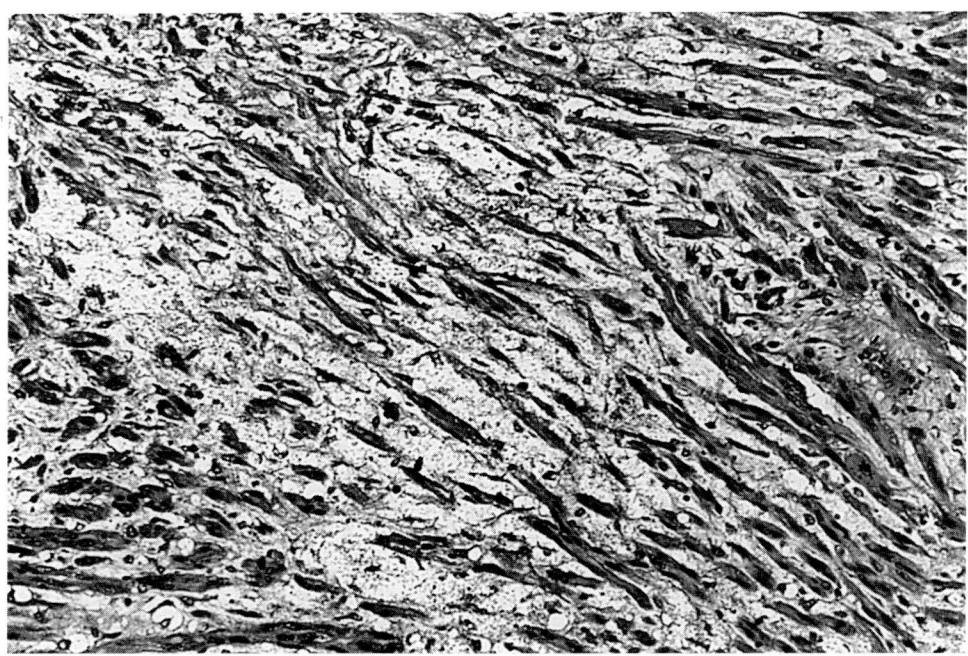

Fig. 19-125 Myxoid leiomyosarcoma of uterus. Fascicles of neoplastic smooth muscle cells are widely separated by granular myxoid material. Mitotic activity was minimal.

CATEGORIZATION OF PROBLEMATIC SMOOTH MUSCLE UTERINE TUMORS

Group I: Tumors with mitotic index ranging from five to ten per ten high-power fields with coagulative tumor cell necrosis (CTCN) and with no more than mild atypia; all but one of these tumors behaved in a benign fashion, and the authors propose to call them leiomyomas with increased mitotic index (MI).

Group IIA: Tumors with no CTCN, diffuse moderate to severe atypia, and MI ≥, ten per ten high-power fields; these are leimyosarcomas.

Group III: Tumors with diffuse moderate to severe atypia and CTCN; these are leiomyosarcomas regardless of the MI.

Group IV: Tumors with insignificant mitotic atypia but CTCN; the authors suggest that these be called leiomyosarcomas when the MI exceeds ten per ten high-power fields.

Group V: Tumors with no CTCN and atypia which was moderate to severe but focal or multifocal rather than diffuse. These had a favorable outcome even if occasionally the MI was high.

Adapted from Bell SW, Kempson RL, Hendrickson MR: Problematic uterine smooth muscle neoplasms. A clinicopathologic study of 213 cases. Am J Surg Pathol **18**:535-558, 1994.

smooth muscle nature of the spindle cells distinguishes this tumor from malignant fibrous histiocytoma and malignant giant cell tumor.

Immunohistochemically, markers of smooth muscle differentiation are present. Reactivity for keratin may also be seen, particularly in the epithelioid tumors.[477a] Overexpression of p53 is common, in contrast to leiomyomas.[476a] Overexpression of *c-myc* oncogene is frequent in leiomyosarcomas (as well as in malignant mixed müllerian tumors), but it also occurs in half of the leiomyomas.[471a]

There is no consistent correlation between survival and histologic grade of the tumor. Extension outside the confines of the uterus is a finding of ominous prognosis.[478] Of twenty patients studied by Bartsich et al.[462] in whom this occurred, no survivors were recorded beyond 29 months. The most common manifestation of malignancy is local recurrence in the pelvis. However, distant metastases (particularly to the lungs) can occur unaccompanied by local recrudescence. Lymph node involvement is exceptional.

There is recent evidence that DNA ploidy patterns as determined by flow cytometry may be of prognostic significance in leiomyosarcomas.[484]

Other tumors and tumorlike conditions

Postoperative spindle cell nodules similar to those occurring in the vagina have been observed in the endometrium.[491]

Extramedullary hematopoiesis can occur in the endometrium in the absence of any hematologic disorder or systemic disease.[513]

Adenomatoid tumors identical to those more commonly seen in the fallopian tube are sometimes found in the uterine wall, usually beneath the serosa and close to the cornua.[519]

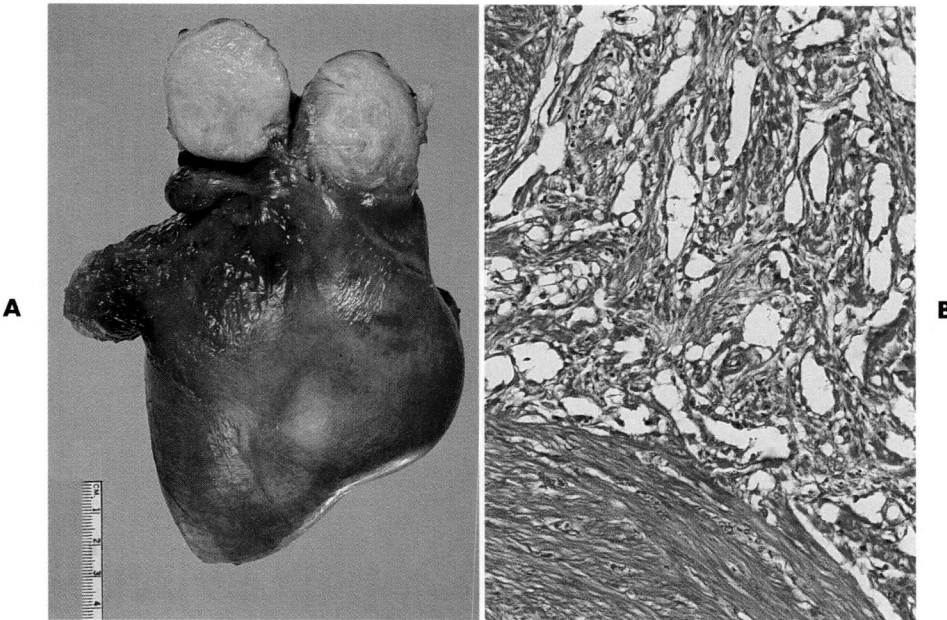

Fig. 19-126 Adenomatoid tumor of uterus. **A,** Gross appearance. The location at one of the cornua is characteristic. **B,** Microscopic appearance showing gland-like formations lined by flattened mesothelial cells.

Exceptionally, they will be apparent in a curetting specimen. These tumors are usually small (mean diameter, 2 cm) and characterized microscopically by adenoid, angiomatoid, solid, and cystic patterns occurring singly or in combination[509,511] (Fig. 19-126). The most cystic examples can simulate lymphangiomas. They are often accompanied by smooth muscle hypertrophy and can be confused with leiomyomas.[525] Their mesothelial nature seems established on the basis of ultrastructural and immunohistochemical findings.[515,516]

Arteriovenous fistula in the wall of the uterus may produce large pulsating masses. The vascular connections are demonstrated by angiography.[506]

Chondrosarcomas, rhabdomyosarcomas, leiomyosarcomas, osteosarcomas, and *angiosarcomas** of the uterus have been described as types of pure heterologous sarcoma, some following radiation therapy for cervical carcinoma.[508a] They are regarded as belonging to the same general category of mixed müllerian tumors, from which they are distinguished microscopically by the absence of an epithelial component. Needless to say, a thorough sampling of these tumors is necessary before making a diagnosis of uterine heterologous sarcoma.

Interestingly, some of the reported angiosarcomas have been of epithelioid type, immunohistochemically positive for keratin, and located within benign smooth muscle nodules with the features of leiomyomas.[517]

Malignant fibrous histiocytomas[489] and *alveolar soft part sarcomas*[497] have also been described in the uterine corpus.

Malignant lymphomas can present initially in the endometrium, myometrium, or both.[488,498] The patients typically present with bleeding and a subepithelial mass. Most tumors are of diffuse large cell type.[485] Cases of Hodgkin's disease[501] and angiotropic lymphoma[492] with primary uterine involvement have also been described. Malignant lymphomas should be distinguished from florid but reactive immunoproliferative conditions involving the endometrium[522] and from *inflammatory pseudotumor.*[496] In these benign conditions, the large lymphoid cells are usually accompanied by plasma cells, small lymphocytes, and/or neutrophils.[495] *Granulocytic sarcomas* can also present initially in the uterus.[498,504]

Other exceptionally rare primary uterine tumors include *lymphangiomyomama(tosis)* (associated with tuberous sclerosis),[497a,502] *Brenner tumor*[486] (microscopically identical to its ovarian counterpart), *glioma,*[523] *primitive neuroectodermal tumor,*[493,500] *carcinoid tumor,*[487] *paraganglioma,*[524] *pigmented paraganglioma,*[518] and *yolk sac (endodermal sinus) tumor.*[503]

Metastatic carcinoma from extrapelvic sites may cause uterine bleeding as the presenting symptom. The breast, gastrointestinal tract, kidney, and skin (melanoma) are the most frequent primary sites.[505,507,514] The myometrium is more often involved than the endometrium, and sometimes the leiomyomas present contain metastatic tumor; however, it is not rare for the malignancy to be present in material from endometrial curettings, especially in cases of lobular carcinoma of the breast.[518a]

REFERENCES
NORMAL ANATOMY

1 Arias-Stella J: A topographic study of uterine epithelia atypia associated with chorionic tissue. Demonstration of alteration in the endocervix. Cancer **12**:782-790, 1959.

2 Arias-Stella J: Atypical endometrial changes produced by chorionic tissue. Hum Pathol **3**:450-453, 1972.

*References 490, 494, 499, 508, 510, 512, 520, 521.

2a Arias-Stella J Jr, Arias-Velasquez A, Arias-Stella J: Normal and abnormal mitoses in the atypical endometrial change associated with chorionic tissue effect. Am J Surg Pathol **18:**694-701, 1994.

3 Azzopardi JC, Zayid I: Synthetic progestogen-oestrogen therapy and uterine changes. J Clin Pathol **20:**731-738, 1967.

4 Banks ER, Mills SE, Frierson HF Jr: Uterine intravascular menstrual endometrium simulating malignancy. Am J Surg Pathol **15:**407-412, 1991.

5 Clement PB, Scully RE: Idiopathic postmenopausal decidual reaction of the endometrium. A clinicopathologic analysis of four cases. Int J Gynecol Pathol **7:**152-161, 1988.

6 Dallenbach-Hellweg G: Histopathology of the endometrium (English translation by FD Dallenbach). New York, 1971, Springer-Verlag, New York, Inc.

7 Ehrmann RL: Histologic dating of the endometrium. J Reprod Med **3:**179-200, 1969.

8 Ferenczy A, Bertrand G, Gelfand MM: Proliferation kinetics of human endometrium during the normal menstrual cycle. Am J Obstet Gynecol **133:**859-867, 1979.

9 Hertig AT: Gestational hyperplasia of the endometrium. A morphologic correlation of ova, endometrium, and corpora lutea during early pregnancy. Lab Invest **13:**1153-1191, 1964.

9a Huettner PC, Gersell DJ: Arias-Stella reaction in nonpregnant women. A clinicopathologic study of nine cases. Int Gynecol Pathol **13:**241-247, 1994.

10 Mazur MT, Hendrickson MR, Kempson RL: Optically clear nuclei. An alteration of endometrial epithelium in the presence of trophoblast. Am J Surg Pathol **7:**415-423, 1983.

11 Norris HJ, Hertig AT, Abell MR: The uterus. Baltimore, 1973, Williams & Wilkins.

12 Noyes RW: Uniformity of secretory endometrium. Study of multiple sections from 100 uteri removed at operation. Fertil Steril **7:**103-109, 1956.

13 Noyes RW, Haman JO: Accuracy of endometrial dating. Fertil Steril **4:**504-517, 1954.

14 Noyes RW, Hertig AT, Rock J: Dating the endometrial biopsy. Fertil Steril **1:**3-25, 1950.

15 Poropatich C, Rojas M, Silverberg SG: Polymorphonuclear leukocytes in the endometrium during the normal menstrual cycle. Int J Gynecol Pathol **6:**230-234, 1987.

16 Sahin AA, Silva EG, Landon G, Ordonez NG, Gershenson DM: Endometrial tissue in myometrial vessels not associated with menstruation. Int J Gynecol Pathol **8:**139-146, 1989.

16a Sickel JZ, di Sant'Agnese PA: Anomalous immunostaining of 'optically clear' nuclei in gestational endometrium. A potential pitfall in the diagnosis of pregnancy-related herpesvirus infection. Arch Pathol Lab Med **118:**831-833, 1994.

17 Yokoyama S, Kashima K, Inoue S, Daa T, Nakayama I, Moriuchi A: Biotin-containing intranuclear inclusions in endometrial glands during gestation and puerperium. Am J Clin Pathol **99:**13-17, 1993.

CURETTAGE AND BIOPSY

18 Baitlon D, Hadley JO: Endometrial biopsy. Pathologic findings in 3600 biopsies from selected patients. Am J Clin Pathol **63:**9-15, 1975.

19 Carmichael DE: Asherman's syndrome. Obstet Gynecol **36:**933-928, 1970.

19a Chambers JT, Chambers SK: Endometrial sampling. When? Where? Why? With what? Clin Obstet Gyn **35:**28-39, 1992.

20 Foix A, Bruno RO, Davison T, Lema B: The pathology of postcurettage intrauterine adhesions. Am J Obstet Gynecol **96:**1027-1033, 1966.

21 Hofmeister FJ, Vondrak B, Barbo DM: The value of the endometrial biopsy. A study of 14,655 office endometrial biopsies. Am J Obstet Gynecol **95:**91-98, 1966.

22 Kahler VL, Creasy RK, Morris JA: Value of the endometrial biopsy. Obstet Gynecol **34:**91-95, 1969.

23 Lampe B, Kürzl R, Hantschmann P: Reliability of tumor typing of endometrial carcinoma in prehysterectomy curettage. Int J Gynecol Pathol **14:**2-6, 1995.

24 McLennan CE: Endometrial regeneration after curettage. Am J Obstet Gynecol **104:**185-194, 1969.

EFFECTS OF HORMONE ADMINISTRATION

25 Antunes CM, Strolley PD, Rosenshein NB, Davies JL, Tonascia JA, Brown C, Burnett L, Rutledge A, Pokempner M, Garcia R: Endometrial cancer and estrogen use. Report of a large case-control study. N Engl J Med **300:**9-13, 1979.

26 Azzopardi JG, Zayid I: Synthetic progestogen-oestrogen therapy and uterine changes. J Clin Pathol **20:**731-738, 1967.

27 Charles D: Iatrogenic endometrial patterns. J Clin Pathol **17:**205-212, 1964.

28 Cohen CJ, Deppe G: Endometrial carcinoma and oral contraceptive agents. Obstet Gynecol **49:**390-392, 1977.

29 Deligdisch L: Effects of hormone therapy on the endometrium. Mod Pathol **6:**94-106, 1993.

30 Dockerty MB, Smith RA, Symmonds RE: Pseudomalignant endometrial changes induced by administration of new synthetic progestins. Mayo Clin Proc **34:**321-328, 1959.

31 Goldzieher JW, Rice-Wray E, Schulz-Contreras M, Aranda-Rosell A: Fertility following termination of contraception with norethindrone. Am J Obstet Gynecol **84:**1474-1477, 1962.

32 Gordon J, Reagan JW, Finkle WD, Ziel HK: Estrogen and endometrial carcinoma. An independent pathology review supporting original risk estimate. N Engl J Med **297:**570-571, 1977.

33 Irey NS, Manion WC, Taylor HB: Vascular lesions in women taking oral contraceptives. Arch Pathol **89:**1-8, 1970.

34 Maqueo M, Becerra C, Munguia H, Goldzieher JW: Endometrial histology and vaginal cytology during oral contraception with sequential estrogen and progestin. Am J Obstet Gynecol **90:**396-400, 1964.

35 Ober WB: Synthetic progestogen-oestrogen preparations and endometrial morphology. J Clin Pathol **19:**138-147, 1966.

36 Ober WB: Effects of oral and intrauterine administration of contraceptives on the uterus. Hum Pathol **8:**513-527, 1977.

37 Rice-Wray E, Aranda-Rosell A, Maqueo M, Goldzieher JW: Comparison of the long-term endometrial effects of synthetic progestins used in fertility control. Am J Obstet Gynecol **87:**429-433, 1963.

38 Roland M, Clyman MJ, Decker A, Ober WB: Classification of endometrial response to synthetic progestogen-estrogen compounds. J Clin Pathol **15:**143-163, 1964.

39 Sartwell PE, Masi AT, Arthes FG, Greene GR, Smith HE: Thromboembolism and oral contraceptives. An epidemiological case-control study. Am J Epidemiol **90:**365-380, 1969.

40 Silverberg SG, Makowski EL: Endometrial carcinoma in young women taking oral contraceptive agents. Obstet Gynecol **46:**503-506, 1975.

41 Silverberg SG, Makowski EL, Roche WD: Endometrial carcinoma in women under 40 years of age. Comparison of cases in oral contraceptive users and non-users. Cancer **39:**592-598, 1977.

42 Silverberg SG, Mullen D, Faraci JA, Makowski EL, Miller A, Finch JL, Sutherland JV: Endometrial carcinoma. Clinical-pathologic comparison of cases in post-menopausal women receiving and not receiving exogenous estrogens. Cancer **45:**3018-3026, 1980.

43 Smith DC, Prentice R, Thompson DJ, Herrmann WL: Association of exogenous estrogen and endometrial carcinoma. N Engl J Med **293:**1164-1166, 1975.

44 Studd JWW, Thom MH, Paterson MEL, Wade-Evans T: The prevention and treatment of endometrial pathology in postmenopausal women receiving exogenous estrogens. In Pasetto N, Paoletti R, Ambrus JL, eds: The menopause and postmenopause. Lancaster, 1980, MTP Press, pp. 127-139.

45 Vessey MP, Doll R: Investigation of relation between use of oral contraceptives and thromboembolic disease. A further report. Br Med J **2:**651-657, 1969.

46 Whitehead MI, King RJB, McQueen J, Campbell S: Endometrial histology and biochemistry in climacteric women during oestrogen and oestrogen/progestogen therapy. J R Soc Med **72:**322-327, 1979.

47 Whitehead MI, Townsend PT, Pryse-Davies J, Ryder TA, King RJB: Effects of estrogens and progestins on the biochemistry and morphology of the postmenopausal endometrium. N Engl J Med **305:**1599-1605, 1981.

48 Ziel HK, Finkle WD: Increased risk of endometrial carcinoma among users of conjugated estrogens. N Engl J Med **293:**1167-1170, 1975.

ENDOMETRITIS

49 Ashworth MT, Moss CI, Kenyon WE: Granulomatous endometritis following hysteroscopic resection of the endometrium. Histopathology **18:**185-187, 1991.

50 Bell DA, Mondschein M, Scully RE: Giant cell arteritis of the female genital tract. A report of three cases. Am J Surg Pathol **10:**696-701, 1986.

51 Bhagavan BS, Gupta PK: Genital actinomyosis and intrauterine contraceptive devices. Cytopathologic diagnosis and clinical significance. Hum Pathol **9:**567-578, 1978.

52 Bhagavan BS, Ruffier J, Shinn B: Pseudoactinomycotic radiate granules in the lower female genital tract. Relationship to the Splendore-Hoeppli phenomenon. Hum Pathol **13:**898-904, 1982.

53 Buckley CH, Fox H: Histiocytic endometritis. Histopathology **4:**105-110, 1980.

54 Burkman R, Schlesselman S, McCaffrey L, Gupta PK, Spence M: The relationship of genital tract *Actinomyces* and the development of pelvic inflammatory disease. Am J Obstet Gynecol **143:**585-589, 1982.

55 Bylund DJ, Nanfro JJ, Marsh WL: Coccidioidomycosis of the female genital tract. Arch Pathol Lab Med **110:**232-235, 1986.

56 Corfman PA, Segal SJ: Biologic effects of intrauterine devices. Am J Obstet Gynecol **100:**448-459, 1968.

57 Crum CP, Egawa K, Fenoglio CM, Richart RM: Chronic endometritis. The role of immunohistochemistry in the detection of plasma cells. Am J Obstet Gynecol **147:**812-815, 1983.

58 Dehner LP, Askin FB: Cytomegalovirus endometritis. Obstet Gynecol **45**:211-214, 1975.

59 Di Carlo FJ Jr, Di Carlo JP, Robboy SJ, Lyons MM: Sarcoidosis of the uterus. Arch Pathol Lab Med **113**:941-943, 1989.

60 Dumoulin JG, Hughesdon PE: Chronic endometritis. J Obstet Gynaecol Br Commonw **58**:222-235, 1951.

61 Frank TS, Himebaugh KS, Wilson MD: Granulomatous endometritis associated with histologically occult cytomegalovirus in a healthy patient. Am J Surg Pathol **16**:716-720, 1992.

62 Govan ADT: Tuberculous endometritis. J Pathol Bacteriol **83**:363-372, 1962.

63 Gupta PK: Intrauterine contraceptive devices. Vaginal cytology, pathologic changes and clinical implications. Acta Cytol (Baltimore) **26**:571-613, 1982.

64 Hart WR, Prins RP, Tsai JC: Isolated coccidioidomycosis of the uterus. Hum Pathol **7**:235-239, 1976.

65 Ho K-L: Sarcoidosis of the uterus. Hum Pathol **10**:219-222, 1978.

66 Ismail SM: Follicular myometritis. A previously undescribed component of pelvic inflammatory disease. Histopathology **16**:91-93, 1990.

67 Israel SL, Roitman HB, Clancy E: Infrequency of unsuspected endometrial tuberculosis. Histologic and bacteriologic study. JAMA **183**:63-65, 1963.

68 Jessen DA, Lane RE, Greene RR: Intrauterine foreign body. A clinical and histopathologic study on use of Graefenberg ring. Am J Obstet Gynecol **85**:1023-1032, 1963.

69 Keebler C, Chatwani A, Schwartz R: Actinomycosis infection associated with intrauterine contraceptive devices. Am J Obstet Gynecol **145**:596-599, 1983.

70 Kiviat NB, Wolner-Hanssen P, Eschenbach DA, Wasserheit JN, Paavonen JA, Bell TA, Critchlow CW, Stamm WE, Moore DE, Holmes KK: Endometrial histopathology in patients with culture-proved upper genital tract infection and laparoscopically diagnosed acute salpingitis. Am J Surg Pathol **14**:167-175, 1990.

71 Lombard CM, Moore MH, Seifer DB: Diagnosis of systemic polyarteritis nodosa following total abdominal hysterectomy and bilateral salpingo-oophorectomy. A case report. Int J Gynecol Pathol **5**:63-68, 1986.

72 Molnar JJ, Poliak A: Recurrent endometrial malakoplakia. Am J Clin Pathol **80**:762-764, 1983.

73 Müller-Holzner E, Ruth NR, Abfalter E, Schröcksnadel H, Dapunt O, Martin-Sances L, Nogales FF: IUD-associated pelvic actinomycosis. A report of five cases. Int J Gynecol Pathol **14**:70-74, 1995.

74 Ober WB, Sobrero AJ, Kurman R, Gold S: Endometrial morphology and polyethylene intrauterine devices. A study of 200 endometrial biopsies. Obstet Gynecol **32**:782-793, 1968.

75 Paavonen J, Aine R, Teisala K, Heinonen PK, Punnonen R: Comparison of endometrial biopsy and peritoneal fluid cytologic testing with laparoscopy in the diagnosis of acute pelvic inflammatory disease. Am J Obstet Gynecol **151**:645-650, 1985.

76 Paavonen J, Kiviat N, Brunham RC, Stevens CE, Kuo C-C, Stamm WE, Miettinen A, Soules M, Eschenbach DA, Holmes KK: Prevalence and manifestations of endometritis among women with cervicitis. Am J Obstet Gynecol **152**:280-286, 1985.

77 Poropatich C, Rojas M, Silverberg SG: Polymorphonuclear leukocytes in the endometrium during the normal menstrual cycle. Int J Gynecol Pathol **6**:230-234, 1987.

78 Risse EKJ, Beerthuizen RJCM, Vooijs GP: Cytologic and histologic findings in women using an IUD. Obstet Gynecol **58**:569-573, 1981.

79 Rotterdam H: Chronic endometritis. A clinicopathologic study. Pathol Annu **13**(Pt 2):209-231, 1978.

80 Russack V, Lammers RJ: Xanthogranulomatous endometritis. Report of six cases and a proposed mechanism of development. Arch Pathol Lab Med **114**:929-932, 1990.

81 Schmidt WA: IUDs, inflammation, and infection. Assessment after two decades of IUD use. Hum Pathol **13**:878-881, 1982.

82 Sen DK, Fox H: The lymphoid tissue of the endometrium. Gynaecologia (Basel) **163**:371-378, 1967.

83 Shintaku M, Sasaki M, Baba Y: Ceroid-containing histiocytic granuloma of the endometrium. Histopathology **18**:169-172, 1991.

84 Silverberg SG, Haukkamaa M, Arko H, Nilsson CG, Luukkainen T: Endometrial morphology during long-term use of levonorgestrel-releasing intrauterine devices. Int J Gynecol Pathol **5**:235-241, 1986.

85 Taylor ES, McMillan JH, Greer BE, Droegemueller W, Thompson HE: The intrauterine device and tubo-ovarian abscess. Am J Obstet Gynecol **123**:338-347, 1975.

86 Venkataseshan VS, Woo TH: Diffuse viral papillomatosis (condyloma) of the uterine cavity. Int J Gynecol Pathol **4**:370-377, 1985.

87 Westrom L, Bengtsson LP, Mardh P: The risk of pelvic inflammatory disease in women using intrauterine contraceptive devices as compared to non-users. Lancet **2**:221-224, 1976.

88 Whiteley PF, Hamlett JD: Pyometra—a reappraisal. Am J Obstet Gynecol **109**:108-112, 1971.

89 Winkler B, Reumann W, Mitao M, Gallo L, Richart RM, Crum CP: Chlamydial endometritis. A histological and immunohistochemical analysis. Am J Surg Pathol **8**:771-778, 1984.

METAPLASIA

90 Abell MR: Endometrial biopsy. Normal and abnormal diagnostic characteristics. In Gold JJ, ed: Gynecologic endocrinology. New York, 1975, Harper & Row, Publishers, Inc., pp. 156-190.

91 Bhatia NN, Hoshiko MG: Uterine osseous metaplasia. Obstet Gynecol **60**:256-259, 1982.

92 Bird CC, Willis RA: The production of smooth muscle by the endometrial stroma of the adult human uterus. J Pathol Bacteriol **90**:75-81, 1965.

93 Blaustein A: Morular metaplasia misdiagnosed as adenoacanthoma in young women with polycystic ovarian disease. Am J Surg Pathol **6**:223-228, 1982.

94 Bomze EJ, Friedman NB: Squamous metaplasia and adenoacanthosis of the endometrium. Obstet Gynecol **30**:619-625, 1967.

95 Crum CP, Richart RM, Fenoglio CM: Adenoacanthosis of the endometrium. A clinicopathologic study in premenopausal women. Am J Surg Pathol **5**:15-20, 1981.

96 Demopoulos RI, Greco MA: Mucinous metaplasia of the endometrium. Ultrastructural and histochemical characteristics. Int J Gynecol Pathol **1**:383-390, 1983.

97 Dutra FR: Intraglandular morules of the endometrium. Am J Clin Pathol **31**:60-65, 1959.

98 Fluhmann CF: The histogenesis of squamous metaplasia in the cervix and endometrium. Surg Gynecol Obstet **97**:45-58, 1953.

99 Gersell DJ: Endometrial papillary syncytial change. Another perspective. Am J Clin Pathol **99**:656-657, 1993.

100 Hendrickson MR, Kempson RL: Surgical pathology of the uterine corpus. Bennington JL, ed: Major problems in pathology, vol. 12. Philadelphia, 1980, WB Saunders Co.

101 Hendrickson MR, Kempson RL: Endometrial epithelial metaplasias. Proliferations frequently misdiagnosed as adenocarcinoma. Report of 89 cases and proposed classification. Am J Surg Pathol **4**:525-542, 1980.

102 Kaku T, Silverberg SG, Tsukamoto N, Tsuruchi N, Kamura T, Saito T, Nakano H: Association of endometrial epithelial metaplasias with endometrial carcinoma and hyperplasia in Japanese and American women. Int J Gynecol Pathol **12**:297-300, 1993.

102a Miranda MC, Mazur MT: Endometrial squamous metaplasia. An unusual response to progestin therapy of hyperplasia. Arch Pathol Lab Med **119**:458-460, 1995.

103 Rorat E, Wallach RC: Papillary metaplasia of the endometrium. Clinical and histopathologic considerations. Obstet Gynecol **64**:90S-92S, 1984.

104 Roth E, Taylor HB: Heterotopic cartilage in the uterus. Obstet Gynecol **27**:838-844, 1966.

105 Salm R: Mucin production of the normal and abnormal endometrium. Arch Pathol **73**:30-39, 1962.

106 Schueller EF: Ciliated epithelia of the human uterine mucosa. Obstet Gynecol **31**:215-223, 1968.

107 Tyagi SP, Saxena K, Rizvi R, Langley FA: Foetal remnants in the uterus and their relation to other uterine heterotopia. Histopathology **3**:339-345, 1979.

108 Wells M, Tiltman A: Intestinal metaplasia of the endometrium. Histopathology **15**:431-433, 1989.

109 Zaman SS, Mazur MT: Endometrial papillary syncytial change. A nonspecific alteration associated with active breakdown. Am J Clin Pathol **99**:741-745, 1993.

ADENOMYOSIS AND ENDOMETRIOSIS

110 Ahn GH, Scully RE: Clear cell carcinoma of the inguinal region arising from endometriosis. Cancer **67**:116-120, 1991.

111 Barbieri RL: Etiology and epidemiology of endometriosis. Am J Obstet Gynecol **162**:565-567, 1990.

112 Bergqvist A, Ljungberg O, Myhre E: Human endometrium and endometriotic tissue obtained simultaneously. A comparative histological study. Int J Gynecol Pathol **3**:135-145, 1984.

113 Brooks JJ, Wheeler JE: Malignancy arising in extragonadal endometriosis. A case report and summary of the world literature. Cancer **40**:3065-3073, 1977.

114 Chumas JC, Thanning L, Mann WJ: Malignant mixed müllerian tumor arising in extragenital endometriosis. Report of a case and review of the literature. Gynecol Oncol **23**:227-233, 1986.

115 Clement PB: Pathology of endometriosis. Pathol Annu **25**(Pt 1):245-295, 1990.

115a Clement PB, Granai CO, Young RH, Scully RE: Endometriosis with myxoid change. A case simulating pseudomyxoma peritonei. Am J Surg Pathol **18**:849-853, 1994.

116 Emge LA: The elusive adenomyosis of the uterus. Its historical past and its present stage of recognition. Am J Obstet Gynecol **83**:1541-1563, 1962.

117 Ferguson BR, Bennington JL, Haber SL: Histochemistry of mucosubstances and histology of mixed müllerian pelvic lymph node glandular inclusions. Evidence for histogenesis by müllerian metaplasia of coelomic epithelium. Obstet Gynecol **33**:617-625, 1969.

117a Goldblum JR, Clement PB, Hart WR: Adenosarcomamyosis with sparse glands. A potential mimic of low-grade endometrial stromal. Am J Clin Pathol **103**:218-223, 1995.

118 Hall JB, Young RH, Nelson JH: The prognostic significance of adenomyosis in endometrial carcinoma. Gynecol Oncol **17**:32-40, 1984.

119 Heaps JM, Nieberg RK, Berek JS: Malignant neoplasms arising in endometriosis. Obstet Gynecol **75**:1023-1028, 1990.

120 Javert CJ: Pathogenesis of endometriosis based on endometrial homeoplasia, direct extension, exfoliation and implantation, lymphatic and hematogenous metastasis. Cancer **2**:399-410, 1949.

121 Karp LA, Czernobilsky B: Glandular inclusions in pelvic and abdominal para-aortic lymph nodes. Am J Clin Pathol **52**:212-218, 1969.

122 Li SF, Nakayama K, Masuzawa H, Fujii S: The number of proliferating cell nuclear antigen positive cells in endometriotic lesions differs from that in the endometrium. Analysis of PCNA positive cells during the menstrual cycle and in post-menopause. Virchows Arch [A] **423**:257-263, 1993.

122a Lu PY, Ory SJ: Endometriosis. Current management. Mayo Clin Proc **70**:453-463, 1995.

123 Mathur BBL, Shah BS, Bhende YM: Adenomyosis uteri. Am J Obstet Gynecol **84**:1820-1829, 1962.

124 Molitor JJ: Adenomyosis. A clinical and pathological appraisal. Am J Obstet Gynecol **110**:275-284, 1971.

125 Mostoufizadeh M, Scully RE: Malignant tumors arising in endometriosis. Clin Obstet Gynecol **23**:951-963, 1980.

125a Nakayama K, Masuzawa H, Li SF, Yoshikawa F, Toki T, Nikaido T, Silverberg SG, Fujii S: Immunohistochemical analysis of the peritoneum adjacent to endometriotic lesions using antibodies to Ber-EP4 antigen, estrogen receptors, and progesterone receptors. Implication of peritoneal metaplasia in the pathogenesis of endometriosis. Int J Gynecol Pathol **13**:348-358, 1994.

126 Olive DL, Schwartz LB: Endometriosis. N Engl J Med **328**:1759-1769, 1993.

127 Prade M, Spatz A, Bentledy R, Duvillard P, Bognel C, Robboy SJ: Borderline and malignant serous tumor arising in pelvic lymph nodes. Evidence of origin in benign glandular inclusions. Int J Gynecol Pathol **14**:87-91, 1995.

128 Roth LM: Endometriosis with perineural involvement. Am J Clin Pathol **59**:807-809, 1973.

129 Steck WD, Helwig EB: Cutaneous endometriosis. JAMA **191**:167-170, 1965.

130 Telium G, Madsen V: Endometriosis ovarii et peritonaei caused by hysterosalpingography (contribution to the pathogenesis of endometriosis). J Obstet Gynaecol Br Emp **57**:10-17, 1950.

131 Tornquist B: Endometriosis in vaginal, vulvar and perineal scars. Acta Obstet Gynecol Scand **29**:485-489, 1949.

132 Winkelman J, Robinson R: Adenocarcinoma of endometrium involving adenomyosis. Report of an unusual case and review of the literature. Cancer **19**:901-908, 1966.

DYSFUNCTIONAL UTERINE BLEEDING AND HYPERPLASIA

133 Abell MR: Adenocarcinoma (gland-cell carcinoma) in situ of endometrium. Pathol Res Pract **174**:221-236, 1982.

134 Ausems EWMA, van der Kamp J-K, Baak JPA: Nuclear morphometry in the determination of the prognosis of marked atypical endometrial hyperplasia. Int J Gynecol Pathol **4**:180-185, 1985.

135 Baak JPA, Kurver PHJ, Diegenbach PC, Delemarre JFM, Brekelmans ECM, Nieuwlaat JE: Discrimination of hyperplasia and carcinoma of the endometrium by quantitative microscopy—a feasibility study. Histopathology **5**:61-68, 1981.

136 Baak JP, Wisse-Brekelmans EC, Fleege JC, van der Putten HW, Bezemer PD: Assessment of the risk on endometrial cancer in hyperplasia, by means of morphological and morphometrical features. Pathol Res Pract **188**:856-859, 1992.

137 Bell CD, Ostrezega E: The significance of secretory features and coincident hyperplastic changes in endometrial biopsy specimens. Hum Pathol **18**:830-838, 1987.

137a Beutler HK, Dockerty MB, Randall L: Precancerous lesions of the endometrium. Am J Obstet Gynecol **86**:433-443, 1963.

138 Campbell PE, Barter RA: The significance of atypical endometrial hyperplasia. J Obstet Gynaecol Br Commonw **68**:668-672, 1961.

139 Castelbaum AJ, Wheeler J, Coutifaris CB, Mastroianni L Jr, Lessey BA: Timing of the endometrial biopsy may be critical for the accurate diagnosis of luteal phase deficiency. Fertil Steril **61**:443-447, 1994.

140 Chamlian LD, Taylor HB: Endometrial hyperplasia in young women. Obstet Gynecol **36**:659-666, 1970.

141 Choo YC, Mak KC, Hsu C, Wong TS, Ma HK: Postmenopausal uterine bleeding of nonorganic cause. Obstet Gynecol **66**:225-228, 1985.

142 Contreras F, Segura A, Nistal M, Patron M, Agustin P de, Larrauri J, Sanchez J, Schwarz A, Arguello MC, Calvo M, Claver M, Gutierrez M, Capdevila A, Lopez-Barea F, Lopez-Rubio F, Picazo ML, Ruiz A, Valbuena L: Patologia no tumoral del endometrio. Patologia (Spain) **4**:127-182, 1971.

143 Dallenbach-Hellweg G: The endometrium of infertility. Pathol Res Pract **178**:527-537, 1984.

144 Dallenbach-Hellweg G: Histopathology of the endometrium (English translation by FD Dallenbach), ed. 3. New York, 1985, Springer-Verlag, Inc.

145 Feichter GE, Hoffken H, Heep J, Haag D, Heberling D, Brandt H, Rummel H, Goerttler KL: DNA-flow-cytometric measurements on the normal, atrophic, hyperplastic and neoplastic human endometrium. Virchows Arch [A] **398**:53-65, 1982.

146 Fenoglio CM, Crum CP, Ferenczy A: Endometrial hyperplasia and carcinoma. Are ultrastructural, biochemical and immunocytochemical studies useful in distinguishing between them? Pathol Res Pract **174**:257-284, 1982.

147 Ferenczy A: Cytodynamics of endometrial hyperplasia and neoplasia. II. In vitro DNA histoautoradiography. Hum Pathol **14**:77-82, 1983.

148 Fox H, Buckley CH: The endometrial hyperplasias and their relationship to endometrial neoplasia. Histopathology **6**:493-510, 1982.

149 Gal D: Hormonal therapy for lesions of the endometrium. Semin Oncol **13**:33-36, 1986.

150 Gillam JS: Study of the inadequate secretion phase endometrium. Fertil Steril **6**:18-36, 1955.

151 Gordon MD, Ireland K: Pathology of hyperplasia and carcinoma of the endometrium. Semin Oncol **21**:64-70, 1994.

152 Gore H, Hertig AT: Carcinoma in situ of the endometrium. Am J Obstet Gynecol **94**:135-155, 1966.

153 Greenblatt RB, Hammond DO, Clark SL: Membranous dysmenorrhea. Studies in etiology and treatment. Am J Obstet Gynecol **68**:835-844, 1954.

154 Gusberg SB, Kaplan AL: Precursors of corpus cancer. IV. Adenomatous hyperplasia as stage 0 carcinoma of the endometrium. Am J Obstet Gynecol **87**:662-676, 1963.

155 Hendrickson MR, Kempson RL: Surgical pathology of the uterine corpus. In Bennington JL, ed: Major problems in pathology, vol. 12. Philadelphia, 1980, WB Saunders Co., pp. 285-318.

156 Hendrickson MR, Ross JC, Kempson RL: Toward the development of morphologic criteria for well-differentiated adenocarcinoma of the endometrium. Am J Surg Pathol **7**:819-838, 1983.

157 Hertig AT, Sommers SC: Genesis of endometrial carcinoma. I. Study of prior biopsies. Cancer **2**:946-956, 1949.

157a Jacques SM, Qureshi F, Lawrence WD: Surface epithelial changes in endometrial adenocarcinoma. Diagnostic pitfalls in curettage specimens. Int J Gynecol Pathol **14**:191-197, 1995.

158 Kurman RJ, Kaminski PF, Norris HJ: The behavior of endometrial hyperplasia. A long-term study of "untreated" hyperplasia in 170 patients. Cancer **56**:403-412, 1985.

159 Kurman RJ, Norris HJ: Evaluation of criteria for distinguishing atypical endometrial hyperplasia from well-differentiated carcinoma. Cancer **49**:2547-2559, 1982.

160 Kurman RJ, Norris HJ: Endometrium. In Henson DE, Albores-Saavedra J, eds: The pathology of incipient neoplasia. Philadelphia, 1986, WB Saunders Co., pp. 265-277.

161 Lee KR, Scully RE: Complex endometrial hyperplasia and carcinoma in adolescents and young women 15 to 20 years of age. A report of 10 cases. Int J Gynecol Pathol **8**:201-213, 1989.

162 McBride JM: Pre-menopausal cystic hyperplasia and endometrial carcinoma. J Obstet Gynaecol Br Emp **66**:288-296, 1959.

163 McElin TW, Bird CC, Reeves BD, Scott RC: Diagnostic dilation and curettage. A 20-year survey. Obstet Gynecol **33**:807-812, 1969.

164 McLennan CE: Current concepts of prolonged or irregular endometrial shedding. Am J Obstet Gynecol **64**:988-998, 1952.

165 McLennan CE, Rydell AH: Extent of endometrial shedding during normal menstruation. Obstet Gynecol **26**:605-621, 1965.

166 Meyer WC, Malkasian GD, Dockerty MB, Decker DG: Postmenopausal bleeding from atrophic endometrium. Obstet Gynecol **38**:731-738, 1971.

167 Moszkowski E, Woodruff JD, Jones GES: The inadequate luteal phase. Am J Obstet Gynecol **83**:363-372, 1962.

167a Mutter GL, Chaponot ML, Fletcher JA: A polymerase chain reaction assay for non-random X chromosome inactivation identifies monoclonal endometrial cancers and precancers. Am J Pathol **146**:501-508, 1995.

168 Norris HJ, Becker RL, Mikel UV: A comparative morphometric and cytophotometric study of endometrial hyperplasia, atypical hyperplasia, and endometrial carcinoma. Hum Pathol **20**:219-223, 1989.

169 Norris HJ, Tavassoli FA, Kurman RJ: Endometrial hyperplasia and carcinoma. Diagnostic considerations. Am J Surg Pathol **7**:839-847, 1983.

170 Noyes RW: The underdeveloped secretory endometrium. Am J Obstet Gynecol **83**:363-372, 1962.

171 Pacheco JC, Kempers RD: Etiology of postmenopausal bleeding. Obstet Gynecol **32**:40-46, 1968.

172 Picoff RC, Luginbuhl WH: Fibrin in the endometrial stroma. Its relation to uterine bleeding. Am J Obstet Gynecol **88**:642-646, 1964.

173 Rome M, Brown JB, Mason T, Smith MA, Laverty C, Cortune D: Oestrogen excretion and ovarian pathology in postmenopausal women with atypical hyperplasia, adenocarcinoma, and mixed adenosquamous carcinoma of the endometrium. Br J Obstet Gynaecol **84**:88-97, 1977.

174 Schwartz AM, Silverberg SG, Fu YS, Nozawa S, Huang S, Tsukasaki K, Williams KR: Use of monoclonal antibodies MSN-1 and B72.3 in the prediction of the natural history of endometrial hyperplasia. Int J Gynecol Pathol **12**:253-258, 1993.

175 Scully RE: Definition of precursors in gynecologic cancer. Cancer **48**:531-537, 1981.

176 Silverberg SG: Hyperplasia and carcinoma of the endometrium. Semin Diagn Pathol **5**:135-153, 1988.

177 Sinykin MB, Goodlin RC, Barr MM: Irregular shedding of the endometrium. Am J Obstet Gynecol **71**:990-1000, 1956.

178 Söderström K-O: Lectin binding to human endometrial hyperplasias and adenocarcinoma. Int J Gynecol Pathol **6**:356-365, 1987.

179 Sommers SC: Defining the pathology of endometrial hyperplasia, dysplasia and carcinoma. Pathol Res Pract **174**:175-197, 1982.

180 Steiner G, Kistner RW, Craig JM: Histological effects of progestins on hyperplasia and carcinoma in situ of the endometrium—further observations. Metabolism **14**:356-386, 1965.

181 Tavassoli F, Kraus FT: Endometrial lesions in uteri resected for atypical endometrial hyperplasia. Am J Clin Pathol **70**:770-779, 1978.

182 Vellios F: Endometrial hyperplasias, precursors of endometrial carcinoma. Pathol Annu **7**:201-229, 1972.

183 Welch WR, Scully RE: Precancerous lesions of the endometrium. Hum Pathol **8**:503-512, 1977.

184 Winkler B, Alvarez S, Richart RM, Crum CP: Pitfalls in the diagnosis of endometrial neoplasia. Obstet Gynecol **64**:185-194, 1984.

TUMORS
Endometrial polyps

185 Clement PB, Young RH: Atypical polypoid adenomyoma of the uterus associated with Turner's syndrome. A report of three cases, including a review of "estrogen-associated" endometrial neoplasms and neoplasms associated with Turner's syndrome. Int J Gynecol Pathol **6**:104-113, 1987.

185a Corley D, Rowe J, Curtis MT, Hogan WM, Noumoff JS, Livolsi VA: Postmenopausal bleeding from unusual endometrial polyps in women on chronic tamoxifen therapy. Obstet Gynecol **79**:111-116, 1992.

185b Creagh TM, Krausz T, Flanagan AM: Atypical stromal cells in a hyperplastic endometrial polyp. Histopathology **27**:386-387, 1995.

186 Duggan MA, Rowlands C, Kneafsey PD, Nation JG, Stuart GCE: Uterine atypical polypoid adenomyoma and ovarian endometrioid carcinoma. Metastatic disease or dual primaries? Int J Gynecol Pathol **14**:81-86, 1995.

186a Fukunaga M, Endo Y, Ushigome S, Ishikawa E: Atypical polypoid adenomyomas of the uterus. Histopathology **27**:35-42, 1995.

187 Mazur MT: Atypical polypoid adenomyomas of the endometrium. Am J Surg Pathol **5**:473-482, 1981.

187a Mittal KR, Peng XC, Wallach RC, Demopoulos RI: Coexistent atypical polypoid adenomyoma and endometrial adenocarcinoma. Hum Pathol **26**:574-575, 1995.

188 Peterson WF, Novak ER: Endometrial polyps. Obstet Gynecol **8**:40-49, 1956.

189 Staros EB, Shilkitus WF: Atypical polypoid adenomyoma with carcinomatous transformation. A case report. Surg Pathol **4**:157-166, 1991.

190 Young RH, Treger T, Scully RE: Atypical polypoid adenomyoma of the uterus. A report of 27 cases. Am J Clin Pathol **86**:139-145, 1986.

Endometrial carcinoma
General and clinical features

191 Beckner ME, Mori T, Silverberg SG: Endometrial carcinoma. Nontumor factors in prognosis. Int J Gynecol Pathol **4**:131-145, 1985.

192 Clement PB, Young RH: Atypical polypoid adenomyoma of the uterus associated with Turner's syndrome. A report of three cases, including a review of "estrogen-associated" endometrial neoplasms and neoplasms associated with Turner's syndrome. Int J Gynecol Pathol **6**:104-113, 1987.

192a Dallenbach-Hellweg G, Hahn U: Mucinous and clear cell adenocarcinomas of the endometrium in patients receiving antiestrogens (tamoxifen) and gestagens. Int J Gynecol Pathol **14**:7-15, 1995.

193 Deligdisch L, Cohen CJ: Histologic correlates and virulence implications of endometrial carcinoma associated with adenomatous hyperplasia. Cancer **56**:1452-1455, 1985.

194 Fechner RE, Kaufman RH: Endometrial adenocarcinoma in Stein-Leventhal syndrome. Cancer **34**:444-452, 1974.

195 Fisher B, Costantino JP, Redmond CK, Fisher ER, Wickerham DL, Cronin WM: Endometrial cancer in tamoxifen-treated breast cancer patients. Findings from the National Surgical Adjuvant Breast and Bowel Project (NSABP) B-14. J Natl Cancer Inst **86**:527-537, 1994.

196 Geisler HE, Huber CP, Rogers S: Carcinoma of the endometrium in premenopausal women. Am J Obstet Gynecol **104**:657-663, 1969.

197 Gusberg SB: The changing nature of endometrial cancer. N Engl J Med **302**:709-732, 1980.

198 Gusberg SB, Hall RE: Precursors of corpus cancer. III. The appearance of cancer of the endometrium in estrogenically conditioned patients. Obstet Gynecol **17**:397-412, 1961.

199 Kaufman RH, Abbott JP, Wall JA: The endometrium before and after wedge resection of the ovaries in the Stein-Leventhal syndrome. Am J Obstet Gynecol **77**:1271-1285, 1959.

200 Magriples U, Naftolin F, Schwartz PE, Carcangiu ML: High-grade endometrial carcinoma in tamoxifen-treated breast cancer patients. J Clin Oncol **11**:485-490, 1993.

201 McCarty KS Jr, Barton TK, Peete CH Jr, Creasman WT: Gonadal dysgenesis with adenocarcinoma of the endometrium. An electron microscopic and steroid receptor analyses with a review of the literature. Cancer **42**:512-520, 1978.

202 Reagan JW: Endometrial cancer. I. Rising incidence. Kalamazoo, MI, 1972, The Upjohn Co.

203 Robboy SJ, Miller AW III, Kurman RJ: The pathologic features and behavior of endometrial carcinoma associated with exogenous estrogen administration. Pathol Res Pract **174**:237-256, 1982.

204 Rodriguez J, Hart WR: Endometrial cancers occurring 10 or more years after pelvic irradiation for carcinoma. Int J Gynecol Pathol **1**:135-144, 1982.

205 Shapiro S, Kelly JP, Rosenberg L, Kaufman DW, Helmrich SP, Rosenshein NB, Lewis JL, Knapp RC, Stolley PD, Schottenfeld D: Risk of localized and widespread endometrial cancer in relation to recent and discontinued use of conjugated estrogens. N Engl J Med **313**:969-972, 1985.

206 Silva EG, Tornos CS, Follen-Mitchell M: Malignant neoplasms of the uterine corpus in patients treated for breast carcinoma. The effects of tamoxifen. Int J Gynecol Pathol **13**:248-258, 1994.

206a Spiegel GW: Endometrial carcinoma in situ in postmenopausal women. Am J Surg Pathol **19**:417-432, 1995.

207 Voigt LF, Weiss NS: Epidemiology of endometrial cancer. Cancer Treat Res **49**:1-21, 1989.

208 Weiss NS, Szekely DR, Austin DF: Increasing incidence of endometrial cancer in the United States. N Engl J Med **294**:1259-1262, 1976.

Pathologic features

209 Ambros RA, Ballouk F, Malfetano JH, Ross JS: Significance of papillary (villoglandular) differentiation in endometrioid carcinoma of the uterus. Am J Surg Pathol **18**:569-575, 1994.

210 Chen JL, Trost DC, Wilkinson EJ: Endometrial papillary adenocarcinomas. Two clinicopathological types. Int J Gynecol Pathol **4**:279-288, 1985.

211 Clement PB: Pathology of the uterine corpus. Hum Pathol **22**:776-791, 1991.

212 Fanning J, Alvarez PM, Tsukada Y, Piver MS: Cervical implantation metastasis by endometrial adenocarcinoma. Cancer **68**:1335-1339, 1991.

213 Fechner RE, Bossart MI, Spjut HJ: Ultrastructure of endometrial stroma foam cells. Am J Clin Pathol **72**:628-633, 1979.

214 Frauenhoffer EE, Zaino RJ, Wolff TV, Whitney CE: Value of endocervical curettage in the staging of endometrial carcinoma. Int J Gynecol Pathol **6**:195-202, 1987.

215 Gospel C: Ultrastructure of endometrial carcinoma. Review of fourteen cases. Cancer **28**:745-754, 1971.

216 Hall JB, Young RH, Nelson JH: The prognostic significance of adenomyosis in endometrial carcinoma. Gynecol Oncol **17**:32-40, 1984.

217 Isaacson PG, Pilot LM Jr, Gooselaw JG: Foam cells in the stroma in carcinoma of the endometrium. Obstet Gynecol **23**:9-11, 1964.

218 Jacques SM, Lawrence WD: Endometrial adenocarcinoma with variable-level myometrial involvement limited to adenomyosis. A clinicopathologic study of 23 cases. Gynecol Oncol **37**:401-407, 1990.

219 Kadar NRD, Kohorn EI, LiVolsi VA, Kapp DS: Histologic variants of cervical involvement by endometrial carcinoma. Obstet Gynecol **59**:85-93, 1982.

220 Larson DM, Copeland LJ, Gallagher HS, Gershenson DM, Freedman RS, Wharton JT, Kline RC: Nature of cervical involvement in endometrial carcinoma. Cancer **59**:959-962, 1987.

220a Longacre TA, Chung MH, Jensen DN, Hendrickson MR: Proposed criteria for the diagnosis of well-differentiated endometrial carcinoma. A diagnostic test for myoinvasion. Am J Surg Pathol **19**:371-406, 1995.

221 Risberg B, Grontoft O, Westholm B: Origin of carcinoma in secretory endometrium—a study using a whole-organ sectioning technique. Gynecol Oncol **15**:32-41, 1983.

222 Salm R: Macrophages in endometrial lesions. J Pathol Bacteriol **83**:405-409, 1962.

222a Zaino RJ, Kurman RJ, Diana KL, Morrow CP: The utility of the revised International Federation of Gynecology and Obstetrics histologic grading of endometrial adenocarcinoma using a defined nuclear grading system. A Gynecologic Oncology Group study. Cancer **75**:81-86, 1995.

Variants and other microscopic types

223 Abeler V, Kjorstad KE: Endometrial squamous cell carcinoma. Report of three cases and review of the literature. Gynecol Oncol **36**:321-326, 1990.

224 Abeler VM, Kjorstad KE, Nesland JM: Undifferentiated carcinoma of the endometrium. A histopathologic and clinical study of 31 cases. Cancer **68**:98-105, 1991.

225 Aguirre P, Scully RE, Wolfe HJ, DeLellis RA: Endometrial carcinoma with argyrophil cells. A histochemical and immunohistochemical analysis. Hum Pathol **15**:210-217, 1984.

226 Alberhasky RC, Connelly PJ, Christopherson WM: Carcinoma of the endometrium. IV. Mixed adenosquamous carcinoma. A clinical-pathological study of 68 cases with long-term follow-up. Am J Clin Pathol **77**:655-664, 1982.

227 Bannatyne P, Russell P, Wills EJ: Argyrophilia and endometrial carcinoma. Int J Gynecol Pathol **2**:235-254, 1983.

228 Carcangiu ML, Chambers JT: Early pathologic stage clear cell carcinoma and uterine papillary serous carcinoma of the endometrium. Comparison of clinicopathologic features and survival. Int J Gynecol Pathol **14**:30-38, 1995.

229 Carcangiu ML, Chambers JT: Uterine papillary serous carcinoma. A study on 108 cases with emphasis on the prognostic significance of associated endometrioid carcinoma, absence of invasion, and concomitant ovarian carcinoma. Gynecol Oncol **47**:298-305, 1992.

230 Christopherson WM, Alberhasky RC, Connelly PJ: Carcinoma of the endometrium. I. A clinicopathologic study of clear cell carcinoma and secretory carcinoma. Cancer **49**:1511-1523, 1982.

231 Christopherson WM, Alberhasky RC, Connelly PJ: Glassy cell carcinoma of the endometrium. Hum Pathol **13**:418-421, 1982.

232 Deligdisch L, Gil J, Heller D, Cohen CJ: Two types of endometrial papillary neoplasm. A morphometric study. Pathol Res Pract **188**:473-477, 1992.

233 Fechner RE: Endometrium with pattern of mesonephroma. Report of a case. Obstet Gynecol **31**:485-490, 1968.

233a Gitsch G, Friedlander ML, Wain GV, Hacker NF: Uterine papillary serous carcinoma. A clinical study. Cancer **75**:2239-2243, 1995.

234 Hachisuga T, Sugimori H, Kaku T, Matsukuma K, Tsukamoto N, Nakano H: Glassy cell carcinoma of the endometrium. Gynecol Oncol **36**:134-138, 1990.

235 Haqqani MT, Fox H: Adenosquamous carcinoma of the endometrium. J Clin Pathol **29**:959-966, 1976.

236 Hendrickson MR, Kempson RL: Ciliated carcinoma—a variant of endometrial adenocarcinoma. A report of 10 cases. Int J Gynecol Pathol **2**:1-12, 1983.

237 Hendrickson M, Ross J, Eifel P, Martinez A, Kempson R: Uterine papillary serous carcinoma. A highly malignant form of endometrial adenocarcinoma. Am J Surg Pathol **6**:93-108, 1982.

238 Hopkin ID, Harlow RA, Stevens PJ: Squamous carcinoma of the body of the uterus. Br J Cancer **24**:71-76, 1970.

239 Huntsman DG, Clement PB, Gilks CB, Scully RE: Small-cell carcinoma of the endometrium. A clinicopathological study of sixteen cases. Am J Surg Pathol **18**:364-375, 1994.

240 Inoue M, DeLellis RA, Scully RE: Immunohistochemical demonstration of chromogranin in endometrial carcinomas with argyrophil cells. Hum Pathol **17**:841-847, 1986.

241 Jeffers MD, McDonald GS, McGuinness EP: Primary squamous cell carcinoma of the endometrium. Histopathology **19**:177-179, 1991.

242 Jeffrey JF, Krepart GV, Lotocki RJ: Papillary serous adenocarcinoma of the endometrium. Obstet Gynecol **67**:670-674, 1986.

243 Jones MA, Young RH, Scully RE: Endometrial adenocarcinoma with a component of giant cell carcinoma. Int J Gynecol Pathol **10**:260-270, 1991.

243a Kalir T, Seijo L, Deligdisch L, Cohen C: Endometrial adenocarcinoma with choriocarcinomatous differentiation in an elderly virginal woman. Int J Gynecol Pathol **14**:266-269, 1995.

244 Kuebler DL, Nikrui N, Bell DA: Cytologic features of endometrial papillary serous carcinoma. Acta Cytol **33**:120-126, 1989.

245 Kurman RJ, Scully RE: Clear cell carcinoma of the endometrium. An analysis of 21 cases. Cancer **37**:872-882, 1976.

246 Lauchlan SC: Tubal (serous) carcinoma of the endometrium. Arch Pathol Lab Med **105**:615-618, 1981.

246a Malpica A, Tornos C, Burke TW, Silva EG: Low-stage clear-cell carcinoma of the endometrium. Am J Surg Pathol **19**:769-774, 1995.

246b McCluggage WG, Roberts N, Bharucha H: Enteric differentiation in endometrial adenocarcinomas. A mucin histochemical study. Int J Gynecol Pathol **14**:255-260, 1995.

247 Melhem MF, Tobon H: Mucinous adenocarcinoma of the endometrium. A clinico-pathological review of 18 cases. Int J Gynecol Pathol **6**:347-355, 1987.

248 Ng ABP: Mixed carcinoma of the endometrium. Am J Obstet Gynecol **102**:506-515, 1968.

249 Ng ABP, Reagan JW, Storassli JP, Wentz WB: Mixed adenosquamous carcinoma of the endometrium. Am J Clin Pathol **59**:765-781, 1973.

250 Parkash V, Carcangiu ML: Uterine papillary serous carcinoma after radiation therapy for carcinoma of the cervix. Cancer **69**:496-501, 1992.

251 Paz RA, Frigerio B, Sundblad AS, Eusebi V: Small-cell (oat cell) carcinoma of the endometrium. Arch Pathol Lab Med **109**:270-272, 1985.

252 Pesce C, Merino MJ, Chambers JT, Nogales F: Endometrial carcinoma with trophoblastic differentiation. An aggressive form of uterine cancer. Cancer **68**:1799-1802, 1991.

252a Pitman MB, Young RH, Clement PB, Dickersin GR, Scully RE: Endometrioid carcinoma of the ovary and endometrium, oxyphilic cell type. A report of nine cases. Int J Gynecol Pathol **13**:290-301, 1994.

253 Rorat E, Ferenczy A, Richart RM: The ultrastructure of clear cell adenocarcinoma of endometrium. Cancer **33**:880-887, 1974.

254 Ross JC, Eifel PJ, Cox RS, Kempson RL, Hendrickson MR: Primary mucinous adenocarcinoma of the endometrium. A clinicopathologic and histochemical study. Am J Surg Pathol **7**:715-729, 1983.

255 Roth LM: Clear-cell adenocarcinoma of the female genital tract. A light and electron microscopic study. Cancer **33**:990-1001, 1974.

256 Ryder DE: Verrucous carcinoma of the endometrium—a unique neoplasm with long survival. Obstet Gynecol **59**:78S-80S, 1982.

257 Salazar OM, DePapp EW, Bonfiglio TA, Feldstein ML, Rubin P, Rudolph JH: Adenosquamous carcinoma of the endometrium. An entity with an inherent poor prognosis? Cancer **40**:119-130, 1977.

258 Salm R: Mucin production of abnormal endometrium. Arch Pathol **73**:30-39, 1962.

259 Sherman ME, Bitterman P, Rosenshein NB, Delgado G, Kurman RJ: Uterine serous carcinoma. A morphologically diverse neoplasm with unifying clinicopathologic features. Am J Surg Pathol **16**:600-610, 1992.

260 Silva EG, Jenkins R: Serous carcinoma in endometrial polyps. Mod Pathol **3**:120-128, 1990.

261 Silverberg SG, DeGiorgi LS: Clear cell carcinoma of the endometrium. Cancer **31**:1127-1140, 1973.

262 Sivridis E, Buckley CH, Fox H: Argyrophil cells in normal, hyperplastic, and neoplastic endometrium. J Clin Pathol **37**:378-381, 1984.

263 Sorvari TE: A histochemical study of epithelial mucosubstances in endometrial and cervical adenocarcinomas. With reference to normal endometrium and cervical mucosa. Acta Pathol Microbiol Scand **207**(Suppl):56-60, 1969.

264 Tobon H, Watkins GJ: Secretory adenocarcinoma of the endometrium. Int J Gynecol Pathol **4**:328-335, 1985.

264a Usadi RS, Bentley RC: Endometrioid carcinoma of the endometrium with sertoliform differentiation. Int J Gynecol Pathol **14**:360-364, 1995.

265 van Hoeven KH, Hudock JA, Woodruff JM, Suhrland MJ: Small cell neuroendocrine carcinoma of the endometrium. Int J Gynecol Pathol **14**:21-29, 1995.

266 Warhol MJ, Rice RH, Pinkus GS, Robboy SJ: Evaluation of squamous epithelium in adenoacanthoma and adenosquamous carcinoma of the endometrium. Immunoperoxidase analysis of involucrin and keratin localization. Int J Gynecol Pathol **3**:82-91, 1984.

267 Yamamoto Y, Izumi K, Otsuka H, Kishi Y, Mimura T, Okitsu O: Primary squamous cell carcinoma of the endometrium. A case report and a suggestion of new histogenesis. Int J Gynecol Pathol **14**:75-80, 1995.

268 Yamashina M, Kobara TY: Primary squamous cell carcinoma with its spindle cell variant in the endometrium. A case report and review of literature. Cancer **57**:340-345, 1986.

269 Young RH, Scully RE: Uterine carcinomas simulating microglandular hyperplasia. A report of six cases. Am J Surg Pathol **16**:1092-1097, 1994.

270 Zaino RJ, Kurman RJ: Squamous differentiation in carcinoma of the endometrium. A critical appraisal of adenoacanthoma and adenosquamous carcinoma. Semin Diagn Pathol **5**:154-171, 1988.

271 Zaino RJ, Kurman R, Herbold D, Gliedman J, Bundy BN, Voet R, Advani H: The significance of squamous differentiation in endometrial carcinoma. Data from a Gynecologic Oncology Group study. Cancer **68**:2293-2302, 1991.

Cytology

272 Bibbo M, Shanklin DR, Wied L: Endometrial cytology on jet wash material. J Reprod Med **8**:90-96, 1972.

273 Burk JR, Lehman HF, Wolf FS: Inadequacy of Papanicolaou smears in the detection of endometrial cancer. N Engl J Med **291**:191-192, 1974.

274 Christopherson WM, Mendez WM, Ahuja EM, Lundin FE, Parker JE: Cervix cancer control in Louisville, Kentucky. Cancer **26**:29-38, 1970.

275 Gravlee LC: Jet-irrigation method for the diagnosis of endometrial adenocarcinoma. Obstet Gynecol **34**:168-173, 1969.

276 Gusberg SB, Milano C: Detection of endometrial carcinoma and its precursors. Cancer **47**:1173-1175, 1981.

277 Hibbard LT, Schwinn CP: Diagnosis of endometrial jet washings. Am J Obstet Gynecol **111**:1039-1042, 1971.

278 Isaacs JH, Wilmoite RW: Aspiration cytology of the endometrium. Office and hospital sampling procedures. Am J Obstet Gynecol **118**:679-687, 1974.

279 Kanbour A, Klionsky B, Cooper R: Cytohistologic diagnosis of uterine jet wash preparations. Acta Cytol (Baltimore) **18**:51-57, 1974.

280 Ng ABP, Reagan JW, Hawliczek CT, Wentz BW: Significance of endometrial cells in the detection of endometrial carcinoma and its precursors. Acta Cytol (Baltimore) **18**:356-361, 1974.

281 Reagan JW: Can screening for endometrial cancer be justified? [editorial]. Acta Cytol (Baltimore) **24**:87-89, 1980.

282 Reagan JW: Cytologic aspects of endometrial neoplasia. Acta Cytol **24**:488-489, 1980.

283 Reagan JW, Ng ABP: The cells of uterine adenocarcinoma. Baltimore, 1965, Williams & Wilkins.

284 Rodrigues MA, Rubin A, Koss LG, Harris J: Evaluation of endometrial jet wash technique (Gravlee) in 303 patients in a community hospital. Obstet Gynecol **43**:392-399, 1974.

285 Vuopala S: Diagnostic accuracy and clinical applicability of cytological and histological methods for investigating endometrial carcinoma. Acta Obstet Gynecol Scand **70**(Suppl):1-72, 1977.

Immunohistochemical and other special techniques

286 Brustein S, Fruchter R, Greene GL, Pertschuk LP: Immunocytochemical assay of progesterone receptors in paraffin-embedded specimens of endometrial carcinoma and hyperplasia. A preliminary evaluation. Mod Pathol **2**:449-455, 1989.

287 Bur ME, Perlman C, Edelmann L, Fey E, Rose PG: p53 expression in neoplasms of the uterine corpus. Am J Clin Pathol **98**:81-87, 1992.

288 Carcangiu ML, Chambers JT, Voynick IM, Pirro M, Schwartz PE: Immunohistochemical evaluation of estrogen and progesterone receptor content in 183 patients with endometrial carcinoma. Part I. Clinical and histologic correlations. Am J Clin Pathol **94**:247-254, 1990.

289 Dabbs DJ, Geisinger KR, Norris HT: Intermediate filaments in endometrial and endocervical carcinomas. The diagnostic utility of vimentin patterns. Am J Surg Pathol **10**:568-576, 1986.

290 Deligdisch L, Holinka CF: Progesterone receptors in two groups of endometrial carcinoma. Cancer **57**:1385-1388, 1986.

291 Geisinger KR, Marshall RB, Kute TE, Homesley HD: Correlation of female sex steroid hormone receptors with histologic and ultrastructural differentiation in adenocarcinoma of the endometrium. Cancer **58**:1506-1517, 1986.

292 Ikeda M, Watanabe Y, Nanjoh T, Noda K: Evaluation of DNA ploidy in endometrial cancer. Gynecol Oncol **50**:25-29, 1993.

293 Kohler MF, Berchuck A, Davidoff AM, Humphrey PA, Dodge RK, Iglehart JD, Soper JT, Clarke-Pearson DL, Bast RC Jr, Marks JR: Overexpression and mutation of p53 in endometrial carcinoma. Cancer Res **52**:1622-1627, 1992.

294 Koshiyama M, Konishi I, Wang DP, Mandai M, Komatsu T, Yamamoto S, Nanbu K, Naito MF, Mori T: Immunohistochemical analysis of p53 protein over-expression in endometrial carcinomas. Inverse correlation with sex steroid receptor status. Virchows Arch [A] **423**:265-271, 1993.

295 McCarty KS Jr, Barton TK, Fetter BF, Creasman WT, McCarty KS Sr: Correlation of estrogen and progesterone receptors with histologic differentiation in endometrial adenocarcinoma. Am J Pathol **96**:171-183, 1979.

296 Moll R, Levy R, Czernobilsky B, Hohlweg-Majert P, Dallenbach-Hellweg G, Franke WW: Cytokeratins of normal epithelia and some neoplasms of the female genital tract. Lab Invest **49**:599-610, 1983.

297 Moll R, Pitz S, Levy R, Weikel W, Franke WW, Czernobilsky B: Complexity of expression of intermediate filament proteins, including glial filament protein, in endometrial and ovarian adenocarcinomas. Hum Pathol **22**:989-1001, 1991.

298 Pertschuk LP, Beddoe AM, Gorelic LS, Shain SA: Immunocytochemical assay of estrogen receptors in endometrial carcinoma with monoclonal antibodies. Comparison with biochemical assay. Cancer **57**:1000-1004, 1986.

299 Podczaski E, Kaminski PF, Zaino R: CA 125 and CA 19-9 immunolocalization in normal, hyperplastic, and carcinomatous endometrium. Cancer **71**:2551-2556, 1993.

299a Prat J, Oliva E, Lerma E, Vaquero M, Matias-Guiu X: Uterine papillary serous adenocarcinoma. A 10-case study of p53 and c-*erb*B-2 expression and DNA content. Cancer **74**:1778-1783, 1994.

300 Puts JJG, Moesker O, Aldeweireldt J, Vooijs GP, Ramaekers FCS: Application of antibodies to intermediate filament proteins in simple and complex tumors of the female genital tract. Int J Gynecol Pathol **6**:257-274, 1987.

301 Sasano H, Comerford J, Wilkinson DS, Schwartz A, Garrett CT: Serous papillary adenocarcinoma of the endometrium. Analysis of proto-oncogene amplification, flow cytometry, estrogen and progesterone receptors, and immunohistochemistry. Cancer **65**:1545-1551, 1990.

302 Takeda A, Matsuyama M, Kuzuya K, Chihara T, Ariyoshi Y, Suchi T, Kato K: Secretory component and IgA in endometrial adenocarcinomas. An immunohistochemical study. Acta Pathol Jpn **33**:725-732, 1983.

302a Tsuda H, Jiko K, Yajima M, Yamada T, Tanemura K, Tsunematsu R, Ohmi K, Sonoda T, Hirohashi S: Frequent occurrence of c-Ki-*ras* rene mutations in well differentiated endometrial adenocarcinoma showing infiltrative local growth with fibrosing stromal response. Int J Gynecol Pathol **14**:255-259, 1995.

303 Ueda S, Tsubura A, Izumi H, Sasaki M, Morii S: Immunohistochemical studies on carcinoembryonic antigen in adenocarcinomas of the uterus. Acta Pathol Jpn **33**:59-69, 1983.

304 Ueda G, Yamasaki M, Inoue M, Tanaka Y, Inoue Y, Nishino T, Ogawa M: Immunohistochemical demonstration of amylase in endometrial carcinomas. Int J Gynecol Pathol **5**:47-51, 1986.

Spread and metastases

305 Boronow RC, Morrow CP, Creasman WT, Disaia PJ, Silverberg SG, Miller A, Blessing JA: Surgical staging in endometrial cancer. Clinical-pathologic findings of a prospective study. Obstet Gynecol **63**:825-832, 1984.

306 Chen KTK, Kostich ND, Rosai J: Peritoneal foreign body granulomas to keratin in uterine adenoacanthoma. Arch Pathol Lab Med **102**:174-177, 1978.

307 Creasman WI, Morrow CP, Bundy BN, Homesley HD, Graham JE, Heller PB: Surgical pathologic spread patterns of endometrial cancer. Cancer **60**:2035-2041, 1987.

308 Kim KR, Scully RE: Peritoneal keratin granulomas with carcinomas of endometrium and ovary and atypical polypoid adenomyoma of endometrium. A clinicopathological analysis of 22 cases. Am J Surg Pathol **14**:925-932, 1990.

309 Prat J, Matias-Guiu X, Barreto J: Simultaneous carcinoma involving the endometrium and the ovary. A clinicopathologic, immunohistochemical, and DNA flow cytometric study of 18 cases. Cancer **68**:2455-2459, 1991.

310 Schink JC, Rademaker AW, Miller DS, Lurain JR: Tumor size in endometrial cancer. Cancer **67**:2791-2794, 1991.

311 Young RH, Johnston WH: Serous adenocarcinoma of the uterus metastatic to the urinary bladder mimicking primary bladder neoplasia. A report of a case. Am J Surg Pathol **14**:877-880, 1990.

Therapy

312 Aalders JG, Abeler V, Kolstad P: Recurrent adenocarcinoma of the endometrium. A clinical and histopathological study of 379 patients. Gynecol Oncol **17**:85-103, 1984.

313 Frank AH, Tseng PC, Haffty BG, Papadopoulos DP, Kacinski BM, Dowling SW, Carcangiu ML, Kohorn EI, Chambers JT, Chambers SK, et al: Adjuvant whole-abdominal radiation therapy in uterine papillary serous carcinoma. Cancer **68**:1516-1519, 1991.

314 Price FV, Chambers SK, Carcangiu ML, Kohorn EI, Schwartz PE, Chambers JT: Intravenous cisplatin, doxorubicin, and cyclophosphamide in the treatment of uterine papillary serous carcinoma (UPSC). Gynecol Oncol **51**:383-389, 1993.

314a Sears JD, Greven KM, Hoen HM, Randall ME: Prognostic factors and treatment outcome for patients with locally recurrent endometrial cancer. Cancer **74**:1303-1308, 1994.

315 Silverberg SG, DeGiorgi LS: Histopathologic analysis of preoperative radiation therapy in endometrial carcinoma. Am J Obstet Gynecol **119**:698-704, 1974.

Prognosis

316 Ambros RA, Kurman RJ: Combined assessment of vascular and myometrial invasion as a model to predict prognosis in stage I endometrioid adenocarcinoma of the uterine corpus. Cancer **69**:1424-1431, 1992.

317 Ambros RA, Kurman RJ: Identification of patients with stage I uterine endometrioid adenocarcinoma at high risk of recurrence by DNA ploidy, myometrial invasion, and vascular invasion. Gynecol Oncol **45:**235-239, 1992.

317a Ambros RA, Vigna PA, Figge J, Kallakury BV, Mastrangelo A, Eastman AY, Malfetano J, Figge HL, Ross JS: Observations on tumor and metastatic suppressor gene status in endometrial carcinoma with particular emphasis on p53. Cancer **73:**1686-1692, 1994.

318 Beckner ME, Mori T, Silverberg SG: Endometrial carcinoma. Nontumor factors in prognosis. Int J Gynecol Pathol **4:**131-145, 1985.

319 Boronow RC: Advances in diagnosis, staging, and management of cervical and endometrial cancer, stages I and II. Cancer **65:**648-659, 1990.

320 Boronow RC, Morrow CP, Creasman WT, DiSaia PJ, Silverberg SG, Miller A, Blessing JA: Surgical staging in endometrial cancer. Clinical-pathologic findings of a prospective study. Obstet Gynecol **63:**825-832, 1984.

321 Britton LC, Wilson TO, Gaffey TA, Cha SS, Wieand HS, Podratz KC: DNA ploidy in endometrial carcinoma. Major objective prognostic factor. Mayo Clin Proc **65:**643-650, 1990.

322 Chambers JT, Carcangiu ML, Voynick IM, Schwartz PE: Immunohistochemical evaluation of estrogen and progesterone receptor content in 183 patients with endometrial carcinoma. Part II. Correlation between biochemical and immunohistochemical methods and survival. Am J Clin Pathol **94:**255-260, 1990.

323 Christopherson WM, Connelly PJ, Alberhasky RC: Carcinoma of the endometrium. V. An analysis of prognosticators in patients with favorable subtypes and stage I disease. Cancer **51:**1705-1709, 1983.

324 Creasman WT: Prognostic significance of hormone receptors in endometrial cancer. Cancer **71:**1467-1470, 1993.

325 Fanning J, Alvarez PM, Tsukada Y, Piver MS: Prognostic significance of the extent of cervical involvement by endometrial cancer. Gynecol Oncol **40:**46-47, 1991.

326 Greven KM, Lanciano RM, Corn B, Case D, Randall ME: Pathologic stage III endometrial carcinoma. Prognostic factors and patterns of recurrence. Cancer **71:**3697-3702, 1993.

327 Hanson MB, Van Nagell JR, Powell DE, Donaldson ES, Gallion H, Merhige M, Pavlik EJ: The prognostic significance of lymph-vascular space invasion in stage I endometrial cancer. Cancer **55:**1753-1757, 1985.

328 Hendrickson M, Ross J, Eifel PJ, Cox RS, Martinez A, Kempson R: Adenocarcinoma of the endometrium. Analysis of 256 cases with carcinoma limited to the uterine corpus. Pathology review and analysis of prognostic variables. Gynecol Oncol **13:**373-392, 1982.

329 Hetzel DJ, Wilson TO, Keeney GL, Roche PC, Cha SS, Podratz KC: HER-2/neu expression. A major prognostic factor in endometrial cancer. Gynecol Oncol **47:**179-185, 1992.

330 Homesley HD, Zaino R: Endometrial cancer. Prognostic factors. Semin Oncol **21:**71-78, 1994.

331 Ikeda M, Watanabe Y, Nanjoh T, Noda K: Evaluation of DNA ploidy in endometrial cancer. Gynecol Oncol **50:**25-29, 1993.

332 Kempson RL, Pokorny GE: Adenocarcinoma of the endometrium in women aged forty and younger. Cancer **21:**650-662, 1968.

333 Larson DM, Copeland LJ, Gallagher HS, Gershenson DM, Freedman RS, Wharton JT, Kline RC: Nature of cervical involvement in endometrial carcinoma. Cancer **59:**959-962, 1987.

334 Lukes AS, Kohler MF, Pieper CF, Kerns BJ, Bentley R, Rodriguez GC, Soper JT, Clarke-Pearson DL, Bast RC Jr, Berchuck A: Multivariable analysis of DNA ploidy, p53, and HER-2/neu as prognostic factors in endometrial cancer. Cancer **73:**2380-2385, 1994.

335 Malkasian GD Jr: Carcinoma of the endometrium. Effect of stage and grade on survival. Cancer **41:**996-1001, 1978.

336 Mikuta JJ: International Federation of Gynecology and Obstetrics staging of endometrial cancer 1988. Cancer **71:**1460-1463, 1993.

337 Ng ABP, Reagan JW: Incidence and prognosis of endometrial carcinoma by histologic grade and extent. Obstet Gynecol **35:**437-443, 1970.

337a Niikura H, Sasano H, Matsunaga G, Watanabe K, Ito K, Sato S, Yajima A: Prognostic value of epidermal growth factor receptor expression in endometrioid endometrial carcinoma. Hum Pathol **26:**892-896, 1995.

337b Reinartz JJ, George E, Lindgren BR, Niehans GA: Expression of p53, transforming growth factor alpha, epidermal growth factor receptor, and c-*erb*B-2 in endometrial carcinoma and correlation with survival and known predictors of survival. Hum Pathol **25:**1075-1083, 1994.

338 Robboy SJ, Miller AW III, Kurman RJ: The pathologic features and behavior of endometrial carcinoma associated with exogenous estrogen administration. Pathol Res Pract **174:**237-256, 1982.

338a Sasano H, Watanabe K, Ito K, Sato S, Yajima A: New concepts in the diagnosis and prognosis of endometrial carcinoma. Pathol Annu **29**(Pt 2):31-49, 1995.

339 Sidawy MK, Silverberg SG: Endometrial carcinoma. Pathologic factors of therapeutic and prognostic significance. Pathol Annu **27:**153-185, 1992.

340 Stendahl U, Strang P, Wagenius G, Bergstrom R, Tribukait B: Prognostic significance of proliferation in endometrial adenocarcinomas. A multivariate analysis of clinical and flow cytometric variables. Int J Gynecol Pathol **10:**271-284, 1991.

341 Tobon H, Watkins GJ: Secretory adenocarcinoma of the endometrium. Int J Gynecol Pathol **4:**328-335, 1985.

342 Tornos C, Silva EG, el-Naggar A, Burke TW: Aggressive stage I grade 1 endometrial carcinoma. Cancer **70:**790-798, 1992.

342a Zaino RJ: Pathologic indicators of prognosis in endometrial adenocarcinoma. Selected aspects emphasizing the GOG experience. Gynecologic Oncology Group. Pathol Annu **30**(Pt 1):1-28, 1995.

343 Zaino RJ, Kurman R, Herbold D, Gliedman J, Bundy BN, Voet R, Advani H: The significance of squamous differentiation in endometrial carcinoma. Data from a Gynecologic Oncology Group study. Cancer **68:**2293-2302, 1991.

344 Zaino RJ, Silverberg SG, Norris HJ, Bundy BN, Morrow CP, Okagaki T: The prognostic value of nuclear versus architectural grading in endometrial adenocarcinoma. A Gynecologic Oncology Group study. Int J Gynecol Pathol **13:**29-36, 1994.

Endometrial stromal tumors

345 Abrams J, Talcott J, Corson JM: Pulmonary metastases in patients with low-grade endometrial stromal sarcoma. Clinicopathologic findings with immunohistochemical characterization. Am J Surg Pathol **13:**133-140, 1989.

346 Akhtar M, Kim PY, Young I: Ultrastructure of endometrial stromal sarcoma. Cancer **35:**406-412, 1975.

347 August CZ, Bauer KD, Lurain J, Murad T: Neoplasms of endometrial stroma. Histopathologic and flow cytometric analysis with clinical correlation. Hum Pathol **20:**232-237, 1989.

348 Balaton AJ, Vuong PN, Vaury P, Baviera EE: Plexiform tumorlet of the uterus. Immunohistological evidence for a smooth muscle origin. Histopathology **10:**749-754, 1986.

349 Chang KL, Crabtree GS, Lim-Tan SK, Kempson RL, Hendrickson MR: Primary uterine endometrial stromal neoplasms. A clinicopathologic study of 117 cases. Am J Surg Pathol **14:**415-438, 1994.

350 Clement PB, Scully RE: Uterine tumors resembling ovarian sex-cord tumors. A clinicopathologic analysis of fourteen cases. Am J Clin Pathol **66:**512-525, 1976.

351 Clement PB, Scully RE: Endometrial stromal sarcomas of the uterus with extensive endometrioid glandular differentiation. A report of three cases that caused problems in differential diagnosis. Int J Gynecol Pathol **11:**163-173, 1992.

352 De Fusco PA, Gaffey TA, Malkasian GD Jr, Long HJ, Cha SS: Endometrial stromal sarcoma. Review of Mayo Clinic experience, 1945-1980. Gynecol Oncol **35:**8-14, 1989.

353 Devaney K, Tavassoli FA: Immunohistochemistry as a diagnostic aid in the interpretation of unusual mesenchymal tumors of the uterus. Mod Pathol **4:**225-231, 1991.

354 Dickersin GR, Scully RE: Role of electron microscopy in metastatic endometrial stromal tumors. Ultrastruct Pathol **17:**377-403, 1993.

355 el-Naggar AK, Abdul-Karim FW, Silva EG, McLemore D, Garnsey L: Uterine stromal neoplasms. A clinicopathologic and DNA flow cytometric correlation. Hum Pathol **22:**897-903, 1991.

356 Evans HL: Endometrial stromal sarcoma and poorly differentiated endometrial sarcoma. Cancer **50:**2170-2182, 1982.

357 Farhood AI, Abrams J: Immunohistochemistry of endometrial stromal sarcoma. Hum Pathol **22:**224-230, 1991.

358 Fekete PS, Vellios F: The clinical and histologic spectrum of endometrial stromal neoplasms. A report of 41 cases. Int J Gynecol Pathol **3:**198-212, 1984.

359 Fisher ER, Paulson JD, Gregorio RM: The myofibroblastic nature of the uterine plexiform tumor. Arch Pathol Lab Med **102:**477-480, 1978.

360 Franquemont DW, Frierson HF Jr, Mills SE: An immunohistochemical study of normal endometrial stroma and endometrial stromal neoplasms. Evidence for smooth muscle differentiation. Am J Surg Pathol **15:**861-870, 1991.

361 Goodhue WW, Susin M, Kramer EE: Smooth muscle origin of uterine plexiform tumors. Ultrastructural and histochemical evidence. Arch Pathol **97:**263-268, 1974.

362 Hitchcock CL, Norris HJ: Flow cytometric analysis of endometrial stromal sarcoma. Am J Clin Pathol **97:**267-271, 1992.

363 Kaminski PF, Tavassoli FA: Plexiform tumorlet. A clinical and pathologic study of 15 cases with ultrastructural observations. Int J Gynecol Pathol **3:**124-134, 1984.

364 Kempson RL, Bari W: Uterine sarcomas. Classification, diagnosis, and prognosis. Hum Pathol **1:**331-349, 1970.

365 Larbig GG, Clemmer JJ, Koss LG, Foote FW: Plexiform tumorlets of endometrial stromal origin. Am J Clin Pathol **44:**32-35, 1965.

366 Lillemoe TJ, Perrone T, Norris HJ, Dehner LP: Myogenous phenotype of epithelial-like areas in endometrial stromal sarcomas. Arch Pathol Lab Med **115**:215-219, 1991.

367 Lloreta J, Prat J: Ultrastructure of an endometrial stromal nodule with skeletal muscle. Ultrastruct Pathol **17**:405-410, 1993.

368 Mazur MT, Askin FB: Endolymphatic stromal myosis. Unique presentation and ultrastructural study. Cancer **42**:2661-2667, 1978.

369 Norris HJ, Taylor HB: Mesenchymal tumors of the uterus. I. A clinical and pathological study of 53 endometrial stromal tumors. Cancer **19**:755-766, 1966.

370 Roth LM, Senteny GE: Stromomyoma of the uterus. Ultrastruct Pathol **9**:137-143, 1985.

371 Sabini G, Chumas JC, Mann WJ: Steroid hormone receptors in endometrial stromal sarcomas. A biochemical and immunohistochemical study. Am J Clin Pathol **97**:381-386, 1992.

372 Shiraki M, Otis CN, Powell JL: Endometrial stromal sarcoma arising from ovarian and extraovarian endometriosis—report of two cases and review of the literature. Surg Pathol **4**:333-343, 1991.

373 Silverberg SG, Willson MA, Board JA: Hemangiopericytoma of the uterus. An ultrastructural study. Am J Obstet Gynecol **110**:397-404, 1971.

374 Tang C-K, Toker C, Ances IG: Stromomyoma of the uterus. Cancer **43**:308-316, 1979.

375 Tavassoli FA, Norris HJ: Mesenchymal tumours of the uterus. VII. A clinicopathological study of 60 endometrial stromal nodules. Histopathology **5**:1-10, 1981.

376 Thatcher SS, Woodruff JD: Uterine stromatosis. A report of 33 cases. Obstet Gynecol **59**:428-434, 1982.

377 Tsukamoto N, Kamura T, Matsukuma K, Imachi M, Uchino H, Saito T, Ono M: Endolymphatic stromal myosis. A case with positive estrogen and progesterone receptors and good response to progestins. Gynecol Oncol **20**:120-128, 1985.

378 Ulbright TM, Kraus FT: Endometrial stromal tumors of extra-uterine tissue. Am J Clin Pathol **76**:371-377, 1981.

379 Yoonessi M, Hart WR: Endometrial stromal sarcomas. Cancer **40**:898-906, 1977.

Malignant mixed müllerian tumor (mixed mesodermal tumor)

380 Barwick KW, LiVolsi VA: Malignant mixed müllerian tumors of the uterus. Am J Surg Pathol **3**:125-135, 1979.

381 Bitterman P, Chun B, Kurman RJ: The significance of epithelial differentiation in mixed mesodermal tumors of the uterus. a clinicopathologic and immunohistochemical study. Am J Surg Pathol **4**:317-328, 1990.

381a Costa MJ, Vogelsan J, Young LJ: p53 gene mutation in female genital tract carcinosarcomas (malignant mixed müllerian tumors). A clinicopathologic study of 74 cases. Mod Pathol **7**:619-627, 1994.

382 Chuang JT, Van Velden DJJ, Graham JB: Carcinosarcoma and mixed mesodermal tumor of the uterine corpus. Review of 49 cases. Obstet Gynecol **35**:769-780, 1970.

383 Chumas JC, Mann WJ, Tseng L: Malignant mixed müllerian tumor of the endometrium in a young woman with polycystic ovaries. Cancer **52**:1478-1481, 1983.

384 de Brito PA, Silverberg SG, Orenstein JM: Carcinosarcoma (malignant mixed müllerian [mesodermal] tumor) of the female genital tract. Immunohistochemical and ultrastructural analysis of 28 cases. Hum Pathol **24**:132-142, 1993.

385 Dellers EA, Valente PT, Edmonds PR, Balsara G: Extrauterine mixed mesodermal tumors. An immunohistochemical study. Arch Pathol Lab Med **115**:918-920, 1991.

386 Doss LL, Llorens AS, Henriquez EM: Carcinosarcoma of the uterus. A 40-year experience from the state of Missouri. Gynecol Oncol **18**:43-53, 1984.

387 Fehr PE, Prem KA: Malignancy of the uterine corpus following irradiation therapy for squamous cell carcinoma of the cervix. Am J Obstet Gynecol **119**:685-692, 1974.

388 Gagne E, Tetu B, Blondeau L, Raymond PE, Blais R: Morphologic prognostic factors of malignant mixed müllerian tumor of the uterus. A clinicopathologic study of 58 cases. Mod Pathol **2**:433-438, 1989.

389 George E, Lillemoe TJ, Twiggs LB, Perrone T: Malignant mixed müllerian tumor versus high-grade endometrial carcinoma and aggressive variants of endometrial carcinoma. A comparative analysis of survival. Int J Gynecol Pathol **14**:39-44, 1995.

390 George E, Manivel JC, Dehner LP, Wick MR: Malignant mixed müllerian tumors. An immunohistochemical study of 47 cases, with histogenetic considerations and clinical correlation. Hum Pathol **22**:215-223, 1991.

391 Gersell DJ, Duncan DA, Fulling KH: Malignant mixed müllerian tumor of the uterus with neuroectodermal differentiation. Int J Gynecol Pathol **8**:169-178, 1989.

392 Hasiuk AS, Petersen RO, Hanjani P, Griffin TD: Extragenital malignant mixed müllerian tumor. Case report and review of the literature. Am J Clin Pathol **81**:102-105, 1984.

393 Kempson RL, Bari W: Uterine sarcomas. Classification, diagnosis, and prognosis. Hum Pathol **1**:331-349, 1970.

394 Kohorn EI, Schwartz PE, Chambers JT, Peschel RE, Kapp DS, Merino M: Adjuvant therapy in mixed müllerian tumors of the uterus. Gynecol Oncol **23**:212-221, 1986.

394a Krigman HR, Coogan AC, Marks JR: Simultaneous endometrial malignant mixed mesodermal tumor and ovarian serous adenocarcinoma. Arch Pathol Lab Med **119**:99-103, 1995.

395 Mayall P, Rutty K, Campbell F, Goddard H: p53 immunostaining suggests that uterine carcinosarcomas are monoclonal. Histopathology **24**:211-214, 1994.

396 Meis JM, Lawrence WD: The immunohistochemical profile of malignant mixed müllerian tumor. Overlap with endometrial adenocarcinoma. Am J Clin Pathol **94**:1-7, 1990.

396a Mount SL, Lee KR, Taatjes DJ: Carcinosarcoma (malignant mixed müllerian tumor) of the uterus with a rhabdoid tumor component. An immunohistochemical, ultrastructural, and immunoelectron microscopic case study. Am J Clin Pathol **103**:235-239, 1995.

397 Mukai K, Varela-Duran J, Nochomovitz LE: The rhabdomyoblast in mixed müllerian tumors of the uterus and ovary. An immunohistochemical study of myoglobin in 25 cases. Am J Clin Pathol **74**:101-104, 1980.

398 Norris HJ, Roth E, Taylor HB: Mesenchymal tumors of the uterus. II. A clinical and pathologic study of 31 mixed mesodermal tumors. Obstet Gynecol **28**:57-63, 1966.

399 Norris HJ, Taylor HB: Postirradiation sarcomas of the uterus. Obstet Gynecol **26**:689-694, 1965.

400 Norris NJ, Taylor HB: Mesenchymal tumors of the uterus. III. A clinical and pathologic study of 31 carcinosarcomas. Cancer **19**:1459-1465, 1966.

401 Press MF, Scully RE: Endometrial "sarcomas" complicating ovarian thecoma, polycystic ovarian disease and estrogen therapy. Gynecol Oncol **21**:135-154, 1985.

402 Schaepman-van Geuns EJ: Mixed tumors and carcinosarcomas of the uterus evaluated five years after treatment. Cancer **25**:72-77, 1970.

403 Silverberg SG, Major FJ, Blessing JA, Fetter B, Askin FB, Liao SY, Miller A: Carcinosarcoma (malignant mixed mesodermal tumor) of the uterus. A Gynecologic Oncology Group pathologic study of 203 cases. Int J Gynecol Pathol **9**:1-19, 1990.

404 Spanos WJ, Peters LJ, Oswald MJ: Patterns of recurrence in malignant mixed müllerian tumor of the uterus. Cancer **57**:155-159, 1986.

405 Spanos WJ, Wharton JT, Gomez L, Fletcher GH, Oswald MJ: Malignant mixed müllerian tumors of the uterus. Cancer **53**:311-316, 1984.

405a Sreenan JJ, Hart WR: Carcinosarcomas of the female genital tract. A pathologic study of 29 metastatic tumors—further evidence for the dominant role of the epithelial component and the conversion theory of histogenesis. Am J Surg Pathol **19**:666-674, 1995.

406 Varela-Duran J, Nochomovitz LE, Prem KA, Dehner LP: Postirradiation mixed müllerian tumors of the uterus. A comparative clinicopathologic study. Cancer **45**:1625-1631, 1980.

Müllerian adenosarcoma and related tumors

407 Chen KTK: Rhabdomyosarcomatous uterine adenosarcoma. Int J Gynecol Pathol **4**:146-152, 1985.

408 Clement PB: Müllerian adenosarcomas of the uterus with sarcomatous overgrowth. A clinicopathological analysis of 10 cases. Am J Surg Pathol **13**:28-38, 1989.

409 Clement PB, Scully RE: Müllerian adenosarcoma of the uterus. A clinicopathologic analysis of ten cases of a distinctive type of müllerian mixed tumor. Cancer **34**:1138-1149, 1974.

410 Clement PB, Scully RE: Extrauterine mesodermal (müllerian) adenosarcoma. A clinicopathologic analysis of five cases. Am J Clin Pathol **69**:276-283, 1978.

411 Clement PB, Scully RE: Müllerian adenosarcomas of the uterus with sex cord-like elements. A clinicopathologic analysis of eight cases. Am J Clin Pathol **91**:664-672, 1989.

412 Clement PB, Scully RE: Müllerian adenosarcoma of the uterus. A clinicopathologic analysis of 100 cases with a review of the literature. Hum Pathol **21**:363-381, 1990.

413 Clement PB, Scully RE: Müllerian adenofibroma of the uterus with invasion of myometrium and pelvic veins. Int J Gynecol Pathol **9**:363-371, 1990.

414 Fox H, Harilal KR, Youell A: Müllerian adenosarcoma of the uterine body. A report of nine cases. Histopathology **3**:167-180, 1979.

415 Gloor E: Müllerian adenosarcoma of the uterus. Am J Surg Pathol **3**:203-209, 1979.

416 Grimalt M, Arguelles M, Ferenczy A: Papillary cyst-adenofibroma of endometrium. a histochemical and ultrastructural study. Cancer **36**:137-144, 1975.

417 Hirschfield L, Kahn LB, Chen S, Winkler B, Rosenberg S: Müllerian adenosarcoma with ovarian sex cord-like differentiation. A light and electron-microscopic study. Cancer **57**:1197-1200, 1986.

417a Horie Y, Ikawa S, Kadowaki K, Minagawa Y, Kigawa J, Terakawa N: Lipoadenofibroma of the uterine corpus. Report of a new variant of adenofibroma (benign müllerian mixed tumor). Arch Pathol Lab Med 119:274-276, 1995.

418 Kaku T, Silverberg SG, Major FJ, Miller A, Fetter B, Brady MF: Adenosarcoma of the uterus. A Gynecologic Oncology Group clinicopathologic study of 31 cases. Int J Gynecol Pathol 11:75-88, 1992.

419 Katzenstein AA, Askin FB, Feldman PS: Müllerian adenosarcoma of the uterus. An ultrastructural study of four cases. Cancer 40:2233-2242, 1977.

420 Kempson RL, Bari W: Uterine sarcomas. Classification, diagnosis, and prognosis. Hum Pathol 1:331-349, 1970.

421 Lack EE, Bitterman P, Sundeen JT: Müllerian adenosarcoma of the uterus with pure angiosarcoma. Case report. Hum Pathol 22:1289-1291, 1991.

422 Miller KN, McClure SP: Papillary adenofibroma of the uterus. Report of a case involved by adenocarcinoma and review of the literature. Am J Clin Pathol 97:806-809, 1992.

423 Peters WM, Wells MJ, Bryce FC: Müllerian clear cell carcinofibroma of the uterine corpus. Histopathology 8:1069-1078, 1984.

424 Silverberg SG: Adenomyomatosis of endometrium and endocervix. A hamartoma? Am J Clin Pathol 64:192-199, 1975.

425 Valdez VA, Planas AT, Lopez VF, Goldberg M, Herrera NE: Adenosarcoma of uterus and ovary. A clinicopathologic study of two cases. Cancer 43:1439-1447, 1979.

426 Vellios F: Papillary adenofibroma-adenosarcoma. The uterine cystosarcoma phyllodes. In Fenoglio CM, Wolff M, eds: Progress in surgical pathology. New York, 1980, Masson Publishing USA, Inc., pp. 205-219.

427 Vellios F, Ng ABP, Reagan JW: Papillary adenofibroma of the uterus. A benign mesodermal mixed tumor of müllerian origin. Am J Clin Pathol 60:543-551, 1973.

428 Zaloudek CJ, Norris HJ: Adenofibroma and adenosarcoma of the uterus. A clinicopathologic study of 35 cases. Cancer 48:354-366, 1981.

Leiomyoma

429 Brescia RJ, Tazelaar HD, Hobbs J, Miller AW: Intravascular lipoleiomyomatosis. A report of two cases. Hum Pathol 20:252-256, 1989.

430 Brown JM, Malkasian GD Jr, Symmonds RE: Abdominal myomectomy. Am J Obstet Gynecol 99:126-129, 1967.

430a Canzonieri V, D'Amore ES, Bartoloni G, Piazza M, Blandamura S, Carbone A: Leiomyomatosis with vascular invasion. A unified pathogenesis regarding leiomyoma with vascular microinvasion, benign metastasizing leiomyoma and intravenous leiomyomatosis. Virchows Arch 425:541-545, 1994.

431 Clement PB, Young RH: Diffuse leiomyomatosis of the uterus. A report of four cases. Int J Gynecol Pathol 6:332-330, 1987.

432 Clement PB, Young RH, Scully RE: Diffuse, perinodular, and other patterns of hydropic degeneration within and adjacent to uterine leiomyomas. Problems in differential diagnosis. Am J Surg Pathol 16:26-32, 1992.

433 Colgan TJ, Pendergast S, Le Blanc M: The histopathology of uterine leiomyomas following treatment with gonadotropin-releasing hormone analogues. Hum Pathol 24:1073-1077, 1993.

434 Cramer SF, Patel A: The frequency of uterine leiomyomas. Am J Clin Pathol 94:435-438, 1990.

434a Cramer SF, Patel A: Myometrial hyperplasia. Proposed criteria for a discrete morphological entity. Mod Pathol 8:71-77, 1995.

435 Fechner RE: Atypical leiomyomas and synthetic progestin therapy. Am J Clin Pathol 49:697-703, 1968.

436 Ferry JA, Harris NL, Scully RE: Uterine leiomyomas with lymphoid infiltration simulating lymphoma. A report of seven cases. Int J Gynecol Pathol 8:263-270, 1989.

437 Friedman AJ, Hoffman DI, Comite F, Browneller RW, Miller JD: Treatment of leiomyomata uteri with leuprolide acetate depot. A double-blind, placebo-controlled, multicenter study. The Leuprolide Study Group. Obstet Gynecol 77:720-725, 1991.

438 Gilks CB, Taylor GP, Clement PB: Inflammatory pseudotumor of the uterus. Int J Gynecol Pathol 6:275-286, 1987.

439 Gutmann JN, Thornton KL, Diamond MP, Carcangiu ML: Evaluation of leuprolide acetate treatment on histopathology of uterine myomata. Fertil Steril 61:622-626, 1994.

440 Harper RS, Scully RE: Intravenous leiomyomatosis of the uterus. Am J Clin Pathol 4:45-51, 1965.

441 Hu J, Surti U: Subgroups of uterine leiomyomas based on cytogenetic analysis. Hum Pathol 22:1009-1016, 1991.

442 Hyde KE, Geisinger KR, Marshall RB, Jones TL: The clear-cell variant of uterine epithelioid leiomyoma. An immunohistologic and ultrastructural study. Arch Pathol Lab Med 113:551-553, 1989.

443 Jacobs DS, Cohen H, Johnson JS: Lipoleiomyomas of the uterus. Am J Clin Pathol 44:45-51, 1965.

444 Konishi I, Fujii S, Ban C, Okuda Y, Okamura H, Tojo S: Ultrastructural study of minute uterine leiomyomas. Int J Gynecol Pathol 2:113-120, 1983.

445 Kurman RJ, Norris HJ: Mesenchymal tumors of the uterus. VI. Epithelioid smooth muscle tumors including leiomyoblastoma and clear-cell leiomyoma. A clinical and pathologic analysis of 26 cases. Cancer 37:1853-1865, 1976.

445a Lascano EF: Mast cells in human tumors. Cancer 11:1110-1114, 1958.

446 Lemis PL, Lee ABH, Easler RE: Myometrial hypertrophy. A clinical pathologic study and review of the literature. Am J Obstet Gynecol 84:1032-1041, 1962.

446a Maluf HM, Gersell DJ: Uterine leiomyomas with high content of mast cells. Arch Pathol Lab Med 118:712-714, 1994.

447 Martin-Reay DG, Christ ML, La Pata RE: Uterine leiomyoma with skeletal muscle differentiation. Report of a case. Am J Clin Pathol 96:344-347, 1991.

448 Mazur MT: Clear cell leiomyoma (leiomyoblastoma) of the uterus. Ultrastructural observations. Ultrastruct Pathol 10:249-255, 1986.

449 Mazur MT, Kraus FT: Histogenesis of morphologic variations in tumors of the uterine wall. Am J Surg Pathol 4:59-74, 1980.

449a Mulvany NJ, Ostör AG, Ross I: Diffuse leiomyomatosis of the uterus. Histopathology 27:175-179, 1995.

449b Mulvany NJ, Slavin JL, Ostor AG, Fortune DW: Intravenous leiomyomatosis of the uterus. A clinicopathologic study of 22 cases. Int J Gynecol Pathol 13:1-9, 1994.

450 Myles JL, Hart HR: Apoplectic leiomyomas of the uterus. Am J Surg Pathol 9:798-805, 1985.

451 Nedwich A, Frumin A, Meranze DR: Erythrocytosis associated with uterine myomas. Am J Obstet Gynecol 84:174-178, 1962.

452 Nilbert M, Heim S, Mandahl N, Flodérus UM, Willén H, Mitelman F: Karyotypic rearrangements in 20 uterine leiomyomas. Cytogenet Cell Genet 49:300-304, 1988.

453 Nogales FF, Novano N, Martinez de Victoria JM, Contreras F, Redondo C, Herraiz MA, Seco MA, Velasco A: Uterine intravascular leiomyomatosis. An update and report of seven cases. Int J Gynecol Pathol 6:331-339, 1987.

454 Norris HJ, Parmley T: Mesenchymal tumors of the uterus. V. Intravenous leiomyomatosis. A clinical and pathologic study of 14 cases. Cancer 36:2164-2178, 1975.

455 O'Connor DM, Norris HJ: Mitotically active leiomyomas of the uterus. Hum Pathol 21:223-227, 1990.

455a Oliva E, Young RH, Clement PB, Bhan AK, Scully RE: Cellular benign mesenchymal tumors of the uterus. A comparative morphologic and immunohistochemical analysis of 33 highly cellular leiomyomas and six endometrial stromal nodules, two frequently confused tumors. Am J Surg Pathol 19:769-774, 1995.

456 Parazzini F, La Vecchia C, Negri E, Cecchetti G, Fedele L: Epidemiologic characteristics of women with uterine fibroids. A case-control study. Obstet Gynecol 72:853-857, 1988.

457 Persaud V, Arjoon PD: Uterine leiomyoma. Incidence of degenerative change and a correlation of associated symptoms. Obstet Gynecol 35:432-436, 1970.

458 Pounder DJ: Fatty tumours of the uterus. J Clin Pathol 35:1380-1383, 1982.

459 Prakash S, Scully RE: Sarcoma-like pseudopregnancy. Changes in uterine leiomyomas. Report of a case resulting from prolonged norethindrone therapy. Obstet Gynecol 24:106-110, 1964.

460 Prayson RA, Hart WR: Mitotically active leiomyomas of the uterus. Am J Clin Pathol 97:14-20, 1992.

460a Resta L, Maiorano E, Piscitelli D, Botticella MA: Lipomatous tumors of the uterus. Clinico-pathological features of 10 cases with immunocytochemical study of histogenesis. Pathol Res Pract 190:378-383, 1994.

Leiomyosarcoma

461 Abell MR, Littler ER: Benign metastasizing uterine leiomyoma. Multiple lymph nodal metastases. Cancer 36:2206-2213, 1975.

462 Bartsich EG, Bowe ET, Moore JG: Leiomyosarcoma of the uterus. A 50-year review of 42 cases. Obstet Gynecol 32:101-106, 1968.

463 Bell SW, Kempson RL, Hendrickson MR: Problematic uterine smooth muscle neoplasms. A clinicopathologic study of 213 cases. Am J Surg Pathol 18:535-558, 1994.

464 Buscema J, Carpenter SE, Rosenshein NB, Woodruff JD: Epithelioid leiomyosarcoma of the uterus. Cancer 7:1192-1196, 1986.

465 Cho KR, Woodruff JD, Epstein JI: Leiomyoma of the uterus with multiple extrauterine smooth muscle tumors. A case report suggesting multifocal origin. Hum Pathol 20:80-83, 1989.

466 Christopherson WM, Williamson EO, Gray LA: Leiomyosarcoma of the uterus. Cancer 29:70-75, 1972.

467 Darby AJ, Papadaki L, Beilby JOW: An unusual leiomyosarcoma of the uterus containing osteoclast-like giant cells. Cancer 36:495-504, 1975.

468 Donhuijsen K: Mitosis counts. Reproducibility and significance in grading of malignancy. Hum Pathol 17:1122-1125, 1986.

469 Editorials: Mitosis counting—I. (Scully RE et al) Mitosis counting—II. (Kempson RL) Mitosis counting—III. (Norris HJ) Hum Pathol **7**:481-484, 1976.

470 Evans N: Mitotic figures in malignant tumors as affected by time before fixation of tissues. Arch Pathol **1**:894-898, 1926.

471 Hart WR, Billman JK Jr: A reassessment of uterine neoplasms originally diagnosed as leiomyosarcomas. Cancer **41**:1902-1910, 1978.

471a Jeffers MD, Richmond JA, Macaulay EM: Overexpression of the *c-myc* proto-oncogene occurs frequently in uterine sarcomas. Mod Pathol **8**:701-704, 1995.

471b Jones MW, Norris HJ: Clinocopathologic study of 28 uterine leiomyosarcomas with metastasis. Int J Gynecol Pathol **14**:243-249, 1995.

472 Kempson RL, Bari W: Uterine sarcomas. Classification, diagnosis, and prognosis. Hum Pathol **1**:331-349, 1970.

473 King E, Dickersin GR, Scully RE: Myxoid leiomyosarcoma of the uterus. Am J Surg Pathol **6**:589-598, 1982.

474 Kurman RJ, Norris HJ: Mesenchymal tumors of the uterus. VI. Epithelioid smooth muscle tumors including leiomyoblastoma and clear cell leiomyoma. A clinical and pathologic analysis of 26 cases. Cancer **37**:1853-1865, 1976.

475 Marshall RJ, Braye SG: Alpha-1-antitrypsin, alpha-1-antichymotrypsin, actin, and myosin in uterine sarcomas. Int J Gynecol Pathol **4**:346-354, 1985.

476 Marshall RJ, Braye SG, Jones DB: Leiomyosarcoma of the uterus with giant cells resembling osteoclasts. Int J Gynecol Pathol **5**:260-268, 1986.

476a Niemann TH, Raab SS, Lenel JC, Rodgers JR, Robinson RA: p53 protein overexpression in smooth muscle tumors of the uterus. Hum Pathol **26**:375-379, 1995.

477 Pounder DJ, Iyer PV: Uterine leiomyosarcoma with myxoid stroma. Arch Pathol Lab Med **109**:762-764, 1985.

477a Rizeq MN, van de Rijn M, Hendrickson MR, Rouse RV: A comparative immunohistochemical study of uterine smooth muscle neoplasms with emphasis on the epithelioid variant. Hum Pathol **25**:671-677, 1994.

478 Salazar OM, Bonfiglio TA, Patten SF, Keller BE, Feldstein M, Dunne ME, Rudolph J: Uterine sarcomas. Natural history, treatment and prognosis. Cancer **42**:1152-1160, 1978.

479 Seidman JD, Yetter RA, Papadimitriou JC: Epithelioid component of uterine leiomyosarcoma simulating metastatic carcinoma. Arch Pathol Lab Med **116**:287-290, 1992.

480 Silverberg SG: Reproducibility of the mitosis count in the histologic diagnosis of smooth muscle tumors of the uterus. Hum Pathol **7**:451-454, 1976.

481 Spiro RH, McPeak CJ: On the so-called metastasizing leiomyoma. Cancer **19**:544-548, 1966.

482 Taylor HB, Norris HJ: Mesenchymal tumors of the uterus. IV. Diagnosis and prognosis of leiomyosarcomas. Arch Pathol **82**:40-44, 1966.

483 Tench WD, Dail D, Gmelich JT, Matani N: Benign metastasizing leiomyomas. A review of 21 cases (abstract). Lab Invest **38**:367, 1978.

484 Tsushima K, Stanhope CR, Gaffey TA, Lieber MM: Uterine leiomyosarcomas and benign smooth muscle tumors. Usefulness of nuclear DNA patterns studied by flow cytometry. Mayo Clin Proc **63**:248-255, 1988.

Other tumors and tumorlike conditions

485 Aozasa K, Saeki K, Ohsawa M, Horiuchi K, Mishima K, Tsujimoto M: Malignant lymphoma of the uterus. Report of seven cases with immunohistochemical study. Cancer **72**:1959-1964, 1993.

486 Arhelger RB, Bocian JJ: Brenner tumor of the uterus. Cancer **38**:1741-1743, 1976.

487 Chetty R, Clark SP, Bhathal PS: Carcinoid tumor of the uterine corpus. Virchows Arch A Pathol Anat Histopathol **422**:93-95, 1993.

488 Chorlton I, Karnei RF Jr, Norris HJ: Primary malignant reticuloendothelial disease involving the vagina, cervix, and corpus uteri. Obstet Gynecol **44**:735-748, 1974.

489 Chou S-T, Fortune D, Beischer NA, McLeish G, Castles LA, McKelvie BA, Planner RS: Primary malignant fibrous histiocytoma of the uterus—ultrastructural and immunocytochemical studies of two cases. Pathology **17**:36-40, 1985.

490 Clement PB: Chondrosarcoma of the uterus. Report of a case and review of the literature. Hum Pathol **9**:726-732, 1978.

491 Clement PB: Postoperative spindle-cell nodule of the endometrium. Arch Pathol Lab Med **112**:566-568, 1988.

492 Davey DD, Munn R, Smith LW, Cibull ML: Angiotropic lymphoma. Presentation in uterine vessels with cytogenetic studies. Arch Pathol Lab Med **114**:879-882, 1990.

493 Daya D, Lukka H, Clement PB: Primitive neuroectodermal tumors of the uterus. A report of four cases. Hum Pathol **23**:1120-1129, 1992.

494 De Young B, Bitterman P, Lack EE: Primary osteosarcoma of the uterus. Report of a case with immunohistochemical study. Mod Pathol **5**:212-215, 1992.

495 Ferry JA, Young RH: Malignant lymphoma, pseudolymphoma, and hematopoietic disorders of the female genital tract. Pathol Annu **26**:227-263, 1991.

496 Gilks CB, Taylor GP, Clement PB: Inflammatory pseudotumor of the uterus. Int J Gynecol Pathol **6**:275-286, 1987.

497 Gray GF, Glick AD, Kurtin PJ, Jones HW III: Alveolar soft part sarcoma of the uterus. Hum Pathol **17**:297-300, 1986.

497a Gyure KA, Hart WR, Kennedy AW: Lymphangiomyomatosis of the uterus associated with tuberous sclerosis and malignant neoplasia of the female genital tract. A report of two cases. Int J Gynecol Pathol **14**:344-351, 1995.

498 Harris NL, Scully RE: Malignant lymphoma and granulocytic sarcoma of the uterus and vagina. Cancer **53**:2530-2545, 1984.

499 Hart WR, Craig JR: Rhabdomyosarcomas of the uterus. Am J Clin Pathol **70**:217-223, 1978.

500 Hendrickson MR, Scheithauer BW: Primitive neuroectodermal tumor of the endometrium. Report of two cases, one with electron microscopic observations. Int J Gynecol Pathol **5**:249-259, 1986.

501 Hung LHY, Kurtz DM: Hodgkin's disease of the endometrium. Arch Pathol Lab Med **109**:952-953, 1985.

502 Jameson CF: Angiomyoma of the uterus in a patient with tuberous sclerosis. Histopathology **16**:202-203, 1990.

503 Joseph MG, Fellows FG, Hearn SA: Primary endodermal sinus tumor of the endometrium. A clinicopathologic, immunocytochemical, and ultrastructural study. Cancer **65**:297-302, 1990.

504 Kapadia SB, Krause JR, Kanbour AI, Hartsock RJ: Granulocytic sarcoma of the uterus. Cancer **41**:687-691, 1978.

505 Kumar NB, Hart WR: Metastases to the uterine corpus from extragenital cancers. Cancer **50**:2163-2169, 1982.

506 Liggins GC: Uterine arteriovenous fistula. Obstet Gynecol **23**:214-217, 1964.

507 Mazur MT, Hsueh S, Gersell DJ: Metastases to the female genital tract. Cancer **53**:1978-1984, 1984.

508 Milne DS, Hinshaw K, Malcolm AJ, Hilton P: Primary angiosarcoma of the uterus. A case report. Histopathology **16**:203-205, 1994.

508a Morrel B, Mulder AF, Chadha S, Tjokrowardojo AJ, Wijnen JA: Angiosarcoma of the uterus following radiotherapy for squamous cell carcinoma of the cervix. Eur J Obstet Gynecol Reprod Biol **49**:193-197, 1993.

509 Palacios J, Suarez Manrique A, Ruiz Villaespesa A, Burgos Lizaldez E, Gamallo Amat C: Cystic adenomatoid tumor of the uterus. Int J Gynecol Pathol **10**:296-301, 1991.

510 Podczaski E, Sees J, Kaminski P, Sorosky J, Larson JE, De Geest K, Zaino RJ, Mortel R: Rhabdomyosarcoma of the uterus in a postmenopausal patient. Gynecol Oncol **37**:439-442, 1990.

511 Quigley JC, Hart WR: Adenomatoid tumors of the uterus. Am J Clin Pathol **76**:627-635, 1981.

512 Siegal GP, Taylor LL III, Nelson KG, Reddick RL, Frazelle M, Siegfried JM, Walton LA, Kaufman DG: Characterization of a pure heterologous sarcoma of the uterus. Rhabdomyosarcoma of the corpus. Int J Gynecol Pathol **2**:303-315, 1983.

513 Sirgi KE, Swanson PE, Gersell DJ: Extramedullary hematopoiesis in the endometrium. Report of four cases and review of the literature. Am J Clin Pathol **101**:643-646, 1994.

514 Stemmermann GN: Extrapelvic carcinoma metastatic to the uterus. Am J Obstet Gynecol **82**:1261-1266, 1961.

515 Stephenson TJ, Mill PM: Adenomatoid tumours. An immunohistochemical and ultrastructural appraisal of their histogenesis. J Pathol **148**:327-335, 1986.

516 Suzuki T, Yoshida Y, Kaku T, Kikuchi K, Mori M: Adenomatoid tumor of the uterus. Ultrastructural, histochemical, and immunohistochemical analysis. Arch Pathol Lab Med **109**:1049-1051, 1985.

517 Tallini G, Price FV, Carcangiu ML: Epithelioid angiosarcoma arising in uterine leiomyomas. Am J Clin Pathol **100**:514-518, 1993.

518 Tavassoli FA: Melanotic paraganglioma of the uterus. Cancer **58**:942-948, 1986.

518a Taxy JB, Trujillo YP: Breast cancer metastatic to the uterus. Clinical manifestations of a rare event. Arch Pathol Lab Med **118**:819-821, 1994.

519 Tiltman AJ: Adenomatoid tumours of the uterus. Histopathology **4**:437-443, 1980.

520 Vakiani M, Mawad J, Talerman A: Heterologous sarcomas of the uterus. Int J Gynecol Pathol **1**:211-219, 1982.

521 Witkin B, Askin FB, Geratz JD, Reddick RL: Angiosarcoma of the uterus. A light microscopic, immunohistochemical and ultrastructural study. Int J Gynecol Pathol **6**:176-184, 1987.

522 Young RH, Harris NL, Scully RE: Lymphoma-like lesions of the lower female genital tract. A report of 16 cases. Int J Gynecol Pathol **4**:289-299, 1985.

523 Young RH, Kleinman GM, Scully RE: Glioma of the uterus. Am J Surg Pathol **5**:695-699, 1981.

524 Young TW, Thrasher TV: Nonchromaffin paraganglioma of the uterus. Arch Pathol Lab Med **106**:608-609, 1982.

525 Youngs LA, Taylor HB: Adenomatoid tumors of the uterus and fallopian tube. Am J Clin Pathol **48**:537-545, 1967.

Fallopian tube

NORMAL ANATOMY

The fallopian tube or salpinx is a tubular hollow structure measuring 11 to 12 cm in length that runs throughout the apex of the broad ligament and spans the distance between the uterine cornus and the ovary. It is divided into four segments: intramural (inside the uterine wall), isthmus (2 to 3 cm, thick-walled), ampulla (a thin-walled expanded area), and infundibulum (a trumpet-shaped ending that opens into the peritoneal cavity and is fringed by the fimbriae). One of the latter structures, known as the ovarian fimbria, attaches to the ovary.

The inner aspect of the tube is lined by mucosa arranged in the shape of longitudinal, branching folds (known as plicae), which merge with the fimbriae. There is good correlation between the microscopic features of this mucosa and its salpingoscopic appearance.[31] Microscopically, the epithelium is composed of three distinct cell types: secretory, ciliated, and intercalated (peg). Amylase is secreted by the epithelium, and its presence can be demonstrated immunohistochemically.[10] Endocrine cells have been found only exceptionally. A low degree of proliferative activity takes place normally in the tubal epithelium, apparently not synchronized with the menstrual cycle. At the time of menstruation, as well as a few days postpartum, the tubal mucosa may be normally infiltrated by neutrophils, probably as a reaction to blood and necrotic debris. It is accompanied by negative cultures and should not be confused with a bacterial salpingitis.[54,66]

The muscular wall (myosalpinx) is composed of an inner circular layer and an outer longitudinal layer; the isthmus near the uterotubal junction also possesses an inner longitudinal layer.

The lymphatics of the fallopian tube leave the tubal wall within the mesosalpinx, where they join efferent lymphatics from the ovary and uterus and follow the ovarian vessels to terminate in the aortic lymph nodes. Other lymphatics course within the broad ligament and drain into the interiliac nodes; a separate lymphatic channel from the ampulla of the tube follows the broad ligament to terminate in the superior gluteal lymph nodes.

The broad ligament and adjacent areas contain a variety of tubular structures that may give rise to grossly evident cysts. Most of these are lined by müllerian-type epithelium and have been variously referred to—depending on their location—as parovarian cyst, paratubal cyst (hydatid of Morgagni), subserosal müllerian cyst, Kobelt's cyst (appendix vesiculosa), cyst of the paroöphoron, and cyst of the rete ovarii.[22a] Remnants of mesonephric ducts are also constantly present in this location. Walthard's nests are mentioned on p. 1463.

INFLAMMATION

Bacterial infection of the fallopian tube is a common disease, and its incidence keeps increasing. It may follow invasive procedures such as curettage or the insertion of intrauterine devices, but in most cases it is due to an ascending infection, often sexually transmitted.[84] The inflammation results in fusion of tubal plicae and obliteration of the ostium. Obstruction of the fimbriated end and, less commonly, of the transmural and isthmic portion leads subsequently to infertility.[21] Microscopically, the trapped epithelial spaces produce a complicated gland-like pattern that can simulate malignancy[14] (Fig. 19-127).

The lumen is often distended and filled with secretions or pus *(pyosalpinx)* (Fig. 19-128). Massive intraluminal hemorrhage may lead to the formation of **hematosalpinx,** a rare condition that needs to be distinguished from the much more common form secondary to ruptured tubal pregnancy. In chronic inflammatory cases, the wall is markedly fibrotic, and serosal adhesions are numerous. The inflammatory exudate often spreads to the ovary, resulting in the formation of a **tubo-ovarian abscess** and obliteration of the pelvic anatomic relationships. The rupture of such an abscess may lead to localized or generalized peritonitis and requires prompt surgical intervention.[49,58] **Hydrosalpinx** is generally regarded as the end stage of a purulent salpingitis in which pus has been reabsorbed and replaced by a transudate of plasma.[16] The external gross appearance has been likened to that of a retort. Exceptionally, the involvement is limited to the intrauterine portion of the tube. The wall is thin and fibrotic, with atrophy or even disappearance of the smooth muscle wall. The epithelium is flat and focally absent. **Pelvic inflammatory disease** (PID) is the generic term used for inflammatory processes of this region in which the fallopian tube is the epicenter and presumably the source of the inflammation.[47,89]

Eschenbach et al.[20] recovered *Neisseria gonorrhoeae* from 91 of 204 cases of acute PID in patients with cervical gonococcal infections. Chlamydial infection is also common, accounting for over 20% and perhaps as many as half of the cases.[88,90] This etiology should be suspected in cases of chronic salpingitis with marked lymphofollicular hyperplasia.[88] Polymicrobial tuboperitoneal infection (resulting from *Bacteroides fragilis,* peptostreptococci, peptococci, and other organisms) is responsible for most others. In established tubo-ovarian abscesses, the most common agents recovered are coliform organisms. *N. gonorrhoeae* was isolated only once in a series of ninety-three such cases studies by Mickal et al.,[49] although this finding does not rule out its role as a possible initiating factor before superinfection has occurred, in view of the fact that isolation of *N. gon-*

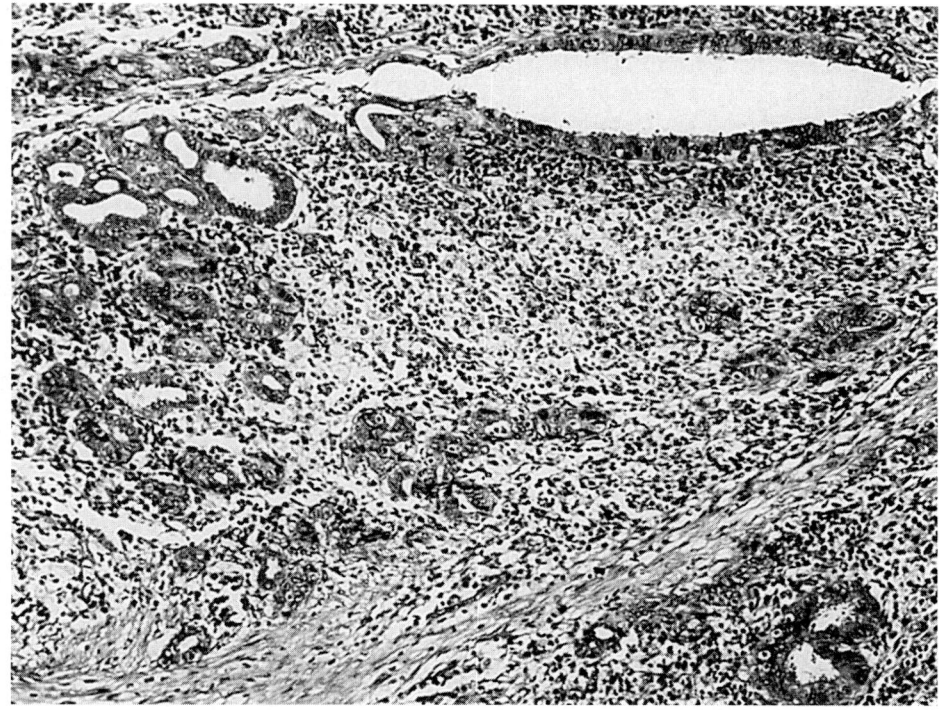

Fig. 19-127 Chronic salpingitis. Fusion of plicae produces pseudoglandular pattern.

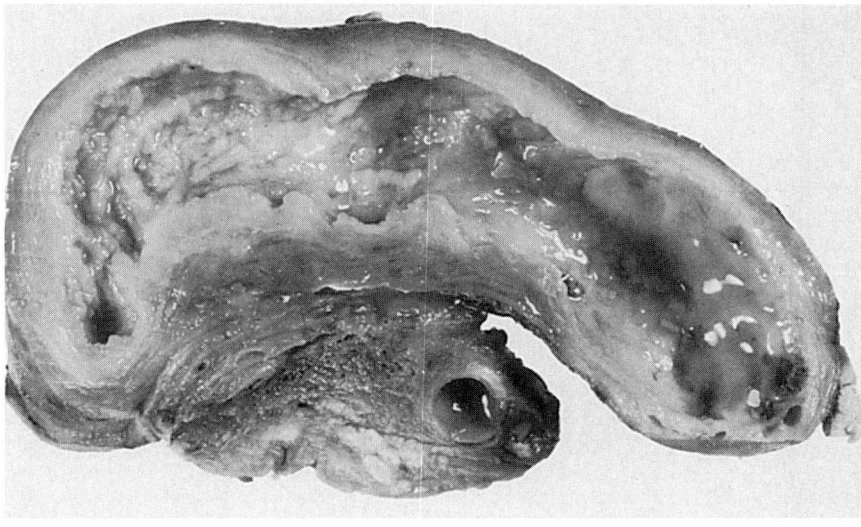

Fig. 19-128 Large dilated fallopian tube with shaggy lining and thick scarred wall, result of chronic inflammation.

orrhoeae is inversely proportional to the number of episodes of salpingitis.[80]

Tuberculosis of the tube is hematogenous. In advanced cases, both tubes are replaced by caseous tuberculous masses. There is often extreme adenomatous proliferation of the tubal mucosa in association with granulomatous inflammation, and this may lead to a mistaken diagnosis of carcinoma (Fig. 19-129). Most patients with pelvic tuberculosis are young. Infertility is common.[22,30] The endometrium is involved in about 80% of the cases.[55]

Granulomatous inflammation of the tubes can also be produced by *Schistosoma, Oxyuris vermicularis, Actinomyces, Coccidioides immitis,* and other organisms. *Sarcoidosis* and *Crohn's disease* may be accompanied by tubal involvement.

Foreign bodies introduced for diagnostic or therapeutic measures can induce a bizarre granulomatous response. Reaction to *Lipiodol* following the Rubin test may be so proliferative as to resemble a neoplasm. The push of a uterine sound may drive lubricant into the tube, causing *lipoid granulomas.*[19]

Giant cell arteritis is occasionally found in the tubes, ovary, and uterus of postmenopausal patients, as an isolated finding or as a manifestation of a generalized autoimmune disease.[6]

TORSION

Torsion of the fallopian tube and ovary is usually secondary to inflammation or tumor, but occasionally it develops in a previously normal organ, the appearance at surgery being that of a hemorrhagic infarct. This phenomenon can occur in adults[29] as well as in infants and children.[28,38] In children, torsion of the normal adnexa is about a third as common as torsion of an ovarian cyst or tumor. If the operation is done early enough, untwisting of the adnexa may lead to full recovery. Nonoperated cases may resolve spontaneously or result in a necrotic and calcified mass, which may later detach from the uterus. It has been suggested that this complication, when occurring in previously normal adnexa, is due to the fact that the infundibulopelvic ligament extends along the edge of the ovarian ligament so that the tube and ovary hang on a very narrow stalk.

TUBAL PREGNANCY

The incidence of tubal pregnancy (eccyesis) has increased markedly in recent times.[57] It is often the consequence of chronic salpingitis, which leads to inflammatory destruction of the lining folds and retention of the ovum.[25] Congenital tubal abnormalities, functional tubal disturbances, and salpingitis isthmica nodosa are also responsible for a minority of the cases.[25,44] A history of infertility is associated with an

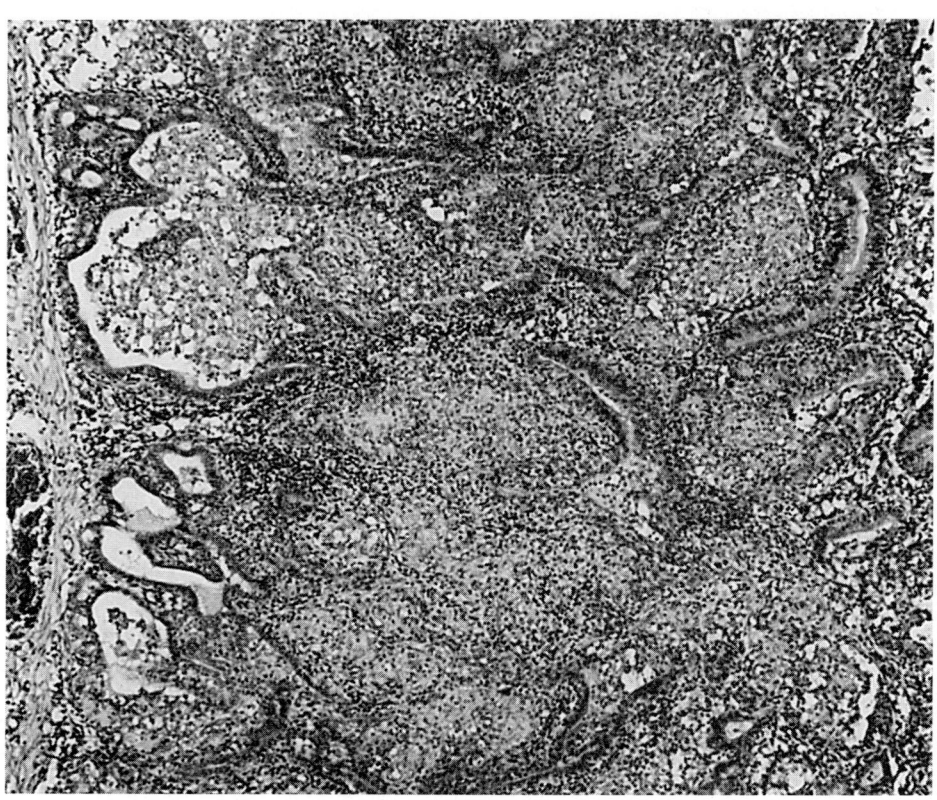

Fig. 19-129 Tuberculosis of fallopian tube involving chiefly mucosal layers. Glands become hyperplastic, and their borders may be indistinct as result of inflammatory reaction in which characteristic tubercles are often inconspicuous.

increased risk of tubal pregnancy,[92] whereas induced abortion has no apparent effect on a woman's risk of tubal pregnancy in subsequent pregnancies.[34]

In tubal pregnancy the gestational sac is completely made up of tubal tissue, with no participation from the ovarian or intraligamentary tissues. Following implantation of the ovum in the tubal epithelium (usually in the ampullo-isthmic or midtubal portion), chorionic villi and extravillous (intermediate) trophoblast can grow predominantly intraluminally[79] or penetrate deeply into the wall, just as they do in the uterus.[25,60] Trophoblastic invasion of muscle and vessels is a common finding of no clinical significance (Fig. 19-130). Changes resembling atherosclerosis may be seen in tubal arteries at the site of implantation, analogous to those occurring in the uterus in orthotopic pregnancy.[8] Although a few tubal pregnancies have gone to term,[15] the usual outcome is abortion. The maternal vessels rupture into the gestational sac and cause hematosalpinx (Figs. 19-131 and 19-132). In the presence of a large hematosalpinx, it may be difficult to identify the products of gestation; numerous blocks *from the intratubal blood clot* should be taken. Tubal rupture can occur (usually near the end of the second month) because of destruction of the tubal wall by the invading trophoblast, and this may result in severe intra-abdominal hemorrhage. This rupture may result in a brisk reactive proliferation of the mesothelium, with formation of papillae and psammoma bodies. These changes should be recognized as reactive and not misinterpreted as metastases or implants from an ovarian serous neoplasm. The usual treatment for tubal pregnancy is salpingectomy. It is possible to conserve the ovary in about 80% of the cases. Segmental tubal resec-

tion may be appropriate in selected cases; some of these individuals may develop recurrent tubal pregnancy, which is more related to the pre-existing disease than the operation.[78]

Uterine curettings in the presence of a *viable* tubal pregnancy show gestational hyperplasia, sometimes associated

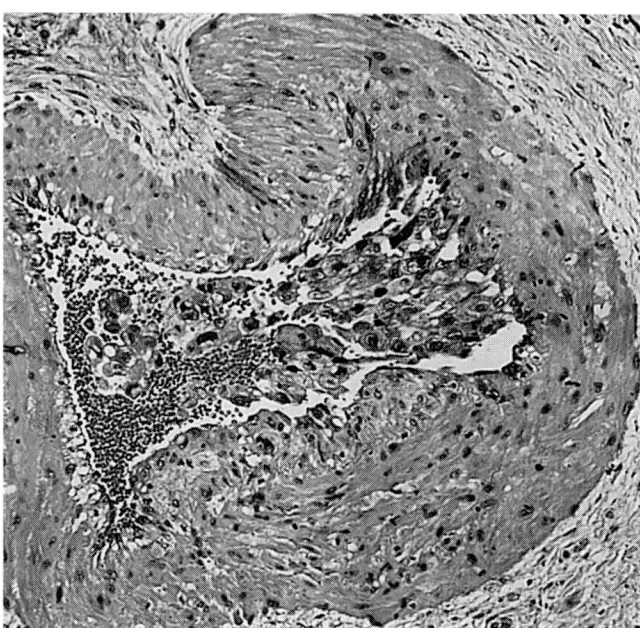

Fig. 19-130 Trophoblastic vascular invasion in tubal pregnancy, a common finding of no clinical significance.

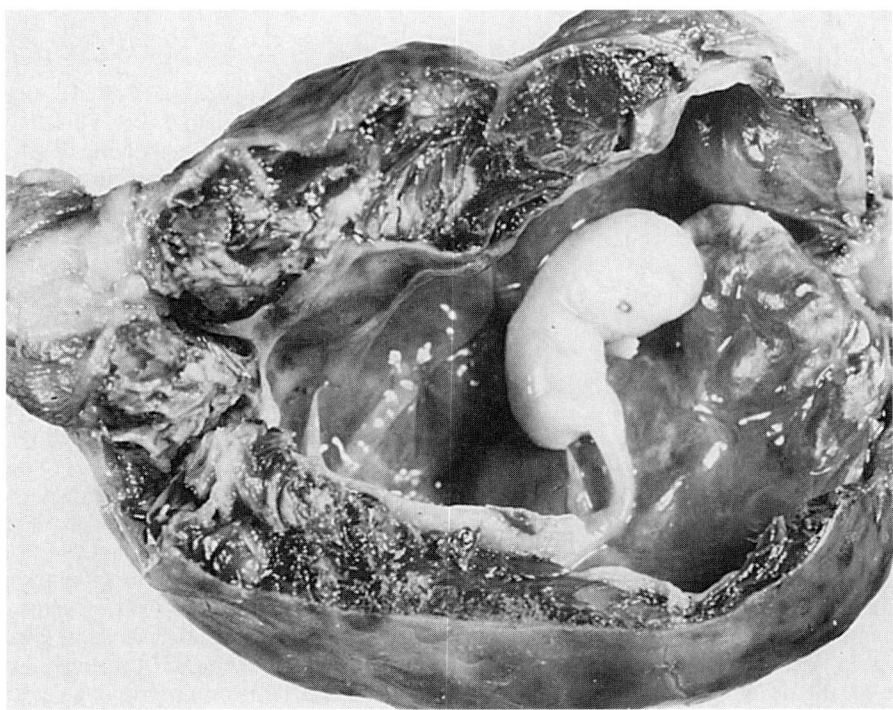

Fig. 19-131 Tubal pregnancy that ruptured at about third month in 34-year-old woman.

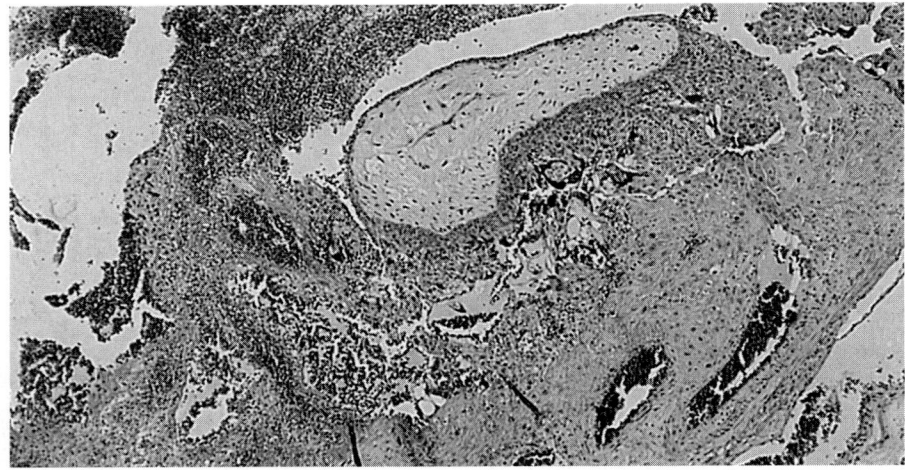

Fig. 19-132 Implantation site of placenta in fallopian tube. Chorionic villus can be seen. Placenta is firmly attached to edematous wall of tube, which was filled with blood.

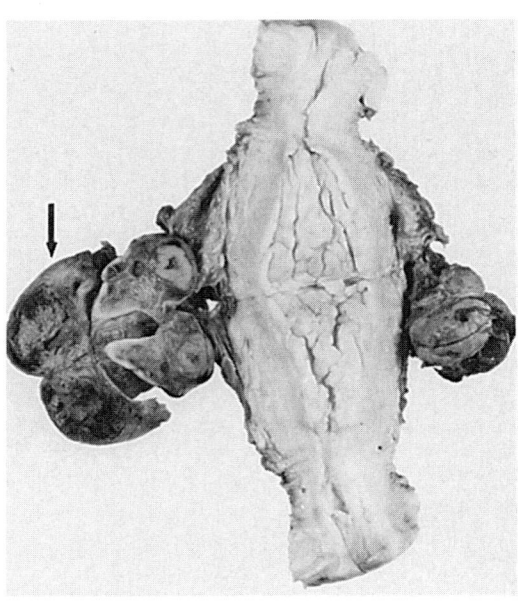

Fig. 19-133 Ruptured tubal pregnancy *(arrow).* Note gestational hyperplasia of endometrium and corpus luteum of pregnancy in homolateral ovary.

with the Arias-Stella reaction (Fig. 19-133). The key feature in the differential diagnosis between ectopic pregnancy and missed or incomplete abortion is the absence of fetal parts, chorionic villi, or trophoblastic cells in the latter (except for the extraordinarily rare occurrence of simultaneous intrauterine and ectopic pregnancy). Enlarged hyalinized spiral arteries and a fibrinoid matrix are not seen in the endometrium in cases of ectopic pregnancy, and therefore their presence is a strong indicator of intrauterine implantation.[56]

When trophoblastic elements are not obvious in routinely stained sections from the curettings, further search can be made with immunocytochemical stains for hCG, human placental lactogen (HPL), and keratin.[2,56] If none are found and a tubal mass is present, laparotomy under the presumptive diagnosis of tubal pregnancy is indicated. Death of the embryo or fetus often results in expulsion of the endometrial decidual cast, regeneration of the epithelium, and re-establishment of the cyclic pattern. Therefore the presence of a proliferative, secretory, or menstrual endometrium in a patient with an adnexal mass does not rule out the possibility of an ectopic pregnancy.

OTHER NON-NEOPLASTIC PROCESSES

Walthard cell nests are small, glistening, round collections of flat to cuboidal cells with the appearance of transitional epithelium located on the tubal serosa. They probably are the result of focal mesothelial hyperplasia or metaplasia.[83] They should not be mistaken for serosal implants in patients with ovarian neoplasms.

Paratubal cysts, generally known as *hydatids of Morgagni,* are commonly seen as small round cysts attached by a pedicle to the fimbriated end of the tube. Their wall is paper-thin and their content is clear. Occasionally, they attain a large size and may undergo torsion. Most are lined by tubal columnar epithelium containing both ciliated and secretory cells, sometimes projecting in a papillary fashion into the lumen and covered by a thin layer of smooth muscle.[9] Other paratubal cysts, lined by flat cells and surrounded by a thin fibrous wall, are regarded as of mesothelial origin.[70]

Endometriosis frequently involves the tube in the form of nodules located in the wall or serosa.[75] In this context, it should be mentioned that the most common manifestation of ectopic endometrium in the tube is focal replacement of tubal epithelium by uterine mucosa[67]; however, it is questionable whether this abnormality should be equated with conventional tubal endometriosis, as previously described.

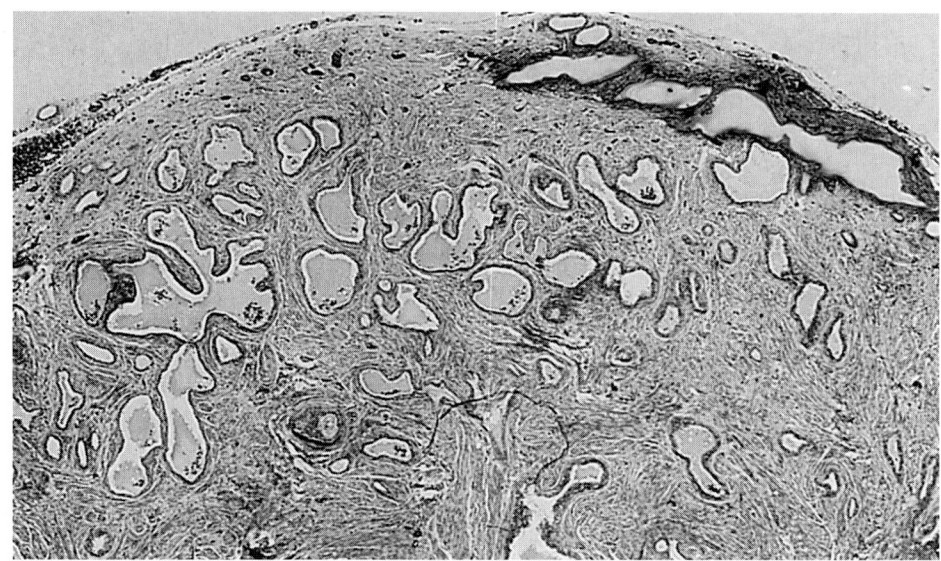

Fig. 19-134 Salpingitis isthmica nodosa. There is outpouching of tubal mucosa and prominent myohypertrophy.

Pseudoxanthomatous salpingiosis is characterized by a localized deposition of lipofuscin-laden macrophages in the lamina propria of the fallopian tubes; this is thought to represent the result of hemorrhage in endometriotic foci, possibly induced by an episode of acute salpingitis.[74]

Endosalpingiosis refers to the presence of tubal epithelium outside the tube proper, a concept somewhat analogous to endometriosis. The most common location is the ovarian surface close to the fimbria, suggesting that it may be secondary to extension of tubal epithelium over the inflammatory adhesions. Sometimes these changes are seen following surgical interventions, such as vaginal hysterectomy. Following the report of Burmeister et al.,[11] the term is more commonly used for a peritoneal process of different pathogenesis, probably representing a proliferative disorder of the mesothelium and subjacent tissue (more often in the pelvic region) in which small cystic structures lined by an epithelium of tubal appearance form. Since this disorder is often associated with ovarian serous tumors, it is discussed in more detail in the next section of this chapter.

Decidual reaction of the tubal mucosa is a common finding in specimens of tubal ligation obtained at the time of cesarean section; it appears as small nodular collections of decidual cells covered by a flattened, sometimes inflamed epithelium. Similar changes have been documented following hormonal therapy.[51]

Arias-Stella reaction can occur in the fallopian tube epithelium in association with either orthotopic or tubal pregnancy.[50]

Salpingitis isthmica nodosa is a usually bilateral tubal lesion that presents grossly as a well-delimited nodular enlargement of the isthmic portion. Microscopically, cystically dilated gland-like formations are seen surrounded by hypertrophic muscle (Fig. 19-134). Radiographic and tridimensional reconstructive studies have shown that the cystic formations are connected to the lumen of the tube.[71] Although classically regarded as the result of inflammation (hence its name), convincing evidence has been presented that its pathogenesis is analogous to that of uterine adenomyosis.[7] It is accompanied by infertility in approximately one half of the patients, and it may also lead to ectopic pregnancy.[44]

Tubal sterilization procedures lead to a sequence of morphologic alterations, which include proximal luminal dilatation, plical attenuation, chronic inflammation with pseudopolyp formation, and plical thickening in the distal segment.[66] The appearance varies depending on the length of time from the sterilization procedure.[77]

Metaplastic papillary tumor is a distinctive lesion characterized by eosinophilic and mucinous metaplasia of the mucosa resulting in a sharply outlined papillary configuration, occasionally encountered in tubes removed in the immediate postpartum period[5,68] (Fig. 19-135). Their behavior is benign. We favor the interpretation that this lesion is of non-neoplastic nature.

Proliferative epithelial lesions are occasionally found during the microscopic examination of a specimen from tubal ligation or salpingectomy. They may show one or more of the following features: nuclear crowding, stratification, loss of polarity, mild to moderate atypia, occasional mitoses, acidophilic metaplasia, and papillary formations[52,76,91] (Fig. 19-136). Invasion is absent. An association with salpingitis, exogenous or endogenous estrogen stimulation, and serous borderline tumors of the ovary has been described.[63,76] The latter association suggests the existence of a field effect in müllerian carcinogenesis.[63,91a] Some of these lesions have been designated as *adenomatous hyperplasia* and are regarded as the precursor stage of tubal carcinoma. Although this may well be the case for some of them, progression of these proliferative lesions to invasive

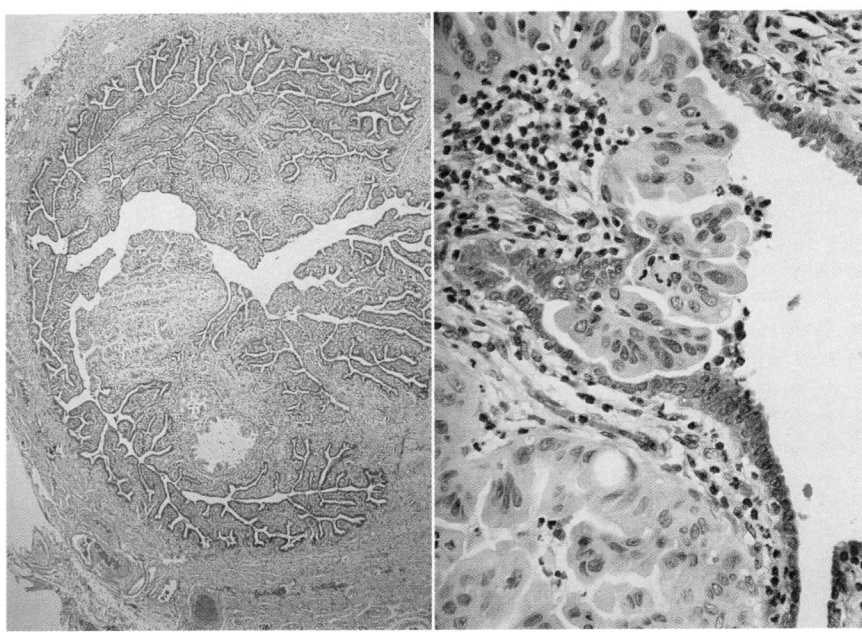

Fig. 19-135 So-called metaplastic papillary tumor. This lesion, which occurred in a pregnant woman, is characterized by a papillary proliferation of acidophilic epithelium. This process is probably of non-neoplastic nature.

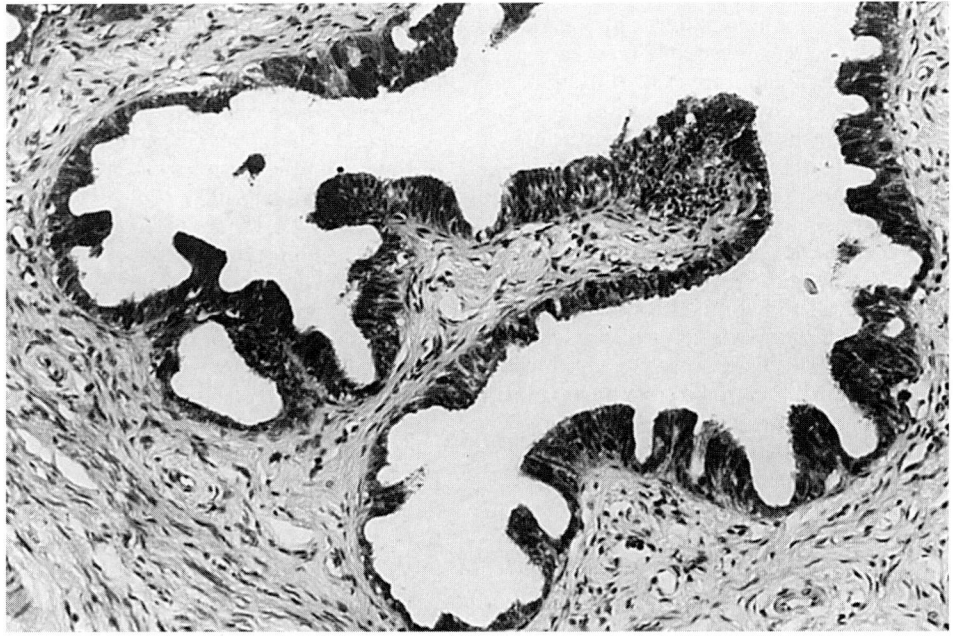

Fig. 19-136 Focal proliferative lesion in epithelium of fallopian tube. There is marked pseudostratification and some degree of nuclear atypicality.

tubal carcinoma has not been documented.[76] Therefore their presence in a specimen from tubal ligation does not justify additional surgical therapy.

CARCINOMA

Primary carcinoma of the fallopian tube is rare, accounting for about 1% of primary genital tract malignancies.[65] Most patients are postmenopausal, and the preoperative diagnosis is rarely correct. The tumor may be bilateral, but more often the contralateral tube is either normal or the site of a hydrosalpinx. Atypical vaginal bleeding is the most common form of presentation.[32] The classical triad of the disease, represented by pain, vaginal discharge, and a palpable adnexal mass, occurs in less than half of the cases. Cervicovaginal cytology is positive in only a minority of patients,[42] but an endometrial smear will reveal malignant cells in a high percentage of cases.[81] Grossly, the tube is enlarged and has fibrous adhesions, the outer appearance resembling that of chronic salpingitis. The cut surface shows a solid or papillary tumor filling the lumen (Fig. 19-137, *A*). Microscopically, the appearance is usually that of an invasive papillary adenocarcinoma of varying degrees of differentiation (Figs. 19-137, *B,* to 19-139). The light and electron microscopic appearance is often very similar to that of ovarian papillary serous adenocarcinoma.[82] Endometrioid, adenoacanthomatous, adenosquamous, squamous, seromucinous, mucinous, transitional cell, and clear cell variants have been reported.[13,41,84,85,87] The endometrioid carcinomas typically present as intraluminal masses and may resemble microscopically the so-called female adnexal tumor of probable wolffian origin.[17] Isolated cases of carcinoma in situ and of borderline serous tumors are also on record.[76]

The criteria for the diagnosis of primary tubal carcinoma should be very rigid because the frequency of this tumor is only a tenth of that of direct tubal extensions by uterine or ovarian carcinoma. By convention, a carcinoma extensively involving both endometrium and tube is classified as an endometrial tumor, and one extensively involving both ovary and tube is regarded as an ovarian neoplasm. In primary tubal carcinoma, the uterus and ovaries should appear largely normal on gross examination; the foci of malignancy in these organs, when present, should have the appearance of metastases or independent primaries by virtue of their size and distribution.[64]

The prognosis of tubal carcinoma depends more on staging than histologic grade. The staging system currently used is adapted from the FIGO staging system for ovarian carcinoma (Table 19-6).

Involvement of the tubal serosa, of the ovary or corpus uteri, or of other pelvic and abdominal structures indicates a poor prognosis.[72] Interestingly, the tumors of all five of the survivors studied by Green and Scully[26] were confined to a tube with fimbriated ends sealed by previous inflammatory disease. Five-year survival rates are as high as 77% for stage I lesions, approximately 40% for stage II, and about 20% for stage III.[18,48,59,62,64] The initial tumor recurrence is intraabdominal in over 80% of the cases, its pattern of spread mirroring that of ovarian carcinoma.

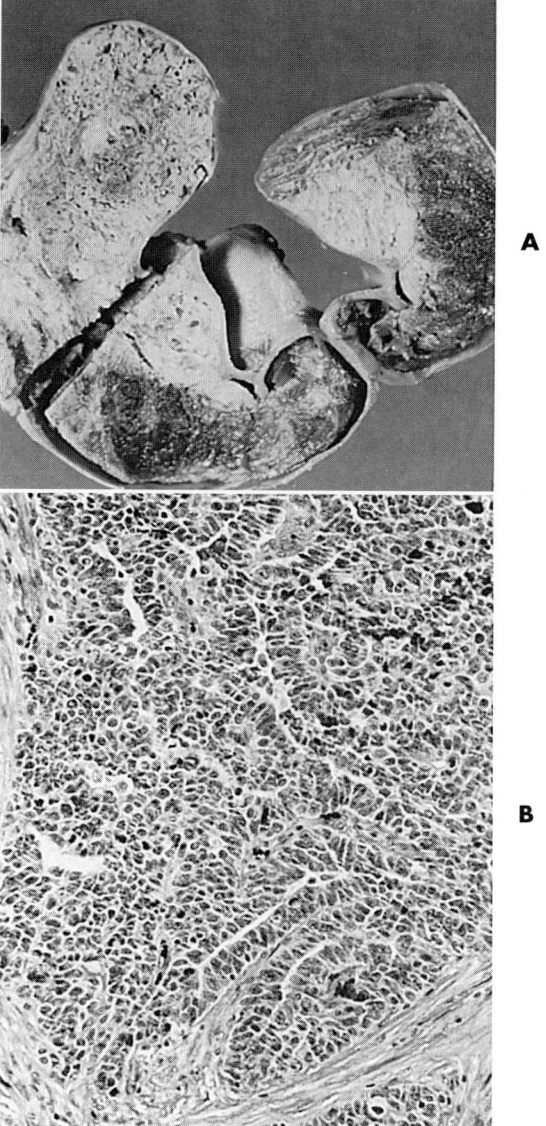

Fig. 19-137 A, Carcinoma of fallopian tube with extensive replacement of organ. Uterus and ovaries were normal. **B,** Primary adenocarcinoma of fallopian tube. Tumor is poorly differentiated and highly cellular.

OTHER TUMORS

Adenomatoid tumor is a benign, usually small lesion that may be found within the wall of the tube or beneath the uterine serosa near a cornu. The gross and microscopic features are identical to those of its epididymal counterpart (see Chapter 18). The ill-defined, seemingly infiltrating margins may lead to a mistaken diagnosis of carcinoma.[93] A marked degree of smooth muscle hyperplasia may be present and obscure the true nature of the lesion. There is now general agreement on the basis of ultrastructural and immunohistochemical findings that this entity is of mesothelial (rather than wolffian, müllerian, or endothelial) derivation and that

Table 19-6 FIGO staging for carcinoma of the fallopian tube

Stage O	Carcinoma in situ (limited to tubal mucosa).
Stage I	Growth limited to fallopian tubes.
Stage IA	Growth limited to one tube with extension into submucosa and/or muscularis but not penetrating serosal surface; no ascites.
Stage IB	Growth limited to both tubes with extension into submucosa and/or muscularis but not penetratingserosal surface; no ascites.
Stage IC	Tumor either Stage IA or Stage IB but with extension through or onto tubal serosa or with ascites containing malignant cells or with positive peritoneal washings.
Stage II	Growth involving one or both fallopian tubes with pelvic extension.
Stage IIA	Extension and/or metastasis to uterus and/or ovaries.
Stage IIB	Extension to other pelvic tissues.
Stage IIC	Tumor either Stage IIA or IIB and with ascites containing malignant cells or with positive peritoneal washings.
Stage III	Tumor involving one or both fallopian tubes with peritoneal or inguinal nodes. Superficial liver metastasis equals Stage III. Tumor appears limited to true pelvis but with historically proved malignant extension to small bowel or omentum.
Stage IIIA	Tumor grossly limited to true pelvis with negative nodes but with historically confirmed microscopic seeding of abdominal peritoneal surfaces.
Stage IIB	Tumor involving one or both tubes with historically confirmed implants of abdominal peritoneal surfaces, none exceeding 2 cm in diameter. Lymph nodes are negative.
Stage IIIC	Abdominal implants >2 cm in diameter and/or positive retroperitoneal or inguinal nodes.
Stage IV	Growth involving one or both fallopian tubes with distant metastases. If pleural effusion is present, cytologic fluid must be positive for malignant cells to be Stage IV. Parenchymal liver metastasis equals Stage IV.

NOTE: Staging for fallopian tube carcinoma is by the surgical pathologic system. Operative findings designating stage are determined before tumor debulking.
From SGO handbook. Staging of gynecologic malignancies. Chicago, 1994, Society of Gynecologic Oncologists.
See also Appendix G.

it represents a unique variant of benign mesothelioma largely restricted to the genital region,[43,69] as originally postulated by Masson. However, the alternative should be considered of at least some of these lesions representing examples of nodular mesothelial hyperplasia of a reactive nature.

Papillary cystadenoma of the mesosalpinx has been seen in patients with von Hippel–Lindau disease.[23]

Mucinous lesions of the fallopian tubes comprise a wide variety of processes, which include mucinous metaplasia, mucinous cystadenoma, mucinous tumors of low malignant potential ("borderline mucinous tumors"), and the already mentioned mucinous adenocarcinoma. Some of these lesions have occurred in patients with the Peutz-Jeghers syndrome, others in association with in situ or invasive adenocarcinoma of other portions of the female genital tract, and still others in conjunction with mucinous neoplasms of the appendix.[37,73]

About 50 cases of tubal *teratomas* have been published, all but one cystic and benign[35] (Fig. 19-140); one of them contained a carcinoid tumor and another was entirely composed of mature thyroid tissue (struma salpingis).[33] Other benign tubal tumors, all very rare, are *leiomyoma, hemangioma, adenofibroma,*[39] *sex-cord tumor with annular tubules* (associated with endometriosis),[27] and *papilloma.*[24] The latter should be distinguished from the more common papillary hyperplasia associated with inflammation and hyperestrinism. Malignant tumors other than carcinoma include *malignant mixed müllerian tumor*[12,36,45,53] (some bilateral[86]) (Fig. 19-141), *leiomyosarcoma,* and *choriocarcinoma.*[61] The latter is of gestational origin. All three tumor types resemble grossly and microscopically their more common uterine counterparts; tubal extension from the latter should always be considered in the differential diagnosis. Tubal involvement by *malignant lymphoma* is always the expression of systemic disease. *Secondary tubal invasion* by carcinoma of the ovary and uterus is a much more common event than primary tubal carcinoma. Most *metastases* to the tube also originate from genital organs, with very few exceptions.[46]

TUMORS AND TUMORLIKE CONDITIONS OF BROAD AND ROUND LIGAMENTS

Cystic formations derived from mesonephric or paramesonephric rests that can be found in or around the broad ligament were mentioned on p. 1452.

Female adnexal tumor of probable wolffian origin is a distinctive lesion of the broad ligament, although it has also been described in the ovary (see p. 1519). In its most typical form, it is seen within the leaves of the broad ligament or hanging on a pedicle from it or the fallopian tube. Grossly, it is predominantly solid. Microscopically, it is composed of epithelial cells growing in diffuse, trabecular, and tubular patterns. Mitotic activity and capsular invasion may be present, but the prognosis is generally good.[39a,59a]

Other tumors that can be found in the broad ligament unassociated with either uterine or ovarian disease are borderline serous papillary tumors[3]; serous, endometrioid, clear cell, and mucinous carcinomas[1,4]; papillary cystadenomas associated with von Hippel–Lindau disease[40]; ependymoma[6a]; smooth muscle tumors; and other nonspecific mesenchymal neoplasms. Some of the carcinomas of this region are thought to arise from foci of endometriosis.[4]

The *round ligament* is only rarely the site of primary disease. Striated muscle heteroplasia is an inconsequential incidental finding, thought to represent aberrant persistence of gubernacular rhabdomyoblasts.[34a] Cases of leiomyomas (including the epithelioid variety), "fibromas," and benign mesenchymomas (angiomyolipomas) have been reported.[22b,55a]

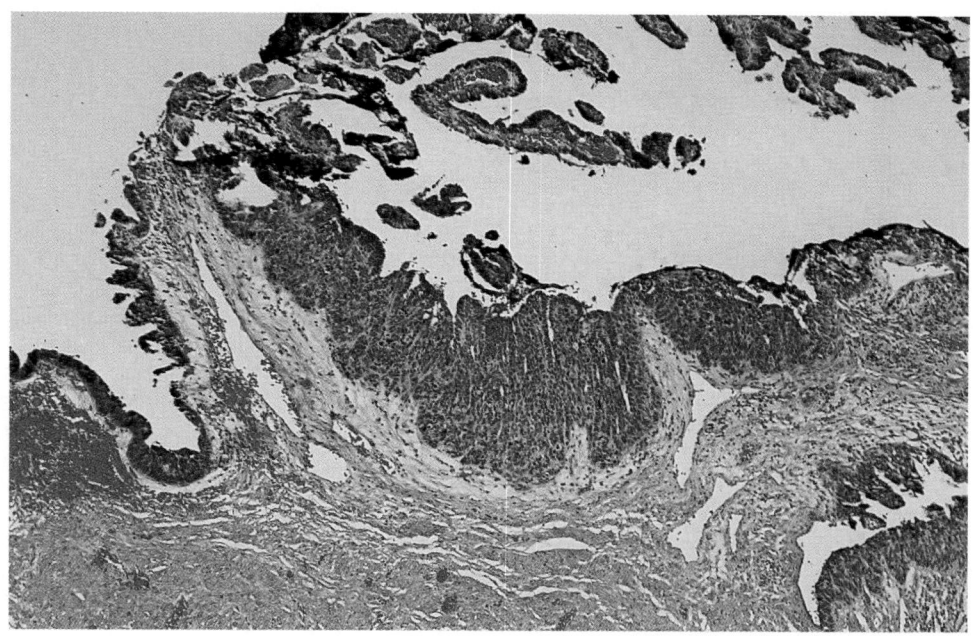

Fig. 19-138 Carcinoma of fallopian tube. Low-power microscopic appearance showing continuity between the mucosa and the tumor.

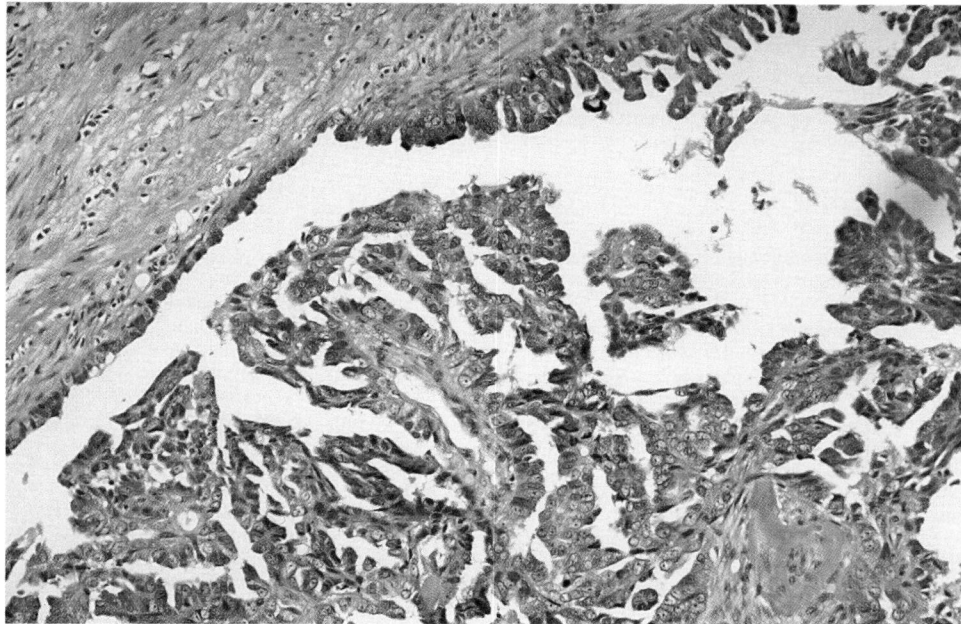

Fig. 19-139 High-power view showing the complex papillary architecture that is characteristic of tumors of this organ.

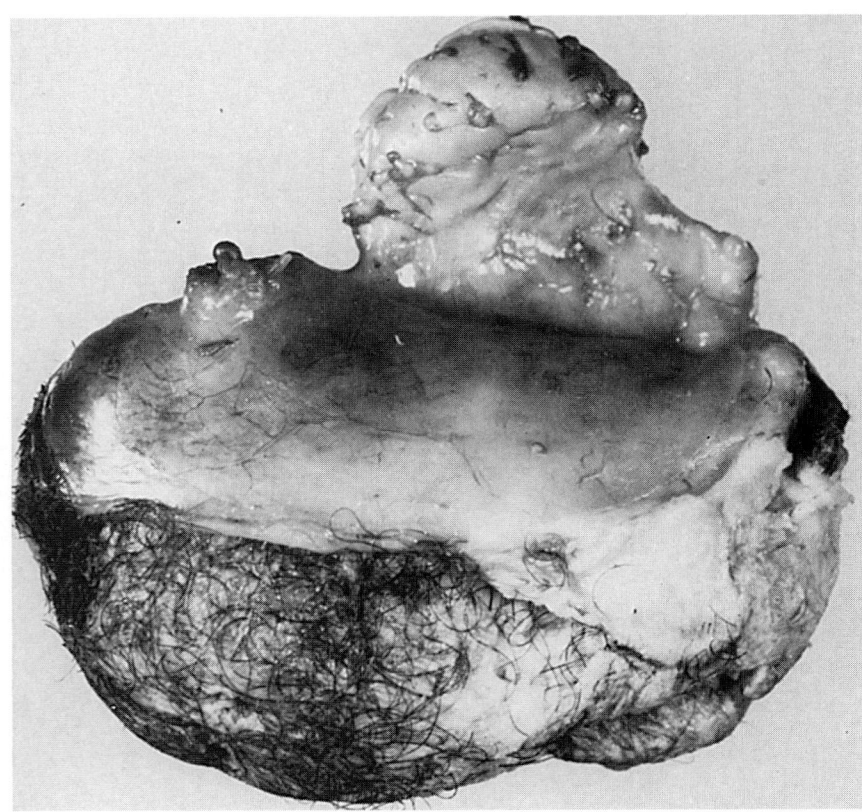

Fig. 19-140 Benign teratoma of fallopian tube in 41-year-old woman.

REFERENCES

1 Altaras MM, Jaffe R, Corduba M, Holtzinger M, Bahary C: Primary paraovarian cystadenocarcinoma. Clinical and management aspects and literature review. Gynecol Oncol **38:**268-272, 1990.

2 Angel E, Davis JR, Nagle RB: Immunohistochemical demonstration of placental hormones in the diagnosis of uterine versus ectopic pregnancy. Am J Clin Pathol **84:**705-709, 1985.

3 Aslani M, Ahn GH, Scully RE: Serous papillary cystadenoma of borderline malignancy of broad ligament. A report of 25 cases. Int J Gynecol Pathol **7:**131-138, 1988.

4 Aslani M, Scully RE: Primary carcinoma of the broad ligament. Report of four cases and review of the literature. Cancer **64:**1540-1545, 1989.

5 Bartnik J, Powell WS, Moriber-Katz S, Amenta PS: Metaplastic papillary tumor of the fallopian tube. Case report, immunohistochemical features, and review of the literature. Arch Pathol Lab Med **113:**545-547, 1989.

6 Bell DA, Mondschein M, Scully RE: Giant cell arteritis of the female genital tract. A report of three cases. Am J Surg Pathol **10:**696-701, 1986.

6a Bell DA, Woodruff JM, Scully RE: Ependymoma of the broad ligament. A report of two cases. Am J Surg Pathol **8:**203-209, 1984.

7 Benjamin CL, Beaver DC: Pathogenesis of salpingitis isthmica nodosa. Am J Clin Pathol **21:**212-222, 1951.

8 Blaustein A, Shenker L: Vascular lesions of the uterine tube in ectopic pregnancy. Obstet Gynecol **30:**551-555, 1967.

9 Bransilver BR, Ferenczy A, Richart RM: Female genital tract remnants. An ultrastructural comparison of hydatid of Morgagni and mesonephric ducts and tubules. Arch Pathol **96:**255-261, 1973.

10 Bruns DE, Mills SE, Savory J: Amylase in fallopian tube and serous ovarian neoplasms. Immunohistochemical localization. Arch Pathol Lab Med **106:**17-20, 1982.

11 Burmeister RE, Fechner RE, Franklin RR: Endosalpingiosis of the peritoneum. Obstet Gynecol **34:**310-318, 1969.

12 Carlson J, Ackerman B, Wheeler J: Malignant mixed mullerian tumor of the fallopian tube. Cancer **71:**187-192, 1993.

13 Cheung A, So K, Ngan H, Wong L: Primary squamous cell carcinoma of fallopian tube. Int J Gynecol Pathol **13:**92-95, 1994.

14 Cheung ANY, Young RH, Scully RE: Pseudocarcinomatous hyperplasia of the fallopian tube associated with salpingitis. A report of 14 cases. Am J Surg Pathol **18:**1125-1130, 1994.

15 Chokroverty M, Caballes RL, Gear PE: An unruptured tubal pregnancy at term. Arch Pathol Lab Med **110:**250-251, 1986.

16 David A, Garcia C-S, Czernobilsky B: Human hydrosalpinx. Histologic study and chemical composition of fluid. Am J Obstet Gynecol **105:**400-411, 1969.

17 Daya D, Young RH, Scully RE: Endometrioid carcinoma of the fallopian tube resembling an adnexal tumor of probable wolffian origin. A report of six cases. Int J Gynecol Pathol **11:**122-130, 1992.

18 Eddy GL, Copeland LJ, Gershenson DM, Atkinson EN, Wharton JT, Rutledge FN: Fallopian tube carcinoma. Obstet Gynecol **64:**546-552, 1984.

19 Elliott GB, Brody H, Elliott KA: Implications of "lipoid salpingitis." Fertil Steril **16:**541-548, 1965.

20 Eschenbach DA, Buchanan TM, Pollock HM, Forsyth PS, Alexander ER, Lin I-S, Wang SP, Wentworth BB, McCormack WM, Holmes KK: Polymicrobial etiology of acute pelvic inflammatory disease. N Engl J Med **29:**166-171, 1975.

21 Fortier KJ, Haney AF: The pathologic spectrum of uterotubal junction obstruction. Obstet Gynecol **65:**93-98, 1985.

22 Francis WAJ: Female genital tuberculosis. A review of 135 cases. J Obstet Gynaecol Br Commonw **71:**418-428, 1964.

22a Gardner GH, Greene RR, Peckham B: Normal and cystic structures of the broad ligament. Am J Obstet Gynecol **55:**917-939, 1948.

22b Gardner GH, Greene RR, Peckham B: Tumors of the broad ligament. Am J Obstet Gynecol **73:**536-555, 1957.

23 Gersell DJ, King TC: Papillary cystadenoma of the mesosalpinx in von Hippel–Lindau disease. Am J Surg Pathol **12:**145-149, 1988.

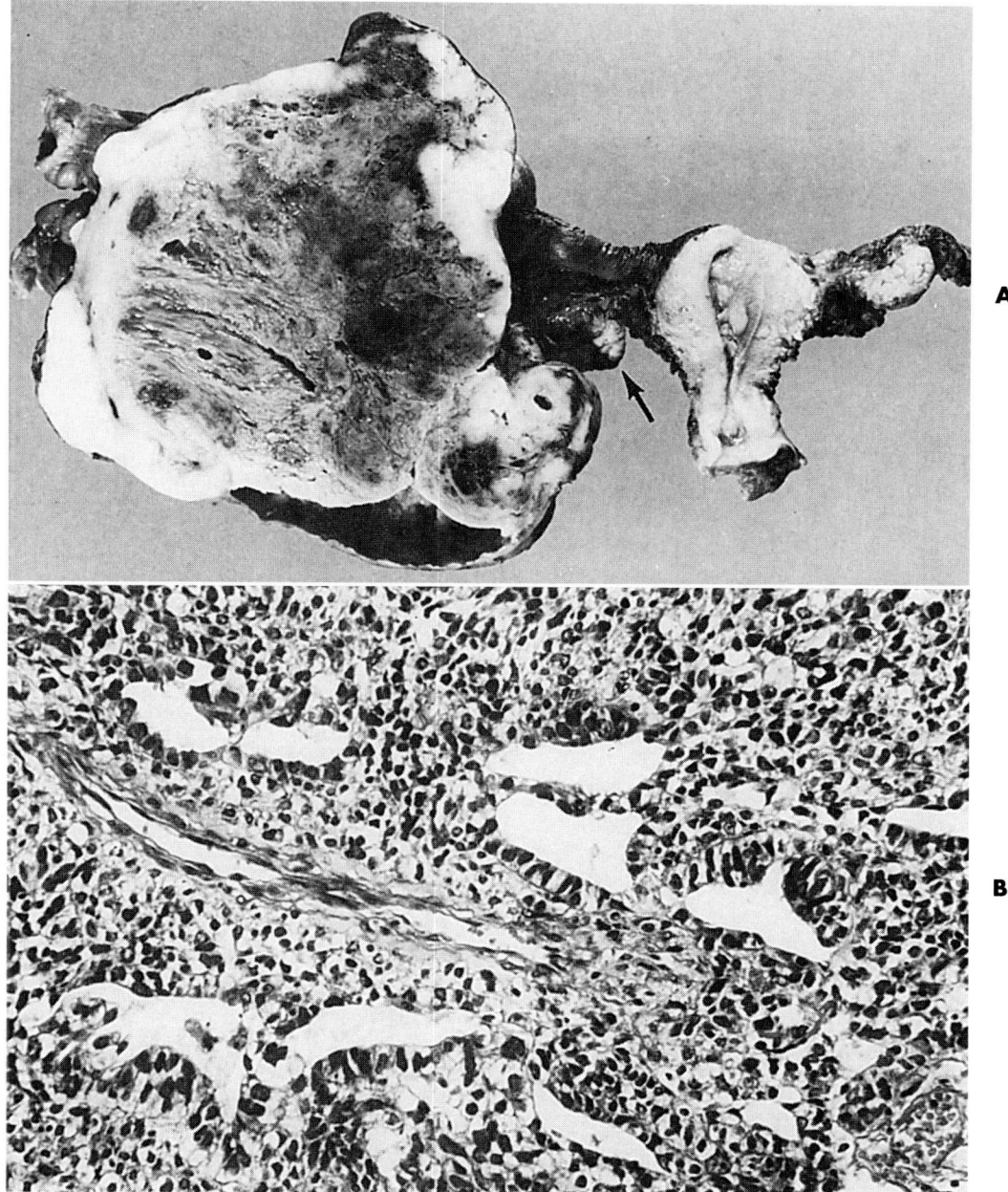

Fig. 19-141 Malignant mixed müllerian tumor of fallopian tube. **A,** Large tumor, partially necrotic and hemorrhagic, totally obliterates the organ. Ovary is not involved *(arrow).* **B,** Photomicrograph showing areas of adenocarcinoma and undifferentiated stromal sarcoma. There were also areas of osteosarcoma. (Courtesy Dr. H. Rodriguez-Martinez, Mexico City.)

24 Gisser SD: Obstructing fallopian tube papilloma. Int J Gynecol Pathol 5:179-182, 1986.

25 Green LK, Kott ML: Histopathologic findings in ectopic tubal pregnancy. Int J Gynecol 8:255-262, 1989.

26 Green TH, Scully RE: Tumors of the fallopian tube. Clin Obstet Gynecol 5:886-906, 1962.

27 Griffith LM, Carcangiu ML: Sex cord tumor with annular tubules associated with endometriosis of the fallopian tube. Am J Clin Pathol 96:259-262, 1991.

28 Grosfeld JL: Torsion of normal ovary in the first two years of life. Am J Surg 117:726-727, 1969.

29 Hansen OH: Isolated torsion of the fallopian tube. Acta Obstet Gynecol Scand 49:3-6, 1970.

30 Henderson DN, Harkins JL, Stitt JF: Pelvic tuberculosis. Am J Obstet Gynecol 94:630-633, 1966.

31 Hershlag A, Seifer DB, Carcangiu ML, Patton DL, Diamond MP, De Cherney AH: Salpingoscopy. Light microscopic and electron microscopic correlations (published erratum appears in Obstet Gynecol 1991 May; 77[5]:809-10). Obstet Gynecol 77:399-405, 1991.

32 Hirai Y, Kaku S, Teshima H, Shimizu Y, Chen JT, Hamada T, Fujimoto I, Yamauchi K, Sakamoto A, Hasumi K, et al: Clinical study of primary carcinoma of the fallopian tube. Experience with 15 cases. Gynecol Oncol 34:20-26, 1989.

33 Hoda SA, Huvos AG: Struma salpingis associated with struma ovarii. Am J Surg Pathol 17:1187-1189, 1993.

34 Holt VL, Daling JR, Voigt LF, McKnight B, Stergachis A, Chu J, Weiss NS: Induced abortion and the risk of subsequent ectopic pregnancy. Am J Public Health 79:1234-1238, 1989.

34a Honore LH, Manickavel V: Striated muscle heteroplasia in the uterine round ligament. A report of 30 cases. Arch Pathol Lab Med 115:223-225, 1991.

35 Horn T, Jao W, Keh PC: Benign cystic teratoma of the fallopian tube (Letter to the Editor). Arch Pathol Lab Med 107:48, 1983.

36 Imachi M, Tsukamoto N, Shigematsu T, Watanabe T, Uehira K, Amada S, Umezu T, Nakano H: Malignant mixed Mullerian tumor of the fallopian tube. Report of two cases and review of literature. Gynecol Oncol 47:114-124, 1992.

37 Jackson-York GL, Ramzy I: Synchronous papillary mucinous adenocarcinoma of the endocervix and fallopian tubes. Int J Gynecol Pathol 10:394-401, 1991.

38 James DF, Barber HRK, Graber EA: Torsion of normal uterine adnexa in children. Report of three cases. Obstet Gynecol 35:226-230, 1970.

39 Kanbour AI, Burgess F, Salazar H: Intramural adenofibroma of the fallopian tube. Light and electron microscopy. Cancer 31:1433-1439, 1973.

39a Kariminejad MH, Scully RE: Female adnexal tumor of probable wolffian origin. A distinctive pathologic entity. Cancer 31:671-677, 1973.

40 Korn WT, Schatzki SC, Di Sciullo AJ, Scully RE: Papillary cystadenoma of the broad ligament in von Hippel–Lindau disease. Am J Obstet Gynecol 163:596-598, 1990.

41 Koshiyama M, Konishi I, Yoshida M, Wang D-P, Mandal M, Mori T, Fuji S: Transitional cell carcinoma of the fallopian tube. A light and electron microscopic study. Int J Gynecol Pathol 13:175-180, 1994.

42 Lehto L: Cytology of the human fallopian tube. Acta Obstet Gynecol Scand 42(Suppl 14):1-95, 1963.

43 Mackay B, Bennington JL, Skoglund RW: The adenomatoid tumor. Fine structural evidence for a mesothelial origin. Cancer 27:109-115, 1971.

44 Majmudar B, Henderson PH, Semple E: Salpingitis isthmica nodosa. A high-risk for tubal pregnancy. Obstet Gynecol 62:73-78, 1983.

45 Manes JL, Taylor HB: Carcinosarcoma and mixed müllerian tumors of the fallopian tube. Report of four cases. Cancer 38:1687-1693, 1976.

46 Mazur MT, Hsueh S, Gersell DJ: Metastases to the female genital tract. Analysis of 325 cases. Cancer 53:1978-1984, 1984.

47 McCormack WM: Pelvic inflammatory disease. N Engl J Med 330:115-119, 1994.

48 McMurray EH, Jacobs AJ, Perez CA, Camel HM, Kao M-S, Galakatos A: Carcinoma of the fallopian tube. Management and sites of failure. Cancer 58:2070-2075, 1986.

49 Mickal A, Sellmann AH, Beebe JL: Ruptured tuboovarian abscess. Am J Obstet Gynecol 100:432-436, 1968.

50 Milchgrub S, Sandstad J: Arias-Stella reaction in fallopian tube epithelium. A light and electron microscopic study with a review of the literature. Am J Clin Pathol 95:892-895, 1991.

51 Mills SE, Fechner RE: Stromal and epithelial changes in the fallopian tube following hormonal therapy. Hum Pathol 11:583-584, 1980.

52 Moore SW, Enterline HT: Significance of proliferative epithelial lesions of the uterine tube. Obstet Gynecol 45:385-390, 1975.

53 Muntz HG, Rutgers JL, Tarraza HM, Fuller AF Jr: Carcinosarcomas and mixed Mullerian tumors of the fallopian tube. Gynecol Oncol 34:109-115, 1989.

54 Nassberg S, McKay DG, Hertig AT: Physiologic salpingitis. Am J Obstet Gynecol 67:130-137, 1954.

55 Nogales-Ortiz F, Tarancón I, Nogales FF Jr: The pathology of female genital tuberculosis. Obstet Gynecol 53:422-428, 1979.

55a Nuovo MA, Nuovo GJ, Smith D, Lewis SH: Benign mesenchymoma of the round ligament. A report of two cases with immunohistochemistry. Am J Clin Pathol 93:421-424, 1990.

56 O'Connor DM, Kurman RJ: Intermediate trophoblast in uterine curettings in the diagnosis of ectopic pregnancy. Obstet Gynecol 72:665-670, 1988.

57 Pauerstein CJ, Croxatto HB, Eddy CA, Ramzy I, Walters MD: Anatomy and pathology of tubal pregnancy. Obstet Gynecol 67:301-308, 1986.

58 Pedowitz R, Bloomfield RD: Ruptured adnexal abscess (tuboovarian) with generalized peritonitis. Am J Obstet Gynecol 88:721-729, 1964.

59 Podratz KC, Podczaski ES, Gaffey TA, O'Brien PC, Schray MF, Malkasian GD: Primary carcinoma of the fallopian tube. Am J Obstet Gynecol 154:1319-1326, 1986.

59a Rahilly MA, Williams AR, Krausz T, al Nafussi A: Female adnexal tumour of probable Wolffian origin. A clinicopathological and immunohistochemical study of three cases. Histopathology 26:69-74, 1995.

60 Randall S, Buckley CH, Fox H: Placentation in the fallopian tube. Int J Gynecol Pathol 6:132-139, 1987.

61 Riggs JA, Wainer AS, Hahn GA, Farell MD: Extrauterine tubal choriocarcinoma. Am J Obstet Gynecol 88:637-641, 1964.

62 Roberts JA, Lifshitz S: Primary adenocarcinoma of the fallopian tube. Gynecol Oncol 13:301-308, 1982.

63 Robey SS, Silva EG: Epithelial hyperplasia of the fallopian tube. Its association with serous borderline tumors of the ovary. Int J Gynecol Pathol 8:214-220, 1989.

64 Rose PG, Piver MS, Tsukada Y: Fallopian tube cancer. The Roswell Park experience. Cancer 66:2661-2667, 1990.

65 Rosenblatt KA, Weiss NS, Schwartz SM: Incidence of malignant fallopian tube tumors. Gynecol Oncol 35:236-239, 1989.

66 Rubin A, Czernobilsky B: Tubal ligation. A bacteriologic, histologic and clinical study. Obstet Gynecol 36:199-203, 1970.

67 Rubin IC, Lisa JR, Trinidad S: Further observations of ectopic endometrium of fallopian tube. Surg Gynecol Obstet 103:469-474, 1956.

68 Saffos RO, Rhatigan RM, Scully RE: Metaplastic papillary tumor of the fallopian tube—a distinctive lesion of pregnancy. Am J Clin Pathol 74:232-236, 1980.

69 Salazar H, Kanbour A, Burgess F: Ultrastructure and observations on the histogenesis of mesotheliomas "adenomatoid tumors" of the female genital tract. Cancer 29:141-152, 1972.

70 Samaha M, Woodruff JD: Paratubal cysts. Frequency, histogenesis, and associated clinical features. Obstet Gynecol 65:691-694, 1985.

71 Schencken JR, Burns EL: A study and classification of nodular lesions of the fallopian tube. Am J Obstet Gynecol 45:624-636, 1943.

72 Schiller HM, Silverberg SG: Staging and prognosis in primary carcinoma of the fallopian tube. Cancer 28:389-395, 1971.

73 Seidman JD: Mucinous lesions of the fallopian tube. A report of seven cases. Am J Surg Pathol 18:1205-1212, 1994.

74 Seidman JD, Oberer S, Bitterman P, Aisner SC: Pathogenesis of pseudoxanthomatous salpingiosis. Mod Pathol 6:53-55, 1993.

75 Sheldon RS, Wilson RB, Dockerty MB: Serosal endometriosis of fallopian tubes. Am J Obstet Gynecol 99:882-884, 1967.

76 Stern J, Buscema J, Parmley T, Woodruff JD, Rosenshein NB: Atypical epithelial proliferations in the fallopian tube. Am J Obstet Gynecol 140:309-312, 1981.

77 Stock RJ: Histopathologic changes in fallopian tubes subsequent to sterilization procedures. Int J Gynecol Pathol 2:13-27, 1983.

78 Stock RJ: Histopathology of fallopian tubes with recurrent tubal pregnancy. Obstet Gynecol 75:9-14, 1990.

79 Stock RJ: Tubal pregnancy. Associated histopathology. Obstet Gynecol Clin North Am 18:73-94, 1991.

80 Sweet RL, Draper DL, Hadley WK: Etiology of acute salpingitis. Influence of episode number and duration of symptoms. Obstet Gynecol 58:62-68, 1981.

81 Takashina T, Ito E, Kudo R: Cytologic diagnosis of primary tubal cancer. Acta Cytol (Baltimore) 29:367-372, 1984.

82 Talamo TS, Bender BL, Ellis LD, Scioscia EA: Adenocarcinoma of the fallopian tube. An ultrastructural study. Virchows Arch [A] 397:363-368, 1982.

83 Teoh TB: The structure and development of Walthard nests. J Pathol Bacteriol 66:433-439, 1953.

84 Thor AD, Young RH, Clement PB: Pathology of the fallopian tube, broad ligament, peritoneum, and pelvic soft tissues. Hum Pathol 22:856-867, 1991.

85 Uehira K, Hashimoto H, Tsuneyoshi M, Enjoji M: Transitional cell carcinoma pattern in primary carcinoma of the fallopian tube. Cancer 72:2447-2456, 1993.

86 van Dijk CM, Kooijman CD, van Lindert AC: Malignant mixed mullerian tumor of the fallopian tube. Histopathology 16:300-302, 1990.

87 Voet RL, Lifshitz S: Primary clear cell adenocarcinoma of the fallopian tube. Light microscopic and ultrastructural findings. Int J Gynecol Pathol 1:292-298, 1982.

88 Wallace TM, Hart WR: Acute chlamydial salpingitis with ascites and adnexal mass simulating a malignant neoplasm. Int J Gynecol Pathol 10:394-401, 1991.

89 Washington AE, Aral SO, Wolner-Hanssen P, Grimes DA, Holmes KK: Assessing risk for pelvic inflammatory disease and its sequelae. JAMA 266:2581-2586, 1991.

90 Winkler B, Reumann W, Mitao M, Gallo L, Richart RM, Crum CP: Immunoperoxidase localization of chlamydial antigens in acute salpingitis. Am J Obstet Gynecol 152:275-278, 1985.

91 Woodruff JD, Pauerstein CJ: The fallopian tube. Structure, function, pathology, and management. Baltimore, 1969, The Williams & Wilkins Co.

91a Yanai-Inbar I, Siriaunkgul S, Silverberg SG: Mucosal epithelial proliferation of the fallopian tube. A particular association with ovarian serous tumor of low malignant potential? Int J Gynecol Pathol 14:107-113, 1995.

92 Yang CP, Chow WH, Daling JR, Weiss NS, Moore DE: Does prior infertility increase the risk of tubal pregnancy? Fertil Steril 48:62-66, 1987.

93 Youngs LA, Taylor HB: Adenomatoid tumors of the uterus and fallopian tube. Am J Clin Pathol 48:537-545, 1967.

Ovary

NORMAL ANATOMY

The ovaries are paired pelvic organs located on the sides of the uterus close to the lateral pelvic wall, behind the broad ligament and anterior to the rectum. They are connected to the broad ligament by the mesovarium (a double fold of peritoneum), to the uterine cornu by the ovarian (or utero-ovarian) ligament, and to the lateral pelvic wall by the infundibulopelvic (or suspensory) ligament. During the reproductive period, their average size is $4 \times 2 \times 1$ cm, and their average weight is 5 to 8 g; after menopause, they shrink to one half or less of this size.

The ovarian lymph vessels drain to large trunks that form a plexus at the hilus, from which they travel through the mesovarium to drain into the para-aortic nodes; others drain into the internal iliac, external iliac, interaortic, common iliac, and inguinal nodes.

The ovary is covered by a single layer of modified mesothelium variously known as *surface, celomic,* or *germinal epithelium*. The close embryologic and functional relationship of this structure with the lining epithelium of the müllerian ducts (i.e., the progenitor of the tubal, endometrial, and endocervical mucosa) probably explains the marked similarities among these tissues and the tumors arising from them. Indeed, the entire pelvic and lower abdominal mesothelium and the subjacent mesenchyme of females are referred to as the secondary müllerian system.

The *ovarian stroma* is divided into a cortical and a medullary region, but the boundaries between them are indistinct. It is composed mainly of spindle-shaped stromal cells resembling fibroblasts, typically arranged in whorls or a storiform pattern. The cells may contain cytoplasmic lipid and are surrounded by a dense network of reticulin fibers. Some of these cells have myofibroblastic features and acquire immunoreactivity for smooth muscle actin and desmin.[3,6] Other cells that may be found in the ovarian stroma are luteinized stromal cells (singly or in small nests, mainly in the medulla), so-called enzymatically active stromal cells, decidual cells, bundles of smooth muscle, nests of cells resembling endometrial stromal cells, mature fat cells, and neuroendocrine cells.[1,4]

The life cycle of the *ovarian follicle* includes primordial, maturing (primary, secondary, tertiary, and graafian), and atretic, together with corpora lutea and corpora albicantia for those that have reached full maturation. Primordial follicles contain germ cells that have originated from the yolk sac endoderm and migrated into the ovary, where they develop into oogonia and oocytes.[2] These remain arrested at the dictyate stage of mitotic prophase at the time of birth, entering an interphase period at the time of follicular maturation prior to ovulation. The maturing follicle is composed of the oocyte, the granulosa layer, and the theca layers. *Granulosa cells* lack a reticulum around them and are immunoreactive for vimentin, keratin, and desmoplakin. They feature small rosette-like formations known as Call-Exner bodies, which contain at their center a deeply eosinophilic filamentous material consisting of excess basal lamina. Whether the granulosa cells derive from the ovarian stroma or from the *sex cords* (structures that first appear beneath the surface epithelium of the gonadal anlage and later converge toward the hilus of the gland) is still unre-

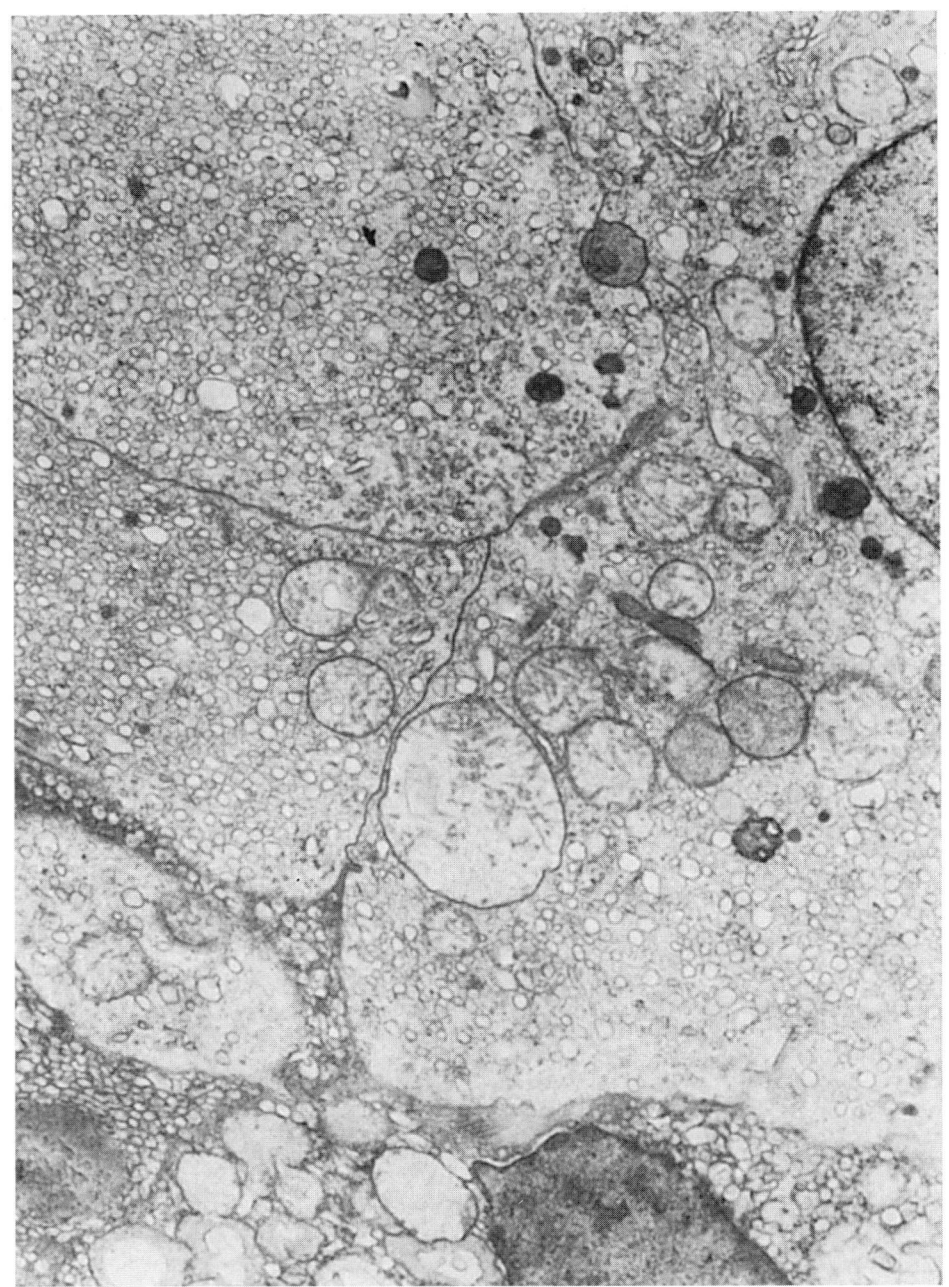

Fig. 19-142 Normal ovarian hilus cells. They have ultrastructural characteristics of steroid-producing cells such as those of adrenal cortex, Leydig cells of testis, and cells of corpus luteum. Cells have cytoplasm filled with microtubular forms of smooth endoplasmic reticulum and mitochondria with tubular cristae. (×10,500.)

solved. The stroma-derived *theca cells* form an internal layer (which is typically luteinized) and an external layer (which is very cellular and can simulate a neoplastic process when cut tangentially). Internal theca cells are an important site of sex steroid production, as determined indirectly by the immunohistochemical detection of enzymes involved in steroid hormone biosynthesis.[7,7a]

The mature *corpus luteum* is a 1.5 to 2.5 cm round yellow structure with lobulated outlines and a cystic center. Both

the granulosa and the theca cells that form it show prominent luteinization. Morphologic criteria for the dating of the corpus luteum have been established.[10] The corpus luteum of pregnancy is characterized by its larger size, bright yellow color, and prominent central cavity and the presence of hyaline droplets and calcification.[2]

At the ovarian hilus, there are clusters of cells analogous to testicular Leydig cells known as *ovarian hilus cells*. They are closely associated with large hilar veins and lymph ves-

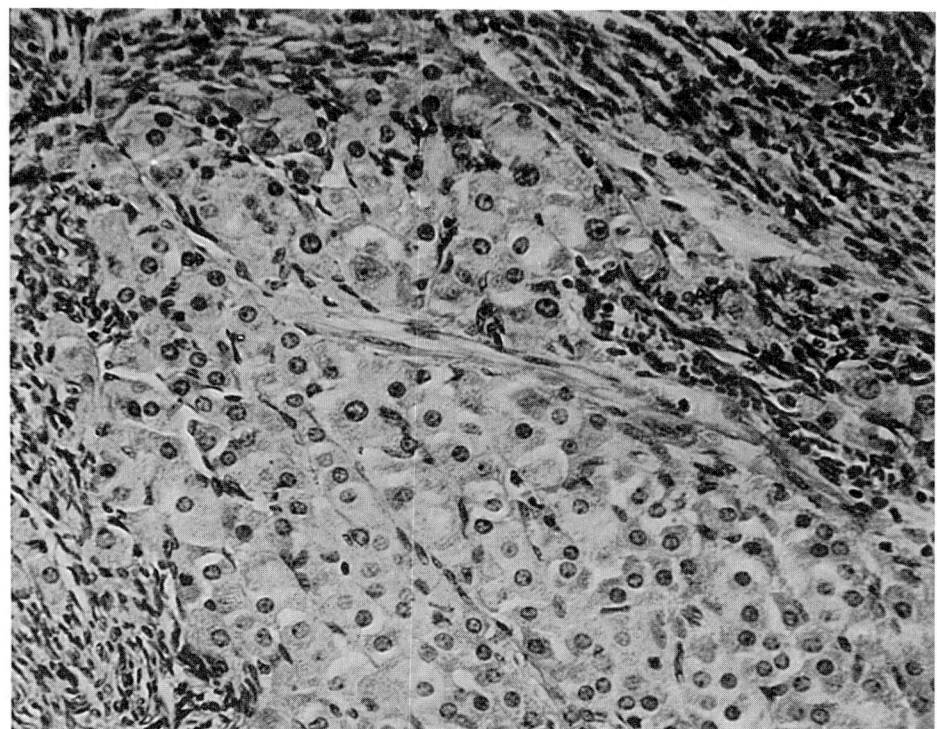

Fig. 19-143 Ovarian Leydig (hilus) cell hyperplasia. Note poorly circumscribed masses of large cells separated by ovarian stroma.

sels and may form nodular protrusions within their lumina. They also exhibit an intimate relationship with the nonmedullated nerves of the region[5,8] (Fig. 19-142). They may contain Reinke's crystalloids, lipids, and lipochrome pigment. Hyperplasia of these cells is found following the administration of chorionic gonadotropin, in pregnancy, and in the presence of choriocarcinoma[9] (Fig. 19-143).

The *rete ovarii,* present in the ovarian hilus, represents the ovarian counterpart of the rete testis. It consists of a network of clefts, tubules, cysts, and papillae lined by an epithelium of variable height and surrounded by a cuff of spindle-cell stroma.

Walthard cell nests may be cystic or solid; they are composed of urothelial-type epithelium (sometimes mucin-producing) and are located in the mesovarium, in the adjacent mesosalpinx, or within the ovarian hilus.

The previous description mainly pertains to the fully developed ovary in women of child-bearing age. The many modifications exhibited by the prepuberal and postmenopausal ovary are beyond the scope of this chapter. It should be mentioned, however, that prominent cystic follicles are normally seen during the first few months of life and at puberty and that the shrunken postmenopausal ovary "ovarium gyratum") has thick-walled medullary and hilar vessels (which should not be mistaken for hemangiomas). These atrophic ovaries may also contain granulomas and hyaline scars.[2]

GONADAL DYSGENESIS

Patients with gonadal dysgenesis have abnormally developed gonads and infantile sexual development; sex chromosome abnormalities are often found. Sometimes, gonadal tissue is biopsied or removed in the course of evaluation of these malformations.[23,24] In patients with **gonadal dysgenesis,** either *"pure"* (with a 46,XX or 46,XY karyotype) or associated with the somatic features of **Turner's syndrome** (with a 45,XO karyotype), both gonads are represented by a streak of fibrous tissue that vaguely resembles ovarian stroma.[14,25] These patients do not seem to have an increased incidence of gonadal tumors,[26] but various types of nongonadal neoplasms (such as atypical polypoid adenomyoma of uterus, leukemia, and soft tissue tumors) have been reported in patients with the syndrome.[11,16] Also, several cases of Turner's syndrome have been reported in association with endometrial adenocarcinoma; in some of these, prolonged estrogen therapy had been administered.[18] In **mixed gonadal dysgenesis,** one gonad is represented by a streak gonad or a streak testis and a contralateral testis (that is typically cryptorchid) or bilateral streak-testis. Individuals with this condition are particularly prone to the development of gonadoblastomas, a complication prevented by early removal of the gonads.[22] The tumors may totally obliterate the testicular elements and thus lead to an incorrect typing of the dysgenesis. **True hermaphrodites** may have ovotestes containing both ova and immature seminiferous tubules or other combinations of ovary and testis.[12,15] Multiple tumors can occur in these gonads.[21]

The familial syndrome of **testicular feminization** is a type of male pseudohermaphroditism occurring in genetic males with well-developed female secondary sex characteristics (Fig. 19-144). These patients consult a gynecologist because of amenorrhea or sterility. They are found to have a vagina,

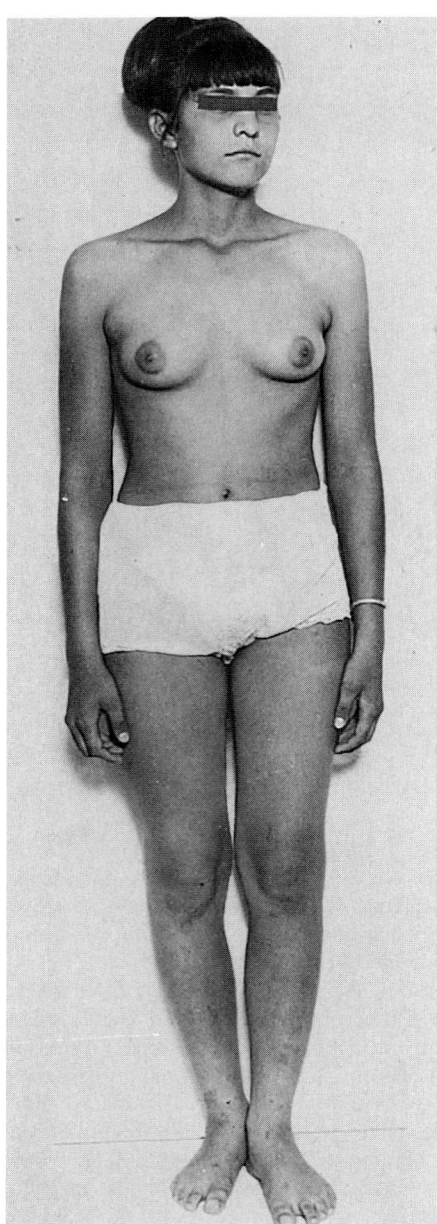

Fig. 19-144 Testicular feminization. Note female development of secondary sex characteristics and absence of axillary hair. Patient had no uterus and short vagina. There were testes in each inguinal area. (Coutesy Dr. W.J. Pepler, Pretoria, South Africa.)

no uterus, and bilateral cryptorchid testes. The latter often contain nodular masses of immature tubules that should not be confused with Sertoli–Leydig cell tumor[13,20] (Fig. 19-145). The syndrome is of further clinical importance because of the eventual occurrence of malignant tumors in the cryptorchid testes of about 9% of these patients.[19] For this reason, the testes should be removed after puberty and supplemental estrogen therapy given.

Márquez-Monter et al.[17] correlated the histology of the gonads with the cytogenetic findings in twenty cases of gonadal dysgenesis; they found a good correlation between the presence of ova and mosaics involving X chromosomes, whereas XO cases had dysgenetic gonads without ova.

A classification of disorders of sexual development is presented in Table 19-7.

CYSTS, STROMAL HYPERPLASIA, AND OTHER NON-NEOPLASTIC LESIONS

Ovarian diseases of surgical importance can be broadly divided into non-neoplastic cysts, inflammations, and neoplasms. Non-neoplastic cysts are unfortunately too commonly seen as surgical specimens. It has been said that if the ovaries were placed externally, their removal would be undertaken with more hesitation. The general surgeon exploring the abdomen may find a mildly cystic or nodular ovary in an otherwise normal abdominal cavity and remove it with the hope that a pathologic process will be found to justify the patient's symptoms and the surgery. More often than not, the microscopic diagnosis will be that of "cystic follicle" or "mature corpus luteum," but then it will be too late to replace the organ. Realizing that the ovary is normally a partially cystic structure and that the risk of carcinoma developing in these cystic structures is negligible should help avoid many of these excisions.

Inclusion cysts ("germinal inclusion cysts") are common in older women; they are generally small and multiple and have no clinical significance. Most of them probably arise from invaginations of the surface epithelium, with subsequent loss of the connection with the surface.[29] Microscopically, they are lined by a flattened, cuboidal, or columnar epithelium; tubal metaplasia is frequent. Psammoma bodies may be seen in their lumen or in the adjacent stroma.

Follicular cysts form by distention of developing or atretic follicles and usually do not exceed 10 cm in diameter. It has been proposed that cystic follicular structures be designated as (normal) cystic follicles when measuring less than 2.5 cm and as follicular cysts when exceeding this diameter. The latter may occur at any age from infancy to menopause and are asymptomatic in the majority of cases. Occasionally, twisting of the pedicle occurs, with the resulting hemorrhagic infarct. In children, the cysts may be seen in conjunction with precocious puberty.[27,58] During reproductive life, they may be associated with endometrial hyperplasia and metrorrhagia.[48] The cyst fluid may contain estrogens.

The cyst wall is lined by theca with or without an inner granulosa layer. The theca layer is frequently luteinized. The granulosa layer may be luteinized after puberty but not before. *Multiple luteinized follicular cysts* (theca-lutein cysts; hyperreactio luteinalis) are common in cases of hydatidiform mole and choriocarcinoma but also have been seen in twin pregnancies and, exceptionally, in uncomplicated single pregnancies[59] (Fig. 19-146). *Large solitary luteinized follicular cyst* is a rare lesion presenting during pregnancy and puerperium, unaccompanied by endocrine abnormalities. The median diameter of the cyst is 25 cm.[33] Marked focal atypia is often seen in the luteinized cells of this lesion.[32]

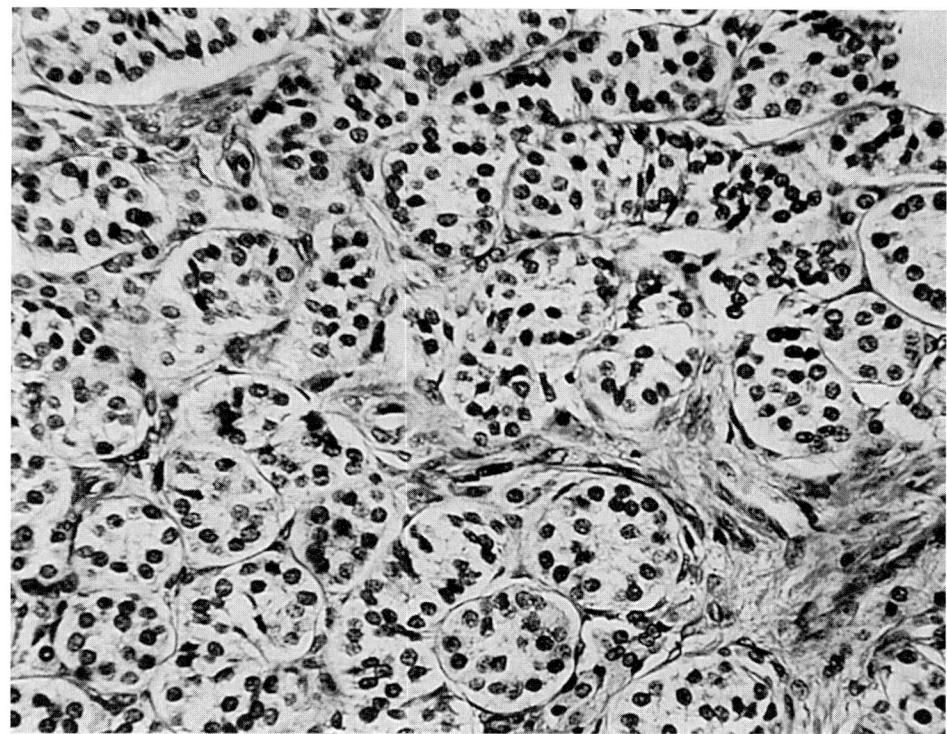

Fig. 19-145 Nodular masses of immature tubules in cryptorchild testis in patient with testicular feminization. Both testes were removed. Patient was given replacement therapy and is now a happily married woman. (Slide contributed by Dr. D.W. Frazier, Jacksonville, FL.)

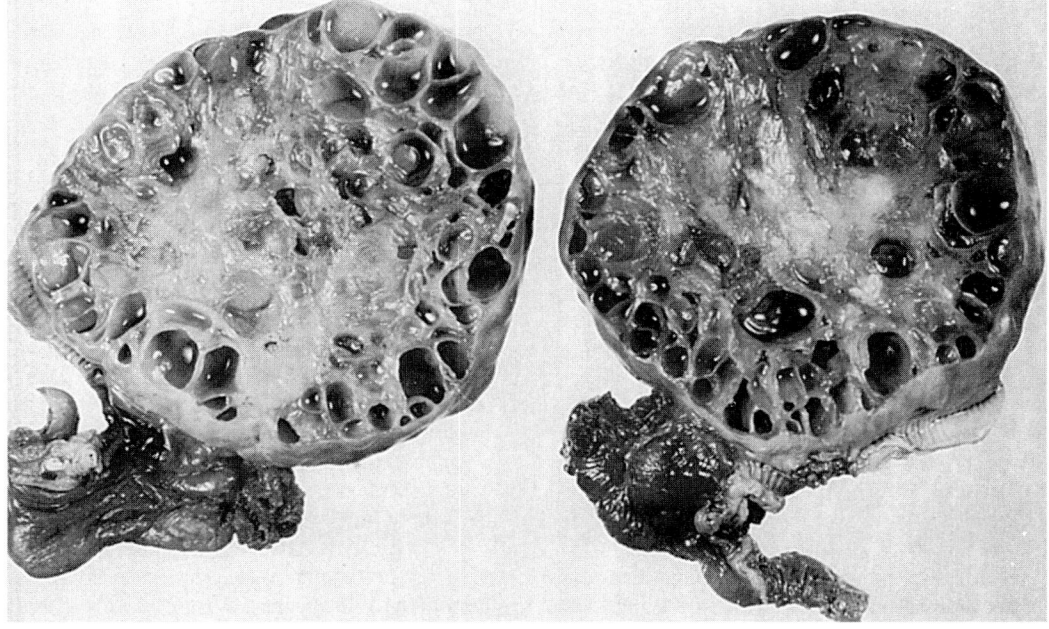

Fig. 19-146 Marked bilateral ovarian enlargement secondary to multiple theca-lutein cysts associated with normal pregnancy. Changes were misinterpreted as representing neoplasms and both ovaries were excised.

Table 19-7 Disorders of sexual development*

Syndrome	Gonad	Ducts	External genitalia	Puberty
Klinefelter's	Testis with hyalinized sclerotic tubules and clumped Leydig cells	Male	Male	Normal penis with small testes; partial androgen lack
Turner's	Streak gonad with whorled stroma	Female	Female	No pubertal development; rare cases show mild virilization
True hermaphrodite	Ovary and testis	All have uterus, most have tubes too, a few have vasa	Ambiguous but 80% favor the male	80% have gynecomastia; 50% menstruate
Mixed gonadal dysgenesis	Streak plus testis or tumor	Female; vas found occasionally	Vary from female (often with clitoromegaly) to male with hypospadias to normal male	Virilization, sometimes complete; breast development only with tumors
Dysgenetic male pseudo-hermaphroditism	Dysgenetic testis	Mixed male and/or female	Variably virilized	Rarely patients may be fertile
Familial male pseudo-hermaphroditism that ranges from testicular feminization to	Immature infertile testis	No uterus, ± rudimentary vas	Female with short, blind vagina	Breasts develop but sexual hair is missing
Reifenstein's syndrome	Infertile testis	Male	Male with hypospadias ± cleft scrotum	Androgen lack is evident in incomplete virilization
Female pseudo-hermaphroditism				
1. Congenital adrenal hyperplasia	Ovary	Female	Variably virilized	Amenorrhea with virilization
2. Nonadrenal	Ovary	Female	Variably virilized	Normal

From Federman DD: Abnormal sexual development. A genetic and endocrine approach to differential diagnosis. Philadelphia, 1967, W.B. Saunders Co.
*The summaries under the several headings are necessarily brief; the text should be consulted for details, qualifications, and crucial exceptions.
↑, Increased; ↑↑, markedly increased; ↓ N, normal.

Polycystic (sclerocystic) ovaries are characterized by multiple follicular cysts or cystic follicles with varying degrees of luteinization of the theca interna, covered by a dense fibrous capsule[56] (Figs. 19-147 and 19-148). Various clinical syndromes may develop in patients with polycystic ovaries, including the Stein-Leventhal syndrome (characterized by amenorrhea and sterility), so-called metropathia hemorrhagica (typically accompanied by endometrial hyperplasia), and frank virilism. These syndromes tend to overlap considerably, as do the pathologic findings.[38] The pathogenesis of Stein-Leventhal syndrome is poorly understood.[40,47] These patients have "masculinizing" pituitary and ovarian responses to stimulation by the specific gonadotropin-releasing hormone agonist nafarelin, suggesting that the regulation of the ovarian 17-hydroxylase and C-17,20-lyase activities is abnormal.[28] Dysregulation of 11ß-hydroxysteroid dehydrogenase, causing increased oxidation of cortisol to cortisone, has also been documented.[52]

In general, the ovaries of patients with Stein-Leventhal syndrome have the features of polycystic ovaries just described. Corpora lutea and corpora albicantia are almost always absent. Residua of atretic follicles should not be misinterpreted as corpora albicantia. Rarely, typical polycystic ovaries associated with the clinical features of the Stein-Leventhal syndrome have been found associated with con-genital adrenal hyperplasia and ovarian neoplasms.[44,46,61] Polycystic ovaries have also been observed in association with primary hypothyroidism.[45]

Most patients with Stein-Leventhal syndrome will respond favorably with restoration of the menstrual cycle to medical treatment with cortisone or clomiphene citrate.[47] Wedge resection of the ovary, regarded for many years as the standard therapy for this condition, is rarely if ever carried out nowadays. The endometrium of patients with Stein-Leventhal syndrome is usually hyperplastic, sometime markedly so. Exceptionally, an endometrial carcinoma develops against this background, the tumor being typically well-differentiated and superficial.[34,41,55]

Stromal hyperplasia is characterized by a diffuse or nodular proliferation of plump ovarian cortical stromal cells encroaching on the medulla.[30] Patchy luteinization of these cells may be present; when extensive, terms such as *(stromal) hyperthecosis, diffuse thecomatosis,* or *stromal luteinization* have been employed (Fig. 19-149). Stromal luteomas and thecomas may develop against this background (see p. 1509). Hyperthecosis may be associated with estrogenic or androgenic effects, obesity, hypertension, and an abnormal glucose tolerance test or even frank diabetes.[31] The onset of symptoms may be abrupt, thus simulating a virilizing ovarian tumor. Immunohistochemical studies have

Barr	Chromosomes	Hormones			Remarks
		FSH	17-KS	Estrogen	
"True" are chromatin positive, a few are 2+ or 3+	All chromatin positive have 2 Xs and a Y in at least some cells. Chromatin negative are 46,XY	↑↑	N or ↓	N	Affects 1:400 newborn males
50% chromatin negative	Second sex chromosome missing or abnormal in some or all of the cells	↑↑	↓	↓	1:7000 newborns, more common in abortuses; short stature
80% chromatin positive	~60% are 46,XX in blood cells only; Y present in most of the others	N	N	N	
Chromatin negative	Almost all are mosaics including XO stem; many have Y-bearing stem as well	↑	N	?	
Chromatin negative	Some are XO/XY	↑	N	?	
Chromatin negative	46,XY	↑ or N	↑ or N	N	Sex-linked recessive or sex-limited autosomal dominant
Chromatin negative	46,XY	↑ or N	↑ or N	?	
Chromatin positive	46,XX	N	↑↑	N	Autosomal recessive
Chromatin positive	46,XX	N	N	N	Consider maternal exposure to progestins or androgens

shown androgen production by the luteinized stromal cells, suggesting that estrogenic effects in these cases are mediated through peripheral aromatization of these androgens.[54]

The boundaries between polycystic disease and stromal hyperplasia are ill-defined.[42,56] However, typical stromal hyperplasia lacks cysts and is usually more refractory to therapy.

Corpus luteum cysts are single and usually less than 6 cm in diameter. They may develop at the end of the menstrual cycle or may occur in pregnancy (Fig. 19-150). The cyst wall is composed of luteinized granulosa and theca cell layers. Hyaline bodies and foci of calcification may be found in the cysts associated with pregnancy. The fluid content often is bloody. If the cyst ruptures, hemorrhage into the peritoneal cavity occurs (sometimes over 500 ml), and an erroneous diagnosis of ruptured ectopic pregnancy may be made.[39] It should be remembered that the corpus luteum is normally a cystic structure. The arbitrary diameter of 2.5 cm has been proposed to distinguish the (normal) cystic corpus luteum from a corpus luteum cyst, in a manner analogous to that employed for follicle-related cystic formations.

Ectopic decidual reaction can occur in the ovary during pregnancy and occasionally even in the absence of current or recent pregnancy. A functioning corpus luteum that has undergone destruction is present in most instances.[51]

So-called *luteomas of pregnancy* are yellow or orange solid nodules that may reach sizable proportions[32] (Fig. 19-151). They have been typically encountered during cesarean section in multiparous women. If left undisturbed, they will regress after delivery.[57] A mild degree of virilization can be present.[35,50] Microscopically, the lesions are composed of masses of uniform theca-lutein cells (Fig. 19-152). Ultrastructurally, the proliferating cells exhibit abundant smooth endoplasmic reticulum, dispersed Golgi apparatus, and tubular cristae in the mitochondria, in keeping with their function as steroid hormone–producing cells.[36] All of the reported lesions have been benign. It is reasonable to regard them as nodular hyperplasias of theca-lutein cells rather than true neoplasms.[50] If pregnancy luteoma is correctly identified by frozen section biopsy, no further surgery is necessary.

Developmental cysts derived from mesonephric and paramesonephric remnants are common in the region of the ovarian hilus. These are discussed on p. 1452. Suffice it to say here that, according to some authors, it is possible to distinguish mesonephric from paramesonephric tissues—and sometimes the cysts derived from them—on microscopic grounds.[37] Mesonephric structures are lined by cuboidal, predominantly nonciliated epithelium resting on a well-developed basement membrane; paramesonephric forma-

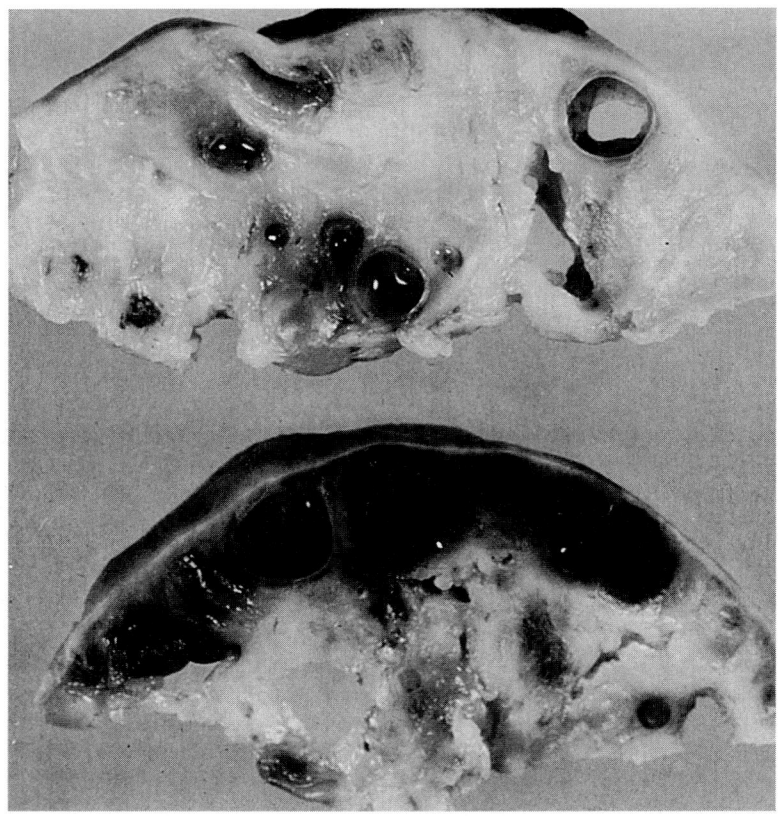

Fig. 19-147 Wedges of ovarian tissue resected from 21-year-old woman with Stein-Leventhal syndrome. Multiple cystic follicles, dense outer capsule, and abundant pale gray stroma are characteristic features.

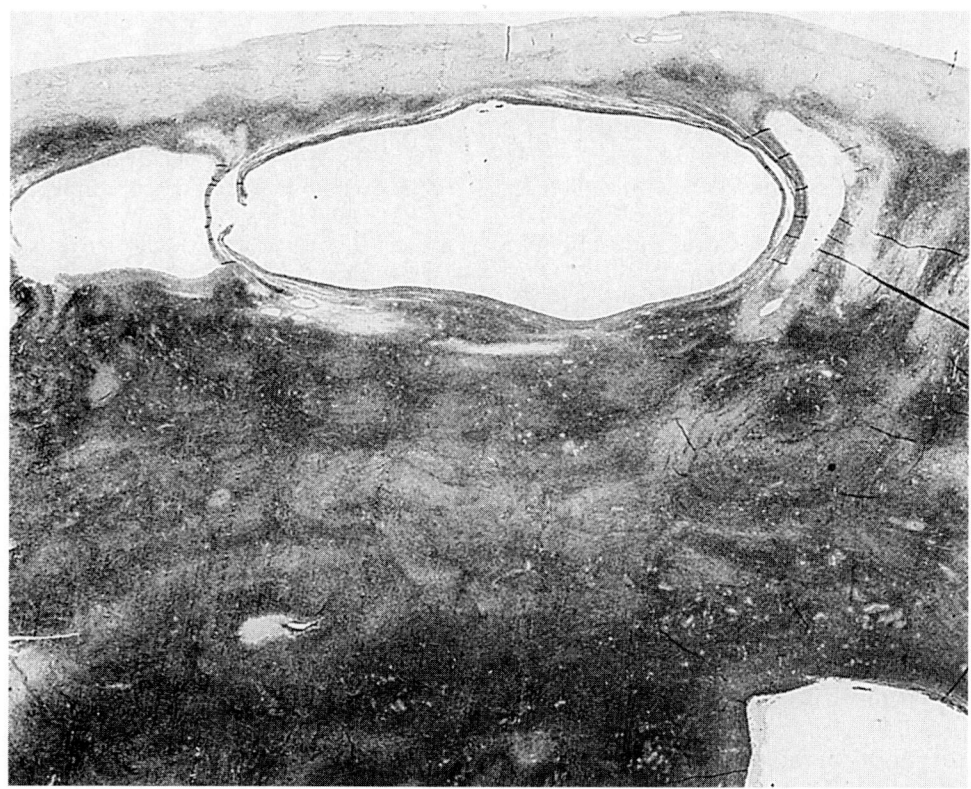

Fig. 19-148 Ovary from patient with Stein-Leventhal syndrome showing dense outer fibrous coat, multiple follicular cysts and atretic follicles, and abundant cortical stroma. Theca interna is well developed.

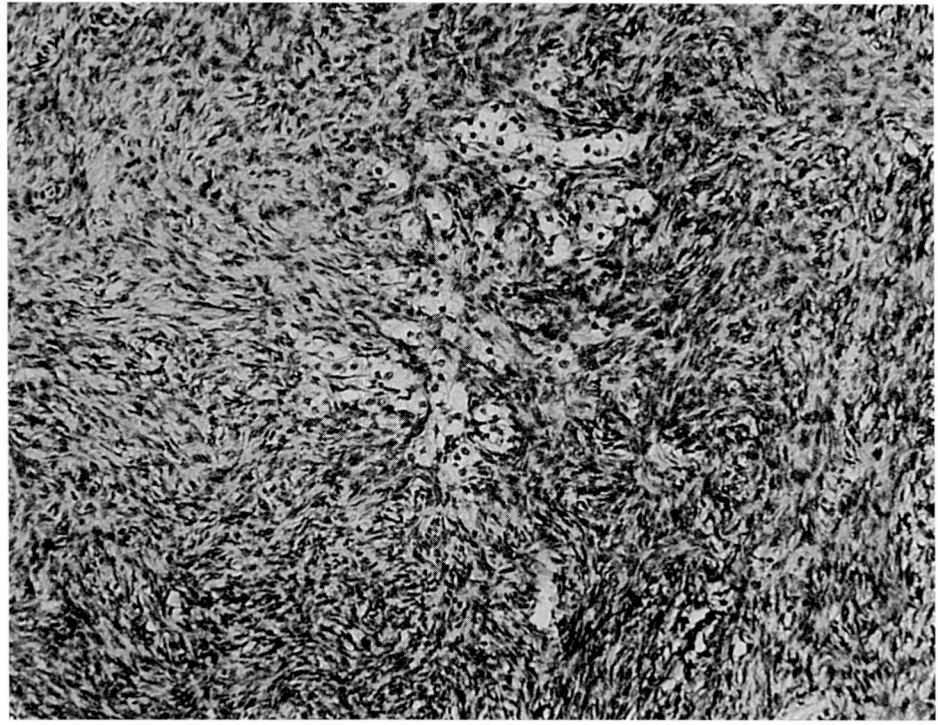

Fig. 19-149 Ovarian stromal hyperplasia with focal stroma luteinization ("hyperthecosis") associated with amenorrhea, hypertension, and virilization syndrome in 40-year-old woman. Ovaries were symmetrically enlarged and solid. There was no improvement following wedge resection.

A

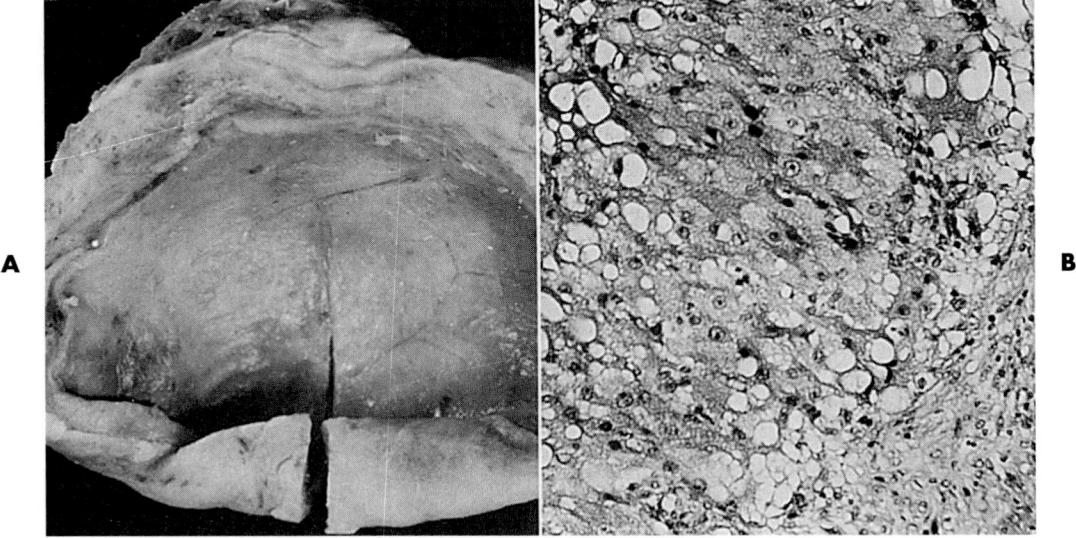

B

Fig. 19-150 Corpus luteum cyst. It was found at time of exploration for another condition, and surgeon incorrectly removed ovary. **B,** Wall of cyst shown in **A** composed of luteinized granulosa.

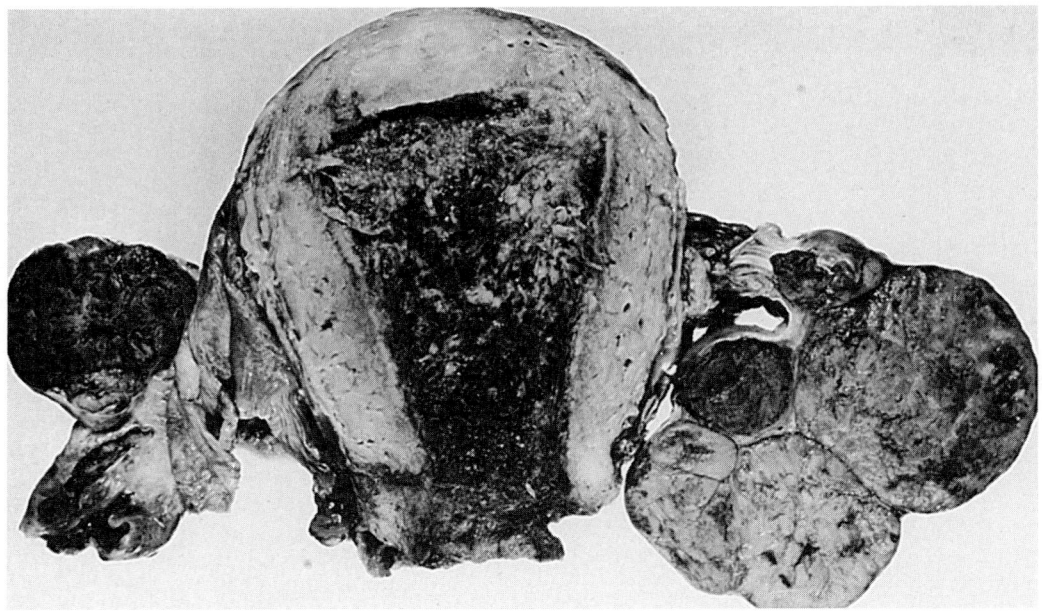

Fig. 19-151 Bilateral pregnancy luteomas in 29-year-old woman that were discovered incidentally at time of cesarean section performed for cord prolapse. Tumors bled excessively on manipulation by surgeon and had to be removed.

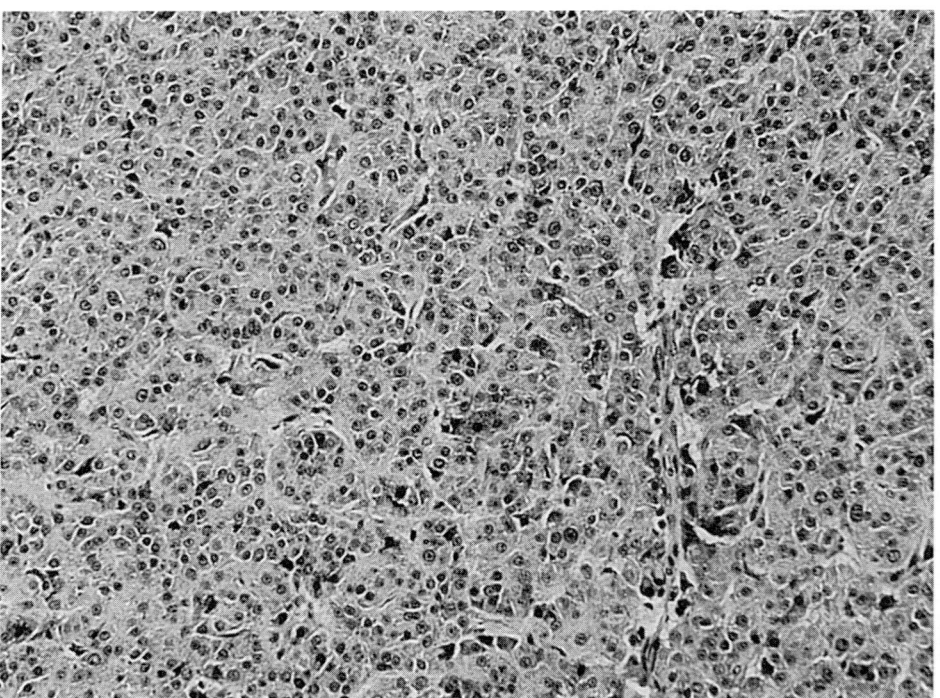

Fig. 19-152 Luteoma of pregnancy showing small clusters and masses of uniform luteinized theca cells.

tions are lined by generally taller, ciliated and nonciliated epithelium with larger nuclei and resting on an inconspicuous basement membrane. Both may have a smooth muscle coat. According to these criteria and some ultrastructural differences,[31] *hydatids of Morgagni* (pedunculated cysts at the fimbriated end of the fallopian tube) are believed to be of paramesonephric origin, whereas most *parovarian* and *paratubal cysts* (in the tubo-ovarian ligament) and *Gartner's duct cysts* (in the vaginal wall) are thought to arise from mesonephric remnants.

Cysts of the rete ovarii are characterized by a hilar position, an epithelial lining of variable height that is usually nonciliated, crevices along the inner surfaces, and a fibromuscular wall that often contains hyperplastic hilus cells.[53]

Epidermoid cysts, exceptionally rare, are thought to be related to Walthard cell nests, but some may well represent mature monodermal teratomas.[49,60]

Supernumerary ovaries are extremely rare. Most of the reported cases have measured less than 1 cm. They should be distinguished from *accessory ovaries,* which are small portions of ovarian tissue situated near—and sometimes connected to—the normally placed ovary.[43]

INFLAMMATION

Nonspecific inflammation of the ovary usually spreads from the endometrium and is practically always associated with tubal involvement. A large, loculated cystic mass filled with pus or secretion is often the result, the ovarian stroma forming part of the cystic wall (tubo-ovarian abscess or cyst). Exceptionally, a solid mass rich in foamy macrophages develops in long-standing cases ("xanthogranulomatous oophoritis").[68]

Granulomatous infections such as tuberculosis occur in the ovary. Invariably this is hematogenous in origin and often also involves the tube and endometrium. In time, the infection may subside and leave a large tubo-ovarian cystic mass. Other infectious agents responsible for granulomatous oophoritis are *Actinomyces* (particularly common after the introduction of intrauterine devices), *Schistosoma,* and *Enterobius vermicularis.* Rarely, sarcoidosis and Crohn's disease involve the ovary, the latter as a result of direct extension from the bowel. Foreign body granulomas can occur in the ovarian surface secondarily to talc, cornstarch, other foreign materials,[67] and keratin; the latter may originate from a ruptured ovarian cystic teratoma or may have spilled through the fallopian tube from an endometrial adenoacanthoma. *Palisading granulomas* of unknown etiology have also been reported, most of them in patients with previous pelvic surgery.[64]

Autoimmune oophoritis is a poorly understood disorder characterized microscopically by lymphocytic and plasma cell infiltration in relation to developing follicles but not primordial follicles.[63] It results in primary ovarian failure with either primary or secondary amenorrhea.[62] Many of the reported cases have been associated with adrenal failure (Addison's disease), hypothyroidism, or both conditions.[62,65]

Eosinophilic perifolliculitis is characterized by a predominantly eosinophilic infiltrate around the follicles; it is not clear how this rare disorder relates to autoimmune oophoritis.[66]

Giant cell arteritis occasionally involves the ovary of elderly women; it may occur as an isolated finding or as a component of generalized giant cell arteritis.

ENDOMETRIOSIS

The ovary is the most common site of endometriosis, as defined by the presence of endometrial glands *and* stroma outside the uterus (see p. 1401).[75] Ovarian endometriosis is usually associated with infertility, and it remains active during the child-bearing years.[72,77] Pain is the most common symptom; infrequently, the disease is complicated by massive ascites or perforation into the peritoneal cavity.[76] Grossly, it usually presents as small, slightly raised, blueberry-like spots on the ovarian surface, often accompanied by fibrous adhesions.[73] In cases with extensive involvement, the entire ovary may be converted into a "chocolate cyst" as a result of repeated hemorrhages (Fig. 19-153). Microscopically, the typical lesions are composed of endometrial glands, endometrial stroma, and hemorrhagic foci (Figs. 19-154 and 19-155).[69] The endometrial stroma is responsible for the bleeding; it has cells with "naked nucleus" surrounded by reticulin and typical spiral arterioles, in conjunction with old and recent hemorrhage. Unfortunately, this diagnostic combination of findings is not always present. The more advanced the endometrial lesion, the more difficult the diagnosis and the greater the number of sections required to make it. Not infrequently, the repeated hemorrhages have totally destroyed the endometrial tissue, the cyst being lined by several layers of hemosiderin-laden macrophages. Under these circumstances, the most the pathologist can do is to report the case as a hemorrhagic cyst and comment that the changes are "consistent" with those of endometriosis. Sometimes, the lesion is entirely composed of *necrotic pseudoxanthomatous nodules,* to be distinguished from infectious granulomas and necrotic neoplasms.[70]

Ectopic endometrial tissue is subject to most of the influences that affect intrauterine endometrium. Consequently, it may be the site of reactive atypia (sometimes referred to as "atypical endometriosis"), glandular hyperplasia, or malignancy, of which endometrioid carcinoma is the most common form[68a,71,74] (see p. 1482).

OVARIAN BIOPSY

Ovarian biopsy obtained by either laparotomy or surgical culdoscopy used to be carried out for the evaluation of selected patients with amenorrhea and sterility resulting from anovulation. The specimen, which corresponds to about one fifth of the organ, was evaluated for the presence and quantity of follicles, evidence of ovulation (corpora lutea and albicantia), and the character of the stroma.[81,82]

Mori[78] attempted to correlate the morphologic findings in the ovarian biopsy with a series of endocrinologic analyses. He found that the ovaries of patients with hypergonadotropic ovarian failure contained no follicles, whereas in those of patients with normogonadotropic or hypogonadotropic ovarian failure, many developing follicles were present. The results were somewhat different in the series of nineteen patients reported by Russell et al.,[80] all of whom had premature (before 35 years of age) hypergonadotropic ovarian failure. There were fourteen cases classified as pre-

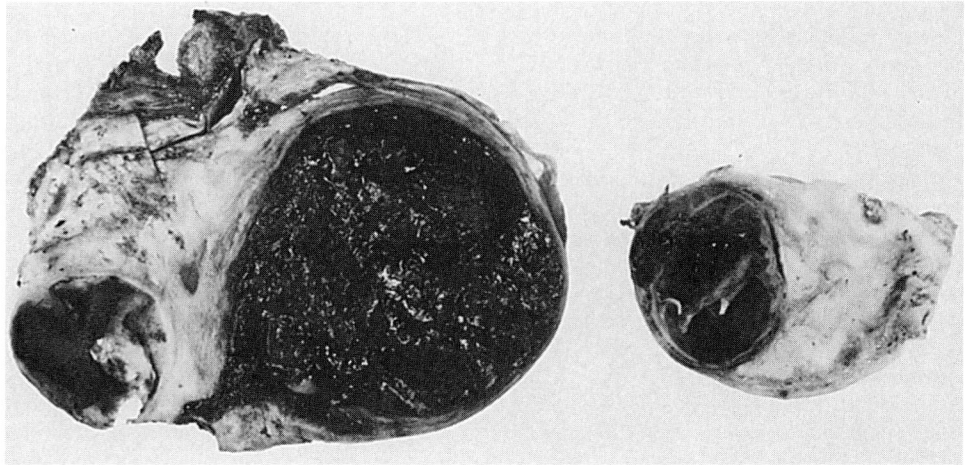

Fig. 19-153 Bilateral "chocolate cysts" of ovary resulting from endometriosis.

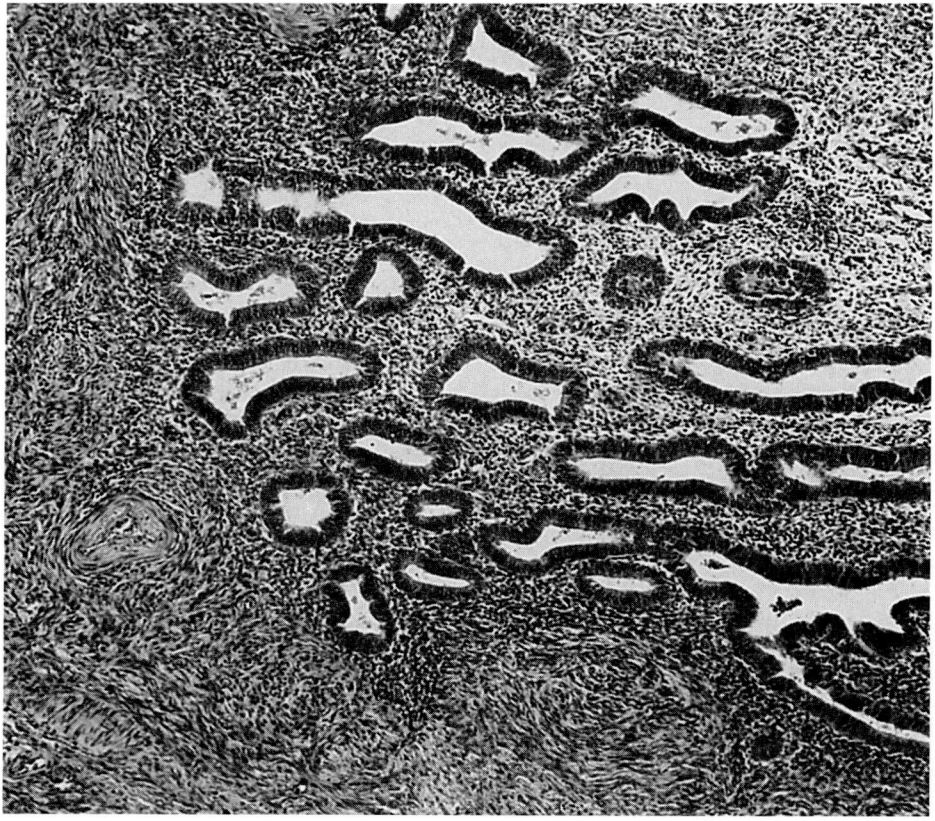

Fig. 19-154 Ovarian endometriosis composed of narrow proliferative glands surrounded by endometrial stroma, which contrasts with ovarian stroma at lower left.

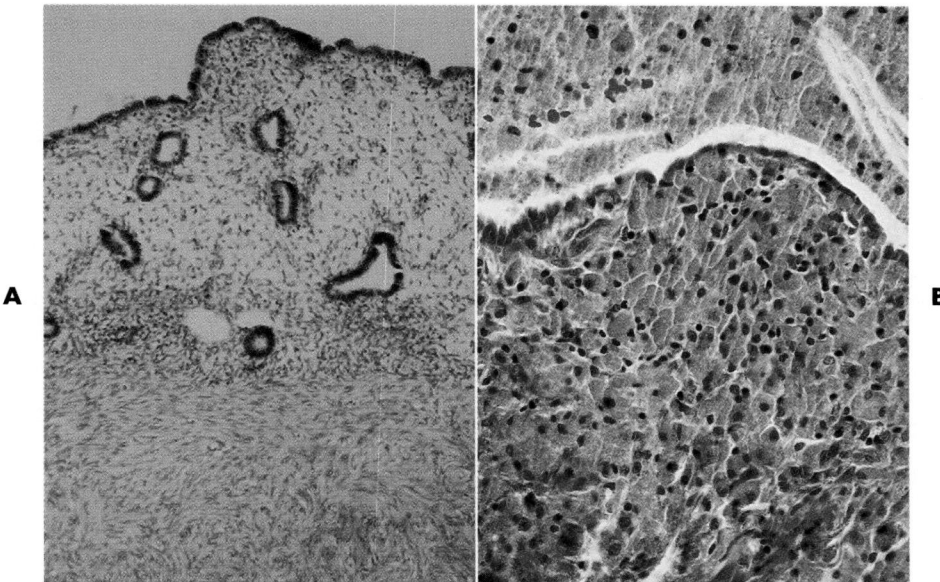

Fig. 19-155 Ovarian endometriosis. **A,** In this area the endometrial tissue faithfully reproduces the appearance of that of the normal organ, both in terms of glands and stroma. **B,** A more common appearance resulting from repeated hemorrhage and accumulation of hemosiderin-laden macrophages.

mature menopause, characterized by the absence of primordial follicles; three designated as "resistant ovary syndrome," having primordial follicles but little or no follicular development; and two cases of chronic—presumably autoimmune—oophoritis, characterized by a granulomatous reaction centered in the theca of the developing follicles.

Nowadays, ovarian biopsies are rarely if ever performed in women with premature ovarian failure and a normal karyotype. The reasons for this reluctance are the realization that they can provide misleading information (i.e., cases with no oocytes in the biopsy in which the patients eventually become pregnant) and the fact that affected patients generally require estrogen replacement regardless of the results of the biopsy.[79]

TUMORS
Classification

The classification of ovarian tumors is primarily morphologic but is intended to reflect current concepts of embryogenesis and histogenesis of this complex organ.[83-89] Since many of these concepts are still controversial, it should be viewed as a working compromise, subject to changes and improvements. It is based on the premise that the ovary contains four major types of tissues, all of which can give rise to a variety of neoplasms:

1 Surface, celomic, or germinal epithelium
2 Germ cells
3 Sex cords
4 Specialized ovarian stroma

The vast majority of malignant ovarian tumors arise from the surface epithelium. It has been speculated that the rapid cycles of cell division associated with wound repair at the time of follicular rupture may contribute to the development of ovarian carcinoma.[85]

Listed in the box on pp. 1474-1475 is the classification used in this text for ovarian tumors. It is largely adapted from the World Health Organization (WHO) scheme and is modified to include newer concepts and recently described entities.

Surface epithelial tumors

This group of neoplasms, numerically the most important, is thought to derive from the epithelium that normally lines the outer aspect of the ovary, variously referred to as *surface, celomic, or germinal*.[91] This epithelium is continuous with the mesothelium that covers the peritoneal cavity, representing a modification of it and sharing with it a common origin and many morphologic features.[92] Some authors have therefore suggested that ovarian tumors arising from this structure should be regarded as mesotheliomas, a proposal that has not met with general acceptance. Clear-cut histochemical, enzymatic, and biologic differences between ovarian surface epithelium and extraovarian peritoneal mesothelium exist.[93] Furthermore, ovarian epithelial tumors differ significantly as a group from peritoneal mesotheliomas on morphologic and behavioral grounds, these differences being highlighted by two rare but notable occurrences: the ovarian tumor with a bona fide mesotheliomatous appearance[90] and the existence of intra-abdominal extraovarian malignancies having more resemblance to ovarian carcinomas than to peritoneal mesotheliomas (see p. 1489).

The ovarian surface epithelium, when involved in metaplastic or neoplastic conditions, often undergoes a "müllerian differentiation"; as a result, it may produce any of the adult structures formed by the müllerian ducts, including tubal, endometrial, and endocervical mucosa, singly or in combination.[99] This plasticity is also evident at the immunohistochemical level.[103]

WHO HISTOLOGIC CLASSIFICATION OF OVARIAN TUMORS
(1995)

Surface epithelial–stromal tumors

Serous tumors

Benign
  Cystadenoma and papillary cystadenoma
  Surface papilloma
  Adenofibroma and cystadenofibroma
Of borderline malignancy (of low malignant potential)
  Cystic tumor and papillary cystic tumor
  Surface papillary tumor
  Adenofibroma and cystadenofibroma
Malignant
  Adenocarcinoma, papillary adenocarcinoma, and papillary
    cystadenocarcinoma
  Surface papillary adenocarcinoma
  Adenocarcinofibroma and cystadenocarcinofibroma

Mucinous tumors, endocervical-like and intestinal-type

Benign
  Cystadenoma
  Adenofibroma and cystadenofibroma
Of borderline malignancy (of low malignant potential)
  Cystic tumor
  Adenofibroma and cystadenofibroma
Malignant
  Adenocarcinoma and cystadenocarcinoma
  Adenocarcinofibroma and cystadenocarcinofibroma

Endometrioid tumors

Benign
  Cystadenoma with squamous differentiation
  Adenofibroma and cystadenofibroma
  Adenofibroma and cystadenofibroma with squamous
    differentiation
Malignant
  Adenocarcinoma and cystadenocarcinoma
  Adenocarcinoma and cystadenocarcinoma with
    squamous differentiation
  Adenocarcinofibroma and cystadenocarcinofibroma
  Adenocarcinofibroma and cystadenocarcinofibroma with
    squamous differentiation
Epithelial-(endometrioid) stromal and (endometrioid) stromal
  Adenosarcoma, homologous and heterologous
  Mesodermal (müllerian) mixed tumor (carcinosarcoma),
    homologous and heterologous
  Stromal sarcoma

Clear cell tumors

Benign
  Cystadenoma
  Adenofibroma and cystadenofibroma
Of borderline malignancy (of low malignant potential)
  Cystic tumor
  Adenofibroma and cystadenofibroma
Malignant
  Adenocarcinoma
  Adenocarcinofibroma and cystadenocarcinofibroma

Transitional cell tumors
  Brenner tumor
  Brenner tumor of borderline malignancy (proliferating)
  Malignant Brenner tumor
  Transitional cell carcinoma (non-Brenner type)

Squamous cell tumors

Mixed epithelial tumors (specify types)
  Benign
  Of borderline malignancy (of low malignant potential)
  Malignant

Undifferentiated carcinoma

Unclassified

Sex–cord stromal tumors

Granulosa–stromal cell tumors
  Granulosa cell tumor
    Juvenile
    Adult
  Tumors in the thecoma-fibroma group
    Thecoma
      Typical
      Luteinized*
    Fibroma
    Cellular fibroma
    Fibrosarcoma
    Stromal tumor with minor sex–cord elements
    Sclerosing stromal tumor
    (Stromal luteoma) see steroid (lipid) cell tumors
    Unclassified (fibrothecoma)
    Others

Sertoli–stromal cell tumors; androblastomas
  Well differentiated
    Sertoli cell tumor; tubular androblastoma
    Sertoli-Leydig cell tumor
    (Leydig cell tumor) see steroid (lipid) cell tumors
  Of intermediate differentiation
    Variant—with heterologous elements (specify types)
  Retiform
  Mixed (specify types)

Sex–cord tumor with annular tubules

Gynandroblastoma

Steroid (lipid) cell tumors
  Stromal luteoma
  Leydig cell tumor (Hilus cell tumor)†
  Unclassified

Germ cell tumors

Dysgerminoma
  Variant—with syncytiotrophoblast cells

Yolk sac tumor (endodermal sinus tumor)
  Variants—Polyvesicular vitelline tumor
    —Hepatoid
    —Glandular‡

*A rare tumor has the features of luteinized thecoma and additionally, crystals of Reinke in the steroid cell component. This tumor has been called "stromal Leydig cell tumor."

† A rare tumor does not arise from hilus cells but within the ovarian stroma. This tumor has been called "Leydig cell tumor, non-hilar type."

‡Some glandular yolk sac tumors resemble endometrioid adenocarcinoma and have been called "endometrioid-like."

WHO HISTOLOGIC CLASSIFICATION OF OVARIAN TUMORS
(1995)—cont'd

Embryonal carcinoma
Polyembryoma
Choriocarcinoma
Teratomas
  Immature
  Mature
    Solid
    Cystic (dermoid cyst)
    With secondary tumor formation (specify type)
    Fetiform (homunculus)
  Monodermal and highly specialized
    Struma ovarii
      Variant—with thyroid tumor (specify type)
    Carcinoid
      Insular
      Trabecular
    Strumal carcinoid
    Mucinous carcinoid
    Neuroectodermal tumors
    Sebaceous tumors
    Others
  Mixed (specify types)
Mixed (specify types)
Gonadoblastoma
  Variant—with dysgerminoma or other germ cell tumor
Germ cell–sex-cord–stromal tumor
  Variant—with dysgerminoma or other germ cell tumor
Tumors of rete ovarii
  Adenoma and cystadenoma
  Carcinoma
Mesothelial tumors
  Adenomatoid tumor
  Others

Tumors of uncertain origin
  Small cell carcinoma
  Tumor of probable wolffian origin
  Hepatoid carcinoma
  Oncocytoma
Gestational trophoblastic diseases
Soft tissue tumors not specific to ovary
Malignant lymphomas
Unclassified tumors
Secondary (metastatic) tumors
Tumorlike lesions
  Solitary follicle cyst
  Multiple follicle cysts (polycystic diseases) (sclerocystic ovaries)
  Large solitary luteinized follicle cyst of pregnancy and puerperium
  Hyperreactio luteinalis (multiple luteinized follicle cysts)
    Variant—with corpora lutea
  Corpus luteum cyst
  Pregnancy luteoma
  Ectopic pregnancy
  Hyperplasia of stroma
  Stromal hyperthecosis
  Massive edema
  Fibromatosis
  Endometriosis
  Cyst, unclassified (simple cyst)
  Inflammatory lesions
    Xanthogranuloma
    Malakoplakia
    Others

It seems likely that the majority of surface tumors of the ovary arise not from the outer epithelium itself, but rather from the portion of this epithelium that has invaginated to produce surface epithelial glands and cysts. This is supported by some immunohistochemical similarities,[98] the overexpression of p53,[97a] and the occasional finding of atypical proliferation (dysplasia) or carcinoma in situ in these structures.[97,101] Ovarian endometriosis may also give rise to these tumors, but this is probably true for only a small minority of them, even if they are of endometrioid type.

Surface epithelial ovarian tumors are classified according to the following parameters:

1 Cell type: serous, mucinous, endometrioid, etc.
2 Pattern of growth: cystic, solid, surface
3 Amount of fibrous stroma
4 Atypia and invasiveness: benign, borderline, and malignant

Thorough sampling is essential to carry out these important determinations. It has been suggested that one block should be taken for every 1 to 2 cm of maximum tumor diameter.[94] The selection of the site of sampling is actually more important than the total number of blocks: solid foci, areas adjacent to the ovarian surface, and the base of the papillary formations need to be studied with particular care.

It should also be emphasized that, important as these distinctions are, they are sometimes applied only with difficulty to the individual case because of the existence of mixed and hybrid tumors (*mixed epithelial tumors* in the WHO classification).[100] In general, the less differentiated the tumor, the more difficult it is to place it into a specific category in regard to cell type (*undifferentiated and unclassified epithelial tumors* in same classification).[102] The distinction between serous and endometrioid tumors and the identification of borderline tumors are also subject to considerable individual observer variability.[95,96]

Serous tumors

Serous tumors make up about one fourth of all ovarian tumors. Most cases occur in adults. About 30% to 50% are bilateral. Grossly, the better differentiated tumors consist of

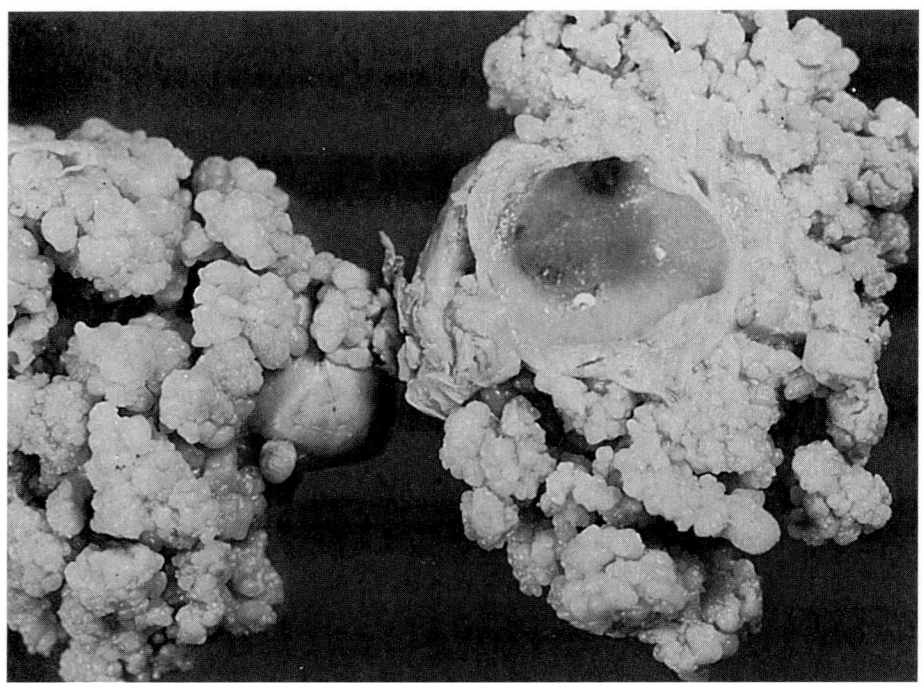

Fig. 19-156 Serous cystadenoma of ovary with papillary projections.

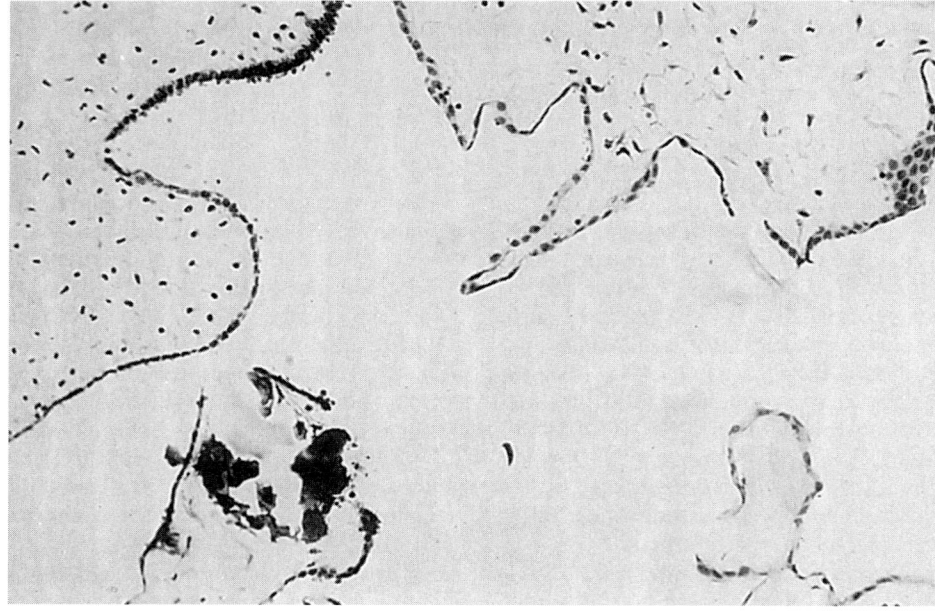

Fig. 19-157 Serous cystadenoma lined by flat or cuboidal layer of epithelial cells.

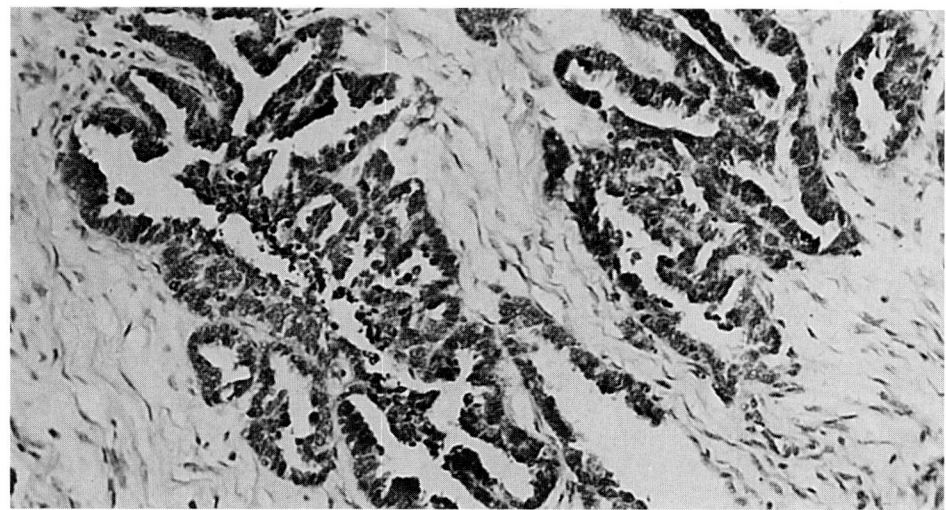

Fig. 19-158 Obviously malignant serous cystadenocarcinoma of ovary.

cystic masses, usually unilocular, containing a clear but sometimes viscous fluid. Papillary formations are often present, most of them protruding into the cavity but some occasionally occur on the outer surface (Fig. 19-156). The more malignant tumors tend to be solid and invasive, with areas of necrosis and hemorrhage.

Microscopically, cuboidal to columnar cells are seen lining the wall of the cysts and the papillae in the better differentiated tumors. They are similar to normal tubal epithelium at both a light and electron microscopic level.[114] In about 30% of the cases, calcific concretions with concentric laminations (psammoma bodies) are present. Ultrastructural studies suggest that the formation of these psammoma bodies is initiated intracellularly in association with autophagocytosis.[115]

It is now accepted that a morphologic spectrum exists in these tumors. At one end is the benign **serous cystadenoma,** in which the cysts and the papillae (if present, in which case the tumor is called serous papillary cystadenoma) are lined by a single layer of cells, without atypia, architectural complexity, or invasion (Fig. 19-157). At the other end are the **serous adenocarcinoma, serous papillary adenocarcinoma,** and **serous papillary cystadenocarcinoma,** characterized by nuclear atypia, high mitotic activity, stratification, glandular complexity, branching papillary fronds, and *stromal invasion* (Fig. 19-158). In between are tumors showing some or all of the features associated with carcinoma but *lacking* definite stromal invasion, i.e., irregular or destructive stromal infiltration by small glands or sheets of cells[111,138] (Fig. 19-159) (but see below). These tumors—known as **borderline, indeterminate, intermediate, of low malignant potential,** or **possibly malignant**—make up about 15% of all serous tumors. In our view they represent low-grade serous (cyst)adenocarcinomas, but it is important to separate them from the obviously invasive tumors because of their vastly better prognosis.[124] The outcome is even more favorable (as a matter of fact, not different from that of cystadenoma) when the "borderline" features are present only focally in an

otherwise benign tumor ("cystadenomas with focally proliferative areas").[124] It should be pointed out that the decision as to whether an ovarian serous neoplasm is of malignant or borderline nature should be made purely on the basis of the morphologic features of the primary tumor, regardless of whether or not peritoneal lesions, lymph node metastases, or even lung metastases exist.[134,136a] Allegedly, there are differences in nuclear features between these two tumor types that can be appreciated in a more consistent and reproducible fashion by the use of computerized interactive morphometric analysis.[121,126]

The proposal has recently been made that tumors should still be placed into the borderline category even if they show foci of stromal microinvasion, as long as they are otherwise typical of that category. The microinvasive foci appear as individual cells or clusters of cells with abundant eosinophilic cytoplasm ("eosinophilic metaplastic cells") or, less commonly, as small confluent nests with a cribriform pattern; these tumors have a prognosis similar to that of the usual noninvasive serous borderline tumor[105] (Plate XIV-A).

In contrast to endometrioid neoplasms, squamous metaplasia is exceptional in serous tumors; however, well-documented cases of this occurrence are on record.[139]

In some serous neoplasms, the fibroblastic stromal component is unduly prominent, appearing grossly as solid, white, nodular foci in an otherwise typical cystic neoplasm. These, too, can be separated into *benign* (**adenofibroma** and **cystadenofibroma),** *borderline,* and *malignant* (**adenofibrocarcinoma** and **cystadenofibrocarcinoma)** types[112,113] (Fig. 19-160). The benign type is much more frequent than the others. The borderline category of this neoplasm, extremely rare, has been documented by Kao and Norris[123]; none of their ten cases developed a recurrence following excision of the neoplasm. Exceptionally, osseous metaplasia develops in these stroma-rich tumors.[106]

Other serous neoplasms grow exophytically on the surface of the ovary, with little if any involvement of the underlying organ, the normal shape of which is maintained. These

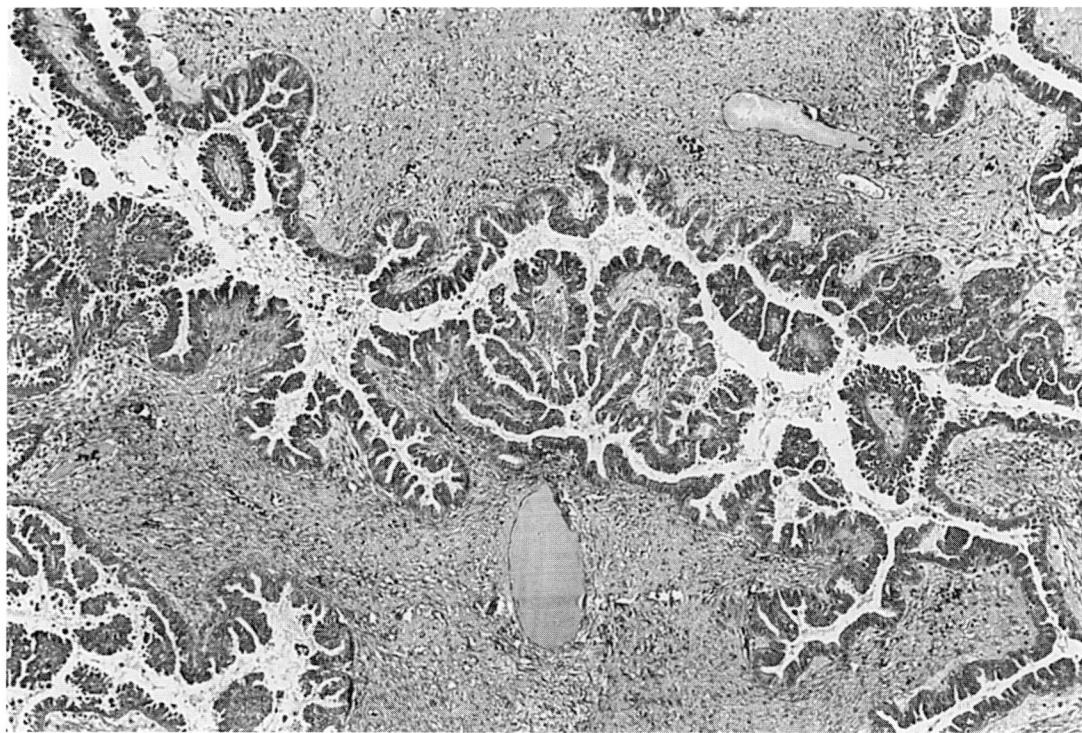

Fig. 19-159 Serous papillary tumor of borderline type. There is marked proliferation and complexity of papillae, but stromal invasion is absent.

are referred to as *surface papillomas* when benign, *borderline surface papillary tumors* when intermediate, and *serous surface papillary (adeno)carcinomas* when malignant. Most of the latter are bilateral, highly aggressive, and usually associated with peritoneal spread at the time of surgery[118,133,141] (Fig. 19-161).

An altogether different type of tumor predominantly involving the ovarian surface is so-called *serous psammocarcinoma,* a rare variant of serous carcinoma characterized by massive psammoma body formation and low-grade cytologic features; the behavior of these tumors more closely resembles that of borderline serous tumors than of serous carcinomas.[117]

Ovarian serous tumors are positive immunohistochemically for epithelial markers, such as keratin (mainly types 7, 8, 18, and 19), EMA, and B 72.3.[107,119,132] They are also often immunoreactive for S-100 protein (particularly in the case of the borderline tumors).[127] Some malignant tumors also contain vimentin[130] and glial fibrillary acidic protein.[132] These tumors also express HLA and Ia histocompatibility antigens[122] and contain glycoconjugates that result in a pattern of lectin binding that is different from that of mucinous tumors.[135] Interestingly, one quarter of the serous and endometrioid tumors (but *not* the mucinous tumors) produce amylase, which can be demonstrated in the tumor cells (by immunohistochemistry), in the cyst fluid, and sometimes in elevated levels in the peripheral blood.[137,140] CEA stain is negative, in contrast to the mucinous tumors.[110] The beta subunit of hCG has been detected in a minority of cases.[131] Various monoclonal antibodies have been produced against epithelial ovarian tumors, of which CA 125 is the most used[110,116,125,128,129]; at the present time, their ability to distinguish benign from malignant and primary from metastatic tumors remains to be determined. Receptors for estrogens, progesterone, and androgens can be demonstrated biochemically or immunohistochemically in over half of ovarian serous tumors[104,109,120,136]; they do not seem to relate to grade or prognosis but may be of value in predicting the response to hormonal therapy.

A continuous basement membrane (as detected immunohistochemically with antibodies to laminin or type IV collagen) is present in benign cystadenomas and borderline tumors without microinvasion; disruption of this structure occurs in areas of microinvasion (in the borderline tumors) or frank invasion (in the cystadenocarcinomas).[108]

Mucinous tumors

Mucinous neoplasms are less common than the serous neoplasms and are bilateral in only 10% to 20% of the cases. As with their serous counterpart, they can be divided into *benign (mucinous cystadenoma), borderline,* and *malignant (mucinous adenocarcinoma* and *cystadenocarcinoma).* Grossly, they tend to grow larger than the serous types and are partially or completely cystic, often multiloculated. A fluid to viscous material of mucoid nature is present in the lumen (Figs. 19-162 and 19-163). In the past, these tumors have been designated as *pseudomucinous;* however, since the material secreted by the tumor cells has all the histochemical features of a mucosubstance, the designation of *mucinous* is more appropriate.[169a] The malignant types are

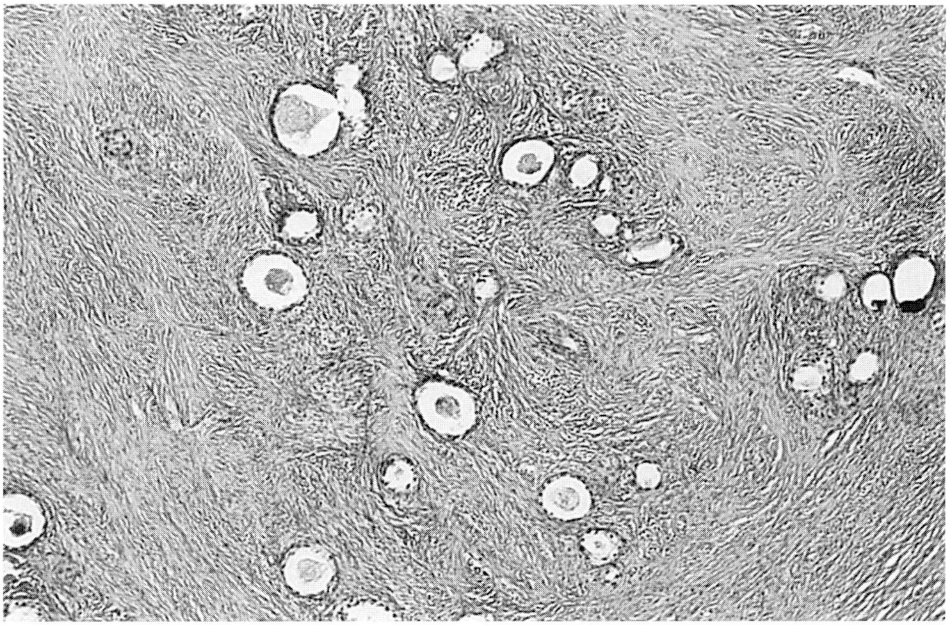

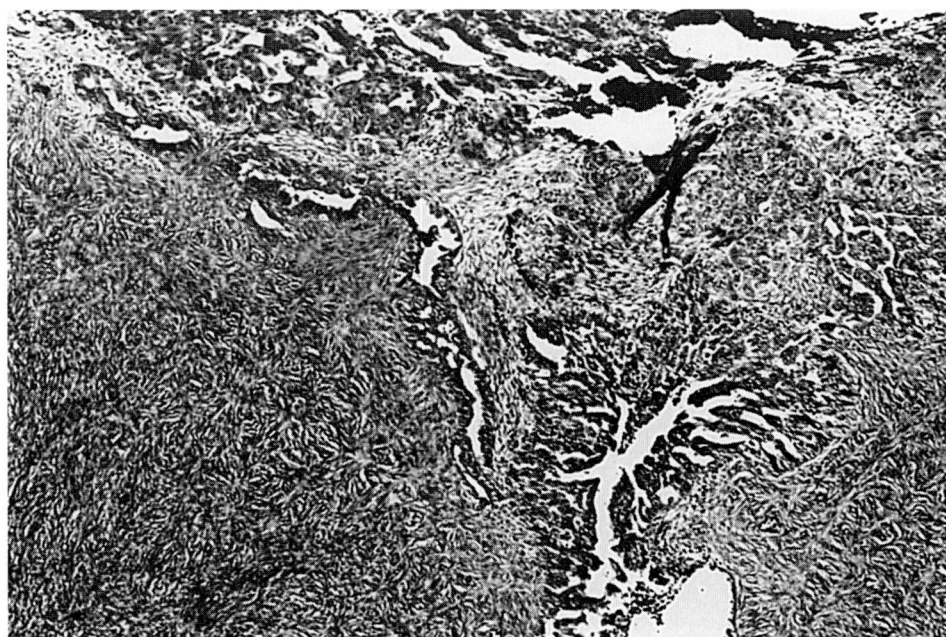

Fig. 19-160 Cystadenofibroma. Small round glands lined by cuboidal epithelium are irregularly distributed in dense fibrous stroma.

Fig. 19-161 Serous surface papillary carcinoma. Poorly differentiated epithelial neoplasm of serous type is seen covering surface of ovary, associated with only minimal stromal invasion.

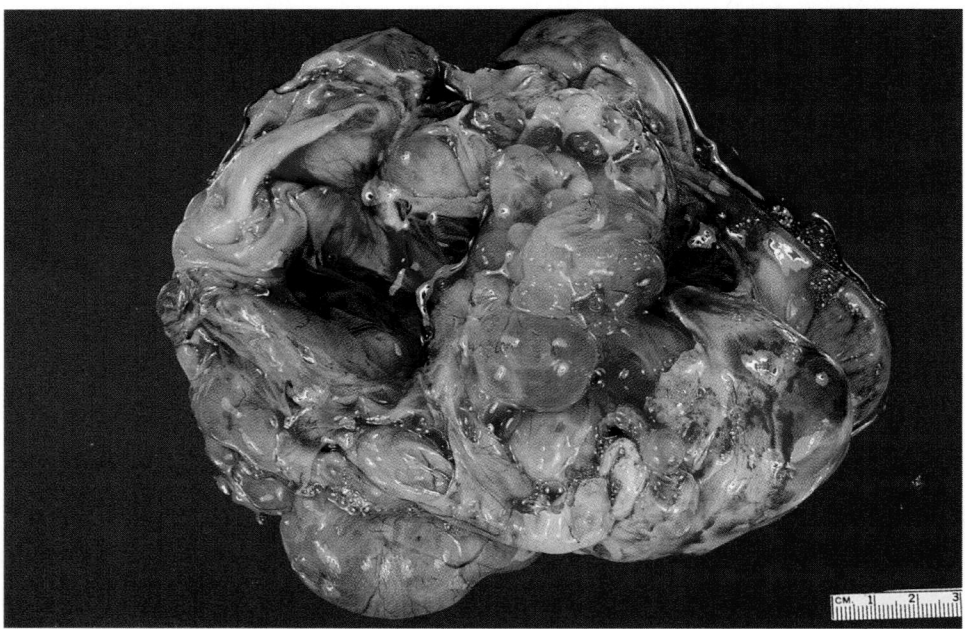

Fig. 19-162 Mucinous cystadenoma. The lesion is multilocular, and the cysts contain mucinous material in their lumen.

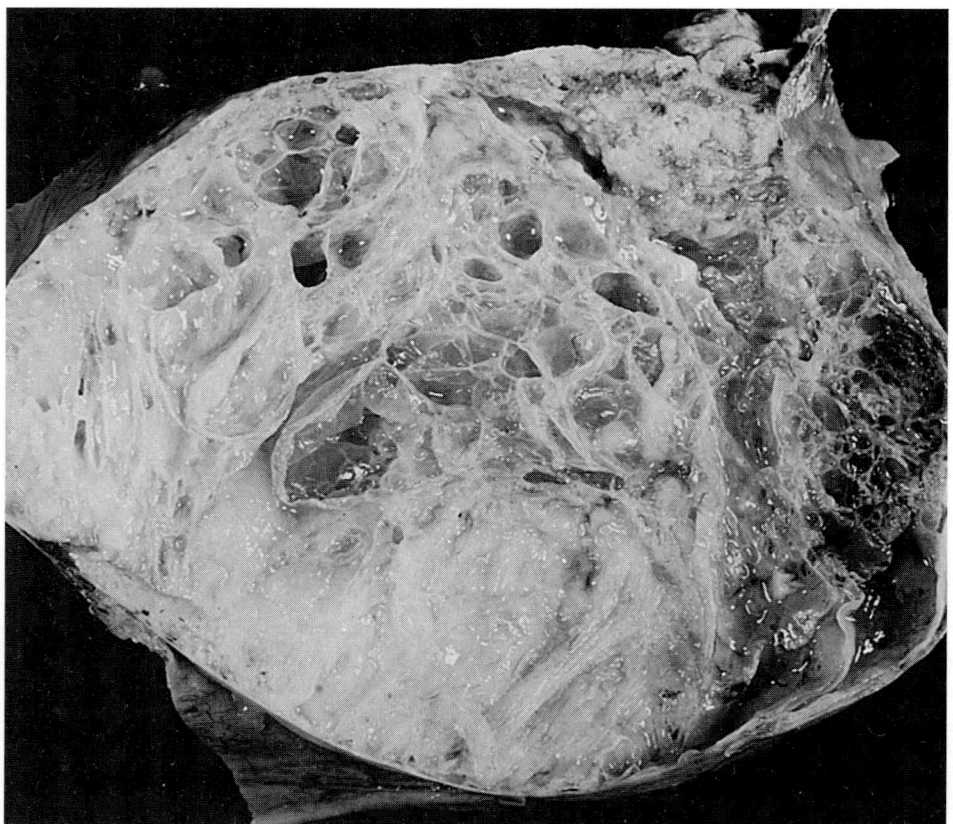

Fig. 19-163 Huge mucinous cystadenoma in 59-year-old woman. Note characteristic multilocular spaces.

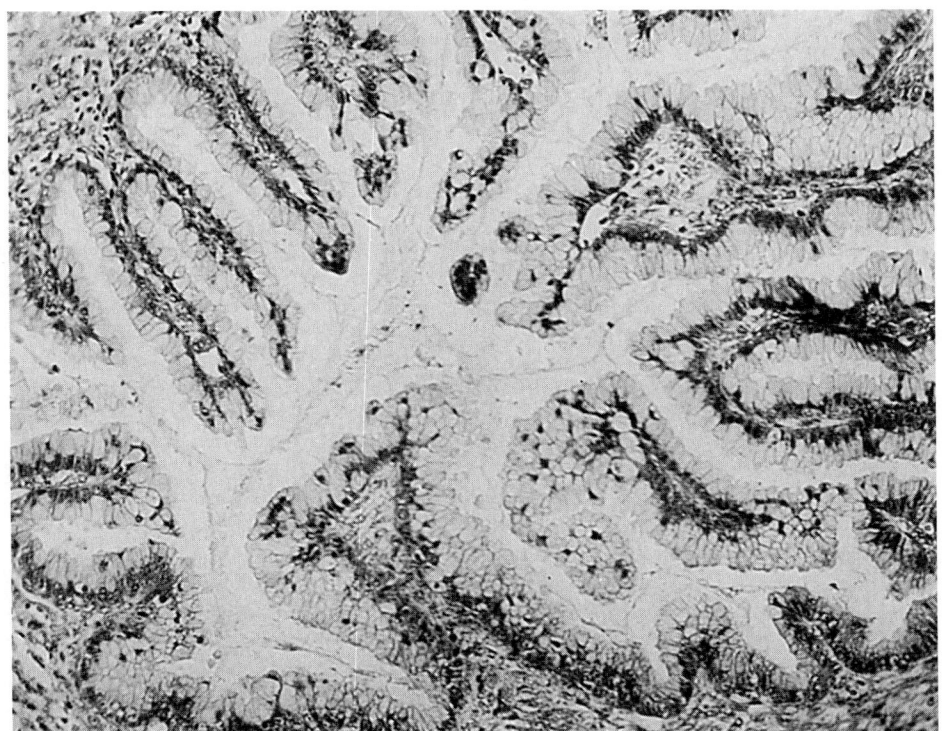

Fig. 19-164 Ovarian mucinous cystadenoma composed of well-differentiated mucinous glands resembling endocervix.

more apt to have papillae, solid areas, necrosis, and hemorrhage. Stromal invasion may be apparent. Since this may involve only a small portion of the tumor, thorough sampling for microscopic examination is necessary.

Microscopically, the benign mucinous neoplasms are lined by tall, columnar, nonciliated cells with basally situated nuclei and abundant intracellular mucin. The appearance in most cases is highly reminiscent of endocervical epithelium at both a light and electron microscopic level[151,157] ("endocervical type") (Fig. 19-164). Others have an epithelium with an intestinal appearance ("intestinal type") and still others show an admixture of both types ("mixed").[177] Intestinal-type epithelium is characterized by a "picket fence" appearance, goblet cells, Paneth cells, endocrine cells, the secretion of gastrointestinal and pancreatobiliary type mucin, and the production of intestinal enzymes such as lipase, trypsin, amylase, and sucrase.[175,178] The endocrine cells, which are more common in the borderline category, are argyrophil and sometimes argentaffin.[156] Serotonin, ACTH, gastrin, somatostatin, and other peptide hormones have been detected immunohistochemically in them.[142,160,172,173,176] There is usually no clinical evidence of hormone excess, but cases associated with Zollinger-Ellison syndrome have been described.[145] Furthermore, mucinous tumors have been found in association with carcinoid tumors in the same ovary.[169] On the basis of these findings, some authors have postulated a monodermal teratomatous derivation for these tumors; most evidence, however, favors a metaplastic origin from the surface epithelium.[151] Indeed, some have been found to coexist with endocervical adenocarcinoma.[159,183] The stroma can be hypercellular, particularly in the area

immediately beneath the neoplastic epithelium; on occasions, it may show signs of luteinization and be accompanied by hormonal manifestations.[162] Exceptionally, the appearance is that of a ***mucinous adenofibroma*** or ***cystadenofibroma,*** a lesion not to be confused with low-grade metastatic adenocarcinoma.[144] Immunohistochemically, the epithelial tumor cells express CEA (particularly if of intestinal type and/or malignant),[170] keratin, epithelial membrane antigen, and amylase (benign neoplasms, 20%; malignant, 75%).[147,153]

The *malignant* type of mucinous tumor is characterized by cell atypia, increased layering of cells, greater complexity of the glands and papillae (budding, bridging, appearance of solid foci), and areas of stromal invasion[181] (Fig. 19-165). Stroma-rich variants are referred to as ***mucinous adenocarcinofibroma*** and ***cystadenocarcinofibroma.*** K-*ras* activation is common in malignant mucinous tumors, in contrast with the serous epithelial neoplasms.[150]

The existence and clinical significance of a *borderline* category in the mucinous tumors is not as well-defined as for their serous counterpart.[175a] One of the problems is that stromal invasion is difficult to evaluate in cases with a complex interaction of glands and stroma. Hart and Norris[154] proposed the following rules for the distinction between borderline and malignant mucinous tumors: If there is unquestionable invasion, the tumor is classified as a carcinoma; if invasion is uncertain, the tumor is classified as borderline when the atypical epithelium is less than four cells in thickness and as carcinoma when it is four cells or greater. Some independent studies have confirmed the prognostic utility of this arbitrary and biologically unsound criterion,[146] but oth-

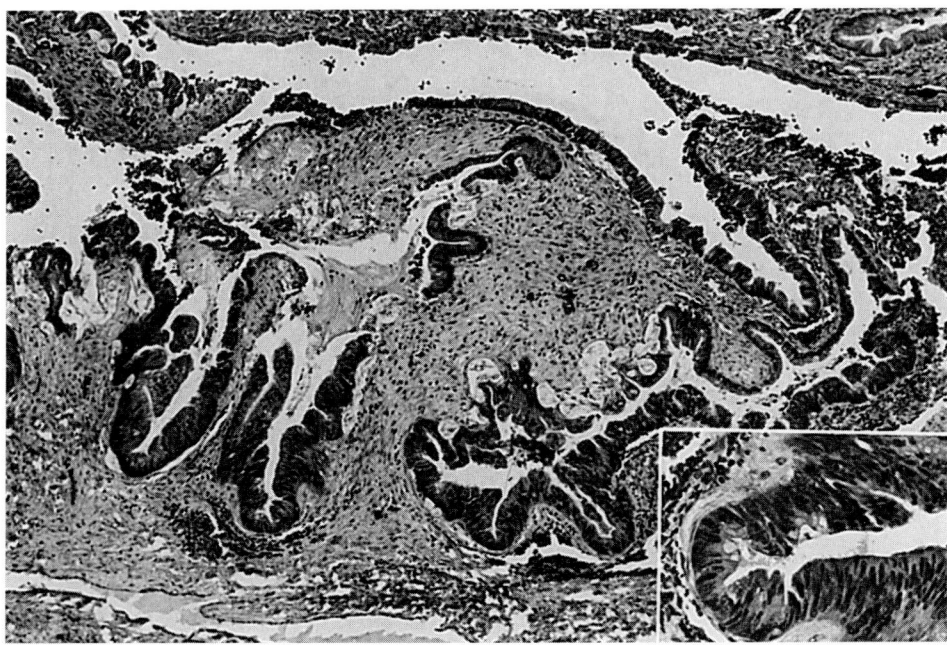

Fig. 19-165 Low-grade mucinous cystadenocarcinoma. There is marked complexity in glandular formations, which are lined by a stratified epithelium with marked nuclear atypia. Epithelial stratification can be particularly well appreciated in **inset**.

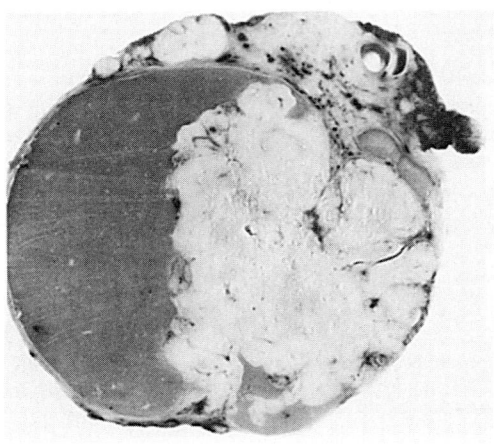

Fig. 19-166 Gross appearance of endometrioid carcinoma. Tumor is half solid and half cystic and extends to surface of ovary.

ers have not.[180] Some of these borderline mucinous tumors have papillae similar to those of serous tumors.[171] Like the benign mucinous tumors, intestinal and endocervical types of borderline mucinous neoplasms exist.[149]

Exceptionally, ovarian mucinous tumors have been found to contain foci of (1) *sarcoma-like nodules,* with a configuration and cytologic composition similar to those of giant cell tumor of soft parts,[166] and lack of reactivity for keratin[161]; (2) *sarcoma,* usually spindle-shaped and sometimes with heterologous features[165,179]; and (3) *anaplastic carcinoma,* with pleomorphic round-to-spindle cells that are

immunoreactive for keratin.[164,167] The distinction between the latter two lesions is very tenuous, both on microscopic and histogenetic grounds (as it is in the pancreas or thyroid under similar circumstances), and both are associated with a very poor prognosis. Actually, we favor the interpretation that the sarcoma-like nodules themselves are also of neoplastic nature and related histogenetically to the other two processes, a possibility also expressed by others[148] and supported by occasional coexistence of these various lesions. However, it is important to consider the sarcoma-like nodules separately because of their excellent prognosis.[143,166,167] On occasion, the appearance of the mural nodule is that of a benign leiomyomatous growth.[158]

Mucinous cystadenocarcinomas tend to implant on and locally invade neighboring tissues such as the bowel, abdominal wall, and bladder. Metastases to distant areas are infrequent. At times, ovarian mucinous neoplasms are seen in association with *pseudomyxoma peritonei,* in which gelatinous masses within a distended abdomen cause intestinal obstruction, and peritonitis frequently supervenes.[152,153a,155,163] In such cases, a mucinous neoplasm of the appendix is nearly always present.[168] Whether the ovarian and appendiceal lesions represent independent primaries or whether one is yet another implant from the other remains a controversial issue.[168,174,182] The factor that they both express keratin 7[153a] and that they have an identical pattern of c-Ki-*ras* mutations[147a] supports a common origin.

Endometrioid tumors

Endometrioid carcinoma comprises 10% to 25% of all primary ovarian carcinomas.[196,197] Coexistent endometriosis can be demonstrated in 10% to 20% of the cases,[187,199] and

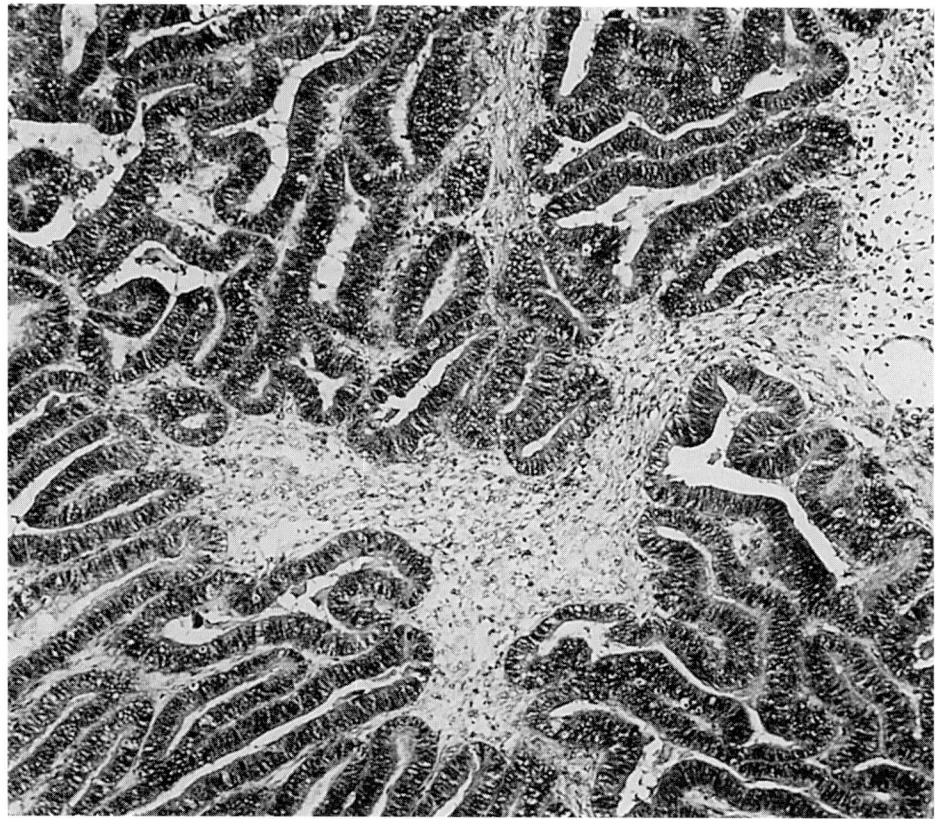

Fig. 19-167 Endometrioid carcinoma of ovary. Pattern of glands exactly resembles that of usual endometrial carcinoma.

some of the tumors can be seen actually arising from these endometriotic cysts. However, the identification of endometriosis is not a prerequisite for the diagnosis of endometrioid carcinoma, inasmuch as the majority of these tumors are thought to originate de novo from the ovarian surface epithelium. The occasional admixture of endometrioid with serous and/or mucinous patterns would seem to support this interpretation.

Grossly, endometrioid carcinoma may present as a cystic or solid mass (Fig. 19-166). The content tends to be hemorrhagic rather than serous or mucinous. Visible papillary formations are usually absent or inconspicuous. Microscopically, the tumors resemble greatly the appearance of the ordinary type of endometrial adenocarcinoma— hence their name[188,189] (Fig. 19-167). Most are well differentiated, with or without papillary formations. Half of the tumors have foci of squamous metaplasia, some of these having been reported in the past as adenoacanthomas.[194] As in uterine adenoacanthomas, the keratin produced by these ovarian neoplasms can result in the formation of peritoneal keratin granulomas.[193] It seems likely that at least some of the reported cases of primary *squamous cell carcinomas* of the ovary represent the extreme expression of this metaplastic tendency of endometrioid carcinoma.[198,204,206]

About 10% of the endometrioid carcinomas are accompanied by luteinized stromal cells. Mucin may be present in the glandular lumina and in the apical border of the tumor cells but not in the cytoplasm. CEA, CA 19-9, and human placental lactogen can be demonstrated immunohistochemically in some of the cases.[186,190] Scattered argyrophil cells are seen in almost half of the cases[205]; curiously, these have been found to be negative for neuron-specific enolase.[192] Psammoma bodies are exceptional. Ultrastructurally, the two most distinctive features (also shared with endometrial adenocarcinoma) are paranuclear collections of microfilaments and nucleoli with a "mesh basket" appearance (Fig. 19-168).

In some endometrioid carcinomas, the neoplastic glands are small and tubular or solid and elongated, simulating the pattern of sex cord–stromal tumors, particularly of Sertoli– Leydig cell type.[202,207] Features that favor a diagnosis of endometrioid carcinoma in such cases are the older age of the patients, the usual absence of endocrine manifestations, and the occurrence elsewhere in the tumor of larger tubular glands, foci of squamous metaplasia, luminal mucin accumulation, adenofibromatous components, and immunohistochemical positivity for keratin.[184] Two cases of endometrioid carcinoma containing yolk sac elements have been described.[203] Other endometrioid carcinomas have been found to be composed of oxyphilic epithelium.[200a]

Benign, atypical (proliferating), and borderline types of endometrioid ovarian tumors exist.[185,191] Most of these have a prominent stromal component and have been traditionally included with the adenofibromas or cystadenofibromas,

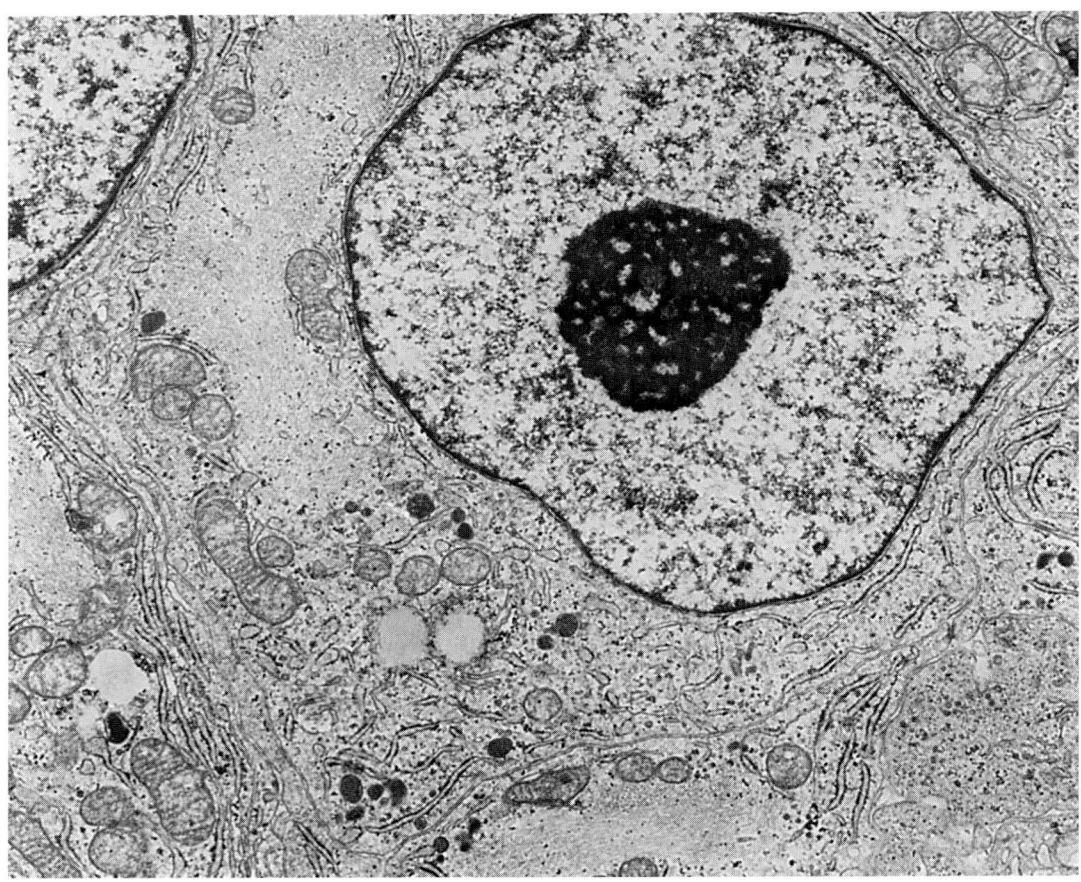

Fig. 19-168 Endometrioid adenocarcinoma of ovary. Most typical features are presence of paranuclear collections of microfilaments and nucleoli with mesh basket appearance.

Table 19-8 Differential characteristics of serous, mucinous, and endometrioid carcinomas

Characteristic	Serous	Mucinous	Endometrioid
Relative frequency	60%-80%	5%-15%	10%-25%
Bilaterality	30%-50%	10%-20%	15%-30%
Size	Moderate	Often huge	Moderate
Usual character of fluid	Clear	Slimy, viscous	Hemorrhagic
Coexistent endometrial hyperplasia or carcinoma	Exceptional	Exceptional	15%-30%
Epithelium	Cuboidal	Columnar, with basally located nucleus	Columnar, with centrally located nucleus
Mucin	Only in luminal border	Often abundant, intracytoplasmic	Only in luminal border
Squamous metaplasia	Exceptional	Exceptional	50%
Cilia	Frequent	Absent	Rare
Psammoma bodies	30%	Exceptional	Exceptional

depending on the degree of cystic change. Sometimes, benign and malignant areas coexist in the same case.[191,201] In the atypical category, the epithelial changes are equivalent to those of atypical endometrial hyperplasia; in the borderline category, they are akin to well-differentiated endometrial adenocarcinoma *without stromal invasion.*[185,200] Oophorectomy is generally curative for all of these forms.

As a group, endometrioid carcinoma has a prognosis twice as good as that of serous or mucinous carcinoma.[195] However, this seems to be mainly a function of the fact that many of these tumors are stage I and well differentiated. When these various tumor types are evaluated stage for stage, the outcome is not significantly different.[188]

Some patients with endometrioid carcinoma of the ovary have either endometrial hyperplasia or a synchronous endo-

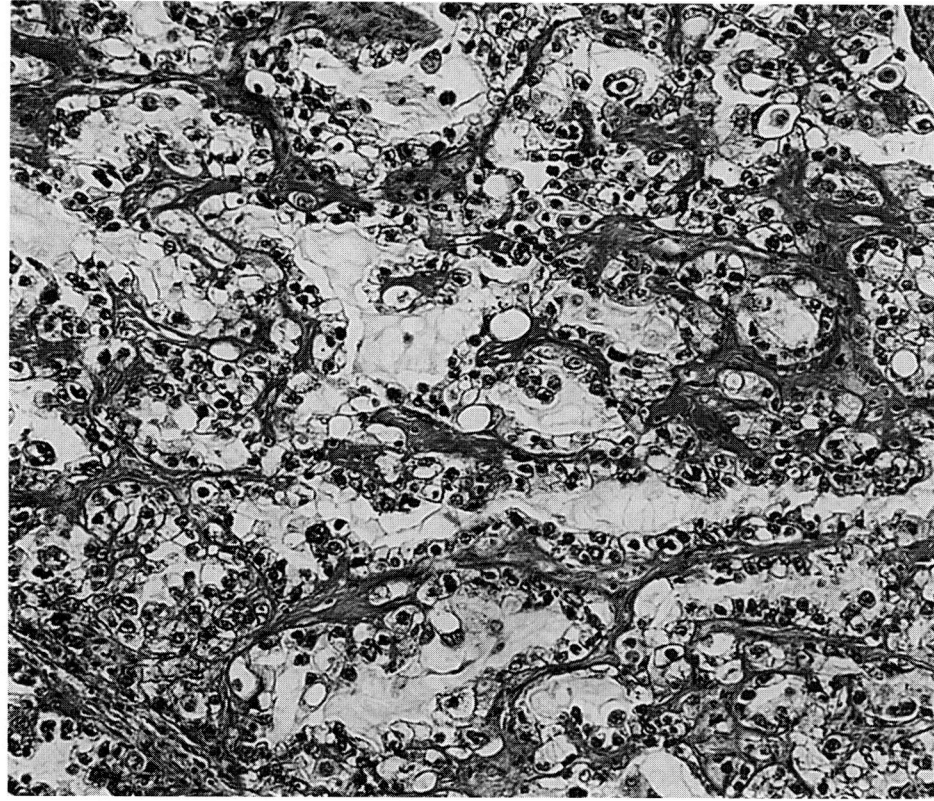

Fig. 19-169 Clear cell (mesonephroid) adenocarcinoma showing characteristic peg cells supported by delicate fibrous trabeculae forming small cystic spaces.

metrial adenocarcinoma, often well differentiated and superficial and sometimes exhibiting squamous metaplasia (so-called adenoacanthoma).[208] There is a wide disparity in the reported incidence of the latter occurrence (largely because of different diagnostic criteria), with most series ranging between 15% to 30%.[189,208] This is discussed further on p. 1489.

The most important differences among serous, mucinous, and endometrioid carcinomas are listed in Table 19-8.

Clear cell (mesonephroid) tumors

Clear cell (mesonephroid) adenocarcinoma is a distinctive ovarian tumor with a grossly spongy, often cystic appearance, which microscopically grows in tubular-cystic, papillary, and solid-sheet fashion.[214] The cores of the papillae often exhibit prominent hyalinization. Stroma-rich variants are known as clear cell adenocarcinofibroma and cystadenocarcinofibroma.

The tumor cells are large. Some of the nuclei protrude into the lumina, resulting in a "hobnail" configuration (Fig. 19-169). Their cytoplasm is clear; it often contains glycogen, mucin, and fat, and it may exhibit PAS-positive, diastase-resistant hyaline globules, which are negative for alpha-fetoprotein (the latter unassociated to the hyaline globules).[213] In some of the tumor cells, the cytoplasm may appear oxyphilic rather than clear.[220] Immunohistochemically, the tumor cells are always reactive for keratin, often for Leu-M1, and occasionally for alpha-fetoprotein.[221]

This tumor type was included in Schiller's original description of mesonephroma and regarded as of mesonephric rest derivation[217]; however, convincing evidence has been brought forward to indicate that it is of surface epithelial type and specifically related to endometrioid carcinoma, of which it should be regarded as a variant.[218,219] This interpretation is supported by the high association with pelvic endometriosis, the origin in some cases from endometriotic cysts, the frequent admixture with typical endometrioid carcinoma, and the ultrastructural similarities with müllerian endometrioid epithelium.[209,218]

Patients with clear cell adenocarcinoma are usually in the fifth or sixth decades. The incidence of bilaterality is less than 10%, and the 5-year survival rate ranges from 37% to 47%.[210,211,215] Stage for stage, their prognosis is similar to that of other epithelial ovarian carcinomas.[210,212]

Benign and *borderline* (low malignant potential) ovarian clear cell tumors are very rare. Their growth pattern may be that of a cystadenoma, an adenofibroma, or a cystadenofibroma. The borderline tumors are identified because of moderate to marked degrees of epithelial proliferation and atypia in the absence of recognizable stromal invasion.[216]

Brenner tumor and transitional cell carcinoma

Brenner tumors constitute between 1% and 2% of all ovarian neoplasms.[226,242] The average age at presentation is about 50 years, 71% of the patients being over 40 years of age. Some cases are accompanied by signs of hyperestrin-

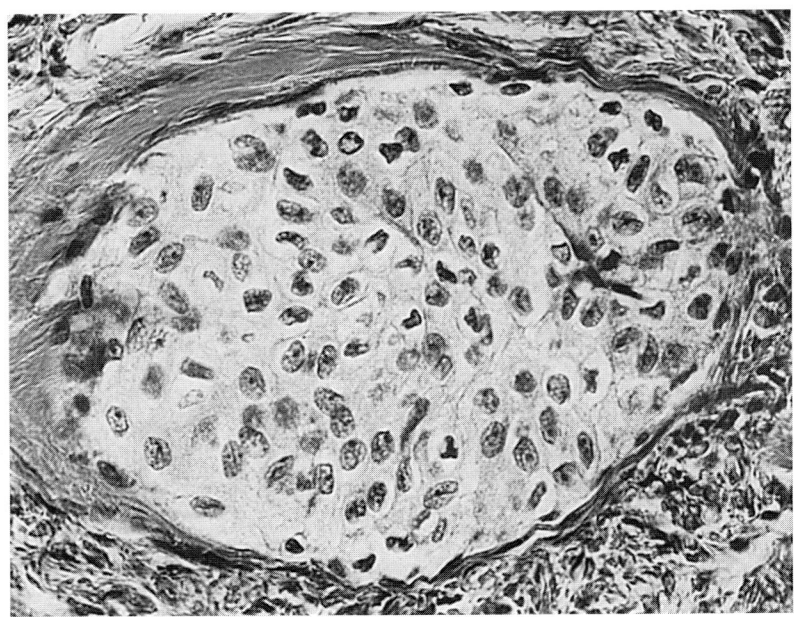

Fig. 19-170 Characteristic collection of closely packed cells with clear cytoplasm and deeply staining nuclei seen in Brenner tumor. Longitudinal groove is seen in several nuclei.

ism, such as uterine bleeding from endometrial hyperplasia in the postmenopausal woman.[231] The rate of growth is slow, and ascites is rare. Grossly, these tumors vary greatly in size; they are usually unilateral, firm, and white or yellowish white. They closely resemble fibromas or thecomas, except for the frequent presence of small cystic areas filled with opaque, viscous, yellowish brown fluid. Microscopically, they consist of solid and cystic nests of epithelial cells resembling transitional epithelium (urothelium) surrounded by an abundant stromal component of dense, fibroblastic nature.[225] The epithelial cells have sharply defined outlines; those lining the cysts may be flattened, cuboidal, or columnar. The nuclei of the tumor cells are oval, with a small but distinct nucleolus and longitudinal grooves similar to those seen in granulosa cell tumors (Fig. 19-170). The cytoplasm is clear and immunoreactive for keratin, EMA, and CEA (the latter also present in the lumen of the cysts).[227] It may contain glycogen, mucin, and lipid.[231,237,241] The latter is found in larger amounts in the stromal cells in the cases accompanied by hyperestrinism. Scattered argyrophilic cells are present in 39% of the cases; they are positive for chromogranin and serotonin, have dense core granules at the ultrastructural level, and are similar to those seen in normal urothelium.[223] Steroidogenic enzymes as detected immunohistochemically are usually absent.[238]

Sometimes the cystic formations within the tumor are unduly prominent and accompanied by florid mucinous changes (a lesion analogous to cystitis glandularis); Roth et al.[235] refer to this pattern as *metaplastic* Brenner tumor as long as papillary fronds and nuclear atypia are absent. If the latter two features are present (the pattern thus resembling that of a low-grade [grades I or II] transitional carcinoma of the urinary bladder), they designate it as a *proliferating* Brenner tumor[230,235] (Fig. 19-171). When this pattern is

associated with a greater degree of atypia (equivalent to a grade III transitional cell carcinoma) but stromal invasion cannot be demonstrated, the terms *borderline* or *low malignant potential* have been suggested.[235] Typical, metaplastic, proliferating, and borderline Brenner tumors have been found to follow a benign clinical course after oophorectomy. The latter three types are sometimes grouped under the term *intermediate Brenner tumor.*[236] Cytologically malignant neoplasms associated with *stromal invasion* are referred to as *malignant Brenner tumors* (Plate XIV-B). Some of these cases have been bilateral.[222,228,230,239] They are recognized mainly because of their association with a typical benign, metaplastic, proliferating, or borderline component.[234] The appearance may be that of a transitional cell, squamous, or undifferentiated carcinoma, or an admixture of these.

Adenocarcinomatous foci may also be present.[234] Austin and Norris[224] pointed out that malignant Brenner tumors with an associated benign component have a better prognosis than morphologically similar tumors in which such a component was absent. The latter are referred to as *transitional cell carcinomas* (non-Brenner type). It has been claimed that the presence of a transitional cell pattern in high-grade ovarian carcinomas is an indicator of favorable response to chemotherapy.[233]

Brenner tumors can be seen in association with mucinous cystadenoma (Fig. 19-172) and, exceptionally, struma ovarii.[232] They have also been found to coexist with transitional cell tumors of the urinary bladder.[243,244] We have seen a case of benign Brenner tumor of the ovary associated with transitional cell carcinoma of the endometrium.

Although the histogenesis of Brenner tumors remains controversial, most authors favor an origin from surface epithelium or the cysts derived from them, through a process of transitional cell metaplasia.[240] The continuity that has

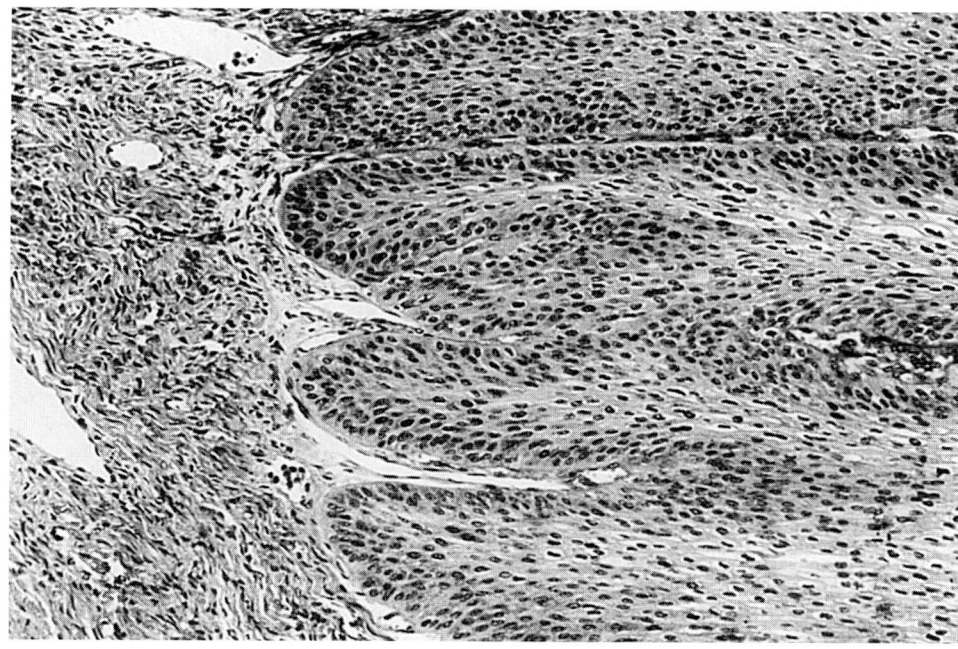

Fig. 19-171 Proliferating Brenner tumor. Both cytologic composition and architectural pattern closely simulate appearance of a transitional cell tumor of bladder.

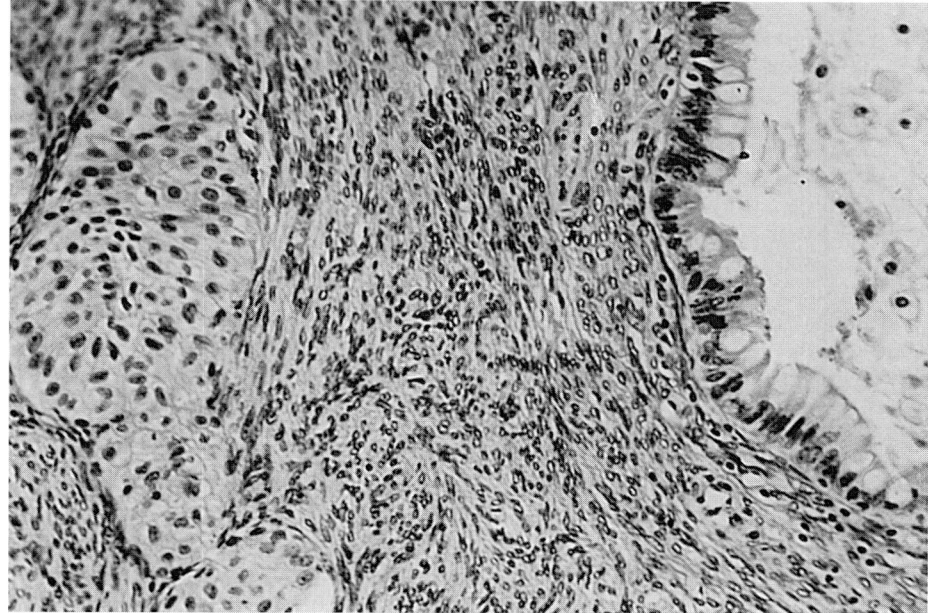

Fig. 19-172 Mucinous cystadenoma and Brenner tumor. Mucinous tumor with typical lining epithelium is at right, and Brenner tumor with its characteristic collection of cells is at left. (Slide contributed by Dr. R. Johnson, Columbia, MO.)

been demonstrated between the epithelial nests of Brenner tumor and the ovarian surface supports this concept, which is currently preferred over the alternatives of an origin from Walthard cell nests (microscopically similar but usually located in the mesosalpinx rather than the ovary), granulosa cells, rete ovarii, or germ cells.

Brenner tumors have been exceptionally seen to occur in accessory ovaries or in other female genital tract sites, such as the uterine cervix.[229]

Mixed müllerian tumors

The gross and microscopic features of *malignant mixed müllerian tumor* resemble in every respect those of its more common uterine counterpart. Thus a *homologous* variety (with nonspecific malignant stroma; also called *carcinosarcoma*) and a *heterologous* variety (with malignant heterologous elements, particularly cartilage) occur.[250] The carcinomatous component may appear serous, endometrioid, squamous, or clear cell (mesonephroid). Hyaline droplets containing alpha-1-antitrypsin are often present in the cytoplasm of the tumor cells.[249] Although some response to chemotherapy has been noted,[254] the prognosis remains extremely poor.[248] The most reliable prognostic criterion is the initial tumor stage.[245,246,253] Unfortunately, most tumors have already extended outside the ovary at the time of surgery.[252] The most important differential diagnosis is with immature (malignant) teratoma. Almost all malignant mixed müllerian tumors are seen in postmenopausal patients (often with history of low parity), whereas immature teratomas are typically tumors of children and adolescents. Furthermore, the former lack the neural and other germ cell elements of teratomas. However, a case of malignant mixed müllerian tumor featuring prominent neuroectodermal differentiation has been described, its appearance being reminiscent of teratoid carcinosarcoma of the upper respiratory tract.[251]

Müllerian adenosarcoma, regarded as a low-grade variant of mixed müllerian tumor and more commonly seen in the endometrium and cervix, also can occur in the ovary.[247] The morphologic appearance and behavior are again similar to those of its uterine counterpart, which is fully discussed earlier in this chapter (see Uterus—Corpus).

Adenoid cystic and basaloid carcinomas

Exceptionally, surface epithelial carcinomas of ovary show a pattern resembling that of salivary gland carcinomas of adenoid cystic type or that of cutaneous basal cell carcinomas. These may be seen in pure form or in association with conventional serous, endometrioid, or clear cell patterns. The tumors with an adenoid cystic carcinoma–like appearance are more aggressive than the basaloid neoplasms.[254a]

Ovarian carcinoma—overview
General and clinical features

Ovarian carcinoma accounts for the greatest number of deaths from malignancies of the female genital tract and is the fifth leading cause of cancer fatalities in women.[265] The incidence remains constant. It is predominantly a disease of older white women of northern European extraction, but it is seen in all ages and ethnic groups.[255,256,262,267,269] Pregnancy (especially if before age 25 years) and use of oral contraceptives are associated with a diminished risk.[257,259,266,268] A

cohort of infertile women treated wth clomiphene has been found to be at an increased risk for borderline and invasive ovarian tumors.[267a] Familial predisposition has been noted in a small percentage of patients.[258,260,261,264] Recently, the gene for hereditary breast and ovarian cancer, BRCA1 (located on 17q), was discovered, and its complete nucleotide sequence was reported. Unfortunately, there is a huge number of mutations that can destroy this gene, a fact that will render it very difficult to screen women on a large scale.[263]

Clinically, ovarian carcinomas usually present with lower abdominal pain, abdominal enlargement, and signs of increased pressure on neighboring organs.

"Early" and in situ carcinoma

The concept of carcinoma in situ or ovarian intraepithelial neoplasia distinct from the borderline tumors has only recently begun to gain some accceptance.[271] As in other organs, one of the criteria for its recognition is its occurrence in the remainder of an ovary affected by a primary invasive carcinoma[273] or in the contralateral ovary.[272] Bell and Scully[270] studied 14 "early de novo" carcinomas detected as microscopic findings in grossly normal ovaries. All were unilateral, and four were multifocal. Most cases involved the superficial cortex only. The large majority were of serous type. Severe atypia of the noncarcinomatous surface epithelium or its inclusion cysts was present in three cases. In six of the cases, tumor spread developed, indicating an aggressive behavior despite their minute dimensions.

Special techniques

Cytogenetically, ovarian carcinomas have been found to have complex numerical and structural anomalies. Rearrangements of chromosomes 1, 3, 6, 11, and 19 have been recognized. There is increasing evidence suggesting that genes located on the short arm of chromosome 11 play an important role in the development of this tumor.[279] However, in one series the most consistent change was a 19p+ marker.[281] In another, frequent allele losses were observed on chromosomes 13q, 17p, 17q, and Xp.[284] In a further study using the FISH technique, a relative loss of chromosomes 17 and X and a relative gain of chromosomes 12 and 8 were the most common findings.[282] As already mentioned, the long arm of chromosome 17 contains BRCA1, the gene responsible for a form of hereditary breast and ovarian carcinoma. Trisomy 12 is sometimes the only chromosomal abnormality found in benign and borderline serous tumors.[285]

Activation of several genes has been described in ovarian carcinomas. This includes HER-2/*neu, myc, ras,* and p53.[274-276,283] In addition, epidermal growth factor receptor and the M-CSF receptor are expressed along with the respective ligands (peptide growth factors) in some cases.[274,277,278]

DNA ploidy analyses have shown that benign and borderline tumors are usually diploid, whereas a majority of the invasive carcinomas are aneuploid.[280]

Spread and metastases

The pattern of metastatic spread in ovarian carcinoma is similar regardless of the microscopic type.[291] The most common sites of involvement are the contralateral ovary, peritoneal cavity (further discussed in the next section), para-aortic and pelvic lymph nodes, and liver. With intra-abdominal spread, there are often ascites and involvement of the omentum.[292] Invasion of the intestinal wall may result in obstruction.[287] Ureteral involvement is usually associated with hydronephrosis. An umbilical metastasis ("sister Joseph's nodule") may be the first manifestation of the disease.[286,290] Lung and pleura are the most common sites of extra-abdominal spread.[288] Most lung metastases have a subpleural location. Metastases can also occur in unusual sites, such as the breast.[289]

Coexistence with uterine carcinoma

The simultaneous presence of carcinoma in the ovary and uterus is an uncommon but well-recognized event. The two tumors may have a similar appearance (usually endometrioid but sometimes papillary, clear cell, or mucinous) or be of different histologic types.[293] Theoretically, this phenomenon could be the result of (1) metastasis from an endometrial carcinoma into the ovary, (2) two independent primary tumors, or (3) metastasis from an ovarian carcinoma to the endometrium. All three events probably occur, the third being by far the least common. A distinction between the first two possibilities is often difficult and may be impossible to make. Ovarian metastasis from an endometrial tumor should be favored in the presence of multiplicity, bilaterality, and/or very small size of the ovarian tumor, involvement of the tubal lumen, and presence of deep myometrial invasion and/or vascular invasion in the uterine tumor.[293] Most neoplasms with an endometrioid appearance in both sites are probably independent neoplasms, and their prognosis is excellent; most of those with histologies other than endometrioid probably represent a single primary tumor with metastases, and their prognosis is correspondingly poor.[293,296]

Immunohistochemical and DNA flow studies may offer some help in this distinction, but at present the differential diagnosis must rely largely on the conventional clinicopathologic criteria previously listed.[295]

Sometimes, the uterine tumor involves the cervix rather than the corpus; interestingly, a high proportion of these cervical tumors are of endometrioid type.[294] The lesion should be regarded as an ovarian metastasis from a cervical primary if there is bilateral ovarian involvement and extensive extracervical disease and if the microscopic type is one unusual for an ovarian primary (such as squamous cell carcinoma or small cell carcinoma).[297]

The association between ovarian and uterine neoplasms is also discussed in connection with the individual types.

Related peritoneal lesions

Lesions primarily involving the peritoneal surface rather than the ovary but discussed here because of their relationship with ovarian tumor pathology include implants and endosalpingiosis. The latter is thought to arise from the so-called secondary müllerian system (i.e., the pelvic and lower abdominal mesothelium and the subjacent mesenchyme of females); whether or not some of the "implants" have a similar origin remains controversial. Some are clearly metastatic from the ovarian primary, as shown by molecular analyses of loss of heterozygosity.[310]

Implants. One of the most common patterns of spread of ovarian carcinoma—particularly the serous type—is in the form of tumor deposits on the peritoneal surfaces. Sites of early peritoneal spread are the lateral gutters and diaphragmatic surface (predominantly on the right side) and omentum. Involvement of abdominal viscera (bowel, liver, spleen) is generally by direct spread from the underlying peritoneum. There is a tendency for concentration of tumor nodules close to the primary tumor, so the pelvic peritoneum, sigmoid colon, cecum, and terminal ileum are most frequently involved. Sometimes, the entire peritoneal cavity is covered by implants measuring less than 1 cm in diameter and grossly simulating miliary tuberculosis.

Peritoneal implants are present in 16% to 47% of borderline serous tumors and are associated with a mortality rate of 13% to 30%.[301] Although generically designated as "implants," it is possible and indeed likely that some arise in situ from the peritoneal mesothelium.[309] The large majority of ovarian borderline neoplasms associated with peritoneal implants have an exophytic pattern of growth.[315] The most common sites for these implants are the pelvic peritoneum, omentum, uterine serosa, and fallopian tube serosa.[307] Their microscopic appearance is similar to that of the ovarian tumor and is therefore characterized by tufting, stratification, cytologic atypia, and psammoma bodies[299,313] (Fig. 19-173). They can be predominantly cystic or papillary. Some have been known to regress spontaneously, sometimes leaving a shower of psammoma bodies behind. It has been shown that infiltration of underlying tissues (referred to as "destructive invasion" and to be distinguished from desmoplastic response in noninvasive tumors) and marked cytologic atypia are associated with a high probability of disease progression.[312] These patients may benefit from additional therapy, whereas such an approach is probably unnecessary in patients without these adverse prognostic features.[301]

Peritoneal implants should be distinguished from endosalpingiosis (as described later) and from florid mesothelial hyperplasia, of a type similar to that most commonly seen in hernia sacs and around ruptured tubal pregnancies.[304]

Occasionally, one or multiple peritoneal nodules with features of ovarian serous borderline or malignant tumors are seen in the presence of minimal or no ovarian involvement. The malignant-appearing lesions have been generally regarded as ovarian carcinomas with widespread metastases if the ovary was affected, however focally and superficially (see discussion of serous surface papillary carcinomas on p. 1477), and as *extraovarian serous carcinomas* or *papillary tumors of the peritoneum* in the absence of ovarian abnormalities.[298,305,306,311,314a] Their immunohistochemical and ultrastructural profile and their natural history are closer to ovarian serous carcinoma than to diffuse peritoneal mesothelioma[316,317]; they should therefore be viewed as *carcinomas* composed of cells analogous to those lining the ovarian surface. Notably, some of these tumors have developed after prophylactic oophorectomy in women with a family history of ovarian carcinoma.[314]

Immunohistochemical evaluation is useful in their differential diagnosis with conventional malignant mesothelioma; diffuse reactivity for LeuM1, B72.3, PLAP, or CEA is indicative of extraovarian serous papillary carcinoma.[303,308]

The borderline lesions, which have also been designated as *peritoneal serous micropapillomatosis of low malignant potential,*[302] have a natural history equivalent to that of their ovarian counterpart (i.e., characterized by a good long-term prognosis).[300,318]

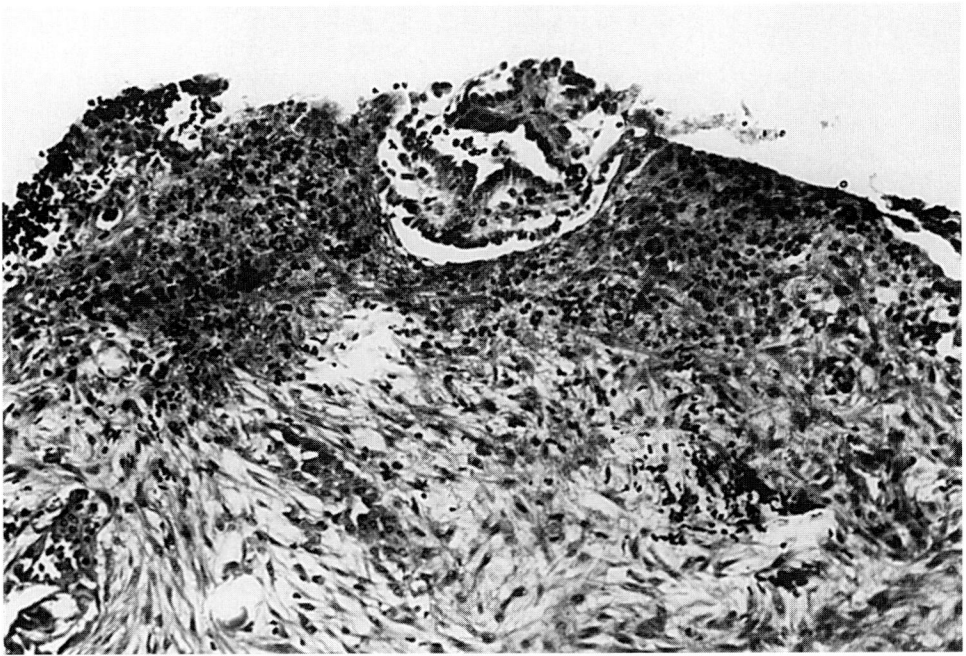

Fig. 19-173 Peritoneal implants from ovarian serous papillary carcinoma. Implant shows some degree of cellular atypia and has elicited marked inflammatory and desmoplastic response from stroma.

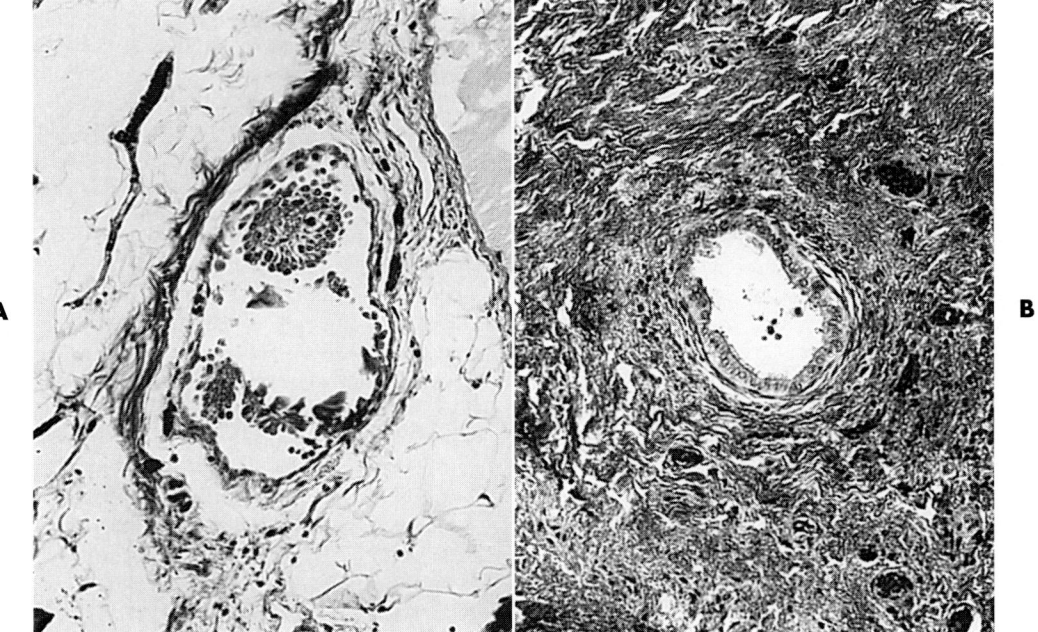

Fig. 19-174 So-called endosalpingiosis of peritoneum. Structure shown in **A** is lined by discontinuous flattened epithelium with some protrusions into lumen. There is also focal calcification. Structure shown in **B** is lined by low columnar ciliated epithelium and is surrounded by dense fibrous tissue.

Table 19-9 FIGO staging for carcinoma of the ovary

Staging of ovarian carcinoma is based on findings at clinical examination and by surgical exploration. The histologic findings are to be considered in the staging, as are the cytologic findings as fas as effusions are concerned. It is desirable that a biopsy be taken from suspicious areas outside of the pelvis.

Stage I	Growth llimited to the ovaries.
Stage IA	Growth limited to one ovary, no ascites present containing malignant cells. No tumor on the external surface; capsule intact.
Stage IB	Growth limited to both ovaries; no ascites present containing malignant cells. No tumor on the external surfaces; capsules intact.
Stage IC*	Tumor classified as either Stage IA or IB but with tumor on the surface of one or both ovaries; or with ruptured capsule(s); or with ascites containing malignant cells or with positive peritoneal washings.
Stage II	Growth involving one or both ovaries, with pelvic extension.
Stage IIA	Extension and/or metastases to the uterus and/or tubes.
Stage IIB	Extension to other pelvic tissues.
Stage IIC*	Tumor either Stage IIA or IIB but with tumor on the surface of one or both ovaries; or with capsule(s) ruptured; or with ascites containing malignant cells present or with positive peritoneal washings.
Stage III	Tumor involving one or both ovaries with peritoneal implants outside the pelvis and/or positive retroperitoneal or inguinal nodes. Superficial liver metastasis equals Stage III. Tumor is limited to the true pelvis but with histologically proven malignant extension to small bowel or omentum.
Stage IIIA	Tumor grossly limited to the true pelvis with negative nodes but with histologically confirmed microscopic seeding of abdominal peritoneal surfaces.
Stage IIIB	Tumor of one or both ovaries with histologically confirmed implants of abdominal peritoneal surfaces none exceeding 2 cm in diameter; nodes are negative.
Stage IIIC	Abdominal implants greater than 2 cm in diameter and/or positive retroperitoneal or inguinal nodes.
Stage IV	Growth involving one or both ovaries, with distant metastases. If pleural effusion is present, there must be positive cytologic findings to allot a case to Stage IV. Parenchymal liver metastasis equals Stage IV.

Notes about the staging: To evaluate the impact on prognosis of the different criteria for allotting cases to Stage IC or IIC, it would be of value to know whether the rupture of the capsule was spontaneous or caused by the surgeon and if the source of malignant cells detected was peritoneal washings or ascites.
From SGO handbook. Staging of gynecologic malignancies. Chicago, 1994, Society of Gynecologic Oncologists.
See also Appendix G.

Endosalpingiosis. The term *endosalpingiosis,* originally coined for a presumably inflammatory condition of the fallopian tube characterized by attachment of the fimbria to the ovarian surface (see p. 1448), is now more commonly applied to the presence beneath the peritoneal surface of glands and tubules (sometimes containing papillae and psammoma bodies), lined by cuboidal to low columnar cells, which are sometimes ciliated. Some resemble the endosalpingeal mucosa, hence the name (Fig. 19-174). They are thought to be the result of müllerian differentiation or metaplasia of the celomic mesothelium. Endosalpingiosis is generally seen in association with ovarian serous tumors, usually of borderline type (alone or in conjunction with implants), but it may occur in the absence of ovarian abnormalities.[318]

The distinction between endosalpingiosis and implants is not as sharp morphologically or as well documented pathogenetically as these two terms seem to imply. Therefore it may be preferable to modify the terminology to indicate that fact as well as to emphasize that presence of invasion is the key feature from a prognostic standpoint. One such scheme would be the following: (1) benign (so-called endosalpingiosis), (2) noninvasive, and (3) invasive.[307] Only mature,

benign-appearing structures should be placed in the first category. Formations exhibiting atypia, stratification, and tufting (although conceivably developing from endosalpingiosis in some of the cases) should be placed in one of the other two categories depending on whether they exhibit invasion or not.[318]

Cytology

The main role of diagnostic cytology in ovarian carcinoma is the identification of malignant cells in the peritoneal cavity. The value of peritoneal washing cytology to detect the microscopic spread of ovarian carcinoma has been acknowledged by the fact that the FIGO staging system incorporates the results of the washing in its scheme[322] (Table 19-9). This technique is useful during the initial surgical staging and during second-look operations for the evaluation of therapy effect. Serous and endometrioid carcinomas are more often positive than carcinomas of other types and high-grade tumors more than low-grade tumors.[321] Specifically, a high positive rate is related to advanced stage of disease, involvement of the ovarian surface, a moderate to large amount of fluid, and nonbloody serous ascites.[320]

Patients with positive fluids have a worse prognosis than others, but at least some of the difference is related to the stage of the disease; analysis of a large number of patients with stage I and II tumors is needed to determine the prognostic significance of a positive cytology independently of other prognostic factors.[321]

The interpretation of peritoneal washings can be made difficult by the admixture of reactive mesothelial cells and problems in distinguishing cytologically borderline from malignant tumors.[319]

Therapy

The primary form of therapy of surface epithelial tumors is surgical.[323,332] Benign tumors are cured by a conservative operation in the form of unilateral salpingo-oophorectomy. Although in occasional small benign tumors (some surface papillomas and cystadenofibromas) the uninvolved portion of the ovary can be preserved, the majority require the excision of the entire gonad. Most borderline tumors in young females can also be treated conservatively with safety, the results following salpingo-oophorectomy being equivalent to those seen following more extensive procedures.[339] As a matter of fact, some cases have been treated with cystectomy only, the overall outcome being excellent; however, presence of tumor at the margin is a strong predictor of tumor recurrence.[330]

Carcinomas require bilateral salpingo-oophorectomy with total abdominal hysterectomy, with the possible exception of grade I mucinous cystadenocarcinoma, for which a conservative approach has been suggested by some in selected young patients.[340] The role of pelvic lymphadenectomy remains controversial.[325]

It is important to examine carefully the peritoneal cavity and to biopsy selected sites to properly stage the disease for future therapy.[341] This surgical staging includes sampling from pelvic and abdominal peritoneal surfaces, diaphragm, omentum, and lymph nodes (pelvic and para-aortic).[329] If ascitic fluid is present, it should be examined cytologically; if not, peritoneal washings should be taken.[324] Adjuvant therapy (radiation therapy and/or chemotherapy) is said to be particularly important for high-grade stage I tumors, for tumors accompanied by positive ascitic fluid, and for minimal stage III disease.[327,335,337,342]

In some institutions, "second-look" operations have become a standard procedure for patients with ovarian carcinomas treated with surgery and chemotherapy who are clinically free of disease, to determine prognosis and decide whether chemotherapy should be continued, discontinued, or changed. However, the practical value of this procedure is being increasingly questioned on the grounds that the sub group of patients whose condition can be salvaged by a second-line therapy is small (about 8%) and that an effective salvage therapy still remains to be identified.[328,334]

The second-look operation includes direct visual inspection of the abdominal cavity, cytologic examination of peritoneal washings, and multiple biopsies of peritoneum, omentum, and lymph nodes. Residual tumor has been found pathologically in over 40% of the patients in most series.[333,336,338] This tends to be found in the same sites as the initial tumor. The microscopic interpretation can be complicated by the presence of mesothelial hyperplasia, psammoma bodies without accompanying epithelium, foreign

body giant cell reaction, focal fibroblastic proliferation, fat necrosis, and other changes.[326] Immunohistochemical staining for CEA, LeuM1, and other markers can be helpful in the differential diagnosis.[331]

Prognosis

The overall prognosis of ovarian carcinoma remains poor, a direct result of its rapid growth rate and the lack of early symptoms. The survival rate is approximately 35% at 5 years, 28% at 10 years, and 15% at 25 years.[351] Factors known to influence prognosis are listed below.

1 *Age.* As a group, younger patients have a better outcome. This is at least partially due to the fact that there is a higher percentage of borderline, well-differentiated, and stage I tumors in this group.[343,362]

2 Presence and extent of *tumor spread* beyond the ovary, as expressed by clinical staging (Table 19-9). For the carcinomas (as opposed to the borderline tumors, see later section), this is the most important prognostic determinator.

3 *Ascites.* This clinical finding constitutes, by itself, an unfavorable prognostic sign.[346]

4 *Borderline versus invasive tumor.* This is a distinction of utmost significance for prognostic purposes.[353] The incidence of recurrence is nearly zero for borderline mucinous and endometrioid tumors and about 20% for borderline serous or seromucinous tumors.[344] The prognosis in borderline tumors is still very good even in the presence of involvement of the peritoneal cavity, microinvasion, or tumor recrudescence in the abdominal cavity. In one series, the survival was 99% for stage I tumor and an astonishing 92% for advanced stage disease.[350] Because of these figures, some authors have questioned whether it is justified to keep labeling these tumors as of low-grade malignant potential or even borderline.[350]

5 *Tumor grade and type.* Among the carcinomas, tumor grade correlates closely with survival.[351,360,361] The microscopic type (serous, mucinous, endometrioid, or other) is of less significance in this regard, particularly among the lesser differentiated tumors.[351] However, as a group, endometrioid carcinomas do better when pure than when mixed with papillary serous or undifferentiated components.[362a]

6 *Psammoma bodies.* Serous tumors containing numerous such structures have a better prognosis.[359] This may be related to the fact that most of these tumors are well differentiated.

7 *Rupture of tumor capsule.* There is no convincing evidence that this occasional intraoperative complication has any influence on survival rates.[357]

8 *DNA ploidy.* DNA analysis with flow cytometry (using either fresh tissue or paraffin-embedded material) has proved a strong prognostic indicator, in the sense that aneuploid tumors belong to a higher grade and behave in a much more aggressive fashion than the diploid tumors.[347,348,355,363] Correlation has also been found between tumor DNA ploidy and response to chemotherapy.[345]

9 *CA 125.* This serum marker has been found of great value in the initial evaluation of these patients (particu-

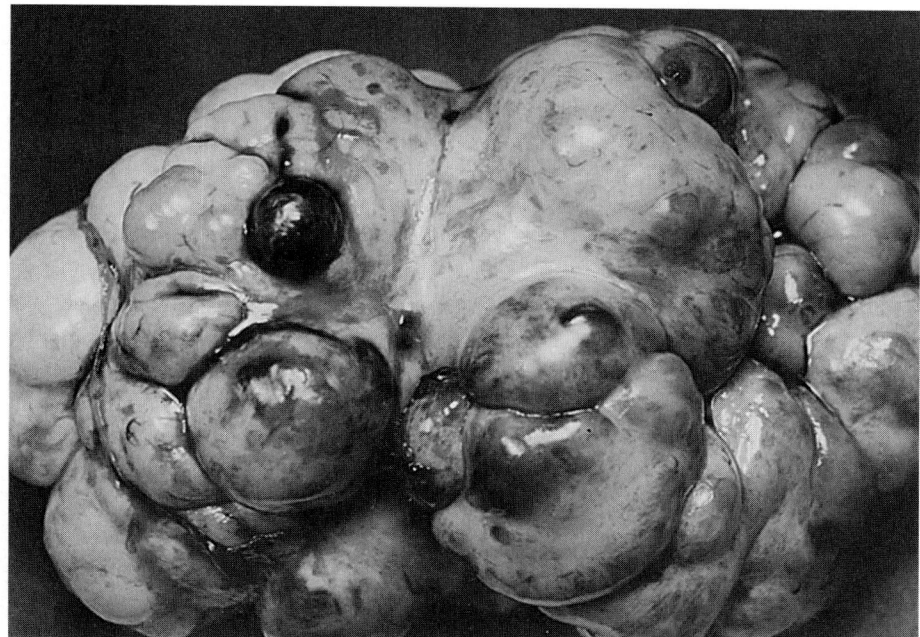

Fig. 19-175 Large dysgerminoma with external surface suggesting convolutions of cerebral cortex. (From Potter EB: Dysgerminoma of the ovary. Am J Pathol **22**:551-563, 1946.)

larly in stage II and beyond) and in the follow-up of recurrent disease.[356,358]

10 *Other markers.* Overexpression of p53,[349,350a] c-*erb*B-2,[352] and concentration of colony-stimulating factor-1[354] in ascites have all been found to be associated with aggressive behavior in ovarian carcinoma, but their value as independent prognostic factors needs to be established.

Ovarian tumors in children

Germ cell tumors are the most common tumors in children, accounting for 60% to 70% of all ovarian tumors in this age group.[367] Whereas mature cystic teratomas predominate, the proportion of malignant germ cell tumors (especially immature teratomas, yolk sac tumors, and dysgerminomas) is much greater than in adults.[365,366,369-372]

Sex cord–stromal tumors constitute 10% to 25% of the cases and are largely represented by the juvenile form of granulosa cell tumor and fibrothecomas.[374] Tumors of surface epithelium represent only 15% to 20% of ovarian tumors in children, and the vast majority are benign.[368] Indubitable cases of cystadenocarcinomas occur, particularly of the mucinous type[364]; however, some cases reported as serous carcinomas actually represent yolk sac tumors or retiform Sertoli–Leydig cell tumors with a prominent papillary component. It has been estimated that only 3% of ovarian carcinomas develop in patients younger than 20 years of age.

As in adults, primary malignant ovarian tumors in children need to be distinguished from metastatic neoplasms. The latter include neuroblastoma, adnexal gland carcinoma, rhabdomyosarcoma, Ewing's sarcoma/PNET, and intraabdominal desmoplastic small cell tumor.[373]

Germ cell tumors

Germ cell tumors constitute about 20% of all ovarian tumors. Most of them are seen in children and young adults. About 95% of these tumors are benign cystic teratomas; the younger the patient, the more likely the germ cell tumor will be malignant.[378]

In the sections that follow, the tumors are discussed as individual types; however, it should be recognized that a combination of various elements occurs in about 8% of the cases. These are referred to as *mixed germ cell tumors*[376,377]; the most common combination is that of dysgerminoma with yolk sac tumor, but many others occur.[380]

One of the most successful and exciting advances in oncology is represented by the therapy of ovarian germ cell tumors. Chemotherapeutic regimens consisting of a combination of bleomycin, etoposide, and cisplatin have resulted in overall disease-free survival rates greater than 95%.[375,379]

Dysgerminoma

Dysgerminoma constitutes less than 1% of all ovarian tumors and about 5% of malignant ovarian tumors.[385,398] Most patients are young. In Santesson's series of 299 cases, 81% of the patients were under 30 years of age and 44% were under 20 years of age.[400] Dysgerminoma made up 6% of 188 childhood ovarian neoplasms collected by Abell et al.[381] About 5% of dysgerminomas arise in abnormal gonads: pure or mixed gonadal dysgenesis (from a gonadoblastoma, see p. 1521) or androgen insensitivity (testicular germinization) syndrome. Exceptionally, the tumor is associated with hypercalcemia.[388]

Dysgerminoma is somewhat more common on the right side and is bilateral in 15% of the cases.[400] It is often large (it may reach over 1000 g) and encapsulated, with a smooth,

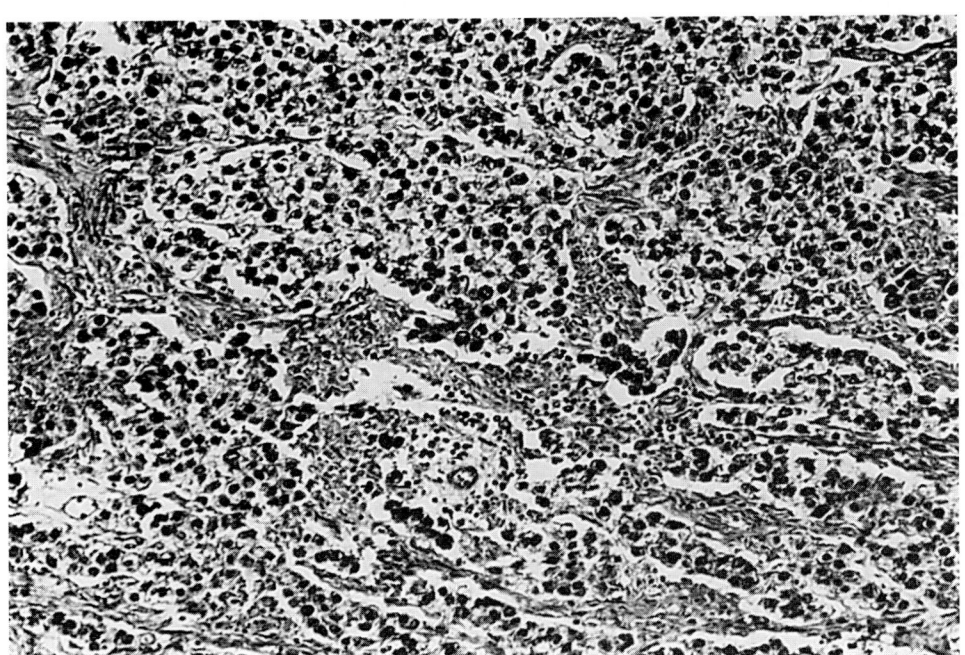

Fig. 19-176 Dysgerminoma of ovary. Well-defined nests of tumor cells are separated by fibrous strands containing numerous lymphocytes. Tumor cells have clear cytoplasm and well-defined cell membranes. Nuclei are large and hyperchromatic.

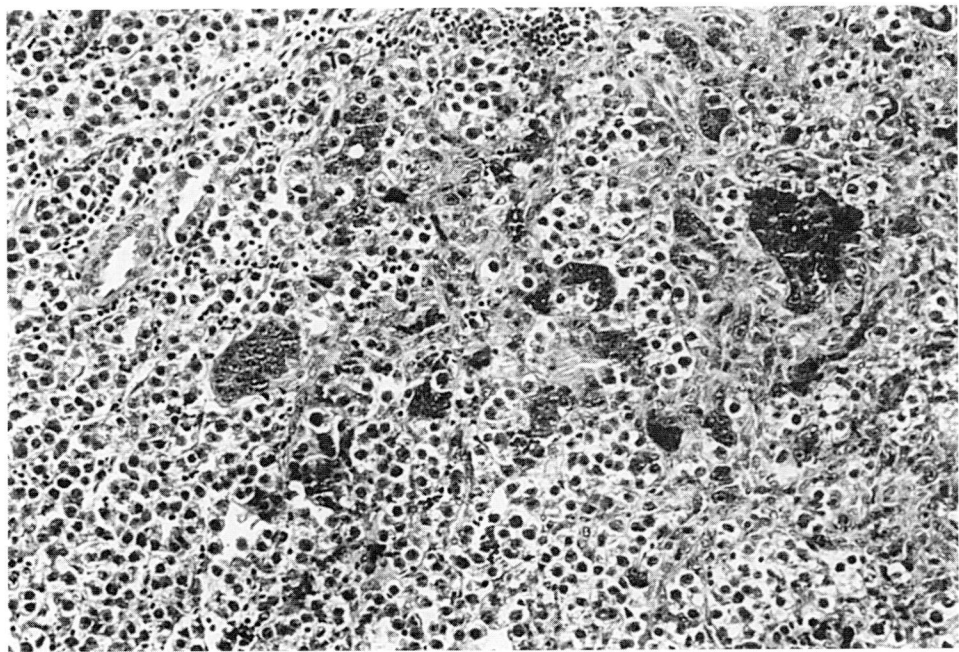

Fig. 19-177 Dysgerminoma with multinucleated giant cells of trophoblastic type. These cells are arranged in ill-defined clusters and are often associated with red blood cells.

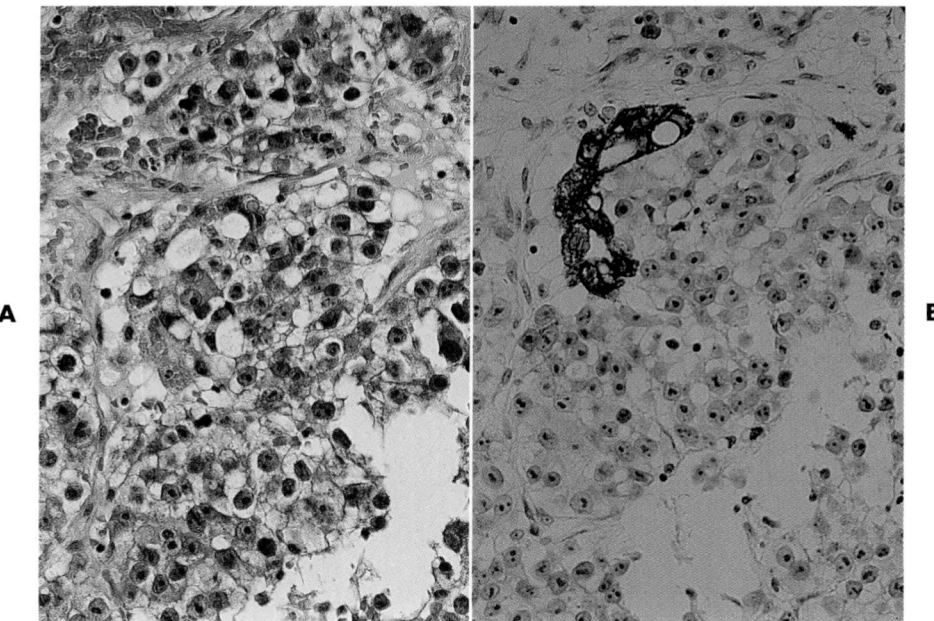

Fig. 19-178 Ovarian dysgerminoma with early yolk sac differentiation. **A,** H&E appearance. The foci of early yolk sac differentiation are represented by the small gland-like structures near the center. **B,** This formation is strongly immunoreactive for keratin, in contrast with the rest of the neoplasm. (Courtesy Dr. Vinita Parkash, New Haven, CT.)

often convoluted surface reminiscent of cerebral cortex (Fig. 19-175). The cut surface is solid and gray; foci of hemorrhage and necrosis can occur, but they are not as common or prominent as in other malignant germ cell tumors. Microscopically, the tumor cells usually group themselves in well-defined nests separated by fibrous strands infiltrated by lymphocytes (most of which are of T-cell type[387]). Occasionally, a pseudotubular or cord-like arrangement may be seen (particularly at the tumor periphery), which may be quite confusing. Focal necrosis, hyaline changes in vessels, germinal centers, and granulomatous foci may be present. The individual tumor cells are uniform and have large nuclei, *one or more prominent elongated nucleoli,* and abundant clear to finely granular cytoplasm that contains glycogen and sometimes fine droplets of fat (Fig. 19-176). The cell membrane is prominent; large amounts of alkaline phosphatase can be demonstrated with enzymatic or immunohistochemical techniques.[383,396] The microscopic pattern, ultrastructural appearance, immunohistochemical and cytogenetic profiles, clinical behavior, and probable histogenesis (from indifferent or primordial germ cells) are the same as for classical seminoma of the testis.[389,391,393,394] Like the latter, it may exhibit signs of early differentiation toward other types of germ cell elements.[399] These include:

1 Scattered hCG-positive syncytiotrophoblastic cells, often in close proximity to blood vessels or to hemorrhagic foci[401] (Fig. 19-177). This change, seen in about 3% of all dysgerminomas, may be accompanied by serum elevation of hCG and tissue immunoreactivity for this marker.

2 "Early carcinomatous differentiation" accompanied by increased mitotic activity (over thirty mitoses per ten HPF), a change sometimes designated—by analogy with its testicular counterpart—*anaplastic dysgerminoma.*[392] This change may be accompanied by increased immunoreactivity for keratin, although it should be noted that positivity for this marker is not unusual in the ordinary dysgerminoma.[396]

3 Abortive yolk sac elements, accompanied by serum elevation of AFP and tissue immunoreactivity for this marker[399] (Fig. 19-178).

In addition, variable immunoreactivity for GFAP and desmin has been detected in these tumors.[396]

As with the equivalent testicular examples, it is not clear whether any of these changes alters the prognosis of dysgerminoma, and it is therefore important to distinguish them from the dysgerminoma admixed with choriocarcinoma, embryonal carcinoma, or yolk sac tumor (Fig. 19-178), a phenomenon that occurs in about 10% of the cases and that affects prognosis significantly.

Metastases of dysgerminoma occur more commonly in the contralateral ovary, retroperitoneal nodes, and peritoneal cavity, the latter being associated with a decreased survival.[386]

The survival rate of pure dysgerminoma is 95%. The initial treatment of unilateral dysgerminoma is oophorectomy.[382,397] Until recently, radiation therapy was also recommended. In some institutions this was carried out in all cases, whereas in others it was reserved for the unfavorable ones (i.e., tumors larger than 10 cm and/or if ruptured dur-

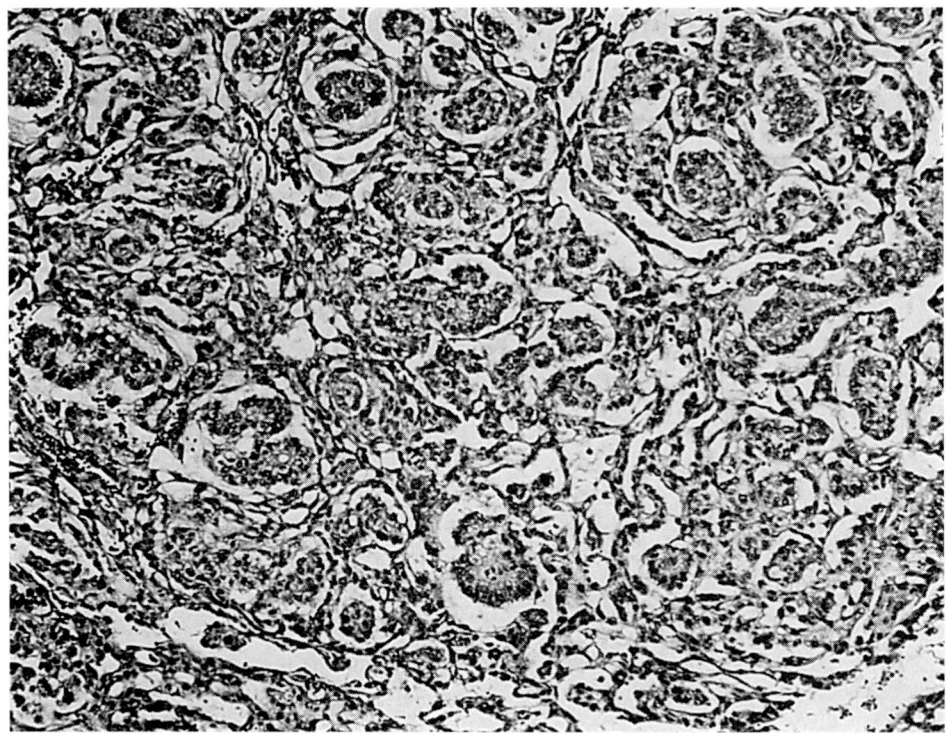

Fig. 19-179 Yolk sac tumor of ovary. Loose reticular pattern and rounded papillary processes with central capillary are typical.

ing removal).[384-386,395] At present, multidrug chemotherapy is regarded as the method of choice for this tumor following its removal.[390]

Yolk sac tumor (endodermal sinus tumor) and embryonal carcinoma

The history of these two germ cell neoplasms of the ovary is replete with confusing, contradictory, and often erroneous statements as to their origin, relationship, and natural history. Yolk sac tumor was included in Schiller's original description of mesonephroma,[426] together with the ovarian tumor presently designated as clear cell carcinoma.[428] Once it was realized that the latter has a different histogenesis, morphologic appearance, and natural history, the analogy became no longer tenable.[410,420] The next generation of articles on the subject clearly separated these two neoplasms but used more or less interchangeably the terms *yolk sac tumor* and *embryonal carcinoma*.[420] Since both of these neoplasms are of germ cell derivation and share many morphologic features, this is not entirely inappropriate.[418] However, enough differences exist between the two to justify their separation.

Yolk sac tumor (endodermal sinus tumor) is a neoplasm of children and young adults (median age, 19 years). In the series of Kurman and Norris,[416] 23% of the patients were prepuberal at the time of diagnosis. None of the patients presented with precocious puberty, amenorrhea, or hirsutism. Vaginal bleeding occurred in only 1%. The serum alpha-fetoprotein level was invariably elevated, whereas the chorionic gonadotropin levels were normal, resulting in consistently negative pregnancy tests. Grossly, the tumors had an

average diameter of 15 cm, a smooth and glistening external surface, and a variegated cut surface, partially cystic and often containing large foci of hemorrhage and necrosis. A component of benign cystic teratoma was identified in ten of the seventy-one cases. Exceptionally, a yolk sac tumor will be found in the pelvis (in close proximity to the uterus) or mesentery, unattached to the ovary.[405,412]

Microscopically, the appearance of yolk sac tumors is very variable.[409] There are reticular or microcystic areas formed by a loose meshwork lined by flat or cuboidal cells (Fig. 19-179), rounded or festooning pseudopapillary processes with central vessels (Schiller-Duval bodies), and solid "undifferentiated" areas. The mesenchyme-like component of these tumors has pluripotential properties; it usually presents in the form of spindle cells in a well-vascularized myxoid background, but it exhibits keratin immunoreactivity as a sign of early epithelial differentiation and may contain heterologous elements such as skeletal muscle.[419]

Intracytoplasmic and extracellular PAS-positive hyaline droplets are nearly always present. Their chemical composition is heterogeneous; they usually stain for alpha-fetoprotein, but they may also contain alpha-1-antitrypsin and basement membrane components (type IV collagen and laminin).[402] DNA ploidy studies have shown that these tumors are almost invariably aneuploid.[415]

A fourth of the yolk sac tumors have vesicular structures with eccentric constrictions surrounded by a dense spindle cell stroma; this has been referred to as a *polyvesicular vitelline pattern* and is said to be associated with a good prognosis when present in a pure form.[423] Others show a scattered hCG-positive syncytiotrophoblast component. Still

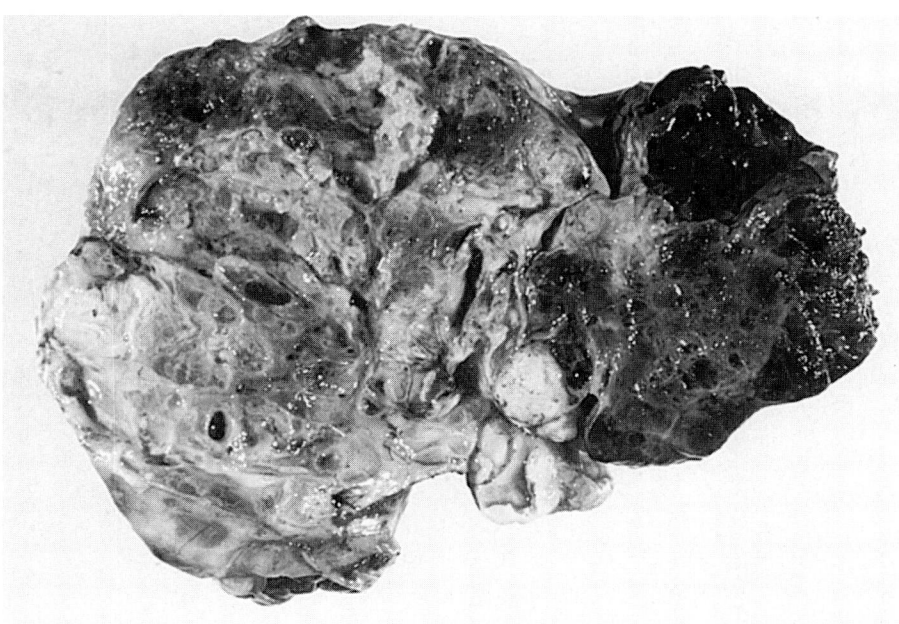

Fig. 19-180 Gross appearance of ovarian embryonal carcinoma. Tumor is predominantly solid, with extensive areas of necrosis and hemorrhage. (Courtesy Dr. J. Costa, Lausanne, Switzerland.)

others exhibit evidence of differentiation toward hepatic, intestinal,[406] and parietal yolk sac structures. The latter are recognized by the presence of thick layers of intercellular basement membrane.[429] The *hepatoid* component, which can predominate almost to the exclusion of the others, is composed of masses, nests, and broad bands of large polyhedral cells with occasional glandular formations and numerous hyaline bodies. Alpha-1-antitrypsin can be identified immunohistochemically.[425] These hepatoid yolk sac tumors are distinguished by Ishikura and Scully from *hepatoid carcinomas,* rare tumors of probable surface epithelial origin.[411] In some yolk sac tumors, the presence of *glandular* formations may simulate the appearance of endometrioid carcinoma.[404]

Areas of luteinized stromal cells may be present and may sometimes be responsible for virilization.

Teilum's brilliant hypothesis that this tumor recapitulates normal yolk sac elements has been amply confirmed by histochemical and ultrastructural studies.[421,422,424]

In the series of Kurman and Norris,[416] written only twenty years ago, the actuarial survival at 3 years was only 13%; although 71% of the patients were thought to have stage I tumors, subclinical metastases were present in 84%. The introduction of multidrug chemotherapy has dramatically improved survival rates: twenty-one of forty-one patients treated at M.D. Anderson Hospital were alive and well at the time of the last follow-up.[408] Clinical stage is the most important prognostic indicator.[414] Serial determinations of serum alpha-fetoprotein are useful in monitoring the tumor course.[413,427]

Embryonal carcinoma also occurs in a young age group (median age, 15 years). In one series, 47% of the patients were prepubertal at the time of diagnosis, and 43% of them presented with precocious puberty.[417] Vaginal bleeding was

recorded in 33%, amenorrhea in 7%, and hirsutism in 7%. Serum alpha-fetoprotein levels are often (but not always) elevated, whereas chorionic gonadotropin levels are invariably high, to a level that results in consistently positive pregnancy tests.

Grossly, the median diameter of these neoplasms is 17 cm. Their external surface is smooth and glistening, and their cut surface is predominantly solid and variegated, with extensive areas of necrosis and hemorrhage (Fig. 19-180). Microscopically, this tumor has a similar appearance to the embryonal carcinoma of the adult testis. As such, it is composed of solid sheets and nests of large primitive cells, occasionally forming papillae and abortive glandular structures. Syncytiotrophoblast-like tumor cells frequently are seen scattered among the smaller cells. These have been shown to contain chorionic gonadotropin by immunocytochemical techniques. In the Kurman and Norris series,[417] the prognosis was somewhat better than for yolk sac tumor, but current multidrug chemotherapeutic regimens have erased these differences.[403,407]

Embryonal carcinomas largely composed of embryoid bodies are referred to as *polyembryomas* (Plate XIV-C).

Choriocarcinoma

Most choriocarcinomas involving the ovary represent metastases from uterine tumors. The exceedingly rare primary ovarian choriocarcinomas can develop from an ovarian pregnancy (gestational type, which is the most common) or as a form of germ cell neoplasm (nongestational).[433] The latter can be pure or, more frequently, be a component of a mixed germ cell tumor. Microscopically, they show the typical admixture of syncytial and cytotrophoblastic elements in a necrotic and hemorrhagic background. Immunohistochemical reactivity for hCG is the rule; in

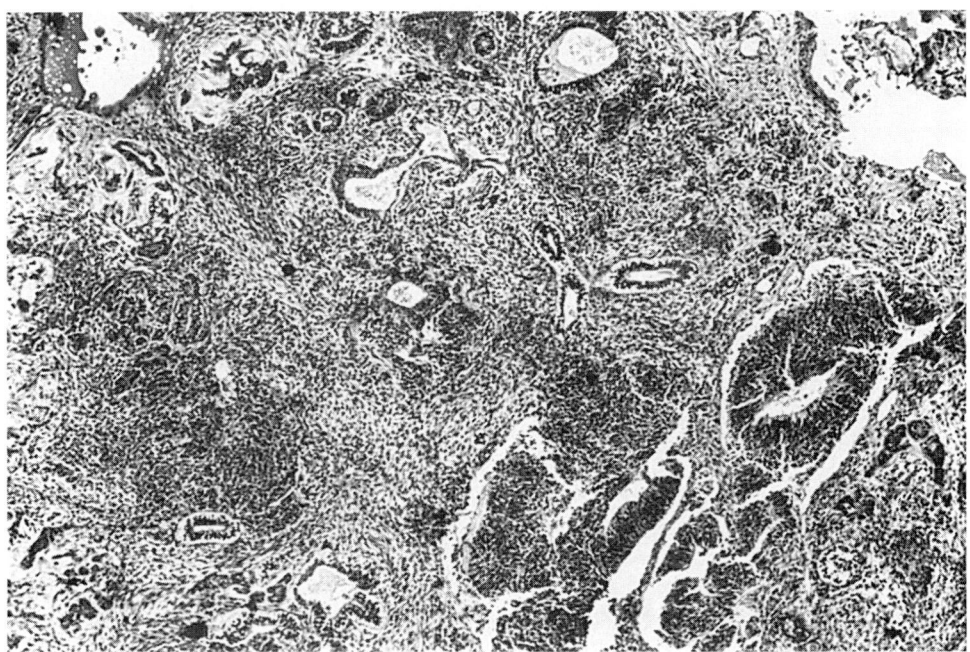

Fig. 19-181 Immature teratoma of ovary. Most of neoplasm is composed of immature neuroepithelial elements.

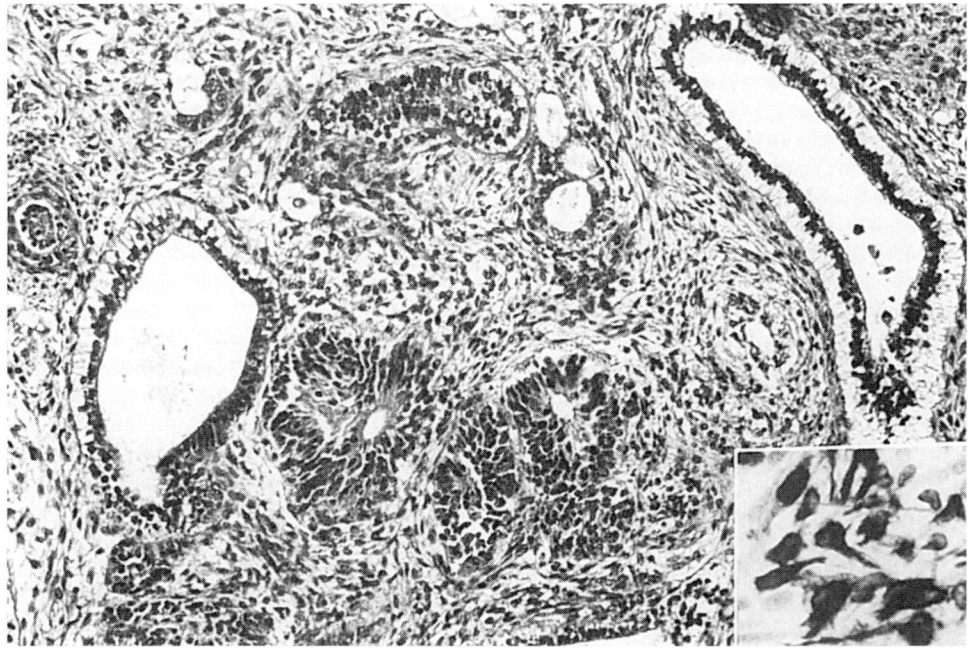

Fig. 19-182 Immature teratoma of ovary. Rosettes of neuroepithelial type are apparent. Glandular formations with prominent subnuclear vacuolization are also seen. **Inset** shows immunocytochemical positivity for GFAP in glial elements of tumor.

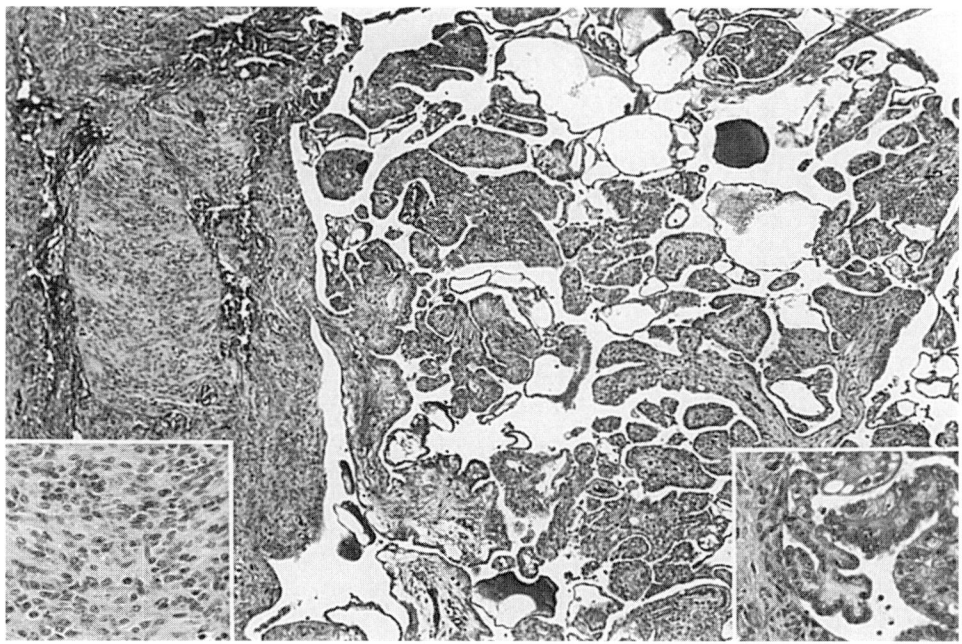

Fig. 19-183 Ependymoma of ovary. Papillary formations simulating appearance of serous papillary tumor alternate with solid tumor nests. **Insets** show papillary and solid areas on higher magnification. This tumor was focally positive for GFAP.

addition, keratin 7 is said to represent a marker for a subset of trophoblastic cells in these tumors.[431] LK26 is also consistently expressed, but this can also be found in other ovarian malignancies.[432]

Ovarian choriocarcinomas of either gestational or nongestational type should be distinguished from the exceptionally rare ovarian carcinomas of surface epithelial origin exhibiting choriocarcinomatous differentiation, a phenomenon analogous to that sometimes seen in carcinomas of the lung, breast, endometrium, and other sites.[435]

Ovarian gestational choriocarcinomas have a better prognosis than their nongestational counterparts.[434,436] Among the latter, pure choriocarcinomas are often lethal; conversely, good survival rates have been obtained with the mixed types.[430]

Immature (malignant) teratoma

Immature teratoma is the currently preferred term for the malignant ovarian teratoma composed of a mixture of embryonal and adult tissues derived from all three germ layers, regardless of its gross appearance. Any type of tissue may be represented. The main component is usually neurogenic, but mesodermal elements are also common[448] (Figs. 19-181 and 19-182). Some tumors are predominantly composed of endodermal derivatives, including esophagus, liver, and intestinal structures.[450]

Staining for glial fibrillary acidic protein (GFAP) is helpful in the identification of mature and immature glial tissue[454] (Fig. 19-177, *inset*). Interestingly, GFAP is detectable also in chondrocytes, together with S-100 protein immunoreactivity.[452] Another marker of both immature and mature neural tissue is represented by the long-chain polysialic acid moiety of the neural cell adhesion molecule.[447]

Grossly, immature teratoma may be solid throughout, solid with multiple minute cysts, or predominantly cystic. It is a tumor of children and adolescents. The prognosis depends a great deal on the nature and amount of the embryonal component.[438] It is best when the latter is predominantly made up of neural tissue. Norris et al.[451] have shown that the size and stage of the teratomas were related to survival but that it was the microscopic grade of the primary tumor that best determined the likelihood of extraovarian spread; similarly, the grade of the metastases correlated best with the subsequent course.

Interestingly, higher microscopic grades correlate with various types of karyotype abnormalities.[441] The grading system of Norris et al.[451] is as follows:

> *Grade I* Abundance of mature tissues, intermixed with loose mesenchymal tissue with occasional mitoses; immature cartilage; tooth anlage
> *Grade II* Fewer mature tissues; rare foci of neuroepithelium with common mitoses, *not exceeding* three low-magnification (×40) fields in any one slide
> *Grade III* Few or no mature tissues; numerous neuroepithelial elements, merging with a cellular stroma *occupying* four or more low-magnification fields.

Obviously, a thorough tumor sampling is necessary for this grading system to be accurate. The amount of immature neuroepithelial tissue may also be expressed as an estimated percentage of all the tissue examined microscopically.[452a,454]

It is important to separate from this group the teratomas that also have a yolk sac tumor pattern, since the prognosis substantially decreases under these circumstances.[438] On occasion, an ovarian immature teratoma can be predominantly or exclusively composed of one type of tissue, such

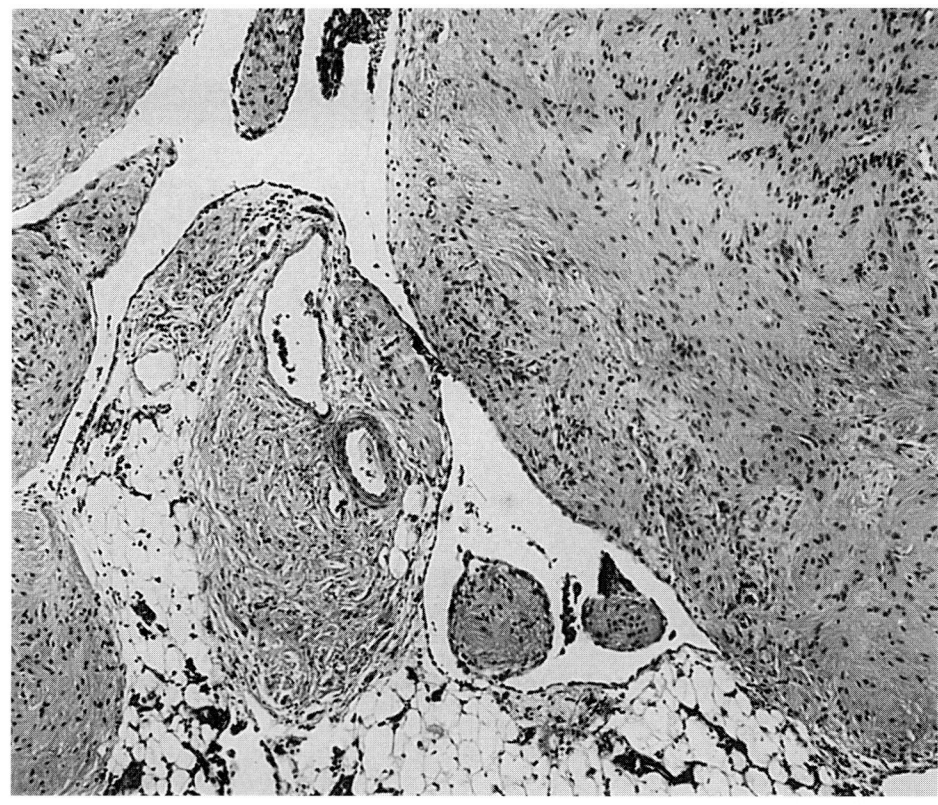

Fig. 19-184 Omental implants composed of glial tissue in child. Multiple tumor masses were removed from peritoneal cavity 18 months following oophorectomy for rather well-differentiated solid teratoma in which all three germ layers were represented. Maturation of tissues had apparently occurred in intervening time. Child was living and well 12 years following original oophorectomy.

as renal (metanephrogenic),[449] retinal anlage,[443] primitive neuroectoderm, or ependyma.

Neoplasms with an exclusive or almost exclusive malignant neuroectodermal composition are designated ***malignant neuroectodermal tumor*** and are generally regarded as a form of monodermal teratoma.[437,445] A further variation in the theme is the ovarian ***ependymoma,*** in which this neuroectodermal component is made up entirely of primitive ependymal structures[440,444,445] (Fig. 19-183).

The treatment of immature teratoma consists of surgery plus multidrug chemotherapy[442,446]; sometimes, only mature tissue is found in metastatic sites following chemotherapy, a sign of excellent prognosis.[453] It is interesting, however, that the abnormal karyotype of the original immature teratoma is maintained in the area of chemotherapy-induced maturation.[439]

Mature solid teratoma

Mature solid teratoma has a predominantly solid gross appearance, but multiple small cystic areas also are present. Because of this, some authors prefer the descriptively more accurate designation of *polycystic.* By definition, the tumor should be *composed entirely of adult tissues* derived from all three germ layers.[456,457]

Clearly, extensive sampling is needed to separate this tumor from a grade I immature teratoma. The two tumors

are closely related, and the distinction is somewhat subjective; as a matter of fact, some authors refer to mature solid teratoma as grade 0 immature teratoma.

This rare neoplasm occurs in young women, predominantly in the second decade. The prognosis is excellent, even if peritoneal implants (also mature and for the most part glial in composition) are present[455] (see p. 1502) (Fig. 19-184).

Mature cystic teratoma, benign and with secondary tumor formation

Mature cystic teratomas make up almost 20% of all ovarian neoplasms. They constitute the most common ovarian tumor in childhood.[466] They are unilateral in 88% of the cases and provoke only symptoms relating to the mass. Occasionally they are accompanied by hemolytic anemia.[483] Grossly, they are usually multiloculated. The cystic content is greasy, largely composed of keratin, sebum, and hairs (Fig. 19-185, Plate XIV-D, and Fig. 2-8).

Sometimes teratomas rupture into the peritoneal cavity, this material provoking a prominent foreign body reaction that can simulate metastatic carcinoma grossly and tuberculosis microscopically.[458] The teratoma often contains teeth.[465] Sometimes, it may feature an imperfectly formed mandible or even a partial human body–like structure (homunculus); the latter are referred to as *fetiform teratoma.*[478] The teeth tend to be located in a well-defined nip-

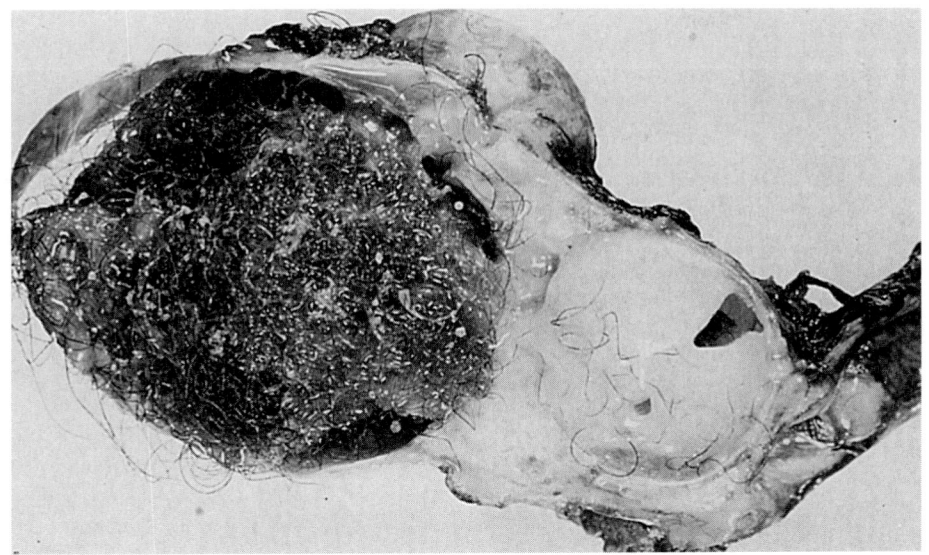

Fig. 19-185 Mature cystic teratoma of ovary showing greasy contents and hair.

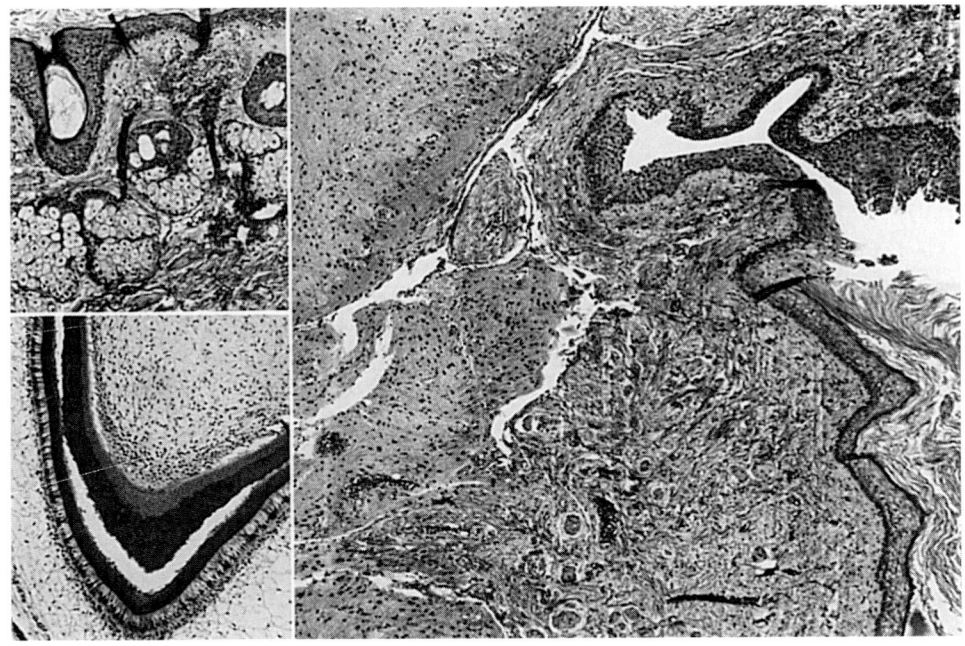

Fig. 19-186 Mature cystic teratoma of ovary. The various components include neural tissue, squamous epithelium, skin adnexae, and developing tooth.

ple-like structure covered with hair, known as *Rokitansky's protuberance*. This structure should be selected for microscopic examination (even if decalcification may be required) because it will exhibit the greatest variety of tissue types.

Microscopically, Blackwell et al.[459] found ectodermal derivatives in 100% of the tumors, mesodermal structures in 93%, and endodermal derivatives in 71%. The cystic cavities are lined by mature epidermis. Skin appendages and neural (particularly glial) tissue are extremely common, followed by cartilage, respiratory tissue, and gastrointestinal tract tissue (Fig. 19-186). The gastric mucosa can be so well developed anatomically and functionally as to be accompanied by peptic ulcer formation.[489] Other tissues include thyroid (10% of the cases), anterior pituitary,[476] other endocrine cells,[461] prostate,[460,477] pancreas, and cavernous blood vessels.

Immunohistochemically, the phenotype of the epidermal lining may be mature (epidermis-like) or immature (resembling stratified nonkeratinizing and metaplastic squamous epithelium).[464]

A female nuclear sex chromatin pattern is present in all cases; chromosomal analyses have shown a 46,XX pat-

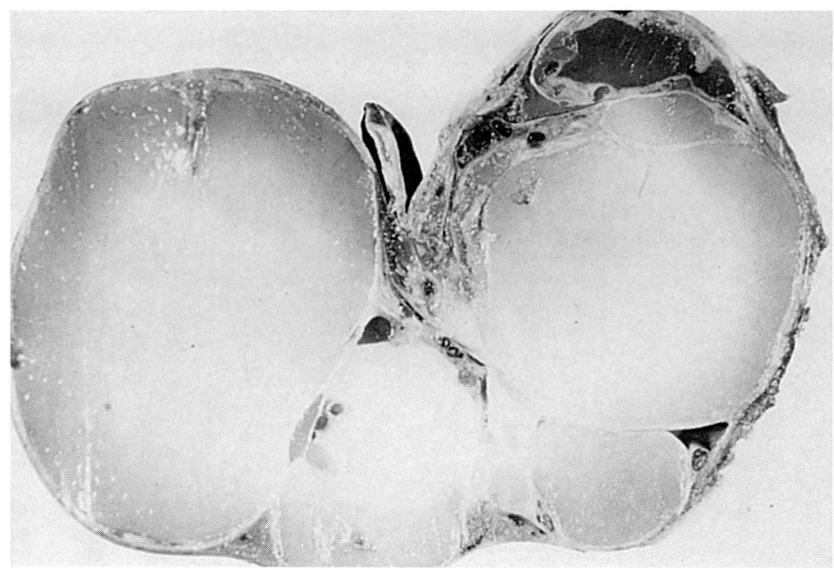

Fig. 19-187 Teratoma of ovary demonstrating typical gross appearance of struma ovarii. Tumor was composed almost entirely of thyroid tissue. (Contributed by Dr. R. Johnson, Columbia, MO.)

tern.[485] Linder et al.[474] have elegantly shown by chromosome-banding studies that these tumors are of parthenogenetic origin and probably arise from a single germ cell after the first meiotic division. Riley and Sutton[487] have proposed a possible mechanism to account for the fact that most ovarian germ cell tumors are benign, whereas most of the testicular ones are malignant, based on the different development of the germ cells in the male and in the female.

The most common malignant change in cystic teratoma is squamous cell carcinoma, followed by carcinoid tumor and adenocarcinoma.[463,470,472,484] Other types include malignant melanoma,[468,493] Paget's disease,[490] sarcomas of various types, carcinosarcoma, and neuroblastoma/PNET.[471,486] Benign tumors have also been described, such as blue nevus,[473,492] sebaceous adenoma,[462] sweat gland adenoma,[480] epithelioid (histiocytoid) hemangioma,[475] and prolactinoma.[482] Cystic teratomas containing microscopic foci of immature tissue also occur, their behavior being usually benign.[495] These should be distinguished from immature teratomas.

Adult ovarian and extraovarian teratomas of both the cystic and solid variety—as well as immature teratomas—may be accompanied by peritoneal implants exclusively composed of mature glial tissue (gliomatosis peritonei).[469,488,494] This is a benign condition *as long as the tissue is entirely mature and other teratomatous elements are absent.*[467,481,491] The implants appear grossly as miliary grayish white nodules in the peritoneal surface or omentum and may be accompanied by fibrosis and chronic inflammation.

The rare ***epidermoid cyst*** of the ovary possibly arises from epithelial cell nests, of the type encountered in Brenner tumors.[496] It is distinguished from mature cystic teratoma on thorough sampling by the absence of skin adnexae and other tissues.

Mature cystic teratoma may coexist with mucinous cystadenoma, Brenner tumor, and thecoma.[479]

Struma ovarii

Struma ovarii represents the dominant growth of thyroid tissue in a teratoma and sometimes occurs in the absence of other components (Figs. 19-187 and 19-188). Grossly, the mass has the color and consistency of thyroid tissue, but it is often cystic. The thyroid nature of the lesion has been substantiated by biologic and immunohistochemical studies for thyroid hormones.[498,499] The tissue may show any of the pathologic changes seen in a normally placed gland, including diffuse or nodular hyperplasia (which may lead to hyperthyroidism), thyroiditis, carcinoma (sometimes associated with metastases), and malignant lymphoma.[497,498,501] Cystic changes can be prominent and obscure the diagnosis.[501a] The opposite phenomenon, just as baffling diagnostically, is represented by the cases having a predominantly solid or trabecular pattern.[501b]

We have seen a case of follicular variant of papillary carcinoma developing in struma ovarii that contained numerous intraluminal crystalloids, and a similar case has been reported.[500]

Struma ovarii can be seen combined with mucinous cystadenoma, Brenner tumor, or carcinoid tumor. The latter combination, known as strumal carcinoid, is discussed in the following section.

Carcinoid tumor and strumal carcinoid

Carcinoid tumor can be seen in the ovary as a metastasis of a tumor located in the gastrointestinal tract or elsewhere,[511] as a component of adult cystic teratoma, or as a primary pure neoplasm of this organ. Approximately one third of the latter are associated with the carcinoid syndrome, even in the absence of liver metastases[510]; the larger the tumor, the more likely that the carcinoid syndrome will develop. Some cases present with severe constipation, presumably because of secretion of peptide YY.[507] Small

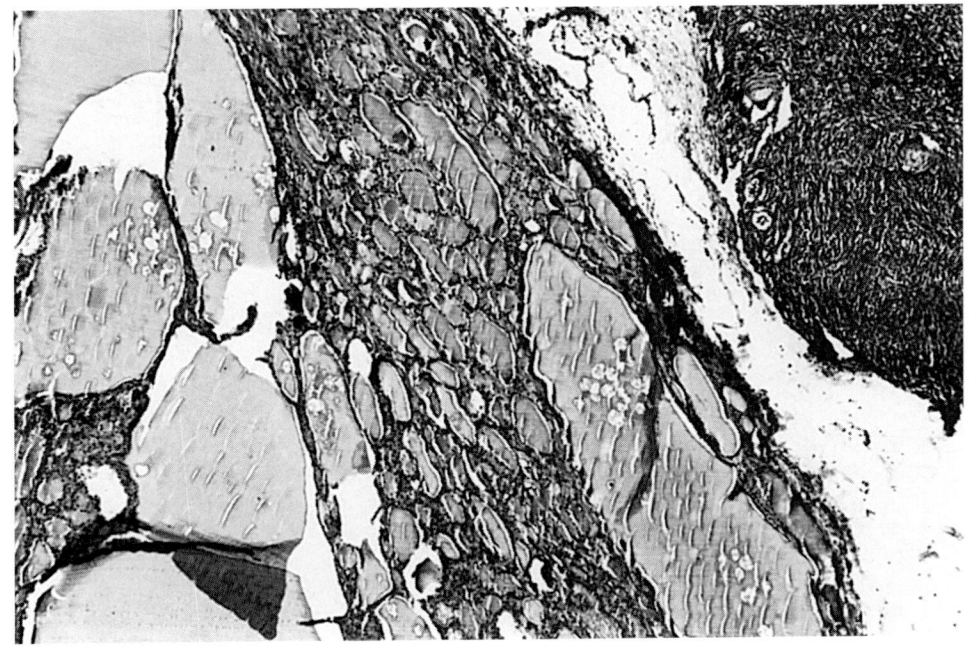

Fig. 19-188 Struma ovarii. Thyroid tissue with relatively normal microscopic appearance except some follicular dilatation is seen surrounded by ovarian stoma.

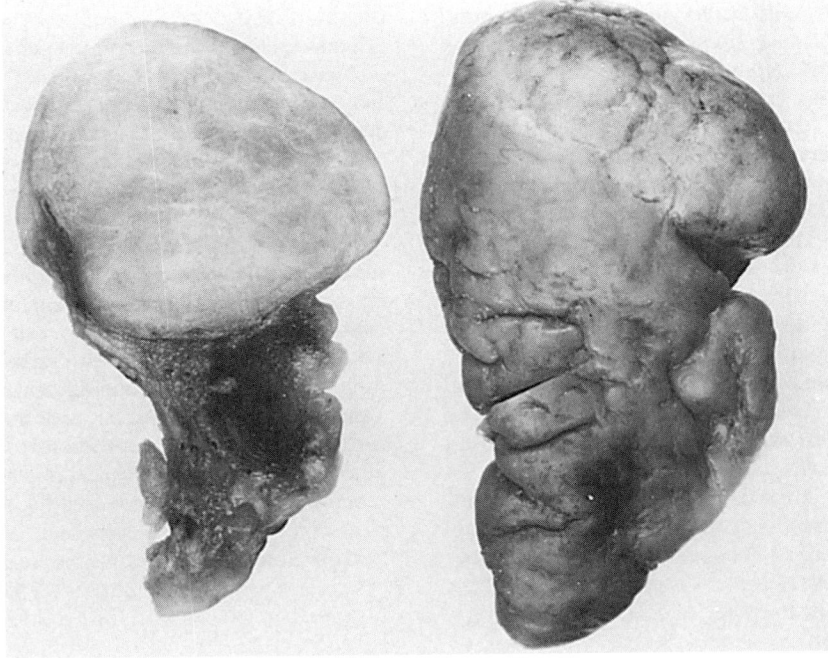

Fig. 19-189 Primary carcinoid tumor of ovary. Tumor is solid, homogeneous, firm, and associated with abundant fibrous tissue. (Courtesy Dr. E. Segal, Minneapolis.)

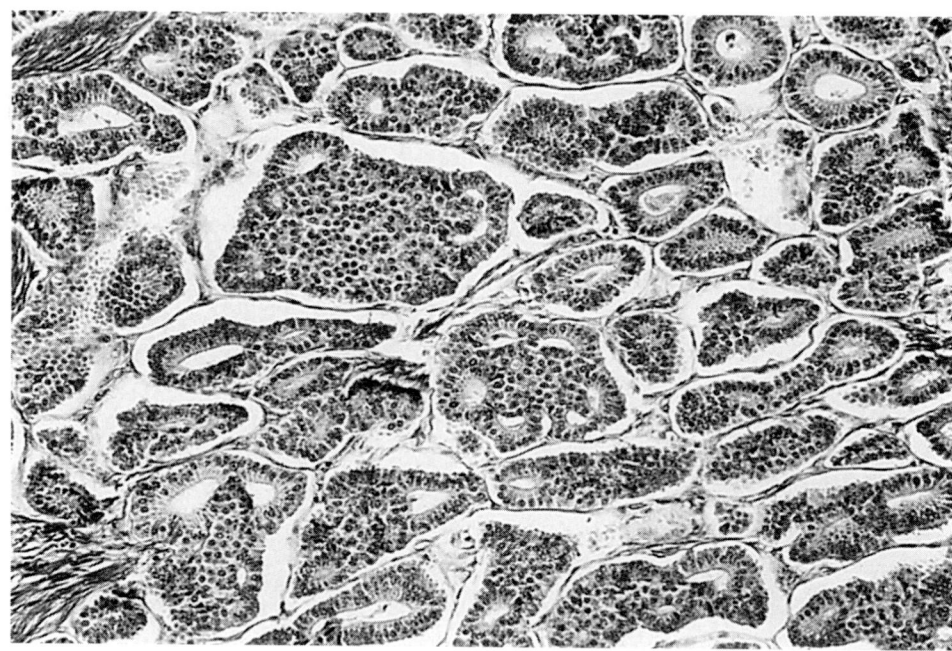

Fig. 19-190 Ovarian carcinoid tumor of predominantly insular type. Well-defined nests of tumor cells with artifactual retraction from stroma are evident. In some of these nests there are well-defined tubular formations with central lumen.

tumors arising in cystic teratomas are nearly always asymptomatic. The large majority of primary ovarian carcinoid tumors are unilateral, but in 16% of the cases the contralateral ovary is involved by a cystic teratoma or a mucinous neoplasm.[509] In contrast, most metastatic carcinoid tumors to the ovary are bilateral and associated with peritoneal metastases. The prognosis in primary ovarian carcinoid tumors (whether pure or as a component of cystic teratoma) is very good, whereas metastatic carcinoids have a poor outcome.

Grossly, pure primary carcinoid tumors have a mean diameter of 10 cm; their external surface is smooth or bosselated, and the cut surface is predominantly solid, firm, tan to yellow, and homogeneous (Fig. 19-189). Microscopically, the appearance is similar to that of carcinoid tumors elsewhere: solid masses of small round cells alternate with ribbons and acinar formations (Fig. 19-190). Those resembling carcinoid tumors arising from midgut derivatives (such as the appendix) are called *insular,* and those resembling carcinoid tumors of the foregut (i.e., stomach) and hindgut (i.e., rectum) derivatives are known as *trabecular.*[512] Fibrous stroma can be abundant and lead to a mistaken diagnosis of granulosa–theca cell tumor or Brenner tumor. The argentaffin reaction is usually positive, and ultrastructural examination consistently reveals the presence of neurosecretory granules.[513]

Neuron-specific enolase, chromogranin, serotonin, and a large variety of peptide hormones (including peptide YY) have been demonstrated immunohistochemically, particularly in tumors of the trabecular type.[507,516]

It is not possible to separate primary from metastatic carcinoid tumors on morphologic grounds; however, if the ovarian carcinoid is admixed with areas of teratoma, the chances are overwhelming that it is of primary origin. Occasionally, a primary ovarian carcinoid will exhibit prominent pleomorphism[503] or a *mucinous* or *signet ring* pattern analogous to that more commonly seen in the appendix.[518,521]

Strumal carcinoid is an ovarian neoplasm combining the features of carcinoid tumor and struma ovarii[505,509] (Fig. 19-191 and Plate XIV-E). Some authors have questioned the thyroidal nature of the latter element on the basis of ultrastructural studies,[506,508] but the immunohistochemical demonstration of thyroglobulin has settled the issue.[520] Others have suggested that the carcinoid-like component represents a medullary carcinoma arising from thyroid C cells,[502] but the morphologic appearance and immunohistochemical profile of the tumor are more akin to those of a trabecular carcinoid of hindgut derivation[515,517] (Fig. 19-192); specifically, calcitonin and amyloid are only rarely demonstrated.[504] It is of interest that these tumors also exhibit immunoreactivity for prostatic acid phosphatase in the carcinoid component, as further evidence of their similarity to rectal carcinoids.[514] Exceptionally, the carcinoid component is of mucinous type.[506a]

Other teratomatous elements are found in over 50% of the cases of strumal carcinoid.[510] This lesion has also been observed in association with multiple endocrine neoplasia type IIA (III).[519]

Sex cord–stromal tumors

This category, which comprises about 5% of all ovarian neoplasms, is made up of tumors that differentiate in the direction of sex cords and/or the specialized ovarian stroma.[532] This includes female-type cells (granulosa and

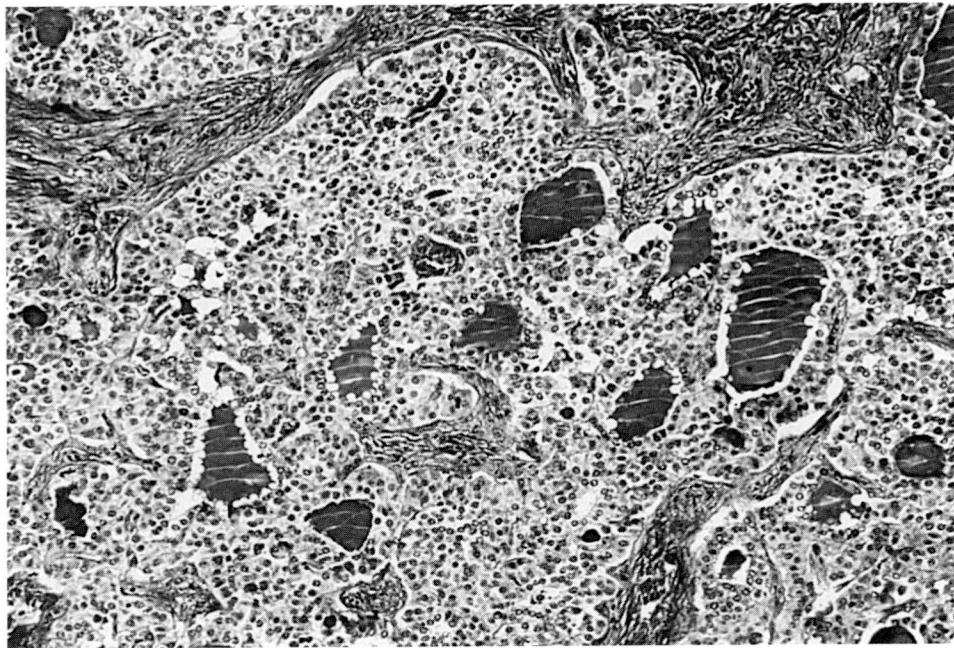

Fig. 19-191 Strumal carcinoid of ovary. This neoplasm combines carcinoid pattern of growth with formations of follicles containing colloid. Immunohistochemically, there was positivity for both thyroglobulin and neuroendocrine markers, such as chromogranin.

theca cells), male-type cells (Sertoli and Leydig cells), and indifferent elements.[523,529,531] These various elements can occur in combination and exhibit a wide range of differentiation, which often seems to recapitulate the patterns produced during embryogenesis of both the ovary and testis.[530] Secondary changes, such as luteinization, may also develop. As a result, a wide array of tumor types may be seen, some of which do not fit easily into a rigid classification system. In general, a relationship exists between the morphologic appearance of the tumor and the presence and type of clinically evident hormonal activity.[527a,529a] However, there may be no demonstrable endocrine effects, and rare examples of hormonal effects opposite to those expected from the morphologic features also occur.[524,527] Along similar lines, there is general agreement between the cytoarchitectural features of the tumor and the presence of various steroid hormones, hormone precursors, and related enzymes, as demonstrated by immunohistochemical techniques.[522,526,528] However, it is important to emphasize that the classification of ovarian neoplasms is primarily based on their morphologic appearance, rather than on the presence or type of hormonal activity or their immunohistochemical profile. The latter is plagued with so many conceptual and technical difficulties when evaluated in formalin-fixed, paraffin-embedded material (hormone loss from organic solvents, tissue diffusion of the lipid-soluble hormones, hormone-binding to receptors, etc.) as to make it unwise to classify an ovarian tumor as belonging to the sex cord–stromal category solely on this basis.[526] Recently, müllerian inhibiting substance has been proposed as an additional generic marker for this family of neoplasms.[525]

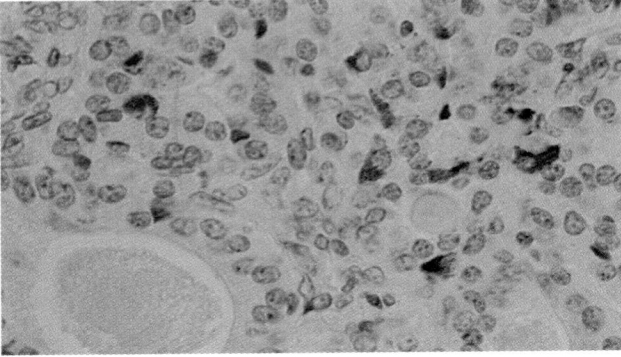

Fig. 19-192 Strumal carcinoid of ovary with scattered insulin-reactive cells (insulin).

Granulosa cell tumor

Granulosa cell tumor is an ovarian neoplasm showing differentiation toward follicular granulosa cells. Whether it actually arises from granulosa cells in pre-existing follicles or from the specialized ovarian stroma is debatable. Two distinct types exist, known respectively as adult and juvenile. *Adult granulosa cell tumor* is usually diagnosed during child-bearing age, but it can occur after menopause and sometimes even before puberty. Three fourths of cases are associated with hyperestrinism; the excessive production of estrogens can lead to isosexual precocious puberty in children[544] and to metrorrhagia in adults, including postmenopausal patients[538] (Fig. 19-193). Other tumors are hormonally inactive, and a very few are androgenic.[548]

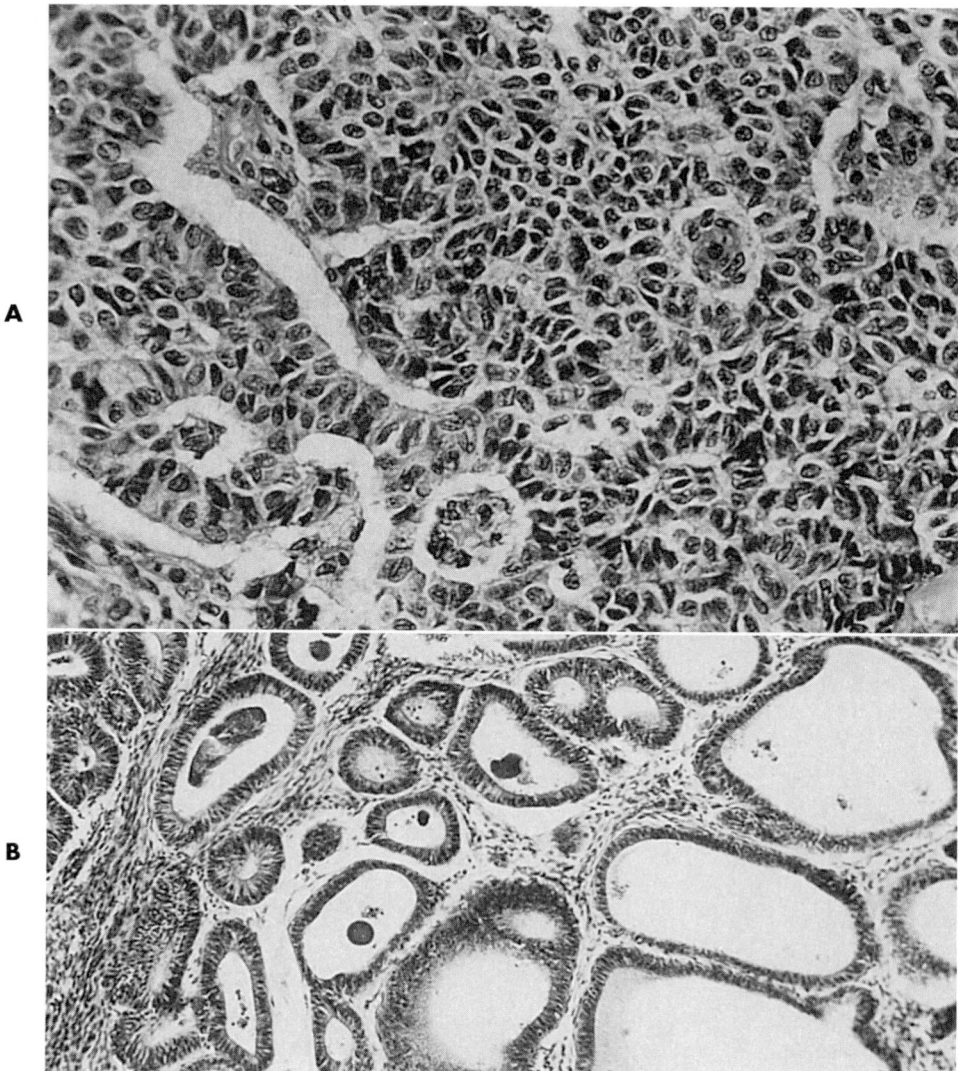

Fig. 19-193 A, Typical granulosa cell tumor of ovary with folliculoid pattern. **B,** Prominent endometrial hyperplasia occurring in association with tumor shown in **A.**

Grossly, adult granulosa cell tumors are usually encapsulated, with a smooth, lobulated outline and a predominantly solid cut surface (Fig. 19-194). The color is usually gray, but it may be yellow in areas of luteinization. Cysts filled with straw-colored or mucoid fluid may be present. Sometimes the cysts are so prominent as to simulate grossly the appearance of a cystadenoma. Interestingly, a disproportionate number of androgenic granulosa cell tumors are large and cystic, either unilocular or multilocular.[548,551] The microscopic appearance of granulosa cell tumor is extremely variable, even within the same neoplasm.[552] Patterns of growth include microfollicular (with Call-Exner bodies), macrofollicular, trabecular, insular, watered-silk, solid, and diffuse (sarcomatoid)[557] (Figs. 19-193 and 19-195). A theca cell component may also be present. Focal luteinization of either the granulosa or the theca cell component may occur[563a]; it is particularly prominent in those tumors associated with

pregnancy, together with edema and disorderly arrangement.[563] An important diagnostic feature is the presence of folds or grooves in the nuclei, resulting in a "coffee-bean" appearance[550] (Fig. 19-196). Occasionally, bizarre nuclei and multinucleated giant cells (sometimes of the "floret" type) are seen; this change is not a sign of malignancy *per se* but is rather of a degenerative nature.[565] A case of granulosa cell tumor has been reported associated with hepatocytic differentiation.[549]

Traditionally, secretion of steroid hormones has been related to theca cells rather than granulosa cells, both in normal follicles and tumors[546]; however, immunohistochemical studies have shown steroid production in both cells, with predominance of estradiol in the granulosa cells and progesterone in luteinized theca cells.[543] Other consistent immunohistochemical markers of granulosa cell tumors include vimentin and desmoplakin (desmosomal plaque pro-

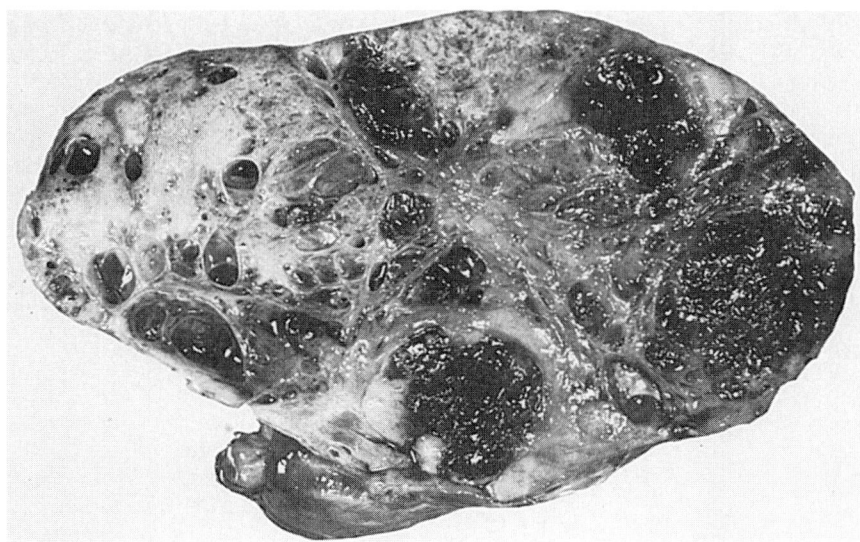

Fig. 19-194 Large cystic and hemorrhagic granulosa cell tumor of ovary.

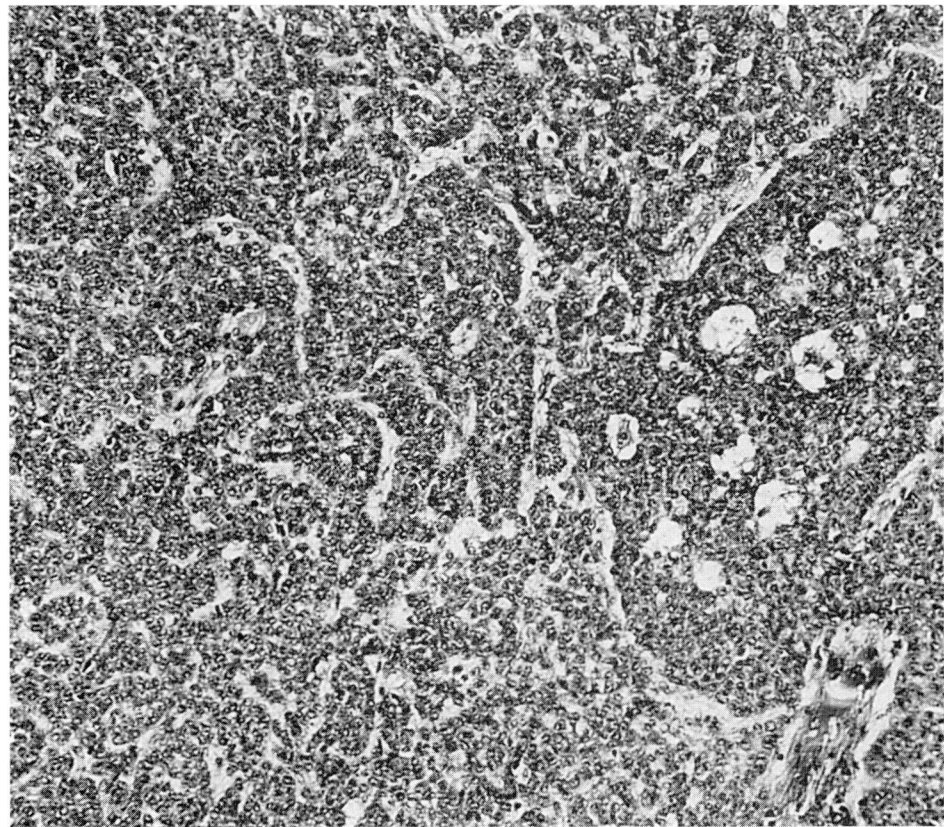

Fig. 19-195 Granulosa cell tumor of less well-differentiated pattern. Note Call-Exner bodies in small mass of cells on right.

tein).[537,547] Keratin is present in one third to one half of the cases; it has a typical dot-like distribution and is consistent with the expression of keratins 8 and 18.[536,553] Smooth muscle actin is seen in nearly all cases, but desmin less commonly so.[555a] About 50% of the cases react for S-100 protein, whereas none are immunoreactive for EMA.[536] The peptide hormone inhibin and follicle regulatory proteins, two substances normally produced by ovarian granulosa

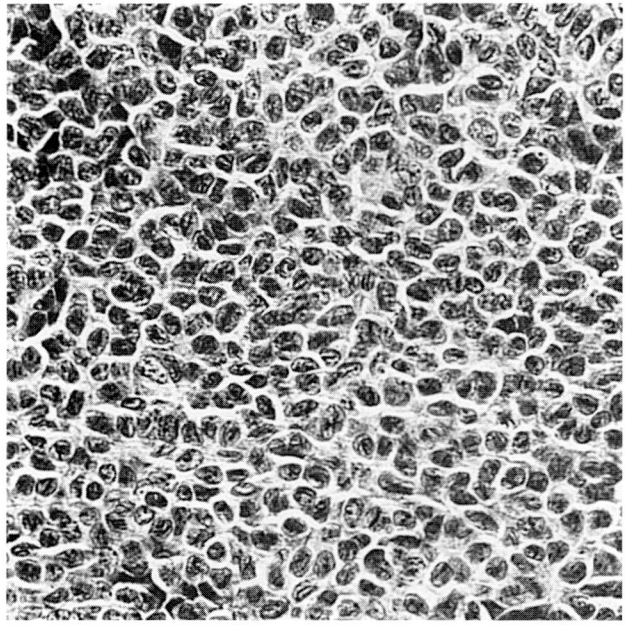

Fig. 19-196 High-power view of granulosa cell tumor of ovary with solid pattern of growth. Oval shape of nuclei and prominent nuclear grooves, resulting in "coffee bean" appearance, are evident.

cells, have been found to be elevated in the serum of patients with granulosa cell tumor[545,554]; inhibin has also been demonstrated immunohistochemically.[538b] Curiously, granulosa cell tumors have also been found to be often immunoreactive for O13, a marker associated with Ewing's sarcoma/PNET (see Chapter 25).[545a]

Ultrastructurally, the neoplastic granulosa cells have abundant intermediate filaments and specialized cell junctions, some of the latter having the appearance of typical desmosomes.[537] Cytogenetically, there is consistent trisomy for chromosome 12.[539,540] Flow cytometry studies have shown that the large majority of adult granulosa cell tumors are diploid or near-diploid; there is no convincing evidence that DNA ploidy analysis has independent prognostic value.[534,538a,541,558]

Juvenile granulosa cell tumor is diagnosed in nearly 80% of the cases during the first two decades of life, most patients presenting with isosexual precocity. A few cases have been associated with enchondromatosis (Ollier's disease)[560] and Maffucci's syndrome.[561] Typical morphologic features include diffuse or macrofollicular patterns of growth (the former predominating), mucin-positive intrafollicular secretion, larger tumor cells with extensive luteinization, paucity of nuclear grooves, presence of a thecal component, nuclear atypia, and variable but often high mitotic activity[555,562,567] (Figs. 19-197 and 19-198). Like their adult counterpart, they show consistent trisomy for chromosome 12.[556]

DNA ploidy analysis has shown a greater percentage of aneuploidy in juvenile granulosa cell tumors than in the adult variety; however, the prognostic value of this determination still needs to be demonstrated.[542,559]

• • •

The differential diagnosis of granulosa cell tumor (particularly of the adult variety) includes poorly differentiated

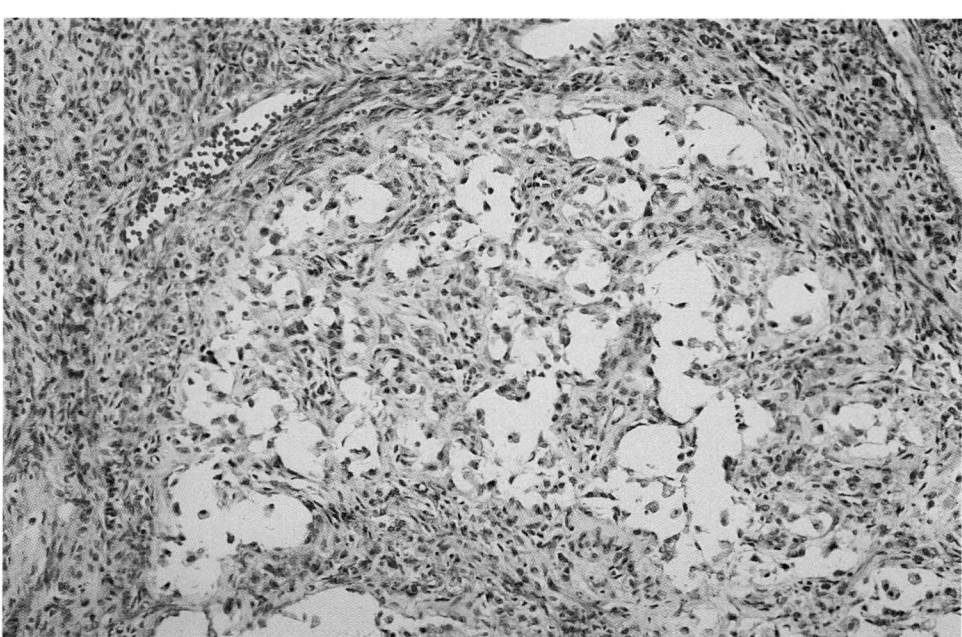

Fig. 19-197 Low-power microscopic view of juvenile granulosa cell tumor.

(predominantly solid) carcinoma of surface epithelial origin, carcinoid tumor, and the very rare tumors of endometrial stromal type.[566] The nuclear features are of crucial importance in this regard. Some early series describing a poor prognosis for granulosa cell tumors are probably contaminated with solid ovarian carcinomas of surface origin. Strong and widespread positivity for keratin should point toward the direction of carcinoma in a controversial case, especially if this positivity is diffuse cytoplasmic rather than dot-like. The differential diagnosis also includes the non-neoplastic proliferation of ovarian granulosa cells occurring during pregnancy; this change is usually microscopic, multiple, and associated with atretic follicles.[535]

The prognosis of granulosa cell tumors is largely related to the clinical staging. It also depends on size, tumor rupture, and presence of nuclear atypia.[564] The effect of the histologic pattern on prognosis is not clear-cut. Some authors have claimed that tumors with follicular or trabecular patterns have a better prognosis than those with a sarcomatoid pattern, but most studies have failed to demonstrate a convincing relationship.[533] In the series of Norris and Taylor,[550] 12 of 187 patients had persistent tumor after surgery, and 10 died as a result. Most deaths occurred more than 5 years after the original diagnosis and treatment, indicating that 5-year survival figures are not accurate predictors of permanent cure.[540]

Thecoma, fibroma, and related tumors

Thecoma presents after menopause in 65% of patients. It is usually unilateral and varies considerably in size. It has a well-defined capsule and a firm consistency. The cut surface is largely or entirely solid, but cysts may be present (Fig. 19-199). It has a yellow color, an important feature in the differential diagnosis with fibroma. Microscopically, it is com-posed of fascicles of spindle cells with centrally placed nuclei and a moderate amount of pale cytoplasm (Fig. 19-200). The intervening tissue may show considerable collagen deposition and focal hyaline plaque formation. The degree of cellularity varies considerably. Some tumors are heavily calcified.[596]

With oil red O, the cells of thecoma show abundant intracytoplasmic neutral fat, and silver stains usually demonstrate reticulin fibers surrounding individual cells (as opposed to granulosa cell tumor, in which the reticulin surrounds clusters of cells). However, islands may occur in the thecoma that are devoid of reticulin, especially in areas of luteinization. Immunohistochemical localization of estradiol is usually limited to a small number of tumor cells.[575]

Thecomas may be associated with prominent stromal hyperplasia, particularly in postmenopausal patients. In such cases, transitions may be seen from focal stromal hyperplasia through diffuse thecomatosis (hyperthecosis) to thecomas, suggesting a pathogenetic continuum.[590] It is likely that the small tumors designated as **stromal luteomas**[576,588] are yet another manifestation of this spectrum.

Sometimes, ovarian tumors otherwise typical of thecoma contain cells with the features of steroid hormone–secreting cells (lutein, Leydig, and adrenal cortical).[599] This tumor has generally been designated as **luteinized thecoma,**[585] the terms *stromal–Leydig cell tumor* or *Leydig cell–containing thecoma* being reserved for the rare examples in which Reinke's crystalloids are identified in the cytoplasm of these cells.[591,599] These variants tend to occur in younger women and may have an androgenic rather than estrogenic effect on the host.

Thecomas are typically associated with estrogenic manifestations, although some (particularly those containing steroid cells) may be androgenic. They are nearly always

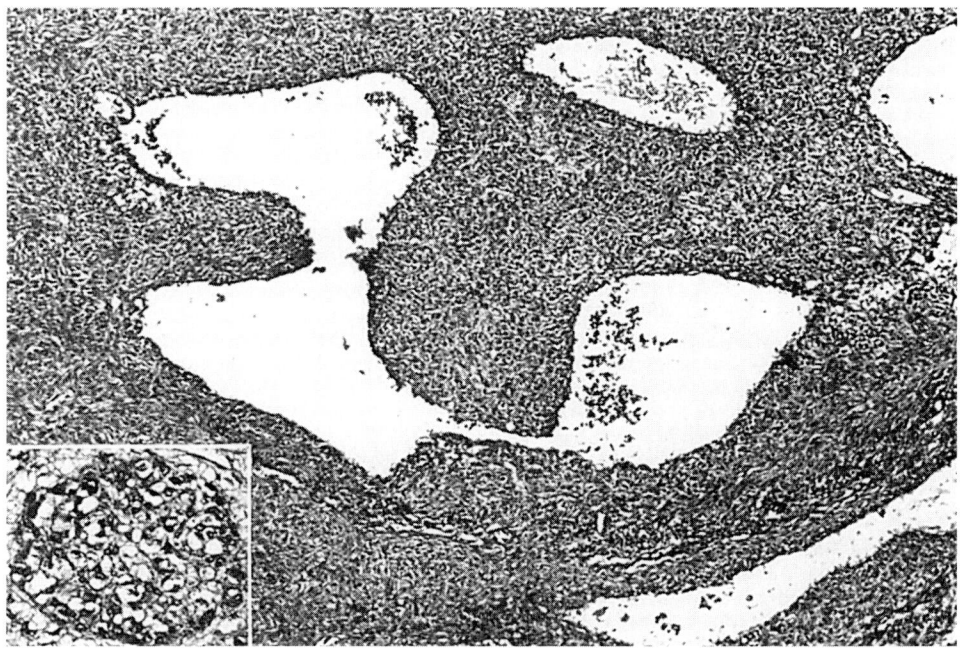

Fig. 19-198 Juvenile granulosa cell tumor. Follicular structures are present in predominantly solid neoplasm. **Inset** shows luteinized appearance of most tumor cells.

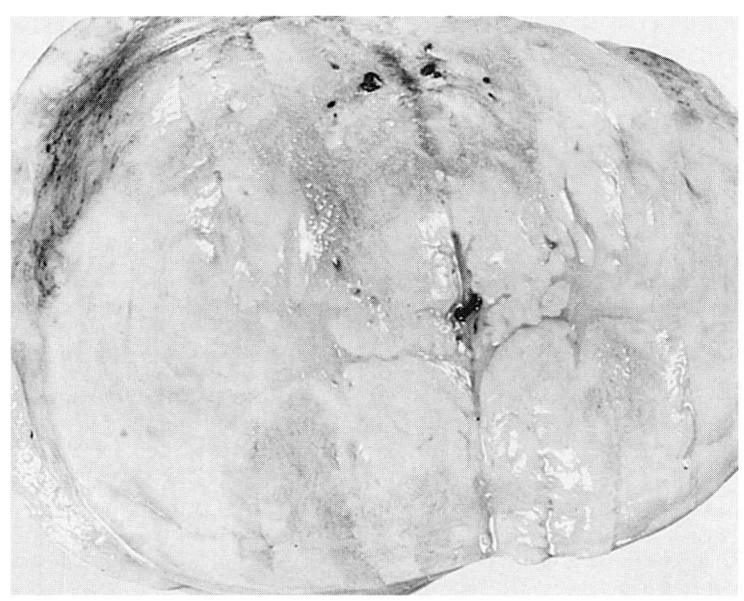

Fig. 19-199 Large thecoma that has small yellow areas.

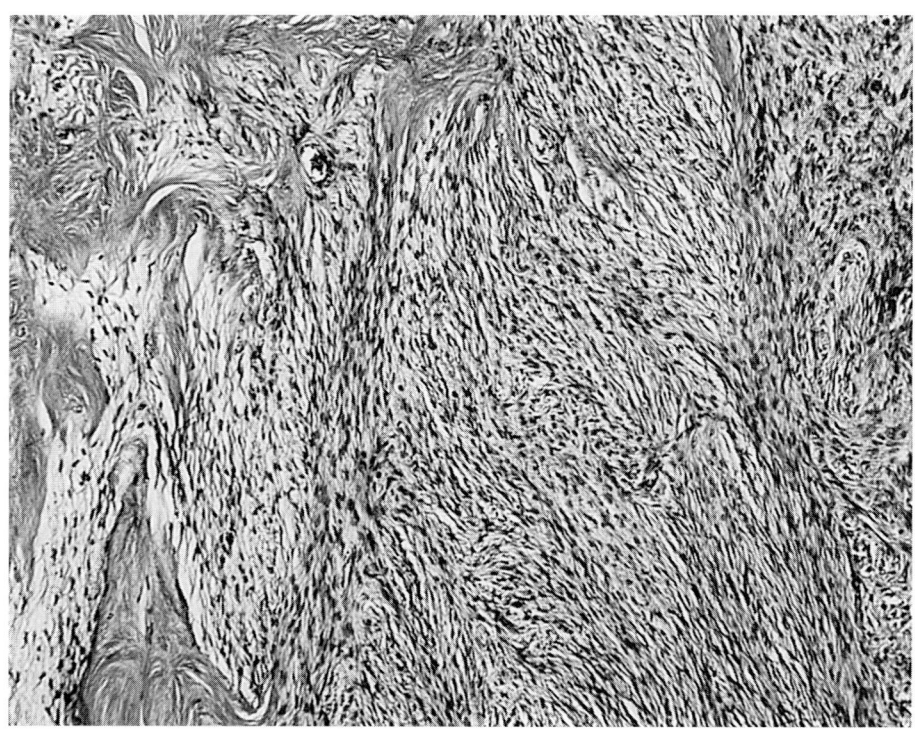

Fig. 19-200 Thecoma composed of spindle-shaped cells intermixed with dense hyaline plaques. Fat stains showed cytoplasmic lipid. Patient, 59-year-old woman, had endometrial hyperplasia.

benign, but a few malignant examples have been documented.[595] Some luteinized thecomas have been found to be associated with sclerosing peritonitis.[569]

Fibromas are common ovarian tumors, usually unilateral, which occur almost invariably after puberty.[574] They are solid, lobulated, firm, uniformly white, and usually not accompanied by adhesions (Fig. 19-201, *A*). The average

diameter is 6 cm.[572] Myxoid changes may be seen, sometimes resulting in cystic degeneration. Grossly, fibromas need to be distinguished mainly from thecoma, Brenner tumor, and Krukenberg tumor.

Microscopically, fibromas are composed of closely packed spindle stromal cells arranged in a "feather-stitched" or storiform pattern (Fig. 19-200, *B*). Hyaline bands and

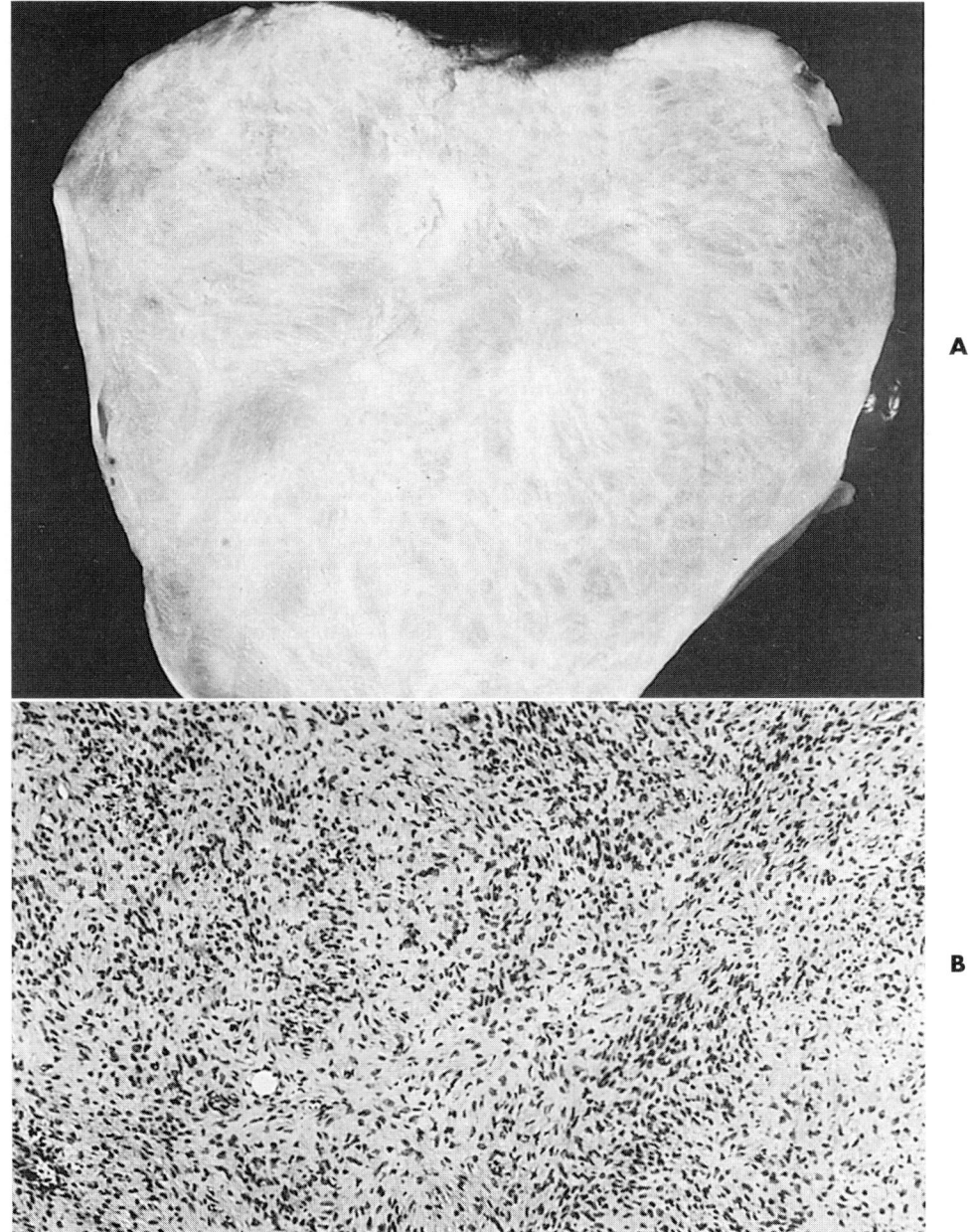

Fig. 19-201 A, Typical cut surface of ovarian fibroma showing interlacing bands of dense fibrous tissue. **B,** Fibroma with well-differentiated fibroblasts separated by hyaline stroma. (From Kraus FT: Gynecologic pathology, St. Lous, 1967, Mosby.)

edema may be present. Some fibromas occur in young women with the basal cell nevus (Gorlin's) syndrome; these are calcified, usually bilateral, and often multinodular.[583] Fibromas exhibiting a great deal of cellularity are referred to as *cellular fibromas* if the mitotic activity does not exceed three per ten high-power fields; mitotically more active tumors are regarded as fibrosarcomas.[582] Some otherwise typical fibromas have a minor component of sex-cord elements.[597]

Cytogenetically, both thecomas and fibromas have been found to exhibit trisomy of chromosome 12 in a minority of the tumor cells.[581a,592]

Ovarian fibroma (especially if large) can be associated with ascites, sometimes in combination with right-sided pleural effusion (Meigs' syndrome).[581,587] This may lead to a mistaken impression of inoperable ovarian neoplasm, but removal of the tumor leads to the disappearance of these manifestations. The mechanism for the pleural effusion is

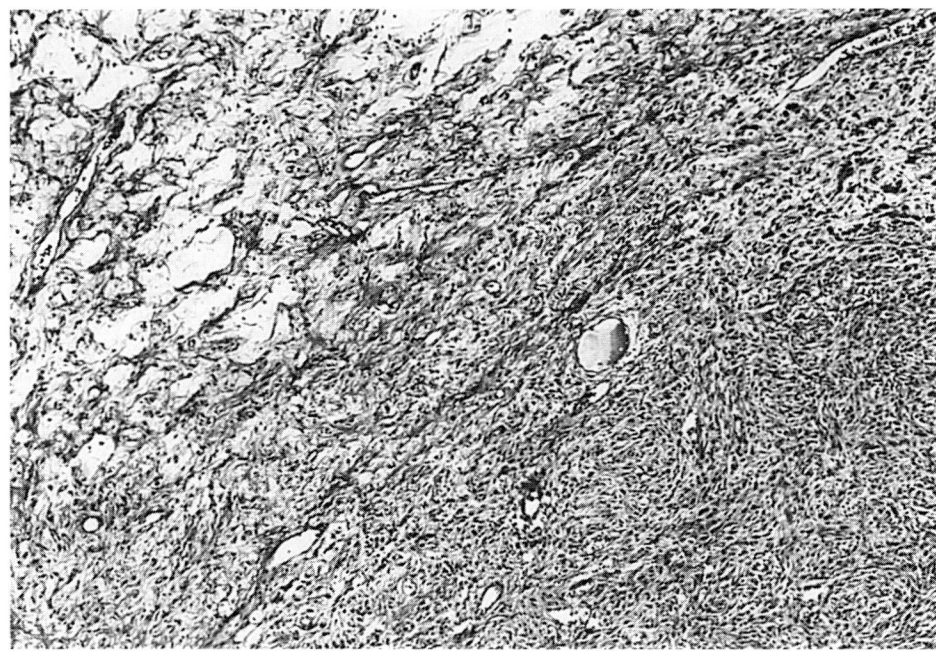

Fig. 19-202 Sclerosing stromal tumor of ovary. Areas of hypercellularity alternate with hypocellular foci exhibiting prominent edema.

said to be related to intrathoracic negative pressure and transdiaphragmatic passage of fluid through peritoneal "pores" or lymphatics. Meigs' syndrome can also occur in association with other ovarian tumors.[580]

Fibromas are benign, and oophorectomy is curative. Cellular fibromas may recur or be associated with peritoneal implants.[582]

Sclerosing stromal tumor is a benign ovarian neoplasm that shares many features with fibroma-thecoma. However, it occurs in a younger age group, has a less homogeneous gross appearance, and is characterized microscopically by a lobular pattern of growth, interlobular fibrosis, marked vascularity, and the presence of a dual cell population: collagen-producing spindle cells and lipid-containing round or oval cells (Fig. 19-202). Some of the latter may have a signet ring appearance and thus simulate a Krukenberg tumor.[568] Endocrine manifestations are rarely present, and *ligandin* (a probable indicator of steroidogenesis) has been demonstrated immunohistochemically.[594] The tumor cells are also immunoreactive for desmin and smooth muscle actin.[586] Evidence of differentiation along smooth muscle lines is also seen at the ultrastructural level.[589]

Massive edema of the ovary is probably not a neoplasm but is discussed here because of its gross similarities with fibroma. Most patients present with pain, abdominal mass, and/or menstrual irregularities; virilization, precocious puberty, and Meigs' syndrome have also been described.[577,579,584] Partial torsion of the mesoovarium with interference in the venous and lymphatic drainage has been suggested as the pathogenetic mechanism.[577,584] The cut surface has been described as watery. Microscopically, there is marked edema of the stroma surrounding follicles and other

structures (Fig. 19-203). Clusters of luteinized cells are often present.[578]

Fibromatosis is the term proposed by Young and Scully[598] for a disorder that they believe is possibly related to massive edema. The patients usually present because of menstrual irregularities. Grossly, the ovaries show a firm, white, cut surface. Microscopically, a diffuse proliferation of spindle cells separated by dense collagen is seen surrounding normal follicular structures. Luteinized cells may be present. The fact that some cases of massive ovarian edema are accompanied by small cellular foci of fibromatosis lends support to their interpretation. The term *fibromatosis,* although descriptively correct, should not be equated with the similarly named lesion of soft tissues.

Myxoma of ovary presents as a solid and cystic mass, some of the cysts being occasionally filled with blood. Microscopically, scattered cells with fibroblastic/myofibroblastic features are seen in a well-vascularized myxoid background.[573,593] Some authors regard this as a distinct type of ovarian neoplasm, whereas others view it as part of the spectrum of differentiation in the thecoma-fibroma group.[570,571]

Endometrial abnormalities associated with granulosa cell tumor, thecoma, and related tumors. The endometrium of patients with granulosa cell tumors or thecomas exhibits various degrees of hyperplasia in about a quarter of the cases,[602] even when the tumors are of minute size. In the remaining cases, the endometrium shows a normal proliferative or secretory pattern, and it may even be atrophic. Some of the hyperplasias are so florid as to closely resemble the appearance of an endometrial adenocarcinoma. This fact is at the heart of the controversy as to how often an endometrial adenocarcinoma occurs in the setting of these ovarian

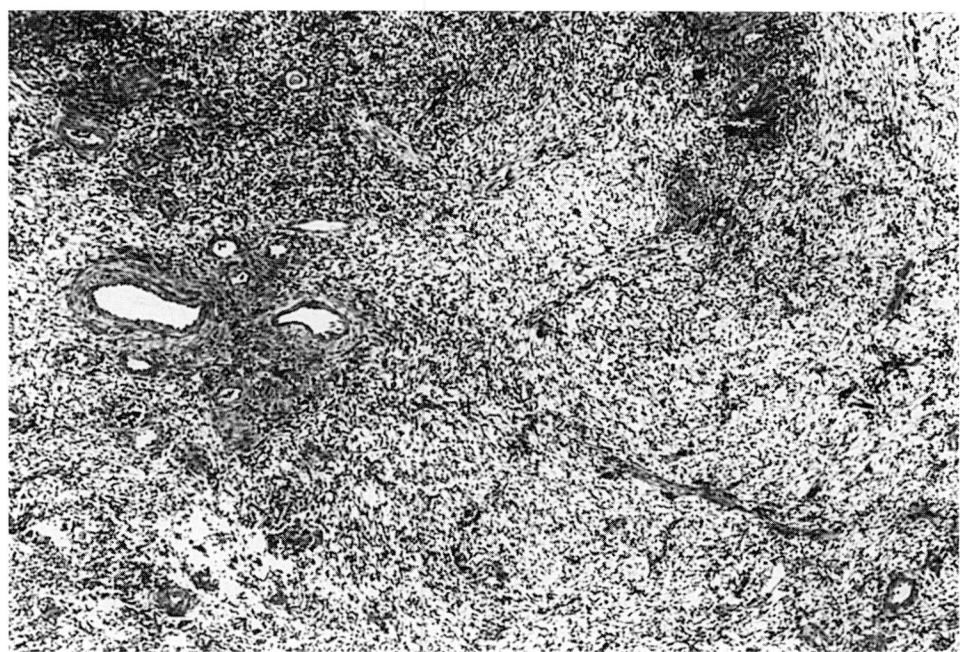

Fig. 19-203 Massive edema of ovary. Only stroma immediately surrounding blood vessels retains a normal appearance.

neoplasms. The quoted incidence varies from 3% to 21%,[600,602] this wide range strongly suggesting the lack of uniform diagnostic criteria. Some of the lesions are undoubtedly hyperplasias, proved by the fact that they have been found to regress following excision of the ovarian tumors. The bona fide carcinomas are nearly always well differentiated and superficial, and this explains the excellent prognosis associated with them. A case of endometrial adenocarcinoma has been reported in association with ovarian sclerosing stromal tumor.[601]

Rarely thecomas have been found to be associated with endometrial sarcomas of one type or another.[603]

Small cell carcinoma

Small cell carcinoma is a high-grade ovarian malignancy that may be confused with granulosa cell tumor.[605,610,611a] It occurs in young females (average age, 23 years) and is nearly always bilateral. Some familial cases have been reported.[608a] The tumor is associated with hypercalcemia in two thirds of the cases, which disappears following removal of the tumor. Grossly, the tumor is large and solid, with areas of necrosis and hemorrhage. Microscopically, a diffuse proliferation of small, closely packed cells of carcinomatous appearance with scant cytoplasm and small nuclei is seen (Fig. 19-204). Clusters of larger and more pleomorphic cells may be present, some of them resembling luteinized cells.[606] Cytoplasmic hyaline globules may also be seen. Tumors containing a large number of these cells have been referred to, tongue-in-cheek, as the large variant of small cell carcinoma. There may also be islands, cords, trabeculae, mucinous glands, and *follicle-like structures* (Fig. 19-205). The latter are an important clue to the diagnosis.

The tumor cells may express keratin, vimentin, EMA, chromogranins and laminin, but not B 72.3 or S-100 protein.[604,611] Immunoreactivity has also been found for human parathyroid hormone–related protein, although the correlation between the degree of staining and the serum calcium level is poor.[609] Ultrastructurally, the cells have a poorly differentiated appearance, with relatively abundant dilated rough endoplasmic reticulum and specialized cell junctions; neurosecretory-type granules are generally absent.[606] Most surprisingly, this tumor has been found to have a diploid DNA pattern.[607]

The prognosis is very poor because of frequent extra-ovarian spread. The histogenesis is unknown. Germ cell, sex cord–stromal, and neuroendocrine origins have been suggested; the frequent immunoreactivity for chromogranin speaks in favor of the latter.[604]

Small cell carcinoma as previously described should be distinguished from the tumor type resembling small cell (neuroendocrine) carcinoma of the lung and other organs and referred to as **ovarian small cell carcinoma of pulmonary type**.[608] Such tumors may be associated with endometrioid carcinoma or other patterns. Immunohistochemically, there is reactivity for keratin, EMA, NSE, and (rarely) for chromogranin and Leu7. In contrast to the small cell carcinoma associated with hypercalcemia, the DNA pattern is often aneuploid.[608] The prognosis is poor.

Sertoli–Leydig cell tumor (arrhenoblastoma; androblastoma)

As the name indicates, Sertoli–Leydig cell tumors are composed of a mixture in variable proportions of cells morphologically resembling male Sertoli and Leydig cells. Pure

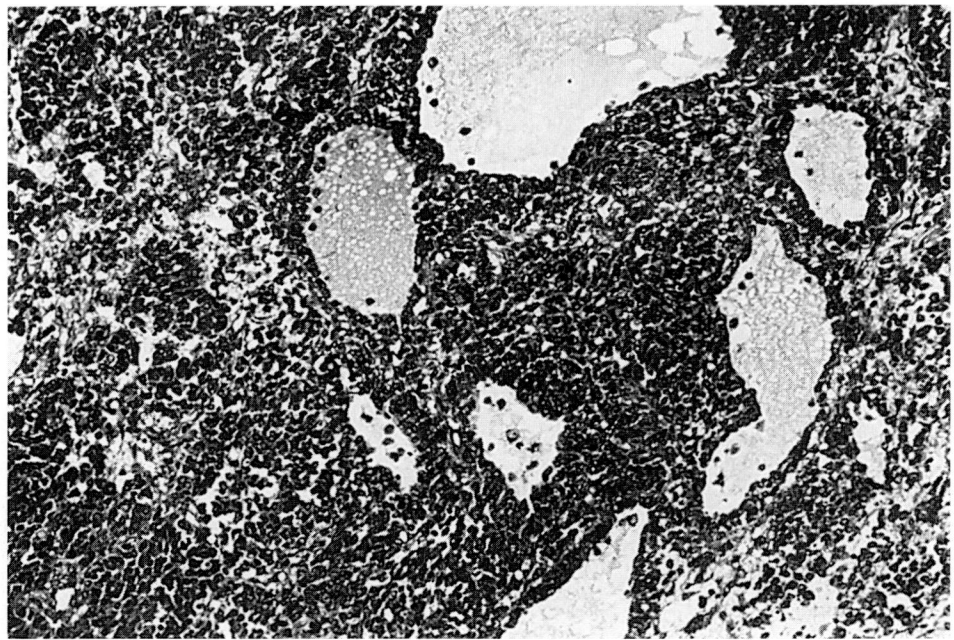

Fig. 19-204 Small cell carcinoma of ovary. Tumor is composed of small cells with scanty cytoplasm, which grow in predominantly solid pattern but which also exhibit formation of follicle-like structures.

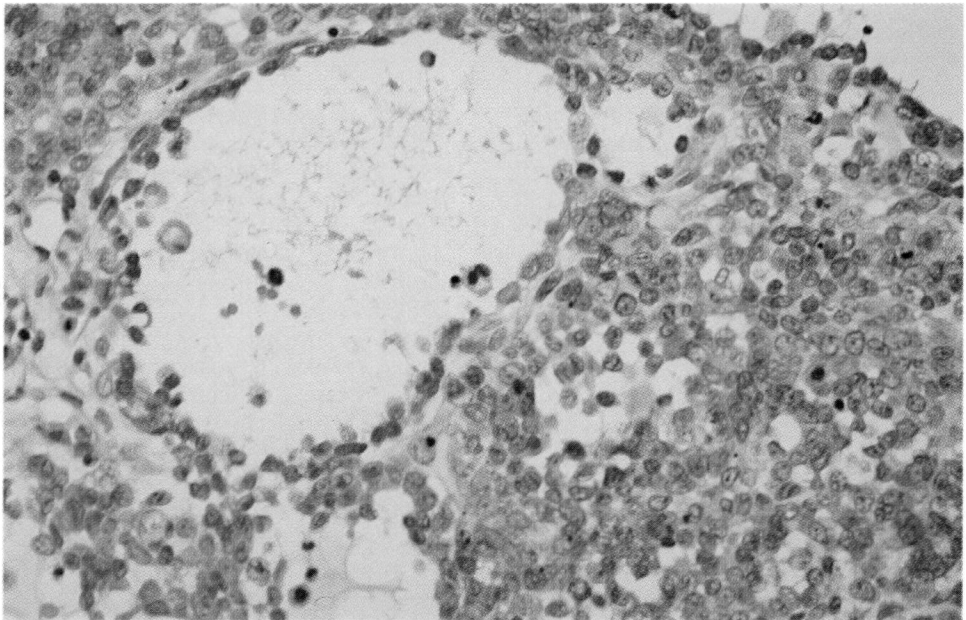

Fig. 19-205 Small cell carcinoma. The presence of follicle-like formations is an important diagnostic clue.

Sertoli cell tumors are also included in this group, but pure Leydig cell tumors are included with the lipid cell tumors.[615] Meyer[621,635] championed the concept that male-directed cells persisting from the primitive testis-like structure that develops during embryogenesis in the ovarian medulla near the hilus are the origin of this tumor. However, by electron microscopy, the Sertoli-like cells resemble ovarian granulosa cells more than they do male Sertoli cells.[618] Furthermore, both tumor cell types contain female sex chromatin.[623] It is perhaps more logical to think of these tumors as derived directly from specialized ovarian stromal cells through different pathways of differentiation.[633] They are uncommon,

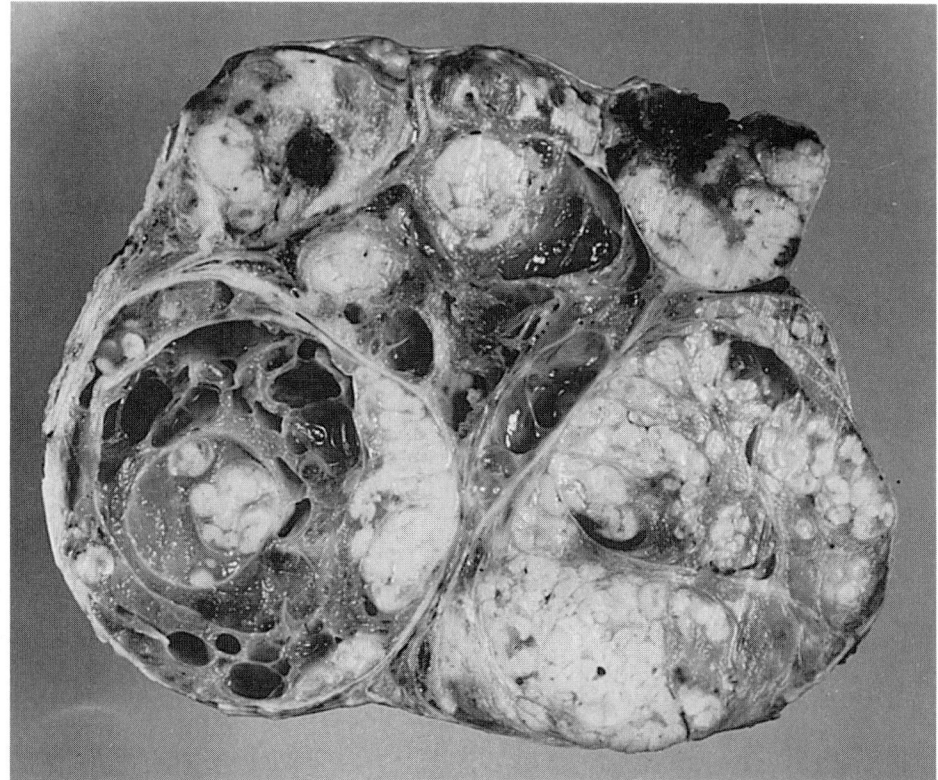

Fig. 19-206 Large Sertoli–Leydig cell tumor in 17-year-old girl. Patient had amenorrhea and increased body and facial hair.

comprising less than 0.1% of ovarian neoplasms. Grossly they are predominantly solid, but cystic areas may also be present (Fig. 19-206).

The microscopic pattern is extremely variable. Several major categories have been described; these may coexist in the same tumor:

1 ***Well-differentiated (Meyer's type I)*** (11%). Composed of tubules lined by Sertoli-like cells separated by variable numbers of Leydig-like cells[642] (Fig. 19-207).

2 ***Intermediate (Meyer's type II)*** (54%). Characterized by the formation of cords, sheets, and aggregates of Sertoli-like cells, separated by spindle stromal cells and recognizable Leydig cells (Fig. 19-208).

3 ***Poorly differentiated (sarcomatoid; undifferentiated; Meyer's type III)*** (13%). Composed of masses of spindle-shaped cells arranged in a "sarcomatoid" pattern.

4 ***Pure Sertoli cell tumors (tubular androblastoma).*** Essentially identical to well-differentiated Sertoli–Leydig cell tumors but lacking Leydig cells and primitive stromal elements.[641] Abundant lipid may be present in the cytoplasm. The microscopic pattern can be tubular or have the configuration of *folliculoma lipidique.*[643] Amyloid-like material can be present, and cytoplasmic crystalline structures have been found by electron microscopy.[632] Some Sertoli cell tumors are composed of cells with oxyphilic cytoplasm.[614a]

5 ***With heterologous elements (teratoid androblastoma)*** (22%). Associated with tissues such as mucinous epithelium of gastrointestinal type, liver,[637] skeletal muscle, or cartilage[624,626] (Fig. 19-209). The epithelial portion of this neoplasm contains a variety of endocrine cells[612] and can give rise to microscopic carcinoid tumors.[629,638]

6 ***Retiform*** (15%). In this category, typical elements of Sertoli–Leydig cell tumor coexist with formations resembling the rete of the ovary or testis. These appear as irregular cleft-like spaces lined by low cuboidal cells; blunt papillae with hyalinized or edematous cores are often present. Sometimes the retiform formations predominate almost to the exclusion of the Sertoli–Leydig cell component[627,639] (Fig. 19-210).

• • •

As in the case of granulosa cell tumor, the cells of a few Sertoli–Leydig cell tumors may contain bizarre and/or multiple nuclei, a change of no apparent prognostic significance.[640]

Immunohistochemically, testosterone and estradiol are found in both Sertoli and Leydig cells and less frequently in primitive stromal cells.[619,620] The areas of Sertoli cell differentiation stain for keratin, but not for EMA, PLAP, CEA, CA 19-9, CA 125, or S-100 protein; knowledge of this profile is useful in the differential diagnosis between Sertoli–Leydig cell tumors with heterologous elements (in which this profile is maintained) and carcinosarcoma.[614]

Most Sertoli–Leydig cell tumors are seen in young patients (average age, 25 years) and are relatively rare after

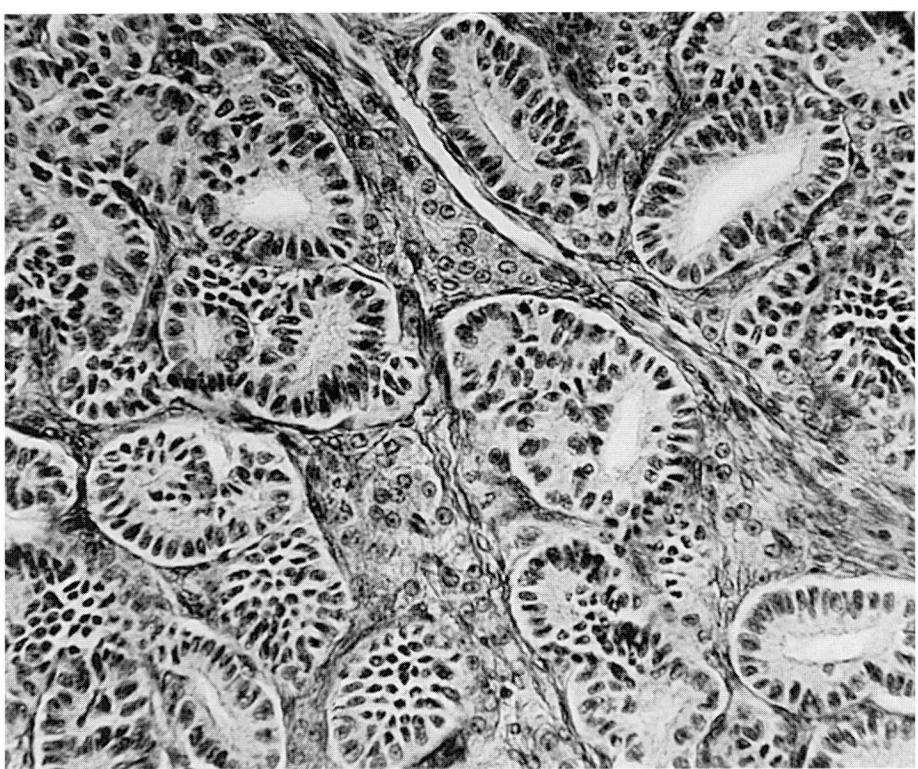

Fig. 19-207 Well-differentiated tubular type of Sertoli–Leydig cell tumor (type I). This pattern usually is not associated with masculinization. Note clusters of Leydig cells in trabeculae between tubules. (Slide contributed by Dr. W. Ober, New York.)

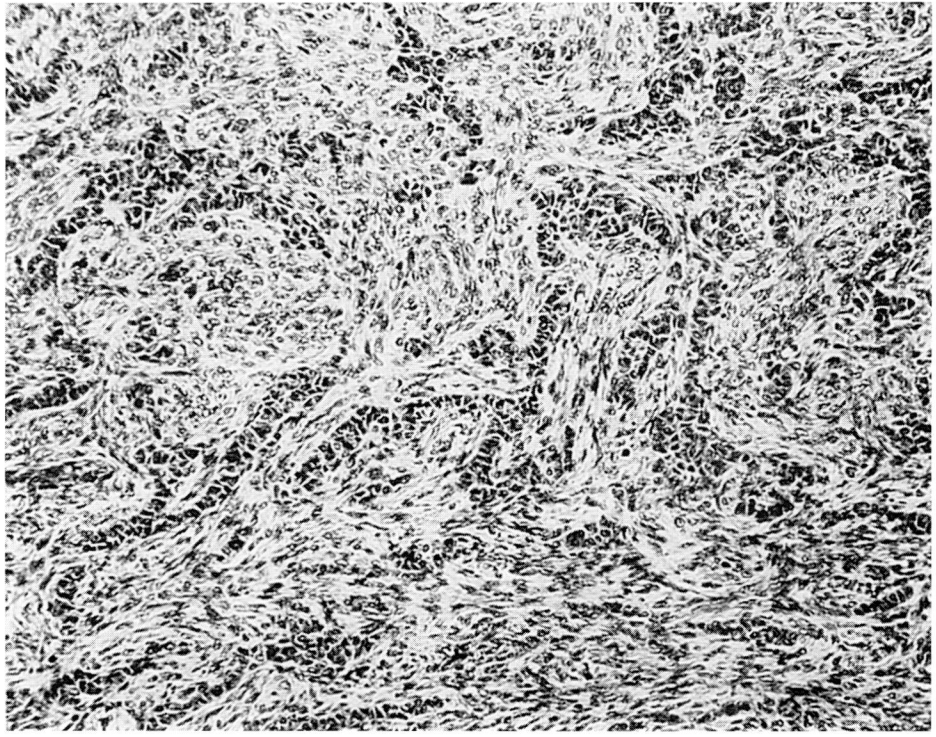

Fig. 19-208 Ovarian Sertoli–Leydig cell tumor (arrhenoblastoma, type II of Meyer). This pattern of irregular branching rows of Sertoli cells mimics sex cord formation in embryonic testis prior to formation of lumina. Virilization syndrome occurs most frequently in this group, which is also most common.

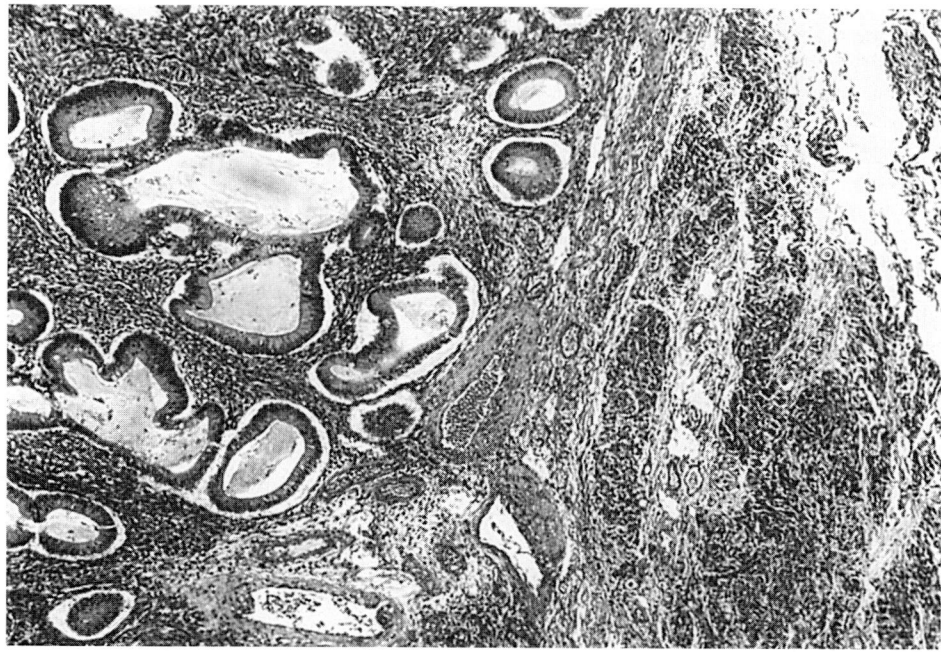

Fig. 19-209 Sertoli–Leydig cell tumor with formation of heterologous elements. Latter component is represented by well-differentiated mucin-producing glands.

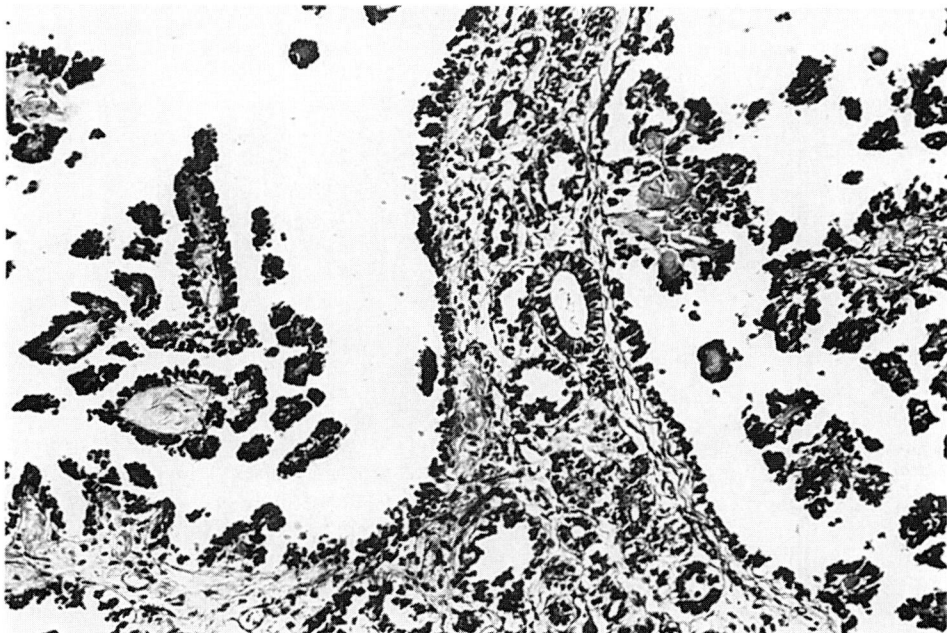

Fig. 19-210 Retiform variant of Sertoli–Leydig cell tumor. In this area only retiform elements are present. Micropapillary formations alternate with tubular structures lined by low cylindric epithelium. Patient was 12-year-old child.

menopause. Some are diagnosed during pregnancy.[636] These tend to exhibit prominent intercellular edema.[635] Bilateral involvement is seen in fewer than 2% of the cases. Cases have been reported in association with mature cystic teratoma.[630] Nearly half of the cases are accompanied by signs of androgen excess. This is manifested first by *defeminization* (amenorrhea, breast atrophy, loss of subcutaneous tissue deposits) and later by *masculinization* (clitoral hypertrophy, deeping of the voice, hirsutism). Usually prompt return of feminine characteristics follows excision of the tumor, but the manifestations of masculinization disappear more slowly. Urinary 17-ketosteroids are frequently normal, but elevations have been recorded. Tumor tissue incubated with progesterone or pregnenolone causes a synthesis of various hormones (androstenedione, 17-hydroxyprogesterone, testosterone), but the final aromatizing reaction to estrogens does not occur.[628,631]

Some Sertoli–Leydig cell tumors do not have demonstrable endocrine effect, whereas others are accompanied by secretion of estrogen or progesterone. The latter is often the case for pure Sertoli cell tumors.[634] It is opportune to mention again that the diagnosis of these neoplasms should be based on their morphologic appearance rather than on the nature of their hormonal manifestations; terms such as "feminizing mesenchymoma" should be avoided. Curiously, some cases of Sertoli–Leydig cell tumor have been associated with serum elevation of alpha-fetoprotein[613,622]; this marker has been detected immunohistochemically in areas of hepatocytic differentiation[637] and in the more conventional Leydig and Sertoli cell–like component.[616]

The prognosis of Sertoli–Leydig cell tumor, which is usually good, correlates with the stage and degree of differentiation of the tumor.[623,625,644] The overall incidence of clinical malignancy in one large series was 18%; all the well-differentiated tumors were benign, but 11% of those with intermediate differentiation, 59% of those with poor differentiation, and 19% of those with heterologous elements were malignant.[637] In one series of twenty-eight cases of pure Sertoli cell tumor, there were two recurrences.[632] Conservative surgery is indicated in young women for Sertoli–Leydig cell tumors grossly confined to the ovary.[617,643,644]

Lipid (lipoid, steroid) cell tumor

A small group of ovarian tumors is composed entirely of cells with morphologic features indicative of steroid hormone secretion. These are manifested by an abundant eosinophilic or vacuolated cytoplasm that is often positive for fat stains and that at the ultrastructural level is shown to contain well-developed smooth endoplasmic reticulum and mitochondria with tubulovesicular cristae.[645,648] Normal steroid hormone–secreting cells can be of lutein (thecal or stromal), Leydig (hilus), and adrenal cortical type.[650] Theoretically, these tumors could arise from any of these sources. In the few cases in which Reinke's crystalloids are found, the tumor can be categorized as Leydig or hilus cell tumor.[649,650,652] In a few others, an ectopic adrenal origin has been suggested on the basis of their hormonal profile (presence of Cushing's syndrome)[655] and the fact that adrenal cortical rests can be found in the hilus of the ovary and the broad ligament (although not within the adult ovary itself). In the majority of the cases, however, the exact origin of this

tumor remains undecided; the descriptive terms *lipid, lipoid,* and—more recently—*steroid cell tumor* have therefore been proposed for the entire group, with the added designations *Leydig cell type* or *adrenal cortical type* whenever indicated.[654,655] This is preferable to terms such as *luteoma, hypernephroma,* or *masculinovoblastoma.*

Enzymatic conversion studies performed on freshly excised tumors have demonstrated that a variety of androgenic hormones are produced by these tumors in vitro[653]; occasionally large amounts of adrenal corticoids have been found.

Lipid cell tumors are usually unilateral and are composed of yellow or yellowish brown nodules separated by fibrous trabeculae (Fig. 19-211, *A*). Microscopically, they are characterized by masses of large rounded or polyhedral cells with the morphologic and ultrastructural features previously described for their normal counterparts (Fig. 19-211, *B*). Immunohistochemically, there is reactivity for vimentin in three fourths of the cases, for keratin in one half, and for actin in about one third.[653a]

This neoplasm can occur at any age.[654] Most are associated with a virilizing syndrome (with defeminization and amenorrhea),[646] and a few of the cases meet the criteria for Cushing's syndrome.[655] Some of the tumors are biologically inactive, at least at the clinical level, and others are associated with estrogenic or progestagenic manifestations. A few cases have been associated with endometrioid carcinoma.[647] The incidence of clinical malignancy is about 25%.[646,654] Malignant tumors tend to be larger (7 cm in diameter or greater), with foci of necrosis and hemorrhage, and to exhibit nuclear atypia and mitotic activity.[646,654] Tumors containing Reinke's crystalloids are almost invariably benign.[649,654] The malignant tumors can be associated with peritoneal implants.[654]

Lipid cell tumors should be distinguished from lesions in which proliferation of steroid hormone–producing cells occurs as a secondary event. These include stromal luteoma (although the position of this lesion in the scheme of ovarian neoplasms remains controversial), luteinized granulosa cell tumor (particularly the juvenile type), thecoma-fibroma, stromal–Leydig cell tumor, and the non-neoplastic proliferation of steroid cells that may be seen at the periphery of other tumors, such as struma ovarii, strumal carcinoid, surface epithelial tumors, and metastatic carcinoma.[651]

Other types

Gynandroblastoma is the term used for the sex cord–stromal tumor composed of a mixture *in similar amounts* of clearly identifiable granulosa-theca cell and Sertoli–Leydig cell elements. When thus defined, this entity is extremely rare, to the point that some authors doubt its existence. Reported cases of this entity have been accompanied by androgenic, estrogenic, or no hormonal effects.[664,665]

Sex-cord tumor with annular tubules is a distinctive ovarian tumor that is associated in one third of the cases with the Peutz–Jeghers syndrome.[661,666,671] This lesion combines features suggestive of a granulosa cell tumor with a pattern of growth reminiscent of Sertoli cells.[657,666] Its morphologic hallmark is the presence of simple and complex annular tubules containing eosinophilic hyaline bodies, often calcified (Fig. 19-212). The appearance is similar to

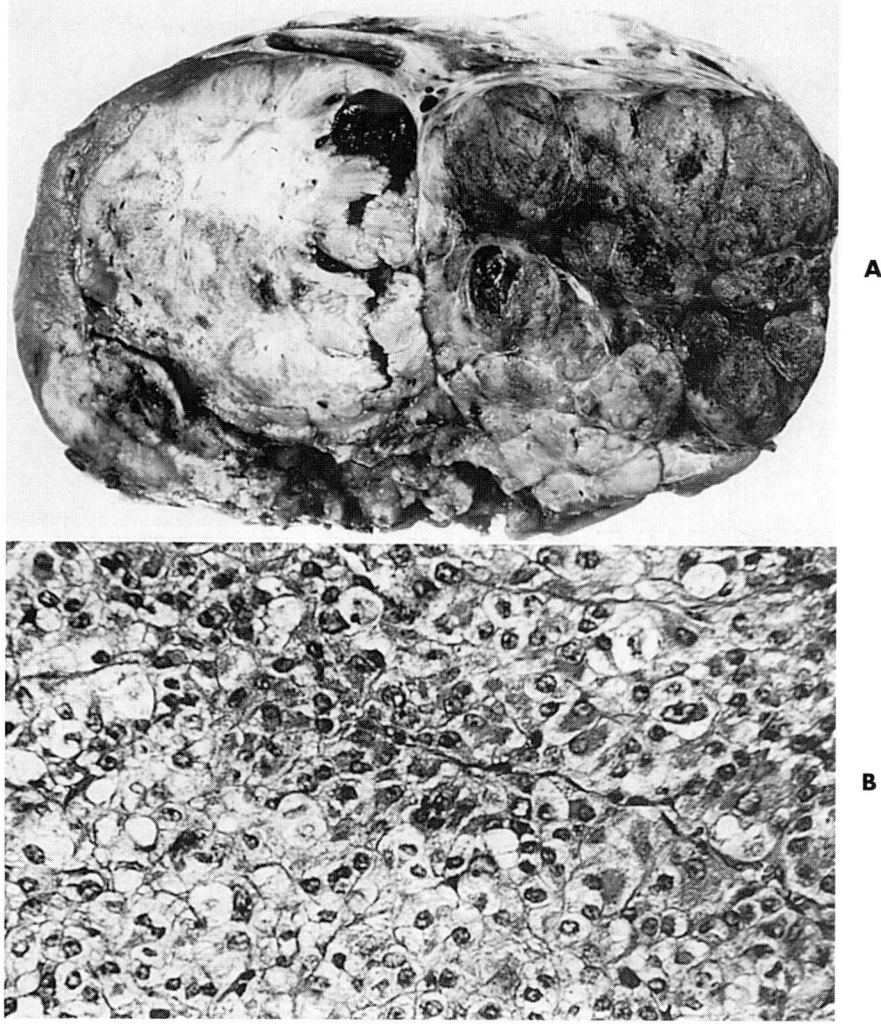

Fig. 19-211 A, Cross section of large malignant lipid cell tumor removed from right ovary of 75-year-old woman with mild hirsutism and marked elevation of blood testosterone level. Bright yellow areas alternate with darker foci. Ragged edge at lower margin corresponds to site of attachment to pelvic wall. **B,** Microscopic appearance of same tumor. Large cells with abundant lipid-containing cytoplasm alternate with smaller cells of deeply acidophilic cytoplasm.

that of gonadoblastoma, from which it differs because of the clinical/genetic background and the presence of a germ cell component in the latter.

The ambiguous or biphasic nature of the tumor cells is also apparent on ultrastructural examination: Features consistent with granulosa cell or nonspecialized ovarian stroma[659,662] alternate with features indicative of Sertoli cell differentiation, notably the presence of Charcot-Bottcher filaments.[656] Symptoms suggestive of hyperestrinism have been described in about 50% of the cases. Tumors associated with the Peutz–Jeghers syndrome are typically multifocal, bilateral, small (or even microscopic), calcified, and usually benign. Those unassociated with the syndrome are unilateral, often large, and clinically malignant in about 22% of the cases.[660,671]

It should be mentioned here that Peutz–Jeghers syndrome can be associated with other neoplasms of the female genital tract, such as other sex cord–stromal ovarian tumors,[669] mucinous ovarian tumors, and well-differentiated adenocarcinoma (adenoma malignum) of the cervix.

Ovarian tumor of probable wolffian origin is the name proposed for a neoplasm originally described as occurring in the broad ligament[663] and subsequently in the retroperitoneum[667] and the ovary itself.[665a,670] It is thought to be of wolffian (mesonephric) derivation, the first term being chosen to avoid confusion with tumors formerly regarded as of mesonephric nature (such as clear cell carcinoma) and now included in other categories. If this interpretation is correct, these neoplasms are *not* of sex cord–stromal nature, but they are discussed here because of their resemblance to them and the fact that their exact histogenesis is still unclear. Grossly, they may be either solid or solid and cystic. Microscopically, epithelial cells are seen growing in the form of cystic structures, solid or hollow tubules, and diffuse sheets (Fig. 19-

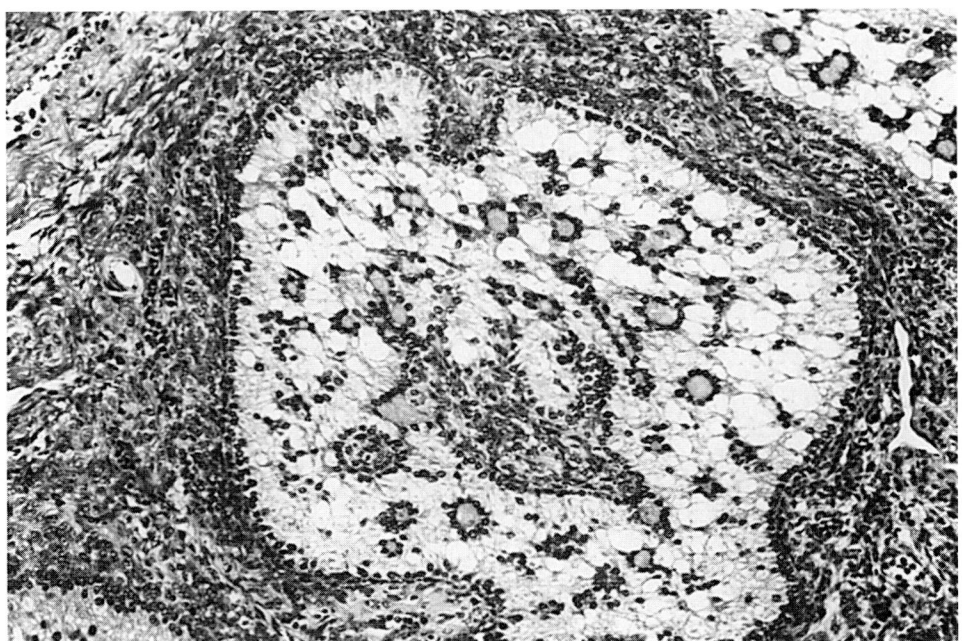

Fig. 19-212 Sex-cord tumor with annular tubules. Sharply outlined lobular structure surrounded by cellular stroma contains round tubules with hyaline homogeneous material in center.

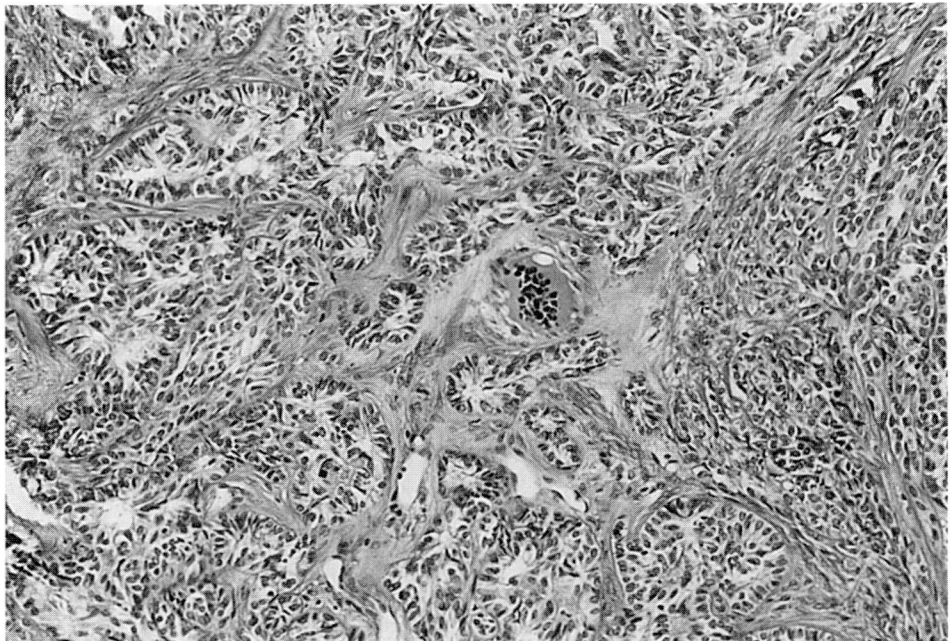

Fig. 19-213 Ovarian tumor of probably wolffian origin. Lesion is formed by ducts and solid nests composed of cells with oval nuclei, without atypia or mitotic activity.

213). The sieve-like appearance on low-power examination is a useful diagnostic feature. PAS-positive basement membranes are prominent around the epithelial aggregates. These tumors lack stromal cells of steroid hormone–secreting type and are unaccompanied by hormonal manifestations. Mucin stains are negative. The behavior is generally benign, but a few have recurred or metastasized.[658,668,670]

Sex cord–stromal tumor, indeterminate or unclassified type, is a justifiable designation for ovarian tumors in which the cytologic and/or architectural features are consistent with a sex cord–stromal origin but which cannot be assigned to any specific category.

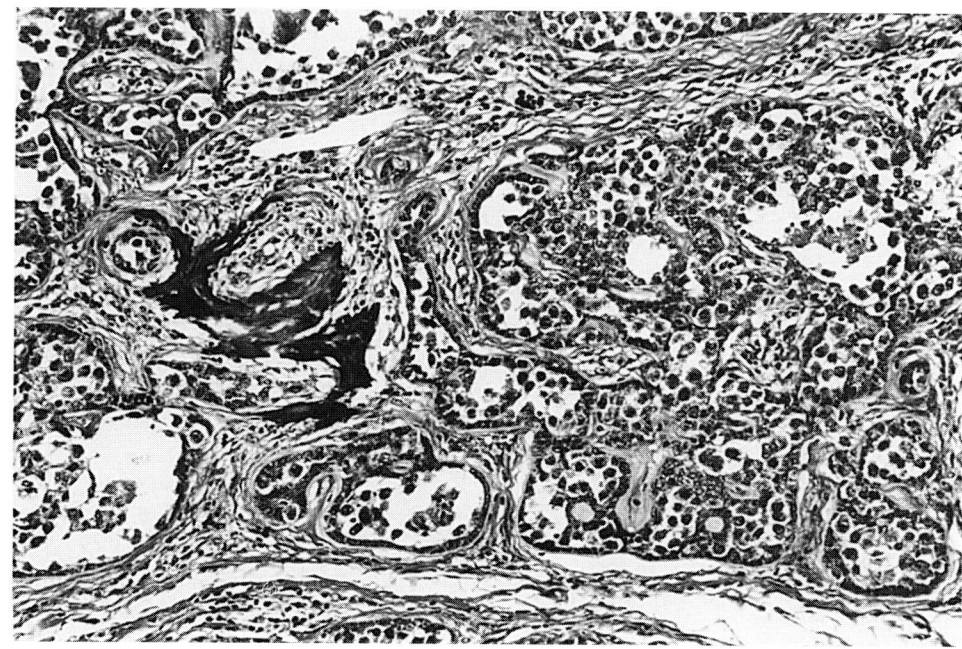

Fig. 19-214 Gonadoblastoma of ovary showing biphasic population of stromal and germ cells. Focus of stromal calcification is also present.

Germ cell–sex cord–stromal tumors

The most distinctive member of the group of tumors composed of a combination of germ cells and sex cord–stromal cells is **gonadoblastoma,** also known as *dysgenetic gonadoma* and included among the gonocytomas in Teter's elaborate classification.[685] This tumor occurs practically always in sexually abnormal individuals, most commonly affected by gonadal dysgenesis and carrying the Y chromosome (i.e., XY gonadal dysgenesis and XO-XY mosaicism but not XX gonadal dysgenesis).[672] The risk of neoplasia in these dysgenetic gonads is estimated to be 25%. However, gonadoblastomas have also been documented in phenotypically and chromosomally normal females, even during pregnancy.[679,680] They have has also been seen in association with ataxia-telangiectasia.[673] It is often impossible to determine the nature of the gonad bearing the tumor. In some cases it has been identified as a streak and in others as a cryptorchid testis, but never as a normal ovary.

About 36% of the tumors are bilateral. They are usually small, and many become apparent only on microscopic examination[683] (Plate XIV-F). The key microscopic feature is the admixture of primitive germ cells (resembling those of dysgerminoma) with sex cord–stromal cells resembling immature Sertoli and granulosa cells[676,683] (Fig. 19-214). Steroid hormone–producing cells may also be present, especially after puberty; their capacity for steroidogenesis has been demonstrated by their in vitro production of androgens and estrogens.[678] Hyalinization and calcification are common. The hyaline material reacts strongly with anti-laminin antibodies, indicating basement membrane deposition.[681] When abundant, this material can become obvious on plain abdominal roentgenograms. The germ cell component may overgrow the stromal elements and result in the formation of a dysgerminoma or, exceptionally, another type of germ cell tumor.[674,675] Only under these circumstances is the tumor endowed with a malignant potential.

Microscopic structures resembling gonadoblastoma and sex-cord tumor with annular tubules are sometimes found incidentally in the ovaries of *normal* infants and children in association with follicular cysts; it has been suggested that they represent the precursor of these tumors.[682]

Rare *germ cell–sex cord–stromal tumors* not fulfilling the diagnostic criteria for gonadoblastoma have been described in normal females[684]; some of them also contain retiform structures.[686] These tumors can be hormonally active and clinically malignant.[677] Like gonadoblastoma, they can be accompanied by dysgerminoma or other germ cell tumors.

Tumors not specific to ovary
Malignant lymphoma and leukemia

Secondary ovarian involvement by generalized lymphoma or leukemia is well recognized.[689] Much more rarely, malignant lymphoma involves the ovaries as the primary manifestation of the disease[688,693,695] (Fig. 19-215). This is also true for granulocytic leukemia (granulocytic sarcoma).[687,691,694]

Nearly all ovarian lymphomas are of non-Hodgkin's type.[690] In children, undifferentiated (small, noncleaved) lymphomas predominate; in adults, most are large cell diffuse (either noncleaved or immunoblastic) or follicular.[690] Immunophenotypically, practically all of the cases are of B-cell nature.[690] In the series of Osborne and Robboy,[692] 55% were bilateral, and 64% also involved extragonadal sites (usually the omentum, fallopian tubes, or lymph nodes); only nine of their forty-two patients survived more than 5 years, and two subsequently died of lymphoma.

Exceptionally, ovarian lymphoma has been found to coexist with a borderline serous tumor.[696]

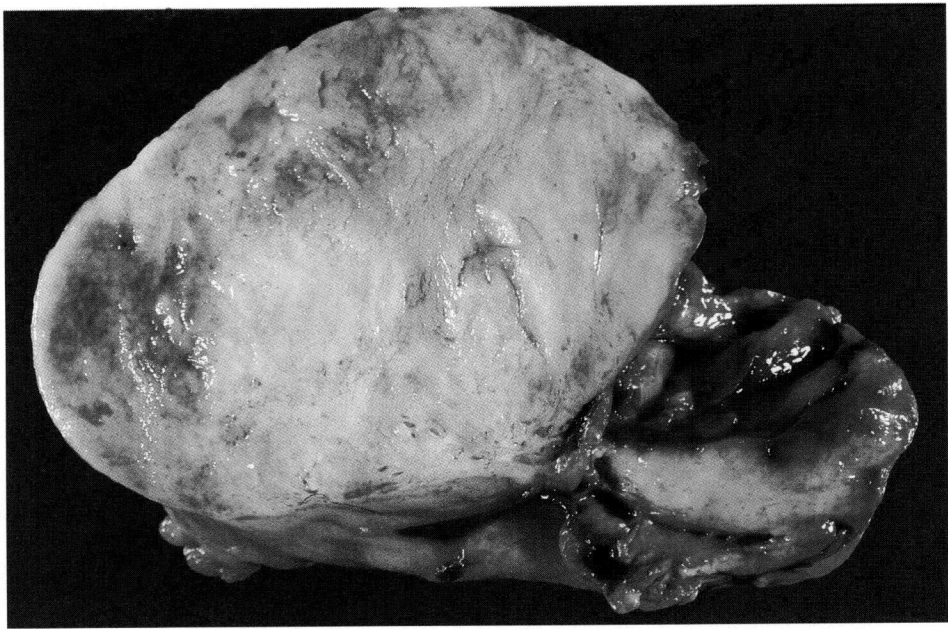

Fig. 19-215 Malignant lymphoma of ovary of Burkitt type massively replacing the organ.

Sarcoma

Primary sarcomas of the ovary are extremely rare. They need to be distinguished from undifferentiated carcinomas, mixed müllerian tumors, "sarcomatoid" forms of sex cord–stromal tumors, Krukenberg's tumors associated with brisk stromal reaction, and cellular fibromas.

Fibrosarcomas are separated from cellular fibromas mainly on the basis of their mitotic activity (four or more per ten high-power fields) (see p. 1510). They tend to be large, solid, and accompanied by adhesions. The clinical course is aggressive.[701] One case has been diagnosed in the context of the nevus–basal cell carcinoma syndrome.[699]

Endometrial (endometrioid) stromal sarcomas, both of the low-grade and high-grade variety, can present as primary ovarian neoplasms; the low-grade tumors closely simulate the pattern of growth of the diffuse type of granulosa tumor.[706] They are recognized because of the presence of plump oval cells arranged around vessels of the spiral arteriole type.[703]

Other sarcomas of the adult ovary, all exceptionally rare, are *leiomyosarcoma, chondrosarcoma,*[705] *osteosarcoma,*[698,702] *malignant peripheral nerve sheath tumor,*[704] *angiosarcoma,*[700] and *rhabdomyosarcoma.*[697]

Other primary tumors

About twenty cases of ovarian *hemangioma* have been reported.[707] Most are small, found incidentally, unilateral, and cavernous in type. Rarely, they are bilateral and/or associated with hemangiomas elsewhere in the body. Ovarian hemangiomas should be distinguished from lipid cell tumors having a prominent vascular component. *Leiomyomas* can exceptionally develop in the ovary, usually in association with uterine leiomyomas; some are mitotically active and need to be distinguished from leiomyosarcomas.[709-712]

Isolated examples of ovarian *pheochromocytoma*[708] and *hydatidiform mole*[713] have also been described. *Adenomatoid tumors* can occur in an intra- or juxta-ovarian location; they can simulate the appearance of yolk sac tumor.[714]

Metastatic tumors

The ovary is a common site of involvement for metastases. About 7% of lesions presenting clinically as primary ovarian tumors are of metastatic origin. Over half are bilateral. The most common sources are the stomach, large bowel, appendix, breast, uterus (corpus and cervix), lung,[742] and skin (melanoma)* (Fig. 19-216). The difficult situation resulting from the simultaneous presence of carcinoma in ovary and uterus is discussed on p. 1489. Metastatic carcinomas from the breast tend to be small (often microscopic) and may be found incidentally in specimens from therapeutic oophorectomies. Most have either an Indian file or ductal pattern of growth.[720] Immunoreactivity for GCDFP-15 is the rule, a fact of importance in the differential diagnosis with primary ovarian carcinoma, which is generally negative.[728]

Appendiceal tumors may have the appearance of mucinous adenocarcinoma or adenocarcinoid.[727] Those from the large bowel are particularly prone to be mistaken for primary ovarian carcinoma of the mucinous or endometrioid type.[716,731] Many are cystic, well differentiated, and mucin producing, associated with necrosis and hemorrhage. They tend to rupture spontaneously or at the time of the operation. The primary tumors are always advanced (Dukes' B or C). In some cases, the ovarian metastases are associated with luteinization of the surrounding stroma, which may lead to masculinization and other endocrine changes.[730] The most characteristic features are garland and cribriform growth

---

*References 717, 719, 726, 731, 736, 746, 747.

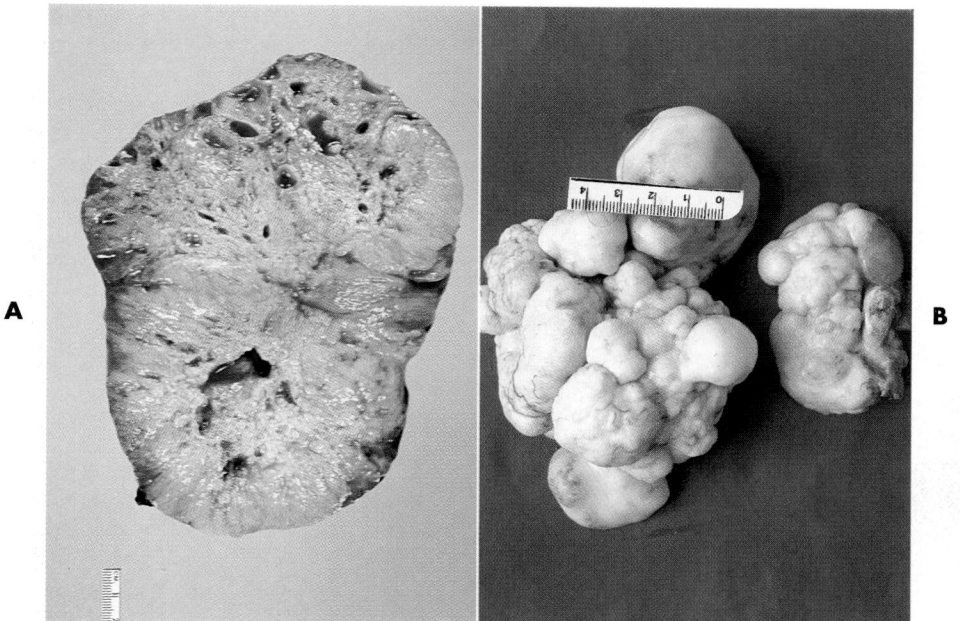

Fig. 19-216 Carcinoma metastatic to ovary. **A,** Metastatic colonic carcinoma. **B,** Metastatic mammary lobular carcinoma. The multinodular quality of the ovarian metastasis is typical of Krukenberg tumor.

patterns, intraluminal ("dirty") necrosis, segmental destruction of glands, and lack of squamous metaplasia.[716,724] Mucin stains have not been found helpful in distinguishing them from primary mucinous neoplasms. Conversely, immunostains for keratins 7 and 20 have been found to be of value in that they are often positive in metastatic adenocarcinomas but not in primary carcinomas.[732a]

Metastatic carcinoid tumors to the ovary are discussed on p. 1502. Small cell (neuroendocrine) carcinomas from the lung, gastrointestinal tract, thymus, and other sites can metastasize to the ovary; these should be distinguished from primary small cell carcinoma associated with hypercalcemia and (with much more difficulty) from the "pulmonary" type of primary ovarian small cell carcinoma (see p. 1513).[718]

The eponym ***Krukenberg tumor*** is used to designate an ovarian neoplasm, usually bilateral and nearly always of metastatic origin, characterized grossly by moderate solid multinodular enlargement of the ovaries and microscopically by a diffuse infiltration by signet ring cells containing abundant neutral and acidic (sialo-)mucins[725,734,735] (Figs. 19-216, *B,* and 19-217). Tumor emboli are found in over half of the cases.[722] Marked stromal proliferation with storiform pattern of growth and variable degree of luteinization are common and may obscure the diagnosis.[735] Another difficult problem is represented by the variant of this tumor referred to as *tubular,* in which a prominent tubular pattern, stromal luteinization, and occasional associated virilization may lead to a mistaken diagnosis of Sertoli–Leydig cell tumor[715]; the presence of typical mucin-positive signet ring cells should point toward the correct diagnosis.

Most examples of Krukenberg tumors occur after the age of 40 years, but younger patients can also be affected. In the latter instance, a mistaken diagnosis of granulosa cell tumor or lipid cell tumor is often made.

The usual primary sources are stomach (by far the most common), large bowel, and breast.[722,732] The ovarian deposits can be accompanied by retroperitoneal lymph node metastases and peritoneal implants.

Exceptionally, an extraovarian primary tumor is not found at autopsy in a patient harboring a Krukenberg tumor. In such an instance, the lesion is assumed to be primary in the ovary.[723] Before such an occurrence is accepted, a meticulous gross and microscopic study of the gastrointestinal tract, breast, and other organs should be carried out.[722] In the only case that we were almost ready to accept as primary Krukenberg tumor of the ovaries, a random section through a grossly unremarkable gastric antrum revealed diffuse infiltration by signet ring cells. It should be emphasized here that the diagnosis of Krukenberg tumor requires the histochemical identification of intracytoplasmic mucin, inasmuch as signet ring cells (negative with mucicarmine stains) are occasionally seen in other ovarian conditions.[729]

Other tumors that can metastasize to the ovary and give rise to difficult diagnostic problems are pancreatobiliary carcinomas (which can simulate mucinous tumors),[739,744] renal cell carcinoma (which mimics ovarian clear cell adenocarcinoma),[740] thyroid carcinoma (which can be confused with struma ovarii),[741] hepatocellular carcinoma and hepatoblastoma (not to be mistaken for hepatoid yolk sac tumor or hepatoid carcinoma),[721,738] intra-abdominal desmoplastic small cell tumor,[737,747a] and a variety of sarcomas, including alveolar rhabdomyosarcoma, leiomyosarcoma, and chordoma.[743,745,748] We have also seen three cases of ovarian metastases from malignant thymoma.

Malignant melanomas are usually easy to recognize because of their pigmentation, nodular pattern of growth, and cytologic features; however, some can be confused with primary ovarian tumors (particularly juvenile granulosa cell

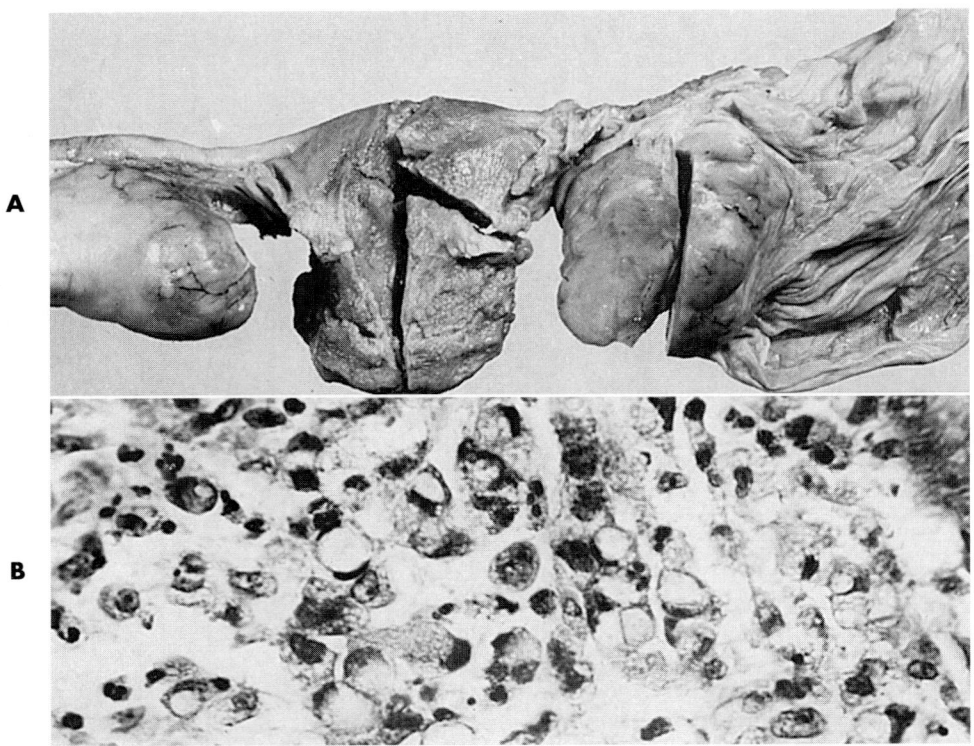

Fig. 19-217 A, Bilateral metastatic carcinoma of ovary (Krukenberg tumor) appearing in young woman. Primary tumor was in stomach. **B,** Signet-ring cells in metastatic carcinoma (Krukenberg tumor) of ovary.

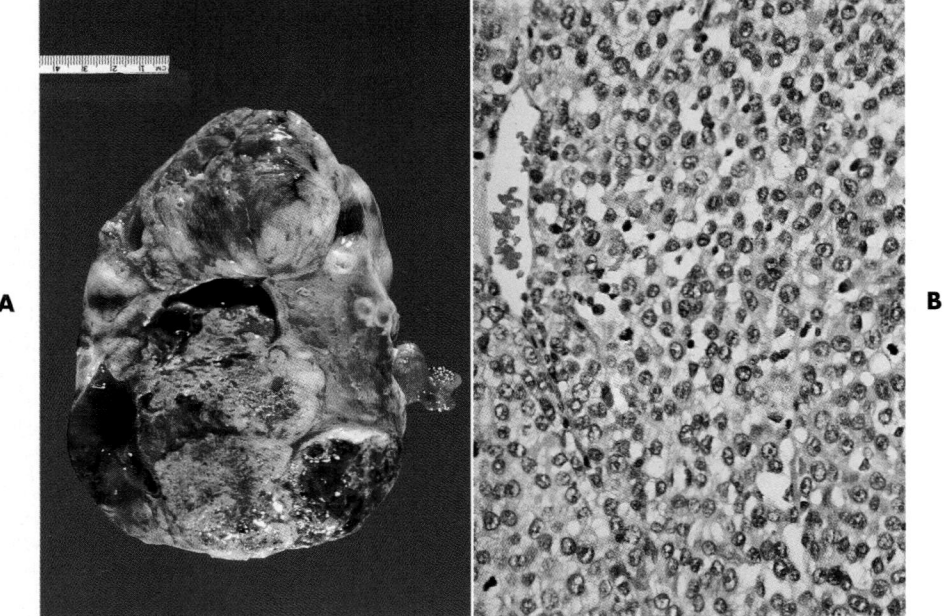

Fig. 19-218 Malignant melanoma metastatic to ovary. **A,** Gross appearance. **B,** Microscopic appearance. The homogeneous solid quality of the tumor may induce confusion with a primary sex-cord tumor.

tumor and small cell carcinoma) because of their tendency to form follicle-like spaces[746] (Fig. 19-218).

Not surprisingly, carcinoma metastatic to the ovary is associated with a very poor prognosis. Factors influencing survival in these patients are the site of the primary tumor, degree of differentiation, menstrual status, and type of treatment.[733]

REFERENCES
NORMAL ANATOMY

1 Boss JH, Scully RE, Wegner KH, Cohen RB: Structural variations in the adult ovary. Clinical significance. Obstet Gynecol **25**:747-764, 1965.
2 Clement PB: Histology of the ovary. Am J Surg Pathol **11**:277-303, 1987.
3 Czernobilsky B, Shezen E, Lifschitz-Mercer B, Fogel M, Luzon A, Jacob N, Skalli O, Gabbiani G: Alpha smooth muscle actin (alpha-SM actin) in normal human ovaries, in ovarian stromal hyperplasia and in ovarian neoplasms. Virchows Arch [Cell Pathol] **57**:55-61, 1989.
4 Fetissof F, Dubois MP, Heitz PU, Lansac J, Arbeille-Brassart B, Jobard P: Endocrine cells in the female genital tract. Int J Gynecol Pathol **5**:75-87, 1986.
5 Laffargue P, Benkoël L, Laffargue F, Casanova P, Chamlian A: Ultrastructural and enzyme histochemical study of ovarian hilar cells in women and their relationships with sympathetic nerves. Hum Pathol **9**:649-659, 1978.
6 Lastarria D, Sachdev RK, Babury RA, Yu HM, Nuovo GJ: Immunohistochemical analysis for desmin in normal and neoplastic ovarian stromal tissue. Arch Pathol Lab Med **114**:502-505, 1990.
7 Sasano H, Okamoto M, Mason JI, Simpson ER, Mendelson CR, Sasano N, Silverberg SG: Immunolocalization of aromatase, 17 alpha-hydroxylase and side-chain cleavage cytochromes P-450 in the human ovary. J Reprod Fertil **85**:163-169, 1989.
7a Sasano H, Sasano N: What's new in the localization of sex steroids in the human ovary and its tumors? Pathol Res Pract **185**:942-948, 1989.
8 Sternberg WH: The morphology, androgenic function, hyperplasia and tumors of the human ovarian hilus cells. Am J Pathol **25**:493-521, 1949.
9 Sternberg WH, Segaloff A, Gaskill CJ: Influence of chorionic gonadotrophin on human ovarian hilus cells (Leydig-like cells). J Clin Endocrinol **13**:139-153, 1953.
10 Visfeldt J, Starup J: Dating of the human corpus luteum of menstruation using histological parameters. Acta Pathol Microbiol Scand (A) **82**:137-144, 1974.

GONADAL DYSGENESIS

11 Clement PB, Young RH: Atypical polypoid adenomyoma of the uterus associated with Turner's syndrome. A report of three cases, including a review of "estrogen-associated" endometrial neoplasms and neoplasms associated with Turner's syndrome. Int J Gynecol Pathol **6**:104-113, 1987.
12 Federman DD: Abnormal sexual development. A genetic and endocrine approach to differential diagnosis. Philadelphia, 1967, W.B. Saunders Co.
13 Ferenczy A, Richart RM: The fine structure of the gonads in the complete form of testicular feminization syndrome. Am J Obstet Gynecol **113**:399-409, 1972.
14 Jones HW, Ferguson-Smith MA, Heller RH: The pathology and cytogenetics of gonadal agenesis. Am J Obstet Gynecol **87**:578-600, 1963.
15 Jones HW, Ferguson-Smith MA, Heller RH: Pathologic and cytogenetic findings in true hermaphroditism. Report of 6 cases and review of 23 cases from the literature. Obstet Gynecol **25**:435-447, 1962.
16 Males JL, Lain KC: Epithelioid sarcoma in XO/XX Turner's syndrome. Arch Pathol **94**:214-216, 1972.
17 Márquez-Monter H, Armendares S, Buentello L, Villegas J: Histopathologic study with cytogenetic correlation in 20 cases of gonadal dysgenesis. Am J Clin Pathol **57**:449-456, 1972.
18 McCarty KS Jr, Barton TK, Peete CH Jr, Creasman WT: Gonadal dysgenesis with adenocarcinoma of the endometrium. An electron microscopic and steroid receptor analyses with a review of the literature. Cancer **42**:512-520, 1978.
19 Morris JM: The syndrome of testicular feminization in male pseudohermaphrodites. Am J Obstet Gynecol **65**:1192-1211, 1953.
20 Neubecker RD, Theiss EA: Sertoli cell adenomas in patients with testicular feminization. Am J Clin Pathol **38**:52-59, 1962.
21 Radhakrishnan S, Sivaraman L, Natarajan PS: True hermaphrodite with multiple gonadal neoplasms. Report of a case with cytogenetic study. Cancer **42**:2726-2732, 1978.
22 Robboy SJ, Miller T, Donahoe PK, Jahre C, Welch WR, Haseltine FP, Miller WA, Atkins L, Crawford JD: Dysgenesis of testicular and streak gonads in the syndrome of mixed gonadal dysgenesis. Perspective derived from a clinico-pathologic analysis of twenty-one cases. Hum Pathol **13**:700-716, 1982.

23 Rutgers JL: Advances in the pathology of intersex conditions. Hum Pathol **22**:884-891, 1991.
24 Scully RE: Gonadal pathology of genetically determined diseases. Monogr Pathol **33**:257-285, 1991.
25 Sohval AR: The syndrome of pure gonadal dysgenesis. Am J Med **38**:615-625, 1965.
26 Taylor H, Barter RH, Jacobson CB: Neoplasms of dysgenetic gonads. Am J Obstet Gynecol **96**:816-823, 1966.

CYSTS, STROMAL HYPERPLASIA, AND OTHER NON-NEOPLASTIC LESIONS

27 Adelman S, Benson CD, Hertzler JH: Surgical lesions of the ovary in infancy and childhood. Surg Gynecol Obstet **141**:219-222, 1975.
28 Barnes RB, Rosenfield RL, Burstein S, Ehrmann DA: Pituitary-ovarian responses to nafarelin testing in the polycystic ovary syndrome. N Engl J Med **320**:559-565, 1989.
29 Blaustein A: Surface cells and inclusion cysts in fetal ovaries. Gynecol Oncol **12**:222-233, 1981.
30 Boss JH, Scully RE, Wegner KH, Cohen RB: Structural variations in the adult ovary—clinical significance. Obstet Gynecol **25**:747-764, 1965.
31 Bransilver BR, Ferenczy A, Richart RM: Female genital tract remnants. An ultra-structural comparison of hydatid of Morgagni and mesonephric ducts and tubules. Arch Pathol **96**:255-261, 1973.
32 Clement PB: Tumor-like lesions of the ovary associated with pregnancy. Int J Gynecol Pathol **12**:108-115, 1993.
33 Clement PB, Scully RE: Large solitary luteinized follicle cyst of pregnancy and puerperium. A clinicopathological analysis of eight cases. Am J Surg Pathol **4**:431-438, 1980.
34 Fechner RE, Kaufman RH: Endometrial adenocarcinoma in Stein-Leventhal syndrome. Cancer **34**:444-452, 1974.
34a Franks S: Polycystic ovary syndrome. N Engl J Med **333**:853-861, 1995.
35 Garcia-Bunuel R, Berek JS, Woodruff JD: Luteomas of pregnancy. Obstet Gynecol **45**:407-414, 1975.
36 Garcia-Bunuel R, Brandes D: Luteoma of pregnancy. Ultrastructural features. Hum Pathol **7**:205-214, 1976.
37 Gardner GH, Greene RR, Peckham B: Normal and cystic structures of broad ligament. Am J Obstet Gynecol **55**:917-939, 1948.
38 Goldzieher JW, Green JA: The polycystic ovary. I. Clinical and histologic features. J Clin Endocrinol **22**:325-338, 1962.
39 Hallatt JG, Steele CH Jr, Snyder M: Ruptured corpus luteum with hemoperitoneum. A study of 173 surgical cases. Am J Obstet Gynecol **149**:5-9, 1984.
40 Insler V, Lunenfeld B: Pathophysiology of polycystic ovarian disease. New insights. Hum Reprod **6**:1025-1029, 1991.
41 Jackson RL, Dockerty MB: The Stein-Leventhal syndrome. Analysis of 43 cases with special reference to association with endometrial carcinoma. Am J Obstet Gynecol **73**:161-173, 1957.
42 Judd HL, Scully RE, Herbst AL, Yen SSC, Ingersol FM, Kliman B: Familial hyperthecosis. Comparison of endocrinologic and histologic findings with polycystic ovarian disease. Am J Obstet Gynecol **117**:976-982, 1973.
43 Lee B, Gore BZ: A case of supernumerary ovary. Obstet Gynecol **64**:738-740, 1984.
44 Leventhal ML: Functional and morphologic studies of the ovaries and suprarenal glands in the Stein-Leventhal syndrome. Am J Obstet Gynecol **84**:154-164, 1962.
45 Lindsay AN, Voorhess ML, MacGillivray MH: Multicystic ovaries in primary hypothyroidism. Obstet Gynecol **61**:433-437, 1983.
46 Lucis OJ, Hobkirk R, Hollenberg CH, MacDonald SA, Blahey P: Polycystic ovaries associated with congenital adrenal hyperplasia. Can Med Assoc J **94**:1-7, 1966.
47 McKenna TJ: Pathogenesis and treatment of polycystic ovary syndrome. N Engl J Med **318**:558-562, 1988.
48 Morris JM, Scully RE: Endocrine pathology of the ovary. St. Louis, 1958, The C.V. Mosby Co.
49 Nogales FF, Silverberg SG: Epidermoid cysts of the ovary. A report of five cases with histogenetic considerations and ultrastructural findings. Am J Obstet Gynecol **124**:523-528, 1976.
50 Norris HJ, Taylor HB: Nodular theca-lutein hyperplasia of pregnancy (so-called "pregnancy luteoma"). Am J Clin Pathol **47**:557-566, 1967.
51 Ober WB, Grady HG, Schoenbucher AK: Ectopic ovarian decidua without pregnancy. Am J Pathol **33**:199-217, 1957.
52 Rodin A, Thakkar H, Taylor N, Clayton R: Hyperandrogenism in polycystic ovary syndrome. Evidence of dysregulation of 11ß-hydroxysteroid dehydrogenase. N Engl J Med **330**:460-465, 1994.

53   Rutgers JL, Scully RE: Cysts (cystadenomas) and tumors of the rete ovarii. Int J Gynecol Pathol **7:**330-342, 1988.

54   Sasano H, Fukunaga M, Rojas M, Silverberg SG: Hyperthecosis of the ovary. Clinicopathologic study of 19 cases with immunohistochemical analysis of steroidogenic enzymes. Int J Gynecol Pathol **8:**311-320, 1989.

55   Smyczek-Gargya B, Geppert M: Endometrial cancer associated with polycystic ovaries in young women. Pathol Res Pract **188:**946-948, 1992.

56   Sommers SC: Polycystic ovaries revisited. In Fenoglio CM, Wolfe M, eds: Progress in surgical pathology. New York, 1980, Masson Publishing USA, Inc., pp. 221-232.

57   Sternberg WH, Barclay DL: Luteoma of pregnancy. Am J Obstet Gynecol **95:**165-184, 1966.

58   Towne BH, Mahour GH, Woolley MM, Isaacs H: Ovarian cysts and tumors in infancy and childhood. J Pediatr Surg **10:**311-320, 1975.

59   Wajda KJ, Lucas JG, Marsh WL Jr: Hyperreactio luteinalis. Benign disorder masquerading as an ovarian neoplasm. Arch Pathol Lab Med **113:**921-925, 1989.

60   Young RH, Prat J, Scully RE: Epidermoid cyst of the ovary. A report of three cases with comments on histogenesis. Am J Clin Pathol **73:**272-276, 1980.

61   Zourlas PA, Jones HW Jr: Stein-Leventhal syndrome with masculinizing ovarian tumors. Report of 3 cases. Obstet Gynecol **34:**861-866, 1969.

INFLAMMATION

62   Bannatyne P, Russell P, Shearman RP: Autoimmune oophoritis. A clinicopathologic assessment of 12 cases. Int J Gynecol Pathol **9:**191-207, 1990.

63   Gloor E, Hurlimann J: Autoimmune oophoritis. Am J Clin Pathol **81:**105-109, 1984.

64   Herbold DR, Frable WJ, Kraus FT: Isolated noninfectious granulomas of the ovary. Int J Gynecol Pathol **2:**380-391, 1984.

65   Irvine WJ, Barnes EW: Addison's disease and autoimmune ovarian failure. J Reprod Fertil **21**(Suppl):1-31, 1974.

66   Lewis J: Eosinophilic perifolliculitis. A variant of autoimmune oophoritis. Int J Gynecol Pathol **12:**360-364, 1993.

67   Mostafa SAM, Bargeron CB, Flower RW, Rosenshein NB, Parmley TH, Woodruff JD: Foreign body granulomas in normal ovaries. Obstet Gynecol **66:**701-702, 1985.

68   Pace EH, Voet RL, Melancon JT: Xanthogranulomatous oophoritis. An inflammatory pseudotumor of the ovary. Int J Gynecol Pathol **3:**398-402, 1984.

ENDOMETRIOSIS

68a   Ballouk F, Ross JS, Wolf BC: Ovarian endometriotic cysts. An analysis of cytologic atypia and DNA ploidy patterns. Am J Clin Pathol **102:**415-419, 1994.

69   Clement PB: Pathology of endometriosis. Pathol Annu **25:**245-295, 1990.

70   Clement PB, Young RH, Scully RE: Necrotic pseudoxanthomatous nodules of ovary and peritoneum in endometriosis. Am J Surg Pathol **12:**390-397, 1988.

71   Czernobilsky B, Morris WJ. A histologic study of ovarian endometriosis with emphasis on hyperplastic and atypical changes. Obstet Gynecol **53:**318-323, 1979.

72   Devereux WP: Endometriosis. Long-term observation with particular reference to incidence of pregnancy. Obstet Gynecol **22:**444-450, 1963.

73   Fallon J. Brosnan JT. Moran WG: Endometriosis. N Engl J Med **235:**669-673. 1946.

74   La Grenade A. Silverberg SG: Ovarian tumors associated with atypical endometriosis. Hum Pathol **19:**1080-1084, 1988.

75   Olive DL, Schwartz LB: Endometriosis. N Engl J Med **328:**1759-1769, 1993.

76   Pratt JH, Shamblin WR: Spontaneous rupture of endometrial cysts of the ovary presenting as an acute abdominal emergency. Am J Obstet Gynecol **108:**56-62, 1970.

77   Young RH, Scully RE: Ovarian pathology of infertility. Monogr Pathol **33:**104-139, 1991.

OVARIAN BIOPSY

78   Mori T: Histological and histochemical studies of human anovulatory ovaries correlated with endocrinological analysis. Acta Obstet Gynaecol Jpn **16:**156-164, 1969.

79   Reber RW, Erickson GF, Coulam CB: Premature ovarian failure. In Gondos B, Riddick DH, eds: Pathology of infertility; clinical correlations in the male and female. New York, 1987, Thieme Medical Publishers, Inc., pp. 123-141.

80   Russell P, Bannatyne P, Shearman RP, Fraser IS, Corbett P: Premature hypergonadotropic ovarian failure. Clinicopathological study of 19 cases. Int J Gynecol Pathol **1:**185-201, 1982.

81   Steele SJ, Beilbui JOW, Papadaki L: Visualization and biopsy of the ovary in the investigation of amenorrhea. Obstet Gynecol **36:**899-902, 1970.

82   Stevenson CS: The ovaries in infertile women. A clinical and pathologic study of 81 women having ovarian surgery at laparotomy. Fertil Steril **21:**411-425, 1970.

TUMORS
Classification

83   Fox H, Langley FA: Tumours of the ovary. London, 1976, William Heinemann Medical Books Ltd.

84   Gillman J: The development of the gonads in man, with a consideration of the role of fetal endocrines and the histogenesis of ovarian tumors. Contrib Embryol **32:**83-131, 1948 (Carnegie Institute of Washington).

85   Godwin AK, Testa JR, Hamilton TC: The biology of ovarian cancer development. Cancer **71**(Suppl 2):530-536, 1993.

86   Scully RE: Tumors of the ovary and maldeveloped gonads. In Atlas of tumor pathology, Second Series, Fasc. 16. Washington, D.C., 1979, Armed Forces Institute of Pathology.

87   Teilum G: Classification of ovarian tumours. Acta Obstet Gynecol Scand **31:**292-312, 1952.

88   Van Wagenen G, Simpson ME: Embryology of the ovary and testis, *Homo sapiens* and *Macaca mulatta.* New Haven, 1965, Yale University Press.

89   Witschi E: Migration of the germ cells of human embryos from the yolk sac to the primitive gonadal folds. Contrib Embryol **32:**69-80, 1948 (Carnegie Institute of Washington).

Surface epithelial tumors

90   Addis BJ, Fox H: Papillary mesothelioma of ovary. Histopathology **7:**287-298, 1983.

91   Bell DA: Ovarian surface epithelial-stromal tumors. Hum Pathol **22:**750-762, 1991.

92   Blaustein A: Peritoneal mesothelium and ovarian surface cells—shared characteristics. Int J Gynecol Pathol **3:**361-375, 1984.

93   Clement PB: Histology of the ovary. Am J Surg Pathol **11:**277-303, 1987.

94   Colgan TJ, Norris HJ: Ovarian epithelial tumors of low malignant potential. A review. Int J Gynecol Pathol **1:**367-382, 1983.

95   Cramer SF, Roth LM, Mills SE, Ulbright TM, Gersell DJ, Nunez CA, Kraus FT: Sources of variability in classifying common ovarian cancers using the World Health Organization classification. Application of the pathtracking method. Pathol Annu **28**(Pt 2):243-286, 1993.

96   Cramer SF, Roth LM, Ulbright TM, Mazur MT, Nunez CA, Gersell DJ. Mills SE, Kraus FT: Evaluation of the reproducibility of the World Health Organization classification of common ovarian cancers. With emphasis on methodology. Arch Pathol Lab Med **111:**819-829, 1987.

97   Gusberg SB, Deligdisch L: Ovarian dysplasia. A study of identical twins. Cancer **54:**1-4, 1984.

97a   Hutson R, Ramsdale J, Wells M: p53 protein expression in putative precursor lesions of epithelioid ovarian cancer. Histopathology **27:**367-371, 1995.

98   Nouwen EJ, Pollet DE, Schelstraete JB, Eerdekens MW, Hansch C, Van de Voorde A, De Broe ME: Human placental alkaline phosphatase in benign and malignant ovarian neoplasia. Cancer Res **45:**892-902, 1985.

99   Russell P: Common epithelial tumours of the ovary—a new look. Pathology **17:**555-557, 1985.

100   Rutgers JL, Scully RE: Ovarian mixed-epithelial papillary cystadenomas of borderline malignancy of Müllerian type. A clinicopathologic analysis. Cancer **61:**546-554, 1988.

101   Scully RE: Ovary. In Henson DE, Albores-Saavedra J, eds: The pathology of incipient neoplasia. Philadelphia, 1986, W.B. Saunders Co., pp. 279-293.

102   Silva EG, Tornos C, Bailey MA, Morris M: Undifferentiated carcinoma of the ovary. Arch Pathol Lab Med **115:**377-381, 1991.

103   van Niekerk CC, Boerman OC, Ramaekers FC, Poels LG: Marker profile of different phases in the transition of normal human ovarian epithelium to ovarian carcinomas. Am J Pathol **138:**455-463, 1991.

Serous tumors

104   Al-Timimi A, Buckley CH, Fox H: An immunohistochemical study of the incidence and significance of sex steroid hormone binding sites in normal and neoplastic human ovarian tissue. Int J Gynecol Pathol **4:**24-41, 1985.

105   Bell DA, Scully RE: Ovarian serous borderline tumors with stromal microinvasion. A report of 21 cases. Hum Pathol **21:**397-403, 1990.

106   Bosscher J, Barnhill D, O'Connor D, Doering D, Nash J, Park R: Osseous metaplasia in ovarian papillary serous cystadenocarcinoma. Gynecol Oncol **39:**228-231, 1990.

107   Cajigas HE, Fariza E, Scully RE, Thor AD: Enhancement of tumor-associated glycoprotein-72 antigen expression in hormone-related ovarian serous borderline tumors. Cancer **68:**348-354, 1991.

108   Campo E, Merino MJ, Tavassoli FA, Charonis AS, Stetler-Stevenson WG, Liotta LA: Evaluation of basement membrane components and the 72 kDa type IV collagenase in serous tumors of the ovary. Am J Surg Pathol **16:**500-507, 1992.

109 Chadha S, Rao BR, Slotman BJ, van Vroonhoven CC, van der Kwast TH: An immunohistochemical evaluation of androgen and progesterone receptors in ovarian tumors. Hum Pathol **24**:90-95, 1993.

110 Charpin C, Bhan AK, Zurawski VR Jr, Scully RE: Carcinoembryonic antigen (CEA) and carbohydrate determinant 19-9 (CA 19-9) localization in 121 primary and metastatic ovarian tumors. An immunohistochemical study with the use of monoclonal antibodies. Int J Gynecol Pathol **1**:231-245. 1982.

111 Colgan TJ, Norris HJ: Ovarian epithelial tumors of low malignant potential. A review. Int J Gynecol Pathol **1**:367-382, 1983.

112 Compton HL, Finck FM: Serous adenofibroma and cystadenofibroma of the ovary. Obstet Gynecol **36**:636-645, 1970.

113 Czernobilsky B, Bornstein R, Lancet M: Cystadenofibroma of the ovary. A clinicopathologic study of 34 cases and comparison with serous cystadenoma. Cancer **34**:1971-1981, 1974.

114 Fenoglio CM: Ultrastructural features of the common epithelial tumors of the ovary. Ultrastruct Pathol **1**:419-444, 1980.

115 Ferenczy A, Talens M, Zoghby M, Hussain SS: Ultrastructural studies on the morphogenesis of psammoma bodies in ovarian serous neoplasia. Cancer **39**:2451-2459, 1977.

116 Ferguson AM, Fox H. A study of the Ca antigen in epithelial tumours of the ovary. J Clin Pathol **37**:6-9, 1984.

117 Gilks CB, Bell DA, Scully RE: Serous psammocarcinoma of the ovary and peritoneum. Int J Gynecol Pathol **9**:110-121, 1990.

118 Gooneratne S, Sassone M, Blaustein A, Talerman A: Serous surface papillary carcinoma of the ovary. A clinicopathologic study of 16 cases. Int J Gynecol Pathol **1**:258-269, 1982.

119 Hanselaar AG, Vooijs GP, Mayall B, Ras-Zeijlmans GJ, Chadha-Ajwani S: Epithelial markers to detect occult microinvasion in serous ovarian tumors. Int J Gynecol Pathol **12**:20-27, 1993.

120 Harding M, Cowan S, Hole D, Cassidy L, Kitchener H, Davis J, Leake R: Estrogen and progesterone receptors in ovarian cancer. Cancer **65**:486-491, 1990.

121 Hytiroglou P, Harpaz N, Heller DS, Zhiyuan L, Deligdisch L, Gil J: Differential diagnosis of borderline and invasive serous cystadenocarcinomas of the ovary by computerized interactive morphometric analysis of nuclear features. Cancer **69**:988-992, 1992.

122 Kabawat SE, Bast RC Jr, Welch WR, Knapp RC, Bhan AK: Expression of major histocompatibility antigens and nature of inflammatory cellular infiltrate in ovarian neoplasms. Int J Cancer **32**:547-554, 1983.

123 Kao GF, Norris HJ: Cystadenofibromas of the ovary with epithelial atypia. Am J Surg Pathol **2**:357-363, 1978.

124 Katzenstein AL, Mazur MT, Morgan TE, Kao MS: Proliferative serous tumors of the ovary. Histologic features and prognosis. Am J Surg Pathol **2**:339-355, 1978.

125 Koelma IA, Nap M, Rodenburg GJ, Fleuren GJ: The value of tumour marker CA 125 in surgical pathology. Histopathology **11**:287-294, 1987.

126 Komitowski D, Janson C, Szamaborski J, Czernobilsky B: Quantitative nuclear morphology in the diagnosis of ovarian tumors of low malignant potential (borderline). Cancer **64**:905-910, 1989.

127 Lin M, Hanai J, Wada A, Ozaki M, Nasu K, Okamoto S, Matsumoto K: S-100 protein in ovarian tumors. A comparative immunohistochemical study of 135 cases. Acta Pathol Jpn **41**:233-239, 1991.

128 Mariani-Costantini R, Agresti R, Colnaghi MI, Menard S: Characterization of the specificity by immunohistology of a monoclonal antibody to a novel epithelial antigen of ovarian carcinomas. Pathol Res Pract **180**:169-180, 1985.

129 Mettler L, Radzun HJ, Salmassi A, Kochling W, Parwaresch MR: Six new monoclonal antibodies to serous, mucinous, and poorly differentiated ovarian adenocarcinomas. Cancer **65**:1525-1532, 1990.

130 Miettinen M, Lehto V-P, Virtanen I: Expression of intermediate filaments in normal ovaries and ovarian epithelial, sex cord-stromal, and germinal tumors. Int J Gynecol Pathol **2**:64-71, 1983.

131 Mohabeer J, Buckley CH, Fox H: An immunohistochemical study of the incidence and significance of human chorionic gonadotrophin synthesis by epithelial ovarian neoplasms. Gynecol Oncol **16**:78-84, 1983.

132 Moll R, Pitz S, Levy R, Weikel W, Franke WW, Czernobilsky B: Complexity of expression of intermediate filament proteins, including glial filament protein, in endometrial and ovarian adenocarcinomas. Hum Pathol **22**:989-1001, 1991.

133 Mulhollan TJ, Silva EG, Tornos C, Guerrieri C, Fromm GL, Gershenson D: Ovarian involvement by serous surface papillary carcinoma. Int J Gynecol Pathol **13**:120-126, 1994.

134 Rice LW, Berkowitz RS, Mark SD, Yavner DL, Lage JM: Epithelial ovarian tumors of borderline malignancy. Gynecol Oncol **39**:195-198, 1990.

135 Sasano H, Saito Y, Nagura H, Kudo R, Rojas M, Silverberg SG: Lectin histochemistry in mucinous and serous ovarian neoplasms. Int J Gynecol **10**:252-259, 1991.

136 Schwartz PE, LiVolsi VA, Hildreth N, MacLusky NJ, Naftolin FN, Eisenfeld AJ: Estrogen receptors in ovarian epithelial carcinoma. Obstet Gynecol **59**:229-238, 1982.

136a Tan LK, Flynn SD, Carcangiu ML: Ovarian serous borderline tumors with lymph node involvement. Clinicopathologic and DNA content study of seven cases and review of the literature. Am J Surg Pathol **18**:904-912, 1994.

137 Ueda G, Yamasaki M, Inoue M, Tanaka Y, Abe Y, Ogawa M: Immunohistochemical study of amylase in common epithelial tumors of the ovary. Int J Gynecol Pathol **4**:240-244, 1985.

138 Ulbright TM, Roth LM: Common epithelial tumors of the ovary. Proliferating and of low malignant potential. Semin Diagn Pathol **2**:2-15, 1985.

139 Ulbright TM, Roth LM, Sutton GP: Papillary serous carcinoma of the ovary with squamous differentiation. Int J Gynecol Pathol **9**:86-94, 1990.

140 Van Kley H, Cramer S, Bruns DE: Serous ovarian neoplastic amylase (SONA). A potentially useful marker for serous ovarian tumors. Cancer **48**:1444-1449, 1981.

141 White PF, Merino MJ, Barwick KW: Serous surface papillary carcinoma of the ovary. A clinical, pathologic, ultrastructural, and immunohistochemical study of 11 cases. Pathol Annu **20**(Pt 1):403-418, 1985.

Mucinous tumors

142 Aguirre P, Scully RE, Dayal Y, DeLellis RA: Mucinous tumors of the ovary with argyrophil cells. An immunohistochemical analysis. Am J Surg Pathol **8**:345-356, 1984.

143 Baergen RN, Rutgers JL: Mural nodules in common epithelial tumors of the ovary. Int J Gynecol Pathol **13**:62-72, 1994.

144 Bell DA: Mucinous adenofibromas of the ovary. A report of 10 cases. Am J Surg Pathol **15**:227-232, 1991.

145 Bhagavan BS, Slavin RE, Goldberg J, Rao RN: Ectopic gastrinoma and Zollinger-Ellison syndrome. Hum Pathol **17**:584-592, 1986.

146 Chaitin BA, Gershenson DM, Evans HL: Mucinous tumors of the ovary. A clinicopathologic study of 70 cases. Cancer **55**:1958-1962, 1985.

147 Charpin C, Bhan AK, Zurawski VR, Scully RE: Carcinoembryonic antigen (CEA) and carbohydrate determinant 19-9 (CA 19-9) localization in 121 primary and metastatic ovarian tumors. An immunohistochemical study with the use of monoclonal antibodies. Int J Gynecol Pathol **1**:231-245, 1982.

147a Cuatrecasas M, Matias-Guiu X, Prat J: Synchronous mucinous tumors of the appendix and the ovary associated with pseudomyxoma peritonei. A clinicopathologic study of six cases with comparative analysis of c-Ki-*ras*-mutations. Am J Surg Pathol (in press).

148 Czernobilsky B, Dgani R, Roth LM: Ovarian mucinous cystadenocarcinoma with mural nodule of carcinomatous derivation. A light and electron microscopic study. Cancer **51**:141-148, 1983.

149 de Nictolis M, Montironi R, Tommasoni S, Valli M, Pisani E, Fabris G, Prat J: Benign, borderline, and well-differentiated malignant intestinal mucinous tumors of the ovary. A clinicopathologic, histochemical, immunohistochemical, and nuclear quantitative study of 57 cases. Int J Gynecol Pathol **13**:10-21, 1994.

150 Enomoto T, Weghorst CM, Inoue M, Tanizawa O, Rice JM: K-*ras* activation occurs frequently in mucinous adenocarcinomas and rarely in other common epithelial tumors of the human ovary. Am J Pathol **139**:777-785, 1991.

151 Fenoglio CM, Ferenczy A, Richart RM: Mucinous tumors of the ovary. Ultrastructural studies of mucinous cystadenomas with histogenetic considerations. Cancer **36**:1709-1722, 1975.

152 Fernandez RN, Daly JM: Pseudomyxoma peritonei. Arch Surg **115**:409-414, 1980.

153 Griffin NR, Wells M: Immunolocalization of alpha-amylase in ovarian mucinous tumours. Int J Gynecol Pathol **9**:41-46, 1990.

153a Guerrieri C, Hogberg T, Wingren S, Fristedt S, Simonsen E, Boeryd B: Mucinous borderline and malignant tumors of the ovary. A clinicopathologic and DNA ploidy study of 92 cases. Cancer **74**:2329-2340, 1994.

154 Hart WR, Norris HJ: Borderline and malignant mucinous tumors of the ovary. Cancer **31**:1031-1045, 1973.

155 Kahn MA, Demopoulos RI: Mucinous ovarian tumors with pseudomyxoma peritonei. A clinicopathological study. Int J Gynecol Pathol **11**:15-23, 1992.

156 Klemi PJ: Pathology of mucinous ovarian cystadenomas. I. Argyrophil and argentaffin cells and epithelial mucosubstances. Acta Pathol Microbiol Scand (A) **86**:465-470, 1978.

157 Klemi PJ, Nevalainen TJ: Pathology of mucinous ovarian cystadenomas. II. Ultrastructural findings. Acta Pathol Microbiol Scand (A) **86**:471-481, 1978.

158 Lifschitz-Mercer B, Dgani R, Jacob N, Fogel M, Czernobilsky B: Ovarian mucinous cystadenoma with leiomyomatous mural nodule. Int J Gynecol Pathol **9**:80-85, 1990.

159 LiVolsi VA, Merino MJ, Schwartz PE: Coexistent endocervical adenocarcinoma and mucinous adenocarcinoma of ovary. A clinicopathologic study of four cases. Int J Gynecol Pathol **1**:391-402, 1983.

160 Louwerens JK, Schaberg A, Bosman FT: Neuroendocrine cells in cystic mucinous tumours of the ovary. Histopathology 7:389-398, 1983.

161 Matias-Guiu X, Aranda I, Prat J: Immunohistochemical study of sarcoma-like mural nodules in a mucinous cystadenocarcinoma of the ovary. Virchows Arch [A] 419:89-92, 1991.

162 Matias-Guiu X, Prat J: Ovarian tumors with functioning stroma. An immunohistochemical study of 100 cases with human chorionic gonadotropin monoclonal and polyclonal antibodies. Cancer 65:2001-2005, 1990.

163 Michael H, Sutton G, Roth LM: Ovarian carcinoma with extracellular mucin production. Reassessment of "pseudomyxoma ovarii et peritonei." Int J Gynecol Pathol 6:298-312, 1987.

164 Nichols GE, Mills SE, Ulbright TM, Czernobilsky B, Roth LM: Spindle cell mural nodules in cystic ovarian mucinous tumors. A clinicopathologic and immunohistochemical study of five cases. Am J Surg Pathol 15:1055-1062, 1991.

165 Prat J, Scully RE: Sarcomas in ovarian mucinous tumors. A report of two cases. Cancer 44:1327-1331, 1979.

166 Prat J, Scully RE: Ovarian mucinous tumors with sarcoma-like nodules. A report of seven cases. Cancer 44:1332-1344, 1979.

167 Prat J, Young RH, Scully RE: Ovarian mucinous tumors with foci of anaplastic carcinoma. Cancer 50:300-304, 1982.

168 Prayson RA, Hart WR, Petras RE: Pseudomyxoma peritonei. A clinicopathologic study of 19 cases with emphasis on site of origin and nature of associated ovarian tumors. Am J Surg Pathol 18:591-603, 1994.

169 Robboy SJ: Insular carcinoid of ovary associated with malignant mucinous tumors. Cancer 54:2273-2276, 1984.

169a Rutgers JL, Baergen RN: Mucin histochemistry of ovarian borderline tumors of mucinous and mixed-epithelial types. Mod Pathol 7:825-828, 1994.

170 Rutgers JL, Bell DA: Immunohistochemical characterization of ovarian borderline tumors of intestinal and mullerian types. Mod Pathol 5:367-371, 1992.

171 Rutgers JL, Scully RE: Ovarian Müllerian mucinous papillary cystadenomas of borderline malignancy. A clinicopathologic analysis. Cancer 61:340-348, 1988.

172 Sasaki E, Sasano N, Kimura N, Andoh N, Yajima A: Demonstration of neuroendocrine cells in ovarian mucinous tumors. Int J Gynecol Pathol 8:189-200, 1989.

173 Scully RE, Aguirre P, DeLellis RA: Argyrophilia, serotonin, and peptide hormones in the female genital tract and its tumors. Int J Gynecol Pathol 3:51-70, 1984.

174 Seidman JD, Elsayed AM, Sobin LH, Tavassoli FA: Association of mucinous tumors of the ovary and appendix. A clinicopathologic study of 25 cases. Am J Surg Pathol 17:22-34, 1993.

175 Shiozawa T, Tsukahara Y, Ishii K, Ota H, Nakayama J, Katsuyama T: Histochemical demonstration of gastrointestinal mucins in ovarian mucinous cystadenoma. Acta Pathol Jpn 42:104-110, 1992.

175a Siriaunkgul S, Robbins KM, McGowan L, Silverberg SG: Ovarian mucinous tumors of low malignant potential. A clinicopathologic study of 54 tumors of intestinal and Mullerian type. Int J Gynecol Pathol 14:198-208, 1995.

176 Sporrong B, Alumets J, Clase L, Falkmer S, Hakanson R, Ljungberg O, Sundler F: Neurohormonal peptide immunoreactive cells in mucinous cystadenomas and cystadenocarcinomas of the ovary. Virchows Arch [A] 392:271-280, 1981.

177 Szymanska K, Szamborski J, Miechowiecka N, Czerwinski W: Malignant transformation of mucinous ovarian cystadenomas of intestinal epithelial type. Histopathology 7:497-509, 1983.

178 Tenti P, Aguzzi A, Riva C, Usellini L, Zappatore R, Bara J, Samloff M, Solcia E: Ovarian mucinous tumors frequently express markers of gastric, intestinal, and pancreatobiliary epithelial cells. Cancer 69:2131-2142, 1992.

179 Tsujimura T, Kawano K: Rhabdomyosarcoma coexistent with ovarian mucinous cystadenocarcinoma. A case report. Int J Gynecol Pathol 11:58-62, 1992.

180 Watkin W, Silva EG, Gershenson DM: Mucinous carcinoma of the ovary. Pathologic prognostic factors. Cancer 69:208-212, 1992.

181 Woodruff JD, Perry H, Genadry R, Parmley T: Mucinous cystadenocarcinoma of the ovary. Obstet Gynecol 51:483-489, 1978.

182 Young RH, Gilks CB, Scully RE: Mucinous tumors of the appendix associated with mucinous tumors of the ovary and pseudomyxoma peritonei. A clinicopathological analysis of 22 cases supporting an origin in the appendix. Am J Surg Pathol 15:415-429, 1991.

183 Young RH, Scully RE: Mucinous ovarian tumors associated with mucinous adenocarcinomas of the cervix. A clinicopathological analysis of 16 cases. Int J Gynecol Pathol 7:99-111, 1988.

Endometrioid tumors

184 Aguirre P, Thor AD, Scully RE: Ovarian endometrioid carcinomas resembling sex cord-stromal tumors. An immunohistochemical study. Int J Gynecol Pathol 8:364-373, 1989.

185 Bell DA, Scully RE: Atypical and borderline endometrioid adenofibromas of the ovary. A report of 27 cases. Am J Surg Pathol 9:205-214, 1985.

186 Casper S, van Nagell JR Jr, Powell DF, Dubilier LD, Donaldson ES, Hanson MB, Pavlik EJ: Immunohistochemical localization of tumor markers in epithelial ovarian cancer. Am J Obstet Gynecol 149:154-158, 1984.

187 Corner GW Jr, Hu CY, Hertig AT: Ovarian carcinoma arising in endometriosis. Am J Obstet Gynecol 59:760-774, 1950.

188 Czernobilsky B: Endometrioid neoplasia of the ovary. A reappraisal. Int J Gynecol Pathol 1:203-210, 1982.

189 Czernobilsky B, Silverman BB, Mikuta JJ: Endometrioid carcinoma of the ovary. A clinicopathologic study of 75 cases. Cancer 26:1141-1152, 1970.

190 Helle M, Helin H, Ashorn P, Putkinen EL, Krohn K, Wahlstrom T: The expression of CEA, CA 19-9 and HMFG antigens in ovarian clear-cell and endometrioid carcinomas. Pathol Res Pract 188:74-77, 1992.

191 Hughesdon PE: Benign endometrioid tumours of the ovary and the müllerian concept of ovarian epithelial tumours. Histopathology 8:977-990, 1984.

192 Inoue M, Ueda G, Nakajima T: Immunohistochemical demonstration of neuron-specific enolase in gynecologic malignant tumors. Cancer 55:1686-1690, 1985.

193 Kim KR, Scully RE: Peritoneal keratin granulomas with carcinomas of endometrium and ovary and atypical polypoid adenomyoma of endometrium. A clinicopathological analysis of 22 cases. Am J Surg Pathol 14:925-932, 1990.

194 Kistner RW, Hertig AT: Primary adenoacanthoma of the ovary. Cancer 5:1134-1145, 1952.

195 Klemi PJ, Gronroos M: Endometrioid carcinoma of the ovary. Obstet Gynecol 53:572-579, 1979.

196 Kline RC, Wharton JT, Atkinson EN, Burke TW, Gershenson DM, Edwards CL: Endometrioid carcinoma of the ovary. Retrospective review of 145 cases. Gynecol Oncol 39:337-346, 1990.

197 Long ME, Taylor HC Jr: Endometrioid carcinoma of the ovary. Am J Obstet Gynecol 90:936-950, 1964.

198 Macko MB, Johnson LA: Primary squamous ovarian carcinoma. A case report and review of the literature. Cancer 52:1117-1119, 1983.

199 Mostoufizadeh M, Scully RE: Malignant tumors arising in endometriosis. Clin Obstet Gynecol 23:951-963, 1980.

200 Norris HJ: Proliferative endometrioid tumors and endometrioid tumors of low malignant potential of the ovary. Int J Gynecol Pathol 12:134-140, 1993.

200a Pitman MB, Young RH, Clement PB, Dickersin GR, Scully RE: Endometrioid carcinoma of the ovary and endometrium, oxyphilic cell type. A report of nine cases. Int J Gynecol Pathol 13:290-301, 1994.

201 Roth LM, Czernobilsky B, Langley FA: Ovarian endometrioid adenofibromatous and cystadenofibromatous tumors. Benign, proliferating, and malignant. Cancer 48:1838-1845, 1981.

202 Roth LM, Liban E, Czernobilsky B: Ovarian endometrioid tumors mimicking Sertoli and Sertoli–Leydig cell tumors. Sertoliform variant of endometrioid carcinoma. Cancer 50:1322-1331, 1984.

203 Rutgers JL, Young RH, Scully RE: Ovarian yolk sac tumor arising from an endometrioid carcinoma. Hum Pathol 18:1296-1299, 1987.

204 Tetu B, Silva EG, Gershenson DM: Squamous cell carcinoma of the ovary. Arch Pathol Lab Med 111:864-866, 1987.

205 Ueda G, Yamasaki M, Inoue M, Tanaka Y, Hiramatsu K, Inoue Y, Saito O, Nishino T, Kurachi K: Argyrophil cells in the endometrioid carcinoma of the ovary. Cancer 54:1569-1573, 1984.

206 Yetman TJ, Dudzinski MR: Primary squamous carcinoma of the ovary. A case report and review of the literature. Gynecol Oncol 34:240-243, 1989.

207 Young RH, Prat J, Scully RE: Ovarian endometrioid carcinomas resembling sex cord-stromal tumors. A clinicopathological analysis of 13 cases. Am J Surg Pathol 6:513-522, 1982.

208 Zaino RJ, Unger ER, Whitney C: Synchronous carcinomas of the uterine corpus and ovary. Gynecol Oncol 19:329-335, 1984.

Clear cell (mesonephroid) tumors

209 Brescia RJ, Dubin N, Demopoulos RI: Endometrioid and clear cell carcinoma of the ovary. Factors affecting survival. Int J Gynecol Pathol 8:132-138, 1989.

210 Crozier MA, Copeland LJ, Silva EG, Gershenson DM, Stringer CA: Clear cell carcinoma of the ovary. A study of 59 cases. Gynecol Oncol 35:199-203, 1989.

211 Czernobilsky B, Silverman BB, Enterline HT: Clear cell carcinoma of the ovary. A clinicopathologic analysis of pure and mixed forms and comparison with endometroid carcinoma. Cancer 25:762-772, 1970.

212 Kennedy AW, Biscotti CV, Hart WR, Tuason LJ: Histologic correlates of progression-free interval and survival in ovarian clear cell adenocarcinoma. Gynecol Oncol 50:334-338, 1993.

213 Klemi PJ, Meurman L, Gronroos M, Talerman A: Clear cell (mesonephroid) tumors of the ovary with characteristics resembling endodermal sinus tumor. Int J Gynecol Pathol 1:95-100, 1982.

214 Montag AG, Jenison EL, Griffiths CT, Welch WR, Lavin PT, Knapp RC: Ovarian clear cell carcinoma. A clinicopathologic analysis of 44 cases. Int J Gynecol Pathol **8**:85-96, 1989.

215 Norris HJ, Robinowitz M: Ovarian adenocarcinoma of mesonephric type. Cancer **28**:1074-1081, 1971.

216 Roth LM, Langley FA, Fox H, Wheeler JE, Czernobilsky B: Ovarian clear cell adenofibromatous tumors. Benign, of low malignant potential, and associated with invasive clear cell carcinoma. Cancer **53**:1156-1163, 1984.

217 Schiller W: Mesonephroma ovarii. Am J Cancer **35**:1-21, 1939.

218 Scully RE, Barlow JF: Mesonephroma of the ovary. Tumor of müllerian nature related to the endometrioid carcinoma. Cancer **20**:1405-1417, 1967.

219 Shevchuk MM, Winkler-Monsanto B, Fenoglio CM, Richart RM: Clear cell carcinoma of the ovary. A clinicopathologic study with review of the literature. Cancer **47**:1344-1351, 1981.

220 Young RH, Scully RE: Oxyphilic clear cell carcinoma of the ovary. A report of nine cases. Am J Surg Pathol **11**:661-667, 1987.

221 Zirker TA, Silva EG, Morris M, Ordonez NG: Immunohistochemical differentiation of clear-cell carcinoma of the female genital tract and endodermal sinus tumor with the use of alpha-fetoprotein and Leu-M1. Am J Clin Pathol **91**:511-514, 1989.

Brenner tumor and transitional cell carcinoma

222 Abell MR: Malignant Brenner tumors of the ovary. Cancer **10**:1263-1274, 1957.

223 Aguirre P, Scully RE, Wolfe HJ, DeLellis RA: Argyrophil cells in Brenner tumors. Histochemical and immunohistochemical analysis. Int J Gynecol Pathol **5**:223-234, 1986.

224 Austin RM, Norris HJ: Malignant Brenner tumor and transitional cell carcinoma of the ovary. A comparison. Int J Gynecol Pathol **6**:29-39, 1987.

225 Bransilver BR, Ferenczy A, Richart RM: Brenner tumors and Walthard cell nests. Arch Pathol **98**:76-86, 1974.

226 Ehrlich CE, Roth LM: The Brenner tumor. A clinicopathologic study of 75 cases. Cancer **27**:332-342, 1971.

227 Ganjei P, Nadji M, Penneys NS, Averette HE, Morales AR: Immunoreactive prekeratin in Brenner tumors of the ovary. Int J Gynecol Pathol **1**:353-358, 1983.

228 Hallgrimsson J, Scully RE: Borderline and malignant Brenner tumours of the ovary. A report of 15 cases. Acta Pathol Microbiol Scand **233**(Suppl):56-66, 1972.

229 Heller DS, Harpaz N, Breakstone B: Neoplasms arising in ectopic ovaries. A case of Brenner tumor in an accessory ovary. Int J Gynecol Pathol **9**:185-189, 1990.

230 Miles PA, Norris HJ: Proliferative and malignant Brenner tumors of the ovary. Cancer **30**:174-186, 1972.

231 Ming SC, Goldman H: Hormonal activity of Brenner tumors in postmenopausal women. Am J Obstet Gynecol **83**:666-673, 1962.

232 Moon S, Waxman M: Mixed ovarian tumor composed of Brenner and thyroid elements. Cancer **38**:1997-2001, 1976.

233 Robey SS, Silva EG, Gershenson DM, McLemore D, el-Naggar A, Ordonez NG: Transitional cell carcinoma in high-grade high-stage ovarian carcinoma. An indicator of favorable response to chemotherapy. Cancer **63**:839-847, 1989.

234 Roth LM, Czernobilsky B: Ovarian Brenner tumors. II. Malignant. Cancer **56**:592-601, 1985.

235 Roth LM, Dallenbach-Hellweg G, Czernobilsky B: Ovarian Brenner tumors. I. Metaplastic, proliferating, and of low malignant potential. Cancer **56**:582-591, 1985.

236 Roth LM, Gersell DJ, Ulbright TM: Ovarian Brenner tumors and transitional cell carcinoma. Recent developments. Int J Gynecol Pathol **12**:128-133, 1993.

237 Santini D, Gelli MC, Mazzoleni G, Ricci M, Severi B, Pasquinelli G, Pelusi G, Martinelli G: Brenner tumor of the ovary. A correlative histologic, histochemical, immunohistochemical, and ultrastructural investigation. Hum Pathol **20**:787-795, 1989.

238 Sasano H, Wargotz ES, Silverberg SG, Mason JI, Simpson ER: Brenner tumor of the ovary. Immunoanalysis of steroidogenic enzymes in 23 cases. Hum Pathol **20**:1103-1107, 1989.

239 Seldenrijk CA, Willig AP, Baak JPA, Kuhnel R, Rao BR, Burger CW, van der Harten JJ, Dijkhuizen GH, Meijer CJLM: Malignant Brenner tumor. A histologic, morphometrical, immunohistochemical, and ultrastructural study. Cancer **58**:754-760, 1986.

240 Shevchuk MM, Fenoglio CM, Richart RM: Histogenesis of Brenner tumors. I. Histology and ultrastructure. Cancer **46**:2607-2616, 1980.

241 Shevchuk MM, Fenoglio CM, Richart RM: Histogenesis of Brenner tumors. II. Histochemistry and CEA. Cancer **46**:2617-2622, 1980.

242 Silverberg SG: Brenner tumor of the ovary. A clinicopathologic study of 60 tumors in 54 women. Cancer **28**:588-596, 1971.

243 Svenes KB, Eide J: Proliferative Brenner tumor or ovarian metastases? A case report. Cancer **53**:2692-2697, 1984.

244 Young RH, Scully RE: Urothelial and ovarian carcinomas of identical cell types. Problems in interpretation. A report of three cases and review of the literature. Int J Gynecol Pathol **7**:197-211, 1988.

Mixed müllerian tumors

245 Barwick KW, LiVolsi VA: Malignant mixed mesodermal tumors of the ovary. A clinicopathologic assessment of 12 cases. Am J Surg Pathol **4**:37-42, 1980.

246 Boucher D, Tetu B: Morphologic prognostic factors of malignant mixed mullerian tumors of the ovary. A clinicopathologic study of 15 cases. Int J Gynecol Pathol **13**:22-28, 1994.

247 Clement PB, Scully RE: Extrauterine mesodermal (müllerian) adenosarcoma. A clinicopathologic analysis of five cases. Am J Clin Pathol **69**:276-283, 1978.

248 Dehner LP, Norris HJ, Taylor HB: Carcinosarcomas and mixed mesodermal tumors of the ovary. Cancer **27**:207-216, 1971.

249 Dictor M: Ovarian malignant mixed mesodermal tumor. The occurrence of hyaline droplets containing alpha-1-antitrypsin. Hum Pathol **13**:930-933, 1982.

250 Dictor M: Malignant mixed mesodermal tumor of the ovary. A report of 22 cases. Obstet Gynecol **65**:720-724, 1985.

251 Ehrmann RL, Weidner N, Welch WR, Gleiberman I: Malignant mixed mullerian tumor of the ovary with prominent neuroectodermal differentiation (teratoid carcinosarcoma). Int J Gynecol Pathol **9**:272-282, 1990.

252 Fenn ME, Abell MR: Carcinosarcoma of the ovary. Am J Obstet Gynecol **110**:1066-1074, 1971.

253 Morrow CP, d'Ablaing G, Brady LW, Blessing JA, Hreshchyshyn MM: A clinical and pathologic study of 30 cases of malignant mixed müllerian epithelial and mesenchymal ovarian tumors. A gynecologic oncology group study. Gynecol Oncol **18**:278-292, 1984.

254 Plaxe SC, Dottino PR, Goodman HM, Deligdisch L, Idelson M, Cohen CJ: Clinical features of advanced ovarian mixed mesodermal tumors and treatment with doxorubicin- and *cis*-platinum–based chemotherapy. Gynecol Oncol **37**:244-249, 1990.

Adenoid cystic and basaloid carcinomas

254a Eichhorn JH, Scully RE: "Adenoid cystic" and basaloid carcinomas of the ovary. Evidence for a surface epithelial lineage. A report of 12 cases. Mod Pathol **8**:731-740, 1995.

Ovarian carcinoma—overview
General and clinical features

255 Cannistra SA: Cancer of the ovary. N Engl J Med **329**:1550-1559, 1993.

256 Carter J, Fowler J, Carlson J, Carson L, Twiggs LB: Borderline and invasive epithelial ovarian tumors in young women. Obstet Gynecol **82**:752-756, 1993.

257 Greene MH, Clark JW, Blayney DW: The epidemiology of ovarian cancer. Semin Oncol **11**:209-226, 1984.

258 Greggi S, Genuardi M, Benedetti-Panici P, Cento R, Scambia G, Neri G, Mancuso S: Analysis of 138 consecutive ovarian cancer patients. Incidence and characteristics of familial cases. Gynecol Oncol **39**:300-304, 1990.

259 Harlow BL, Weiss NS, Roth GJ, Chu J, Daling JR: Case-control study of borderline ovarian tumors. Reproductive history and exposure to exogenous female hormones. Cancer Res **48**:5849-5852, 1988.

260 Heintz APM, Hacker NF, Lagasse LD: Epidemiology and etiology of ovarian cancer. A review. Obstet Gynecol **66**:127-135, 1985.

261 Lynch HT, Watson P, Bewtra C, Conway TA, Hippee CR, Kaur P, Lynch JF, Ponder BA: Hereditary ovarian cancer. Heterogeneity in age at diagnosis. Cancer **67**:1460-1466, 1991.

262 Markman M, Lewis JL Jr, Saigo P, Hakes T, Jones W, Rubin S, Reichman B, Barakat R, Curtin J, Almadrones L, et al: Epithelial ovarian cancer in the elderly. The Memorial Sloan-Kettering Cancer Center experience. Cancer **71**:634-637, 1993.

263 Miki Y, Swensen J, Shattuck-Eidens D et al: A strong candidate for the breast and ovarian cancer susceptibility gene BRCA1. Science **266**:66-71, 1994.

264 Piver MS, Baker TR, Jishi MF, Sandecki AM, Tsukada Y, Natarajan N, Mettlin CJ, Blake CA: Familial ovarian cancer. A report of 658 families from the Gilda Radner Familial Ovarian Cancer Registry, 1981-1991. Cancer **71**:582-588, 1993.

265 Piver MS, Baker TR, Piedmonte M, Sandecki AM: Epidemiology and etiology of ovarian cancer. Semin Oncol **18**:177-185, 1991.

266 Richardson GS, Scully RE, Nikrui N, Nelson JH: Common epithelial cancer of the ovary. N Engl J Med **312**:415-424, 474-483, 1985.

267 Rodriguez M, Nguyen HN, Averette HE, Steren AJ, Penalver MA, Harrison T, Sevin BU: National survey of ovarian carcinoma. XII. Epithelial ovarian malignancies in women less than or equal to 25 years of age. Cancer **73**:1245-1250, 1994.

267a Rossing MA, Daling JR, Weiss NS, Moore DE, Self SG: Ovarian tumors in a cohort of infertile women. N Engl J Med **331:**771-776, 1994.

268 Weiss NS: Measuring the separate effects of low parity and its antecedents on the incidence of ovarian cancer. Am J Epidemiol **128:**451-455, 1988.

269 Yancik R: Ovarian cancer. Age contrasts in incidence, histology, disease stage at diagnosis, and mortality. Cancer **71:**517-523, 1993.

"Early" and in situ carcinoma

270 Bell DA, Scully RE: Early de novo ovarian carcinoma. A study of fourteen cases. Cancer **73:**1859-1864, 1994.

271 Fox H: Pathology of early malignant change in the ovary. Int J Gynecol Pathol **12:**153-155, 1993.

272 Mittal KR, Zeleniuch-Jacquotte A, Cooper JL, Demopoulos RI: Contralateral ovary in unilateral ovarian carcinoma. A search for preneoplastic lesions. Int J Gynecol Pathol **12:**59-63, 1993.

273 Plaxe SC, Deligdisch L, Dottino PR, Cohen CJ: Ovarian intraepithelial neoplasia demonstrated in patients with stage I ovarian carcinoma. Gynecol Oncol **38:**367-372, 1990.

Special techniques

274 Berchuck A, Kohler MF, Boente MP, Rodriguez GC, Whitaker RS, Bast RC Jr: Growth regulation and transformation of ovarian epithelium. Cancer **71:**545-551, 1993.

275 Bosari S, Viale G, Radaelli U, Bossi P, Bonoldi E, Coggi G: p53 accumulation in ovarian carcinomas and its prognostic implications. Hum Pathol **24:**1175-1179, 1993.

276 Frank TS, Bartos RE, Haefner HK, Roberts JA, Wilson MD, Hubbell GP: Loss of heterozygosity and overexpression of the p53 gene in ovarian carcinoma. Mod Pathol **7:**3-8, 1994.

277 Huettner PC, Weinberg DS, Lage JM: Assessment of proliferative activity in ovarian neoplasms by flow and static cytometry. Correlation with prognostic features. Am J Pathol **141:**699-706, 1992.

278 Kacinski BM, Carter D, Mittal K, Yee LD, Scata KA, Donofrio L, Chambers SK, Wang KI, Yang-Feng T, Rohrschneider LR, et al: Ovarian adenocarcinomas express fms-complementary transcripts and fms antigen, often with coexpression of CSF-1. Am J Pathol **137:**135-147, 1990.

279 Kiechle-Schwarz M, Bauknecht T, Wienker T, Walz L, Pfleiderer A: Loss of constitutional heterozygosity on chromosome 11p in human ovarian cancer. Positive correlation with grade of differentiation. Cancer **72:**2423-2432, 1993.

280 Lage JM, Weinberg DS, Huettner PC, Mark SD: Flow cytometric analysis of nuclear DNA content in ovarian tumors. Association of ploidy with tumor type, histologic grade, and clinical stage. Cancer **69:**2668-2675, 1992.

281 Pejovic T, Heim S, Mandahl N, Baldetorp B, Elmfors B, Flodérus U-M, Furgyik S, Göran H, Himmelmann A, Willén H, Mitelman F: Chromosome aberrations in 35 primary ovarian carcinomas. Genes Chromosom Cancer **4:**58-68, 1992.

282 Persons DL, Hartmann LC, Herath JF, Borell TJ, Cliby WA, Keeney GL, Jenkins RB: Interphase molecular cytogenetic analysis of epithelial ovarian carcinomas. Am J Pathol **142:**733-741, 1993.

283 Slamon DJ, Godolphin W, Jones LA, Holt JA, Wong SG, Keith DE, Levin WJ, Stuart SG, Udove J, Ullrich A, et al: Studies of the HER-2/*neu* proto-oncogene in human breast and ovarian cancer. Science **244:**707-712, 1989.

284 Yang-Feng TL, Han H, Chen KC, Li SB, Claus EB, Carcangiu ML, Chambers SK, Chambers JT, Schwartz PE: Allelic loss in ovarian cancer. Int J Cancer **54:**546-551, 1993.

285 Yang-Feng TL, Li SB, Leung WY, Carcangiu ML, Schwartz PE: Trisomy 12 and K-*ras*-2 amplification in human ovarian tumors. Int J Cancer **48:**678-681, 1991.

Spread and metastases

286 Brustman L, Seltzer V: Sister Joseph's nodule. Seven cases of umbilical metastases from gynecologic malignancies. Gynecol Oncol **19:**155-162, 1984.

287 Dvoretsky PM, Richards KA, Bonfiglio TA: The pathology and biologic behavior of ovarian cancer. An autopsy review. Pathol Annu **24**(Pt 1):1-24, 1989.

288 Kerr VE, Cadman E: Pulmonary metastases in ovarian cancer. Analysis of 357 patients. Cancer **56:**1209-1213, 1985.

289 Loredo DS, Powell JL, Reed WP, Rosenbaum JM: Ovarian carcinoma metastatic to breast. A case report and review of the literature. Gynecol Oncol **37:**432-436, 1990.

290 Majmudar B, Wiskind AK, Croft BN, Dudley AG: The Sister (Mary) Joseph nodule. Its significance in gynecology. Gynecol Oncol **40:**152-159, 1991.

291 Rose PG, Piver MS, Tsukada Y, Lau TS: Metastatic patterns in histologic variants of ovarian cancer. An autopsy study. Cancer **64:**1508-1513, 1989.

292 Steinberg JJ, Demopoulos RI, Bigelow B: The evaluation of the omentum in ovarian cancer. Gynecol Oncol **24:**327-330, 1986.

Coexistence with uterine carcinoma

293 Eifel P, Hendrickson M, Ross J, Ballon S, Martinez A, Kempson R: Simultaneous presentation of carcinoma involving the ovary and the uterine corpus. Cancer **50:**163-170, 1982.

294 Kaminski PF, Norris HJ: Coexistence of ovarian neoplasms and endocervical adenocarcinoma. Obstet Gynecol **64:**553-556, 1984.

295 Prat J, Matias-Guiu X, Barreto J: Simultaneous carcinoma involving the endometrium and the ovary. A clinicopathologic, immunohistochemical, and DNA flow cytometric study of 18 cases. Cancer **68:**2455-2459, 1991.

296 Ulbright TM, Roth LM: Metastatic and independent cancers of the endometrium and ovary. A clinicopathologic study of 34 cases. Hum Pathol **16:**28-34, 1985.

297 Young RH, Gersell DJ, Roth LM, Scully RE: Ovarian metastases from cervical carcinomas other than pure adenocarcinomas. A report of 12 cases. Cancer **71:**407-418, 1993.

Related peritoneal lesions

298 August CZ, Murad TM, Newton M: Multiple focal extraovarian serous carcinoma. Int J Gynecol Pathol **4:**11-23, 1985.

299 Bell DA, Scully RE: Benign and borderline serous lesions of the peritoneum in women. Pathol Annu **24:**1-21, 1989.

300 Bell DA, Scully RE: Serous borderline tumors of the peritoneum. Am J Surg Pathol **14:**230-239, 1990.

301 Bell DA, Weinstock MA, Scully RE: Peritoneal implants of ovarian serous borderline tumors. Histologic features and prognosis. Cancer **62:**2212-2222, 1988.

302 Biscotti CV, Hart WR: Peritoneal serous micropapillomatosis of low malignant potential (serous borderline tumors of the peritoneum). A clinicopathologic study of 17 cases. Am J Surg Pathol **16:**467-475, 1992.

303 Bollinger DJ, Wick MR, Dehner LP, Mills SE, Swanson PE, Clarke RE: Peritoneal malignant mesothelioma versus serous papillary adenocarcinoma. A histochemical and immunohistochemical comparison. Am J Surg Pathol **13:**659-670, 1989.

304 Clement PB, Young RH: Florid mesothelial hyperplasia associated with ovarian tumors. A potential source of error in tumor diagnosis and staging. Int J Gynecol Pathol **12:**51-58, 1993.

305 Dalrymple JC, Bannatyne P, Russell P, Solomon HJ, Tattersall MH, Atkinson K, Carter J, Duval P, Elliott P, Friedlander M, et al: Extraovarian peritoneal serous papillary carcinoma. A clinicopathologic study of 31 cases. Cancer **64:**110-115, 1989.

306 Foyle A, Al-Jabi M, McCaughey WTE: Papillary peritoneal tumors in women. Am J Surg Pathol **5:**241-249, 1981.

307 Gershenson DM, Silva EG: Serous ovarian tumors of low malignant potential with peritoneal implants. Cancer **65:**578-585, 1990.

308 Khoury N, Raju U, Crissman JD, Zarbo RJ, Greenawald KA. A comparative immunohistochemical study of peritoneal and ovarian serous tumors, and mesotheliomas. Hum Pathol **21:**811-819, 1990.

309 Lauchlan SC: Non-invasive ovarian carcinoma. Int J Gynecol Pathol **9:**158-169, 1990.

310 Li S, Han H, Resnik E, Carcangiu ML, Schwartz PE, Yang-Feng TL: Advanced ovarian carcinoma. Molecular evidence of unifocal origin. Gynecol Oncol **51:**21-25, 1993.

311 McCaughey WTE: Papillary peritoneal neoplasms in females. Pathol Annu **20**(Pt 2):387-404, 1985.

312 McCaughey WTE, Kirk ME, Lester W, Dardick I: Peritoneal epithelial lesions associated with proliferative serous tumours of ovary. Histopathology **8:**195-208, 1984.

313 Michael H, Roth LM: Invasive and noninvasive implants in ovarian serous tumors of low malignant potential. Cancer **57:**1240-1247, 1986.

314 Piver MS, Jishi MF, Tsukada Y, Nava G: Primary peritoneal carcinoma after prophylactic oophorectomy in women with a family history of ovarian cancer. A report of the Gilda Radner Familial Ovarian Cancer Registry. Cancer **71:**2751-2755, 1993.

314a Rothacker D, Möbius G: Varieties of serous surface papillary carcinoma of the peritoneum in Northern Germany. A thirty-year autopsy study. Int J Gynecol Pathol **14:**310-318, 1995.

315 Segal GH, Hart WR: Ovarian serous tumors of low malignant potential (serous borderline tumors). The relationship of exophytic surface tumor to peritoneal "implants." Am J Surg Pathol **16:**577-583, 1992.

316 Warhol MJ, Hunter NJ, Corson JM: An ultrastructural comparison of mesotheliomas and adenocarcinomas of the ovary and endometrium. Int J Gynecol Pathol **1:**125-134, 1982.

317 Wick MR, Mills SE, Dehner LP, Bollinger DJ, Fechner RE: Serous papillary carcinomas arising from the peritoneum and ovaries. A clinicopathologic and immunohistochemical comparison. Int J Gynecol Pathol **8:**179-188, 1989.

318 Zinsser KR, Wheeler JE: Endosalpingiosis in the omentum. A study of autopsy and surgical material. Am J Surg Pathol **6:**109-117, 1982.

Cytology

319 Covell JL, Carry JB, Feldman PS: Peritoneal washings in ovarian tumors. Potential sources of error in cytologic diagnosis. Acta Cytol (Baltimore) **29:**310-316, 1984.

320 Yoshimura S, Scully RE, Bell DA, Taft PD: Correlation of ascitic fluid cytology with histologic findings before and after treatment of ovarian cancer. Am J Obstet Gynecol **148:**716-721, 1984.

321 Yoshimura S, Scully RE, Taft PD, Herrington JB: Peritoneal fluid cytology in patients with ovarian cancer. Gynecol Oncol **17:**161-167, 1984.

322 Ziselman EM, Harkavy SE, Hogan M, West W, Atkinson B: Peritoneal washing cytology. Uses and diagnostic criteria in gynecologic neoplasms. Acta Cytol (Baltimore) **28:**105-110, 1983.

Therapy

323 Averette HE, Donato DM: Ovarian carcinoma. Advances in diagnosis, staging, and treatment. Cancer **65:**703-708, 1990.

324 Barber HRK: Ovarian cancer. Diagnosis and management. Am J Obstet Gynecol **150:**910-916, 1984.

325 Burghardt E, Pickel H, Lahousen M, Stettner H: Pelvic lymphadenectomy in operative treatment of ovarian cancer. Am J Obstet Gynecol **155:**315-319, 1986.

326 Coffin CM, Adcock LL, Dehner LP: The second-look operation for ovarian neoplasms. A study of 85 cases emphasizing cytologic and histologic problems. Int J Gynecol Pathol **4:**97-109, 1985.

327 Dembo AJ: Radiotherapeutic management of ovarian cancer. Semin Oncol **11:**238-250, 1984.

328 Friedman JB, Weiss NS: Second thoughts about second-look laparotomy in advanced ovarian cancer. N Engl J Med **322:**1079-1082, 1990.

329 Helewa ME, Krepart GV, Lotocki R: Staging laparotomy in early epithelial ovarian carcinoma. Am J Obstet Gynecol **154:**282-286, 1986.

330 Lim-Tan SK, Cajigas HE, Scully RE: Ovarian cystectomy for serous borderline tumors. A follow-up study of 35 cases. Obstet Gynecol **72:**775-781, 1988.

331 Manivel JC, Wick MR, Coffin CM, Dehner LP: Immunohistochemistry in the differential diagnosis in the second-look operation for ovarian carcinomas. Int J Gynecol Pathol **8:**103-113, 1989.

332 McGuire WP: Primary treatment of epithelial ovarian malignancies. Cancer **71:**1541-1550, 1993.

333 Miller DS, Ballon SC, Teng NNH, Seifer DB, Soriero OM: A critical reassessment of second-look laparotomy in epithelial ovarian carcinoma. Cancer **57:**530-535, 1986.

334 Miller DS, Spirtos NM, Ballon SC, Cox RS, Soriero OM, Teng NN: Critical reassessment of second-look exploratory laparotomy for epithelial ovarian carcinoma. Minimal diagnostic and therapeutic value in patients with persistent cancer. Cancer **69:**502-510, 1992.

335 Ozols RF, Young RC: Chemotherapy of ovarian cancer. Semin Oncol **11:**251-263, 1984.

336 Podratz KC, Malkasian GD, Hilton JF, Harris EA, Gaffey TA: Second-look laparotomy in ovarian cancer. Evaluation of pathologic variables. Am J Obstet Gynecol **152:**230-238, 1985.

337 Richardson GS, Scully RE, Nikrui N, Nelson JH: Common epithelial cancer of the ovary. N Engl J Med **312:**415-424, 474-483, 1985.

338 Smirz LR, Stehman FB, Ulbright TM, Sutton GP, Ehrlich CE: Second-look laparotomy after chemotherapy in the management of ovarian malignancy. Am J Obstet Gynecol **152:**661-668, 1985.

339 Tazelaar HD, Bostwick DG, Ballon SC, Hendrickson MR, Kempson RL: Conservative treatment of borderline ovarian tumors. Obstet Gynecol **66:**417-422, 1985.

340 Thigpen JT, Lambuth BW, Vance RB: Management of stage I and II ovarian carcinoma. Semin Oncol **18:**596-602, 1991.

341 Young RC: Initial therapy for early ovarian carcinoma. Cancer **60:**2042-2049, 1987.

342 Young RC, Walton LA, Ellenberg SS, Homesley HD, Wilbanks GD, Decker DG, Miller A, Park R, Major F Jr: Adjuvant therapy in stage I and stage II epithelial ovarian cancer. Results of two prospective randomized trials. N Engl J Med **322:**1021-1027, 1990.

Prognosis

343 Beller U, Bigelow B, Beckman EM, Brown B, Demopoulos RI: Epithelial carcinoma of the ovary in the reproductive years. Clinical and morphological characterization. Gynecol Oncol **15:**422-427, 1983.

344 Bostwick DG, Tazelaar HD, Ballon SC, Hendrickson MR, Kempson RL: Ovarian epithelial tumors of borderline malignancy. A clinical and pathologic study of 109 cases. Cancer **58:**2052-2065, 1986.

345 Brescia RJ, Barakat RA, Beller U, Frederickson G, Suhrland MJ, Dubin N, Demopoulos RI: The prognostic significance of nuclear DNA content in malignant epithelial tumors of the ovary. Cancer **65:**141-147, 1990.

346 Demopoulos RI, Bigelow B, Blaustein A, Chait J, Gutman E, Dubin N: Characterization and survival of patients with serous cystadenocarcinoma of the ovaries. Obstet Gynecol **64:**557-563, 1984.

347 Erhardt K, Auer G, Bjorkholm E, Forsslund G, Moberger B, Silfversward C, Wicksell G, Zetterberg A: Combined morphologic and cytochemical grading of serous ovarian tumors. Am J Obstet Gynecol **151:**356-361, 1985.

348 Feichter GE, Kuhn W, Czernobilsky B, Muller A, Heep J, Abel U, Haag D, Kaufmann M, Rummel HH, Kubli F, Goerttler K: DNA flow cytometry of ovarian tumors with correlation to histopathology. Int J Gynecol Pathol **4:**336-345, 1985.

349 Hartmann LC, Podratz KC, Keeney GL, Kamel NA, Edmonson JH, Grill JP, Su JQ, Katzmann JA, Roche PC: Prognostic significance of p53 immunostaining in epithelial ovarian cancer. J Clin Oncol **12:**64-69, 1994.

350 Kurman RJ, Trimble CL: The behavior of serous tumors of low malignant potential. Are they ever malignant? Int J Gynecol Pathol **12:**120-127, 1993.

350a Levesque MA, Katsaros D, Yu H, Zola P, Sismondi P, Giardina G, Diamandis EP: Mutant p53 protein overexpression is associated with poor outcome in patients with well or moderately differentiated ovarian carcinoma. Cancer **75:**1327-1338, 1995.

351 Malkasian GD, Melton LJ, O'Brien PC, Greene MH: Prognostic significance of histologic classification and grading of epithelial malignancies of the ovary. Am J Obstet Gynecol **149:**274-284, 1984.

352 Meden H, Marx D, Rath W, Kron M, Fattahi-Meibodi A, Hinney B, Kuhn W, Schauer A: Overexpression of the oncogene c-*erb*B2 in primary ovarian cancer. Evaluation of the prognostic value in a Cox proportional hazards multiple regression. Int J Gynecol Pathol **13:**45-53, 1994.

353 Nikrui N: Survey of clinical behavior of patients with borderline epithelial tumors of the ovary. Gynecol Oncol **12:**107-119, 1981.

354 Price FV, Chambers SK, Chambers JT, Carcangiu ML, Schwartz PE, Kohorn EI, Stanley ER, Kacinski BM: Colony-stimulating factor-1 in primary ascites of ovarian cancer is a significant predictor of survival. Am J Obstet Gynecol **168:**520-527, 1993.

355 Rodenburg CJ, Cornelisse CJ, Heintz PAM, Hermans J, Fleuren GJ: Tumor ploidy as a major prognostic factor in advanced ovarian cancer. Cancer **59:**317-323, 1987.

356 Saksela E: Prognostic markers in epithelial ovarian cancer. Int J Gynecol Pathol **12:**156-161, 1993.

357 Sevelda P, Dittrich C, Salzer H: Prognostic value of the rupture of the capsule in stage I epithelial ovarian carcinoma. Gynecol Oncol **35:**321-322, 1989.

358 Sevelda P, Schemper M, Spona J: CA 125 as an independent prognostic factor for survival in patients with epithelial ovarian cancer. Am J Obstet Gynecol **161:**1213-1216, 1989.

359 Sorbe B, Frankendal BO: Prognostic importance of psammoma bodies in adenocarcinomas of the ovaries. Gynecol Oncol **14:**6-14, 1982.

360 Sorbe B, Frankendal BO, Veress B: Importance of histologic grading in the prognosis of epithelial ovarian carcinoma. Obstet Gynecol **59:**576-582, 1982.

361 Swenerton KD, Hislop TG, Spinelli J, LeRiche JC, Yang N, Boyes DA: Ovarian carcinoma. A multivariate analysis of prognostic factors. Obstet Gynecol **65:**264-270, 1985.

362 Thigpen T, Brady MF, Omura GA, Creasman WT, McGuire WP, Hoskins WJ, Williams S: Age as a prognostic factor in ovarian carcinoma. The Gynecologic Oncology Group experience. Cancer **71:**606-614, 1993.

362a Tornos C, Silva EG, Khorana SM, Burke TW: High-stage endometrioid carcinoma of the ovary. Prognostic significance of pure versus mixed histologic types. Am J Surg Pathol **18:**687-693, 1994.

363 Volm M, Kleine W, Pfleiderer A: Flow-cytometric prognostic factors for the survival of patients with ovarian carcinoma. A 5-year follow-up study. Gynecol Oncol **35:**84-89, 1989.

Ovarian tumors in children

364 Blom GP, Torkidensen EM: Ovarian cystadenocarcinoma in a 4-year-old girl. Report of a case and review of the literature. Gynecol Obstet **13:**242-246, 1982.

365 Breen JL, Neubecker RD: Ovarian malignancy in children with special reference to the germ cell tumors. Ann NY Acad Sci **142:**658-674, 1967.

366 Ein SH, Darte JMM, Stephens CA: Cystic and solid ovarian tumors in children. A 44-year review. J Pediatr Surg **5:**148-156, 1970.

367 Lack EE, Young RH, Scully RE: Pathology of ovarian neoplasms in childhood and adolescence. Pathol Annu **27**(Pt 2):281-356, 1992.

368 Morris HB, La Vecchia C, Draper GJ: Malignant epithelial tumors of the ovary in childhood. A clinicopathological study of 13 cases in Great Britain 1962-1978. Gynecol Oncol 19:290-297, 1984.

369 Morris HB, La Vecchia C, Draper GJ: Endodermal sinus tumor and embryonal carcinoma of the ovary in children. Gynecol Obstet 21:7-17, 1985.

370 Norris HJ, Jensen RD: Relative frequency of ovarian neoplasms in children and adolescents. Cancer 30:713-719, 1972.

371 Thompson JP, Dockerty MB, Symmonds RE, Hayles AB: Ovarian and para-ovarian tumors in infants and children. Am J Obstet Gynecol 97:1059-1065, 1967.

372 Wollner N, Exelby PR, Woodruff JM, Cham WC, Murphy L, Lewis JL: Malignant ovarian tumors in childhood. Prognosis in relation to initial therapy. Cancer 37:1953-1964, 1976.

373 Young RH, Kozakewich HP, Scully RE: Metastatic ovarian tumors in children. A report of 14 cases and review of the literature. Int J Gynecol Pathol 12:8-19, 1993.

374 Zaloudek C, Norris HJ: Granulosa tumors of the ovary in children. A clinical and pathologic study of 32 cases. Am J Surg Pathol 6:513-522, 1982.

Germ cell tumors

375 Gershenson DM: Update on malignant ovarian germ cell tumors. Cancer 71:1581-1590, 1993.

376 Gershenson DM, Del Junco G, Copeland LJ, Rutledge FN: Mixed germ cell tumors of the ovary. Obstet Gynecol 64:200-206, 1984.

377 Kurman RJ, Norris HJ: Malignant mixed germ cell tumors of the ovary. A clinical and pathologic analysis of 30 cases. Obstet Gynecol 48:579-589, 1976.

378 Kurman RJ, Norris HJ: Malignant germ cell tumors of the ovary. Hum Pathol 8:551-564, 1977.

379 Pfleiderer A: Therapy of ovarian malignant germ cell tumors and granulosa tumors. Int J Gynecol Pathol 12:162-165, 1993.

380 Young RH: New and unusual aspects of ovarian germ cell tumors. Am J Surg Pathol 17:1210-1224, 1993.

Dysgerminoma

381 Abell MR, Johnson VJ, Holtz F: Ovarian neoplasms in childhood and adolescence. Am J Obstet Gynecol 92:1059-1081, 1965.

382 Asadourian LA, Taylor HB: Dysgerminoma. An analysis of 105 cases. Obstet Gynecol 33:370-379, 1969.

383 Beckstead JH: Alkaline phosphatase histochemistry in human germ cell neoplasms. Am J Surg Pathol 7:341-349, 1983.

384 Bjorkholm E, Lundell M, Gyftodimos A, Silfversward C: Dysgerminoma. The Radiumhemmet series 1927-1984. Cancer 65:38-44, 1990.

385 Creasman WT, Fetter BF, Hammond CB, Parker RT: Germ cell malignancies of the ovary. Obstet Gynecol 53:226-230, 1979.

386 De Palo G, Pilotti S, Kenda R, Ratti E, Musumeci R, Mangioni C, Di Re F, Lattuada A, Conti U, Cefis F, Recanatini L, Carinelli S, Rossi G: Natural history of dysgerminoma. Am J Obstet Gynecol 143:799-807, 1982.

387 Dietl J, Horny HP, Ruck P, Kaiserling E: Dysgerminoma of the ovary. An immunohistochemical study of tumor-infiltrating lymphoreticular cells and tumor cells. Cancer 71:2562-2568, 1993.

388 Fleischhacker DS, Young RH: Dysgerminoma of the ovary associated with hypercalcemia. Gynecol Oncol 52:87-90, 1994.

389 Freel JH, Cassir JF, Pierce VK, Woodruff J, Lewis JL Jr: Dysgerminoma of the ovary. Cancer 43:798-805, 1979.

390 Gershenson DM: Update on malignant ovarian germ cell tumors. Cancer 71:1581-1590, 1993.

391 Gibas Z, Talerman A: Analysis of chromosome aneuploidy in ovarian dysgerminoma by flow cytometry and fluorescence in situ hybridization. Diagn Mol Pathol 2:50-56, 1993.

392 Gillespie JJ, Arnold LK: Anaplastic dysgerminoma. Cancer 42:1886-1889, 1978.

393 Gondos B: Comparative studies of normal and neoplastic ovarian germ cells. II. Ultrastructure and pathogenesis of dysgerminoma. Int J Gynecol Pathol 6:124-131, 1987.

394 Kay S, Silverberg SG, Schatzki PF: Ultrastructure of an ovarian dysgerminoma. Am J Clin Pathol 58:458-468, 1972.

395 Krepart G, Smith JP, Rutledge F, Delclos L: The treatment for dysgerminoma of the ovary. Cancer 41:986-990, 1978.

396 Lifshitz-Mercer B, Walt H, Kushnir I, Jacob N, Diener PA, Moll R, Czernobilsky B: Differentiation potential of ovarian dysgerminoma. An immunohistochemical study of 15 cases. Hum Pathol 26:62-66, 1995.

397 Malkasian GD, Symmonds RE: Treatment of the unilateral encapsulated ovarian germinoma. Am J Obstet Gynecol 90:379-382, 1964.

398 Morris JM, Scully RE: Endocrine pathology of the ovary. St. Louis, 1958, The C.V. Mosby Co.

399 Parkash V, Carcangiu ML: Transformation of ovarian dysgerminoma to yolk sac tumor. Evidence for a histogenetic continuum. Mod Pathol 8:881-887, 1995.

400 Santesson L: Clinical and pathological survey of ovarian tumors treated at the Radium-hemmet. Acta Radiol (Stockh) 28:643-668, 1947.

401 Zaloudek CJ, Tavassoli FA, Norris HJ: Dysgerminoma with syncytiotrophoblastic giant cells. A histologically and clinically distinctive subtype of dysgerminoma. Am J Surg Pathol 5:361-367, 1981.

Yolk sac tumor (endodermal sinus tumor) and embryonal carcinoma

402 Barsky SH, Hannah JB: Extracellular hyaline bodies are basement membrane accumulations. Am J Clin Pathol 87:455-460, 1987.

403 Cangir A, Smith J, van Eys J: Improved prognosis in children with ovarian cancers following modified VAC (vincristine sulfate, dactinomycin, and cyclophosphamide) chemotherapy. Cancer 42:1234-1238, 1978.

404 Clement PB, Young RH, Scully RE: Endometrioid-like variant of ovarian yolk sac tumor. A clinicopathological analysis of eight cases. Am J Surg Pathol 11:767-778, 1987.

405 Clement PB, Young RH, Scully RE: Extraovarian pelvic yolk sac tumors. Cancer 62:620-626, 1988.

406 Cohen MB, Friend DS, Molnar JJ: Gonadal endodermal sinus (yolk sac) tumor with pure intestinal differentiation. A new histologic type. Pathol Res Pract 182:609-616, 1987.

407 Creasman WT, Soper JT: Assessment of the contemporary management of germ cell malignancies of the ovary. Am J Obstet Gynecol 153:828-834, 1985.

408 Gershenson DM, Del Junco G, Herson J, Rutledge FN: Endodermal sinus tumor of the ovary. The M.D. Anderson experience. Obstet Gynecol 61:194-202, 1983.

409 Gonzalez-Crussi F: The human yolk sac and yolk sac (endodermal sinus) tumors. A review. Persp Pediatr Pathol 5:179-215, 1979.

410 Huntington RW, Bullock WK: Yolk sac tumors of the ovary. Cancer 25:1357-1367, 1970.

411 Ishikura H, Scully RE: Hepatoid carcinoma of the ovary. A newly described tumor. Cancer 60:2775-2784, 1987.

412 Jones MA, Clement PB, Young RH: Primary yolk sac tumors of the mesentery. A report of two cases. Am J Clin Pathol 101:42-47, 1994.

413 Kawai M, Furuhashi Y, Kano T, Misawa T, Nakashima N, Hattori S, Okamoto Y, Kobayashi I, Ohta M, Arii Y, et al: Alpha-fetoprotein in malignant germ cell tumors of the ovary. Gynecol Oncol 39:160-166, 1990.

414 Kawai M, Kano T, Furuhashi Y, Mizuno K, Nakashima N, Hattori SE, Kazeto S, Iida S, Ohta M, Arii Y, et al: Prognostic factors in yolk sac tumors of the ovary. A clinicopathologic analysis of 29 cases. Cancer 67:184-192, 1991.

415 Kommoss F, Bibbo M, Talerman A: Nuclear deoxyribonucleic acid content (ploidy) of endodermal sinus (yolk sac) tumor. Lab Invest 62:223-231, 1990.

416 Kurman RJ, Norris HJ: Endodermal sinus tumor of the ovary. A clinical and pathologic analysis of 71 cases. Cancer 38:2404-2419, 1976.

417 Kurman RJ, Norris HJ: Embryonal carcinoma of the ovary. A clinicopathologic entity distinct from endodermal sinus tumor resembling embryonal carcinoma of the adult testis. Cancer 38:2420-2433, 1976.

418 Langley FA, Govan ADT, Anderson MC, Gowing NFC, Woodcock AS, Harilal KR: Yolk sac and allied tumours of the ovary. Histopathology 5:389-401, 1981.

419 Michael H, Ulbright TM, Brodhecker CA: The pluripotential nature of the mesenchyme-like component of yolk sac tumor. Arch Pathol Lab Med 113:1115-1119, 1989.

420 Neubecker RD, Breen JL: Embryonal carcinoma of the ovary. Cancer 15:546-556, 1962.

421 Nogales FF: Embryologic clues to human yolk sac tumors. A review. Int J Gynecol Pathol 12:101-107, 1993.

422 Nogales FF, Beltran E, Pavcovich M, Bustos M: Ectopic somatic endoderm in secondary human yolk sac. Hum Pathol 23:921-924, 1992.

423 Nogales FF Jr, Matilla A, Nogales-Ortiz F, Galera-Davidson HL: Yolk sac tumors with pure and mixed polyvesicular vitelline patterns. Hum Pathol 9:553-566, 1978.

424 Nogales-Fernandez G, Silverberg SG, Bloustein PA, Martinez-Hernandez A, Pierce GB: Yolk sac carcinoma (endodermal sinus tumor). Ultrastructure and histogenesis of gonadal and extragonadal tumors in comparison with normal human yolk sac. Cancer 39:1462-1474, 1977.

425 Prat J, Bhan AK, Dickersin GR, Robboy SJ, Scully RE: Hepatoid yolk sac tumor of the ovary (endodermal sinus tumor with hepatoid differentiation). A light microscopic, ultrastructural and immunohistochemical study of seven cases. Cancer 50:2355-2368, 1982.

426 Schiller W: Mesonephroma ovarii. Am J Cancer 35:1-21, 1939.

427 Talerman A, Haije WG, Baggerman L: Serum alphafetoprotein (AFP) in diagnosis and management of endodermal sinus (yolk sac) tumor and mixed germ cell tumor of the ovary. Cancer 41:272-278, 1978.

428 Teilum G: Endodermal sinus tumors of the ovary and testis. Comparative morphogenesis of the so-called mesonephroma ovarii (Schiller) and extraembryonic (yolk-sac-allantoic) structures of the rat's placenta. Cancer **12:**1092-1105, 1959.

429 Ulbright TM, Roth LM, Brodhecker CA: Yolk sac differentiation in germ cell tumors. A morphologic study of 50 cases with emphasis on hepatic, enteric, and parietal yolk sac features. Am J Surg Pathol **10:**151-164, 1986.

Choriocarcinoma

430 Axe SR, Klein VR, Woodruff JD: Choriocarcinoma of the ovary. Obstet Gynecol **66:**111-114, 1985.

431 Damjanov I, Osborn M, Miettinen M: Keratin 7 is a marker for a subset of trophoblastic cells in human germ cell tumors. Arch Pathol Lab Med **114:**81-83, 1990.

432 Garin-Chesa P, Campbell I, Saigo PE, Lewis JL Jr, Old LJ, Rettig WJ: Trophoblast and ovarian cancer antigen LK26. Sensitivity and specificity in immunopathology and molecular identification as a folate-binding protein. Am J Pathol **142:**557-567, 1993.

433 Gerbie MV, Brewer JI, Tamini H: Primary choriocarcinoma of the ovary. Obstet Gynecol **46:**720-723, 1975.

434 Marrubini G: Primary chorionepithelioma of the ovary. Acta Obstet Gynecol Scand **28:**251-284, 1949.

435 Oliva E, Andrada E, Pezzica E, Prat J: Ovarian carcinomas with choriocarcinomatous differentiation. Cancer **72:**2441-2446, 1993.

436 Vance RP, Geisinger KR: Pure nongestational choriocarcinoma of the ovary. Report of a case. Cancer **56:**2321-2325, 1985.

Immature (malignant) teratoma

437 Aguirre P, Scully RE: Malignant neuroectodermal tumor of the ovary, a distinctive form of monodermal teratoma. Report of five cases. Am J Surg Pathol **6:**283-292, 1982.

438 Beilby JOW, Parkinson C: Features of prognostic significance in solid ovarian teratoma. Cancer **36:**2147-2159, 1975.

439 Gibas Z, Talerman A, Faruqi S, Carlson J, Noumoff J: Cytogenetic analysis of an immature teratoma of the ovary and its metastasis after chemotherapy-induced maturation. Int J Gynecol Pathol **12:**276-280, 1993.

440 Guerrieri C, Jarlsfelt I: Ependymoma of the ovary. A case report with immunohistochemical, ultrastructural, and DNA cytometric findings, as well as histogenetic considerations. Am J Surg Pathol **17:**623-632, 1993.

441 Ihara T, Ohama K, Satoh H, Fujii TV, Nomura K, Fujiwara A: Histologic grade and karyotype of immature teratoma of the ovary. Cancer **54:**2988-2994, 1984.

442 Kawai M, Kano T, Furuhashi Y, Iwata M, Nakashima N, Imai N, Kuzuya K, Hayashi H, Ohta M, Arii Y, et al: Immature teratoma of the ovary. Gynecol Oncol **40:**133-137, 1991.

443 King ME, Micha JP, Allen SL, Mouradian JA, Chaganti RSK: Immature teratoma of the ovary with predominant malignant retinal anlage component. A parthenogenically derived tumor. Am J Surg Pathol **9:**221-231, 1985.

444 Kleinman GM, Young RH, Scully RE: Ependymoma of the ovary. Report of three cases. Hum Pathol **15:**632-638, 1984.

445 Kleinman GM, Young RH, Scully RE: Primary neuroectodermal tumors of the ovary. A report of 25 cases. Am J Surg Pathol **17:**764-778, 1993.

446 Koulos JP, Hoffman JS, Steinhoff MM: Immature teratoma of the ovary. Gynecol Oncol **34:**46-49, 1989.

447 Metzman RA, Warhol MJ, Gee B, Roth J: Polysialic acid as a marker of both immature and mature neural tissue in human teratomas. Mod Pathol **4:**491-497, 1991.

448 Nogales FF Jr, Favara BE, Major FJ, Silverberg SG: Immature teratoma of the ovary with a neural component ("solid" teratoma). Hum Pathol **7:**625-642, 1976.

449 Nogales FF Jr, Ortega I, Rivera F, Armas JR: Metanephrogenic tissue in immature ovarian teratoma. Am J Surg Pathol **4:**297-299, 1980.

450 Nogales FF, Ruiz Avila I, Concha A, del Moral E: Immature endodermal teratoma of the ovary. Embryologic correlations and immunohistochemistry. Hum Pathol **24:**364-370, 1993.

451 Norris HJ, Zirkin HJ, Benson WL: Immature (malignant) teratoma of the ovary. A clinical and pathologic study of 58 cases. Cancer **37:**2359-2372, 1976.

452 Notohara K, Hsueh CL, Awai M: Glial fibrillary acidic protein immunoreactivity of chondrocytes in immature and mature teratomas. Acta Pathol Jpn **40:**335-342, 1990.

452a O'Connor DM, Norris HJ: The influence of grade on the outcome of stage I ovarian immature (malignant) teratomas and the reproducibility of grading. Int J Gynecol Pathol **13:**283-289, 1994.

453 Schwartz PE, Merino MJ, LiVolsi VA: Immature ovarian teratomas. Maturation following chemotherapy. Am J Diagn Gynecol Obstet **1:**361-366, 1979.

454 Steeper TA, Mukai K: Solid ovarian teratomas. An immunocytochemical study of thirteen cases with clinicopathologic correlation. Pathol Annu **19**(Pt 1):81-92, 1984.

Mature solid teratoma

455 Benirschke K, Easterday C, Abramson D: Malignant solid teratoma of the ovary. Report of three cases. Obstet Gynecol **15:**512-521, 1960.

456 Peterson WF: Solid, histologically benign teratomas of the ovary. A report of four cases and review of the literature. Am J Obstet Gynecol **72:**1094-1102, 1956.

457 Thurlbeck WM, Scully RE: Solid teratoma of the ovary. A clinicopathological analysis of 9 cases. Cancer **13:**804-811, 1960.

Mature cystic teratoma, benign and with secondary tumor formation

458 Auer EA, Dockerty MB, Mayo CW: Ruptured dermoid cyst of the ovary simulating abdominal carcinomatosis. Mayo Clin Proc **26:**489-497, 1951.

459 Blackwell WJ, Dockerty MB, Masson JC, Mussey RD: Dermoid cysts of the ovary. Their clinical and pathologic significance. Am J Obstet Gynecol **51:**151-172, 1946.

460 Brumback RA, Brown BS, di Sant'Agnese A: Unique finding of prostatic tissue in a benign cystic ovarian teratoma. Arch Pathol Lab Med **109:**675-677, 1985.

461 Calame J, Bosman FT, Schaberg A, Louwerens JWK: Immunocytochemical localization of neuroendocrine hormones and oncofetal antigens in ovarian teratomas. Int J Gynecol Pathol **3:**92-100, 1984.

462 Chumas JC, Scully RE: Sebaceous tumors arising in ovarian dermoid cysts. Int J Gynecol Pathol **10:**356-363, 1991.

463 Climie ARW, Heath LP: Malignant degeneration of benign cystic teratomas of the ovary. Review of the literature and report of a chondrosarcoma and carcinoid tumor. Cancer **22:**824-832, 1968.

464 Czernobilsky B, Lifschitz-Mercer B, Luzon A, Jacob N, Ben-Hur H, Gorbacz S, Fogel M: Cytokeratin patterns in the epidermis of human ovarian mature cystic teratomas. Hum Pathol **20:**185-192, 1989.

465 Dick HM, Honoré LH: Dental structures in benign ovarian cystic teratomas (dermoid cysts). A study of ten cases with a review of the literature. Oral Surg **60:**299-307, 1985.

466 Ein SH, Darte JMM, Stephens CA: Cystic and solid ovarian tumors in children. A 44-year review. J Pediatr Surg **5:**148-156, 1970.

467 Fortt RW, Mathie IK: Gliomatosis peritonei caused by ovarian teratoma. J Clin Pathol **22:**348-353, 1969.

468 Gregg RH: Primary malignant melanoma arising in an ovarian dermoid cyst. Am J Obstet Gynecol **143:**25-28, 1982.

469 Harms D, Janig U, Gobel U: Gliomatosis peritonei in childhood and adolescence. Clinicopathological study of 13 cases including immunohistochemical findings. Pathol Res Pract **184:**422-430, 1989.

470 Hirakawa T, Tsuneyoshi M, Enjoji M: Squamous cell carcinoma arising in mature cystic teratoma of the ovary. Clinicopathologic and topographic analysis. Am J Surg Pathol **13:**397-405, 1989.

471 Kanbour-Shakir A, Sawaday J, Kanbour AI, Kunschner A, Stock RJ: Primitive neuroectodermal tumor arising in an ovarian mature cystic teratoma. Immunohistochemical and electron microscopic studies. Int J Gynecol Pathol **12:**270-275, 1993.

472 Kelley RR, Scully RE: Cancer developing in dermoid cysts of the ovary. Cancer **14:**989-1000, 1961.

473 Kudo M: The nature of "blue nevus" in cystic teratomas of the ovary. An ultrastructural evidence for Schwann cell origin. Acta Pathol Jpn **35:**693-698, 1985.

474 Linder D, McCaw BK, Hecht F: Parthenogenic origin of benign ovarian teratomas. N Engl J Med **292:**63-66, 1975.

475 Madison JF, Cooper PH: A histiocytoid (epithelioid) vascular tumor of the ovary. Occurrence within a benign cystic teratoma. Mod Pathol **2:**55-58, 1989.

476 McKeel DW Jr, Askin FB: Ectopic hypophyseal hormonal cells in benign cystic teratoma of the ovary. Light microscopic histochemical dye staining and immunoperoxidase cytochemistry. Arch Pathol Lab Med **102:**122-128, 1978.

477 McLachlin CM, Srigley JR: Prostatic tissue in mature cystic teratomas of the ovary. Am J Surg Pathol **16:**780-784, 1992.

478 Miyake J, Ireland K: Ovarian mature teratoma with homunculus coexisting with an intrauterine pregnancy. Arch Pathol Lab Med **110:**1192-1194, 1986.

479 Morimitsu Y, Nakashima O, Kage M, Kojiro M, Kawano K, Koga T: Coexistence of mature teratoma and thecoma in an ovary. A report of two cases. Acta Pathol Jpn **41:**922-926, 1991.

480 Morimitsu Y, Nakashima O, Nakashima Y, Kojiro M, Shimokobe T: Apocrine adenocarcinoma arising in cystic teratoma of the ovary. Arch Pathol Lab Med **117:**647-649, 1993.

481 Nielsen SNJ, Scheithauer BW, Gaffey TA: Gliomatosis peritonei. Cancer **56:**2499-2503, 1985.

482 Palmer PE, Bogojavlensky S, Bhan AK, Scully RE: Prolactinoma in wall of ovarian dermoid cyst with hyperprolactinemia. Obstet Gynecol **75:**540-543, 1990.

483 Payne D, Muss HB, Homesley HD, Jobson VW, Baird FG: Autoimmune hemolytic anemia and ovarian dermoid cysts. Case report and review of the literature. Cancer **48:**721-724, 1981.

484 Peterson WF: Malignant degeneration of benign cystic teratomas of the ovary. A collective review of the literature. Obstet Gynecol Survey **12:**793-830, 1957.

485 Rashad MH, Fathalla MF, Kerr MG: Sex chromatin and chromosome analysis in ovarian teratomas. Am J Obstet Gynecol **96:**461-465, 1966.

486 Reid H, van der Walt JD, Fox H: Neuroblastoma arising in a mature cystic teratoma of the ovary. J Clin Pathol **36:**68-73, 1983.

487 Riley PA, Sutton PM: Why are ovarian teratomas benign whilst teratomas of the testis are malignant? Lancet **1:**1360-1362, 1975.

488 Robboy SJ, Scully RE: Ovarian teratoma with glial implants on the peritoneum. An analysis of 12 cases. Hum Pathol **1:**644-653, 1970.

489 Sahin AA, Ro JY, Chen J, Ayala AG: Spindle cell nodule and peptic ulcer arising in a fully developed gastric wall in a mature cystic teratoma. Arch Pathol Lab Med **114:**529-531, 1990.

490 Shimizu S, Kobayashi H, Suchi T, Torii Y, Narita K, Aoki S: Extramammary Paget's disease arising in mature cystic teratoma of the ovary. Am J Surg Pathol **15:**1002-1006, 1991.

491 Truong LD, Jurco S III, McGavran MH: Gliomatosis peritonei. Report of two cases and review of literature. Am J Surg Pathol **6:**443-449, 1982.

492 Tsang P, Berman L, Kasznica J: Adnexal tumor and a pigmented nevoid lesion in a benign cystic ovarian teratoma. Arch Pathol Lab Med **117:**846-847, 1993.

493 Ueda Y, Kimura A, Kawahara E, Kitagawa H, Nakanishi I: Malignant melanoma arising in a dermoid cyst of the ovary. Cancer **67:**3141-3145, 1991.

494 Wheeler JE: Extraovarian teratoma with peritoneal gliomatosis. Hum Pathol **9:**232-234, 1978.

495 Yanai-Inbar I, Scully RE: Relation of ovarian dermoid cysts and immature teratomas. An analysis of 350 cases of immature teratoma and 10 cases of dermoid cyst with microscopic foci of immature tissue. Int J Gynecol Pathol **6:**203-212, 1987.

496 Young RH, Prat J, Scully RE: Epidermoid cyst of the ovary. A report of three cases with comments on histogenesis. Am J Clin Pathol **73:**272-276, 1980.

Struma ovarii

497 Emge LA: Functional and growth characteristics of struma ovarii. Am J Obstet Gynecol **40:**738-750, 1940.

498 Hasleton PS, Kelehan P, Wittaker JS, Turner L, Burslem RW: Benign and malignant struma ovarii. Arch Pathol Lab Med **102:**180-184, 1978.

499 Plaut A: Ovarian struma. A morphologic, pharmacologic, and biologic examination. Am J Obstet Gynecol **25:**351-360, 1933.

500 Ro JY, Sahin AA, el-Naggar AK, Ordonez NG, Mackay B, Llamas LL, Ayala AG: Intraluminal crystalloids in struma ovarii. Immunohistochemical, DNA flow cytometric, and ultrastructural study. Arch Pathol Lab Med **115:**145-149, 1991.

501 Seifer DB, Weiss LM, Kempson RL: Malignant lymphoma arising within thyroid tissue in a mature cystic teratoma. Cancer **58:**2459-2461, 1986.

501a Szyfelbein WM, Young RH, Scully RE: Cystic struma ovarii. A frequently unrecognized tumor. A report of 20 cases. Am J Surg Pathol **18:**785-788, 1994.

501b Szyfelbein WM, Young RH, Scully RE: Struma ovarii simulating ovarian tumors of other types. A report of 30 cases. Am J Surg Pathol **19:**21-29, 1995.

Carcinoid tumor and strumal carcinoid

502 Arhelger RB, Kelly B: Strumal carcinoid. Report of a case with electron microscopical observations. Arch Pathol **97:**323-325, 1974.

503 Czernobilsky B, Segal M, Dgani R: Primary ovarian carcinoid with marked heterogeneity of microscopic features. Cancer **54:**585-589, 1984.

504 Dayal Y, Tashjian H Jr, Wolfe HJ: Immunocytochemical localization of calcitonin-producing cells in a strumal carcinoid with amyloid stroma. Cancer **43:**1331-1338, 1979.

505 Greco MA, LiVolsi VA, Pertschuk LP, Bigelow B: Strumal carcinoid of the ovary. Cancer **43:**1380-1388, 1979.

506 Livnat EJ, Scommegna A, Recant W, Jao W: Ultrastructural observations of the so-called strumal carcinoid of the ovary. Arch Pathol Lab Med **101:**585-589, 1977.

506a Matias-Guiu X, Forteza J, Prat J: Mixed strumal and mucinous carcinoid tumor of the ovary. Int J Gynecol Pathol **14:**179-183, 1995.

507 Motoyama T, Katayama Y, Watanabe H, Okazaki E, Shibuya H: Functioning ovarian carcinoids induce severe constipation. Cancer **70:**513-518, 1992.

508 Ranchod M, Kempson RL, Dorgeloh JR: Strumal carcinoid of the ovary. Cancer **37:**1913-1922, 1976.

509 Robboy SJ, Norris HJ, Scully RE: Insular carcinoid primary in ovary—a clinicopathologic analysis of 48 cases. Cancer **36:**406-420, 1975.

510 Robboy SJ, Scully RE: Strumal carcinoid of the ovary. An analysis of 50 cases of a distinctive tumor composed of thyroid tissue and carcinoid. Cancer **46:**2019-2034, 1980.

511 Robboy SJ, Scully RE, Norris HJ: Carcinoid metastatic to ovary. A clinicopathologic analysis of 35 cases. Cancer **33:**798-811, 1974.

512 Robboy SJ, Scully RE, Norris HJ: Primary trabecular carcinoid of the ovary. Obstet Gynecol **49:**202-207, 1977.

513 Serratoni FT, Robboy SJ: Ultrastructure of primary and metastatic ovarian carcinoids. Analysis of 11 cases. Cancer **36:**157-160, 1975.

514 Sidhu J, Sanchez RL: Prostatic acid tase in strumal carcinoids of the ovary. An immunohistochemical study. Cancer **72:**1673-1678, 1993.

515 Snyder RR, Tavassoli FA: Ovarian strumal carcinoid. Immunohistochemical, ultrastructural, and clinicopathologic observations. Int J Gynecol Pathol **3:**187-201, 1984.

516 Sporrong B, Falkmer S, Robboy SJ, Alumets J, Hakanson R, Ljungberg O, Sundler F: Neurohormonal peptides in ovarian carcinoids. An immunohistochemical study of 81 primary carcinoids and of intraovarian metastases from six mid-gut carcinoids. Cancer **49:**68-74, 1982.

517 Stagno PA, Petras RE, Hart WR: Strumal carcinoids of the ovary. An immunohistologic and ultrastructural study. Arch Pathol Lab Med **111:**440-446, 1987.

518 Talerman A: Carcinoid tumors of the ovary. J Cancer Res Clin Oncol **107:**125-135, 1984.

519 Tamsen A, Mazur MT: Ovarian strumal carcinoid in association with multiple endocrine neoplasia, type IIA. Arch Pathol Lab Med **116:**200-203, 1992.

520 Ulbright TM, Roth LM, Ehrlich CE: Ovarian strumal carcinoid. An immunocytochemical and ultrastructural study of two cases. Am J Clin Pathol **77:**622-631, 1982.

521 Wolpert HR, Fuller AF, Bell DA: Primary mucinous carcinoid tumor of the ovary. A case report. Int J Gynecol Pathol **8:**156-162, 1989.

Sex cord–stromal tumors

522 Costa MJ, Morris R, Sasano H: Sex steroid biosynthesis enzymes in ovarian sex-cord stromal tumors. Int J Gynecol Pathol **13:**109-119, 1994.

523 Fox H: Sex cord–stromal tumours of the ovary. J Pathol **145:**127-148, 1985.

524 Freeman DA: Steroid hormone-producing tumors of the adrenal, ovary, and testes. Endocrinol Metab Clin North Am **20:**751-766, 1991.

525 Gustafson ML, Lee MM, Scully RE, Moncure AC, Hirakawa T, Goodman A, Muntz HG, Donahoe PK, Mac Laughlin DT, Fuller AF Jr: Mullerian inhibiting substance as a marker for ovarian sex-cord tumor. N Engl J Med **326:**466-471, 1992.

526 Kurman RJ, Ganjei P, Nadji M: Contributions of immunocytochemistry to the diagnosis and study of ovarian neoplasms. Int J Gynecol Pathol **3:**3-26, 1984.

527 Lobo RA: Ovarian hyperandrogenism and androgen-producing tumors. Endocrinol Metab Clin North Am **20:**773-805, 1991.

527a Sasano H: Functional pathology of human ovarian steroidogenesis. Normal cycling ovary and steroid-producing neoplasms. Endocr Pathol **5:**81-89, 1994.

528 Sasano H, Okamoto M, Mason JI, Simpson ER, Mendelson CR, Sasano N, Silverberg SG: Immunohistochemical studies of steroidogenic enzymes (aromatase, 17 alpha-hydroxylase and cholesterol side-chain cleavage cytochromes P-450) in sex cord-stromal tumors of the ovary. Hum Pathol **20:**452-457, 1989.

529 Sternberg WH, Dhurandhar HN: Functional ovarian tumors of stromal and sex cord origin. Hum Pathol **8:**565-582, 1977.

529a Tavassoli FA: Ovarian tumors with functioning manifestations. Endocr Pathol **5:**137-148, 1994.

530 Teilum G: Estrogen-producing Sertoli cell tumors (androblastoma tubular lipoides) of the human testis and ovary. Homologous ovarian and testicular tumors. J Clin Endocrinol **9:**301-318, 1949.

531 Young RH, Scully RE: Ovarian sex cord-stromal tumors. Recent progress. Int J Gynecol Pathol **1:**101-123, 1982.

532 Young RH, Scully RE: Ovarian sex cord-stromal tumors. Problems in differential diagnosis. Pathol Annu **23**(Pt 1):273-296, 1988.

Granulosa cell tumor

533 Bjorkholm E, Silfversward C: Prognostic factors in granulosa-cell tumors. Gynecol Oncol **11:**261-274, 1981.

534 Chadha S, Cornelisse CJ, Schaberg A: Flow cytometric DNA ploidy analysis of ovarian granulosa cell tumors. Gynecol Oncol **36:**240-245, 1990.

535 Clement PB, Young RH, Scully RE: Ovarian granulosa cell proliferations of pregnancy. A report of nine cases. Hum Pathol **19:**657-662, 1988.

536 Costa MJ, De Rose PB, Roth LM, Brescia RJ, Zaloudek CJ, Cohen C: Immunohistochemical phenotype of ovarian granulosa cell tumors. Absence of epithelial membrane antigen has diagnostic value. Hum Pathol **25:**60-66, 1994.

537 Czernobilsky B, Moll R, Leppien G, Schweikhart G, Franke WW: Desmosomal plaque-associated vimentin filaments in human ovarian granulosa cell tumors of various histologic patterns. Am J Pathol **126**:476-486, 1987.

538 Evans AT III, Gaffey TA, Malkasian GD Jr, Annegers JF: Clinicopathologic review of 118 granulosa and 82 theca cell tumors. Obstet Gynecol **55**:231-238, 1980.

538a Evans MP, Webb MJ, Gaffey TA, Katzmann JA, Suman VJ, Hu TC: DNA ploidy of ovarian granulosa cell tumors. Lack of correlation between DNA index or proliferative index and outcome in 40 patients. Cancer **75**:2295-2298, 1995.

538b Flemming P, Wellmann A, Maschjek H, Lang H, Georgii A: Monoclonal antibodies against inhibin represent key markers of adult granulosa cell tumors of the ovary even in their metastases. A report of three cases with late metastasis, being previously misinterpreted as hemangiopericytoma. Am J Surg Pathol **19**:927-933, 1995.

539 Fletcher JA, Gibas Z, Donovan K, Perez-Atayde A, Genest D, Morton CC, Lage JM: Ovarian granulosa-stromal cell tumors are characterized by trisomy 12. Am J Pathol **138**:515-520, 1991.

540 Fox H, Agrawal K, Langley FA: A clinicopathologic study of 92 cases of granulosa cell tumor of the ovary with special reference to the factors influencing prognosis. Cancer **35**:231-241, 1975.

540a Halperin D, Visscher DW, Wallis T, Lawrence WD: Evaluation of chromosome 12 copy number in ovarian granulosa cell tumors using interphase cytogenetics. Int J Gynecol Pathol **14**:319-323, 1995.

541 Hitchcock CL, Norris HJ, Khalifa MA, Wargotz ES: Flow cytometric analysis of granulosa tumors. Cancer **64**:2127-2132, 1989.

542 Jacoby AF, Young RH, Colvin RB, Flotte TJ, Preffer F, Scully RE, Swymer CM, Bell DA: DNA content in juvenile granulosa cell tumors of the ovary. A study of early- and advanced-stage disease. Gynecol Oncol **46**:97-103, 1992.

543 Kurman RJ, Goebelsmann U, Taylor CR: Steroid localization in granulosa-theca tumors of the ovary. Cancer **43**:2377-2384, 1979.

544 Lack EE, Perez-Atayde AR, Murthy ASK, Goldstein DP, Crigler JF, Vawter GF: Granulosa theca cell tumors in premenarchal girls. A clinical and pathologic study of ten cases. Cancer **48**:1846-1854, 1981.

545 Lappohn RE, Burger HG, Bouma J, Bangah M, Krans M, de Bruijn HW: Inhibin as a marker for granulosa-cell tumors. N Engl J Med **321**:790-793, 1989.

545a Loo KT, Leung AKF, Chan JKC: Immunohistochemical staining of ovarian granulosa cell tumours with MIC2 antibody. Histopathology **27**:388-390, 1995.

546 McKay DG, Robinson D, Hertig AT: Histochemical observations on granulosa cell tumors, thecomas and fibromas of the ovary. Am J Obstet Gynecol **58**:625-639, 1949.

547 Miettinen M, Wahlstrom T, Virtanen I, Talerman A, Astengo-Osuna C: Cellular differentiation in ovarian sex cord–stromal and germ-cell tumors studied with antibodies to intermediate-filament proteins. Am J Surg Pathol **9**:640-651, 1985.

548 Nakashima N, Young RH, Scully RE: Androgenic granulosa cell tumors of the ovary. A clinicopathologic analysis of 17 cases and review of the literature. Arch Pathol Lab Med **108**:786-791, 1984.

549 Nogales FF, Concha A, Plata C, Ruiz-Avila I: Granulosa cell tumor of the ovary with diffuse true hepatic differentiation simulating stromal luteinization. Am J Surg Pathol **17**:85-90, 1993.

550 Norris HJ, Taylor HB: Prognosis of granulosa-theca tumors of the ovary. Cancer **21**:255-263, 1968.

551 Norris HJ, Taylor HB: Virilization associated with cystic granulosa tumors. Obstet Gynecol **34**:629-635, 1969.

552 Novak ER, Kutchmeshgi J, Mupas RS, Woodruff JD: Feminizing gonadal stromal tumors. Analysis of the granulosa-theca cell tumors of the ovarian tumor registry. Obstet Gynecol **38**:701-713, 1971.

553 Otis CN, Powell JL, Barbuto D, Carcangiu ML: Intermediate filamentous proteins in adult granulosa cell tumors. An immunohistochemical study of 25 cases. Am J Surg Pathol **16**:962-968, 1992.

554 Rodgers KE, Marks JF, Ellefson DD, Yanagihara DL, Tonetta SA, Vasilev SA, Morrow CP, Montz FJ, di Zerega GS: Follicle regulatory protein. A novel marker for granulosa cell cancer patients. Gynecol Oncol **37**:381-387, 1990.

555 Roth LM, Nicholas TR, Ehrlich CE: Juvenile granulosa cell tumor. A clinicopathologic study of three cases with ultrastructural observations. Cancer **44**:2194-2205, 1979.

555a Santini D, Ceccarelli C, Leone O, Pasquinelli G, Piana S, Marabini A, Martinelli GN: Smooth muscle differentiation in normal human ovaries, ovarian stromal hyperplasia and ovarian granulosa-stromal cells tumors. Mod Pathol **8**:25-30, 1995.

556 Schofield DE, Fletcher JA: Trisomy 12 in pediatric granulosa–stromal cell tumors. Demonstration by a modified method of fluorescence in situ hybridization on paraffin-embedded material. Am J Pathol **141**:1265-1269, 1992.

557 Scully RE: Ovarian tumors. A review. Am J Pathol **87**:686-720, 1977.

558 Suh KS, Silverberg SG, Rhame JG, Wilkinson DS: Granulosa cell tumor of the ovary. Histopathologic and flow cytometric analysis with clinical correlation. Arch Pathol Lab Med **114**:496-501, 1990.

559 Swanson SA, Norris HJ, Kelsten ML, Wheeler JE: DNA content of juvenile granulosa tumors determined by flow cytometry. Int J Gynecol Pathol **9**:101-109, 1990.

560 Tamimi HK, Bolen JW: Enchondromatosis (Ollier's disease) and ovarian juvenile granulosa cell tumor. A case report and review of the literature. Cancer **53**:1605-1608, 1984.

561 Tanaka Y, Sasaki Y, Nishihira H, Izawa T, Nishi T: Ovarian juvenile granulosa cell tumor associated with Maffucci's syndrome. Am J Clin Pathol **97**:523-527, 1992.

562 Young RH, Dickersin GR, Scully RE: Juvenile granulosa cell tumor of the ovary. A clinicopathologic analysis of 125 cases. Am J Surg Pathol **8**:575-596, 1984.

563 Young RH, Dudley AG, Scully RE: Granulosa cell, Sertoli–Leydig cell, and unclassified sex cord–stromal tumors associated with pregnancy. A clinico-pathological analysis of thirty-six cases. Gynecol Oncol **18**:181-205, 1984.

563a Young RH, Oliva E, Scully RE: Luteinized adult granulosa cell tumors of the ovary. A report of four cases. Int J Gynecol Pathol **13**:302-310, 1994.

564 Young RH, Scully RE: Ovarian sex cord–stromal tumors. Recent progress. Int J Gynecol Pathol **1**:101-123, 1982.

565 Young RH, Scully RE: Ovarian sex cord–stromal tumors with bizarre nuclei. A clinicopathologic analysis of 17 cases. Int J Gynecol Pathol **1**:325-335, 1983.

566 Young RH, Scully RE: Ovarian sex cord–stromal tumors. Problems in differential diagnosis. Pathol Annu **23**(Pt 1):237-296, 1988.

567 Zaloudek C, Norris HJ: Granulosa tumors of the ovary in children. A clinical and pathologic study of 32 cases. Am J Surg Pathol **6**:513-522, 1982.

Thecoma, fibroma, and related tumors

568 Chalvardjian A, Scully RE: Sclerosing stromal tumors of the ovary. Cancer **31**:664-670, 1973.

569 Clement PB, Young RH, Hanna W, Scully RE: Sclerosing peritonitis associated with luteinized thecomas of the ovary. A clinicopathological analysis of six cases. Am J Surg Pathol **18**:1-13, 1994.

570 Costa MJ, Morris R, De Rose PB, Cohen C: Histologic and immunohistochemical evidence for considering ovarian myxoma as a variant of the thecoma-fibroma group of ovarian stromal tumors. Arch Pathol Lab Med **117**:802-808, 1993.

571 Costa MJ, Thomas W, Majmudar B, Hewan-Lowe K: Ovarian myxoma. Ultrastructural and immunohistochemical findings. Ultrastruct Pathol **16**:429-438, 1992.

572 Dockerty MB, Masson JC: Ovarian fibromas. A clinical and pathologic study of two hundred and eighty-three cases. Am J Obstet Gynecol **47**:741-752, 1944.

573 Eichhorn JH, Scully RE: Ovarian myxoma. Clinicopathologic and immunocytologic analysis of five cases and a review of the literature. Int J Gynecol Pathol **10**:156-169, 1991.

574 Fox H: Sex cord-stromal tumours of the ovary. J Pathol **145**:127-148, 1985.

575 Gaffney EF, Majmudar B, Hewan-Lowe K: Ultrastructure and immunohistochemical localization of estradiol of three thecomas. Hum Pathol **15**:153-160, 1984.

576 Hayes MC, Scully RE: Stromal luteoma of the ovary. A clinicopathological analysis of 25 cases. Int J Gynecol Pathol **6**:313-321, 1987.

577 Kalstone CE, Jaffe RB, Abell MR: Massive edema of the ovary simulating fibroma. Obstet Gynecol **34**:564-571, 1969.

578 Kanbour AI, Salazar H, Tobon H: Massive ovarian edema. A non-neoplastic pelvic mass of young women. Arch Pathol Lab Med **103**:42-45, 1979.

579 Lacson AG, Alrabeeah A, Gillis DA, Salisbury S, Grantmyre EB: Secondary massive ovarian edema with Meigs' syndrome. Am J Clin Pathol **91**:597-603, 1989.

580 Meigs JV: Pelvic tumors other than fibromas of the ovary with ascites and hydrothorax. Obstet Gynecol **3**:471-486, 1954.

581 Meigs JV, Cass JW: Fibroma of the ovary with ascites and hydrothorax. Am J Obstet Gynecol **33**:249-266, 1937.

581a Persons DL, Hartmann LC, Herath JF, Keeney GL, Jenkins RB: Fluorescence in situ hybridization analysis of trisomy 12 in ovarian tumors. Am J Clin Pathol **102**:775-779, 1994.

582 Prat J, Scully RE: Cellular fibromas and fibrosarcomas of the ovary. A comparative clinicopathologic analysis of seventeen cases. Cancer **47**:2663-2670, 1981.

583 Raggio M, Kaplan AL, Harberg JF: Recurrent ovarian fibromas with basal cell nevus syndrome (Gorlin syndrome). Obstet Gynecol **61**:95S-96S, 1983.

584 Roth LM, Deaton RL, Sternberg WH: Massive ovarian edema. A clinicopathologic study of five cases including ultrastructural observations and review of the literature. Am J Surg Pathol **3**:11-21, 1979.

585 Roth LM, Sternberg WH: Partly luteinized theca cell tumor of the ovary. Cancer **51:**1697-1704, 1983.

586 Saitoh A, Tsutsumi Y, Osamura RY, Watanabe K: Sclerosing stromal tumor of the ovary. Immunohistochemical and electron-microscopic demonstration of smooth-muscle differentiation. Arch Pathol Lab Med **113:**372-376, 1989.

587 Samanth KK, Black WC III: Benign ovarian stromal tumors associated with free peritoneal fluid. Am J Obstet Gynecol **107:**538-545, 1970.

588 Scully RE: Stromal luteoma of the ovary. A distinctive type of lipoid-cell tumor. Cancer **17:**769-778, 1964.

589 Shaw JA, Dabbs DJ, Geisinger KR: Sclerosing stromal tumor of the ovary. An ultrastructural and immunohistochemical analysis with histogenetic considerations. Ultrastruct Pathol **16:**363-377, 1992.

590 Sternberg WH, Gaskill CJ: Theca-cell tumors. Am J Obstet Gynecol **59:**575-587, 1950.

591 Sternberg WH, Roth LM: Ovarian stromal tumors containing Leydig cells. I. Stromal–Leydig cell tumor and non-neoplastic transformation of ovarian stroma to Leydig cells. Cancer **32:**940-951, 1973.

592 Taruscio D, Carcangiu ML, Ward DC: Detection of trisomy 12 on ovarian sex cord stromal tumors by fluorescence in situ hybridization. Diagn Mol Pathol **2:**94-98, 1993.

593 Tetu B, Bonenfant JL: Ovarian myxoma. A study of two cases with long-term follow-up. Am J Clin Pathol **95:**340-346, 1991.

594 Tiltman AJ: Sclerosing stromal tumor of the ovary. Demonstration of ligandin in three cases. Int J Gynecol Pathol **4:**362-369, 1985.

595 Waxman M, Vuletin JC, Urcuyo R, Belling CG: Ovarian low-grade stromal sarcoma with thecomatous features. A critical reappraisal of the so-called "malignant thecoma." Cancer **44:**2206-2217, 1979.

596 Young RH, Clement PB, Scully RE: Calcified thecomas in young women. A report of four cases. Int J Gynecol Pathol **7:**343-350, 1988.

597 Young RH, Scully RE: Ovarian stromal tumors with minor sex-cord elements. A report of seven cases. Int J Gynecol Pathol **2:**227-234, 1983.

598 Young RH, Scully RE: Fibromatosis and massive edema of the ovary, possibly related entities. A report of 14 cases of fibromatosis and 11 cases of massive edema. Int J Gynecol Pathol **3:**153-178, 1984.

599 Zhang J, Young RH, Arseneau J, Scully RE: Ovarian stromal tumors containing lutein or Leydig cells (luteinized thecomas and stromal Leydig cell tumors). A clinicopathologic analysis of fifty cases. Int J Gynecol Pathol **1:**270-285, 1982.

Endometrial abnormalities associated with granulosa cell tumor and thecoma

600 Gusberg SB, Kardon P: Proliferative endometrial response to theca-granulosa cell tumors. Am J Obstet Gynecol **111:**633-643, 1971.

601 Katsube Y, Iwaoki Y, Silverberg SG, Fujiwara A: Sclerosing stromal tumor of the ovary associated with endometrial adenocarcinoma. A case report. Gynecol Oncol **29:**392-398, 1988.

602 Norris HJ, Taylor HB: Prognosis of granulosa-theca tumors of the ovary. Cancer **21:**255-263, 1968.

603 Press MF, Scully RE: Endometrial "sarcomas" complicating ovarian thecoma, polycystic ovarian disease and estrogen therapy. Gynecol Oncol **21:**135-154, 1985.

Small cell carcinoma

604 Aguirre P, Thor AD, Scully RE: Ovarian small cell carcinoma. Histogenetic considerations based on immunohistochemical and other findings. Am J Clin Pathol **92:**140-149, 1989.

605 Dickersin GR, Kline IW, Scully RE: Small cell carcinoma of the ovary with hypercalcemia. A report of eleven cases. Cancer **49:**188-197, 1982.

606 Dickersin GR, Scully RE: An update on the electron microscopy of small cell carcinoma of the ovary with hypercalcemia. Ultrastruct Pathol **17:**411-422, 1993.

607 Eichhorn JH, Bell DA, Young RH, Swymer CM, Flotte TJ, Preffer RI, Scully RE: DNA content and proliferative activity in ovarian small cell carcinomas of the hypercalcemic type. Implications for diagnosis, prognosis, and histogenesis. Am J Clin Pathol **98:**579-586, 1992.

608 Eichhorn JH, Young RH, Scully RE: Primary ovarian small cell carcinoma of pulmonary type. A clinicopathologic, immunohistologic, and flow cytometric analysis of 11 cases. Am J Surg Pathol **16:**926-938, 1992.

608a Lamovec J, Bracko M, Cerar O: Familial occurrence of small-cell carcinoma of the ovary. Arch Pathol Lab Med **119:**551-554, 1995.

609 Matias-Guiu X, Prat J, Young RH, Capen CC, Rosol TJ, DeLellis RA, Scully RE: Human parathyroid hormone-related protein in ovarian small cell carcinoma. An immunohistochemical study. Cancer **73:**1878-1881, 1994.

610 Scully RE: Small cell carcinoma of hypercalcemic type. Int J Gynecol Pathol **12:**148-152, 1993.

611 Ulbright TM, Roth LM, Stehman FB, Talerman A, Senekjian EK: Poorly differentiated (small cell) carcinoma of the ovary in young women. Evidence supporting a germ cell origin. Hum Pathol **18:**175-184, 1987.

611a Young RH, Oliva E, Scully RE: Small cell carcinoma of the ovary, hypercalcemic type. A clinicopathological analysis of 150 cases. Am J Surg Pathol **18:**1102-1116, 1994.

Sertoli–Leydig cell tumor (arrhenoblastoma; androblastoma)

612 Aguirre P, Scully RE, DeLellis RA: Ovarian heterologous Sertoli–Leydig cell tumors with gastrointestinal-type epithelium. An immunohistochemical analysis. Arch Pathol Lab Med **110:**528-533, 1986.

613 Chadha S, Honnebier WJ, Schaberg A: Raised serum alphafetoprotein in Sertoli–Leydig cell tumor (androblastoma) of ovary. Report of two cases. Int J Gynecol Pathol **6:**82-88, 1987.

614 Costa MJ, Morris RJ, Wilson R, Judd R: Utility of immunohistochemistry in distinguishing ovarian Sertoli–stromal cell tumors from carcinosarcomas. Hum Pathol **23:**787-797, 1992.

614a Ferry JA, Young RH, Engel G, Scully RE: Oxyphilic Sertoli cell tumor of the ovary. A report of three cases, two in patients with the Peutz-Jeghers syndrome. Int J Gynecol Pathol **13:**259-266, 1994.

615 Fox H, Langley FA: Tumours of the ovary. London, 1976, Heinemann Medical Books, Ltd., pp. 156-157.

616 Gagnon S, Tetu B, Silva EG, McCaughey WT: Frequency of alpha-fetoprotein production by Sertoli–Leydig cell tumors of the ovary. An immunohistochemical study of eight cases. Mod Pathol **2:**63-67, 1989.

617 Hughesdon PE, Fraser IT: Arrhenoblastoma of ovary. Acta Obstet Gynecol Scand **32:**1-78, 1953.

618 Jenson AB, Fechner RE: Ultrastructure of an intermediate Sertoli–Leydig cell tumor. A histogenetic misnomer. Lab Invest **21:**527-535, 1969.

619 Kurman RJ, Andrade D, Goebelsmann U, Taylor CR: An immunohistological study of steroid localization in Steroli–Leydig tumors of the ovary and testis. Cancer **42:**1772-1783, 1978.

620 Kurman RJ, Ganjei P, Nadji M: Contributions of immunocytochemistry to the diagnosis and study of ovarian neoplasms. Int J Gynecol Pathol **3:**3-26, 1984.

621 Meyer R: Tubuläre (testikuläre) und solide Foramen des Andreiblastoma ovarii und ihre Beziehung zur Vermännlickung. Beitr Pathol Anat **84:**485-520, 1930.

622 Motoyama I, Watanabe H, Gotoh A, Takeuchi S, Tanabe N, Nashimoto I: Ovarian Sertoli–Leydig cell tumor with elevated serum alpha-fetoprotein. Cancer **63:**2047-2053, 1989.

623 O'Hern TM, Neubecker RD: Arrhenoblastoma of the ovary. Obstet Gynecol **19:**758-770, 1962.

624 Prat J, Young RH, Scully RE: Ovarian Sertoli–Leydig cell tumors with heterologous elements. II. Cartilage and skeletal muscle. A clinicopathologic analysis of twelve cases. Cancer **50:**2465-2475, 1982.

625 Roth LM, Anderson MC, Govan ADT, Langley FA, Gowing NFC, Woodcock AS: Sertoli–Leydig cell tumors. A clinicopathologic study of 34 cases. Cancer **48:**187-197, 1981.

626 Roth LM, Cleary RE, Rosenfield RL: Sertoli–Leydig cell tumor of the ovary, with an associated mucinous cystadenoma. An ultrastructural and endocrine study. Lab Invest **31:**648-657, 1974.

627 Roth LM, Slayton RE, Brady LW, Blessing JA, Johnson G: Retiform differentiation in ovarian Sertoli–Leydig cell tumors. A clinicopathologic study of six cases from a gynecologic oncology group study. Cancer **55:**1093-1098, 1985.

628 Savard K, Gut M, Dorfman RI, Gabrilove JL, Soffer LJ: Formation of androgens by human arrhenoblastoma tissue in vitro. J Clin Endocrinol **21:**165-174, 1961.

629 Scully RE: Ovarian tumors. A review. Am J Pathol **87:**686-720, 1977.

630 Seidman JD, Patterson JA, Bitterman P: Sertoli–Leydig cell tumor associated with a mature cystic teratoma in a single ovary. Mod Pathol **2:**687-692, 1989.

631 Stegner H-E, Lisboa BP: Steroid metabolism in an androblastoma (Sertoli–Leydig cell tumor). A histopathological and biochemical study. Int J Gynecol Pathol **2:**410-425, 1984.

632 Tavassoli FA, Norris HJ: Sertoli tumors of the ovary. A clinicopathologic study of 28 cases with ultrastructural observations. Cancer **46:**2281-2297, 1980.

633 Taylor HB: Functioning ovarian tumors and related conditions. Pathol Annu **1:**127-147, 1966.

634 Tracy SL, Askin FB, Reddick RL, Jackson B, Kurman RJ: Progesterone-secreting Sertoli cell tumor of the ovary. Gynecol Oncol **22:**85-96, 1985.

635 Young RH: Sertoli-Leydig cell tumors of the ovary. Review with emphasis on historical aspects and unusual variants. Int J Gynecol Pathol **12:**141-147, 1993.

636 Young RH, Dudley AG, Scully RE: Granulosa cell, Sertoli–Leydig cell and unclassified sex cord-stromal tumors associated with pregnancy. A clinico-pathological analysis of thirty-six cases. Gynecol Oncol **18**:181-205, 1984.

637 Young RH, Perez-Atayde AR, Scully RE: Ovarian Sertoli–Leydig cell tumor with retiform and heterologous components. Report of a case with hepatocytic differentiation and elevated serum alpha-fetoprotein. Am J Surg Pathol **8**:709-718, 1984.

638 Young RH, Prat J, Scully RE: Ovarian Sertoli–Leydig cell tumors with heterologous elements. I. Gastrointestinal epithelium and carcinoid. A clinicopathologic analysis of thirty-six cases. Cancer **50**:2448-2456, 1982.

639 Young RH, Scully RE: Ovarian Sertoli–Leydig cell tumors with a retiform pattern. A problem in histopathologic diagnosis. A report of 25 cases. Am J Surg Pathol **7**:755-771, 1983.

640 Young RH, Scully RE: Ovarian sex cord–stromal tumors with bizarre nuclei. A clinicopathologic analysis of 17 cases. Int J Gynecol Pathol **1**:325-335, 1983.

641 Young RH, Scully RE: Ovarian Sertoli cell tumors. A report of 10 cases. Int J Gynecol Pathol **2**:349-363, 1984.

642 Young RH, Scully RE: Well-differentiated ovarian Sertoli–Leydig cell tumors. A clinicopathological analysis of 23 cases. Int J Gynecol **3**:277-290, 1984.

643 Young RH, Scully RE: Ovarian Sertoli–Leydig cell tumors. A clinicopathological analysis of 207 cases. Am J Surg Pathol **9**:543-569, 1985.

644 Zaloudek C, Norris HJ: Sertoli–Leydig tumors of the ovary. A clinicopathologic study of 64 intermediate and poorly differentiated neoplasms. Am J Surg Pathol **8**:405-418, 1984.

Lipid (lipoid, steroid) cell tumor

645 Dunnihoo DR, Grieme DL, Woolf RB: Hilar cell tumors of the ovary. Report of 2 new cases and a review of the world literature. Obstet Gynecol **27**:703-713, 1966.

646 Hayes MC, Scully RE: Ovarian steroid cell tumors (not otherwise specified). A clinicopathological analysis of 63 cases. Am J Surg Pathol **11**:835-845, 1987.

647 Ichinohasama R, Teshima S, Kishi K, Mukai K, Tsunematsu R, Ishii-Ohba H, Shimosato Y: Leydig cell tumor of the ovary associated with endometrial carcinoma and containing 17 beta-hydroxysteroid dehydrogenase. Int J Gynecol Pathol **8**:64-71, 1989.

648 Ishida T, Okagaki T, Tagatz GE, Jacobson ME, Doe RP: Lipid cell tumor of the ovary. An ultrastructural study. Cancer **40**:234-243, 1977.

649 Paraskevas M, Scully RE: Hilus cell tumor of the ovary. A clinicopathological analysis of 12 Reinke crystal-positive and nine crystal-negative cases. Int J Gynecol Pathol **8**:299-310, 1989.

650 Roth LM, Sternberg WH: Ovarian stromal tumors containing Leydig cells. II. Pure Leydig cell tumor, nonhilar type. Cancer **32**:952-960, 1973.

651 Rutgers JL, Scully RE: Functioning ovarian tumors with peripheral steroid cell proliferation. A report of twenty-four cases. Int J Gynecol Pathol **5**:319-337, 1986.

652 Salm R: Ovarian hilus-cell tumours. Their varying presentations. J Pathol **113**:117-127, 1974.

653 Sandberg AA, Slaunwhite WR, Jackson JE, Frawley TF: Androgen biosynthesis by an ovarian lipoid cell tumor. J Clin Endocrinol **22**:929-934, 1962.

653a Seidman JD, Abbondanzo SL, Bratthauer GL: Lipid cell (steroid cell) tumor of the ovary. Immunophenotype with analysis of potential pitfall due to endogenous biotin-like activity. Int J Gynecol Pathol **14**:331-338, 1995.

654 Taylor HB, Norris HJ: Lipid cell tumors of the ovary. Cancer **20**:1953-1962, 1967.

655 Young RH, Scully RE: Ovarian steroid cell tumors associated with Cushing's syndrome. A report of three cases. Int J Gynecol Pathol **6**:40-48, 1987.

Other types

656 Ahn GH, Chi JG, Lee SK: Ovarian sex cord tumor with annular tubules. Cancer **57**:1066-1073, 1986.

657 Anderson MC, Govan ADT, Langley FA, Woodcock AS, Tyagi SP: Ovarian sex cord tumours with annular tubules. Histopathology **4**:137-145, 1980.

658 Brescia RJ, Cardoso De Almeida PC, Fuller AF, Dickersin GR, Robboy SJ: Female adnexal tumor of probable wolffian origin with multiple recurrences over 16 years. Cancer **56**:1456-1461, 1985.

659 Crissman JD, Hart WR: Ovarian sex cord tumors with annular tubules. An ultrastructural study of three cases. Am J Clin Pathol **75**:11-17, 1981.

660 Gloor E: Ovarian sex-cord tumor with annular tubules. Clinicopathologic report of two benign and one malignant cases with long follow-ups. Virchows Arch [A] **384**:185-193, 1979.

661 Hart WR, Kumar N, Crissman JD: Ovarian neoplasms resembling sex cord tumors with annular tubules. Cancer **45**:2352-2363, 1980.

662 Hertel BF, Kempson RL: Ovarian sex cord tumors with annular tubules. An ultrastructural study. Am J Surg Pathol **1**:145-153, 1977.

663 Kariminejad MH, Scully RE: Female adnexal tumor of probable wolffian origin—a distinctive pathological entity. Cancer **31**:671-677, 1973.

664 Neubecker RD, Breen JL: Gynandroblastoma. A report of five cases, with a discussion of the histogenesis and classification of ovarian tumors. Am J Clin Pathol **38**:60-69, 1962.

665 Novak ER: Gynandroblastoma of the ovary. Review of 8 cases from the Ovarian Tumor Registry. Obstet Gynecol **30**:709-715, 1967.

665a Rahilly MA, Williams ARW, Krausz T, al Nafussi A: Female adnexal tumour of probable Wolffian origin. A clinicopathological and immunohistochemical study of three cases. Histopathology **26**:69-74, 1995.

666 Scully RE: Sex cord tumor with annular tubules. A distinctive ovarian tumor of the Peutz-Jeghers syndrome. Cancer **25**:1107-1121, 1970.

667 Sivathondan Y, Salm R, Hughesdon PE, Faccini JM: Female adnexal tumour of probably wolffian origin. J Clin Pathol **32**:616-624, 1979.

668 Taxy JB, Battifora H: Female adnexal tumor of probable wolffian origin. Evidence for a low grade malignancy. Cancer **37**:2349-2354, 1976.

669 Young RH, Dickersin GR, Scully RE: A distinctive ovarian sex cord–stromal tumor causing sexual precocity in the Peutz-Jeghers syndrome. Am J Surg Pathol **7**:233-243, 1983.

670 Young RH, Scully RE: Ovarian tumors of probable wolffian origin. A report of 11 cases. Am J Surg Pathol **7**:125-135, 1983.

671 Young RH, Welch WR, Dickersin GR, Scully RE: Ovarian sex cord tumor with annular tubules. Review of 74 cases including 27 with Peutz-Jeghers syndrome and four with adenoma malignum of the cervix. Cancer **50**:1384-1402, 1982.

Germ cell–sex cord–stromal tumors

672 Bjersing L, Cajander S: Ultrastructure of gonadoblastoma and dysgerminoma (seminoma) in a patient with XY gonadal dysgenesis. Cancer **40**:1127-1137, 1977.

673 Goldsmith CI, Hart WR: Ataxia-telangiectasia with ovarian gonadoblastoma and contralateral dysgerminoma. Cancer **36**:1838-1842, 1975.

674 Govan ADT, Woodcock AS, Gowing NFC, Langley FA, Neville AM, Anderson MC: A clinico-pathological study of gonadoblastoma. Br J Obstet Gynecol **84**:222-228, 1977.

675 Hart WR, Burkons DM: Germ cell neoplasms arising in gonadoblastomas. Cancer **43**:669-678, 1979.

676 Hou-Jensen K, Kempson RL: The ultrastructure of gonadoblastoma and dysgerminoma. Hum Pathol **5**:79-91, 1974.

677 Lacson AG, Gillis DA, Shawwa A: Malignant mixed germ-cell-sex cord-stromal tumors of the ovary associated with isosexual precocious puberty. Cancer **61**:2122-2133, 1988.

678 Mackay AM, Pettigrew N, Symington T, Neville AM: Tumors of dysgenetic gonads (gonadoblastoma). Ultrastructural and steroidogenic aspects. Cancer **34**:1108-1125, 1974.

679 Nakashima N, Nagasaka T, Fukata S, Oiwa N, Nara Y, Fukatsu T, Takeuchi J: Ovarian gonadoblastoma with dysgerminoma in a woman with two normal children. Hum Pathol **20**:814-816, 1989.

680 Pratt-Thomas HR, Cooper JM: Gonadoblastoma with tubal pregnancy. Am J Clin Pathol **65**:121-125, 1976.

681 Roth LM, Eglen DE: Gonadoblastoma. Immunohistochemical and ultrastructural observations. Int J Gynecol Pathol **8**:72-81, 1989.

682 Safneck JR, deSa DJ: Structures mimicking sex cord-stromal tumours and gonadoblastomas in the ovaries of normal infants and children. Histopathology **10**:909-920, 1986.

683 Scully RE: Gonadoblastoma. A review of 74 cases. Cancer **25**:1340-1356, 1970.

684 Talerman A, van der Harten JJ. A mixed germ cell-sex cord-stromal tumor of the ovary associated with isosexual precocious puberty in a normal girl. Cancer **40**:889-894, 1977.

685 Teter J: The mixed germ tumours with hormonal activity. Acta Pathol Microbiol Scand (A) **58**:306-320, 1963.

686 Tokuoka S, Aoki Y, Hayashi Y, Yokoyama T, Ishii T: A mixed germ cell-sex cord-stromal tumor of the ovary with retiform tubular structure. A case report. Int J Gynecol Pathol **4**:161-170, 1985.

Tumors not specific to ovary
Malignant lymphoma and leukemia

687 Ballon SC, Donaldson RC, Berman ML, Swanson GA, Byron RL: Myeloblastoma (granulocytic sarcoma) of the ovary. Arch Pathol Lab Med **102**:474-476, 1978.

688 Chorlton I, Norris HJ, King FM: Malignant reticuloendothelial disease involving the ovary as a primary manifestation. A series of 19 lymphomas and 1 granulocytic sarcoma. Cancer **34**:397-407, 1974.

689 Ferry JA, Young RH: Malignant lymphoma, pseudolymphoma, and hematopoietic disorders of the female genital tract. Pathol Annu **26**(Pt 1):227-263, 1991.

690 Monterroso V, Jaffe ES, Merino MJ, Medeiros LJ: Malignant lymphomas involving the ovary. A clinicopathologic analysis of 39 cases. Am J Surg Pathol **17**:154-170, 1992.

691 Morgan ER, Labotka RJ, Gonzalez-Crussi F, Wiederhold M, Sherman JO: Ovarian granulocytic sarcoma as the primary manifestation of acute infantile myelomonocytic leukemia. Cancer **48**:1819-1824, 1981.

692 Osborne BM, Robboy SJ: Lymphomas or leukemias presenting as ovarian tumors. An analysis of 42 cases. Cancer **52**:1933-1943, 1983.

693 Paladugu RR, Bearman RM, Rappaport H: Malignant lymphoma with primary manifestation in the gonad. A clinicopathologic study of 38 patients. Cancer **45**:561-571, 1980.

694 Pressler H, Horny HP, Wolf A, Kaiserling E: Isolated granulocytic sarcoma of the ovary. Histologic, electron microscopic, and immunohistochemical findings. Int J Gynecol Pathol **11**:68-74, 1992.

695 Rotmensch J, Woodruff JD: Lymphoma of the ovary. Report of twenty new cases and update of previous series. Am J Obstet Gynecol **143**:870-875, 1982.

696 Skodras G, Fields V, Kragel PJ: Ovarian lymphoma and serous carcinoma of low malignant potential arising in the same ovary. A case report with literature review of 14 primary ovarian lymphomas. Arch Pathol Lab Med **118**:647-650, 1994.

Sarcoma

697 Guerard MJ, Arguelles MA, Ferenczy A: Rhabdomyosarcoma of the ovary. Ultrastructural study of a case and review of literature. Gynecol Oncol **15**:325-339, 1983.

698 Hines JF, Compton DM, Stacy CC, Potter ME: Pure primary osteosarcoma of the ovary presenting as an extensively calcified adnexal mass. A case report and review of the literature. Gynecol Oncol **39**:259-263, 1990.

699 Kraemer BB, Silva EG, Sneige N: Fibrosarcoma of ovary. A new component in the nevoid basal-cell carcinoma syndrome. Am J Surg Pathol **8**:231-236, 1984.

700 Ongkasuwan C, Taylor JE, Tang C-K, Prempree T: Angiosarcomas of the uterus and ovary. Clinicopathologic report. Cancer **49**:1469-1475, 1982.

701 Prat J, Scully RE: Cellular fibromas and fibrosarcomas of the ovary. A comparative clinicopathologic analysis of seventeen cases. Cancer **47**:2663-2670, 1981.

702 Sakata H, Hirahara T, Ryu A, Sawada T, Yamamoto M, Sakurai I: Primary osteosarcoma of the ovary. A case report. Acta Pathol Jpn **41**:311-317, 1991.

703 Silverberg SG, Fernandez FN: Endolymphatic stromal myosis of the ovary. A report of three cases and literature review. Gynecol Oncol **12**:129-138, 1981.

704 Stone GC, Bell DA, Fuller A, Dickersin GR, Scully RE: Malignant schwannoma of the ovary. Report of a case. Cancer **58**:1575-1582, 1986.

705 Talerman A, Auerbach WM, Van Meurs AJ: Primary chondrosarcoma of the ovary. Histopathology **5**:319-324, 1981.

706 Young RH, Prat J, Scully RE: Endometrioid stromal sarcomas of the ovary. A clinicopathologic analysis of 23 cases. Cancer **53**:1143-1155, 1984.

Other primary tumors

707 Alvarez M, Cerezo L: Ovarian cavernous hemangioma. Arch Pathol Lab Med **110**:77-78, 1986.

708 Fawcett FJ, Kimbell NKB: Phaeochromocytoma of the ovary. J Obstet Gynaecol Br Commonw **78**:458-459, 1971.

709 Friedman HD, Mazur MT: Primary ovarian leiomyosarcoma. An immunohistochemical and ultrastructural study. Arch Pathol Lab Med **115**:941-945, 1991.

710 Kandalaft PL, Esteban JM: Bilateral massive ovarian leiomyomata in a young woman. A case report with review of the literature. Mod Pathol **5**:586-589, 1992.

711 Nogales FF, Ayala A, Ruiz-Avila I, Sirvent JJ: Myxoid leiomyosarcoma of the ovary. Analysis of three cases. Hum Pathol **22**:1268-1273, 1991.

712 Prayson RA, Hart WR: Primary smooth-muscle tumors of the ovary. A clinicopathologic study of four leiomyomas and two mitotically active leiomyomas. Arch Pathol Lab Med **116**:1068-1071, 1992.

713 Yenen E, Inanc FA, Babuna C: Primary ovarian hydatidiform mole. Report of a case. Obstet Gynecol **26**:721-724, 1966.

714 Young RH, Silva EG, Scully RE: Ovarian and juxtaovarian adenomatoid tumors. A report of six cases. Int J Gynecol Pathol **10**:364-371, 1991.

Metastatic tumors

715 Bullon A Jr, Arseneau J, Prat J, Young RH, Scully RE: Tubular Krukenberg tumor. A problem in histopathologic diagnosis. Am J Surg Pathol **5**:225-232, 1981.

716 Daya D, Nazerali L, Frank GL: Metastatic ovarian carcinoma of large intestinal origin simulating primary ovarian carcinoma. A clinicopathologic study of 25 cases. Am J Clin Pathol **97**:751-758, 1992.

717 Demopoulos RI, Touger L, Dubin N: Secondary ovarian carcinoma. A clinical and pathological evaluation. Int J Gynecol Pathol **6**:166-175, 1987.

718 Eichhorn JH, Young RH, Scully RE: Nonpulmonary small cell carcinomas of extragenital origin metastatic to the ovary. Cancer **71**:177-186, 1993.

719 Fitzgibbons PL, Martin SE, Simmons TJ: Malignant melanoma metastatic to the ovary. Am J Surg Pathol **11**:959-964, 1987.

720 Gagnon Y, Tetu B: Ovarian metastases of breast carcinoma. A clinicopathologic study of 59 cases. Cancer **64**:892-898, 1989.

721 Green LK, Silva EG: Hepatoblastoma in an adult with metastasis to the ovaries. Am J Clin Pathol **92**:110-115, 1989.

722 Holtz F, Hart WR: Krukenberg tumors of the ovary. A clinicopathologic analysis of 27 cases. Cancer **50**:2438-2447, 1982.

723 Joshi VV: Primary Krukenberg tumor of ovary. Review of literature and case report. Cancer **22**:1199-1207, 1968.

724 Lash RH, Hart WR: Intestinal adenocarcinomas metastatic to the ovaries. A clinicopathologic evaluation of 22 cases. Am J Surg Pathol **11**:114-121, 1987.

725 Leffel JM, Masson JC, Dockerty MB: Krukenberg's tumors. Ann Surg **115**:102-113, 1942.

726 Mazur MT, Hsueh S, Gersell DJ: Metastases to the female genital tract. Analysis of 325 cases. Cancer **53**:1978-1984, 1984.

727 Merino MJ, Edmonds P, LiVolsi V: Appendiceal carcinoma metastatic to the ovaries and mimicking primary ovarian tumors. Int J Gynecol Pathol **4**:110-120, 1985.

728 Monteagudo C, Merino MJ, La Porte N, Neumann RD: Value of gross cystic disease fluid protein-15 in distinguishing metastatic breast carcinomas among poorly differentiated neoplasms involving the ovary. Hum Pathol **22**:368-372, 1991.

729 Ramzy I: Signet-ring stromal tumor of ovary. Histochemical, light, and electron microscopic study. Cancer **38**:166-172, 1976.

730 Scully RE, Richardson GS: Luteinization of the stroma of metastatic cancer involving the ovary and its endocrine significance. Cancer **14**:827-840, 1961.

731 Ulbright TM, Roth LM, Stehman FB: Secondary ovarian neoplasia. A clinicopathologic study of 35 cases. Cancer **53**:1164-1174, 1984.

732 Warren S, Macomber WB: Tumor metastasis. IV. Ovarian metastasis of carcinoma. Arch Pathol **19**:75-82, 1935.

732a Wauters CCAP, Smedts F, Gerrits LGM, Bosman FT, Ramaekers FCS: Keratins 7 and 20 as diagnostic markers of carcinomas metastatic to the ovary. Hum Pathol **26**:852-855, 1995.

733 Webb MJ, Decker DG, Mussey E: Cancer metastatic to the ovary. Factors influencing survival. Obstet Gynecol **45**:391-396, 1975.

734 Wong PC, Ferenczy A, Fan L-D, McCaughey E: Krukenberg tumors of the ovary. Ultrastructural, histochemical, and immunohistochemical studies of 15 cases. Cancer **57**:751-760, 1986.

735 Woodruff JD, Novak ER: The Krukenberg tumor. Study of 48 cases from the Ovarian Tumor Registry. Obstet Gynecol **15**:351-360, 1960.

736 Yazigi R, Sandstad J: Ovarian involvement in extragenital cancer. Gynecol Oncol **34**:84-87, 1989.

737 Young RH, Eichhorn JH, Dickersin GR, Scully RE: Ovarian involvement by the intra-abdominal desmoplastic small round cell tumor with divergent differentiation. A report of three cases. Hum Pathol **23**:454-464, 1992.

738 Young RH, Gersell DJ, Clement PB, Scully RE: Hepatocellular carcinoma metastatic to the ovary. A report of three cases discovered during life with discussion of the differential diagnosis of hepatoid tumors of the ovary. Hum Pathol **23**:574-580, 1992.

739 Young RH, Hart WR: Metastases from carcinomas of the pancreas simulating primary mucinous tumors of the ovary. A report of seven cases. Am J Surg Pathol **13**:748-756, 1989.

740 Young RH, Hart WR: Renal cell carcinoma metastatic to the ovary. A report of three cases emphasizing possible confusion with ovarian clear cell adenocarcinoma. Int J Gynecol Pathol **11**:96-104, 1992.

741 Young RH, Jackson A, Wells M: Ovarian metastasis from thyroid carcinoma 12 years after partial thyroidectomy mimicking struma ovarii. Report of a case. Int J Gynecol Pathol **13**:181-185, 1994.

742 Young RH, Scully RE: Ovarian metastases from cancer of the lung. Problems in interpretation—a report of seven cases. Gynecol Oncol **21**:337-350, 1985.

743 Young RH, Scully RE: Alveolar rhabdomyosarcoma metastatic to the ovary. A report of two cases and a discussion of the differential diagnosis of small cell malignant tumors of the ovary. Cancer **64**:899-904, 1989.

744 Young RH, Scully RE: Ovarian metastases from carcinoma of the gallbladder and extrahepatic bile ducts simulating primary tumors of the ovary. A report of six cases. Int J Gynecol Pathol **9:**60-72, 1990.

745 Young RH, Scully RE: Sarcomas metastatic to the ovary. A report of 21 cases. Int J Gynecol Pathol **9:**231-252, 1990.

746 Young RH, Scully RE: Malignant melanoma metastatic to the ovary. A clinicopathologic analysis of 20 cases. Am J Surg Pathol **15:**849-860, 1991.

747 Young RH, Scully RE: Metastatic tumors in the ovary. A problem-oriented approach and review of the recent literature. Semin Diagn Pathol **8:**250-276, 1991.

747a Zaloudek C, Miller TR, Stern JL: Desmoplastic small cell tumor of the ovary. A unique polyphenotypic tumor with an unfavorable prognosis. Int J Gynecol Pathol **14:**260-265, 1995.

748 Zukerberg LR, Young RH: Chordoma metastatic to the ovary. Arch Pathol Lab Med **114:**208-210, 1990.

Placenta

NORMAL ANATOMY

The normal-term placenta measures 15 to 20 cm in diameter and 1.5 to 3 cm in thickness and weighs 450 to 600 g.[5] The main components are the umbilical cord, membranes (amnion and chorion), villous parenchyma, and maternal decidual tissue.

The umbilical cord at term measures 55 to 65 cm in length.[13] It has an outer layer of amniotic epithelium, which becomes stratified at the fetal end. The bulk of the cord is made up of highly mucoid connective tissue known as Wharton's jelly. Embedded within its substance are the umbilical vessels, represented by two arteries and a single vein. The arteries have a double-layered muscular wall but no internal elastic lamina. The vein has a larger diameter and a thinner wall, consisting of a single layer of circular smooth muscle, and an internal elastic lamina. The umbilical cord may insert in the placenta in a central or eccentric fashion. Insertion at the margin is referred to as *battledore placenta*. Whereas it is easy to distinguish microscopically the arteries from the vein in the cord itself, this becomes difficult or impossible once those vessels branch into the chorionic plate.

The placental membranes consist of the amnion and chorion. The amnion, which represents the innermost covering of the amniotic cavity, is lined by a single layer of flat epithelial cells resting on a basement membrane.[6,14a] Squamous metaplasia is common in them, especially near the insertion of the cord. The chorion is composed of a connective tissue membrane that carries the fetal vasculature. Its inner aspect is bounded by the outer layer of the amnion, and the outer aspect is associated with villi that sprout from the surface. The chorion associated with the membrane is referred to as *chorion laeve* and is distinguished from the *chorion frondosum* located in the placenta proper.[11,15] Some of the trophoblast located in the chorion laeve has a characteristic vacuolated appearance.[17]

The trophoblastic villi that arise from the trophoectoderm following formation of the blastocyst constitute the functional unit of the placenta. During the first trimester, they are composed of an outer syncytiotrophoblastic layer and an inner cytotrophoblastic layer, which surround a central mesenchymal core containing primitive fibroblasts and scattered macrophages (Hofbauer cells).

The syncytiotrophoblast is composed of multinucleated giant cells with abundant acidophilic cytoplasm that is strongly immunoreactive for hCG. The cytotrophoblast, which is the progenitor of the syncytiotrophoblast, is made up of hCG-negative mononuclear cells with clear cytoplasm and a well-defined cell membrane. In the term placenta, the cytotrophoblast is inconspicuous, and the syncytiotrophoblast is clumped in the form of "syncytial knots."

The third trophoblastic type is represented by the intermediate trophoblast, also known as interstitial extravillous trophoblast and X cells.[10] This type is present in the villi and in the membranes but is particularly numerous in the extravillous region that forms the deepest structural component of the implantation site. Its most distinctive immunohistochemical property is a strong reactivity for human placental lactogen. All three types of trophoblast are immunoreactive for keratin. They have also been shown to produce and secrete parathyroid hormone–related protein, and this is also true for their neoplastic counterparts.[6a]

The villous vessels become apparent at 6 weeks. At about 8 weeks they contain only nucleated red blood cells, but by weeks 10 to 12 the percentage of nucleated cells has dropped to 10%, and after week 12 they are virtually absent.

Decidual tissue is present both in the placental disk (from which, however, it may be denuded during delivery) and on the chorionic side of the membranes.

The placenta is best examined in the fresh state immediately after delivery.[1,14,16] A thorough evaluation of this organ can disclose abnormalities of clinical significance, contribute to the understanding of disabilities among surviving children, and be of great importance in the resolution of medicolegal cases.[2,3,7-9,12]

Gross inspection of a *twin placenta* provides important information in regard to the type of twinning (Fig. 19-219). A monochorionic placenta (whether monoamnionic or diamnionic) is indicative of monozygotic twins. Instead, dichorionic placentas (whether fused or separated) are compatible with either monozygotic or dizygotic twinning. In a monochorionic placenta, stripping of the amnion reveals a continuous chorionic plate beneath the septum and major vascular anastomoses between the twins. In contrast, dichorionic fused placentas have a rough chorionic ridge at the base of the septum and lack vascular anastomoses.[4]

ABORTION

The clinical incidence of spontaneous abortion is about 15%, but the real incidence may be as high as 40% to 80%. The etiologic factors are many. They include infections (particularly rubella, *Campylobacter, Listeria,* syphilis, toxoplasmosis, and cytomegalovirus), mechanical disturbances (uterine leiomyomas, cervical incompetence), endocrine disease, immunologic mechanisms (autoimmune disease, ABO incompatibility), and inherited chromosomal abnormalities.[41]

Possible combination of fetal membranes in monozygotic twin placenta (identical twins)

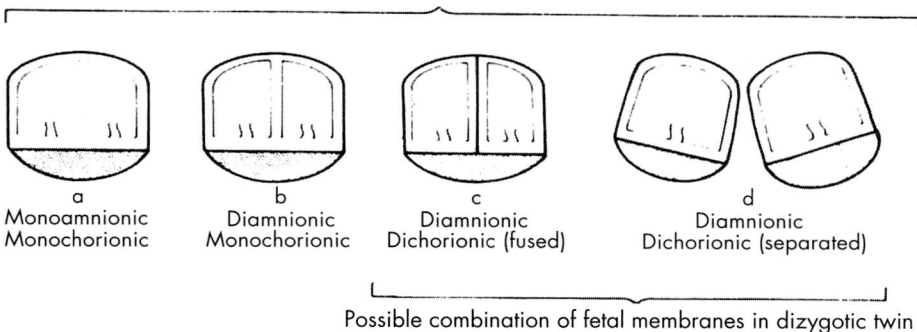

a	b	c	d
Monoamnionic Monochorionic	Diamnionic Monochorionic	Diamnionic Dichorionic (fused)	Diamnionic Dichorionic (separated)

Possible combination of fetal membranes in dizygotic twin placenta (fraternal twins)

Fig. 19-219 Diagrammatic representation of common variations possible in monochorionic and dichorionic twin placentation. Types **a** and **b** of monochorionic twin placenta are seen only with identical twins. Variations **c** and **d** are common to both identical and fraternal twins. Hence, identification of dichorionic twin placenta does not distinguish between identical and fraternal twins. (From Kraus FT: Gynecologic pathology, St. Louis, 1967, Mosby.)

The morphologic confirmation of the occurrence of a pregnancy is one of the most common determinations performed by the pathologist.[18] When fetal parts, gestational sac, or viable chorionic villi are present, the task is easy (Fig. 19-220, *A*). In the presence of an identifiable fetus, determination should be made whether it is macerated or not and whether it appears normal, grossly disorganized, or focally abnormal.* There is a good correlation between cytogenetic abnormalities and embryonic growth disorganization leading to early death, usually before the fetal stage (30 mm) is reached.[26a,47] Occasionally, only a type of tissue from the embryo survives, such as glial tissue.[48,53] When the gestational sac is identified, a statement should be made as to whether it is intact or ruptured and—for the latter—whether it contains a cord stump or not. The chorionic villi may be already apparent grossly to the gynecologist by the simple procedure of examining contents from the curettage in saline solution after rinsing the blood.[32] In other instances, they are impossible to identify grossly, and numerous paraffin blocks may be necessary to identify them microscopically.

Necrotic ("ghost") villi are particularly difficult to recognize, since clumps of fibrin may closely simulate them. The overall configuration and the presence of shadows of stromal cells and trophoblast are the main identifying criteria (Fig. 19-220, *B*). In the absence of chorionic villi, a search should be made for trophoblastic cells, whether isolated or in clumps (Fig. 19-221). Care should be exercised not to confuse these trophoblastic cells—particularly those of intermediate type—with decidual cells. Intermediate trophoblastic cells infiltrate the decidua surrounding the blastocyst to form the trophoblastic shell, invade the spiral arterioles of the placental bed, and infiltrate the myometrium beneath the implantation site. They are usually mononuclear, of variable shape (round, polygonal, or spindled), with amphophilic or eosinophilic granular cytoplasm and indis-

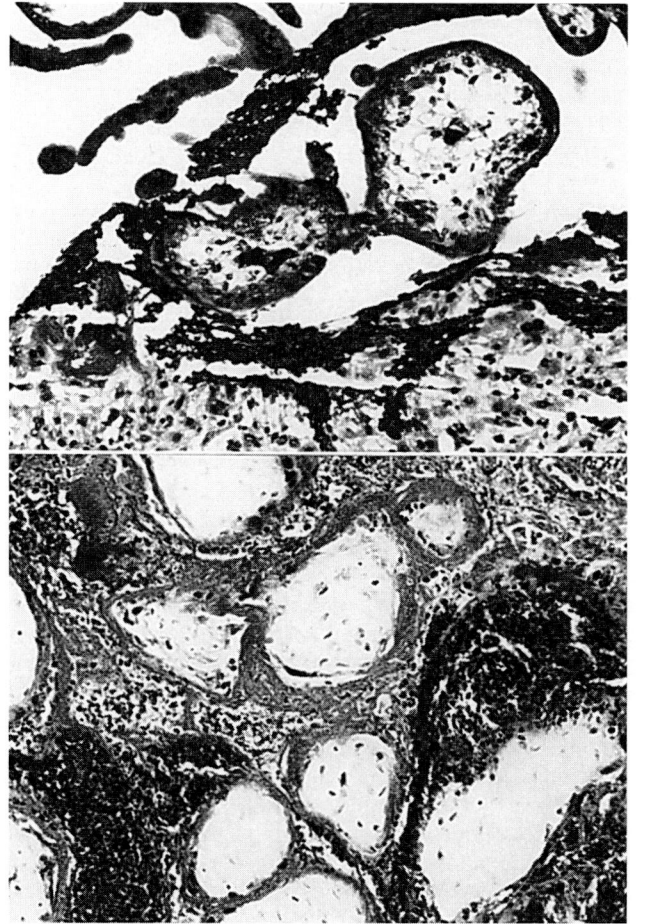

A

B

Fig. 19-220 Chorionic villi in D&C specimen. Villi shown in **A** are well preserved and accompanied by sheets of syncytiotrophoblasts. Villi shown in **B** are necrotic but still identifiable.

*References 18, 19, 31a, 34, 38, 39, 43, 44, 52.

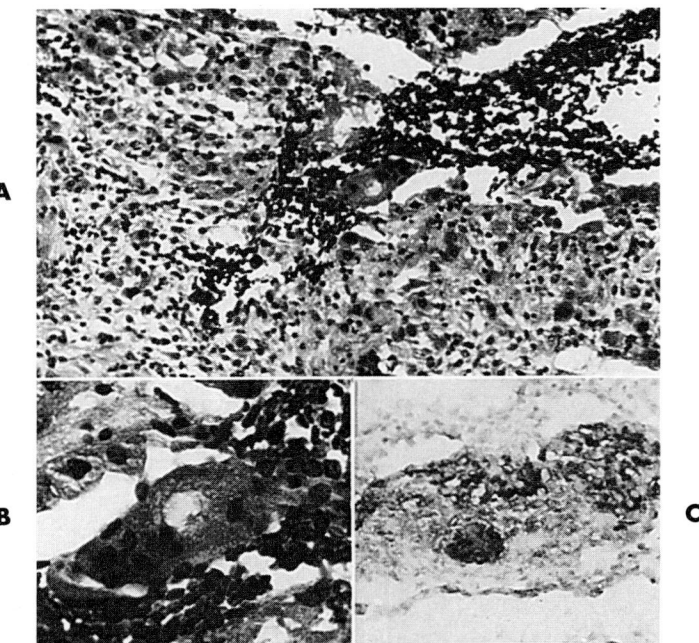

Fig. 19-221 Isolated syncytiotrophoblastic cells in a D&C specimen. **A** is panoramic view, **B** is high-power magnification, and **C** shows positive immunocytochemical staining for hCG.

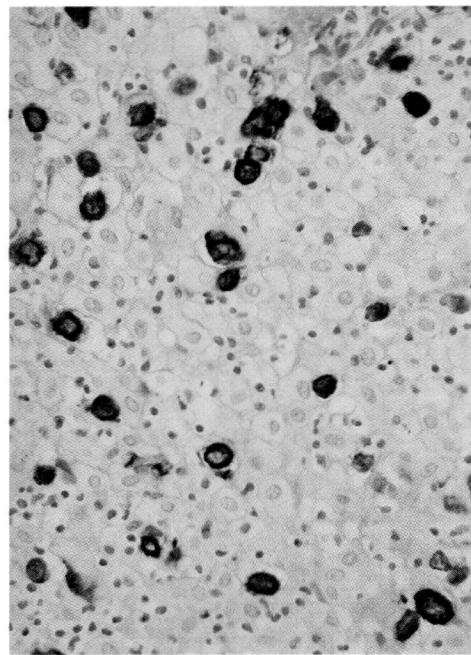

Fig. 19-222 Isolated intermediate trophoblast cells strongly staining for keratin.

tinct cell borders. Their nuclei are round or lobulated, sometimes multiclefted, and frequently hyperchromatic.[51] In contrast, decidual cells have distinct cell borders, pale homogeneous cytoplasm, and round uniform nuclei with fine chromatin.

When it is impossible to determine on the basis of routinely stained sections whether trophoblastic cells of any type are present or not and this determination is of clinical importance (as in the differential diagnosis between intrauterine and ectopic pregnancy), immunocytochemical stains for hCG, human placental lactogen (hPL), pregnancy-specific beta-1-glycoprotein (SP1), and keratin should be employed (Figs. 19-221, *C,* and 19-222).*

In the absence of fetal parts, villi, or trophoblast (as detected morphologically or immunohistochemically), the diagnosis of intrauterine pregnancy cannot be made with absolute certainty, although enlarged hyalinized spiral arterioles and the presence of a fibrinoid matrix are features associated with intrauterine implantation.[35] There are other endometrial patterns that are strongly suggestive that a gestation has occurred, but they do not establish its site (intrauterine versus ectopic) and are not pathognomonic.[21] These include decidual reaction, gestational hyperplasia, and Arias-Stella reaction. The microscopic appearance of the decidua of pregnancy can be closely simulated by the deciduoid changes secondary to the use of oral contraceptives, even if the latter usually lack the dilated vascular channels of true decidua and have a more inactive glandular pattern.

Gestational hyperplasia is characterized by the *simultaneous* presence in the endometrial mucosa of glandular secre-

---

*References 20, 23, 28, 30, 40, 45, 46.

tion, stromal edema, and deciduoid changes.[27] The basal glandular cells show strong immunoreactivity for S-100 protein.[33] The Arias-Stella reaction (discussed earlier in this chapter in the section on Uterus—Corpus) is a physiologic response to viable trophoblastic tissue[36]; it characteristically develops during pregnancy, but it may also occur following the use of progestational agents and other exogenous hormones.[29]

In some institutions, frozen sections of curetted endometrial material are requested in an attempt to distinguish intrauterine from ectopic pregnancy. If fetal parts or well-developed chorionic villi are present, the task is easy. However, the identification of trophoblast—particularly of the intermediate type—is difficult enough in formalin-fixed paraffin-embedded material (as previously discussed) to expect for this to be reliably achieved in frozen section material, no matter how experienced the observer. The use of laparoscopy and ultrasonography (particularly after the advent of the vaginal transducer) should obviate the need for this intrinsically unreliable procedure.[37]

Septic abortion is usually caused by coliform organisms or anaerobic streptococci. The pathologist should identify the microorganisms in the tissue sections before making a diagnosis of septic abortion. The presence of polymorphonuclear neutrophils, even in large numbers, is not necessarily an indication of infection, since it may simply represent an inflammatory reaction to the necrotic decidua and fetal tissues.

Herpes simplex infection was detected immunohistochemically by Robb et al.[42] in material from abortion in several cases, suggesting the existence of a latent subclinical infection that produced transplacental infection of the fetus.

Most patients who have had a miscarriage should undergo a uterine dilatation and curettage in order to remove residual trophoblastic tissue. This material should always be examined microscopically in order to rule out early gestational trophoblastic disease.

Hydropic changes may be seen in the chorionic villi of abortion material ("hydropic abortus") and need to be distinguished from those accompanying a complete or a partial mole. In the hydropic abortus, *gross* villous swelling and cistern formation are not seen. More important, these villi are typically surrounded by *attenuated* trophoblast. If trophoblastic proliferation is present, it has an orderly, centrifugal, and polar quality and lacks significant nuclear atypia.

Lately, flow cytometric DNA analysis has been applied as an adjunct to this differential diagnosis. A correlation between DNA values, karyotypic abnormalities, and microscopic changes exists, but this is not as close as one might have wished.[22,31,49] As a matter of fact, the degree of interobserver variability and the lack of predictive value of the microscopic evaluation are such as to have led some experts to conclude that a classification of abortion material on morphologic grounds—beyond documenting the fact that a pregnancy has occurred and ruling out gestational trophoblastic disease—is a valueless exercise.[24,50] Admittedly, hydropic villi are more likely to have a nondiploid DNA content than nonhydropic ones.[26] However, of the abortuses with a triploid DNA pattern, only half show the morphologic features of a partial mole, most of the others being morphologically unremarkable.[26]

Examination of placental tissue from second-trimester abortions (whether spontaneous, surgically induced, or prostaglandin-induced) consistently shows degenerative changes consisting of focal decidual necrosis, intradecidual hemorrhage, and congestion and thrombosis of maternal vessels.[25]

GESTATIONAL TROPHOBLASTIC DISEASE

There is a group of diseases related to normal or abnormal gestation that have as a common feature the proliferation of trophoblast and that are generically designated as (gestational) trophoblastic disease. The individual disorders differ remarkably in appearance and clinical significance; they include hydatidiform mole, placental site trophoblastic tumor, and choriocarcinoma. In hydatidiform moles, the trophoblastic proliferation is associated with swelling of the villi. They are subdivided into complete, partial, and invasive.

Hydatidiform mole
Complete mole

Complete hydatidiform mole is caused by abnormal gametogenesis and fertilization. The nuclei of the trophoblastic cells in this disease contain only paternal chromosomes and are therefore androgenetic in origin.[70] The chromosomal number is normal; 85% of the cases are 46,XX, and 15% are 46,XY. It has been hypothesized that in the 46,XX cases, the process is fertilization of an "empty" ovum with no effective genome by a haploid sperm that duplicates without cytokinesis, whereas in the 46,XY cases there might be fertilization of the "empty" ovum by two haploid sperms with subsequent fusion and replication. This

hypothesis is supported by the genetic analysis of molar mitochondrial DNA.[55]

There is a striking geographic variation in the frequency of complete mole. The incidence of 1 in 2000 deliveries reported in the classic studies by Hertig[65] represents an average for young healthy women in the United States. In Southeast Asia, the reported incidence is at least four to five times greater.[67,68] Yet higher incidences have been reported from Mexico (1:200), the Philippines (1:173), India (1:160), Taiwan (1:125), and Indonesia (1:82).[78,80] Patients with complete mole tend to be older than 30 years of age and more likely to have diets deficient in vitamin A precursors (which may explain some of the geographic differences previously mentioned).[56] The risk is reduced by increased consumption of carotene. A history of previous term birth reduces the risk of molar pregnancy, whereas a history of a previous mole greatly increases the probability of developing another.[69,82] "Repetitive" moles are usually of complete type, but they can be of partial type, or a complete mole may be followed by a partial mole.[81]

Clinically, the uterus involved by a complete mole is disproportionately large for the stage of pregnancy.[54] Serum hCG levels continue to rise after the fourteenth week, as opposed to the drop typically seen in the course of normal gestation. Evidence of toxemia of pregnancy (hypertension, edema, albuminuria) is frequently found, and this typically occurs during the early stages of the pregnancy. Exceptionally, hyperthyroidism develops as a result of a thyroid stimulator secreted by the molar tissue, perhaps residing in the hCG molecule itself.[59,64] At the time of the medical consultation there may be vaginal bleeding, a sign that the mole has begun to abort spontaneously.

Grossly, the complete mole has been typically described as a "bunch of grapes," with all or nearly all the villi showing hydropic degeneration. The individual vesicles measure anywhere from 1 to 30 mm in diameter, and the total weight is usually over 200 g. In a hysterectomy specimen, these swollen villi are seen to fill and distend the uterus (Fig. 19-223). There are no identifiable embryo, cord, or amniotic membranes. The exceptional cases of bona fide complete mole in which an embryo is present almost invariably represent a twin gestation.[84a]

Microscopically, the two constant features of a complete mole are trophoblastic hyperplasia and vesicular swelling, the latter probably representing a secondary phenomenon. The severity of the changes varies considerably from case to case and from villus to villus. Some of the villi are surrounded by an attenuated layer of degenerating trophoblast. In others, the trophoblast forms large hyperplastic sheets of cells (Fig. 19-224). The distended core of the villus is traversed by widely separated, broken strands of fibrillar material ("cistern" formation). Vessels are usually absent or are very sparse. The trophoblastic hyperplasia characteristically has a circumferential but haphazard arrangement around the individual villi, as opposed to the polar proliferation seen in normal first-trimester villi. The plexiform pattern of intermixed syncytiotrophoblast and cytotrophoblast seen in choriocarcinoma does not occur. At the implantation site of a molar pregnancy, there is an increased number of lymphocytes, most of which are of T-cell type (with a predominance of CD4+ cells).

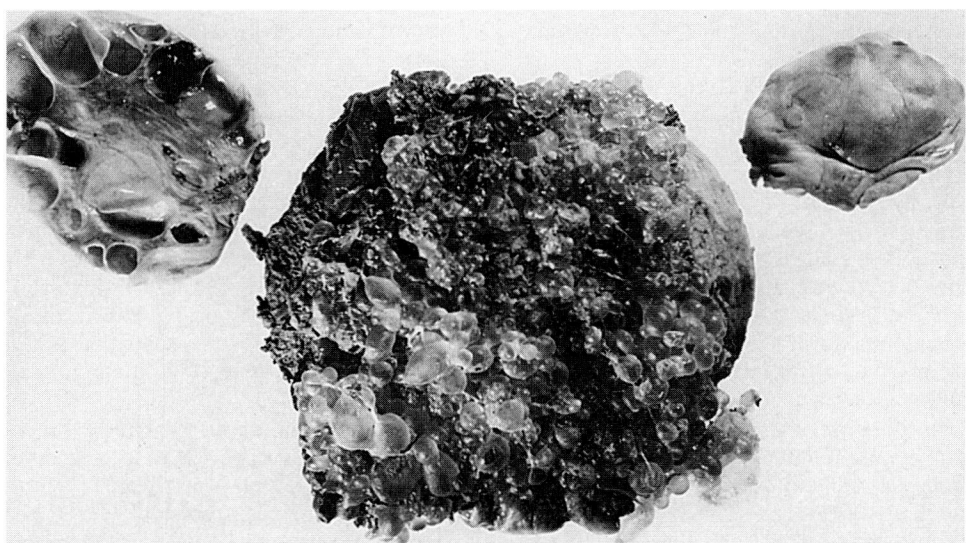

Fig. 19-223 Classic example of hydatidiform mole almost obscuring wall of uterus. Note multiple theca-lutein cysts in ovaries. (Courtesy Dr. M. Carter Houston.)

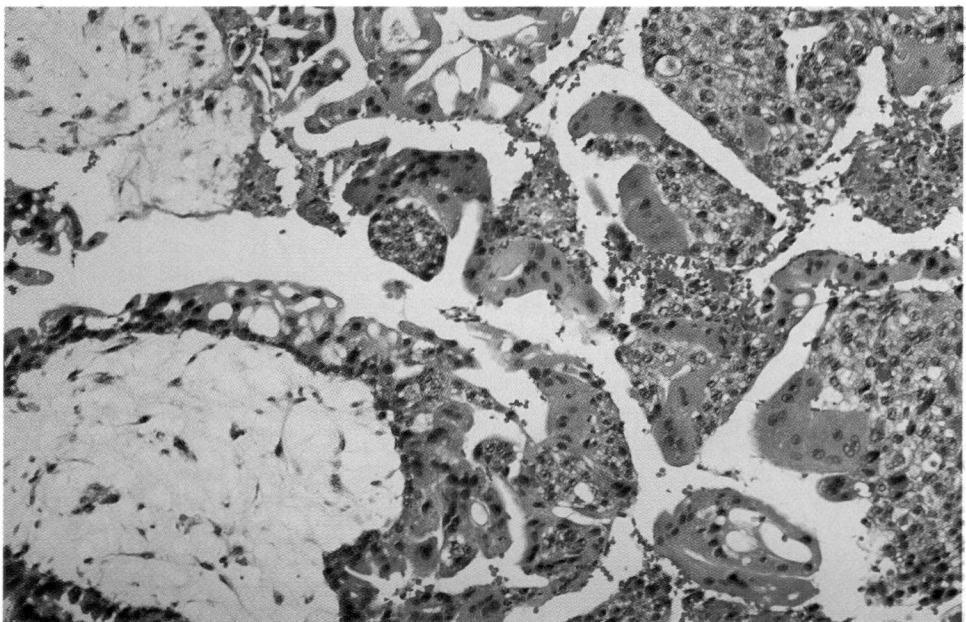

Fig. 19-224 Complete mole showing large villi with stromal edema and marked trophoblastic proliferation.

Ultrastructurally, the molar trophoblast closely resembles that seen during the first trimester of a normal pregnancy.[79]

Immunohistochemically, hCG is widely distributed and placental alkaline phosphatase is patchily distributed in the molar syncytiotrophoblast regardless of gestational age, whereas human placental lactogen tends to increase with increased gestational age.[57,62] The tumor suppressor gene p53 is expressed in direct relation to the proliferative activity of the trophoblast (mainly cytotrophoblast). Thus the intensity of staining in complete mole is higher than in partial mole and lower than in choriocarcinoma.[75a] Interestingly, some staining is also present in the normal trophoblast of early pregnancy.[84b]

Expression of *myc, ras,* and *sis* oncogenes has been demonstrated in complete moles by in situ hybridization, and epidermal growth factor has been detected immunohistochemically.

By flow cytometry, 50% of complete moles are diploid, 43% are tetraploid, 3.6% are polyploid, and 1.7% are triploid.[73-75] The claim has been made that the more pronounced the trophoblastic hyperplasia, the higher the chance of the development of a choriocarcinoma. However, the number of exceptions renders this evaluation of little if any practical utility, especially after the advent of highly sensitive techniques for monitoring serum hCG levels.[61,63] According to Driscoll,[61] molar lesions characterized by the interposition of fibrin-like material at the tumor-host interphase and by the presence of abundant syncytiotrophoblast respond very well to chemotherapy, whereas those having a compact growth of cytotrophoblast with little differentiation tend to be relatively resistant. Heterozygous (dispermic) moles, including dispermic heterozygous XY moles, are associated with a higher incidence of persistent trophoblastic disease than homozygous (monospermic) moles. The proliferation index and DNA ploidy have not been found to be statistically associated with outcome.[73]

The initial therapy of complete mole consists of evacuation of the uterus by curettage.[81a] This is followed by sequential quantitative determination by radioimmunoassay of the beta subunit of hCG (which is different from that of the closely related pituitary luteinizing hormone).[60,66,83,84] The standard recommendation has been to measure the serum level of hCG at 10, 20, 30, 45, and 60 days after termination of the molar gestation.[58] In about 80% of the cases, normal levels will be reached by day 60.[58] If there is rising titer between day 45 and day 60 or the level is still elevated by day 60, chemotherapy is administered; this is necessary in about 20% of the cases.[76]

Other authors recommend the administration of chemotherapy to those patients who have a plateau of three high values of hCG over a 2-week period after evacuation of the mole (about 20% to 30% of the cases). Still others recommend waiting for 4 weeks or even 2 months before initiating chemotherapy, especially if the hCG levels are low.[71,72] In a series of 738 patients with mole, spontaneous regression occurred in 81%. Of the remaining patients, 17% developed an invasive mole, and 2% developed choriocarcinoma.[77] The presence of villi or atypical trophoblast following the evacuation of a molar pregnancy indicates "persistent trophoblastic disease," but the decision whether to give chemotherapy or not still largely depends on the hCG levels.

Partial mole

About 15% to 35% of all moles are of the partial type.[89] In contrast to complete mole, the condition is often associated with the presence of an embryo, although this is usually abnormal ("blighted ovum"). The volume of placental tissue is relatively normal, and the grossly vesicular villi are mixed with normal appearing ones (Fig. 19-225). The former often show focal edema leading to central "cisternal" formation and stromal inclusions of trophoblast (Fig. 19-226). Many of the villi have an irregular, scalloped outline and contain vessels with fetal (nucleated) red blood cells.[102] Fibrosis of the villous stroma is common. Trophoblastic proliferation is present, although generally in lesser degree than in complete mole; cytoplasmic vacuolization of the syncytium is prominent. Immunohistochemically, some differences in localization of hCG and hPL when compared with complete moles have been described.[88]

Most partial moles are triploid (69,XXX or 69,XXY) and a few show trisomy 16.[87,102,104,105,105a]

Because of the generally small size of the lesion, the uterine size is nearly always small or appropriate for the gestational age. Serum hCG levels—although elevated—tend to be relatively low, and the ovarian theca-lutein cysts that commonly accompany complete moles do not occur.[86] The risk for the development of choriocarcinoma following a partial mole is very low, but a few well-documented cases are on record.[92,103] Furthermore, some series document a 5% to 10% incidence of persistent disease, indicating that follow-up of these patients is mandatory.[95,97,99] Some of the recurrences have been in the form of invasive mole.[91,93,98,100]

It should be noted that not all placentas of triploid conceptuses show partial molar transformation; as already indicated (see p. 1543), some have a normal morphologic appearance.[90] The triploid fetuses in both groups tend to die at about 8 weeks menstrual age.[101]

Partial moles should be distinguished not only from complete moles but also from the hydropic villi seen in 15% to 40% of spontaneous abortions.[85,94] In the latter, gross villous swelling and cistern formation are not present. As already stated, the villous trophoblast in spontaneous abortions either is attenuated or—if proliferating—has a polar distribution. Furthermore, trophoblastic atypia is absent or minimal. Flow cytometry studies can be of utility in the evaluation of this problem.[95,96]

Invasive mole

The term *invasive mole (chorioadenoma destruens)* refers to a hydatidiform mole (nearly always of the complete type but occasionally of the partial type) in which villi penetrate the myometrium and/or its blood vessels[111,112] (Figs. 19-227 and 19-228). This phenomenon, which occurs in 16% of all complete moles, is an exaggerated expression of the capacity of normal trophoblast for invasion, a necessary property for implantation. Placenta accreta (see p. 1556) is another manifestation of this phenomenon; the common demonstration of microscopic trophoblastic emboli in the lungs after normal pregnancy is yet another.[106]

The myometrial permeation in invasive mole may be extensive and may lead to persistent hemorrhage, but the serosa is usually intact. However, uterine perforation may

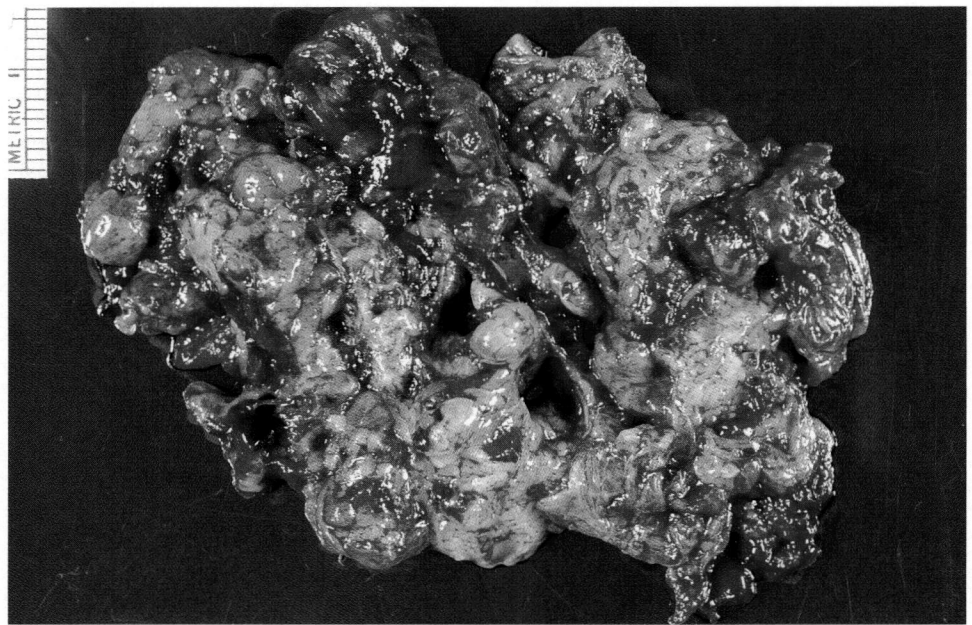

Fig. 19-225 Gross appearance of partial mole. The hydropic degeneration of the villi is not as pronounced as in the classical complete mole.

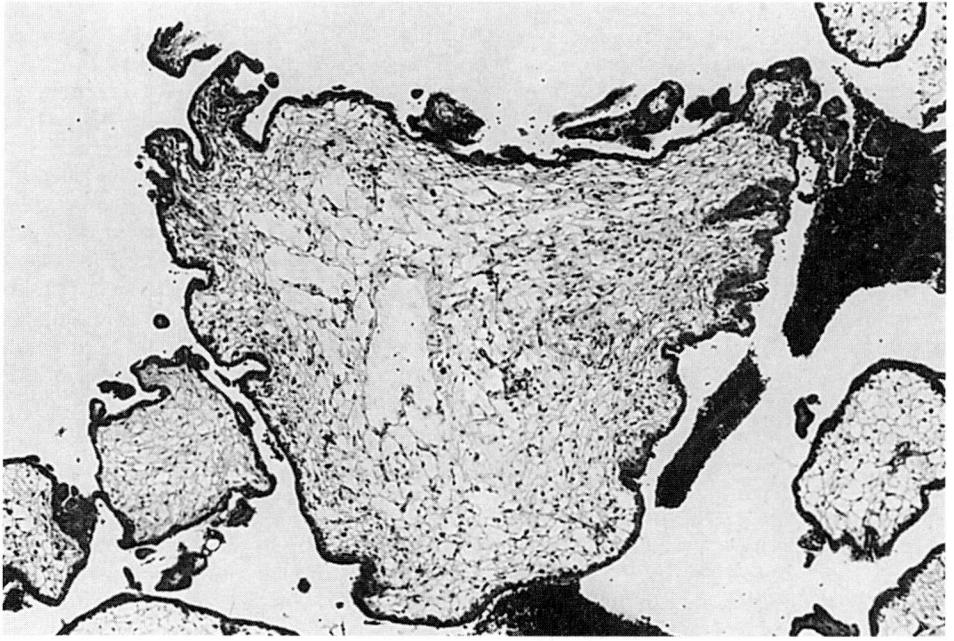

Fig. 19-226 Partial hydatidiform mole. There is marked enlargement of villi with edema and beginning central "cistern" formation. Trophoblastic proliferation is minimal.

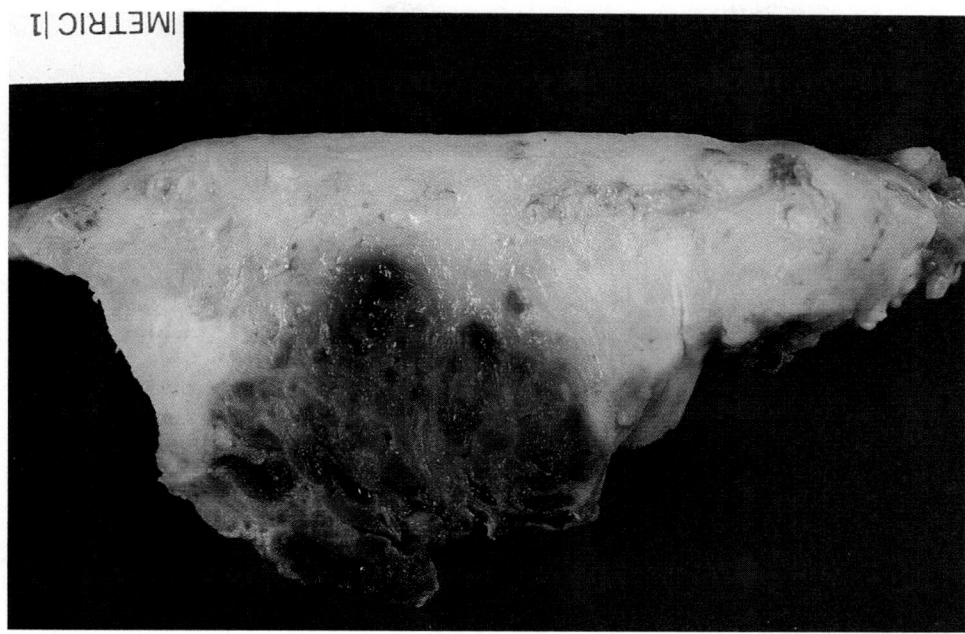

Fig. 19-227 Gross appearance of invasive mole. A hemorrhagic mass has permeated half of the thickness of the myometrial wall.

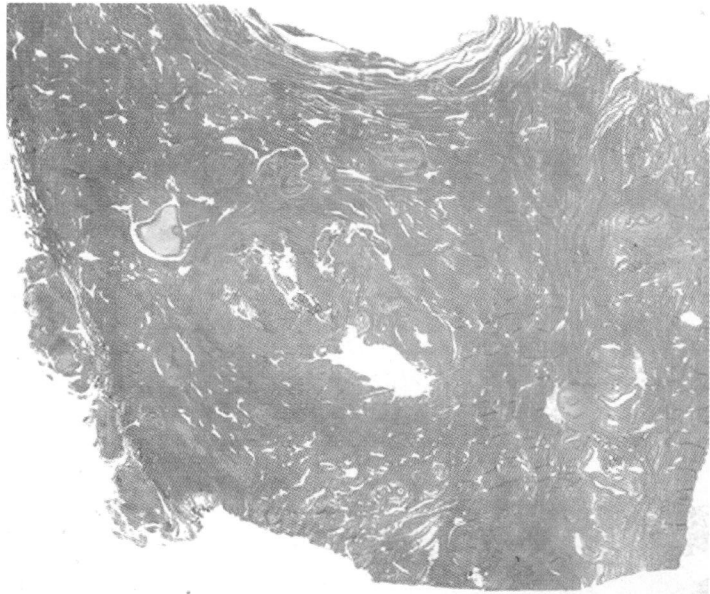

Fig. 19-228 Whole-mount view of invasive mole. Abnormal villi are seen permeating the thickened myometrium.

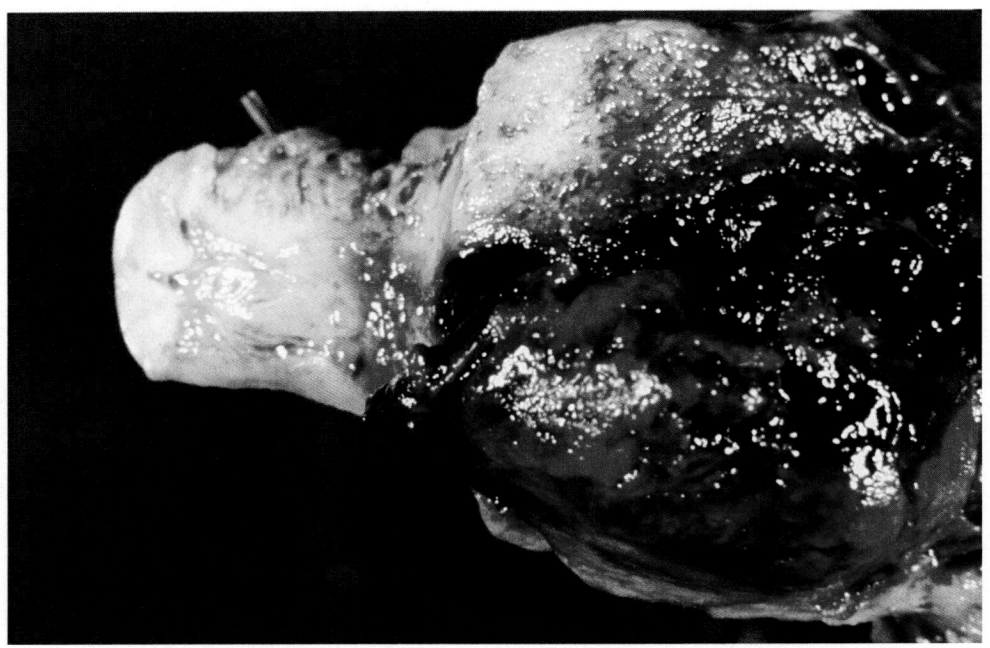

Fig. 19-229 Gross appearance of placental site trophoblastic tumor. A polypoid mass is seen filling the endometrial cavity. Most cases of this tumor are not as hemorrhagic as the example shown here.

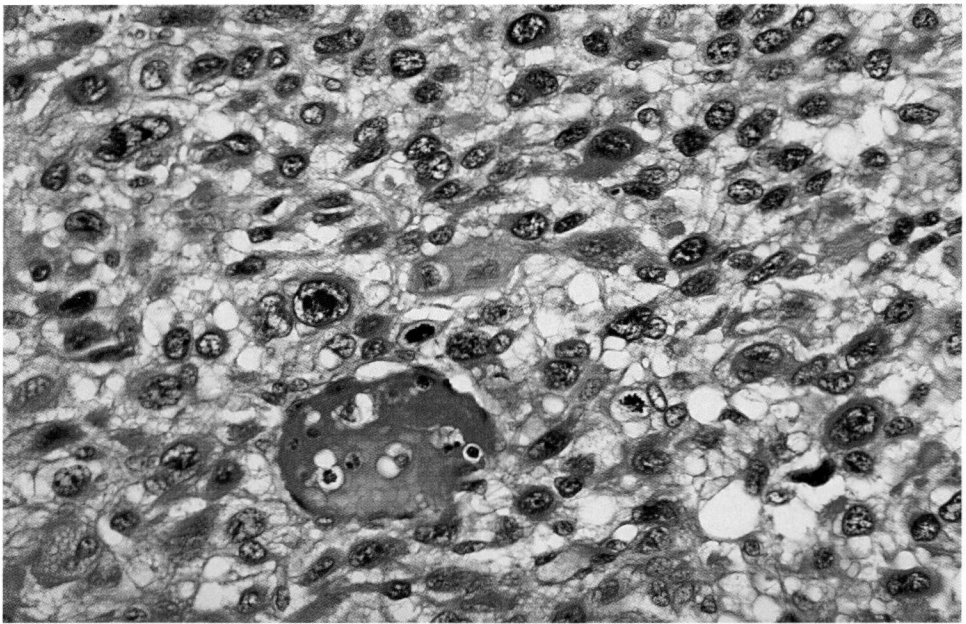

Fig. 19-230 Placental site trophoblastic tumor showing medium-sized cells with moderate atypia growing in a diffuse fashion in the myometrium. The biphasic pattern resulting from the admixture of cytotrophoplast and syncytiotrophoblast, which is typical of choriocarcinoma, is absent.

occur. The vascular invasion may result in trophoblastic nodules in sites outside the uterus, such as the vagina, lung, brain, and spinal cord.[110,113] The lung nodules have a characteristic radiographic appearance[107,108]; they continue to produce hCG and have a similar tendency for hemorrhagic complications. The clinical manifestations depend on the site involved: A sizable mass in the lung may regress spontaneously without ever causing symptoms, whereas a deposit in the brain may produce fatal hemorrhage.[109,115]

Invasive mole is distinguished from the usual mole by its invasiveness and from choriocarcinoma by the presence of villi, which are also present in the "metastatic" foci. The degree of trophoblastic proliferation in invasive mole does not differ significantly from that of its ordinary counterpart. Patients with invasive mole are primarily treated with chemotherapy, but hysterectomy may be indicated in some circumstances.[112,114]

Placental site trophoblastic tumor

Placental site trophoblastic tumor is the term currently preferred for a rare form of trophoblastic disease formerly described as *atypical choriocarcinoma* and *trophoblastic pseudotumor*.[124,130,135] About 75% of the cases follow a normal pregnancy, with only 5% of the reported patients having had a preceding molar pregnancy.[131] It presents grossly as a myometrial mass that can be well localized or ill defined. Hemorrhage is not as conspicuous as in invasive mole or choriocarcinoma (Fig. 19-229). The uterine penetration may be deep, and perforation may result, either spontaneously or following curettage.

Microscopically, large trophoblastic cells with abundant eosinophilic cytoplasm and nuclear pleomorphism are seen invading the myometrium and vessel lumina (Fig. 19-230). The morphologic, ultrastructural, and immunohistochemical features of these cells correspond to those of intermediate trophoblast.[117,122,123,128,133] As such, the immunoreactivity for hPL is strong and widespread, whereas that for hCG tends to be focal.[116,125] There is also cytoplasmic positivity for keratin. The DNA pattern, as determined by flow cytometry, is usually diploid.[119,121]

Although this condition was initially considered to be an exuberant form of syncytial endometritis,[124] additional experience has shown that it is instead a neoplastic process with a 10% to 20% mortality rate.[126] Some cases have resulted in widespread metastases[119,129]; these have generally shown a high mitotic count in the primary tumor, extensive necrosis, and/or a preponderance of cells with clear cytoplasm.[130]

Serum hCG levels in placental site trophoblastic tumor are usually not as high as in choriocarcinoma and may not accurately reflect the extent of the disease. Sometimes the tumor is totally resistant to chemotherapy.[118,120] A distinctive renal glomerular lesion accompanied by proteinuria and hematuria and characterized by occlusive eosinophilic deposits in the glomerular capillary lumina has been observed in connection with this neoplasm.[136]

The differential diagnosis of placental site trophoblastic tumor includes other gestational trophoblastic diseases as well as nonneoplastic placental proliferations of intermediate trophoblast. The distinction with choriocarcinoma is made because of a lack of a dimorphic population of cytotrophoblast and syncytiotrophoblast (although scattered multinucleated cells may be present), lack or paucity of hemorrhage, and the presence of an interdigitating pattern of muscle invasion.

Non-neoplastic proliferations of intermediate trophoblast include so-called syncytial endometritis and placental site nodules and plaques. *Syncytial endometritis* (a double misnomer because the condition neither is composed of syncytiotrophoblast nor is primarily of inflammatory nature) is the result of excessive but otherwise normal infiltration of the implantation site by intermediate trophoblast. Exaggerated placental site reaction is a more accurate designation for this process.

Placental site nodules and plaques appear as single or multiple, mostly well-circumscribed, variably cellular round or flat lesions that tend to be extensively hyalinized[120a,130a] (Fig. 19-231). The cells have abundant amphophilic or acidophilic cytoplasm, irregularly shaped nuclei, and very scanty mitotic activity. Mallory bodies (representing abnormal cytoplasmic aggregates of keratin filaments) may be present.[132] These nodules and plaques are distinguished from placental site trophoblastic tumor because of their smaller size, better circumscription, extensive hyalinization, degenerative appearance, and paucity of mitotic activity.[127,134]

The differential diagnosis between placental site trophoblastic tumor and the non-neoplastic proliferations previously mentioned may not be always possible in a curettage specimen. In such cases, subsequent curettings and monitoring of serum levels of hCG and hPL become imperative.[135]

Choriocarcinoma

Choriocarcinoma is the most aggressive form of gestational trophoblastic disease. Most cases occur following a complete hydatidiform mole; consequently, this malignant tumor is more common in areas of the world in which hydatidiform mole is prevalent. It has been estimated that 1% to 2% of complete moles are followed by choriocarcinoma.[139]

Choriocarcinoma can also be preceded by a partial mole (a very unusual event), ectopic pregnancy, nonmolar intrauterine abortion, or term pregnancy[140,151,166] (Fig.19-232). In the latter instance, which is exceptionally rare, the tumor may appear as one or more masses in an otherwise normal placenta or develop following the delivery.[141,156]

In cases of choriocarcinoma following abortion—whether molar or not—the latent period is almost always less than 1 year, although it can be considerably longer.[146] At the time of the diagnosis of the malignancy, the average age of the patient is 29 years. When reviewing the microscopic sections of a nonmolar abortion in women who subsequently developed choriocarcinoma, it is not unusual to find foci of increased trophoblastic proliferation. These foci, although not diagnostic of trophoblastic disease even in retrospect, suggest the existence of a precursor lesion.

Bagshawe et al.[137,138] have shown a striking relationship between the incidence and prognosis of choriocarcinoma and the ABO groups of both the woman and her husband. The highest risk is for women of group A married to men of the same group. The relative risk of the two extreme groups was 10.4:1. Women married to men of their own ABO group

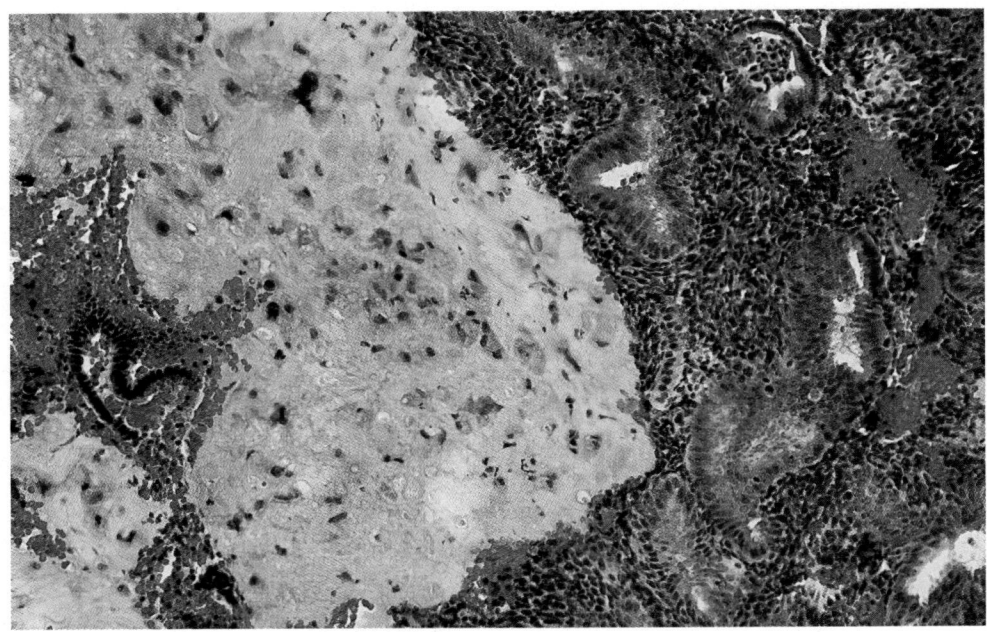

Fig. 19-231 Placental plaque in the endometrium. The lesion is well circumscribed, and it has a characteristic eosinophilic staining quality.

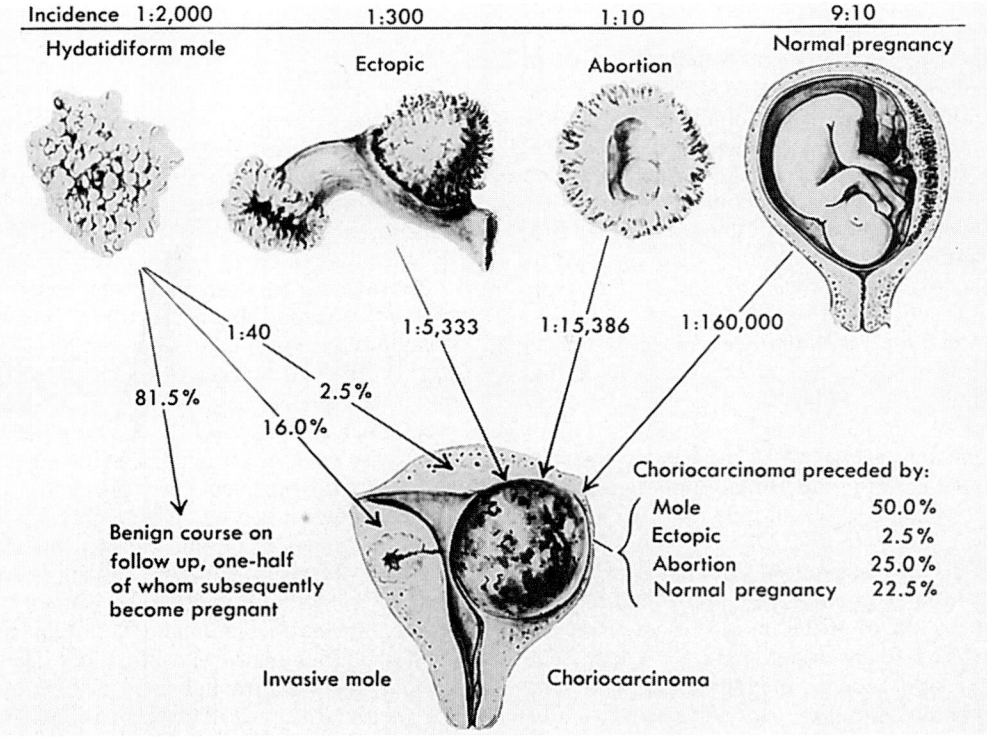

Fig. 19-232 Origin and incidence of choriocarcinoma. (Modified from Hertig AT: Hydatidiform mole and chorionepithelioma. In Meigs JV, Sturgis SH, eds: Progress in gynecology. New York, 1950, Grune & Stratton, Inc.)

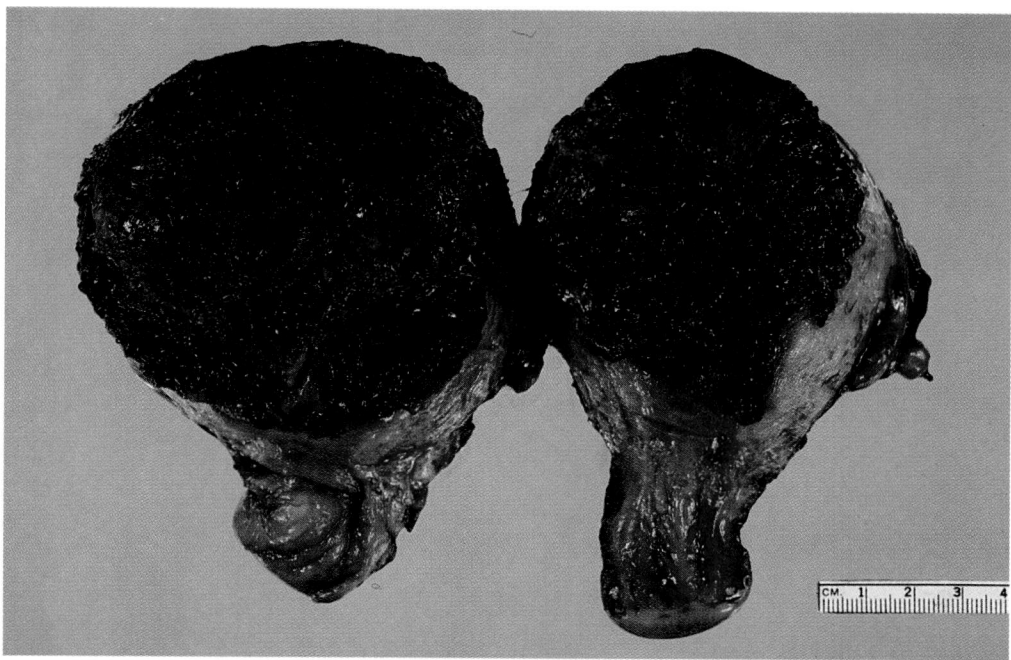

Fig. 19-233 Uterine choriocarcinoma showing typical highly hemorrhagic appearance.

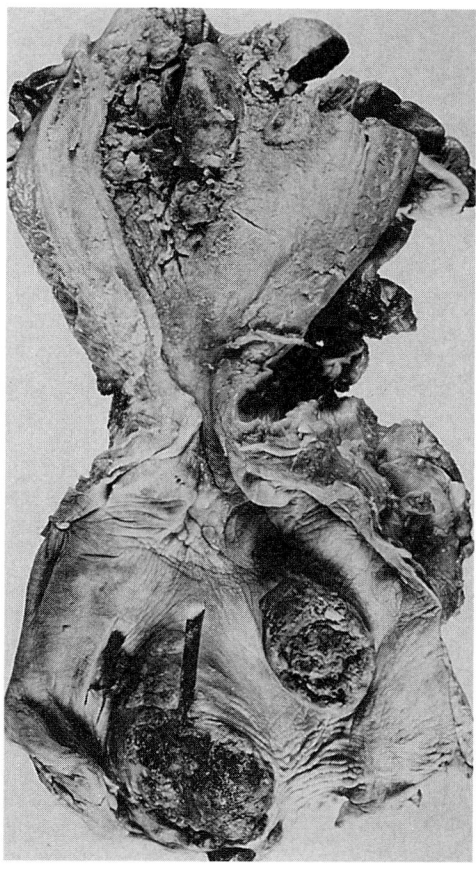

Fig. 19-234 Uterus and vagina showing large masses of hemorrhagic choriocarcinoma within uterus and metastatic to vagina.

had the highest incidence of spontaneous regression of trophoblast after evacuation of a hydatidiform mole.

Grossly, choriocarcinoma characteristically forms soft, dark red, hemorrhagic, round nodular tumor masses (Figs. 19-233 and 19-234). Microscopically, the tumor is composed of clusters of cytotrophoblast separated by streaming masses of syncytiotrophoblast, resulting in a characteristic dimorphic plexiform pattern[166a] (Fig. 19-235). Hemorrhage and necrosis are usually present but have no real diagnostic significance, since they are also commonly found in spontaneous abortions. Villi are characteristically absent; as a matter of fact, their presence is said to rule out the diagnosis of choriocarcinoma no matter how atypical the trophoblastic cells may be.[147] The rationale for this criterion is hard to accept. After all, if such choriocarcinomas arise from complete moles, there should be a point in time in which both molar and choriocarcinomatous tissue are simultaneously present. Yet, there is no question that it represents a useful parameter at the practical level.

Immunohistochemically, choriocarcinoma cells are positive for hCG and keratin. There may also be reactivity for hPL, pregnancy-specific beta-1-glycoprotein, and CEA.[158]

Microscopic grading of choriocarcinoma is of little value. Some attempts at correlating various patterns of growth with prognosis have been recorded[145,164]; of these, the most convincing are those showing an improved prognosis in the presence of an intense inflammatory infiltrate at the interphase between tumor and stroma.[148,149a,153,162]

The natural history of untreated choriocarcinoma is characterized by the development of early hematogenous metastases, the most common sites being the lung, brain, liver, kidney, and bowel.[152,161,167] They can be clinically solitary, may occur in the most unusual places, and often present

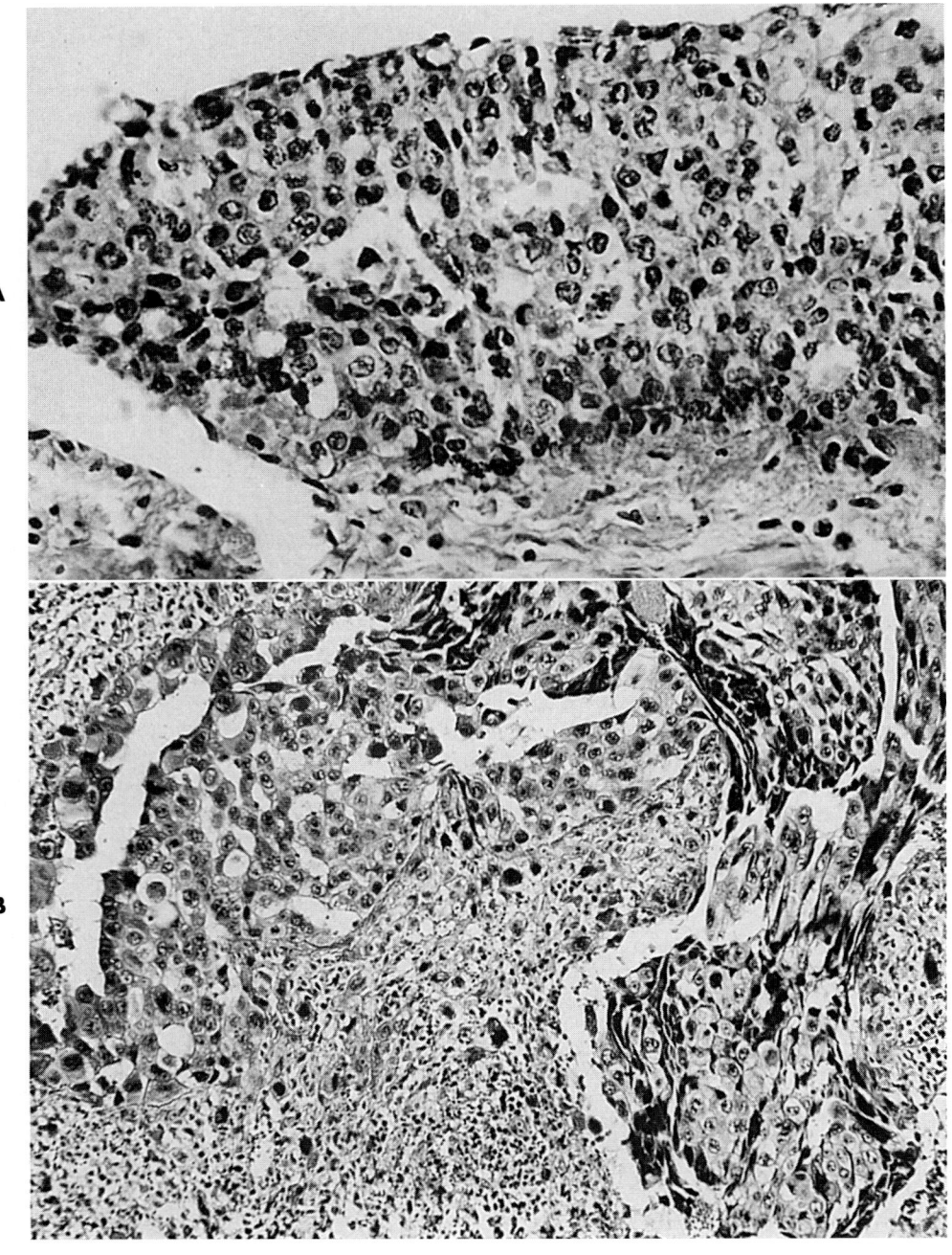

Fig. 19-235 A, Choriocarcinoma in large vein within uterus. Cytotrophoblasts predominate. Patient died with pulmonary metastases. **B,** Choriocarcinoma invading myometrial wall, accompanied by extensive inflammatory response. Cytotrophoblastic and syncytiotrophoblastic elements can easily be identified. Chorionic villi are absent.

with massive hemorrhage.[150] Interestingly, the fetus is rarely involved, even in cases of widespread metastatic disease.[168] Residual tumor in the uterus of patients dying of disseminated choriocarcinoma may be inconspicuous or altogether absent.[165]

Many of the morphologic changes seen in other organs in patients with choriocarcinoma are the result of increased secretion of hCG and other hormones by the tumor cells. These include hyperplasia of endocervical glands, decidual reaction (both endometrial and ectopic), Arias-Stella phenomenon, bilateral enlargement of the ovaries by theca-lutein cysts ("hyperreactio luteinalis"), and hyperplasia of mammary lobules. The detection of ovarian theca-lutein cysts long after a case of choriocarcinoma has been treated should be taken as presumptive evidence of persistent dis-

ease.[155] In the endometrial decidual reaction of patients with choriocarcinoma, the spiral arterioles fail to develop as they do in the normal cycle, the appearance of the mucosa being similar to that seen after the administration of progestogens.[165]

The evolution of the treatment of choriocarcinoma (and of gestational trophoblastic disease in general) is one of the greatest success stories in medical oncology. When treated by surgery alone, the cure rate was only 40% for tumors apparently restricted to the uterus and less than 20% for those accompanied by metastases.[142] With the use of the chemotherapeutic agents methotrexate, actinomycin D, and chlorambucil (a combination usually referred to as MAC), the survival rate is close to 100% for cases restricted to the uterus and about 83% for patients with metastatic disease.[154,159] These figures are impressive indeed, although in all fairness it should be pointed out that in most series they apply not just to choriocarcinoma as strictly defined on pathologic terms but to gestational trophoblastic disease (or to "metastatic" gestational trophoblastic disease) in a more generic sense. Low- and high-risk patient groups have been identified on the basis of location of metastases, hCG, and duration of the disease[163] (Tables 19-10 and 19-11 and box).

In most cases, the uterus can be preserved. Hysterectomy is performed in those patients in whom preservation of the reproductive function is not desired and/or who are unresponsive to chemotherapy alone. Surgery also remains useful in controlling life-threatening hemorrhage from metastatic lesions.[144,157]

Some metastases of choriocarcinomas that are surgically excised after chemotherapy show a monomorphic mononu-

Table 19-10 FIGO staging for trophoblastic tumor

Stage I	Disease confined to uterus.
Stage IA	Disease confined to uterus with no risk factors.
Stage IB	Disease confined to uterus with one risk factor.
Stage IC	Disease confined to uterus with two risk factors.
Stage II	Gestational trophoblastic tumor extending outside uterus but limited to genital structures (adnexa, vagina, broad ligament).
Stage IIA	Gestational trophoblastic tumor involving genital structures without risk factors.
Stage IIB	Gestational trophoblastic tumor extending outside uterus but limited to genital structures with one risk factor.
Stage IIC	Gestational trophoblastic tumor extending outside uterus but limited to genital structures with one risk factor.
Stage III	Gestational trophoblastic tumor extending to lungs with or without known genital tract involvement.
Stage IIIA	Gestational trophoblastic tumor extending to lungs with or without genital tract involvement and with no risk factors.
Stage IIIB	Gestational trophoblastic tumor extending to lungs with or without genital tract involvement and with one risk factor.
Stage IIIC	Gestational trophoblastic tumor extending to lungs with or without genital tract involvement and with two risk factors.
Stage IV	All other metastatic sites.
Stage IVA	All other metastatic sites without risk factors.
Stage IVB	All other metastatic sites with one risk factor.
Stage IVC	All other metastatic sites with two risk factors.

Notes on staging:

Risk factors affecting staging include the following: (1) serum human chorionic gonadotropin >100,000 mIU/ml and (2) duration of disease >6 months from termination of antecedent pregnancy.

The following factors should be considered and noted in reporting: (1) Prior chemotherapy has been given for known gestational trophoblastic tumor; (2) placental site tumors should be reported separately; and (3) histologic verification of disease is not required.

From SGO handbook. Staging of gynecologic malignancies. Chicago, 1994, Society of Gynecologic Oncologists.

See also Appendix G.

Table 19-11 World Health Organization Prognostic Index Score for Gestational Trophoblastic Disease

	SCORE*			
Prognostic Factor	**0**	**1**	**2**	**4**
Age (y)	≤39	>39	—	—
Antecedent pregnancy	Hydatidiform mole	Abortion	Term	—
Interval (mo)†	4	4-6	7-12	>12
β-hCG (IU/L)	<10^3	10^3-10^4	10^4-10^5	>10^5
ABO groups (female x male)	—	OxA,AxO	B, AB	—
Largest tumor, including uterine tumor	—	3-5 cm	>5 cm	—
Site of metastases	—	Spleen, kidney	GI tract, liver	Brain
Number of metastases identified	—	1-4	4-8	>8
Prior chemotherapy	—	—	Single drug	Two or more drugs

From SGO handbook. Staging of gynecologic malignancies. Chicago, 1994, Society of Gynecologic Oncologists.

*The total score for a patient is obtained by adding the individual scores for each prognostic factor. Low risk = 0-4, intermediate risk = 5-7, high risk ≥8.

†Interval is time between end of antecedent pregnancy and start of chemotherapy.

NIH CLASSIFICATION OF GESTATIONAL TROPHOBLASTIC DISEASE

I. Benign GTD
  A. Complete hydatidiform mole
  B. Partial hydatidiform mole
II. Malignant GTD
  A. Nonmetastatic GTD
  B. Metastatic GTD
    1. Good prognosis, low risk—absence of any risk factor
    2. Poor prognosis, high risk—presence of any risk factor
      a. Duration >4 months
      b. Pretherapy level of β-hCG in serum >40,000 mIU/ml
      c. Brain or liver metastases
      d. GTD after term gestation
      e. Prior to failed therapy

From SGO handbook. Staging of gynecologic malignancies. Chicago, 1994, Society of Gynecologic Oncologists.

clear cell composition accompanied by a paucity of multinucleated syncytiotrophoblasts, resulting in a picture that can be difficult to distinguish from that of a carcinoma.[160]

The importance of early diagnosis, prompt institution of therapy, and monitoring of the effects of treatment with sequential quantitative determination of hCG production cannot be overemphasized. In regard to the latter, it should be mentioned that hCG secretion is by no means restricted to gestational choriocarcinomas. It can also occur in nongestational choriocarcinoma; other ovarian and testicular germ cell tumors; melanoma; malignant lymphoma; and carcinomas of the esophagus, stomach, pancreas, kidney, liver, lung, urinary bladder, uterus, adrenal gland, breast, and other sites. A feature common to many of these tumors is the presence of tumor giant cells shown to contain hCG by immunocytochemical techniques.[143]

Cytogenetic studies using locus-specific minisatellite probes to identify restriction fragment length polymorphisms in DNA from tumor tissue are useful in distinguishing gestational from nongestational (germ cell) choriocarcinoma and in documenting the tumor derivation from an antecedent complete mole (by establishing the androgenetic nature of the tumor).[149]

NON-NEOPLASTIC LESIONS OF TERM PLACENTA

Abnormally large placentas are frequently seen in association with polyhydramnios. They accompany conditions leading to fetal anemia or cardiac failure, such as erythroblastosis fetalis; infections, such as syphilis, toxoplasmosis, or cytomegalovirus; tumors of the placenta and fetus; or fetal renal vein thrombosis.[173] Histologically, these enlarged placentas retain immature features.

Abnormally small placentas are seen in prematurely born infants and in many growth-retarded ("small for dates")

infants. Causes of the latter include maternal vascular disease and fetal malformations,[199,218] but many remain of undetermined etiology.

Placenta accreta refers to a condition in which placental villi adhere to the underlying myometrium, without an intervening layer of decidua.[184] Morphologic subtypes of this condition are designated as *placenta increta* when the villi invade the myometrium and *placenta percreta* when the villous infiltration extends through the whole thickness of the myometrium.

Placenta circummarginata and *placenta circumvallata* are two morphologic variants of extrachorial placenta (i.e., a placenta in which the chorionic plate is smaller than its basal plate). In placenta circummarginata, the transition from the membranous to the villous chorion is flat, whereas in placenta circumvallata the marginal membrane is folded or folded back on itself. Wentworth[216] examined 895 placentas and found 25.5% to be circummarginate and 6.5% circumvallate. He considered these two malformations of no clinical significance. Others have reported an increased incidence of antepartum bleeding, particularly with circumvallation.[174]

Amnion nodosum is the result of fetal renal agenesis and is associated with oligohydramnios. It presents as small plaques on the amniotic surface, formed by squamous cells and fibrin. Ultrastructural and other studies suggest that amnion nodosum originates from the apposition of desquamated fetal skin elements on the amnion epithelium in the presence of oligohydramnios.[210]

Malformations of umbilical cord of clinical importance include *velamentous insertion* and the *absence of one umbilical artery*. The former is seen in 1% of all placentas and may result in massive fetal hemorrhage if located at the cervical opening. The latter, also present in approximately 1% of all cords, is associated with congenital abnormalities of the infant in 30% of the cases.[177,189] The abnormalities may involve the cardiac, renal, skeletal, or other systems. There is also an increased incidence of prematurity (16.5%) and of small size for dates (34%).[177] The absence of one umbilical artery can be detected by gross inspection of the cross section of the cord, but it should always be confirmed microscopically.

Other malformations of the umbilical cord are represented by persistence of embryonic structures. The large majority of these are of no clinical significance and show no particular association with congenital malformations or perinatal complications. Most are located at the fetal end of the cord and are represented by remnants of the allantoic duct, omphalomesenteric duct, and embryonic vessels.[192]

Infection of the placenta is due most commonly to organisms that ascend from the maternal vaginal tract.[173,176] It shows a good correlation with prematurity and sepsis during the first 2 days of life.[207] Overall estimates of its frequency range from 5.4%[92] to 24.4%.[185] It is manifested morphologically by an inflammatory infiltrate of predominantly neutrophilic nature that is contributed by both the maternal and fetal circulation. The former is primarily located in the peripheral membranes and chorionic plate, whereas the latter is concentrated in the umbilical and fetal surface vessels (Fig. 19-236). Grossly, the placental surface may appear

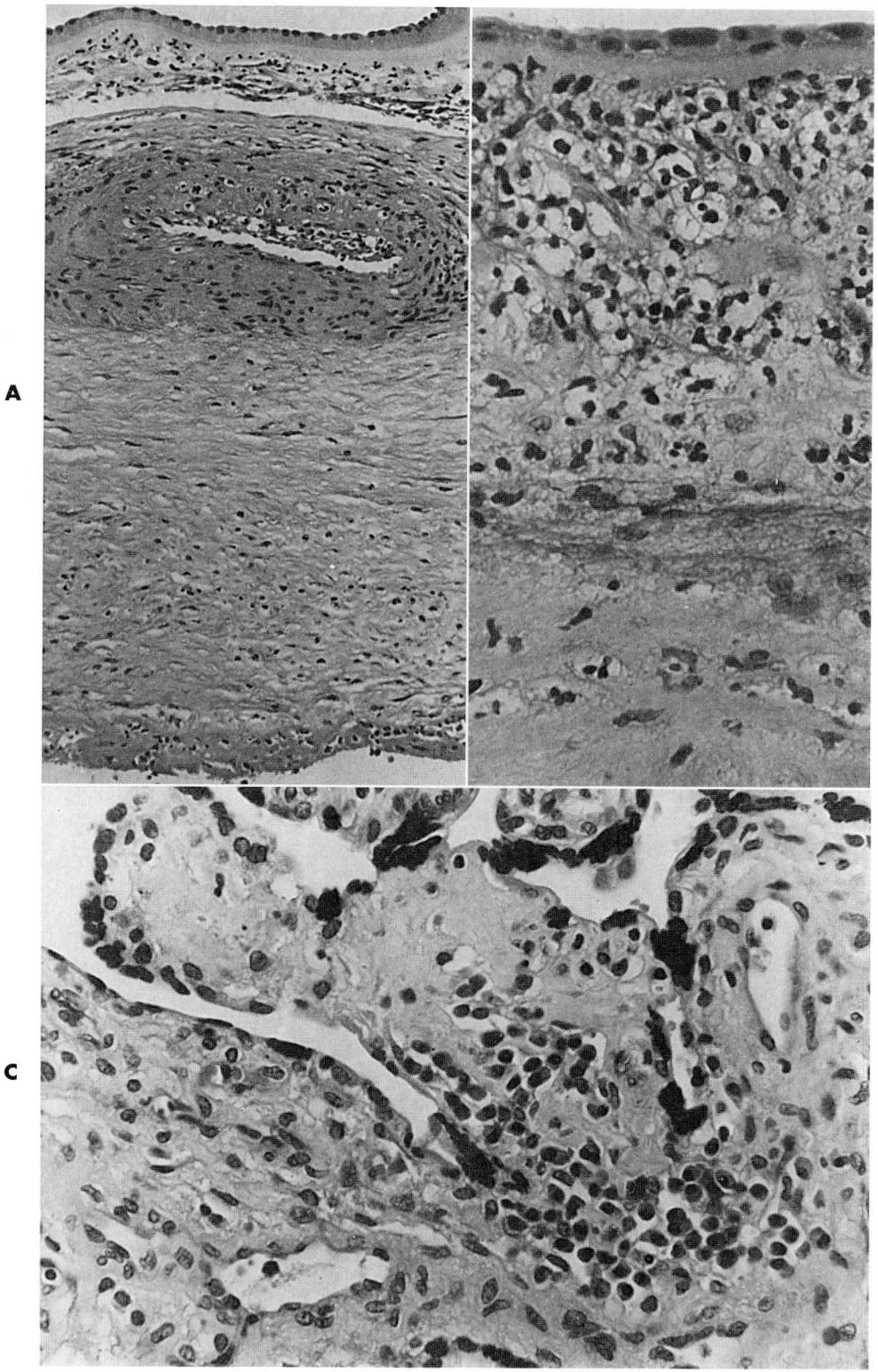

Fig. 19-236 **A,** Early chorioamnionitis. Note neutrophils in subchorionic fibrin at bottom that pass through chorion toward amnion at surface. Neutrophils also emanate from large fetal surface vessel toward amnionic cavity. **B,** More pronounced chorioamnionitis with neutrophils throughout fetal membranes. **C,** Cytomegalovirus villitis. Note numerous plasma cell and vascular villi. Small granules of hemosiderin were present. Such a morphologic pattern should suggest diagnosis. Inclusions may be present but are often difficult to find or not diagnostic. (Courtesy Dr. C. Kaplan, Long Island, NY; photos by Media Services, SUNY at Stony Brook).

cloudy and dull; however, in most cases the inflammation is detectable only microscopically. Infection may also reach the placenta through the maternal bloodstream, leading to inflammatory infiltrates within the villi.[171] These may be of acute, chronic, or granulomatous nature and may be associated with hemorrhagic vasculitis or vascular obliteration.[171,211] It should be mentioned here that fetal anoxia or meconium staining of the membranes *does not* result in inflammatory changes in the placenta.[197]

The most common cause of placental infection acquired from an ascending route is bacterial (including fusobacteria),[170] but other vaginal inhabitants such as *herpes virus* or *Candida* may be implicated.[206] Herpetic infection of placental tissues may be accompanied by necrotizing funisitis.[190] The diagnosis of herpetic infection can be confirmed by immunohistochemical stains or in situ hybridization.[212]

The organisms implicated in placentitis acquired through the hematogenous route are very numerous. They include cytomegalovirus, *Listeria,* rubella, syphilis, toxoplasmosis, tuberculosis, coccidioidomycosis, and cryptococcosis[193-195,198,204] (Fig. 19-237). In cytomegalovirus infection, diagnostic viral inclusions are only rarely found (Fig. 19-236, *C*).[200,213] However, immunohistochemical staining for CMV antigens is often positive, the infected cells being usually located in the villous stroma.[202] The diagnosis can also be made by detecting CMV genetic material by the PCR technique; these studies have shown that about 10% of the cases of chronic villitis are caused by CMV infection.[203] In syphilis, the characteristic changes include vascular proliferation, chronic villitis, and relative villous immaturity; in some instances, acute villitis is also present.[203,213a,214]

Placentas from HIV-infected patients do not have specific gross or microscopic alterations, although there is an increased incidence of chorioamnionitis in them.[211a]

Chronic villitis is a nonspecific inflammatory process involving the villi that is morphologically similar to that seen in rubella but unaccompanied by serologic evidence of this infection.[171,208,209] The etiology of this condition, which may be associated with intrauterine growth retardation and occasional unexplained stillbirths, remains unknown; infection by unidentified organisms and abnormal immune reactions have been implicated.[175] It is found in 1% to 9% of all placentas, depending on the degree of sampling, diagnostic criteria, and patient population studied, and is sometimes seen in subsequent pregnancies of the same individual.[205]

Chronic villitis may be associated with **chronic chorioamnionitis**[187]; in some instances the latter may dominate the microscopic picture.[188] The chorioamnionitis can be graded microscopically into mild, moderate, or severe; its frequency and severity are inversely related to gestational age at preterm birth.[201,219]

In **chronic intervillositis,** the inflammatory infiltrate is mainly histiocytic and predominantly located in the intervillous space; these rare cases have been found to be associated with poor fetal outcome.[191]

Placental infarct represents an area of villous necrosis secondary to local obstruction of the *maternal* uteroplacental circulation. Grossly, the fresh infarct is dark red and of firmer consistency than the surrounding tissue (Fig. 19-238, *A*). Microscopically, it is characterized by crowding of villi, virtual obliteration of the intervillous space, and marked congestion of the villous vessels. When old, it appears grossly as a hard, white mass of granular appearance and microscopically as a mass of crowded "ghost" villi. True infarcts should be distinguished from hematomas, subchorionic fibrin plaques, foci of intervillous fibrin deposition, and intervillous laminated thrombi.[215] Wigglesworth[217] demonstrated by injection studies that infarcts and hematomas have

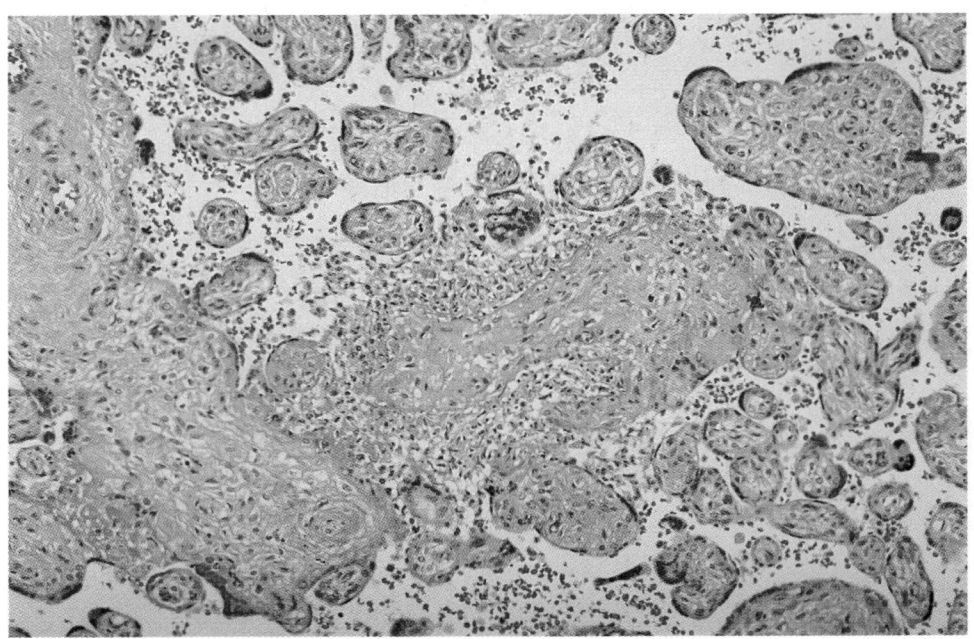

Fig. 19-237 Necrotizing villitis resulting from *Listeria*. (Courtesy Dr. Maria L. Carcangiu, New Haven, CT.)

a lobular distribution, thrombi occur in either the arterial or venous regions of the intervillous space, and perivillous fibrin deposits are predominantly venous lesions.

Minor degrees of infarction are seen in about 25% of placentas from uncomplicated term pregnancies and can therefore be regarded as an inconsequential phenomenon. A significant increase in the incidence and severity of infarcts in pregnancies has been found associated with preeclamptic toxemia, essential hypertension, Rh incompatibility, and nontoxic antepartum hemorrhage.[180] However, the fact that more than half the placentas from pregnancies associated with preeclamptic toxemia show no infarcts indicates that the infarct per se is not necessarily the cause of the clinical manifestations of this disease. In most instances, the infarcts are the result of a retroplacental hematoma (abruptio placentae) or a thrombosed maternal vessel. Extensive degrees of placental infarcts are associated with a high incidence of neonatal asphyxia, low birth weight, and intrauterine death.[180]

Thrombosis of fetal arteries should be distinguished from placental infarcts (which, as already stated, are always secondary to occlusion of the maternal uteroplacental circulation).[196] The placental changes resulting from thrombosis of fetal arteries appear grossly as roughly triangular or hemispheric pale areas, otherwise indistinguishable from the surrounding normal placenta. They are better seen after formalin fixation. Microscopically, the villi are fibrosed and avascular, except for occasional small, thickened vessels. A thrombosed fetal artery is present at the apex of the lesion. Fox[179] found this lesion in 3.6% of 715 placentas examined. It was particularly frequent in diabetic women, and it did not seem to result in any deleterious effect on the fetus (Fig. 19-238, *B*). It should be mentioned here that, in addition to fetal artery thrombosis, placentas of diabetic women often show an increased number of syncytial knots, fibrotic villi, Langhans cells, and foci of villous fibrinoid necrosis.[181-183]

Placental iron deposits are normal in the form of granular structures along the trophoblastic basement membrane; their presence in 7.5% or more of the villi is said to be abnormal and to be associated with fetal growth anomalies.[178]

Decidual vascular lesions of a necrotizing or inflammatory nature were found by Abramowsky et al.[169] in five of eleven patients with lupus erythematosus.

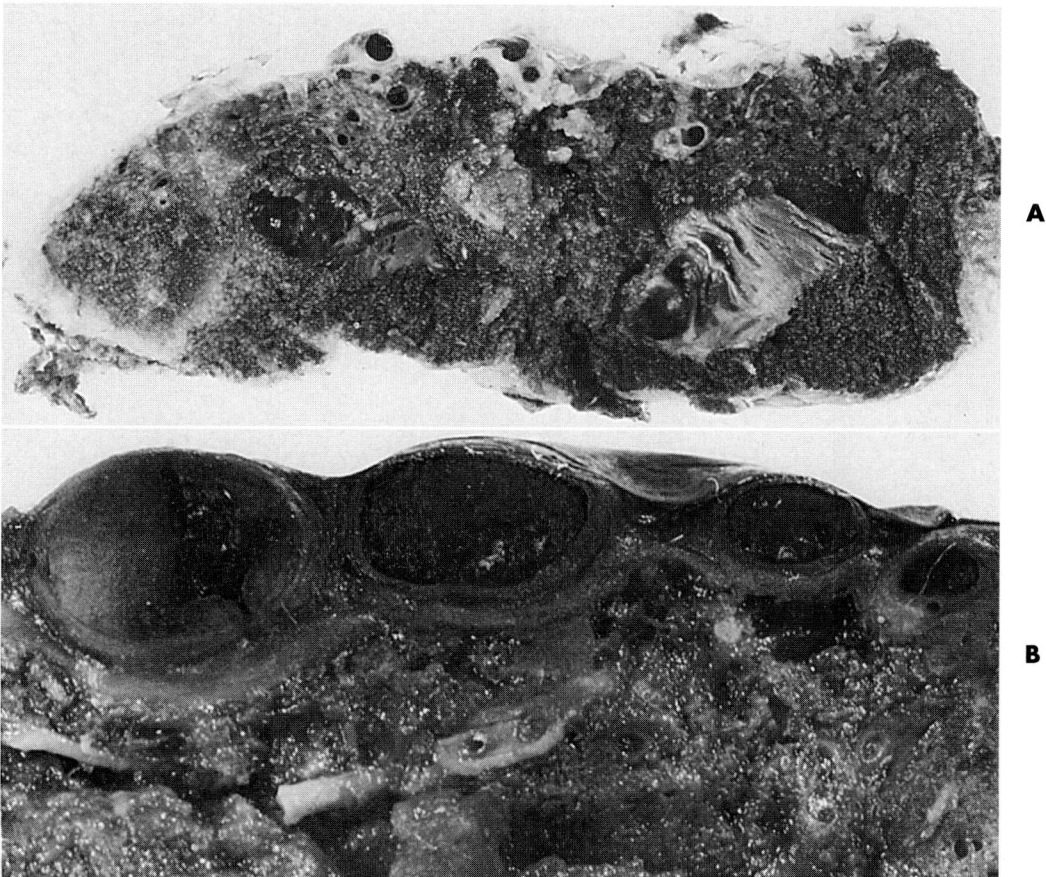

Fig. 19-238 **A,** Infarct contrasted with intervillous thrombus in adjacent areas of placenta. Infarct *(left)* is marginal and basal at maternal surface. Villous granular character is still apparent. Intervillous thrombus *(right)* shows layers of blood and fibrin. It is located within villous tissue, separating placental substance. **B,** Organizing thrombi within fetal surface vessels associated with stillborn fetus at term. (Courtesy Dr. C. Kaplan, Long Island, NY; photos by Media Services, SUNY at Stony Brook.)

Table 19-12 Correlation between morphologic changes in placenta and variety of clinical situations

	Normal pregnancy	Prolonged pregnancy	Premature onset of labor	Rh Incompatibility	Diabetes	Essential hypertension	Toxemia
Infarct	±	±	±	±	+	+ +	+ +
Thrombosis of fetal arteries	±	±	±	±	+ +	±	±
Fibrinoid necrosis of villi	±	−	+ +	+ +	+ +	±	+
Immaturity of villi	±	±	±	+ +	+ +	±	±
Senescence of villi	±	+ +	±	±	±	±	+
Basement membrane thickening in villi	±	+	±	+	+	+ +	+ + +
Fibrosis of villi	±	+ + +	±	±	+ +	±	±

Based almost entirely on the gross and microscopic examination of placentas by Fox[64-69] and Fox and Langley.[70]

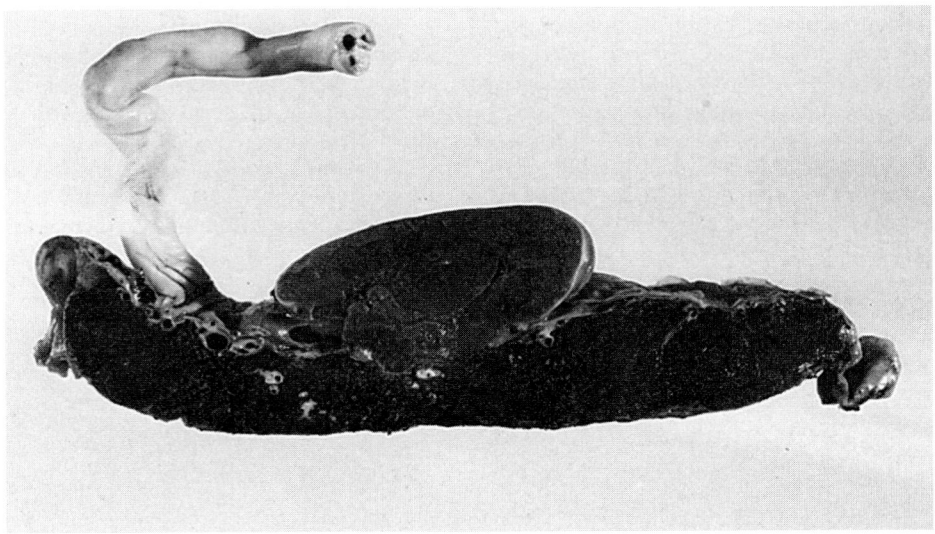

Fig. 19-239 Placental hemangioma (so-called chorangioma). Well-circumscribed reddish mass of spongy consistency is seen protuding in amniotic cavity.

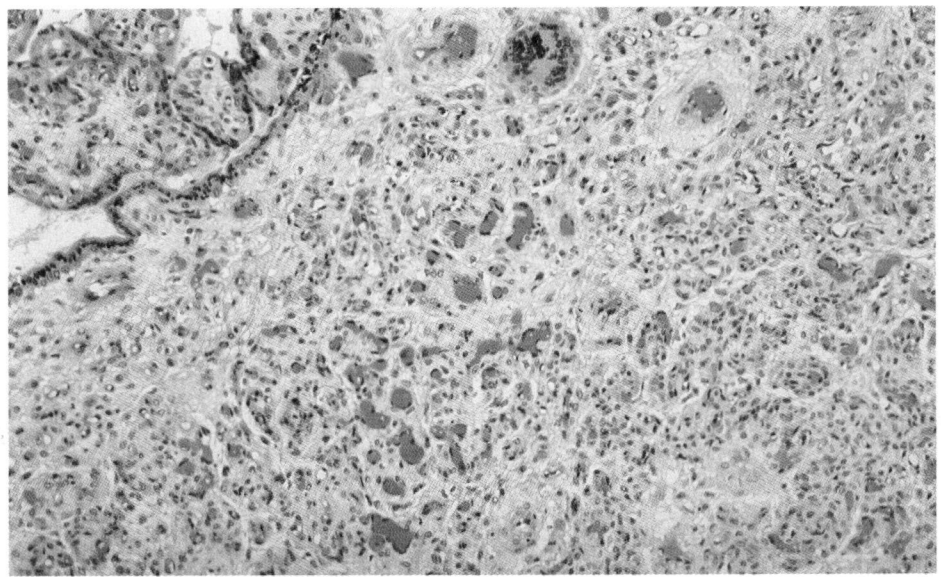

Fig. 19-240 Microscopic appearance of chorangioma. A complex network of capillaries distends the stroma of the placenta.

Sickle cell anemia can often be diagnosed by microscopic examination of the placenta, the deformation in the red blood cells developing as a result of the hypoxia created by the separation of the placenta from the uterine wall. Fujikura and Froehlich[186] found this change in 9.4% of 2117 placentas from black women.

Table 19-12 shows the correlation between morphologic changes in the placenta and a variety of clinical situations.

Placental site subinvolution may result in vaginal bleeding several weeks after delivery of the placenta, even in the absence of retained placental tissue. Curettage specimens from such cases contain large maternal vessels from the placental site partly filled with thrombi. In the normal state, these thrombi become organized and remain as scars in the endometrium or adjacent myometrium. Some differences in deposition of immunoglobulins and complement factors have been detected immunohistochemically between subinvoluted and normal vessels. These have been interpreted as indicating that immunologic factors are necessary for the process of normal involution of uteroplacental arteries and that these may be deficient in subinvoluted vessels.[172]

TUMORS OF TERM PLACENTA

Hemangiomas of placenta (chorangiomas) are found in approximately 1 of every 100 term specimens if a careful gross examination is performed.[227] Grossly, they are well circumscribed and purplish red. They may protrude on the fetal surface or be located entirely in the placental substance (Fig. 19-239). Microscopically, they are composed of a network of proliferating capillaries (Fig. 19-240). Mitoses may be present. Degenerative changes are common. Small hemangiomas (which represent the majority of the cases) are almost always asymptomatic, but the larger ones (more than 5 cm) may be associated with hydramnios, hemorrhage, premature delivery, premature placental separation, and placenta previa.[221] These manifestations may result in severe fetal distress and intrauterine death. The left-to-right shunting of blood across the tumor may lead to transient congestive heart failure in the infant.[222] There is apparently no relationship between placental hemangioma and toxemia.

Immunohistochemically, the tumor cells show focal staining for cytokeratin 18, a finding that suggests origin from blood vessels of the chorionic plate and anchoring villi.[230]

Chorangiosis (villous vascular proliferation) is a condition characterized by an increase in the number of vascular channels per villus, and allegedly associated with neonatal morbidity and mortality.[220]

Teratomas of the placenta are very rare; their typical location is between the amnion and corium.[228,228a,239] A reported case of *hepatocellular adenoma* of the placenta may have represented a monodermal teratoma.[223] *Heterotopic tissue* such as adrenal cortex has also been described.[224]

Umbilical cord tumors are even less common than placental neoplasms. Hemangiomas occur, and may lead to nonimmune hydrops fetalis.[235] A few cases of teratoma[236] and angiomyxoma[240] have also been reported.

Metastatic tumors of maternal origin can lodge in the placenta and form distinct nodules. This phenomenon has been seen most often with malignant melanoma and malignant lymphoma/leukemia[229,232,233,238] but can also occur with carcinoma of lung and other organs.[225,234] Metastases to the fetus may or may not be present. Awareness of this dramatic event should not obscure the fact that in the large majority of pregnant women with widespread metastatic disease from any source, the placenta and fetus are totally spared from the effects of the neoplasia. An even stranger and rarer phenomenon is that of placental spread from congenital tumors in the fetus; this has been observed with leukemia and neuroblastoma.[231] *Giant pigmented nevi* of the newborn can be accompanied by clusters of melanocytes in the placenta; this should not be taken as evidence that the tumor is malignant and that it has metastasized.[226,237]

REFERENCES
NORMAL ANATOMY

1 Altshuler G: The placenta, how to examine it, its normal growth and development. In Naeye RL, Kissane JM, Kaufman N, eds: Perinatal diseases, IAP Monograph (22). Baltimore, 1981, Williams & Wilkins, pp 5-22.

2 Altshuler G: A conceptual approach to placental pathology and pregnancy outcome. Semin Diagn Pathol **10**:204-221, 1993.

3 Benirschke K, Kaufmann P: The pathology of the human placenta, ed 2. New York, 1990, Springer-Verlag.

4 Bleisch VR: Diagnosis of monochorionic twin placentation. Am J Clin Pathol **42**:277-284, 1964.

5 Boyd JD, Hamilton WJ: The human placenta. Cambridge, 1970, W. Heffer & Sons, Ltd.

6 Danforth DM, Hull RW: The microscopic anatomy of the fetal membranes with particular reference to the detailed structure of the amnion. Am J Obstet Gynecol **75**:536-550,1958.

6a Deftos LJ, Burton DW, Brandt DW, Pinar H, Rubin LP: Neoplastic hormone–producing cells of the placenta produce and secrete parathyroid hormone–related protein. Studies by immunohistology, immunoassay, and polymerase chain reaction. Lab Invest **71**:847-852, 1994.

7 Driscoll SG: Placental examination in a clinical setting. Arch Pathol Lab Med **115**:668-671, 1991.

8 Fox H: Pathology of placenta. Philadelphia, 1978, W.B. Saunders, pp 343-367.

9 Kaplan C: Placental pathology for the nineties. Pathol Annu **28**(Pt 1):15-72, 1993.

10 Kurman RJ, Main CS, Chen H-C: Intermediate trophoblast. A distinctive form of trophoblast with specific morphological, biochemical and functional features. Placenta **5**:349-370, 1984.

11 Lewis SH, Benirschke K: Placenta. In Sternberg SS, ed: Histology for pathologists. New York, 1992, Raven Press.

12 Macpherson T: Fact and fancy. What can we really tell from the placenta? Arch Pathol Lab Med **115**:672-681, 1991.

13 Naeye RL: Umbilical cord length. Clinical significance. J Pediatr **107**:278-281, 1985.

14 Naeye RL: Functionally important disorders of the placenta, umbilical cord, and fetal membranes. Hum Pathol **18**:680-691, 1987.

14a Naeya RL: Disorders of the placenta, fetus, and neonate. Diagnosis and clinical significance. St. Louis, 1991, Mosby.

15 Novak RF: A brief review of the anatomy, histology, and ultrastructure of the full-term placenta. Arch Pathol Lab Med **115**:654-659, 1991.

16 Sander CH: The surgical pathologist examines the placenta. Pathol Annu **20**(Pt 2):235-288, 1985.

17 Yeh I-T, O'Connor DM, Kurman RJ: Vacuolated cytotrophoblast: a subpopulation of trophoblast in the chorion laeve. Placenta **10**:429-438, 1989.

ABORTION

18 Abaci F, Aterman K: Changes of the placenta and embryo in early spontaneous abortion. Am J Obstet Gynecol **102**:252-263, 1968.

19 Berry CL: The examination of embryonic and fetal material in diagnostic histopathology laboratories. J Clin Pathol **33**:317-326, 1980.

20 Clark RK, Damjanov I: Intermediate filaments of human trophoblast and choriocarcinoma cell lines. Virchows Arch [A] **407**:203-208, 1985.

21 Clement PB, Young RH, Scully RE: Nontrophoblastic pathology of the female genital tract and peritoneum associated with pregnancy. Semin Diagn Pathol **6**:372-406, 1989.

22 Conran RM, Hitchcock CL, Popek EJ, Norris HJ, Griffin JL, Geissel A, McCarthy WF: Diagnostic considerations in molar gestations. Hum Pathol **24**:41-48, 1993.

23 Daya D, Sabet L: The use of cytokeratin as a sensitive and reliable marker for trophoblastic tissue. Am J Clin Pathol **95**:137-141, 1991.

24 Fox H: Histological classification of tissue from spontaneous abortions. A valueless exercise? Histopathology **22**:599-600, 1993.

25 Fox H, Herd ME, Harilal KR: Morphological changes in the placenta and decidua after induction of abortion by extra-amniotic prostaglandin. Histopathology **2**:145-151, 1978.

26 Fukunaga M, Ushigome S, Fukunaga M: Spontaneous abortions and DNA ploidy. An application of flow cytometric DNA analysis in detection of nondiploidy in early abortions. Mod Pathol **6**:619-624, 1993.

26a Genest DR, Roberts D, Boyd T, Bieber FR: Fetoplacental histology as a predictor of karyotype. A controlled study of spontaneous first trimester abortions. Hum Pathol **26**:201-209, 1995.

27 Hertig AT: Gestational hyperplasia of endometrium. A morphologic correlation of ova, endometrium, and corpora lutea during pregnancy. Lab Invest **13**:1153-1191, 1964.

28 Horne CH, Rankin R, Bremner RD: Pregnancy-specific proteins as markers for gestational trophoblastic disease. Int J Gynecol Pathol **3**:27-40, 1984.

29 Huettner PC, Gersell DJ: Arias-Stella reaction in nonpregnant women. A clinicopathologic study of nine cases. Int J Gynecol Pathol **13**:241-247, 1994.

30 Inaba N, Ishige H, Ijichi M, Satoh N, Katoh T, Sekiya S, Shirotake S, Ohkawa R, Takamizawa H, Nitoh A, Renk T, Bohn H: Possible new markers in trophoblastic disease. Am J Obstet Gynecol **143**:973-974, 1982.

31 Jauniaux E, Hustin J: Histological examination of first trimester spontaneous abortions. The impact of materno-embryonic interface features. Histopathology **21**:409-414, 1992.

31a Klatt EC: Pathologic examination of fetal specimens from dilation and evacuation procedures. Am J Clin Pathol **103**:415-418, 1995.

32 Lindahl B, Ahlgren M: Identification of chorion villi in abortion specimens. Obstet Gynecol **67**:79-81, 1986.

33 Nakamura Y, Moritsuka Y, Ohta Y, Itoh S, Haratake A, Kage M, Kawano K: S-100 protein in glands within decidua and cervical glands during early pregnancy. Hum Pathol **20**:1204-1209, 1989.

34 Novak RW, Malone JM, Robinson HB: The role of the pathologist in the evaluation of first trimester abortions. Pathol Annu **25**(Pt 1):297-311, 1990.

35 O'Connor DM, Kurman RJ: Intermediate trophoblast in uterine curettings in the diagnosis of ectopic pregnancy. Obstet Gynecol **72**:665-670, 1988.

36 Oertel YC: The Arias-Stella reaction revisited. Arch Pathol Lab Med **102**:651-654, 1978.

37 Ory SJ: Ectopic pregnancy: current evaluation and treatment. Mayo Clin Proc **64**:874-877, 1989.

38 Poland BJ, Miller JR, Harris M, Livingston J: Spontaneous abortion. A study of 1961 women and their conceptuses. Acta Obstet Gynecol Scand **102**(Suppl), 1981.

39 Potter EL, Craig JM: Pathology of the fetus and the infant. London, 1976, Lloyd-Luke.

40 Rettig WJ, Cordon-Cardo C, Koulos JP, Lewis JL, Oettgen HF: Cell surface antigens of human trophoblast and choriocarcinoma defined by monoclonal antibodies. Int J Cancer **35**:469-475, 1985.

41 Risch HA, Weiss NS, Clarke EA, Miller AB: Risk factors for spontaneous abortion and its recurrence. Am J Epidemiol **128**:420-420, 1988.

42 Robb JA, Benirschke K, Barmeyer R: Intrauterine latent herpes simplex virus infection. I. Spontaneous abortion. Hum Pathol **17**:1196-1209, 1986.

43 Rushton DI: Examination of products of conception from previable human pregnancies. J Clin Pathol **34**:819-835, 1981.

44 Rushton DI: Examination of abortions. In Barson AJ, ed: Fetal and neonatal pathology. Eastbourne, 1982, Praeger Scientific, pp 27-64.

45 Sasagawa M, Watanabe S, Ohmono Y, Honma S, Kanazawa K, Takeuchi S: Reactivity of two monoclonal antibodies (Troma 1 and CAM 5.2) on human tissue sections. Analysis of their usefulness as a histologic trophoblast marker in normal pregnancy and trophoblastic disease. Int J Gynecol Pathol **5**:345-356, 1986.

46 Strom J, Bewtra C, Monif GRG: Immunohistochemical localization of placental hormones as markers for differentiating uterine abortion vs ectopic pregnancy. Int J Surg Pathol **1**:51-56, 1993.

47 Szulman AE: Examination of the early conceptus. Arch Pathol Lab Med **115**:696-700, 1991.

48 Tyagi SP, Saxena M, Rizvi R, Langley FA: Foetal remnants in the uterus and their relation to other uterine heterotopia. Histopathology **3**:339-345, 1979.

49 van Lijnschoten G, Arends JW, De La Fuente AA, Schouten HJ, Geraedts JP: Intra- and inter-observer variation in the interpretation of histological features suggesting chromosomal abnormality in early abortion specimens. Histopathology **22**:25-29, 1993.

50 van Lijnschoten G, Arends JW, Leffers P, De La Fuente AA, Van Der Looij HJ, Geraedts JP: The value of histomorphological features of chorionic villi in early spontaneous abortion for the prediction of karyotype. Histopathology **22**:557-563, 1993.

51 Wan SK, Lam PW, Pau MY, Chan JK: Multiclefted nuclei. A helpful feature for identification of intermediate trophoblastic cells in uterine curetting specimens. Am J Surg Pathol **16**:1226-1232, 1992.

52 Wigglesworth JS: Perinatal pathology. Major problems in pathology, vol 15. Philadelphia, 1984, W.B. Saunders Co.

53 Zettergren L: Glial tissue in the uterus. Am J Pathol **71**:419-426, 1973.

GESTATIONAL TROPHOBLASTIC DISEASE
Hydatidiform mole
Complete mole

54 Atrash HK, Hogue CJR, Grimes DA: Epidemiology of hydatidiform mole during early gestation. Am J Obstet Gynecol **154**:906-909, 1986.

55 Azuma C, Saji F, Tokugawa Y, Kimura T, Nobunaga T, Takemura M, Kameda T, Tanizawa O: Application of gene amplification by polymerase chain reaction to genetic analysis of molar mitochondrial DNA. The detection of anuclear empty ovum as the cause of complete mole. Gynecol Oncol **40**:29-33, 1991.

56 Berkowitz RS. Recent advances in the biology and treatment of gestational trophoblastic diseases and germ cell tumors. Curr Opin Oncol **2**:901-905, 1990.

57 Brescia RJ, Kurman RJ, Main CS, Surti U, Szulman AE: Immunocytochemical localization of chorionic gonadotropin, placental lactogen, and placental alkaline phosphatase in the diagnosis of complete and partial hydatidiform moles. Int J Gynecol Pathol **6**:213-229, 1987.

58 Brewer JI, Torok EE, Webster A, Dolkart RE: Hydatidiform mole. A follow-up regimen for identification of invasive mole and choriocarcinoma and for selection of patients for treatment. Am J Obstet Gynecol **101**:557-563, 1968.

59 Cave WT Jr, Dunn JT: Choriocarcinoma with hyperthyroidism. Probable identity of the thyrotropin with human chorionic gonadotropin. Ann Intern Med **85**:60-63, 1976.

60 Dehner LP: Gestational and non-gestational trophoblastic neoplasia. A historic and pathobiologic survey. Am J Surg Pathol **4**:43-58, 1980.

61 Driscoll SG: Gestational trophoblastic neoplasms. Morphologic considerations. Hum Pathol **8**:529-539, 1977.

62 Fukunaga M, Miyazawa Y, Sugishita M, Ushigome S: Immunohistochemistry of molar and non-molar placentas with special reference to their differential diagnosis. Acta Pathol Jpn **43**:683-689, 1993.

63 Genest DR, Laborde O, Berkowitz RS, Goldstein DP, Bernstein MR, Lage J: A clinicopathologic study of 153 cases of complete hydatidiform mole (1980-1990). Histologic grade lacks prognostic significance. Obstet Gynecol **78**:402-409, 1991.

64 Hershman JM, Higgins HP: Hydatidiform mole—a cause of clinical hyperthyroidism. Report of two cases with evidence that the molar tissue secreted a thyroid stimulator. N Engl J Med **284**:573-577, 1971.

65 Hertig AT: Hydatidiform mole and chorionepithelioma. In Meigs JV, Sturgis SH, eds: Progress in gynecology. New York, 1950, Grune & Stratton, Inc.

66 Hertz R: Choriocarcinoma and related gestational trophoblastic tumors in women. New York, 1978, Raven Press Books Ltd.

67 Hsu CT, Chen TY, Chiu WH, Yang C-C, Lai C-H, Chancheng C-H, Tung PH, Chen CC: Some aspects of trophoblastic diseases peculiar to Taiwan. Am J Obstet Gynecol **90**:308-316, 1964.

68 Joint Project for Study of Choriocarcinoma and Hydatidiform Mole in Asia. Geographic variation in the occurrence of hydatidiform mole and choriocarcinoma. Ann NY Acad Sci **80**:178-195, 1959.

69 Jones WB: Gestational trophoblastic disease. What have we learned in the past decade? Am J Obstet Gynecol **162**:1286-1295, 1990.

70 Kajii T, Ohama K: Androgenetic origin of hydatidiform mole. Nature **268**:633-634, 1977.

71 Kohorn EI: Criteria toward the definition of nonmetastatic gestational trophoblastic disease after hydatidiform mole. Am J Obstet Gynecol **142**:416-419, 1982.

72 Kohorn EI: Hydatidiform mole and gestational trophoblastic disease in southern Connecticut. Obstet Gynecol **59**:78-84, 1982.

73 Lage JM, Mark SD, Roberts DJ, Goldstein DP, Bernstein MR, Berkowitz RS: A flow cytometric study of 137 fresh hydropic placentas: correlations between types of hydatidiform moles and nuclear DNA ploidy. Obstet Gynecol **79**:403-410, 1992.

74 Lage JM, Popek EJ: The role of DNA flow cytometry in evaluation of partial and complete hydatidiform moles and hydropic abortions. Semin Diagn Pathol **10**:267-274, 1993.

75 Lage JM, Weinberg DS, Yavner DL, Bieber FR: The biology of tetraploid hydatidiform moles. Histopathology, cytogenetics, and flow cytometry. Hum Pathol **20**:419-425, 1989.

75a Lee Y-S: p53 expression in gestational trophoblastic disease. Int J Gynecol Pathol **14**:119-124, 1995.

76 Lewis JL Jr: Diagnosis and management of gestational trophoblastic disease. Cancer **71:**1639-1647, 1993.

77 Lurain JR, Brewer JI, Torok EE, Halpern B: Natural history of hydatidiform mole after primary evacuation. Am J Obstet Gynecol **145:**591-595, 1983.

78 McGregor C, Ontiveros E, Vargas LE, Valenzuela LS: Hydatidiform mole. Analysis of 145 patients. Obstet Gynecol **33:**343-351, 1969.

79 Okudaira Y, Strauss L: Ultrastructure of molar trophoblast. Observations on hydatidiform mole and chorioadenoma destruens. Obstet Gynecol **30:**172-187, 1967.

80 Park WW: Choriocarcinoma. A study of its pathology. Philadelphia, 1971, F.A. Davis Co.

81 Rice LW, Lage JM, Berkowitz RS, Goldstein DP, Bernstein MR: Repetitive complete and partial hydatidiform mole. Obstet Gynecol **74:**217-219, 1989.

81a Rose PG: Hydatidiform mole. Diagnosis and management. Semin Oncol **22:**149-156, 1995.

82 Sand PK, Lurain JR, Brewer JI: Repeat gestational trophoblastic disease. Obstet Gynecol **63:**140-144, 1984.

83 Tyrey L: Human chorionic gonadotropin. Structural, biologic, and immunologic aspects. Semin Oncol **9:**163-173, 1982.

84 Vaitukaitus J, Braunstein GD, Ross GT: A radioimmunoassay which specifically measures human chorionic gonadotropin in the presence of human LH. Am J Obstet Gynecol **113:**751-758, 1972.

84a Van de Kaa CA, Robben JC, Hopman AH, Hanselaar AG, Vooijs GP: Complete hydatidiform mole in twin pregnancy. Differentiation from partial mole with interphase cytogenetic and DNA cytometric analyses on paraffin embedded tissues. Histopathology **26:**123-129, 1995.

84b Yasuda M, Kawai K, Serizawa A, Tang X, Osamura Y: Immunohistochemical analysis of expression of p53 protein in normal placentas and trophoblastic diseases. Appl Immunohistochem **3:**132-136, 1995.

Partial mole

85 Abaci F, Aterman K: Changes of the placenta and embryo in early spontaneous abortion. Am J Obstet Gynecol **102:**252-263, 1968.

86 Berkowitz RS, Goldstein DP, Bernstein MR: Natural history of partial molar pregnancy. Obstet Gynecol **66:**677-681, 1983.

87 Boue J, Boue A: Chromosomal anomalies in early spontaneous abortion. In Gropp A, Benirschke K, eds: Current topics in pathology. 62. Developmental biology and pathology. Berlin, 1977, Springer-Verlag.

88 Brescia RJ, Kurman RJ, Main CS, Surti U, Szulman E: Immunocytochemical localization of chorionic gonadotropin, placental lactogen, and placental alkaline phosphatase in the diagnosis of complete and partial hydatidiform moles. Int J Gynecol Pathol **6:**213-229, 1987.

89 Czernobilsky B, Barash A, Lancet M: Partial moles. A clinicopathologic study of 25 cases. Obstet Gynecol **59:**75-78, 1982.

90 Doshi N, Surti U, Szulman AE: Morphologic anomalies in triploid liveborn fetuses. Hum Pathol **14:**716-723, 1983.

91 Gaber LW, Redline RW, Mostoufi-zadeh M, Driscoll SG: Invasive partial mole. Am J Clin Pathol **85:**722-724, 1986.

92 Gardner HA, Lage JM: Choriocarcinoma following a partial hydatidiform mole. A case report. Hum Pathol **23:**468-471, 1992.

93 Goto S, Yamada A, Ishizuka T, Tomoda Y: Development of postmolar trophoblastic disease after partial molar pregnancy. Gynecol Oncol **48:**165-170, 1993.

94 Hertig AT: Hydatidiform mole and chorionepithelioma. In Meigs JV, Sturgis SH, eds: Progress in gynecology. New York, 1950, Grune & Stratton, Inc.

95 Jeffers MD, O'Dwyer P, Curran B, Leader M, Gillan JE: Partial hydatidiform mole. A common but underdiagnosed condition. A 3-year retrospective clinico-pathological and DNA flow cytometric analysis. Int J Gynecol Pathol **12:**315-323, 1993.

96 Koenig C, Demopoulos RI, Vamvakas EC, Mittal KR, Feiner HD, Espiritu EC: Flow cytometric DNA ploidy and quantitative histopathology in partial moles. Int J Gynecol Pathol **12:**235-240, 1993.

97 Lage JM, Berkowitz RS, Rice LW, Goldstein DP, Bernstein MR, Weinberg DS: Flow cytometric analysis of DNA content in partial hydatidiform moles with persistent gestational trophoblastic tumor. Obstet Gynecol **77:**111-115, 1991.

98 Lurain JR, Brewer JI: Invasive mole. Semin Oncol **9:**174-180, 1982.

99 Mostoufi-zadeh M, Berkowitz RS, Driscoll SG: Persistence of partial mole. Am J Clin Pathol **87:**377-380, 1987.

100 Rice LW, Berkowitz RS, Lage JM, Goldstein DP, Bernstein MR: Persistent gestational trophoblastic tumor after partial hydatidiform mole. Gynecol Oncol **36:**358-362, 1990.

101 Szulman AE, Philippe E, Boue JG, Boue A: Human triploidy. Association with partial hydatidiform moles and nonmolar conceptuses. Hum Pathol **12:**1016-1021, 1981.

102 Szulman AE, Surti U: The syndromes of hydatidiform mole. I. Cytogenetic and morphologic correlations. Am J Obstet Gynecol **131:**665-671, 1978.

103 Szulman AE, Surti U: The clinicopathologic profile of the partial hydatidiform mole. Obstet Gynecol **59:**597-602, 1982.

104 Vassilakos P, Riotton G, Kajii T: Hydatidiform mole. Two entities. A morphologic and cytogenetic study with some clinical considerations. Am J Obstet Gynecol **127:**167-170, 1977.

105 Vejerslev LO, Fisher RA, Surti U, Walke N: Hydatidiform mole. Cytogenetically unusual cases and their implications for the present classification. Am J Obstet Gynecol **157:**180-184, 1987.

105a Wolf NG, Lage JM: Genetic analysis of gestational trophoblastic disease. A review. Semin Oncol **22:**113-120, 1995.

Invasive mole

106 Attwood HD, Park WW: Embolism to the lungs by trophoblast. J Obstet Gynaecol Br Commonw **68:**611-617, 1961.

107 Bagshawe KD, Garnett ES: Radiological changes in the lungs of patients with trophoblastic tumours. Br J Radiol **36:**673-679, 1963.

108 Evans KT, Cockshott WP, Hendrickse P de V: Pulmonary changes in malignant trophoblastic disease. Br J Radiol **38:**161-171, 1965.

109 Greene RR: Chorioadenoma destruens. Ann NY Acad Sci **80:**143-148, 1959.

110 Haines M: Hydatidiform mole and vaginal nodules. J Obstet Gynaecol Br Emp **62:**6-11, 1955.

111 Kurman RJ: Pathology of trophoblast. Monogr Pathol **33:**195-227, 1991.

112 Lurain JR, Brewer JI: Invasive mole. Semin Oncol **9:**174-180, 1982.

113 Ring AM: The concept of benign metastasizing hydatidiform moles. Am J Clin Pathol **58:**111-117, 1972.

114 Takeuchi S: Nature of invasive mole and its rational management. Semin Oncol **9:**181-186, 1982.

115 Wilson RB, Hunter JS Jr, Dockerty MB: Chorioadenoma destruens. Am J Obstet Gynecol **81:**546-559, 1961.

Placental site trophoblastic tumor

116 Berger G, Verbaere J, Feroldi J: Placental site trophoblastic tumor of the uterus. An ultrastructural and immunohistochemical study. Ultrastruct Pathol **6:**319-329, 1984.

117 Duncan DA, Mazur MT: Trophoblastic tumors. Ultrastructural comparison of choriocarcinoma and placental-site trophoblastic tumor. Hum Pathol **20:**370-381, 1989.

118 Eckstein RP, Paradinas FJ, Bagshawe KD: Placental site trophoblastic tumour (trophoblastic pseudotumour). A study of four cases requiring hysterectomy including one fatal case. Histopathology **6:**211-226, 1982.

119 Fukunaga M, Ushigome S: Metastasizing placental site trophoblastic tumor. An immunohistochemical and flow cytometric study of two cases. Am J Surg Pathol **17:**1003-1010, 1993.

120 Gloor E, Dialdas J, Hurlimann J, Ribolzi J, Barrelet L: Placental site trophoblastic tumor (trophoblastic pseudotumor) of the uterus with metastases and fetal outcome. Clinial and autopsy observations of a case. Am J Surg Pathol **7:**483-486, 1983.

120a Huettner PC, Gersell DJ: Placental site nodules. A clinicopathologic study of 38 cases. Int J Gynecol Pathol **13:**191-198, 1994.

121 Kotylo PK, Michael H, Davis TE, Sutton GP, Mark PR, Roth LM: Flow cytometric DNA analysis of placental-site trophoblastic tumors. Int J Gynecol Pathol **11:**245-252, 1992.

122 Kurman RJ: The morphology, biology, and pathology of intermediate trophoblast. A look back to the present. Hum Pathol **22:**847-855, 1991.

123 Kurman RJ, Main CS, Chen H-C: Intermediate trophoblast. A distinctive form of trophoblast with specific morphological, biochemical and functional features. Placenta **5:**349-370, 1984.

124 Kurman RJ, Scully RE, Norris HJ: Trophoblastic pseudotumor of the uterus. An exaggerated form of "syncytial endometritis" simulating a malignant tumor. Cancer **38:**1214-1226, 1976.

125 Kurman RJ, Young RH, Norris HJ, Main CS, Lawrence WD, Scully RE: Immunocytochemical localization of placental lactogen and chorionic gonadotropin in the normal placenta and trophoblastic tumors, with emphasis on intermediate trophoblast and the placental site trophoblastic tumor. Int J Gynecol Pathol **3:**101-121, 1984.

126 Lathrop JC, Lauchlan S, Nayak R, Ambler M: Clinical characteristics of placental site trophoblastic tumor (PSTT). Gynecol Oncol **31:**32-42, 1988.

127 Lee KC, Chan JK: Placental site nodule. Histopathology **16:**193-195, 1988.

128 Motoyama T, Ohta T, Ajioka Y, Watanabe H: Neoplastic and non-neoplastic intermediate trophoblasts. An immunohistochemical and ultrastructural study. Pathol Int **44:**57-65, 1994.

129 Orrell JM, Sanders DS: A particularly aggressive placental site trophoblastic tumour. Histopathology 18:559-561, 1991.

130 Scully RE, Young RH: Trophoblastic pseudotumor. A reappraisal. Am J Surg Pathol 5:75-76, 1981.

130a Shitabata PK, Rutgers JL: The placental site nodule. An immunohistochemical study. Hum Pathol 25:1295-1301, 1994.

131 Silva EG, Tornos C, Lage J, Ordonez NG, Morris M, Kavanagh J: Multiple nodules of intermediate trophoblast following hydatidiform moles. Int J Gynecol Pathol 12:324-332, 1993.

132 Tsang WY, Chum NP, Tang SK, Tse CC, Chan JK: Mallory's bodies in placental site nodule. Arch Pathol Lab Med 117:547-550, 1993.

133 Yeh IT, O'Connor DM, Kurman RJ: Intermediate trophoblast. Further immunocytochemical characterization. Mod Pathol 3:282-287, 1990.

134 Young RH, Kurman RJ, Scully RE: Placental site nodules and plaques. A clinicopathologic analysis of 20 cases. Am J Surg Pathol 14:1001-1009, 1990.

135 Young RH, Scully RE: Placental-site trophoblastic tumor. Current status. Clin Obstet Gynecol 27:248-258, 1984.

136 Young RH, Scully RE, McCluskey RT: A distinctive glomerular lesion complicating placental site trophoblastic tumor. Report of two cases. Hum Pathol 16:35-42, 1985.

Choriocarcinoma

137 Bagshawe KD: Risk and prognostic factors in trophoblastic neoplasia. Cancer 38:1373-1385, 1976.

138 Bagshawe KD, Rawlins G, Pike MC, Lawler SD: ABO blood groups in trophoblastic neoplasia. Lancet 1:553-557, 1971.

139 Benirschke K, Driscoll SG: The pathology of the human placenta. New York, 1967, Springer-Verlag, New York, Inc.

140 Berkowitz RS, Goldstein DP, Bernstein MR: Choriocarcinoma following term gestation. Gynecol Oncol 17:52-57, 1984.

141 Brewer JI, Mazur MT: Gestational choriocarcinoma. Its origin in the placenta during seemingly normal pregnancy. Am J Surg Pathol 5:267-277, 1981.

142 Brewer JI, Smith RT, Pratt GB: Choriocarcinoma. Absolute 5-year survival rates of 122 patients treated by hysterectomy. Am J Obstet Gynecol 85:841-843, 1963.

143 Civantos F, Rywlin AM: Carcinomas with trophoblastic differentiation and secretion of chorionic gonadotrophins. Cancer 29:789-798, 1972.

144 Clayton LA, Barnard DE, Weed JC Jr, Hammond CB: The role of surgery in the management of gestational trophoblastic disease. Semin Oncol 9:213-220, 1982.

145 Deligdisch L, Driscoll SG, Goldstein P: Gestational trophoblastic neoplasms. Morphologic correlates of therapeutic response. Am J Obstet Gynecol 130:801-806, 1978.

146 Dyke PC, Fink LM: Latent choriocarcinoma. Cancer 20:150-154, 1967.

147 Elston CW, Bagshawe KD: The diagnosis of trophoblastic tumours from uterine curettings. J Clin Pathol 25:111-118, 1972.

148 Elston CW, Bagshawe KD: Cellular reaction to trophoblastic tumors. Br J Cancer 28:245-255, 1973.

149 Fisher RA, Newlands ES, Jeffreys AJ, Boxer GM, Begent RH, Rustin GJ, Bagshawe KD: Gestational and nongestational trophoblastic tumors distinguished by DNA analysis. Cancer 69:839-845, 1992.

149a Greenfield AW: Gestational trophoblastic disease. Prognostic variables and staging. Semin Oncol 22:142-148, 1995.

150 Heaton GE, Matthews TH, Christopherson WM: Malignant trophoblastic tumors with massive hemorrhage presenting as liver primary. A report of two cases. Am J Surg Pathol 10:342-347, 1986.

151 Hertig AT: Hydatidiform mole and chorionepithelioma. In Meigs JV, Sturgis SH, eds: Progress in gynecology. New York, 1950, Grune & Stratton, Inc.

152 Ishizuka T, Tomoda Y, Kaseki S, Goto S, Hara T, Kobayashi T: Intracranial metastasis of choriocarcinoma. A clinicopathologic study. Cancer 52:1896-1903, 1983.

153 Ito H, Sekine T, Komuro N, Tanaka T, Yokoyama S, Hosokawa T: Histologic stromal reaction of the host with gestational choriocarcinoma and its relation to clinical stage classification and prognosis. Am J Obstet Gynecol 140:781-786, 1981.

154 Kaseki S: Prognosis and treatment of trophoblastic diseases. Excerpta Medica, 1980, International Congress Series no. 512:566-570.

155 Kohorn EI: Theca lutein ovarian cyst may be pathognomonic for trophoblastic neoplasia. Obstet Gynecol 62:80S-81S, 1983.

156 Lage J, Roberts DJ: Choriocarcinoma in a term placenta. Pathologic diagnosis of tumor in an asymptomatic patient with metastatic disease. Int J Gynecol Pathol 12:80-85, 1993.

157 Lewis J, Ketcham AS, Hertz R: Surgical intervention during chemotherapy of gestational trophoblastic neoplasms. Cancer 19:1517-1522, 1966.

158 Lind HM, Haghighi P: Carcinoembryonic antigen staining in choriocarcinoma. Am J Clin Pathol 86:538-540, 1986.

159 Lurain JR, Brewer JI, Torok EE, Halpern B: Gestational trophoblastic disease. Treatment results at the Brewer Trophoblastic Disease Center. Obstet Gynecol 60:354-360, 1982.

160 Mazur MT: Metastatic gestational choriocarcinoma. Unusual pathologic variant following therapy. Cancer 63:1370-1377, 1989.

161 Mazur MT, Lurain JR, Brewer JI: Fatal gestational choriocarcinoma. Clinicopathologic study of patients treated at a trophoblastic disease center. Cancer 50:1833-1846, 1982.

162 Mogensen B, Olsen S: Cellular reaction to gestational choriocarcinoma and invasive mole. Acta Pathol Microbiol Scand (A) 81:453-456, 1973.

163 Mortakis AE, Braga CA: "Poor prognosis" metastatic gestational trophoblastic disease. The prognostic significance of the scoring system in predicting chemotherapy failures. Obstet Gynecol 76:272-277, 1990.

164 Nishikawa Y, Kaseki S, Tomoda Y, Ishizuka T, Asai Y, Susuki T, Ushijima H: Histopathologic classification of uterine choriocarcinoma. Cancer 55:1044-1051, 1985.

165 Ober WB, Edgcomb JH, Price EB Jr. The pathology of choriocarcinoma. Ann NY Acad Sci 172:299-321, 1971.

166 Olive DL, Lurain JR, Brewer JI: Choriocarcinoma associated with term gestation. Am J Obstet Gynecol 148:711-716, 1984.

166a Redline RW, Abdul-Karim FW: Pathology of gestational trophoblastic disease. Semin Oncol 22:96-108, 1995.

167 Soper JT, Mutch DG, Chin N, Clarke-Pearson DL, Hammond CB: Renal metastases of gestational trophoblastic disease. A report of eight cases. Obstet Gynecol 72:796-798, 1988.

168 Tsukamoto N, Matsumura M, Matsukuma K, Kamura T, Baba K: Choriocarcinoma in mother and fetus. Gynecol Oncol 24:113-119, 1986.

NON-NEOPLASTIC LESIONS OF TERM PLACENTA

169 Abramowsky CR, Vegas ME, Swinehart G, Gyves MT: Decidual vasculopathy of the placenta in lupus erythematosus. N Engl J Med 303:668-672, 1980.

170 Altshuler G, Hyde S: Fusobacteria. An important cause of chorioamnionitis. Arch Pathol Lab Med 109:739-743, 1985.

171 Altshuler G, Russell P: The human placental villitides. A review of chronic intrauterine infection. Curr Top Pathol 60:63-112, 1975.

172 Andrew A, Bulmer JN, Morrison L, Wells M, Buckley CH: Subinvolution of the uteroplacental arteries. An immunohistochemical study. Int J Gynecol Pathol 12:28-33, 1993.

173 Benirschke K, Driscoll SG: The pathology of the human placenta. New York, 1967, Springer-Verlag, New York, Inc.

174 Benson RC, Fujikura T: Circumvallate and circummarginate placenta. Unimportant clinical entities. Obstet Gynecol 34:799-804, 1969.

175 Bjoro K Jr., Myhre E: The role of chronic nonspecific inflammatory lesions of the placenta in intrauterine growth retardation. Acta Pathol Microbiol Immunol Scand (A) 92:133-137, 1984.

176 Blanc WA: Pathways of fetal and early neonatal infection. Viral placentitis, bacterial and fungal chorioamnionitis. J Pediatr Surg 59:473-496, 1961.

177 Bryan EM, Kohler HG: The missing umbilical artery. I. Prospective study based on a maternity unit. Arch Dis Child 49:844-852, 1974.

178 Drachenberg CB, Papadimitriou JC: Placental iron deposits: significance in normal and abnormal pregnancies. Hum Pathol 25:379-385, 1994.

179 Fox H: Thrombosis of foetal arteries in the human placenta. J Obstet Gynaecol Br Commonw 73:961-965, 1966.

180 Fox H: The significance of placental infarction in perinatal morbidity and mortality. Biol Neonate 11:87-105, 1967.

181 Fox H: Fibrinoid necrosis of placental villi. J Obstet Gynaecol Br Commonw 75:448-452, 1968.

182 Fox H: Fibrosis of placental villi. J Pathol Bacteriol 95:573-579, 1968.

183 Fox H: Pathology of the placenta in maternal diabetes mellitus. Obstet Gynecol 34:792-798, 1969.

184 Fox H: Placenta accreta, 1945-1969. Obstet Gynecol Surv 27:475-490, 1972.

185 Fox H, Langley FA: Leukocytic infiltration of the placenta and umbilical cord. A clinicopathologic study. Obstet Gynecol 37:451-458, 1971.

186 Fujikura T, Froehlich LA: Diagnosis of sickling by placental examination. Geographic differences in incidence. Am J Obstet Gynecol 100:1122-1124, 1968.

187 Gersell DJ: Chronic villitis, chronic chorioamnionitis, and maternal floor infarction. Semin Diagn Pathol 10:251-266, 1993.

188 Gersell DJ, Phillips NJ, Beckerman K: Chronic chorioamnionitis. A clinicopathologic study of 17 cases. Int J Gynecol Pathol 10:217-229, 1991.

189 Heifetz, SA: Single umbilical artery. A statistical analysis of 237 autopsy cases and review of the literature. Perspect Pediatr Pathol 8:345-378, 1984.

190 Heifetz SA, Bauman M: Necrotizing funisitis and herpes simplex infection of placental and decidual tissues. Study of four cases. Hum Pathol 25:715-722, 1994.

191 Jacques SM, Qureshi F: Chronic intervillositis of the placenta. Arch Pathol Lab Med 117:1032-1035, 1993.

192 Jauniaux E, De Munter C, Vanesse M, Wilkin P, Hustin J: Embryonic remnants of the umbilical cord: morphologic and clinical aspects. Hum Pathol 20:458-462, 1989.

193 Kaplan C: The placenta and viral infections. Semin Diagn Pathol 10:232-250, 1993.

194 Kaplan C, Benirschke K, Tarzy B: Placental tuberculosis in early and late pregnancy. Am J Obstet Gynecol 137:858-860, 1980.

195 Kida M, Abramowsky CR, Santoscoy C: Cryptococcosis of the placenta in a woman with acquired immunodeficiency syndrome. Hum Pathol 20:920-921, 1989.

196 Kraus FT: Placental thrombi and related problems. Semin Diagn Pathol 10:275-283, 1993.

197 Lauweryns J, Bernat R, Lerut A, Detournay G: Intrauterine pneumonia. An experimental study. Biol Neonate 22:301-318, 1978.

198 McCaffree MA, Altshuler G, Benirschke K: Placental coccidioidomycosis without fetal disease. Arch Pathol Lab Med 102:512-514, 1978.

199 Morris ED: Placental insufficiency. Br Med Bull 24:76-79, 1968.

200 Mostoufi-zadeh M, Driscoll SG, Biano SA, Kundsin RB: Placental evidence of cytomegalovirus infection of the fetus and neonate. Arch Pathol Lab Med 108:403-406, 1984.

201 Mueller-Heubach E, Rubinstein DN, Schwarz SS: Histologic chorioamnionitis and preterm delivery in different patient populations. Obstet Gynecol 75:622-626, 1990.

202 Muhlemann K, Miller RK, Metlay L, Menegus MA: Cytomegalovirus infection of the human placenta: an immunocytochemical study. Hum Pathol 23:1234-1237, 1992.

203 Nakamura Y, Sakuma S, Ohta Y, Kawano K, Hashimoto T: Detection of the human cytomegalovirus gene in placental chronic villitis by polymerase chain reaction. Hum Pathol 25:815-818, 1994.

204 Qureshi F, Jacques SM, Reyes MP: Placental histopathology in syphilis. Hum Pathol 24:779-784, 1993.

205 Redline RW, Abramowsky CR: Clinical and pathologic aspects of recurrent placental villitis. Hum Pathol 16:727-731, 1985.

206 Robb JA, Benirschke K, Mannino F, Voland J: Intrauterine latent herpes simplex virus infection. II. Latent neonatal infection. Hum Pathol 17:1210-1217, 1986.

207 Russell P: Inflammatory lesions of the human placenta. I. Clinical significance of acute chorioamnionitis. Am J Diagn Gynecol Obstet 1:127-137, 1979.

208 Russell P: Inflammatory lesions of the human placenta. II. Villitis of unknown etiology in perspective. Am J Diagn Gynecol Obstet 1:339-346, 1979.

209 Russell P, Atkinson K, Krishnan L: Recurrent reproductive failure due to severe placental villitis of unknown etiology. J Reprod Med 24:93-98, 1980.

210 Salazar H, Kanbour AI: Amnion nodosum. Ultrastructure and histopathogenesis. Arch Pathol 98:39-46, 1974.

211 Sander CH, Stevens NG: Hemorrhagic endovasculitis of the placenta. An in-depth morphologic appraisal with initial clinical and epidemiologic observations. Pathol Annu 19(Pt 1):37-79, 1984.

211a Sander CM: What's new in placental pathology. Pathol Annu 30(Pt 1):59-93, 1995.

212 Schwartz DA, Caldwell E: Herpes simplex virus infection of the placenta. The role of molecular pathology in the diagnosis of viral infection of placental-associated tissues. Arch Pathol Lab Med 115:1141-1144, 1991.

213 Schwartz DA, Khan R, Stoll B: Characterization of the fetal inflammatory response to cytomegalovirus placentitis. An immunohistochemical study. Arch Pathol Lab Med 116:21-27, 1992.

213a Schwartz DA, Larsen SA, Beck-Sague C, Fears M, Rice RJ: Pathology of the umbilical cord in congenital syphilis. Analysis of 25 specimens using histochemistry and immunofluorescent antibody to *treponema pallidum.* Hum Pathol 26:784-791, 1995.

214 Walter P, Blot P, Ivanoff B: The placental lesions in congenital syphilis. A study of six cases. Virchows Arch [A] 397:313-326, 1982.

215 Wentworth P: Placental infarction and toxemia of pregnancy. Am J Obstet Gynecol 99:318-326, 1967.

216 Wentworth P: Circumvallate and circummarginate placentas. Their incidence and clinical significance. Am J Obstet Gynecol 102:44-47, 1968.

217 Wigglesworth JS: Vascular anatomy of the human placenta and its significance for placental pathology. J Obstet Gynaecol Br Commonw 76:979-989, 1969.

218 Younoszai MK, Haworth JC: Placental dimensions and relations in preterm, term, and growth-retarded infants. Am J Obstet Gynecol 103:265-271, 1969.

219 Zlatnik FJ, Gellhaus TM, Benda JA, Koontz FP, Burmeister LF: Histologic chorioamnionitis, microbial infection, and prematurity. Obstet Gynecol 76:355-359, 1990.

TUMORS OF TERM PLACENTA

220 Altshuler G: Chorangiosis. An important placental sign of neonatal morbidity and mortality. Arch Pathol Lab Med 108:71-74, 1984.

221 Asadourian LA, Taylor HB: Clinical significance of placental hemangiomas. Obstet Gynecol 31:551-555, 1968.

222 Cash JB, Powell DE: Placental chorioangioma. Presentation of a case with electron-microscopic and immunochemical studies. Am J Surg Pathol 4:87-92, 1980.

223 Chen KTK, Ma CK, Kassel SH: Hepatocellular adenoma of the placenta. Am J Surg Pathol 10:436-440, 1986.

224 Cox JN, Chavrier F: Heterotopic adrenocortical tissue within a placenta. Placenta 1:131-133, 1980.

225 Delerive C, Locquet F, Mallart A, Janin A, Gosselin B: Placental metastasis from maternal bronchial oat cell carcinoma. Arch Pathol Lab Med 113:556-558, 1989.

226 Demian SDE, Donnelly WH, Frias JL, Monif GRG: Placental lesions in congenital giant pigmented nevi. Am J Clin Pathol 61:438-442, 1974.

227 Fox H: Vascular tumors of the placenta. Obstet Gynecol Surv 22:697-711, 1967.

228 Fox H: Pathology of the placenta. Philadelphia, 1978, W.B. Saunders Co., pp. 343-367.

228a Kreczy A, Alge A, Menardi G, Gassner I, Gschwendtner A, Mikuz G: Teratoma of the umbilical cord. Case report with review of the literature. Arch Pathol Lab Med 118:934-937, 1994.

229 Kurtin PJ, Gaffey TA, Habermann TM: Peripheral T-cell lymphoma involving the placenta. Cancer 70:2963-2968, 1992.

230 Lifschitz-Mercer B, Fogel M, Kushnir I, Czernobilsky B: Chorangioma. A cytoskeletal profile. Int J Gynecol Pathol 8:349-356, 1989.

231 Perkins DG, Kopp CM, Haust MD: Placental infiltration in congenital neuroblastoma. A case study with ultrastructure. Histopathology 4:383-389, 1980.

232 Potter JF, Schoeneman M: Metastasis of maternal cancer to the placenta and fetus. Cancer 25:380-388, 1970.

233 Read EJ Jr, Platzer PB: Placental metastasis from maternal carcinoma of the lung. Obstet Gynecol 58:387-391, 1981.

234 Schmitt FC, Zelandi Filho C, Bacchi MM, Castilho ED, Bacchi CE: Adenoid cystic carcinoma of trachea metastatic to the placenta. Hum Pathol 20:193-195, 1989.

235 Seifer DB, Ferguson JE II, Behrens CM, Zemel S, Stevenson DK, Ross JC: Nonimmune hydrops fetalis in association with hemangioma of the umbilical cord. Obstet Gynecol 66:283-286, 1985.

236 Smith D, Majmudar B: Teratoma of the umbilical cord. Hum Pathol 16:190-193, 1985.

237 Sotelo-Avila C, Graham M, Hanby DE, Rudolph AJ: Nevus cell aggregates in the placenta. A histochemical and electron microscopic study. Am J Clin Pathol 89:395-400, 1988.

238 Tsujimura T, Matsumoto K, Aozasa K: Placental involvement by maternal non-Hodgkin's lymphoma. Arch Pathol Lab Med 117:325-327, 1993.

239 Unger JL: Placental teratoma. Am J Clin Pathol 92:371-373, 1989.

240 Yavner DL, Redline RW: Angiomyxoma of the umbilical cord with massive cystic degeneration of Wharton's jelly. Arch Pathol Lab Med 113:935-937, 1989.

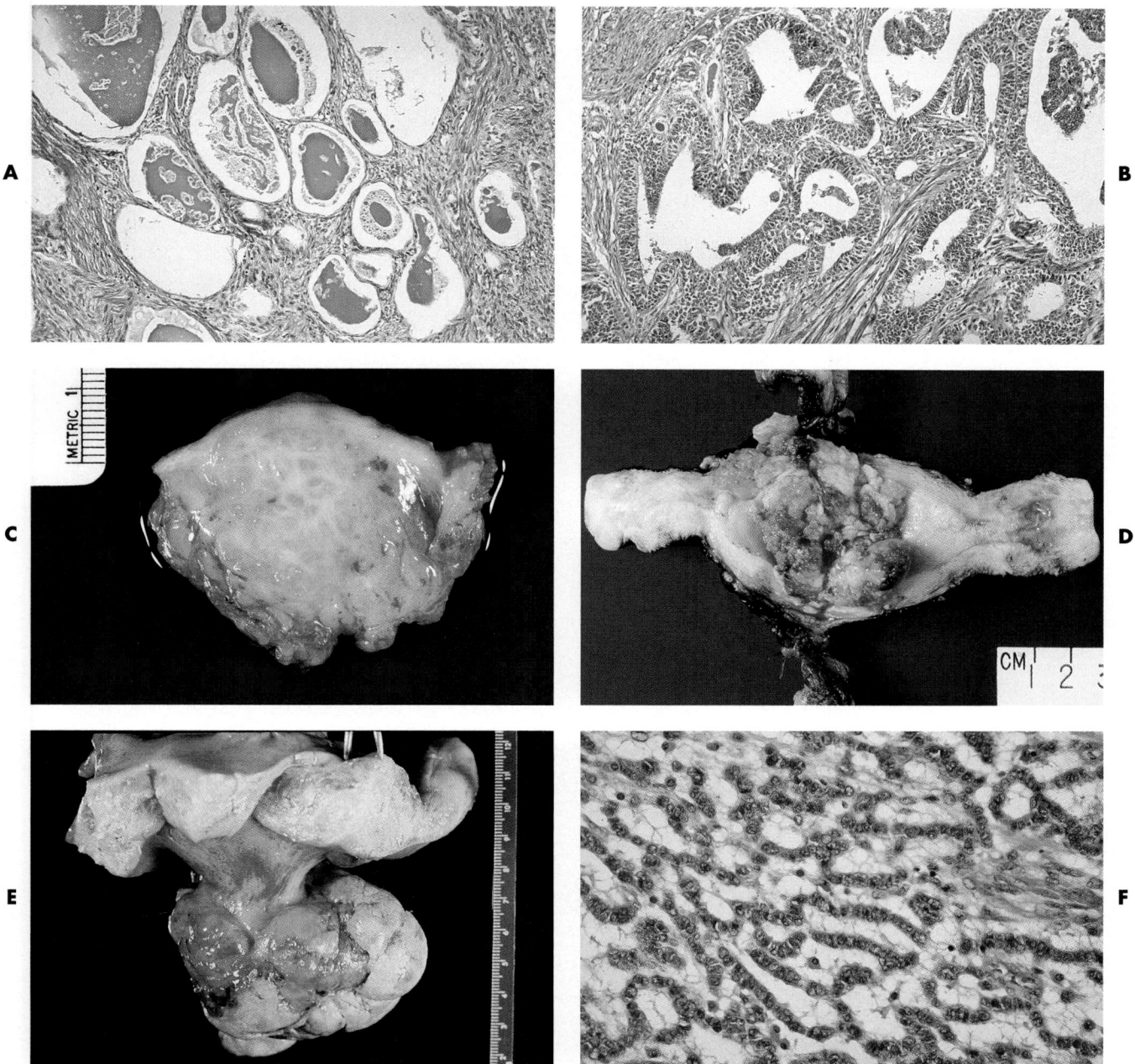

Plate XIII A, Mesonephric glands embedded within the stroma of the uterine cervix exhibiting cystic dilatation. The presence of a dense eosinophilic secretion is characteristic. **B,** Carcinoma arising from mesonephric rests (same case as **A**). **C,** Gross appearance of endometriosis involving the anterior abdominal wall. A few hemorrhagic cystic spaces are seen in an otherwise fibrous mass located in the dermis and subcutaneous tissue. **D,** Gross appearance of a papillary serous carcinoma of endometrium. The neoplasm is filling the endometrial cavity. **E,** Low-grade endometrial stromal sarcoma presenting as a huge polypoid mass within the endometrial cavity. This pattern of growth is unusual in this tumor type. **F,** So-called plexiform tumor of the uterus. This lesion is probably related to endometrial stromal neoplasms, but its histogenesis is still controversial. (**A, B,** and **D** courtesy Dr. Maria L. Carcangiu, New Haven, CT.)

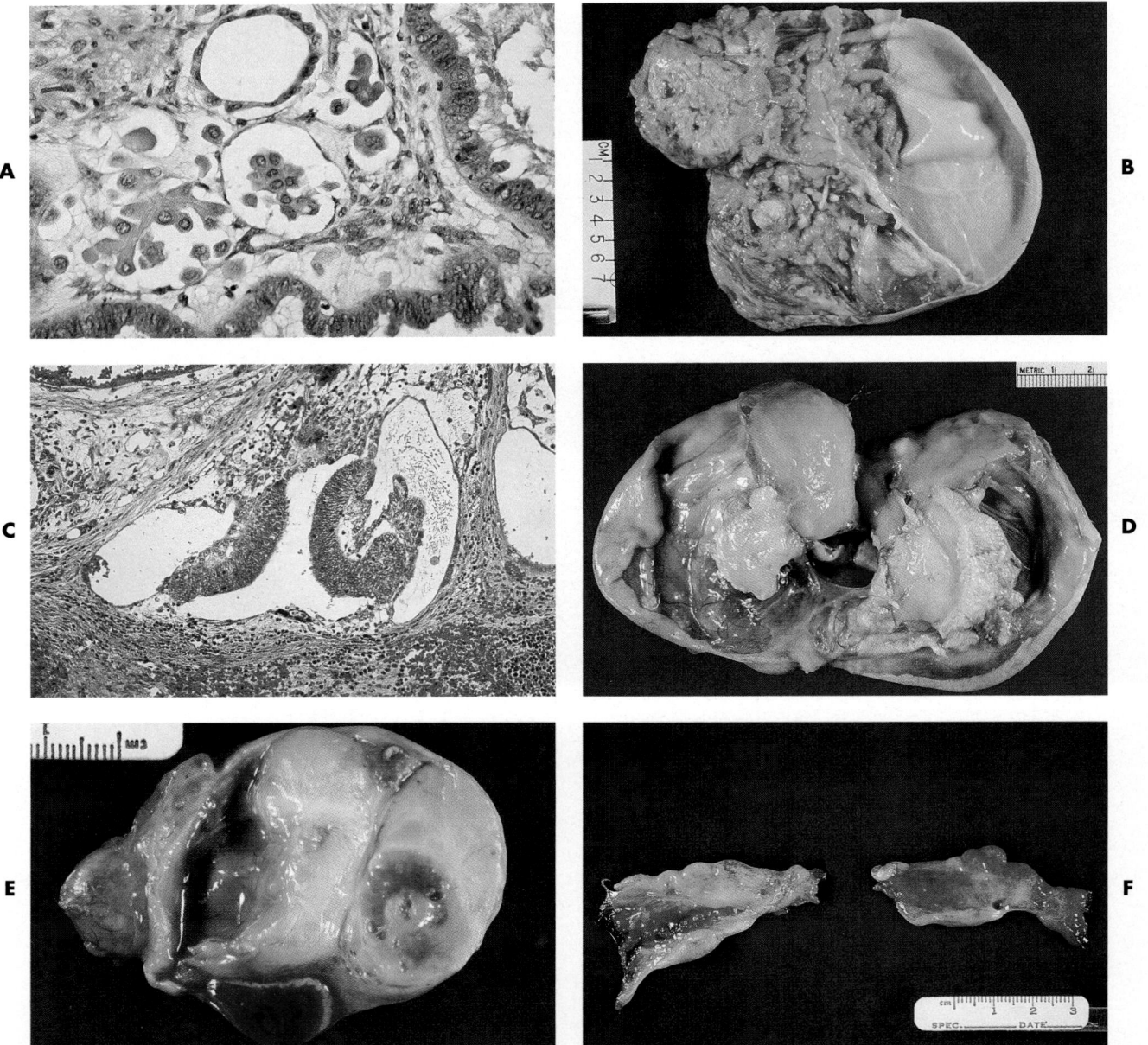

Plate XIV **A,** Borderline serous neoplasm with foci of microinvasion represented by clusters of cells with abundant eosinophilic cytoplasm. **B,** Malignant Brenner's tumor showing solid area with papillary formations, associated with a large cystic space. **C,** Mature cystic teratoma showing fat, skin, skin adnexum, and other tissues. **D,** Polyembryoma of ovary showing well-formed embryoid bodies. **E,** Gross appearance of strumal carcinoid showing a variegated appearance resulting from the admixture of carcinoid tumor and struma ovarii. **F,** Bilateral gonadoblastomas arising in streak gonads. The tumors were apparent only on microscopic examination. (**A, B, D,** and **F** courtesy Dr. Maria L. Carcangiu, New Haven, CT.)

20 Breast

Normal Anatomy

The breast is a modified sweat gland covered by skin and subcutaneous tissue. It rests on the pectoralis muscle, from which it is separated by a fascia. The morphofunctional unit of the organ is the single gland, a complex branching structure that is composed of two major parts: the terminal duct–lobular unit (TDLU) and the large duct system. The TDLU is formed by the lobule and terminal ductule and represents the secretory portion of the gland. It connects with the subsegmental duct, which in turn leads to a segmental duct, and this to a collecting (lactiferous or galactophorous) duct, which empties into the nipple. A fusiform dilatation located beneath the nipple between the collecting and the segmental duct is known as the lactiferous sinus (Fig. 20-1, A and B).

The TDLU is recognized because of its distinctly lobular architecture; the presence of a mantle of specialized, myxoid-appearing hormone-responsive connective tissue; and the absence of elastic fibers. The development of the breast is dependent on the close interaction of these specialized epithelial and mesenchymal tissues.[8] The large ducts have a lesser amount of specialized stroma and are enveloped by a continuous and well-developed layer of elastic tissue.

The entire ductal-lobular epithelial system of the breast is covered by a specialized two-cell–type epithelial lining: the inner epithelium with secretory and absorptive functions (often simply called epithelium), and the outer myoepithelial cells. These two cell types have distinctive ultrastructural and immunohistochemical features that differ considerably from each other. The most reliable markers for the epithelial cells are the various keratins, EMA (but see later discussion), the related milk fat globule membrane antigen, and alpha-lactalbumin[6,13,14] (Fig. 20-2, A). The best markers for the myoepithelial cells are actin, other types of keratin (see later discussion), and—to a lesser extent—S-100 protein[9,10,14,30] (Fig. 20-2, B). EMA reacts strongly with the apical region of active secretory cells but may be faint or negative in other epithelial cells. Pankeratin antibodies react

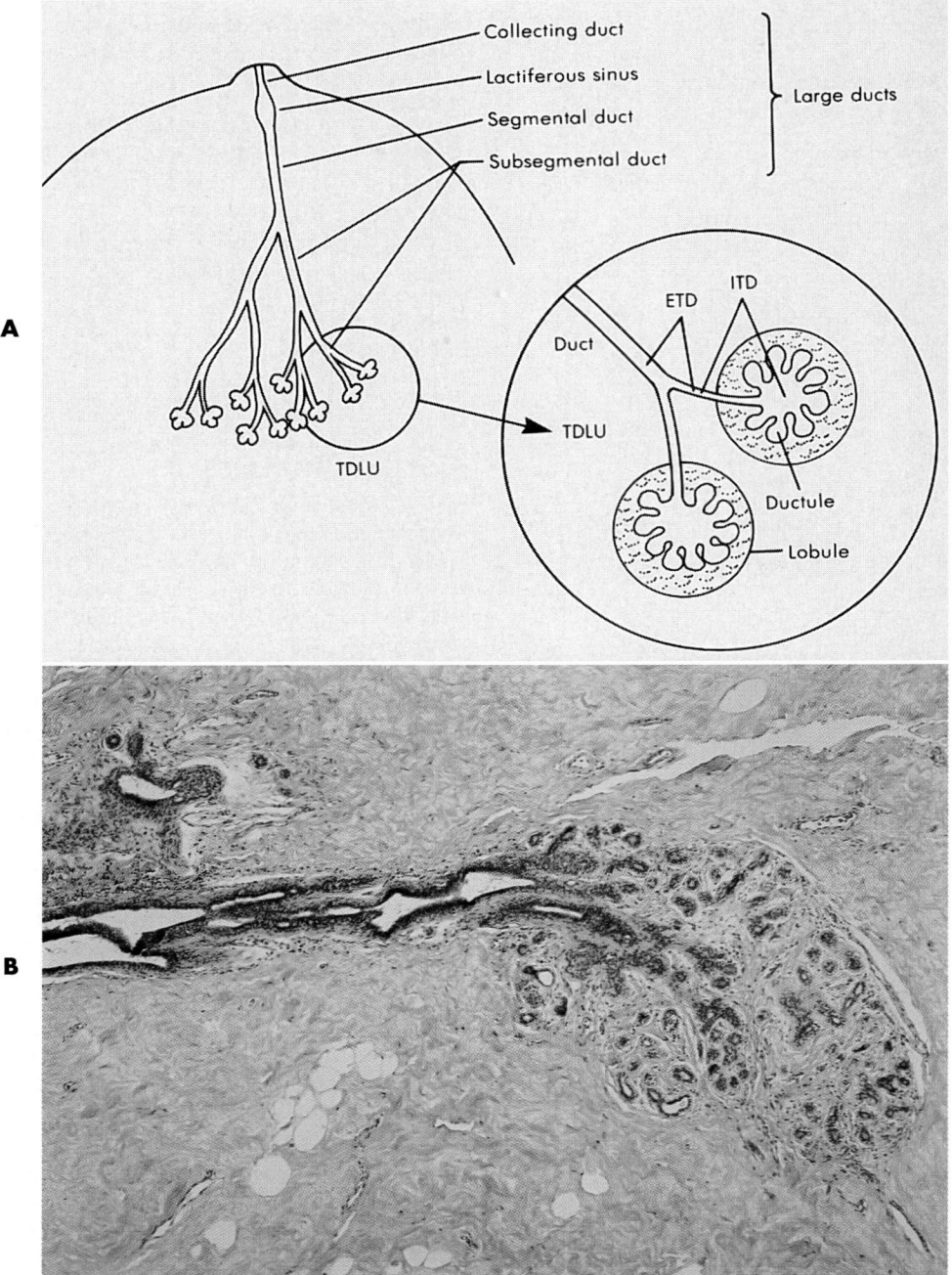

Fig. 20-1 Terminal duct-lobular unit (TDLU). **A,** Diagrammatic representation of this structure. *ETD,* Extralobular terminal duct; *ITD,* intralobular terminal duct. **B,** Photomicrograph of this unit as seen in normal adult female.

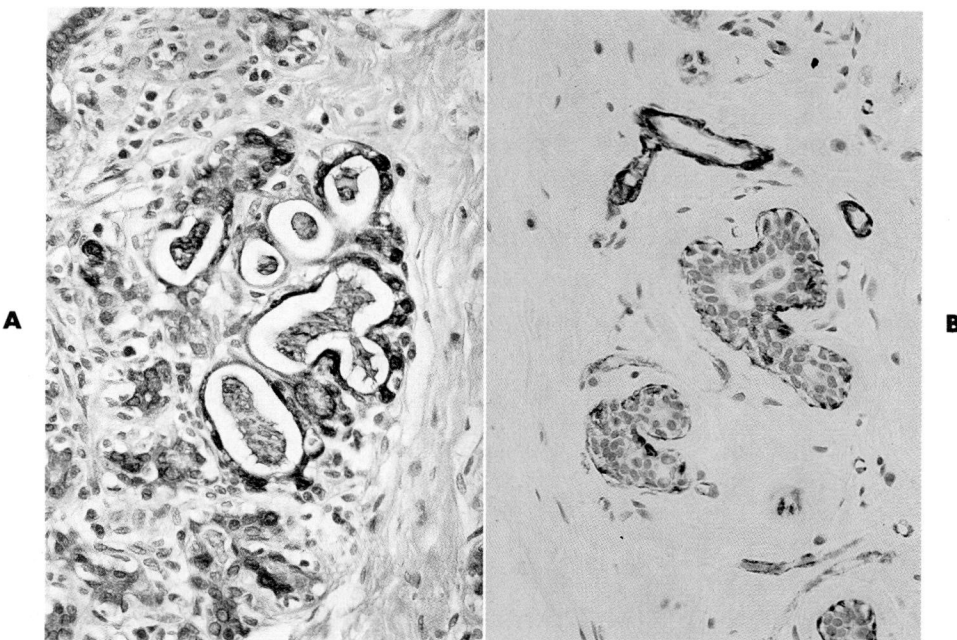

Fig. 20-2 Immunocytochemical markers of mammary lobule. **A,** Lactalbumin showing positivity in secretory epithelium and intraglandular lumina. **B,** Actin showing positivity in outer myoepithelial cell component. Smooth muscle cells present in adjacent vessel walls serve as built-in controls.

with both epithelial and myoepithelial cells. The acidic cytokeratins 18 and 19 react with the epithelial cells throughout the system but not with the myoepithelial cells, whereas the reverse is true for cytokeratin 14, as demonstrated by the monoclonal antibody KA1.[14]

Some studies mention a type of epithelial cell variously named intermediate, indeterminate, or basal clear cell; although the exact identity of these cells vis-à-vis the epithelial-myoepithelial cell binomium is not fully understood, the favored hypothesis is that they are myoepithelial cell precursors.[26]

A sparse population of endocrine cells has been shown in the normal breast with the use of chromogranin stain.[4,24]

The entire glandular epithelial system rests on a continuous basement membrane. This can be demonstrated with reticulin stains, ultrastructurally,[21] or with immunohistochemical reactions for laminin or type IV collagen[5] (see Plate I-C). Type IV collagenase (an enzyme involved in basement membrane turnover) is strongly expressed in myoepithelial cells and to a lesser degree in epithelial cells of terminal ducts.[20]

The nipple has a very characteristic microscopic appearance. In addition to the large collecting ducts opening into the surface, it contains numerous sebaceous glands that open independently of hair follicles and a dense fibrous stroma into which erectile smooth muscle tissue is embedded. Montgomery's tubercles are areolar protuberances, usually between ten and twenty in number, which become prominent during pregnancy; microscopically, they are formed by a collecting (lactiferous) duct associated with a sebaceous apparatus.[27] The epidermis of the nipple and areola resembles that of the skin elsewhere, except for an increase in melanin content in the basal layer and the occasional presence of basally located clear cells, which may be related histogenetically to Paget's disease[29] (see p. 1616). The irregular corrugated appearance of the lactiferous sinus as seen in a tangential cut should not be confused with a pathologic condition. In about 17% of the cases, normal breast lobules are present in the nipple region.[22]

Breast tissue responds markedly to hormonal and other influences throughout life, and as a result, it may display a wide range of "normal" appearances: the immature and largely resting breast before puberty; the developed breast of reproductive life, which exhibits changes depending on the time of the menstrual cycle[19,31]; the actively secreting breast of lactation; and the involuted postmenopausal breast.[7] In the resting breast, cellular proliferation is largely confined to epithelial cells[16]; during pregnancy and lactation, all cell types show a high level of proliferative activity.[3,15,18] Nodularity and spillage of milk into the stroma can occur; exaggerated expressions of these phenomena have been designated as lactation adenoma and milk granuloma, respectively (see p. 1576).[23,25]

Painful engorgement of the breasts occurs not infrequently during the first cycles of contraceptive therapy. This is usually a mild and transient symptom. Microscopically, the only definite mammary change that can be ascribed to the medication is the development of true acini resembling lactating breast.[12]

The process of normal senile involution is more apparent in the TDLU, and it involves both epithelium and special-

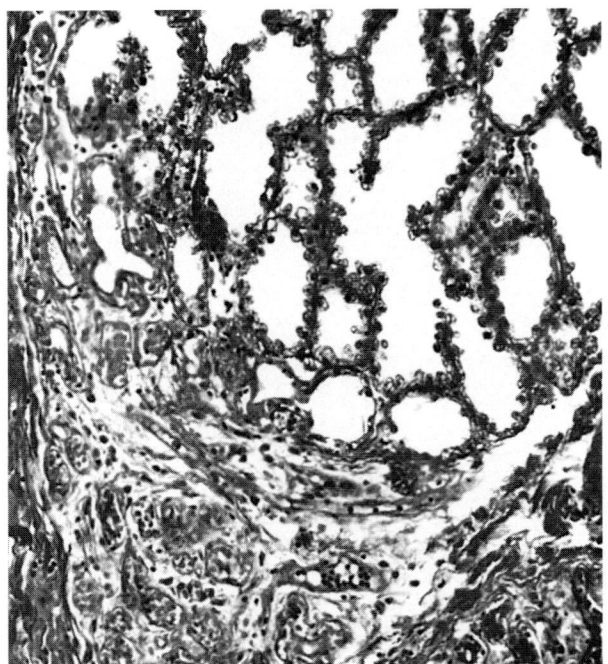

Fig. 20-3 Pregnancy-like changes. Affected lobule is markedly dilated, and lining cells show prominent vacuolization. Morphologic changes are indistinguishable from those seen in normal pregnancy.

ized stroma; it may acquire a microcystic quality (*cystic lobular involution*), not to be confused with fibrocystic disease. Deposits of elastic tissue in the stroma *(elastosis)* are found in nearly half of all women over age 50. They may be located diffusely in the stroma, around vessels, and around ducts.[11]

There are two morphologic curiosities of the breast worth knowing about, not because of their clinical significance (they have none) but because they can simulate other conditions of greater consequence. One is the *pregnancy-like change* seen in one or several lobules in the absence of pregnancy or hormonal manipulation.[17,28] The cells have an abundant vacuolated cytoplasm, the nuclei are large and sometimes apically located (giving the lesion an appearance that resembles the Arias-Stella reaction), and the lumina are dilated (Fig. 20-3). The cause is unknown.

The other process is a *clear cell change* of the ductal or lobular epithelium, in which the cytoplasm acquires a finely granular, finely vacuolated, or totally clear appearance.[2,28] The mechanism of this change is also unknown.

• • •

The main importance of the division of the mammary gland unit into two major portions resides in its relation to diseases of this organ. As Wellings et al.[32] convincingly showed and Azzopardi[1] strongly emphasized, the site of origin of fibrocystic disease (including that accompanied by the formation of large cysts), so-called ductal hyperplasia (epitheliosis or papillomatosis), and most carcinomas (including those of so-called ductal type) is the TDLU and

not the large duct system. The latter is the primary site of most single solitary papillomas, duct ectasia, and a few rare types of ductal carcinoma.

Ectopia

The mammary gland is not a sharply demarcated organ; as a result, isolated mammary lobules can sometimes be seen outside the standard anatomic confines of the breast parenchyma, such as in the nipple or in the axilla. The latter may explain the occurrence of some seemingly primary breast carcinomas in the axilla.

Ectopic breast tissue has also been reported within axillary lymph nodes (although with extreme rarity)[33,35] and along the "milk line" that runs from the axilla to the inguinal region, the most common sites being the chest wall and the vulva.[34]

Ectopic breast parenchyma is subject to changes similar to those of the orthotopic organ, including lactational changes, benign tumors, and carcinomas.[34] It seems likely that papillary hydradenoma of the vulva is not a sweat gland neoplasm, as traditionally believed, but an intraductal papilloma arisen from ectopic breast parenchyma (see Chapter 19, vulva).

Inflammatory and Related Lesions
MAMMARY DUCT ECTASIA

Mammary duct ectasia has also been referred to as varicocele tumor, comedomastitis, periductal mastitis, stale milk mastitis, chemical mastitis, granulomatous mastitis, and mastitis obliterans.[36] Most of the cases are seen in premenopausal parous women and probably represent a localized response to different components of stagnant colostrum. Clinically, the disease may produce retraction or inversion of the nipple and thus simulate invasive carcinoma. Nipple discharge is present in 20% of the cases. Microscopically, there is dilatation of large ducts, with accumulation of fatty detritus in the lumen and fibrous thickening of the wall, which contains an increased amount of elastic fibers (Fig. 20-4).

Calcification is common, producing tubular, annular, and linear shadows on the mammogram. There is no epithelial hyperplasia or apocrine metaplasia. If the luminal material escapes from the duct, a florid inflammatory reaction rich in macrophages and plasma cells may ensue (see p. 1583). It is likely that at least some of the cases categorized in the older literature as plasma cell mastitis belong to this category. In advanced stages, fibrous obliteration of the ducts can occur.

Mammary duct ectasia is probably unrelated to fibrocystic disease, although it is often confused with it.

FAT NECROSIS

A process with the microscopic features of fat necrosis (i.e., foamy macrophages infiltrating partially necrotic adipose tissue) can be seen in the breast under two disparate circumstances; the distinction between the two has not been made clear in many of the articles on the subject. One is as a secondary and relatively minor event in mammary duct ectasia and—to a lesser extent—fibrocystic disease with large cyst formation. In these cases, the rupture of the dilated or cystic structures leads to extravasation of the luminal content, some degree of tissue necrosis, and a secondary

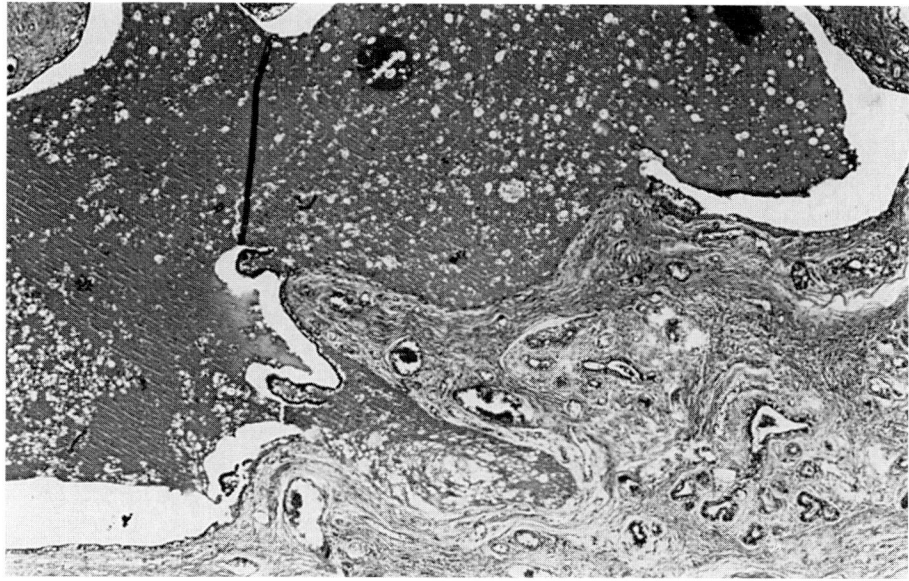

Fig. 20-4 Mammary duct ectasia. There is pronounced dilatation of a large duct, which contains inspissated secretion in its lumen. Epithelium does not show hyperplasia. There is some periductal fibrosis and chronic inflammation.

inflammatory reaction in which foamy macrophages can be numerous. Parenthetically, small collections of foamy cells are seen not infrequently within duct lumina or in cohesive masses along duct walls in cases of fibrocystic disease; their immunohistochemical profile is that of histiocytes rather than epithelial cells.[38]

The other circumstance, which perhaps is the only one that deserves to be called fat necrosis, is of the traumatic (either accidental or surgical) type and often involves the superficial subcutaneous tissue rather than the breast parenchyma itself (Fig. 20-5). A history of trauma can be elicited in about half of the cases, usually 1 to 2 weeks before the time of diagnosis. The disease can simulate carcinoma clinically because of skin retraction (Fig. 20-6). In long-standing cases, the nodule is harder and more fibrotic; it has an orange-brown color because of the deposition of hemoglobin-derived pigments. The microscopic diagnosis is usually easy, but the frozen section may cause some perplexity. A somewhat unorthodox clue to the diagnosis is the fact that a satisfactory frozen section is very difficult to obtain because this tissue is largely made up of liquefied fat.

Cases of mammary fat necrosis have also been reported following radiation therapy for breast carcinoma,[37] and as a local manifestation of Weber-Christian disease.

OTHER INFLAMMATORY DISEASES

Abscess of the breast usually results from rupture of mammary ducts, occurring most often during lactation but also independently from it.[45,62] It may be located deep within the parenchyma or periareolar region.[69] Microscopically, a central cavity filled with neutrophils and secretion is surrounded by inflamed and eventually fibrotic breast parenchyma, with obliteration of the lobular pattern. Clini-

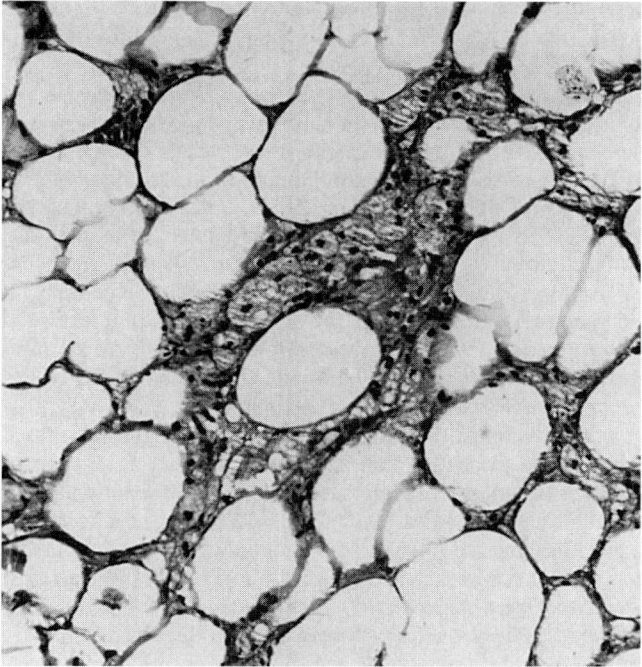

Fig. 20-5 Fat necrosis involving adipose tissue of breast. Clusters of foamy macrophages are seen between necrotic fat lobules. This rare disorder should be distinguished from inflammatory changes seen in fibrocystic disease.

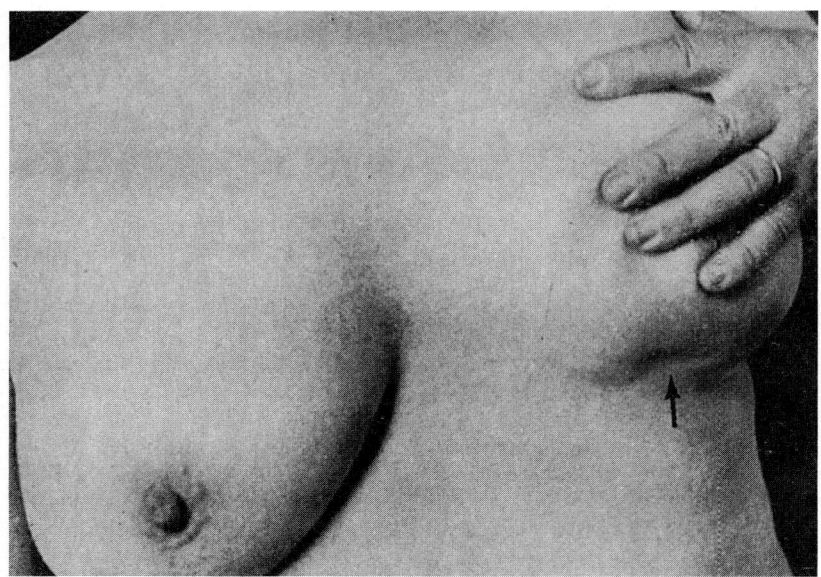

Fig. 20-6 Retraction of skin in patient with fat necrosis *(arrow)*. (From Lee BJ, Adair F: Traumatic fat necrosis of the female breast and its differentiation from carcinoma. Ann Surg **80**:670-691, 1924.)

cally, a localized abscess may simulate carcinoma. *Periareolar abscess* associated with squamous metaplasia of lactiferous ducts is referred to as Zuska's disease.[64,69]

Lymphocytic mastitis is an unusual breast lesion of probable immune-mediated pathogenesis consisting microscopically of dense intralobular, perilobular, and perivascular lymphocytic infiltrates associated with lobular atrophy and sclerosis.[63] When the latter is intense, the term sclerosing lymphocytic mastitis has sometimes been employed.[55] The lymphocytes are mainly of the B-cell type. Sometimes, the lymphocytic infiltrate is accompanied by a stromal infiltrate of epithelioid cells that can lead to a mistaken diagnosis of invasive carcinoma or granular cell tumor. These cells appear to be of a fibroblastic or myofibroblastic nature.[40] Lymphocytic mastitis can result clinically in a palpable mass; most cases are seen in association with diabetes (hence the proposed synonym diabetic mastopathy[56a,67]), but can also occur in the absence of this disorder.[40,65] On occasion, it has been associated with intraductal carcinoma.[44a]

Granulomatous mastitis (lobular granulomatous mastitis; granulomatous lobulitis) is a term that has been proposed for a granulomatous inflammatory process of the breast characterized by the presence of noncaseating granulomas, confined to breast lobules, in which no micro-organisms are found; the suggestion has been made that the disease may be immunologically mediated and therefore analogous to granulomatous thyroiditis or granulomatous orchitis.[49,54,68]

Tuberculosis of the breast is rare; it may be secondary to bloodstream dissemination or to extension from an adjacent tuberculous process. Grossly, multiple sinuses and areas of caseation necrosis occur. Microscopically, typical granulomas are identified in most cases. The lesion may be mistaken clinically for advanced breast carcinoma. The regional nodes are often involved; occasionally, these nodes are intramammary.[39]

Actinomycosis, coccidioidomycosis, and *histoplasmosis* of the breast can cause necrotizing granulomatous masses and multiple sinus tracts.[42,59]

Sarcoidosis can begin in the breast and remain localized in this organ for long periods.[41,48]

Foreign body reaction to polyvinyl plastic or silicone used for mammoplasty can result in tumorlike masses and sinus tracts.[50,66]

Breast infarct can complicate a large variety of conditions, including intraductal papilloma, fibroadenoma, phylloides tumor, hyperplastic lobules during pregnancy, syphilis, and Wegener's granulomatosis.[46,53,56,60] It also has been reported in association with anticoagulant therapy,[58] postpartum abscess and gangrene, thrombophlebitis migrans disseminata, and mitral stenosis with heart failure.[61]

Mondor's disease is the eponymic term given to a peculiar thrombophlebitis involving the breast and contiguous thoracoabdominal wall.[47] The condition, which may simulate clinically a malignant neoplasm, often has a sudden onset and appears as a firm, slightly nodular cord beneath the skin. Ecchymosis may or may not be present. Microscopically, the process is one of phlebitis with thrombosis.[52] With time, the thrombus recanalizes completely. The condition is self-limited and practically never recurs. It may be related to mechanical injury. In eight of the fifteen cases reported by Herrmann,[51] the disease appeared a few months following a radical mastectomy. A few cases have been found to be associated with breast carcinoma.[43]

Rheumatoid nodules and *periarteritis nodosa* may present as single or multiple breast masses.[44,57]

Benign Proliferative Breast Disease

This is an extremely complex and interrelated group of proliferative disorders of the breast parenchyma, most of which are probably not true neoplasms but rather hormonally induced

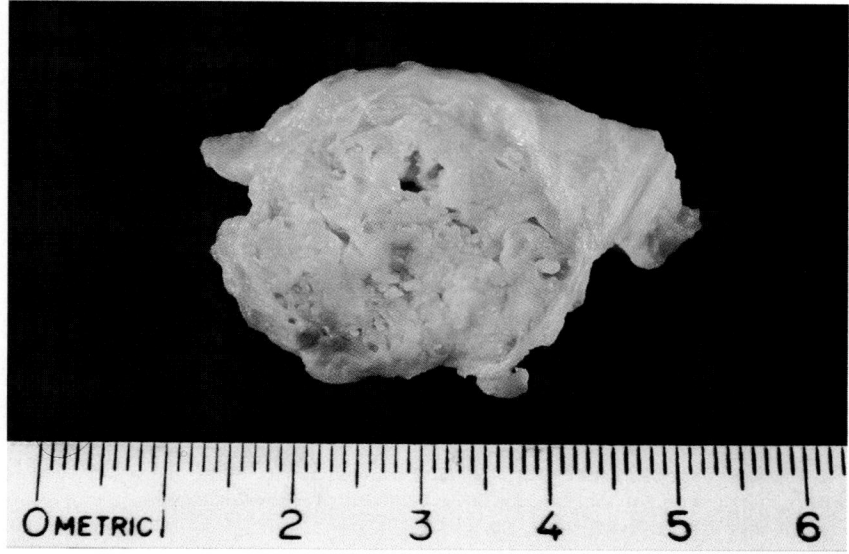

Fig. 20-7 Gross appearance of fibroadenoma. The lesion is sharply circumscribed and perfectly round, and it contains numerous slits.

hyperplastic processes. Some, like typical fibroadenoma, are recognized at a glance. Others raise the differential diagnosis of carcinoma at the clinical, gross, or microscopic level, and some of them are probably related to the development of malignancy but in a fashion that remains ill defined and highly controversial.

FIBROADENOMA

Fibroadenoma is a common benign breast lesion usually occurring in patients between the ages of 20 and 35 years. It increases in size during pregnancy and tends to regress as the age of the patient increases. It is usually single, but in 20% of the cases there are multiple lesions in the same breast or bilaterally. A lineage-restricted cytogenetic analysis of nine fibroadenomas revealed clonal chromosomal aberrations of the stromal cells in four, suggesting that this component is neoplastic.[79]

Grossly, the usual fibroadenoma is a sharply demarcated, firm mass, usually no more than 3 cm in diameter. The cut surface is solid, grayish white, and bulging, with a whorl-like pattern and slit-like spaces. Necrosis is absent (Fig. 20-7).

Microscopically, fibroadenomas vary in appearance from case to case depending on the relative amounts of glandular and connective tissue and the configuration of the former (Fig. 20-8). They are labeled intracanalicular (a misnomer) when the connective tissue invaginates into the glandular spaces so that it appears to be within them, and pericanalicular when the regular round or oval glandular configuration of the glands is maintained. Often, both types of growth are seen in the same lesion. The distinction has no practical connotations. The tubules are composed of cuboidal or low columnar cells with round uniform nuclei resting on a myoepithelial cell layer. The stroma is usually made up of loose connective tissue rich in acid mucopolysaccharides, but it may be partially or totally composed of dense fibrous

type. Elastic tissue is absent, in keeping with the presumed TDLU origin of the lesion. The cellularity of the stroma varies from case to case, but in any unduly hypercellular lesion the alternative diagnosis of phylloides tumor should be considered (see p. 1629).

Morphologic variations in fibroadenoma are plentiful, some of more significance than others:

1 Hyalinization, calcification, and/or ossification of the stroma. These changes are more commonly seen in older patients and can be appreciated radiographically (Fig. 20-9).

2 Presence in the stroma of multinucleated giant cells of reactive nature, similar to those seen in polypoid lesions of nasal cavity and other sites.[72]

3 Presence in the stroma of mature adipose tissue, smooth muscle, or metaplastic cartilage.[80,83] Some of the lesions described as hamartoma or choristoma of the breast probably belong to this category[70,81,85] (see p. 1630).

4 Prominent myxoid changes. Most of these fibroadenomas are not otherwise different from the others. However, whenever multiple highly myxoid fibroadenomas are found, the possibility that they are a component of the syndrome that also includes endocrine hyperactivity, cardiac myxoma, cutaneous hyperpigmentation, and other abnormalities (Carney's syndrome) should be investigated.[89] Other breast abnormalities that can be seen in the syndrome are lobular and nodular myxoid changes,[73] and ductal adenoma with tubular features (see p. 1576).

5 Peculiar fibrocellular stroma. Azzopardi[71] has pointed out the existence of a fibroadenoma variant in which the stroma is simultaneously highly collagenous and cellular, has a somewhat laminated appearance, and is sometimes accompanied by a mononuclear infiltrate.

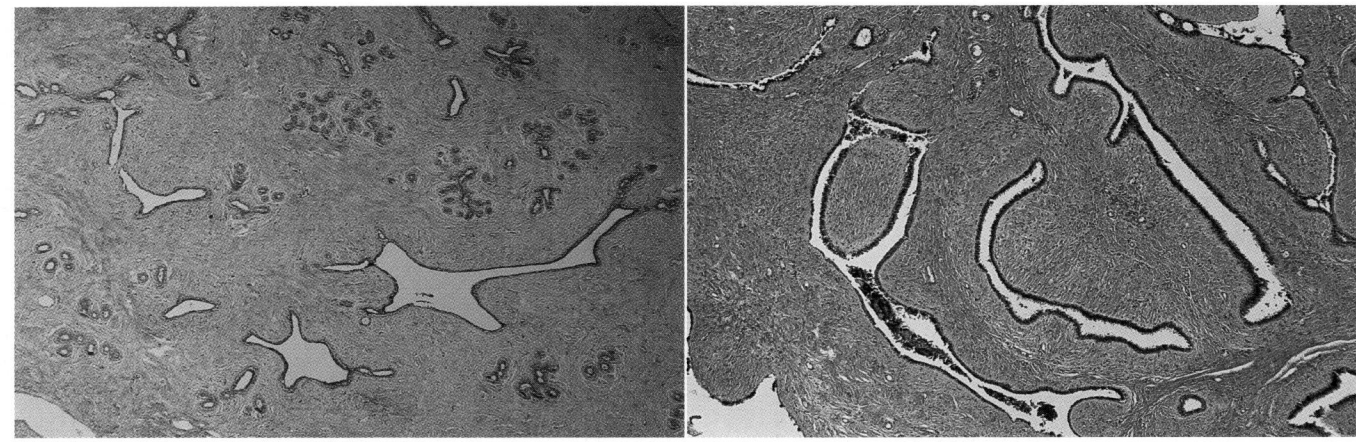

Fig. 20-8 Microscopic appearance of fibroadenoma. The tumor shown in **B** has a slightly hypercellular stroma but not to a degree that would justify a diagnosis of phylloides tumor.

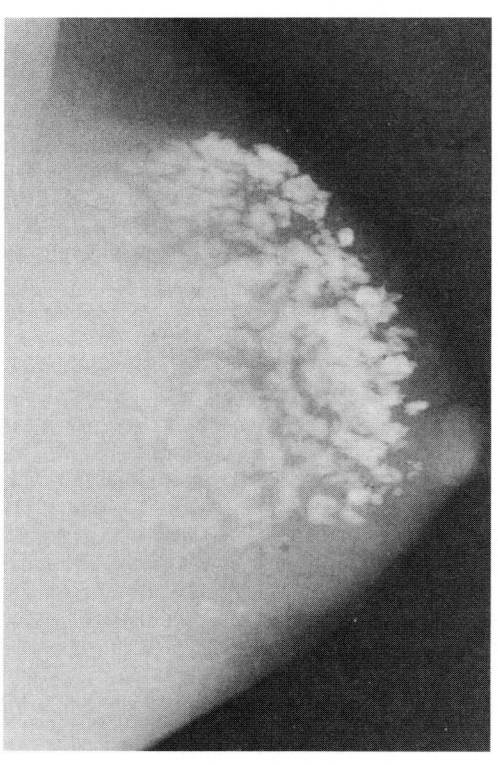

Fig. 20-9 Heavy, coarse calcification in large breast fibroadenoma as seen in mammogram.

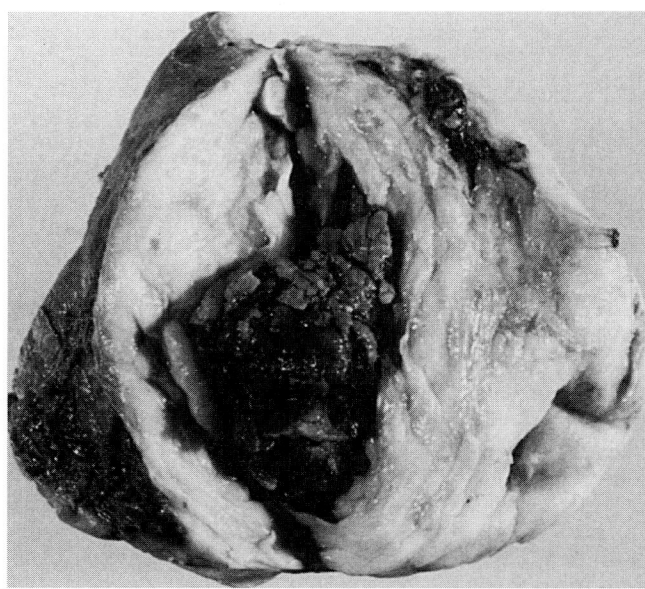

Fig. 20-10 Fibroadenoma with hemorrhagic infarction involving central region.

6 Hemorrhagic infarction. Fibroadenomas with this complication show grossly a bulging red appearance that can be quite perplexing. This complication is more likely to occur during pregnancy (Fig. 20-10).

7 Ill-defined margins blending with a surrounding breast that shows the features of fibrocystic disease. This form, which has been designated *fibroadenomatosis* or *fibroadenomatoid hyperplasia*, shares the features of fibroadenoma and fibrocystic disease and suggests a pathogenetic link between the two.

8 Apocrine metaplasia. This change is found in about 15% of the cases.[71] In retrospect, it would seem that the change originally described as endocrine neoplasia in fibroadenoma[76] represents a morphologic variation on the theme of apocrine metaplasia; in the cases we have studied, the endocrine-like cells stained strongly for GCDFP-15 but were negative for chromogranin (Figs. 20-11 and 20-12).

9 Sclerosing adenosis. This occurs in less than 10% of the cases.[71] Fibroadenomas with cysts, sclerosing adenosis, calcifications, or papillary apocrine changes are sometimes referred to as "complex."[75]

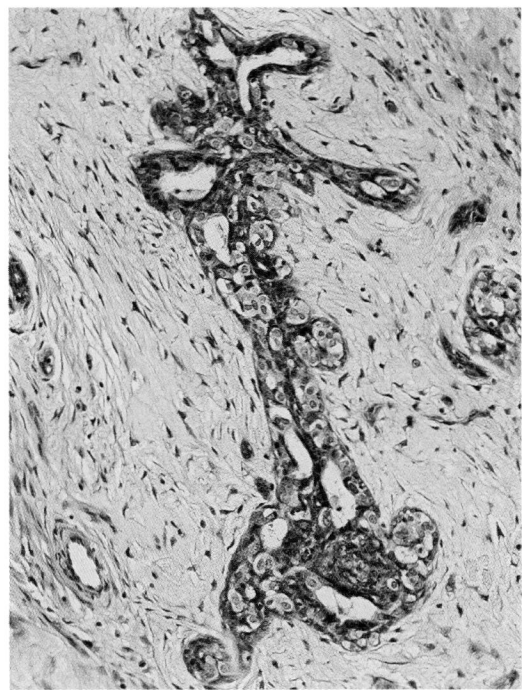

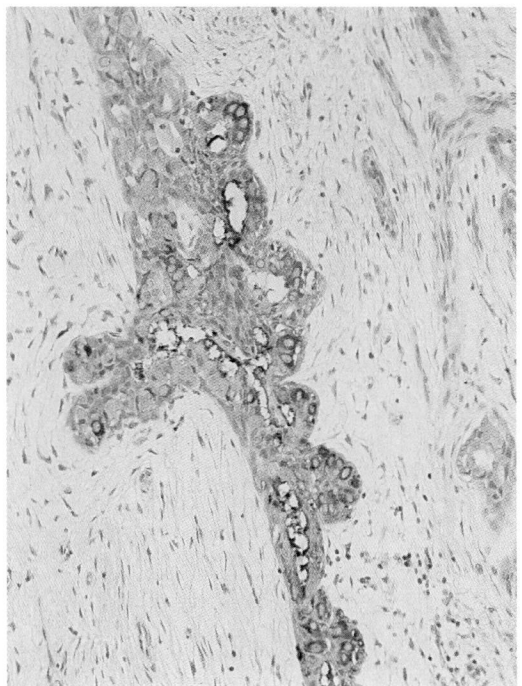

Fig. 20-11 Fibroadenoma with apocrine metaplasia. Hematoxylin-eosin section showing prominent discontinuous layer of plump eosinophilic cells at the base of the gland. These should not be confused with neuroendocrine cells.

Fig. 20-12 Same case as Fig. 20-11. Immunostain for GCDFP-15.

10 Squamous metaplasia. This is a rare finding; its presence in abundance should suggest the alternative possibility of phylloides tumor.

11 Lactational changes. These are manifested by an increase in the amount of cytoplasm in the epithelial cells, which appear vacuolated, and by dilatation of the glandular lumina by secretion.[84]

12 Young age, large size, and hypercellularity. There is a reasonably distinct type of fibroadenoma that tends to occur in adolescents (often in blacks and sometimes involving both breasts), reach a large size (over 10 cm), and show hypercellularity of glands and/or stroma (Fig. 20-13). These attributes can be found independently from each other, but there is clearly a link between them. A plethora of names exists to designate these lesions, depending on which feature predominates or which has impressed the writer the most. There are age-related terms, such as juvenile fibroadenoma[82,86]; size-related terms, such as giant or massive fibroadenoma; and cellularity-related terms, such as fetal or cellular fibroadenoma.[86] When the cellularity is mainly epithelial and very florid, they have also been called fibroadenomas with atypical epithelial hyperplasia[82]; when the stroma is prominent, they have been designated fibroadenomas with stromal cellularity.[78] It is easy to imagine the difficulty one may encounter in selecting a name for the fibroadenoma that at the same time is very large, is hypercellular, and occurs in an adolescent, not an

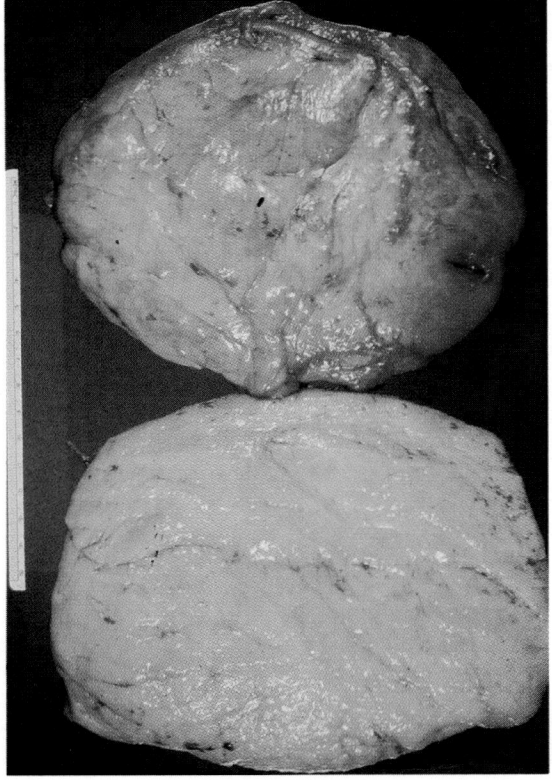

Fig. 20-13 Giant fibroadenoma occurring in an adolescent female.

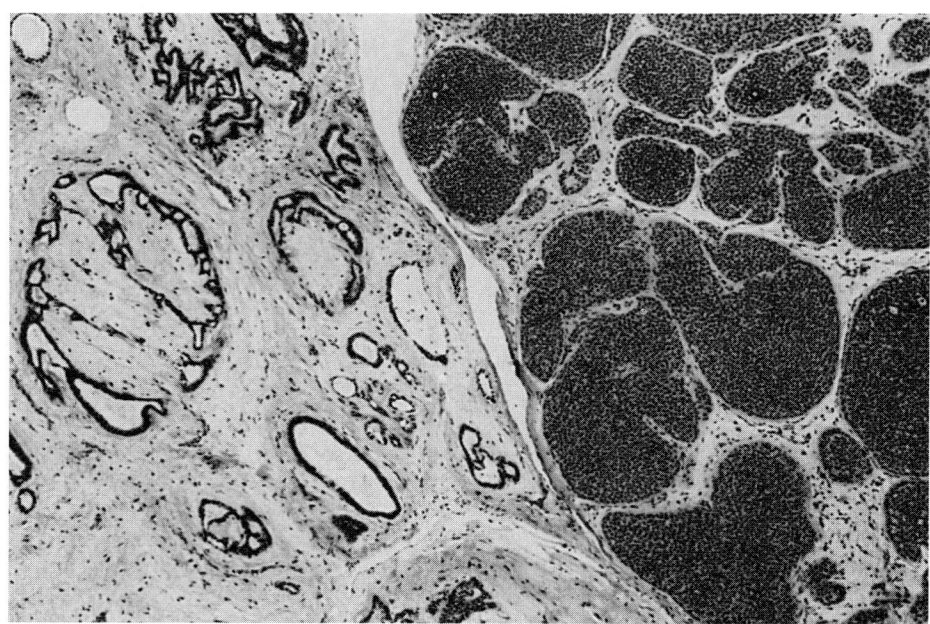

Fig. 20-14 Fibroadenoma with malignant transformation manifested by lobular carcinoma in situ.

infrequent occurrence. Of course, the choice of term is not very important. What matters is to recognize that the lesion is a fibroadenoma and not to confuse it with virginal hypertrophy or—more cogently—phylloides tumor. The epithelial hypercellularity can be dismissed as clinically inconsequential (unless it has the cytoarchitectural features of carcinoma). The stromal hypercellularity should be evaluated more carefully in terms of degree and atypicality; it is good to remember, however, that it is very rare for phylloides tumors to occur in young patients.

• • •

No differences have been found in the incidence, gross appearance, and microscopic configuration of fibroadenomas removed in patients taking oral contraceptives and those in control cases, except for the occasional formation of acini in the former.[77]

Ultrastructurally, the most interesting feature of fibroadenomas is the constant presence of a multilayered basal lamina around the epithelial and endothelial cells.[74,90] The stromal cells have features of fibroblasts.[88] Biochemical studies have shown that most fibroadenomas have a progesterone receptor but lack an estrogen receptor.[87]

A recent epidemiologic study suggests that fibroadenoma represents a long-term risk for breast carcinomas and that this risk is increased in women with complex fibroadenomas, ductal hyperplasias, or a family history of breast carcinoma.[75]

Malignant transformation

Malignant changes in fibroadenomas are found in only 0.1% of the cases.[91,95,96] They usually involve the epithelial component, and the large majority are in situ lesions[93,94,97]

(Fig. 20-14). In some cases the malignant tumor is entirely within the confines of the fibroadenoma, and in others it involves the surrounding breast as well. The latter may simply represent extension into the fibroadenoma by a carcinoma originating elsewhere in the breast. In a series of 105 fibroadenomas containing carcinoma, 95% of the cases were in situ lesions, and lobular and ductal types occurred with equal frequency. Nine of ten fibroadenomas harboring an invasive carcinoma also contained CIS, supporting the origin of the invasive component in the fibroadenoma. CIS within the fibroadenoma was associated with CIS in the surrounding breast in 21% of the cases. The prognosis for the entire group was excellent.[93]

Sarcomatous transformation of the stroma of a fibroadenoma is an even rarer phenomenon.[92] We have seen only one possible case in which a well-circumscribed small nodule had in some areas the appearance of an osteosarcoma, whereas in others it was composed of hyaline stroma enclosing slit-like glandular spaces, a configuration strongly reminiscent of an ancient fibroadenoma.

ADENOMA

Adenomas of the breast (exclusive of those having a salivary or sweat gland appearance and so-called nipple adenoma, discussed on pp. 1626 and 1577, respectively) can be divided into the following categories.[100]

Tubular adenoma presents in young adults as a solitary, well-circumscribed, firm mass that is tan-yellow. Microscopically, a close packing of uniform small tubules lined by a single layer of epithelial cells and an attenuated layer of myoepithelial cells is seen; the stroma is characteristically sparse (Fig. 20-15). Sometimes this pattern is seen combined with that of a fibroadenoma, suggesting that the two processes are closely related.[102] A type of *ductal adenoma*

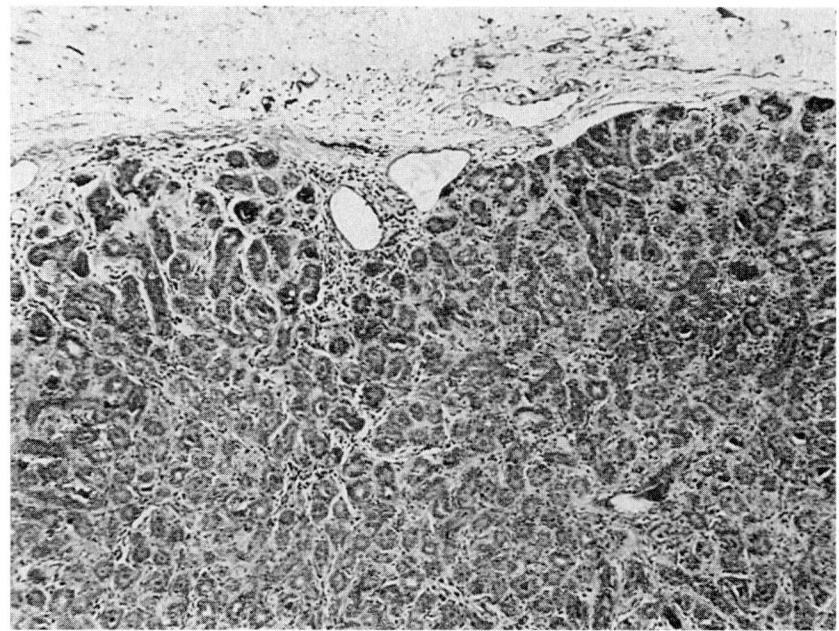

Fig. 20-15 Tubular adenoma of breast. Small uniform ducts are present with only minimal intervening stroma. (From Hertel BF, Zaloudek C, Kempson RL: Breast adenomas. Cancer **37:**2891-2905, 1976.)

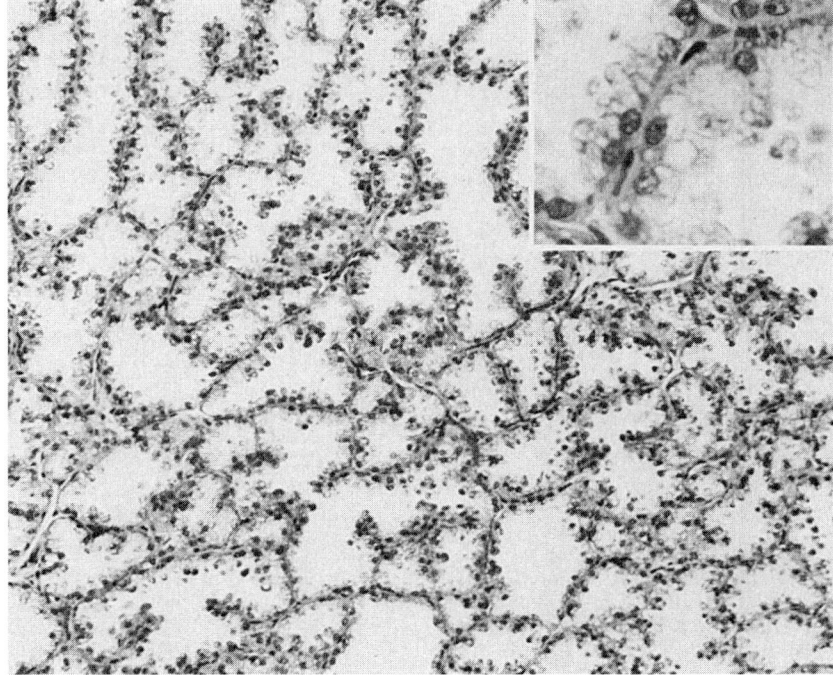

Fig. 20-16 Lactating adenoma. Lumen is large, and cytoplasm is actively secreting. **Inset** shows abundant secretory cytoplasm in greater detail. (Courtesy Dr. B.F. Hertel, Woodruff, WI.)

with tubular features has been found to be associated with Carney's syndrome. Microscopically, it presents as an encapsulated solid intraductal tumor composed of arrays of long, narrow tubules composed of a dual population of epithelial and myoepithelial cells and a modest amount of fibrous tissue. Because of their complexity and cellularity, they can be mistaken for carcinoma.[99] The subject of *ductal adenoma* is further discussed on p. 1577.

Lactating adenoma presents as a solitary or multiple freely movable breast mass during pregnancy or puerperium. The lesion is actually a localized focus of hyperplasia in the lactating breast, which may also develop in ectopic locations such as the axilla, chest wall, or vulva.[103] Grossly, the lesion is well circumscribed and lobulated. The cut sur-

face is gray or tan, in contrast to the white color of fibroadenoma (Plate XV-A). Necrotic changes are frequent.[101] Microscopically, proliferated glands are seen lined by actively secreting cuboidal cells (Fig. 20-16). This lesion should be distinguished from the proliferative and secretory changes brought on by pregnancy in a pre-existing fibroadenoma.[103]

Apocrine adenoma is a form of adenoma composed exclusively of apocrine cells. This exceptionally rare lesion should be distinguished from fibrocystic disease with focally prominent apocrine changes and from well-differentiated apocrine carcinoma.[98]

INTRADUCTAL PAPILLOMA

Papilloma of the breast occurs at an average age of 48 years. It can arise in large or small ducts; consequently, it can be identified grossly as a polypoid intraluminal mass or be found only on microscopic examination.[108] The grossly visible papilloma can give rise to bloody nipple discharge and may be palpable in a subareolar location, but its diameter rarely exceeds 3 cm, a point of importance in the differential diagnosis with papillary carcinoma. The lesion is soft and fragile, and it may have areas of hemorrhage in it. The duct that contains the papilloma may be dilated (Fig. 20-17). About 90% of the cases are solitary.[108] Multiple papillomas are seen in slightly younger patients, arise in smaller ducts, are usually not associated with nipple discharge, and are bilateral in one fourth of the cases.

Microscopically, papillomas are complex, cellular, and often intricately arborescent (Fig. 20-18, *A*). Features favoring benignancy in a papillary breast lesion are a well-developed stroma in the papillary folds, the presence of two cell types, normochromatic and often oval nuclei, scanty mitotic activity, the presence of apocrine metaplasia, and a lack of cribriform or trabecular patterns[109] (Fig. 20-18, *B*). Tumor necrosis is nearly always absent. The presence of a prominent myoepithelial cell component can be highlighted with actin or S-100 protein stains.[106,112,114] Clonal analysis using

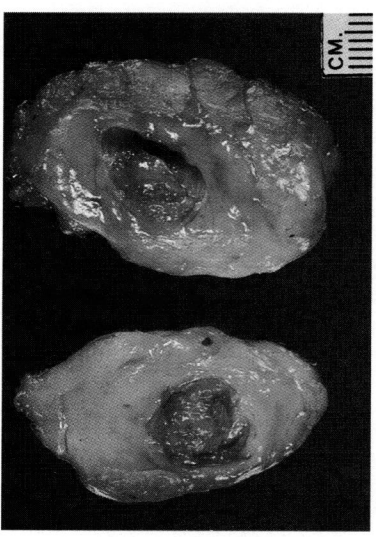

Fig. 20-17 Gross appearance of intraductal papilloma. A polypoid tumor mass is seen protruding within the lumen of a markedly dilated duct.

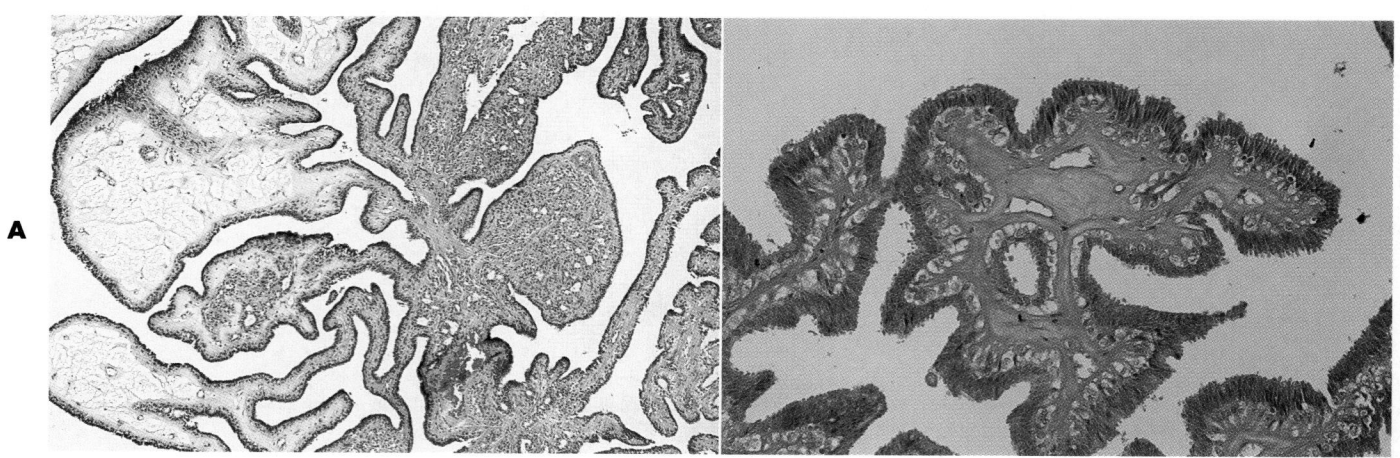

Fig. 20-18 Intraductal papilloma. **A,** Low-power appearance showing complex arborizing architecture. **B,** High-power view showing dual cell composition, with a well-defined row of myoepithelial cells.

PCR technology has shown that intraductal papilloma is a clonal lesion, a fact that supports its neoplastic nature and suggests the existence of a common cell precursor that can differentiate into both luminal epithelial and myoepithelial lines.[111]

Morphologic variations sometimes encountered in intraductal papilloma include:

1 Location within a large cystic ("tension") duct. This variant has been designated intracystic papilloma, papillary cystadenoma, and multiradicular papilloma.

2 Partial or total hemorrhagic infarct. This change, which is probably caused by interruption of the blood supply, is entirely different from the tumor necrosis seen in carcinoma.

3 Squamous metaplasia. This change is probably secondary to focal necrosis and is quite rare. The presence of an extensive squamous component in a mammary lesion should raise the suspicion of malignancy.

4 Pseudo-infiltration at the base of the papilloma. This is the result of fibrosis perhaps secondary to hemorrhage, which leads to a marked distortion of the glandular component and sometimes to the presence of isolated tubules embedded in dense fibrous tissue (Plate XV-B). Preservation of the two-cell layer in these areas and an accompaniment of hemosiderin deposits and cholesterol clefts are supporting diagnostic features. This pseudomalignant change blends with the lesion designated as infiltrating epitheliosis by Azzopardi[104] and is represented by at least some of the cases described as sclerosing papillary proliferations by Fenoglio and Lattes[107] (see p. 1587).

5 The lesion designated as ductal adenoma.[105,110] Although this lacks the arborescent papillary quality of the typical papilloma, its intraductal location, the distorted epithelial proliferation composed of two cell types, the frequent occurrence of apocrine metaplasia, and the benign behavior speak of a link between the two processes. Ductal adenoma with tubular features can be seen as a component of Carney's syndrome (see p. 1576).

• • •

Papilloma is a benign lesion that is curable by local excision.[108] There is no indication that patients so treated have a higher incidence of carcinoma at a later date.[115] Instead, multiple grossly detectable papillomas have been found to be associated with or to develop into carcinoma at a frequency higher than that expected from chance alone.[108,113]

NIPPLE ADENOMA

Nipple adenoma, also known as florid papillomatosis of the nipple ducts and erosive adenomatosis, usually occurs in the fourth or fifth decade, is nearly always unilateral, and is often accompanied by serous or bloody discharge from the nipple.[119,121] Clinically, the nipple may appear eroded, and the disease may be confused with Paget's disease.[117]

Microscopically, there are marked papillomatous changes of ductal elements, often associated with distortion induced by the dense stroma present (Fig. 20-19, *A* and *B*). This is referred to by Rosen et al.[120] as the sclerosing papillomatosis pattern, the other patterns being papillomatosis (without sclerosis) and adenosis (the least common of the three). The features used to identify this lesion as benign are to a large extent analogous to those seen in ductal papilloma and include the presence of two cell types, a dual population of epithelial and myoepithelial cells (confirmed by immunohistochemical evaluation[118]), an oval nuclear shape, a lack of atypia, streaming, the formation of peripheral clefts, and the absence of a cribriform pattern (Fig. 20-19, *B*). However, some minor differences between the two lesions exist. One is secondary to the close interaction of the glandular epithelium of the mammary ducts and the squamous epithelium from the epidermis, resulting in formation of adenosquamous nests that may be incorrectly diagnosed. The other difference is that otherwise typical nipple adenomas can exhibit small necrotic foci in the center of the prolifer-

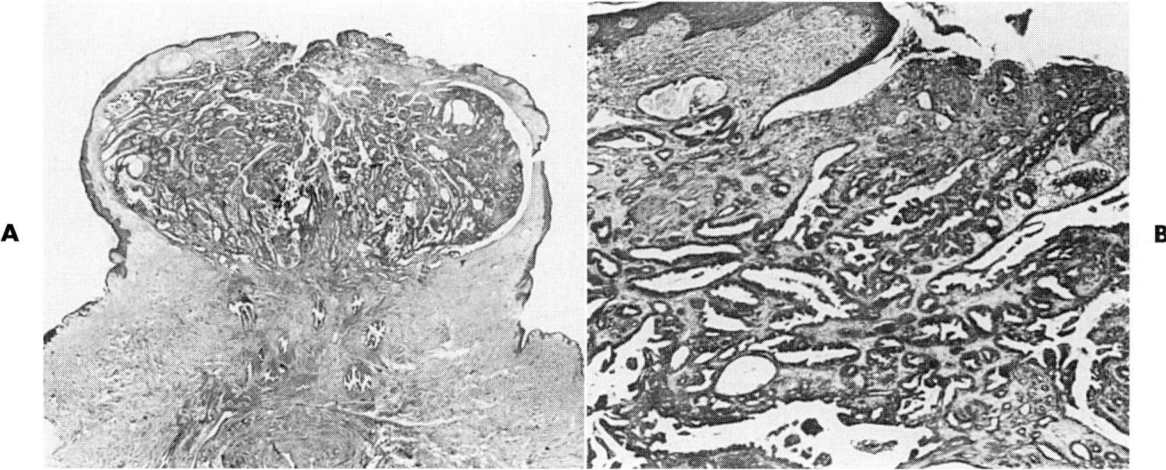

A

B

Fig. 20-19 Nipple adenoma. **A,** Panoramic view of lesion. **B,** Intricate glandular pattern merging with overlying squamous epithelium.

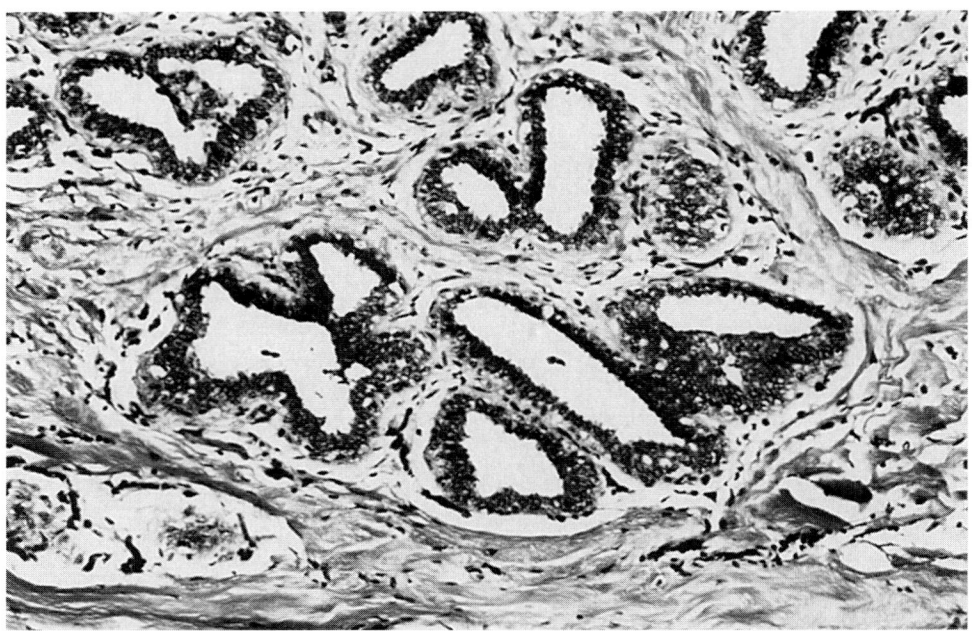

Fig. 20-20 Blunt duct adenosis. Individual lobule is markedly enlarged, and there is dilatation and some cellular proliferation of individual components.

ating ducts, a feature that in a more deeply located papillary lesion would be strongly suggestive of malignancy.[120]

A note of warning is in order. Just because an intraductal papillary lesion is located in or close to the nipple, it does not necessarily mean that it is a nipple adenoma and therefore benign. Intraductal papillary carcinomas and ordinary invasive ductal carcinomas can also occur in this location, some of them apparently arising within a nipple adenoma.[116,116a,120]

The treatment of uncomplicated nipple adenoma is local excision.[119,120]

ADENOSIS

The term adenosis can be applied to any hyperplastic process that primarily involves the glandular component of the breast; it should therefore be used with a qualifier in order to acquire a specific clinicopathologic connotation.

Blunt duct adenosis

In this very common alteration of the breast lobule, the involved components are lined by two cell types and show blunting of both the lateral outlines and the tips, hence the name.[123] There is an accompanying increase in the surrounding specialized connective tissue (Fig. 20-20). Minor morphologic variations have been described as organoid, microcystic, and nonorganoid forms of the disease.[122] Blunt duct adenosis can be secondarily involved by duct hyperplasia.

Sclerosing adenosis

Sclerosing adenosis is the better known form of adenosis, mainly because of the high likelihood of it being misdiagnosed as carcinoma by the beginner. The average age of the patient is about 30 years. Grossly, it is small, has a disklike

and somewhat multinodular configuration, and cuts with increased resistance; in some cases, its overall appearance is quite reminiscent of invasive carcinoma.

Microscopically, the most important diagnostic feature of the lesion is its architecture as seen at very low magnification. The nodule retains a round or oval lobular configuration and is more cellular centrally than peripherally (Fig. 20-21). The elongated and compressed proliferating tubules are lined by two cell types that are themselves elongated along the tubular axis. The myoepithelial component predominates in some lesions and may even acquire spindle-shaped "myoid" features. Trabecular formations, pleomorphism, and necrosis are absent. The stroma is dense and may show foci of elastosis, although not as commonly as in radial scar or invasive carcinoma.

Morphologic variations of sclerosing adenosis that further complicate it are the very florid changes that accompany pregnancy, the presence of apocrine metaplasia (which is accompanied by nuclear and nucleolar enlargement), and the occasional occurrence of permeation of perineurial spaces[129] and the walls of veins[124] (Fig. 20-22).

The marked participation of myoepithelial cells in this process can be dramatically demonstrated with an immunohistochemical stain for actin and the presence of a basement membrane around the tubules by electron microscopy or with stains for laminin or type IV collagen.

The risk of subsequent invasive carcinoma in patients with sclerosing adenosis seems to be the same as for ordinary fibrocystic disease.[127] On rare occasions the foci of sclerosing adenosis may be secondarily involved by lobular carcinoma in situ[128] (Fig. 20-21, *D*). In these cases, the distortion already present because of the sclerosing adenosis may result in a mistaken diagnosis of invasive lobular carci-

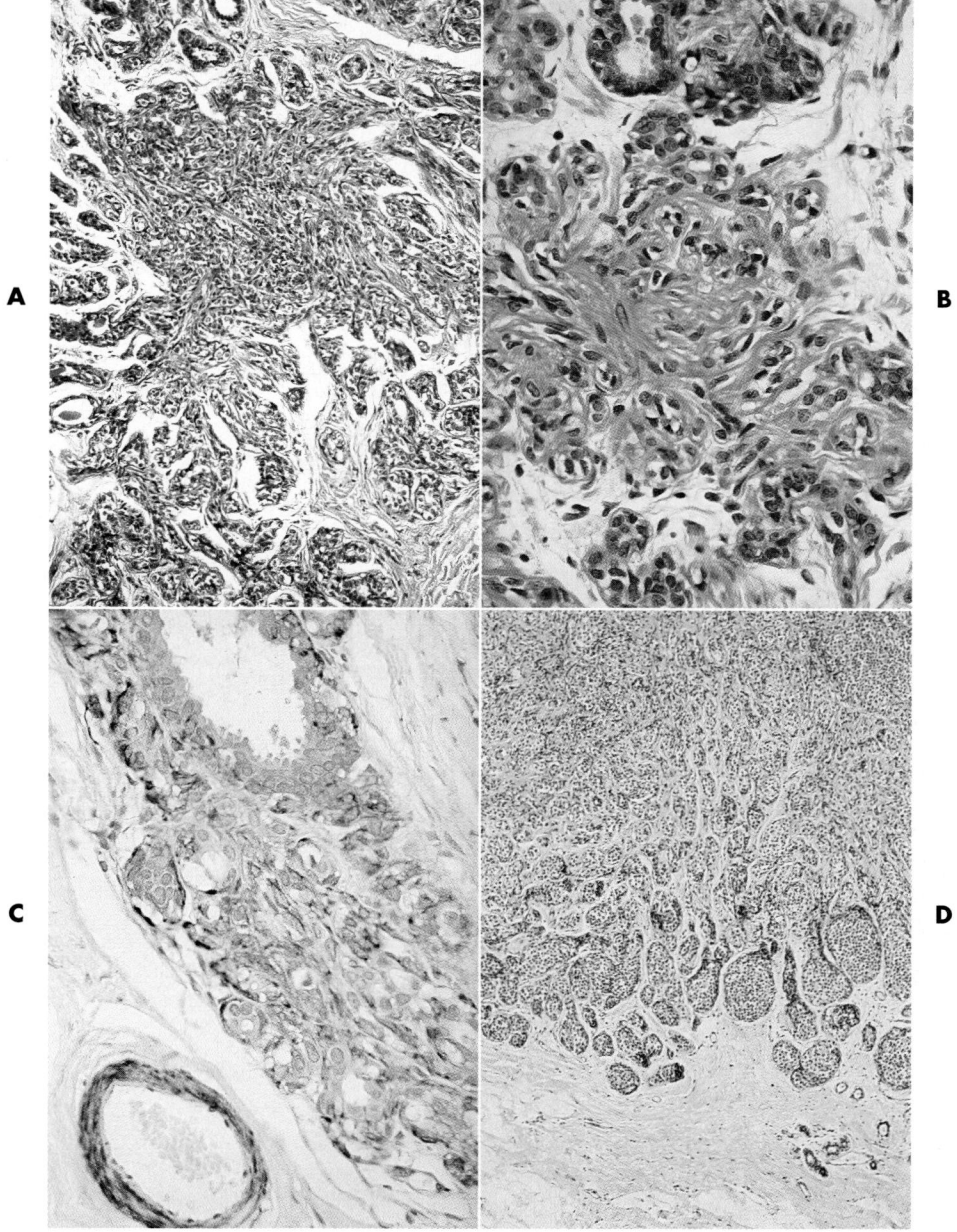

Fig. 20-21 Sclerosing adenosis. **A,** Low-power view. The lobular configuration of the lesion is obvious. **B,** Medium-power view. Note the spindle shape of the proliferating cells in the center of the lobule and the cells' fibrillary cytophilic cytoplasm, indicative of myoepithelial nature. **C,** Immunocytochemical stain for actin showing strong immunoreactivity in the myoepithelial cell component. **D,** Sclerosing adenosis with lobular carcinoma in situ. Note the regularity of the edge and absence of infiltrative features. (Courtesy Dr. Robert E. Fechner, Charlottesville, VA.)

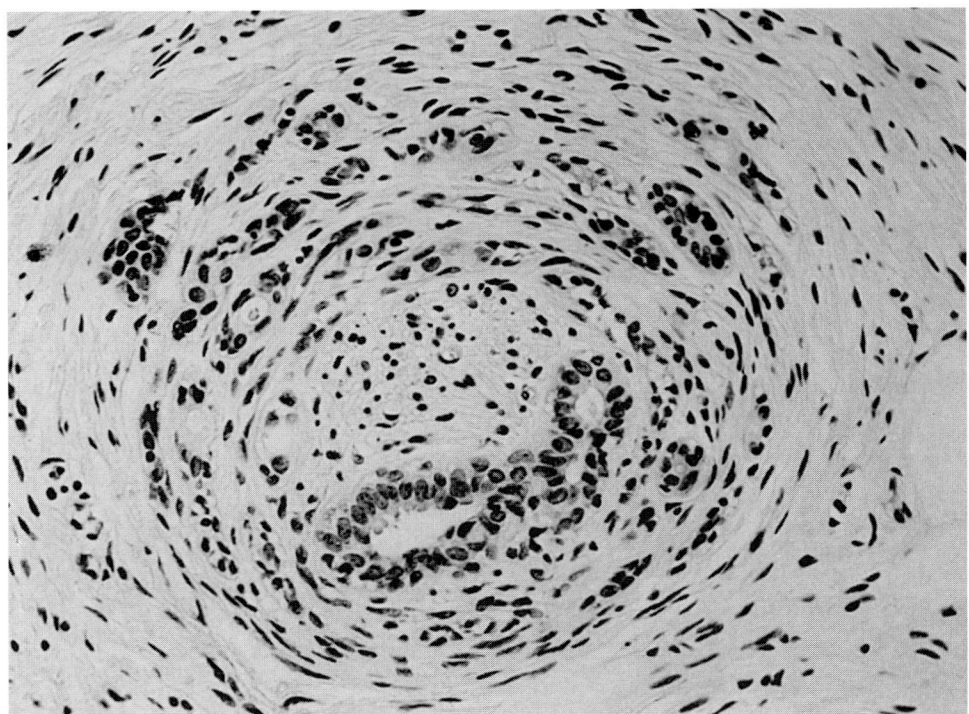

Fig. 20-22 Perineurial involvement in sclerosing adenosis. Nests of well-differentiated glands are present. This finding is not evidence of malignancy.

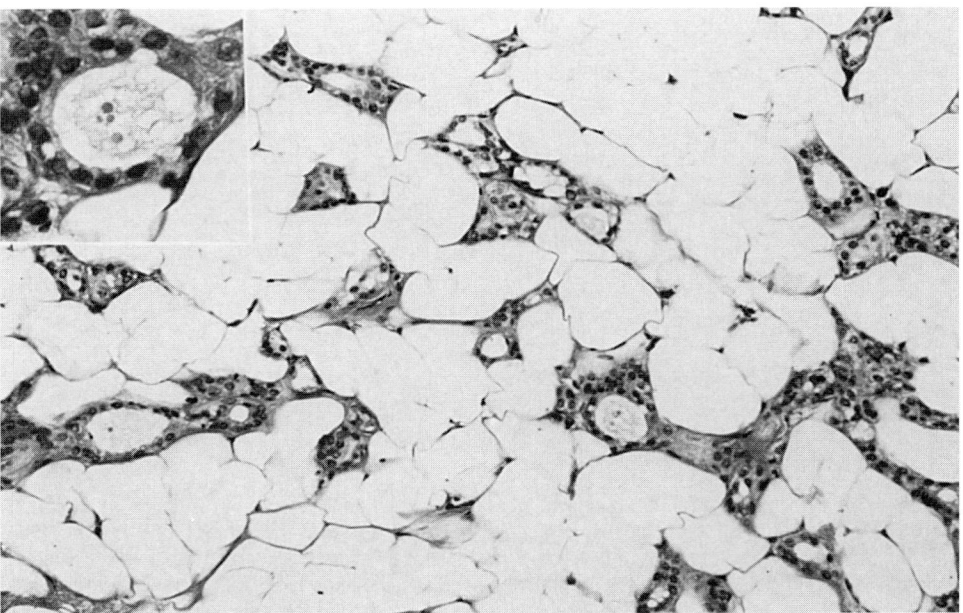

Fig. 20-23 Microglandular adenosis. Small uniform glands are seen distributed in an irregular fashion in adipose tissue. Their lumina are wide open and contain granular eosinophilic secretion, better seen in **inset.**

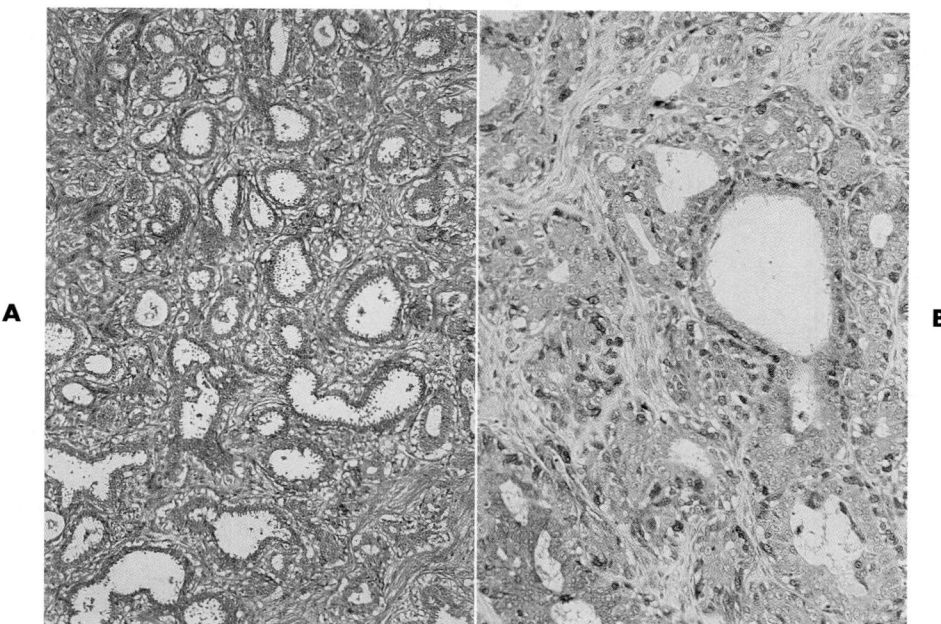

Fig. 20-24 **A** and **B,** Adenomyoepithelial adenosis. The glands are relatively large, with a wide, open lumen and apocrine metaplasia. The cellular component in between is composed of myoepithelial cells. **B,** S-100 Protein stain highlights the prominent myoepithelial component.

noma. Fechner[126] points out that the differential diagnosis should be made at low power; the foci of sclerosing adenosis (with or without carcinoma in situ) have dilated ductules peripherally and narrow ones centrally, whereas invasive lobular carcinoma has no overall organization. Immunohistochemical evaluation can be of assistance in the recognition of this lesion.[125]

Nodular adenosis

Nodular adenosis combines features of blunt duct adenosis and sclerosing adenosis. The proliferating nodules are much more cellular than in blunt duct adenosis but better circumscribed than in sclerosing adenosis and without the fibrosis and distortion of the latter. Some authors regard nodular adenosis as the early nonsclerotic phase of sclerosing adenosis.

Adenosis tumor is simply a form of nodular or sclerosing adenosis of larger dimensions than usual, which therefore becomes palpable and more tumorlike clinically.[130] The term *florid adenosis* has been applied to lesions of nodular or sclerosing adenosis that are unduly cellular and proliferative. Neither of these two forms of adenosis represents a distinct entity.

Microglandular adenosis

Microglandular adenosis, also known as microglandular hyperplasia, is a rare form of adenosis in which small uniform glands with open lumina containing an eosinophilic secretion are distributed in an irregular fashion within fibrous tissue or fat[131,137,140] (Fig. 20-23). There is no trabecular bar formation. The glands are lined by a single layer of small uniform cuboidal or flat cells with vacuolated or gran-

ular cytoplasm, lacking apocrine-type "snouts." In contrast to other forms of adenosis, the myoepithelial layer may be absent.[131,136a] However, there is a thick basement membrane that can be well appreciated ultrastructurally.[140] The stroma may be hyalinized but is not cellular or elastotic. The main differential diagnosis of this lesion is with tubular carcinoma.[131] Microglandular hyperplasia is a benign condition and should be treated conservatively; however, enough cases have been reported in continuity with carcinoma to suggest that it may evolve into malignancy with a frequency greater than the other forms of adenosis described in this section.[134,138]

Adenomyoepithelial (apocrine) adenosis is a form of adenosis closely related to microglandular adenosis and perhaps representing a variant of it, in which the glands are larger, the lining epithelium is taller and has apocrine metaplasia, and the myoepithelial cells are present and even prominent[132,133,135,139] (Fig. 20-24). The most interesting aspect of this lesion is that it can give rise to a biphasic breast tumor that has been designated as adenomyoepithelioma[132,141] (see p. 1628).

Tubular adenosis is also related to microglandular adenosis, from which it differs by the tubular configuration and the presence of a myoepithelial component. Like microglandular adenosis, it may be accompanied by carcinoma.[136]

FIBROCYSTIC DISEASE

Fibrocystic disease of the breast is an extremely important lesion because of its high frequency; the ability of some of its subtypes to simulate the clinical, radiographic, gross, and microscopic appearance of carcinoma; and the possible relationship of some of its forms to carcinoma.[147] Many other names have been proposed over the years for this disorder;

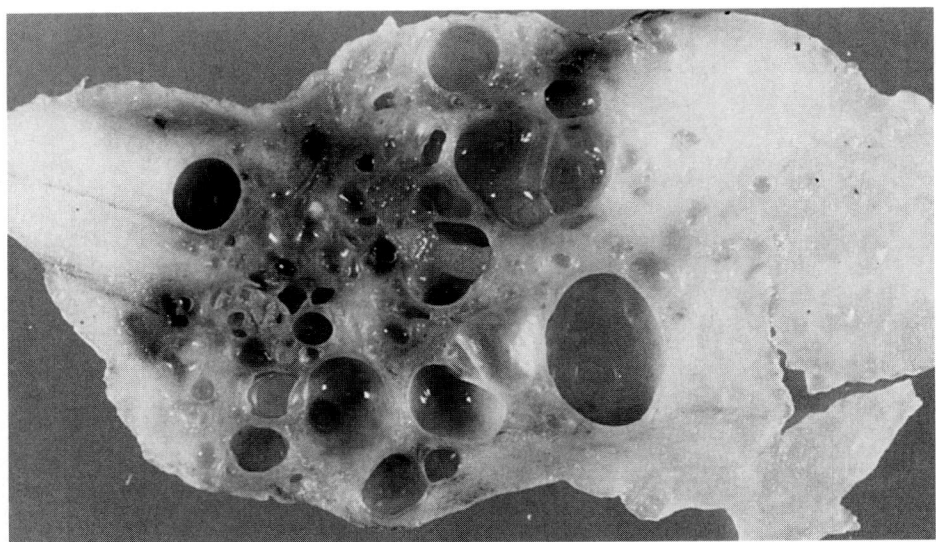

Fig. 20-25 Fibrocystic disease showing variously sized, smooth-walled cysts with tendency for clustering. (Courtesy Dr. J. Costa, Lausanne, Switzerland.)

none of them is entirely satisfactory, and some are highly objectionable: cystic disease, cystic mastopathy, cystic hyperplasia, mammary dysplasia, Reclus' disease, Schimmelbusch's disease, mazoplasia, chronic cystic mastitis, benign breast disease, and others. Fibrocystic disease is the name most commonly used in the United States and is likely to remain in use even though it has at least two drawbacks: (1) It overemphasizes the fibrous component of the disorder, and (2) it is linked in the mind of many physicians, patients, and life insurance agents with a precancerous condition, which in most instances it is not. To avoid the potentially serious problems related to the latter situation, a group convened by the College of American Pathologists recommended the use of alternative terms such as fibrocystic changes or fibrocystic condition, followed by specification of the component lesions either in the body of the pathology report or in the diagnosis.[148]

Fibrocystic disease is most frequently seen, at least at the clinical level, between the ages of 25 and 45. The most proliferative forms of the disease are more common in Anglo-Saxon than in Latin-American, American Indian, or Japanese women.[145,161] The real incidence of this disease is difficult to estimate because the diagnosis depends a great deal on the liberality of the individual clinician or pathologist.[150,154,160] Hormones obviously play a role in its development, but the exact pathogenesis remains obscure.[143,151,165] There is no evidence that administration of oral contraceptives increases the degree of epithelial proliferation[149,152]; on the contrary, there are statistical data indicating a lower frequency of fibrocystic disease (at least of those forms without epithelial atypia[153]) among long-term users of contraceptives.[159] Epidemiologic evidence has been presented suggesting a relationship between coffee consumption and the development of fibrocystic disease, but this has not been confirmed in other studies.[142,155]

The process is most often bilateral, but one breast may be much more diseased than the other and appear clinically to be the only one involved.

It is important to realize that fibrocystic disease primarily affects the TDLU, although the epithelial hyperplasia can also extend to larger ducts. There is a great degree of variability in the gross and microscopic appearance depending on which manifestation of the disease predominates. The basic morphologic changes are as follows:

1 *Formation of cysts.* These can be microscopic or grossly visible, and sometimes reach large proportions (Fig. 20-25). They usually contain a cloudy yellow or clear fluid. Some of these cysts have a bluish cast when seen from the outside ("blue dome cysts" of Bloodgood). Often, numerous small thin-walled cysts are seen in the breast parenchyma surrounding a large cyst. Microscopically, the epithelial lining of most cysts, especially the larger ones, is flattened or altogether absent, the cyst having only a thick fibrous wall. Frequently these cysts rupture and elicit an inflammatory response in the stroma, with abundant foamy macrophages and cholesterol clefts (see discussion following). Azzopardi[144] has remarked that these cysts—no matter how large—arise from the TDLU rather than from ducts.

2 *Apocrine metaplasia.* This is a very common change. It is most often seen in dilated and cystic structures, but it may appear in normal-sized tubules as well. Cysts lined by apocrine-type epithelium containing fluid under pressure are known as *tension cysts.* The appearance of the lining is indistinguishable from the lining of apocrine sweat glands. The individual cells have an abundant granular acidophilic cytoplasm, often containing supranuclear vacuoles and yellow-brown pigment, some of which contains iron. The apical portion

of the cytoplasm shows the typical "apocrine snout." The nucleus is medium sized, and the nucleolus can be very prominent. PAS stain shows a crescent of coarse glycolipid granules on the luminal side, and immuno-histochemical stain for GCDFP-15 shows strong cyto-plasmic reactivity.[156] Transitional or poorly developed phases of this process exist; these have been termed *partial* or *incomplete* apocrine metaplasia. In some of these cases, the apocrine metaplasia has atypical cyto-logic features and is accompanied by sclerosis. There is no evidence that patients with *atypical apocrine meta-plasia* as thus defined are at an increased risk for the development of carcinoma.[146]

3 *Fibrosis of the stroma.* This change is often present, but its degree varies markedly. It is probably a sec-ondary event to the rupture of the cysts and it may pro-ceed to hyalinization. The terms *fibrous disease* of the breast and *fibrous mastopathy* have been used by some authors to designate a breast condition in which the main change seems to be a more or less localized stro-mal fibrosis[158] (Fig. 20-26); it is not clear whether this is related to fibrocystic disease or even whether it rep-resents a distinct clinicopathologic entity, although the latter seems more likely.

4 *Calcification.* This is less common than in duct ectasia or carcinoma; it tends to have a coarse, highly irregular pattern. Chemically, it may be composed of calcium phosphate or calcium oxalate. On mammography, the latter is of an amorphous, low to medium density (in contrast to the medium to high density of calcium phosphate) and is nearly always associated with benign disease.[166] Calcium phosphate deposition is usually easily detectable on H&E sections and is highlighted by the von Kossa stain, which may be necessary to identify minute foci.[162] Instead, calcium oxalate crys-tals can be easily missed with these techniques; they are better seen with polarized lenses (because of their birefringent quality) or after silver nitrate–rubeanic acid with 5% acetic acid pretreatment.[164]

5 *Chronic inflammation.* This is another common but secondary feature of fibrocystic disease. It is related not to infection but rather to the rupture of cysts with release of secretion in the stroma. Lymphocytes, plasma cells, and foamy histiocytes are the predominant ele-ments. Fibrocystic disease with intense chronic inflam-mation should not be confused with duct ectasia (see p. 1568).

6 *Epithelial hyperplasia.* This is the most important and troublesome component of fibrocystic disease. It is also the most significant because of its possible relationship to carcinoma and the fact that it is responsible for most difficulties in the differential diagnosis between fibro-cystic disease and carcinoma. In most cases it is only of minimal degree, as confirmed by the fact that the degree of cell proliferation as measured by thymidine labeling is generally not significantly higher in fibrocystic disease than in the normal breast.[157] Epithelial hyper-plasia is discussed in detail in the next section.

7 *Fibroadenomatoid change.* This is the least common abnormality seen as a component of fibrocystic dis-

ease. The stromal proliferation and slit-like epithelial formations result in a picture reminiscent of fibroade-noma but lacking the sharp circumscription of the lat-ter (see p. 1571).

8 *Intranuclear helioid inclusions.* These rare structures appear as round, intranuclear eosinophilic bodies that—when large—may simulate viral inclusions. Ultrastruc-turally, they are single membrane–bound structures con-taining a laminated or homogeneously electron-dense core with a corona of radiating filaments.[163]

Ductal and lobular hyperplasia

Epithelial hyperplasia of **ductal** type, when florid, has been traditionally designated as papillomatosis, particularly in the United States. Azzopardi[167] has rightly objected to the term on grounds that in most instances the lesion does not form true papillae. He prefers the term epitheliosis, but this has not been widely accepted. Perhaps the more general term epithelial hyperplasia is the best compromise, followed by an indication of its degree: *mild* (when made up of three or four epithelial cells in thickness), *moderate to florid* (when more pronounced), and *atypical* (see following dis-cussion). In the most proliferative cases, the entire lumen can be filled by the proliferation. Some forms of hyperpla-sia have true papillary qualities (Fig. 20-27). The features that we have found most helpful in the identification of the benign nature of the proliferation are the following:

1 Nuclei that are oval (rather than round, except when cut transversely), normochromatic (rather than hyperchromatic), and with slight overlap; small, single, indistinct nucleoli; scanty or no mitotic activity (Figs. 20-28 and 20-29).

2 Cytoplasm that is acidophilic and finely granular rather than pale and homogeneous.

3 Indistinct cytoplasmic borders, so that the nuclei seem to lie in a syncytial mass rather than within sharply outlined cell membranes.

4 Streaming effect, induced by the oval cells being vaguely arranged in parallel bundles (see Fig. 20-29).

5 "Tufts" and "mounds" projecting into the lumen.

6 Presence of peripheral elongated clefts, bound on one side by a single layer of basally located cells and on the other by a solid intraluminal formation; some-times this cleft spans almost the entirety of the cir-cumference, with the retracted solid ball of epithelial cells hanging from the wall like the vascular tuft of a renal glomerulus (see Fig. 20-28). The intratubular lumina of ductal hyperplasia tend to be irregular in size, shape (elongated rather than round), and location (predominating at the periphery) as opposed to regu-lar in all three parameters as seen in the cribriform pattern of intraductal carcinoma.

7 Presence of irregularly shaped bridges connecting opposite portions of the wall. The cells in these bridges have oval nuclei arranged parallel to the long axis of the bridge (Fig. 20-30). Their appearance is very different from that seen in the rigid trabecular bars and Roman bridges of intraductal carcinoma.

8 Complete or incomplete apocrine metaplasia; cyto-plasmic blebbing.

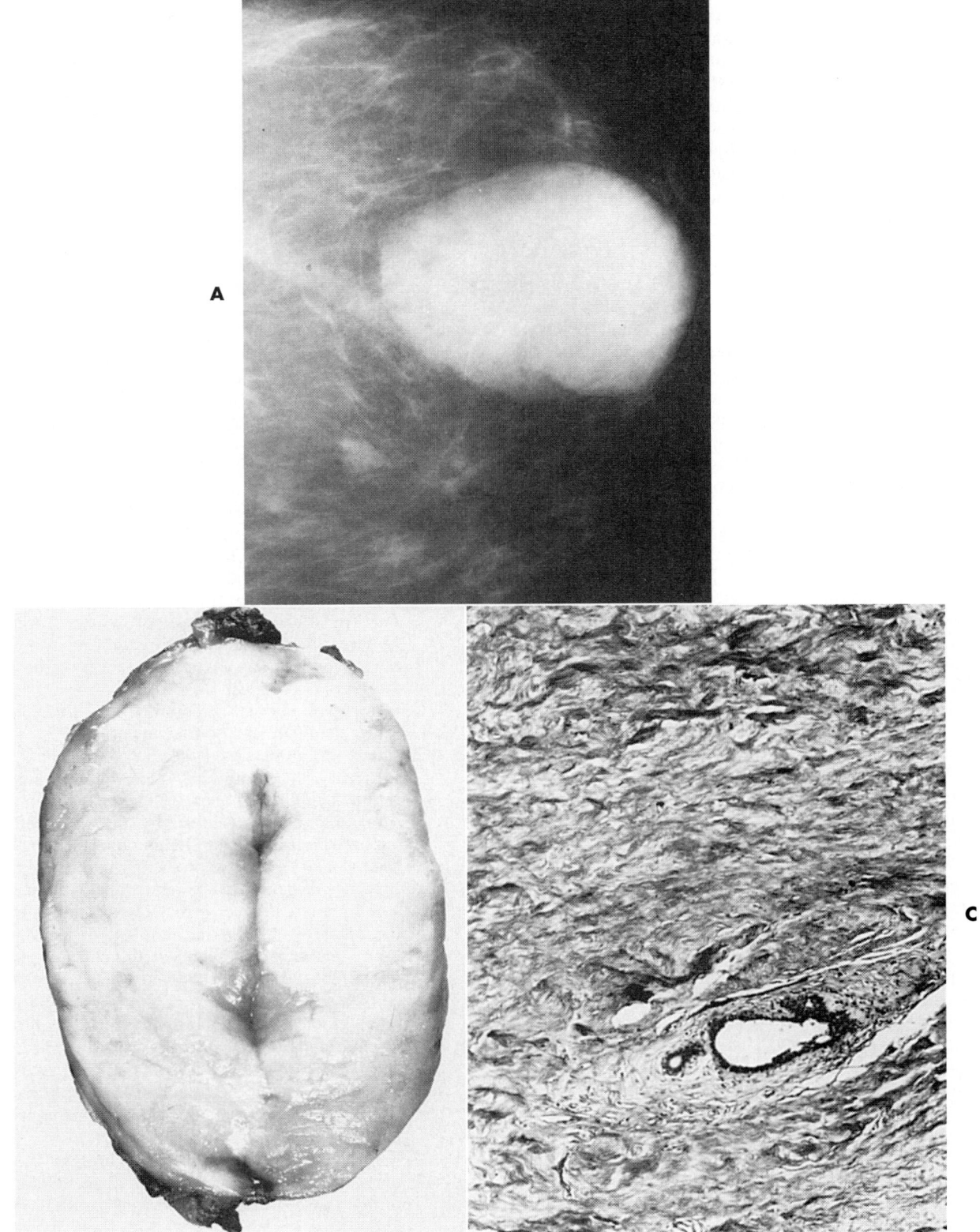

Fig. 20-26 Fibrous disease of breast. **A,** Mammographic appearance. **B,** Well-circumscribed gross appearance. **C,** Microscopic appearance. Some entrapped epithelial tissue is seen at edge of lesion, which is largely composed of dense fibrous tissue. (Mammograms courtesy Dr. P. Kornguth, New Haven, CT.)

9 Presence of myoepithelial cells, whether scattered or as a continuous row, and clear, acidophilic, or elongated and smooth muscle–like ("myoid").

10 Presence of foamy macrophages, both in the lumen and intimately admixed with the proliferating epithelial cells.

11 Frequent intraluminal or stromal calcification but absence of calcific spherules or psammoma bodies between epithelium and stroma.

12 Absence of necrosis.

•   •   •

As important as these features are, none of them is diagnostic by itself. They need to be weighed against each other, sometimes modified depending on the nature of the case, and occasionally ignored altogether. For instance, very prominent nucleoli and structures reminiscent of Roman bridges are strongly suggestive of intraductal carcinoma under ordinary circumstances but lose much of their significance when occurring in apocrine epithelium. The myoepithelial cell layer may be preserved in intraductal carcinoma. Focal necrosis may be found in benign disease, particularly in nipple adenoma. Furthermore, proliferative benign breast disease and carcinoma can and often do coexist, which means that an area may be diagnostic of intraductal carcinoma even if the immediately surrounding glands show features indicative of benign disease.

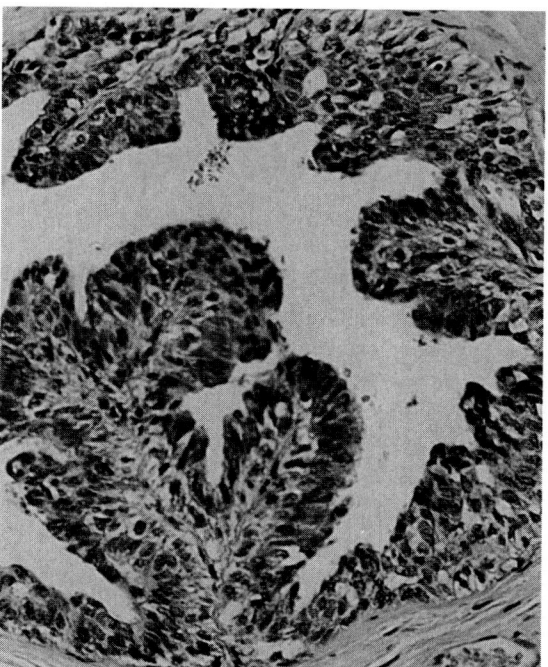

Fig. 20-27 Intraductal epithelial hyperplasia with true papillary pattern.

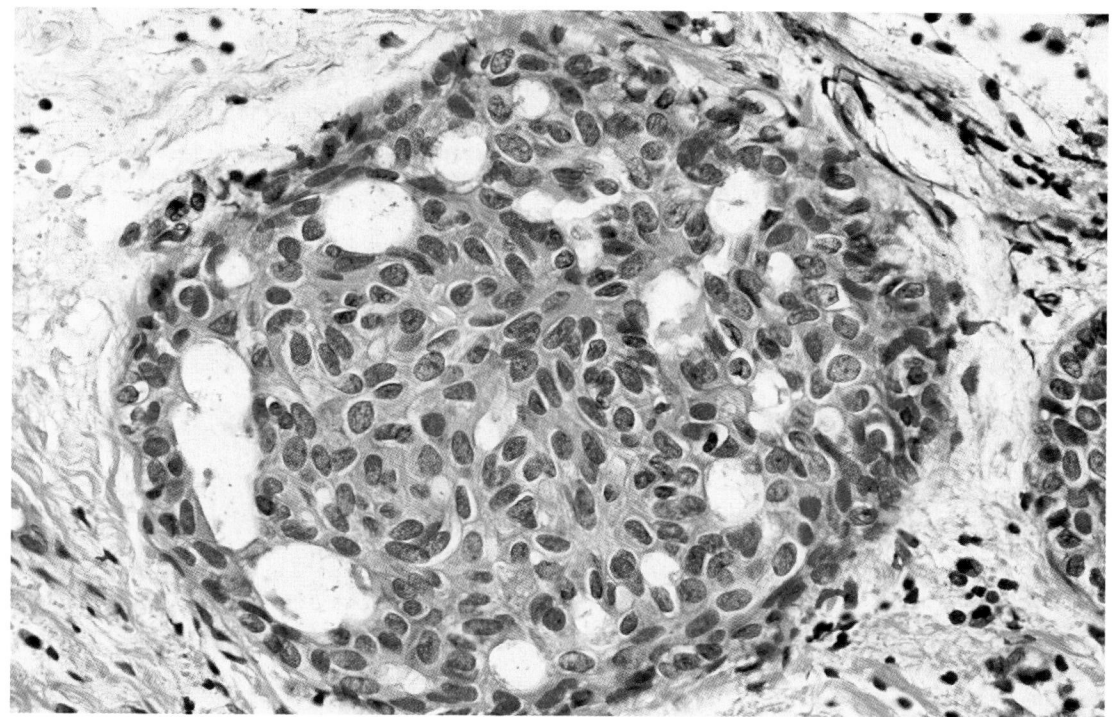

Fig. 20-28 Photomicrograph demonstrating florid epithelial hyperplasia within dilated duct. There is no evidence of necrosis, and individual cells are well supported by their stroma. Prominent cleft has formed between solid intraluminal proliferation and outer epithelial row. In our experience, this feature is usually indicative of a benign condition.

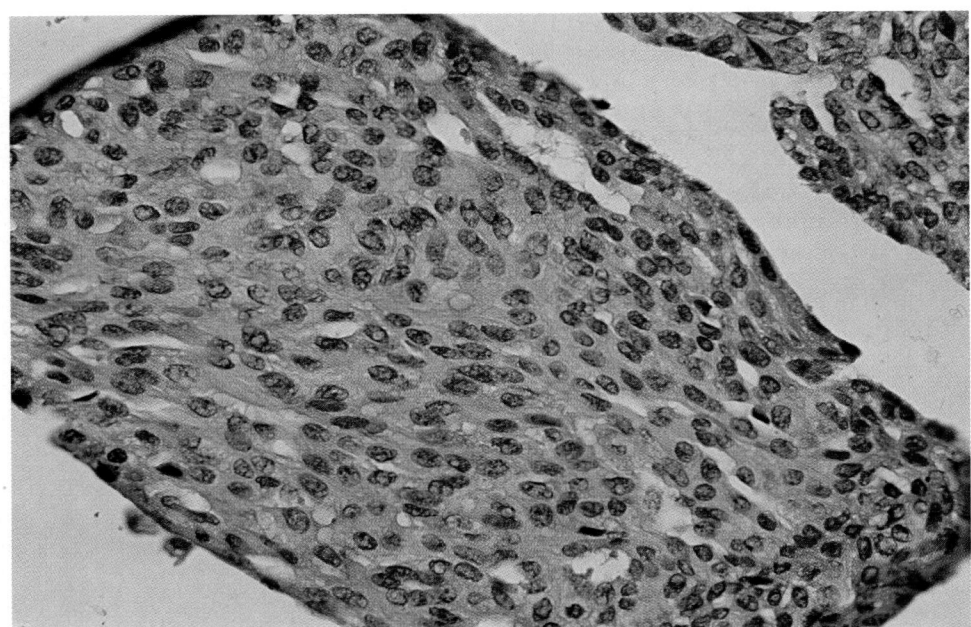

Fig. 20-29 Florid ductal hyperplasia. Note the oval shape of the nuclei and the parallel arrangement, resulting in "streaming" effect.

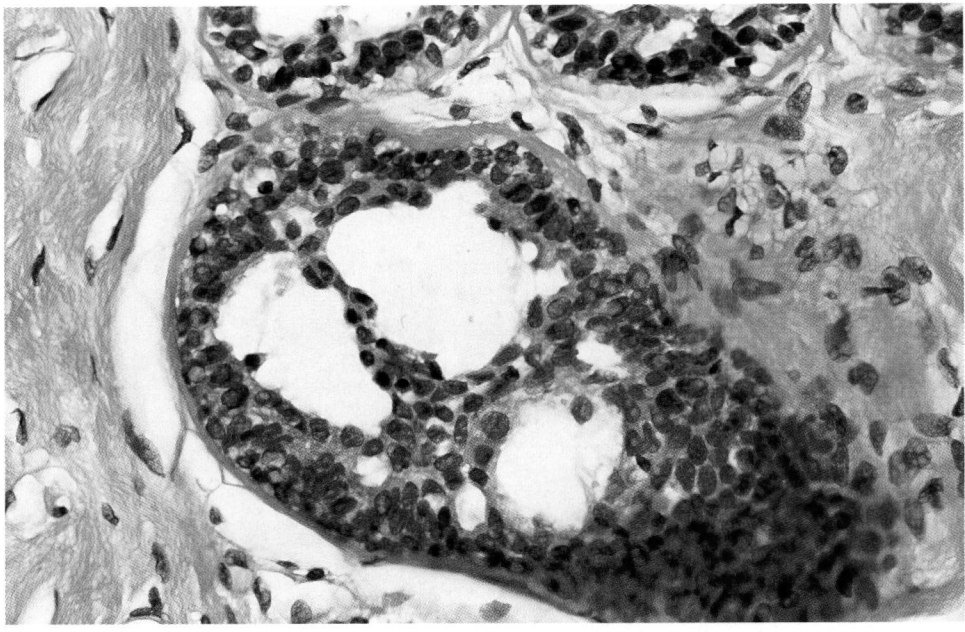

Fig. 20-30 Ductal hyperplasia showing irregularly shaped ridges connecting opposite portions of the wall. Note the fact that the oval nuclei are arranged parallel to the long axis of the ridge.

Immunohistochemically, ductal hyperplasia is characterized by strong immunoreactivity for high-molecular-weight keratin associated with weak S-100 protein expression.[172]

Rare morphologic variants of ductal hyperplasia have been described. One, which can also be seen in association with intraductal papilloma and sclerosing adenosis, has been designated as *collagenous spherulosis*.[168] It is characterized by the presence of intraluminal clusters of eosinophilic, collagen-rich spherules that seem to arise within the spaces between epithelial and myoepithelial cells[169] (Plate XV-C). This curious lesion, which may also be seen in salivary gland tumors,[171] should not be confused with adenoid cystic carcinoma or with signet ring carcinoma.

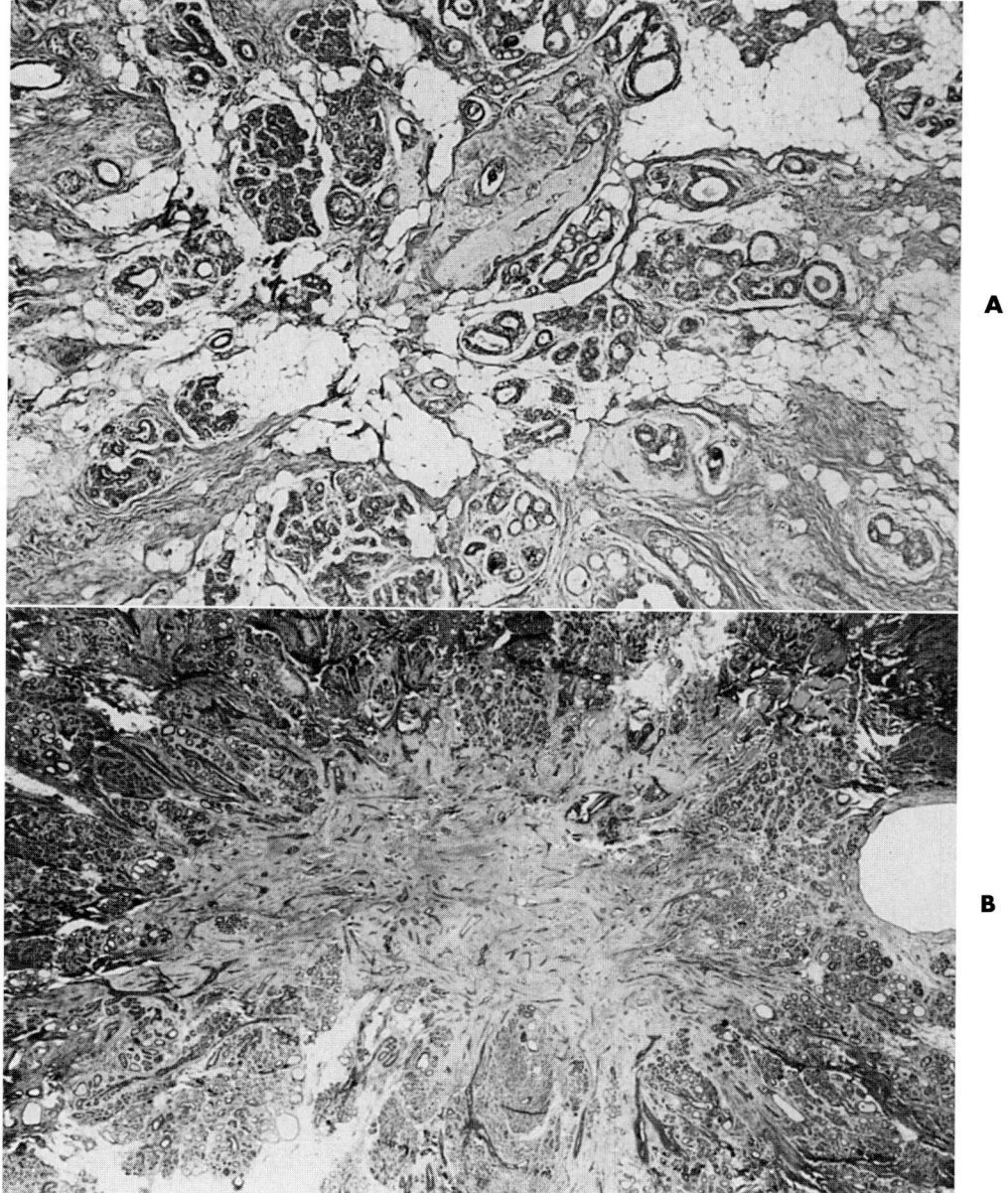

Fig. 20-31 Sclerosing ductal lesion. Process in **A** is a radial scar with focally prominent elastosis associated with only minimal degree of epithelial proliferation. Lesion shown in **B** has intense epithelial proliferation around central scar.

Another variant is represented by *cystic hypersecretory hyperplasia,* in which cystically dilated ducts form containing a colloid-like material; this lesion should be distinguished from cystic hypersecretory carcinoma (see p. 1601).[170]

Yet another variant, which may be accompanied by atypical features, has a *gynecomastia-like* appearance.[173]

• • •

As far as **lobular hyperplasia** is concerned, the term could be used whenever—in the absence of pregnancy, puerperium, or exogenous hormone stimulation—the lobules appear larger and more cellular than usual but do not fulfill the criteria for lobular carcinoma in situ or even for atypical lobular hyperplasia. Since the definition of the latter is rather vague itself, it follows that the diagnosis of lobular hyperplasia is of dubious reproducibility and significance.

The special variant of ductal hyperplasia known as juvenile papillomatosis or Swiss cheese disease is discussed on p. 1636.

Sclerosing ductal lesions

This is a group of breast lesions characterized by a generally small size, stellate shape, central fibrous and often elastotic core, and variable degree of epithelial distortion and proliferation[174,184,188] (Fig. 20-31, *A* and *B*). They are usually

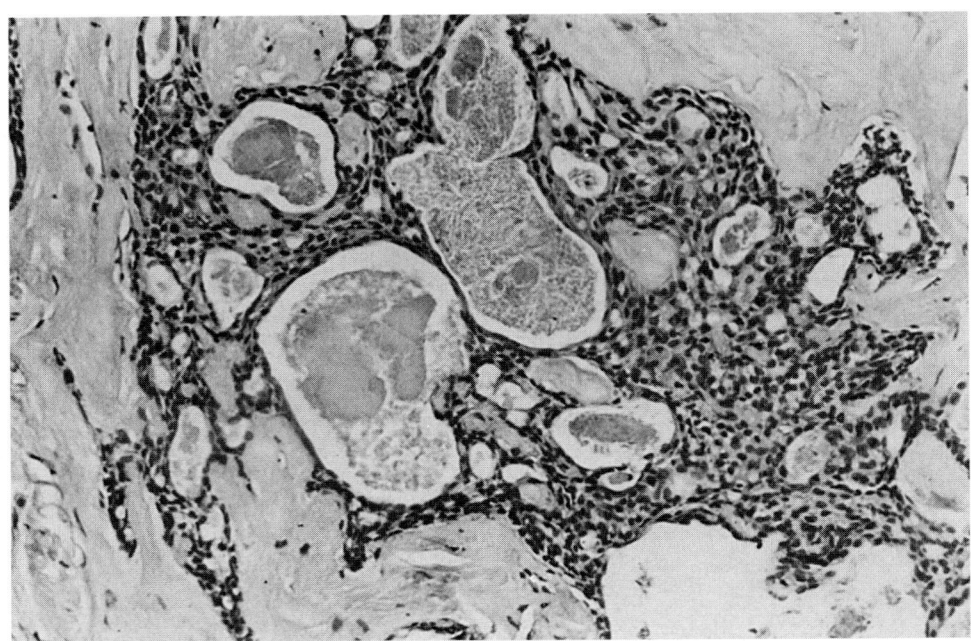

Fig. 20-32 Complicated pattern resulting from epithelial proliferation and stromal fibrosis. Lesion belongs to general group of sclerosing ductal lesions, and its appearance can simulate that of invasive carcinoma.

seen within the context of fibrocystic disease and have been variously designated as radial scar, nonencapsulated sclerosing lesion, indurative mastopathy, infiltrating epitheliosis, benign sclerosing ductal proliferation, sclerosing papillary proliferation, scleroelastotic lesion, and sclerosing adenosis with pseudoinfiltration.[178,179,185,187] Some are thought to represent primary proliferative diseases (ductal hyperplasias or even intraductal papillomas) in which the stromal change and epithelial distortion occur as a secondary and often focal event (Fig. 20-32); others are viewed as a primary obliterative disease of the terminal duct (perhaps induced by inflammation) with secondary epithelial proliferation of their branches. Cases exist in which a strong point can be made in favor of one or the other of these postulated mechanisms, such as the otherwise typical ductal hyperplasia (epitheliosis) with a small focus of fibroelastosis or—at the other extreme—the fibroelastotic lesion with almost no epithelial proliferation.[177,187] In many lesions, however, it is difficult or impossible to establish with certainty whether the fibrosis or the epithelial proliferation was the primary event. They are therefore described here as a group. On mammography and gross examination, their irregularly stellate shape results in a great resemblance to invasive ductal carcinoma of either conventional or tubular type.[181] Microscopically, the connective tissue center is densely fibrotic, only occasionally cellular. Clumps of basophilic material, strongly reactive for elastic tissue stain, are seen in the walls of oblit-erated ducts and elsewhere, sometimes in abundance. Embedded within this stroma are small ductular for-mations that are disorganized but still composed of two cell types; at the periphery of the spokes are larger duct-like structures that may be dilated and/or may exhibit epithelial hyperplastic changes having the features described on p. 1583.

The most important aspects of the sclerosing ductal lesion are the differential diagnosis and possible relationship with ductal carcinoma. As far as the former problem is concerned, suffice it to say that the diagnostic criteria for the identification of carcinoma should be the same whether a central scar is present or not. They include the usual cytoarchitectural criteria as seen in H&E-stained section, as well as the evaluation of myoepithelial cell participation in immunocytochemical preparations.[180]

As for the latter problem, the issue is not settled; some authors believe that most tubular carcinomas arise from radial scars; most others do not.[174,182] We have seen enough cases showing continuity between the central elastotic area, the surrounding benign ductal hyperplasia, and foci of tubular carcinoma to favor the interpretation that at least some cases of this type of carcinoma originate on the basis of this sequence. However, if the sclerosing ductal lesion does not show recognizable features of carcinoma, it should not be regarded as indicating a propensity for the subsequent development of invasive carcinoma unless the proliferating epithelial component has the features of atypical hyperplasia[176,183,186] (see next section). Accordingly, the treatment should be local excision, and follow-up should be instituted.[175]

Atypical ductal and lobular hyperplasia

As already mentioned, there is a wide range in the degree of epithelial proliferation in fibrocystic disease. It has been postulated that there is a correlation between the degree of this proliferation and the likelihood of subsequent development of invasive carcinoma, and various attempts have been made to quantify both the degree of the change and the magnitude of the risk.[189,194,203] The most ambitious and success-

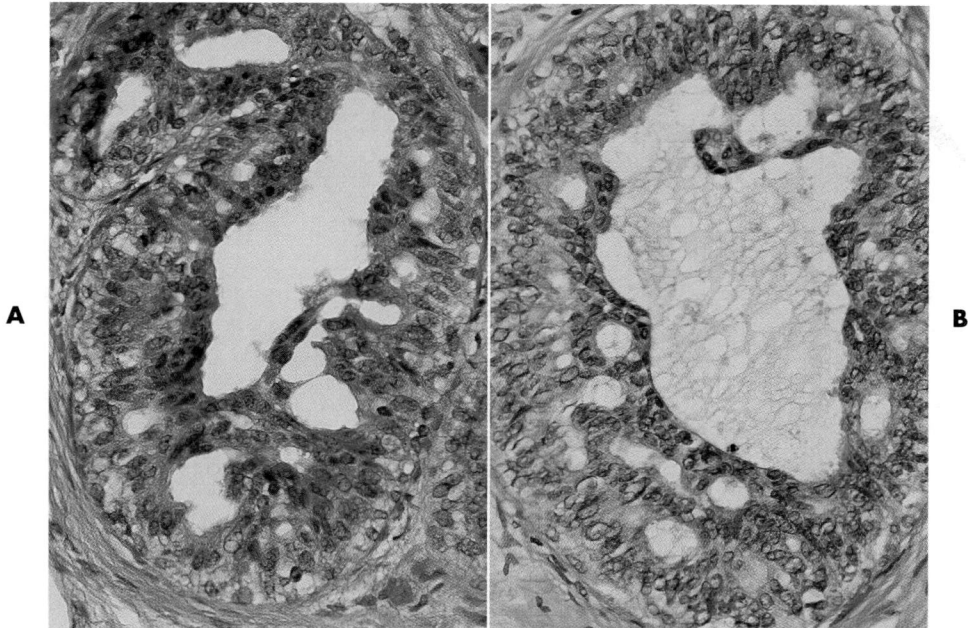

Fig. 20-33 A and **B,** Two different breast lesions diagnosed as atypical ductal hyperplasia by two fore-most experts in breast pathology. There is marked epithelial proliferation in structures of ductal type associated with atypia, but they were felt not to fulfill all criteria for carcinoma in situ.

ful attempts are those of Dupont et al.[193] and Page et al.,[198,199] who have proposed the terms atypical ductal hyperplasia (ADH) and atypical lobular hyperplasia (ALH) for prolifer-ative lesions in which some but not all of the features of intraductal carcinoma or lobular carcinoma in situ, respec-tively, are present (Figs. 20-33 and 20-34). Using these cri-teria in a retrospective study, they diagnosed ADH and/or ALH in 3.6% of the cases and concluded that these patients had a risk of invasive breast carcinoma that was four to five times that of the general population (i.e., about half of that of ductal or lobular carcinoma in situ). Largely on the basis of this study, a group convened by the College of American Pathologists[191a] recommended grouping patients with "fibrocystic disease" in the following three categories:

  I No or mild hyperplasia: no increased risk for subsequent invasive
     carcinoma.
  II Moderate or florid hyperplasia: 1.5 to 2 times the risk.
  III Atypical ductal or lobular hyperplasia: 5 times the risk.

For completeness and comparison purposes, Page[197] added to this list the following category:

  III H IV Ductal or lobular carcinoma in situ: 8 to 10 times the risk.

The Dupont-Page studies represent an extremely impor-tant contribution to the study of fibrocystic disease vis-à-vis breast carcinoma and have had a great impact on clinicians and pathologists. However, additional work needs to be done before this concept is fully accepted and widely applied. The definitions of ADH and ALH need to be defined in a more precise way (not just on negative terms), tests of inter- and intra-observer reproducibility need to be carried out, and the results obtained need to be confirmed in other populations. Several studies have shown an unacceptably high level of observer variability in estimating the type and degree of epithelial hyperplasia,[190,191,201] although there is some evi-

dence that strict adherence to a standardized set of criteria might lead to more consistent results.[202] Proposals to include cytologic parameters[200] and the size of the lesion (as mea-sured on the slide)[204] as criteria for the differential diagnosis between atypical hyperplasia and carcinoma in situ have been made. We find the former more appealing than the lat-ter. Special techniques such as morphometry, DNA ploidy studies, and immunohistochemical stains for various anti-gens have so far failed to establish a consistent separation among the various groups.[192,195,196]

Since an element of subjectivity in the microscopic inter-pretation persists and is unlikely to be completely elimi-nated and in view of the fact that the current terminology suggests a sharper separation than what the evidence seems to indicate, we believe that consideration should be given to adopting a terminology such as mammary intraepithelial neoplasia (MIN) of either ductal or lobular type, followed by a grading system.[201]

Relationship with carcinoma and treatment

A possible relationship between fibrocystic disease and breast carcinoma has been suggested over the years on the basis of the following evidence:

  1 The observation that breasts excised for carcinoma usu-ally also exhibit changes of fibrocystic disease[213] and that this fibrocystic disease seems to have a greater degree of epithelial proliferation than the one found in a population without carcinoma.[211]
  2 The fact that retrospectively studied breast biopsies in patients who subsequently developed invasive carci-noma often show very florid and even atypical prolifer-ative changes rather than the usual pattern of prolifera-tive disease.[212,219]

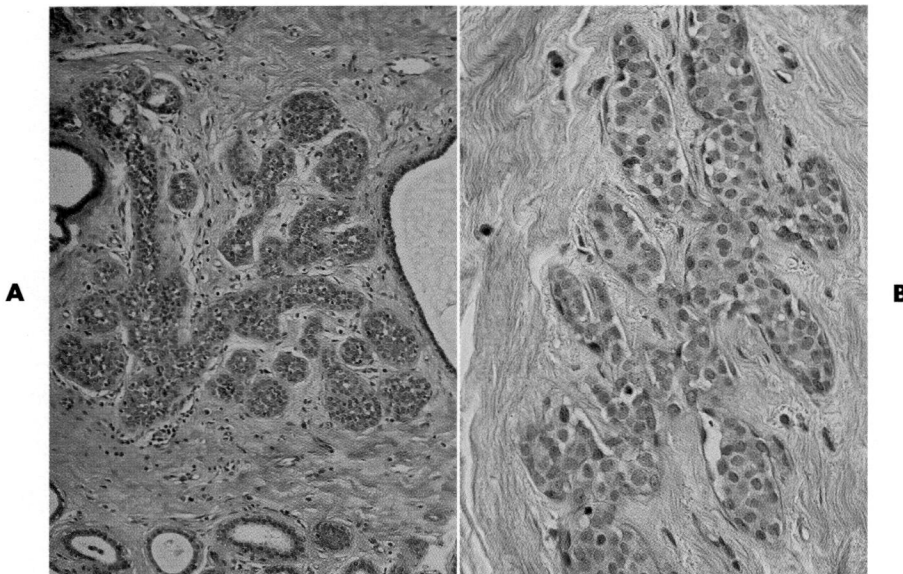

Fig. 20-34 A and **B,** Two different breast lesions diagnosed as atypical lobular hyperplasia by four experts in breast pathology. There is lobular enlargement and proliferation, but some lumina are preserved, and there is only minimal distention of individual units.

3 The parallelism in the incidence of breast carcinoma and benign proliferative breast lesions in the various populations,[217] including the fact that kindreds susceptible to breast carcinoma also inherit a predisposition to proliferative breast disease.[218]

4 The presence of karyotypic and molecular alterations in benign proliferative breast lesions that parallel those of breast carcinoma.[213a,213b,220a]

5 The claim that patients with fibrocystic disease treated conservatively and subjected to long-term follow-up are found to develop invasive carcinoma at a rate that is two to four times higher than the control population.

A quantitative leap has been made by the realization that it is not the fibrocystic disease per se but rather the presence and type of proliferative epithelial disease that determine the risk for subsequent carcinoma and that this risk seems to range from one to five times that of the control population, as indicated in the section on atypical and ductal hyperplasia.[210,214] This fact, which has been confirmed in independent studies,[205,206,220] indicates that evaluation of epithelial hyperplasia is an important gauge in deciding on the best approach to these patients.[215] Naturally, several other factors need to be taken into consideration, including the length of time since the diagnosis of atypical hyperplasia was made.[207-209] In general, a conservative approach to fibrocystic disease (i.e., local excision and follow-up) is amply justified.[216] However, extensive and/or recurrent disease, atypical hyperplasia, a strong family history of breast carcinoma, or cancerophobia may well justify the performance of a simple mastectomy in the individual case, particularly if two or more of these factors are present together.

Carcinoma
GENERAL FEATURES
Incidence

Breast carcinoma is the most common malignant tumor and the leading cause of carcinoma death in women. In the United States, each year about 100,000 new cases are diagnosed and about 30,000 patients die from the disease. The incidence is high in North America and northern Europe, intermediate in southern European and Latin American countries, and low in most Asian and African countries. In the United States, there has been a sharp increase in the detection of breast carcinoma, largely due to the widespread use of mammography.[246] Most of these cases have been localized, measuring less than 2 cm in diameter and/or in situ.[230] However, no significant decrease in the mortality from breast cancer has yet been noted; actually this has changed very little since the 1930s.[230]

Risk factors

Several risk factors for the development of breast carcinoma have been established, whereas many others remain questionable.[234,240] It has been proposed that the common denominator for most of these factors is strong and/or prolonged estrogen stimulation, operating on a genetically susceptible background.[237]

1 Country of birth. This has already been mentioned in the paragraph on incidence.

2 Family history. Women who have a first-degree relative with breast carcinoma have a risk two or three times that of the general population, a risk further increased if the relative was affected at an early age and/or had bilateral disease.[245] The long-sought gene responsible for the hereditary form of breast carcinoma has been identified on chromosome 17q and named BRCA1.[229a,236] A second gene that predisposes to breast carcinoma has been localized to chromosome 13q12-13 and named BRCA2.[250a] These two genes together probably account for about two thirds of familial breast carcinoma, or roughly 5% of all cases.[240a] BRCA1 also predisposes to ovarian carcinoma. Interestingly, it has been recently reported that in many cases of sporadic breast carcinoma (unassociated with mutations of BRCA 1 gene), an apparently normal BRCA 1 protein is found *in the cytoplasm* of the tumor cells, in addition to (or instead of) its normal nuclear site (i.e., the place where it exerts its regulatory function). [235]

3 Menstrual and reproductive history. Breast carcinoma is rare in women who have been castrated; oophorectomy before 35 years of age reduces the risk to one third. Women who have their first child before the age of 18 years have only one third the risk compared with those whose first child is delayed until age 30.[249] A reduction in the risk of breast carcinoma among premenopausal women who have lactated has been documented, but no such effect was detected among postmenopausal women.[238]

4 Fibrocystic disease and epithelial hyperplasia. The controversial relationship between these changes and breast carcinoma was discussed in the preceding section.

5 Exogenous estrogens. In some series, there has been an overall risk increase (2½-fold), [234,242] whereas in others an increased risk (2- to 9-fold) was observed only in patients with a previous diagnosis of fibrocystic disease. [232]

6 Contraceptive agents. The various epidemiologic studies that have been done in this regard have shown no increased risk,[224,241] or a possible very low increase among young long-term users.[234,250] The tumors that have developed in this population have not differed qualitatively from those seen in control cases.[227,228]

7 Ionizing radiation. An increased risk of breast carcinoma has also been documented with exposure to ionizing radiation.[231,243,244]

8 Breast augmentation. Breast carcinomas (mainly of in situ types) are sometimes detected in women who have undergone augmentation mammoplasty.[225] However, a re-analysis of a recently published linkage study has shown that the incidence of breast carcinoma in that cohort was neither higher nor lower than that among the general population.[222,223b]

9 Others. A peculiar association between breast carcinoma and meningioma has been repeatedly noted.[223] Even more peculiar is that fact that sometimes the breast carcinoma is found to metastasize within the meningioma.

Patients with ataxia-telangiectasia syndrome have an excess risk of breast cancer.[247]

Location

The location of breast carcinoma is usually indicated in relation to the breast quadrants: About 50% are in the upper outer quadrant, 15% in the upper inner quadrant, 10% in the lower outer quadrant, 5% in the lower inner quadrant, 17% in the central region (within 1 cm of the areola), and 3% are diffuse (massive or multifocal). The marked difference in the carcinoma frequency depending on the quadrant, surprising at first, becomes easily explainable when one realizes that it matches closely the amount of breast parenchyma in each quadrant. Several studies have documented the peculiar fact that unilateral breast carcinoma is slightly more frequent in the left breast than in the right. In one recent series, the excess for the left side was 13%.[248]

Multicentricity

Multicentricity (as defined by presence of carcinoma in a breast quadrant other than the one containing the dominant mass) was detected by Fisher et al.[229] in 121 (13.4%) of 904 cases of invasive carcinomas; one third of the smaller foci were invasive and the rest were in situ. Multicentricity was more common in lobular than in ductal carcinomas. A higher incidence of multicentricity was reported in studies in which whole organ preparations were examined by radiography and light microscopy.[233] Clonal analysis studies suggest that these tumors do not arise independently but rather that a single primary carcinoma spreads throughout the breast.[239]

Bilaterality

The incidence of bilaterality in invasive breast carcinoma is about five times that of the general population and is even higher if there is a family history of breast carcinoma.[221,226] It is particularly high in lobular carcinoma in situ, reaching figures of 25% to 50% in some series. The tumors may be synchronous or metachronous. They may result either from intramammary spread or from independent events; the latter mechanism seems the most frequent.[226,226a] The use of adjuvant chemotherapy significantly decreases the risk of metachronous contralateral breast carcinoma.[223a] It is doubtful whether a biopsy of the opposite breast should be taken routinely in patients with breast carcinoma; it seems more logical to limit this practice only to those patients in whom an abnormality is suspected on clinical or mammographic grounds or to those with types of carcinoma for which the incidence of bilaterality is particularly high.[235]

DIAGNOSIS

Clinical examination

Clinical examination, particularly palpation, is the time-honored method for the detection and evaluation of breast disease. It remains an extremely useful and practical technique, whether carried out by the physician or by the patient herself. However, both its sensitivity and discriminatory power are limited. Only 60% of the tumors detected by mammography are palpable. The clinical impression is incorrect in about 15% of the cases thought to be benign and about 10% of those thought to be malignant. The clinical evaluation of axillary lymph nodes is also fraught with error. In patients with a palpable mass, nodes clinically thought to be negative will be found to be involved microscopically by tumor in over 40% of the cases; nodes clinically thought to be negative will be found to be involved microscopically by tumor in over 40% of the cases; nodes clinically thought to be positive will be found free of metastases microscopically in 15% of the cases. The overall error in axillary palpation is 30%.

Mammography

The widespread use of mammography has radically changed the diagnostic approach to breast cancer.[251,259] Extremely small tumors (1 to 2 mm) can be detected with this technique, which relies primarily on the presence of calcification. The incidence of calcification in breast carcinoma is about 50% to 60%, and the incidence in benign breast disease is 20%.[252,260] There are also important qualitative differences in the appearance of the calcification.

It should be kept in mind that a negative mammogram does not rule out the possibility of the presence of carcinoma, since about 20% of palpable tumors are not detectable with this technique. The incidence of false positivity is in the neighborhood of 1%.

The proper handling of breast lesions detected by mammography requires close cooperation between radiologist, surgeon, and pathologist.[252,254,264,266] Once the radiologist identifies the abnormal area on mammography, he should provide the surgeon with a "map" showing the relative position of the suspicious area within the breast. Once the appropriate area is excised, the cephalad and lateral margins should be marked by sutures, and an x-ray study should be taken of the specimen. If no lesion is seen, the surgeon should obtain additional tissue. If the abnormal area is present in the specimen, this can be accurately located by slicing the specimen, identifying the slices with a lead number, taking another x-ray study, and selecting for frozen sections the slice (and the specific area within the slice) containing the abnormal area. The whole procedure takes no more than 15 minutes and is well worth the small delay. Otherwise, small carcinomas can be entirely missed.[257,263] The highest yield is obtained from histologic examination of the areas of radiographic calcification and fibrous parenchymas.[261]

X-ray studies can even be taken of the paraffin blocks to document the fact that the area seen in the mammogram has been embedded (Fig. 20-35). An important source of discrepancy between mammographic and microscopic findings is represented by calcium oxalate crystals, which are easily identified radiographically but easily missed on histologic examination.[256]

It should be obvious from the preceding comments that every attempt should be made to identify in the microscopic slide the area regarded by the radiologist as "suspicious" of carcinoma. However, if this is satisfactorily accomplished and the pathologist still fails to find carcinoma, neither he nor the radiologist should be overly surprised. Only 20% of the lesions labeled "suspicious" mammographically are malignant, and the large majority of these are carcinomas in situ. McDivitt[258] estimated that the chances for the pathologist of finding an invasive carcinoma in a biopsy from a nonpalpable lesion that was interpreted "suspicious" by mammography is less than 2%. On the other hand, "nonpalpable" should not be viewed as synonymous for inconsequential. In a series of 558 patients with nonpalpable invasive carcino-

mas detected by mammography and subjected to axillary dissection, 27% had at least one positive node.[265]

Wolfe[267] has divided breasts into four groups on the basis of the mammographic appearance, which he believes correlates with the risk for development of carcinoma. This correlation might well exist, but it is perplexing that, if this is the case, no correlation seems to exist between these four patterns and the types of histologic alterations.[253]

The available information suggests that the newer radiographic technique of nuclear magnetic resonance is not likely to replace mammography as the imaging modality of choice, largely because of its inability to detect microcalcifications.[262] Instead, breast ultrasonography has emerged as a valuable examination, particularly for determining whether a mass lesion is cystic or solid.[255]

Cytology

The two methods that have been used to obtain cytologic material from breast lesions are aspiration of nipple secretion and aspiration of the lesion with a fine needle.

Nipple secretion aspiration cytology is, in our opinion, of very little value, whether for the diagnosis of a clinically or mammographically detectable breast lesion or for screening purposes. Some carcinomas will undoubtedly be found, but the number of false-positive results is so high as to render this technique of only marginal value. As a matter of fact, its use as a screening procedure may have a deleterious effect because a negative cytologic diagnosis may give a false sense of security and delay recognition of the carcinoma.

The situation with fine-needle aspiration is quite different, as already shown in the early attempts at Memorial Sloan-Kettering Cancer Center in the 1930s (Fig. 20-36). There is no longer any question that in experienced hands the technique is highly reliable[275,281,284,287] (Figs. 20-37 and 20-38). The average sensitivity is about 87%, the specificity close to 100%, the predictive value of a positive diagnosis nearly 100%, and the predictive value of a negative diagnosis between 60% and 90%.* Most benign lesions misinterpreted cytologically as possibly malignant belong to the fibrocystic disease category with marked epithelial proliferation.[270a,274] The cytologic distinction between atypical ductal hyperplasia and intraductal carcinoma has been attempted, both in mammographically detected lesions and to screen women with a family history of breast carcinoma.[268,278,288,289b] Since the differential diagnosis between these two conditions is based not only on cytologic but also on architectural criteria as seen on tissue sections, it is not surprising to find that such attempts have not been very successful.[273a,288] Along similar lines, it is generally not possible to distinguish between in situ and invasive ductal carcinoma on fine-needle aspiration biopsy.[268]

The most significant variables in the accuracy of the procedure are size of the lesion and proficiency of the individual performing the aspiration.[269] Material from fine-needle aspiration is also suitable for hormone receptor determination,[282,286] kinetic studies,[279,283] and oncoprotein expression.[277]

Fine-needle aspiration is less than ideal for some types of breast carcinoma. These include those associated with very

---

*References 270, 272, 273, 280, 285, 289, 290, 292.

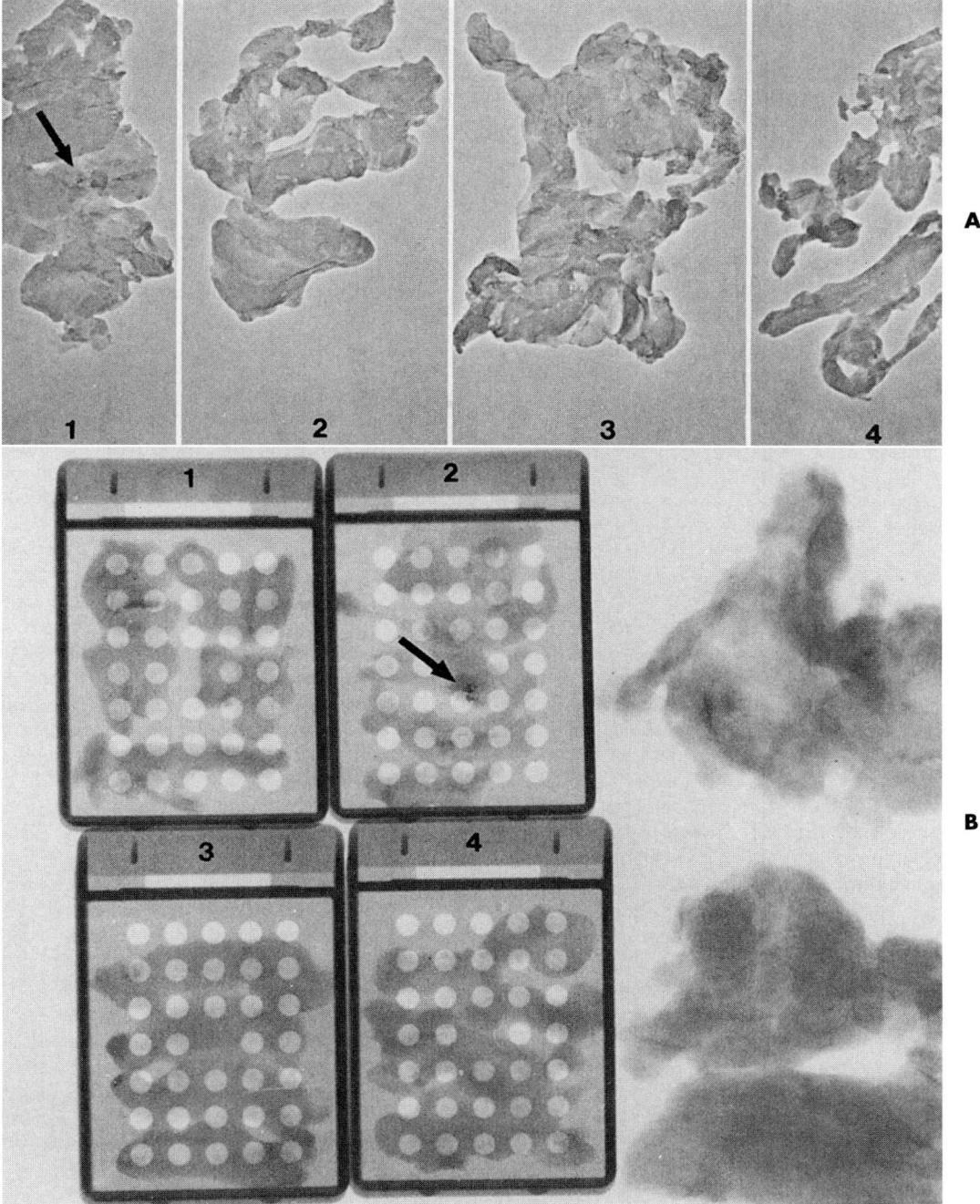

Fig. 20-35 Demonstration of use of specimen radiography. All photographs were taken with Polaroid camera and film.Mammographically detected breast lesion was excised. **A,** Specimen was sliced in four portions and radiograph taken. Pattern of calcification identical to that seen in original mammography was detected in slice 1 *(arrow).* **B,** Portion corresponding to this area of calcification was further divided in four fragments, and all four were embedded in paraffin. Radiograph of cassettes show that suspicious area is in cassette 2 *(arrow).* Remainder of slide (two fragments at right) shows no calcification.

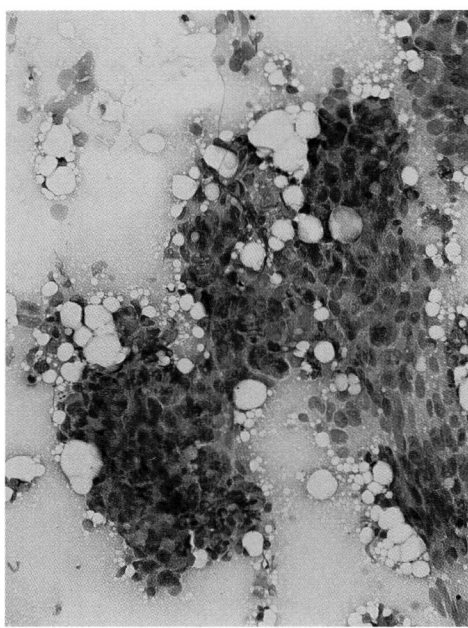

Fig. 20-36 Fine-needle aspiration biopsy performed at Memorial Sloan-Kettering Cancer Center in 1935. This was diagnosed as breast carcinoma and followed by the performance of a mastectomy, which confirmed the cytologic interpretation. (Courtesy Dr. Maureen Zakowski, Memorial Sloan-Kettering Cancer Center.)

extensive fibrosis, intraductal carcinoma, tubular and cribriform carcinoma, and, in general, the very small tumors. As Kline et al.[275] wisely indicated, this technique should be used to supplement, and not compete with, histologic examination. Most important, it should be always remembered that negative or inconclusive cytologic findings are not to be regarded as a definitive diagnosis if there is clinical suspicion of a malignant neoplasm.[271]

The performance of the fine-needle aspiration procedures may lead to mechanical displacement of epithelium, hemorrhage, necrosis, and other changes.[276,291,291a] The former is particularly troublesome, because it can mimic stromal and vascular invasion.[289a,291] The frequency of this complication is probably related to the type of needle used and the skill of the operator.

Core needle biopsy

Core needle biopsy can be very useful for documenting the malignant nature of a true neoplasm.[296] As one would expect, the larger the lesion, the higher the sensitivity of the method; for lesions greater than 2.5 cm in diameter, the sensitivity is over 90%.[295] The overall sensitivity rate in the various series has ranged between 75% and 90%.[293-295] The use of core needle biopsy has increased proportionally in recent years to the decrease in the use of open biopsy with frozen section.

Open biopsy and frozen section

Open biopsies from breast lesions are usually of excisional type when the tumor measures 2.5 cm or less and of incisional type for larger neoplasms. Performance of an open biopsy followed by frozen section and mastectomy if the diagnosis is carcinoma has been the standard approach for breast nodules for many years. The procedure is highly accurate; the false-positive rate is essentially zero, the false-negative rate is less than 1%, and the number of deferred diagnoses is less than 5%.[297,302] The greatest difficulties in frozen section are found with evaluation of papillary proliferations, and it has therefore been routine policy to defer the diagnosis on these lesions until the permanent sections are available.

Much has changed in recent years concerning the indications for frozen section as a result of several factors: the wish to discuss with the patient the therapeutic options after the diagnosis has been made; the realization that a delay of days or weeks between biopsy and mastectomy does not affect prognosis; the increasing alternative use of core needle biopsy and fine-needle aspiration biopsy; and the fact that a large number of cases involve small, nonpalpable lesions. Indeed, the need for performing this time-honored procedure is being increasingly questioned, one of the powerful reasons being that the final interpretation of the lesion may become difficult or impossible if the entire biopsy has been frozen.[303a] The following recommendations have been made depending on the setting[299-301]:

1 A palpable mass, which usually measures over 1 cm in diameter, provides ample tissue for frozen section, permanent section, and hormone receptors. Therefore not much harm results from doing the frozen section even if the medical indication is questionable.

2 A nonpalpable mass identified on a mammogram is often less than 1.0 cm in diameter. This *should not* be submitted for frozen section. If it turns out to be an invasive carcinoma, hormone receptor determinations can be done immunohistochemically on the paraffin-embedded material. Parenthetically, a close correlation is known to exist between tumor grade and hormone receptor status.

3 A biopsy carried out only for calcifications without a mass *should not* be frozen. Instead it should be examined by specimen radiography as already indicated (see p. 1592).

• • •

It should be added here that intraoperative cytologic examination can be very useful and that this procedure is used routinely by some authors in conjunction with (or instead of) the frozen section procedure. When interpreted by experienced individuals, the smears are as accurate as the frozen sections.[298]

Finally, frozen sections have been used effectively in evaluating reexcision lumpectomy margins.[303]

MICROSCOPIC TYPES

The two key determinations to make in the morphologic study of breast carcinoma are (1) whether the tumor is confined to the glandular component of the organ (in situ carcinoma) or whether it has invaded the stroma (invasive carcinoma) and (2) whether it is of ductal or lobular type. The first criterion, whose prognostic significance far outweighs that of the second, is self-explanatory, but it may be appro-

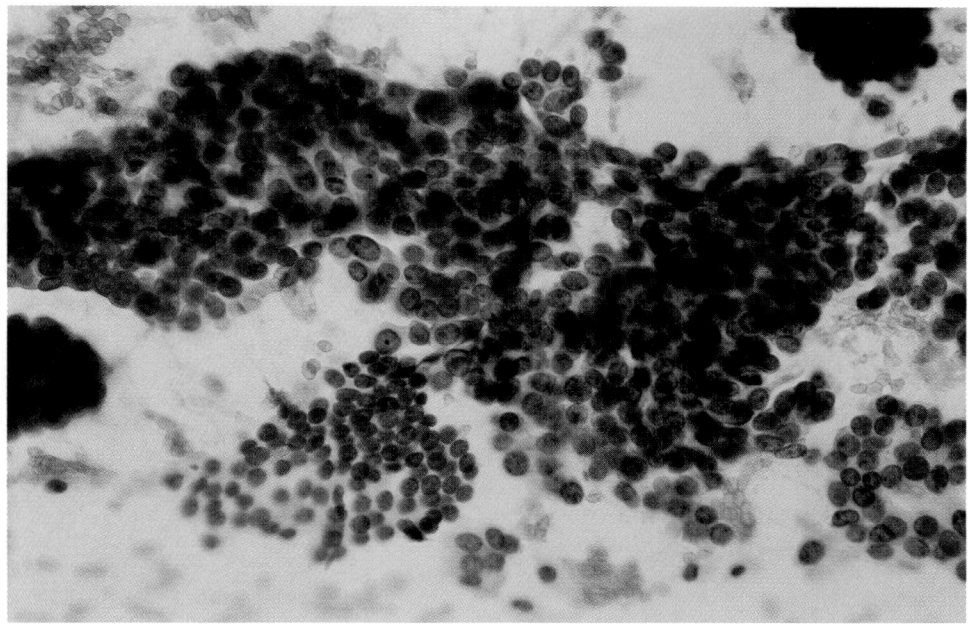

Fig. 20-37 Cytologic preparation of invasive ductal carcinoma as seen in a fine-needle aspiration specimen. The clusters of tumor cells are cohesive and have irregular margins. (Courtesy Dr. Maureen Zakowski, Memorial Sloan-Kettering Cancer Center.)

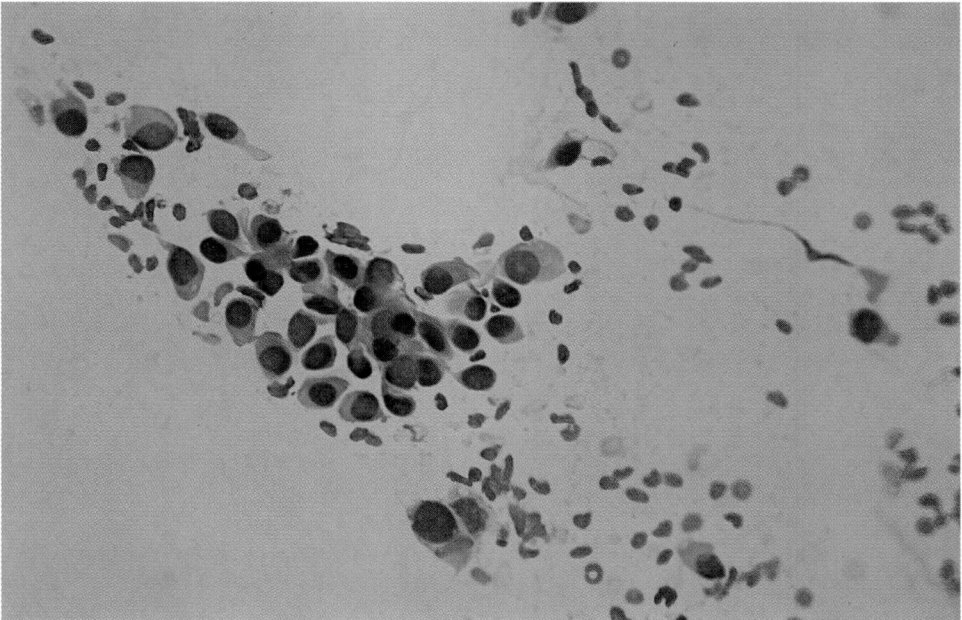

Fig. 20-38 Cluster of malignant cells from an invasive breast carcinoma of ductal type, as seen in a high-power view from a fine-needle aspiration specimen. (Courtesy Dr. Paul P. Rosen, Memorial Sloan-Kettering Cancer Center.)

priate to elaborate about the second. The term ductal carcinoma may be taken to imply that the tumor is either arising from or involving a duct, and an analogous assumption could be made about lobular carcinoma. The evidence obtained from the classic study of Wellings et al.[305] and several others indicates instead that both tumor types (and, for that matter, most benign proliferative breast diseases) arise from the same segment of the mammary gland (i.e., the TDLU). As far as location is concerned, it is certainly true that many ductal carcinomas involve preferentially structures with the appearance of ducts and that most lobular carcinomas involve preferentially lobules. However, numerous exceptions in both directions exist. It has been hypothesized that these cases represent—respectively—ductal carcinomas with secondary extension ("cancerization" of lobules), or lobular carcinomas with secondary extension into ducts, but there is no convincing indication that this is indeed the case.[304] Be that as it may, it should be made clear that it is the type of tumor as defined by cytoarchitectural features that establish its identity rather than its precise location within the breast. Therefore it may be more accurate and less confusing to refer to these tumors as ductal type and lobular type, respectively. For the sake of brevity and tradition, the conventional nomenclature of ductal and lobular will be used instead in this chapter.

IN SITU CARCINOMA
Ductal carcinoma in situ (DCIS)

Several morphologic variants of DCIS exist: papillary, comedocarcinoma, solid, cribriform, micropapillary, clinging, and cystic hypersecretory. Papillary carcinoma is a very distinct type, thought to arise from large ducts. The others, believed to originate in the TDLU (although usually extending to larger ducts) have been traditionally divided into comedocarcinoma (characterized by large pleomorphic cells associated with necrosis) and the solid/cribriform/micropapillary group (composed of smaller uniform cells unassociated with necrosis), with the "clinging" lesions being included in one or another of these two categories depending on their cytologic features.[307,315] Recently, a proposal has been made to regard these tumors as part of a continuum and to divide them in a three-grade system largely on the basis of cytologic criteria. According to this scheme, a classic comedocarcinoma becomes a grade 3 DCIS, classic solid/cribriform/micropapillary lesions become grade 1 DCIS, and those showing intermediate cytologic features are reported as grade 2 DCIS. These criteria apply whether the proliferation is solid, cribriform, micropapillary, or flat (i.e., "clinging"). They also apply independently of the presence or absence of necrosis and/or calcification,[312] although there is a relationship between the type of calcification when present and the type of carcinoma in situ.[311b]

Comedocarcinoma

Comedocarcinoma may reach a relatively large size and become palpable. In one series 28% were over 5 cm in diameter, and another 33% were between 2 and 5 cm.[318] Over half of these tumors are centrally located, whereas this is true for less than 20% of invasive tumors.[328] The incidence of multicentricity is 32% to 33%,[309,314] and the incidence of bilaterality is 10%.[309]

Grossly, the tumor presents as a cluster of thick-walled ducts with normal breast parenchyma between them. When these ducts are compressed, plugs of necrotic tumor reminiscent grossly of those seen in comedos extrude from them, hence the name comedocarcinoma. If the duct walls are not thickened, the tumor may not be apparent grossly. Microscopically, the ducts show a solid growth of large pleomorphic tumor cells accompanied by generally abundant mitotic activity and lacking connective tissue support. Necrosis is always present and constitutes an important diagnostic sign, whether in the form of a large central focus or of individual tumor cells (Fig. 20-39). The mean diameter of the ducts containing necrosis is significantly larger than for those lacking this feature, suggesting the existence of a "hypoxic compartment" in these tumors.[317] Coarse calcification often supervenes in these necrotic areas, and this can be identified by mammography. Myoepithelial cells are usually absent in ducts involved by comedocarcinoma, but their presence in no way invalidates the diagnosis. The stroma around the involved ducts shows a characteristic concentric fibrosis accompanied by a mild to moderate mononuclear inflammatory reaction.

Tumors with the classical comedocarcinoma appearance (or the grade 3 DCIS of other classifications) are characterized by aneuploidy, negativity for hormone receptors, metallothionein expression, c-erbB-2 overexpression, and a high frequency of p53 mutations.*

Once the diagnosis of comedocarcinoma has been established, two other important determinations need to be made. The first is the degree of intraductal spread, which in some cases may be very extensive and even reach the nipple, resulting in Paget's disease.[319,352a] The other is to search for areas of definite stromal invasion and, if these are present, to estimate the relative amounts of in situ and invasive components.[326] The term *extensive intraductal carcinoma* (EIC) has been proposed for tumors in which the intraductal component comprises 25% or more of the area encompassed by the infiltrating tumor and is also present in the surrounding breast tissue.[325] Interestingly, no correlation exists between the size of the tumor and the degree of invasion present in it.[326] Lagios et al.[314] found occult foci of invasion in 21% of their cases. Even if no definite invasion is detected in the sections examined, the possibility always exists with comedocarcinoma—more than with any other form of DCIS—that a minute focus of invasion is present elsewhere.[310] This may explain the fact that some patients have axillary lymph node metastases in the absence of an identifiable invasive component.[323] Another possible explanation is that the comedocarcinomatous areas themselves are actually invasive in a "pushing" fashion, as suggested by the large size they sometimes attain, the ultrastructural demonstration of basement membrane defects,[321] the prominent fibrosis associated with stromal metachromasia found around them,[324] and the fact that neural invasion has been exceptionally demonstrated in them.[327] Although we find this possibility rather appealing, for practical purposes we would advise designating these tumors as invasive only when irregular ("destructive") infiltration of the stroma is detected in them.

---

*References 306, 308, 308a, 311a, 313, 314a, 316, 320, 322.

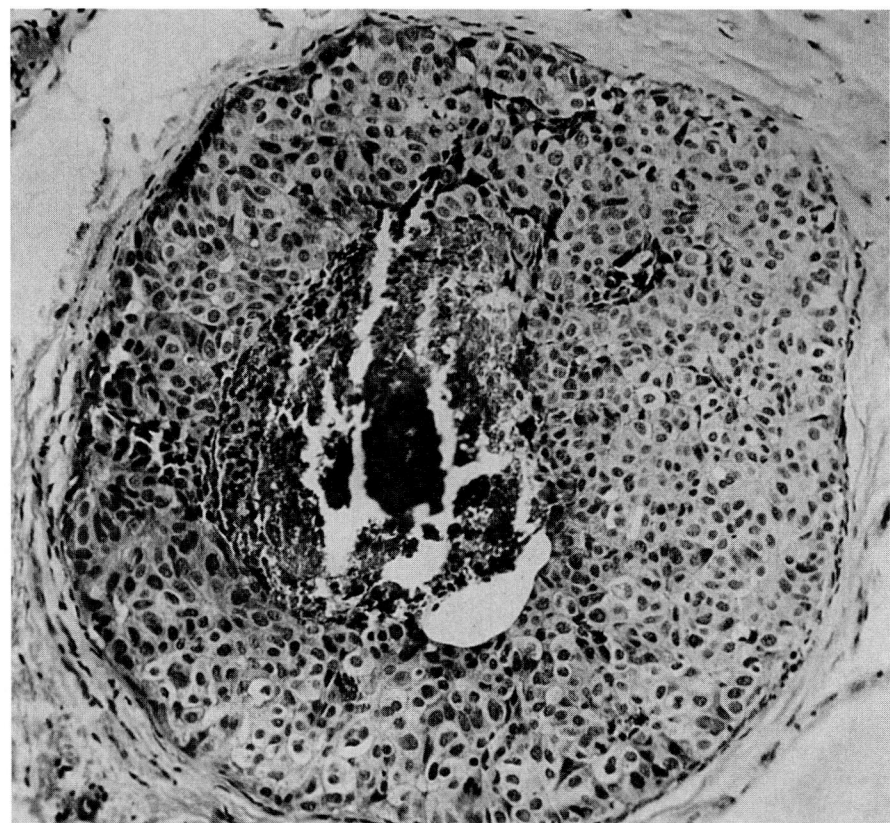

Fig. 20-39 Ductal carcinoma in situ of so-called comedocarcinoma type. There is central necrosis and calcification.

Rarely, the foci of microinvasion are accompanied by a granulomatous tissue response.[311]

(In situ) papillary carcinoma

Papillary carcinoma makes up only a small percentage of breast carcinomas. Grossly, it may present as a well-circumscribed mass or it may ramify within several ducts to involve an entire breast segment. In the variant known as *intracystic papillary carcinoma,* the tumor appears as a mural nodule within a large cystic space supposedly representing a dilated duct[330,332] (Plate XV-D). The microscopic criteria for the diagnosis must be strict, because most papillary breast lesions are benign. The most important differential features were listed in the classic study by Kraus and Neubecker[331] and further elaborated (and somewhat modified) by Azzopardi.[329] As a group, papillary carcinomas occur in an older age group and are larger than papillomas. Microscopically, features favoring carcinoma are (paradoxically) uniformity in size and shape of the epithelial cells (whether round, oval, or spindle, the latter arranged perpendicularly to the duct axis), presence of one cell type only (i.e., lack of myoepithelial cells), nuclear hyperchromasia and high nucleocytoplasmic ratio, high mitotic activity, lack of apocrine metaplasia, cribriform and trabecular patterns, scanty or absent stroma, and lack of benign proliferative disease in the adjacent breast[329,331] (Fig. 20-40). It should

be realized that no feature among those just listed is sufficient in itself to establish the distinction between papilloma and papillary carcinoma. The amount of stroma present could serve as an example of this fact; although scanty or nil in most papillary carcinomas, it may be bulky and well developed in others, prompting a mistaken diagnosis of benignancy (Fig. 20-41). Another diagnostic trap is provided by the presence of scattered large pale eosinophilic cells (known as clear or globoid cells) concentrated in the basilar portion, which can be mistaken for myoepithelial cells.[331,333] In general, special techniques are not of great help in this differential diagnosis; the only notable exception is actin stain, which highlights the presence or absence of myoepithelial cells.[333]

It seems likely that most papillary carcinomas arise de novo. In some cases, however, there is convincing morphologic and immunohistochemical evidence for the carcinoma arising within the context of multiple papillomas.[334]

Papillary carcinoma with invasion is discussed on p.1611.

Other forms

In the *solid* form of DCIS, the glandular lumen is filled by the proliferation of medium-sized cells, which are larger than those of LCIS but smaller and more uniform than those of comedocarcinoma (Fig. 20-42). Azzopardi[336] pointed out the sharp cell edges (as opposed to a "syncytial" quality) and

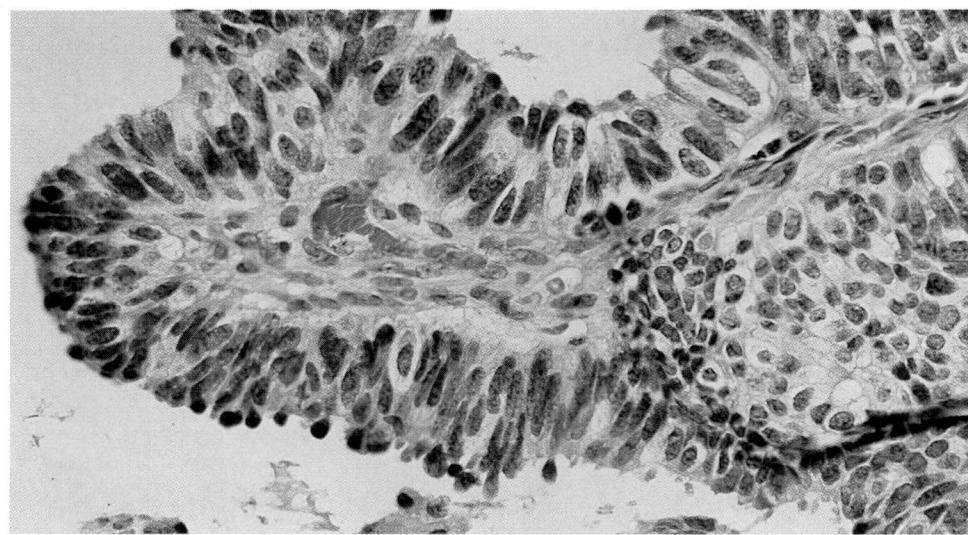

Fig. 20-40 High-power view of an in situ papillary papilloma. Note the layering of cells, loss of nuclear polarity, marked hyperchromasia, and lack of a myoepithelial component.

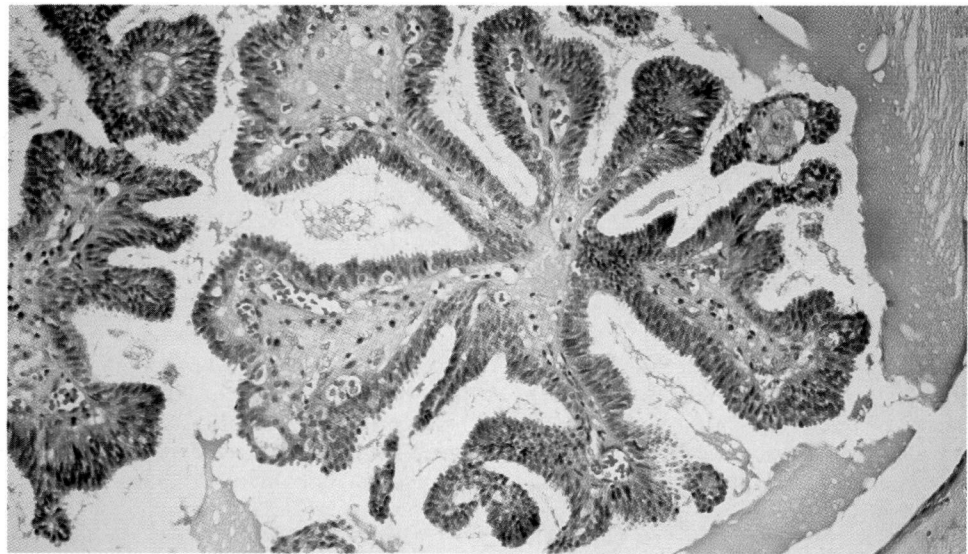

Fig. 20-41 In situ papillary carcinoma. The arborizing nature of this tumor and the stout fibrovascular core are not too different from those of a benign papilloma.

pallor of the cytoplasm (as opposed to prominent aci-dophilia) often exhibited by these cells. In the *cribriform* variety, round regular spaces are formed within the glands; the more regular these spaces are in terms of distribution, size, and shape, the more likely the lesion is to be malignant (Fig. 20-43). These spaces are often associated with two formations of similar pathogenesis, designated by Azzopardi[336] as trabecular bars and Roman bridges, respectively. Trabecular bars are rigid rows of cells with their long axes arranged more or less perpendicular (or at least not parallel) to the long axis of the bar; these should be distinguished from partial detachments of the duct lining (Plate XV-E). Roman bridges are curvilinear trabecular bars connecting two portions of the epithelial lining. The cribriform pattern of DCIS should not be equated with that of adenoid cystic carcinoma (see p. 1627).

The *micropapillary* variety (more closely connected to the preceding types of DCIS than to papillary carcinoma) shows elongated epithelial projections projecting into the glandular lumen; these lack connective tissue support, may have a cavity at the base, and often show a bulbous expansion at the tip (Plate XV-F). This variant is more likely than others to involve multiple quadrants of the breast.[337]

Clinging carcinoma, the more controversial member of this family, shows one or two layers of malignant cells lining a glandular formation with a large empty lumen.[336] In the more easily recognizable cases, the tumor cells are large,

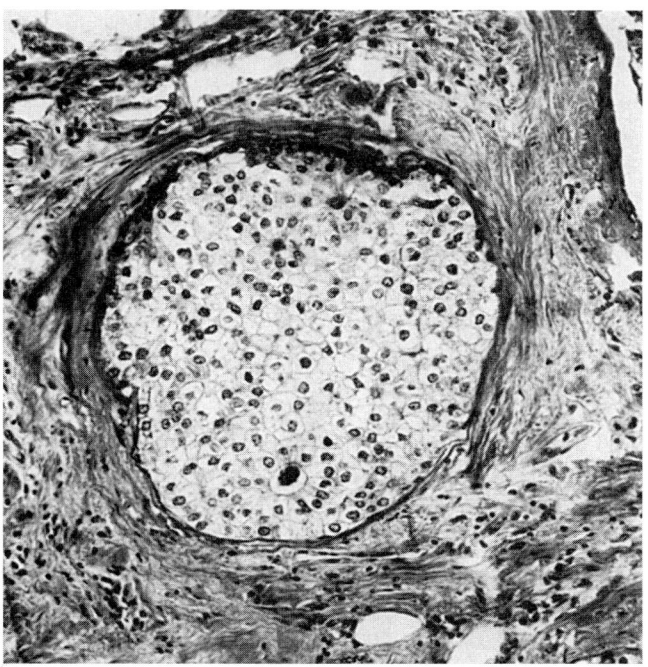

Fig. 20-42 Ductal carcinoma in situ of solid type. Uniformity of cell population, cytoplasmic pallor, and sharply outlined cell borders are important diagnostic clues.

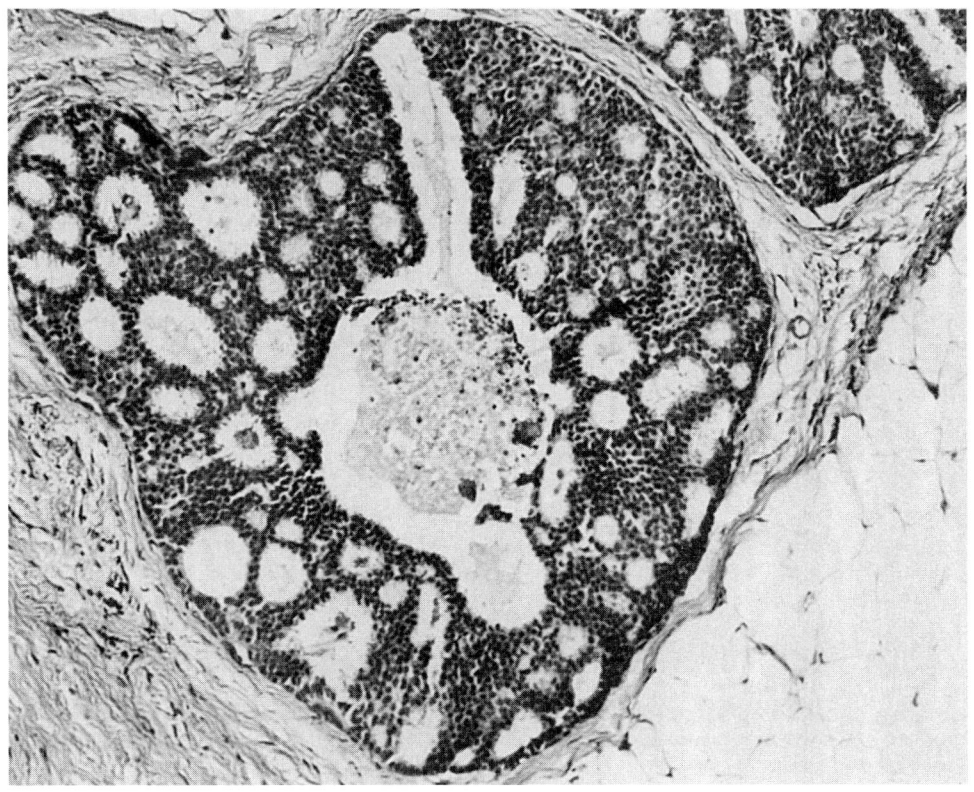

Fig. 20-43 Ductal carcinoma in situ of cribriform type. Note regular round shape of glandular formations and central necrosis.

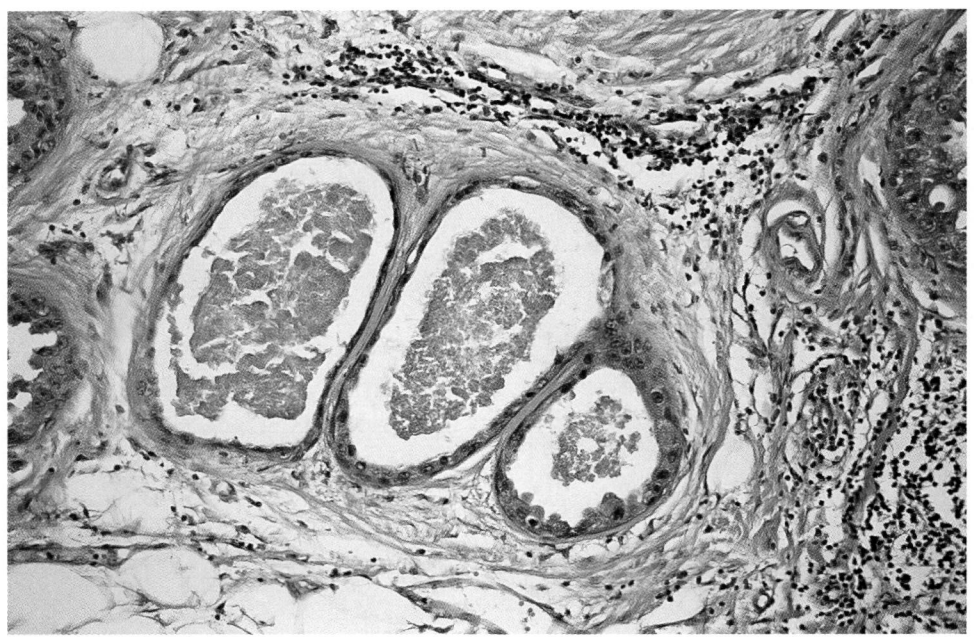

Fig. 20-44 Ductal carcinoma in situ of so-called clinging type. One or two layers of atypical cells line dilated glandular structures containing granular intraluminal material in which ghosts of tumor cells are identified.

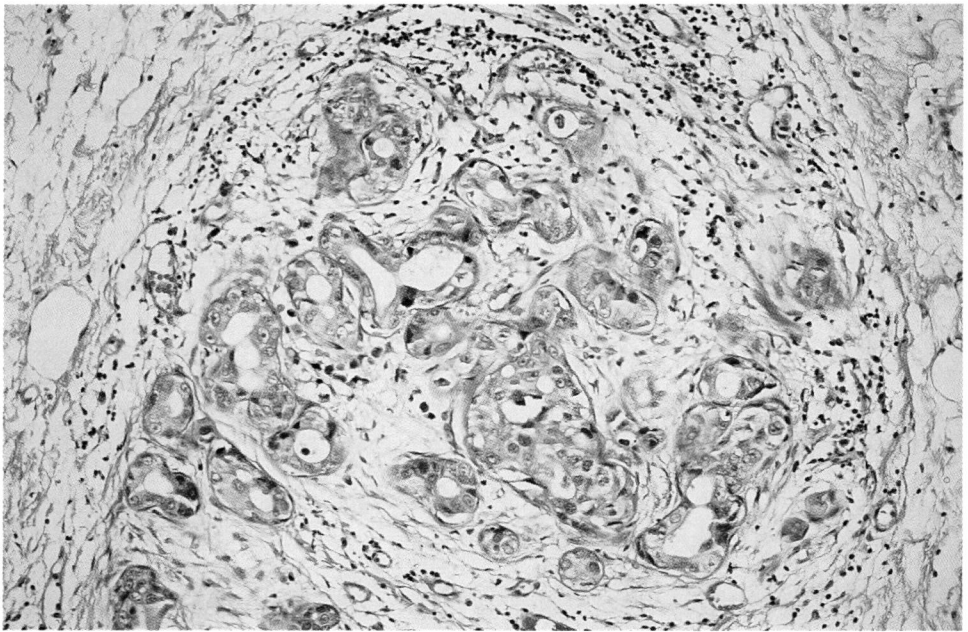

Fig. 20-45 So-called lobular cancerization. Lobule is markedly expanded and composed of relatively large tumor cells with appearance of ductal-type carcinoma. Typical ductal carcinoma was present elsewhere in specimen.

highly atypical, and associated with individual cell necrosis, these features suggesting a link with comedocarcinoma (Fig. 20-44). In other instances, the tumor cells are smaller and more regular; these have been interpreted as being related to the "noncomedo" form of intraductal carcinoma, particularly the micropapillary variety. Indeed, some authors refer to this as the "flat" variant of micropapillary in situ carcinoma.

The *cystic hypersecretory* form is a variation of DCIS characterized by the cystic formations induced by the abundant secretory material present; although hardly a distinct entity, it deserves mention because of the ease with which it can be confused with a benign process.[341,344]

Adding to the complexity of the situation is the pattern traditionally known as *lobular cancerization*.[335,339] The term refers to the presence, in a structure easily identifiable as a lobule, of carcinoma with the cytoarchitectural features of any of the forms of DCIS (Fig. 20-45). As the name indicates, the original assumption was that this represented a secondary extension into a lobule of a carcinoma of ductal origin, particularly when this was found associated with a conventional DCIS such as comedocarcinoma. The interpretation is probably erroneous. The available evidence suggests that this phenomenon represents instead a variation in the growth pattern of DCIS in which the structure involved is still easily recognizable as belonging to a lobule. Further evidence for the basic unity of these various manifestations comes from the occasional occurrence of DCIS and LCIS in the same TDLU.[343]

Rare additional morphologic variations of DCIS include cases with signet ring cells[340] with apocrine-type cytology,[342,345] and those with evidence of endocrine differentiation[338] (see p. 1611). The latter are often accompanied by adjacent intraductal papillomas with pagetoid involvement by the carcinoma.[346]

In closing, it could be said that a feature of diagnostic importance common to all forms of DCIS (although better developed in the comedocarcinoma type) is the appearance of the luminal content. As Azzopardi[336] pointed out, the presence of nuclear debris, ghosts of dead cell outlines, granular and fragmented products, and inspissated densely stained material should raise suspicion and stimulate a thorough search for more diagnostic areas.

Evolution

The often assumed implication of the diagnosis of DCIS is that, if left untreated, the lesion will inevitably progress to an invasive carcinoma of similar morphologic features. This is a gross and inaccurate oversimplification of a very complex situation. These are some of the reasonably established facts:

1 The transformation to an invasive phenotype does not occur in all cases, at least during the normal life span of an individual.[354]

2 When such a transformation occurs, the process usually evolves over a period of years if not decades.[354]

3 There is a substantial difference in the frequency with which this phenomenon occurs depending on the type of DCIS: high for comedocarcinoma and low for all the others.[350,357] This can also be expressed by saying that

the risk for the development of invasive carcinoma is directly proportional to the cytologic grade of the tumors.[352a]

4 There is a definite relationship between the microscopic type of the DCIS and the invasive component, much more so than for lobular CIS; however, numerous exceptions occur.[351]

5 Not all invasive breast carcinomas go through the sequence just described; some (perhaps the majority) have a very short intraductal stage and become invasive long before being detectable by any technique. It is this very fact that takes some of the value away from screening techniques such as mammography, which are much more likely to detect slow-growing carcinomas with a prolonged in situ stage.

The most informative data on which these conclusions are based derive from retrospective studies on DCIS that were treated by biopsy only.[349,352,356] In the series of Page et al.,[353] seven of twenty-five patients with DCIS of non-comedocarcinoma type whose cases had been followed for over 3 years developed homolateral invasive breast carcinoma. In an earlier and smaller series by Betsill et al.,[347] invasive carcinoma had developed in six of the ten patients for whom follow-up information was available. In a large series of patients treated with biopsy and local breast irradiation, it was found that comedo-type necrosis and uncertain/involved surgical margins were the best predictors of recurrence.[350a]

When mastectomy is done within 6 months after the identification of DCIS by biopsy, the incidence of invasive carcinoma in the mastectomy specimen has been 6% in one series[355] and 18% in another.[348] Interestingly, residual DCIS was found in 60% of the specimens, a different quadrant being involved in 33% of them.[355]

Lobular carcinoma in situ (LCIS)

Lobular carcinoma in situ (LCIS), also known as lobular neoplasia, has no distinguishing features on gross examination and is usually found incidentally in breasts removed for other reasons. It is multicentric in about 70% of the cases[378] and bilateral in about 30% to 40%.[364] Most cases are found within 5 cm of the nipple from the skin surface in the outer and inner upper quadrants.[374,375] Residual tumor foci are found in 60% of breasts removed following a diagnosis of LCIS made from a biopsy specimen.[376]

Microscopically, the lobules are distended and completely filled by relatively uniform, round, small to medium-sized cells with round and normochromatic (or only mildly hyperchromatic) nuclei. In general, atypia, pleomorphism, mitotic activity, and necrosis are minimal or absent[359,373,379] (Fig. 20-46). Any of the following minor morphologic variations can occur, singly or in combination: moderate nuclear pleomorphism, larger nuclear size, loss of cohesiveness, appreciable mitotic activity, scattered signet ring cells (relatively common), apocrine changes (exceptional), focal necrosis, and variations in the shape of the involved lobules.[362,366,372,376] The neighboring terminal ducts often exhibit proliferation of cells similar to those involving the lobules. These cells may form a continuous row beneath the secretory epithelium, a pattern that has been referred to as mural or pagetoid (Fig. 20-47); they can also grow in a solid,

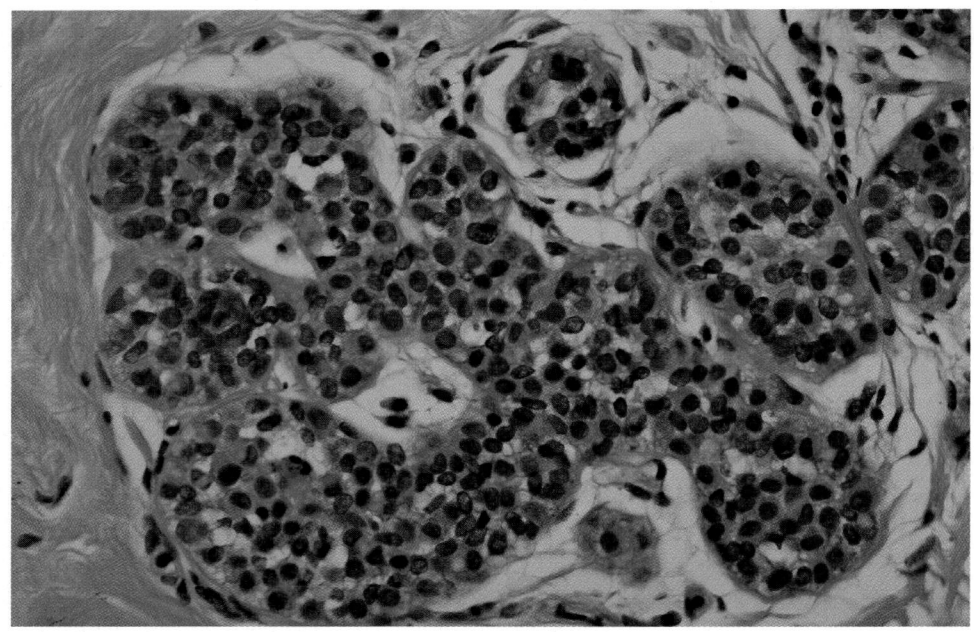

Fig. 20-46 Lobular carcinoma in situ. Note lobular pattern, small size of tumor cells, and lack of necrosis.

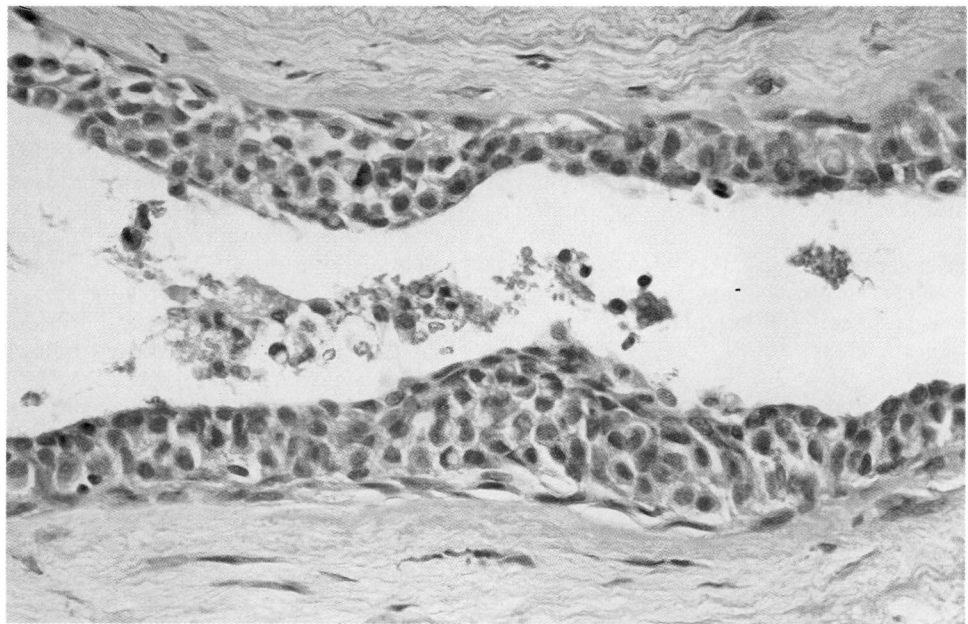

Fig. 20-47 Involvement of duct by lobular carcinoma in situ. In presence of such change, a thorough search for typical areas of lobular involvement should be undertaken.

cribriform, or micropapillary fashion.[369,378] Although occasionally this change extends to larger (lactiferous) ducts, true Paget's disease of the nipple has not been reported as a result of lobular carcinoma. The presence of these ductal changes is of histogenetic interest and sometimes the first clue for the existence of typical LCIS nearby, but it does not carry prognostic implications of its own.[360]

LCIS can also be found in fibroadenomas[371] and in foci of sclerosing adenosis.[370] The diagnosis of LCIS (or whatever equivalent term one might like to use) should be made only in those cases in which the cellular proliferation has resulted in the formation of solid nests that have expanded the lobules, whereas the designation of lobular hyperplasia (usually preceded by the qualifier "atypical") is to be given to those lesions accompanied by normal-sized lobules in which central lumina are still identifiable. LCIS should also be distinguished from DCIS, particularly the form traditionally known as lobular cancerization and already discussed on p. 1596. The latter is identified by the fact that its cytoarchitectural features are those of one of the forms of DCIS, usually comedocarcinoma. When the latter is the case, there is obvious cellular pleomorphism, atypical nuclear configuration, formation of small lumina, and necrosis.[358,368]

The only conventional special stains of some significance for the evaluation of LCIS are those for mucin, which show positivity in scattered tumor cells in about three quarters of the cases.[361,362] Immunohistochemically, the tumor cells show positivity for keratin, EMA, and milk fat globule membrane antigen.[367] S-100 protein is demonstrable in 60% of the cases.[365] Stains for actin or electron microscopy show residual myoepithelial cells, which may lie flat on the basement membrane, perpendicular to it, or admixed with the tumor cells; the latter do not have myoepithelial features themselves.[363,377] Laminin and collagen type IV can be demonstrated in the underlying basement membrane.

Evolution

One of the most controversial aspects of breast pathology is the nature of LCIS, specifically in regard to the probability of development of invasive carcinoma following a biopsy diagnosis of LCIS without additional therapy. Although the figures obtained in the various reported series[380,382-387] are not exactly superimposable, it seems safe to conclude from them that (1) about 20% to 30% of patients will develop invasive carcinoma, a risk about eight to ten times higher than for a control population; (2) the risk seems greater in well-developed LCIS ("histologically flagrant") than in atypical lobular hyperplasia ("histologically subtle"); (3) this increased risk applies to both breasts, although it is greater on the side of the biopsy; (4) the invasive carcinoma may be of either lobular or ductal type; (5) the amount of LCIS or its morphologic variations bears little or no relation to the magnitude of the risk; and (6) if a patient with a biopsy diagnosis of LCIS is examined periodically, the chances of her dying as a result of breast carcinoma are minimal.

Most investigators agree that careful lifelong follow-up appears to be a safe and rational option for this lesion.[381,382] The performance of a simple mastectomy can be considered in the presence of a strong family history of carcinoma, extensive fibrocystic disease, or excessive apprehension on the part of the patient or if a prolonged follow-up evaluation cannot be assured.

INVASIVE CARCINOMA

Tumors included in this category are all those in which stromal invasion is detectable, whether an in situ component is identifiable or not and regardless of the relative proportion of the two components. Like the in situ lesions, most of these tumors can be divided into two major categories—ductal type and lobular type—acknowledging the existence of mixed and undetermined forms. It should be emphasized that the type of invasive carcinoma should be determined from its appearance, rather than deduced from the type of in situ component present, if any.

The classification of invasive breast carcinoma has evolved over a long period of time and, as a result, has incorporated into it a wide range of criteria, such as cell type (as in apocrine carcinoma), type and amount of secretion (as in mucinous carcinoma), architectural features (as in papillary carcinoma), and pattern of spread (as in inflammatory carcinoma). Not surprisingly, this has resulted in a considerable degree of confusion.

Invasive ductal carcinoma

For purposes of discussion, invasive ductal carcinomas are here divided according to two major criteria: cytoarchitecture and pattern of spread.

Cytoarchitectural variants

The morphologic variations in the theme of invasive ductal carcinoma are innumerable. Some of them are distinctive enough to deserve recognition as special types, especially when associated with a particular behavior. The others, which represent about 75% of all the cases, are generically designated as invasive ductal carcinomas of classic, ordinary, or not-otherwise-specified (NOS) type.[390b]

Classic (NOS) invasive ductal carcinoma. This lesion represents the prototypic expression of breast carcinoma, and it is the tumor type usually implied when the term "breast carcinoma" is used without further qualification. The size, shape, consistency, and type of margins are highly variable; some of these factors depend on the relative amounts of tumor cells and stroma. Grossly, the typical case is firm and poorly circumscribed, cuts with a resistant gritty sensation, and shows a yellowish gray cut surface, with trabeculae radiating through the surrounding parenchyma into the fat, resulting in the notorious stellate or crab-like configuration from which the word "cancer" has originated (Figs. 20-48, A and B, and 20-49, A). Sometimes these strands are seen connecting with other tumor nodules located at some distance from the primary tumor. Areas of necrosis, hemorrhage, and cystic degeneration may be present, particularly in the larger neoplasms. The tumor may have invaded overlying skin or underlying fascia and pectoralis muscle. Tumors that are particularly hard because of the large amounts of stroma were traditionally referred to as "scirrhous carcinomas," a term no longer used. It is common for these neoplasms to exhibit "chalky streaks" on the cut surface, a feature not caused by necrosis

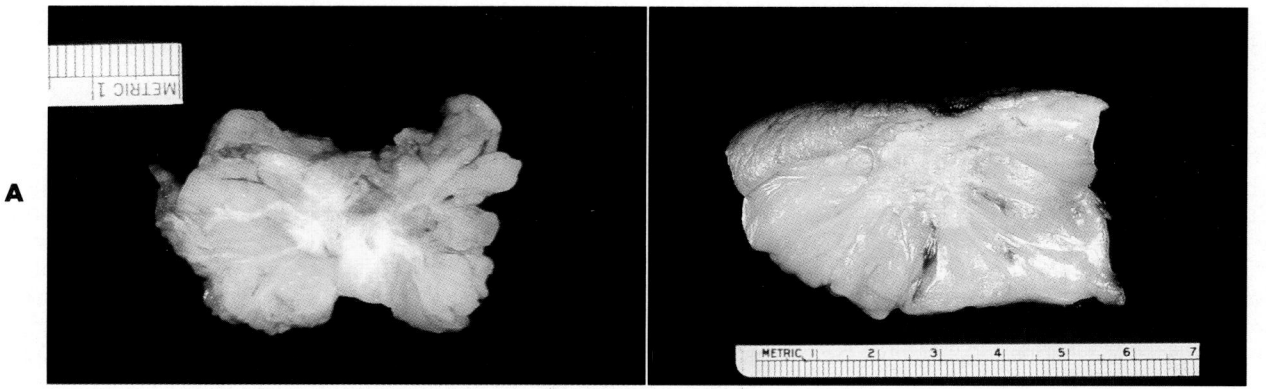

Fig. 20-48 **A** and **B,** Typical gross appearance of invasive ductal carcinoma. Note the irregular (crab-like) shape of the tumor, white fibrous appearance, and chalky streaks. Retraction of the overlying skin is obvious in the specimen shown in **B.**

as generally believed but by duct elastosis[405] (Fig. 20-49, *B*). When this occurs, the appearance of the lesion has an uncanny resemblance to an unripe pear, further accentuated by the consistency and the sensation one has while cutting it.

Other tumors are better delineated, softer, rounded, and lobulated. These have been variously designated as circumscribed, multinodular, or knobby carcinomas. In the past, they were also known as medullary carcinomas, a practice that should be avoided at all costs to avoid confusion with the specific variant of breast carcinoma bearing that name (see p. 1609).

Microscopically the variations are also legion.[400] The tumor can grow in diffuse sheets, well-defined nests, cords, or as individual cells. Glandular/tubular differentiation may be well developed, barely detectable, or altogether absent. Parenthetically, this is the reason why the term adenocarcinoma is not advisable as a synonym for invasive ductal carcinoma (Fig. 20-50). The tumor cells vary in size and shape, but by definition they are larger and more pleomorphic than those of invasive lobular carcinomas, their nuclei and nucleoli are more prominent, and mitotic figures are more numerous. Areas of necrosis occur in about 60% of the cases.[401] Foci of squamous metaplasia, apocrine metaplasia, or clear cell changes may be seen. The amount of stroma ranges from none to abundant, and its appearance from densely fibrotic to cellular ("desmoplastic"). In cases with abundant stroma, it may be difficult to identify the tumor cells. Bulky masses of elastic tissue are present in about 90% of the cases; this "elastosis," which can involve the wall of the ducts and the vessels (mainly veins), is responsible for the chalky streaks seen on gross examination.[388] Calcification can be detected in about 60% of the cases, either as coarse or fine granules or, rarely, as psammoma bodies.[400] A mononuclear inflammatory infiltrate of variable intensity is usually present at the interphase between tumor and stroma. Granulomatous inflammation is rarely seen.[416]

Definite invasion of the perineurial spaces, lymph vessels, and blood vessels was found by Fisher et al.[400] in 28%, 33%, and 5%, respectively. Lymph vessel invasion may be difficult to distinguish from artifactual tissue retraction. Features used to document the presence of lymphatic tumor emboli are the following: (1) the occurrence of the area in question

outside the margin of the carcinoma, (2) the fact that the tumor emboli do not conform exactly to the space in which they lie, (3) the presence of an endothelial cell lining, and (4) the presence of blood vessels in the immediate vicinity.[421] If doubts persist, a stain with *Ulex europaeus* I lectin, FVIII-related antigen, or other endothelial cell markers might prove helpful[410,413,422] (Fig. 20-51). These reactions can even be carried out in the H&E-stained preparations after removing the coverslip and decolorizing the slide.[418]

The mucin amount present in these tumors, as evaluated by Fisher et al.[400] in over 900 cases with the Alcian blue–PAS stain, was judged to be nil in 47% of the cases, slight in 34%, moderate in 12%, and marked in 7%. In the same study, intracytoplasmic glycogen was found after PAS stain with diastase control in 62% of the cases.[400] Focal argyrophilia is found in about 5% of the cases, a feature further discussed on p. 1613.[393]

Ultrastructurally, the tumor cells exhibit, in greater or lesser degree, features of glandular differentiation such as microvilli and terminal bars on their luminal side.[399] A particularly characteristic feature, although not as specific for breast carcinoma as originally suggested, is the presence of intracytoplasmic lumina bordered by microvilli.[390,423] These formations, when sufficiently large, appear as "bull's-eyes" at the light microscopic level. Early claims that the ultrastructural features of some ductal carcinomas were indicative of myoepithelial cell origin have been disproved. The desmoplastic stroma accompanying breast carcinomas is formed by cells having the ultrastructural features of fibroblasts and myofibroblasts.[417]

Immunohistochemically, the tumor cells show reactivity for low-molecular-weight keratin (particularly types 8, 18, and 19) and EMA.[406] Some of the tumors (particularly those with foci of squamous metaplasia) are also immunoreactive for high-molecular-weight (epidermal-type) keratin.[425] In addition to EMA (which also stains carcinomas of most other sites), the cells of breast carcinoma are reactive for an apparently more organ-specific antigen obtained from milk fat globule membrane.[403] Close to 70% of the cases are positive for lactalbumin, another marker almost entirely restricted to mammary epithelium.[396,409] CEA, B72.3, and BCA-225 are positive in the majority of the cases.[408,411,419,420,424] Vimentin

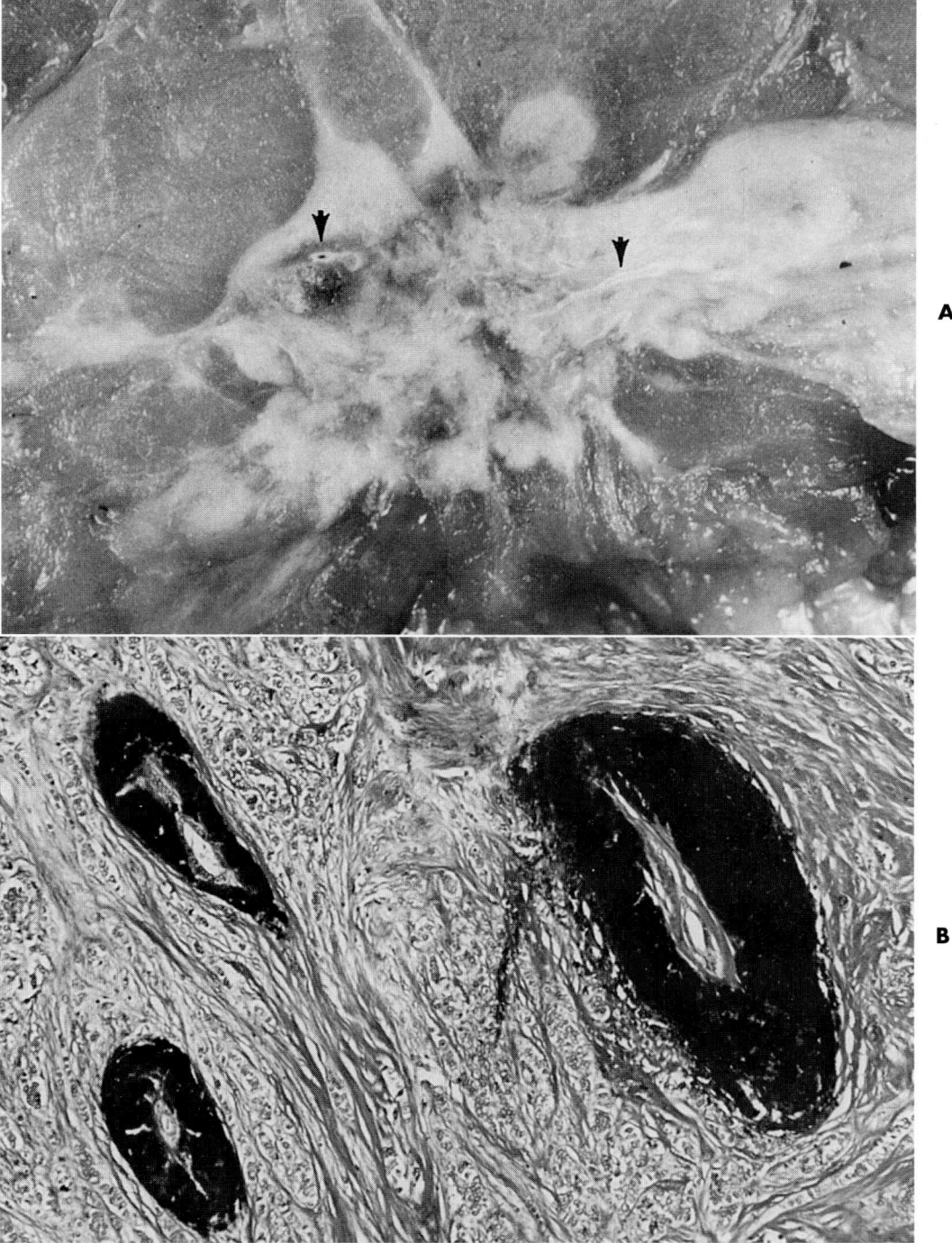

Fig. 20-49 A, Gross appearance of typical invasive ductal carcinoma. "Chalky streaks" can be seen throughout tumor. Central space can be identified in some of them *(arrows).* **B,** Elastic tissue stain of lesion illustrated in **A** showing that "chalky streaks" correspond to markedly thickened elastic layer in wall of non-neoplastic ducts crossing tumor. (**B** Verhoeff–van Gieson.)

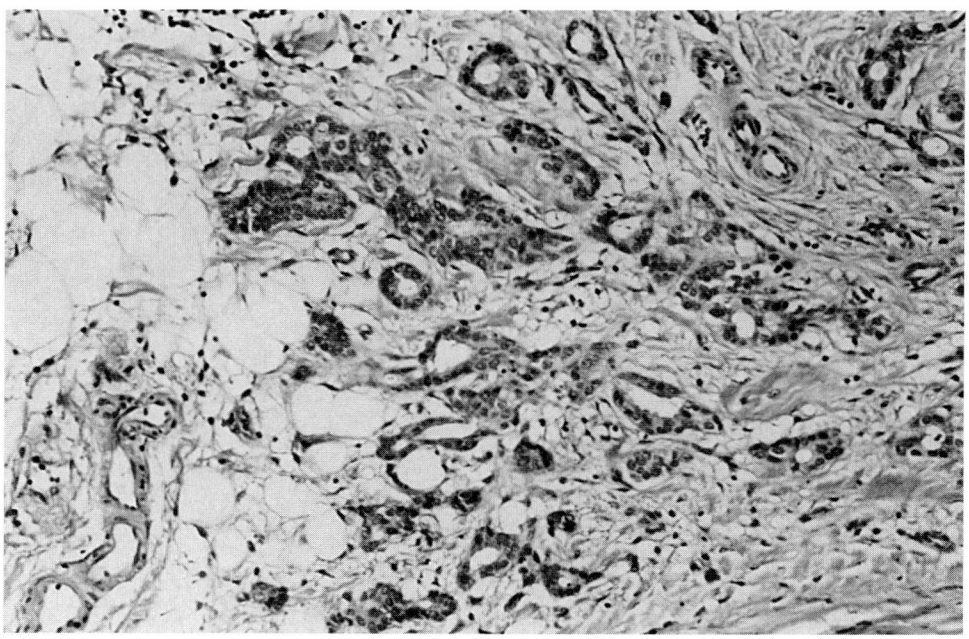

Fig. 20-50 Invasive ductal carcinoma of classic (NOS) type. Small glands of irregular shape are seen infiltrating cellular stroma. Tumor is relatively well differentiated but is not a tubular carcinoma.

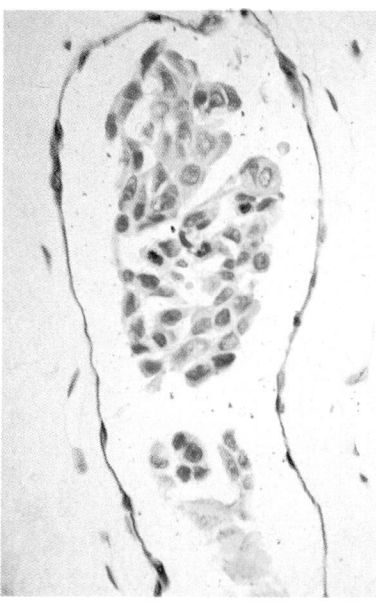

Fig. 20-51 Vascular invasion by breast carcinoma demonstrated by positivity of endothelial cells for *Ulex europaeus* lectin I.

may be expressed,[397] sometimes together with GFAP.[402] Breast carcinomas can be immunoreactive for S-100 protein, the number ranging from 10% to 45% in the various reported series[398,412]; this is a fact to remember in the differential diagnosis of metastatic tumors to axillary nodes, lest a breast carcinoma be mislabeled as metastatic melanoma. Even more treacherous is the fact that some cases show a granular reactivity for HMB-45.[392] An increased expression of the bone matrix proteins osteonectin and osteopontin

has been documented, with the added suggestion that this may play a role in the bone homing of breast carcinoma metastases.[390a,403a] The basement membrane components laminin and collagen IV show a discontinuous linear pattern or are altogether absent, in contrast to the continuous pattern they exhibit in the intraductal lesions.[395,426,428] An increased amount of type V collagen is found in the desmoplastic stroma.[389] Actin stains are negative, confirming the absence of myoepithelial cells around the tumor nests. A small number of carcinomas show focal reactivity for hCG, SP-1 or other placental proteins,[407] chromogranin[393] (see p. 1614), GCDFP-15[414,427] (see p. 1613), or lactoferrin.[394]

Breast carcinomas have also shown an increased expression of T and Tn antigens (precursors to the MN blood group system), as detected by normal human sera[404] or peanut lectins.[391] In about half of the cases they also express an antigen that is cross-reactive with a major glycoprotein of the mouse mammary tumor virus.[415]

Tubular carcinoma. Tubular carcinoma has also been designated as well-differentiated carcinoma, but the latter term is not advisable because it has also been used for other well-differentiated tumors with other patterns of growth. The average age of the patients is about 50 years.[443] Grossly, tubular carcinoma suggests malignancy by virtue of its poorly circumscribed margins and hard consistency. It is characteristically small, with a mean diameter of about 1 cm.[437,440] Microscopically, it simulates a benign condition (particularly radial scar and microglandular adenosis) because of the well-differentiated nature of the glands, absence of necrosis or mitoses, and scanty pleomorphism.[438] The clues to the diagnosis are the haphazard arrangement of the glands in the stroma with absence of any organoid configuration; frequent invasion of fat at the periphery of the lesion; cellular (but often also elastotic[442]) nature of the

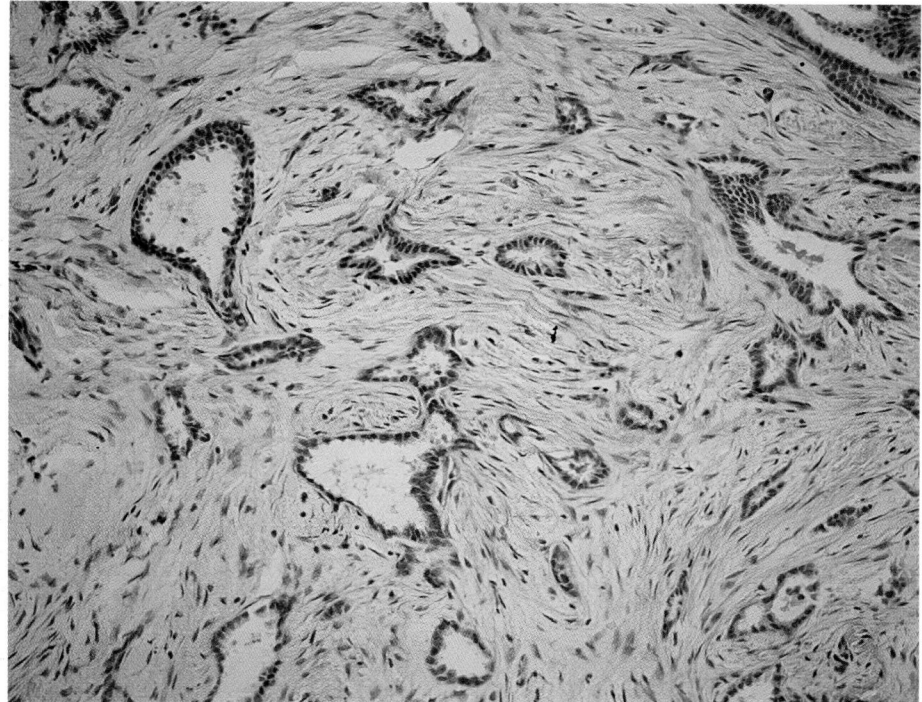

Fig. 20-52 Tubular carcinoma of breast. The angulated shape of the glands and the cellular stroma are characteristic of this lesion.

stroma; irregular and often angulated contours of the glands; open lumina with basophilic secretion; apocrine-type "snouts" in the apical cytoplasm; formation of trabecular bars; lack of a myoepithelial cell component (well appreciated in actin-stained preparations); lack of basement membrane (well seen with a PAS stain); and occurrence in two thirds or more of the cases of typical intraductal carcinoma in ducts within or outside the lesion, nearly always of micropapillary or cribriform type[430,434,437,443] (Fig. 20-52).

Because of the marked degree of cellular differentiation, it is not unusual for these tumors to be underdiagnosed as fibroadenoma or some other benign process on FNA material.[431]

Ultrastructurally, the degree of ductal differentiation is striking, but myoepithelial cells and basal lamina are lacking.[433,435] A high incidence of multicentricity (56%), history of bilateral breast carcinoma (38%), and family history of breast carcinoma (40%) were found by Lagios et al.[436] in a series of seventeen tubular carcinomas.

Metastases to axillary nodes occur in about 10% of the cases,[430,432,437] and the prognosis is excellent. In the series of McDivitt et al.,[437] only 4% of their 135 patients developed recurrent or metastatic disease during a mean follow-up period of 72 years. Local excision has been suggested by some as the therapy of choice; however, in one series this was followed by a recurrence rate of 50%.[432]

Sometimes, a tubular carcinoma pattern is seen in association with an ordinary invasive ductal carcinoma. The prognosis of these "mixed" tumors is substantially worse than for

pure tubular carcinoma,[429,432,439] although better than for the ordinary invasive ductal carcinoma when the tubular component represents the dominant element.[429,432] It is likely that series of tubular carcinomas in which the incidence of nodal metastases is high include a high proportion of "mixed" carcinomas.[441]

Cribriform carcinoma. Invasive cribriform carcinoma is a rare form of breast malignancy closely related to tubular carcinoma and sharing with it an excellent prognosis.[444,445] As the name indicates, the tumor has a cribriform appearance similar to that seen in the more common in situ counterpart, but it also exhibits stromal invasion (Fig. 20-53). This pattern is often seen in association with tubular formations, the relative proportion of the two elements determining the term used, according to the scheme proposed by Page et al.[444] The most important aspect of this concept is the realization that a breast carcinoma can be cribriform throughout yet invasive; we have seen examples of this tumor extensively invading the breast and beyond and being called in situ tumors simply because they had a cribriform pattern.

Mucinous carcinoma. Mucinous carcinoma, also known as mucoid, colloid, or gelatinous carcinoma, usually occurs in postmenopausal women.[447,453] Grossly, it is well circumscribed, crepitant to palpation, and formed by a currant jelly–like mass held together by delicate septa (Fig. 20-54). Foci of hemorrhage are frequent. Microscopically, the classic and often quoted description is that of small clusters of tumor cells "floating in a sea of mucin" (Fig. 20-55, *A*).

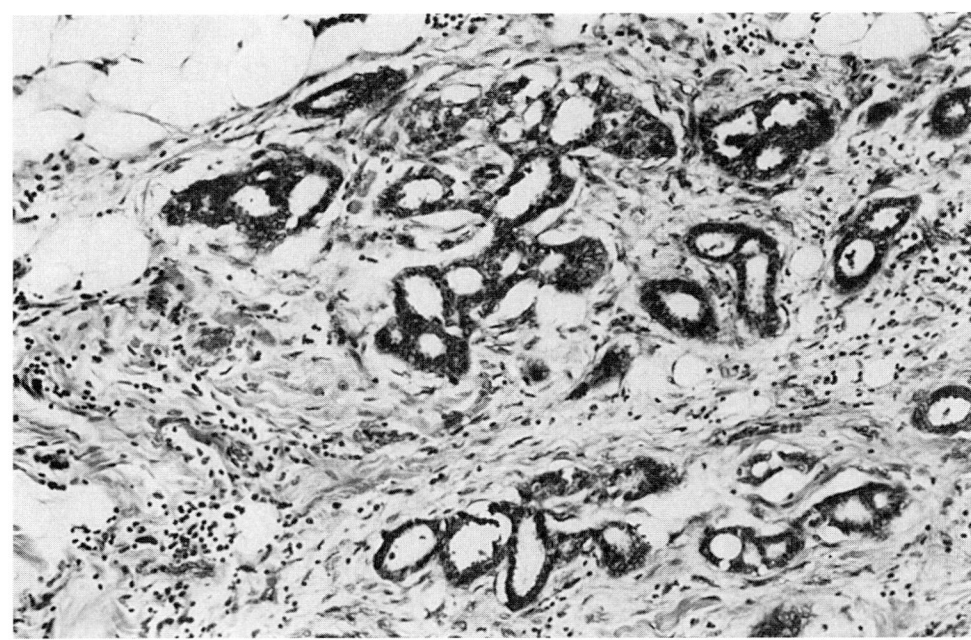

Fig. 20-53 Invasive cribriform carcinoma. Relatively well-differentiated small glands with cribriform appearance are seen infiltrating stroma. Tumor is closely related to tubular carcinoma.

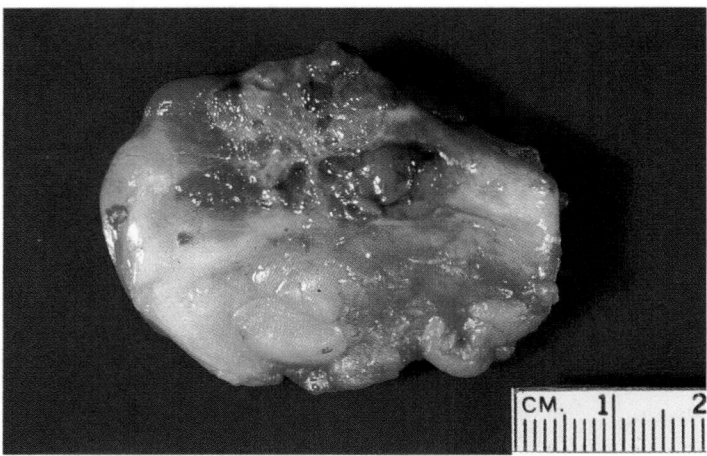

Fig. 20-54 Gross appearance of pure mucinous carcinoma of the breast. The well-circumscribed character and the gelatinous cut surface are evident.

These clusters may be solid or exhibit acinar formations. The mucin is almost entirely extracellular, and it may be of acid or neutral type.[462] Occasionally, mucinous carcinoma will consist almost entirely of mucin, and a thorough sampling will be necessary to detect the neoplastic epithelium.[458] An easily recognizable in situ component is usually absent or inconspicuous (but see later section).

Interestingly, about a fourth to nearly half of mucinous carcinomas show features suggestive of endocrine differentiation, such as argyrophilia, NSE immunoreactivity, and the presence of dense-core secretory granules by ultrastructural examination[446,450,451,456] (Fig. 20-55, *B*). This unexpected finding has raised the possibility of a link between mucinous carcinoma and so-called carcinoid tumor of the breast (see p. 1613).[450] Some authors have suggested the existence of two types of mucinous carcinoma, which they have designated as A and B, respectively.[446] Others have found that the variability of morphologic and ultrastructural features within these tumors precludes a sharp segregation,[448,449] or that such segregation has no influence on survival.[460]

It is important for prognostic reasons, and perhaps useful histogenetically, to restrict the term mucinous carcinoma to

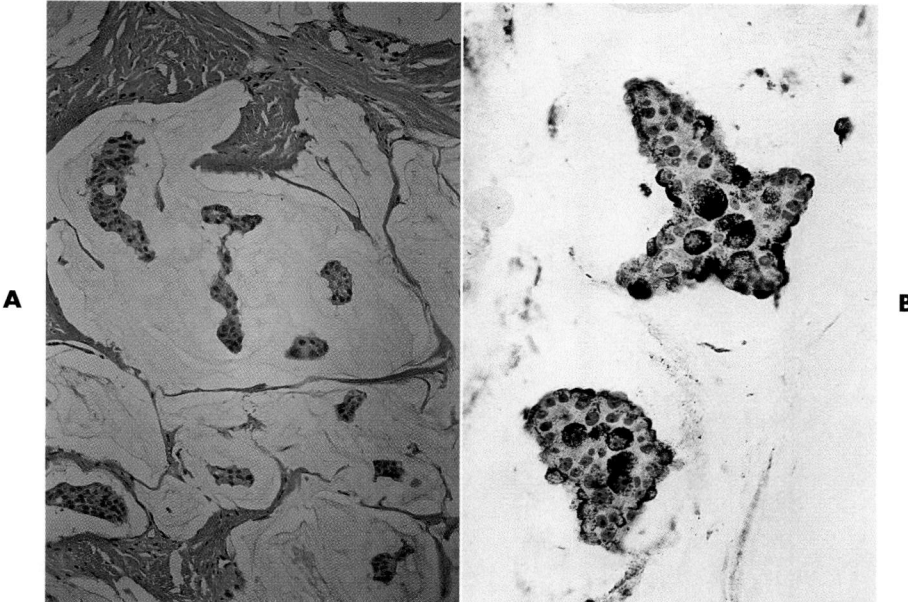

Fig. 20-55 Microscopic appearance of mucinous carcinoma of the breast. **A,** Clusters of well-differentiated tumor cells are seen floating in a sea of mucin. **B,** Argyrophilic cells present in mucinous carcinoma of the breast, indicative of neuroendocrine differentiation. (Sevier-Munger stain.)

breast neoplasms exhibiting this feature throughout ("pure" mucinous carcinomas) and to exclude (1) the "impure" or "mixed" tumors in which the mucinous pattern is admixed with an ordinary invasive ductal carcinoma[454,461] (these having a prognosis analogous to the latter) and (2) signet ring carcinomas (see p. 1619), even if technically speaking these are just as mucinous as the others. Along these lines, it should be pointed out that some degree of mucin production can be identified in over 60% of breast carcinomas. The distinctiveness of signet ring carcinoma resides in the fact that nearly all of it remains within the cell (possibly because of a blockage in secretion), and the uniqueness of mucinous carcinoma is that most of it is extracellular (see later section). In contrast to large bowel and other sites, a combination of these two patterns is very rare in the breast.

Pure mucinous carcinoma is associated with a very low incidence (2% to 4%) of nodal metastases.[453,455] The larger incidence reported in other series is probably attributable to the inclusion of "mixed" mucinous tumors. Consequently, the pure form of mucinous carcinoma carries an excellent short-term prognosis, particularly when the tumor measures less than 3 cm (or even less than 5 cm) in diameter.[447,453] However, it has been shown that deaths from this tumor can occur 12 years or more after therapy, indicating the need for long-term follow-up.[447,459] There seems to be no prognostic difference between the mucinous carcinomas with endocrine-like features and those without it.[456]

Pure mucinous carcinoma is generally regarded as an invasive type of tumor. We would like to offer an alternative point of view, i.e., that this neoplasm is partially—and sometimes entirely—a form of in situ ductal carcinoma in which some component of the mucin secretion detaches the epithelium from the underlying stroma, breaks it up in strips and nests, and engulfs it (Fig. 20-56). This process may be facilitated by an "inversion of polarity" of the mucin secretion toward the base of the cell rather than the luminal border, as shown ultrastructurally. The implication is that it is the mucin, rather than the tumor cells, that is "invading" the stroma, in a fashion analogous to that often seen in mucinous tumors of the appendix. This would explain not only the excellent prognosis of pure mucinous carcinoma, but also the seemingly paradoxic fact that nearly all the mucin produced by this tumor is extracellular. Along these lines, it should be pointed out that not all mucin-containing breast nodules represent carcinomas. Papillomas, papillary carcinomas, and ductal hyperplasia of either the florid or atypical type can also be accompanied by focal or sometimes abundant mucin secretion, which may accumulate in large extracellular pools.[452,457] Some of these lesions have been referred to as "mucocele-like tumors,"[458] but we feel that the term should be used in a descriptive rather than diagnostic sense. As in the appendix and other sites, the formation of a "mucocele" is nearly always the expression of mucin hyperproduction and extravasation by a proliferative epithelial process, which may be hyperplastic or neoplastic, benign or malignant, in situ or invasive. The key determination is the nature of that process, rather than the spectacular but relatively inconsequential presence of the "mucocele." Specifically, a thorough sampling is always mandatory.[457]

Medullary carcinoma. Medullary carcinoma usually appears in patients under 50 years of age and is said to be particularly common in Japanese women. Grossly, it is well circumscribed and may become large; it can be mistaken clinically and grossly for a fibroadenoma, but it lacks the trabeculation or whorling of the latter. Its cut surface is solid, homogeneous, and gray, sometimes exhibiting small

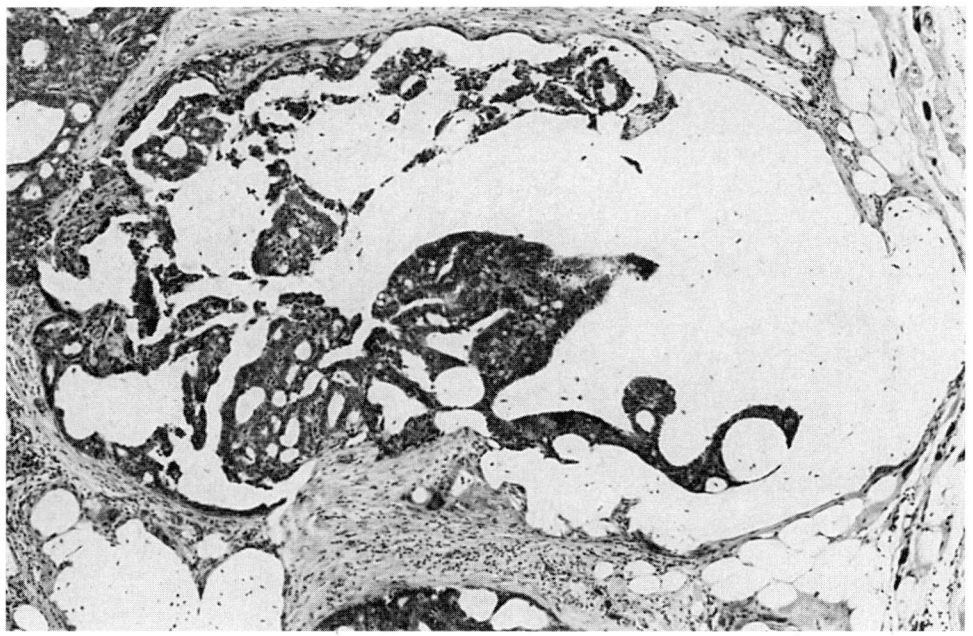

Fig. 20-56 Mucinous carcinoma. Tumor in this case is predominantly intraductal, but intraluminal mucin is detaching epithelium from underlying stroma, giving an impression of stromal invasion.

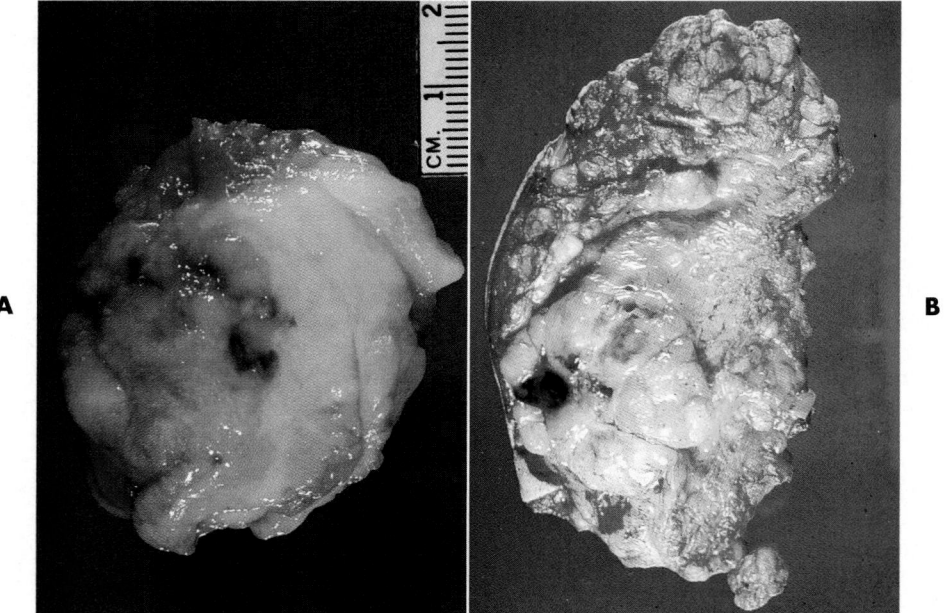

Fig. 20-57 A and **B,** Gross appearance of medullary carcinoma. Note the well-circumscribed character and fleshy appearance.

foci of necrosis (Fig. 20-57, *A* and *B*). Rare examples are partially or predominantly cystic.[468] Microscopically, the borders are always of the "pushing" type. The pattern of growth is diffuse, with minimal or no glandular differentiation or intraductal growth and absence of mucin secretion. The tumor cells are large and pleomorphic, with large nuclei and prominent nucleoli and numerous mitoses (some of them atypical). The cell borders are indistinct, giving the tumor a syncytial or sheet-like appearance somewhat reminiscent of a germ cell tumor of the embryonal carcinoma type. This is accentuated by the fact that the tumor cells located at the periphery of the clusters are more elongated and have a denser, more acidophilic cytoplasm, acquiring a vague resemblance to syncytiotrophoblast. Spindle cell metaplasia, bizarre tumor giant cells, extensive necrosis, and the absence of calcification are other common features.

A constant microscopic component is a prominent lymphoplasmacytic infiltrate at the periphery of the tumor, which is thought to represent a reaction of the host tissues to the neoplasm (Fig. 20-58). Most of the lymphocytes are of the peripheral T-cell type and do not differ phenotypically from those seen in ordinary ductal carcinomas[463,466]; most of the plasma cells are of the IgA-producing type; some of the tumor cells also stain for IgA and for secretory component.[469] Ultrastructurally, the cells of medullary carcinoma do not seem to have distinctive features, despite early statements to the contrary.[467] Immunohistochemically, they share the markers of ordinary invasive ductal carcinoma but are more commonly positive for S-100 protein.[465] The interesting observation has been made that medullary carcinomas lack keratin 19, in contrast to ordinary ductal carcinoma; however, this is also true for poorly differentiated tumors of nonmedullary type.[464a] Another interesting feature is the frequent expression of HLA-DR antigen, this being a possible reason for the prominent lymphocytic infiltration.[478]

Axillary lymph node metastases are common, but they are usually few in number and limited to the low axillary group. The prognosis for medullary carcinoma is better than for the ordinary invasive ductal carcinoma, a fact already apparent in the early reports on this tumor.[464,472,474] In the series of Ridolfi et al.,[475] the 10-year survival rate was 84% as opposed to 63% for ordinary ductal carcinomas. The prognosis was particularly good for tumors that were smaller than 3 cm, and it remained better than for ductal carcinoma even when nodal metastases were present.

The terms atypical medullary carcinoma and invasive ductal carcinoma with medullary features have been used for tumors that depart somewhat from the foregoing definition, but the delineation of criteria for their recognition remains imprecise.[475,477] We have too often seen the term medullary carcinoma misused for highly cellular breast carcinomas that behaved in a very aggressive fashion, and we caution the reader to use this term only when all the pathologic features necessary for this diagnosis are present.[473] As a matter of fact, we wonder whether medullary carcinoma constitutes a bona fide subtype of breast carcinoma as currently defined.[466a,476] We are particularly concerned about the lack of precise boundaries between it and the following tumors: the predominantly solid (undifferentiated) form of

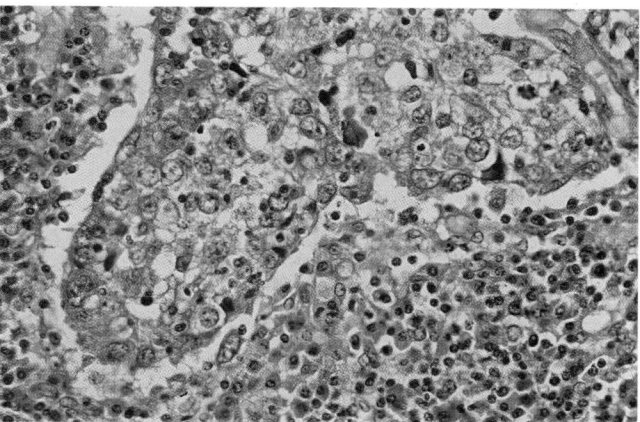

Fig. 20-58 Medullary carcinoma. The large tumor cells grow in a "syncytial" fashion and are sharply separated from the surrounding stroma, which is heavily infiltrated by lymphocytes and plasma cells.

invasive ductal carcinoma; carcinoma with germ cell–like features, as also seen in the lung, the gastrointestinal tract, and other sites; and so-called lymphoepithelioma-like carcinoma.[470] In regard to the latter, it should be noted that no evidence of EBV participation has been found in medullary carcinoma.[471a]

Invasive papillary carcinoma. Most papillary carcinomas of the breast are entirely or predominantly in situ lesions; these have been discussed on p. 1597. The invasive component of a papillary carcinoma also may be papillary or have the features of an ordinary ductal-type carcinoma; the prognosis is substantially better for the former. This tumor is said to occur more frequently among whites and postmenopausal women,[481] but, on the whole, it remains a very rare entity. Part of the problem may be that although the recognition of an ordinary ductal-type carcinoma offers no difficulties, the documentation of invasion in tumors that maintain a well-differentiated pattern may not be as clearcut. For instance, some of the cases reported as intracystic papillary carcinomas[479] may well represent invasive papillary carcinomas with a "pushing" pattern of growth. The distinctive features of these tumors can be appreciated on FNA specimens.[480]

Apocrine carcinoma. Apocrine carcinoma is a very rare form of breast malignancy (ranging from 1% to 4% of all cases), at least when defined as composed entirely or predominantly of apocrine-type epithelium.[482] The large tumor cells have an abundant acidophilic, somewhat granular cytoplasm, which may contain eosinophilic or golden brown granules that are strongly PAS positive. The nuclei are vesicular and nucleoli are prominent. Glandular differentiation is usually found, the luminal portion of the tumor having a characteristic bulbous expansion ("apocrine snout"). Some of these tumors present as mural nodules within a cyst lined by benign apocrine-type epithelium. Ultrastructurally, the cells of apocrine carcinoma show prominent mitochondria (some with abnormal cristae) and a variable number of large

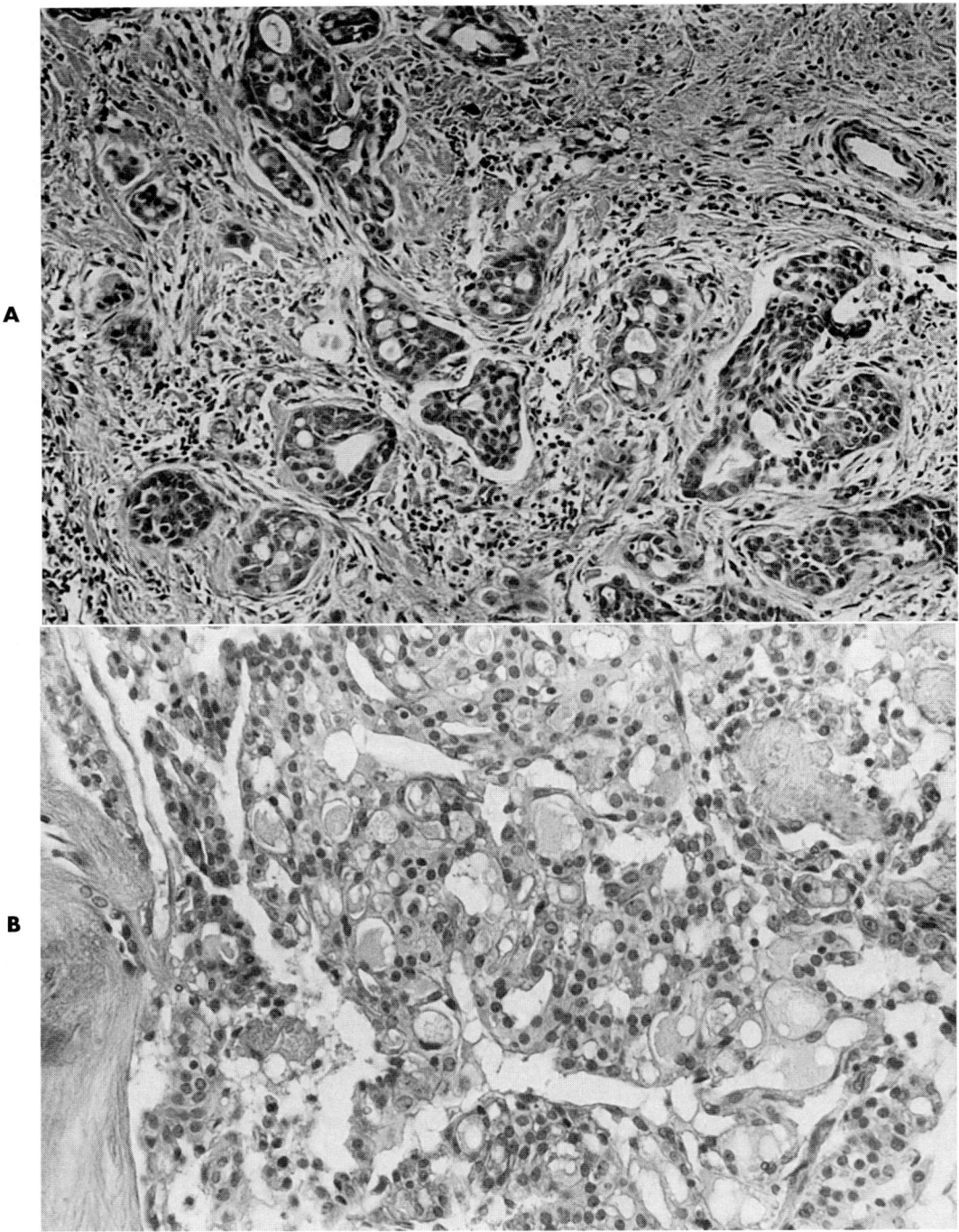

Fig. 20-59 **A,** Breast carcinoma in 10-year-old girl. Small glands composed of atypical cell infiltrate mammary stroma. Total mastectomy was performed. Patient is alive and well 6 years later. **B,** Secretory carcinoma of breast. Note well-differentiated nature of neoplastic cells and large amount of intracellular and extracellular secretory material. This tumor occurred in 16-year-old girl, and regional lymph nodes were negative. (**A** Courtesy Dr. W.S. Medart, Savannah, GA. **B** Courtesy Dr. L. Beauchesne and Dr. C. Beauchesne, Sherbrooke, Canada.)

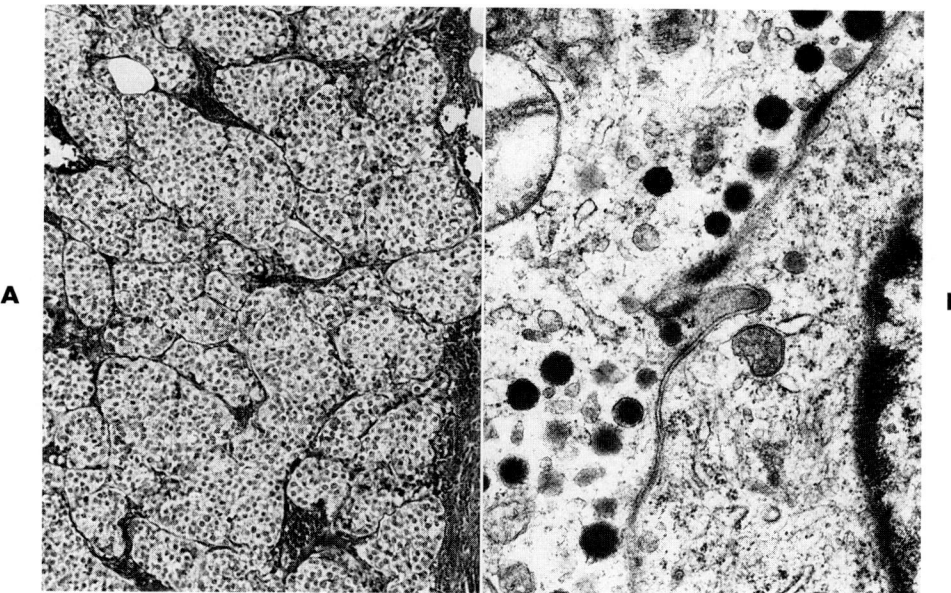

Fig. 20-60 A, So-called carcinoid tumor of breast. Sharply outlined nests of tumor cells are separated by fibrovascular stroma. Cells are relatively uniform in size and shape, and their cytoplasm has fine granularity. Tumor was positive for argyrophilic stains. **B,** Electron microscopic appearance of breast carcinoma with neuroendocrine differentiation. Primarily ectoplasmic dense core neurosecretory type granules ranging in size from 140 to 225 nm are seen. (×29,400.) (Courtesy Dr. Robert A. Erlandson, Memorial Sloan-Kettering Cancer Center.)

(400 to 600 nm) membrane-bound vesicles with dense homogeneous osmophilic cores.[485] Immunohistochemically, there is reactivity for GCDFP-15.[484] The gene coding for this marker is located in chromosome 7q and is identical to the gene of the prolactin-inducible protein (PIP); the expression of this gene in apocrine carcinoma has been demonstrated with in situ hybridization techniques.[484a,486]

Since apocrine changes in the breast are usually indicative of benignancy (even when the cells exhibit prominent nucleolar enlargement), the diagnosis of apocrine carcinoma should be made only when the architectural features are clearly those of a malignant tumor. It is also important to limit the diagnosis of apocrine carcinoma to malignant tumors in which the apocrine change is widespread, in view of the fact that focal apocrine differentiation (as detected by GCDFP-15) can be detected in close to 10% of ordinary carcinomas.[484] Finally, it should be noted that although apocrine carcinoma is usually a variant of either in situ or invasive ductal carcinoma, apocrine differentiation has also been described in in situ and invasive lobular carcinoma.[483]

Juvenile (secretory) carcinoma. This rare form of breast carcinoma is seen primarily in children, but it can also occur in adults.[488,491,493] Grossly, it is well circumscribed and usually small. The microscopic appearance is distinctive. The margins are of the "pushing" type, and prominent hyalinization is often present in the central portion. The microscopic appearance is distinctive. Tubuloalveolar and focally papillary formations lined by cells with a vacuolated (sometimes hypernephroid) cytoplasm are seen forming lumina filled by an eosinophilic PAS-positive secretion.[490,493] Nucleoli may be prominent, but mitoses are very scanty. Ultrastructurally, the tumor cells contain numerous membrane-bound intracytoplasmic secretory vacuoles[487] (Fig. 20-59).

Immunohistochemically, there is strong reactivity for alpha-lactalbumin and S-100 protein. accompanied by variable expression of GCDF-15 and CEA.[489]

The overall prognosis is excellent, most series quoting a 5-year survival rate close to 100%.[490] Local recurrences and nodal metastases can develop, sometimes very late in the course of the disease.[488,492,493] Death resulting from disseminated tumor has been recorded only exceptionally.[493]

Carcinomas with neuroendocrine features (including so-called carcinoid tumor). The term carcinoid tumor was originally proposed for a type of invasive ductal carcinoma exhibiting features consistent with endocrine differentiation.[500] In general, the clinical presentation is no different from that of the ordinary breast carcinoma, although a case with bilateral tumors in a male has been reported associated with norepinephrine and ACTH secretion.[502] Specifically, none of the patients has had carcinoid syndrome, even in the presence of widespread disease. Multicentricity and bilaterality can occur.[500] There are no distinctive gross features.

Microscopically, the tumor cells are small, arranged in solid nests separated by fibrous tissue (Fig. 20-60, A). Ribbons and rosette-like formations may be formed. Mitoses are generally rare. The presence of an intraductal component and of mucin secretion has been detected in a minority of the cases.[500] The microscopic diagnosis includes lobular carci-

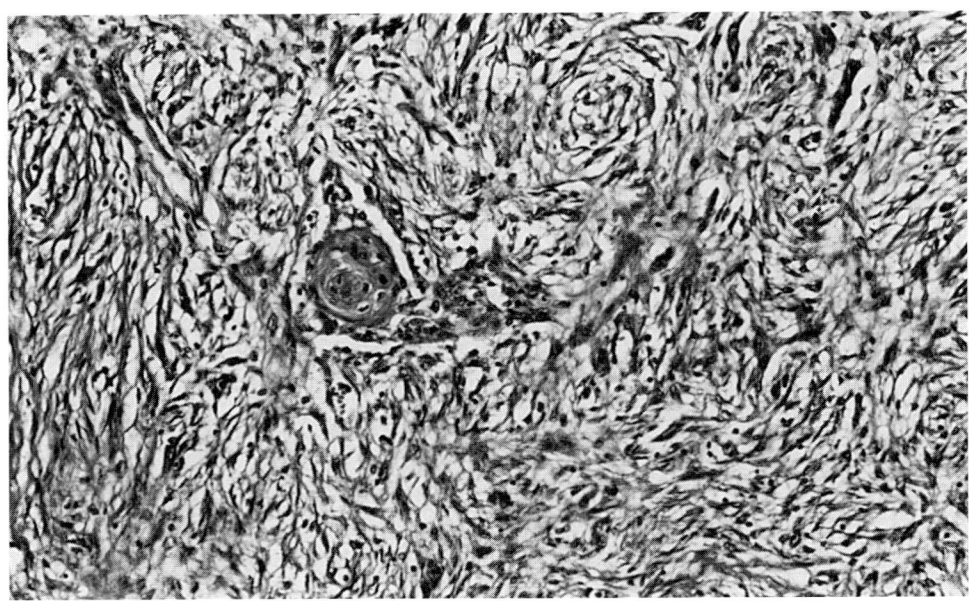

Fig. 20-61 Metaplastic carcinoma. Small area of squamous cell carcinoma close to center of photograph merges with spindle-cell component of mesenchymal appearance.

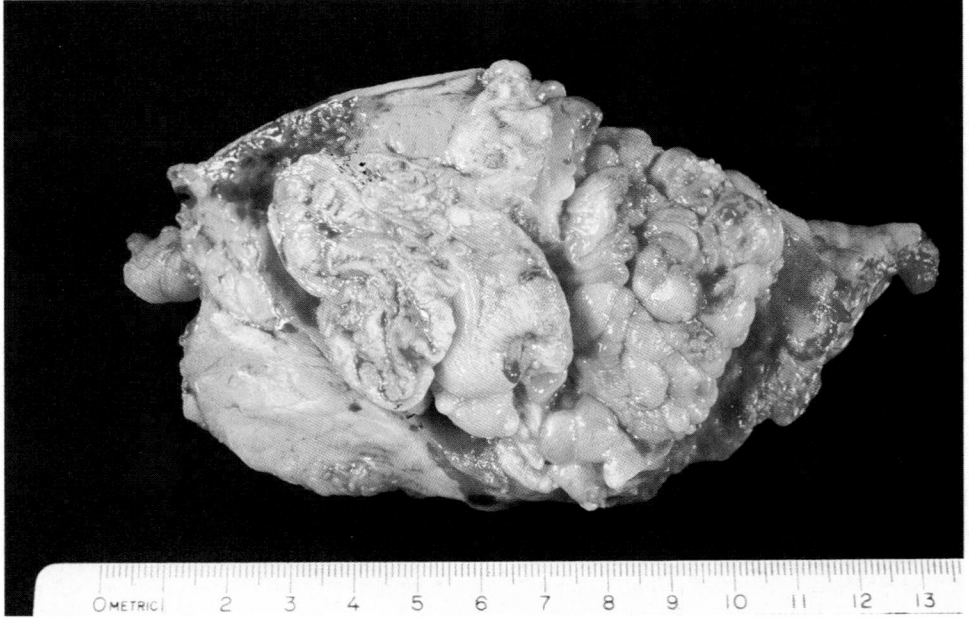

Fig. 20-62 Gross appearance of metaplastic carcinoma. A large, fleshy mass is seen protruding inside a cystic cavity. Microscopically, this tumor showed an admixture of squamous and spindle elements.

noma and a metastasis to the breast of a carcinoid tumor located elsewhere.

The tumor cells of carcinoid tumor of the breast are argyrophilic but not argentaffin and are found to contain dense-core secretory granules of various types ultrastructurally[497,500] (Fig. 20-60, *B*).

The nature of this neoplasm has been controversial from the very first description.[503,509] It has even been suggested

that the argyrophilia and the dense-core secretory granules are not an indication of neuroendocrine differentiation at all but rather of lactalbumin secretion by the tumor cells.[498] To be sure, not all membrane-bound dense core cytoplasmic granules are of neurosecretory type.[495] However, the immunohistochemical positivity that has been obtained for chromogranin, synaptophysin, and neuron-specific enolase,[496,506,511,513] and in some instances for specific hormone peptides,[505,508] would

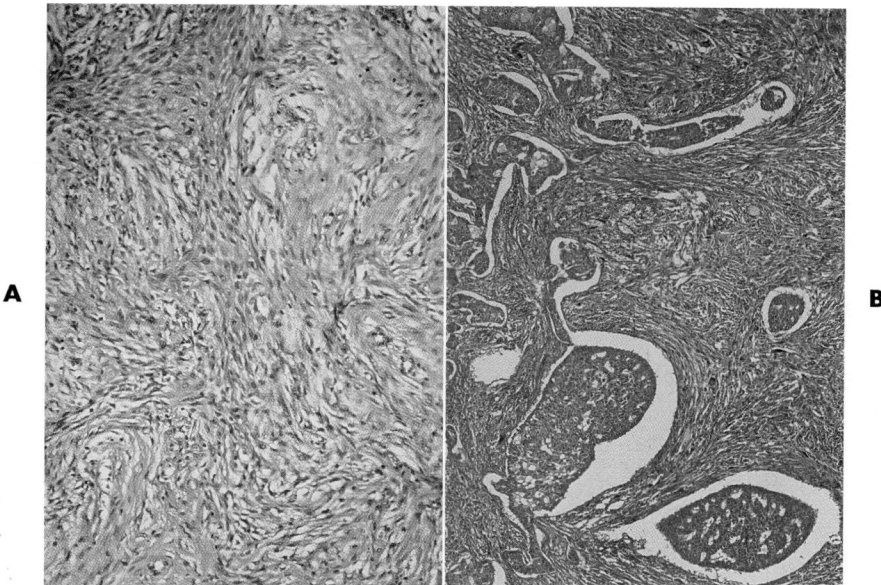

Fig. 20-63 Metaplastic carcinoma. The tumor shown in **A** contains only spindle cells. The tumor shown in **B** has a biphasic appearance that has led to terms such as carcinosarcoma.

seem to verify that these tumors do indeed exhibit signs of endocrine differentiation. Whether this justifies calling them carcinoid tumors is another matter. It seems to us that they are the example of a phenomenon similar to that described in practically all other organs (i.e., that of a carcinoma arising from primitive epithelial cells with the capacity to differentiate focally or extensively towards an endocrine line).[503] Such carcinomas otherwise resemble ordinary ductal-type carcinoma in most other ways: occasional presence of an in situ component, frequent positivity for estrogen receptors, pattern of metastases, and outcome.[507] Therefore we like to view and designate this tumor as invasive ductal carcinoma with (neuro) endocrine differentiation or features, a term we prefer to the alternative designation argyrophilic carcinoma.[494,510] According to Azzopardi et al.,[494] this tumor constitutes about 5% of all breast carcinomas.

It should be mentioned here that there are breast carcinomas of other morphologic patterns in which endocrine features have been found: the already mentioned mucinous carcinoma[501] (see p. 1607), small cell (oat cell) carcinoma,[512] invasive ductal-type carcinomas of ordinary type,[504,510] and a variant of in situ ductal carcinoma.[499] Interestingly, carcinoid tumors of the conventional type are virtually nonexistent in the breast. We have seen only one case that had morphologic and histochemical features (argentaffinity) identical to those of classic (insular) carcinoid tumors of midgut derivation; remarkably, it was associated with the presence of argentaffin cells in the adjacent breast epithelium.

Metaplastic carcinoma. Metaplastic carcinoma is a generic term for breast carcinoma of ductal type in which the predominant component of the neoplasm has an appearance other than epithelial and glandular and more in keeping with another cell type (Figs. 20-61 to 20-63). As such, the

designation is too encompassing and imprecise and should not be used without a qualifier. It includes the following categories:

1 A tumor equivalent to the one designated in other sites (notably the upper aerodigestive tract and lung) as *sarcomatoid carcinoma,* carcinoma with sarcoma-like stroma, and carcinosarcoma (Fig. 20-61). Grossly, it tends to be well circumscribed. Microscopically, the sarcoma-like component may resemble fibrosarcoma, malignant fibrous histiocytoma, chondrosarcoma, osteosarcoma, rhabdomyosarcoma, angiosarcoma, or a combination of these various patterns.[515,519,521,522] There may be a gradual transition from carcinomatous to sarcoma-like elements,[518] or the separation between them can be sharp (Fig. 20-63, *B*). When the latter is the case, the term *carcinosarcoma* tends to be used.[528,532] Tumors having overt carcinomas with direct transition to a cartilaginous and/or osseous matrix without an intervening spindle-cell zone or osteoclastic giant cells have been referred to as "matrix-producing carcinomas,"[531] but the distinction seems to be of little clinical value and dubious biologic significance.[517,525]

Immunohistochemically, the sarcoma-like elements of these tumors have usually acquired vimentin positivity and other features of a mesenchymal nature ("phenotypical switch") but occasionally still retain epithelial markers.[516,527]

2 *Spindle-cell carcinoma.* The overt carcinomatous component of these tumors, when present, may have invasive or in situ ductal features, and it may be entirely squamous.[530] The spindle-cell component, which may be deceptively bland, forms abundant fibrocollagenous stroma with feathered, myxoid, angioid, and storiform patterns[533a] (Fig. 20-63, *A*). Areas of merging between the epithelial and the spindle component are common. The latter foci

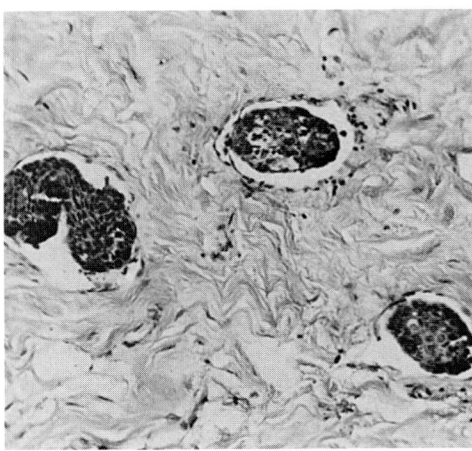

Fig. 20-64 Widespread invasion of dermal lymphatics in inflammatory carcinoma.

are usually immunoreactive for keratin. A myoepithelial participation in the genesis of these tumors has been suggested.[526]

3 *Carcinoma with osteoclastic giant cells.*[514,529,533] When these cells appear in conjunction with sarcoma-like elements, the tumor should be regarded as a variant of the first category listed. When they are seen in the stroma of what is otherwise a typical invasive ductal-type carcinoma lacking sarcomatoid foci, the tumor should be placed in a category of its own but closer to ordinary ductal carcinoma. All available evidence suggests that the osteoclast-like elements are of histiocytic nature and that they form from fusion of mononuclear precursors.[520,523]

4 *Squamous cell carcinoma.* Although technically speaking this represents a form of tumor metaplasia, it differs so substantially from the others that we thought of discussing it separately (see next section).

• • •

The differential diagnosis of these tumor types (particularly the first two categories) includes phylloides tumor and primary breast sarcoma.

On the whole, the behavior of metaplastic carcinoma seems to be more aggressive than that of ordinary invasive ductal-type carcinoma.[521,524] The differences in survival among the various subgroups are rather minor, although some authors have suggested a worse prognosis for the "carcinosarcoma" subgroup. Metastases tend to be hematogenous rather than to lymph nodes, in keeping with the sarcomatous phenotype.[521] The size of the neoplasm at the time of initial excision is one of the best predictors of survival.[524]

Squamous cell carcinoma and related tumors. Squamous cell carcinoma is an extremely rare variant of breast tumor.[535,543] Tumors of cutaneous origin and those in which the squamous component is a portion of an otherwise typical phylloides tumor should be excluded. It is also important not to misinterpret the syncytial areas of medullary carcinoma or the partial apocrine changes sometimes seen in other tumors as representing squamous changes.

The gross appearance of squamous cell carcinoma differs little from that of the usual breast carcinomas, although sometimes a large central cyst filled with keratin can be identified. Microscopically, most cases seem to represent instances of squamous metaplasia in ductal carcinoma, indicating that squamous cell carcinoma could be viewed as a special type of metaplastic carcinoma.[541] This view is reinforced by the existence of so-called spindle-cell carcinoma, in which a well-differentiated squamous component merges with a prominent spindle-cell sarcomatoid component[534,540] (see p. 1615). Occasionally, the tumor is accompanied by a prominent myxoid stroma.[539]

Two further variants are *acantholytic squamous cell carcinoma,* in which the lack of cohesiveness of tumor cells results in a pseudovascular or pseudoglandular appearance,[537] and *adenosquamous carcinoma.*[542,545] Some examples of the latter tumor type have been designated as mucoepidermoid carcinoma,[538] a term that should be avoided except for those tumors having cytoarchitectural features analogous to those of their salivary gland counterparts (see p. 1628).

It is difficult to ascertain what the prognosis of squamous cell carcinoma is, in view of the differences in diagnostic criteria from series to series and the rarity of the disease. In the series of Wargotz et al.,[544] the 5-year disease-specific survival rate was 63%. On the whole, the behavior of this tumor does not seem to be substantially different from that of ordinary ductal-type invasive carcinoma.[534,536] This may not hold true for the acantholytic variant, which seems to be associated with a very aggressive course,[537] or for the low-grade adenosquamous carcinoma, which is said to have a favorable prognosis.[542]

Spread-related variants
Inflammatory carcinoma. The term inflammatory carcinoma was originally used in a clinical sense for a type of breast carcinoma in which the entire breast was reddened and warm, with widespread edema of the skin, thus simulating the appearance of mastitis. Pathologic studies in some of those cases revealed the lesion to be an undifferentiated carcinoma with widespread carcinomatosis of the dermal lymphatic vessels (Fig. 20-64). This led to the belief that an "inflammatory" clinical appearance always corresponded pathologically to dermal lymphatic permeation and vice versa. This assumption is not always correct. Patients may have inflammatory carcinoma clinically in the absence of dermal invasion; conversely, widespread permeation of dermal lymphatics can be seen in the absence of the clinical features of inflammatory carcinoma (so-called "occult" inflammatory carcinoma[551]). From a prognostic standpoint, the presence of dermal lymphatic permeation on microscopic examination is a sign of ominous prognosis, whether the clinical appearance is that of an inflammatory carcinoma or not.[548,549,551] The clinical recognition of this entity by an experienced observer is also reliable and associated with a poor prognosis, but ideally it should be accompanied by a skin biopsy showing dermal lymphatic involvement before the tumor is deemed inoperable.[550] Some authors have recommended discarding the term inflammatory carcinoma altogether.[548] The choice of therapy for this neoplasm remains highly controversial.[546,547,552]

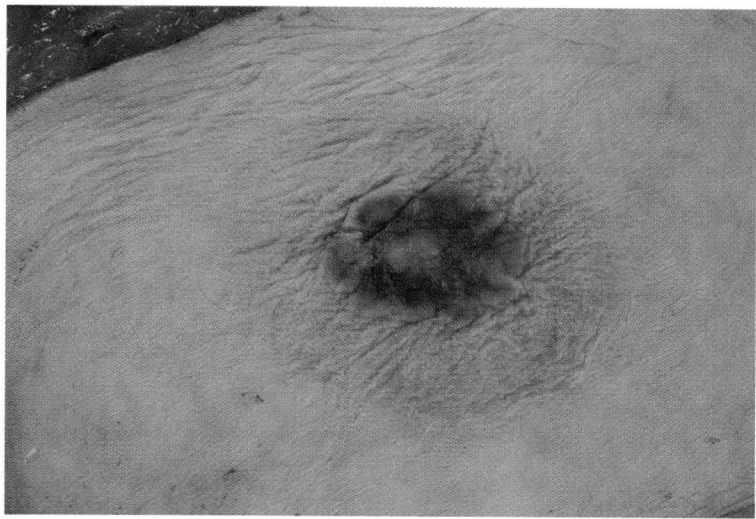

Fig. 20-65 Gross appearance of Paget's disease of the nipple. There was underlying carcinoma.

Paget's disease. Paget's disease is the name given to a crusted lesion of the nipple caused by breast carcinoma, as originally described by Sir James Paget in 1874.[566] It is accompanied in nearly all instances by an underlying breast carcinoma of in situ ductal type, with or without associated stromal invasion. In this regard, the presence of Paget's disease is only a secondary, albeit dramatic, feature of the tumor. The management and prognosis depend largely on the intraductal versus invasive nature of the underlying carcinoma and on the presence or absence of axillary lymph node involvement, rather than on the presence or appearance of the intraepithelial component in the nipple.[567]

Clinically, these weeping, eczema-like lesions are centered in the nipple (Fig. 20-65). Later they may involve the areola and surrounding epidermis, but they rarely extend more than a few centimeters. If a definite mass can be palpated beneath the diseased nipple, the underlying tumor will have an invasive component in over 90% of the cases. Conversely, 66% of the cases without a palpable mass are exclusively intraductal.[553]

Microscopically, large clear cells with atypical nuclei are seen within the epidermis, usually concentrated along the basal layer but also permeating the malpighian layer (Fig. 20-66, A). The cells can be isolated or in clusters, and sometimes they form small glandular structures. In rare instances they have an anaplastic appearance.[568] Occasionally, intracytoplasmic melanin granules are present, a feature that may result in a mistaken diagnosis of malignant melanoma; these granules have probably been transferred from neighboring melanocytes by the process of cytocrinia[554] (Plate XVI-A). The underlying breast carcinoma is always of ductal type and is composed of cells similar to those present within the nipple. If enough sections are taken, a connection between the carcinoma within the duct and the Paget's disease will be demonstrated in most instances. However, in some cases the underlying tumor is found 2 cm or more from the nipple.[567]

Mucin stains may or may not be positive, in contrast to their almost universal presence in extramammary Paget's

disease.[564,570] Ultrastructurally, the tumor cells have microvilli and other features indicative of glandular differentiation.[569] Immunohistochemically, they show reactivity for EMA and the related milk fat globule membrane antigen, CEA (at least when using polyclonal antibodies), low-molecular-weight keratin, and (in half of the cases) GCDFP-15[555,559,565,572] (Fig. 20-66, B). In general, they are negative for S-100 protein and involucrin.[565]

The main differential diagnosis is with Bowen's disease and malignant melanoma. Examples of these disorders located in the nipple have been reported,[573] and there is no reason why they could not involve this structure. We can only say that, in our experience, whenever this differential diagnosis was considered for a lesion of the nipple (because of pigmentation, transepidermal atypia, or any other reason), the definitive diagnosis invariably turned out to be Paget's disease.

The heated controversies in the past regarding the glandular versus keratinocytic versus melanocytic origin of Paget's disease have subsided. There can no longer be any doubt that Paget's cells exhibit glandular differentiation.[563] However, a point still unsettled is whether the Paget's cells in the nipple have migrated there from deeper ductal structures (probably as a result of keratinocyte-induced chemotaxis[557]) or whether they represent an in situ malignant transformation either of the intraepidermal portion of the mammary ducts or of basally located multipotential epithelial cells capable of glandular differentiation. The similarities in immunohistochemical profile and oncogene expression (such as c-*erb* B-2 or *ras* 21) favor the former.[556,558,561,562,574] On the other hand, the existence of rare cases of Paget's disease without underlying ductal carcinoma or with very limited in situ carcinoma of the most distal lactiferous ducts suggests that in some cases the latter mechanism may be operating.[560] In this regard, the observation made by Toker[571] about the presence of clear cells in nipples without clinical evidence of Paget's disease and without microscopic evidence of breast carcinoma is of

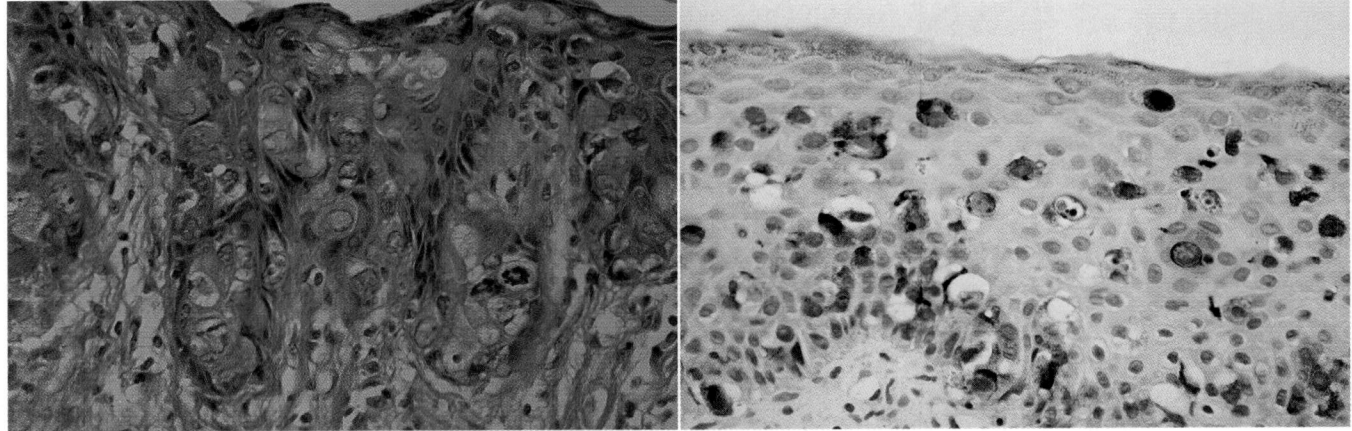

Fig. 20-66 Paget's disease of the breast. **A,** Large acidophilic cells are present in an intraepidermal location, clearly distinguishable from adjacent keratinocytes. **B,** Strong immunoreactivity of Paget's cells for epithelial membrane antigen.

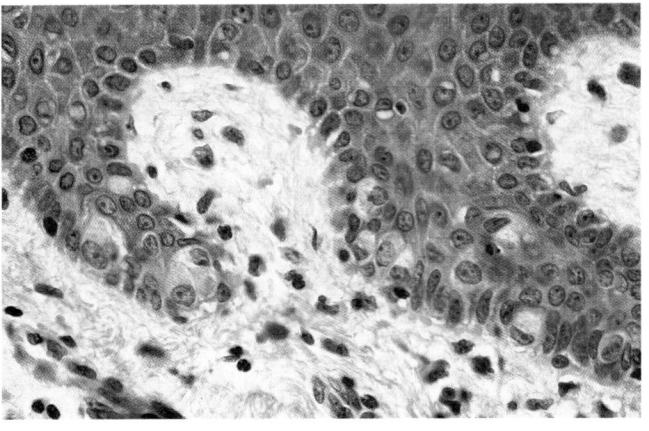

Fig. 20-67 Biopsy of nipple showing scattered clear cells in the basal layer. These cells show a mild degree of nuclear atypia and were immunohistochemically similar to the cells of Paget's disease.

great interest. We have also observed these cells (although not nearly with that frequency) and found not only that they react immunohistochemically like Paget's cells but also that they may exhibit mild nuclear atypical changes, suggesting the possibility of a dysplastic or "pre-Paget's" change (Fig. 20-67). From a practical standpoint, these cells are distinguished from those of Paget's disease because of the lack of eczema-like changes clinically and the absence of clear-cut cytologic features of malignancy.

Invasive lobular carcinoma (ILC)

Classic type. In its most characteristic form, invasive lobular carcinoma (ILC) is characterized by the presence of small and relatively uniform tumor cells growing singly, in Indian file, and in a concentric ("pagetoid") fashion around lobules involved by in situ lobular neoplasia[575] (Figs. 20-68 and 20-69). Most of the breast tumors designated in the past as small cell carcinomas belong to this category. Gland formation is not a feature of classic ILC. The stroma is usually abundant, is of dense fibrous type, and contains foci of periductal and perivenous elastosis in virtually every case. A lymphocytic infiltrate may be present, sometimes so intense as to obscure the neoplastic component.[580]

It is currently accepted that the diagnosis of ILC can be made in the presence of these cytoarchitectural features even if an in situ component is absent.[577,579] Conversely, an invasive tumor should not be called ILC simply because it is associated with in situ lobular neoplasia; rather, it should have the features of lobular carcinoma in the invasive component itself in order to deserve this designation.

The histochemical, ultrastructural, and immunohistochemical features of ILC are analogous to those described for its in situ counterpart. In contrast to invasive ductal carcinoma, ILC usually shows no accumulation of p53 protein.[576]

The main differential diagnosis of ILC is with IDC. The small size and uniformity of the cells and their lack of cohesiveness are the most important distinguishing features. It should be remarked, however, that in many cases the distinction is difficult and to a large extent subjective, as borne out by the fact that the incidence of ILC ranges from 0.7% to 20% in the published series.[578] Other entities that can be confused with ILC are so-called carcinoid tumor and malignant lymphoma. The latter possibility arises more often when ILC metastasizes to axillary nodes and other sites, particularly the eyelid; we have seen several cases misdiagnosed as large cell malignant lymphoma or malignant histiocytosis because of their diffuse pattern of growth and the histiocyte-like appearance of the tumor cells. Reactions for keratin, EMA, CEA, LCA, and an old-fashioned mucicarmine stain should eliminate any problems not resolved by the examination of the routinely stained slides.

Histiocytoid carcinoma. Histiocytoid carcinoma is characterized by a diffuse pattern of growth by tumor cells dis-

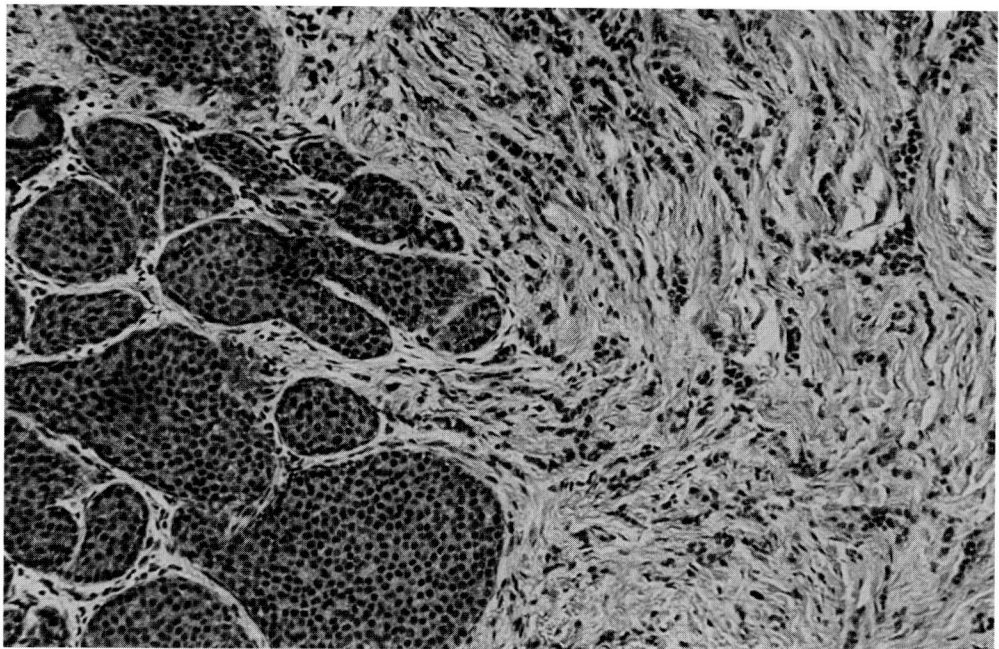

Fig. 20-68 Lobular carcinoma in situ with areas of invasive lobular carcinoma of small cell type. In situ areas demonstrate complete packing of individual lobules by uniform cells.

playing abundant granular, foamy cytoplasm.[583] It may simulate the appearance of a granular cell tumor, hence the recently proposed synonym *myoblastoid carcinoma*.[581] This tumor type is currently viewed as a variant of invasive lobular carcinoma exhibiting apocrine differentiation, as evidenced by immunohistochemical reactivity for GCDFP-15 and the demonstration of mRNA for the related prolactin-inducible protein (PIP) by in situ hybridization.[581,585a]

Histiocytoid carcinoma should also be distinguished from *lipid-rich carcinoma*. The latter is simply a form of breast carcinoma showing lipid accumulation in the cytoplasm of the tumor cells.[582,584,585]

Signet ring carcinoma. Signet ring carcinoma is a type of breast carcinoma in which a significant number of tumor cells show intracytoplasmic mucin accumulation, resulting in the typical signet ring appearance.[588] Unfortunately, the term "significant" is used differently by different people. Some will place a tumor into this category only if the majority of the cells have a signet ring morphology, whereas others would settle for a much lesser number.[586,587a] In any event, it is important to sharply separate this tumor from mucinous carcinoma because of their vastly different prognoses, even if occasionally the two types have been found to coexist (see p. 1607).

Most cases of signet ring carcinoma show cytoarchitectural features (such as small cell size, uniformity, and dissociation) similar to those of classic ILC and sometimes coexist with it.[590] Furthermore, it is not rare for in situ or invasive lobular carcinoma to contain scattered signet ring cells.[591] Because of these reasons, most cases of signet ring carcinoma are regarded as variants of ILC.[589,592] Some, however,

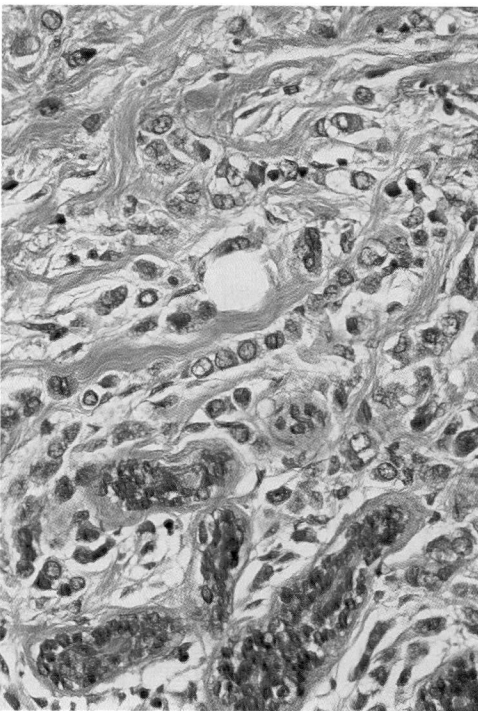

Fig. 20-69 Invasive lobular carcinoma. The tumor cells are small and uniform with round nuclei and grow in an Indian-file fashion.

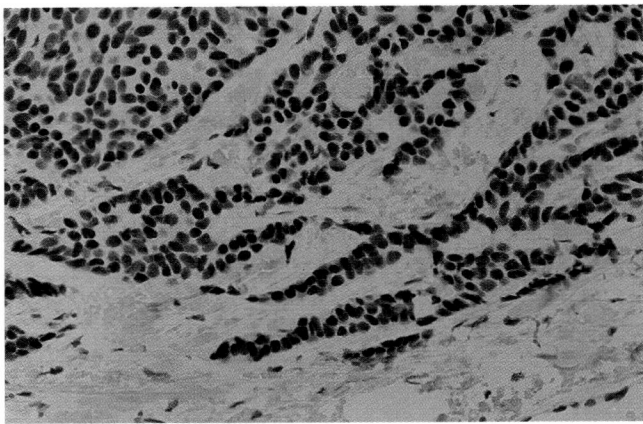

Fig. 20-70 Immunocytochemical stain for estrogen receptors in invasive breast carcinoma. The strong nuclear positivity in tumor cells is shown against a negative cytoplasmic and stromal background.

are probably more closely related to ductal carcinoma of either invasive[588] or in situ type.[587]

The intracellular mucin accumulation resulting in the signet ring appearance is probably the result of a blockage in secretion resulting from deletion of one or more of the enzymes needed for this extremely complex process. Ultrastructurally it is manifested in its more extreme form by a large membrane-bound vacuole of varying but usually low electron density.[593] This is a different process from that of intracellular lumen formation, which is characterized ultrastructurally by a microvillus-coated cavity and which appears as a bull's-eye on light microscopic examination.

Other types. Some authors restrict their diagnosis of ILC to tumors having the features described for the classic type and for some of the signet ring carcinomas. Others have expanded considerably the concept and include in this category tumors that traditionally have been placed into the IDC category.[594,597,599] Cases having closely aggregated cells, solid pattern, trabecular pattern, loose alveolar pattern, and spindle-cell chains have been accepted as ILC, *as long as the relatively bland and homogeneous cytologic appearance was maintained.* Perhaps the most distinctive of these forms is the alveolar variant, in which the tumor cells are arranged in sharply outlined groups separated by fibrous tissue sometimes containing osteoclast-like giant cells.[600,601] Yet another variation is represented by *tubulolobular carcinoma,*[598] in which typical areas of ILC merge with small tubules with a minute or undetectable lumen ("closed" or "almost closed" tubules). A converse approach has been taken more recently, and that consists of including tumors with pleomorphic nuclear features into the ILC *as long as the infiltrating pattern* of classic ILC is maintained. Such tumors have been designated as the *pleomorphic variant* of ILC[602]; the further suggestion has been made that this tumor shows apocrine differentiation.[596]

The cytologic and/or architectural similarities between these various forms and classic ILC are undeniable. The problem, however, is that the more the concept of ILC is

widened and to some extent diluted, the less distinct the entity becomes and the less significant (or at least the less uniform) its clinical connotations are.[595]

Mixed ductal and lobular carcinoma

Biphasic carcinomas composed in part of a component with definite features of invasive ductal carcinoma and in part of a component with definite features of invasive lobular carcinoma do occur, but they are very rare. These tumors, of course, should be distinguished from the cases in which two separate neoplasms of different microscopic appearances are present in the same breast.

Undetermined (unclassified) carcinoma

This category includes all cases of invasive carcinoma in which features of ductal or lobular type are not definite enough to place it into either category. Azzopardi[603] places 3% to 4% of the invasive breast carcinomas in this category.

HORMONE RECEPTORS

A very important development in the evaluation of breast carcinoma is the realization that the presence of hormone receptors in the tumor tissue correlates well with response to hormone therapy and chemotherapy.[613] The hormone (estrogen and progesterone) receptors can be measured by the standard dextran-coated charcoal and sucrose gradient assays or by immunohistochemical techniques using monoclonal antibodies directed against the receptor molecule (Fig. 20-70). Fresh tissue is needed for the biochemical methods, whereas sensitive and reproducible techniques are now available for the immunohistochemical detection of the receptor in formalin-fixed, paraffin-embedded material.* Correlation between the biochemical and the immunohistochemical methods is very good.[604] The latter is preferable when the sample is very small and when the proportion of tumor tissue as opposed to fibrous stroma is reduced. Actually, most evidence suggests that the immunohistochemical assay will become the gold standard if it has not already.[606,606a] The method can be semiquantitated by computer-assisted image analysis.[605,610] Estrogen receptors can also be detected by the in situ hybridization technique, which is actually a more sensitive method than either immunohistochemistry or the biochemical assay.[612]

Not much correlation exists between the cytoarchitectural type of breast carcinoma and presence of hormone receptor protein; specifically, no statistically significant difference has been found between ductal-type and lobular-type tumors. However, most series have shown that most medullary carcinomas and intraductal carcinomas of the comedocarcinoma type are negative,[614,621,624,626] whereas mucinous carcinomas have the highest rates of positivity.[617] In DCIS, a predominance of large cells is the best morphologic predictor of estrogen receptor–negative status.[608]

Generally, estrogen receptor concentrations are lower in tumors of premenopausal women than in those of postmenopausal women.[624] Fisher et al.[611] found the presence

---

*References 615, 616, 618, 619, 620, 622, 623, 625.

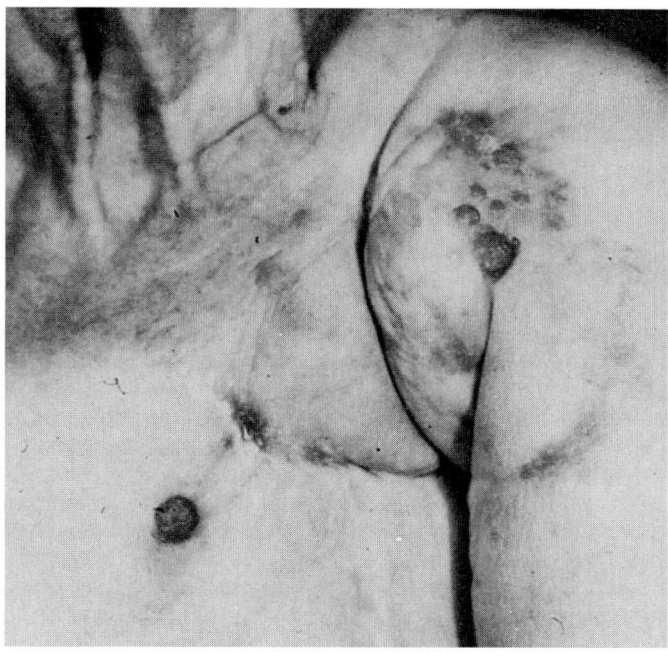

Fig. 20-71 Patient with local recurrence of carcinoma 27 years after original operation.

of estrogen receptors to be significantly associated with high nuclear and low histologic grades, absence of tumor necrosis, presence of marked tumor elastosis, and older patients' age groups. Hormone receptor positivity also correlates with bcl-2 immunoreactivity[607] and absence of p53 mutations,[609] and it correlates inversely with the presence of epidermal growth factor receptors.[626a]

SPREAD AND METASTASES

Breast carcinoma spreads by direct invasion, by the lymphatic route, and by the blood vessel route.[652] Some of these metastases are already present at the time of diagnosis, and others become manifest clinically months, years, or decades after the initial therapy[628] (Fig. 20-71).

Local invasion can occur in the breast parenchyma itself, nipple, skin, fascia, pectoralis muscle, or other structures of the chest wall. The frequency of microscopic invasion in the breast outside the gross confines was evaluated by Rosen et al.[653] by performing a "local excision" with a 2-cm gross margin in specimens of radical mastectomy and studying microscopically the remainder of the breast. Of eighteen mastectomies for carcinoma measuring less than 1 cm, residual invasive carcinoma was found in 11% and residual in situ carcinoma in an additional 22%. The importance of a proper pathologic evaluation of local invasion in breast carcinoma is now greater because of the increasing number of conservative surgical procedures being performed.[631]

A somewhat related problem is that of microscopic involvement of the nipple by breast carcinoma, since this structure would obviously be left in the patient if a local excision of the lump were carried out. Nipple invasion has been found in 23% to 31% of all invasive carcinomas; the large majority are seen in tumors located less than 2.5 cm from the nipple.[641,648,655]

Local recurrence following mastectomy appears as superficial nodules in or near the surgical scar or as subcutaneous parasternal nodules. Their malignant nature should always be documented by biopsy because the condition can be closely simulated by foreign body granulomas and infectious processes. Although women with local recurrences have an increased risk of distant metastases,[639] these seem to represent partially independent events that occur at different times.[654a]

Tumor recurrence following local excision often develops in the same segment, a fact that has led some authors to recommend a primary excision technique that removes en bloc the tumor mass and the associated duct system.[640b]

The most common site of lymph node involvement is the axilla, followed by the supraclavicular and internal mammary region. Axillary node metastases are present in 40% to 50% of the cases and are divided into levels according to their topographic relation with the insertion of the pectoralis minor muscle: low or proximal, medium, and high or distal. When extensive they are clinically detectable, but the margin of error with clinical palpation is high. Careful dissection of the submitted nodes by the pathologist is of importance. The yield of nodes will increase if they are searched for after the axilla is cleared with an organic solvent, but this seems hardly worth the trouble and expense. The yield of microscopic detection of metastatic involvement in these nodes will increase substantially (up to 20% or more) if each node is serially sectioned,[637,650] but this seems to carry no prognostic connotations (see p. 1626).

The second major lymph node drainage area is to the internal mammary chain, which lies at the anterior ends of the intercostal spaces by the side of the internal thoracic artery. The overall incidence of metastatic involvement of this chain is about 22%.[635] It is less than 1% for tumors in the outer half of the breast and negative axillary nodes, about 20% for tumors in the inner half and negative axillary nodes, about 30% in tumors of the outer half and positive axillary nodes, and over 50% for tumors in the inner half and positive axillary nodes.

Supraclavicular lymph node involvement is present in close to 20% of patients with axillary lymph node involvement but is almost zero in cases with negative axillae.[654]

Distant metastases are seen most commonly in the skeletal system, lung and pleura, liver, ovary, adrenal gland, and central nervous system (including leptomeninges and eyes)[630,642,645] (Plate XVI-B). Carcinomatous meningitis is a particularly devastating pattern of spread.[640a] Diffuse metastases to spleen can result in idiopathic thrombocytopenic purpura.[633] Invasive lobular carcinoma (including signet ring carcinoma) has a particular tendency to metastasize to the abdominal cavity, particularly to the gastrointestinal tract, ovaries, and serosal surfaces.[638,644] A peculiar recipient for metastatic breast carcinoma is meningioma; over thirty cases have been reported.[646] Bone marrow examination (particularly biopsy) is very efficient in documenting systemic disease,[640,643] but the incidence of positivity when both bone scan and x-ray studies are normal is too low (4%) to justify its routine use. Techniques using monoclonal antibodies have been developed for the detection of occult breast carcinoma metastases in the bone marrow.[632,651] These are particularly useful in cases of lobular carcinoma, which can be easily missed in H&E-stained sections.[627] Recently reverse transcriptase PCR assays for keratin 19[634] or MUCI[649] have been employed in attempts to detect occult breast carcinomas in bone marrow, lymph nodes, or peripheral blood. MUCI encodes a core protein of polymorphic epithelial mucin, and theoretically offers a greater degree of specificity than the ubiquitous keratin marker.

In the presence of metastatic deposits of unknown source, immunoreactivity for GCDF-15, lactalbumin, estrogen receptors, and zinc-alpha 2-glycoprotein strongly suggests a breast primary, especially when combined.[629,647]

The pattern of metastatic spread of breast carcinoma as evaluated by Fisher et al.[636] in a large randomized series of patients treated with various modalities brought them to the following conclusions: There is no orderly pattern of tumor dissemination; regional nodes are ineffective as barriers to tumor spread and, when positive, are more an indicator of a particular host-tumor relationship than the instigator of distant metastases; the bloodstream is of considerable importance in tumor dissemination; complex host-tumor interrelationships affect every facet of the disease; operable breast carcinoma is a systemic disease; and variations in local-regional therapy are unlikely to substantially affect survival.

Occult breast carcinoma

Sometimes a single enlarged axillary lymph node in an adult female is found to be involved by metastatic tumor in the presence of a clinically and radiographically normal breast, with no evidence of tumor elsewhere.[658] When this situation arises, the diagnosis will be metastatic breast carcinoma or metastatic malignant melanoma in over 90% of the cases. Making the distinction between carcinoma and melanoma should be possible in nearly every case from the combination of morphologic features, immunohistochemical stains for keratin, CEA, vimentin, S-100 protein, HMB-45 and other markers, and (rarely needed at this point) electron microscopy. A note of caution is in order regarding the interpretation of S-100 protein stains, since this marker (originally thought to be very distinctive of melanoma in this situation) is now known to stain a high number of breast carcinomas (see p. 1604).

If this combined approach has shown that the tumor is a carcinoma rather than a melanoma and if the appearance of this carcinoma is compatible with breast origin, removal of the homolateral breast is justified even in the absence of positive findings. A primary malignant tumor, which can be extremely small, will be found in most of the cases.[657] This was true in twenty-three of thirty-four cases reviewed by Ashikari et al.[656] Two thirds of these tumors were less than 2 cm in diameter. Interestingly, the survival rates were the same whether or not a primary tumor was found in the breast. In an updated series from the same institution, a primary tumor was found in 75% of the cases and the disease-free survival rate was 60%.[659]

STAGING

The most widely used clinical staging system for breast carcinoma is the one adopted by both the International Union against Cancer (UICC) and the American Joint Commission on Cancer Staging and End Results Reporting (AJC). It is based on the TNM system (T, tumor; N, nodes; M, metastases) and is shown in Appendix G.[660]

THERAPY

The therapy of breast carcinoma includes surgery, radiation therapy, hormonal therapy, and chemotherapy (the latter sometimes combined with bone marrow transplantation), depending on the type and extent of the disease.[666a]

Surgical therapy, traditionally synonymous with Halsted's radical mastectomy, now comprises a wide variety of options, which include partial mastectomy (lumpectomy or segmentectomy), total (simple) mastectomy, and modified radical mastectomy.[665,667a,670,671,683]

Radiation therapy has been employed as a postoperative adjunct (especially in connection with the more limited operations), sometimes as the primary treatment, and for the control of locally recurrent disease.[672-674,680]

When conservative surgery is employed, microscopic evaluation of the surgical margins becomes necessary. Several studies have shown that patients with positive margins are more likely to develop local recurrence as well as distant failure.[678] Surgical margins are more difficult to evaluate for intraductal tumors,[666,679] and their very utility in this circumstance has been questioned.[682]

Breast implants used for reconstructive purposes usually develop a fibrous capsule around them (Fig. 20-72, *A*). The inside surface of this capsule has a tendency to undergo *synovial metaplasia,* a process that has also been referred to as pseudoepithelization and that is microscopically very similar to "detritic synovitis."[663,664,666b,669,676] Rarely, the capsule is surrounded by benign squamous epithelium.[671a]

Systemic therapy is used for the palliative treatment of generalized disease.[684] Hormonal therapy, which has traditionally included the options of castration, adrenalectomy, and hypophysectomy, is now largely dependent on antiestrogen drugs, of which tamoxifen has emerged as the most important.[661,675]

Chemotherapy has had a significant impact on the survival of patients with metastatic breast carcinoma, the best results having been obtained with combination regimens.[661,661a,673a] In highly selected patients, this has been combined with autologous bone marrow transplantation; it remains to be seen whether the survival benefit justifies the considerably high cost of the procedure.[667,668,681] In addition, chemotherapy is currently used as an adjunct following local treatment with curative intent in patients with positive axillary nodes. The decision as to whether to give chemotherapy or hormonal therapy to node-negative patients is a difficult one and is dependent upon a variety of clinical and pathologic parameters.[677] Chemotherapy has also been used sequentially combined with conservative surgery and radiation in patients with localized large (≥3 cm) tumors in order to avoid mastectomy.[662]

EFFECTS OF THERAPY ON THE TUMOR AND ON NORMAL BREAST

Radiation therapy of breast carcinoma may result in bizarre nuclear changes, formation of giant tumor cells, naked nuclei, and abnormal mitotic figures. Extensive tumor necrosis may develop, which is later surrounded by a thick fibrous wall. These alterations can be very focal. It is important to remember that morphologic viability is not necessarily equivalent to biologic viability (i.e., the capacity of the tumor cell to replicate). In the non-neoplastic breast, the most characteristic irradiation effect is atypia of epithelial cells in the terminal ductules, associated with lobular sclerosis and atrophy.[687] Cases of *pseudosclerodermatous panniculitis* after irradiation have been reported.[688]

Hormonal therapy of responsive tumors leads to prominent stromal fibrosis and hyalinization, an increase in the amount of elastic tissue, and degenerative changes in the tumor cells. The latter are manifested by cytoplasmic vacuolization, rupture of cell membranes, nuclear aberrations, and eventual necrosis. These changes may occur both in the primary tumor and in the metastases and can be very patchy, morphologically unaffected cells lying side by side with highly altered cells.

Chemotherapy can also induce striking morphologic changes in the tumor cells, including a degree of vacuolization such as to simulate histiocytes (Fig. 20-72, *B* and *C*). It also results in atrophy of the terminal duct lobular unit, with occasional atypia.[686] However, in most instances it does not affect the histologic grading of the carcinoma.[685]

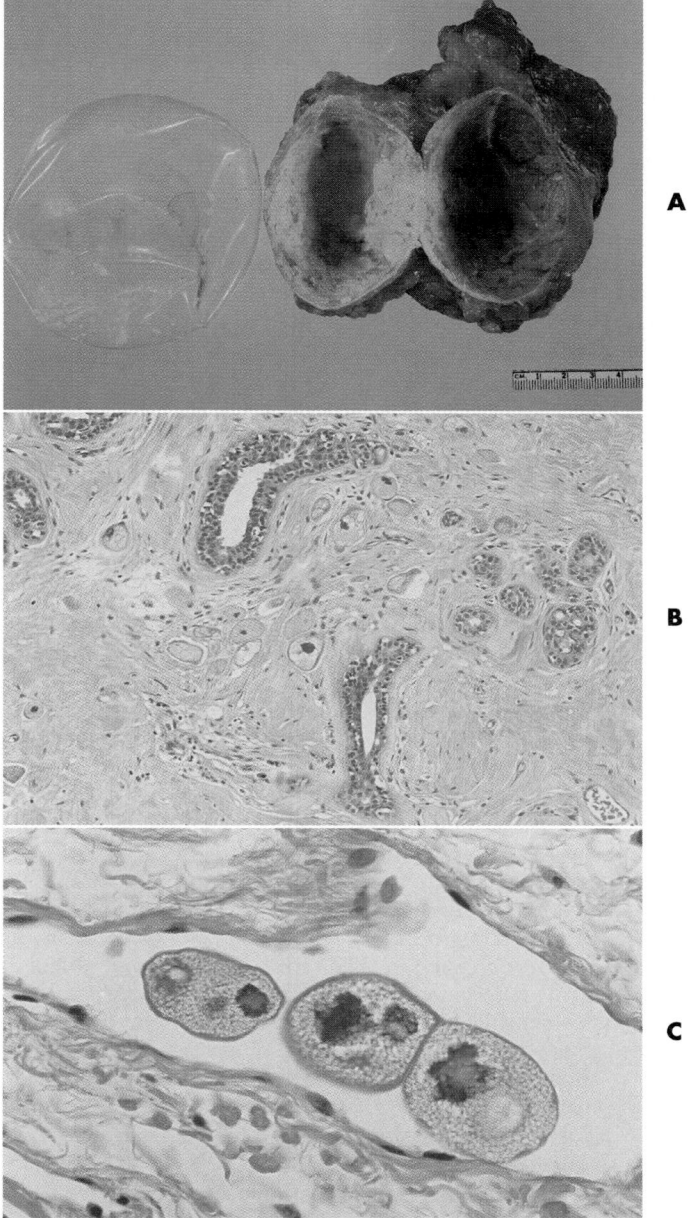

Fig. 20-72 A, Breast implant *(left)* surrounded by thick fibrous wall that has undergone heavy calcification *(right)*. **B** and **C**, Striking vacuolization of breast carcinoma cells induced by chemotherapy. The appearance simulates that of histiocytes. The tumor cells shown in **B** are located within a blood vessel. (Courtesy Dr. Maria J. Merino, Bethesda, MD.)

The microscopic features of the tumor correlate poorly with response to chemotherapy.[689]

PROGNOSIS

The overall 5-year survival rate for invasive breast carcinoma is 60% for clinically localized disease and 34% for regional disease.[769] This figure is modified markedly by a large variety of clinical and pathologic factors.*

1 **Patient's age.** Women who are younger than 50 years of age at the time of diagnosis have the best prognosis. Relative survival declines after the age of 50 years and is particularly low in older women.[691] As far as very young women (≤35 years of age) are concerned, some studies have shown a prognosis similar to that in older patients,[783] whereas others have shown a significantly higher risk for recurrence and distant metastases.[771]

2 **Pregnancy.** There is general agreement that carcinoma of the breast manifesting during pregnancy or lactation is associated with an overall poorer prognosis, the 5-year survival rate in most series ranging from 15% to 35%.[776] However, it has been stated that this difference does not reach statistical significance when evaluated stage by stage.[737,777]

3 **Oral contraceptives.** No convincing evidence has been found that use of oral contraceptive agents has an effect on the evolution or survival of breast carcinoma.[786]

4 **Early diagnosis.** The relative 5-, 8-, and 10-year survival rates for asymptomatic breast carcinomas detected in a large screening project (BCDDP) were 88%, 83%, and 79%, respectively.[792] These figures are much higher than those for the clinically detectable carcinoma and relate to the fact that the tumors were small in most cases, were usually devoid of axillary metastases, and included a high percentage of microscopically favorable types.

5 **Presence or absence of invasiveness.** Needless to say, this is the single most important prognostic determinator in breast carcinoma. For all practical purposes, in situ carcinomas are 100% curable with mastectomy. In tumors of ductal type that have both an in situ and an invasive component, a relationship exists between the proportion of the invasive component and the probability of nodal metastases. The amount of in situ component correlates with the incidence of multicentricity and, indirectly, with the probability of occult invasion.[758,761] It should be noted, however, that sometimes in situ ductal malignancies of the comedocarcinoma type can be associated with metastases in the absence of detectable invasion (see p. 1596).

6 **Size.** The diameter of the primary tumor shows a good correlation with the incidence of nodal metastases and with survival rate.[711,787] As a matter of fact—and despite earlier expressions of skepticism[727]—this easily, quickly and cheaply determined parameter has been found to be one of the strongest predictors of dissemination and rate of relapse in node-negative breast carcinomas.[780a] It should be noted that in tumors having both an in situ and an invasive component, the size of the latter is a better predictor than is the total tumor size.[792a] Tumor size is one of the two criteria for the definition of *minimal breast carcinoma*, which includes all in situ carcinomas regardless of size and invasive carcinomas 1 cm or less in diameter. Saigo and Rosen[790] studied 111 patients with invasive breast carcinoma 1 cm or less in diameter associated with negative nodes who were treated with a minimum of a modified radical mastectomy and fol-

lowed for at least 10 years: 75% were alive with no evidence of disease, 4% were alive with recurrent carcinoma, 6% had died of disease, and 15% had died of other causes.

7 **Site.** No relationship has been found in most studies between prognosis and the quadrant location of the primary tumor.

8 **Cytoarchitectural type.** There is no significant prognostic difference between ordinary invasive ductal and invasive lobular carcinoma. Morphologic variants of invasive ductal carcinoma with a more favorable prognosis are tubular carcinoma, cribriform carcinoma, medullary carcinoma (when strictly defined), pure mucinous carcinoma, papillary carcinoma, adenoid cystic carcinoma, and juvenile (secretory) carcinoma.[718,755] A variant of lobular (and sometimes ductal) carcinoma associated with an extremely bad prognosis is signet ring carcinoma. The prognosis of inflammatory carcinoma is also particularly ominous. Tumors that have been said to be more aggressive than ordinary ductal carcinoma but that actually show little difference in survival rates are squamous cell carcinoma, metaplastic carcinoma, and carcinomas with neuroendocrine features (including so-called carcinoid tumor). The prognostic significance of these and other varieties is further discussed in the section on microscopic types.

9 **Microscopic grade.** The two most widely used systems over the years for the microscopic grading of breast carcinoma have been those of Bloom and Richardson[705] and Black,[704] the first based mainly on architectural features (extent of tubular formation) and the second on the degree of nuclear atypia. These are usually estimated by visual microscopic examination of routinely stained sections, although various attempts at quantitating these changes (particularly the nuclear aberrations) by computer-assisted analysis have been made.[696,697,779,803] Since both architecture and cytology have been found to correlate with prognosis, the sensible proposal has been made to use them in conjunction.[716,760,787] Elston has been the most vocal champion of this approach, which is usually referred to as the Nottingham modification of the Bloom-Richardson system and which also incorporates the evaluation of mitotic activity.[723,736] In this scheme, the grade is obtained by adding up the scores for tubule formation, nuclear pleomorphism, and mitotic count, each of which is given 1, 2, or 3 points. This results in a total score of 3 to 9 points, which is translated into the final grade by the following formula: 3 to 5 points = Grade I; 6 to 7 points = Grade II; and 8 to 9 points = Grade III. The specific criteria for point assignments are described in the box and Table 20-1.

The utility of this and related grading systems has been convincingly and repeatedly proved[733,738,746,795] to the point that incorporation of this information into the routine pathology report is becoming a requirement.[775] This is reinforced by the fact that an acceptable degree of interobserver reproducibility has been achieved.[714,736,781a]

10 **Type of margins.** Tumors with "pushing" margins have a better prognosis than tumors with infiltrating margins. This applies not only to medullary carcinoma, but

also to other types of well-circumscribed neo-plasms.[712,748,756]

11 Tumor necrosis. Tumor necrosis is associated with an increased incidence of lymph node metastases and decreased survival rates,[701,712,740,767], but this feature is usually associated with tumors of high histologic grade.

12 Stromal reaction. Surprisingly, it has been found that tumors with an absence of inflammatory reaction at the periphery have a lesser degree of nodal metastases and presumably a better prognosis.[732] Obviously, these considerations do not apply to the specific case of medullary carcinoma.

13 Microvessel density. The very interesting observation has been recently made that invasive breast carcinomas having a prominent vascular component in the surrounding stroma behave in a more aggressive fashion than the others.[807,807a,808,810] Accordingly, attempts have been made to quantitate the "density" of these vessels and to correlate this feature to other parameters, notably prognosis.[697a] The original proponents of this approach have shown rather impressive results, and these have been corroborated by some independent observers.[708,739] Others have failed to show significant correlations and have commented on the great difficulties encountered in estimating the surface or volume of the intricate vascular network that surrounds these tumors.[694a,774,793a] It should be added that microvessel density is a phenomenon independent from intratumoral endothelial cell proliferation,[804] and that an increase in microvessel density has also been noted in intraductal carcinoma, particularly of the comedo type.[743]

14 Elastosis. It has been claimed that breast carcinomas with no associated elastosis have a lower rate of response to endocrine therapy than those with gross elastosis.[766] In terms of survival rate, no convincing differences have been found between tumors with and without elastosis.[707,742]

15 CEA staining pattern. This immunohistochemical feature has not been found to relate to prognosis.[802]

16 Vimentin staining pattern. The claim has been made that vimentin expression is associated with poor prognosis in node-negative ductal carcinomas.[720]

17 Cathepsin D. Despite original claims to the contrary,[798] assays for neither cathepsin D immunoreactivity in the tumor nor serum levels of this enzyme have proved to have independent prognostic value.[693,721,753,781,789]

18 c-*erb*B-2 (neu/HER-2) oncogene. As already stated, amplification of this oncogene (which encodes a transmembrane glycoprotein with tyrosine kinase activity known as p185) is seen in almost all cases of comedo-type intraductal carcinoma, in 10% to 40% of invasive ductal carcinomas and in only a few cases of invasive lobular carcinoma.[717,718a] It can be detected by immunohistochemical demonstration of the protein product or by in situ hybridization of mRNA.[797] This amplification is believed to identify a subset of patients with poor prognosis, particularly if axillary node metastases are present.[700,722,745] However, in multivariate analyses—and like so many other prognostic indicators in this disease—this feature is overshadowed by the morphologic parameters.[695,783b] Specifically, it correlates closely with the tumor grade.[801] It has also been claimed that patients

with overexpression of c-*erb*B-2 show a better response to adjuvant chemotherapy.[768a]

19 p53 and nm23. Accumulation of p53 protein (presumably as a result of gene mutation) and low expression of the recently discovered nm23 protein have been said to correlate with reduced patient survival.[698,699,749] However, the authors of a large recent study comprising 440 node-negative patients concluded that the immunohistochemical demonstration of p53 was not a reliable prognostic indicator in this population and that it was not associated with any major epidemiologic risk factor.[783a]

20 Bcl-2. A relationship between Bcl-2 protein expression and long-term survival in breast carcinoma has been shown.[749a] Bcl-2 is also correlated with estrogen receptor status.[719,752]

MICROSCOPIC GRADING OF BREAST CARCINOMA: NOTTINGHAM MODIFICATION OF THE BLOOM-RICHARDSON SYSTEM

Tubule formation
   1 point: Tubular formation in >75% of the tumor
   2 points: Tubular formation in 10% to 75% of the tumor
   3 points: Tubular formations in <10% of the tumor
   NOTE: For scoring tubule formations, the overall appearance of the tumor has to be taken into consideration.

Nuclear pleomorphism
   1 point: Nuclei with minimal variation in size and shape
   2 points: Nuclei with moderate variation in size and shape
   3 points: Nuclei with marked variation in size and shape
   NOTE: The tumor areas having cells with greatest atypia should be evaluated.

Mitotic count
   1, 2, or 3 points, according to Table 20-2.
   NOTE: Mitotic figures are to be counted only at the periphery of the tumor. Counting should begin in the most mitotically active area; 10 high-power fields (APF) are to be counted in the same area (but not necessarily contiguous). The fields should be filled with as much tumor as possible; poorly preserved areas are to be avoided. Cells in the prophase should be ignored.

Table 20-1 Assignment of points for mitotic counts according to the field area, using several microscopes

	Leitz Ortholux	Microscope Nikon Labophot	Leitz Diaplan
Objective	×25	×40	×40
Field diameter (mm)	0.59	0.44	0.63
Field area (mm²)	0.274	0.152	0.312
Mitotic count			
1 point	0-9	0-5	0-11
2 points	10-19	6-10	12-22
3 points	>20	>11	>23

21 Skin invasion. Breast carcinomas in which invasion of the overlying skin has occurred are associated with a decreased survival rate.[791] Invasion of dermal lymph vessels as a determinant of the "inflammatory carcinoma" picture is a particularly ominous prognostic sign.

22 Nipple invasion. Involvement of the nipple by carcinoma is associated with a higher incidence of axillary metastases.[811]

23 Lymphatic tumor emboli. The presence of tumor emboli in lymphatic vessels within the breast is associated with an increased risk of tumor recurrence.[715,770,785]

24 Blood vessel emboli. This finding shows a high correlation with tumor size, histologic grade, tumor type, lymph node status, development of distant metastases, and poor prognosis.[709,755,762,780]

25 Paget's disease. The presence or absence of Paget's disease in invasive ductal carcinoma is of no prognostic relevance per se.

26 Estrogen receptors. Several authors have concluded that patients with estrogen receptor–positive tumors— whether determined biochemically or immunohistochemically—have a longer disease-free survival than the others. However, the differences in long-term prognosis are minimal and perhaps not statistically significant.[690,710,747]

27 DNA ploidy. Despite numerous studies evaluating DNA ploidy with this technique, if is yet unclear whether this parameter adds *independent* information of therapeutic or prognostic value once the size of the tumor, microscopic grading, lymph node status, and hormone-receptor status have been taken into account.[*]

28 Cell proliferation. This parameter, whether measured by the old-fashioned mitotic count,[703,757,759] by Ki-67 or analogous immunostain,[768,788,805,809,812] or by determination of S-phase fraction by flow cytometry,[814] has emerged as a very important prognostic determinator.[735,773,793,806] As such, it has been incorporated into the combined grading scheme espoused by Elston (see paragraph 9).

29 Axillary lymph node metastases. This is one of the most important prognostic parameters.[692,750] Not only is there a sharp difference in survival rates between patients with positive and negative nodes, but the survival rate also depends on the level of axillary node involved (low, medium, or high),[702] the absolute number (fewer than four versus four or more),[724,730,796] the amount of metastatic tumor,[751,784] the presence or absence of extranodal spread,[731,742a,762a,764] and the presence or absence of tumor cells in the efferent vessels.[713,744] Interestingly, patients in whom the initial lymph node sections are negative but who are found to have micrometastases on serial sections have the same prognosis as patients in whom no tumor is found.[734,778] For prognostic purposes, the best grouping seems to be the following: negative nodes, one to three positive nodes, and four or more positive nodes.

30 Pattern of lymph node reaction. It has been suggested that the microscopic appearance of the regional node

---

*References 694, 735, 754, 764, 799, 813.

(lymphoid response and/or sinus histiocytosis) is an indication of the type of host response to the tumor and that it relates to prognosis.[800] The issue remains controversial; if there is indeed a correlation, it does not seem to be a statistically significant one.[730,732]

31 Internal mammary lymph node metastases. Survival in patients with involvement of this lymph node group is lower than in those without such involvement, especially if only patients with one to three positive axillary nodes are evaluated.[772]

32 Local recurrence. This is a sign of ominous prognosis. In one series of sixty patients with ipsilateral chest wall recurrence and no detectable distant metastases, all patients eventually died of metastatic breast carcinoma.[741]

33 Type of therapy. This is too complex and multifactorial an issue to be properly addressed here. Suffice to say that all available evidence suggests that the outcome in breast carcinoma depends more on the nature of the individual tumor than on the type of therapy performed. There is certainly a striking similarity in survival rates from different centers employing widely disparate therapeutic approaches.[763] A complicating factor in evaluating therapeutic results is the marked individual variations in the natural life history of the disease, which renders imperative the use of carefully randomized studies. Most of these studies have shown no significant differences in survival among the various groups, which have included the following[725,726,751a]:

a For patients with clinically negative axillary nodes:
  - Radical mastectomy versus total mastectomy with postoperative regional radiation
  - Total mastectomy alone versus segmentectomy with postoperative regional radiation

b For patients with clinically positive axillary nodes:
  - Radical mastectomy versus total mastectomy with postoperative regional radiation

Bloom et al.[706] provided a good baseline on which to judge the effectiveness of therapy by showing that in a series of 250 untreated breast cancers, the 5-year survival rate after diagnosis was 18%.

Salivary and Sweat Gland–Type Tumors

A small proportion of benign and malignant tumors of the breast have an appearance analogous to that more commonly seen in salivary glands or sweat glands. This should not be too surprising, since the breast is a modified sweat gland and a close analogy exists between sweat gland tumors and salivary gland neoplasms.

The benign tumors in this category include *eccrine spiradenoma*,[821] *syringomatous squamous tumors* (to be distinguished from low-grade mucoepidermoid carcinoma),[829,842,848] *papillary syringocystadenoma*,[841] and *benign mixed tumor.* The latter, which is very rare in humans but relatively common in female dogs, has been interpreted by some as an intraductal papilloma,[839] but its appearance is quite similar to that of benign mixed tumor of salivary glands (pleomorphic adenoma) or of cutaneous sweat glands (chondroid syringoma)[815,818,820] (Fig. 20-73, *A* and *B*). This tumor can arise in an otherwise normal breast,

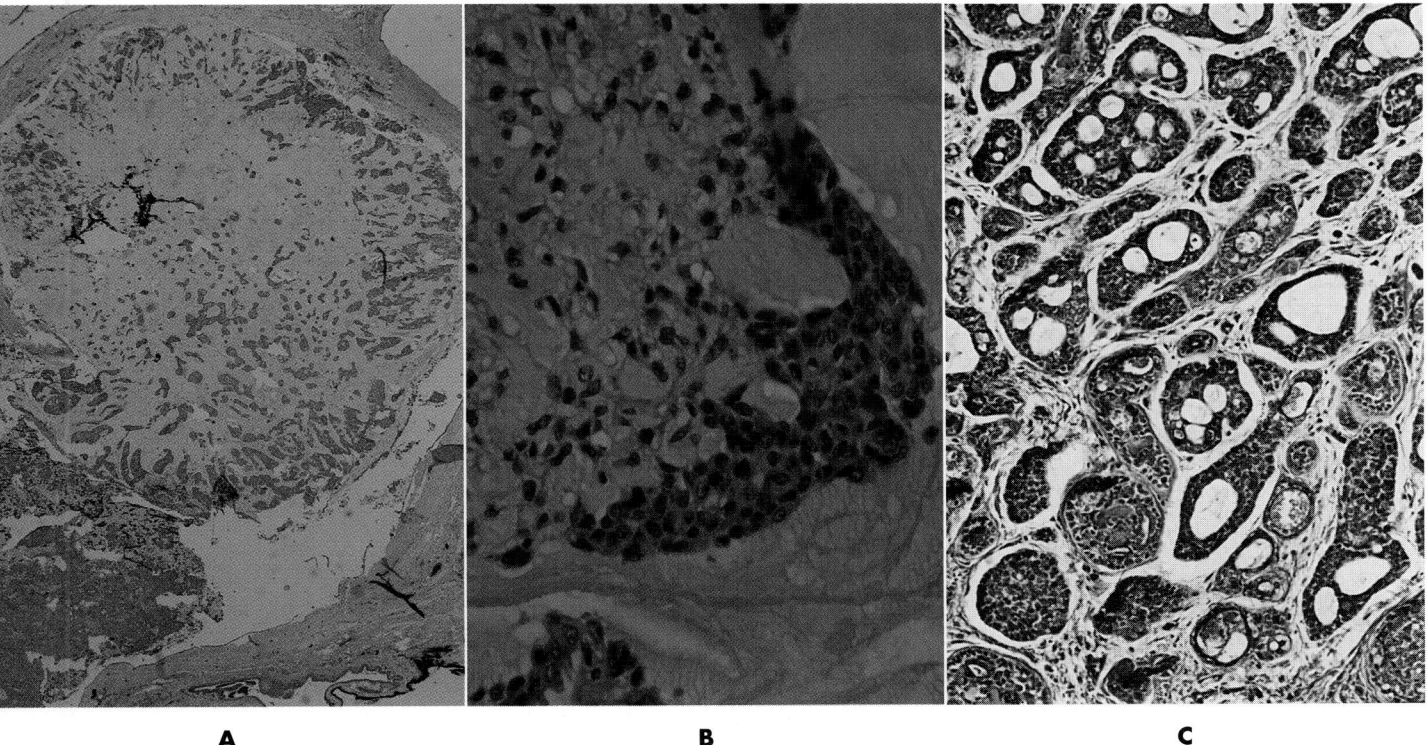

Fig. 20-73 A and **B,** Benign mixed tumor of breast. Clusters of epithelial cells are seen merging with a nonepithelial component, which acquires chondroid features. **C,** Adenoid cystic carcinoma of breast. Appearance is analogous to salivary gland tumor that carries the same name. (**A** and **B** courtesy Dr. Darryl Carter, New Haven, CT.)

as single or multiple nodules against a background of ductal hyperplasia or associated with breast carcinoma.[833]

Adenoid cystic carcinoma is the most important member of the malignant category. It is important not to confuse this very rare neoplasm with the much more common intraductal carcinoma with cribriform pattern, sometimes referred to as pseudoadenoid cystic carcinoma.[827,837] True adenoid cystic carcinoma of the breast shows, as in the salivary glands, two types of cavity formation: true glandular lumina and the well-known eosinophilic "cylinders" containing basement membrane material[830] (Fig. 20-73, *C*). It may also show foci of sebaceous differentiation, indicating a potential to differentiate into skin adnexal structures.[845] Perineural involvement may be present. Axillary lymph node metastases are extremely rare.[835,849] Some of the patients have developed local recurrence of pulmonary metastases many years after initial therapy,[817,823,835] but the prognosis for this tumor as a group is remarkably good; a possible relationship between microscopic grading and prognosis has been suggested.[835]

Other malignant breast tumors that could be included in this category are *mucoepidermoid carcinoma* (see p. 1616) and *apocrine carcinoma* (see p. 1616).

A more complicated issue is represented by the breast tumors of probable myoepithelial nature. First, it should be recognized that myoepithelial participation is an integral component of benign proliferative breast diseases (such as sclerosing adenosis, ductal hyperplasia, intraductal papilloma, and nipple adenoma) and that in some instances it dominates the histologic picture. Such cases, when presenting in the form of multifocal microscopic lesions, have been designated as *myoepitheliosis*.[844]

Second, myoepithelial cells are a normal constituent of the ducts and lobules, and therefore one might question whether these neoplasms should be regarded as of salivary or sweat gland type. They are discussed here because the morphologic variations they exhibit and classification problems they elicit are very similar to those they pose in the salivary glands (see Chapter 12). *Adenomyoepithelioma* is a small (average diameter, 1 cm), firm, well-circumscribed tumor microscopically composed of cells of polygonal shape and optically clear cytoplasm, arranged in nests sometimes centered by gland-forming epithelial cells.[844] The patterns of growth may be spindle-cell (myoid), tubular, or lobulated[836,844,850] (Fig. 20-74). Interestingly, some of these lesions seem to arise on the basis of a peculiar form of adenosis designated as of adenomyoepithelial or apocrine type (see p. 1581). In the series of eighteen adenomyoepitheliomas reported by Rosen,[836] two developed local recurrences but there were no instances of metastatic spread. It seems likely that the cases formerly reported as clear cell hidradenoma[825] belong to this category. *Malignant myoepithelioma (myoepithelial carcinoma)* is purely composed

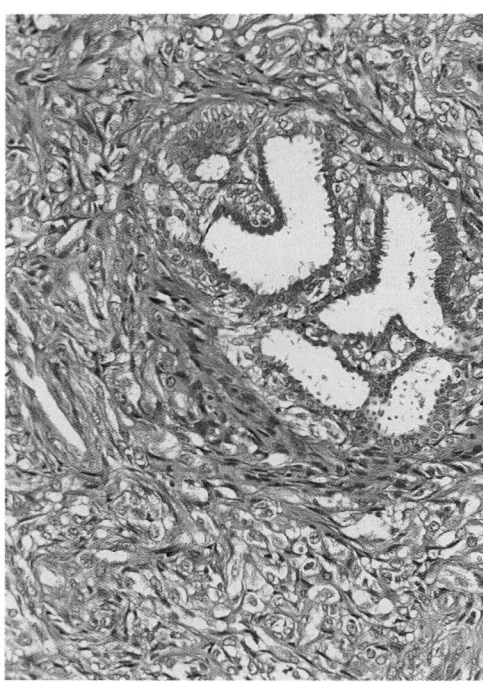

Fig. 20-74 Two patterns of growth of myoepithelial tumors of the breast. Adenomyoepithelioma. In some areas there is a clear relationship between the secretory and the myoepithelial component (similar to that seen in adenomyoepitheliosis), but in others the spindle myoepithelial cells become the exclusive neoplastic element.

of myoepithelial cells and is cytologically malignant.[834a,844] Some of these carcinomas (which may be quite undifferentiated) arise on the basis of an adenomyoepithelioma, the latter providing the best clue for their recognition.[819,832] Intraductal growth may be noted in them.[843]

The spindle cell form of this tumor presents as a nonencapsulated cellular spindle cell tumor that grows in a fascicular pattern in the breast stroma.[816,831] Its light microscopic appearance resembles very much that of a mesenchymal neoplasm; support for the alleged myoepithelial nature of the few reported cases is largely based on ultrastructural observations, and/or the existence of a preceding or coexisting adenomyoepithelioma.[824,838]

Low-grade adenosquamous carcinoma is a well-differentiated tumor with dual glandular and squamous differentiation. Many of the reported cases have originated from an intraductal papillary tumor.[822,847] Local recurrence is common following conservative surgery, but nodal and distant metastases are exceptional.[847] Whether this neoplasm and the related low-grade mucoepidermoid carcinoma[834] are differentiations in the direction of salivary gland or sweat gland–type structures is debatable.

Glycogen-rich (clear cell) carcinoma is composed of large clear cells, which are found to contain abundant glycogen.[826,827a,828,840] The biphasic appearance of adenomyoepithelioma is not apparent. It is possible that some of these tumors are of myoepithelial or apocrine nature, but the evidence for either is not very compelling. These neoplasms are full-blown carcinomas, with a prognosis not better and perhaps worse than that of ordinary invasive ductal carcinoma.[826,846]

Stromal Tumors and Tumorlike Conditions
PHYLLOIDES TUMOR

Phylloides tumor—a better term than the traditional cystosarcoma phylloides coined by Johannes Müller in 1838[857]—occurs in the same age group as breast carcinoma, the median age at the time of diagnosis being 45 years.[853,861] Very few of the patients are younger than 25 years of age, in striking contrast with the age distribution of fibroadenoma. The interesting observation has been made that phylloides tumors are more common in Hispanics than in other ethnic groups, and that this risk is higher among those Hispanics born in Latin America than those born in the United States.[853]

Grossly, the typical phylloides tumor is round, relatively well circumscribed, and firm. The nipple may be flattened, but the overlying skin is almost never attached. The cut surface is solid and gray-white and shows the cleft-like spaces that give the tumor its name (Fig. 20-75, *A*). Areas of necrosis, cystic degeneration, and hemorrhage may be present (Fig. 20-75, *B*). Rarely, the entire tumor undergoes hemorrhagic infarct. Many phylloides tumors are large and some reach huge dimensions, but others measure less than 5 cm in diameter. It follows, then, that the diagnosis of phylloides tumor can be neither made nor ruled out by size alone. A lesion with the microscopic appearance of fibroadenoma should still be diagnosed as such even if it reaches 10 cm or more in diameter (see p. 1573).

Microscopically, the two key features of phylloides tumor are stromal hypercellularity and the presence of benign glandular elements as an integral component of the neoplasm[851] (Figs. 20-76 and 20-77). It is the amount and appearance of

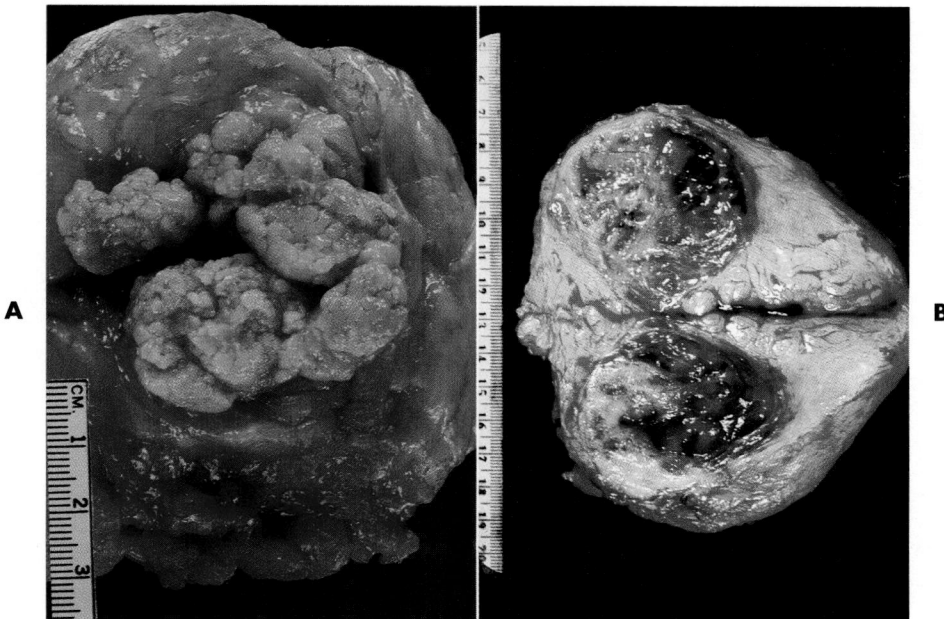

Fig. 20-75 Gross appearance of cystosarcoma phylloides. The tumor shown in **A** exhibits the typical leaf-like appearance of cut surface. The tumor illustrated in **B** has undergone extensive hemorrhagic infarct.

the stromal component that determines whether a breast neoplasm should be called a fibroadenoma or a phylloides tumor and, in the latter instance, what the chances are of the tumor behaving clinically in an aggressive fashion. Although a sharp distinction between benign and malignant forms of phylloides tumor is not always possible, sufficient information is available on the natural history of this neoplasm to allow a statement to be made about the likelihood of metastases and proper management on the basis of the pathologic features.

Tumors with the configuration of fibroadenomas having a cellular stroma without atypical features concentrated in the periductal areas are on the "benign" end of the spectrum; this stromal component has a fibroblastic appearance, with occasional admixture of mature adipose tissue foci. When the latter are prominent, the term *lipophylloides tumor* has been employed.[868] Cytologically, malignant phylloides tumors have marked nuclear atypia, numerous mitoses, and loss of the relationship between glands and stroma. An important diagnostic criterion of malignancy is overgrowth of the glands by the sarcomatous stroma so that low-power views of the tumor show only stroma without epithelial elements.[859,869] The neoplastic stromal component may be monomorphic or highly pleomorphic, and its appearance may be reminiscent of fibrosarcoma, malignant fibrous histiocytoma, or liposarcoma[864]; metaplastic cartilage, bone, or, exceptionally, skeletal muscle may be encountered.[852] Phylloides tumors with stromal elements other than fibromyxoid do worse than the others. Tumor necrosis is also associated with poor prognosis.[855]

We view phylloides tumor as a tumor of the specialized mammary stroma with the capacity for epithelial induction.

This tumor stroma has progesterone receptors but no estrogen receptors.[865] Ultrastructurally, the features of the tumor cells are largely those of fibroblasts, with occasional focal muscle differentiation.[866,870] The epithelial component, although probably not neoplastic, can have a markedly proliferative appearance, as it sometimes also does in fibroadenoma,[861] a finding of no clinical significance. Very rarely, the features of carcinoma of either ductal or lobular type will be present in it.[854,860,861]

The behavior of the better-differentiated phylloides tumors is characterized by a tendency for local recurrence but an extreme rarity of distant metastases. If an enucleation has been done under the clinical impression of fibroadenoma, the patient can be safely followed for the possibility of recurrence. If the latter develops or if this type of phylloides tumor is recognized at the time of initial surgery, local excision with a wide margin of normal tissue is the treatment of choice. Recurrent phylloides tumor, which is the consequence of inadequate excision, may still be cured by wide local excision.[860a]

The cytologically malignant tumors are potentially metastasizing neoplasms, the incidence of metastases ranging from 3% to 12% in the various series. Deposits in the axillary nodes are exceptional. The most common sites of distant involvement are lung and bone, but the central nervous system also can be affected.[858,867] The metastases are of stromal elements only, although entrapping of normal structures in the lung may simulate a biphasic composition.

Simple mastectomy is sufficient therapy for most cytologically malignant phylloides tumors, but if there is any question of invasion of the fascia, the tumor should be removed together with the underlying muscle. There is no

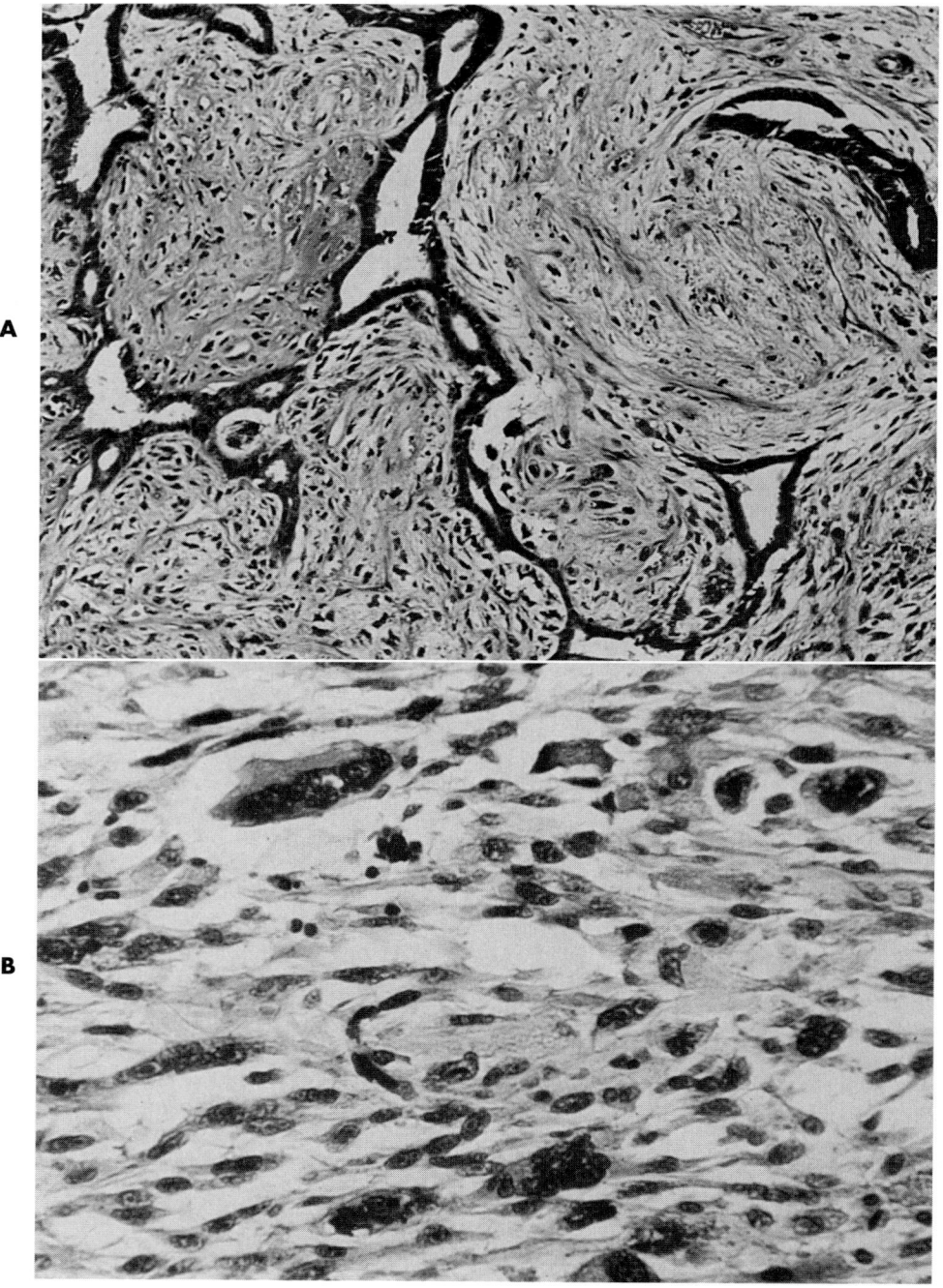

Fig. 20-76 A, Phylloides tumor. Overall architecture is that of fibroadenoma, but there is marked stromal cellularity. **B,** Another area of tumor shown in **A.** Stroma is highly atypical and grows independently from epithelial components, two signs indicative of malignancy.

need for removal of the axillary nodes, except for the exceptional instances in which they are clinically involved.

For the phylloides tumors that do not fall easily into one of these two extreme categories, the prognostic prediction and therapeutic recommendation have to be made on the basis of size, pushing versus peripheral margins, cellular atypia, and mitotic count.[861,863] There is some indication that

DNA ploidy and S-phase fraction analysis may be useful adjuncts to the assessment of this tumor.[856,862]

VASCULAR TUMORS

Angiosarcoma of the breast characteristically occurs in young women. Mammographically, it presents as a solitary mass that is usually uncalcified.[877a] Grossly, the tumor is

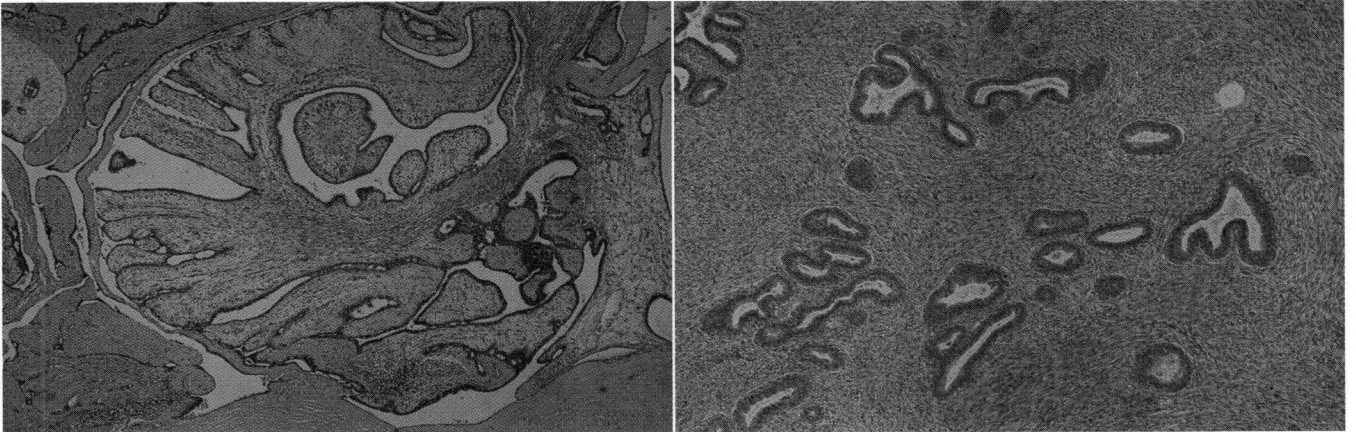

Fig. 20-77 Microscopic appearance of phylloides tumor. The tumor shown in **A** has the more common "intracanalicular" pattern of growth, whereas the tumor illustrated in **B** has a "pericanalicular" configuration.

soft, spongy, and hemorrhagic (Plate XVI-C). Microscopically, the diagnostic areas are characterized by anastomosing vascular channels lined by atypical endothelial cells. The appearance may vary in the same tumor from that of a highly undifferentiated solid neoplasm to one that is extremely bland cytologically, to the point that some early cases were reported as metastasizing hemangiomas.[887] However, close examination will usually reveal that even the better differentiated areas exhibit the telltale sign of angiosarcoma (i.e., freely anastomosing vascular channels) (Fig. 20-78). The tumor is thought to be of blood vessels rather than lymph vessels and is therefore also referred to as hemangiosarcoma. Curiously, some of these cases have been found to contain estrogen receptors.[873] The differential diagnosis of angiosarcoma includes metaplastic carcinoma (see p. 1615), the acantholytic variant of squamous cell carcinoma (see p. 1616), hemangioma (see following discussion), and pseudoangiomatous stromal hyperplasia (see p. 1634).

The overall prognosis of angiosarcoma is poor, most of the patients developing metastases through the bloodstream.[887] Donnell et al.[875] have shown that a good correlation exists between microscopic grade and outcome. In their series, the 5-year disease-free survival was 33%; ten of their thirteen patients with grade I lesions were alive and well. They recommended the use of adjuvant chemotherapy, specifically actinomycin D. The relation of grading with prognosis has been confirmed in other series.[878,883]

Lymphangiosarcoma can develop in the soft tissues of the upper extremity as a result of long-standing postmastectomy lymphedema (Stewart-Treves syndrome) (see Chapter 25). Interestingly, a case has been reported of angiosarcoma of the breast itself following lymphedema resulting from segmental mastectomy.[872] Following radiation therapy for carcinoma of the breast, the overlying skin can develop a variety of vascular proliferative lesions, which range from lymphangioma-like nodules to full-blown angiosarcomas.[875a,880,885a]

* * *

The statement has often been made that nearly all vascular tumors of the breast are malignant. Although the bland microscopic appearance of some angiosarcomas cannot be overemphasized, it is also true that a number of perfectly benign vascular tumors can occur in this area. First of all, hemangiomas of various types that share the features of those seen elsewhere in the body can develop in the overlying skin and subcutaneous fat. The most likely to be overdiagnosed is angiolipoma, because sometimes it can be very cellular and the adipose tissue component can be inconspicuous.[882,888] The encapsulation and presence of hyaline thrombi in the vessels are important diagnostic clues (see Chapter 25).

Benign vascular breast tumors can also develop within the breast parenchyma.[874] *Benign hemangioendothelioma* can occur in children, its microscopic appearance being similar to that of its more common cutaneous counterpart (Fig. 20-79, *A*). *Perilobular hemangioma* is usually detected only microscopically; it is characterized by dilated capillary vessels in a perilobular location, without anastomoses or cellular atypia.[885] Autopsy studies have shown that it is a relatively common lesion, having been found in 11% of all breasts.[877] Other *hemangiomas* are not located perilobularly; they also tend to be small but can reach a diameter of 2 cm.[876] There are also *venous hemangiomas*.[884] A few hemangiomas having a diffuse quality (although without anastomosing channels) have been referred to as *angiomatosis*.[881] Other benign vascular tumors that can exceptionally involve the breast are *hemangiopericytoma*[871,879] and *cystic lymphangioma* (cystic hygroma).[886] We have also seen cases of *epithelioid (histiocytoid) hemangioma* and *Mas-*

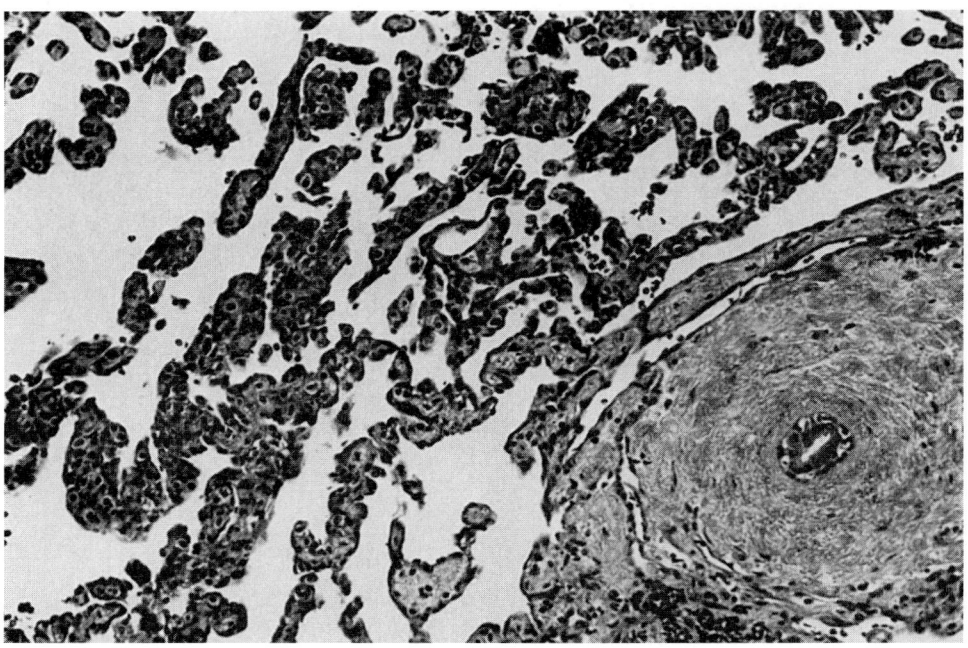

Fig. 20-78 Angiosarcoma of breast. Freely anastomosing vascular channels and papillary structures lined by atypical endothelial cells are seen surrounding small mammary duct.

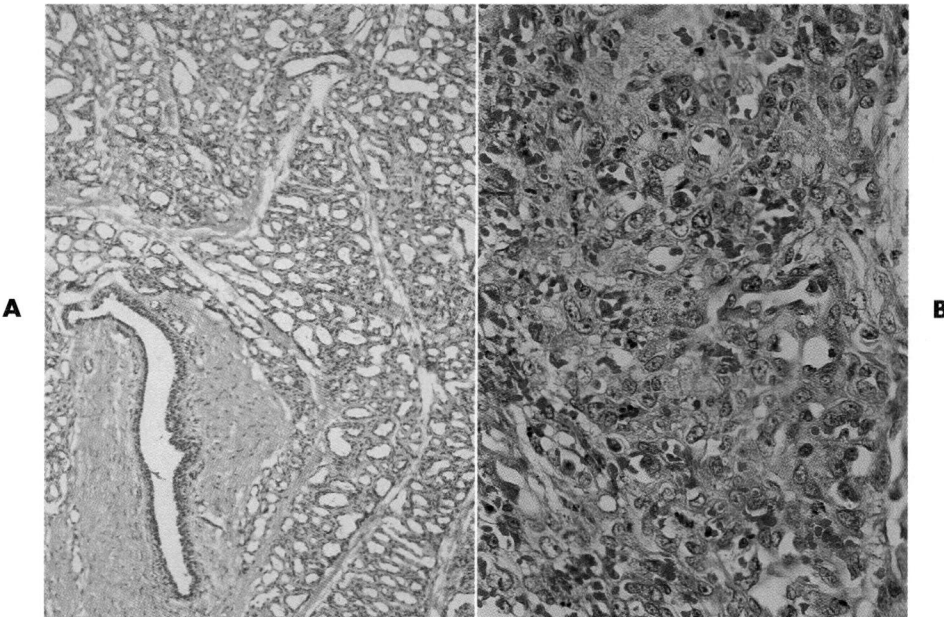

Fig. 20-79 A, Benign hemangioendothelioma of breast in a child. The appearance is identical to that of the homologous tumor seen more commonly in skin or salivary gland. **B,** Epithelioid (histiocytoid) hemangioma located within the breast substance. (**A** courtesy Dr. Louis P. Dehner, St. Louis.)

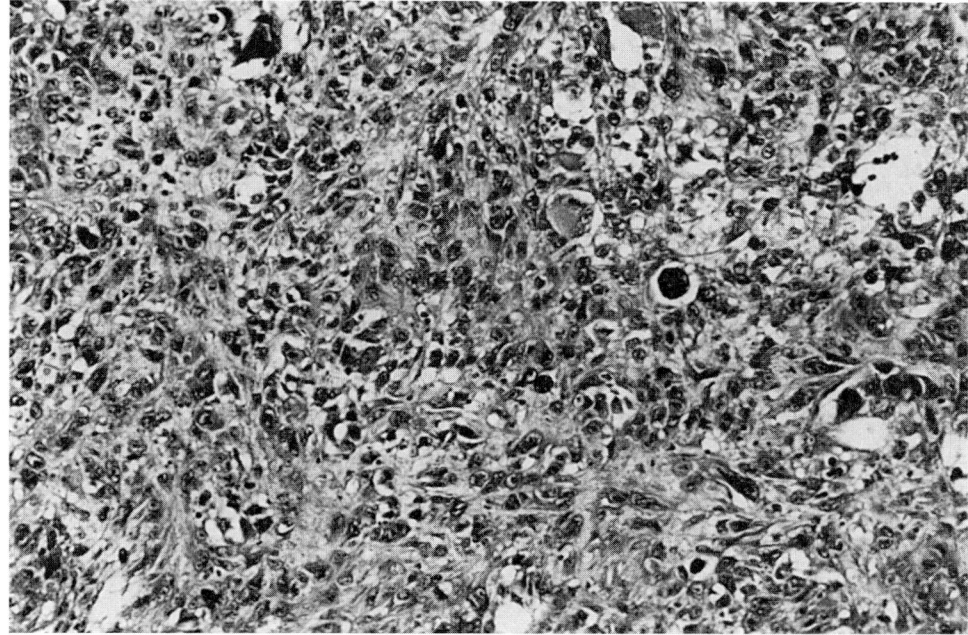

Fig. 20-80 Stromal sarcoma of breast. Neoplasm has mesenchymal appearance and lacks epithelial component of phylloides tumor.

son's hemangioma (papillary endothelial hyperplasia) located inside the breast parenchyma[882] (Fig. 20-79, B).

OTHER MALIGNANT STROMAL TUMORS

Stromal sarcoma is the generic term given to malignant breast tumors thought to arise from the specialized stroma of this organ but lacking the epithelial component of phylloides tumor[892,896] (Fig. 20-80). Grossly, the tumors appear solid, grayish white, and homogeneous. Necrosis may be present. Microscopically, most of them have the features of fibrosarcoma; focal osseous metaplasia can occur. Infiltrative margins and severe atypia indicate a greater tendency for local recurrence and distant metastases.[896]

Stromal tumors with an appearance equivalent to that of various types of sarcomas of somatic soft tissues exist.[897] They include *liposarcoma,*[890] *leiomyosarcoma,*[889,893] *rhabdomyosarcoma, fibrosarcoma,*[895] *malignant fibrous histiocytoma,*[895] *chondrosarcoma,*[891] and *osteosarcoma.*[894] The latter two entities should be distinguished from phylloides tumors with an osseous and/or cartilaginous stromal component and from sarcomatoid carcinomas.[898]

OTHER PRIMARY TUMORS AND TUMORLIKE CONDITIONS

Basal cell carcinomas, squamous cell carcinomas, keratinous cysts, and **sweat gland tumors** may arise in the skin of the nipple or other sites in the breast, but they are not to be considered primary breast tumors.[908,914] The nipple can also be the site of **leiomyomas.** These tumors, which are thought to arise from the muscularis mamillae and areola, are often painful.[921]

Hamartoma has already been mentioned (see p. 1571). The definition of this entity—if it is an entity at all—

remains unsatisfactory. Its identification is said to depend on the combination of clinical, radiologic, and pathologic criteria.[903a,908a] Morphologically, lesions that have been thought to be hamartomas on mammography may exhibit a wide diversity of appearances, the common denominator being the admixture of epithelial and stromal elements, the latter including fat[907,911,916,922] (Plate XVI-D). A reproducible morphologic distinction of this process from circumscribed fibrocystic disease and fibroadenoma has yet to be achieved. *Myoid hamartoma*[906] and *chondrolipoma* (a benign lesion composed of an admixture of fat, cartilage, and sometimes bone)[917,919,920] are two other processes straddling the fence between malformation and benign neoplasia.

Granular cell tumor is important because of its ability to simulate grossly the appearance of invasive carcinoma.[905,909,915] It is usually small, but it may reach a size of 10 cm or more. On section, it is firm, homogeneous, and white or grayish yellow. As a rule, it is not attached to the overlying skin, but it may be fixed to the underlying fascia. The microscopic appearance is described in Chapter 25. The behavior is benign, and the treatment is local excision.

Myofibroblastoma is a benign mesenchymal tumor seen most commonly in the male breast but also occurring in females.[932] This is further described on p. 1639.

Leiomyoma usually involves the nipple but occasionally is seen within the breast substance.[910] Some have been reported having epithelioid features and granular changes.[926]

Benign peripheral nerve tumors of both schwannian[904] and perineurial types[903] have been described.

Fibromatosis and **nodular fasciitis** can involve the breast as primary lesions. Their microscopic appearance and natural history are analogous to those of the respective entities when occurring in the usual somatic soft tissue location.

Thus fibromatosis of the breast is infiltrative, aggressive, and prone to local recurrence,[899,912,924,928,929] whereas nodular fasciitis is self-limited and spontaneously regressing. A type of fibromatosis containing eosinophilic inclusions identical to those seen in infantile digital fibromatosis has been identified.[925] Parenthetically, similar inclusions have been identified in the stromal component of fibroepithelial lesions having a phylloides tumor–like appearance.[902,913]

Pseudoangiomatous stromal hyperplasia (PASH) is characterized by a proliferation of stromal spindle cells of fibroblastic/myofibroblastic nature associated with the formation of probably artefactual clefts that simulate vascular channels[931] (Plate XVI-E). In the more cellular areas the pseudoangiomatous pattern may be absent.[925a] The spindle cells are immunoreactive for vimentin and CD34, and negative for FVIII-related antigen, *Ulex*, and CD31. In addition, they show intense positivity for progesterone receptors. The latter finding suggests that PASH represents a localized form of stromal overgrowth with a hormonal (primarily progestogenic) pathogenesis.[900]

Multinucleated giant cells of reactive appearance are sometimes found incidentally in the normal mammary stroma or in the stroma of fibroadenomas[901,927]; they are of no clinical significance and are probably analogous to those seen in non-neoplastic polypoid stromal lesions located beneath mucosal membranes, such as the nasal cavity, oral cavity, anus, and lower female genital tract[927] (Plate XVI-F).

Amyloidosis can appear as a solitary nodule within the breast parenchyma (so-called amyloid tumor).[923,930]

Sinus histiocytosis with massive lymphadenopathy (Rosai-Dorfman disease) can also present under exceptional circumstances as a breast mass.[918]

Lymphoid Tumors and Tumorlike Conditions

Malignant lymphoma can present as a primary mammary neoplasm or involve the breast as part of a generalized process.[937,948] A few cases have been reported associated with (and perhaps arising from) lymphocytic lobulitis,[947] and a case has been observed surrounding a silicone breast prosthesis.[936a] Grossly, the tumor is soft and grayish white. It is not accompanied by skin retraction or nipple discharge. For some peculiar reason, the right breast is affected more commonly than the left. Multiple nodules are sometimes encountered. The involvement is bilateral in one of every four patients. Primary lymphoma of the breast is almost always of non-Hodgkin's type and usually has a diffuse pattern of growth. In adult patients, the most common lymphoma is the large cell type, followed by small lymphocytic and follicular types; nearly all of these tumors are of B-cell nature.[933,939,943,949,950] Microscopically, the tumor generally grows in a diffuse fashion, with a tendency to surround and invade the wall and lumen of the epithelial structures (so-called lymphoepithelial lesions) in a fashion similar to that seen in other lymphomas arising from so-called mucosa-associated lymphoid tissue.[941,944] Immunohistochemical studies have shown that nearly all of these cases lack evidence of marginal or mantle cell differentiation.[933,934] The targetoid pattern sometimes seen around the ducts may sim-

ulate the appearance of invasive lobular carcinoma; in such cases, stains for LCA and keratin should solve the diagnostic dilemma (Fig. 20-81). The survival of patients with breast lymphoma is related to stage and microscopic type.[936]

In some of the African cases of *Burkitt's lymphoma* in children, involvement of the breast has resulted in huge bilateral masses. Bilateral Burkitt-type lymphomas have also been seen in young women during pregnancy.[934]

Primary *Hodgkin's disease* of the breast is exceptional. Most cases of Hodgkin's disease involving the breast represent secondary involvement in stage IV disease.

Plasmacytoma has seen presenting as a primary breast mass, sometimes associated with a serum monoclonal protein.[940]

Pseudolymphoma, a reactive process better designated as lymphoid hyperplasia, can present as a distinct mass in the breast.[945] It appears grossly as a firm, solid nodule and microscopically as a lymphoid infiltrate often containing germinal centers and accompanied by vascular proliferation. Some of the cases seem to represent an exuberant local reaction to injury.[942] As to be expected from a reactive lesion, both B and T cells are present, the former exhibiting polyclonal features.[938]

As in other organs, the nature and significance of diffuse masses composed of a monotonous proliferation of mature lymphocytes may be difficult to determine, even with cell marker studies. In such cases, the noncommittal diagnosis of "small lymphocytic proliferation" may be the best approach, with recommendation for conservative therapy if no systemic evidence for lymphoma is encountered.

Acute and chronic *myelocytic leukemia* can present as a localized mass ("granulocytic sarcoma") in the breast and be microscopically confused with large cell lymphoma[935a,946] (Fig. 20-82). The most important clue to the diagnosis in H&E sections is the presence of eosinophilic myelocytes or metamyelocytes, identified because of their round or slightly indented nucleus and bright eosinophilic cytoplasmic granules. The diagnosis can be confirmed by performing the Leder's chloroacetate esterase stain.

Exceptionally, a mass of myeloid metaplasia can form in the breast in patients with idiopathic myelofibrosis.[935]

Metastatic Tumors

Metastatic malignant tumors rarely affect the breast except in widely disseminated tumors. They typically appear as superficial, well-defined multinodular masses. Malignant melanoma and carcinoma of the lung, ovary, kidney, and stomach are the most common sources.[952,953,957] Most of the lung tumors are of the small cell type. Metastases can also develop from endocrine tumors, such as bronchial carcinoid and thyroid medullary carcinoma.[954,956] One should not forget in this listing the metastases from contralateral breast carcinoma, which is not an infrequent finding in autopsy series. Azzopardi[951] has made the interesting observation that presence of elastosis has not been documented in association with metastatic disease of the breast.

In children, the most common malignant tumor to metastasize to the breast (hematopoietic malignancies excluded) is rhabdomyosarcoma, particularly of the alveolar type.[955]

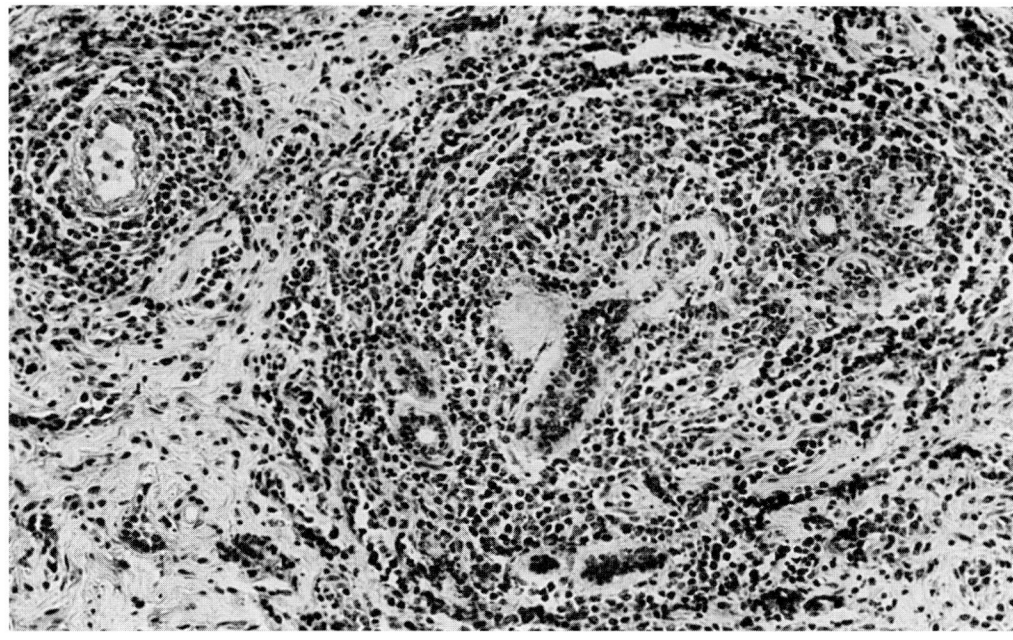

Fig. 20-81 Malignant lymphoma of breast. Concentric arrangement of tumor cells around lobules resembles that of lobular carcinoma in situ. Perivascular arrangement of tumor cells is also evident.

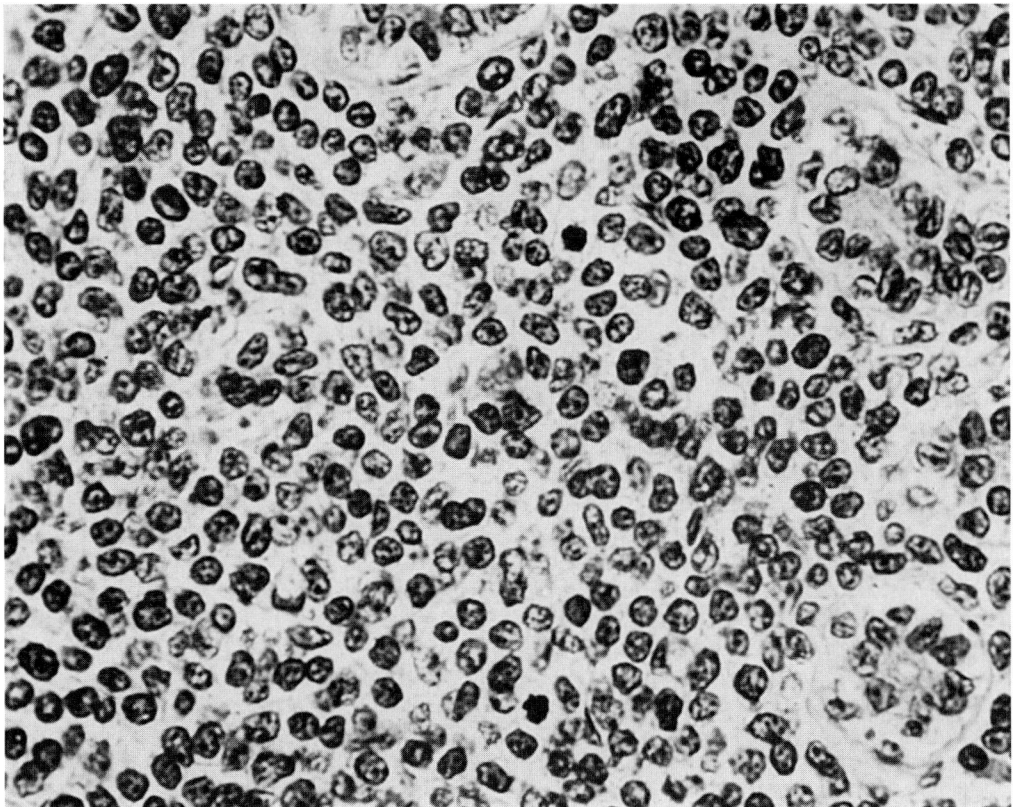

Fig. 20-82 Involvement of breast by myelocytic leukemia. It would be extremely difficult to distinguish this lesion from large cell lymphoma on H&E sections. Leder stain for chloroacetate esterase was positive.

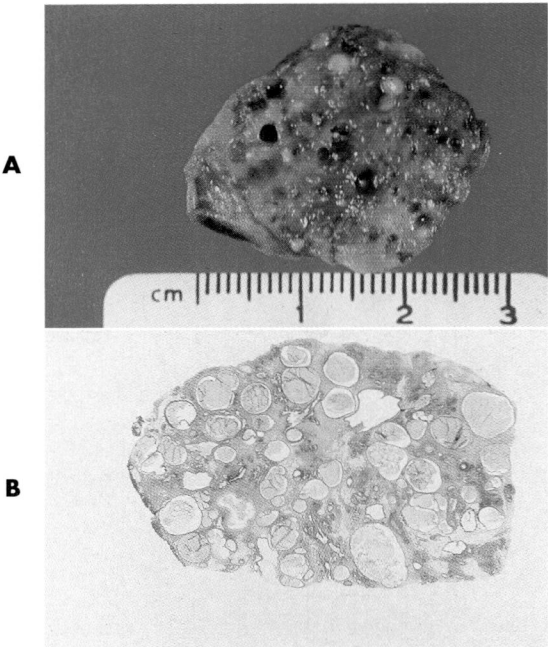

Fig. 20-83 Juvenile papillomatosis (Swiss cheese disease). A, Gross appearance is that of clustered cystic formations. B, Wholemount view showing variously sized cystic formations, alternating with solid epithelial proliferations.

Breast Diseases in Children and Adolescents

The most common breast "mass" for which clinical consultation is sought in this age group is actually not a pathologic condition at all but rather precocious and/or predominantly unilateral breast development.[958] Should such a "mass" be removed, no development of the breast will occur.[966]

Fibroadenoma is the most common pathologic condition of the breast between puberty and 20 years of age, but it is exceptional before puberty.[959]

Virginal hypertrophy (gigantomastia) may result in massive unilateral or bilateral enlargement.[958] Microscopically, it is characterized by a combined proliferation of ducts and stroma with little, if any, lobular participation.[961]

Fibrocystic disease of the conventional type is practically never seen in this age group. However, highly proliferative epithelial lesions can develop. Some of them have the appearance of intraductal papillomas.[960,963] Others resemble duct hyperplasia (epitheliosis) of the adult breast, with or without associated sclerosis and ductular distortion.[963] Wilson et al.[968] studied seventy-four patients with a process they termed *papillary duct hyperplasia,* which they distinguish from the juvenile papillomatosis described later. They found that 28% of the patients had a family history for breast carcinoma but that none of them had developed carcinoma at the time of the last follow-up.

Juvenile papillomatosis (Swiss cheese disease) is a probably related but morphologically somewhat distinct form of ductal-type hyperplasia usually seen in young individuals (average age, 19 years) but occurring in a wide age range (10 to 44 years). Clinically, the localized, multinodular masses simulate the appearance of fibroadenoma. Grossly, the clustering of the cystic formations results in a cut surface appearance reminiscent of Swiss cheese—hence the alternative designation for this entity (Fig. 20-83, A). Microscopically, there is florid epithelial hyperplasia (sometimes with marked atypia and/or focal necrosis), cysts with or without apocrine metaplasia, duct stasis, and sclerosing adenosis[960,964] (Fig. 20-83, B). A family history of breast carcinoma is reported in 58% of the cases, and 10% of the patients subsequently develop breast carcinoma.[965,967]

Carcinoma of the infantile breast is very rare. Most cases are of the so-called juvenile (secretory) type and are discussed on p. 1613. A few tumors have the appearance of ordinary invasive ductal carcinomas.

The other type of malignancy that has been described in the breast of children is a highly undifferentiated solid neoplasm formed by medium-sized round cells without ductular or acinar formation. Some of these cases have been reported as small cell undifferentiated carcinomas.[962] After having personally reviewed some examples, we believe that at least some of them actually represent embryonal or alveolar rhabdomyosarcomas or other types of soft tissue sarcomas of the chest wall.

Breast Diseases in Males
GYNECOMASTIA

Gynecomastia is defined as the enlargement of the male breast resulting from hypertrophy and hyperplasia of both glandular and stromal components. It may result from numerous causes, which share the pathophysiologic feature of a relative increase in estrogenic activity (whether endogenous or exogenous), a decrease in androgenic activity, or both.[970,977] Development of gynecomastia before 25 years of age is usually related to hormonal pubertal changes, whereas development in later years may be caused by hormonally active tumors (Leydig cell tumor of testis, hCG-secreting germ cell tumor, lung carcinoma, or others), cirrhosis, or medications (digitalis, reserpine, Dilantin, and others).[971,976] Many cases remain idiopathic.

Clinically, gynecomastia is usually centered below the nipple, an important point in the differential diagnosis with carcinoma, which tends to be located eccentrically.[970] It may be unilateral (at least at the clinical level, the left breast being more commonly involved than the right) or bilateral. It has been noted that pubertal and hormone-induced gynecomastias tend to be bilateral, whereas idiopathic and nonhormonal drug-induced gynecomastias are usually unilateral.[975]

The gross appearance is characteristic. The mass is oval, disk shaped, of elastic consistency, and with well-circumscribed borders. Microscopically, the ducts show a variable and sometimes very prominent degree of epithelial hyperplasia and are surrounded by a prominent swollen stroma, which results in a typical "halo" effect[975] (Fig. 20-84). This stroma contains large amounts of acid mucopolysaccharides (mainly hyaluronic acid) of a type similar to that seen in fibroadenoma of the female breast.[972] Focal squamous meta-

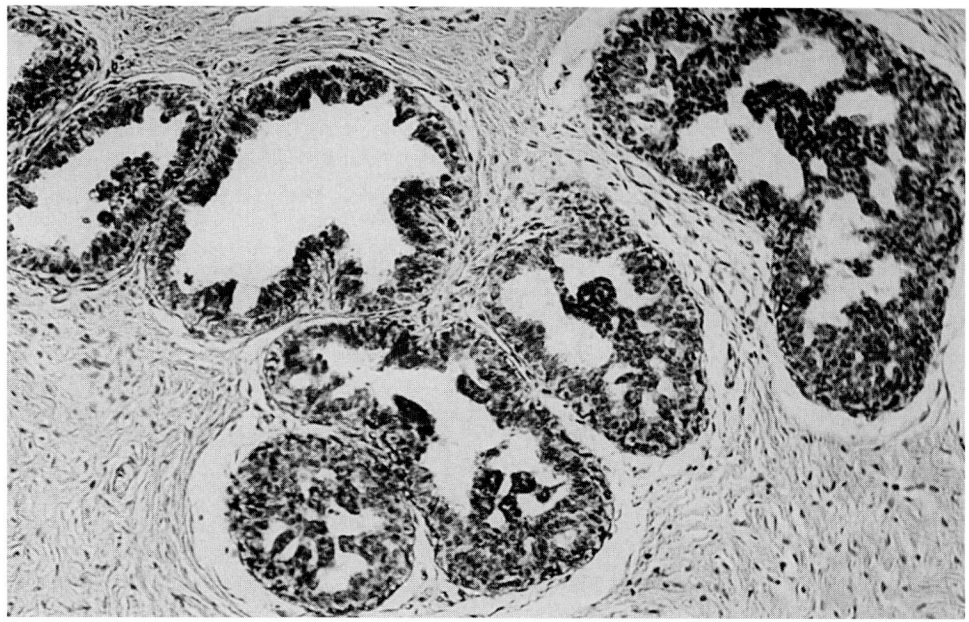

Fig. 20-84 Prominent intraductal hyperplasia and stromal edema in gynecomastia.

plasia and formation of lobules may be observed.[970,973] Exceptionally, a population of clear or globoid cells immunoreactive for GCDFP-15 may be present.[973a]

The microscopic changes are related to the duration of the gynecomastia. Cases of short duration tend to have a prominent hyperplastic epithelial component and stromal edema, whereas those of long duration have prominent stromal fibrosis.[969] In rare cases, the intraductal epithelial hyperplasia is so extreme as to simulate carcinoma. In others, the proliferation has fibroadenoma-like qualities.[974]

The possible relationship between gynecomastia and carcinoma is discussed in the next section.

CARCINOMA

In the United States, only 1% of all breast carcinomas occur in males, but in Egypt and other countries the incidence rises to nearly 10%.[985,986] An increased incidence of breast carcinoma is seen in patients with Klinefelter's syndrome.[997] Familial cases have also been recorded.[984,991] An important and not entirely resolved issue is that of the possible relationship between gynecomastia and breast carcinoma. In one series, microscopic changes consistent with gynecomastia were found in 40% of breast carcinoma cases.[990] Furthermore, cases of primary breast carcinoma have occurred in patients with prostatic carcinoma treated with estrogens.[993] Finally, countries in which the incidence of gynecomastia is high also have a high incidence of breast carcinoma. All these data would seem to point toward a pathogenetic link between the two entities.

Clinically, most breast carcinomas present in elderly individuals as breast nodules, with or without associated nipple abnormalities.[979,983] Nipple discharge in an adult male, espe-

cially if bloody, should arouse a strong suspicion of carcinoma. Skin involvement by fixation and Paget's disease are much more common in males. As in females, the condition can simulate malignant melanoma.[1000]

Grossly and microscopically, carcinomas of the male breast are remarkably similar to those seen in females[985] (Fig. 20-85). As such, they can be in situ or invasive.[981] All of the microscopic types identified in the female breast have been encountered in males, including tumors with neuroendocrine features.[994,998] The least common of the major categories is invasive lobular carcinoma, only a few cases having been observed.[987,997] Other very unusual types include adenomyoepithelioma[1001] and oncocytic carcinoma.[982] We have seen two examples of the latter (Fig. 20-86).

The tumors can be identified by FNA, the most important differential diagnosis using this modality being gynecomastia.[980] The incidence of positivity for estrogen receptors is higher than in females.[989]

The incidence of axillary metastases is the same in men as in women, but the prognosis is slightly worse in males, especially for stage II and III disease.[978,988,992,996] In a series of ninety-seven cases of male breast carcinoma reported by Heller et al.,[990] the 10-year survival rate was 40% for the whole group, 79% for those with negative axillary nodes, and 11% for those with positive nodes.

As in females, the prognosis of breast carcinoma in males is dependent upon clinical stage and microscopic grade.[999,1002] It also correlates with proliferative activity.[995]

OTHER LESIONS

Mammary duct ectasia[1013] and *sclerosing adenosis*[1005] can occur in the male breast. Fibrocystic disease, fibroadenoma, pseudoangiomatous stromal hyperplasia (PASH), and phylloides tumor have also been reported but are vanishingly rare.[1002b,1010]

Nipple adenoma and ***intraductal papilloma*** have been seen on several occasions, in one instance following estrogen therapy for prostatic carcinoma.[1008,1012,1015] There is a single report of ***leiomyosarcoma*** of the nipple,[1009] and another of ***neurofibromatosis*** in a child whose condition simulated gynecomastia.[1011]

Myofibroblastoma (myogenic stromal tumor) is a benign spindle-cell neoplasm that occurs more commonly in the male than in the female breast.[1003,1016] Similar cases had been previously reported by Toker et al. as benign spindle-cell tumors.[1014] Grossly, the well-circumscribed nodules are usually small, but on occasion they can reach a large size.[1002a] Microscopically, uniform, bland-looking spindle cells are haphazardly arranged in fascicles separated by broad bands of hyalinized collagen (Fig. 20-87). The appearance is reminiscent of solitary fibrous tumor, sometimes to a striking degree.[1006] Their similarity is accentuated by the fact that some of these tumors show strong CD34 immunoreactivity. Focal cartilaginous metaplasia can occur. The ultrastructural features are said to be those of myofibroblasts, and immunoreactivity for desmin has been encountered in a few of the cases.[1016] The behavior has invariably been benign.

Metastatic carcinoma to the male breast usually originates from the prostate, is often bilateral, and is almost always seen following estrogen therapy.[1004] As such, it occurs against a background of gynecomastia. Some of these cases have been confused with primary breast carcinoma. Immunohistochemical stains for PSA and prostatic acid phosphatase are helpful in the differential diagnosis.[1007]

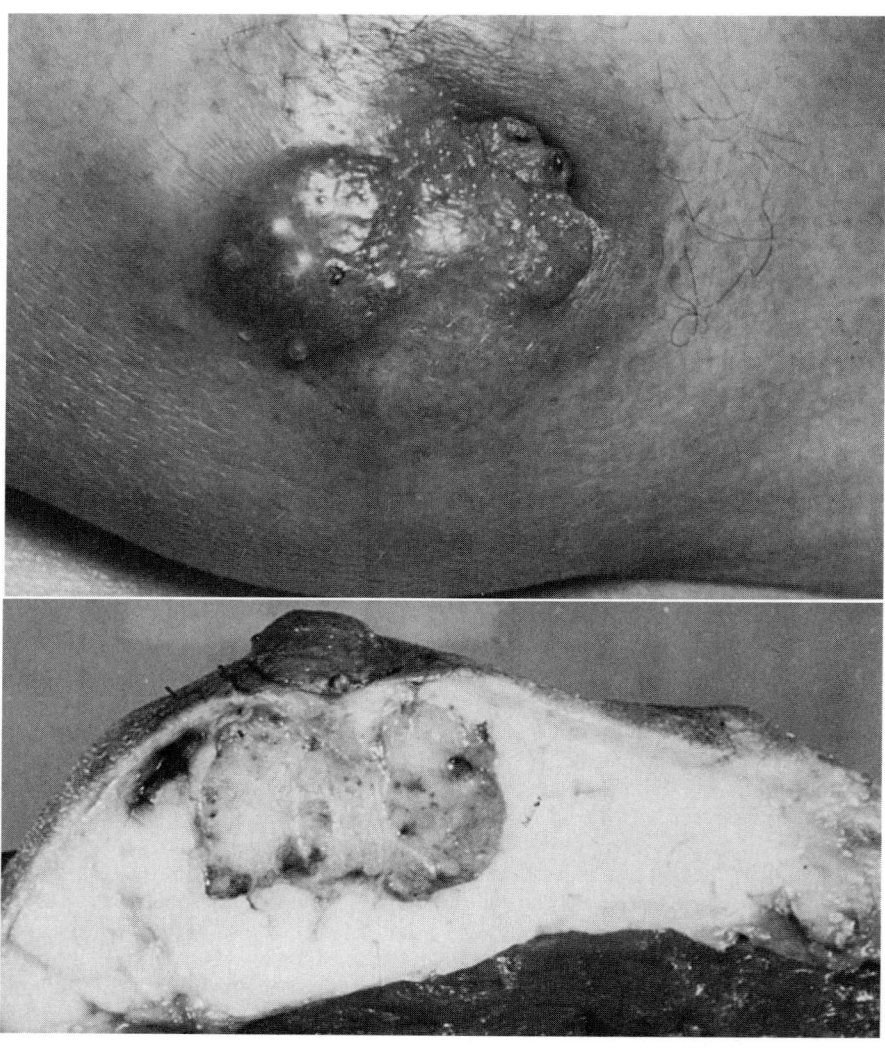

Fig. 20-85 Right breast of 65-year-old man showing marked nipple deformity and ulceration with nodularity of areolar skin secondary to infiltrating duct carcinoma. (Courtesy Dr. J.C. Ashhurst, Tuskegee, AL.)

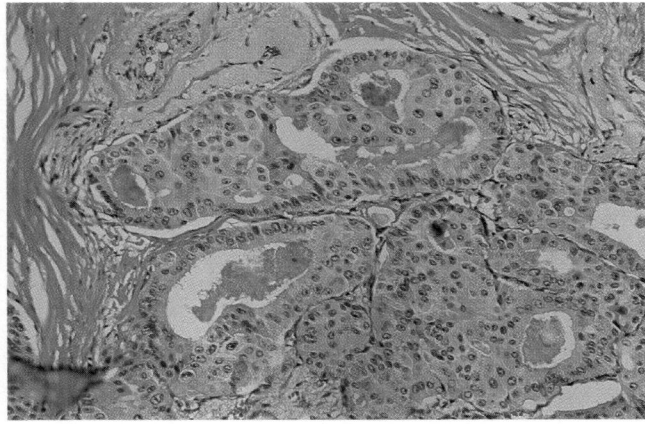

Fig. 20-86 Carcinoma of the male breast composed of well-differentiated tumor cells with abundant granular cytoplasm having oncocytic features.

REFERENCES
Normal anatomy

1 Azzopardi JG: Problems in breast pathology. In Bennington JL, consulting ed: Major problems in pathology, vol 11. Philadelphia, 1979, WB Saunders Co.
2 Barwick KW, Kashgarian M, Rosen PP: "Clear-cell" change within duct and lobular epithelium of the human breast. Pathol Annu 17(Pt 1):319-328, 1982.
3 Battersby S, Anderson TJ: Histological changes in breast tissue that characterize recent pregnancy. Histopathology 15:415-419, 1989.
4 Bussolati G, Gugliotta P, Sapino A, Eusebi V, Lloyd RV: Chromogranin reactive endocrine cells in argyrophilic carcinomas ("carcinoids") and normal tissue of the breast. Am J Pathol 120:186-192, 1985.
5 Charpin C, Lissitzky JC, Jacquemier J, Lavaut MN, Kopp F, Pourreau-Schneider N, Martin PM, Toga M: Immunohistochemical detection of laminin in 98 human breast carcinomas. A light and electron microscopic study. Hum Pathol 17:355-365, 1986.
6 Clayton F, Ordóñez NG, Hanssen GM, Hanssen H: Immunoperoxidase localization of lactalbumin in malignant breast neoplasms. Arch Pathol Lab Med 106:268-270, 1982.
7 Cowan DF, Herbert TA: Involution of the breast in women aged 50 to 104 years. A histological study of 102 cases. Surg Pathol 2:323-334, 1989.
8 Cunha GR: Role of mesenchymal-epithelial interactions in normal and abnormal development of the mammary gland and prostate. Cancer 74:1030-1044, 1994.
9 Dwarakanath S, Lee AKC, DeLellis RA, Silverman ML, Frasca L, Wolfe HJ: S-100 protein positivity in breast carcinomas. A potential pitfall in diagnostic immunohistochemistry. Hum Pathol 18:1144-1148, 1987.
10 Egan MJ, Newman J, Crocker J, Collard M: Immunohistochemical localization of S100 protein in benign and malignant conditions of the breast. Arch Pathol Lab Med 111:28-31, 1987.
11 Farahmand S, Cowan DF: Elastosis in the normal aging breast. A histopathologic study of 140 cases. Arch Pathol Lab Med 115:1241-1246, 1991.
12 Fechner RE: The surgical pathology of the reproductive system and breast during oral contraceptive therapy. Pathol Annu 6:299-319, 1971.
13 Greenwalt DE, Johnson VG, Kuhajda FP, Eggleston JC, Mather IH: Localization of a membrane glycoprotein in benign fibrocystic disease and infiltrating duct carcinomas of the human breast with the use of a monoclonal antibody to guinea pig milk fat globule membrane. Am J Pathol 118:351-359, 1985.

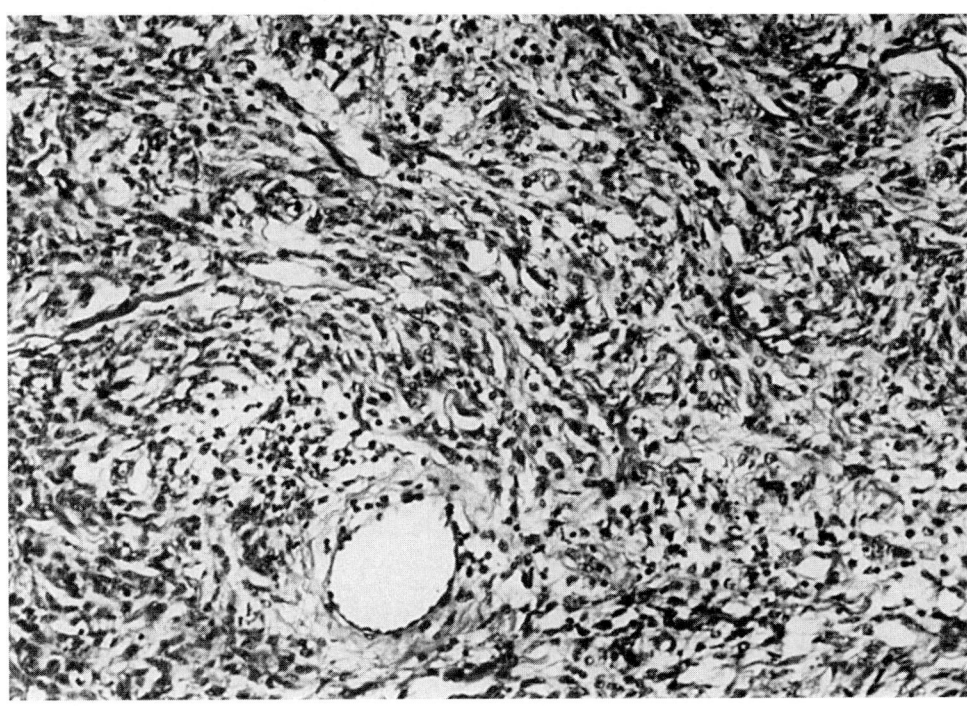

Fig. 20-87 So-called myofibroblastoma of male breast. Cellular tumor composed of spindle to oval cells is set against collagenous background with scattering of prominent vessels.

14　Jarasch E-D, Nagle RB, Kaufmann M, Maurer C, Böcker WJ: Differential diagnosis of benign epithelial proliferations and carcinomas of the breast using antibodies to cytokeratins. Hum Pathol **19:**276-289, 1988.

15　Joshi K, Ellis JTB, Hughes CM, Monaghan P, Neville AM: Cellular proliferation in the rat mammary gland during pregnancy and lactation. Lab Invest **54:**52-61, 1986.

16　Joshi K, Smith JA, Perusinghe N, Monoghan P: Cell proliferation in the human mammary epithelium. Differential contribution by epithelial and myoepithelial cells. Am J Pathol **124:**199-206, 1986.

17　Kiaer HW, Andersen JA: Focal pregnancy-like changes in the breast. Acta Pathol Microbiol Scand (A) **85:**931-941, 1977.

18　Larsen BL, Smith VR, eds: Lactation. A comprehensive treatise. New York, 1974, Academic Press.

19　Longacre TA, Bartow SA: A correlative morphologic study of human breast and endometrium in the menstrual cycle. Am J Surg Pathol **10:**382-393, 1986.

20　Monteagudo C, Merino MJ, San-Juan J, Liotta LA, Stetler-Stevenson WG: Immunohistochemical distribution of type IV collagenase in normal, benign, and malignant breast tissue. Am J Pathol **136:**585-592, 1990.

21　Ozzello L: Epithelial-stromal junction of normal and dysplastic mammary glands. Cancer **25:**586-600, 1970.

22　Rosen PP, Tench W: Lobules in the nipple. Frequency and significance for breast cancer treatment. Pathol Annu **20** (Pt 2):317-322, 1985.

23　Rytina ER, Coady AT, Millis RR: Milk granuloma. An unusual appearance in lactational breast tissue. Histopathology **17:**466-468, 1990.

24　Satake T, Matsuyama M: Endocrine cells in a normal breast and non-cancerous breast lesion. Acta Pathol Jpn **41:**874-878, 1991.

25　Slavin JL, Billson VR, Ostor AG: Nodular breast lesions during pregnancy and lactation. Histopathology **22:**481-485, 1993.

26　Smith CA, Monaghan P, Neville AM: Basal clear cells of the normal human breast. Virchows Arch [A] **402:**319-329, 1984.

27　Smith DM Jr, Peters TG, Donegan WL: Montgomery's areolar tubercle. A light microscopic study. Arch Pathol Lab Med **106:**60-63, 1982.

28　Tavassoli FA, Yeh IT: Lactational and clear cell changes of the breast in nonlactating, nonpregnant women. Am J Clin Pathol **87:**23-29, 1987.

29　Toker C: Clear cells of the nipple epidermis. Cancer **25:**601-610, 1970.

30　Tsubura A, Okada H, Senzaki H, Hatano T, Morii S: Keratin expression in the normal breast and in breast carcinoma. Histopathology **18:**517-522, 1991.

31　Vogel PM, Georgiade NG, Fetter BF, Vogel FS, McCarty KS Jr: The correlation of histologic changes in the human breast with the menstrual cycle. Am J Pathol **104:**23-34, 1981.

32　Wellings SR, Jensen HM, Marcum RG: An atlas of subgross pathology of the human breast with special reference to possible precancerous lesions. JNCI **55:**231-273, 1975.

Ectopia

33　Edlow DW, Carter D: Heterotopic epithelium in axillary lymph nodes. Report of a case and review of the literature. Am J Clin Pathol **59:**666-673, 1973.

34　O'Hara MF, Page DL: Adenomas of the breast and ectopic breast under lactational influences. Hum Pathol **16:**707-712, 1985.

35　Turner DR, Millis RR: Breast tissue inclusions in axillary lymph nodes. Histopathology **4:**631-363, 1980.

Inflammatory and related lesions
MAMMARY DUCT ECTASIA

36　Haagensen CD: Mammary-duct ectasia. A disease that may simulate carcinoma. Cancer **4:**749-761, 1951.

FAT NECROSIS

37　Clarke D, Curtis JL, Martinez A, Fajardo L, Goffinet D: Fat necrosis of the breast simulating recurrent carcinoma after primary radiotherapy in the management of early stage breast carcinoma. Cancer **52:**442-445, 1983.

38　Dabbs DJ: Mammary ductal foam cells. Macrophage immunophenotype. Hum Pathol **24:**977-981, 1993.

OTHER INFLAMMATORY DISEASES

39　Arnaout AH, Shousha S, Metaxas N, Husain OA: Intramammary tuberculous lymphadenitis. Histopathology **17:**91-93, 1990.

40　Ashton MA, Lefkowitz M, Tavassoli FA: Epithelioid stromal cells in lymphocytic mastitis. A source of confusion with invasive carcinoma. Mod Pathol **7:**49-54, 1994.

41　Banik S, Bishop PW, Ormerod LP, O'Brien TE: Sarcoidosis of the breast. J Clin Pathol **39:**446-448, 1986.

42　Bocian JJ, Fahmy RN, Michas CA: A rare case of 'coccidioidoma' of the breast. Arch Pathol Lab Med **115:**1064-1067, 1991.

43　Catania S, Zurrida S, Veronesi P, Galimberti V, Bono A, Pluchinotta A: Mondor's disease and breast cancer. Cancer **69:**2267-2270, 1992.

44　Cooper NE: Rheumatoid nodule in the breast. Histopathology **19:**193-194, 1991.

44a　Coyne JD, Baildam AD, Asbury D: Lymphocytic mastopathy associated with ductal carcinoma in situ of the breast. Histopathology **26:**579-580, 1995.

45　Eckland DA, Zeigler MG: Abscess in the nonlactating breast. Arch Surg **107:**398-401, 1973.

46　Elsner B, Harper FB: Disseminated Wegener's granulomatosis with breast involvement. Report of a case. Arch Pathol **87:**544-547, 1969.

47　Farrow JH: Thrombophlebitis of the superficial veins of the breast and anterior chest wall (Mondor's disease). Surg Gynecol Obstet **101:**63-68, 1955.

48　Fitzgibbons PL, Smiley DF, Kern WH: Sarcoidosis presenting initially as breast mass. Report of two cases. Hum Pathol **16:**851-852, 1985.

49　Fletcher A, Magrath IM, Riddell RH, Talbot IC: Granulomatous mastitis. A report of seven cases. J Clin Pathol **35:**941-945, 1982.

50　Hamit HF: Implantation of plastics in the breast. Arch Surg **75:**224-229, 1957.

51　Herrmann JB: Thrombophlebitis of breast and contiguous thoracicoabdominal wall (Mondor's disease). NY State J Med **66:**3146-3152, 1966.

52　Johnson WC, Wallrich R, Helwig EB: Superficial thrombophlebitis of the chest wall. JAMA **180:**103-108, 1962.

53　Jordan JM, Rowe WT, Allen NB: Wegener's granulomatosis involving the breast. Report of three cases and review of the literature. Am J Med **83:**159-164, 1987.

54　Kessler EI, Katzav JA: Lobular granulomatous mastitis. Surg Pathol **3:**115-120, 1990.

55　Lammie GA, Bobrow LG, Staunton MD, Levison DA, Page G, Millis RR: Sclerosing lymphocytic lobulitis of the breast. Evidence for an autoimmune pathogenesis. Histopathology **19:**13-20, 1991.

56　Lucey JJ: Spontaneous infarction of the breast. J Clin Pathol **28:**937-943, 1975.

56a　Morgan MC, Weaver MG, Crowe JP, Abdul-Karim FW: Diabetic mastopathy. A clinicopathologic study in palpable and nonpalpable breast lesions. Mod Pathol **8:**349-354, 1995.

57　Ng WF, Chow LT, Lam PW: Localized polyarteritis nodosa of breast. Report of two cases and a review of the literature. Histopathology **23:**535-539, 1993.

58　Nudelman HL, Kempson RL: Necrosis of the breast. A rare complication of anticoagulant therapy. Am J Surg **111:**728-733, 1966.

59　Osborne BM: Granulomatous mastitis caused by histoplasma and mimicking inflammatory breast carcinoma. Hum Pathol **20:**47-52, 1989.

60　Rickert RR, Rajan S: Localized breast infarcts associated with pregnancy. Arch Pathol **97:**159-161, 1974.

61　Robitaille Y, Seemayer TA, Thelmo WL, Cumberlidge MC: Infarction of the mammary region mimicking carcinoma of the breast. Cancer **33:**1183-1189, 1974.

62　Scholefield JH, Duncan JL, Rogers K: Review of a hospital experience of breast abscesses. Br J Surg **74:**469-470, 1987.

63　Schwartz IS, Strauchen JA: Lymphocytic mastopathy. An autoimmune disease of the breast? Am J Clin Pathol **93:**725-730, 1990.

64　Sebek B: Periareolar abscess associated with squamous metaplasia of lactiferous ducts (Zuska's disease). Lab Invest **58:**83A, 1988.

65　Seidman JD, Schnaper LA, Phillips LE: Mastopathy in insulin-requiring diabetes mellitus. Hum Pathol **25:**819-824, 1994.

66　Symmers W St C: Silicone mastitis in "topless" waitress and some other varieties of foreign-body mastitis. Br Med J **3:**19-22, 1968.

67　Tomaszewski JE, Brooks JS, Hicks D, Livolsi VA: Diabetic mastopathy. A distinctive clinicopathologic entity. Hum Pathol **23:**780-786, 1992.

68　Vuitch F: Spectrum of granulomatous mastitis (abstract). Lab Invest **58:**99A, 1988.

69　Watt-Boolsen S, Rasmussen NR, Blichert-Toft M: Primary periareolar abscess in the nonlactating breast. Risk of recurrence. Am J Surg **153:**571-573, 1987.

Benign proliferative breast disease
FIBROADENOMA

70　Arrigoni MG, Dockerty MB, Judd ES: The identification and treatment of mammary hamartoma. Surg Gynecol Obstet **133:**577-582, 1971.

71　Azzopardi JG: Problems in breast pathology. In Bennington JL, consulting ed: Major problems in pathology, vol 11. Philadelphia, 1979, WB Saunders Co.

72　Berean K, Tron VA, Churg A, Clement PB: Mammary fibroadenoma with multinucleated stromal giant cells. Am J Surg Pathol **10:**823-827, 1986.

73　Carney JA, Toorkey BC: Myxoid fibroadenoma and allied conditions (myxomatosis) of the breast. A heritable disorder with special associations including cardiac and cutaneous myxomas. Am J Surg Pathol **15:**713-721, 1991.

74　Carstens PHB: Ultrastructure of human fibroadenoma. Arch Pathol **98:**23-32, 1974.

75 Dupont WD, Page DL, Parl FF, Vnencak-Jones CL, Plummer WD Jr, Rados MS, Schuyler PA: Long-term risk of breast cancer in women with fibroadenoma. N Engl J Med **331**:10-15, 1994.

76 Eusebi V, Azzopardi JG: Lobular endocrine neoplasia in fibroadenoma of the breast. Histopathology **4**:413-428, 1980.

77 Fechner RE: Fibroadenomas in patients receiving oral contraceptives. A clinical and pathologic study. Am J Clin Pathol **53**:857-864, 1970.

78 Fekete P, Petrek J, Majmudar B, Someren A, Sandberg W: Fibroadenomas with stromal cellularity. A clinicopathologic study of 21 patients. Arch Pathol Lab Med **111**:427-432, 1987.

79 Fletcher JA, Pinkus GS, Weidner N, Morton CC: Lineage-restricted clonality in biphasic solid tumors. Am J Pathol **138**:1199-1207, 1991.

80 Goodman ZD, Taxy JB: Fibroadenomas of the breast with prominent smooth muscle. Am J Surg Pathol **5**:99-101, 1981.

81 Metcalf JS, Ellis B: Choristoma of the breast. Hum Pathol **16**:739-740, 1985.

82 Mies C, Rosen PP: Juvenile fibroadenoma with atypical epithelial hyperplasia. Am J Surg Pathol **11**:184-190, 1987.

83 Oberman HA, Nosanchuk HS, Finger JE: Periductal stromal tumors of breast with adipose metaplasia. Arch Surg **98**:384-387, 1969.

84 O'Hara MF, Page DL: Adenomas of the breast and ectopic breast under lactational influences. Hum Pathol **16**:707-712, 1985.

85 Petrik PK: Mammary hamartoma. Am J Surg Pathol **11**:234-235, 1987.

86 Pike AM, Oberman HA: Juvenile (cellular) adenofibromas. A clinicopathologic study. Am J Surg Pathol **9**:730-736, 1985.

87 Rao BR, Meyer JS, Fry CG: Most cystosarcoma phyllodes and fibroadenomas have progesterone receptor but lack estrogen receptor. Stromal localization of progesterone receptor. Cancer **47**:2016-2021, 1981.

88 Reddick RL, Shin TK, Sawhney D, Siegal GP: Stromal proliferations of the breast. An ultrastructural and immunohistochemical evaluation of cystosarcoma phyllodes, juvenile fibroadenoma, and fibroadenoma. Hum Pathol **18**:45-49, 1987.

89 Schweizer-Cagianut M, Salomon F, Hedinger CE: Primary adrenocortical nodular dysplasia with Cushing's syndrome and cardiac myxomas. A peculiar familial disease. Virchows Arch **397**:183-192, 1982.

90 Yeh I-T, Francis DJ, Orenstein JM, Silverberg SG: Ultrastructure of cystosarcoma phyllodes and fibroadenoma. A comparative study. Am J Clin Pathol **84**:131-136, 1985.

Malignant transformation

91 Buzanowski-Konakry K, Harrison EG Jr, Payne WS: Lobular carcinoma arising in fibroadenoma of the breast. Cancer **35**:450-456, 1975.

92 Curran RC, Dodge OG: Sarcoma of breast, with particular reference to its origin from fibroadenoma. J Clin Pathol **15**:1-16, 1962.

93 Diaz NM, Palmer JO, McDivitt RW: Carcinoma arising within fibroadenomas of the breast. A clinicopathologic study of 105 patients. Am J Clin Pathol **95**:614-622, 1991.

94 Fondo EY, Rosen PP, Fracchia AA, Urban JA: The problem of carcinoma developing in a fibroadenoma. Recent experience at Memorial Hospital. Cancer **43**:563-567, 1979.

95 Goldman RC, Friedman NB: Carcinoma of the breast arising in fibroadenomas with emphasis on lobular carcinoma. A clinicopathologic study. Cancer **23**:544-550, 1969.

96 McDivitt RW, Stewart FW, Farrow JH: Breast carcinoma arising in solitary fibroadenomas. Surg Gynecol Obstet **125**:572-576, 1967.

97 Pick PW, Iossifides IA: Occurrence of breast carcinoma within a fibroadenoma. A review. Arch Pathol Lab Med **108**:590-594, 1984.

ADENOMA

98 Baddoura FK, Judd RL: Apocrine adenoma of the breast. Report of a case with investigation of lectin binding patterns in apocrine breast lesions. Mod Pathol **3**:373-376, 1990.

99 Carney JA, Toorkey BC: Ductal adenoma of the breast with tubular features. A probable component of the complex of myxomas, spotty pigmentation, endocrine overactivity, and schwannomas. Am J Surg Pathol **15**:722-731, 1991.

100 Hertel BF, Zaloudek C, Kempson RL: Breast adenomas. Cancer **37**:2891-2905, 1976.

101 Le Gal Y: Adenomas of the breast. Relationship of adenofibromas to pregnancy and lactation. Am Surg **27**:14-22, 1961.

102 Morris JA, Kelly JF: Multiple bilateral breast adenomata in identical adolescent Negro twins. Histopathology **6**:539-547, 1982.

103 O'Hara MF, Page DL: Adenomas of the breast and ectopic breast under lactational influences. Hum Pathol **16**:707-712, 1985.

INTRADUCTAL PAPILLOMA

104 Azzopardi JG: Problems in breast pathology. In Bennington JL, consulting ed: Major problems in pathology, vol 11. Philadelphia, 1979, WB Saunders Co.

105 Azzopardi JG, Salm R: Ductal adenoma of the breast. A lesion which can mimic carcinoma. J Pathol **144**:15-23, 1984.

106 Egan MJ, Newman J, Crocker J, Collard M: Immunohistochemical localization of S100 protein in benign and malignant conditions of the breast. Arch Pathol Lab Med **111**:28-31, 1987.

107 Fenoglio C, Lattes R: Sclerosing papillary proliferations in the female breast. A benign lesion often mistaken for carcinoma. Cancer **33**:691-700, 1974.

108 Haagensen CD, Stout AP, Phillips JS: The papillary neoplasms of the breast. Ann Surg **133**:18-36, 1951.

109 Kraus FT, Neubecker RD: The differential diagnosis of papillary tumors of the breast. Cancer **15**:444-455, 1962.

110 Lammie GA, Millis RR: Ductal adenoma of the breast. A review of fifteen cases. Hum Pathol **20**:903-908, 1989.

111 Noguchi S, Motomura K, Inaji H, Imaoka S, Koyama H: Clonal analysis of solitary intraductal papilloma of the breast by means of polymerase chain reaction. Am J Pathol **144**:1320-1325, 1994.

112 Papotti M, Eusebi V, Gugliotta P, Bussolati G: Immunohistochemical analysis of benign and malignant papillary lesions of the breast. Am J Surg Pathol **7**:451-461, 1983.

113 Papotti M, Gugliotta P, Ghiringhello B, Bussolati G: Association of breast carcinoma and multiple intraductal papillomas. An histological and immunohistochemical investigation. Histopathology **8**:963-975, 1984.

114 Raju UB, Lee MW, Zarbo RJ, Crissman JD: Papillary neoplasia of the breast. Immunohistochemically defined myoepithelial cells in the diagnosis of benign and malignant papillary breast neoplasms. Mod Pathol **2**:569-576, 1989.

115 Rosen PP: Arthur Purdy Stout and papilloma of the breast. Comments on the occasion of his 100th birthday. Am J Surg Pathol **10**(Suppl 1):100-107. 1986.

NIPPLE ADENOMA

116 Bhagavan BS, Patchefsky A, Koss LG: Florid subareolar duct papillomatosis (nipple adenoma) and mammary carcinoma. Report of three cases. Hum Pathol **4**:289-295, 1973.

116a Jones MW, Tavassoli FA: Coexistence of nipple duct adenoma and breast carcinoma. A clinicopathologic study of five cases and review of the literature. Mod Pathol **8**:637-642, 1995.

117 Le Gal Y, Gros CM, Bader P: L'adenomatose erosive du mamelon. Ann Acad Pathol (Paris) **4**:292-304, 1959.

118 Myers JL, Mazur MT, Urist MM, Peiper SC: Florid papillomatosis of the nipple. Immunohistochemical and flow cytometric analysis of two cases. Mod Pathol **3**:288-293, 1990.

119 Perzin KH, Lattes R: Papillary adenoma of the nipple (florid papillomatosis, adenoma, adenomatosis). A clinicopathologic study. Cancer **29**:996-1009, 1972.

120 Rosen PP, Caicco JA: Florid papillomatosis of the nipple. A study of 51 patients, including nine with mammary carcinoma. Am J Surg Pathol **10**:87-101, 1986.

121 Taylor HB, Robertson AG: Adenomas of the nipple. Cancer **18**:995-1002, 1966.

ADENOSIS
Blunt duct adenosis

122 Azzopardi JG: Problems in breast pathology. In Bennington JL, consulting ed: Major problems in pathology, vol 11. Philadelphia, 1979, WB Saunders Co.

123 Foote FW, Stewart FW: Comparative studies of cancerous vs. noncancerous breasts. Am Surg **121**:6-79, 1945.

Sclerosing adenosis

124 Eusebi V, Azzopardi JG: Vascular infiltration in benign breast disease. J Pathol **118**:9-16, 1976.

125 Eusebi V, Collina G, Bussolati G: Carcinoma in situ in sclerosing adenosis of the breast. An immunocytochemical study. Semin Diagn Pathol **6**:146-152, 1989.

126 Fechner RE: Lobular carcinoma in situ in sclerosing adenosis. A potential source of confusion with invasive carcinoma. Am J Surg Pathol **5**:233-239, 1981.

127 Jensen RA, Page DL, Dupont WD, Rogers LW: Invasive breast cancer risk in women with sclerosing adenosis. Cancer **64**:1977-1983, 1989.

128 Oberman HA, Markey BA: Noninvasive carcinoma of the breast presenting in adenosis. Mod Pathol **4**:31-35, 1991.

129 Taylor HB, Norris HJ: Epithelial invasion of nerves in benign diseases of the breast. Cancer **20**:2245-2249, 1967.

Nodular adenosis

130 Nielsen BB: Adenosis tumour of the breast. A clinicopathological investigation of 27 cases. Histopathology 11:1259-1275, 1987.

Microglandular adenosis

131 Clement PB, Azzopardi JG: Microglandular adenosis of the breast. A lesion simulating tubular carcinoma. Histopathology 7:169-180, 1983.

132 Eusebi V, Casedei GP, Bussolati G, Azzopardi JG: Adenomyoepithelioma of the breast with a distinctive type of apocrine adenosis. Histopathology 11:305-315, 1987.

133 Eusebi V, Foschini MP, Betts CM, Gherardi G, Millis RR, Bussolati G, Azzopardi JG: Microglandular adenosis, apocrine adenosis, and tubular carcinoma of the breast. An immunohistochemical comparison. Am J Surg Pathol 17:99-109, 1993.

134 James B, Cranor M, Rosen PP: Carcinoma of the breast arising in microglandular adenosis. Am J Clin Pathol 100:507-513, 1993.

135 Kiaer H, Nielsen B, Paulsen S, Soresen IM, Dyreborg V, Blichert-Toft M: Adenomyoepithelial adenosis and low grade malignant adenomyoepithelioma of the breast. Virchows Arch [A] 405:55-67, 1984.

136 Lee KC, Chan JKC, Gwi E: Tubular adenosis. A distinctive pseudomalignant lesion of the breast (abstract). Mod Pathol 8:20A, 1995.

136a Millis RR, Eusebi V: Microglandular adenosis of the breast. Adv Anat Pathol 2:10-18, 1995.

137 Rosen PP: Microglandular adenosis. A benign lesion simulating invasive mammary carcinoma. Am J Surg Pathol 7:137-144, 1983.

138 Rosenblum MK, Purrazzella R, Rosen PP: Is microglandular adenosis a precancerous disease? A study of carcinoma arising therein. Am J Surg Pathol 10:237-245, 1986.

139 Simpson JF, Page DL, Dupont WD: Apocrine adenosis. A mimic of mammary carcinoma. Surg Pathol 3:289-299, 1990.

140 Tavassoli FA, Norris NJ: Microglandular adenosis of the breast. A clinicopathologic study of 11 cases with ultrastructural observations. Am J Surg Pathol 7:731-737, 1983.

141 Tsuda H, Mukai K, Fukutomi T, Hirohashi S: Malignant progression of adenomyoepithelial adenosis of the breast. Pathol Int 44:475-479, 1994.

FIBROCYSTIC DISEASE

142 Allen SS, Froberg DG: The effect of decreased caffeine consumption on benign proliferative breast disease. A randomized clinical trial. Surgery 101:720-730, 1987.

143 Angeli A, Bradlow HL, Dogliotti L, eds: Endocrinology of the breast. Basic and clinical aspects. Turin, Italy, September 19-22, 1984. Ann NY Acad Sci 464:1-640, 1986.

144 Azzopardi JG: Problems in breast pathology. In Bennington JL, consulting ed: Major problems in pathology, vol 11. Philadelphia, 1979, WB Saunders Co.

145 Bartow SA, Black WC, Waeckerlin RW, Mettler FA: Fibrocystic disease. A continuing enigma. Pathol Annu 17(Pt 2):93-111, 1982.

146 Carter DJ, Rosen PP: Atypical apocrine metaplasia in sclerosing lesions of the breast. A study of 51 patients. Mod Pathol 4:1-5, 1991.

147 Connolly JL, Schnitt SJ: Benign breast disease. Resolved and unresolved issues. Cancer 71:1187-1189, 1993.

148 Consensus Meeting, Oct 3 to 5, 1985, New York, Cancer Committee of the College of American Pathologists: Is 'fibrocystic disease' of the breast precancerous? Arch Pathol Lab Med 110:171-173, 1986.

149 Fechner RE: Fibrocystic disease in women receiving oral contraceptive hormones. Cancer 25:1332-1339, 1970.

150 Frantz VK, Pickren JW, Melcher GW, Auchincloss H Jr: Incidence of chronic cystic disease in so-called "normal breast." Cancer 4:762-783, 1951.

151 Golinger RC: Hormones and the pathophysiology of fibrocystic mastopathy. Surg Gynecol Obstet 146:273-285, 1978.

152 Hislop TG, Threlfall WJ: Oral contraceptives and benign breast disease. Am J Epidemiol 120:273-280, 1984.

153 LiVolsi VA, Stadel BV, Kelsey JL, Holford TR, White C: Fibrocystic breast disease in oral-contraceptive users. A histopathological evaluation of epithelial atypia. N Engl J Med 299:381-385, 1978.

154 Love SM, Gelman RS, Silen W: Fibrocystic "disease" of the breast. A nondisease? N Engl J Med 307:1010-1014, 1982.

155 Lubin F, Ron E, Wax Y, Black M, Funaro M, Shitrit A: A case-control study of caffeine and methylxanthines in benign breast disease. JAMA 253:2388-2392, 1985.

156 Mazoujian G, Pinkus GS, Davis S, Haagensen DE Jr: Immunohistochemistry of a gross cystic disease fluid protein (GCDFP-15) of the breast. A marker of apocrine epithelium and breast carcinomas with apocrine features. Am J Pathol 110:105-112, 1983.

157 Meyer JS, Connor RE: Cell proliferation in fibrocystic disease and postmenopausal breast ducts measured by thymidine labeling. Cancer 50:746-751, 1982.

158 Minkowitz S, Hedayati H, Hiller S, Gardner B: Fibrous mastopathy. A clinical histopathologic study. Cancer 32:913-916, 1973.

159 Ory H, Cole P, MacMahon B, Hoover R: Oral contraceptives and reduced risk of benign breast diseases. N Engl J Med 294:419-422, 1976.

160 Sandison AT: An autopsy study of the adult human breast. With special reference to proliferative epithelial changes of importance in the pathology of the breast. Natl Cancer Inst Monogr 8:1-145, 1962.

161 Schuerch C III, Rosen PP, Hirota T, Itabashi M, Yamamoto H, Kinne DW, Beattie EJ Jr: A pathologic study of benign breast disease in Tokyo and New York. Cancer 50:1899-1903, 1982.

162 Symonds DA: Use of the von Kossa stain in identifying occult calcifications in breast biopsies. Am J Clin Pathol 94:44-48, 1990.

163 Tavassoli FA, Majeste RM, Snyder RC: Intranuclear helioid inclusions in mammary intraductal hyperplasias. Ultrastruct Pathol 15:267-279, 1991.

164 Tornos C, Silva E, el-Naggar A, Pritzker KP: Calcium oxalate crystals in breast biopsies. The missing microcalcifications. Am J Surg Pathol 14:961-968, 1990.

165 Vorherr H: Fibrocystic breast disease. Pathophysiology, pathomorphology, clinical picture, and management. Am J Obstet Gynecol 154:161-179, 1986.

166 Winston JS, Yeh IT, Evers K, Friedman AK: Calcium oxalate is associated with benign breast tissue. Can we avoid biopsy? Am J Clin Pathol 100:488-492, 1993.

Ductal and lobular hyperplasia

167 Azzopardi JG: Problems in breast pathology. In Bennington JL, consulting ed: Major problems in pathology, vol 11. Philadelphia, 1979, WB Saunders Co.

168 Clement PB, Young RH, Azzopardi JG: Collagenous spherulosis of the breast. Am J Surg Pathol 11:411-417, 1987.

169 Grignon DJ, Ro JY, Mackay BN, Ordóñez NG, Ayala AG: Collagenous spherulosis of the breast. Immunohistochemical and ultrastructural studies. Am J Clin Pathol 91:386-392, 1989.

170 Guerry P, Erlandson RA, Rosen PP: Cystic hypersecretory hyperplasia and cystic hypersecretory duct carcinoma of the breast. Pathology, therapy, and follow-up of 39 patients. Cancer 61:1611-1620, 1988.

171 Michal M, Skalova A: Collagenous spherulosis. A comment on its histogenesis. Pathol Res Pract 186:365-370, 1990.

172 Raju U, Crissman JD, Zarbo RJ, Gottlieb C: Epitheliosis of the breast. An immunohistochemical characterization and comparison to malignant intraductal proliferations of the breast. Am J Surg Pathol 14:939-947, 1990.

173 Tham K, Dupont WD, Page DL, Gray GF, Rogers LW: Micro-papillary hyperplasia with atypical features in female breasts, resembling gynecomastia. Progr Surg Pathol 10:101-110, 1989.

Sclerosing ductal lesions

174 Andersen JA, Carter D, Linell F: A symposium on sclerosing duct lesions of the breast. Pathol Annu 21(Pt 2):144-179, 1986.

175 Andersen JA, Gram JB: Radial scar in the female breast. A long-term follow-up study of 32 cases. Cancer 53:2557-2560, 1984.

176 Consensus Meeting, Oct 3 to 5, 1985, New York, Cancer Committee of the College of American Pathologists: Is 'fibrocystic disease' of the breast precancerous? Arch Pathol Lab Med 110:171-173, 1986.

177 Davies JD: Hyperelastosis, obliteration and fibrous plaques in major ducts of the human breast. J Pathol 110:13-26, 1973.

178 Fenoglio C, Lattes R: Sclerosing papillary proliferations in the female breast. A benign lesion often mistaken for carcinoma. Cancer 33:691-700, 1974.

179 Fisher ER, Palekar AS, Kotwal N, Lipana N: A non-encapsulated sclerosing lesion of the breast. Am J Clin Pathol 71:240-246, 1979.

180 Gottlieb C, Raju U, Greenwald KA: Myoepithelial cells in the differential diagnosis of complex benign and malignant breast lesions. An immunohistochemical study. Mod Pathol 3:135-140, 1990.

181 Keen ME, Murad TM, Cohen MI, Matthies HJ: Benign breast lesions with malignant clinical and mammographic presentations. Hum Pathol 16:1147-1152, 1985.

182 Linell F, Ljungberg O, Andersson I: Breast carcinoma. Aspects of early stages, progression and related problems. Acta Pathol Microbiol Scand (A) 272(Suppl):1-233, 1980.

183 Nielsen M, Christensen L, Andersen J: Radial scars in women with breast cancer. Cancer 59:1019-1025, 1987.

184 Nielsen M, Jensen J, Andersen JA: An autopsy study of radial scar in the female breast. Histopathology 9:287-295, 1985.

185 Rickert RR, Kalisher L, Hutter RVP: Indurative mastopathy. A benign sclerosing lesion of breast with elastosis which may simulate carcinoma. Cancer 47:561-571, 1981.

186 Sloane JP, Mayers MM: Carcinoma and atypical hyperplasia in radial scars and complex sclerosing lesions. Importance of lesion size and patient age. Histopathology **23:**225-231, 1993.

187 Tremblay G, Buell RH, Seemayer TA: Elastosis in benign sclerosing ductal proliferation of the female breast. Am J Surg Pathol **1:**155-159, 1977.

188 Wellings SR, Alpers CE: Subgross pathologic features and incidence of radial scars in the breast. Hum Pathol **15:**475-479, 1984.

Atypical ductal and lobular hyperplasia

189 Ashikari R, Huvos AG, Snyder RE, Lucas JC, Hutter RVP, McDivitt RW, Schottenfeld D: A clinicopathologic study of atypical lesions of the breast. Cancer **33:**310-317, 1974.

190 Beck JS: Observer variability in reporting of breast lesions. J Clin Pathol **38:**1358-1365, 1985.

191 Bodian CA, Perzin KH, Lattes R, Hoffmann P: Reproducibility and validity of pathologic classifications of benign breast disease and implications for clinical applications. Cancer **71:**3908-3913, 1993.

191a Consensus Meeting, Oct 3 to 5, 1985, New York, Cancer Committee of the College of American Pathologists: Is 'fibrocystic disease' of the breast precancerous? Arch Pathol Lab Med **110:**171-173, 1986.

192 Crissman JD, Visscher DW, Kubus J: Image cytophotometric DNA analysis of atypical hyperplasias and intraductal carcinomas the breast. Arch Pathol Lab Med **114:**1249-1253, 1990.

193 Dupont WD, Page DL: Risk factors for breast cancer in women with proliferative breast disease. N Engl J Med **312:**146-151, 1985.

194 Kern WH, Brooks RN: Atypical epithelial hyperplasia associated with breast cancer and fibrocystic disease. Cancer **24:**668-675, 1969.

195 King EB, Chew KL, Hom JD, Duarte LA, Mayall B, Miller TR, Neuhaus JM, Wrensch MR, Petrakis NL: Characterization by image cytometry of duct epithelial proliferative disease of the breast. Mod Pathol **4:**291-296, 1991.

196 Ohuchi N, Page DL, Merino MJ, Viglione MJ, Kufe DW, Schlom J: Expression of tumor-associated antigen (DF3) in atypical hyperplasias and in situ carcinomas of the human breast. JNCI **79:**109-117, 1987.

197 Page DL: Cancer risk assessment in benign breast biopsies. Hum Pathol **17:**871-874, 1986.

198 Page DL, Dupont WD, Rogers LW, Rados MS: Atypical hyperplastic lesions of the female breast. A long-term follow-up study. Cancer **55:**2698-2708, 1985.

199 Page DL, Kidd TE, Dupont WD, Rogers LW: Lobular neoplasia of the breast (LN) has varying magnitudes of risk for subsequent invasive carcinoma (IBC) (abstract). Lab Invest **58:**69A, 1988.

200 Page DL, Rogers LW: Combined histologic and cytologic criteria for the diagnosis of mammary atypical ductal hyperplasia. Hum Pathol **23:**1095-1097, 1992.

201 Rosai J: Borderline epithelial lesions of the breast. Am J Surg Pathol **15:**209-221, 1991.

202 Schnitt SJ, Connolly JL, Tavassoli FA, Fechner RE, Kempson RL, Gelman R, Page DL: Interobserver reproducibility in the diagnosis of ductal proliferative breast lesions using standardized criteria. Am J Surg Pathol **16:**1133-1143, 1992.

203 Steinhoff NG, Black WC: Florid cystic disease preceding mammary cancer. Ann Surg **171:**501-508, 1970.

204 Tavassoli FA, Norris HJ: A comparison of the results of long-term follow-up for atypical intraductal hyperplasia and intraductal hyperplasia of the breast. Cancer **65:**518-529, 1990.

Relationship with carcinoma and treatment

205 Bianchi S, Palli D, Galli M, Zampi G: Benign breast disease and cancer risk. Crit Rev Oncol Hematol **15:**221-242, 1993.

206 Bodian CA, Perzin KH, Lattes R, Hoffmann P, Abernathy TG: Prognostic significance of benign proliferative breast disease. Cancer **71:**3896-3907, 1993.

207 Connolly JL, Schnitt SJ: Benign breast disease. Resolved and unresolved issues. Cancer **71:**1187-1189, 1993.

208 Dupont WD, Page DL: Relative risk of breast cancer varies with time since diagnosis of atypical hyperplasia. Hum Pathol **20:**723-725, 1989.

209 Dupont WD, Page DL, Rogers LW, Parl FF: Influence of exogenous estrogens, proliferative breast disease, and other variables on breast cancer risk. Cancer **63:**948-957, 1989.

210 Dupont WD, Parl FF, Hartmann WH, Brinton LA, Winfield AC, Worrell JA, Schuyler PA, Plummer WD: Breast cancer risk associated with proliferative breast disease and atypical hyperplasia. Cancer **71:**1258-1265, 1993.

211 Frantz VK, Pickren JW, Melcher GW, Auchincloss H Jr: Incidence of chronic cystic disease in so-called "normal breast." Cancer **4:**762-783, 1951.

212 Kern WH, Brooks RN: Atypical epithelial hyperplasia associated with breast cancer and fibrocystic disease. Cancer **24:**668-675, 1969.

213 McDivitt RW: Breast carcinoma. Hum Pathol **9:**3-21, 1978.

213a Micale MA, Visscher DW, Gulino SE, Wolman SR: Chromosomal aneuploidy in proliferative breast disease. Hum Pathol **25:**29-35, 1994.

213b Millikan R, Hulka B, Thor A, Zhang Y, Edgerton S, Zhang X, Pei H, He M, Wold L, Melton LJ, Ballard D, Conway K, Liu ET: p53 mutations in benign breast tissue. J Clin Oncol **13:**2293-2300, 1995.

214 Page DL: Cancer risk assessment in benign breast biopsies. Hum Pathol **17:**871-874, 1986.

215 Page DL, Dupont WD: Anatomic markers of human premalignancy and risk of breast cancer. Cancer **66:**1326-1335, 1990.

216 Rosen PP: Proliferative breast "disease." An unresolved diagnostic dilemma. Cancer **71:**3798-3807, 1993.

217 Schnitt SJ, Jimi A, Kojiro M: The increasing prevalence of benign proliferative breast lesions in Japanese women. Cancer **71:**2528-2531, 1993.

218 Skolnick MH, Cannon-Albright LA, Goldgar DE, Ward JH, Marshall CJ, Schumann GB, Hogle H, McWhorter WP, Wright EC, Tran TD, et al.: Inheritance of proliferative breast disease in breast cancer kindreds. Science **250:**1715-1720, 1990.

219 Steinhoff NG, Black WC: Florid cystic disease preceding mammary cancer. Ann Surg **171:**501-508, 1970.

220 Tavassoli FA, Norris HJ: A comparison of the results of long-term follow-up for atypical intraductal hyperplasia and intraductal hyperplasia of the breast. Cancer **65:**518-529, 1990.

220a Younes M, Lebovitz RM, Bommer KE, Cagle PT, Morton D, Khan S, Laucirica R: p53 accumulation in benign breast biopsy specimens. Hum Pathol **26:**155-158, 1995.

Carcinoma
GENERAL FEATURES

221 Anastassiades O, Iakovou E, Stavridou N, Gogas J, Karameris A: Multicentricity in breast cancer. A study of 366 cases. Am J Clin Pathol **99:**238-243, 1993.

222 Berkel H, Birdsell DC, Jenkins H: Breast augmentation. A risk factor for breast cancer? N Engl J Med **326:**1649-1653, 1992.

223 Bonito D, Giarelli L, Falconieri G, Bonifacio-Gori D, Tomasic G, Vielh P: Association of breast cancer and meningioma. Report of 12 new cases and review of the literature. Pathol Res Pract **189:**399-404, 1993.

223a Broët P, de la Rochefordière A, Scholl SM, Fourquet A, Massen V, Durand J-C, Pouillart P, Asselain B: Contralateral breast cancer. Annual incidence and risk parameters. J Clin Oncol **13:**1578-1583, 1995.

223b Bryant H, Brasher P: Breast implants and breast cancer. Reanalysis of a linkage study. N Engl J Med **332:**1535-1539, 1995.

224 The Centers for Disease Control Cancer and Steroid Hormone Study: Long-term oral contraceptive use and the risk of breast cancer. JAMA **249:**1591-1595, 1983.

225 Clark CP, Peters GN, O'Brien KM: Cancer in the augmented breast. Diagnosis and prognosis. Cancer **72:**2170-2174, 1993.

225a Colditz GA, Hankinson SE, Hunter DJ, Willett WC, Manson JE, Stampfer MJ, Hennekens C, Rosner B, Speizer FE: The use of estrogens and progestins and the risk of breast cancer in postmenopausal women. N Engl J Med **332:**1589-1593, 1995.

226 Dawson PJ: What is new in our understanding of multifocal breast cancer. Pathol Res Pract **189:**111-116, 1993.

226a Dawson PJ, Baekey PA, Clark RA: Mechanisms of multifocal breast cancer. An immunocytochemical study. Hum Pathol **26:**965-969, 1995.

227 Fechner RE: Breast cancer during oral contraceptive therapy. Cancer **26:**1204-1211, 1970.

228 Fechner RE: The surgical pathology of the reproductive system and breast during oral contraceptive therapy. Pathol Annu **6:**299-319, 1971.

229 Fisher ER, Gregorio R, Redmond C, Vellios F, Sommers SC, Fisher B: Pathologic findings from the National Surgical Adjuvant Breast Project (Protocol no. 4). I. Observations concerning the multicentricity of mammary cancer. Cancer **35:**247-254, 1975.

229a Futreal PA, Liu Q, Shattuck-Eidens D, Cochran C, Harshman K, Tavtigian S, Bennett LM, Haugen-Strano A, Swensen J, Miki Y, Eddington K, McClure M, Frye C, Weaver-Feldhaus J, Ding W, Gholami Z, Söderkvist P, Terry L, Jhanwar S, Berchuck A, Iglehart JD, Marks J, Ballinger DG, Barrett JC, Skolnick MH, Kamb A, Wiseman R: BRCA 1 mutations in primary breast and ovarian carcinomas. Science **266:**120-122, 1994.

230 Garfinkel L, Boring CC, Heath CW Jr: Changing trends. An overview of breast cancer incidence and mortality. Cancer **74:**222-227, 1994.

231 Hildreth NG, Shore RE, Hempelmann LH: Risk of breast cancer among women receiving radiation treatment in infancy for thymic enlargement. Lancet **2**:273, 1983.

232 Hoover R, Gray LA Sr, Cole P, MacMahon B: Menopausal estrogens and breast cancer. N Engl J Med **295**:401-405, 1976.

233 Hutter RVP, Kim DU: The problem of multiple lesions of the breast. Cancer **28**:1591-1607, 1971.

234 Kelsey JL, Gammon MD: The epidemiology of breast cancer. CA Cancer J Clin **41**:146-165, 1991.

235 King RE, Terz JJ, Lawrence W Jr: Experience with opposite breast biopsy in patients with operable breast cancer. Cancer **37**:43-45, 1976.

236 Miki Y, Swensen J, Shattuck-Eidens D, Futreal PA, Harshman K, Tavtigian S, Liu Q, Cochran C, Bennett LM, Ding W, et al.: A strong candidate for the breast and ovarian cancer susceptibility gene BRCA1. Science **266**:66-71, 1994.

237 Moore DH, Moore DH II, Moore CT: Breast carcinoma etiological factors. Adv Cancer Res **40**:189-253, 1983.

238 Newcomb PA, Storer BE, Longnecker MP, Mittendorf R, Greenberg ER, Clapp RW, Burke KP, Willett WC, MacMahon B: Lactation and a reduced risk of premenopausal breast cancer. N Engl J Med **330**:81-87, 1994.

239 Noguchi S, Aihara T, Koyama H, Motomura K, Inaji H, Imaoka S: Discrimination between multicentric and multifocal carcinomas of the breast through clonal analysis. Cancer **74**:872-877, 1994.

240 Ottman R, Pike MC, King M, Henderson BE: Practical guide for estimating risk for familial breast cancer. Lancet **2**:556-558, 1983.

240a Ponder B: Breast cancer genes. Searches begin and end (editorial). Nature **371**:279, 1994.

241 Romieu I, Berlin JA, Colditz G: Oral contraceptives and breast cancer. Review and meta-analysis. Cancer **66**:2253-2263, 1990.

242 Ross RK, Paganini-Hill A, Gerkins VR, Mack TM, Pfeffer R, Arthur M, Henderson BE: A case-control study of menopausal estrogen therapy and breast cancer. JAMA **243**:1635-1639, 1980.

243 Shore RE, Hempelmann LH, Kowaluk E, Mansur PS, Pasternack BS, Albert RE, Haughie GE: Breast neoplasms in women treated with x-rays for acute postpartum mastitis. JNCI **59**:813-822, 1977.

244 Simon N, Silverstone SM: Radiation as a cause of breast cancer. Bull NY Acad Sci **52**:741-751, 1976.

245 Skolnick MH, Cannon-Albright LA: Genetic predisposition to breast cancer. Cancer **70**:1747-1754, 1992.

246 Sondik EJ: Breast cancer trends. Incidence, mortality, and survival. Cancer **74**:995-999, 1994.

247 Swift M, Morrell D, Massey RB, Chase CL: Incidence of cancer in 161 families affected by ataxia-telangiectasia. N Engl J Med **325**:1831-1836, 1991.

248 Tulinius H, Sigvaldason H, Olafsdottir G: Left and right sided breast cancer. Pathol Res Pract **186**:92-94, 1990.

249 Wang DY, Rubens RD, Allen DS, Millis RR, Bulbrook RD, Chaudary MA, Hayward JL: Influence of reproductive history of age at diagnosis of breast cancer and prognosis. Int J Cancer **36**:427-432, 1985.

250 White E, Malone KE, Weiss NS, Daling JR: Breast cancer among young U.S. women in relation to oral contraceptive use. J Natl Cancer Inst **86**:505-514, 1994.

250a Wooster R, Neuhausen Susan L, Mangion J, Quirk Y, Ford D, Collins N, Nguyen K, Seal S, Tran T, Averill D, Fields P, Marshall G, Narod S, Lenoir GM, Lynch H, Feunteun J, Devilee P, Cornelisse CJ, Menko FH, Daly PA, Ormiston W, McManus R, Pye C, Lewis CM, Cannon-Albright LA, Peto J, Ponder BAJ, Skolnick MH, Easton DF, Goldgar DE, Stratton MR: Localization of a breast cancer susceptibility gene, BRCA2, to chromosome 13q12-13. Science **265**:2088-2090, 1994.

DIAGNOSIS
Mammography

251 Bassett LW, Gambhir S: Breast imaging for the 1990s. Semin Oncol **18**:80-86, 1991.

252 Charpin C, Bonnier P, Khouzami A, Andrac L, Habib M, Vacheret H, Lavaut MN, Piana L: Non palpable breast carcinomas. Histological and immunohistochemical studies of 160 cases. Pathol Res Pract **189**:267-274, 1993.

253 Fisher ER, Palekar A, Kim WS, Redmond C: The histopathology of mammographic patterns. Am J Clin Pathol **69**:421-426, 1978.

254 Gallager HS: Breast specimen radiography. Obligatory, adjuvant and investigative. Am J Clin Pathol **64**:749-766, 1975.

255 Gisvold JJ: Imaging of the breast. Techniques and results. Mayo Clin Proc **65**:56-66, 1990.

256 Gonzalez JE, Caldwell RG, Valaitis J: Calcium oxalate crystals in the breast. Pathology and significance. Am J Surg Pathol **15**:586-591, 1991.

257 Koehl RH, Snyder RE, Hutter RVP, Foote FW Jr: The incidence and significance of calcifications within operative breast specimens. Am J Clin Pathol **53**:3-14, 1970.

258 McDivitt RW: Breast carcinoma. Hum Pathol **9**:3-21, 1978.

259 McLelland R: Screening mammography. Cancer **67**:1129-1131, 1991.

260 Millis RR, Davis R, Stacey AJ: The detection and significance of calcification in the breasts. A radiological and pathological study. Br J Radiol **49**:12-26, 1976.

261 Owings DV, Hann L, Schnitt SJ: How thoroughly should needle localization breast biopsies be sampled for microscopic examination? A prospective mammographic/pathologic correlative study. Am J Surg Pathol **14**:578-583, 1990.

262 Powell DE, Stelling CB: Magnetic resonance imaging of the human female breast. Current status and pathologic correlations. Pathol Annu **23**(Pt 1):159-194, 1988.

263 Rosen P, Snyder RE, Foote FW, Wallace T: Detection of occult carcinoma in the apparently benign breast biopsy through specimen radiography. Cancer **26**:944-952, 1970.

264 Rosen PP, Snyder RE, Robbins G: Specimen radiography for nonpalpable breast lesions found by mammography. Procedures and results. Cancer **34**:2028-2033, 1974.

265 Schwartz GF, Carter DL, Conant EF, Gannon FH, Finkel GC, Feig SA: Mammographically detected breast cancer. Nonpalpable is not a synonym for inconsequential. Cancer **73**:1660-1665, 1994.

266 Stevens GM, Jamplis RW: Mammographically directed biopsy of nonpalpable breast lesions. Arch Surg **102**:292-295, 1971.

267 Wolfe JN: Breast patterns as an index of risk for developing breast cancer. Am J Roentgenol **126**:1130-1139, 1976.

Cytology

268 Abendroth CS, Wang HH, Ducatman BS: Comparative features of carcinoma in situ and atypical ductal hyperplasia of the breast on fine-needle aspiration biopsy specimens. Am J Clin Pathol **96**:654-659, 1991.

269 Barrows GH, Anderson TJ, Lamb JL, Dixon JM: Fine-needle aspiration of breast cancer. Relationship of clinical factors to cytology results in 689 primary malignancies. Cancer **58**:1493-1498, 1986.

270 Bell DA, Hajdu SI, Urban JA, Gaston JP: Role of aspiration cytology in the diagnosis and management of mammary lesions in office practice. Cancer **51**:1182-1189, 1983.

270a Dawson AE, Mulford DK, Sheils LA: The cytopathology of proliferative breast disease. Am J Clin Pathol **103**:438-442, 1995.

271 Eisenberg AJ, Hajdu SI, Wilhelmus J, Melamed MR, Kinne D: Preoperative aspiration cytology of breast tumors. Acta Cytol (Baltimore) **30**:135-146, 1986.

272 Frable WJ: Needle aspiration of the breast. Cancer **53**:671-676, 1984.

273 Grant CS, Goellner JR, Welch JS, Martin JK: Fine-needle aspiration of the breast. Mayo Clin Proc **61**:377-381, 1986.

273a Jeffrey PB, Ljung BM: Benign and malignant papillary lesions of the breast. A cytomorphologic study. Am J Clin Pathol **101**:500-507, 1994.

274 Kline TS: Masquerades of malignancy. A review of 4,241 aspirates from the breast. Acta Cytol (Baltimore) **25**:263-266, 1981.

275 Kline TS, Joshi LP, Neal HS: Fine-needle aspiration of the breast. Diagnoses and pitfalls. A review of 3545 cases. Cancer **44**:1458-1464, 1979.

276 Lee KC, Chan JK, Ho LC: Histologic changes in the breast after fine-needle aspiration. Am J Surg Pathol **18**:1039-1047, 1994.

277 Ljung BM, Chew K, Deng G, Matsumura K, Waldman F, Smith H: Fine needle aspiration techniques for the characterization of breast cancers. Cancer **74**:1000-1005, 1994.

278 Marshall CJ, Schumann GB, Ward JH, Riding JM, Cannon-Albright L, Skolnick M: Cytologic identification of clinically occult proliferative breast disease in women with a family history of breast cancer. Am J Clin Pathol **95**:157-165, 1991.

279 Nordenskjold B, Skoog L, Wallgren A, Silfversward C, Gustafsson S, Ljung B-M, Westerberg H, Gustafsson J-A, Wrange O: Measurements of DNA synthesis and estrogen receptor in needle aspirates as powerful methods in the management of mammary carcinoma. Adv Enzyme Regul **19**:489-496, 1981.

280 Norton LW, Davis JR, Wiens JL, Trego DC, Dunnington GL: Accuracy of aspiration cytology in detecting breast cancer. Surgery **96**:806-811, 1984.

281 Oertel YC: Fine needle aspiration of the breast. Stoneham, MA, 1987, Butterworths.

282 Reiner A, Spona J, Reiner G, Schemper M, Kolb R, Kwasny W, Függer R, Jakesz R, Holzner JH: Estrogen receptor analysis on biopsies and fine-needle aspirates from human breast carcinoma. Correlation of biochemical and immunohistochemical methods using monoclonal antireceptor antibodies. Am J Pathol **125:**443-449, 1986.

283 Remvikos Y, Magdelenat H, Zajdela A: DNA flow cytometry applied to fine needle sampling of human breast cancer. Cancer **61:**1629-1634, 1988.

284 Rosen P, Najdu SI, Robbins G, Foote FW: Diagnosis of carcinoma of the breast by aspiration biopsy. Surg Gynecol Obstet **134:**837-838, 1972.

285 Rosenthal DL: Breast lesions diagnosed by fine needle aspiration. Pathol Res Pract **181:**645-656, 1986.

286 Silfversward C, Gustafsson J-A, Gustafsson SA, Nordenskjold B, Wallgren A, Wrange O: Estrogen receptor analysis on fine needle aspirates and on histologic biopsies from human breast cancer. Eur J Cancer **16:**1351-1357, 1980.

287 Sneige N, Singletary SE: Fine-needle aspiration of the breast. Diagnostic problems and approaches to surgical management. Pathol Annu **29**(Pt 1):281-301, 1994.

288 Sneige N, Staerkel GA: Fine-needle aspiration cytology of ductal hyperplasia with and without atypia and ductal carcinoma in situ. Hum Pathol **25:**485-492, 1994.

289 Strawbridge HTG, Bassett AA, Foldes I: Role of cytology in management of lesions of the breast. Surg Gynecol Obstet **152:**1-7, 1981.

289a Tavassoli FA, Pestaner JP: Pseudoinvasion in intraductal carcinoma. Mod Pathol **8:**380-383, 1995.

289b Thomas PA, Cangiarella J, Raab SS, Waisman J: Fine needle aspiration biopsy of proliferative breast disease. Mod Pathol **8:**130-136, 1995.

290 Thomas PA, Vazquez MF, Waisman J: Comparison of fine-needle aspiration and frozen section of palpable mammary lesions. Mod Pathol **3:**570-574, 1990.

291 Youngson BJ, Cranor M, Rosen PP: Epithelial displacement in surgical breast specimens following needling procedures. Am J Surg Pathol **18:**896-903, 1994.

291a Youngson BJ, Liberman L, Rosen PP: Displacement of carcinomatous epithelium in surgical breast specimens following stereotaxic core biopsy. Am J Clin Pathol **103:**598-602, 1995.

292 Wanebo HJ, Feldman PS, Wilhelm MC, Covell JL, Binns RL: Fine needle aspiration cytology in lieu of open biopsy in management of primary breast cancer. Ann Surg **199:**569-578, 1984.

Core needle biopsy

293 Elston CW, Cotton RE, Davies CJ, Blamey RW: A comparison of the use of the "TRU-CUT" needle and fine needle aspiration cytology in the pre-operative diagnosis of carcinoma of the breast. Histopathology **2:**239-254, 1978.

294 Fentiman IS, Millis RR, Hayward JL: Value of needle biopsy in outpatient diagnosis of breast cancer. Arch Surg **115:**652-653, 1980.

295 Minkowitz S, Moskowitz R, Khafif RA, Alderete MN: TRU-CUT needle biopsy of the breast. An analysis of its specificity and sensitivity. Cancer **57:**320-323, 1986.

296 Saltzstein SL: Histologic diagnosis of breast carcinoma with the Silverman needle biopsy. Surgery **48:**366-374, 1960.

Open biopsy and frozen section

297 Bianchi S, Palli D, Ciatto S, Galli M, Giorgi D, Vezzosi V, Rosselli del Turco M, Cataliotti L, Cardona G, Zampi G: Accuracy and reliability of frozen section diagnosis in a series of 672 nonpalpable breast lesions. Am J Clin Pathol **103:**199-205, 1993.

298 Esteban JM, Zaloudek C, Silverberg SG: Intraoperative diagnosis of breast lesions. Comparison of cytologic with frozen section technics. Am J Clin Pathol **88:**681-688, 1987.

299 Fechner RE: Frozen section examination of breast biopsies. Practice parameter. Am J Clin Pathol **103:**6-7, 1995.

300 Oberman HA: A modest proposal (editorial). Am J Surg Pathol **16:**69-70, 1992.

301 Recommendations of the Association of Directors of Anatomic and Surgical Pathology. Part I. Immediate management of mammographically detected breast lesions. Hum Pathol **24:**689-690, 1993.

302 Rosen PP: Frozen section diagnosis of breast lesions. Recent experience with 556 consecutive biopsies. Ann Surg **187:**17-19, 1978.

303 Sauter ER, Hoffman JP, Ottery FD, Kowalyshyn MJ, Litwin S, Eisenberg BL: Is frozen section analysis of reexcision lumpectomy margins worthwhile? Margin analysis in breast reexcisions. Cancer **73:**2607-2612, 1994.

303a Speights VO Jr: Evaluation of frozen sections in grossly benign breast biopsies. Mod Pathol **7:**762-765, 1994.

MICROSCOPIC TYPES

304 Ishige H, Komatsu T, Kondo Y, Sugano I, Horinaka E, Okui K: Lobular involvement in human breast carcinoma. Acta Pathol Jpn **41:**227-232, 1991.

305 Wellings SR, Jensen HM, Marcum RG: An atlas of subgross pathology of the human breast with special reference to possible precancerous lesions. JNCI **55:**231-273, 1975.

IN SITU CARCINOMA
Ductal carcinoma in situ (DCIS)
Comedocarcinoma

306 Bacus SS, Ruby SG, Weinberg DS, Chin D, Ortiz R, Bacus JW: HER-2/neu oncogene expression and proliferation in breast cancers. Am J Pathol **137:**103-111, 1990.

307 Bellamy CD, McDonald C, Salter DM, Chetty U, Anderson TJ: Noninvasive ductal carcinoma of the breast. The relevance of histologic categorization. Hum Pathol **24:**16-23, 1993.

308 Bobrow LG, Happerfield LC, Gregory WM, Springall RD, Millis RR: The classification of ductal carcinoma in situ and its association with biological markers. Semin Diagn Pathol **11:**199-207, 1994.

308a Bose S, Lesser ML, Norton L, Rosen PP: Immunophenotype of intraductal carcinoma. Arch Pathol (in press).

309 Brown PW, Silverman J, Owens E, Tabor DC, Terz JJ, Lawrence W Jr: Intraductal "noninfiltrating" carcinoma of the breast. Arch Surg **111:**1063-1067, 1976.

310 Carter D, Smith RRL: Carcinoma in situ of the breast. Cancer **40:**1189-1193, 1977.

311 Coyne J, Haboubi NY: Micro-invasive breast carcinoma with granulomatous stromal response. Histopathology **20:**184-185, 1992.

311a Douglas-Jones AG, Schmid KW, Bier B, Horgan K, Lyons K, Dallimore ND, Moneypenny IJ, Jasani B: Metallothionein expression in duct carcinoma in situ of the breast. Hum Pathol **26:**217-222, 1995.

311b Holland R, Hendriks JH: Microcalcifications associated with ductal carcinoma in situ. Mammographic-pathologic correlation. Semin Diagn Pathol **11:**181-192, 1994.

312 Holland R, Peterse JL, Millis RR, Eusebi V, Faverly D, van de Vijver MJ, Zafrani B: Ductal carcinoma in situ. A proposal for a new classification. Semin Diagn Pathol **11:**167-180, 1994.

313 Killeen JL, Namiki H: DNA analysis of ductal carcinoma in situ of the breast. A comparison with histologic features. Cancer **68:**2602-2607, 1991.

314 Lagios MD, Westdahl PR, Margolin FR, Rose MR: Duct carcinoma in situ. Relationship of extent of noninvasive disease to the frequency of occult invasion, multicentricity, lymph node metastases, and short-term treatment failures. Cancer **50:**1309-1314, 1982.

314a Leal CB, Schmitt FC, Bento MJ, Maia NC, Lopes CS: Ductal carcinoma in situ of the breast. Histologic categorization and its relationship to ploidy and immunohistochemical expression of hormone receptors, p53, and c-*erb*B-2 protein. Cancer **75:**2123-2131, 1995.

315 Lennington WJ, Jensen RA, Dalton LW, Page DL: Ductal carcinoma in situ of the breast. Heterogeneity of individual lesions. Cancer **73:**118-124, 1994.

316 Lodato RF, Maguire HC Jr, Greene MI, Weiner DB, Li Volsi VA: Immunohistochemical evaluation of c-*erb*B-2 oncogene expression in ductal carcinoma in situ and atypical ductal hyperplasia of the breast. Mod Pathol **3:**449-454, 1990.

317 Mayr NA, Staples JJ, Robinson RA, Vanmetre JE, Hussey DH: Morphometric studies in intraductal breast carcinoma using computerized image analysis. Cancer **67:**2805-2812, 1991.

318 Millis RR, Thynne GSJ: In situ intraduct carcinoma of the breast. A long-term follow-up study. Br J Surg **62:**957-962, 1975.

319 Ohuchi N, Furuta A, Mori S: Management of ductal carcinoma in situ with nipple discharge. Intraductal spreading of carcinoma is an unfavorable pathologic factor for breast-conserving surgery. Cancer **74:**1294-1302, 1994.

320 O'Malley FP, Vnencak-Jones CL, Dupont WD, Parl F, Manning S, Page DL: p53 mutations are confined to the comedo type ductal carcinoma in situ of the breast. Immunohistochemical and sequencing data. Lab Invest **71:**67-72, 1994.

321 Ozzello I, Sanpitak P: Epithelial-stromal junction of intraductal carcinoma of the breast. Cancer **26:**1186-1198, 1970.

322 Poller DN, Silverstein MJ, Galea M, Locker AP, Elston CW, Blamey RW, Ellis IO: Ideas in pathology. Ductal carcinoma in situ of the breast. A proposal for a new simplified histological classification association between cellular proliferation and c-*erb*B-2 protein expression. Mod Pathol **7:**257-262, 1994.

323 Rosen PP: Axillary lymph node metastases in patients with occult noninvasive breast carcinoma. Cancer **46:**1298-1306, 1980.

324 Sandstad E, Hartveit F: Stromal metachromasia. A marker for areas of incipient invasion in ductal carcinoma of the breast? Histopathology **11:**73-80, 1987.

325 Schnitt SJ, Connolly JL, Khettry U, Mazoujian G, Brenner M, Silver B, Recht A, Beadle G, Harris JR: Pathologic findings on re-excision of the primary site in breast cancer patients considered for treatment by primary radiation therapy. Cancer **59:**675-681, 1987.

326 Silverberg SG, Chitale AR: Assessment of significance of proportions of intraductal and infiltrating tumor growth in ductal carcinoma of the breast. Cancer **32:**830-837, 1973.

327 Tsang WY, Chan JK: Neural invasion in intraductal carcinoma of the breast. Hum Pathol **23:**202-204, 1992.

328 Westbrook KC, Gallager HS: Intraductal carcinoma of the breast. A comparative study. Am J Surg **130:**667-670, 1975.

(In situ) papillary carcinoma

329 Azzopardi JG: Problems in breast pathology. In Bennington JL, consulting ed: Major problems in pathology, vol 11. Philadelphia, 1979, WB Saunders Co.

330 Carter D, Orr SL, Merino MJ: Intracystic papillary carcinoma of the breast. After mastectomy, radiotherapy or excisional biopsy alone. Cancer **52:**14-19, 1983.

331 Kraus FT, Neubecker RD: The differential diagnosis of papillary tumors of the breast. Cancer **15:**444-455, 1962.

332 Lefkowitz M, Lefkowitz W, Wargotz ES: Intraductal (intracystic) papillary carcinoma of the breast and its variants. A clinicopathological study of 77 cases. Hum Pathol **25:**802-809, 1994.

333 Papotti M, Eusebi V, Gugliotta P, Bussolati G: Immunohistochemical analysis of benign and malignant papillary lesions of the breast. Am J Surg Pathol **7:**451-461, 1983.

334 Papotti M, Gugliotta P, Ghiringhello B, Bussolati G: Association of breast carcinoma and multiple intraductal papillomas. An histological and immunohistochemical investigation. Histopathology **8:**963-975, 1984.

Other forms

335 Andersen JA: Invasive breast carcinoma with lobular involvement. Frequency and location of lobular carcinoma in situ. Acta Pathol Microbiol Scand (A) **82:**719-729, 1974.

336 Azzopardi JG: Problems in breast pathology. In Bennington JL, consulting ed: Major problems in pathology, vol 11. Philadelphia, 1979, WB Saunders Co.

337 Bellamy CO, McDonald C, Salter DM, Chetty U, Anderson TJ: Noninvasive ductal carcinoma of the breast. The relevance of histologic categorization. Hum Pathol **24:**16-23, 1993.

338 Cross AS, Azzopardi JG, Krausz T, Van Noorden S, Polak JM: A morphological and immunocytochemical study of a distinctive variant of ductal carcinoma in-situ of the breast. Histopathology **9:**21-37, 1985.

339 Fechner RE: Ductal carcinoma involving the lobule of the breast. A source of confusion with lobular carcinoma in situ. Cancer **28:**274-281, 1971.

340 Fisher ER, Brown R: Intraductal signet ring carcinoma. A hitherto undescribed form of intraductal carcinoma of the breast. Cancer **55:**2533-2537, 1985.

341 Guerry P, Erlandson RA, Rosen PP: Cystic hypersecretory hyperplasia and cystic hypersecretory duct carcinoma of the breast. Pathology, therapy, and follow-up of 39 patients. Cancer **61:**1611-1620, 1988.

342 O'Malley FP, Page DL, Nelson EH, Dupont WD: Ductal carcinoma in situ of the breast with apocrine cytology. Definition of a borderline category. Hum Pathol **25:**164-168, 1994.

343 Rosen PP: Coexistent lobular carcinoma in situ and intraductal carcinoma in a single lobular-duct unit. Am J Surg Pathol **4:**241-246, 1980.

344 Rosen PP, Scott M: Cystic hypersecretory duct carcinoma of the breast. Am J Surg Pathol **8:**31-41, 1984.

345 Tavassoli FA, Norris HJ: Intraductal apocrine carcinoma. A clinicopathologic study of 37 cases. Mod Pathol **7:**813-818, 1994.

346 Tsang WYW, Chan JKC: Endocrine ductal carcinoma-in-situ (E-DCIS) of the breast. A subset of DCIS with distinctive clinicopathologic features (abstract). Mod Pathol **8:**27A, 1995.

Evolution

347 Betsill WL, Rosen PP, Robbins GF: Intraductal carcinoma. Long term follow-up after treatment by biopsy only. JAMA **239:**1863-1867, 1978.

348 Carter D, Smith RRL: Carcinoma in situ of the breast. Cancer **40:**1189-1193, 1977.

349 Eusebi V, Feudale E, Foschini MP, Micheli A, Conti A, Riva C, Di Palma S, Rilke F: Long-term follow-up of in situ carcinoma of the breast. Semin Diagn Pathol **11:**220-235, 1994.

350 Eusebi V, Foschini MP, Cook MG, Berrino F, Azzopardi JG: Long-term follow-up of in situ carcinoma of the breast with special emphasis on clinging carcinoma. Semin Diagn Pathol **6:**165-173, 1989.

350a Fisher ER, Costantino J, Fisher B, Palekar AS, Redmond C, Mamounas E, for the National Surgical Adjuvant Breast and Bowel Project Collaborating Investigators: Pathologic findings from the national surgical adjuvant breast project (NSABP) protocol B-17. Intraductal carcinoma (ductal carcinoma in situ). Cancer **75:**1310-1319, 1995.

351 Lampejo O, Barnes DM, Smith P, Millis RR: Evaluation of infiltrating ductal carcinomas with a DCIS component. Correlation of the histologic type of the in situ component with grade of the infiltrating component. Semin Diagn Pathol **11:**215-222, 1994.

352 McDivitt RW, Holleb AI, Foote FW: Prior breast disease in patients treated for papillary carcinoma. Arch Pathol **85:**117-124, 1968.

352a Moriya T, Silverberg SG: Intraductal carcinoma (ductal carcinoma in situ) of the breast. A comparison of pure noninvasive tumors with those including different proportions of infiltrating carcinoma. Cancer **74:**2972-2978, 1994.

353 Page DL, Dupont WD, Rogers LW, Landenberger M: Intraductal carcinoma of the breast. Follow-up after biopsy only. Cancer **49:**751-758, 1982.

354 Rosen PP, Braun DW Jr, Kinne DE: The clinical significance of pre-invasive breast carcinoma. Cancer **46:**919-925, 1980.

355 Rosen PP, Senie R, Schottenfeld D, Ashikari R: Noninvasive breast carcinoma. Ann Surg **189:**377-382, 1979.

356 Schnitt SJ, Silen W, Sadowsky NL, Connolly JL, Harris JR: Ductal carcinoma in situ (intraductal carcinoma) of the breast. N Engl J Med **318:**898-903, 1988.

357 Silverstein MJ, Waisman JR, Gamagami P, Gierson ED, Colburn WJ, Rosser RJ, Gordon PS, Lewinsky BS, Fingerhut A: Intraductal carcinoma of the breast (208 cases). Clinical factors influencing treatment choice. Cancer **66:**102-108, 1990.

Lobular carcinoma in situ (LCIS)

358 Andersen JA: Invasive breast carcinoma with lobular involvement. Frequency and location of lobular carcinoma in situ. Acta Pathol Microbiol Scand (A) **82:**719-729, 1974.

359 Andersen JA: Lobular carcinoma in situ. A histological study of 52 cases. Acta Pathol Microbiol Scand (A) **82:**735-741, 1974.

360 Andersen JA: Lobular carcinoma in situ of the breast with ductal involvement. Frequency and possible influence on prognosis. Acta Pathol Microbiol Scand (A) **82:**655-662, 1974.

361 Andersen JA, Vendelboe ML: Cytoplasmic mucous globules in lobular carcinoma in situ. Diagnosis and prognosis. Am J Surg Pathol **5:**251-255, 1981.

362 Breslow A, Brancaccio ME: Intracellular mucin production by lobular breast carcinoma cells. Arch Pathol Lab Med **100:**620-621, 1976.

363 Bussolati G, Micca FB, Eusebi V, Betts CM: Myoepithelial cells in lobular carcinoma in situ of the breast. A parallel immunocytochemical and ultrastructural study. Ultrastruct Pathol **2:**219-230, 1981.

364 Carter D, Smith RRL: Carcinoma in situ of the breast. Cancer **40:**1189-1193, 1977.

365 Dwarakanath S, Lee AKC, DeLellis RA, Silverman ML, Frasca L, Wolfe HJ: S-100 protein positivity in breast carcinomas. A potential pitfall in diagnostic immunohistochemistry. Hum Pathol **18:**1144-1148, 1987.

366 Eusebi V, Betts C, Haagensen DE Jr, Gugliotta P, Bussolati G, Azzopardi JG: Apocrine differentiation in lobular carcinoma of the breast. A morphologic, immunologic, and ultrastructural study. Hum Pathol **15:**134-140, 1984.

367 Eusebi V, Pich A, Macchiorlatti E, Bussolati G: Morpho-functional differentiation in lobular carcinoma of the breast. Histopathology **1:**301-314, 1977.

368 Fechner RE: Ductal carcinoma involving the lobule of the breast. A source of confusion with lobular carcinoma in situ. Cancer **28:**274-281, 1971.

369 Fechner RE: Epithelial alterations in the extralobular ducts of breasts with lobular carcinoma in situ. Arch Pathol **93:**164-171, 1972.

370 Fechner RE: Lobular carcinoma in situ in sclerosing adenosis. A potential source of confusion with invasive carcinoma. Am J Surg Pathol **5:**233-239, 1981.

371 Fondo EY, Rosen PP, Fracchia AA, Urban JA: The problem of carcinoma developing in a fibroadenoma. Recent experience at Memorial Hospital. Cancer **43:**563-567, 1979.

372 Haagensen CD, Lane N, Bodian C: Coexisting lobular neoplasia and carcinoma of the breast. Cancer **51:**1468-1482, 1983.

373 Haagensen CD, Lane N, Lattes R: Neoplastic proliferation of the epithelium of the mammary lobules. Adenosis, lobular neoplasia and small cell carcinoma. Surg Clin North Am **52:**497-524, 1972.

374 Lambird PA, Shelley WM: The spatial distribution of lobular in situ mammary carcinoma. Implications for size and site of breast biopsy. JAMA **210:**689-693, 1969.

375 Newman W: Lobular carcinoma of the female breast. Ann Surg **164:**305-314, 1966.

376 Rosen PP, Lieberman PH, Braun DW Jr, Kosloff C, Adair F: Lobular carcinoma in situ of the breast. Detailed analysis of 99 patients with average follow-up of 24 years. Am J Surg Pathol 2:225-251, 1978.

377 Tobon H, Price HM: Lobular carcinoma in situ. Some ultrastructural observations. Cancer 39:1082-1091, 1972.

378 Warner NE: Lobular carcinoma of the breast. Cancer 23:840-846, 1969.

379 Wheeler JE, Enterline HT: Lobular carcinoma of the breast in situ and infiltrating. Pathol Annu 11:161-188, 1976.

Evolution

380 Andersen JA: Lobular carcinoma in situ. A long-term follow-up in 52 cases. Acta Pathol Microbiol Scand (A) 82:519-533, 1974.

381 Andersen JA: Lobular carcinoma in situ of the breast. An approach to rational treatment. Cancer 39:2597-2602, 1977.

382 Haagensen CD, Lane N, Lattes R, Bodian C: Lobular neoplasia (so-called lobular carcinoma in situ) of the breast. Cancer 42:737-769, 1978.

383 Ottesen GL, Graversen HP, Blichert-Toft M, Zedeler K, Andersen JA: Lobular carcinoma in situ of the female breast. Short-term results of a prospective nationwide study. The Danish Breast Cancer Cooperative Group. Am J Surg Pathol 17:14-21, 1993.

384 Page DL, Kidd TE Jr, Dupont WD, Simpson JF, Rogers LW: Lobular neoplasia of the breast. Higher risk for subsequent invasive cancer predicted by more extensive disease. Hum Pathol 22:1232-1239, 1991.

385 Rosen PP, Lieberman PH, Braun DW Jr, Kosloff C, Adair F: Lobular carcinoma in situ of the breast. Detailed analysis of 99 patients with average follow-up of 24 years. Am J Surg Pathol 2:225-251, 1978.

386 Wheeler JE, Enterline HT: Lobular carcinoma of the breast in situ and infiltrating. Pathol Annu 11:161-188, 1976.

387 Wheeler JE, Enterline HT, Roseman JM, Tomasulo JP, McIlraine CH, Fitts WT Jr, Kirshenbaum J: Lobular carcinoma in situ of the breast. Long-term follow-up. Cancer 34:554-563, 1974.

INVASIVE CARCINOMA
Invasive ductal carcinoma
Cytoarchitectural variants
Classic (NOS) invasive ductal carcinoma

388 Azzopardi JG, Laurini RN: Elastosis in breast cancer. Cancer 33:174-183, 1974.

389 Barsky SH, Grotendorst GR, Liotta LA: Increased content of type V collagen in desmoplasia of human breast carcinoma. Am J Pathol 108:276-283, 1982.

390 Battifora H: Intracytoplasmic lumina in breast carcinoma. A helpful histopathologic feature. Arch Pathol 99:614-617, 1975.

390a Bellahcène A, Castronovo V: Increased expression of osteonectin and osteopontin, two bone matrix proteins, in human breast cancer. Am J Pathol 146:95-100, 1995.

390b Berg JW, Hutter RV: Breast cancer. Cancer 75:257-269, 1995.

391 Bocker W, Klaubert A, Bahnsen J, Schweikhart G, Pollow K, Mitze M, Kreienberg R, Beck T, Stegner H-E: Peanut lectin histochemistry of 120 mammary carcinomas and its relation to tumor type, grading, staging, and receptor status. Virchows Arch [A] 403:149-161, 1984.

392 Bonetti F, Colombari R, Manfrin E, Zamboni G, Martignoni G, Mombello A, Chilosi M: Breast carcinoma with positive results for melanoma marker (HMB-45). HMB-45 immunoreactivity in normal and neoplastic breast. Am J Clin Pathol 92:491-495, 1989.

393 Bussolati G, Papotti M, Sapino A, Gugliotta P, Ghiringhello B, Azzopardi JG: Endocrine markers in argyrophilic carcinomas of the breast. Am J Surg Pathol 11:248-256, 1987.

394 Charpin C, Lachard A, Pourreau-Schneider N, Jacquemier J, Lavaut MN, Andonian C, Martin PM, Toga M: Localization of lactoferrin and nonspecific cross-reacting antigen in human breast carcinomas. An immunohistochemical study using the avidin-biotin-peroxidase complex method. Cancer 55:2612-2617, 1985.

395 Charpin C, Lissitzky JC, Jacquemier J, Lavaut MN, Kopp F, Pourreau-Schneider N, Martin PM, Toga M: Immunohistochemical detection of laminin in 98 human breast carcinomas. A light and electron microscopic study. Hum Pathol 17:355-365, 1986.

396 Clayton F, Ordóñez NG, Hanssen GM, Hanssen H: Immunoperoxidase localization of lactalbumin in malignant breast neoplasms. Arch Pathol Lab Med 106:268-270, 1982.

397 Domagala W, Wozniak L, Lasota J, Weber K, Osborn M: Vimentin is preferentially expressed in high-grade ductal and medullary, but not in lobular breast carcinomas. Am J Pathol 137:1059-1064, 1990.

398 Dwarakanath S, Lee AKC, DeLellis RA, Silverman ML, Frasca L, Wolfe HJ: S-100 protein positivity in breast carcinomas. A potential pitfall in diagnostic immunohistochemistry. Hum Pathol 18:1144-1148, 1987.

399 Fisher ER: Ultrastructure of the human breast and its disorders. Am J Clin Pathol 66:291-374, 1976.

400 Fisher ER, Gregorio RM, Fisher B, with the assistance of Redmond C, Vellios F, Sommers SC, and cooperating investigators: The pathology of invasive breast cancer. A syllabus derived from findings of the National Surgical Adjuvant Breast Project (Protocol No. 4). Cancer 36:1-85, 1975.

401 Fisher ER, Palekar AS, Gregorio RM, Redmond C, Fisher B: Pathological findings from the National Surgical Adjuvant Breast Project (Protocol No. 4). IV. Significance of tumor necrosis. Hum Pathol 9:523-530, 1978.

402 Gould VE, Koukoulis GK, Jansson DS, Nagle RB, Franke WW, Moll R: Coexpression patterns of vimentin and glial filament protein with cytokeratins in the normal, hyperplastic, and neoplastic breast. Am J Pathol 137:1143-1155, 1990.

403 Greenwalt DE, Johnson VG, Kuhajda FP, Eggleston JC, Mather IH: Localization of a membrane glycoprotein in benign fibrocystic disease and infiltrating duct carcinomas of the human breast with the use of a monoclonal antibody to guinea pig milk fat globule membrane. Am J Pathol 118:351-359, 1985.

403a Hirota S, Ito A, Nagoshi J, Takeda M, Kurata A, Takatsuka Y, Kohri K, Nomura S, Kitamura Y: Expression of bone matrix protein messenger ribonucleic acids in human breast cancers. Possible involvement of osteopontin in development of calcifying foci. Lab Invest 72:64-69, 1995.

404 Howard DR, Taylor CR: A method for distinguishing benign from malignant breast lesions utilizing antibody present in normal human sera. Cancer 43:2279-2287, 1979.

405 Jackson JG, Orr JW: The ducts of carcinomatous breasts, with particular reference to connective-tissue changes. J Pathol Bacteriol 74:265-273, 1957.

406 Jarasch E-D, Nagle RB, Kaufmann M, Maurer C, Bocker WJ: Differential diagnosis of benign epithelial proliferations and carcinomas of the breast using antibodies to cytokeratins. Hum Pathol 19:276-289, 1988.

407 Kuhajda FP, Bohn H, Mendelsohn G: Pregnancy-specific beta-1 glycoprotein (SP-1) in breast carcinoma. Pathologic and clinical considerations. Cancer 54:1392-1396, 1984.

408 Kuhajda FP, Offutt LE, Mendelsohn G: The distribution of carcinoembryonic antigen in breast carcinoma. Diagnostic and prognostic implications. Cancer 52:1257-1264, 1983.

409 Lee AK, DeLellis RA, Rosen PP, Herbert-Stanton T, Tallberg K, Garcia C, Wolfe HJ: Alpha-lactalbumin as an immunohistochemical marker for metastatic breast carcinomas. Am J Surg Pathol 8:93-100, 1984.

410 Lee AKC, DeLellis RA, Wolfe HJ: Intramammary lymphatic invasion in breast carcinomas. Evaluation using ABH isoantigens as endothelial markers. Am J Surg Pathol 10:589-594, 1986.

411 Loy TS, Chapman RK, Diaz-Arias AA, Bulatao IS, Bickel JT: Distribution of BCA-225 in adenocarcinomas. An immunohistochemical study of 446 cases. Am J Clin Pathol 96:326-329, 1991.

412 Lunde S, Nesland JM, Holm R, Johannessen JV: Breast carcinomas with protein S-100 immunoreactivity. An immunocytochemical and ultrastructural study. Pathol Res Pract 182:627-631, 1987.

413 Martin SA, Perez-Reyes N, Mendelsohn G: Angioinvasion in breast carcinoma. An immunohistochemical study of factor VIII-related antigen. Cancer 59:1918-1922, 1987.

414 Mazoujian G, Bodian C, Haagensen DE Jr, Haagensen CD: Expression of GCDFP-15 in breast carcinomas. Relationship to pathologic and clinical factors. Cancer 63:2156-2161, 1989.

415 Mesa-Tejada R, Oster MW, Fenoglio CM, Magidson J, Spiegelman S: Diagnosis of primary breast carcinoma through immunohistochemical detection of antigen related to mouse mammary tumor virus in metastatic lesions. A report of two cases. Cancer 49:261-268, 1982.

416 Oberman HA: Invasive carcinoma of the breast with granulomatous response. Am J Clin Pathol 88:718-721, 1987.

417 Ohtani H, Sasano N: Myofibroblasts and myoepithelial cells in human breast carcinoma. An ultrastructural study. Virchows Arch [A] 385:247-261, 1980.

418 Ordóñez NG, Brooks T, Thompson S, Batsakis JG: Use of *Ulex europaeus* agglutinin I in the identification of lymphatic and blood vessel invasion in previously stained microscopic slides. Am J Surg Pathol 11:543-550, 1987.

419 Prey MU, Bedrossian CW, Masood S: The value of monoclonal antibody B72.3 for the diagnosis of breast carcinoma. Experience with the first commercially available source. Hum Pathol 22:598-602, 1991.

420 Robertson JF, Ellis IO, Bell J, Todd JH, Robins A, Elston CW, Blamey RW: Car-cinoembryonic antigen immunocytochemistry in primary breast cancer. Cancer 64:1638-1645, 1989.

421 Rosen PP: Tumor emboli in intramammary lymphatics in breast carcinoma. Pathologic criteria for diagnosis and clinical significance. Pathol Annu 18(Pt 2):215-232, 1983.

422 Saigo PE, Rosen PP: The application of immunohistochemical stains to identify endothelial-lined channels in mammary carcinoma. Cancer **59:**51-54, 1987.

423 Sobrinho-Simões M, Johannessen JV, Gould VE: The diagnostic significance of intracytoplasmic lumina in metastatic neoplasms. Ultrastruct Pathol**2:**327-335, 1981.

424 Tavassoli FA, Jones MW, Majeste RM, Bratthauer GL, O'Leary TJ: Immuno-histochemical staining with monoclonal Ab B72.3 in benign and malignant breast disease. Am J Surg Pathol **14:**128-133, 1990.

425 Tsubura A, Okada H, Senzaki H, Hatano T, Morii S: Keratin expression in the normal breast and in breast carcinoma. Histopathology **18:**517-522, 1991.

426 Wetzels RH, Holland R, van Haelst UJ, Lane EB, Leigh IM, Ramaekers FC: Detection of basement membrane components and basal cell keratin 14 in non-invasive and invasive carcinomas of the breast. Am J Pathol **134:**571-579, 1989.

427 Wick MR, Lillemoe TJ, Copland GT, Swanson PE, Manivel JC, Kiang DT: Gross cystic disease fluid protein-15 as a marker for breast cancer. Immunohistochemical analysis of 690 human neoplasms and comparison with alpha-lactalbumin. Hum Pathol **20:**281-287, 1989.

428 Willebrand D, Bosman FT, De Goeij AFPM: Patterns of basement membrane deposition in benign and malignant breast tumours. Histopathology **10:**1231-1241, 1986.

Tubular carcinoma

429 Carstens PHB, Greenberg RA, Francis D, Lyon H: Tubular carcinoma of the breast. A long term follow-up. Histopathology **9:**271-280, 1985.

430 Carstens PHB, Huvos AG, Foote FW Jr, Ashikari R: Tubular carcinoma of the breast. A clinicopathologic study of 35 cases. Am J Clin Pathol **58:**231-238, 1972.

431 Dawson AE, Logan-Young W, Mulford DK: Aspiration cytology of tubular car-cinoma. Diagnostic features with mammographic correlation. Am J Clin Pathol **101:**488-492, 1994.

432 Deos PH, Norris HJ: Well-differentiated (tubular) carcinoma of the breast. A clinicopathologic study of 145 pure and mixed cases. Am J Clin Pathol **78:**1-7, 1982.

433 Erlandson RA, Carstens PHB: Ultrastructure of tubular carcinoma of the breast. Cancer **29:**987-995, 1972.

434 Flotte TJ, Bell DA, Greco MA: Tubular carcinoma and sclerosing adenosis. The use of basal lamina as a differential feature. Am J Surg Pathol **4:**75-77, 1980.

435 Jao W, Recant W, Swerdlow MA: Comparative ultrastructure of tubular carci-noma and sclerosing adenosis of the breast. Cancer **38:**180-186, 1976.

436 Lagios MD, Rose MR, Margolin FR: Tubular carcinoma of the breast. Associa-tion with multicentricity, bilaterality, and family history of mammary carci-noma. Am J Clin Pathol **73:**25-30, 1980.

437 McDivitt RW, Boyce W, Gersell D: Tubular carcinoma of the breast. Clinical and pathological observations concerning 135 cases. Am J Surg Pathol **6:**401-411, 1982.

438 Oberman HA, Fidler WJ Jr: Tubular carcinoma of the breast. Am J Surg Pathol **3:**387-395, 1979.

439 Parl FF, Richardson LD: The histologic and biologic spectrum of tubular carci-noma of the breast. Hum Pathol **14:**694-698, 1983.

440 Peters GN, Wolff M, Haagensen CD: Tubular carcinoma of the breast. Clinical pathologic correlations based on 100 cases. Ann Surg **193:**138-149, 1981.

441 Taylor HB, Norris HJ: Well-differentiated carcinoma of the breast. Cancer **25:**687-692, 1970.

442 Tremblay G: Elastosis in tubular carcinoma of the breast. Arch Pathol **98:**302-307, 1974.

443 van Bogaert L-J: Clinicopathologic hallmarks of mammary tubular carcinoma. Hum Pathol **13:**558-562, 1982.

Cribriform carcinoma

444 Page DL, Dixon JM, Anderson TJ, Lee D, Stewart HJ: Invasive cribriform car-cinoma of the breast. Histopathology **7:**525-536, 1983.

445 Venable JG, Schwartz AM, Silverberg SG: Infiltrating cribriform carcinoma of the breast. A distinctive clinicopathologic entity. Hum Pathol **21:**333-338, 1990.

Mucinous carcinoma

446 Capella C, Eusebi V, Mann B, Azzopardi JG: Endocrine differentiation in mucoid carcinoma of the breast. Histopathology **4:**613-630, 1980.

447 Clayton F: Pure mucinous carcinomas of breast. Morphologic features and prog-nostic correlates. Hum Pathol **17:**34-38, 1986.

448 Coady AT, Shousha S, Dawson PM, Moss M, James KR, Bull TB: Mucinous carcinoma of the breast. Further characterization of its three subtypes. Histopathology **15:**617-626, 1989.

449 Ferguson DJP, Anderson TJ, Wells CA, Battersby S: An ultrastructural study of mucoid carcinoma of the breast. Variability of cytoplasmic features. His-topathology **10:**1219-1230, 1986.

450 Fisher ER, Palekar AS, NSABP collaborators: Solid and mucinous varieties of so-called mammary carcinoid tumors. Am J Clin Pathol **72:**909-916, 1979.

451 Hull MT, Warfel KA: Mucinous breast carcinomas with abundant intracyto-plasmic mucin and neuroendocrine features. Light microscopic, immunohisto-chemical, and ultrastructural study. Ultrastruct Pathol **11:**29-38, 1987.

452 Komaki K, Sakamoto G, Sugano H, Kasumi F, Watanabe S, Nishi M, Morimoto T, Monden Y: The morphologic feature of mucus leakage appearing in low pap-illary carcinoma of the breast. Hum Pathol **22:**231-236, 1991.

453 Norris HJ, Taylor HB: Prognosis of mucinous (gelatinous) carcinoma of the breast. Cancer **18:**879-885, 1965.

454 Rasmussen BB: Human mucinous breast carcinomas and their lymph node metastases. A histological review of 247 cases. Pathol Res Pract **180:**377-382, 1985.

455 Rasmussen BB, Rose C, Christensen IB: Prognostic factors in primary muci-nous breast carcinoma. Am J Clin Pathol **87:**155-160, 1987.

456 Rasmussen BB, Rose C, Thorpe SM, Andersen KW, Hou-Jensen K: Argy-rophilic cells in 202 human mucinous breast carcinomas. Relation to histopathologic and clinical factors. Am J Clin Pathol **84:**737-740, 1985.

457 Ro JY, Sneige N, Sahin AA, Silva EG, del Junco GW, Ayala AG: Mucocele-like tumor of the breast associated with atypical ductal hyperplasia or mucinous carcinoma. A clinicopathologic study of seven cases. Arch Pathol Lab Med **115:**137-140, 1991.

458 Rosen PP: Mucocele-like tumors of the breast. Am J Surg Pathol **10:**464-469, 1986.

459 Rosen PP, Wang T-Y: Colloid carcinoma of the breast. Analysis of 64 patients with long-term follow-up (abstract). Am J Clin Pathol **73:**304, 1980.

460 Scopsi L, Andreola S, Pilotti S, Bufalino R, Baldini MT, Testori A, Rilke F: Mucinous carcinoma of the breast. A clinicopathologic, histochemical, and immunocytochemical study with special reference to neuroendocrine differen-tiation. Am J Surg Pathol **18:**702-711, 1994.

461 Toikkanen S, Kujari H: Pure and mixed mucinous carcinomas of the breast. A clinicopathologic analysis of 61 cases with long-term follow-up. Hum Pathol **20:**758-764, 1989.

462 Walker RA: Mucoid carcinomas of the breast. A study using mucin histochem-istry and peanut lectin. Histopathology **6:**571-579, 1982.

Medullary carcinoma

463 Ben-Ezra J, Sheibani K: Antigenic phenotype of the lymphocytic component of medullary carcinoma of the breast. Cancer **59:**2037-2041, 1987.

464 Bloom HJG, Richardson WW, Fields JR: Host resistance and survival in carcinoma of breasts. A study of 104 cases of medullary carcinoma in a series of 1,411 cases of breast cancer followed for 20 years. Br Med J **3:**181-188, 1970.

464a Dalal P, Shousha S: Keratin 19 in paraffin sections of medullary carcinoma and other benign and malignant breast lesions. Mod Pathol **8:**413-416, 1995.

465 Dwarakanath S, Lee AKC, DeLellis RA, Silverman ML, Frasca L, Wolfe HJ: S-100 protein positivity in breast carcinomas. A potential pitfall in diagnostic immunohistochemistry. Hum Pathol **18:**1144-1148, 1987.

466 Gaffey MJ, Frierson HF Jr, Mills SE, Boyd JC, Zarbo RJ, Simpson JF, Gross LK, Weiss LM: Medullary carcinoma of the breast. Identification of lympho-cyte subpopulations and their significance. Mod Pathol **6:**721-728, 1993.

466a Gaffey MJ, Mills SE, Frierson HF Jr, Zarbo RJ, Boyd JC, Simpson JF, Weiss LM: Medullary carcinoma of the breast. Interobserver variability in histopatho-logic diagnosis. Mod Pathol **8:**31-38, 1995.

467 Harris M, Lessells AM: The ultrastructure of medullary, atypical medullary and non-medullary carcinomas of the breast. Histopathology **10:**405-414, 1986.

468 Howell LP, Kline TS: Medullary carcinoma of the breast. An unusual cytologic finding in cyst fluid aspirates. Cancer **65:**277-282, 1990.

469 Hsu S-M, Raine L, Nayak RN: Medullary carcinoma of breast. An immunohis-tochemical study of its lymphoid stroma. Cancer **48:**1368-1376, 1981.

470 Kumar S, Kumar D: Lymphoepithelioma-like carcinoma of the breast. Mod Pathol **7:**129-131, 1994.

471 Larsimont D, Lespagnard L, Degeyter M, Heimann R: Medullary carcinoma of the breast. A tumour lacking keratin 19. Histopathology **24:**549-552, 1994.

471a Lespagnard L, Cochaux P, Larsimont D, Degeyter M, Velu T, Heimann R: Absence of Epstein-Barr virus in medullary carcinoma of the breast as demon-strated by immunophenotyping, *in situ* hybridization and polymerase chain reaction. Am J Clin Pathol **103:**449-452, 1995.

472 Moore OS Jr, Foote FW Jr: The relatively favorable prognosis of medullary car-cinoma of the breast. Cancer **2:**635-642, 1949.

473 Rapin V, Contesso G, Mouriesse H, Bertin F, LaCombe MJ, Piekarski JD, Travagli JP, Gadenne C, Friedman S: Medullary breast carcinoma. A reevaluation of 95 cases of breast cancer with inflammatory stroma. Cancer **61**:2503-2510, 1988.

474 Richardson WW: Medullary carcinoma of the breast. A distinctive tumour type with a relatively good prognosis following radical mastectomy. Br J Cancer **10**:415-423, 1956.

475 Ridolfi RL, Rosen PP, Port A, Kinne D, Miké V: Medullary carcinoma of the breast. A clinicopathologic study with 10 year follow-up. Cancer **40**:1365-1385, 1977.

476 Rigaud C, Theobald S, Noel P, Badreddine J, Barlier C, Delobelle A, Gentile A, Jacquemier J, Maisongrosse V, Peffault de Latour M, et al.: Medullary carcinoma of the breast. A multicenter study of its diagnostic consistency. Arch Pathol Lab Med **117**:1005-1008, 1993.

477 Wargotz ES, Silverberg SG: Medullary carcinoma of the breast. A clinicopathologic study with appraisal of current diagnostic criteria (abstract). Lab Invest **58**:100A, 1988.

478 Yazawa T, Kamma H, Ogata T: Frequent expression of HLA-DR antigen in medullary carcinoma of the breast. A possible reason for its prominent lymphocytic infiltration and favorable prognosis. Appl Immunohistochem **1**:289-296, 1993.

Invasive papillary carcinoma

479 Carter D, Orr SL, Merino MJ: Intracystic papillary carcinoma of the breast. After mastectomy, radiotherapy or excisional biopsy alone. Cancer **52**:14-19, 1983.

480 Corkill ME, Sneige N, Fanning T, el-Naggar A: Fine-needle aspiration cytology and flow cytometry of intracystic papillary carcinoma of breast. Am J Clin Pathol **94**:673-680, 1990.

481 Fisher ER, Palekar AS, Redmond C, Barton B, Fisher B: Pathologic findings from the National Surgical Adjuvant Breast Project (Protocol No. 4). VI. Invasive papillary cancer. Am J Clin Pathol **73**:313-322, 1980.

Apocrine carcinoma

482 Abati AD, Kimmel M, Rosen PP: Apocrine mammary carcinoma. A clinicopathologic study of 72 cases. Am J Clin Pathol **94**:371-377, 1990.

483 Eusebi V, Betts C, Haagensen DE Jr, Gugliotta P, Bussolati G, Azzopardi JG: Apocrine differentiation in lobular carcinoma of the breast. A morphologic, immunologic, and ultrastructural study. Hum Pathol **15**:134-140, 1984.

484 Eusebi V, Millis RR, Cattani MG, Bussolati G, Azzopardi JG: Apocrine carcinoma of the breast. A morphologic and immunocytochemical study. Am J Pathol **123**:532-541, 1986.

484a Losi L, Lorenzini R, Eusebi V, Bussolati G: Apocrine differentiation in invasive carcinoma of the breast. Comparison of monoclonal and polyclonal gross cystic disease fluid protein-15 antibodies with prolactin-inducible protein mRNA gene expression. Appl Immunohistochem **3**:91-98, 1995.

485 Mossler JA, Barton TK, Brinkhous AD, McCarty KS, Moylan JA, McCarty KS Jr: Apocrine differentiation in human mammary carcinoma. Cancer **46**:2463-2471, 1980.

486 Pagani A, Sapino A, Eusebi V, Bergnolo P, Bussolati G: PIP/GCDFP-15 gene expression and apocrine differentiation in carcinomas of the breast. Virchows Arch [A] **425**:459-465, 1994.

Juvenile (secretory) carcinoma

487 Akhtar M, Robinson C, Ali MA, Godwin JT: Secretory carcinoma of the breast in adults. Light and electron microscopic study of three cases with review of the literature. Cancer **51**:2245-2254, 1983.

488 Krausz T, Jenkins D, Grontoft O, Pollock DJ, Azzopardi JG: Secretory carcinoma of the breast in adults. Emphasis on late recurrence and metastasis. Histopathology **14**:25-36, 1989.

489 Lamovec J, Bracko M: Secretory carcinoma of the breast. Light microscopical, immunohistochemical and flow cytometric study. Mod Pathol **7**:475-479, 1994.

490 McDivitt RW, Stewart FW: Breast carcinoma in children. JAMA **195**:388-390, 1966.

491 Oberman HA: Secretory carcinoma of the breast in adults. Am J Surg Pathol **4**:465-470, 1980.

492 Rosen PP, Cranor ML: Secretory carcinoma of the breast. Arch Pathol Lab Med **115**:141-144, 1991.

493 Tavassoli FA, Norris HJ: Secretory carcinoma of the breast. Cancer **45**:2404-2413, 1980.

Carcinomas with neuroendocrine features (including so-called carcinoid tumor)

494 Azzopardi JG, Muretto P, Goddeeris P, Eusebi V, Lauweryns JM: 'Carcinoid' tumours of the breast. The morphological spectrum of argyrophil carcinomas. Histopathology **6**:549-569, 1982.

495 Battersby S, Dely CJ, Hopkinson HE, Anderson TJ: The nature of breast dense core granules. Chromogranin reactivity. Histopathology **20**:107-114, 1992.

496 Bussolati G, Papotti M, Sapino A, Gugliotta P, Ghiringhello B, Azzopardi JG: Endocrine markers in argyrophilic carcinomas of the breast. Am J Surg Pathol **11**:248-256, 1987.

497 Capella C, Usellini L, Papotti M, Macri L, Finzi G, Eusebi V, Bussolati G: Ultrastructural features of neuroendocrine differentiated carcinomas of the breast. Ultrastruct Pathol **14**:321-334, 1990.

498 Clayton F, Sibley RK, Ordóñez NG, Hanssen G: Argyrophilic breast carcinomas. Evidence of lactational differentiation. Am J Surg Pathol **6**:323-333, 1982.

499 Cross AS, Azzopardi JG, Krausz T, Van Noorden S, Polak JM: A morphological and immunocytochemical study of a distinctive variant of ductal carcinoma in-situ of the breast. Histopathology **9**:21-37, 1985.

500 Cubilla AL, Woodruff JM: Primary carcinoid tumor of the breast. A report of eight patients. Am J Surg Pathol **1**:283-292, 1977.

501 Fisher ER, Palekar AS, NSABP Collaborators: Solid and mucinous varieties of so-called mammary carcinoid tumors. Am J Clin Pathol **72**:909-916, 1979.

502 Kaneko H, Hôjô H, Ishikawa S, Yamanouchi H, Sumida T, Saito R: Norepinephrine-producing tumors of bilateral breasts. A case report. Cancer **41**:2002-2007, 1978.

503 Maluf HM, Koerner FC: Carcinomas of the breast with endocrine differentiation. A review. Virchows Archiv **425**:449-457, 1994.

504 Nesland JM, Holm R, Johannessen JV, Gould VE: Neurone specific enolase immunostaining in the diagnosis of breast carcinomas with neuroendocrine differentiation. Its usefulness and limitations. J Pathol **148**:35-43, 1986.

505 Nesland JM, Memoli VA, Holm R, Gould VE, Johannessen JV: Breast carcinomas with neuroendocrine differentiation. Ultrastruct Pathol **8**:225-240, 1985.

506 Pagani A, Papotti M, Hofler H, Weiler R, Winkler H, Bussolati G: Chromogranin A and B gene expression in carcinomas of the breast. Correlation of immunocytochemical, immunoblot, and hybridization analyses. Am J Pathol **136**:319-327, 1990.

507 Papotti M, Macri L, Finzi G, Capella C, Eusebi V, Bussolati G: Neuroendocrine differentiation in carcinomas of the breast. A study of 51 cases. Semin Diagn Pathol **6**:174-188, 1989.

508 Scopsi L, Balslev E, Brunner N, Poulsen HS, Andersen J, Rank F, Larsson LI: Immunoreactive opioid peptides in human breast cancer. Am J Pathol **134**:473-479, 1989.

509 Taxy JB, Tischler AS, Insalaco SJ, Battifora H: "Carcinoid" tumor of the breast. A variant of conventional breast cancer? Hum Pathol **12**:170-179, 1981.

510 Toyoshima S: Mammary carcinoma with argyrophil cells. Cancer **52**:2129-2138, 1983.

511 Uccini S, Monardo F, Paradiso P, Masciangelo R, Marzullo A, Ruco LP, Baroni CD: Synaptophysin in human breast carcinomas. Histopathology **18**:271-273,1991.

512 Wade PM Jr, Mills SE, Read M, Cloud W, Lambert MJ III, Smith RE: Small cell neuroendocrine (oat cell) carcinoma of the breast. Cancer **52**:121-125, 1983.

513 Wilander E, Páhlman S, Sällström J, Lindgren A: Neuron-specific enolase expression and neuroendocrine differentiation in carcinomas of the breast. Arch Pathol Lab Med **111**:830-832, 1987.

Metaplastic carcinoma

514 Agnantis NT, Rosen PP: Mammary carcinoma with osteoclast-like giant cells. A study of eight cases with follow-up data. Am J Clin Pathol **72**:383-389, 1979.

515 Banerjee SS, Eyden BP, Wells S, McWilliam LJ, Harris M: Pseudoangiosarcomatous carcinoma. A clinicopathological study of seven cases. Histopathology **21**:13-23, 1992.

516 Eusebi V, Cattani MG, Ceccarelli C, Lamovec J: Sarcomatoid carcinomas of the breast. An immunohistochemical study of 14 cases. Progr Surg Pathol **10**:83-100, 1989.

517 Foschini MP, Dina RE, Eusebi V: Sarcomatoid neoplasms of the breast. Proposed definitions for biphasic and monophasic sarcomatoid mammary carcinomas. Semin Diagn Pathol **10**:128-136, 1993.

518 Harris M, Persaud V: Carcinosarcoma of the breast. J Pathol **112**:99-105, 1974.

519 Herrington CS, Tarin D, Buley I, Athanasou N: Osteosarcomatous differentiation in carcinoma of the breast. A case of 'metaplastic' carcinoma with osteoclasts and osteoclast-like giant cells. Histopathology **24**:282-285, 1994.

520 Holland R, van Haelst UJGM: Mammary carcinoma with osteoclast-like giant cells. Additional observations on six cases. Cancer **53**:1963-1973, 1984.

521 Kaufman MW, Marti JR, Gallager HS, Hoehn JL: Carcinoma of the breast with pseudosarcomatous metaplasia. Cancer **53:**1908-1917, 1984.

522 Llombart-Bosch A, Peydro A: Malignant mixed osteogenic tumours of the breast. An ultrastructural study of two cases. Virchows Arch [A] **366:**1-14, 1975.

523 Nielsen BB, Kiaer HW: Carcinoma of the breast with stromal multinucleated giant cells. Histopathology **9:**183-193, 1985.

524 Oberman HA: Metaplastic carcinoma of the breast. A clinicopathologic study of 29 patients. Am J Surg Pathol **11:**918-929, 1987.

525 Pitts WC, Rojas VA, Gaffey MJ, Rouse RV, Esteban J, Frierson HF, Kempson RL, Weiss LM: Carcinomas with metaplasia and sarcomas of the breast. Am J Clin Pathol **95:**623-632, 1991.

526 Raju GC, Wee A: Spindle cell carcinoma of the breast. Histopathology **16:**497-499, 1990.

527 Santeusanio G, Pascal RR, Bisceglia M, Costantino AM, Bosman C: Metaplastic breast carcinoma with epithelial phenotype of pseudosarcomatous components. Arch Pathol Lab Med **112:**82-85, 1988.

528 Tavassoli FA: Classification of metaplastic carcinomas of the breast. Pathol Annu **27**(Pt 2):89-119, 1992.

529 Tavassoli FA, Norris HJ: Breast carcinoma with osteoclastlike giant cells. Arch Pathol Lab Med **110:**636-639, 1986.

530 Wargotz ES, Deos PH, Norris HJ: Metaplastic carcinomas of the breast. II. Spindle cell carcinoma. Hum Pathol **20:**732-740, 1989.

531 Wargotz ES, Norris HJ: Metaplastic carcinomas of the breast. I. Matrix-producing carcinoma. Hum Pathol **20:**628-635, 1989.

532 Wargotz ES, Norris HJ: Metaplastic carcinomas of the breast. III. Carcinosarcoma. Cancer **64:**1490-1499, 1989.

533 Wargotz ES, Norris HJ: Metaplastic carcinomas of the breast. V. Metaplastic carcinoma with osteoclastic giant cells. Hum Pathol **21:**1142-1150, 1990.

533a Weidner N: Malignant breast lesions that may mimic benign tumors. Semin Diagn Pathol **12:**2-13, 1995.

Squamous cell carcinoma and related tumors

534 Bauer TW, Rostock RA, Eggleston JC, Baral E: Spindle cell carcinoma of the breast. Four cases and review of the literature. Hum Pathol **15:**147-152, 1984.

535 Cornog JL, Mobini J, Steiger E, Enterline HT: Squamous carcinoma of the breast. Am J Clin Pathol **55:**410-417, 1971.

536 Eggers JW, Chesney TM: Squamous cell carcinoma of the breast. A clinicopathologic analysis of eight cases and review of the literature. Hum Pathol **15:**526-531, 1984.

537 Eusebi V, Lamovec J, Cattani MG, Fedeli F, Millis RR: Acantholytic variant of squamous-cell carcinoma of the breast. Am J Surg Pathol **10:**855-861, 1986.

538 Fisher ER, Palekar AS, Gregorio RM, Paulson JD: Mucoepidermoid and squamous cell carcinomas of breast with reference to squamous metaplasia and giant cell tumors. Am J Surg Pathol **7:**15-27, 1983.

539 Foschini MP, Fulcheri E, Baracchini P, Ceccarelli C, Betts CM, Eusebi V: Squamous cell carcinoma with prominent myxoid stroma. Hum Pathol **21:**859-865, 1990.

540 Gersell DJ, Katzenstein A-LA: Spindle cell carcinoma of the breast. A clinicopathologic and ultrastructural study. Hum Pathol **12:**550-561, 1981.

541 Oberman HA: Metaplastic carcinoma of the breast. A clinicopathologic study of 29 patients. Am J Surg Pathol **11:**918-929, 1987.

542 Rosen PP, Ernsberger D: Low-grade adenosquamous carcinoma. A variant of metaplastic mammary carcinoma. Am J Surg Pathol **11:**351-358, 1987.

543 Toikkanen S: Primary squamous cell carcinoma of the breast. Cancer **48:**1629-1632, 1981.

544 Wargotz ES, Norris HJ: Metaplastic carcinomas of the breast. IV. Squamous cell carcinoma of ductal origin. Cancer **65:**272-276, 1990.

545 Woodard BH, Brinkhous AD, McCarty KS Sr, McCarty KS Jr: Adenosquamous differentiation in mammary carcinoma. An ultrastructural and steroid receptor study. Arch Pathol Lab Med **104:**130-133, 1980.

Spread-related variants
Inflammatory carcinoma

546 Buzdar AU, Montague ED, Barker JL, Hortobagyi GN, Blumenschein GR: Management of inflammatory carcinoma of breast with combined modality approach. An update. Cancer **47:**2537-2542, 1981.

547 Chu AM, Wood WC, Doucette JA: Inflammatory breast carcinoma treated by radical radiotherapy. Cancer **45:**2730-2737, 1980.

548 Ellis DL, Teitelbaum SL: Inflammatory carcinoma of the breast. A pathological definition. Cancer **33:**1045-1047, 1974.

549 Fields JN, Kuske RR, Perez CA, Fineberg BB, Bartlett N: Prognostic factors in inflammatory breast cancer. Univariate and multivariate analysis. Cancer **63:**1225-1232, 1989.

550 Lucas FV, Perez-Mesa C: Inflammatory carcinoma of the breast. Cancer **41:**1595-1605, 1978.

551 Saltzstein SL: Clinically occult inflammatory carcinoma of the breast. Cancer **34:**382-388, 1974.

552 Schafer P, Alberto P, Forni M, Obradovic D, Pipard G, Krauer F: Surgery as part of a combined modality approach for inflammatory breast carcinoma. Cancer **59:**1063-1067, 1987.

Paget's disease

553 Ashikari R, Park K, Huvos AG, Urban JA: Paget's disease of the breast. Cancer **26:**680-685, 1970.

554 Azzopardi JG, Eusebi V: Melanocyte colonization and pigmentation of breast carcinoma. Histopathology **1:**21-30, 1977.

555 Bussolati G, Pich A: Mammary and extramammary Paget's disease. An immunocytochemical study. Am J Pathol **80:**117-127, 1975.

556 Cohen C, Guarner J, De Rose PB: Mammary Paget's disease and associated carcinoma. An immunohistochemical study. Arch Pathol Lab Med **117:**291-294, 1993.

557 de Potter CR, Eeckhout I, Schelfhout AM, Geerts ML, Roels HJ: Keratinocyte induced chemotaxis in the pathogenesis of Paget's disease of the breast. Histopathology **24:**349-356, 1994.

558 Keatings L, Sinclair J, Wright C, Corbett IP, Watchorn C, Hennessy C, Angus B, Lennard T, Horne CH: c-erbB-2 oncoprotein expression in mammary and extramammary Paget's disease. An immunohistochemical study. Histopathology **17:**243-247, 1990.

559 Kirkham N, Berry N, Jones DB, Taylor-Papadimitriou J: Paget's disease of the nipple. Immunohistochemical localization of milk fat globule membrane antigens. Cancer **55:**1510-1512, 1985.

560 Lagios MD, Westdahl PR, Rose MR, Concannon S: Paget's disease of the nipple. Alternative management in cases without or with minimal extent of underlying breast carcinoma. Cancer **54:**545-551, 1984.

561 Meissner K, Riviere A, Haupt G, Loning T: Study of neu-protein expression in mammary Paget's disease with and without underlying breast carcinoma and in extramammary Paget's disease. Am J Pathol **137:**1305-1309, 1990.

562 Mori O, Hachisuka H, Nakano S, Sasai Y, Shiku H: Expression of *ras* p21 in mammary and extramammary Paget's disease. Arch Pathol Lab Med **114:**858-861, 1990.

563 Nagle RB, Lucas DO, McDaniel KM, Clark VA, Schmalzel GM: New evidence linking mammary and extramammary Paget cells to a common cell phenotype. Am J Clin Pathol **83:**431-438, 1985.

564 Neubecker RD, Bradshaw RP: Mucin, melanin, and glycogen in Paget's disease of the breast. Am J Clin Pathol **36:**40-53, 1961.

565 Ordóñez NG, Awalt H, Mackay B: Mammary and extramammary Paget's disease. An immunocytochemical and ultrastructural study. Cancer **59:**1173-1183, 1987.

566 Paget J: On disease of the mammary areola preceding cancer of the mammary gland. St Barth Hosp Rep **10:**87-89, 1874.

567 Paone JF, Baker RR: Pathogenesis and treatment of Paget's disease of the breast. Cancer **48:**825-829, 1981.

568 Rayne SC, Santa Cruz DJ: Anaplastic Paget's disease. Am J Surg Pathol **16:**1085-1091, 1992.

569 Sagebiel RW: Ultrastructural observations on epidermal cells in Paget's disease of the breast. Am J Pathol **57:**49-64, 1969.

570 Sitakalin C, Ackerman AB: Mammary and extramammary Paget's disease. Am J Dermatopathol **7:**335-340, 1985.

571 Toker C: Clear cells of the nipple epidermis. Cancer **25:**601-610, 1970.

572 Vanstapel M-J, Gatter KC, DeWolf-Peeters C, Millard PR, Desmet VJ, Mason DY: Immunohistochemical study of mammary and extra-mammary Paget's disease. Histopathology **8:**1013-1023, 1984.

573 Venkataseshan VS, Budd DC, Kim DU, Hutter RVP: Intraepidermal squamous carcinoma (Bowen's disease) of the nipple. Hum Pathol **25:**1371-1374, 1994.

574 Wolber RA, Dupuis BA, Wick MR: Expression of c-erbB-2 oncoprotein in mammary and extramammary Paget's disease. Am J Clin Pathol **96:**243-247, 1991.

Invasive lobular carcinoma (ILC)
Classic type

575 Di Costanzo D, Rosen PP, Gareen I, Franklin S, Lesser M: Prognosis in infiltrating lobular carcinoma. An analysis of "classical" and variant tumors. Am J Surg Pathol **14:**12-23, 1990.

576 Domagala W, Harezga B, Szadowska A, Markiewski M, Weber K, Osborn M: Nuclear p53 protein accumulates preferentially in medullary and high-grade ductal but rarely in lobular breast carcinomas. Am J Pathol **142:**669-674, 1993.

577 Fechner RE: Infiltrating lobular carcinoma without lobular carcinoma in situ. Cancer 29:1539-1545, 1972.

578 Martinez V, Azzopardi JG: Invasive lobular carcinoma of the breast. Incidence and variants. Histopathology 3:467-488, 1979.

579 Silverstein MJ, Lewinsky BS, Waisman JR, Gierson ED, Colburn WJ, Senofsky GM, Gamagami P: Infiltrating lobular carcinoma. Is it different from infiltrating duct carcinoma? Cancer 73:1673-1677, 1994.

580 Vitsky JL, Page DL, Bluth RF: Lymphoid infiltrates in the breast may obscure infiltrating lobular carcinoma (abstract). Mod Pathol 8:28A, 1995.

Histiocytoid carcinoma

581 Eusebi V, Foschini MP, Bussolati G, Rosen PP: Myoblastomatoid (histiocytoid) carcinoma of the breast. A type of apocrine carcinoma. Am J Surg Pathol 19:553-562, 1995.

582 Fisher ER, Gregorio R, Kim WS, Redmond C: Lipid in invasive cancer of the breast. Am J Clin Pathol 68:558-561, 1977.

583 Hood CI, Font RL, Zimmerman LE: Metastatic mammary carcinoma in the eyelid with histiocytoid appearance. Cancer 31:793-800, 1973.

584 Ramos CV, Taylor HB: Lipid-rich carcinoma of the breast. Cancer 33:812-819, 1974.

585 van Bogaert LJ, Maldague P: Histologic variants of lipid-secreting carcinoma of the breast. Virchows Arch [A] 375:345-353, 1977.

585a Walford N, ten Velden J: Histiocytoid breast carcinoma. An apocrine variant of lobular carcinoma. Histopathology 14:515-522, 1989.

Signet ring carcinoma

586 Eltorky M, Hall JC, Osborne PT, el Zeky F: Signet-ring cell variant of invasive lobular carcinoma of the breast. A clinicopathologic study of 11 cases. Arch Pathol Lab Med 118:245-248, 1994.

587 Fisher ER, Brown R: Intraductal signet ring carcinoma. A hitherto undescribed form of intraductal carcinoma of the breast. Cancer 55:2533-2537, 1985.

587a Frost AR, Terahata S, Yeh IT, Siegel RS, Overmoyer B, Silverberg SG: The significance of signet ring cells in infiltrating lobular carcinoma of the breast. Arch Pathol Lab Med 119:64-68, 1995.

588 Hull MT, Seo IS, Battersby JS, Csicsko JF: Signet-ring cell carcinoma of the breast. A clinicopathologic study of 24 cases. Am J Clin Pathol 73:31-35, 1980.

589 Martinez V, Azzopardi JG: Invasive lobular carcinoma of the breast. Incidence and variants. Histopathology 3:467-488, 1979.

590 Merino MJ, LiVolsi VA: Signet ring carcinoma of the female breast. A clinicopathologic analysis of 24 cases. Cancer 48:1830-1837, 1981.

591 Quincey C, Raitt N, Bell J, Ellis IO: Intracytoplasmic lumina—a useful diagnostic feature of adenocarcinomas. Histopathology 19:83-87, 1991.

592 Steinbrecher JS, Silverberg SG: Signet-ring cell carcinoma of the breast. The mucinous variant of infiltrating lobular carcinoma? Cancer 37:828-840, 1976.

593 Yoshida H, Hatanaka S, Oneda S, Yoshida H: Signet ring cells in breast carcinoma. An immunohistochemical and ultrastructural study. Acta Pathol Jpn 42:523-528, 1992.

Other types

594 Azzopardi JG: Problems in breast pathology. In Bennington JL, consulting ed: Major problems in pathology, vol 11. Philadelphia, 1979, WB Saunders Co.

595 Dixon JM, Anderson TJ, Page DL, Lee D, Duffy SW: Infiltrating lobular carcinoma of the breast. Histopathology 6:149-161, 1982.

596 Eusebi V, Magalhaes F, Azzopardi JG: Pleomorphic lobular carcinoma of the breast. An aggressive tumor showing apocrine differentiation. Hum Pathol 23:655-662, 1992.

597 Fechner RE: Histologic variants of infiltrating lobular carcinoma of the breast. Hum Pathol 6:373-378, 1975.

598 Fisher ER, Gregorio RM, Redmond C, Fisher B: Tubulolobular invasive breast cancer. A variant of lobular invasive cancer. Hum Pathol 8:679-683, 1977.

599 Martinez V, Azzopardi JG: Invasive lobular carcinoma of the breast. Incidence and variants. Histopathology 3:467-488, 1979.

600 Pettinato G, Manivel JC, Picone A, Petrella G, Insabato L: Alveolar variant of infiltrating lobular carcinoma of the breast with stromal osteoclast-like giant cells. Pathol Res Pract 185:388-386, 1989.

601 Shousha S, Backhous CM, Alaghband-Zadeh J, Burn I: Alveolar variant of invasive lobular carcinoma of the breast. A tumor rich in estrogen receptors. Am J Clin Pathol 85:1-5, 1986.

602 Weidner N, Semple JP: Pleomorphic variant of invasive lobular carcinoma of the breast. Hum Pathol 23:1167-1171, 1992.

Undetermined (unclassified) carcinoma

603 Azzopardi JG: Problems in breast pathology. In Bennington JL, consulting ed: Major problems in pathology, vol 11. Philadelphia, 1979, WB Saunders Co.

HORMONE RECEPTORS

604 Allred DC, Bustamante MA, Daniel CO, Gaskill HV, Cruz AB Jr: Immunocytochemical analysis of estrogen receptors in human breast carcinomas. Evaluation of 130 cases and review of the literature regarding concordance with biochemical assay and clinical relevance. Arch Surg 125:107-113, 1990.

605 Baddoura FK, Cohen C, Unger ER, De Rose PB, Chenggis M: Image analysis for quantitation of estrogen receptor in formalin-fixed paraffin-embedded sections of breast carcinoma. Mod Pathol 4:91-95, 1991.

606 Battifora H, Mehta P, Ahn C, Esteban J: Estrogen receptor immunohistochemical assay in paraffin-embedded tissue. A better gold standard? Appl Immunohistochem 1:39-45, 1993.

606a Battifora H: Immunocytochemistry of hormone receptors in routinely processed tissues. The new gold standard (editorial). Appl Immunohistochem 2:143-145, 1994.

607 Bhargava V, Kell DL, van de Rijn M, Warnke RA: Bcl-2 immunoreactivity in breast carcinoma correlates with hormone receptor positivity. Am J Pathol 145:535-540, 1994.

608 Bur ME, Zimarowski MJ, Schnitt SJ, Baker S, Lew R: Estrogen receptor immunohistochemistry in carcinoma in situ of the breast. Cancer 69:1174-1181, 1992.

609 Caleffi M, Teague MW, Jensen RA, Vnencak-Jones CL, Dupont WD, Parl FF: p53 gene mutations and steroid receptor status in breast cancer. Clinicopathologic correlations and prognostic assessment. Cancer 73:2147-2156, 1994.

610 Esteban JM, Ahn C, Battifora H, Felder B: Predictive value of estrogen receptors evaluated by quantitative immunohistochemical analysis in breast cancer. Am J Clin Pathol 102:S9-12, 1994.

611 Fisher ER, Redmond CK, Liu H, Rockette H, Fisher B, and collaborating NSABP investigators: Correlation of estrogen receptor and pathologic characteristics of invasive breast cancer. Cancer 45:349-353, 1980.

612 Graham DM, Jin L, Lloyd RV: Detection of estrogen receptor in paraffin-embedded sections of breast carcinoma by immunohistochemistry and in situ hybridization. Am J Surg Pathol 15:475-485, 1991.

613 Hawkins RA, Roberts MM, Forrest APM: Oestrogen receptors and breast cancer. Current status. Br J Surg 67:162-165, 1980.

614 Lee SH: Cancer cell estrogen receptor of human mammary carcinoma. Cancer 44:1-12, 1979.

615 Masood S, Dee S, Goldstein JD: Immunocytochemical analysis of progesterone receptors in breast cancer. Am J Clin Pathol 96:59-63, 1991.

616 McCarty KS Jr, Miller LS, Cox EB, Konrath J, McCarty KS Sr: Estrogen receptor analyses. Correlation of biochemical and immunohistochemical methods using monoclonal antireceptor antibodies. Arch Pathol Lab Med 109:716-721, 1985.

617 Mohammed RH, Lakatua DJ, Haus E, Yasmineh WJ: Estrogen and progesterone receptors in human breast cancer. Correlation with histologic subtype and degree of differentiation. Cancer 58:1076-1081, 1986.

618 Pascal RR, Santeusanio G, Sarrell D, Johnson CE: Immunohistologic detection of estrogen receptors in paraffin-embedded breast cancers. Correlation with cytosol measurements. Hum Pathol 17:370-375, 1986.

619 Pertschuk LP, Eisenberg KB, Carter AC, Feldman JG: Immunohistologic localization of estrogen receptors in breast cancer with monoclonal antibodies. Correlation with biochemistry and clinical endocrine response. Cancer 55:1513-1518, 1985.

620 Pertschuk LP, Kim DS, Nayer K, Feldman JG, Eisenberg KB, Carter AC, Rong ZT, Thelmo WL, Fleisher J, Greene GL: Immunocytochemical estrogen and progestin receptor assays in breast cancer with monoclonal antibodies. Histopathologic, demographic, and biochemical correlations and relationship to endocrine response and survival. Cancer 66:1663-1670, 1990.

621 Rosen PP, Menendez-Botet CJ, Nisselbaum JS, Urban JA, Miké V, Fracchia A, Schwartz MK: Pathological review of breast lesions analyzed for estrogen receptor protein. Cancer Res 35:3187-3194, 1975.

622 Shimizu M, Wajima O, Miura M, Katayama I: PAP immunoperoxidase method demonstrating endogenous estrogen in breast carcinomas. Cancer 52:486-492, 1983.

623 Shintaku IP, Said JW: Detection of estrogen receptors with monoclonal antibodies in routinely processed formalin-fixed paraffin sections of breast carcinoma. Use of DNase pretreatment to enhance sensitivity of the reaction. Am J Clin Pathol 87:161-167, 1987.

624 Silfverswärd C, Gustafsson JÅ, Gustafsson SA, Humla S, Nordenskjöld B, Wallgren A, Wrange Ö: Estrogen receptor concentrations in 269 cases of histologically classified human breast cancer. Cancer 45:2001-2005, 1980.

625 Taylor CR, Cooper CL, Kurman RJ, Goebelsmann U, Markland FS Jr: Detection of estrogen receptor in breast and endometrial carcinoma by the immunoperoxidase technique. Cancer 47:2634-2640, 1981.

626 Terenius L, Johansson H, Rimsten A, Thorén L: Malignant and benign human mammary disease. Estrogen binding in relation to clinical data. Cancer **33**:1364-1368, 1974.

626a van Agthoven T, Timmermans M, Foekens JA, Dorssers LC, Henzen-Logmans SC: Differential expression of estrogen, progesterone, and epidermal growth factor receptors in normal, benign, and malignant human breast tissues using dual staining immunohistochemistry. Am J Pathol **144**:1238-1246, 1994.

SPREAD AND METASTASES

627 Bitter MA, Fiorito D, Corkill ME, Huffer WE, Stemmer SM, Shpall EJ, Archer PG, Franklin WA: Bone marrow involvement by lobular carcinoma of the breast cannot be identified reliably by routine histological examination alone. Hum Pathol **25**:781-788, 1994.

628 Brinkley D, Haybittle JL: The curability of breast cancer. Lancet **2**:95-97, 1975.

629 Chaubert P, Hurlimann J: Mammary origin of metastases. Immunohistochemical determination. Arch Pathol Lab Med **116**:1181-1188, 1992.

630 Cifuentes N, Pickren JW: Metastases from carcinoma of mammary gland. An autopsy study. J Surg Oncol **11**:193-205, 1979.

631 Connolly JL, Schnitt SJ: Evaluation of breast biopsy specimens in patients considered for treatment by conservative surgery and radiation therapy for early breast cancer. Pathol Annu **23**(Pt 1):1-23, 1988.

632 Cote RJ, Rosen PP, Hakes TB, Sedira M, Bazinet M, Kinne DW, Old LJ, Osborne MP: Monoclonal antibodies detect occult breast carcinoma metastases in the bone marrow of patients with early stage disease. Am J Surg Pathol **12**:333-340, 1988.

633 Cummings OW, Mazur MT: Breast carcinoma diffusely metastatic to the spleen. A report of two cases presenting as idiopathic thrombocytopenic purpura. Am J Clin Pathol **97**:484-489, 1992.

634 Datta YH, Adams PT, Drobyski WR, Ethier SP, Terry VH, Roth MS: Sensitive detection of occult breast cancer by the reverse-transcriptase polymerase chain reaction. J Clin Oncol **12**:475-482, 1994.

635 Donegan WL: The influence of untreated internal mammary metastases upon the course of mammary cancer. Cancer **39**:533-538, 1977.

636 Fisher B, Montague E, Redmond C, Barton B, Borland D, Fisher ER, Deutsch M, Schwarz G, Margolese R, Donegan W, Volk H, Honvolinka C, Gardner B, Cohn I Jr, Lesnick G, Cruz AB, Lawrence W, Nealon T, Butcher H, Lawton R: Comparison of radical mastectomy with alternative treatments for primary breast cancer. A first report of results from a prospective randomized clinical trial. Cancer **39**:2827-2839, 1977.

637 Fisher ER, Swamidoss S, Lee CH, Rockette H, Redmond C, Fisher B: Detection and significance of occult axillary node metastases in patients with invasive breast cancer. Cancer **42**:2025-2031, 1978.

638 Gagnon Y, Tetu B: Ovarian metastases of breast carcinoma. A clinicopathologic study of 59 cases. Cancer **64**:892-898, 1989.

639 Gilliland MD, Barton RM, Copeland EM III: The implications of local recurrence of breast cancer as the first site of therapeutic failure. Ann Surg **197**:284-287, 1983.

640 Ingle JN, Tormey DC, Tan HK: The bone marrow examination in breast cancer. Diagnostic considerations and clinical usefulness. Cancer **41**:670-674, 1978.

640a Jayson GC, Howell A, Harris M, Morgenstern G, Chang J, Ryder WD: Carcinomatous meningitis in patients with breast cancer. An aggressive disease variant. Cancer **74**:3135-3141, 1994.

640b Johnson JE, Page DL, Winfield AC, Reynolds VH, Sawyers JL: Recurrent mammary carcinoma after local excision. A segmental problem. Cancer **75**:1612-1618, 1995.

641 Lagios MD, Gates EA, Westdahl PR, Richards V, Alpert BS: A guide to the frequency of nipple involvement in breast cancer. A study of 149 consecutive mastectomies using a serial subgross and correlated radiographic technique. Am J Surg **138**:135-142, 1979.

642 Lamovec J, Zidar A: Association of leptomeningeal carcinomatosis in carcinoma of the breast with infiltrating lobular carcinoma. An autopsy study. Arch Pathol Lab Med **115**:507-510, 1991.

643 Landys K: Prognostic value of bone marrow biopsy in breast cancer. Cancer **49**:513-518, 1982.

644 Merino MJ, LiVolsi VA: Signet ring carcinoma of the female breast. A clinicopathologic analysis of 24 cases. Cancer **48**:1830-1837, 1981.

645 Merrill CF, Kaufman DI, Dimitrov NV: Breast cancer metastatic to the eye is a common entity. Cancer **68**:623-627, 1991.

646 Miller RE: Breast cancer and meningioma. J Surg Oncol **31**:182-183, 1986.

647 Monteagudo C, Merino MJ, La Porte N, Neumann RD: Value of gross cystic disease fluid protein-15 in distinguishing metastatic breast carcinomas among poorly differentiated neoplasms involving the ovary. Hum Pathol **22**:368-372, 1991.

648 Morimoto T, Komaki K, Inui K, Umemoto A, Yamamoto H, Harada K, Inoue K: Involvement of nipple and areola in early breast cancer. Cancer **55**:2459-2463, 1985.

649 Noguchi S, Aihara T, Nakamori S, Motomura K, Inaji H, Imaoka S, Koyama H: The detection of breast carcinoma micrometastases in axillary lymph nodes by means of reverse transcriptase-polymerase chain reaction. Cancer **74**:1595-1600, 1994.

650 Pickren JW: Significance of occult metastases. A study of breast cancer. Cancer **14**:1266-1273, 1961.

651 Porro G, Menard S, Tagliabue E, Orefice S, Salvadori B, Squicciarini P, Andreola S, Rilke F, Colnaghi MI: Monoclonal antibody detection of carcinoma cells in bone marrow biopsy specimens from breast cancer patients. Cancer **61**:2407-2411, 1988.

652 Price JE: The biology of metastatic breast cancer. Cancer **66**:1313-1320, 1990.

653 Rosen PP, Fracchia AA, Urban JA, Schattenfeld D, Robbins GF: "Residual" mammary carcinoma following simulated partial mastectomy. Cancer **35**:739-747, 1975.

654 Veronesi U, Cascinelli N, Bufalino R, Morabito A, Greco M, Galluzzo D, Donne VD, DeLellis R, Piotti P, Sacchini V, Conti R, Clemente C: Risk of internal mammary lymph node metastases and its relevance on prognosis of breast cancer patients. Ann Surg **198**:681-684, 1983.

654a Veronesi U, Marubini E, Del Vecchio M, Manzari A, Andreola S, Greco M, Luini A, Merson M, Saccozzi R, Rilke F, Salvadori B: Local recurrences and distant metastases after conservative breast cancer treatments: partly independent events. J Natl Cancer Inst **87**:19-27, 1995.

655 Wertheim U, Ozzello L: Neoplastic involvement of nipple and skin flap in carcinoma of the breast. Am J Surg Pathol **4**:543-549, 1980.

Occult breast carcinoma

656 Ashikari R, Rosen PP, Urban JA, Senoo T: Breast cancer presenting as an axillary mass. Ann Surg **183**:415-417, 1976.

657 Fitts WT Jr, Steiner GC, Enterline HT: Prognosis of occult carcinoma of the breast. Am J Surg **106**:460-463, 1963.

658 Merson M, Andreola S, Galimberti V, Bufalino R, Marchini S, Veronesi U: Breast carcinoma presenting as axillary metastases without evidence of a primary tumor. Cancer **70**:504-508, 1992.

659 Rosen PP, Kimmel M: Occult breast carcinoma presenting with axillary lymph node metastases. A follow-up study of 48 patients. Hum Pathol **21**:518-523, 1990.

STAGING

660 Kinne DW: Staging and follow-up of breast cancer patients. Cancer **67**:1196-1198, 1991.

THERAPY

661 Bonadonna G, Valagussa P, Brambilla C, Moliterni A, Zambetti M, Ferrari L: Adjuvant and neoadjuvant treatment of breast cancer with chemotherapy and/or endocrine therapy. Semin Oncol **18**:515-524, 1991.

661a Bonadonna G, Valagussa P, Moliterni A, Zambetti M, Brambilla C: Adjuvant cyclophosphamide, methotrexate, and fluorouracil in node-positive breast cancer. The results of 20 years of follow-up. N Engl J Med **332**:901-906, 1995.

662 Bonadonna G, Veronesi U, Brambilla C, Ferrari L, Luini A, Greco M, Bartoli C, Coopmans de Yoldi G, Zucali R, Rilke F, et al.: Primary chemotherapy to avoid mastectomy in tumors with diameters of three centimeters or more. J Natl Cancer Inst **82**:1539-1545, 1990.

663 Chase DR, Oberg KC, Chase RL, Malott RL, Weeks DA: Pseudoepithelialization of breast implant capsules. Int J Surg Pathol **1**:151-154, 1994.

664 Emery J, Spanier SS, Kasnic G Jr, Hardt NS: The synovial structure of breast-implant associated bursae. Mod Pathol **7**:728-722, 1994.

665 Fisher B: Breast-cancer management. Alternatives to radical mastectomy. N Engl J Med **301**:326-328, 1979.

666 Frykberg ER, Bland KI: Overview of the biology and management of ductal carcinoma in situ of the breast. Cancer **74**:350-361, 1994.

666a Goldhirsch A, Wood WC, Senn H-J, Glick JH, Gelber RD: Meeting highlights. International consensus panel on the treatment of primary breast cancer. J Natl Cancer Inst **87**:1441-1445, 1995.

666b Hameed MR, Erlandson R, Rosen PP: Capsular synovial-like hyperplasia around mammary implants similar to detritic synovitis. A morphologic and immunohistochemical study of 15 cases. Am J Surg Pathol **19**:433-438, 1995.

667 Hillner BE, Smith TJ, Desch CE: Efficacy and cost-effectiveness of autologous bone marrow transplantation in metastatic breast cancer. Estimates using decision analysis while awaiting clinical trial results. JAMA **267**:2055-2061, 1992.

667a Jacobson JA, Danforth DN, Cowan KH, D'Angelo T, Steinberg SM, Pierce L, Lippman ME, Lichter AS, Glatstein E, Okunieff P: Ten-year results of a comparison of conservation with mastectomy in the treatment of stage I and II breast cancer. New Engl J Med, 332:907-911, 1995.

668 Jones RJ: Autologous bone marrow transplantation. Curr Opin Oncol **5:**270-275, 1993.

669 Kasper CS: Histologic features of breast capsules reflect surface configuration and composition of silicone bag implants. Am J Clin Pathol **102:**655-659, 1994.

670 Kinne DW: Surgical management of stage I and stage II breast cancer. Cancer **66:**1373-1377, 1990.

671 Kinne DW: Primary treatment for breast cancer. Semin Surg Oncol **7:**271-277, 1991.

671a Kitchen SB, Paletta CE, Shehadi SI, Bauer WC: Epithelialization of the lining of a breast implant capsule. Possible origins of squamous cell carcinoma associated with a breast implant capsule. Cancer **73:**1449-1452, 1994.

672 Mansfield CM, Krishnan L, Komarnicky LT, Ayyangar KM, Kramer CA: A review of the role of radiation therapy in the treatment of patients with breast cancer. Semin Oncol **18:**525-535, 1991.

673 Marcial VA: Primary therapy for limited breast cancer. Radiation therapy techniques. Cancer **65:**2159-2164, 1990.

673a Olivotto IA, Bajdik CD, Plenderleith IH, Coppin CM, Gelmon KA, Jackson SM, Ragaz J, Wilson KS, Worth A: Adjuvant systemic therapy and survival after breast cancer. N Engl J Med **330:**805-810, 1994.

674 Pierguin B, Owen R, Maylin C, Otmezguine Y, Raynal M, Mueller W, Hannoun S: Radical radiation therapy of breast cancer. Int J Radiat Oncol Biol Phys **6:**17-24, 1980.

675 Plowman PN: Tamoxifen as adjuvant therapy in breast cancer. Current status. Drugs **46:**819-833, 1993.

676 Raso DS, Greene WB, Metcalf JS: Synovial metaplasia of a periprosthetic breast capsule. Arch Pathol Lab Med **118:**249-251, 1994.

677 Rosner D, Lane WW: Should all patients with node-negative breast cancer receive adjuvant therapy? Identifying additional subsets of low-risk patients who are highly curable by surgery alone. Cancer **68:**1482-1494, 1991.

678 Schnitt SJ, Abner A, Gelman R, Connolly JL, Recht A, Duda RB, Eberlein TJ, Mayzel K, Silver B, Harris JR: The relationship between microscopic margins of resection and the risk of local recurrence in patients with breast cancer treated with breast-conserving surgery and radiation therapy. Cancer **74:**1746-1751, 1994.

679 Silverstein MJ, Gierson ED, Colburn WJ, Cope LM, Furmanski M, Senofsky GM, Gamagami P, Waisman JR: Can intraductal breast carcinoma be excised completely by local excision? Clinical and pathologic predictors. Cancer **73:**2985-2989, 1994.

680 Solin LJ, Recht A, Fourquet A, Kurtz J, Kuske R, McNeese M, McCormick B, Cross MA, Schultz DJ, Bornstein BA, et al.: Ten-year results of breast-conserving surgery and definitive irradiation for intraductal carcinoma (ductal carcinoma in situ) of the breast. Cancer **68:**2337-2344, 1991.

681 Vaughan WP: Autologous bone marrow transplantation in the treatment of breast cancer. Clinical and technologic strategies. Semin Oncol **20:**55-58, 1993.

682 Veronesi U: How important is the assessment of resection margins in conservative surgery for breast cancer? Cancer **74:**1660-1661, 1994.

683 Veronesi U, Saccozzi R, Del Vecchio M, Banfi A, Clemente C, De Lena M, Gallus G, Greco M, Luini A, Marubini E, Mucolino G, Rilke F, Salvadori B, Zecchini A, Zucali R: Comparing radical mastectomy with quadrantectomy, axillary dissection and radiotherapy in patients with small cancers of the breast. N Engl J Med **305:**6-11, 1981.

684 Wong K, Henderson IC: Management of metastatic breast cancer. World J Surg **18:**98-111, 1994.

EFFECTS OF THERAPY ON THE TUMOR AND ON NORMAL BREAST

685 Frierson HF Jr, Fechner RE: Histologic grade of locally advanced infiltrating ductal carcinoma after treatment with induction chemotherapy. Am J Clin Pathol **102:**154-157, 1994.

686 Kennedy S, Merino MJ, Swain SM, Lippman ME: The effects of hormonal and chemotherapy on tumoral and nonneoplastic breast tissue. Hum Pathol **21:**192-198, 1990.

687 Schnitt SJ, Connolly JL, Harris JR, Cohen RB: Radiation-induced changes in the breast. Hum Pathol **15:**545-550, 1984.

688 Winkelmann RK, Grado GL, Quimby SR, Connolly SM: Pseudosclerodermatous panniculitis after irradiation. An unusual complication of megavoltage treatment of breast carcinoma. Mayo Clin Proc **68:**122-127, 1993.

689 Ziegler LD, Connelly JH, Frye D, Smith TL, Hortobagyi GN: Lack of correlation between histologic findings and response to chemotherapy in metastatic breast cancer. Cancer **68:**628-633, 1991.

PROGNOSIS

690 Aamdal S, Bormer O, Jorgensen O, Host H, Eliassen G, Kaalhus O, Pihl A: Estrogen receptors and long-term prognosis in breast cancer. Cancer **53:**2525-2529, 1984.

691 Adami H-O, Malker B, Holmberg L, Persson I, Stone B: The relation between survival and age at diagnosis in breast cancer. N Engl J Med **315:**559-563, 1986.

692 Alderson MR, Hamlin I, Staunton MD: The relative significance of prognostic factors in breast carcinoma. Br J Cancer **25:**646-655, 1971.

693 Armas OA, Gerald WL, Lesser ML, Arroyo CD, Norton L, Rosen PP: Immunohistochemical detection of cathepsin D in T2N0M0 breast carcinoma. Am J Surg Pathol **18:**158-166, 1994.

694 Auer G, Eriksson E, Azavedo E, Caspersson T, Wallgren A: Prognostic significance of nuclear DNA content in mammary adenocarcinomas in humans. Cancer Res **44:**394-396, 1984.

694a Axelsson K, Ljung B-M, Moore DH II, Thor AD, Chew KL, Edgerton SM, Smith HS, Mayall BH: Tumor angiogenesis as a prognostic assay for invasive ductal breast carcinoma. J Natl Cancer Inst **87:**997-1008, 1995.

695 Baak JP, Chin D, van Diest PJ, Ortiz R, Matze-Cok P, Bacus SS: Comparative long-term prognostic value of quantitative HER-2/neu protein expression, DNA ploidy, and morphometric and clinical features in paraffin-embedded invasive breast cancer. Lab Invest **64:**215-223, 1991.

696 Baak JPA, Kurver PHJ, de Snoo-Niewlaat AJE, de Graef S, Makkink B, Boon ME: Prognostic indicators in breast cancer. Morphometric methods. Histopathology **6:**327-339, 1982.

697 Baak JPA, Van Dop H, Kurver PHJ, Hermans J: The value of morphometry to classic prognosticators in breast cancer. Cancer **56:**374-382, 1985.

697a Barbareschi M, Weidner N, Gasparini G, Morelli L, Forti S, Ercher C, Fina P, Caffo O, Leonardi E, Mauri F, Bevilacqua P, Dalla Palma P: Microvessel density quantification in breast carcinomas. Assessment by light microscopy vs. a computer-aided image analysis system. Appl Immunohistochem **3:**75-84, 1995.

698 Barnes DM, Dublin EA, Fisher CJ, Levison DA, Millis RR: Immunohistochemical detection of p53 protein in mammary carcinoma. An important new independent indicator of prognosis? Hum Pathol **24:**469-476, 1993.

699 Barnes R, Masood S, Barker E, Rosengard AM, Coggin DL, Crowell T, King CR, Porter-Jordan K, Wargotz ES, Liotta LA, et al.: Low nm23 protein expression in infiltrating ductal breast carcinomas correlates with reduced patient survival. Am J Pathol **139:**245-250, 1991.

700 Battifora H, Gaffey M, Esteban J, Mehta P, Bailey A, Faucett C, Niland J: Immunohistochemical assay of neu/c-erbB-2 oncogene product in paraffin-embedded tissues in early breast cancer. Retrospective follow-up study of 245 stage I and II cases. Mod Pathol **4:**466-474, 1991.

701 Bauer TW, O'Ceallaigh D, Eggleston JC, Moore GW, Baker RR: Prognostic factors in patients with stage I, estrogen receptor-negative carcinoma of the breast. A clinicopathologic study. Cancer **52:**1423-1431, 1983.

702 Berg JW, Robbins GF: Factors influencing short and long-term survival of breast cancer patients. Surg Gynecol Obstet **122:**1311-1316, 1966.

703 Biesterfield S, Noll I, Noll E, Wohltmann D, Blocking A: Mitotic frequency as a prognostic factor in breast cancer. Hum Pathol **26:**47-52, 1995.

704 Black MM, Barclay THC, Hankey BF: Prognosis in breast cancer utilizing histologic characteristics of the primary tumor. Cancer **36:**2048-2055, 1975.

705 Bloom HJG, Richardson WW: Histological grading and prognosis in breast cancer. A study of 1409 cases of which 359 have been followed for 15 years. Br J Cancer **11:**359-377, 1957.

706 Bloom HJG, Richardson WW, Harris ED: Natural history of untreated breast cancer. Comparison of untreated cases according to histological grade of malignancy. Br Med J **2:**213-221, 1962.

707 Bogomoletz WV: Elastosis in breast cancer. Pathol Annu **21**(Pt 2):345-366, 1986.

708 Bosari S, Lee AK, De Lellis RA, Wiley BD, Heatley GJ, Silverman ML: Microvessel quantitation and prognosis in invasive breast carcinoma. Hum Pathol **23:**755-761, 1992.

709 Breast Cancer Study Group: Identification of breast cancer patients with high risk of early recurrence after radical mastectomy. II. Clinical and pathological correlations. Cancer **42:**2809-2826, 1978.

710 Butler JA, Bretsky S, Menendez-Botet C, Kinne DW: Estrogen receptor protein of breast cancer as a predictor of recurrence. Cancer **55:**1178-1181, 1985.

711 Carter CL, Allen C, Henson DE: Relation of tumor size, lymph node status, and survival in 24,740 breast cancer cases. Cancer **63:**181-187, 1989.

712 Carter D, Pipkin RD, Shepard RH, Elkins RC, Abbey H: Relationship of necrosis and tumor border to lymph node metastases and 10-year survival in carcinoma of the breast. Am J Surg Pathol **2:**39-46, 1978.

713 Clemente CG, Boracchi P, Andreola S, Del Vecchio M, Veronesi P, Rilke FO: Peritumoral lymphatic invasion in patients with node-negative mammary duct carcinoma. Cancer **69:**1396-1403, 1992.

714 Dalton LW, Page DL, Dupont WD: Histologic grading of breast carcinoma. A reproducibility study. Cancer **73:**2765-2770, 1994.

715 Davis BW, Gelber R, Goldhirsch A, Hartmann WH, Hollaway L, Russell I, Rudenstam CM: Prognostic significance of peritumoral vessel invasion in clinical trials of adjuvant therapy for breast cancer with axillary lymph node metastasis. Hum Pathol **16:**1212-1218, 1985.

716 Davis BW, Gelber RD, Goldhirsch A, Hartmann WH, Locher GW, Reed R, Golouh R, Save-Soderbergh J, Holloway L, Russell I, Rudenstam CM: Prognostic significance of tumor grade in clinical trials of adjuvant therapy for breast cancer with axillary lymph node metastasis. Cancer **58:**2662-2670, 1986.

717 Dawkins HJ, Robbins PD, Smith KL, Sarna M, Harvey JM, Sterrett GF, Papadimitriou JM: What's new in breast cancer? Molecular perspectives of cancer development and the role of the oncogene c-erbB-2 in prognosis and disease. Pathol Res Pract **189:**1233-1252, 1993.

718 Dawson PJ, Ferguson DJ, Karrison T: The pathologic findings of breast cancer in patients surviving 25 years after radical mastectomy. Cancer **50:**2131-2138, 1982.

718a De Potter CR, Schelfhout A-M: The neu-protein and breast cancer. Virchows Archiv **426:**107-115, 1995.

719 Doglioni C, Dei Tos AP, Laurino L, Chiarelli C, Barbareschi M, Viale G: The prevalence of BCL-w immunoreactivity in breast carcinomas and its clinicopathological correlates with particular reference to oestrogen receptor status. Virchows Arch **424:**47-52, 1994.

720 Domagala W, Lasota J, Dukowicz A, Markiewski M, Striker G, Weber K, Osborn M: Vimentin expression appears to be associated with poor prognosis in node-negative ductal NOS breast carcinomas. Am J Pathol **137:**1299-1304, 1990.

721 Domagala W, Striker G, Szadowska A, Dukowicz A, Weber K, Osborn M: Cathepsin D in invasive ductal NOS breast carcinoma as defined by immunohistochemistry. No correlation with survival at 5 years. Am J Pathol **141:**1003-1012, 1992.

722 Ellis GK, Gown AM: New applications of monoclonal antibodies to the diagnosis and prognosis of breast cancer. Pathol Annu **25** (Pt 2):193-235, 1990.

723 Elston CW, Ellis IO: Pathological prognostic factors in breast cancer. I. The value of histological grades in breast cancer. Experience from a large study with long-term follow-up. Histopathology **19:**403-410, 1991.

724 Fisher B, Bauer M, Wickerham L, Redmond CK, Fisher ER: Relation of number of positive axillary nodes to the prognosis of patients with primary breast cancer. An NSABP update. Cancer **52:**1551-1557, 1983.

725 Fisher B, Montague E, Redmond C, Barton B, Borland D, Fisher ER, Deutsch M, Schwarz G, Margolese R, Donegan W, Volk H, Honvolinka C, Gardner B, Cohn I Jr, Lesnick G, Cruz AB, Lawrence W, Nealon T, Butcher H, Lawton R: Comparison of radical mastectomy with alternative treatments for primary breast cancer. A first report of results from a prospective randomized clinical trial. Cancer **39:**2827-2839, 1977.

726 Fisher B, Redmond C, Poisson R, Margolese R, Wolmark N, Wickerham L, Fisher E, Deutsch M, Caplan R, Pilch Y, et al.: Eight-year results of a randomized clinical trial comparing total mastectomy and lumpectomy with or without irradiation in the treatment of breast cancer. N Engl J Med **320:**822-828, 1989.

727 Fisher B, Slack NH, Bross IDJ: Cancer of the breast. Size of neoplasm and prognosis. Cancer **24:**1071-1080, 1969.

728 Fisher ER, Anderson S, Redmond C, Fisher B: Pathologic findings from the National Surgical Adjuvant Breast Project protocol B-06. 10-year pathologic and clinical prognostic discriminants. Cancer **71:**2507-2514, 1993.

729 Fisher ER, Costantino J, Fisher B, Redmond C: Pathologic findings from the National Surgical Adjuvant Breast Project (Protocol 4). Discriminants for 15-year survival. National Surgical Adjuvant Breast and Bowel Project Investigators. Cancer **71:**2141-2150, 1993.

730 Fisher ER, Gregorio R, Redmond C, Dekker A, Fisher B: Pathologic findings from the National Surgical Adjuvant Breast Project (Protocol No. 4). II. The significance of regional node histology other than sinus histiocytosis in invasive mammary cancer. Am J Clin Pathol **65:**21-30, 1976.

731 Fisher ER, Gregorio RM, Redmond C, Kim WS, Fisher B: Pathologic findings from the National Surgical Adjuvant Breast Project (Protocol No. 4). III. The significance of extranodal extension of axillary metastases. Am J Clin Pathol **65:**439-444, 1976.

732 Fisher ER, Kotwal N, Hermann C, Fisher B: Types of tumor lymphoid response and sinus histiocytosis. Arch Pathol Lab Med **107:**222-227, 1983.

733 Fisher ER, Redmond C, Fisher B, Bass G: Pathologic findings from the National Surgical Adjuvant Breast and Bowel Projects (NSABP). Prognostic discriminants for 8-year survival for node-negative invasive breast cancer patients. Cancer **65:**2121-2128, 1990.

734 Fisher ER, Swamidoss S, Lee CH, Rockette H, Redmond C, Fisher B: Detection and significance of occult axillary node metastases in patients with invasive breast cancer. Cancer **42:**2025-2031, 1978.

735 Frierson HF Jr: Ploidy analysis and S-phase fraction determination by flow cytometry of invasive adenocarcinomas of the breast. Am J Surg Pathol **15:**358-367, 1991.

736 Frierson HF Jr, Wolber RA, Berean KW, Franquemont DW, Gaffey MJ, Boyd JC, Wilbur DC: Interobserver reproducibility of the Nottingham modification of the Bloom and Richardson histologic grading scheme for infiltrating ductal carcinoma. Am J Clin Pathol **103:**195-198, 1995.

737 Gallenberg MM, Loprinzi CL: Breast cancer and pregnancy. Semin Oncol **16:**369-376, 1989.

738 Garne JP, Aspegren K, Linell F, Rank F, Ranstam J: Primary prognostic factors in invasive breast cancer with special reference to ductal carcinoma and histologic malignancy grade. Cancer **73:**1438-1448, 1994.

739 Gasparini G, Weidner N, Bevilacqua P, Maluta S, Dalla Palma P, Caffo O, Barbareschi M, Boracchi P, Marubini E, Pozza F: Tumor microvessel density, p53 expression, tumor size, and peritumoral lymphatic vessel invasion are relevant prognostic markers in node-negative breast carcinoma. J Clin Oncol **12:**454-466, 1994.

740 Gilchrist KW, Gray R, Fowble B, Tormey DC, Taylor SG 4th: Tumor necrosis is a prognostic predictor for early recurrence and death in lymph node-positive breast cancer. A 10-year follow-up study of 728 Eastern Cooperative Oncology Group patients. J Clin Oncol **11:**1929-1935, 1993.

741 Gilliland MD, Barton RM, Copeland EM III: The implications of local recurrence of breast cancer as the first site of therapeutic failure. Ann Surg **197:**284-287, 1983.

742 Glaubitz LC, Bowen JH, Cox EB, McCarty KS Jr: Elastosis in human breast cancer. Correlation with sex steroid receptors and comparison with clinical outcome. Arch Pathol Lab Med **108:**27-30, 1984.

742a Goldstein NS: The significance of extracapsular axillary lymph node extension by metastatic breast cancer. Int J Surg Pathol **3:**65-66, 1995.

743 Guidi AJ, Fischer L, Harris JR, Schnitt SJ: Microvessel density and distribution in ductal carcinoma in situ of the breast. J Natl Cancer Inst **86:**614-619, 1994.

744 Hartveit F, Skjaerven R, Maehle BO: Prognosis in breast cancer patients with tumour cells in the efferent vessels of their axillary nodes. Pathology **139:**379-382, 1983.

745 Heintz NH, Leslie KO, Rogers LA, Howard PL: Amplification of the c-erb B-2 oncogene and prognosis of breast adenocarcinoma. Arch Pathol Lab Med **114:**160-163, 1990.

746 Henson DE, Ries L, Freedman LS, Carriaga M: Relationship among outcome, stage of disease, and histologic grade for 22,616 cases of breast cancer. The basis for a prognostic index. Cancer **68:**2142-2149, 1991.

747 Hilf R, Feldstein ML, Gibson SL, Savlov ED: The relative importance of estrogen receptor analysis as a prognostic factor for recurrence or response to chemotherapy in women with breast cancer. Cancer **45:**1993-2000, 1980.

748 Hultborn KA, Tornberg B: Mammary carcinoma. The biologic character of mammary carcinoma studied in 517 cases by a new form of malignancy grading. Acta Radiol (Stockh) **196:**1-143, 1960.

749 Hurlimann J: Prognostic value of p53 protein expression in breast carcinomas. Pathol Res Pract **189:**996-1003, 1993.

749a Hurlimann J, Larrinaga B, Vala DLM: bcl-2 protein in invasive ductal breast carcinomas. Virchows Archiv **426:**163-168, 1995.

750 Hutter RVP: The influence of pathologic factors on breast cancer management. Cancer **46:**961-976, 1980.

751 Huvos AG, Hutter RVP, Berg JW: Significance of axillary macrometastases and micrometastases in mammary cancer. Ann Surg **173:**44-46, 1971.

751a Jacobson JA, Danforth DN, Cowan KH, d'Angelo T, Steinberg SM, Pierce L, Lippman ME, Lichter AS, Glatstein E, Okunieff P: Ten-year results of a comparison of conservation with mastectomy in the treatment of stage I and II breast cancer. N Engl J Med **332:**907-911, 1995.

752 Joensuu H, Pylkkanen L, Toikkanen S: Bcl-2 protein expression and long-term survival in breast cancer. Am J Pathol **145:**1191-1198, 1994.

753 Kandalaft PL, Chang KL, Ahn CW, Traweek ST, Mehta P, Battifora H: Prognostic significance of immunohistochemical analysis of cathepsin D in low stage breast cancer. Cancer **71:**2756-2763, 1993.

754 Keyhani-Rofagha S, O'Toole RV, Farrar WB, Sickle-Santanello B, De Cenzo J, Young D: Is DNA ploidy an independent prognostic indicator in infiltrative node-negative breast adenocarcinoma? Cancer **65:**1577-1582, 1990.

755 Kister SJ, Sommers SC, Haagensen CD, Cooley E: Re-evaluation of blood vessel invasion as a prognostic factor in carcinoma of the breast. Cancer **19:**1213-1216, 1966.

756 Kouchoukos NT, Ackerman LV, Butcher HR Jr: Prediction of axillary nodal metastases from the morphology of primary mammary carcinomas. A guide to operative therapy. Cancer **20:**948-960, 1967.

757 Kujari HP, Collan YUI, Atkin NB: Use of the mitotic counts for the prognosis and grading of breast cancer. Pathol Res Pract **190:**593-599, 1994.

758 Lagios MD, Westdahl PR, Margolin FR, Rose MR: Duct carcinoma in situ. Relationship of extent of noninvasive disease to the frequency of occult invasion, multicentricity, lymph node metastases, and short-term treatment failures. Cancer 50:1309-1314, 1982.

759 Laroye GJ, Minkin S: The impact of mitotic index on predicting outcome in breast carcinoma. A comparison of different counting methods in patients with different lymph node status. Mod Pathol 4:456-460, 1991.

760 Lash RH, Bauer TW, Hermann RE, Esselstyn CB: Partial mastectomy. Pathologic findings and prognosis. Hum Pathol 17:813-822, 1986.

761 Lash RH, Bauer TW, Medendorp SV: Prognostic significance of the proportion of intraductal and infiltrating ductal carcinoma in women treated by partial mastectomy. Surg Pathol 3:47-58, 1990.

762 Lee AKC, DeLellis RA, Silverman ML, Wolfe HJ: Lymphatic and blood vessel invasion in breast carcinoma. A useful prognostic indicator? Hum Pathol 17:984-987, 1986.

762a Leonard C, Corkill M, Tompkin J, Zhen B, Waitz D, Norton L, Kinzie J: Are axillary recurrence and overall survival affected by axillary extranodal tumor extension in breast cancer? Implications for radiation therapy. J Clin Oncol 13:47-53, 1995.

763 Lewison EF, Montague ACW, Kuller L: Breast cancer treated at The Johns Hopkins Hospital, 1951-1956. Review of international ten-year survival rates. Cancer 19:1359-1368, 1966.

764 Mambo NC, Gallager HS: Carcinoma of the breast. The prognostic significance of extranodal extension of axillary disease. Cancer 39:2280-2285, 1977.

765 Mansour EG, Ravdin PM, Dressler L: Prognostic factors in early breast carcinoma. Cancer 74:381-400, 1994.

766 Masters JRW, Millis RR, King RJB, Rubens RD: Elastosis and response to endocrine therapy in human breast cancer. Br J Cancer 39:536-539, 1979.

767 Mate TP, Carter D, Fischer DB, Hartman PV, McKhann C, Merino M, Prosnitz LR, Weissberg JB: A clinical and histopathologic analysis of the results of conservation surgery and radiation therapy in stage I and II breast carcinoma. Cancer 58:1995-2002, 1986.

768 Mauri FA, Girlando S, Dalla Palma P, Buffa G, Perrone G, Doglioni C, Kreipe H, Barbareschi M: Ki-67 antibodies (Ki-S5, MIB-1, and Ki-67) in breast carcinomas. A brief quantitative comparison. Appl Immunohistochem 2:171-176, 1994.

768a Muss HB, Thor AD, Berry DA, Kute T, Liu ET, Koerner F, Cirrincione CT, Budman DR, Wood WC, Barcos M et al.: c-erbB-2 expression and response to adjuvant therapy in women with node-positive early breast cancer. N Engl J Med 330:1260-1266, 1994.

769 Nemoto T, Vana J, Bedwani RN, Baker HW, McGregor FH, Murphy GP: Management and survival of female breast cancer. Results of a national survey by the American College of Surgeons. Cancer 45:2917-2924, 1980.

770 Nime FA, Rosen PP, Thaler HT, Ashikari R, Urban JA: Prognostic significance of tumor emboli in intramammary lymphatics in patients with mammary carcinoma. Am J Surg Pathol 1:25-30, 1977.

771 Nixon AJ, Neuberg D, Hayes DF, Gelman R, Connolly JL, Schnitt S, Abner A, Recht A, Vicini F, Harris JR: Relationship of patient age to pathologic features of the tumor and prognosis for patients with stage I or II breast cancer. J Clin Oncol 12:888-894, 1994.

772 Noguchi M, Ohta N, Koyasaki N, Taniya T, Miyazaki I, Mizukami Y: Reappraisal of internal mammary node metastases as a prognostic factor in patients with breast cancer. Cancer 68:1918-1925, 1991.

773 Page DL: Prognosis and breast cancer. Recognition of lethal and favorable prognostic types. Am J Surg Pathol 15:334-349, 1991.

774 Page DL, Dupont WD. Breast cancer angiogenesis. Through a narrow window. JNCI 84:1850-1851, 1992.

775 Page DL, Ellis IO, Elston CW: Histologic grading of breast cancer. Let's do it (editorial). Am J Clin Pathol 103:123-124, 1995.

776 Peters MV: The effect of pregnancy on breast cancer. In Forrest APM, Kunkler PB, eds: Prognostic factors in breast carcinoma. Baltimore, 1968, Williams & Wilkins.

777 Petrek JA, Dukoff R, Rogatko A: Prognosis of pregnancy-associated breast cancer. Cancer 67:869-872, 1991.

778 Pickren JW: Significance of occult metastases. A study of breast cancer. Cancer 14:1266-1273, 1961.

779 Pienta KJ, Coffey DS: Correlation of nuclear morphometry with progression of breast cancer. Cancer 68:2012-2016, 1991.

780 Pinder SE, Ellis IO, Galea M, O'Rouke S, Blamey RW, Elston CW: Pathological prognostic factors in breast cancer. III. Vascular invasion. Relationship with recurrence and survival in a large study with long-term follow-up. Histopathology 24:41-47, 1994.

780a Quiet CA, Ferguson DJ, Weichselbaum RR, Hellman S: Natural history of node-negative breast cancer. A study of 826 patients with long-term follow-up. J Clin Oncol 13:1144-1151, 1995.

781 Ravdin PM, Tandon AK, Allred DC, Clark GM, Fuqua SA, Hilsenbeck SH, Chamness GC, Osborne CK: Cathepsin D by Western blotting and immunohistochemistry. Failure to confirm correlations with prognosis in node-negative breast cancer. J Clin Oncol 12:467-474, 1994.

781a Robbins P, Pinder S, de Klerk N, Dawkins H, Harvey J, Sterrett G, Ellis I, Elston C: Histological grading of breast carcinomas. A study of interobserver agreement. Hum Pathol 26:873-879, 1995.

782 Rosen PP, Groshen S, Kinne DW, Norton L: Factors influencing prognosis in node-negative breast carcinoma. Analysis of 767 T1N0M0/T2N0M0 patients with long-term follow-up. J Clin Oncol 11:2090-2100, 1993.

783 Rosen PP, Lesser ML, Kinne DW, Beattie EJ: Breast carcinoma in women 35 years of age or younger. Ann Surg 199:133-142, 1984.

783a Rosen PP, Lesser ML, Arroyo CD, Cranor M, Borgen P, Norton L: p53 in node-negative breast carcinoma. An immunohistochemical study of epidemiologic risk factors, histologic features, and prognosis. J Clin Oncol 13:821-830, 1995.

783b Rosen PP, Lesser ML, Arroyo CD, Cranor M, Borgen P, Norton L: Immunohistochemical detection of HER2/neu in patients with axillary lymph node–negative breast carcinoma. A study of epidemiologic risk factors, histologic features, and prognosis. Cancer 75:1320-1326, 1995.

784 Rosen PP, Saigo PE, Braun DW, Weathers E, Fracchia AA, Kinne DW: Axillary micro- and macrometastases in breast cancer. Prognostic significance of tumor size. Ann Surg 196:585-591, 1981.

785 Roses DF, Bell DA, Flotte TJ, Taylor R, Ratech H, Dubin N: Pathologic predictors of recurrence in stage 1 (T1N0M0) breast cancer. Am J Clin Pathol 78:817-820, 1982.

786 Rosner D, Lane WW: Oral contraceptive use has no adverse effect on the prognosis of breast cancer. Cancer 57:591-596, 1986.

787 Russo J, Frederick J, Ownby HE, Fine G, Hussain M, Kirckstein HI, Robbins TO, Rosenberg B: Predictors of recurrence and survival of patients with breast cancer. Am J Clin Pathol 88:123-131, 1987.

788 Sahin AA, Ro J, Ro JY, Blick MB, el-Naggar AK, Ordonez NG, Fritsche HA, Smith TL, Hortobagyi GN, Ayala AG: Ki-67 immunostaining in node-negative stage I/II breast carcinoma. Significant correlation with prognosis. Cancer 68:549-557, 1991.

789 Sahin AA, Sneige N, Ordonez NG, Singletary SE, Ro JY, El Naggar AK, Ayala AG: Immunohistochemical assessment of cathepsin D in stages I and II node-negative breast cancer. Appl Immunohistochem 2:15-21, 1994.

790 Saigo P, Rosen PP: Prognostic factors in invasive mammary carcinomas 1.0 cm or less in diameter (abstract). Am J Clin Pathol 73:303-304, 1980.

791 Sears HF, Janus C, Levy W, Hopson R, Creech R, Grotzinger P: Breast cancer without axillary metastases. Are there high-risk biologic subpopulations? Cancer 50:1820-1827, 1982.

792 Seidman H, Gelb SK, Silverberg E, LaVerda N, Lubera JA: Survival experience in the breast cancer detection demonstration project. Cancer J Clin 37:258-290, 1987.

792a Seidman JD, Schnaper LA, Aisner SC: Relationship of the size of the invasive component of the primary breast carcinoma to axillary lymph node metastasis. Cancer 75:65-71, 1995.

793 Sigurdsson H, Baldetorp B, Borg A, Dalberg M, Ferno M, Killander D, Olsson H: Indicators of prognosis in node-negative breast cancer. N Engl J Med 322:1045-1053, 1990.

793a Siitonen SM, Haapasalo HK, Rantala IS, Helin HJ, Isola JJ: Comparison of different immunohistochemical methods in the assessment of angiogenesis. Lack of prognostic value in a group of 77 selected node-negative breast carcinomas. Mod Pathol 8:745-752, 1995.

794 Simpson J, Page D: Prognostic value of histopathology in the breast. Semin Oncol 19:254-262, 1992.

794a Simpson JF, Page DL: Status of breast cancer prognostication based on histopathologic data. Am J Clin Pathol 102:S3-S8, 1994.

795 Simpson JF, Page DL: Cellular proliferation and prognosis in breast cancer. Statistical purity versus clinical utility. Hum Pathol 25:331-332, 1994.

796 Smith JA III, Gamez-Araujo J, Gallager HS, White EC, McBride CM: Carcinoma of the breast. Analysis of total lymph node involvement versus level of metastasis. Cancer 39:527-532, 1977.

797 Smith KL, Robbins PD, Dawkins HJ, Papadimitriou JM, Redmond SL, Carrello S, Harvey JM, Sterrett GF: c-erbB-2 amplification in breast cancer. Detection in formalin-fixed, paraffin-embedded tissue by in situ hybridization. Hum Pathol 25:413-418, 1994.

798 Tandon AK, Clark GM, Chamness GC, Chirgwin JM, McGuire WL: Cathepsin D and prognosis in breast cancer. N Engl J Med 322:297-302, 1990.

799 Toikkanen S, Joensuu H, Klemi P: Nuclear DNA content as a prognostic factor in T1-2N0 breast cancer. Am J Clin Pathol 93:471-479, 1990.

800 Tsakraklides V, Olson P, Kersey JH, Good RA: Prognostic significance of the regional lymph node histology in cancer of the breast. Cancer 34:1259-1266, 1974.

801 Tsuda H, Hirohashi S, Shimosato Y, Hirota T, Tsugane S, Watanabe S, Terada M, Yamamoto H: Correlation between histologic grade of malignancy and copy number of c-erbB-2 gene in breast carcinoma. A retrospective analysis of 176 cases. Cancer 65:1794-1800, 1990.

802 van der Linden JC, Baak JPA, Lindeman J, Smeulders AWM, Meyer CJLM: Carcinoembryonic antigen expression and peanut agglutinin binding in primary breast cancer and lymph node metastases. Lack of correlation with clinical, histopathological, biochemical and morphometric features. Histopathology 9:1051-1059, 1985.

803 van Diest PJ, Baak JP: The morphometric prognostic index is the strongest prognosticator in premenopausal lymph node-negative and lymph node-positive breast cancer patients. Hum Pathol 22:326-330, 1991.

804 Vartanian RK, Weidner N: Correlation of intratumoral endothelial cell proliferation with microvessel density (tumor angiogenesis) and tumor cell proliferation in breast carcinoma. Am J Pathol 144:1188-1194, 1994.

805 Vielh P, Chevillard S, Mosseri V, Donatini B, Magdelenat H: Ki67 index and S-phase fraction in human breast carcinomas. Comparison and correlations with prognostic factors. Am J Clin Pathol 94:681-686, 1990.

806 Visscher DW, Zarbo RJ, Greenawald KA, Crissman JD: Prognostic significance of morphological parameters and flow cytometric DNA analysis in carcinoma of the breast. Pathol Annu 25(Pt 1):171-210, 1990.

807 Weidner N: Tumor angiogenesis. Review of current applications in tumor prognostication. Semin Diagn Pathol 10:302-313, 1993.

807a Weidner N: Intratumor microvessel density as a prognostic factor in cancer. Am J Pathol 147:9-19, 1995.

808 Weidner N, Folkman J, Pozza F, Bevilacqua P, Allred EN, Moore DH, Meli S, Gasparini G: Tumor angiogenesis. A new significant and independent prognostic indicator in early-stage breast carcinoma. J Natl Cancer Inst 84:1875-1887, 1992.

809 Weidner N, Moore DH, Vartanian R: Correlation of Ki-67 antigen expression with mitotic figure index and tumor grade in breast carcinomas using the novel "paraffin"-reactive MIB1 antibody. Hum Pathol 25:337-342, 1994.

810 Weidner N, Semple JP, Welch WR, Folkman J: Tumor angiogenesis and metastasis—correlation in invasive breast carcinoma. N Engl J Med 324:1-8, 1991.

811 Wertheim U, Ozzello L: Neoplastic involvement of nipple and skin flap in carcinoma of the breast. Am J Surg Pathol 4:543-549, 1980.

812 Wintzer HO, Zipfel I, Schulte-Monting J, Hellerich U, von Kleist S: Ki-67 immunostaining in human breast tumors and its relationship to prognosis. Cancer 67:421-428, 1991.

813 Witzig TE, Gonchoroff NJ, Therneau T, Gilbertson DT, Wold LE, Grant C, Grande J, Katzmann JA, Ahmann DL, Ingle JN: DNA content flow cytometry as a prognostic factor for node-positive breast cancer. Cancer 68:1781-1788, 1991.

814 Witzig TE, Ingle JN, Cha SS, Schaid DJ, Tabery RL, Wold LE, Grant C, Gonchoroff NJ, Katzmann JA: DNA ploidy and the percentage of cells in S-phase as prognostic factors for women with lymph node negative breast cancer. Cancer 74:1752-1761, 1994.

814a Wold LE, Ingle JN, Pisansky TM, Johnson RE, Donohue JH: Prognostic factors for patients with carcinoma of the breast. Mayo Clin Proc 70:678-679, 1995.

Salivary and sweat gland–type tumors

815 Ballance WA, Ro JY, el-Naggar AK, Grignon DJ, Ayala AG, Romsdahl MG: Pleomorphic adenoma (benign mixed tumor) of the breast. An immunohistochemical, flow cytometric, and ultrastructural study and review of the literature. Am J Clin Pathol 93:795-801, 1990.

816 Begin LR, Mitmaker B, Bahary J-P: Infiltrating myofibroblastoma of the breast. Surg Pathol 2:151-156, 1989.

817 Cavanzo FJ, Taylor HB: Adenoid cystic carcinoma of the breast. An analysis of 21 cases. Cancer 24:740-745, 1969.

818 Chen KT: Pleomorphic adenoma of the breast. Am J Clin Pathol 93:792-794, 1990.

819 Chen PC, Chen CK, Nicastri AD, Wait RB: Myoepithelial carcinoma of the breast with distant metastasis and accompanied by adenomyoepitheliomas. Histopathology 24:543-548, 1994.

820 Diaz NM, McDivitt RW, Wick MR: Pleomorphic adenoma of the breast. A clinicopathologic and immunohistochemical study of 10 cases. Hum Pathol 22:1206-1214, 1991.

821 Draheim JH, Neubecker RD, Sprinz H: An unusual tumor of the breast resembling eccrine spiradenoma. Am J Clin Pathol 31:511-516, 1959.

822 Drudis T, Arroyo C, Van Hoeven K, Cordon-Cardo C, Rosen PP: The pathology of low-grade adenosquamous carcinoma of the breast. An immunohistochemical study. Pathol Annu 29(Pt 2):181-197, 1994.

823 Elsner B: Adenoid cystic carcinoma of the breast. Review of the literature and clinicopathologic study of seven patients. Pathol Eur 5:357-364, 1970.

824 Erlandson RA, Rosen PP: Infiltrating myoepithelioma of the breast. Am J Surg Pathol 6:785-793, 1982.

825 Finck FM, Schwinn CP, Keasby LE: Clear cell hidradenoma of the breast. Cancer 22:125-135, 1968.

826 Fisher ER, Tavares J, Bulatao IS, Sass R, Fisher B, collaborating NSABP investigators: Glycogen-rich, clear cell breast cancer. With comments concerning other clear cell variants. Hum Pathol 16:1085-1090, 1985.

827 Harris M: Pseudoadenoid cystic carcinoma of the breast. Arch Pathol Lab Med 101:307-309, 1977.

827a Hayes MMM, Seidman JD, Ashton MA: Glycogen-rich clear cell carcinoma of the breast. A clinicopathologic study of 21 cases. Am J Surg Pathol 19:904-911, 1995.

828 Hull MT, Warfel KA: Glycogen-rich clear cell carcinomas of the breast. A clinicopathologic and ultrastructural study. Am J Surg Pathol 10:553-559, 1986.

829 Jones MW, Norris HJ, Snyder RC: Infiltrating syringomatous adenoma of the nipple. A clinical and pathological study of 11 cases. Am J Surg Pathol 13:197-201, 1989.

830 Koss LG, Brannan CD, Ashikari R: Histologic and ultrastructural features of adenoid cystic carcinoma of the breast. Cancer 26:1271-1279, 1970.

831 Maiorano E, Ricco R, Virgintino D, Lastilla G: Infiltrating myoepithelioma of the breast. Appl Immunohistochem 2:130-136, 1994.

832 Michal M, Baumruk L, Burger J, Manhalova M: Adenomyoepithelioma of the breast with undifferentiated carcinoma component. Histopathology 24:274-276, 1994.

833 Moran CA, Suster S, Carter D: Benign mixed tumors (pleomorphic adenomas) of the breast. Am J Surg Pathol 14:913-921, 1990.

834 Patchefsky AS, Frauenhoffer CM, Krall RA, Cooper HS: Low-grade mucoepidermoid carcinoma of the breast. Arch Pathol Lab Med 103:196-198, 1979.

834a Pauwels C, De Potter C: Adenomyoepithelioma of the breast with features of malignancy. Histopathology 24:94-96, 1994.

835 Ro JY, Silva EG, Gallager HS: Adenoid cystic carcinoma of the breast. Hum Pathol 18:1276-1281, 1987.

836 Rosen PP: Adenomyoepithelioma of the breast. Hum Pathol 18:1232-1237, 1987.

837 Rosen PP: Adenoid cystic carcinoma of the breast. A morphologically heterogeneous neoplasm. Pathol Annu 24(Pt 2):237-254, 1989.

838 Schürch W, Potvin C: Malignant myoepithelioma (myoepithelial carcinoma) of the breast. An ultrastructural and immunocytochemical study. Ultrastruct Pathol 8:1-11, 1985.

839 Smith BH, Taylor HB: The occurrence of bone and cartilage in mammary tumors. Am J Clin Pathol 51:610-618, 1969.

840 Storensen FB, Paulsen SM: Glycogen-rich clear cell carcinoma of the breast. A solid variant with mucus. A light microscopic, immunohistochemical and ultrastructural study of a case. Histopathology 11:857-869, 1987.

841 Subramony C: Bilateral breast tumors resembling syringocystadenoma papilliferum. Am J Clin Pathol 87:656-659, 1987.

842 Suster S, Moran CA, Hurt MA: Syringomatous squamous tumors of the breast. Cancer 67:2350-2355, 1991.

843 Tamai M: Intraductal growth of malignant mammary myoepithelioma. Am J Surg Pathol 16:1116-1125, 1992.

844 Tavassoli FA: Myoepithelial lesions of the breast. Myoepitheliosis, adenomyoepithelioma, and myoepithelial carcinoma. Am J Surg Pathol 15:554-568, 1991.

845 Tavassoli FA, Norris HJ: Mammary adenoid cystic carcinoma with sebaceous differentiation. A morphologic study of the cell types. Arch Pathol Lab Med 110:1045-1053, 1986.

846 Toikkanen S, Joensuu H: Glycogen-rich clear-cell carcinoma of the breast. A clinicopathologic and flow cytometric study. Hum Pathol 22:81-83, 1991.

847 Van Hoeven KH, Drudis T, Cranor ML, Erlandson RA, Rosen PP: Low-grade adenosquamous carcinoma of the breast. A clinicopathologic study of 32 cases with ultrastructural analysis. Am J Surg Pathol 17:248-258, 1993.

848 Ward BE, Cooper PH, Subramony C: Syringomatous tumor of the nipple. Am J Clin Pathol 92:692-696, 1989.

849 Wells CA, Nicoll S, Ferguson DJP: Adenoid cystic carcinoma of the breast. A case with axillary lymph node metastasis. Histopathology 10:415-424, 1986.

850 Zarbo RJ, Oberman HA: Cellular adenomyoepithelioma of the breast. Am J Surg Pathol 7:863-870, 1983.

Stromal tumors and tumorlike conditions
PHYLLOIDES TUMOR

851 Azzopardi JG: Problems in breast pathology. In Bennington JL, consulting ed: Major problems in pathology. Philadephia, 1979, WB Saunders Co.

852 Barnes L, Pietruszka M: Rhabdomyosarcoma arising within a cystosarcoma phyllodes. Case report and review of the literature. Am J Surg Pathol **2:**423-429, 1978.

853 Bernstein L, Deapen D, Ross RK: The descriptive epidemiology of malignant cystosarcoma phyllodes tumors of the breast. Cancer **71:**3020-3024, 1993.

854 Christensen L, Nielsen M, Madsen PM: Cystosarcoma phyllodes. A review of 19 cases with emphasis on the occurrence of associated breast carcinoma. Acta Pathol Microbiol Immunol Scand (A) **94:**35-41, 1986.

855 Cohn-Cedermark G, Rutqvist LE, Rosendahl I, Silfversward C: Prognostic factors in cystosarcoma phyllodes. A clinicopathologic study of 77 patients. Cancer **68:**2017-2022, 1991.

856 el-Naggar AK, Ro JY, McLemore D, Garnsy L: DNA content and proliferative activity of cystosarcoma phyllodes of the breast. Potential prognostic significance. Am J Clin Pathol **93:**480-485, 1990.

857 Fiks A: Cystosarcoma phyllodes of the mammary gland. Müller's tumor. For the 180th birthday of Johannes Müller. Virchows Arch [A] **392:** 1-6, 1981.

858 Grimes MM, Lattes R, Jaretzki A III: Cystosarcoma phyllodes. Report of an unusual case, with death due to intraneural extension to the central nervous system. Cancer **56:**1691-1695, 1985.

859 Hart WR, Bauer RC, Oberman HA: Cystosarcoma phyllodes. A clinicopathologic study of twenty-six hypercellular periductal stromal tumors of the breast. Am J Clin Pathol **70:**211-216, 1978.

860 Knudsen PJT, Ostergaard J: Cystosarcoma phylloides with lobular and ductal carcinoma in situ. Arch Pathol Lab Med **111:**873-875, 1987.

860a Moffat CJC, Pinder SE, Dixon AR, Elston CW, Blarney RW, Ellis IO: Phyllodes tumours of the breast. A clinicopathological review of thirty-two cases. Histopathology **27:**205-218, 1995.

861 Norris HJ, Taylor HB: Relationship of histologic features to behavior of cystosarcoma phyllodes. Analysis of ninety-four cases. Cancer **20:**2090-2099, 1967.

862 Palko MJ, Wang SE, Shackney SE, Cottington EM, Levitt SB, Hartsock RJ: Flow cytometric S fraction as a predictor of clinical outcome in cystosarcoma \phyllodes. Arch Pathol Lab Med **114:**949-952, 1990.

863 Pietruszka M, Barnes L: Cystosarcoma phyllodes. A clinicopathologic analysis of 42 cases. Cancer **41:**1974-1983, 1978.

864 Powell CM, Rosen PP: Adipose differentiation in cystosarcoma phyllodes. A study of 14 cases. Am J Surg Pathol **18:**720-727, 1994.

865 Rao BR, Meyer JS, Fry CG: Most cystosarcoma phyllodes and fibroadenomas have progesterone receptor but lack estrogen receptor. Stromal localization of progesterone receptor. Cancer **47:**2016-2021, 1981.

866 Reddick RL, Shin TK, Sawhney D, Siegal GP: Stromal proliferations of the breast. An ultrastructural and immunohistochemical evaluation of cystosarcoma phyllodes, juvenile fibroadenoma, and fibroadenoma. Hum Pathol **18:**45-49, 1987.

867 Rhodes RH, Frankel KA, Davis RL, Tatter D: Metastatic cystosarcoma phyllodes. A report of 2 cases presenting with neurological symptoms. Cancer **41:**1179-1187, 1978.

868 Rosen PP, Romain K, Liberman L: Mammary cystosarcoma with mature adipose stromal differentiation (lipophyllodes tumor) arising in a lipomatous hamartoma. Arch Pathol Lab Med **118:**91-94, 1994.

869 Ward RM, Evans HL: Cystosarcoma phyllodes. A clinicopathologic study of 26 cases. Cancer **58:**2282-2289, 1986.

870 Yeh I-T, Francis DJ, Orenstein JM, Silverberg SG: Ultrastructure of cystosarcoma phyllodes and fibroadenoma. A comparative study. Am J Clin Pathol **84:**131-136, 1985.

VASCULAR TUMORS

871 Arias-Stella J Jr, Rosen PP: Hemangiopericytoma of the breast. Mod Pathol **2:**98-103, 1988.

872 Benda JA, Al-Jurf AS, Benson AB III: Angiosarcoma of the breast following segmental mastectomy complicated by lymphedema. Am J Clin Pathol **87:**651-655, 1987.

873 Brentani MM, Pacheco MM, Oshima CTF, Nagai MA, Lemos LB, Góes JCS: Steroid receptors in breast angiosarcoma. Cancer **51:**2105-2111, 1983.

874 Chen KTK: Rare variants of benign vascular tumors of the breast. Surg Pathol **4:**309-316,1991.

875 Donnell RM, Rosen PP, Lieberman PH, Kaufman RJ, Kay S, Braun DW Jr, Kinne DW: Angiosarcoma and other vascular tumors of the breast. Pathologic analysis as a guide to prognosis. Am J Surg Pathol **5:**629-642, 1981.

875a Fineberg S, Rosen PP: Cutaneous angiosarcoma and atypical vascular lesions of the skin and breast after radiation therapy for breast carcinoma. Am J Clin Pathol **102:**757-763, 1994.

876 Jozefczyk MA, Rosen PP: Vascular tumors of the breast. II. Perilobular hemangiomas and hemangiomas. Am J Surg Pathol **9:**491-503, 1985.

877 Lesueur GC, Brown RW, Bhathal PS: Incidence of perilobular hemangioma in the female breast. Arch Pathol Lab Med **107:**308-310, 1983.

877a Liberman L, Dershaw DD, Kaufman RJ, Rosen PP: Angiosarcoma of the breast. Radiology **183:**649-654, 1992.

878 Merino MJ, Carter D, Berman M: Angiosarcoma of the breast. Am J Surg Pathol **7:**53-60, 1983.

879 Mittal KR, Gerald W, True LD: Hemangiopericytoma of the breast. Report of a case with ultrastructural and immunohistochemical findings. Hum Pathol **17:**1181-1183, 1986.

880 Otis CN, Peschel R, McKhann C, Merino MJ, Duray PH: The rapid onset of cutaneous angiosarcoma after radiotherapy for breast carcinoma. Cancer **57:**2130-2134, 1986.

881 Rosen PP: Vascular tumors of the breast. III. Angiomatosis. Am J Surg Pathol **9:**652-658, 1985.

882 Rosen PP: Vascular tumors of the breast. V. Nonparenchymal hemangiomas of mammary subcutaneous tissues. Am J Surg Pathol **9:**723-729, 1985.

883 Rosen PP, Ernsberger DL: Grading mammary angiosarcoma. Prognostic study of 62 cases (abstract). Lab Invest **58:**78A, 1988.

884 Rosen PP, Jozefczyk MA, Boram LH: Vascular tumors of the breast. IV. The venous hemangioma. Am J Surg Pathol **9:**659-665, 1985.

885 Rosen PP, Ridolfi RL: The perilobular hemangioma. A benign microscopic vascular lesion of the breast. Am J Clin Pathol **68:**21-23, 1977.

885a Rosso R, Gianelli U, Carnevali L: Acquired progressive lymphangioma of the skin following radiotherapy for breast carcinoma. J Cutan Pathol **22:**164-167, 1995.

886 Sieber PR, Sharkey FE: Cystic hygroma of the breast. Arch Pathol Lab Med **110:**353, 1986.

887 Steingaszner LC, Enzinger FM, Taylor HB: Hemangiosarcoma of the breast. Cancer **18:**352-361, 1965.

888 Yu GH, Fishman SJ, Brooks JS: Cellular angiolipoma of the breast. Mod Pathol **6:**497-499, 1993.

OTHER MALIGNANT STROMAL TUMORS

889 Arista-Nasr J, Gonzalez-Gomez I, Angeles-Angeles A, Illanes-Baz E, Brandt-Brandt H, Larriva-Sahd J: Primary recurrent leiomyosarcoma of the breast. Case report with ultrastructural and immunohistochemical study and review of the literature. Am J Clin Pathol **92:**500-505, 1989.

890 Austin RM, Dupree WB: Liposarcoma of the breast. A clinicopathologic study of 20 cases. Hum Pathol **17:**906-913, 1986.

891 Beltaos E, Banerjee TK: Chondrosarcoma of the breast. Report of two cases. Am J Clin Pathol **71:**345-349, 1979.

892 Callery CD, Rosen PP, Kinne DW: Sarcoma of the breast. A study of 32 patients with reappraisal of classification and therapy. Ann Surg **201:**527-532, 1985.

893 Chen KTK, Kuo T-T, Hoffmann KD: Leiomyosarcoma of the breast. A case of long survival and late hepatic metastasis. Cancer **47:**1883-1886, 1981.

894 Going JJ, Lumsden AB, Anderson TJ: A classical osteogenic sarcoma of the breast. Histology, immunohistochemistry and ultrastructure. Histopathology **10:**631-641, 1986.

895 Jones MW, Norris HJ, Wargotz ES, Weiss SW: Fibrosarcoma-malignant fibrous histiocytoma of the breast. A clinicopathological study of 32 cases. Am J Surg Pathol **16:**667-674, 1992.

896 Norris HJ, Taylor HB: Sarcomas and related mesenchymal tumors of the breast. Cancer **22:**22-28, 1968.

897 Pollard SG, Marks PV, Temple LN, Thompson HH: Breast sarcoma. A clinicopathologic review of 25 cases. Cancer **66:**941-944, 1990.

898 Smith BH, Taylor HB: The occurrence of bone and cartilage in mammary tumors. Am J Clin Pathol **51:**610-618, 1969.

OTHER PRIMARY TUMORS AND TUMORLIKE CONDITIONS

899 Ali M, Fayemi AO, Braun EV, Remy R: Fibromatosis of the breast. Am J Surg Pathol **3:**501-505, 1979.

900 Anderson C, Ricci A Jr, Pedersen CA, Cartun RW: Immunocytochemical analysis of estrogen and progesterone receptors in benign stromal lesions of the breast. Evidence for hormonal etiology in pseudoangiomatous hyperplasia of mammary stroma. Am J Surg Pathol **15:**145-149, 1991.

901 Berean K, Tron VA, Churg A, Clement PB: Mammary fibroadenoma with multinucleated stromal giant cells. Am J Surg Pathol **10:**823-827, 1986.

902 Bittesini L, Dei Tos AP, Doglioni C, Della Libera D, Laurino L, Fletcher CD: Fibroepithelial tumor of the breast with digital fibroma-like inclusions in the stromal component. Case report with immunocytochemical and ultrastructural analysis. Am J Surg Pathol **18:**296-301, 1994.

903 Carneiro F, Brandao O, Correia AC, Sobrinho-Simoes M: Spindle cell tumor of the breast. Ultrastruct Pathol **13:**593-598, 1989.

903a Charpin C, Mathoulin MP, Andrac L, Barberis J, Boulat J, Sarradour B, Bonnier P, Piana L: Reappraisal of breast hamartomas. A morphological study of 41 cases. Pathol Res Pract **190:**362-371, 1994.

904 Cohen MB, Fisher PE: Schwann cell tumors of the breast and mammary region. Surg Pathol **4:**47-56, 1991.

905 Damiani S, Koerner FC, Dickersin GR, Cook MG, Eusebi V: Granular cell tumour of the breast. Virchows Arch [A] **420:**219-226, 1992.

906 Daroca PJ Jr, Reed RJ, Love GL, Kraus SD: Myoid hamartomas of the breast. Hum Pathol **16:**212-219, 1985.

907 Davies JD, Kulka J, Mumford AD, Armstrong JS, Wells CA: Hamartomas of the breast. Six novel diagnostic features in three-dimensional thick sections. Histopathology **24:**161-168, 1994.

908 Davis AB, Patchefsky AS: Basal cell carcinoma of the nipple. Case report and review of the literature. Cancer **40:**1780-1781, 1977.

908a Daya D, Trus T, D'Souza TJ, Minuk T, Yemen B: Hamartoma of the breast, an underrecognized breast lesion. A clinicopathologic and radiographic study of 25 cases. Am J Clin Pathol **103:**685-689, 1995.

909 DeMay RM, Kay S: Granular cell tumor of the breast. Pathol Annu **19**(Pt 2):121-148, 1982.

910 Diaz-Arias AA, Hurt MA, Loy TS, Seeger RM, Bickel JT: Leiomyoma of the breast. Hum Pathol **20:**396-399, 1989.

911 Fisher CJ, Hanby AM, Robinson L, Millis RR: Mammary hamartoma—a review of 35 cases. Histopathology **20:**99-106, 1992.

912 Hanna WM, Jambrosic J, Fish E: Aggressive fibromatosis of the breast. Arch Pathol Lab Med **109:**260-262, 1985.

913 Hiraoka N, Mukai M, Hosoda Y, Hata J: Phyllodes tumor of the breast containing the intracytoplasmic inclusion bodies identical with infantile digital fibromatosis. Am J Surg Pathol **18:**506-511, 1994.

914 Ilie B: Neoplasms in skin and subcutis over the breast, simulating breast neoplasms. Case reports and literature review. J Surg Oncol **31:**191-198, 1986.

915 Ingram DL, Mossler JA, Snowhite J, Leight GS, McCarty KS Jr: Granular cell tumors of the breast. Steroid receptor analysis and localization of carcinoembryonic antigen, myoglobin, and S100 protein. Arch Pathol Lab Med **108:**897-901, 1984.

916 Jones MW, Norris HJ, Wargotz ES: Hamartomas of the breast. Surg Gynecol Obstet **173:**54-56, 1991.

917 Kaplan L, Walts AE: Benign chondrolipomatous tumor of the human female breast. Arch Pathol Lab Med **101:**149-151, 1977.

918 Lai FM-M, Lam WY, Chin CW, Ng WL: Cutaneous Rosai-Dorfman disease presenting as a suspicious breast mass. J Cutan Pathol **21:**377-382, 1994.

919 Lugo M, Reyes JM, Putong PB: Benign chondrolipomatous tumors of the breast. Arch Pathol Lab Med **106:**691-692, 1982.

920 Marsh WL Jr, Lucas JG, Olsen J: Chondrolipoma of the breast. Arch Pathol Lab Med **113:**369-371, 1989.

921 Nascimento AG, Karas M, Rosen PP, Caron AG: Leiomyoma of the nipple. Am J Surg Pathol **3:**151-154, 1979.

922 Oberman HA: Hamartomas and hamartoma variants of the breast. Semin Diagn Pathol **6:**135-145, 1989.

923 O'Connor CR, Rubinow A, Cohen AS: Primary (AL) amyloidosis as a cause of breast masses. Am J Med **77:**981-986, 1984.

924 Pang JS, Alagaratnam TT: Fibromatosis of the breast. Case report and review of the literature. Pathology **14:**477-480, 1982.

925 Pettinato G, Manivel JC, Gould EW, Albores-Saavedra J: Inclusion body fibromatosis of the breast. Two cases with immunohistochemical and ultrastructural findings. Am J Clin Pathol **101:**714-718, 1994.

925a Powell CM, Cranor ML, Rosen PP: Pseudoangiomatous stromal hyperplasia (PASH). A mammary stromal tumor with myofibroblastic differentiation. Am J Surg Pathol **19:**270-277, 1995.

926 Roncaroli F, Rossi R, Severi B, Martinelli GN, Eusebi V: Epithelioid leiomyoma of the breast with granular cell change: A case report. Hum Pathol **24:**1260-1263, 1993.

927 Rosen PP: Multinucleated mammary stromal giant cells. A benign lesion that simulates invasive carcinoma. Cancer **44:**1305-1308, 1979.

928 Rosen PP, Ernsberger D: Mammary fibromatosis. A benign spindle-cell tumor with significant risk for local recurrence. Cancer **63:**1363-1369, 1989.

929 Rosen Y, Papasozomenos SC, Gardner B: Fibromatosis of the breast. Cancer **41:**1409-1413, 1978.

930 Silverman JF, Dabbs DJ, Norris HT, Pories WJ, Legier J, Kay S: Localized primary (AL) amyloid tumor of the breast. Cytologic, histologic, immunocytochemical and ultrastructural observations. Am J Surg Pathol **10:**539-545, 1986.

931 Vuitch MF, Rosen PP, Erlandson RA: Pseudoangiomatous hyperplasia of mammary stroma. Hum Pathol **17:**185-191, 1986.

932 Wargotz ES, Weiss SW, Norris HJ: Myofibroblastoma of the breast. Sixteen cases of a distinctive benign mesenchymal tumor. Am J Surg Pathol **11:**493-502, 1987.

Lymphoid tumors and tumorlike conditions

933 Arber DA, Simpson JF, Weiss LM, Rappaport H: Non-Hodgkin's lymphoma involving the breast. Am J Surg Pathol **18:**288-295, 1994.

934 Bobrow LG, Richards MA, Happerfield LC, Diss TC, Isaacson PG, Lammie GA, Millis RR: Breast lymphomas. A clinicopathologic review. Hum Pathol **24:**274-278, 1993.

935 Brooks JJ, Krugman DT, Damjanov I: Myeloid metaplasia presenting as a breast mass. Am J Surg Pathol **4:**281-285, 1980.

935a Byrd JC, Edenfield WJ, Shields DJ, Dawson NA: Extramedullary myeloid cell tumors in acute nonlymphocytic leukemia. A clinical review. J Clin Oncol **13:**1800-1816, 1995.

936 Cohen PL, Brooks JJ: Lymphomas of the breast. A clinicopathologic and immunohistochemical study of primary and secondary cases. Cancer **67:**1359-1369, 1991.

936a Cook PD, Osborne BM, Connor RL, Strauss JF: Follicular lymphoma adjacent to foreign body granulomatous inflammation and fibrosis surrounding silicone breast prosthesis. Am J Surg Pathol **19:**712-717, 1995.

937 De Cosse JJ, Berg JW, Fracchia AA, Farrow JH: Primary lymphosarcoma of the breast. A review of 14 cases. Cancer **15:**1264-1268, 1962.

938 Fisher ER, Palekar AS, Paulson JD, Golinger R: Pseudolymphoma of breast. Cancer **44:**258-263, 1979.

939 Hugh JC, Jackson FI, Hanson J, Poppema S: Primary breast lymphoma. An immunohistologic study of 20 new cases. Cancer **66:**2602-2611, 1990.

940 Kirshenbaum G, Rhone DP: Solitary extramedullary plasmacytoma of the breast with serum monoclonal protein. A case report and review of the literature. Am J Clin Pathol **83:**230-232, 1985.

941 Lamovec J, Jančar J: Primary malignant lymphoma of the breast. Lymphoma of the mucosa-associated lymphoid tissue. Cancer **60:**3033-3041, 1987.

942 Lin JJ, Farha GJ, Taylor RJ: Pseudolymphoma of the breast. I. In a study of 8,654 consecutive tylectomies and mastectomies. Cancer **45:**973-978, 1980.

943 Mambo NC, Burke JS, Butler JJ: Primary malignant lymphomas of the breast. Cancer **39:**2033-2040, 1977.

944 Mattia AR, Ferry JA, Harris NL: Breast lymphoma. A B-cell spectrum including the low grade B-cell lymphoma of mucosa associated lymphoid tissue. Am J Surg Pathol **17:**574-587, 1993.

945 Oberman HA: Primary lymphoreticular neoplasms of the breast. Surg Gynecol Obstet **123:**1047-1051, 1966.

946 Pascoe HR: Tumors composed of immature granulocytes occurring in the breast in chronic granulocytic leukemia. Cancer **25:**697-704, 1970.

947 Rooney N, Snead D, Goodman S, Webb AJ: Primary breast lymphoma with skin involvement arising in lymphocytic lobulitis. Histopathology **24:**81-84, 1994.

948 Schouten JT, Weese JL, Carbone PP: Lymphoma of the breast. Ann Surg **194:**749-753, 1981.

949 Telesinghe PU, Anthony PP: Primary lymphoma of the breast. Histopathology **9:**297-307, 1985.

950 Wiseman C, Liao KT: Primary lymphoma of the breast. Cancer **29:**1705-1712, 1972.

Metastatic tumors

951 Azzopardi JG: Problems in breast pathology. In Bennington JL, consulting ed: Major problems in pathology, vol 11. Philadelphia, 1979, WB Saunders Co.

952 Di Bonito L, Luchi M, Giarelli L, Falconieri G, Viehl P: Metastatic tumors to the female breast. An autopsy study of 12 cases. Pathol Res Pract **187:**432-436, 1991.

953 Hajdu SI, Urban JA: Cancers metastatic to the breast. Cancer **22:**1691-1696, 1968.

954 Harrist TJ, Kalisher L: Breast metastasis. An unusual manifestation of a malignant carcinoid tumor. Cancer **40:**3102-3106, 1977.

955 Howarth CB, Caces JN, Pratt CB: Breast metastases in children with rhabdomyosarcoma. Cancer **46:**2520-2524, 1980.

956 Warner TFCS, Seo IS: Bronchial carcinoid appearing as a breast mass. Arch Pathol Lab Med **104**:531-534, 1980.

957 Yamasaki H, Saw D, Zdanowitz J, Faltz LL: Ovarian carcinoma metastasis to the breast case report and review of the literature. Am J Surg Pathol **17**:193-197, 1993.

Breast diseases in children and adolescents

958 Bauer BS, Jones KM, Talbot CW: Mammary masses in the adolescent female. Surg Gynecol Obstet **165**:63-65, 1987.

959 Farrow JH, Ashikari H: Breast lesions in young girls. Surg Clin North Am **49**:261-269, 1969.

960 Kiaer HW, Kiaer WW, Linell F, Jacobsen S: Extreme duct papillomatosis of the juvenile breast. Acta Pathol Microbiol Scand (A) **87**:353-359, 1979.

961 Pettinato G, Manivel JC, Kelly DR, Wold LE, Dehner LP: Lesions of the breast in children exclusive of typical fibroadenoma and gynecomastia. A clinicpatho-logic study of 113 cases. Pathol Annu **24**(Pt 2):296-328, 1989.

962 Ramirez G, Ansfield FJ: Carcinoma of the breast in children. Arch Surg **96**:222-225, 1968.

963 Rosen PP: Papillary duct hyperplasia of the breast in children and young adults. Cancer **56**:1611-1617, 1985.

964 Rosen PP, Cantrell B, Mullen DL, DePalo A: Juvenile papillomatosis (Swiss cheese disease) of the breast. Am J Surg Pathol **4**:3-12, 1980.

965 Rosen PP, Kimmel M: Juvenile papillomatosis of the breast. A follow-up study of 41 patients having biopsies before 1979. Am J Clin Pathol **93**:599-603, 1990.

966 Steiner MW: Enlargement of the breast during childhood. Pediatr Clin North Am **2**:575-593, 1955.

967 Taffurelli M, Santini D, Martinelli G, Mazzoleni G, Rossati U, Giosa F, Grassigli A, Marrano D: Juvenile papillomatosis of the breast. A multidisciplinary study. Pathol Annu **26**(Pt 1):25-35, 1991.

968 Wilson M, Cranor ML, Rosen PP: Papillary duct hyperplasia of the breast in children and young women. Mod Pathol **6**:570-574, 1993.

Breast diseases in males
GYNECOMASTIA

969 Andersen JA, Gram JB: Gynecomasty. Histological aspects in a surgical mate-rial. Acta Pathol Microbiol Immunol Scand (A) **90**:185-190, 1982.

970 Bannayan GA, Hajdu SI: Gynecomastia. Clinicopathologic study of 351 cases. Am J Clin Pathol **57**:431-437, 1972.

971 Coen P, Kulin H, Ballantine T, Zaino R, Frauenhoffer E, Boal D, Inkster S, Brodie A, Santen R: An aromatase-producing sex-cord tumor resulting in pre-pubertal gynecomastia. N Engl J Med **324**:317-322, 1991.

972 Fisher ER, Creed DL: Nature of the periductal stroma in gynecomastia. Lab Invest **5**:267-275, 1956.

973 Gottfried MR: Extensive squamous metaplasia in gynecomastia. Arch Pathol Lab Med **110**:971-973, 1986.

973a Guillou L, Gebhard S: Gynecomastia with unusual intraductal "clear cell" changes mimicking pagetoid ductal spread of lobular neoplasia. Path Res Pract **191**:156-163, 1995.

974 Nielsen BB: Fibroadenomatoid hyperplasia of the male breast. Am J Surg Pathol **14**:774-777, 1990.

975 Sirtori C, Veronesi U: Gynecomastia. A review of 218 cases. Cancer **10**:645-654, 1957.

976 Wheeler CE, Cawley EP, Curtis AC: Gynecomastia. A review and an analysis of 160 cases. Ann Intern Med **40**:985-1004, 1954.

977 Wilson JD, Aiman J, MacDonald PC: The pathogenesis of gynecomastia. Adv Intern Med **25**:1-32, 1980.

CARCINOMA

978 Adami HO, Hakulinen T, Ewertz M, Tretli S, Holmberg L, Karjalainen S: The survival pattern in male breast cancer. An analysis of 1429 patients from the Nordic countries. Cancer **64**:1177-1182, 1989.

979 Bavafa S, Reyes CV, Choudhury AM: Male breast carcinoma. An updated experience at a Veterans Administration hospital and review of the literature. J Surg Oncol **24**:41-45, 1983.

980 Bhagat P, Kline TS: The male breast and malignant neoplasms. Diagnosis by aspiration biopsy cytology. Cancer **65**:2338-2341, 1990.

981 Camus MG, Joshi MG, Mackarem G, Lee AK, Rossi RL, Munson JL, Buyske J, Barbarisi LJ, Sanders LE, Hughes KS: Ductal carcinoma in situ of the male breast. Cancer **74**:1289-1293, 1994.

982 Costa MH, Silverberg SG: Oncocytic carcinoma of the male breast. Arch Pathol **113**:1396-1398, 1989.

983 Cunha F, Andre S, Soares J: Morphology of male breast carcinoma in the eval-uation of prognosis. Pathol Res Pract **186**:745-750, 1990.

984 Demeter JG, Waterman NG, Verdi GD: Familial male breast carcinoma. Cancer **65**:2342-2343, 1990.

985 Donegan WL: Cancer of the breast in men. CA Cancer J Clin **41**:339-354, 1991.

986 El-Gazayerli M, Abdel-Aziz AS: On bilharziasis and male breast cancer in Egypt. A preliminary report and review of the literature. Br J Cancer **17**:566-571, 1963.

987 Giffler RF, Kay S: Small-cell carcinoma of the male mammary gland. A tumor resembling infiltrating lobular carcinoma. Am J Clin Pathol **66**:715-722, 1976.

988 Guinee VF, Olsson H, Moller T, Shallenberger RC, van den Blink JW, Peter Z, Durand M, Dische S, Cleton FJ, Zewuster R, et al.: The prognosis of breast can-cer in males. A report of 335 cases. Cancer **71**:154-161, 1993.

989 Hecht JR, Winchester DJ: Male breast cancer. Am J Clin Pathol **102**:S25-30, 1994.

990 Heller KS, Rosen PP, Schottenfeld D, Ashikari R, Kinne DW: Male breast cancer. A clinicopathologic study of 97 cases. Ann Surg **188**:60-65, 1978.

991 Kozak FK, Hall JG, Baird PA: Familial breast cancer in males. A case report and review of the literature. Cancer **58**:2736-2739, 1986.

992 Norris HJ, Taylor HB: Carcinoma of the male breast. Cancer **23**:1428-1435, 1969.

993 O'Grady WP, McDivitt RW: Breast cancer in a man treated with diethylstilbe-strol. Arch Pathol **88**:162-165, 1969.

994 Papotti M, Tanda F, Bussolati G, Pugno F, Bosincu L, Massareli G: Argy-rophilic neuroendocrine carcinoma of the male breast. Ultrastruct Pathol **17**:115-121, 1993.

995 Pich A, Margaria E, Chiusa L: Proliferative activity is a significant prognostic factor in male breast carcinoma. Am J Pathol **145**:481-489, 1994.

996 Ribeiro GG: Carcinoma of the male breast. A review of 200 cases. Br J Surg **64**:381-383, 1977.

997 Sanchez AG, Villanueva AG, Redondo C: Lobular carcinoma of the breast in a patient with Klinefelter's syndrome. A case with bilateral, synchronous, his-tologically different breast tumors. Cancer **57**:1181-1183, 1986.

998 Scopsi L, Andreola S, Saccozzi R, Pilotti S, Boracchi P, Rosa P, Conti AR, Manzari A, Huttner WB, Rilke F: Argyrophilic carcinoma of the male breast. A neuroendocrine tumor containing predominantly chromogranin B (secre-togranin I). Am J Surg Pathol **15**:1063-1071, 1991.

999 Spence RAJ, Mackenzie G, Anderson JR, Lyons AR, Bell M: Long-term sur-vival following cancer of the male breast in Northern Ireland. A report of 81 cases. Cancer **55**:648-652, 1985.

1000 Stretch JR, Denton KJ, Millard PR, Horak E: Paget's disease of the male breast clinically and histopathologically mimicking melanoma. Histopathol-ogy **19**:470-472, 1991.

1001 Tamura G, Monma N, Suzuki Y, Satodate R, Abe H: Adenomyoepithelioma (myoepithelioma) of the breast in a male. Hum Pathol **24**:678-681, 1993.

1002 Visfeldt J, Scheike O: Male breast cancer. I. Histologic typing and grading of 187 Danish cases. Cancer **32**:985-990, 1973.

OTHER LESIONS

1002a Ali S, Teichberg S, De Risi DC, Urmacher C: Giant myofibroblastoma of the male breast. Am J Surg Pathol **18**:1170-1176, 1994.

1002b Badve S, Sloane JP: Pseudoangiomatous hyperplasia of male breast. Histopathology **26**:463-466, 1995.

1003 Begin LR: Myogenic stromal tumor of the male breast (so-called myofibro-blastoma). Ultrastruct Pathol **15**:613-622, 1991.

1004 Benson WR: Carcinoma of the prostate with metastases to breast and testis. Cancer **10**:1235-1245, 1957.

1005 Bigotti G, Kasznica J: Sclerosing adenosis in the breast of a man with pulmonary oat cell carcinoma. Report of a case. Hum Pathol **17**:861-863, 1986.

1006 Damiani S, Miettinen M, Peterse JL, Eusebi V: Solitary fibrous tumour (myofibroblastoma) of the breast. Virchows Arch **425**:89-92, 1994.

1007 Green LK, Klima M: The use of immunohistochemistry in metastatic prostatic adenocarcinoma to the breast. Hum Pathol **22**:242-246, 1991.

1008 Hassan MO, Gogate PA, Al-Kaisi N: Intraductal papilloma of the male breast. An ultrastructural and immunohistochemical study. Ultrastruct Pathol **18**:601-610, 1994.

1009 Hernandez FJ: Leiomyosarcoma of male breast originating in the nipple. Am J Surg Pathol **2**:299-304, 1978.

1010 Hilton DA, Jameson JS, Furness PN: A cellular fibroadenoma resembling a benign phyllodes tumour in a young male with gynaecomastia. Histopathology **18:**476-477, 1991.

1011 Lipper S, Willson CF, Copeland KC: Pseudogynecomastia due to neurofibromatosis. A light microscopic and ultrastructural study. Hum Pathol **12:**755-79, 1981.

1012 Sara AS, Gottfried MR: Benign papilloma of the male breast following chronic phenothiazine therapy. Am J Clin Pathol **87:**649-650, 1987.

1013 Tedeschi LG, McCarthy PE: Involutional mammary duct ectasia and periductal mastitis in a male. Hum Pathol **5:**232-236, 1974.

1014 Toker C, Tang C-K, Whitely JF, Berkheiser SW, Rachman R: Benign spindle cell breast tumor. Cancer **48:**1615-1622, 1981.

1015 Waldo ED, Sidhu GS, Hu AW: Florid papillomatosis of the male nipple after diethylstilbestrol therapy. Arch Pathol **99:**364-366, 1975.

1016 Wargotz ES, Weiss SW, Norris HJ: Myofibroblastoma of the breast. Sixteen cases of a distinctive benign mesenchymal tumor. Am J Surg Pathol **11:**493-502, 1987.

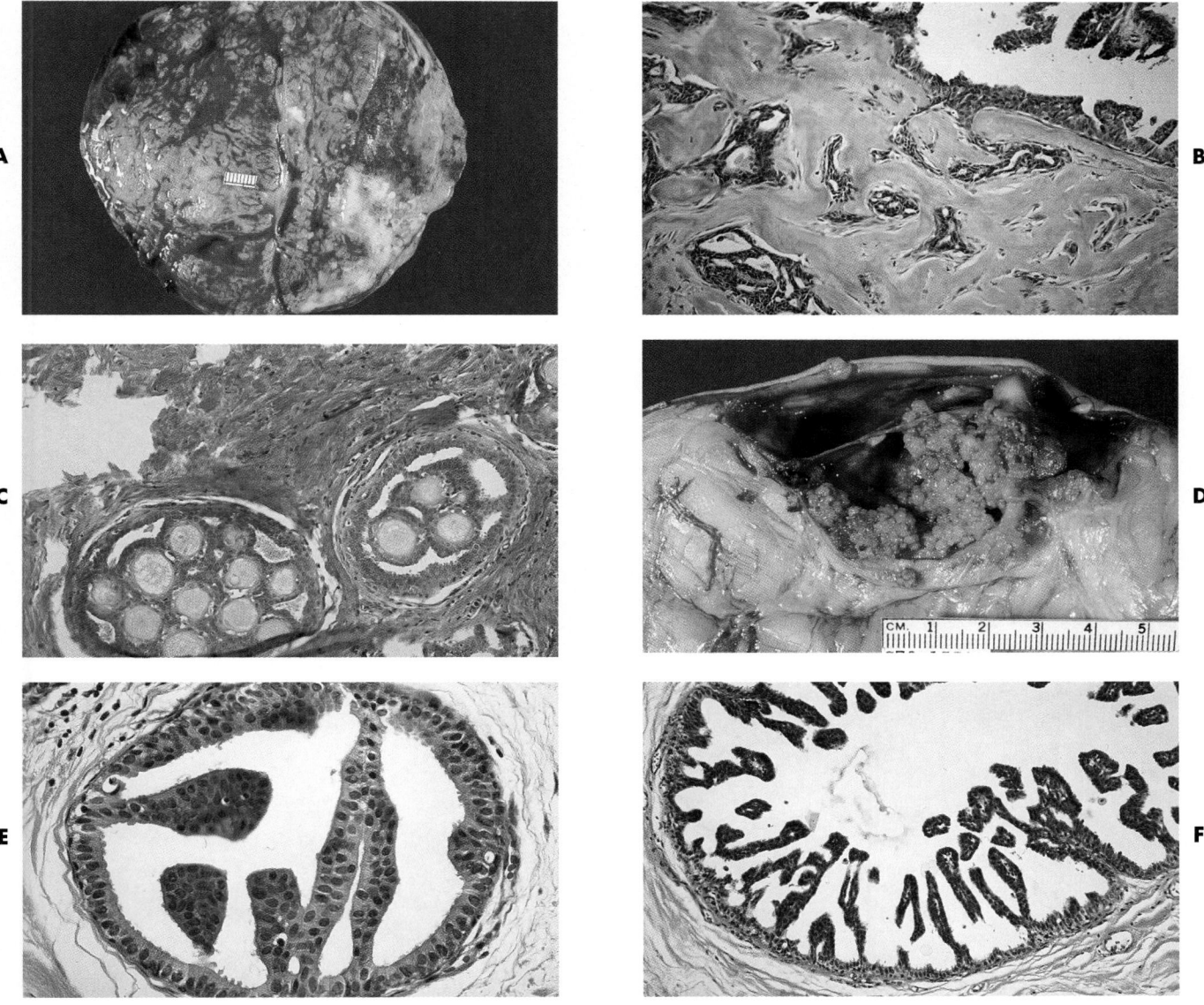

Plate XV A, Gross appearance of lactating adenoma. The mass has a distinct lobular configuration, yellowish color, and marked vascularization. B, Papilloma of breast showing entrapment of epithelial structures by fibrohyaline stroma, resulting in a pseudoinvasive appearance. C, So-called collagenous spherulosis. This morphologic variant of ductal hyperplasia should not be confused with adenoid cystic carcinoma. D, Intracystic carcinoma of the breast. The papillary configuration of the tumor is already appreciable grossly. E, Trabecular bars in intraductal carcinoma. Note the perpendicular arrangement of the nuclei in relation to the long axis of the bars. F, Micropapillary carcinoma of breast. Most of the papillae lack a central fibrovascular core.

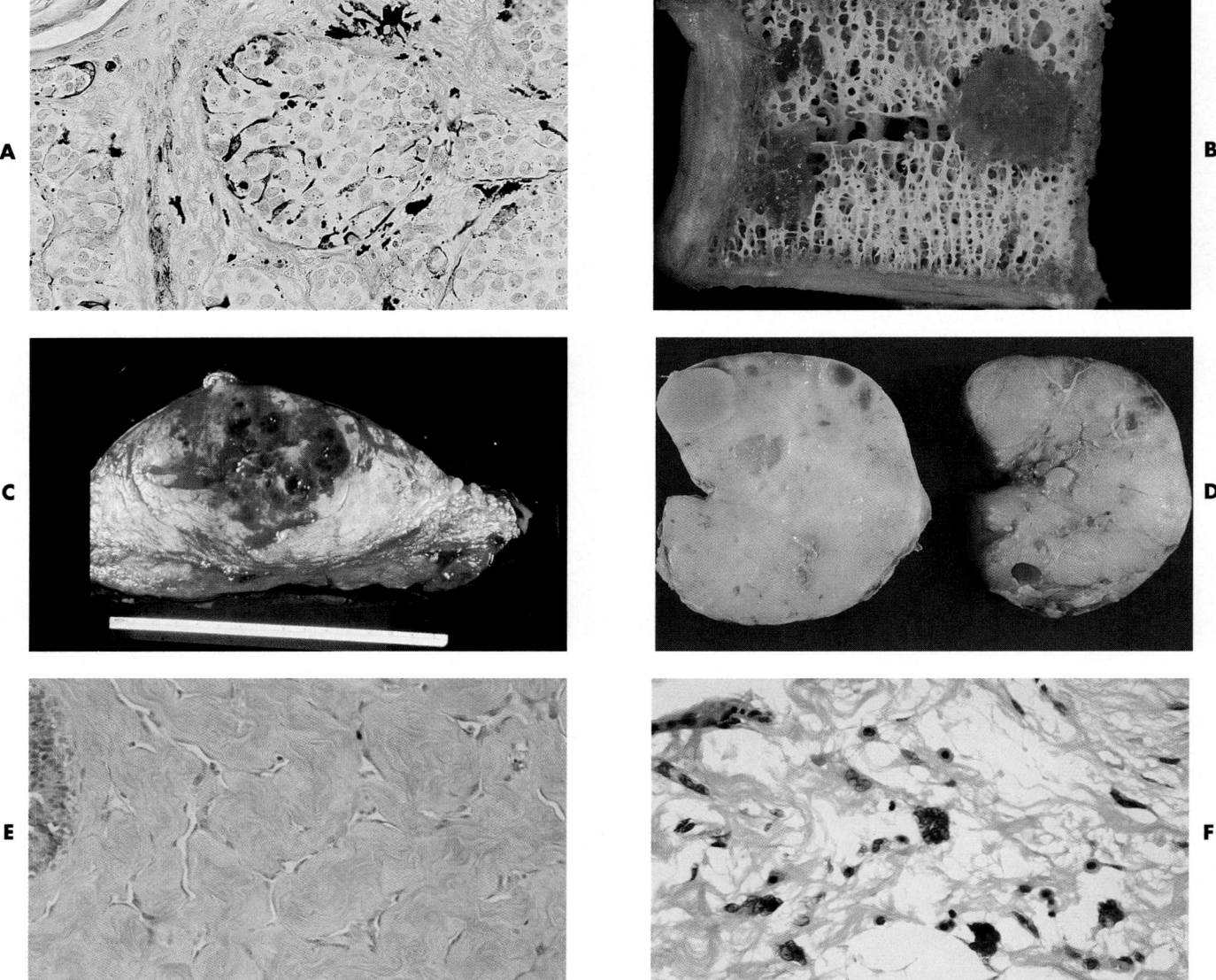

Plate XVI **A,** Melanin colonization in breast carcinoma as seen with argentaffin stain. **B,** Breast carcinoma metastatic to vertebra. The normal bone marrow has been flushed out by placing a thin slice of tissue under a strong jet of water. **C,** Gross appearance of angiosarcoma of the breast. The tumor has a markedly hemorrhagic appearance. **D,** Gross appearance of so-called hamartoma of breast. There is a combination of cystic dilatation of ducts, fibrosis, and entrapment of adipose tissue. This lesion is more distinctive and impressive grossly than microscopically. **E,** Pseudoangiomatous stromal hyperplasia. Thin channels lined by spindle cells are seen scattered within a hyalinized stroma. **F,** Bizarre multinucleated cells in mammary stroma. This neoplastic change is analogous to that more often seen in the stroma of the upper aerodigestive tract and in the genital tract. (**A** slide prepared by Dr. Pierre Masson, University of Montreal, and sent by him to Dr. Fred W. Stewart, Memorial Sloan-Kettering Cancer Center.)

21 Lymph nodes

NORMAL ANATOMY

The three major regions of a lymph node are the cortex, paracortex, and medulla. The cortex is situated beneath the capsule and contains the largest number of follicles. The medulla, close to the hilum, is rich in lymph sinuses, arteries, and veins but contains only a minor lymphocytic component. Both cortex and medulla represent B zones and are therefore associated with humoral types of immune response.[3] The appearance of the follicles varies according to their state of activity. Primary follicles appear as round aggregates of lymphocytes; secondary follicles appear following antigenic stimulation and are characterized by the presence of germinal centers.[2] The cells present in these formations are B lymphocytes known as follicular center cells (centroblasts and centrocytes or small and large cleaved and noncleaved cells), macrophages, and follicular dendritic cells. The germinal center shows polarization toward the side of antigen stimulation and is surrounded by a mantle of small B lymphocytes.[3] Proliferated germinal centers are always indicative of humoral antibody production. Under conditions of intense antigenic stimulation, they also can appear within the medullary cords.[4]

The paracortex is the zone situated between the cortex and the medulla, which contains the mobile pool of T lymphocytes responsible for cell-mediated immune responses.[3] A characteristic feature is the presence of postcapillary venules, which are identifiable by their lining of high endothelial cells and the presence of lymphocytes in their walls. Another cell type present in the paracortex is the interdigitating dendritic cell. Expansion of the paracortex is indicative of a cell-mediated immunologic reaction. The number of lymphocytes within the lumen and wall of postcapillary venules gives a rough indication of the degree of lymphocyte recirculation.[1]

Afferent lymph vessels penetrate the nodal capsule to open into the marginal sinus; this communicates with an intricate intranodal sinus network that merges into efferent lymph vessels exiting the node at the hilum. The endothelial lining of the outer (subcapsular) side of the marginal sinus is nonphagocytic and similar to that of the afferent and efferent vessels; the lining of the intranodal sinuses has strong phagocytic properties (littoral cells or sinus-lining histiocytes). The main arteries and veins pass through the hilum and radiate to the medulla, paracortex, and inner part of the cortex; other blood vessels penetrate the capsule to supply the superficial cortex and a small area surrounding the trabecula.

LYMPH NODE EVALUATION

The proper examination of a lymph node is a complicated task that may require the performance of a variety of specialized procedures depending on the nature of the case.

Biopsy

Selection of the lymph node to be biopsied is of great importance. Inguinal nodes are to be avoided whenever possible because of the high frequency of chronic inflammatory and fibrotic changes present in them. Axillary or cervical nodes are more likely to be informative in cases of generalized lymphadenopathy. Whenever possible, the largest lymph node in the region should be biopsied. Small superficial nodes may show only nonspecific hyperplasia, whereas a deeper node of the same group may show diagnostic features.

The surgeon biopsying intra-abdominal nodes or large cervical or axillary masses should have a frozen section performed to be certain that the tissue is representative—*not* to obtain a specific diagnosis at this point. This may save a second biopsy.

Adherence to a strict technique for the preparation of lymph nodes in the pathology laboratory is of paramount importance[5-7] (see Appendix E). The specimen should be received fresh in the laboratory immediately after excision, bisected as soon as it is received, and sampled for the appropriate studies. The portion to be embedded in paraffin (which should not exceed 3 mm in thickness) can be placed in 10% buffered formalin or, preferably, in B5 or analogous mercury-containing fixative. The alcohols and xylenes should be changed frequently. Sections should be cut with a sharp knife without distortion at 5 μm or less. As a routine, satisfactory results can be attained with hematoxylin-eosin staining.[5,8,11]

A technique that complements the study of tissue sections and that is too often neglected is the examination of touch preparations from the cut surface of the fresh lymph node stained with Giemsa or Wright's solution.[9,10] (see Appendix E). This is particularly useful in the evaluation of lymphoma and leukemia. Granulocytic leukemia can closely simulate large cell lymphoma in a hematoxylin-eosin–stained section, but an imprint will readily distinguish the two conditions.

Bacteriologic examination

If there is a possibility that the node contains an infectious process, an adequate sample of the biopsied lymph node must be sent directly for bacteriologic study or at least be placed in a sterile Petri dish in the refrigerator. If permanent sections show an inflammatory process, the material can then be retrieved and studied bacteriologically (see Appendix E).

Needle biopsy

Core needle biopsy is adequate for the diagnosis of metastatic carcinoma but is rarely used for the evaluation of primary lymphoid disorders.

Fine-needle aspiration of lymph nodes is particularly useful for the documentation of metastatic carcinoma, especially in cervical lymph nodes[14] but also in other locations, including intra-abdominal and retroperitoneal regions.[12] The cytologic diagnosis of malignant lymphoma can be made in 50% to 75% of the cases, the accuracy being greatest in the high-grade lesions.[13,15,16] The technique has been found most useful for the selection of a representative node for biopsy, for the diagnosis of recurrent lymphoma, for staging the extent of the disease, and for monitoring treatment.[18] Hemorrhage, necrosis, and myofibroblastic proliferation may develop along the needle tract; the latter should not be confused with Kaposi's sarcoma or other neoplasms.[17]

Electron microscopy

Ultrastructural examination of lymph nodes can be of use in some specific diseases, such as Langerhans' cell granulomatosis (histiocytosis X) and various metastatic tumors. Its role in the evaluation of primary lymphoid disorders is relatively small, especially after the advent of immunocytochemical and molecular biology techniques.[19,20]

Immunophenotyping

Phenotyping of lymphoid disorders has evolved into a highly complex field in the past few years, as a result of the enormous cellular diversity within the immune system and the huge number (over 1000) of markers that have become available for this purpose.

Rosetting tests with coated or uncoated red blood cells and polyclonal antibodies, which have been so useful for the early characterization of lymphomas, have been all but replaced by the use of monoclonal antibodies. These have received a multitude of designations, which are more dependent on the manufacturer's source than the features of the antibody.[21-31] Fortunately, an internationally agreed-upon nomenclature (the CD system, which stands for cluster designation) has evolved, and this has allowed for better communication among the various laboratories. Many of these monoclonal antibodies are now applicable to paraffin sections (Table 21-1), whereas others can be employed only in fresh cells (from suspension, cytospin preparations, or frozen section) (Table 21-2). A detailed discussion of these tests is clearly outside the scope of this book.

Text continued on p. 1668.

Table 21-1 Principal antibodies employed in immunohistochemical staining of paraffin tissue sections

CD antigen and/or antibody	Predominant normal cell reactivity	Reactivity in neoplasms	Comment/caution
Leukocytes			
CD45RB (PD7) Leukocyte common antigen*	B cells and most T cells, macrophages, myeloid cells	Most lymphomas and leukemias	Plasma cell neoplasms and Reed-Sternberg cells usually unreactive; some lymphoblastic and anaplastic large cell lymphomas unreactive
B lymphocytes			
Immunoglobulin (polyclonal)	B cells and plasma cells	B-cell and plasma cell neoplasms	Diffuse cytoplasmic staining for both light chains seen in macrophages, Reed-Sternberg cells, and degenerated cells (attributed to passive uptake); cytoplasmic Ig often detectable in paraffin sections; surface Ig often requires frozen tissue
CD79 (MB1/B29) (Ig associated)	B cells (B29 absent in plasma cells)	Most B lymphomas, B leukemias from pre–B-cell stage	Associated with antigen receptor (Ig) on B-cells in a similar manner as CD3 on T-cells; antibodies cross react with all mammalian species tested
CD20 (L26)	B-cells, sometimes macrophages	Most B-cell lymphomas, L&H cells in nLPHD, some Reed-Sternberg cells in ≈20% of classic Hodgkin's disease, rare T-cell lymphomas	Does not work well in acid-decalcified tissues, particularly if Bouin fixed, (unless microwaved); plasma cell neoplasms usually unreactive, some thymomas may stain
CD45RA (4KB5, MB1)	B-cells and subpopulation of T-cells	Most B-cell lymphomas, few T-cell lymphomas, L&H cells in nLPHD, some myeloid leukemias	Plasma cell neoplasms usually ureactive
CDw75 (LN1)	B-cells (mainly germinal center cells)	Many B-cell lymphomas, some T-cell lymphomas, L&H cells in nLPHD; Reed-Sternberg cells in classic Hodgkin's disease (some cases)	Works better in mercuric chloride–containing fixatives
CD74 (LN2 and MB3)	B-cells, interdigitating dendritic cells, some macrophages, Langerhans' cells	Many B-cell lymphomas, some T-cell lymphomas, Reed-Sternberg cells, many myeloid leukemias, Langerhans' cell histiocytosis	Works better in mercuric chloride–containing fixatives
MB2	B-cells, some macrophages	Most B-cell lymphomas, some T-cell lymphomas, some myeloid leukemias	Plasma cell neoplasms unreactive, many nonhematolymphoid neoplasms reactive
T lymphocytes			
CD3 (polyclonal)	T-cells	Many T-cell lymphomas	May require prolonged proteolytic digestion or wet heat pretreatment; may see nonspecific cytoplasmic staining in macrophages and plasma cells
bF1 (TCR beta chain)	T-cells	Many T-cell lymphomas	Requires proteolytic digestion; more sensitive in frozen sections
CD43 (Leu-22, MTI, LIFT1)	T-cells, plasma cells, some macrophages, granulocytes, erythroid cells, Langerhans' cells	Most T-cell lymphomas, 1/3 B-cell lymphomas, myeloid leukemias, many plasma cell neoplasms, Langerhans' cell histiocytosis	Can be exploited especially for diagnosis of small B-cell lymphoma/leukemia
CD45RO (UCHL1, A6, OPD4)	Major T-cell subset. some macrophages, granulocytes	Many T-cell lymphomas, few B-cell lymphomas, myeloid leukemias, some plasma cell neoplasms	May see nonspecific cytoplasmic staining
CD57 (Leu-7, HNK1)	Subset of germinal center T cells, some natural killer cells	Few lymphoblastic lymphomas, some natural killer cell neoplasms	CD56 in frozen sections better marker for natural killer cells; IgM isotype may benefit from isotype-specific detection; subset of reactive T-cells ring L&H cells in nLPHD

Continued.

Table 21-1 Principal antibodies employed in immunohistochemical staining of paraffin tissue sections—cont'd

CD antigen and or antibody	Predominant normal cell reactivity	Reactivity in neoplasms	Comment/caution
Hodgkin's disease–associated			
CD15 (LeuMl)	Granulocytes, some macrophages	Reed-Sternberg cells in most cases of classic Hodgkin's disease, large cells in some B- and T-cell lymphomas, some myeloid leukemias	Many carcinomas reactive, CMV-infected cells reactive; IgM isotype may benefit from isotype-specific detection; L&H cells usually unreactive in paraffin sections
CD30 (BerH2)	Some activated B and T cells, some plasma cells	Reed-Sternberg cells in most cases of Hodgkin's disease, most cases anaplastic large cell lymphomas, some B- and T-cell lymphomas, many plasma cell neoplasms; L&H cells usually unreactive in paraffin sections	Less sensitive in mercuric chloride–containing fixatives; embryonal carcinomas and few other non-hematolymphoid neoplasms reactive; cytoplasmic staining (nonspecific) of plasma cells may be abolished by prior wet heat treatment (such as microwave)
Accessory cells			
CD68 (KP1)	Macrophages, myeloid cells	True histiocytic neoplasms, many myeloid leukemias, dot-like staining in some small cell B-lymphomas and leukemias, especially hairy cell leukemia, mastocytosis	Reactive in granular cell tumors, some melanomas, malignant fibrous histiocytomas, and renal cell carcinomas; PGM (CD68) does not stain myeloid cells
Lysozyme (polyclonal)	Macrophages, myeloid cells	True histiocytic lymphomas, myeloid leukemias	Reactive with many non-hematolymphoid neoplasms
S-100 protein (polyclonal/monoclonal)	Langerhans' cells, interdigitating (IDRC) and some-times dendritic follicular cells	Langerhans' cell histiocytosis, IDRC tumors, rare T-cell lymphomas, true histiocytic lymphomas, myeloid leukemias, Rosai-Dorfman disease	Reactive with many non-hematolymphoid neoplasms
Mac-387	Macrophages, myeloid cells	True histiocytic lymphomas, myeloid leukemias	Reactive with some squamous cell carcinomas
Miscellaneous			
bcl-2	Nongerminal center B cells, most T cells, plasma cells	Overexpressed in most follicular lymphomas and some diffuse large B-cell lymphomas; also expressed in many other lymphomas and leukemias	Works best in B5 and Bouin 1-fixed tissues (unless microwaved); most useful in differentiating benign from malignant follicular lesions, i. e., non-neoplastic germinal center B-cells unreactive
EBV-latent membrane protein (LMP-1)	EBV-infected cells	Reed-Sternberg cells in some cases of classic Hodgkin's disease, i.e., those containing EBV DNA; most immunodeficiency-associated lymphomas	
Myeloperoxi-dase (polyclonal)	Myeloid cells	Myeloid leukemias	Most sensitive and specific marker for myeloid neoplasms
Epithelial membrane antigen	Plasma cells	In Hodgkin's disease, mainly nLPHD type; plasma cell neoplasms, many anaplastic large cell lymphomas and some other B and T large cell lymphomas	Many epithelial tumors reactive

*CMV, Cytomegalovirus; EBV, Epstein-Barr virus; nLPHD, nodular lymphocyte predominance Hodgkin's disease.
All of these markers produce cell membrane and/or Golgi staining except (1) CD74 (LN2): nuclear membrane staining; (2) S-100 protein: nuclear +/− cytoplasmic staining; and (3) Mbw,CD68 (KP1), Mac-387, Ig, lysozyme, bcl-2m, and myeloperoxidase: diffuse cytoplasmic staining.
From Warnke RA, Weiss LM, Chan JKC, Cleary ML, Dorfman RF: Tumors of the lymph nodes and spleen. Atlas of tumor pathology, 3rd Series, Fascicle 14. Washington, DC, 1995, Armed Forces Institute of Pathology.

Table 21-2 Principal antibodies employed in staining fresh cells in suspension or in cytospins and frozen sections

CD-antigen or antibody	Predominant normal cell reactivity	Reactivity in neoplasms	Comment/caution
Leukocytes			
CD45 (2D1, L3B12, T29/33)	Hemato-lymphoid cells	Nearly all lymphomas and leukemias	Some plasma cell neoplasms unreactive, few precursor cell neoplasms unreactive, some anaplastic large cell lymphomas unreactive
CD11A/18 (LFA-1α and b)	Hemato-lymphoid cells	Many lymphomas and leukemias	Many intermediate and high-grade B lineage lymphomas lack expression of the alpha and/or beta chain of LFA-1
B lymphocytes			
Immuno-globulins (Ig)	B-cells (Ig staining of normal germ-inal center cells weak to absent)	Most B-cell lymphomas and leukemias, plasma cell neoplasms	Precursor B-cell lymphomas and leukemias do not express Ig except for cytoplasmic mu chains in pre-B-cell tumors; some follicular and diffuse large cell lymphomas of B-cell lineage lack expression; monoclonal anti-Ig reagents less sensitive than polyclonal reagents; detection of cyto-plasmic Ig often better in fixed and processed tissues; neoplasms show Ig light chain expression restricted to either kappa or lambda chains
CD79 (MB1/B29) (Ig associated)	B cells (B29 absent in plasma cells)	Most B-cell lymphomas, B-cell leukemias from pre–B-cell stage	Associated with antigen receptor (Ig) on B-cells in a similar manner as CD3 on T-cells; anti-bodies cross react with all mammalian species tested
CD19 (B4, Leu-12)	B cells	More B-cell lymphomas, and leukemias, few myeloid leukemias	Earliest expressed B-cell differentiation antigen; most plasma cell neoplasms unreactive
CD20 (B1, Leu-16, L26)	B cells	Most B-cell lymphomas, B-cell leukemias, Reed-Sternberg cells in some cases of classic Hodgkin's disease	Most plasma cell neoplasms unreactive; cytoplasmic reactivity may be seen in macrophages
CD22 (Leu-14)	B cells	Most B-cell lymphomas, most B-cell leukemias	Expressed early in B-cell differentiation in the cytoplasm and arrives at the cell membrane at about the same time as Ig; may be undetectable on the surface in some chronic lymphocytic leukemias; most plasma cell neoplasms unreactive
CD24 (BA1)	B cells	Most B-cell lymphomas, most B-cell leukemias	Most plasma cell neoplasms unreactive; granulocytes reactive; nonhematolymphoid neoplasms may be reactive
CD37	B cells	Most B-cell lymphomas, many B-cell leukemias, some T-cell lymphomas	Most plasma cell neoplasms unreactive; reactivity with subset of T-cell lymphomas may be useful in diagnosis
B-lymphocyte subsets			
CD10 (J5) (CALLA)	Precursor B cells, germinal center B-cells	Many precursor B leu-kemias, some precursor T leukemias, many follicular lymphomas subset of the other	May be useful in separating follicular from other low-grade B-cell lymphomas; expressed by subset of myeloma; reactive with some non-hematolymphoid neoplasms, e.g., Ewing's sarcoma and malignant fibrous histiocytoma
CD21 (B2)	Mantle and marginal zone B-cells, follicular dendritic cells	Most lymphomas of mantle and marginal zone B-cells, follicular dendritic cell tumors	C3d (CR2) complement receptor; receptor for EBV
CD23	Mantle zone B-cells, subset of follicular dendritic cells	CLL/small lymphocytic lymphoma often reactive; mantle cell lymphomas often unreactive	Low-affinity Fc receptor for IgE; upregulated by EBV infection

Continued.

Table 21-2 Principal antibodies employed in staining fresh cells in suspension or in cytospins and frozen sections—cont'd

CD-antigen or antibody	Predominant normal cell reactivity	Reactivity in neoplasms	Comment/caution
B-lymphocyte subsets—cont'd			
CD32	Mantle zone B-cells, many macrophages, plasma cells	Most lymphomas of mantle zone B-cells, subset of follicular and other B-cell lymphomas, myeloid leukemias, plasma cell neoplasms	Low-affinity Fc receptor for IgG; reactivity with many follicular lymphomas may be useful in diagnosis
CD35 (TO5)	Mantle and marginal zone B cells, follicular dendritic cells, some macrophages	Most lymphomas of mantle and marginal zone B cells, follicular dendritic cell tumors	C3b (CR1) complement receptor
CD38 (OKT10, Leu-17)	Lymphoid progenitor cells, NK cells, plasma cells	Some B and T lymphomas, especially of progenitor cells, plasma cell neoplasms	One of few markers commonly expressed by plasma cell neoplasms
T lymphocytes			
CD2 (OKT11, Leu-5)	T cells, NK cells	Most T-cell lymphomas and leukemias, few myeloid leukemias	Sheep erythrocyte receptor
CD3 (OKT3, Leu-4)	T cells	Most T-cell lymphomas and leukemias	Associated with antigen receptor in a multimolecular complex; T-lymphoblastic lymphomas and leukemias more often show cytoplasmic rather than surface expression
CD5 (OKT1, Leu-1)	T cells, weak expression by small B-cell subset	Most T-cell lymphomas and leukemias, many diffuse small B-cell neoplasms	CD5-reactive B-cells may be elevated in autoimmune disorders; expression of CD5 by many diffuse small B-cell neoplasms useful in diagnosis
CD7 (3A1, Leu-9)	Most T cells, NK cells	Many T-cell lymphomas and leukemias, some myeloid leukemias	Earliest expressed antigen in T-cell ontogeny and one of best T-cell markers for lymphoblastic neoplasms; most commonly deleted antigen in post-thymic T-cell malignancy, particularly mycosis fungoides
T-cell receptor beta chain (WT1, βF1)	T cells	Most T-cell lymphomas leukemias	Some T-cell lymphomas, especially thymic ones, lack expression; few of the cases that lack expression show the alternative γδ receptor
T-lymphocyte subsets			
CD1A (NA134, OKT6, Leu-3)	Cortical thymocytes, Langerhans' cells	Many thymic T-cell lymphomas and leukemias, Langerhans' cell histiocytosis	Reliable marker for many precursor T-cell neoplasms; thymomas are rich in CD1A-positive thymocytes
CD4 (OKT4. Leu-3)	Most helper/inducer T cells, class II MHC restricted T cells, many macrophages, many dendritic cells including follicular dendritic and Langerhans' cells	Many post-thymic T-cell lymphomas, often lacking or expressed together with CD8 on T-precursor neoplasms; many accessory cell neoplasms; some myeloid leukemias	HIV receptor generally predominates; reactive and neoplastic disorders may be one of myelomonocytic markers; expressed in some plasma cell neoplasms
CD8 (OKT8, Leu-2)	Most cytotoxic/suppressor T cells, class I MHC restricted, subset of NK cells splenic sinus lining cells	Minority of post-thymic T-cell lymphomas, often lacking or expressed together with CD4 on T-precursor neoplasms	Generally minority of T-subset neoplasms, but may predominate in early phase of some viral infections and in late phase of HIV infection
T-cell receptor delta chain	Few T cells	Few T-cell lymphomas and leukemias (predominantly thymic ones)	Reactive and neoplastic γδ T cells generally lack expression of both CD4 and CD8

Table 21-2 Principal antibodies employed in staining fresh cells in suspension or in cytospins and frozen sections—cont'd

CD-antigen or antibody	Predominant normal cell reactivity	Reactivity in neoplasms	Comment/caution
Myelomonocytic cells			
CD11c (Leu-M5)	Myelomonocytic cells	Hairy cell leukemia, monocytoid B-cell lymphoma, few small B-cell lymphomas/leukemias, few T-cell lymphomas, some myeloid leukemias especially M4 and M5, Langerhans' cell histiocytosis	Sensitive but not totally specific marker for hairy cell leukemia or monocytoid B-cell lymphoma
CD13 (My7)	Myelomonocytic cells, many macrophages, interdigitating dendritic cells	Most myeloid leukemias from M1-M5, few B-lymphoblastic leukemias, rare T-lymphoblastic leukemias	Some nonhematolymphoid cells
CD14 (Mo2, Leu-M3)	Monocytes and macrophages, dendritic cells, including follicular, interdigitating, and Langerhans' cells	Many M4 or M5 leukemias	My4 antibody but not others such as Leu-M3 reacts with some B-cell lymphomas and rare T-cell lymphomas
CD33 (My 9)	Early myeloid cells and all monocytes	Most myeloid leukemias	B-cell and T-cell lymphomas unreactive
Natural killer cells			
CD16 (Leu-11)	NK cells, granulocytes	Many NK proliferative disorders	IgG Fc receptor III
CD56 (Leu-19, NKH1)	NK cells, few T cells	Many NK proliferative disorders, many nasal non–B-lymphomas, plasma cell neoplasms	Reactivity with neoplastic but not reactive plasma cells may be useful for diagnosis; reacts with neural and neuroendocrine cells and their neoplasms
Miscellaneous			
CD25 (TAC)	Activated T cells, B-cells, and monocytes	Adult T-cell lymphoma/leukemia, hairy cell leukemia, most anaplastic large cell lymphomas, Reed-Sternberg cells in many cases of Hodgkin's disease, some other B-cell and T-cell lymphomas	Low-affinity interleukin-2 receptor
CD34 (HPCA1)	Progenitor cells, endothelial cells	Some myeloid leukemias, some lymphoblastic leukemias	Useful in identifying some difficult-to-classify hematolymphoid neoplasms; useful for diagnosis of vascular tumors
Ki-67	Cells not in G0 phase of cell cycle (proliferating cells)	Cells not in G0 phase of cell cycle	General correlation with grade of lymphoma; most consistent correlation in lymphomas as is between high proliferation fraction and adverse survival in low-grade B-cell lymphoma; may be useful in differentiating proliferating tumor cells from nonproliferating host cells
TdT	Precursor cells in marrow, cortical thymocytes	Most lymphoblastic lymphomas and leukemias of a T- or B-lineage, some myeloid leukemias	Useful as marker of precursor cell lymphoma/leukemia

EBV, Epstein-Barr virus; *HIV,* human immunodeficiency virus; *MHC,* major histocompatibility complex; *NK,* natural killer.
From Warnke RA, Weiss LM, Chan JKC, Cleary ML, Dorfman RF: Tumors of the lymph nodes and spleen. Atlas of tumor pathology, 3rd Series, Fascicle 14, Washington, DC, 1995, Armed Forces Institute of Pathology.

Table 21-3 Recurrent chromosomal abnormalities in lymphomas

Chromosomal abnormality	Most frequent types of lymphoma	Antigen receptor gene	Oncogene
t(8;14)(q24;q32)	Small noncleaved cell lymphoma	IgH	c-*myc*
t(2;8)(2p12;q24)	(Burkitt's and non-Burkitt's); some	Igκ	c-*myc*
t(8;22)(q24;q11)	diffuse large cell lymphomas (B-cell type)	Igλ	c-*myc*
t(14;18)(q32;q21)	Follicular lymphoma, subset of large B-cell lymphomas	IgH	bcl-2
t(11;14)(q13;q32)	Mantle cell lymphoma	IgH	bcl-1 (PRAD 1)
t(3;v)(q27;v)*	Large cell lymphoma	IgH, Igκ, Igλ, others	bcl-6 (LAZ 3)
t(14;v)(q11;v)	Lymphoblastic lymphoma, adult T-cell leukemia/lymphoma	TCRα/TCRδ	Several
t(14;v)(q32;v)	Occasional small lymphocytic lymphoma, diffuse large cell lymphoma, others	IgH	bcl-3, unknown
t(7;v)(q35;v)	Lymphoblastic lymphoma (T-cell type)	TCRβ	Several
t(2;5)(p23;q35)	Anaplastic large cell lymphoma, others	NA†	NPM-ALK fusion gene

*Variable.
†NA = Not applicable.
From Warnke RA, Weiss LM, Chan JKC, Cleary ML, Dorfman RF: Tumors of the lymph nodes and spleen. Atlas of tumor pathology, 3rd Series, Fascicle 14. Washington DC, 1995, Armed Forces Institute of Pathology.

Chromosomal studies

Several nonrandom chromosomal translocations have been detected in malignant lymphoma (Table 21-3).[32-36] Remarkably, most of these translocations are associated with specific lymphoma subtypes even if exceptions occur. Many result from errors in the rearrangement of antigen receptor genes in progenitor B or T lymphocytes; they lead to deregulated expression of cellular oncogenes following their juxtaposition with antigen receptor genes. Probes for some of these oncogenes (such as bcl-2, bcl-1, bcl-6, and *myc*) may be used for molecular genetic studies. Since rearrangement of the bcl-2 gene is the molecular marker of the t(14;18) chromosomal translocation, its detection by Southern blot techniques can be used as a substitute for conventional cytogenetic analysis.

Gene rearrangement analysis

Antigen receptor genes code for immunoglobulin and T-cell receptor protein molecules. B-cells express immunoglobulins in both a membrane and soluble form, whereas T-cells express T-cell receptors, which are membrane-bound molecules. These two kinds of molecules have significant functional and structural similarities and are involved in the specific recognition of antigens by lymphocytes.

Both molecules are multisubunit glycoproteins. Each subunit can be divided roughly into two parts: a constant region and a variable region. Variable regions of two subunits collaborate to form highly specific antigen-binding sites. A given lymphocyte, throughout its lifetime, can express only one type of variable region for each of two (or in the case of T-cells, at most three) antigen receptor subunits.

Genetic rearrangements that occur within the genes of these subunits determine which variable region is expressed for a given subunit (Fig. 21-1). During the lifetime of a lyphocyte, rearrangement generally occurs only once per allele or twice for a given gene, since there are two alleles for each gene. The rearrangement can be detected by Southern blot or polymerase chain reaction (PCR).[40] The Southern blot hybridization procedure is used to assess the size of rearranged fragments using a radiolabeled DNA hybridization probe specific for DNA sequences in or around the constant region. This procedure results in an autoradiogram in which a rearranged fragment can be identified as a dark band. In practice, detecting a rearrangement of antigen receptor DNA in a biopsy specimen requires that 1% or greater of the total number of cells within the specimen carry uniform rearrangements within their genome.

Three general types of applications of gene rearrangements to the diagnosis of lymphoid neoplasms exist: (1) for the differential diagnosis between benign and malignant lesions, (2) as markers for B- or T-cell derivation, and (3) as markers for the presence of multiple lymphocytic clones in a single patient (Tables 21-4 and 21-5).[37,39,41,42]

Application for the primary diagnosis of malignancy assumes that clonal proliferations of lymphocytes correlate with neoplasia, an assumption that remains controversial. However, even if clonal antigen receptor gene rearrangements were not absolutely specific for neoplasia, they can still be confidently used for the staging or detection of relapse in lymphoid cases with established diagnosis.

Applications of antigen receptor gene rearrangements for determining the B- or T-cell derivation of a given tumor rely on the fact that rearrangements of these genes occur only in lymphoid tissues. Immunoglobulin gene rearrangements are largely limited to cells of B lineage, and T-cell receptor rearrangements are generally restricted to cells of T lineage, although exceptions occur.

The technique can be adapted to fine-needle aspiration material and to formalin-fixed, paraffin-embedded material.[38]

DNA ploidy studies

Examination of DNA ploidy by flow cytometry of cell suspensions from fluids or material from fine-needle aspiration or from tissue sections has shown a good correlation

Table 21-4 Usual antigen receptor gene status in various lymphoproliferative lesions

Abnormality	IgH	Igκ	Igλ	TCRβ	TCRγ	TCRδ
Normal lymphoid tissue	G	G	G	G	Rp	Rp
Reactive lymphoid tissue	G	G	G	G	Rp	Rp
Lymphoid hyperplasia in a setting of immunodeficiency	G/R	Rp	G	G	Rp	Rp
B-cell lymphoma	R	R	G/R	G/R	G/Rp	G/Rp
T-cell lymphoma	G/R	G	G	R	R	R
Hodgkin's disease	G/R	G	G	G	Rp	Rp
Hodgkin's disease lymphocyte predominance	G	G	G	G	Rp	Rp

G, Germline band; R, rearranged band; Rp, polyclonal rearranged bands.
Some T-cell lymphomas may lack detectable TCR gene rearrangements. AILD-like T-cell lymphomas show a fairly high frequency of simultaneous IgH gene rearrangements (30% to 40%).
From Warnke RA, Weiss LM, Chan JKC, Cleary ML, Dorfman RF: Tumors of the lymph nodes and spleen. Atlas of tumor pathology, 3rd Series, Fascicle 14. Washington, DC, 1995, Armed Forces Institute of Pathology.

Table 21-5 Commonly encountered gene rearrangement patterns and their interpretation

Antigen receptor gene status					Most probable interpretation
IgH	Igκ	Igλ	TCRβ	TCRγ	
R	R	G	G	G	B-cell neoplasms
R	R	R	G	G	B-cell neoplasms
G	G	G	R	R	T-cell neoplasm
R	G	G	R	R	T-cell neoplasm
G	G	G	G	G	No molecular support for lymphoma

R, Rearranged band; G, germline band.
From Warnke RA, Weiss LM, Chan JKC, Cleary ML, Dorfman RF: Tumors of the lymph nodes and spleen. Atlas of tumor pathology, 3rd Series, Fascicle 14. Washington, DC, 1995, Armed Forces Institute of Pathology.

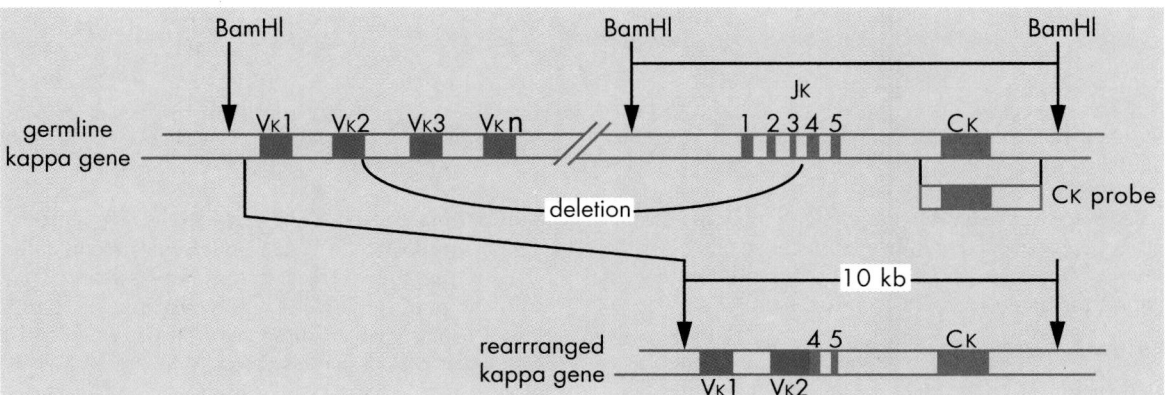

Fig. 21-1 Schematic representation of immunoglobulin gene rearrangement. The germline configuration of the kappa light chain gene *(upper line)* consists of numerous variable gene segments (V-kappa, 1-n), five joining gene segments (J-kappa, 1-5), and a single constant region gene segment (C-kappa). To assemble a functional light chain gene *(lower line),* select V and J segments are juxtaposed with each other by deletion of the intervening DNA. The deletion reconfigures restriction enzyme cutting sites upstream of J-kappa, changing the size of the BamH1 fragment detected with a C-kappa hybridization probe (12 kb germline verus 10kb rearranged in figure). (From Warnke RA, Weiss LM, Chan JKC, Cleary ML, Dorfman RF: Tumors of the lymph nodes and spleen. Atlas of tumor pathology, 3rd Series, Fascicle 14, Washington, DC, 1995 Armed Forces Institute of Pathology.)

Table 21-6 Differential diagnosis based upon recognition of predominant pattern in lymph node at low magnification

Follicular/ nodular	Interfollicular/ paracortical	Diffuse	Sinus	Mixed/other
Non-neoplastic				
Reactive follicular hyperplasia	Immunoblastic proliferations	Immunoblastic proliferations	Sinus hyperplasia	Mixed hyperplasia
Explosive follicular hyperplasia (HIV)	Viral lymphadenitis (EBV, CMV, herpes)	Viral lymphadenitis (EBV, CMV, herpes)	Rosai-Dorfman disease	Dermatopathic lymphadenopathy
Progressive trans-formation of germinal centers	Post-vaccination lymphadenitis	Post-vaccination lymphadenitis	Lymphangiogram effect	Toxoplasmosis
Castleman's disease	Drug sensitivity, e.g., Dilantin	Drug sensitivity e.g., Dilantin	Whipple's disease	Cat-scratch disease
Rheumatoid lymphadenopathy			Vascular transfor-mation of sinuses	Systemic lupus erythematosus
Luetic lymphadenitis			Hemophagocytic syndrome	Kawasaki's disease
Kimura's disease				Kikuchi's lymph-adenitis
				Granulomatosis lymphadenitis
				Inflammatory pseudotumor
Uncertain if neoplastic				
Nodular lymphocyte predominance HD		Angioimmuno-blastic lympha-denopathy	Langerhans' cell histiocytosis	Systemic Castle-man's disease
Neoplastic				
Nodular sclerosing HD	Interfollicular HD	Mixed cellularity HD	Sinusoidal large cell lymphoma	Mucosa-associated lymphoid tissue lymphoma
Follicular lymphoma	T-zone lymphoma	Small cell B/T lym-phoma/leukemia	Mastocytosis	Monocytoid B-cell lymphoma
Mantle cell lymphoma	Mixed cellularity HD	Large cell B/T lym-phoma	Nonlymphoid leu-kemia	
Monocytoid B-cell lymphoma	Small cell B/T lym-phoma/leukemia	Lymphoblastic lym-phoma/leukemia	Histiocytic neoplasms	
CLL/SLL with pro-liferation centers	Large cell B/T lym-phoma	Burkitt's lymphoma	Non-hematolymph-oid neoplasms	
	Lymphoblastic lym-phoma/leukemia	Plasmacytoma		
	Burkitt's lymphoma	Anaplastic large cell lymphoma		
	Plasmacytoma	Nonlymphoid leukemia		
	Nonlymphoid leukemia	Mastocytosis		
	Mastocytosis	Histiocytic neoplasms		
	Histiocytic neoplasms	Non-hematolymph-oid neoplasms		
	Non-hematolymph-oid neoplasms			

From Warnke RA, Weiss LM, Chan JKC, Cleary ML, Dorfman RF: Tumors of the lymph nodes and spleen. Atlas of tumor pathology, 3rd Series, Fascicle 14. Washington, DC, 1995, Armed Forces Institute of Pathology.

with the microscopic grades of malignant lymphoma.[43,44,46] Whether it provides prognostic information above and beyond that obtainable from conventional morphology and immuno-phenotyping of the tumors remains controversial.[43,45]

PRIMARY IMMUNODEFICIENCIES

The many varieties of primary immunodeficiencies can be broadly divided in three major categories according to the type of the immunologic deficit: humoral, cell-mediated, and combined.[47,51] The diagnosis of these disorders is based on a variety of laboratory tests, including qualitative and quan-titative immunoglobulin determinations, delayed-type skin reactions, and in vitro stimulation of lymphocytes. Some-times lymph nodes are biopsied to assess the amount and composition of the lymphoid tissue. In immune diseases of the humoral type, cortical reactive centers and medullary plasma cells are scanty or absent.[50] In diseases of cell-medi-

ated immunity, the thickness of the paracortical area is greatly diminished.[50] When both humoral and cell-mediated types of immunities are defective, the lymphocyte and plasma cell content of the node is practically nil. The lymph node is reduced to a mass of connective tissue and blood vessels.[49] If an antigen such as diphtheria or tetanus toxoid is injected into the medial aspect of the thigh and an ipsilateral inguinal node is biopsied 5 to 7 days later, its capacity to react to the antigenic stimulus can be evaluated.[48]

The increased susceptibility of patients with primary immunodeficiencies to the development of malignant lym-phoma is discussed on p. 1736.

PATTERNS OF HYPERPLASIA

The various components of the lymph node react to vari-ous known and unknown stimuli by undergoing reactive changes, some related to an inflammatory reaction and some

Table 21-7 Architectural and cytologic features of follicular lymphoma and of reactive follicular hyperplasia

Follicular lymphoma	Reactive follicular hyperplasia
Architectural features	
Complete effacement of normal architecture	Preservation of nodal architecture
Even distribution of follicles throughout cortex and medulla	Follicles more prominent in cortical portion of lymph node
Slight or moderate variations in size and shape of follicles	Marked variations in size and shape of follicles with presence of elongated, angulated, and dumbbell-shaped forms
Fading of follicles	Sharply demarcated reaction centers
Massive infiltration of capsule and pericapsular fat with or without formation of neoplastic follicles outside capsule	No, or only moderate, infiltration of capsule and pericapsular fat tissue with inflammatory cells that may be arranged in perivascular focal aggregates (when associated with lymphadenitis)
Condensation of reticulin fibers at periphery of follicles	Little or no alteration of reticular framework
Cytologic features	
Follicles composed of neoplastic cells exhibiting cellular pleomorphism with nuclear irregularities	Centers of follicles (reaction centers) composed of lymphoid cells, histiocytes, and "reticulum cells," with few or no cellular and nuclear irregularities
Lack of phagocytosis	Active phagocytosis in reaction centers
Relative paucity of mitotic figures usually without significant difference in their number inside and outside the follicles; occurrence of atypical mitoses	Moderate to pronounced mitotic activity in reaction centers; rare or no mitoses outside reaction centers; no atypical mitoses
Similarity of cell type inside and outside follicles	Infiltration of tissue between reaction centers with inflammatory cells (when associated with lymphadenitis)

Slightly modified from Rappaport H, Winter WJ, Hicks EB: Follicular lymphoma. A re-evaluation of its position in the scheme of malignant lymphoma, based on a survey of 253 cases. Cancer **9:**792-821, 1956.

to an immune response, the two often being present together. A similar microscopic picture may result from a variety of causes, but some agents produce a characteristic microscopic picture. When the hyperplastic change is very intense, the differential diagnosis with malignant lymphoma may become difficult.[52]

Although most lymph node reactions involve several compartments, it is useful to evaluate these compartments individually, not only because their presence and relative intensity correlates with various specific disorders (thus providing important etiologic clues), but also because each of them raises differential diagnostic problems with different types of malignant processes. From a topographic and functional standpoint, the major patterns of reactive lymphoid proliferations are follicular/nodular, interfollicular/paracortical, diffuse, sinusal, and mixed. These patterns also apply to the various types of malignant lymphoma (Table 21-6).[53]

Follicular hyperplasia

The criteria laid down in the classic article by Rappaport et al.[57] and further developed by Nathwani et al.[56] remain extremely useful and reliable to distinguish reactive follicular hyperplasia from follicular lymphoma (Table 21-7). In general, reactive follicles vary considerably in size and shape; their margins are sharply defined and surrounded by a mantle of small lymphocytes often arranged circumferentially with an onion-skin pattern and sometimes concentrating on one pole of the follicle (corresponding to the side of the antigenic stimulation); the follicles are composed of an admixture of small and large lymphoid cells with irregular (elongated and cleaved) nuclei; mitoses are numerous; and phagocytosis of nuclear debris by histiocytes is prominent. The lymphoid tissue present between the follicles is distinctly different from that of the follicles themselves (although this

also may be true for follicular lymphoma); it is composed of a mixture of small lymphocytes, large lymphoid cells, prominent postcapillary venules, and sometimes, an admixture of mature plasma cells (Fig. 21-2).

If doubts persist, diagnostic assistance can be obtained by performing cell marker studies for immunoglobulin light chains, MT2, and bcl-2[54,55,58] (see p. 1668).

Progressively and regressively transformed germinal centers

Progressively transformed germinal centers is a term that has applied to a morphologically distinct type of reactive germinal center. They usually are seen in conjunction with more typical reactive germinal centers and are often located more centrally within the node (Fig. 21-3). They are large and contain numerous small lymphocytes, the borders are indistinct, and the interphase between the center of large lymphoid cells and the cuff of small lymphocytes is blurred. However, residual "starry sky" macrophages are present, together with scattered large lymphoid cells (cleaved and noncleaved) and occasional collections of epithelioid cells at the periphery.[64] There is an increased network of follicular dendritic cells, a larger number of mantle zone lymphocytes, and a relatively large number of T lymphocytes.[66] Evaluation of these features should allow the differential diagnosis between progressively transformed germinal centers and follicular lymphoma to be made with ease in most instances; however, cases exist in which this is extremely difficult on the basis of routinely stained sections.[62]

Progressively transformed germinal centers can occur as an isolated reactive process, particularly in young men.[60,63] However, they also show an interesting and still poorly understood relation with nodular lymphocyte predominance Hodgkin's disease (NLPHD), which may manifest itself in three ways: they may precede the development of NLPHD, they may accompany NLPHD in involved nodes, or they may appear in the absence of NLPHD in recurrent post-therapy adenopathy[59,61,65] (see p. 1703).

Regressively transformed germinal centers are small, practically devoid of lymphoid cells, and composed of follicular dendritic cells, vascular endothelial cells, and hyalinized PAS-positive intercellular material. These abnormal centers have an onion-skin appearance in low-power examination. Regressively transformed germinal centers are particularly prominent and numerous in Castleman's disease (see p. 1688).

Paracortical hyperplasia

Expansion of the paracortical (interfollicular) region can be nodular or diffuse. The nodular form is characteristic of dermatopathic lymphadenitis (see p. 1693) and of nodal

reactions to malignancy.[67] The diffuse form is a feature of viral lymphadenitis (see p. 1685) and drug reactions (see p. 1693), and of immunoblastic proliferations in general (Fig. 21-4).

Sinus hyperplasia

The sinuses appear dilated and prominent in various disorders. The most common and least significant is *sinus hyperplasia* (sinus histiocytosis, sinus catarrh) seen in nodes draining infectious or neoplastic processes and characterized by an increased number of macrophages in the lumen (Fig. 21-5). Other reactive disorders involving primarily the sinuses are sinus histiocytosis with massive lymphadenopathy (Rosai-Dorfman's disease, see p. 1694), Langerhans' cell granulomatosis (histiocytosis X, see p. 1695), Whipple's disease, vascular transformation of sinuses, and virus-associated hemophagocytic syndrome (see Chapter 23).

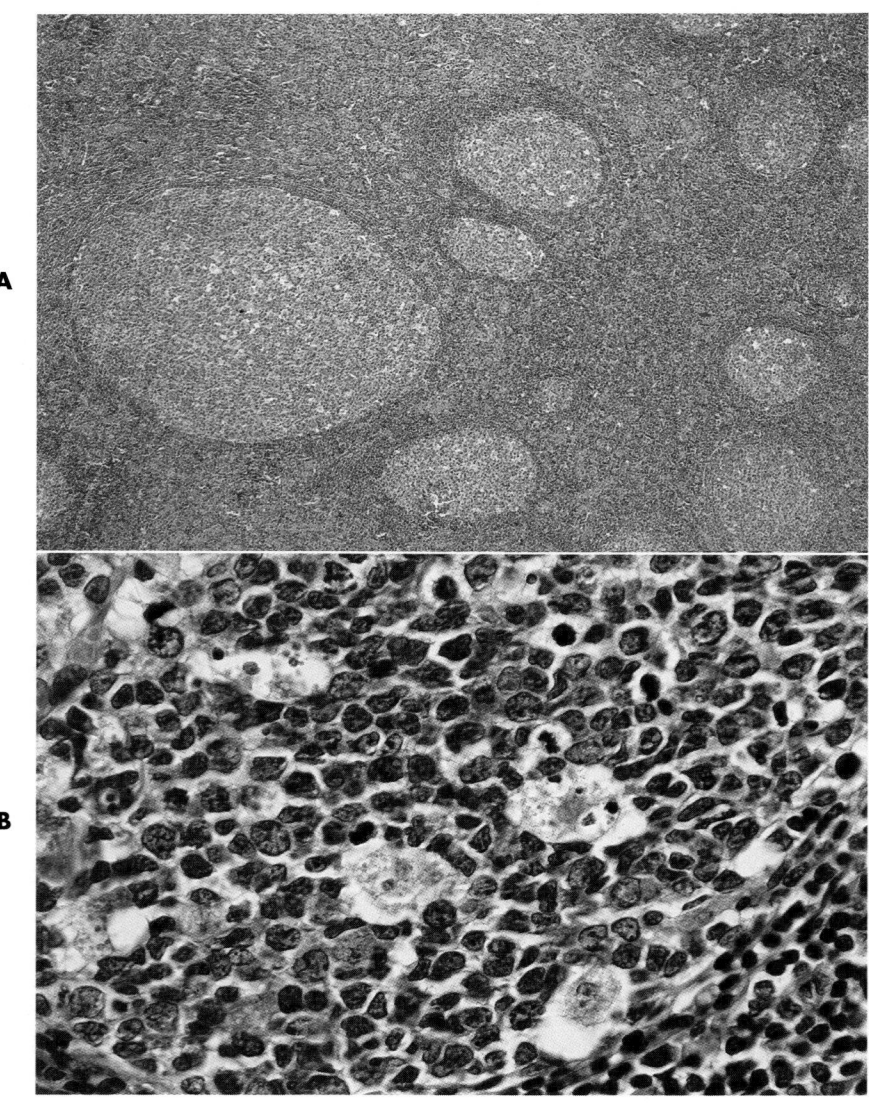

Fig. 21-2 Follicular hyperplasia. **A,** Low-power view showing marked differences in size of germinal centers, their well-circumscribed character, and the fact that they are surrounded by a well-defined mantle. **B,** High-power view showing numerous "tingible-body" macrophages.

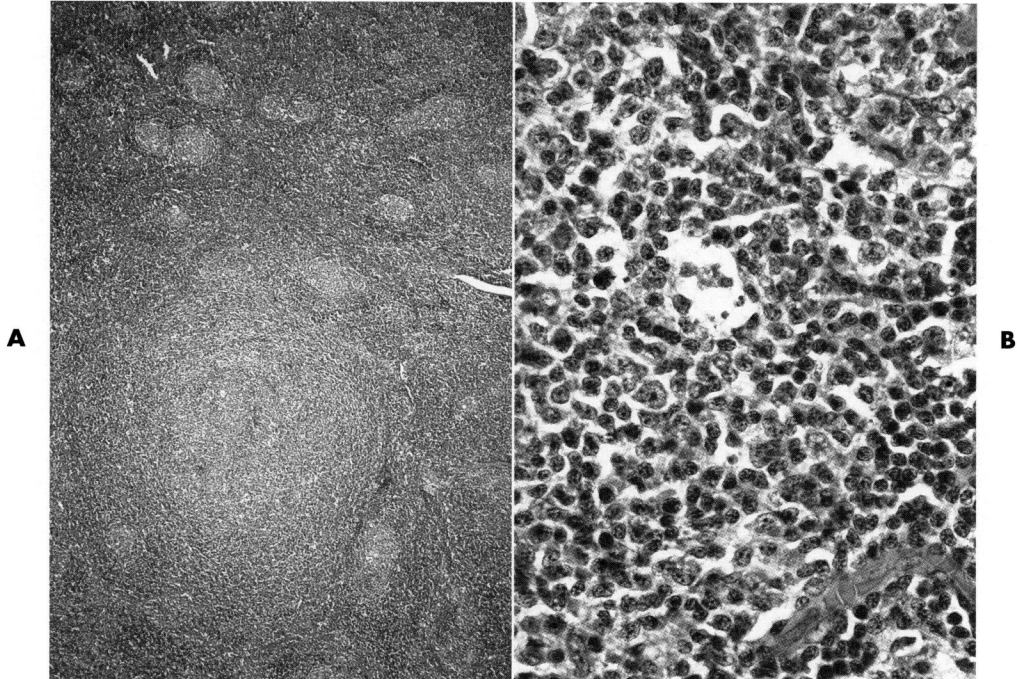

Fig. 21-3 Progressively transformed germinal centers. **A,** Low-power view showing that this formation is larger and less well defined than the adjacent hyperplastic follicles. **B,** High-power view showing cytologic composition not too dissimilar from that of ordinary hyperplastic follicles.

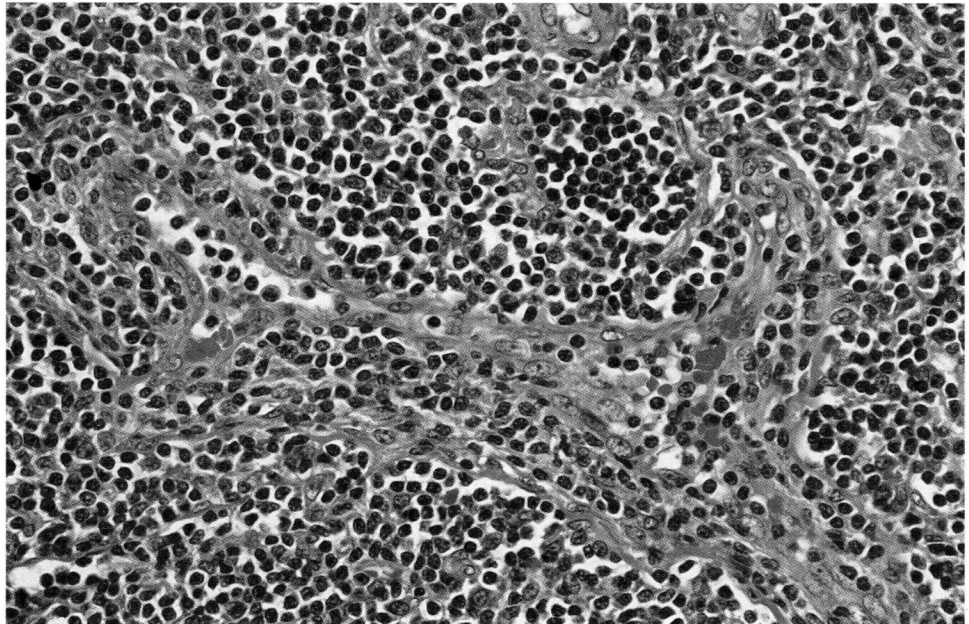

Fig. 21-4 Paracortical hyperplasia, identified by the prominence of postcapillary venules.

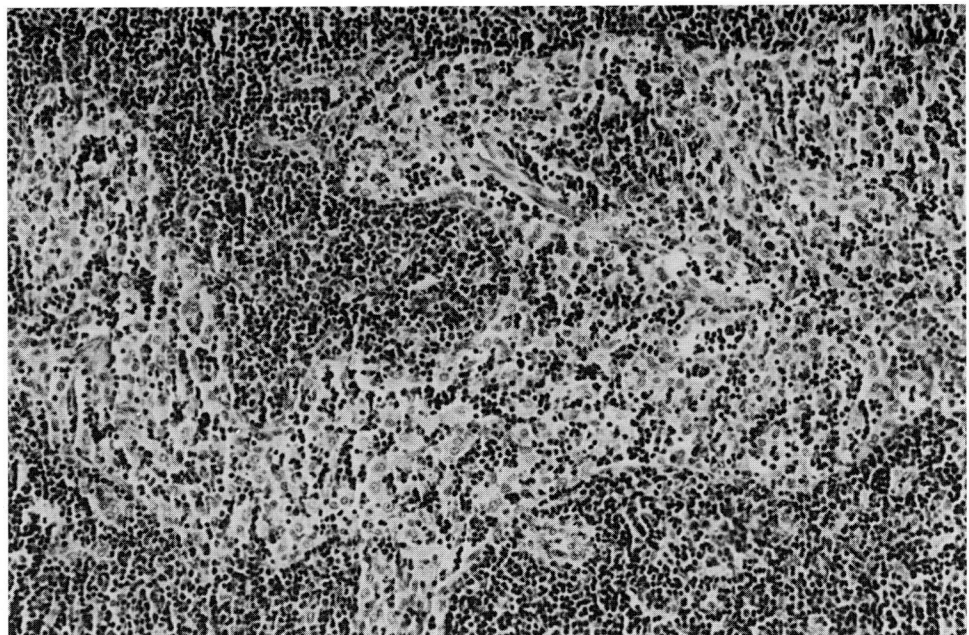

Fig. 21-5 Nonspecific sinus hyperplasia of lymph node. Dilated sinuses contain large number of sinus histiocytes and lymphocytes. This nonspecific reaction should not be equated to entity known as sinus histiocytosis with massive lymphadenopathy.

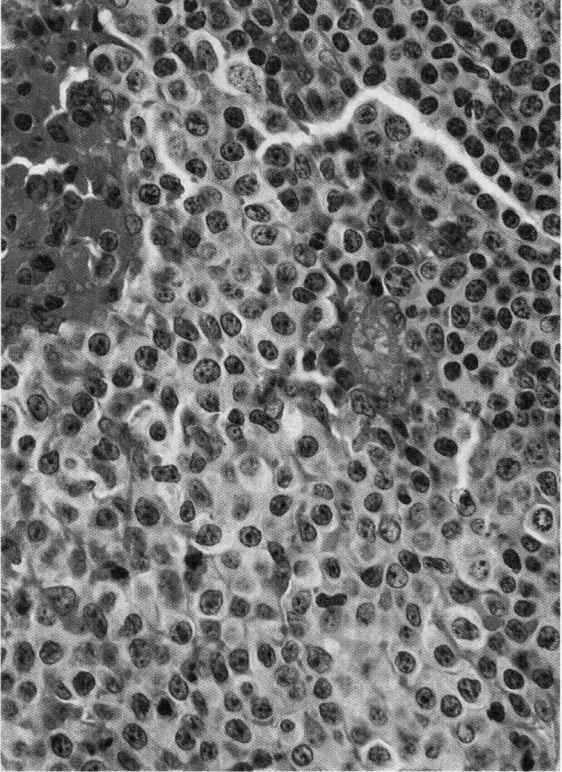

Fig. 21-6 Monocytoid B-cell hyperplasia. These cells are characterized by centrally located nuclei and clear appearance of the cytoplasm.

Granulomatous inflammation

There is a large number of diseases that can result in granulomatous formations in lymph nodes. They include various types of infections, foreign body reactions, and secondary responses in lymph nodes draining carcinoma[68,73] or in patients with Hodgkin's disease and other lymphomas, whether the node is involved by the malignancy or not.[69,70,72] Sometimes the appearance of the granulomas is such that a specific diagnosis can be strongly suggested on the basis of the hematoxylin-eosin–stained slide.[71] Features of importance in this regard are the presence and type of necrosis; presence, number, and size of Langhans' giant cells; size, shape, and distribution of the granulomas; and type of associated changes in the intervening tissue. In most cases, however, a combination of clinical, morphologic, and bacteriologic data is necessary to determine the etiology of the granulomas. It is therefore important that any node suspected of harboring a granulomatous process be sampled for bacteriologic analysis in addition to being subjected to the standard microscopic examination.

Other patterns

Monocytoid B-cell hyperplasia

Monocytoid B-cell hyperplasia is characterized by the filling of the sinuses by small lymphoid cells with round or angulated nuclei and clear cytoplasm, sometimes admixed with neutrophils (Fig. 21-6). A variant characterized by the presence of a larger cell component has also been recognized.[77] It was originally described as immature sinus histiocytosis, but marker studies have shown that these monocytoid clear cells are of B-cell type.[78,80] This alteration occurs

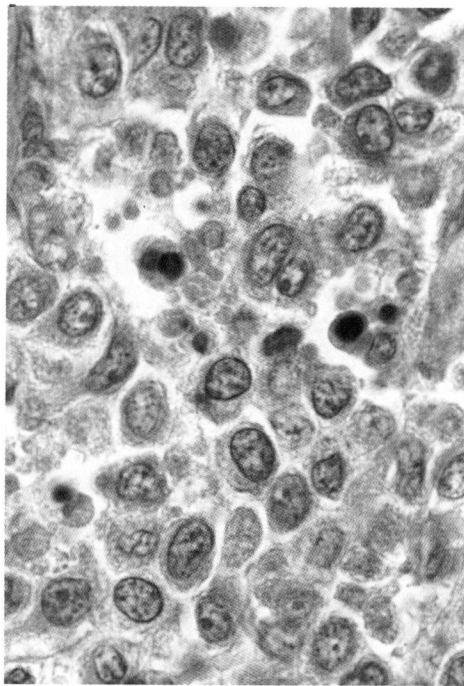

Fig. 21-7 Plasmacytoid monocytes. The nuclear lateralization and the perinuclear halo result in a resemblance to plasma cells. (Courtesy Dr. Glauco Frizzera, New York.)

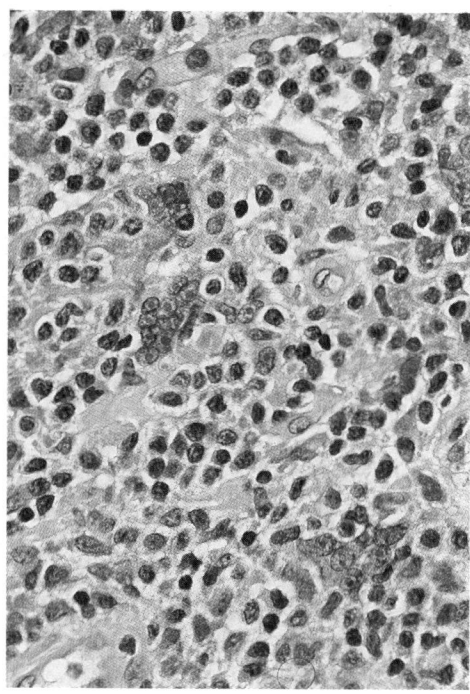

Fig. 21-8 So-called polykaryocytes. These cells are characterized by numerous clustered nuclei and barely identified cytoplasm.

most frequently in toxoplasmosis, but it has also been seen in many other reactive disorders, such as cat-scratch disease,[75] infectious mononucleosis, AIDS, and autoimmune disorders[74]; it may also accompany malignant lymphomas, including Hodgkin's disease.[76] It should be distinguished from other nodal lesions featuring cells with clear cytoplasm (such as peripheral T-cell lymphomas, hairy cell leukemia, and mastocytosis) and also from a type of malignant lymphoma composed of cells with features of monocytoid B-cells (variously known as monocytoid B, MALT-lymphoma, and marginal zone lymphoma) (see p. 1723).[79]

Plasmacytoid monocytes

Clusters of cells with plasmacytoid cytoplasm, fine nuclear chromatin pattern, and small nucleoli are sometimes seen in a variety of reactive nodal lesions (Fig. 21-7). Pyknosis and "starry-sky" pattern may be present.[88] These cells were originally interpreted as T-associated plasma cells and later as a subtype of T cells, but more recent marker studies have shown that they belong to the macrophage/monocyte series. Accordingly, these cells have been renamed plasmacytoid monocytes.[81,85] They are particularly common in necrotizing lymphadenitis and Castleman's disease,[83,84] but they can also be seen in other lymphadenitides.[82] A variety of malignant lymphoma composed of plasmacytoid monocytes has also been described.[86,87] (see p. 1734).

Polykaryocytes

The term *polykaryocyte* is used for a type of multinucleated giant cells found in lymphoid tissues, of which the Warthin-Finkeldey giant cell of measles is the paradigm.

These cells can be found in lymph nodes in association with a variety of reactive and neoplastic disorders. They measure 25 to 150 μm in diameter and have as many as sixty nuclei arranged in grapevine clusters.[90] Their cytoplasm is very scanty (Fig. 21-8). Cell marker studies have shown that these cells are lymphoid rather than histiocytic, and that they display a T-cell phenotype.[89]

INFLAMMATORY/HYPERPLASTIC DISEASES

Acute nonspecific lymphadenitis

The typical case of acute nonspecific lymphadenitis is rarely biopsied. Microscopically, the earliest change is sinus dilatation resulting from increased flow of lymph, followed by accumulation of neutrophils, vascular dilatation, and edema of the capsule. *Suppurative lymphadenitis* is a feature of staphylococcal infections, mesenteric lymphadenitis (see p. 1682), lymphogranuloma venereum (see p. 1683), and cat-scratch disease (see p. 1682). *Necrotizing features* may be seen in bubonic plague, tularemia, anthrax, typhoid fever, melioidosis, and the entity known as necrotizing lymphadenitis (see next section).

Necrotizing lymphadenitis

Necrotizing lymphadenitis (Kikuchi's lymphadenitis) is seen most commonly in Japan and other Asian countries,[92] but it also occurs elsewhere, including the United States and Western Europe. Most patients are young women with a persistent, painless cervical lymphadenopathy of modest dimensions that may be accompanied by fever. Microscopically, the affected nodes show focal, well-circumscribed, paracortical necrotizing lesions. There are abundant karyor-

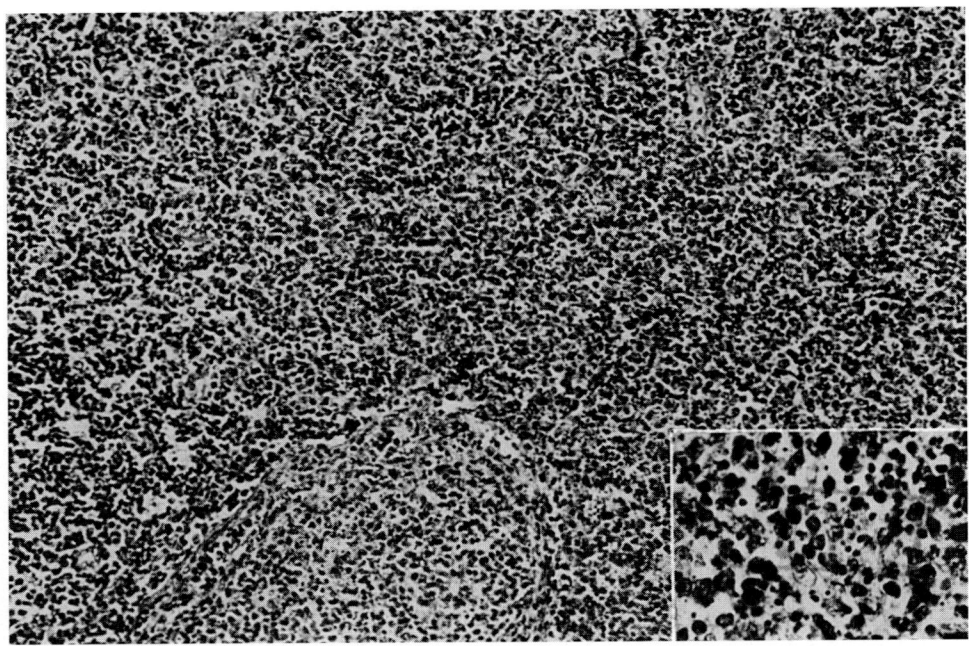

Fig. 21-9 Necrotizing lymphadenitis. Reactive germinal center can be appreciated in lower portion of the illustration, but remainder of lymph node shows extensive necrosis. **Inset** demonstrates large number of nuclear fragments throughout node, some of them within the cytoplasm of macrophages.

rhectic debris, scattered fibrin deposits, and collections of large mononuclear cells[94] (Fig. 21-9). Plasma cells and neutrophils are very scanty, a feature of diagnostic importance.[100,105] Instead, plasmacytoid monocytes are often numerous.[96,102] When the latter cells grow in a diffuse fashion, the appearance may simulate that of malignant lymphoma.[91,104] On occasion, a prominent secondary xanthomatous reaction is seen.[99] Ultrastructurally, tubuloreticular structures and intracytoplasmic rodlets similar to those described in lupus erythematosus are often found.[95]

The diagnosis can be made or at least suspected in material from fine-needle aspiration because of the prominence of phagocytic histiocytes with peripherally placed ("crescentic") nuclei and medium-sized cells with eccentrically placed nuclei consistent with plasmacytoid monocytes.[103]

The evolution is generally benign and self-limited. However, cases have been described with recurrent lymphadenopathy or accompanied by skin lesions.[98] Isolated fatal cases are also on record.[93] The etiology is unknown; an early suggestion that *Toxoplasma* may be involved has not been substantiated. Epstein-Barr virus and human herpes virus type 6 have also been implicated,[101] but the evidence is not conclusive.[97] The most important differential diagnosis is with malignant lymphoma with secondary necrosis.

Chronic nonspecific lymphadenitis

The morphologic features and the very concept of chronic lymphadenitis merge with those of hyperplasia (see p. 1670.) The general features of chronic lymphadenitis are follicular hyperplasia; prominence of postcapillary venules; increased number of immunoblasts, plasma cells, and histiocytes; and fibrosis. The capsule may appear inflamed

and/or fibrotic, and the process may extend into the immediate perinodal tissues. In some cases, one may find an undue predominance in the number of eosinophils, foamy macrophages, and/or mast cells. Terms such as *eosinophilic* or *xanthogranulomatous lymphadenitis* have been sometimes used, depending on the type of the infiltrate.[106] The presence of numerous eosinophils in a lymph node should raise the possibility of Langerhans' cell granulomatosis (histiocytosis X), parasitic infections, Hodgkin's disease, and autoimmune disorders.

Tuberculosis

Lymph nodes involved by tuberculosis may become adherent to each other and form a large multinodular mass that can be confused clinically with metastatic carcinoma (Fig. 21-10). The most common location of clinically apparent lymphadenopathy is the cervical region ("scrofula"), where a draining sinus that communicates with the skin ("scrofuloderma") may form. Microscopically, the appearance ranges from multiple small epithelioid granulomas reminiscent of sarcoidosis to huge caseous masses surrounded by Langhans' giant cells, epithelioid cells, and lymphocytes. Demonstration of the organisms by special stains or cultures is necessary to establish the diagnosis.

Atypical mycobacteriosis

Atypical mycobacteria are a common cause of granulomatous lymphadenitis. A caseating granulomatous disease in a cervical lymph node of a child unaccompanied by pulmonary involvement is more likely to be caused by an atypical organism than by *Mycobacterium tuberculosis*. The process typically involves lateral nodes in the midportion of the

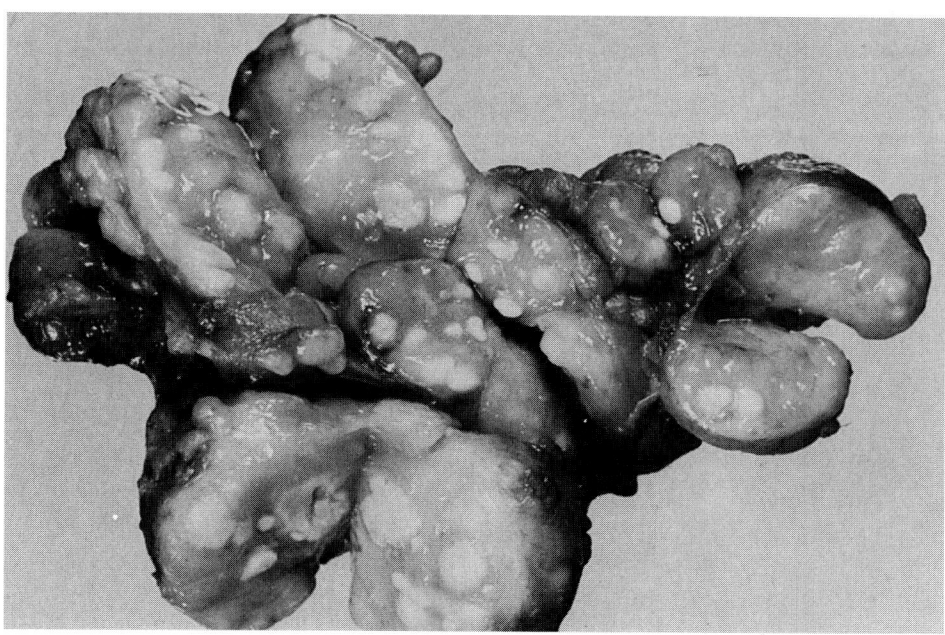

Fig. 21-10 Large adherent tuberculous lymph nodes containing extensive foci of caseation necrosis.

neck. Drainage may continue for months or years in the absence of specific therapy, and healing may result in scarring and contractures. Microscopically, the host reaction may be indistinguishable from that of tuberculosis, but often the granulomatous response is overshadowed by suppurative changes.[107-109] A nontuberculous mycobacterial etiology should also be suspected if the granulomas are ill-defined (nonpalisading), irregularly shaped, or serpiginous.[108] An acid-fast stain should be performed in every granulomatous and suppurative lymphadenitis of unknown etiology, especially if the patient is a child. The final identification of the organism rests on the cultural characteristics.

Sarcoidosis

The diagnosis of sarcoidosis is always one of exclusion. A noncaseating granulomatous inflammation in the lymph nodes or skin microscopically indistinguishable from sarcoidosis can be seen in tuberculosis, atypical mycobacteriosis (including swimming pool granuloma), fungous diseases, leprosy, syphilis, leishmaniasis, brucellosis, tularemia, chalazion, zirconium granuloma, berylliosis, Crohn's disease, Hodgkin's disease; in nodes draining a carcinoma; and in several other conditions.[112] Only when all these possibilities have been excluded and the clinical picture is characteristic is there justification in labeling a case as sarcoidosis. Whether this is a specific disease or a peculiar granulomatous reaction to a variety of agents remains a moot point.[128] Scandinavian countries are particularly affected.[127] In the United States, the disease is ten to fifteen times more common in blacks than in whites. Practically every organ can be involved, but the ones most commonly affected are the lung, lymph nodes, eyes, skin,

and liver.[111,114,117] Erythema nodosum often precedes or accompanies the disease. Functional hypoparathyroidism is the rule, although a few cases of sarcoidosis co-existing with primary hyperparathyroidism have been reported.[113,132]

Microscopically, the basic lesion is a small granuloma mainly composed of epithelioid cells, with scattered Langhans' giant cells and lymphocytes[125] (Figs. 21-11 and 21-12). Necrosis is either absent or limited to a small central fibrinoid focus. Schaumann bodies, asteroid bodies, and calcium oxalate crystals are sometimes found in the cytoplasm of the giant cells[124] (Fig. 21-13). None of these inclusions are specific for sarcoidosis. Schaumann bodies are round, have concentric laminations, and contain iron and calcium. Ultrastructurally, asteroid bodies are composed of radiating filamentous arms enveloped by "myelonoid" membranes.[121] Elemental analysis has shown a calcium peak and a probable phosphorus peak in these formations.[121] Peculiar PAS-positive inclusions known as Hamazaki-Wesenberg, yellow, or ovoid bodies[131] were claimed to be specific for sarcoidosis, but subsequent histochemical and ultrastructural studies[126] have shown that they have no etiologic or pathogenetic significance. They probably represent large lysosomes containing hemolipofuscin material and are found in a large variety of conditions.[124,129]

Most of the lymphocytes present in the sarcoidal granulomas are T cells with the helper phenotype; both these cells and the epithelioid histiocytes exhibit features of proliferation and/or activation, as shown by their immunocytochemical positivity with the Ki67 antibody and for interleukin-1, respectively.[110,115] Pathogenetically, sarcoidsis is thought to represent a dysfunction of circulat-

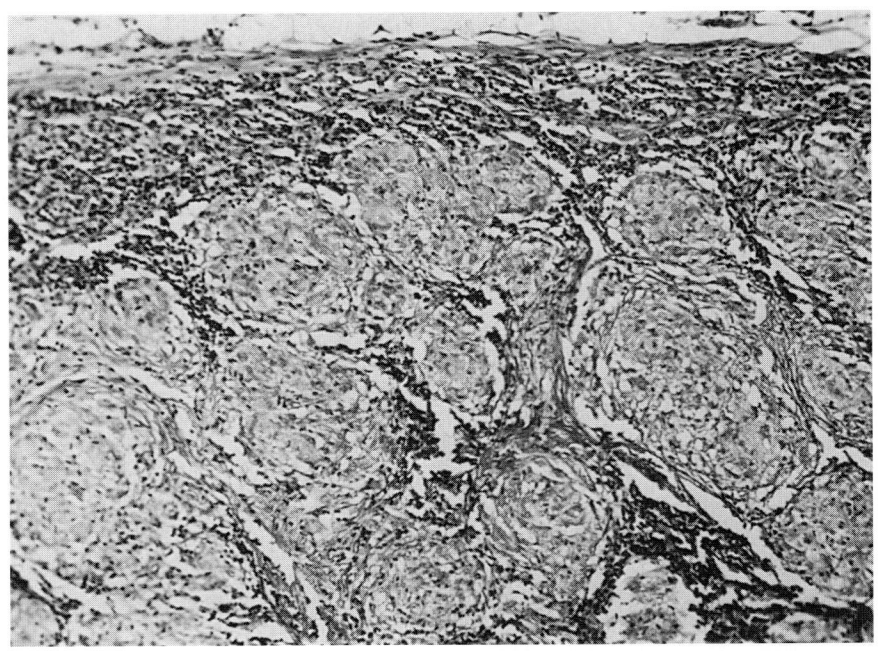

Fig. 21-11 Lymph node involved by sarcoidosis demonstrating noncaseating granulomatous lesions.

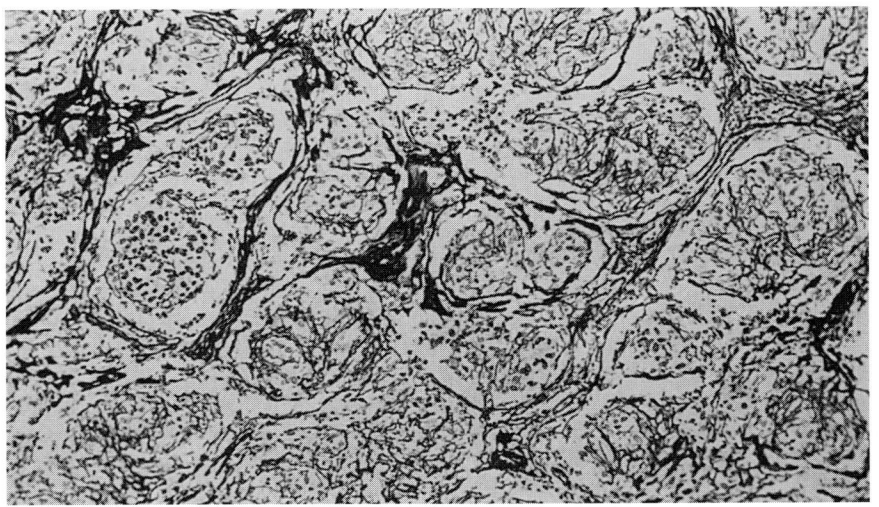

Fig. 21-12 Even distribution of reticulin in sarcoidosis.

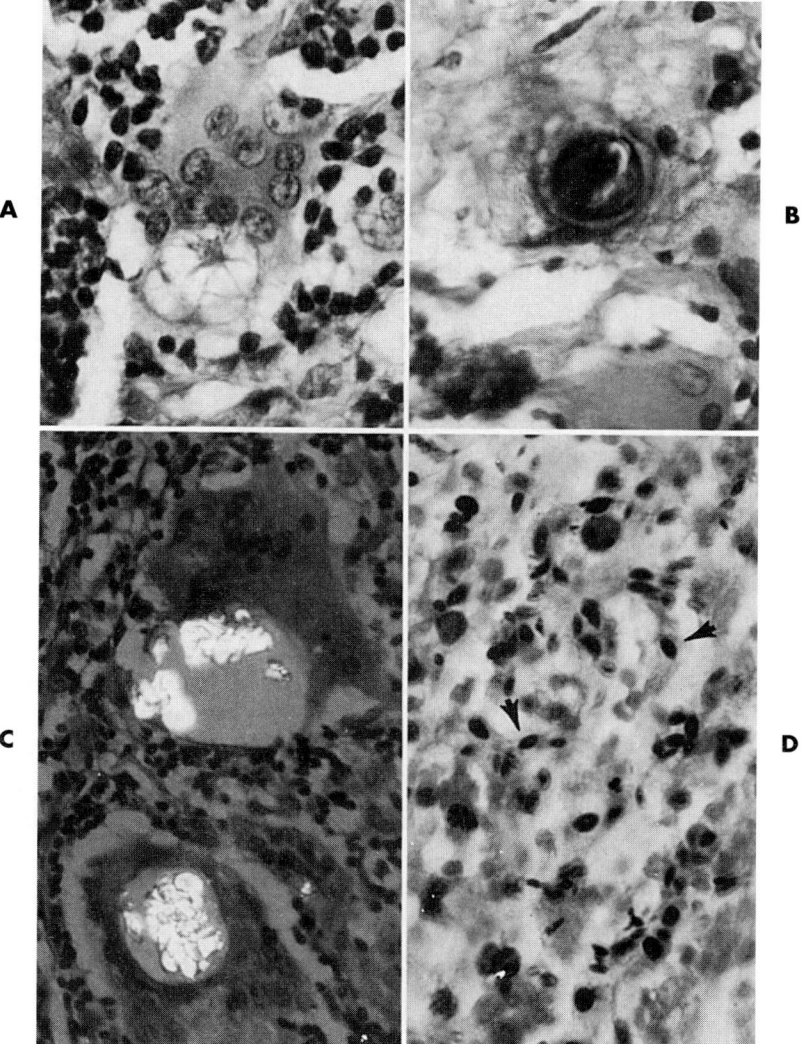

Fig. 21-13 Four types of inclusions that can be found in sarcoidosis. None of them is specific for this condition. **A,** Asteroid body within cytoplasm of multinucleated giant cell. **B,** Schaumann body. Note round shape and concentric lamination. **C,** Calcium oxalate crystals under polarized light. **D,** So-called Wesenberg-Hamasaki bodies concentrated in perivascular location. They are of small size and have oval or needle-like configuration *(arrows)*. All sections are from same case and originated in lymph node involved by disease. (**D** acid-fast stain.) (Slides contributed by Dr. F.B. Johnson, Washington, D.C.)

ing T-cells with overactivity of B-cells.[120] The association of particular HLA antigens with sarcoidosis suggests a role for HLA-linked immune response genes and disease susceptibility.[118]

The Kveim test for sarcoidosis is an intradermal reaction that occurs following inoculation with an extract of human spleen involved with the disease. It is positive in 60% to 85% of patients with sarcoidosis, and the number of false-positive results is small. The test is regarded as positive when a biopsy of the area taken 4 to 6 weeks after inoculation shows microscopically sarcoid-type granuloma. A trial employing a single test suspension among 2400 subjects in thirty-seven countries on six continents showed a similar level of reactivity and microscopic appearance from country to country,

supporting the concept that sarcoidosis is the same disease the world over. The Kveim test is rarely practiced today because of lack of availability of the antigen.

The etiology of sarcoidosis remains elusive. Mycobacterial organisms have long been suspected.[116] Substances like α-diaminopimelic acid and mycolic acid, which occur in mycobacteria but are foreign to human tissue, have been identified in sarcoid lesions.[123] In several careful microscopic and cultural studies performed on morphologically typical cases of sarcoidosis, acid-fast organisms have been identified in a significant number.[122,130] However, and despite some statements to the contrary, PCR studies have failed to demonstrate mycobacterial DNA in lesions of sarcoidosis.[119]

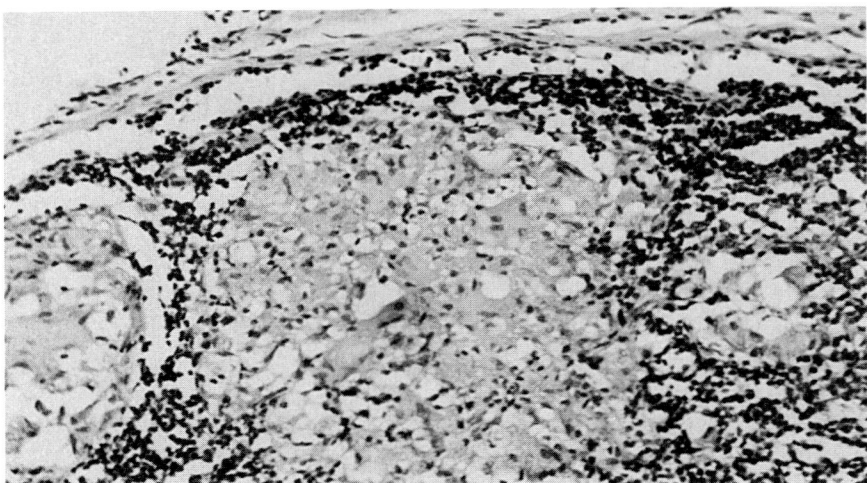

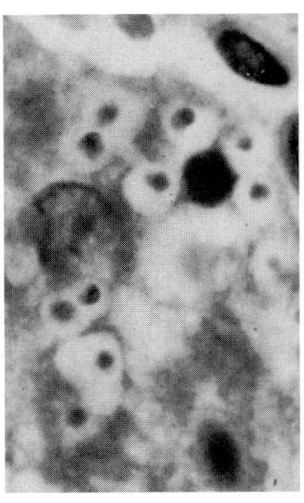

Fig. 21-14 Noncaseating lesion in axillary lymph node. No organisms could be identified. At postmortem examination it was discovered that patient had disseminated histoplasmosis.

Fig. 21-15 Histoplasmosis. Note well-defined bodies surrounded by clear area.

Fungal infections

Fungal infections of lymph nodes may present as chronic suppurative lesions, as granulomatous processes, or as a combination of the two. The most important fungal lymphadenitis is *histoplasmosis*, which in addition to the previously mentioned patterns can also result in widespread nodal necrosis and in marked diffuse hyperplasia of sinus histiocytes (Figs. 21-14 and 21-15). Other fungal diseases known to result in lymphadenitis are blastomycosis, paracoccidioidomycosis, coccidioidomycosis, and sporotrichosis. To these, one should add opportunistic infections such as cryptococcosis, aspergillosis, mucormycosis, and candidiasis.

The fungal organisms can usually be demonstrated with Gomori methenamine-silver (GMS) or PAS-Gridley stains, but sometimes their number is so small that they can be detected only in cultures.

Toxoplasmosis

Toxoplasmic lymphadenitis, in its most typical form, involves the posterior cervical nodes of young women (so-called Piringer-Kuchinka lymphadenitis).[137] On palpation, the nodes are firm and only moderately enlarged. Microscopically, the nodal architecture is rather well preserved. The triad of the disease, which, however, is not present in all cases, is constituted by (1) marked follicular hyperplasia, associated with intense mitotic activity and phagocytosis of nuclear debris; (2) small granulomas composed almost entirely of epithelioid cells, located within the hyperplastic follicles and at the periphery, encroaching on and blurring their margins (Fig. 21-16); these granulomas rarely exhibit necrosis or more than an occasional Langhans' giant cell; and (3) distention of marginal and cortical sinuses by monocytoid B cells. An additional feature is the presence of immunoblasts and plasma cells in the medullary cords.[138]

It is extremely rare to find *Toxoplasma* organisms by morphologic examination and just as difficult to detect the *Tox-*

oplasma gondii genome by PCR.[139] The latter finding contrasts sharply with the results obtained in toxoplasmic encephalitis and myocarditis.[139] However, the combination of microscopic features described correlates remarkably well with serologic studies. Of thirty-one cases studied by Dorfman and Remington,[134] the Sabin-Feldman dye test was positive in all, and the IgM immunofluorescent antibody test was positive in 97% of the cases.

If the diagnosis of toxoplasmic lymphadenitis is suspected from the microscopic pattern, it should be confirmed serologically, keeping in mind that these tests may be normal in the early stages of the disease.[135]

The differential diagnosis of toxoplasmosis includes other infectious diseases and the lymphocyte predominance form of Hodgkin's disease. In this regard, Miettinen et al.[136] have made the interesting point that occurrence of collections of epithelioid cells *within* germinal centers seems to be a nearly specific feature for toxoplasmosis.

Syphilis

Generalized lymphadenopathy is a common finding in secondary syphilis, whereas localized node enlargement can be seen in the primary and tertiary stages of the disease. In secondary syphilis, the changes are those of a florid follicular hyperplasia. In primary syphilis, the combination of changes may result in a mistaken diagnosis of malignant lymphoma. Most of the cases have presented as solitary inguinal lymphadenopathy.[141] There are capsular and pericapsular inflammation and extensive fibrosis, diffuse plasma cell infiltration, proliferation of blood vessels with endothelium swelling and inflammatory infiltration of their wall (phlebitis and endarteritis), and follicular hyperplasia[141] (Fig. 21-17). Rarely, noncaseating granulomas and abscesses are present. Spirochetes can be identified in most cases by the Warthin-Starry or Levaditi stains or by immunofluorescence techniques applied to imprint preparations.[140] The organisms are most frequently found in the wall of blood vessels.

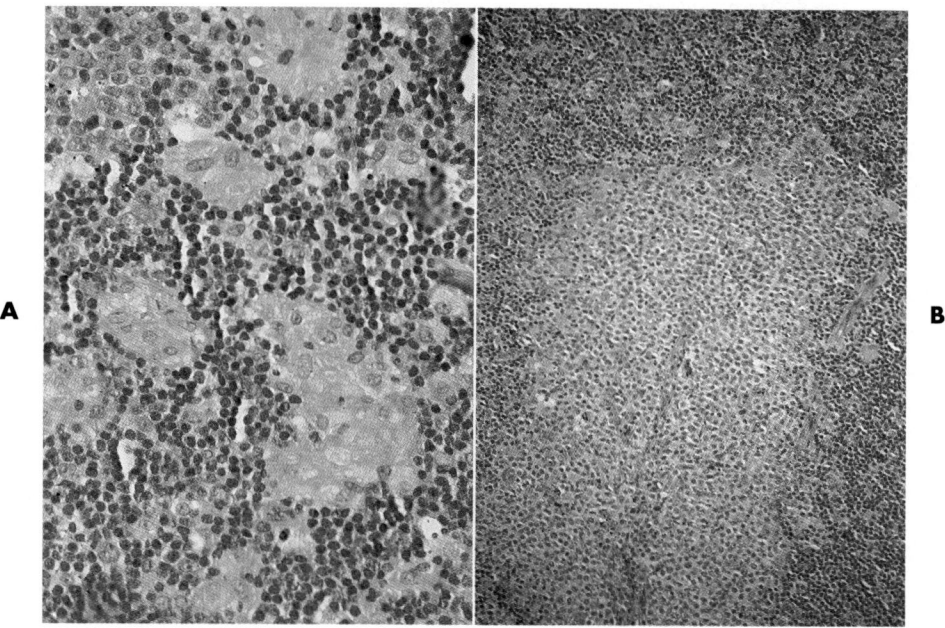

Fig. 21-16 Toxoplasmosis of lymph node. **A,** Small noncaseating granulomas composed of epithelioid cells, located at the periphery of hyperplastic follicle. This picture is almost pathognomonic of this disease. **B,** Area of massive monocytoid B-cell hyperplasia.

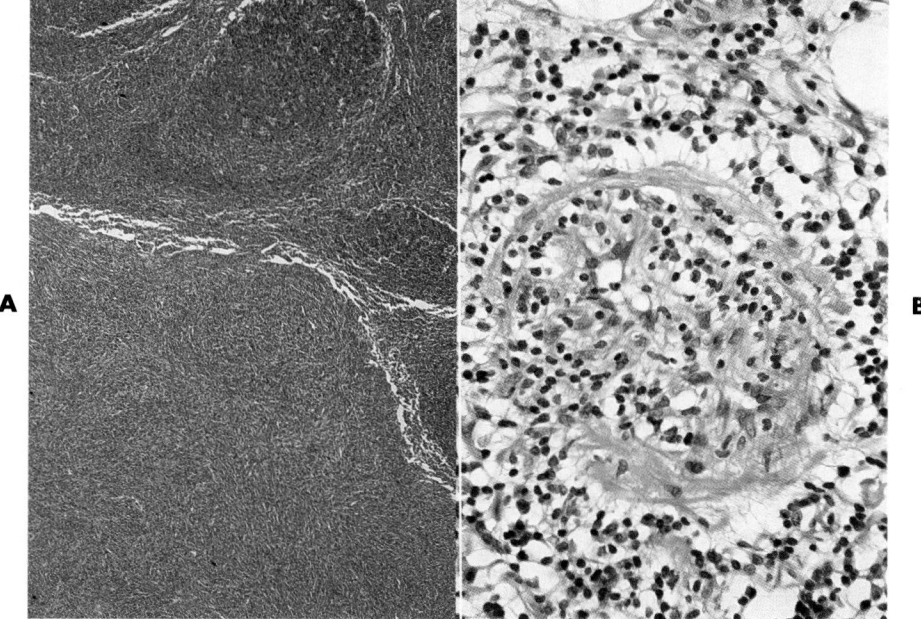

Fig. 21-17 Syphilis of lymph node. **A,** Follicular hyperplasia associated with striking pericapsular inflammatory fibrosis. **B,** The prominent vasculitis seen in this field is an important clue to the diagnosis.

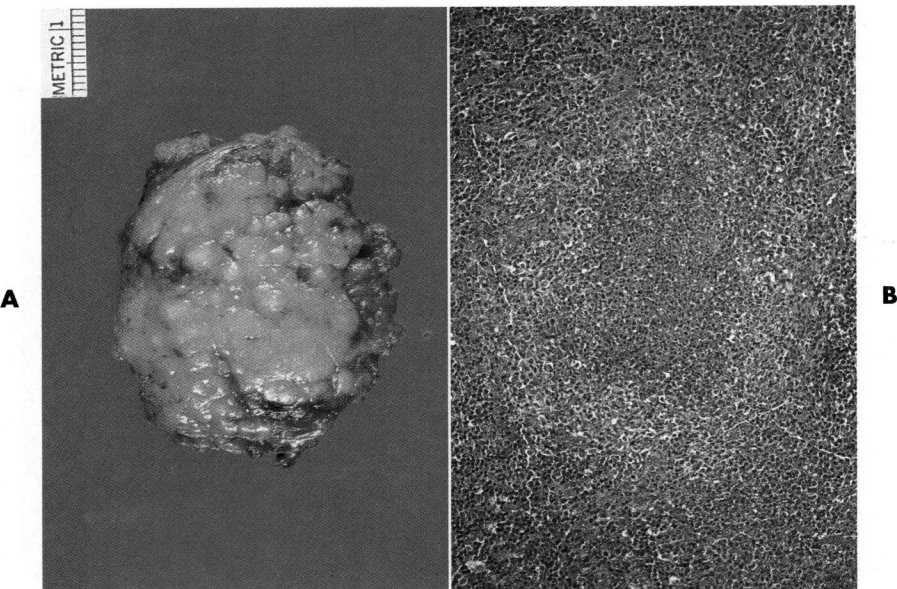

Fig. 21-18 A, Lymph node involved by cat-scratch disease. A large area of necrosis is present in the center. **B,** Area of stellate necrosis in proven case of cat-scratch disease.

Leprosy

Lymph nodes involved by the lepromatous type of leprosy have a very characteristic microscopic appearance. The main change is the progressive accumulation of large, pale, rounded histiocytes ("lepra" or "Virchow" cells), without granuloma formation and with minimal or no necrosis. Wade-Fite and File-Farasco stains (modified Ziehl-Neelsen reactions) demonstrate packing of the cytoplasm by acid-fast organisms.

Mesenteric lymphadenitis

Mesenteric (Masshoff's) lymphadenitis is produced by *Yersinia pseudotuberculosis* or *Yersinia enterocolitica,* two gram-negative polymorphic coccoid or ovoid motile organisms.[143-146] It is a benign, self-limited disease that can clinically simulate acute appendicitis. Microscopically, there are capsular thickening and edema, increase of immunoblasts and plasma cells in the cortical and paracortical region, dilatation of sinuses with accumulation of large lymphocytes within, and germinal center hyperplasia.[142,147] In the lymphadenitis produced by *Yersinia pseudotuberculosis,* small granulomas and abscesses are commonly present, but this is unusual in infection caused by *Yersinia enterocolitica.*[147] These nodal changes are sometimes accompanied by inflammatory changes of the terminal ileum and cecum. Ideally, the diagnosis should be confirmed with cultures. Too often, the diagnosis of mesenteric lymphadenitis is made on normal or mildly hyperplastic nodes in an attempt to explain why a patient with the clinical picture of acute appendicitis has a normal appendix.

Cat-scratch disease

Cat-scratch disease is characterized by a primary cutaneous lesion and enlargement of regional lymph nodes, usually axillary or cervical.[149] The changes in the nodes vary with time. Early lesions have histiocytic proliferation and follicular hyperplasia, intermediate lesions have granulomatous changes, and late lesions have abscesses of various sizes.[161] These abscesses are very suggestive of the diagnosis because of their pattern of central, sometimes stellate necrosis with neutrophils, surrounded by a palisading of histiocytes.[156] However, similar abscesses can be seen in lymphogranuloma venereum. Another common feature of lymph nodes with cat-scratch disease is the packing of sinuses by monocytoid B cells, which together with the follicular hyperplasia, may simulate toxoplasmosis.[155] However, clusters of perifollicular and intrafollicular epithelioid cells are absent[151] (Fig. 21-18).

The primary lesion is a red papule in the skin at the site of inoculation, usually appearing between 7 and 12 days following contact. It may become pustular or crusted. Microscopically, there are foci of necrosis in the dermis surrounded by a mantle of histiocytes. Multinucleated giant cells, lymphocytes, and eosinophils are also present.[154]

The agent of cat-scratch disease is a coccobacillary pleomorphic extracellular bacterium that can be identified with the Warthin-Starry silver stain, particularly in those cases exhibiting extensive necrosis.[152,153,157,160] This organism, which has also been detected ultrastructurally,[159] is thought to belong to the *Rochalimaea* species[148] and has been named *Afipia felis,*[162] even if some questions remain about its taxonomy. The diagnosis of cat-scratch disease can be confirmed by skin testing and by immunocytochemical labeling.[158,162]

Rare complications of the disease include granulomatous conjunctivitis ("oculoglandular syndrome of Parinaud"), thrombocytopenic purpura, and central nervous system manifestations.[150]

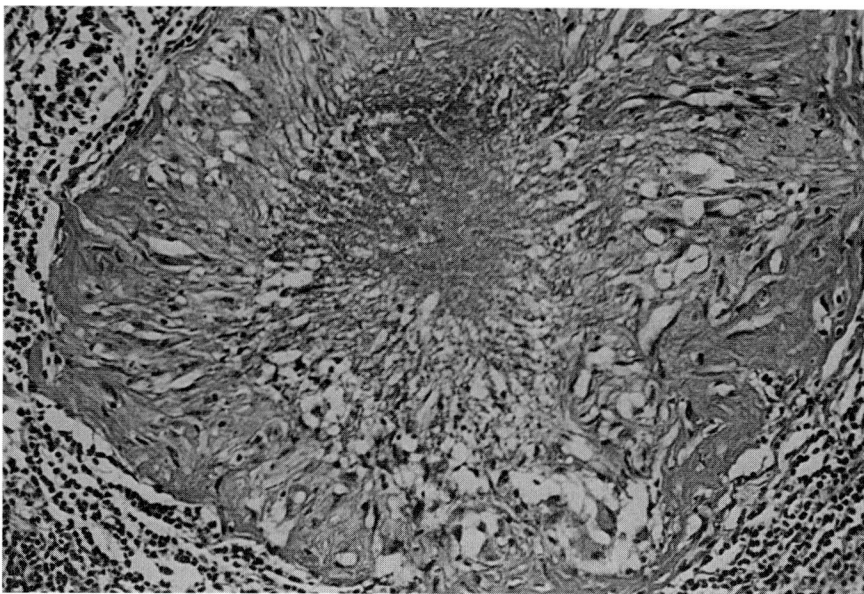

Fig. 21-19 Stellate abscess in lymphogranuloma venereum.

Lymphogranuloma venereum

This sexually transmitted disease (not to be confused with granuloma inguinale) is caused by *Chlamydia* organisms corresponding to serotypes L1, L2, and L3. The initial lesion is a small (2 to 3 mm), painless genital vesicle or ulcer which often goes unnoticed and heals in a few days. This is followed by inguinal adenopathy, which can be very prominent. The earliest microscopic change in an affected node is represented by tiny necrotic foci infiltrated by neutrophils. These enlarge and coalesce to form the stellate abscess that is the most characteristic feature of this disease (Fig. 21-19). In later stages, epithelioid cells, scattered Langhans' giant cells, and fibroblasts are seen to line the walls. Confluence of these abscesses is common, and cutaneous sinus tracts may develop. The healing stage is represented by nodules with dense fibrous walls surrounding amorphous material.[165]

The microscopic picture just described is not pathognomonic of this disease. Similar changes can occur in cat-scratch disease, atypical mycobacteriosis, and tularemia. Therefore a presumptive diagnosis of lymphogranuloma venereum should be confirmed with the Frei test (a delayed hypersensitivity skin test using purified "lygranum" chlamydial antigen), complement fixation, or immunofluorescent testing.[163,166] A monoclonal antibody that has been recently raised against the causative agent may prove useful in the diagnosis of the disease.[164]

Tularemia

Tularemia is a bacterial disease produced by *Francisella tularensis,* an extremely virulent pathogen.[167] In the ulceroglandular form of the disease, prominent lymphadenopathy occurs; this predominates in the axillary region when mammalian vectors are involved and in cervical or inguinal regions with arthropod vectors.[168] A history of handling rabbits suggests the diagnosis in the first instance. The diagnosis is supported by a rise in hemagglutinin titers.[167,169]

Microscopically, the picture in the acute phase is that of an intense lymphadenitis with widespread necrosis. In the more chronic forms, there is a granulomatous reaction that in some cases may have a frankly tuberculoid appearance.[170]

Brucellosis

Brucellosis is caused by *Brucella abortus, melitensis,* or *suis.*[172] In this country it has evolved from an occupational to a foodborne illness related to consumption of milk and cheese.[171] Lymphadenopathy is uncommon and, when present, usually of modest dimensions. Microscopically, there may be nonspecific follicular hyperplasia and clusters of epithelioid histiocytes sometimes forming large noncaseating granulomas. This is accompanied by a polymorphic infiltrate containing eosinophils, plasma cells, and immunoblasts. When the latter are numerous, the microscopic picture may show a vague resemblance to Hodgkin's disease.

A definitive diagnosis can only be made by recovery of the organism or the detection of a high agglutination titer.[173]

AIDS-related lymphadenopathy

The lymph node abnormalities in AIDS patients can be of various types. They include opportunistic infections (some resulting in spindle cell pseudotumors),[185] Kaposi's sarcoma, malignant lymphomas of either Hodgkin's or non-Hodgkin's type, and *florid reactive hyperplasia.*[175,183] The latter change is the most common (Fig. 21-20). It may be accompanied by collections of monocytoid B-cells in the sinuses, neutrophils, and features of dermatopathic lymphadenopathy. In many of the cases, the reactive germinal

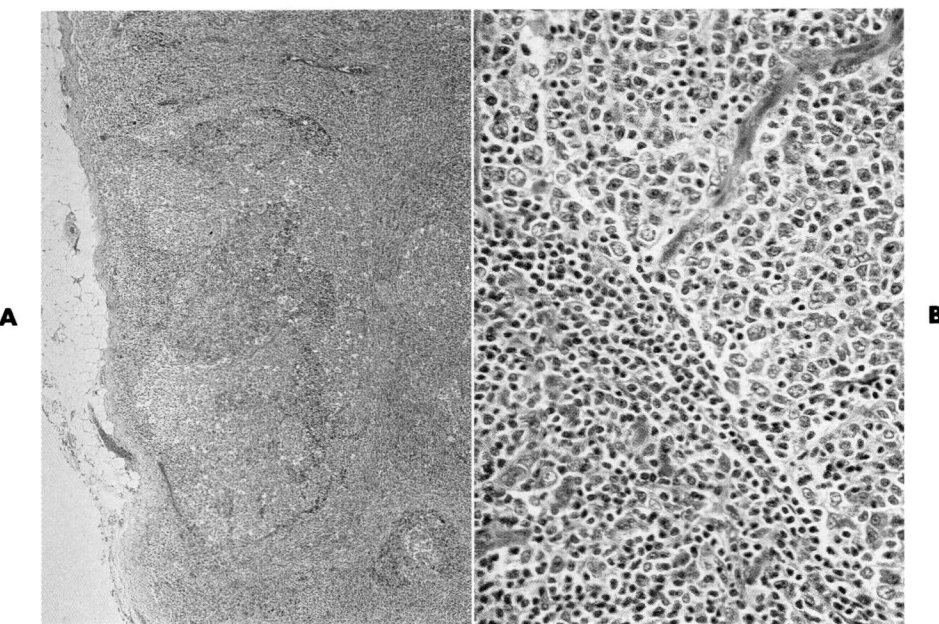

Fig. 21-20 Low-power **(A)** and high-power **(B)** microscopic views AIDS-related lymphadenopathy. The depicted germinal center shows disruption of its architecture by intrusion of small lymphocytes from mantle zone. This is a common but not pathognomonic feature of this disease.

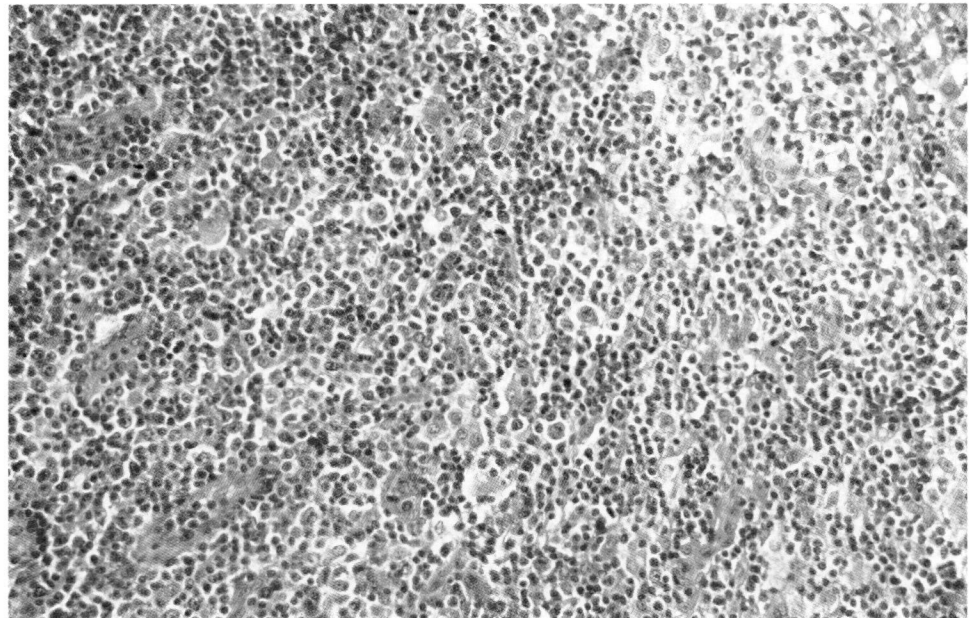

Fig. 21-21 Lymph node involved by infectious mononucleosis. There is a marked effacement of the architecture by a polymorphic lymphoid infiltrate.

centers show a feature termed *follicle lysis,* characterized by invagination of mantle lymphocytes into the germinal centers. This is associated with disruption of these centers ("moth-eaten appearance") and a distinctive clustering of large follicular center cells,[176,187] resulting in an appearance that has been termed *explosive follicular hyperplasia.* Ultrastructurally, a prominence of follicular dendritic cells exhibiting alterations of their fine processes has been described[184]; it has been suggested that the AIDS virus preferentially infects these cells. Immunohistochemically, positive stain for the HIV core protein P24 has been documented within the abnormal germinal centers.[182]

This combination of follicular changes is not pathognomonic of AIDS, but the possibility of this disease should be considered and investigated whenever they are found.

Some lymph nodes in AIDS patients may also show advanced lymphocyte depletion, with or without abnormal (regressively transformed) germinal centers.[176,184]

The interfollicular tissue may show prominent vascular proliferation, the resulting picture acquiring a vague resemblance to Castleman's disease. It is important to search in these areas and in the subcapsular region for the earliest signs of development of Kaposi's sarcoma.[180] These changes should be distinguished from those of vascular transformation of the sinuses (see p. 1745).

A rough relationship has been found among the pattern of nodal reaction, the cell suspension immunophenotypic data, and the patient's HIV status.[177,186]

The term *chronic lymphadenopathy syndrome* has been defined as an unexplained enlargement of nodes of at least 3 months' duration at two or more extrainguinal sites in an individual at risk for AIDS.[174] The microscopic picture is similar to that described previously.[181] Overall, up to a fourth of the patients have developed AIDS on follow-up, cachexia and weight loss being the clinical signs of this progression.[178,179]

Infectious mononucleosis

It is rare for the pathologist to see a lymph node from a patient with a typical clinical picture of infectious mononucleosis because in most instances the presumptive clinical diagnosis is confirmed by examination of the peripheral blood and serologic evaluation. It is in the atypical case, presenting with lymphadenopathy without fever, sore throat, or splenomegaly, that the clinician will perform a lymph node biopsy to rule out the possibility of malignant lymphoma.

Microscopically, nodes and other lymphoid organs affected by infectious mononucleosis can be confused with malignant lymphoma because of the effacement of the architecture; infiltration of the trabecula, capsule, and perinodal fat; and the marked proliferation of immunoblasts, immature plasma cells, and mature plasma cells ("polymorphic B-cell hyperplasia") (Fig. 21-21). These features are particularly prominent when the disease develops in transplant recipients or other immunosuppressed patients.[188] Necrosis may also be present; this is usually only focal but in immunodeficient children may be massive.

Features of importance in the differential diagnosis with lymphoma include predominantly sinusal distribution of the large lymphoid cells, follicular hyperplasia with marked mitotic activity and phagocytosis (these follicles being usually small), increase in the number of plasma cells, and vascular proliferation.[191] Another important feature is the fact that, although the nodal architecture may appear effaced, the sinusal pattern remains intact or even focally accentuated, a fact appreciated particularly well with reticulin stains. Sier-

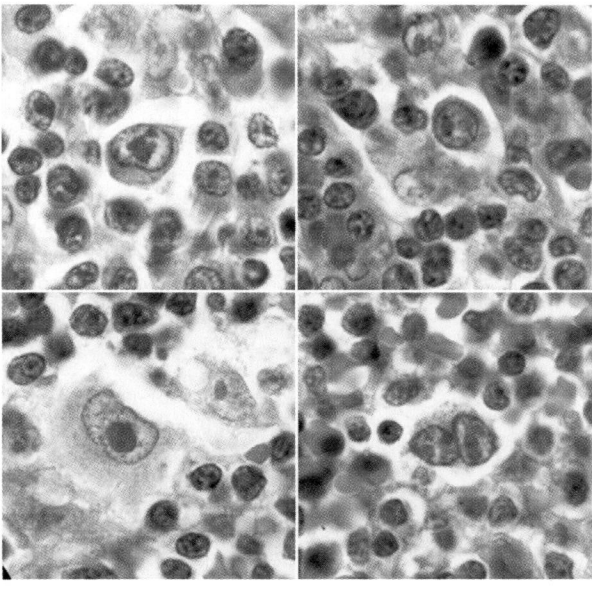

Fig. 21-22 Various types of immunoblasts seen in a lymph node involved by infectious mononucleosis. The binucleated form *(lower right)* can stimulate Reed-Sternberg cells. Note the basophilic character of the nucleus and the presence of a paranuclear hof.

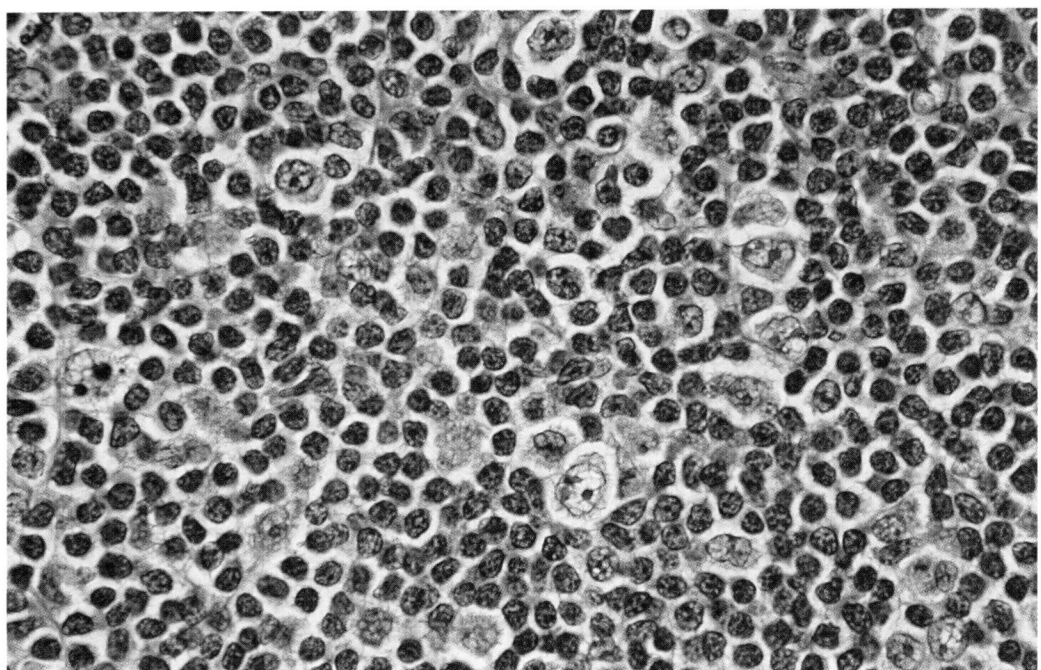

Fig. 21-23 Viral lymphadenitis showing scattered immunoblasts resulting in a "salt-and-pepper" appearance.

acki and Fisher[193] described as a characteristic feature of this disease the presence in the sinuses of clusters or "colonies" of lymphocytes in graduated sizes, from the small lymphocyte to the large lymphoid cell or immunoblast. The latter cell usually has only one large vesicular nucleus with a thin nuclear membrane and one or two prominent amphophilic or basophilic nucleoli. A paranuclear "hof" is often seen. When binucleated, this cell may closely resemble a Reed-Sternberg cell and result in a mistaken diagnosis of Hodgkin's disease[189,195] (Fig. 21-22). Immunophenotyping evaluation should resolve the issue in most cases, despite the existence of an overlap that may be providing a pathogenetic insight into the nature and possible relationship of these two disorders.[190] The diagnosis of infectious mononucleosis can be supported by in situ hybridization techniques.[192,194]

Other viral (including postvaccinial) lymphadenitides

Lymph nodes draining an area of the skin subjected to smallpox vaccination can enlarge and become painful. If removed and examined microscopically, they can be easily confused with lymphoma, especially if the history of vaccination is overlooked. Of twenty cases reported by Hartsock,[199] thirteen were located in the supraclavicular region on the side of the vaccination. The largest node measured 6 cm in diameter. The interval between the vaccination and the biopsy varied between 1 week and 3 months.

Microscopically, the changes are those of a diffuse or nodular paracortical expansion, with mixed cellular proliferation, consisting of eosinophils, plasma cells, and a large number of immunoblasts. The alterations are accompanied by vascular and sinusal changes and focal discrete necrosis. The most important histologic feature of postvaccinal hyperplasia is the presence of numerous immunoblasts scattered among the lymphocytes and imparting to the lymphoid tissue a mottled appearance (Fig. 21-23). Hartsock[199] noted that follicular hyperplasia was present only in those nodes removed more than 15 days after vaccination. These changes have been reproduced experimentally.[199]

Viral lymphadenitis resulting from herpes simplex infection may be localized[202] or generalized.[200] The morphologic features are similar to those of postvaccinial lymphadenitis, particularly in reference to the marked immunoblastic proliferation.[201,203] Intranuclear viral inclusions may be found, especially at the edge of necrotic areas.[196,198] The nodal changes seen in herpes zoster lymphadenitis and infectious mononucleosis are of similar nature; the latter are discussed under a separate heading (see preceding section). It is likely that analogous morphologic changes occurring in the absence of these clinical conditions are, in most cases, the result of some unidentified viral infection.

Prominent regional lymphadenopathy also may follow the administration of live attenuated measles virus vaccine. Microscopically, the typical multinucleated giant cell of Warthin-Finkeldey (polykaryocytes) may be found[197] (see Fig. 11-114).

Mucocutaneous lymph node syndrome

Mucocutaneous lymph node syndrome, also known as Kawasaki's syndrome, is a febrile disorder of unknown eti-

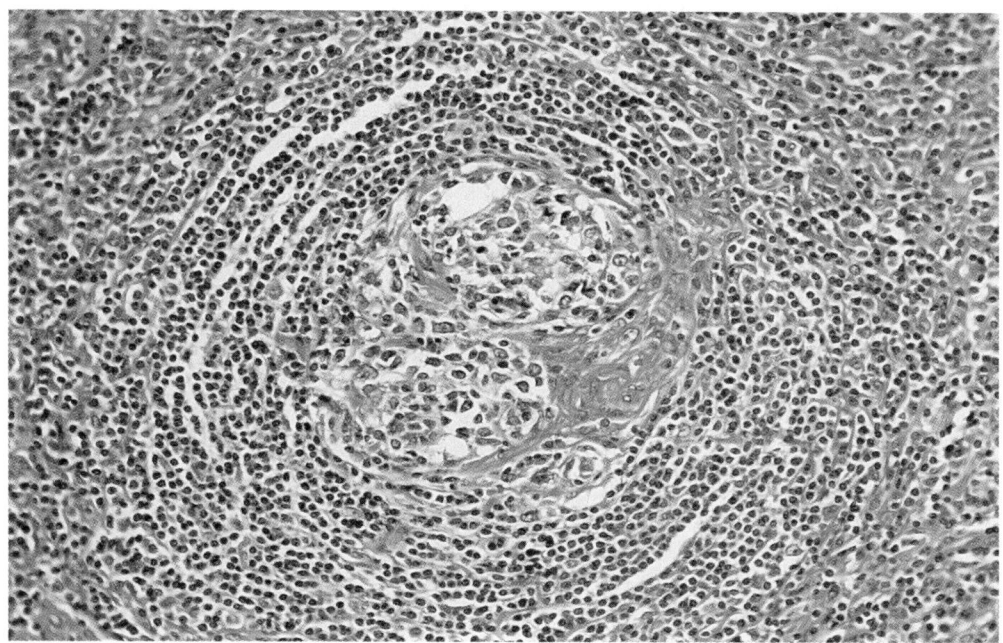

Fig. 21-24 Castleman's disease of vascular hyaline type. There is a prominent germinal center show-ing well-developed vascular hyaline changes.

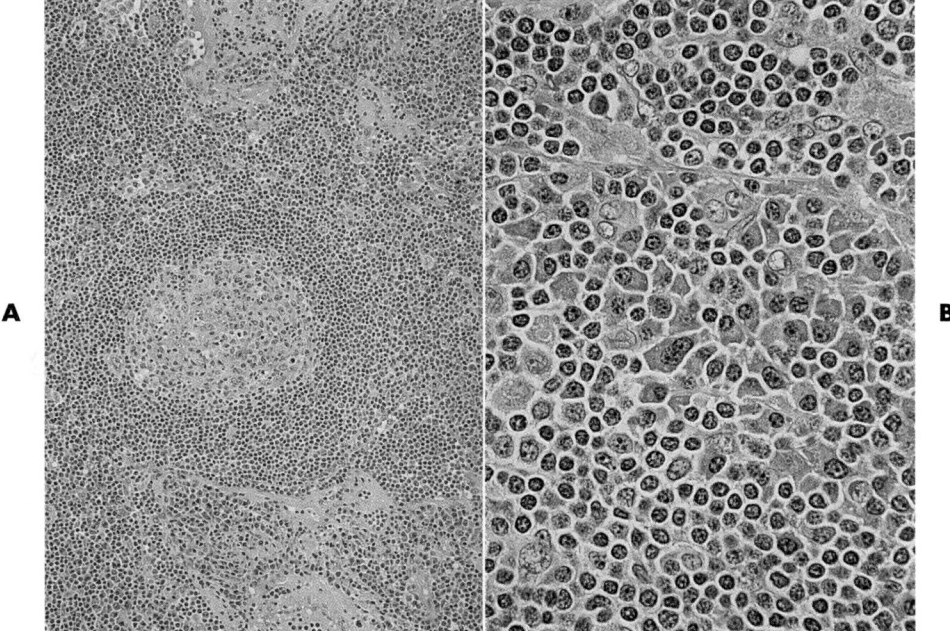

Fig. 21-25 Castleman's disease of plasma cell type. **A,** Low-power view showing follicular hyperplasia without vascular hyaline changes. **B,** High-power view of the interfollicular region showing a massive infiltration by plasma cells. Some of these plasma cells show multinucleation and mild nuclear atypia.

ology usually affecting children, originally described in the Japanese literature but having a worldwide distribution.[204] Fever, cervical lymphadenopathy, pharyngeal and conjunctival inflammation, and erythematous skin rashes are the most common clinical symptoms. Sometimes lymphadenopathy represents the dominant manifestation of the disease.[206] Arthritis is present in about 40% of the cases. Coronary arteritis may lead to fatal complications. The etiology is unknown, but an infectious agent is suspected.

Microscopically, the affected lymph nodes may show fibrin thrombi in the smaller vessels accompanied by patchy infarcts.[205,207]

Lupus erythematosus

The lymph node changes in lupus erythematosus are generally of a nonspecific nature and consist of moderate follicular hyperplasia associated with increased vascularization and scattered immunoblasts and plasma cells; some of the latter contain PAS-positive cytoplasmic bodies that represent sites of immunoglobulin production. Occasionally, one encounters a peculiar form of necrosis characterized by the deposition of hematoxyphilic material in the stroma, in the sinuses, and on the wall of blood vessels.[209] These have been found to be composed of DNA derived from karyorrhectic nuclear material, presumably from lymphocytes. Similar changes have been seen in cases of necrotizing lymphadenitis (see p. 1675). In other instances, Warthin-Findeldey–like polykaryocytes have been numerous.[208] The immunophenotype of lupus lymphadenitis is nonspecific.[209]

Rheumatoid arthritis

Most patients with rheumatoid arthritis have generalized lymphadenopathy at some time during their illness.[212,214] The lymph node enlargement may precede the arthritis and raise the clinical suspicion of lymphoma.

Microscopically, the most important changes are follicular hyperplasia and plasma cell proliferation, with formation of Russell bodies.[213] Vascular proliferation is also a consistent finding. The appearance may be quite similar to that of the plasma cell type of Castleman's disease. Small foci of necrosis and clumps of neutrophils are seen in some instances. The capsule is often infiltrated by lymphocytes.

Immunohistochemically, the plasma cell proliferation is of polyclonal nature.[211] Other collagen-vascular diseases, such as lupus erythematosus, polyarteritis nodosa, and scleroderma, are usually not associated with this type of lymph node abnormality.

Patients with rheumatoid arthritis treated with gold compounds can develop gold-associated lymphadenopathy.[215] They are also said to have a slightly increased incidence of malignant lymphomas[210] (see p. 1738).

Castleman's disease

Castleman's disease (giant lymph node hyperplasia, lymph nodal hamartoma) represents a morphologically distinct form of lymph node hyperplasia rather than a neoplasm or a hamartoma. Microscopically, two major categories have been described.[220,230] The first, designated as *hyaline-vascular type* or angiofollicular, shows large follicles scattered in

a mass of lymphoid tissue. The follicles show marked vascular proliferation and hyalinization of their abnormal germinal centers; they have been confused with Hassall's corpuscles and with splenic white pulp, prompting in the first case a mistaken diagnosis of thymoma and in the second of ectopic spleen. Their appearance corresponds to that of regressively transformed germinal centers (see p. 1672). Many of the large cells with vesicular nuclei present in the hyaline center are follicular dendritic cells, as evidenced by their strong immunoreactivity for CD21 and CD35.[237] There is a tight concentric layering of lymphocytes at the periphery of the follicles (corresponding to the mantle zone), resulting in an onion-skin appearance. The interfollicular stroma is also prominent, with numerous hyperplastic vessels of the postcapillary venule type and an admixture of plasma cells, eosinophils, immunoblasts, and KP1-positive plasmacytoid monocytes[219,236] (Fig. 21-24). Sinuses are characteristically absent. In the variant of the hyaline-vascular type described as the *lymphoid subtype,* the follicles have a marked expansion of the mantle zone and small, relatively inconspicuous germinal centers. This variant of Castleman's disease merges with the process designated as *mantle zone hyperplasia,* and it is the more likely to be confused with malignant lymphoma of either follicular or mantle cell type. Immunohistochemically, there is polyclonal immunoglobulin production by plasma cells, and large numbers of suppressor T cells are found in the interfollicular areas. Strong positivity for FVIII-related antigen is seen in the endothelium of the interfollicular vessels, but only a weak and focal reaction for this marker is found in the hyalinized vessels located in the center of the follicles.[229]

The second major morphologic category of Castleman's disease is known as the *plasma cell type.*[230] It is characterized by a diffuse plasma cell proliferation in the interfollicular tissue, sometimes accompanied by numerous Russell bodies. The hyaline-vascular changes in the follicles are inconspicuous or absent; instead, one often encounters in the center of these follicles a deposition of an amorphous acidophilic material that probably contains fibrin and immune complexes. The overall appearance is reminiscent of that seen in the lymph nodes from patients with rheumatoid arthritis (Fig. 21-25). The abundant expression of interleukin-6 that has been detected in this condition is thought to be responsible for the marked plasma cell infiltration.[227]

From the point of view of clinical presentation, Castleman's disease has been divided into a solitary and a multicentric form. The *solitary form* presents as a mass located most commonly in the mediastinum but also described in the neck, lung, axilla, mesentery, broad ligament, retroperitoneum, soft tissues of the extremities, and nasopharynx.[218] Grossly, it is round, well-circumscribed, with a solid gray cut surface, and can measure 15 cm or more in diameter (Fig. 21-26). Although this form by definition presents as a single mass, microscopic changes suggesting an early stage of the same process are sometimes seen in adjacent nodes. Microscopically, over 90% of the cases are of the hyaline-vascular type (including the lymphoid subtype), and the remainder are of the plasma cell type. The former is usually asymptomatic, whereas the plasma cell type is often associated with fever, anemia, elevated erythrosedimentation rate,

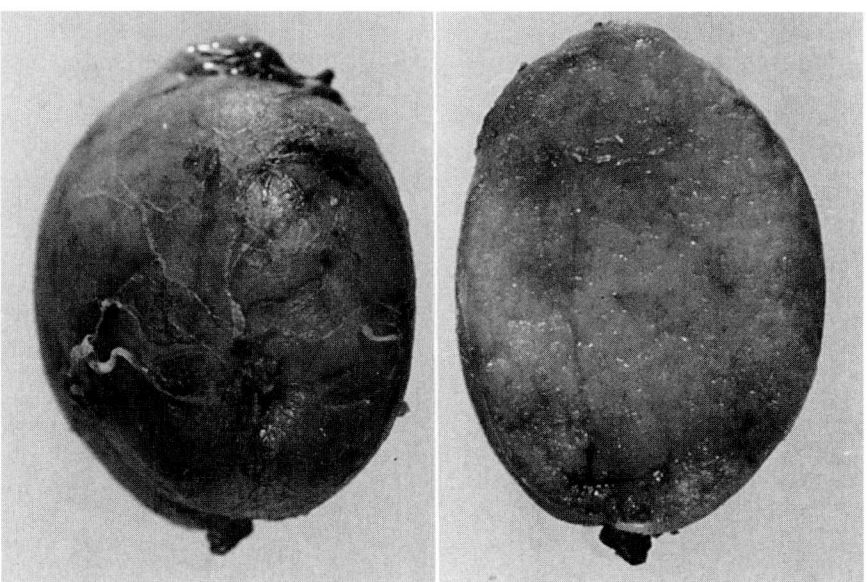

Fig. 21-26 Gross appearance of Castleman's disease. Both outer aspect and cut surface are shown. Lesion, which is surrounded by a capsule, shows granular, vaguely nodular appearance. (Courtesy Dr. J. Costa, Lausanne, Switzerland.)

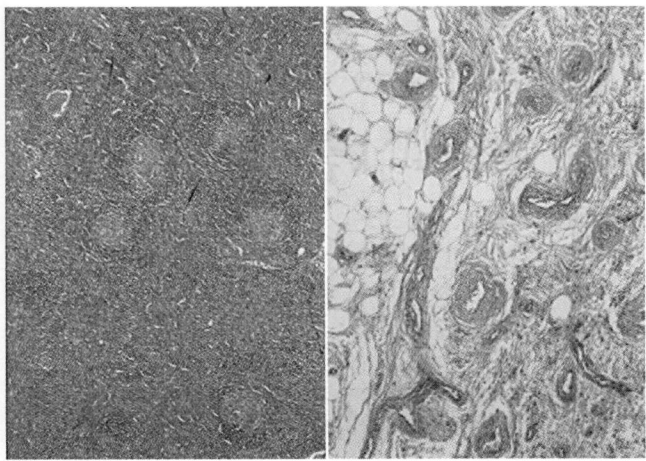

Fig. 21-27 Castleman's disease associated with vascular polifera-tion in the surrounding soft tissues. (Courtesy Dr. Pietro Muretto, Pesaro, Italy.)

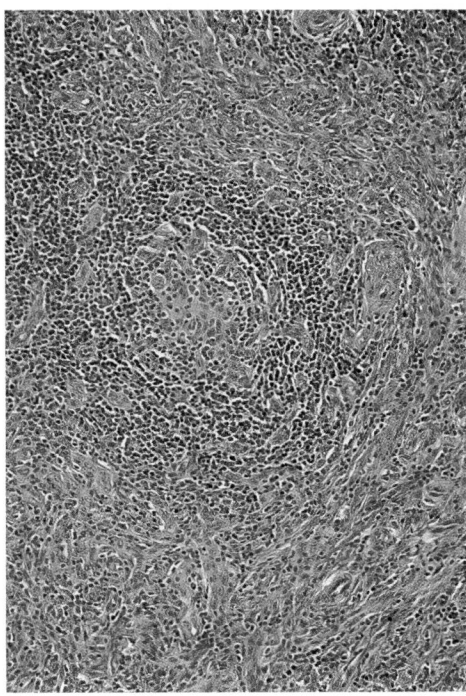

Fig. 21-28 Castleman's disease of vascular hyaline type associated with marked vascular proliferation in the interfollicular tissue.

hypergammaglobulinemia, and hypoalbuminemia. The treatment of solitary Castleman's disease is surgical excision, which has been found to result in rapid regression of the associated abnormalities whenever present.

The *multicentric* or *systemic form* is nearly always of the plasma cell type.[234] It presents with generalized lymphadenopathy and may also involve the spleen.[221,222,245] The clinical and laboratory features are similar to those of angioimmunoblastic lymphadenopathy, suggesting a related pathogenesis resulting from an abnormal immune response.[228] Sometimes the disease is seen in association with the POEMS syndrome, an acronymic designation for polyneuropathy, organomegaly, endocrinopathy, M-protein, and skin changes.[233,235] The latter include a distinctive vascular lesion known as glomeruloid hemangioma.[216] In other instances, Castleman's disease has been reported in association with amyloid deposits.[239]

The long-term prognosis of systemic Castleman's disease is poor; the disease tends to persist for months or years and to result sometimes in renal or pulmonary complications.[240] Furthermore, some of the patients have been found to have Kaposi's sarcoma, and others have developed large cell lymphomas of immunoblastic type. Evidence of clonal rearrangement for immunoglobulin and T-cell receptor genes has been found in cases of systemic Castleman's disease together with copies of the EBV genome, no such features having been detected in the solitary form of the disease.[225,226,238,241] This suggests that multicentric Castleman's disease is a disorder different from the classic localized type and one that may evolve into a clonal lymphoproliferation.

In some cases of Castleman's disease of the vascular-hyaline type, there are scattered atypical ("dysplastic") cells with large hyperchromatic nuclei, both within the abnormal germinal centers and in the intervening tissue.[243] Many of these cells have the phenotypical features of follicular dendritic cells, and it has been suggested that a dysfunction of these antigen-presenting cells is at the core of the pathogenesis of this disorder.[237,243] We have seen a case of follicular dendritic cell tumor occurring in a lymph node with Castleman's disease, and a similar case has been reported.[217]

In other cases of Castleman's disease of the vascular-hyaline type—particularly those located in the retroperitoneum—there is an undue prominence of stromal elements (stroma-rich variant).[219] This includes proliferation of actin-positive cells (consistent with fibroblastic reticulum cells or "myoid cells") and vessel-related elements. The latter may acquire the features of an angiomatous hamartoma[231] (Fig. 21-27), a highly cellular spindle cell proliferation resembling Kaposi's sarcoma or hemangiopericytoma[217] (Fig. 21-28) or a frank spindle cell sarcoma.[223] (Fig. 21-29, *A* and *B*). It is possible that some of these vascular proliferative lesions are the result of the secretion of angiogenic factors by the lymphoid elements.

Finally, cases of vascular-hyaline Castleman's disease have been reported in association with plasmacytoma[224,242] and follicular lymphoma.[244]

Hodgkin's disease may be accompanied or preceded by lymph node changes that greatly resemble those of Castleman's disease of either the plasma cell or the vascular-hyaline type.[232,246]

Angioimmunoblastic lymphadenopathy

Angioimmunoblastic lymphadenopathy (AILD, immunoblastic lymphadenopathy) occurs almost exclusively in adults and elderly individuals and is characterized clinically by fever, anemia (usually hemolytic), polyclonal hypergammaglobulinemia, and generalized lymphadenopathy.[252,253,261] Other common manifestations include hepatomegaly, splenomegaly, constitutional symptoms, and skin rash.[248,254,265] In 27% of the patients studied by Lukes and Tindle,[261] the disease occurred abruptly after administration of drugs, particularly penicillin.

Microscopically, the disease is systemic, with lesions in the lymph nodes, spleen, liver, bone marrow, and skin. The lymph node changes are characterized by obliteration of the nodal architecture (with focal preservation of sinuses) by a polymorphic cellular infiltrate and by an extensive proliferation of finely arborizing vessels of the caliber of postcapillary venules (Fig. 21-30). The cellular infiltrate is composed of small lymphocytes, plasma cells, numerous immunoblasts, frequent and sometimes abundant eosinophils, and, occasionally, multinucleated giant cells. Normal germinal centers are consistently absent; what one may find instead are germinal centers composed of loose aggregates of pale histiocytes, rare immunoblasts, or large epithelioid cells; these are referred to as "burnt-out germinal centers" and can closely resemble the appearance of granulomas. An amorphous, eosinophilic PAS-positive intercellular material may be found scattered throughout the node. Extension of the infiltrate in the capsule and pericapsular tissue is common. Methyl green–pyronine stain shows that most of the large lymphoid cells are pyroninophilic, and immunoperoxidase stain reveals a polyclonal pattern of immunoglobulin production.

The nature of AILD has been controversial since the time of its first description and remains so today. It was originally regarded as a non-neoplastic hyperimmune proliferation of the B-cell system with an exaggerated transformation of lymphocytes into immunoblasts and plasma cells, possibly induced by a primary abnormality of the T-cell system (such as a loss of suppressor T cells).[249,250,258,263] However, subsequent studies revealed the existence of cases having the AILD pattern but also exhibiting features suggesting the presence of a neoplastic lymphoid component. Thus Nathwani et al.[262] described cases of AILD characterized by the appearance of "clones" (clusters or islands) of tightly packed immunoblasts, followed by a diffuse replacement of the node by these elements. Several Japanese groups described cases with the AILD pattern that also exhibited cytologic atypia in the small and large lymphoid cells (clear cells and/or convoluted cells).[266] In many of these cases, the existence of a clonal population of T lymphocytes was documented by molecular techniques.[260,267] Although these cases were initially interpreted as AILD-like T-cell lymphomas and an attempt was made to separate them from "true" AILD, it has become increasingly apparent that a sharp separation among these lesions is impossible. AILD should be viewed as an arbitrarily defined morphologic portion of a spectrum of atypical immunoproliferative disorders (also known as lymphogranulomatosis X in some circles)[256] that range from the probably reactive and reversible to the

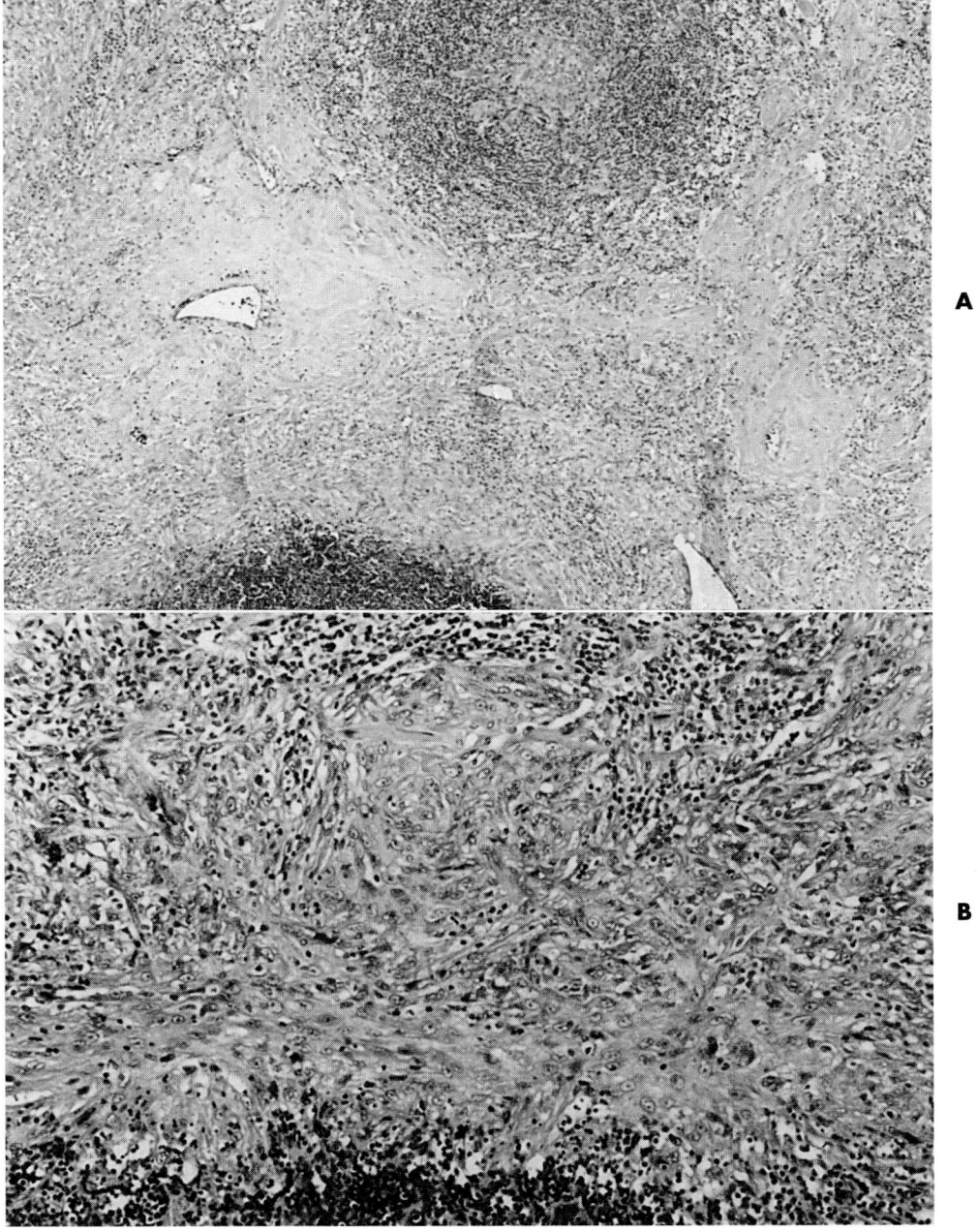

Fig. 21-29 Castleman's disease associated with vascular sarcoma. **A,** Panoramic view of lesion. It shows characteristic vascular hyaline changes of Castleman's disease at top and spindle cell proliferation at bottom, separated by areas of dense fibrosis. **B,** Vascular spindle cell neoplasm that has developed against background of Castleman's disease.

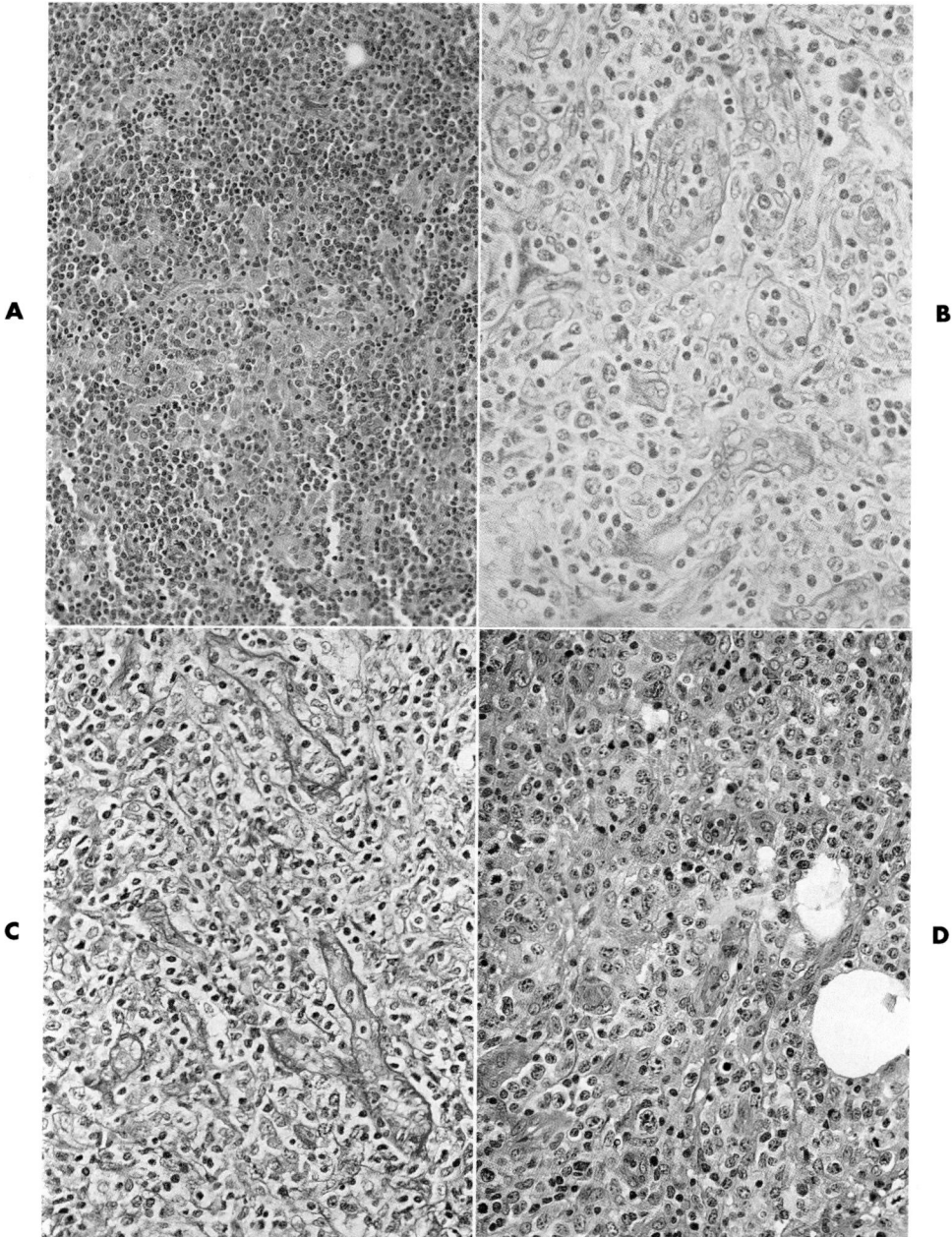

Fig. 21-30 Lymph node involvement by angioimmunoblastic lymphadenopathy. **A,** Low-power view showing a moderate effacement of the architecture by a polymorphic infiltrate composed of lymphocytes, plasma cells, and histiocytes. There is also marked vascular proliferation. **B** and **C,** The PAS stain highlights the prominence of the postcapillary venules. **D,** Atypical lymphoid cells are present in this polymorphic infiltrate. There are also scattered eosinophils.

clearly neoplastic and highly aggressive. The issue is further complicated by the fact that some cases show a clonal population of B cells *in addition* to a clonal population of T cells.[251] The possible role of a viral agent in the genesis of this disorder has been repeatedly proposed but not yet conclusively demonstrated.[255,257,264]

From a practical standpoint, the presence of atypical lymphoid cells (whether immunoblastic "clones," clear cells, or small cells with convoluted nuclei) correlates with a more aggressive clinical course.[247,262] In retrospect, we believe that the cases that we described many years ago as "malignant histiocytosis with cutaneous involve-

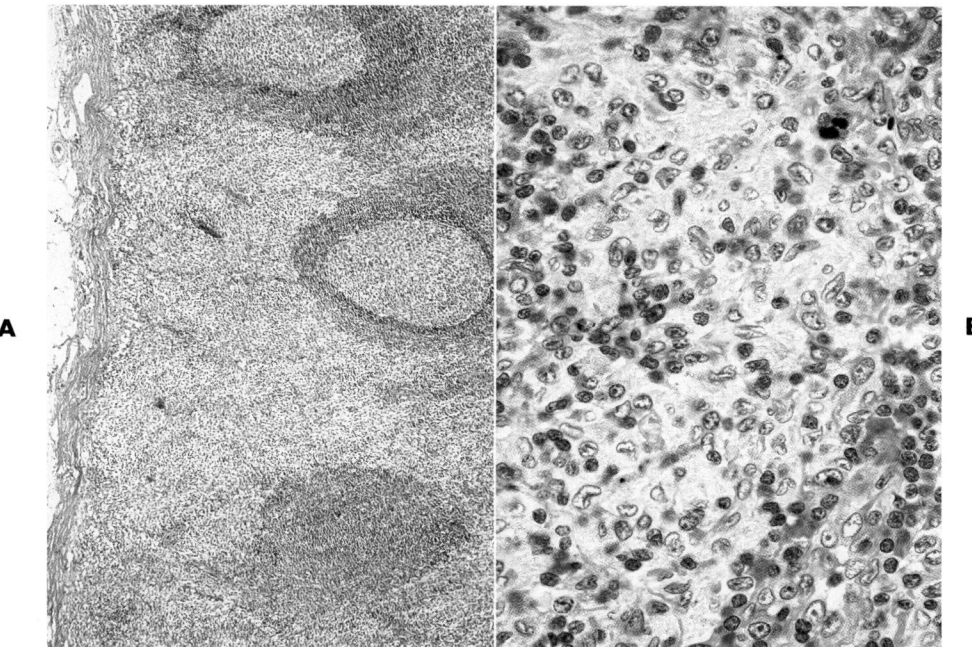

Fig. 21-31 Dermatopathic lymphadenopathy. **A,** Massive expansion of the paracortical region, resulting in a wide, pale area between the capsule and the lymphoid follicles. **B,** High-power view of the para-cortical region showing numerous cells with oval vesicular nuclei, which correspond to an admixture of interdigitating dendritic cells and Langerhans' cells.

ment and eosinophilia"[259] belong to this general cate-gory as representatives of the more aggressive and neo-plastic type. Similar cases have been described recently.[250a]

Drug hypersensitivity

Antiepileptic drugs derived from hydantoin, such as diphenylhydantoin (Dilantin) and mephenytoin (Mesan-toin), can result in a hypersensitivity reaction manifested by skin rash, fever, generalized lymphadenopathy (mainly cer-vical), and peripheral eosinophilia. The reaction, which is quite uncommon, tends to occur within the first few months of therapy. The changes disappear if the drug is discontin-ued. The nodal enlargement can occur in the absence of some of the other manifestations of the drug reaction.

Microscopically, partial effacement of the architecture by a polymorphic cellular infiltration is seen.[268] Histiocytes, immunoblasts, eosinophils, neutrophils, and plasma cells are all present. Some of the immunoblasts have atypical nuclear features, but Reed-Sternberg cells are absent. Foci of necrosis are common.[269] In some of the cases, the micro-scopic appearance is indistinguishable from that of AILD. The problem may simply be one of semantics, since one could interpret these cases as examples of AILD induced by the anticonvulsant therapy.

Dermatopathic lymphadenitis

Dermatopathic lymphadenitis (lipomelanosis reticularis of Pautrier) is a form of nodal hyperplasia usually secondary to various forms of generalized dermatitis, particularly those with exfoliative features. Pathogenetically, it represents a T-

cell response to skin antigens processed and presented by interdigitating dendritic cells. It may occur in any skin dis-order in which itching and scratching are prominent; this includes inflammatory dermatoses such as psoriasis and neoplastic diseases such as mycosis fungoides. Rarely, the morphologic changes of dermatopathic lymphadenitis are seen in the absence of clinical skin disease.[272]

Grossly, the lymph node is enlarged, the cut surface bulging, and the color pale yellow. Sometimes, black linear areas are seen in the periphery, representing clumps of melanin pigment and simulating the appearance of malig-nant melanoma.

Microscopically, the nodal architecture is preserved. The main change is represented by a marked pale widening of the thymic-dependent paracortical zone, which stands out prominently on low-power examination[274] (Fig. 21-31). The cells occupying this area are thought to be of three types: histiocytes, Langerhans' cells, and interdigitating dendritic cells.[270,273] Many of the histiocytes contain phagocytosed melanin and neutral fat in their cytoplasm. Plasma cell infil-tration and follicular hyperplasia are often present. A scat-tering of eosinophils also may be seen.

Nodes affected by dermatopathic lymphadenitis may be confused with Hodgkin's disease, mycosis fungoides, monocytic leukemia, or Langerhans' cell granulomatosis (histiocytosis X). The differential diagnosis with mycosis fungoides is of particular concern because of the fact that mycosis fungoides is one of the cutaneous disorders that can be associated with dermatopathic lymphadenitis.[271] Diag-nostic assistance can be obtained from immunohistochem-

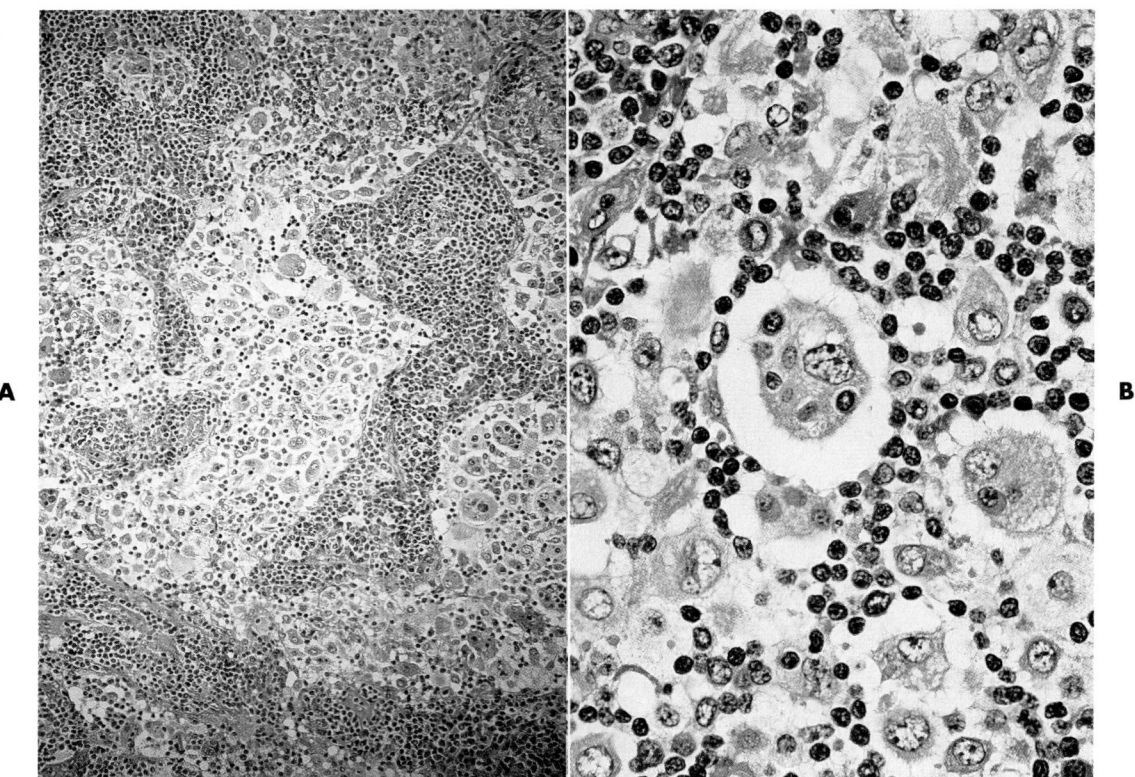

Fig. 21-32 Sinus histiocytosis with massive lymphadenopathy (Rosai-Dorfman disease). **A,** Low-power view showing massive distention of the sinuses by the histiocytic infiltrate. **B,** High-power view showing lymphocytophagocytosis by the sinus histiocytes.

istry and molecular pathology. Dermatopathic lymph nodes that are also involved by mycosis fungoides may show loss of Leu9 and Leu8 expression, and sometimes also loss of the pan–T-cell markers Leu1, Leu4, and Leu5.[276] At the molecular level, clonal rearrangements of T-cell receptor genes may be demonstrated.[275]

Sinus histiocytosis with massive lymphadenopathy (Rosai-Dorfman's disease)

Sinus histiocytosis with massive lymphadenopathy (SHML, Rosai-Dorfman disease) presents in its most typical form as massive, painless, bilateral lymph node enlargement in the neck, associated with fever, leukocytosis, elevated erythrosedimentation rate, and polyclonal hypergammaglobulinemia.[285,299] Most cases occur during the first or second decade of life, but any age group can be affected. A few cases have affected two members of the same family.[292] There is a predisposition for the condition in blacks. Although the disease has a widespread geographic distribution and most of the reported cases have been from the United States and Western Europe, there is a disproportionally high number of cases from Africa and the Caribbean region in our SHML registry, which now contains close to 600 cases.[285] Although the cervical region is by far the most common and most prominent site of involvement, other peripheral or central lymph node groups can be affected, with or without cervical disease.

Grossly, the nodes are matted together by prominent perinodal fibrosis. Their cut surface varies from gray to golden yellow, depending on the amount of fat present.

Microscopically, there is a pronounced dilatation of the lymph sinuses, resulting in partial or complete architectural effacement (Fig. 21-32, *A*). These sinuses are occupied by lymphocytes, plasma cells, and—most importantly—by numerous histiocytes with a large vesicular nucleus and abundant clear cytoplasm that may contain large amounts of neutral lipids. Many of these histiocytes have within their cytoplasm numerous intact lymphocytes, a feature that has been designated as emperipolesis or lymphocytophagocytosis. Although not specific, this is a constant feature of SHML and is therefore of great diagnostic significance (Fig. 21-32, *B*). Sometimes other cell types are present within the cytoplasm of the histiocytes, such as plasma cells and red blood cells.

The intersinusal tissue exhibits a variable but sometimes impressive number of mature plasma cells, some of which may contain Russell's bodies. Capsular and pericapsular inflammation and fibrosis are common. In a minority of cases, small microabscesses or foci of necrosis are found within the dilated sinuses. Ultrastructurally, the sinus histiocytes have extensive pseudopodia and lack Birbeck's granules; viral particles or other evidence of infection is consistently lacking. The sinus histiocytes contain cytoplasmic fat (Fig. 21-33, *A*) and are strongly reactive for S-100 protein[293] (Fig. 21-33, *B*); some of them are also positive for immunoglobulin, presumably phagocytosed from the surroundings. Their immunohistochemical profile suggests that they are monocytes that have been recently recruited from the circulation.[278,280,298] The plasma cells show a polyclonal pattern of immunoglobulin expression. The lymphocytes present are an admixture of B and T cells. A pathogenetic role for interleukin-6 has been suggested.[279]

In over one fourth of the cases, the disease involves extranodal sites.[285] This usually occurs in the presence of massive lymphadenopathy, and the disease is therefore easily recognized. However, in some cases these extranodal manifestations represent the predominant or even exclusive manifestation of the disease. The most common sites are eyes and ocular adnexae (especially orbit),[283] head and neck region,[304] upper respiratory tract,[282,290] skin and subcutaneous tissue,[294,302] and central nervous system.[286,300] However, the disease has been reported in many other sites, including gastrointestinal tract,[296] genitourinary tract, thyroid,[289] and uterine cervix.[295] In some instances, widespread nodal and extranodal dissemination is found.[307] Two organs that stand out because of their almost universal sparing by the disorder are the spleen and bone marrow. The histopathologic features of SHML in extranodal sites are similar to the nodal disease except for the facts that fibrosis tends to be more pronounced and lymphocytophagocytosis less conspicuous.

The etiology of SHML remains unknown, the two most likely possibilities (not mutually exclusive) being infection by a virus or some other microorganism and the manifestation of a subtle undefined immunologic defect. Despite some suggestive early data derived from serologic tests, the histiocytes of this disease are not infected by Epstein-Barr virus.[303] Human herpes virus 6 (HHV-6) has been detected in SHML tissues, but this organism is so commonly present in lymphoid tissue that the significance of this finding remains dubious.[291] Molecular studies done on involved tissue have failed to show evidence of clonality, in keeping with their presumed reactive nature.[291a] This contrasts with the findings in Langerhans' cell granulomatosis, a disease that it otherwise resembles in many clinical, morphologic,[306] and phenotypical aspects.[297]

SHML is relatively unaffected by therapy, although chemotherapy has proved effective in some cases.[288,301] In many cases, SHML undergoes quick and complete spontaneous resolution. In others, it follows a protracted clinical course for years or decades. The latter is particularly true in cases with widespread extranodal involvement. Some patients have died as a result of SHML, either because of extensive disease affecting vital organs or because of complications related to the immunologic abnormalities that may be present.[284,287]

The differential diagnosis of SHML includes nonspecific sinus hyperplasia (in which the cells lack emperipolesis and are S-100 protein negative), Langerhans' cell granulomatosis, leprosy, and metastatic malignant melanoma. Perhaps the condition that resembles it most is the sinus histiocytosis induced by cobalt-chromium and titanium that can occur in pelvic lymph nodes after hip replacement.[277]

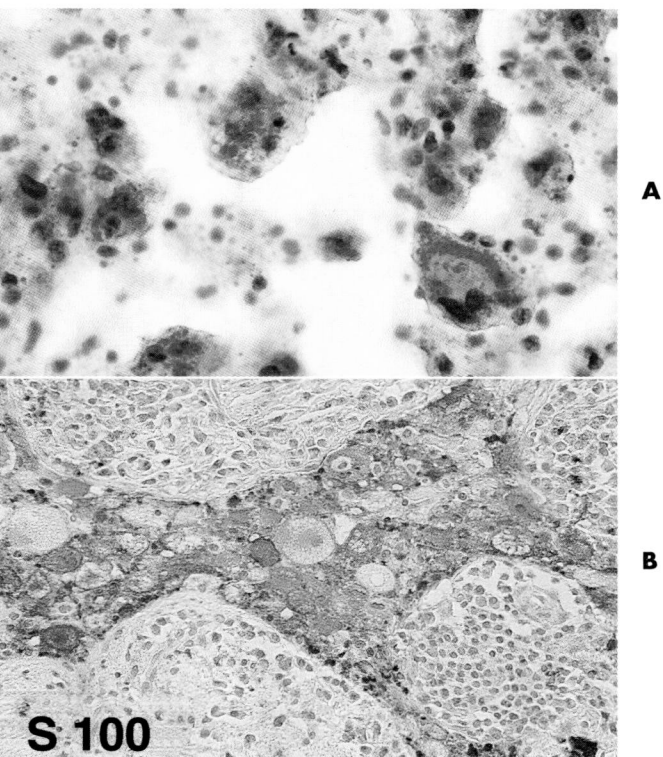

Fig. 21-33 Sinus histiocytosis with massive lymphadenopathy (Rosai-Dorfman disease). **A**, Oil red O stain showing abundant neutral lipid in the cytoplasm of the histiocytes. **B**, Strong immunoreactivity of the sinus histiocytes for S-100 protein.

It should also be noted that SHML-like changes can sometimes be seen in lymph nodes involved by other processes, such as Hodgkin's disease.[281]

Langerhans' cell granulomatosis (histiocytosis X)

The terms Langerhans' cell granulomatosis (LCG), Langerhans' cell histiocytosis, histiocytosis X, differentiated histiocytosis, and eosinophilic granuloma are applied to a specific, although remarkably variable, clinicopathologic entity characterized and defined by the proliferation of Langerhans' cells.[309,315] These cells are regarded as a distinct type of immune "accessory" cells that are involved in the capturing of some antigens and their presentation to the lymphoid cells. Contrary to a formerly held belief, these cells are not primarily phagocytic in nature. Their nuclei are highly characteristic: irregular, usually elongated, with prominent grooves and folds that traverse them in all directions. The cytoplasm is abundant and acidophilic, sometimes to the point that an embryonal rhabdomyosarcoma is simulated. Most Langerhans' cells are mononuclear, but occasional ones contain several nuclei while still maintaining the aforementioned nuclear and cytoplasmic features. Histochemically, they show weak acid phosphatase and nonspecific esterase activity but considerable leucyl-β-naphtylamidase activity and membrane-bound ATPase activity.[310]

PATHOLOGIC STAGING OF LANGERHANS' CELL HISTIOCYTOSIS (HISTIOCYTE SOCIETY)

A. Bone only or bone with involvement of first echelon lymph nodes in drainage field (osteolymphatic disease) and/or contiguous soft tissue involvement.
    A1. Monostotic
    A2. Monostotic with osteolymphatic disease
    A3. Monostotic with contiguous soft tissue involvement
    A4. Polyostotic
    A5. Polyostotic with osteolymphatic disease
    A6. Polyostotic with contiguous soft tissue involvement
B. Skin and/or other squamous mucous membranes only or with involvement of related superficial lymph nodes.
    B1. Nodular disease; neonatal period without nodal disease
    B2. Nodular disease; neonatal period with nodal disease
    B3. Multiple nodules or diffuse maculopapular disease without nodal disease
    B4. Multiple nodules or diffuse maculopapular disease with nodal disease
C. Soft tissue and viscera only excluding above and multisystem disease. Specify tissue involved, e.g., lung, lymph node, brain.
D. Multisystem disease with any combination of above. Specify each organ/tissue involved, e.g., skin, bone marrow, bone.

From Warnke RA, Weiss LM, Chan JKC, Cleary ML, Dorfman RF: Tumors of the lymph nodes and spleen. Atlas of tumor pathology, 3rd Series, Fascicle 14. Washington, DC, 1995, Armed Forces Institute of Pathology.

In paraffin sections, both Langerhans' cells and the cells of LCG are reactive for S-100 protein, vimentin, CD1a (O10), CD74, and HLA-DR in most cases.[331,336] They also tend to be positive for peanut agglutinin lectin and the macrophage-associated antigens CD68, cathepsin D, and cathepsin E.[317,330,332] They generally do not express CD45RA, CD45 RB, CDw75, alpha-1-antitrypsin, EMA, or CD15. The most useful of these formalin-resistant epitopes are S-100 protein and CD1a(O10).[314]

In frozen sections, these cells are positive for CD45 but negative for CD45 RA, CD4B, and CD45RD. In addition, they express CD1, CD4, CD11b, CD11c, CD14, CD16, CD25, CDw32, CD71, and HLA-A, -B, -C, and -DR, and they lack expression of most B- and T-cell markers.[328]

CD1 is the most useful marker in frozen sections in view of the fact that other histiocytic and dendritic/reticulum cells lack it. Interestingly, the cells of LCG—but not normal Langerhans' cells—may also be positive for cytoplasmic CD2 and CD3. At the molecular level, these cells show no rearrangement of the T-cell receptor gene.[342]

By electron microscopy, they contain a highly characteristic and apparently diagnostic organelle: the Birbeck's or Langerhans' granule. This is an elongated, zipper-like cytoplasmic structure of unknown function, sometimes continuous with the cell membrane.[324]

Scattered Langerhans' cells are normally present in the skin, lymph node, thymus, and other organs. Therefore the identification of a few cells with this feature in one of these sites is not necessarily indicative that the patient has LCG.[338] Rather, the infiltrate should have a sizable number of these cells before such a diagnosis is entertained. Conversely, the

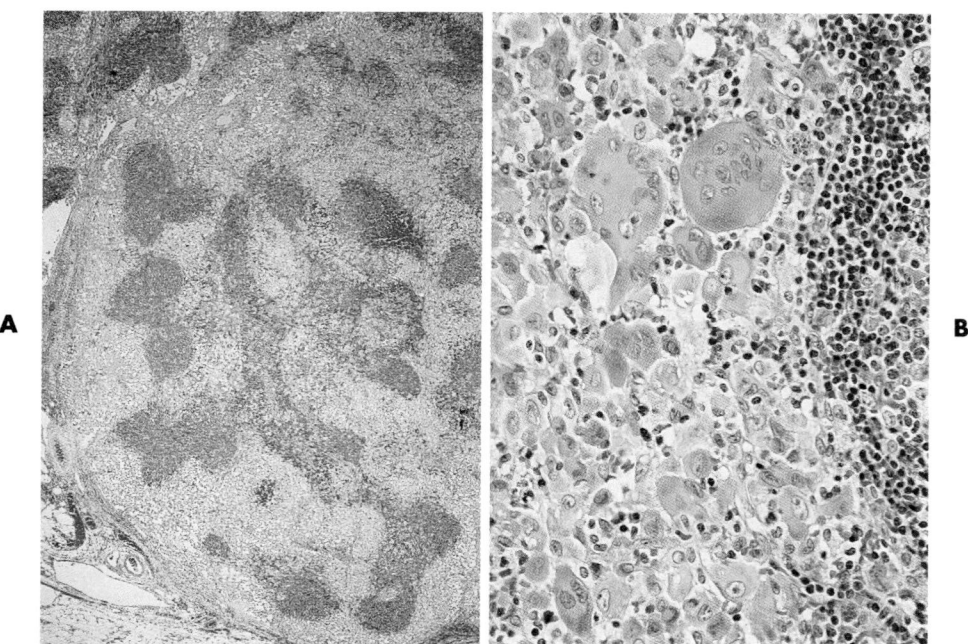

Fig. 21-34 Lymph node involvement by histiocytosis X. **A,** The infiltrate has a predominantly sinusal distribution. **B,** High-power view showing mononuclear and multinucleated Langerhans' cells. There are also numerous eosinophils.

identification of Langerhans' cells is necessary for the diagnosis of LCG. There is already too much confusion in the literature stemming from the fact that cases have been given this label only because a widespread proliferation of histiocytes was associated with a compatible clinical picture.

LCG can present as solitary or multiple lesions in one organ system (bone being the most common; see Chapter 24) or as a disseminated disease.[327] The treatment, prognosis, and terminology used largely depend on the extent (staging) of the disease (see box) rather than microscopic features or pattern of DNA ploidy.[320,321,335] The term Letterer-Siwe's disease was used in the past for the systemic form occurring in infants, and Hand-Schüller-Christian's disease for the less widespread and more indolent type seen in older children and adults.[312] A self-healing, congenital form is known as Hashimoto-Pritzker's disease.[318]

Lymph node involvement can be seen as a component of the systemic form, or it may represent the initial and sometimes exclusive manifestation of the disease.[325,333,339] The microscopic appearance is characteristic. There is distention of the sinuses by an infiltrate of mononuclear and multinuclear Langerhans' cells, admixed with a variable number of eosinophils (Fig. 21-34); foci of necrosis are common, often surrounded by a rim of eosinophils (so-called eosinophilic microabscesses), and always confined to the sinuses.

Sometimes, incidental foci of LCG are seen in lymph nodes involved by non-Hodgkin's lymphoma or Hodgkin's disease, a sharp separation existing between the two processes.[313,319] In most of these cases, the Langerhans' cell proliferation is limited to the node and may represent a reaction to the lymphoma, but in others it is an expression of generalized LCG.[326] Follow-up studies have shown a broad spectrum of involvement, embracing all those syndromes that have been associated with LCG. However, the prognosis is usually excellent. Focal LCG-like changes have also been seen in association with malignant melanoma.[334]

In addition to bone and lymph nodes, solitary LCG has been described in the lung, thymus, skin, central nervous system, and many other sites, including the stomach, anus, female genital tract, and thyroid[308,316,329,337] (see respective chapters).

The etiology of LCG remains unknown. A viral cause has been suggested but not substantiated.[322,323] Molecular studies have shown that the proliferation of Langerhans' is of a clonal nature.[340]

Exceptionally, a morphologically malignant process is seen in which the tumor cells have the ultrastructural and immunohistochemical features of Langerhans' cells.[311,341]

Kimura's disease

Kimura's disease is an inflammatory disorder of unknown etiology seen in an endemic form in the Orient.[346] It usually presents as a mass lesion in the subcutaneous tissue of the head and neck region or the major salivary glands, often associated with regional lymphadenopathy. Sometimes lymph node enlargement is the only manifestation of the disease.

Microscopically, the involved nodes show marked hyperplasia of germinal centers, a few of which may be of the progressively transformed type. These germinal centers are often well vascularized and contain polykaryocytes, interstitial fibrosis, and deposition of a proteinaceous material. There is also extensive infiltration by mature eosinophils, with occasional formation of eosinophilic abscesses (Fig. 21-35). Hyalinized vessels are often seen in the paracortical region, and there is a variable degree of sinusal

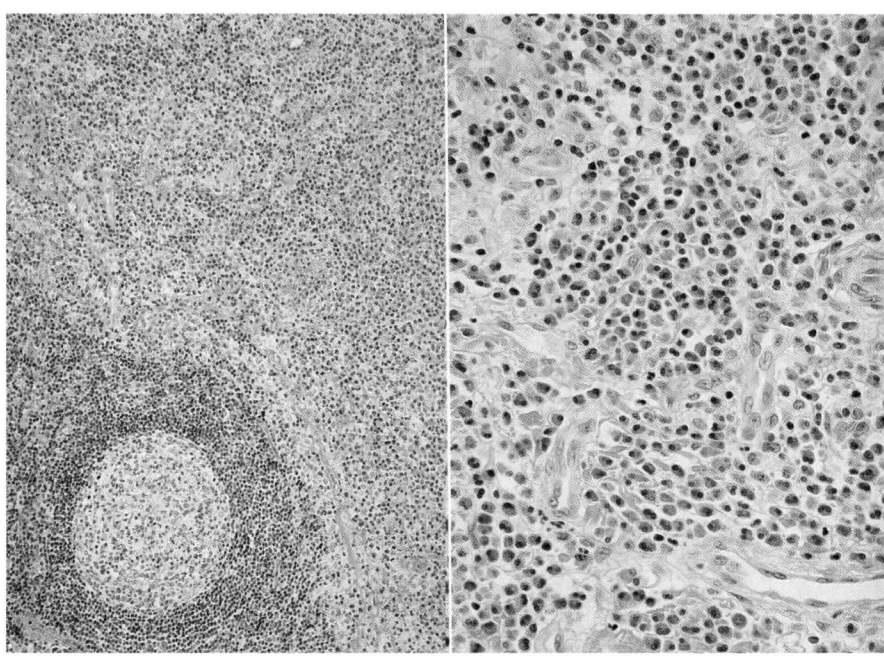

Fig. 21-35 Lymph node involvement by Kimura's disease. There is follicular hyperplasia and massive perinodal infiltration, which is predominantly composed of eosinophils. (Courtesy Dr. T-T Kuo, Taipei, Taiwan.)

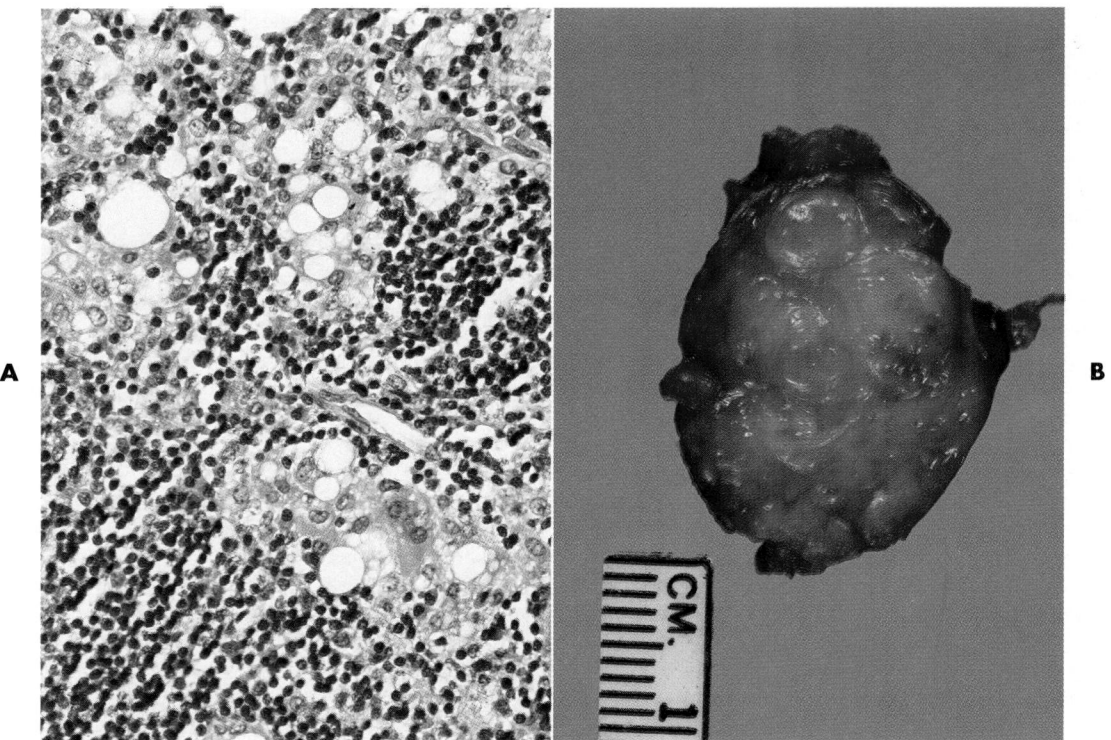

Fig. 21-36 Lymph node containing lipophagic granulomas. The change is manifested by the presence of mononuclear and multinucleated histiocytes located in the sinuses and containing large cytoplasmic vacuoles.

and paracortical sclerosis. An increase in the number of plasma cells and mast cells has been noted in the paracortex.[345]

Despite early statements to the contrary, current evidence strongly suggests that Kimura's disease and the disease known to dermatologists as angiolymphoid hyperplasia with eosinophilia are different entities (see Chapter 4); specifically, the former disorder lacks the epithelioid (histiocytoid) endothelial cells that are the morphologic hallmark of the latter.[343,344,346-349]

Chronic granulomatous disease

Chronic granulomatous disease is the result of a genetically determined enzymatic defect of granulocytes and monocytes.[356] These cells ingest microorganisms but are unable to destroy them because of their inability to generate superoxide anion (O_2^-). This is due to a defect in any one of four components of NADPH oxidases, the enzyme responsible for the generation of the antimicrobial oxidants. A pattern of Y-linked inheritance is seen in about 65% of the patients and results from mutations in the gene that encodes the g91-phox subunit of the cytochrome b558 component of the oxidase. The remaining 35% of patients inherit the disease in an autosomal recessive manner resulting from mutations in the genes that encode the other three oxidase components.[352,355,357] The traditional laboratory technique for the detection of the disease is the nitro blue tetrazolium test.[350]

The main clinical features are recurrent lymphadenitis, hepatosplenomegaly, skin rash, pulmonary infiltrates, ane-

mia, leukocytosis, and hypergammaglobulinemia.[351,353] Microscopically, granulomas with necrotic purulent centers are seen in lymph nodes and other organs. They closely simulate the appearance of cat-scratch disease and lymphogranuloma venereum.[353] Collections of histiocytes containing a lipofuscin-like pigment are also commonly observed.[354]

Lipophagic reactions

There are several conditions that result in the accumulation of phagocytosed fat within foamy histiocytes and multinucleated giant cells in the lymph node sinuses. The most common is the type seen in periportal and mesenteric nodes in asymptomatic individuals, probably the result of mineral oil ingestion[360] (Fig. 21-36, *A*). Boitnott and Margolis[358] found this change in 78% of a series of forty-nine autopsied adults. Their chemical and histochemical studies showed that the oil droplets represent deposits of liquid-saturated hydrocarbons. Mineral oil is extensively used in the food processing industry, as a release agent and lubricant in capsules, tablets, bakery products, and dehydrated fruits and vegetables.

Whipple's disease can result in marked enlargement of mesenteric lymph nodes, with formation of numerous lipophagic granulomas. Collections of histiocytes containing a PAS-positive glycoprotein are also present.[359] Under oil immersion with electron microscopy, the characteristic bacillary bodies can be identified. Collections of PAS-positive histiocytes can also develop in peripheral nodes and may be the first clue to the diagnosis in a patient with gradual weight loss, weakness, and polyarthritis. Steatorrhea, the other classic symptom of the disease, may appear only in a later stage. Unfortunately, the peripheral lymph node changes are not pathognomonic unless bacillary bodies can be demonstrated. All that the pathologist can do is to suggest the possibility and request a small bowel biopsy.

Lymphangiography induces a lipophagic granulomatous reaction that may persist for several months. The sinuses are markedly distended and lined by histiocytes, many of which are multinucleated. Eosinophils may be present in appreciable numbers in the medullary cords. This is preceded by a predominantly neutrophilic infiltration.[361]

MALIGNANT LYMPHOMA

Malignant lymphoma is the generic term given to tumors of the lymphoid system and specifically of lymphocytes and their precursor cells, whether of T, B, or null phenotypes.[362] Although traditionally tumors presumed to be composed of histiocytes and "reticulum cells" have also been included in the category of malignant lymphoma, it would seem more appropriate to regard them separately for both conceptual and practical reasons. Such tumors undoubtedly exist, and they are discussed later in this chapter. One should be aware, however, that the large majority of tumors that were designated in the past as histiocytic lymphomas or reticulum cell sarcomas are in reality of lymphocytic nature and therefore true malignant lymphomas.

Although some overlapping exists, the term *malignant lymphoma* is reserved for those neoplastic processes that initially present as localized lesions and are characterized by the formation of gross tumor nodules. Conversely, neoplastic lymphoid proliferations that are systemic and diffuse from their inception are included among the leukemias (see Chapter 23).

The malignant lymphomas can be divided into two major categories: Hodgkin's disease and all the others, which, for lack of a better term, are known collectively as non-Hodgkin's lymphomas.[361a,363-366] Both groups are further subdivided into several more or less distinct subcategories.

Hodgkin's disease

The term Hodgkin's disease has been traditionally used for a type of malignant lymphoma in which Reed-Sternberg cells are present in a "characteristic background" of reactive inflammatory cells of various types, accompanied by fibrosis of a variable degree. Thus identification of typical Reed-Sternberg cells is necessary for the initial diagnosis of Hodgkin's disease. As far as the "characteristic background" or "appropriate milieu" is concerned, it is highly variable, but it always lacks the monomorphic appearance of most other malignant lymphomas. Mature lymphocytes, eosinophils, plasma cells, and histiocytes may all be present in greater or lesser amount, depending on the microscopic type.

The etiology of Hodgkin's disease remains unknown, but there is considerable evidence to suggest that the Epstein-Barr virus (EBV) plays an important role. Individuals with a history of infectious mononucleosis have an increased incidence of Hodgkin's disease[368]; patients with Hodgkin's disease have an altered antibody pattern to EBV prior to diagnosis[371]; marked phenotypic similarities exist between infectious mononucleosis and Hodgkin's disease[373]; and EBV genomes have been identified in Reed-Sternberg cells in up to half of the cases (particularly in the mixed cellularity subtype, in young patients, and/or in developing countries).[367,369,372,374,375] There is also evidence for a genetic susceptibility factor.[370]

Gross features

Except for the very early stages, lymph nodes involved by Hodgkin's disease are enlarged, sometimes massively so. The gross appearance is somewhat dependent on the microscopic subtypes (see later section). The consistency varies from soft to hard depending on the amount of fibrosis. Some degree of nodularity is often appreciated, particularly in the nodular sclerosis form (Fig. 21-36, *B*). Foci of necrosis may be present. Except for lymphocyte-predominance Hodgkin's disease, the cut surface of the node has a more heterogeneous appearance than most non-Hodgkin's lymphoma. In advanced cases, several nodes from the same group become matted together, a feature spectacularly demonstrated in the drawing that accompanied Hodgkin's classic article.

Reed-Sternberg cell

The classic Reed-Sternberg cell is a large cell (20 to 50 μm in diameter or more) with abundant weakly acidophilic or amphophilic cytoplasm, which may appear homogeneous or granular and which lacks a pale zone in the Golgi area. The nucleus is bilobed or polylobed so that the cell appears binucleated or multinucleated; it is possible that in some cases bona fide binucleation or multinucleation actually occurs (Fig. 21-37, *A* and *B*). The nuclear membrane is thick and sharply defined. The nuclear pattern is usually vesicular but with some coarse chromatin clumps scattered throughout. There is a very large, variously shaped, but usually rounded, highly acidophilic central nucleolus surrounded by a clear halo. In the most typical example of the Reed-Sternberg cell, the two nuclear lobes face each other ("mirror image"), resulting in the oft-cited "owl eye" appearance. When multilobation occurs, the appearance has been likened to that of an "egg basket." Cells with this set of features but lacking nuclear lobation have been referred to as mononuclear variants of Reed-Sternberg cells or Hodgkin's cells (Fig. 21-37, *C*). Although their presence should suggest the possibility of Hodgkin's disease, they are not diagnostic by themselves. It has been stated that the minimal requirement for a diagnostic Reed-Sternberg cell is a bilobed nucleus in which at least one of the lobes has a prominent acidophilic nucleolus. At the other end of this spectrum is the Reed-Sternberg cell of giant size and highly pleomorphic hyperchromatic nuclei, having an appearance such as to simulate the cells of anaplastic carcinoma or one of the pleomorphic sarcomas. Another type of Reed-Sternberg cell, characterized by a darkly staining and retracted quality, is referred to as the mummified or necrobiotic variant and appears to be the morphologic expression of apoptosis (Fig. 21-37, *D*). Additional morphologic variations of Reed-Sternberg cells exist, and these will be discussed with the various types of Hodgkin's disease.

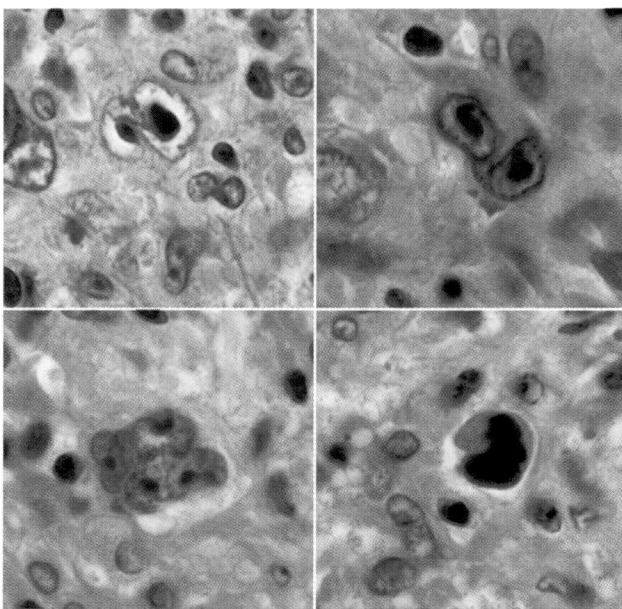

Fig. 21-37 Various appearances of Reed-Sternberg cell. The cell located in the right lower corner has a "mummified" appearance.

The Reed-Sternberg cell of Hodgkin's disease needs to be distinguished from other multinucleated cells that may be present in lymph nodes. Megakaryocytes can simulate it closely in hematoxylin-eosin–stained sections, but they can be identified by the presence of a strongly PAS-positive substance in their cytoplasm[383] and their different immunophenotype, which includes positivity for factor VIII–related antigen. Cells morphologically very similar to Reed-Sternberg cells, representing pleomorphic immunoblasts, can be seen in infectious mononucleosis and other viral diseases.[402] The most important morphologic differences between these two cells are summarized in Table 21-8. Neoplastic cells from a variety of epithelial and mesenchymal tumors also can resemble Reed-Sternberg cells.[399] Finally, some malignant lymphomas of non-Hodgkin's type may be accompanied by cells with the appearance of Reed-Sternberg cells, a fact that raises some questions about the very definition of Hodgkin's disease and its existence as an entity. In all of these disorders—and especially in the lymphomas—it is of the utmost importance to examine not only the putative Reed-Sternberg cells but also the background in which they are situated. The more cytologically atypical the lymphoid population, the less likely the diagnosis of Hodgkin's disease.

The requirement for the presence of classic Reed-Sternberg cells, which is absolute for the initial diagnosis of Hodgkin's disease, can be lessened somewhat in subsequent biopsies from patients with documented Hodgkin's disease. Under these circumstances, the presence of a polymorphic infiltrate *with atypical mononuclear cells* but not classic Reed-Sternberg cells in a biopsy of bone marrow, liver, or some other organ can be taken as evidence of involvement by Hodgkin's disease; however, a note of caution should be interjected. Atypical large lymphoid cells *need* to be present; an infiltrate of eosinophils, lymphocytes, and plasma cells or a collection of epithelioid granulomas is not enough.

The nature of the Reed-Sternberg cell remains controversial. Practically all the cells present in the normal node (and even some that are not) have been proposed at one time or another as possible progenitors: B cells, T cells, histiocytes, follicular dendritic cells, and interdigitating dendritic cells.[388]

The immunocytochemical profile of the Reed-Sternberg cell is yet to be totally agreed upon because of the discrepancies among the various laboratories. The most important findings in paraffin-embedded material have been the following*:

- CD15 (Leu-M1): This is expressed in over 80% of the cases; the pattern may be paranuclear (corresponding to the Golgi region), diffuse cytoplasmic, and/or corresponding to the cell membrane.
- CD30 (Ki-1): As recognized by the monoclonal antibody Be-Hz, this is found in about 90% of the cases.
- CD45 RB (LCA): This is expressed in less than 10% of the cases.
- CD45 RO and CD43 (T-lineage–related antigens): These are expressed in less than 10% of the cases.
- CD20 (L26, B-lineage antigen): This is expressed in 10% to 20% of the cases.
- CD40 (a protein present in B cells and nerve growth factor receptor): This is expressed in approximately 70%.
- CD74: This is expressed in over 75%.

---

*References 376-380, 382, 384, 386, 387, 389, 394, 396, 397, 404.

Table 21-8 Major morphologic differences between the pleomorphic immunoblast (Reed-Sternberg–like cell) of infectious mononucleosis and the Reed-Sternberg cell of Hodgkin's disease

Feature	Immunoblast	Reed-Sternberg cell
Nucleolus		
Stain pattern	Basophilic	Acidophilic
Contours	Irregular	Regular, with clear halo (inclusion-like)
Position	Adjacent to nuclear membrane	More centrally located
Cytoplasm		
Staining pattern	Usually amphophilic	Usually acidophilic
Pyroninophilia	Invariably strong	Variable
Paranuclear hof	Prominent	Inconspicuous
Surrounding cells	Mononuclear immunoblasts and plasmacytoid cells	Lymphocytes and histiocytes

Compiled from data in Dorfman RF, Warnke R: Lymphadenopathy simulating the malignant lymphomas. Hum Pathol **5**:519-550.

Table 21-9 Comparison between the different classification of Hodgkin's disease

Jackson and Parker (1947)[416]	Smetana and Cohen's modification (1956)[437]	Lukes (1963)[419]	Rye Conference (1966)[421]
Paragranuloma	Paragranuloma	Lymphocytic and histiocytic, diffuse Lymphocytic and histiocytic, nodular	Lymphocyte predominance
	Nodular sclerosis	Nodular sclerosis	Nodular sclerosis
Granuloma	Granuloma	Mixed cellularity	Mixed cellularity
Sarcoma	Sarcoma	Diffuse fibrosis Reticular	Lymphocyte depletion

Note the close correspondence between Smetana and Cohen's modification of Jackson and Parker's classification and the currently used Rye classification.

- Restin (an intermediate filament-associated protein): This is present in about 80%. The same is true for anaplastic large cell lymphoma but not for other types of non-Hodgkin's lymphoma.
- Peanut agglutinin and *Bauhinia purpurea* lectins: They are expressed in over 60% of the cases, in contrast to their near universal absence in non-Hodgkin's lymphoma.

In frozen sections, a large percentage of Reed-Sternberg cells have been found to exhibit reactivity for one or more pan–T-cell or pan–B-cell antigens, including the framework antigen of the T-cell receptor beta chain. They also express polyclonal IgG (probably representing passive uptake via the Fc receptor), HLA-DR, CD25 (the interleukin-2 receptor), and CD71 (the transferrin receptor).

Molecular studies have also given rise to controversial results. Most cases of Hodgkin's disease yield a germ line configuration for immunoglobulin heavy and light chain genes and the beta T-cell receptor genes, but this may simply result from a dilution factor by the non-neoplastic cells; indeed, some studies suggest that an increased number of Reed-Sternberg cells and their variants is associated with a detectable increase in clonal rearrangements of either gene.[381,385,390,403] Recently, Reed-Sternberg cells of B-cell immunophenotype were isolated from 12 cases of "classic" Hodgkin's disease (see p. 1703) and found to have rearranged immunoglobulin variable-region heavy-chain (V_H) genes, indicating their origin from B cells. In half of the

cases the population of Reed-Sternberg cells was polyclonal, and in the other half it was monoclonal or mixed.[386a]

The karyotype of these cells is generally hyperdiploid and with structural abnormalities, but no recurring chromosomal abnormalities have yet been detected.[395,400,401]

Another unresolved issue is the prevalence of t(14;18) in Hodgkin's disease, the reported figures ranging from zero to over 30%; perhaps of significance in this regard is the fact that the bcl-2 protein (a hallmark of the 14;18 translocation) is never overexpressed, except in those exceptional instances of Hodgkin's disease that arise in the setting of follicular lymphoma.[391-393,398]

Microscopic types

For many years, Jackson and Parker's classification of Hodgkin's disease into granuloma, paragranuloma, and sarcoma variants[416] was widely used because of its reproducibility and clear-cut prognostic implications, the major objection being that too many of the cases (about 80%) fell into one of the categories—i.e., Hodgkin's granuloma. The concept of a sclerosing type of Hodgkin's disease associated with a very good prognosis was first introduced by Smetana and Cohen in 1956[437] and was incorporated into a new classification proposed by Lukes et al.[419,420] In this scheme, six categories were included: lymphocytic and/or histiocytic (L&H) nodular, L&H diffuse, nodular sclerosis, mixed cellularity, diffuse fibrosis, and reticular. This classification, somewhat simplified and with some changes in nomenclature (not always for the better), was adopted by the Nomen

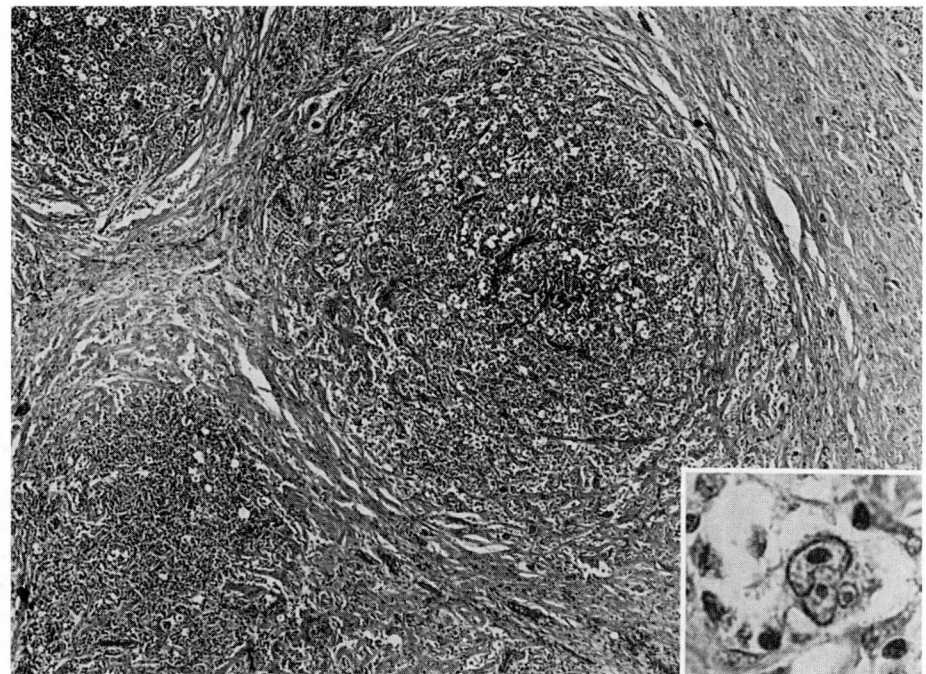

Fig. 21-38 Hodgkin's disease of nodular sclerosing type. Bands of collagen separate nodules. **Inset** shows lacunar Reed-Sternberg cell.

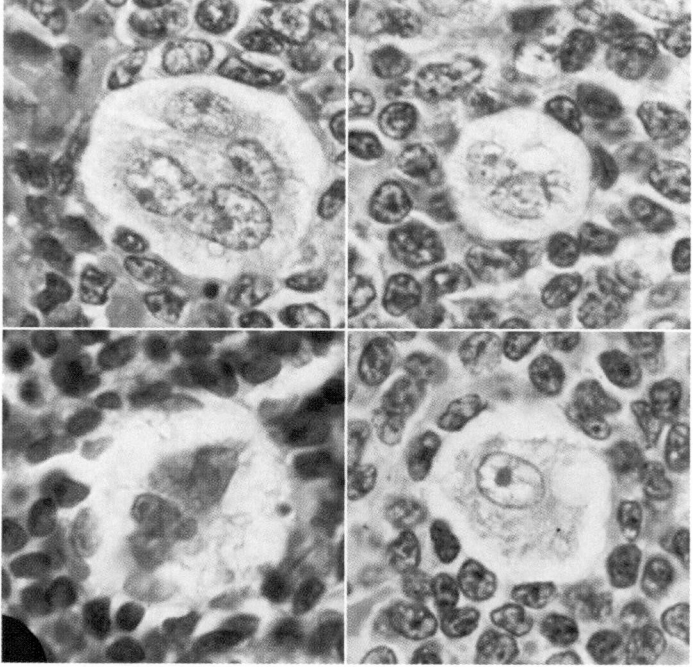

Fig. 21-39 Various appearances of lacunar cells in nodular sclerosis Hodgkin's diesase.

clature Committee at the Rye Conference[421] on Hodgkin's disease and has gained widespread recognition. Other classifications that were proposed during this period failed to achieve general acceptance.[413] The relationship between these classifications is shown in Table 21-9.

Four major categories are currently accepted.

Nodular sclerosis Hodgkin's disease is characterized in its fully developed staged by broad collagen bands separating the lymphoid tissue in well-defined nodules (Fig. 21-38). These fibrous bands, which have a birefringent quality when examined under polarized light, often center around blood vessels. In addition to the classic Reed-Sternberg cell, nodular sclerosis Hodgkin's disease also displays a variant known as *lacunar* or *cytoplasmic* (Fig. 21-39). This cell type is quite large (40 to 50 µm in diameter), with an abundant clear cytoplasm and multilobulated nuclei having complicated infoldings and nucleoli of smaller size than those of the classic Reed-Sternberg cell. The "frail" cytoplasm of these cells is retracted close to the nuclear membrane so that the cell appears to be floating in a "lacuna." This is the result of an artifact induced by formalin fixation, inasmuch as it is absent in tissues fixed in Zenker or B-5. In some cases, there is clustering of these lacunar cells, particularly around areas of necrosis. They form sheets and cohesive nests, to the point that a mistaken diagnosis of large cell non-Hodgkin's lymphoma, carcinoma, germ cell tumor, or thymoma can be made. Cases of nodular sclerosis Hodgkin's disease showing prominence of this feature have been referred to as the *syncytial, sarcomatoid,* or *sarcomatous* variant.[440]

Some workers regard the lacunar variant of Reed-Sternberg cell as more typical of this type of Hodgkin's disease than the fibrosis itself and make the diagnosis of nodular sclerosis Hodgkin's disease in the presence of lacunar cells even if fibrosis is totally lacking (so-called *cellular phase*)[440]; however, it should be remarked that lacunar cells are not pathognomonic of this condition. They can also be seen in mixed cellularity Hodgkin's disease and even in reactive disorders.[423]

The composition of the non-neoplastic infiltrate varies widely, to the point that some authors have proposed to subdivide nodular sclerosis Hodgkin's disease into lymphocyte predominance, mixed cellularity, and lymphocyte depletion categories and have claimed that this subdivision carries some prognostic implications. Along similar lines, the British National Lymphoma Investigation group has proposed to divide cases of nodular sclerosis Hodgkin's disease into two grades. In their scheme, cases are assigned to the allegedly more aggressive grade II if any of these features are present: (1) a "reticular" or "pleomorphic" pattern of lymphocytic depletion in over 25% of the cellular nodules, (2) a "fibrohistiocytic" pattern of lymphocyte depletion in over 80% of the cellular nodules, and (3) the presence of numerous bizarre and highly anaplastic Reed-Sternberg and Hodgkin's cells without lymphocyte depletion in over 25% of the nodules.[422] Grade II lesions include the "syncytial" variant of other authors already mentioned.

By electron microscopy, nodular sclerosis Hodgkin's disease shows abundant collagen fibers together with myofibroblasts[436]; it has been suggested that the latter contribute to the retraction seen in this condition. In regard to the fibro-sis, it should be kept in mind that practically all types of Hodgkin's disease can exhibit some degree of this change, particularly after therapy. If the pathologist is too liberal in the criteria for diagnosis of nodular sclerosis, the clinical and prognostic connotations associated with this microscopic type will lose most of their meaning.

In ***lymphocyte predominance*** Hodgkin's disease, the predominant cell is a small B lymphocyte, with or without an accompanying population of benign-appearing histiocytes.[432,442] Postcapillary venules with high endothelium may be prominent.[425,438] The lymph node architecture is patially or totally effaced, and the infiltrate may have a diffuse or nodular pattern of growth.[431] The latter may be so pronounced as to simulate on low power the appearance of follicular lymphoma; however, the nodules of Hodgkin's disease are more irregular in size and staining quality, and the admixture of lymphocytes and epithelioid cells gives them a mottled appearance (Fig. 21-40, *A*). A rim of uninvolved or hyperplastic lymphoid tissue may be present. Progressively transformed germinal centers may be seen adjacent to the lesion.[414] Eosinophils, plasma cells, and foci of fibrosis are scanty or absent. Classic Reed-Sternberg cells are difficult to find or altogether absent. One sees instead a variable but usually large number of a type of Reed-Sternberg cell (the L&H cell or "popcorn" cell) characterized by a folded, multilobed nucleus with smaller nucleoli (Fig. 21-40, *B*). If numerous diagnostic Reed-Sternberg cells are found in a node with a lymphocyte predominance background, the case should probably be classified as one of mixed cellularity. Occasionally, the L&H cells predominate at the margins of the nodules, creating a "wreath" around them. In others, they cluster in large confluent sheets resembling diffuse large cell lymphoma.

Poppema et al.[428-430] first proposed that cases of lymphocyte predominance Hodgkin's disease having a nodular pattern of growth (the L&H nodular type of the classification of Lukes et al.[420]) arise from B-cell regions of the node and specifically from progressively transformed germinal centers (see p. 1671). They supported their theory by showing that the L&H cell that is characteristic of this condition is of B-cell lineage, and this has been confirmed by many others.* L&H cells express the pan–B-cell markers CD19, CD20, CD22, CD74, CDw75, and CD45 RA. They are also positive for CD45 RB (LCA) but consistently negative for T-cell markers. They may express CD30 or EMA, and they generally lack CD15 expression. J chain, a protein associated with immunoglobulin synthesis, has been demonstrated in these cells, but expression of immunoglobulin heavy or light chains has been generally lacking.[434,435] However, evidence that lymphocyte predominance Hodgkin's disease is a κ light chain–restricted monotypic B-cell neoplasm has been recently presented.[439] No Epstein-Barr virus or bcl-2 protein overexpression has been encountered.[405]

The evidence discussed, plus a wealth of epidemiologic and clinical data, has led to the current trend of segregating nodular L&H from all other types of Hodgkin's disease,[424] even if occasional cases are seen to coexist.[415] According to

---

*References 406, 407, 411, 417, 426, 427, 430, 433.

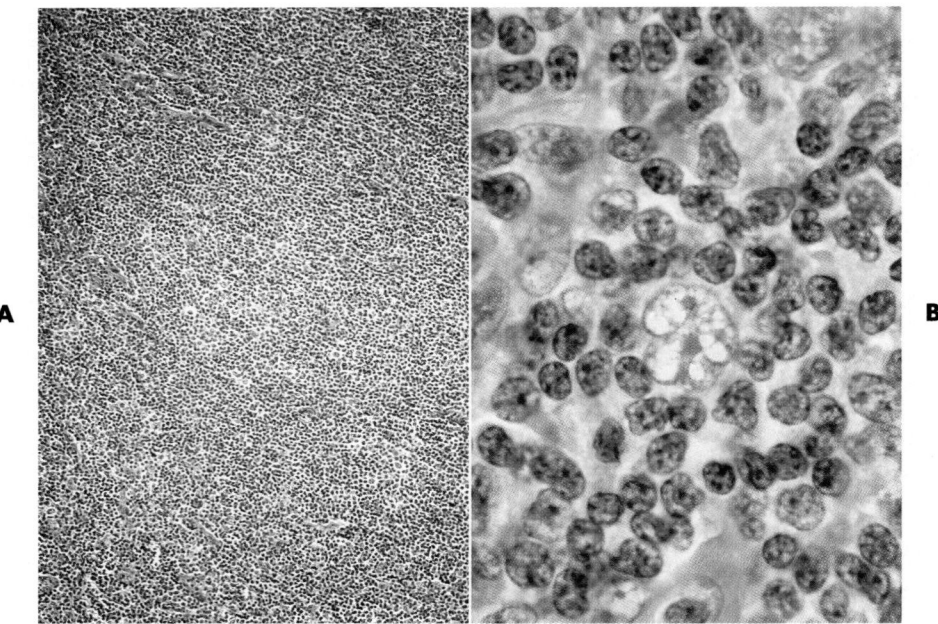

Fig. 21-40 Lymphocyte-predominance Hodgkin's disease. **A,** Low-power view showing a mottled appearance of the node. **B,** High-power view showing the L&H type of cell ("popcorn" cell) that is characteristic of this condition.

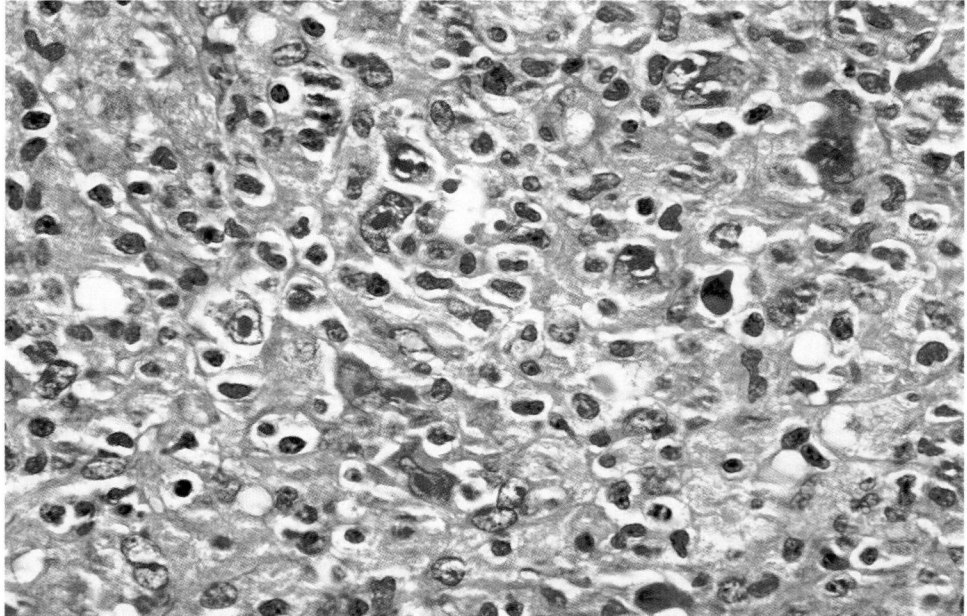

Fig. 21-41 Lymphocyte depletion type of Hodgkin's disease. Numerous atypical cells are present in a densely fibrotic stroma. Lymphocytes are scanty.

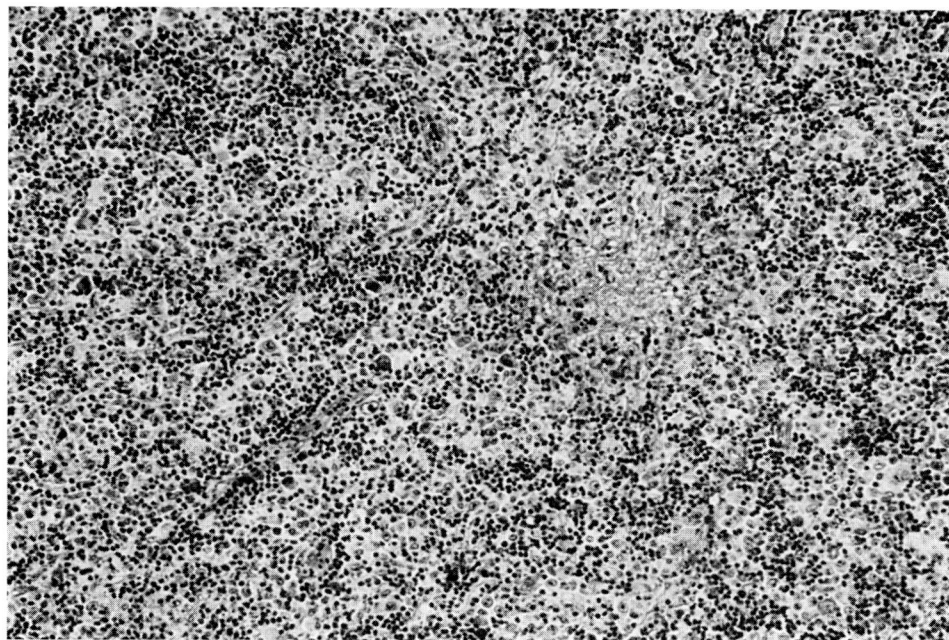

Fig. 21-42 Hodgkin's disease of mixed cellularity type. Mixed cell infiltrate containing numerous Reed-Sternberg cells is present. Small focus of necrosis is seen close to center of illustration.

this emerging scheme, Hodgkin's disease *minus* the nodular L&H form is to be renamed *classic* Hodgkin's disease.

And what of the diffuse L&H form? Some such cases become forms of nodular L&H in which the nodularity is minimal or has been lost, whereas others are viewed as a *lymphocyte-rich* subtype of classic Hodgkin's disease.

The **lymphocyte depletion** group, which comprises less than 5% of all cases of Hodgkin's disease, includes two morphologically different subtypes, designated as "diffuse fibrosis" and "reticular" in the original Lukes classification. In the diffuse fibrosis subtype, the number of lymphocytes and other cells progressively decreases as the result of heavy deposition of collagen fibers. The reticular subtype is characterized by a very large number of diagnostic Reed-Sternberg cells (many of them of bizarre configuration) among atypical mononuclear cells and other elements (Fig. 21-41). Areas of necrosis are more common than in other types. The "reticular" subtype of lymphocyte depletion Hodgkin's disease needs to be distinguished from non-Hodgkin's lymphoma of large cell type (including the pleomorphic Ki-1+ type) and from the variant of nodular sclerosis Hodgkin's disease with aggregates of lacunar cells.

In **mixed cellularity** Hodgkin's disease, a large number of eosinophils, plasma cells, and atypical mononuclear cells are admixed with classic Reed-Sternberg cells, which tend to be numerous. Focal necrosis may be present, but fibrosis should be minimal or absent (Fig. 21-42). It is somewhat ironic that mixed cellularity Hodgkin's disease, which fits more closely the histopathologic picture of the disease as depicted in the classical textbooks, has now almost become a diagnosis of exclusion.

• • •

The histologic types of Hodgkin's disease remain constant over long follow-up periods in most cases, particularly for the nodular sclerosis form.[441] In patients who have relapses in a site *not included* in the radiation field (and who have not received chemotherapy), the same histologic appearance is often maintained in the relapse biopsies.[409] When change occurs, it usually is toward a histologically more malignant form. It also should be remembered that patients with Hodgkin's disease may develop non-Hodgkin's lymphoma or leukemia,[410,418] either spontaneously or as a result of therapy.

The microscopic typing of Hodgkin's disease should always be made on examination of a biopsy obtained before the institution of treatment. Radiation therapy and chemotherapy result in focal necrosis, fibrosis, and profound nuclear aberrations—features that may render impossible a proper pathologic evaluation. These alterations may be seen in post-therapy biopsy material or at autopsy.[408]

The currently used classification of Hodgkin's disease is useful but far from ideal. Its nomenclature, for instance, is such that there is very little relation between the names given and the microscopic picture observed. A case with lymphocyte predominance or mixed cellularity will be diagnosed as nodular sclerosis if bands of fibrous tissue are present. A case with marked predominance of lymphocytes will be categorized as mixed cellularity if there are numerous Reed-Sternberg cells. In lymphocyte depletion Hodgkin's disease, lymphocytes are still the numerically more abundant cells, more so than in the mixed cellularity type.[423]

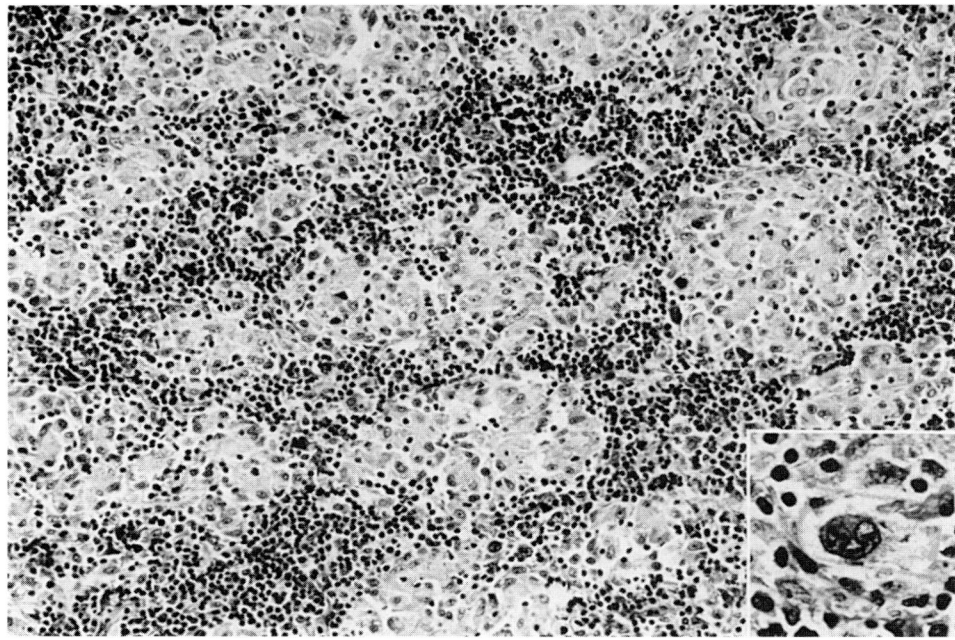

Fig. 21-43 Hodgkin's disease in which associated granulomatous sarcoid-like reaction simulates inflammatory process. **Inset** shows one of several Reed-Sternberg cells present in lymphoid tissue between granulomas.

An alternative approach has been tried by Coppleson et al.[412] and consists of evaluating individually the frequencies of the different cell types. They found that a large number of lymphocytes was associated with a good prognosis, whereas malignant and mononuclear cells and benign-appearing histiocytes independently influenced the prognosis adversely. Reed-Sternberg cells had no prognostic effect independent of the malignant mononuclear cells, and eosinophils and plasma cells had no prognostic value. However, these authors concluded that the Rye classification of Hodgkin's disease furnished more prognostic information than any estimates of individual cell frequencies.

Other microscopic features

There are some microscopic variations on the theme of Hodgkin's disease worth mentioning, mainly because lack of knowledge of their occurrence may result in mistaken diagnoses. Some of these are associated with one or another of the subtypes of Hodgkin's disease, but others are not.

1 *Foamy macrophages.* Clumps of foamy macrophages resulting in a xanthogranulomatous appearance may be found, particularly in the nodular sclerosis form.[454]

2 *Eosinophils.* In some instances, the intensity of eosinophilic infiltration is massive and accompanied by so-called eosinophilic microabscesses. Such cases may be confused with Langerhans' cell granulomatosis (eosinophilic granuloma), hypersensitivity reaction, or "allergic granulomatosis."

3 *Other inflammatory cells.* S-100 protein–positive follicular dendritic cells,[443] mast cells,[445] and monocytoid B cells[448] may be very numerous.

4 *Focal interfollicular involvement.* In the early stages of the disease, only focal involvement of a lymph node may be encountered,[453] often restricted to the paracortical region between florid hyperplastic follicles; this pattern, which has been referred to as *interfollicular Hodgkin's disease,* should not be regarded as a specific subtype.[446]

5 *Castleman's disease–like features.* Cases of Hodgkin's disease may be accompanied or preceded by a plasmacytic infiltrate and abnormalities of germinal centers closely resembling those seen in Castleman's disease (see p. 1688).

6 *Fibrosis.* In cases of nodular sclerosis Hodgkin's disease but sometimes also in other types, the amount of fibrosis can be such as to simulate the appearance of one of the inflammatory fibroscleroses (such as sclerosing mediastinitis or retroperitoneal fibrosis).

7 *Spindle cell proliferation.* In rare cases of Hodgkin's disease, there is a proliferation of oval to spindle cells of such a degree as to simulate fibrosarcoma, malignant fibrous histiocytoma, or a follicular dendritic cell tumor; such lesions have been referred to as fibrosarcomatous or fibroblastic Hodgkin's disease. Some of these spindle cells have a degree of nuclear atypia such as to indicate their neoplastic nature and relationship with Reed-Sternberg's and Hodgkin's cells; indeed, most of these lesions would be included in the grade II category of nodular sclerosis Hodgkin's disease proposed by the British National Lymphoma Investigation group (see p. 1703). Others are of a reactive nature and stromal derivation (i.e., made up of fibroblasts and myofibroblasts).[444]

8 *Noncaseating granulomas.* These formations are sometimes present in nodes and other organs involved by Hodgkin's disease. Occasionally they are so numerous as to obscure the diagnostic features of the disease (Fig. 21-43). In other instances, these granulomas may be seen within otherwise uninvolved organs of patients with Hodgkin's disease.[447] Their significance is unknown. Perhaps they represent an expression of delayed hypersensitivity. Others are reactions to the contrast material used in lymphangiography.[449] Their presence does not indicate involvement of that organ by Hodgkin's disease and should therefore not influence the staging criteria. Actually, it has been suggested that, within a given stage, the presence of these granulomas is associated with a better prognosis.[451]

9 *Vascular invasion.* Blood vessel infiltration has been detected microscopically in 6% to 14% of the cases of Hodgkin's disease by the use of elastic tissue stains.[452] This finding is said to be associated with an increased incidence of extranodal organ involvement.[450]

General and clinical features

Hodgkin's disease comprises about 20% to 30% of all malignant lymphomas in the United States and Western Europe but a much lower percentage in Japan and other Oriental countries.[455] There is a wide range in age incidence, which varies according to geographic location. In the United States, there is a bimodal distribution, with a peak at 15 to 40 years and a second, smaller peak in the seventh decade. In Japan, the peak in young adulthood is absent. In poorly developed countries, there is a high incidence in children, a relatively low incidence in the 15- to 40-year age group, and a third peak later in life.[456,459] There is a male preponderance (about 1.5 to 1) in all microscopic types except nodular sclerosis. The disease may present in a variety of ways, the most common (about 90% of the cases) being painless enlargement of superficial (usually cervical) lymph nodes. Fever, night sweats, and loss of weight (so-called B symptoms) occur in approximately 25% of the cases; their presence influences the clinical staging. Pruritus is also frequent.

Important clinical differences exist related to the microscopic types. The typical patient with lymphocyte predominance Hodgkin's disease is a man in his 40s with involvement of the high cervical nodes. This microscopic form practically never involves the spleen, liver, or bone marrow except when it changes to a more aggressive histologic pattern.[461,464]

Nodular sclerosis is by far the most common type of Hodgkin's disease in the United States. It characteristically presents in the neck and/or mediastinum of young females.[457]

Lymphocyte depletion Hodgkin's disease may present in adults or elderly patients as a febrile illness with pancytopenia or lymphocytopenia, hepatomegaly, abnormal liver function tests, and no peripheral lymphadenopathy,[462] or it may manifest the usual clinical presentation of Hodgkin's disease.[458] This form is extremely rare in children, in whom nodular sclerosis and lymphocyte predominance predominate greatly.[463,467]

Mediastinal involvement is the rule in nodular sclerosis, inconstant in mixed cellularity and lymphocyte depletion, and exceptional in lymphocyte predominance. The risk of abdominal involvement is greater in patients with B symptoms and in lymphocyte depletion or mixed cellularity types; the lowest risk is for asymptomatic females with nodular sclerosis histology (6%).[465]

The diagnosis of Hodgkin's disease should be questioned for any lymphoma involving Waldeyer's ring, the skin, and the gastrointestinal tract, especially if this happens to be the first manifestation of the disease. Most of these cases are examples of non-Hodgkin's lymphomas with Reed-Sternberg–like cells.

Patients with Hodgkin's disease often have defects in cellular immunity, which leads to an increased susceptibility to some infections.[460] However, a diagnosis of Hodgkin's disease also should be viewed with suspicion if it presents as a complication of a natural immune deficiency, immunosuppression, or other immune diseases. Although indubitable cases of this association exist (particularly in patients with ataxia-telangiectasia and with AIDS),[466] most of these cases actually represent immunoblastic sarcomas containing binucleated immunoblasts morphologically similar to Reed-Sternberg cells.

Spread

Most cases of Hodgkin's disease begin in lymph nodes and spread from there to other lymph node groups and to extranodal sites. Important information has been acquired in regard to the frequency and significance of this spread as a result of an aggressive diagnostic approach, particularly with the use of laparotomy as a routine staging procedure.[469,470]

1 *Direct extension.* The disease may spread to the perinodal tissues, sometimes extensively, and result in a fusion of the involved nodes. In advanced cases, direct invasion of skin, skeletal muscle, and other sites can occur. Mediastinal Hodgkin's disease can extend by continuity into the large vessels, lung, and chest wall.[472]

2 *Other lymph node groups.* Most cases of Hodgkin's disease spread by involvement of adjacent lymph node groups.[471] This contiguous manner of spread is particularly common in the nodular sclerosis and lymphocytic predominance types.[472] Nodal spread can be evaluated with lymphangiogram, CT scan, and staging laparotomy (Fig. 21-44). In competent hands, lymphangiography has an overall diagnostic accuracy in excess of 90%; it is more effective in detecting involvement below the level of the second lumbar vertebra but inconsistent for nodes situated higher in the periaortic area. About 30% of patients with negative lymphangiograms in whom the para-aortic nodes are left untreated will later demonstrate disease below the diaphragm.[468] Of the nodes biopsied at laparotomy during the course of a staging procedure, the most likely to be involved are those located in the splenic hilum and retroperitoneum. Mesenteric nodes are almost always spared.

3 *Spleen.* A spleen weighing 400 g or more is practically always histologically positive. The converse is not true: spleens below this weight are involved in a high proportion of cases. The focal nature of the disease calls for a careful gross examination of this organ. The spec-

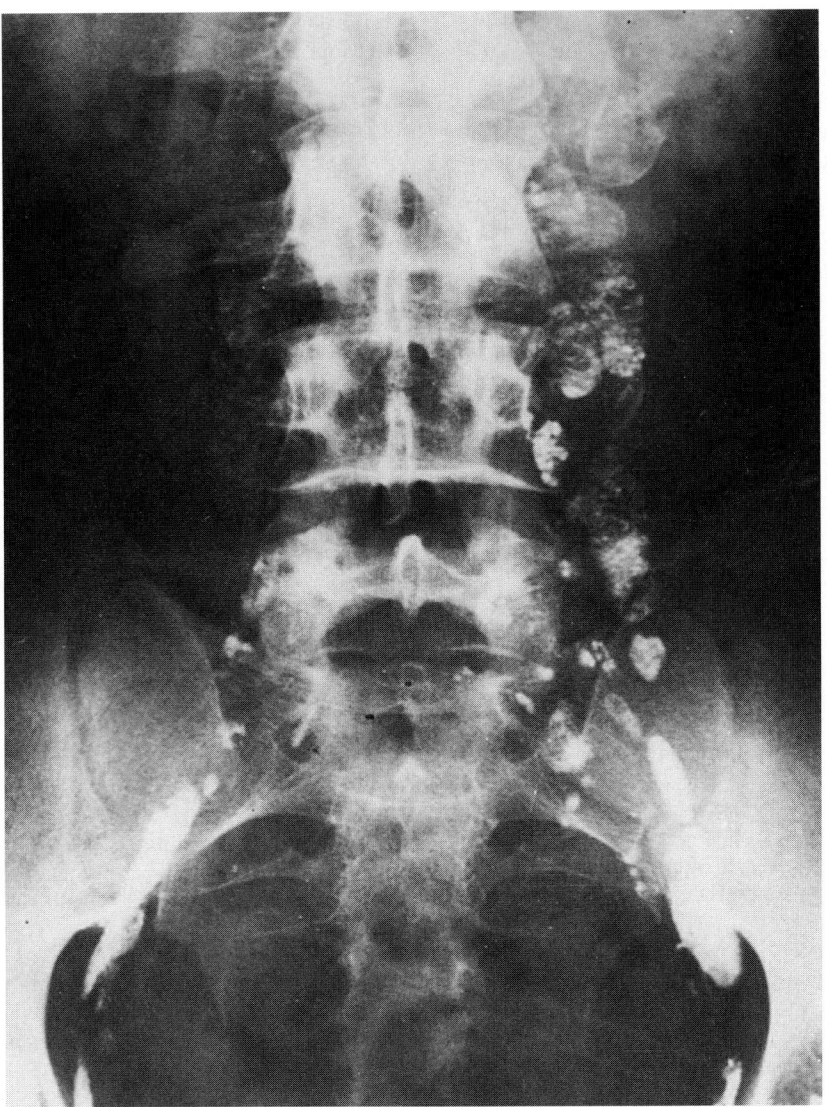

Fig. 21-44 Positive retroperitoneal lymphangiogram in patient with Hodgkin's disease. Lymph nodes are enlarged and have coarse reticulated appearance.

imens should be sectioned throughout in thin slices, and every suspicious area should be examined microscopically. If no nodules are detected on gross inspection, the chances of finding Hodgkin's disease in random microscopic sections are negligible. Splenic involvement is thought to represent a critical stage in the spread of Hodgkin's disease and is an early manifestation of blood vessel dissemination. The approximate number of tumor nodules present in the spleen should be indicated because of their relation to prognosis; specifically, it should be stated whether there are five or more. It is not important to subclassify the disease in the spleen into the specific type.

4 *Liver.* Hepatic disease is almost invariably associated with splenic and retroperitoneal lymph node involve-

ment and with so-called B symptoms. Clinical assessment of liver involvement is quite unreliable. Care should be exercised in distinguishing involvement by Hodgkin's disease from benign lymphoid aggregates, some of which may show mild atypia.[473]

5 *Bone marrow.* This is discussed in Chapter 23.

6 *Others.* Practically any other organ can show secondary involvement by Hodgkin's disease, such as the lung, skin, gastrointestinal tract, and central nervous system (see respective chapters).

Staging

The current staging classification for Hodgkin's disease was established by the Ann Arbor Workshop in 1971 and modified at Cotswolds in 1989[474,476,477] (see box). Clinical staging refers to all procedures short of laparotomy. It includes physical examination, bone marrow aspiration and biopsy, clinical laboratory evaluation, and numerous radiographic studies. Chest x-ray and thoracic and abdominal CT studies have become the norm, and these are supplemented in some centers by bipedal lymphangiogram and gallium scans. Pathologic staging used to refer to the findings at staging laparotomy during which liver, splenectomy, and biopsies of retroperitoneal lymph nodes, liver, and bone marrow were performed. Although much important information has been obtained from the performance of routine staging laparotomy in patients with Hodgkin's disease, the procedure is now used only sparingly, the reasons being the increased diagnostic power of radiographic techniques, the high efficiency of current therapies, and the occurrence of postsurgical complications, particularly in the pediatric population.[475,476]

Treatment

The two pillars of therapy in Hodgkin's disease are radiation therapy and chemotherapy, the choice being largely dependent on the stage of the disease and the bias of the individual centers.[481,482,484] Bone marrow transplantation is used in selected cases.[478,480]

Successful therapy results in disappearance of the tumor foci, some of which are still detectable on post-therapy biopsy or at autopsy as fibrous nodules.[479] Sometimes Hodgkin's disease persists for a long time following therapy, even if it has been controlled on clinical grounds. Of nineteen autopsied patients who died after having survived Hodgkin's disease for 10 years or more, Strum and Rappaport[483] found residual disease in sixteen.

Prognosis

The current overall 5-year survival rate of Hodgkin's disease is approximately 75%.

Many clinical and morphologic parameters have been found to correlate with prognosis.[496] These parameters follow, but only after a comment about the spectacular advances in the therapy of this disease that have blurred the differences, to the point that most of them are no longer significant.

1 *Clinical stage.* This remains by far the most important prognostic parameter, although the differences between the various stages have greatly diminished. According to Kaplan,[493] only stage IV disease and constitutional symptoms continue to present serious therapeutic problems.
2 *Age.* Patients over 50 years of age have a worsened prognosis.[490]
3 *Sex and race.* In some series, males and blacks with nodular sclerosis disease have had a less favorable course than females and whites, respectively.
4 *Pregnancy.* This appears to have no effect on the course of the disease.
5 *Location, number, and size of tumor masses.* A large mediastinal mass (greater than one third of the maximum intrathoracic diameter), multiple nodules in the spleen, or multiple extranodal sites of involvement are unfavorable prognostic factors. The latter feature

ANN ARBOR STAGING CLASSIFICATION FOR HODGKIN'S DISEASE (as modified at Cotswolds)

Stage I
Involvement of a single lymph node region (I) or a single extralymphatic organ or site (Ig)
Stage II
Involvement of two or more lymph node regions on the same side of the diaphragm (II) or localized involvement of an extralymphatic organ or site (IIg)
Stage III
Involvement of lymph node regions on both sides of the diaphragm (III) or localized involvement of an extralymphatic organ or site (IIIg) or spleen (IIIg) or both (IIIse)
Stage IV
Diffuse or disseminated involvement of one or more extralymphatic organs with or without associated lymph node involvement. The organ(s) involved should be identified by a symbol.*

*A, Asymptomatic; B, fever >38° previous month, sweats previous month, weight loss >10% of body weight previous 6 months; X, bulk (>10 cm for lymph node, >1/3 of internal transverse diameter of thorax at >5/6 on a posteroanterior chest radiograph).
From Warnke RA, Weiss LM, Chan JKC, Cleary ML, Dorfman RF: Tumors of the lymph nodes and spleen. Atlas of tumor pathology, 3rd Series, Fascicle 14. Washington, DC, 1995, Armed Forces Institute of Pathology.

relates directly to the staging and is of great prognostic import.[497] There is, however, a substantial difference depending on whether the involvement is at a distance ("metastatic") or whether it represents spread in contiguity from a nodal site. For instance, direct extension from mediastinal nodes of lung or chest wall in nodular sclerosis Hodgkin's disease does not result in an appreciable decrease in survival.[494]

6 *Laboratory findings.* Decreased hematocrit, elevated levels of lactate dehydrogenase, increased erythrosedimentation rate, increased beta-2-microglobulin, and elevated serum levels of CD30 and soluble CD25 have all been claimed to have a negative impact on survival in high-stage patients.[489,492,495]
7 *Microscopic types.* Traditionally, lymphocyte predominance and nodular sclerosis have been the most favorable forms, mixed cellularity has been intermediate, and the lymphocyte depletion form has had the worst prognosis.[487,488] The long-term prognosis of lymphocyte predominance Hodgkin's disease is so good that some authors have referred to it as "the benign form" of Hodgkin's disease, and have even doubted that it represents a neoplastic process.[499] A stark contrast is offered by lymphocyte depletion Hodgkin's disease; in the series of Bearman et al.,[486] the median survival was 25.1 months, with only eight (21%) patients surviving 4 years or longer. In general, no prognostic differences have been found between

the subtypes of nodular sclerosis or lymphocyte depletion[498]; however, the suggestion has been made that nodular sclerosis cases belonging to what the British have called grade II lesions (which include the so-called syncytial variant of other authors) are somewhat more aggressive[491] (see p. 1703).

It has been pointed out that at least some of the prognostic significance of the various microscopic types depends on the clinical stage, in view of the fact that a definite correlation between the two exists. Thus most lymphocyte predominance and nodular sclerosis cases are in stages I and II, whereas most lymphocyte depletion cases are in stages III and IV; however, until relatively recently the prognostic differences among microscopic types were maintained even within staging groups.[494] This is no longer the case. At present, only lymphocyte depletion histology carries an unfavorable significance, and in some series even this difference has been erased.

8 *Noncaseating granulomas.* The presence of these formations may be associated with a slightly better prognosis within a given stage.

9 *Follicular dendritic cells.* Cases with an extensive network of these cells are said to have a better prognosis than the others.[485]

10 *Epstein-Barr virus.* No differences in survival have been found between EBV-positive and EBV-negative cases.

Non-Hodgkin's lymphoma

The classification of non-Hodgkin's lymphoma that was most widely used until the early 1980s in the United States and many other countries was that proposed by Rappaport in 1966[519] (Table 21-10). This represented a slight modification of the classification that Gall and Rappaport had presented at a Seminar of the American Society of Clinical Pathologists held in New Orleans, Louisiana, in 1963. This, in turn, was based on the classification proposed by Gall and Mallory[506] as part of their comprehensive critical study of 618 lymphomas. Rappaport's classification was, of necessity, based entirely on morphologic grounds. Numerous independent clinicopathologic studies have shown its reproducibility, usefulness, and clinical relevance.[501] However, application of the remarkable advances in the fields of immunology, cytogenetics, and molecular pathology in the past years to the study of lymphomas has shown that these can be viewed as clonal expansions of the normal anatomic and functional components of the immune system. Most of them have been studied using immunologic markers and, as a result, have been "typed" as to their normal counterparts, from which presumably they arose. This "functional" approach, championed by Lukes[500,514] in this country and by Lennert in Germany, incorporated a number of entities and showed that a functional classification of lymphoma was possible to some extent on the basis of morphologic interpretation of routinely stained sections[511,513] (Table 21-10). Independent of this, aggressive clinical investigations coupled with staging laparotomies provided a wealth of new [infor]mation on the sites of predilection and spread of the [lymp]homas according to type.[504,507,520] The results obtained [from] these investigations pointed to some inaccuracies and

other deficiencies of Rappaport's classification and the need to revise it, taking into account all these new data.

Five new classifications were proposed,[503,509,515,516] which, needless to say, resulted in a confusing state of affairs for both pathologists and clinicians.

Since there was no clear-cut evidence that one classification was clearly superior to the others, the National Cancer Institute sponsored a retrospective study of 1175 cases of non-Hodgkin's lymphoma, which were classified according to the different categories by the investigators who proposed them, as well as by a panel of "control" pathologists.[517,518] Analysis of the data showed that all six classifications were successful in predicting the prognosis in a large number of lymphoma patients and that no classification appeared superior to any other in this respect.[517] It also confirmed that lymphomas with a follicular pattern of growth (a feature consistently identified by all reviewers) had a more favorable prognosis than those with diffuse patterns within the same cytologic subtypes. This was true whether the nodularity was extensive or only partial. Finally, it confirmed the suspicion that within the "histiocytic lymphoma" category of Rappaport there was a variety of morphologically recognizable neoplasms with a somewhat different natural history. As a result of the analysis of these 1175 cases, the investigators involved in this study proposed a new classification ("Working Formulation") of non-Hodgkin's malignant lymphomas, based primarily on light microscopic differences, as seen in sections stained with hematoxylin-eosin, that showed a correlation with survival. Ten major types plus a miscellaneous group were identified, and these we subdivided into three major prognostic groups that were of favorable, intermediate, and unfavorable prognosis, respectively.

Although this classification has gained some degree of acceptability, it was viewed by many as a compromise rather than a conceptual advance, just as the Rye classification of Hodgkin's disease was seen as a compromise (not necessarily for the better) over the Lukes-Butler classification.[505] It was pointed out from the very beginning that the Working Formulation did not take into account all the entities that had been recognized at that time. This, plus the continuing advances that have been made in the field, has led to additions and other changes to the scheme.[517]

Lately, an international group of hematopathologists has prepared a list of lymphoid neoplasms that they felt could be recognized with available techniques and which appeared to be clinically distinctive.[502,508] The approach was strictly pragmatic, in the sense that the list included only those categories that appeared reasonably identifiable as such, without attempting to always relate them to normal stages of lymphoid differentiation. Whether this listing (see box) will become the basis for a new classification of lymphoma remains to be seen.[510]

The individual descriptions that follow generally employ the terminology proposed in the Working Formulation, modified whenever indicated.

Small lymphocytic lymphoma

Small lymphocytic lymphoma preferentially occurs in middle-aged and elderly individuals.[523,539] The symptoms

Table 21-10 Major classifications of non-Hodgkin's lymphoma as modified by the respective authors for use in the National Cancer Institute–sponsored study on the subject and in the new International Formulation[518]

Rappaport	Lukes and Collins	Kiel
Nodular	Undefined cell type	Low-grade malignancy
Lymphocytic, well differentiated	T-cell type	Lymphocytic
Lymphocytic, poorly differentiated	Small lymphocytic	Chronic lymphocytic leukemia
Mixed (lymphocytic and histiocytic)	Sézary–mycosis fungoides (cerebriform)	Other
Histiocytic	Convoluted lymphocytic	Lymphoplasmacytoid
Diffuse	Immunoblastic sarcoma (T-cell)	Centrocytic
Lymphocytic, well differentiated	Small lymphocytic	Centroblastic-centrocytic
Without plasmacytoid features	B-cell type	Follicular, without sclerosis
With plasmacytoid features	Small lymphocytic	Follicular, with sclerosis
Lymphocytic, poorly differentiated	Plasmacytoid lymphocytic	Follicular and diffuse, without sclerosis
Without plasmacytoid features	Follicular center cell*	Follicular and diffuse, with sclerosis
With plasmacytoid features	Small cleaved	Diffuse
Lymphoblastic	Large cleaved	Unclassified
Convoluted	Small noncleaved	High-grade malignancy
Nonconvuluted	Large noncleaved	Centroblastic
Mixed (lymphocytic and histiocytic)	Immunoblastic sarcoma (B-cell)	Lymphoblastic
Histiocytic	Histiocytic	Burkitt's type
Without sclerosis	Unclassified	Convoluted cell type
With sclerosis	Composite	Other (unclassified)
Burkitt's tumor		Immunoblastic
Undifferentiated		Unclassified
Unclassified		Unclassified
Composite		Composite

International Formulation		

Low grade
  ML,† small lymphocytic
    Consistent with chronic lymphocytic leukemia
    Plasmacytoid
  ML, follicular, predominantly small cleaved cell
    With diffuse areas
    With sclerosis
  ML, follicular, mixed (small cleaved and large cell)
    With diffuse areas
    With sclerosis
Intermediate grade
  ML, follicular, predominantly large cell
    With diffuse areas
    With sclerosis
  ML, diffuse, small cleaved cell
    With sclerosis
  ML, diffuse, mixed (small and large cell)
    With sclerosis
    With epithelioid cell component
  ML, diffuse, large cell
    Cleaved cell
    Noncleaved cell
    With sclerosis

High grade
  ML, large cell, immunoblastic
    Plasmacytoid
    Clear cell
    Polymorphous
    With epithelioid cell component
  ML, lymphoblastic
    Convoluted
    Nonconvoluted
  ML, small noncleaved cell
    Burkitt's
    With follicular areas
Miscellaneous
  Composite
  Mycosis fungoides
  Histiocytic
  Extramedullary plasmacytoma
  Unclassifiable
  Other

*Subdivided into (1) follicular, follicular and diffuse, and diffuse and (2) without sclerosis and with sclerosis.
†ML, Malignant lymphoma.

LIST OF LYMPHOID NEOPLASMS RECOGNIZED BY THE INTERNATIONAL LYMPHOMA STUDY GROUP

B-cell neoplasms

I. Precursor B-cell neoplasm: B-precursor lymphoblastic leukemia/lymphoma
II. Peripheral B-cell neoplasms
   1. B-cell chronic lymphocytic leukemia/prolymphocytic leukemia/small lymphocytic lymphoma
   2. Lymphoplasmacytoid lymphoma/immunocytoma
   3. Mantle cell lymphoma
   4. Follicle center lymphoma, follicular
      Provisional cytologic grades: Small cell, mixed small and large cell, large cell
      Provisional subtype: Diffuse, predominantly small cell type
   5. Marginal zone B-cell lymphoma
      Extranodal (MALT type ± monocytoid B cells)
      Provisional category: Nodal (± monocytoid B cells)
      Provisional category: Splenic (± villous lymphocytes)
   6. Hairy cell leukemia
   7. Plasmacytoma/myeloma
   8. Diffuse large cell B-cell lymphoma
      Subtype: Primary mediastinal (thymic) B-cell lymphoma
   9. Burkitt's lymphoma
   10. Provisional category: High-grade B-cell lymphoma, Burkitt's-like

T-cell and putative NK-cell* neoplasms

I. Precursor T-cell neoplasm: T-precursor lymphoblastic lymphoma/leukemia
II. Peripheral T-cell and NK-cell neoplasms
   1. T-cell chronic lymphocytic leukemia/prolymphocytic leukemia
   2. Large granular lymphocytic leukemia (LGL)
   3. Mycosis fungoides/ Sézary's syndrome
   4. Peripheral T-cell lymphoma provisional subtypes: Medium-sized cell, mixed medium and large cell, large cell, lymphoepithelioid cell
   5. Angioimmunoblastic T-cell lymphoma (AILD)
   6. Angiocentric lymphoma
   7. Intestinal T-cell lymphoma (± enteropathy associated)
   8. Adult T-cell lymphoma/leukemia (ATL/L)
   9. Anaplastic large cell lymphoma (ALCL), CD30+, T- and null-cell types
   10. Provisional subtype: Anaplastic large-cell lymphoma, Hodgkin's-like

Unclassifiable

1. B-cell lymphoma, unclassifiable (low grade/high grade)
2. T-cell lymphoma, unclassifiable (low grade/high grade)
3. Malignant lymphoma, unclassifiable

*NK, Natural killer.
From Warnke RA, Weiss LM, Chan JKC, Cleary ML, Dorfman RF: Tumors of the lymph nodes and spleen. Atlas of tumor pathology. 3rd Series, Fascicle 14. Washington, DC, 1995, Armed Forces Institute of Pathology.

---

are scanty, the evolution is prolonged, and the survival is very good.

The architecture of the node in small lymphocytic lymphoma is massively and monotonously effaced by a population of small round lymphocytes with clumped chromatin, inconspicuous nucleoli, barely visible cytoplasm, and scanty mitotic activity (Figs. 21-45 and 21-46). Extranodal extension is seen in about one third of the cases. In some, there are numerous residual lymphoid follicles (so-called interfollicular small lymphocytic lymphoma).[530] In others, there is selective involvement of the B zones of the node.[527] Yet other cases may show a propensity for infiltration of veins.[534] Ultrastructurally, the cells of small lymphocytic lymphoma are extremely well differentiated.

Cases of small lymphocytic lymphomas can be divided into three categories: (1) those with absolute lymphocytosis (i.e., chronic lymphocytic leukemia), (2) those associated with monoclonal gammopathy (50% of which have bone marrow involvement), and (3) those with neither; the latter are often accompanied by hypogammaglobulinemia.[523,532,537,540] There are no statistical differences in survival between these three groups and no appreciable morphologic differences between the first and the third groups.[522] In the cases associated with monoclonal gammopathy, some or most of the neoplastic lymphocytes may exhibit morphologic signs of plasmacytoid differentiation (as evidenced by oval shape, lateralization of the nucleus, appearance of a perinuclear halo, and pyroninophilia) and admixture of plasma cells (Fig. 21-47). Effacement of the nodal architecture is generally not as complete as with the usual type. These cases are referred to as *small lymphocytic lymphoma with plasmacytic differentiation* and are discussed further in the section on lymphoma and dysproteinemia.

Immunohistochemically, small lymphocytic lymphomas are nearly always of B-cell type.[543] Monoclonal immunoglobulins, usually of the IgM type, are consistently found on their surface (see Fig. 21-48). They differ from the B lymphocytes of follicular lymphoma in the intensity and appearance of the reaction (brighter and more clumped in the latter), as well as by their lesser content of complement receptors. They are usually reactive for the B-cell–related antigens CD5, CD23 (in contrast to mantle cell lymphoma),[529,544] and CD43. At the molecular level, Ig heavy and light chain genes are rearranged. Cytogenetically, trisomy 12 has been reported in one third of the cases, and abnormalities of 13q in up to one quarter.[533] In a small number of cases of chronic lymphocytic leukemia, the lymphocytes have T- rather than B-cell markers and differ clinically and cytologically from the rest[526,536] (see Chapter 23). The cells are somewhat larger, have numerous azurophilic granules, and contain large amounts of acid phosphatase and β-glucuronidase.

Not infrequently, cases of small lymphocytic lymphoma with or without leukemia (but particularly the latter) show, in addition to the well-differentiated lymphocytes, an admixture of larger cells (prolymphocytes or paraimmunoblasts) with vesicular nuclei and prominent nucleoli, singly or in small aggregates that simulate germinal cen-

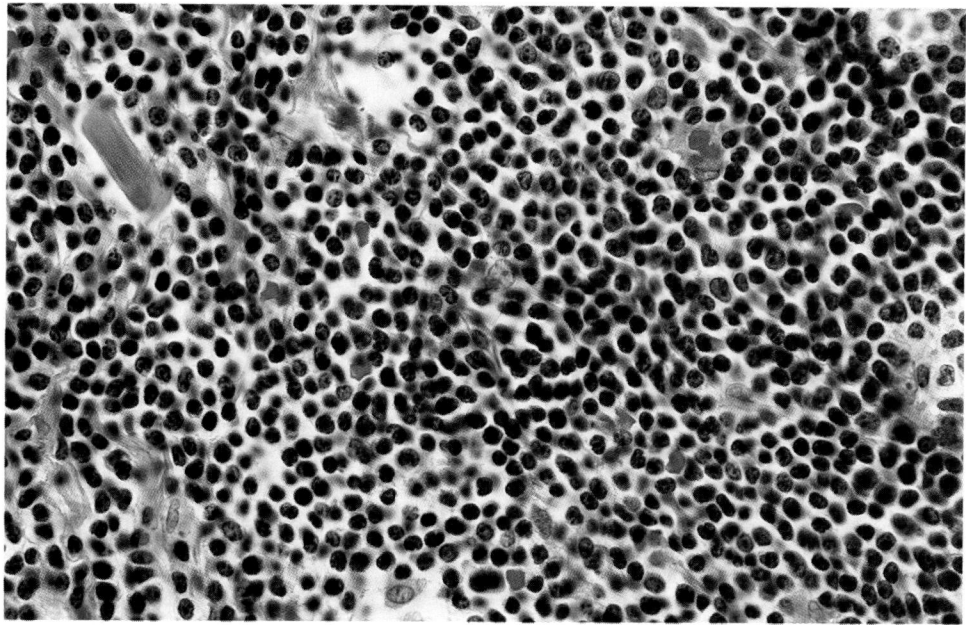

Fig. 21-45 Low-power view of small lymphocytic lymphoma. A monotonous proliferation of small lymphocytes effaces the architecture of the node.

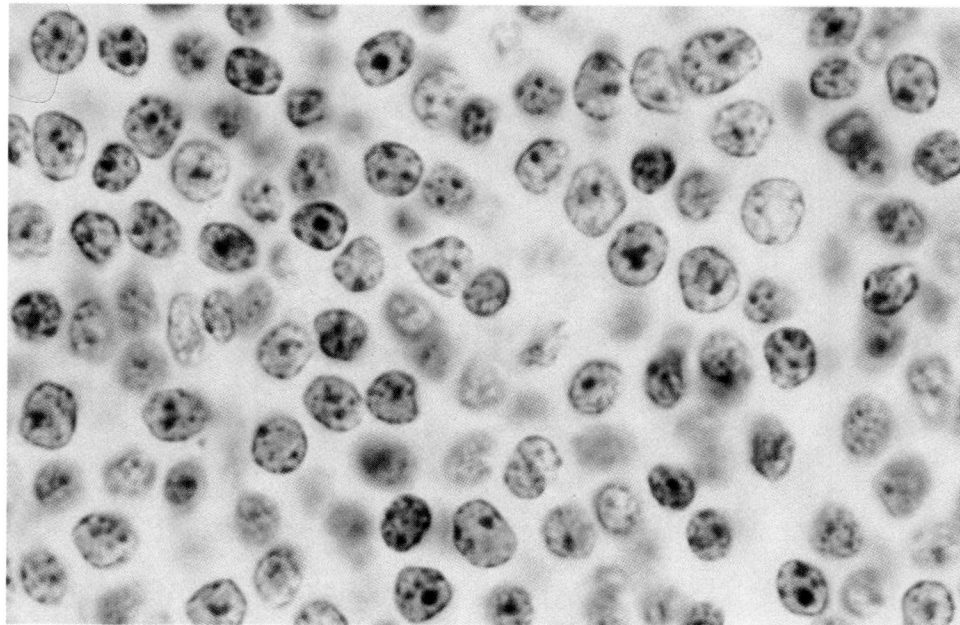

Fig. 21-46 High-power view of small lymphocytic lymphoma. The nuclear contours are regular, the chromatin is clumped, and nucleoli are inconspicuous.

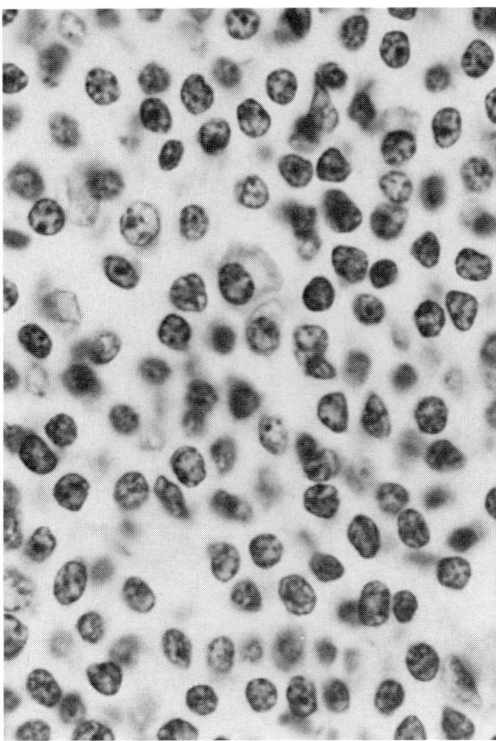

Fig. 21-47 Small lymphocytic lymphoma accompanied by Waldenstrom's macroglobulinemia. Proliferation is composed of lymphocytes and plasmacytoid lymphocytes. (From Mann RB, Jaffe ES, Berard CW: Malignant lymphomas. A conceptual understanding of morphologic diversity. A review. Am J Pathol **94:**105-191, 1979.)

ters[528,540,541] (Fig. 21-49). These formations (known as proliferative centers, growth centers, or pseudofollicles) have an increased number of Ki-67–positive cells.[537] This feature, which is apparently of no prognostic significance, should not lead to confusion with follicular lymphoma or lymphocyte predominance Hodgkin's disease. It should be noted, however, that on occasion one sees cases of small lymphocytic lymphoma with typical Reed-Sternberg cells, suggesting a possible transformation to Hodgkin's disease; it has been hypothesized that such a transformation may be mediated by the Epstein-Barr virus.[538] Another development of great clinical significance is the transformation of a small lymphocytic lymphoma (or a chronic lymphocytic leukemia) into a "blastic," "histiocytic," or large cell neoplasm.[521] This occurrence, when developing in the background of chronic lymphocytic leukemia, is known as *Richter's syndrome*[535] and is accompanied by a precipitous decline in the clinical course. Fever, increasing lymphadenopathy, weight loss, and abdominal pain are frequent,[545] sometimes accompanied by hepatomegaly and splenomegaly. The earliest infiltrates may be detected in the lymph nodes or in the bone marrow.[531] Cell surface studies in these cases have shown that the large cells generally possess the same type of immunoglobulin heavy and light chain as the pre-existing small lymphocytes, indicating that they represent dedifferentiation of the original tumor rather than a second neoplasm. However, exceptions to this rule have been reported, some of the pleomorphic cells having the immunocytochemical features of Reed-Sternberg cells.[525,542,546]

Lymphoma and dysproteinemia. In view of the fact that most malignant lymphomas arise from B lymphocytes (i.e.,

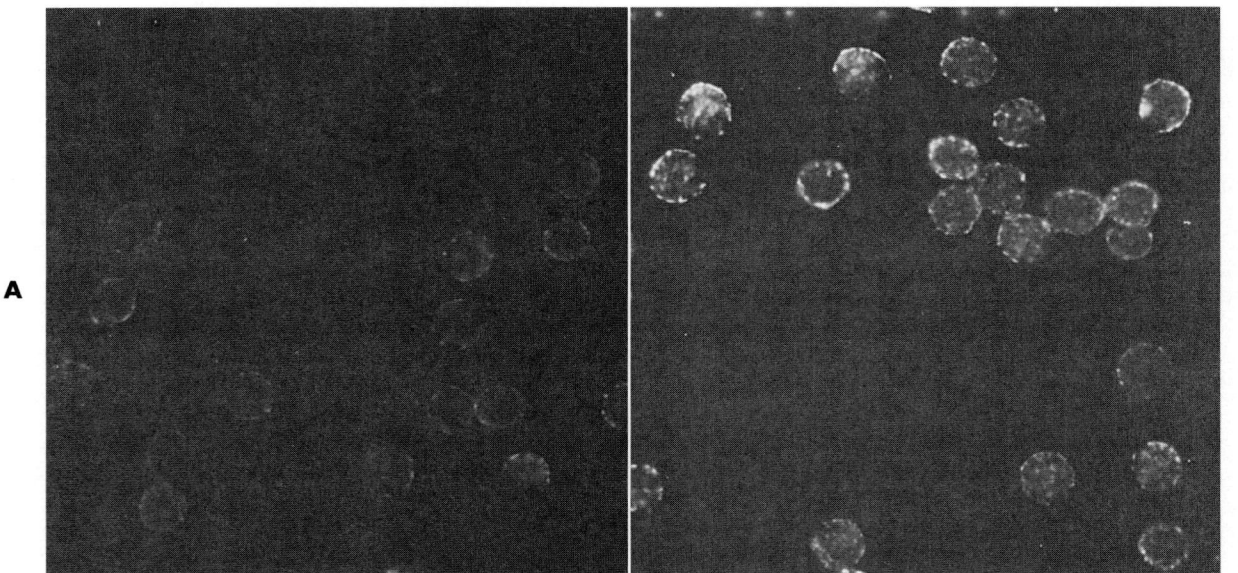

Fig. 21-48 Surface immunoglobulin demonstration in neoplastic lymphocytes by immunofluorescence using antibodies against μ heavy chain. **A,** Chronic lymphocytic leukemia. Faint but definite staining may be seen in all cells. **B,** Malignant lymphoma associated with Waldenstrom's macroglobulinemia. Staining is more intense. Cells of follicular lymphoma stain with similar degree of intensity, although not all cells will be stained. (Courtesy Dr. K. Gaji-Peczalska, Minneapolis.)

cells normally engaged in humoral immune responses) it is not surprising that in some of them the tumor cells express their potentialities by producing immunoglobulins of one sort or another.[548,559] Ranging in between the typical malignant lymphoma without immunoglobulin abnormalities and the typical plasma cell myeloma with monoclonal peak and Bence Jones proteinuria, all types of morphologic and biochemical hybrids have been encountered.[524] Tumors have been described that secrete completely assembled immunoglobulins of the IgG, IgA, IgM, IgD, or IgE type (with or without concomitant production of isolated light chains), isolated light chains to the almost total exclusion of complete immunoglobulin molecules, and "heavy chains" (or, more accurately, Fc fragments) of IgG, IgM, or IgA specificity. Some of these immunoglobulins have the physicochemical properties of cryoglobulins and can result in necrotizing vasculitis.[549] This remarkably diverse expression of function has led to the introduction of such names as Waldenström's macroglobulinemia, light chain disease, α-chain disease, and Franklin's heavy chain disease and even to the proposal of grouping all immunoglobulin-secreting lymphoid and plasmacytic tumors under the term *immunocytoma.*[551,554]

This practice has led to considerable confusion as happens whenever morphologic and functional parameters are mixed in a common terminology. For instance, the serum picture of macroglobulinemia can be associated with a microscopic picture of small lymphocytic lymphoma, small lymphocytic lymphoma with plasmacytic differentiation, plasma cell myeloma, and large cell lymphoma. It is obvious that by giving a tissue diagnosis "consistent with macroglobulinemia," the pathologist is not rendering an accurate account of the situation. We believe that these neoplasms should be classified according to conventional morphologic criteria rather than by the biochemical findings in the patient's serum—i.e., a small lymphocytic lymphoma should be designated as such whether it produces macroglobulins, heavy chains, light chains, or no detectable globulins. Four main cytologic patterns are observed in these immunoglobulin-secreting neoplasms:

1 Malignant lymphomas of conventional appearance, usually of small lymphocytic type, indistinguishable from those not associated with immunoglobulin abnormalities.

2 Plasma cytomas, in which most of the tumor cells have the characteristic light and electron microscopic features of plasma cells.

3 Tumors having the overall appearance of a malignant lymphoma of small lymphocytic type but in which a certain proportion of the tumor cells has undergone a plasmacytic differentiation, as evidenced light microscopically by lateralization of the nucleus, coarse chromatin clumping, appearance of a perinuclear clear halo, and/or increased basophilic cytoplasm and ultrastructurally by prominence of the Golgi apparatus and abundance of granular endoplasmic reticulum.[555] Some of the tumor cells may be PAS positive. Immunoperoxidase stains will often show monoclonal immunoglobulin in the cytoplasm of the plasmacytoid cells much more frequently than in ordinary small lymphocytic

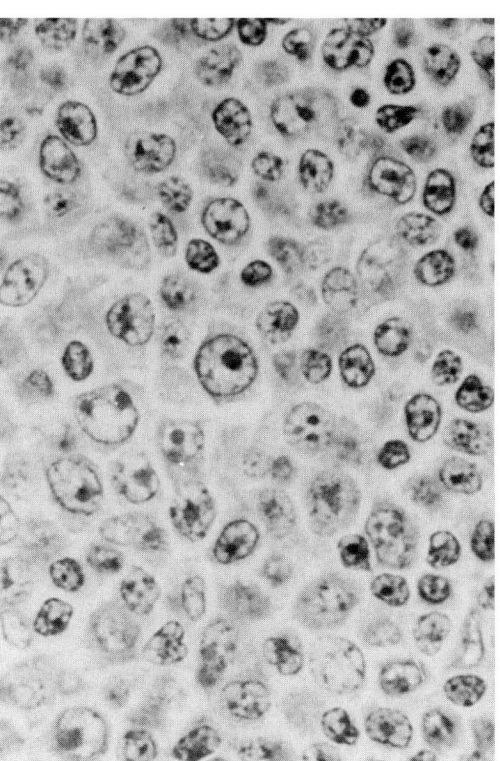

Fig. 21-49 Diffuse lymphoma of small lymphocytic type exhibiting pseudofollicular foci referred to as "growth centers." These foci contain large cells with vesicular nuclei and prominent, often central, nucleoli. Tumors exhibiting these features should not be confused with large cell or undifferentiated lymphoma. (From Mann RB, Jaffe ES, Berard CW: Malignant lymphomas. A conceptual understanding of morphologic diversity. A review. Am J Pathol **94**:105-191, 1979.)

lymphomas or chronic lymphocytic leukemias.[562,563] These tumors have been designated as small lymphocytic malignant lymphomas with plasmacytic differentiation, lymphoplasmacytoid lymphomas, or immunocytomas, lymphoplasmacytic type. Their cell marker profile is similar to that of ordinary small lymphocytic lymphomas except for the presence of *cytoplasmic* immunoglobulin in some of the cells and a lesser percentage and degree of reactivity for CD5.[567]

4 Large cell lymphomas predominantly or exclusively composed of B-immunoblasts. These cases are better designated as immunoblastic sarcomas.

5 Lymphomas composed of an admixture of immunoblasts, large plasmacytoid cells, and mature plasma cells. These cases have sometimes been designated *pleomorphic immunocytomas.* Some of the reported cases of primary plasmacytomas of lymph nodes[547,553] belong to this or to one or another of the previous categories. The term *plasmacytoma* of lymph nodes should be restricted to those rare cases having typical bone marrow involvement by plasmacytoma and/or cases in which nearly all of the malignant cells have plasmacytoid features, and in which a lymphocytic component is absent.

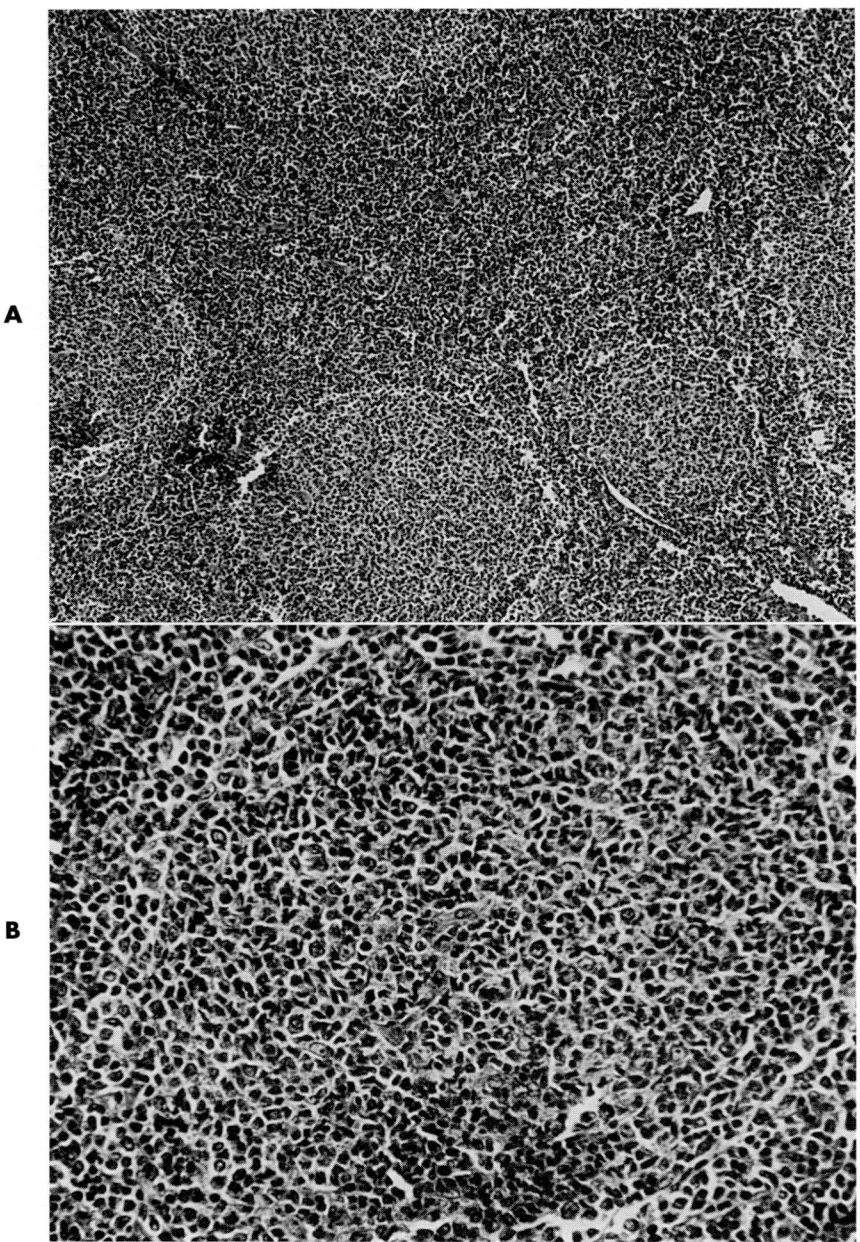

Fig. 21-50 Follicular lymphoma of small cleaved cell type occurring in 51-year-old man with generalized lymphadenopathy. **A,** Large nodules scattered throughout. **B,** Large nodule in which cells inside are streaming outside follicle. There is no evidence of phagocytosis.

Attempts to correlate the microscopic appearance with the secretory activity of these tumors have been made by several authors. The results have been largely discouraging, although a few more or less distinctive patterns have emerged.[556,558] In general, tumors producing IgM globulin or "heavy chains" have the anatomic distribution and cytologic appearance of malignant lymphoma, whereas most of those secreting IgG globulin or a light chain are clinically and microscopically classifiable as plasma cell myeloma. Intranuclear and cytoplasmic inclusions are not specific for any type of immunoglobulin.[564] However, those composed of IgM or IgA are often PAS positive because of their high carbohydrate content, whereas those composed of IgG are not.[550,552] The immunoglobulin inclusions may appear as round eosinophilic bodies or crystals.[561] The former may be so abundant and prominent (perhaps resulting from a blockage in secretion) as to displace the nucleus laterally, creating a signet-ring effect.[557] Tumors that have been reported as secreting IgA "heavy chains" have involved the gastrointestinal tract[566] or, much less commonly, the respiratory tract.[565] The former is discussed in Chapter 11. Production of IgM heavy chains, an exceptionally rare event, occurs in

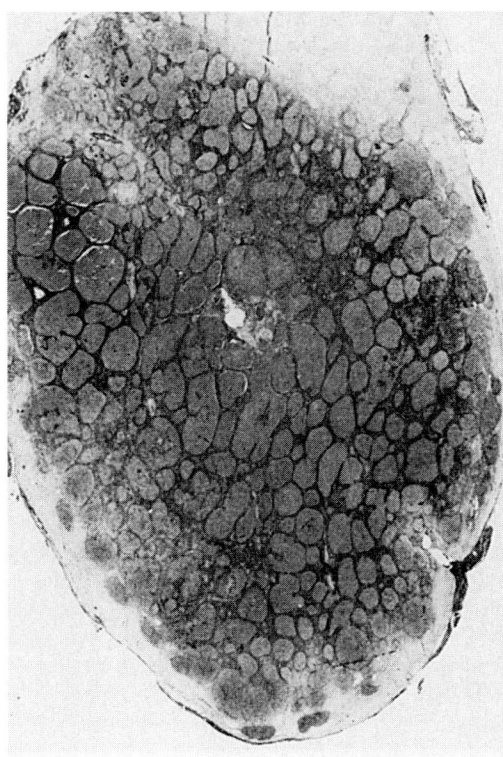

Fig. 21-51 Low-power view of follicular lymphoma. Nodules of relatively uniform size and shape efface nodal architecture. (From Mann RB, Jaffe ES, Berard CW: Malignant lymphomas. A conceptual understanding of morphologic diversity. A review. Am J Pathol **94:**105-191, 1979.)

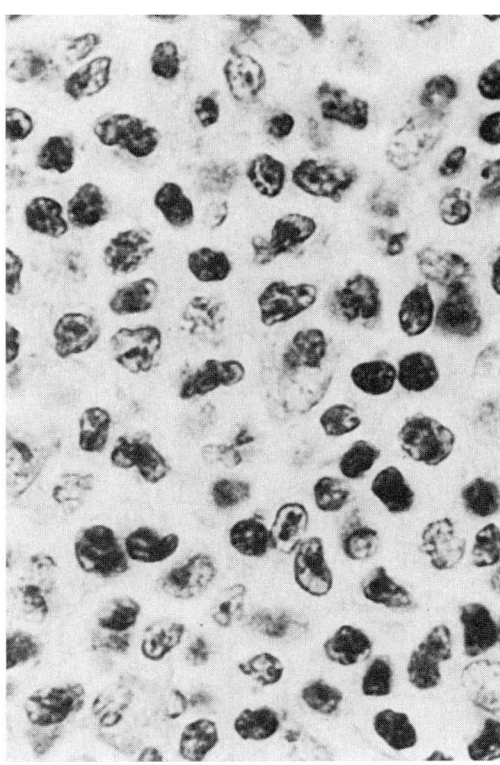

Fig. 21-52 Follicular lymphoma of small cleaved cell type. Note cleaved and indented nuclei with coarsely clumped chromatin. Mitoses are rare. (From Mann RB, Jaffe ES, Berard CW: Malignant lymphomas. A conceptual understanding of morphologic diversity. A review. Am J Pathol **94:**105-191, 1979.)

elderly patients who present with chronic lymphocytic leukemia.[560]

Of all the anatomic varieties of malignant lymphoma, Hodgkin's disease and lymphomas with follicular pattern of growth are the least likely to be associated with immunoglobulin serum abnormalities. The more obvious the plasmacytic differentiation, the higher the chances of immunoglobulin alterations. However, it should be remembered that even fully differentiated plasma cell tumors may sometimes be associated with complete lack of detectable immunoglobulin production.

Follicular lymphoma

Follicular (nodular) lymphoma is a B-cell neoplasm that recapitulates the architectural and cytologic features of the normal secondary lymphoid follicle. This tumor comprises up to 40% of all adult non-Hodgkin's lymphomas in the United States, but in other countries the relative incidence is much lower. Most cases occur in elderly individuals. It is very unusual under 20 years of age and relatively uncommon in blacks.[586] Most of the cases diagnosed in the past as follicular lymphomas in children actually represent nodular types of lymphocyte-predominance Hodgkin's disease or reactive follicular hyperplasia. However, well-documented cases of follicular lymphoma in children are on record.[603,612]

At low-power examination, the most distinctive feature of these tumors is the nodular pattern of growth (Figs. 21-50 and 21-51). Rappaport et al.[604] have carefully outlined in a classic article the differential points between these neoplastic nodules and the reactive follicles of follicular hyperplasia (see Table 21-17). With progression of the disease, this distinct nodularity becomes blurred, and eventually most of the proliferation acquires a diffuse pattern. The cytologic composition of the neoplastic nodules is characterized by a mixture in different proportions of small and large lymphoid cells, both of which resemble their normal follicular counterparts.[594] The small cells have scanty cytoplasm and an irregular, elongated, cleaved nucleus with prominent indentations and infoldings; the size is similar or slightly larger than that of normal lymphocytes, the chromatin is coarse, and the nucleolus is inconspicuous (Fig. 21-52). These cells have been variously referred to as germinocytes, centrocytes, poorly differentiated lymphocytes, and small cleaved follicular center cells. The large cells are two or three times the size of normal lymphocytes; they have a distinct rim of cytoplasm and a vesicular nucleus with one or three nucleoli often adjacent to the nuclear membrane. These cells, which have a rapid turnover rate and probably represent the proliferating component of the tumor, have been designated over the years as germinoblasts, centroblasts, histiocytes, large

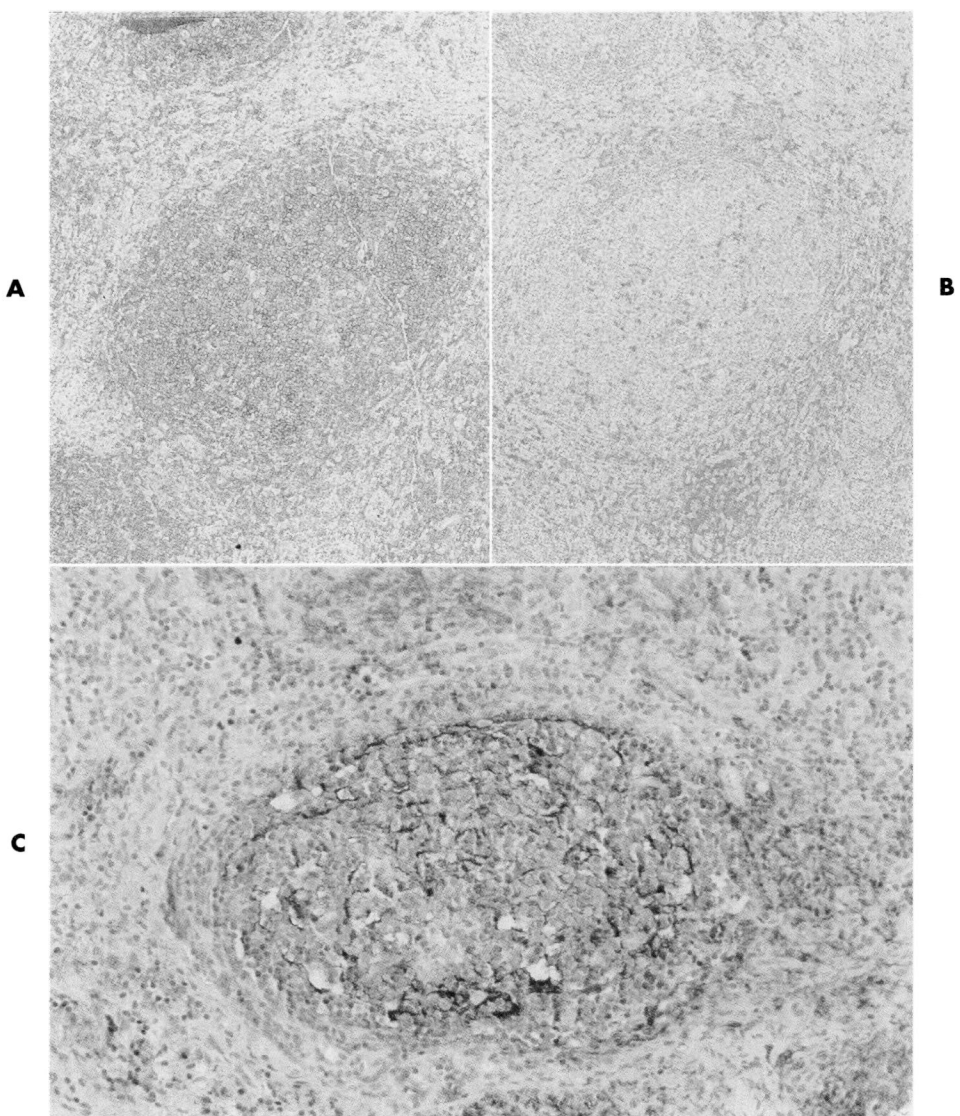

Fig. 21-53 Follicular lymphoma. **A,** CD20 stain decorates the neoplastic nodule and identifies the cells as of B-cell nature. **B,** CD3 stain shows a rim of non-neoplastic T cells around the follicles. **C,** CD21 stain shows a large number of dendritic follicular cells within the neoplastic follicle. (Courtesy Dr. Glauco Frizzera, New York.)

(cleaved or noncleaved) follicular center cells, large lymphoid cells, and lymphoblasts. Some may be binucleated and simulate Reed-Sternberg cells.[596]

Immunohistochemically, the follicles of follicular lymphoma (including all its variants) are composed of a monoclonal population of B cells admixed with a non-neoplastic population representing all the elements normally present in a normal germinal center, including follicular center B cells, small T cells, macrophages, and follicular dendritic cells[607,609] (Fig. 21-53). The tumor cells express pan B-antigens, such as CD19, CD20, CD22, and CD79a, in addition to HLA-DR, CDw75 (LN1), and CD74 (LN2). They also express surface and/or cytoplasmic immunoglobulins (usually of the IgM type) with light chain restriction and stain with monoclonal antibody MT2 (Fig. 21-54, *A*). CD10 (CALLA) has been detected in about 60% of the

cases; CD5 and CD43 are usually negative.[613] Cytogenetically, over 85% of the cases have the 5(14;18) (q32;q21) translocation. This results in the bcl-2 gene being translocated from its normal position on chromosome 18 to chromosome 14, in juxtaposition with the J region of the immunoglobulin heavy chain gene.[577,585,599] The bcl-2 gene product is an integral membrane protein located in the inner mitochondrial membrane and acting as a suppressor of apoptosis.[583,590] The bcl-2 rearrangements can be identified by Southern blot and PCR techniques.[592] They can also be detected in the bone marrow and peripheral circulation, thus allowing for the monitoring of these patients for evidence of residual disease following therapy.[593,602] The bcl-2 protein can be identified immunohistochemically; it is present in about 85% of the follicular lymphomas while being absent in follicular hyperplasia.[581,609,610a] (Fig. 21-54, *B*). Other

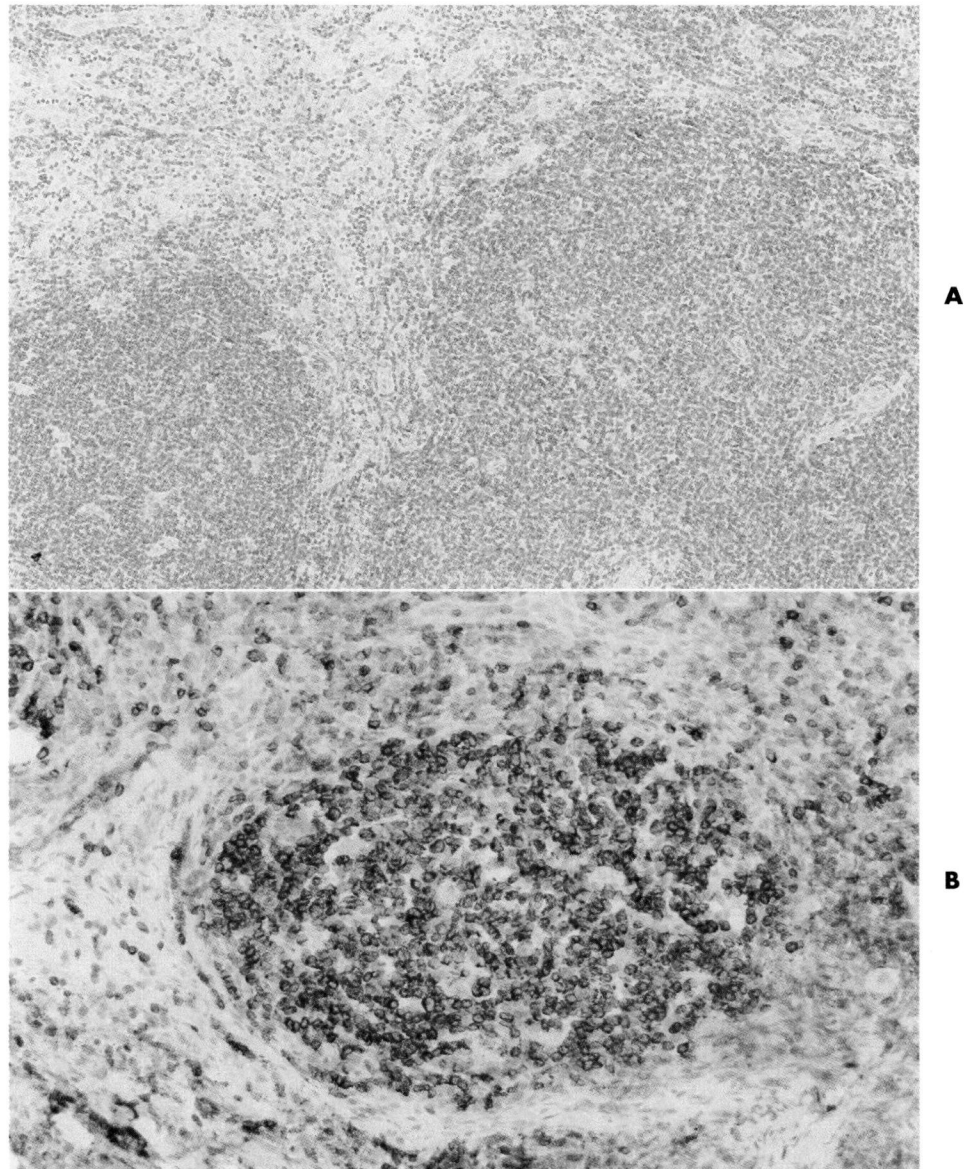

Fig. 21-54 Follicular lymphoma stained for MT2 **(A)** and bcl-2 **(B)**. (Courtesy Dr. Glauco Frizzera, New York.)

types of translocations have been described in follicular lymphoma, such as t(8;14).[591]

Rearrangements of immunoglobulin heavy and light chain genes are present in virtually all cases of follicular lymphoma.

• • •

Depending on the relative proportion of small and large cells, follicular lymphomas are subdivided into three categories, respectively designated in the International Formulation as follows:

1 Predominantly small cleaved cells, when the population of large cells in the nodules is less than 20%
2 Mixed, small cleaved, and large cells, when the proportion of large cells is between 20% and 50%
3 Predominantly large cell, when the proportion of large cells is more than 50%

A rare fourth category has been described, in which the neoplastic follicles are *entirely* composed of small lymphocytes.[573]

In the first category, which is the most common, mitotic activity is infrequent. Conversely, the appearance of large cells is often accompanied by a parallel increase in the number of mitoses.

Several important clinical differences exist between these groups, whether one uses this or a different terminology.[574,610] Patients in the first category are often asymptomatic, usually have generalized disease (often involving extranodal sites, such as the liver and bone marrow), and

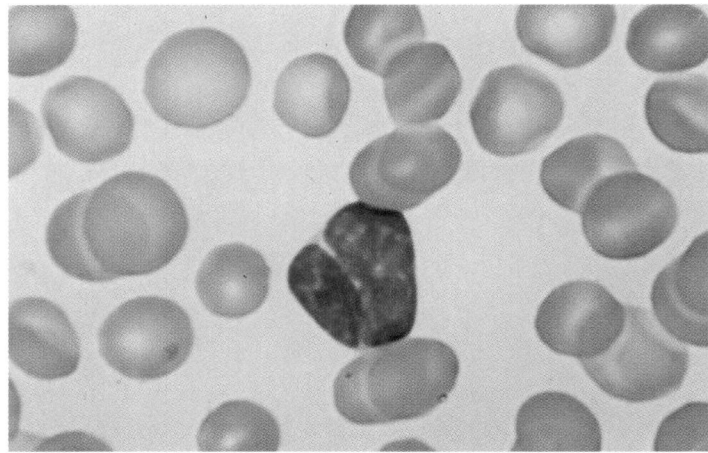

Fig. 21-55 Blood smear from patient with follicular lymphoma showing so-called "notched nucleus cell" or "buttock cell."

have a good prognosis, to the point that some authors advise against aggressive treatment for them.* Tumors in the third category are more commonly localized at the time of presentation but run a more aggressive clinical course[584,586] and are more likely to lose their nodular pattern of growth and become diffuse. The prognosis of tumors in the second category is intermediate between these two but closer to the first. As a matter of fact, in an early series it was associated with an even longer survival.[568] Because of this fact, the first two categories are sometimes grouped under the term *low-grade follicular lymphoma,* the implication being that the predominantly large cell lymphoma is a high-grade tumor. Another morphologic parameter that has been evaluated in this tumor is the relative degree of nodularity. Warnke et al.[611] have shown that among the predominantly small cleaved cell and mixed lymphomas, the survival rate is similar in patients with purely follicular tumors and those with tumors of a follicular and diffuse pattern. However, in the predominantly large cell category, patients with tumors of both follicular and diffuse patterns have a worse prognosis than those with tumors of a pure follicular pattern.

The extranodal spread of follicular lymphoma is quite predictable. In the spleen, it tends to affect the B-derived lymphoid follicles located eccentrically in the white pulp. In the liver, the infiltrate is predominantly periportal. The bone marrow infiltrates tend to have a paratrabecular location. In the skin, there is an extensive dermal infiltrate without particular relation to vessels or adnexa.

In some cases of follicular lymphoma (particularly of the predominantly small cleaved cell type), malignant cells are found in the peripheral blood; hematologists refer to them by the inelegant term "buttock" cells because of their prominent nuclear cleft (Fig. 21-55). No prognostic significance has been assigned to this finding.

Specimens from subsequent biopsies or autopsy from patients with predominantly small cleaved cell lymphomas

may show a similar microscopic appearance or a progression to a large cell type.[580,601] A more ominous development is represented by the occasional "blastic" transformation of follicular lymphoma, in which the tumor cells acquire the morphologic features of markedly atypical cells; this is accompanied by a highly aggressive clinical course.[576]

Several morphologic variations in the theme of follicular lymphoma have been described. They include the following:

1 Presence of fine or coarse bands of fibrosis that accentuate even more the nodular character of the lesion but, in so doing, may induce confusion with carcinoma. This feature is more commonly seen in the large cell type[570]; it is particularly frequent in the retroperitoneum, but it also occurs in the cervical region, mediastinum, and other locations.

2 Deposition of proteinaceous material in the center of the nodules, similar to that seen in some reactive conditions, particularly the plasma cell variant of Castleman's disease. The material is amorphous, acellular, brightly eosinophilic, and PAS positive.[574,606] Ultrastructurally, it is composed of membranous structures, membrane-bound vesicles, and electron-dense bodies.[574] It can appear both in predominantly small cleaved cell and mixed follicular lymphomas.[606]

3 Presence of large cytoplasmic eosinophilic globules—presumably immunoglobulins—that push the nucleus laterally and result in a signet ring effect[589] (Fig. 21-56).

4 Clear-cut plasmacytic differentiation in some or many of the neoplastic follicular center cells.[578,587]

5 Presence of cells with cerebriform nuclei (similar to those of T-cell lymphoma)[598] or multilobated nuclei.[572]

6 Permeation of the tumor follicles by small round lymphocytes of presumably mantle zone origin, the appearance simulating that of progressively transformed germinal center ("floral" variant).[582,600]

*References 569, 575, 588, 595, 605, 614.

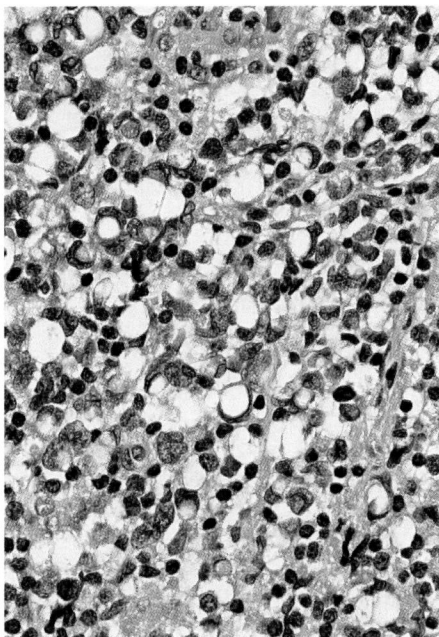

Fig. 21-56 Malignant lymphoma featuring signet ring changes in some of the tumor cells.

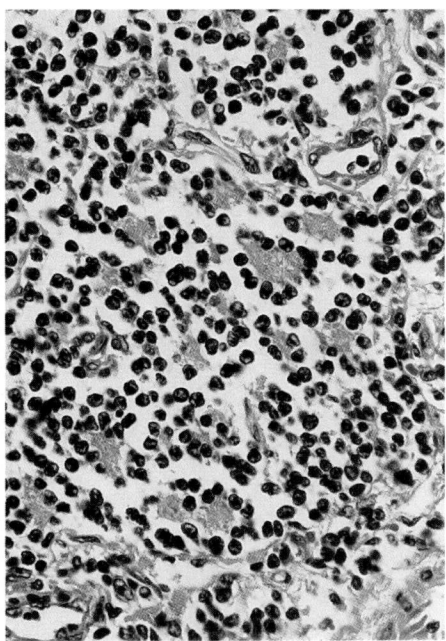

Fig. 21-57 Malignant lymphoma showing rosette formation by some of the lymphoid cells.

7 Presence of rosettes made up of cytoplasm and cytoplasmic processes of the lymphoid tumor cells and simulating the appearance of a neuroendocrine neoplasm (Fig. 21-57).[579]

8 Presence of hyaline vascular follicles similar to those seen in the vascular-hyaline type of Castleman's disease.

9 Inversion of the usual staining pattern as seen on low-power examination so that the neoplastic follicles appear darker than the surrounding lymphoid tissue. This pattern, which is referred to as the "reverse" or "inverse" variant of follicular lymphoma, carries no prognostic significance.[571]

10 Monocytoid B-cell differentiation, presenting as pale collars of variable widths around the neoplastic follicles.[597]

Mantle cell lymphoma

Mantle cell lymphoma is a low-grade neoplasm also known as intermediate lymphocytic, mantle zone, centrocytic, and diffuse small cleaved cell lymphoma.[615,619,625] Like follicular lymphoma, it usually occurs in middle-aged and elderly individuals and runs an indolent course.[617,621] The low-power appearance is largely that of a diffuse lymphoma, although there may be a suggestion of nodularity accentuated by the occasional presence of small germinal center–like structures (Fig. 21-58, A). Most of the cells are small lymphocytes similar to those of small lymphocytic lymphoma, but others show slightly irregular and indented nuclear contours approaching those seen in small cleaved cell follicular lymphoma[625] (Figs. 21-58, B, and 21-59). In some cases, the tumor cells have larger nuclei with more

dispersed chromatin and a higher proliferative factor ("blastic" or "lymphomatoid" variant).[618]

The immunocytochemical profile suggests that this is a distinct type of malignant lymphoma having the features of the lymphocytes of primary follicles and/or the mantle zones of secondary follicles.[623,624] The tumor cells are positive for immunoglobulins (IgM and often also IgD), B-cell–associated antigen, and CD5.[615,616] The absence of CD23 is useful in distinguishing mantle cell lymphoma from small lymphocytic lymphoma, and the presence of CD5 is useful in the differential diagnosis with follicular and marginal zone lymphomas. Cytogenetically, the t(11;14) translocation is present in about 70% of the cases. This involves the immunoglobulin heavy chain locus and the bcl-1 locus.[622,626] It results in overexpression of the PRAD1 gene, which encodes for cyclin D1.[619,620] Overexpression of cyclin D1 protein may be present without detectable rearrangement of the gene.[623a] Mantle cell lymphoma may be difficult to distinguish from foliclar hyperplasia with a prominence of mantle zone cells ("mantle zone hyperplasia") and Castleman's disease. Determination of clonality of the infiltrate by immunocytochemical techniques is of importance in this regard. The differential diagnosis also includes follicular lymphoma. The fact that centroblasts and immunoblast-like cells are totally absent in mantle cell lymphoma is an important differential feature.

Monocytoid B-cell lymphoma, MALT-lymphoma, and marginal zone lymphoma

Numerous reports have appeared in recent years describing a category of low-grade lymphoma that is distinct from small lymphocytic lymphoma (with or without plasmacy-

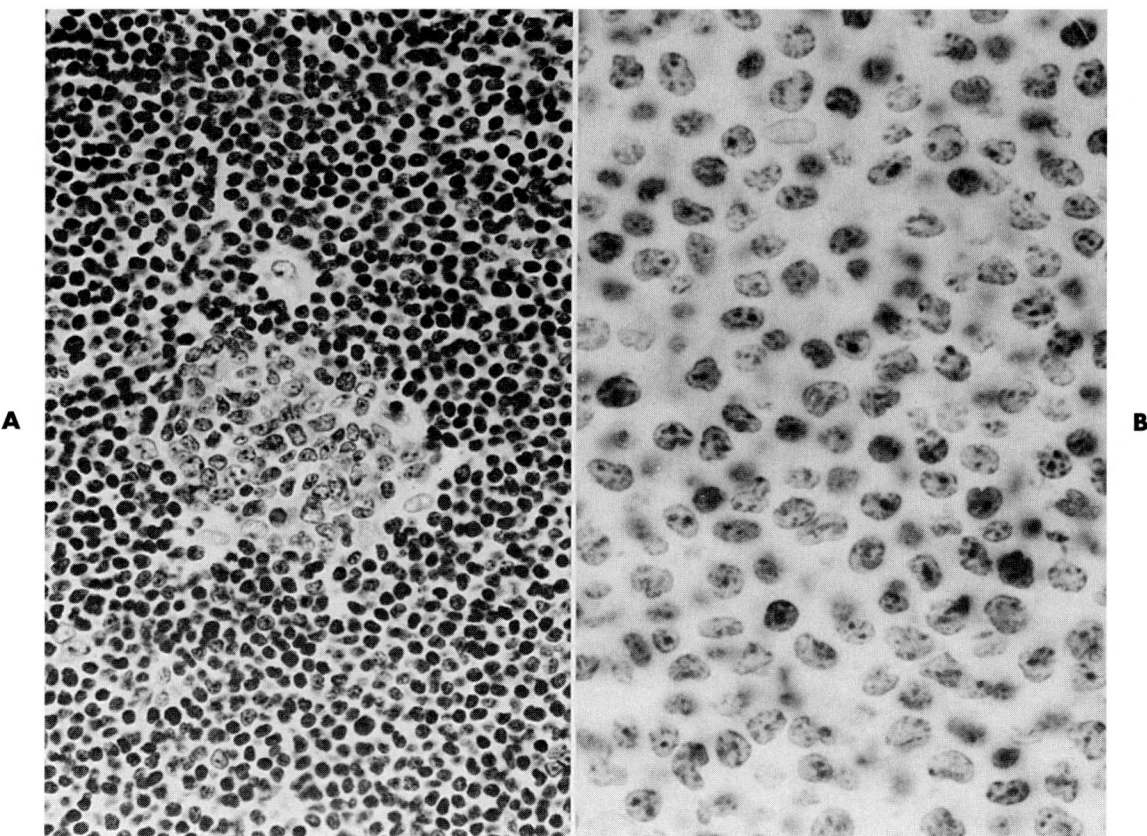

Fig. 21-58 Lymphocytic lymphoma of intermediate differentiation. **A,** Diffuse infiltrate with small germinal center–like structure in center of field. **B,** High-power view of same case illustrated in **A** shows that proliferation consists of small round lymphocytes admixed with irregular lymphoid cells. (From Mann RB, Jaffe ES, Berard CW: Malignant lymphoma. A conceptual understanding of morphologic diversity. A review. Am J Pathol **94:**105-191, 1979.)

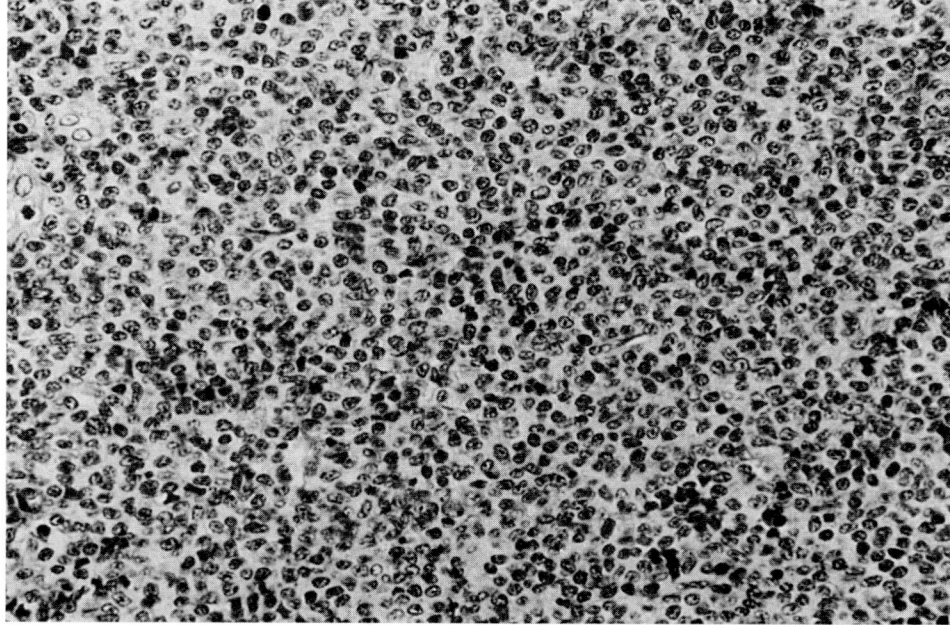

Fig. 21-59 Diffuse small cleaved (centrocytic) lymphoma. There is monotonous proliferation of small cleaved cells without follicular formation. This tumor entity blends with intermediate lymphocytic lymphoma and mantle zone lymphoma.

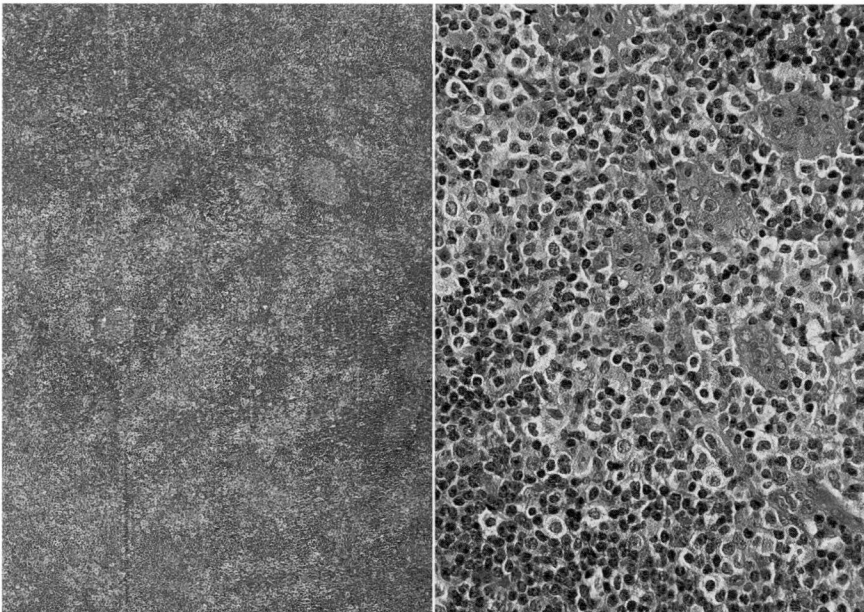

Fig. 21-60 Lymph node involvement by malignant lymphoma of so-called MALT type. This tumor also affected the thymus gland. (Courtesy Dr. John Chan, Hong Kong.)

toid features), follicular lymphoma, and mantle zone lymphoma. This category includes the following separately described entities:

1 *Monocytoid B-cell lymphoma.* This term has been used for a tumor of small to medium-sized lymphocytes with round or slightly indented nuclei and relatively abundant clear cytoplasm.[632,634] These cells have been regarded as the neoplastic counterpart of the monocytoid B lymphocytes found in lymph node sinuses in toxoplasmosis and other reactive disorders[637] (see p. 1674). Plasmacytoid features are prominent in some cases. The pattern of involvement is predominantly sinusal and interfollicular,[630] but cases have been seen with "follicular colonization." Clinically, the disease is more common in women and is often localized at presentation.[629] Some patients have suffered from autoimmune disorders such as Sjögren's disease. Histologic transformation to large cell lymphoma occurred in some cases.

2 *Low-grade lymphoma of mucosa-associated lymphoid tissue* (usually abbreviated as MALT-lymphoma).[631a] This is a neoplasm in which the cell population—all of small size—includes small round lymphocytes, monocytoid B cells, cells with slightly irregular nuclei (centrocyte-like), plasmacytoid cells, and plasma cells. Occasional large lymphoid cells may also be seen (Fig. 21-60).

   This tumor was originally described at extranodal sites in relation to mucosae or glandular epithelia, such as gastrointestinal tract, salivary and lacrimal glands, lung, thyroid, conjunctiva, bladder, and skin. It characteristically remains localized for a long time and has a tendency to relapse in the same or other epithelium-containing extranodal sites. It is now believed that many of the extranodal processes described years ago as pseudolymphomas of the lung, stomach, skin, and other sites are examples of this process. Patients may suffer from autoimmune disorders such as Sjögren's disease and Hashimoto's thyroiditis. Transformation to large cell lymphoma can occur.[628]

   Immunohistochemically, the cell of MALT-lymphoma are nearly always B-cells expressing immunoglobulin light chain restriction. There are no specific cell marker differences that separate MALT lymphoma from the other low-grade B-cell lymphomas listed at the beginning of this section. However, as a group they are less likely to express CD5 and CD25 and more likely to express CD11C. At the molecular level, they show rearranged heavy and light immunoglobulin genes,[640] but there is no rearrangement of the bcl-2 gene.[627] In some cases, trisomy 3 has been reported.[639]

3 *Splenic marginal zone lymphoma.* Several cases of lymphoma involving the marginal zone of the spleen have been reported, sometimes in association with bone marrow and peripheral blood involvement.[633,636] The disease is probably related if not identical to that reported under the term "splenic lymphoma with villous lymphocytes."

• • •

There appears to be considerable clinical, morphologic immunohistochemical overlap among the three entities just described.[631] Consequently, the proposal has been made that they represent a related family of neoplasms showing morphologic evidence of differentiation into cells of marginal zone type.[635,638] These cells are thought to have the capacity to mature into both monocytoid B cells and plasma cells, and to display tissue-specific homing patterns. A

Table 21-11 Summary of various types of diffuse mixed cell lymphoma

Type	Lineage	Clinical features	Histologic features	Immunohisto-chemical features	Behavior
Follicular center cell type (diffuse centroblastic-centrocytic)	B	Adults, usually presenting with lymphadenopathy; may have known history of follicular lymphoma or arising de novo; disease often at high stage at presentation; extranodal involvement is common	Small cells with angulated (cleaved) or elongated nuclei, fairly condensed chromatin, and scanty cytoplasm; large cells with round or folded nuclei, vesicular chromatin, and multiple distinct nucleoli; neoplastic follicles should be absent; sclerosis common	Pan-B+; CD5−; CD10+/−; CD23+/−; may have irregular loose meshworks of follicular dendritic cells	No reliable data in literature on its behavior; some studies suggest that it is low-grade neoplasm, but prognosis is less favorable than for follicular lymphoma
Post-thymic T-cell lymphoma	T	Usually adults; nodal or extranodal presentation; disease often at high stage at presentation	Prominent high endothelial venules; continuous spectrum of small, medium-sized, and large lymphoid cells; nuclear irregularities chromatin pattern often granular; clear cytoplasm commonly seen in some cells; may show rich component of inflammatory cells (such as eosinophils, histiocytes, and epithelioid cells)	Pan-T+ (often with loss of one or more pan T-antigens; usually CD4+, sometimes CD8+, CD4+CD8+ or CD4− CD8−)	Generally aggressive neoplasm
Lymphoplasmacytic/cytoid immunocytoma with increased blasts (polymorphic subtype)	B	Usually older adults; nodal or extranodal presentation; may have monoclonal gammopathy (20%-40%); disease often disseminated at presentation; occasional cases may have circulating lymphoma cells	Small lymphocytes; lymphoplasmacytoid cells; plasma cells; immunoblasts; rare follicular center cells; Dutcher bodies (nuclear pseudoinclusions of immunoglobulin) may be found; specific lymphoma types should be excluded (e.g., follicular lymphoma, low-grade B-cell lymphoma of MALT)	Pan B+; CD5−; CD10−; CD23−; sIg+, cIg+ (usually IgM type)	Low-grade neoplasm, but prognosis is worse than that of B-SLL/CLL or conventional LP immunocytoma; median survival 55 months; may rarely transform to diffuse large cell lymphoma
T-cell–rich large B-cell lymphoma	B	Older adults, usually presenting with lymphadenopathy; disease often disseminated at presentation	Small lymphocytes with round or irregular nuclei; scattered atypical large cells with round to folded nuclei, distinct nucleoli, and amphophilic cytoplasm; may show rich vascularity and component of inflammatory cells	Large atypical cells; pan-B+; small cells; pan-T+	Aggressive neoplasm; prognosis probably similar to conventional diffuse large cell lymphoma
Low-grade B-cell lymphoma of mucosa-associated lymphoid tissue (MALT)	B	Any age; tumor often localized to mucosal site and/or regional lymph nodes at presentation	Small lymphoid cells with round or irregular nuclei and pale to clear cytoplasm; scattered large blast cells with vesicular nuclei and distinct nucleoli; glandular invasion (lymphoepithelial lesions) common; plasma cells common	Pan-B+; CD5−; CD10−; CD23−	Low-grade neoplasm, with median survival of 8 years; may show late relapse locally or in other mucosal sites; may transform to diffuse large cell lymphoma

From Warnke RA, Weiss LM, Chan JKC, Cleary ML, Dorfman RF: Tumors of the lymph nodes and spleen. Atlas of tumor pathology. 3rd Series, Fascicle 14. Washington, DC, 1995, Armed Forces Institute of Pathology.

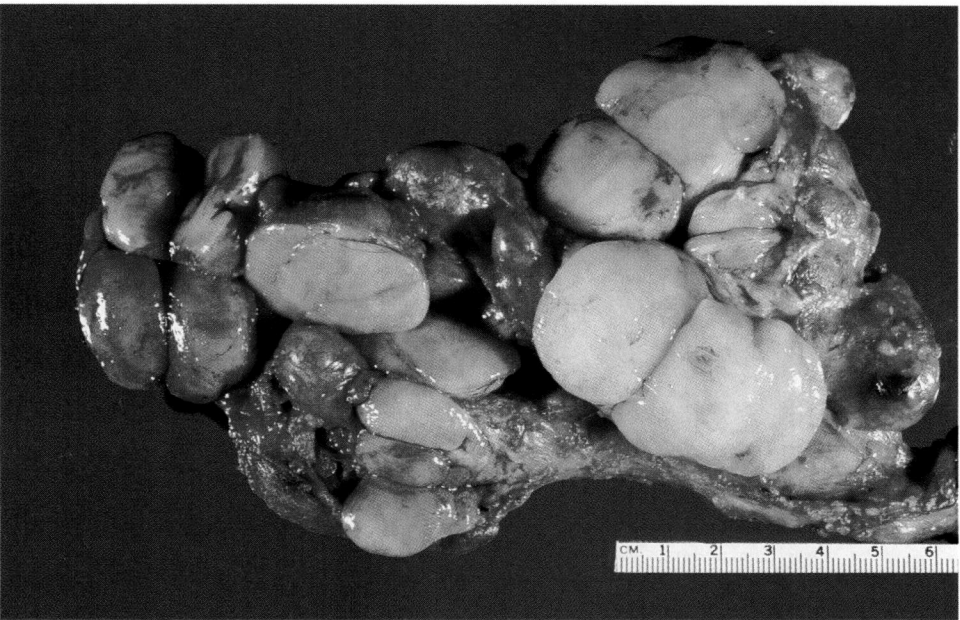

Fig. 21-61 Gross appearance of lymph nodes involved by non-Hodgkin's lymphoma. The nodes are enlarged and show a homogenous tan cut surface.

corollary of this proposal is that the various clinical syndromes may be the result of the homing pattern of the specific neoplastic clone. Accordingly, the recommendation has been made to use the term *marginal zone lymphoma* to encompass all tumors in this group and to subdivide them into extranodal, nodal, and splenic subtypes.

Diffuse mixed (small and large cell) lymphoma

Diffuse mixed lymphoma is not a specific lymphoma type but a heterogeneous category composed of lymphomas of various types that share a mixed composition of large and small lymphoid cells.[641-643] It includes (1) the diffuse mixed cell form of follicular lymphoma, (2) peripheral (postthymic) T-cell lymphoma, (3) lymphoplasmacytic lymphoma with increased number of immunoblasts (also known as pleomorphic immunocytoma), (4) the recently described T-cell–rich large B-cell lymphoma, and (5) some examples of MALT/marginal zone lymphoma with an admixture of large cells. The differential diagnosis among these various entities is based on a combination of clinical, morphologic, and immunohistochemical criteria (Table 21-11).

Diffuse large cell lymphoma

Large cell lymphoma is the most complex and heterogeneous of all the non-Hodgkin's lymphomas.[676] It corresponds to the old histiocytic lymphoma and the older reticulum cell sarcoma and is morphologically defined by the large size of the cells, their vesicular nuclei with prominent nucleoli, and their relatively abundant cytoplasm.

As a group, large cell lymphoma occurs both in children and adults, but mostly in the latter.[677] In comparison with other lymphomas, it has a greater tendency for extranodal

presentation and for being localized at the time of presentation. The progression is rapid and the prognosis is poor if untreated, but excellent responses have been obtained with aggressive chemotherapy.[645,654] In more than half of the cases, the tumor is limited to one side of the diaphragm (40%, as opposed to 90% for follicular lymphoma).[650] Involvement of the bone marrow or liver is less common than in the small cleaved or small lymphocytic tumors.[680] About 40% of the cases present in extranodal sites, such as the digestive system, skin, and skeletal system.[650] When the liver or spleen is involved, it is usually in the form of scattered large tumor masses instead of the multiple smaller nodules or miliary type seen with the small cleaved or small lymphocytic types. The involved nodes are usually markedly enlarged, homogeneous, individualized, and with little or no necrosis (Fig. 21-61). Immunologic studies performed in these tumors have shown a significant heterogeneity.[646,683] This indicates that large cell lymphoma is not a specific entity like the others but rather a common denominator for all the highly anaplastic or "blastic" lymphomas, just as large cell undifferentiated carcinoma of the lung represents the end of the spectrum for all major microscopic types of pulmonary carcinoma. About 50% to 60% of the large cell lymphomas exhibit B-cell markers, 5% to 15% have T-cell markers, a few have features consistent with true histiocytes, and as many as a third of the cases have no markers at all ("null" lymphoma).[663] Gene rearrangement studies have shown that most tumors in the latter group are of B-cell nature.[651]

The distinction between the various subtypes of large cell lymphoma is of some practical importance because of differences in occurrence, location, and prognosis.

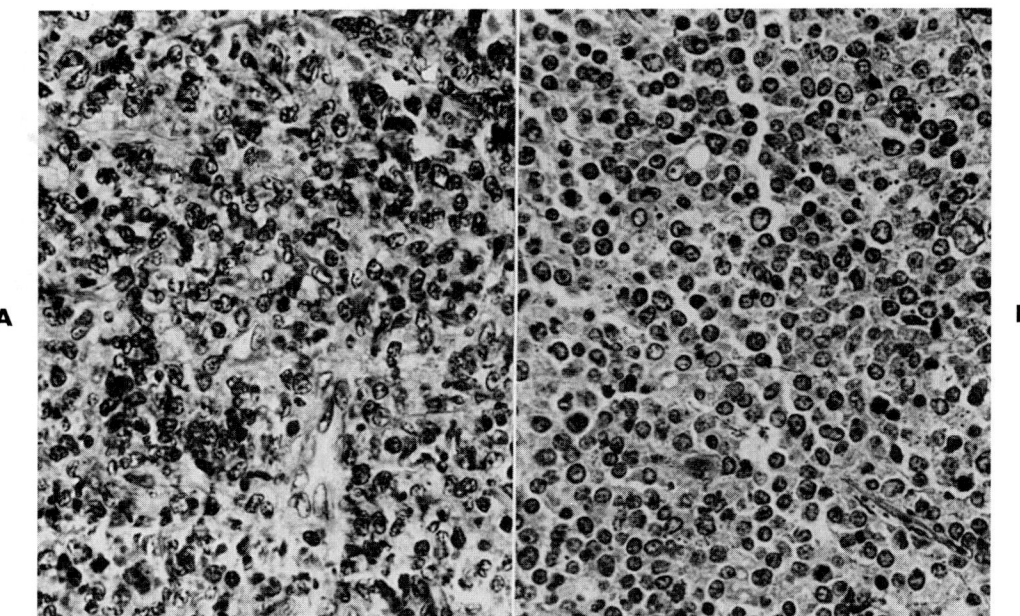

Fig. 21-62 Large cell malignant lymphoma. Tumor in **A** is predominantly composed of large cleaved cells, and tumor in **B** is predominantly composed of large noncleaved cells. Both types are of B-cell nature and follicular center cell origin.

Diffuse large cell lymphoma (cleaved and noncleaved). When the term diffuse large cell lymphoma is used without a qualifier, the assumption is that the tumor is of B-cell origin and follicular center cell derivation. As such, it is regarded as the diffuse counterpart of the follicular (or follicular *and* diffuse) lymphoma of the corresponding cell type. When totally diffuse, the behavior of this tumor is more aggressive than when some nodularity is present.[682]

Two morphologic subtypes are recognized: large cleaved cell and large noncleaved cell (Fig. 21-62). The latter, which is by far the more common, may be difficult to distinguish from B-cell immunoblastic sarcoma. The subtle differences are the lighter-staining and less pyroninophilic cytoplasm, the more peripheral location of the nucleoli, the absence of plasmacytoid differentiation, the occasional admixture with small and large cleaved cells, and the fact that a vaguely follicular pattern may still be discerned.[661] Mitoses are numerous, and a "starry sky" pattern may be present.

Immunoblastic sarcoma. Immunoblastic sarcoma is the term applied to large cell malignant lymphomas composed of cells having the morphologic features of immunoblasts (transformed lymphocytes).[675] There are two categories, corresponding to the two major lymphocyte types (Fig. 21-63).

In ***B-cell immunoblastic sarcoma*** ("malignant lymphoma, large cell, immunoblastic plasmacytoid type" in the International Formulation), the predominant cell has the appearance of an immunoblast: large vesicular nucleus with prominent central nucleoli and thick nuclear membrane and deeply staining amphophilic and pyroninophilic cytoplasm with a distinct nuclear hof. Some of the cells are binucleated or multinucleated and simulate Reed-Sternberg cells, and

others acquire plasmacytoid features (cartwheel chromatin, larger perinuclear hof). Immunoperoxidase staining often shows intracytoplasmic immunoglobulin. This is the most common type of lymphoma arising on the basis of natural immunodeficiency, immunosuppression, immunoproliferative states (such as angioimmunoblastic lymphadenopathy), and other immune diseases, such as Hashimoto's thyroiditis, Sjögren's disease, α-chain disease, and lupus erythematosus. This was true for 30% of the thirty-three patients studied by Lichtenstein et al.[659] The prognosis is poor; the disease disseminates early and progresses rapidly.[673] In the series of Lichtenstein et al.,[659] the median survival was 14 months.

T-cell immunoblastic sarcoma (probably equivalent to the "malignant lymphoma, large cell, immunoblastic, clear cell type" in the International Formulation) is less common than its B-cell counterpart, and the morphologic distinction between the two is difficult. The tumor cells differ from those of the B-cell type by having irregular, contorted nuclei and a pale, water-clear cytoplasm with well-defined interlocking plasma membranes, giving the tumor a cohesive appearance.[665] The chromatin is finely dispersed, and the nucleoli are smaller. A wide size range exists among cells exhibiting these features. The neighboring cells are atypical lymphocytes, rather than plasmacytoid cells as in the B-cell type. Reactive histiocytes may be present in large numbers. High endothelial venules are prominent. The initial lymph node involvement is in the paracortical region, with sparing of the follicles.[675] A prominent inflammatory component may be present, with a predominance of eosinophils. In contrast to the B-cell immunoblastic sarcoma, the T-cell variety is usually not preceded by an abnormal immune disorder.

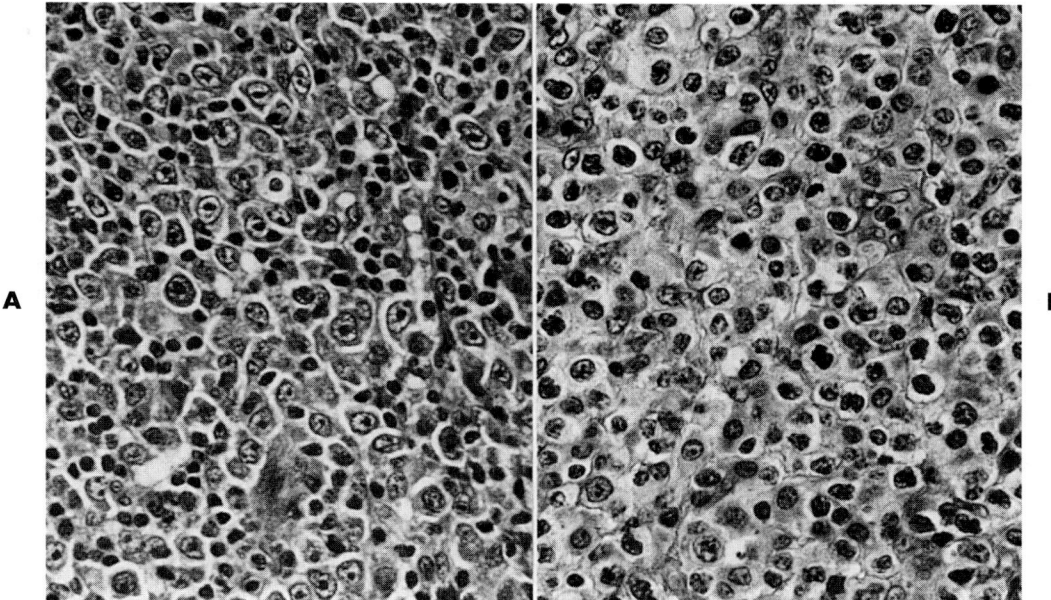

Fig. 21-63 Immunoblastic sarcoma. Tumor in **A** is of B-cell type. Note central location of large nucleoli and perinuclear hof present in some tumor cells. **B** is example of T-immunoblastic sarcoma. Note clear appearance of cytoplasm and nuclear irregularities.

However, it can be superimposed on mycosis fungoides (a T-cell malignancy). It may be seen in children and in adults and is usually associated with generalized lymphadenopathy and polyclonal hypergammaglobulinemia. Some authors claim that T-cell lymphoma has a worse prognosis than B-cell lymphoma,[652] but others have found no differences.[658]

Histiocytic lymphoma. Although it has become obvious that the large majority of tumors formerly called histiocytic lymphomas are in reality of lymphoid origin, some evidence exists for a malignant neoplasm that exhibits immunocytochemical evidence of monocyte-histiocyte differentiation (see p. 1743).

• • •

The karyotypic and molecular abnormalities found in diffuse large cell lymphoma are varied, as one would expect from the previous discussion. Large B-cell lymphoma usually shows rearrangements of the immunoglobulin heavy and light chain genes, whereas large T-cell lymphomas usually shows rearrangements of the beta or chain T-cell receptor genes. Rearrangements of bcl-2 are found in 20% to 30% of the cases, suggesting a relationship with follicular lymphoma.[644] About one third of diffuse large lymphomas show rearrangements of bcl-6, this feature being more common in extranodal sites.[652,653,660,667,686] It is extremely rare for a lymphoma to show concomitant rearrangement of bcl-2 and bcl-6.

Variants. Numerous morphologic variations on the theme of large cell malignant lymphoma have been described, some of a cytologic and others of an architectural/topographic nature. Some of them relate to the lymphoma subtypes described and others do not. Most of these variations do not have an impact on therapy or prognosis, but they are important because they may result in a mistaken diagnosis. They include the following:

1 *Sclerosis.* Diffuse large cell lymphomas can undergo marked sclerosing changes, similar to those seen in follicular lymphomas.[648,672,674,681] This material is mainly composed of types I, III, and V collagen and fibronectin.[664] Sclerosis is a common feature of mediastinal (thymic) large cell lymphomas.

2 *Spindling of tumor cells.* This phenomenon, which is probably related to the aforementioned variations, seems to be more common in large cell lymphomas of mediastinum and bone, but it can be seen in any location, including lymph nodes.

3 Presence of a *myxoid stroma* that can simulate the appearance of myxoid malignant fibrous histiocytoma or myxoid chondrosarcoma.[656,679]

4 *Rosette formation.* This peculiar change, originally described in follicular lymphoma, has also been seen in large cell lymphoma. Ultrastructural studies have shown that the material in the center of the rosettes is made up of complex cell prolongations.[678]

5 *Filiform cell prolongations.* This phenomenon, which is probably related to that described in the previous paragraph, is appreciable in ultrastructural preparations and is similar to that sometimes seen in carcinomas, mesotheliomas, and other neoplasms. Large cell lymphomas exhibiting this spectacular feature have been designated anemone cell, microvillous, filiform cell, villiform cell, and porcupine lymphomas.[649,669]

6 *Signet ring features.* This alteration, which is more common in follicular lymphoma, is rarely seen in large cell lymphoma and may simulate metastatic adenocarcinoma.[685]

7 *Sinusal pattern of spread,* in which the tumor cells are predominantly or entirely confined to the lymph node sinuses, resulting in an appearance closely

simulating that of metastatic carcinoma or malignant melanoma.[670]

8 *Interfollicular pattern of growth.* This is more common in T-cell tumors but has also been described in B-cell neoplasms.[666]

9 *Nuclear multilobation.* Although originally thought to be a feature of T-cell tumors, this alteration is now known to be more common in B-cell neoplasms.[668,684]

10 *Lymphohistiocytic lymphoma.* The tumor cells are usually of T-cell type and immunoreactive for CD30. As a matter of fact, this entity was originally described as a type of anaplastic large cell lymphoma. Its distinctiveness results from the presence of a large number of reactive (nonepithelioid) histiocytes. Most cases have occurred in young patients presenting with systemic symptoms and superficial lymphadenopathy.[671]

11 *T-cell–rich large B-cell lymphoma.* This is a type of large B-cell lymphoma associated with a component of T lymphocytes that makes up more than 50% of the entire cellular population.[647,655,657,662] The main differential diagnosis is with diffuse L&H Hodgkin's disease; it is believed that the presence of numerous CD57 (Leu7)–positive cells rosetting around the large tumor cells favors the latter diagnosis.

Peripheral (post-thymic) T-cell lymphoma

Peripheral (post-thymic) T-cell lymphoma is the generic group given to a family of tumors composed of neoplastic lymphocytes with phenotypic and genotypic features of peripheral T-cells.[688,708] This is a heterogeneous and poorly understood group of lesions having morphologic and histogenetic links with several other types of lymphoma.* They comprise mycosis fungoides–Sézary syndrome (see Chapter 4), lymphomatoid granulomatosis and some forms of lethal midline granuloma (see Chapter 7), T-cell chronic lymphocytic leukemia and prolymphocytic leukemia[691] (see Chapter 23), T-cell immunoblastic sarcoma (see preceding section), T-cell lymphoma with multilobated nuclei,[701] T-zone lymphoma, erythrophagocytic T-cell lymphoma,[689,694] paracortical nodular T-cell lymphoma,[696] angioimmunoblastic lymphadenopathy–like T-cell lymphoma,[698] pleomorphic T-cell lymphoma (occurring in an endemic form in Japan),[704] anaplastic large cell lymphoma, and lymphoepithelioid T-cell lymphoma (Lennert's lymphoma)[697,706] (Fig. 21-64). To this long and impressive list one should perhaps add Hodgkin's disease, the T-cell nature of which has been suggested by several observers. A common feature of these varieties, together with the atypia of the T-cells, is prominence of the vascular network.[695]

Immunohistochemically, all peripheral T-cell lymphomas show—by definition—the markers of the mature T-cell.[687] In paraffin sections, they are positive for CD45 RB in about 90% of the cases, and for the T-cell–associated markers CD45 R0, CD43, and CD3 in a similar percentage. CD15 positivity is seen in 10% to 15% of the cases, but with a cytoplasmic granular quality that is generally different from

that seen in Hodgkin's disease.[702,711] In frozen sections, the tumor cells often show aberrant phenotypes, such as absence of CD2, CD3, CD5, and/or CD7. Most tumors express the alpha/beta T-cell receptor, but aberrant absence of the beta-f-1′ antigen has been documented in one quarter of the cases.[699]

Most cases of peripheral T-cell lymphoma express a CD4+/CD8− mature helper phenotype; about 20% express a CD4−/CD8+ cytotoxic/suppressor phenotype, with rare cases having CD4−/DC8− or CD4+/CD8+ phenotypes.

At the molecular level, most peripheral T-cell lymphomas exhibit clonal rearrangements of the beta T-cell receptor gene, with a minority showing rearrangement of the gamma or delta T-cell receptor genes.[709] The clonality of these tumors has also been shown through the demonstration of a single episomal configuration of the Epstein-Barr viral terminal repeat. About 10% of peripheral T-cell lymphomas show clonal rearrangements of the immunoglobulin heavy chain gene in addition to clonal rearrangements of the beta T-cell receptor gene.[703]

Karyotypically, the pattern is complex, but no consistent abnormality has yet been detected.

From an etiologic standpoint, evidence of a specific viral agent (HTLV-1) has been found for T-cell leukemia/lymphoma endemic to certain regions, such as Japan and the Caribbean.[705] Cases of T-cell lymphomas containing EB-viral DNA have been reported in the United States.[693] This is particularly true for the angiocentric lymphomas of upper respiratory tract (see Chapter 7).

Lymphoepithelioid T-cell lymphoma. Lymphoepithelioid T-cell lymphoma (Lennert's lymphoma) is a type of peripheral T-cell lymphoma accompanied by a high number of non-neoplastic epithelioid histiocytes.[713,716,717] It occurs in adults, it is often generalized (74% of the patients have stage IV disease at presentation), and the prognosis is poor.[714,718] Microscopically, there is effacement of the architecture by a lymphohistiocytic infiltrate, often accompanied by plasma cells and eosinophils and by proliferation of small vessels with plump endothelial cells. The polymorphic nature of the infiltrate and the occasional presence of Reed-Sternberg–like cells often elicits a mistaken diagnosis of Hodgkin's disease. The key to the diagnosis resides in the atypical appearance of the small lymphocytes located between the reactive histiocytes (Fig. 21-65). In addition to Hodgkin's disease, the differential diagnosis includes atypical lymphoepithelioid hyperplasia and angioimmunoblastic lymphadenopathy. Some cases of Lennert's lymphoma have been seen to undergo a "blastic" transformation into a large cell lymphoma.[715] According to Lennert, lymphoepithelioid T-cell lymphoma is at the interphase between Hodgkin's disease and non-Hodgkin's lymphoma.[717]

Anaplastic large cell lymphoma

Anaplastic large cell lymphoma is also known as Ki-1 lymphoma and as pleomorphic histiocytoid lymphoma.[732,745] It occurs in all age groups, about 20% of the patients being under age 20 years.[719,746] Most cases arise de novo, but a few have been reported as engrafted on mycosis fungoides or Hodgkin's disease or developing in HIV-infected patients.[758] Clinically, two types of presentation are

---

*References 690,692,700,707,710,712.

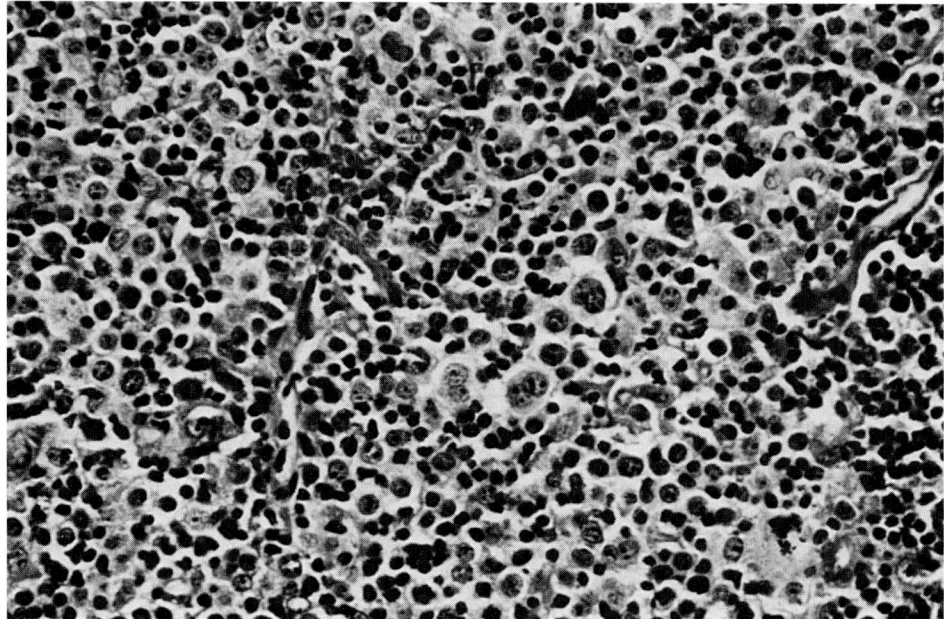

Fig. 21-64 Pleomorphic peripheral T-cell lymphoma. Appearance closely resembles that of Hodgkin's disease, but these are not diagnostic. Reed-Sternberg cells, and small lymphocytes show atypical nuclear features.

recognized: a systemic form (which may involve nodes or extranodal sites, including skin) and a primary cutaneous form (without extracutaneous involvement at the time of presentation).[720,730,734] The systemic form can involve sites such as the bone marrow, bone, respiratory tract, and gastrointestinal tract.[731,759] It can occur in children or adults and is rather aggressive.[744,757] The cutaneous form occurs predominantly in adults and has an indolent course, with some of the individual lesions regressing spontaneously.[722,739] In retrospect, it seems likely that the cases originally reported as *regressive atypical histiocytosis* belong to this category.[737,742,752,754]

Microscopically, the infiltrate has a polymorphic appearance, with a variable admixture of neutrophils, lymphocytes, histiocytes, and large highly atypical cells showing marked pleomorphism. The nuclei of these cells are often horseshoe shaped and multiple, and nucleoli are prominent. Cells indistinguishable from Reed-Sternberg cells may be seen. The cytoplasm is abundant and eosinophilic. It is characteristic for these tumor cells to form in a cohesive fashion and to involve preferentially the lymph node sinuses. When the latter feature is very prominent, the lesion is likely to be diagnosed as malignant histiocytosis. A *small cell variant* and a *neutrophil-rich variant* have been described.[747,750] Anaplastic large cell lymphoma can simulate malignant melanoma, undifferentiated carcinoma, and various types of soft tissue sarcoma.[729]

Immunohistochemically, the tumor cells are by definition CD30+ (Ki-1) positive, both in frozen and in paraffin sections. The latter material requires the use of monoclonal antibody BerH2.[741] There is also consistent positivity for EMA and interleukin-2 receptor, particularly in the systemic cases.[735] Pan-lymphoid and some T-cell related markers are found in about half of the cases, and B-cell related markers in 10% to 15% (Fig. 21-66). Some histiocytic markers can also be expressed.[721,727,738,756] Some observers have also reported occasional reactivity for keratin.[740] At the molecular level, about half of the cases show rearrangement of one of the T-cell receptor genes.[743,753]

Cytogenically, several of the cases have shown a t(2;5) (p23; q35) translocation.[723,724,728,751] This results in the juxtaposition of the nucleophosmin gene (which codes for a nucleolar phosphoprotein) on chromosome 5q35 with the "anaplastic lymphoma kinase" gene (a novel tyrosine kinase gene) on chromosome 2p23.[726,747a]

A complex and as yet not fully understood relationship seems to exist between anaplastic large cell lymphoma and Hodgkin's disease, to the point that some authors view these two diseases as part of a continuous spectrum.[733,748,755] It has also been suggested that anaplastic large cell lymphoma represents the link between peripheral (post-thymic) T-cell lymphoma and Hodgkin's disease. However, in contrast to Hodgkin's disease, most cases of anaplastic large cell lymphoma lack evidence of EBV genomes.[725,736,749]

Lymphoblastic lymphoma

Lymphoblastic lymphoma is seen primarily in children and adolescents, but it also occurs in adults.[767,770] It has a distinctive clinical presentation. In approximately half of the cases there is a mediastinal mass in the thymic region. The clinical course of the untreated disease is extremely aggressive, with rapid multisystem dissemination, leukemic blood

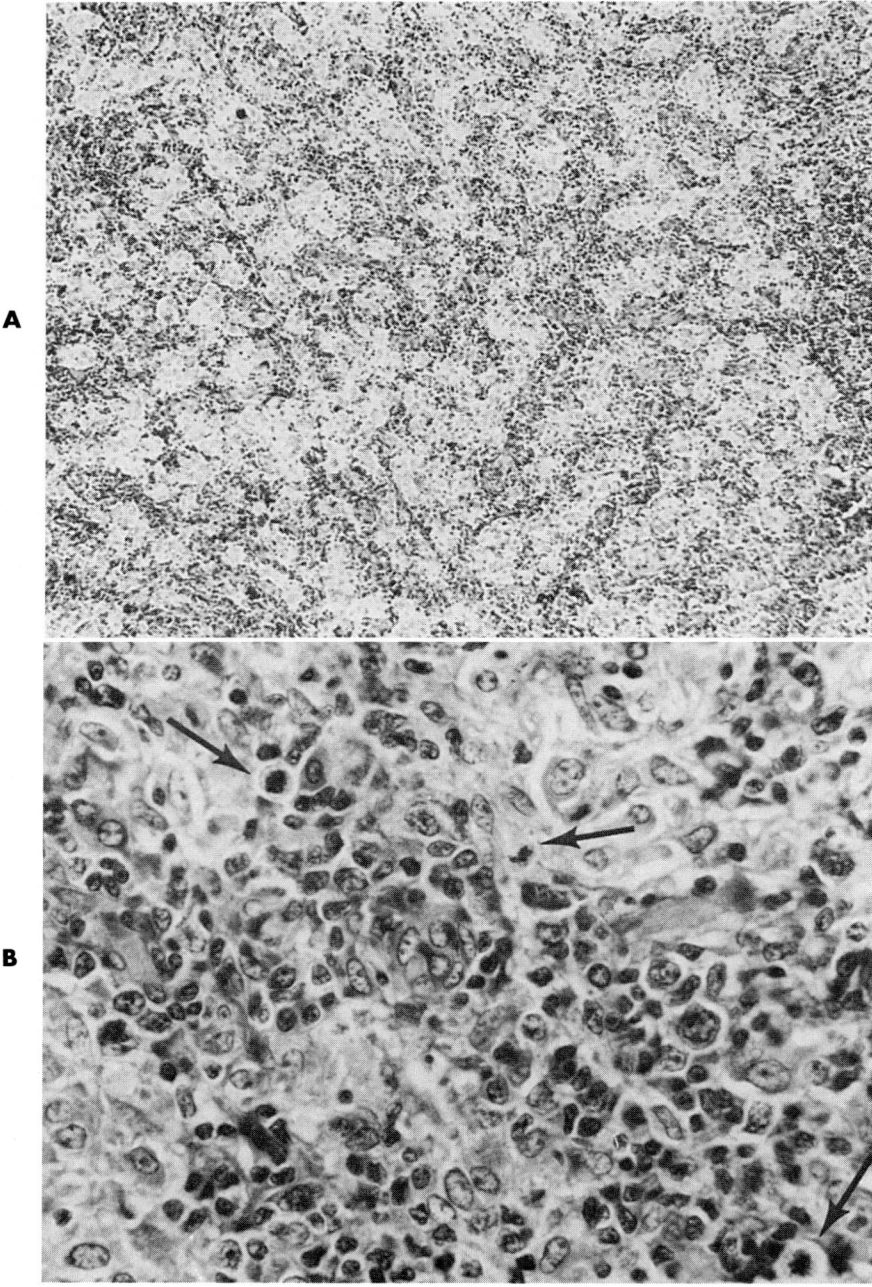

Fig. 21-65 Low-power **(A)** and high-power **(B)** views of so-called Lennert's lymphoma. Extensive infiltrate of epithelioid histiocytes may be seen closely admixed with small lymphocytes (some of them atypical) and scattered large lymphoid cells; several mitotic figures are present *(arrows)*. (From Kim H, Jacobs C, Warnke RA, Dorfman RF: Malignant lymphoma with a high content of epithelioid histiocytes. A distinct clinicopathologic entity and a form of the so-called "Lennert's lymphoma." Cancer **41:**620-635, 1978.)

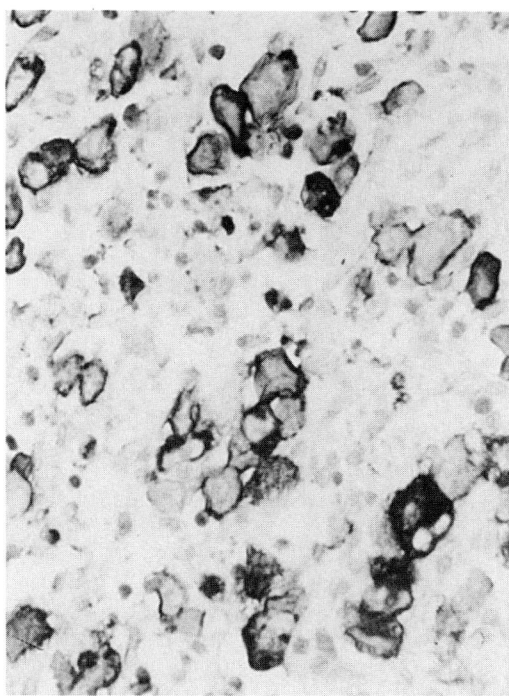

Fig. 21-66 EMA positivity in case of large cell malignant lymphoma. This finding may lead to diagnostic confusion with metastatic carcinoma.

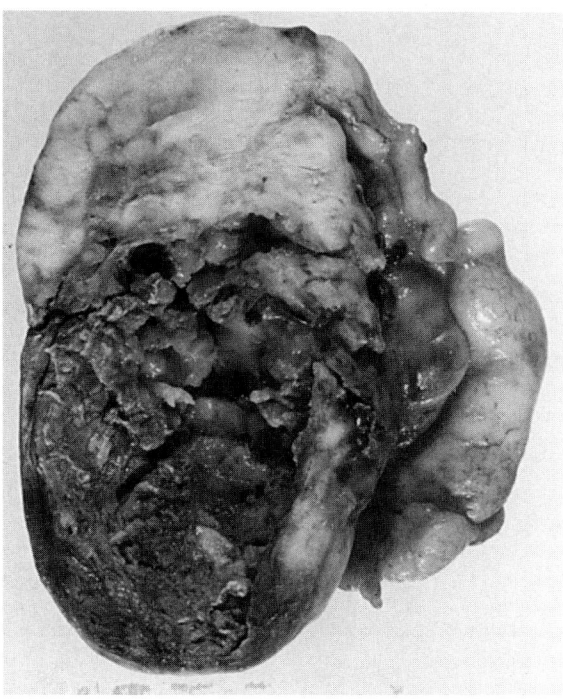

Fig. 21-67 Gross appearance of lymphoblastic lymphoma located in intraabdominal region. Homogeneous whitish areas with a fish-flesh appearance alternate with areas of hemorrhage and necrosis. Fallopian tube is seen on one side of tumor. Ovary could not be identified. (Courtesy Dr. J. Costa, Lausanne, Switzerland.)

picture, and death after a few months.[764] Grossly, the tumor is whitish and soft and often exhibits foci of hemorrhage and necrosis (Fig. 21-67). Microscopically, there is a diffuse and relatively monomorphic pattern of proliferation, broken only by a focal "starry sky" appearance in some of the cases. The tumor often extends outside the node or thymus to invade the adipose tissue in a diffuse fashion. Permeation of the wall of blood vessels in a targetoid fashion is another characteristic feature. The neoplastic cells have scanty cytoplasm and a nucleus that has a round contour (instead of the angulated shape typical of follicular lymphoma) but that shows, on close examination, the presence of delicate convolutions resulting from multiple small invaginations of the nuclear membrane. Oil-immersion examination of well-prepared, very thin sections is necessary to demonstrate this feature, which may be present in only a small percentage of the tumor cells. The chromatin is finely stippled, and nucleoli are inconspicuous. Mitotic activity is extremely high. These convoluted cells are similar to the cerebroid cells of mycosis fungoides–Sézary's syndrome (as one might assume from their similar names) but differ from the latter because the nuclear membrane is thinner, the chromatin more disperse, and the invaginations more delicate. Actually, the need for distinction between these two cell types is more theoretical than real because of the fact that the two diseases are vastly different in their clinical presentation.

In some cases (up to 50% in the series of Nathwani et al.[764]), nuclear convolutions are not appreciated despite the fact that all the other morphologic and clinical features are the same as for the cases that exhibit them. An *atypical* or *large cell* variant of lymphoblastic lymphoma has been described, and is said to comprise about 10% of the cases.[762]

Remnants of thymus often are found in the mediastinal mass, and this may lead to a mistaken diagnosis of thymoma; in this regard, it should be remembered that thymoma is very infrequent in children and that, when it occurs, it is characterized by a population of small or activated lymphocytes but not convoluted ones. When lymphoblastic lymphoma spreads to lymph nodes, it preferentially involves the paracortical (thymic-dependent) zone.

At the histochemical level, features of the cells of lymphoblastic lymphoma include the presence of acid phosphatase (focally strong in a paranuclear location, as in normal thymocytes), β-glucuronidase, α-naphthyl acetate esterase,[768] and terminal deoxynucleotidyl transferase (TdT), a marker of thymocytes.[761,763] The latter can also be demonstrated immunohistochemically in paraffin-embedded material.[765,771]

About 80% to 85% of lymphoblastic lymphomas show T-cell markers. Their phenotypes correspond to those of the various stages of intrathymic T-cell differentiation. In about 90% of the cases, these tumors express all of the panT-antigens, such as CD1, CD2, CD7, cytoplasmic CD3, and CD43. The latter two markers can be evaluated in paraffin sections. Practically all cases express CD71 (the transferrin receptor antigen), 20% express HLA-DR, and 20% express

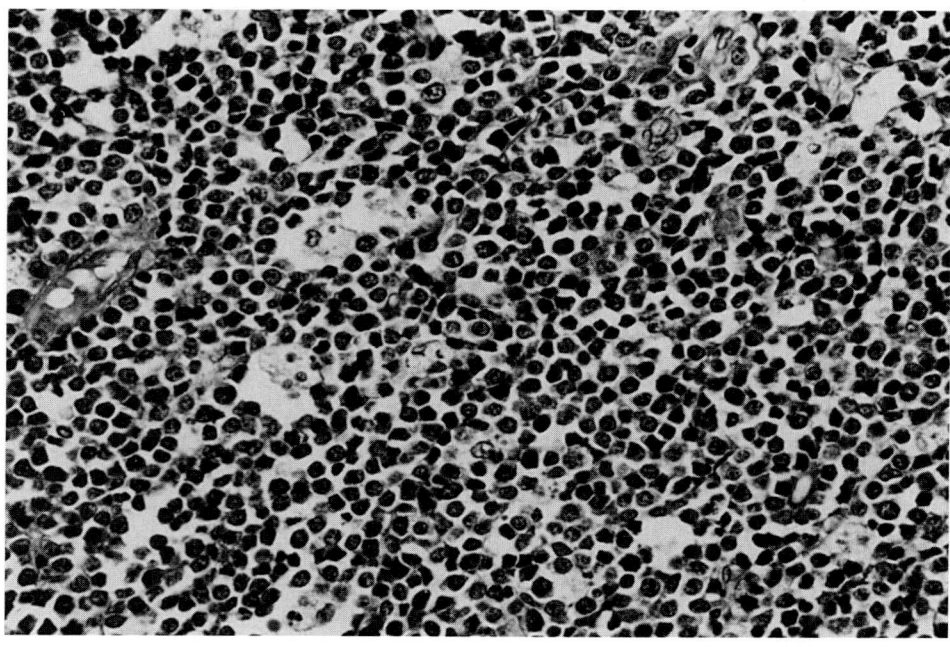

Fig. 21-68 Burkitt's lymphoma. Neoplasm, which is composed of small noncleaved cells, shows characteristic "starry sky" pattern resulting from presence of macrophages containing nuclear debris.

markers for natural killer cells, such as CD16 and CD57. Positivity is also consistently encountered for O13 (Ewing sarcoma antigen).

In about 15% to 20% of the cases, the tumor cells express B-cell rather than T-cell markers.[772] These include CD19, CD20, CD21, and CD24. However, these tumors do not generally express surface immunoglobulin and therefore are viewed as having a pre-pre–B-cell phenotype (when cytoplasmic immunoglobulin is absent) or a pre–B-cell phenotype (when present).

At the molecular level, lymphoblastic lymphomas generally exhibit rearrangements of the T-cell receptor β-chain gene. Cytogenetically, no consistent translocations have been identified; however, up to 30% of the cases show alterations of chromosome band 14q11 or 7q35, which are known to be the site of the T-cell receptor α/δ and β gene complexes, respectively.[769]

The close clinical, immunologic, and morphologic relationship between lymphoblastic lymphoma and acute lymphoblastic leukemia (particularly the T-cell variety) has been extensively discussed, although not completely elucidated.[766]

The main differential diagnosis of lymphoblastic lymphoma is with small noncleaved cell lymphoma. The distinction is usually possible on morphologic grounds and is also clear-cut in most cases by immunophenotypic analysis if fresh material is available.[760]

Small noncleaved cell lymphoma

Small noncleaved cell lymphoma (SNCL) is the term used in the International Formulation for a type of high-grade malignant lymphoma also known as undifferentiated lymphoma.[779] Two major categories have been described, the differences between them being relatively minor.[786]

Burkitt's lymphoma. Burkitt's lymphoma is a malignant tumor with distinct epidemiologic, clinical, and microscopic features. It is endemic in the equatorial strip of Africa, but it has been reported in a sporadic form throughout the world.[780,788] Most cases occur in childhood. The African patients characteristically present with jaw lesions, whereas the sporadic cases most often manifest with abdominal masses (ileocecal region, ovaries, abdominal lymph nodes, and retroperitoneum).[780] Peripheral lymphadenopathy is rare and, when present, usually limited to a single group.[773,774] Bone marrow involvement is common in the late stages of the disease, but leukemic manifestations are very rare.[784,785]

Microscopically, the pattern of growth is usually diffuse, although early cases may show preferential involvement of germinal centers.[783] The tumor cells are small (10 to 25 μm) and round. The nuclei are round or oval and have *several* prominent basophilic nucleoli. The chromatin is coarse and the nuclear membrane is rather thick. The cytoplasm is easily identifiable; it is amphophilic in hematoxylin-eosin–stained preparations and strongly pyroninophilic. Fat-containing small vacuoles are prominent; these are particularly well appreciated in touch preparations. Mitoses are numerous, and a prominent "starry sky" pattern is the rule, although by no means pathognomonic[775] (Fig. 21-68). In well-fixed material, the cytoplasm of individual cells "squares off," forming acute angles in which the membranes of adjacent cells abut on each other. Ultrastructurally, the

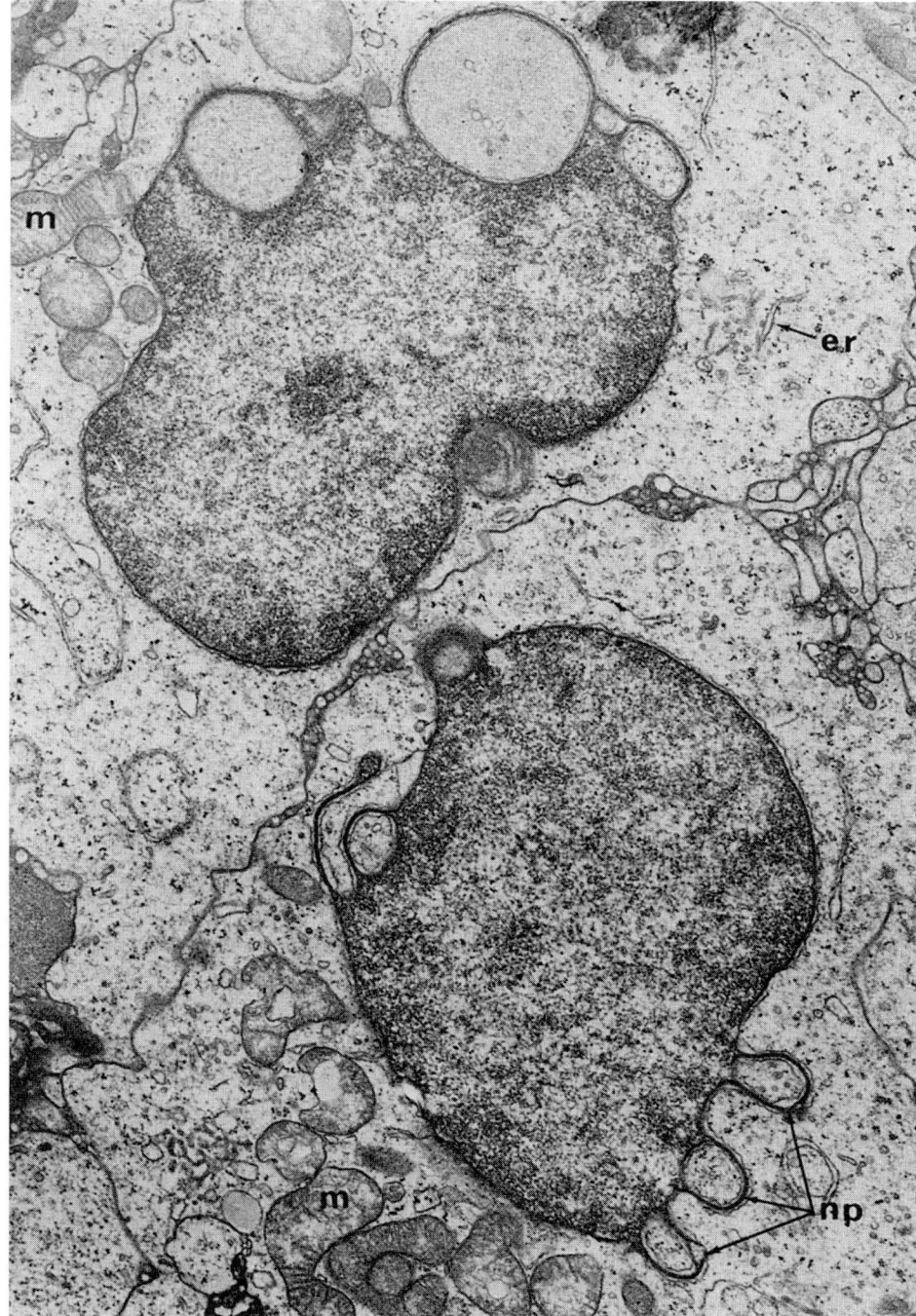

Fig. 21-69 These neoplastic lymphocytic cells from patient with Burkitt's lymphoma have numerous peculiar, though not unique, nuclear projections *(np)*, polar aggregation of mitochondria *(m)*, sparse endoplasmic reticulum *(er)*, and scattered ribosomes.

main features are abundant ribosomes, frequent lipid inclusions, lack of glycogen particles, and presence of nuclear pockets or projections[776] (Fig. 21-69).

Pleomorphic (non-Burkitt's) lymphoma. In pleomorphic (non-Burkitt's) lymphoma, the tumor cells are somewhat intermediate in size between small cleaved cells and large cells. A distinct pleomorphism is evident, which sets

this tumor apart from Burkitt's lymphoma.[781] Most of the cells have a well-defined rim of cytoplasm; their nucleus contains a large, eosinophilic nucleolus. Binucleated and multinucleated cells are common, and phagocytosis of nuclear debris by reactive histiocytes is frequently observed, resulting in a "starry sky" appearance. The pattern of growth is generally diffuse, but areas of minimal nodularity may be encountered. Clinically, gastrointestinal involvement is less common and bone marrow involvement more frequent than in the Burkitt's type. The clinical course is said to be more aggressive[773,774,781] although the response to therapy is similar.[787]

• • •

Immunohistochemically, it has been shown that virtually all cases of SNCL are of B-cell lineage. They express immunoglobulins (predominantly IgM), invariably associated with light chain restriction.[779] B-cell–specific antigens (such as CD19, CD20, and CD22) and B-cell–associated antigens (such as CD24 and HLA-DR) are present. Most cases also feature CD10. They are negative for the activation markers CD25 and CD30. In contrast to lymphoblastic lymphoma, they do not express TdT.

Cytogenetically, over 80% of SNCL of the Burkitt's subtype carry the t(8;14)(q23;q21) translocation.[778] This results in the juxtaposition of the *myc* gene (located in 8q23) with one of the Ig heavy or light chain genes.[777,778] This results in a deregulation of *myc* gene expression and increased cell proliferation. In sporadic cases of Burkitt's lymphomas, the breakpoint shows a different distribution pattern, suggesting that the tumor develops at a later stage of B-cell differentiation. Most Burkitt's lymphomas (especially of the endemic form) harbor latent EBV genomes; these have been found to be clonally homogeneous within the tumor, in keeping with their presence in the lymphoid cells *prior* to their clonal expansion.[782]

Other non-Hodgkin's lymphomas

Types of non-Hodgkin's malignancies of the lymphoid system other than those already described include the following:

1 *Mycosis fungoides–Sézary's syndrome* (see Chapter 4).
2 *Leukemias* (see Chapter 23).
3 *Lymphomatoid granulomatosis* and some of the *lethal midline granulomas* (see Chapter 7).
4 So-called *malignant angioendotheliomatosis*. This systemic malignant disease, originally regarded as a multicentric malignant transformation of endothelial cells, is now known to be a type of malignant lymphoma with a remarkable tropism for blood vessels.[791] Accordingly, it has been renamed *angiotropic lymphoma* or intravascular lymphomatosis (see Chapter 4).
5 *Hairy cell leukemia.* This entity is fully discussed in Chapter 23. Suffice it to say here that the lymph nodes can be involved by the disease and that this involvement is characterized by diffuse infiltration of the subcapsular sinuses, cortex, and medullary cords by typical small mononuclear cells having nuclei slightly larger than those of lymphocytes, fine chromatin pattern, relatively abundant cytoplasm, and essentially no mitotic activity. Despite the extensiveness of the infiltrate, the nodal architecture is partially preserved.[789]
6 *Lymphoma of plasmacytoid monocytes.* These were formerly known as plasmacytoid T-cell lymphomas.[790,792]

Composite and discordant lymphomas

In general, there is constancy within the various types of malignant lymphoma, so that a patient with a certain type of lymphoma at a given site will have the same type at other sites and will maintain it during the entire evolution of the disease. However, on occasion one encounters two distinct types of lymphoma in the same patient, either sequentially or simultaneously, even in the same lymph node. The occurrence of two different and well-delineated varieties of lymphoma occurring in a single anatomic site or mass is known as *composite lymphoma,* and the occurrence of two different types of lymphoma at separate anatomic sites has been referred to as *discordant lymphoma.*[795,807] Some of these combinations may represent the occurrence of two unrelated neoplasms, either spontaneously or as a result of the therapy given for one of them. The majority, however, are probably the expression of different biologic and morphologic manifestations of the same lesion, the more malignant one representing the morphologic expression of tumor progression.[811]

The most important manifestations of this phenomenon are the following:

1 Low-grade B-cell lymphoma (small lymphocytic, follicular small cleaved, or follicular mixed) that transforms into a diffuse large cell lymphoma.[796,810,815]
2 Low-grade T-cell lymphoma (such as mycosis fungoides) that transforms into a diffuse large cell lymphoma (see Chapter 4).[793,798,801,808,812]
3 Combination of nodular L&H Hodgkin's disease and other lymphomas, particularly diffuse large cell lymphoma.[800,802-804]
4 Combination of "classic" Hodgkin's disease and large cell lymphoma of B-cell type (Fig. 21-70). We have seen this combination several times in the thymic region.[797,800,805] The Hodgkin's disease may coexist with, follow, or precede the non-Hodgkin's lymphoma.[806,813,814]
5 Combination of "classic" Hodgkin's disease and peripheral (post-thymic) T-cell lymphoma.[794,799,805]
6 Combination of "classic" Hodgkin's disease and chronic lymphocytic leukemia.[809]

So-called malignant histiocytosis

Malignant histiocytosis is a term first proposed by Rappaport[834] for a disease characterized by a systemic, neoplastic proliferation histologically resembling histiocytes and their precursors. It can affect any age group, but has a predilection for children and young adults.[838,842a] Fever, lymph node enlargement, and constitutional symptoms appear early in the course of the disease. Hepatomegaly, splenomegaly, and skin involvement also are common.[816,830] In some patients, pulmonary symptoms dominate the clinical presentation.[819] It is typical of the disease for the patient to be acutely ill when first seen by the physician. Common laboratory findings are anemia, leukopenia, and thrombocytopenia.[840] There is also elevation of serum ferritin levels.[821] Microscopically, the distinctive feature in the involved lymph nodes is the proliferation of atypical cells with the appearance of histiocytes within the subcapsular or medullary sinuses and/or within the lymphoid parenchyma (Fig. 21-71). The degree of atypia varies greatly from case to case.[841a] The tumor cells often surround lymphoid follicles in a concentric fashion. A variable number of cells within the infiltrate exhibit phagocytosis (especially of red blood cells), but it is sometimes difficult to decide whether

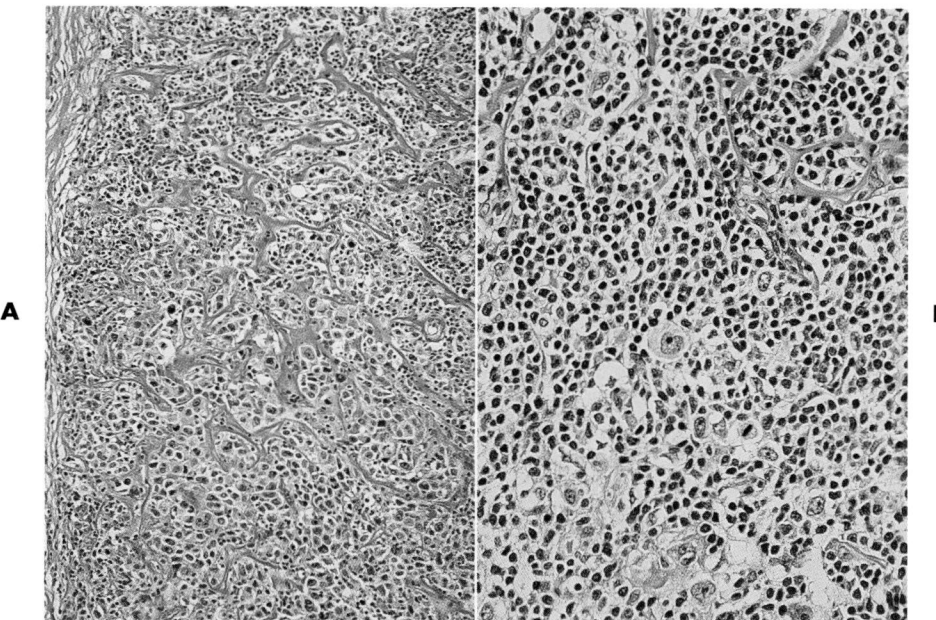

Fig. 21-70 Composite lymphoma of mediastinum. **A** corresponds to large cell lymphoma with sclerosis (which had a B immunophenotype), and **B** corresponds to nodular sclerosis Hodgkin's disease (which had the typical phenotype of Reed-Sternberg cells). (Slide contributed by Dr. Kiyoshi Mukai, Tokyo.)

this phagocytosis is occurring in neoplastic cells or in accompanying reactive histiocytes. This feature is better demonstrated in bone marrow smears and touch preparations of lymph nodes than in tissue sections.[839] Plasma cells are usually present in small numbers but may be abundant. Capsular invasion is rare; even when present, the peripheral sinuses tend to be preserved. The tumor cells themselves exhibit a pattern of individual cell infiltration rather than the cohesive masses of large cell lymphoma. Their cytoplasm is more abundant and eosinophilic, to the point that some cases that we have seen were originally misinterpreted as metastatic malignant melanoma or carcinoma.

Most of the cases are rapidly progressive and fatal, two thirds of the patients dying within the first months after diagnosis.[820,833] At autopsy, widespread organ involvement is found, usually without formation of large tumor masses but rather growing diffusely in the interstitium. In the skin, the infiltrate is periadnexal and perivascular, in contrast to the diffuse dermal infiltration with epidermal involvement observed in Langerhans' cell granulomatosis (histiocytosis X).

The differential diagnosis includes atypical reactive hyperplasia induced by viral and parasitic agents,[828] sinus histiocytosis with massive lymphadenopathy, Langerhans' cell granulomatosis, Hodgkin's disease, metastatic melanoma or carcinoma, large cell lymphoma, and malignant fibrous histiocytoma. The latter possibility arises because some cases of malignant histiocytosis have been reported exhibiting marked pleomorphism[841] and spindle-cell metaplasia.[827]

The entity described by Scott and Robb-Smith[837] as *histiocytic medullary reticulosis* needs to be discussed in this context.[835,836] This has been described clinically as characterized by hepatosplenomegaly, jaundice, and rapidly fatal

outcome and pathologically by prominent erythrophagocytosis by more or less atypical histiocytes. Probably some of these cases are equivalent to malignant histiocytosis as just described[817]; as a matter of fact, some authors use the two terms synonymously.[840] Other cases might have been examples of the virus-associated hemophagocytic syndrome (see Chapter 23). Along similar lines, it is possible that so-called familial hemophagocytic reticulosis is a viral infection occurring in a family with an immune defect that makes them susceptible to the virus.[832] Similarly, it is possible that some of the reported cases of lymphoma, leukemia, or myeloproliferative diseases terminating in histiocytic medullary reticulosis[822,825] represent overwhelming viral infections in a compromised host.

Some of the above considerations apply to the concept of malignant histiocytosis in a more global sense. The original definition of the disease was based on clinicomorphologic criteria; subsequent enzyme histochemical, immunohistochemical, and ultrastructural studies claimed to have found support for the histiocytic nature of the cellular proliferation,[824,826,829] and it was further suggested that the t(2;5) translocation was characteristic of the disease.[831] However, cell marker and molecular analysis studies have shown that most cases are actually examples of large cell lymphoma, especially anaplastic large cell (Ki-1+) lymphoma and peripheral T-cell lymphoma[818,842] (with or without a hemophagocytic syndrome component). Malignant histiocytosis of the small bowel has been reinterpreted as a T-cell lymphoma (enteropathy associated, see Chapter 11). In view of these findings, the current view is that "malignant histiocytosis" is a syndrome rather than a single disease entity and that every effort should be made to classify each case according to current terminology based on a thorough

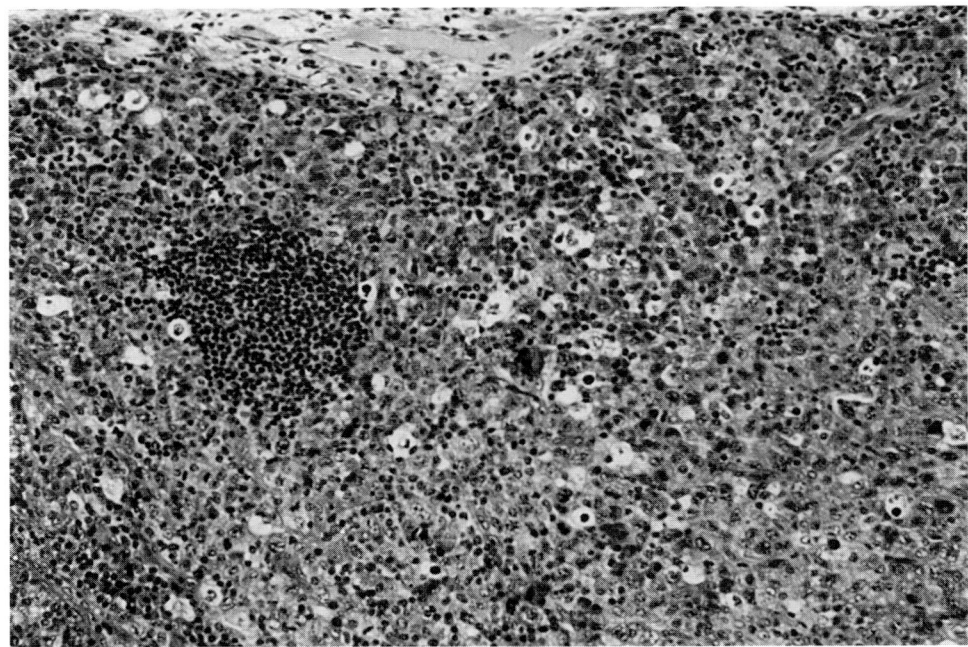

Fig. 21-71 Malignant histiocytosis. Pleomorphic infiltrate is present in expanded sinuses, with resulting compression and atrophy of intervening lymphoid tissue. This pattern of growth closely simulates that of metastatic carcinoma.

immunohistochemical and molecular evaluation of the case.[823]

Lymphoma in immunodeficiency states

An increase in the incidence of malignant lymphoma has been documented in most types of congenital and acquired immunodeficiency.[860] Chronic antigenic stimulation—possibly by oncogenic viruses—and perhaps loss of antibody feedback inhibition of the lymphoid proliferation may account for the high rate of lymphoid malignancies. The Epstein-Barr virus in particular has been repeatedly implicated.[869]

1 *Primary immunodeficiencies.* Patients with genetically determined immune deficiencies have an increased incidence of malignant tumors, especially lymphomas.[863,884] This includes ataxia-telangiectasia, Wiskott-Aldrich syndrome, X-linked lymphoproliferative syndrome, common variable immunodeficiency, and severe combined immunodeficiency syndrome.[880]

Patients with *ataxia-telangiectasia* and the *Wiskott-Aldrich syndrome* are particularly prone to this complication, about 10% of the reported patients having died from it.[871] An interesting correlation exists between the type of immune deficiency and the type of lymphoma. In a series from the University of Minnesota, all the lymphomas arising in Wiskott-Aldrich syndrome were of non-Hodgkin's type (predominantly B-cell immunoblastic sarcoma) presenting as localized extranodal masses, whereas those arising in patients with ataxia-telangiectasia were of both Hodgkin's and non-Hodgkin's types, with a more conventional organ distribution. Surprisingly for this age group, half of the

cases of Hodgkin's disease belonged to the lymphocyte depletion type. Most of the non-Hodgkin's lymphomas in ataxia-telangiectasia were of the histologic types associated with the 14q+ chromosomal abnormality.[853] Parenthetically, a gene for ataxia-telangiectasia (ATM) that codes a product similar to PI-3 kinase has been recently cloned.[862a,881] Also, mutations of Jak-3 gene have been detected in severe combined immunodeficiency syndrome.[870a]

The microscopic diagnosis of the lymphoma can be extremely difficult in early cases; sometimes, the only morphologic diagnosis of the lymphoma possible is that of an atypical lymphoproliferative process.

Several members of families affected by the *X-linked lymphoproliferative syndrome* (believed to result from an immunodeficiency to the Epstein-Barr virus)[875] have developed sporadic Burkitt's lymphoma, immunoblastic sarcoma of B cells, fatal infectious mononucleosis, or "plasmacytoma."

2 *Organ transplant recipients.* The incidence of malignancy after renal transplantation is in the order of 4% to 6%.[851] Skin tumors, malignant lymphomas, Kaposi's sarcoma, and cervical carcinoma are the most common neoplasms. The frequency of lymphoma has been estimated to be 350 times higher than in the age-matched general population.[850,866,874] The incidence is particularly high in adult cardiac transplant patients treated with OKT-3–containing regimens.[847,885] In about half of the reported cases, the central nervous system is involved, compared with less than 1% in lymphoma patients in general. In 30% of the cases, the allograft is also involved. The clinical course is usually very

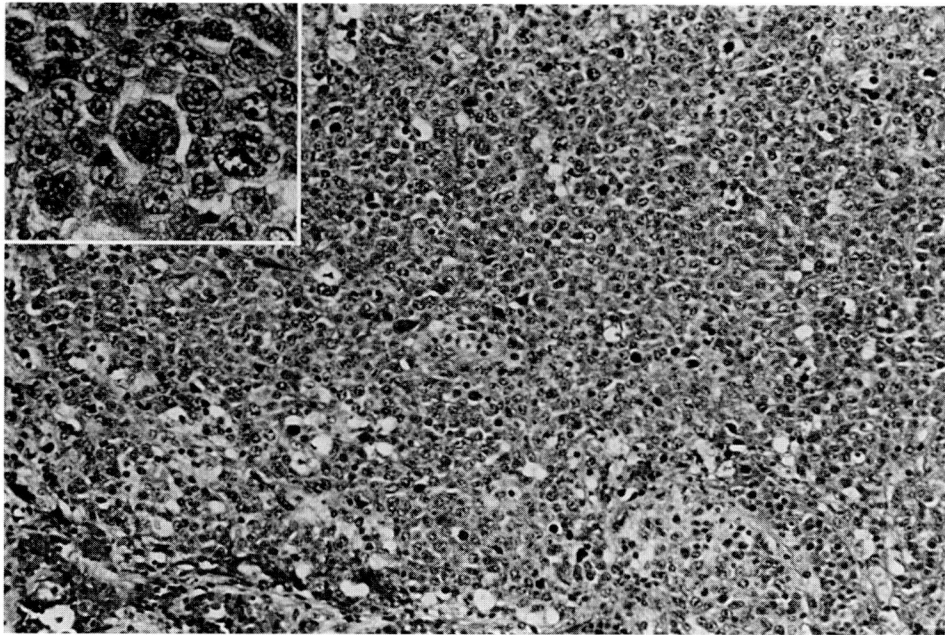

Fig. 21-72 Large cell lymphoma developing in transplant recipient. Note marked pleomorphism of tumor cells, better shown in **inset.**

rapid.[877] Microscopically, most of these lymphomas show marked cytologic polymorphism (small and large follicular center cells and immunoblasts), atypia of the immunoblasts, and extensive necrosis (Fig. 21-72). The initial infiltrate has polyclonal B-cell features, in keeping with a reactive origin.[857,858] The development of lymphoma is signaled by the appearance of a monoclonal component with chromosomal aberrations.[852] The term "polymorphic B-cell lymphoma" has been suggested for this tumor type. A transition has been observed from a polyclonal activation of B-cells to an oligoclonal B-cell proliferation and finally to a monoclonal B-cell lymphoma.[858,883] Immunoglobulin rearrangement studies have shown the existence of a monoclonal population in early stages of the process, before the malignancy is recognizable morphologically.[847,868] Virtually all cases of post-transplant lymphoproliferative disorders harbor EBV genomic DNA and RNA.[876] In most cases, these genomes are clonal, indicating the presence of EBV in the progenitor B-cell that originated the neoplastic population.[872] In contrast to AIDS-associated lymphoma, *myc* rearrangements are uncommon in post-transplant lymphoma. A minority of these tumors have been found to be of T-cell type.[855,867]

Treatment of post-transplant lymphoproliferative disorders consists of a combination of immunosuppression reduction and standard lymphoma therapy (chemotherapy and radiation).[843a]

3 *AIDS.* Patients with AIDS are at a high risk for developing malignant tumors, principally Kaposi's sarcoma and malignant lymphoma.* It has been estimated that about 3% of AIDS patients develop non-Hodgkin's lymphoma, and that the risk of developing a lymphoma in this population is sixty-fold greater than in the normal population. The incidence of lymphoma is highest in hemophiliacs and lowest in individuals born in the Caribbean or Africa who have acquired the disease by heterosexual contact. The majority of the cases present with multiple sites of extranodal involvement, with a high incidence of involvement of the gastrointestinal tract, central nervous system, bone marrow, liver, and heart.[861] Practically all cases are of B-cell lineage and —as such—show clonal immunoglobulin gene rearrangements.[848,870] Morphologically, most cases are of small noncleaved, plasmacytoid, immunoblastic, or diffuse large cell type.[846,878]

The molecular and cytogenetic features of Burkitt's lymphoma seen in the AIDS population are similar to those of sporadic Burkitt's lymphoma, especially in regard to rearrangements of the *myc* gene. The bcl-2 and T-cell receptor genes are unaffected. Evidence of EBV infection is often present.[856,873]

The incidence of Hodgkin's disease in HIV-infected patients does not seem to be increased, but the disease presents several differences with that seen in the immunocompetent population. Almost all cases are clinical stage III or IV at presentation, with frequent involvement of unusual sites such as the liver and skin; spread often occurs in a noncontiguous fashion; mixed cellularity is the predominant histologic subtype; Reed-Sternberg cells and (especially) their variants are more numerous and more atypical; there is an increased

*References 845, 848, 854, 861, 864, 887.

number of nonlymphoid stromal cells; and there is a much higher incidence of presence of the EBV genomes in Reed-Sternberg cells (reaching almost 100% in some series).[843,844,859,879,886]

4 *Others.* Acquired diseases of the immune system in which an increased incidence of lymphoma has been recorded include rheumatoid arthritis,[849,862] Sjögren's syndrome,[882] Hashimoto's thyroiditis, and other autoimmune diseases.[844a] This includes the ill-defined group of disorders variously designated as abnormal immune reactions or atypical immunoproliferative processes, of which angioimmunoblastic lymphadenopathy is a prime example.[865]

LYMPH NODE INCLUSIONS

Inclusions of various types of benign tissue can occur within lymph nodes. Lack of awareness of this phenomenon can lead to a mistaken diagnosis of metastatic carcinoma. These include the following:

1 *Salivary gland tissue.* This is an extremely common finding in high cervical nodes, to the point that it should be regarded as a normal event related to the embryology of the region.[892] Both ducts and acini are usually present. These inclusions may undergo neoplastic changes. Warthin's tumor is the most common type, but many other types have been reported, including benign mixed tumor, monomorphic adenoma, mucoepidermoid carcinoma, and acinic cell carcinoma (see Chapter 12).

2 *Squamous epithelium.* Microscopic cystic structures lined by well-differentiated squamous epithelium are sometimes seen in the upper cervical lesion. They are thought to represent an anomaly related to the aforementioned one, in the sense of being composed of branchial pouch derivatives. The term "benign lymphoepithelial cyst" is sometimes applied to them (see Chapter 12). Similar formations have been described in peripancreatic lymph nodes.[888] The obvious differential diagnosis is metastatic well-differentiated squamous cell carcinoma, which in the cervical region is notorious for its tendency to undergo marked cystic changes.[903]

3 *Thyroid follicles.* These can be found within the marginal sinus of a midcervical node in the absence of pathologic changes of the thyroid gland. The differential diagnosis with metastatic thyroid carcinoma can be very difficult (see Chapter 9).

4 *Decidual reaction.* During pregnancy, *decidual reaction* may occur within pelvic nodes and mimic metastatic carcinoma[893] (Fig. 21-73). The decidual reaction can occur in the stromal cells of endometriosis or in hormonally receptive cells of the region, in a fashion similar to that seen in peritoneal decidual reaction.

5 *Müllerian-type epithelium.* Glandular inclusions lined by cuboidal cells with a müllerian or coelomic appearance are commonly found in the capsule of the pelvic lymph nodes of females and sometimes within the node itself.[899,902] Their appearance and pathogenesis are similar to those of the peritoneal lesions generally known as endosalpingiosis (Fig. 21-74). Like the latter, these lymph node inclusions may be difficult to distinguish

from metastases originating in low-grade ovarian neoplasms, since they may grow into the peripheral sinuses, form papillae, be accompanied by psammoma bodies, and even proliferate as small sheets of cells.[895] These are thought to give origin to the rare primary borderline and serous tumors of pelvic nodes.[904] Morphologically similar inclusions have been seen in the mediastinal nodes of males.[901]

Nodal glandular inclusions of similar appearance but surrounded by endometrial-type stroma occur less frequently and represent *nodal endometriosis.*

6 *Nevus cells.* Clusters of normal-appearing nevus cells are occasionally found in the capsule of lymph nodes, without involvement of the nodal parenchyma (Fig. 21-75). Most of the reported cases have occurred in axillary lymph nodes.[898] A related lesion is the *blue nevus* that has been reported in the lymph node capsule.[889]

7 *Mesothelial cells.* Occasionally, mesothelial cells are found within lymph nodes in the apparent absence of a malignant mesothelioma. Brooks et al.[891] reported two cases in mediastinal lymph nodes in patients with pleuritis associated with pleural effusion; they suggested that the mesothelial cells may have traveled from the pleura to the node via lymph channels that freely communicated with the inflamed pleural surface. We have seen similar cases in mediastinal and retroperitoneal lymph nodes, and others have been reported.[905] The obvious differential diagnosis is with metastatic malignant mesothelioma from an occult primary in the peritoneal cavity or pleura.[906]

8 *Breast tissue.* One of the most unusual forms of ectopia is represented by normal mammary lobules within axillary lymph nodes.[894,907] A slightly more common occurrence is the presence in axillary nodes of tubules lined by a single layer of cuboidal cells (sometimes with a hobnail appearance), located in the nodal capsule or immediately beneath. These formations are similar to the müllerian-type epithelial inclusions in pelvic lymph nodes previously described. Since some of these cases occur in patients with breast carcinoma, the distinct possibility exists of mistaking them for metastatic tumor.[890,896,897]

OTHER NON-NEOPLASTIC LESIONS

Adipose metaplasia of lymph nodes, when extensive, may lead to the formation of large masses, up to 10 cm or more in diameter. These nodes are sometimes referred to as *lipolymph nodes;* the external iliac and obturator groups are the sites most commonly involved.[914]

Ectopic thymus sometimes seen in supraclavicular lymph node biopsies should be mentioned here for the sake of completeness, even if it is not a lymph node lesion. The pathologist unaware of this occurrence might easily interpret the Hassall's corpuscles as islands of metastatic squamous cell carcinoma.

Vasculitis involving lymph nodes may be seen in a large number of disorders: polyarteritis nodosa (necrotizing, rarely biopsied), Henoch-Schönlein purpura (leukocytoclastic, rarely biopsied), Wegener's granulomatosis (sometimes accompanied by extensive infarct but rarely biopsied), sys-

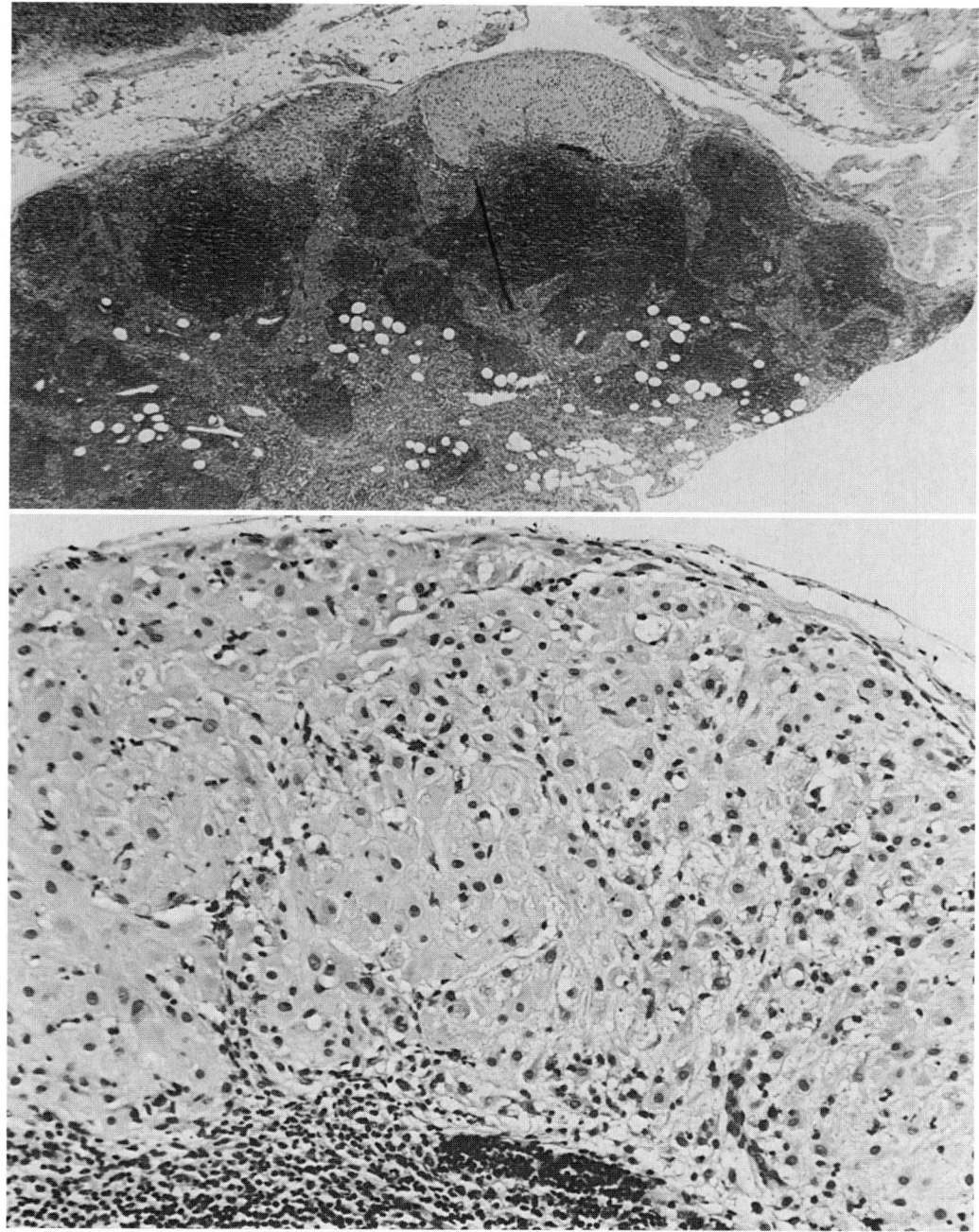

Fig. 21-73 Decidual change in pelvic lymph node of 27-year-old pregnant woman operated on for postirradiation persistence of cervical carcinoma. Subserial sections of nodes did not reveal any glandular elements. (Slides courtesy Dr. R. Fechner, Charlottesville, VA; photos by Media Services, SUNY at Stony Brook.)

temic lupus erythematosus, drug hypersensitivity (see p. 1693), and mucocutaneous lymph node syndrome (see p. 1686). Some nodes otherwise showing the typical features of angioimmunoblastic lymphadenopathy may also show extensive vasculitis. One should also mention the obliterative vasculitis often seen in syphilitic lymphadenitis (see p. 1680).

Infarction of the lymph nodes presents with painful swelling, usually located in a superficial lymph node chain.

Microscopically, there is extensive necrosis of medullary and cortical lymphoid cells, with marked reactive perinodal inflammation and a layer of granulation tissue. A thin rim of viable subcapsular lymphoid tissue may be present.[911] Thrombosis of veins within the substance and the hilum of the nodes has been suggested as the pathogenesis.[911] Similar changes can be seen in mesenteric lymph nodes in patients with intestinal volvulus.[915] Other cases are the result of embolism, arterial occlusion in cases of polyarteritis nodosa

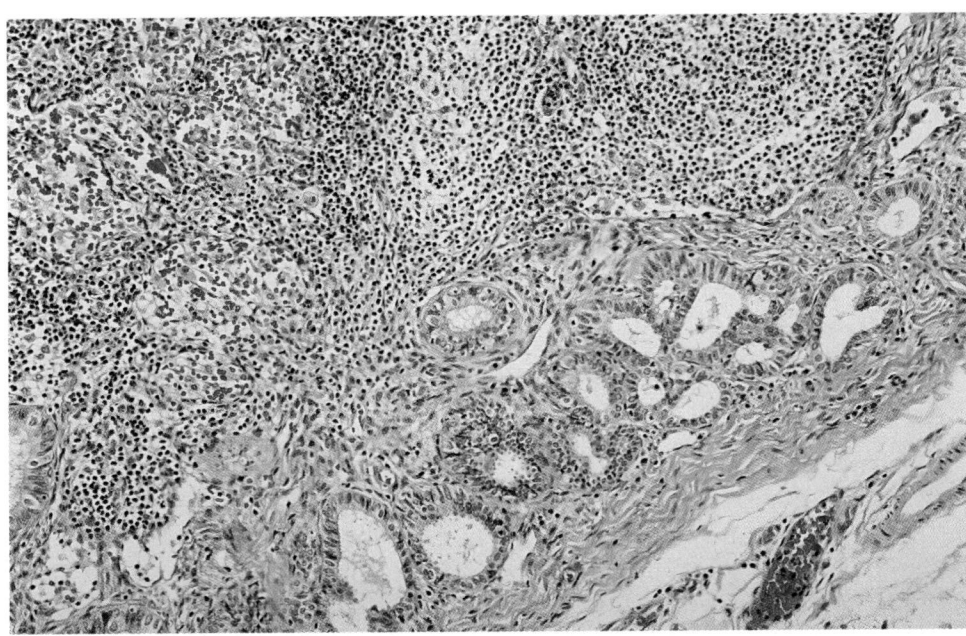

Fig. 21-74 Pelvic lymph node involved by endosalpingiosis. Glands lined by cuboidal cells with a müllerian appearance and lacking atypical figures are present in the capsule of the node.

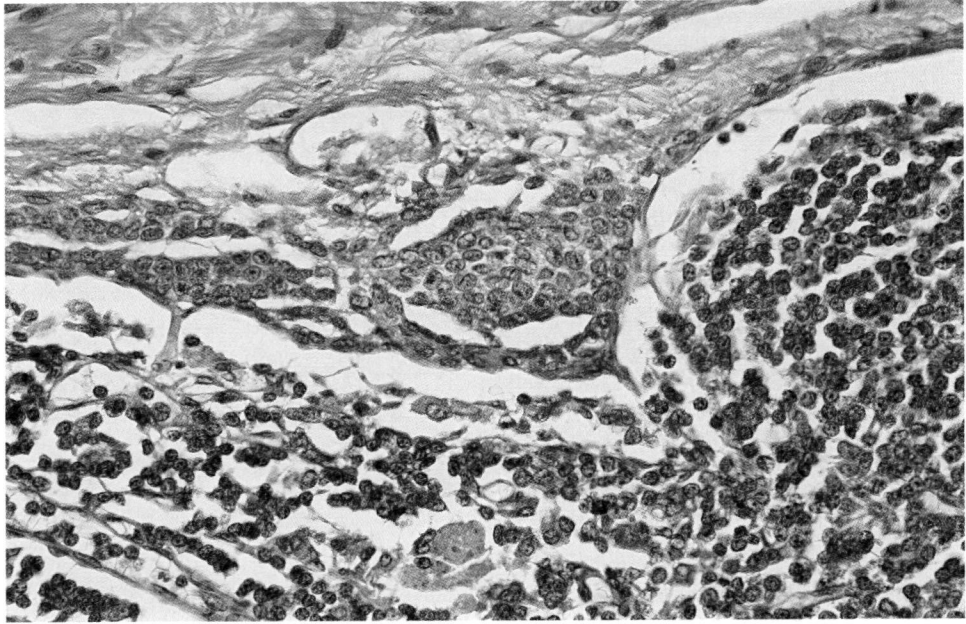

Fig. 21-75 Nevus cells in the capsule of an axillary lymph node. These inconsequential formations should not be mistaken for metastatic melanoma or metastatic carcinoma.

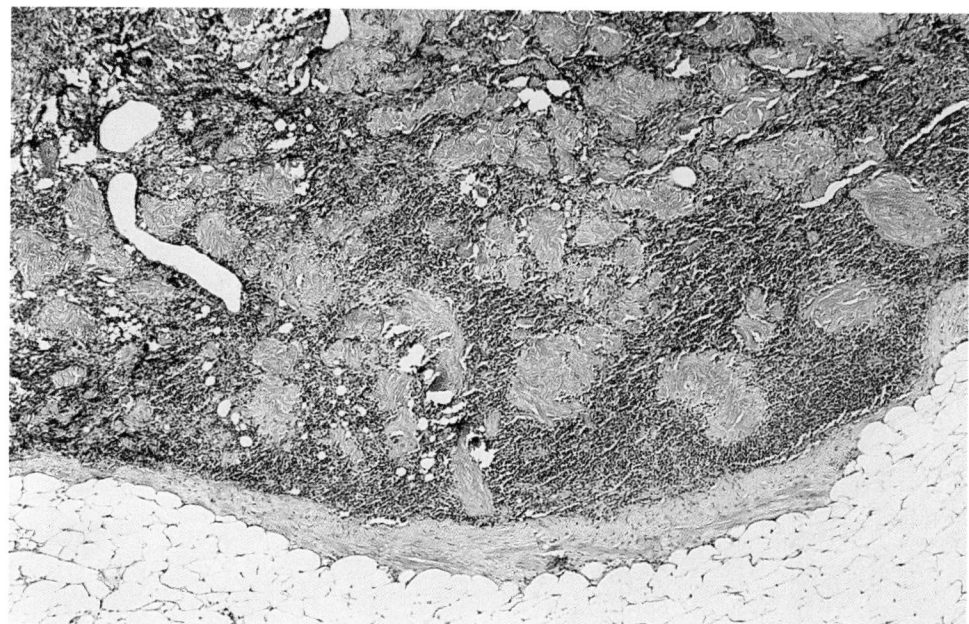

Fig. 21-76 Hyaline deposits in pelvic lymph node. This change is of no clinical significance.

and related disorders, or fine-needle aspiration[913,918]; in these instances, the nodal infarct tends to have a segmental quality. The differential diagnosis of lymph node infarction includes necrotizing lymphadenitis (see p. 1675), mucocutaneous lymph node syndrome (see p. 1686), necrotizing granulomatous inflammation, and necrotic malignant tumors. Two types of malignancies that have been occasionally found to undergo extensive and sometimes massive infarct-type necrosis when involving lymph nodes are malignant lymphoma[910,916] and metastatic malignant melanoma. Therefore thorough examination of the infarcted node, the extranodal region, and other nodes submitted is mandatory in order to exclude a concomitant or underlying malignancy.[916] As a general rule, the possibility of an underlying malignancy should be suspected if the infarcted node is markedly enlarged.

Hyaline material sometimes accumulates in the stroma of lymph nodes, particularly in those situated in the aorto-iliac region (Fig. 21-76). This material can undergo secondary calcification. Because of its homogeneous eosinophilic appearance, it can be confused with amyloid and has been referred to in the past as para-amyloid. It should also be distinguished from the hyaline material deposited in nodes in cases of hemorrhagic spindle cell tumor with amianthoid fibers (see p. 1747). The presence of hyaline material in pelvic nodes has no clinical significance.

Proteinaceous lymphadenopathy is the name given by Osborne et al.[917] to a lymph node abnormality in which an eosinophilic extracellular material of proteinaceous nature is deposited in lymph nodes. This material simulates the appearance of amyloid but is histochemically and ultrastructurally distinct from it. The few patients that have been described with this nodal abnormality had hypergammaglobulinemia, and the hyaline material itself has been shown to contain precipitated immunoglobulin.[909]

Foreign material of various types can accumulate in lymph nodes. One example is the *silicone lymphadenopathy* developing as a side effect of mammary augmentation produced by injection of liquid silicone or by placement of a bag-gel prosthesis. Microscopically, a nonbirefrigent refractive material is present in the sinuses, together with variously sized vacuoles and multinucleated giant cells[919] (Fig. 21-77).

Another example is the already mentioned sinus histiocytosis of pelvic lymph nodes, which is induced by the cobalt-chromium and titanium contained in a hip prosthesis and which closely simulates the appearance of sinus histiocytosis with massive lymphadenopathy (Rosai-Dorfman's disease).[908]

TUMORS OF DENDRITIC CELLS AND MACROPHAGES

The histiocytic system includes two major categories of cells: antigen-presenting cells (dendritic cells) and antigen-processing cells (macrophages). The dendritic cells belong to the group of non-lymphoid elements classically designated as reticulum cells, which have been divided into four subtypes on the basis of location, enzyme histochemical, ultrastructural, and immunohistochemical features. These are:

1 **Dendritic reticulum cells.** These elements, now renamed *dendritic follicular cells,* are associated with the B zones of the node and specifically with the germinal centers. Ultrastructurally, they have complex cell prolongations joined by complex desmosomes. Immunohistochemically, they exhibit reactivity for CD21, CD35, Ki-M4p, and Ki-FDRC1p.[920,926,934]
2 **Interdigitating reticulum cells.** These cells, renamed *dendritic interdigitating cells,* are associated with the T zones of the nodes. They also have complex cell pro-

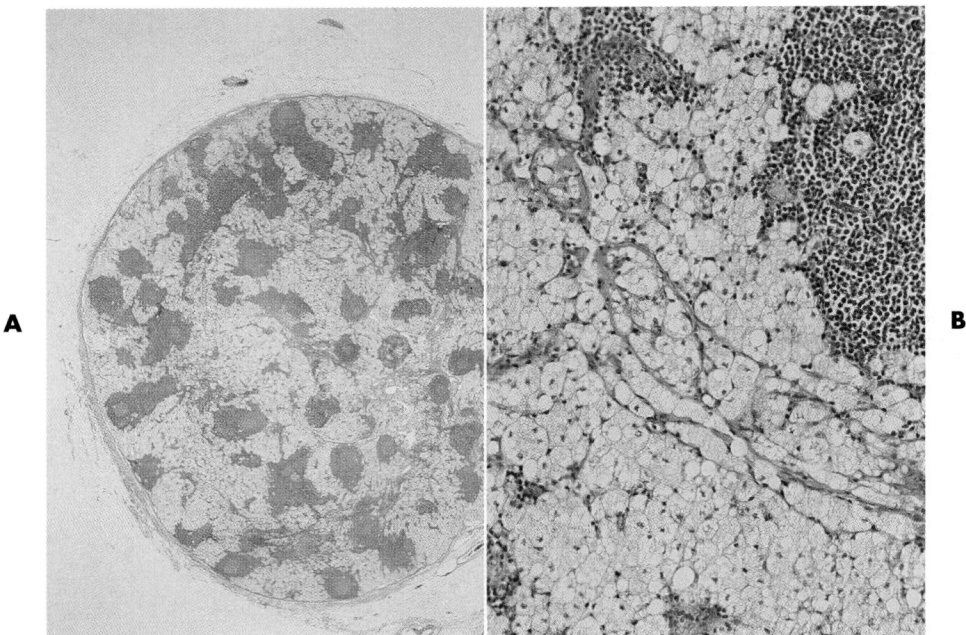

Fig. 21-77 Low-power **(A)** and medium-power **(B)** appearances of silicon lymphadenitis. The sinuses are massively enlarged by a histiocytic infiltrate, which simulates the appearance of sinus histiocytosis with massive lymphadenopathy.

longations that interdigitate with each other, but desmosomes are absent. Immunohistochemically, they are reactive for S-100 protein.[924,931]

3 **Fibroblastic reticulum cells.** These are located in the capsule, hilus, and other stromal-rich areas of the node. They have a high content of alkaline phosphatase, exhibit filaments with focal condensations at the ultrastructural level, and probably correspond to the *myoid cells* described by other authors.

4 **Histiocytic reticulum cells.** These elements, which contain large amounts of hydrolytic enzymes, are very similar to macrophages.

5 Other types of "reticulum" cells probably exist, including a population that is keratin positive.[923]

Rare tumors have been described having phenotypic features corresponding to several of these cell categories.

Dendritic follicular cell tumor (follicular dendritic cell sarcoma; dendritic reticulum cell sarcoma) often presents as a solitary mass in a cervical lymph node, but can involve other lymph node sites and extranodal locations, such as the bowel, oral cavity, and spleen[920,927,933] (Fig. 21-78, *A*). Microscopically, it is characterized by a proliferation of oval to spindle cells that form fascicles and whorls[938] (Figs. 21-78, *B*, and 21-79). Sometimes there is a suggestion of storiform pattern.[926,933] The appearance at low power may simulate that of meningioma. The nuclei are generally oval, with a vesicular chromatin pattern, small nucleoli, and scanty mitotic activity. Pseudonuclear inclusions and multinucleated giant cells may be present. A characteristic feature is the presence of small lymphocytes scattered throughout the tumor cells, resulting in a thymoma-like appearance. The ultrastructural and immunohistochemical features correspond to those of dendritic follicular cells (Fig. 21-80).

Markers that are particularly useful for their identification in paraffin-embedded material are CD21, CD35, Ki-M4P, and Ki-FDRC1p.[934]

The tumor cells are negative or equivocal for CD45RB and inconstantly positive for S-100 protein. In frozen sections, they also stain for the dendritic follicular cell marker R4/23, HLA-DR, and the lymphocyte adhesion markers CD11a and CD18.[920] At the molecular level, they show a germline configuration for both the immunoglobulin heavy chain gene and the beta T-cell receptor gene.[938]

The behavior is that of a low-grade malignancy, with capacity for local recurrence and distant metastases to sites such as the liver and lung.[934] The pattern of spread resembles that of a soft tissue sarcoma more than it does that of a malignant lymphoma. Recurrent and metastatic lesions may show increased atypia and pleomorphism.[934]

Interdigitating dendritic cell tumor (interdigitating reticulum cell sarcoma) is even more unusual. Most of the reported cases have arisen in lymph nodes,[921,923] but extranodal sites such as the skin and bowel have been recorded.[929,931] The microscopic appearance can be indistinguishable from that of dendritic follicular cell tumor, but there is more tendency to spindling and pleomorphism.[937,939] The diagnosis is dependent on the immunohistochemical profile. The tumor cells are positive for CD45RB, S-100 protein, and the macrophage marker CD68 but are negative for CD21 and CD35. The behavior seems more aggressive than for the dendritic cell tumor.

Tumors corresponding to other subtypes of "reticulum cells" have not yet been characterized, although we have seen a case that we interpreted as a primary keratin-positive spindle-cell tumor of the node that may correspond to one such subtype.

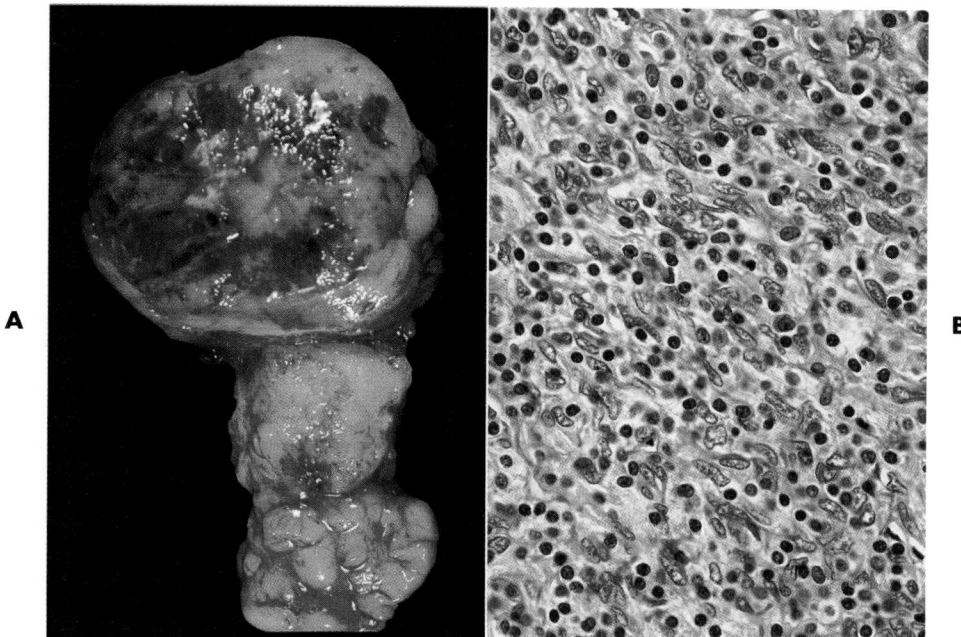

Fig. 21-78 Dendritic follicular cell tumor. **A,** Gross appearance. **B,** Microscopic appearance. The admixture of tumor cells with oval to spindle nuclei and mature lymphocytes results in a picture reminiscent of thymoma.

True histiocytic lymphomas (sarcomas) remain rare and controversial. The issue is complicated by the fact that the majority of neoplasms to which the term "histiocytic" was applied in the past (such as Rappaport's histiocytic lymphoma, malignant histiocytosis, and regressing atypical histiocytosis) were later shown to be of lymphoid nature in the overwhelming majority of the cases. However, it would seem that tumors of true histiocytes do exist.[930] Their presentation is highly variable, with a high proportion of extranodal involvement in sites such as the spleen, skin, bone, and bowel.[922,932,936] Microscopically, the tumor cells are large, with irregularly shaped nuclei and abundant, generally acidophilic cytoplasm. Immunohistochemically, the tumor cells lack by definition B-cell– and T-cell–related markers and show reactivity for histiocytic markers, such as CD63, CD11c, CD13, CD14, CD15, CD32, CD33, Mac-387, and lysozyme.[925,928,935] At the molecular level, some authors require the lack of rearrangement of immunoglobulin and T-cell receptor genes to retain a tumor in this category, whereas others accept the presence of such rearrangements.

VASCULAR TUMORS AND TUMORLIKE CONDITIONS

Hemangioma and ***lymphangioma*** involving nodes usually represent extension by contiguity of primary soft tissue lesions. However, rare cases of primary nodal hemangioma and lymphangioma have been described.[940,951]

Epithelioid (histiocytoid) vascular neoplasms of lymph nodes include epithelioid hemangioma, epithelioid hemangioendothelioma, spindle and epithelioid hemangioendothelioma, and polymorphous hemangioendothelioma.[942,958,960,961] The differential diagnosis includes (1) epithelioid hemangioma of soft tissue with a peripheral rim of germinal centers resulting in a node-like appearance on low power (a much more common occurrence than true nodal epithelioid hemangioma),[963] (2) Kimura's disease (an altogether different process lacking epithelioid endothelial cells (see p. 1697), and (3) bacillary angiomatosis.

Bacillary angiomatosis, which occurs almost exclusively in the setting of immunodeficiency (especially in patients with AIDS), presents as multiple coalescent intranodal clusters of proliferating vessels. These vessels are lined by plump, somewhat epithelioid endothelial cells (hence the original term epithelioid angiomatosis for this condition). A feature of great diagnostic importance is the presence of abundant eosinophilic to amphophilic, amorphous, or granular material in the interstitium. When stained with the Warthin-Starry technique, this material is shown to be composed of aggregated bacillary organisms that are indistinguishable from those of cat-scratch disease. Another helpful feature is the presence of neutrophils, sometimes forming microabscesses.[943,945,957]

Vascular transformation of the sinuses is characterized by a conversion of lymph node sinuses into a complex network of anastomosing endothelial-lined channel (Fig. 21-81).[952] Fibrosis and reactive stromal changes are commonly present.[956] *Nodal angiomatosis* probably refers to a more cellular form of this condition[948,953] (Fig. 21-82). In the nodular spindle-cell variant, spindle-cell nodules composed of interlacing fascicles alternate with the vascular clefts.[944] This variant is likely to be misdiagnosed as Kaposi's sarcoma. It is distinguished from the latter because it is confined to the sinus (with sparing of the capsule and parenchyma), there is no cellular atypia, the fascicles blend with well-formed vascular channels, fibrosis is common,

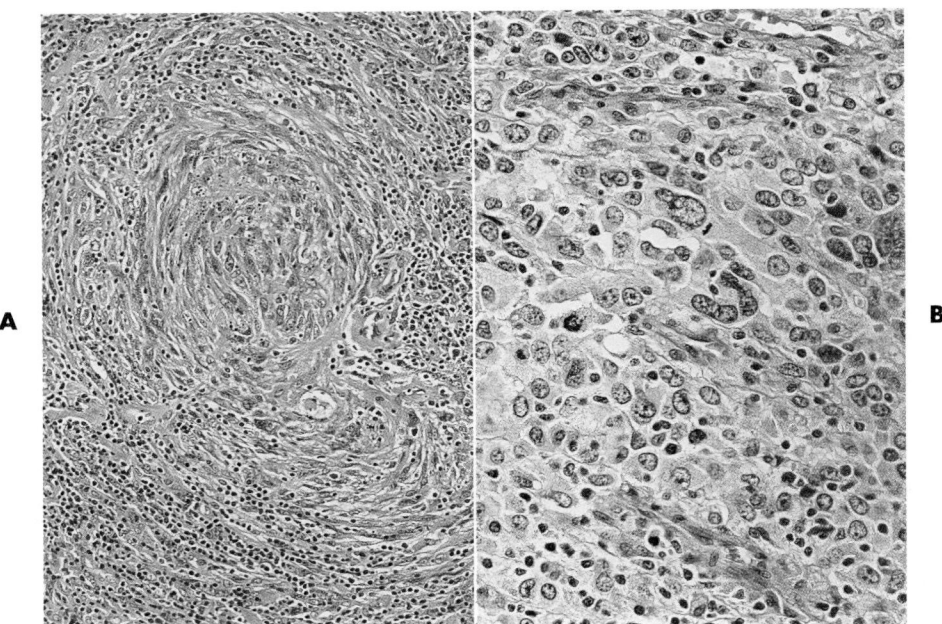

Fig. 21-79 Dendritic follicular cell tumor. **A,** In this area the prominent whorling configuration resembles the appearance of a meningioma. **B,** This recurrent tumor shows a marked degree of pleomorphism.

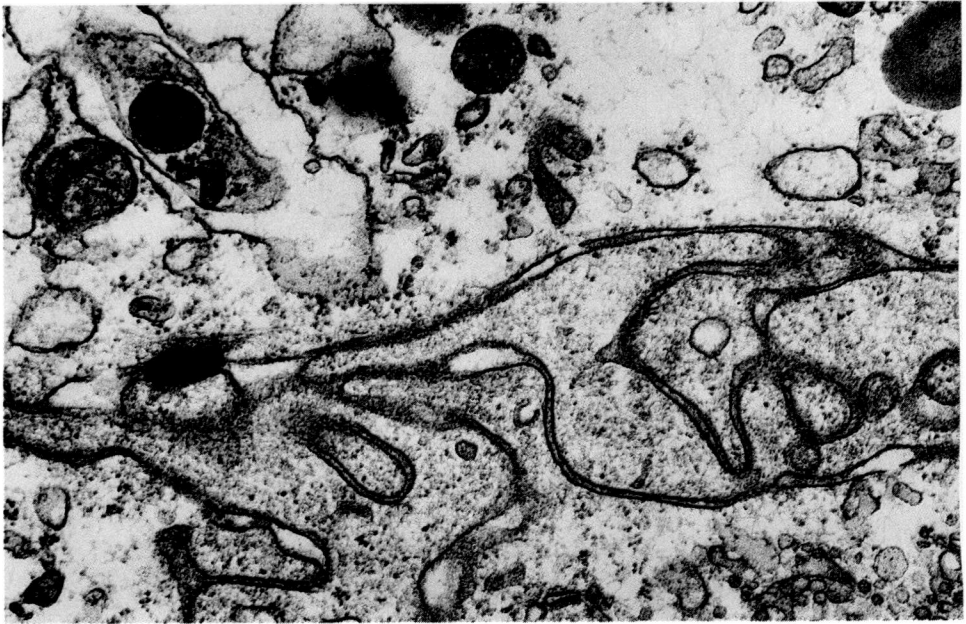

Fig. 21-80 Electron microscopic appearance of dendritic follicular cell tumor. A characteristic feature includes the presence of well-developed cytoplasmic prolongations joined by desmosomes.

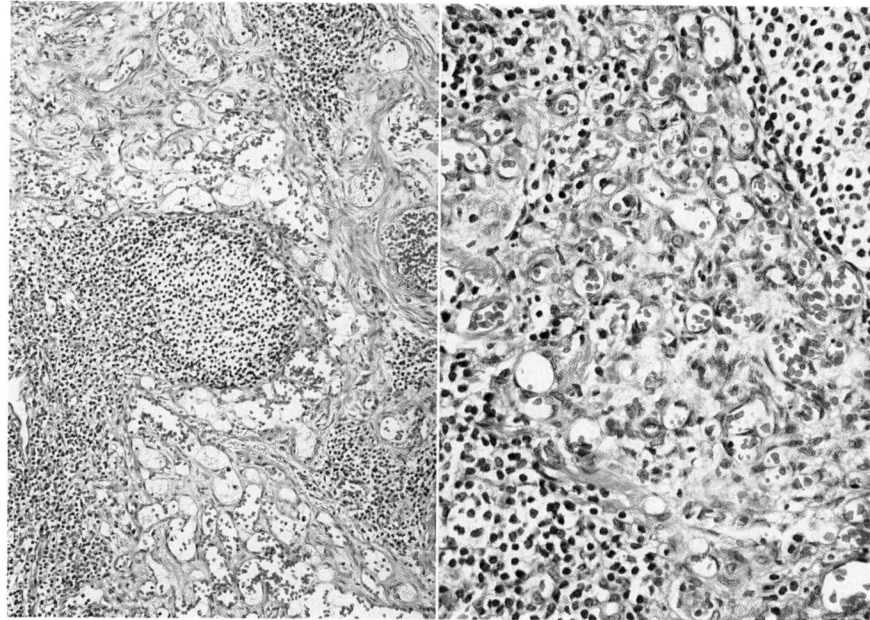

Fig. 21-81 Vascular transformation of lymph nodes. The process involves the sinuses, and it has a reactive appearance.

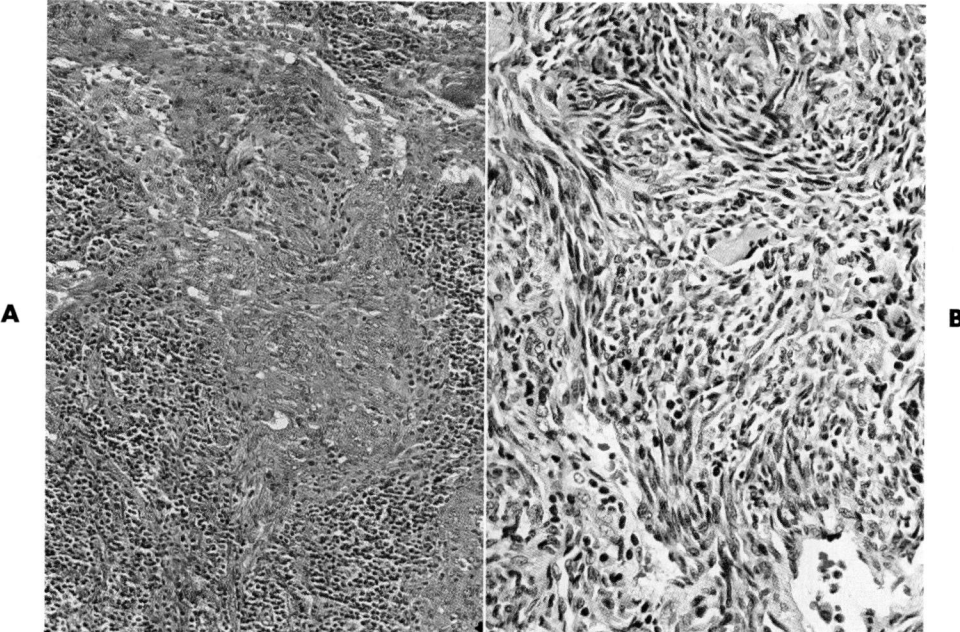

Fig. 21-82 Solid form of vascular transformation of lymph nodes. This process has also been designated as nodal angiomatosis. The example shown in **B** occurred in a retroperitoneal lymph node in a patient with renal cell carcinoma.

and PAS-positive hyaline globules are almost invariably absent. We have seen cases of this nodular spindle-cell variant in retroperitoneal lymph nodes draining renal cell carcinomas and have speculated about the possibility of its being the result of secretion of angiogenic factor by the carcinoma cells[946] (Fig. 21-82, *B*). Other cases of vascular transforma-

tion may result from proximal obstruction of the efferent vessels; indeed, the process has been reproduced experimentally by complete occlusion of these vessels.[959]

Kaposi's sarcoma of the lymph nodes may be associated with typical skin lesions or be present in their absence.[955] The latter occurrence is seen mainly in African children, but it also occurs in adults affected by AIDS.[947] Microscopically, the involved nodes show proliferation of spindle cells separated by slit-like spaces containing red blood cells (Fig. 21-83).[941] The earliest changes are seen in the subcapsular and trabecular sinuses, but eventually there is involvement of the entire node and extension into the perinodal tissues. Cytoplasmic and extracellular hyaline globules that are positive for PAS and PTAH are almost always present.[950] Recognition of early nodal involvement by Kaposi's sarcoma is an extremely difficult task; often, only a diagnosis of "atypical vascular proliferation suggestive of early Kaposi's disease" can be made. In well-developed cases, the tumor may grow in a diffuse fashion or as discrete deposits. The spindle-cell lesion is often accompanied by a lymphoid proliferation with a prominent component of plasma cells and immunoblasts. Sometimes, this reactive lymphoid process acquires the features of Castleman's disease of the plasma cell type.[949,954] In this context, it should be mentioned that sometimes cases of Castleman's disease of the vascular hyaline type are associated with angiolipomatous hamartomas and various forms of vascular neoplasia (see p. 1688). In other instances, nodal Kaposi's sarcoma co-exists with malignant lymphoma or leukemia.[962]

If a lymph node is involved by a malignant tumor with the morphologic features of *angiosarcoma*, there is a high probability that the tumor is metastatic.

OTHER PRIMARY TUMORS AND TUMORLIKE CONDITIONS

Mastocytosis of the diffuse (systemic) type often involves lymph nodes, resulting in a partial or complete effacement of the architecture by a monotonous proliferation of round or polygonal cells.[967,979] Clues as to the nature of the proliferation include the regular contours of the round or oval nucleus, the clear or granular cytoplasm, the well-defined cell outlines, and the admixture of eosinophils. Special techniques that allow the identification of mast cells include Giemsa, metachromatic stains (i.e., toluidine blue, polychrome methylene blue), chloroacetate esterase (Leder), and immunohistochemical demonstration of tryptase (Fig. 21-84).[971,976] Monoclonal antibodies allegedly specific for mast cell antigens have also been described.[983]

It should be remembered that occasional mast cells are normally present in small number in lymph nodes. Their number is increased in some parasitoses, in Waldenström macroglobulinemia, and in several types of lymphadenitis.[978]

Granulocytic leukemia can first be seen in a lymph node biopsy and misdiagnosed as malignant lymphoma. Clues to the diagnosis include a patchy or sinusal type of nodal involvement, sometimes associated with a single-file pattern of infiltration in the capsule; fine granularity of the cytoplasm; and presence of eosinophilic myelocytes.

Smooth muscle proliferations of a primary nature can be seen within lymph nodes in the following situations:

1 *Smooth muscle proliferation in the hilum.* This is often accompanied by fibrosis and prominent vascularity.[969] It is most common in the inguinal region and is of no clinical significance.

2 *Angiomyolipoma.* The most common location is the retroperitoneal region, usually in conjunction with a renal tumor of the same type (see Chapter 17).[966]

3 *Lymphangiomyomatosis.* This is seen exclusively in women, often in association with pulmonary involvement.[970]

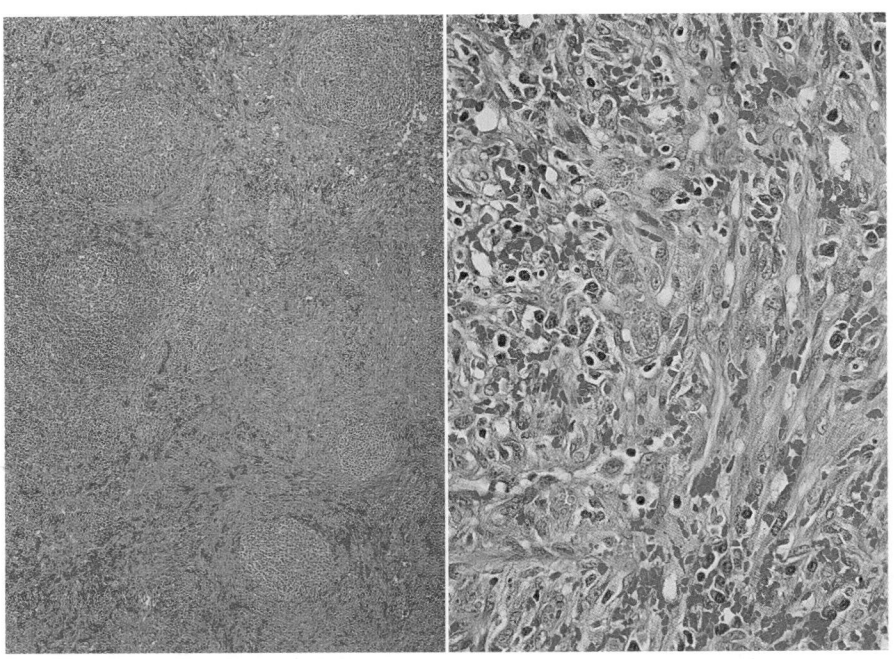

Fig. 21-83 Lymph node involvement by Kaposi's sarcoma. The infiltrate is predominantly sinusal and is characterized by a proliferation of spindle cells forming slits containing red blood cells.

4 *Leiomyomatosis.* This has been reported mainly in intra-abdominal nodes, sometimes in association with uterine leiomyomas or leiomyomatosis peritonealis disseminata.[975,980]

5 *Angiomatous hamartoma.* This is a distinctive form of smooth muscle proliferation that seems to occur only in the inguinal region. It is characterized by a proliferation of thick-walled hilar blood vessels that sometimes extends into the nodal parenchyma.[968]

6 *Intranodal leiomyoma.* Some of the reported cases have occurred in the setting of HIV infection.[985]

Hemorrhagic spindle-cell tumor with amianthoid fibers (also known as palisaded myofibroblastoma) is a distinctive benign neoplasm that occurs preferentially in inguinal lymph nodes but that can involve other sites, such as the

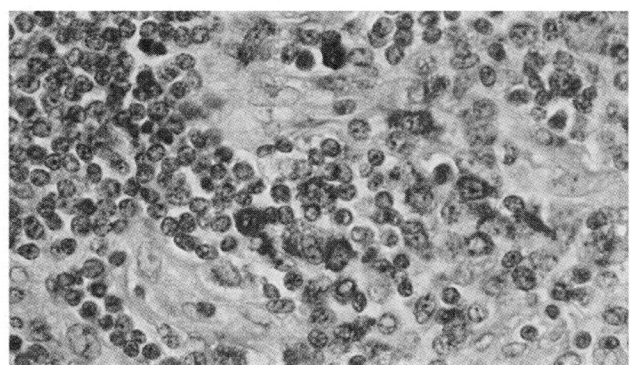

Fig. 21-84 Lymph node involved by systemic mastocytosis. The myeloid precursors stain an intense red color. (Leder's chloroacetate esterase.)

neck and mediastinum.[964,965,974,986,988] The main microscopic features are the proliferation of bland-looking spindle cells, sometimes in a palisading fashion; extensive foci of recent and old hemorrhage; and giant rosette-like collections of collagen fibers (so-called amianthoid fibers)[981,984,985,987] (Fig. 21-85). The differential diagnosis includes Kaposi's sarcoma and intranodal schwannoma. Immunohistochemically, the spindle cells are reactive for vimentin and actin, particularly around the rosette-like formations. The staining qualities and ultrastructural features are more in favor of a smooth muscle than a myofibroblastic derivation.[989] The behavior has been benign in all reported cases.

Inflammatory pseudotumor is an inflammatory disorder of lymph nodes having a morphologic appearance similar to that of similarly named lesions in the lung and other organs.[972,973,982] The process may be localized or affect several lymph node groups and may be accompanied by fever, anemia, elevated erythrosedimentation rate, and hypergammaglobulinemia.[977] Microscopically, the process involves primarily the fibrous stroma of the node, with secondary spread into the lymphoid tissue and perinodal tissues. It is characterized by a storiform pattern of growth, vascular proliferation, and a polymorphic infiltrate composed of fibroblasts, plasma cells, immunoblasts, small lymphocytes, histiocytes, and neutrophils (Fig. 21-86). The etiology is unknown, but EBV is frequently present. The behavior is benign.[982]

METASTATIC TUMORS

Lymph nodes are the most common site of metastatic malignancy, and sometimes constitute the first clinical manifestation of the disease.[993,997,1004] The task of the pathologist is to identify the presence of a malignant process in the node, to establish whether it is metastatic or not, and—if

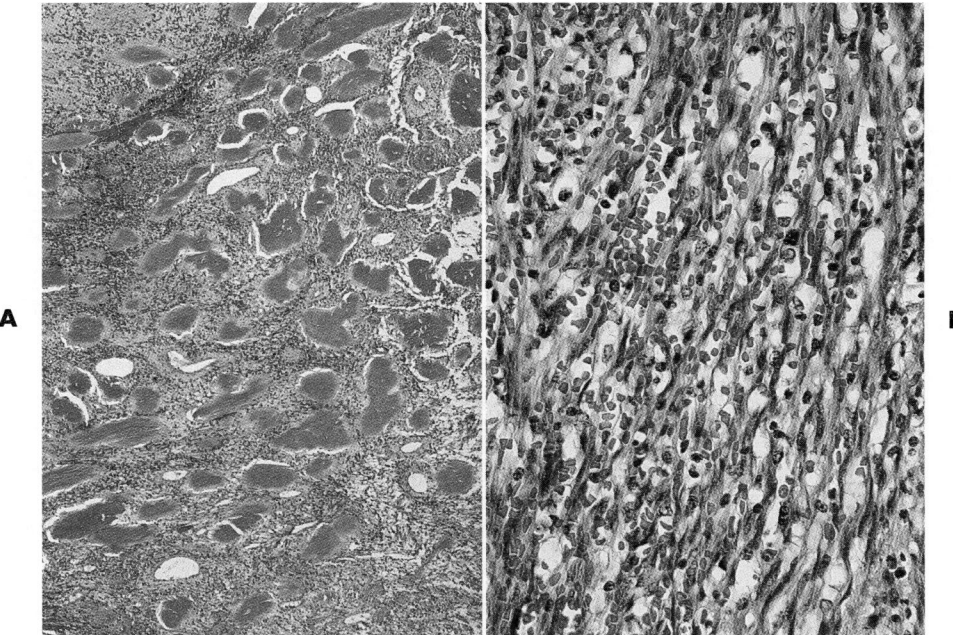

Fig. 21-85 Hemorrhagic spindle-cell tumor with amianthoid fibers. **A,** Prominent deposition of "amianthoid" collagen throughout the tumor. **B,** The admixture of neoplastic spindle cells and extravasated red blood cells results in a Kaposi's sarcoma–like appearance.

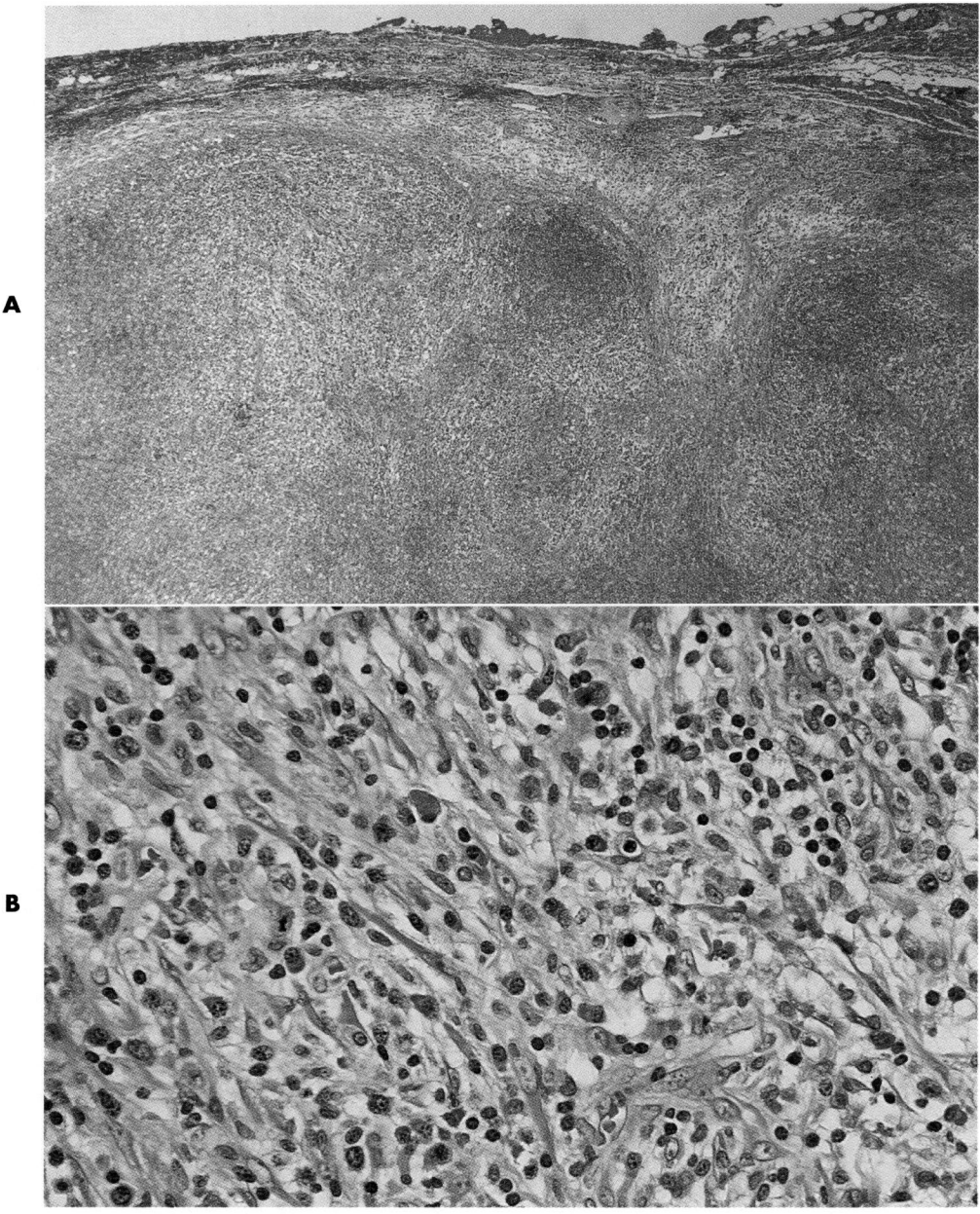

Fig. 21-86 Inflammatory pseudotumor of lymph node. **A,** Low-power appearance showing partial effacement of architecture and expansion of the sinusal and perinodal regions by a reactive proliferation. **B,** High-power view showing a polymorphic infiltrate composed of lymphocytes, plasma cells, and myofibroblasts.

metastatic—to provide an estimate of its amount, microscopic type, and possible source.[999] If malignant cells are identified within the efferent lymph vessels and/or extranodal adipose tissue, this should also be noted in the report because of the possible prognostic significance of these findings.

Any malignant tumor can give rise to lymph node metastases, but the incidence varies greatly depending on the tumor type. It is common with carcinomas, malignant melanomas, and germ cell tumors and rare with sarcomas and central nervous system tumors. It should also be noted that large cell lymphomas primary in an organ (such as stomach or thyroid) sometimes involve the regional nodes in a pattern consistent with metastatic spread (see p. 1728).

An additional diagnosis to consider in a lymph node involvement by metastatic tumor is *malignant mesothelioma* (Fig. 21-87). We have seen several examples of this tumor type presenting initially with lymphadenopathy in the cervical or inguinal region; most of the primary tumors were located in the peritoneum rather than the pleura, regardless of the location of the nodes.[1003]

It is very rare for soft tissue sarcomas to present initially as a lymph node metastasis. The outstanding exception is alveolar rhabdomyosarcoma (particularly the solid variant), which can be confused with malignant lymphoma not only on morphologic grounds but also because it may involve several lymph node groups (so-called lymphadenopathic form) (Fig. 21-88). Other sarcomas that have a greater than average tendency to metastasize to regional nodes are embryonal rhabdomyosarcoma, angiosarcoma, epithelioid sarcoma, synovial sarcoma, and—in some series—malignant fibrous histiocytoma.

The differential diagnosis between metastatic undifferentiated carcinoma and diffuse large cell lymphoma in routine sections may be difficult or even impossible in some cases. Features favoring lymphoma are suggestive of focal nodularity not induced by fibrosis and diffuse permeation of walls of veins (as opposed to tumor thrombi) and adipose tissue if an extranodal component is present. Features favoring metastatic tumor are focal nodal involvement, definite nesting, extensive necrosis, predominantly sinusal distribution, and solid tumor plugs in lymphatic vessels. The types of malignant lymphoma most likely to be misdiagnosed as metastatic carcinoma are anaplastic large cell lymphoma, large cell lymphoma with sclerosis resulting in prominent nesting, large cell lymphoma with a predominantly sinusal pattern of growth, nodular sclerosis Hodgkin's disease with concentration of large mononuclear variants of Reed-Sternberg cells around areas of necrosis, and signet ring lymphoma. Yet another type is the composite lymphoma made up of follicular small cleaved and diffuse large cell components, the double error consisting in diagnosing the latter component as metastatic carcinoma and the former as follicular hyperplasia.

The metastatic carcinomas that most closely simulate a malignant lymphoid process are nasopharyngeal lymphoepithelioma and lobular carcinoma of the breast (Figs. 21-89 and 21-90). The first may masquerade clinically and pathologically as Hodgkin's disease because of its common presentation in a young adult with painless unilateral cervical lymphadenopathy and the presence of a polymorphic population (including eosinophils) on microscopic examination.[996] The second may be confused with large cell lymphoma or malignant histiocytosis. Metastatic small cell car-

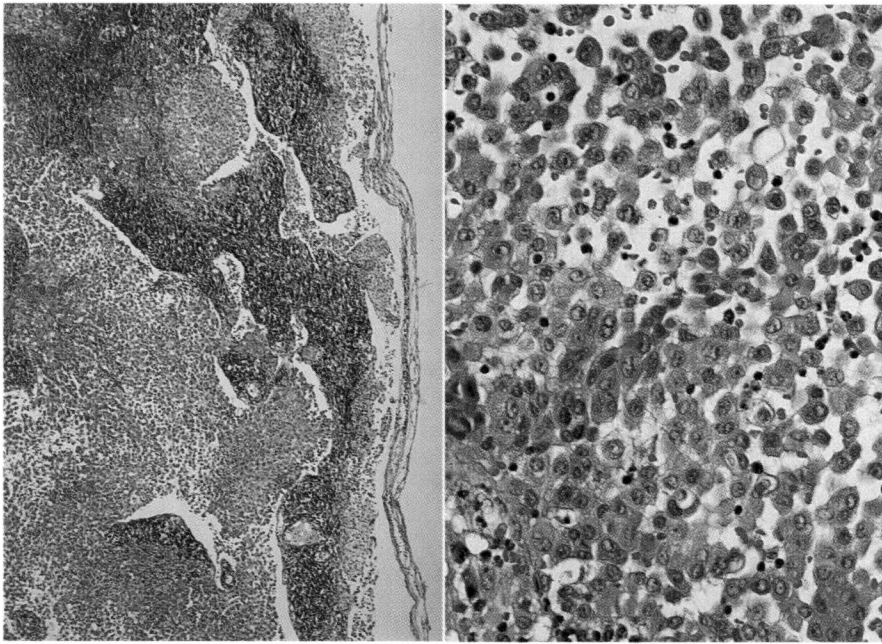

Fig. 21-87 Lymph node involved by metastatic mesothelioma. The tumor massively expands the sinuses and is composed of cuboidal cells with central nucleus and acidophilic cytoplasm. The primary tumor was located in the peritoneal cavity.

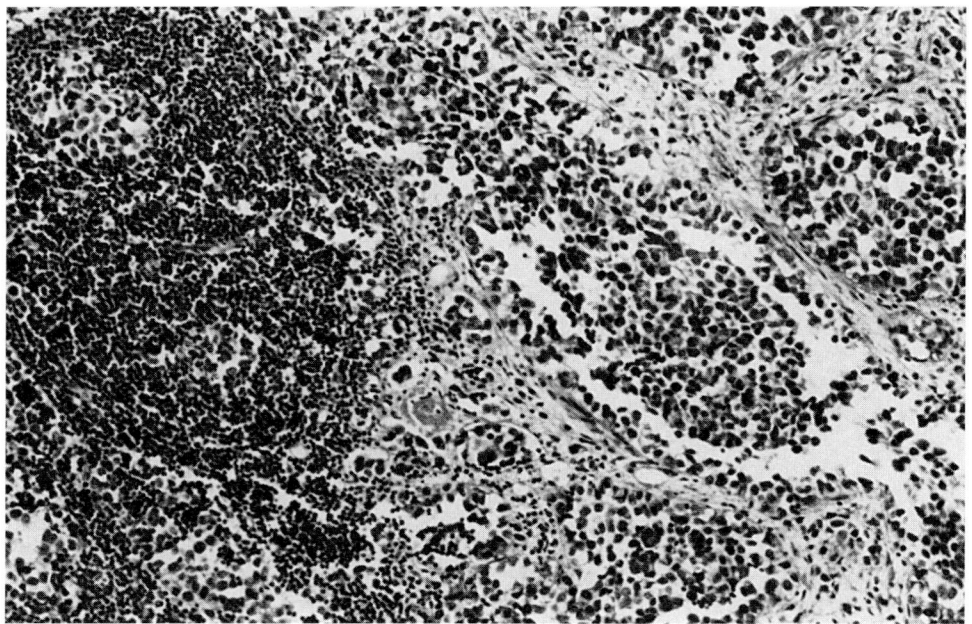

Fig. 21-88 Alveolar rhabdomyosarcoma metastatic to lymph node. Predominantly solid pattern of this tumor may induce confusion with other malignancies, including malignant lymphoma.

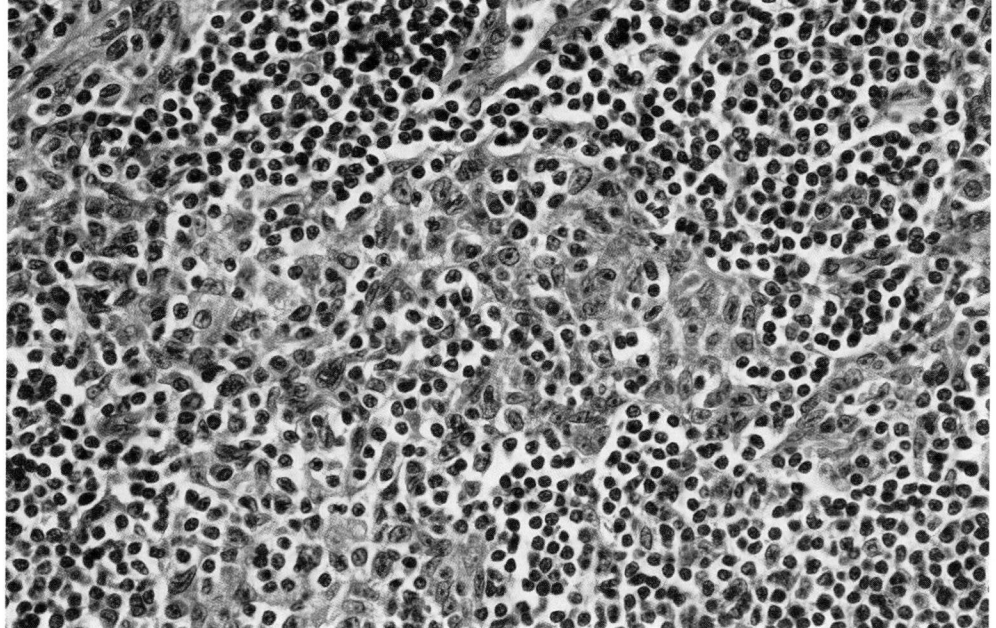

Fig. 21-89 Lymph node involved by metastatic lymphoepithelioma from the nasopharynx. The relatively diffuse pattern of the proliferation may result in a mistaken diagnosis of malignant lymphoma.

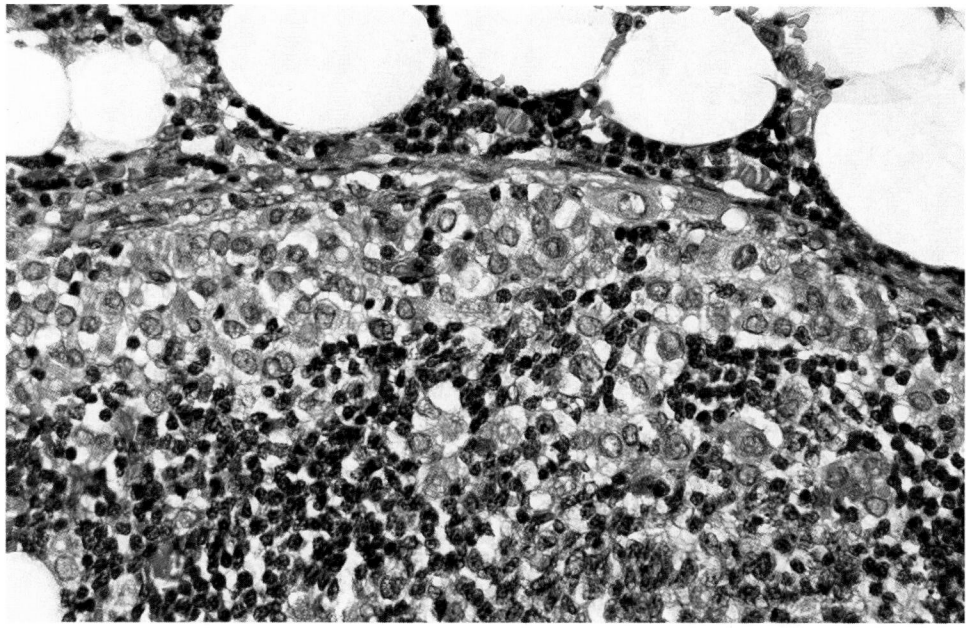

Fig. 21-90 Breast carcinoma of lobular type metastatic to the sinuses of a lymph node. The cytologic appearance may be confused with that of large cell lymphoma or malignant histiocytosis.

cinoma from the lung or other sites can be difficult to distinguish from lymphoma; dense nuclear chromatin pattern, nuclear molding, focal areas of necrosis, and hematoxyphilic staining of vessel walls favor a diagnosis of small cell carcinoma. Somewhat similar considerations pertain to the diagnosis of metastatic Merkel cell tumor. Metastatic melanoma can closely simulate on cytologic grounds the appearance of large cell lymphoma and plasmacytoma. One should also not forget that metastases can develop in a node already involved by lymphoma or leukemia.

Among the conventional special stains, the two most likely to help in the differential diagnosis between metastatic carcinoma and lymphoma are PAS and mucin stains. In general, positivity for the latter will establish the diagnosis of adenocarcinoma. The presence of abundant glycogen and/or diastase-resistant mucosubstances in the cytoplasm of a large cell tumor on a PAS stain will also rule out, for all practical purposes, a diagnosis of lymphoma. We have found reticulin stains of only limited value in this differential diagnosis. Instead, touch preparations can be of great diagnostic utility by showing clumping of the tumor cells in carcinoma and the absence of clumping in lymphoma. Ultrastructural examination is also likely to be useful because it will usually demonstrate epithelial markers such as complex desmosomes, tonofibrils, and extracellular or intracellular glandular lumina.[994] However, the special technique that is clearly the top choice for the efficient resolution of this problem is immunocytochemistry. The "basic kit" with which to approach an obviously malignant tumor involving a lymph node is LCA, keratin, and S-100 protein, as markers for lymphoid, epithelial, and melanocytic cells, respectively. A second line of reagents could include EMA,

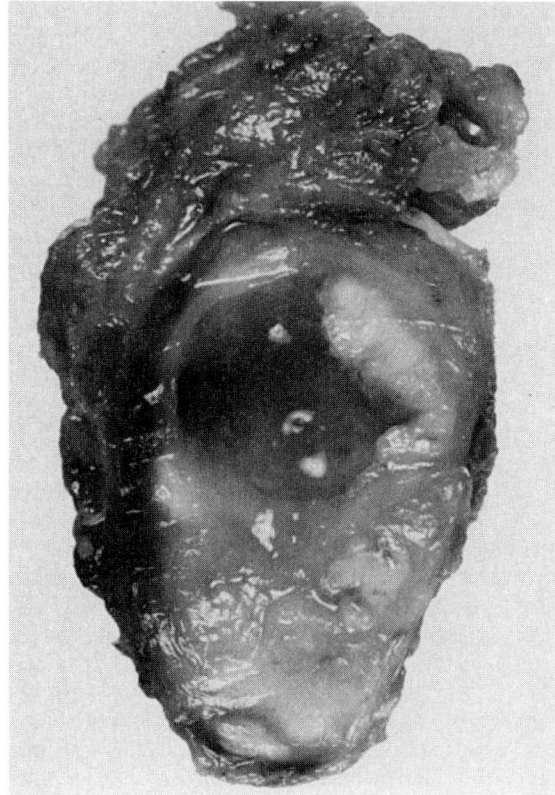

Fig. 21-91 Metastatic squamous cell carcinoma in lymph node. Cavitation resulting from necrosis is evident.

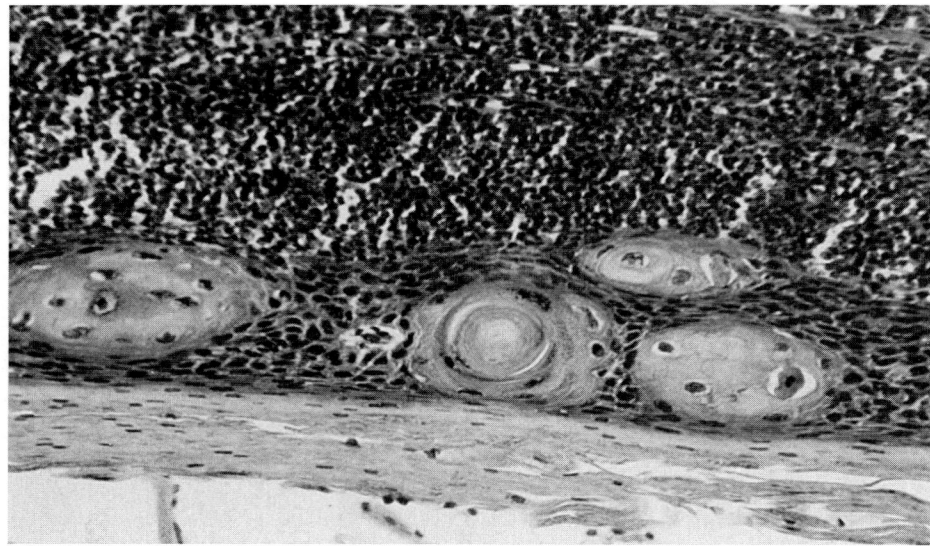

Fig. 21-92 Margin of cystic node replaced by metastatic, well-differentiated epidermoid carcinoma. This pattern can easily be mistaken for branchial cleft cyst because inner layer consists of keratin and squamous cells and next layer is composed of lymphoid tissue.

CEA, vimentin, and—depending on the circumstances—GCDFP-15 and lactalbumin (for breast), chromogranin (for endocrine tumors), and PSA/PAP (for prostate). When properly applied and interpreted, the performance of these reactions should solve all but a very small minority of cases.

Nodal metastases of squamous cell carcinoma have a particular tendency to undergo cystic changes. When these are prominent in a node located in the neck, a mistaken diagnosis of branchial cleft cyst may ensue (Figs. 21-91 and 21-92).

The location of a node involved by metastatic carcinoma gives important clues about the possible site of the primary. The large majority of tumors metastatic to *upper cervical* lymph nodes originate from the upper aerodigestive tract. Sites well known for harboring small, clinically undetectable primaries in the presence of cervical adenopathy are nasopharynx and retrotonsillar pillar.[990,998,1000] *Midcervical* nodes containing papillary carcinoma are usually examples of metastatic thyroid carcinoma, a possibility that becomes a virtual certainty in the presence of psammoma bodies. However, these papillary tumors may also originate from salivary gland or ovary, and we have seen one arising from the thymus. Squamous cell carcinomas in lymph nodes of this region usually arise in the upper aerodigestive tract, particularly pharynx and larynx.[1002] Most carcinomas metastatic to *supraclavicular* lymph nodes originate in the lung or breast. Other sources of metastases to this nodal group, particularly if located on the left side, are carcinoma of stomach, pancreas, prostate, and testis.[998,1001] These reach the node through the terminal collecting lymphatic trunks. Supraclavicular nodes involved by intra-abdominal carcinomas are sometimes referred to as Virchow's or Troisier's

nodes.[990a] The large majority of metastatic tumors in *axillary* nodes of an adult female are breast carcinoma and malignant melanoma.[992,995] Lung carcinoma should also be considered, especially in older patients with a smoking history.[991] *Inguinal* nodes are often the recipients of carcinomas from the external genital organs (usually evident on clinical examination) or malignant melanomas of the lower extremities but only rarely from the internal abdominal organs (ovary, uterine cervix, anal canal) and even less commonly from the testis, unless direct extension to the scrotal skin has occurred.[1005]

REFERENCES
NORMAL ANATOMY

1 Cottier H, Turk J, Sobin L: A proposal for a standardized system of reporting human lymph node morphology in relation to immunological function. Bull WHO **47**:375-408, 1972.
2 Liu YJ, Zhang J, Lane PJ, Chan EY, MacLennan IC: Sites of specific B cell activation in primary and secondary responses to T cell-dependent and T cell-independent antigens. Eur J Immunol **21**:2951-2962, 1991.
3 Stein H, Bonk A, Tolksdorf G, Lennert K, Rodt H, Gerdes J: Immunohistologic analysis of the organization of normal lymphoid tissue and non-Hodgkin's lymphomas. J Histochem Cytochem **28**:746-760, 1980.
4 Szakal AK, Kosco MH, Tew JG: Microanatomy of lymphoid tissue during humoral immune responses. Structure function relationships. Annu Rev Immunol **7**:91-109, 1989.

LYMPH NODE EVALUATION
Biopsy

5 Banks PM: Technical factors in the preparation and evaluation of lymph node biopsies. In Knowles DM, ed: Neoplastic hematopathology. Baltimore, 1992, Williams & Wilkins.
6 Banks PM, Long JC, Howard CA: Preparation of lymph node biopsy specimens. Hum Pathol **10**:617-621, 1979.

7   Beard C, Nabers K, Bowling MC, Berard CW: Achieving technical excellence in lymph node specimens. An update. Lab Med 16:468-475, 1985.

8   Butler JJ: Non-neoplastic lesions of lymph nodes of man to be differentiated from lymphomas. NCI Monogr 32:233-255, 1969.

9   Moore RD, Weisberger AS, Bowerfind ES Jr: An evaluation of lymphadenopathy in systemic disease. Arch Intern Med 99:751-759, 1957.

10 Velez-Garcia E, Fradera J, Grillo AJ, Velazquez J, Maldonado N: A study of lymph node and tumor imprints and aspirations. Bol Assoc Med PR 63:188-203, 1971.

11 Weiss LM, Dorfman RF, Warnke RA: Lymph node work-up. In: Fenoglio-Preiser C, ed: Advances in pathology, vol. 1. Chicago, 1988, Year Book Medical Publishers.

Needle biopsy

12 Cafferty LL, Katz RL, Ordonez NG, Carrasco CH, Cabanillas FR: Fine needle aspiration diagnosis of intraabdominal and retroperitoneal lymphomas by a morphologic and immunocytochemical approach. Cancer 65:72-77, 1990.

13 Frable WJ, Kardos TF: Fine needle aspiration biopsy. Applications in the diagnosis of lymphoproliferative diseases. Am J Surg Pathol 12(Suppl 1):62-72, 1988.

14 Kardos TF, Maygarden SJ, Blumberg AK, Wakely PE Jr, Frable WJ: Fine needle aspiration biopsy in the management of children and young adults with peripheral lymphadenopathy. Cancer 63:703-707, 1989.

15 Kern WH: Exfoliative and aspiration cytology of malignant lymphomas. Semin Diagn Pathol 3:211-218, 1986.

16 Pitts WC, Weiss LM: Fine needle aspiration biopsy of lymph nodes. Pathol Annu 23(Pt 2):329-360, 1988.

17 Tsang WY, Chan JK: Spectrum of morphologic changes in lymph nodes attributable to fine needle aspiration. Hum Pathol 23:562-565, 1992.

18 van Heerde P, Go DMDS, Koolman-Schellekens MA, Peterse JL: Cytodiagnosis of non-Hodgkin's lymphoma. A morphological analysis of 215 biopsy proven cases. Virchows Arch [A] 403:213-233, 1984.

Electron microscopy

19 Mackay B: Ultrastructural diagnosis of lymphomas and leukemias. Ultrastruct Pathol 9:209-214, 1985.

20 Peiper SC, Kahn LB: Ultrastructural comparison of Hodgkin's and non-Hodgkin's lymphomas. Histopathology 6:93-109, 1982.

Immunophenotyping

21 Andrade RE, Wick MR, Frizzera G, Gajl-Peczalska KJ: Immunophenotyping of hematopoietic malignancies in paraffin sections. Hum Pathol 19:394-402, 1988.

22 Davey FR, Gatter KC, Ralfkiaer E, Pulford KAF, Krissansen GW, Mason DY: Immunophenotyping of non-Hodgkin's lymphomas using a panel of antibodies on paraffin-embedded tissues. Am J Pathol 129:54-63, 1987.

23 Knowles DM, Chadburn A, Inghirami G: Immunophenotypic markers useful in the diagnosis and classification of hematopoietic neoplasms. In Knowles DM, ed: Neoplastic hematopathology. Baltimore, 1992, Williams & Wilkins.

24 Linder J, Ye Y, Harrington DS. Armitage JO, Weisenburger DD: Monoclonal antibodies marking T lymphocytes in paraffin-embedded tissue. Am J Pathol 127:1-8, 1987.

25 Norton AJ, Isaacson PG: An immunocytochemical study of T-cell lymphomas using monoclonal and polyclonal antibodies effective in routinely fixed wax embedded tissues. Histopathology 10:1243-1260, 1986.

26 Norton AJ, Isaacson PG: Detailed phenotypic analysis of B-cell lymphoma using a panel of antibodies reactive in routinely fixed wax-embedded tissue. Am J Pathol 128:225-240, 1987.

27 Picker LJ, Weiss LM, Medeiros LJ, Wood GS, Warnke RA: Immunophenotypic criteria for the diagnosis of non-Hodgkin's lymphoma. Am J Pathol 128:181-201, 1987.

28 Roholl PJM, Kleyne J, Prins MEF, Hooijkaas H, Vroom TM, Van Unnik JAM: Immunologic marker analysis of normal and malignant histiocytes. A comparative study of monoclonal antibodies for diagnostic purposes. Am J Clin Pathol 89:187-194, 1988.

29 Strickler JG, Weiss LM, Copenhaver CM, Bindl J, McDaid R, Buck D, Warnke R: Monoclonal antibodies reactive in routinely processed tissue sections of malignant lymphoma, with emphasis on T-cell lymphomas. Hum Pathol 18:808-814, 1987.

30 Tubbs RR, Sheibani K: Immunohistology of lymphoproliferative disorders. Semin Diagn Pathol 1:272-284, 1984.

31 Warnke RA, Gatter KC, Falini B, Hildreth P, Woolston RE, Pulford K, Cordell JL, Cohen B, De Wolf-Peeters C, Mason DY: Diagnosis of human lymphoma with monoclonal antileukocyte antibodies. N Engl J Med 309:1275-1281, 1983.

Chromosomal studies

32 LeBeau M: The role of cytogenetics in the diagnosis and classification of hematopoietic neoplasms. In Knowles DM, ed: Neoplastic hematopathology. Baltimore, 1992, Williams & Wilkins.

33 Ngan BY, Chen-Levy Z, Weiss LM, Warnke RA, Cleary ML: Expression in non-Hodgkin's lymphoma of the bcl-2 protein associated with the t(14;18) chromosomal translocation. N Engl J Med 318:1638-1644, 1988.

34 Testa JR, Arthur DC: Cytogenetics of leukemia and lymphoma. In Wiernik PH, ed: Contemporary issues in clinical oncology. Leukemias and lymphomas. New York, 1985, Churchill-Livingstone, pp. 155-182.

35 Weiss LM, Warnke RA, Sklar J, Cleary ML: Molecular analysis of the t(14;18) chromosomal translocation in malignant lymphomas. N Engl J Med 317:1185-1189, 1987.

36 Yunis JJ, Frizzera G, Oken MM, McKenna J, Theologides A, Arnesen M: Multiple recurrent genomic defects in follicular lymphoma. A possible model for cancer. N Engl J Med 316:79-84, 1987.

Gene rearrangement analysis

37 Davis RE, Warnke RA, Dorfman RF, Cleary ML: Utility of molecular genetic analysis for the diagnosis of neoplasia in morphologically and immunophenotypically equivocal hematolymphoid lesions. Cancer 67:2890-2899, 1991.

38 Dubeau L, Weinberg K, Jones PA, Nichols PW: Studies on immunoglobulin gene rearrangement in formalin-fixed, paraffin-embedded pathology specimens. Am J Pathol 130:588-594, 1988.

39 Henni T, Gaulard P, Divine M, Le Couedic JP, Rocha D, Haioun C, Henni Z, Marolleau JP, Pinaudeau Y, Goossens M, et al.: Comparison of genetic probe with immunophenotype analysis in lymphoproliferative disorders. A study of 87 cases. Blood 72:1937-1943, 1988.

40 Ilyas M, Jalal H, Linton C, Rooney N: The use of the polymerase chain reaction in the diagnosis of B-cell lymphomas from formalin-fixed paraffin-embedded tissue. Histopathology 26:333-338, 1995.

41 Kamat D, Laszewski MJ, Kemp JD, Goeken JA, Lutz CT, Platz CE, Dick FR: The diagnostic utility of immunophenotyping and immunogenotyping in the pathologic evaluation of lymphoid proliferations. Mod Pathol 3:105-112, 1990.

42 Medeiros LJ, Bagg A, Cossman J: Application of molecular genetics to the diagnosis of hematopoietic neoplasms. In Knowles DM, ed: Neoplastic hematopathology. Baltimore, 1992, Williams & Wilkins.

DNA ploidy studies

43 Braylan RC: Flow-cytometric DNA analysis in the diagnosis and prognosis of lymphoma. Am J Clin Pathol 99:374-380, 1993.

44 Duque RE: Flow cytometric analysis of lymphomas and acute leukemias. Ann NY Acad Sci 677:309-325, 1993.

45 Duque RE, Andreeff M, Braylan RC, Diamond LW, Peiper SC: Consensus review of the clinical utility of DNA flow cytometry in neoplastic hematopathology. Cytometry 14:492-496, 1993.

46 Zander DS, Iturraspe JA, Everett ET, Massey JK, Braylan RC: Flow cytometry. In vitro assessment of its potential application for diagnosis and classification of lymphoid processes in cytologic preparations from fine-needle aspirates. Am J Clin Pathol 101:577-586, 1994.

PRIMARY IMMUNODEFICIENCIES

47 Fudenberg H: Primary immunodeficiencies. Report of a World Health Organization Committee. Pediatrics 47:927-946, 1971.

48 Gitlin D, Janeway CA, Apt L, Craig JM: Agammaglobulinemia. In Lawrence H, ed: Cellular and humoral aspects of hypersensitivity states. New York, 1959, Paul B Hoeber, Inc, pp 375-441.

49 Heymer B, Niethammer D, Spanel R, Galle J, Kleihauer E, Haferkamp O: Pathomorphology of humoral, cellular and combined primary immunodeficiencies. Virchows Arch [A] 374:87-103, 1977.

50 Huber J, Zegers BJ, Schuurman HJ: Pathology of congenital immunodeficiencies. Semin Diagn Pathol 9:31-62, 1992.

51 Stiehm ER, Fulginiti VA: Immunologic disorders in infants and children. Philadelphia, 1973, WB Saunders Co.

PATTERNS OF HYPERPLASIA

52 Dorfman RF, Warnke R: Lymphadenopathy simulating the malignant lymphomas. Hum Pathol 5:519-550, 1974.

53 Warnke RA, Weiss LM, Chan JKC, Cleary ML, Dorfman RF: Tumors of the lymph nodes and spleen. Atlas of tumor pathology, 3rd Series, Fascicle 14, Washington, DC, 1995, Armed Forces Institute of Pathology.

Follicular hyperplasia

54 Browne G, Tobin B, Carney DN, Dervan PA: Aberrant MT2 positivity distinguishes follicular lymphoma from reactive follicular hyperplasia in B5- and formalin-fixed paraffin sections. Am J Clin Pathol **96**:90-94, 1991.

55 Chilosi M, Mombello A, Menestrina F, Gilioli E, Manfrin E, Pizzolo G, Fiore-Donati L: Immunohistochemical differentiation of follicular lymphoma from florid reactive hyperplasia with monoclonal antibodies reactive on paraffin sections. Cancer **65**:1562-1569, 1990.

56 Nathwani BN, Winberg CD, Diamond LW, Bearman RM, Kim H: Morphologic criteria for the differentiation of follicular lymphoma from florid reactive hyperplasia. A study of 80 cases. Cancer **48**:1794-1806, 1981.

57 Rappaport H, Winter WJ, Hicks EB: Follicular lymphoma. A reevaluation of its position in the scheme of malignant lymphoma, based on a survey of 253 cases. Cancer **9**:792-821, 1956.

58 Utz GL, Swerdlow SH: Distinction of follicular hyperplasia from follicular lymphoma in B5-fixed tissues. Comparison of MT2 and bcl-2 antibodies. Hum Pathol **24**:1155-1158, 1993.

Progressively and regressively transformed germinal centers

59 Burns BF, Colby TV, Dorfman RF: Differential diagnostic features of nodular L&H Hodgkin's disease, including progressive transformation of germinal centers. Am J Surg Pathol **8**:253-261, 1984.

60 Ferry JA, Zukerberg LR, Harris NL: Florid progressive transformation of germinal centers. A syndrome affecting young men, without early progression to nodular lymphocyte predominance Hodgkin's disease. Am J Surg Pathol **16**:252-258, 1992.

61 Hansmann ML, Fellbaum C, Hui PK, Moubayed P: Progressive transformation of germinal centers with and without association to Hodgkin's disease. Am J Clin Pathol **93**:219-226, 1990.

62 Osborne BM, Butler JJ: Follicular lymphoma mimicking progressive transformation of germinal centers. Am J Clin Pathol **88**:264-269, 1987.

63 Osborne BM, Butler JJ, Gresik MV: Progressive transformation of germinal centers. Comparison of 23 pediatric patients to the adult population. Mod Pathol **5**:135-140, 1992.

64 Poppema S, Kaiserling E, Lennert K: Hodgkin's disease with lymphocytic predominance, nodular type (nodular paragranuloma) and progressively transformed germinal centers. A cytohistological study. Histopathology **3**:295-308, 1979.

65 Poppema S, Kaiserling E, Lennert K: Nodular paragranuloma and progressively transformed germinal centers. Ultrastructural and immunohistologic findings. Virchows Arch [Cell Pathol] **31**:211-225, 1979.

66 Stein H, Gerdes J, Mason DY: The normal and malignant germinal centre. Clin Hematol **11**:531-559, 1982.

Paracortical hyperplasia

67 van den Oord JJ, de Wolf-Peeters C, Desmet VJ, Takahashi K, Ohtsuki Y, Akagi T: Nodular alteration of the paracortical area. An in situ immunohistochemical analysis of primary, secondary, and tertiary T-nodules. Am J Pathol **120**:55-66, 1985.

Granulomatous inflammation

68 Gorton G, Linell F: Malignant tumours and sarcoid reactions in regional lymph nodes. Acta Radiol (Stockh) **47**:381-392, 1957.

69 Hall PA, Kingston J, Stansfeld AG: Extensive necrosis in malignant lymphoma with granulomatous reaction mimicking tuberculosis. Histopathology **13**:339-346, 1988.

70 Hollingsworth HC, Longo DL, Jaffe ES: Small noncleaved cell lymphoma associated with florid epithelioid granulomatous response. A clinicopathologic study of seven patients. Am J Surg Pathol **17**:51-59, 1993.

71 Ioachim HL, ed: Pathology of granulomas. New York, 1983, Raven Press.

72 Kadin ME, Donaldson SS, Dorfman RF: Isolated granulomas in Hodgkin's disease. N Engl J Med **283**:859-861, 1970.

73 Nadel E, Ackerman LV: Lesions resembling Boeck's sarcoid. Am J Clin Pathol **20**:952-957, 1952.

Other patterns
Monocytoid B-cell hyperplasia

74 Aozasa K, Ohsawa M, Horiuchi K, Saeki K, Katayama S, Matsuzuka F, Yamamura T: The occurrence of monocytoid B-lymphocytes in autoimmune disorders. Mod Pathol **6**:121-124, 1993.

75 Kojima M, Hosomura Y, Itoh H, Johshita T, Ohno Y, Yoshida K, Asano S, Wakasa H, Nakamura S, Suchi T: Monocytoid B lymphocytes and epithelioid cell clusters in abscess-forming granulomatous lymphadenitis. With special reference to cat scratch disease. Acta Pathol Jpn **41**:363-368, 1991.

76 Ohsawa M, Kanno H, Naka N, Aozasa K: Occurrence of monocytoid B-lymphocytes in Hodgkin's disease. Mod Pathol **7**:540-543, 1994.

77 Plank L, Hansmann ML, Fischer R: The cytological spectrum of the monocytoid B-cell reaction. Recognition of its large cell type. Histopathology **23**:425-431, 1993.

78 Sheibani K, Fritz RM, Winberg CD, Burke JS, Rappaport H: "Monocytoid" cells in reactive follicular hyperplasia with and without multifocal histiocytic reactions. An immunohistochemical study of 21 cases including suspected cases of toxoplasmic lymphadenitis. Am J Clin Pathol **81**:453-458, 1984.

79 Shin SS, Sheibani K: Monocytoid B-cell lymphoma. Am J Clin Pathol **99**:421-425, 1993.

80 van den Oord JJ, de Wolf-Peeters C, De Vos R, Desmet VJ: Immature sinus histiocytosis. Light- and electron-microscopic features, immunologic phenotype, and relationship with marginal zone lymphocytes. Am J Pathol **118**:266-277, 1985.

Plasmacytoid monocytes

81 Facchetti F, de Wolf-Peeters C, Mason DY, Pulford K, van den Oord JJ, Desmet VJ: Plasmacytoid T cells. Immunohistochemical evidence for their monocyte/macrophage origin. Am J Pathol **133**:15-21, 1988.

82 Facchetti F, de Wolf-Peeters C, de Vos R, van den Oord JJ, Pulford KA, Desmet VJ: Plasmacytoid monocytes (so-called plasmacytoid T cells) in granulomatous lymphadenitis. Hum Pathol **20**:588-593, 1989.

83 Facchetti F, de Wolf-Peeters C, van den Oord JJ, de Vos R, Desmet VJ: Plasmacytoid monocytes (so-called plasmacytoid T-cells) in Kikuchi's lymphadenitis. An immunohistologic study. Am J Clin Pathol **92**:42-50, 1989.

84 Hansmann ML, Kikuchi M, Wacker HH, Radzun HJ, Nathwani BN, Hesse K, Parwaresch MR: Immunohistochemical monitoring of plasmacytoid cells in lymph node sections of Kikuchi-Fujimoto disease by a new panmacrophage antibody Ki-M1P. Hum Pathol **23**:676-680, 1992.

85 Koo CH, Mason DY, Miller R, Ben-Ezra J, Sheibani K, Rappaport H: Additional evidence that "plasmacytoid T-cell lymphoma" associated with chronic myeloproliferative disorders is of macrophage/monocyte origin. Am J Clin Pathol **93**:822-827, 1990.

86 Müller-Hermelink HK, Stein H, Steinmann G, Lennert K: Malignant lymphoma of plasmacytoid T-cells. Morphologic and immunologic studies characterizing a special type of T-cell. Am J Surg Pathol **7**:849-862, 1983.

87 Prasthofer EF, Grizzle WE, Prchal JT, Grossi CE: Plasmacytoid T-cell lymphoma associated with chronic myeloproliferative disorder. Am J Surg Pathol **9**:380-387, 1985.

88 Vollenweider R, Lennert K: Plasmacytoid T-cell clusters in non-specific lymphadenitis. Virchows Arch [Cell Pathol] **44**:1-14, 1983.

Polykaryocytes

89 Kamel OW, Le Brun DP, Berry GJ, Dorfman RF, Warnke RA: Warthin-Finkeldey polykaryocytes demonstrate a T-cell immunophenotype. Am J Clin Pathol **97**:179-183, 1992.

90 Kjeldsberg CR, Kim H: Polykaryocytes resembling Warthin-Finkeldey giant cells in reactive and neoplastic lymphoid disorders. Hum Pathol **12**:267-272, 1981.

INFLAMMATORY/HYPERPLASTIC DISEASES
Necrotizing lymphadenitis

91 Chamulak GA, Brynes RK, Nathwani BN: Kikuchi-Fujimoto disease mimicking malignant lymphoma. Am J Surg Pathol **14**:514-523, 1990.

92 Chan JKC, Saw D: Histiocytic necrotizing lymphadenitis (Kikuchi's disease). A clinicopathologic study of 9 cases. Pathology **18**:22-28, 1986.

93 Chan JK, Wong KC, Ng CS: A fatal case of multicentric Kikuchi's histiocytic necrotizing lymphadenitis. Cancer **63**:1856-1862, 1989.

94 Dorfman RF, Berry GJ: Kikuchi's histiocytic necrotizing lymphadenitis. An analysis of 108 cases with emphasis on differential diagnosis. Semin Diagn Pathol **5**:329-345, 1988.

95 Eimoto T, Kikuchi M, Mitsui T: Histiocytic necrotizing lymphadenitis. An ultrastructural study in comparison with other types of lymphadenitis. Acta Pathol Jpn **33**:863-879, 1983.

96 Facchetti F, de Wolf-Peeters C, van den Oord JJ, de Vos R, Desmet VJ: Plasmacytoid monocytes (so-called plasmacytoid T-cells) in Kikuchi's lymphadenitis. An immunohistologic study. Am J Clin Pathol **92**:42-50, 1989.

97 Hollingsworth HC, Peiper SC, Weiss LM, Raffeld M, Jaffe ES: An investigation of the viral pathogenesis of Kikuchi-Fujimoto disease. Lack of evidence for Epstein-Barr virus or human herpesvirus type 6 as the causative agents. Arch Pathol Lab Med **118**:134-140, 1994.

98 Kuo TT: Cutaneous manifestation of Kikuchi's histiocytic necrotizing lymphadenitis. Am J Surg Pathol 14:872-876, 1990.

99 Kuo TT: Kikuchi's disease (histiocytic necrotizing lymphadenitis). A clinicopathologic study of 79 cases with an analysis of histologic subtypes, immunohistology, and DNA ploidy. Am J Surg Pathol 19:798-809, 1995.

100 Pileri S, Kikuchi M, Lennert K: Histiocytic necrotizing lymphadenitis without granulocytic infiltration. Virchows Arch [A] 395:257-271, 1982.

101 Sumiyoshi Y, Kikuchi M, Ohshima K, Yoneda S, Kobari S, Takeshita M, Eizuru Y, Minamishima Y: Human herpesvirus-6 genomes in histiocytic necrotizing lymphadenitis (Kikuchi's disease) and other forms of lymphadenitis. Am J Clin Pathol 99:609-614, 1993.

102 Sumiyoshi Y, Kikuchi M, Takeshita M, Ohshima K, Masuda Y, Parwaresch MR: Immunohistologic studies of Kikuchi's disease. Hum Pathol 24:1114-1119, 1993.

103 Tsang WY, Chan JK: Fine-needle aspiration cytologic diagnosis of Kikuchi's lymphadenitis. A report of 27 cases. Am J Clin Pathol 102:454-458, 1994.

104 Tsang WY, Chan JK, Ng CS: Kikuchi's lymphadenitis. A morphologic analysis of 75 cases with special reference to unusual features. Am J Surg Pathol 18:219-231, 1994.

105 Turner RR, Martin J, Dorfman RF: Necrotizing lymphadenitis. A study of 30 cases. Am J Surg Pathol 7:115-123, 1983.

Chronic nonspecific lymphadenitis

106 Cozzutto C, Soave F: Xanthogranulomatous lymphadenitis. Virchows Arch [A] 385:103-108, 1979.

Atypical mycobacteriosis

107 Mackellar A, Hilton HB, Masters PL: Mycobacterial lymphadenitis in childhood. Arch Dis Child 42:70-74, 1967.

108 Pinder SE, Colville A: Mycobacterial cervical lymphadenitis in children. Can histological assessment help differentiate infections caused by non-tuberculous mycobacteria from Mycobacterium tuberculosis? Histopathology 22:59-64, 1993.

109 Reid JD, Wolinsky E: Histopathology of lymphadenitis caused by atypical mycobacteria. Am Rev Respir Dis 99:8-12, 1969.

Sarcoidosis

110 Chilosi M, Menestrina F, Capelli P, Montagna L, Lestani M, Pizzolo G, Cipriani A, Agostini C, Trentin L, Zambello R, Semenzato G: Immunohistochemical analysis of sarcoid granulomas. Evaluation of Ki67+ and interleukin-1+ cells. Am J Pathol 131:191-198, 1988.

111 Collison JM, Miller NR, Green WR: Involvement of orbital tissues by sarcoid. Am J Ophthalmol 102:302-307, 1986.

112 Cunningham JA: Sarcoidosis. Pathol Annu 2:31-46, 1967.

113 Cushard WG Jr, Simon AB, Caterbury JM, Reiss E: Parathyroid function in sarcoidosis. N Engl J Med 286:395-398, 1972.

114 Devaney K, Goodman ZD, Epstein MS, Zimmerman HJ, Ishak KG: Hepatic sarcoidosis. Clinicopathologic features in 100 patients. Am J Surg Pathol 17:1272-1280, 1993.

115 Devergne O, Emilie D, Peuchmaur M, Crevon MC, D'Agay MF, Galanaud P: Production of cytokines in sarcoid lymph nodes. Preferential expression of interleukin-1 beta and interferon-gamma genes. Hum Pathol 23:317-323, 1992.

116 Fidler HM: Mycobacteria and sarcoidosis. Recent advances. Sarcoidosis 11:66-68, 1994.

117 Fink SD, Kremer JM: Cutaneous and musculoskeletal features, diagnostic modalities, and immunopathology in sarcoidosis. Curr Opin Rheumatol 6:78-81, 1994.

118 Gardner J, Kennedy HG, Hamblin A, Jones E: HLA associations in sarcoidosis. A study of two ethnic groups. Thorax 39:19-22, 1984.

119 Ghossein RA, Ross DG, Salomon RN, Rabson AR: A search for mycobacterial DNA in sarcoidosis using the polymerase chain reaction. Am J Clin Pathol 101:733-737, 1994.

120 James DG, Williams WJ: Immunology of sarcoidosis. Am J Med 72:5-8, 1982.

121 Kirkpatrick CJ, Curry A, Bisset DL: Light- and electron-microscopic studies on multinucleated giant cells in sarcoid granuloma. New aspects of asteroid and Schaumann bodies. Ultrastruct Pathol 12:581-597, 1988.

122 Määtta KT: Histological study of mediastinal lymph nodes in clinical sarcoidosis. A report of 86 cases. Ann Acad Sci Fenn (Med.) 138:1-106, 1968.

123 Nethercott SE, Strawbridge WG: Identification of bacterial residues in sarcoid lesions. Lancet 2:1132, 1956.

124 Reid JD, Andersen ME: Calcium oxalate in sarcoid granulomas. With particular reference to the small ovoid body and a note on the finding of dolomite. Am J Clin Pathol 90:545-558, 1988.

125 Rosen Y, Vuletin JC, Pertschuk LP, Silverstein E: Sarcoidosis. From the pathologist's vantage point. Pathol Annu 14(Pt 1):405-439, 1979.

126 Sieracki JC, Fisher ER: The ceroid nature of the so-called "Hamazaki-Wesenberg bodies." Am J Clin Pathol 59:248-253, 1973.

127 Siltzbach LE: Geographic aspects of sarcoidosis. Trans NY Acad Sci 29(Series II):364-374, 1967.

128 Thomas PD, Hunninghake GW: Current concepts of the pathogenesis of sarcoidosis. Am Rev Respir Dis 135:747-760, 1987.

129 Tudway AJC: Yellow bodies in superficial and deep lymph nodes. J Clin Pathol 32:52-55, 1979.

130 Vanék J, Schwarz J: Demonstration of acid-fast rods in sarcoidosis. Am Rev Respir Dis 101:395-400, 1970.

131 Wesenberg W: Saurefeste, Spindelkorper Hamazaki bei Sarkoidose. Arch Klin Exp Med 227:101-112, 1966.

132 Winnacker JL, Becker KL, Friedlander M, Higgins GA, Moore CF: Sarcoidosis and hyperparathyroidism. Am J Med 46:305-312, 1969.

Toxoplasmosis

134 Dorfman RF, Remington JS: Value of lymph-node biopsy in the diagnosis of acute acquired toxoplasmosis. N Engl J Med 289:878-881, 1973.

135 Frenkel JK: Toxoplasmosis. Mechanisms of infection, laboratory diagnosis and management. Curr Top Pathol 54:28-75, 1971.

136 Miettinen M, Franssila K: Malignant lymphoma simulating lymph node toxoplasmosis. Histopathology 6:129-140, 1982.

137 Piringer-Kuchinka A, Martin I, Thalhammer O: Ueber die vorzuglich cerviconuchale Lymphadenitis mit kleinherdiger Epitheloid-zellwucherung. Virchows Arch [A] 331:522-535, 1958.

138 Saxen L, Saxen E, Tenhunen A: The significance of histological diagnosis in glandular toxoplasmosis. Acta Pathol Microbiol Scand 56:284-294, 1962.

139 Weiss LM, Chen YY, Berry GJ, Strickler JG, Dorfman RF, Warnke RA: Infrequent detection of Toxoplasma gondii genome in toxoplasmic lymphadenitis. A polymerase chain reaction study. Hum Pathol 23:154-158, 1992.

Syphilis

140 Choi YJ, Reiner L: Syphilitic lymphadenitis. Immunofluorescent identification of spirochetes from imprints. Am J Surg Pathol 3:553-555, 1979.

141 Hartsock RJ, Halling W, King FM: Luetic lymphadenitis. A clinical and histologic study of 20 cases. Am J Clin Pathol 53:304-314, 1970.

Mesenteric lymphadenitis

142 Ahlqvist J, Ahvohen P, Rasanen JA, Wallgren GR: Enteric infection with Yersinia enterocolitica. Large pyroninophilic cell reaction in mesenteric lymph nodes associated with early production of specific antibodies. Acta Pathol Microbiol Scand (A) 79:109-122, 1971.

143 Cover TL, Aber RC: Yersinia enterocolitica. N Engl J Med 321:16-24, 1989.

144 Jansson E, Wallgren GR, Ahvenen P: Y. enterocolitica as a cause of acute mesenteric lymphadenitis. Acta Paediatr Scand 57:448-450, 1968.

145 Knapp W: Mesenteric adenitis due to Pasteurella pseudotuberculosis in young people. N Engl J Med 259:776-778, 1958.

146 Nilthn B: Studies on Yersinia enterocolitica with special reference to bacterial diagnosis and occurrence in human enteric disease. Acta Pathol Microbiol Scand (Suppl) 206:1-48, 1969.

147 Schapers RFM, Reif R, Lennert K, Knapp W: Mesenteric lymphadenitis due to Yersinia enterocolitica. Virchows Arch [A] 390:127-138, 1981.

Cat-scratch disease

148 Adal KA, Cockerell CJ, Petri WA Jr: Cat scratch disease, bacillary angiomatosis, and other infections due to Rochalimaea. N Engl J Med 330:1509-1515, 1994.

149 Carithers HA: Cat-scratch disease. An overview based on a study of 1,200 patients. Am J Dis Child 139:1124-1133, 1985.

150 Carithers HA, Carithers CM, Edwards RO, Jr.: Cat-scratch disease. Its natural history. JAMA 207:312-316, 1969.

151 Dorfman RF, Warnke R: Lymphadenopathy simulating the malignant lymphomas. Hum Pathol 5:519-550, 1974.

152 English CK, Wear DJ, Margileth AM, Lissner CR, Walsh GP: Cat-scratch disease. Isolation and culture of the bacterial agent. JAMA 259:1347-1352, 1988.

153 Gerber MA, MacAlister TM, Ballow M, Sedgwick AK, Gustafson KB, Tilton RC: The aetiological agent of cat-scratch disease. Lancet 1:1236-1239, 1985.

154 Johnson WT, Helwig EB: Cat-scratch disease. Histopathologic changes in the skin. Arch Dermatol 100:148-154, 1969.

155 Kojima M, Hosomura Y, Itoh H, Johshita T, Ohno Y, Yoshida K, Asano S, Wakasa H, Nakamura S, Suchi T: Monocytoid B lymphocytes and epithelioid cell clusters in abscess-forming granulomatous lymphadenitis. With special reference to cat scratch disease. Acta Pathol Jpn 41:363-368, 1991.

156 Kojima M, Nakamura S, Hosomura Y, Shimizu K, Kurabayashi Y, Itoh H, Yoshida K, Ohno Y, Kaneko A, Asano S, et al.: Abscess-forming granulomatous lymphadenitis. Histological typing of suppurative granulomas and clinicopathological findings with special reference to cat scratch disease. Acta Pathol Jpn **43:**11-17, 1993.

157 Miller-Catchpole R, Variakojis D, Vardiman JW, Loew JM, Carter J: Cat scratch disease. Identification of bacteria in seven cases of lymphadenitis. Am J Surg Pathol **10:**276-281, 1986.

158 Min KW, Reed JA, Welch DF, Slater LN: Morphologically variable bacilli of cat scratch disease are identified by immunocytochemical labeling with antibodies to *Rochalimaea henselae.* Am J Clin Pathol **101:**607-610, 1994.

159 Osborne BM, Butler JJ, Mackay B: Ultrastructural observations in cat scratch disease. Am J Clin Pathol **87:**739-744, 1987.

160 Wear DJ, Hadfield TL, Fisher FW, Schlagel CJ, King FM: Cat scratch disease. A bacterial infection. Science **221:**1403-1405, 1983.

161 Winship T: Pathologic changes in so-called cat-scratch fever. Review of findings in lymph nodes of 29 patients and cutaneous lesions in 2 patients. Am J Clin Pathol **23:**1012-1018, 1953.

162 Yu X, Raoult D: Monoclonal antibodies to *Afipia felis*—a putative agent of cat scratch disease. Am J Clin Pathol **101:**603-606, 1994.

Lymphogranuloma venereum

163 Joseph AK, Rosen T: Laboratory techniques used in the diagnosis of chancroid, granuloma inguinale, and lymphogranuloma venereum. Dermatol Clin **12:**1-8, 1994.

164 Mittal A, Sachdeva KG: Monoclonal antibody for the diagnosis of lymphogranuloma venereum. A preliminary report. Br J Biomed Sci **50:**3-7, 1993.

165 Smith EB, Custer RP: The histopathology of lymphogranuloma venereum. J Urol **63:**546-563, 1950.

166 Van Dyck E, Piot P: Laboratory techniques in the investigation of chancroid, lymphogranuloma venereum and donovanosis. Genitourin Med **68:**130-133, 1992.

Tularemia

167 Evans ME, Gregory DW, Schaffner W, McGee ZA: Tularemia. A 30-year experience with 88 cases. Medicine (Baltimore) **64:**251-267, 1985.

168 Ohara Y, Sato T, Fujita H, Ueno T, Homma M: Clinical manifestations of tularemia in Japan—analysis of 1,355 cases observed between 1924 and 1987. Infection **19:**14-17, 1991.

169 Sato T, Fujita H, Ohara Y, Homma M: Microagglutination test for early and specific serodiagnosis of tularemia. J Clin Microbiol **28:**2372-2374, 1990.

170 Sutinen S, Syrjala H: Histopathology of human lymph node tularemia caused by *Francisella tularensis* var *palaearctica.* Arch Pathol Lab Med **110:**42-46, 1986.

Brucellosis

171 Chomel BB, De Bess EE, Mangiamele DM, Reilly KF, Farver TB, Sun RK, Barrett LR: Changing trends in the epidemiology of human brucellosis in California from 1973 to 1992. A shift toward foodborne transmission. J Infect Dis **170:**1216-1223, 1994.

172 Trujillo IZ, Zavala AN, Caceres JG, Miranda CQ: Brucellosis. Infect Dis Clin North Am **8:**225-241, 1994.

173 Weed LA, Dahlin DC: Bacteriologic examination of tissues removed for biopsy. Am J Clin Pathol **20:**116-132, 1950.

AIDS-related lymphadenopathy

174 Abrams DI: Lymphadenopathy syndrome in male homosexuals. Adv Host Def Mechan **5:**75-97, 1985.

175 Baroni CD, Uccini S: The lymphadenopathy of HIV infection. Am J Clin Pathol **99:**397-401, 1993.

176 Burns BF, Wood GS, Dorfman RF: The varied histopathology of lymphadenopathy in the homosexual male. Am J Surg Pathol **9:**287-297, 1985.

177 Chadburn A, Metroka C, Mouradian J: Progressive lymph node histology and its prognostic value in patients with acquired immunodeficiency syndrome and AIDS-related complex. Hum Pathol **20:**579-587, 1989.

178 Fishbein DB, Kaplan JE, Spira TJ, Miller B, Schonberger LB, Pinsky PF, Getchell JP, Kalyanaraman VS, Braude JS: Unexplained lymphadenopathy in homosexual men. A longitudinal study. JAMA **254:**929-935, 1985.

179 Groopman JE: Clinical symptomatology of the acquired immunodeficiency syndrome (AIDS) and related disorders. Prog Allergy **37:**182-193, 1986.

180 Harris NL: Hypervascular follicular hyperplasia and Kaposi's sarcoma in patients at risk for AIDS. N Engl J Med **310:**462-463, 1984.

181 Ioachim HL, Cronin W, Roy M, Maya M: Persistent lymphadenopathies in people at high risk for HIV infection. Clinicopathologic correlations and long-term follow-up in 79 cases. Am J Clin Pathol **93:**208-218, 1990.

182 O'Hara CJ, Groopman JE, Federman M: The ultrastructural and immunohistochemical demonstration of viral particles in lymph nodes from human immunodeficiency virus-related and non-human immunodeficiency virus-related lymphadenopathy syndromes. Hum Pathol **19:**545-549, 1988.

183 Said JW: AIDS-related lymphadenopathies. Semin Diagn Pathol **5:**365-375, 1988.

184 Schuurman H-J, Kluin PM, Gmelig Meijling FHJ, Van Unnik JAM, Kater L: Lymphocyte status of lymph node and blood in acquired immunodeficiency syndrome (AIDS) and AIDS-related complex disease. J Pathol **147:**269-280, 1985.

185 Umlas J, Federman M, Crawford C, O'Hara CJ, Fitzgibbon JS, Modeste A: Spindle cell pseudotumor due to *Mycobacterium avium-intracellulare* in patients with acquired immunodeficiency syndrome (AIDS). Positive staining of mycobacteria for cytoskeleton filaments. Am J Surg Pathol **15:**1181-1187, 1991.

186 Westermann CD, Hurtubise PE, Linnemann CC, Swerdlow SH: Comparison of histologic nodal reactive patterns, cell suspension immunophenotypic data, and HIV status. Mod Pathol **3:**54-60, 1990.

187 Wood GS, Garcia CF, Dorfman RF, Warnke RA: The immunohistology of follicle lysis in lymph node biopsies from homosexual men. Blood **66:**1092-1097, 1985.

Infectious mononucleosis

188 Frizzera G, Hanto DW, Gajl-Peczalska KJ, Rosai J, McKenna RW, Sibley RK, Holahan KP, Lindquist LL: Polymorphic diffuse B-cell hyperplasias and lymphomas in renal transplant recipients. Cancer Res **41:**4262-4279, 1981.

189 McMahon NJ, Gordon HW, Rosen RB: Reed-Sternberg cells in infectious mononucleosis. Am J Dis Child **120:**148-150, 1970.

190 Reynolds DJ, Banks PM, Gulley ML: New characterization of infectious mononucleosis and a phenotypic comparison with Hodgkin's disease. Am J Pathol **146:**379-388, 1995.

191 Salvador AH, Harrison EG, Kyle RA: Lymphadenopathy due to infectious mononucleosis. Its confusion with malignant lymphoma. Cancer **27:**1029-1040, 1971.

192 Shin SS, Berry GJ, Weiss LM: Infectious mononucleosis. Diagnosis by in situ hybridization in two cases with atypical features. Am J Surg Pathol **15:**625-631, 1991.

193 Sieracki JC, Fisher ER: Diagnostic problems involving nodal lymphomas. Pathol Annu **5:**91-124, 1970.

194 Strickler JG, Fedeli F, Horwitz CA, Copenhaver CM, Frizzera G: Infectious mononucleosis in lymphoid tissue. Histopathology, in situ hybridization, and differential diagnosis. Arch Pathol Lab Med **117:**269-278, 1993.

195 Tindle BH, Parker JW, Lukes RJ: "Reed-Sternberg cells" in infectious mononucleosis? Am J Clin Pathol **58:**607-617, 1972.

Other viral (including postvaccinial) lymphadenitides

196 Audouin J, Le Tourneau A, Aubert J-P, Diebold J: Herpes simplex virus lymphadenitis mimicking tumoral relapse in a patient with Hodgkin's disease in remission. Virchows Arch [A] **408:**313-321, 1985.

197 Dorfman RF, Herweg JC: Live, attenuated measles virus vaccine. Inguinal lymphadenopathy complicating administration. JAMA **198:**320-321, 1966.

198 Gaffey MJ, Ben-Ezra JM, Weiss LM: Herpes simplex lymphadenitis. Am J Clin Pathol **95:**709-714, 1991.

199 Hartsock, RJ: Postvaccinial lymphadenitis. Hyperplasia of lymphoid tissue that simulates malignant lymphomas. Cancer **21:**632-649, 1968.

200 Howat AJ, Campbell AR, Stewart DJ: Generalized lymphadenopathy due to herpes simplex virus type I. Histopathology **19:**563-564, 1991.

201 Lapsley M, Kettle P, Sloan JM: Herpes simplex lymphadenitis. A case report and review of the published work. J Clin Pathol **37:**1119-1122, 1984.

202 Miliauskas JR, Leong AS: Localized herpes simplex lymphadenitis. Report of three cases and review of the literature. Histopathology **19:**355-360, 1991.

203 Tamaru J, Mikata A, Horie H, Itoh K, Asai T, Hondo R, Mori S: Herpes simplex lymphadenitis. Report of two cases with review of the literature. Am J Surg Pathol **14:**571-577, 1990.

Mucocutaneous lymph node syndrome

204 Beitz LO, Barron KS: Kawasaki syndrome. Curr Opin Dermatol 114-122, 1995.

205 Giesker DW, Krause PJ, Pastuszak WT, Hine P, Forouhar FA: Lymph node biopsy for early diagnosis in Kawasaki disease. Am J Surg Pathol **6:**493-501, 1982.

206 Stamos JK, Corydon K, Donaldson J, Shulman ST: Lymphadenitis as the dominant manifestation of Kawasaki disease. Pediatrics **93:**525-528, 1994.

207 Marsh WL, Bishop JW, Koenig HM: Bone marrow and lymph node findings in a fatal case of Kawasaki's disease. Arch Pathol Lab Med **104**:563-567, 1980.

Lupus erythematosus

208 Kubota K, Tamura J, Kurabayashi H, Yanagisawa T, Shirakura T, Mori S: Warthin-Finkeldey-like giant cells in a patient with systemic lupus erythematosus. Hum Pathol **19**:1358-1359, 1988.

209 Medeiros LJ, Kaynor B, Harris NL: Lupus lymphadenitis. Report of a case with immunohistologic studies on frozen sections. Hum Pathol **20**:295-299, 1989.

Rheumatoid arthritis

210 Kamel OW, van de Rijn M, Le Brun DP, Weiss LM, Warnke RA, Dorfman RF: Lymphoid neoplasms in patients with rheumatoid arthritis and dermatomyositis. Frequency of Epstein-Barr virus and other features associated with immunosuppression. Hum Pathol **25**:638-643, 1994.

211 Kojima M, Hosomura Y, Itoh H, Johshita T, Yoshida K, Nakamura S, Suchi T: Reactive proliferative lesions in lymph nodes from rheumatoid arthritis patients. A clinicopathological and immunohistological study. Acta Pathol Jpn **40**:249-254, 1990.

212 Motulsky OG, Weinberg S, Saphir O, Rosenberg E: Lymph nodes in rheumatoid arthritis. Arch Intern Med **90**:660-676, 1952.

213 Nosanchuk JS, Schnitzer B: Follicular hyperplasia in lymph nodes from patients with rheumatoid arthritis. A clinicopathologic study. Cancer **24**:343-354, 1969.

214 Robertson MDJ, Hart FD, White WF, Nuki G, Boardman PL: Rheumatoid lymphadenopathy. Ann Rheum Dis **27**:253-260, 1968.

215 Rollins SD, Craig JP: Gold-associated lymphadenopathy in a patient with rheumatoid arthritis. Histologic and scanning electron microscopic features. Arch Pathol Lab Med **115**:175-177, 1991.

Castleman's disease

216 Chan JK, Fletcher CD, Hicklin GA, Rosai J: Glomeruloid hemangioma. A distinctive cutaneous lesion of multicentric Castleman's disease associated with POEMS syndrome. Am J Surg Pathol **14**:1036-1046, 1990.

217 Chan JK, Tsang WY, Ng CS: Follicular dendritic cell tumor and vascular neoplasm complicating hyaline-vascular Castleman's disease. Am J Surg Pathol **18**:517-525, 1994.

218 Chen TC, Kuo T: Castleman's disease presenting as a pedunculated nasopharyngeal tumour simulating angiofibroma. Histopathology **23**:485-488, 1993.

219 Danon AD, Krishnan J, Frizzera G: Morpho-immunophenotypic diversity of Castleman's disease, hyaline-vascular type. With emphasis on a stroma-rich variant and a new pathogenetic hypothesis. Virchows Arch [A] **423**:369-382, 1993.

220 Frizzera G: Castleman's disease and related disorders. Semin Diagn Pathol **5**:346-364, 1988.

221 Frizzera G, Banks PM, Massarelli G, Rosai J: A systemic lymphoproliferative disorder with morphologic features of Castleman's disease. Pathological findings in 15 patients. Am J Surg Pathol **7**:211-231, 1983.

222 Frizzera G, Peterson BA, Bayrd ED, Goldman A: A systemic lymphoproliferative disorder with morphologic features of Castleman's disease. Clinical findings and clinicopathologic correlations in 15 patients. J. Clin Oncol **3**:1202-1216, 1985.

223 Gerald W, Kostianovsky M, Rosai J: Development of vascular neoplasia in Castleman's disease. Report of seven cases. Am J Surg Pathol **14**:603-614, 1990.

224 Gould SJ, Diss T, Isaacson PG: Multicentric Castleman's disease in association with a solitary plasmacytoma. A case report. Histopathology **17**:135-140, 1990.

225 Hall PA, Donaghy M, Cotter FE, Stansfeld AG, Levison DA: An immunohistological and genotypic study of the plasma cell form of Castleman's disease. Histopathology **14**:333-346, 1989.

226 Hanson CA, Frizzera G, Patton DF, Peterson BA, McClain KL, Gajl-Peczalska KJ, Kersey JH: Clonal rearrangement for immunoglobulin and T-cell receptor genes in systemic Castleman's disease. Association with Epstein-Barr virus. Am J Pathol **131**:84-91, 1988.

227 Hsu SM, Waldron JA, Xie SS, Barlogie B: Expression of interleukin6 in Castleman's disease. Hum Pathol **24**:833-839, 1993.

228 Isaacson PG: Commentary: Castleman's disease. Histopathology **14**:429-432, 1989.

229 Jones EL, Crocker J, Gregory J, Guibarra M, Curran RC: Angiofollicular lymph node hyperplasia (Castleman's disease). An immunohistochemical and enzyme-histochemical study of the hyaline-vascular form of lesion. J Pathol **144**:131-147, 1984.

230 Keller AR, Hochholzer L, Castleman, B: Hyaline-vascular and plasma-cell types of giant lymph node hyperplasia of mediastinum and other locations. Cancer **29**:670-683, 1972.

231 Madero S, Oñate JM, Garzón A: Giant lymph node hyperplasia in an angiolipomatous mediastinal mass. Arch Pathol Lab Med **110**:853-855, 1986.

232 Maheswaran PR, Ramsay AD, Norton AJ, Roche WR: Hodgkin's disease presenting with the histological features of Castleman's disease. Histopathology **18**:249-253, 1991.

233 Mandler RN, Kerrigan DP, Smart J, Kuis W, Villiger P, Lotz M: Castleman's disease in POEMS syndrome with elevated interleukin-6. Cancer **69**:2697-2703, 1992.

234 Menke DM, Camoriano JK, Banks PM: Angiofollicular lymph node hyperplasia. A comparison of unicentric, multicentric, hyaline vascular, and plasma cell types of disease by morphometric and clinical analysis. Mod Pathol **5**:525-530, 1992.

235 Munoz G, Geijo P, Moldenhauer F, Perez-Moro E, Razquin J, Piris MA: Plasmacellular Castleman's disease and POEMS syndrome. Histopathology **17**:172-174, 1990.

236 Nagai K, Sato I, Shimoyama N: Pathohistological and immunohistochemical studies on Castleman's disease of the lymph node. Virchows Arch [A] **409**:287-297, 1986.

237 Nguyen DT, Diamond LW, Hansmann ML, Alavaikko MJ, Schroder H, Fellbaum C, Fischer R: Castleman's disease. Differences in follicular dendritic network in the hyaline vascular and plasma cell variants. Histopathology **24**:437-443, 1994.

238 Ohyashiki JH, Ohyashiki K, Kawakubo K, Serizawa H, Abe K, Mikata A, Toyama K: Molecular genetic, cytogenetic, and immunophenotypic analyses in Castleman's disease of the plasma cell type. Am J Clin Pathol **101**:290-295, 1994.

239 Ordi J, Grau JM, Junque A, Nomdedeu B, Palacin A, Cardesa A: Secondary (AA) amyloidosis associated with Castleman's disease. Report of two cases and review of the literature. Am J Clin Pathol **100**:394-397, 1993.

240 Peterson BA, Frizzera G: Multicentric Castleman's disease. Semin Oncol **20**:636-647, 1993.

241 Radaszkiewicz T, Hansmann ML, Lennert K: Monoclonality and polyclonality of plasma cells in Castleman's disease of the plasma cell variant. Histopathology **14**:11-24, 1989.

242 Rolon PG, Audouin J, Diebold J, Rolon PA, Gonzalez A: Multicentric angiofollicular lymph node hyperplasia associated with a solitary osteolytic costal IgG lambda myeloma. POEMS syndrome in a South American (Paraguayan) patient. Pathol Res Pract **185**:468-469, 1989.

243 Ruco LP, Gearing AJ, Pigott R, Pomponi D, Burgio VL, Cafolla A, Baiocchini A, Baroni CD: Expression of ICAM-1, VCAM-1 and ELAM-1 in angiofollicular lymph node hyperplasia (Castleman's disease). Evidence for dysplasia of follicular dendritic reticulum cells. Histopathology **19**:523-528, 1991.

244 Vasef M, Katzin WE, Mendelsohn G, Reydman M: Report of a case of localized Castleman's disease with progression to malignant lymphoma. Am J Clin Pathol **98**:633-636, 1992.

245 Weisenburger DD, Nathwani BN, Winberg CD, Rappaport H: Multicentric angiofollicular lymph node hyperplasia. A clinicopathologic study of 16 cases. Hum Pathol **16**:162-172, 1985.

246 Zarate-Osorno A, Medeiros LJ, Danon AD, Neiman RS: Hodgkin's disease with coexistent Castleman-like histologic features. A report of three cases. Arch Pathol Lab Med **118**:270-274, 1994.

Angioimmunoblastic lymphadenopathy

247 Aozasa K, Ohsawa M, Fujita MQ, Kanayama Y, Tominaga N, Yonezawa T, Matsubuchi T, Hirata M, Uda H, Kanamaru A, et al.: Angioimmunoblastic lymphadenopathy. Review of 44 patients with emphasis on prognostic behavior. Cancer **63**:1625-1629, 1989.

248 Bernengo MG, Levi L, Zina G: Skin lesions in angioimmunoblastic lymphadenopathy. Histological and immunological studies. Br J Dermatol **104**:131-139, 1981.

249 Bluming AZ, Cohen HG, Saxon A: Angioimmunoblastic lymphadenopathy with dysproteinemia. A pathogenetic link between physiologic lymphoid proliferation and malignant lymphoma. Am J Med **67**:421-428, 1979.

250 Cullen MH, Stansfeld AG, Oliver RTD, Lister TA, Malpas JS: Angioimmunoblastic lymphadenopathy. Report of ten cases and review of the literature. Q J Med **48**:151-177, 1979.

250a Dargent JL, Jacobovitz D, Pradier O, Velu T, Martiat P, Delplace J, Neve P, Diebold J: A case of pleomorphic T-cell lymphoma with a high content of reactive histiocytes presented with hypereosinophilia. Pathol Res Pract **191**:463-468, 1995.

251 Feller AC, Griesser H, Schilling CV, Wacker HH, Dallenbach F, Bartels H, Kuse R, Mak TW, Lennert K: Clonal gene rearrangement patterns correlate with immunophenotype and clinical parameters in patients with angioimmunoblastic lymphadenopathy. Am J Pathol **133**:549-556, 1988.

252 Freter CE, Cossman J: Angioimmunoblastic lymphadenopathy with dysproteinemia. Semin Oncol **20**:627-635, 1993.

253 Frizzera G, Moran EM, Rappaport H: Angio-immunoblastic lymphadenopathy with dysproteinaemia. Lancet **1:**1070-1073, 1974.

254 Frizzera G, Moran EM, Rappaport H: Angio-immunoblastic lymphadenopathy. Diagnosis and clinical course. Am J Med **59:**803-818, 1975.

255 Khan G, Norton AJ, Slavin G: Epstein-Barr virus in angioimmunoblastic T-cell lymphomas. Histopathology **22:**145-149, 1993.

256 Knecht H, Schwarze E-W, Lennert K: Histological, immunohistological and autopsy findings in lymphogranulomatosis X (including angioimmunoblastic lymphadenopathy). Virchows Arch [A] **406:**105-124, 1985.

257 Kon S, Sato T, Onodera K, Satoh M, Kikuchi K, Imai S, Osato T: Detection of Epstein-Barr virus DNA and EBV-determined nuclear antigen in angioimmunoblastic lymphadenopathy with dysproteinemia type T cell lymphoma. Pathol Res Pract **189:**1137-1144, 1993.

258 Kosmidis PA, Axelrod AR, Palacas C, Stahl M: Angioimmunoblastic lymphadenopathy. A T-cell deficiency. Cancer **42:**447-452, 1978.

259 Liao DT, Rosai J, Daneshbod K: Malignant histocytosis with cutaneous involvement and eosinophilia. Am J Clin Pathol **57:**438-448, 1972.

260 Lorenzen J, Li G, Zhao-Hohn M, Wintzer C, Fischer R, Hansmann ML: Angioimmunoblastic lymphadenopathy type of T-cell lymphoma and angioimmunoblastic lymphadenopathy. A clinicopathological and molecular biological study of 13 Chinese patients using polymerase chain reaction and paraffin-embedded tissues. Virchows Arch **424:**593-600, 1994.

261 Lukes RJ, Tindle BH: Immunoblastic lymphadenopathy. A hyperimmune entity resembling Hodgkin's disease. N Engl J Med **292:**1-8, 1975.

262 Nathwani BN, Rappaport H, Moran EM, Pangalis GA, Kim H: Malignant lymphoma arising in angioimmunoblastic lymphadenopathy. Cancer **41:**578-606, 1978.

263 Neiman RS, Dervan P, Haudenschild C, Jaffe R: Angioimmunoblastic lymphadenopathy. An ultrastructural and immunologic study with review of the literature. Cancer **41:**507-518, 1978.

264 Ohshima K, Takeo H, Kikuchi M, Kozuru M, Uike N, Masuda Y, Yoneda S, Takeshita M, Shibata T, Akamatsu M: Heterogeneity of Epstein-Barr virus infection in angioimmunoblastic lymphadenopathy type T-cell lymphoma. Histopathology **25:**569-580, 1994.

265 Seehafer JR, Goldberg NC, Dicken CH, Su WPD: Cutaneous manifestations of angioimmunoblastic lymphadenopathy. Arch Dermatol **116:**41-45, 1980.

266 Shimoyama M, Minato K, Saito H, Takenaka T, Watanabe S, Nagatani T, Naruto M: Immunoblastic lymphadenopathy (IBL)-like T-cell lymphoma. Jpn J Clin Oncol **9**(Suppl 1):347-356, 1979.

267 Weiss LM, Strickler JG, Dorfman RF, Horning SJ, Warnke RA, Sklar J: Clonal T-cell populations in angioimmunoblastic lymphadenopathy and angioimmunoblastic lymphadenopathy-like lymphoma. Am J Pathol **122:**392-398, 1986.

Drug hypersensitivity

268 Abbondanzo SL, Irey NS, Frizzera G: Dilantin-associated lymphadenopathy. Spectrum of histopathologic patterns. Am J Surg Pathol **19:**675-686, 1995.

269 Saltzstein SL, Ackerman LV: Lymphadenopathy induced by anticonvulsant drugs clinically and pathologically mimicking malignant lymphomas. Cancer **12:**164-182, 1959.

Dermatopathic lymphadenitis

270 Asano S, Muramatsu T, Kanno H, Wakasa H: Dermatopathic lymphadenopathy. Electronmicroscopic, enzyme-histochemical and immunohistochemical study. Acta Pathol Jpn **37:**887-900, 1987.

271 Burke JS, Colby TV: Dermatopathic lymphadenopathy. Comparison of cases associated and unassociated with mycosis fungoides. Am J Surg Pathol **5:**343-352, 1981.

272 Gould E, Porto R, Albores-Saavedra J, Ibe MJ: Dermatopathic lymphadenitis. The spectrum and significance of its morphologic features. Arch Pathol Lab Med **112:**1145-1150, 1988.

273 Rausch E, Kaiserling E, Goos M: Langerhans cells and interdigitating reticulum cells in the thymus-dependent region in human dermatopathic lymphadenitis. Virchows Arch [Cell Pathol] **25:**327-343, 1977.

274 Ree H, Fanger H: Paracortical alteration in lymphadenopathic and tumor-draining lymph nodes. Histologic study. Hum Pathol **6:**363-372, 1975.

275 Weiss LM, Hu E, Wood GS, Moulds C, Cleary ML, Warnke R, Sklar J: Clonal rearrangements of T-cell receptor genes in mycosis fungoides and dermatopathic lymphadenopathy. N Engl J Med **313:**539-544, 1985.

276 Weiss LM, Wood GS, Warnke RA: Immunophenotypic differences between dermatopathic lymphadenopathy and lymph node involvement in mycosis fungoides. Am J Pathol **120:**179-185, 1985.

Sinus histiocytosis with massive lymphadenopathy (Rosai-Dorfman's disease)

277 Albores-Saavedra J, Vuitch F, Delgado R, Wiley E, Hagler H: Sinus histiocytosis of pelvic lymph nodes after hip replacement. A histiocytic proliferation induced by cobalt-chromium and titanium. Am J Surg Pathol **18:**83-90, 1994.

278 Bonetti F, Chilosi M, Menestrina F, Scarpa A, Pelicci PG, Amorosi E, Fiore-Donati L, Knowles DM: Immunohistological analysis of Rosai-Dorfman histiocytosis. A disease of S-100 + CD1-histiocytes. Virchows Arch [A] **411:**129-135, 1987.

279 Brown RE, Danville PA: Personal communication, 1994.

280 Eisen RN, Buckley PJ, Rosai J: Immunophenotypic characterization of sinus histiocytosis with massive lymphadenopathy (Rosai-Dorfman disease). Semin Diagn Pathol **7:**74-82, 1990.

281 Falk S, Stutte HJ, Frizzera G: Hodgkin's disease and sinus histiocytosis with massive lymphadenopathy-like changes. Histopathology **19:**221-224, 1991.

282 Foucar E, Rosai J, Dorfman RF: Sinus histiocytosis with massive lymphadenopathy. Ear, nose, and throat manifestations. Arch Otolaryngol **104:**687-693, 1978.

283 Foucar E, Rosai J, Dorfman RF: The ophthalmologic manifestations of sinus histiocytosis with massive lymphadenopathy. Am J Ophthalmol **87:**354-367, 1979.

284 Foucar E, Rosai J, Dorfman RF: Sinus histiocytosis with massive lymphadenopathy. An analysis of 14 deaths occurring in a patient registry. Cancer **54:**1834-1840, 1984.

285 Foucar E, Rosai J, Dorfman R: Sinus histiocytosis with massive lymphadenopathy (Rosai-Dorfman disease). Review of the entity. Semin Diagn Pathol **7:**19-73, 1990.

286 Foucar E, Rosai J, Dorfman RF, Brynes RK: The neurologic manifestations of sinus histiocytosis with massive lymphadenopathy. Neurology **32:**365-371, 1982.

287 Foucar E, Rosai J, Dorfman RF, Eyman JM: Immunologic abnormalities and their significance in the pathogenesis of sinus histiocytosis with massive lymphadenopathy. Am J Clin Pathol **82:**515-525, 1984.

288 Komp DM: The treatment of sinus histiocytosis with massive lymphadenopathy (Rosai-Dorfman disease). Semin Diagn Pathol **7:**83-86, 1990.

289 Larkin DFP, Dervan PA, Munnelly J, Finucane J: Sinus histiocytosis with massive lymphadenopathy simulating subacute thyroiditis. Hum Pathol **17:**321-324, 1986.

290 Leighton SE, Gallimore AP: Extranodal sinus histiocytosis with massive lymphadenopathy affecting the subglottis and trachea. Histopathology **24:**393-394, 1994.

291 Levine PH, Jahan N, Murari P, Manak M, Jaffe ES: Detection of human herpesvirus 6 in tissues involved by sinus histiocytosis with massive lymphadenopathy (Rosai-Dorfman disease). J Infect Dis **166:**291-295, 1992.

291a Marmaduke DP, Rosai J, Warnke R, Foucar K, Emmert-Buck MR, Liotta LA, Willman CL: Molecular assessment of clonality in sinus histiocytosis with massive lymphadenopathy (SHML). A reactive disorder of polyclonal histiocytes (abstract). Mod Pathol (in press).

292 Marsh WL Jr, McCarrick JP, Harlan DM: Sinus histiocytosis with massive lymphadenopathy. Occurrence in identical twins with retroperitoneal disease. Arch Pathol Lab Med **112:**298-301, 1988.

293 Miettinen M, Paljakka P, Haveri P, Saxén E: Sinus histiocytosis with massive lymphadenopathy. A nodal and extranodal proliferation of S-100 protein positive histiocytes? Am J Clin Pathol **88:**270-277, 1987.

294 Montgomery EA, Meis JM, Frizzera G: Rosai-Dorfman disease of soft tissue. Am J Surg Pathol **16:**122-129, 1992.

295 Murray J, Fox H: Rosai-Dorfman disease of the uterine cervix. Int J Gynecol Pathol **10:**209-213, 1991.

296 Osborne BM, Hagemeister FB, Butler JJ: Extranodal gastrointestinal sinus histiocytosis with massive lymphadenopathy. Clinically presenting as a malignant tumor. Am J Surg Pathol **5:**603-611, 1981.

297 Paulli M, Feller AC, Boveri E, Kindl S, Berti E, Rosso R, Merz H, Facchetti F, Gambini C, Bonetti F, et al.: Cathepsin D and E co-expression in sinus histiocytosis with massive lymphadenopathy (Rosai-Dorfman disease) and Langerhans' cell histiocytosis. Further evidences of a phenotypic overlap between these histiocytic disorders. Virchows Arch **424:**601-606, 1994.

298 Paulli M, Rosso R, Kindl S, Boveri E, Marocolo D, Chioda C, Agostini C, Magrini U, Facchetti F: Immunophenotypic characterization of the cell infiltrate in five cases of sinus histiocytosis with massive lymphadenopathy (Rosai-Dorfman disease). Hum Pathol **23:**647-654, 1992.

299 Rosai J, Dorfman RF: Sinus histiocytosis with massive lymphadenopathy. A pseudolymphomatous benign disorder. Analysis of 34 cases. Cancer **30:**1174-1188, 1972.

300 Song SK, Schwartz IS, Strauchen JA, Huang YP, Sachdev V, Daftary DR, Vas CJ: Meningeal nodules with features of extranodal sinus histiocytosis with massive lymphadenopathy. Am J Surg Pathol 13:406-412, 1989.

301 Suarez CR, Zeller WP, Silberman S, Rust G, Messmore H: Sinus histiocytosis with massive lymphadenopathy. Remission with chemotherapy. Am J Pediatr Hematol Oncol 5:235-241, 1983.

302 Thawerani H, Sanchez RL, Rosai J, Dorfman RF: The cutaneous manifestations of sinus histiocytosis with massive lymphadenopathy. Arch Dermatol 114:191-197, 1978.

303 Tsang WY, Yip TT, Chan JK: The Rosai-Dorfman disease histiocytes are not infected by Epstein-Barr virus. Histopathology 25:88-90, 1994.

304 Wenig BM, Abbondanzo SL, Childers EL, Kapadia SB, Heffner DR: Extranodal sinus histiocytosis with massive lymphadenopathy (Rosai-Dorfman disease) of the head and neck. Hum Pathol 24:483-492, 1993.

305 Willman CL: Personal communication, 1995.

306 Willman CL, Busque L, Griffith BB, Favara BE, McClain KL, Duncan MH, Gilliland DG: Langerhans-cell histiocytosis (histiocytosis X). A clonal proliferative disease. N Engl J Med 331:154-160, 1994.

307 Wright DH, Richards DB: Sinus histiocytosis with massive lymphadenopathy (Rosai-Dorfman disease). Report of a case with widespread nodal and extra nodal dissemination. Histopathology 5:697-709, 1981.

Langerhans' cell granulomatosis (histiocytosis X)

308 Axiotis CA, Merino MJ, Duray PH: Langerhans cell histiocytosis of the female genital tract. Cancer 67:1650-1660, 1991.

309 Basset F, Nezelof C, Ferrans VJ: The histiocytoses. Pathol Annu 18(Pt 2):27-78, 1983.

310 Beckstead JH, Wood GS, Turner RR: Histiocytosis X cells and Langerhans cells. Enzyme histochemical and immunologic similarities. Hum Pathol 15:826-833, 1984.

311 Ben-Ezra J, Bailey A, Azumi N, Delsol G, Stroup R, Sheibani K, Rappaport H: Malignant histiocytosis X. A distinct clinicopathologic entity. Cancer 68:1050-1060, 1991.

312 Bingham EA, Bridges JM, Kelly AMT, Burrows D, Nevins NC: Letterer-Siwe disease. A study of thirteen cases over a 21-year period. Br J Dermatol 106:205-209, 1982.

313 Burns BF, Colby TV, Dorfman RF: Langerhans cell granulomatosis (histiocytosis X) associated with malignant lymphomas. Am J Surg Pathol 7:529-533, 1983.

314 Emile J-F, Wechsler J, Brousse N, Boulland ML, Cologon R, Freitag S, Voisin M-C, Gaulard P, Boumsell L, Zafrani E-S: Langerhans' cell histiocytosis. Definitive diagnosis with the use of monoclonal antibody O10 on routinely paraffin-embedded samples. Am J Surg Pathol 19:636-641, 1995.

315 Favara BE: Langerhans' cell histiocytosis pathobiology and pathogenesis. Semin Oncol 18:3-7, 1991.

316 Groisman GM, Rosh JR, Harpaz N: Langerhans cell histiocytosis of the stomach. A cause of granulomatous gastritis and gastric polyposis. Arch Pathol Lab Med 118:1232-1235, 1994.

317 Hage C, Willman CL, Favara BE, Isaacson PG: Langerhans' cell histiocytosis (histiocytosis X). Immunophenotype and growth fraction. Hum Pathol 24:840-845, 1993.

318 Hashimoto K, Griffin D, Kohbaki M: Self-healing reticulohistiocytosis. A clinical, histologic, and ultrastructural study of the fourth case in the literature. Cancer 49:331-337, 1982.

319 Kjedlsberg CR, Kim H: Eosinophilic granuloma as an incidental finding in malignant lymphoma. Arch Pathol Lab Med 104:137-140, 1980.

320 Komp DM: Concepts in staging and clinical studies for treatment of Langerhans' cell histiocytosis. Semin Oncol 18:18-23, 1991.

321 Lahey ME: Prognostic factors in histiocytosis X. Am J Pediatr Hematol/Oncol 3:57-65, 1981.

322 Leahy MA, Krejci SM, Friednash M, Stockert SS, Wilson H, Huff JC, Weston WL, Brice SL: Human herpesvirus 6 is present in lesions of Langerhans cell histiocytosis. J Invest Dermatol 101:642-645, 1993.

323 McClain K, Jin H, Gresik V, Favara B: Langerhans cell histiocytosis. Lack of a viral etiology. Am J Hematol 47:16-20, 1994.

324 Mierau GW, Favara BE, Brenman JM: Electron microscopy in histiocytosis X. Ultrastruct Pathol 3:137-142, 1982.

325 Motoi M, Helbron D, Kaiserling E, Lennert K: Eosinophilic granuloma of lymph nodes. A variant of histiocytosis X. Histopathology 4:585-606, 1980.

326 Neumann MP, Frizzera G: The coexistence of Langerhans' cell granulomatosis and malignant lymphoma may take different forms. Report of seven cases with a review of the literature. Hum Pathol 17:1060-1065, 1986.

327 Ornvold K, Nielsen MH, Clausen N: Disseminated histiocytosis X. A clinical and immunohistochemical retrospective study. Acta Pathol Microbiol Immunol Scand (A) 93:311-316, 1985.

328 Ornvold K, Ralfkiaer E, Carstensen H: Immunohistochemical study of the abnormal cells in Langerhans cell histiocytosis (histiocytosis X). Virchows Arch [A] 416:403-410, 1990.

329 Otis CN, Fischer RA, Johnson N, Kelleher JF, Powell JL: Histiocytosis X of the vulva. A case report and review of the literature. Obstet Gynecol 75:555-558, 1990.

330 Paulli M, Feller AC, Boveri E, Kindl S, Berti E, Rosso R, Merz H, Facchetti F, Gambini C, Bonetti F, et al. Cathepsin D and E co-expression in sinus histiocytosis with massive lymphadenopathy (Rosai-Dorfman disease) and Langerhans' cell histiocytosis. Further evidences of a phenotypic overlap between these histiocytic disorders. Virchows Arch 424:601-606, 1994.

331 Rabkin MS, Kjeldsberg CR, Wittwer CT, Marty J: A comparison study of two methods of peanut agglutinin staining with S100 immunostaining in 29 cases of histiocytosis X (Langerhans' cell histiocytosis). Arch Pathol Lab Med 114:511-515, 1990.

332 Ree HJ, Kadin ME: Peanut agglutinin. A useful marker for histiocytosis X and interdigitating reticulum cells. Cancer 57:282-287, 1986.

333 Reid H, Fox H, Whittaker JS: Eosinophilic granuloma of lymph nodes. Histopathology 1:31-37, 1977.

334 Richmond I, Eyden BP, Banerjee SS: Intranodal Langerhans' cell histiocytosis associated with malignant melanoma. Histopathology 26:380-382, 1995.

335 Risdall RJ, Dehner LP, Duray P, Kobrinsky N, Robison L, Nesbit ME Jr: Histiocytosis X (Langerhans' cell histiocytosis). Prognostic role of histopathology. Arch Pathol Lab Med 107:59-63, 1983.

336 Santamaria M, Llamas L, Ree HJ, Sheibani K, Ho YS, Su I-J, Hsu S-M: Expression of sialylated leu-M1 antigen in histiocytosis X. Am J Clin Pathol 89:211-219, 1988.

337 Tsang WY, Lau MF, Chan JK: Incidental Langerhans' cell histiocytosis of the thyroid. Histopathology 24:397-399, 1994.

338 Vernon ML, Fountain L, Krebs HM, Barbosa LH, Fuccillo DA, Sever JL: Birbeck granules (Langerhan's cell granules) in human lymph nodes. Am J Clin Pathol 60:771-779, 1973.

339 Williams JW, Dorfman RF: Lymphadenopathy as the initial manifestation of histiocytosis X. Am J Surg Pathol 3:405-421, 1979.

340 Willman CL, Busque L, Griffith BB, Favara BE, McClain KL, Duncan MH, Gilliland DG: Langerhans'-cell histiocytosis (histiocytosis X)—a clonal proliferative disease. N Engl J Med 331:154-160, 1994.

341 Wood C, Wood GS, Deneau DG, Oseroff A, Beckstead JH, Malin J: Malignant histiocytosis X. Report of a rapidly fatal case in an elderly man. Cancer 54:347-352, 1984.

342 Yu RC, Chu AC: Lack of T-cell receptor gene rearrangements in cells involved in Langerhans' cell histiocytosis. Cancer 75:1162-1166, 1995.

Kimura's disease

343 Chan JK, Hui PK, Ng CS, Yuen NW, Kung IT, Gwi E: Epithelioid haemangioma (angiolymphoid hyperplasia with eosinophilia) and Kimura's disease in Chinese. Histopathology 15:557-574, 1989.

344 Googe PB, Harris NL, Mihm MC Jr: Kimura's disease and angiolymphoid hyperplasia with eosinophilia. Two distinct histopathological entities. J Cutan Pathol 14:263-271, 1987.

345 Hui PK, Chan JK, Ng CS, Kung IT, Gwi E: Lymphadenopathy of Kimura's disease. Am J Surg Pathol 13:177-186, 1989.

346 Kung ITM, Gibson JB, Bannatyne PM: Kimura's disease. A clinico-pathologic study of 21 cases and its distinction from angiolymphoid hyperplasia with eosinophilia. Pathology 16:39-44, 1984.

347 Kuo TT, Shih LY, Chan HL: Kimura's disease. Involvement of regional lymph nodes and distinction from angiolymphoid hyperplasia with eosinophilia. Am J Surg Pathol 12:843-854, 1988.

348 Rosai J, Gold J, Landy R: The histiocytoid hemangiomas. A unifying concept embracing several previously described entities of skin, soft tissue, large vessels, bone, and heart. Hum Pathol 10:707-730, 1979.

349 Urabe A, Tsuneyoshi M, Enjoji M: Epithelioid hemangioma versus Kimura's disease. A comparative clinicopathologic study. Am J Surg Pathol 11:758-766, 1987.

Chronic granulomatous disease

350 Baehner RL, Nathan DG: Quantitative nitroblue tetrazolium test in chronic granulomatous disease. N Engl J Med 278:971-976, 1968.

351 Carson MJ, Chadwick DL, Brubaker CA, Cleland RS, Landing BH: Thirteen boys with progressive septic granulomatosis. Pediatrics 35:405-412, 1965.

352 Curnutte JT: Chronic granulomatous disease: The solving of a clinical riddle at the molecular level. Clin Immunol Immunopathol 67:S2-15, 1993.

353 Johnston RB, McMurry JS: Chronic familial granulomatosis. Am J Dis Child 114:370-378, 1967.

354 Landing BH, Shirkey NS: A syndrome of recurrent infection and infiltration of viscera by pigmented lipid histiocytes. Pediatrics 20:431-438, 1957.

355 Roos D: The genetic basis of chronic granulomatous disease. Immunol Rev 138:121-157, 1994.

356 Thrasher AJ, Keep NH, Wientjes F, Segal AW: Chronic granulomatous disease. Biochim Biophys Acta 1227:1-24, 1994.

357 Umeki S: Mechanisms for the activation/electron transfer of neutrophil NADPH-oxidase complex and molecular pathology of chronic granulomatous disease. Ann Hematol 68:267-277, 1994.

Lipophagic reactions

358 Boitnott JK, Margolis S: Mineral oil in human tissues. II. Oil droplets in lymph nodes of the porta hepatis. Bull Hopkins Hosp 118:414-422, 1966.

359 Fisher ER: Whipple's disease. Pathogenetic considerations. Electron microscopic and histochemical observations. JAMA 181:396-403, 1962.

360 Kelsall GR, Blackwell JB: The occurrence and significance of lipophage clusters in lymph nodes and spleen. Pathology 1:211-220, 1969.

361 Ravel R: Histopathology of lymph nodes after lymphangiography. Am J Clin Pathol 46:335-355, 1966.

MALIGNANT LYMPHOMA

361a Aisenberg AC: Coherent view of non-Hodgkin's lymphoma. J Clin Oncol 13:2656-2675, 1995.

362 Berard CW, Dorfman RF: Histopathology of malignant lymphomas. Clin Haematol 3:39-76, 1974.

363 Jaffe ES, Raffeld M, Medeiros LJ, Stetler-Stevenson M: An overview of the classification of non-Hodgkin's lymphomas. An integration of morphological and phenotypical concepts. Cancer Res 52:5447s-5452s, 1992.

364 Jaffe ES: Surgical pathology of the lymph nodes and related organs, ed 2. Philadelphia, 1995, WB Saunders.

365 Lennert K, Feller AC: Histopathology of non-Hodgkin's lymphomas, ed 2. New York, 1992, Springer-Verlag.

366 Warnke RA, Weiss LM, Chan JKC, Cleary ML, Dorfman RF: Tumors of the lymph nodes and spleen. Atlas of tumor pathology. 3rd Series, Fascicle 14, Washington, DC, Armed Forces Institute of Pathology.

Hodgkin's disease

367 Chang KL, Albujar PF, Chen YY, Johnson RM, Weiss LM: High prevalence of Epstein-Barr virus in the Reed-Sternberg cells of Hodgkin's disease occurring in Peru. Blood 81:496-501, 1993.

368 Gutensohn N, Cole P: Childhood social environment and Hodgkin's disease. N Engl J Med 304:135-140, 1981.

369 Jarrett RF, Gallagher A, Jones DB, Alexander FE, Krajewski AS, Kelsey A, Adams J, Angus B, Gledhill S, Wright DH, et al.: Detection of Epstein-Barr virus genomes in Hodgkin's disease. Relation to age. J Clin Pathol 44:844-848, 1991.

370 Mack TM, Cozen W, Shibata DK, Weiss LM, Nathwani BN, Hernandez AM, Taylor CR, Hamilton AS, Deapen DM, Rappaport EB: Concordance for Hodgkin's disease in identical twins suggesting genetic susceptibility to the young adult form of the disease. N Engl J Med 332:413-418, 1995.

371 Mueller N, Evans A, Harris NL, Comstock GW, Jellum E, Magnus K, Orentreich N, Polk BF, Vogelman J: Hodgkin's disease and Epstein-Barr virus. Altered antibody pattern before diagnosis. N Engl J Med 320:689-695, 1989.

372 Pallesen G, Hamilton-Dutoit SJ, Rowe M, Young LS: Expression of Epstein-Barr virus latent gene products in tumour cells of Hodgkin's disease. Lancet 337:320-322, 1991.

373 Reynolds DJ, Banks PM, Gulley ML: New characterization of infectious mononucleosis and a phenotypic comparison with Hodgkin's disease. Am J Pathol 146:379-388, 1995.

374 Weiss LM, Chang KL: Molecular biologic studies of Hodgkin's disease. Semin Diagn Pathol 9:272-278, 1992.

375 Weiss LM, Chen YY, Liu XF, Shibata D: Epstein-Barr virus and Hodgkin's disease. A correlative in situ hybridization and polymerase chain reaction study. Am J Pathol 139:1259-1265, 1991.

Reed-Sternberg cell

376 Agnarsson BA, Kadin ME: The immunophenotype of Reed-Sternberg cells. A study of 50 cases of Hodgkin's disease using fixed frozen tissues. Cancer 63:2083-2087, 1989.

377 Carbone A, Gloghini A, Gruss H-J, Pinto A: CD40 antigen expression on Reed-Sternberg cells. A reliable diagnostic tool for Hodgkin's disease. Am J Pathol 146:780-781, 1995.

378 Casey TT, Olson SJ, Cousar JB, Collins RD: Immunophenotypes of Reed-Sternberg cells. A study of 19 cases of Hodgkin's disease in plastic-embedded sections. Blood 74:2624-2628, 1989.

379 Chang KL, Curtis CM, Momose H, Lopategui J, Weiss LM: Sensitivity and specificity of *Bauhinia purpurea* as a paraffin section marker for the Reed-Sternberg cells of Hodgkin's disease. Appl Immunohistochem 1:208-212, 1993.

380 Chittal SM, Caveriviere P, Schwarting R, Gerdes J, Al Saati T, Rigal-Huguet F, Stein H, Delsol G: Monoclonal antibodies in the diagnosis of Hodgkin's disease. The search for a rational panel. Am J Surg Pathol 12:9-21, 1988.

381 Dallenbach FE, Stein H: Expression of T-cell-receptor beta chain in Reed-Sternberg cells. Lancet 2:828-830, 1989.

382 Delabie J, Shipman R, Bruggen J, De Strooper B, van Leuven F, Tarcsay L, Cerletti N, Odink K, Diehl V, Bilbe G, et al.: Expression of the novel intermediate filament-associated protein restin in Hodgkin's disease and anaplastic large-cell lymphoma. Blood 80:2891-2896, 1992.

383 Fisher ER, Hazard JB: Differentiation of megakaryocyte and Reed-Sternberg cell. Lab Invest 3:261-269, 1954.

384 Foss H-D, Hummel M, Gottstein S, Ziemann K, Falini B, Herbst H, Stein H: Frequent expression of IL-7 gene transcripts in tumor cells of classical Hodgkin's disease. Am J Pathol 146:33-39, 1995.

385 Griesser H, Feller AC, Mak TW, Lennert K: Clonal rearrangements of T-cell receptor and immunoglobulin genes and immunophenotypic antigen expression in different subclasses of Hodgkin's disease. Int J Cancer 40:157-160, 1987.

386 Hsu S-M, Yang K, Jaffe ES: Phenotypic expression of Hodgkin's and Reed-Sternberg cells in Hodgkin's disease. Am J Pathol 118:209-217, 1985.

386a Hummel M, Ziemann K, Lammert H, Pileri S, Sabattini E, Stein H: Hodgkin's disease with monoclonal and polyclonal populations of Reed-Sternberg cells. N Engl J Med 333:901-906, 1995.

387 Hyder DM, Schnitzer B: Utility of Leu M1 monoclonal antibody in the differential diagnosis of Hodgkin's disease. Arch Pathol Lab Med 110:416-419, 1986.

388 Kadin ME: A reappraisal of the Reed-Sternberg cell. A commentary. Blood Cells 6:525-532, 1980.

389 Kadin ME, Muramoto L, Said J: Expression of T-cell antigens on Reed-Sternberg cells in a subset of patients with nodular sclerosing and mixed cellularity Hodgkin's disease. Am J Pathol 130:345-353, 1988.

390 Knowles DM, Neri A, Pelicci PG, Burke JS, Wu A, Winberg CD, Sheibani K, Dalla-Favera R: Immunoglobulin and T-cell receptor beta-chain gene rearrangement analysis of Hodgkin's disease. Implications for lineage determination and differential diagnosis. Proc Natl Acad Sci USA 83:7942-7946, 1986.

391 Le Brun DP, Ngan BY, Weiss LM, Huie P, Warnke RA, Cleary ML: The bcl-2 oncogene in Hodgkin's disease arising in the setting of follicular non-Hodgkin's lymphoma. Blood 83:223-230, 1994.

392 Louie DC, Kant JA, Brooks JJ, Reed JC: Absence of t(14; 18) major and minor breakpoints and of Bcl-2 protein overproduction in Reed-Sternberg cells of Hodgkin's disease. Am J Pathol 139:1231-1237, 1991.

393 Nolte M, Werner M, Spann W, Schnabel B, von Wasielewski R, Wilkens L, Hubner K, Fischer R, Georgii A: The bcl/2/JH gene rearrangement is undetectable in Hodgkin's lymphomas. Results from the German Hodgkin trial. Virchows Arch 426:37-42, 1995.

394 O'Grady JT, Stewart S, Lowrey J, Howie SE, Krajewski AS: CD40 expression in Hodgkin's disease. Am J Pathol 144:21-26, 1994.

395 Poppema S, Kaleta J, Hepperle B: Chromosomal abnormalities in patients with Hodgkin's disease. Evidence for frequent involvement of the 14q chromosomal region but infrequent bcl-2 gene rearrangement in Reed-Sternberg cells. J Natl Cancer Inst 84:1789-1793, 1992.

396 Sarker AB, Akagi T, Jeon HJ, Miyake K, Murakami I, Yoshino T, Takahashi K, Nose S: *Bauhinia purpurea*—a new paraffin section marker for Reed-Sternberg cells of Hodgkin's disease. A comparison with Leu-M1 (CD15), LN2 (CD74), peanut agglutinin, and Ber-H2 (CD30). Am J Pathol 141:19-23, 1992.

397 Schmid C, Pan L, Diss T, Isaacson PG: Expression of B-cell antigens by Hodgkin's and Reed-Sternberg cells. Am J Pathol 139:701-707, 1991.

398 Stetler-Stevenson M, Crush-Stanton S, Cossman J: Involvement of the bcl-2 gene in Hodgkin's disease. J Natl Cancer Inst 82:855-858, 1990.

399 Strum SB, Park JK, Rappaport H: Observation of cells resembling Sternberg-Reed cells in conditions other than Hodgkin's disease. Cancer 26:176-190, 1977.

400 Thangavelu M, Le Beau MM: Chromosomal abnormalities in Hodgkin's disease. Hematol Oncol Clin North Am 3:221-236, 1989.

401 Tilly H, Bastard C, Delastre T, Duval C, Bizet M, Lenormand B, Dauce JP, Monconduit M, Piguet H: Cytogenetic studies in untreated Hodgkin's disease. Blood 77:1298-1304, 1991.

Microscopic types

402 Tindle BH, Parker JW, Lukes RJ: "Reed-Sternberg cells" in infectious mononu-cleosis? Am J Clin Pathol **58:**607-617, 1972.
403 Weiss LM, Strickler JG, Hu E, Warnke RA, Sklar J: Immunoglobulin gene rear-rangements in Hodgkin's disease. Hum Pathol **17:**1009-1014, 1986.
404 Zukerberg LR, Collins AB, Ferry JA, Harris NL: Coexpression of CD15 and CD20 by Reed-Sternberg cells in Hodgkin's disease. Am J Pathol **139:**475-483, 1991.

Microscopic types

405 Alkan S, Ross CW, Hanson CA, Schnitzer B: Epstein-Barr virus and bcl-2 pro-tein overexpression are not detected in the neoplastic cells of nodular lymphocyte predominance Hodgkin's disease. Mod Pathol **8:**544-547, 1995.
406 Chittal SM, Alard C, Rossi JF, al Saati T, Le Tourneau A, Diebold J, Delsol G: Further phenotypic evidence that nodular, lymphocyte-predominant Hodgkin's disease is a large B-cell lymphoma in evolution. Am J Surg Pathol **14:**1024-1035, 1990.
407 Cibull ML, Stein H, Gatter KC, Mason DY: The expression of the CD3 antigen in Hodgkin's disease. Histopathology **15:**599-605, 1989.
408 Colby TV, Hoppe RT, Warnke RA: Hodgkin's disease at autopsy. 1972-1977. Cancer **47:**1852-1862, 1981.
409 Colby TV, Warnke RA: The histology of the initial relapse of Hodgkin's disease. Cancer **45:**289-292, 1980.
410 Coleman CN, Williams CJ, Flint A, Glatstein EJ, Rosenberg SA, Kaplan HS: Hematologic neoplasia in patients treated for Hodgkin's disease. N Engl J Med **297:**1249-1252, 1977.
411 Coles FB, Cartun RW, Pastuszak WT: Hodgkin's disease, lymphocyte-predomi-nant type. Immunoreactivity with B-cell antibodies. Mod Pathol **1:**274-278, 1988.
412 Coppleson LW, Rappaport H, Strum SB, Rose J: Analysis of the Rye classifica-tion of Hodgkin's disease. The prognostic significance of cellular composition. J Natl Cancer Inst **51:**379-390, 1973.
413 Cross RM: Hodgkin's disease. Histological classification and diagnosis. J Clin Pathol **22:**165-182, 1969.
414 Ferry JA, Zukerberg LR, Harris NL: Florid progressive transformation of germi-nal centers. A syndrome affecting young men, without early progression to nodu-lar lymphocyte predominance Hodgkin's disease. Am J Surg Pathol **16:**252-258, 1992.
415 Gelb AB, Dorfman RF, Warnke RA: Coexistence of nodular lymphocyte pre-dominance Hodgkin's disease and Hodgkin's disease of the usual type. Am J Surg Pathol **17:**364-374, 1993.
416 Jackson H, Parker F: Hodgkin's disease. 1. General considerations. N Engl J Med **230:**1-8, 1944.
417 Kamel OW, Gelb AB, Shibuya RB, Warnke RA: Leu 7 (CD57) reactivity distin-guishes nodular lymphocyte predominance Hodgkin's disease from nodular scle-rosing Hodgkin's disease, T-cell-rich B-cell lymphoma and follicular lymphoma. Am J Pathol **142:**541-546, 1993.
418 Krikorian JG, Burke JS, Rosenberg SA, Kaplan HS: Occurrence of non-Hodgkin's lymphoma after therapy for Hodgkin's disease. N Engl J Med **300:**452-458, 1979.
419 Lukes RJ: Relationship of histologic features to clinical stages in Hodgkin's dis-ease. Am J Roentgenol **90:**944-955, 1963.
420 Lukes RJ, Butler JJ, Hicks EB: Natural history of Hodgkin's disease as related to its pathologic picture. Cancer **19:**317-344, 1966.
421 Lukes RJ, Craver LF, Hall TC, Rappaport H, Ruben P: Report of Nomenclature Committee. Cancer Res **16:**1311, 1966.
422 MacLennan KA, Bennett MH, Tu A, Hudson BV, Easterling MJ, Hudson GV, Jelliffe AM: Relationship of histopathologic features to survival and relapse in nodular sclerosing Hodgkin's disease. A study of 1659 patients. Cancer **64:**1686-1693, 1989.
423 Marshall AHE, Matilla A, Pollock DJ: A critique and case study of nodular scle-rosing Hodgkin's disease. J Clin Pathol **29:**923-930, 1976.
424 Mason DY, Banks PM, Chan J, Cleary ML, Delsol G, de Wolf Peeters C, Falini B, Gatter K, Grogan TM, Harris NL, et al.: Nodular lymphocyte predominance Hodgkin's disease. A distinct clinicopathological entity (editorial). Am J Surg Pathol **18:**526-530, 1994.
425 Möller P, Lennert K: On the angiostructure of lymph nodes in Hodgkin's disease. An immunohistochemical study using the lectin I of *Ulex europaeus* as endothe-lial marker. Virchows Arch [A] **403:**257-270, 1984.
426 Momose H, Chen YY, Ben-Ezra J, Weiss LM: Nodular lymphocyte-predominant Hodgkin's disease. Study of immunoglobulin light chain protein and mRNA expression. Hum Pathol **23:**1115-1119, 1992.
427 Nicholas DS, Harris S, Wright DH: Lymphocyte predominance Hodgkin's dis-ease—an immunohistochemical study. Histopathology **16:**157-165, 1990.
428 Poppema S: Lymphocyte-predominance Hodgkin's disease. Semin Diagn Pathol **9:**257-264, 1992.

429 Poppema S, Kaiserling E, Lennert K: Epidemiology of nodular paragranuloma (Hodgkin's disease with lymphocytic predominance, nodular). J Cancer Res Clin Oncol **95:**57-63, 1979.
430 Poppema S, Kaiserling E, Lennert K: Hodgkin's disease with lymphocytic pre-dominance, nodular type (nodular paragranuloma) and progressively transformed germinal centers. A cytohistological study. Histopathology **3:**295-308, 1979.
431 Regula DP Jr, Hoppe RT, Weiss LM: Nodular and diffuse types of lymphocyte predominance Hodgkin's disease. N Engl J Med **318:**214-219, 1988.
432 Regula DP Jr, Weiss LM, Warnke RA, Dorfman RS: Lymphocyte predominance Hodgkin's disease. A reappraisal based upon histological and immunophenotyp-ical findings in relapsing cases. Histopathology **11:**1107-1120, 1987.
433 Ruprai AK, Pringle JH, Angel CA, Kind CN, Lauder I: Localization of immunoglobulin light chain mRNA expression in Hodgkin's disease by in situ hybridization. J Pathol **164:**37-40, 1991.
434 Said JW, Sassoon AF, Shintaku IP, Kurtin PJ, Pinkus GS: Absence of bcl-2 major breakpoint region and JH gene rearrangement in lymphocyte predomi-nance Hodgkin's disease. Results of Southern blot analysis and polymerase chain reaction. Am J Pathol **138:**261-264, 1991.
435 Schmid C, Sargent C, Isaacson PG: L and H cells of nodular lymphocyte pre-dominant Hodgkin's disease show immunoglobulin light-chain restriction. Am J Pathol **139:**1281-1289, 1991.
436 Seemayer TA, Lagace R, Schürch W: On the pathogenesis of sclerosis and nodu-larity in nodular sclerosing Hodgkin's disease. Virchows Arch [A] **385:**283-291, 1980.
437 Smetana HF, Cohen BM: Mortality in relation to histologic type in Hodgkin's disease. Blood **11:**211-224, 1956.
438 Soderstrom N, Norberg B: Observations regarding the specific postcapillary venules of lymph nodes in malignant lymphomas. Acta Pathol Microbiol Scand (A) **82:**71-79, 1974.
439 Stoler MH, Nichols GE, Symbula M, Weiss LM: Lymphocyte predominance Hodgkin's disease. Evidence for a k light chain-restricted monotypic B-cell neo-plasm. Am J Pathol **146:**810-818, 1995.
440 Strickler JG, Michie SA, Warnke RA, Dorfman RF: The "syncytial variant" of nodular sclerosing Hodgkin's disease. Am J Surg Pathol **10:**470-477, 1986.
441 Strum SB, Rappaport H: Interrelations of the histologic types of Hodgkin's dis-ease. Arch Pathol **91:**127-134, 1971.
442 Trudel MA, Krikorian JG, Neiman RS: Lymphocyte predominance Hodgkin's disease. A clinicopathologic reassessment. Cancer **59:**99-106, 1987.

Other microscopic features

443 Alavaikko MJ, Hansmann ML, Nebendahl C, Parwaresch MR, Lennert K: Fol-licular dendritic cells in Hodgkin's disease. Am J Clin Pathol **95:**194-200, 1991.
444 Colby TV, Hoppe RT, Warnke RA: Hodgkin's disease. A clinicopathologic study of 659 cases. Cancer **49:**1848-1858, 1982.
445 Crocker J, Smith PJ: A quantitative study of mast cells in Hodgkin's disease. J Clin Pathol **37:**519-522, 1984.
446 Doggett RS, Colby TV, Dorfman RF: Interfollicular Hodgkin's disease. Am J Surg Pathol **7:**145-149, 1983.
447 Kadin ME, Donaldson SS, Dorfman RF: Isolated granulomas in Hodgkin's dis-ease. N Engl J Med **283:**859-861, 1970.
448 Mohrmann RL, Nathwani BN, Brynes RK, Sheibani K: Hodgkin's disease occur-ring in monocytoid B-cell clusters. Am J Clin Pathol **95:**802-808, 1991.
449 Pak HY, Friedman NB: Pseudosarcoid granulomas in Hodgkin's disease. Hum Pathol **12:**832-837, 1981.
450 Rappaport H, Strum SB, Hutchison G, Allen LW: Clinical and biological signif-icance of vascular invasion in Hodgkin's disease. Cancer Res **31:**1794-1798, 1971.
451 Sacks EL, Donaldson SS, Gordon J, Dorfman RF: Epithelioid granulomas asso-ciated with Hodgkin's disease. Clinical correlations in 55 previously untreated patients. Cancer **41:**562-567, 1978.
452 Strum SB, Hutchison GB, Park JK, Rappaport H: Further observations on the biologic significance of vascular invasion in Hodgkin's disease. Cancer **27:**1-6, 1971.
453 Strum SB, Rappaport H: Significance of focal involvement of lymph nodes for the diagnosis and staging of Hodgkin's disease. Cancer **25:**1314-1319, 1970.
454 Variakojis D, Strum SB, Rappaport H: The foamy macrophages in Hodgkin's disease. Arch Pathol **93:**453-456, 1971.

General and clinical features

455 Akazaki K, Wakasa H: Frequency of lymphoreticular tumors and leukemias in Japan. J Natl Cancer Inst **52:**339-343, 1974.
456 Correa P, O'Conor GT: Epidemiologic patterns of Hodgkin's disease. Int J Can-cer **8:**192-201, 1971.
457 Cross RM: A clinicopathological study of nodular sclerosing Hodgkin's disease. J Clin Pathol **21:**303-310, 1968.

458 Greer JP, Kinney MC, Cousar JB, Flexner JM, Dupont WD, Graber SE, Greco FA, Collins RD, Stein RS: Lymphocyte-depleted Hodgkin's disease. Clinicopathologic review of 25 patients. Am J Med **81**:208-214, 1986.

459 Grufferman S, Delzell E: Epidemiology of Hodgkin's disease. Epidemiol Rev **6**:76-106, 1984.

460 Levy R, Kaplan HS: Impaired lymphocyte function in untreated Hodgkin's disease. N Engl J Med **290**:181-186, 1974.

461 Neiman RS: Current problems in the histopathologic diagnosis and classification of Hodgkin's disease. Pathol Annu **13**(Pt 2):289-328, 1978.

462 Neiman RS, Rosen PJ, Lukes RJ: Lymphocyte-depletion Hodgkin's disease. A clinicopathologic entity. N Engl J Med **288**:751-755, 1973.

463 Poppema S, Lennert K: Hodgkin's disease in childhood. Histopathologic classification in relation to age and sex. Cancer **45**:1443-1447, 1980.

464 Siebert JD, Stuckey JH, Kurtin PJ, Banks PM: Extranodal lymphocyte predominance Hodgkin's disease. Clinical and pathologic features. Am J Clin Pathol **103**:485-491, 1995.

465 Trotter MC, Cloud GA, Davis M, Sanford SP, Urist MM, Soong S-J, Halpern NB, Maddox WA, Balch CM: Predicting the risk of abdominal disease in Hodgkin's lymphoma. A multifactorial analysis of staging laparotomy results in 255 patients. Ann Surg **201**:465-469, 1985.

466 Unger PD, Strauchen JA: Hodgkin's disease in AIDS complex patients. Report of four cases and tissue immunologic marker studies. Cancer **58**:821-825, 1986.

467 White L, McCourt BA, Isaacs H, Siegel SE, Stowe SM, Higgins GR: Patterns of Hodgkin's disease at diagnosis in young children. Am J Pediatr Hematol Oncol **5**:251-257, 1983.

Spread

468 Aisenberg AC: Malignant lymphoma. N Engl J Med **288**:883-890, 935-941, 1973.

469 Glatstein E, Trueblood HW, Enright LP, Rosenberg SA, Kaplan HS: Surgical staging of abdominal involvement in unselected patients with Hodgkin's disease. Radiology **97**:425-432, 1970.

470 Kadin ME, Glatstein E, Dorfman RF: Clinicopathologic studies of 117 untreated patients subjected to laparotomy for the staging of Hodgkin's disease. Cancer **27**:1277-1294, 1971.

471 Kaplan HS: Contiguity and progression in Hodgkin's disease. Cancer Res **31**:1811-1813, 1971.

472 Keller AR, Kaplan HS, Lukes RJ, Rappaport H: Correlation of histopathology with other prognostic indicators in Hodgkin's disease. Cancer **22**:487-499, 1968.

473 Leslie KO, Colby TV: Hepatic parenchymal lymphoid aggregates in Hodgkin's disease. Hum Pathol **15**:808-809, 1984.

Staging

474 Carbone PP, Kaplan HS, Musshoff K, Smithers DW, Tubiana M: Report of the committee on Hodgkin's disease staging classification. Cancer Res **31**:1860-1861, 1971.

475 Hays DM, Ternberg JL, Chen TT, Sullivan MP, Fuller LM, Tefft M, Kung F, Gilchrist G, Fryer C, Heller RN, Wharam M, White L, Jenkins DL, Higgins G, Gehan EA: Complications related to 234 staging laparotomies performed in the Intergroup Hodgkin's Disease in Childhood Study. Surgery **96**:471-478, 1984.

476 Lacher MJ: Routine staging laparotomy for patients with Hodgkin's disease is no longer necessary. Cancer Invest **1**:93-99, 1983.

477 Lister TA, Crowther D, Sutcliffe SB, Glatstein E, Canellos GP, Young RC, Rosenberg SA, Coltman CA, Tubiana M: Report of a committee convened to discuss the evaluation and staging of patients with Hodgkin's disease. Cotswolds meeting. J Clin Oncol **7**:1630-1636, 1989.

Treatment

478 Anderson JE, Litzow MR, Appelbaum FR, Schoch G, Fisher LD, Buckner CD, Petersen FB, Crawford SW, Press OW, Sanders JE, et al.: Allogeneic, syngeneic, and autologous marrow transplantation for Hodgkin's disease. The 21-year Seattle experience. J Clin Oncol **11**:2342-2350, 1993.

479 Colby TV, Hoppe RT, Warnke RA: Hodgkin's disease at autopsy. 1972-1977. Cancer **47**:1852-1862, 1981.

480 Jones RJ, Piantadosi S, Mann RB, Ambinder RF, Seifter EJ, Vriesendorp HM, Abeloff MD, Burns WH, May WS, Rowley SD, et al.: High-dose cytotoxic therapy and bone marrow transplantation for relapsed Hodgkin's disease. J Clin Oncol **8**:527-537, 1990.

481 Rosenberg SA, Kaplan HS: The evolution and summary results of the Stanford randomized clinical trials of the management of Hodgkin's disease. 1962-1984. Int J Radiat Oncol Biol Phys **11**:5-22, 1985.

482 Straus DJ: Strategies in the treatment of Hodgkin's disease. Semin Oncol **13**:26-34, 1985.

483 Strum SB, Rappaport H: The persistence of Hodgkin's disease in long-term survivors. Am J Med **51**:222-240, 1971.

484 Urba WJ, Longo DL: Hodgkin's disease. N Engl J Med **326**:678-687, 1992.

Prognosis

485 Alavaikko MJ, Blanco G, Aine R, Lehtinen T, Fellbaum C, Taskinen PJ, Sarpola A, Hansmann ML: Follicular dendritic cells have prognostic relevance in Hodgkin's disease. Am J Clin Pathol **101**:761-767, 1994.

486 Bearman RM, Pangalis GA, Rappaport H: Hodgkin's disease, lymphocyte depletion type. A clinicopathologic study of 39 patients. Cancer **41**:293-302, 1978.

487 Butler JJ: Relationship of histologic findings to survival in Hodgkin's disease. Gann Monogr Cancer Res **15**:275-286, 1973.

488 Colby TV, Hoppe RT, Warnke RA: Hodgkin's disease. A clinicopathologic study of 659 cases. Cancer **49**:1848-1858, 1981.

489 Dimopoulos MA, Cabanillas F, Lee JJ, Swan F, Fuller L, Allen PK, Hagemeister FB: Prognostic role of serum beta 2-microglobulin in Hodgkin's disease. J Clin Oncol **11**:1108-1111, 1993.

490 Eghbali H, Hoerni-Simon G, de Mascarel I, Durand M, Chauvergne J, Hoerni B: Hodgkin's disease in the elderly. A series of 30 patients aged older than 70 years. Cancer **53**:2191-2193, 1984.

491 Ferry JA, Linggood RM, Convery KM, Efird JT, Eliseo R, Harris NL: Hodgkin disease, nodular sclerosis type. Implications of histologic subclassification. Cancer **71**:457-463, 1993.

492 Gause A, Roschansky V, Tschiersch A, Smith K, Hasenclever D, Schmits R, Diehl V, Pfreundschuh M: Low serum interleukin-2 receptor levels correlate with a good prognosis in patients with Hodgkin's lymphoma. Ann Oncol **2**(Suppl):43-47, 1991.

493 Kaplan HS: Hodgkin's disease, ed 2. Cambridge, Mass, 1980, Harvard University Press.

494 Keller AR, Kaplan HS, Lukes RJ, Rappaport H: Correlation of histopathology with other prognostic indicators in Hodgkin's disease. Cancer **22**:487-499, 1968.

495 Pizzolo G, Vinante F, Chilosi M, Dallenbach F, Josimovic-Alasevic O, Diamantstein T, Stein H: Serum levels of soluble CD30 molecule (Ki-1 antigen) in Hodgkin's disease. Relationship with disease activity and clinical stage. Br J Haematol **75**:282-284, 1990.

496 Straus DJ, Gaynor JJ, Myers J, Merke DP, Caravelli J, Chapman D, Yahalom J, Clarkson BD: Prognostic factors among 185 adults with newly diagnosed advanced Hodgkin's disease treated with alternating potentially non-cross-resistant chemotherapy and intermediate-dose radiation therapy. J Clin Oncol **8**:1173-1186, 1990.

497 Torti FM, Portlock CS, Rosenberg SA, Kaplan HS: Extralymphatic Hodgkin's disease. Prognosis and response to therapy. Am J Med **70**:487-492, 1981.

498 Trudel MA, Krikorian JG, Neiman RS: Lymphocyte predominance Hodgkin's disease. A clinicopathologic reassessment. Cancer **59**:99-106, 1987.

499 Wright CJE: Prospects of cure in lymphocyte-predominant Hodgkin's disease. Am J Clin Pathol **67**:507-511, 1977.

Non-Hodgkin's lymphoma

500 Alavaikko M, Aine R: The Lukes and Collins classification on non-Hodgkin's lymphomas. 1. A histological reappraisal of 301 cases. Acta Pathol Microbiol Immunol Scand (A) **90**:241-249, 1982.

501 Byrne GE Jr: Rappaport classification of non-Hodgkin's lymphoma. Histologic features and clinical significance. Cancer Treat Rep **61**:935-944, 1977.

502 Chan JKC, Banks PM, Cleary ML, Delsol G, De Wolf-Peeters C, Falini B, Gatter KC, Grogan TM, Harris NL, Isaacson PG, Jaffe ES, Knowles DM, Mason DY, Muller-Hermelink HK, Pileri SA, Piris MA, Ralfkiaer E, Stein H, Warnke RA: A revised European-American classification of lymphoid neoplasms proposed by the International Lymphoma Study Group. A summary version. Am J Clin Pathol **103**:543-560, 1995.

503 Dorfman RF: Classification of the malignant lymphomas. Am J Surg Pathol **1**:167-170, 1977.

504 Dorfman RF, Kim H: Relationship of histology to site in the non-Hodgkin's lymphomata. A study based on surgical staging procedures. Br J Cancer **31**:217-220, 1975.

505 Ersboll J, Schultz HB, Hougaard P, Nissen NI, Hou-Jensen K: Comparison of the working formulation of non-Hodgkin's lymphoma with the Rappaport, Kiel, and Lukes & Collins classifications. Translational value and prognostic significance based on review of 658 patients treated at a single institution. Cancer **55**:2442-2458, 1985.

506 Gall EA, Mallory TB: Malignant lymphoma. A clinicopathologic survey of 618 cases. Am J Pathol **18**:381-429, 1942.

507 Goffinet DR, Warnke R, Dunnick NR, Castellino R, Glatstein E, Nelsen TS, Dorfman RF, Rosenberg SA, Kaplan AS: Clinical and surgical (laparotomy) evaluation of patients with non-Hodgkin's lymphomas. Cancer Treat Rep **61:**981-992, 1977.

508 Harris NL, Jaffe ES, Stein H, Banks PM, Chan JK, Cleary ML, Delsol G, De Wolf-Peeters C, Falini B, Gatter KC, et al.: A revised European-American classification of lymphoid neoplasms. A proposal from the International Lymphoma Study Group. Blood **84:**1361-1392, 1994.

509 Lennert K: Classification of non-Hodgkin's lymphomas. In Lennert K, et al: Malignant lymphomas other than Hodgkin's disease. Histology, cytology, ultrastructure, immunology. Berlin, 1978, Springer-Verlag, pt 3, 1978, pp. 83-110.

510 Lennert K: The proposal for a revised European American lymphoma classification—a new start of a transatlantic discussion. Histopathology **26:**481-484, 1995.

511 Lennert K, Collins RD, Lukes RJ: Concordance of the Kiel and Lukes-Collins classifications of non-Hodgkin's lymphomas. Histopathology **7:**549-559, 1983.

512 Lennert K, Feller AC: Histopathology of non-Hodgkin's lymphomas, New York, 1992, Springer-Verlag.

513 Lukes RJ, Collins RD: Immunologic characterization of human malignant lymphomas. Cancer **34:**1488-1503, 1974.

514 Lukes RJ, Parker JW, Taylor CR, Tindle BH, Cramer AD, Lincoln TL: Immunologic approach to non-Hodgkin lymphomas and related leukemias. Analysis of the results of multiparameter studies of 425 cases. Semin Hematol **15:**322-351, 1978.

515 Nathwani BN: A critical analysis of the classifications of non-Hodgkin's lymphomas. Cancer **44:**347-384, 1979.

516 Nathwani BN, Kim H, Rappaport H, Solomon J, Fox M: Non-Hodgkin's lymphomas. A clinicopathologic study comparing two classifications. Cancer **41:**303-325, 1978.

517 NCI Non-Hodgkin's Classification Project Writing Committee: Classification of non-Hodgkin's lymphomas. Reproducibility of major classification systems. Cancer **55:**91-95, 1985.

518 Non-Hodgkin's Lymphoma Pathologic Classification Project: National Cancer Institute sponsored study of classifications of non-Hodgkin's lymphoma. Summary and description of a working formulation for clinical usage. Cancer **49:**2112-2135, 1982.

519 Rappaport H: Tumors of the hematopoietic system. In Atlas of tumor pathology. Sect. 3, Fasc. 8. Washington, DC, 1966, Armed Forces Institute of Pathology.

520 Rosenberg SA, Dorfman RF, Kaplan HS: A summary of the results of a review of 405 patients with non-Hodgkin's lymphoma at Stanford University. Br J Cancer **31:**168-173, 1975.

Small lymphocytic lymphoma

521 Armitage JO, Dick FR, Corder MP: Diffuse histiocytic lymphoma complicating chronic lymphocytic leukemia. Cancer **41:**422-427, 1978.

522 Batata A, Shen B: Relationship between chronic lymphocytic leukemia and small lymphocytic lymphoma. A comparative study of membrane phenotypes in 270 cases. Cancer **70:**625-632, 1992.

523 Ben-Ezra J, Burke JS, Swartz WG, Brownell MD, Brynes RK, Hill LR, Nathwani BN, Oken MM, Wolf BC, Woodruff R, et al.: Small lymphocytic lymphoma. A clinicopathologic analysis of 268 cases. Blood **73:**579-587, 1989.

524 Berger F, Felman P, Sonet A, Salles G, Bastion Y, Bryon PA, Coiffier B: Non-follicular small B-cell lymphomas. A heterogeneous group of patients with distinct clinical features and outcome. Blood **83:**2829-2835, 1994.

525 Brecher M, Banks PM: Hodgkin's disease variant of Richter's syndrome. Report of eight cases. Am J Clin Pathol **93:**333-339, 1990.

526 Brouet J-C, Sasportes M, Flandrin G, Preud'Homme J-L, Seligmann M: Chronic lymphocytic leukaemia of T-cell origin. Immunological and clinical evaluation in eleven patients. Lancet **2:**890-893, 1975.

527 Carbone A, Pinto A, Gloghini A, Volpe R, Zagonel V: B-zone small lymphocytic lymphoma. A morphologic, immunophenotypic, and clinical study with comparison to "well-differentiated" lymphocytic disorders. Hum Pathol **23:**438-448, 1992.

528 Dick FR, Maca RD: The lymph node in chronic lymphocytic leukemia. Cancer **41:**283-292, 1978.

529 Dorfman DM, Pinkus GS: Distinction between small lymphocytic and mantle cell lymphoma by immunoreactivity for CD23. Mod Pathol **7:**326-331, 1994.

530 Ellison DJ, Nathwani BN, Cho SY, Martin SE: Interfollicular small lymphocytic lymphoma. The diagnostic significance of pseudofollicles. Hum Pathol **20:**1108-1118, 1989.

531 Foucar C, Rydell RE: Richter's syndrome in chronic lymphocytic leukemia. Cancer **46:**118-134, 1980.

532 Harris NL, Bhan AK: B-cell neoplasms of the lymphocytic, lymphoplasmacytoid, and plasma cell types. Immunohistologic analysis and clinical correlation. Hum Pathol **16:**829-837, 1985.

533 Knuutila S, Elonen E, Teerenhovi L, Rossi L, Leskinen R, Bloomfield CD, de la Chapelle A: Trisomy 12 in B cells of patients with B-cell chronic lymphocytic leukemia. N Engl J Med **314:**865-869, 1986.

534 Lennert K: Malignant lymphomas other than Hodgkin's disease. Histology. Cytology. Ultrastructure. Immunology. Berlin, 1978, Springer-Verlag.

535 Long JC, Aisenberg AC: Richter's syndrome. A terminal complication of chronic lymphocytic leukemia with distinct clinicopathologic features. Am J Clin Pathol **63:**786-795, 1975.

536 McKenna RW, Parkin J, Kersey JH, Gajl-Peczalska KJ, Peterson L, Brunning RD: Chronic lymphoproliferative disorder with unusual clinical, morphologic, ultrastructural and membrane surface marker characteristics. Am J Med **62:**588-596, 1977.

537 Medeiros LJ, Strickler JG, Picker LJ, Gelb AB, Weiss LM, Warnke RA: "Well-differentiated" lymphocytic neoplasms. Immunologic findings correlated with clinical presentation and morphologic features. Am J Pathol **129:**523-535, 1987.

538 Momose H, Jaffe ES, Shin SS, Chen YY, Weiss LM: Chronic lymphocytic leukemia/small lymphocytic lymphoma with Reed-Sternberg-like cells and possible transformation to Hodgkin's disease. Mediation by Epstein-Barr virus. Am J Surg Pathol **16:**859-867, 1992.

539 Morrison WH, Hoppe RT, Weiss LM, Picozzi VJ Jr, Horning SJ: Small lymphocytic lymphoma. J Clin Oncol **7:**598-606, 1989.

540 Pangalis GA, Nathwani BN, Rappaport H: Malignant lymphoma, well differentiated lymphocytic. Its relationship with chronic lymphocytic leukemia and macroglobulinemia of Waldenström. Cancer **39:**999-1010, 1977.

541 Schmid C, Isaacson PG: Proliferation centres in B-cell malignant lymphoma, lymphocytic (BCLL). An immunophenotypic study. Histopathology **24:**445-451, 1994.

542 Sheibani K, Nathwani BN, Winberg CD, Scott EP, Teplitz RR, Rappaport H: Small lymphocytic lymphoma. Morphologic and immunologic progression. Am J Clin Pathol **84:**237-243, 1985.

543 Spier CM, Grogan TM, Fielder K, Richter L, Rangel C: Immunophenotypes in "well-differentiated" lymphoproliferative disorders, with emphasis on small lymphocytic lymphoma. Hum Pathol **17:**1126-1136, 1986.

544 Sundeen JT, Longo DL, Jaffe ES: CD5 expression in B-cell small lymphocytic malignancies. Correlations with clinical presentation and sites of disease. Am J Surg Pathol **16:**130-137, 1992.

545 Trump DL, Mann RB, Phelps R, Roberts H, Conley CL: Richter's syndrome. Diffuse histiocytic lymphoma in patients with chronic lymphocytic leukemia. A report of five cases and review of the literature. Am J Med **68:**539-548, 1980.

546 Williams J, Schned A, Cotelingam JD, Jaffe ES: Chronic lymphocytic leukemia with coexistent Hodgkin's disease. Implications for the origin of the Reed-Sternberg cell. Am J Surg Pathol **15:**33-42, 1991.

Lymphoma and dysproteinemia

547 Addis BJ, Isaacson P, Billings JA: Plasmacytoma of lymph nodes. Cancer **46:**340-346, 1980.

548 Alexanian R: Monoclonal gammopathy in lymphoma. Arch Intern Med **135:**62-66, 1975.

549 Brouet J-C, Clauvel J-P, Danon F, Klein M, Seligmann M: Biologic and clinical significance of cryoglobulins. A report of 86 cases. Am J Med **57:**775-788, 1974.

550 Brunning RD, Parkin J: Intranuclear inclusions in plasma cells and lymphocytes from patients with monoclonal gammopathies. Am J Clin Pathol **66:**10-21, 1976.

551 Cohen RJ, Bohannon RA, Wallterstein RO: Waldenstrom's macroglobulinemia. A study of ten cases. Am J Med **41:**274, 1966.

552 Dutcher TF, Fahey JL: The histopathology of the macroglobulinemia of Waldenstrom. J Natl Cancer Inst **22:**887-917, 1959.

553 Fishkin BG, Spiegelberg HL: Cervical lymph node metastasis as the first manifestation of localized extramedullary plasmacytoma. Cancer **38:**1641-1644, 1976.

554 Franklin EC, Lowenstein J, Bigelow B, Meltzer M: Heavy chain disease. A new disorder of serum gamma-globulins. Report of the first case. Am J Med **37:**332-350, 1964.

555 Harris NL, Bhan AK: B-cell neoplasms of the lymphocytic, lymphoplasmacytoid, and plasma cell types. Immunohistologic analysis and clinical correlation. Hum Pathol **16:**829-837, 1985.

556 Harrison CV: The morphology of the lymph node in the macroglobulinaemia of Waldenstrom. J Clin Pathol **25:**12-16, 1972.

557 Kim H, Dorfman RF, Rappaport H: Signet ring cell lymphoma. A rare morphologic and functional expression of nodular (follicular) lymphoma. Am J Surg Pathol **2:**119-132, 1978.

558 Kim H, Heller P, Rappaport H: Monoclonal gammopathies associated with lymphoproliferative disorders. A morphologic study. Am J Clin Pathol **59:**282-294, 1973.

559 Krauss S, Sokal JE: Paraproteinemia in the lymphomas. Am J Med **40**:400-413, 1966.

560 Lee SL, Rosner F, Ruberman W,Glasberg S: μ-Chain disease. Ann Intern Med **75**:407-414, 1971.

561 Mennemeyer R, Hammar SP, Cathey WJ: Malignant lymphoma with intracytoplasmic IgM crystalline inclusions. N Engl J Med **291**:960-963, 1974.

562 Pangalis GA, Nathwani BN, Rappaport H: Detection of cytoplasmic immunoglobulin in well-differentiated lymphoproliferative diseases by the immunoperoxidase method. Cancer **45**:1334-1339, 1980.

563 Papadimitriou CS, Müller-Hermelink U, Lennert K: Histologic and immunohistochemical findings in the differential diagnosis of chronic lymphocytic leukemia of B-cell type and lymphoplasmacytic/lymphoplasmacytoid lymphoma. Virchows Arch [A] **384**:149-158, 1979.

564 Peters O, Thielemans C, Steenssens L, De Waele M, Hijmans W, Van Camp B: Intracellular inclusion bodies in 14 patients with B cell lymphoproliferative disorders. J Clin Pathol **37**:45-50, 1984.

565 Seligmann M: Immunochemical, clinical, and pathological features of a-chain disease. Arch Intern Med **135**:78-82, 1975.

566 Seligmann M, Danon F, Hurez D, Mihaesco E, Preud'homme J-L: Alpha-chain disease. A new immunoglobulin abnormality. Science **162**:1396-1397, 1968.

567 Zukerberg LR, Medeiros LJ, Ferry JA, Harris NL: Diffuse low-grade B-cell lymphomas. Four clinically distinct subtypes defined by a combination of morphologic and immunophenotypic features. Am J Clin Pathol **100**:373-385, 1993.

Follicular lymphoma

568 Anderson T, Bender RA, Fisher RI, DeVita VT, Chabner BA, Berard CW, Norton L, Young RC: Combination chemotherapy in non-Hodgkin's lymphoma. Results of long-term followup. Cancer Treat Rep **61**:1057-1066, 1977.

569 Bastion Y, Berger F, Bryon PA, Felman P, Ffreuch M, Coiffier B: Follicular lymphomas. Assessment of prognostic factors in 127 patients followed for 10 years. Ann Oncol **2**:123-129, 1991.

570 Bennett MH: Sclerosis in non-Hodgkin's lymphomata. Br J Cancer **31**:44-52, 1975.

571 Chan JK, Ng CS, Hui PK: An unusual morphological variant of follicular lymphoma. Report of two cases. Histopathology **12**:649-658, 1988.

572 Chan JK, Ng CS, Tung S: Multilobated B-cell lymphoma, a variant of centroblastic lymphoma. Report of four cases. Histopathology **10**:601-612, 1986.

573 Chang KL, Arber DA, Shibata D, Rappaport H, Weiss LM: Follicular small lymphocytic lymphoma. Am J Surg Pathol **18**:999-1009, 1994.

574 Chittal SM, Caverivière P, Voigt J-J, Dumont J, Bénévent B, Fauré P, Bordessoule GD, Delsol G: Follicular lymphoma with abundant PAS-positive extracellular material. Immunohistochemical and ultrastructural observations. Am J Surg Pathol **11**:618-624, 1987.

575 Coiffier B, Bastion Y, Berger F, Felman P, Bryon PA: Prognostic factors in follicular lymphomas. Semin Oncol **20**:89-95, 1993.

576 Come SE, Jaffe ES, Anderson JC, Mann RB, Johnson BL, DeVita VT, Young RC: Non-Hodgkin's lymphomas in leukemic phase. Clinicopathologic correlations. Am J Med **69**:667-674, 1980.

577 Crisan D, Anstett MJ: Bcl-2 gene rearrangements in follicular lymphomas. Lab Med **24**:579-588, 1993.

578 Frizzera G, Anaya JS, Banks PM: Neoplastic plasma cells in follicular lymphomas. Clinical and pathologic findings in six cases. Virchows Arch [A] **409**:149-162, 1986.

579 Frizzera G, Gajl-Peczalska K, Sibley RK, Rosai J, Cherwitz D, Hurd DD: Rosette formation in malignant lymphoma. Am J Pathol **119**:351-356, 1985.

580 Garvin AJ, Simon RM, Osborne CK, Merrill J, Young RC, Berard CW: An autopsy study of histologic progression in non-Hodgkin's lymphomas. 192 cases from the National Cancer Institute. Cancer **52**:393-398, 1983.

581 Gaulard P, d'Agay MF, Peuchmaur M, Brousse N, Gisselbrecht C, Solal-Celigny P, Diebold J, Mason DY: Expression of the bcl-2 gene product in follicular lymphoma. Am J Pathol **140**:1089-1095, 1992.

582 Goates JJ, Kamel OW, Le Brun DP, Benharroch D, Dorfman RF: Floral variant of follicular lymphoma. Immunological and molecular studies support a neoplastic process. Am J Surg Pathol **18**:37-47, 1994.

583 Hockenbery D, Nunez G, Milliman C, Schreiber RD, Korsmeyer SJ: Bcl-2 is an inner mitochondrial membrane protein that blocks programmed cell death. Nature **348**:334-336, 1990.

584 Horning SJ, Weiss LM, Nevitt JB, Warnke RA: Clinical and pathologic features of follicular large cell (nodular histiocytic) lymphoma. Cancer **59**:1470-1474, 1987.

585 Horsman DE, Gascoyne RD, Coupland RW, Coldman AJ, Adomat SA: Comparison of cytogenetic analysis, Southern analysis, and polymerase chain reaction for the detection of t(14;18) in follicular lymphoma. Am J Clin Pathol **103**:472-478, 1995.

586 Jones SE, Fuks Z, Bull M, Kadin ME, Dorfman RF, Kaplan HS, Rosenberg SA, Kim H: Non-Hodgkin's lymphomas. IV. Clinicopathologic correlation in 405 cases. Cancer **31**:806-823, 1973.

587 Keith TA, Cousar JB, Glick AD, Vogler LB, Collins RD: Plasmacytic differentiation in follicular center cell (FCC) lymphomas. Am J Clin Pathol **84**:283-290, 1985.

588 Kim H, Dorfman RF: Morphological studies of 84 untreated patients subjected to laparotomy for the staging of non-Hodgkin's lymphomas. Cancer **33**:657-674, 1974.

589 Kim H, Dorfman RF, Rappaport H: Signet ring cell lymphoma. A rare morphologic and functional expression of nodular (follicular) lymphoma. Am J Surg Pathol **2**:119-132, 1978.

590 Korsmeyer SJ: Bcl-2 initiates a new category of oncogenes. Regulators of cell death. Blood **80**:879-886, 1992.

591 Ladanyi M, Offit K, Parsa NZ, Condon MR, Chekka N, Murphy JP, Filippa DA, Jhanwar SC, Dalla-Favera R, Chaganti RS: Follicular lymphoma with t(8; 14)(q24; q32). A distinct clinical and molecular subset of t(8; 14)-bearing lymphomas. Blood **79**:2124-2130, 1992.

592 Ladanyi M, Wang S: Detection of rearrangements of the bcl-2 major breakpoint region in follicular lymphomas. Correlation of polymerase chain reaction results with Southern blot analysis. Diagn Mol Pathol **1**:31-35, 1992.

593 Lambrechts AC, Hupkes PE, Dorssers LC, van't Veer MB: Clinical significance of t(14; 18)-positive cells in the circulation of patients with stage III or IV follicular non-Hodgkin's lymphoma during first remission. J Clin Oncol **12**:1541-1546, 1994.

594 Levine GD, Dorfman RF: Nodular lymphoma. An ultrastructural study of its relationship to germinal centers and a correlation of light and electron microscopic findings. Cancer **35**:148-164, 1975.

595 Lister TA: The management of follicular lymphoma. Ann Oncol **2**(suppl 2):131-135, 1991.

596 McKenna RW, Brunning RD: Reed-Sternberg-like cells in nodular lymphoma involving the bone marrow. Am J Clin Pathol **63**:779-785, 1975.

597 Mollejo M, Menarguez J, Cristobal E, Algara P, Sanchez-Diaz E, Fraga M, Piris MA: Monocytoid B cells. A comparative clinical pathological study of their distribution in different types of low-grade lymphomas. Am J Surg Pathol **18**:1131-1139, 1994.

598 Nathwani BN, Sheibani K, Winberg CD, Burke JS, Rappaport H: Neoplastic B cells with cerebriform nuclei in follicular lymphomas. Hum Pathol **16**:173-180, 1985.

599 Ngan BY, Chen-Levy Z, Weiss LM, Warnke RA, Cleary ML: Expression in non-Hodgkin's lymphoma of the bcl-2 protein associated with the t(14; 18) chromosomal translocation. N Engl J Med **318**:1638-1644, 1988.

600 Osborne BM, Butler JJ: Follicular lymphoma mimicking progressive transformation of germinal centers. Am J Clin Pathol **88**:264-269, 1987.

601 Oviatt DL, Cousar JB, Collins RD, Flexner JM, Stein RS: Malignant lymphomas of follicular center cell origin in humans. V. Incidence, clinical features, and prognostic implications of transformation of small cleaved cell nodular lymphoma. Cancer **53**:1109-1114, 1984.

602 Pezzella F, Gatter K: What is the value of bcl-2 protein detection for histopathologists? Histopathology **26**:89-94, 1995.

603 Pinto A, Hutchison RE, Grant LH, Trevenen CL, Berard CW: Follicular lymphomas in pediatric patients. Mod Pathol **3**:308-313, 1990.

604 Rappaport H, Winter WJ, Hicks EB: Follicular lymphoma. A re-evaluation of its position in the scheme of malignant lymphoma, based on a survey of 253 cases. Cancer **9**:792-821, 1956.

605 Rohatiner AZ, Lister TA: New approaches to the treatment of follicular lymphoma. Br J Haematol **79**:349-354, 1991.

606 Rosas-Uribe A, Variakojis D, Rappaport H: Proteinaceous precipitate in nodular (follicular) lymphomas. Cancer **31**:534-542, 1973.

607 Scoazec JY, Berger F, Magaud JP, Brochier J, Coiffier B, Bryon PA: The dendritic reticulum cell pattern in B cell lymphomas of the small cleaved, mixed, and large cell types. An immunohistochemical study of 48 cases. Hum Pathol **20**:124-131, 1989

608 Swerdlow SH, Murray LJ, Habeshaw JA, Stansfeld AG: B- and T-cell subsets in follicular centroblastic/centrocytic (cleaved follicular center cell) lymphoma. An immunohistologic analysis of 26 lymph nodes and three spleens. Hum Pathol **16**:339-352, 1985.

609 Utz GL, Swerdlow SH: Distinction of follicular hyperplasia from follicular lymphoma in B5-fixed tissues. Comparison of MT2 and bcl-2 antibodies. Hum Pathol **24**:1155-1158, 1993.

610 van den Berg HM, Molenaar WM, Poppema S, Halie MR: The heterogeneity of follicular follicle center cell tumors. II. Clinical follow-up of 30 patients. Cancer **52**:2264-2268, 1983.

610a Veloso JD, Rezuke WN, Cartun RW, Abernathy EC, Pastuszak WT: Immuno-histochemical distinction of follicular lymphoma from follicular hyperplasia in formalin-fixed tissues using monoclonal antibodies MT2 and bcl-2. Appl Immunohistochem **3**:153-159, 1995.

611 Warnke RA, Kim H, Fuks D, Dorfman RF: The coexistence of nodular and dif-fuse patterns in nodular non-Hodgkin's lymphomas. Significance and clinico-pathologic correlation. Cancer **40**:1229-1233, 1977.

612 Winberg CD, Nathwani BN, Bearman RM, Rappaport H: Follicular (nodular) lymphoma during the first two decades of life. A clinicopathologic study of 12 patients. Cancer **48**:2223-2235, 1981.

613 Wood BL, Bacchi MM, Bacchi CE, Kidd P, Gown AM: Immunocytochemical differentiation of reactive hyperplasia from follicular lymphoma using mono-clonal antibodies to cell surface and proliferation-related markers. Diagn Immunohistochem **2**:48-53, 1994.

614 Young RC, Longo DL, Glatstein E, Ihde DC, Jaffe ES, DeVita VT Jr: The treat-ment of indolent lymphomas. Watchful waiting *V* aggressive combined modal-ity treatment. Semin Hematol **25**:11-16, 1988.

Mantle cell lymphoma

615 Banks PM, Chan J, Cleary ML, Delsol G, De Wolf-Peeters C, Gatter K, Grogan TM, Harris NL, Isaacson PG, Jaffe ES, et al.: Mantle cell lymphoma. A proposal for unification of morphologic, immunologic, and molecular data. Am J Surg Pathol **16**:637-640, 1992.

616 Bookman MA, Lardelli P, Jaffe ES, Duffey PL, Longo DL: Lymphocytic lym-phoma of intermediate differentiation. Morphologic, immunophenotypic, and prognostic factors. J Natl Cancer Inst **82**:742-748, 1990.

617 Duggan MJ, Weisenburger DD, Ye YL, Bast MA, Pierson JL, Linder J, Armitage JO: Mantle zone lymphoma. A clinicopathologic study of 22 cases. Cancer **66**:522-529, 1990.

618 Ellison DJ, Turner RR, Van Antwerp R, Martin SE, Nathwani BN: High-grade mantle zone lymphoma. Cancer **60**:2717-2720, 1987.

619 Jaffe ES, Bookman MA, Longo DL: Lymphocytic lymphoma of intermediate differentiation—mantle zone lymphoma. A distinct subtype of B-cell lymphoma. Hum Pathol **18**:877-880, 1987.

620 Motokura T, Bloom T, Kim HG, et al.: A novel cyclin encoded by a bcl-1 linked candidate oncogene. Nature **350**:512-515, 1991.

621 Pittaluga S, Wlodarska I, Stul MS, Thomas J, Verhoef G, Cassiman JJ, van den Berghe H, De Wolf-Peeters C: Mantle cell lymphoma. A clinicopathological study of 55 cases. Histopathology **26**:17-24, 1995.

622 Rimokh R, Berger F, Cornillet P, Wahbi K, Rouault JP, Ffrench M, Bryon PA, Gadoux M, Gentilhomme O, Germain D, et al.: Break in the BCL1 locus is closely associated with intermediate lymphocytic lymphoma subtype. Genes Chromosom Cancer **2**:223-226, 1990.

623 Strickler JG, Medeiros, LJ, Copenhaver CM, Weiss LM, Warnke RA: Interme-diate lymphocytic lymphoma. An immunophenotypic study with comparison to small lymphocytic lymphoma and diffuse small cleaved cell lymphoma. Hum Pathol **19**:550-554, 1988.

623a Swerdlow SH, Yang W-I, Zukerberg LR, Harris NL, Arnold A, Williams ME: Expression of cyclin D1 protein in centrocytic/mantle cell lymphomas with and without rearrangement of the bc11/cyclin D1 gene. Hum Pathol **26**:999-1004, 1995.

624 van den Oord, de Wolf-Peeters C, Pulford KAF, Mason DY, Desmet VJ: Mantle zone lymphoma. Immuno- and enzyme-histochemical studies on the cell of ori-gin. Am J Surg Pathol **10**:780-788, 1986.

625 Weisenburger DD, Nathwani BN, Diamond LW, Winberg BD, Rappaport H: Malignant lymphoma, intermediate lymphocytic type. A clinicopathologic study of 42 cases. Cancer **48**:1415-1425, 1981.

626 Withers DA, Harvey RC, Faust JB, Melnyk O, Carey K, Meeker TC: Character-ization of a candidate bcl-1 gene. Mol Cell Biol **11**:4846-4853, 1991.

Monocytoid B-cell lymphoma, MALT-lymphoma, and marginal zone lymphoma

627 Ashton-Key M, Biddolph SC, Stein H, Gatter KC, Mason DY: Heterogeneity of bcl-2 expression in MALT lymphoma. Histopathology **26**:75-78, 1995.

628 Chan JK, Ng CS, Isaacson PG: Relationship between high-grade lymphoma and low-grade B-cell mucosa-associated lymphoid tissue lymphoma (MALToma) of the stomach. Am J Pathol **136**:1153-1164, 1990.

629 Cogliatti SB, Lennert K, Hansmann ML, Zwingers TL: Monocytoid B cell lym-phoma. Clinical and prognostic features of 21 patients. J Clin Pathol **43**:619-625, 1990.

630 Cousar JB, McGinn DL, Glick AD, List AF, Collins RD: Report of an unusual lymphoma arising from parafollicular B-lymphocytes (PBLs) or so-called "monocytoid" lymphocytes. Am J Clin Pathol **87**:121-128, 1987.

631 Isaacson PG, Spencer J: Monocytoid B-cell lymphomas. Am J Surg Pathol **14**:888-891, 1990.

631a Mori N, Yatabe Y, Asai J: Mucosa-associated lymphoid tissue (MALT) lym-phoma. Pathol Int **45**:544-551, 1995.

632 Nathwani BN, Mohrmann RL, Brynes RK, Taylor CR, Hansmann ML, Sheibani K: Monocytoid B-cell lymphomas. An assessment of diagnostic criteria and a perspective on histogenesis. Hum Pathol **23**:1061-1071, 1992.

633 Neiman RS, Sullivan AL, Jaffe R: Malignant lymphoma simulating leukemic reticuloendotheliosis. A clinicopathologic study of ten cases. Cancer **43**:329-342, 1979.

634 Ngan BY, Warnke RA, Wilson M, Takagi K, Cleary ML, Dorfman RF: Mono-cytoid B-cell lymphoma. A study of 36 cases. Hum Pathol **22**:409-421, 1991.

635 Piris MA, Rivas C, Morente M, Cruz MA, Rubio C, Oliva H: Monocytoid B-cell lymphoma, a tumour related to the marginal zone. Histopathology **12**:383-392, 1988.

636 Schmid C, Kirkham N, Diss T, Isaacson PG: Splenic marginal zone cell lym-phoma. Am J Surg Pathol **16**:455-466, 1992.

637 Sheibani K, Burke JS, Swartz WG, Nademanee A, Winberg CD: Monocytoid B-cell lymphoma. Clinicopathologic study of 21 cases of a unique type of low-grade lymphoma. Cancer **62**:1531-1538, 1988.

638 van Krieken JH, von Schilling C, Kluin PM, Lennert K: Splenic marginal zone lymphocytes and related cells in the lymph node. A morphologic and immuno-histochemical study. Hum Pathol **20**:320-325, 1989.

639 Wotherspoon AC, Finn T, Isaacson PG: Numerical abnormalities of chromo-somes 3 and 7 in lymphomas of mucosa associated lymphoid tissue and the splenic marginal zone (abstract). Lab Invest **7**:124A, 1994.

640 Wotherspoon AC, Pan LX, Diss TC, Isaacson PG: A genotypic study of low grade B-cell lymphomas, including lymphomas of mucosa associated lymphoid tissue (MALT). J Pathol **162**:135-140, 1990.

Diffuse mixed (small and large cell) lymphoma

641 Hu E, Weiss LM, Hoppe RT, Horning SJ: Follicular and diffuse mixed small-cleaved and large-cell lymphoma—a clinicopathologic study. J Clin Oncol **3**:1183-1187, 1985.

642 Katzin WE, Linden MD, Fishleder AJ, Tubbs RR: Immunophenotypic and geno-typic characterization of diffuse mixed non-Hodgkin's lymphomas. Am J Pathol **135**:615-621, 1989.

643 Medeiros LJ, Lardelli P, Stetler-Stevenson M, Longo DL, Jaffe ES: Genotypic analysis of diffuse mixed cell lymphomas. Comparison with morphologic and immunophenotypic findings. Am J Clin Pathol **95**:547-555, 1991.

Diffuse large cell lymphoma

644 Aisenberg AC, Wilkes BM, Jacobson JO: The bcl-2 gene is rearranged in many diffuse B-cell lymphomas. Blood **71**:969-972, 1988.

645 Armitage JO: Treatment of non-Hodgkin's lymphoma. N Engl J Med **328**:1023-1030, 1993.

646 Azar HA, Jaffe ES, Berard CW, Callihan TR, Braylan RR, Cossman J, Triche TJ: Diffuse large cell lymphomas (reticulum cell sarcomas, histiocytic lymphomas). Correlation of morphologic features with functional markers. Cancer **46**:1428-1441, 1980.

647 Baddoura FK, Chan WC, Masih AS, Mitchell D, Sun NC, Weisenburger DD: T-cell-rich B-cell lymphoma. A clinicopathologic study of eight cases. Am J Clin Pathol **103**:65-75, 1995.

648 Bennett MH: Sclerosis in non-Hodgkins's lymphoma. Br J Cancer **31**:44-52, 1975.

649 Bernier V, Azar HA: Filiform large-cell lymphomas. An ultrastructural and immunohistochemical study. Am J Surg Pathol **11**:387-396, 1987.

650 Chabner BA, Johnson RE, Young RC, Canellos GP, Hubbard SP, Johnson SK, DeVita VT Jr: Sequential nonsurgical and surgical staging of non-Hodgkin's lymphoma. Ann Intern Med **85**:149-154, 1976.

651 Cleary ML, Trela MJ, Weiss LM, Warnke R, Sklar J: Most null large cell lym-phomas are B lineage neoplasms. Lab Invest **53**:521-525, 1985.

652 Coiffier B, Brousse N, Peuchmaur M, Berger F, Gisselbrecht C, Bryon PA, Diebold J: Peripheral T-cell lymphomas have a worse prognosis than B-cell lym-phomas. A prospective study of 361 immunophenotyped patients treatedwith the LNH-84 regimen. The GELA (Groupe d'Etude des Lymphomes Agressives). Ann Oncol **1**:45-50, 1990.

653 Dalla-Favera R, Ye RH, Lo Coco F, Gaidano G, Lista F, Knowles DM, Louie DC, Offitt K, Chaganti RSK: Identification of genetic lesions associated with dif-fuse large-cell lymphoma. Ann Oncol **5**:S55-60, 1994.

654 DeVita VT Jr, Hubbard SM, Young RC, Longo DL: The role of chemotherapy in diffuse aggressive lymphomas. Semin Hematol **25**:2-10, 1988.

655 De Wolf-Peeters C, Pittaluga S: T-cell rich B-cell lymphoma. A morphological variant of a variety of non-Hodgkin's lymphomas or a clinicopathological entity? Histopathology 26:383-386, 1995.

656 Fung DT, Chan JK, Tse CC, Sze WM: Myxoid change in malignant lymphoma. Pathogenetic considerations. Arch Pathol Lab Med 116:103-105, 1992.

657 Greer JP, Macon WR, Lamar RE, Wolff SN, Stein RS, Flexner JM, Collins RD, Cousar JB: T-cell-rich B-cell lymphomas. Diagnosis and response to therapy of 44 patients. J Clin Oncol 13:1742-1750, 1995.

658 Kwak LW, Wilson M, Weiss LM, Doggett R, Dorfman RF, Warnke RA, Horning SJ: Similar outcome of treatment of B-cell and T-cell diffuse large-cell lymphomas. The Stanford experience. J Clin Oncol 9:1426-1431, 1991.

659 Lichtenstein A, Levine AM, Lukes RJ, Cramer AD, Taylor CR, Lincoln TL, Feinstein DI: Immunoblastic sarcoma. A clinical description. Cancer 43:343-352, 1979.

660 Lo Coco F, Ye BH, Lista F, Corradini P, Offit K, Knowles DM, Chaganti RS, Dalla-Favera R: Rearrangements of the BCL6 gene in diffuse large cell non-Hodgkin's lymphoma. Blood 83:1757-1759, 1994.

661 Lukes RJ, Parker JW, Taylor CR, Tindle BH, Cramer AD, Lincoln TL: Immunologic approach to non-Hodgkin lymphomas and related leukemias. Analysis of the results of multiparameter studies of 425 cases. Semin Hematol 15:322-351, 1978.

662 Macon WR, Williams ME, Greer JP, Stein RS, Collins RD, Cousar JB: T-cell-rich B-cell lymphomas. A clinicopathologic study of 19 cases. Am J Surg Pathol 16:351-363, 1992.

663 Mann RB, Jaffe ES, Berard CW: Malignant lymphoma. A conceptual understanding of morphologic diversity. A review. Am J Pathol 94:105-191, 1979.

664 McCurley TL, Gay RE, Gay S, Glick AD, Haralson MA, Collins RD: The extracellular matrix in "sclerosing" follicular center cell lymphomas. An immunohistochemical and ultrastructural study. Hum Pathol 17:930-938, 1986.

665 Nakamine H, Masih AS, Strobach RS, Duggan MJ, Bast MA, Armitage JO, Weisenburger DD: Immunoblastic lymphoma with abundant clear cytoplasm, a comparative study of B- and T- cell types. Am J Clin Pathol 96:177-183, 1991.

666 Ng CS, Chan JKC, Hui PK: Heterogeneity of interfollicular lymphomas (abstract). Surg Pathol 4:372, 1991.

667 Offit K, Lo Coco F, Louie DC, Parsa NZ, Leung D, Portlock C, Ye BH, Lista F, Filippa DA, Rosenbaum A, et al.: Rearrangement of the bcl-6 gene as a prognostic marker in diffuse large-cell lymphoma. N Engl J Med 331:74-80, 1994.

668 O'Hara CJ, Said JW, Pinkus GS: Non-Hodgkin's lymphoma, multilobated B-cell type. Report of nine cases with immunohistochemical and immunoultrastructural evidence for a follicular center cell derivation. Hum Pathol 17:593-599, 1986.

669 Osborne BM, Mackay B, Butler JJ, Ordonez NG: Large cell lymphoma with microvillus-like projections. An ultrastructural study. Am J Clin Pathol 79:443-450, 1983.

670 Osborne BM, Butler JJ, Mackay B: Sinusoidal large cell ("histiocytic") lymphoma. Cancer 46:2484-2491, 1980.

671 Pileri S, Falini B, Delsol G, Stein H, Baglioni P, Poggi S, Martelli MF, Rivano MT, Mason DY, Stansfeld AG: Lymphohistiocytic T-cell lymphoma (anaplastic large cell lymphoma CD301 /Ki1 1 with a high content of reactive histiocytes). Histopathology 16:383-391, 1990.

672 Ree HJ, Leone LA, Crowley JP: Sclerosis in diffuse histiocytic lymphoma. A clinicopathologic study of 25 cases. Cancer 49:1636-1648, 1982.

673 Reed RJ, Dhurandhar HN: Stem cell (immunoblastic) lymphoma. A variant of B lymphocytic lymphoma. Am J Clin Pathol 68:8-16, 1977.

674 Rosas-Uribe A, Rappaport H: Malignant lymphoma, histiocytic type with sclerosis (sclerosing reticulum cell sarcoma). Cancer 29:946-953, 1972.

675 Schneider DR, Taylor CR, Parker JW, Cramer AC, Meyer PR, Lukes RJ: Immunoblastic sarcoma of T- and B-cell types. Morphologic description and comparison. Hum Pathol 16:885-900, 1985.

676 Strauchen JA, Young RC, DeVita VT Jr, Anderson T, Fantone JC, Berard CW: Clinical relevance of the histopathological subclassification of diffuse "histiocytic" lymphoma. N Engl J Med 299:1382-1387, 1978.

677 Straus DJ, Filippa DA, Lieberman PH, Koziner B, Thaler HT, Clarkson BD: The non-Hodgkin's lymphomas. I. A retrospective clinical and pathologic analysis of 499 cases diagnosed between 1958 and 1969. Cancer 51:101-109, 1983.

678 Tsang WY, Chan JK, Tang SK, Tse CC, Cheung MM: Large cell lymphoma with fibrillary matrix. Histopathology 20:80-82, 1992.

679 Tse CC, Chan JK, Yuen RW, Ng CS: Malignant lymphoma with myxoid stroma. A new pattern in need of recognition. Histopathology 18:31-35, 1991.

680 Veronesi U, Musumeci R, Pizzetti F, Gennari L, Bonadonna G: The value of staging laparotomy in non-Hodgkin's lymphomas (with emphasis on the histiocytic type). Cancer 33:446-459, 1974.

681 Waldron JA Jr, Newcomer LN, Katz ME, Cadman E: Sclerosing variants of follicular center cell lymphomas presenting in the retroperitoneum. Cancer 52:712-720, 1983.

682 Warnke RA, Kim H, Fuks Z, Dorfman RE: The coexistence of nodular and diffuse patterns in nodular non-Hodgkin's lymphomas. Significance and clinicopathologic correlation. Cancer 40:1229-1233, 1977.

683 Warnke R, Miller R, Grogan T, Pederson M, Dilley J, Levy R: Immunologic phenotype in 30 patients with diffuse large-cell lymphoma. N Engl J Med 303:293-300, 1980.

684 Weiss RL, Kjeldsberg CR, Colby TV, Marty J: Multilobated B cell lymphomas. A study of 7 cases. Hematol Oncol 3:79-86, 1985.

685 Weiss LM, Wood GS, Dorfman RF: T-cell signet-ring cell lymphoma. A histologic, ultrastructural, and immunohistochemical study of two cases. Am J Surg Pathol 9:273-280, 1985.

686 Ye BH, Rao PH, Chaganti RSK, Dalla-Favera R: Cloning of bcl-6, the locus involved in chromosomal translocations affecting band 3q27 in B-cell lymphoma. Cancer Res 43:2732-2735, 1993.

Peripheral (post-thymic) T-cell lymphoma

687 Borowitz MJ, Reichert TA, Brynes RK, Cousar JB, Whitcomb CC, Collins RD, Crissman JD, Byrne GE Jr: The phenotypic diversity of peripheral T-cell lymphomas. The Southeastern Cancer Study Group experience. Hum Pathol 17:567-574, 1986.

688 Cabecadas JM, Isaacson PG: Phenotyping of T-cell lymphomas in paraffin sections—which antibodies? Histopathology 19:419-424, 1991.

689 Falini B, Pileri S, De Solas I, Martelli MF, Mason DY, Delsol G, Gatter KC, Fagioli M: Peripheral T-cell lymphoma associated with hemophagocytic syndrome. Blood 75:434-444, 1990.

690 Grogan TM, Fielder K, Rangel C, Jolley CJ, Wirt DP, Hicks MJ, Miller TP, Brooks R, Greenberg B, Jones S: Peripheral T-cell lymphoma. Aggressive disease with heterogeneous immunotypes. Am J Clin Pathol 83:279-288, 1985.

691 Haratake J, Horie A, Oda S, Chiba S, Kobori K, Sato H: A clinicopathological review of 12 autopsied cases of adult T-cell leukemia. Acta Pathol Jpn 36:349-362, 1986.

692 Hastrup N, Hamilton-Dutoit S, Ralfkiaer E, Pallesen G: Peripheral T-cell lymphomas. An evaluation of reproducibility of the updated Kiel classification. Histopathology 18:99-105, 1991.

693 Jones JF, Shurin S, Abramowsky C, Tubbs RR, Sciotto CG, Wahl R, Sands J, Gottman D, Katz BZ, Sklar J: T-cell lymphomas containing Epstein-Barr viral DNA in patients with chronic Epstein-Barr virus infections. N Engl J Med 318:733-741, 1988.

694 Kadin ME, Kamoun M, Lamberg J: Erythrophagocytic T-gamma lymphoma. A clinicopathologic entity resembling malignant histiocytosis. N Engl J Med 304:648-653, 1981.

695 Kittas C, Hansmann M-L, Borisch B, Feller AC, Lennert K: The blood microvasculature in T-cell lymphomas. A morphological, ultrastructural and immunohistochemical study. Virchows Arch [A] 405:439-452, 1985.

696 Macon WR, Williams ME, Greer JP, Cousar JB: Paracortical nodular T-cell lymphoma. Identification of an unusual variant of peripheral T-cell lymphoma. Am J Surg Pathol 19:297-303, 1995.

697 Nakamura S, Suchi T: A clinicopathologic study of node-based, low-grade, peripheral T-cell lymphoma. Angioimmunoblastic lymphoma, T-zone lymphoma, and lymphoepithelioid lymphoma. Cancer 67:2566-2578, 1991.

698 Patsouris E, Noel H, Lennert K: Angioimmunoblastic lymphadenopathy-type of T-cell lymphoma with a high content of epithelioid cells. Histopathology and comparison with lymphoepithelioid cell lymphoma. Am J Surg Pathol 13:262-275, 1989.

699 Picker LJ, Brenner MB, Weiss LM, Smith SD, Warnke RA: Discordant expression of CD3 and T-cell receptor beta-chain antigens in T-lineage lymphomas. Am J Pathol 129:434-440, 1987.

700 Pinkus GS, O'Hara CJ, Said JW: Peripheral/post-thymic T-cell lymphomas. A spectrum of disease. Clinical, pathologic, and immunologic features of 78 cases. Cancer 65:971-998, 1990.

701 Pinkus GS, Said JW, Hargreaves H: Malignant lymphoma, T-cell type. A distinct morphologic variant with large multilobulated nuclei, with a report of four cases. Am J Clin Pathol 72:540-550, 1979.

702 Sheibani K, Battifora H, Burke JS, Rappaport H: Leu-M1 antigen in human neoplasms. An immunohistologic study of 400 cases. Am J Surg Pathol 10:227-236, 1986.

703 Sheibani K, Wu A, Ben-Ezra J, Stroup R, Rappaport H, Winberg C: Rearrangement of kappa-chain and T-cell receptor b-chain genes in malignant lymphomas of "T-cell" phenotype. Am J Pathol 129:201-207, 1987.

704 Su I-J, Wang CH, Cheng A-L, Chen Y-C, Hsieh H-C, Chen C-J, Tien H-F, Woei-Tsay, Huang S-S, Hu C-Y, Chen P-J, Chen J-Y, Hsu H-C, Chuang S-M, Shen M-C, Kadin ME: Characterization of the spectrum of postthymic T-cell malignancies in Taiwan. A clinicopathologic study of HTLV-1-positive and HTLV-1-negative cases. Cancer **61**:2060-2070, 1988.

705 Tajima K, Kuroishi T: Estimation of rate of incidence of ATL among ATLV (HTLV-I) carriers in Kyushu, Japan. Jpn J Clin Oncol **15**:423-430, 1985.

706 Takagi N, Nakamura S, Ueda R, Osada H, Obata Y, Kitoh K, Suchi T, Takahashi T: A phenotypic and genotypic study of three node-based, low-grade peripheral T-cell lymphomas. Angioimmunoblastic lymphoma, T-zone lymphoma, and lymphoepithelioid lymphoma. Cancer **69**:2571-2582, 1992.

707 van der Valk P, Willemze R, Meijer CJLM: Peripheral T-cell lymphoma. A clinicopathological and immunological study of 10 cases. Histopathology **10**:235-249, 1986.

708 van Krieken JH, Elwood L, Andrade RE, Jaffe ES, Cossman J, Medeiros LJ: Rearrangement of the T-cell receptor delta chain gene in T-cell lymphomas with a mature phenotype. Am J Pathol **139**:161-168, 1991.

709 Waldmann TA, Davis MM, Bongiovanni KD, Korsmeyer SJ: Rearrangements of genes for the antigen receptor on T-cells as markers of lineage and clonality in human lymphoid neoplasms. N Engl J Med **313**:776-783, 1985.

710 Weis JW, Winter MW, Phyliky RL, Banks PM: Peripheral T-cell lymphomas. Histologic, immunohistologic, and clinical characterization. Mayo Clin Proc **61**:411-426, 1986.

711 Wieczorek R, Burke JS, Knowles DM II: Leu-M1 antigen expression in T-cell neoplasia. Am J Pathol **121**:374-380, 1985.

712 Winberg CD, Krance R, Sheibani K, Rappaport H: Peripheral T-cell lymphoma. Cancer **57**:2329-2342, 1986.

Lymphoepithelioid T-cell lymphoma

713 Burke JS, Butler JJ: Malignant lymphoma with a high content of epithelioid histiocytes (Lennert's lymphoma). Am J Clin Pathol **66**:1-9, 1976.

714 Kim H, Jacobs C, Warnke RA, Dorfman RF: Malignant lymphoma with a high content of epithelioid histiocytes. A distinct clinicopathologic entity and a form of so-called "Lennert's lymphoma." Cancer **41**:620-635, 1978.

715 Klein MA, Jaffe R, Neiman RS: "Lennert's lymphoma" with transformation to malignant lymphoma, histiocytic type (immunoblastic sarcoma). Am J Clin Pathol **68**:601-605, 1977.

716 Lennert K, Mestdagh J: Lymphogranulomatosen mit konstant hohem Epithelioidzellgehalt. Virchows Arch [A] **344**:1-20, 1968.

717 Patsouris E, Noël H, Lennert K: Histological and immunohistological findings in lymphoepithelioid cell lymphoma (Lennert's lymphoma). Am J Surg Pathol **12**:341-350, 1988.

718 Spier CM, Lippman SM, Miller TP, Grogan TM: Lennert's lymphoma. A clinicopathologic study with emphasis on phenotype and its relationship to survival. Cancer **61**:517-524, 1988.

Anaplastic large cell lymphoma

719 Agnarsson BA, Kadin ME: Ki-1 positive large cell lymphoma. A morphologic and immunologic study of 19 cases. Am J Surg Pathol **12**:264-274, 1988.

720 Banerjee SS, Heald J, Harris M: Twelve cases of Ki-1 positive anaplastic large cell lymphoma of skin. J Clin Pathol **44**:119-125, 1991.

721 Banks PM, Metter J, Allred DC: Anaplastic large cell (Ki-1) lymphoma with histiocytic phenotype simulating carcinoma. Am J Clin Pathol **94**:445-452, 1990.

722 Beljaards RC, Kaudewitz P, Berti E, Gianotti R, Neumann C, Rosso R, Paulli M, Meijer CJ, Willemze R: Primary cutaneous CD30-positive large cell lymphoma. Definition of a new type of cutaneous lymphoma with a favorable prognosis. A European Multicenter Study of 47 patients. Cancer **71**:2097-2104, 1993.

723 Benz-Lemoine E, Brizard A, Huret JL, Babin P, Guilhot F, Couet D, Tanzer J: Malignant histiocytosis. A specific t(2; 5)(p23; q35) translocation? Review of the literature. Blood **72**:1045-1047, 1988.

724 Bitter MA, Franklin WA, Larson RA, McKeithan TW, Rubin CM, Le Beau MM, Stephens JK, Vardiman JW: Morphology in Ki-1(CD30)-positive non-Hodgkin's lymphoma is correlated with clinical features and the presence of a unique chromosomal abnormality, t(2; 5)(p23; q35). Am J Surg Pathol **14**:305-316, 1990.

725 Brousset P, Rochaix P, Chittal S, Rubie H, Robert A, Delsol G: High incidence of Epstein-Barr virus detection in Hodgkin's disease and absence of detection in anaplastic large-cell lymphoma in children. Histopathology **23**:189-191, 1993.

726 Bullrich F, Morris SW, Hummel M, Pileri S, Stein H, Croce CM: Nucleophosmin (NPM) gene rearrangements in Ki-1-positive lymphomas. Cancer Res **54**:2873-2877, 1994.

727 Carbone A, Gloghini A, De Re V, Tamaro P, Boiocchi M, Volpe R: Histopathologic, immunophenotypic, and genotypic analysis of Ki-1 anaplastic large cell lymphomas that express histiocyte-associated antigens. Cancer **66**:2547-2556, 1990.

728 Chan JK: CD30+ (Ki-1) lymphoma. t(2;5) translocation, the implicated genes, and more. Adv Anat Pathol (in press).

729 Chan JK, Buchanan R, Fletcher CD: Sarcomatoid variant of anaplastic large-cell Ki-1 lymphoma. Am J Surg Pathol **14**:983-988, 1990.

730 Chan JK, Ng CS, Hui PK, Leung TW, Lo ES, Lau WH, McGuire LJ: Anaplastic large cell Ki-1 lymphoma. Delineation of two morphological types. Histopathology **15**:11-34, 1989.

731 Chan JK, Ng CS, Hui PK, Leung WT, Sin VC, Lam TK, Chick KW, Lam WY: Anaplastic large cell Ki-1 lymphoma of bone. Cancer **68**:2186-2191, 1991.

732 Chott A, Kaserer K, Augustin I, Vesely M, Heinz R, Oehlinger W, Hanak H, Radaszkiewicz T: Ki-1-positive large cell lymphoma. A clinicopathologic study of 41 cases. Am J Surg Pathol **14**:439-448, 1990.

733 Cohen PL, Butmarc J, Kadin ME: Expression of Hodgkin's disease associated antigen BLA. 36 in anaplastic large cell lymphomas and lymphomatoid papulosis primarily of T-cell origin. Am J Clin Pathol **104**:50-53, 1995.

734 de Bruin PC, Beljaards RC, van Heerde P, Van Der Valk P, Noorduyn LA, Van Krieken JH, Kluin-Nelemans JC, Willemze R, Meijer CJ: Differences in clinical behaviour and immunophenotype between primary cutaneous and primary nodal anaplastic large cell lymphoma of T-cell or null cell phenotype. Histopathology **23**:127-135, 1993.

735 Delsol G, Al Saati T, Gatter KC, Gerdes J, Schwarting R, Caveriviere P, Rigal-Huguet F, Robert A, Stein H, Mason DY: Coexpression of epithelial membrane antigen (EMA), Ki-1, and interleukin-2 receptor by anaplastic large cell lymphomas. Diagnostic value in so-called malignant histiocytosis. Am J Pathol **130**:59-70, 1988.

736 DiGiuseppe JA, Wu T-Z, Zehnbauer BA, McDowell PR, Barletta JM, Ambinder RF, Mann RB: Epstein-Barr virus and progression of non-Hodgkin's lymphoma to Ki-1-positive, anaplastic large cell phenotype. Mod Pathol **8**:553-559, 1995.

737 Flynn KJ, Dehner LP, Gajl-Peczalska KJ, Dahl MV, Ramsay N, Wang N: Regressing atypical histiocytosis. A cutaneous proliferation of atypical neoplastic histiocytes with unexpectedly indolent biologic behavior. Cancer **49**:959-970, 1982.

738 Falini B, Pileri S, Stein H, Dieneman D, Dallenbach F, Delsol G, Minelli O, Poggi S, Martelli MF, Pallesen G, et al.: Variable expression of leucocyte-common (CD45) antigen in CD30 (Ki1)-positive anaplastic large-cell lymphoma. Implications for the differential diagnosis between lymphoid and nonlymphoid malignancies. Hum Pathol **21**:624-629, 1990.

739 Greer JP, Kinney MC, Collins RD, Salhany KE, Wolff SN, Hainsworth JD, Flexner JM, Stein RS: Clinical features of 31 patients with Ki-1 anaplastic large-cell lymphoma. J Clin Oncol **9**:539-547, 1991.

740 Gustmann C, Altmannsberger M, Osborn M, Griesser H, Feller AC: Cytokeratin expression and vimentin content in large cell anaplastic lymphomas and other non-Hodgkin's lymphomas. Am J Pathol **138**:1413-1422, 1991.

741 Hansmann ML, Fellbaum C, Bohm A: Large cell anaplastic lymphoma. Evaluation of immunophenotype on paraffin and frozen sections in comparison with ultrastructural features. Virchows Arch [A] **418**:427-433, 1991.

742 Headington JT, Roth MS, Schnitzer B: Regressing atypical histiocytosis. A review and critical appraisal. Semin Diagn Pathol **4**:28-37, 1987.

743 Herbst H, Tippelmann G, Anagnostopoulos I, Gerdes J, Schwarting R, Boehm T, Pileri S, Jones DB, Stein H: Immunoglobulin and T-cell receptor gene rearrangements in Hodgkin's disease and Ki-1-positive anaplastic large cell lymphoma. Dissociation between phenotype and genotype. Leuk Res **13**:103-116, 1989.

744 Kadin ME: Ki-1/CD30+ (anaplastic) large-cell lymphoma. Maturation of a clinicopathologic entity with prospects of effective therapy (editorial). J Clin Oncol **12**:884-887, 1994.

745 Kaudewitz P, Greer JP, Glick AD, Salhany KE, Collins RD: Anaplastic large-cell Ki-1 malignant lymphomas. Recognition, biological and clinical implications. Pathol Annu **26**(Pt 1):1-24, 1991.

746 Kaudewitz P, Stein H, Dallenbach F, Eckert F, Bieber K, Burg G, Braun-Falco O: Primary and secondary cutaneous Ki-1+ (CD30+) anaplastic large cell lymphomas. Morphologic, immunohistologic, and clinical characteristics. Am J Pathol **135**:359-367, 1989.

747 Kinney MC, Collins RD, Greer JP, Whitlock JA, Sioutos N, Kadin ME: A small-cell-predominant variant of primary Ki-1 (CD30)+ T-cell lymphoma. Am J Surg Pathol **17**:859-868, 1993.

747a Ladanyi M, Cavalchire G: Detection of the NPM-ALK genomic rearrangement of Ki-1 lymphoma and isolation of the involved NPM and ALK introns. Diagn Mol Pathol (in press).

748 Leoncini L, Del Vecchio MT, Kraft R, Megha T, Barbini P, Cevenini G, Poggi S, Pileri S, Tosi P, Cottier H: Hodgkin's disease and CD30-positive anaplastic large cell lymphomas—a continuous spectrum of malignant disorders. A quantitative morphometric and immunohistologic study. Am J Pathol 137:1047-1057, 1990.

749 Lopategui JR, Gaffey MJ, Chan JK, Frierson HF, Sun LH, Bellafiore FJ, Chang KL, Weiss LM: Infrequent association of Epstein-Barr virus with CD30-positive anaplastic large cell lymphomas from American and Asian patients. Am J Surg Pathol 19:42-49, 1995.

750 Mann KP, Hall B, Kamino H, Borowitz MJ, Ratech H: Neutrophil-rich, Ki-1-positive anaplastic large-cell malignant lymphoma. Am J Surg Pathol 19:407-416, 1995.

751 Mason DY, Bastard C, Rimokh R, Dastugue N, Huret JL, Kristoffersson U, Magaud JP, Nezelof C, Tilly H, Vannier JP, et al.: CD30-positive large cell lymphomas ('Ki-1 lymphoma') are associated with a chromosomal translocation involving 5q35. Br J Haematol 74:161-168, 1990.

752 Motley RJ, Jasani B, Ford AM, Poynton CH, Calonje-Daly JE, Holt PJ: Regressing atypical histiocytosis, a regressing cutaneous phase of Ki-1-positive anaplastic large cell lymphoma. Immunocytochemical, nucleic acid, and cytogenetic studies of a new case in view of current opinion. Cancer 70:476-483, 1992.

753 O'Connor NT, Stein H, Gatter KC, Wainscoat JS, Crick J, Al Saati T, Falini B, Delsol G, Mason DY: Genotypic analysis of large cell lymphomas which express the Ki-1 antigen. Histopathology 11:733-740, 1987.

754 Pileri S, Bocchia M, Baroni CD, Martelli M, Falini B, Sabattini E, Gherlinzoni F, Amadori S, Poggi S, Mazza P, et al.: Anaplastic large cell lymphoma (CD30 +/Ki-1+). Results of a prospective clinico-pathological study of 69 cases. Br J Haematol 86:513-523, 1994.

755 Rosso R, Paulli M, Magrini U, Kindl S, Boveri E, Volpato G, Poggi S, Baglioni P, Pileri S: Anaplastic large cell lymphoma, CD30/Ki-1 positive, expressing the CD15/Leu-M1 antigen. Immunohistochemical and morphological relationships to Hodgkin's disease. Virchows Arch [A] 416:229-235, 1990.

756 Sakurai S, Nakajima T, Oyama T, Sano T, Hosomura Y: Anaplastic large cell lymphoma with histiocytic phenotypes. Acta Pathol Jpn 43:142-145, 1993.

757 Shulman LN, Frisard B, Antin JH, Wheeler C, Pinkus G, Magauran N, Mauch P, Nobles E, Mashal R, Canellos G, et al.: Primary Ki-1 anaplastic large-cell lymphoma in adults. Clinical characteristics and therapeutic outcome. J Clin Oncol 11:937-942, 1993.

758 Tirelli U, Vaccher E, Zagonel V, Talamini R, Bernardi D, Tavio M, Gloghini A, Merola MC, Monfardini S, Carbone A: CD30 (Ki1)-positive anaplastic large-cell lymphomas in 13 patients with and 27 patients without human immunodeficiency virus infections. The first comparative clinicopathologic study from a single institution that also includes 80 patients with other human immunodeficiency virus-related systemic lymphomas. J Clin Oncol 13:373-380, 1995.

759 Wong KF, Chan JK, Ng CS, Chu YC, Lam PW, Yuen HL: Anaplastic large cell Ki-1 lymphoma involving bone marrow. Marrow findings and association with reactive hemophagocytosis. Am J Hematol 37:112-119, 1991.

Lymphoblastic lymphoma

760 Brownell MD, Sheibani K, Battifora H, Winberg CD, Rappaport H: Distinction between undifferentiated (small noncleaved) and lymphoblastic lymphoma. An immunohistologic study on paraffin-embedded, fixed tissue sections. Am J Surg Pathol 11:779-787, 1987.

761 Donlon JA, Jaffe ES, Braylan RC: Terminal deoxynucleotidyl transferase activity in malignant lymphomas. N Engl J Med 297:461-464, 1977.

762 Griffith RC, Kelly DR, Nathwani BN, Shuster JJ, Murphy SB, Hvizdala E, Sullivan MP, Berard CW: A morphologic study of childhood lymphoma of the lymphoblastic type. The pediatric Oncology Group experience. Cancer 59:1126-1131, 1987.

763 Jaffe ES, Braylan RC, Frank MM, Green I, Berard CW: Heterogeneity of immunologic markers and surface morphology in childhood lymphoblastic lymphoma. Blood 48:213-222, 1976.

764 Nathwani BN, Kim H, Rappaport H: Malignant lymphoma, lymphoblastic. Cancer 38:964-983, 1976.

765 Orazi A, Cattoretti G, John K, Neiman RS: Terminal deoxynucleotidyl transferase staining of malignant lymphomas in paraffin sections. Mod Pathol 7:582-586, 1994.

766 Pangalis GA, Nathwani BN, Rappaport H, Rosen RB: Acute lymphoblastic leukemia. The significance of nuclear convolutions. Cancer 43:551-557, 1979.

767 Picozzi VJ Jr, Coleman CN: Lymphoblastic lymphoma. Semin Oncol 17:96-103, 1990.

768 Pinkus GS, Hargreaves HK, McLeod JA, Nadler LM, Rosenthal DS, Said JW: α-Naphthyl acetate esterase activity. A cytochemical marker for T lymphocytes. Correlation with immunologic studies of normal tissues, lymphocytic leukemias, non-Hodgkin's lymphomas, Hodgkin's disease, and other lymphoproliferative disorders. Am J Pathol 97:17-42, 1979.

769 Raimondi SC, Behm FG, Roberson PK, Pui CH, Rivera GK, Murphy SB, Williams DL: Cytogenetics of childhood T-cell leukemia. Blood 72:1560-1566, 1988.

770 Rosen PJ, Feinstein DI, Pattengale PK, Tindle BH, Williams AH, Cain MJ, Bonorris JB, Parker JW, Lukes RJ: Convoluted lymphocytic lymphoma in adults. A clinicopathologic entity. Ann Intern Med 89:319-324, 1978.

771 Said JW, Shintaku IP, Pinkus GS: Immunohistochemical staining for terminal deoxynucleotidyl transferase (TDT). An enhanced method in routinely processed formalin-fixed tissue sections. Am J Clin Pathol 89:649-652, 1988.

772 Sheibani K, Nathwani BN, Winberg CD, Burke JS, Swartz WG, Blayney D, van de Velde S, Hill LR, Rappaport H: Antigenically defined subgroups of lymphoblastic lymphoma. Relationship to clinical presentation and biologic behavior. Cancer 60:183-190, 1987.

Small noncleaved cell lymphoma

773 Arseneau JC, Canellos GP, Banks PM, Berard CW, Gralnick HR, DeVita VT Jr: American Burkitt's lymphoma. A clinicopathologic study of 30 cases. I. Clinical factors relating to prolonged survival. Am J Med 58:314-321, 1975.

774 Banks PM, Arseneau JC, Gralnick HR, Cannellos GP, DeVita VT Jr, Berard CW: American Burkitt's lymphoma. A clinicopathologic study of 30 cases. II. Pathologic correlations. Am J Med 58:322-329, 1975.

775 Berard CB, O'Connor GT, Thomas LB, Torloni H: Histopathologic definition of Burkitt's tumor. Bull WHO 40:601-608, 1969.

776 Bernhard W: Fine structure of Burkitt's lymphoma. In Burkitt DP, Wright DH, eds: Burkitt's lymphoma. Edinburgh and London, 1970, E & S Livingstone, pp 103-117.

777 Dalla-Favera R: Chromosomal translocations involving the c-myc oncogene and their role in the pathogenesis of B cell neoplasia. In Brugge J, Curran T, Harlow E, McCormick F, eds: Origin of human cancer. Cold Spring Harbor, NY, 1991, Cold Spring Harbor Laboratory Press.

778 Dalla-Favera R, Bregni M, Erikson J, Patterson D, Gallo RC, Croce CM: Human c-myc oncogene is located on the region of chromosome 8 that is translocated in Burkitt lymphoma cells. Proc Natl Acad Sci USA 79:7824-7827, 1982.

779 Garcia CF, Weiss LM, Warnke RA: Small noncleaved cell lymphoma. An immunophenotypic study of 18 cases and comparison with large cell lymphoma. Hum Pathol 17:454-461, 1986.

780 Levine PH, Kamaraju LS, Connelly RR, Berard CW, Dorfman RF, Magrath I, Easton JM: The American Burkitt's Lymphoma Registry. Eight years' experience. Cancer 49:1016-1022, 1982.

781 Levine AM, Pavlova Z, Pockros AW, Parker JW, Teitelbaum AH, Paganini-Hill A, Powars DR, Lukes RJ, Feinstein DI: Small noncleaved follicular center cell (FCC) lymphoma. Burkitt and non-Burkitt variants in the United States. Cancer 52:1073-1079, 1983.

782 Magrath IT: The pathogenesis of Burkitt's lymphoma. In Van de Woude GF, Klein G, eds: Advances of cancer research. San Diego, 1990, Academic Press.

783 Mann RB, Jaffe ES, Braylan RC, Nanba K, Frank MM, Ziegler JL, Berard CW: Non-endemic Burkitt's lymphoma. A B cell tumor related to germinal centers. N Engl J Med 295:685-691, 1976.

784 Minerbrook M, Schulman P, Budman DR, Teichberg S, Vinciguerra V, Kardon N, Degnan TJ: Burkitt's leukemia. A re-evaluation. Cancer 49:1444-1448, 1982.

785 Nkrumah FK, Perkins IV: Burkitt's lymphoma. A clinical study of 100 patients. Cancer 37:671-676, 1976.

786 Yano T, van Krieken JH, Magrath IT, Longo DL, Jaffe ES, Raffeld M: Histogenetic correlations between subcategories of small noncleaved cell lymphomas. Blood 79:1282-1290, 1992.

787 Ziegler JL: Treatment results of 54 American patients with Burkitt's lymphoma are similar to the African experience. N Engl J Med 297:75-80, 1977.

788 Ziegler JL: Burkitt's lymphoma. N Engl J Med 305:735-745, 1981.

Other non-Hodgkin's lymphomas

789 Burke JS, Byrne GE Jr, Rappaport H: Hairy cell leukemia (leukemic reticuloendotheliosis). I. A clinical pathologic study of 21 patients. Cancer 33:1399-1410, 1974.

790 Müller-Hermelink HK, Stein H, Steinmann G, Lennert K: Malignant lymphoma of plasmacytoid T-cells. Morphologic and immunologic studies characterizing a special type of T-cell. Am J Surg Pathol 7:849-862, 1983.

791 Nakamura S, Suchi T, Koshikawa T, Kitoh K, Koike K, Komatsu H, Iida S, Kagami Y, Ogura M, Katoh E, Kurita S, Suzuki H, Kobashi Y, Yamabe H, Hirabayashi N, Ueda R, Takahashi T: Clinicopathologic study of CD56 (NCAM)-positive angiocentric lymphoma occurring in sites other than the upper and lower respiratory tract. Am J Surg Pathol 19:284-296, 1995.

792 Prasthofer EF, Grizzle WE, Prchal JT, Grossi CE: Plasmacytoid T-cell lymphoma associated with chronic myeloproliferative disorder. Am J Surg Pathol 9:380-387, 1985.

Composite and discordant lymphoma

793 Cerroni L, Rieger E, Hodl S, Kerl H: Clinicopathologic and immunologic features associated with transformation of mycosis fungoides to large-cell lymphoma. Am J Surg Pathol **16**:543-552, 1992.

794 Chan WC, Griem ML, Grozea PN, Freel RJ, Variakojis D: Mycosis fungoides and Hodgkin's disease occurring in the same patient. Report of three cases. Cancer **44**:1408-1413, 1979.

795 Cossman J, Schnitzer B, Deegan MJ: Coexistence of two lymphomas with distinctive histologic, ultrastructural, and immunologic features. Am J Clin Pathol **70**:409-415, 1978.

796 Cullen MH, Lister TA, Brearley RI, Shand WS, Stansfield AG: Histological transformation of non-Hodgkin's lymphoma. A prospective study. Cancer **44**:645-651, 1979.

797 Damotte D, Le Tourneau A, Audouin J, Duval C, Martin-Bastenaire F, Villain O, Delobelle-Deroide A, Diebold J: Discordant malignant lymphoma synchronous or successive high-grade B lymphoma associated with Hodgkin's disease. A clinicopathologic and immunophenotypic study of 4 cases. Pathol Res Pract **191**:8-15, 1995.

798 Dmitrovsky E, Matthews MJ, Bunn PA, Schechter GP, Makuch RW, Winkler CF, Eddy J, Sausville EA, Ihde DC: Cytologic transformation in cutaneous T cell lymphoma. A clinicopathologic entity associated with poor prognosis. J Clin Oncol **5**:208-215, 1987.

799 Donald D, Green JA, White M: Mycosis fungoides associated with nodular sclerosing Hodgkin's disease. A case report. Cancer **46**:2505-2508, 1980.

800 Gonzalez CL, Medeiros LJ, Jaffe ES: Composite lymphoma. A clinicopathologic analysis of nine patients with Hodgkin's disease and B-cell non-Hodgkin's lymphoma. Am J Clin Pathol **96**:81-89, 1991.

801 Greer JP, Salhany KE, Cousar JB, Fields JP, King LE, Graber SE, Flexner JM, Stein RS, Collins RD: Clinical features associated with transformation of cerebriform T-cell lymphoma to a large cell process. Hematol Oncol **8**:215-227, 1990.

802 Grossman DM, Hanson CA, Schnitzer B: Simultaneous lymphocyte predominant Hodgkin's disease and large-cell lymphoma. Am J Surg Pathol **15**:668-676, 1991.

803 Hansmann ML, Fellbaum C, Hui PK, Lennert K: Morphological and immunohistochemical investigation of non-Hodgkin's lymphoma combined with Hodgkin's disease. Histopathology **15**:35-48, 1989.

804 Hansmann ML, Stein H, Fellbaum C, Hui PK, Parwaresch MR, Lennert K: Nodular paragranuloma can transform into high-grade malignant lymphoma of B type. Hum Pathol **20**:1169-1175, 1989.

805 Harris NL: The relationship between Hodgkin's disease and non-Hodgkin's lymphoma. Semin Diagn Pathol **9**:304-310, 1992.

806 Jaffe ES, Zarate-Osorno A, Medeiros LJ: The interrelationship of Hodgkin's disease and non-Hodgkin's lymphomas—lessons learned from composite and sequential malignancies. Semin Diagn Pathol **9**:297-303, 1992.

807 Kim H, Hendrickson MR, Dorfman RF: Composite lymphoma. Cancer **40**:959-976, 1977.

808 Salhany KE, Cousar JB, Greer JP, Casey TT, Fields JP, Collins RD: Transformation of cutaneous T cell lymphoma to large cell lymphoma. A clinicopathologic and immunologic study. Am J Pathol **132**:265-277, 1988.

809 Weisenberg E, Anastasi J, Adeyanju M, Variakojis D, Vardiman JW: Hodgkin's disease associated with chronic lymphocytic leukemia. Eight additional cases, including two of the nodular lymphocyte predominant type. Am J Clin Pathol **103**:479-484, 1995.

810 Weiss LM, Warnke RA: Follicular lymphoma with blastic conversion. A report of two cases with confirmation by immunoperoxidase studies on bone marrow sections. Am J Clin Pathol **83**:681-686, 1985.

811 Woda BA, Knowles DM II: Nodular lymphocytic lymphoma eventuating into diffuse histiocytic lymphoma. Immunoperoxidase demonstration of monoclonality. Cancer **43**:303-307, 1979.

812 Wood GS, Bahler DW, Hoppe RT, Warnke RA, Sklar JL, Levy R: Transformation of mycosis fungoides. T-cell receptor beta gene analysis demonstrates a common clonal origin for plaque-type mycosis fungoides and CD30+ large-cell lymphoma. J Invest Dermatol **101**:296-300, 1993.

813 Zarate-Osorno A, Medeiros LJ, Kingma DW, Longo DL, Jaffe ES: Hodgkin's disease following non-Hodgkin's lymphoma. A clinicopathologic and immunophenotypic study of nine cases. Am J Surg Pathol **17**:123-132, 1993.

814 Zarate-Osorno A, Medeiros LJ, Longo DL, Jaffe ES: Non-Hodgkin's lymphomas arising in patients successfully treated for Hodgkin's disease. A clinical, histologic, and immunophenotypic study of 14 cases. Am J Surg Pathol **16**:885-895, 1992.

815 Zelenetz AD, Chen TT, Levy R: Histologic transformation of follicular lymphoma to diffuse lymphoma represents tumor progression by a single malignant B cell. J Exp Med **173**:197-207, 1991.

So-called malignant histiocytosis

816 Aozasa K, Tsujimoto M, Inoue A: Malignant histiocytosis. Report of twenty five cases with pulmonary, renal and/or gastro-intestinal involvement. Histopathology **9**:39-49, 1985.

817 Byrne GE Jr, Rappaport H: Malignant histiocytosis. Gann Monogr Cancer Res **15**:145-162, 1973.

818 Cattoretti G, Villa A, Vezzoni P, Giardini R, Lombardi L, Rilke F: Malignant histiocytosis. A phenotypic and genotypic investigation. Am J Pathol **136**:1009-1019, 1990.

819 Colby TV, Carrington CB, Mark GJ: Pulmonary involvement in malignant histiocytosis. A clinicopathologic spectrum. Am J Surg Pathol **5**:61-73, 1981.

820 Ducatman BS, Wick MR, Morgan TW, Banks PM, Pierre RV: Malignant histiocytosis. A clinical, histologic and immunohistochemical study of 20 cases. Hum Pathol **15**:368-377, 1984.

821 Esumi N, Ikushima S, Hibi S, Todo S, Imashuku S: High serum ferritin level as a marker of malignant histiocytosis and virus-associated hemophagocytic syndrome. Cancer **61**:2071-2076, 1988.

822 Griffin JD, Ellman L, Long JC, Dvorak AM: Development of a histiocytic medullary reticulosis-like syndrome during the course of acute lymphocytic leukemia. Am J Med **64**:851-858, 1978.

823 Hsu SM, Ho YS, Hsu PL: Lymphomas of true histiocytic origin. Expression of different phenotypes in so-called true histiocytic lymphoma and malignant histiocytosis. Am J Pathol **138**:1389-1404, 1991.

824 Huhn D, Meister P: Malignant histiocytosis. Morphologic and cytochemical findings. Cancer **42**:1341-1349, 1978.

825 Karcher DS, Head DR, Mullins JD: Malignant histiocytosis occurring in patients with acute lymphocytic leukemia. Cancer **41**:1967-1973, 1978.

826 Lombardi L, Carbone A, Pilotti S, Rilke F: Malignant histiocytosis. A histological and ultrastructural study of lymph nodes in six cases. Histopathology **2**:315-328, 1978.

827 Macgillivray JB, Duthie JS: Malignant histiocytosis (histiocytic medullary reticulosis) with spindle cell differentiation and tumour formation. J Clin Pathol **30**:120-125, 1977.

828 Matzner Y, Behar A, Beeri E, Gunders AE, Hershko C: Systemic leishmaniasis mimicking malignant histiocytosis. Cancer **43**:398-402, 1979.

829 Mendelsohn G, Eggleston JC, Mann RB: Relationship of lysozyme (muramidase) to histiocytic differentiation in malignant histiocytosis. An immunohistochemical study. Cancer **45**:273-279, 1980.

830 Morgan NE, Fretzin D, Variakojis D, Caro WA: Clinical and pathologic cutaneous manifestations of malignant histiocytosis. Arch Dermatol **119**:367-372, 1983.

831 Nezelof C, Barbey S, Gogusev J, Terrier-Lacombe MJ: Malignant histiocytosis in childhood. A distinctive CD30-positive clinicopathological entity associated with a chromosomal translocation involving 5q35. Semin Diagn Pathol **9**:75-89, 1992.

832 Perry MC, Harrison EG Jr, Burgert EO, Gilchrist GS: Familial erythrophagocytic lymphohistiocytosis. Report of two cases and clinicopathologic review. Cancer **38**:209-218, 1976.

833 Pileri S, Mazza P, Rivano MT, Martinelli G, Cavazzini G, Gobbi M, Taruscio D, Lauria F, Tura S: Malignant histiocytosis (true histiocytic lymphoma) clinicopathological study of 25 cases. Histopathology **9**:905-920, 1985.

834 Rappaport H: Tumors of the hematopoietic system. In Atlas of tumor pathology, Sect. III, Fasc. 8. Washington, DC, 1966, Armed Forces Institute of Pathology, pp 91-206.

835 Reiner AP, Spivak JL: Hematophagic histiocytosis. A report of 23 new patients and a review of the literature. Medicine (Baltimore) **67**:369-388, 1988.

836 Robb-Smith AH: Before our time. Half a century of histiocytic medullary reticulosis. A T-cell teaser? Histopathology **17**:279-283, 1990.

837 Scott RB, Robb-Smith AH: Histiocytic medullary reticulosis. Lancet **2**:194-198, 1939.

838 Sonneveld P, van Lom K, Kappers-Klunne M, Prins ME, Abels J: Clinicopathological diagnosis and treatment of malignant histiocytosis. Br J Haematol **75**:511-516, 1990.

839 Takeshita M, Kikuchi M, Ohshima K, Nibu K, Suzumiya J, Hisano S, Miyamoto Y, Okamura T: Bone marrow findings in malignant histiocytosis and/or malignant lymphoma with concurrent hemophagocytic syndrome. Leuk Lymphoma **12**:79-89, 1993.

840 Warnke RA, Kim H, Dorfman RF: Malignant histiocytosis (histiocytic medullary reticulosis). I. Clinicopathologic study of 29 cases. Cancer **35**:215-230, 1975.

841 Watanabe S, Mikata A, Toyama K, Kitamura K, Minato K: Sarcomatous variant of malignant histiocytosis. A case report and review of the literature. Acta Pathol Jpn **28**:963-978, 1978.

841a Weiss LM, Azzi R, Dorfman RF, Warnke RA: Sinusoidal hematolymphoid malignancy ("malignant histiocytosis") presenting as atypical sinusoidal proliferation. A study of nine cases. Cancer **58**:1681-1688, 1986.

842 Wilson MS, Weiss LM, Gatter KC, Mason DY, Dorfman RF, Warnke RA: Malignant histiocytosis. A reassessment of cases previously reported in 1975 based on paraffin section immunophenotyping studies. Cancer **66:**530-536, 1990.

842a Zucker JM, Caillaux JM, Vanel D, Gerard-Marchant R: Malignant histiocytosis in childhood. Clinical study and therapeutic results in 22 cases. Cancer **45:**2821-2829, 1980.

Lymphoma in immunodeficiency states

843 Arber DA, Shibata D, Chen YY, Weiss LM: Characterization of the topography of Epstein-Barr virus infection in human immunodeficiency virus-associated lymphoid tissues. Mod Pathol **5:**559-566, 1992.

843a Armitage J, Kornos R, Stuart R, et al.: Posttransplant lymphoproliferative disease in thoracic organ transplant patients. Ten years of cyclosporine-based immunosuppression. J Heart Lung Transplant **10:**877-887, 1991.

844 Audouin J, Diebold J, Pallesen G: Frequent expression of Epstein-Barr virus latent membrane protein-1 in tumour cells of Hodgkin's disease in HIV-positive patients. J Pathol **167:**381-384, 1992.

844a Banks PM, Witrak GA, Conn DL: Lymphoid neoplasia following connective tissue disease. Mayo Clin Proc **54:**104-108, 1979.

845 Beral V, Peterman T, Berkelman R, Jaffe H: AIDS-associated non-Hodgkin lymphoma. Lancet **337:**805-809, 1991.

846 Carbone A, Gloghini A, Gaidano G, Cilia AM, Bassi P, Polito P, Vaccher E, Saglio G, Tirelli U: AIDS-related Burkitt's lymphoma. Morphologic and immunophenotypic study of biopsy specimens. Am J Clin Pathol **103:**561-567, 1995.

847 Cleary ML, Warnke R, Sklar J: Monoclonality of lymphoproliferative lesions in cardiac-transplant recipients. Clonal analysis based on immunoglobulin-gene rearrangements. N Engl J Med **310:**477-482, 1984.

848 Di Carlo EF, Amberson JB, Metroka CE, Ballard P, Moore A, Mouradian JA: Malignant lymphomas and the acquired immunodeficiency syndrome. Evaluation of 30 cases using a working formulation. Arch Pathol Lab Med **110:**1012-1016, 1986.

849 Ellman MH, Hurwitz H, Thomas C, Kozloff M: Lymphoma developing in a patient with rheumatoid arthritis taking low dose weekly methotrexate. J Rheumatol **18:**1741-1743, 1991.

850 Ferry JA, Jacobson JO, Conti D, Delmonico F, Harris NL: Lymphoproliferative disorders and hematologic malignancies following organ transplantation. Mod Pathol **2:**583-592, 1989.

851 Filipovich AH, Mathur A, Kamat D, Shapiro RS: Primary immunodeficiencies: genetic risk factors for lymphoma. Cancer Res **52:**5465s-5467s, 1992.

852 Frizzera G, Hanto DW, Gajl-Peczalska KJ, Rosai J, McKenna RW, Sibley RK, Holahan KP, Lindquist LL: Polymorphic diffuse B-cell hyperplasias and lymphomas in renal transplant recipients. Cancer Res **41:**4262-4279, 1981.

853 Frizzera G, Rosai J, Dehner LP, Spector BD, Kersey JH: Lymphoreticular disorders in primary immunodeficiencies. New findings based on an up-to-date histologic review of 35 cases. Cancer **46:**692-699, 1980.

854 Gail MH, Pluda JM, Rabkin CS, Biggar RJ, Goedert JJ, Horm JW, Sondik EJ, Yarchoan R, Broder S: Projections of the incidence of non-Hodgkin's lymphoma related to acquired immunodeficiency syndrome. J Natl Cancer Inst **83:**695-701, 1991.

855 Garvin AJ, Self S, Sahovic EA, Stuart RK, Marchalonis JJ: The occurrence of a peripheral T-cell lymphoma in a chronically immunosuppressed renal transplant patient. Am J Surg Pathol **12:**64-70, 1988.

856 Hamilton-Dutoit SJ, Raphael M, Audouin J, et al.: In situ demonstration of Epstein-Barr virus small RNAs (EBER 1) in acquired immunodeficiency syndrome-related lymphomas. Correlation with tumor morphology and primary site. Blood **92:**610-624, 1993.

857 Hanto DW, Birkenbach M, Frizzera G, Gajl-Peczalska KJ, Simmons RL, Schubach WH: Confirmation of the heterogeneity of posttransplant Epstein-Barr virus-associated B cell proliferations by immunoglobulin gene rearrangement analyses. Transplantation **47:**458-464, 1989.

858 Hanto DW, Frizzera G, Gajl-Peczalska KJ, Sakamoto K, Purtilo DT, Balfour HH Jr, Simmons RL, Najarian JS: Epstein-Barr virus induced B-cell lymphoma after renal transplantation. Acyclovir therapy and transition from polyclonal to monoclonal B-cell proliferation. N Engl J Med **306:**913-918, 1982.

859 Herndier B, Sanchez H, Chang KC, Chen YY, Weiss LM: High prevalence of detection of EBV RNA in the Reed-Sternberg cells of HIV-associated Hodgkin's disease. Am J Pathol **142:**1073-1079, 1993.

860 Ioachim HL: Neoplasms associated with immune deficiencies. Pathol Annu **22**(Pt 2):177-222, 1987.

861 Ioachim HL, Cooper MC, Hellman GC: Lymphomas in men at high risk for acquired immune deficiency syndrome (AIDS). A study of 21 cases. Cancer **56:**2831-2842, 1985.

862 Kamel OW, van de Rijn M, Weiss LM, Del Zoppo GJ, Hench PK, Robbins BA, Montgomery PG, Warnke RA, Dorfman RF: Brief report. Reversible lymphomas associated with Epstein-Barr virus occurring during methotrexate therapy for rheumatoid arthritis and dermatomyositis. N Engl J Med **328:**1317-1321, 1993.

862a Kastan M: Ataxia-telangiectasia. Broad implications for a rare disorder. N Engl J Med **333:**662-663, 1995.

863 Kersey JH, Spector BD, Good RA: Primary immunodeficiency diseases and cancer. The Immunodeficiency-Cancer Registry. Int J Cancer **12:**333-347, 1973.

864 Knowles DM: Acquired immunodeficiency syndrome-related lymphoma. Blood **80:**8-20, 1992.

865 Koo CH, Nathwani BN, Winberg CD, Hill LR, Rappaport H: Atypical lymphoplasmacytic and immunoblastic proliferation in lymph nodes of patients with autoimmune disease (autoimmune-disease-associated lymphadenopathy). Medicine (Baltimore) **63:**274-290, 1984.

866 Leblond V, Sutton L, Dorent R, Davi F, Bitker M-O, Gabarre J, Charlotte F, Ghoussoub J-J, Fourcase C, Fischer A, Gandjbakhch I, Binet J-L, Raphael M: Lymphoproliferative disorders after organ transplantation. A report of 24 cases observed in a single center. J Clin Oncol **13:**961-968, 1995.

867 Lippman SM, Grogan TM, Carry P, Pgden DA, Miller TP: Post-transplantation T cell lymphoblastic lymphoma. Am J Med **82:**814-816, 1987.

868 Locker J, Nalesnik M: Molecular genetic analysis of lymphoid tumors arising after organ transplantation. Am J Pathol **135:**977-987, 1989.

869 Louie S, Schwartz RS: Immunodeficiency and the pathogenesis of lymphoma and leukemia. Semin Hematol **15:**117-138, 1978.

870 Lowenthal DA, Straus DJ, Campbell SW, Gold JWM, Clarkson BD, Koziner B: AIDS-related lymphoid neoplasia. The Memorial Hospital experience. Cancer **61:**2325-2337, 1988.

870a Macchi P, Villa A, Gillani S, Sacco MG, Frattini A, Porta F, Ugazio AG, Johnston JR, Candotti F, O'Shea JJ, Vezzoni P, Notarangelo LD: Mutations of Jak-3 gene in patients with autosomal severe combined immune deficiency (SCID). Nature **377:**65-68, 1995.

871 Morrell D, Cromartie E, Swift M: Mortality and cancer incidence in 263 patients with ataxia-telangiectasia. J Natl Cancer Inst **77:**89-92, 1986.

871a Pathmanathan R, Prasad U, Sadler R, Flynn K, Raab-Traub N: Clonal proliferations of cells infected with Epstein-Barr virus in preinvasive lesions related to nasopharyngeal carcinoma. N Engl J Med **333:**693-698, 1995.

872 Patton DF, Wilkowski CW, Hanson CA, Shapiro R, Gajl-Peczalska KJ, Filipovich AH, McClain KL: Epstein-Barr virus–determined clonality in posttransplant lymphoproliferative disease. Transplantation **49:**1080-1084, 1990.

873 Pedersen C, Gerstoft J, Lundgren JD, Skinhoj P, Bottzauw J, Geisler C, Hamilton-Dutoit SJ, Thorsen S, Lisse I, Ralfkiaer E, et al.: HIV-associated lymphoma. Histopathology and association with Epstein-Barr virus genome related to clinical, immunological and prognostic features. Eur J Cancer **27:**1416-1423, 1991.

874 Penn I: Tumor incidence in human allograft recipients. Transplant Proc **11:**1047-1051, 1979.

875 Purtilo DT, DeFlorio D Jr, Hutt LM, Bhawan J, Yang JP, Otto R, Edwards W: Variable phenotypic expression of an X-linked recessive lymphoproliferative syndrome. N Engl J Med **297:**1077-1081, 1977.

876 Randhawa PS, Jaffe R, Demetris AJ, Nalesnik M, Starzl TE, Chen YY, Weiss LM: The systemic distribution of Epstein-Barr virus genomes in fatal post-transplantation lymphoproliferative disorders. An in situ hybridization study. Am J Pathol **138:**1027-1033, 1991.

877 Randhawa PS, Yousem SA, Paradis IL, Dauber JA, Griffith BP, Locker J: The clinical spectrum, pathology, and clonal analysis of Epstein-Barr virus-associated lymphoproliferative disorders in heart-lung transplant recipients. Am J Clin Pathol **92:**177-185, 1991.

878 Raphael M, Gentilhomme O, Tulliez M, Byron PA, Diebold J: Histopathologic features of high-grade non-Hodgkin's lymphomas in acquired immunodeficiency syndrome. The French Study Group of Pathology for Human Immunodeficiency Virus-Associated Tumors. Arch Pathol Lab Med **115:**15-20, 1991.

879 Ree HJ, Strauchen JA, Khan AA, Gold JE, Crowley JP, Kahn H, Zalusky R: Human immunodeficiency virus-associated Hodgkin's disease. Clinicopathologic studies of 24 cases and preponderance of mixed cellularity type characterized by the occurrence of fibrohistiocytoid stromal cells. Cancer **67:**1614-1621, 1991.

880 Sander CA, Medeiros LJ, Weiss LM, Yano T, Sneller MC, Jaffe ES: Lymphoproliferative lesions in patients with common variable immunodeficiency syndrome. Am J Surg Pathol **16:**1170-1182, 1992.

881 Savitsky K, Bar-Shira A, Gilad S, Rotman G, Ziv Y, Vanagaite L, Tagle DA, Smith S, Uziel T, Sfez S, Ashkenazi M, Pecker I, Frydman M, Harnik R, Patanjali SR, Simmons A, Clines GA, Sartiel A, Gatti RA, Chessa L, Sanal O, Lavin MF, Jaspers NGJ, Taylor AMR, Arlett CF, Miki T, Weissman SM, Lovett M, Collins FS, Shiloh Y: A single ataxia telangiectasia gene with a product similar to PI-3 kinase. Science **268:**1749-1753, 1995.

882 Schmid U, Helbron D, Lennert K: Development of malignant lymphoma in myoepithelial sialadenitis (Sjögren's syndrome). Virchows Arch [A] **395**:11-43, 1982.

883 Shearer WT, Ritz J, Finegold MJ, Guerra IC, Rosenblatt HM, Lewis DE, Pollack MS, Taber LH, Sumaya CV, Grumet FC, Cleary ML, Warnke R, Sklar J: Epstein-Barr virus-associated B-cell proliferations of diverse clonal origins after bone marrow transplantation in a 12-year-old patient with severe combined immunodeficiency. N Engl J Med **312**:1151-1159, 1985.

884 Spector BD, Perry GS III, Kersey JH: Genetically determined immunodeficiency diseases (GDID) and malignancy. Report from the Immunodeficiency-Cancer Registry. Clin Immunol Immunopathol **11**:12-29, 1978.

885 Swinnen LJ, Costanzo-Nordin MR, Fisher SG, O'Sullivan EJ, Johnson MR, Heroux AL, Dizikes GJ, Pifarre R, Fisher RI: Increased incidence of lymphoproliferative disorder after immunosuppression with the monoclonal antibody OKT3 in cardiac-transplant recipients. N Engl J Med **323**:1723-1728, 1990.

886 Tirelli U, Errante D, Dolcetti R, Gloghini A, Serraino D, Vaccher E, Franceschi S, Boiocchi M, Carbone A: Hodgkin's disease and human immunodeficiency virus infection. Clinicopathologic and virologic features of 114 patients from the Italian Cooperative Group on AIDS and Tumors. J Clin Oncol **13**:1758-1767, 1995.

887 Wang C-Y, Snow JL, Su WPD: Lymphoma associated with human immunodeficiency virus infection. Mayo Clin Proc **70**:665-672, 1995.

LYMPH NODE INCLUSIONS

888 Arai T, Kino I, Nakamura S, Ogawa H: Epidermal inclusions in abdominal lymph nodes. Report of two cases studied immunohistochemically. Acta Pathol Jpn **42**:126-129, 1992.

889 Azzopardi JG, Ross CMD, Frizzera G: Blue naevi of lymph node capsule. Histopathology **1**:451-461, 1977.

890 Bramlett CB, Laucirica R, Page DL, Bluth RF: Differentiation between metastatic low grade carcinoma of the breast and benign epithelial inclusions in axillary lymph nodes (abstract). Mod Pathol **8**:15A, 1995.

891 Brooks JS, Li Volsi VA, Pietra GG: Mesothelial cell inclusions in mediastinal lymph nodes mimicking metastatic carcinoma. Am J Clin Pathol **93**:741-748, 1990.

892 Brown RB, Gaillard RA, Turner JA: The significance of aberrant or heterotopic parotid gland tissue in lymph nodes. Ann Surg **138**:850-856, 1953.

893 Covell LM, Disciullo AJ, Knapp RC: Decidual change in pelvic lymph nodes in the presence of cervical squamous cell carcinoma during pregnancy. Am J Obstet Gynecol **127**:674-676, 1977.

894 Edlow DW, Carter D: Heterotopic epithelium in axillary lymph nodes. Am J Clin Pathol **59**:666-673, 1973.

895 Ehrmann RL, Federschneider JM, Knapp RC: Distinguishing lymph node metastases from benign glandular inclusions in low-grade ovarian carcinoma. Am J Obstet Gynecol **136**:737-746, 1980.

896 Fisher CJ, Hill S, Millis RR: Benign lymph node inclusions mimicking metastatic carcinoma. J Clin Pathol **47**:245-247, 1994.

897 Holdsworth PJ, Hopkinson JM, Leveson SH: Benign axillary epithelial lymph node inclusions—a histological pitfall. Histopathology **13**:226-228, 1988.

898 Johnson WT, Helwig EB: Benign nevus cells in the capsule of lymph nodes. Cancer **23**:747-753, 1969.

899 Karp LA, Czernobilsky B: Glandular inclusions in pelvic and abdominal paraaortic lymph nodes. Am J Clin Pathol **52**:212-218, 1969.

900 Koss LG: Miniature adenoacanthoma arising in an endometriotic cyst in an obturator lymph node. Report of first case. Cancer **16**:1369-1372, 1963.

901 Longo S: Benign lymph node inclusions. Hum Pathol **7**:349-354, 1976.

902 Maassen V, Hiller K: Glandular inclusions in lymph nodes: Pattern of distribution and metaplastic transformation. Arch Gynecol Obstet **255**:1-8, 1994.

903 Micheau C, Cachin Y, Caillou B: Cystic metastases in the neck revealing occult carcinoma of the tonsil. A report of six cases. Cancer **33**:228-233, 1974.

904 Prade M, Spatz A, Bentler R, Duvillar P, Bognel C, Robboy SJ: Borderline and malignant serous tumor arising in pelvic lymph nodes. Evidence of origin in benign glandular inclusions. Int J Gynecol Pathol **14**:87-91, 1995.

905 Rutty GN, Lauder I: Mesothelial cell inclusions within mediastinal lymph nodes. Histopathology **25**:483-488, 1994.

906 Sussman J, Rosai J: Lymph node metastasis as the initial manifestation of malignant mesothelioma. Report of six cases. Am J Surg Pathol **14**:819-828, 1990.

907 Turner DR, Millis RR: Breast tissue inclusions in axillary lymph nodes. Histopathology **4**:631-636, 1980.

OTHER NON-NEOPLASTIC LESIONS

908 Albores-Saavedra J, Vuitch F, Delgado R, Wiley E, Hagler H: Sinus histiocytosis of pelvic lymph nodes after hip replacement. A histiocytic proliferation induced by cobalt-chromium and titanium. Am J Surg Pathol **18**:83-90, 1994.

908a Arber DA, Kamel OW, van de Rijn M, Davis E, Medeiros LJ, Jaffe ES, Weiss LM: Frequent presence of the Epstein-Barr virus in inflammatory pseudotumor. Hum Pathol **26**:1093-1098, 1995.

909 Banerjee D, Mills DM, Hearn SA, Meek M, Turner KL: Proteinaceous lymphadenopathy due to monoclonal nonamyloid immunoglobulin deposit disease. Arch Pathol Lab Med **114**:34-39, 1990.

910 Cleary KR, Osborne BM, Butler JJ: Lymph node infarction foreshadowing malignant lymphoma. Am J Surg Pathol **6**:435-442, 1982.

911 Davies JD, Stansfeld AG: Spontaneous infarction of superficial lymph nodes. J Clin Pathol **25**:689-696, 1972.

913 Davies JD, Webb AJ: Segmental lymph-node infarction after fine-needle aspiration. J Clin Pathol **35**:855-857, 1982.

914 Magrina JF, Symmonds RE, Dahlin DC: Pelvic "lipolymph nodes." A consideration in the differential diagnosis of pelvic masses. Am J Obstet Gynecol **136**:727-731, 1980.

915 Mahy NJ, Davies JD: Ischaemic changes in human mesenteric lymph nodes. J Pathol **144**:257-267, 1984.

916 Maurer R, Schmid U, Davies JD, Mahy NJ, Stansfeld AG, Lukes RJ: Lymph-node infarction and malignant lymphoma. A multicentre survey of European, English and American cases. Histopathology **10**:571-588, 1986.

917 Osborne BM, Butler JJ, Mackay B: Proteinaceous lymphadenopathy with hypergammaglobulinemia. Am J Surg Pathol **3**:137-145, 1979.

918 Shah KH, Kisilevsky R: Infarction of the lymph nodes. A cause of a palisading macrophage reaction mimicking necrotizing granulomas. Hum Pathol **9**:597-599, 1978.

919 Truong LD, Cartwright J Jr, Goodman MD, Woznicki D: Silicone lymphadenopathy associated with augmentation mammaplasty. Morphologic features of nine cases. Am J Surg Pathol **12**:484-491, 1988.

TUMORS OF DENDRITIC CELLS AND MACROPHAGES

920 Chan JK, Tsang WY, Ng CS, Tang SK, Yu HC, Lee AW: Follicular dendritic cell tumors of the oral cavity. Am J Surg Pathol **18**:148-157, 1994.

921 Feltkamp CA, van Heerde P, Feltkamp-Vroom TM, Koudstaal J: A malignant tumor arising from interdigitating cells; light microscopical, ultrastructural, immuno- and enzyme-histochemical characteristics. Virchows Arch [A] **393**:183-192, 1981.

922 Franchino C, Reich C, Distenfeld A, Ubriaco A, Knowles DM: A clinicopathologically distinctive primary splenic histiocytic neoplasm. Demonstration of its histiocyte derivation by immunophenotypic and molecular genetic analysis. Am J Surg Pathol **12**:398-404, 1988.

923 Gould VE, Bloom KJ, Franke WW, Warren WH, Moll R: Increased numbers of cytokeratin-positive interstitial reticulum cells (CIRC) in reactive, inflammatory and neoplastic lymphadenopathies. Hyperplasia or induced expression? Virchows Arch **425**:617-630, 1995.

924 Hammar SP, Rudolph RH, Bockus DE, Remington FL: Interdigitating reticulum cell sarcoma with unusual features. Ultrastruct Pathol **15**:631-645, 1991.

925 Hanson CA, Jaszcz W, Kersey JH, Astorga MG, Peterson BA, Gajl-Peczalska KJ, Frizzera G: True histiocytic lymphoma. Histopathologic, immunophenotypic and genotypic analysis. Br J Haematol **73**:187-198, 1989.

926 Hollowood K, Pease C, Mackay AM, Fletcher CD: Sarcomatoid tumours of lymph nodes showing follicular dendritic cell differentiation. J Pathol **163**:205-216, 1991.

927 Hollowood K, Stamp G, Zouvani J, Fletcher CDM: Extranodal follicular dendritic cell sarcoma of the gastrointestinal tract. Morphologic, immunohistochemical and ultrastructural analysis of two cases. Am J Clin Pathol **103**:90-97, 1995.

928 Hsu SM, Ho YS, Hsu PL: Lymphomas of true histiocytic origin. Expression of different phenotypes in so-called true histiocytic lymphoma and malignant histiocytosis. Am J Pathol **138**:1389-1404, 1991.

929 Hui PK, Feller AC, Kaiserling E, Hesse G, Rodermund OE, Haneke E, Weber L, Lennert K: Skin tumor of T accessory cells (interdigitating reticulum cells) with high content of T lymphocytes. Am J Dermatopathol **9**:129-137, 1987.

930 Kamel O, Kell D, Gocke C, Warnke R: True histiocytic lymphoma. A study of 12 cases based on current definition (abstract). Mod Pathol **7**:112A, 1994.

931 Miettinen M, Fletcher CD, Lasota J: True histiocytic lymphoma of small intestine. Analysis of two S-100 protein-positive cases with features of interdigitating reticulum cell sarcoma. Am J Clin Pathol **100**:285-292, 1993.

932 Milchgrub S, Kamel OW, Wiley E, Vuitch F, Cleary ML, Warnke RA: Malignant histiocytic neoplasms of the small intestine. Am J Surg Pathol **16**:11-20, 1992.

933 Monda L, Warnke R, Rosai J: A primary lymph node malignancy with features suggestive of dendritic reticulum cell differentiation. A report of 4 cases. Am J Pathol **122**:562-572, 1986.

934 Perez-Ordóñez B, Erlandson RA, Rosai J: Dendritic follicular cell tumor. Report of 13 additional cases of a distinctive entity. Am J Surg Pathol (in press).

935 Ralfkiaer E, Delsol G, O'Connor NT, Brandtzaeg P, Brousset P, Vejlsgaard GL, Mason DY: Malignant lymphomas of true histiocytic origin. A clinical, histological, immunophenotypic and genotypic study. J Pathol 160:9-17, 1990.

936 Soria C, Orradre JL, Garcia-Almagro D, Martinez B, Algara P, Piris MA: True histiocytic lymphoma (monocytic sarcoma). Am J Dermatopathol 14:511-517, 1992.

937 van den Oord JJ, de Wolf-Peeters C, de Vos R, Thomas J, Desmet VJ: Sarcoma arising from interdigitating reticulum cells. Report of a case, studied with light and electron microscopy, and enzyme- and immunohistochemistry. Histopathology 10:509-523, 1986.

938 Weiss LM, Berry GJ, Dorfman RF, Banks P, Kaiserling E, Curtis J, Rosai J, Warnke RA: Spindle cell neoplasms of lymph nodes of probable reticulum cell lineage. True reticulum cell sarcoma? Am J Surg Pathol 14:405-414, 1990.

939 Yamakawa M, Matsuda M, Imai Y, Arai S, Harada K, Sato T: Lymph node interdigitating cell sarcoma. A case report. Am J Clin Pathol 97:139-146, 1992.

VASCULAR TUMORS AND TUMORLIKE CONDITIONS

940 Almagro UA, Choi H, Rouse TM: Hemangioma in a lymph node. Arch Pathol Lab Med 109:576-578, 1985.

941 Bonzanini M, Togni R, Barabareschi M, Parenti A, Dalla Palma P: Primary Kaposi's sarcoma of intraparotid lymph node. Histopathology 21:489-491, 1992.

942 Chan JK, Frizzera G, Fletcher CD, Rosai J: Primary vascular tumors of lymph nodes other than Kaposi's sarcoma. Analysis of 39 cases and delineation of two new entities. Am J Surg Pathol 16:335-350, 1992.

943 Chan JK, Lewin KJ, Lombard CM, Teitelbaum S, Dorfman RF: Histopathology of bacillary angiomatosis of lymph node. Am J Surg Pathol 15:430-437, 1991.

944 Chan JK, Warnke RA, Dorfman R: Vascular transformation of sinuses in lymph nodes. A study of its morphological spectrum and distinction from Kaposi's sarcoma. Am J Surg Pathol 15:732-743, 1991.

945 Cockerell CJ, Whitlow MA, Webster GF, Friedman-Kien AE: Epithelioid angiomatosis. A distinct vascular disorder in patients with the acquired immunodeficiency syndrome or AIDS-related complex. Lancet 2:654-656, 1987.

946 Cook PD, Czerniak B, Chan JKC, Mackay B, Ordóñez NG, Ayala AG, Rosai J: Nodular spindle-cell vascular transformation of lymph nodes. A benign process occurring predominantly in retroperitoneal lymph nodes draining carcinomas that can simulate Kaposi's sarcoma or metastatic tumor. Am J Surg Pathol 19:1010-1020, 1995.

947 Dorfman RF: Kaposi's sarcoma revisited. Hum Pathol 15:1013-1017, 1984.

948 Fayemi AO, Toker C: Nodal angiomatosis. Arch Pathol 99:170-172, 1975.

949 Frizzera G, Banks PM, Massarelli G, Rosai J: A systemic lymphoproliferative disorder with morphologic features of Castleman's disease. Pathological findings in 15 patients. Am J Surg Pathol 7:211-231, 1983.

950 Fukunaga M, Silverberg SG: Hyaline globules in Kaposi's sarcoma. A light microscopic and immunohistochemical study. Mod Pathol 4:187-190, 1991.

951 Goldstein JED, Bartal N: Hemangioendothelioma of the lymph node. A case report. J Surg Oncol 23:314-317, 1985.

952 Haferkamp O, Rosenau W, Lennert K: Vascular transformation of lymph node sinuses due to venous obstruction. Arch Pathol Lab Med 92:81-83, 1971.

953 Lott MF, Davies JD: Lymph node hypervascularity. Haemangiomatoid lesions and pan-nodal vasodilatation. J Pathol 140:209-219, 1983.

954 Lubin J, Rywlin AM: Lymphoma-like lymph node changes in Kaposi's sarcoma. Arch Pathol 92:338-341, 1971.

955 O'Connell KM: Kaposi's sarcoma in lymph nodes. Histological study of lesions from 16 cases in Malawi. J Clin Pathol 30:696-703, 1977.

956 Ostrowski ML, Siddiqui T, Barnes RE, Howton MJ: Vascular transformation of lymph node sinuses. A process displaying a spectrum of histologic features. Arch Pathol Lab Med 114:656-660, 1990.

957 Perez-Piteira J, Ariza A, Mate JL, Ojanguren I, Navas-Palacios JJ: Bacillary angiomatosis. A gross mimicker of malignancy. Histopathology 26:476-478, 1995.

958 Silva EG, Phillips MJ, Langer B, Ordonez NG: Spindle and histiocytoid (epithelioid) hemangioendothelioma. Primary in lymph node. Am J Clin Pathol 85:731-735, 1986.

959 Steinmann G, Földi E, Földi M, Racz P, Lennert K: Morphologic findings in lymph nodes after occlusion of their efferent lymphatic vessels and veins. Lab Invest 47:43-50, 1982.

960 Suster S: Nodal angiolymphoid hyperplasia with eosinophilia. Am J Clin Pathol 88:236-239, 1987.

961 Tsang WY, Chan JK, Dorfman RF, Rosai J: Vasoproliferative lesions of the lymph node. Pathol Annu 29(Pt 1):63-133, 1994.

962 Weshler Z, Leviatan A, Krasnokuki D, Kopolovitch J: Primary Kaposi's sarcoma in lymph nodes concurrent with chronic lymphatic leukemia. Am J Clin Pathol 71:234-237, 1979.

963 Wright DH, Padley NR, Judd MA: Angiolymphoid hyperplasia with eosinophilia simulating lymphadenopathy. Histopathology 5:127-140, 1981.

OTHER PRIMARY TUMORS AND TUMORLIKE CONDITIONS

964 Alguacil-Garcia A: Intranodal myofibroblastoma in a submandibular lymph node. A case report. Am J Clin Pathol 97:69-72, 1992.

965 Barbareschi M, Mariscotti C, Ferrero S, Pignatiello U: Intranodal haemorrhagic spindle cell tumour. A benign Kaposi-like nodal tumour. Histopathology 17:93-96, 1990.

966 Brecher ME, Gill WB, Straus FH: Angiomyolipoma with regional lymph node involvement and long-term follow-up study. Hum Pathol 17:962-963, 1986.

967 Brunning RD, McKenna RW, Rosai J, Parkin JL, Risdall R: Systemic mastocytosis. Extracutaneous manifestations. Am J Surg Pathol 7:425-438, 1983.

968 Chan JK, Frizzera G, Fletcher CD, Rosai J: Primary vascular tumors of lymph nodes other than Kaposi's sarcoma. Analysis of 39 cases and delineation of two new entities. Am J Surg Pathol 16:335-350, 1992.

969 Channer JL, Davies JD: Smooth muscle proliferation in the hilum of superficial lymph nodes. Virchows Arch [A] 406:261-270, 1985.

970 Corrin B, Liebow AA, Friedman PJ: Pulmonary lymphangiomyomatosis. Am J Pathol 79:348-382, 1975.

971 Craig SS, DeBlois G, Schwartz LB: Mast cells in human keloid, small intestine, and lung by an immunoperoxidase technique using a murine monoclonal antibody against tryptase. Am J Pathol 124:427-435, 1986.

972 Davis RE, Warnke RA, Dorfman RF: Inflammatory pseudotumor of lymph nodes. Additional observations and evidence for an inflammatory etiology. Am J Surg Pathol 15:744-756, 1991.

973 Facchetti F, De Wolf Peeters C, De Wever I, Frizzera G: Inflammatory pseudotumor of lymph nodes. Immunohistochemical evidence for its fibrohistiocytic nature. Am J Pathol 137:281-289, 1990.

974 Fletcher CD, Stirling RW: Intranodal myofibroblastoma presenting in the submandibular region. Evidence of a broader clinical and histological spectrum. Histopathology 16:287-293, 1990.

975 Horie A, Ishii N, Matsumoto M, Hashizume Y, Kawakami M, Sato Y: Leiomyomatosis in the pelvic lymph node and peritoneum. Acta Pathol Jpn 34:813-819, 1984.

976 Hudock C, Chatten J, Miettinen M: Immunohistochemical evaluation of myeloid leukemia infiltrates (granulocytic sarcomas) in formaldehyde-fixed, paraffin-embedded tissue. Am J Clin Pathol 102:55-60, 1994.

977 Kemper CA, Davis RE, Deresinski SC, Dorfmann RF: Inflammatory pseudotumor of intra-abdominal lymph nodes manifesting as recurrent fever of unknown origin. A case report. Am J Med 90:519-523, 1991.

978 Lennert K, Illert E: Die Häufigkeit der Gewebsmastzellen im Lymphknoten bei verschiedenen Erkrankungen. Frankf Z Pathol 70:121-131, 1959.

979 Lennert K, Parwaresch MR: Mast cells and mast cell neoplasia. A review. Histopathology 3:349-365, 1979.

980 Mazzoleni G, Salerno A, Santini D, Marabini A, Martinelli G: Leiomyomatosis in pelvic lymph nodes. Histopathology 21:588-589, 1992.

981 Michal M, Chlumska A, Povysilova V: Intranodal "amianthoid" myofibroblastoma. Report of six cases immunohistochemical and electron microscopical study. Pathol Res Pract 188:199-204, 1992.

982 Perrone T, De Wolf-Peeters C, Frizzera G: Inflammatory pseudotumor of lymph nodes. A distinctive pattern of nodal reaction. Am J Surg Pathol 12:351-361, 1988.

983 Rimmer EF, Turberville C, Horton M: Human mast cells detected by monoclonal antibodies. J Clin Pathol 37:1249-1255, 1984.

984 Skalova A, Michal M, Chlumska A, Leivo I: Collagen composition and ultrastructure of the so-called amianthoid fibres in palisaded myofibroblastoma. Ultrastructural and immunohistochemical study. J Pathol 167:335-340, 1992.

985 Starasoler L, Vuitch F, Albores-Saavedra J: Intranodal leiomyoma. Another distinctive primary spindle cell neoplasm of lymph node. Am J Clin Pathol 95:858-862, 1991.

986 Suster S, Rosai J: Intranodal hemorrhagic spindle-cell tumor with "amianthoid" fibers. Report of six cases of a distinctive mesenchymal neoplasm of the inguinal region that simulates Kaposi's sarcoma. Am J Surg Pathol 13:347-357, 1989.

987 Tanda F, Massarelli G, Cossu A, Bosincu L, Cossu S, Ibba M: Primary spindle cell tumor of lymph node with "amianthoid" fibers. A histological, immunohistochemical and ultrastructural study. Ultrastruct Pathol **17:**195-205, 1993.

988 Weiss SW, Gnepp DR, Bratthauer GL: Palisaded myofibroblastoma. A benign mesenchymal tumor of lymph node. Am J Surg Pathol **13:**341-346, 1989.

989 White JET, Chan YF, Miller MV: Intranodal leiomyoma or myofibroblastoma. An identical lesion? Histopathology **26:**188-189, 1995.

METASTATIC TUMORS

990 Batsakis JG: The pathology of head and neck tumors. The occult primary and metastases to the head and neck, part 10. Head Neck Surg **3:**409-423, 1981.

990a Cervin JR, Silverman JF, Loggie BW, Geisinger KR: Virchow's node revisited. Analysis with clinicopathologic correlation of 152 fine-needle aspiration biopsies of supraclavicular lymph nodes. Arch Pathol Lab Med **119:**727-730, 1995.

991 Clary CF, Michel RP, Wang N-S, Hanson RE: Metastatic carcinoma. The lung as the site for the clinically undiagnosed primary. Cancer **51:**362-366, 1983.

992 Copeland EM, McBride CM: Axillary metastases from unknown primary sites. Ann Surg **178:**25-27, 1973.

993 Didlolker MS, Fanous N, Elias EG, et al.: Metastatic carcinomas from occult primary tumours. A study of 254 patients. Ann Surg **186:**628-630, 1977.

994 Dvorak AM, Monahan RA: Metastatic adenocarcinoma of unknown primary site. Diagnostic electron microscopy to determine the site of tumor origin. Arch Pathol Lab Med **106:**21-24, 1982.

995 Feigenberg Z, Zer M, Dintsman M: Axillary metastases from an unknown primary source. Isr J Med Sci **12:**1153-1158, 1976.

996 Giffler RF, Gillespie JJ, Ayala AG, Newland JR: Lymphoepithelioma in cervical lymph nodes of children and young adults. Am J Surg Pathol **1:**293-302, 1977.

997 Haagensen CD, Feind CR, Herter FP, Slanetz CA Jr, Weinberg JA: The lymphatics in cancer. Philadelphia, 1972, WB Saunders Co.

998 Lindbergh R: Distribution of cervical lymph node metastases from squamous cell carcinoma of the upper respiratory and digestive tracts. Cancer **29:**1446-1449, 1972.

999 Mackay B, Ordoñez NG: The role of the pathologist in the evaluation of poorly differentiated tumors and metastatic tumors of unknown origin. In Fer MF, Greco FA, Oldham RK, eds: Poorly differentiated neoplasms and tumors of unknown origin, New York, 1986, Grune & Stratton, Inc.

1000 Mancuso AA, Hanafee WN: Elusive head and neck carcinomas beneath intact mucosa. Laryngoscope **93:**133-139, 1983.

1001 Markman M: Metastatic adenocarcinoma of unknown primary site. Analysis of 245 patients seen at the Johns Hopkins Hospital from 1965-1979. Med Pediatr Oncol **10:**569-574, 1982.

1002 Silverman CL, Marks JE: Metastatic cancer of unknown origin. Epidermoid and undifferentiated carcinomas. Semin Oncol **9:**435-441, 1982.

1003 Sussman J, Rosai J: Lymph node metastases as the initial manifestation of malignant mesothelioma. Report of six cases. Am J Surg Pathol **14:**819-828, 1990.

1004 Willis RA: The spread of tumours in the human body, ed 3. Stoneham, Mass, 1973, Butterworth Publishers.

1005 Zaren HA, Copeland EM: Inguinal node metastases. Cancer **41:**919-923, 1978.

22 Spleen

NORMAL ANATOMY

The spleen performs a variety of functions, most of which have been correlated with specific anatomic compartments.[2,4,5,10] The most important are (1) hematopoiesis (erythrocytes, granulocytes, megakaryocytes, lymphocytes, and macrophages), (2) reservoir (storage or sequestration of platelets and other formed elements), (3) phagocytosis (removal of particulate matter, red blood cell destruction, pitting, and erythroclasis), and (4) immunity (trapping and processing of antigen, "homing" of lymphocytes, lymphocyte transformation and proliferation, and antibody production).[2,4] The first two functions are not important in normal adult humans.

Anatomically, the spleen is divided into two compartments —white pulp and red pulp—separated by an ill-defined interphase known as the marginal zone.[3,7,9,10] The white pulp is made up of T and B lymphocytes, the former located in the periarteriolar lymphoid sheath and the latter eccentrically to this sheath in the form of primary lymphoid follicles.[6] These lymphoid follicles contain germinal centers, particularly in children.[5]

The red pulp consists of a complex network of venous sinuses and cords. The latter contain most of the splenic macrophages, which are responsible for the important phagocytic function of this organ. The sinuses are lined by a particular type of endothelial cell (known as littoral cell) and have a discontinuous wall, which allows traffic of blood cells between cords and sinuses.[1,8,11]

BIOPSY AND FINE-NEEDLE ASPIRATION

Biopsy of the spleen is rarely attempted because of the possibility of hemorrhage and the preconceived notion that the biopsy will not be of diagnostic help. Obviously, the procedure should not be performed on patients with a bleeding tendency. A few authors in this country and abroad have used it routinely, either with the Vim-Silverman–type needle to obtain a core of tissue or with a fine needle to obtain an aspirate.[12,14-16] These authors claim that morbidity is nil and that in some instances the technique results in a definitive diagnosis that is not easily obtainable by other means. Cavanna et al.[13] performed ultrasonically guided percutaneous splenic tissue core biopsy in 46 patients with malignant lymphoma (in most instances as a staging or restaging procedure) and were able to obtain adequate material in all but one of the cases. There were no complications in any of the patients.

RUPTURE AND SPLENECTOMY

Blunt trauma to the abdomen and surgical intervention within the abdominal cavity are the two most common factors responsible for rupture of the normal spleen.[31] In most instances, hemoperitoneum is an immediate consequence, leading to an emergency splenectomy. In about 15% of the cases, the rupture is "delayed" anywhere from 48 hours to several months.[25] Examination of the excised spleen will reveal the ruptured area, which, in many cases, is limited to a deceptively small capsular tear. Microscopically, leukocytic infiltration often is seen along the edges of the tear.

Following traumatic rupture, splenic tissue in small nodules may grow as implants on the peritoneal surface, abdominal wall, and even within the pleural cavity, a process known as *splenosis*[18,19] (Fig. 22-1). These nodules are surrounded by a capsule. Some are poorly developed architecturally,[24] but others show a full complement of red and white pulp, resulting in an appearance similar to that of accessory spleen.[20]

The diseases most commonly associated with *spontaneous rupture* of the spleen are infectious mononucleosis,[17] malaria, typhoid fever, subacute bacterial endocarditis, peliosis lienis[26,27] (see p. 1782), malignant lymphomas (including those occurring in HIV-infected patients),[23] leukemias, and primary nonlymphoid splenic neoplasms.[34] In every case of ruptured spleen without history of trauma or in which the trauma seems insignificant, a careful microscopic study should be performed in order to rule out all these possibilities. Rupture of the spleen with resulting hemoperitoneum is the most frequent cause of death in infectious mononucleosis. This complication usually occurs from 10 to 21 days after the onset of the disease.[32] In rare cases, "spontaneous" rupture may occur in a perfectly normal spleen, particularly during pregnancy.[29]

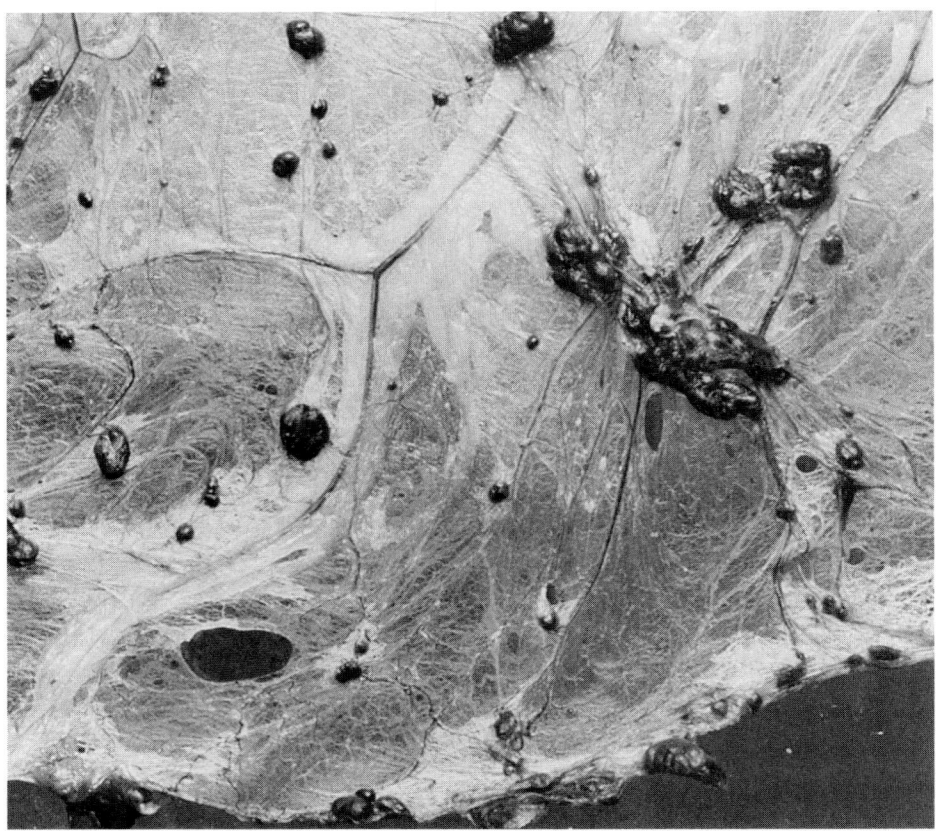

Fig. 22-1 Splenosis presenting as multiple, small nodules on peritoneal surface. Patient previously had ruptured spleen.

Splenectomy performed in adults for traumatic rupture of the spleen usually does not result in any sequelae of significance.[30] Conversely, an increased incidence and severity of infections have been reported following splenectomy in young children.[28] It has been shown that this is the result of a decrease in immunoglobulin production and phagocytic activity during episodes of transient bacteremia.[21,22] Overwhelming infection may occur days to years after removal of the spleen; it begins abruptly, frequently lacks an identifiable focus, and usually progresses rapidly despite appropriate antibiotic therapy, resulting in a mortality of 50% to 80%.[33] Because of this, an attempt is now made to save splenic function in children by performing repair of the laceration or by partial splenectomy. If a total splenectomy is necessary, spleen autotransplant has been recommended.[33] The patient's immune function is better preserved by any of these measures than by splenectomy alone.[35]

Whenever splenectomy is performed for hematologic disorders, a thorough search should be made for accessory spleens in order to excise them if present.

CONGENITAL ANOMALIES

Accessory (supernumerary) spleen is found in about 10% of individuals. It may be solitary or multiple, usually measures no more than 4 cm in diameter, and has a gross and microscopic appearance similar to that of the parent organ. Its most common location is the hilum of the spleen, and it is sometimes seen in contiguity with the tail of the pancreas. It should be distinguished from lymph nodes (especially when involved by Castleman's disease) and splenosis (see p. 1775). Accessory spleens may contain epithelial cysts within them (see p. 1777).

Congenital absence of the spleen ***(asplenia)*** is associated in more than 80% of the cases with malformations of the heart, nearly always involving the atrioventricular endocardial cushion and the ventricular outflow tracts.[41] Anomalies of the blood vessels, lung, and abdominal viscera also are frequent.[37] In ***polysplenia,*** the cardiac anomalies are less severe and the prognosis is therefore more favorable.[43] A hereditary form of splenic ***hypoplasia*** has been reported.[39]

Splenic-gonadal fusion occurs in two forms. One is *continuous,* in which the main spleen is connected by a cord of splenic and fibrous tissue to the gonadal (usually testicular) mesonephric structures; the other is *discontinuous,* in which discrete masses of splenic tissue are found fused to these same structures.[40,42] Of the fifty-two cases reviewed by Watson,[44] only four were in females. Eleven were associated with other congenital defects, such as peromelus and micrognathia. Various degrees of testicular ectopia and inguinal hernias are common. All of the reported cases have been on the left side.[42]

Cases of ***splenohepatic*** and ***splenorenal fusion*** have also been recorded.[36,38]

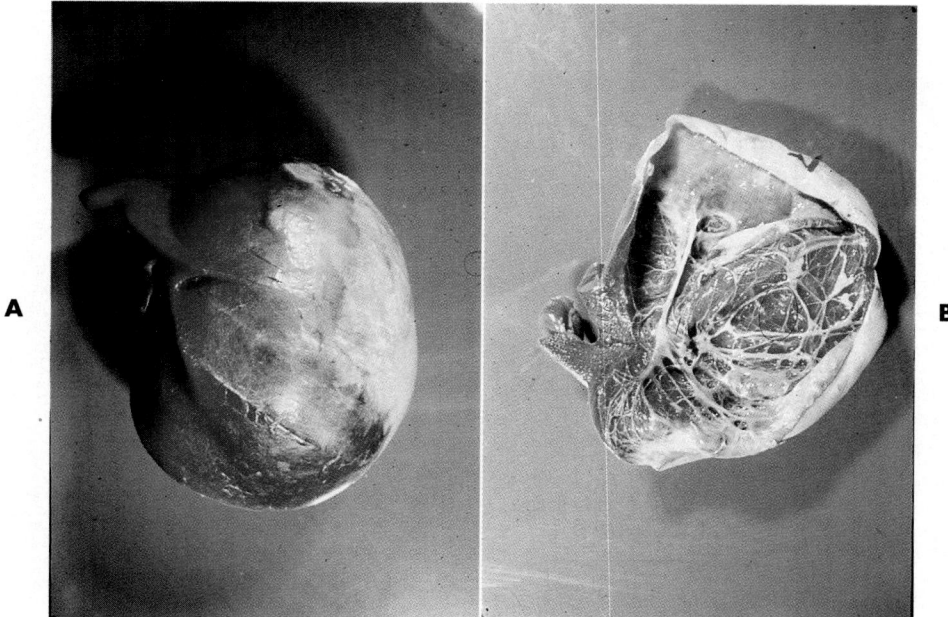

Fig. 22-2 False (secondary) cyst. **A,** Outer aspect. **B,** Inner surface. Notice the white trabeculation.

CYSTS

False (secondary) cysts constitute approximately 75% of the nonparasitic cysts of the spleen (Fig. 22-2).[47,48,52] Their wall is composed of dense fibrous tissue, often calcified, with no epithelial lining. The content is a mixture of blood and necrotic debris. If the cyst ruptures, massive hemoperitoneum may result. The majority of these cysts are solitary and asymptomatic. Trauma is the most likely etiologic factor, although it is possible that some are epithelial cysts of the type described below in which part or all of the lining has been destroyed.

Epithelial (epidermoid or primary) cysts are mainly seen in children or young adults.[45,53,54] They are usually solitary, but can be multiple. Cases have also been described in accessory spleens.[50] Grossly, a glistening inner surface with marked trabeculation is often seen (Fig. 22-3). Microscopically, the wall is lined by columnar, cuboidal (mesothelial-like), or squamous epithelium. Skin adnexae are absent. The histogenesis is unknown; embryonic inclusions of epithelial cells from adjacent structures and invagination of capsular surface mesothelium have been proposed.[46,51] The immunohistochemical profile is more in keeping with a teratomatous derivation or origin from fetal squamous epithelium than from squamous mesothelial hyperplasia or inclusions of mature squamous epithelium.[49] Most cases of epithelial splenic cysts are large and require splenectomy. If enough parenchyma is preserved, the performance of a partial splenectomy should be attempted, particularly in children.

INFLAMMATION

Reactive follicular hyperplasia of the spleen can be seen as an acute phenomenon in response to a systemic infection, associated with variable degrees of congestion, diffuse immunoblastic and plasmacytic proliferation, and outpouring of neutrophils in the red pulp (so-called septic spleen or acute septic splenitis); measles and typhoid fever are the two better known examples. It also occurs in a chronic form in a large number of infectious diseases—including AIDS[61,65]—and in immune-mediated diseases, such as idiopathic thrombocytopenic purpura, acquired hemolytic anemia, rheumatoid arthritis (including Felty's syndrome), and the systemic form of Castleman's disease,[62,76] as well as in hemodialyzed patients.[70]

Diffuse lymphoid hyperplasia with production of immunoblasts and plasma cells can be the result of infection (particularly viral), graft rejection, or a component of angioimmunoblastic lymphadenopathy (see Chapter 21). In infectious mononucleosis, the splenic involvement is mainly in the red pulp.

Bagshawe[55] compared the clinical and laboratory features of hypersplenism among forty-six patients with congestive splenomegaly and twenty-nine with reactive splenomegaly and found no significant differences between them. Massive splenomegaly of a reactive nature is commonly seen in inhabitants of several tropical countries, such as Zaire, Malagasy Republic, Nigeria, and New Guinea.[60] Spleens removed for this *tropical splenomegaly syndrome* are often extremely heavy (mean, 3270 g) and exhibit a uniform dark red, cut surface. Microscopically, there is marked dilatation of the sinuses and foci of extramedullary hematopoiesis but no significant fibrosis or hemosiderin deposition.[71] Signs of hypersplenism are the rule. Epidemiologic and therapeutic studies suggest a causal relationship with malaria.[71,73] In this regard, it is interesting that the cases of idiopathic splenomegaly reported by Banti in 1883[66] were from an area of central Italy that at the time was endemic for malaria (see p. 1782).

Abscess of the spleen, an extremely rare condition, can be the result of trauma or metastatic spread of infection from another site.[58,59] Septic abscesses of the spleen secondary to

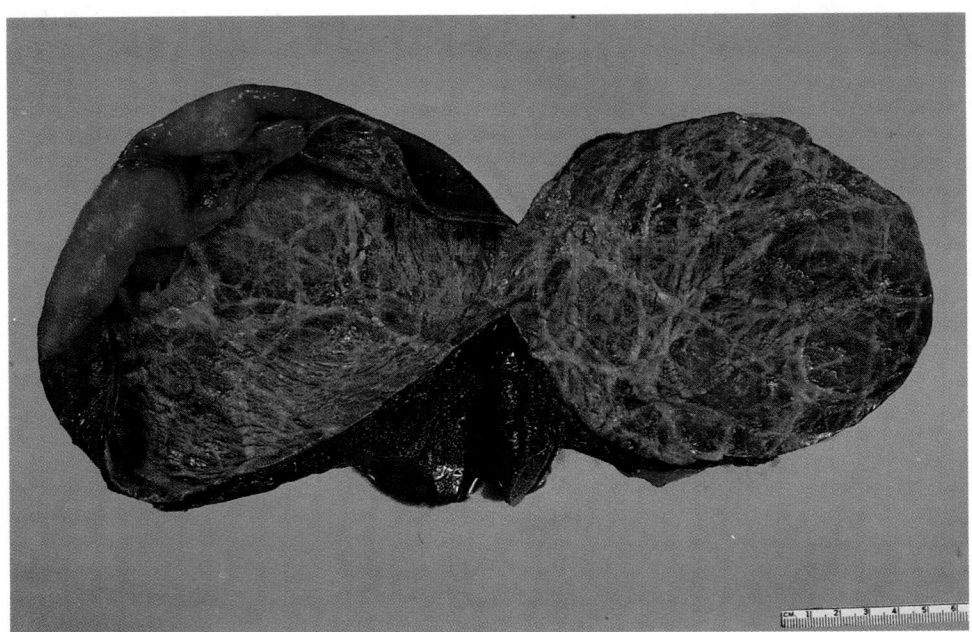

Fig. 22-3 Epithelial cyst. Grossly, it is very difficult, if not impossible, to distinguish this lesion from a false cyst.

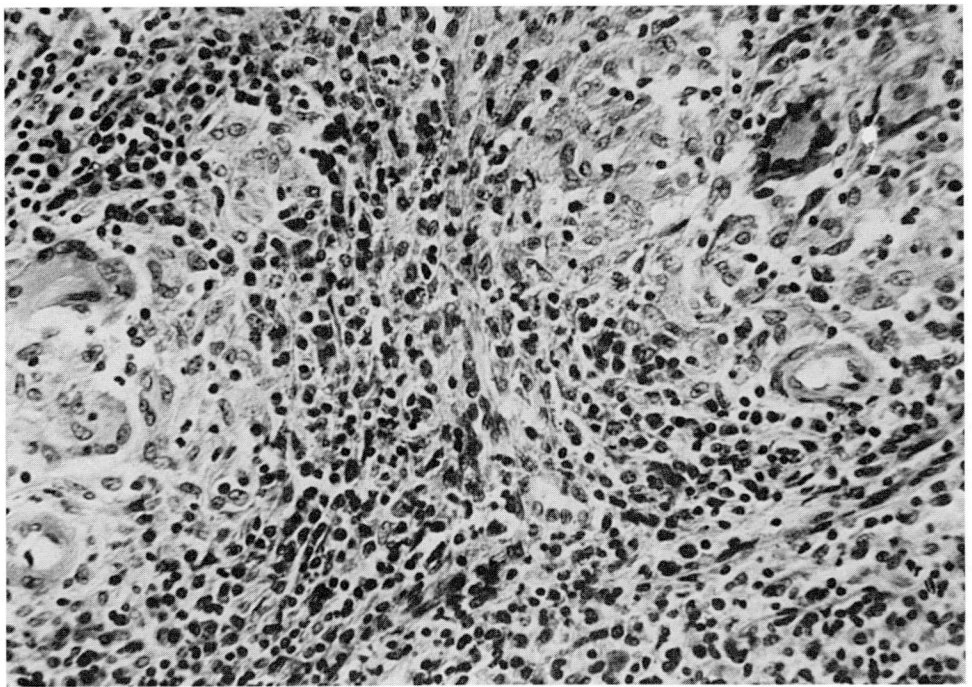

Fig. 22-4 Section of spleen weighing 750 g removed from 31-year-old woman with fever and hepatosplenomegaly. These granulomatous lesions with giant cells were proved to be reaction to *Histoplasma capsulatum.*

subacute bacterial endocarditis may lead to surgical intervention.[63]

Granulomatous inflammation is a relatively common finding in splenectomy specimens. The granulomas can be roughly divided into three major types: (1) large active granulomas containing epithelioid and Langhans' type of giant cells, with or without central necrosis; (2) small, widespread, sarcoid-like epithelioid granulomas with scanty giant cells and no necrosis (not to be equated with "epithelioid" germinal centers)[68]; and (3) old inactive granulomas, with fibrosis and calcification. A variant of the first type, characterized by extensive necrotizing changes, has been seen as a complication of leukemia in childhood.[75]

The third type of granuloma, which can be solitary or found scattered throughout the spleen, is particularly common in areas of endemic histoplasmosis.[77] We have evaluated twenty cases of splenectomy done for splenomegaly and/or hypersplenism in which the only major pathologic finding was the presence of active granulomas of either the first or second type.[67] All of the patients were adults. Fever, weight loss, hepatosplenomegaly, and the various manifestations of hypersplenism were the most common symptoms, and these were markedly ameliorated with splenectomy. The splenic granulomas were nearly always the expression of a generalized disease, which also often involved lymph nodes, liver, and bone marrow. Despite the performance of special stains and cultures, the etiology remained unknown in all but three cases. In these, the organisms identified were *Histoplasma capsulatum,* an *atypical Mycobacterium,* and *Sporotrichum schenkii,* respectively (Fig. 22-4). None of the patients developed malignant lymphoma on follow-up.

Sarcoid-like granulomas can be seen in the spleen of patients with Hodgkin's disease[64] and, less commonly, non-Hodgkin's lymphoma or hairy cell leukemia,[56] with or without involvement of the spleen by tumor. In some cases of non-Hodgkin's lymphoma, the number of granulomas is such as to obscure the diagnosis of lymphoma if present.[57] It should be emphasized that the presence of splenic granulomas in patients with lymphoma is not an indication per se that the spleen is involved by tumor. Actually, some authors have suggested that in patients with Hodgkin's disease, this finding is associated with an improved prognosis.[72] Neiman[69] found sarcoid-like granulomas in 24 of 412 splenectomy specimens; in addition to the conditions previously listed, he found them in chronic uremia and in a single case of IgA deficiency. He pointed out that in all cases the granulomas appeared to arise in the periarteriolar lymphoid sheath, suggesting that they are the result of abnormal or defective processing of antigen presented to the spleen. Granulomas have also been described in spleens affected by infectious mononucleosis.[74]

HYPERSPLENISM

Hypersplenism (dysplenism) is the generic term used for the group of disorders in which the removal of hematopoietic elements by the spleen increases to a pathologic degree.[78] Any of the cellular elements of the blood may be affected, singly or in combination. Thus neutropenia, thrombocytopenia, hemolytic anemia, or pancytopenia may all be present. In some conditions, such as spherocytic hemolytic anemia

or idiopathic thrombocytopenic purpura, the basic abnormality resides in the blood elements themselves. In others, the hypersplenism results from widening of the splenic cords with an increase in macrophages and/or connective tissue fibers and premature destruction of the normal elements of the blood. Hypersplenism resulting from this mechanism can be seen with congestive splenomegaly, Gaucher's disease (Fig. 22-5, *A*), malignant lymphoma, leukemia, Langerhans' cell granulomatosis (histiocytosis X), hemangioma, hamartoma, angiosarcoma, and practically any condition involving more or less diffusely the splenic parenchyma.[80]

A syndrome of hypersplenism developing in uremic hemodialyzed patients has also been recognized.[79] Splenectomy resulted in a marked improvement; a striking degree of lymphoid hyperplasia was found in the excised spleens.

Thrombocytopenic purpuras

Idiopathic (immuno)thrombocytopenic purpura is caused by the presence of an antiplatelet IgG, which is produced largely in the spleen.[92-94] Occasionally, thrombocytopenic purpura is seen as a manifestation of lupus erythematosus, viral infection, drug hypersensitivity,[81] chronic lymphocytic leukemia,[87] or Hodgkin's disease.[95] The antibody-coated platelets have a short life span because they are rapidly removed by the cells of the reticuloendothelial system, particularly in the spleen and liver. There is some evidence that the number of antibody molecules bound to the platelets may determine the main site of removal. Heavily coated platelets are removed by the liver phagocytes, whereas lightly coated platelets pass through the liver but are sequestered in the spleen.[98]

Grossly, the spleen is of normal size or only mildly enlarged[89]; malpighian follicles may be prominent. Microscopically, there is formation of secondary follicles with well-developed germinal centers (containing the platelet antigen CD34),[90] prominence of histiocytes in the red pulp, dilatation of sinuses, variable numbers of perivascular plasma cells in the marginal zone, and infiltration with neutrophils of the red pulp.[85] Mild myeloid metaplasia, usually in the form of megakaryocytes, is present in most cases.[84,85,89] The germinal centers, which usually show phagocytosis of nuclear debris and periarterial fibrosis,[82] are no longer prominent in cases previously treated with steroids.[88]

Collections of foamy macrophages containing phospholipid deposits are present in the red pulp in some of the cases[86,96] (Fig. 22-5, *B*). They are the result of phagocytosis of platelets and of incompletely degraded membrane-derived phospholipids,[91,99] as supported by the fact that the platelet antigen CD41 has been detected immunohistochemically in them.[90] The phagocytosis of platelets by splenic histiocytes can be better appreciated in touch preparations. It should be noted that the presence of foamy macrophages in the spleen is not pathognomonic of this disorder (see p. 1782).

Splenectomy in idiopathic thrombocytopenic purpura is reserved for the patients unresponsive to steroid or immunosuppressive therapy.[83] It achieves sustained remission in 50% to 80% of the cases. It is difficult to predict what effect the splenectomy will have in an individual case. However,

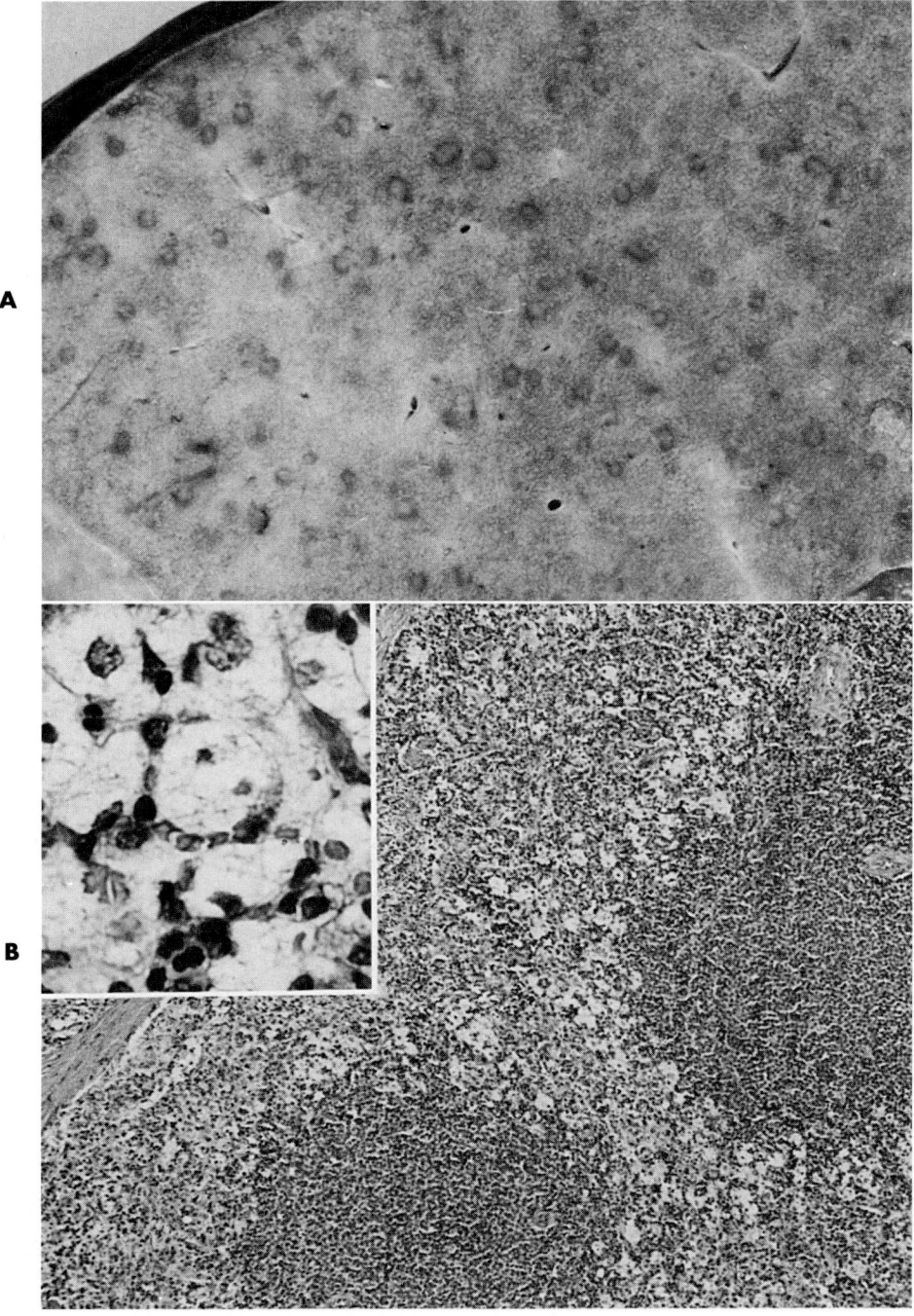

Fig. 22-5 **A,** Huge spleen in Gaucher's disease. White pulp is widely separated by expanded red pulp replaced by cells of Gaucher's disease. **B,** Idiopathic thrombocytopenic purpura. Lipid-filled macrophages in splenic white pulp immediately around malpighian corpuscles. **Inset,** High-power view demonstrates foamy nature of cytoplasm. Patient had no platelets before splenectomy.

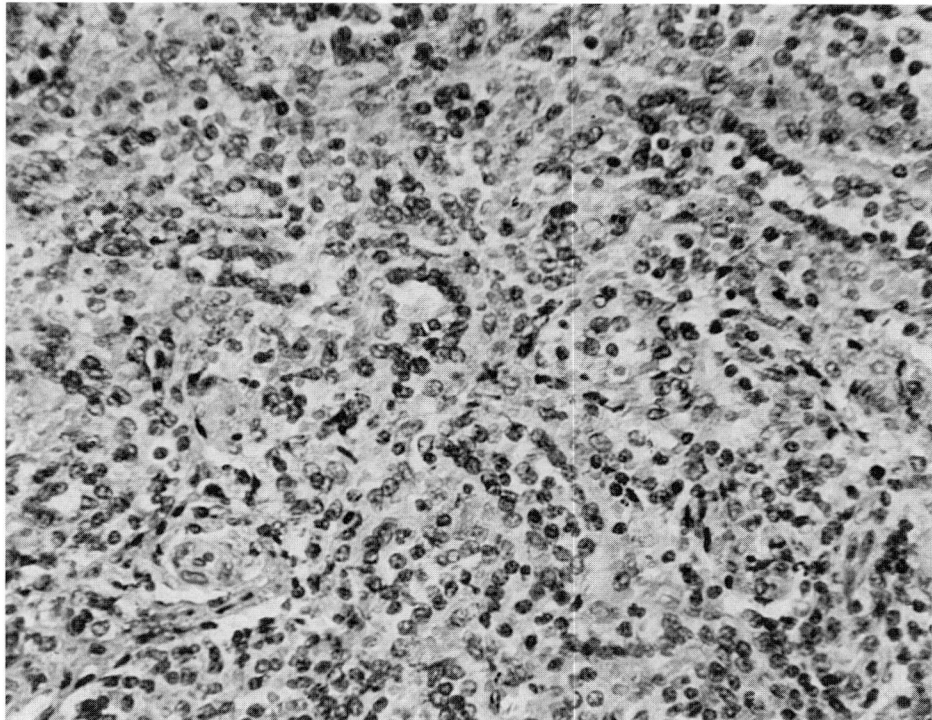

Fig. 22-6 Spleen of 4-year-old girl with hereditary spherocytosis. Splenic cords are congested, but sinusoids as seen on light microscopy seem practically empty.

Chang et al.[85] have shown that patients with prominent secondary follicles have a higher rate of antiplatelet antibody production and exhibit a better initial response, with a great increase in platelets postoperatively.

Thrombotic thrombocytic purpura may be accompanied by splenic enlargement. The most important pathologic change is the presence of thrombi in arteries and arterioles without associated inflammation. Periodic acid–Schiff–positive hyaline subendothelial deposits are present. Other changes include hyperplasia of B cells and germinal centers, periarteriolar concentric fibrosis, hemosiderin-laden macrophages, hemophagocytosis, and extramedullary hematopoiesis.[97]

Hemolytic anemia

Congenital hemolytic anemia (hereditary spherocytosis) is a genetically determined disease in which the red blood cells acquire a spheric shape (spherocytes).[102] The abnormality lies in the cell membrane of the red blood cell. The responsible genes have not been identified yet, but consistent molecular alterations of spectrin and ankyrin have been detected.[103,106,108] As a result, the erythrocytes lack the plasticity of normal red blood cells and become trapped in the interstices of the spleen.[110] The splenic function itself is normal.

Acquired hemolytic anemia can be caused by toxins (bacterial hemolysins), plasma lipid abnormalities, parasites that invade red blood cells, and most important, immune reactions that result in deposition of immune complexes on red blood cell membranes.[105] About one half of the cases of immune hemolytic anemias are unassociated with other significant pathologic abnormalities. The remaining cases are seen as a manifestation of a large variety of diseases, such as various forms of acute and chronic leukemia, Hodgkin's disease, sarcoidosis, lupus erythematosus, tuberculosis, and brucellosis. The Coombs test is the classic method to distinguish between the acquired and congenital types of hemolytic anemia. A positive Coombs test, as seen in the former disease, consists of agglutination of the patient's washed red blood cells following mixture with antihuman globulin rabbit serum.

Grossly, the spleen of both congenital and acquired hemolytic anemia is fairly firm and deep red, has a thin capsule and no grossly discernible malpighian follicles, and ranges in weight from 100 to 1000 g. In congenital hemolytic anemia, the splenic cords are congested, whereas the sinusoids appear relatively empty because of the presence of ghost red blood cells[111] (Fig. 22-6). The lining cells of the sinuses are prominent, sometimes resulting in a gland-like appearance. Hemosiderin deposition and erythrophagocytosis are present in both conditions but are usually more pronounced in the acquired variety. Ultrastructural studies have shown that the splenic cords are not empty but rather contain red blood cells that have lost their electron density, thus corresponding to the red cell ghosts of light microscopy.[104]

In acquired hemolytic anemia, the congestion may predominate in the cords or sinuses or be equally prominent in both. A high correlation exists between spherocytosis and increased osmotic fragility on one hand and the degree of cord congestion on the other. Foci of extramedullary hematopoiesis may be present. Splenic infarcts are found in one fourth of the cases.[107]

Hereditary spherocytosis is the hematologic disease that most benefits from splenectomy.[109] The clinical cure rate is almost 100%, although the intrinsic red cell abnormality persists.[101] In acquired hemolytic anemia, splenectomy is usually reserved for cases that cannot be controlled by steroid or immunosuppressive therapy. A sustained remission rate is obtained in about 50% of the cases and an objective improvement is obtained in an additional 25% of the cases. Studies of splenic sequestration using Cr^{51}-tagged red cells give a rough estimation of the benefit to be expected from splenectomy.[100]

Congestive splenomegaly

Congestive splenomegaly is a direct consequence of portal hypertension. It may be caused by cirrhosis (by far the most common pathogenesis); thrombosis of hepatic veins (Budd-Chiari syndrome); thrombosis of the splenic veins; or occlusive thrombosis, cavernous transformation (recanalized thrombosis), sclerosis, or stenosis of the portal vein. Portal vein thrombosis may be the result of inflammation, trauma, or extrinsic pressure by inflammatory or neoplastic tissue.[112] Stenotic or sclerotic changes may be the result of extension into the main portal vein of the physiologic obliterative process that takes place at birth in the umbilical vein and the ductus venosus as they empty into the left portal vein. Cases of portal hypertension accompanied by congestive splenomegaly in which no apparent cause is discernible either in the liver or in the hepatic or portal veins are referred to as *idiopathic portal hypertension*. This condition was originally described by Guido Banti at the University of Florence, Italy, and is generally known as *Banti's syndrome*. It has been regarded by many with skepticism, but cases with similar features are still being seen today, particularly in Japan.[113] The main changes in the liver are papillary dilatation, phlebosclerosis, and fibroelastosis in the portal tracts and disturbance of the acinar architecture[113] (see also p. 1777).

Congestive splenomegaly may be accompanied by signs of hypersplenism, such as anemia, leukopenia, and/or thrombocytopenia. Grossly, the spleen is large, firm, and dark. Fibrous thickening of the capsule is frequent.[115] Microscopically, there is marked dilatation of the veins and sinuses, fibrosis of the red pulp, and accumulation of hemosiderin-containing macrophages. Lymphoid follicles are inconspicuous. Iron incrustation of the connective tissue and sclerosiderotic nodules ("Gamna-Gandy bodies") develop as a result of focal hemorrhages. Because fibrosis is commonly present in advanced cases, the condition is also known as *fibrocongestive splenomegaly*.

Splenectomy without shunt is successful when the coronary vein joins the portal system central to the point of obstruction. Otherwise, shunt is indicated. Various types have been done, including anastomosis of the splenic vein to the renal vein and anastomosis of the portal vein to the vena cava. These operations have been successful as a means of controlling repetitive hemorrhage from esophageal varices but do not seem to prolong life.[114]

OTHER NON-NEOPLASTIC DISORDERS

Foamy macrophages can be found in the spleens of patients with idiopathic thrombocytopenic purpura, as already indicated (see p. 1779). They also occur, as an incidental finding without clinical significance, in the malpighian follicles of normal individuals (so-called follicular lipidosis) in association with similar changes in the liver and intra-abdominal lymph nodes.[130] They are much more common in North American than in Latin American or African populations.[117,118] Biochemical studies have demonstrated the presence of saturated hydrocarbons, which imply the ingestion of exogenous mineral oil. The most common source seems to be material related to the packaging and display of foodstuff.[117,124]

Foamy histiocytes have also been described in Gaucher's disease, Niemann-Pick disease,[120] Tay-Sachs disease, chronic granulomatous disease, thalassemia,[122] and hyperlipemic stages.[127] Histochemical techniques usually allow for a distinction among these various conditions.[126] It is now accepted that the process originally designated as *sea-blue histiocyte syndrome*[128] is not a specific entity and that histiocytes with a sea-blue appearance can be present in any of the disorders previously mentioned[125] and also in chronic myelocytic leukemia.

Infarction of the spleen (peliosis lienis) may result from thrombosis of the splenic vein, a phenomenon not always associated with a detectable etiology. Splenic infarcts are also common in cases of massive splenomegaly, regardless of its cause.

Peliosis of the spleen is characterized by widespread, blood-filled cystic spaces. Most reported cases have been associated with peliosis hepatis,[123] but it may occur independently from it.[129] The most common location for the lesions is the parafollicular region.[129] Cases have been reported in which splenic involvement led to rupture[121] and death[129] (see p. 1775). Most cases have occurred in patients with wasting diseases, such as tuberculosis and carcinomatosis, or in patients who have received anabolic-androgenic steroids.[131] They have also been seen in association with chronic leukemia.[121]

Radiation injury to the spleen, usually produced in the course of therapy for lymphoma, results in an organ with a wrinkled, thick capsule and parenchymal collapse, with diffuse fibrosis of the red pulp and lymphocyte depletion.[119]

Amyloidosis of the spleen is nearly always an expression of the "secondary" form of the disease. "Sago spleen" and "lardaceous spleen" are the classic descriptions, depending respectively on the follicular versus diffuse locations of the deposits. Exceptional cases of localized splenic amyloid nodules ("amyloid tumor") have also been described.[116]

HEMATOLYMPHOID TUMORS AND TUMORLIKE CONDITIONS
Benign lymphoid processes

Reactive lymphoid hyperplasia can present in the spleen as a solitary nodule that may be confused grossly with lym-

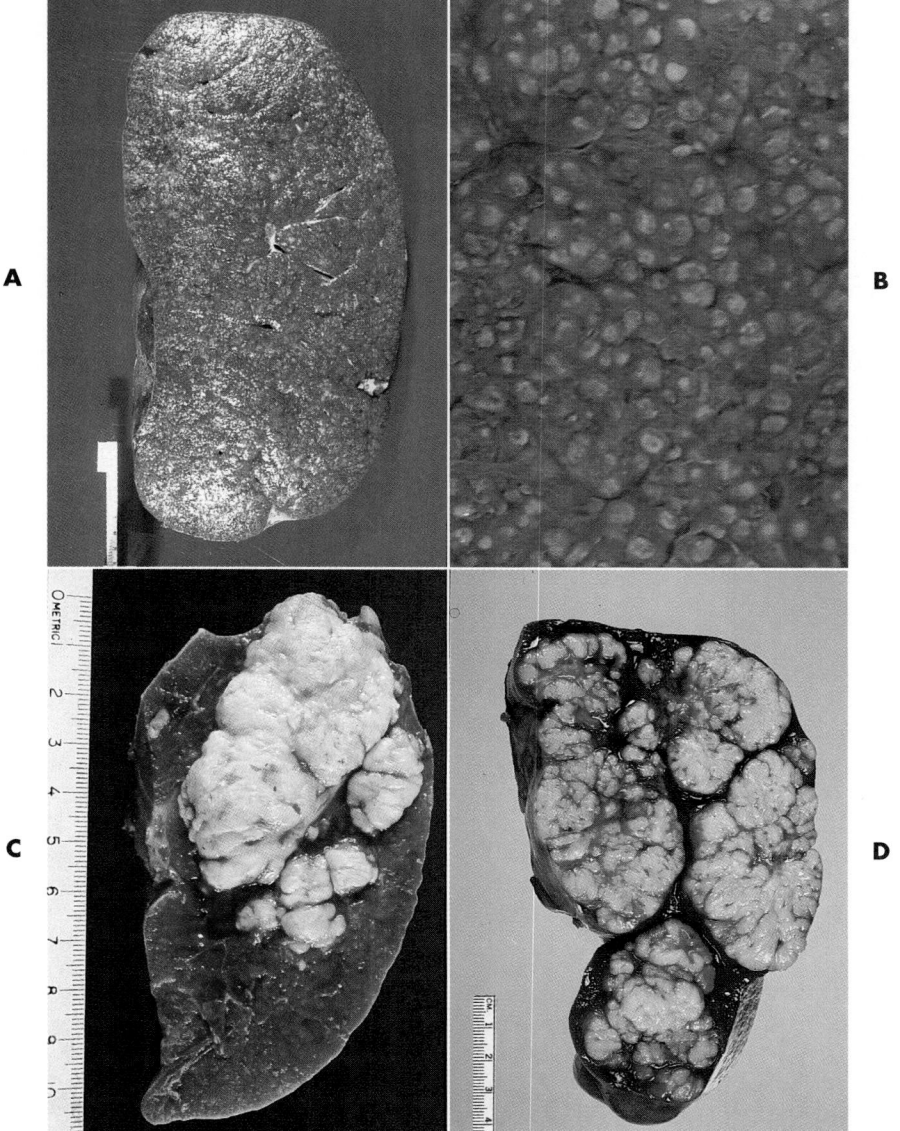

Fig. 22-7 Gross appearances of various types of malignant lymphoma involving the spleen. **A,** Small lymphocytic lymphoma. **B,** Follicular lymphoma. **C** and **D,** Large cell lymphoma.

phoma, especially if the splenectomy specimen has been obtained at staging laparotomy for that disease. Microscopically, the nodule is formed either by aggregates of reactive germinal centers or by a localized proliferation of lympho cytes, immunoblasts, and plasma cells.[132,133]

Inflammatory pseudotumor is another reactive tumorlike condition; it may be an incidental finding at laparotomy or present as a symptomatic splenic mass.[135] Grossly, there is a great size range, with some lesions reaching 11 cm. The lesions are usually solitary and may be multinodular.[137] Microscopically, there is a variable mixture of lymphocytes, plasma cells, eosinophils, histiocytes, and spindle cells. The

predominant pattern may be sclerotic, xanthogranuloma-tous, or plasma cell granuloma–type.[134,136,137] Central coag-ulative necrosis is often present, usually in association with a neutrophilic infiltrate. Most of the small lymphocytes are of the T-cell type.[137] The evolution following splenectomy is benign.

Non-Hodgkin's lymphoma

Malignant lymphoma is by far the most common malig-nant tumor involving the spleen. Although usually affected as part of a generalized process, in some cases the spleen represents the only detectable site of disease. Splenic

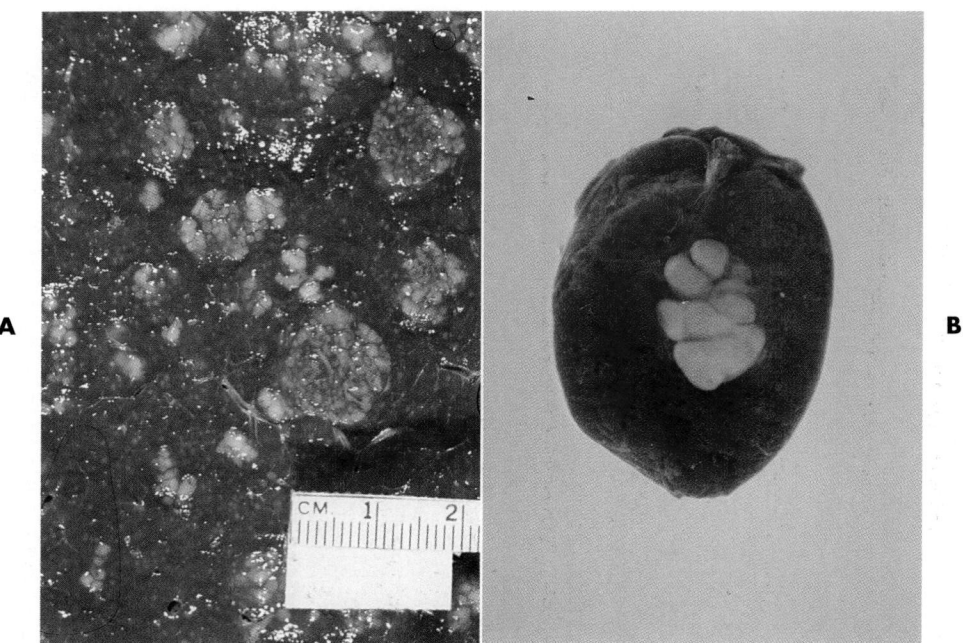

Fig. 22-8 A and **B,** Gross appearance of Hodgkin's disease involving the spleen.

involvement by malignant lymphoma may present as an asymptomatic splenomegaly or result in a picture of hypersplenism.[158] Ahmann et al.[138] described four gross patterns of involvement: homogeneous, miliary, multiple masses, and solitary masses, which correspond closely to the various microscopic types (Figs. 22-7 and 22-8).

The most common malignant lymphoma of the spleen is of low-grade type, showing the phenotypic features of B cells.[151,155,159] This includes small lymphocytic lymphoma, follicular (small-cleaved) lymphoma, and a subtype variously designated as intermediate differentiation, mantle zone, and monocytoid.[154] It has been suggested that most of the tumors in the latter category arise from splenic marginal zone lymphocytes and that these *marginal zone cell lymphomas* are the splenic equivalent of MALT lymphomas of other sites.[148,155a,156,157]

Low-grade splenic small lymphocytic lymphoma usually presents grossly as nodules measuring a few millimeters in diameter ("miliary" nodules) scattered throughout the organ. The low-power appearance is also distinctly nodular because of the preferential involvement of the white pulp. In this regard, it is important to point out that a nodular pattern of growth is common to several types of lymphoproliferative diseases of the spleen (including chronic lymphocytic leukemia) and that its presence should not be equated with a diagnosis of follicular center cell lymphoma.[138,140]

In the early stages, the diagnosis of small lymphocytic lymphoma can be easily missed. Clues to the diagnosis in these cases include prominent enlargement and coalescence of follicles; presence of a marked expansion of their mantle zone; germinal centers that are absent, inconspicuous, or overrun by small cells; and presence of clusters of small lymphoid cells protruding beneath the endothelium of tra-

becular veins[146] (Fig. 22-9). The only other condition in which we have seen the latter change in a prominent degree in an adult has been infectious mononucleosis. We have also seen the subendothelial space occupied by red cell precursors in infants with erythroblastosis fetalis and (together with granulocyte precursors) in adults with myelofibrosis. Another helpful measure for the diagnosis of lymphoma is to carefully dissect and examine the lymph nodes in the splenic hilum since they may show obvious lymphoma when the changes in the spleen are only equivocal.

An "entity" that exemplifies the difficulties sometimes encountered in the recognition of splenic small lymphocytic lymphoma is so-called *idiopathic nontropical splenomegaly.* Although originally regarded as a benign and probably reactive form of splenomegaly,[142] a follow-up study by the same group showed that half of these cases actually represented malignant lymphoma.[143]

The second most common lymphoma of the spleen is the large-cell type, which characteristically presents as solitary or multiple tumor masses. These patients often present with left-upper-quadrant pain, fever, weight loss, and an elevated erythrosedimentation rate.[147] Some of these cases have been seen in association with HIV infection.[139] Grossly, transgression of the splenic capsule is common, sometimes accompanied by invasion of adjacent structures. Hilar and retroperitoneal lymph nodes are often involved. Microscopically, most of these tumors fall into the large noncleaved cell category, followed by the immunoblastic group. Immunophenotypically, B-cell neoplasms predominate over T-cell tumors.[144] Morphologic features favoring a B-cell phenotype are multiple discrete nodules in the white pulp, large coalescing nodules, co-existence of small lymphocytic lymphoma, and plasmacytoid features. Features favor-

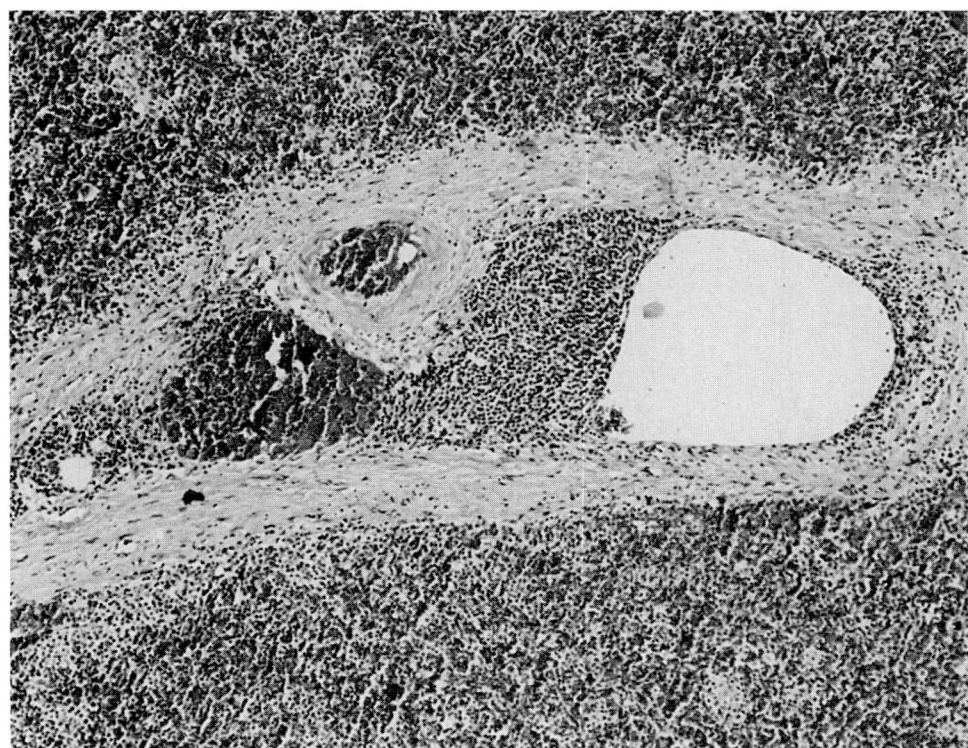

Fig. 22-9 Involvement of subendothelial space of large splenic vein in small lymphocytic lymphoma. This is an important diagnostic sign.

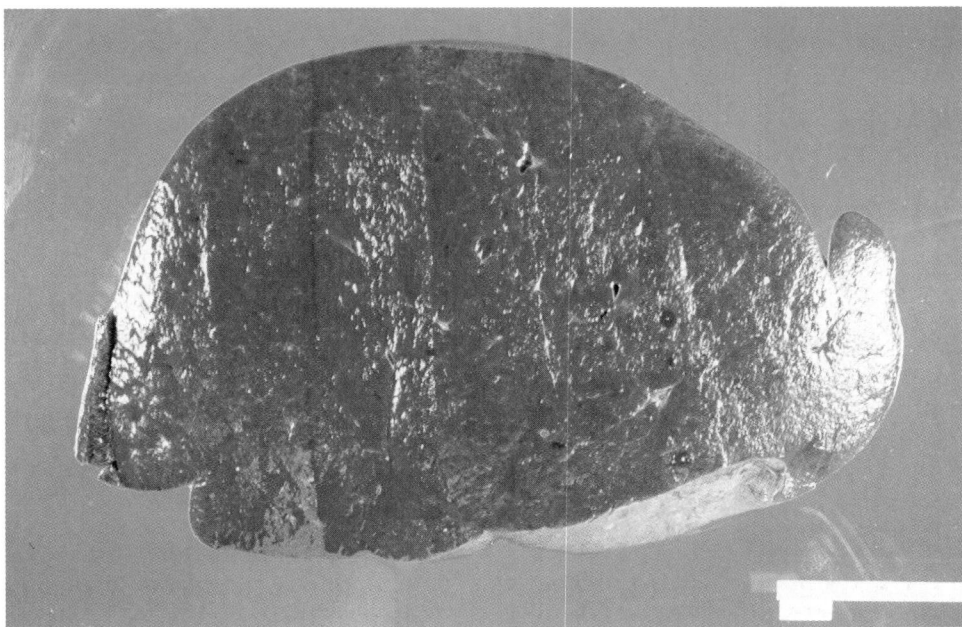

Fig. 22-10 Gross appearance of hairy cell leukemia. Notice the diffuse involvement, lack of nodularity, and dark red color.

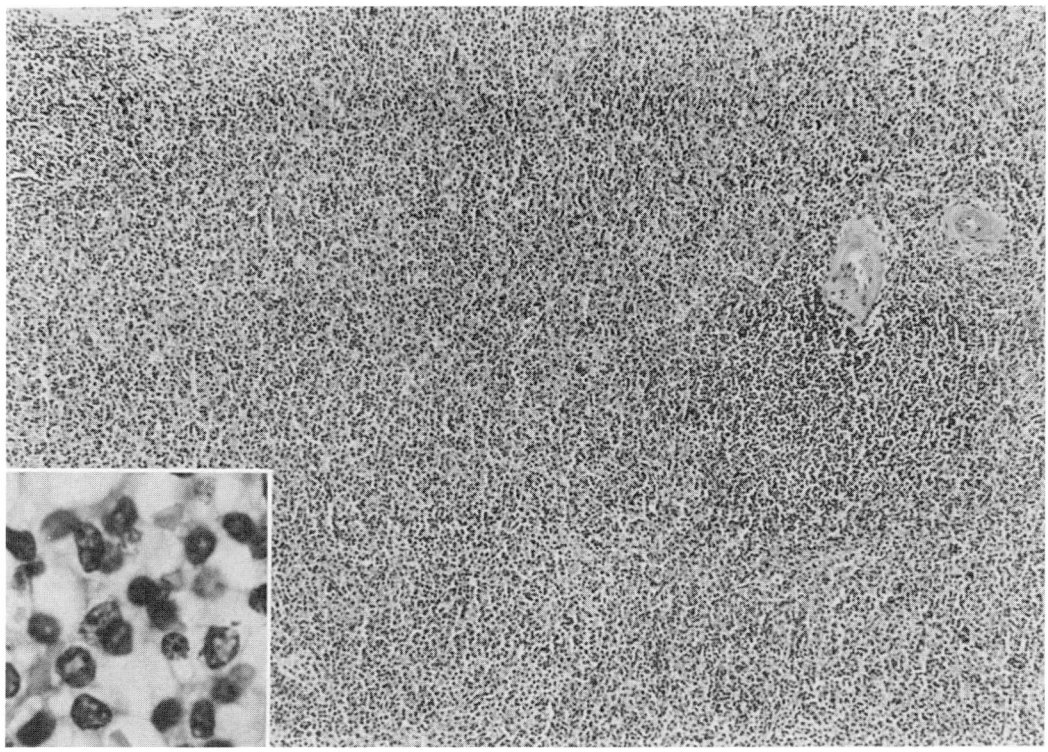

Fig. 22-11 Hairy cell leukemia in spleen. There is massive involvement of red pulp. **Inset** shows monotonous cells with scanty cytoplasm and no mitoses.

ing a T-cell phenotype are epithelioid histiocytic reaction, tumor confinement to the periarteriolar lymphoid sheath and marginal zone, and clear cell or polymorphous cytologic features.[160,161] Some of the T-cell splenic lymphomas have been shown to express the rare γδ T-cell receptor, along with a double negative CD4/CD8 phenotype; these have been characterized by an associated liver involvement, a sinusal/sinusoidal distribution, and an aggressive clinical course.[143a,162a] A few of the large cell lymphomas represent true histiocytic tumors of this organ[145] (see also p. 1791).

Rarely, malignant lymphomas (and chronic lymphocytic leukemias) preferentially affect the red pulp; as a result, they can be confused with hairy cell leukemia when composed of small cells[152,155] or malignant histiocytosis when composed of large cells. In regard to the latter, one should mention here the cases interpreted by Vardiman et al.[162] as a possible chronic form of *malignant histiocytosis* with predominant splenic involvement on the basis of phagocytotic activity, lysozyme positivity, and clinical evolution.[141] It is likely that these cases instead represent variants of large cell lymphoma, possibly of T-cell type. Exceptionally, large cell lymphomas are seen in a predominant intrasinusal location, as a variation on the theme of angiotropic lymphoma.[150]

The treatment of malignant lymphoma involving exclusively or preferentially the spleen includes splenectomy, followed by chemotherapy.[153]

The prognosis is directly related to the microscopic type and the clinical stage, in the sense that it is distinctly better for small lymphocytic tumors and for stage I and II disease.[138,148,151] Patients with localized splenic non-Hodgkin's lymphoma seem to have the same rate of survival as other Stage I non-Hodgkin's lymphoma patients.[149]

Hodgkin's disease

The morphologic features of Hodgkin's disease in the spleen are discussed in Chapter 21. Grossly the involvement is in the form of one or multiple nodules, sometimes indistinguishable from those of large cell lymphoma. By far the most common type is nodular sclerosis, but others may be seen as well, including lymphocyte predominance.[164] Some cases have initially presented with spontaneous splenic rupture.[163]

Leukemias

Any type of leukemia can involve the spleen.[165,169]

Chronic lymphocytic leukemia may appear grossly as a diffuse or miliary enlargement. From a morphologic standpoint, it is not possible to distinguish it from small lymphocytic lymphoma.

Prolymphocytic leukemia shows a similar type of involvement, but the lymphocytes have nuclei that are larger, often indented, and with distinct nucleoli.[173] Massive splenomegaly is the predominant clinical finding.

Chronic myelocytic leukemia preferentially affects the red pulp and results grossly in a large, dark red, diffusely involved organ in which malpighian follicles are inconspicuous or absent. In rare cases, blastic transformation of chronic

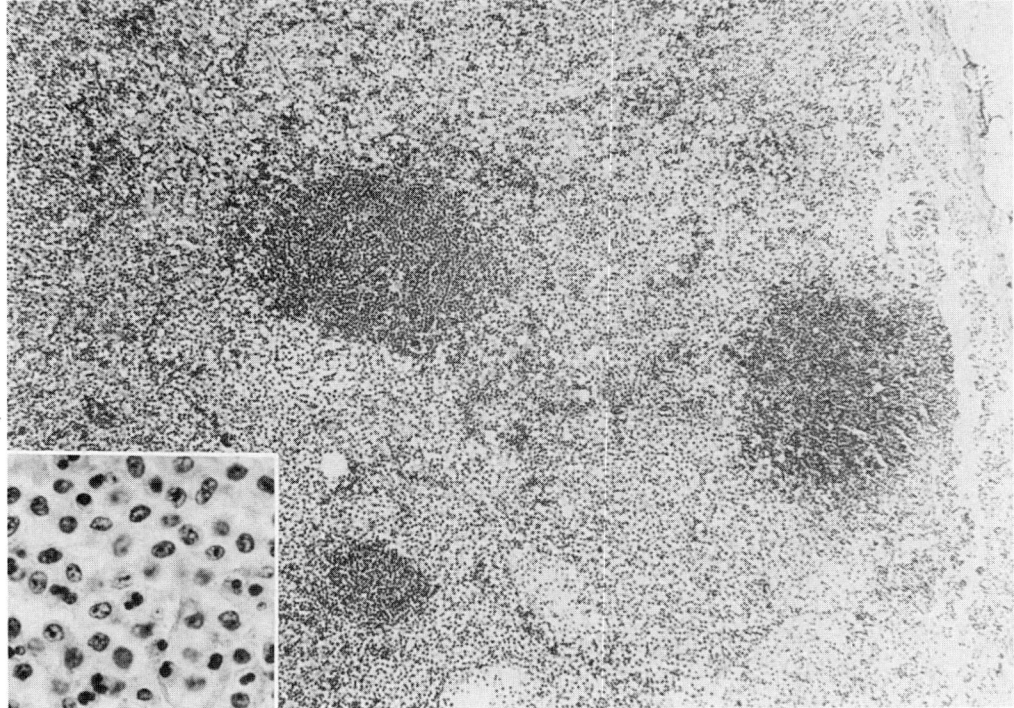

Fig. 22-12 Lymph node involvement by hairy cell leukemia. T-cell regions are preferentially affected. **Inset** shows uniformity of proliferation and irregular nuclear contour.

leukemia (known as Richter's syndrome in cases of chronic lymphocytic leukemia) is first seen in a splenectomy specimen.

Hairy cell leukemia, also known as leukemic reticuloendotheliosis, is a specific subtype of B-cell malignancy[170]; it is further discussed in Chapter 23. Grossly the spleen shows diffuse and usually marked enlargement without formation of nodules, except in the very early stages of the disease (Fig.22-10).[172] Microscopically, hairy cell leukemia *is a disease of the red pulp,* which shows diffuse infiltration by a monotonous population of small mononuclear cells with very scanty mitotic activity and practically no phagocytosis[166,175] (Fig. 22-11). The initial involvement occurs around the fibrous trabeculae. The nuclei of the hairy cells are small, round, or oval, with irregular contours, occasional deep indentations ("coffee beans"), and inconspicuous nucleoli. Rarely, the nuclei have a multilobular appearance simulating those of T-cell lymphoma.[171] The cytoplasm is usually scanty, although in some cells it is moderate to abundant and lightly stained. Ultrastructurally, prominent cytoplasmic villous projections are evident.[167] The predominant antigenic phenotype of hairy cells is CD45+, CD45RA+, L26+, CDw75+, CD74+, LN3+, MB2+, CD45RO−, MT1−, CD15−, and CD30−.[178,179] The splenic vasculature is abnormal in the sense of showing an absolute increase in the volume, surface, and length of pulp arterial vessels, as well as enlargement of pulp cords and sinuses.[177] Pools of blood in the red pulp, lined by hairy cells and simulating dilated sinuses or even hemangiomas, are commonly seen and constitute an important diagnostic feature.[174] It has been

suggested that this results from the hairy cells adhering to the sinus surface, producing endothelial cell injury and impeding the venous blood flow.[176] In what is perhaps the preceding stage of this process, some of the tumor cells are seen to aggregate in the subendothelial spaces of trabecular veins; sometimes this is the only recognizable site of involvement.[168]

The lymph nodes in the splenic hilum are often involved, the pattern of permeation being interfollicular (Fig. 22-12).

Splenectomy is the treatment of choice, and long survivals are common.[180]

Myelofibrosis

Myelofibrosis (agnogenic myeloid metaplasia) is discussed in Chapter 23. Spleen involvement in this disease is the rule, the average weight being 2 kg.[184] Grossly, the spleen is diffusely dark red and moderately firm, with frequent areas of hemorrhage. Microscopically, the diagnostic feature is the presence in the red pulp of all three hematopoietic cell lines: megakaryocytes, erythroid precursors, and granulocyte precursors (Fig. 22-13). The latter are made evident with Leder's chloroacetate esterase stain. The megakaryocytes often have atypical nuclear features and can be confused with Reed-Sternberg cells; in contrast with the latter, their cytoplasm is strongly PAS positive.[182] They are immunohistochemically reactive for factor VIII–related antigen and negative for CD30 and Leu-M1.

It has been suggested that the hematopoietic cells result from filtration of circulating cells from the peripheral blood rather than arising de novo from splenic stem cells.[183,187]

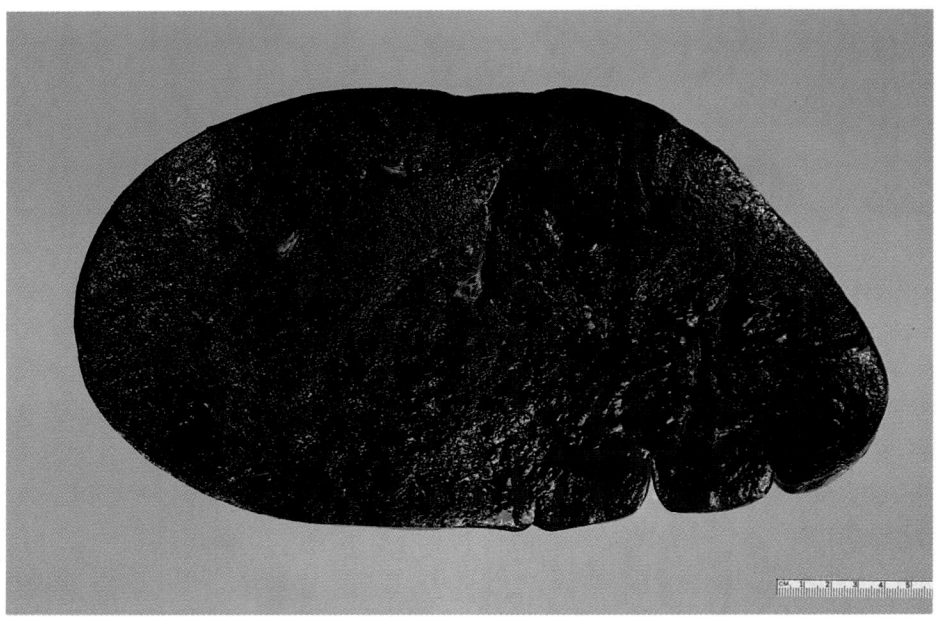

Fig. 22-13 Diffuse involvement of the spleen by myelofibrosis.

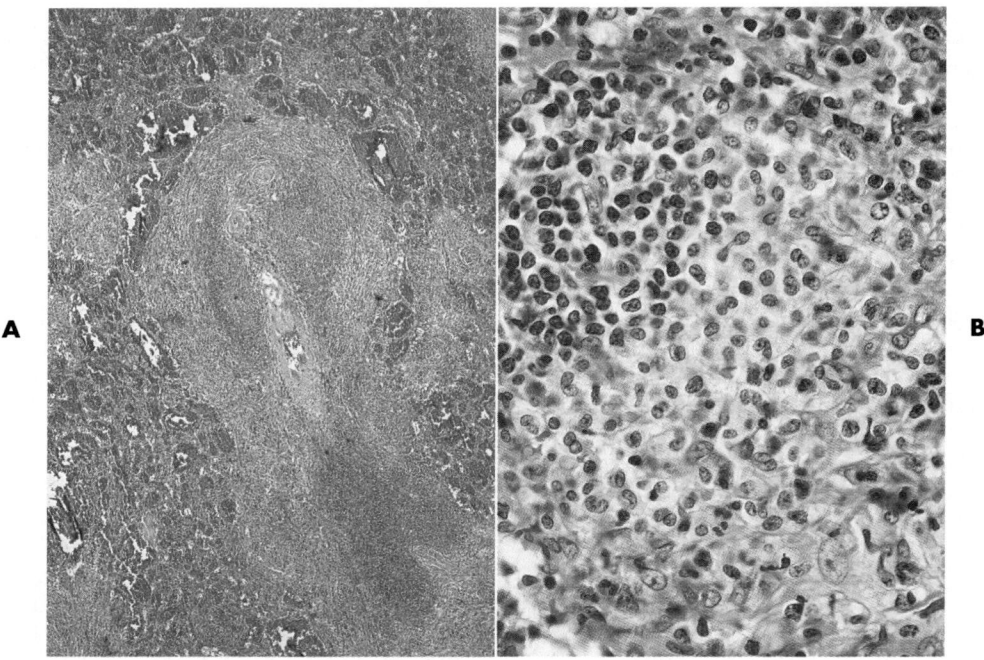

Fig. 22-14 Involvement of the spleen by systemic mastocytosis. **A,** Low-power view showing the perimalpighian and perivascular arrangement of the infiltrate. **B,** High-power view showing clusters of mast cells.

Other splenic changes in myelofibrosis include congestion, hemosiderosis, and paucity of lymphoid follicles.[185,186]

Splenectomy is sometimes carried out for this disease, especially when hemolytic phenomena or thrombocytopenia is severe. The results are not spectacular, but in some cases a moderate improvement has been noted.

Splenic extramedullary hematopoiesis as seen in myelofibrosis should be distinguished from the rare *myelolipomas* occurring within or adjacent to the spleen.[181]

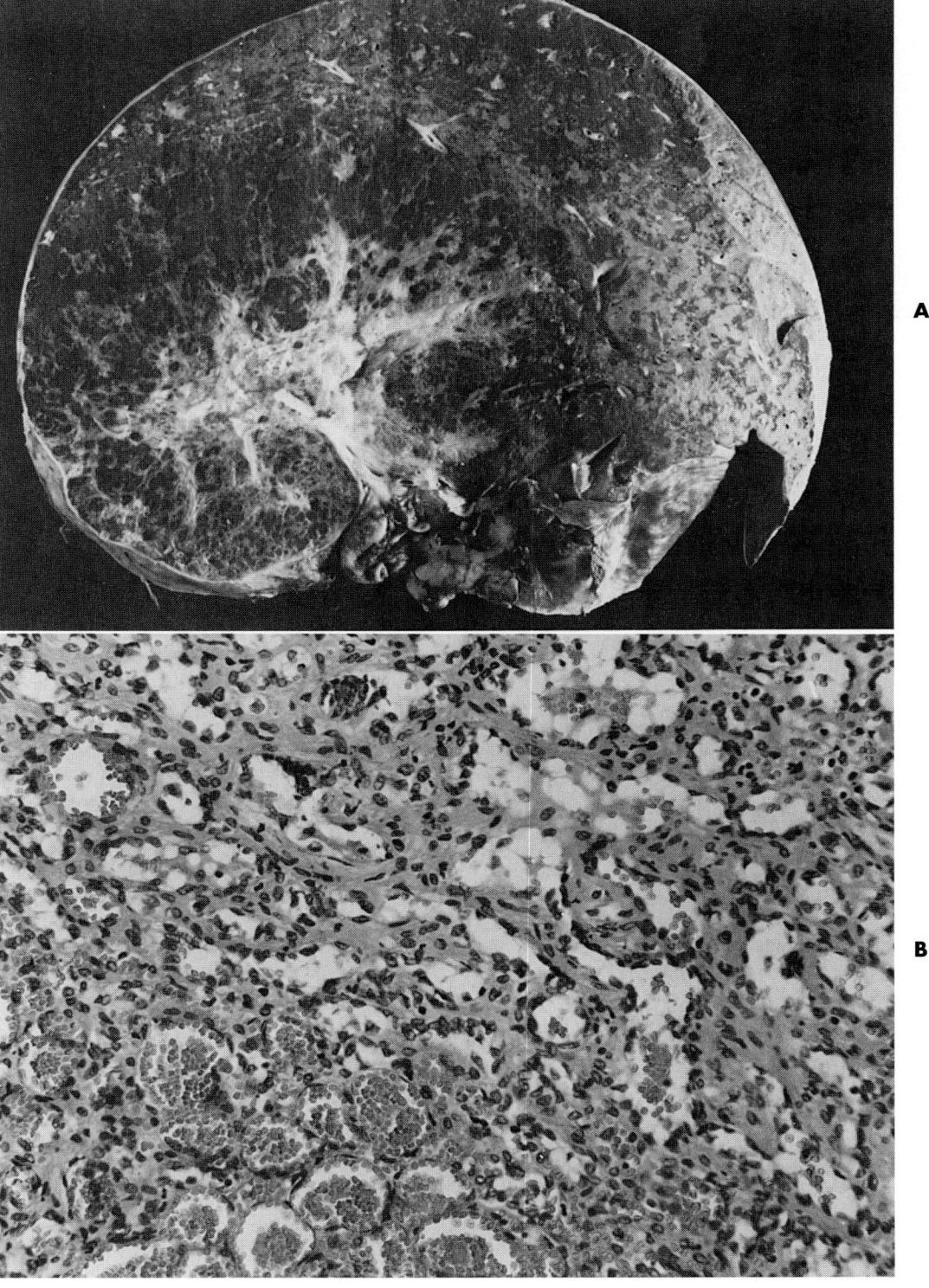

Fig. 22-15 A, Large hemangioma of spleen in 44-year-old man who presented with mild anemia and leukopenia. Tumor weighed over 3000 g. Patient had no other vascular lesions. **B,** Microscopic appearance of same lesion. Dilated vascular channels filled with red blood cells may be seen. (Courtesy Dr. B.W. Sharpe, Jackson, TN.)

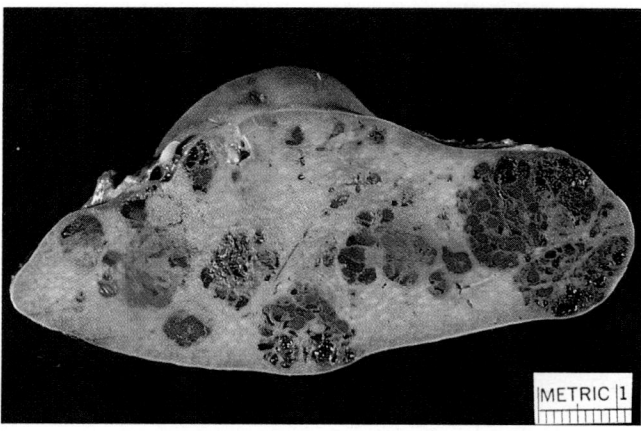

Fig. 22-16 Gross appearance of littoral cell angioma. Numerous hemorrhagic lesions with a lobular configuration are seen.

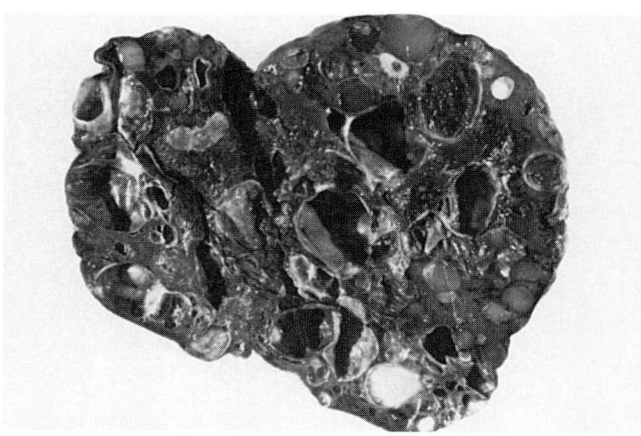

Fig. 22-17 Cystic lymphangioma of spleen. Cut surface shows multiple large cystic spaces lined by shiny surface. (Courtesy Dr. J. Costa, Lausanne, Switzerland.)

Mastocytosis

The general features of systemic mastocytosis are discussed in Chapter 23. The spleen is always involved, but the morphologic changes can be very confusing.[188] Grossly, ill-defined granuloma-like nodules having a fibrotic appearance are scattered throughout the organ (Fig. 22-14). Microscopically, these highly fibrotic foci are often centered by a vessel, an important diagnostic clue.[188,190] The diagnosis depends on the identification of mast cells, which usually appear as small clusters embedded in fibrous tissue, accompanied by a variable number of eosinophils, lymphocytes, or histiocytes. The nucleus is centrally located and of regular outline; the cytoplasm is light staining, with a variable degree of granularity; the cell borders tend to be sharply outlined. Confirmation of the diagnosis is obtained by staining the cytoplasmic granules with metachromatic dyes, with Leder's chloroacetate esterase reaction, or by the immunohistochemical demonstration of tryptase, chymase, and carboxypeptidase.[188,189,191]

The lymph nodes in the splenic hilum are often involved; the diagnosis may be easier on them than on the spleen. The foci of involvement in the lymph nodes are usually perifollicular and may also show a perivascular distribution.

Other hematolymphoid conditions

Langerhans' cell granulomatosis (histiocytosis X) of the spleen is nearly always an expression of systemic disease and is therefore rarely seen as a surgical specimen. The red pulp is preferentially affected.[192]

Follicular dendritic tumor has been reported presenting as a large multinodular tumor mass in the spleen.[192a]

OTHER PRIMARY TUMORS AND TUMORLIKE CONDITIONS

Hemangioma is the most common primary tumor of the spleen.[200] It is often of the *cavernous* variety. Most are under 2 cm in diameter and present as incidental findings. Rarely, they are large and/or multiple, and they may involve the entire spleen (Fig. 22-15). They may be associated with

hemangiomas of other sites (angiomatosis). The most common complication is rupture and bleeding.[204] Cases associated with anemia, thrombocytopenia, and consumption coagulopathy have been reported.[212]

Other types of splenic hemangiomas include venous hemangioma, capillary hemangioma, benign (infantile) hemangioendothelioma,[205] diffuse sinusoidal hemangiomatosis (in which the entire spleen is permeated by blood vessels),[210] epithelioid (histiocytoid) hemangioendothelioma (which can be associated with functional hyposplenism),[194a] and epithelioid and spindle-cell hemangioendothelioma.[216]

Littoral cell angioma varies in size from minute foci to large nodules almost completely replacing the splenic tissue (Fig. 22-16). Microscopically, it is composed of anastomosing vascular channels resembling splenic sinuses. These channels have irregular lumina often featuring papillary projections and cyst-like spaces. They are lined by tall endothelial cells which sometimes show hemophagocytosis. Immunohistochemically, the neoplastic cells express both endothelial (factor VIII) and histiocytic (KP-1, lysozyme) markers and occasionally also S-100 protein, reflecting the dual differentiation potential of the reticuloendothelial cells lining the sinuses.[199] This entity blends conceptually, morphologically, and immunohistochemically with epithelioid hemangioendothelioma. We have seen several cases in which the distinctly multinodular quality of the proliferation on low-power examination simulated the appearance of a granulomatous inflammatory process.

Hemangiopericytoma is an exceptionally rare tumor in this location.[207]

Lymphangioma tends to be located in the subcapsular region but may involve the entire organ (diffuse lymphangiomatosis)[211] (Fig. 22-17). Most cases have been reported in children, sometimes in association with lymphangiomas in other organs.[202]

Hamartoma (splenadenoma or splenoma) is the term proposed for a nodular lesion of the spleen composed exclusively of red pulp elements.[208,214,220] It does not contain fol-

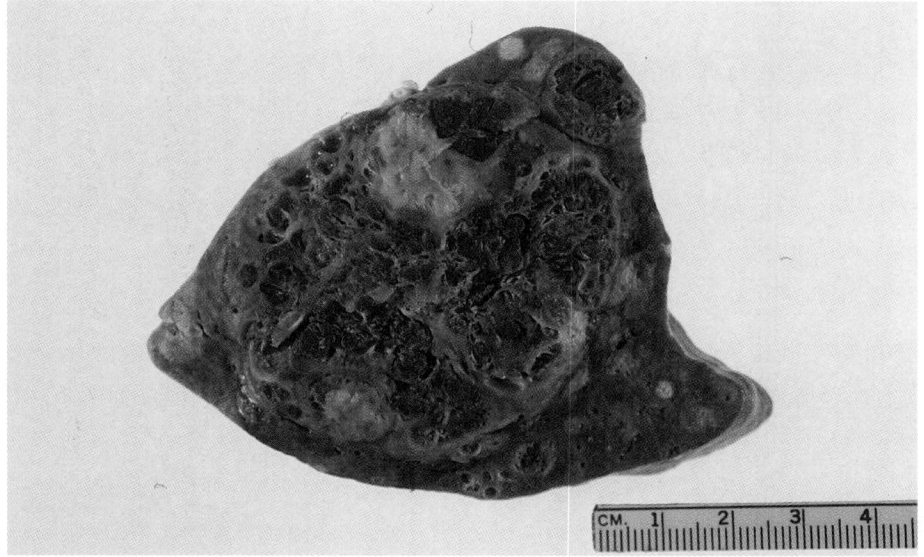

Fig. 22-18 Angiosarcoma of spleen. The tumor is markedly hemorrhagic and necrotic.

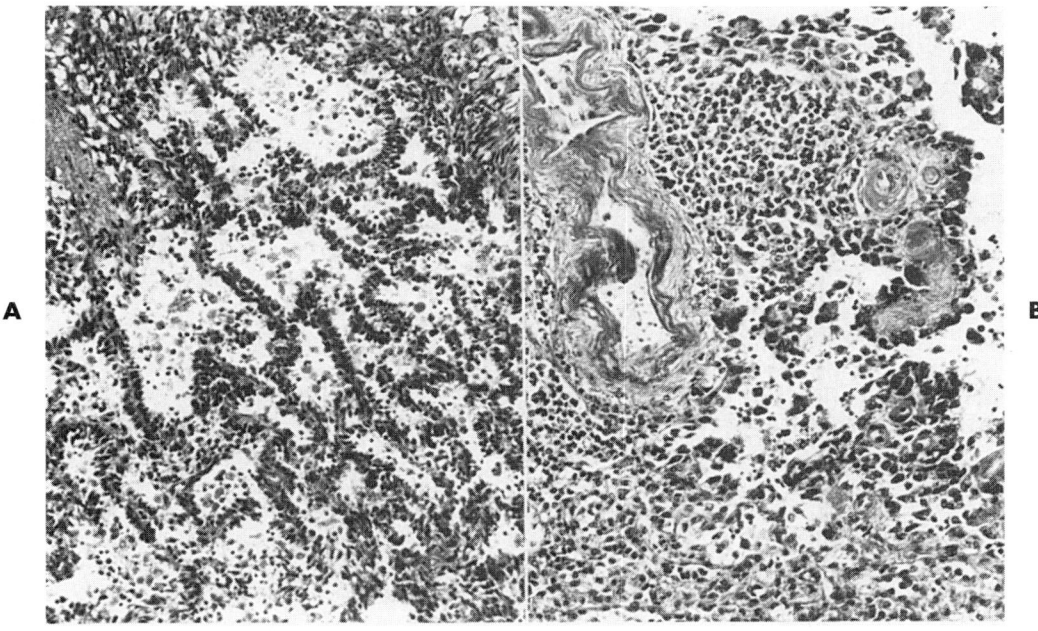

Fig. 22-19 Angiosarcoma of spleen. **A** and **B** show a malignant tumor composed of atypical endothelial cells lining vascular sinuses. Tumor in **A** is well differentiated, and tumor in **B** is poorly differentiated.

licles or dendritic follicular cells, and fibrous trabeculae are scanty; foci of extramedullary hematopoiesis may be present.[198] This lesion may be large and accompanied by thrombocytopenia and other signs of hypersplenism.[209]

Lipoma can occur as an intrasplenic mass.[196]

Angiosarcoma is the most common malignant primary nonlymphoid tumor of the spleen.[215] It may present as a well-defined hemorrhagic nodule or involve the spleen diffusely and may lead to spontaneous rupture of the organ[194,195] (Figs. 22-18 and 22-19). It may also be accompanied by microangiopathic anemia, thrombocytopenia, and consumption coagulopathy.[203] The clinical course is rapid and almost invariably fatal, with widespread metastases occurring frequently.[193,197]

Malignant fibrous histiocytoma has also been described as a primary splenic tumor.[201,219] In some cases with this morphologic appearance, cell marker studies have shown a histiocytic phenotype.[213]

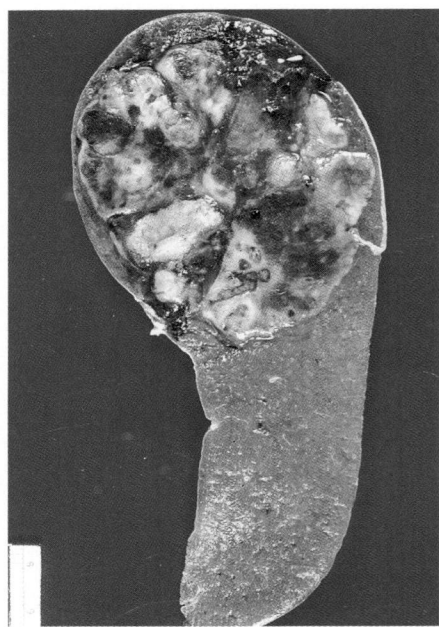

Fig. 22-20 Gross appearance of inflammatory pseudotumor of the spleen. The cut surface has a variegated color resulting from a combination of necrosis, hemorrhage, and cellular infiltration.

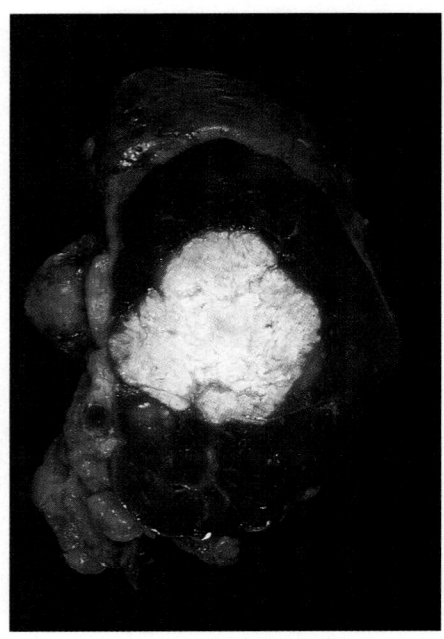

Fig. 22-21 Metastatic endometrial carcinoma to the spleen presenting as a single well-circumscribed nodule.

Carcinosarcoma apparently primary in the spleen has been interpreted as a probable extragenital type of malignant mixed müllerian tumor.[218]

Radiographically, the most useful techniques to detect and evaluate splenic tumors are CT scan, ultrasonography, and angiography.[206]

Tumorlike conditions of the spleen include the already mentioned hamartoma (see p. 1790) and inflammatory pseudotumor (Fig. 22-20) (see p. 1783). Spindle-cell pseudoneoplastic nodules resulting from mycobacteria have been reported in the spleen of HIV-infected patients.[217]

METASTATIC TUMORS

Metastatic carcinoma of the spleen is a very uncommon clinical problem[225] but not too unusual at autopsy if a thorough examination of the organ is carried out.[221] Malignant melanoma, breast carcinoma, and lung carcinoma are the most common sites for the primary tumor, but many others have been described, including carcinoid tumor of the ileum[224] (Fig. 22-21). Breast carcinoma diffusely metastatic to the spleen may present as idiopathic thrombocytopenic purpura.[222] Occasionally, metastases in the spleen result in a nodular configuration that simulates follicular lymphoma on low-power examination.[223] The metastases can be superimposed on pre-existent diseases of the spleen, such as hairy cell leukemia.[226]

REFERENCES
NORMAL ANATOMY

1 Bishop MB, Lansing LS: The spleen. A correlative overview of normal and pathologic anatomy. Hum Pathol **13:**334-342, 1982.
2 Enriquez P, Neiman RS: The pathology of the spleen. A functional approach. Chicago, 1976, American Society of Clinical Pathology.

3 Ham AW: The structure of the spleen. In Blaustein A, ed: The spleen. New York, 1963, McGraw-Hill Book Co.
4 Lennert K, Harms D, eds: Die Milz. Berlin, 1970, Springer-Verlag.
5 Millikin PD: The nodular white pulp of the human spleen. Arch Pathol **87:**247-258, 1969.
6 van Krieken JHJM, te Velde J: Immunohistology of the human spleen. An inventory of the localization of lymphocyte subpopulations. Histopathology **10:**285-294, 1986.
7 van Krieken JH, te Velde J: Normal histology of the human spleen. Am J Surg Pathol **12:**777-785, 1988.
8 van Krieken JHJM, te Velde J, Hermans J, Welvaart K: The splenic red pulp. A histomorphometrical study in splenectomy specimens embedded in methylmethacrylate. Histopathology **9:**401-416, 1985.
9 van Krieken JHJM, te Velde J, Kleiverda K, Leenheers-Binnendijk L, Van de Velde CJH: The human spleen. A histological study in splenectomy specimens embedded in methylmethacrylate. Histopathology **9:**571-585, 1985.
10 Weiss L: The structure of the normal spleen. Semin Hematol **2:**205-228, 1965.
11 Weiss L, Tavassoli M: Anatomical hazards to the passage of erythrocytes through the spleen. Semin Hematol **7:**372-380, 1970.

BIOPSY AND FINE-NEEDLE ASPIRATION

12 Block M, Jacobson LO: Splenic puncture. JAMA **142:**641-647, 1950.
13 Cavanna L, Civardi G, Fornari F, Di Stasi M, Sbolli G, Buscarini E, Vallisa D, Rossi S, Tansini P, Buscarini L: Ultrasonically guided percutaneous splenic tissue core biopsy in patients with malignant lymphomas. Cancer **69:**2932-2936, 1992.
14 Ferris DO, Hargraves MM: Splenic puncture. Arch Surg **67:**402-407, 1953.
15 Moeschlin S: Spleen puncture. London, 1951, William Heinemann, Ltd.
16 Soderström N: Cytologie der Milz in Punktaten. In Lennert K, Harms D, eds: Die Milz. Berlin, 1970, Springer-Verlag.

RUPTURE AND SPLENECTOMY

17 Aldrete JS: Spontaneous rupture of the spleen in patients with infectious mononucleosis (editorial). Mayo Clin Proc **67:**910-912, 1992.
18 Baack BR, Varsa EW, Burgdorf WH, Blaugrund AC: Splenosis. A report of subcutaneous involvement. Am J Dermatopathol **12:**585-588, 1990.
19 Carr NJ, Turk EP: The histological features of splenosis. Histopathology **21:**549-553, 1992.
20 Dalton ML Jr, Strange WH, Downs EA: Intrathoracic splenosis. Case report and review of the literature. Am Rev Respir Dis **103:**827-830, 1971.

21 Editorial: Infective hazards of splenectomy. Lancet **1:**1167-1168, 1976.
22 Ellis EF, Smith RT: The role of the spleen in immunity. Pediatrics **37:**111-119, 1966.
23 Fausel R, Sun NC, Klein S: Splenic rupture in a human immunodeficiency virus–infected patient with primary splenic lymphoma. Cancer **66:**2414-2416, 1990.
24 Fleming CR, Dickson ER, Harrison EG Jr: Splenosis. Autotransplantation of splenic tissue. Am J Med **61:**414-419, 1976.
25 Foster RP: Delayed haemorrhage from the ruptured spleen. Br J Surg **57:**189-192, 1970.
26 Gabor S, Back F, Csiffary D: Peliosis lienis. Uncommon cause of rupture of the spleen. Pathol Res Pract **188:**380-383, 1992.
27 Kubosawa H, Konno A, Komatsu T, Ishige H, Kondo Y: Peliosis hepatis. An unusual case involving the spleen and lymph nodes. Acta Pathol Jpn **39:**212-215, 1989.
28 Nordøy A: The spleenless state in man. In Lennert K, Harms D, eds: Die Milz. Berlin, 1970, Springer-Verlag.
29 Orloff MJ, Peskin GW: Spontaneous rupture of the normal spleen. A surgical enigma. Int Abstr Surg **106:**1-11, 1958.
30 Pedersen B, Videbaek A: On the late effects of removal of the normal spleen. A follow-up study of 40 persons. Acta Chir Scand **131:**89-98, 1966.
31 Pratt DB, Andersen RC, Hitchcock CR: Splenic rupture. A review of 114 cases. Minn Med **54:**177-184, 1971.
32 Rawsthorne GB, Cole TP, Kyle J: Spontaneous rupture of the spleen in infectious mononucleosis. Br J Surg **57:**396-398, 1970.
33 Sherman R: Management of trauma to the spleen. Adv Surg **17:**37-71, 1984.
34 Stites TB, Ultmann JE: Spontaneous rupture of the spleen in chronic lymphocytic leukemia. Cancer **19:**1587-1590, 1966.
35 Traub A, Giebink GS, Smith C, Kuni CC, Brekke ML, Edlund D, Perry JF: Splenic reticuloendothelial function after splenectomy, spleen repair, and spleen autotransplantation. N Engl J Med **317:**1559-1564, 1987.

CONGENITAL ANOMALIES

36 Cotelingam JD, Saito R: Hepatolienal fusion. Case report of an unusual lesion. Hum Pathol **9:**234-236, 1978.
37 Esterly JR, Oppenheimer EH: Lymphangiectasis and other pulmonary lesions in the asplenia syndrome. Arch Pathol **90:**553-560, 1970.
38 Gonzalez-Crussi F, Raibley S, Ballantine TVN, Grosfeld JL: Splenorenal fusion. Heterotopia simulating a renal neoplasm. Am J Dis Child **131:**994-996, 1977.
39 Kevy SV, Tefft M, Vawter GF, Rosen FS: Hereditary splenic hypoplasia. Pediatrics **42:**752-757, 1968.
40 Meneses MF, Ostrowski ML: Female splenic-gonadal fusion of the discontinuous type. Hum Pathol **20:**486-488, 1989.
41 Putschar WGJ, Manion WC: Congenital absence of the spleen and associated anomalies. Am J Pathol **26:**429-470, 1956.
42 Putschar WGJ, Manion WC: Splenic-gonadal fusion. Cancer **32:**15-34, 1956.
43 Rose V, Izukawa T, Moës CAF: Syndromes of asplenia and polysplenia. A review of cardiac and noncardiac malformations in 60 cases with special reference to diagnosis and prognosis. Br Heart J **37:**840-852, 1975.
44 Watson RJ: Splenogonadal fusion. Surgery **63:**853-858, 1968.

CYSTS

45 Blank E, Campbell JR: Epidermoid cysts of the spleen. Pediatrics **51:**75-84, 1973.
46 Bürring K-F: Epithelial (true) splenic cysts. Pathogenesis of the mesothelial and so-called epidermoid cyst of the spleen. Am J Surg Pathol **12:**275-281, 1988.
47 Fowler RH: Nonparasitic benign cystic tumors of the spleen. Surg Gynecol Obstet **96**(Suppl):209-227, 1953.
48 Garvin DF, King FM: Cysts and nonlymphomatous tumors of the spleen. Pathol Annu **16**(Pt 1):61-80, 1981.
49 Lifschitz-Mercer B, Open M, Kushnir I, Czernobilsky B: Epidermoid cyst of the spleen. A cytokeratin profile with comparison to other squamous epithelia. Virchows Arch **424:**213-216, 1994.
50 Morohoshi T, Hamamoto T, Kunimura T, Yoshida E, Kanda M, Funo K, Nagayama T, Maeda M, Araki S: Epidermoid cyst derived from an accessory spleen in the pancreas. A case report with literature survey. Acta Pathol Jpn **41:**916-921, 1991.
51 Ough YD, Nash HR, Wood DA: Mesothelial cysts of the spleen with squamous metaplasia. Am J Clin Pathol **76:**666-669, 1981.
52 Park JY, Song KT: Splenic cyst. A case report and review of literature. Am Surg **37:**544-547, 1971.
53 Talerman A, Hart S: Epithelial cysts of the spleen. Br J Surg **57:**201-204, 1970.
54 Tsakraklikes V, Hadley TW: Epidermoid cysts of the spleen. A report of five cases. Arch Pathol **96:**251-254, 1973.

INFLAMMATION

55 Bagshawe A: A comparative study of hypersplenism in reactive and congestive splenomegaly. Br J Haematol **19:**729-737, 1970.
56 Bendix-Hansen K, Kristensen IB: Granulomas of spleen and liver in hairy cell leukaemia. Acta Pathol Microbiol Immunol Scand (A) **92:**157-160, 1984.
57 Braylan RC. Long J, Jaffe ES, Greco FA, Orr SL, Berard CW: Malignant lymphoma obscured by concomitant extensive epithelioid granulomas. Report of three cases with similar clinicopathologic features. Cancer **39:**1146-1155, 1977.
58 Briggs RD, Davidson AI, Fletcher BRG: Solitary abscesses of the spleen. J R Coll Surg Edinb **22:**345-347, 1977.
59 Chun CH, Raff MJ, Contreras L, Varghese R, Waterman N, Daffner R, Melo JC: Splenic abscess. Medicine (Baltimore) **59:**50-65, 1980.
60 Editorial: Tropical splenomegaly syndrome. Lancet **1:**1058-1059, 1976.
61 Falk S, Muller H, Stutte HJ: The spleen in acquired immunodeficiency syndrome (AIDS). Pathol Res Pract **183:**425-433, 1988.
62 Gaba AR, Stein RS, Sweet DL, Variakojis D: Multicentric giant lymph node hyperplasia. Am J Clin Pathol **69:**86-90, 1978.
63 Hermann RE, Deltaven KE, Hawk WA: Splenectomy for the diagnosis of splenomegaly. Ann Surg **168:**896-900, 1968.
64 Kadin ME, Donaldson SS, Dorfman RF: Isolated granulomas in Hodgkin's disease. N Engl J Med **283:**859-861, 1970.
65 Klatt EC, Meyer PR: Pathology of the spleen in the acquired immunodeficiency syndrome. Arch Pathol Lab Med **111:**1050-1053, 1987.
66 Klemperer P: The pathologic anatomy of splenomegaly. Am J Clin Pathol **6:**99-159, 1936.
67 Kuo T, Rosai J: Granulomatous inflammation in splenectomy specimens. Clinicopathologic study of 20 cases. Arch Pathol **98:**261-268, 1974.
68 Millikin PD: Epithelioid germinal centers in the human spleen. Arch Pathol **89:**314-320, 1970.
69 Neiman RS: Incidence and importance of splenic sarcoid-like granulomas. Arch Pathol **101:**518-521, 1977.
70 Neiman RS, Bischel MD, Lukes RJ: Hypersplenism in the uremic hemodialyzed patient. Pathology and proposed pathophysiologic mechanisms. Am J Clin Pathol **60:**502-511, 1973.
71 Pitney WR: The tropical splenomegaly syndrome. Trans R Soc Trop Med Hyg **62:**717-728, 1968.
72 Sacks EL, Donaldson SS, Gordon J, Dorfman RF: Epithelioid granulomas associated with Hodgkin's disease. Clinical conditions in 55 previously untreated patients. Cancer **41:**562-567, 1978.
73 Sagoe AS: Tropical splenomegaly syndrome. Long-term proguanil therapy correlated with spleen size, serum IgM, and lymphocyte transformation. Br Med J **3:**378-382, 1970.
74 Thomas DM, Akosa AB, Lampert IA: Granulomatous inflammation of the spleen in infectious mononucleosis. Histopathology **17:**265-267, 1990.
75 Walker DA, Howat AJ, Shannon RS, Bouch DC, Lilleyman JS: Necrotizing granulomatous splenitis complicating leukemia in childhood. Cancer **56:**371-373, 1985.
76 Weisenburger DD: Multicentric angiofollicular lymph node hyperplasia. Pathology of the spleen. Am J Surg Pathol **12:**176-181, 1988.
77 Young JM, Bills RJ, Ulrich E: Discrete splenic calcification in necropsy material. Am J Pathol **33:**189-197, 1957.

HYPERSPLENISM

78 Bowdler AJ: Splenomegaly and hypersplenism. Clin Haematol **12:**467-488, 1983.
79 Neiman RS, Bischel MD, Lukes RJ: Hypersplenism in the uremic hemodialyzed patient. Pathology and proposed pathophysiologic mechanisms. Am J Clin Pathol **60:**502-511, 1973.
80 Rappaport H: The pathologic anatomy of the splenic red pulp. In Lennert K, Harms D, eds: Die Milz. Berlin, 1970, Springer-Verlag.

Thrombocytopenic purpuras

81 Baldini M: Idiopathic thrombocytopenic purpura. N Engl J Med **274:**1245-1251, 1301-1306, 1360-1367, 1966.
82 Berendt HL, Mant MJ, Jewell LD: Periarterial fibrosis in the spleen in idiopathic thrombocytopenic purpura. Arch Pathol Lab Med **110:**1152-1154, 1986.
83 Bowdler AJ: The role of the spleen and splenectomy in autoimmune hemolytic disease. Semin Hematol **13:**335-348, 1976.
84 Bowman HE, Pettit VD, Caldwell FT, Smith EB: Morphology of the spleen in idiopathic thrombocytopenic purpura. Lab Invest **4:**206-216, 1955.

85 Chang CS, Li CY, Cha SS: Chronic idiopathic thrombocytopenic purpura. Splenic pathologic features and their clinical correlation. Arch Pathol Lab Med 117:981-985, 1993.

86 Cohn J, Tygstrup I: Foamy histiocytosis of the spleen in patients with chronic thrombocytopenia. Scand J Hematol 16:33-37, 1976.

87 Ebbe S, Wittels B, Dameshek W: Autoimmune thrombocytopenic purpura ("ITP" type) with chronic lymphocytic leukemia. Blood 19:23-27, 1962.

88 Hassan NMR, Neiman RS: The pathology of the spleen in steroid-treated immune thrombocytopenic purpura. Am J Clin Pathol 84:433-438, 1985.

89 Hayes MM, Jacobs P, Wood L, Dent DM: Splenic pathology in immune thrombocytopenia. J Clin Pathol 38:985-988, 1985.

90 Jiang DY, Li C-Y: Immunohistochemical study of the spleen in chronic immune thrombocytopenic purpura with special reference to hyperplastic follicles and foamy macrophages. Arch Pathol Lab Med 119:533-537, 1995.

91 Luk SC. Musclow E, Simon GT: Platelet phagocytosis in the spleen of patients with idiopathic thrombocytopenic purpura (ITP). Histopathology 4:127-136, 1980.

92 McMillan R: Chronic idiopathic thrombocytopenic purpura. N Engl J Med 304:1135-1147, 1981.

93 McMillan R, Longmire RL, Yelenosky R, Donnell RL, Armstrong S: Quantitation of platelet-binding IgG produced in vitro by spleens from patients with idiopathic thrombocytopenic purpura. N Engl J Med 291:812-817, 1974.

94 McMillan R, Longmire RL, Yelenosky BS, Smith RS, Craddock CG: Immunoglobulin synthesis in vitro by splenic tissue in idiopathic thrombocytopenic purpura. N Engl J Med 286:681-684, 1972.

95 Rudders RA, Aisenberg AC, Schiller AL: Hodgkin's disease presenting as "idiopathic" thrombocytopenic purpura. Cancer 30:220-230, 1972.

96 Saltzstein SL: Phospholipid accumulation in histiocytes of splenic pulp associated with thrombocytopenic purpura. Blood 18:73-88, 1961.

97 Saracco SM, Farhi DC: Splenic pathology in thrombotic thrombocytopenic purpura. Am J Surg Pathol 14:223-229, 1990.

98 Shulman NR, Marder VJ, Hiller MC, Collier EM: Platelet and leukocyte isoantigens and their antibodies. Serologic, physiologic, and clinical studies. Prog Hematol 4:222-304, 1964.

99 Tavassoli M, McMillan R: Structure of the spleen in idiopathic thrombocytopenic purpura. Am J Clin Pathol 64:180-191, 1975.

Hemolytic anemia

100 Amorosi EL: Hypersplenism. Semin Hematol 2:249-285, 1965.

101 Crosby WH: Splenectomy in hematologic disorders. N Engl J Med 286:1252-1254, 1972.

102 Jacob HS: The defective red blood cell in hereditary spherocytosis. Annu Rev Med 20:41-46, 1969.

103 Miraglia del Giudice E, Iolascon A, Pinto L, Nobili B, Perrotta S: Erythrocyte membrane protein alterations underlying clinical heterogeneity in hereditary spherocytosis. Br J Haematol 88:52-55, 1994.

104 Molnar Z, Rappaport H: Fine structure of the red pulp of the spleen in hereditary spherocytosis. Blood 39:81-98, 1972.

105 Pattern E: Immunohematologic diseases. JAMA 258:2945-2951, 1987.

106 Peters LL, Lux SE: Ankyrins. Structure and function in normal cells and hereditary spherocytes. Semin Hematol 30:85-118, 1993.

107 Rappaport H, Crosby WH: Autoimmune hemolytic anemia. II. Morphologic observations and clinicopathologic correlation. Am J Pathol 33:429-458, 1957.

108 Saad ST, Costa FF, Vicentim DL, Salles TS, Pranke PH: Red cell membrane protein abnormalities in hereditary spherocytosis in Brazil. Br J Haematol 88:295-299, 1994.

109 Sandusky WR, Leavell BS, Burton IB: Splenectomy. Indications and results in hematologic disorders. Ann Surg 159:695-710, 1964.

110 Weed RI: The importance of erythrocyte deformability. Am J Med 49:147-150, 1970.

111 Wiland OK, Smith EB: The morphology of the spleen in congenital hemolytic anemia (hereditary spherocytosis). Am J Clin Pathol 26:619-629, 1956.

Congestive splenomegaly

112 Bowder AJ: Splenomegaly and hypersplenism. Clin Haematol 12:467-488, 1983.

113 Ludwig J, Hashimoto E, Obata H, Baldus WP: Idiopathic portal hypertension. A histopathological study of 26 Japanese cases. Histopathology 22:227-234, 1993.

114 Satterfield JV, Mulligan LV, Butcher HR Jr: Bleeding esophageal varices. Arch Surg 90:667-672, 1965.

115 Wanless IR, Bernier V: Fibrous thickening of the splenic capsule. A response to chronic splenic congestion. Arch Pathol Lab Med 107:595-599, 1983.

OTHER NON-NEOPLASTIC DISORDERS

116 Chen KTK, Flam MS, Workman RD: Amyloid tumor of the spleen. Am J Surg Pathol 11:723-725, 1987.

117 Cruickshank B: Follicular (mineral oil) lipidosis. I. Epidemiologic studies of involvement of the spleen. Hum Pathol 15:724-730, 1984.

118 Cruickshank B, Thomas MJ: Mineral oil (follicular) lipidosis. II. Histologic studies of spleen, liver, lymph nodes, and bone marrow. Hum Pathol 15:731-737, 1984.

119 Dailey MO, Coleman CN, Fajardo LF: Splenic injury caused by therapeutic irradiation. Am J Surg Pathol 5:325-331, 1981.

120 Dawson PJ, Dawson G: Adult Niemann-Pick disease with sea-blue histiocytes in the spleen. Hum Pathol 13:1115-1120, 1982.

121 Diebold J, Audouin J: Peliosis of the spleen. Report of a case associated with chronic myelomonocytic leukemia, presenting with spontaneous splenic rupture. Am J Surg Pathol 7:197-204, 1983.

122 Gupta PC, Chatterjea JB, Mukherjee AM, Chatterji A: Observations on the foam cell in thalassemia. Blood 16:1039-1044, 1960.

123 Lacson A, Berman LD, Neiman RS: Peliosis of the spleen. Am J Clin Pathol 71:586-590, 1979.

124 Liber A, Rose HG: Saturated hydrocarbons in follicular lipidosis of the spleen. Arch Pathol 83:116-122, 1967.

125 Parker AC, Bain AD, Brydon WG, Harkness RA, Smith AF, Smith II, Boyd DHA: Sea-blue histiocytosis associated with hyperlipidemia. J Clin Pathol 29:634-638, 1976.

126 Reidbord HR, Branimir LH, Fisher ER: Splenic lipidoses. Histochemical and ultrastructural differentiation with special reference to the syndrome of the sea-blue histiocyte. Arch Pathol 93:518-524, 1972.

127 Rywlin AM, Lopez-Gomez A, Tachimes P, Pardo V: Ceroid histiocytosis of the spleen in hyperlipemia. Relationship to the syndrome of the sea-blue histiocyte. Am J Clin Pathol 56:572-579, 1971.

128 Silverstein MN, Ellefson RD, Ahern EJ: The syndrome of the sea-blue histiocyte. N Engl J Med 282:1-4, 1970.

129 Tada T, Wakabayashi T, Kishimoto H: Peliosis of the spleen. Am J Clin Pathol 79:708-713, 1983.

130 Wanless IR, Geddie WR: Mineral oil lipogranulomata in liver and spleen. A study of 465 autopsies. Arch Pathol Lab Med 109:283-286, 1985.

131 Warfel KA, Ellis GH: Peliosis of the spleen. Report of a case and review of the literature. Arch Pathol Lab Med 106:99-100, 1982.

HEMATOLYMPHOID TUMORS AND TUMORLIKE CONDITIONS
Benign lymphoid processes

132 Burke JS: Splenic lymphoid hyperplasias versus lymphomas/leukemias. A diagnostic guide. Am J Clin Pathol 99:486-493, 1993.

133 Burke JS, Osborne BM: Localized reactive lymphoid hyperplasia of the spleen simulating malignant lymphoma. A report of seven cases. Am J Surg Pathol 7:373-380, 1983.

134 Cotelingam JD, Jaffe ES: Inflammatory pseudotumor of the spleen. Am J Surg Pathol 8:375-380, 1984.

135 Monforte-Munoz H, Ro JY, Manning JT Jr, Landon G, Del Junco G, Carlson TS, Ayala AG: Inflammatory pseudotumor of the spleen. Report of two cases with a review of the literature. Am J Clin Pathol 96:491-495, 1991.

136 Sheahan K, Wolf BC, Neiman RS: Inflammatory pseudotumor of the spleen. A clinicopathology study of three cases. Hum Pathol 19:1024-1029, 1988.

137 Thomas RM, Jaffe ES, Zarate-Osorno A, Medeiros LJ: Inflammatory pseudotumor of the spleen. A clinicopathologic and immunophenotypic study of eight cases. Arch Pathol Lab Med 117:921-926, 1993.

Non-Hodgkin's lymphoma

138 Ahmann DL, Kiely JM, Harrison EG Jr, Payne S: Malignant lymphoma of the spleen. Cancer 19:461-469, 1966.

139 Bellamy CO, Krajewski AS: Primary splenic large cell anaplastic lymphoma associated with HIV infection. Histopathology 24:481-483, 1994.

140 Burke JS: Surgical pathology of the spleen. An approach to the differential diagnosis of splenic lymphomas and leukemias. I. Diseases of the white pulp. Am J Surg Pathol 5:551-563, 1981.

141 Burke JS: Surgical pathology of the spleen. An approach to the differential diagnosis of splenic lymphomas and leukemias. II. Diseases of the red pulp. Am J Surg Pathol 5:681-694, 1981.

142 Dacie JV, Brain MC, Harrison CV, Lewis SM, Worlledge SM: Non-tropical idiopathic splenomegaly (primary hypersplenism). A review of ten cases and their relationship to malignant lymphomas. Br J Haematol 17:317-333, 1969.

143 Dacie JV, Galton DAG, Gordon-Smith EC, Harrison CV: Non-tropical 'idiopathic splenomegaly.' A follow-up study of ten patients described in 1969. Br J Haematol 38:185-193, 1978.

143a Dommann-Scherrer CC, Baumann Kurer S, Zimmermann DR, Odermatt BF, Dours-Zimmermann MT, Briner J, Heitz PU: Occult hepatosplenic T-γδ lymphoma. Value of genotypic analysis in the differential diagnosis. Virchows Arch **426:**629-634, 1995.

144 Falk S, Stutte HJ: Primary malignant lymphomas of the spleen. A morphologic and immunohistochemical analysis of 17 cases. Cancer **66:**2612-2619, 1990.

145 Franchino C, Reich C, Distenfeld A, Ubriaco A, Knowles DM: A clinicopathologically distinctive primary splenic histiocytic neoplasm. Demonstration of its histiocytic derivation by immunophenotypic and molecular genetic analysis. Am J Surg Pathol **12:**398-404, 1988.

146 Goldberg GM: A study of malignant lymphomas and leukemias. VII. Lymphogenous leukemia and lymphosarcoma involvement of the lymphatic and hemic bed, with reference to differentiating criteria. Cancer **17:**277-287, 1964.

147 Harris NL, Aisenberg AC, Meyer JE, Ellman L, Elman A: Diffuse large cell (histiocytic) lymphoma of the spleen. Clinical and pathologic characteristics of ten cases. Cancer **54:**2460-2467, 1984.

148 Hollema H, Visser L, Poppema S: Small lymphocytic lymphomas with predominant splenomegaly. A comparison of immunophenotypes with cases of predominant lymphadenopathy. Mod Pathol **4:**712-717, 1991.

149 Kehoe J, Straus DJ: Primary lymphoma of the spleen. Clinical features and out come after splenectomy. Cancer **62:**1433-1438, 1988.

150 Kobrich U, Falk S, Karhoff M, Middeke B, Anselstetter V, Stutte HJ: Primary large cell lymphoma of the splenic sinuses. A variant of angiotropic B-cell lymphoma (neoplastic angioendotheliomatosis)? Hum Pathol **23:**1184-1187, 1992.

151 Kraemer BB, Osborne BM, Butler JJ: Primary splenic presentation of malignant lymphoma and related disorders. Cancer **54:**1606-1619, 1984.

152 Melo JV, Hedge U, Parreira A, Thompson I, Lampert IA, Catovsky D: Splenic B cell lymphoma with circulating villous lymphocytes. Differential diagnosis of B cell leukaemias with large spleens. J Clin Pathol **40:**642-651, 1987.

153 Morel P, Dupriez B, Gosselin B, Fenaux P, Estienne MH, Facon T, Jouet JP, Bauters F: Role of early splenectomy in malignant lymphomas with prominent splenic involvement (primary lymphomas of the spleen). A study of 59 cases. Cancer **71:**207-215, 1993.

154 Narang S, Wolf BC, Neiman RS: Malignant lymphoma presenting with prominent splenomegaly. A clinicopathologic study with special reference to intermediate cell lymphoma. Cancer **55:**1948-1957, 1985.

155 Neiman RS, Sullivan AL, Jaffe R: Malignant lymphoma simulating leukemic reticuloendotheliosis. Cancer **43:**329-342, 1979.

155a Pawade J, Wilkins BS, Wright DH: Low-grade B-cell lymphomas of the splenic marginal zone. A clinicopathological and immunohistochemical study of 14 cases. Histopathology **17:**129-137, 1995.

156 Rosso R, Neiman RS, Paulli M, Boveri E, Kindl S, Magrini U, Barosi G: Splenic marginal zone cell lymphoma. Report of an indolent variant without massive splenomegaly presumably representing an early phase of the disease. Hum Pathol **26:**39-46, 1995.

157 Schmid C, Kirkham N, Diss T, Isaacson PG: Splenic marginal zone cell lymphoma. Am J Surg Pathol **16:**455-466, 1992.

158 Skarin AT, Davey FR, Moloney WC: Lymphosarcoma of the spleen. Arch Intern Med **127:**259-265, 1971.

159 Spier CM, Kjeldsberg CR, Eyre HJ, Behm FG: Malignant lymphoma with primary presentation in the spleen. A study of 20 patients. Arch Pathol Lab Med **109:**1076-1080, 1985.

160 Stroup RM, Burke JS, Sheibani K, Ben-Ezra J, Brownell M, Winberg CD: Splenic involvement by aggressive malignant lymphomas of B-cell and T-cell types. A morphologic and immunophenotypic study. Cancer **69:**413-420, 1992.

161 van Krieken JH, Feller AC, te Velde J: The distribution of non-Hodgkin's lymphoma in the lymphoid compartments of the human spleen. Am J Surg Pathol **13:**757-765, 1989.

162 Vardiman JW, Byrne GE Jr, Rappaport H: Malignant histiocytosis with massive splenomegaly in asymptomatic patients. A possible chronic form of the disease. Cancer **36:**419-427, 1975.

162a Wong KF, Chan JK, Matutes E, McCarthy K, Ng CS, Chan CH, Ma SK: Hepatosplenic gamma delta T-cell lymphoma. A distinctive aggressive lymphoma type. Am J Surg Pathol **19:**718-726, 1995.

Hodgkin's disease

163 Brissette M, Dhru RD: Hodgkin's disease presenting as spontaneous splenic rupture. Arch Pathol Lab Med **116:**1077-1079, 1992.

164 Siebert JD, Stuckey JH, Kurtin PJ, Banks PM: Extranodal lymphocyte predominance Hodgkin's disease. Clinical and pathologic features. Am J Clin Pathol **103:**485-491, 1995.

Leukemias

165 Burke JS: Surgical pathology of the spleen. An approach to the differential diagnosis of splenic lymphomas and leukemias. II. Diseases of the red pulp. Am J Surg Pathol **5:**681-694, 1981.

166 Burke JS, Byrne GE Jr, Rappaport H: Hairy cell leukemia (leukemic reticuloendotheliosis). I. A clinical pathologic study of 21 patients. Cancer **33:**1399-1410, 1974.

167 Burke JS, Mackay B, Rappaport H: Hairy cell leukemia. II. Ultrastructure of the spleen. Cancer **37:**2267-2274, 1976.

168 Burke JS, Sheibani K, Winberg CD, Rappaport H: Recognition of hairy cell leukemia in a spleen of normal weight. The contribution of immunohistologic studies. Am J Clin Pathol **87:**276-281, 1987.

169 Butler JJ: Pathology of the spleen in benign and malignant conditions. Histopathology **7:**453-474, 1983.

170 Chang KL, Stroup R, Weiss LM: Hairy cell leukemia. Current status. Am J Clin Pathol **97:**719-738, 1992.

171 Hanson CA, Ward PC, Schnitzer B: A multilobular variant of hairy cell leukemia with morphologic similarities to T-cell lymphoma. Am J Surg Pathol **13:**671-679, 1989.

172 Hogan SF, Osborne BM, Butler JJ: Unexpected splenic nodules in leukemic patients. Hum Pathol **20:**62-68, 1989.

173 Lampert I, Catovsky D, Marsh GW, Child JA, Galton DAG: The histopathology of prolymphocytic leukaemia with particular reference to the spleen. A comparison with chronic lymphocytic leukaemia. Histopathology **4:**3-19, 1980.

174 Nanba K, Soban EJ, Bowling MC, Berard CW: Splenic pseudosinuses and hepatic angiomatous lesions. Distinctive features of hairy cell leukemia. Am J Clin Pathol **67:**415-426, 1977.

175 Pilon VA, Davey FR, Gordon GB: Splenic alterations in hairy cell leukemia. Arch Pathol Lab Med **105:**577-581, 1981.

176 Pilon VA, Davey FR, Gordon GB, Jones DB: Splenic alterations in hairy-cell leukemia. II. An electron microscopic study. Cancer **49:**1617-1623, 1982.

177 Re G, Pileri S, Cau R, Bucchi ML, Casali AM, Cavalli G: Histometry of splenic microvascular architecture in hairy cell leukaemia. Histopathology **13:**425-434, 1988.

178 Strickler JG, Schmidt CM, Wick MR: Immunophenotype of hairy cell leukemia in paraffin sections. Mod Pathol **3:**518-523, 1990.

179 Stroup R, Sheibani K: Antigenic phenotypes of hairy cell leukemia and monocytoid B-cell lymphoma. An immunohistochemical evaluation of 66 cases. Hum Pathol **23:**172-177, 1992.

180 Van Norman AS, Nagorney DM, Martin JK, Phyliky RL, Ilstrup DM: Splenectomy for hairy cell leukemia. A clinical review of 63 patients. Cancer **57:**644-648, 1986.

Myelofibrosis

181 Cina SJ, Gordon BM, Curry NS: Ectopic adrenal myelolipoma presenting as a splenic mass. Arch Pathol Lab Med **119:**561-563, 1995.

182 Fisher ER, Hazard JB: Differentiation of megakaryocyte and Reed-Sternberg cell. Lab Invest **3:**261-269, 1954.

183 O'Keane JC, Wolf BC, Neiman RS: The pathogenesis of splenic extramedullary hematopoiesis in metastatic carcinoma. Cancer **63:**1539-1543, 1989.

184 Pitcock JA, Reinhard EH, Justus BW, Mendelsohn RA: A clinical and pathological study of seventy cases of myelofibrosis. Ann Intern Med **57:**73-84, 1962.

185 Söderström N, Bandmann U, Lundh B: Patho-anatomical features of the spleen and liver. In Videbaek A, ed: Polycythaemia and myelofibrosis. Clin Haematol **4:**309-329, 1975.

186 Varki A, Lottenberg R, Griffith R, Reinhard E: The syndrome of idiopathic myelofibrosis. A clinicopathologic review with emphasis on the prognostic variables predicting survival. Medicine (Baltimore) **62:**353-371, 1983.

187 Wilkins BS, Green A, Wild AE, Jones DB: Extramedullary haemopoiesis in fetal and adult human spleen. A quantitative immunohistological study. Histopathology **24:**241-247, 1994.

Mastocytosis

188 Brunning RD, Parkin JL, McKenna RW, Risdall R, Rosai J: Systemic mastocytosis. Extracutaneous manifestations. Am J Surg Pathol **7:**425-438, 1983.

189 Craig SS, DeBlois G, Schwartz LB: Mast cells in human keloid, small intestine, and lung by an immunoperoxidase technique using a murine monoclonal antibody against tryptase. Am J Pathol **124:**427-435, 1986.

190 Travis WD, Li C-Y: Pathology of the lymph node and spleen in systemic mast cell disease. Mod Pathol **1:**4-14, 1988.

191 Weidner N, Horan RF, Austen KF: Mast-cell phenotype in indolent forms of mastocytosis. Ultrastructural features, fluorescence detection of avidin binding, and immunofluorescent determination of chymase, tryptase, and carboxypeptidase. Am J Pathol **140:**847-857, 1992.

Other hematolymphoid conditions

192 Burke JS: Surgical pathology of the spleen. An approach to the differential diagnosis of splenic lymphomas and leukemias. II. Diseases of the red pulp. Am J Surg Pathol **5:**681-694, 1981.

192a Perez-Ordóñez B, Erlandson RA, Rosai J: Dendritic follicular cell tumor: report of 15 additional cases of a distinctive entity. Am J Surg Pathol (in press).

OTHER PRIMARY TUMORS AND TUMORLIKE CONDITIONS

193 Aranha GV, Gold J, Grage TB: Hemangiosarcoma of the spleen. Report of a case and review of previously reported cases. J Surg Oncol **8:**481-487, 1976.

194 Autry JR, Weitzner S: Hemangiosarcoma of spleen with spontaneous rupture. Cancer **35:**534-539, 1975.

194a Budke HL, Breitfeld PP, Neiman RS: Functional hyposplenism due to a primary epithelioid hemangioendothelioma of the spleen. Arch Pathol Lab Med **119:**755-757, 1995.

195 Chen TK, Bolles J, Gilbert EF: Angiosarcoma of the spleen. Arch Pathol Lab Med **103:**122-124, 1979.

196 Easler RE, Dowlin WM: Primary lipoma of the spleen. Report of a case. Arch Pathol **88:**557-559, 1969.

197 Falk S, Krishnan J, Meis JM: Primary angiosarcoma of the spleen. A clinicopathologic study of 40 cases. Am J Surg Pathol **17:**959-970, 1993.

198 Falk S, Stutte HJ: Hamartomas of the spleen. A study of 20 biopsy cases. Histopathology **14:**603-612, 1989.

199 Falk S, Stutte HJ, Frizzera G: Littoral cell angioma. A novel splenic vascular lesion demonstrating histiocytic differentiation. Am J Surg Pathol **15:**1023-1033, 1991.

200 Garvin DF, King FM: Cysts and nonlymphomatous tumors of the spleen. Pathol Annu **16**(Pt 1):61-80, 1981.

201 Govoni E, Bazzocchi F, Pileri S, Martinelli G: Primary malignant fibrous histiocytoma of the spleen. An ultrastructural study. Histopathology **6:**351-361, 1982.

202 Hamoudi AB, Vassy LE, Morse TS: Multiple lymphangioendothelioma of the spleen in a 13-year-old girl. Arch Pathol **99:**605-606, 1975.

203 Hermann GG, Fogh J, Graem N, Hansen OP, Hippe E: Primary hemangiosarcoma of the spleen with angioscintigraphic demonstration of metastases. Cancer **53:**1682-1685, 1984.

204 Husni EA: The clinical course of splenic hemangioma with emphasis on spontaneous rupture. Arch Surg **83:**681-688, 1961.

205 Kaw YT, Duwaji MS, Knisley RE, Esparza AR: Hemangioendothelioma of the spleen. Arch Pathol Lab Med **116:**1079-1082, 1992.

206 Kishiwara T, Numaguchi Y, Watanabe K, Matsuura K: Angiographic diagnosis of benign and malignant splenic tumors. AJR **130:**339-344, 1978.

207 Neill JS, Park HK: Hemangiopericytoma of the spleen. Am J Clin Pathol **95:**680-683, 1991.

208 Rappaport H: The pathologic anatomy of the splenic red pulp. In Lennert K, Harms D, eds: Die Milz. Berlin, 1970, Springer-Verlag.

209 Ross CS, Schiller KFR: Hamartoma of spleen associated with thrombocytopenia. J Pathol **105:**62-64, 1971.

210 Ruck P, Horny HP, Xiao JC, Bajinski R, Kaiserling E: Diffuse sinusoidal hemangiomatosis of the spleen. A case report with enzyme-histochemical, immunohistochemical, and electron-microscopic findings. Pathol Res Pract **190:**708-714, 1994.

211 Schmid C, Beham A, Uranus S, Melzer G, Aubock L, Seewann HL, Klimpfinger M: Non-systemic diffuse lymphangiomatosis of spleen and liver. Histopathology **18:**478-480, 1991.

212 Shanberge JN, Tanaka K, Grouhl MC: Chronic consumption coagulopathy due to hemangiomatous transformation of the spleen. Am J Clin Pathol **56:**723-729, 1971.

213 Sieber SC, Lopez V, Rosai J, Buckley PJ: Primary tumor of spleen with morphologic features of malignant fibrous histiocytoma. Immunohistochemical evidence for a macrophage origin. Am J Surg Pathol **14:**1061-1070, 1990.

214 Silverman ML, LiVolsi VA: Splenic hamartoma. Am J Clin Pathol **70:**224-229, 1978.

215 Smith VC, Eisenberg BL, McDonald EC: Primary splenic angiosarcoma. Case report and literature review. Cancer **55:**1625-1627, 1985.

216 Suster S: Epithelioid and spindle-cell hemangioendothelioma of the spleen. Report of a distinctive splenic vascular neoplasm of childhood. Am J Surg Pathol **16:**785-792, 1992.

217 Suster S, Moran CA, Blanco M: Mycobacterial spindle-cell pseudotumor of the spleen. Am J Clin Pathol **101:**539-542, 1994.

218 Westra WH, Anderson BO, Klimstra DS: Carcinosarcoma of the spleen. An extragenital malignant mixed müllerian tumor? Am J Surg Pathol **18:**309-315, 1994.

219 Wick MR, Scheithauer BW, Smith SL, Beart RW Jr: Primary nonlymphoreticular malignant neoplasms of the spleen. Am J Surg Pathol **6:**229-242, 1982.

220 Zukerberg LR, Kaynor BL, Silverman ML, Harris NL: Splenic hamartoma and capillary hemangioma are distinct entities. Immunohistochemical analysis of CD8 expression by endothelial cells. Hum Pathol **22:**1258-1261, 1991.

METASTATIC TUMORS

221 Berge T: Splenic metastases. Frequencies and patterns. Acta Pathol Microbiol Scand (A) **82:**499-506, 1974.

222 Cummings OW, Mazur MT: Breast carcinoma diffusely metastatic to the spleen. A report of two cases presenting as idiopathic thrombocytopenic purpura. Am J Clin Pathol **97:**484-489, 1992.

223 Fakan F, Michal M: Nodular transformation of splenic red pulp due to carcinomatous infiltration. A diagnostic pitfall. Histopathology **25:**175-178, 1994.

224 Falk S, Stutte HJ: Splenic metastasis in an ileal carcinoid tumor. Pathol Res Pract **185:**238-242, 1994.

225 Klein B, Stein M, Kuten A, Steiner M, Barshalom D, Robinson E, Gal D: Splenomegaly and solitary spleen metastasis in solid tumors. Cancer **60:**100-102, 1987.

226 Sharpe RW, Rector JT, Rushin JM, Garvin DF, Cotelingam JD: Splenic metastasis in hairy cell leukemia. Cancer **71:**2222-2226, 1993.

23 Bone marrow

Richard D. Brunning, M.D.

Trephine biopsy of the bone marrow has wide application in clinical medicine; its greatest utility is in the evaluation of patients with malignant lymphoma, leukemia, metastatic tumor, granulomatous disorders, myelofibrosis, aplastic anemia, and plasma cell dyscrasias.[3-5,7,8] It also serves as the most reliable method for assessing marrow cellularity following the administration of antineoplastic drugs and in assessing the status of engraftment following bone marrow transplantation. Marrow biopsy is also utilized in the investigation of patients with infectious disease and metabolic disorders.

The trephine biopsy should be viewed as one component of the bone marrow specimen that ideally includes smears and particle crush preparations from aspirated marrow and touch imprint preparations of the core biopsy specimen. In some instances, because of marrow fibrosis, the trephine biopsy specimen will be the only marrow tissue available for examination. Marrow biopsy can usually be done with relatively little discomfort to the patient and is accompanied by very low morbidity when performed by experienced individuals with the biopsy needles now available.[12] The posterior superior iliac spines are the preferred sites. In general, severe thrombocytopenia is not a contraindication to marrow biopsy. Whenever a marrow biopsy is performed, careful attention should be directed to preventing hematoma formation by applying an adequate pressure bandage on the biopsy site following the procedure.

Paraffin embedding is the preferred method for the routine processing of bone marrow biopsies,[9] and the observations described in this chapter are based primarily on examination of specimens prepared in this manner. Plastic embedding offers some advantages over the paraffin method, such as excellent cytology and the ability to perform numerous histochemical reactions; it may also be useful in special situations, as will be noted in the section on mastocytosis.[1,2] The use of plastic embedding has been facilitated by the introduction of resins such as glycol methacrylate. However, the technique is more time-consuming than the processing of paraffin-embedded tissue, and with careful attention to technical detail, excellent results can be obtained with specimens processed in paraffin.

Considerable discussion has occurred about the relative merits of trephine biopsy of the bone marrow as opposed to sections of particles obtained by aspiration biopsy.[6,10,11,13] Particle sections are of limited value in marrow disorders that are accompanied by fibrosis; these frequently result in inadequately aspirated specimens. In addition, assessment of cellularity, determination of the extent of marrow involvement by neoplastic processes, and the relationship of lesions to marrow structures such as bone trabeculae and vasculature can be accurately assessed only in trephine biopsies. Nevertheless, any particles obtained in a marrow aspirate should be processed for histologic examination.

Myelofibrosis is one of the more vexing problems in bone marrow histopathology because of the wide range of disorders that may cause marrow fibrosis and the usual difficulty in obtaining satisfactory aspirates for cytologic studies.[14] Although marrow fibrosis occurs as an idiopathic or primary disorder, it is usually a secondary phenomenon; the most common causes are metastatic tumor and malignant lymphoma. Fibrosis also occurs relatively frequently in the evolution of chronic myeloproliferative disorders, such as chronic myeloid leukemia and polycythemia vera. In general, fibrosis that occurs as a component of hematopoietic proliferations is characterized by the deposition of increased reticulin fibers; with metastatic tumors such as breast or prostate, there may be a severe desmoplastic reaction with collagenous fibrosis.

In those instances in which the reason for the marrow fibrosis is not apparent, several techniques may be used in an attempt to determine the cause. Immunohistology, using paraffin-embedded specimens and the several antibodies described in the section on immunohistology, may be particularly helpful in identifying lymphoma or metastatic tumor; antibodies to myeloperoxidase or CD68 are particularly useful for identifying cells of granulocytic or monocytic origin. An additional procedure that may be useful in hematopoietic disorders associated with marrow fibrosis is the preparation of particle crush preparations from trephine biopsy specimens. This approach may necessitate a second biopsy unless the problem of fibrosis is anticipated before the initial procedure. As soon as possible after the trephine specimen is obtained and before it is placed in a fixative, small portions of the biopsy are cut away with a sharp scalpel blade and used for particle crush preparations in the same manner as particles from aspirated specimens. These crush preparations can be used for routine stains, cytochemistry, and immunocytochemistry. Portions of the biopsy specimen obtained in this manner may also be processed for routine electron microscopic studies and ultrastructural cytochemistry.

The use of special stains in bone marrow pathology should be determined following review of the routinely stained biopsy and the patient's clinical history.

BIOPSY PROCEDURE AND PROCESSING OF THE SPECIMEN

Several instruments are available for the bone marrow trephine biopsy procedure. The most satisfactory from the standpoint of safety, ease of performance, and overall quality of specimen obtained is the Jamshidi-type biopsy needle; several such instruments, both reusable and disposable, are commercially available.[18] These instruments are produced in several sizes for both adult and pediatric patients. The 11-gauge needle is the most commonly used for routine procedures in adults and older children. The 8-gauge instruments are preferred by some for lymphoma staging procedures; this size may result in more postbiopsy discomfort. If diffi-

culty is encountered with the 11-gauge needle in obtaining adequate specimens from patients with severe osteoporosis, an 8- or 9-gauge instrument should be used.

The importance of proper technique in performing the biopsy procedure cannot be overemphasized. Instructions for the use of the biopsy needles are included with the instruments, and some manufacturers provide audiovisual aids that illustrate proper technique. Accurate identification of body landmarks is crucial in obtaining satisfactory specimens; an improperly positioned needle may cause considerable discomfort to the patient and frequently yields an inadequate biopsy specimen. Individuals not acquainted with the biopsy technique are advised to familiarize themselves with the procedure on cadavers.

Optimally, the biopsy specimen should be at least 1.5 cm in length and should be free of distortion caused by crushing or other damage. Crush artifact and the deposition of fibrin in torn biopsies may render accurate interpretation difficult or impossible. In such instances the biopsy should be repeated. Aspiration through the biopsy needle prior to obtaining the trephine biopsy specimen should be discouraged because of the possibility of introducing hemorrhage or another artifact in the biopsy specimen.

Imprint preparations should be routinely made from the biopsy specimen immediately after it is removed from the biopsy needle. These can be used for Romanovsky stains and special cytochemical and immunocytochemical procedures. Following the preparation of imprints, the specimen is placed in an appropriate fixative; the most satisfactory are Zenker's acetic acid, B5, or 10% buffered neutral formalin.[15,19] In laboratories where bone marrow is processed with other tissues, buffered neutral formalin may be the preferred fixative. The other fixatives require special handling and are more suitable for laboratories dedicated to the processing of hematopoietic tissue. As noted in the section on immunohistochemistry, reactivity with some antibodies may be ablated by some fixatives, and the choice of fixative may be determined by the reason for the biopsy. Following fixation for an appropriate period of time, the biopsy is decalcified. Several appropriate decalcification solutions are commercially available. Most biopsy specimens will be adequately decalcified following 45 to 60 minutes in a rapid decalcifying solution. Details of the processing methodology, including decalcification, have been published.[15]

The biopsies should be sectioned at 3 to 4 μm with a sharp knife that is checked frequently for the presence of defects. In those patients being evaluated for the extent of lymphomatous involvement, metastatic tumor, or granulomatous disease, the specimens should be completely sectioned and stepwise serial sections mounted for hematoxylin-eosin staining.[16,17] The remaining ribbon should be retained and stored in a manner that will facilitate the ready and accurate mounting of additional sections for special stains and immunocytochemical reactions. Most of the stains used for other fixed tissues are also applicable to bone marrow sections. However, tissue processed with acid fixatives such as B5 and Zenker's or with acid decalcifiers will yield unsatisfactory results with the chloroacetate esterase stain.

Optimally, when interpreting the trephine biopsy, the pathologist should examine the trephine imprints, bone marrow aspirate, blood smears, and other pathology specimens. Knowledge of the patient's clinical history, hematology profile, immunoelectrophoretic studies, and x-ray findings may be of considerable importance and may greatly facilitate the interpretation of the biopsy specimen.

IMMUNOHISTOLOGY

As in other areas of pathology, immunohistology is an important resource in the evaluation of proliferative processes involving the marrow. The availability of antibodies reactive in paraffin-embedded tissue and the use of microwave methodology and enzyme digestion have been of considerable importance in the application of immunohistology in bone marrow pathology.* Although cryostat sections of marrow may be used for immunohistology, the procedure is difficult and is essentially limited to specialized laboratories.[25] In addition, cytologic preservation in cryostat sections is frequently of marginal quality.

Although decalcification with rapid acid decalcifiers may result in ablation of some antigens, there are several antibodies to membrane antigens and cytoplasmic constituents that are reactive in parafffin-embedded decalcified marrow biopsies that can be of considerable aid in identifying the lineage of immature cell populations in the marrow; these include antibodies to kappa and lambda light chains, myeloperoxidase, hemoglobin A, CD68, CD20 (L26), CD3, CD45, and tumor-related antigens[20,21,23,24,26-35] (Figs. 23-1 to 23-4). Antibodies to kappa and lambda immunoglobulin light chains are particularly useful for determining the relative proportions of kappa- and lambda-containing cells in immunoproliferative disorders such as multiple myeloma.[29] Reactivity with these antibodies is generally restricted to processes in which the cells contain cytoplasmic immunoglobulin. The technique is not sufficiently sensitive to detect surface immunoglobulin on the lymphocytes in most lymphoproliferative diseases. Occasionally the lymphocytes in a B-cell lymphocytic lymphoma contain cytoplasmic immunoglobulin that may be detected by this method (see Fig. 23-1). The antibodies to lymphocyte antigens are useful in determining the B- or T-cell origin of the lymphoproliferative processes and the extent of marrow involvement (see Fig. 23-4). These antibodies are not determinants of clonality. Polyclonal antibody to myeloperoxidase is a highly specific and sensitive antibody for cells of neutrophil origin that reacts with the myeloblasts in acute myeloid leukemia.[30] Diagnostic kits for the avidin-biotin complex, peroxidase-antiperoxidase, and alkaline phosphatase–antialkaline phosphastase methods are commercially available.

It is important that the reactivity pattern of all antibodies be determined by each laboratory. The range of reactivity attributed to an antibody by the manufacturer should be confirmed with lesions of known antigenicity. The pattern of reactivity of the antibodies to lymphoid cells is generally based on studies of lymph nodes fixed in B5 or neutral buffered formalin. The same reactivity pattern may not be applicable to marrow biopsies fixed in Zenker's fixative or B5 and decalcified in a rapid acid decalcifier; L26, an excel-

lent antibody to CD20, a pan B-cell antigen, works well in bone marrow biopsies fixed in B5 and decalcified with a rapid acid decalcifier, but does not react in Zenker fixed tissue decalcified in the same manner. Antibody to CD74 (LN2) and MB_2 reacts with both Zenker and B5 fixed specimens. The effects of decalcification on antibody reactivity should be determined by subjecting lymph node tissue to the same decalcification procedure employed for bone marrow biopsies.

In the experience of the author, B5 fixative generally yields superior lymphoid antigen preservation in marrow biopsies and appears to be the fixative of choice for marrow biopsies performed for evaluation of lymphoproliferative disorders. As noted, Zenker's fixative, which results in superior cytomorphology, appears to hinder reactivity with some antibodies, including L26 (CD20) and antibody to common leukocyte antigen. Some antibodies that are particularly useful in the evaluation of bone marrow disorders appear to be equally reactive in Zenker and B5 fixed tissue decalcified in rapid acid decalcifiers; these include antibodies to kappa and lambda light chains, myeloperoxidase, lysozyme, hemoglobin A, and mast cell tryptase. Monoclonal antibody to glycophorin C on the erythrocyte membrane reacts in paraffin-embedded sections fixed in acidic formalin; megakaryocytes react with monoclonal antibody to CD 61 (platelet glycoprotein III_a) in biopsies fixed in acidic formalin.[22]

NORMOCELLULAR BONE MARROW

Assessment of marrow cellularity must take into account the age of the patient because the amount of hematopoietic tissue in bone marrow from normal individuals varies with age.[36] In the first decade, the mean marrow cellularity is 79%; the mean cellularity in the eighth decade is 29%. In the first three decades of life more than half of the marrow is composed of hematopoietic cells. During this period, there is a gradual decrease in the amount of hematopoietic tissue with an increase in fat cells. From the fourth to the seventh decade, there is relative stabilization of the number of hematopoietic cells (Fig. 23-5); beginning in the eighth decade, there is a renewed decrease.

The immediate subcortical area of the bone marrow may normally be more hypocellular than the deeper medullary areas. As a result, specimens that contain a substantial amount of subcortical bone may be inadequate for estimating cellularity. In addition, the immediate paratrabecular areas may be preferentially hypocellular.

ALTERATIONS IN CELLULARITY
Aplastic anemia

Aplastic or hypoplastic marrow, referred to as aplastic anemia, occurs as both acquired and congenital forms. Acquired aplastic anemia may be idiopathic or result from known exposure to drugs, chemicals, viral infections, or ionizing radiation.[37,38,44-46,48] Bone marrow aplasia also has been observed in paroxysmal nocturnal hemoglobinuria.[49] The term *constitutional aplastic anemia* is used collectively for all congenital forms of aplastic anemia, familial and nonfamilial, with and without associated malformations of body structures.[39,42] Fanconi's anemia is a syndrome of familial

---

*References 20, 22, 24, 27, 28, 31.

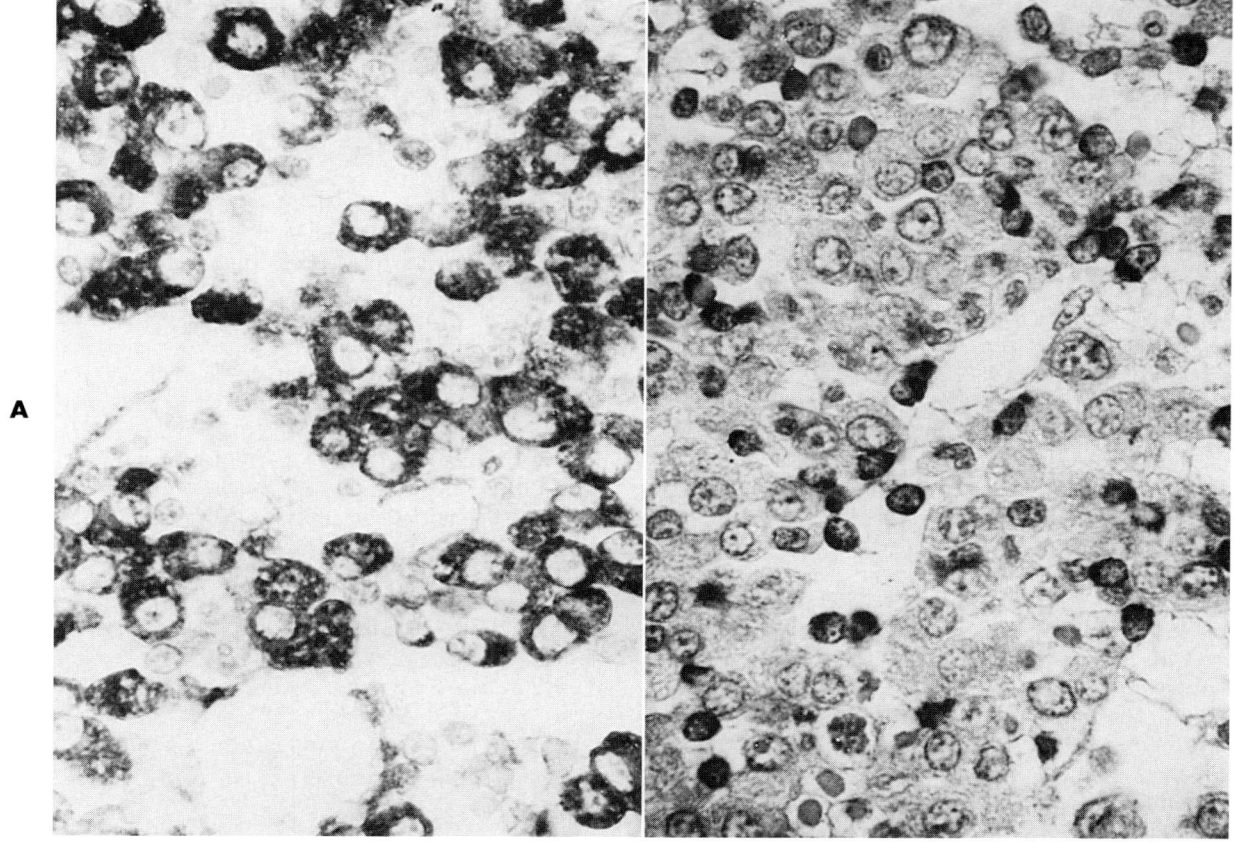

Fig. 23-1 A, Marrow biopsy from 57-year-old male with 2-year history of multiple myeloma reacted with polyclonal antibody to kappa light chain using peroxidase-antiperoxidase (PAP) technique. Plasma cells show positive reaction. **B,** Same biopsy specimen as in A reacted with anti-lambda antibody. Plasma cells are negative, but population of positively reacting small lymphocytes is present. Additional studies documented well-differentiated lymphocytic lymphoma of lambda light chain type in addition to multiple myeloma. (**A** and **B** Immunoperoxidase.)

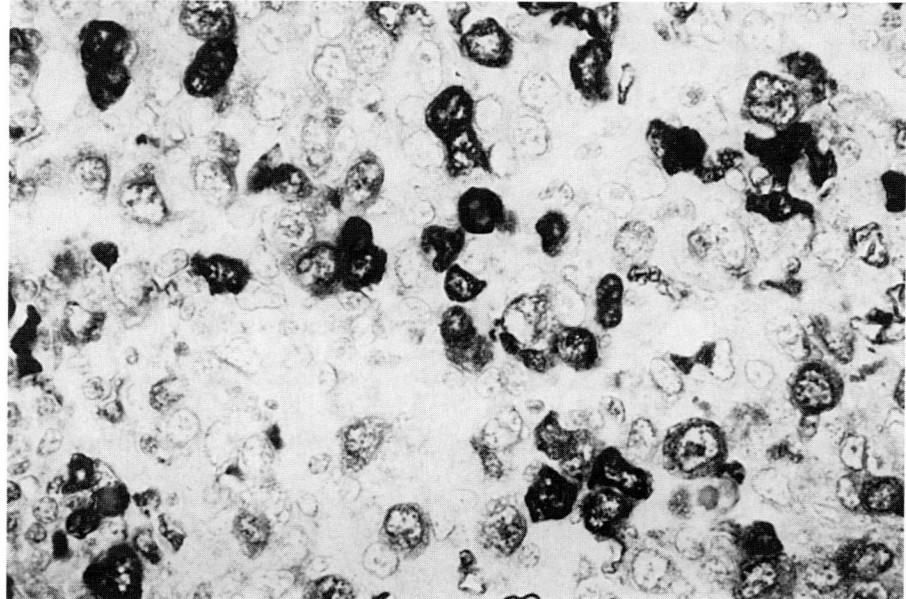

Fig. 23-2 Marrow from patient with erythroleukemia (AML-M6) reacted with antihemogloblin A antibody using the avidin-biotin complex (ABC) immunoperoxidase technique. Many of the cells show a positive cytoplasmic reaction. Intensity of reaction varies from very slight to marked. (Immunoperoxidase.)

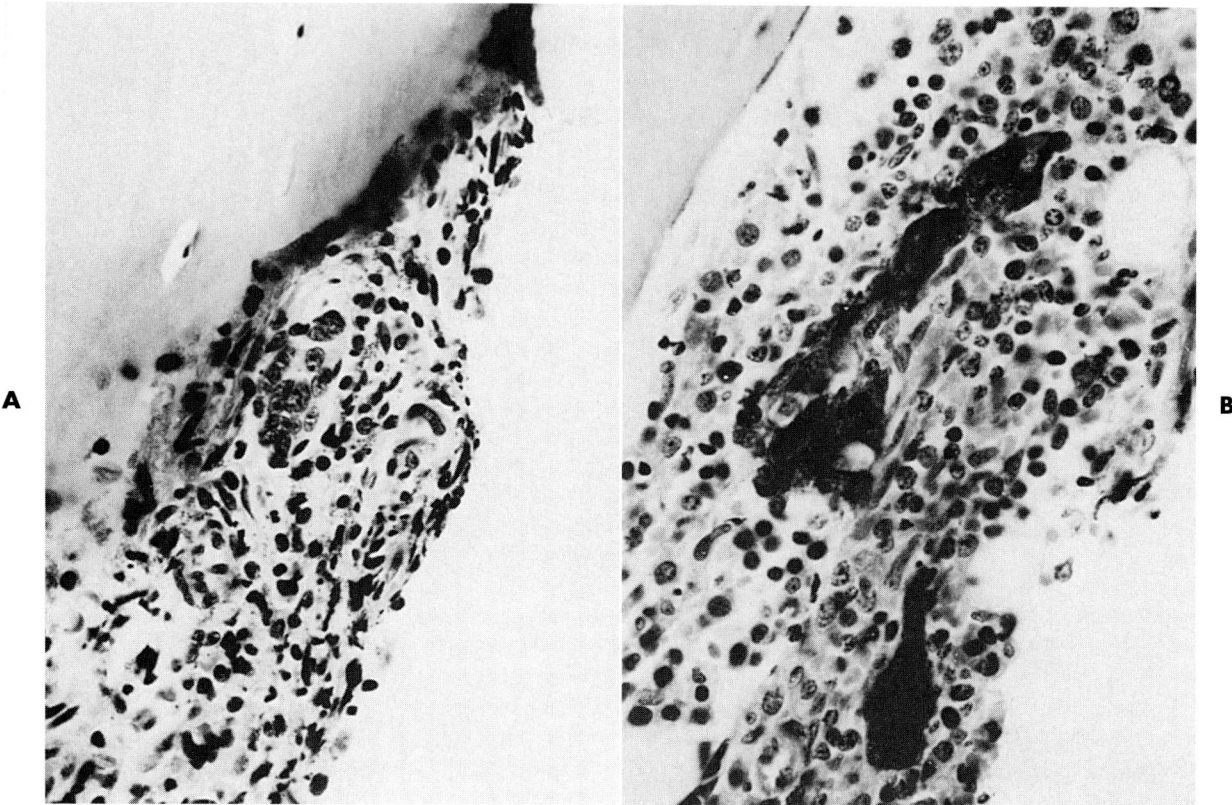

Fig. 23-3 A, Isolated focus of tumor cells in marrow of 11-year-old child with neuroblastoma. **B,** Same area as in **A** reacted with antibody to neuron-specific enolase shows several positive cells. (**B** Immunoperoxidase.)

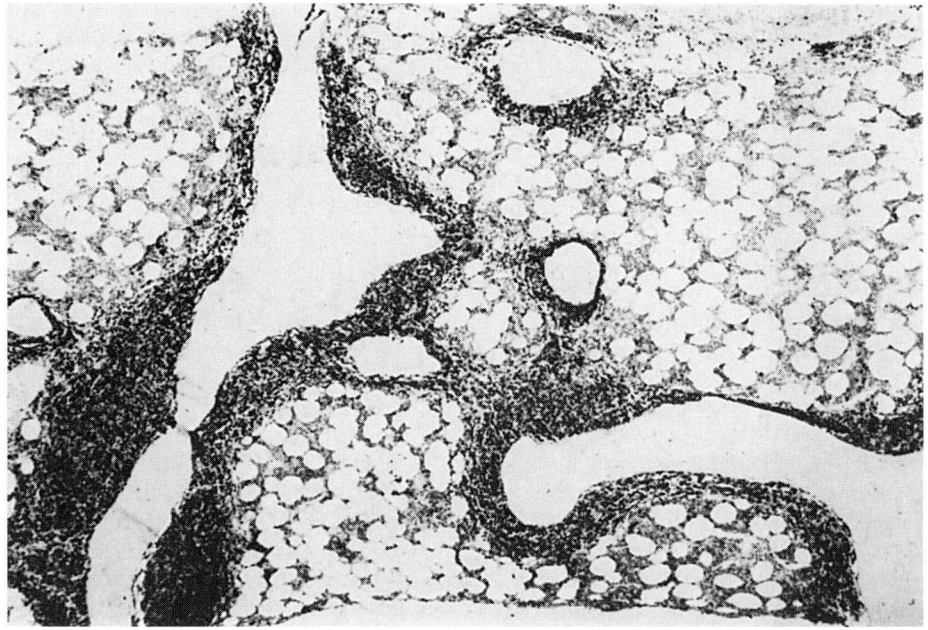

Fig. 23-4 Marrow section from patient with small cleaved cell lymphoma reacted with monoclonal antibody to CD74 (LN2). Antibody markedly accentuates the paratrabecular lymphoma involvement. (Immunoperoxidase.)

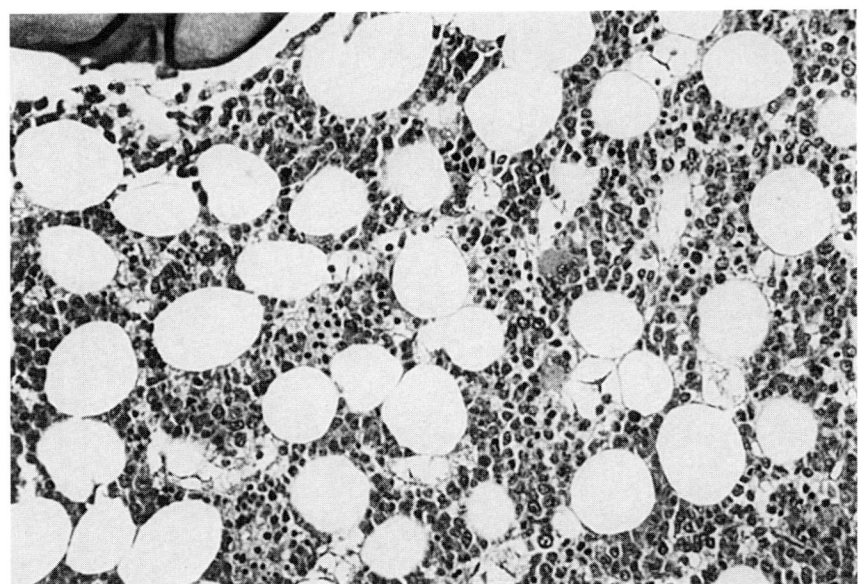

Fig. 23-5 Normocellular bone marrow from 42-year-old man obtained as part of evaluation as potential donor for bone marrow transplant. Hematopoietic cells and adipose tissue are present in approximately equal quantities.

hypoplastic anemia occurring in the first decade of life that is associated with multiple organ malformations, including hypoplasia of the kidneys and absent or hypoplastic thumbs or radii.[39,41,43] An association of hypoplastic bone marrow and pancreatic dysfunction (Shwachman syndrome) is a rare disorder occurring in children.[52]

In the most severe form of aplastic anemia, the intertrabecular marrow space is occupied predominantly by adipose tissue with scattered lymphocytes, plasma cells, tissue mast cells, and hemosiderin-laden macrophages (Fig. 23-6). In less severe processes, there are an increased amount of fat tissue and scattered small collections of erythroblasts, granulocytes, and megakaryocytes; in some instances the decrease in megakaryocytes is disproportionate to other cell types. In occasional cases of aplastic anemia, the marrow contains prominent lymphocytic aggregates. The blood findings in aplastic anemia are characterized by varying degrees of pancytopenia.

Uncommonly, the marrow biopsy in a patient with aplastic anemia contains aggregates of well-differentiated lymphocytes similar to the lesions that occur in a variety of immune disorders; these are described in this chapter as polymorphous lymphoid aggregates.

The use of bone marrow transplantation as a therapeutic approach to aplastic anemia has gained wide acceptance. Evidence of marrow reconstitution usually is present in biopsies obtained 2 to 3 weeks following transplantation and consists of foci or islands of hematopoietic cells.[47] Sequential marrow biopsies in the subsequent 5- to 10-week period show increasing numbers of erythroid precursors, granulocytes, and megakaryocytes in patients with engraftment. Impending rejection of engraftment may be heralded by a decrease in one myeloid cell line. An association between high mast cell counts in post–marrow transplant specimens from patients with aplastic anemia and marrow rejection

has been reported, but this has not been a uniform observation.[47,51]

Immunosuppressive and antibiotic therapy may alter the morphology of the proliferating engrafted cells, and evidence of dyserythropoiesis and dysgranulopoiesis may be present. At times, agranulocytosis with a "maturation arrest" of the proliferating neutrophil precursors at the promyelocyte stage may occur as a result of antibiotic or other drug therapy. The use of recombinant granulocyte growth factor may result in a marked shift to immaturity in the developing neutrophils. Selective hypoplasias of myeloid cell lines may occur and are frequently related to specific drug- or viral-related immune mechanisms.[40,50]

Serous degeneration (gelatinous transformation)

In patients who are extremely malnourished for a variety of reasons, including anorexia nervosa, the bone marrow may show hypocellularity with serous degeneration of the adipose tissue.[53] This finding may also be one of the changes noted in marrow biopsies from patients with acquired immune deficiency syndrome (AIDS). The fat cells in serous degeneration decrease in size, and serous fluid accumulates in the interstices. The serous fluid stains lightly eosinophilic and has a fine granular appearance in sections stained with hematoxylin-eosin; it is pale pink with the PAS stain. Studies have indicated that the intercellular substance is primarily hyaluronic acid. The changes may be present with intervening areas of normal hematopoiesis or the entire marrow biopsy may manifest the changes of serous degeneration (Fig. 23-7).

Marrow hyperplasia

Hyperplasia of one or more myeloid cell lines may be found in several hematopoietic disorders. Several benign hematologic disorders are characterized by hypercellularity;

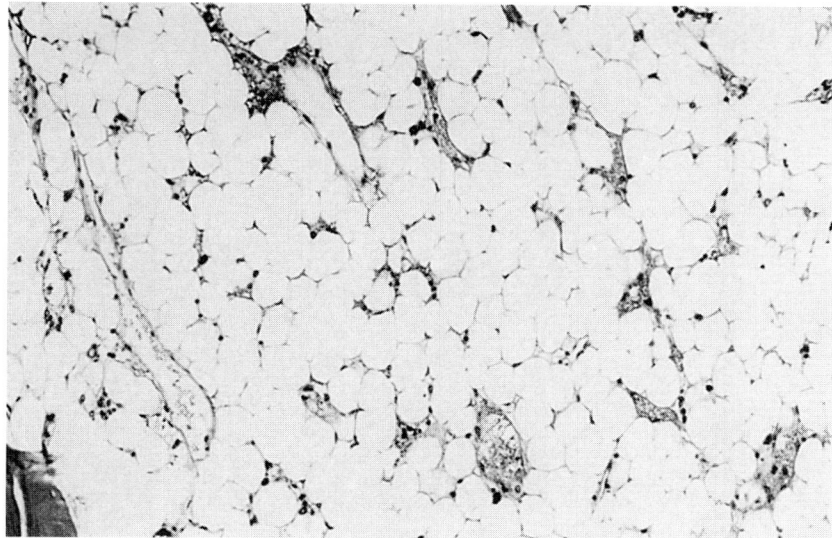

Fig. 23-6 Bone marrow section from 7-year-old girl with idiopathic acquired aplastic anemia. Hematopoietic cells are almost totally absent. Sinuses and capillaries are prominent.

these include cell maturation defects such as the megaloblastic and sideroblastic anemias or disorders with increased rates of destruction or utilization of various cell types in which the hypercellularity is due to compensatory hyperplasia. Hemolytic anemias are generally characterized by a marked erythroid hyperplasia. In immune thrombocytopenia in which there is an increased rate of platelet destruction, the megakaryocytes are normal to increased in number. The major problem in evaluation of marrow from patients with benign disorders, such as megaloblastic anemia in which the marrow may be very hypercellular and precursor cells may show striking nuclear changes, is that the proliferating erythroblasts or other myeloid cells may be misinterpreted as a leukemic proliferation; examination of the blood and marrow smears will obviate the possibility of this type of error.

OSTEOPETROSIS

Osteopetrosis, also known as marble bones or Albers-Schönberg disease, is an uncommon disorder in which the bone trabeculae are markedly thickened, resulting in decreased marrow space with a reduction in hematopoietic tissue.[55,56] The disease appears to occur in both hereditary and sporadic forms. The underlying defect is defective osteoclast function that results in impaired bone resorption. The decreased marrow hematopoiesis leads to extramedullary hematopoiesis with splenomegaly and a leukoerythroblastic blood picture.

The autosomal recessive form of the disease, which is observed in infants and young children, is accompanied by high morbidity and frequently death in the first 5 years of life; it is potentially reversible with allogeneic bone marrow transplantation with engraftment of normal functioning osteoclasts.[54]

Posterior iliac spine biopsies may be performed prior to and following bone marrow transplantation. The diagnostic features include marked thickening of the bone trabeculae and marked reduction in the medullary cavity. The bone structures contain cartilaginous plates, which in nondecalcified specimens show calcium deposition (Fig. 23-8). Osteo-

clasts are frequently numerous along the endosteal surface. Following successful allogeneic bone marrow transplant, there are gradual resorption of the abnormal bone structure, regression of the cartilaginous plates, and expansion of the medullary space with growth of hematopoietic cells. This is accompanied by regression of splenomegaly and reversal of the leukoerythroblastic blood picture.

BONE MARROW NECROSIS

Bone marrow necrosis unrelated to chemotherapy or radiation therapy occurs occasionally in patients with acute leukemia, malignant lymphoma, and metastatic tumor[57,58,60-62]; it also has been observed in patients with sickle cell anemia, infectious processes, systemic lupus erythematosus, caisson disease, and megaloblastic anemia complicated by infection.[58,59,63] The process may be accompanied by severe and generalized bone pain.

The aspirated marrow specimens from these patients frequently have a gelatinous consistency. The microscopic picture in the trephine section reflects the stage of necrosis; different stages are frequently found in the same biopsy specimen. In the early stages, the nuclei show pyknosis and karyorrhexis, and the cells have a granular appearance; this is followed by karyolysis. In advanced stages, all cell outlines disappear, and the marrow space is replaced by an amorphous, granular, eosinophilic debris. The trabeculae may be involved and show loss of osteocytes. The necrosis may be patchy or involve virtually all of the cells in the biopsy specimen (Fig. 23-9).

INFLAMMATORY DISORDERS
Granulomatous inflammation

The inflammatory diseases that are most readily identified in marrow biopsies are those associated with a granulomatous reaction; the etiologic bases include fungi, *Mycobacterium tuberculosis, Mycobacterium avium-intracellulare*, sarcoidosis,[64,68,77,78] *Mycoplasma pneumoniae,*

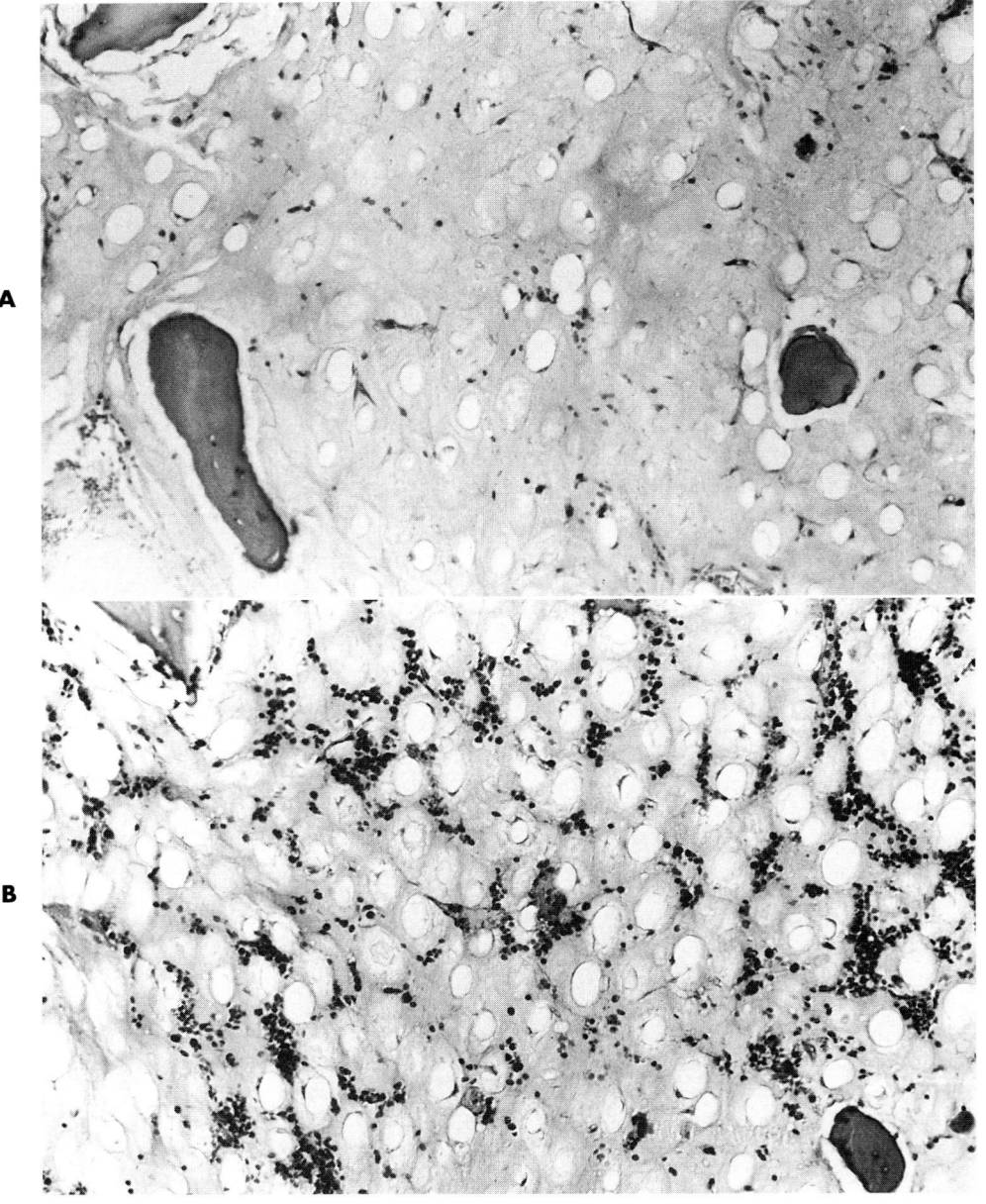

Fig. 23-7 **A,** Bone marrow section from 27-year-old woman with anorexia nervosa and severe weight loss, showing marked serous degeneration (gelatinous transformation). There is marked reduction in hematopoietic and fat cells with accumulation of an amorphous, eosinophilic substance. **B,** Another area of biopsy illustrated in **A** showing scattered foci of hematopoiesis.

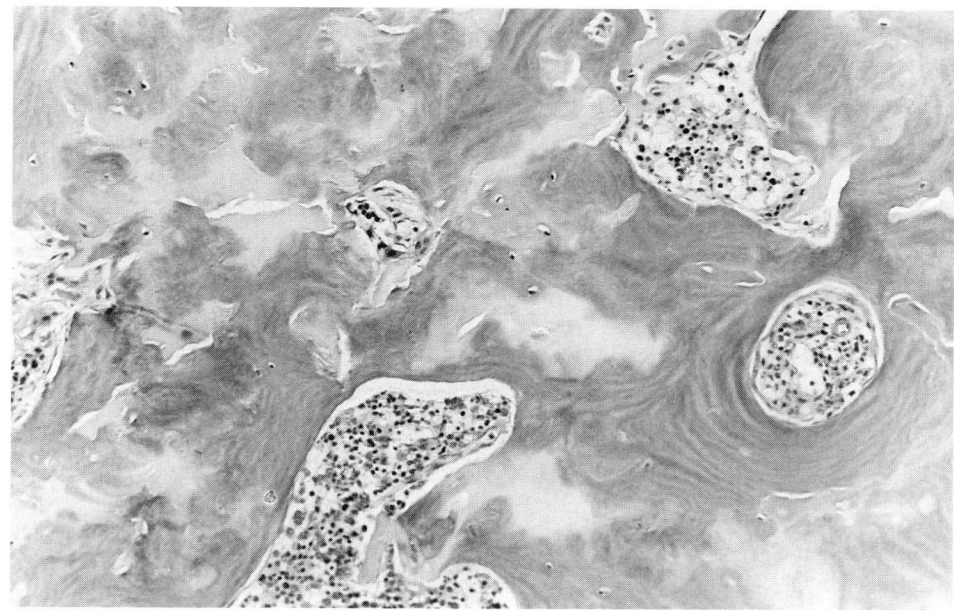

Fig. 23-8 Decalcified posterior iliac spine bone marrow trephine biopsy from 8-month-old girl with osteopetrosis. Marrow space is markedly reduced as consequence of widely expanded bone structure. Lighter areas in bone structure represent cartilaginous plates. Numerous osteoclasts are present in some areas along endosteal surface.

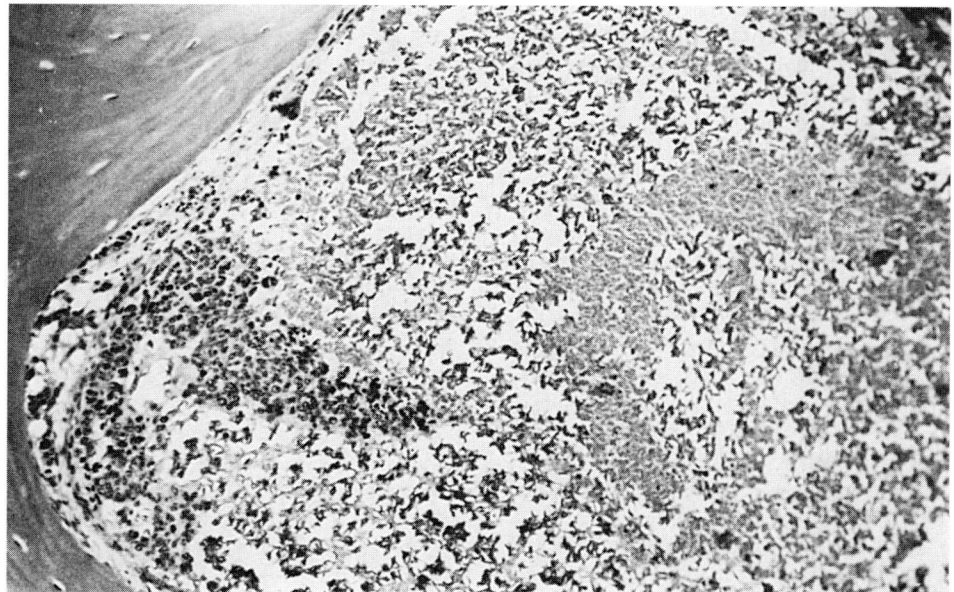

Fig. 23-9 Marrow biopsy from 17-year-old male with acute lymphoblastic leukemia and severe generalized bone pain. Large areas of marrow illustrated here are undergoing necrosis.

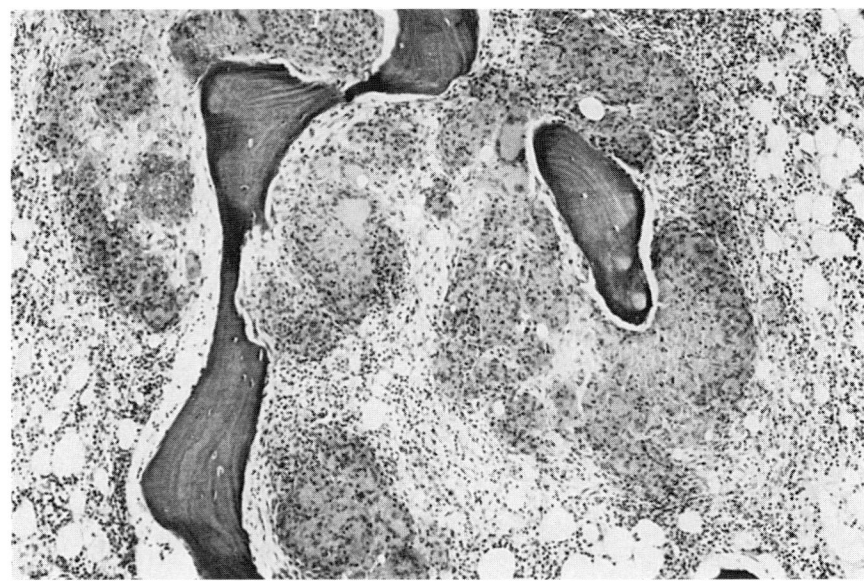

Fig. 23-10 Multiple noncaseating granulomas in marrow biopsy of 33-year-old male admitted with marked hypercalcemia. Clinical diagnosis of sarcoidosis was established.

and viral infections such as infectious mononucleosis. Granulomas may also be found in patients with Hodgkin's disease and non-Hodgkin's lymphomas with or without marrow involvement by the lymphoma.[65,69,77] Perivascular granulomas may be related to hypersensitivity states. In approximately 80% of the cases with bone marrow granulomas, no etiologic basis for the lesions is identified.[73]

Granulomas in the marrow are similar to those in other sites; the most commonly encountered are composed only of a collection of epithelioid histiocytes that may be surrounded by a rim of well-differentiated lymphocytes. The number may range from a single lesion to numerous and confluent granulomas (Fig. 23-10). An unusual granulomatous lesion referred to as "doughnut" or ring granuloma, because of a central clear area or lumen, has been described in the bone marrow of some patients with Q fever.[67,72,76] The appearance of these lesions, which is similar to those in other organs, varies from vascular structures or fat globules encircled by a rim of fibrinoid material, polymorphonuclear leukocytes, and monocytes to a collection of epithelioid histiocytes surrounding a clear space[72] (Fig. 23-11). In addition to Q fever, these lesions may be observed in marrows from patients with a variety of diseases, both neoplastic and nonneoplastic.[74] The vascular-associated granulomas observed in hypersensitivity states are similar in appearance.

Cells with prominent intranuclear inclusions may be found in granulomas in the marrow of patients with cytomegalovirus or other viral infection.[71] In rare cases, cells with intranuclear viral inclusions may be found scattered among normal hematopoietic cells without granuloma formation (Fig. 23-12).

Parvovirus B19 infection may be associated with marked erythroblast hypoplasia and giant erythroblasts, some of which may contain viral inclusions[80] (Fig. 23-13). Recovery from the erythroid hypoplasia may be marked by a wave of regeneration with a large number of erythroblasts at an early stage of

maturation, analogous to the proliferation of promyelocytes and myelocytes that occurs in agranulocytosis (Fig. 23-14).

As with other tissues, stains for acid-fast bacilli and fungi should be performed in all cases of marrow granulomas. Failure to detect acid-fast bacilli does not exclude infection with *M. tuberculosis;* organisms are found in approximately 25% of marrow specimens from patients with documented disease.[77] The need for culture of a portion of the bone marrow aspirate for acid-fast bacilli and fungi should be anticipated in all patients suspected of having a granulomatous disorder, particularly those with AIDS or patients being investigated for a fever of undermined etiology.

The presence of infection-related granulomas in the bone marrow sections may occasionally be accompanied by macrophages containing microorganisms in the bone marrow smears or trephine imprints. The morphology of the organisms in these preparations is usually sufficient to establish a diagnosis.

Bone marrow biopsies performed on immunosuppressed patients should always be thoroughly examined for opportunistic infections (Fig. 23-15). Typical granuloma formation may not be present in the marrows of some patients with disseminated fungal or mycobacterial disease. Marrow biopsies from patients with AIDS may contain scattered macrophages containing acid-fast bacilli in the absence of granuloma formation (Fig. 23-16). Uncommonly, *Pneumocytis carinii* may be observed in scattered macrophages in sections stained with periodic acid–Schiff or methenamine silver (Fig. 23-17). Increased numbers of macrophages with or without evident phagocytosis are sufficient reason to perform special stains for micro-organisms.

Lipid granulomas, which have been reported to be the most frequent type of granuloma in bone marrow, are similar to those found in the liver, spleen, and lymph node.[66,75] These granulomas range from 0.2 to 0.8 µm in size and usually are associated with lymphocytic aggregates or sinu-

Text continued on p. 1812.

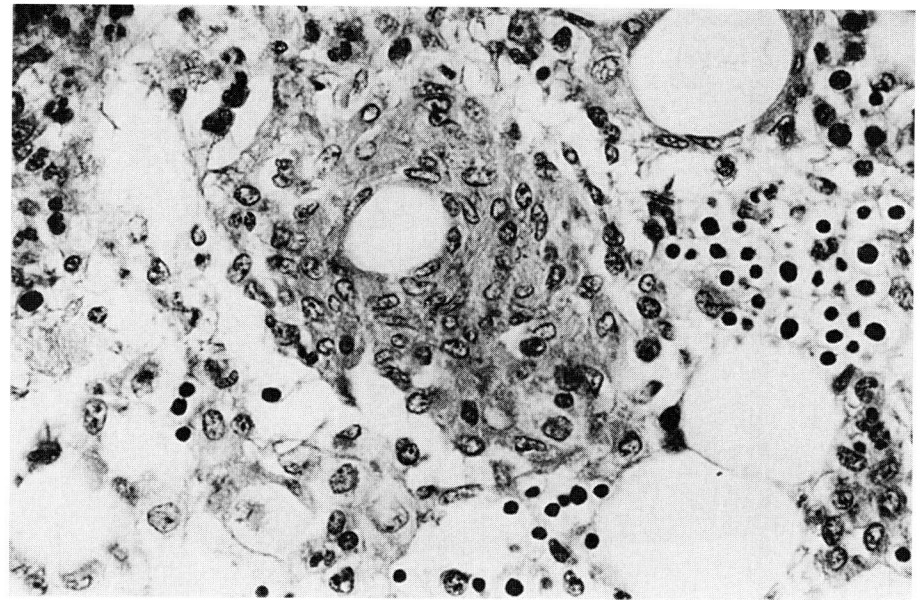

Fig. 23-11 Granuloma with central lumen (ring or donut granuloma) in marrow biopsy from patient undergoing chemotherapy for lymphoblastic lymphoma who developed a hypersensitivity reaction to penicillin. Several similar structures were scattered throughout marrow biopsy: Some were associated with vascular structures; others appeared to be surrounding fat cells. All microbiologic cultures were negative, and lesions were not present in biopsy performed 21 days later.

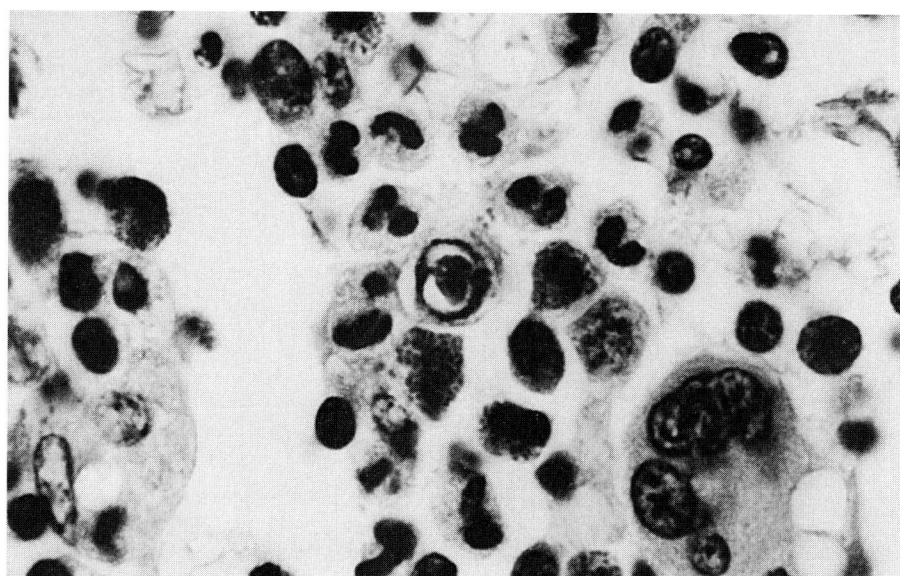

Fig. 23-12 Cell with prominent intranuclear inclusion in marrow of 4-year-old child being evaluated as marrow transplant donor; numerous similar cells were scattered throughout biopsy specimen. There is no evidence of related inflammatory reaction. Subsequent serologic studies documented cytomegalovirus infection.

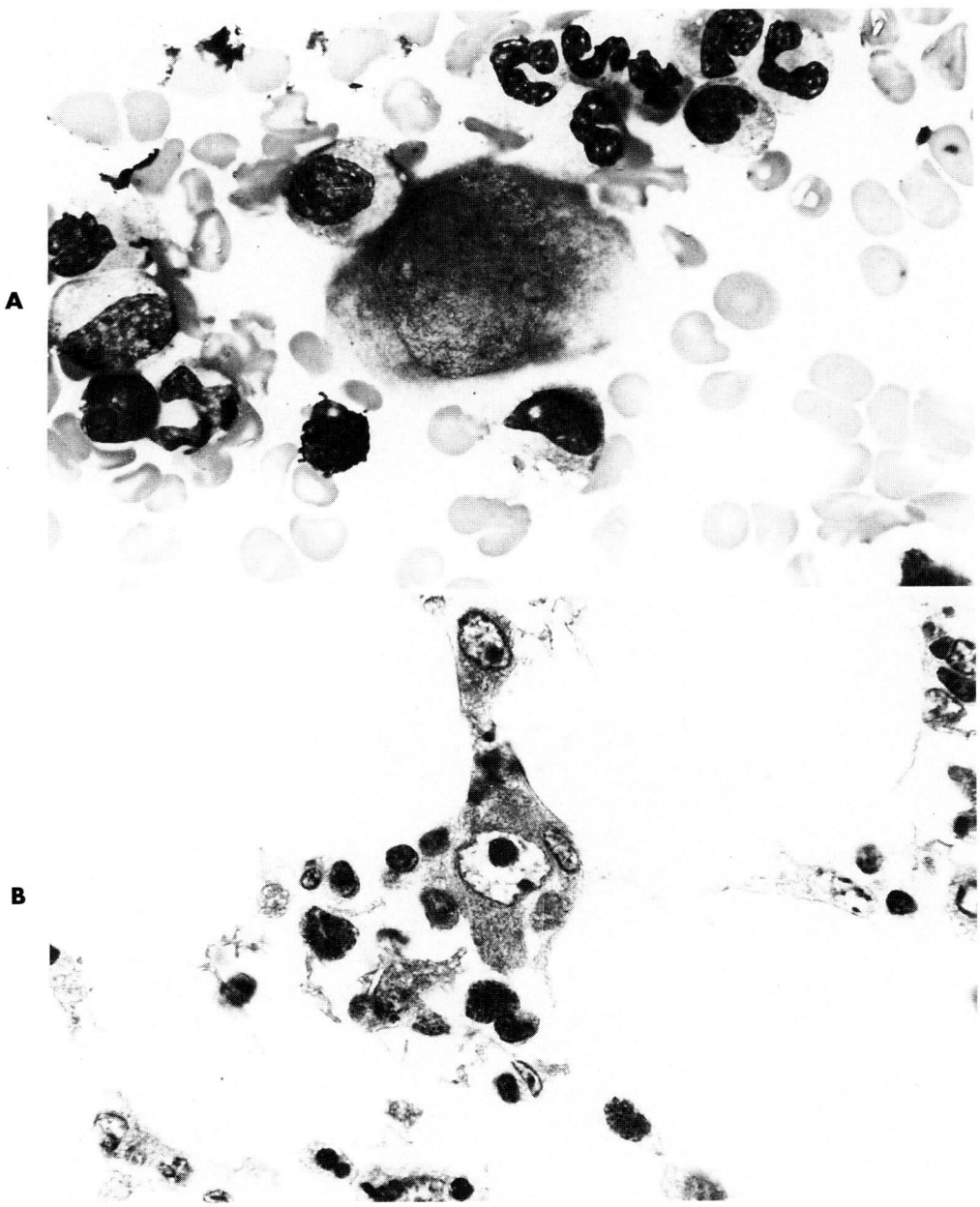

Fig. 23-13 A, Bone marrow smear from 17-year-old patient being treated for metastatic tumor. Marrow showed marked hypoplasia of erythroid precursors. Occasional giant erythroid precursors, as illustrated, were present. Serologic studies were positive for parvovirus B19 infection. **B,** Marrow biopsy from case in **A.** Occasional, very large erythroblasts with abundant cytoplasm and very prominent nucleoli were present. (**A** Wright-Giemsa.)

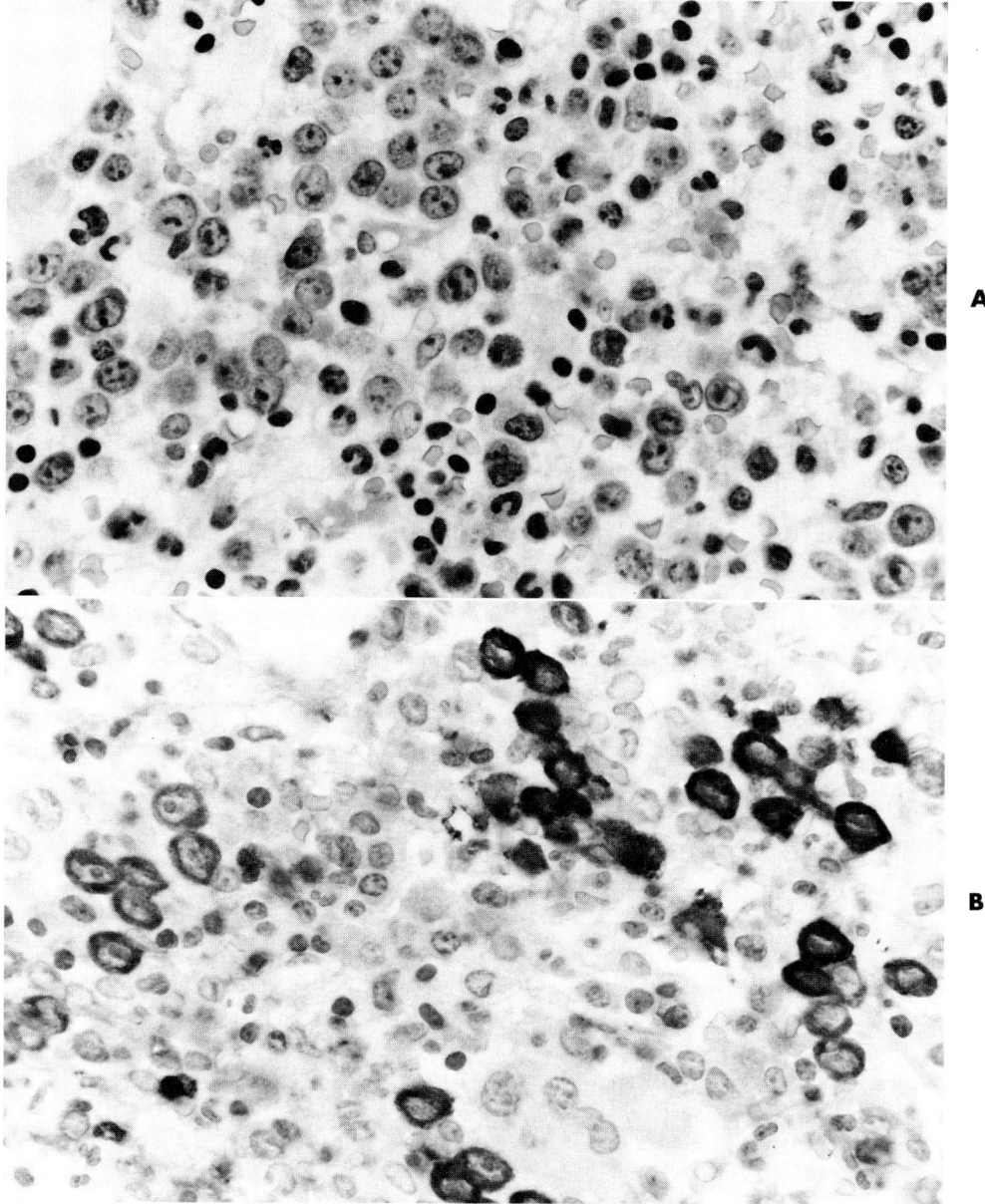

Fig. 23-14 **A,** Bone marrow biopsy from 33-year-old woman with hereditary spherocytosis and par-vovirus B19 infection. Patient presented with hemoglobin level of 7 g/dl. Previous hemoglobin levels had been in normal range. Bone marrow smear contained numerous erythroblasts at pronormoblast and basophilic normoblast stages of maturation with no evidence of more mature erythroid precursors. Serologic studies confirmed parvovirus B19 infection. There is marked hyperplasia of erythroid precursors, and findings were interpreted as early recovery phase of parvovirus infection. Hemoglobin level rose to 11 g/dl 2 weeks following this biopsy. **B,** Biopsy specimen in **A** reacted with polyclonal antibody to hemoglobin A. Large number of immature cells is reactive, confirming erythroid origin. (**B** Peroxidase-antiperoxidase.)

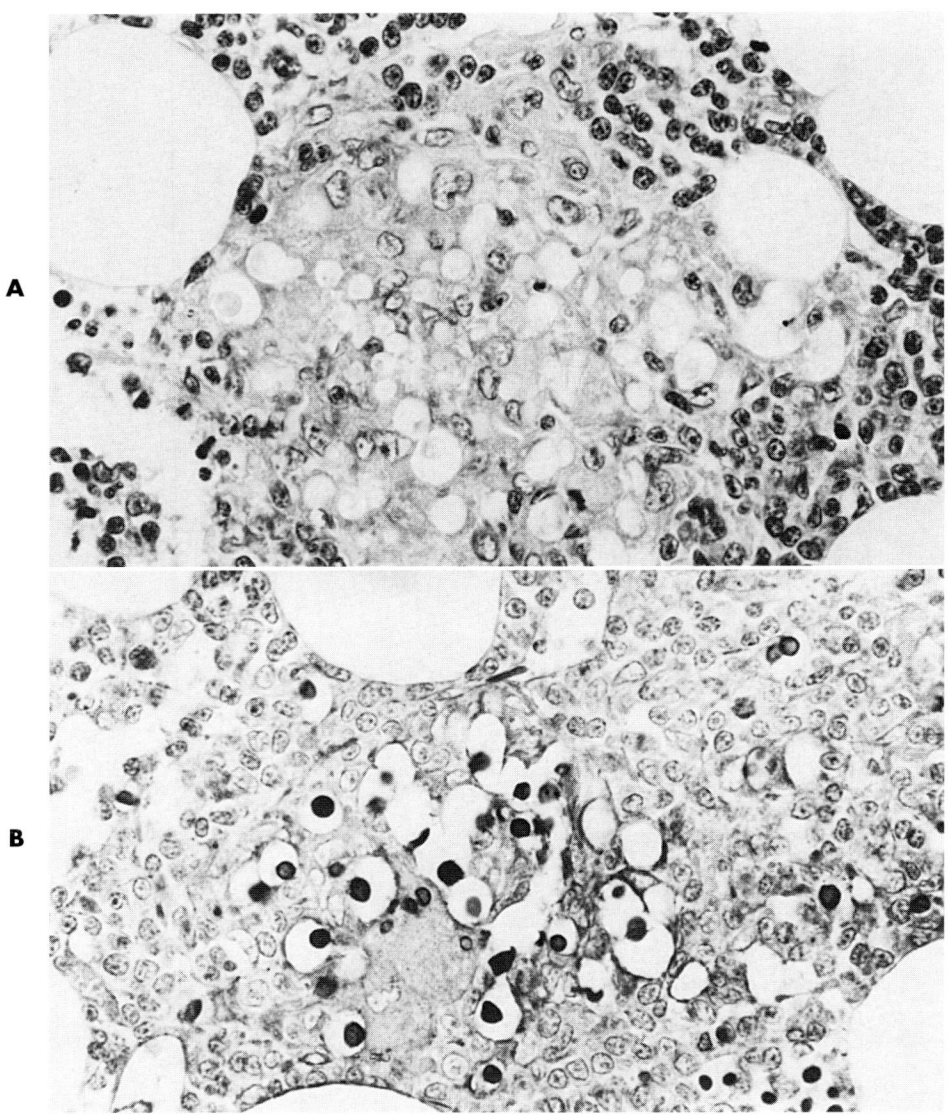

Fig. 23-15 **A,** Postchemotherapy marrow biopsy from patient with marrow involvement by intermediate differentiated lymphocytic lymphoma. One of several clusters of macrophages containing microorganisms is shown. **B,** Same lesion as in **A** showing numerous cryptococci. (**B** Gomori's methenamine silver.)

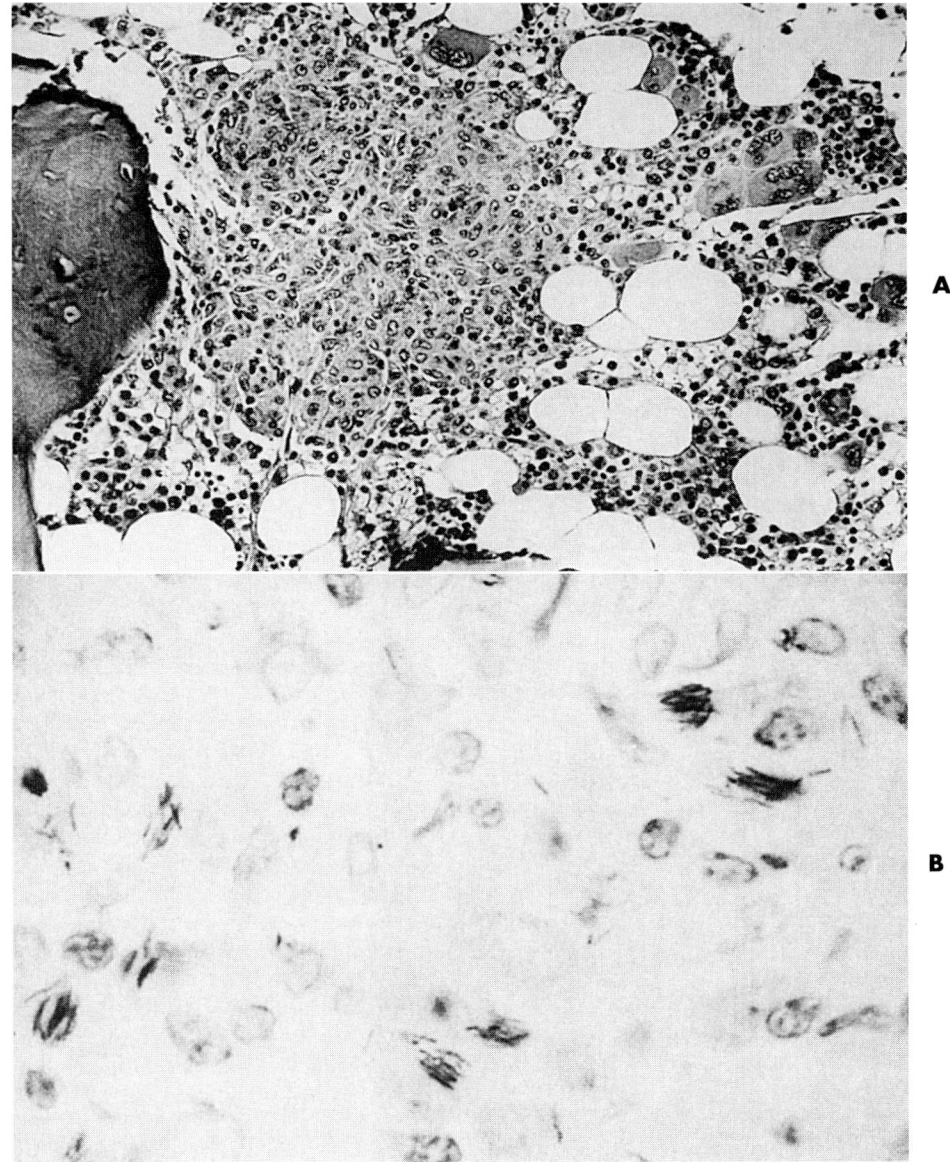

Fig. 23-16 A, Marrow biopsy from patient with AIDS showing granuloma without evident necrosis. **B,** One of granulomas in **A** showing numerous intracellular acid-fast bacilli. (**B** Fite.)

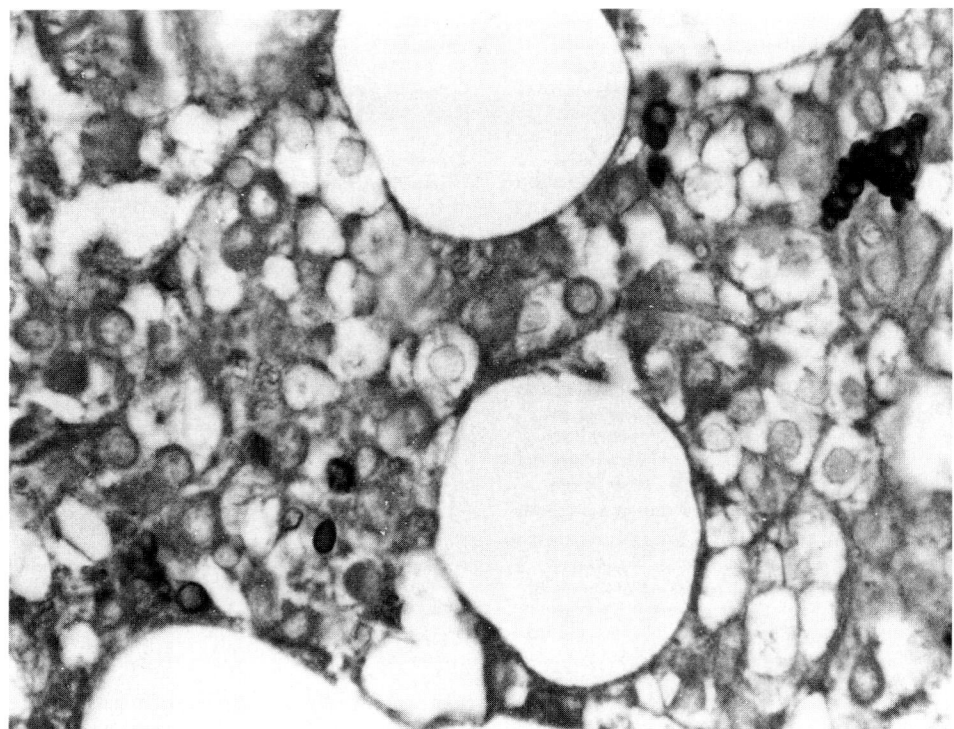

Fig. 23-17 Marrow from patient with AIDS with scattered *Pneumocystis carinii* micro-organisms occurring both singly and in small clusters. Micro-organisms are not associated with any recognizable tissue response. (Gomori's methenamine silver.)

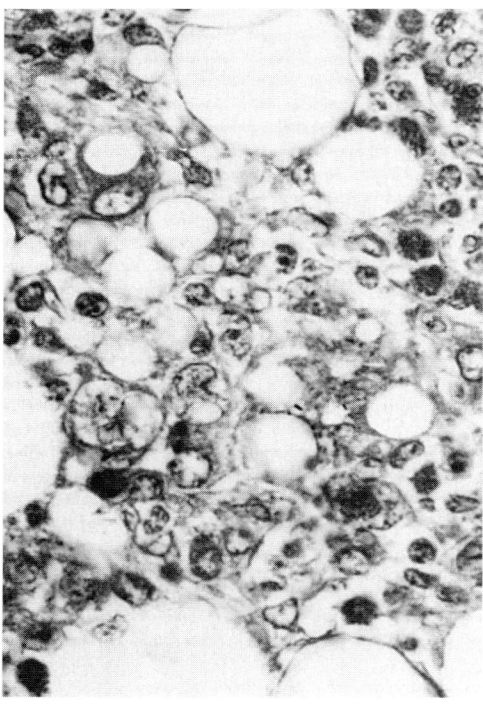

Fig. 23-18 Lipid granuloma in bone marrow section. Several fat vacuoles are present both intracellularly in macrophages and extracellulary. This granuloma is associated with small aggregate of well-differentiated lymphocytes.

soids. The loosely spaced macrophages contain fat vacuoles of varying size (Fig. 23-18). The lesions also contain admixed lymphocytes, plasma cells, and eosinophils; giant cells are found in approximately 5% of cases. Some of these granulomas resemble those found in sarcoidosis.

An unusual form of granulomatous reaction can be found in the bone marrow of patients with the genetic disorder of glyoxalate metabolism, primary hyperoxaluria.[70,79] This finding is secondary to the deposition of calcium oxalate crystals. The crystals, which have a slightly yellowish tinge, form a radial pattern, are encircled or engulfed by epithelioid and giant cells, and are doubly refractile with polarized light (Fig. 23-19). Substantial portions of the marrow biopsy may be replaced by these lesions, which are similar to those found in the kidneys and other tissues.

Nonspecific inflammatory reactions

Nonspecific inflammatory alterations may be noted in the marrow from patients with a variety of systemic disorders, including acute infection, malignancy, connective tissue disease, and immune disorders, most notably AIDS (Fig. 23-20). These alterations generally are characterized by changes in both the vascular structures and parenchyma. The terms *tumor myelopathy* and myelitis have been applied to the nonspecific marrow changes that are observed in a high percentage of patients with malignant lymphoma.[82] These changes include edema of the vessel walls, plasma cell and mast cell proliferations in the adventitia, protein deposits adjacent to the vessels, patchy edema, depressed erythro-

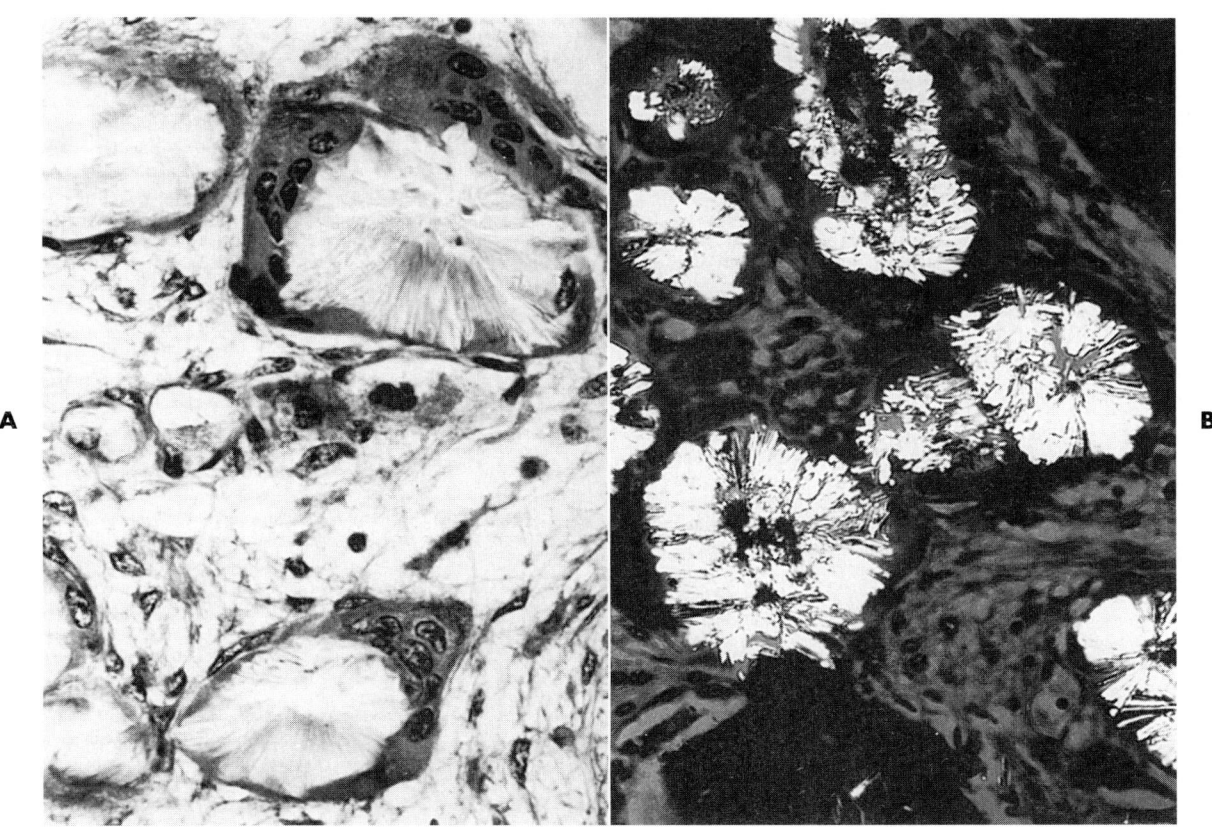

Fig. 23-19 A, Section of bone marrow trephine biopsy from child with hereditary oxalosis. Calcium oxalate crystals form radial pattern and appear to be encircled by giant cells. **B,** Calcium oxalate crystals are doubly refractile in polarized light.

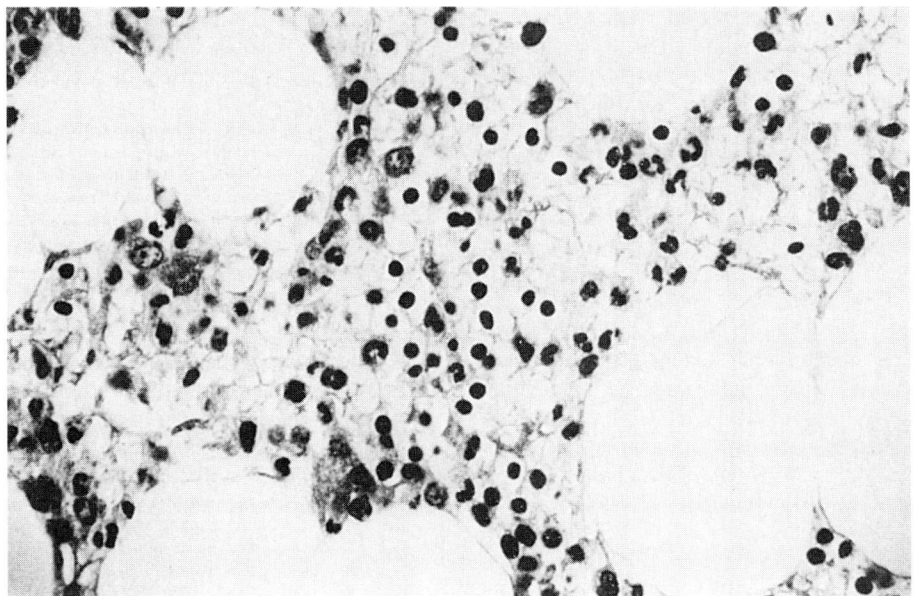

Fig. 23-20 Marrow biopsy from patient with AIDS illustrating reduced interstitial cellularity.

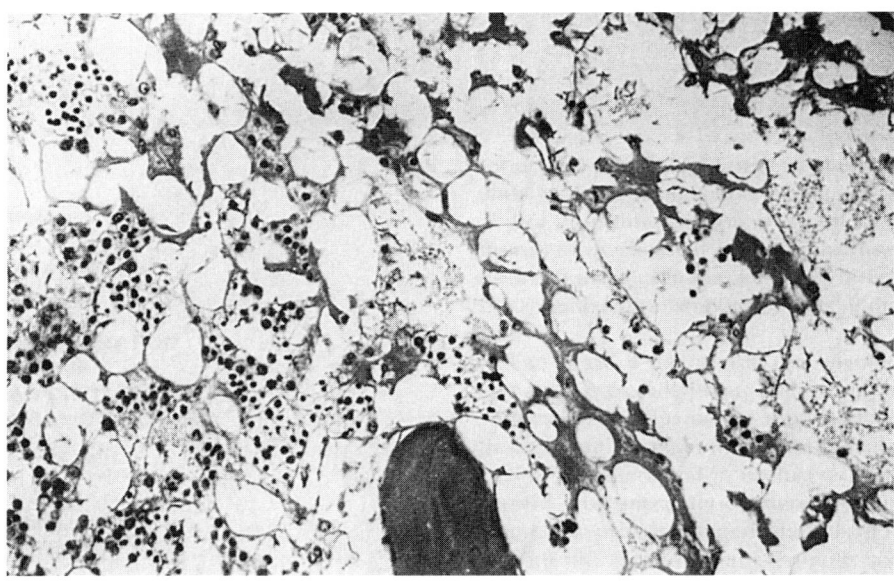

Fig. 23-21 Marrow biopsy from patient with AIDS showing hypocellularity and prominent serous degeneration.

poiesis, and increased granulopoiesis and megakaryocytopoiesis. Acute necrosis of bone marrow tissue is reported in patients with tuberculosis and typhoid fever.[81]

ACQUIRED IMMUNE DEFICIENCY SYNDROME (AIDS)

Marrow biopsies from patients with AIDS have been generally reported to be hypercellular, although normocellular and hypocellular specimens may be observed; several nonspecific findings, including marrow damage, increased plasma cells, myelodysplasia, serous degeneration, lymphocytic infiltration, and increased reticulin, may be present.* Opportunistic organisms, including acid-fast bacilli and *P. carinii,* may be present with or without granuloma formation (see Fig. 23-17). Immune thrombocytopenia may be observed.[83,88,92] Persistent parvovirus B19 infection may be an important causative factor of anemia.[85]

The marrow damage that may be present in AIDS patients is characterized principally by a loosely structured, hypocellular interstitium (see Fig. 23-20). Areas of fibrinoid necrosis may be present. The changes resemble those found in marrows from patients recovering from chemotherapy with myelotoxic agents and are distinct from serous atrophy, which usually occurs in severely malnourished individuals and which may also be present in marrow biopsies from patients with AIDS (Fig. 23-21). Both of these alterations may be accompanied by an increase in plasma cells.

As noted previously, one of the problems in the evaluation of marrow biopsies from patients with AIDS is poorly formed or no granulomas in opportunistic infections. Marrow with only mild nonspecific alterations may contain scattered macrophages with mycobacteria. These macrophages may resemble pseudo-Gaucher cells in hematoxylin-eosin stained specimens. Scattered macrophages containing *P. carinii* may be present in a background of essentially normal-appearing or only slightly altered marrow. As a result, it is prudent to routinely stain marrows from AIDS patients for acid-fast bacilli and fungi, regardless of the appearance of the marrow with routine stains.

Lymphocytic aggregates of varying size occur in the marrow of a relatively high percentage of patients with AIDS.[84,90] These are randomly distributed without any preferential paratrabecular distribution; in some cases the lesions appear to be preferentially perisinusoidal. The composition is primarily small lymphocytes, some of which may have irregularly shaped nuclei. There are usually associated plasma cells, histiocytes, and increased vascular structures; eosinophils may be increased (Fig. 23-22). Occasional immunoblasts may be noted. This type of lymphocyte proliferation, which we refer to as polymorphous reactive lymphoid hyperplasia, is not unique to patients with AIDS and may be observed in marrow biopsies in a wide range of immunologic disorders. Because of the large size and cellular composition, these aggregates may be difficult to distinguish from the lesions of peripheral T-cell lymphoma; the latter lesions are frequently accompanied by more numerous epithelioid histiocytes and scattered large transformed cells. In some instances, the distinction between the two processes based on morphologic criteria may not be possible.[90] Peripheral T-cell lymphoma in AIDS patients, however, is quite rare, and such a diagnosis should be established with considerable caution and only after review of all pathology specimens. Molecular studies for T-cell receptor rearrangement should be performed if the distinction will influence patient management.

*References 84, 86, 87, 89, 90, 93-96.

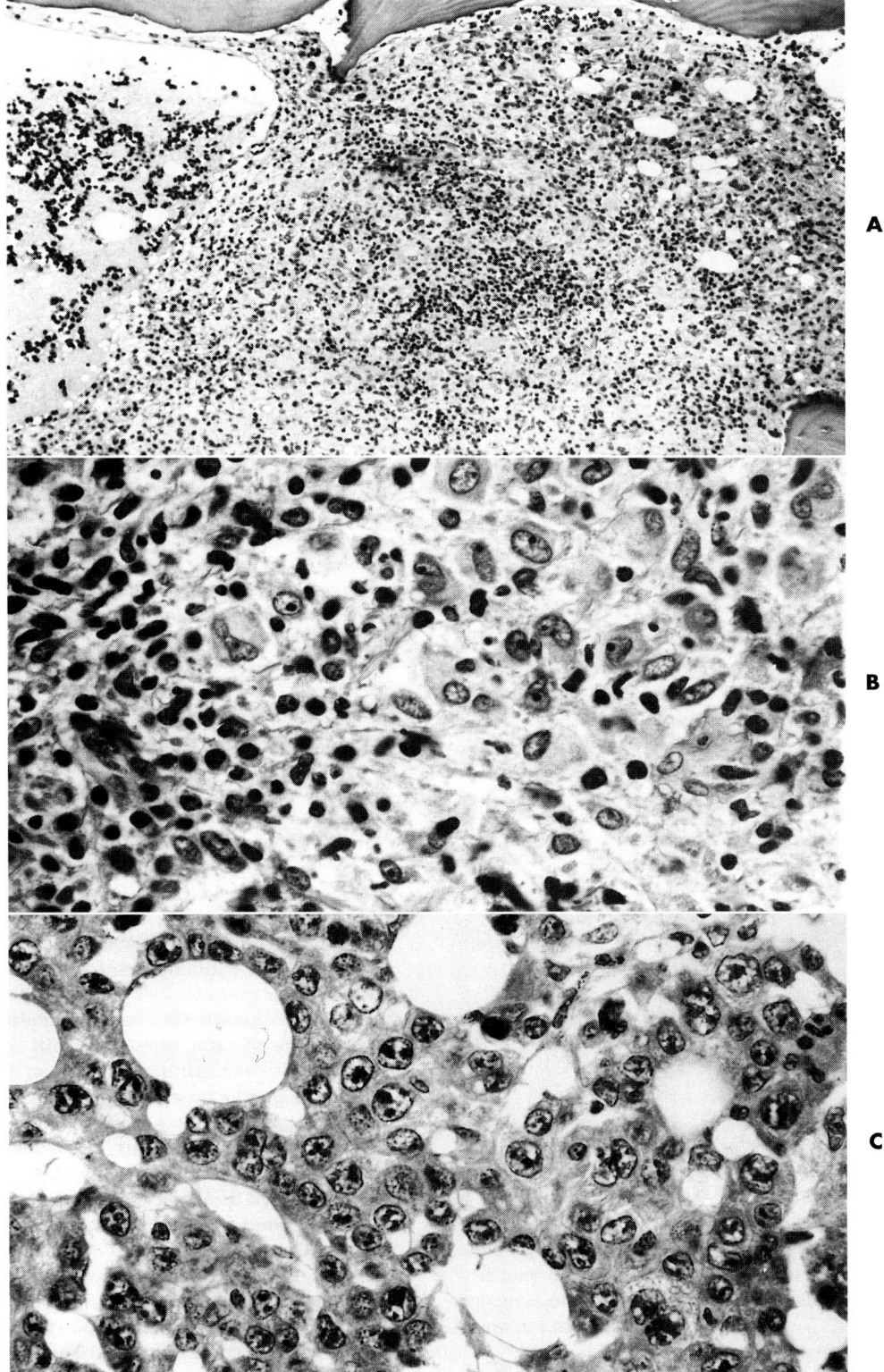

Fig. 23-22 A, One of several lymphocytic-histiocytic aggregates in marrow biopsy from patient with advanced AIDS. Acid-fast bacilli were identified in this specimen. **B,** High magnification of specimen in **A** illustrating polycellular characteristics of lesion. **C,** Small noncleaved cell lymphoma infiltrate in same biopsy section as the specimen in **A.** Cytogenetic studies of specimen showed a t(8;14) abnormality. Within 24 hours of this biopsy patient died of cryptococcal meningitis.

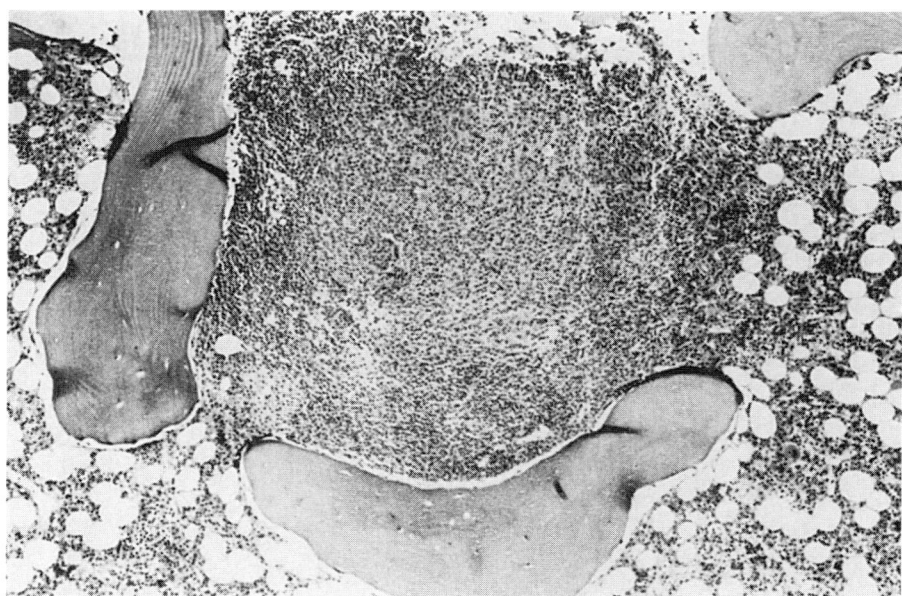

Fig. 23-23 Marrow biopsy from 27-year-old male with persistent generalized lymphadenopathy and positive serology for human immunodeficiency virus. Biopsy shows a large lymphoid aggregate with germinal center.

Occasionally, marrow specimens from patients with AIDS contain germinal centers (Fig. 23-23).

In addition to reactive lymphocytic lesions, the marrow biopsies from AIDS patients may exhibit a florid immunocytic reaction. In rare cases, this may be accompanied by a proliferation of immunoblasts and may resemble a neoplastic process because of the degree of replacement of marrow. The use of immunocytochemical reactions with anti-kappa and anti-lambda antibodies can be very useful in demonstrating the polyclonal nature of these lesions. In equivocal cases immunoglobulin gene rearrangement studies may be necessary for determination of the biology of these lesions.

Although it is important to recognize that marrow biopsies from patients with AIDS may show a variety of reactive lymphocytic proliferations, it is equally important to appreciate that these patients may develop a malignant lymphoma, either non-Hodgkin's or Hodgkin's type, and the marrow biopsy may be the initial diagnostic specimen. A single biopsy may contain both reactive lymphocytic lesions and malignant lymphoma (see Fig. 23-22). In suspected cases of Hodgkin's disease, adherence to established criteria for marrow involvement by Hodgkin's disease should be observed.

Patients with AIDS who are receiving zidovudine (AZT) may develop evidence of marrow suppression such as anemia and neutropenia. Marrow hypoplasia may be present.[91] Abnormal megakaryocytes with sparse cytoplasm, "naked" megakaryocyte nuclei, may be numerous; this finding is not specific for AIDS and may be present in other disorders, including the myeloproliferative diseases.

LEUKEMIAS AND RELATED DISORDERS
Acute leukemia

The diagnosis and classification of the acute leukemias are optimally established from examination of Romanovsky-stained blood and bone marrow smears in conjunction with appropriate cytochemical techniques; this approach forms the basis for the French American British (FAB) Cooperative Group classification.[97,102] Chromosome analysis also has an important role in the evaluation of cases of acute leukemia, primarily in regard to prognostic significance.[104,105] Although smears and imprint preparations are generally superior to sections in classifying the majority of cases of acute leukemia, there are some types of acute leukemia, most notably acute megakaryoblastic leukemia (M7), in which the bone marrow sections may show more clear evidence of the differentiation pattern than is evident from examination of routinely stained smears (Fig. 23-24). In addition, as noted in the section on immunohistology, the development of antibodies reactive in paraffin-embedded tissue, most notably antimyeloperoxidase, has enhanced the recognition of myeloid leukemia in trephine biopsy sections.

In the majority of cases of acute leukemia, both myeloid and lymphoblastic, in children and adults, the marrow is markedly hypercellular because of the proliferation of leukemic cells; normal hematopoietic cells are markedly reduced. In a small minority of patients, particularly older individuals, acute myeloid leukemia and, rarely, acute lymphoblastic leukemia may present with a hypocellular marrow (i.e., hypoplastic or hypocellular acute leukemia).[98,99,101] The marrow biopsies in these patients may, on low magnification, suggest the diagnosis of aplastic anemia (Fig. 23-25). In contrast to aplastic anemia, the cell population in the interstitium is principally blasts; some normal cells may be present but are markedly reduced. The diagnosis is confirmed by examination of blood and bone marrow smears and the use of appropriate cytochemical reactions. In rare instances, acute lymphoblastic leukemia in children is preceded by an aplastic or hypocellular phase.

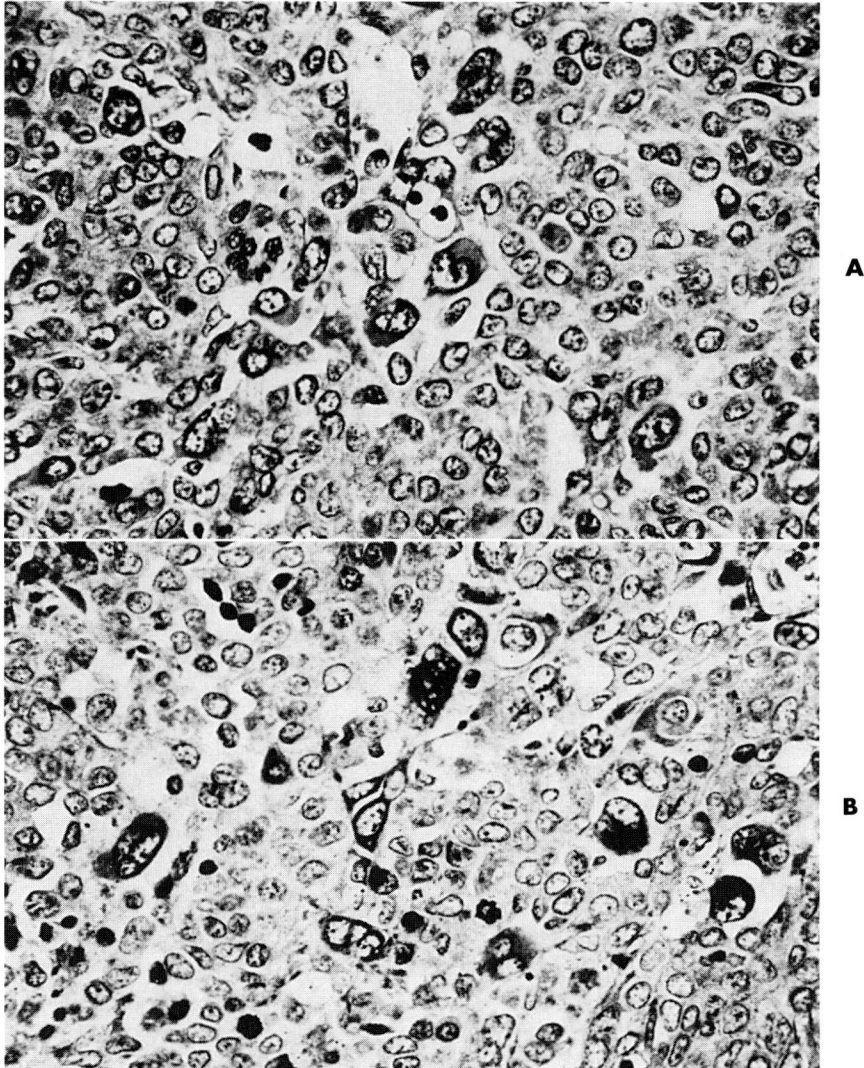

Fig. 23-24 A, Marrow from patient with acute megakaryoblastic leukemia (AML-M7). Predominant cell population consists of blasts and numerous megakaryocytes at varying stages of maturation. Megakaryocytes have more abundant cytoplasm that is uniformly eosinophilic. **B,** PAS stain of specimen in **A** accentuates intensely positive megakaryocytes.

Myelofibrosis with a slight-to-moderate increase in reticulin fibers may be present in the initial or late stages of acute leukemia in a minority of cases; it may occur in both acute lymphoblastic and acute myeloid leukemia.[103] The presence of myelofibrosis in acute leukemia may result in difficult and inadequate marrow aspiration and an erroneous diagnosis of aplastic anemia if trephine biopsy sections are not available. This problem is more prevalent in pediatric than in adult patients and emphasizes the importance of obtaining adequate biopsies. The long-held view that difficult aspirations in acute leukemia are caused by "packed" marrows has little basis in fact. The vast majority of hypercellular marrows in acute leukemia are readily aspirated. If aspiration is difficult, it is probably a result of poor biopsy technique or an increase in reticulin fibers.

The trephine biopsy provides the only accurate assessment of marrow cellularity and is of considerable importance in monitoring changes following treatment for leukemia. The rapidity of development and degree of necrosis and aplasia following the institution of therapy will vary with the different chemotherapeutic agents or combination of agents used. In general, the sequence of histopathologic events is marked initially by nuclear karyorrhexis followed by karyolysis; the cells then disintegrate into a relatively uniform granular, eosinophilic debris. Subsequently the marrow shows a somewhat irregular, loosely structured appearance with scattered fat cells, vessels, stromal elements, and distended sinusoids (Fig. 23-26). Regeneration of fat cells is followed by regeneration of normal hematopoietic cells in the successfully treated patient. The ery-

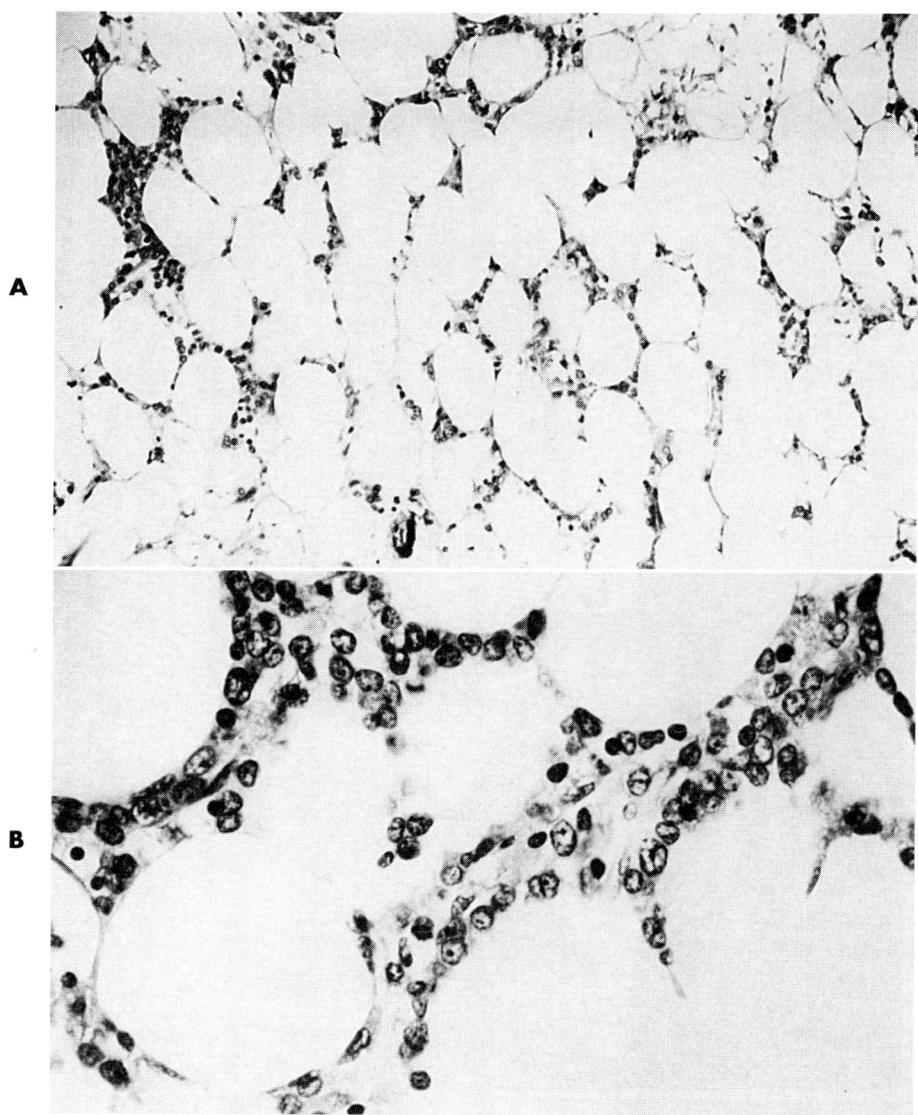

Fig. 23-25 A, Marrow section from 67-year-old male with acute myeloid leukemia with markedly hypocellular marrow. **B,** Higher magnification of same specimen showing numerous blast cells in interstitium.

throid cells are usually the first to recover and frequently manifest dyserythropoietic changes as the result of chemotherapeutic drugs[100] (Fig. 23-27). The regeneration of the erythroid cells is followed in sequence by that of the granulocytes and megakaryocytes. This sequence may be altered with different drug regimens. The marrow from patients receiving recombinant granulocyte growth factor may show an early marked increase in neutrophil promyelocytes and myelocytes.

As noted, the course of events described in the preceding discussion is characteristic of effective therapy. In those patients in whom there has been partial or no response to treatment, the marrow will show varying numbers of leukemic cells. In the totally nonresponsive patient, the findings are essentially those of the pretreatment specimen; scattered isolated areas of necrosis may be present. In a partial response the areas of residual leukemia will be intermixed with necrotic or regenerating normal marrow cells. In some patients, the areas of residual leukemia may be very small and difficult to distinguish from foci of regenerating normal cells, particularly early erythroblasts and promyelocytes. Careful comparison of suspicious foci with the cytologic pattern in the initial diagnostic biopsy should always be performed. Distinguishing foci of normal regenerative promyelocytes from the foci of leukemic promyelocytes in patients being treated for acute promyelocytic leukemia may be particularly troublesome. Normal promyelocyte regeneration is usually accentuated along the endosteal surface of the bone trabecelae and in perivascular locations. Acute promyelocytic leukemia in marrows with partial response may manifest as large or small focal lesions unrelated to bone trabeculae or vascular structures (Fig. 23-28). The cytoplasm of

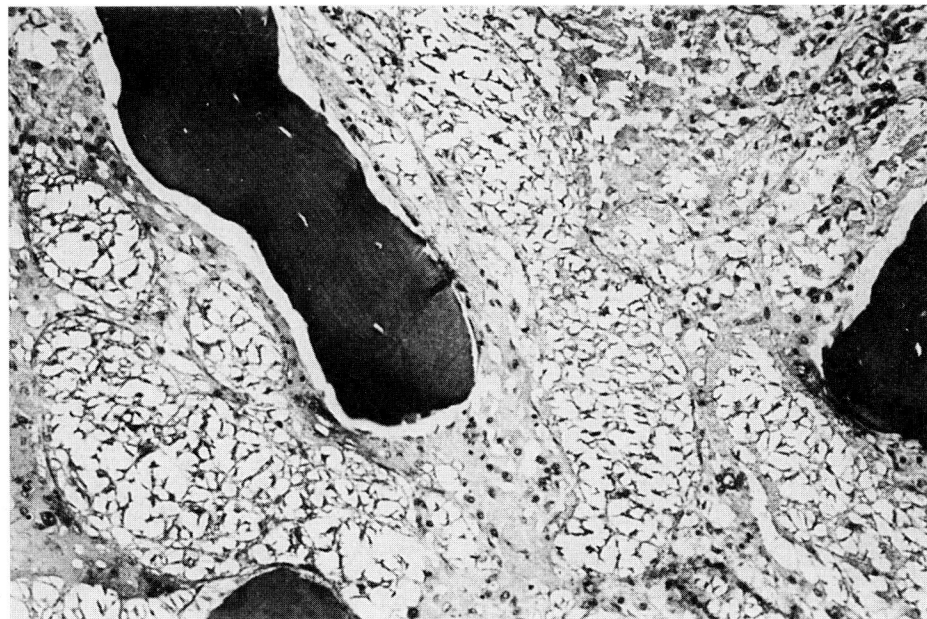

Fig. 23-26 Marrow biopsy 14 days after institution of therapy with daunorubicin and cytosine arabi-noside for acute myeloid leukemia. Marrow is markedly hypocellular with dilated sinuses. Interstitial areas contain lightly eosinophilic, proteinaceous debris that represents residue of leukemic cell necrosis.

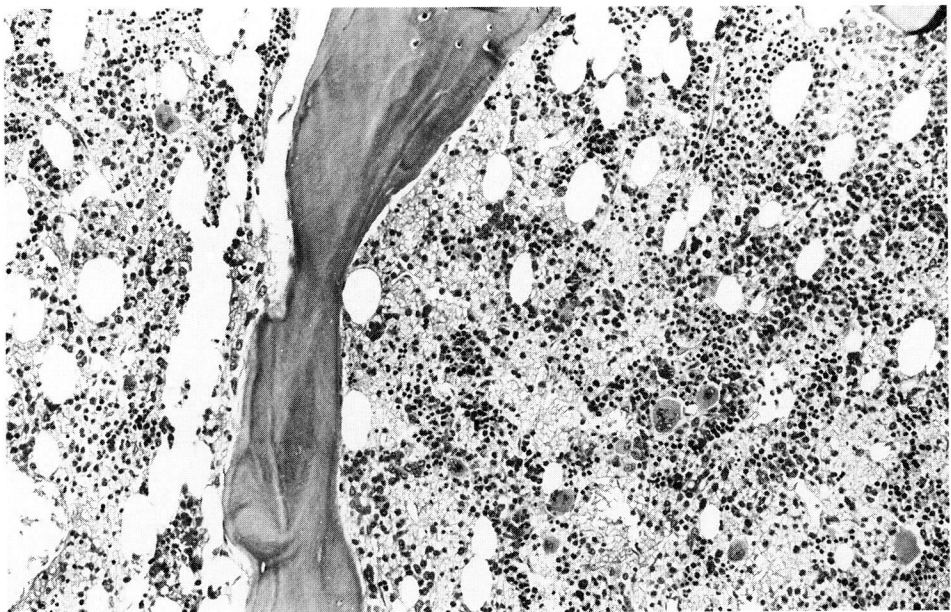

Fig. 23-27 Bone marrow biopsy from adult woman 28 days following completion of chemotherapy for acute myeloid leukemia. Marrow is variably cellular with large areas of interstitial cell depletion. Ery-throid precursors predominate, megakaryocytes are normal in number, and neutrophils are reduced.

the leukemic promyelocyte may be more abundant than in normal promyelocytes.

In addition to assessment of the effects of chemotherapy, postchemotherapy biopsy specimens should always be carefully evaluated for the presence of granulomas or other evidence of infection. In some instances, a focus of microorganisms may be present only as an area of nonspecific necrosis with a few histiocytes. These foci may be very difficult to recognize in a marrow biopsy showing cell necrosis as a result of chemotherapy (Fig. 23-29). Any suspicious lesion should be studied with special stains. Proliferation of histiocytes, with and without hemophagocytosis, may be prominent in infected patients. The histiocytes are widely dispersed throughout the interstitium and in the sinusoids; in some patients this may be a very prominent feature.

Patients being monitored for the effects of chemotherapy will usually have sequential marrow biopsies at relatively short time intervals. If a specimen is from the area of a recent biopsy procedure, there may be evidence of granulation tissue and new bone formation (Fig. 23-30). The biopsy repair site will usually be relatively well demarcated from the remainder of the biopsy specimen but at times may lead to difficulties in interpretation.

Acute myelofibrosis

Although idiopathic myelofibrosis (agnogenic myeloid metaplasia) is usually a chronic disorder, an entity that is characterized by idiopathic marrow fibrosis and a rapid clinical course has been recognized. Several terms have been used for this process, including *acute myelofibrosis, acute myelosclerosis, malignant myelosclerosis,* and *acute myelodysplasia* with *myelofibrosis.*[106-109] This entity is distinguished from chronic idiopathic myelofibrosis by little or no red cell poikilocytosis, absence of or minimal splenomegaly, and a rapid clinical course. Cases of acute myelofibrosis have also been reported as part of a spectrum of therapy-related leukemia occurring in patients previously treated with chemotherapy, primarily alkylating agents, and/or radiotherapy for a variety of tumors and occasionally benign conditions.[109]

In acute myelofibrosis there is hyperplasia of all three myeloid cell lines: erythroblasts, granulocytes, and megakaryocytes (Fig. 23-31). The megakaryocytes, because of their size, developmental characteristics, and tendency to occur in clusters, may be particularly conspicuous; there may be considerable size variation from very small megakaryocytes with nonlobulated nuclei to large cells with bizarre nuclear shapes. The nuclear chromatin is usually finely stippled in contrast to the megakaryocytes in chronic idiopathic myelofibrosis in which the chromatin is more dense. The PAS stain may be particularly useful in accentuating the megakaryocytes. The granulocytes and erythroid cells in acute myelofibrosis are predominantly immature, but some evidence of maturation is usually present. The more immature cells may be difficult to categorize in routinely stained sections. Giemsa-stained sections and sections imunocytochemically reacted with antibodies to myeloperoxidase, CD68, lysozyme, and hemoglobin may be of considerable help in distinguishing granulocyte and monocyte precursors and erythroblasts. The reticulin stain in acute myelofibrosis shows an increase in reticulin fibers; the fibers may be dense and confluent. Stains for collagen are usually negative, although an occasional case may show collagen fibrosis.

The relationship of acute myelofibrosis to acute megakaryoblastic leukemia has been the subject of considerable

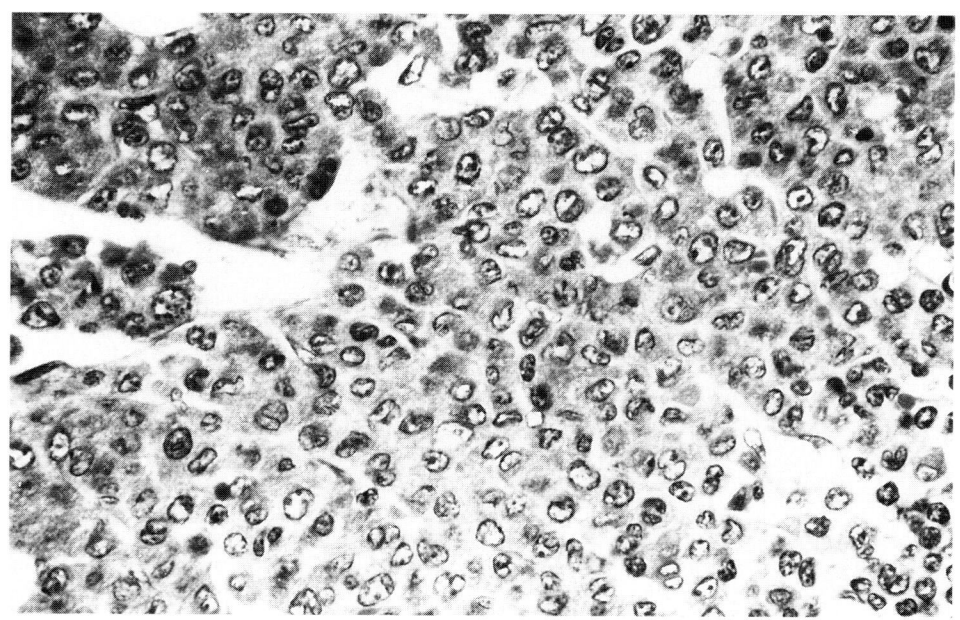

Fig. 23-28 Marrow biopsy from adult woman with acute promyelocytic leukemia following two courses of chemotherapy. Large areas of marrow are replaced by leukemic promyelocytes.

discussion, and some observers have equated the two disorders. Some cases of acute megakaryoblastic leukemia present with myelofibrosis; however, this is not an invariant finding, and myelofibrosis is not a feature of all cases of acute megakaryoblastic leukemia. Acute myelofibrosis is essentially a panmyeloid disorder, although in some instances the megakaryoblastic component may be the most obvious because of the prominent and bizarre features of the developing megakaryocytes.

Acute myelofibrosis is distinguished from cases of acute myeloid leukemia presenting with marrow fibrosis by the predominance of one cell line in most cases of acute leukemia and the essentially trilineage proliferation in acute myelofibrosis. This distinction, however, may not be possible in all instances and the therapeutic importance of the distinction is not completely clear.

The therapy-related acute panmyeloses have marrow findings that are generally similar to the de novo processes.

Granulocytic sarcoma (chloroma)

Granulocytic sarcoma is an unusual variant of myeloid malignancy in which there is an extramedullary tumor mass composed of myeloblasts or myeloblasts and more mature neutrophils.[113,115,117-124] An association of granulocytic sar-

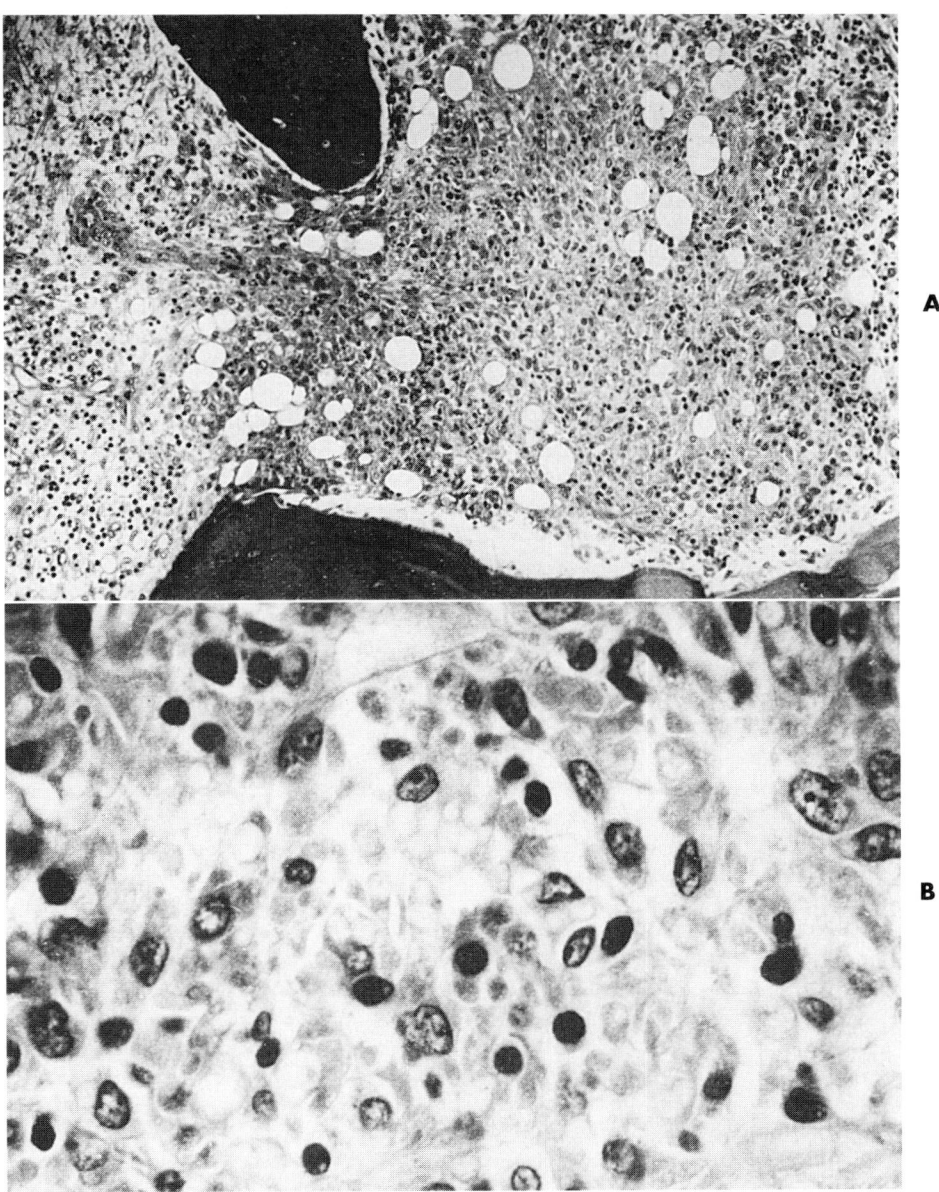

Fig. 23-29 A, Marrow biopsy following chemotherapy from patient with acute lymphoblastic leukemia. On right is poorly defined collection of histiocytes, interspersed mature lymphocytes, and necrotic debris. **B,** Higher magnification of same lesion showing several macrophages with cytoplasmic vacuoles.   *Continued.*

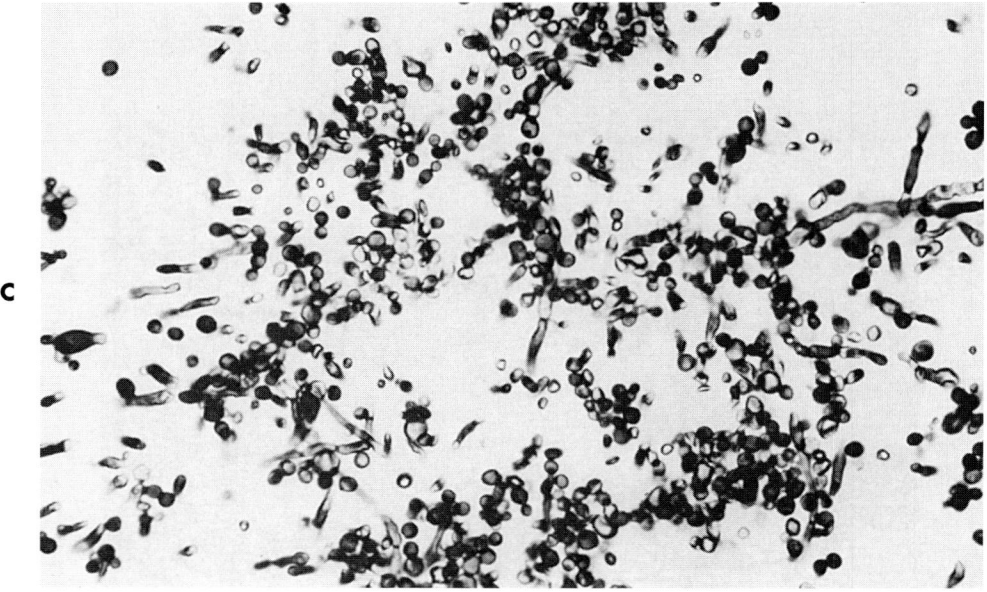

C

Fig. 23-29, cont'd **C,** Same lesion showing numerous *Candida* hyphae. (**C,** Gomori's methenamine silver.)

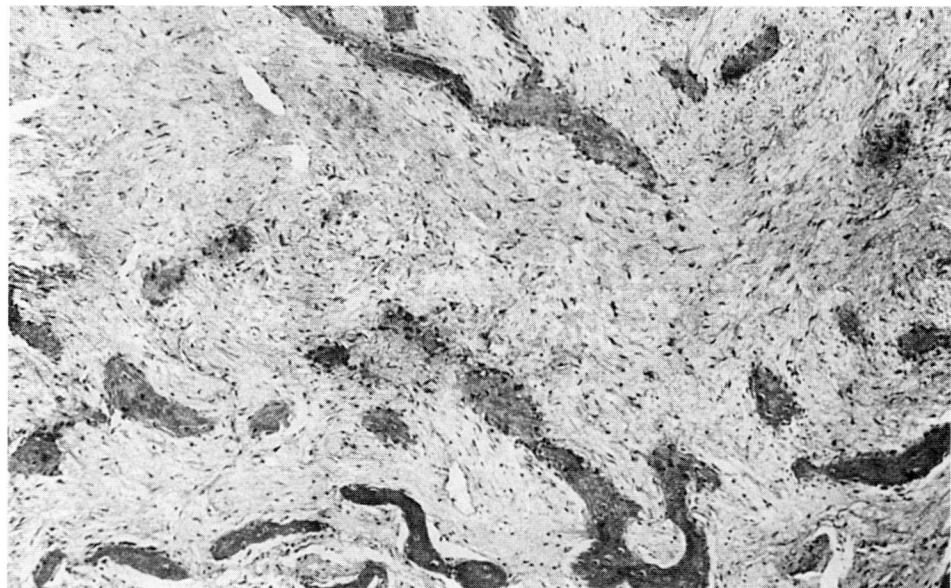

Fig. 23-30 Marrow section from patient biopsied in same location 14 days earlier; area of earlier biopsy shows new bone formation and characteristic granulation tissue.

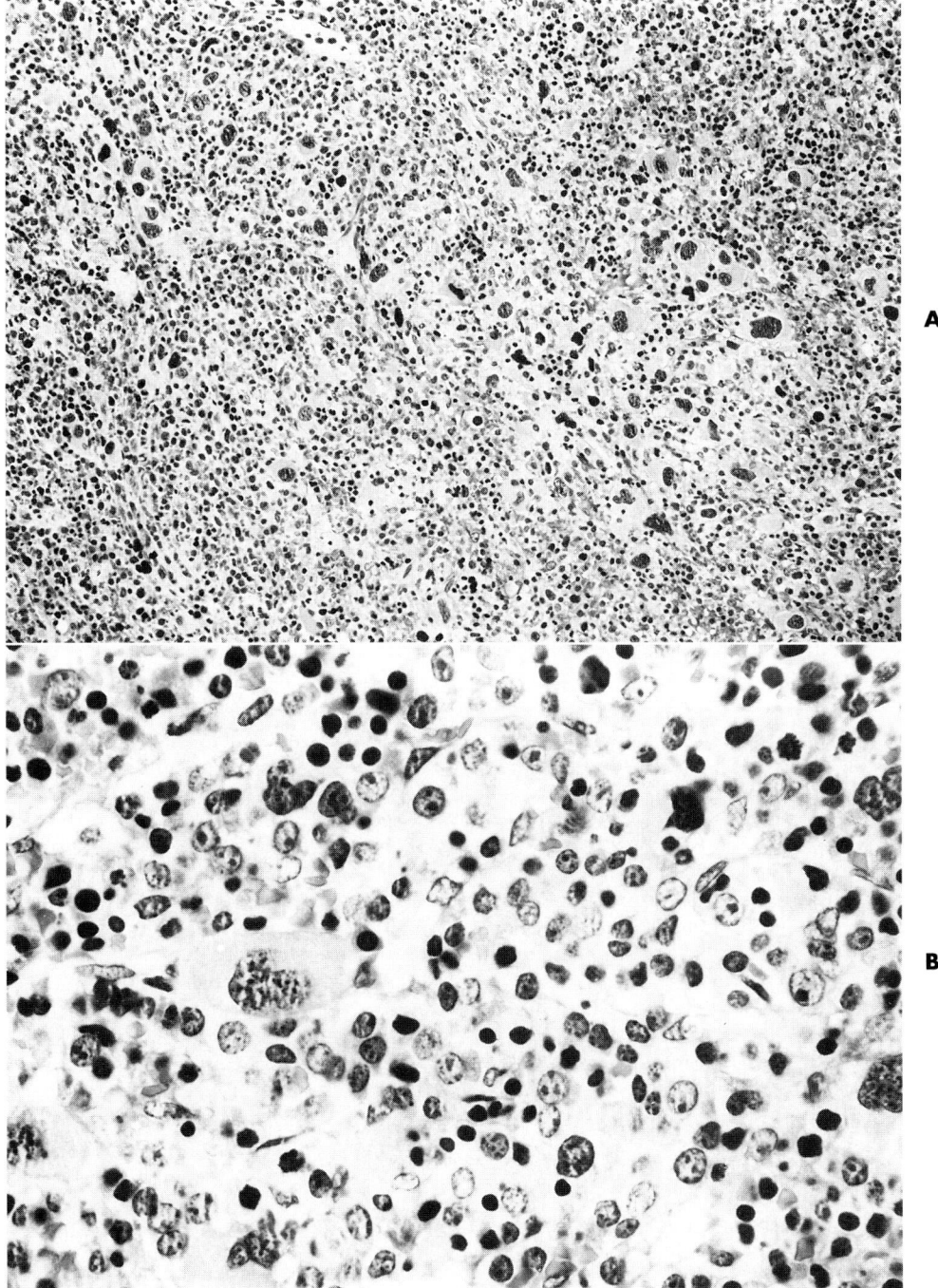

Fig. 23-31 A, Bone marrow biopsy from adult male with acute myelofibrosis. Marrow is markedly hypercellular as a result of panmyeloid hyperplasia. Megakaryocytes are numerous and vary markedly in size. **B,** High magnification of the specimen in **A.** There is predominance of blasts and promyelocytes. Erythroid cells show more complete maturation sequence.   *Continued.*

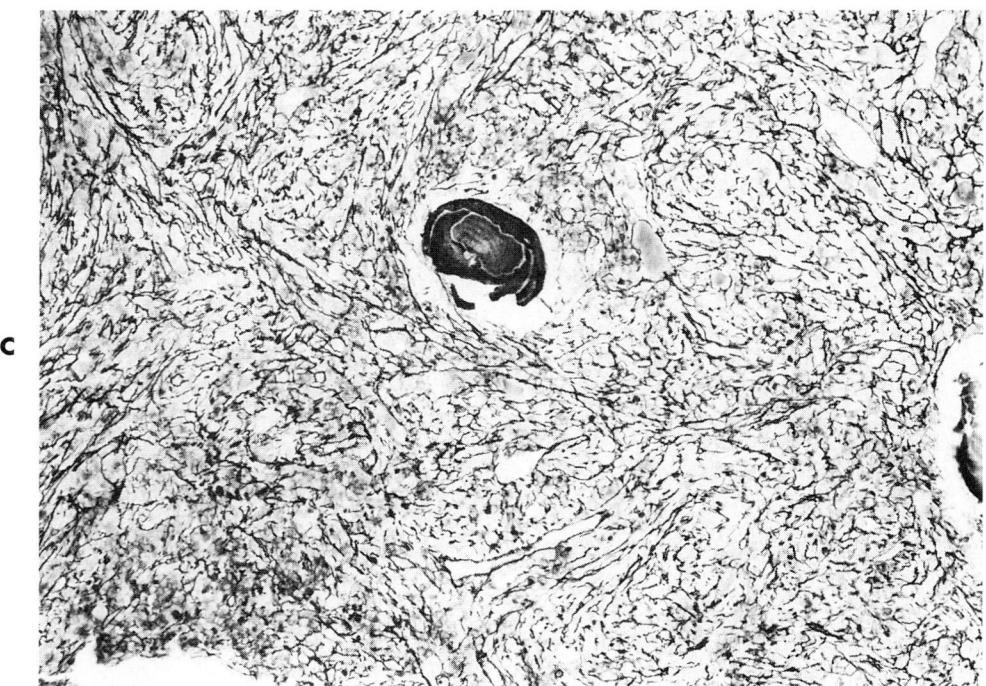

Fig. 23-31, cont'd **C,** Reticulin stain of biopsy in **A** and **B** showing marked increase in coarse reticulin fibers. (**C** Wilder's reticulin).

coma and acute myeloid leukemia with the t(8;21) chromosome abnormality has been reported.[123] The tumor may occur as an isolated finding or may be associated with acute myeloid leukemia, chronic myeloid leukemia, chronic idiopathic myelofibrosis, hypereosinophilic syndrome, and polycythemia vera.[110,112,119] In earlier literature, the term *chloroma* was used for these lesions because of the green appearance of the freshly cut surface of the tumor. The green color, which is due to the presence of peroxidase in the leukemic cells, is not present in all tumors of this type, and the less specific designation of granulocytic sarcoma is preferred.[121]

The granulocytic sarcomas are more frequent in children than adults and are most commonly associated with the subperiosteal bone structures; the most common sites are the skull, paranasal sinuses, sternum, ribs, vertebrae, and pelvis; lymph nodes and skin are also relatively frequently involved. Orbital masses leading to proptosis and spinal canal lesions resulting in neurologic manifestations are two of the clinical presentations associated with these tumors (Fig. 23-32). A high incidence of granulocytic sarcomas involving the orbit has been reported in Turkish children with acute myelomonocytic leukemia.[111] Granulocytic sarcomas may present as a mediastinal mass and clinically resemble a mediastinal lymphoma.[110a]

A granulocytic sarcoma may occur simultaneously with a typical blood and bone marrow pattern of acute myeloid leukemia or may antedate leukemia by many months or rarely years.[117] It may be the first evidence of relapse in a patient with acute myeloid leukemia on maintenance chemotherapy and may be the only evidence of recurrence. These tumors may also represent the initial manifestation of a blast crisis of chronic myeloid leukemia, and an isolated tumor mass or enlarged lymph node in a patient with chronic myeloid leukemia should be evaluated for this possibility, including cytogenetic studies for the Ph` chromosome or molecular studies for evidence of the BCR/abl hybrid gene[112,119] (Fig. 23-33).

Histologically the tumor is composed of a relatively uniform population of immature cells and may be misdiagnosed as one of the poorly differentiated malignant lymphomas. Occasionally, the presence of immature eosinophils and maturing neutrophils may indicate the true nature of the lesion. Attempts at histopathologic classification have generally resulted in three levels of differentiation: blastic, immature, and differentiated.[117,119] The blastic type is composed primarily of myeloblasts with little evidence of differentiation to the promyelocyte stage (Fig. 23-34). The myeloblasts have a slight to moderate rim of basophilic cytoplasm, fine nuclear chromatin, and two to four nucleoli. Eosinophil myelocytes are not usually found with this degree of differentiation. The immature type with an intermediate degree of differentiation contains principally myeloblasts and promyelocytes; eosinophil myelocytes are usually present. The differentiated type comprises primarily promyelocytes and later stages of maturation. Eosinophil myelocytes are most abundant in this type. The chloroacetate esterase stain, which stains neutrophils and precursors in formalin-fixed tissue, is of considerable aid in establishing the diagnosis of a granulocytic sarcoma.[114] Immunocytochemistry using anti-myeloperoxidase, anti-lysosome, and anti-CD68 (KP-1) antibodies may be particularly useful[120] (see Fig. 23-34). Although tumors of monocytes are not gen-

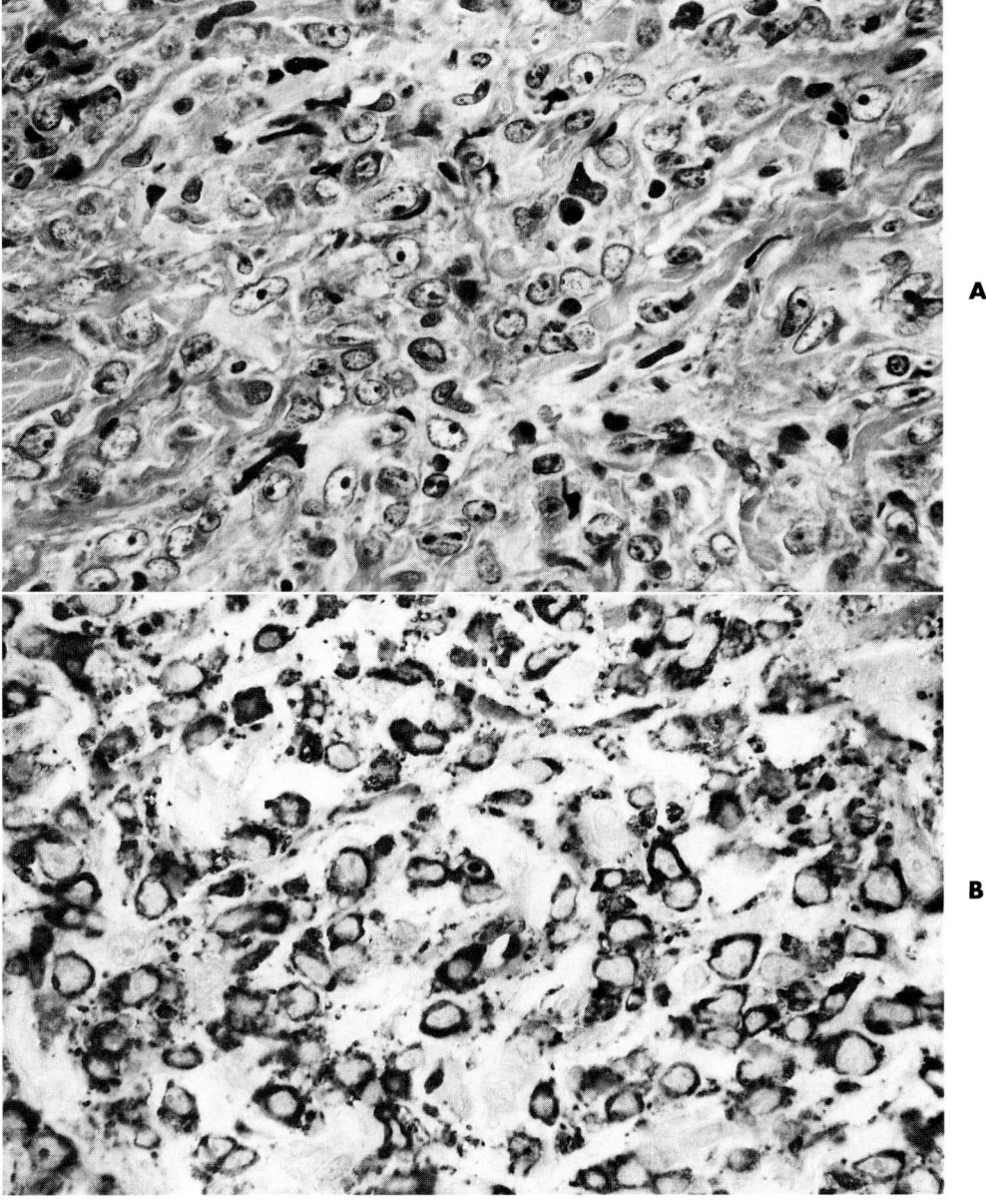

Fig. 23-32 A, Biopsy of orbital granulocytic sarcoma from 6-year-old child who presented with bilateral proptosis. Numerous blasts are present. Chromosome studies of this lesion showed t(8;21) chromosome abnormality. Blood and marrow smears showed acute myeloblastic leukemia with maturation (M2). **B,** Same specimen reacted with antibody to myeloperoxidase. Virtually all blasts are positive. (**B** Peroxidase-antiperoxidase.)

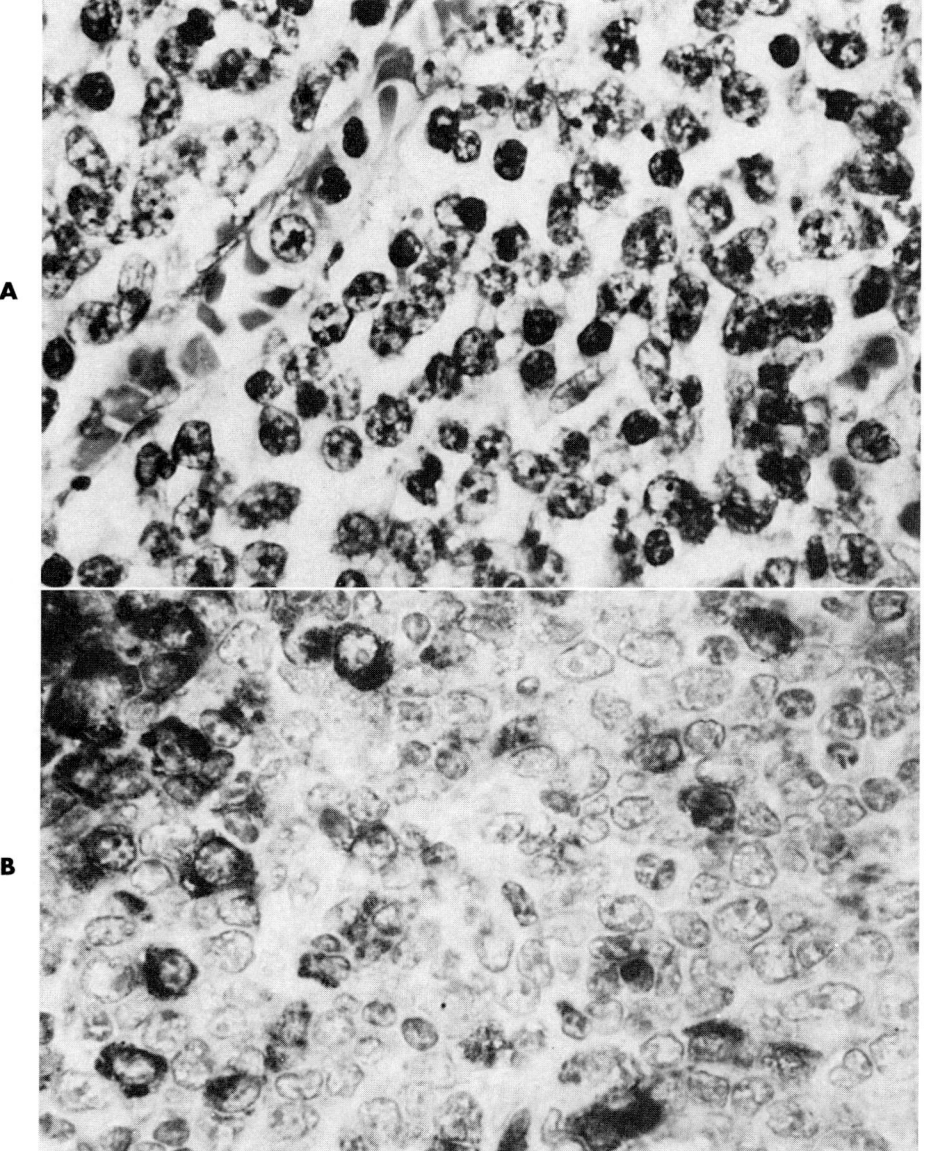

Fig. 23-33 A, Portion of lymph node biopsy from 63-year-old woman with chronic myelogenous leukemia. Lymph node is completely effaced by infiltrate of poorly differentiated blast cells. **B,** Same specimen reacted with anti-lysozyme antibody using peroxidase-antiperoxidase technique. Several of the blast forms react positively, confirming myeloid origin of blast infiltration. (Peroxidase-antiperoxidase.)

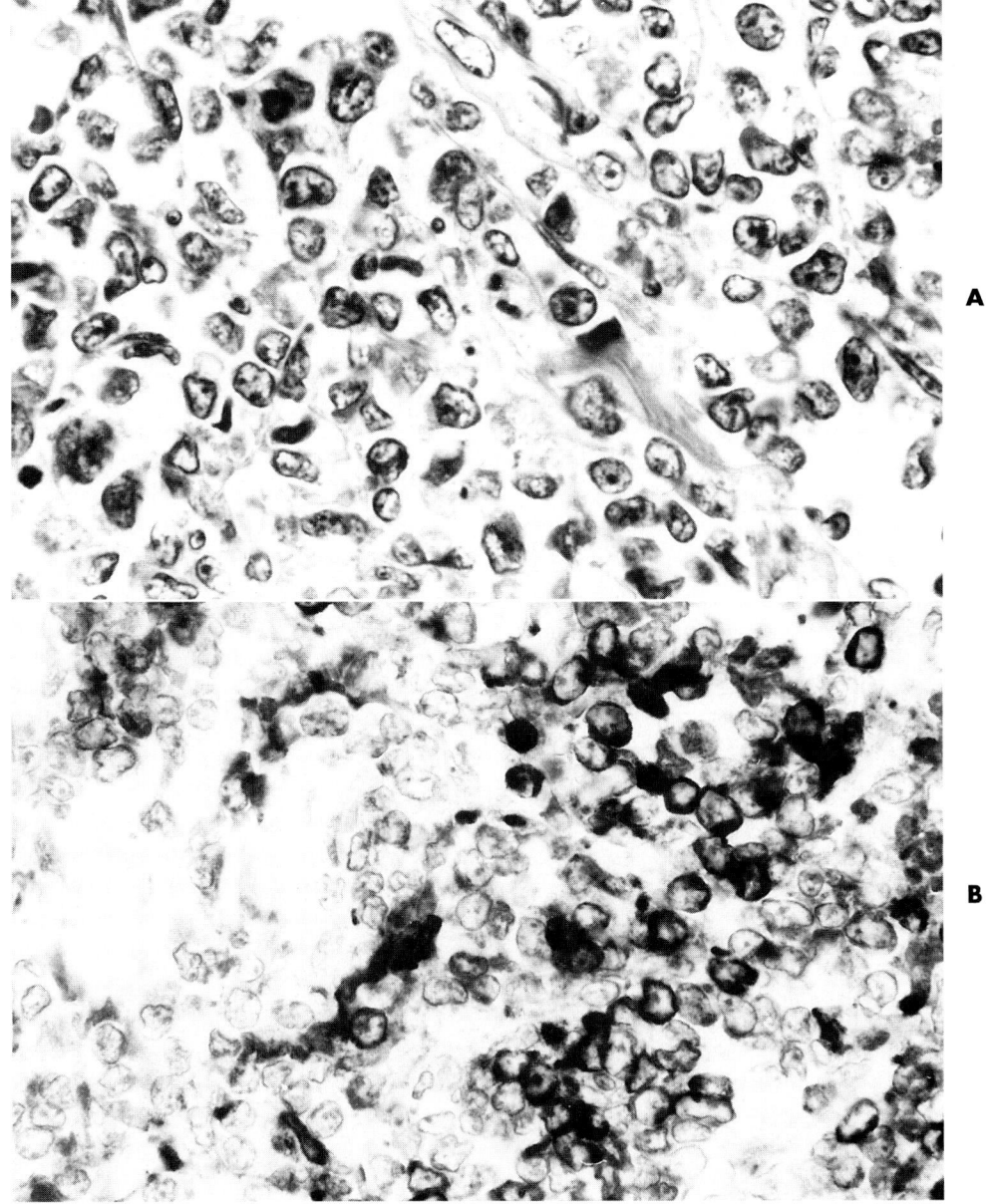

Fig. 23-34 A, Biopsy of a granulocytic sarcoma from subcutaneous tissue of chest wall of 49-year-old man. Tumor is composed of poorly differentiated blast cells interpreted as granulocytic sarcoma. There is essentially no evidence of differentiation. **B,** Same specimen reacted with polyclonal antibody to myeloperoxidase. In this field, there are numerous reacting cells identifying cells as myeloblasts. Blood and marrow showed no evidence of leukemia. (**B** Peroxidase-antiperoxidase.)

erally classified with the granulocytic sarcomas, they represent a similar process with a similar predilection to leukemic evolution, primarily acute monoblastic leukemia.[116] Monocytic lesions react with antibodies to lysozyme and CD68.

Imprint preparations of tumor masses may be particularly useful in identifying the myeloid nature of the cells. Auer rods may be found, and the myeloblasts may show intense staining with the myeloperoxidase cytochemical reaction.

Localized tumor masses occurring in the absence of blood or marrow involvement may respond to local radiation therapy. Eventually the process in the majority of patients will evolve into a form of acute myeloid leukemia or may be associated with additional tumor masses at other sites. The leukemic evolution may be characterized by a gradual increase in myeloblasts in the blood and marrow; frequently, blasts containing Auer rods are identified. In seven of sixteen patients with isolated granulocytic sarcomas reported by Meis et al.,[117] the process did not show a leukemic evolution although three of the seven patients developed granulocytic sarcomas at additional sites and died 2 to 8 months following initial presentation. The other four patients showed no evidence of recurrent disease from 3.5 to 16 years following presentation.

Unlike the granulocytic sarcomas that occur in patients with established hematologic disorders and are usually correctly diagnosed, the predominantly blastic granulocytic sarcomas occurring as isolated lesions may be misdiagnosed as a malignant lymphoma or poorly differentiated tumor because of the lack of diagnostic features.[117] In lymph nodes involved by granulocytic sarcoma, the germinal centers are frequently preserved; the infiltrate is usually present in the sinuses and occasionally in the paracortex and medulla. In other tissues, the cells usually display an infiltrative pattern with the overall architecture remaining intact. The presence of immature eosinophils or cells with lobulated nuclei should evoke suspicion of a granulocytic sarcoma.

Myelodysplastic syndromes

The myelodysplastic syndromes are a heterogenous group of bone marrow disorders with varying degrees of potential for evolution to acute myeloid leukemia.[125,128] Five primary types have been proposed by the FAB Cooperative Group based on features in blood and bone marrow smears: (1) refractory anemia, (2) idiopathic refractory sideroblastic anemia, (3) chronic myelomonocytic leukemia, (4) refractory anemia with excess blasts (RAEB), and (5) refractory anemia with excess of blasts in transformation (RAEB-T).[125] Modifications in the classification have been introduced.[126]

The myelodysplastic syndromes are basically proliferative processes, and the marrow in the majority of cases is hypercellular (Fig. 23-35). In a minority of patients the marrow biopsy is hypocellular. In some instances, the hypocellularity is characterized by the presence of a proteinaceous debris in the interstitium similar to the findings that occur in the marrow biopsies from patients on chemotherapy or with immune-related disorders such as AIDS. This type of change may also be found in marrow biopsies from children with the myelodysplastic syndrome associated with an isolated monosomy 7 cytogenetic abnormality (Fig. 23-36).

The cell population in biopsy specimens varies according to the primary classification.[127] In sideroblastic anemia, there is generally a marked increase in erythroid precursors, with greatly increased iron accumulation in macrophages. In refractory anemia with excess blasts, the marrow is hypercellular in the majority of patients, with an increase in granulocytes and precursors. Refractory anemia with excess of blasts in transformation has histologic features similar to refractory anemia with excess of blasts, but the number of blasts is higher. Chronic myelomonocytic leukemia is characterized by a hypercellular marrow with an increase in both monocytes and granulocytes. In any of these types of myelodysplastic syndrome, the marrow may be hypocellular in a minority of patients.

Increased reticulin fibers may be observed in chronic myelomonocytic leukemia, refractory anemia with excess of blasts, and refractory anemia with excess of blasts in transformation but is not usually a prominent feature.[129] In occasional patients there is marked fibrosis (Fig. 23-37).

A finding referred to as ***abnormal localization of immature precursors (ALIP)***, characterized by clusters of myeloblasts and promyelocytes in central areas of the marrow tissue away from the endosteal surface of the bone trabeculae, has been described in the myelodysplastic syndromes[131] (Fig. 23-38, *A*); this finding has been reported to have predictive value for evolution to leukemia. Apoptosis may be a feature in some cases (Fig. 23-38, *B*).

Although the precise classification of the myelodysplastic syndromes is based principally on the evaluation of blood and marrow smears, there are some forms of myelodysplastic syndromes in which the bone marrow biopsy findings are highly suggestive of a specific process. The de novo 5q− syndrome is a type of myelodysplastic syndrome occurring primarily in older women who present with a macrocytic anemia that is often severe, with normal to increased platelet counts and usually prolonged survival.[130] The hematologic findings are in most cases those of refractory anemia or refractory anemia with excess blasts. The marrow biopsy shows increased megakaryocytes, many with hypolobulated nuclei (Fig. 23-39). Somewhat similar marrow findings may be observed in myelodysplastic syndromes associated with abnormalities of chromosome 3.

Similar to the myeloid leukemias and myeloproliferative disorders, extramedullary granulocytic sarcomas may occur in the course of a myelodysplastic syndrome (Fig. 23-40).

Therapy-related myelodysplastic syndromes occur in patients who have been treated with chemotherapy, radiation, or both for a variety of malignant and nonmalignant conditions. The bone marrow cellularity in these therapy-related myelodysplastic syndromes is more variable than with the de novo myelodysplastic syndromes; in approximately 50% of patients the marrow is hypercellular; in 25%, normocellular; and in 25%, hypocellular.[126] The marrow specimen may show evidence of the initial lesion for which treatment was given, in addition to changes characteristic of the myelodysplastic syndrome.

These processes are frequently panmyelopathies with involvement of all major myeloid cell lines; megakaryocyte abnormalities may be particularly prominent in marrow biopsies[126] (Fig. 23-41). Fibrosis may be marked, and some of

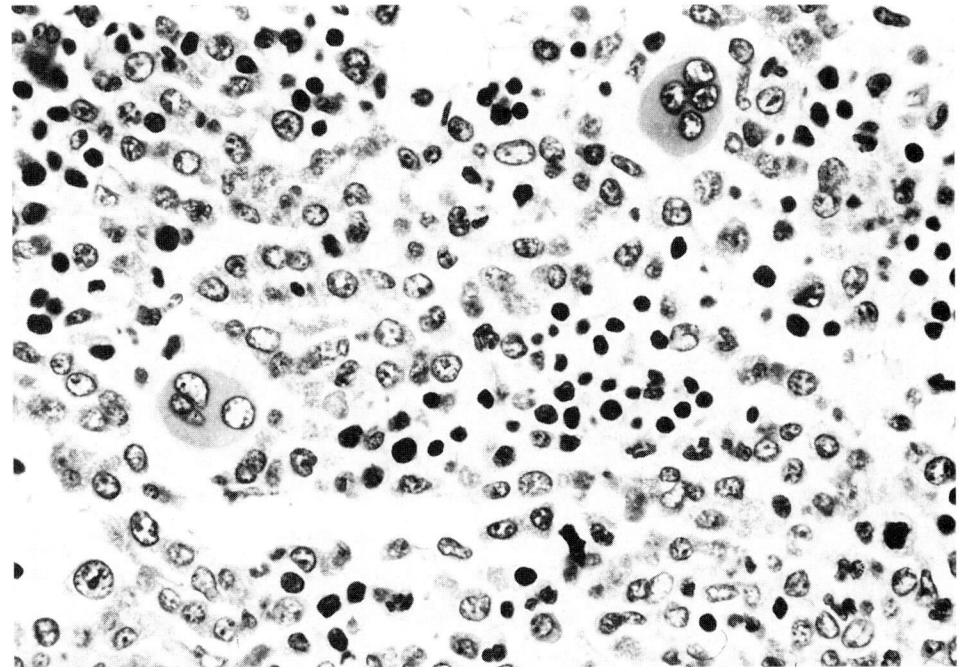

Fig. 23-35 Marrow biopsy from adult with refractory anemia with excess blasts. Marrow is markedly hypercellular. Neutrophils are predominantly promyelocytes and myelocytes. Erythroid precursors are numerous. Two normal megakaryocytes are present.

these cases have been termed acute myelodysplasia with myelofibrosis when there is a pronounced shift to immature cells.

Chronic myeloid leukemia

Chronic myeloid leukemia is generally characterized by an elevated leukocyte count with basophilia, decreased neutrophil alkaline phosphatase, and the presence of the Philadelphia chromosome and/or molecular evidence of the BCR/abl hybrid gene in the hematopoietic cells.[137] The number of myeloblasts in the blood and marrow smears in the chronic phase does not usually exceed 5%. The trephine sections are markedly hypercellular, primarily because of an increase in granulocytes and megakaryocytes.[133] Macrophages resembling Gaucher cells, usually occurring singly, may be present in the bone marrow smears and sections; they are more prominent in perivascular locations.

The natural history of chronic myeloid leukemia includes a chronic phase of 3 to 4 years' duration followed by an accelerated phase that is characterized by a progressive increase in blast cells in the blood and/or marrow and increasing basophilia or myelofibrosis[132,137,139]; the term *blast transformation* is used when the changes occur abruptly and the blasts exceed 30% in the blood or marrow. In some patients, blast transformation may be initially manifest in bone marrow sections as large, irregular, focal collections of blasts. Extramedullary manifestation of blast crisis also occurs, and the diagnosis should be suspected in any patient with chronic myeloid leukemia who develops a tumor mass or lymphadenopathy[140] (see Fig. 23-33).

The development of myelofibrosis in patients with chronic myeloid leukemia usually occurs late in the disease and has been associated with a more aggressive clinical course[136]; exceptions to this generalization have been reported.[134] Myelofibrosis may occur in the early stages of chronic myeloid leukemia with the same prognostic implications as when it occurs late in the disease.[135] The myelofibrosis in chronic myeloid leukemia is usually characterized by an increase in reticulin fibers; collagenous fibrosis is not common but may occasionally occur. Reversal of myelofibrosis may occur following bone marrow transplantation.[138]

Polycythemia vera

Polycythemia vera is classified with the myeloproliferative syndromes; the major diagnostic feature is an increased red cell mass, and there are usually splenomegaly and some degree of leukocytosis and thrombocytosis. The neutrophil alkaline phosphatase is elevated or at the upper range of normal in most patients. Precise criteria for the diagnosis have been established by the Polycythemia Vera Study Group.[155]

The bone marrow in polycythemia vera is usually markedly hypercellular.[142,143] However, this is not an invariant finding; 13% of the patients enrolled in the National Cancer Institute Polycythemia Vera Study had marrow biopsies with cellularity of less than 60%.[141] The cellularity of the marrows from patients in the study ranged from 37% to 100%, with a mean of 82%. The hypercellularity is due to a panhyperplasia of myeloid cells; the increase in megakaryocytes may be particularly striking, and many unusually large megakaryocytes may be present, occasionally in clusters[142,153] (Fig.

Text continued on p. 1834.

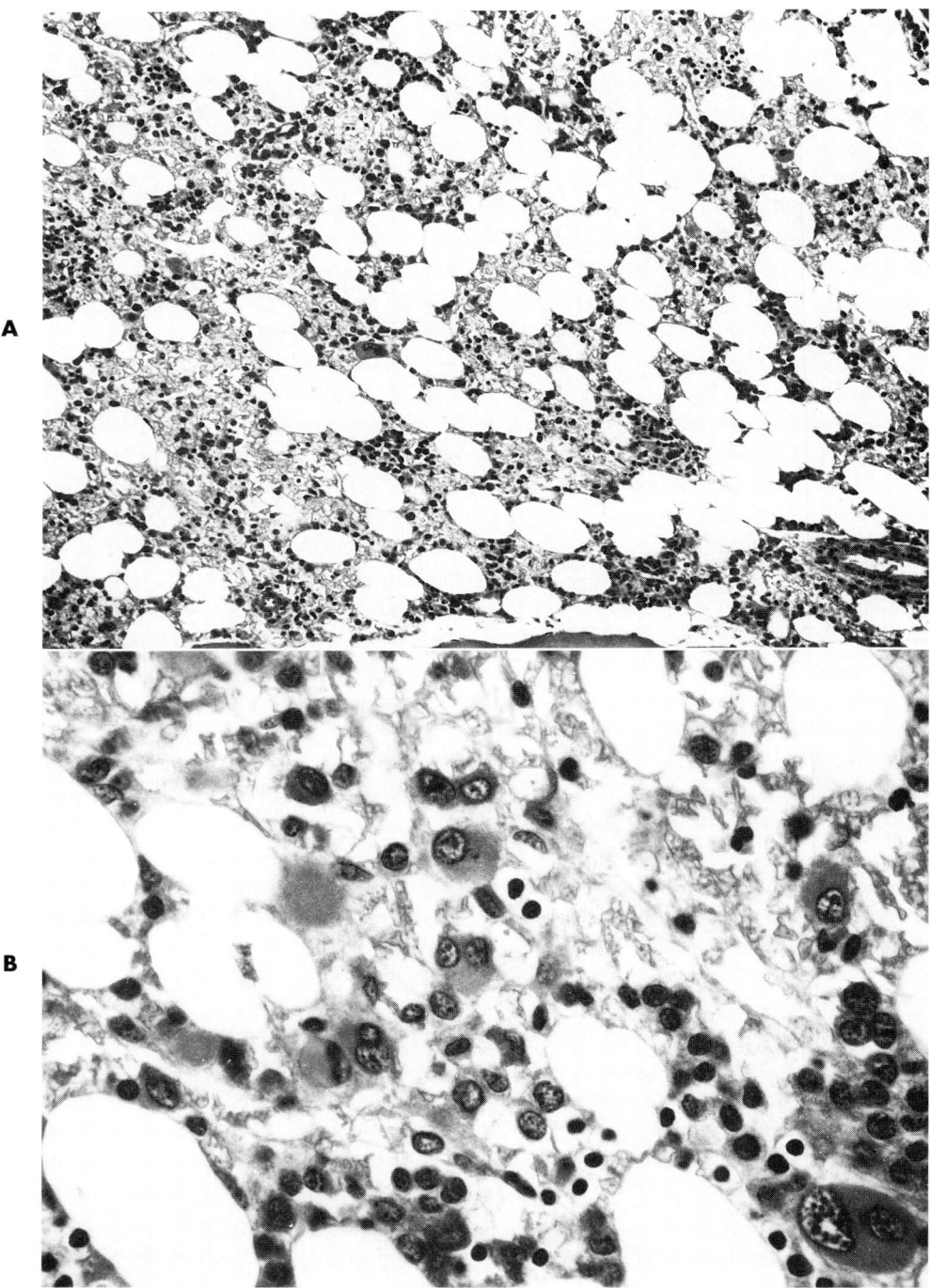

Fig. 23-36 **A,** Marrow biopsy from two-year-old child with myelodysplastic syndrome associated with isolated monosomy 7 cytogenetic abnormality. Marrow is moderately to markedly hypocellular for age with increased fat and interstitial cell depletion. Small megakaryocytes with hypolobulated nuclei are present. **B,** High magnification of specimen in **A** showing interstitial cellular depletion and several hypolobulated megakaryocytes.

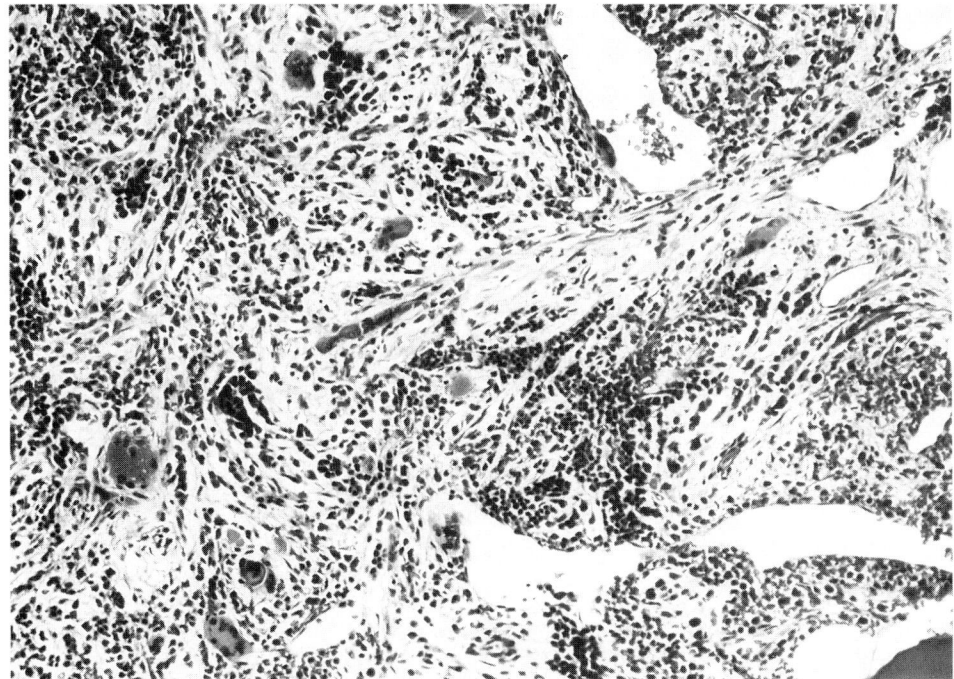

Fig. 23-37 Bone marrow biopsy from adult male with refractory anemia with excess of blasts in transformation based on presence of myeloblasts with Auer rods in blood and marrow touch imprints. There is marked fibrosis with numerous megakaryocytes.

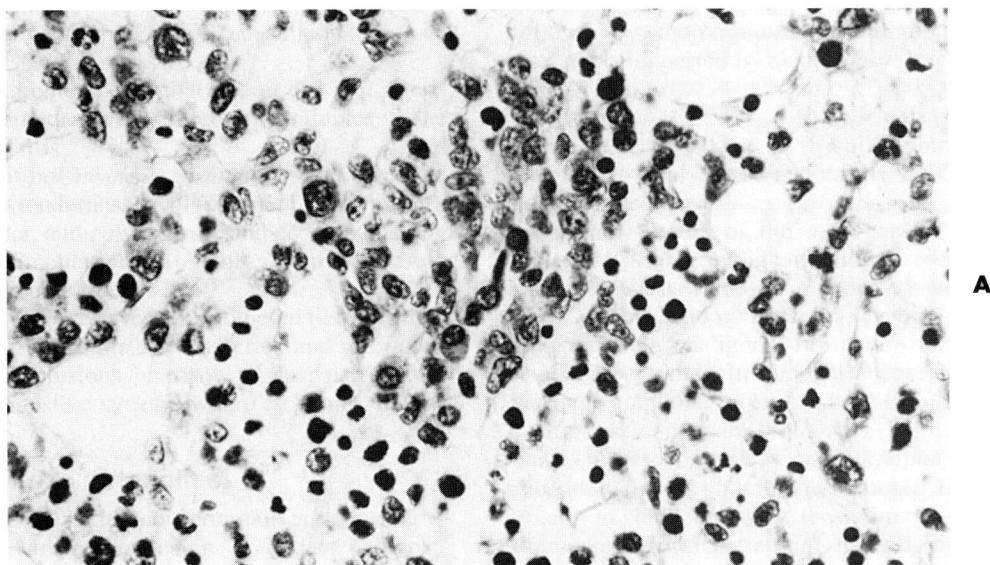

A

Fig. 23-38 A, Marrow biopsy from 67-year-old male with refractory anemia with excess of blast (RAEB), showing abnormal localization of immature precursors (ALIP).   *Continued.*

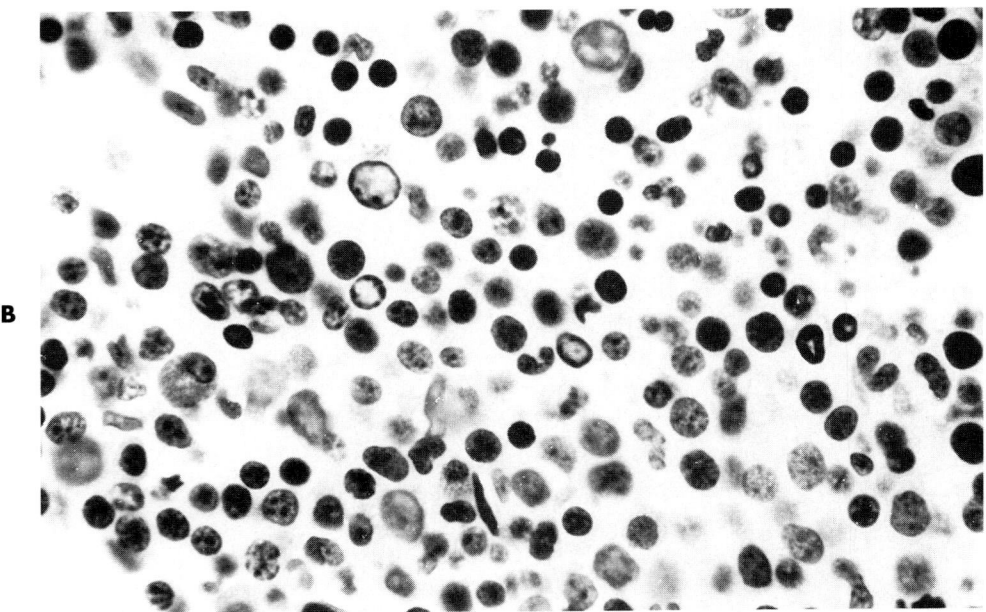

Fig. 23-38, cont'd **B,** Marrow from a patient with refractory anemia with marked erythroid hyperplasia and dyserythropoiesis. Several erythroid precursors with apoptotic nuclei are present.

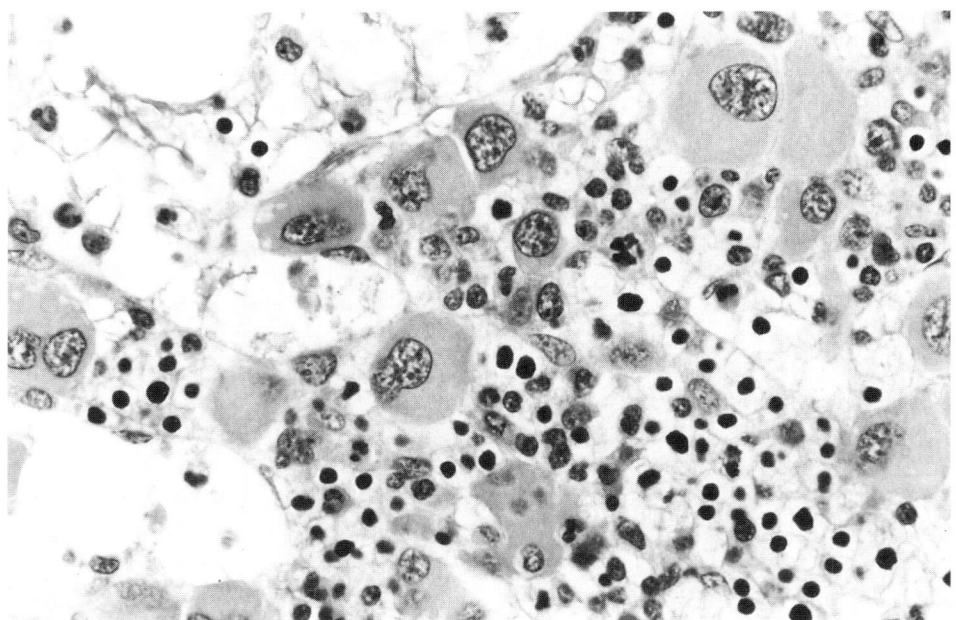

Fig. 23-39 Marrow biopsy from an adult woman with de novo myelodysplastic syndrome associated with 5q- cytogenetic abnormality. There is increase in megakaryocytes, some of which have hypolobulated nuclei. Majority of megakaryocytes are normal in size.

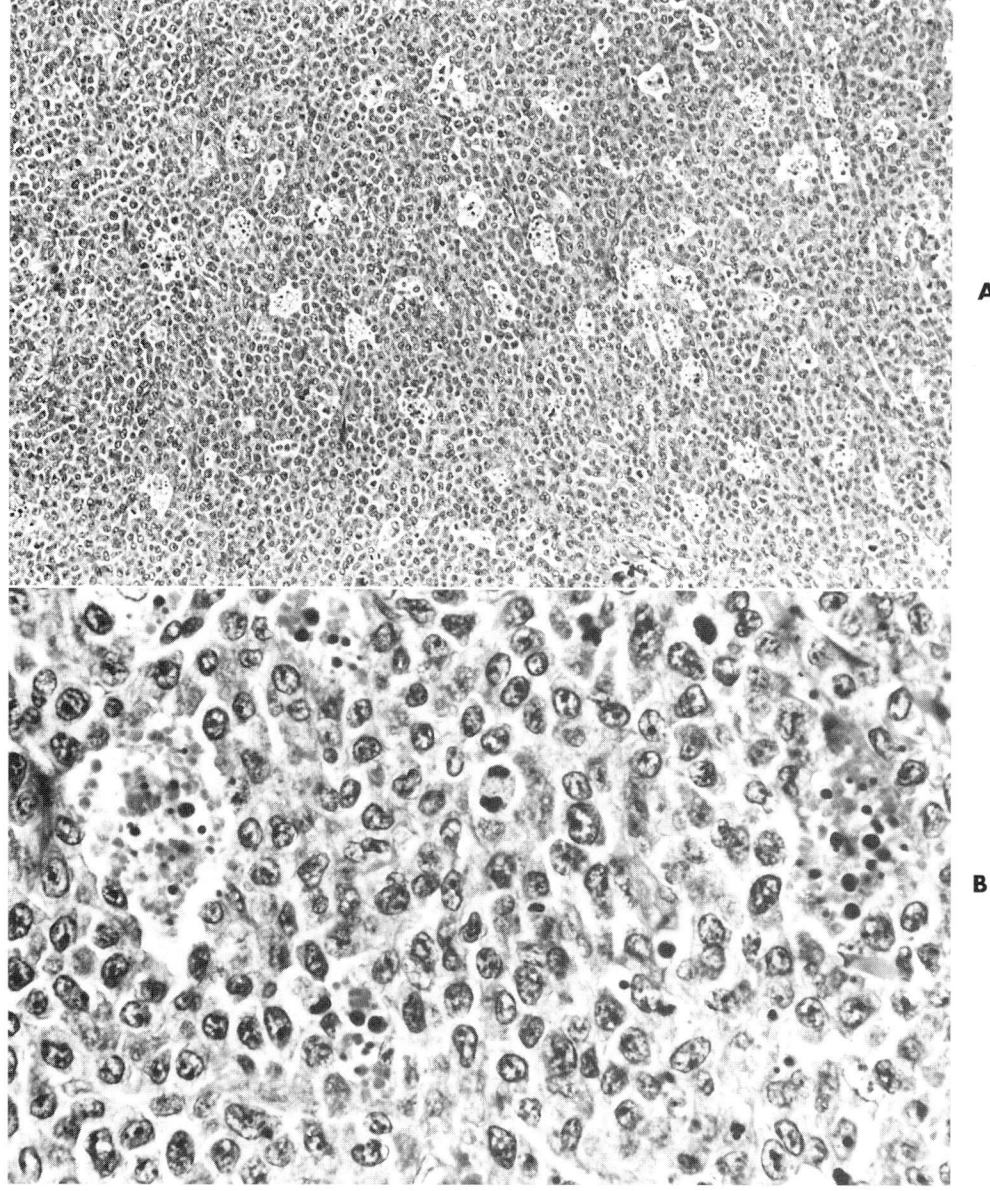

Fig. 23-40 A, Portion of subcutaneous chest wall mass from elderly woman with a 1-year history of chronic myelomonocytic leukemia with less than 5% blasts in marrow and blood. Mass consists of relatively uniform population of blasts; scattered mitotic figures are present. Numerous tingible body macrophages impart "starry sky" appearance to lesion. **B,** High magnification of **A.** Many of blasts reacted with antibody to myeloperoxidase and CD68. Blood and marrow examination at time of appearance of the chest wall mass was essentially unchanged from previous year, with less than 5% blasts.

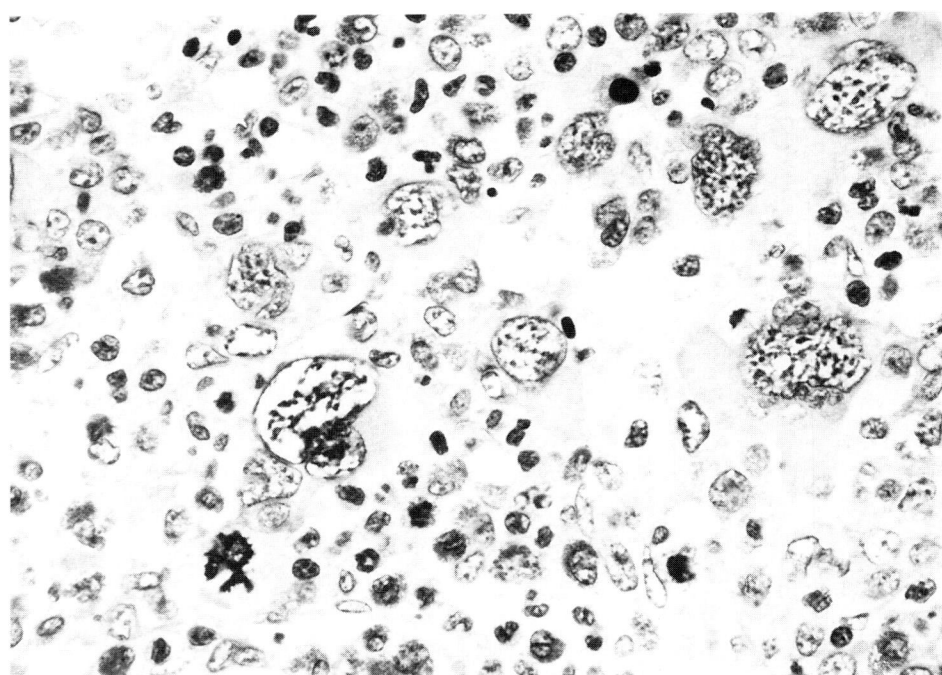

Fig. 23-41 Bone marrow biopsy from patient with therapy-related myelodysplasia with myelofibrosis. There is predominance of neutrophils and megakaryocytes. Megakaryocytes show marked dysplasia.

23-42). Stains for iron usually show decreased or no hemosiderin deposits. A slight increase in reticulin fibers is present at the outset of the disease in 25% of cases; 11% of pretreatment biopsies show a marked increase in reticulin fibers.[141] The increase in reticulin corresponds, in general, to an increase in marrow cellularity.[142] An increase in reticulin fibers in pretreatment marrow biopsies is not necessarily indicative of the spent phase of the disease.[141]

The evolution of polycythemia vera may be marked by a decrease in red cell mass and the development of myelofibrosis with a marked increase in reticulin fibers and collagenous fibrosis; the incidence of this complication, which is referred to as the "spent phase," varies from 9% to 20%[149-151] (Fig. 23-43). An additional complication in some patients is the occurrence of acute myeloid leukemia; the incidence is higher in patients treated with chemotherapy, P[32], or radiation as opposed to those treated only with phlebotomy.[142,143-145,147,152,154]

Essential thrombocythemia

Essential thrombocythemia is a myeloproliferative disorder that is closely related to polycythemia vera but lacks the essential diagnostic criteria of polycythemia vera, most notably an increase of red cell mass.[148] Bone marrow findings of increased and large megakaryocytes are similar to those found in polycythemia.[146]

Chronic idiopathic myelofibrosis (agnogenic myeloid metaplasia)

Chronic idiopathic myelofibrosis (agnogenic myeloid metaplasia) is a disease of undetermined etiology. It occurs pri-

marily in adults; the average age at diagnosis is approximately 60 years.* Rare cases have been reported in the pediatric population.[168] The marrow fibrosis in this disorder is usually accompanied by some degree of detectable hepatosplenomegaly caused by extramedullary hematopoiesis. Chronic idiopathic myelofibrosis may, at times, be confused with chronic myeloid leukemia because of occasional similarities in the blood findings; the important differentiating clinical and laboratory findings have been described in detail.[170] The most important distinguishing biologic feature is the presence of the Philadelphia chromosome or molecular evidence of the BCR/abl hybrid gene in the hematopoietic cells in chronic myeloid leukemia and its absence in the cells from patients with chronic idiopathic myelofibrosis. In addition, the neutrophil alkaline phosphatase is decreased in approximately 90% of the patients with chronic myeloid leukemia and is normal or increased in the majority of patients with idiopathic myelofibrosis. Marrow fibrosis in chronic myeloid leukemia is generally a late occurrence, and its onset usually heralds a more aggressive evolution, unlike idiopathic myelofibrosis in which marrow fibrosis is present to some extent from the inception and is generally associated with a more prolonged clinical course.[170]

In chronic idiopathic myelofibrosis, the marrow is hypercellular with varying proportions of hematopoietic cells and connective tissue elements, although there may be considerable variation in the relative proportions of hematopoietic cells and fibrous connective tissue in a single biopsy specimen because of the patchy nature of the disorder. Some

_____

*References 159, 160, 162, 163, 165-167, 169-172.

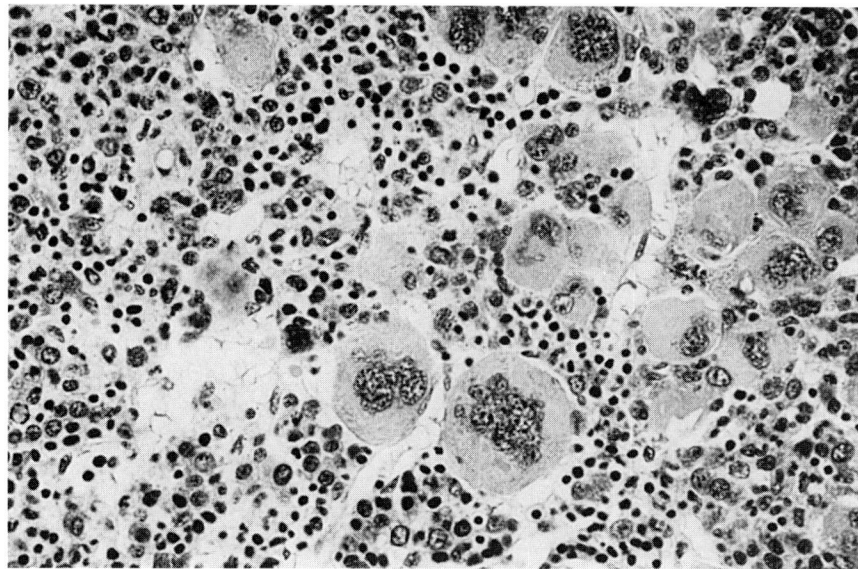

Fig. 23-42 Hyperplastic bone marrow from patient with polycythemia vera. All cellular elements are increased. Megakaryocytes are prominent and show considerable variation in size; many are unusually large.

areas of a biopsy specimen show primarily hematopoietic cells with only a slight increase in reticulin fibrosis, whereas other areas show depletion of hematopoietic cells with a more marked increase in reticulin (Fig. 23-44). In the more cellular areas, all three major myeloid cell lines are present, although one cell line tends to predominate. Clusters of megakaryocytes are usually present and may be the only recognizable hematopoietic cells in areas of dense fibrosis. The megakaryocytes usually are dysplastic in appearance, with marked nuclear chromatin condensation. The marrow sinusoids are usually distended and contain hematopoietic cells; megakaryocytes may be particularly prominent (Fig. 23-45). Widening of bone trabeculae may be present. The number and character of the reticulin fibers may vary substantially.[161] In sections with abundant hematopoietic cells, there is a slight to moderate increase in reticulin. In acellular areas, the fibers are abundant, are greatly thickened, and may appear as intertwining bundles. The reaction for collagen is usually less than anticipated from routine-stained sections but is usually present in the densely fibrotic areas. In approximately 40% of the patients with chronic idiopathic myelofibrosis, osteosclerotic changes can be demonstrated by x-ray examination, most notably in the bones of the axial skeleton and the proximal portions of the long bones.[170] The relative proportion of hematopoietic cells and fibrous tissue has been generally assumed to vary with the stage of disease, the amount of fibrous connective tissue progressively increasing, with the end stage characterized by marked marrow fibrosis and marked splenomegaly. Studies have been reported that show no correlation between extent of marrow fibrosis and duration of disease and spleen size.[172]

Similar to chronic myeloid leukemia, extramedullary tumors of hematopoietic tissue may occur in patients with long-standing chronic idiopathic myelofibrosis.[158] The lesions occur most frequently in the retroperitoneum, pelvis, mesentery, and pleura; lymph node and skin may also be involved. The tumors are usually composed primarily of hematopoietic cells with varying degrees of stromal reaction. The megakaryocytes may be particularly prominent because of their number and frequently bizarre appearance. Rarely, marked fibrosis may be present.

The majority of patients with chronic idiopathic myelofibrosis have a relatively long clinical course, with an estimated median survival of approximately 5 years from the onset of disease. A minor population of patients with this disorder has a more rapid course with a median survival of approximately 2 years.[157,164,167] Amyloidosis has been reported as a complicating condition.[156]

Chronic lymphocytic leukemia

B-cell chronic lymphocytic leukemia (CLL) is characterized by a persistent increase in monoclonal, well-differentiated B lymphocytes in the blood and marrow.[174,181,182,191] T-cell CLL is rare.[177] The diagnosis of B-cell CLL is usually established when there is a persistent absolute lymphocytosis in excess of 15,000, although the disease should be suspected in adults with a persistent absolute lymphocyte count exceeding 5,000. Chronic lymphocytic leukemia is usually accompanied by some degree of lymphadenopathy and hepatosplenomegaly. The morphology of the proliferating cells in CLL and well-differentiated lymphocytic lymphoma is similar.[190] The distinction between these two closely related entities is based on arbitrary criteria; if the marrow shows a pattern of infiltration by small lymphocytes and the absolute lymphocyte count in the blood is less than $5 \times 10^9/L$, the diagnosis of well-differentiated lymphocytic lymphoma is more appropriate.

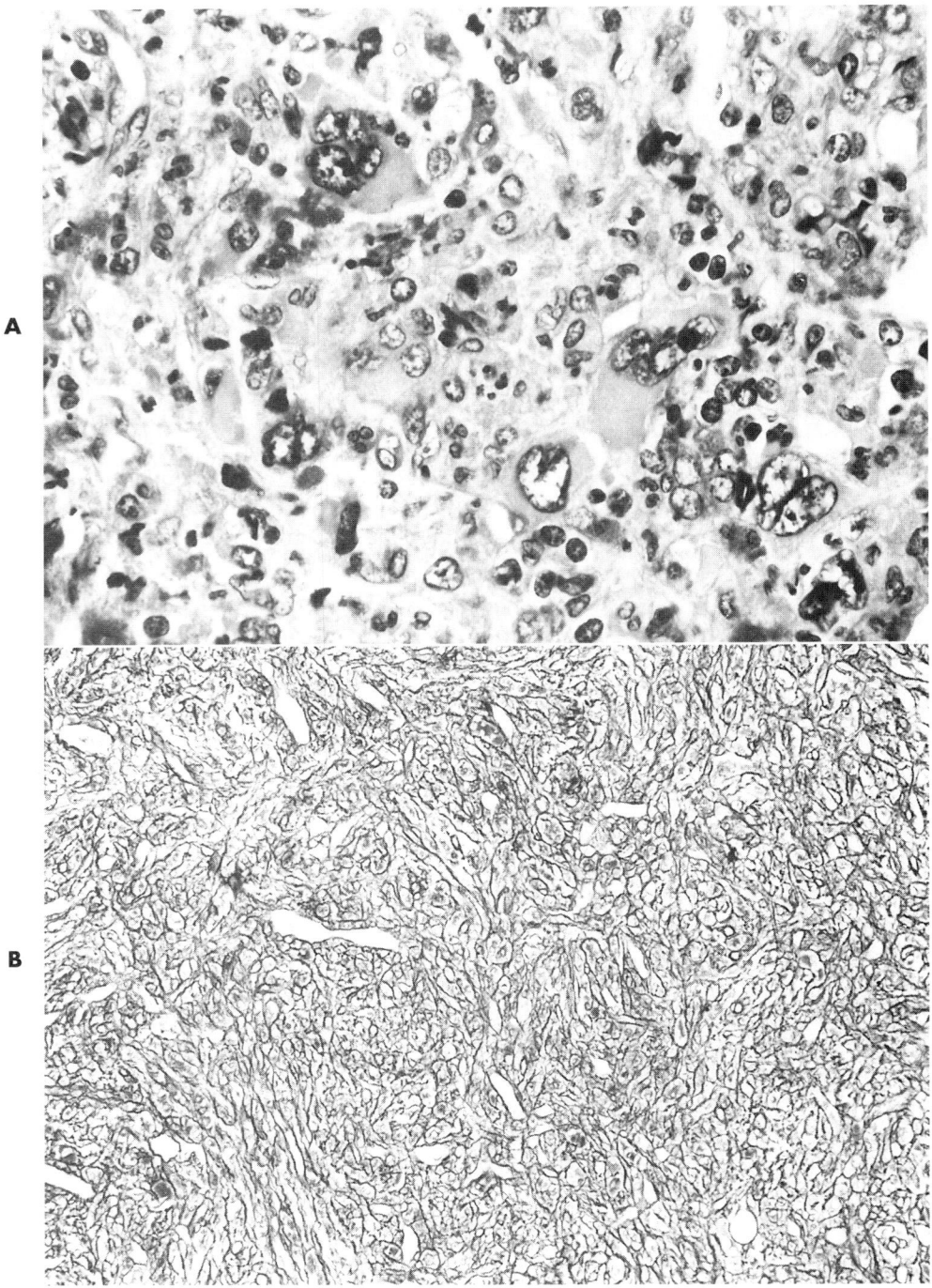

Fig. 23-43 A, Marrow biopsy from patient with long history of polycythemia vera. Marrow is markedly hypercellular as a result of panmyeloid hyperplasia. Megakaryocytes show dysplastic features. **B,** Reticulin stain shows marked increase in coarse reticulin fibers. (**B** Wilder's reticulin.)

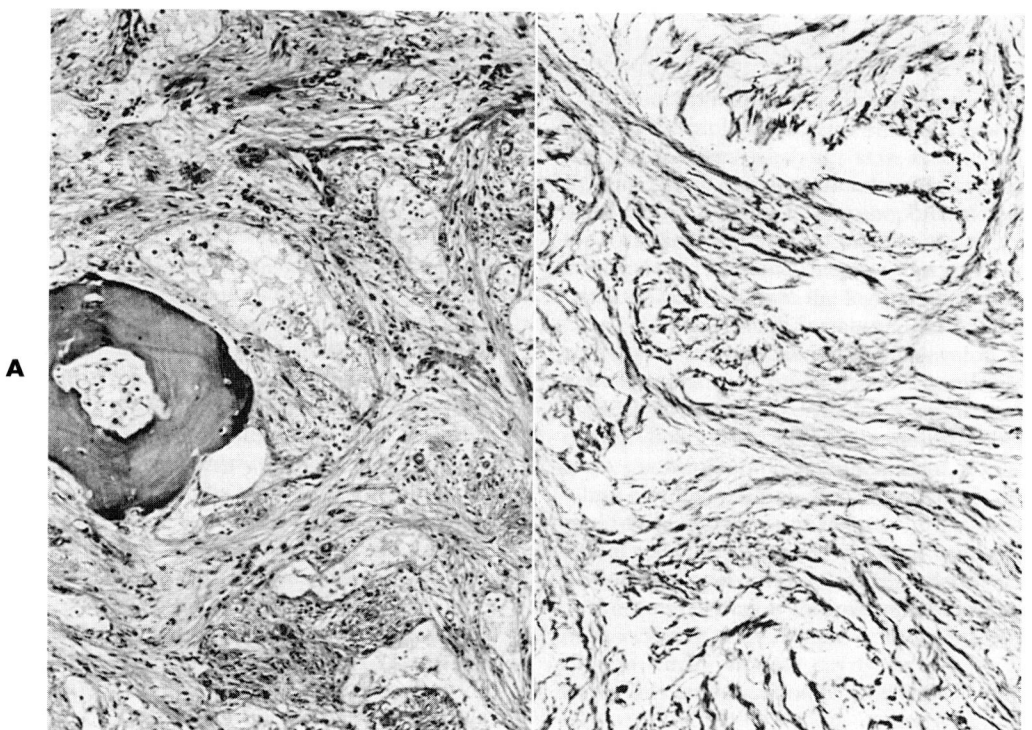

Fig. 23-44 A, Trephine biopsy from adult with 7-year history of chronic idiopathic myelofibrosis (agnogenic myeloid metaplasia). There is extensive marrow fibrosis with marked reduction in hematopoietic tissue. **B,** Same specimen illustrated in **A** shows marked increase in reticulin fibers, which are thickened and have wavy pattern. (**B** Wilder's reticulin.)

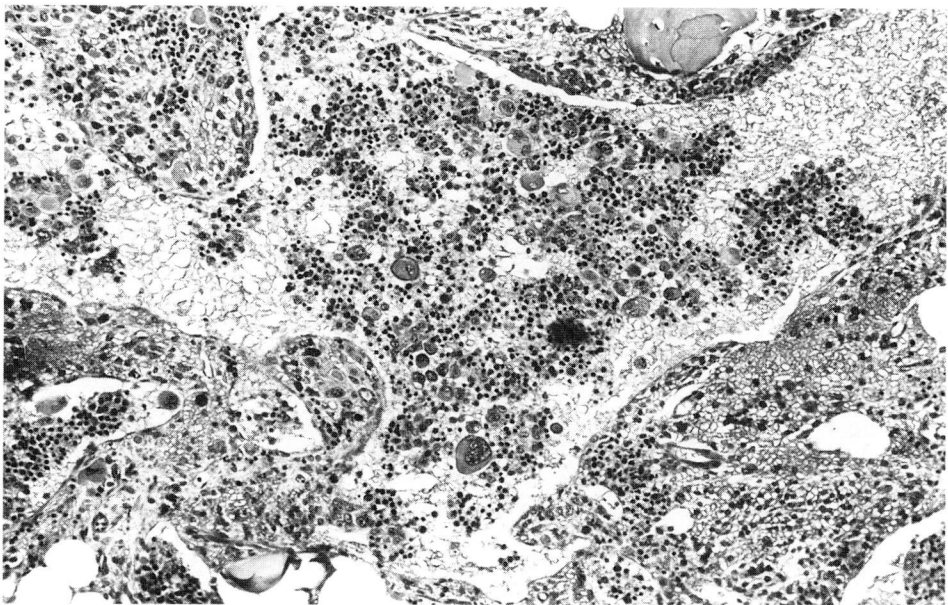

Fig. 23-45 Bone marrow biopsy from patient with chronic idiopathic myelofibrosis showing prominent intrasinusoidal hematopoiesis. Predominant cells in sinusoid are erythroid precursors and megakaryocytes.

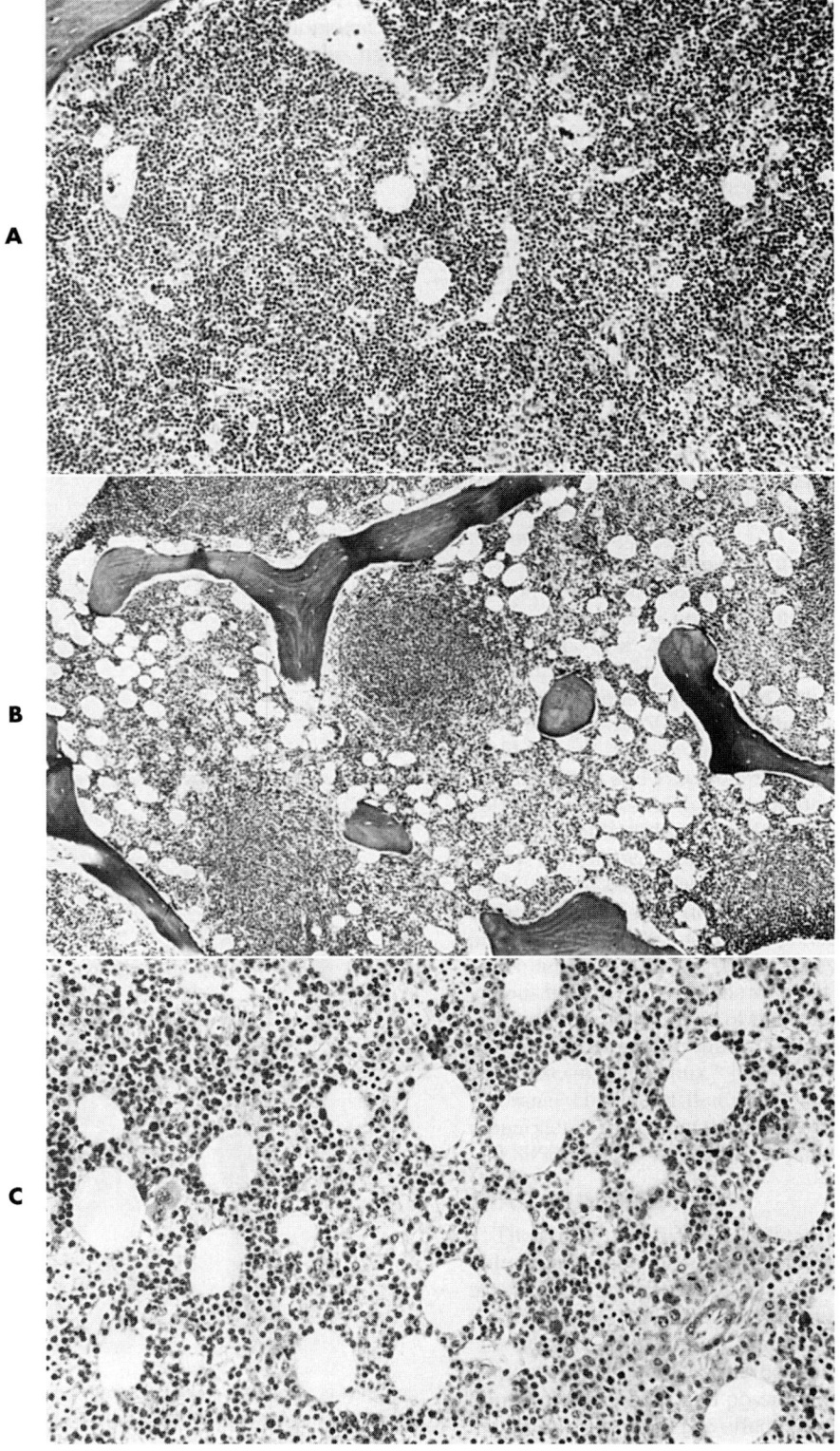

Fig. 23-46 **A,** Marrow biopsy from patient with CLL showing diffuse pattern of involvement. Leukemic cells completely replace normal marrow cells. **B,** Marrow biopsy from patient with CLL with focal involvement. Leukemic cells occur in relatively well-demarcated foci, which are surrounded by normal-appearing marrow. **C,** Marrow section from patient with CLL illustrating an interstitial pattern of involvement; overall marrow architecture is preserved.

Clinical staging systems based on both laboratory and clinical features have been introduced; the higher the stage, the greater the tumor mass.[175,181,192] The system proposed by Rai et al.[192] includes five stages: 0, lymphocytosis in blood and marrow; I, lymphocytosis and lymphadenopathy; II, lymphocytosis and hepatomegaly and/or splenomegaly; III, lymphocytosis and anemia; and IV, lymphocytosis and thrombocytopenia. The system introduced by Binet has three stages.[175,181]

Histopathologic staging of CLL is based on the pattern of involvement in bone marrow sections.[186,187,189,190,194] Five possible patterns are generally recognized: focal, diffuse, interstitial, focal and interstitial, and focal and diffuse (Fig. 23-46). The patients with focal, intersitital, or a combination of focal and interstitial involvement are in predominantly low clinical stages. The diffuse or focal and diffuse patterns generally occur in patients with advanced clinical stages. The diffuse pattern of marrow involvement has been found to have adverse prognostic significance in several studies.[186,189,190,194]

Marrow biopsies from approximately 25% of patients with CLL demonstrate a slight increase in reticulin fibers.

In some patients with CLL, there is a dedifferentiation or transformation of the proliferating cell type; this usually occurs late in the course of the disease in approximately 5% of the patients and has been referred to as "prolymphocytoid" transformation.[179] In these patients, the marrow infiltration may contain foci of prolymphocytoid lymphocytes and paraimmunoblasts (Fig. 23-47). The prolymphocytoid lymphocytes have a moderate amount of basophilic-to-amphophilic cytoplasm, coarsely reticular nuclear chromatin, and relatively prominent single nucleoli. The paraimmunoblast is larger, with more abundant cytoplasm, more dispersed nuclear chromatin, and a single prominent eosinophilic nucleolus. These foci may be circumscribed by more well-differentiated lymphocytes and are similar to the immature foci noted in the lymph nodes of some patients with this process.[178,179,193] Concurrence of CLL and other B-cell neoplasms has been reported.[176]

Difficulties may occur in distinguishing foci of transformation in CLL from poorly differentiated lymphocytic lymphoma. An important feature in CLL is the residual population of well-differentiated lymphocytes. In most instances, examination of the blood and marrow smears aids considerably in distinguishing these two disorders. The concurrence of CLL and mutliple myeloma has been reported.[176]

Prolymphocytic leukemia

Prolymphocytic leukemia (PL), described by Galton et al.,[180] occurs primarily in older individuals and is characterized by a predominant proliferation of more immature lymphocytes referred to as prolymphocytes. Approximately 80% of the cases of this type of leukemia are of B-cell origin; the remainder are of T-cell type.[183] The lymphocyte count is usually markedly elevated and the number of prolymphocytes in the blood exceeds 55% of lymphocytes. The patients with B-cell PL usually have massive splenomegaly without prominent peripheral lymphadenopathy.[184,185] The prolymphocytes in PL are more uniform in appearance than the prolymphocytoid cells in prolymphocytic transforma-

tion of CLL. In PL the prolymphocytes are medium to large in size, with a moderate amount of basophilic cytoplasm (Fig. 23-48). There is usually a single prominent nucleolus. The marrow infiltration may be focal or focal and interstitial; in those with focal involvement the prolymphocytes may be surrounded by well-differentiated lymphocytes. There may be intermixed paraimmunoblasts, larger cells with more prominent nucleoli, and more abundant cytoplasm (Fig. 23-49). Mitotic activity is reported as low, although cases with increased mitotic activity have been observed.[173,188] Prolymphocytic leukemia is usually marked by an aggressive clinical course; occasionally patients have a prolonged survival.

A type of CLL intermediate to typical CLL and PL and referred to as chronic lymphocytic leukemia/prolymphocytic leukemia has been described; it is distinguished by the presence of 11% to 55% prolymphocytes in the blood.[184,185] Typical CLL has less than 11% prolymphocytes in the blood; PL is distinguished by more than 55% prolymphocytes. The degree of splenomegaly in patients with chronic lymphocytic leukemia/prolymphocytic leukemia is disproportionate to the degree of lymphadenopathy. Two major clinical patterns are described in this variant; one is characterized by a course similar to typical CLL and the other by a more rapidly progressive clinical evolution.

Richter's syndrome

Richter's syndrome is the occurrence of a pleomorphic lymphoma in a patient with a prior history of CLL[197-203,207] or another low-grade B lymphoproliferative disorder such as plasmacytoid lymphoma. The reported incidence in CLL is reported as less than 1% to 10%.[207] The syndrome is usually characterized by an abrupt change in clinical course with the onset of fever, weight loss, localized adenopathy, dysglobulinemia, and histopathologic evidence of a pleomorphic lymphoma frequently containing multinucleated giant cells.[207] The focus of transformation is not restricted to hematopoietic organs.[197] A high incidence of lytic bone lesions has been reported.[207] The bone marrow may be involved by the pleomorphic lymphoma; evidence of CLL and the supervening lymphoma may be present in the same biopsy specimen (Fig. 23-50). The blood usually shows no involvement by the pleomorphic cells, and there may be lymphocytopenia. The disorder is marked by an aggressive clinical course and rapid deterioration. The term *Richter's transformation* has been used to describe a somewhat broader spectrum of pathologic findings in patients with CLL who present with a similar clinical evolution.[199]

The biologic events resulting in Richter's transformation are not completely understood, but a dedifferentiation or transformation of the well-differentiated lymphocyte has been suggested.[204] This theory is supported by evidence in some cases of similar surface markers on the cells of the original CLL cells and those of the pleomorphic lymphoma.[196] However, instances in which the cells of the leukemic process and the cells of the pleomorphic lymphoma had dissimilar membrane light chain markers also have been described.[205]

Cases of non-Hodgkin's lymphoma, including small non-cleaved cell lymphoma with the same light chain rearrange-

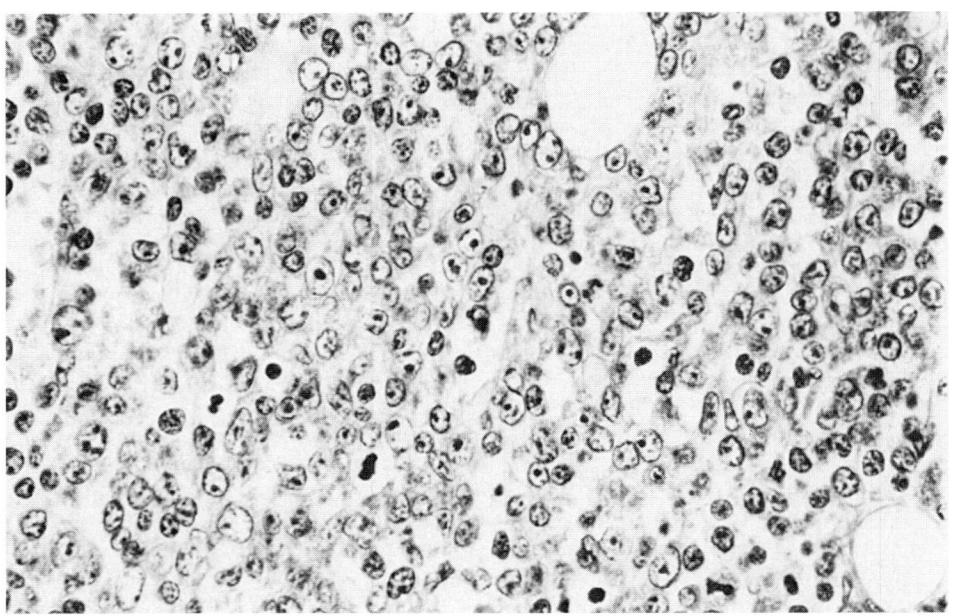

Fig. 23-47 Marrow biopsy from 62-year-old female with 4-year history of untreated chronic lymphocytic leukemia. Biopsy illustrates prolymphocytoid and paraimmunoblastic transformation. There is minor population of interspersed mature lymphocytes.

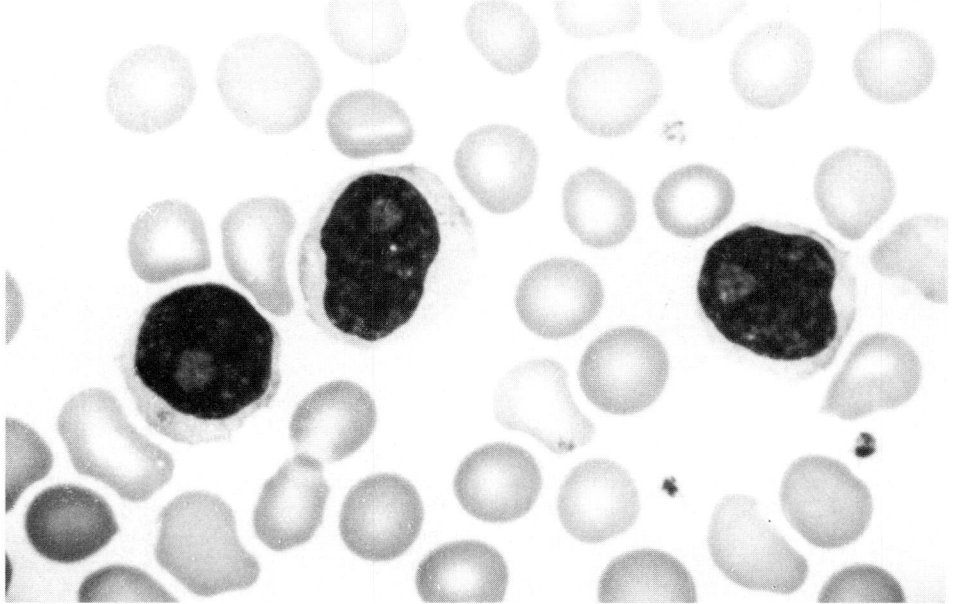

Fig. 23-48 Prolymphocytes in a blood smear from elderly male with B-prolymphocytic leukemia. Cells have single prominent nucleoli and coarse chromatin. (Wright-Giemsa.)

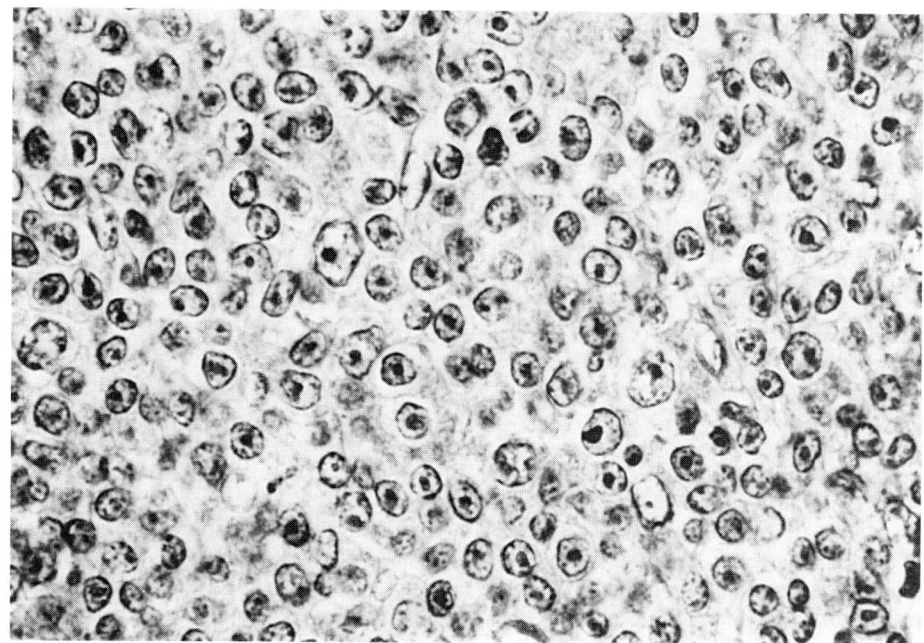

Fig. 23-49 Marrow biopsy from 61-year-old male with PL. Majority of cells have dispersed nuclear chromatin and single, prominent nucleolus. Mitotic figures are sparse.

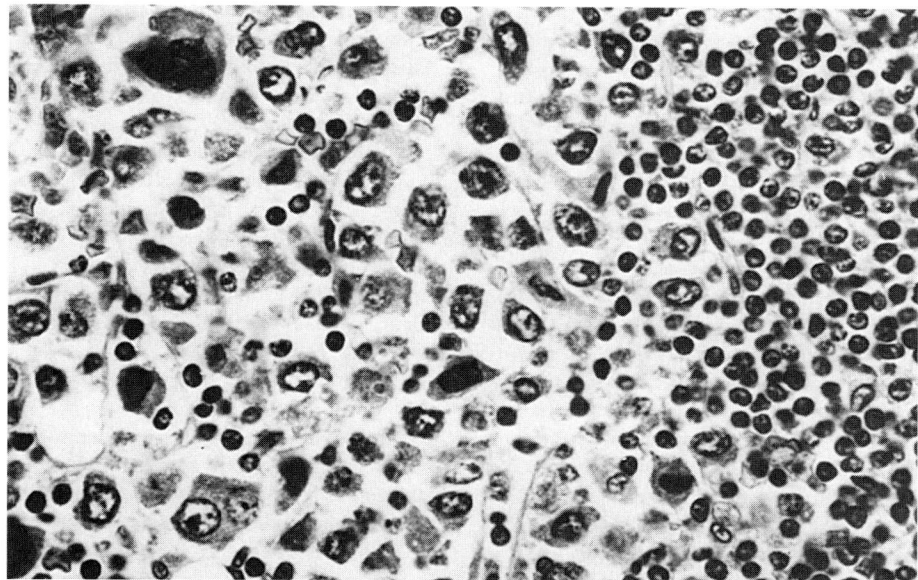

Fig. 23-50 Bone marrow trephine biopsy from patient with history of CLL who developed a pleomorphic lymphoma (B-immunoblastic lymphoma) and a clinical picture typical of Richter's syndrome. Biopsy contains two distinct cell populations, small lymphocytes, and large pleomorphic cells, some of which are multinucleated.

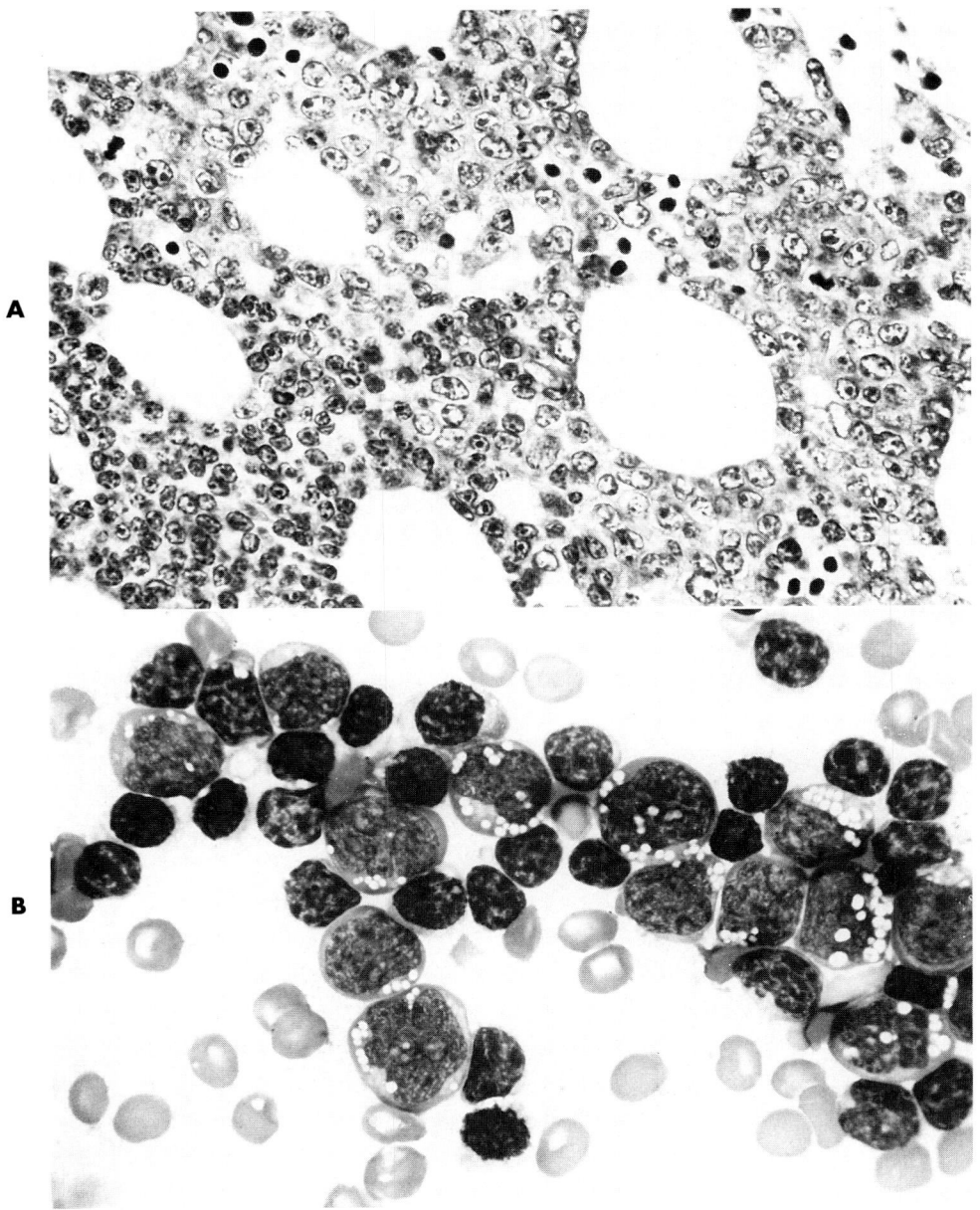

Fig. 23-51 A, Marrow biopsy from adult male with nine-year history of B-cell chronic lymphocytic leukemia. Patient had recent onset of fever, night sweats, myalgia, and axillary, cervical, and inguinal adenopathy. Population of small lymphocytes is at lower left. Small noncleaved lymphoma cells predominate. **B,** Smears contained population of small well-differentiated lymphocytes and small noncleaved lymphoma cells. Cytogenetic studies of the marrow specimen showed t(8;22) (q24;q11) cytogenetic abnormality.

ment on genotypic studies as the lymphocytes of CLL, have been observed[201,206] (Fig. 23-51).

The occurrence of a diffuse histiocytic lymphoma in patients with a prior history of CLL who do not manifest the findings of Richter's syndrome has been reported.[195] In addition, true histiocytic proliferations with no apparent relationship to the B-lymphocyte system may rarely occur in patients with CLL.[208] The clinical course in these patients is very similar to that observed in Richter's syndrome.

Hairy cell leukemia (leukemic reticuloendotheliosis)

Hairy cell leukemia is a chronic lymphoproliferative disorder of B-cell origin that is manifest primarily in blood, marrow, and spleen. It has a male predominance.[210,215,224,226] The age range is 20 to 80 years with a median of approximately 50 years. The patients generally have cytopenias or pancytopenia and splenomegaly without prominent peripheral lymphadenopathy; there is usually an associated monocytopenia. The majority of patients present with leukopenia, and only occasional leukemic cells may be found in the blood. Some 5% to 10% of patients have white blood cell counts exceeding 10×10^9/L; the hairy cells usually comprise the majority of the blood leukocytes in these patients.

The typical hairy cell measures 10 to 14 μm (Fig. 23-52). The clear to lightly basophilic cytoplasm is variable in amount. The surface of the cell is marked by numerous delicate and broad projections; this finding is particularly striking in specimens examined by phase and electron microscopy[219,228] (Fig. 23-53). Vacuoles and occasionally delicate azurophilic granules may be identified in the cytoplasm. The nucleus is oval, folded, or indented; the chromatin is coarsely reticular, and nucleoli are inconspicuous.

Aspiration biopsy of the marrow in patients with hairy cell leukemia is unsuccessful in 30% to 50% of cases

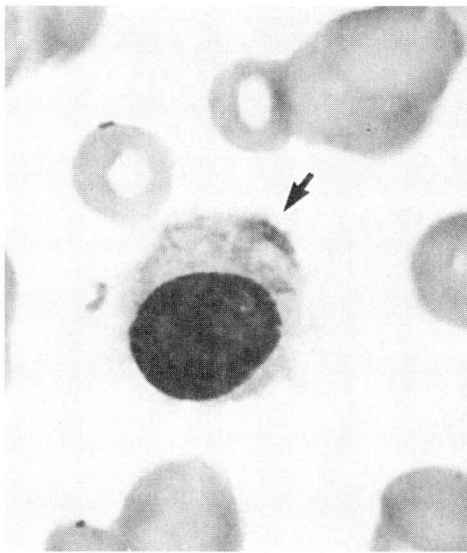

Fig. 23-52 Leukemic cell in blood smear of patient with hairy cell leukemia. Cytoplasm is marked by delicate projections; ribosome lamella complexes are noted in one area of cytoplasm (arrow). (Wright-Giemsa.)

because of increased reticulin fibrosis.[215,224] The pattern of marrow infiltration is virtually diagnostic in most patients.[211,212,214,230,232] The involvement may be diffuse or partial; the diffuse type is more common (Fig. 23-54). The marrow in the majority of patients is hypercellular; in 10% to 15% of patients the involved marrow is hypocellular.[221] Leukemic infiltrates in partial involvement are irregular in outline and poorly demarcated from the normal marrow cells (Fig. 23-55). In very early stages of the disease, partial involvement may take the form of relatively small, indistinctly outlined foci of leukemic cells. Reactivity with B-cell antibodies accentuates the marrow infiltrations[216] (Fig. 23-56). In formalin-fixed tissue, there is frequently a halo-like effect or clear area around the nucleus because of the abundant cytoplasm.[212] The cell borders have an interlocking appearance. With some fixatives, such as Zenker's, the cytoplasm of the hairy cells is retracted with a resultant loosely structured appearance (see Fig. 23-54). The loosely structured appearance and widely spaced nuclei in hairy cell leukemia contrast to the marrow infiltrates in the lymphocytic lymphomas and CLL in which the nuclei of the cells are in close apposition. The nuclear chromatin of the hairy cells is relatively fine. Nucleoli are distinct but not usually prominent, and mitotic figures are infrequent. In an occasional case, the hairy cells have a spindled or fusiform appearance and may resemble the marrow lesions in systemic mastocytosis (Fig. 23-57). A morphologic variant with hyperlobated nuclei resembling T-cell lymphoma has been described.[217] Marrow uninvolved by the leukemic process may be hypocellular or hypercellular. Morphologic subtypes of hairy cell leukemia based on histopathology have been reported to have prognostic significance.[209]

Reticulin stain shows increased deposition of thickened reticulin fibers in the areas of the infiltrates; the reticulin fibers often appear to encircle individual cells (see Fig. 23-54). The reticulin fibers frequently extend into the adjacent normal-appearing marrow.

An important diagnostic procedure in hairy cell leukemia is the demonstration of tartrate-resistant acid phosphatase in the leukemic cells.[218,224] Other lymphoproliferative disorders in which the proliferating cells have tartrate-resistant acid phosphatase have been described; however, these cases are uncommon and do not negate the diagnostic importance of this finding for hairy cell leukemia. Nonspecific esterase positivity also has been demonstrated.[231]

Hairy cells express light chain–restricted cytoplasmic and surface immunoglobulin and pan–B-cell antibodies, including CD19 and CD20.[227] In addition, they express CD11c, which is expressed on myeloid cells; CD25; interleukin-2 receptor; and B-LY-7. They are negative for CD5, a T-cell antigen, which is expressed on the lymphocytes in the majority of cases of B-cell chronic lymphocytic leukemia.

A vascular lesion marked by perivascular and mural leukemia infiltrate has been reported in hairy cell leukemia.[220] This lesion is found in the medium- and large-sized vessels and may involve multiple organs.

Treatment of hairy cell leukemia with the nucleoside analogs results in durable complete or partial remissions in the majority of cases.[225,226,229] The bone marrow biopsies from these patients generally show a return to normal with

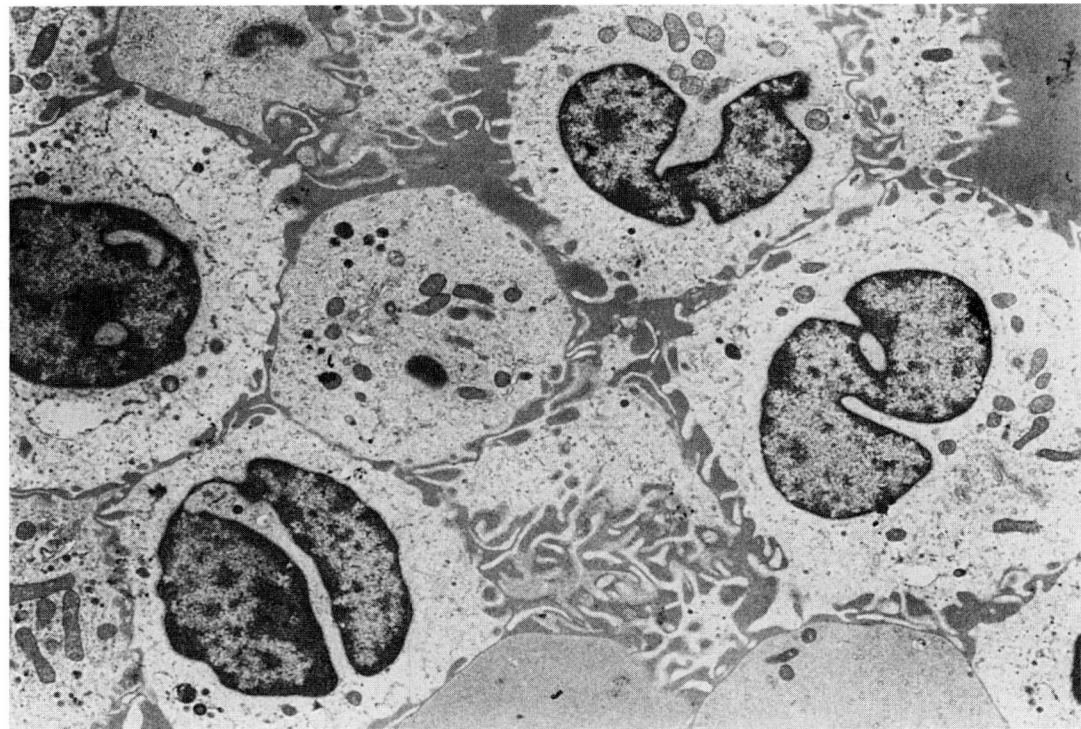

Fig. 23-53 Electron micrograph of several cells from blood of patient with hairy cell leukemia. Numerous delicate cytoplasmic strands project from cell surfaces. Nuclei are irregular in outline and show margination of chromatin. Nucleoli are relatively inconspicuous. (Uranyl acetate–lead citrate; ×5000.)

normal marrow hematopoiesis. Recognition of residual leukemia is facilitated with the use of pan–B-cell monoclonal antibodies reactive in paraffin-embedded biopsies.[216] Treatment with the interferons frequently results in characteristic marrow changes.[223]

Hairy cell leukemia variant

Hairy cell leukemia variant is a lymphoproliferative disorder usually presenting with a marked leukocytosis and lymphocytes with morphologic characteristics intermediate to hairy cells and prolymphocytes.[210,213,222,224] The cells are large with basophilic cytoplasm with villous projections and relatively prominent nucleoli. The disease is rare and occurs primarily in older individuals. In contrast to typical hairy cell leukemia, there is no associated neutropenia and monocytopenia. The cells may be TRAP positive. The cells in some cases express CD11c but are negative for CD25.[210] The pattern of splenic infiltration is similar to hairy cell leukemia, with a predominantly red pulp involvement. Hairy cell leukemia variant has a prolonged clinical course. Unlike typical hairy cell leukemia, the patients may not respond to treatment with interferons or nucleoside analogs.

Splenic lymphoma with villous lymphocytes

Splenic lymphoma with villous lymphocytes is a proliferation of small B lymphocytes with clinical and hematologic features similar to hairy cell leukemia.[234,235] The disease is more common in males; the mean age at presentation is 72 years. There is a slight to moderate lymphocytosis; the leuko-

cyte count is less than $25 \times 10^9/L$ in the majority of patients. Anemia and thrombocytopenia are present in approximately 50% of cases. Most patients have marked splenomegaly.

The lymphocytes in the blood have short villous projections that may have a polar distribution. Villi may not be present on all of the lymphoma cells, and there may be considerable variation in the appearance of the cells. Some have a distinct but not prominent nucleolus (Fig. 23-58, *A*). Plasmacytoid lymphocytes may be present.

The lymphocytes express moderate to intense surface immunoglobulin and pan–B-lymphocyte markers CD19, CD22, and CD24.[233] The cells express CD5 and CD25 in 19% and 25% of cases, respectively. In approximately half of the cases the lymphocytes express CD11c. The cells may be TRAP positive. Approximately 50% to 60% of cases have a modest IgM monoclonal gammopathy.[234] Some 25% of cases are reported to have an associated t(11;14) chromosome abnormality.[235]

The extent of marrow involvement varies. It is usually focal and may be paratrabecular or nonparatrabecular (Fig. 23-58, *B*). The spleen shows primarily white pulp involvement with involvement of the red pulp in some cases. A predominantly marginal zone pattern may be present. The cytologic features may resemble those of a plasmacytoid lymphoma.

Patients with splenic lymphoma with villous lymphocytes generally have a prolonged clinical course. Splenectomy is frequently beneficial in patients with severe anemia, neutropenia, and thrombocytopenia.

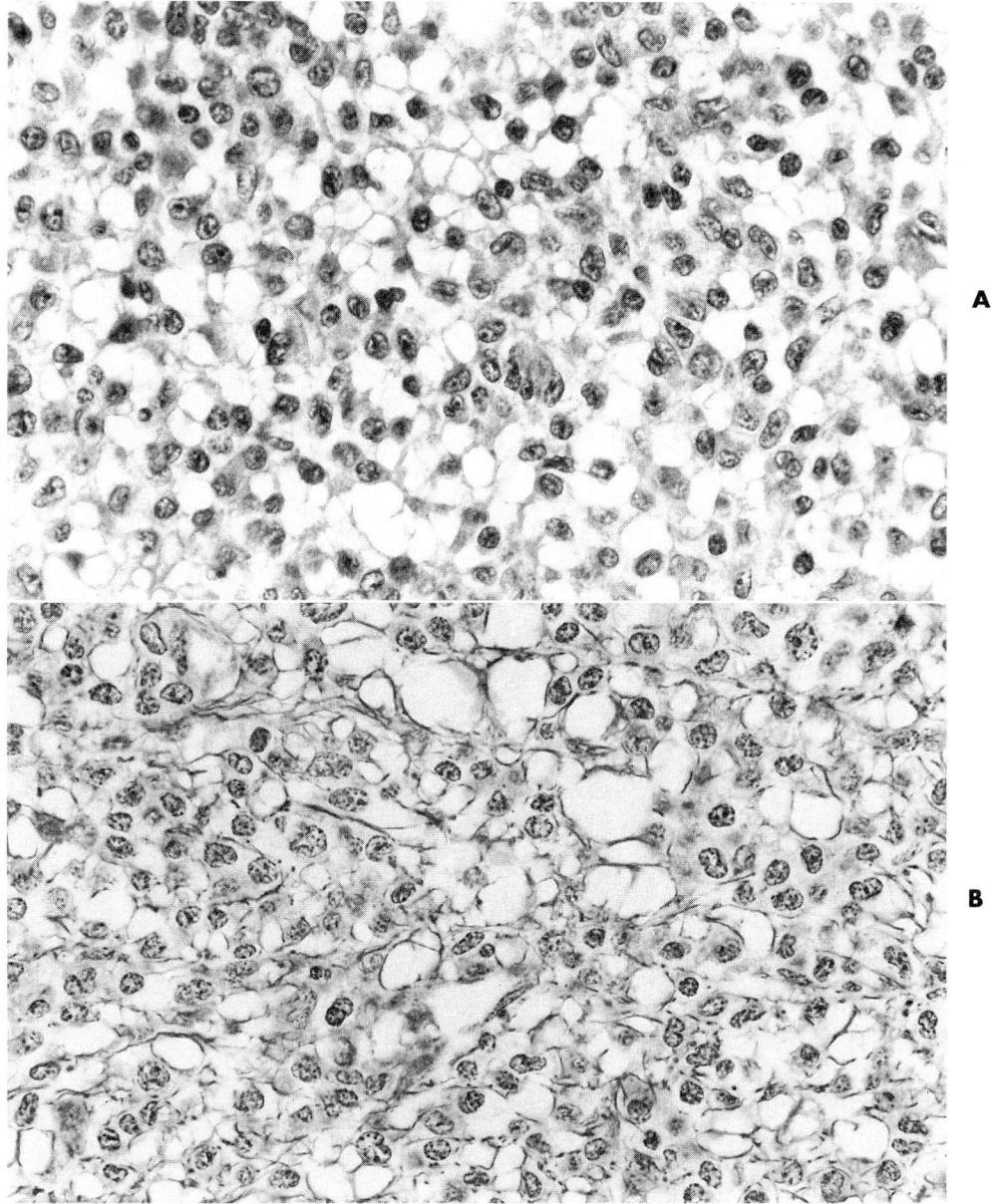

Fig. 23-54 A, Bone marrow section from patient with hairy cell leukemia. Hairy cells are loosely spaced in contrast to aggregates of lymphocytes in chronic lymphocytic leukemia and small lymphocyte lymphomas. Many of nuclei are folded or irregular in outline. Nucleoli are inconspicuous. Mitotic figures are rare. Halo effect around nuclei, characteristic of formalin-fixed tissue, is not prominent in this specimen fixed with Zenker's. **B,** Reticulin stain of bone marrow section from patient with hairy cell leukemia. Thickened and increased reticulin fibers are present. (**B** Wilder's reticulin.)

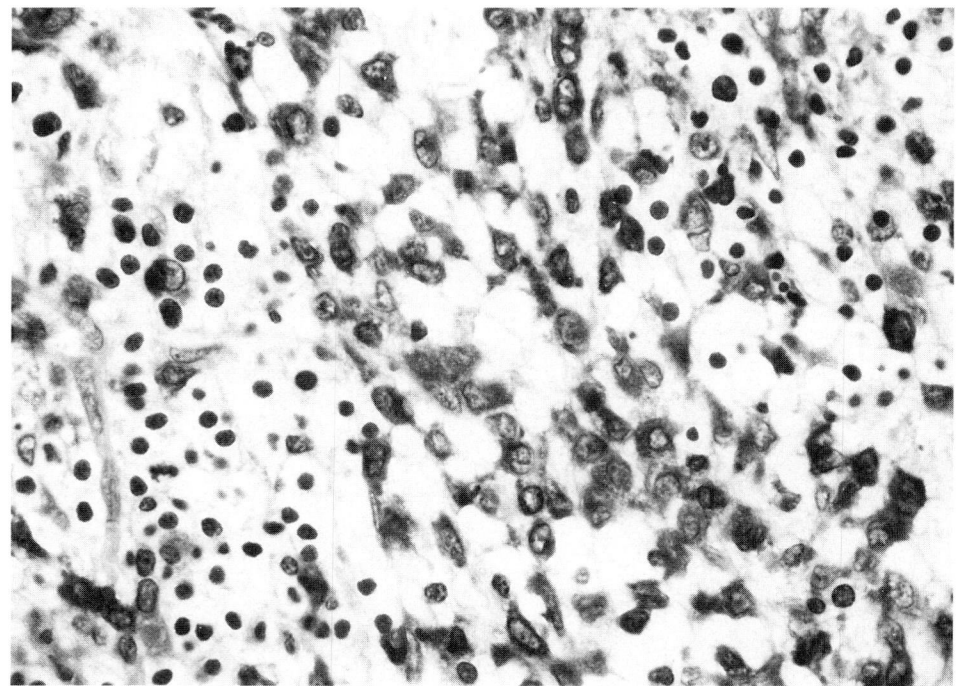

Fig. 23-55 Focus of hairy cell leukemia in marrow with partial involvement. Hairy cell infiltrate is poorly demarcated from adjacent normal marrow cells, predominantly erythroid precursors.

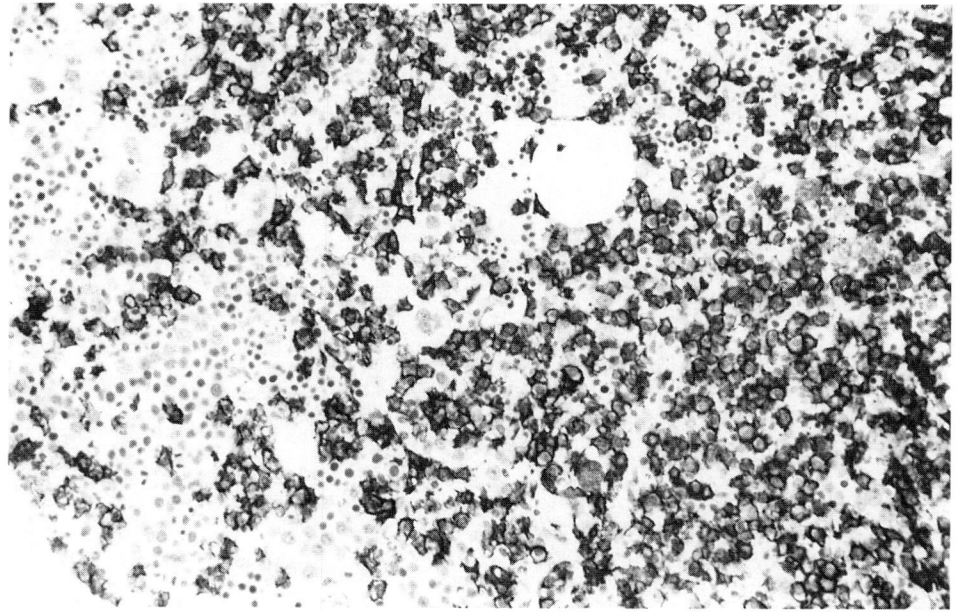

Fig. 23-56 Bone marrow biopsy from patient with hairy cell leukemia reacted with antibody to CD20 (L26). Reactivity accentuates leukemic infiltrate. Scattered normal myeloid cells, principally erythroid precursors, are present. (Peroxidase-antiperoxidase.)

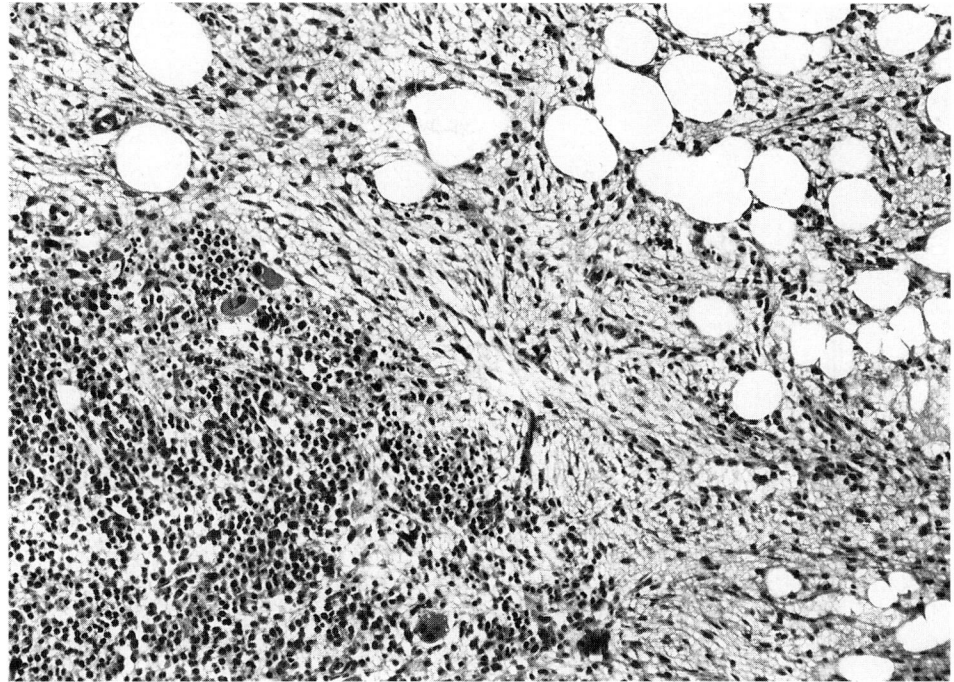

Fig. 23-57 Marrow biopsy from patient with hairy cell leukemia with partial marrow involvement. Many of leukemia cells have elongated spindle shape.

Sézary syndrome

Sézary syndrome is a lymphoproliferative disorder of T helper cells characterized by erythrodema and abnormal lymphoid cells in the blood.[236,239,241] The leukocyte count may be normal or markedly elevated with a high percentage of Sézary cells. The Sézary cells, as observed in Romanovsky-stained blood smears, have distinctive features. The nucleus frequently has an unusual configuration that has been characterized as cerebriform (Fig. 23-59). Cytoplasmic vacuoles, which stain positively with the PAS reaction, may be present in a perinuclear location. Large and small cell variants have been described.[237] Ultrastructurally, the cells show marked nuclear convolutions[237,238,240] (Fig. 23-60). The bone marrow sections in the majority of patients appear normal; scattered Sézary cells randomly infiltrate the interstitium. Obvious marrow infiltration with replacement of normal hematopoietic cells is very uncommon. Rarely small aggregates of Sézary cells may be observed.[236]

NON-HODGKIN'S LYMPHOMA

The incidence of marrow involvement in non-Hodgkin's lymphoma at the time of initial diagnosis varies with the different histopathologic subtypes; the incidence in aggregate for all types ranges from 40% to 55% in most of the larger studies of adults, using the Working Formulation, Rappaport, and Lukes and Collins' classifications.* The incidence of marrow involvement is substantially higher, approximately 70%, in studies using the Kiel classification, which includes CLL and hairy cell leukemia, diseases in which marrow involvement is always present. The incidence is higher in the low-grade lymphomas than in many of the high-grade lymphomas. Approximately 60% to 70% of the cases of small cleaved cell lymphoma have marrow involvement at the time of initial diagnosis in contrast to 33% for T-immunoblastic sarcoma and 25% for B-immunoblastic sarcoma.[262] Intermediate differentiated lymphocytic lymphoma has a 70% incidence of marrow involvement.[260] Bone marrow involvement in monocytoid B-cell lymphoma is reported in 20% to 25% of cases.[257] The incidence of marrow involvement in peripheral T-cell or node-based T-cell lymphoma varies from 30% to 70% in different series.[251,252] Blood involvement may occur with all types of lymphoma.[242,249,253,254]

The pattern of marrow involvement may be diffuse, focal paratrabecular, focal nonparatrabecular, or interstitial (Fig. 23-61). The diffuse and focal nonparatrabecular patterns may occur with all types of lymphoma of both B- and T-cell origin. The focal paratrabecular pattern occurs principally but not exclusively in the follicular center cell lymphomas, predominantly small cleaved cell type; these lymphomas may also involve the marrow in a focal nonparatrabecular pattern (Figs. 23-62 to 23-64). The marrow biopsies from patients with mantle cell lymphoma (lymphoma of intermediate differentiation) and monocytoid B-cell lymphoma may also show both focal paratrabecular and nonparatrabecular lesions (Fig. 23-65). The infiltrate in an occasional case of mantle cell lymphoma may contain a naked germinal center (Fig. 23-65, *B* and *C*).

*References 247, 249, 250, 255, 256, 258.

Text continued on p. 1852.

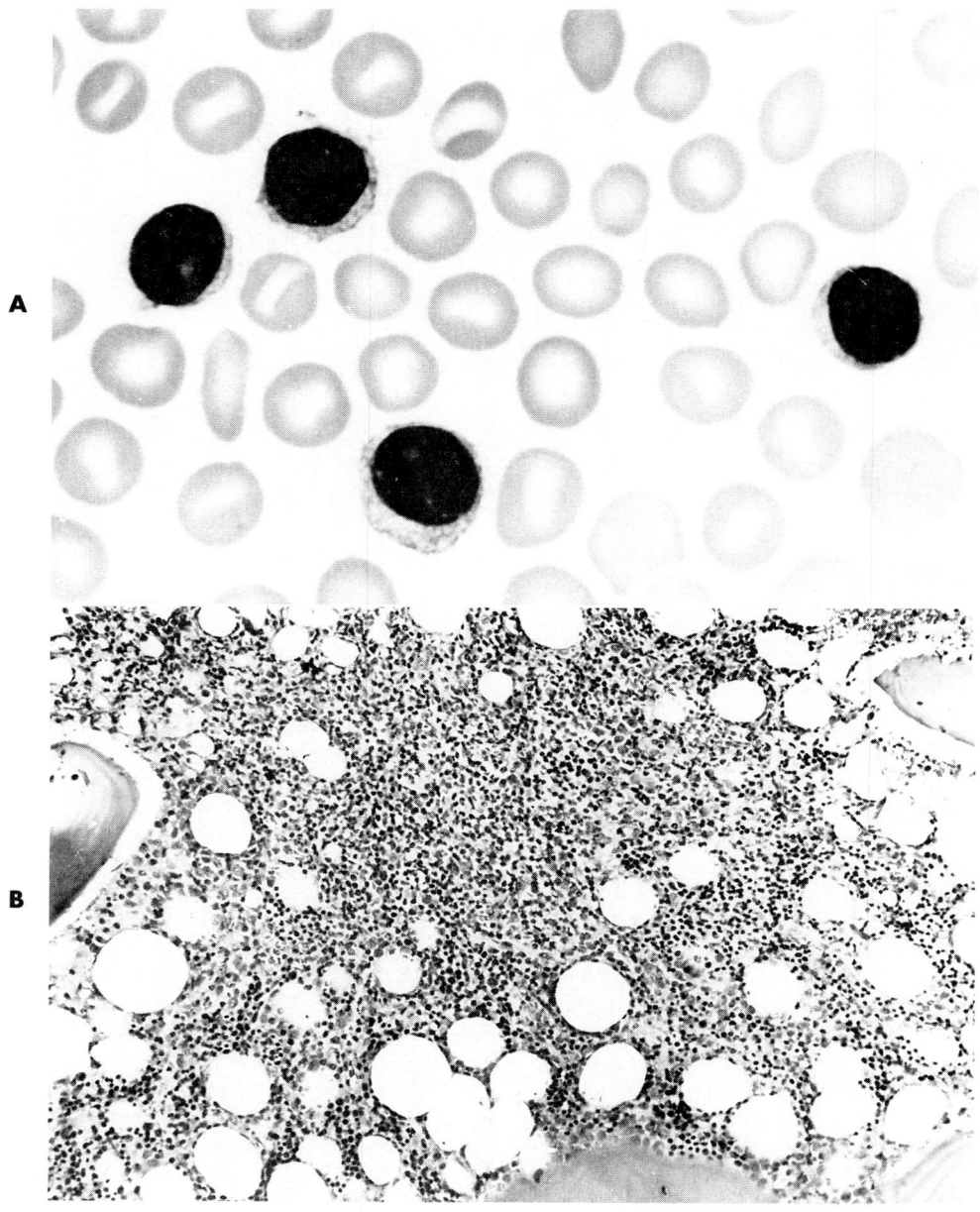

Fig. 23-58 A, Lymphocytes in blood smear from adult male with splenic lymphoma with villous lymphocytes. Cytoplasm of two of lymphocytes in upper left has small villous projections. Nuclear chromatin is coarse. Two cells have distinct but not prominent nucleoli. (Wright-Giemsa.) **B,** Bone marrow biopsy from patient with splenic lymphoma with villous lymphocytes showing nonparatrabecular, poorly demarcated aggregate of lymphocytes.

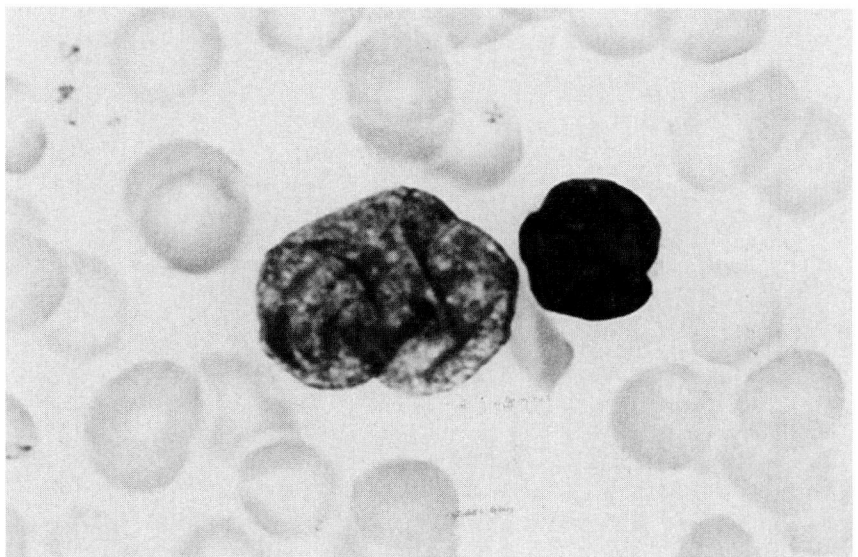

Fig. 23-59 Large Sézary cell with "cerebriform" nucleus in peripheral blood of patient with erythroderma. Nucleus of this Sézary cell shows striking degree of convolution. Smaller lymphocyte also has convoluted nucleus. (Wright-Giemsa.)

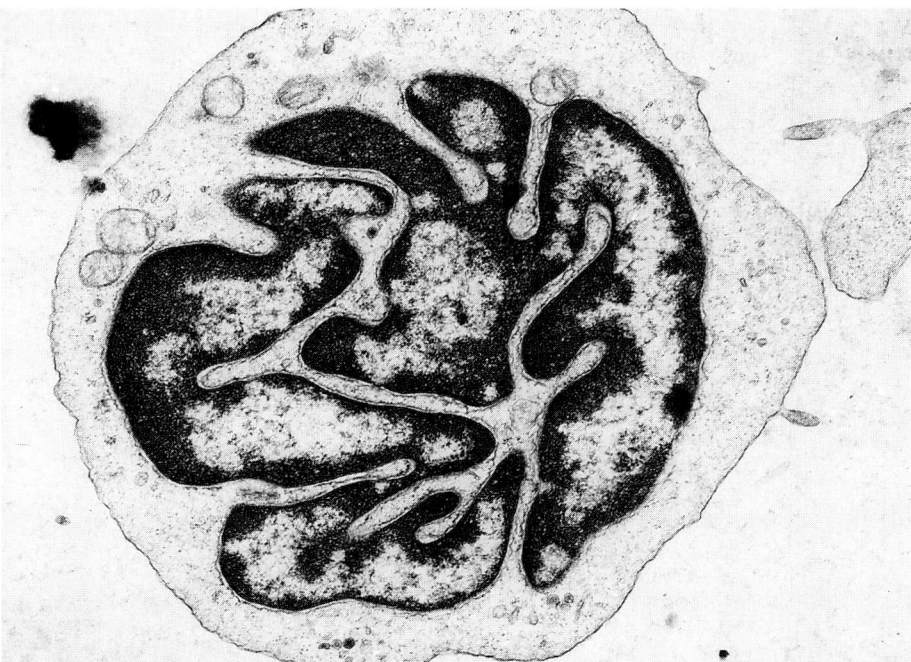

Fig. 23-60 Electron micrograph of Sézary cell. Extreme convolution of nucleus is characteristic ultrastructural feature of Sézary cells. (Uranyl acetate–lead citrate; ×22,000.)

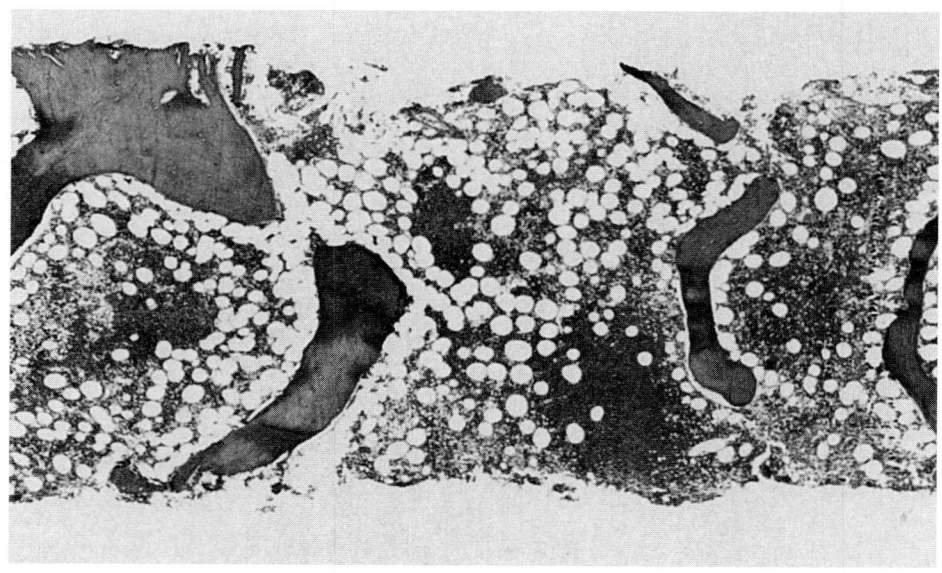

Fig. 23-61 Several focal aggregates of lymphocytes in marrow in patient with well-differentiated lymphocytic lymphoma. Foci of lymphocytes vary in size and have irregular, poorly circumscribed outlines.

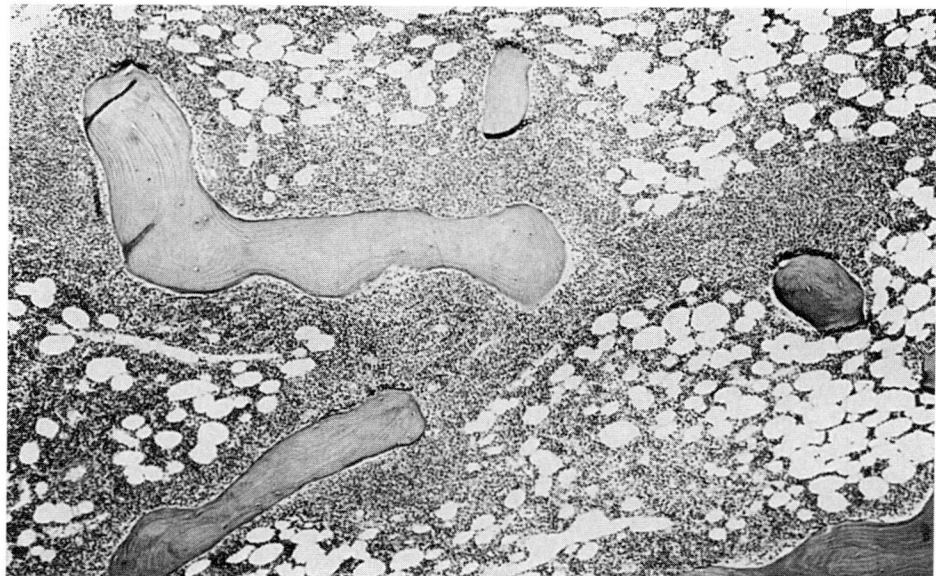

Fig. 23-62 Bone marrow section from patient with follicular small cleaved cell lymphoma illustrating prominent paratrabecular distribution of infiltrate.

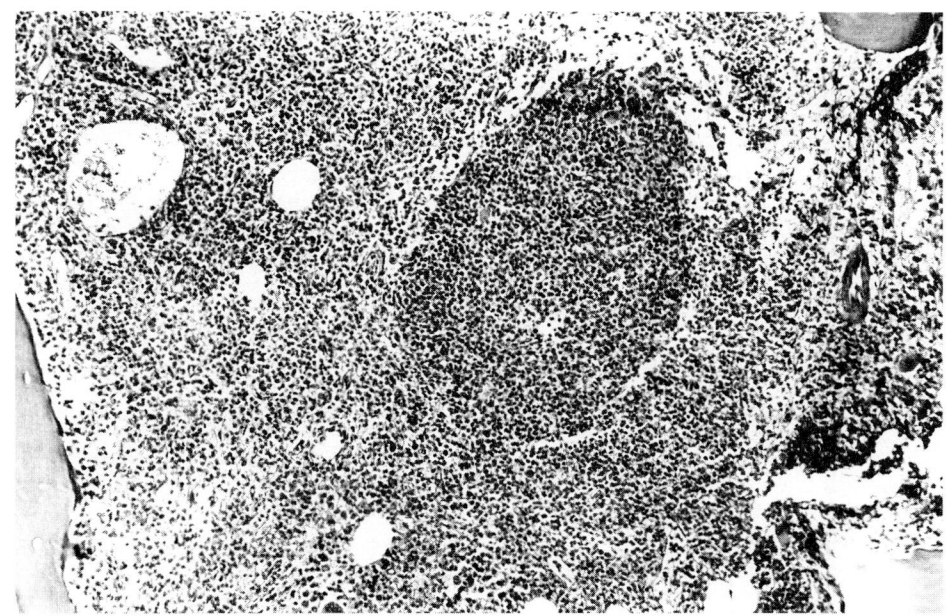

Fig. 23-63 Marrow from patient with extensive blood and marrow involvement by small cleaved cell lymphoma. Lymphoma cells diffusely infiltrate the interstitium and form cluster resembling neoplastic follicle.

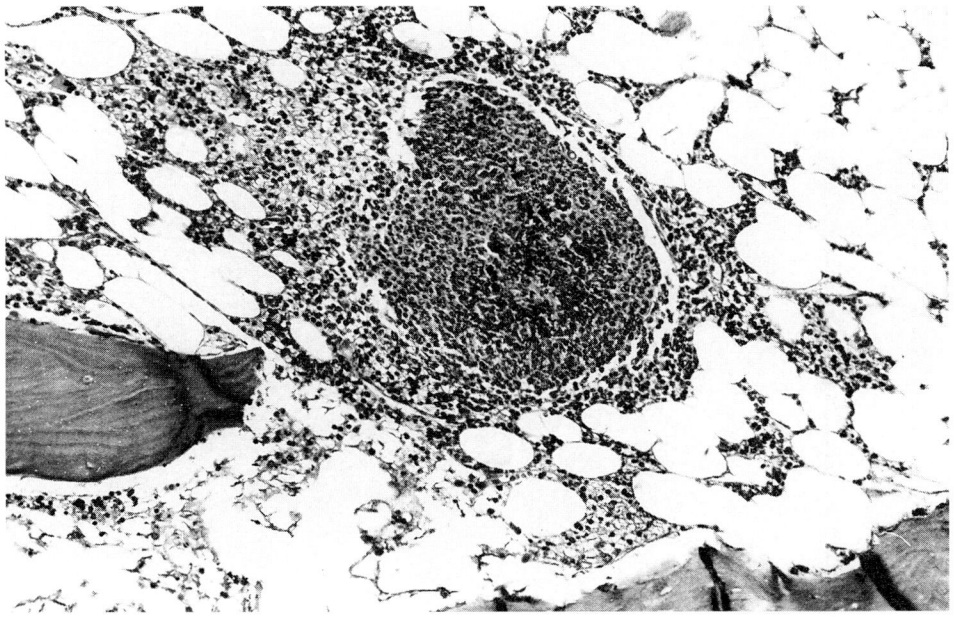

Fig. 23-64 Marrow biopsy from patient with small cleaved cell lymphoma with focal paratrabecular and nonparatrabecular involvement. Few of the nonparatrabecular foci, as illustrated, appear to recapitulate neoplastic follicles. Amorphous eosinophilic proteinaceous debris is deposited in central portion of lesion.

The interstitial pattern of involvement, in which the lymphoma cells infiltrate the interstitium of the marrow with preservation of the overall marrow architecture with some sparing of normal hematopoiesis, is uncommon but may occur with all types of non-Hodgkin's lymphoma. The bone marrow in this type of involvement may be deceptively normal appearing at low magnification (Fig. 23-66). This pattern of infiltration may be present at the time of initial diagnosis or in patients who have received chemotherapy.

The extent of lymphomatous infiltration varies considerably; it is less than 30% in more than half of cases with involvement.[250] In general, the small lymphocytic and small cleaved cell lymphomas are characterized by substantial sparing of normal bone marrow. In post-chemotherapy specimens, paratrabecular lesions may have a loosely structured hypocellular appearance.[259]

The cytopathology of the lesions in the marrow sections usually parallels the cytologic characteristics in the lymph node; this is particularly true for the T-cell lymphomas and small noncleaved cell lymphoma.[243,244] In approximately 20% to 25% of lymphomas there may be discordance between the predominant cell type in the lymph node and the predominant cell type in the marrow.[246,248,261] In these cases, the marrow lesions usually consist of small cleaved cells, and the lymph node findings are a mixed or large cell type; the converse occurs but is less frequent. In either instance, the cytologic characteristics in both sites are usually those of follicular center cell lymphoma. Similar to the findings in lymph nodes, lymphomas of predominantly small lymphocytes in the marrow may show foci of transformation. In occasional cases of small cleaved cell lymphoma, the transformed cells may resemble Reed-Sternberg cells or Reed-Sternberg mononuclear variants[255] (Fig. 23-67).

The follicular pattern of follicular or nodular lymphoma as seen in lymph nodes is uncommonly reflected in the marrow lesions (see Figs. 23-63 and 23-64). Occasionally foci of transformation may mimic follicle formation. As noted, naked germinal centers may be found in occasional cases of intermediate differentiated lymphocytic lymphoma (see Fig. 23-65). In some marrow lesions of small cleaved cell lymphoma, the margins of the lymphomatous focus may be composed of transforming cells, imparting a somewhat reverse germinal center character to the lesion. The paratrabecular lesions may show a zoning phenomenon with a less differentiated population of cells immediately adjacent to the endosteal surface.

There is no relationship between a diffuse or follicular pattern in the lymph node and the presence of focal or diffuse lesions in the marrow. Cases in which the lymph node has a diffuse pattern of involvement such as small lymphocytic lymphoma may manifest as focal lesions in the marrow. Granulomas may be found in all types of lymphomas in the marrow, with and without marrow involvement.[245]

Unusual variants of non-Hodgkin's lymphoma involving marrow may lead to diagnostic problems because of the unusual morphology of the lymphoma cells or because of an accompanying proliferation of reactive cells. In anaplastic large cell lymphoma, the lymphoma cells may by virtue of size and nuclear irregularity mimic megakaryocytes. The problem is accentuated when the foci of lymphoma are small and indistinctly demarcated from the surrounding normal marrow tissue or when the lymphoma cells are intermingled with normal marrow cells (Fig. 23-68). Appropriate antibody studies including CD30 and CD45 expression are important in clarifying the origin of the abnormal cells.[250a] The lymphoma cells in histiocyte-rich B-cell lymphoma and

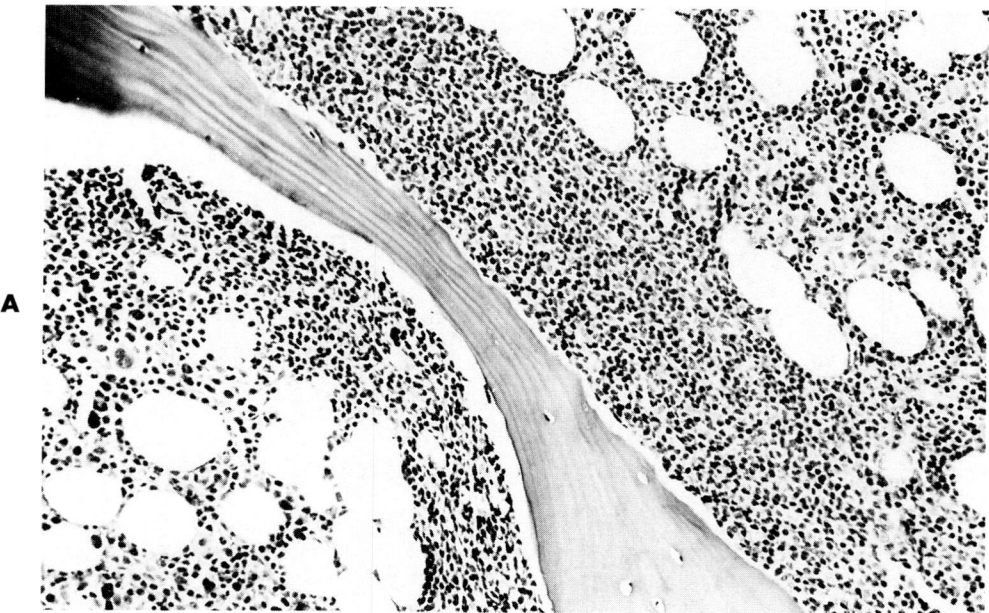

Fig. 23-65 A, Bone marrow biopsy from adult male with extensive blood and marrow involvement by mantle cell lymphoma. Lymphoma cells expressed pan–B-cell markers, CD5, and intense surface immunoglobulin. In areas, lymphoma marginates along the bone trabecula.   *Continued.*

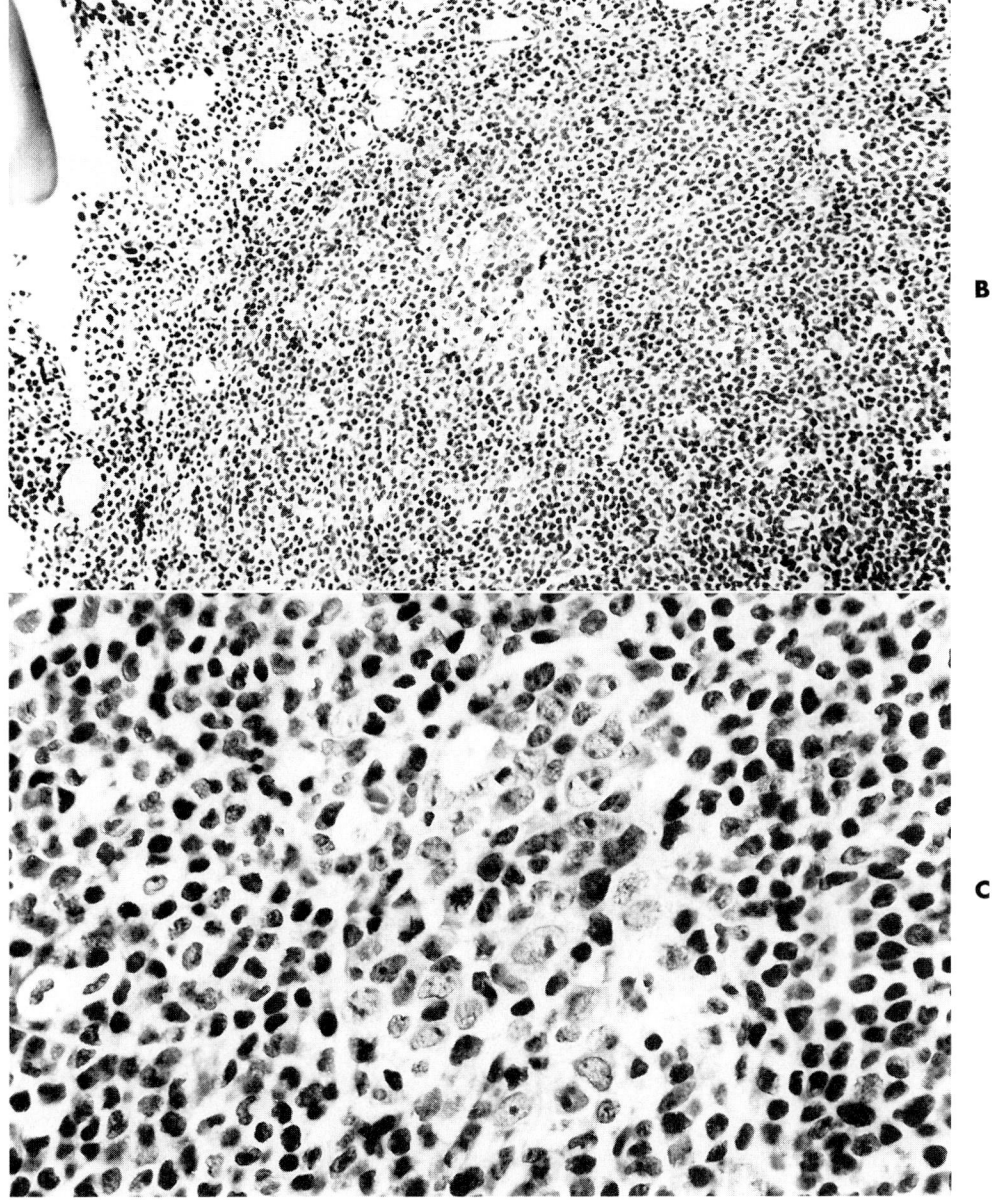

Fig. 23-65, cont'd **B,** Focus of marrow involvement from same biopsy showing structure with characteristics of naked germinal center. **C,** High magnification of naked germinal center.

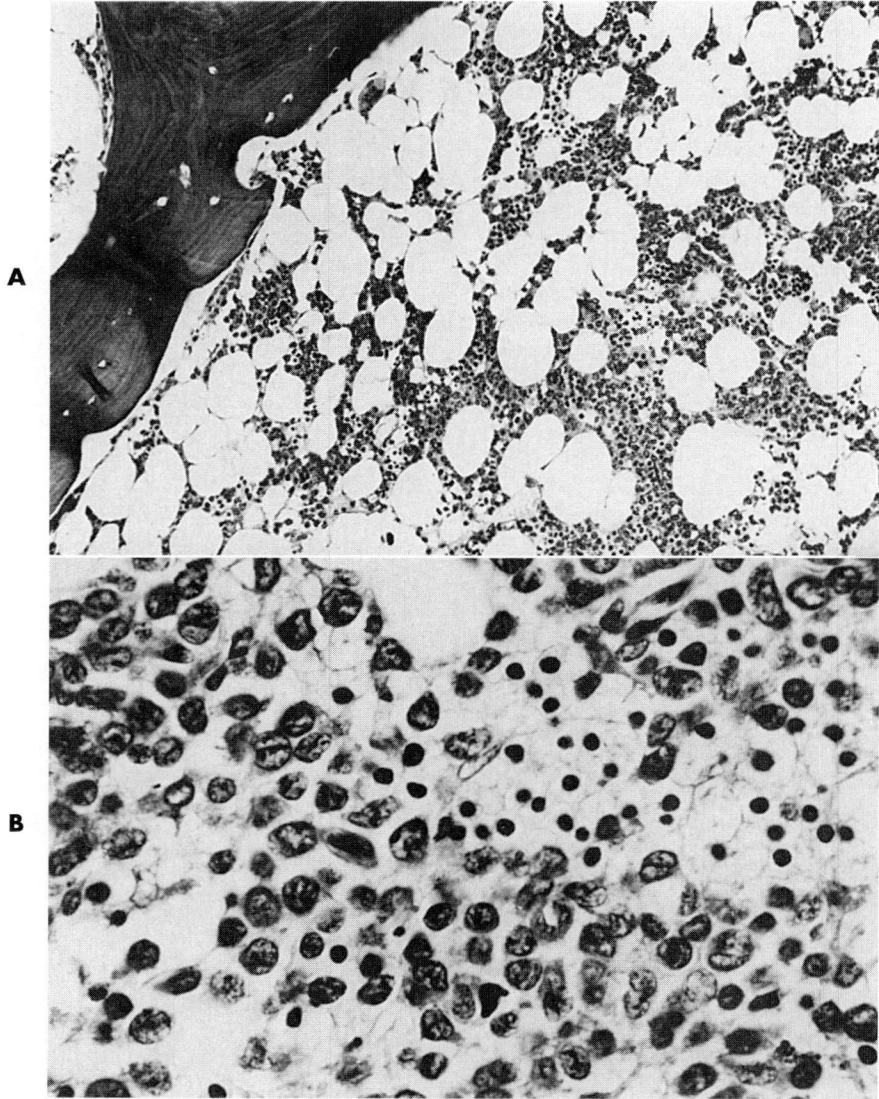

Fig. 23-66 A, Marrow biopsy from patient being treated for small cleaved cell lymphoma. At this magnification, marrow architecture appears normal. **B,** Higher magnification of specimen in **A** shows diffuse infiltration of interstitium by population of small lymphocytes, several of which have irregular and cleaved nuclei.

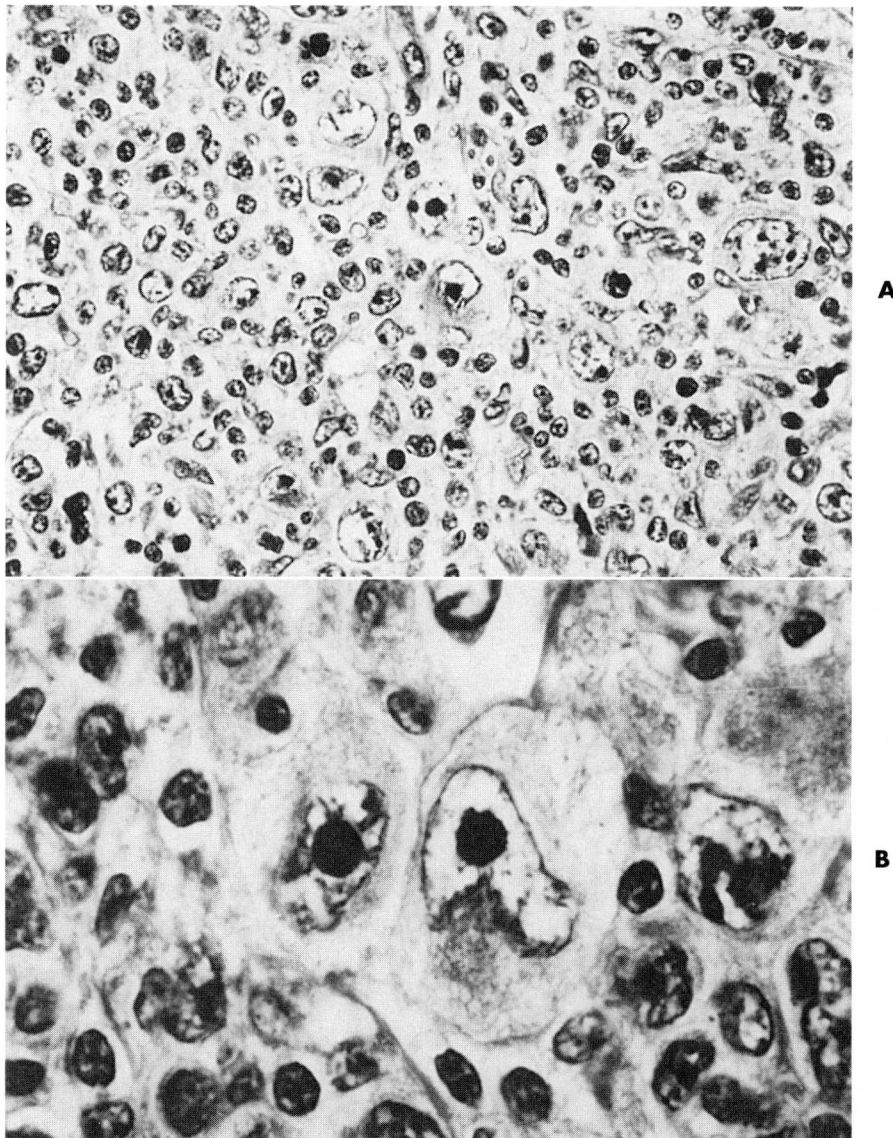

Fig. 23-67 A, Focus of large, poorly differentiated cells in marrow of patient with follicular small cleaved cell lymphoma. Numerous small cells, more typical of this lesion, are also present. **B,** Bone marrow section from patient with 6-year history of follicular small cleaved cell lymphoma. Two large cells resembling Reed-Sternberg mononuclear variants are present.

T-cell–rich B-cell lymphoma may be partially obscured by the non malignant cell proliferation.[246a] In T-cell–rich B-cell lymphoma, antibody studies may accentuate the problem because of the large number of lymphocytes reacting with antibodies to T cells; demonstration of light chain restriction by flow cytometry or genotype studies for immunoglobulin gene arrangement may be necessary to establish clonal B-cell lineage. In histiocyte-rich B-cell lymphoma, reactions with antibodies to B lymphocytes such as L26 (CD20) and histiocytes (CD68) are useful in delineating the two cell populations (Fig. 23-69).

Peripheral T-cell lymphoma

Peripheral T-cell (post-thymic or node-based T-cell) lymphoma (PTCL) has such unusual features in bone marrow biopsies as to warrant separate consideration.[264,265] This type of lymphoma is characterized by a high incidence of marrow involvement at time of initial diagnosis, up to 60% to 70% in some studies.[263] The marrow lesions are diffuse in approximately 60% of involved cases and focal in 40%. The focal lesions are usually randomly distributed in contrast to the preferential paratrabecular involvement in follicular center cell lymphomas; occasional cases present with a paratra-

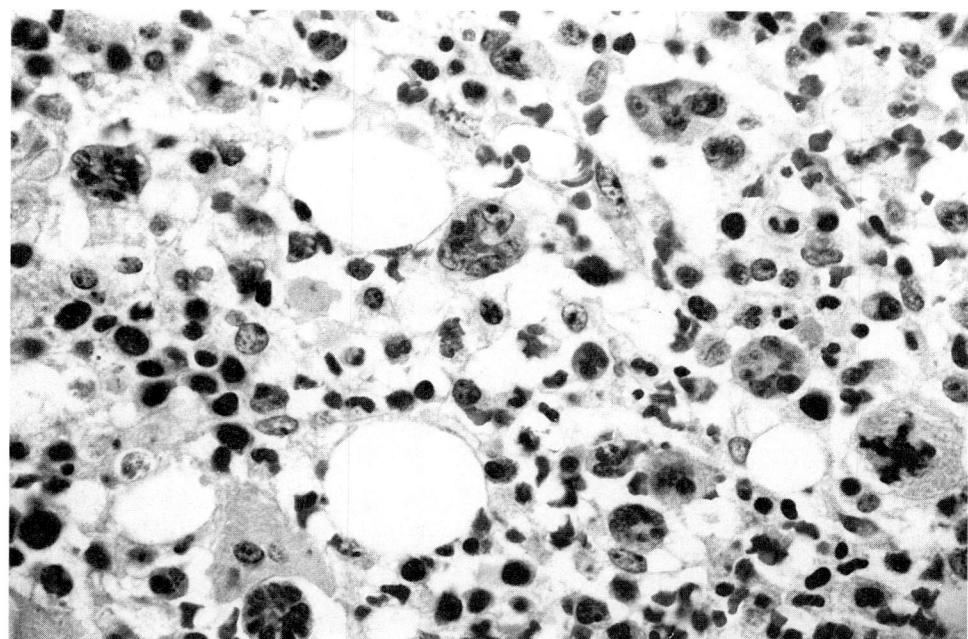

Fig. 23-68 Area of marrow biopsy from a patient with CD30-positive anaplastic large cell lymphoma. The lymphoma cells are intermixed with normal marrow cells.

becular pattern. The infiltrates vary substantially in size and are usually irregular in configuration with poorly demarcated margins; in many instances the lesions appear to extend almost imperceptibly into adjacent normal marrow (Fig. 23-70). The diffuse lesions are characterized by complete intertrabecular replacement of marrow; in some instances the entire biopsy specimen is replaced (Fig. 23-71). Increased reticulin fibers are present in the area of lymphomatous involvement, and reticulin fibers frequently extend into the adjacent normal-appearing marrow.

The predominant cytologic pattern in the marrow lesions usually corresponds to the pattern in lymph node or other tissue biopsies and can generally be categorized into one of three primary histopathologic types: small lymphocytic, mixed cell, and large cell/immunoblastic. The mixed cell type is the most frequent. In some instances there is a relatively distinct demarcation between large and small cells. Large lymphoid cells with abundant amphophilic cytoplasm and prominent eosinophilic nucleoli (see Fig 23-71), cells resembling Reed-Sternberg cells, and mononuclear Reed-Sternberg variants may be present. The small- and medium-sized lymphocytes have nuclei with condensed chromatin and vary from regular to irregular in outline. The mixed cell and large cell/immunoblastic types usually have an associated polycellular infiltrate consisting of histiocytes, plasma cells, eosinophils, and neutrophils. Epithelioid histiocytes are frequently noted either in focal clusters or scattered throughout the lesions. The focal collections frequently have a granulomatous appearance. Increased vascularity is a prominent feature of the mixed and large cell types; the vascular component is primarily an endothelial cell proliferation with straight-lined channels.

The differential diagnosis of PTCL in marrow includes Hodgkin's disease, systemic mastocytosis, angioimmunoblastic lymphadenopathy, and polymorphous reactive lymphoid hyperplasia.[263] The most difficult problem relates to the last lesion, which may be present in marrow from patients with a wide variety of immunologic disorders, including AIDS. Polymorphous reactive lymphoid hyperplasia has many histopathologic features similar to PTCL, including a heterogenous population of lymphocytes with intermixed plasma cells, immunoblasts, eosinophils, endothelial cells, and epithelioid histiocytes. Distinction between the focal lesion of PTCL and the polymorphous reactive lymphoid lesions may not be possible solely on morphologic features. Markedly atypical cells with prominent nucleoli are more compatible with lymphoma. The size of the lesions is not always a reliable distinguishing feature; reactive lesions may show extensive marrow replacement, particularly in patients with AIDS. The lesions of PTCL may be relatively small.

Hodgkin's disease in the marrow may appear similar to the lesions of PTCL. The presence of classic Reed-Sternberg cells and the lack of atypia in the lymphocyte population is evidence of Hodgkin's disease. Multinucleated immunoblasts resembling Reed-Sternberg cells may be present in PTCL; in these instances, review of lymph nodes and other tissue biopsies and immunologic studies are critical in distinguishing PTCL from Hodgkin's disease.

The lesions of PTCL in the marrow may be virtually indistinguishable from AILD. The distinction in these instances must be based on the findings in the lymph node biopsy.

The lesions of systemic mastocytosis may be distinguished from PTCL by the reactivity of mast cells with

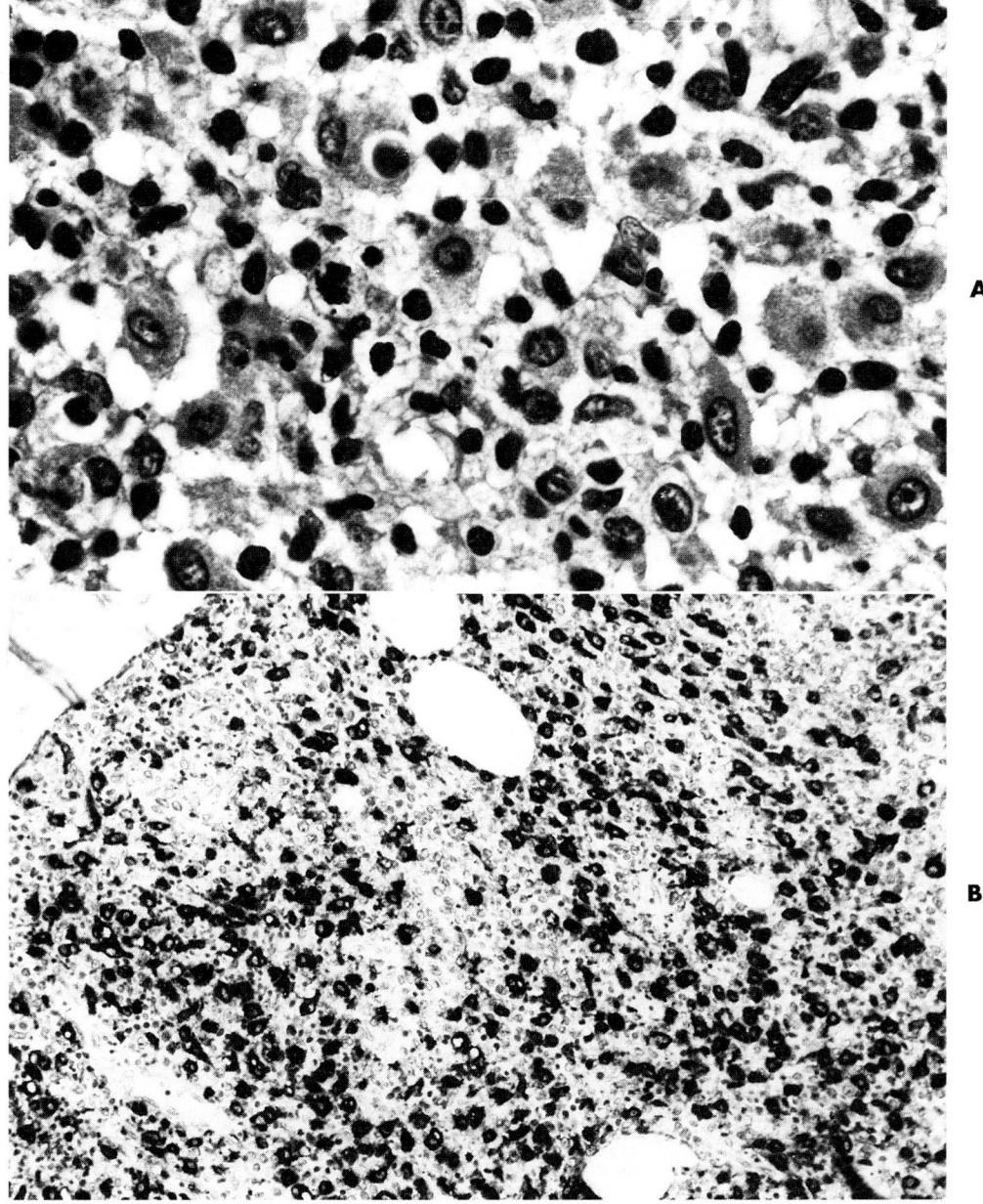

Fig. 23-69 **A,** Marrow from a patient with histiocyte-rich B-cell lymphoma. Histiocytes predominate in this area. **B,** The marrow biopsy in **A,** reacted with antibody to CD68 (KP-1). The numerous positively reacting histiocytes in this area contrast with the negatively reacting lymphoma cells. (Immunoperoxidase.)   *Continued.*

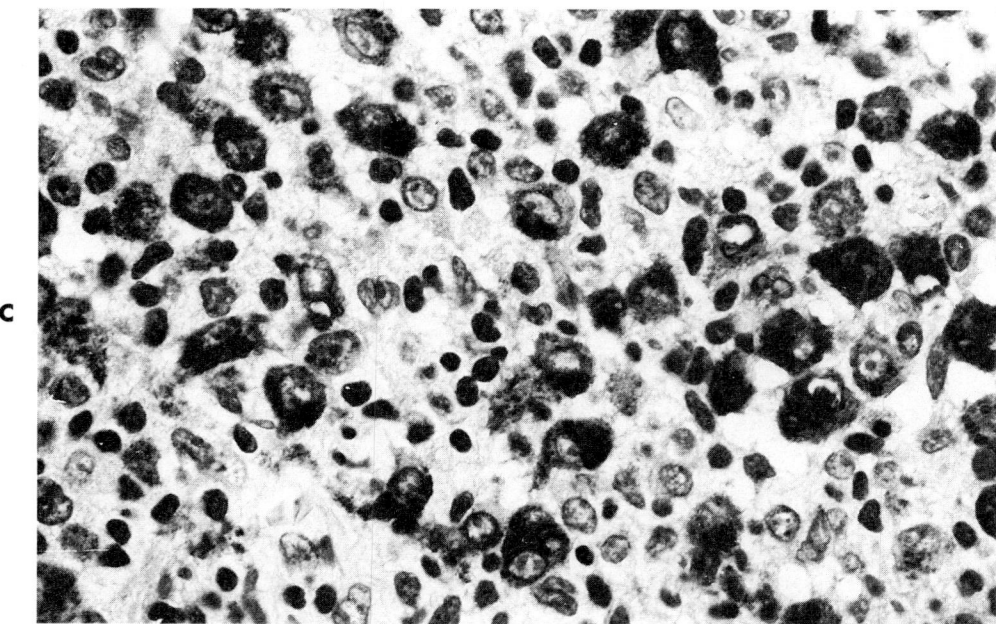

Fig. 23-69, con't **C,** High magnification of the specimen in **B**. (Immunoperoxidase.)

metachromatic stains such as toluidine blue and antibody to mast cell tryptase.

Genotypic studies to determine T-cell clonality are an important advance in distinguishing PTCL in marrow biopsies or other tissues from the disorders considered in the differential diagnosis. Clonal rearrangement of one of the T-cell receptors is substantial evidence of a malignant process.

Adult T-cell leukemia/lymphoma

Adult T-cell leukemia/lymphoma is an unusual form of post-thymic lymphoma occurring primarily in Japan that is associated with the human retrovirus HTLV-1.[266,267] The highest incidence of this disease is in the Kyushu region of Japan; other endemic areas include the Caribbean basin and parts of western Africa. Blood and marrow involvement occurs in a substantial number of patients. Hypercalcemia is present in 28% of patients at diagnosis and in 50% of patients at some time during the course of the disease. The vast majority of patients with hypercalcemia show marrow involvement by lymphoma and evidence of increased osteoclastic activity and bone resorption[266,267] (Fig. 23-72). Increased osteoclastic activity may be present in the absence of marrow involvement.

ANGIOIMMUNOBLASTIC LYMPHADENOPATHY

Angioimmunoblastic lymphadenopathy (AILD) as originally described is primarily a disease of lymph nodes in that all patients have either diffuse or localized adenopathy.[268,269,271] The reported incidence of marrow involvement is 50% to 70%.[270,272,273] These figures antedate the changing concepts of AILD vis-à-vis PTCL. The blood may show several abnormalities, including reactive lymphocytes, immunoblasts, and eosinophilia. In occasional patients the leukocyte count may

be markedly elevated; findings of an immune hemolytic anemia may be present.

The lesions of AILD in bone marrow sections may be diffuse or focal.[270,272,273] Focal involvement is more common. The margins of the focal lesions are usually somewhat indistinct, with poor demarcation from the surrounding hematopoietic tissue. In some cases, confluent multifocal lesions replace extensive areas of normal marrow. The lesions of AILD are somewhat loosely structured and contain varying proportions of lymphocytes, immunoblasts, plasma cells, and histiocytes; neutrophils and eosinophils are also present (Fig. 23-73). Vascular proliferation, endothelial cells, and fibroblasts are frequently identified. Stains for reticulin show a marked increase in reticulin fibers in the involved areas. Collections of epithelioid histiocytes, imparting a granulomatoid appearance to some of the lesions, are reported. The amorphous PAS-positive material found in lymph node biopsies is less frequently encountered in bone marrow lesions. Immunocytochemical reactions with antibodies to kappa and lambda light chains show a polyclonal proliferation of immunoblasts and plasma cells. The uninvolved marrow is frequently hypercellular. The hypercellularity may be a result of panhyperplasia or principally erythroid hyperplasia. The bone marrow and blood smears may contain varying numbers of immunocytes at varying stages of development, including immunoblasts and mature plasma cells. Reactive lymphocytes and eosinophils may be observed.

The significance of marrow involvement in regard to clinical outcome is unclear. Some, but not all, studies have indicated that patients with marrow involvement have a shorter survival than patients without marrow involvement.[268,273]

The differential diagnosis of AILD is one of the most difficult problems in bone marrow pathology. The disorders

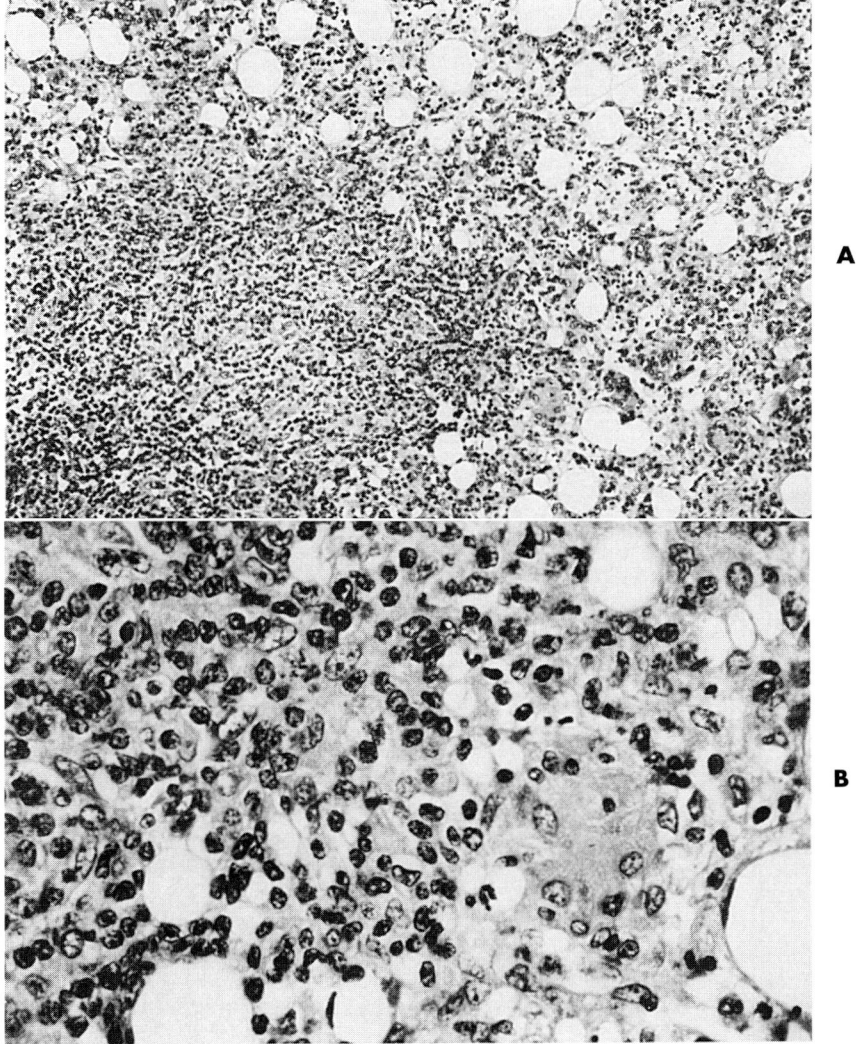

Fig. 23-70 A, Marrow section from patient with focal involvement by peripheral T-cell lymphoma. Lesion is large and poorly demarcated from surrounding marrow tissue. **B,** High magnification of lesion in **A** showing predominant population of small lymphocytes with few admixed larger cells, endothelial cells, and small cluster of epithelioid histiocytes.

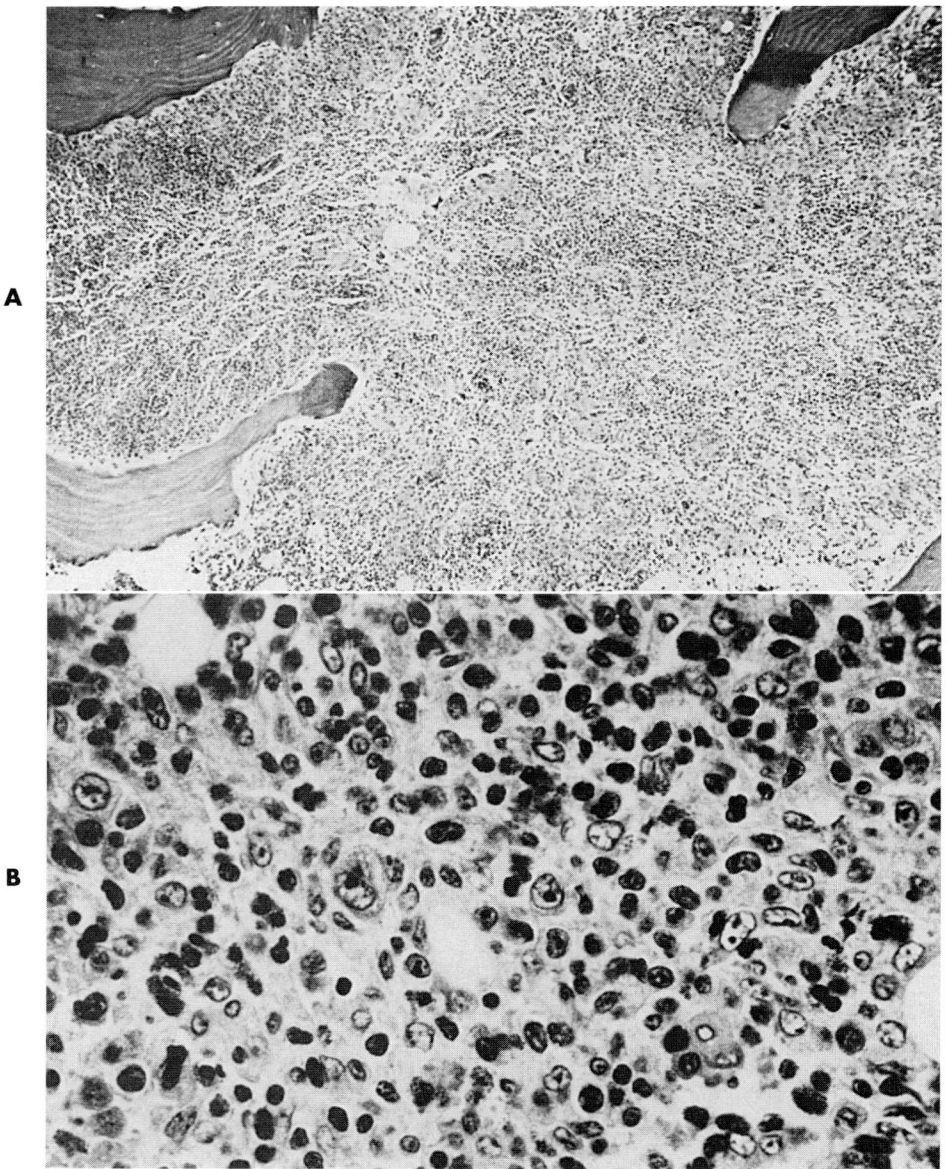

Fig. 23-71 A, Marrow biopsy from patient with PTCL, showing extensive diffuse marrow involvement. **B,** High magnification of lesion illustrated in **A** showing polycellular composition of this tumor. The predominant population consists of small lymphocytes with numerous interspersed larger cells that have prominent nucleoli.
Continued.

from which it must be distinguished include Hodgkin's disease, systemic mastocytosis, and polymorphous reactive lymphoid hyperplasia, which occurs in a variety of immune reactions. The lesions of AILD in the marrow may be virtually indistinguishable from those of PTCL, underscoring the relationship of these two entities. The distinction in these instances should be based on the evaluation of the lymph node biopsy, immunologic markers, genotypic studies, and clinical history. The distinction from Hodgkin's disease is based on the lack of classic Reed-Sternberg cells or mononuclear variants in the typical cellular milieu for Hodgkin's disease. In systemic mastocytosis the mast cells

can be recognized with the Giemsa stain and antibodies to mast cell tryptase.

LYMPHOMA/LEUKEMIA

There are lymphomas involving marrow and frequently blood that may present terminology problems because of their close relationship to leukemic processes; these include well-differentiated lymphocytic lymphoma (WDLL), small noncleaved cell lymphoma, and lymphoblastic lymphoma. The term *lymphosarcoma cell leukemia* has been used for blood involvement by a malignant lymphoma particularly of the small cleaved cell type. This term lacks specificity;

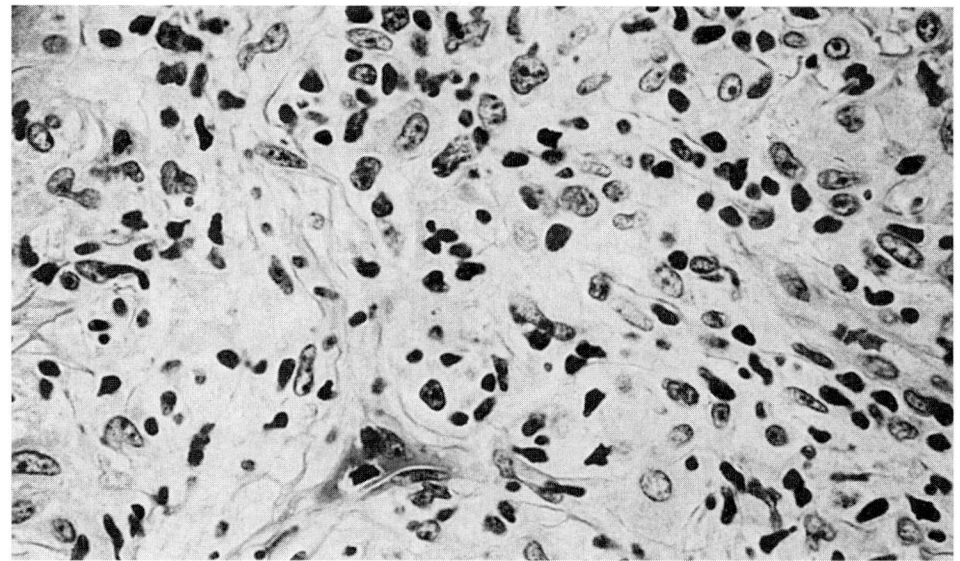

Fig. 23-71, cont'd **C,** Numerous epithelioid histiocytes impart a granulomatous appearance to this area of lesion.

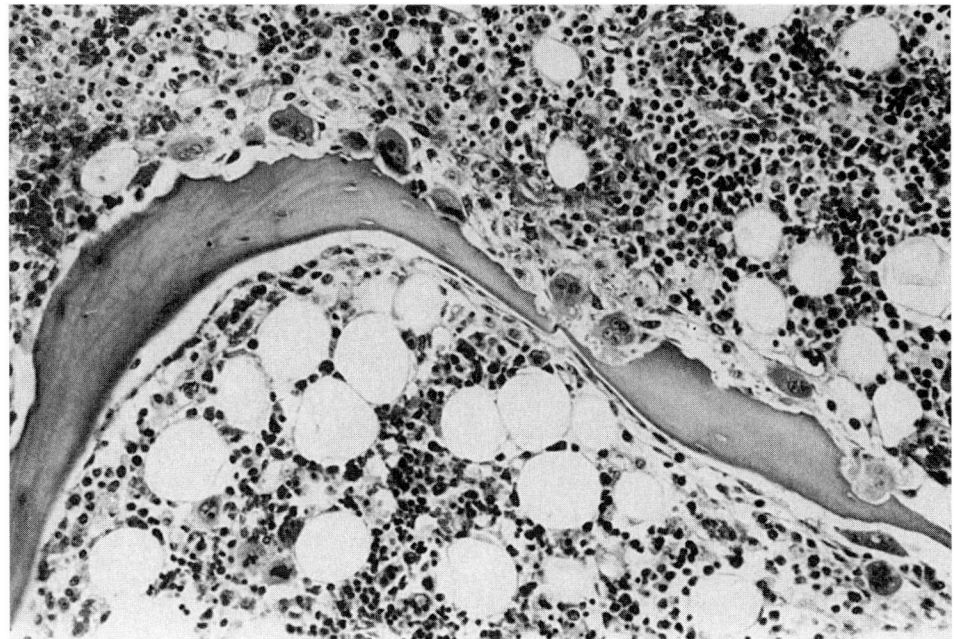

Fig. 23-72 Marrow biopsy from patient with adult T-cell leukemia and hypercalcemia. Marked osteo-clastic activity with bone resorption is present.

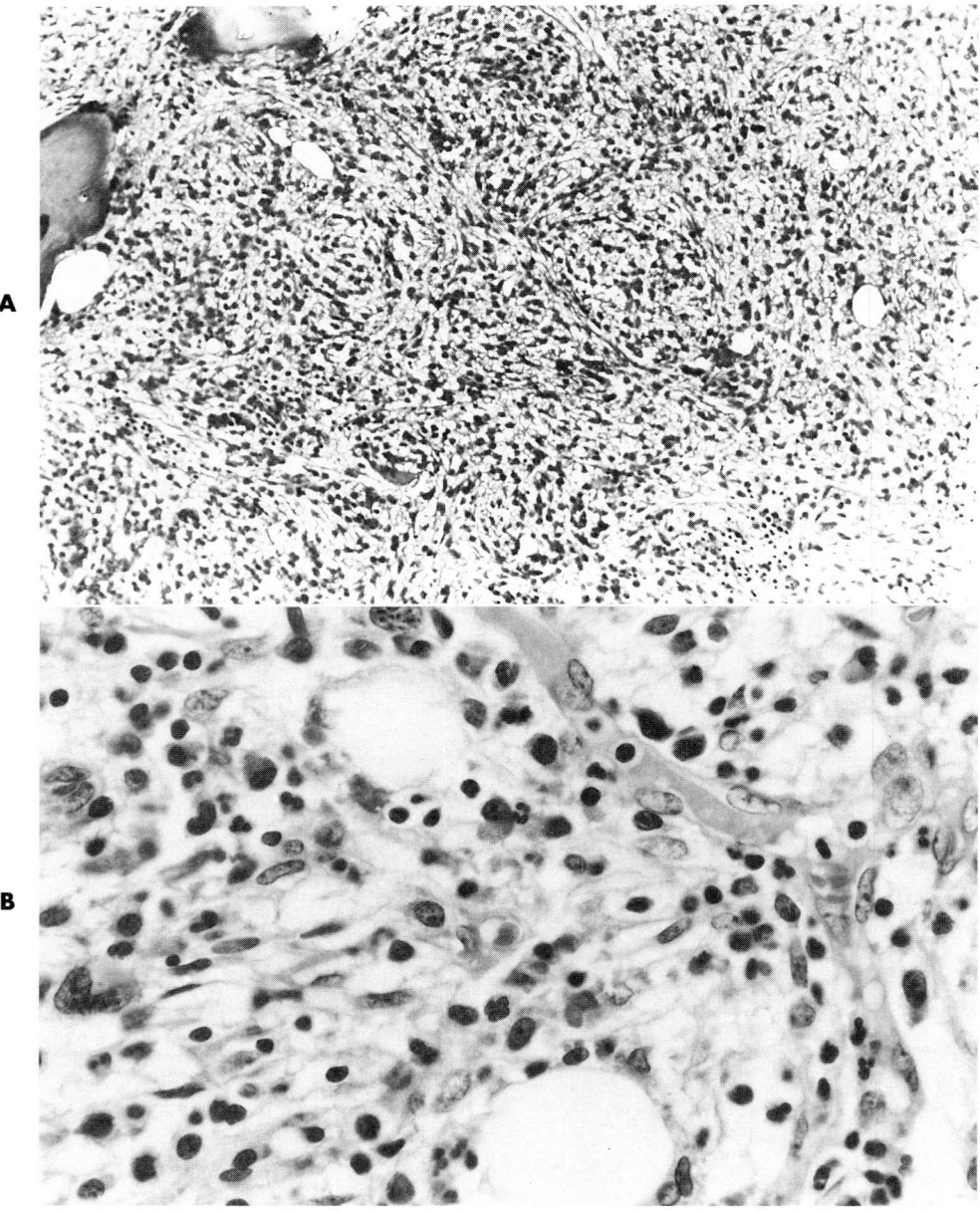

Fig. 23-73 A, Bone marrow biopsy from patient with lymph node diagnosis of AILD. Marrow is diffusely involved by process. **B,** Heterogenous cell population is loosely distributed. Numerous fibroblasts and endothelial cells are present.

appropriate terminology should specify the cytologic type of lymphoma.

WDLL or small B-lymphocytic lymphoma represents a proliferation of well-differentiated lymphocytes; some observers consider this to be the tissue counterpart of CLL.[293,294] It is characterized by a proliferation of small or well-differentiated lymphocytes in lymph nodes and bone marrow without the requisite blood findings of CLL. The distinction from CLL is generally based on the number of lymphocytes in the blood; if there is an absolute monoclonal B-cell lymphocytosis of more than 5000/μl, the diagnosis of CLL is preferred; if the absolute B-lymphocyte count is less than 5000 μl, the term *small lymphocyte lymphoma* is used.[293,294] The immunophenotype of the lymphocytes in B-cell CLL and B-cell WDLL is the same.[277,286,287] The pattern of marrow involvement in WDLL and CLL may be similar: diffuse, focal, interstitial, or a combination of these patterns. In WDLL the focal pattern is the most common, whereas in CLL the pattern is usually interstitial, mixed interstitial and focal, or diffuse. WDLL may progress to blood involvement, but the magnitude of the leukocytosis does not generally reach the levels observed in CLL.

Small noncleaved cell lymphoma, both Burkitt's and non-Burkitt's types, presents with marrow involvement in 15% to 30% of patients.* In some of these cases, varying numbers of lymphoma cells are present in the blood. Acute lymphoblastic leukemia (ALL), L3 type, is cytologically identical to small noncleaved cell lymphoma and is frequently associated with small noncleaved cell lymphoma involving the ileocecal region of the small bowel.[274,275,285] L3 ALL and small noncleaved cell lymphoma are B-cell tumors assoicated with a t(8;14) or variant chromosome translocation and are marked by an aggressive biologic course; both are terminal deoxynucleotidyl transferase (TdT) negative.[283] The diagnostic terminology used in these cases should reflect the status of the marrow and blood. If tumor cells are present in the blood and the marrow is diffusely replaced, L3 ALL is an appropriate designation. If few or no tumor cells are present in the blood and the marrow is partially involved with substantial sparing of normal hematopoiesis, a diagnosis of lymphoma is more appropriate. The therapeutic approach in these situations is similar. Marrow involvement in small noncleaved cell lymphoma is usually characterized by diffuse infiltration of the interstitium with some preservation of adipose tissue. The "starry sky" appearance characteristic of lymph nodes in Burkitt's lymphoma is not usually present on bone marrow biopsies. In contrast to the majority of cases of B-cell precursor ALL in which mitotic figures are sparse, there is prominent mitotic activity in small noncleaved cell lymphoma and L3 ALL (Fig. 23-74).

Malignant lymphoma, lymphoblastic, which is of T-cell origin in approximately 80% of cases and B-cell precursor type in 20%, has a high incidence of mediastinal mass, occurs in young adults, and has a predilection for early blood and marrow involvement; it is observed more commonly in males than in females.[276,291,296] Similar to the lymphoblasts in T-cell ALL, the lymphoma cells in T-

lymphoblastic lymphoma are TdT positive.[280] The blood and marrow may be involved at the time of initial diagnosis and the distinction between T-lymphoblastic lymphoma and T-cell ALL may be difficult. The presence of extramedullary tumor masses and evidence of sparing of marrow function as indicated by a normal platelet count, hemoglobin levels greater than 10 g/dl, and a normal number of neutrophils in the blood are more compatible with a diagnosis of lymphoma with marrow involvement as opposed to ALL. The Children's Cancer Study Group arbitrarily distinguishes leukemia from lymphoblastic lymphoma on the basis of the percentage of lymphoblasts in the marrow.[290] If there are less than 25% lymphoblasts the case is classified as lymphoma; if there are more than 25% lymphoblasts the case is classified as leukemia. In the cases of lymphoma, there may be substantial residual normal marrow with the lymphoma cells diffusely scattered in the interstitium. In other instances the marrow is completely replaced. In T-cell ALL, the marrow is diffusely replaced. In both lymphoblastic lymphoma and T-cell ALL, mitotic activity is usually prominent (Fig. 23-75). The therapeutic approach in these two related processes is the same.

Other types of lymphoma with marrow involvement may present with blood involvement. Approximately 40% of the cases of small cleaved cell lymphoma with lymphoma in the marrow have lymphoma cells in the blood[289] (Fig. 23-76). This is the type most frequently referred to as lymphosarcoma cell leukemia. In some instances, the count may be very high and resemble CLL. The distinction is based on the presence of lymphocytes with cleaved nuclei and the characteristic pattern of focal paratrabecular involvement in small cleaved cell lymphoma. Expression of CD5 and weak surface immunoglobulin on the lymphocytes supports a diagnosis of CLL; lack of CD5 and expression of CD10 and intense surface immunoglobulin are more compatible with small cleaved cell lymphoma.[288,297]

Mantle cell lymphoma, which may manifest as mantle zone lymphoma or diffuse intermediate differentiated lymphocytic lymphoma in the lymph node, may present with marked involvement of the marrow and blood; leukocyte counts of 270 × 10^9/L have been reported.[288,295] The blood findings may resemble both CLL and small cleaved cell lymphoma. The lymphocytes in the blood in mantle cell lymphoma are more pleomorphic than the lymphocytes in CLL or small cleaved cell lymphoma. The cells vary in size, nuclear cytoplasmic ratio, degree of nuclear irregularity, and prominence of nucleoli (Fig. 23-77). The lymphocytes express pan–B-cell antigens, CD5, and strong surface immunoglobulin. The lymphocytes usually do not express CD23 and are usually CD10 negative. The bone marrow involvement may be diffuse or focal; the focal involvement may be paratrabecular or nonparatrabecular. Rarely, naked germinal centers may be observed in the marrow lesions (see Fig. 23-65). The lymphoma cells express bcl-1 and in approximately 50% to 60% of cases show a t(11;14) chromosome abnormality.

The evaluation of blood and marrow samples from patients whose disease is being staged for lymphoma has been advanced substantially by antibodies reactive in paraffin-embedded tissue and genotypic and cytogenetic studies.

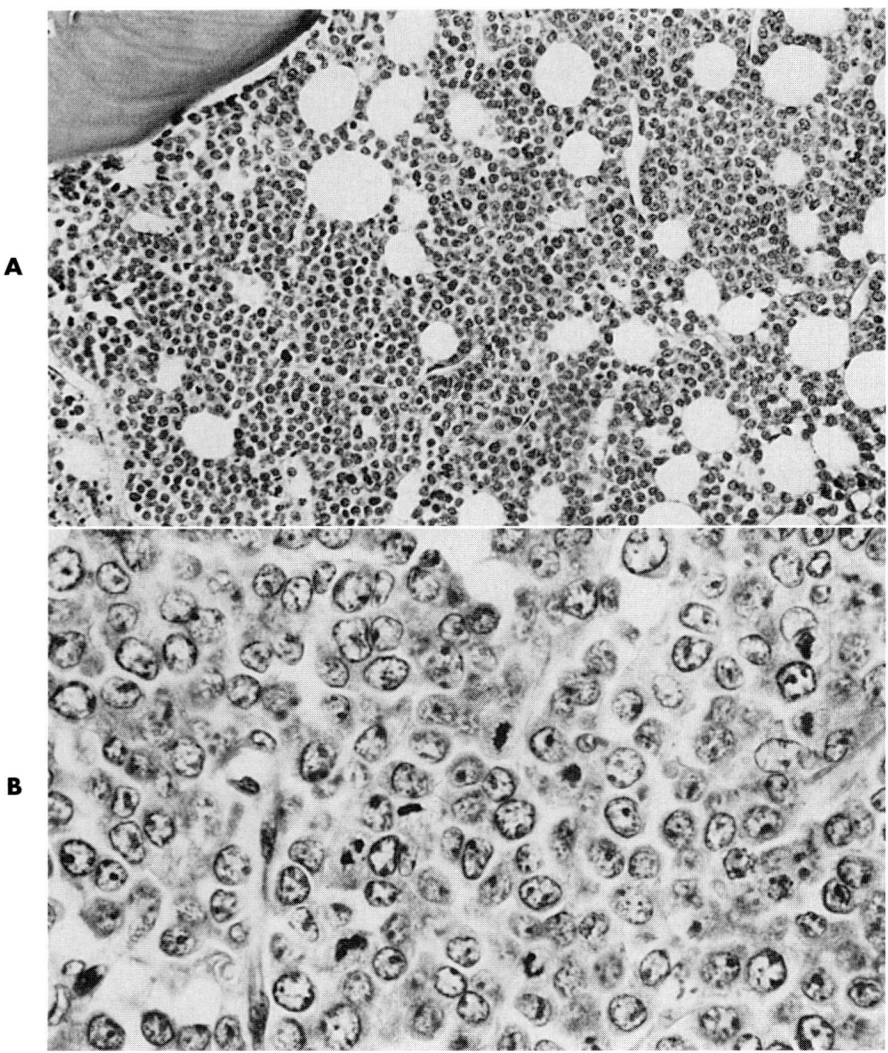

Fig. 23-74 **A,** Marrow biopsy from 8-year-old male with small noncleaved cell lymphoma involving ileal cecal area of gut. Marrow is almost completely replaced by tumor. **B,** Higher magnification of lesion illustrated in **A.** Mitotic figures are numerous.

The genotypic and cytogenetic studies may provide evidence of clonality and cell lineage in equivocal cases.

BENIGN LYMPHOCYTIC AGGREGATES

Benign lymphocytic aggregates are a relatively common finding in bone marrow trephine and particle sections. The incidence in biopsy specimens varies from 3% to 47%.[300,301,303] The reported incidence in autopsy specimens is 26% to 62%. The incidence appears to increase with age and is higher in females than males. The aggregates occur in patients with a wide range of disorders, and the number and size in individual specimens vary considerably. Although lesions up to 1000 μm have been reported, the majority of aggregates are relatively small and well circumscribed.[304] Unusually large aggregates may occur in the marrows of patients with diseases related to the immune system such as AIDS and rheumatoid arthritis. Large and numerous lymphoid aggregates, sometimes with obvious germinal center formation, may be observed in the marrow of patients receiving immunotherapy. These lesions may be paratrabecular (Fig. 23-78). The biologic significance of marrow lymphocytic aggregates in the majority of patients is unknown.[299]

The morphologic distinction between benign lymphocytic aggregates and malignant lymphoma small cell type in marrow biopsies from adults may be very difficult. Although general guidelines for making this distinction are proposed, it is important to recognize that exceptions to these generalizations occur with distressing frequency.

Benign aggregates are usually few in number, well-circumscribed, and loosely structured and contain histiocytes and plasma cells in addition to lymphocytes. The lymphocytes are usually small with generally round nuclei that have condensed chromatin and inconspicuous or no evident nucleoli. Occasional nuclei may have irregular outlines. Vascular structures are frequently present. Germinal centers are uncommon in lymphocytic lesions in the marrow but when

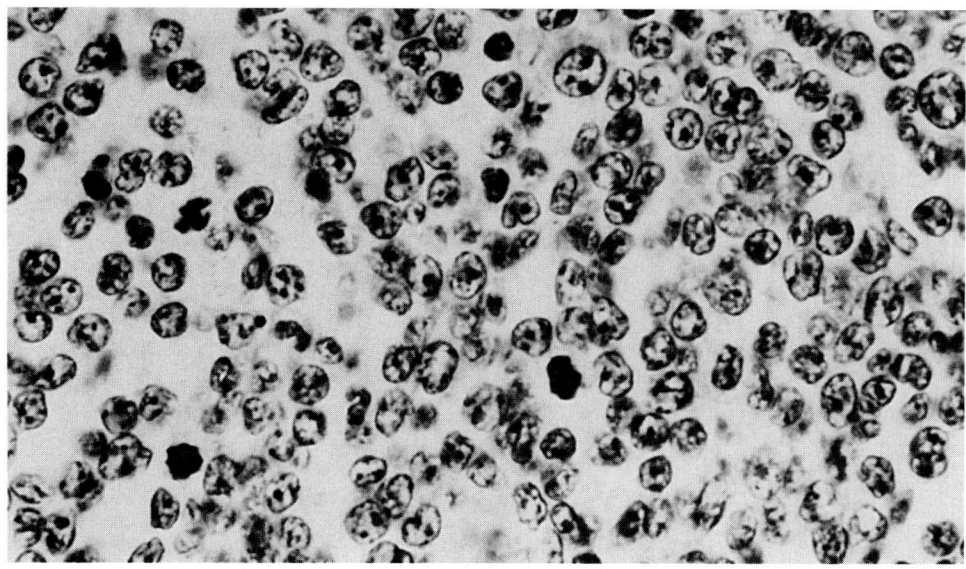

Fig. 23-75 Marrow biopsy from 25-year-old male with mediastinal mass and leukocyte count of 464,000, primarily lymphoblasts expressing T-cell antigens. Convoluted nuclei and increased mitoses are characterisitc of T-cell lymphoblastic lymphoma/leukemia.

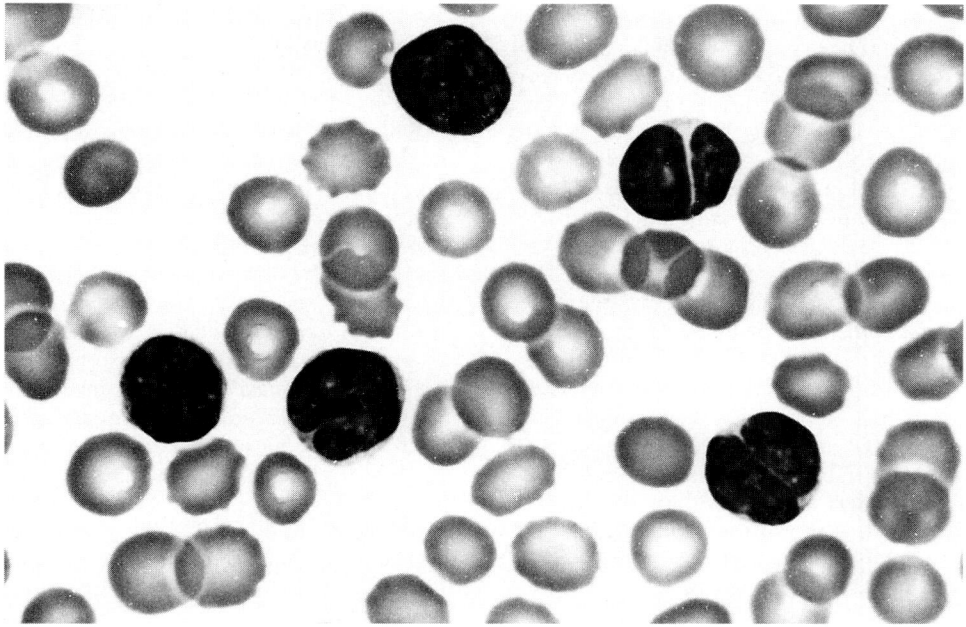

Fig. 23-76 Lymphoma cells in blood smear of adult male with small cleaved cell lymphoma; leukocyte count was 49 × 10⁹/L. Lymphoma cells have very high nuclear cytoplasmic ratio, coarse nuclear chromatin, and no evident nucleoli. Three cells have deeply cleft nuclei. (Wright-Giemsa.)

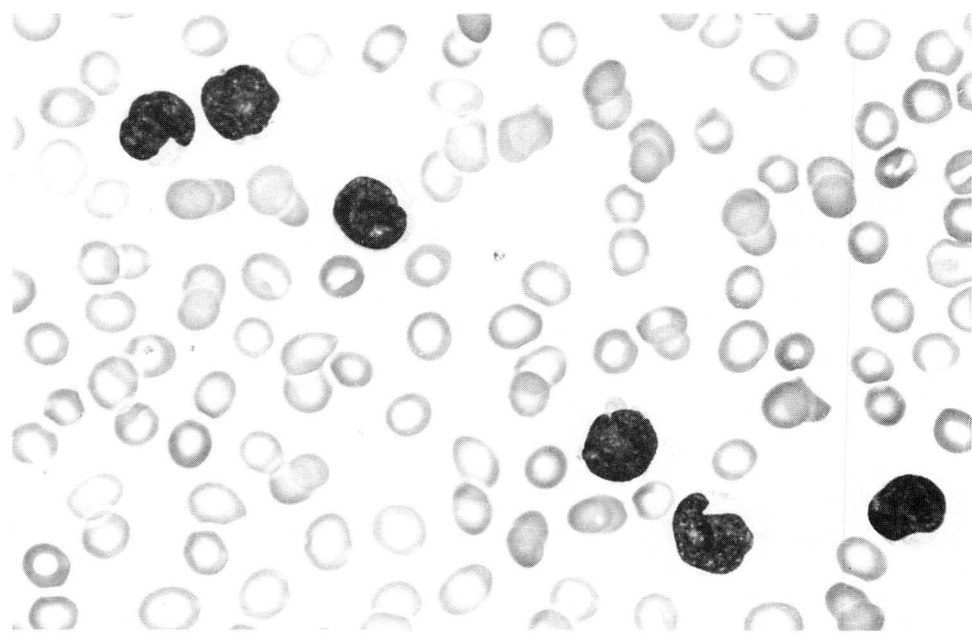

Fig. 23-77 Blood involvement by mantle cell lymphoma (intermediate differentiated lymphocytic lymphoma). Lymphoma cells are variable in size; nuclear outlines vary.

present are evidence of a benign process. Uncommonly, a naked germinal center may be found in marrow involved by mantle cell lymphoma. Areas of transformation that occur in many types of B-cell lymphoma may mimic germinal centers. Unequivocal germinal center formation should be interpreted as benign. A preferential paratrabecular margination of a lymphoid infiltrate is evidence for a diagnosis of lymphoma. A random distribution of lymphoid aggregates has no diagnostic specificity, since this pattern may occur with benign or malignant lesions.

A particularly difficult diagnostic problem is the lymphocytic lesion referred to as *polymorphous reactive lymphoid hyperplasia* (see Fig. 23-22). These lymphoid aggregates are usually focal, poorly circumscribed, and randomly distributed. The lymphocytes are generally well differentiated; the nuclei of some and sometimes of many of the lymphocytes may be irregular. The infiltrate may be predominantly lymphocytes or have associated populations of plasma cells, immunoblasts, eosinophils, endothelial cells, phagocytic histiocytes, and epithelioid histiocytes. This lesion may occur in the marrow in any age group and is frequently associated with immune disorders such as immune cytopenias, collagen vascular disease, and most notably, AIDS. The aggregates may be very large and in certain instances be virtually indistinguishable from the lesions of PTCL. Lesions of this type in marrow specimens from patients with AIDS are almost invariably reactive. In other instances in which the clinical or other tissue findings are equivocal, genotypic studies for clonality may be necessary.

It is important to recognize that benign lymphocytic aggregates may be present in marrow of patients with a prior diagnosis of marrow involvement by lymphoma; lymphoid aggregates in marrow specimens following chemotherapy should be evaluated as critically as those in the initial staging marrow biopsy. Marrow involvement by lymphoma in a patient with no other manifestation of the disease is very uncommon, and the diagnosis in such a situation should be approached with considerable caution.

The application of antibodies that react with lymphocytes in paraffin-embedded, decalcified specimens may aid in distinguishing benign from malignant lymphocytic aggregates.[298,302] Careful analysis of both lymph node and bone marrow specimens with the same panel of antibodies is necessary. The presence of a mixed reactivity pattern (i.e., lymphocyte populations expressing both T and B surface antigens) has been found to be more consistent with reactive lesions. There are exceptions to this generalization, and caution should be observed in the interpretation of immunocytochemical reactivity. Genotypic studies should be performed in those instances in which the marrow findings are indeterminate and a therapeutic decision is contingent on the presence or absence of marrow involvement. Even with this approach, difficulties in distinguishing benign from malignant lesions persist and continued observation is the most prudent course in some patients.

HODGKIN'S DISEASE

The incidence of bone marrow involvement in Hodgkin's disease varies from 2% to 29% in previously untreated patients.[305,311,313,315] The demonstration of bone marrow involvement appears in part to be related to the amount of tissue available for examination. Marrow involvement is in most instances the result of widely disseminated disease; in rare cases, marrow may be involved by direct extension from contiguously involved lymph nodes.

The majority of patients with Hodgkin's disease in the marrow at the time of diagnosis have mixed cellularity or nodular sclerosis type in the lymph node; marrow involve-

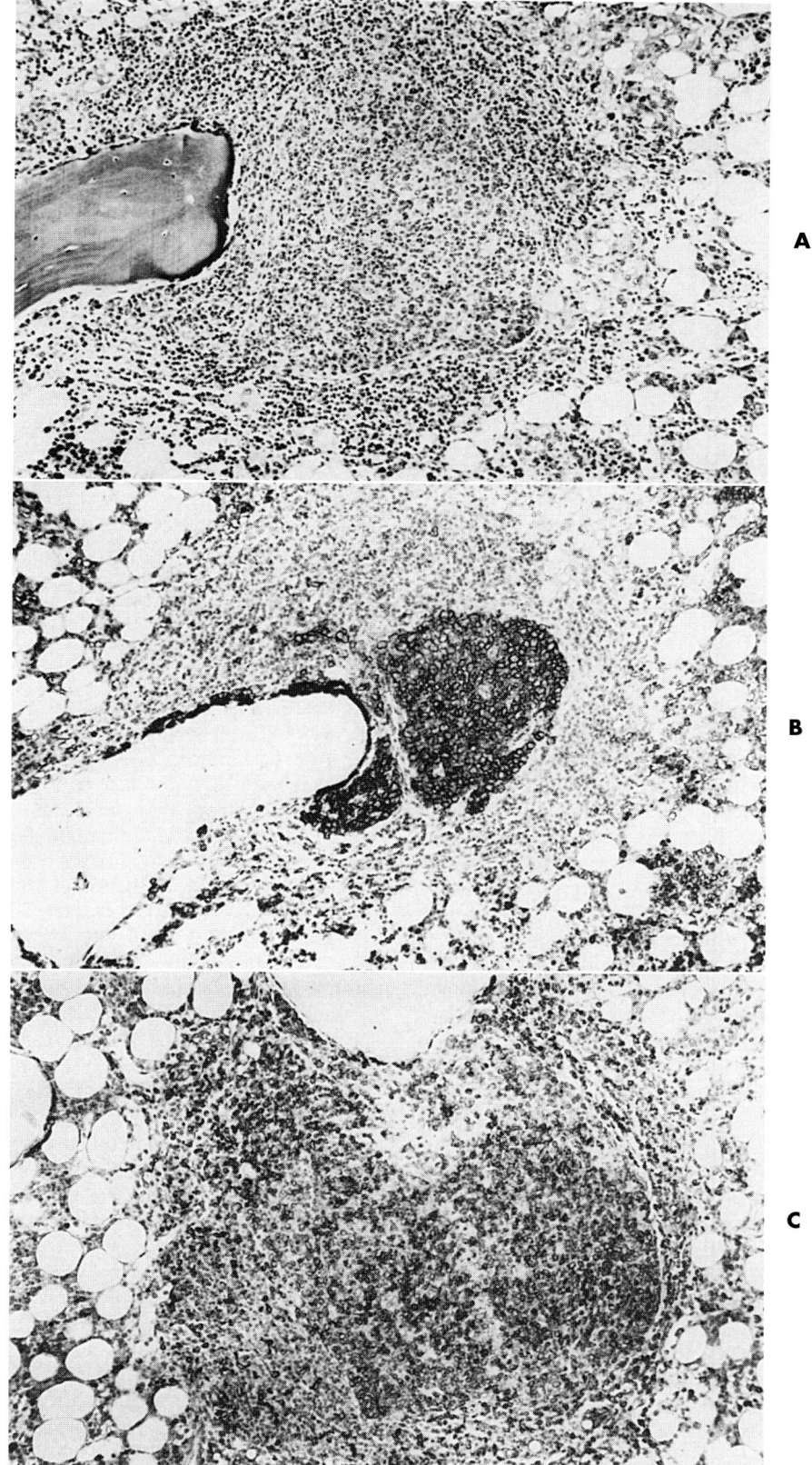

Fig. 23-78 A, Paratrabecular germinal center formation in marrow of patient receiving interleukin-2 therapy for metastatic melanoma. Several vacuolated macrophages are present at margin of lesion. **B,** Lesion illustrated in **A** reacted with monoclonal antibody LN1. Follicular center lymphocytes are intensely positive. **C,** Same lesion as in **A** and **B** reacted with antibody to CD74 (LN2). High percentage of lymphocytes in lesion react with this antibody. (**B** and **C** Immunoperoxidase.)

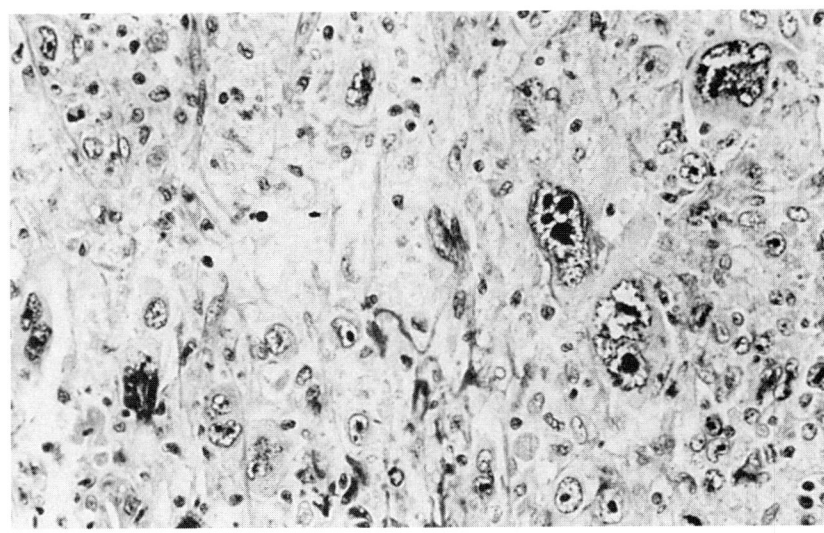

Fig. 23-79 Bone marrow biopsy from patient with mixed-cellularity Hodgkin's disease. Several unusually large Reed-Sternberg–like cells and several mononuclear variants are present. Scattered lymphocytes, plasma cells, histiocytes, and fibroblasts are present.

ment is most unusual in the lymphocyte predominant type[314a] (Fig. 23-79). The lymphocyte-depletion type, which has a high incidence of marrow involvement (approximately 50%), is an uncommon form of Hodgkin's disease.[307,312] Because the clinical presentation in some patients with lymphocyte-depletion Hodgkin's disease is characterized by little or no peripheral lymphadenopathy, the initial diagnostic specimen may be the bone marrow biopsy. The histopathologic classification of Hodgkin's disease should not be based on examination of involved bone marrow because of the different manifestations of the disease in lymph node and bone marrow tissue. Fibrosis is a common finding in Hodgkin's lesions in the marrow and is not limited to the nodular sclerosis and lymphocyte-depletion types.

Definitive histopathologic criteria for the diagnosis of marrow involvement in Hodgkin's disease include typical Reed-Sternberg cells in a cellular background characteristic of Hodgkin's disease or mononuclear Reed-Sternberg variants in a cellular background typical of Hodgkin's disease if typical Reed-Sternberg cells are identified in other specimens (Fig. 23-80).[306,309,314] The presence of atypical cells lacking the features of Reed-Sternberg cells or mononuclear variants in a characteristic Hodgkin's environment in a patient with histopathologically proven disease should be considered suspicious for involvement. Foci of fibrosis in the absence of Reed-Sternberg cells or mononuclear variants in a patient with an established diagnosis of Hodgkin's disease is not in itself sufficient evidence for a definitive diagnosis of marrow involvement but should be viewed as highly suspicious. In these cases repeat biopsies should be performed.

Hodgkin's lesions in the marrow may be diffuse or focal. The extent of marrow involvement ranges from a single, small lesion to complete replacement of multiple biopsy specimens. Diffuse involvement is found in approximately 70% to 80% of positive marrow biopsies; the Hodgkin's tissue in these cases replaces entire areas between trabeculae.[313] Focal lesions are variable in size and may be surrounded by normal hematopoietic tissue or scattered in a hypocellular background (Fig. 23-81); the latter pattern is more frequent following chemotherapy. The focal lesions tend to be polycellular, with a predominant population of small lymphocytes with admixed neutrophils, eosinophils, plasma cells, histiocytes, Reed-Sternberg cells, and mononuclear variants. The diffuse lesions may manifest in several patterns. In the majority of cases the Hodgkin's tissue is hypercellular with a population of cells characteristic of mixed cellularity Hodgkin's disease in the lymph node (see Fig. 23-80). In some patients the marrow shows extensive hypocellularity characterized by a generally loose, sparsely cellular connective tissue with scattered, variably sized hypercellular areas containing lymphocytes, histiocytes, and Reed-Sternberg cells and variants (see Fig. 23-81). Areas of necrosis may be present and are more common in post-therapy specimens than at initial diagnosis. Varying degrees of fibrosis may be present. In some cases, entire biopsy specimens show replacement by dense fibrous connective tissue with few identifiable lymphocytes or histiocytes (Fig. 23-82). In others, scattered islands of cells are interspersed among the collagen fibers; some of these cells show features suggestive of Hodgkin's cells; others are too distorted for accurate identification. In some instances the Hodgkin's lesions are very hypercellular with a predominant population of Reed-Sternberg cells or mononuclear variants (Fig. 23-83). Various combinations of these patterns may be present in the same biopsy specimen or in different specimens from the same patient. Necrosis and hypocellularity are more common in marrow from treated patients than untreated patients. In marrow involvement with lymphocyte-depletion

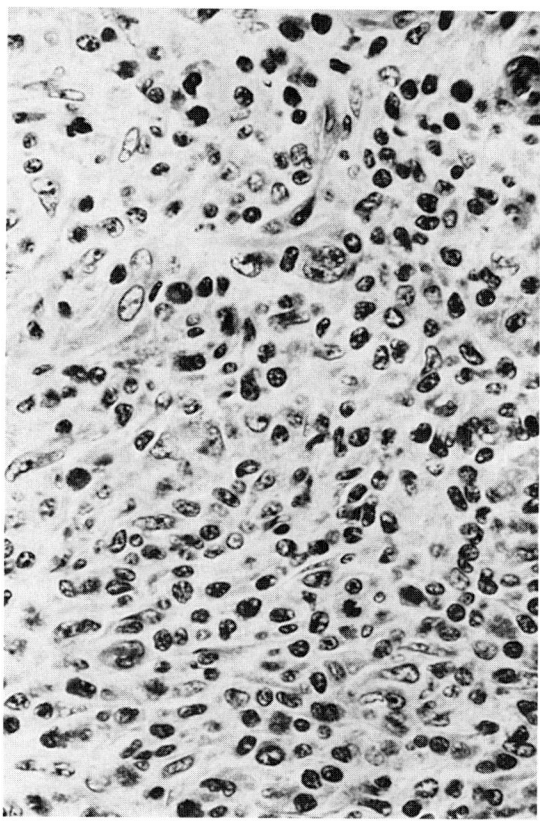

Fig. 23-80 Marrow biopsy with extensive replacement by Hodgkin's tissue. There is polycellular infiltrate of lymphocytes, eosinophils, histiocytes, and occasional Reed-Sternberg cells.

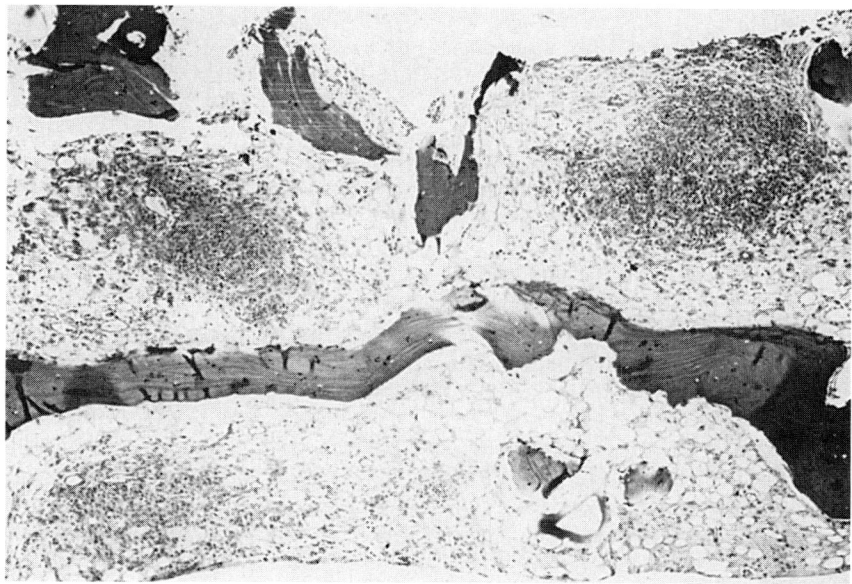

Fig. 23-81 Three densely cellular focal lesions in overall markedly hypocellular bone marrow from patient with Hodgkin's disease.

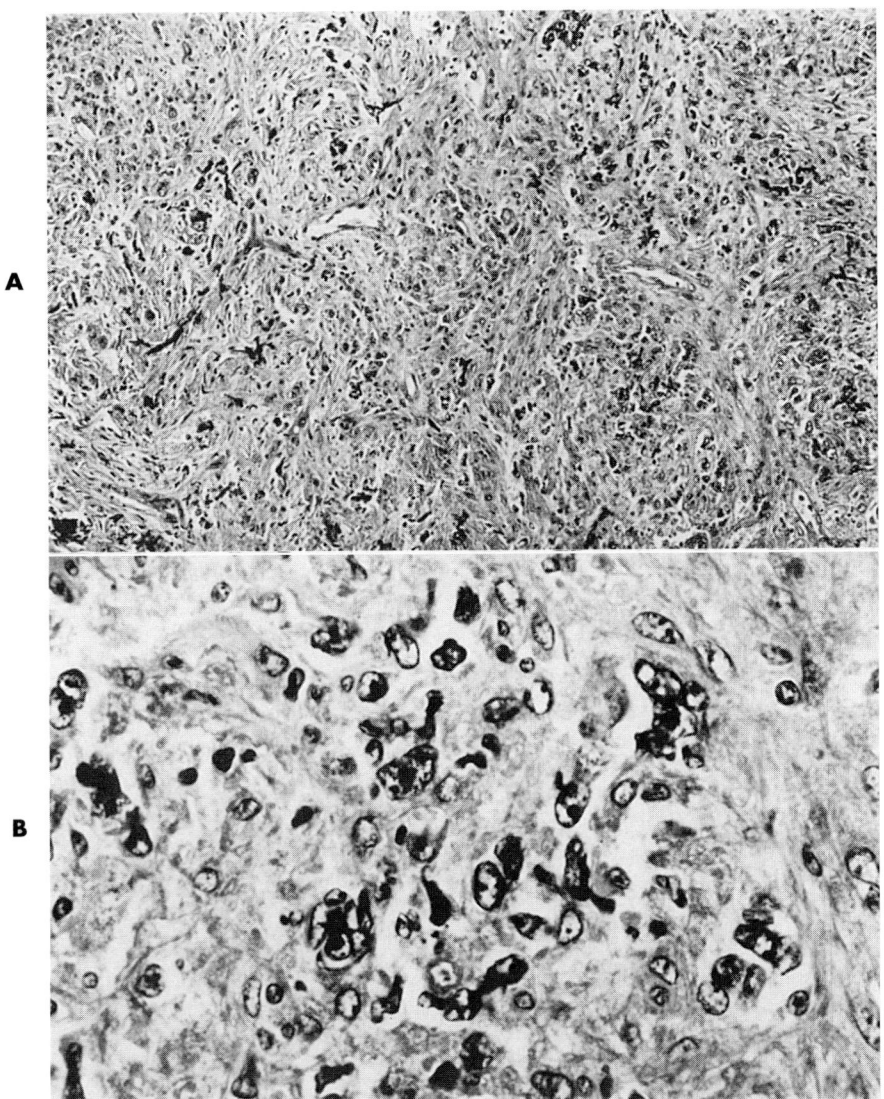

Fig. 23-82 A, Portion of marrow biopsy from patient with Hodgkin's disease. Marrow space is completely replaced by dense fibrous connective tissue. Numerous vascular structures and small foci of distorted cells are present. **B,** High magnification of specimen **A** showing several focal collections of cells that resemble distorted Reed-Sternberg cells and mononuclear variants.

Hodgkin's disease, a typical consolidated lesion characterized by an inflammatory cellular infiltrate accompanied by a distinct amorphous deposition of eosinophilic background substance and Reed-Sternberg cells has been described.[307]

The presence of Reed-Sternberg cells or their mononuclear variants is of critical importance to the recognition of Hodgkin's disease in the marrow, and a definitive diagnosis should not be established without their identification in the appropriate cellular milieu. Several serial sections of the marrow biopsies may have to be examined before satisfactory Reed-Sternberg cells or mononuclear variants are detected. It is important not to misinterpret megakaryocytes as forms of Reed-Sternberg cells; this problem can be avoided by strict adherence to the principle of identifying

Reed-Sternberg cells or variants only in the appropriate cellular background. Reed-Sternberg–like cells may be observed in marrow specimens with involvement by follicular center cell lymphoma, PTCL,[310] and anaplastic large cell lymphoma (see Fig. 23-68); the clinical history, membrane surface marker studies, and characteristic tissue changes of Hodgkin's disease should aid in distinguishing these disorders. In some instances, genotypic studies may be necessary.

The uninvolved areas of marrow in specimens with involvement by Hodgkin's disease may be hypercellular, normocellular, or hypocellular. Nonspecific alterations, including stromal damage, inflammatory cell infiltration, and disturbed hematopoiesis, may be present.[305] These alterations may occur singly or in combination.

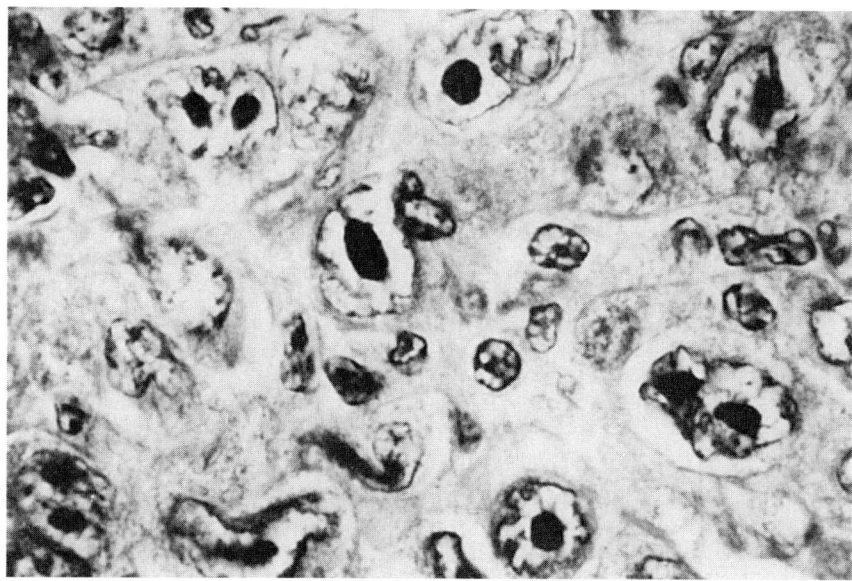

Fig. 23-83 Marrow biopsy with predominance of Reed-Sternberg cells and mononuclear variants from patient with nodular sclerosis type of Hodgkin's disease.

Similar to the spleen, liver, and lymph node, benign granulomatous lesions may be present in the bone marrow sections in patients with Hodgkin's disease.[313] The bone marrow is the least likely organ in this group to contain the granulomas, but their presence may lead to diagnostic difficulty. The lack of typical Reed-Sternberg cells or mononuclear variants is an important feature in distinguishing these lesions from Hodgkin's disease. The presence of granulomas does not constitute evidence of involvement. Granulomas in post-therapy patients should always be evaluated for the possibility of an infectious agent.[308,313] Benign lymphocytic aggregates may also be present.

Rarely a patient whose disease is being staged for marrow involvement by Hodgkin's disease has a concurrent parvovirus B19 infection. The presence of very large erythroid precursors may lead to consideration of marrow Hodgkin's (see Fig. 23-13). The lack of a characteristic cellular environment and marked erythroid hypoplasia are strong evidence of parvovirus infection.

HISTIOCYTIC DISORDERS
Malignant histiocytosis

The term *malignant histiocytosis* was introduced by Rappaport[319] to describe an entity characterized by a systemic, neoplastic proliferation of histiocytes and precursors.[316-324] The diagnosis of marrow involvement by malignant histiocytosis should be made with considerable caution. The disorder is very rare. Other poorly differentiated neoplasms of the hematopoietic system may have morphologic features that have been associated with malignant histiocytosis.[326] The demonstration of nonspecific esterase reactivity in poorly differentiated cells is not sufficiently specific to establish a diagnosis. Cell marker studies for B- and T-cell lineage should be done to exclude poorly differentiated lymphomas. Histiocytes should express markers of monocyte histiocyte lineage. Poorly differentiated carcinomas and plasmablastic tumors must also be excluded.

In marrow biopsies, the infiltration by malignant histiocytes may be focal or diffuse. Bone marrow involvement may be extremely difficult to recognize in sections that contain only scattered malignant cells. In smear preparations, the cells occur singly or in small groups scattered among the normal hematopoietic cells or at the edges of the smears. The malignant histiocyte varies in size; cells up to 40 to 50 μm or larger may be found. The cytoplasm is usually abundant, with evidence of pseudopod formation and fragmentation; it is variably basophilic with numerous small, sharply defined vacuoles in some cells. Very small azurophilic granules may be found in the cytoplasm of some of the larger cells. Occasional malignant histiocytes may show evidence of phagocytosis; prominent hemophagocytosis is a relatively uncommon finding in unequivocally malignant-appearing cells. The nucleus may be round or contorted; the larger cells generally have more contorted nuclei. The chromatin is coarsely reticular. Nucleoli may be very prominent or inconspicuous. Stains for nonspecific esterase and acid phosphatase are positive. The proliferation of the malignant histiocytes may be accompanied by a proliferation of benign-appearing histiocytes with abundant cytoplasm and prominent hemophagocytosis; this probably represents a reaction to the malignant cell proliferation.

Although most cases of malignant histiocytosis present without prior history of a hematologic disorder, cases occurring subsequent to CLL have been reported.[325] The relationship of this phenomenon to Richter's transformation is unclear.

Hemophagocytic syndromes

The hemophagocytic syndromes are a group of disorders with the unifying features of a proliferation of phagocytic histiocytes that may be present in all hematopoietic organs.

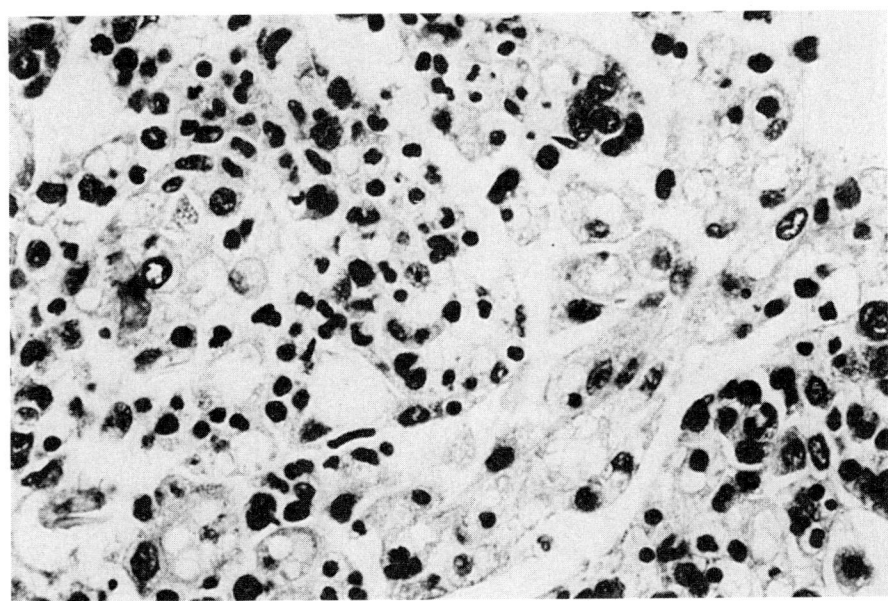

Fig. 23-84 Marrow biopsy from 47-year-old renal transplant recipient receiving immunosuppressive therapy who developed hemophagocytic syndrome associated with EBV infection. Numerous macrophages, some showing hemophagocytosis, are present in sinusoid and interstitium.

These processes usually have systemic manifestations and may be accompanied by a fulminant clinical course and high mortality. Because of the multiorgan involvement and the associated high mortality, these disorders frequently have been interpreted as cases of malignant histiocytosis. The hemophagocytic syndromes appear to be epiphenomena that are triggered by a variety of causes, including but not limited to viral infections and some T-cell lymphomas.[327-347] Viruses associated with this disorder include cytomegalovirus, Epstein-Barr virus (EBV), adenovirus, and parvovirus B19.[345,345a] The process may be observed with bacterial infections, including the protozoan infection, *Babesia microti.* Patients with immune deficiency, either hereditary or acquired, appear to be at increased risk for this problem.[334]

The hemophagocytic syndromes frequently have an abrupt onset. Evidence of multisystem disease is usually present, particularly in patients with viral infections.[345] A high percentage of patients have coagulative abnormalities. The blood is usually marked by cytopenias, frequently pancytopenia. The marrow smears contain numerous histiocytes, many showing evidence of phagocytosis of erythroid cells (both mature and nucleated), platelets, and granulocytes. There is frequently an accompanying depression of erythroid precursors, granulocyte precursors, or both; megakaryocytes may be normal or increased in number. In biopsy sections, the increased histiocytes are dispersed throughout the interstitium and sinuses; occasional clusters may be present (Fig. 23-84). The evidence of phagocytic activity may be less prominent in sections compared with smear preparations (Fig. 23-85). In addition to the histiocytic proliferation, granulomas may be noted, and areas of necrosis are frequently present. The bone marrow findings

may change substantially over a period of days, with fluctuations in the number of granulocyte and erythroid precursors and megakaryocytes. Lymph nodes may show a marked increase in histiocytes in the sinusoidal spaces; evidence of hemophagocytosis may be much less marked than in the bone marrow. The spleen may be markedly enlarged with prominent histiocytic infiltration in the red pulp. Areas of nonsuppurative necrosis have been observed in lymph nodes and spleen.[343]

Evidence of multi-system involvement is usually present, particularly in patients with a viral infection, and a high percentage of patients have abnormalities of the coagulation system.[345] A florid immunoblastic reaction has been reported as an antecedent event in a case of EBV-associated hemophagocytic syndrome.[330]

Patients with EBV-related hemophagocytic syndrome have been reported to show evidence of a permissive viral infection.[346] Cytotoxic T cells, which normally lyse EBV-infected B cells, have been reported to be absent from the peripheral blood of these patients, suggesting an immunoregulatory deficiency. Treatment with antiviral agents has been beneficial in some patients.

The clinical pathologic features of VAHS have been reported in 80% of a group of patients with fatal infectious mononucleosis.[341] The VAHS phase was preceded by features of a viral-like illness. Sequential changes were present in the marrows of these patients; initially there was infiltration by atypical lymphoid cells with areas of necrosis, followed by depletion of normal hematopoietic cells and histiocytic activation with prominent hemophagocytosis; the end stage was marked by marrow aplasia. A similar sequence of histopathologic changes was found in the lymph nodes, spleen, and thymus gland.

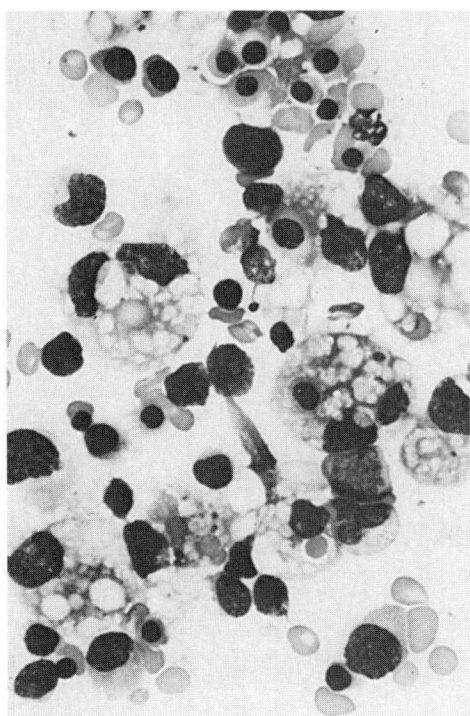

Fig. 23-85 Bone marrow smear from patient with virus-associated hemophagocytic syndrome. Numerous macrophages with ingested red cells and erythroblasts are present. (Wright-Giemsa.)

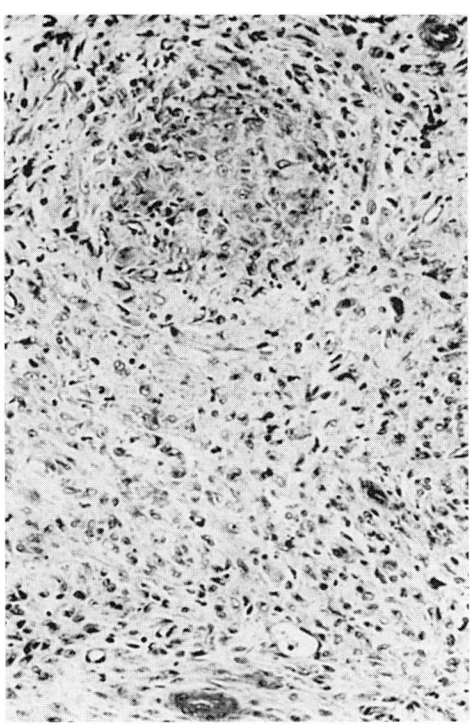

Fig. 23-86 Bone marrow section from child with histiocytosis X. Large portion of marrow is replaced by differentiated histiocytosis that assume granuloma-like arrangement.

Hemophagocytic histiocytosis has been reported as a terminal event in patients with lymphoblastic lymphomas and PTCL.[331,335] The pathologic findings are similar to those in VAHS. The production of macrophage-activating cytokines by the malignant cells has been suggested as a causative mechanism of the histocyte proliferation. The hemophagocytic syndrome may be associated with other types of lymphoma including Ki-1 (CD30)–positive lymphomas with an associated t(2;5) chromosome abnormality.

The distinction between the benign hemophagocytic syndrome and malignant histiocytosis may be difficult because of similarities in clinical presentation.[329,336,337] The cells in the benign histiocytic proliferations are morphologically distinct; they have a low nuclear/cytoplasmic ratio and abundant lightly staining cytoplasm containing large vacuoles of varying sizes and phagocytosed cells or cellular products. Nucleoli, when present, are not prominent, and mitotic figures are rare. The malignant histiocyte has a high nuclear/cytoplasmic ratio and usually an intensely basophilic cytoplasm; nucleoli are frequently prominent, and mitotic figures may be numerous. Phagocytosis by obviously malignant histiocytes is uncommon. Although benign histiocytic hyperplasia may coexist with malignant histiocytosis or a malignant lymphoma, there is no evidence of a transition from the obviously malignant cells to the benign histiocytes.

Serologic studies for viral infection in patients with the picture of a benign hemophagocytic syndrome may not be reliable because impaired immune function may preclude a detectable antibody response. In these cases, molecular hybridization studies may be useful in documenting an EBV infection.[333,337] In addition to studies for a viral infection, it is important that patients with a hemophagocytic process be carefully evaluated for immune suppression and non-Hodgkin's lymphoma. Patients with a hemophagocytic syndrome with both an EBV infection and a malignant lymphoproliferative lesion may be observed. The clinical and morphologic findings in patients with the entity described as familial lymphohistiocytosis may be virtually indistinguishable from patients with a hemophagocytic process associated with a viral infection or T-cell lymphoma.

Histiocytosis X (Langerhans' cell histiocytosis)

Marrow involvement in histiocytosis X is usually a late manifestation of the disease[349]; detection appears to be increased with the use of trephine biopsies as opposed to bone marrow clot section.[348] The lesions of histiocytosis X in the marrow are generally focal and have a granulomatous appearance (Fig. 23-86). Confluent lesions may replace substantial portions of the medullary space. Similar to these lesions in other organs, the histiocytes have a low nuclear/cytoplasmic ratio and mature nuclei without prominent nucleoli. Nuclear folding or clefting may be present. Hemosiderin granules may be present in the cytoplasm. The lesions may be relatively monomorphous or contain a mixture of multinucleate giant cells, lymphocytes, plasma cells, eosinophils, and neutrophils. Stains for reticulin show an increased number of reticulin fibers.

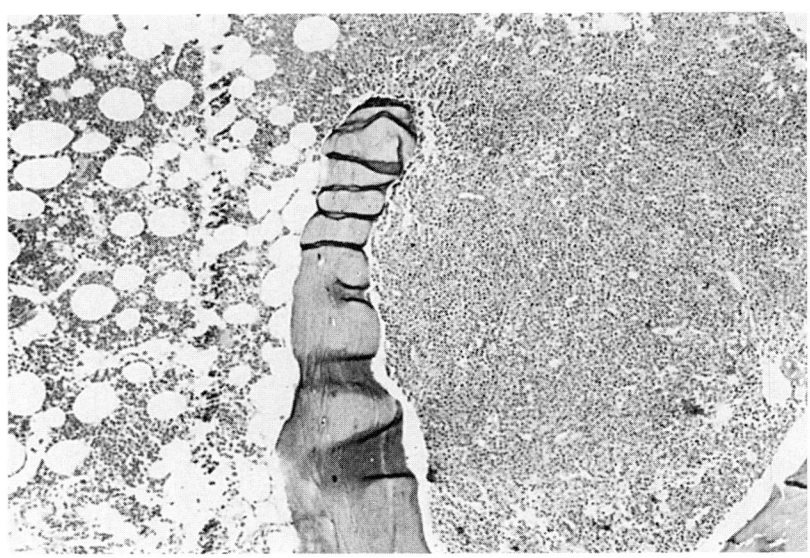

Fig. 23-87 Bone marrow section from patient with multiple myeloma illustrating large, dense focal collection of myeloma cells on one side of bone spicule and interstitial infiltration on other side.

PLASMA CELL DYSCRASIAS
Multiple myeloma

Multiple myeloma is a neoplastic proliferation of plasma cells accompanied by the production of a monoclonal immunoglobulin detectable in the serum, urine, or both.* The peak incidence is in the seventh decade; the disease is slightly more frequent in males than females. Osteolytic lesions in the skull, ribs, sternum, vertebrae, and pelvis are usually present; in rare cases, x-ray films reveal osteosclerotic lesions.

Marrow involvement in myeloma may be patchy, and the percentage of plasma cells may vary in aspirates and biopsies from different sites. In trephine sections, the distribution of plasma cells may be diffuse, focal, interstitial, or a combination of these patterns[353,354,357,361,390a] (Fig. 23-87). There is variability in the appearance of the plasma cells in different cases from very immature plasma cells with a blast-like appearance to mature-appearing plasma cells[358,366,370,371] (Fig. 23-88). Nucleoli may be very prominent in some of the more immature types, and binucleate cells resembling Reed-Sternberg cells may be found. Nuclear and cytoplasmic inclusions of varying types may be noted; these are usually related to immunoglobulin production (Fig. 23-89). The marrow in approximately 10% to 20% of cases shows an associated fibrosis[359,376] (Fig. 23-90).

Several approaches to the staging of myeloma have been introduced; these have included the correlation of myeloma cell mass with presenting laboratory findings, including hemoglobin, monoclonal immunoglobulin, and calcium levels and the presence of osteolytic bone lesions.[363,364,367] The measurement of beta 2 microglobulin in the serum has been found to have prognostic significance in that levels greater than 4 ng/µl are associated with a shorter survival than levels less than 1 ng/µl.[355,369]

Histopathologic staging of myeloma in bone marrow biopsies based on cytologic features of the myeloma cells and the degree of plasma cell infiltration has been shown to have prognostic significance.* The more immature or poorly differentiated the myeloma cells and the more extensive the marrow involvement, the more unfavorable the prognosis. An anaplastic evolution of myeloma may occur, and some of these cases have the histopathologic features of immunoblastic lymphoma.[365] Studies comparing anaplastic myeloma with B-immunoblastic lymphoma have demonstrated clinical and immunologic differences.[389,390] The plasma cells in anaplastic myeloma are usually of the IgG or IgA heavy chain class in contrast to B-immunoblastic lymphoma in which the cells are IgM. The cells in immunoblastic lymphoma usually express pan–B-cell antigens; the plasma cells in approximately 80% of cases of myeloma do not express pan–B-cell antigens. Exceptions to these generalizations occur. All clinical and laboratory findings should be considered. Histopathologic staging of myeloma in the marrow, using an approach similar to that used for CLL, has shown good correlation between pattern of marrow involvement and clinical stage; a diffuse pattern of involvement is usually associated with a more advanced clinical stage.[353,390a] In some patients, the pattern of marrow involvement may be somewhat inconsistent from biopsy to biopsy, and focal involvement may be associated with an advanced clinical stage. Immunohistologic studies on paraffin-embedded biopsy specimens utilizing antibodies to kappa and lambda light chains are very useful in identifying myeloma cells and determining the extent of involvement.[383-385,392]

---

*References 350, 352, 353, 363, 368, 377, 379, 388, 390a.

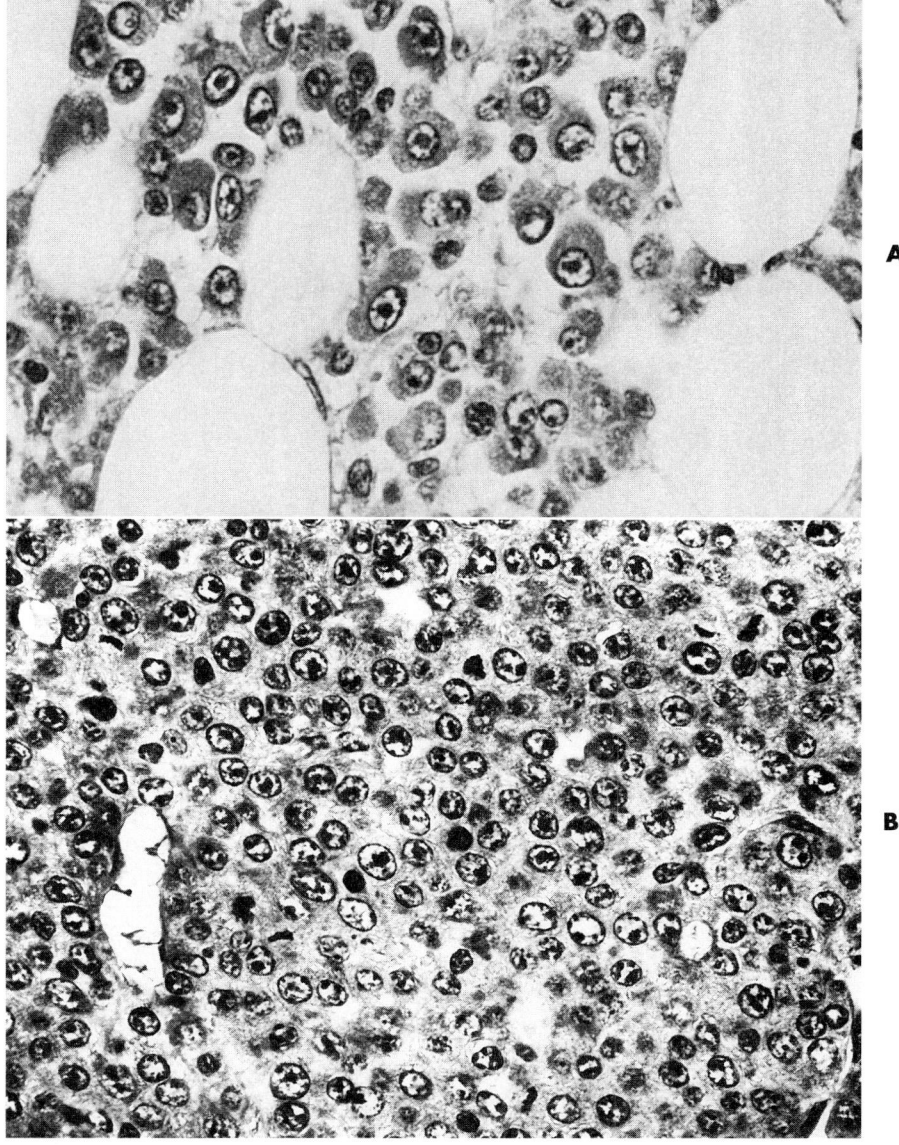

Fig. 23-88 A, Biopsy of marrow from patient with multiple myeloma with an interstial pattern of involvement. Myeloma cells are immature with unusually prominent nucleoli. **B,** Marrow biopsy with diffuse involvement by plasmablastic myeloma. Many of the plasma cells are poorly differentiated with a single prominent nucleolus or multiple nucleoli.

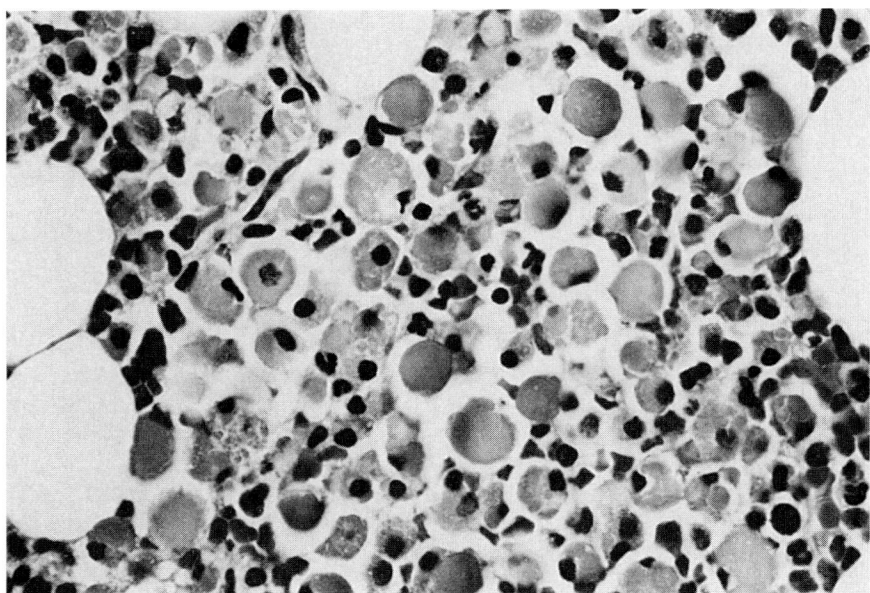

Fig. 23-89 Portion of marrow biopsy from 63-year-old patient with multiple myeloma with hypogam-maglobulinema and kappa light chain Bence Jones proteinuria. Cytoplasm of myeloma cells is distended by numerous, frequently confluent Russell bodies.

In rare cases, a patient with the clinical, x-ray, and histopathologic features of multiple myeloma will have no evidence of monoclonal immunoglobulin production in the serum or urine. These cases have been referred to as "nonsecretory" myeloma.[351,372,386,387] Considerable caution should be exercised in the use of this term, since striking reactive plasmacytosis may be observed with nonmalignant conditions, including liver disease, connective tissue disorders, chronic granulomatous disorders, hypersensitivity states, and drug-related agranulocytosis.[373] When a nonsecretory myeloma is suspected, the monoclonal nature of the proliferating plasma cells should be confirmed by immunoperoxidase or immunofluorescent techniques that will demonstrate kappa or lambda light chain restriction.[372,383,392] An increase in reactive plasma cells will be characterized by a relatively balanced population of kappa- and lambda-containing cells.

Multiple myeloma or amyloidosis may occur in patients with the adult Fanconi's syndrome; the renal abnormalities may precede the overt manifestations of the plasma cell dyscrasia by several years. Bence Jones proteinuria of kappa light chain type is a common finding. A high percentage of the patients with this variant of myeloma manifest crystalline inclusions in the cytoplasm of the proliferating plasma cells and renal tubular cells.[379,381]

The term *plasma cell leukemia* is applied to those processes in which a patient presents with a plasma cell proliferation in the blood; the plasma cells exceed 20% of the blood leukocytes, or the absolute plasma cell count exceeds $20 \times 10^9/L$.[375,380,393] The term should be reserved for cases with this finding at initial presentation. The marrow in plasma cell leukemia usually shows a diffuse and extensive replacement of normal hematopoietic cells by the plasma cells. Patients with plasma cell leukemia have a higher incidence of organomegaly than those with other forms of myeloma, and the disease is frequently associated with an unfavorable prognosis.

Osteosclerotic myeloma

Osteosclerotic myeloma is a form of plasma cell dyscrasia characterized by sclerotic bone lesions and progressive demyelinating polyneuropathology.[360,362,374,382,391] The bone marrow aspirate usually contains less than 10% plasma cells. The plasma cell proliferation is usually evident as a plasmacytoma in the sclerotic lesions or in lymph nodes (Fig. 23-91, *A*). The marrow from areas uninvolved by the sclerotic process may show typical myeloma cell infiltration. The megakaryocytes may be increased and large with hyperlobulated nuclei (see Fig. 23-91). The involved lymph nodes may show hyperplasia of the follicles with a parafollicular infiltration of monoclonal plasma cells.[356] A high percentage of patients with osteosclerotic myeloma have multiorgan involvement, including polyneuropathy, organomegaly, endocrinopathy, and skin changes, the so-called **POEMS syndrome.** Approximately 75% of patients have a thrombocytosis. Polycythemia and leukocytosis are present in about one third of cases. There is usually a low level of monoclonal protein of IgG or IgA class, with a predominance of lambda light chain type.

The median age of onset is 51 years compared with 64 years for typical myeloma; median survival is 97 months in contrast with 30 to 35 months for typical myeloma. The disease appears to be more common in Japan than the United States or Europe.

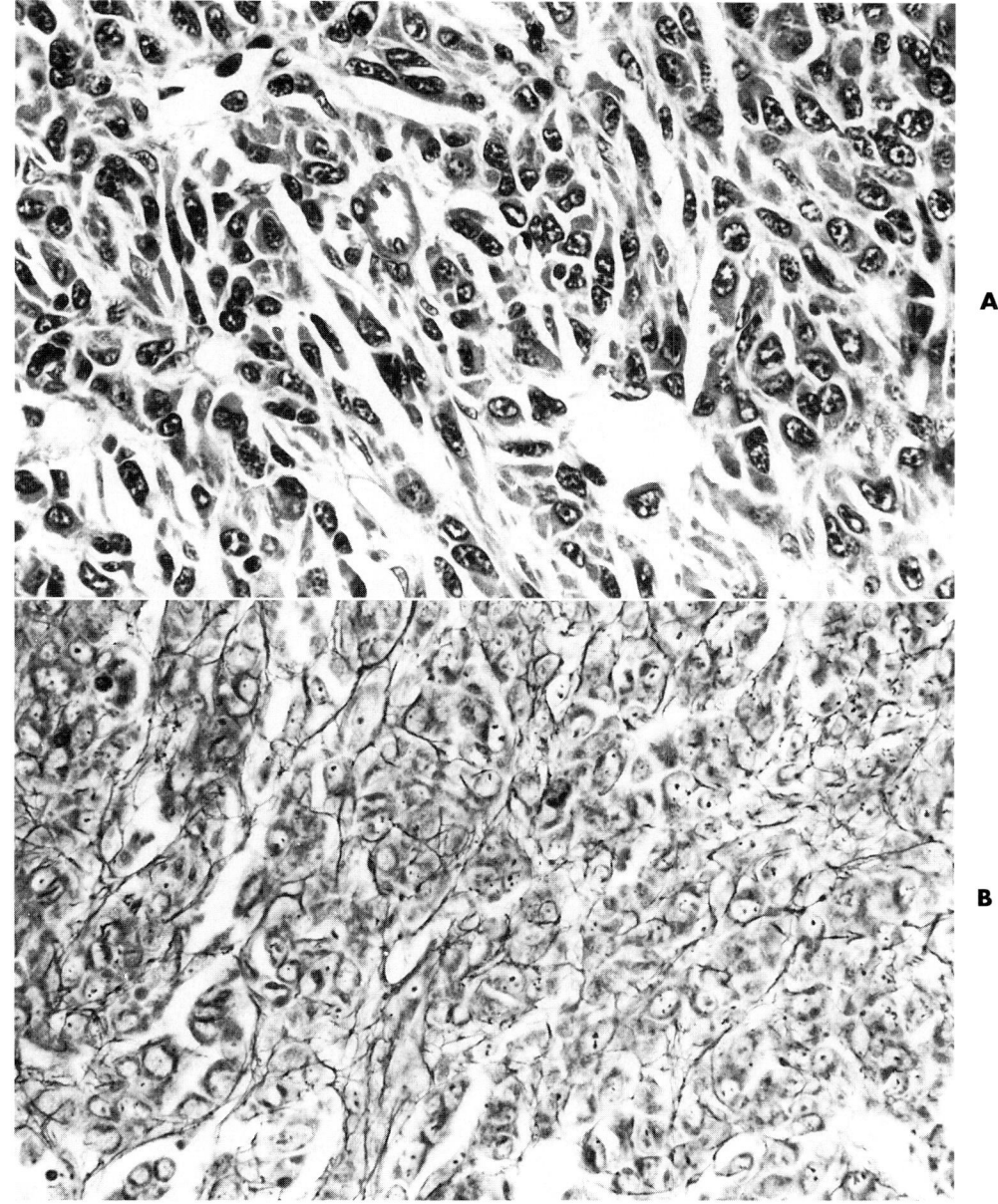

Fig. 23-90 A, Marrow biopsy showing complete replacement by myeloma cells. Cells show considerable distortion. **B,** Reticulin stain of the specimen in **A** showing moderate diffuse increase in coarse reticulin fibers. (**B** Wilder's reticulin.)

An association of giant lymph node hyperplasia with osteoblastic bone lesions and the POEMS syndrome has been reported.[356,360]

Monoclonal gammopathy of undetermined significance

Approximately 1% to 2% of individuals over the age of 50 and 2% to 3% of patients over age 65 have a serum monoclonal gammopathy without other evidence of a plasma cell dyscrasia.[378,378a,379] The monoclonal protein in these individuals is usually less than 3 g/dl; there are usually no or minimal kappa or lambda light chains in the urine. There is no associated hypercalcemia, anemia, renal impairment, or bone lesions on radiographic examination. The bone marrow in these patients may be entirely normal or may manifest a slight increase in mature-appearing plasma cells; this increase is less than 5%. Some of these cases represent incipient myeloma or another type of plasma cell dyscrasia or lymphoproliferative disorder; others continue for several years without undergoing an obvious neoplastic evolution. The term *monoclonal gammopathy of undetermined significance* has been applied to this condition.[378,378a] If the morphologic findings are suspicious for but not diagnostic of myeloma, the patient should be followed with marrow

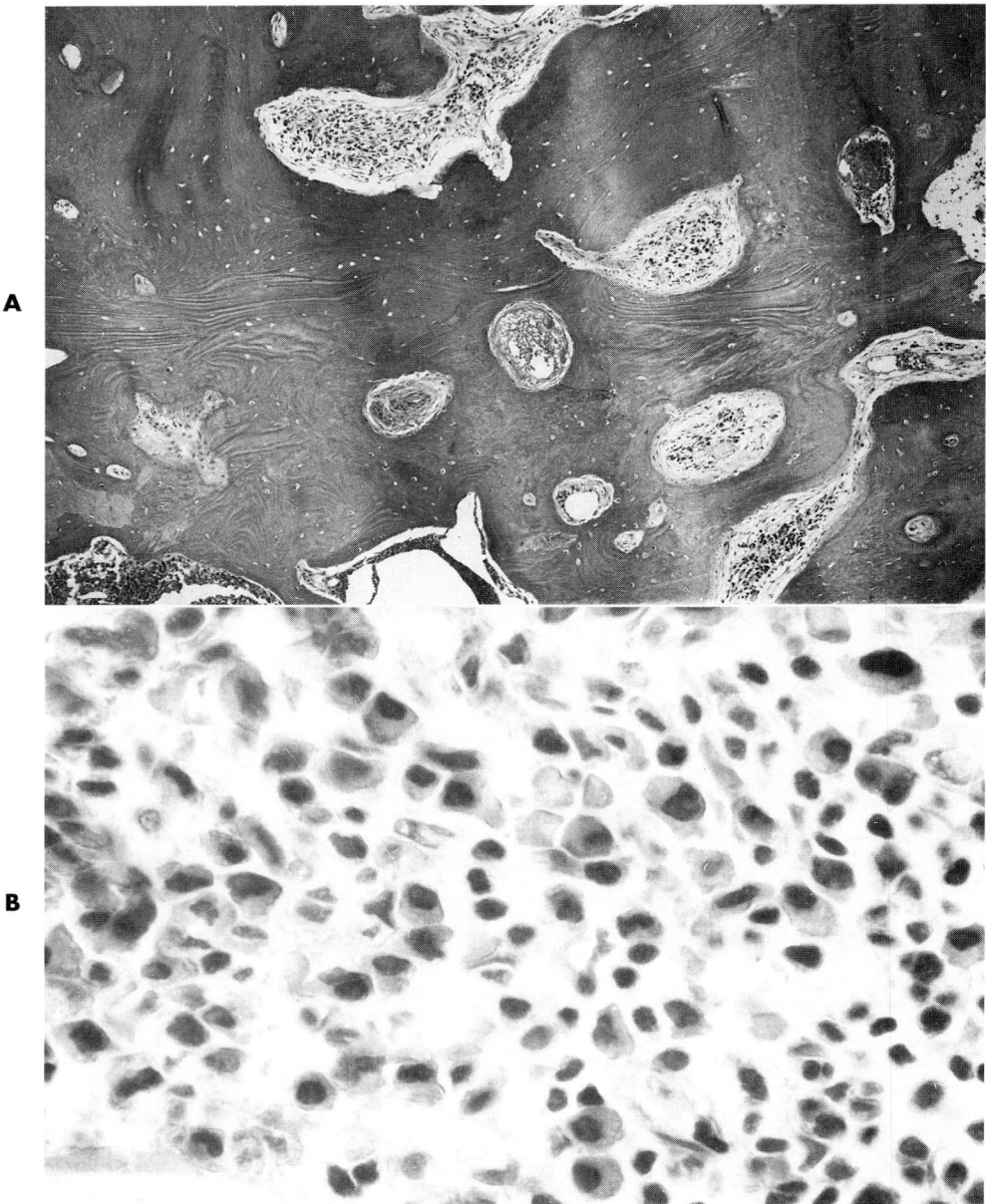

Fig. 23-91 A, Osteosclerotic bone lesion from patient with osteosclerotic myeloma. **B,** High magnification of the marrow in specimen in **A.** This area shows large number of plasma cells that were lambda light chain restricted on immunohistochemical study.   *Continued.*

examination and repeat protein electrophoresis at 6-month intervals. An increase in the number of abnormal plasma cells or light chain–restricted plasma cells and an increase in the amount of monoclonal immunoglobulin suggest a neoplastic process. A stable immunoglobulin level and plasma cell percentage are more reflective of a benign monoclonal gammopathy. The plasma cell labeling index as described by Greipp and Kyle[370] has been helpful in distinguishing monoclonal gammopathy of undetermined significance and smoldering myeloma from overt multiple myeloma. Ultimately, approximately 25% of patients with monoclonal gammopathy of undetermined significance develop a plasma cell

dyscrasia or related process; the interval to the occurrence ranges up to 29 years.[378]

Immunocytochemistry on paraffin-embedded specimens using antibodies to kappa and lambda light chains can be a very important approach to the study of myeloma and related disorders.[383] The primary use of the technique in this group of diseases is to determine the relative proportion of kappa- or lambda-reacting cells; a predominant population of plasma cells reacting with a single light chain antibody is evidence for a monoclonal proliferation (see Fig. 23-1). A balanced proliferation of kappa- and lambda-reacting plasma cells indicates a benign process. A light chain ratio determined by

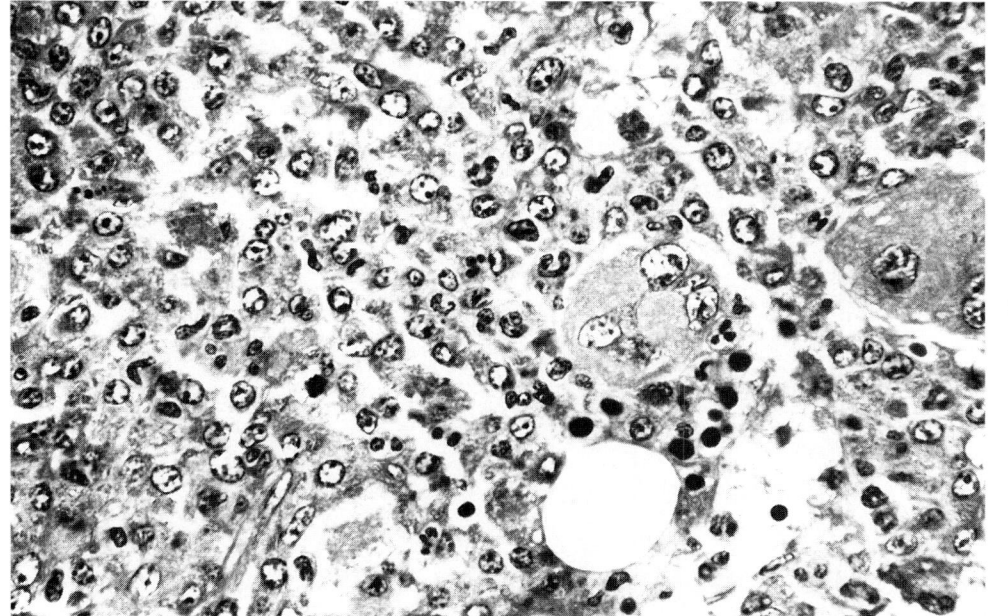

Fig. 23-91, cont'd **C,** Marrow biopsy from a nonsclerotic area from a patient with osteosclerotic myeloma with POEMS syndrome. There was a thrombocytosis. The marrow in this area shows an infiltration by immature plasma cells. There was also an increase in large megakaryocytes, two of which are at right.

dividing the number of positively reacting plasma cells for the predominant light chain by the number of positively reacting cells for the other light chain has been suggested as an aid in the distinction of myeloma from monoclonal gammopathy of undetermined significance or a reactive increase in plasma cells.[383] Patients with overt myeloma generally have values above 16; patients with monoclonal gammopathy of undetermined significance or a reactive process have values less than 16.

Plasmacytoma

A solitary plasmacytoma, in contrast to the disseminated proliferation of plasma cells in multiple myeloma, is a single focus of plasma cells occurring in either bone or soft tissue.[394,395,397-403] Solitary plasmacytomas are more frequent in males than females and have a peak incidence in the sixth decade, slightly earlier than multiple myeloma. Plasmacytomas are generally divided into two broad groups based on location: plasmacytoma of bone and extramedullary or soft tissue plasmacytoma. Evidence for the different biologic behaviors of these two types has been reported; plasmacytoma of bone has been reported to have a greater predilection to progress to multiple myeloma than soft tissue plasmacytoma. Other studies have shown no significant difference between these two locations and the incidence of evolution to myeloma.[397] The solitary plasmacytoma of bone may occur in both the flat and long bones; the most common sites are the vertebrae, ilium, and skull.[398] Soft tissue extension from bone lesions may occur. The majority of plasmacytomas of bone show osteolytic change on radiologic examination, although osteolytic/

osteoblastic lesions may occur.[403] The most frequent sites of extramedullary or soft tissue plasmacytomas are the nasal fossa, maxillary sinus, and nasopharynx.[396,397] Extension into adjacent bone tissue may occur, and multiple lesions may be present.

On microscopic examination the plasmacytoma is frequently very vascular with a minimal stromal component and consists of sheets of plasma cells of varying degrees of differentiation[397] (Fig. 23-92). The plasmacytic nature of the proliferating cells is readily recognized in the more well-differentiated lesions. In plasmacytomas with a predominant population of more immature cells with a fine nuclear chromatin and single prominent nucleolus, there usually is a minor population of more differentiated plasma cells. Amyloid may be present and was noted in 25% of the lesions in one series.[397]

Immunocytochemical study with antibodies to kappa and lambda light chains is an important approach to the evaluation of a suspected plasmacytoma. A kappa or lambda light chain–restricted population confirms a diagnosis of plasmacytoma (Fig. 23-93). There is a predominance of IgG heavy chain type in solitary plasmacytoma of bone and IgA heavy chain type in plasmacytomas from the upper respiratory tract.

Patients with an apparent solitary plasmacytoma should be carefully evaluated for the presence of disseminated disease; studies should include bilateral iliac crest bone marrow biopsies, radiologic survey, and immunoelectrophoretic examination of the serum and urine. The patient with a solitary plasmacytoma usually has a normal hemoglobin level and no hypercalcemia. Approximately 50% of patients have a monoclonal protein in the urine and/or serum; the level almost

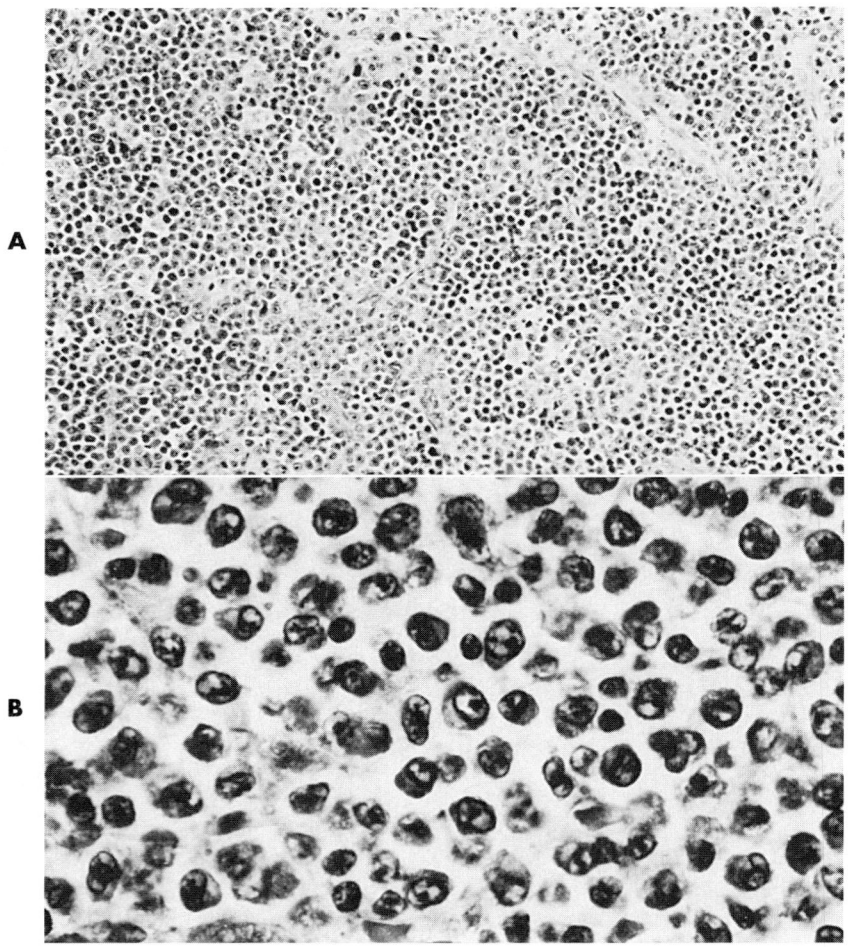

Fig. 23-92 **A,** Extramedullary plasmacytoma from region of nasopharynx. Prominent vascular structures interrupt sheets of plasma cells. **B,** High magnification of lesion in **A.** Minority of cells show distinct plasma cell differentiation.

invariably is less than 2 g/dl, and the non-monoclonal immunoglobulins are normal in contrast to multiple myeloma, in which they are generally decreased. A marked reduction or disappearance in the monoclonal immunoglobulin will usually occur following tumoricidal radiation; the maximum reduction may not occur for several years.[397]

Bone marrow biopsies performed on patients with a solitary plasmacytoma should be studied immunohistochemically with anti-kappa and anti-lambda antibodies to exclude the presence of a light chain–restricted population of plasma cells. Serum beta 2 microglobulin levels should be determined. The diagnosis of a solitary plasmacytoma should be made only if studies for disseminated disease are negative.

Approximately 35% of patients with a solitary plasmacytoma who receive treatment, including radiation, chemotherapy, and surgical excision, will eventually develop multiple myeloma; this evolution may occur up to 12 years after initial diagnosis.[397] The presence of nuclear immaturity with prominent nucleoli appears to have some positive predictive value for the development of multiple myeloma. The presence of a monoclonal protein in serum, urine, or both does not predict the development of disseminated disease. Local recurrence of the lesion is uncommon.

The differential diagnosis of a plasmacytoma includes plasma cell granuloma, plasmacytoid lymphoma, and large cell lymphoma of immunoblastic type. The plasma cell granuloma shows a balanced proliferation of kappa- and lambda-reacting cells on immunocytochemical evaluation. The plasmacytoid lymphoma comprises a mixture of lymphocytes and plasma cells. Some of the large cell lymphomas, particularly the B-immunoblastic lymphoma, may be difficult to distinguish from a plasmacytoma. The immunoblastic lymphoma will usually involve lymph nodes in contrast to a plasmacytoma. Immunophenotypic studies of plasmacytoma and immunoblastic lymphoma using a panel of monoclonal antibodies have shown significant immunophenotypic differences between these two processes.[401] The immunoblastic lymphomas have cytoplasmic IgM heavy chain and express pan–B-cell surface antigens such as CD19 and CD20. The plasmacytomas contain IgA or IgG heavy

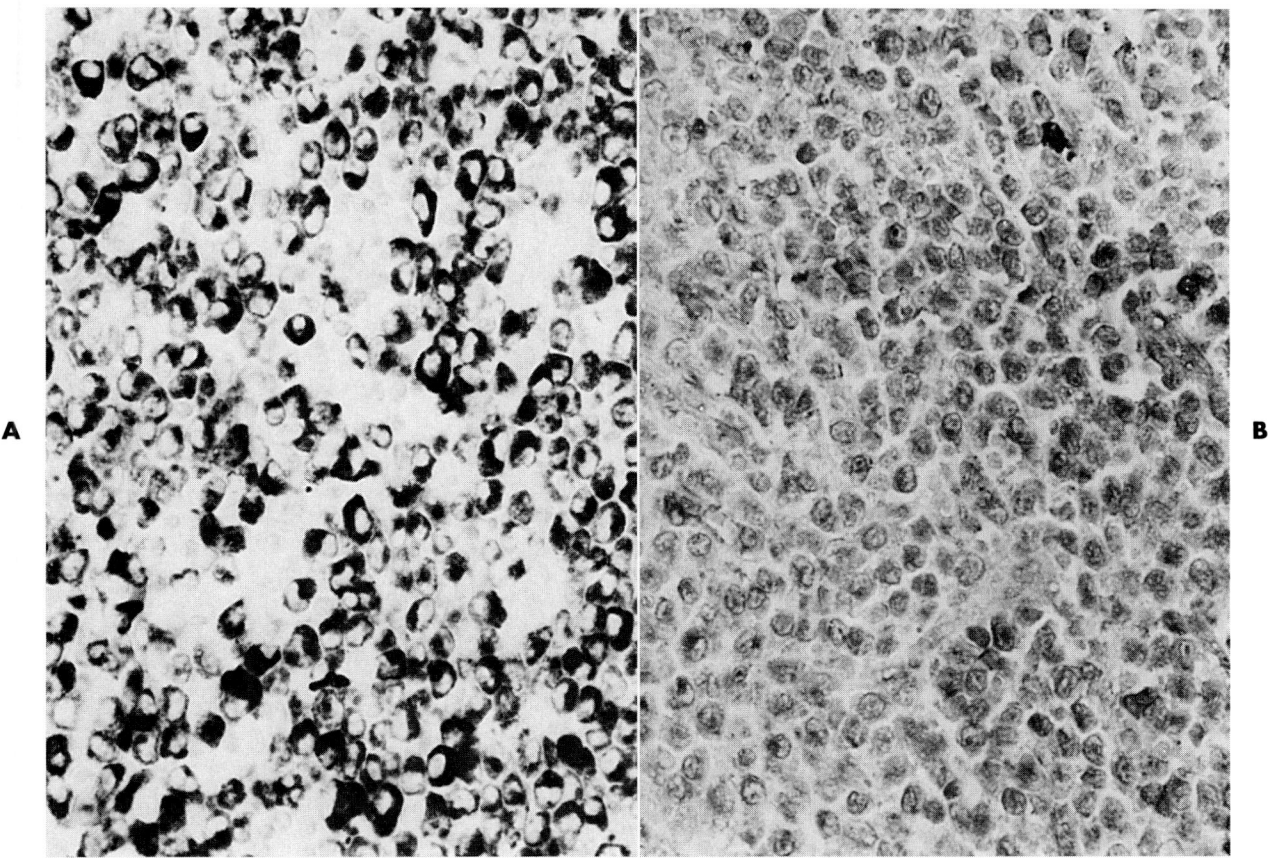

Fig. 23-93 A, Specimen in Fig. 23-92 reacted with anti-kappa light chain antibody using peroxidase-antiperoxidase-immunoperoxidase technique; plasma cells are uniformly intensely reactive. **B,** Same specimen reacted with anti-lambda light chain antibody; plasma cells are negative. (Immunoperoxidase.)

chain and are generally negative for pan–B-surface antigens; approximately 20% of plasmacytomas and myelomas are positive with pan–B-cell antibodies.

Plasmacytoid lymphoma (Waldenström's macroglobulinemia)

In 1944, Waldenström described a clinical syndrome characterized by hyperglobulinemia, increased serum viscosity, and a proliferation of lymphocytes in hematopoietic tissue as well as other organs.[420] This syndrome is usually referred to as Waldenström's macroglobulinemia in recognition of the original description and identification of the globulin as a macroglobulin in the majority of patients. This syndrome has a median age of onset of 60 years and a slight male predominance. Hepatosplenomegaly, lymphadenopathy, and neurologic abnormalities are frequent findings; anemia and hyperviscosity are commonly noted laboratory abnormalities.[412,413,420] The lymphoproliferative process associated with this syndrome usually involves the small B lymphocyte or the small B lymphocyte and plasmacytoid lymphocyte (i.e., small lymphocytic or plasmacytoid lymphoma in the Working Formulation, plasmacytoid lymphocytic in the Lukes-Collins' classification, and lymphoplas-

macytoid or lymphoplasmacytic immunocytoma in the Kiel terminology).[411,414,416,418] Although commonly used to describe the histopathologic lesion occurring in patients with this syndrome, the term *Waldenström's macroglobulinemia* should be reserved for those patients with the clinical syndrome associated with an IgM paraproteinemia and the presence of a lymphoma with well-differentiated lymphocytes or a plasmacytoid lymphoma. Cases of plasmacytoid lymphoma may also be associated with paraprotein of IgG and IgA type.[419] A substantial number of cases of plasmacytoid lymphoma have no associated gammopathy.[419] IgM gammopathy may be associated with lymphomas other than plasmacytoid and has been reported in cases of multiple myeloma.[404,418]

The peripheral blood shows a leukemic picture in approximately 30% of cases; the predominant cells are well-differentiated lymphocytes or a mixture of lymphocytes and plasmacytoid lymphocytes.[412,413] A similar population of cells predominates in the bone marrow[409,410,415,417] (Fig. 23-94). Mature plasma cells, tissue mast cells, and histiocytes may also be increased. In some cases, plasma cells predominate.[405] In marrow sections, the infiltrate may be focal or diffuse; with focal involvement the infiltrate may be

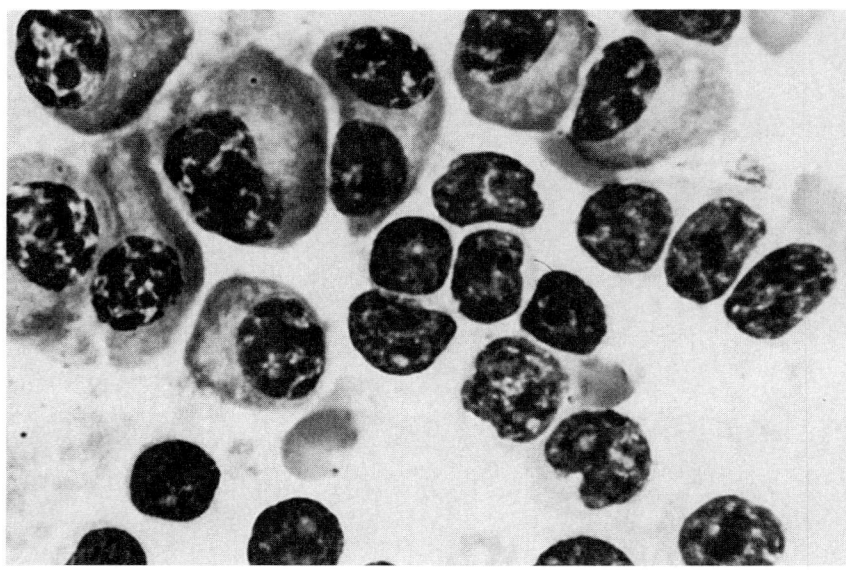

Fig. 23-94 Bone marrow smear from patient with marrow involvement by plasmacytoid lymphoma associated with IgM monoclonal gammopathy. Lymphocytic cells have characteristics of well-differentiated lymphocytes; plasma cells have clumped nuclear chromatin without prominent nucleoli. (Wright-Giemsa.)

preferentially paratrabecular. Marrow involvement may be very extensive, with a marked decrease in normal hematopoietic cells. Intranuclear inclusions, frequently referred to as *Dutcher bodies,* may be observed in some of the lymphocytes and plasma cells[409]; these inclusions, which are variably PAS-positive, may be observed in other lymphomas, multiple myeloma, and reactive proliferations, and are not diagnostic of plasmacytoid lymphoma.[406,407] In some cases of plasmacytoid lymphoma, the plasma cells and plasmacytoid lymphocytes contain abundant cytoplasmic inclusions. These inclusions may be numerous, and some of these cells resemble histiocytes; the inclusions are usually intensely PAS positive (Fig. 23-95). Plasma cells with similar inclusions may occasionally predominate in multiple myeloma. Like other small lymphocytic lymphomas, the plasmacytoid lymphoma associated with Waldenström's macroglobulinemia may terminate with a clinical pathologic picture of Richter's syndrome.[408]

Heavy chain disease

The heavy chain diseases are clinical syndromes that are associated with the production of heavy chain fragments of the immunoglobulin molecule.[421,423] *Gamma-chain disease* has more of the features of a malignant lymphoma than of multiple myeloma. The median age for this disease is 61 years, but it has been reported in individuals younger than 20.[424] Weakness, fatigue, fever, and lymphadenopathy are common symptoms; hepatomegaly, splenomegaly, and peripheral lymphadenopathy are each present in slightly more than half of the cases. There are frequently anemia, leukopenia, and thrombocytopenia. Atypical lymphocytes and plasma cells may be found in the peripheral blood. The bone marrow is usually abnormal and shows an increase in lymphocytes, plasma cells, or both. Occasionally the mar-

row is normal. There may be an accompanying eosinophilia. There are no significant changes in the bone marrow in *alpha-chain disease.*[425] Most of the reported cases of *mu-chain disease* have had long histories of CLL.[422,423] The marrow in several of the reported cases contained vacuolated plasma cells. The occurrence of tumors composed of undifferentiated lymphoid cells in patients with heavy chain disease has been reported.[423,426]

Amyloidosis

Amyloid is present in the marrow of approximately 30% of patients with systemic amyloidosis and is usually detected in biopsies of patients being evaluated for Bence Jones proteinuria or some other form of monoclonal gammopathy; in rare cases it may be found in the marrows of patients without any clinical indication of the disorder.[428,429] Marrow involvement may manifest either as small focal lesions or as extensive marrow replacement.[427,430] Early involvement is characterized by focal deposits of amyloid in the medullary vessels; these range from small deposits in the media to large accumulations that greatly expand the vessel walls, resulting in narrowing of the lumen (Fig. 23-96). With more extensive involvement, the accumulation of amyloid is present in the perivascular tissue and marrow substance (see Fig. 23-96).

SYSTEMIC POLYCLONAL B-IMMUNOBLASTIC PROLIFERATION

A florid polyclonal proliferation of B immunoblasts may occur in patients with a variety of immune disorders and involve blood, bone marrow, and lymph nodes.[431,432,434,435] The leukocyte count may be elevated with a high percentage of B immunoblasts, cells with deeply basophilic cytoplasm, coarse nuclear chromatin, and distinct nucleoli. There fre-

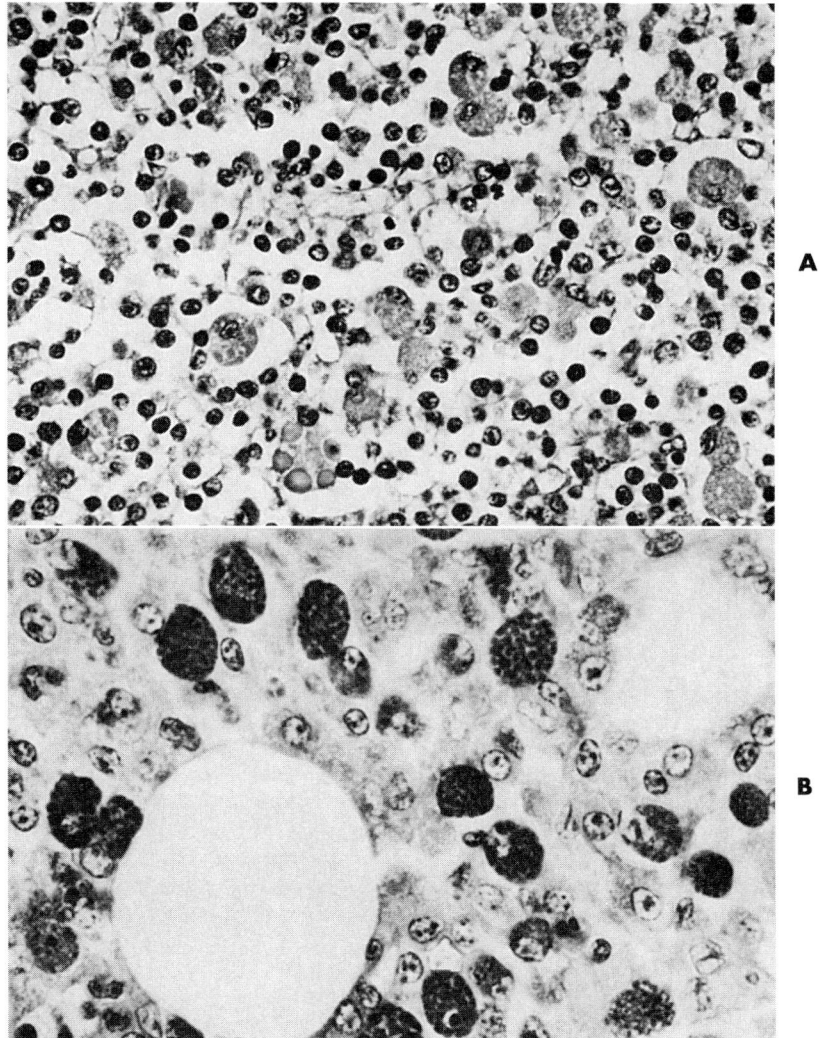

Fig. 23-95 A, Marrow section from patient with plasmacytoid lymphoma associated with serum IgM monoclonal gammopathy. Marrow is replaced by infiltrate of lymphocytes and plasma cells; many of plasma cells contain numerous cytoplasmic inclusions. **B,** Specimen illustrated in **A** reacted with PAS stain. Inclusions in plasma cells are strongly positive.

quently is some evidence of maturation of these cells to plasma cells. The bone marrow may show extensive infiltration and may resemble lymphoma or plasmablastic myeloma with immunoblasts, plasma cells, and intermediate forms (Fig. 23-97). Lymph nodes may show a similar infiltrate, with complete effacement of the normal architecture. Immunologic studies are critical in the evaluation of these lesions. The polyclonal nature of the infiltrate is demonstrated with immunocytochemical reactions that show essentially a balanced population of kappa- and lambda-reacting cells[433-435] (see Fig. 23-97).

The biology of this process is not completely clear; in some patients it appears to represent an acute immune reaction, and it has been observed in patients with laboratory findings of acute lupus erythematosus. It may in some instances be analogous to the polymorphous lymphoid lesions observed

in transplant patients. There may be dramatic regression following steroid therapy.[434,435]

SYSTEMIC MASTOCYTOSIS

Systemic mastocytosis is a relatively rare disorder characterized by mast cell proliferation in several organs.* It usually occurs with urticaria pigmentosa but may present in patients without cutaneous involvement. Whereas the median age for patients with systemic mastocytosis with urticaria pigmentosa is 45 years, the median age for patients presenting without urticaria pigmentosa is around 75 years.[436] The clinical symptoms are varied and include diarrhea, weakness, fractures, weight loss, arthralgia, flushing episodes, and bronchospasm. Splen-

*References 436-438, 440, 442-445, 449, 450, 452-455.

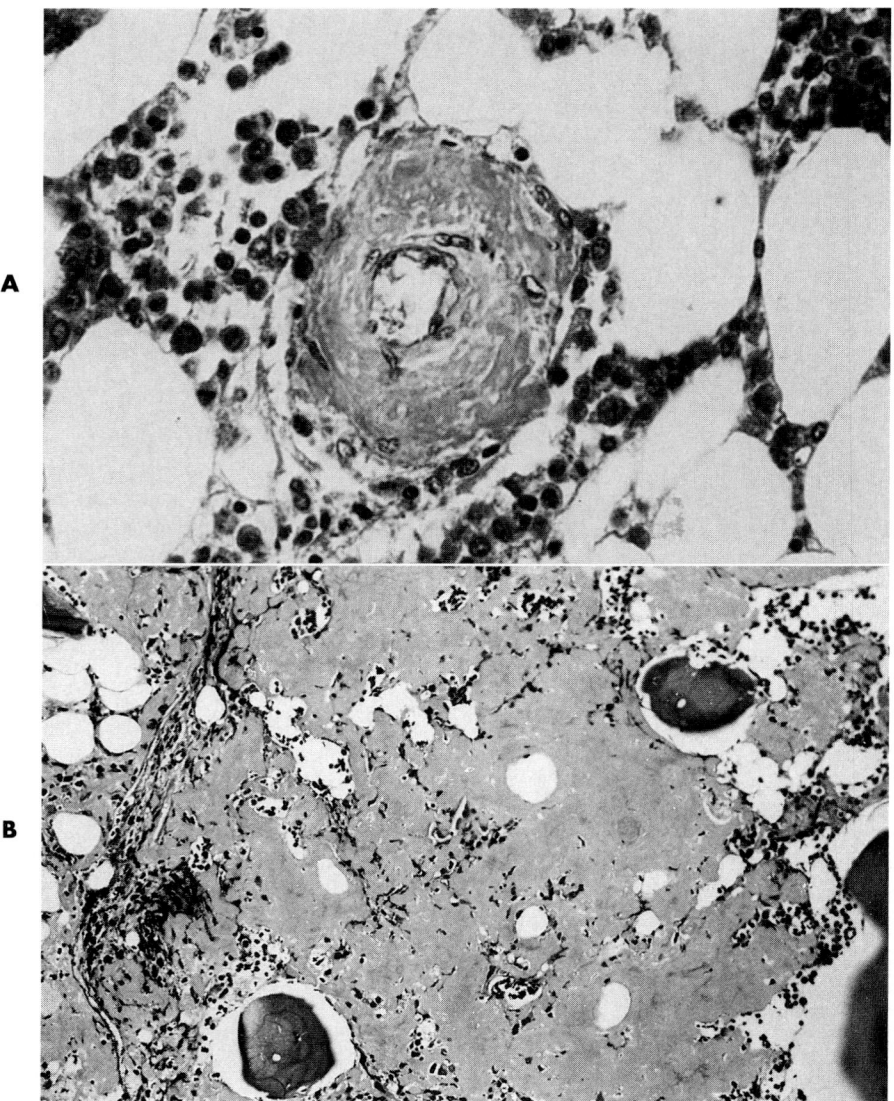

Fig. 23-96 **A,** Marrow vessel with amyloid accumulation in media. Specimen is from patient with primary amyloidosis. **B,** Marrow with diffuse involvement by amyloid.

omegaly may be present. Osteoblastic, osteolytic, or concurrent ostetoblastic-osteolytic lesions may be found on radiologic examination; generalized osteoporosis may also occur (Fig. 23-98).

The bone marrow is the most frequent site of noncutaneous involvement in systemic mastocytosis; lesions may be found as a result of a specific search or may be detected in a biopsy performed for some purpose unrelated to suspected mastocytosis. In the latter instance, when there is no clinical suspicion of the disease, the lesions may be overlooked or misinterpreted because of the difficulty in identifying mast cells in routine sections and because of the changes inherent in the mast cells in this disease; the cells are frequently large and have lobulated nuclei and decreased granules that may be much smaller than normal mast cell granules.[441] Smears obtained by bone marrow aspirate may suggest the diagnosis of mastocytosis if large numbers of atypical mast cells

are present; however, up to 7% mast cells have been reported in aspirate preparations in patients without mast cell disease.[448] In many instances, the mast cells in the marrow in mastocytosis are associated with reticulin fibrosis and are not readily aspirated.

The mast cell lesions in bone marrow sections may be focal or diffuse. Focal lesions are more common and may be paratrabecular, perivascular, or randomly distributed.[436,438,455] The paratrabecular lesions frequently are marked by a margination of the infiltrate along the endosteal surface of the bone structure or juxtaposition of a lesion to a bone spicule (Fig. 23-99). The perivascular lesions may be associated with prominent medial and adventitial hypertrophy and collagen fibrosis.

The focal lesions are variable in appearance but generally can be classified into two primary types based on cell composition: polycellular and monocellular. Both types may be

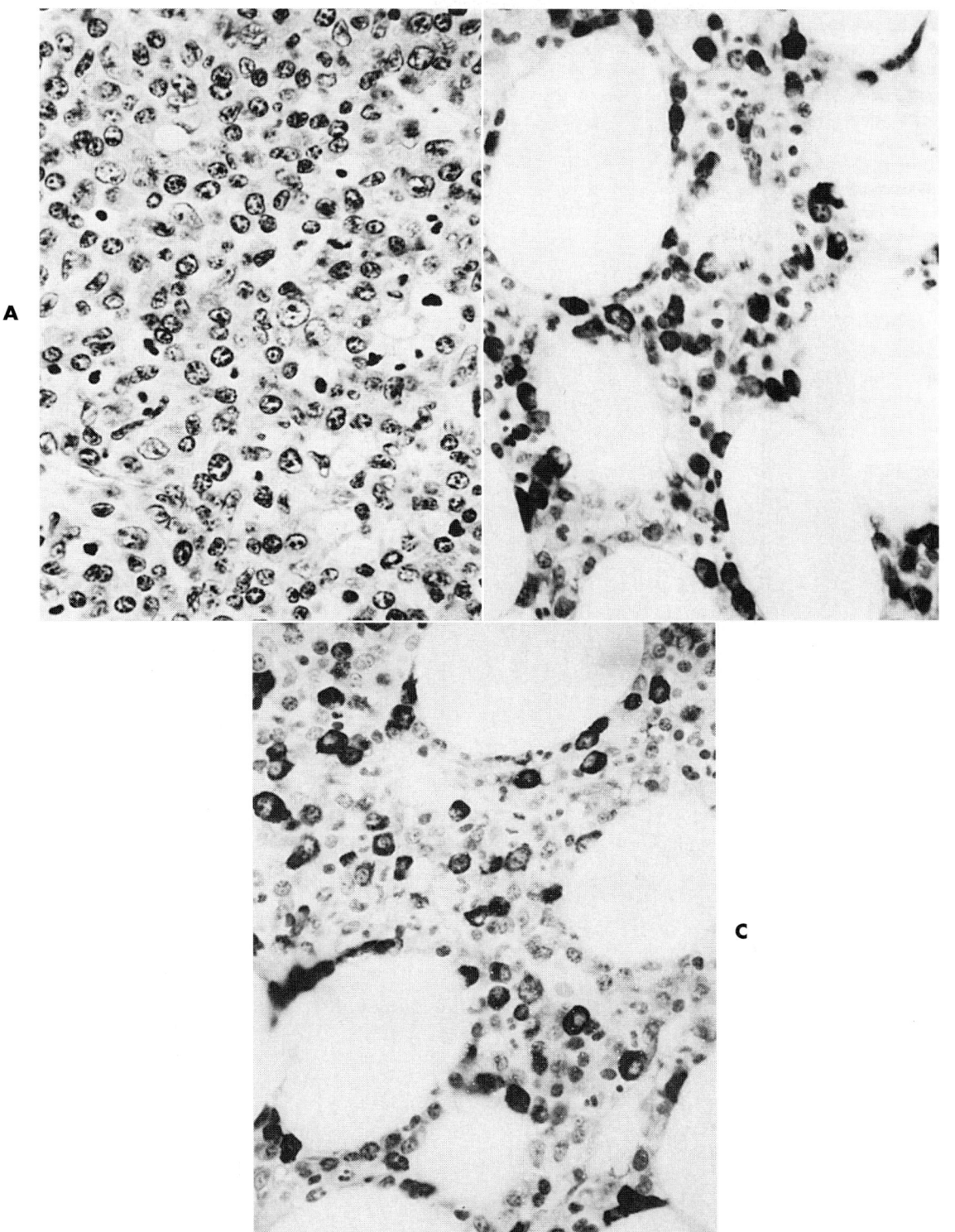

Fig. 23-97 A, Marrow biopsy from 38-year-old woman with autoimmune disorder characterized by extensive infiltration of marrow by plasma cells and B immunoblasts. **B** and **C,** Specimen illustrated in **A** reacted with anti-kappa **(B)** and anti-lambda **(C)** antibodies using peroxidase-antiperoxidase-immunoperoxidase technique. There is balanced proliferation of kappa- and lambda-reacting cells. **(B** and **C** Peroxidase-antiperoxidase.)

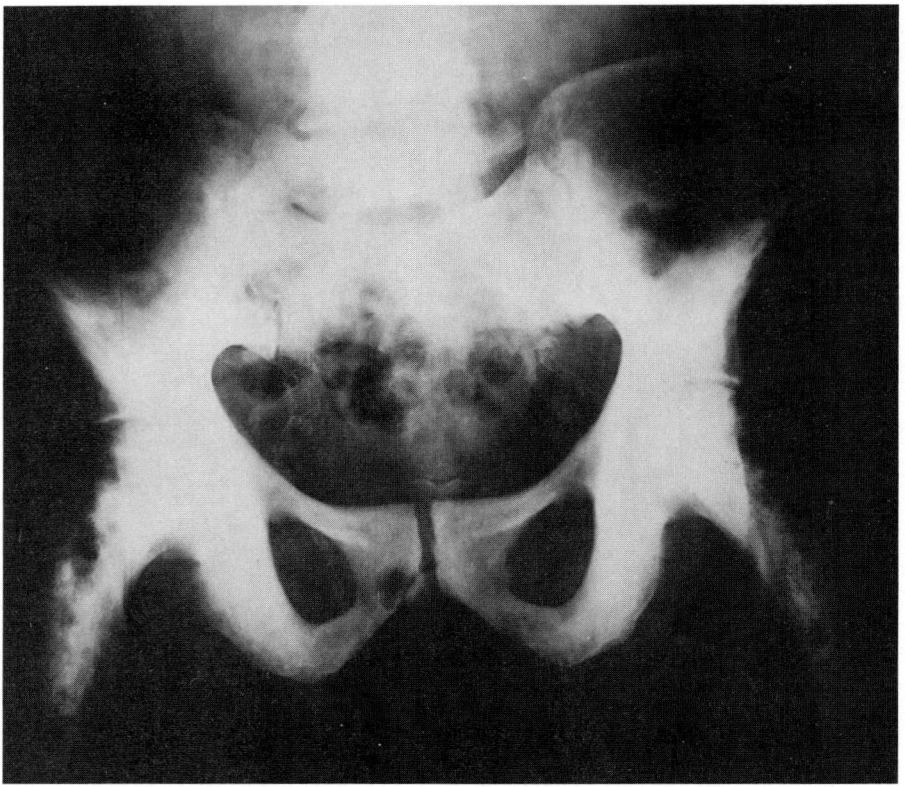

Fig. 23-98 Radiograph of pelvis and upper femurs from patient with systemic mastocytosis; both osteosclerotic and osteolytic changes are prominent.

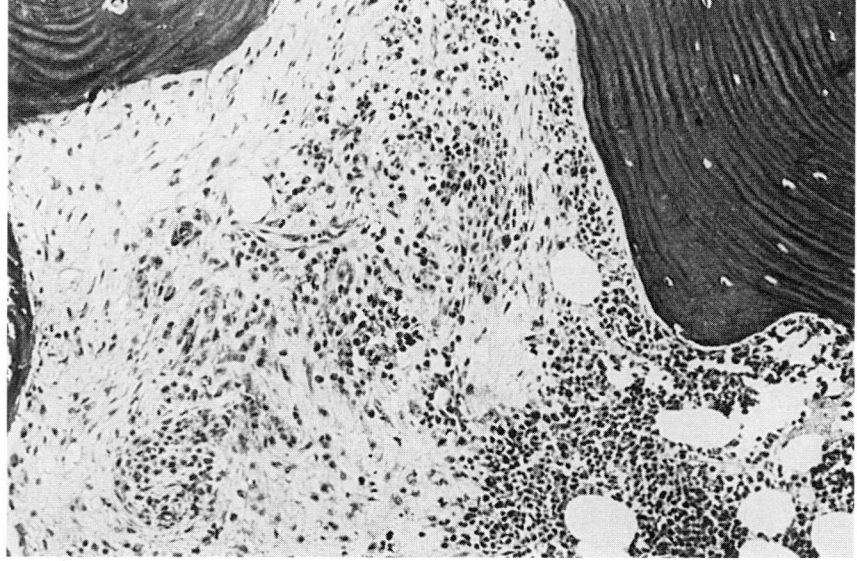

Fig. 23-99 Paratrabecular fibrosis in marrow of patient with systemic mastocytosis. Numerous mast cells, occurring in groups and singly, are enmeshed in fibrous connective tissue. Many mast cells are enlongated and have histiocytic appearance.

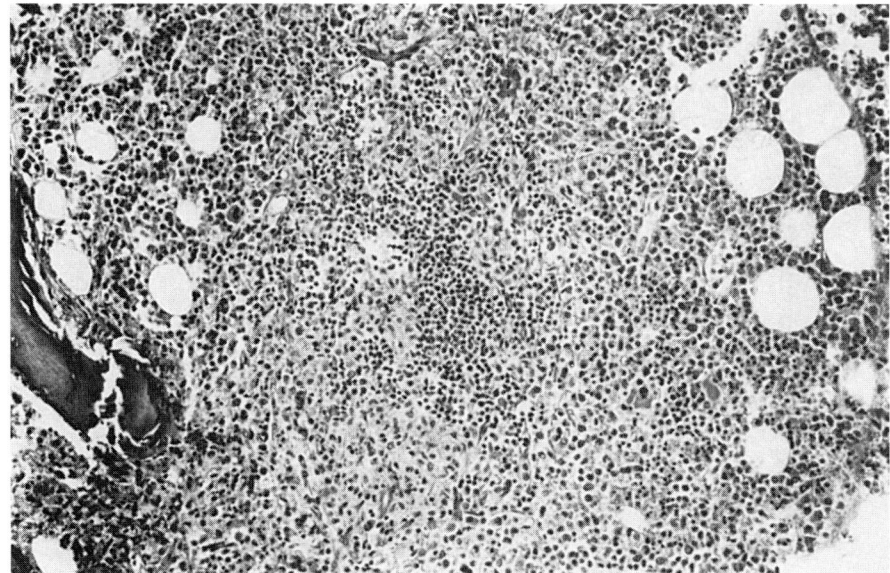

Fig. 23-100 Lesion in bone marrow from patient with systemic mastocytosis. Central collection of well-differentiated lymphocytes is surrounded by lighter-staining mast cells.

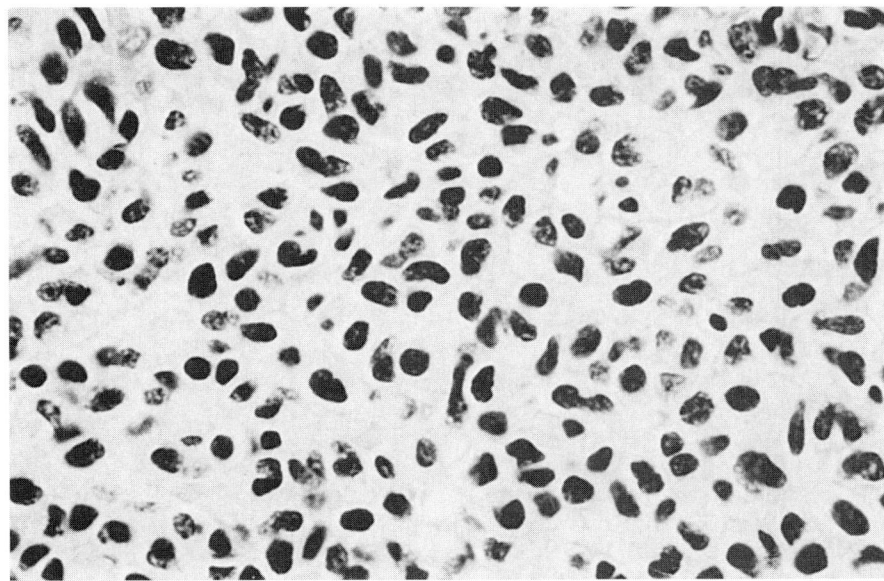

Fig. 23-101 Monomorphous pattern in marrow biopsy from 78-year-old woman with systemic mastocytosis. The mast cells have round-to-monocytoid nuclei and moderate amount of clear cytoplasm, imparting somewhat histiocytic appearance.

observed in the same specimen. The polycellular lesions are characterized by mast cells, lymphocytes, histiocytes, eosinophils, neutrophils, fibroblasts, and endothelial cells in varying numbers; the eosinophils are frequently more numerous at the margins of the lesion. In some cases the different cell types appear to be randomly distributed; in others; the mast cells occur in a central aggregate and are surrounded by well-differentiated lymphocytes, or the mast cells encircle a focus of lymphocytes (Fig. 23-100). The

mast cells in these lesions are frequently atypical and characterized by abundant eosinophilic cytoplasm with very fine granules. In the monomorphic lesions, the cellular composition is predominantly mast cells with only scattered lymphocytes and eosinophils (Fig. 23-101). The mast cells in these lesions may appear as intertwining bundles and vary in shape from round in cross section to spindle shaped in longitudinal cut. The cytoplasm is pale to lightly eosinophilic. The nuclei are round or oval; occasionally the nuclei have a

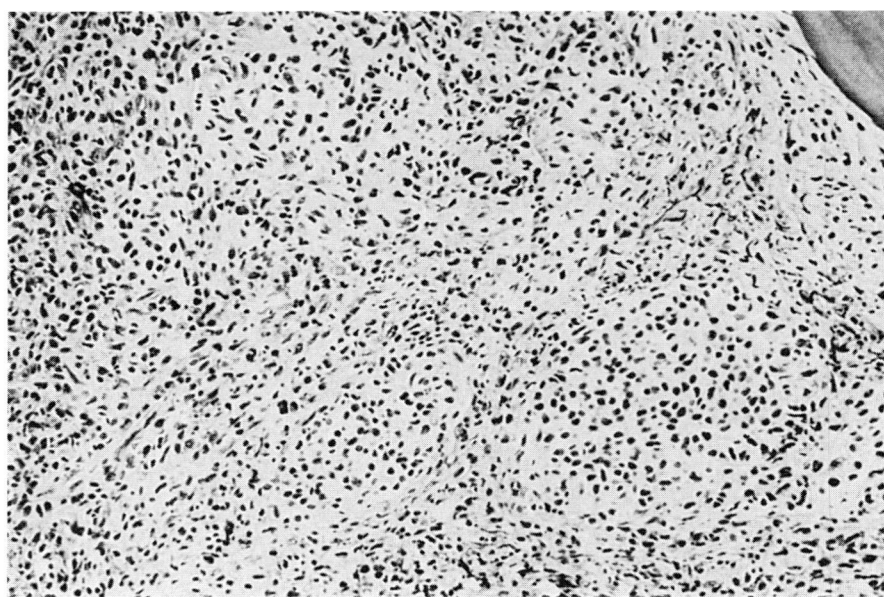

Fig. 23-102 Marrow biopsy from 62-year-old woman with systemic mastocytosis. Patient had history of diarrhea and arthralgia but no evidence of urticaria pigmentosa. Medullary space of entire biopsy specimen is replaced by intertwining bundles of spindle-shaped mast cells.

monocytoid configuration. Nucleoli are inconspicuous, and mitotic figures are infrequent. Some of these lesions may resemble aggregates of histiocytes or granulomas. The marrow exclusive of the mast cell lesions is usually hypercellular or normocellular with a granulocytic hyperplasia.[436,443] The diffuse lesions are characterized by the same cell types as the focal lesions (Fig. 23-102). Changes in the bone trabeculae may be present; both widening and erosion of the trabeculae may be observed. Rarely, evidence of new bone formation may be present (Fig. 23-103). Reticulin stains show varying degrees of reticulin fibrosis.

Horny et al.[438] have described three histopathologic patterns of mastocytosis in the bone marrow: type I, focal lesions with normal-appearing, noninvolved marrow; type II, focal lesions with marked granulocytic hyperplasia in noninvolved marrow; and type III, diffuse mastocytic infiltration. Type I disease in the reported series was always associated with urticaria pigmentosa and a low incidence of associated organomegaly. Types II and III lesions were not associated with cutaneous involvement. The type II pattern was accompanied by an increased incidence of myeloproliferative disorders, both acute and chronic (Fig. 23-104). Type III was associated with mast cell leukemia. Survival studies showed a correlation with histopathology; type I was characterized by a prolonged course in the majority of patients. Types II and III patterns were generally associated with a more aggressive clinical course than type I. The increased incidence of myeloid and monocytic leukemia in systemic mastocytosis also has been observed in other studies.[440,453] In contrast to the results reported, the author has observed type I lesions in patients without urticaria pigmentosa.

Because the mast cells in mastocytosis may be very atypical and possess very abundant cytoplasm without evident granules or have a fibroblastic appearance, there may be considerable difficulty in recognizing the true nature of the cells. Mast cell granules react with both toluidine blue and Giemsa stains. The granules are metachromatic and appear reddish purple. Considerable variability in degree of positivity and number of positive granules may be observed among different cells. The reactivity of the granules can be enhanced in decalcified tissue by treatment of the sections with potassium permanganate followed by oxalic acid before the staining procedure.[448] Zenker's and B5 fixatives may interfere with reactivity with both Giemsa and toluidine blue stains. Mast cells also react with chloroacetate esterase in formalin-fixed tissue decalcified with EDTA; this stain may not work satisfactorily in specimens decalcified in rapid acid decalcifier or biopsy specimens processed with acid fixatives such as Zenker's or B5.

A highly specific antibody to human mast cell tryptase that may be used on decalcified and B5-fixed paraffin-embedded specimens is very accurate for identification of mast cell lesions[454] (Fig. 23-105). Other antibodies that react with mast cells include antibodies to alpha-antitrypsin, alpha-antichymotrypsin, and CD68.[439]

The differential diagnosis of mast cell lesions in the marrow includes AILD, Hodgkin's disease, PTCL, and chronic idiopathic myelofibrosis. The eosinophilic fibrohistiocytic lesion described by Rywlin and colleagues has many of the histopathologic characteristics of mastocytosis lesions and in most instances is a form of mast cell disease.[446,447,451] The primary distinction of mastocytosis from the other disorders is based on the immunohistochemical demonstration of mast cells with antibody to mast cell tryptase.

METASTATIC TUMORS

Bone marrow biopsies frequently are used for the staging of patients with histologically documented malignancies;

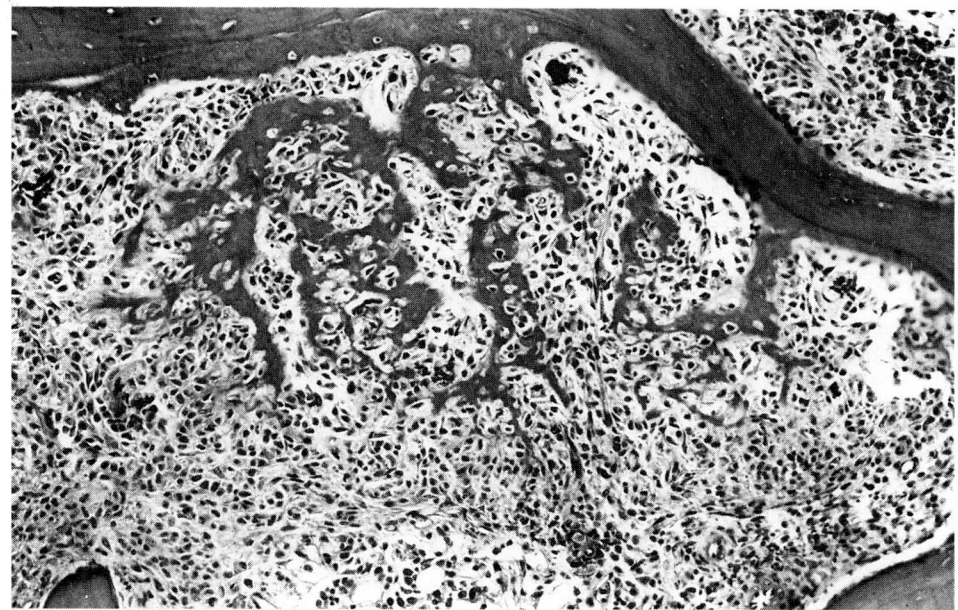

Fig. 23-103 Bone marrow biopsy from patient with concurrent acute myeloblastic leukemia and systemic mastocytosis. Mast cell infiltration in this area of biopsy was associated with new bone formation. No other areas in bilateral biopsies show this finding. This was patient's first marrow biopsy.

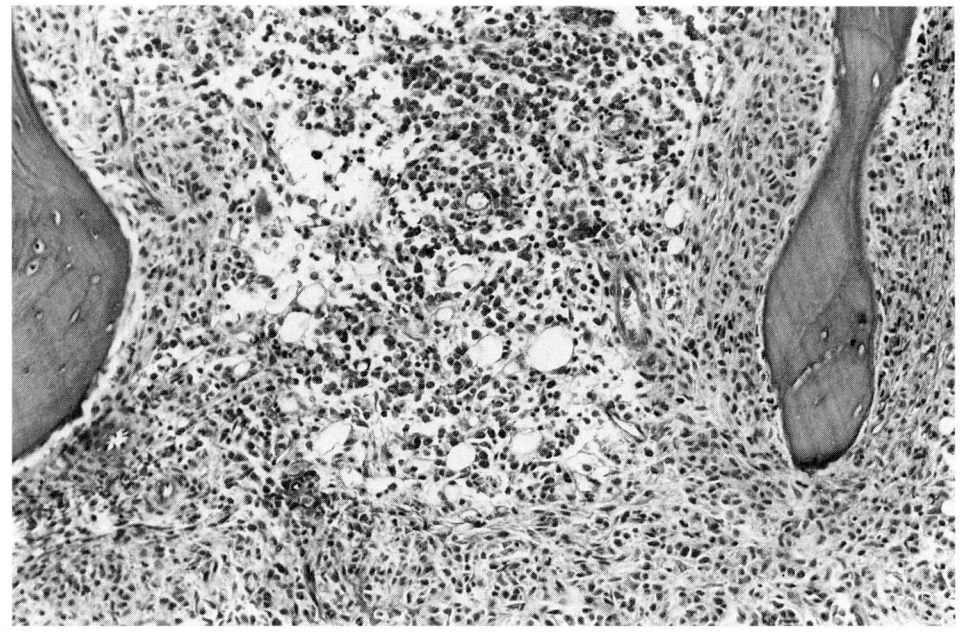

A

Fig. 23-104 A, Bone marrow from patient presenting with concurrent acute myeloblastic leukemia and systemic mastocytosis. Mast cell lesions in this field are predominantly paratrabecular.   *Continued.*

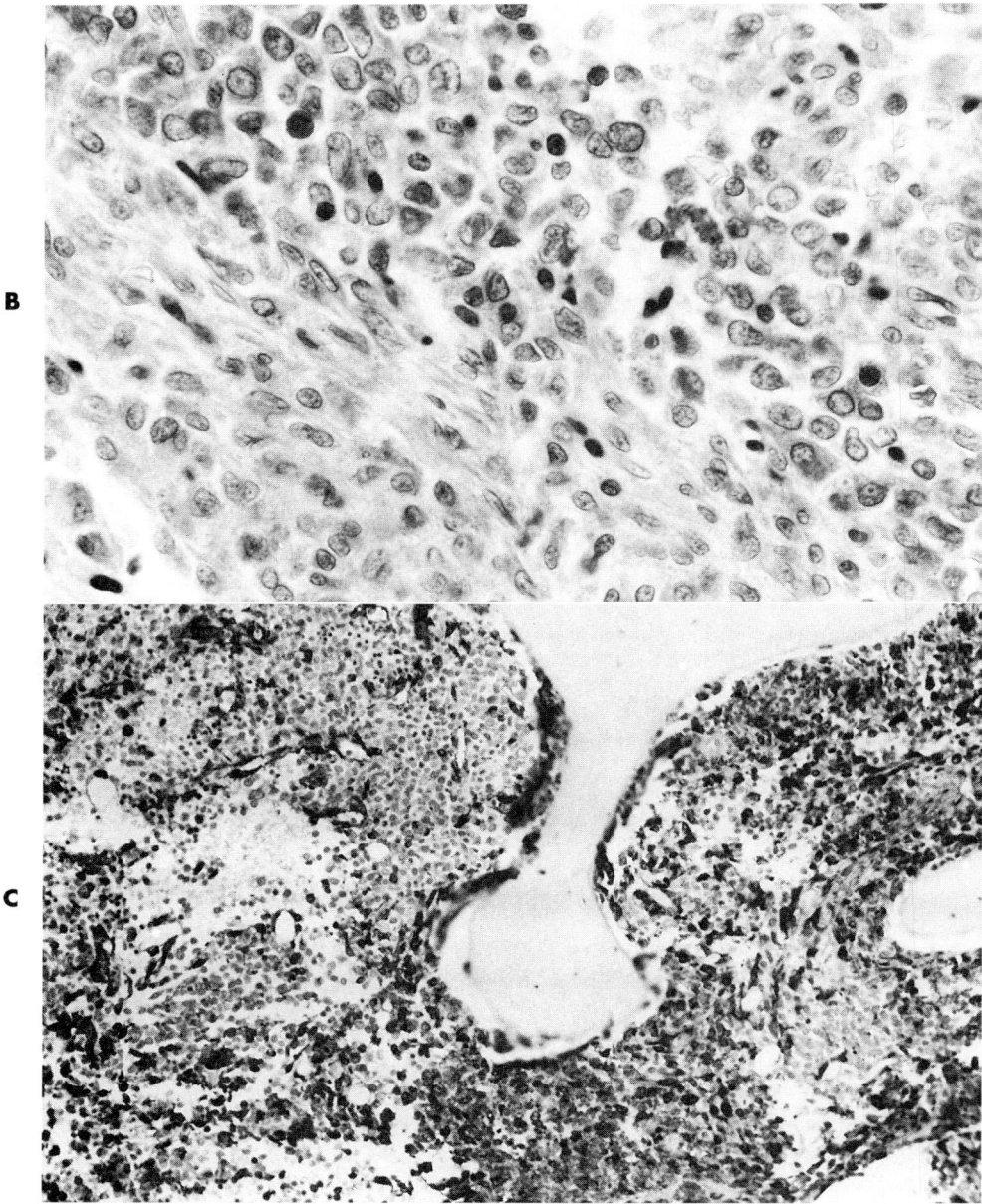

Fig. 23-104, cont'd **B,** High magnification of specimen in **A.** Lower left portion of field shows infiltration of mast cells, some of which are spindly in appearance. Right upper portion of micrograph is predominantly myeloblasts. Patient was treated for acute myeloid leukemia and achieved complete remission of leukemic process. Mast cell lesions were unaffected by therapy. **C,** Marrow biopsy in **A** and **B** reacted with antibody to alpha 1-antitrypsin. Mast cells show intense reactivity. Myeloblasts are negative. Myeloblasts reacted with anti-myeloperoxidase; mast cells were negative. (Peroxidase-antiperoxidase.)

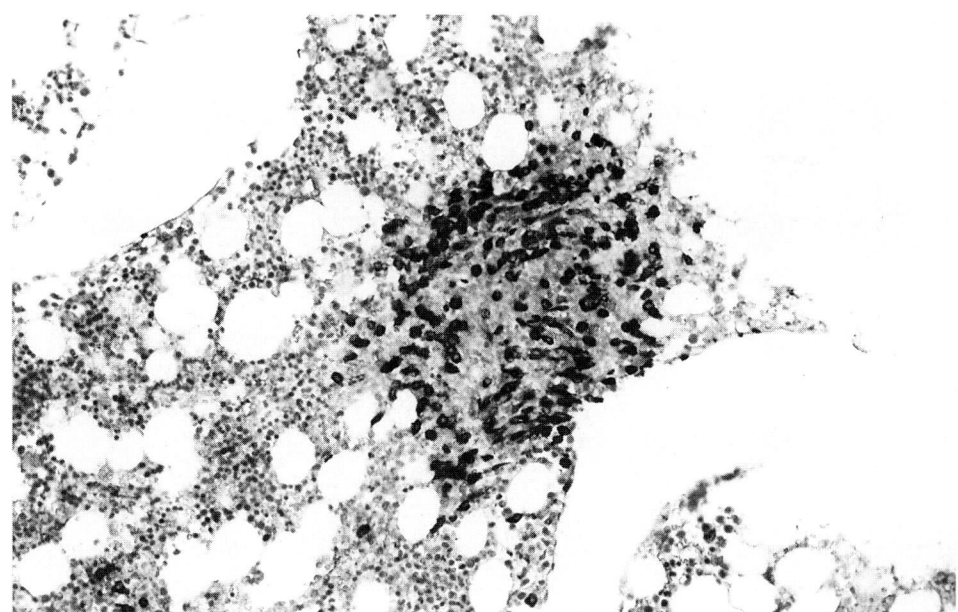

Fig. 23-105 Focal paratrabecular mast cell lesion reacted with antibody to mast cell tryptase. (Peroxidase-antiperoxidase).

they also may be performed on patients with suspected malignancy in an attempt to obtain material for a histologic diagnosis.[461,464,476,480,482] The tumors most frequently detected in bone marrow biopsies in adults are carcinoma of the breast, prostate, lung, stomach, colon, kidney, and thyroid gland. The bone marrow biopsy is widely used for staging small cell carcinoma of the lung.[456,457,462,467-475] Sarcomas have a relatively low incidence of marrow metastasis in adults.[459] In the pediatric age group, neuroblastoma is the most common metastatic lesion, followed by rhabdomyosarcoma, Ewing's sarcoma, and retinoblastoma.[466,478,481] Wilms' tumor metastatic to marrow is extremely uncommon.

In smears, tumor cells frequently, but not invariably, occur in clusters (Fig. 23-106). This may be an important diagnostic feature because tumors of hematopoietic origin generally do not occur in cohesive aggregates. In marrows with extensive involvement, both clusters and individual cells may be present. In some small cell tumors the individual cells may resemble malignant lymphoid cells. In trephine sections, metastatic tumor may occur as small focal lesions surrounded by normal hematopoietic cells, or it may replace virtually the entire specimen. In focal lesions or those occupying only a portion of the biopsy, the tumor foci may be sharply demarcated from the adjacent hematopoietic tissue or may be associated with an irregularly shaped area of fibrosis (Fig. 23-107). Many tumors, most notably breast and prostate, may be associated with a marked desmoplastic reaction, and attempts at aspiration may be unsuccessful. These tumors also may be accompanied by an increase in new bone formation. In the unusual occurrence of a metastatic sarcoma in the marrow, the lesion may resemble primary myelofibrosis.

In the majority of cases of metastatic tumor in marrow smears and aspirates, the tumor cells have characteristics that clearly distinguish them from normal hematopoietic cells. This distinction is aided by the frequent desmoplastic reaction that accompanies some of the tumors that most commonly metastasize to the marrow. In some instances the metastatic tumor cells may have features suggesting a hematopoietic origin, particularly megakaryocytes (Figs. 23-108 and 23-109). This may be a particular problem with some cases of rhabdomyosarcoma in which the tumor cells may react with antibodies to platelet glycoproteins.

The approach to determining the site of origin of a metastatic tumor in a patient without a known primary lesion should be the same as for determining metastatic lesions in other sites. Immunocytochemical techniques may be particularly useful both for determining the possible site of origin and for detecting small lesions. Antibodies to the common leukocyte antigen are useful in distinguishing a metastatic carcinoma or sarcoma from a malignant lymphoma. As with other tissue, it is important to use a panel of antibodies that has the capacity to recognize all reasonable possibilities. In instances in which small foci are identified with the immunocytochemical reaction, the tumor should be found in adjacent sections stained with H & E. Electron microscopic studies may provide definitive evidence of cell origin in some cases.

Detection of micrometastasis from lung and breast carcinoma in bone marrow is increased with the use of immunologic markers applied to smears prepared from Ficoll Hypaque–separated specimens of bone marrow aspirate.[463-465,477]

Special note is made here of **neuroblastoma** because the bone marrow biopsy may serve as the primary diagnostic specimen in patients with neuroblastoma if the aspirate or

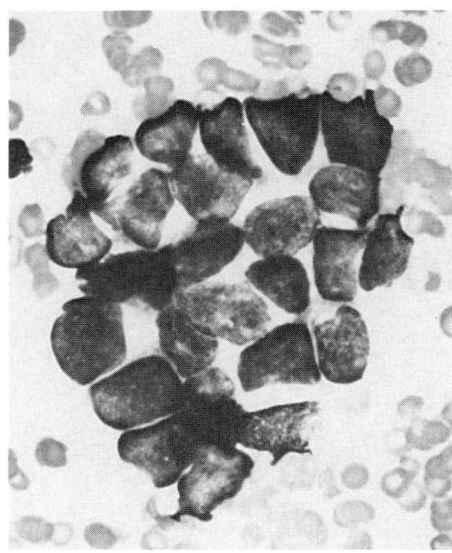

Fig. 23-106 Bone marrow smear from 8-month-old infant with diagnosis of neuroblastoma, showing a cluster of metastatic tumor cells. Cohesive character of tumor cells in this illustration would be unusual for malignant hematopoietic cells. (Wright-Giemsa.)

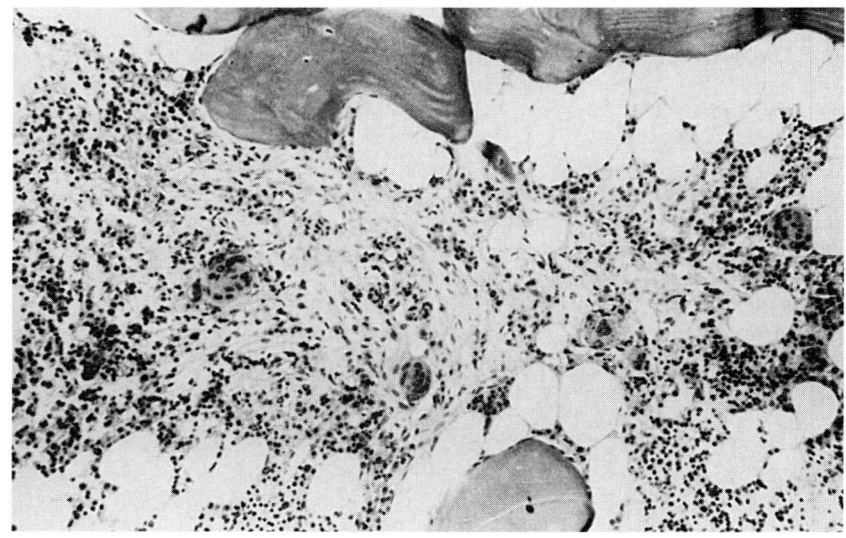

Fig. 23-107 Marrow biopsy from patient with small cell carcinoma of lung. There are four small foci of tumor cells associated with mild desmoplastic reaction.

trephine biopsy specimen contains unequivocal tumor cells and there is significantly increased serum or urinary catecholamines or metabolites.[458,460,479] Two aspirates and two trephine biopsy specimens from each posterior iliac crest are recommended for assessment of marrow involvement. Patients with stage 4S disease have less than 10% involvement; if there is more than 10%, the disease is stage 4.[460]

Tumor cells may be detected in bone marrow smears, particle sections, trephine imprints, or trephine biopsies. The

relative merits of these various techniques for detecting tumor have been the subject of considerable discussion. The yield of positive results has increased with the performance of multiple trephine biopsies.

Immunologic markers may be used for the identification of neuroblastoma cells; antibodies to neuron-specific enolase, synaptophysin, and chromogranin have been recommended by the Second International Neuroblastoma Staging System Conference.[460]

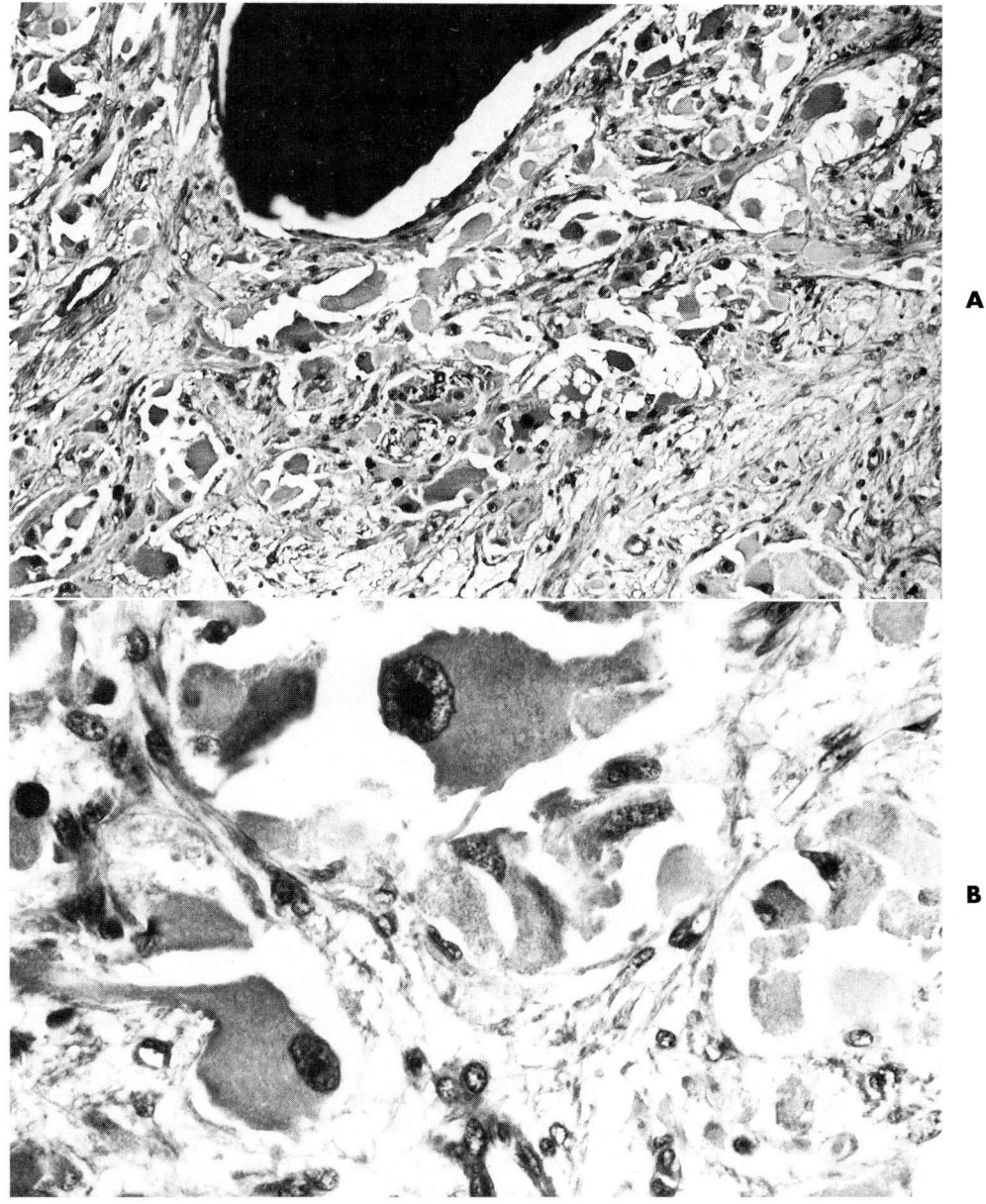

Fig. 23-108 A, Marrow biopsy from child with metastatic ganglioneuroblastoma. **B,** High magnification of specimen in **A** showing marked variability in size of tumor cells. In contrast to megakaryocytes, some tumor cells contain single very prominent nuclei.

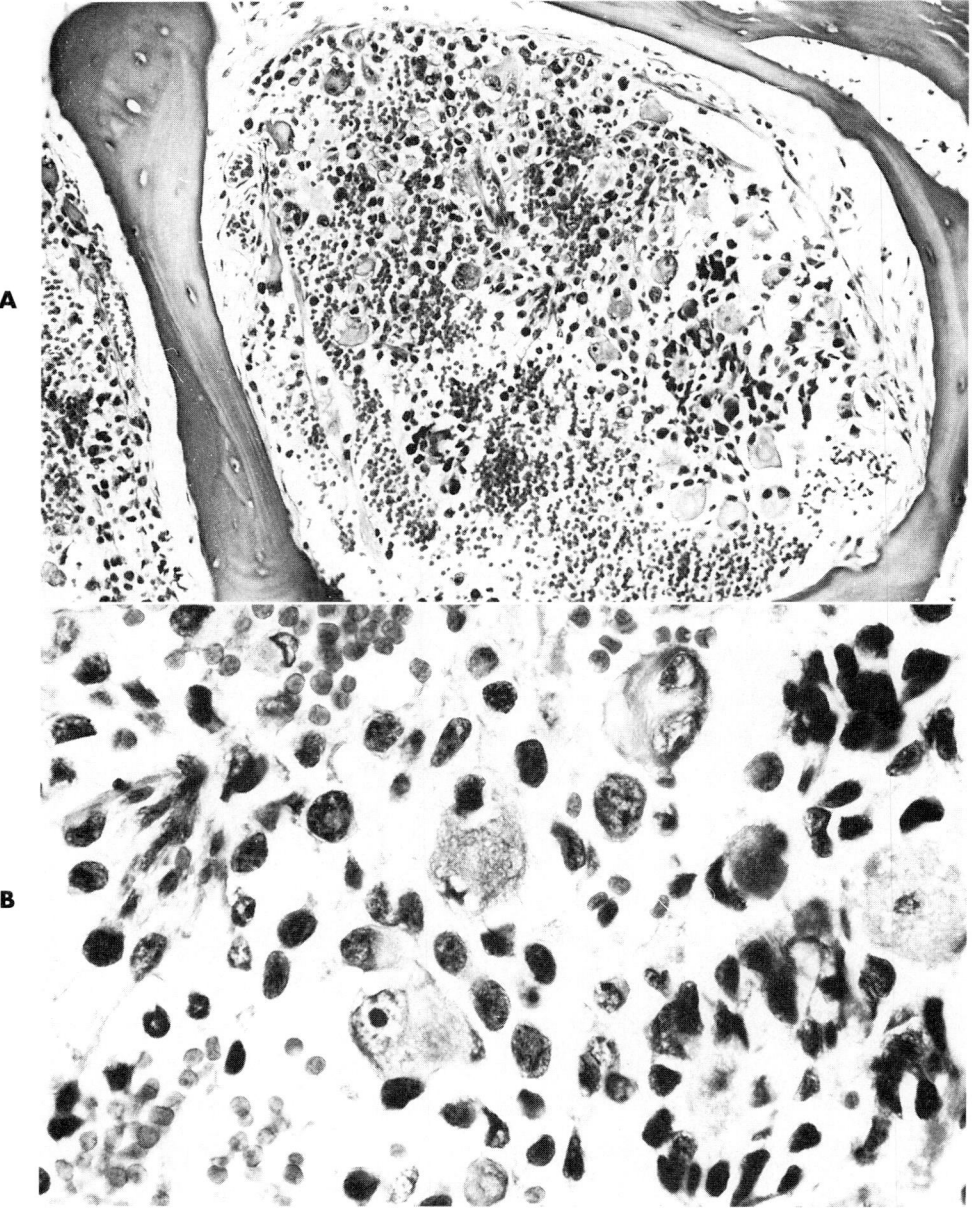

Fig. 23-109 A, Bone marrow biopsy from 17-year-old male with partial replacement of marrow by pleomorphic population of cells, some of which are large with very abundant cytoplasm. **B,** High magnification of specimen in **A** showing marked variation in size of malignant cells. Larger cells have one or two nuclei with distinct and frequently prominent nucleoli. Majority of cells reacted with antibodies to actin and desmin; cytogenetic studies of cells show t(2;13) (q35,q14) abnormality, characteristic cytogenetic finding in alveolar rhabdomyosarcoma. (**A** and **B** H & E.)

LIPID STORAGE DISEASE
Gaucher's disease

Gaucher's disease is an autosomal recessive sphingolipid storage disorder caused by the accumulation of glucosylceramide in organs and tissues as a result of a deficiency in lysosomal glucocerebrosidase.[483,484] It occurs in three forms: type I, chronic non-neuropathic (adult) type; type II, acute neuropathic type; and type III, subacute neuropathic (juvenile) type.

The characteristic diagnostic morphologic feature of the disorder is the presence of Gaucher cells in the bone marrow, spleen, liver, and lymph node.

In the bone marrow sections, Gaucher cells may be found in small focal accumulations or may replace large segments of a biopsy. There is an associated increase in reticulin fibers. In imprint and smear preparations, the Gaucher cell is large, 30 to 100 μm in diameter, and has one or more centrally or eccentrically located nuclei.[485,488] The cytoplasm has a characteristic fibrillary or striated pattern and is pale blue-gray in color. In sections stained with H & E, the cytoplasm is slightly eosinophilic; a fibrillary pattern may be very prominent (Fig. 23-110). The Gaucher cells are variably and often intensely positive with the PAS reaction. The cells also stain positively for iron in older children and adults. Cells similar to Gaucher cells may be found in the marrow of some patients with chronic myelogenous leukemia,[486-489] type II congenital dyserythropoietic anemia,[492] and thalassemia.[493]

A monoclonal gammopathy may be present in patients with chronic Gaucher's disease and may be associated with a marrow plasmacytosis.[490] The coincidence of multiple myeloma, plasmacytoid lymphoma, and Gaucher's disease has been reported.[491]

Niemann-Pick disease

Niemann-Pick disease comprises a group of autosomal recessive sphingomyelin-cholesterol lipidoses characterized by organomegaly and the accumulation of sphingomyelin and other lipids throughout the body as a result of a deficiency of lysosomal sphingomyelinase.[494,497] Three major clinical types are recognized: acute neuronopathic form (A), a chronic form without nervous system involvement (B), and a chronic neuronopathic form (C). The foam cell as seen in the bone marrow in Niemann-Pick disease does not have diagnostic specificity and may be found in other disorders of lipid metabolism such as hypercholesterolemia and Tangier disease.[495] In Romanovsky-stained smears, the cell measures 20 to 50 μm; the cytoplasm is filled with clear vacuoles of varying sizes.[495,496] In sections, the cells are randomly scattered. The cytoplasm of the Niemann-Pick cell is marked by confluent clear vacuoles of varying size. Because of the very light staining cytoplasm, the cells may be difficult to appreciate. The nucleus is randomly located (Fig. 23-111).

Fabry's disease

Fabry's disease is an X-linked inborn error of glycosphingolipid metabolism.[499] The characteristic storage cells in bone marrow specimens in this disease are filled with small globular inclusions that stain blue in Romanovsky-stained smears and lightly eosinophilic in sections stained with H & E.[498,499] The cytoplasmic substance reacts intensely with the PAS and Sudan black B stains.

Sea-blue histiocyte syndrome

The macrophages of the sea-blue histiocyte syndrome[500-502] contain a substance that stains blue in Romanovsky-stained smears and yellow to tan in sections stained with H & E. Positive reactions occur with the PAS and Sudan black B stains. In some instances, the substance appears to be ceroid; in others the material has not been well characterized. Macrophages containing blue pigment may be observed in several unrelated disorders and lack diagnostic specificity. This cell type has been reported in some cases of Niemann-Pick disease.

BONE MARROW TRANSPLANTATION

Bone marrow transplantation is being increasingly used as a therapeutic approach in patients with primary bone marrow disease. The objective of bone marrow transplantation is reconstitution of normal hematopoiesis in marrows that are aplastic; the aplasia may be the result of aplastic anemia, or the marrow is rendered aplastic with chemotherapy and radiation in the preparative regimen employed prior to marrow transplantation.

The source of the marrow graft may be the patient's own marrow that has been harvested prior to the preparatory regimen (*autologous*) or from another individual (*allogeneic*). Autologous marrow in some cases is "purged" with chemotherapeutic agents and/or monoclonal antibodies to eradicate malignant cells. In some patients with marrow involvement by tumor, stem cells harvested from the patient's blood may be used. Sibling umbilical cord blood cells are also being used.

Bone marrow transplant involves preparing the patient for transplant with a regimen utilizing chemotherapy with or without total body radiation therapy. The preparative regimen has two purposes: to immunosuppress the patient and to eradicate malignant cells that may be present in the recipient. For patients with severe aplastic anemia, cyclophosphamide alone or cyclophosphamide plus antithymocyte globulin or cyclophosphamide plus total lymphoid irradiation has been utilized most commonly and now provides long-term success rates of over 80% in matched sibling donor patients. For patients with leukemia, regimens with chemotherapy and total body irradiation have most commonly been used; the combination of busulfan and cyclophosphamide has been successful in the preparation of patients with acute myeloid leukemia.

The major complications associated with bone marrow transplantation involve infection in the severely immunosuppressed host, graft rejection, and graft-versus-host disease. Recurrent disease is also a cause of failure in patients with malignant diseases. Infection continues to be a major cause of peritransplant morbidity and, in some cases, mortality. The use of better antibiotics and growth factors to accelerate white blood cell production has decreased but not

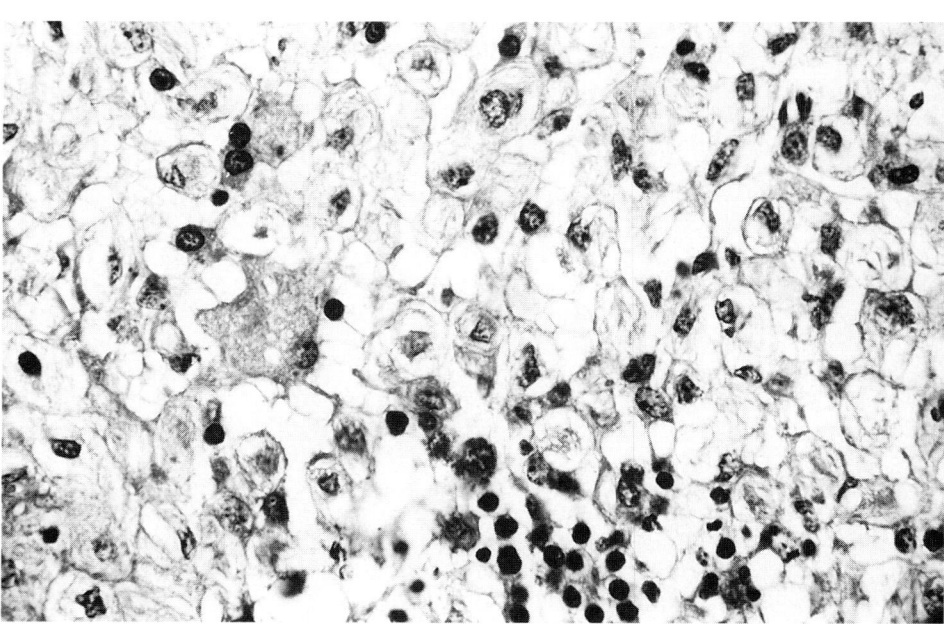

Fig. 23-110 Bone marrow section from adult with type I chronic non-neuropathic Gaucher's disease. Cytoplasm of many of Gaucher cells has fibrillary or granular appearance. Nuclei are small and usually eccentric in location. Group of erythroblasts is present.

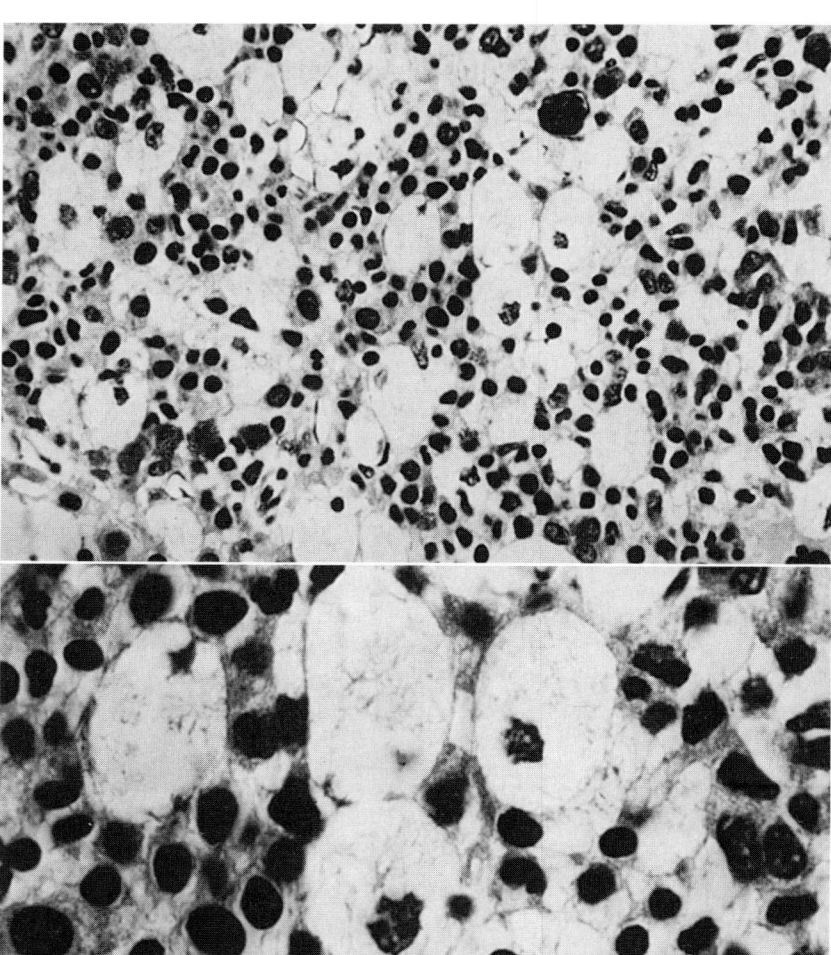

Fig. 23-111 A, Biopsy from 14-month-old child with Niemann-Pick disease. Characteristic foam cells are scattered among normal hematopoietic cells. **B,** Cytoplasm of cells is clear, with suggestion of numerous confluent vacuoles.

eliminated infectious complications. Graft rejection is an infrequent complication of matched sibling donor transplant; however, it is a significant complication in patients undergoing unrelated donor transplant, especially for diseases such as aplastic anemia. Certain methods of graft-versus-host disease prophylaxis, specifically T-cell depletion, may be associated with an increased risk of graft rejection.

The rate of engraftment following bone marrow transplantation is influenced by several factors, and although some generalizations can be made about reconstitution of hematopoiesis, there are frequent exceptions.[504,506,507] The amount of marrow damage incurred prior to the transplant from chemotherapy and radiation used for treatment of the disease for which the transplant is necessary may influence the success rate. Autologous marrow specimens that have been purged with antibodies or chemotherapeutic agents may reconstitute less quickly than allogeneic marrow grafts. The disease for which the transplant was performed may recur early in the transplant period.

Marrow biopsies are not usually performed in the first 7 days following transplantation. However, the marrow biopsies performed during this period show marked hypocellularity with hemorrhage and proteinaceous debris. Scattered fat cells and macrophages are present. The findings are similar to those in patients treated with myelotoxic agents for acute leukemia.[503-505] During the second week, adipose tissue is reconstituted. The appearance of the marrow in the second to third week is variable; there may be evidence of hematopoiesis, or the marrow may be markedly hypocellular (Figs. 23-112 to 23-115). The initial stages of engraftment are usually characterized by foci of hematopoietic cells scattered throughout the adipose tissue in what appears to be a random distribution. These foci initially are usually monolineage and composed of tight clusters of erythroid precursors followed by aggregates of promyelocytes and myelocytes (Fig. 23-116). Blasts are not increased. There is usually no preferential paratrabecular distribution of the promyelocyte and myelocyte islands in this period. Megakaryocytes are usually sparse. Following this stage there is progressive spreading of the hematopoietic cells throughout the interstitium and gradual regression of adipose tissue; the foci of hematopoiesis are usually multilineage, although predominantly monolineage proliferation may persist (Fig. 23-117). Megakaryocyte reconstitution may lag behind the granulocytic and erythroid cells for prolonged periods. In some patients, megakaryocytes appear early in the engraftment period and may form small aggregates. There may be considerable variability in the amount of hematopoietic tissue in different areas of a large biopsy specimen; small specimens or fragmented specimens may be misleading (Fig. 23-118).

There may be a marked shift to promyelocytes and myelocytes early in the post-transplant period; this is accentuated by the administration of recombinant granulocyte growth factor (Fig. 23-118). This shift to immaturity is not usually accompanied by an increase in blasts. During this period, patients frequently receive a large number of drugs, some of which may be associated with agranulocytosis. This factor should be considered in patients who manifest prolonged neutropenia with a morphologic appearance of "maturation arrest" of neutrophils in the marrow specimen.

Granulomas occur with greater frequency in post-transplant marrows than in marrows from other groups of patients; these granulomas usually consist of only a small collection of epithelioid histiocytes. In some cases, giant cells are present (Fig. 23-119). Phagocytic histiocytes may be increased

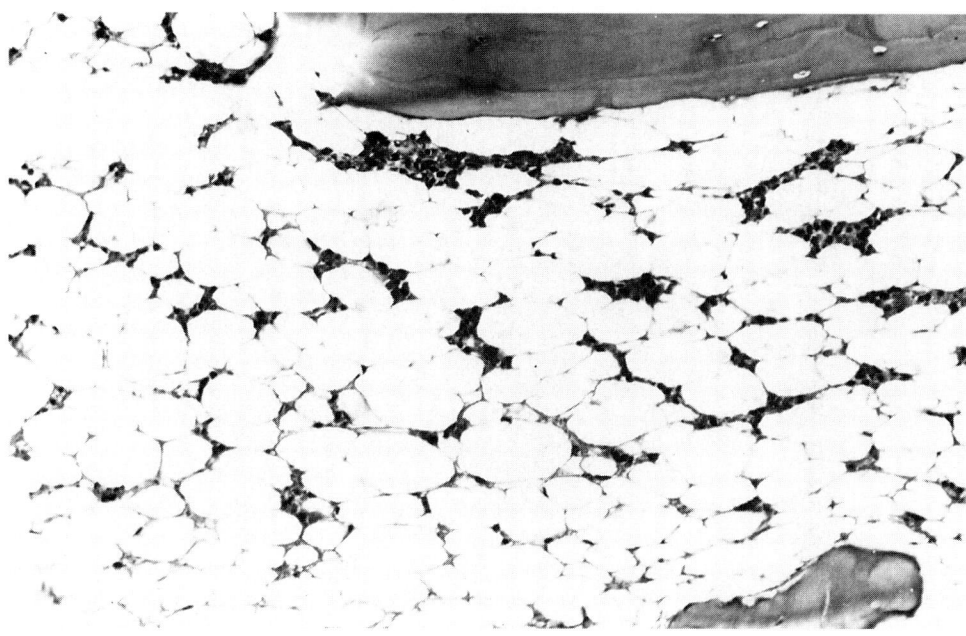

Fig. 23-112 Markedly hypocellular marrow from child 19 days following elutriated allogeneic bone marrow transplant for acute lymphoblastic leukemia. Majority of cells are lymphocytes and plasma cells, with only occasional scattered myeloid cells.

and diffusely scattered throughout the marrow. The histio-cytes may manifest marked phagocytic activity; this finding warrants evaluation for an infectious process.

The rate of growth of the graft varies substantially in the first 3 to 4 weeks. In some cases the marrow may remain hypocellular for many months or years; in other cases one of the major myeloid cell lines remains depressed (Figs. 23-120 to 23-122).

Loss of graft is reflected by decreasing marrow cellular-ity and progressive cytopenias. This may occur gradually or abruptly. In some instances, there is a dissociation between the blood counts and marrow cellularity, with very hypocel-lular marrows and normal blood counts or normocellular marrows and blood cytopenias. Marrow sampling may be the basis of the discrepancy when normal blood counts

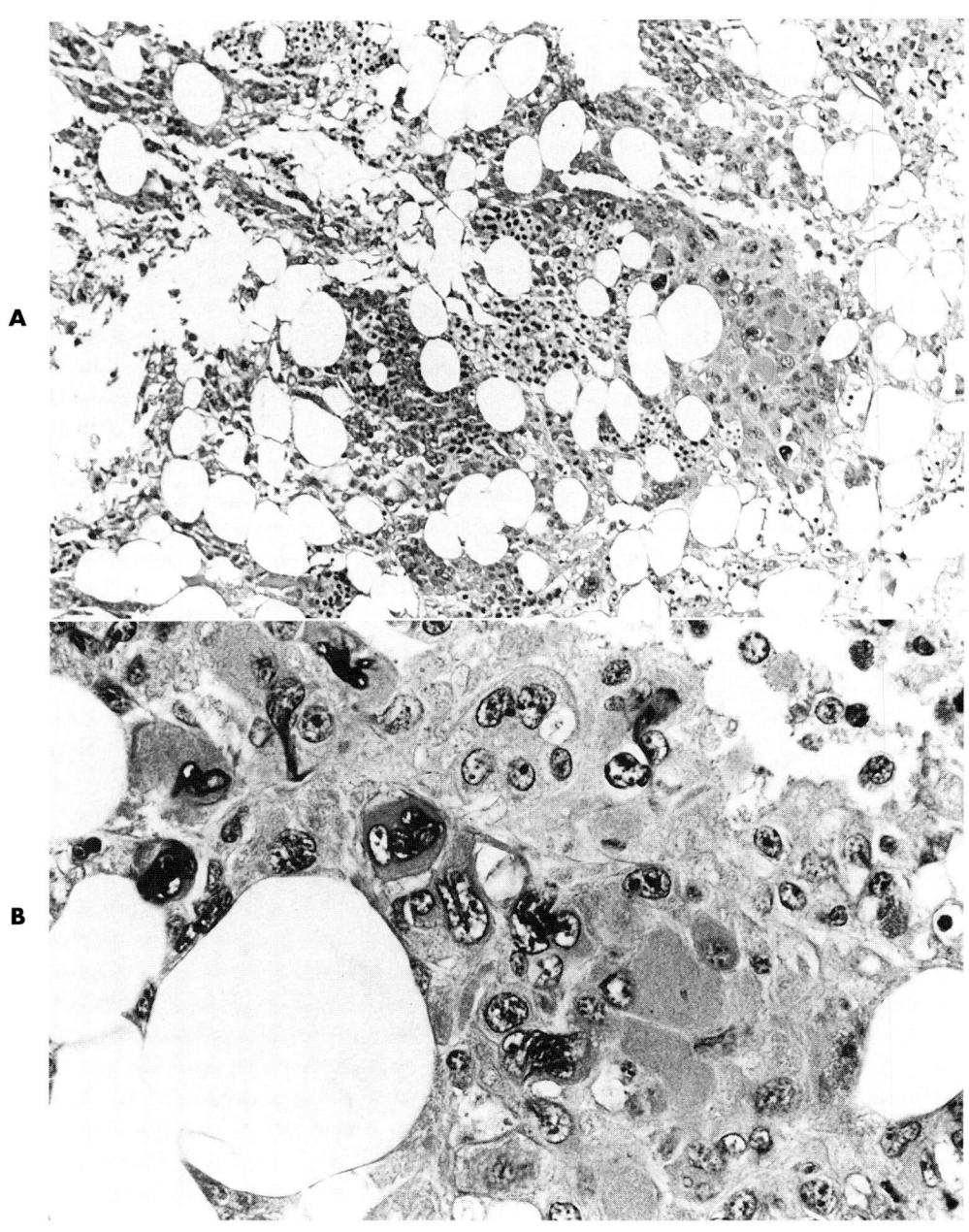

Fig. 23-113 A, Marrow biopsy from adult man 14 days after autologous bone marrow transplant for chronic myeloid leukemia. Marrow is variably cellular, with evidence of trilineage hematopoiesis. Cluster of megakaryocytes is at right. **B,** High magnification of specimen in **A** showing tight cluster of mature megakaryocytes. Cytogenetic studies of this specimen showed Philadelphia chromosome in 20 of 20 cells studied.

occur with hypocellular marrow. There are no specific marrow findings reflecting graft-versus-host disease.

Marrow transplants in patients with leukemia present the additional problem of recognition of recurrent disease. Cytogenetics, membrane surface markers, and molecular studies are very important adjuncts to morphology in the evaluation of these patients. Fluorescent in situ hybridiza-

tion studies using probes for the X and Y chromosomes may be used to determine graft and host cell populations in gender-mismatched transplants. This technique may also be used to identify recurrent leukemic cells in instances in which a specific cytogenetic defect has been identified and for which a probe is available.

Text continued on p. 1906.

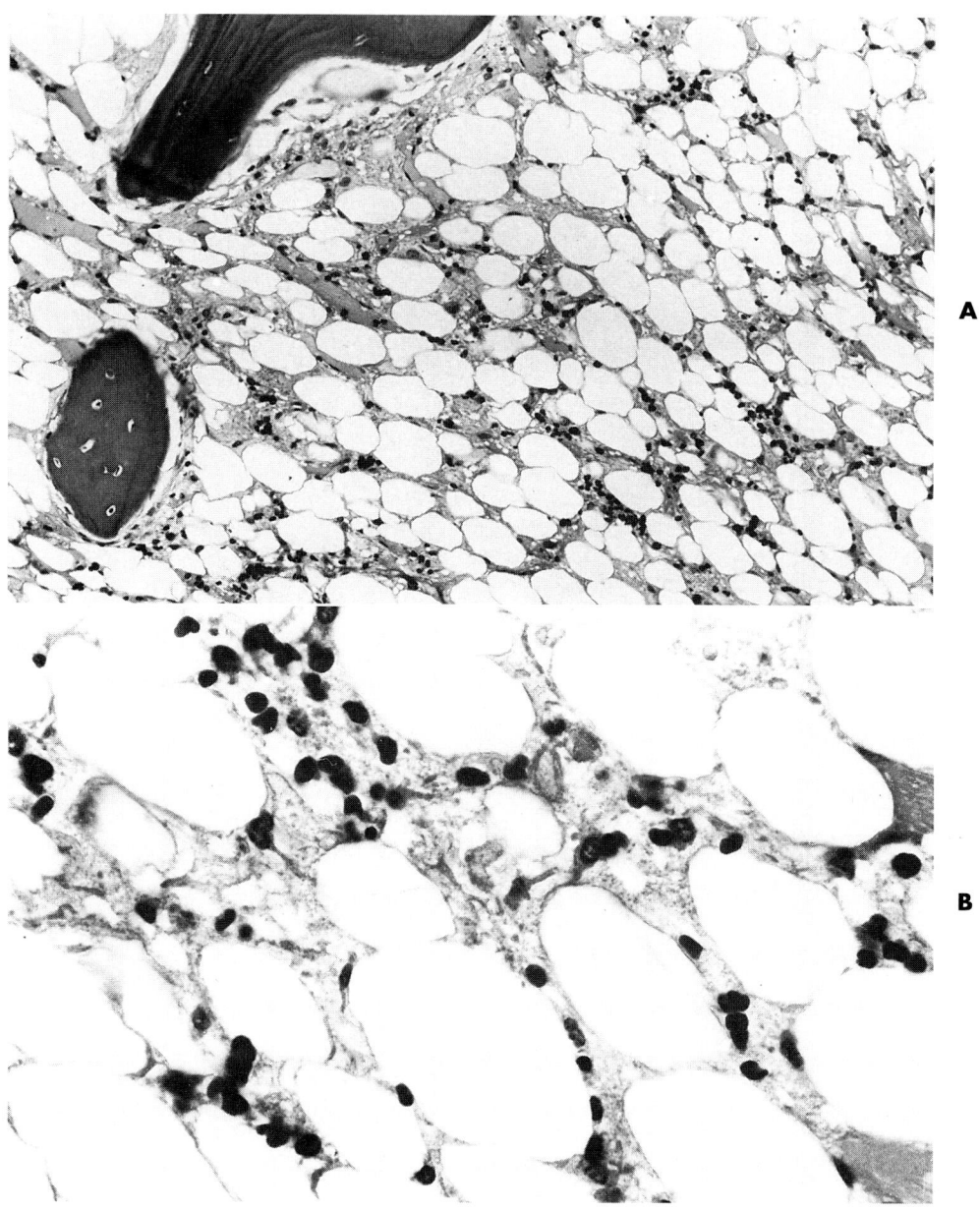

Fig. 23-114 A, Markedly hypocellular marrow from 3-year-old child 21 days following allogeneic bone marrow transplant for acute lymphoblastic leukemia. Interstitium contains proteinaceous debris and scattered lymphocytes, plasma cells, and histiocytes. Myeloid cells are virtually absent. Marrow remained essentially acellular until patient died 5 months following transplant. **B,** High magnification of specimen in **A.**

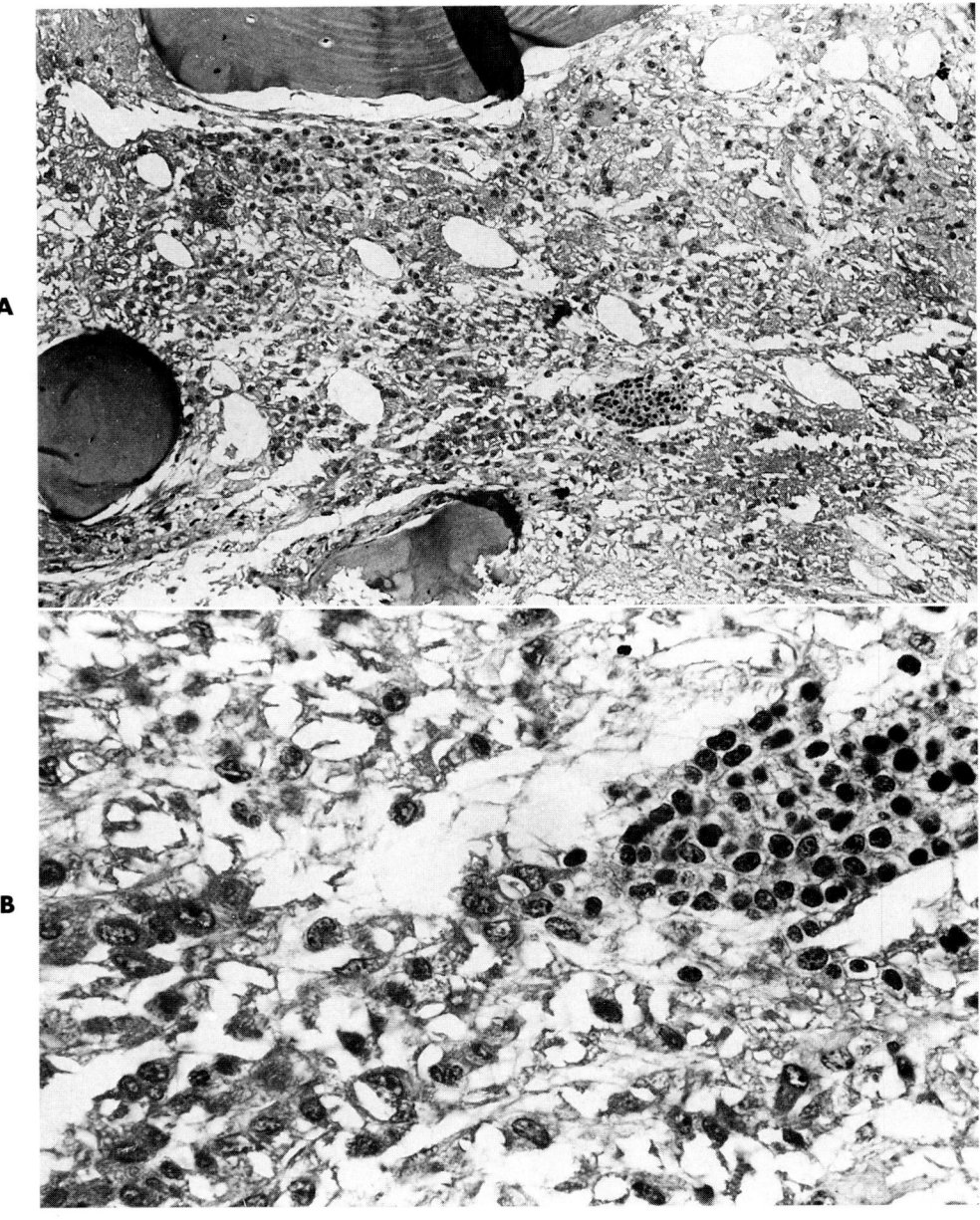

Fig. 23-115 **A,** Hypocellular marrow from adult patient 20 days following allogeneic bone marrow transplant for chronic myeloid leukemia. Patient had evidence of graft-versus-host reaction at time of biopsy. There is abundant eosinophilic proteinaceous debris in interstitium. There are neutrophil precursors scattered throughout marrow and rare megakaryocytes. Scattered small foci of maturing erythroid precursors are present. **B,** High magnification of portion of specimen in **A,** showing focus of late-stage erythroid precursors on right. Loosely structured interstitium contains proteinaceous debris and scattered neutrophil precursors and monocytes.

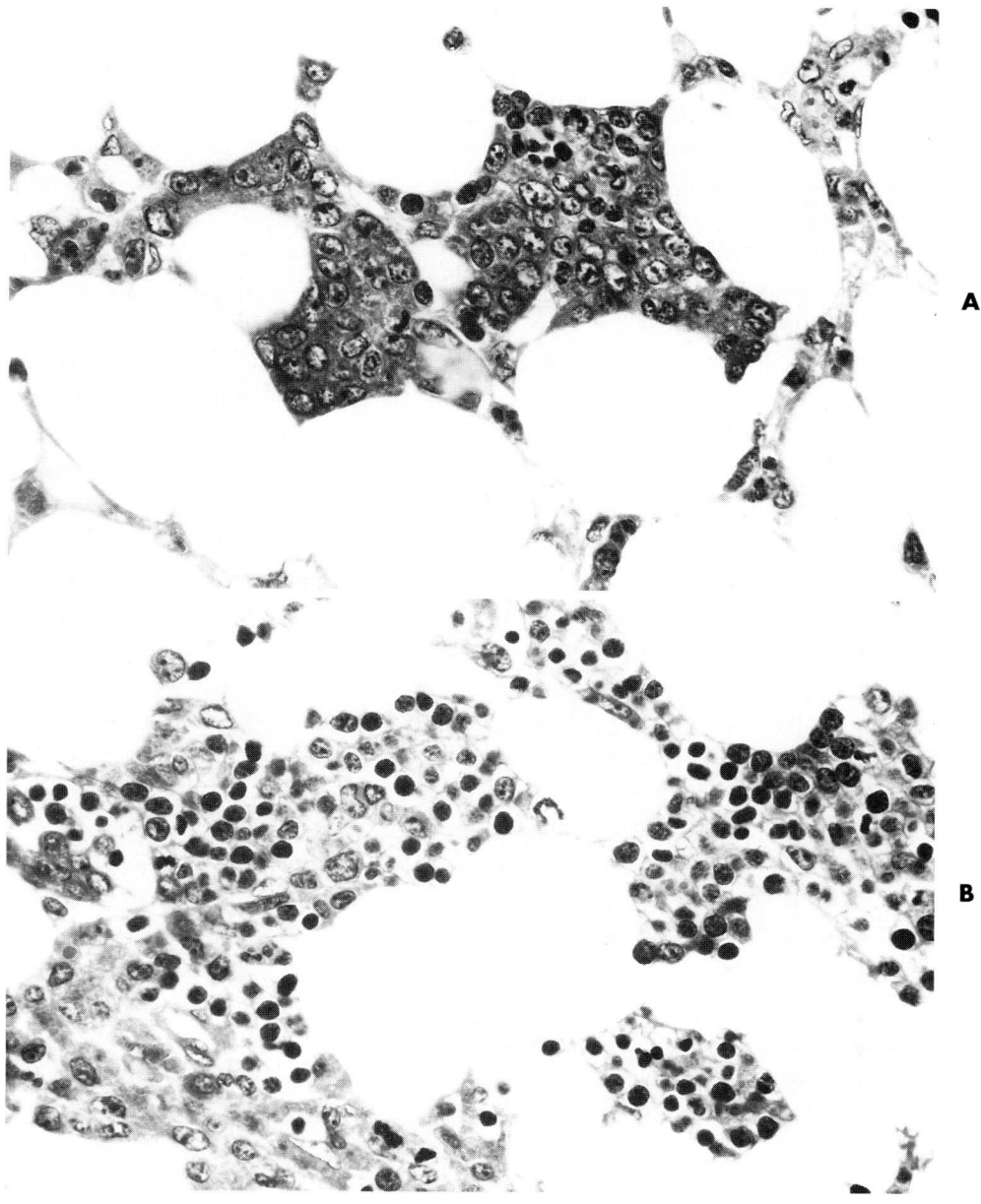

Fig. 23-116 A, Focus of erythroid precursors in marrow 21 days after allogeneic transplant for neu-roectodermal tumor. This illustrates common finding of monolineage cell islands that occurs in imme-diate post-transplant period. **B,** Spreading focus of erythroid precursors from another area of biopsy illustrated in **A.** Majority of erythroid precursors are at later stage than those in **A.** Lower left shows sev-eral neutrophil myelocytes that have more abundant cytoplasm than erythroid precursors. (H & E.)

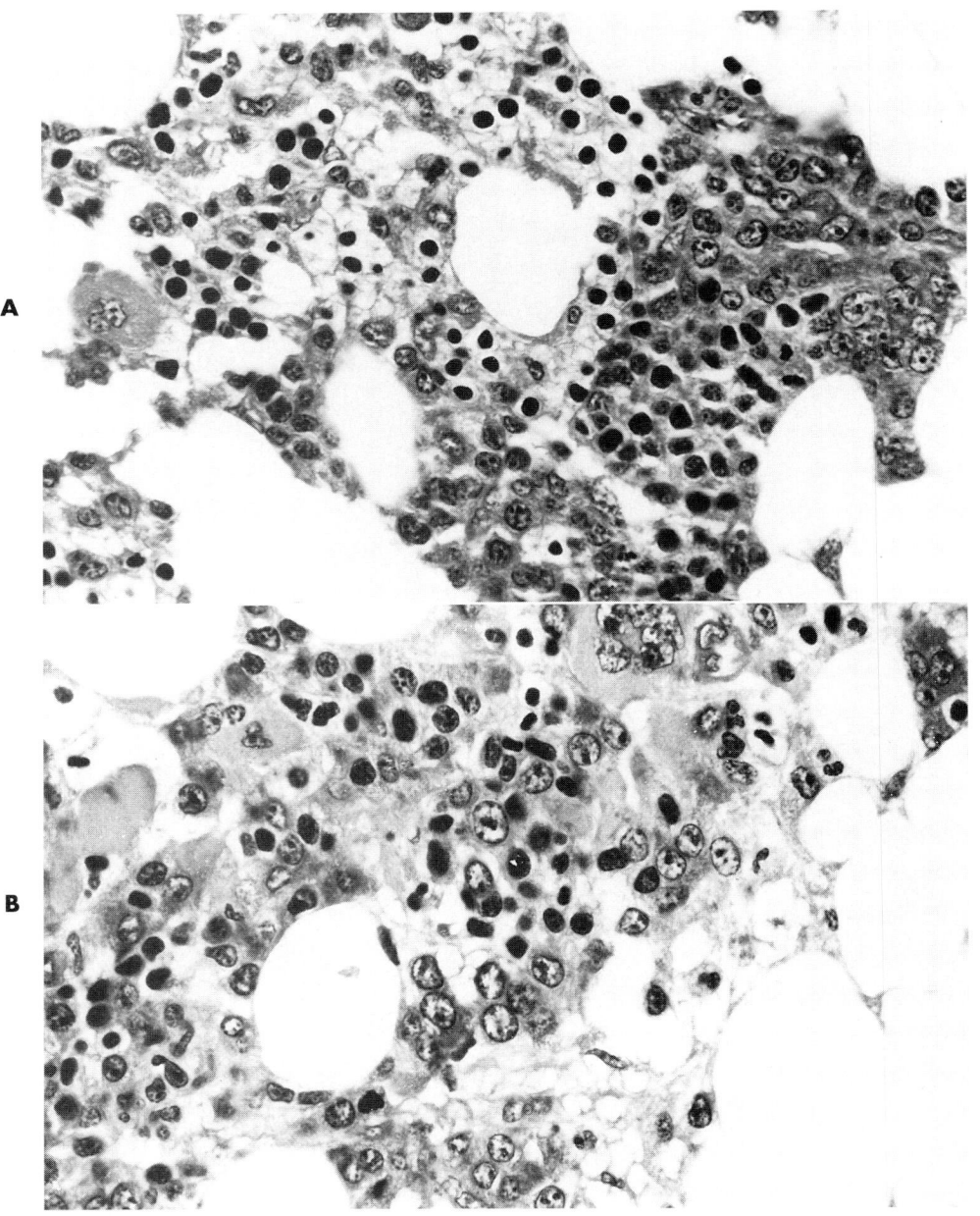

Fig. 23-117 A, Bone marrow biopsy 33 days after autologous bone marrow transplant for acute myeloid leukemia. This area of biopsy shows trilineage myeloid hematopoiesis. Late-stage erythroid precursors are prominent in central portion of photomicrograph. Promyelocytes and myelocytes are prominent on right and lower portion of field. Megakaryocyte is at left. **B,** Another area of the same biopsy showing several mature megakaryocytes in addition to erythroid precursors and small number of immature neutrophils.

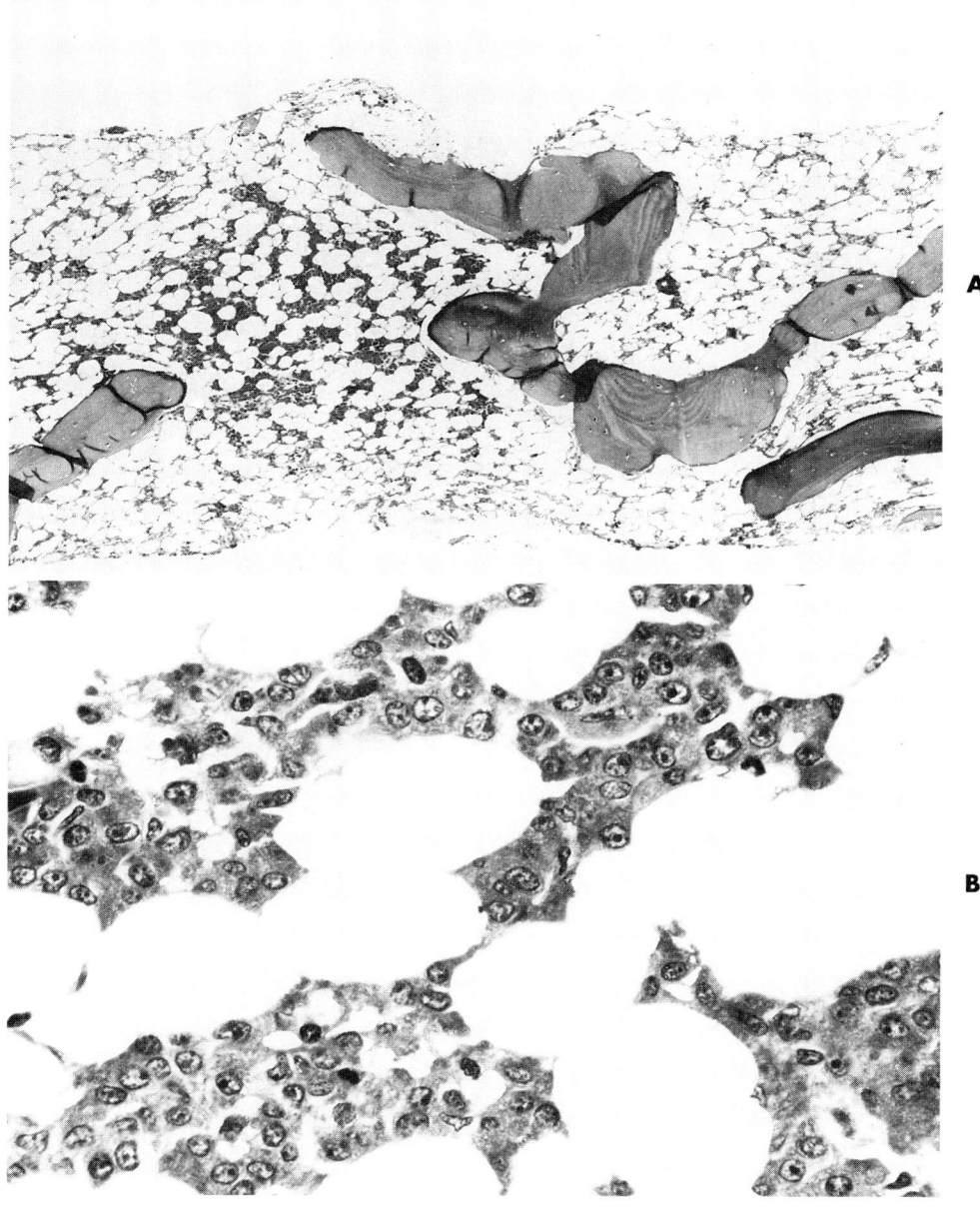

Fig. 23-118 A, Moderately to markedly hypocellular marrow 20 days following allogeneic sibling marrow transplant for acute lymphoblastic leukemia. Patient was receiving recombinant granulocyte
growth factor. There is focal cellular area in which interstitium is populated by numerous immature neutrophils. **B,** High magnification of cellular area in **A** showing relatively homogenous population of
neutrophils at promyelocyte-myelocyte stage of maturation, characteristic feature of early stage of
response to growth factor therapy.

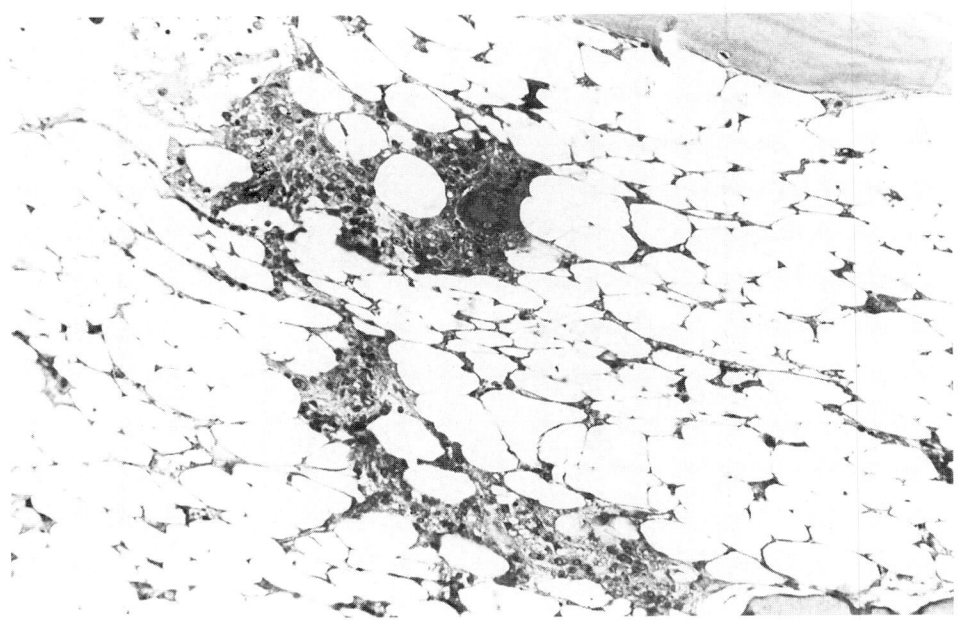

Fig. 23-119 Markedly hypocellular marrow 42 days following allogeneic bone marrow transplant for acute myeloblastic leukemia. Single granuloma with multinucleated giant cell is present. Stains for micro-organisms were negative.

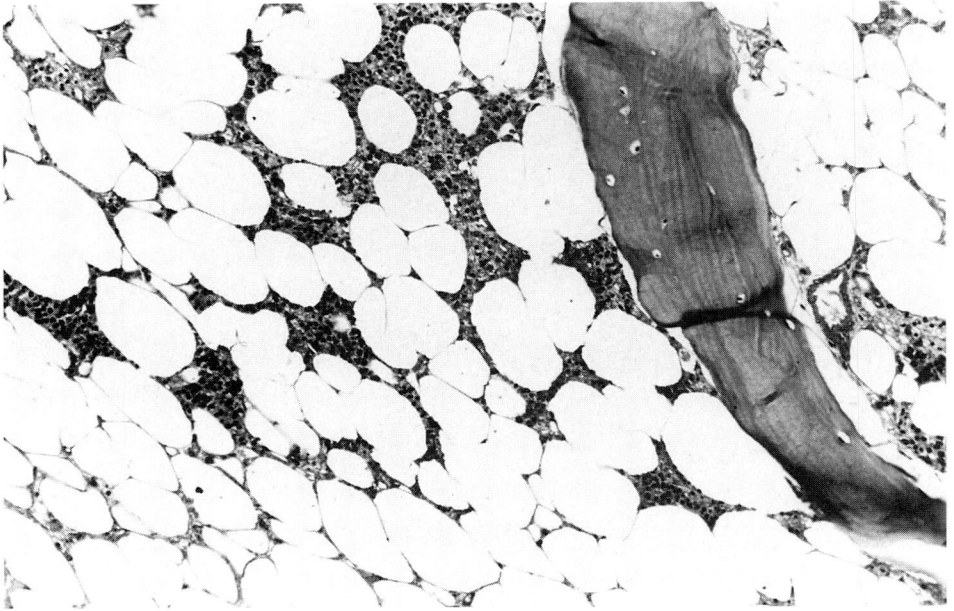

Fig. 23-120 Hypocellular bone marrow biopsy 100 days after autologous bone marrow transplant for chronic myeloid leukemia. Marrow is markedly hypocellular, with scattered foci of hematopoiesis, primarily erythroid.

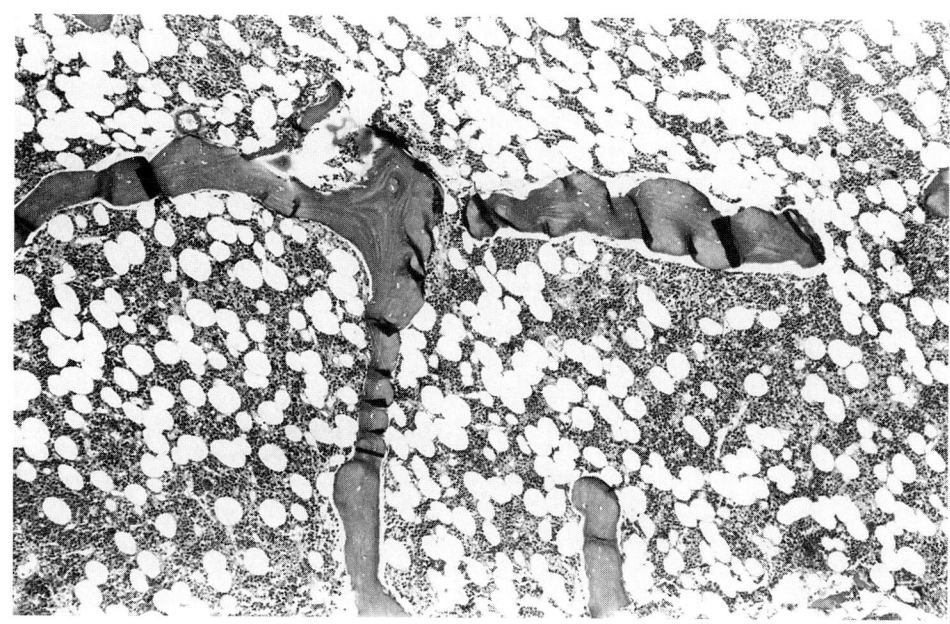

Fig. 23-121 Bone marrow from 32-year-old adult 1 year following unrelated donor marrow transplant for chronic myeloid leukemia. Cellularity is at lower range of normal with normal myelopoiesis.

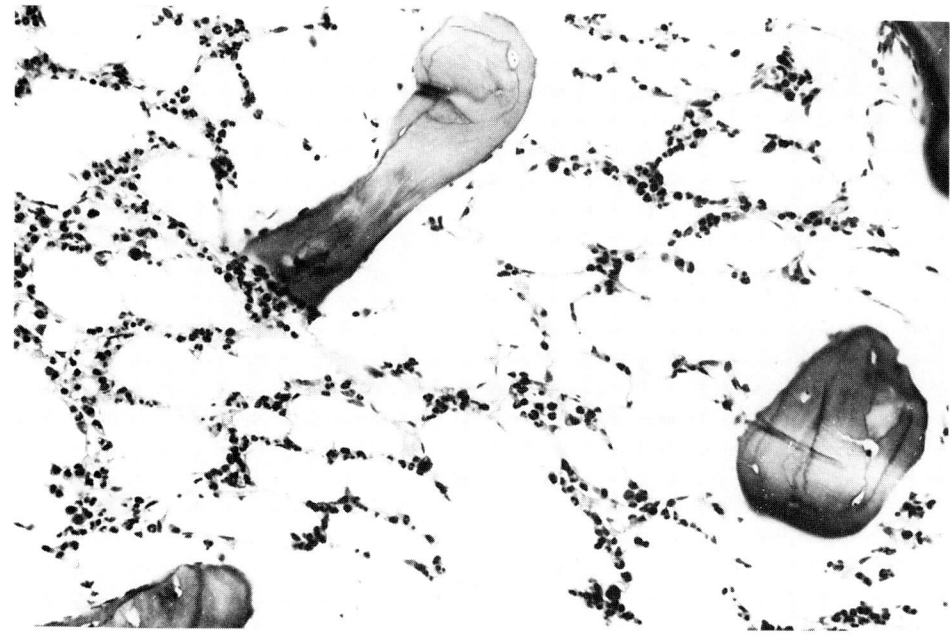

Fig. 23-122 Markedly hypocellular marrow 16 months following unrelated allogeneic marrow transplant for familial lymphohistiocytosis. All myeloid cell lines are reduced, megakaryocytes most severely. (H & E.)

REFERENCES

1 Beckstead JH, Bainton DF: Enzyme histochemistry on bone marrow biopsies. Reactions useful in the differential diagnosis of leukemia and lymphoma applied to 2-micron plastic sections. Blood 55:386-394, 1980.

2 Brinn NT, Pickett JP: Glycol methacrylate for routine, special stains, histochemistry, enzyme histochemistry and immunohistochemistry. A simplified method for surgical biopsy tissue. J Histotechnol 2:125-130, 1979.

3 Brunning RD, Bloomfield CD, McKenna RW, Peterson L: Bilateral trephine bone marrow biopsies in lymphoma and other neoplastic diseases. Ann Intern Med 82:365-366, 1975.

4 Burkhardt R, Frisch B, Bartl R: Bone biopsy in haematological disorders. J Clin Pathol 35:257-284, 1982.

5 Contreras E, Ellis LD, Lee RE: Value of the bone marrow biopsy in the diagnosis of metastatic carcinoma. Cancer 29:778-783, 1972.

6 Dee JW, Valdivieso M, Drewinko B: Comparison of the efficacies of closed trephine needle biopsy, aspirated paraffin-embedded clot section, and smear preparation in the diagnosis of bone marrow involvement by lymphoma. Am J Clin Pathol 65:183-194, 1976.

7 Ellman L: Bone marrow biopsy in the evaluation of lymphoma, carcinoma, and granulomatous disorders. Am J Med 60:1-7, 1976.

8 Garrett TJ, Gee TS, Leiberman PH, McKenzie S, Clarkson BD: The role of bone marrow aspiration and biopsy in detecting marrow involvement by non-hematologic malignancies. Cancer 38:2401-2403, 1976.

9 Gatter KC, Heryt A, Brown DC, Mason DY: Is it necessary to embed bone marrow biopsies in plastic for haematological diagnosis? Histopathology 11:1-7, 1987.

10 Grann V, Pool JL, Mayer K: Comparative study of bone marrow aspiration and biopsy in patients with neoplastic disease. Cancer 19:1898-1900, 1966.

11 Gruppo RA, Lampkin BC, Granger S: Bone marrow cellularity determination. Comparison of the biopsy, aspirate and buffy coat. Blood 49:29-31, 1977.

12 Jamshidi K, Swaim WR: Bone marrow biopsy with unaltered architecture. A new biopsy device. J Lab Clin Med 77:335-343, 1971.

13 Liao KT: The superiority of histologic sections of aspirated bone marrow in malignant lymphomas. Cancer 27:618-628, 1971.

14 McCarthy DM: Annotation, fibrosis of the bone marrow. Content and causes. Br J Haematol 59:1-7, 1985.

BIOPSY PROCEDURE AND PROCESSING OF THE SPECIMEN

15 Brunning RD: Bone marrow specimen processing. In: Knowles DM, ed: Neoplastic hematopathology. Baltimore, 1992, Williams & Wilkins, pp. 1081-1096.

16 Brunning RD, Bloomfield CD, McKenna RW, Peterson L: Bilateral trephine bone marrow biopsies in lymphoma and other neoplastic diseases. Ann Intern Med 82:365-366, 1975.

17 Ellman L: Bone marrow biopsy in the evaluation of lymphoma, carcinoma, and granulomatous disorders. Am J Med 60:1-7, 1976.

18 Jamshidi K, Swaim WR: Bone marrow biopsy with unaltered architecture. A new biopsy device. J Lab Clin Med 77:335-342, 1971.

19 Luna LG, ed: Manual of histologic staining methods of the Armed Forces Institute of Pathology, ed. 3. New York, 1958, McGraw-Hill Book Co.

IMMUNOHISTOLOGY

20 Bluth RF, Casey TT, McCurley TL: Differentiation of reactive from neoplastic small-cell lymphoid aggregates in paraffin-embedded marrow particle preparations using L-26 (CD20) and UCHL-1 (CD45RO) monoclonal antibodies. Am J Clin Pathol 99:150, 1993.

21 Brodeur G, Pritchard J, Berthold F, et al: Revisions of the international criteria for neuroblastoma diagnosis staging, and response to treatment. J Clin Oncol 11:1466-1477, 1993.

22 Brown DC, Gatter KC: The bone marrow trephine biopsy. A review of normal histology. Histopathology 22:411-422, 1993.

23 Dhillon AP, Rode J, Leathem A: Neuron specific enolase. An aid to the diagnosis of melanoma and neuroblastoma. Histopathology 5:81-92, 1982.

24 Horny HP, Wehrmann M, Grisser H, Tiemann M, Bultmann B, Kaiserling E: Investigation of bone marrow lymphocyte subsets in normal, reactive, and neoplastic states, using paraffin-embedded biopsy specimens. Am J Clin Pathol 99:142, 1993.

25 Kronland R, Grogan T, Spier C, Wirt D, Rangel C, Richter L, Durie B, Greenberg B, Miller T, Jones S: Immunotopographic assessment of lymphoid and plasma cell malignancies in the bone marrow. Hum Pathol 16:1247-1254, 1985.

26 Kubic VL, Brunning RD: Immunohistochemical evaluation of neoplasms in bone marrow biopsies using monoclonal antibodies reactive in paraffin embedded tissue. Mod Pathol 2:618, 1989.

27 Mason DY, Comans-Bitter WM, Cordell JL, Verhoeven MAJ, von Dongen JJM: Antibody L26 recognizes an intracellular epitope on the B cell associated CD20 antigen. Am J Pathol 136:1215-1222, 1990.

28 Norton AJ, Issacson PG: Monoclonal antibody L26. An antibody that is reactive with normal and neoplastic B lymphocytes in paraffin-embedded tissue. J Clin Pathol 40:1405-1412, 1987.

29 Peterson LC, Brown BA, Crosson JT, Mladenovic J: Application of the immunoperoxidase technic to bone marrow trephine biopsies in the classification of patients with monoclonal gammopathies. Am J Clin Pathol 85:688-693, 1986.

30 Pinkus GS, Pinkus JL: Myeloperoxidase. A specific marker for myeloid cells in paraffin sections. Mod Pathol 4:733-741, 1991.

31 Poje EJ, Soori GS, Weisenburger DS: Systemic polyclonal B-immunoblastic proliferation with marked peripheral blood and bone marrow plasmacytosis. Am J Clin Pathol 98:220-226, 1992.

32 Poppema S, Hollema H, Visser L, Hans VOS: Monoclonal antibodies (MT1, MT2, MB1, MB3) reactive with leukocytes subsets in paraffin-embedded tissue sections. Am J Pathol 127:418-429, 1987.

33 Trojanowski JQ, Lee VM: Monoclonal and polyclonal antibodies against neural antigens. Diagnostic applications for studies of central and peripheral nervous system tumors. Hum Pathol 14:281-285, 1983.

34 Walls AF, Jones DB, Williams JH, Church MK, Holgate ST: Immunohistochemical identification of mast cells in formaldehyde-fixed tissue using monoclonal antibodies specific for tryptase. J Clin Pathol 162:119-126, 1990.

35 Zutter M, Hockenbery D, Silverman GA, Korsmeyer SJ: Immunolocalization of the bcl-2 protein within hematopoietic neoplasms. Blood 78:1062, 1991.

NORMOCELLULAR BONE MARROW

36 Hartsock RJ, Smith EB, Petty CS: Normal variations with aging of the amount of hematopoietic tissue in bone marrow from the anterior iliac crest. Am J Clin Pathol 43:326-331, 1965.

ALTERATIONS IN CELLULARITY

37 Ajlouni K, Doeblin T: The syndrome of hepatitis and aplastic anemia. Br J Haematol 27:345-355, 1974.

38 Alter BP, Potter NU, Li FP: Classification and aetiology of the aplastic anemias. Clin Haematol 7:431-465, 1978.

39 Dawson JP: Congenital pancytopenia associated with multiple congenital anomalies (Fanconi type). Review of the literature and report of a 20-year-old female with a 10-year follow-up and apparently good response to splenectomy. Pediatrics 15:325-333, 1955.

40 Dessypris EN: The biology of pure red cell aplasia. Semin Hematol 28:275-284, 1991.

41 Estren S, Dameshek W: Familial hypoplastic anemia of childhood. Am J Dis Child 73:671-687, 1947.

42 Evans DIK: Congenital defects of the marrow stem cell. Bailliere's Clin Haematol 2:163-191, 1989.

43 Gordon-Smith EC, Rutherford TR: Fanconi anaemia-consitutional, familial aplastic anaemia. Bailliere's Clin Haematol 2:139-153, 1989.

44 Goswitz FA, Andrews GA, Kniseley RM: Effects of local irradiation (Co60 teletherapy) on the peripheral blood and bone marrow. Blood 21:605-619, 1963.

45 Haak HL, Hartgrink-Groeneveld CA, Eernisse JG, Speck B, Van Rood JJ: Acquired aplastic anemia in adults. Acta Haematol 58:257-277, 1977.

46 Kurtzman G, Young N: Viruses and bone marrow failure. Bailliere's Clin Haematol 2:51-67, 1989.

47 Naeim F, Smith GS, Gale RP: Morphologic aspects of bone marrow transplantation in patients with aplastic anemia. Hum Pathol 9:295-308, 1978.

48 Nissen C: The pathophysiology of aplastic anemia. Semin Hematol 28:313-318, 1991.

49 Rosse WF: Paroxysmal nocturnal hemoglobinuria in aplastic anemia. Clin Haematol 7:541-553, 1978.

50 Saarinen UM, Chorba TL, Tattersall P, et al: Human parvovirus B-19 induced epidemic acute red cell aplasia in patients with hereditary hemolytic anemia. Blood 67:1411-1417, 1986.

51 Sale GE, Marmont BS: Marrow mast cell counts do not predict bone marrow graft rejection. Hum Pathol 12:605-608, 1980.

52 Schwachman H, Diamond LK, Oaski FA, Khaw KT: The syndrome of pancreatic insufficiency and bone marrow dysfunction. J Pediatr 65:645-663, 1964.

53 Seaman JP, Kjeldsberg CR, Linker A: Gelatinous transformation of the bone marrow. Hum Pathol 9:685-692, 1978.

OSTEOPETROSIS

54 Coccia PF, Krivit W, Cervenka J, Clawson C, Kersey JH, Nesbit ME, Ramsay MKC, Warkentin PI, Teitelbaum SL, Kahn AJ, Brown DM: Successful bone marrow transplantation for infantile malignant osteopetrosis. N Engl J Med 302:701-708, 1980.

55 Milgram JW, Jasty M: Osteopetrosis. Bone Joint Surg Am 64:912-928, 1982.

56 Shapiro F, Gilmcher MJ, Holtrop ME, Tashjian AH, Brickley-Parsons D, Kenzora JE: Human osteopetrosis. Bone Joint Surg Am 62:384-387, 1980.

BONE MARROW NECROSIS

57 Brown CH: Bone marrow necrosis. A study of seventy cases. Johns Hopkins Med J 131:189-203, 1972.

58 Goodall HB: Atypical changes in the bone marrow in acute infections. In Clark WJ, Howard EB, Hackett PL, eds: Myeloproliferative disorder of animal and man. Oak Ridge, TN, 1970, United States Energy Commission, pp. 314-339.

59 Kahlstron SC, Burton CC, Phemister DB: Infarction of bones in caisson disease. Surg Gynecol Obstet 68:129-146, 1939.

60 Kundel DW, Brecher G, Bodey GP, Brittin GM: Reticulin fibrosis and bone infarction in acute leukemia. Implications for prognosis. Blood 23:526-544, 1964.

61 Niebrugge DJ, Benjamin DR: Bone marrow necrosis preceding acute lymphoblastic leukemia in childhood. Cancer 52:2162-2164, 1983.

62 Pui CH, Stass S, Green A: Bone marrow necrosis in children with malignant disease. Cancer 56:1522-1525, 1985.

63 Smith RR, Spivak JL: Marrow cell necrosis in anorexia nervosa and in voluntary starvation. Br J Haematol 60:525-530, 1985.

INFLAMMATORY DISORDERS
Granulomatous inflammation

64 Browne PM, Sharma OP, Salkin D: Bone marrow sarcoidosis. JAMA 240:2654-2655, 1978.

65 Choe JK, Hyun BH, Salazar GH, Ashton JK, Sung C: Epithelioid granulomas of the bone marrow in non-Hodgkin's lymphoproliferative malignancies. Am J Clin Pathol 80:19-24, 1983.

66 Cruikshank B, Thomas MJ: Mineral oil (follicular) lipidosis. II. Histologic studies of spleen, liver, lymph nodes, and bone marrow. Hum Pathol 15:731-737, 1984.

67 Delsol G, Pellegin M, Familiades J, Auvergnat JC: Bone marrow lesions in Q fever. Blood 52:637-638, 1978.

68 Farhi DC, Mason UG, Horsburgh CR Jr: The bone marrow in disseminated Mycobacterium avium-intracellulare infection. Am J Clin Pathol 83:463-468, 1985.

69 Kadin ME, Donaldson SS, Dorfman RF: Isolated granulomas in Hodgkin's disease. N Engl J Med 283:859-861, 1970.

70 McKenna RW, Dehner, LP: Oxalosis. An unusual cause of myelophthisis in childhood. Am J Clin Pathol 66:991-997, 1976.

71 Nosanchuk JS: Bone marrow granulomas with acute cytomegalovirus infection. Arch Pathol Lab Med 108:93-94, 1984.

72 Okun DB, Sun NCJ, Tanaka KR: Bone marrow granulomas in Q fever. Am J Clin Pathol 71:117-121, 1979.

73 Pease GL: Granulomatous lesions in bone marrow. Blood 11:720-734, 1956.

74 Rywlin AM: A pathologist's view of the bone marrow. J Fla Med Assoc 67:121-124, 1980.

75 Rywlin AM, Ortega R: Lipid granulomas of the bone marrow. Am J Clin Pathol 57:457-462, 1972.

76 Srigley JR, Vellend H, Palmer N, Phillips MJ, Geddie WR, Van Nostrand AWP, Edwards VD: Q-fever. The liver and bone marrow pathology. Am J Surg Pathol 9:752-758, 1985.

77 Swerdlow SH, Collins RD: Marrow granulomas. In: Iochim HE, ed: Pathology of granulomas, New York, 1983, Raven Press, pp.125-150.

78 White RM: Johnston CL: Granulomatous bone marrow disease in Virginia. Study of 50 cases. Va Med 112:316-319, 1985.

79 Williams HE, Smith LH Jr: Primary hyperoxaluria. In Stanbury JB, Wyngaarden JB, Fredrickson DS, Goldstein JL, Brown MS, eds: The metabolic basis of inherited disease. New York, 1983, McGraw-Hill Book Co., pp. 204-228.

80 Young N: Hematologic and hematopoietic consequences of B19 parvovirus infection. Semin Hematol 25:159-172, 1988.

Nonspecific inflammatory reactions

81 Custer RP: An atlas of the blood and bone marrow. Philadelphia, 1974, W.B. Saunders Co.

82 Georgii A, Vykoupil KF: Unspecific mesenchymal reaction in bone marrow in patients with Hodgkin's disease. Recent Results Cancer Res 46:39-44, 1974.

ACQUIRED IMMUNODEFICIENCY SYNDROME (AIDS)

83 Abrams DI, Kirpov DD, Goedert JJ, Sarngadharan MG, Gallo RC, Volberding PA: Antibodies to human T lymphotropic virus type III and development of the acquired immunodeficiency syndrome in homosexual men presenting with immune thrombocytopenia. Ann Intern Med 104:47-50, 1986.

84 Castella A, Croxson TS, Mildvan D, Witt DH, Zalusky R: The bone marrow in AIDS. A histologic, hematologic, and microbiologic study. Am J Clin Pathol 84:425-432, 1985.

85 Frickhofen N, Abkowitz JL, Safford M, Berry M, Antunez-de-Mayolo J, Astrow A, Cohen R, Halperin I, King L, Mintzer D, Cohen B, Young NS: Persistent B19 parvovirus infection in patients infected with human immunodeficiency virus type 1 (HIV-1). A treatable cause of anemia in AIDS. Ann Intern Med 113:986-993, 1990.

86 Geller SA, Muller R, Greenberg ML, Siegal FP: Acquired immunodeficiency syndrome. Distinctive features of bone marrow biopsies. Arch Pathol Lab Med 109:138-141, 1985.

87 Karcher DS, Frost AR: The bone marrow in human immunodeficiency virus (HIV)-related disease. Morphology and clinical correlation. Am J Clin Pathol 95:63-71, 1991.

88 Morris L, Distenfeld A, Amorosi E, Karpatkin S: Autoimmune thrombocytopenic purpura in homosexual men. Ann Intern Med 96:714-717, 1982.

89 Namiki TS, Boone DC, Meyer PR: A comparison of bone marrow findings in patients with acquired immunodeficiency sydrome (AIDS) and AIDS-related conditions. Hematol Oncol 5:99-106, 1987.

90 Osborne BM, Guarda LA, Butler JJ: Bone marrow biopsies in patients with the acquired immunodeficiency sydrome. Hum Pathol 15:1048-1053, 1984.

91 Richman DD, Fischi MA, Grieco MH, Gottlieb MS, Volberding PA, Laskin OL, Leedom JM, Groopman JE, Mildvan D, Hirsch MS, Jackson GG, Durack DT, Nusinoff-Lehrman S, and the AZT Collaborative Working Group: The efficacy of azidothymidine (AZT) in the treatment of patients with AIDS and AIDS related complex. A double-blind, placebo-controlled trial. N Engl J Med 317:192-197, 1987.

92 Savona S, Nardi MA, Lennette ET, Karpatkin S: Thrombocytopenic purpura in narcotics addicts. Ann Intern Med 102:737-741, 1985.

93 Schneider DR, Picker LJ: Myelodysplasia in the acquired immune deficiency syndrome. Am J Clin Pathol 84:144-152, 1985.

94 Spivak JL, Bender BS, Quinn TC: Hematologic abnormalities in the acquired immune deficiency syndrome. Am J Med 77:224-228, 1984.

95 Treacy M, Lai L, Costello C, Clark A: Peripheral blood and bone marrow abnormalities in patients with HIV and related disease. Br J Haematol 65:289-294, 1987.

96 Zon LI, Arkin C, Groopman JE: Haematologic manifestations of the human immune deficiency virus (HIV). Br J Haematol 66:251-256, 1987.

LEUKEMIAS AND RELATED DISORDERS
Acute leukemia

97 Bennett JM, Catovsky D, Daniel MT, Sultan C, Flandrin G, Galton DAG, Gralnick HR: Proposals for the classification of the acute leukaemias. Br J Haematol 33:451-458, 1976.

98 Berdeaux DH, Glasser L, Serokmann R, Moon T, Durie BG: Hypoplastic acute leukemia. Review of 70 cases with multivariate regression analysis. Hematol Oncol 4:291-305, 1986.

99 Breatnach F, Chessells JM, Greaves MF: The aplastic presentation of childhood leukaemia. A feature of common-ALL. Br J Haematol 49:387-393, 1981.

100 Brunning R: The effects of leukemia and lymphoma therapy on hematopoietic cells. Am J Med Technol 39:165-174, 1973.

101 Howe RB, Bloomfield CD, McKenna RW: Hypocellular acute leukemia. Am J Med 72:391-395, 1982.

102 Litz CE, Brunning RD: Acute myeloid leukemias. In DM Knowles, ed: Neoplastic hematopathology, Baltimore, 1992, Williams & Wilkins, pp. 1315-1350.

103 Manoharan A, Horsley R, Pitney WR: The reticulin content of bone marrow in acute leukaemia in adults. Br J Haematol 43:185-190, 1979.

104 Tricot G, Vlietinck R, Boogaerts MA, Hendrickx B, DeWolf-Peeters C, Van den Berghe H, Verwilghen RL: Prognostic factors in the myelodysplastic syndromes. Importance of initial data on peripheral blood counts, bone marrow cytology, trephine biopsy and chromosomal analysis. Br J Haematol 60:19-32, 1985.

105 Yunis JJ, Brunning RD: Prognostic significance of chromosomal abnormalities in acute leukaemias and myelodysplastic syndromes. Clin Haematol 15:597-620, 1986.

Acute myelofibrosis

106 Bain B, Catovsky D, O'Brien M, Prentice HG, Lawlor E, Kumaran TO, McCann SR, Matutes E, Galton DAG: Megakaryoblastic leukemia presenting as acute myelofibrosis. A study of four cases with the platelet-peroxidase reaction. Blood **58**:206-213, 1981.

107 Bearman RM, Pangalis GA, Rappaport H: Acute (malignant) myelosclerosis. Cancer **43**:279-293, 1979.

108 Hruban RH, Kuhajda FP, Mann RB: Acute myelofibrosis. Immunohistochemical study of four cases and comparison with acute megakaryoblastic leukemia. Am J Clin Pathol **88**:578-588, 1987.

109 Sultan C, Sigaux F, Imbert M, Reyes F: Acute myelodysplasia with myelofibrosis. A report of eight cases. Br J Haematol **49**:11-16, 1981.

Granulocytic sarcoma (chloroma)

110 Beckman EN, Oehrle JS: Fibrous hematopoietic tumors arising in agnogenic myeloid metaplasia. Hum Pathol **13**:804-810, 1982.

110a Brunning R, McKenna RW: Atlas of tumor pathology. Tumors of the hematopoietic system. Third Series, Fasc. 9, Armed Forces Institute of Pathology, Washington, DC, 1994, pp 93-100.

111 Cavdar AO, Arcasoy A, Babacan E, Gözdasoglu S, Topuz Ü, Fraumeni JF: Ocular granulocytic sarcoma (chloroma) with acute myelomonocytic leukemia in Turkish children. Cancer **41**:1606-1609, 1978.

112 Garfinkle LS, Bennett DE: Extramedullary myeloblastic transformation in chronic myelocytic leukemia simulating a coexistent malignant lymphoma. Am J Clin Pathol **51**:638-645, 1969.

113 Gralnick HR, Dittmar K: Development of myeloblastoma with massive breast and ovarian involvement during remission in acute leukemia. Cancer **24**:746-749, 1969.

114 Leder LD: The selective enzymochemical demonstration of neutrophilic myeloid cells and tissue mast cells in paraffin sections. Klin Wochenschr **42**:553, 1964.

115 Mason TE, Damaree R, Margolis CI: Granulocytic sarcoma (chloroma) two years preceding myelogenous leukemia. Cancer **31**:423-432, 1973.

116 McKenna RW, Bloomfield CD, Dick F, Nesbit ME, Brunning RD: Acute monoblastic leukemia. Diagnosis and treatment of ten cases. Blood **46**:481-494, 1975.

117 Meis JM, Butler JJ, Osborne BM, Manning JT: Granulocytic sarcoma in non-leukemic patients. Cancer **58**:2697-2709, 1986.

118 Muller S, Sangster G, Crocker J, Nar P, Burnett D, Brown G, Leyland MJ: An immunohistochemical and clinicopathological study of granulocytic sarcoma ('chloroma'). Hematol Oncol **4**:101-112, 1986.

119 Neiman RS, Barcos M, Berard C, Bonner H, Mann R, Rydell RE, Bennett JM: Granulocytic sarcoma. A clinicopathologic study of 61 biopsied cases. Cancer **48**:1426-1437, 1981.

120 Pinkus GS, Pinkus JL: Myeloperoxidase. A specific marker for myeloid cells in paraffin sections. Mod Pathol **4**:733-741, 1991.

121 Rappaport H: Tumors of the hematopoietic system. In Atlas of tumor pathology. Sect III, Fasc. 8. Washington, D.C., 1966, Armed Forces Institute of Pathology.

122 Reardon G, Moloney WC: Chloroma and related myeloblastic neoplasms. Arch Intern Med **108**:864-871, 1961.

123 Tallman MS, Hakamian D, Shaw JM, Lissner GS, Russell EJ, Variakojis D: Granulocyitc sarcoma is associated with the t(8;21) translocation in acute myeloid leukemia. J Clin Oncol **11**:690-697, 1993.

124 Wiernik PH, Serpick AA: Granulocytic sarcoma (chloroma). Blood **35**:361-369, 1970.

Myelodysplastic syndromes

125 Bennett JM, Catovsky D, Daniel MT, Flandrin G, Galton DAG, Gralnick HR, Sultan C: Proposals for the classification of the myelodysplastic syndromes. Br J Haematol **51**:189-199, 1982.

126 Brunning RD: Myelodysplastic syndromes. In DM Knowles, ed: Neoplastic hematopathology. Baltimore, 1992, Williams & Wilkins, pp. 1367-1404.

127 Delacretaz F, Schmidt PM, Piguet D, Bachmann F, Costa J: Histopathology of myelodysplastic syndromes. The FAB classification (proposals) applied to bone marrow biopsy. Am J Clin Pathol **87**:180-186, 1987.

128 List AF, Garewal HS, Sandberg AA: The myelodysplastic syndromes. Biology and implications for management. J Clin Oncol **8**:1424-1441, 1990.

129 Maschek H, Georgii A, Kaloutal V, et al: Myelofibrosis in primary myelodysplastic syndromes. A retrospective study of 352 patients. Eur J Haematol **48**:208-214, 1992.

130 Mathew P, Tefferi A, Dewald GW, et al: The 5-q syndrome. A single institution study of 43 consecutive cases. Blood **81**:1040-1045, 1993.

131 Tricot G, Vlietnick R, Boogaerts MA, Hendrickx B, DeWolf-Peeters C, Van den Berghe H, Verwilghen RL: Prognostic factors in the myelodysplastic syndromes. Importance of initial data on peripheral blood counts, bone marrow, cytology, trephine biopsy and chromosomal analysis. Br J Haematol **60**:19-32, 1985.

Chronic myeloid leukemia

132 Barrton JC, Conrad M: Current status of blastic transformation in chronic myelogenous leukemia. Am J Hematol **4**:281-291, 1978.

133 Burkhardt R, Bartl R, Jager K, Frisch B, Kettner G, Mahl G, Sunds M: Working classification of chronic myeloproliferative disorders based on histological, haematological, and clinical findings. J Clin Pathol **39**:237-252, 1986.

134 Clough V, Geary CG, Hashmi K, Davson J, Knowlson T: Myelofibrosis in chronic granulocytic leukaemia. Br J Haematol **42**:515-526, 1979.

135 Dekmezian R, Kantarjian HM, Keating MJ, Talpaz M, McCredie KB, Freireich EJ: The relevance of reticulin stain-measured fibrosis at diagnosis in chronic myelogenous leukemia. Cancer **59**:1739-1743, 1987.

136 Gralnick HR, Harbor J, Vogel C: Myelofibrosis in chronic granulocytic leukemia. Blood **37**:152-162, 1971.

137 Kantarjian HM, Deisseroth A, Kurzrock R, Estrov Z, Talpaz M: Chronic myelogenous leukemia. A concise update. Blood **82**:691-703, 1993.

138 McGlave PB, Brunning RD, Hurd DD, Kim TH: Reversal of severe bone marrow fibrosis and osteosclerosis following allogenic bone marrow transplantation for chronic granulocytic leukaemia. Br J Haematol **52**:189-194, 1982.

139 Muehleck SD, McKenna RW, Arthur DC, Parkin JL, Brunning RD: Transformation of chronic myelogenous leukemia. Clinical, morphologic and cytogenetic features. Am J Clin Pathol **82**:1-14, 1984.

140 Woodson DL, Bennett DE, Sears DA: Extramedullary myeloblastic transformation of chronic myelocytic leukemia. Arch Intern Med **134**:523-526, 1974.

Polycythemia vera

141 Ellis JT, Peterson P, Geller SA, Rappaport H: Studies of the bone marrow in polychythemia vera and the evolution of myelofibrosis and second hematologic malignancies. Semin Hematol **12**:144-155, 1986.

142 Ellis JT, Silver RT, Coleman M, Geller SA: The bone marrow in polycythemia vera. Semin Hematol **12**:433-444, 1975.

143 Klein H: Morphology of the hematopoietic tissues. In Klein H, ed: Polycythemia, theory and management. Springfield, Ill., 1973, Charles C Thomas Publisher, pp. 201-208.

144 Landaw SA: Acute leukemia in polycythemia vera. Semin Hematol **23**:156-165, 1986.

145 Lawrence JH, Winchell HS, Donald WG: Leukemia in polycythemia vera. Relationship to splenic myeloid metaplasia and therapeutic radiation dose. Ann Intern Med **70**:763-771, 1969.

146 Lazslo J: Myeloproliferative disorders (MPD). Myelofibrosis, myelosclerosis, extramedullary hematopoiesis, undifferentiated MPD and hemorrhagic thrombocythemia. Semin Hematol **12**:409-432, 1975.

147 Modan B, Lilienfield AM: Polycythemia vera and leukemia. The role of radiation treatment. Medicine (Baltimore) **44**:305-344, 1965.

148 Murphy S, Iland H, Rosenthal D, Lazslo J: Essential thrombocythemia. An interim report from the Polycythemia Vera Study Group. Semin Hematol **23**:177-182, 1986.

149 Roberts BE, Miles DW, Woods CG: Polycythaemia vera and myelosclerosis. A bone marrow study. Br J Haematol **16**:75-85, 1969.

150 Silverstein MN: Post-polycythemia myeloid metaplasia. Arch Intern Med **134**:113-115, 1974.

151 Silverstein MN: The evolution into and the treatment of late stage polycythemia vera. Semin Hematol **13**:79-84, 1976.

152 Szur L, Lewis SM: The haematological complications of polycythaemia vera and treatment with radioactive phosphorus. Br J Radiol **39**:122-130, 1966.

153 Vykoupil KF, Thiele J, Stangel W, Krmpotic E, Georgii A: Polycythemia vera. I. Histopathology, ultrastructure and cytogenetics of the bone marrow in comparison with secondary polycythemia. Virchows Arch [A] **389**:307-324, 1980.

154 Vykoupil KF, Thiele J, Stangel W, Krmpotic E, Georgii A: Polycythemia vera. II. Transgression towards leukemia with special emphasis on histological differential diagnosis, cytogenetics and survival. Virchows Arch [A] **389**:325-341,1980.

155 Wasserman LR: The management of polycythaemia vera. Br J Haematol **21**:371-376, 1971.

Chronic idiopathic myelofibrosis (agnogenic myeloid metaplasia)

156 Akikusa B, Komatsu T, Kondo Y, Yokota T, Uchino F, Yonemitsu H: Amyloidosis complicating idiopathic myelofibrosis. Arch Pathol Lab Med **111**:525-529, 1987.

157 Bearman RM, Pangalis GA, Rappaport H: Acute ('malignant') myelosclerosis. Cancer **43**:279-293, 1979.

158 Beckman BN, Oehrle JS: Fibrous hematopoietic tumors arising in agnogenic myeloid metaplasia. Hum Pathol **13**:804-810, 1982.

159 Block M, Burkhardt R, Chelloul N, Demmler K, Duhamel G, Georgii A, Kirsten WH, Lennert K, Nezelof C, Te Velde J: Myelofibrosis-osteosclerosis syndrome. Pathology and morphology. Adv Biosci **16**:219-240, 1975.

160 Burkhardt R, Bartl R, Beil E, Demmler K, Hoffman E, Kronseder A, Irrgang U, Ulrich M, Wieman H, Langecker H, Saar U: Myelofibrosis-osteosclerosis syndrome. Review of literature and histomorphology. Adv Biosci **16**:9-56, 1975.

161 Burston J, Pinniger JL: The reticulin content of bone marrow in haematological disorders. Br J Haematol **9**:172-184, 1963.

162 Dameshek W: Some speculations on the myeloproliferative syndromes. Blood **6**:372-375, 1951.

163 Dameshek W: The myeloproliferative disorders. In Clark WJ, Howard EB, Hackett DL, eds: Myeloproliferative disorders of animal and man. Oak Ridge, TN, 1970, United States Atomic Energy Commission, pp. 413-420.

164 Lubin J, Rozen S, Rwylin AM: Malignant myelosclerosis. Arch Intern Med **136**:141-145, 1976.

165 Nelson B, Knisely RM: Marrow fibrosis in myeloproliferative disorder. In Clark WJ, Howard EB, Hackett DL, eds: Myeloproliferative disorders of animal and man. Oak Ridge, TN, 1970, United States Atomic Energy Commission, pp. 533-555.

166 Rondeau E, Solal-Geligny P, Dhermy D, Vroclans M, Brousse N, Bernard F, Boivin P: Immune disorders in agnogenic myeloid metaplasia. Relations to myelofibrosis. Br J Haematol **53**:467-475, 1983.

167 Thiele J, Zankovich R, Steinberg T, Fischer R, Diehl V: Agnogenic myeloid metaplasia (AMM). Correlation of bone marrow lesions with laboratory data. A longitudinal clinicopathological study on 114 patients. Hematol Oncol **7**:327-343, 1989.

168 Tobin MS, Tan C, Argano SAP: Myelofibrosis in pediatric age group. N Y State J Med **69**:1080-1083, 1969.

169 Varki A, Lottenberg R, Griffith R, Reinhard E: The syndrome of idiopathic myelofibrosis. A clinicopathologic review with emphasis on the prognostic variables predicting survival. Medicine (Baltimore) **62**:353-371, 1983.

170 Ward HP, Block MH: The natural history of agnogenic myeloid metaplasia (AMM) and a critical evaluation of its relationship with the myeloproliferative syndrome. Medicine (Baltimore) **50**:357-420, 1971.

171 Weinstein IM: Idiopathic myelofibrosis. Historical review, diagnosis, and management. Blood Rev **5**:98-104, 1991.

172 Wolf BC, Neiman RS: Myelofibrosis with myeloid metaplasia. Pathophysiologic implications of the correlation between bone marrow changes and progression of splenomegaly. Blood **65**:803-809, 1985.

Chronic lymphocytic leukemia, prolymphocytic leukemia

173 Bearman RM, Pangalis GA, Rappaport H: Prolymphocytic leukemia. Clinical, histological, and cytochemical observations. Cancer **42**:2360-2372, 1978.

174 Bennett JM, Catovsky D, Daniel M-T, Flandrin G, Galton DAG, Gralnick HR, Sultan C: Proposals for the classification of chronic (mature) B and T lymphoid leukaemias. J Clin Pathol **42**:567-584, 1989.

175 Binet L, Catovsky D, Chandra P, Dighiero G, Montserrat E, Rai KR, Sawitsky A: Chronic lymphocytic leukemia. Proposals for a revised prognostic staging system. Br J Haematol **48**:365-367, 1981.

176 Brouet JC, Fermand JP, Laurent G, Grange MJ, Chevalier A, Jacquillat C, Seligmann M: The association of chronic lymphocytic leukemia and multiple myeloma. A study of eleven patients. Br J Haematol **59**:55-66, 1985.

177 Brouet JC, Flandrin G, Sasportes M, Preud'Homme JL, Seligmann M: Chronic lymphocytic leukemia of T-cell origin. Lancet **2**:890-893, 1975.

178 Dick FR, Maca RD: The lymph node in chronic lymphocytic leukemia. Cancer **41**:283-292, 1978.

179 Enno A, Catovsky D, O'Brien M, Cherchi M, Kumaran TO, Galton DAG: "Prolymphocytoid" transformation of chronic lymphocytic leukemia. Br J Haematol **41**:9-18, 1979.

180 Galton DAG, Goldman JM, Wiltshaw E, Catovsky D, Henry K, Goldenberg GJ: Prolymphocytic leukemia. Br J Haematol **27**:7-23, 1974.

181 International Workshop on Chronic Lymphocytic Leukemia. Chronic lymphocytic leukemia. Recommendations for diagnosis, staging, and response criteria. Ann Intern Med **110**:236-238, 1989.

182 Litz CE, Brunning RD: Chronic lymphoproliferative disorders. Classification and prognosis. Bailliere's Clin Haematol **6**:767-783, 1993.

183 Matutes E, Brito-Babapulle V, Swansbury J, et al: Clinical and laboratory features of 78 cases of T-prolymphocytic leukemia. Blood **78**:3269-3274, 1991.

184 Melo JV, Catovsky D, Galton DAG: The relationship between chronic lymphocytic leukemia and prolymphocytic leukemia. I. Clinical and laboratory features of 300 patients and characterization of an intermediate group. Br J Haematol **63**:377-387, 1986.

185 Melo JV, Catovsky D, Galton DAG: The relationship between chronic lymphocytic leukemia and prolymphocytic leukemia. II. Patterns of evolution of "prolymphocytoid" transformation. Br J Haematol **64**:77-86, 1986.

186 Montserrat E, Marques-Pereira JP, Gallart T, Rozman C: Bone marrow histopathologic patterns and immunologic findings in B chronic lymphocytic leukemia. Cancer **54**:447-451, 1984.

187 Montserrat E, Rozman CR: Chronic lymphocytic leukemia. Prognostic factors and natural history. Bailliere's Clin Haematol **6**:849-866, 1993.

188 Owens MR, Strauchen JA, Rowe JM, Bennett JM: Prolymphocytic leukemia. Histologic features in atypical cases. Hematol Oncol **2**:249-257, 1984.

189 Pangalis GA, Roussou PA, Kittas C, Kokkinou S, Fessas P: B chronic lymphocytic leukemia. Prognostic implication of bone marrow histology in 120 patients. Experience from a single hematology unit. Cancer **59**:767-771, 1987.

190 Pangalis GA, Roussou PA, Kittas C, Mitsoulis-Mentzikoff C, Matsouka-Alexandris P, Anagnostopoulos N, Rombos I, Fessas P: Patterns of bone marrow involvement in chronic lymphocytic leukemia and small lymphocytic (well-differentiated) non-Hodgkin's lymphoma. Its clinical significance in relation to their differential diagnosis and prognosis. Cancer **54**:702-708, 1984.

191 Peterson LC, Bloomfield CD, Sundberg RD, Gajl-Peczalska KJ, Brunning RD: Morphology of chronic lymphocytic leukemia and its relationship to survival. Am J Med **59**:316-324, 1975.

192 Rai KB, Sawitsky A, Cronkite EP, Chanana AD, Levy RN, Pasternack BS: Clinical staging of chronic lymphocytic leukemia. Blood **46**:219-234, 1975.

193 Rausig A: Lymphocytic leukemia and malignant lymphoma in the adult. Acta Med Scand **595**(Suppl):1-270, 1976.

194 Rozman C, Hernandez-Nieto L, Montserrat E, Brugues R: Prognostic significance of bone marrow patterns in chronic lymphocytic leukemia. Br J Haematol **47**:529-537, 1981.

Richter's syndrome

195 Armitage JO, Dick FR, Corder M: Diffuse histiocytic lymphoma complicating chronic lymphocytic leukemia. Cancer **41**:422-427, 1978.

196 Brouet JC, Preud'Homme JL, Seligmann M, Bernard J: Blast cells with monoclonal surface immunoglobulin in two cases of acute blast crisis supervening on chronic lymphocytic leukemia. Br Med J **4**:23-24, 1973.

197 Brousse N, Solal-Celigny P, Herrara A, Breil P, Molas G, Glejou JF, Boivin P, Potet F: Gastrointestinal Richter's syndrome. Hum Pathol **16**:854-857, 1985.

198 Case record of the Massachusetts General Hospital (Case 6-1978). N Engl J Med **298**:387-396, 1978.

199 Foucar K, Rydell RE: Richter's syndrome in chronic lymphocytic leukemia. Cancer **46**:118-134, 1980.

200 Goldstein J, Baden J: Richter's syndrome. South Med J **70**:1381-1382, 1977.

201 Litz CE, Arthur DC, Gajl-Peczalska KJ, Rausch D, Copenhaver C, Coad JE, Brunning RD: Transformation of chronic lymphocytic leukemia to small noncleaved cell lymphoma. A cytogenetic, immunological, and molecular study. Leukemia **5**:972-978, 1991.

202 Long JC, Aisenberg AC: Richter's syndrome. A terminal complication of chronic lymphocytic leukemia with distinct clinicopathologic features. Am J Clin Pathol **63**:786-795, 1975.

203 Richter MN: Generalized reticular cell sarcoma of lymph nodes associated with lymphatic leukemia. Am J Pathol **4**:285-292, 1928.

204 Seligmann M, Preud'Homme JL, Brouet JC: Membrane markers in human lymphoid malignancies. Clinicopathologic correlations and insights into the differentiation of normal and neoplastic cells. In Clarkson B, Marks P, Till JR, eds: Differentiation of normal and neoplastic cells. Cold Spring Harbor, NY, 1978, Cold Spring Harbor Laboratory, pp. 859-876.

205 Splinter TA, Bom-van Noorloos A, Van Heerde P: CLL and diffuse histiocytic lymphoma in one patient. Clonal proliferation of two different cells. Scand J Haematol **20**:29-36, 1978.

206 Traweek ST, Liu J, Johnson RM, Winberg CD, Rappaport H: High-grade transformation of chronic lymphocytic leukemia and low-grade non-Hodgkin's lymphoma. Genotypic confirmation of clonal identity. Am J Clin Pathol **100**:519-526, 1993.

207 Trump DL, Mann RB, Phelps R, Roberts H, Conley CL: Richter's syndrome. Diffuse histiocytic lymhoma in patients with chronic lymphocytic leukemia. Am J Med **68**:539-548, 1980.

208 Wick MR, Li C-Y, Ludwig J, Levitt R, Pierre RV: Malignant histiocytosis as a terminal condition in chronic lymphocyte leukemia. Mayo Clin Proc **55**:108-112, 1980.

Hairy cell leukemia (leukemic reticuloendotheliosis), hairy cell leukemia variant

209 Bartl R, Frisch B, Hill W, Burkhardt R, Sommerfiled W, Sund M: Bone marrow histology in hairy cell leukemia. Identification of subtypes and their prognostic significance. Am J Clin Pathol 79:531-545, 1983.

210 Bennett JM, Catovsky D, Daniel M-T, Flandrin G, Galton DAG, Gralnick HR, Sultan C: Proposals for the classification of chronic (mature) B and T lymphoid leukemias. J Clin Pathol 42:567-584, 1989.

211 Burke JS: The value of the bone marrow biopsy in the diagnosis of hairy cell leukemia. Am J Clin Pathol 70:876-884, 1978.

212 Burke JS, Byrne GE Jr, Rappaport H: Hairy cell leukemia (leukemic reticuloendotheliosis). I. A clinical pathologic study of 21 patients. Cancer 33:1399-1410, 1974.

213 Catovsky D, O'Brien M, Melo JV, Wardle J, Brozovic M: Hairy cell leukemia (HCL) variant. An intermediate disease between HCL and B prolymphocytic leukemia. Semin Oncol 11:362-369, 1984.

214 Chang KL, Stroup R, Weiss LM: Hairy cell leukemia. Current status. Am J Clin Pathol 97:719-738, 1992.

215 Golomb HM, Catovsky D, Golde DW: Hairy cell leukemia. A clinical review based on 71 cases. Ann Intern Med 89:677-683, 1978.

216 Hakimian D, Tallman MS, Kiley C, Peterson L: Detection of minimal residual disease by immunostaining of bone marrow biopsies after 2-chlorodeoxyadenosine for hairy cell leukemia. Blood 82:1798-1802, 1993.

217 Hanson CA, Ward PC, Schnitzer B: A multilobular variant of hairy cell leukemia with morphologic similarities to T-cell lymphoma. Am J Surg Pathol 13:671-679, 1989.

218 Janckila AJ, Li C-Y, Lam KW, Yam LT: The cytochemistry of tartrate-resistant acid phosphatase. Technical considerations. Am J Clin Pathol 70:45-55, 1978.

219 Katayama I, Schneider GB: Further ultrastructural characterization of hairy cells of leukemic reticuloendotheliosis. Am J Pathol 86:163-182, 1977.

220 Klima M, Waddell CC: Hairy cell leukemia associated with focal vascular damage. Hum Pathol 15:657-659, 1984.

221 Lee WMF, Beckstead JH: Hairy cell leukemia with bone marrow hypoplasia. Cancer 50:2207-2210, 1982.

222 Naeim F: Clinicopathological subtypes in hairy-cell leukemia. Am J Clin Pathol 78:80-85, 1982.

223 Naeim F, Jacobs AD: Bone marrow changes in patients with hairy cell leukemia treated by recombinant alpha2-interferon. Hum Pathol 16:1200-1205, 1985.

224 Paoletti M, Bitter MA, Vardiman JW: Hairy cell leukemia. Morphologic cytochemical, and immunologic features. Clin Lab Med 8:179-195, 1988.

225 Piro LD, Carrera CJ, Carson DA, Beutler E: Lasting remissions in hairy cell leukemia induced by a single infusion of 2-chlorodeoxyadenosine. N Engl J Med 322:1117-1121, 1990.

226 Platanias LC, Golomb H: Hairy cell leukemia. Bailliere's Clin Haematol 6:887-898, 1993.

227 Robbins BA, Ellison DJ, Spinosa JC, et al: Diagnostic application of two-color flow cytometry in 161 cases of hairy cell leukemia. Blood 82:1277-1287, 1993.

228 Schnitzer B, Kass L: Hairy cell leukemia. Clinicopathologic and ultrastructural study. Am J Clin Pathol 61:176-187, 1974.

229 Spiers AD, Moore D, Cassileth PA, Harrington DP, Cummings FJ, Neimann RS, Bennett JM, O'Connell MJ: Remission in hairy cell leukemia with Pentostatin (2' deoxycoformycin). N Engl J Med 316:825-830, 1987.

230 Turner A, Kjeldsberg CR: Hairy cell leukemia. A review. Medicine (Baltimore) 57:477-499, 1978.

231 Variakojis D, Vardiman JW, Golomb HM: Cytochemistry of hairy cells. Cancer 45:72-77, 1980.

232 Vykoupil KF, Thiele J, Georgii A: Hairy cell leukemia. Bone marrow findings in 24 patients. Virchows Arch [A] 370:273-289, 1976.

Splenic lymphoma with villous lymphocytes

232a Isaacson PG, Matutes E, Burke M, Catovsky D: The histopathology of splenic lymphoma with villous lymphocytes. Blood 84:3828-3834, 1994.

233 Matutes E, Morilla R, Dwusu-Ankomah K, Houlihan A, Catovsky D: The immunophenotype of splenic lymphoma with villous lymphocytes and its relevance to the differential diagnosis with other B-cell disorders. Blood 83:1558-1562, 1993.

234 Melo JV, Hegde U, Parreira A, Thompson I, Lampert IA, Catovsky D: Splenic B cell lymphoma with circulating villous lymphocytes. Differential diagnosis of B cell leukaemias with large spleens. J Clin Pathol 40:642-651, 1987.

235 Oscier D, Matutes E, Gardiner S, Glyde S, Mould S, Brito-Babapulla V, Ellis J, Catovsky D: Cytogenetic studies in splenic lymphoma with villous lymphocytes. Br J Haematol 85:487-491, 1993.

Sézary syndrome

236 Flandrin G, Brouet J: The Sézary cell. Cytologic, cytochemical and immunologic studies. Mayo Clin Proc 49:575-583, 1974.

237 Lutzner MA, Emerit I, Durepaire R, Flandrin G, Grupper Ch, Prunieras M: Cytogenetic, cytophotometric and ultrastructural study of large cerebriform cells of the Sézary syndrome and description of a small cell variant. J Natl Cancer Inst USA 50:1145-1162, 1973.

238 Lutzner MA, Jordan HW: The ultrastructure of an abnormal cell in Sézary's syndrome. Blood 31:719-726, 1968.

239 Taswell HF, Winkelman RK: Sézary syndrome. A malignant reticulemic erythroderma. JAMA 177:465-472, 1961.

240 Variakojis D, Rosas-Uribe A, Rappaport H: Mycosis fungoides. Pathologic findings in staging laparotomies. Cancer 33:1589-1600, 1974.

241 Zucker-Franklin D, Melton JW, Quagliata F: Ultrastructural, immunologic and functional studies on Sézary cells. A neoplastic variant of thymus derived (T) lymphocytes. Proc Natl Acad Sci USA 71:1877-1881, 1974.

NON-HODGKIN'S LYMPHOMA

242 Bain B, Matutes E, Robinson D, Lampert IA, Brito-Babapulle V, Morilla R, Catovsky D: Leukaemia as a manifestation of large cell lymphoma. Br J Haematol 77:301-310, 1991.

243 Bartl R, Frisch B, Burkhardt R, Kettner G, Mahl G, Fateh-Moghadam A, Sund M: Assessment of bone marrow histology in the malignant lymphoma (non-Hodgkin's). Correlation with clinical factors for diagnosis, prognosis, classification and staging. Br J Haematol 51:511-530, 1982.

244 Bartl R, Hansmann ML, Frisch B, Brukhardt R: Comparative histology of malignant lymphomas in lymph node and bone marrow. Br J Haematol 69:229-237, 1988.

245 Choe JK, Hyun BH, Salazar GH, Ashton JK, Sung C: Epithelioid granulomas of the bone marrow in non-Hodgkin's lymphoproliferative malignancies. Am J Clin Pathol 80:19-24, 1983.

246 Conlan MG, Bast M, Armitage JO, Weisenburger DD for the Nebraska Lymphoma Study Group: Bone marrow involvement by non-Hodgkin's lymphoma. The clinical significance of morphologic disordance between the lymph node and bone marrow. J Clin Oncol 8:1163-1172, 1990.

246a Delabie J, Vandenberghe E, Kennes C, et al: Histiocyte rich B-cell lymphoma. A distinct clinicopathologic entity possibly related to lymphocyte predominant Hodgkin's disease, paragranuloma type. Am J Surg Pathol 16:37-48, 1992.

247 Dick F, Bloomfield CD, Brunning RD: Incidence, cytology, and histopathology of non-Hodgkin's lymphomas in the bone marrow. Cancer 33:1382-1398, 1974.

248 Fisher DE, Jacobson JO, Ault KA, Harris NL: Diffuse large cell lymphoma with discordant histology. Clinical features and biologic implications. Cancer 64:1879-1887, 1989.

249 Foucar K, McKenna RW, Frizzera G, Brunning RD: Incidence and patterns of bone marrow and blood involvement by lymphoma in relationship to the Lukes-Collins classification. Blood 54:1417-1422, 1979.

250 Foucar K, McKenna RW, Frizzera G, Brunning RD: Bone marrow and blood involvement by lymphoma in relationship to the Lukes-Collins classification. Cancer 49:888-897, 1982.

250a Fraga M, Brousset P, Schlaifer D, et al: Bone marrow involvement in anaplastic large cell lymphoma. Immunohistochemical detection of minimal disease and its prognostic significance. Am J Clin Pathol 103:82-89, 1995.

251 Gaulard P, Kanavaros P, Farcet JP, et al: Bone marrow histologic and immunohistochemical findings in peripheral T-cell lymphoma. A study of 38 cases. Hum Pathol 22:331-338, 1991.

252 Hanson CA, Brunning RD, Gajl-Peczalska KJ, Frizzera G, McKenna RW: Bone marrow manifestation of peripheral T cell lymphoma. Am J Clin Pathol 86:449-460, 1986.

253 Litz CE, Brunning RD: Chronic lymphoproliferative disorders. Classification and diagnosis. Bailiere's Clin Haematol 6:767-789, 1993.

254 McKenna RW, Bloomfield CD, Brunning RD: Nodular lymphoma. Bone marrow and blood manifestations. Cancer 36:428-440, 1975.

255 McKenna RW, Brunning RD: Reed-Sternberg–like cells in nodular lymphoma involving the bone marrow. Am J Clin Pathol 63:779-785, 1975.

256 McKenna RW, Hernandez JA: Bone marrow in malignant lymphoma. Hematol Oncol Clin North Am 2:617, 1988.

257 Nathwani BN, Mohrmann RL, Brynes RK, Taylor CR, Hansmann ML, Sheibani K: Monocytoid B-cell lymphomas. An assessment of diagnostic criteria and a perspective on histogenesis. Hum Pathol 23:1061-1071, 1992.

258 Non-Hodgkin's Lymphoma Pathologic Classification Project. National Cancer Institute sponsored study of classification of non-Hodgkin's lymphomas. Cancer 49:2112-2135, 1982.

259 Osborne BM, Butler JJ: Hypocellular paratrabecular foci of treated small cleaved cell lymphoma in bone marrow biopsies. Am J Surg Pathol 13:382-388, 1989.

260 Perry DA, Bast MA, Armitage JO, Weisenburger DD: Diffuse intermediate lymphocyte lymphoma. A clinicopathologic study and comparison with small lymphocytic lymphoma and small cleaved cell lymphoma. Cancer 66:1995-2000, 1990.

261 Robertson LE, Redman JR, Butler JJ, Osborne BM, Velasquez WS, McLaughlin P, Swan F, Rodriguez MA, Hagemeister FB, Fuller LM, Cabanillas F: Discordant bone marrow involvement in diffuse large-cell lymphoma. A distinct clinical-pathologic entity associated with a continuous risk of relapse. J Clin Oncol 9:236-242, 1991.

262 Schneider DR, Taylor CR, Parker JW, Cramer AC, Meyer PR, Lukes RJ: Immunoblastic sarcoma of T and B-cell types. Morphologic description and comparison. Hum Pathol 16:885-900, 1985.

Peripheral T-cell lymphoma, adult T-cell leukemia/lymphoma

263 Hanson CA, Brunning RD, Gajl-Peczalska KJ, Frizzera G, McKenna RW: Bone marrow manifestation of peripheral T cell lymphoma. Am J Clin Pathol 86:449-460, 1986.

264 Jaffe ES: Pathologic and clinical spectrum of post-thymic T-cell malignancies. Cancer Invest 2:413-426, 1984.

265 Kim H, Jacobs C, Warnke R, Dorfman RF: Malignant lymphoma with a high content of epithelioid histiocytes. A distinct clinicopathologic entity and a form of so-called "Lennert's lymphoma." Cancer 41:620-635, 1978.

266 Kiyokawa T, Yamaguchi K, Takeya M, Takahashi K, Watanabe T, Matsumoto T, Lee SY, Takatsuki K: Hypercalcemia and osteoclast proliferation in adult T-cell leukemia. Cancer 59:1187-1191, 1987.

267 Yamaguchi K, Takatsuki K: Adult T cell leukemia lymphoma. Bailiere's Clin Haematol 6:899-915, 1993.

ANGIOIMMUNOBLASTIC LYMPHADENOPATHY

268 Frizzera G, Moran EM, Rappaport H: Angio-immunoblastic lymphadenopathy with dysproteinaemia. Lancet 1:1070-1073, 1974.

269 Frizzera G, Moran EM, Rappaport H: Angioimmunoblastic lymphoadenopathy. Diagnosis and clinical course. Am J Med 59:803-818, 1975.

270 Ghani AM, Krause JR: Bone marrow biopsy findings in angioimmunoblastic lymphadenopathy. Br J Haematol 61:203-231, 1985.

271 Lukes RJ, Tindle BH: Immunoblastic lymphadenopathy. A hyperimmune entity resembling Hodgkin's disease. N Engl J Med 292:1-8, 1975.

272 Pangalis GA, Moran EM, Rappaport H: Blood and bone marrow findings in angio-immunoblastic lymphadenopathy. Blood 51:71-83, 1978.

273 Schnaidt U, Vykoupil KF, Thiele J, Georgii A: Angioimmunoblastic lymphadenopathy. Virchows Arch [A] 389:369-380, 1980.

LYMPHOMA/LEUKEMIA

274 Arseneau JG, Canellos GP, Banks PM, Berard CW, Gralnick HR, DeVita VT: American Burkitt's lymphoma. A clincopathologic study of 30 cases. I. Clinical factors related to prolonged survival. Am J Med 58:314-321, 1975.

275 Banks PM, Arseneua JG, Gralnick HR, Canellos GP, DeVita VT, Berard CW: American Burkitt's lymphoma. A clinicopathologic study of 30 cases II. Pathologic correlations. Am J Med 58:322-329, 1975.

276 Barcos MP, Lukes RJ: Malignant lymphomas of convoluted lymphocytes. A new entity of possible T-cell type. In Sinks LR, Godden JO, eds: Conflicts in childhood cancer. An evaluation of current management, vol 4. New York, 1975, Alan R Liss, Inc., pp. 147-178.

277 Bennett JM, Catovsky D, Daniet MT, Flandrin G, Galton DAG, Gralnick HR, Sultan C: Proposals for the classification of the acute leukaemias. Br J Haematol 33:451-458, 1976.

278 Berard CW, O'Connor GT, Thomas LB, Torloni H: Histopathological definition of Burkitt's tumor. Bull WHO 40:601-607, 1969.

279 Bluming AZ, Zielger JL, Carbone PP: Bone marrow involvement in Burkitt's lymphoma. Results of a prospective study. Br J Haematol 22:369-376, 1972.

280 Brunning RD, McKenna RW: Immunologic markers for acute leukemia. A morphologist's perspective. In Berard CW, Dorfman RF, Kaufman N, eds: Malignant lymphoma. Baltimore, 1986, Williams & Wilkins, pp. 124-160.

281 Brunning RD, McKenna RW, Bloomfield CD, Coccia P, Gajl-Peczalska KJ: Bone marrow involvement in Burkitt's lymphoma. Cancer 40:1771-1779, 1977.

282 Burkitt D, Hutt MSR, Wright DH: The African lymphoma. Preliminary observations on response to therapy. Cancer 18:399-410, 1965.

283 Dayton VD, Arthur DC, Gajl-Peczalsak KJ, Brunning RD: Small noncleaved cell lymphoma involving the bone marrow. Am J Clin Pathol 101:130-139, 1994.

284 Dorfman RF: Childhood lymphosarcoma in St. Louis, Missouri, clinically and histologically resembling Burkitt's tumor. Cancer 18:418-430, 1965.

285 Flandrin G, Brouet JC, Daniel MT, Preud'Homme JL: Acute leukemia with Burkitt's tumor cells. A study of six cases with special reference to lymphocyte surface markers. Blood 45:183-188, 1975.

286 Foon KA, Todd RF: Immunologic classification of leukemia and lymphoma. Blood 68:1-31, 1986.

287 Harris NL, Bhan AK: B-cell neoplasms of the lymphocytic, lymphoplasmacy-toid, and plasma cell types. Immunohistologic analysis and clinical correlation. Hum Pathol 16:829-837, 1985.

287a Imamura N, Kusunoki Y, Kawa-Ha K, et al: Aggressive natural killer cell leukemia/lymphoma. Report of four cases and review of the literature. Br J Haematol 75:49-59, 1990.

288 Litz CE., Brunning RD: Chronic lymphoproliferative disorders. Classification and diagnosis. Bailiere's Clin Haematol 6:767-789, 1993.

289 McKenna RW, Bloomfield CD, Brunning RD: Nodular lymphoma. Bone marrow and blood manifestations. Cancer 36:428-440, 1975.

290 Murphy SB, Hustu HO: A randomized trial of combined modality theory of childhood non-Hodgkin's lymphoma. Cancer 45:630-637, 1980.

291 Nathwani BN, Kim H, Rappaport H: Malignant lymphoma, lymphoblastic. Cancer 38:964-983, 1976.

292 O'Connor GT, Rappaport H, Smith EB: Childhood lymphoma resembling "Burkitt tumor" in the United States. Cancer 18:411-417, 1978.

293 Pangalis GA, Nathwanti BN, Rappaport H: Malignant lymphoma, well-differentiated lymphocytic. Its relationship with chronic lymphocytic leukemia and macroglobulinemia of Waldenström. Cancer 39:999-1010, 1977.

294 Pangalis GA, Roussou PA, Kittas C, Mitsoulis-Mentzikoff C, Matsouka-Alex-andidis P, Anagnostopoulos N, Rombos I, Fessas P: Patterns of bone marrow involvement in chronic lymphocytic leukemia and small lymphocytic (well-differentiated) non-Hodgkin's lymphoma. Its clinical significance in relation to their differential diagnosis and prognosis. Cancer 54:702-708, 1984.

295 Pombo De Oliveira MS, Jaffe E, Catovsky D: Leukaemic phase of mantle zone (intermediate) lymphoma. Its characterization in 11 cases. J Clin Pathol 42:962-972, 1989.

296 Weiss LM, Bindl JM, Picozzi VJ, Link MP, Warnke RA: Lymphoblastic lymphoma. An immunophenotype study of 26 cases with comparison to T cell acute lymphoblastic leukemia. Blood 67:474-478, 1986.

297 Zukerberg LR, Medeiros JL, Ferry JA, Harris NL: Diffuse low grade B-cell lymphomas. Four clinically distinct subtypes defined by a combination of morphologic and immunophenotypic features. Am J Clin Pathol 100:373-385, 1993.

BENIGN LYMPHOCYTIC AGGREGATES

298 Bluth RF, Casey TT, McCurley TL: Differentiation of reactive from neoplastic small-cell lymphoid aggregates in paraffin-embedded marrow particle preparations using L-26 (CD20) and UCHL-1 (CD45RO) monoclonal antibodies. Am J Clin Pathol 99:150, 1993.

299 Faulkner-Jones BE, Howie AJ, Boughton BJ, Franklin IM: Lymphoid aggregates in bone marrow; study of eventual outcome. J Clin Pathol 41:768, 1988.

300 Hashimoto H, Hashimoto N: The occurrence of lymph nodules in human bone marrow with particular reference to their number. Kyushu J Med Sci 14:343-354, 1963.

301 Hashimoto M, Higuchi M, Saito T: Lymph nodules in human bone marrow. Acta Pathol Jpn 7:33-52, 1957.

302 Horny HP, Wehrmann M, Grisser H, Tiemann M, Bultmann B, Kaiserling E: Investigation of bone marrow lymphocyte subsets in normal, reactive, and neoplastic states, using paraffin-embedded biopsy specimens. Am J Clin Pathol 99:142, 1993.

303 Maeda K, Hyun BH, Rebuck JW: Lymphoid follicles in bone marrow aspirates. Am J Clin Pathol 67:41-48, 1977.

304 Rywlin AM, Ortega RS, Dominguez CJ: Lymphoid nodules of bone marrow. Normal and abnormal. Blood 43:389-400, 1974.

HODGKIN'S DISEASE

305 Bartl R, Frisch B, Burkhardt R, Huhn D, Pappenberger R: Assessment of bone marrow histology in Hodgkin's disease. Correlation with clinical factors. Br J Haematol 51:345-360, 1982.

306 Dorfman RF: In discussion of Lukes RJ: Criteria for involvement of lymph node, bone marrow, spleen, and liver in Hodgkin's disease. Cancer Res **31:**1768-1769, 1971.

307 Kinney MC, Greer JP, Stein RS, Collins RD, Cousar JB: Lymphocyte depletion Hodgkin's disease. Histopathologic diagnosis of marrow involvement. Am J Surg Pathol **10:**219-226, 1986.

308 Koene-Bogman J: Granulomas and the diagnosis of Hodgkin's disease. N Engl J Med **299:**533, 1978.

309 Lukes RJ: Criteria for involvement of lymph node, bone marrow, spleen and liver in Hodgkin's disease. Cancer Res **31:**1755-1767, 1971.

310 McKenna RW, Brunning RD: Reed-Sternberg–like cells in nodular lymphoma involving the bone marrow. Am J Clin Pathol **63:**779-785, 1975.

311 Musshoff K: Prognostic and therapeutic implications of staging in extranodal Hodgkin's disease. Cancer Res **31:**1814-1821, 1971.

312 Neiman RS, Rosen PJ, Lukes RJ: Lymphocyte depletion Hodgkin's disease. A clinicopathologic entity. N Engl J Med **288:**751-755, 1973.

313 O'Carroll DI, McKenna RW, Brunning RD: Bone marrow manifestations of Hodgkin's disease. Cancer **38:**1717-1728, 1976.

314 Rappaport H, Berard CW, Butler JJ, Dorfman RF, Lukes RJ, Thomas LB: Report of the Committee of Histopathological Criteria contributing to staging of Hodgkin's disease. Cancer Res **31:**1864-1865, 1971.

314a Siebert JD, Stuckey JH, Kurtin PJ, Banks PM: Extranodal lymphocyte predominance Hodgkin's disease. Am J Clin Pathol **103:**485-491, 1995.

315 TeVelde J, Ottolander GJ, Spaander PJ, Van den Berg C, Hartgrink-Groeneveld CA: The bone marrow in Hodgkin's disease. The non-involved marrow. Histopathology **2:**31-46, 1978.

HISTIOCYTIC DISORDERS
Malignant histiocytosis

316 Byrne GE, Rappaport H: Malignant histiocytosis. Gann Monogr Cancer Res **15:**145-162, 1973.

317 Jurco S, Starling K, Hawkins EP: Malignant histiocytosis in childhood. Morphologic considerations. Hum Pathol **14:**1059-1065, 1983.

318 Lampert IA, Catovsky D, Bergier M: Malignant histiocytosis. A clinicopathological study of 12 cases. Br J Haematol **40:**65-77, 1978.

319 Rappaport H: Tumors of the hematopoietic system. In Atlas of tumor pathology. Sect. III. Fasc 8, Washington, DC, 1966, Armed Forces Institute of Pathology.

320 Roholl PJ, Kleyne J, Pijpers HW, Van Unnik JAM: Comparative immunohistochemical investigation of markers for malignant histiocytes. Hum Pathol **16:**763-771, 1985.

321 Rousseau-Merck MF, Jaubert E, Nezelof C: Malignant histiocytosis in childhood. Hum Pathol **16:**321, 1985.

322 Van Heerde P, Feltkamp CA, Hart AAM, Somers R: Malignant histiocytosis and related tumors. A clinicopathologic study of 42 cases using cytological, histochemical, and ultrastructural parameters. Hematol Oncol **2:**13-32, 1984.

323 Warnke RA, Kim H, Dorfman RF: Malignant histiocytosis (histiocytic medullary reticulosis) I. Clinicopathologic study of 29 cases. Cancer **35:**215-230, 1975.

324 Weiss LM, Azzi R, Dorfman RF, Warnke RA; Sinusoidal hematolymphoid malignancy ("malignant histiocytosis") presenting as atypical sinusoidal proliferation. A study of nine cases. Cancer **58:**1681-1688, 1986.

325 Wick MR, Li C-Y, Ludwig J, Levitt R, Pierre RV: Malignant histiocytosis as a terminal condition in chronic lymphocytic leukemia. Mayo Clin Proc **55:**108-112, 1980.

326 Wilson MS, Weiss LM, Gatter KC, DY, Mason DM, Dorfman RF, Warnke RA: Malignant histiocytosis. A reassessment of cases previously reported in 1975 based on paraffin section immunophenotyping studies. Cancer **66:**530-536, 1990.

Hemophagocytic syndromes

327 Ashby MA, Williams CJ, Buchanan RB, Bleehen NM, Arno J: Mediastinal germ cell tumor associated with malignant histiocytosis and high rubella titres. Hematol Oncol **4:**183-194, 1986.

328 Chandra P, Chaudhery SA, Rosner F, Kagen M: Transient histiocytosis with striking phagocytosis of platelets, leukocytes, and erythrocytes. Arch Intern Med **135:**989-991, 1975.

329 Chen R-L, Su I-J, Lin K-H, Lee S-H, Lin D-T, Chuu W-M, Lin K-S, Huang L-M, Lee C-Y: Fulminant childhood hemophagocytic syndrome mimicking histiocytic medullary reticulosis. Am J Clin Pathol **96:**171-176, 1991.

330 Daum GS, Sullivan JL, Ansell J, Mulder C, Woda BA: Virus-associated hemophagocytic syndrome. Identification of an immunoproliferative precursor lesion. Hum Pathol **18:**1071-1074, 1987.

331 Falini B, Pileri S, De Solas I, Martelli MF, Mason DY, Delsol G, Gatter KC, Fagioli M: Peripheral T-cell lymphoma associated with hemophagocytic syndrome. Blood **75:**434-444, 1990.

332 Frizzera G: The clinico-pathological expressions of Epstein-Barr virus infection in lymphoid tissues. Virchows Arch [Cell Pathol] **53:**1-12, 1987.

333 Gaffey MJ, Frierson HF, Medeiros LJ, Weiss LM: The relationship of Epstein-Barr virus (sporadic) and familial hemophagocytic syndrome and secondary (lymphoma-related) hemophagocytosis. An in situ hybridization study. Hum Pathol **24:**657-667, 1993.

334 Henter JI, Elinder G, Ost A: Diagnostic guidelines for hemophagocytic lymphohistiocytosis. Semin Oncol **18:**29-33, 1991.

335 Jaffe ES, Costa J, Fauci AS, Cossman J, Tsosos M: Malignant lymphoma and erythrophagocytosis simulating malignant histiocytosis. Am J Med **75:**741-749, 1983.

336 Jurco S, Starling K, Hawkins EP: Malignant histiocytosis in childhood. Morphologic considerations. Hum Pathol **14:**1059-1065, 1983.

337 Kikuta H, Sakiyama Y, Matsumoto S, Oh-Ishi T, Nakano T, Nagashima T, Oka T, Hironaka T, Hirai K: Fatal Epstein-Barr virus–associated hemophagocytic syndrome. Blood **82:**3259-3264, 1993.

338 Lampert IA, Catovsky D, Bernier M: Malignant histiocytosis. A clinicopathological study of 12 cases. Br J Haematol **40:**65-77, 1978.

339 Liu Yin JA, Kumaran TO, Marsh GW, Rossiter M, Catovsky D: Complete recovery of histiocytic medullary reticulosis–like syndrome in a child with acute lymphoblastic leukemia. Cancer **51:**200-202, 1983.

340 Look, AT, Naegele RF, Callihan T, Herrod HG, Henle W: Fatal Epstein-Barr virus infections in a child with acute lymphoblastic leukemia in remission. Cancer Res **41:**4280-4283, 1981.

341 Mroczek EC, Weisenburger DD, Grierson HL, Markin R, Purtilo DT: Fatal infectious mononucleosis and virus-associated hemophagocytic syndrome. Arch Pathol Lab Med **111:**530-535, 1987.

342 Reiner AP, Spivak JL: Hematophagocytic histiocytosis. A report of 23 new patients and a review of the literature. Medicine (Baltimore) **67:**345-368, 1988.

343 Reisman RP, Greco MA: Virus-associated hemophagocytic syndrome due to Epstein-Barr virus. Hum Pathol **15:**290-293, 1984.

344 Risdall RJ, Brunning RD, Hernandez JI, Gordon DH: Bacteria-associated hemophagocytic syndrome. Cancer **54:**2968-2972, 1984.

345 Risdall RJ, McKenna RW, Nesbit ME, Krivit W, Balfour HH, Simons RL, Brunning RD: Virus associated hemophagocytic syndrome. Cancer **44:**993-1002, 1979.

345a Shirono K, Tsuda H: Parvovirus B19–associated hemophagocytic syndrome in healthy adults. Br J Haematol **89:**923-926, 1995.

346 Sullivan JL, Woda BA, Herrod HG, Koh G, Rivara FP, Mulder C: Epstein-Barr virus-associated hemophagocytic syndrome. Virological and immunopathological studies. Blood **65:**1097-1104, 1985.

347 Woda BA, Sullivan JL: Reactive histiocytic disorders. Am J Clin Pathol **99:**459-463, 1993.

Histiocytosis X (Langerhans' cell histiocytosis)

348 McClain K, Ramsay NKC, Robison L, Sundberg RD, Nesbit M Jr: Bone marrow involvement in histiocytosis X. Med Pediatr Oncol **11:**167-171, 1983.

349 Nesbit ME, Krivit W: Histiocytosis. In Bloom HSG, Deidhardt MK, Lemerk J, Voute PA, eds: Cancer in children. Clinical management. Berlin, 1975, Springer-Verlag, pp. 193-199.

PLASMA CELL DYSCRASIAS
Multiple myeloma, osteosclerotic myeloma, monoclonal gammopathy of undetermined significance

350 Azar HA: Plasma cell myelomatosis and other monoclonal gammopathies. Pathol Annu **7:**1-17, 1977.

351 Azar HA, Zaino EC, Pham TD, Yannopoulos K: Non-secretory plasma cell myeloma. Observations on seven cases with electron microscopic studies. Am J Clin Pathol **58:**618-629, 1972.

352 Barlogie B, Epstein J, Selvanayagam P, Alexanian R: Plasma cell-myeloma. New biologic insights and advances in therapy. Blood **73:**865-879, 1989.

353 Bartl R, Frisch B, Burkhardt R, Fateh-Moghadam A, Mahl G, Gierster P, Sund M, Ketter G: Bone marrow histology in myeloma. Its importance in diagnosis, prognosis, classification and staging. Br J Haematol **51:**361-375, 1982.

354 Bartl R, Frisch B, Fateh-Moghadam A, Kettner G, Jaeger K, Sommerfeld W: Histologic classification and staging of multiple myeloma. A retrospective study of 674 cases. Am J Clin Pathol **87:**342-355, 1987.

355 Bataille R, Durie BGM, Grenier J: Serum beta₂. Microglobulin and survival duration in multiple myeloma. A simple reliable marker for staging. Br J Haematol **55:**439-447, 1983.

356 Bitter MA, Komaiko W, Franklin WA: Giant lymph node hyperplasia with osteoblastic bone lesions and the POEMS (Takatsuki's) syndrome. Cancer **56:**188-194, 1985.

357 Carbone A, Volpe R, Manconi R, Poletti A, Tirelli U, Monfardini S: Bone marrow pattern and clinical staging in multiple myeloma. Br J Haematol **65:**502, 1987.

358 Carter A, Hocherman I, Linn S, Cohen Y, Tatarsky I: Prognostic significance of plasma cell morphology in multiple myeloma. Cancer **60:**1060-1065, 1987.

359 Case record of the Massachusetts General Hospital; Case 4-1992. N Engl J Med **326:**255-263, 1992.

360 Case record of the Massachusetts General Hospital; Case 39-1992: N Engl J Med **327:**1014-1021, 1992.

361 Cavo M, Baccarani M, Gobbi M, Lipizer A, Tura S: Prognostic value of bone marrow plasma cell infiltration in stage I multiple myeloma. Br J Haematol **55:**683-690, 1983.

362 Diego Miralles G, O'Fallon JR, Talley NJ: Plasma-cell dyscrasia with polyneuropathy. The spectrum of POEMS syndrome. N Engl J Med **327:**1919-1923, 1992.

363 Durie BG: Staging and kinetics of multiple myeloma. Semin Oncol **13:**300-309, 1986.

364 Durie BGM, Salmon SE, Moon TE: Pretreatment tumor mass, cell kinetics, and prognosis in multiple myeloma. Blood **55:**364-372, 1980.

365 Falini B, DeSolas I, Levine AM, Parker JW, Lukes RJ, Taylor CR: Emergence of B-immunoblastic sarcoma in patients with multiple myeloma. A clinicopathologic study of 10 cases. Blood **59:**923-933, 1982.

366 Fritz E, Ludwig H, Kundi M: Prognostic relevance of cellular morphology in multiple myeloma. Blood **63:**1072-1079, 1984.

367 Gassman W, Pralle H, Haferlach T, Pandurevic S, Graubner M, Schmitz N, Loffler H: Staging systems for multiple myeloma. A comparison. Br J Haematol **59:**703-711, 1985.

368 Greipp PR: Advances in the diagnosis and management of myeloma. Semin Hematol **29:**24-45, 1992.

369 Greipp PR, Katzmann JA, O'Fallon WM, Kyle RA: Impact of pretreatment ß₂ microglobulin levels on survival in patients with multiple myeloma. Blood **66:**188a, 1985.

370 Greipp PR, Kyle RA: Clinical, morphological and cell kinetic differences among multiple myeloma, monoclonal gammopathy of undetermined significance, and smoldering multiple myeloma. Blood **62:**166-171, 1983.

371 Greipp PR, Raymond NM, Kyle RA, O'Fallon WM: Multiple myeloma. Significance of plasmablastic subtype in morphological classification. Blood **65:**305-310, 1985.

372 Greipp PR, Witzog TE, Gonchoroff NJ, Haberman TM, Katzmann JA, O'Fallon WM, Kyle RA: Immunofluorescence labeling indices in myeloma and related monoclonal gammopathies. Mayo Clin Proc **62:**969-977, 1987.

373 Hyun BK, Kwa D, Gabaldon H, Ashton JK: Reactive plasmacytic lesions of the bone marrow. Am J Clin Pathol **65:**921-928, 1976.

374 Imawari M, Akatsuka N, Beppu H, Suzuki H, Yoshitoshi Y: Syndrome of plasma cell dyscrasia, polyneuropathy, and endocrine disturbances. Ann Intern Med **81:**490-493, 1974.

375 Kosmo MA, Gale RP: Plasma cell leukemia. Semin Hematol **24:**202-208, 1987.

376 Krzyzaniak RL, Buss DH, Cooper R, Wells HB: Marrow fibrosis and multiple myeloma. Am J Clin Pathol **89:**63-68, 1988.

377 Kyle RA: Multiple myeloma. A review of 869 cases. Mayo Clin Proc **50:**29-49, 1975.

378 Kyle RA: "Benign" monoclonal gammopathy. After 20-35 years of follow-up. Mayo Clin Proc **68:**26-36, 1993.

378a Kyle RA, Lust JA: Monoclonal gammopathies of undetermined significance. Semin Hematol **26:**176-200, 1989.

379 Kyle RA, Greipp PR: The laboratory investigation of monoclonal gammopathies. Mayo Clin Proc **53:**719-739, 1978.

380 Kyle RA, Maldonado JE, Baryd ED: Plasma cell leukemia. Report on 17 cases. Arch Intern Med **133:**813-818, 1974.

381 Maldonado J, Velosa JA, Kyle RA, Wagoner RD, Holley KE, Salassa RM: Fanconi syndrome in adults. A manifestation of a latent form of myeloma. Am J Med **58:**354-364, 1974.

382 Miralles GD, O'Fallon JR, Talley NJ: Plasma-cell dyscrasia with polyneuropathy. The spectrum of POEMS syndrome. N Engl J Med **327:**1919-1923, 1992.

383 Peterson LC, Brown BA, Crosson JT, Mladenovic J: Application of the immunoperoxidase technic to bone marrow trephine biopsies in the classification of patients with monoclonal gammopathies. Am J Clin Pathol **85:**688-693, 1986.

384 Petruch UR, Horny HP, Kaiserling E: Frequent expression of haemopoietic and non-haemopoietic antigens by neoplastic plasma cells. An immunohistochemical study using formalin-fixed, paraffin-embedded tissue. Histopathology **20:**35-40, 1992.

385 Pileri S, Poggi S, Baglioni P, et al: Histology and immunohistology of bone marrow biopsy in multiple myeloma. Eur J Haematol **43:**19-26, 1989.

386 Preud'Homme JL, Hurez D, Danon F, Brouet JC, Seligmann M: Intracytoplasmic and surface-bound immunoglobulins in "nonsecretory" and Bence-Jones myeloma. Clin Exp Immunol **25:**428-436, 1976.

387 Smith DB, Harris M, Gowland E, Chang J, Scargge JH: Non-secretory multiple myeloma. A report of 13 cases with a review of the literature. Hematol Oncol **4:**307-313, 1986.

388 Snapper I, Kahn A: Myelomatosis. Baltimore, 1971, University Park Press.

388a Soubrier MJ, Dubost J-J, Sauvezie BJH, et al: POEMS syndrome. A study of 25 cases and a review of the literature. Am J Med **97:**543-553, 1994.

389 Strand WR, Banks PM, Kyle RA: Anaplastic plasma cell myeloma and immunoblastic lymphoma. Clinical, pathologic, and immunologic comparison. Am J Med **76:**861-867, 1984.

390 Strickler JG, Audeh MW, Copenhaver CM, Warnke RA: Immunophenotypic differences between plasmacytoma/multiple myeloma and immunoblastic lymphoma. Cancer **61:**1782-1786, 1988.

390a Sukpanichnant S, Cousar JB, Leelasiri A, Graber SE, Greer JP, Collins RD: Diagnostic criteria and histologic grading in multiple myeloma. Histologic and immunohistologic analysis of 176 cases with clinical correlation. Hum Pathol **25:**308-318, 1994.

391 Takatsuki K, Sanada I: Plasma cell dyscrasia with polyneuropathy and endocrine disorder. Clinical and laboratory features of 109 reported cases. Jpn J Clin Oncol **13:**543-556, 1983.

392 Thiry A, Delvenne P, Fontaine MA, Bonvier J: Comparison of bone marrow sections, smears, and immunohistological staining for immunoglobulin light chains in the diagnosis of benign and malignant plasma cell proliferations. Histopathology **22:**423-428, 1993.

393 Woodruff RK, Malpas JS, Paxton AM, Lister TA: Plasma cell leukemia (PCL). A report on 15 patients. Blood **52:**839-845, 1978.

Plasmacytoma

394 Alexanian R: Localized and indolent myeloma. Blood **56:**521-525, 1980.

395 Corwin J, Lindberg RD: Solitary plasmacytoma of bone vs. extramedullary plasmacytoma and their relationship to multiple myeloma. Cancer **43:**1007-1013, 1979.

396 Kotner LM, Wang CC: Plasmacytoma of the upper air and food passages. Cancer **30:**414-425, 1972.

397 Meis JM, Butler JJ, Osborne BM, Ordonez NG: Solitary plasmacytomas of bone and extramedullary plasmacytomas. A clinicopathologic and immunohistochemical study. Cancer **59:**1475-1485, 1987.

398 Meyer JE, Schultz MD: "Solitary" myeloma of bone. A review of 12 cases. Cancer **34:**438-440, 1974.

399 Mill WB, Griffith R: The role of radiation therapy in the management of plasma cell tumors. Cancer **45:**647-652, 1980.

400 Peterson LC, Brown BA, Crosson JT, Mladenovic J: Application of the immunoperoxidase technic to bone marrow trephine biopsies in the classification of patients with monoclonal gammopathies. Am J Clin Pathol **85:**688-693, 1986.

401 Strickler JG, Audeh MW, Copenhaver CM, Warnke RA: Immunophenotypic differences between plasmacytoma/multiple myeloma and immunoblastic lymphoma. Cancer **61:**1782-1786, 1988.

402 Wiltshaw E: The natural history of extramedullary plasmacytoma and its relation to solitary myeloma of bone and myelomatosis. Medicine (Baltimore) **55:**217-238, 1976.

403 Woodruff RK, Whittle JM, Malplas JS: Solitary plasmacytoma. Extramedullary soft tissue plasmacytoma. Cancer **43:**2340-2343, 1979.

Plasmacytoid lymphoma (Waldenström's macroglobulinemia)

404 Alexanian R: Monoclonal gammopathy in lymphoma. Arch Intern Med **135:**62-66, 1975.

405 Berman HH: Waldenström's macroglobulinemia with bone lesions and plasma cell morphology. Am J Clin Pathol **63:**397-402, 1975.

406 Brittin G, Yanka Y, Brecher G: Intranuclear inclusions in multiple myeloma and macroglobulinemia. Blood **21:**335-351, 1963.

407 Brunning R, Parkin J: Intranuclear inclusions in plasma cells and lymphocytes from patients with monoclonal gammopathies. Am J Clin Pathol **66:**10-21, 1976.

408 Case records of the Massachusetts General Hospital (Case 6-1978). N Engl J Med **298:**387-396, 1978.

409 Dutcher TF, Fahey JL: The histopathology of the macroglobulinemia of Waldenström. J Natl Cancer Inst USA **22:**887-917, 1959.

410 Kim H, Heller P, Rappaport H: Monoclonal gammopathies associated with lymphoproliferative disorders. Am J Clin Pathol **59:**282-294, 1973.

411 Lennert K, Collins RD, Lukes RJ: Concordance of the Kiel and Lukes-Collins classifications of the non-Hodgkin's lymphomas. Histopathology 7:549-559, 1983.

412 MacKenzie MR, Fudenberg HH: Macroglobulinemia. An analysis for forty patients. Blood 39:874-889, 1972.

413 McCallister BD, Bayrd ED, Harrison EG Jr, McGuckin WF: Primary macroglobulinemia. Review with a report on 31 cases and notes on the value of continuous chlorambucil therapy. Am J Med 43:394-434, 1967.

414 Non-Hodgkin's Lymphoma Classification Project: National Cancer Institute Sponsored Study of Classification of Non-Hodgkin's Lymphomas. Summary and description of working formulations for clinical usage. Cancer 49:2112-2135, 1982.

415 Pangalis GA, Nathwanti BN, Rappaport H: Malignant lymphoma, well differentiated lymphocytic. Its relationship with chronic lymphocytic leukemia and macroglobulinemia of Waldenström. Cancer 39:999-1010, 1977.

416 Rappaport H: Tumors of the hematopoietic system. In Atlas of tumor pathology, Sect. III, Fasc. 8. Washington, DC, 1966. Armed Forces Institute of Pathology.

417 Rywlin AW, Civantos F, Ortega RS, Dominguez CJ: Bone marrow histology in monoclonal macroglobulinemia. Am J Clin Pathol 63:769-778, 1975.

418 Tubbs RR, Hoffman GC, Deodhar SD, Hewlett JS: IgM monoclonal gammopathy. Histopathologic and clinical spectrum. Cleve Clin Q 43:217-235, 1976.

419 Tursz T, Brouet J, Flandrin G, Danon F, Clauvel JP, Seligmann M: Clinical and pathologic features of Waldenström's macroglobulinemia in seven patients with serum monoclonal IgG or IgA. Am J Med 63:499-502, 1977.

420 Waldenström J: Incipient myelomatosis or "essential" hypergammaglobulinemia with fibrinogenopenia. A new syndrome. Acta Med Scand 117:216-247, 1944.

Heavy chain disease

421 Frangione B, Franklin ED: Heavy chain diseases. Clinical features and molecular significance of the disordered immunoglobulin structure. Semin Hematol 10:53-64, 1973.

422 Franklin ED: Mu-chain disease. Arch Intern Med 135:71-72, 1975.

423 Jonsson V, Videbaek A, Axelsen NH, Harboe M: Mu-chain disease in a case of chronic lymphocytic leukemia and malignant histiocytoma. I. Clinical aspects. Scand J Haematol 16:209-217, 1976.

424 Kyle RA, Greipp PR, Banks PM: The diverse picture of gamma heavy-chain disease. Report of seven cases and review of literature. Mayo Clin Proc 56:439-451, 1981.

425 Seligmann M: Immunochemical, clinical, and pathologic features of alpha-chain disease. Arch Intern Med 135:78-82, 1975.

426 Seligmann M, Preud'Homme JL, Brouet JC: Membrane markers in human lymphoid malignancies. Clinicopathological correlations and insights into the differentiation of normal and neoplastic cells. In Clarkson B, Marks P, Till JR, eds: Differentiation of normal and neoplastic hematopoietic cells. Cold Spring Harbor, NY, 1978, Cold Spring Harbor Laboratory, pp. 859-876.

Amloidosis

427 Conn RB Jr, Sundberg RD: Amyloid disease of bone marrow. Diagnosis by sternal aspiration biopsy. Am J Pathol 38:61-71, 1961.

428 Gertz MA, Kyle RA: Primary systemic amyloidosis. A diagnostic primer. Mayo Clin Proc 64:1505-1519, 1989.

429 Kyle RA, Greipp PR: Amyloidosis (AL). Clinical and laboratory features in 229 cases. Mayo Clin Proc 58:665-683, 1983.

430 Wolf BC, Kumar A, Vera JC, Nieman RS: Bone marrow morphology and immunology in systemic amyloidosis. Am J Clin Pathol 86:84-88, 1986.

SYSTEMIC POLYCLONAL B-IMMUNOBLASTIC PROLIFERATION

431 Hanto DW, Frizzera G, Purtilo DT, Sakamoto K, Sullivan JL, Saemundsen AK, Klein G, Simmons RL, Najarian JS: Clinical spectrum of lymphoproliferative disorders in renal transplant recipients and evidence for the role of Epstein-Barr virus. Cancer Res 41:4253-4261, 1981.

432 Koo CH, Nathwant BN, Winberg CD, Hill LR, Rappaport H: Atypical lymphoplasmacytic and immunoblastic proliferation in lymph nodes of patients with autoimmune disease (autoimmune disease-associated lymphadenopathy). Medicine (Baltimore) 63:274-290, 1984.

433 Peterson LC, Brown BA, Crosson JT, Mladenovic J: Application of the immunoperoxidase technique to bone marrow trephine biopsies in the classification of patients with monoclonal gammopathies. Am J Clin Pathol 85:688-693, 1986.

434 Peterson LC, Kueck B, Arthur DC, Dedeker K, Brunning RD: Systemic polyclonal immunoblastic proliferations. Cancer 61:1350-1358, 1988.

435 Poje EJ, Soori GS, Weisenburger DD: Systemic polyclonal B-immunoblastic proliferation with marked peripheral blood and bone marrow plasmacytosis. Am J Clin Pathol 98:222-226, 1992.

SYSTEMIC MASTOCYTOSIS

436 Brunning, RD, McKenna RW, Rosai J, Parkin JL, Risdall R: Systemic mastocytosis. Am J Surg Pathol 7:808-814, 1983.

437 Czarentski BM, Kolde G, Schoemann A, Urbanitz S, Urbanitz D: Bone marrow findings in adult patients with urticaria pigmentosa. J Am Acad Dermatol 18:45-51, 1980.

438 Horny HP, Parwaresch MR, Lennert K: Bone marrow findings in systemic mastocytosis. Hum Pathol 16:808-814, 1985.

439 Horny HP, Reimann O, Kaiserling E: Immunoreactivity of normal and neoplastic tissue mast cells. Am J Clin Pathol 89:335-340, 1988.

440 Horny HP, Rick M, Wehrmann M, Kaiserling E: Blood findings in generalized mastocytosis. Evidence of frequent simultaneous occurrence of myeloproliferative disorders. Br J Haematol 76:186-193, 1990.

441 Johnstone JM: The appearance and significance of tissue mast cells in human bone marrow. J Clin Pathol 7:275-280, 1954.

442 Lawrence JB, Friedman BS, Travis WD, Chinchilli VM, Metcalfe DD, Gralnick HR: Hematologic manifestations of systemic mast cell disease. A prospective study of laboratory and morphologic features and their relation to prognosis. Am J Med 91:612-624, 1991.

443 Lennert K, Parwaresch MR: Mast cells and mast cell neoplasia. A review. Histopathology 3:349-365, 1979.

444 Parker C, Jost RG, Bauer E, Haddad J, Garza R: In Cryer PE, Kissane JM, eds: Clinicopathologic conference. Systemic mastocytosis. Am J Med 61:671-680, 1976.

445 Rappaport H: Tumors of the hematopoietic system. In Atlas of tumor pathology. Sect. III, Fasc. 8. Washington, D.C., 1966, Armed Forces Institute of Pathology.

446 Rywlin AM: Mastocytic eosinophilic fibrohistiocytic lesion of the bone marrow. Hematology 24:1-4, 1982.

447 Rywlin AM, Hoffman EP, Ortega RS: Eosinophilic fibrohistiocytic lesion of bone marrow. Distinctive new morphologic finding, probably related to drug hypersensitivity. Blood 40:464-472, 1972.

448 Sagher F, Even-Paz Z: Mastocytosis and the mast cell. Chicago, 1967, Year Book Medical Publishers, Inc.

449 Scully RE, Mark EJ, McNeely BU: Case records of the Massachusetts General Hospital. N Engl J Med 315:816-824, 1986.

450 Szewda JA, Abraham JP, Fine G, Nixon RK, Rupe CE: Systemic mast cell disease. A review and report of three cases. Am J Med 32:227-239, 1962.

451 Te Velde J, Vismans FJFE, Leenheers-Binnendijk L, Vos CJ, Smecnk D, Bijvoet OLM: The eosinophilic fibrohistiocytic lesion of the bone marrow. A mastocellular lesion in bone disease. Virchows Arch [A] 337:277-284, 1978.

452 Tharp MD: The spectrum of mastocytosis. Am J Med Sci 289:117-132, 1985.

453 Travis W, Li C-Y, Bergstralh E, Yam LT, Swee RG: Systemic mast cell disease. Analysis of 58 cases and literature review. Medicine (Baltimore) 67:345-368, 1988.

454 Walls AF, Jones DB, Williams JH, Church MK, Holgate ST: Immunohistochemical identification of mast cells in formalin-fixed tissue using monoclonal antibodies specific for tryptase. J Clin Pathol 42:414-421, 1989.

455 Webb TA, Li C-Y, Yam LT: Systemic mast cell disease. A clinical and hematopathologic study of 26 cases. Cancer 49:927-938, 1982.

METASTATIC TUMORS

456 Anner RM, Drewinko B: Frequency and significance of bone marrow involvement by metastatic solid tumors. Cancer 39:1337-1344, 1977.

457 Bezwoda WR, Lewis D, Livini N: Bone marrow involvement in anaplastic small cell lung cancer. Cancer 58:1762-1765, 1986.

458 Bostrom BB, Nesbitt ME, Brunning RD: The value of bone marrow biopsy in the diagnosis of metastatic neuroblastoma. Am J Pediatr Hematol Oncol 7:301-305, 1985.

459 Bramwell VHC, Littley MB, Chang J, Crowther D: Bone marrow involvement in adult soft tissue sarcoma. Eur J Cancer Clin Oncol 18:1099-1106, 1982.

460 Brodeur GM, Pritchard J, Berthold F, Carlsen NLT, Castel V, Castleberry RP, De Bernardi B, et al: Revisions of the international criteria for neutroblastoma diagnosis, staging, and response to treatment. J Clin Oncol 11:1466-1477, 1993.

461 Ceci G, Franciosi V, Passalacqua R, Di Blasio B, Boni C, Lottici R, De Lisi V, Nizzoli R, Guazzi A, Cocconi G: The value of bone marrow biopsy in breast cancer at the time of first relapse. A prospective study. Cancer 61:1041-1045, 1988.

462 Clamon GH, Edwards WR, Hamous JE, Scupham RK: Patterns of bone marrow involvement with small cell lung cancer. Cancer 54:100-102, 1984.

24 Bone and joints

Bone
NORMAL ANATOMY

Adult bones are classified according to their shape into long (such as femur), flat (such as pelvis), and short (such as bones of hand and feet). Long bones (and some short bones such as metacarpal bones) are divided topographically into three regions: diaphysis, epiphysis, and metaphysis. The diaphysis is the shaft. The epiphysis is at both ends of the bone and is partially covered by articular cartilage. The metaphysis is at the junction of the diaphysis and epiphysis. In the growing bone, it begins at the epiphyseal plate (epiphyseal disk, physis) and represents the area of active bone growth. It is a very important area in bone pathology because it is by far the most common site for the occurrence of most primary bone tumors.

The *epiphyseal plate* of growing bone is the place where endochondral ossification takes place, a process by which longitudinal, regularly spaced columns of vascularized cartilage are replaced by bone.[6] When the bone has reached its adult length, this process ends, and the epiphysis "closes" by becoming totally ossified. The time of closure of the epiphysis differs in various bones and in the sexes. Whether the epiphysis is closed or open influences the extension of pathologic processes. For instance, cartilage is often at least a partial barrier to spreading osteosarcoma. If the epiphysis is closed and cartilage is no longer present, this area is more easily invaded.[3]

Bones are also classified according to their embryologic development. The two main categories are *membranous* (such as the skull), if formed de novo from primitive connective tissue, and *endochondral* (such as long bones), if their formation is preceded by a cartilaginous anlage.

On cross section, mature bones are seen formed by an outer *compact layer* (cortex, cortical bone, compact bone) and a central *spongy region* (spongiosa, medulla, cancellous bone). Compact bone contains vascular channels, which are divided into two types on the basis of their orientation and their relation to the lamellar structure of the surrounding bone: longitudinal (haversian canals) and transverse/oblique

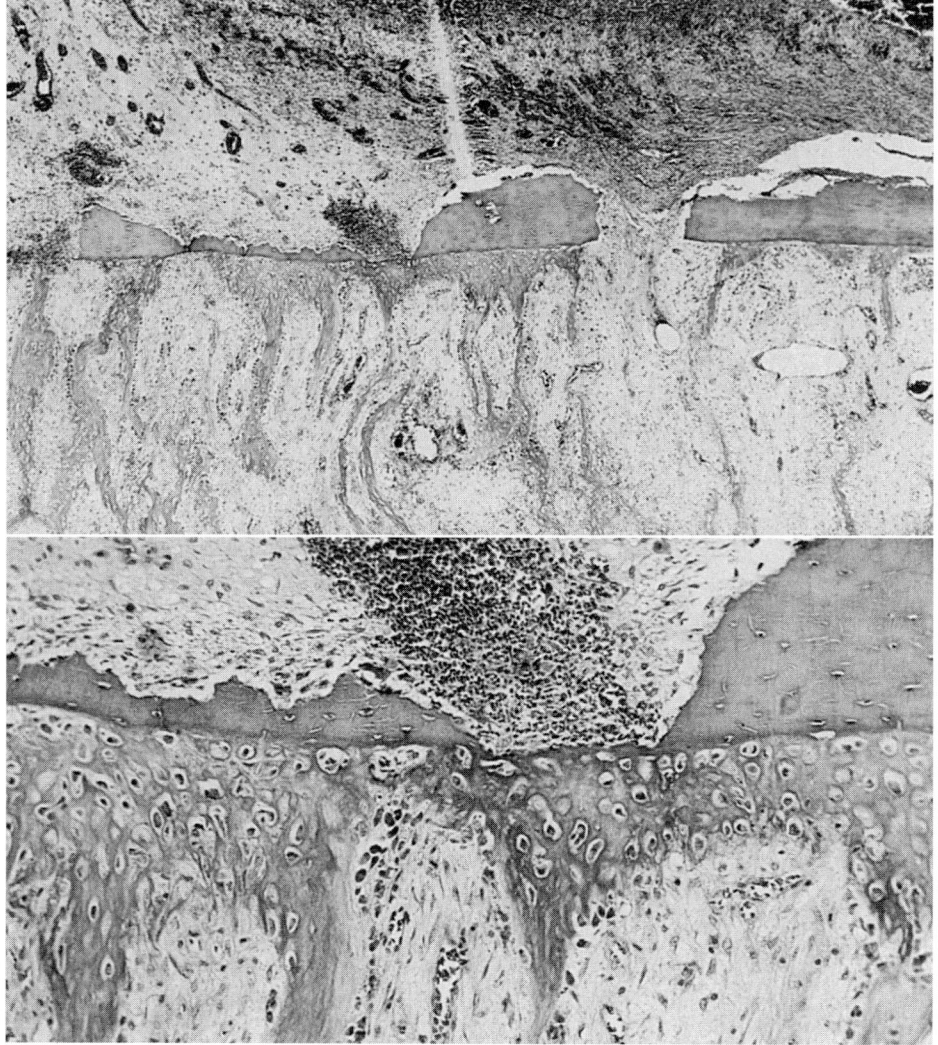

Fig. 24-1 Extreme periosteal new bone formation occurring in mandible after hematoma had almost completely destroyed bone through interference with blood supply. Only fragments of dead mandible remain, but exuberant periosteal bone proliferation is extending from periosteum in long columns.

(Volkmann's canals). Except for the region of the articular cartilage, the cortex is surrounded by the *periosteum,* which consists of an outer fibrous layer and an inner cellular (cambium) layer of osteoprogenitor cells (fibroblasts and osteoblasts). It contains nerve filaments that carry proprioceptive and sensory impulses; small nerve filaments also may pass with the nutrient vessels into the medullary canal. Coarse bundles of collagenous fibers penetrating the outer compact layer from the outer layer of the periosteum are called Sharpey's fibers or perforating fibers.

The periosteum may become detached and elevated from the bone in pathologic processes such as trauma, infection, and primary or secondary malignant tumors. Whenever this happens, new bone formation between the elevated periosteum and the bone will occur. This appears by radiographic examination as fine spicules placed perpendicular to the long axis of the bone. This finding is often considered a manifestation of a primary malignant neoplasm, particularly osteosarcoma and Ewing's sarcoma. However, periosteal bone proliferation also can occur in syphilis, tuberculosis, metastatic carcinoma, and subperiosteal hematoma (Fig. 24-1). In some lesions, such as plasma cell myeloma, the periosteum may be destroyed or encroached upon so that no radiographic changes occur.

An understanding of the blood supply of bone helps to explain the spread and limitation of infection, the healing of fractures, and the involvement of bone by primary or secondary neoplasms. The metaphysis is mainly supplied by end arteries that enter from the diaphysis and terminate at the level of the epiphyseal plate. The epiphyses receive their blood supply from a network of widely anastomosing vessels. The diaphyseal cortex is supplied by vessels that enter through Volkmann's canals and communicate with the haversian system. A nutrient artery enters the medullary canal at

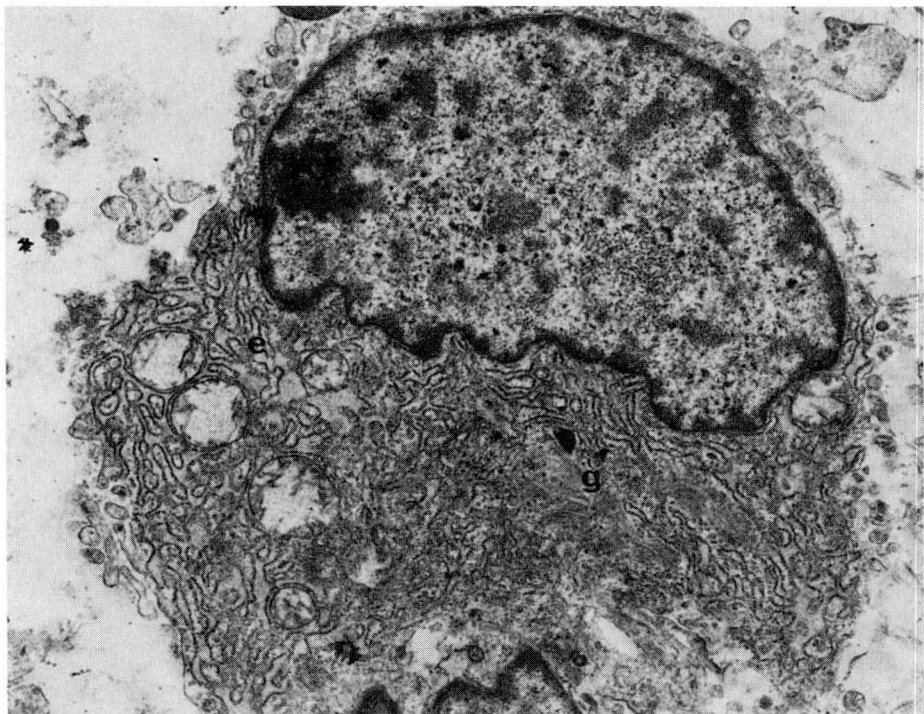

Fig. 24-2 Osteoblast in ossifying fibroma showing prominent Golgi apparatus *(g)* and much ergastoplasm *(e)*. These are features that correlate with osteoid (collagen) synthesis.

about the center of the diaphysis, divides, and extends both distally and proximally. The metabolic exchange of calcium and phosphorus occurs primarily in the metaphysis.

Osteoblasts are bone-producing cells derived from marrow-residing mesenchymal cells. They have a plump appearance and often exhibit a perinuclear halo resulting from a prominent Golgi zone that gives them a resemblance to plasma cells. They have a high cytoplasmic content of alkaline phosphatase. Ultrastructurally, they resemble fibroblasts by virtue of a well-developed rough endoplasmic reticulum and Golgi apparatus (Fig. 24-2). When these are incorporated into the bone matrix and housed in lacunae, they are referred to as osteocytes.

Osteoclasts are multinucleated giant cells involved in bone resorption. As such, they often are found in shallow concavities in the surface of bone called Howship's lacunae. Osteoclasts arise from mononuclear monocyte-macrophage precursors.[15] Osteoclasts contain abundant tartrate-resistant acid phosphatase, respond to osteotropic hormones, and contract under the influence of calcitonin. They express osteoclast-specific antigens (detected by monoclonal antibodies 13c2 and 23c6) and are unreactive for T-cell antigens, most myeloid antigens, and mature macrophage antigens.[9]

Ultrastructurally, the cytoplasm has a very large number of mitochondria and scanty lysosomes; a ruffled edge is present in the area of the cell membrane that is in the process of bone resorption. Various matrix metalloproteinases have been detected immunohistochemically in osteoclasts.[12]

Osteoid is the unmineralized organic precursor matrix of bone. It is composed of a mixture of collagen (mainly type I), acid mucopolysaccharides, and noncollagen proteins.[7] These include osteopontin,[11,14] osteocalcin,[13] and bone morphogenetic protein.[16] The latter is thought to play a critical role in initiating the process that begins with cartilage formation and ends with bone formation.[17] Osteoid is not a homogeneous mass but rather shows a constant, patterned sequence of maturation and organization.[4] It has acidophilic properties in hematoxylin-eosin–stained sections, and it may be difficult to distinguish from hyalinized collagen.

Bone is formed through mineralization of the organic matrix of the osteoid.[5] Extracellular matrix vesicles are present at or near the mineralization front and constitute the initial site of hydroxyapatite mineral deposition.[1] In *woven bone* (fiber bone), there is a haphazard arrangement of collagen fibers within the matrix, which is best appreciated with reticulum stains or under polarized light. Formation of woven bone is the key criterion for the diagnosis of fibrous dysplasia, but it also appears in any condition associated with accelerated bone turnover, such as the callus of a healing fracture and osteitis fibrosa cystica. The difference resides in the fact that in the latter group the woven bone eventually becomes lamellar bone, whereas in fibrous dysplasia it does not. *Lamellar bone* is characterized by concentric parallel lamellae, as seen with examination under polarizing lenses.

Normal skeletal growth results from a balance between the processes of bone matrix synthesis and resorption, these activities being regulated by systemic and local factors.[10] Of these, transforming growth beta factor activity is particularly important for bone matrix production.[2] Vitamin D and parathyroid hormone also play an important role.[8]

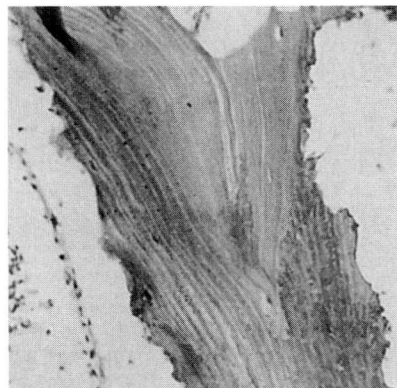

Fig. 24-3 Dead bone with empty lacunae and ragged bone margins.

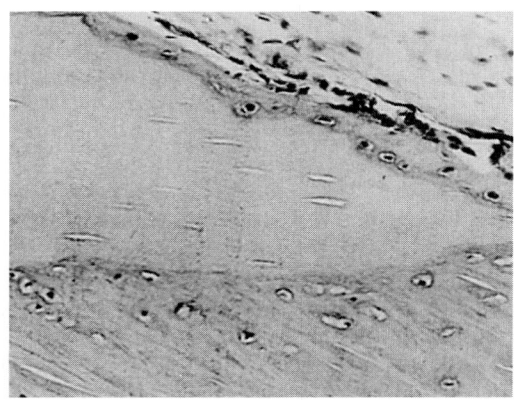

Fig. 24-4 Appositional bone growth proceeding on surface of spicule of dead bone. Living bone is sharply demarcated, and its lacunae contain nuclei.

Bone necrosis can be recognized by the staining quality of the dead bone, which is a deeper blue than normal bone. Lacunar cells are absent, and the margins of the bone are ragged (Fig. 24-3). The presence of osteoclasts on these margins indicates that the bone is already being reabsorbed.

Bone production can be recognized by the presence of well-stained small spicules of bone with cells in their lacunae and osteoblasts along their margins (Fig. 24-4). New bone formation can be found in a variety of physiologic and pathologic processes, such as a healing fracture, Paget's disease, metaplastic ossification, myositis ossificans, and osteitis fibrosa cystica.

Bone resorption (destruction) can be recognized by the presence of numerous osteoclasts in the ragged margins and in Howship's lacunae.

METABOLIC BONE DISEASES

A thorough discussion of metabolic bone diseases is outside the scope of this chapter. Some metabolic bone diseases will be mentioned briefly, but there are entire books, monographs, and excellent articles written on the problem.*

Osteoporosis refers to a decreased mass of normally mineralized bone.[43] It develops when an individual is unable to repair and maintain the mass of bone tissue that has been acquired throughout growth and maturation.[32] Jowsey et al.[29] have demonstrated by quantitative microradiographic studies that the main difference between the bone in most forms of osteoporosis and normal bone is an increase in the amount of resorption, bone formation levels being generally normal. Osteoporosis occurs frequently after menopause, perhaps because of estrogen deficiency.[24] The causes of osteoporosis are multiple.[31] Fluoride consumption has been shown to be important in its prevention.[21,33]

A good biopsy specimen from the iliac crest corresponds well with changes in the spine.[20] However, radiographic examination of the spine is not reliable, since the changes have to be advanced before they can be seen. Studies made at autopsy by Caldwell[22] have helped to clarify the pathology. For instance, he showed that vertebral biconcavity is not a reliable index if osteoporosis.

*References 18, 19, 21a, 23, 26-28, 34-37, 39-41.

Osteomalacia (comparable to rickets in a young person in whom the epiphyses are not yet closed) refers to the accumulation of unmineralized bone matrix resulting from a diminished rate of mineralization. It may result from a wide spectrum of congenital and acquired metabolic abnormalities that result in sufficient decrease in serum calcium, phosphorus, or both to impair mineralization of the skeleton and epiphyseal growth.[30] Some cases have been seen secondary to bone and soft tissue neoplasms (see Chapter 25). In osteomalacia, bone matrix is formed, but its calcification is incomplete, and this gives rise to a noncalcified matrix around the bone trabeculae (Fig. 24-5). These changes can be demonstrated in adequate biopsies from long bones and iliac crests with preparation of nondecalcified specimens and examination with bright-field and phase-contrast microscopes and with the use of fluorescent tetracycline markers.[25]

Sophisticated methods of investigating these metabolic bone processes have been devised, but many of them are difficult to institute in the usual pathology laboratory.[38,42]

FRACTURES

Fractures are breaks in the continuity of bone, usually with severance of periosteum, blood vessels, and sometimes muscles. The speed of return of bone to a normal state following fracture depends on factors such as the age and nutrition of the patient, severity of the fracture, vascularity of the area, and type of treatment (Fig. 24-6). Fractures may fail to heal because of improper immobilization, complete devascularization of the fractured bone segments, persistent infection, and interposition of soft tissue between the ends of the bone (Fig. 24-7).

Following a fracture, a hematoma forms between the two severed ends of bone. Organization of this hematoma begins with the ingrowth of young capillaries. After about 3 days, the devitalized bone fragments begin to be reabsorbed. Intramembranous bone growth makes its appearance from the inner layer of the periosteum, both proximal and distal to the fracture site (Fig. 24-8). The newly formed trabeculae begin to calcify as the cartilage is replaced by bone.[46] This process on each side of the fracture meets at the fracture site to form the primary callus. This is later reabsorbed and

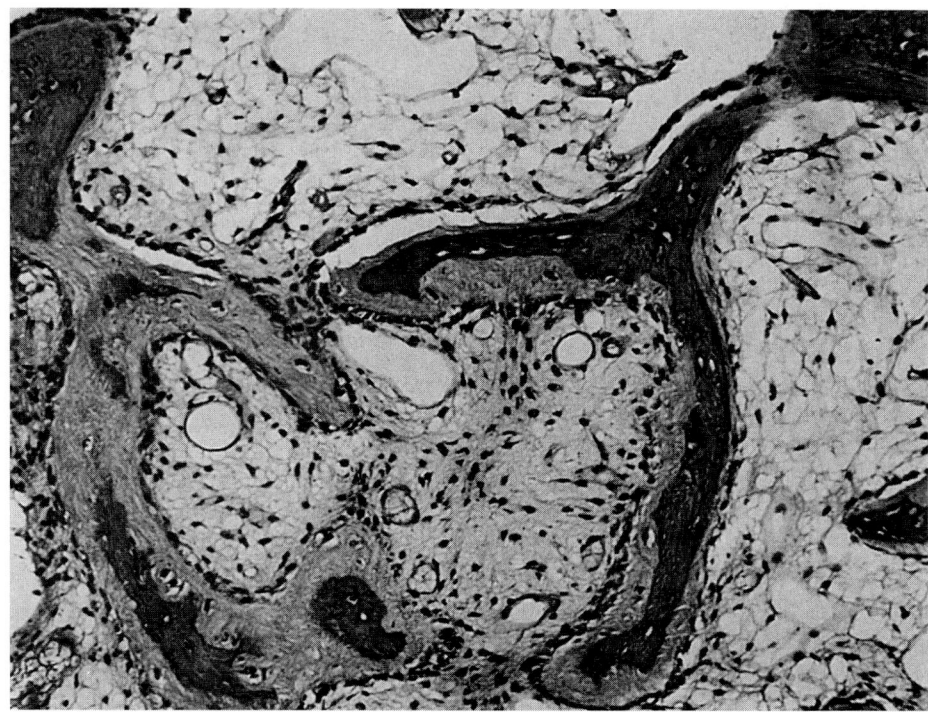

Fig. 24-5 Osteomalacia. Note wide noncalcified matrix around bone trabeculae. Patient has hyperparathyroidism of long duration with profound renal insufficiency.

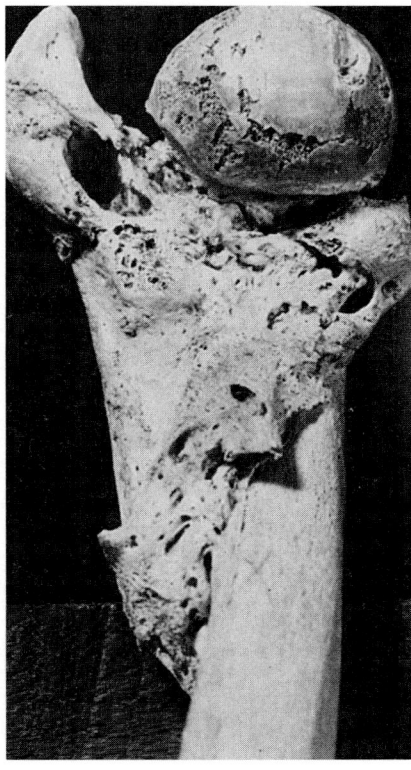

Fig. 24-6 Exuberant callus formation following fracture.

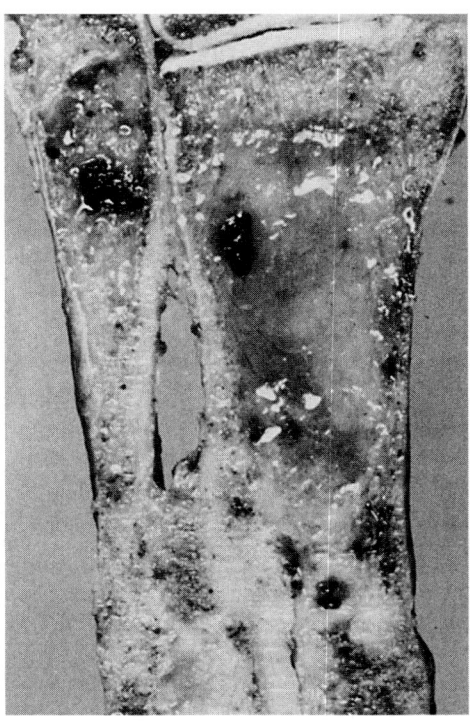

Fig. 24-7 Nonunion of old fracture of tibia and fibula in 53-year-old man. Multiple fractures had occurred 2 years previously and necessitated bone grafting.

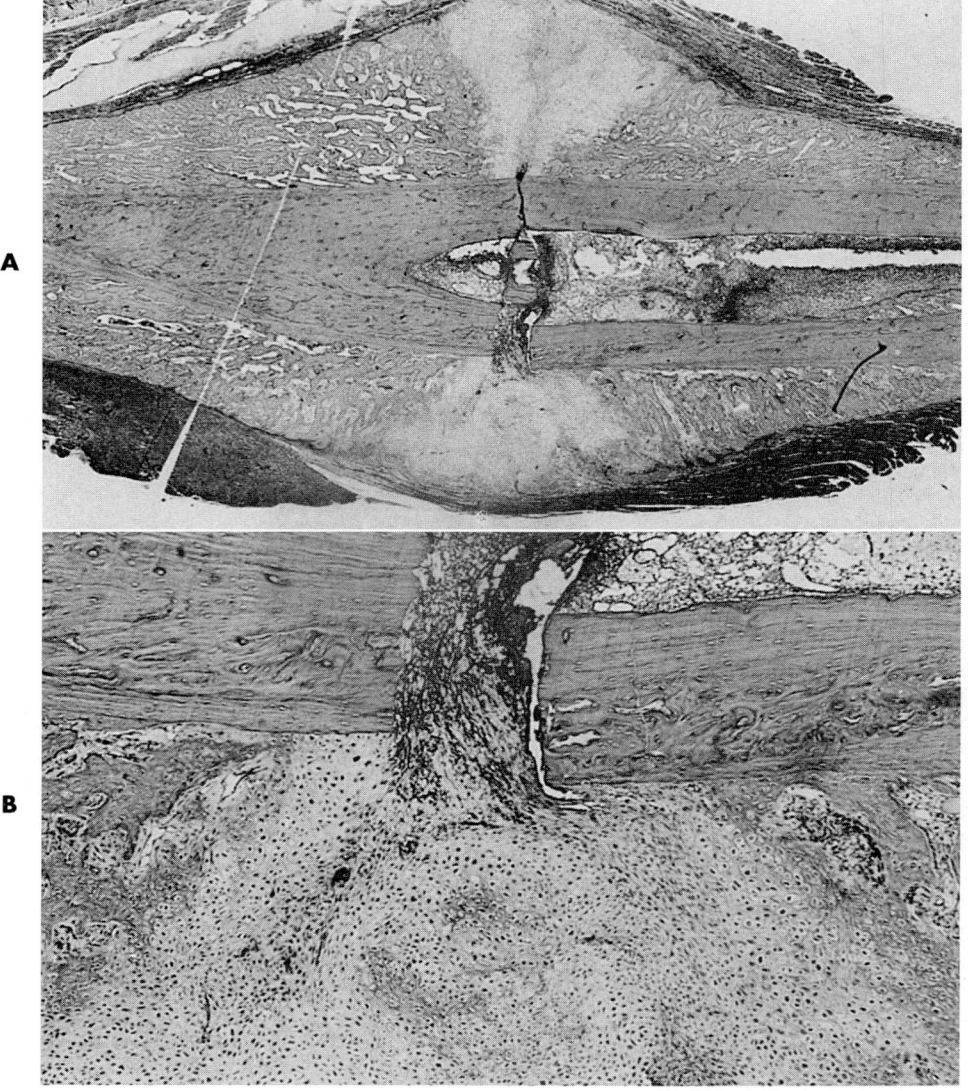

Fig. 24-8 A, Healing fracture of long bone in rat at 7 days. Note intact periosteum and intramembranous bone formation. **B,** Detailed view of point of fracture shown in **A**. Granulation tissue has been replaced with cartilage, and new bone is gradually replacing this cartilage. Fragment of dead bone within marrow cavity is being reabsorbed.

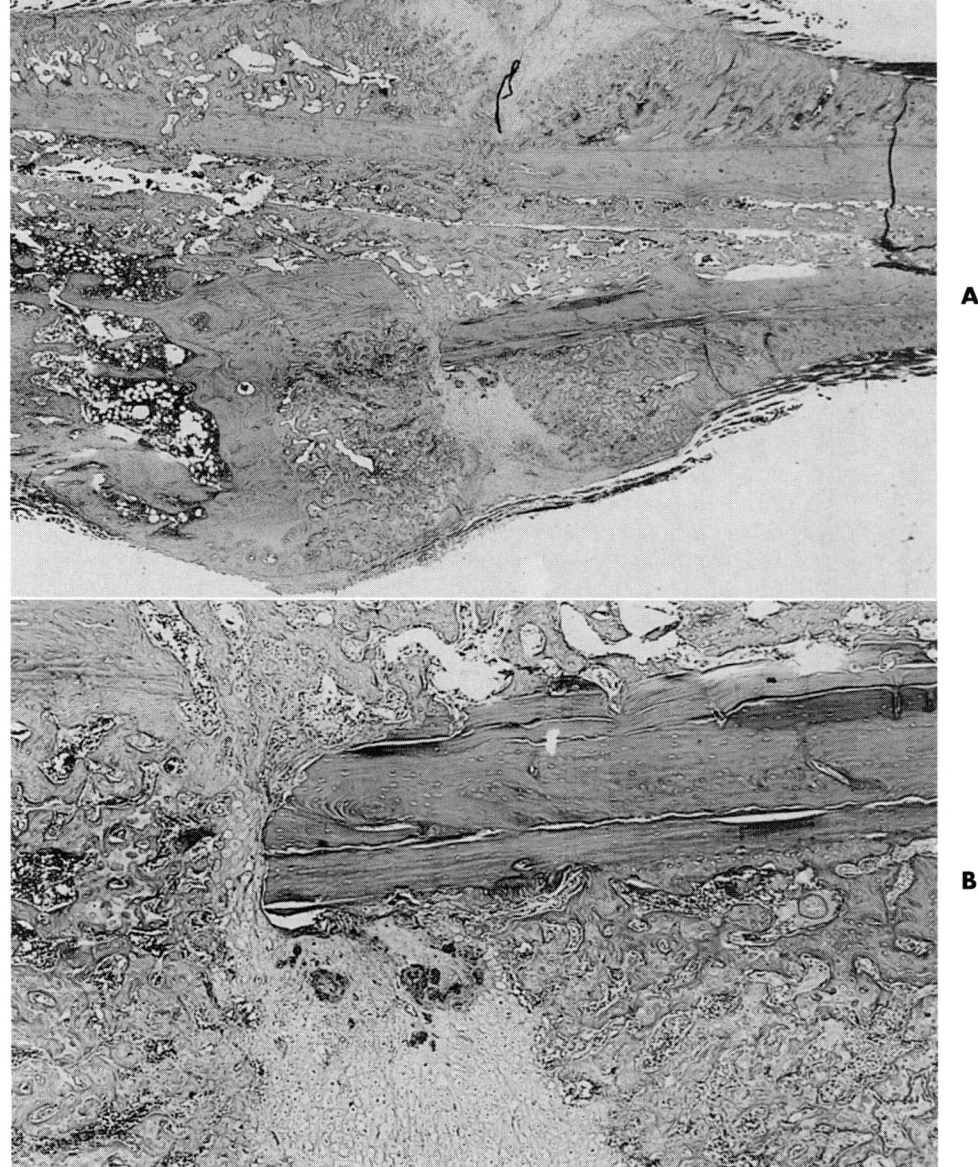

Fig. 24-9 **A,** Healing fracture of long bone in rat at 3 weeks. **B,** Detailed view of fracture site shown in **A.** Bone has almost completely bridged gap. Small amount of cartilage can still be seen near dead bone fragments.

replaced by the secondary callus, which is made up of mature lamellar bone. The new bone is laid down predominantly along lines of stress (Fig. 24-9). The formation and persistence of cartilage largely depend on mechanical factors.[47]

With early proper reduction of the fracture, adequate blood supply, no infection, and normal metabolism, the fracture heals rapidly with little visible callus. Exuberant callus usually means slow fracture healing (Fig. 24-6). In children, even with prominent angulation or deformity, the bone remodels itself to an astonishing degree.[48] For this reason, open reduction and internal fixation of fractures in children are seldom justified. Shortening of a long bone resulting

from overriding of fragments will nearly always correct itself in children by overgrowth of bone.

The formation of exuberant cartilage and disorderly membranous bone in rapidly forming primary callus results in a bewildering microscopic pattern that may be confused with osteosarcoma. Callus formation is particularly luxuriant in osteogenesis imperfecta.[49]

When a noncorrosive nail is driven into a bone to immobilize a fracture, it eventually becomes completely isolated from the bone substance.[44] The nail is separated from the medullary cavity by fibrous tissue that is continuous with the periosteum. Compact-type bone forms adjacent to the fibrous tissue (Fig. 24-10). At a later stage, this becomes

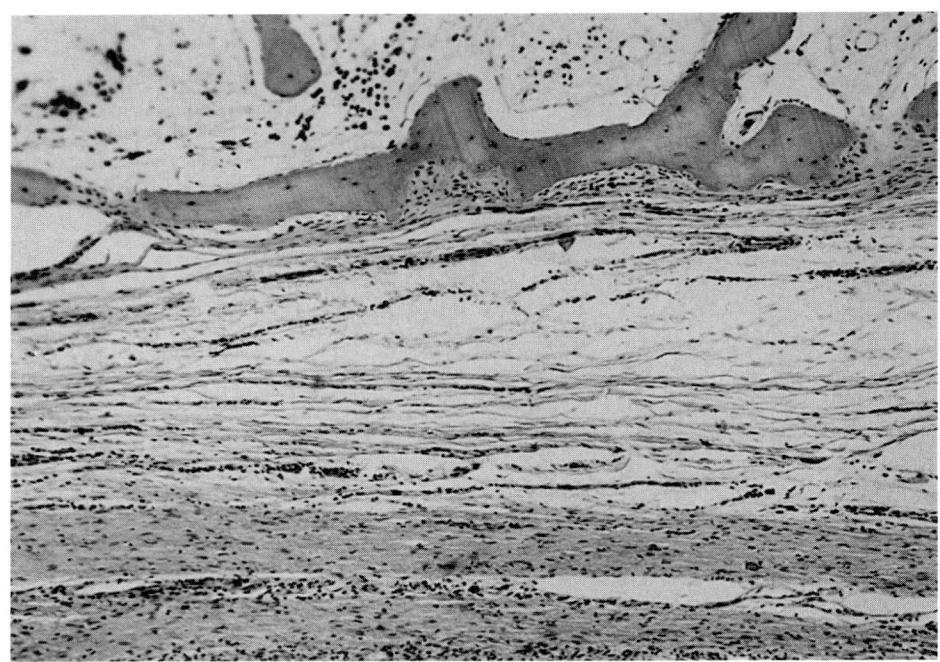

Fig. 24-10 Sequestration within nail tract. Lower margin shows fibrous tissue next to nail tract that is continuous with periosteum. Layer of bone above fibrous tissue is continuous with cortical bone.

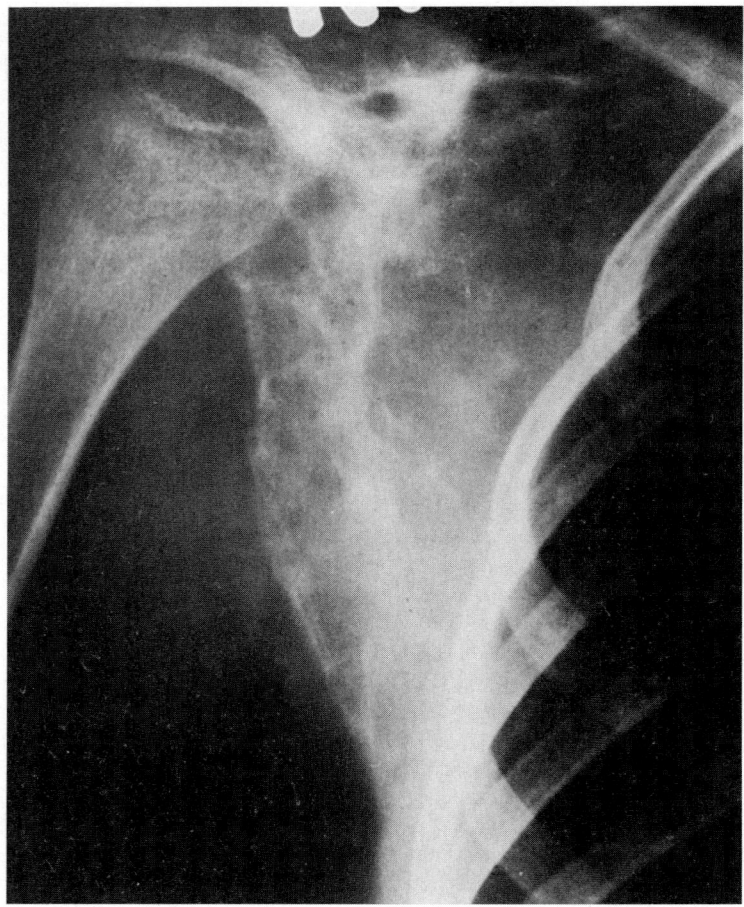

Fig. 24-11 Extensive involvement of scapula by osteomyelitis of staphylococcal origin in 8-year-old child. This was apparently the only bone involved. (Courtesy Dr. P. Flynn, Redding, CA.)

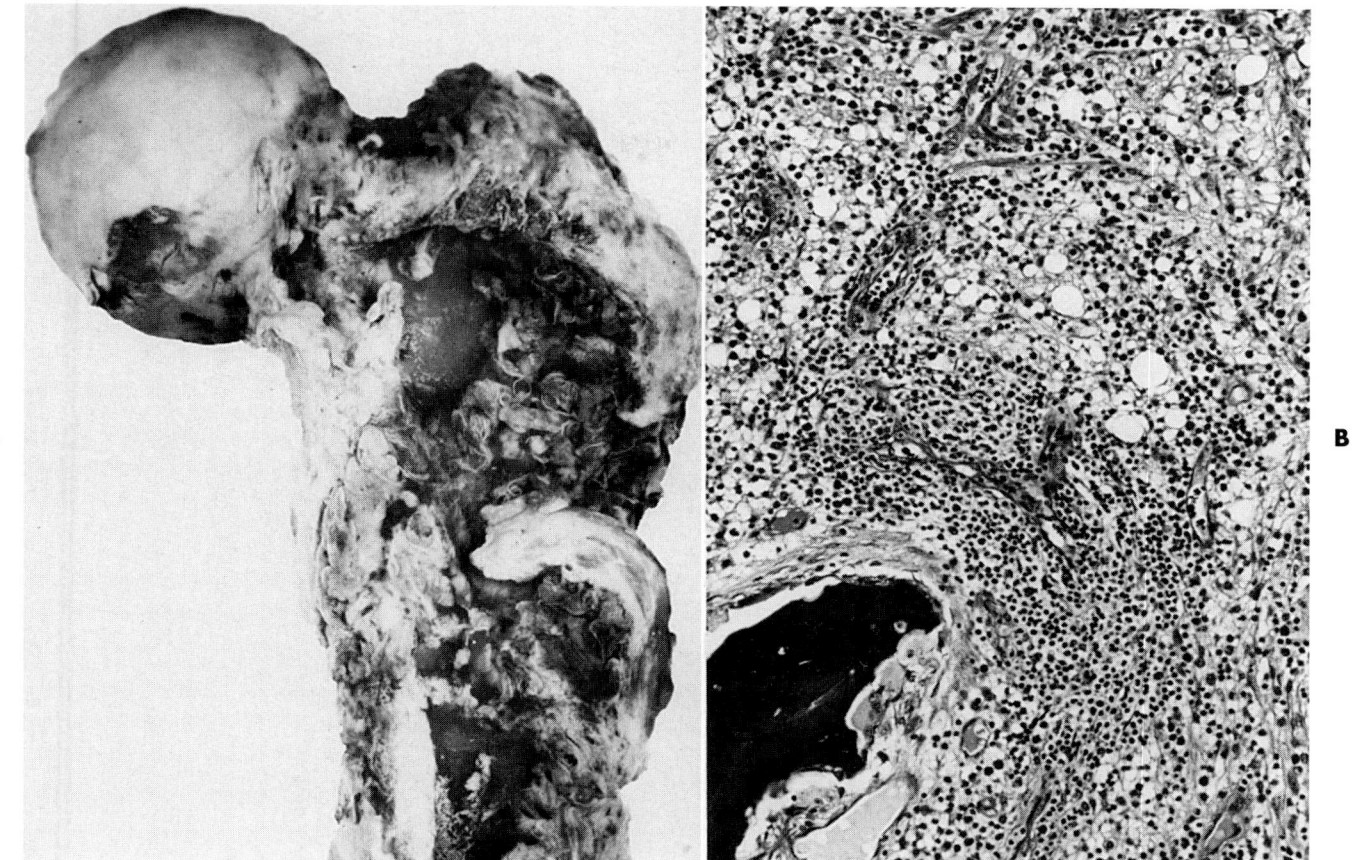

Fig. 25-12 A, Osteomyelitis of upper femur with massive bone destruction and reactive sclerosis. **B,** Chronic osteomyelitis. Heavy inflammatory infiltrate composed of mononuclear cells occupies marrow. Bone trabecula present on one corner shows ragged borders. (Courtesy Dr. H. Rodriguez-Martinez, Mexico City.)

continuous with the original bone cortex. No foreign body giant cell reaction is observed.[45]

OSTEOMYELITIS

Bacterial osteomyelitis may be caused by a large variety of microorganisms. About 70% to 90% of the cases are due to coagulase-positive staphylococci, and their frequency seems to be increasing[63] (Fig. 24-11). Other organisms involved are *Klebsiella, Aerobacter, Proteus, Pseudomonas,* streptococcus, pneumococcus, gonococcus, meningococcus, *Brucella,* and *Salmonella.*[58,65] The latter organism is often involved in the osteomyelitis that affects individuals with abnormal hemoglobin, particularly sickle cell disease.[61]

Osteomyelitis may be due to local or exogenous causes (such as compound fractures)[51] or may develop through the hematogenous route. The latter occurs most often in patients under 20 years of age and involves the bones of the lower extremity in about 75% of cases. It can be acute, subacute, or chronic, these designations referring to the duration of the disease rather than the microscopic composition of the inflammatory infiltrate.

Subacute and chronic osteomyelitis can closely simulate clinically and radiographically a malignant bone tumor (par-

ticularly Ewing's sarcoma, malignant lymphoma, and osteosarcoma) by virtue of the combination of destructive and regenerative bone changes[52] (Fig. 24-12). Hematogenous pyogenic vertebral osteomyelitis is frequently underdiagnosed radiographically because of the subtle nature of the disease.[56] A variant of osteomyelitis characterized by very extensive regenerative bone changes is referred to as Garre's osteomyelitis, sclerosing osteomyelitis, or periostitis ossificans. This form is particularly common in the jawbone.[55]

The morphologic changes in osteomyelitis are conditioned by the age of the patient, bone involved (particularly in regard to its blood supply), virulence of the organism, and resistance of the host.[62] In the infant under 1 year of age, permanent epiphyseal damage and joint infection occur, but there is little damage to the metaphysis or diaphysis. In children over 1 year of age the reverse is true, in the sense that cortical metaphyseal involvement is extensive, whereas permanent damage to cartilage and joints is rare. From its center in the metaphysis, the infection permeates the cortex through the vessels of Volkmann's canals and may spread along the medullary canal to the rest of the bone. If pus accumulates beneath the periosteum, perforation through it

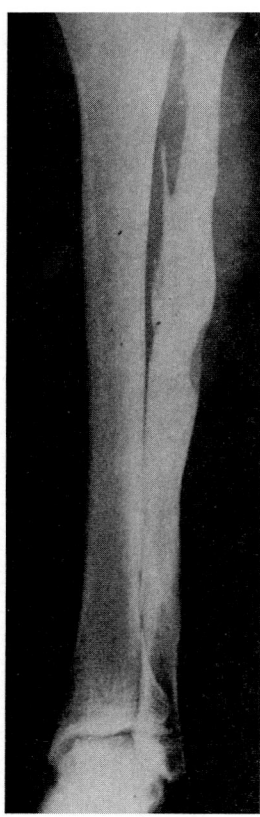

Fig. 24-13 Chronic osteomyelitis of fibula. Note dense, irregular bone.

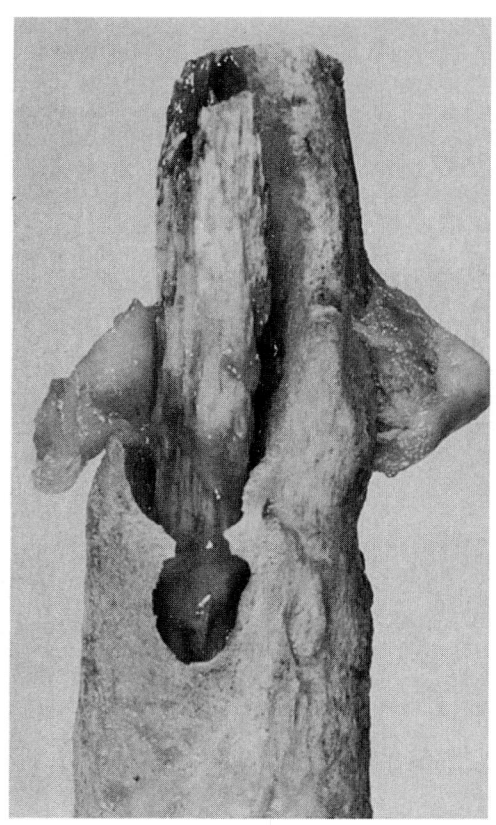

Fig. 24-14 Resected fibula showing dense outer involucrum surrounding loosened sequestrum with its pitted surface.

usually takes place. The dead bone (sequestrum) is later surrounded by new bone laid down by the cambium layer of the periosteum (the involucrum), and this may eventually extend around the entire bone (Figs. 24-13 and 24-14).

Chronic osteomyelitis persists as long as infected dead bone remains. The dead bone is surrounded by granulation tissue that attacks the sequestrum, making it pitted on the surface next to the marrow cavity. The cortical surface remains smooth. Surgical removal of the sequestrum at the proper time usually allows the osteomyelitis to heal. However, the osteomyelitis may recur many years later if bacteria remain within the scar.

In the adult, there is again a high incidence of joint infection, but this time in association with involvement of extensive portions of bone.

Microscopically, the changes of osteomyelitis are represented by an admixture of inflammatory cells (including neutrophils, lymphocytes, and plasma cells), fibrosis, bone necrosis, and new bone formation. When the plasma cell population is particularly prominent, the disease has been designated as *plasma cell osteomyelitis*,[66] and when foamy macrophages are abundant, it has been called *xanthogranulomatous osteomyelitis*.[53] Chronic osteomyelitis may be accompanied by prominent periosteal bone proliferation (Fig. 24-15).

Osteomyelitic sinuses in the adult may become lined by epithelium that extends deeply in the bone and becomes dis-continuous with the cutaneous surface. Despite apparent healing of the overlying skin, large epidermal inclusion cysts slowly develop in the underlying bone. These are filled with keratin-containing debris similar to that in epidermal inclusion cysts of the skin. Rarely, after a long period, squamous cell carcinoma develops within these sinuses. This complication is heralded by the appearance of pain and increasingly malodorous discharge.[54,57]

Tuberculous osteomyelitis as a hematogenous infection is usually seen in young adults or children. The bones most often infected are the vertebrae and bones of the hip, knee, ankle, elbow, and wrist. The areas usually involved are the metaphysis, epiphysis, and synovium.[50]

There has been considerable controversy as to which of these areas is the one first involved. Metaphyseal infection is more common in children, and epiphyseal infection is more common in adults, but with progression of the disease, all zones become affected (Fig. 24-16). Tuberculous granulation tissue forming in the synovia destroys the synovial attachments. The cartilage, no longer nourished from the synovia, undergoes progressive destruction, allowing the inflammation to extend into the epiphysis and finally into the metaphyseal area. If the process begins in the epiphysis, the tuberculous granulation tissue quickly extends into the adjacent joint. When the process begins in the metaphyseal area, extension into the joint may be heralded by the development of fluid in it.

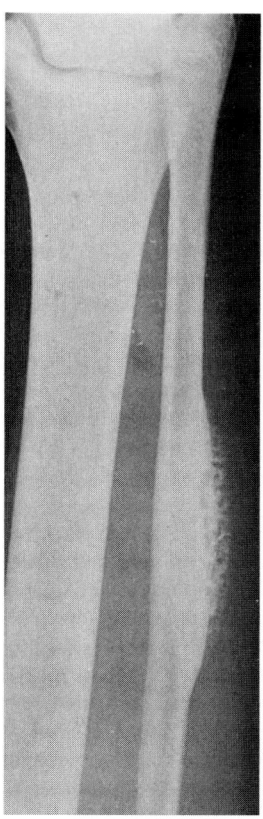

Fig. 24-15 Prominent periosteal bone proliferation in chronic osteomyelitis.

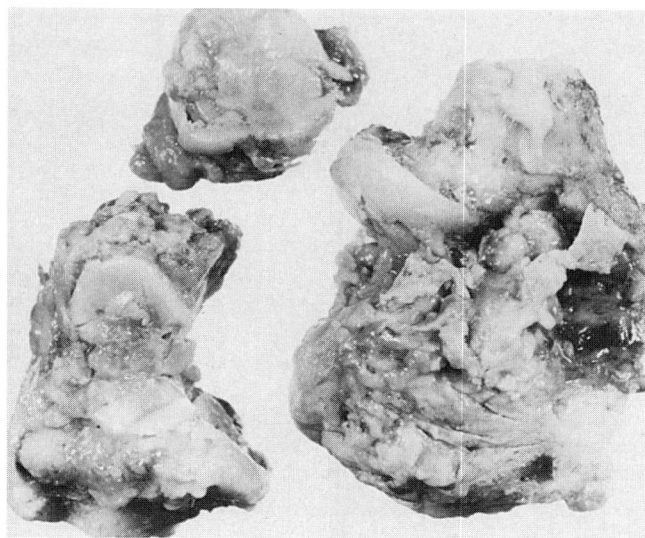

Fig. 24-16 Extensive involvement of synovium of elbow joint by tuberculous granulation tissue.

Cutaneous sinuses may occur in advanced tuberculosis. These sinuses allow entry of secondary bacterial infection that modifies the pathologic changes. When the tuberculous process begins to heal, fusion of the joint may be associated with complete or partial denudation of cartilage and "kissing sequestra." Sequestra are cortical in pyogenic processes, but in tuberculous osteomyelitis they are cancellous.

Fungal infections of bone include blastomycosis, actinomycosis, histoplasmosis, and coccidioidomycosis.[59,60]

Tertiary syphilis may involve the bone and cause both osseous destruction and production, often in association with conspicuous periosteal bone proliferation (Fig. 24-17). The necrotic, well-defined defects are mainly cortical and periosteal and are surrounded by sclerotic bone. They may occur in the vertebrae, flat bones of the hands and feet, and diaphysis of long tubular bones. The radiographic diagnosis is usually apparent if multiple x-ray studies of the bones are taken, but it may be difficult in single or isolated lesions, some of which closely resemble the appearance of osteosarcoma. Biopsy will show a granulomatous process associated with bone destruction and production.

Malakoplakia of bone has been described. As in the bladder and other sites, it probably represents an unusual host reaction to bacterial infection.[64]

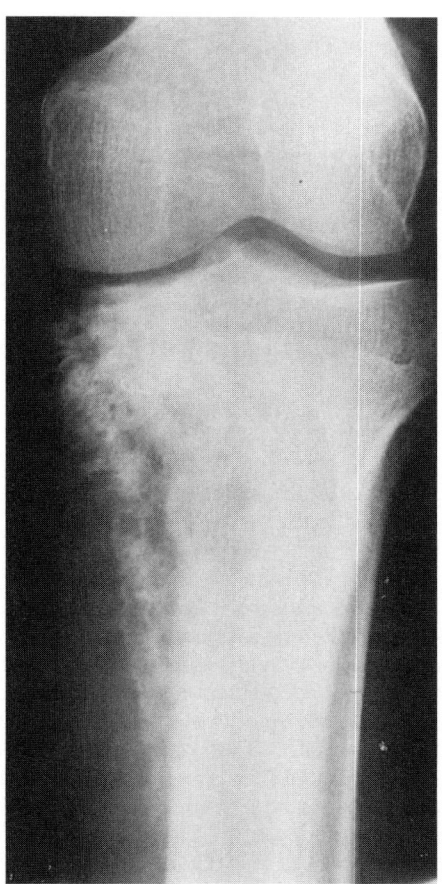

Fig. 24-17 Gummatous involvement of tibia in 45-year-old woman. (Courtesy Dr. R.J. Reed, New Orleans.)

CONDITIONS ASSOCIATED WITH BONE INFARCT

Diaphysometaphyseal infarctions
Caisson disease (decompression sickness)
Gaucher's disease
Sickle cell anemia
Sickle cell trait
Pancreatic disease
   Acute
   Chronic
Occlusive vascular disease
   Arteriosclerosis
   Thromboembolic disease
Periarteritis nodosa (vasculitis)
Pheochromocytoma
Infection
Idiopathic
Epiphysometaphyseal infarctions
Thrombosis
   Sickle cell anemia (SS and SC hemoglobin)
   Corticosteroids
   Thromboembolic disease
Disease of arterial wall
   Lupus erythematosus
   Rheumatoid arthritis
   Boeck's sarcoid
   Arteriosclerosis
Disease of adjacent bone
   Histiocytosis X
   Gaucher's disease
   Osteomyelitis
   Caisson disease
Traumatic and idiopathic
   Fractures and dislocations
   Osteochrondroses

From Libshitz HI, Osborne RL Jr: The diagnosis of bone infarction. Ann Clin Lab Sci **5:**272-275, 1975.

BONE NECROSIS

Infarct

Bone infarct can be the result of a large number of etiologic factors (see box). Radiographically, the changes depend on the age of the lesion and the degree of repair. During the first 1 or 2 weeks, no abnormalities are detected. Resorption of the dead bone results in areas of decreased density, whereas new bone formation growing in apposition to dead trabeculae ("creeping apposition") leads to an increase in bone density. The process of reossification is often irregular, and the combination of incomplete resorption of dead bone and focal deposition of new bone results in a mottled and irregular radiographic appearance (Fig. 24-18).

An increased incidence of primary malignant bone tumors has been seen in association with large infarcts of long bones. Most of the reported cases have occurred in the medulla of the femur or tibia of male adults and have been diagnosed as malignant fibrous histiocytoma, osteosarcoma, or fibrosarcoma.[67-69]

Aseptic (avascular) bone necrosis

Aseptic bone necrosis (avascular necrosis, osteonecrosis) is a common abnormality that has been reported in practically every secondary epiphysis and in many primary epiphyses[72] (Figs. 24-19 and 24-20). Many of these sites have been described separately and given eponymic designations such as Osgood-Schlatter disease (for necrosis of the tibial tuberosity) and Legg-Calvé-Perthes disease (for necrosis of the upper femoral epiphysis).

The pathogenetic mechanism is thought to be interruption of the blood supply induced in most cases by a mechanical disruption, such as fracture or dislocation,[70] but sometimes by thrombosis induced by sickle cell disease.[71] This has been studied particularly well in fractures of the femoral neck.[73]

The initial necrosis of epiphyseal bone is followed by hyperemia of the surrounding tissues. The epiphyseal cartilage may or may not remain viable. The dead bone gradually undergoes resorption by a mechanism of "creeping substitution." This is a slow process that may take months or even years and that results in a dense radiographic appearance, particularly well appreciated in lesions of the femoral neck.[70] Microscopically, it is typical to see osteoclastic activity on one side of the dead trabeculae and osteoblastic activity on the other. The newly formed bone, which is of soft consistency, may flatten because of pressure, resulting in degenerative joint disease.

Osteochondritis dissecans

Osteochondritis dissecans results from a small area of necrosis involving the articular cartilage and subchondral bone that totally or partially separates from the adjacent structures. The etiology is uncertain but is probably related to trauma in most of the cases.[74] It occurs most frequently on the lateral aspect of the medial femoral condyle, near the intercondylar notch (Fig. 24-21). Microscopically, a portion of articular cartilage is always present, often exhibiting secondary calcification; in addition, a fragment of subchondral bone is found in approximately half of the cases.[74] If this osteochondromatous body remains attached to the joint surface or synovium, both components remain viable. If, instead, it becomes completely detached, its osseous portion dies, but the cartilage remains alive, apparently through nutrients obtained from the synovial fluid.

Patients with bilateral symmetric involvement and cases with familial incidence have been described.

Radiation necrosis

Damage to the underlying bone can be a major complication of radiation therapy. Radiation changes resulting in serious complications have been reported in the jaw, ribs, pelvis, spine, humerus, and other bones.[75] In cases of radiation necrosis of the pelvis and femoral neck, the changes usually occur within 3 years of the therapy. Microscopically, these changes consist of necrotic bone, fibrosis of the bone marrow, and neovascularization. Irregular, heavily staining

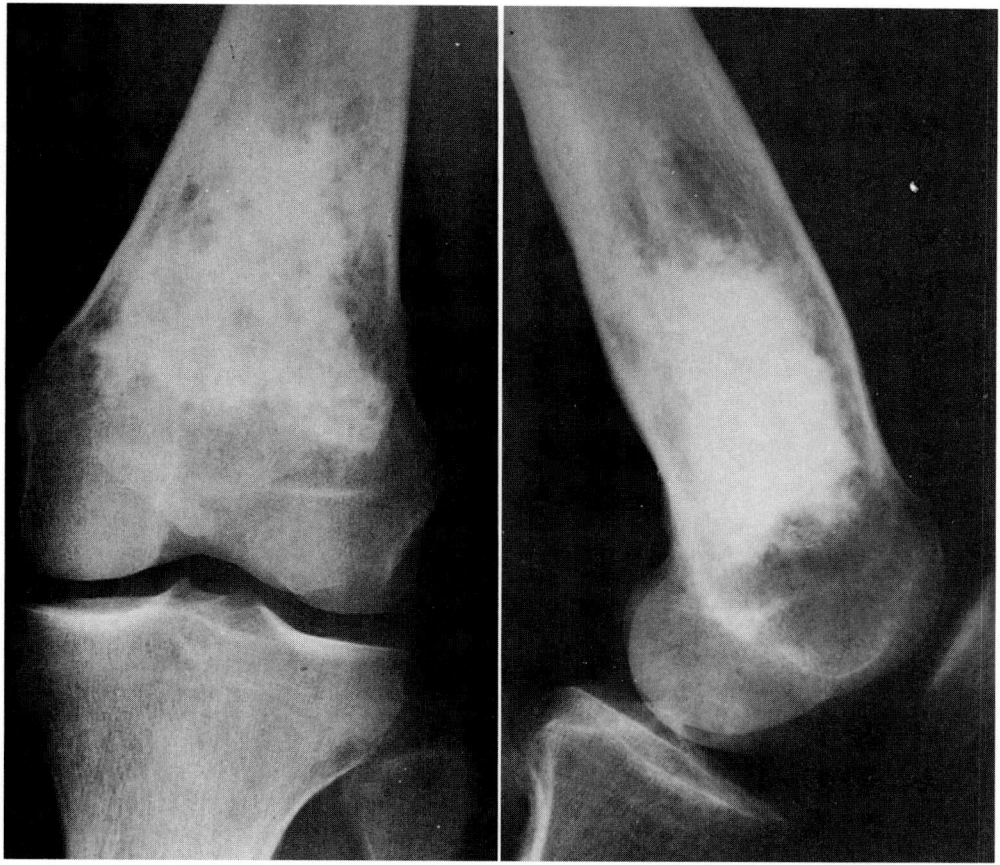

Fig. 24-18 Large diaphysometaphyseal bone infarct of femur. Irregular area of increased radiodensity is indicative of new bone production superimposed on necrosis. (Courtesy Dr. H. Danziger, Welland, Ontario, Canada.)

cement lines may develop and lead to confusion with Paget's disease.

PAGET'S DISEASE

About 90% of the patients with Paget's disease are over 55 years of age. The disease is rare before the age of 40 years and uncommon between the ages of 40 and 55 years, although several cases of precocious onset are on record.[81] It affects men slightly more often than women (4:3). It has a very peculiar geographic distribution. The highest incidence is in England, Australia, and the Western European plain.[76] In an autopsy series from England, about one of every thirty patients over 40 years of age had Paget's disease.[77] The most common sites are the lumbosacral spine, pelvis, and skull. It may also occur in the femur, tibia, clavicle (Fig. 24-22), radius, ulna, fibula, and jaws,[89] but it is extremely rare in the ribs.

The disease is usually polyostotic and accompanied by serum elevations of alkaline phosphatase levels. However, it can also appear as a monostotic process in a long bone, jaw, or vertebra (Fig. 24-23). In such cases, the alkaline phosphatase levels may be normal.

The etiology of Paget's disease is unknown; the suggestion that it might be of viral origin has been raised by the consistent finding of nuclear inclusions resembling viral nucleocapsids of the measles type in the lesional osteoclasts.[80,84,85]

The initial lesion is osteoclastic and therefore lytic.[78,79] Abnormal hyperplasia soon follows, as evidenced by the deposition of primitive coarse-fibered bone in discontinuous trabeculae, which in turn is replaced by thick trabeculae with a disjointed lamellar pattern. This evolution in the morphogenesis of the disease can be better appreciated with reticulin stains than with the use of polarized light. The disorganization in the structure of the lamellar bone leads to the formation of *cement lines*. These are caused by the abrupt interruptions and changes in direction of bone lamellae and fibers resulting from resorption and regeneration of masses of bone during the course of the disease and represent the key to the diagnosis of Paget's disease[88] (Fig. 24-24). However, they are not specific for it; there are many pathologic processes that involve active reparative change accompanied by new bone formation with cement lines. These include irradiation effect, chronic osteomyelitis, reactive bone sur-

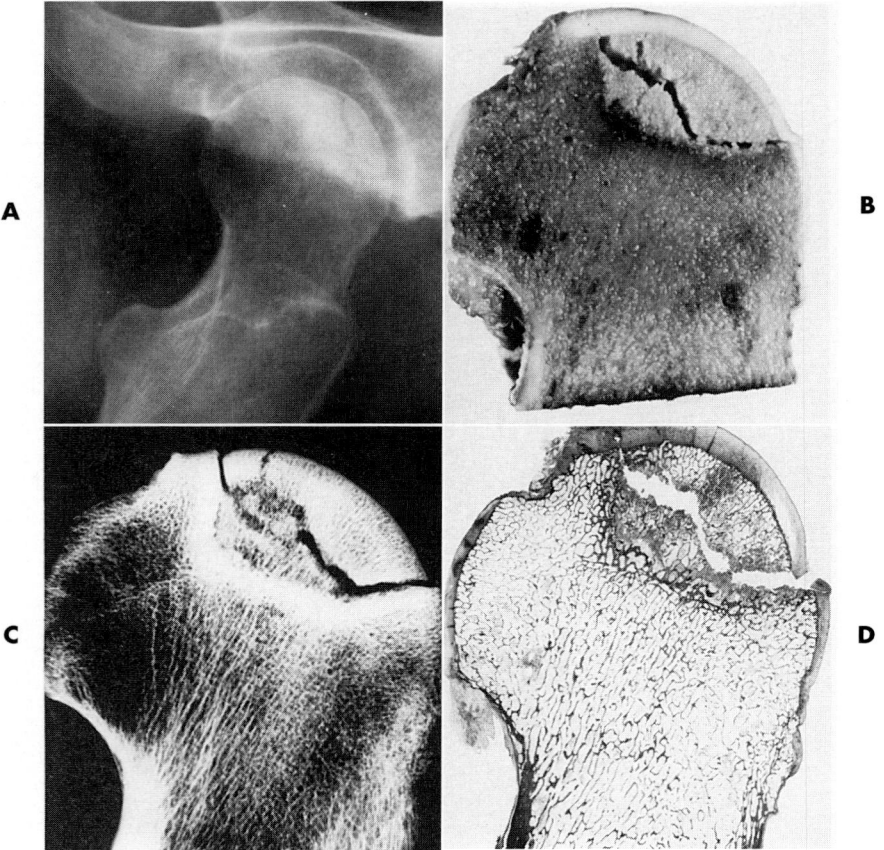

Fig. 24-19 Aseptic necrosis of femoral head with superimposed fracture. **A,** Radiograph. **B,** Cross section of excised specimen. **C,** Radiograph of slice of same specimen, emphasizing peripheral eburnation. **D,** Whole-mount specimen shows well-delimited focus of necrosis.

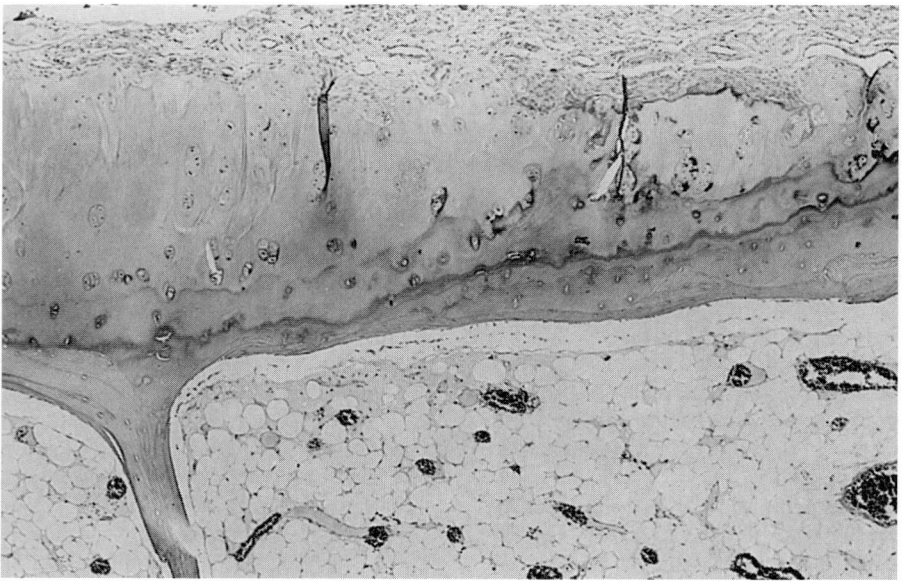

Fig. 24-20 Aseptic bone necrosis in head of femur. Note fibrillation and almost complete absence of cartilage. Subchondral bone is dead with empty lacunae.

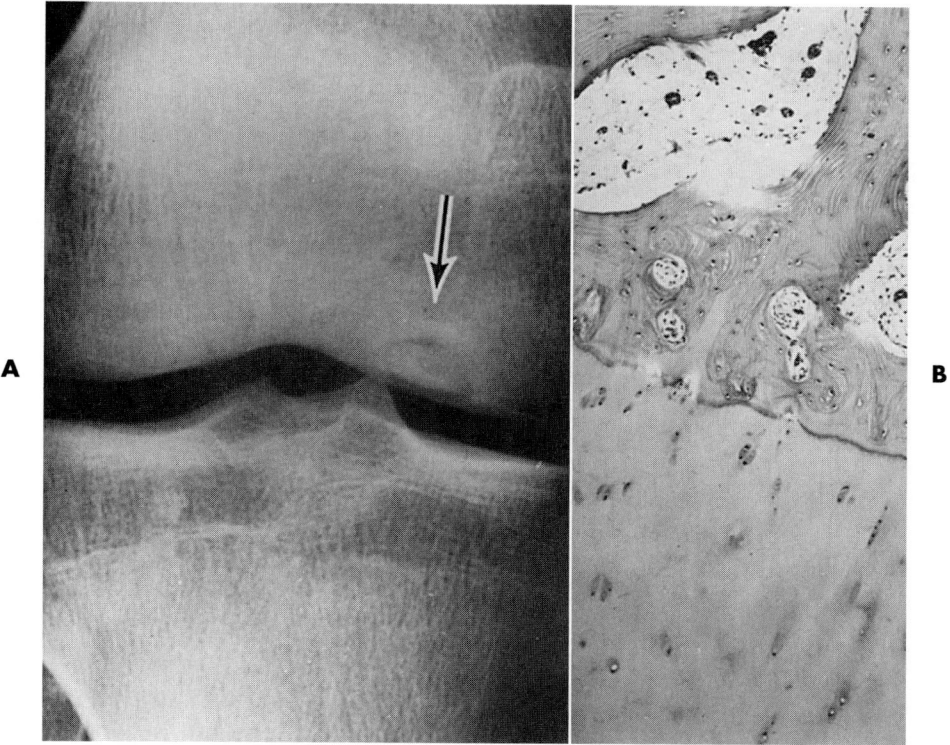

Fig. 24-21 A, Sharply delimited area of osteochrondritis dissecans of medial condyle *(arrow).* This was easily enucleated. **B,** Same lesion shown in **A** demonstrating viability of bone removed from defect. Bone was alive because of its loose attachment of normal adjacent osseous tissue.

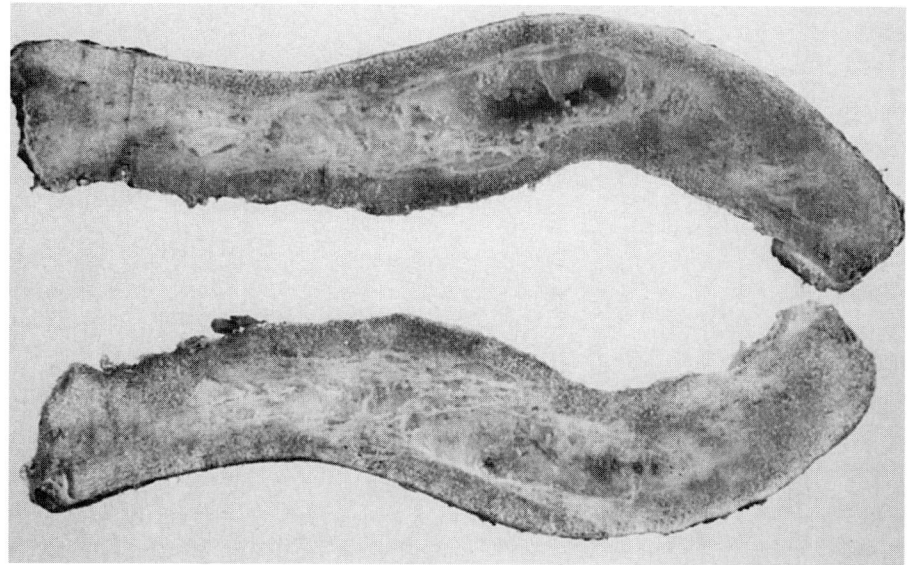

Fig. 24-22 Extensive Paget's disease of clavicle of 60-year-old man. Note distortion and changes in cortex.

rounding metastatic cancer, and polyostotic fibrous dysplasia. In general, the cement lines seen in these conditions are more orderly and structurally better oriented than those of Paget's disease. An additional feature in the differential diagnosis between Paget's disease and polyostotic fibrous

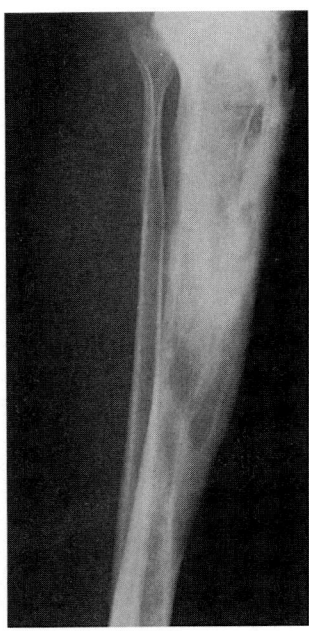

Fig. 24-23 Monostotic Paget's disease of tibia with bone destruction and bone formation. Nature of process was obscure until biopsy.

dysplasia is the consistent presence of *eccentric atrophy* of cortical bone in the latter.[90]

Two important complications of Paget's disease are fractures and development of bone tumors. The fractures are usually of the transverse type.[83] Patients who are immobilized because of long bone fractures may undergo rapid dissolution of bone substance.[87]

The overall incidence of bone sarcoma in Paget's disease is relatively low if one considers the worldwide prevalence of the latter disorder.[77] Osteosarcoma is the most common type, but chondrosarcoma, fibrosarcoma, and giant cell tumors have also been observed.[82,86] Instances of familial or geographic clustering of this complication have been seen. The most common locations of sarcomas arising in Paget's disease are the femur, humerus, pelvis, tibia, and skull.

OSTEOPETROSIS

Osteopetrosis (Albers-Schönberg's disease, marble-bone disease) is thought to represent a defect in bone remodeling secondary to malfunction of osteoclasts resulting from a lysosomal defect. Pathologically, the abnormally deposited tissue is composed of both lamellar bone and calcified cartilage.[92] The disease has been reversed by bone marrow transplantation[91] and has been successfully treated with recombinant human interferon gamma.[91a]

TUMORS
Classification and distribution

The terminology and classification of bone tumors and tumorlike lesions we use are largely those recommended by the WHO International Reference Center for the Histological Definition and Classification of Bone Tumours,[95,96]

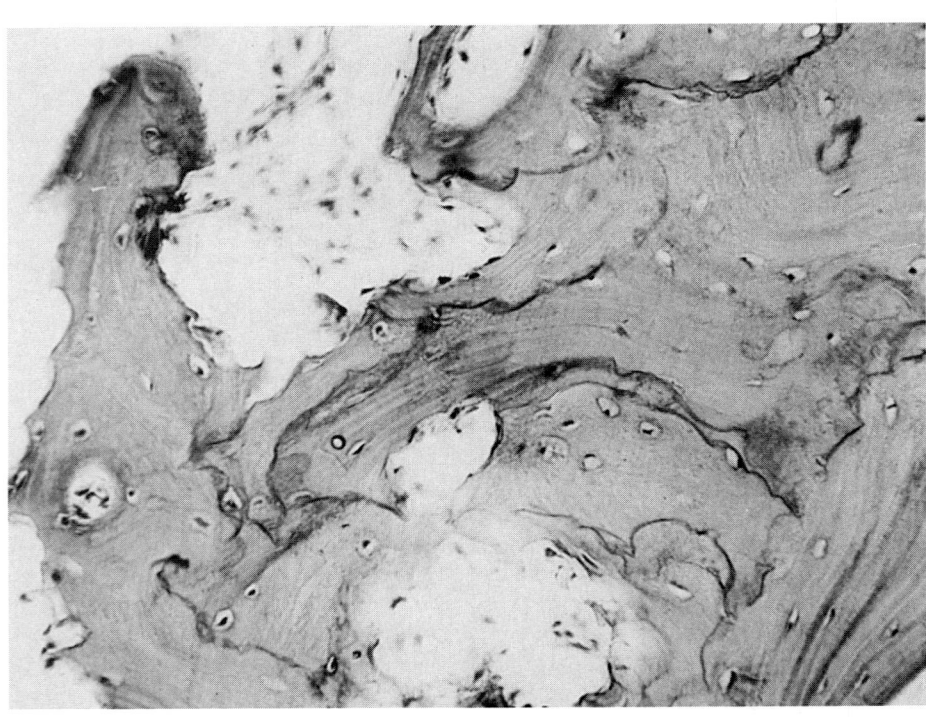

Fig. 24-24 Paget's disease. Note numerous irregular but well-defined mosaic patterns of cement lines.

Table 24-1 Usual age and sex of patient and location and behavior of most common primary bone tumors and tumorlike lesions*

Tumor or tumorlike lesion	Age (yr)	Sex (M : F)	Bones more commonly affected (in order of frequency)	Usual location within long bone	Behavior
Osteoma	40-50	2:1	Skull and facial bones	—	Benign
Osteoid osteoma	10-30	2:1	Femur, tibia, humerus, hands and feet, vertebrae, fibula	Cortex of metaphysis	Benign
Osteoblastoma	10-30	2:1	Vertebrae, tibia, femur, humerus, pelvis, ribs	Medulla of metaphysis	Benign
Osteosarcoma	10-25	3:2	Femur, tibia, humerus, pelvis, jaw, fibula	Medulla of metaphysis	Malignant; 20% 5 yr survival rate
Juxtacortical (parosteal) osteosarcoma	30-60	1:1	Femur, tibia, humerus	Juxtacortical area of metaphysis	Malignant; 80% 5 yr survival rate
Chondroma	10-40	1:1	Hands and feet, ribs, femur, humerus	Medulla of diaphysis	Benign
Osteochondroma	10-30	1:1	Femur, tibia, humerus, pelvis	Cortex of metaphysis	Benign
Chondroblastoma	10-25	2:1	Femur, humerus, tibia, feet, pelvis, scapula	Epiphysis, adjacent to cartilage plate	Practically always benign
Chondromyxoid fibroma	10-25	1:1	Tibia, femur, feet, pelvis	Metaphysis	Benign
Chondrosarcoma	30-60	3:1	Pelvis, ribs, femur, humerus, vertebrae	Central—medulla of diaphysis; peripheral—cortex or periosteum of metaphysis	Malignant; 5 yr survival rate—low grade, 78%; moderate grade, 53%; high grade, 22%
Mesenchymal chondrosarcoma	20-60	1:1	Ribs, skull and jaw, vertebrae, pelvis, soft tissues	Medulla or cortex of diaphysis	Malignant; extremely poor prognosis
Giant cell tumor	20-40	4:5	Femur, tibia, radius	Epiphysis and metaphysis	Potentially malignant; 50% recur; 10% metastasize
Ewing's sarcoma	5-20	1:2	Femur, pelvis, tibia, humerus, ribs, fibula	Medulla of diaphysis or metaphysis	Highly malignant; 20%-30% 5 yr survival rate in recent series
Malignant lymphoma, large cell, and mixed cell types	30-60	1:1	Femur, pelvis, vertebrae, tibia, humerus, jaw, skull, ribs	Medulla of diaphysis or metaphysis	Malignant; 22%-50% 5 yr survival rate
Plasma cell myeloma	40-60	2:1	Vertebrae, pelvis, ribs, sternum, skull	Medulla of diaphysis, metaphysis, or epiphysis	Malignant; diffuse form uniformly fatal, localized form often controlled with radiation therapy
Hemangioma	20-50	1:1	Skull, vertebrae, jaw	Medulla	Benign
Desmoplastic fibroma	20-30	1:1	Humerus, tibia, pelvis, jaw, femur, scapula	Metaphysis	Benign
Fibrosarcoma	20-60	1:1	Femur, tibia, jaw, humerus	Medulla of metaphysis	Malignant; 28% 5 yr survival rate
Chordoma	40-60	2:1	Sacrococcygeal, spheno-occipital, cervical vertebrae	—	Malignant; slow course; locally invasive; 48% distant metastases
Solitary bone cyst	10-20	3:1	Humerus, femur	Medulla of metaphysis	Benign
Aneurysmal bone cyst	10-20	1:1	Vertebrae, flat bones, femur, tibia	Metaphysis	Benign, sometimes secondary to another bone lesion
Metaphyseal fibrous defect	10-20	1:1	Tibia, femur, fibula	Metaphysis	Benign
Fibrous dysplasia	10-30	3:2	Ribs, femur, tibia, jaw, skull	Medulla of diaphysis or metaphysis	Locally aggressive; rarely complicated by sarcoma
Langerhans' cell granulomatosis	5-15	3:2	Skull, jaw, humerus, rib, femur	Metaphysis or diaphysis	Benign

*It should be emphasized that these data correspond to the typical case and they should not be taken in an absolute sense. Isolated exceptions to practically every one of these statements have occurred.

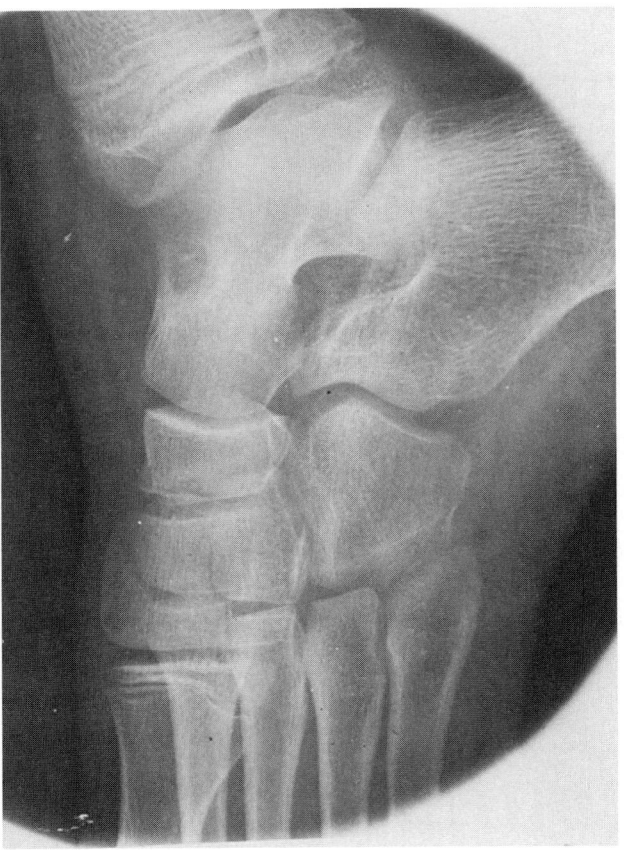

Fig. 24-25 Osteoid osteoma of talus. Note small central osteolytic-nidus surrounded by dense bone.

slightly modified to accommodate some new concepts and entities.[96]

In the WHO classification, most neoplasms are classified as either benign or malignant. Although a sharp separation between these two categories is feasible in most of them, some neoplasms (such as giant cell tumors and some well-differentiated cartilaginous tumors) exhibit borderline or intermediate characteristics. Most malignant bone tumors arise de novo, but there is a small number of benign bone lesions that predispose the patient to the development of skeletal malignancies; these include Paget's disease, chondromatosis, osteochondromatosis, fibrous dysplasia, and osteofibrous dysplasia.[93]

Tumors of the skeletal system, more than tumors arising anywhere else in the body, are relatively constant in their pattern of presentation.[93a] The five basic parameters of importance in this regard are the age of the patient, bone involved, specific area within the bone (epiphysis, metaphysis, or diaphysis; cortex, medulla, or periosteum), radiographic appearance, and microscopic appearance. The pathologist should be fully aware of the first four before trying to evaluate the fifth.[94] Otherwise, serious mistakes may occur. Table 24-1 should help in providing a quick orientation for the pathologist confronted with a bone neoplasm.

Bone-forming tumors
Osteoma

Osteoma is seen almost exclusively in the flat bones of the skull and face. It may protrude inside a paranasal sinus (particularly the frontal and ethmoid) and block the normal drainage from these sinuses.[98] Microscopically, it is composed of dense, mature, predominantly lamellar bone. This lesion is benign and probably not a true neoplasm. Some cases may represent end stages of fibrous dysplasia or related fibro-osseous lesions. Patients with Gardner's syndrome (intestinal polyposis and soft tissue tumors) may have multiple osteomas and other abnormalities.[97] Occasionally, osteomas involve bones other than skull and face. Most of these have a parosteal location and need to be distinguished from parosteal osteosarcoma.[96a]

Osteoid osteoma and osteoblastoma

Osteoid osteoma is a benign bone neoplasm that is found more frequently in patients between 10 and 30 years of age, and that exhibits a 2:1 male-female ratio.[109,118] Intense pain is the most prominent symptom; this is often sharply localized and unaccompanied by clinical or laboratory evidence of infection. Vertebral lesions may be associated with scoliosis.[117]

Osteoid osteoma has been reported in practically every bone but occurs most frequently in the femur, tibia, humerus, bones of the hands and feet, vertebrae, and fibula.[111] Lesions of long bones are usually metaphyseal, but they may be epiphyseal and even juxta- or intra-articular.[100] Most are centered in the cortex (85%), but they may also occur in the spongiosa (13%) or subperiosteal region (2%).[119] Vertebral lesions usually affect the pedicle or the arch.[113]

Radiographically, the typical finding is a radiolucent central nidus that is seldom larger than 1.5 cm and that may or not contain a dense center (Fig. 24-25). This nidus is surrounded by a peripheral sclerotic reaction that may extend for several centimeters along both sides of the cortex and that may lead to a mistaken radiographic diagnosis of Garré's osteomyelitis (Fig. 24-26, *A*).

Microscopically, the sharply delineated central nidus is composed of more or less calcified osteoid lined by plump osteoblasts and growing within highly vascularized connective tissue, without evidence of inflammation (Figs. 24-26, *B*, and 24-27). The appearance is so characteristic that the lesion can still be diagnosed when removed piecemeal. Surrounding the nidus, there is a variably thick layer of dense bone.

The pain associated with osteoid osteoma is characteristically more intense at night, relieved by nonsteroidal anti-inflammatory drugs such as aspirin, and eliminated by the excision of the lesion. It has been attributed by some authors to the effect on nerves and vessels of osteoblast-produced prostaglandin E2, which is typically present in large amounts in these lesions.[108,122] Others believe that the pain is simply related to the presence of nerves within and around the nidus.[107]

Preoperative localization with CT scan and intraoperative monitoring of the location and resection with radioscintigraphy have markedly reduced the recurrence rate.[108,114] The nidus can also be demonstrated by administering tetracy-

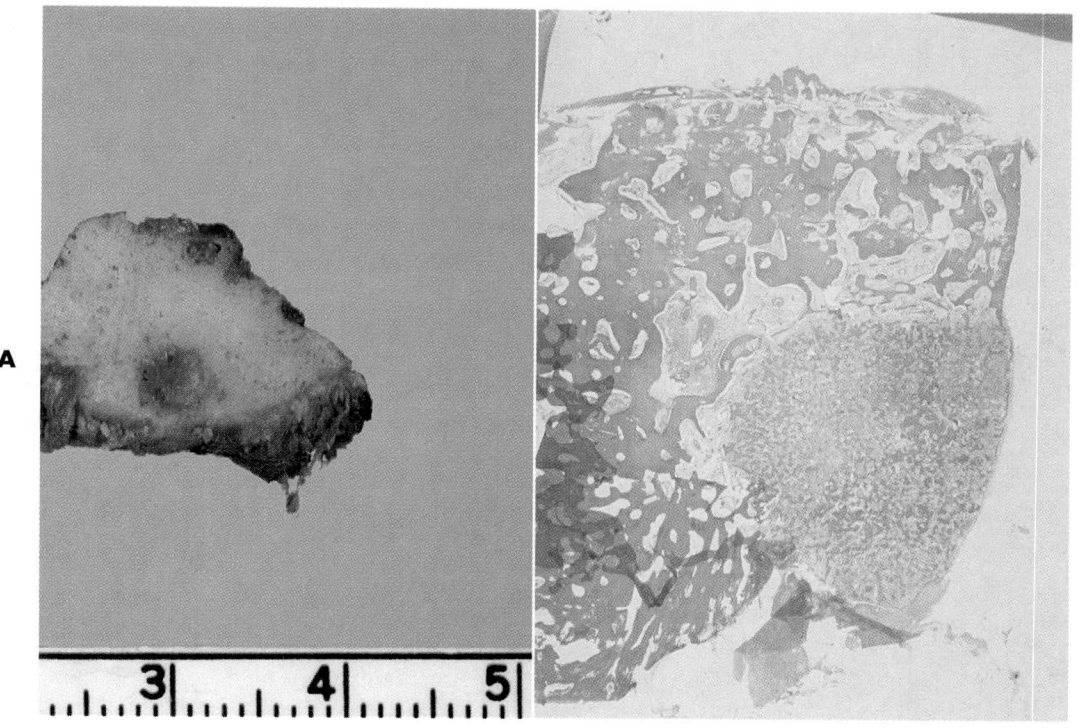

Fig. 24-26 Osteoid osteoma. **A,** Gross appearance. The small, reddish central nidus is surrounded by a thick layer of sclerotic bone. **B,** Low-power microscopic view showing a wedge-shaped nidus slightly protruding over the surface and surrounded by a sclerotic bone.

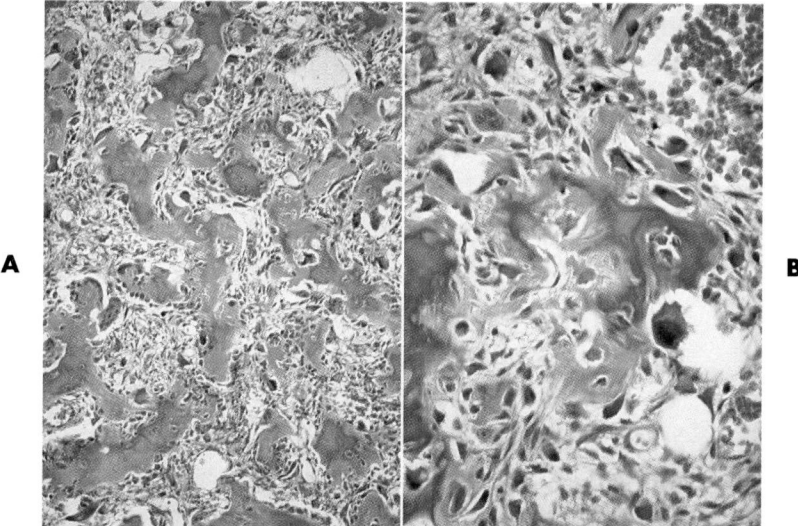

Fig. 24-27 Medium-power **(A)** and high-power **(B)** microscopic views of osteoid osteoma. There is exuberant new osteoid and bone formation by plump osteoblasts. The stroma is cellular and well vascularized.

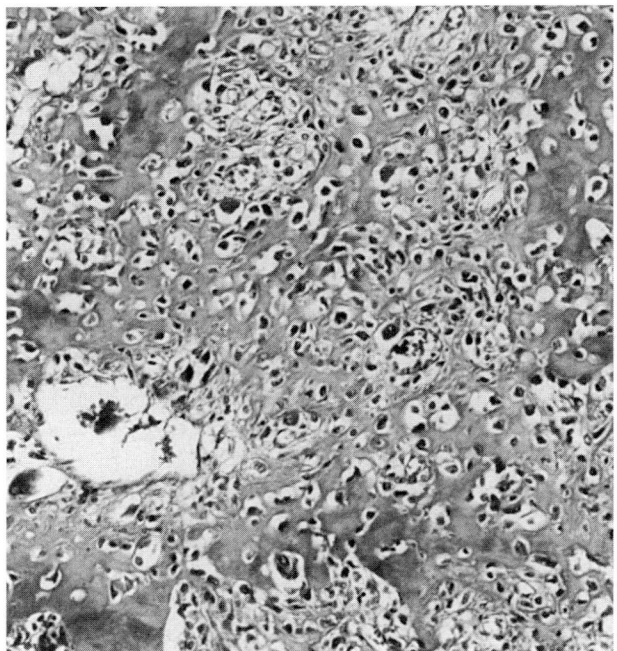

Fig. 24-28 So-called aggressive osteoblastoma. Exuberant new bone formation is evidenced by tumor cells having plump, epithelioid appearance.

cline preoperatively and examining the lesion under ultraviolet light at operation.[99]

Osteoblastoma (benign osteoblastoma, giant osteoid osteoma) is a tumor closely related to osteoid osteoma both microscopically and ultrastructurally.[105,121] It is distinguished from the latter by the larger size of the nidus, the absence or inconspicuousness of a surrounding area of reactive bone formative, and the lack of intense pain.[110] A cartilaginous matrix is present is some cases.[102] Most cases arise in the spongiosa of the bone, but cortical and subperiosteal forms also occur.[119] The majority of the cases are located in the spine or major bones of the lower extremity.[112,116] Osteomalacia can be seen as a complication.[123]

The differential diagnosis between osteoblastoma and osteosarcoma can be extremely difficult because the latter may be very well differentiated and the former is sometimes accompanied by the presence of scattered bizarre tumor cells of probably degenerative nature.[103] As is the case in many other bone tumors, the radiographic pattern is of great assistance in this differential diagnosis. However, in some cases of osteoblastoma, the radiographic picture suggests a malignant neoplasm.[112,115]

Aggressive osteoblastoma and related lesions. Some lesions with the radiographic and architectural features of osteoblastoma show atypical cytologic features that correlate with a tendency for local recurrence. These tumors have been designated as aggressive osteoblastomas. According to Dorfman and Weiss,[106] they are distinguished microscopically from the ordinary osteoblastomas because of the presence of wider or more irregular trabecula, by the focal lack of a trabecular pattern of the osteoid proliferation, and—

most of all—by the fact that the osteoid trabeculae are bordered by epithelioid-appearing osteoblasts (Fig. 24-28). They are distinguished from conventional osteosarcomas because of a low mitotic rate and the absence of the following features: lace-like osteoid, permeation of surrounding intertrabecular spaces, and atypical mitoses. The entity of aggressive osteoblastoma merges with—and may indeed be identical to—tumors described as malignant osteoblastoma,[120] osteosarcoma resembling osteoblastoma,[103] and osteoblastoma-like osteosarcoma,[101] some of which have metastasized. The most reliable signs of malignancy in these lesions are said to be permeation of surrounding tissues and lack of peripheral maturation.[103] To complicate the issue further, there are several reported cases of supposedly ordinary osteoblastomas that have undergone malignant transformation toward osteosarcomas.[104,106]

Osteosarcoma

Generalities. Osteosarcoma is the most frequent primary malignant bone tumor, exclusive of hematopoietic malignancy.[157] It usually occurs in patients between 10 and 25 years of age and is exceptionally rare in preschool children.[127,180] Another peak age incidence occurs after 40, in association with other disorders (see the following discussion). There is a slight male predominance (1.5:1).

Pathogenesis. Most osteosarcomas arise de novo, but others arise within the context of a pre-existing condition:

1 Paget's disease. A high number of osteosarcomas developing in patients over the age of 40 are located in bones affected by Paget's disease[169] (see p. 1929).

2 Radiation exposure. One of the classic cases of human carcinogenesis occurred in a group of factory workers in Illinois who developed osteosarcomas after moistening brushes in their mouths when applying radium paint to create luminous numerals on watches.[192,202] Some cases of osteosarcoma have also been reported years after Thorotrast administration.[219] Many others have been seen, in both adults and children, as a complication of external radiation therapy.[234] The average latency period ranges from 10 to 15 years in the various reported series.[174,237]

3 Chemotherapy. Children treated with alkylating agents for retinoblastoma and other malignancies have an increased risk of osteosarcoma.[227]

4 Pre-existing benign bone lesions. These include fibrous dysplasia, osteochondromatosis, and chondromatosis[220] (see respective sections).

5 Foreign bodies. A few but well-documented cases of osteosarcoma have been reported arising at the site of a total hip replacement.[200]

6 Trauma. Isolated trauma, no matter how intense, does not cause osteosarcoma or other bone tumors.[161] If it did, one would expect to find an increased incidence of bone tumors after fractures, various orthopedic procedures, or other severe injuries. Trauma usually only calls attention to an already present advanced bone tumor.

7 Infectious agent. Some immunologic studies have suggested the presence of an infectious agent, probably a virus, in association with human osteosarcoma,[203] but its pathogenetic role, if any, remains to be determined.

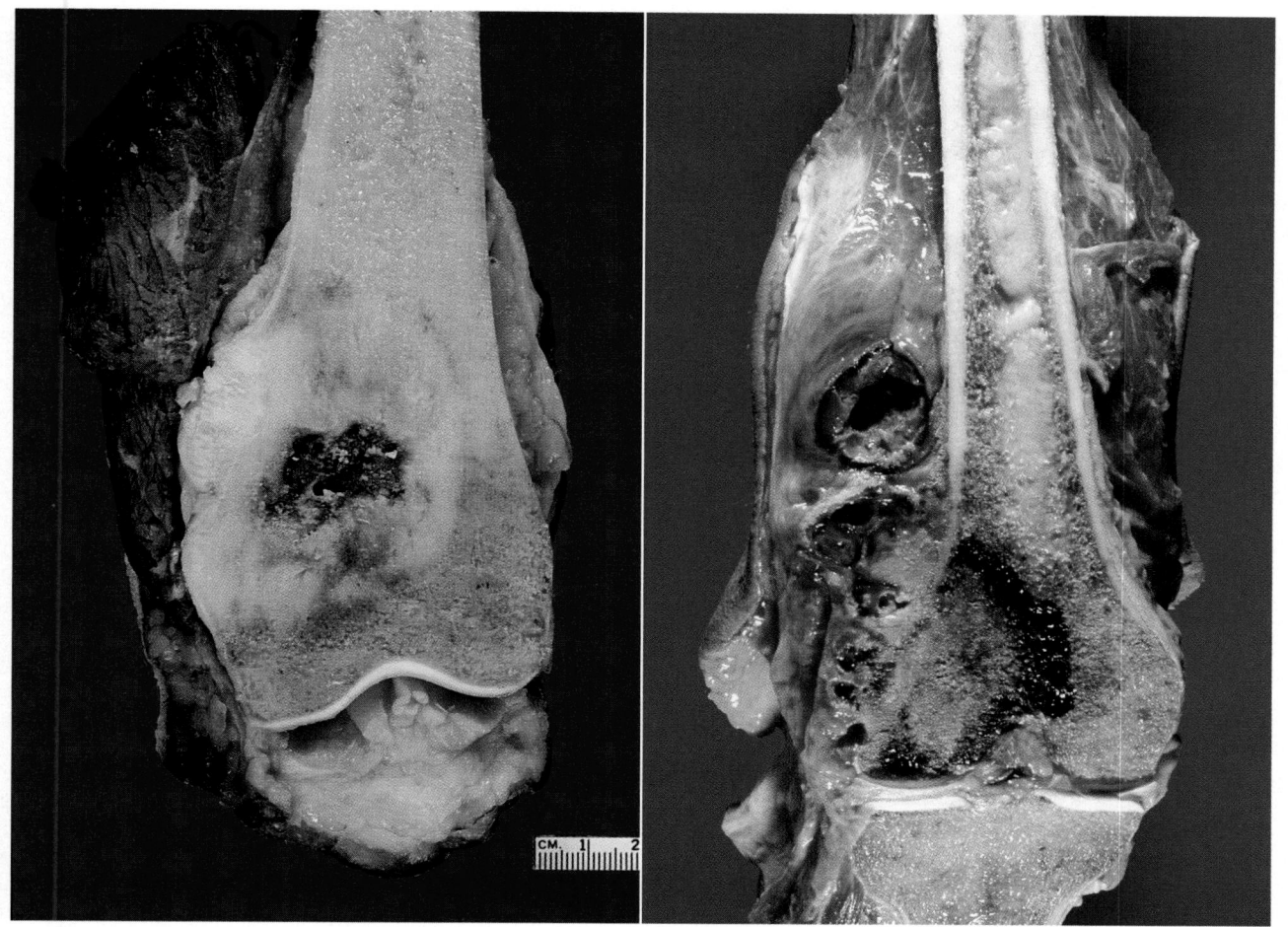

Fig. 24-29 Gross appearances of osteosarcoma of femur. In both instances the tumor is located at the classic metaphyseal site. The tumor shown in **A** is largely restricted to bone, whereas that illustrated in **B** is accompanied by massive soft tissue extension.

Location. Most osteosarcomas arising de novo are located in the metaphyseal area of the long bones, particularly the lower end of the femur, the upper end of the tibia, and the upper end of the humerus.[147] A few cases arise in the diaphyses and an even smaller number in the epiphyses. Less commonly, osteosarcomas are found in flat bones (such as craniofacial bones, pelvis, and scapula)[179] and in short bones.[196] Occasionally, osteosarcomas are multicentric, in either a synchronous or a metachronous fashion; most of these multicentric cases occur in children and tend to be densely sclerotic radiographically and extremely aggressive.[125,199] Germ-line and somatic mutations of p53 have been found in some of these cases.[175]

The large majority of osteosarcomas arise within the medullary cavity, from which they extend into the cortex; only occasionally will they begin within the cortex itself[235]—when they do, they seem to have a predilection for the diaphysis.[183]

Gross appearance and spread. The gross appearance of the cut surface of an osteosarcoma varies a great deal, depending on the relative amounts of bone, cartilage, cellular stroma, and vessels (Figs. 24-29 and 24-30). The range extends from bony hard to cystic, friable, and hemorrhagic. From its usual origin in the metaphysis of a long bone, the tumor may:

1 Spread along the marrow cavity.
2 Invade the adjacent cortex.
3 Elevate or perforate the periosteum. In the latter circumstance, a radiographic sign known as Codman's triangle develops. The two long sides of this triangle are formed by the elevated periosteum and the underlying bone; the space within them is mainly occupied by reactive new bone, arranged perpendicular to the bone surface, but it may also contain malignant tumor. This radiographic sign, although useful, is not specific for osteosarcoma or even for a malignant tumor; it can be

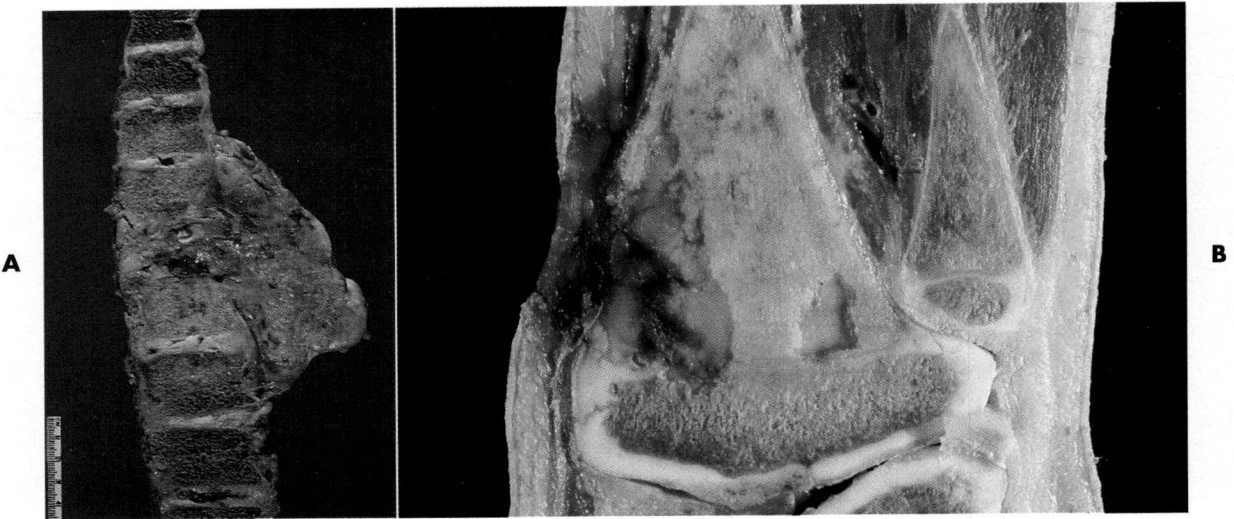

Fig. 24-30 Other gross appearances of osteosarcoma. **A,** Tumor extensively involving spine and producing a large soft tissue mass. **B,** This tumor of the upper tibial metaphysis is being temporarily restrained by the cartilage of the epiphyseal line. The hemorrhagic area represents the biopsy site.

produced by any lesion that elevates the periosteum, including hematoma.

4 Extend into the soft tissues (see Fig. 2-10). It may even reach beneath the skin, although cutaneous ulceration practically never occurs.

5 Extend into the epiphysis. This happens frequently after the epiphysis is closed, but it may also be seen when the epiphyseal growth line is still present.[217]

6 Extend into the joint space. This invasion occurs when the tumor extends under the capsule insertion to involve the margin of the articular cartilage. In the knee, the tumor may extend across or around the osseous-tendinous junction of the cruciate ligaments into the joint space.[218]

7 Form satellite nodules independent from the main tumor mass proximal to the primary lesion, either in the same bone or transarticularly (Plate XVII-A). These have been called "skip" metastases[158] and may be responsible for an increased incidence of local recurrences and subsequent metastases.[187]

8 Metastasize through the bloodstream to distant sites, particularly the lung. In an autopsy series of fifty-four cases, the four main sites of metastases were lung (98%), other bones (37%), pleura (33%), and heart (20%).[231] Conversely, metastases to regional lymph nodes are so rare that they should be disregarded for purposes of therapy. On occasion, the lung metastases present in the form of extensive intraluminal tumor growth in the pulmonary arteries.[236]

Microscopic features. Microscopically, osteosarcoma may destroy the pre-existing bone trabeculae or grow around them in an appositional fashion. The key feature for the diagnosis is the detection, somewhere in the tumor, of osteoid and/or bone (calcified osteoid) produced directly by the tumor cells (Fig. 24-31). Osteoid is recognized by its eosinophilic-staining quality, its glassy appearance, irregular contours, and the fact that it is surrounded by a rim of osteoblasts (Fig. 24-31, *A* to *D*). It may be very difficult to distinguish osteoid from hyalinized collagen; a homogeneous rather than fibrillary appearance, beginning punctate calcification, and a plump appearance of the cells around it favor a diagnosis of osteoid. A different but highly characteristic type of tumor bone is characterized by thin tubular anastomosing "microtrabeculae," which are very basophilic and vaguely reminiscent of the appearance of fungal hyphae (Plate XVII-B).

These osteoblastic areas are often mixed with fibroblastic and chondroblastic foci, the relative proportions among these three components varying a great deal from case to case. Depending on which component predominates, osteosarcomas have been divided into osteoblastic, fibroblastic, and chondroblastic, but there seems to be no prognostic significance to this division. The important fact to remember is that a malignant bone tumor should be designated as osteosarcoma whenever osteoid is seen unconnected with cartilage and being formed directly from the tumor cells, no matter how much neoplastic cartilage (with or without endochondral ossification) or fibrous tissue is present elsewhere.

Morphologic variations in osteosarcoma are plentiful.[148,213,247] The osteoid may be sparse or massive, surrounded by pleomorphic bizarre cells or relatively acellular, irregularly shaped, or with a rosette-like configuration. The tumor cells may grow in diffuse, nesting, or pseudopapillary arrangements. The vessels may be scanty or numerous, sometimes with a dilated or hemangiopericytomatous appearance. The tumor cells may be spindle, oval, or round, and their size may range from small to giant; exceptionally, they have a distinctly epithelial-like appearance.[149,167,181,245] Osteoclast-like multinucleated giant cells are present in one fourth of the cases and may dominate the picture focally (so-

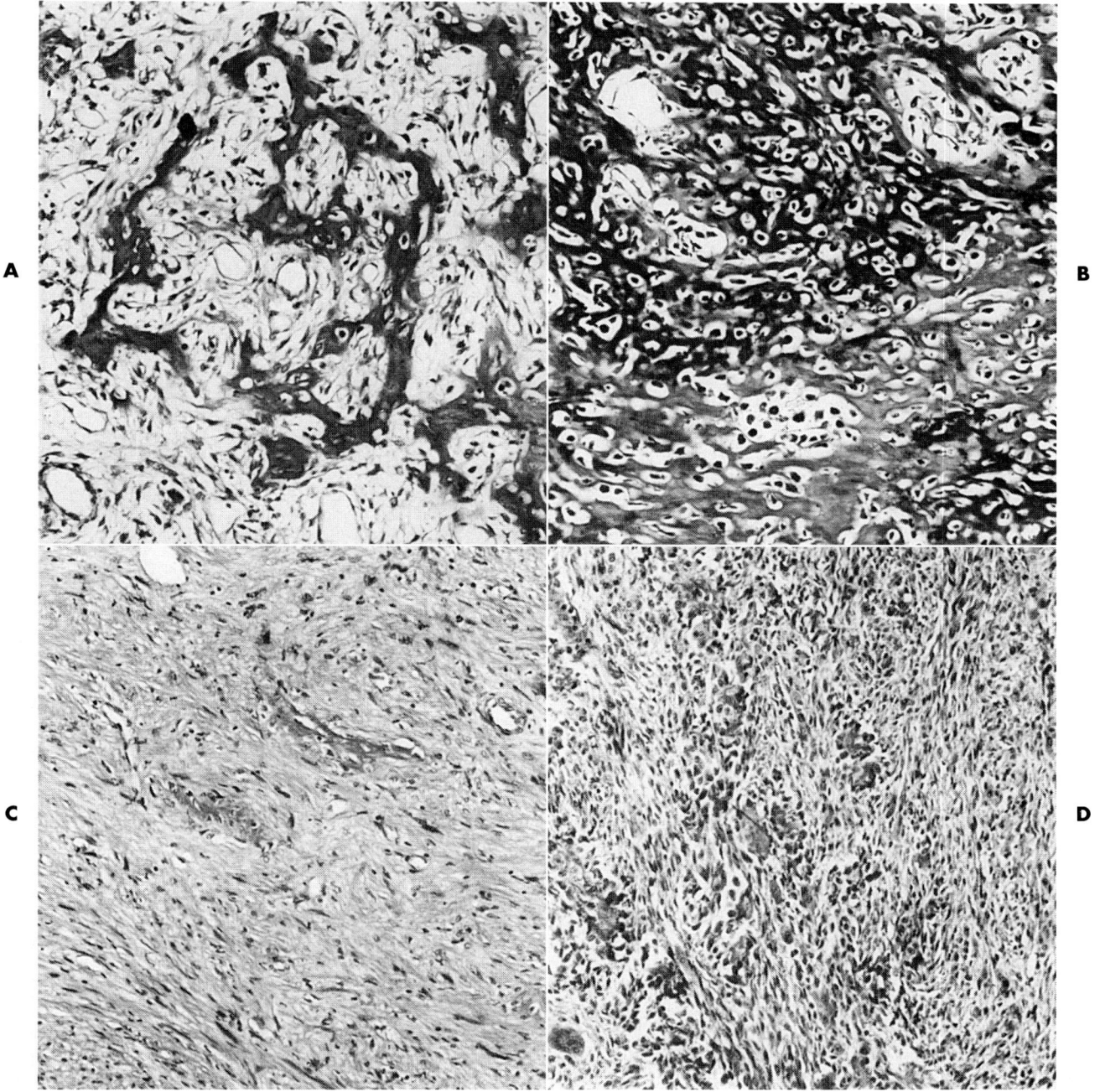

Fig. 24-31 Various morphologic appearances of osteosarcoma. **A,** Thin anastomosing osteoid. **B,** Reticulated osteoid with heavy calcium deposition. **C,** Fibroblastic type of osteosarcoma with only minimal bone formation. **D,** Cellular spindle-cell form with osteoid represented by small rosette-like structures.

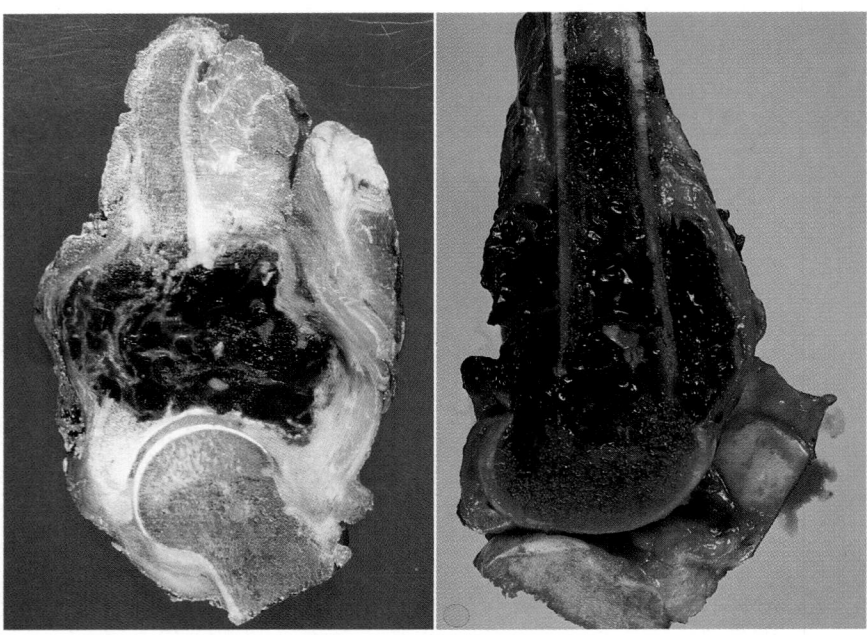

Fig. 24-32 Gross appearances of telangiectatic osteosarcoma.

called giant cell–rich osteosarcoma); the cartilage may be immature, mineralized, or highly myxoid.

Depending on which one of the previously mentioned microscopic patterns happens to be present, the differential diagnosis of osteosarcoma may include a remarkably high number of benign and malignant lesions, such as fracture callus, myositis ossificans, fibrous dysplasia, osteoblastoma, fibrosarcoma, chondrosarcoma, giant cell tumor, malignant lymphoma, and metastatic carcinoma.[247] Exuberant fracture callus is particularly likely to be misdiagnosed as osteosarcoma by the unwary, with disastrous consequences for the patient. This callus may be secondary to a pathologic fracture in a benign lesion such as a metaphyseal fibrous defect or aneurysmal bone cyst, in a metastatic carcinoma, or in osteogenesis imperfecta.[132,178] Myositis ossificans is a reactive lesion pathogenetically closely related to fracture callus and may induce similar diagnostic problems (see p. 1983).

Other entities that need to be considered in the differential diagnosis are discussed in connection with the osteosarcoma variants described in the following section.

Special techniques. Osteosarcoma cells usually exhibit strong alkaline phosphatase activity, regardless of their appearance (osteoblastic or fibroblastic), a feature of diagnostic value.[226,244] Ultrastructurally, the better differentiated tumor cells resemble normal osteoblasts in their abundance of dilated cisternae of granular endoplasmic reticulum and sparse mitochondria.[191,214,223,240] Other cells present are osteocytes, chondroblasts, undifferentiated cells, and myofibroblasts.[206,224,225] The matrix is formed of nonperiodic fibrils, scattered collagen fibers, and focal calcium deposits of hydroxyapatite crystals.[162]

Immunohistochemically, the cells of osteosarcoma consistently express vimentin. In some cases they are also positive for smooth muscle actin and desmin (suggesting myofibroblastic differentiation) and exceptionally for keratin and EMA.[166,177,226a] S-100 protein is always present in foci of chondroid differentiation, but it may also be seen in osteoblastic areas.[166]

Three proteins specifically associated with bone production—osteonectin, bone morphogenetic protein, and bone GLA protein—have been identified immunohistochemically in the cells of osteosarcoma and may be of utility in the differential diagnosis of this tumor.[140,176,212,246,246a] Type I collagen is consistently found in the extracellular material; in addition, type II collagen is present in chondroid foci, and type IV collagen may also be encountered.[185]

The most common cytogenetic abnormalities detected in osteosarcoma involve chromosomes 1, 2, 6, 12, and 17.[198]

Microscopic variants and special types. In addition to the wide range in morphologic appearance already described in osteosarcoma, there are some cases in which the cytoarchitectural characteristics depart enough from the norm to justify recognition as a special category. It should be realized that these variations may be present only focally and that they may occur in combination; their main importance rests on their ability to simulate other bone processes microscopically and also on the fact that some of them carry distinctive prognostic connotations:

1 *Telangiectatic.* Blood-filled cystic formations are prominent, resulting in an appearance similar to that of aneurysmal bone cyst radiographically and pathologically, although the arteriographic pattern is usually

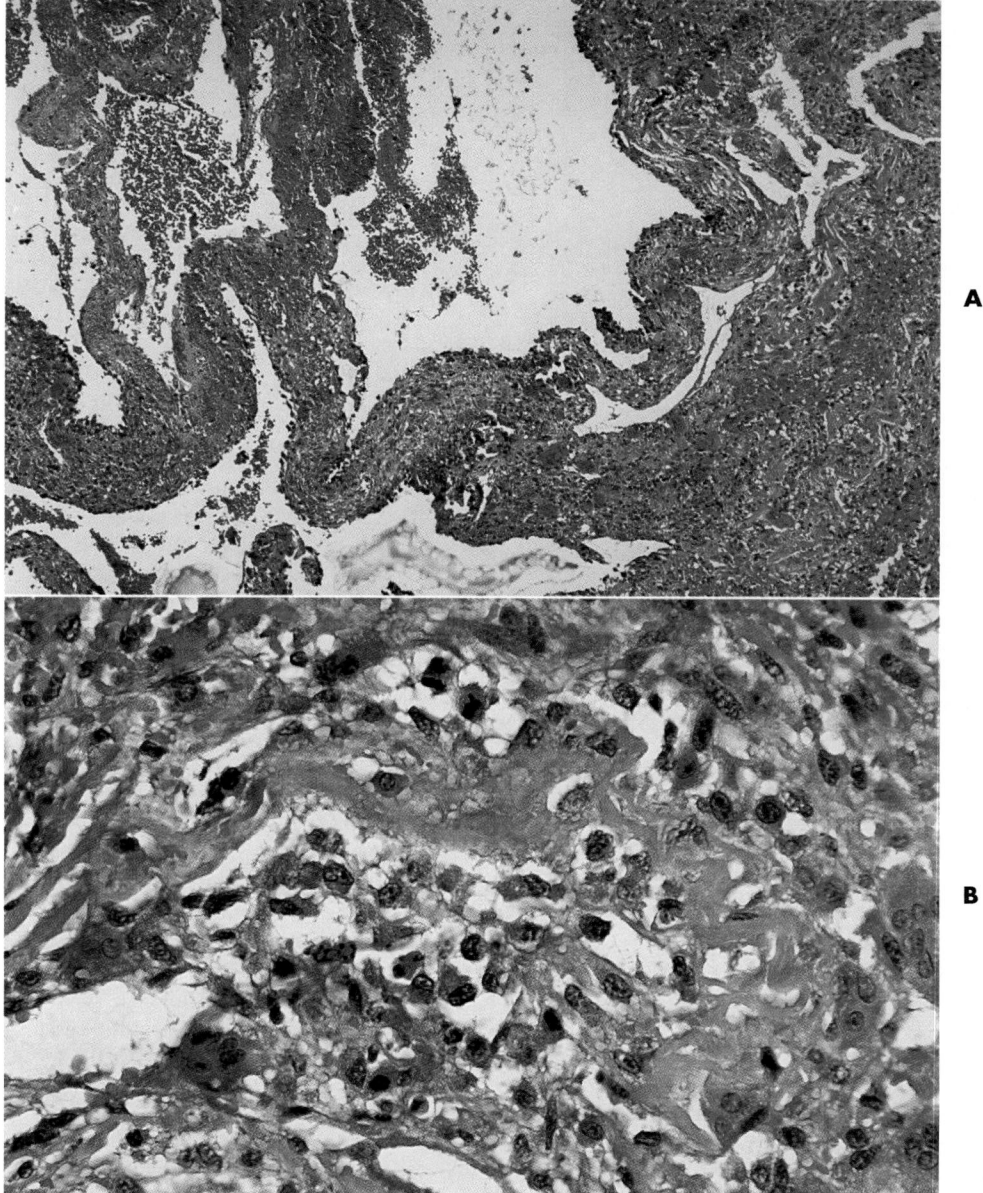

Fig. 24-33 Microscopic appearance of telangiectatic osteosarcoma. **A,** The low-power architecture closely simulates the appearance of an aneurysmal bone cyst. **B,** Malignant osteoid is present in the septa.

different (Fig. 24-32). Pathologic fractures are very frequent.[172] The lesion is identified as osteosarcoma through the detection of malignant stroma in the septa that separate the bloody cysts[137] (Fig. 24-33). Telangiectatic osteosarcoma has been found to be associated with a more aggressive course than the conventional variety in one large series[193] but not in two others.[137,172]

2 *Small cell.* The small size and uniformity of the tumor cells and their diffuse pattern of growth closely simulate the appearance of Ewing's sarcoma and malignant lymphoma. In some cases, these cells are spindle rather than round.[130] Focal production of osteoid (sometimes mixed with cartilage) by these small cells is the distinguishing feature.[138,190,216] Areas of cartilage formation can also be present.[130] In contrast to Ewing's sarcoma/ PNET, most cases of small cell osteosarcoma lack immunoreactivity for O13.[153] There are no pathognomonic ultrastructural features, and it is difficult to distinguish small cell osteosarcoma from Ewing's sarcoma at this level when osteoid is not present in the sample.[154]

3 *Fibrohistiocytic.* The appearance in most areas is indistinguishable from that of malignant fibrous histiocy-

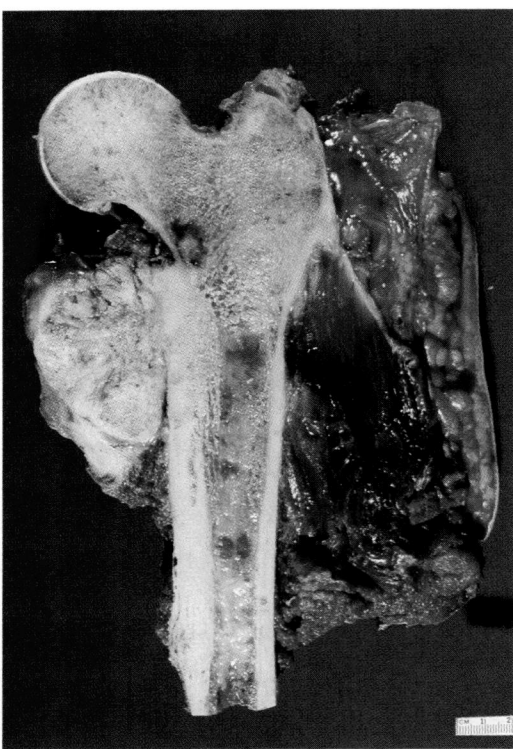

Fig. 24-34 Juxtacortical osteosarcoma of upper femur. There is only minimal involvement of the cortex.

toma, especially in the areas of soft tissue extension and in the distant metastases; however, tumor osteoid is focally present.

4 *Anaplastic.* The tumor is so bizarre and undifferentiated as to raise the possibility of any type of pleomorphic sarcoma or metastatic carcinoma. Once again, the key to the diagnosis is the identification of tumor osteoid.

5 *Well-differentiated (low-grade) intramedullary (intraosseous)* (Plate XVII-C). This tumor is microscopically so bland looking as to be underdiagnosed as a benign lesion, particularly fibrous dysplasia.[230] Other cases resemble histologically parosteal osteosarcoma.[136] Most patients are adults, the femur and tibia being the most commonly affected sites. Spindle cells with minimal atypia and scanty mitoses are seen mixed with abundant osteoid. Recurrences are common, but metastases are very rare (unless the tumor converts in the recurrence into a conventional high-grade osteosarcoma).[182] In contrast to fibrous dysplasia, this tumor shows radiographic evidence of cortical destruction.[182] Microscopically, atypia is minimal but still present. This feature and the invasive growth pattern are helpful in distinguishing this tumor from fibrous dysplasia.[182]

Other variants of osteosarcoma are defined on the basis of topographic, clinical, or radiographic features, or a combination of them:

1 *Juxtacortical (parosteal) osteosarcoma.* This infrequent variant occurs in a slightly older age group than the conventional variety.[228] It usually arises in a juxtacortical position in the metaphyses of long bones (usually the posterior aspect of the lower femoral shaft) and grows very slowly, some cases having a life history of up to 15 years.[208] Eventually, it forms a large lobulated mass with a tendency to encircle the bone (Fig. 24-34). Later in its evolution, it may penetrate into the medullary cavity, a feature associated with a higher microscopic grade and decreased survival.[145] Satellite nodules may be present. Rare cases have been described at other sites, such as the mandible and small bones of the hand.[233] The radiographic appearance is highly characteristic[232] (Fig. 24-35, *A*). Microscopically, there is a disorderly pattern of well-formed bone, osteoid, occasional cartilage, and a highly fibrous spindle-cell stroma (Fig. 24-35, *B*). The cytologic signs of malignancy in the fibrous stroma are often subtle, thus accounting for the great frequency of misdiagnoses made in this tumor.[156] Exceptionally, the tumor is rich in osteoclast-like giant cells.[212a] The most important differential diagnosis is with myositis ossificans, which is distinguished mainly on the basis of its orderly pattern of maturation (see p. 1983). The prognosis for juxtacortical osteosarcoma is very good, even with segmental excision.[155] It should be emphasized that not all osteosarcomas located juxtacortically belong to this variety. Those having morphologic features equivalent to those of the conventional intramedullary osteosarcoma are referred to as high-grade surface osteosarcomas and behave as aggressively as the former.[159,242] This is also true for the conventional intramedullary osteosarcoma with the periosteal spread. Sometimes, features of a high-grade osteosarcoma are seen focally in what is otherwise a typical juxtacortical osteosarcoma, either initially or—more commonly—following repeated tumor recurrences; this phenomenon, which is sometimes referred to as "dedifferentiation," is associated with a markedly decreased survival rate.[124,228,243]

2 *Periosteal osteosarcoma.* This tumor type, which is very different from juxtacortical osteosarcoma despite the similarities in the unfortunate terminology chosen, grows on the surface of long bones.[229] Most of the reported cases have been located in the upper tibial shaft or femur and have presented as small lucent lesions on the bone surface, accompanied by bone spicules arranged perpendicular to the shaft. The lesions are limited to the cortex and only rarely invade the medullary cavity[152,164] (Fig. 24-36, *A*). Microscopically, the tumors are relatively high-grade osteosarcomas, with a prominent cartilaginous component (Fig. 24-36, *B*). The prognosis is better than for conventional osteosarcoma.[222,229] This entity is closely related to, if not identical with, the one discussed on p. 1953 under the term juxtacortical (periosteal) chondrosarcoma.

3 *Osteosarcoma of the jaw.* Gnathic osteosarcoma is distinctive enough to be treated separately from the rest.[146] Patients affected are slightly older (average age, 34 years), and most lesions show a prominent chondroblastic component. The most common sites of involvement are

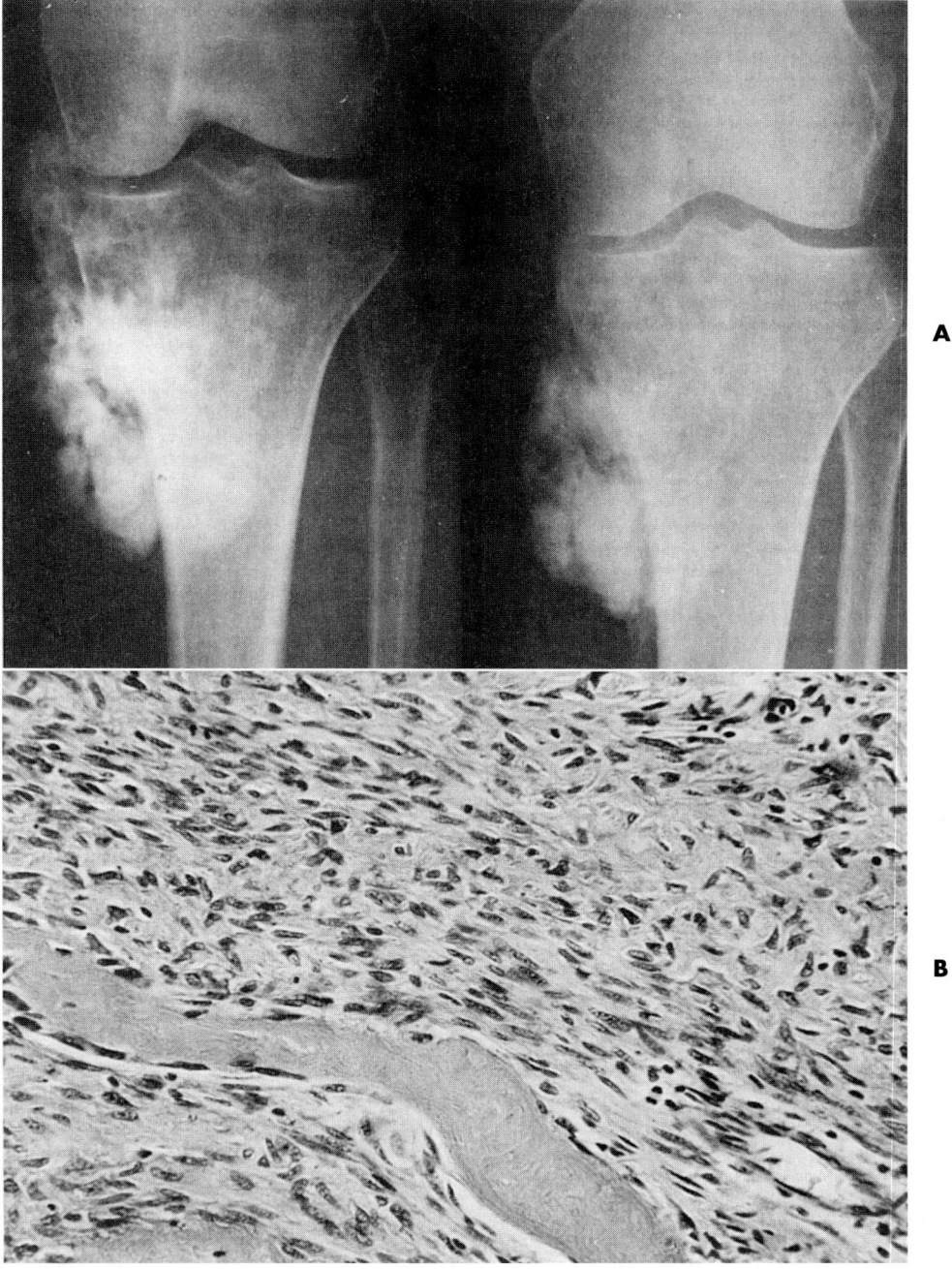

Fig. 24-35 A, Juxtacortical osteosarcoma occurring in 40-year-old woman. Note large extracortical component. **B,** Same lesion shown in **A** demonstrating well-differentiated character of sarcomatous stroma. This lesion has been present for several years.

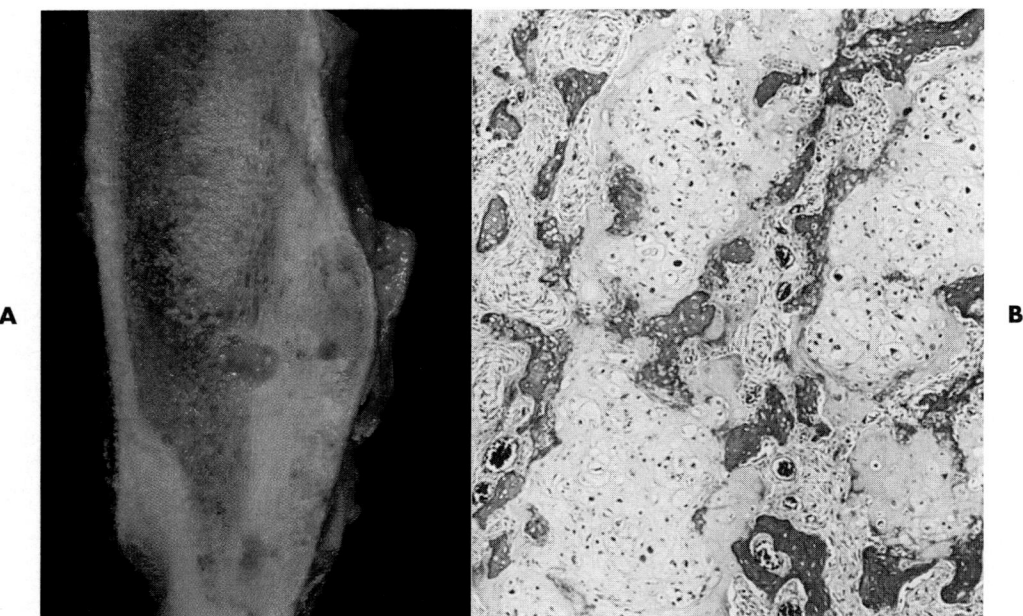

Fig. 24-36 Periosteal osteosarcoma. **A,** Gross appearance. The white shining appearance is due to the high content of cartilage. **B,** Microscopic appearance. There is predominance of neoplastic cartilage, but osteoid is also present.

the body of the mandible and the alveolar ridge of the maxilla. The prognosis is relatively good.[146]

4 *Osteosarcoma in Paget's disease.* Nearly all the cases of Paget's disease complicated by osteosarcoma are of the polyostotic type. The tumors themselves are often multicentric. The most common locations are the pelvis, humerus (Fig. 24-37), femur, tibia, and skull.[170,173,239] According to Schajowicz et al.,[210] these osteosarcomas are characterized microscopically by a large number of osteoclasts alternating with atypical osteoblasts. The prognosis is extremely poor.[170,239]

Diagnosis. Although most osteosarcomas have a very characteristic radiographic appearance, there is sufficient overlap with other malignant bone tumors and with benign conditions to make imperative a pathologic diagnosis before instituting definitive therapy. Depending on the size and location of the tumor and the skill and experience of the diagnostic team, the choice of procedure may be open biopsy, needle biopsy, fine-needle aspiration, or frozen section.[160]

When performing an open biopsy, an attempt should be made to include tumor and adjacent non-neoplastic tissue; excessive trauma should be avoided, and the biopsy incision should be so placed that it will be entirely removed by the subsequent surgical excision.[189] There is no evidence that the performance of an incisional biopsy affects survival in these patients.[141]

Needle biopsy in experienced hands is extremely reliable and is of particular use in locations that are difficult to reach by open biopsy, such as the vertebral column.[129,151,197,209] Fine-needle aspiration has also been used extensively with very good results.[238]

Laboratory tests are of no great value in the diagnosis of osteosarcoma. The only abnormality detected with some frequency is elevation of serum alkaline phosphatase, but this is merely an expression of bone production and, as such, is nonspecific. It can also be elevated in hyperparathyroidism, Paget's disease, and metastatic carcinoma from the breast or prostate. Conversely, it is apt to be negative in a predominantly osteolytic osteosarcoma.

Therapy. Traditionally, the therapy of osteosarcoma of the extremities has consisted of amputation or disarticulation, depending on the location of the tumor. In recent years, more limited forms of surgery (limb-sparing procedures) have been coupled with other therapeutic modalities, particularly preoperative and postoperative neoadjuvant chemotherapy.[131,142,143,204] The preoperative chemotherapy can be administered systemically or intraarterially.[177,241]

Microscopic studies of the tumor following chemotherapy have shown extensive areas of necrosis and hemorrhage[128]; sites where viable tumor was more likely to persist were the soft tissue, cortex and subcortex, ligaments, and areas in contact with cartilage.[201] These morphologic changes correlate well with functional bone imaging, which therefore provides an accurate presurgical assessment of tumor response.[221] The presence of extensive tumor necrosis following chemotherapy constitutes a good prognostic sign[205] (see next section).

Surgical removal of metastatic nodules of osteosarcoma in the lungs appears to prolong survival in selected patients.[135,211]

Prognosis. The overall prognosis for osteosarcoma has significantly improved. For many years, the 5-year survival rate fluctuated very little from the figure of 20% in most series. Lately, many reports listing 5-year disease-free rates of 70% or more have appeared[163,184]; it is not clear how much of this apparent improvement is due to change in treatment (particularly the administration of multidrug chemotherapy following surgery), as opposed to a better selection of surgical candidates through more detailed radiographic studies.[165,207] When making these calculations, it is important to exclude cases of chondrosarcoma or fibrosarcoma, both of which carry a better prognosis than osteosarcoma.

Factors to be considered in regard to prognosis of osteosarcoma are the following:

1 *Age, sex, or pregnancy.* No apparent prognostic differences have been related to any of these parameters.[144,147,171]

2 *Presence of Paget's disease.* These tumors are usually highly malignant; most of the reported cases have proved fatal.[170,239]

3 *History of prior irradiation.* Radiation-induced osteosarcomas do not behave significantly differently from those arising de novo; in one large series, the 5-year survival rate was 28%.[126]

4 *Specific bone involved.* Osteosarcomas of the jaw and distal extremities (below the elbows and knees) have a better prognosis than the others.[147,195] With osteosarcoma of the jaw, survival figures of over 80% have been achieved with current surgical modalities. Instead, osteosarcomas of other craniofacial bones and vertebrae (many of which arise within the context of Paget's disease) have a very poor prognosis.[133,173,194,215]

5 *Multifocal osteosarcoma.* This form is almost uniformly fatal.[199]

6 *Osteoblastic, chondroblastic, and fibroblastic types.* Some authors have claimed a better prognosis for the fibroblastic type, but the difference is so small as to be of no statistical significance.

7 *Microscopic grading.* There is no definite relationship with prognosis[147,195] once the osteosarcoma variants are excluded.

8 *Parosteal and periosteal osteosarcoma.* As already indicated, both of these variants are associated with an improved prognosis, particularly the former.

9 *Microscopic variants.* Telangiectatic osteosarcoma has a worse prognosis (at least in one series), and well-differentiated intramedullary osteosarcoma has a better prognosis than conventional osteosarcoma. Small cell osteosarcoma has a prognosis that is the same or slightly worse than conventional osteosarcoma.[130,138]

10 *Serum elevation of alkaline phosphatase.* In one series, tumors associated with serum elevations of this enzyme were found to have an increased metastatic rate.[186]

11 *Postchemotherapy tumor necrosis.* It has been shown by several independent studies that the amount of tumor necrosis following chemotherapy is directly related to survival rate.[139,205] As a matter of fact, this feature has emerged as the single most important prognostic parameter in conventional osteosarcoma of extremities with no evidence of distant metastases at presentation.[150]

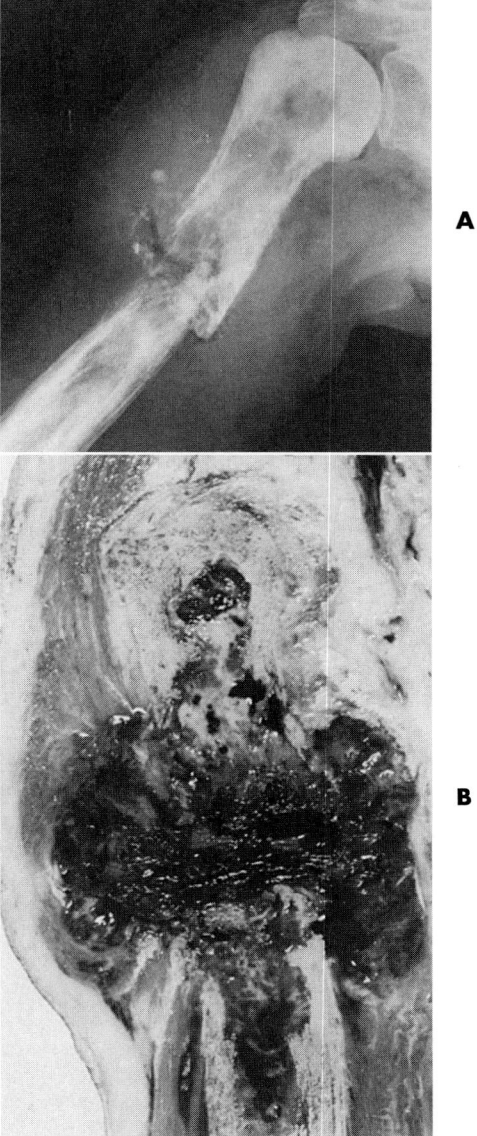

Fig. 24-37 A, Osteosarcoma of upper end of humerus associated with fracture in a patient with Paget's disease. **B,** Point of fracture in humerus shown in **A** demonstrating extension of hemorrhagic neoplasm up shaft and out into soft tissues. Note porous, thickened cortical bone of Paget's disease.

12 *Aneuploidy.* Alteration of DNA ploidy as measured by flow cytometry is correlated with the microscopic grade of the tumor and may prove of prognostic value.[168,188] The technique may also be of help in the differential diagnosis, since most osteosarcomas are hyperploid or aneuploid, whereas the vast majority of benign bone tumors are diploid; however, periosteal and well-differentiated osteosarcomas are also usually diploid.[134]

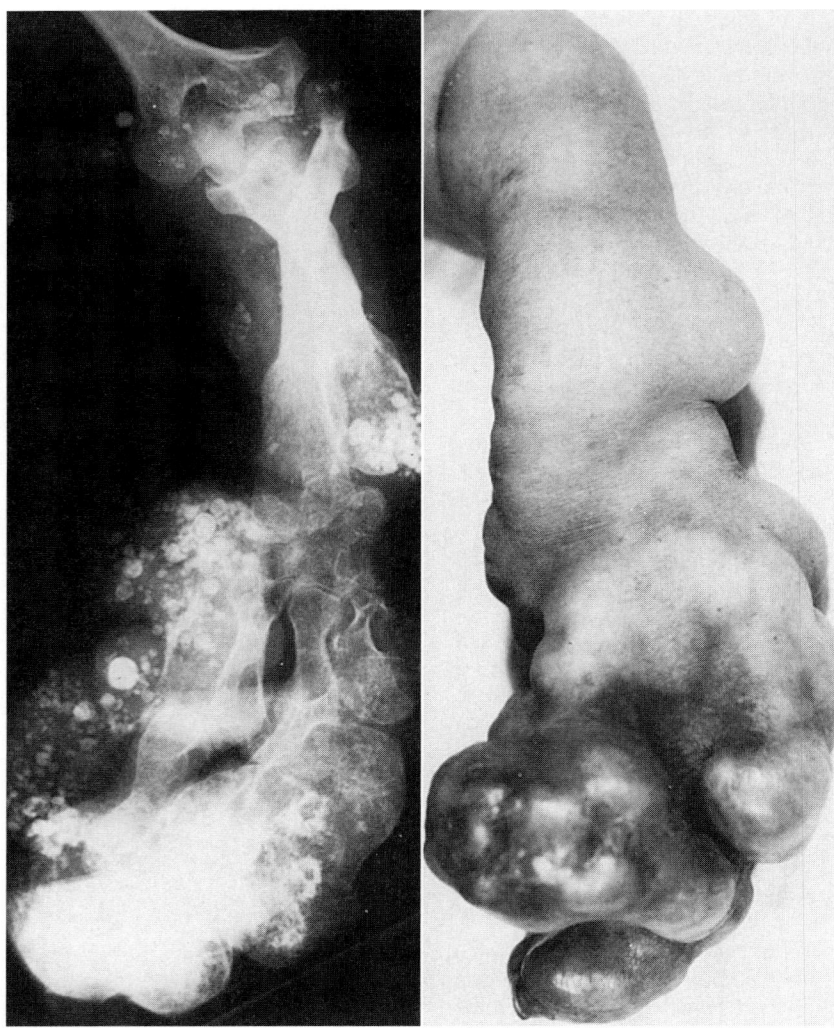

Fig. 24-38 Arm of patient affected by Maffucci's syndrome. Innumerable chondromas are seen concentrated in distal aspect of extremity. Patient developed chondrosarcoma in innominate bone, with pulmonary metastases. (Courtesy Dr. O. Urteaga A, Lima, Peru.)

Cartilage-forming tumors

Chondroma

Chondroma is a common benign cartilaginous tumor that occurs most frequently in the small bones of the hands and feet, particularly the proximal phalanges. Most cases begin in the spongiosa of the diaphysis (enchondromas), from which they expand and thin the cortex. Chondromas of the thumb and terminal phalanges are distinctly uncommon. About 30% of chondromas are multiple.[261]

Multiple enchondromas having a predominantly unilateral distribution are referred to as ***Ollier's disease.*** The association of multiple enchondromas with soft tissue hemangiomas (including spindle cell hemangioendotheliomas) is known as ***Maffucci's syndrome***[254] (Fig. 24-38). In both conditions, there is a significant risk of malignant transformation, usually in the form of chondrosarcoma,[252,256,260] some-

times developing in multiple bones.[251] Ollier's disease is also associated with ovarian sex-cord tumors.[262]

Enchondromas of the ribs and long bones are distinctly unusual. A variant of the latter, presenting in the metaphysis of long bones, is characterized by massive calcification within the neoplasm (calcifying enchondroma)[253] (Fig. 24-39).

Rarely, chondromas arise in a ***juxtacortical*** (periosteal) area of a long bone or a small bone of the hand or foot.[248,255] They characteristically erode and induce sclerosis of the contiguous cortex (Plate XVII-D). Radiographically, juxtacortical chondromas are smaller and better marginated than their malignant counterpart[258] (see p. 1953). Recurrence may follow incomplete excision.[259]

Microscopically, chondromas are composed of mature lobules of hyaline cartilage (Fig. 24-40). Foci of myxoid

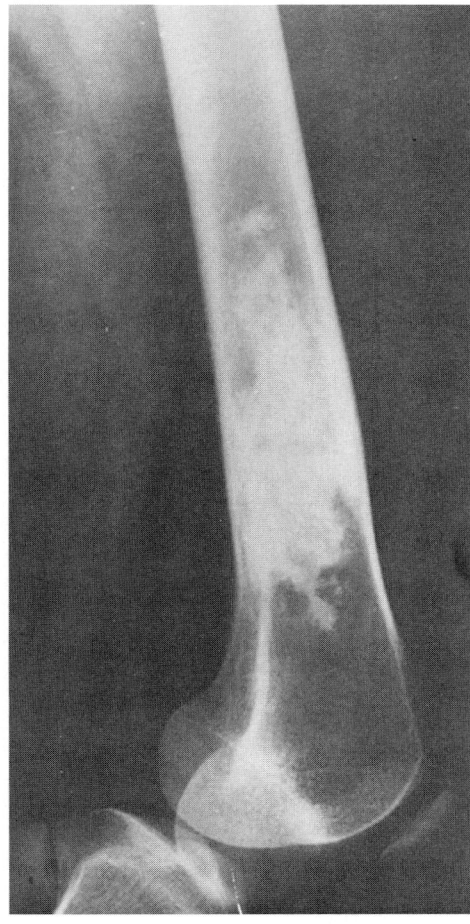

Fig. 24-39 Large asymptomatic enchondroma of femur in 42-year-old woman. Tumor is extensively calcified.

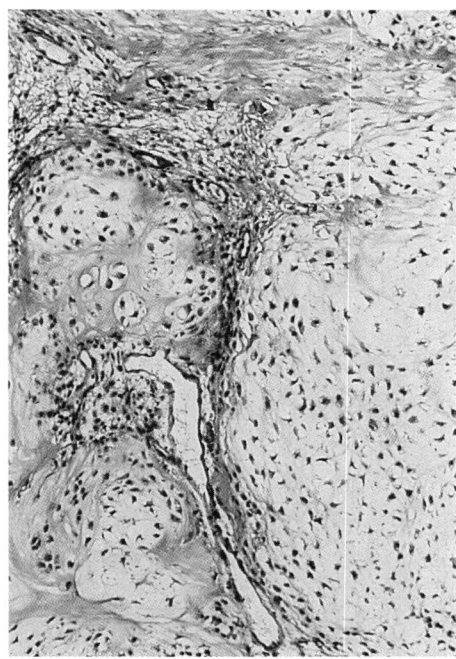

Fig. 24-40 Enchondroma of phalanx. The tumor has a typical lobulated appearance.

degeneration, calcification, and endochondral ossification are common. Juxtacortical chondroma tends to be more cellular than its medullary counterpart and may contain occasional plump or double nuclei.[249]

Although not strictly a chondroma, the peculiar chest wall lesion of infancy known as *cartilaginous and vascular hamartoma (mesenchymoma)* is discussed here because of its benign nature and predominant cartilaginous composition.[249,250,257] These chondroid areas, which often exhibit endochondral ossification, are mixed with spindle areas with an aneurysmal bone cyst–like appearance. Most of the cases are already present at birth, and the behavior is benign.

Osteochondroma

Osteochondroma is the most frequent benign bone tumor. It is usually asymptomatic, but it may lead to deformity or interfere with the function of adjacent structures such as tendons and blood vessels.[266] It may also undergo spontaneous regression.[263] The most common locations are the metaphyses of the lower femur, upper tibia, upper humerus, and pelvis. The radiographic appearance of osteochondroma is very characteristic; one of the most typical features is the fact that the lesions, when located in metaphyses of long bones, grow out in a direction opposite to the adjacent joint.

The average age of the patient at onset is approximately 10 years; in the large majority of the cases, the tumor appears before the patient is 20 years old.

The average greatest diameter is approximately 4 cm, but the tumors may reach sizes of 10 cm or more. The smaller tumors are sessile, and the larger ones are pedunculated. Characteristically, there is a cap of cartilage covered by a fibrous membrane, which is continuous with the periosteum of the adjacent bone. This cap tends to be lobulated in the large lesions (Figs. 24-41 and 24-42). Its average thickness is about 0.6 cm; it is rare for it to exceed 1 cm. Microscopically, the cells resemble those of normal hyaline cartilage. Eosinophilic, PAS-positive inclusions may be seen in the cytoplasm.[264,267] The bulk of the lesion is made up of mature bone trabeculae located beneath the cartilaginous cap and containing normal bone marrow. At the interphase between cartilage and bone, there is active endochondral ossification. In older lesions, the cap thins out and may disappear altogether. A bursa may develop around the head of a long-standing osteochondroma; in turn, this bursa may develop complications such as osteocartilaginous loose bodies, synovial chondrometaplasia, and—exceptionally—chondrosarcoma.[268]

The gross and microscopic appearance of a single lesion of the familial condition known as osteochondromatosis (multiple cartilaginous exostoses, Ehrenfried's hereditary deforming chondrodysplasia, diaphyseal aclasis) cannot be distinguished from solitary osteochondroma.[265,274] A very small proportion of the solitary tumors evolve into chondrosarcomas,[265] but the incidence reaches 10% in the cases with multiple lesions.[273]

Osteochondroma should be distinguished from *bizarre parosteal osteochondromatous proliferations,* which may occur in the bones of the hands and feet[272]; these lesions are radiographically distinctive and can simulate chondrosarcoma because of the presence of enlarged, bizarre, and binucleated chondrocytes.[270,272]

Subungual exostoses (Dupuytren's exostoses) are usually located on the great toe. They are thought to represent a different entity from osteochondromas but also are composed of a proliferating cartilaginous cap that merges into mature trabecular bone at its base. They may recur but are invariably benign.[269,271]

Chondroblastoma

Chondroblastoma occurs predominantly in males under 20 years of age. It usually arises in the epiphyseal end of long bones before the epiphyseal cartilage has disappeared, particularly in the distal end of the femur, proximal end of the humerus, and proximal end of the tibia[293] (Figs. 24-43 and 24-44). Occasionally, it is found in a metaphyseal location or in a small bone.[275]

Radiographically, the tumor usually is fairly well delimited and contains areas of rarefaction. From the epiphysis it may extend into the metaphyseal area or the articular cavity.[296]

Microscopically, this lesion often is confusing because of its extreme cellularity and variability. The occasional scattered collections of giant cells may lead to an erroneous diagnosis of giant cell tumor. The basic tumor cell is an embryonic chondroblast without sufficient differentiation to produce intercellular chondroid. The shape of this cell is usually polyhedral, although spindle elements can also be present. The cell membrane appears thick and sharply defined. The nuclei vary in shape from round to indented and lobulated; some resemble those of Langerhans' cells.[286] Mitoses are exceptional. Intracytoplasmic glycogen granules are present, sometimes in large numbers. Reticulin fibers surround each individual cell. Recurrent lesions may

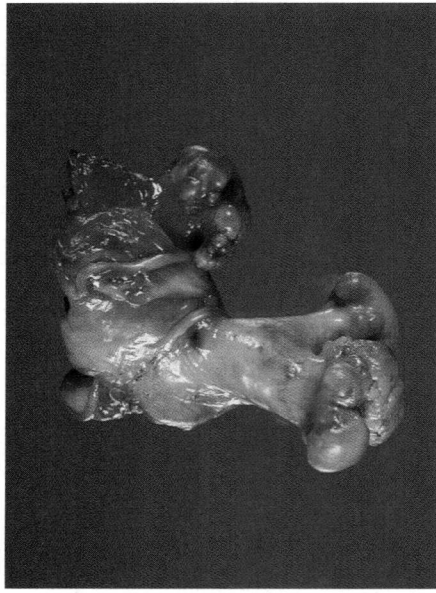

Fig. 24-41 Large osteochondroma of femur with a bilobed appearance.

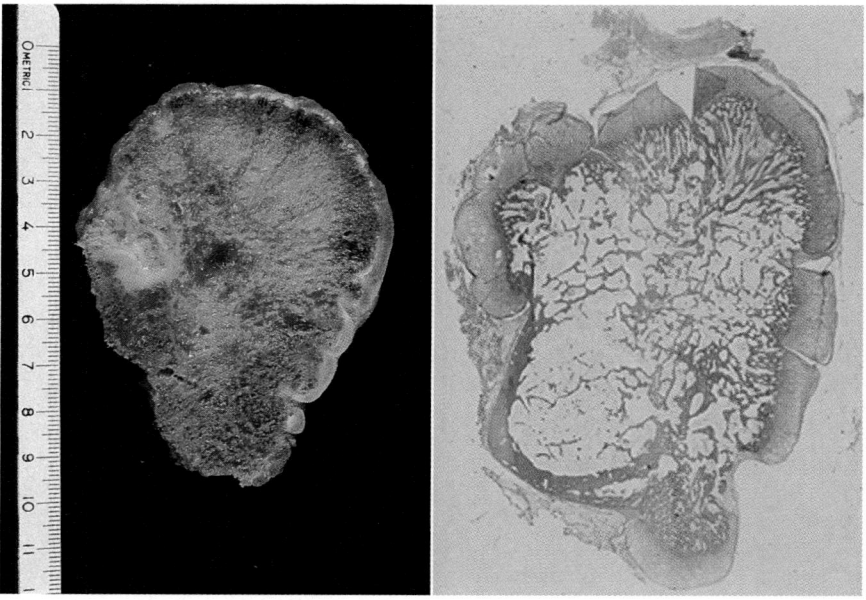

Fig. 24-42 Gross and whole-mount appearance of osteochondroma. Mature bone is covered by a well-differentiated cartilaginous cap.

show some degree of atypia, a feature that should not be interpreted as a sign of malignant change. A distinctive microscopic change is the presence of small zones of focal calcification (Fig. 24-45). These zones range from a network of thin lines ("chicken wire") to obvious deposits surrounded by giant cells.

In approximately one fourth of the cases, areas resembling aneurysmal bone cyst are seen engrafted on the primary bone lesion.[293] In patients with recurrent lesions, the incidence of this phenomenon rises to 50%.

By electron microscopy, the cells of chondroblastoma closely resemble normal epiphyseal cartilage cells grown in tissue culture.[294,297] They often have a prominent "fibrous lamina" lying against the inner aspect of the nuclear membrane, resulting in the membrane thickening seen by light microscopy.[282] Cytoplasmic glycogen is usually abundant. Proteoglycans and calcium have been demonstrated by ultrastructural cytochemistry in the extracellular matrix.[287] Immunohistochemically, the cells of osteoblastoma coexpress vimentin and S-100 protein. They may also be immunoreactive for neuron-specific enolase and low-molecular-weight keratins.[292]

The histogenesis of chondroblastoma has been controversial. It has been variously regarded as a "chondromatous" variant of giant cell tumor,[278] as arising from histiocytic or "reticuloendothelial cells," and as a truly cartilaginous neo-plasm. The frequent areas of calcification, the occasional foci of well-developed cartilaginous stroma, the histochemical and ultrastructural profile, and the immunohistochemical positivity for S-100 protein all point toward a cartilaginous nature.[277,281,286-289]

Clinically, patients with this lesion have pain that may become severe.[293] The diagnosis is possible on the basis of fine-needle aspiration material, which in a typical case will consist of neoplastic chondroblasts, multinucleated osteoclast-like giant cells, and chondroid matrix fragments.[280] Curettement with bone grafting, which is the preferred treatment, provides local control in over 80% of the cases.[279] Local recurrences can be treated similarly.[295]

Several cases of chondroblastoma, microscopically indistinguishable from the rest, have behaved locally in an aggressive fashion, invading the soft tissues and developing tumor thrombi in lymph channels. Most of these aggressive tumors were located in the pelvis.[290] A few others have given rise to distant metastases, usually to the lungs.[276,283,285] In nearly all of the reported cases of this phenomenon, the metastases have occurred after surgical manipulation of the primary tumor.[284,285,291]

Chondromyxoid fibroma and related tumors

Chondromyxoid fibroma of bone is an unusual benign tumor of cartilaginous origin.[301,302] It usually occurs in a

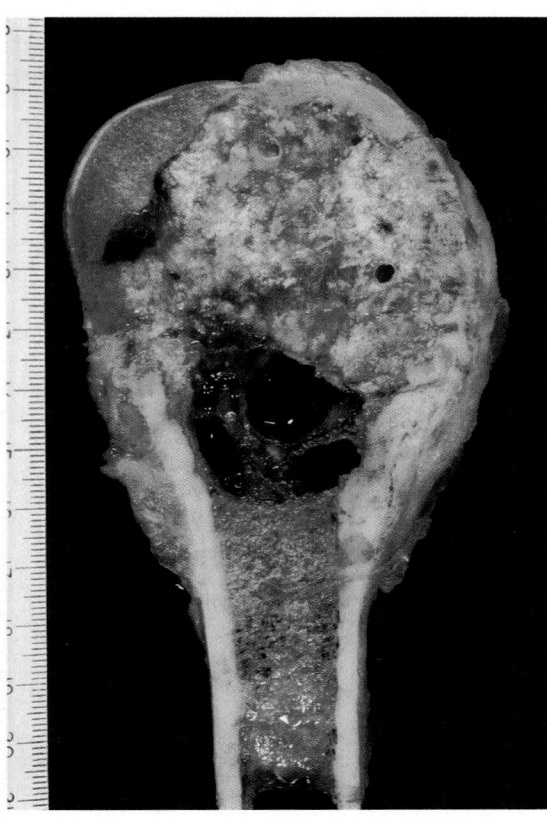

Fig. 24-43 Gross appearance of chondroblastoma of upper end of the humerus, associated with aneurysmal bone cyst-like changes.

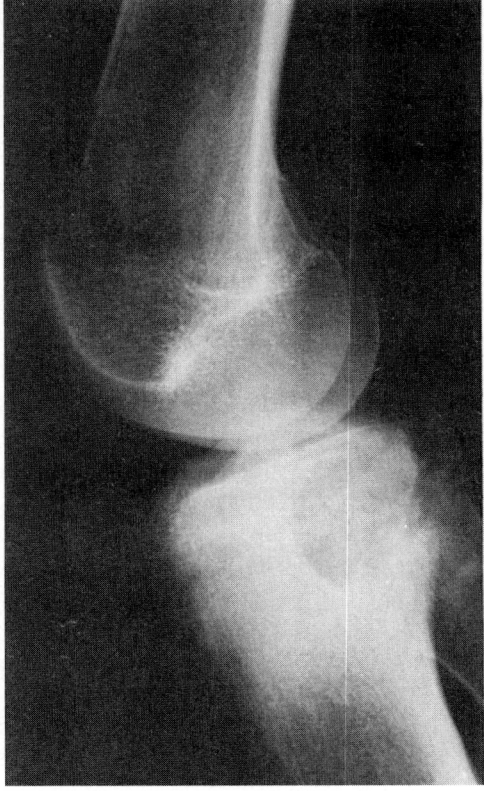

Fig. 24-44 Chondroblastoma of epiphysis of tibia in young man.

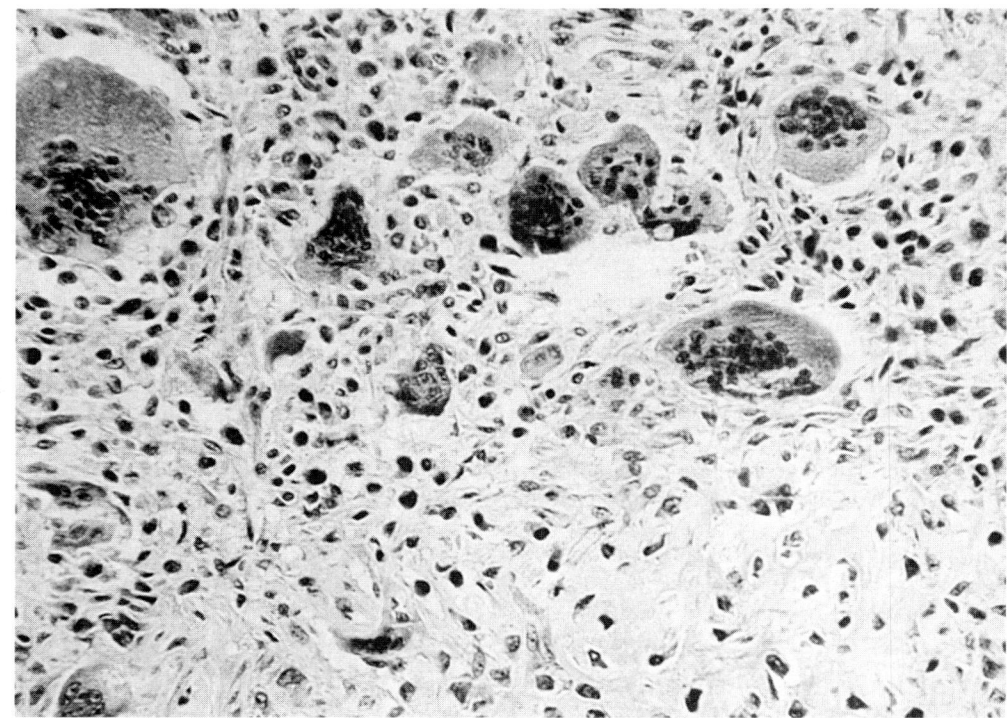

Fig. 24-45 Chondroblastoma showing small cuboidal tumor cells, osteoclasts, and areas of chondroid differentiation.

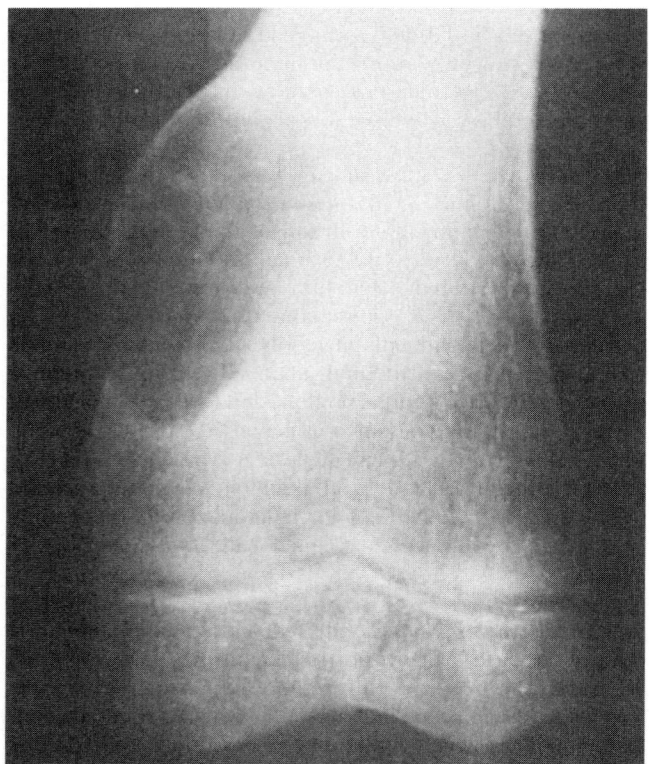

Fig. 24-46 Sharply delimited chondromyxoid fibroma of lower femoral metaphysis in young boy.

long bone of a young adult, but it has also been reported in the small bones of the hands and feet, pelvis, ribs, and vertebrae.

Radiographically, it is sharply defined and may attain a large size (Fig. 24-46). Grossly, it is solid and yellowish white or tan, replaces bone, and thins the cortex. Microscopically, it comprises hypocellular lobules with a myxochondroid appearance, separated by intersecting bands of highly cellular tissue composed of fibroblast-like spindle cells and osteoclasts[300] (Fig. 24-47, *A*).

The occasional presence of large pleomorphic cells may result in an erroneous diagnosis of chondrosarcoma.[307,308] However, mitotic figures are exceptional. Some tumors show a combination of the features of chondroblastoma and chondromyxoid fibroma.[299]

Immunohistochemical reactivity for S-100 protein is the rule, in keeping with its presumed cartilaginous nature.[298]

Local recurrence follows curettage of chondromyxoid fibroma in about 25% of the cases. Because of this, en bloc excision is recommended whenever possible. Soft tissue extension or implantation may occur,[303,308] but distant metastases have not been reported (Fig. 24-47, *B*).

Fibromyxoma is microscopically similar to chondromyxoid fibroma but lacks cartilaginous areas and tends to occur in older individuals.[304,305]

Myxoma of long bones is characterized by an expansile radiographic appearance, distal location, benign behavior, and microscopic appearance similar to soft tissue myxoma.[306]

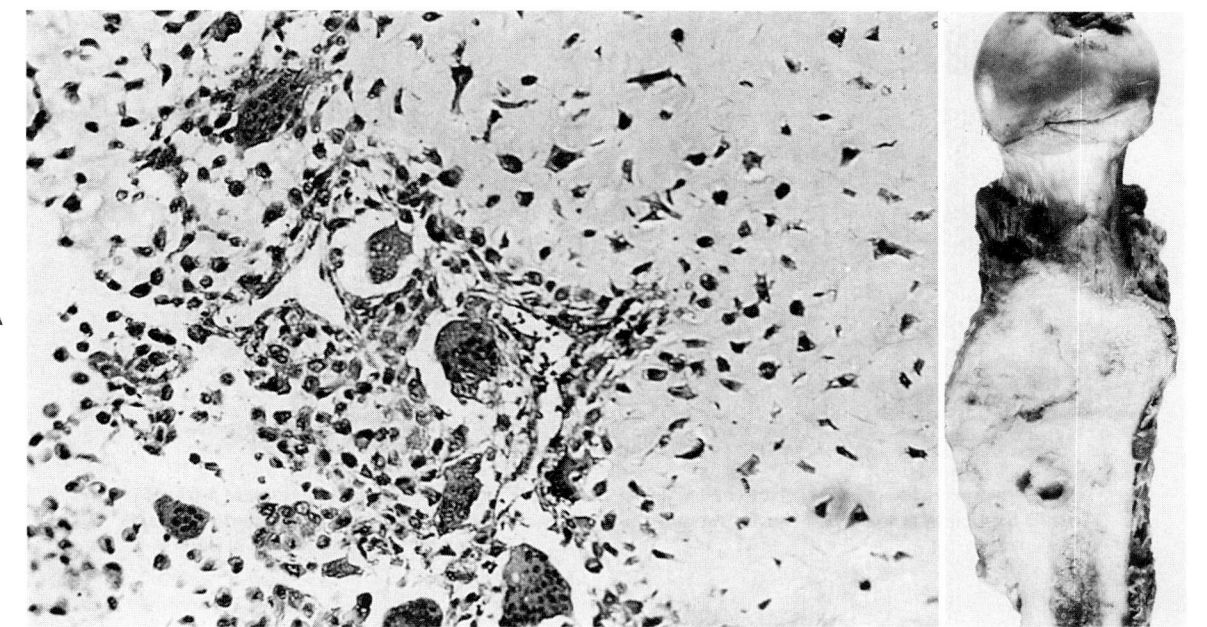

Fig. 24-47 A, Chondromyxoid fibroma showing giant cells, cartilage, and cellular zones. **B,** Chondromyxoid fibroma of proximal femur extending into soft tissue. This rare event should not be regarded as evidence of malignancy.

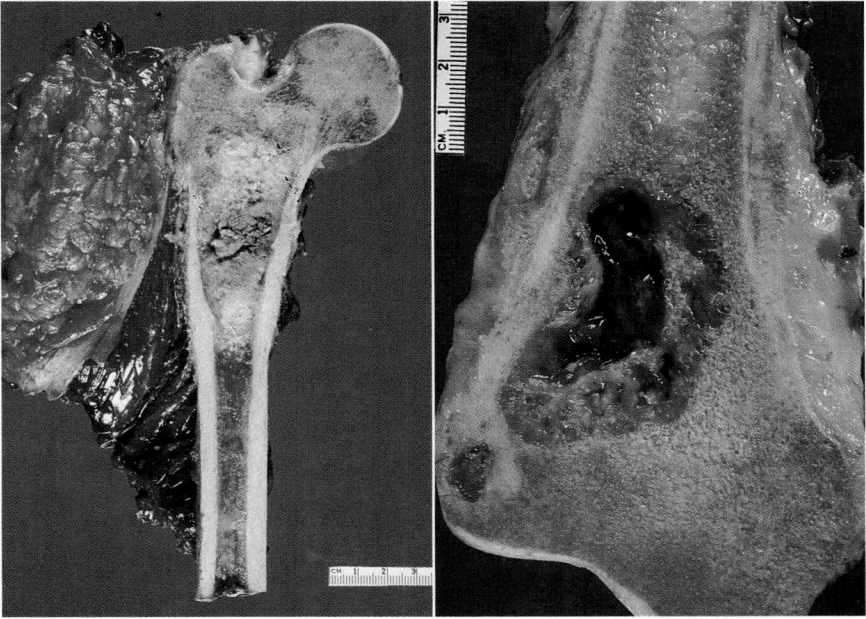

Fig. 24-48 Gross appearances of central chondrosarcoma. Both tumors were located in the femur.

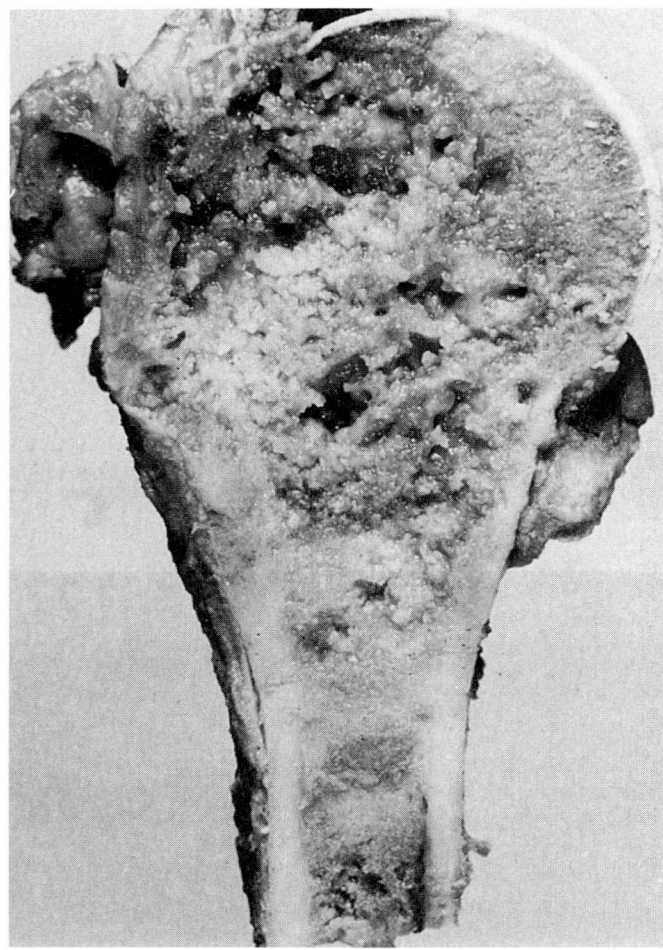

Fig. 24-49 Chondrosarcoma of head of humerus.

Chondrosarcoma

Chondrosarcoma, a malignant tumor of cartilage-forming tissues, is divided into two major categories on the basis of microscopic criteria: conventional chondrosarcoma and chondrosarcoma variants. Each of these categories comprises several distinct types, some defined on microscopic grounds and others on the basis of location within the affected bone.

Conventional chondrosarcoma. The majority of the patients with conventional chondrosarcoma are between 30 and 60 years of age. Chondrosarcoma in childhood is distinctly uncommon[347] and tends more often to be located in the extremities than its adult counterpart[323]; most malignant bone tumors in this age group exhibiting cartilage formation are actually osteosarcomas with a predominant cartilaginous component.

Chondrosarcomas are divided according to location into central, peripheral, and juxtacortical (periosteal) forms.[312] *Central chondrosarcomas* are located in the medullary cavity, usually of a flat or long bone (Figs. 24-48 and 24-49). Radiographically, they present a rather characteristic picture of an osteolytic lesion with splotchy calcification (Fig. 24-50). Ill-defined margins, fusiform thickening of the shaft,

and perforation of the cortex are three important diagnostic signs.[310] In advanced stages, they may break through the cortex but only rarely grow beyond the periosteum. The pelvic bones, ribs (usually at the costochondral junction), and shoulder girdle are the most common locations. Chondrosarcomas of the small bones of the hands and feet are exceptional but have been described by several authors, particularly in the os calcis.[316,328] Chondrosarcoma can also involve the bones of the skull, especially the temporal bone, where the differential diagnosis includes chordoma, meningioma, and glomus jugulare tumor.[314]

Peripheral chondrosarcomas may arise de novo or from the cartilaginous cap of a pre-existing osteochondroma (Fig. 24-51). Osteochondromatosis is particularly prone to this complication, as already indicated. In the 212 cases of chondrosarcoma reported by Dahlin and Henderson,[315] 19 apparently arose from osteochondroma. The risk of malignant transformation in a solitary osteochondroma is believed to be between 1% and 2%. The signs of malignancy in an osteochondroma include increased growth during adolescence, a diameter over 8 cm, and a cartilaginous cap that is irregular and thicker than 3 cm. Radiographically, peripheral chondrosarcomas present as large tumors, with a heavily

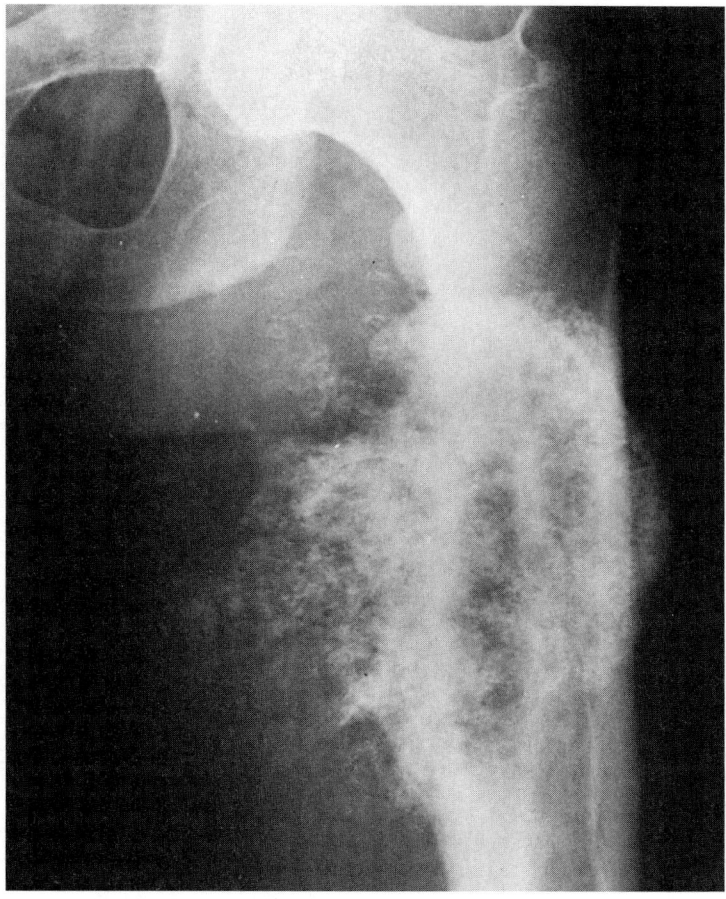

Fig. 24-50 Typical chondrosarcoma of femur showing splotchy calcification and extensive cortical destruction.

calcified center surrounded by a lesser denser periphery with splotchy calcification (Fig. 24-52). Malignant change should be suspected radiographically in an osteochondroma if the cartilage cap has irregular margins or if there are lucent zones within the lesion.[320]

Juxtacortical (periosteal) chondrosarcoma involves the shaft of a long bone (most often the femur) and is characterized by a cartilaginous lobular pattern with areas of spotty calcification and endochondral ossification.[343] This tumor is closely related to the entity reported as periosteal osteosarcoma (see p. 1942). However, some minor differences in location, microscopic grade, and behavior between the two have been described.[311]

Microscopically, conventional chondrosarcomas of central, peripheral, or juxtacortical types show a remarkably wide range of differentiation, the common denominator being the production of a cartilaginous matrix and the lack of direct bone formation by the tumor cells. This range in differentiation is the basis for the grading of these tumors into well, moderately, and poorly differentiated. The differential diagnosis between well-differentiated chondrosar-

coma and chondroma rests on a combination of radiographic, architectural, and cytologic features.[329,344] In well-differentiated chondrosarcoma, the nuclei are plump and hyperchromatic; there may be two or more nuclei per cell and two or more cells per lacuna (Fig. 24-53). Mirra et al.[336] have emphasized permeation of the bone marrow with trapping of host lamellar bone on all sides in well-differentiated chondrosarcoma as an important sign in the differential diagnosis with chondroma. Both the nuclear and architectural abnormalities of chondrosarcoma are often better seen at the growing edge of the tumor. Correlation of the microscopic features with the clinical and especially the radiographic findings is essential. Large tumors of the long bones or ribs or those that begin to grow rapidly over adolescence and reach a size of 8 cm or more are almost invariably malignant.[333] Minor degrees of atypia in the cartilaginous cells under these circumstances justify a diagnosis of chondrosarcoma, whereas similar or even greater atypical changes in cartilaginous tumors of the hands and feet, osteochondromas, synovial osteochondromatosis, and soft tissue neoplasms are much less significant.[329] It also should be

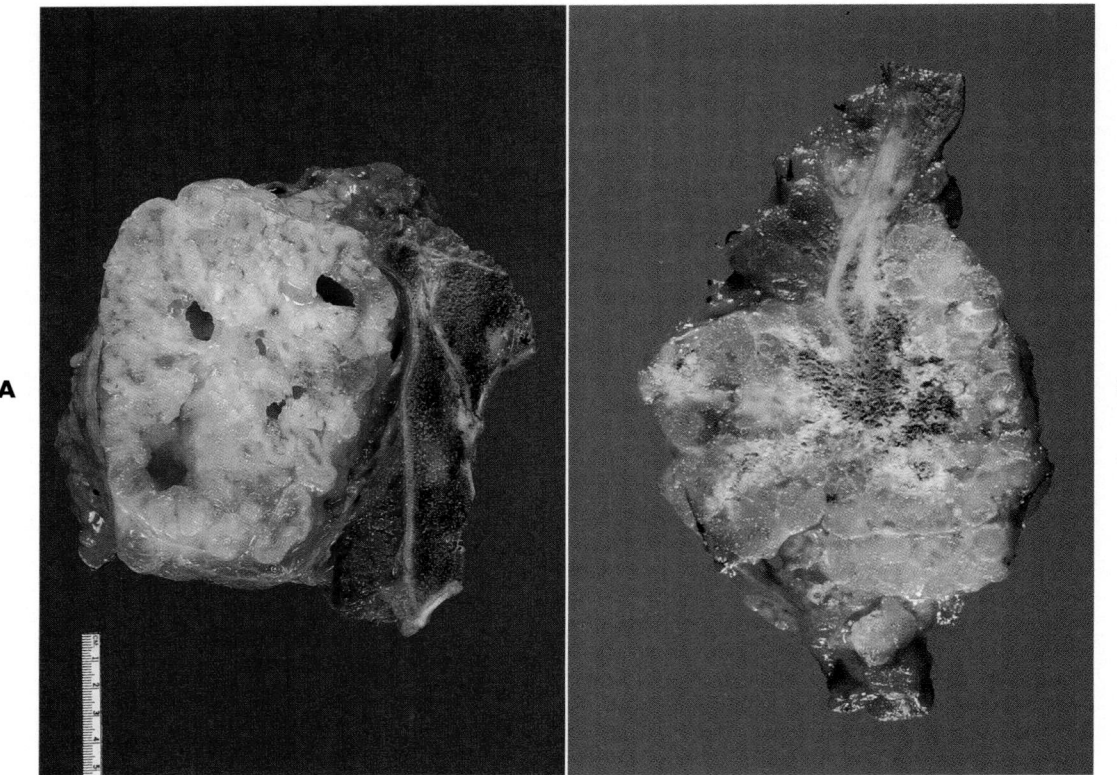

Fig. 24-51 Gross appearance of chondrosarcoma. **A,** Peripheral chondrosarcoma of femur resulting in a huge exophytic mass. **B,** Large expansile chondrosarcoma of sternum. (**A** courtesy Dr. Juan José Segura, San José, Costa Rica.)

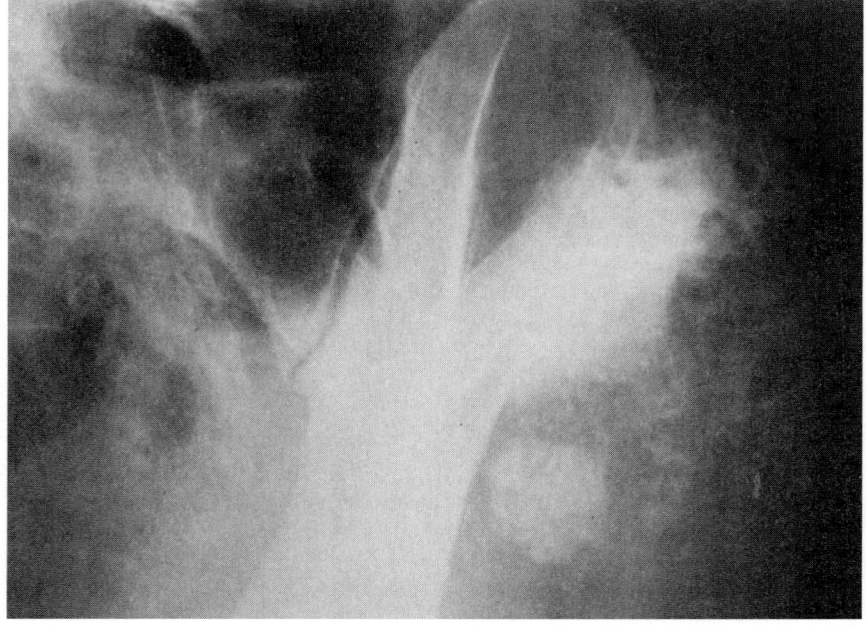

Fig. 24-52 Typical radiographic appearance of peripheral chondrosarcoma of innominate bone. (Courtesy Dr. W.T. Hill, Houston.)

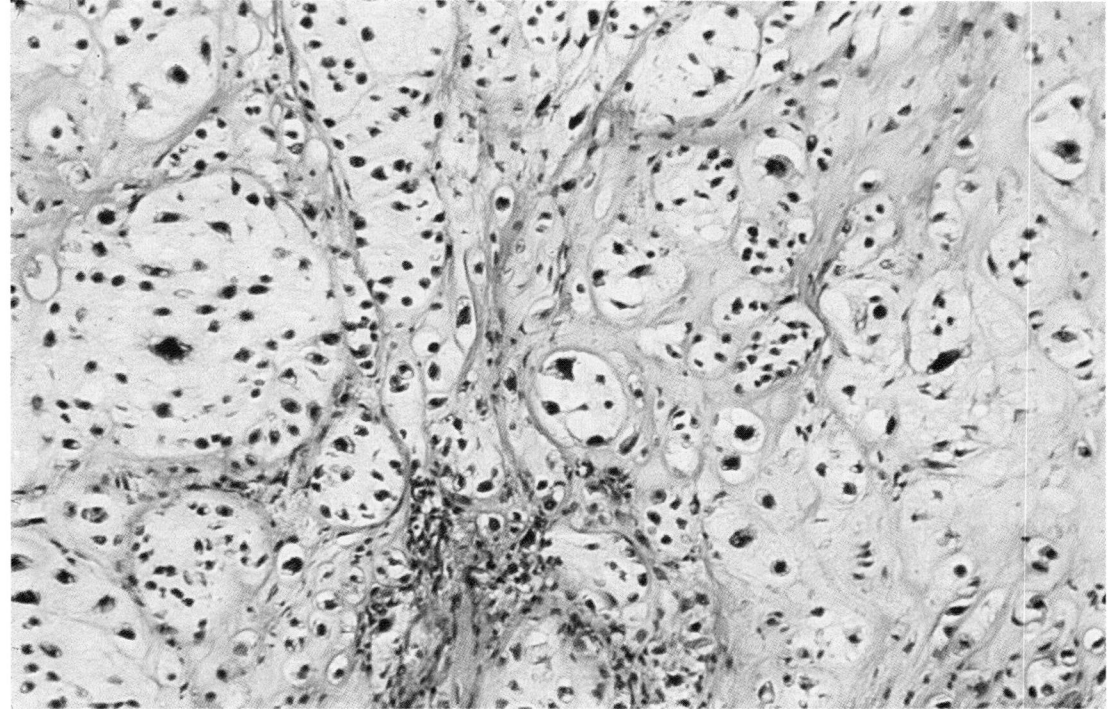

Fig. 24-53 Microscopic appearance of well-differentiated chondrosarcoma. The tumor retains a lobulated appearance, but nuclear atypicality is obvious.

noted that the minor atypical changes on which the diagnosis of malignancy are based are often focal, a point to remember when examining a small sample of a cartilaginous neoplasm.

Chondrosarcoma is distinguished from osteosarcoma by the lack of direct osteoid or bone formation by the tumor cells. Bone can be present in a bona fide chondrosarcoma, but this is non-neoplastic and probably originates from reabsorption of the tumor cartilage by a mechanism of endochondral ossification.

Histochemically, well-differentiated chondrosarcomas have a staining reaction similar to that of adult cartilage, whereas poorly differentiated tumors resemble fetal cartilage.[324] Biochemically, a marked variability in composition has been observed.[331,332] Ultrastructurally, the cells of well-differentiated tumors show cytoplasmic accumulation of glycogen, lipid droplets, and dilated cisternae of granular endoplasmic reticulum.[318] Immunohistochemically, there is reactivity for S-100 protein[337,338] (Fig. 24-54).

Cytogenetically, there is considerable heterogeneity among chondrosarcomas but also evidence that some of the karyotypic anomalies are not random.[330]

Amplification of the c-*myc* oncogene and expression of the c-*erb*B-2 oncogene have been detected in chondrosarcomas.[313,346] Overexpression of p53 is limited to the high-grade (poorly differentiated) types.[317]

Soft tissue implantation following biopsy is a well-known complication of chondrosarcoma. Therefore if a large carti-

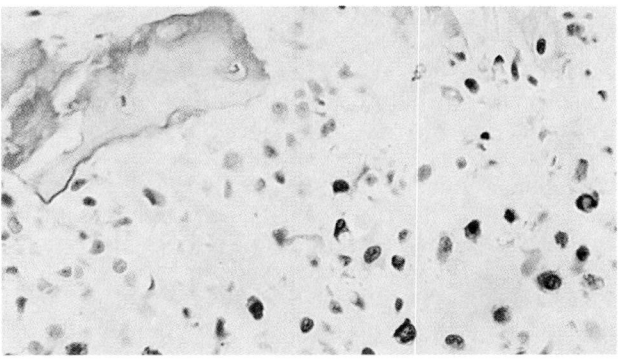

Fig. 24-54 Chondrosarcoma of bone. There is both cytoplasmic and nuclear staining for S-100 protein.

laginous tumor is so located that the biopsy site cannot be entirely excised, the initial excision should be complete. If an extremely large tumor involves the pelvic bone, wide block excision or even hemipelvectomy is justified without prior histologic diagnosis. In about 90% of the patients cured by hemipelvectomy, the tumor was a chondrosarcoma.[340] Chondrosarcomas of the rib should be excised en bloc with the adjacent uninvolved ribs and pleura.[334,335,339] Well-differentiated chondrosarcomas of the extremities are amenable to conservative therapy in the form of segmental resection.[345]

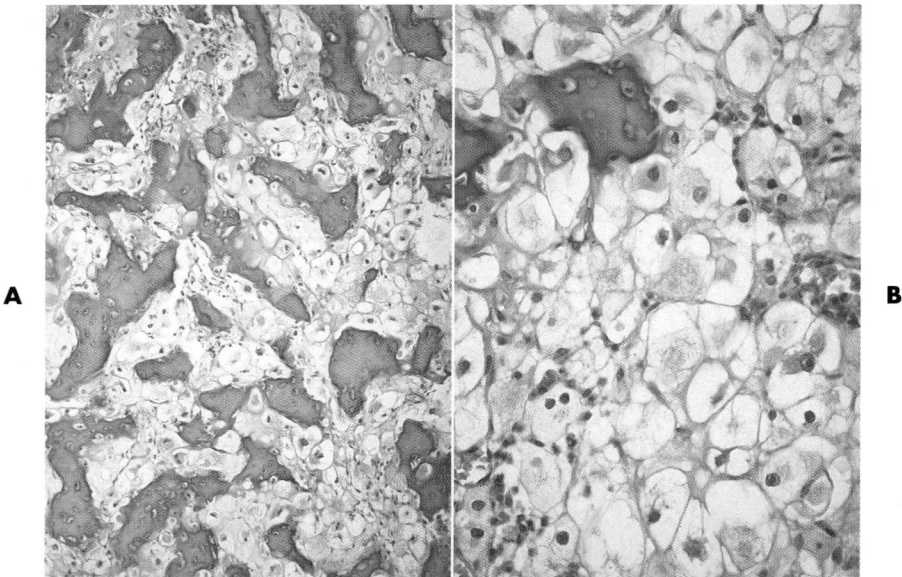

Fig. 24-55 Clear cell chondrosarcoma. **A,** Low-power appearance showing numerous bone trabeculae that may result in a mistaken diagnosis of osteosarcoma. **B,** High-power view showing plump and vacuolated appearance of the tumor cells. S-100 protein was strongly immunoreactive.

In contrast to osteosarcoma, microscopic grading of chondrosarcomas, whether done by a combination of cytoarchitectural features[319,340] or by nuclear grade alone,[326] is of value in predicting the final outcome. In the series reported by McKenna et al.,[335] the 5-year survival rates were 78%, 53%, and 22% for low-, moderate-, and high-grade tumors, respectively. In three more recent series, the overall survival figures were generally better, but the differential between the three grades was still obvious.[319,321,322,341,342] Recurrences often are of a higher microscopic grade than the original tumor.[327] Equally important prognostically is the adequacy of initial therapy.[321] Preliminary results with flow cytometry suggest that determination of DNA ploidy may be an important prognostic determinator.[309,325] High-grade chondrosarcomas metastasize early, particularly to the lungs. Lymph node metastases are practically nonexistent.

Chondrosarcoma variants

Clear cell chondrosarcoma. Clear cell chondrosarcoma is characterized by tumor cells with an abundant clear or ground glass cytoplasm and sharply defined borders, often interspersed with small trabeculae of woven bone. It may be confused with chondroblastoma and may actually represent its malignant counterpart[350] (Fig. 24-55). Ultrastructurally, it shows chondroid cells in various stages of differentiation[349] and, immunohistochemically, exhibits S-100 protein reactivity.[351,352] Most patients are older than those affected by chondroblastoma.[348] Radiographically, the lesion is usually entirely lytic, slightly expansile, and sharply marginated.[348] Most of the cases have involved the proximal end of the femur or humerus, and the behavior has been that of a low-grade malignancy.

Myxoid chondrosarcoma (chordoid sarcoma). This variant of chondrosarcoma can occur in bone or—more commonly —in soft tissue (see Chapter 25). It is morphologically reminiscent of chordoma because of the rows of cuboidal cells separated by a myxoid background.[354] It reacts immunohistochemically for S-100 protein and vimentin but, in contrast to chordoma, is negative for keratin.[355] Ultrastructurally, it is closer in appearance to conventional chondrosarcoma than to chordoma.[356] Whether the tumor reported by Dabska[353] as **parachordoma** is also histogenetically related to myxoid chondrosarcoma remains to be determined.[357]

Dedifferentiated chondrosarcoma. The term dedifferentiated chondrosarcoma refers to the presence of a poorly differentiated sarcomatous component at the periphery of an otherwise typical low-grade chondrosarcoma.[361,366] The chondrosarcoma is usually of the central type, but it can also be peripheral.[359] The dedifferentiation can be found in the initial lesion but occurs more often in specimens from recurrent tumor. The microscopic appearance of this component may be that of malignant fibrous histiocytoma, rhabdomyosarcoma, fibrosarcoma, osteosarcoma, or undifferentiated sarcoma[364] (Fig. 24-56). As such, it is phenotypically different from the pre-existing chondrosarcoma. Accordingly, these areas may acquire immunohistochemical positivity for alpha-1-antichymotrypsin, actin, desmin, myoglobin, and exceptionally even keratin.[362,369] In some cases, however, there is some ultrastructural and immunohistochemical (S-100 protein) preservation of the cartilaginous character of the tumor in the anaplastic portion.[358,363] Simultaneous cytogenetic and immunophenotyping studies indicate that both the differentiated and the "dedifferentiated" components originate from a common primitive mesenchymal cell progenitor, and that the term "dedifferentiated" may be an inaccurate designation.[360]

Regardless of terminology, the development of this component in chondrosarcoma is accompanied by a marked

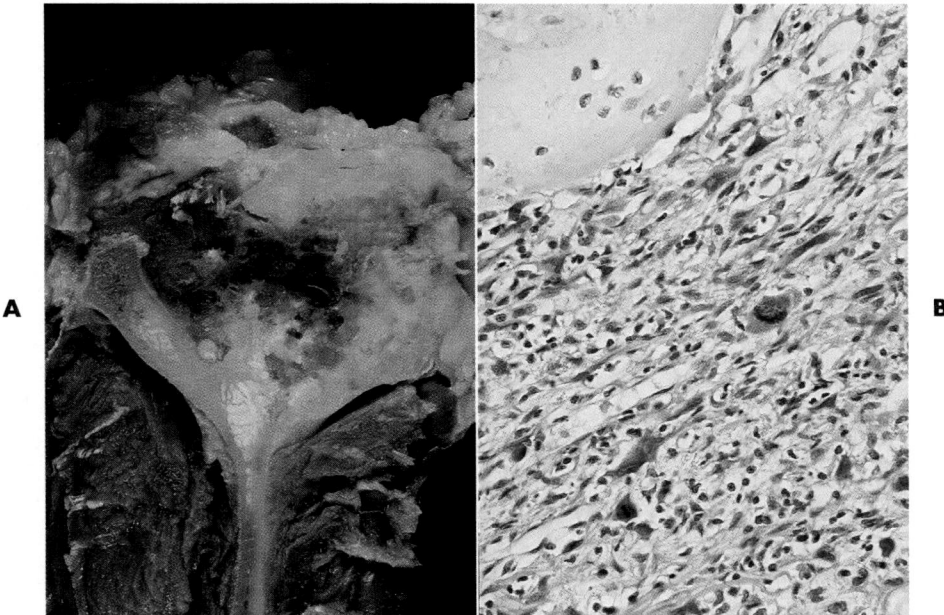

Fig. 24-56 Dedifferentiated chondrosarcoma of pelvic bone. **A,** Gross appearance. **B,** Microscopic appearance. The edge of an island of well-differentiated cartilage *(upper left)* is surrounded by highly pleomorphic sarcoma containing tumor giant cells.

acceleration of the clinical course and a decidedly worsened prognosis.[365,367,368]

Mesenchymal chondrosarcoma. Mesenchymal chondrosarcoma is a specific variant of chondrosarcoma characterized microscopically by a dimorphic pattern, areas of well-differentiated cartilage alternating with undifferentiated stroma[370,372,379,380] (Fig. 24-57). The boundaries between the two components are usually abrupt. The undifferentiated element is composed of small cells and can be confused with malignant lymphoma and hemangiopericytoma. It should be noted that despite the apparently undifferentiated nature of this component at both the light and electron microscopic level, pleomorphism and mitotic activity are remarkably inconspicuous.[380,381] Immunohistochemically, the small cell component is positive for vimentin and Leu7 but not for S-100 protein; the latter is found instead in the chondroid areas.[382]

Most patients are in the second or third decade of life. The radiographic appearance resembles that of conventional chondrosarcomas. The bones most commonly affected are the jaw, pelvis, femur, ribs, and spine.[379] A high percentage of these neoplasms involve extraosseous structures, such as the orbit, paraspinal region, meninges, or soft tissues of the extremities.[374,375] The prognosis is generally poor, although there is great variability in the clinical course.[376,380]

It has been proposed that mesenchymal chondrosarcoma represents a neoplastic caricature of embryonal endochondral osteogenesis.[371] Jacobson[377] postulated that mesenchymal chondrosarcoma is simply one morphologic type of the bone tumor that he proposes to call *polyhistioma.* He defines it as a malignant neoplasm whose basic cells are small and round, like those of Ewing's sarcoma, but that differentiate into various mesenchymal structures, such as bone and car-

tilage, and sometimes even into epithelial tissues. Additional case reports have confirmed the existence of multipotential bone tumors composed of a mixture of mesenchymal (chondrosarcoma) and epithelial (squamous cell carcinoma) elements.[373,378]

Giant cell tumor

Giant cell tumor (osteoclastoma) is usually seen in patients over 20 years of age.[391] It is more common in women than in men and seems to occur more frequently in Oriental than in Western countries.[426]

The classic location is the epiphysis of a long bone, from which it may spread into the metaphyseal area, break through the cortex, invade intermuscular septa, or even cross a joint space. The sites most commonly affected (in order of frequency) are the lower end of the femur, the upper end of the tibia, and the lower end of the radius.[391] It also occurs in the humerus, fibula, and skull, particularly the sphenoid bone.[388,394,429] Occasionally, a giant cell tumor will be seen in a child[415] and/or in a metaphyseal or diaphyseal location.[396,414] Involvement of the bones of the hands and feet, jaw, and vertebrae (other than sacrum) is distinctly unusual. Although giant cell tumor has been documented at these sites,[422,428] the occurrence of a giant cell–containing lesion in any of these locations should suggest an alternative diagnosis.

Radiographically, the typical appearance of a giant cell tumor is that of an entirely lytic, expansile lesion in the epiphysis, usually without peripheral bone sclerosis or periosteal reaction (Fig. 24-58, *A*).

Grossly, the size of the tumor varies considerably; when large, it may be associated with a pathologic fracture. The cut surface is solid and tan or light brown, traversed by

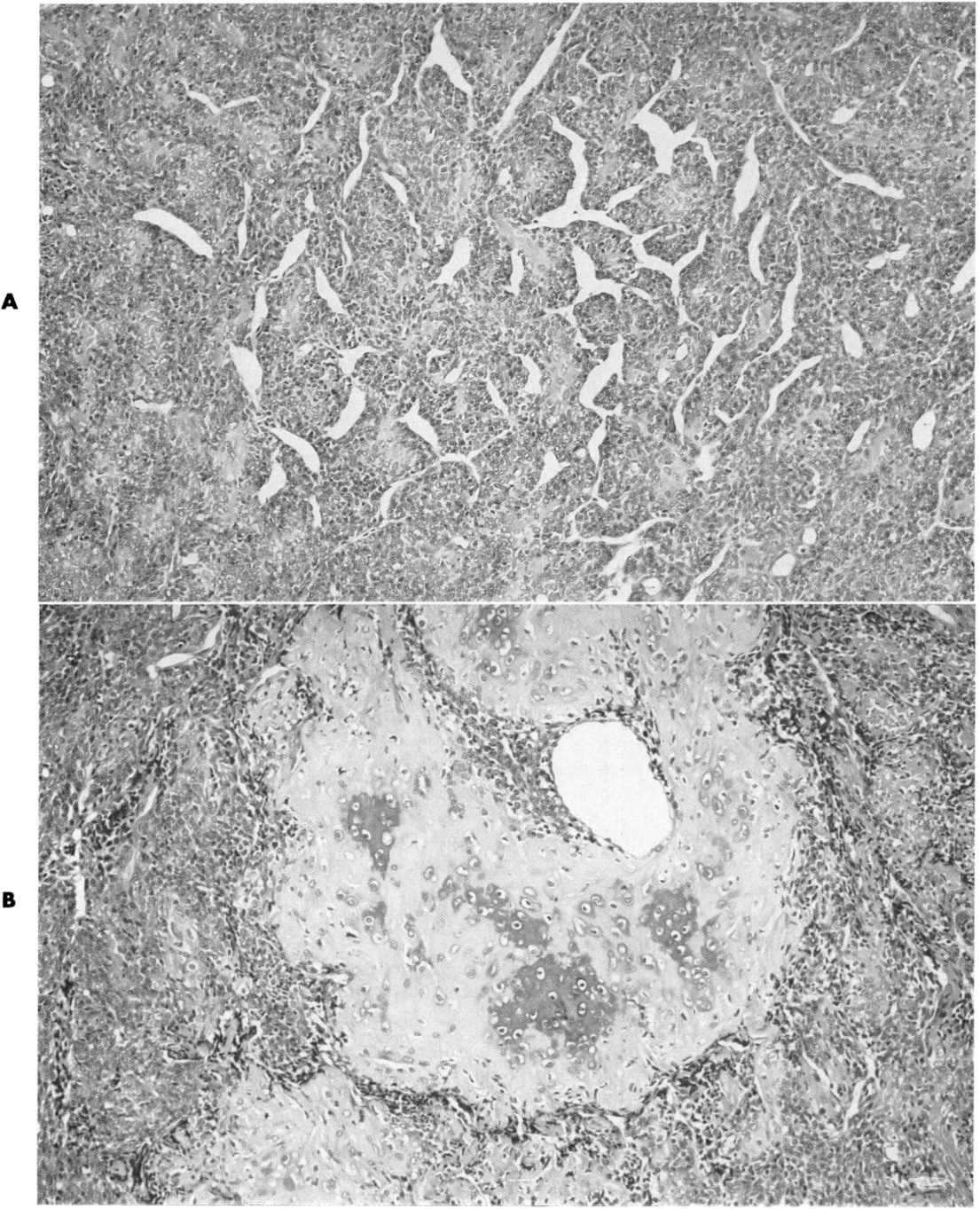

Fig. 24-57 Mesenchymal chondrosarcoma. **A** illustrates cellular, hemangiopericytoma-like component. **B** shows an island of relatively well-differentiated cartilage in the center.

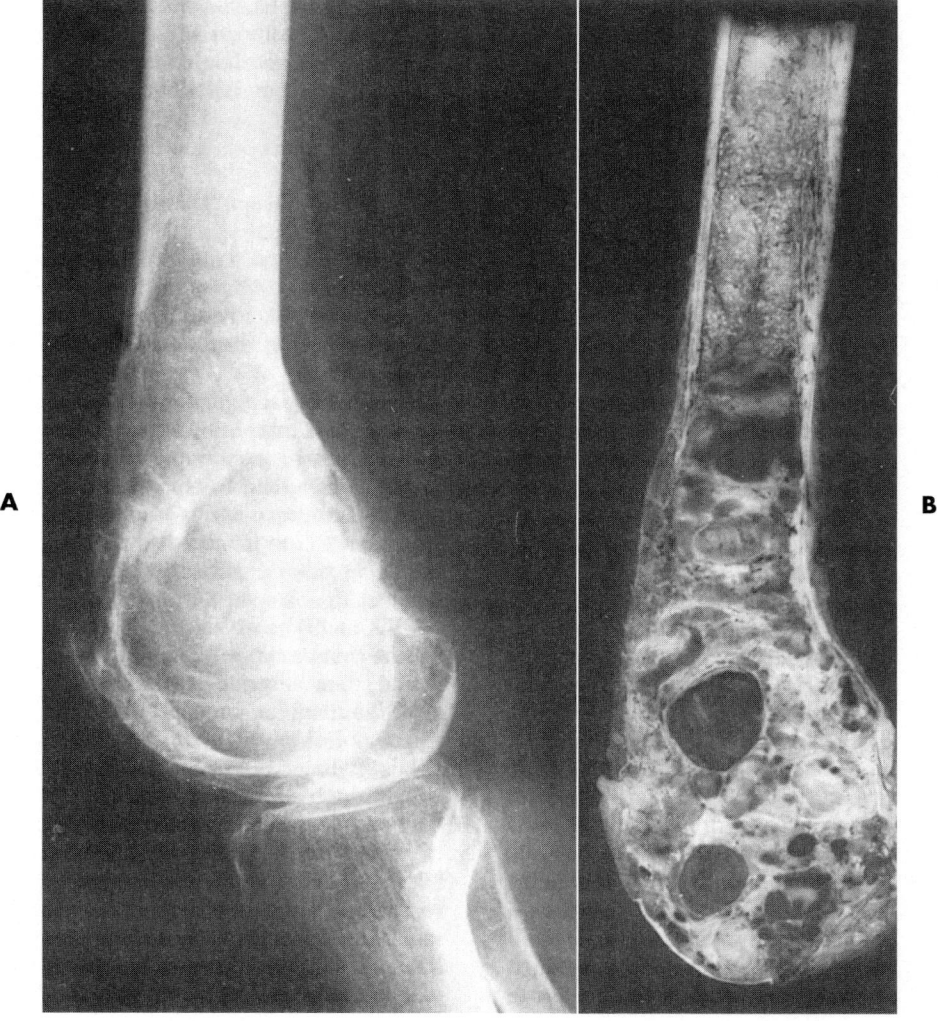

Fig. 24-58 A, Typical radiograph of giant cell tumor of distal end of femur involving epiphysis and metaphyseal area. Lesion was resected surgically. **B,** Gross specimen that faithfully reproduces changes. (From Sissons HA: Malignant tumors of bone and cartilage. In Raven RW, ed: Cancer, vol 2. London, 1958, Butterworth & Co, Ltd.)

fibrous trabeculae, and often contains hemorrhagic areas (Fig. 24-58, *B;* Fig. 2-9; and Plates XVII-E and XVII-F). The cortex is thinned, but periosteal new bone formation is rare.

Microscopically, the two main components of giant cell tumor are the so-called stromal cells and giant cells (Fig. 24-59). The giant cells are usually large and have over twenty or thirty nuclei, most of them arranged toward the center. They resemble osteoclasts at all levels: morphologic, ultrastructural (ruffled border and abundant mitochondria),[400,409,425] enzyme histochemical (abundant acid phosphatase and other hydrolytic enzymes),[430] and immunohistochemical (positivity for lysozyme, alpha-1-antitrypsin, alpha-1-antichymotrypsin, and other histiocytic markers)[386,406,417] (Fig. 24-60). They have also been found to contain receptors for calcitonin, a phenotypic marker for osteoclasts.[399] It is the prominence of these cells that gives the tumor its name. Yet, all evidence indicates that these are not

neoplastic elements but rather the result of fusion of circulating monocytes that have been recruited into the lesion, possibly through an autocrine or paracrine mechanism mediated by transforming growth factor–beta.[431]

By contrast, the mononuclear stromal cell is to be interpreted as neoplastic. It is the only proliferating element in the lesion (as demonstrated by autoradiographic studies)[419] and the one exhibiting atypia in the rare cytologically malignant examples of this tumor[401,411] (see later section). Parenthetically, these changes may be focal, rendering imperative a thorough sampling (Fig. 24-61).

The nature of the neoplastic stromal cell remains controversial. It is clearly mesenchymal rather than hematopoietic in nature, and the ultrastructural features resemble those of fibroblasts or osteoblasts.[383-385] That a close histogenetic relationship with osteoblasts exists is suggested by the fact that focal deposition of osteoid or bone is seen in one third

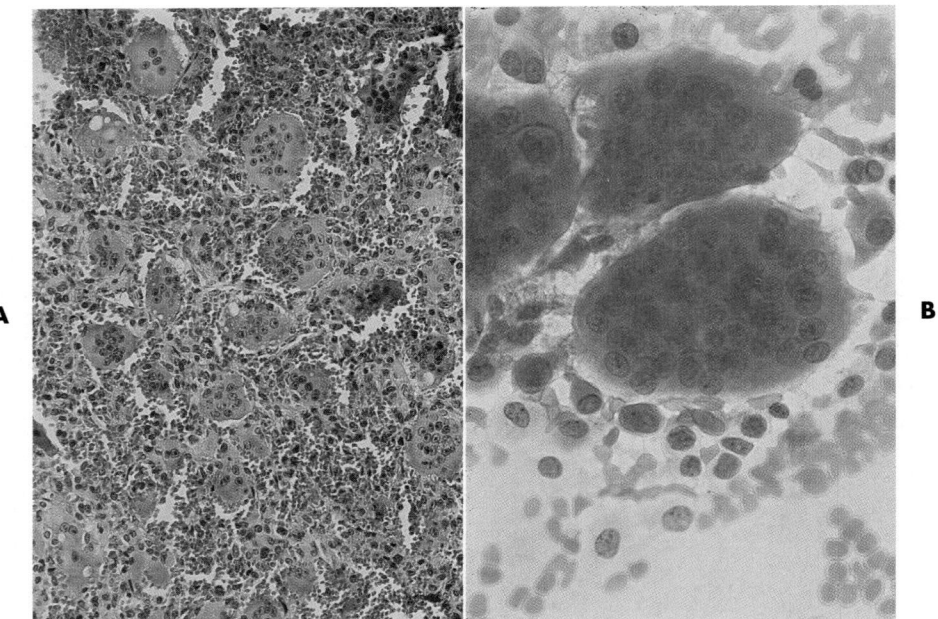

Fig. 24-59 Giant cell tumor of bone. **A,** Microscopic appearance. **B,** Cytologic preparation.

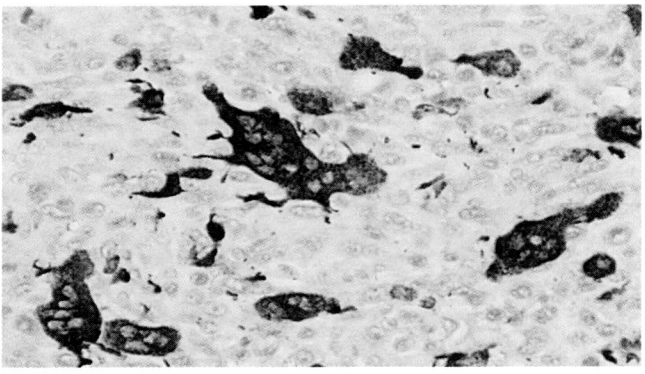

Fig. 24-60 Specimen from giant cell tumor of bone fixed in formalin and embedded in paraffin, stained for acid phosphatase (Duray's technique).

of the cases. This stromal cell produces types I and III collagen and has receptors for parathyroid hormone.[399] It does not express macrophage surface antigen, but it may contain lysozyme and alpha-1-antitrypsin.[389,395] Focal S-100 protein reactivity may also be present.[403] A provocative ultrastructural finding has been the presence of viral-like and other intranuclear inclusions in the cells of giant cell tumor, some of them being similar to those of Paget's disease of bone.[397,412,424]

Many benign lesions with giant cells have been diagnosed as giant cell tumor in the past. These lesions include entities such as metaphyseal fibrous defect and nonossifying fibroma, chondromyxoid fibroma, chondroblastoma, Langerhans' cell granulomatosis, solitary bone cyst, osteitis fibrosa cystica of hyperparathyroidism, aneurysmal bone cyst, osteoid osteoma, and osteoblastoma. So-called giant cell tumors of

tendon sheath are also unrelated to giant cell tumors of bone. One of the main microscopic differences between true giant cell tumor and these so-called variants resides in the spatial relationship between the giant and stromal cells. The former tend to be distributed regularly and uniformly in giant cell tumor, whereas in the lesions that simulate it, foci containing numerous, clumped giant cells alternate with large areas completely lacking this component. The giant cells themselves do not differ significantly in the two groups of disease, morphologically, histochemically, or immunohistochemically.[408,417,423] Statistically, those of giant cell tumor may be larger and have more nuclei than those of the other lesions, but there is enough overlap to render this feature of no differential value. Although exceptions to all of the following statements have been recorded, a diagnosis of a lesion other than giant cell tumor should be favored if (1) the patient is a child; (2) the lesion is located in the metaphysis or diaphysis of a long bone; (3) the lesion is multiple (except if a patient has Goltz's syndrome)[427]; and (4) the lesion is located in the vertebrae (other than sacrum), jaw (except for patients with Paget's disease), or bones of the hands or feet. The distinction is of clinical importance because of the better prognosis associated with most of the giant cell–containing lesions that simulate giant cell tumor.

The treatment of giant cell tumor should be surgical whenever technically feasible. It consists of curettage with bone grafting or en bloc excision with replacement with allograft or artificial material, depending on the location.[393,404,405,413] Special care should be taken to prevent implantation of the tumor into the adjoining soft tissues.

The use of radiation therapy should be reserved only for cases in which surgical removal is impossible, in view of the relatively high number of reported cases of malignant transformation following this therapeutic modality. As a matter

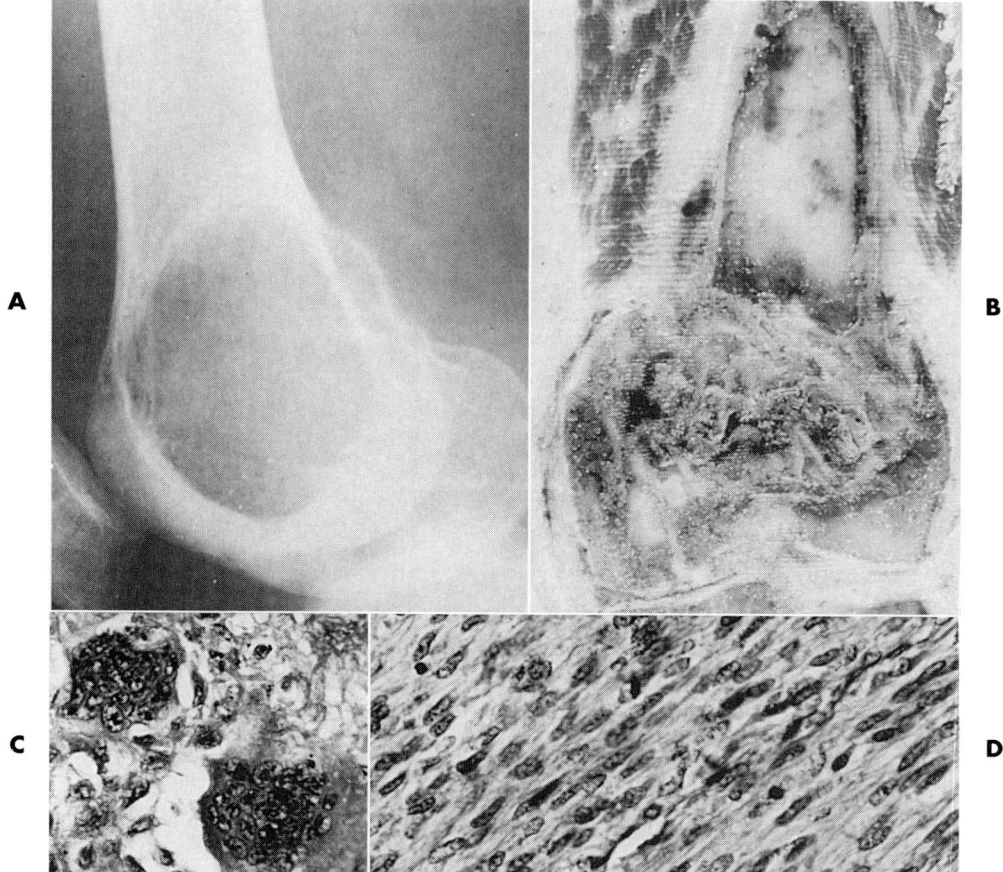

Fig. 24-61 A, Giant cell tumor of distal end of femur. Lesion was curetted and replaced with bone chips. **B,** Giant cell tumor shown in **A** recurred, necessitating amputation. Gross specimen demonstrates bone chips still in place with tumor replacing femur. Review of original sections showed benign giant cell tumor, but recuts of curetted material demonstrated malignant stroma. **C,** Original section of curettings referred to in **B** showing areas of rather innocuous-appearing stroma with typical multinucleated giant cells. These changes were called benign. **D,** Later tissue section of malignant giant cell tumor referred to in **B** and **C** that has appearance of fibrosarcoma. There was no evidence of osteoid formation. Patient died of pulmonary metastases.

of fact, review of series of postradiation sarcoma of bone shows that in a disproportionate number of cases the initial lesion was a giant cell tumor. Giant cell tumors of the spine have been traditionally treated with radiation therapy, but they are also amenable to surgical excision.[422]

The natural history of giant cell tumor is that of a low-grade malignancy. In most reported series, the incidence of clinical malignancy (expressed by uncontrollable local recurrence or metastases) has been in the range of 10%.[392,410] The type of initial surgical removal is the most significant factor in recurrence; in one large series, the recurrence rate was 34% following curettage and 7% following wide resection.[405] A good relation also exists between surgical stage and prognosis[416]; in one series all cases of metastasizing giant cell tumor were deemed to be stage III lesions, with interruption of the cortex and soft tissue extension.[387]

It is also of interest that nearly all cases of metastases of giant cell tumor have occurred after a surgical intervention to the primary tumor, suggesting the possibility of mechanical disruption with access to the bloodstream. However, no relationship has been found between the presence of giant cells in blood vessels and prognosis. Microscopic grading of giant cell tumors is not of great value except for the obviously sarcomatous (grade III) lesions.[420] Indeed, some of these metastases have occurred in tumors with an entirely benign microscopic appearance (1% to 2% of all cases), and the metastases themselves may have a very innocuous look[418]; those developing in the lung, which are by far the most common, are often surrounded by a rim of mature bone.

Nonrandom chromosomal abnormalities have been found in giant cell tumors, particularly in the form of telomeric fusions; these seem to be more common in the clinically more aggressive neoplasms.[390]

DNA ploidy analysis of giant cell tumors has not yet been shown to have prognostic value above and beyond that provided by the more conventional parameters.[398,402,421]

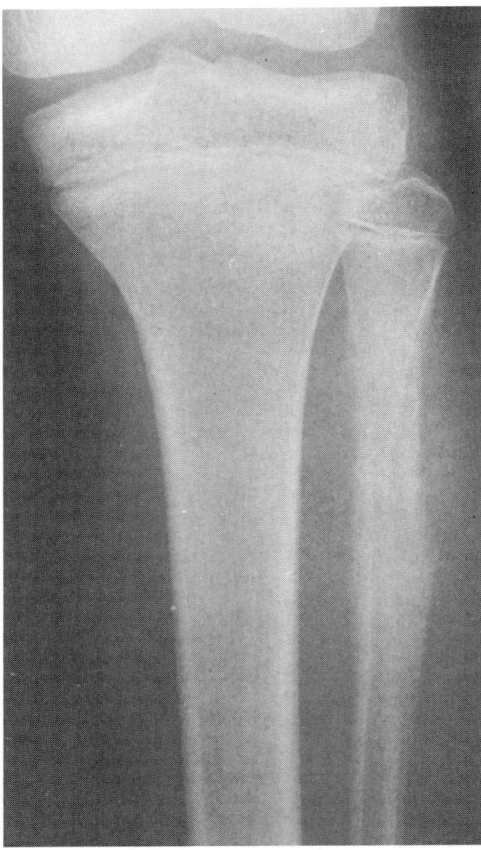

Fig. 24-62 Ewing's sarcoma of fibula. Growth is ill-defined and accompanied by prominent periosteal reaction.

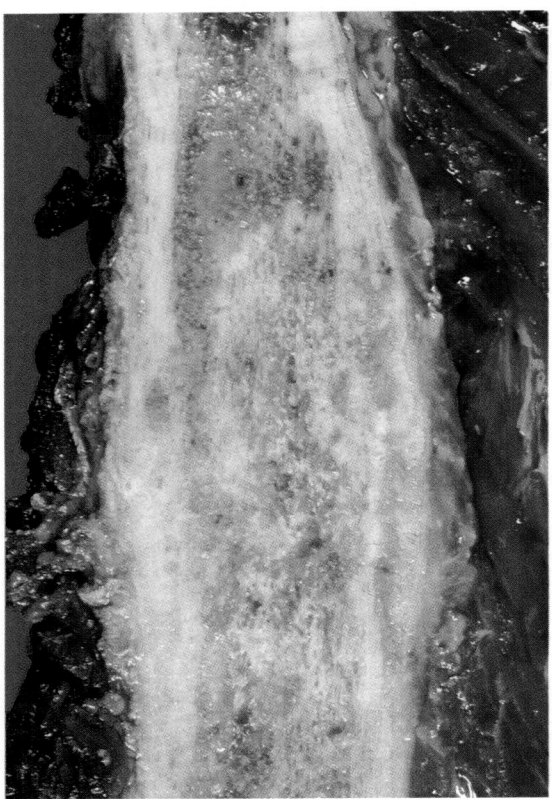

Fig. 24-63 Gross appearance of Ewing's sarcoma. It has a typical ill-defined quality, with extensive involvement of medulla and cortex associated with elevation of periosteum.

Malignant giant cell tumor

As already mentioned, all giant cell tumors of bone should be regarded as potentially low-grade malignancies because of their tendency to recur and their occasional capacity to metastasize regardless of histologic appearance. A contentious issue is the existence of a cytologically malignant giant cell tumor (i.e., a lesion that retains the clinical, topographic, and general microscopic features of giant cell tumor but that exhibits clear-cut evidence of malignancy in the mononuclear stromal component). As such, it is equivalent to a grade III giant cell tumor. It represents a most unusual process, part of the reason being the conceptual and practical difficulties in separating it from other malignant tumors, particularly so-called giant cell–rich osteosarcoma (when osteoid production is present) and malignant fibrous histiocytoma (when osteoid production is absent).

On occasion, a typical benign-appearing giant cell tumor is seen in combination with but sharply segregated from a high-grade sarcoma. This phenomenon has been referred to as dedifferentiation, in analogy to the situation occurring more commonly with chondrosarcoma and chordoma.[407]

Marrow tumors

Ewing's sarcoma

Ewing's sarcoma, originally described as a primary bone tumor of children, is now regarded as a member of the fam-ily of small round cell neoplasms of bone and soft tissue generically known as *primitive neuroectodermal tumor* (PNET), and characterized by a specific molecular alteration to be described later.[438,444,460,472,482] Some authors no longer make a terminologic distinction among the various tumor types within this family and refer to all of them as Ewing's sarcoma/PNET. Others prefer to retain the appellation of Ewing's sarcoma for the tumors of bone and/or those exhibiting no or only a minimal degree of differentiation along the neuroepithelial line (these two characteristics often coexisting) and to designate as PNET those tumors that are localized in the soft tissue and/or that exhibit more obvious evidence of neuroepithelial differentiation (these parameters also being often found together).[483,490] The overlap, however, is considerable, and this is reflected by terms such as extraskeletal Ewing's sarcoma and PNET of bone.[437,455,488,499,500] The link among these tumors is also demonstrated by the fact that neural differentiation can be induced in conventional Ewing's sarcomas by agents such as dibutyryl cyclic AMP and retinoic acid.[475]

Thus defined, Ewing's sarcoma of bone is usually seen in patients between the ages of 5 and 20 years,[459,493,502] with only a minority of cases presenting in infancy or adulthood.[467] The tumor may simulate clinically osteomyelitis because of pain, fever, and leukocytosis. It occurs most often in long bones (femur, tibia, humerus, and fibula) and in bones of the pelvis, rib, vertebra, mandible, and clavicle.[491,497] It generally arises in the medullary canal of the shaft (hence its traditional inclusion among the "marrow tumors"), from which it permeates the cortex and invades the soft tissues (Fig. 24-62). Rarely, it is predominantly periosteal in location.[434]

Occasionally, Ewing's sarcoma presents clinically as a soft tissue neoplasm with a normal appearance of the underlying bone on plain x-ray films. However, CT scans, MRI, and microscopic examination of these cases may reveal that the tumor arose in the medullary canal and that it has diffusely permeated the marrow spaces to extend outside the bone without destroying a significant amount of bone trabeculae, thus remaining undetectable by conventional radiography. This possibility should always be kept in mind before making a diagnosis of primary extraskeletal Ewing's sarcoma[457] (see Chapter 25).

The typical radiographic changes of Ewing's sarcoma are cortical thickening and widening of the medullary canal. With progress of the lesion, reactive periosteal bone may be deposited in layers parallel to the cortex (onion-skin appearance) or at right angles to it (sun-ray appearance) (Fig. 24-63).

Microscopically, Ewing's sarcoma consists of solid sheets of cells divided into irregular masses by fibrous strands. Individual cells are small and uniform. The cell outlines are indistinct, resulting in a "syncytial" appearance. The nuclei are round, with frequent indentations, small nucleoli, and variable but usually brisk mitotic activity (Fig. 24-64). There is a well-developed vascular network. Some of the tumor cells may arrange themselves around the vessels in a pseudorosette fashion. Exceptionally, a few true rosettes (without central lumen) are formed, these having provided some of the earlier evidence for a neuroepithelial pattern of differentiation in these neoplasms.[456] Necrosis is common and may dominate the microscopic picture. Some tumors are composed of larger and more pleomorphic cells exhibiting conspicuous nucleoli.[471] Others feature an organoid pattern characterized by bicellular strands of tissue separated by a "filmy" vascular stroma and referred to as the "filigree pattern."[458]

Ewing's sarcoma cells usually contain large amounts of cytoplasmic glycogen, as demonstrated by a PAS stain with diastase control or by electron microscopy (Figs. 24-65 and 24-66). Traditionally, this has represented an important feature for the differential diagnosis with other small round cell tumors.[486] However, it is far from being specific. Some cases of Ewing's sarcoma show little or no glycogen (at least in routine formalin-fixed and paraffin-embedded preparations), whereas sizable amounts of this substance can be found in metastatic neuroblastoma and malignant lymphoma occasionally and in embryonal rhabdomyosarcoma commonly.[498,503]

Ultrastructurally, the cells of Ewing's sarcoma show a rather primitive appearance. Occasionally, a few dense core granules will be found, either in the cytoplasm or in cell prolongations.[449,450,463,465,466]

Immunohistochemically, the most consistent positivity is for vimentin. However, in ideally processed tissue (and sometimes even in routinely handled tissue) reactivity may be found for low-molecular-weight keratin, neuron-specific

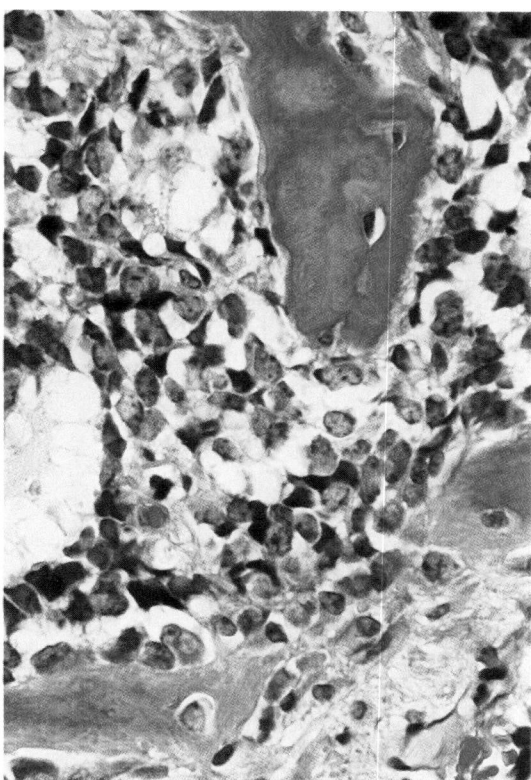

Fig. 24-64 Microscopic appearance of Ewing's sarcoma. Uniform cells with darkly staining nuclei and very scanty cytoplasm infiltrate the marrow spaces around bone trabeculae.

enolase, protein gene product 9.5, Leu7, and neurofilaments, some of these reactions again providing evidence for a neuroepithelial differentiation.*

O13 (HBA 71; p30/32 MIC 2) is a cell membrane protein coded by a gene located on the short arms of the X and Y chromosomes that is consistently expressed by the cells of Ewing's sarcoma/PNET[432,480] (Fig. 24-67). It is, however, not pathognomonic for this family of tumors, inasmuch as occasional expression of this marker has been documented in embryonal rhabdomyosarcoma, other soft tissue sarcomas, and lymphoblastic lymphoma.[446-448,478,495,501] Desmosome-associated proteins are demonstrable immunohistochemically in the areas of cell junctions, but neural cell adhesion molecules are not.[452] Various types of collagen are found in the extracellular matrix.[485]

Practically all cases of Ewing's sarcoma (and PNET) show on cytogenetic examination the reciprocal translocation 11:22 (q24;q12), resulting in the fusion of the EWS (Ewing's sarcoma) and FLI 1 genes.[439,442,461] This translocation can be detected by chromosomal in situ suppression hybridization and by reverse transcriptase PCR reaction; it can be used both for the primary diagnosis and for the detection of metastatic or residual disease.[443,489,492,494]

Ewing's sarcoma has also been found to express the secretogranin II and cholestokinin genes, although rarely to the degree of their respective products being demonstrable with immunohistochemical techniques.[451,476]

_____
*References 436, 441, 462, 464, 469, 470, 473, 479.

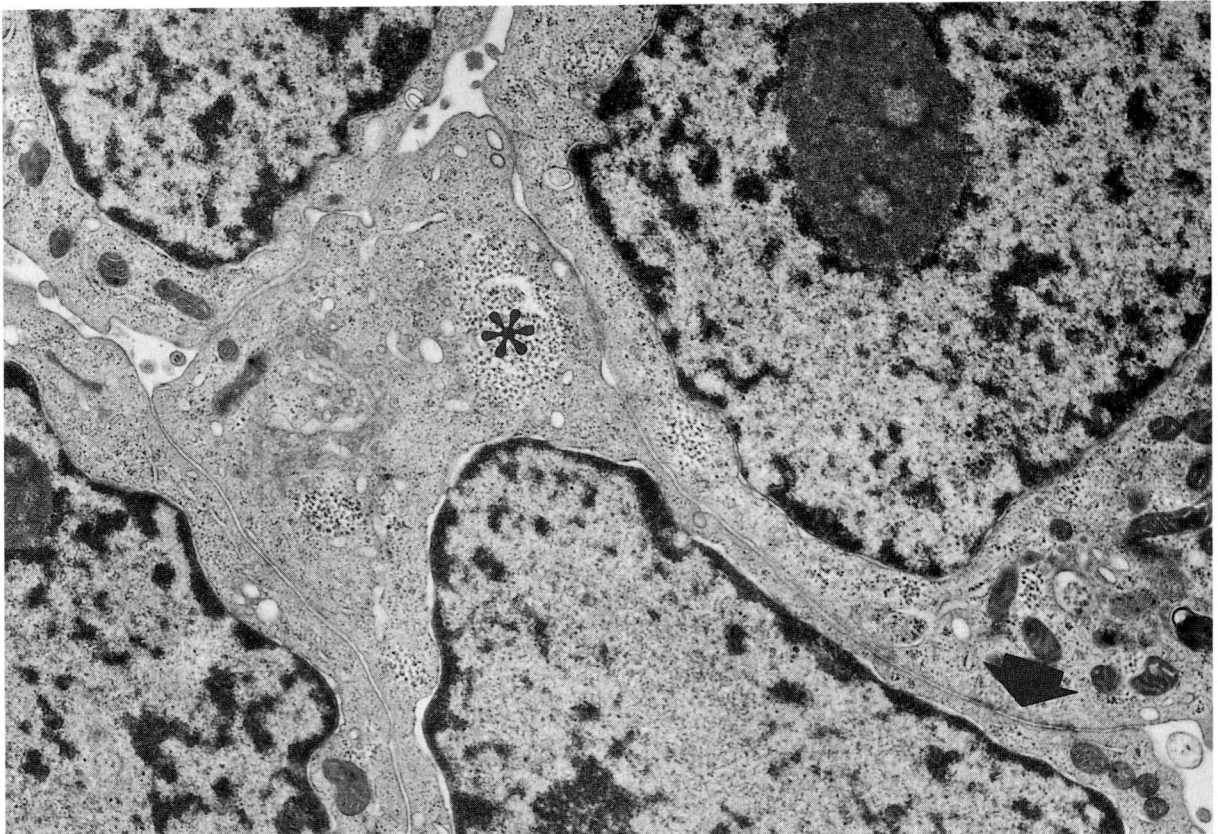

Fig. 24-65 Electron microscopic appearance of Ewing's sarcoma. Undifferentiated tumor cells with multiple small foci of cytoplasmic glycogen *(asterisk)* are joined by two rudimentary cell junctions *(arrow)*. (×12,000.) (Courtesy Dr. Robert A. Erlandson, Memorial Sloan-Kettering Cancer Center.)

The metastatic spread of this tumor is to the lungs and pleura, other bones (particularly the skull), central nervous system, and (rarely) regional lymph nodes. About 25% of the patients have multiple bone and/or visceral lesions at the time of presentation.[435,453]

The treatment of Ewing's sarcoma represents one of the success stories of medical oncology. In the past, surgical excision (including amputation) and radiation therapy resulted in 5-year survival rates of less than 10%, to the point that the pathologist was warned to distrust a previous diagnosis of Ewing's sarcoma in a long-term survivor.[474] The combination of high-dose irradiation and multidrug chemotherapy—sometimes combined with limited surgery—have dramatically changed the picture.[433,481,484] Local control is achieved in over 85% of the cases, and the actuarial 5-year disease-free survival is 75%. Parenthetically, it should be noted that therapy may result in increased pleomorphism and the appearance of bizarre giant cells.[496]

Radiographic evidence of effective treatment consists of reconstitution of the cortical pattern, "periostitis," and regression of the extraosseous soft tissue mass if one was present; any localized lysis at the primary site should be regarded as suspicious for recurrence.[445]

Direct extension of an osseous Ewing's sarcoma into soft tissues is a bad prognostic sign.[468] The claim has been made that classical Ewing's sarcoma of bone has a better prognosis than PNET of soft tissues,[434a,454,487] but it is difficult to separate the relative importance of the osseous versus soft tissue location vis-à-vis the absence or presence of neuroepithelial features in the tumor. A filigree microscopic pattern is also said to represent an unfavorable prognostic indicator, at least with the therapy used at the time that the observation was made.[458] DNA content as determined by flow cytometry or cytophotometry seems to correlate with prognosis in that patients with diploid tumors do better than those with aneuploid ones.[440]

Malignant lymphoma and related lesions

Primary large cell malignant lymphoma of bone is more common in adults than children, 60% of the cases occurring in patients over the age of 30 years. There is no sex predilection.

Grossly, most cases involve the diaphysis or metaphysis of a long bone, producing patchy cortical and medullary destruction. This is associated with minimal to moderate periosteal reaction, usually of the lamellated type. The

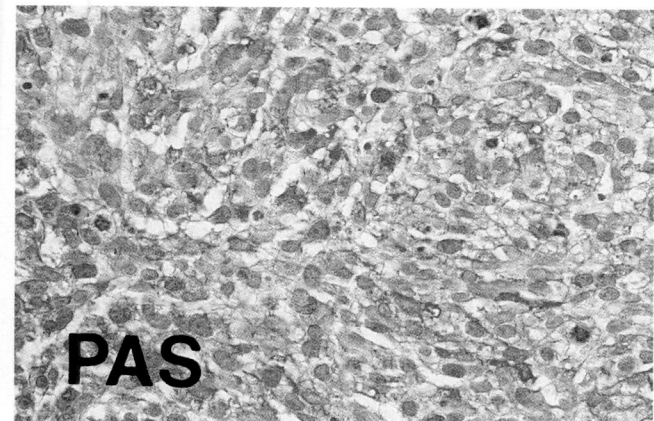

Fig. 24-66 PAS stain in Ewing's sarcoma showing large amounts of cytoplasmic glycogen. The material was entirely removed by diastase treatment.

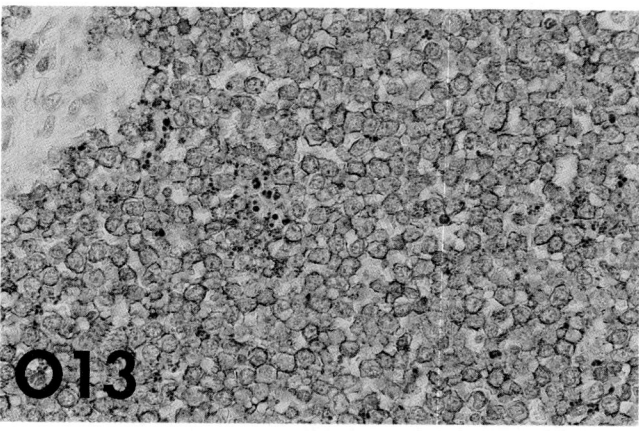

Fig. 24-67 O13 stain in Ewing's sarcoma. All of the tumor cells show strong membrane immunoreactivity for this marker.

tumor, which is pinkish gray and granular, frequently extends into the soft tissues and invades the muscle.

Radiographically, a combination of bone production and bone destruction often involves a wide area of a long bone[510] (Fig. 24-68). This pattern is very suggestive of the diagnosis, but osteosarcoma and chronic osteomyelitis may result in a very similar appearance.

Microscopically, the appearance is similar to that of large cell lymphomas in nodal and other extranodal sites.[506,510,516,523,529] Some cases are accompanied by prominent fibrosis. Traditionally, the main source of diagnostic difficulty has resided in their distinction from Ewing's sarcoma.[515,517,528] The cells of malignant lymphoma are larger, and their nuclei are somewhat pleomorphic, with many indented or horseshoe-shaped forms. They usually have prominent nucleoli, unlike the fine nucleoli of Ewing's sarcoma (Fig. 24-69). Cytoplasmic outlines of large cell lymphoma are well defined, whereas those of Ewing's tumor are indistinct. The cytoplasm is more abundant and often eosinophilic. Reticulin fibers occur between individual cells and groups of cells, whereas in Ewing's sarcoma they are mainly restricted to perivascular areas. Ultrastructurally, the features are analogous to those of nodal and other extranodal lymphomas.[518] Immunohistochemically, there is positivity for LCA and—in the large majority of the cases—for B cell markers.[512,521,522] A few cases have shown an anaplastic appearance and been immunoreactive for the Ki-1 (BerH2) marker.[508]

The 5-year survival rate for localized malignant lymphomas of bone has ranged from 30% to 60% in most series.[505,516,525,530] The stage of the disease is the single most important prognostic determinator,[520] but there is also a definite relation with cell type.[511] The workup of these patients should include skeletal survey and bone marrow examination. The treatment usually consists of a combination of irradiation therapy and chemotherapy.[504]

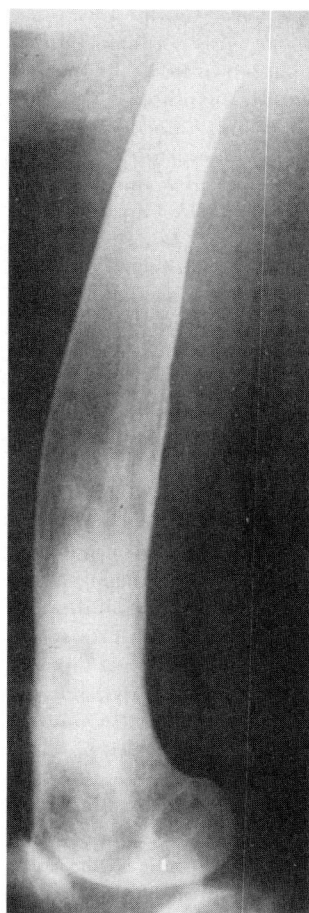

Fig. 24-68 Malignant lymphoma involving lower end of femur demonstrating bone destruction and bone production. Such lesions are often erroneously diagnosed as chronic osteomyelitis.

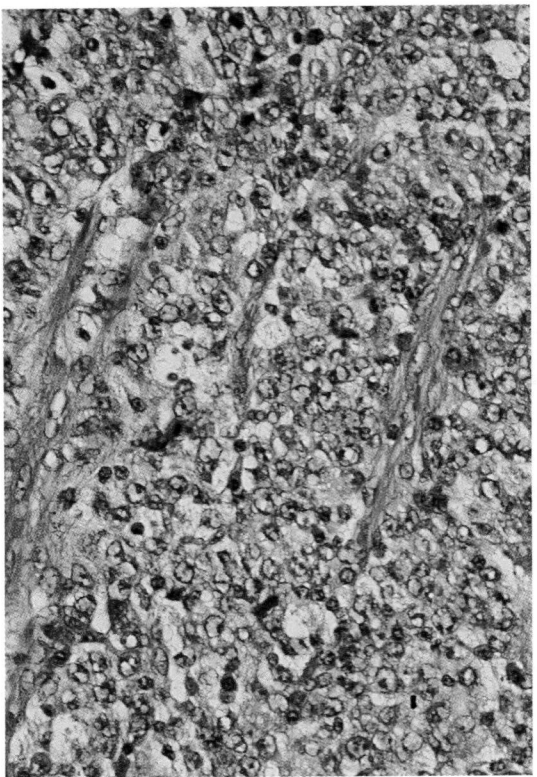

Fig. 24-69 Malignant lymphoma of bone. The tumor is of large cell type and is associated with some fibrosis.

Burkitt's lymphoma as originally reported from Africa typically presented with massive jawbone involvement. It can also result in tumor masses in the long bones and pelvis.[513]

Hodgkin's disease produces radiographically detectable bone lesions in approximately 15% of the patients. The involvement is multifocal in about 60% of the cases, the most frequent sites being vertebrae, pelvis, ribs, sternum, and femur.[514] The osseous lesions of Hodgkin's disease are often asymptomatic and in half of the cases are not demonstrable radiographically. When they become apparent in the x-ray film, the foci may be osteolytic, mixed, or purely osteoblastic. The latter appearance is particularly common in vertebrae. Exceptionally, Hodgkin's disease will present initially as a bone mass.[509] Osteonecrosis of the femoral or humeral head can occur as a complication of therapy for Hodgkin's disease or non-Hodgkin's lymphoma.[524]

Acute leukemia of childhood is associated with radiographic abnormalities in the skeletal system in 70% to 90% of the cases.[519,527] In the large majority of instances, the changes are widespread and therefore unlikely to be confused with a primary bone neoplasm.[526] In contrast, destructive bone lesions are extremely rare in the chronic leukemias. Chabner et al.[507] reported six cases in a series of 205 patients with chronic granulocytic leukemia. In three of the patients, the bone lesion appeared at the time of blastic transformation.

Plasma cell myeloma is discussed in Chapter 23.

Vascular tumors

Hemangiomas of bone are often seen in the vertebrae as an incidental postmortem finding. In 2154 autopsies studied by Töpfer,[551] hemangiomas were detected in 11.9%. They were multiple in 34% of the cases. These lesions should probably be regarded as vascular malformations rather than true neoplasms.

The most common locations of clinically significant osseous hemangiomas are skull, vertebrae, and jawbones.[553,556] Hemangiomas in the long bones are extremely rare. When a lesion involves the flat bones (particularly the skull), sunburst trabeculation occurs because of elevation of the periosteum. Grossly, the cut section of these tumors often has a currant jelly appearance. Microscopically, there is a thick-walled lattice-like pattern of endothelial-lined cavernous spaces filled with blood (Fig. 24-70).

Multiple hemangiomas are mainly seen in children and are associated in about half of the cases with cutaneous, soft tissue, or visceral hemangiomas.[549] Hemangiomas of the sacrum in infants are often accompanied by a variety of congenital abnormalities.[535]

Massive osteolysis (Gorham's disease) is probably not a vascular neoplasm but is included in this discussion because of its microscopic similarities with skeletal angiomatosis. It has a destructive character that the latter lacks. It results in reabsorption of a whole bone or several bones and the filling of the residual spaces by a heavily vascularized fibrous tissue.[536,537]

Lymphangiomas of bone are exceptional.[538] Most cases are multiple and associated with soft tissue tumors of similar appearance; variations on the theme have been termed *cystic angiomatosis* and *hamartomatous hemolymphangiomatosis.*[547]

Glomus tumor of the subungual soft tissues may erode the underlying bone. Much rarer is the occurrence of a purely intraosseous glomus tumor involving the terminal phalanx.[540]

Hemangiopericytoma can present as a primary bone lesion, the most common location being the pelvis[548,558] (Plate XVIII-A). Benign and malignant forms have been described. The differential diagnosis includes metastatic hemangiopericytoma of meninges, which is actually more common than primary hemangiopericytoma of bone.

Phosphaturic mesenchymal tumor is discussed here because it usually exhibits microscopically areas with a hemangiopericytoma-like appearance, combined with foci of giant cells.[542] There is also osteoid production and poorly developed cartilaginous areas. These peculiar tumors of bone or soft tissue cause osteomalacia or rickets through the production of a renal phosphaturic substance that depletes total body phosphates by reducing tubular reabsorption of phosphate.[532] Their behavior is usually benign.[555]

Epithelioid hemangioendothelioma of bone, a distinctive tumor type originally embraced within the histiocytoid hemangioma concept,[546] is a borderline or intermediate type of vascular neoplasm. It is characterized microscopically by the presence of epithelial- or histiocyte-like endothelial cells having abundant acidophilic and often vacuolated cytoplasm, a large vesicular nucleus (sometimes with prominent grooves), scanty mitotic activity, inconspicuous or absent

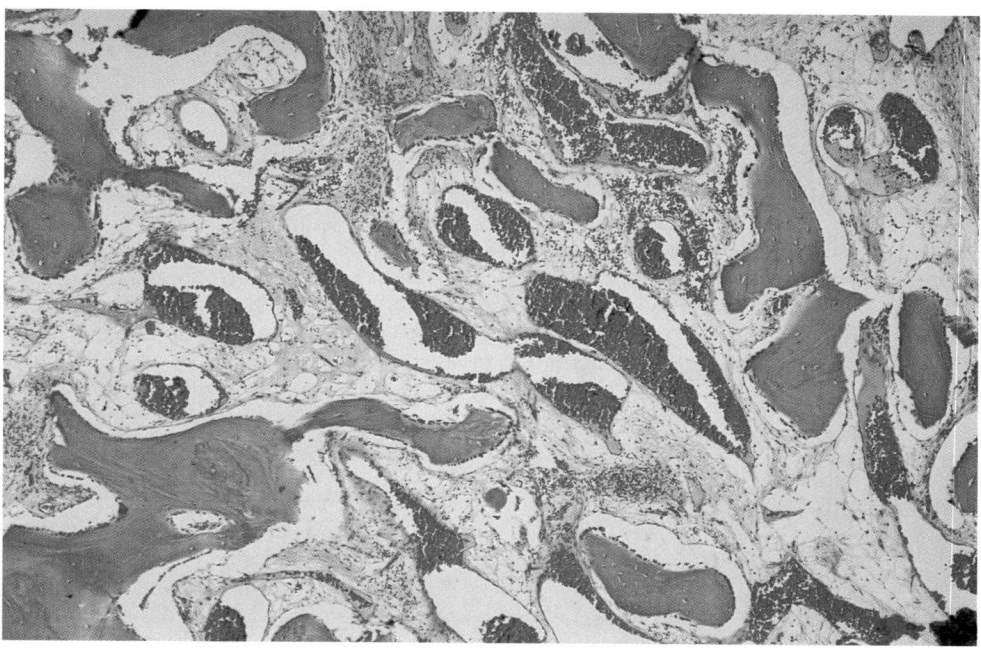

Fig. 24-70 Cavernous hemangioma of bone. Large dilated vessels with thin walls expand marrow spaces and elicit some new bone formation in surrounding trabeculae.

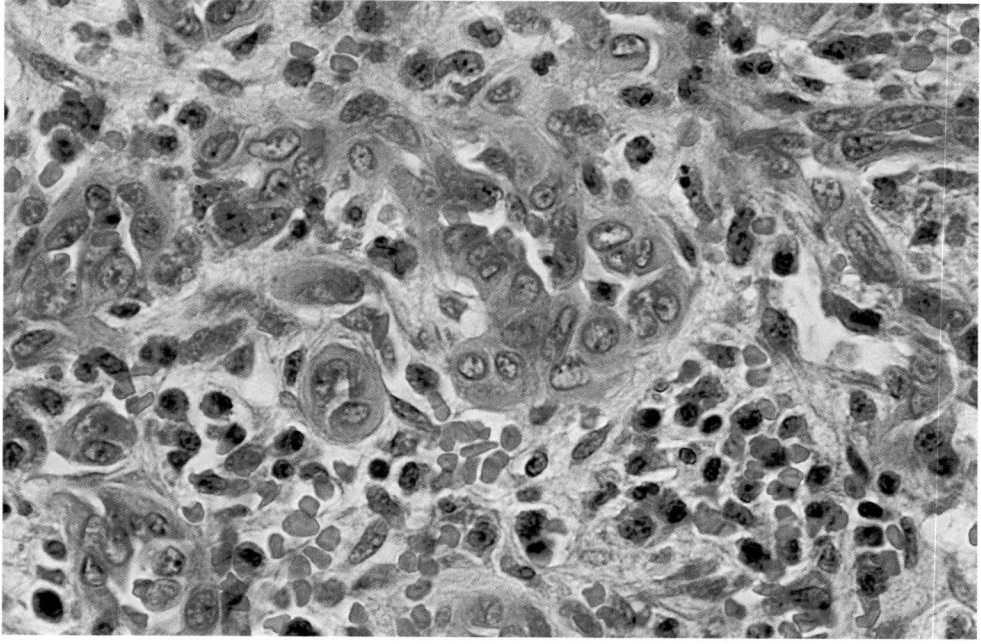

Fig. 24-71 Epithelioid (histiocytoid) hemangioendothelioma. The tumor cells have a plump appearance and acidophilic cytoplasm. The stroma contains inflammatory infiltrate rich in eosinophils.

anastomosing channels, recent and old hemorrhage, and an inconstant but sometimes prominent inflammatory component rich in eosinophils (Figs. 24-71 and 24-72). A myxoid stroma is prominent in some cases and may produce confusion with a cartilaginous neoplasm.[541] Many of the tumors classified as grade I (and perhaps grade II) hemangioendotheliomas of bone in some series[533,545] belong in this category.

In this regard, it should be emphasized that a range of cytologic atypia exists among epithelioid vascular tumors of bone. Those showing only a modest degree of atypia fit better the category of epithelioid hemangioendothelioma and are the most numerous. Those showing little or no atypia could be termed epithelioid hemangiomas, as some authors have done,[543] whereas those exhibiting marked atypia (often accompanied by mitotic activity and necrosis) are better designated as epithelioid angiosarcomas (see later discussion).

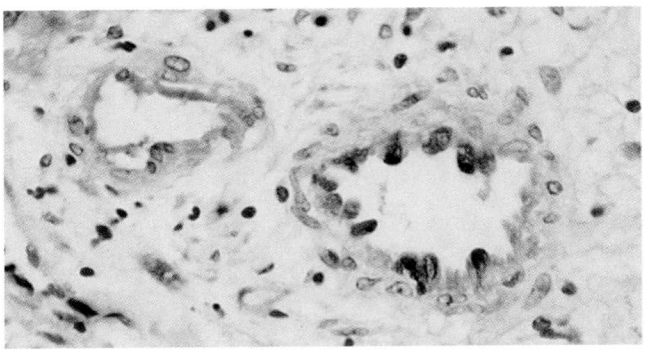

Fig 24-72 Histiocytoid (epithelioid) hemangioendothelioma of bone (FVIII-related antigen).

Unfortunately, the distinction between these categories is not always clear-cut.

Immunohistochemically, the cells of epithelioid hemangioendothelioma display endothelial cell markers, such as factor VIII, CD31, and CD34. However, these antigens can be poorly expressed and/or coexist with epithelial markers such as keratin.[554]

Epithelioid hemangioendothelioma of bone is often multiple[531] and may be associated with similar lesions in the skin or soft tissue, which are characteristically located in close proximity to the osseous foci[544] (Plate XVIII-B). The clinical course is protracted, especially for the multicentric tumors; distant metastases are exceptional.[552]

Angiosarcoma (malignant hemangioendothelioma, hemangioendothelial sarcoma) exhibits obvious atypia of the tumor cells, formation of solid areas alternating with others with anastomosing vascular channels, and foci of necrosis and hemorrhage[534,539] (Fig. 24-73). A wide range of differentiation exists from tumor to tumor and sometimes in the same case.[557] As already mentioned, in some cases the cells have an epithelioid or histiocytoid appearance. Ultrastructurally and immunohistochemically, the large majority of tumor elements have the phenotype of endothelial cells, with only an occasional admixture of pericytes[550] (Plate XVIII-C). Multicentric examples occur. Distant metastases are common, particularly to the lungs. Before a diagnosis of angiosarcoma in a bone lesion is made, the more common possibilities of well-vascularized osteosarcoma and metastatic carcinoma (particularly of renal origin) should be ruled out.[553]

Other connective tissue tumors

Desmoplastic fibroma and related lesions

Desmoplastic fibroma is a rare neoplasm formed by mature fibroblasts separated by abundant collagen.[559,560,567]

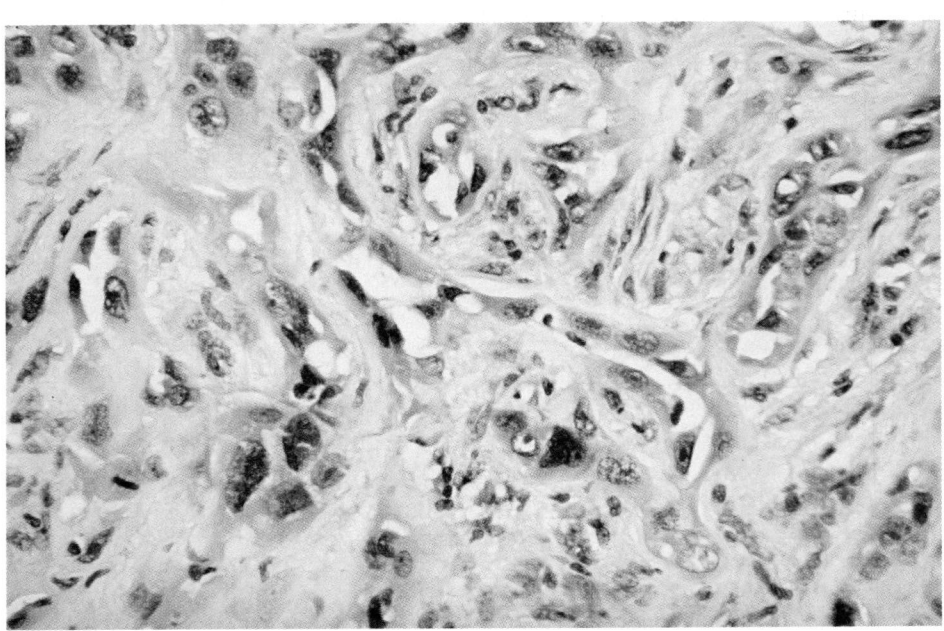

Fig. 24-73 Angiosarcoma of bone. Anastomosing vascular channels lined by highly atypical endothelial cells are seen.

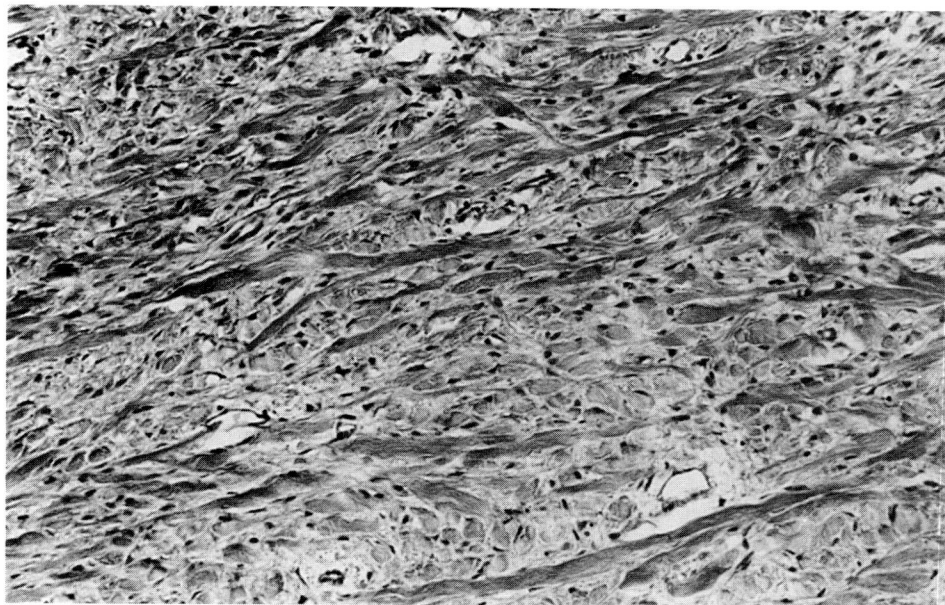

Fig. 24-74 Desmoplastic fibroma. Tumor is hypocellular and accompanied by deposition of thick collagen fibers.

Pleomorphism, necrosis, and mitotic activity are lacking (Fig. 24-74). Ultrastructurally, the predominant cells are myofibroblasts, with a lesser component of fibroblasts and primitive mesenchymal cells.[564] This lesion probably represents the osseous counterpart of soft tissue fibromatosis. It occurs most often in the long bones and jaw.[563] There is a male predominance, and three quarters of the patients are below the age of 30 years.[563] Radiographically, it has a purely lytic, honeycombed appearance. It is destructive locally and often recurs following incomplete excision, but metastases do not occur.[560,566]

Infantile myofibromatosis can present as a solitary lesion in bone. Most of the cases occur in patients 2 years old or younger, and they involve almost always the craniofacial bones.[561,562] The microscopic appearance is the same as for its more common soft tissue counterpart.

Solitary fibrous tumor has been described as a pedunculated periosteal mass.[565]

Fibrosarcoma

Fibrosarcomas of bone often arise in the metaphyseal area of the long bones.[569,571,573] Approximately 50% of these occur in the distal segment of the femur or proximal portion of the tibia.[574] The majority arise in the medullary portion, from where they destroy the cortex and often extend into the soft tissues. A less common location is the periosteum.

Radiographically, these tumors are osteolytic, with a "soap-bubble" appearance. Well-differentiated lesions have well-defined margins, whereas high-grade tumors appear more invasive.[568]

Microscopically, this tumor is similar to its soft tissue counterpart (Figs. 24-75 and 24-76). By definition, it should not contain any areas of tumor osteoid. It has also, somewhat arbitrarily, been agreed that the presence of prominent

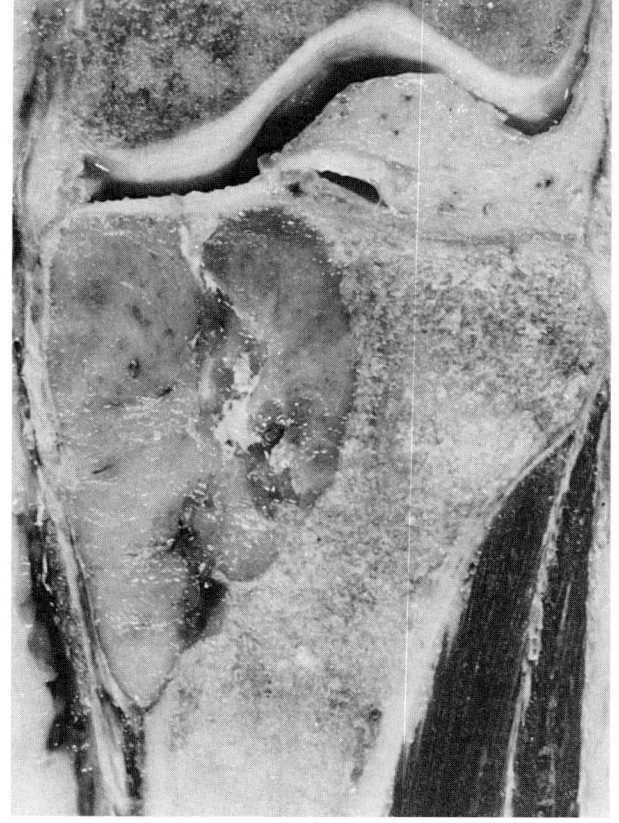

Fig. 24-75 Fibrosarcoma of tibia. Lesion produced osteolytic defect and was confused radiographically with giant cell tumor.

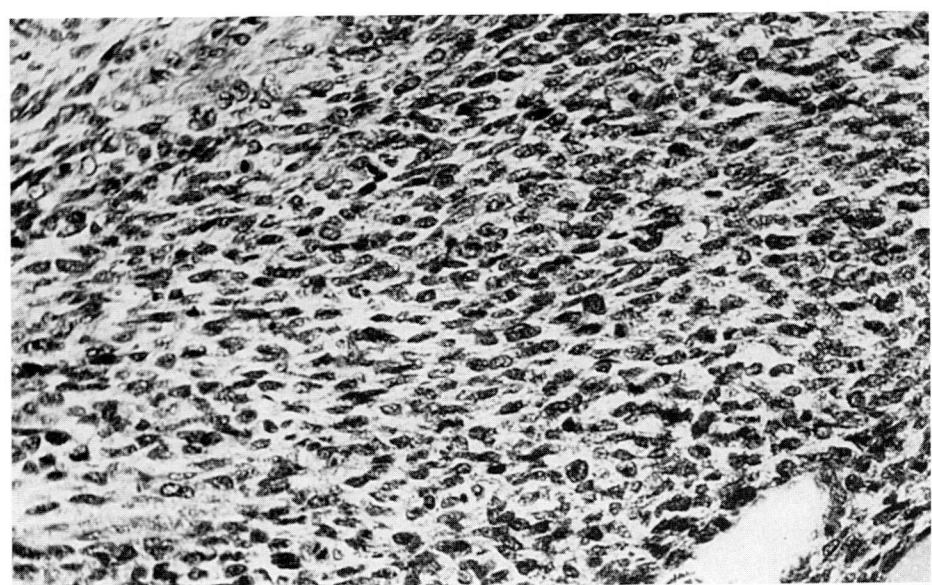

Fig. 24-76 Histologic pattern of this cellular, poorly differentiated fibrosarcoma, primary in right femur, is similar to fibrosarcoma of soft tissues.

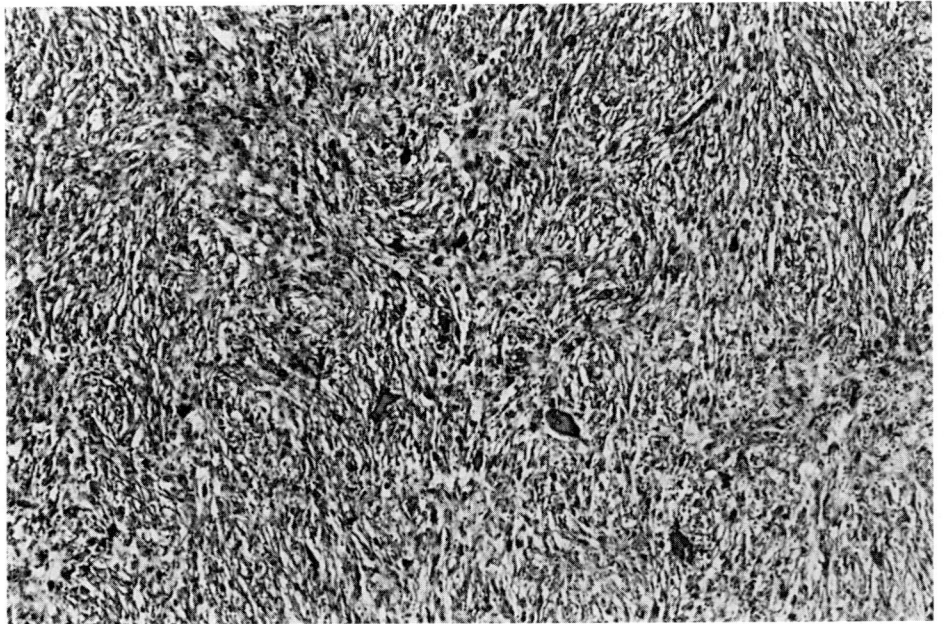

Fig. 24-77 Malignant fibrous histiocytoma of bone. Storiform arrangement is evident. There is no bone formation. Appearance is similar to that of malignant fibrous histiocytoma of soft tissues.

pleomorphism in a lesion of this type removes it from the fibrosarcoma category and places it into the malignant fibrous histiocytoma group.[575]

Extremely well-differentiated fibrosarcomas may be misdiagnosed as benign lesions of fibrous tissue, but the radiographic appearance usually suggests their malignant nature. Microscopically, the presence of cellular areas, mitotic figures, and hyperchromasia are all features that favor a diagnosis of fibrosarcoma over one of desmoplastic fibroma. Fibrosarcoma also should be distinguished from the variety of osteosarcoma mainly composed of fibroblastic elements.[570] Wide local excision and amputation are the two choices of therapy, depending on the location, size, and microscopic grade of the tumor.

A good correlation exists between microscopic grade and prognosis.[568,575] In one recent series, the 10-year survival rate was 83% for low-grade lesions and 34% for high-grade tumors.[568]

Occasionally, fibrosarcoma can present as a multicentric process involving numerous bones.[572] Before this diagnosis is made, the possibility of metastatic sarcomatoid carcinoma (particularly from the kidney) should be ruled out.

Malignant fibrous histiocytoma

A tumor with a microscopic appearance similar to malignant fibrous histiocytoma of the soft tissues (see Chapter 25) can appear in bone[583,585-587,590,592,593] (Fig. 24-77). Many of the reported cases have been located in long bones or the jaw.[576,583] Close to 30% of these tumors arise in bone infarcts,[581,582] around foreign bodies,[577,588] following irradiation,[584] in Paget's disease, or as expression of "dedifferentiation" or anaplastic transformation in chondrosarcoma, chordoma, or giant cell tumor.[578,591] The mean age at the time of presentation is 40 years.[583] The morphologic, ultrastructural, and immunohistochemical features of most tumor cells correspond to those of fibroblasts and myofibroblasts.[589,594]

The histogenesis and differential diagnosis of this tumor when involving bone are just as controversial as for its more common soft tissue counterpart, if not more so. As Dahlin et al.[580] have pointed out, areas indistinguishable from those of malignant fibrous histiocytoma can be found in otherwise typical examples of osteosarcoma or chondrosarcoma. Only when thorough sampling of the tumor reveals no areas suggestive of any of these lesions may a diagnosis of malignant fibrous histiocytoma of bone be justified. Even under these circumstances, it is not clear whether this is a real entity or simply a pleomorphic, poorly differentiated sarcoma. The latter possibility would explain why the overall prognosis is so poor, at least in some series.[579,593] In one series, tumors with marked desmoplasia had a worse prognosis (5-year survival rate of 20%) than those with a prominent chronic inflammatory infiltrate (5-year survival rate of 78%).[595]

Muscle tumors

Malignant smooth muscle tumors of bone are very rare, and *leiomyomas* are virtually nonexistent. The few reported cases of *leiomyosarcoma* have occurred in long bones, particularly the femur.[596,604] The ultrastructural and immunohistochemical features are analogous to those of its soft tissue counterpart.[598] Specifically, the tumor cells are immunoreactive for common and smooth muscle actin and desmin, and they are enveloped by type IV collagen. They may also be positive for keratin and S-100 protein.[597,605] Ultrastructurally, cytoplasmic microfilaments with focal densities are found.[600]

Isolated examples of primary *rhabdomyosarcomas* of bone are on record.[599,601] Some are pure, whereas others are seen as a component of *malignant mesenchymoma*.[599,602,603]

Adipose tissue tumors

Lipoma of bone is a very rare tumor. The few reported cases have occurred in adults and have presented radiographically as sharply outlined lytic lesions. Microscopically, they are composed of mature adipose tissue devoid of hematopoietic elements; dystrophic calcification, fat necrosis, and hemorrhage may be present.[606,607]

Liposarcoma of bone is even more exceptional.[608,609] It is likely that many of the cases reported as such in the past would be reclassified today in other categories.

Other primary tumors
Chordoma

Chordoma is a malignant bone tumor thought to arise from the remnants of the fetal notochord. The latter is normally situated within the vertebral bodies and intervertebral discs and, rarely, in the presacral soft tissues.[629,635,641,647] A benign inconsequential remnant of notochord is the *ecchordosis physaliphora* found incidentally at autopsy as a discrete gelatinous nodule arising from the clivus or overlying the anterior surface of the pons.[646]

Most chordomas arise from notochordal remnants in bone rather than from those located inside the disks. They are more frequent in the fifth and sixth decades but occur at all ages and in both sexes. They grow slowly, the duration of the symptoms before diagnosis usually being over 5 years. A total of 50% arise in the sacrococcygeal area, 35% in the spheno-occipital area, and the remainder along the cervico-thoraco-lumbar ("mobile") spine.[612,624] The sacrococcygeal tumors are more common in the fifth and sixth decades of life, whereas many of the spheno-occipital neoplasms occur in children.[618,656] In the former, a portion of the sacrum is seen destroyed by an osteolytic or rarely an osteoblastic process (Fig. 24-78, *A*). If the tumor encroaches on the spine, symptoms of spinal cord compression arise. The retroperitoneal space is often involved by direct extension. The tumor may grow large enough to narrow the lumen of the large bowel, impinge on the bladder, or invade the skin by direct extension.[622] It can be felt as a firm extrarectal mass. Spheno-occipital chordomas may present with a nasal, paranasal, or nasopharyngeal mass; multiple cranial nerve involvement; and destruction of bone.[614,642] Exceptionally, they may lead to fatal acute pontocerebellar hemorrhage.[621]

Grossly, chordoma is gelatinous and soft and contains areas of hemorrhage (Fig. 24-78, *B*). Microscopically, it closely resembles normal notochord tissue in its different stages of development. It grows in cell cords and lobules separated by a variable but usually extensive amount of mucoid intercellular tissue (Fig. 24-79, *A*). Some of the tumor cells (known as physaliferous) are extremely large,

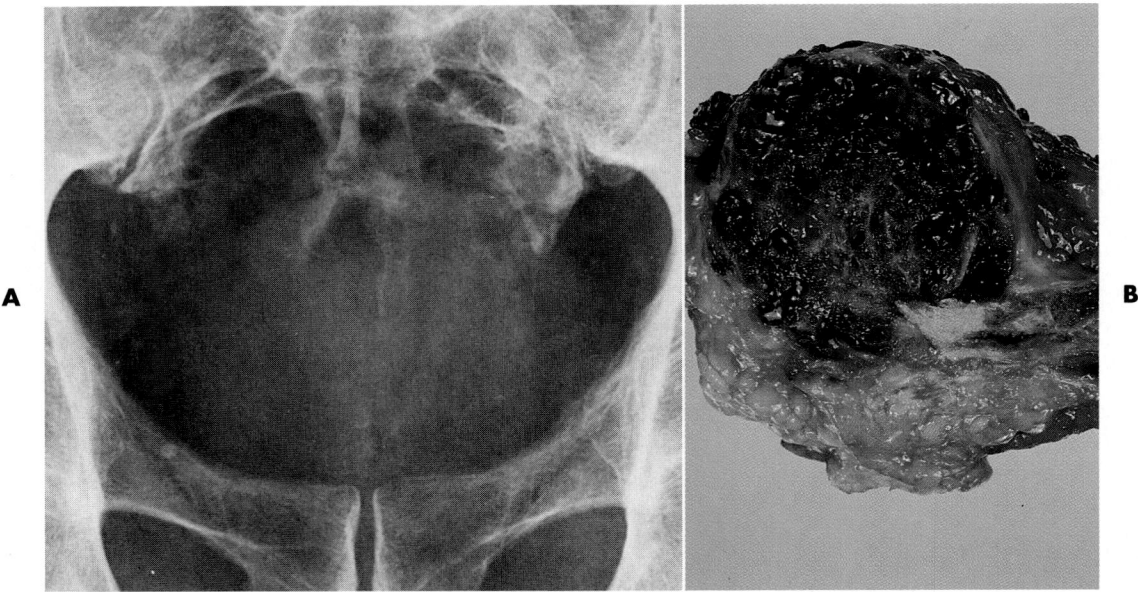

Fig. 24-78 A, Osteolytic destruction of sacrum by chordoma. **B,** Gross appearance of chordoma of sacrum showing a gelatinous tumor with extensive secondary hemorrhage.

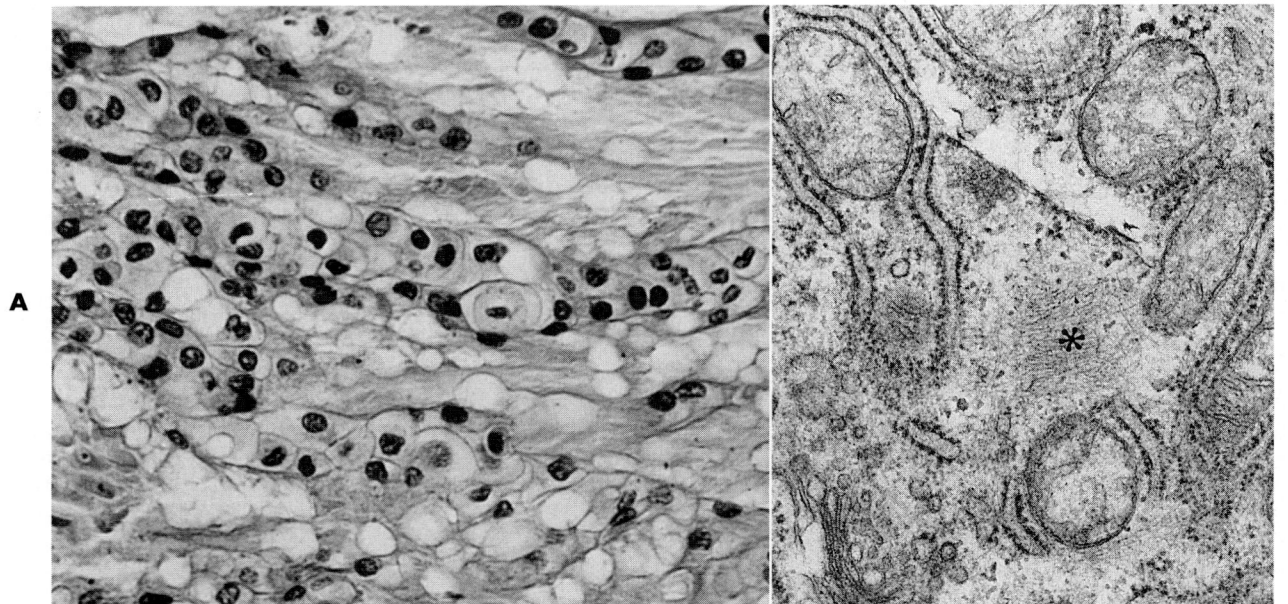

Fig. 24-79 A, Chordoma of spheno-occipital region. Cuboidal and polyhedral cells with central nucleus form row and nests among abundant myxoid matrix. **B,** Electron microscopic appearance of chordoma of sacrum. Mitochondria surrounded by cisternae of rough endoplasmic reticulum and aggregate of cytokeratin filaments *(asterisk)* are illustrated. (×37,000.) (**A** courtesy Dr. J.E. Olvera-Rabiela, Mexico City. **B** courtesy Dr. Robert A. Erlandson, Memorial Sloan-Kettering Cancer Center.)

with vacuolated cytoplasm and prominent vesicular nucleus; some of the cytoplasmic vacuoles contain glycogen, presumably in the process of being broken down.[619,631] Other tumor cells are small, with small nuclei and no visible nucleoli. Mitotic figures are generally scanty or absent. Areas of cartilage and bone may be present.[623] In some areas, the tumor may simulate carcinoma, particularly of renal cell origin. The microscopic differential diagnosis also includes chondrosarcoma, signet cell adenocarcinoma of the rectum, and myxopapillary ependymoma. Ultrastructurally, chordoma cells may contain peculiar mitochondrial–endoplasmic reticulum complexes, as well as parallel bundles of crisscrossing microtubules within the granular endoplasmic reticulum, two interesting albeit nonspecific features[620,628,648] (Fig. 24-79, *B*). They also have desmosomes, in keeping with their epithelial nature.[644] Immunohistochemically, chordoma shows reactivity for S-100 protein, keratin, epithelial membrane antigen, and vimentin* but only rarely for CEA[610] (Fig. 24-80). GFA reactivity is commonly encountered with the use of polyclonal antibodies, less so with their monoclonal counterparts.[654] Strong 5-nucleotidase positivity has been found in the cell membrane of the tumor cells, another feature of potential diagnostic utility.[613] The lectin-binding pattern of chordoma closely recapitulates that of the human fetal notochord.[630] The extracellular material contains collagen of nearly all types (I, II, III, IV, V, and VI); laminin is also present, as evidence of basement membrane deposition.[649]

The characteristic physaliferous cells of chordoma can be identified in material from fine-needle aspiration, which is also amenable to histochemical and immunohistochemical evaluation.[652]

The natural history of chordoma is characterized by repeated episodes of local recurrence and a generally fatal outcome. Recurrences may develop 10 years or longer after the initial therapy.[611] Distant metastases are also late in the evolution of the disease.[615] In one series, the frequency of metastatic disease was 43%.[625] The most common sites are the skin (where they can simulate a sweat gland tumor) and bone, but they can occur in many other places, including the ovary.[622,657]

Treatment is in the form of surgical excision, radiation therapy, or a combination of both modalities.[638,639,641] The recurrence rate is very high following surgery, particularly when the tumor is entered during the procedure.[629]

Foci of high-grade spindle cell and/or pleomorphic sarcoma can be present in conjunction with areas of typical chordoma, either in the primary tumor or in the recurrences.[626] This phenomenon is analogous to that of "dedifferentiated" chondrosarcoma and carries an equally ominous prognostic significance.[633,651] The high-grade foci have an aneuploid-hyperploid pattern on flow cytometry, in stark contrast to that of the conventional chordomatous component.[626]

Chondroid chordoma is a controversial tumor entity, originally defined as a chordoma with prominent cartilaginous foci.[624] It occurs most often in the spheno-occipital region, but it may also be seen in the sacro-coccygeal area.[616] The overall prognosis is better than that of conven-

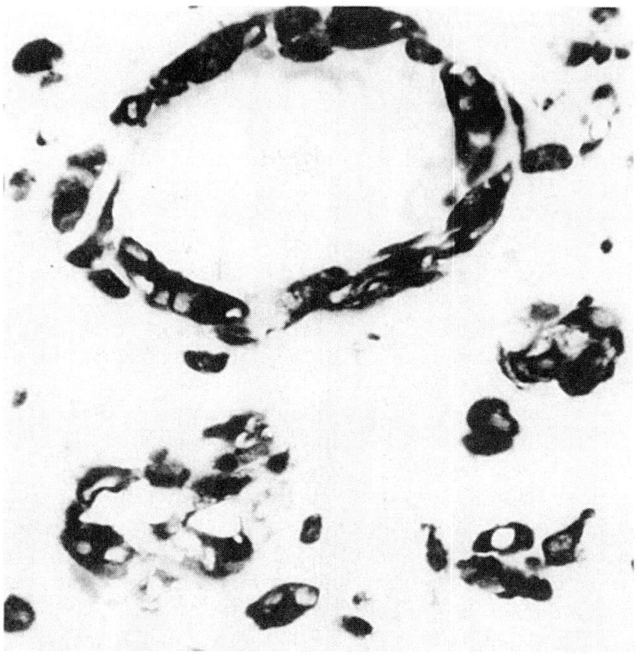

Fig. 24-80 Strong immunocytochemical positivity for keratin in chordoma.

tional chordoma, although the differences in recent series are not as pronounced as in previous work.[636]

Ultrastructurally and immunohistochemically, the tumor seems to share features of chordoma and chondrosarcoma.[650] Immunohistochemically, most authors have found reactivity for S-100 protein, keratin, and—less commonly—EMA and CEA.* Although the two extreme suggestions have been made that this tumor is a chondrosarcoma with no relation to chondroma[653] or a chordoma with no cartilaginous features,[627] most evidence suggests that both components are present.

Adamantinoma of long bones

Adamantinoma of long bones occurs predominantly in the tibia but has been reported in other long bones, such as the femur, ulna, and fibula.[658,665,667,671] Occasionally, adamantinoma of the tibia is seen also involving the adjacent fibula.[673] It may arise in the shaft or in the metaphyseal area of the bone.[660]

Radiographically, it presents as single or multiple lytic areas in the cortex or medulla, surrounded by marked sclerosis. Grossly, it is poorly defined and may extend into the overlying soft tissues.

Microscopically, several patterns of growth have been described. The most common consists of solid nests of basaloid cells with palisading at the periphery and sometimes a stellate configuration in the center. Less frequent forms have been described as spindle, squamoid, and tubular; the latter simulates closely the appearance of a vascular neoplasm[660] (Fig. 24-81, *A*). Electron microscopic and immunohisto-

*References 610, 617, 632, 634, 637, 645.

*References 627, 636, 640, 643, 644, 653, 655.

chemical studies have confirmed the epithelial nature of the tumor cells[664a,668-670,675] (Fig. 24-81, *B*, and Plate XVIII-D). The keratins expressed by adamantinoma are mainly 14 and 19, with lesser representation of keratins 5, 17, 7, and 13.[664] In contrast to other bone and soft tissue tumors with epithelial phenotypes—such as synovial sarcoma, chordoma, and epithelioid sarcoma—it lacks immunoreactivity for keratins 8 and 18.[664]

On occasion the adamantinoma is accompanied by osteofibrous dysplasia, the relative proportions of the two lesions varying greatly from case to case.[661,662,672,674] Of great interest is the fact that the spindle cells of the dysplastic component are also immunoreactive for keratin, suggesting a common histogenesis.[659]

The histogenesis of this tumor remains controversial. Now that the presence of epithelial differentiation has been proved beyond doubt, the two most likely possibilities are origin from intraosseous epithelial rests, possibly of skin adnexal type,[663] or epithelial metaplasia in a primary mesenchymal process. It is of interest that morphologically identical tumors can occur in the soft tissues of the pretibial area in the absence of bone involvement.[666]

Adamantinoma of bone is a low-grade malignant tumor characterized by a tendency for local recurrence and the occasional development of lymph node and distant metastases, particularly to lung.[665] En bloc excision and amputation are the therapeutic choices, depending on the circumstances of the case.[665]

Peripheral nerve tumors

Over sixty cases of intraosseous *schwannoma* have been reported.[676,678] A strong predilection for the mandible has been noted, and origin from the mandibular nerve sometimes has been demonstrated.[682] Schwannomas of the sacrum can reach huge dimensions and present as retrorectal masses; they may simulate a malignant tumor on radiographic grounds (particularly chordoma) and present great technical difficulties for their surgical removal.[681] A few of the reported cases of intraosseous schwannoma have been of the *melanotic* variety.[680]

Recklinghausen's disease often results in several types of skeletal abnormalities (such as scoliosis, bowing, pseudoarthrosis, and other disorders of growth)[679] and may be accompanied by malignant bone tumors such as fibrosarcoma or malignant fibrous histiocytoma[677]; however, intraosseous neurofibromas are extremely rare.

Malignant peripheral nerve sheath tumor has been rarely seen in bone in patients with or without Recklinghausen's disease; several of the cases have involved jawbones.[675a]

Xanthoma

Xanthoma of bone presents in patients over the age of 20 years and has a male:female ratio of 2:1. It is almost always solitary, and the flat bones (pelvis, ribs, skull) are the most frequent sites. Radiographically, it presents as a well-defined, sometimes expansile lytic lesion, often with a sclerotic margin. Microscopically, an admixture of foamy cells, multinucleated giant cells, cholesterol clefts, and fibrosis is seen. The differential diagnosis includes sinus histiocytosis with massive lymphadenopathy (Rosai-Dorfman's disease) and secondary xanthomatous changes in other bone lesions, such as Langerhans' cell granulomatosis and fibrous/posttraumatic dysplasia.[683]

Fibrocartilaginous mesenchymoma

Fibrocartilaginous mesenchymoma is a term that has been applied to a rare benign condition affecting the metaphysis

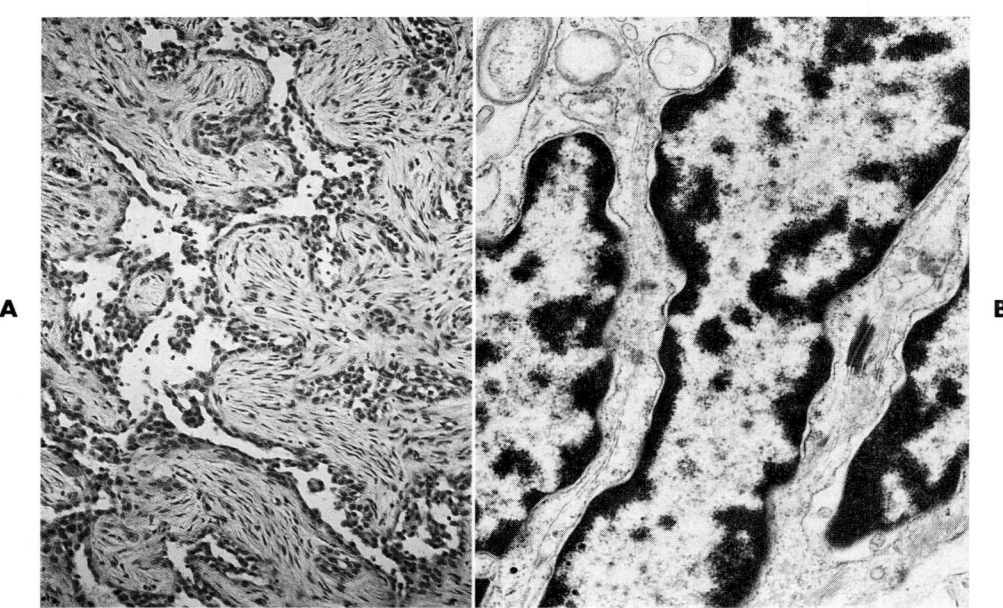

Fig. 24-81 Adamantinoma of tibia. **A,** Microscopic appearance. Lack of cohesiveness of tumor cells in some of the islands results in a pseudovascular appearance. **B,** Electron microscopic appearance showing spindle-shaped epithelial tumor cells joined by desmosomes. (×15,600.) (**B** courtesy Dr. Robert A. Erlandson, Memorial Sloan-Kettering Cancer Center.)

of long bones (particularly the fibula) and characterized microscopically by an admixture of spindle cells, bone trabeculae, and islands of cartilage. Some of the cartilage is in the form of structures resembling epiphyseal plates. Recurrences may supervene, but metastases have not been reported.[684]

Metastatic tumors

Metastatic tumors are the most frequent of all malignant neoplasms of bone[696] (Figs. 24-82 to 24-84). Since in most cases the lesions are multiple and the presence of a tumor elsewhere is known, the diagnosis is obvious. However, solitary metastases from occult primaries can be confused with primary bone tumors. More than 80% of all bone metastases originate in the breast, lung, prostate, thyroid, or kidney; nearly 50% of patients with tumor in any of these sites will develop bone metastases. These metastases can be accompanied by visceral deposits or represent the only apparent site of dissemination.[699] Soft tissue sarcomas rarely metastasize to the skeletal system, the outstanding exception being embryonal rhabdomyosarcoma of the soft tissues in children.[686]

About 70% of bone metastases affect the axial skeleton (cranium, ribs, spine, sacrum), and the remaining involve the appendicular skeleton (long bones) or both compartments. In all bones, metastases are preferentially situated in red bone marrow.[685] When located in long bones, the area usually involved is the metaphysis.

Metastatic bone lesions are usually osteolytic but may be osteoblastic or mixed. Tumors with a tendency to produce pure osteoblastic metastases are prostatic carcinoma, carcinoid tumor and other neuroendocrine neoplasms, and—less commonly—breast carcinoma.[697] If the osteoblastic bone metastases of prostatic carcinoma are extensive, they can be accompanied by osteomalacia, possibly because the organism cannot satisfy the high calcium demand for new bone formation.[687]

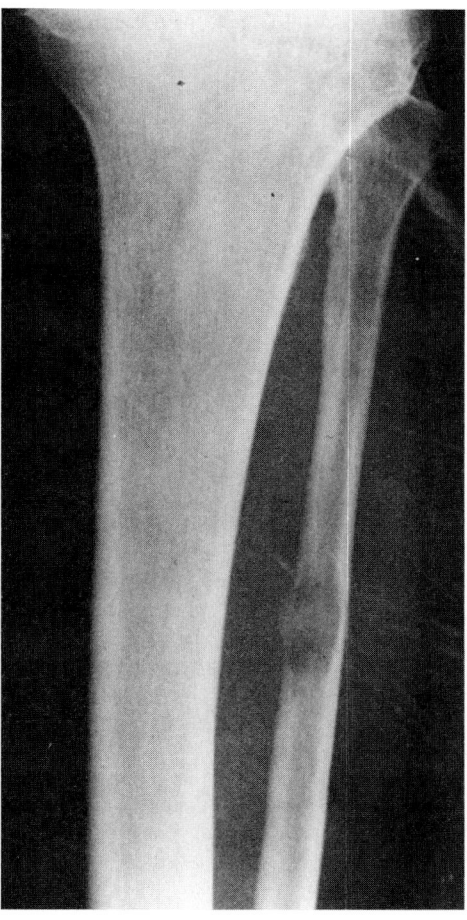

Fig. 24-82 Ill-defined lytic lesion in midshaft of fibula produced by metastasis of lung carcinoma.

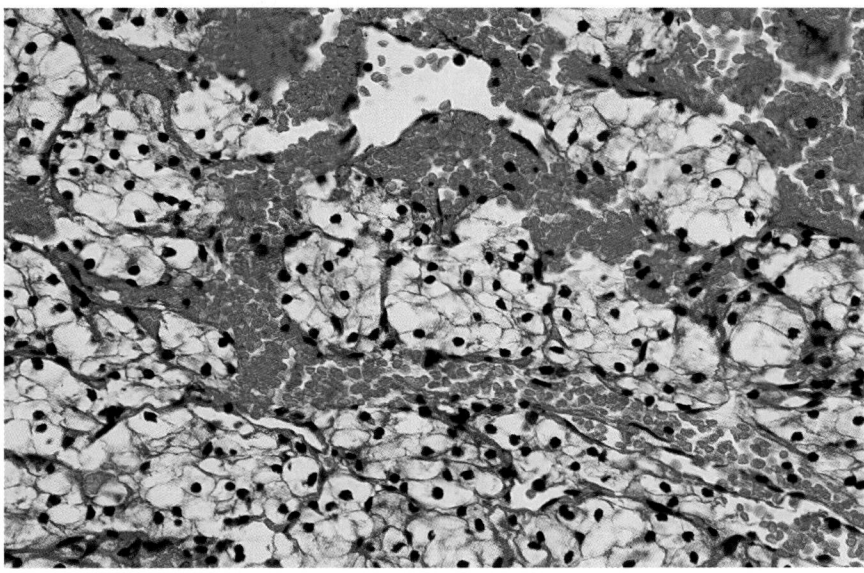

Fig. 24-83 Renal cell carcinoma of clear cell type metastatic to bone. Notice the marked fresh hemorrhage that is a characteristic feature of this tumor.

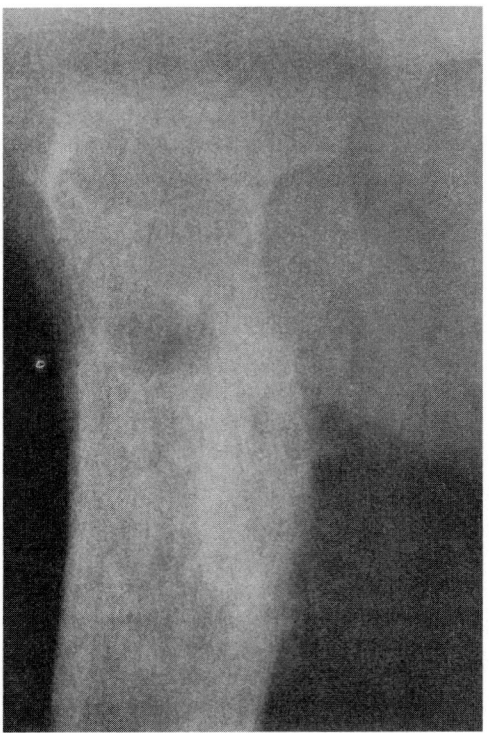

Fig. 24-84 Metastatic carcinoma in femur, with extensive callus formation, which simulated osteosarcoma both radiographically and microscopically. Primary tumor was probably in lung.

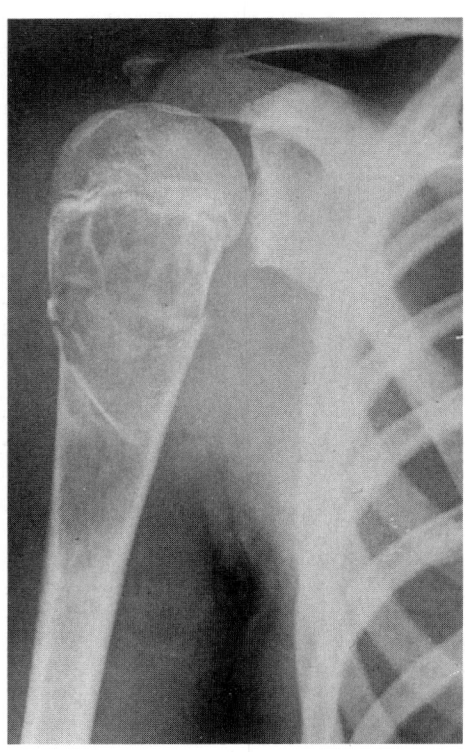

Fig. 24-85 Typical solitary bone cyst of upper end of humerus abutting against epiphyseal plate in 13-year-old boy.

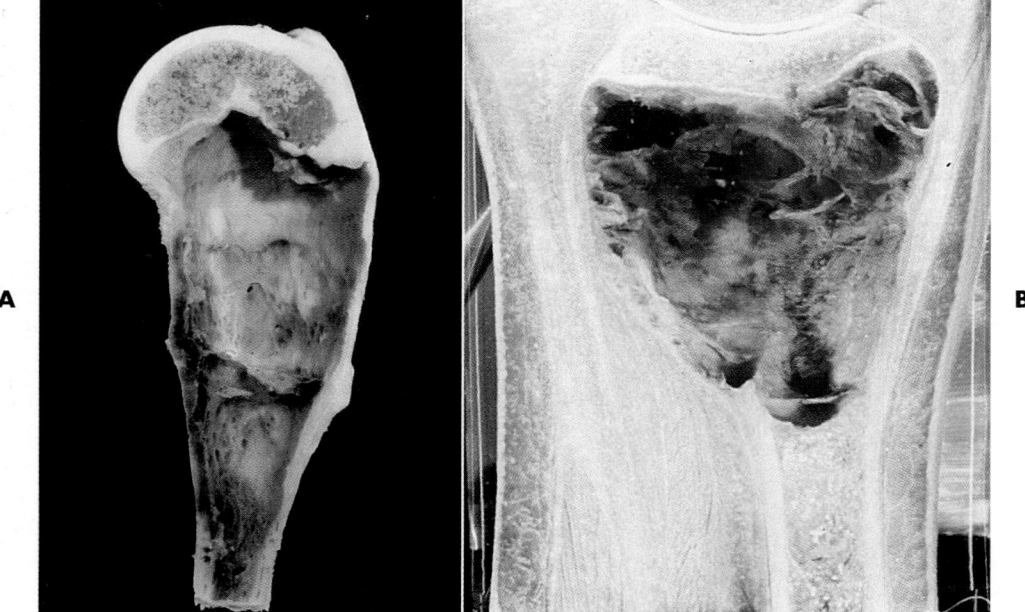

Fig. 24-86 Gross appearances of solitary bone cyst. **A,** Large lesion located in the upper metaphysis of the humerus. **B,** Triangular lesion located in the upper end of the tibia. There has been secondary hemorrhage, leading to an appearance not too dissimilar from that of an aneurysmal bone cyst.

The bone or bones involved and the character of the changes seen radiographically are helpful in predicting the site of the primary neoplasm. Thyroid carcinoma usually metastasizes to the bones of the shoulder girdle, skull, ribs, and sternum. Carcinoma of the kidney tends to involve the skull, sternum, flat bones of the pelvis, upper end of the femur, and scapula.[689] Bone metastases peripheral to the knees or elbows are rare, but they certainly occur, as distally as the terminal phalanges.[690,692,698]

Periosteal bone proliferation may rarely accompany a metastatic lesion.[693] This is more likely to occur in certain sclerosing lesions such as those of the prostate. Exuberant new bone formation can also occur because of a pathologic fracture associated with metastatic carcinoma and lead to diagnostic confusion with osteosarcoma[691] (Fig. 24-84). Metastatic malignant tumors—including carcinoma and melanoma—can be accompanied by a prominent population of osteoclasts and simulate a giant cell tumor.[688] A soft tissue component may be present, particularly in bone metastases from the sternum or spine; sometimes, a pulsating mass will form as a result. Any tumor metastatic to bone, if extensive enough, may lead to hypercalcemia and elevation of serum acid phosphatase.

The mechanism of bone resorption is not well understood but is thought to be related to the transformation of tumor-infiltrating macrophages into osteoclasts.[695]

It is imperative that presumed metastatic lesions to bone be biopsied in order to avoid treatment designed for primary malignant bone tumors. The microscopic recognition usually is simple. The source of the bone metastasis may be suggested microscopically, particularly in cases of carcinoma of the kidney, thyroid gland, or large bowel. Most cases of metastatic squamous cell carcinoma originate from the lung.

Most metastatic bone lesions cause pain. Treatment is for its relief and to prevent fracture of weight-bearing bones. Localized radiation therapy is highly effective, inducing partial or complete relief of pain in over 80% of the cases. When a pathologic fracture supervenes, internal fixation and radiation therapy provide the best results.[694] Palliative measures such as estrogen therapy and/or orchiectomy may afford relief in patients with disseminated metastases from carcinoma of the prostate. The pain of metastatic carcinoma from the breast or prostate is commonly relieved by testosterone, with occasional striking objective improvement in the condition of the bone. Hormonal therapy with estrogens or tamoxifen, or ovarian ablation provides pain relief in 25% to 50% of patients with metastatic breast cancer. Strontium-89 and hormonal manipulation have proved equally successful for pain relief in prostatic carcinoma. In a few instances, a single metastatic focus, particularly from the thyroid or kidney, may be excised with benefit.

TUMORLIKE LESIONS
Solitary bone cyst

Solitary (unicameral) bone cysts usually occur in long bones, most often in the upper portion of the shaft of the humerus and femur[701,704] (Fig. 24-85). They also may be seen in short bones, particularly the calcaneus.[703] Most cases are seen in males, and almost all occur in patients under 20 years of age.

These lesions usually are advanced when first seen. Most are usually metaphyseal in position and do not involve the epiphysis. In time, they tend to migrate away from the epiphysis. The cortex is thinned, but periosteal bone proliferation does not take place except in areas of fracture. Bones affected by these lesions often fracture, usually in the proximal portion of the cystic area.[701]

The cyst contains a clear or yellow fluid and is lined by a smooth fibrous membrane that may be brown (Fig. 24-86). The fluid may be hemorrhagic if a previous fracture has occurred. Microscopically, well-vascularized connective tissue, hemosiderin (often within macrophages), and cholesterol clefts are fre-quent. The bone surrounding the cyst may have a dense quality, with irregular cement lines.[699a,702]

The diagnosis may be difficult in the presence of reparative changes following fracture, in recurrent lesions after bone grafting, and when articular cartilage is included in the curettings, but it becomes clear if the history and the x-ray films are available.

It is believed that this lesion arises on the basis of a local disorder of development and bone growth. A synovial origin has been suggested as an alternative pathogenesis.[702]

The treatment of choice is curettement and replacement of the cyst with bone chips. The results of therapy correlate well with the cyst's "activity" as determined by its location. Good results are obtained when the cyst has migrated away from the epiphyseal line, but recurrences often develop when it has not.[700]

Aneurysmal bone cyst

Aneurysmal bone cyst is seen usually in patients between 10 and 20 years of age.[712,719,729] It occurs mainly in the vertebrae and flat bones but can also arise in the shaft of long bones.[709,726] Multiple involvement is frequent in the vertebral lesions. Exceptionally, a lesion with the features of an osseous aneurysmal bone cyst is seen in a soft tissue location and even within the wall of a major artery.[723,724]

Radiographically, aneurysmal bone cyst shows eccentric expansion of the bone, with erosion and destruction of the cortex and a small peripheral area of periosteal new bone formation (Figs. 24-87 and 24-88). Grossly, it forms a spongy hemorrhagic mass covered by a thin shell of reactive bone, which may extend into the soft tissue. Microscopically, large spaces filled with blood are seen. They do not have an endothelial lining but are rather delimited by cells with the morphologic, ultrastructural, and immunohistochemical features of fibroblasts, myofibroblasts, and histiocytes.[705,706] These cells also occupy the septa that separate the cysts.[706] A row of osteoclasts is often seen beneath the surface (Fig. 24-88, B, and Plate XVIII-E). The septa also contain blood vessels and foci of osteoid and bone. An additional feature of great diagnostic significance is the deposition of a peculiar degenerated calcifying fibromyxoid tissue.[728]

The differential diagnosis includes solitary bone cyst, giant cell tumor, hemangioma, telangiectatic osteosarcoma, and—especially for the lesions located in the jaw—giant cell reparative granuloma.

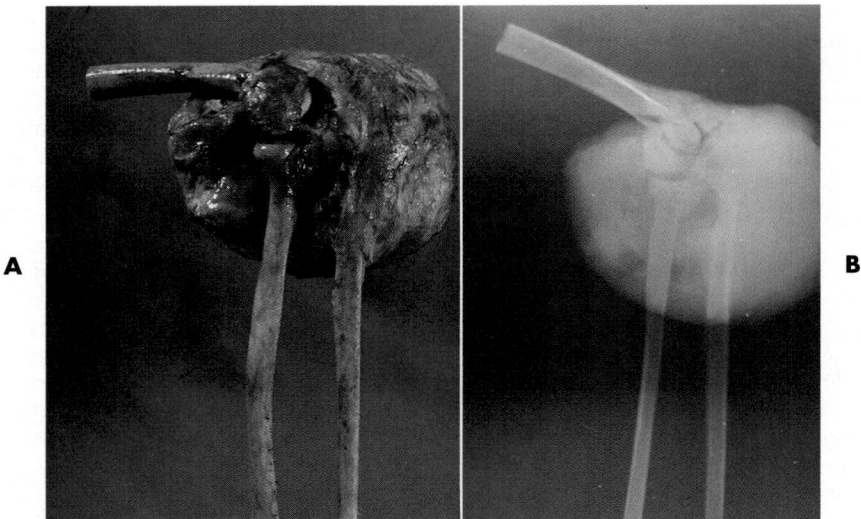

Fig. 24-87 Gross **(A)** and radiographic **(B)** appearances of large aneurysmal bone cyst of ulna. (Courtesy Dr. Juan José Segura, San José, Costa Rica.)

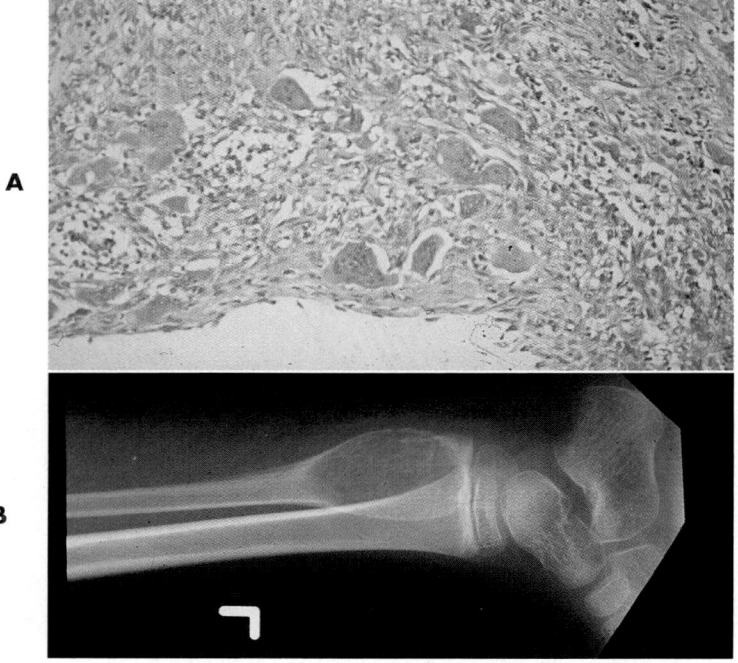

Fig. 24-88 Radiographic **(A)** and microscopic **(B)** appearances of aneurysmal bone cyst of lower end of fibula.

The pathogenesis of aneurysmal bone cyst remains elusive. In a few cases, the lesion is preceded by trauma with fracture or subperiosteal hematoma.[711] In others, it seems to arise in some pre-existing bone lesion as a result of changed hemodynamics.[708,715,718] Areas grossly and microscopically indistinguishable from aneurysmal bone cyst can occur in chondroblastoma, giant cell tumor, fibrous dysplasia, nonossifying fibroma, osteoblastoma, chondrosarcoma, and in the vascular and cartilaginous hamartoma of the chest wall in infants.[720] However, in most aneurysmal bone cysts, an underlying lesion is not encountered.[710,728] Naturally, this might be the result of sampling or the fact that the aneurysmal bone cyst destroyed all evidence of the pre-existing lesion.

Recurrence supervenes in approximately one fourth of the cases treated by curettage alone because of incompleteness of surgical excision.[725,729] En bloc resection or curettage with bone grafting affords better results.[716]

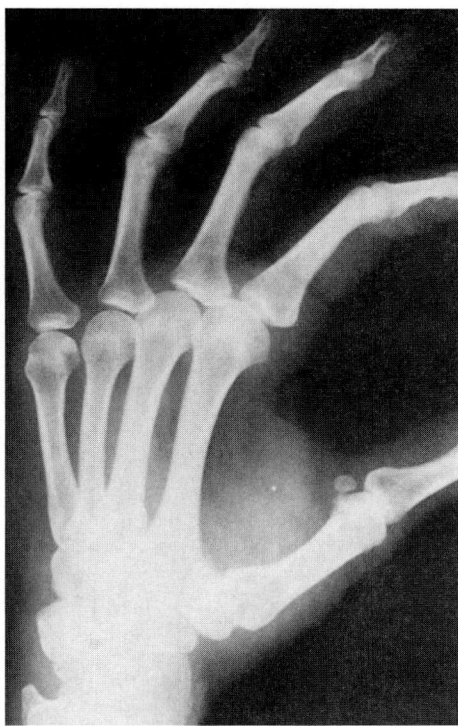

Fig. 24-89 Intraosseous ganglion cyst involving base of first metacarpal. It was associated with larger ganglion of adjacent soft tissue, which is also apparent in radiograph. (Courtesy Dr. G. Davis, St. Louis.)

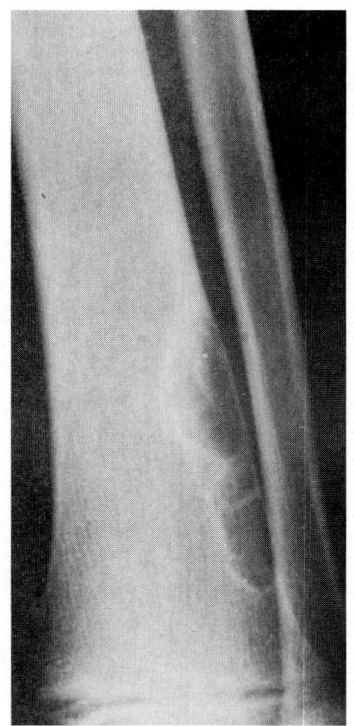

Fig. 24-90 Metaphyseal fibrous defect of lower end of tibia. Note its sharp delineation and sclerotic margins.

A few cases of reasonably convincing malignant transformation of aneurysmal bone cyst into osteosarcoma have been described; this exceptionally rare phenomenon should be distinguished from telangiectatic osteosarcoma and osteosarcoma with aneurysmal cyst-like areas.[717]

Sometimes lesions with the features of aneurysmal bone cysts are seen in association with solid areas composed of an admixture of fibrous tissue, new bone formation, and osteoclasts. In other instances, solid areas with this mixed appearance are seen in the absence of typical aneurysmal bone cyst features. Depending on the location of the lesion, variation in microscopic appearance, and the pathologist's bias, these lesions have been variously referred to as *giant cell reaction, (extragnathic) giant cell reparative granuloma, giant cell–containing fibrous lesion, and solid variant of aneurysmal bone cyst.** Locations include the small bones of the hands and feet, vertebrae, sacrum, and—less commonly—long bones. In the latter locations, they tend to have a metaphyseal location[707] (Plate XVIII-F). Determining whether these lesions are reactive or neoplastic and establishing their exact place in the classification of bone diseases remain to be accomplished.

Ganglion cyst of bone

On rare occasions, ganglion cysts, morphologically indistinguishable from those commonly seen in the periarticular

*References 713, 714, 721, 722, 727, 730.

soft tissue, are found in an intraosseous location, always close to a joint space[731,732] (Fig. 24-89).

The cyst is surrounded by a zone of condensed bone, is often multiloculated, and has a gelatinous content and a wall of attenuated fibrous tissue. The bones of the ankle, particularly the tibia, are those most commonly affected.[733] Intraosseous ganglia need to be distinguished from solitary bone cysts and the periarticular cysts seen in association with degenerative joint diseases.

Metaphyseal fibrous defect (nonossifying fibroma)

Metaphyseal fibrous defects are distinctive lesions of bone that occur in adolescents, most often in long tubular bones, particularly the upper or lower tibia or the lower femur.[736,738] They are eccentric, sharply delimited lesions not too distant from the epiphysis and sometimes accompanied by epiphyseal disorders (Fig. 24-90). When loose and associated with an intramedullary component, they have been designated as nonossifying or nonosteogenic fibromas (Fig. 24-91). There has been a long-standing and still unresolved controversy regarding whether these lesions are neoplastic or whether they represent developmental aberration at the epiphyseal plate.[737]

Grossly, the lesion is granular and brown or dark red. Microscopically, it consists of cellular masses of fibrous tissue often arranged in a storiform pattern (Figs. 24-92 and 24-93). Scattered osteoclasts and collections of foamy and

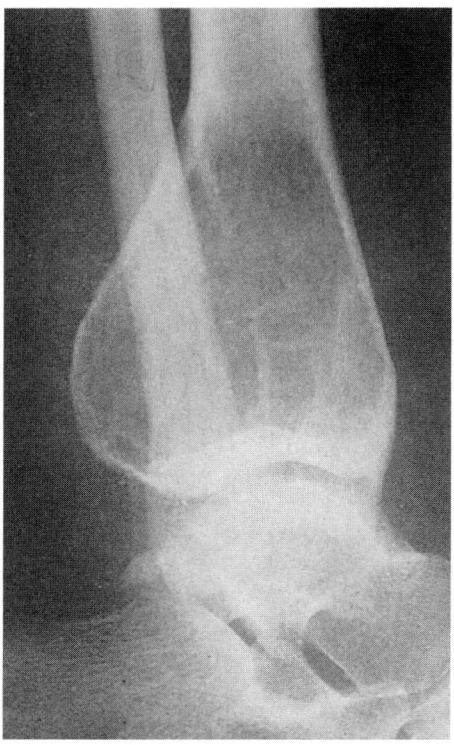

Fig. 24-91 Large metaphyseal fibrous defect expanding lower tibia metaphysis. Lesions of this size are sometimes called nonossifying fibroma.

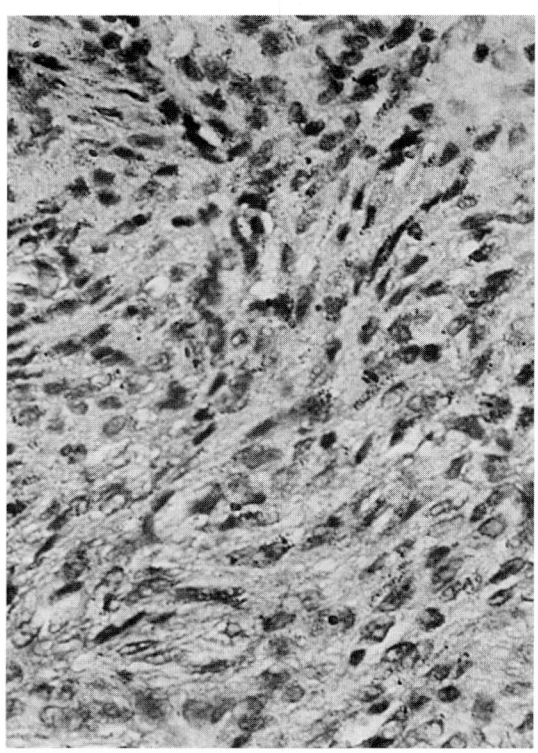

Fig. 24-92 Area of metaphyseal fibrous defect demonstrating cellular whorl-like masses of fibrous tissue.

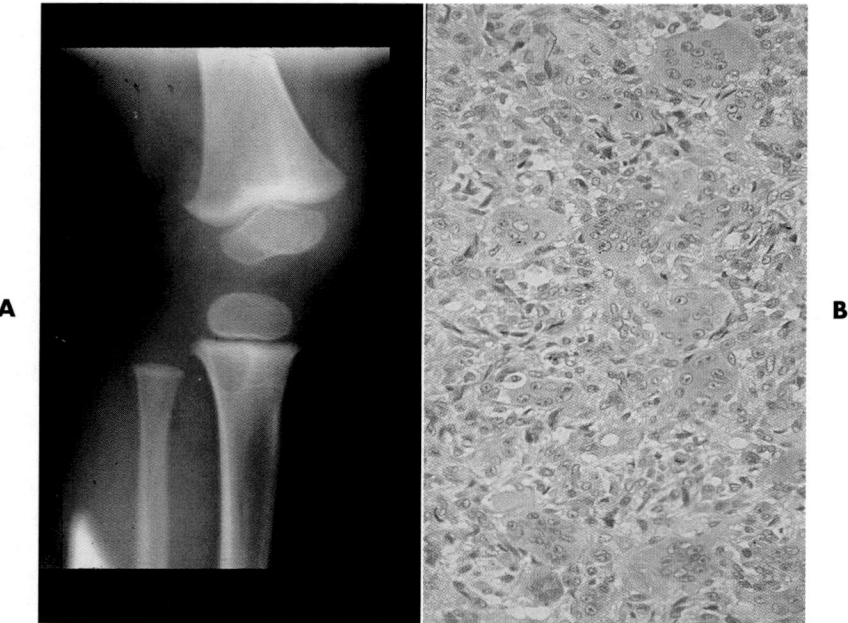

Fig. 24-93 Radiographic (A) and microscopic (B) appearances of metaphyseal fibrous defect involving the upper metaphysis of the tibia.

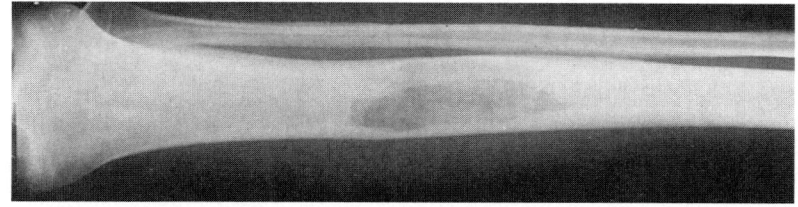

Fig. 24-94 Fibrous dysplasia of tibia forming sharply delimited lesion.

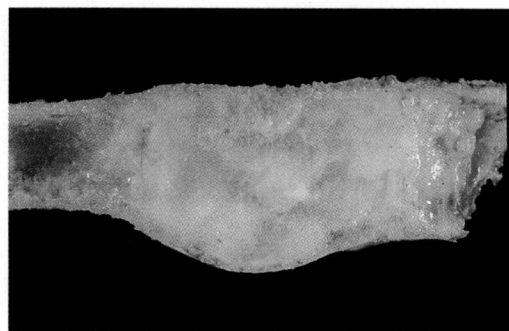

Fig. 24-95 Gross appearance of fibrous dysplasia of the rib. The lesion forms a fusiform, expanded mass that is grayish white.

hemosiderin-laden macrophages are frequent. The microscopic appearance is very reminiscent of a benign fibrous histiocytoma and is designated as such by some authors, especially when it occurs in adult patients in places other than metaphyses of long bones.[735]

Clinically, there are few or no symptoms except pain. The lesion is usually found incidentally on x-ray examination. Fractures can occur through the thinned cortex.[734]

Fibrous dysplasia and related lesions

Fibrous dysplasia is a non-neoplastic condition that can present in two forms: monostotic and polyostotic.[752] The monostotic variety is usually seen in older children and young adults and most commonly affects the rib, femur, and tibia.[747,760] The less common polyostotic type is characterized by a unilateral distribution and is usually associated with endocrine dysfunction, precocious puberty in female individuals, and areas of cutaneous hyperpigmentation (Albright's syndrome).[739] This syndrome is the result of a somatic mutation of the c-*fos* oncogene in affected tissues that results in the activation of the signal-transduction pathway that generates cyclic AMP.[743a,761,764]

Radiographs of these lesions in the rib show a fusiform, expanded mass with thinning of the cortex. In the tibia, a lobulated, sharply delimited lesion of the shaft is formed (Fig. 24-94). This lesion may have a multilocular appearance because of endosteal cortical scalloping. Comparable lesions in membranous bone, particularly in the maxilla or the mandible, may show an overgrowth of dense bone. Occasionally the lesion protrudes far beyond the normal bone contour ("fibrous dysplasia protuberans").[744]

Grossly, the tissue cuts with a gritty consistency and is grayish yellow (Fig. 24-95). The cortical bone often is thinned and expanded.

Microscopically, narrow, curved, and misshaped bone trabeculae, often having a characteristic fishhook configuration, are interspersed with fibrous tissue of variable cellularity[758] (Fig. 24-96). Coarse fiber ("woven") bone never becomes transformed to lamellar bone, suggesting that fibrous dysplasia represents a maturation defect so that the process of bone formation is arrested at an early stage resembling membranous ossification. Rows of cuboidal appositional osteoblasts do not appear on the surface of the trabeculae except as a pattern of reaction following local trauma. Silver stains are helpful in showing this failure of maturation. Ultrastructurally, the immature woven bone trabeculae are lined by abnormal osteoblasts with a fibroblast-like appearance.[746]

If a lesion of fibrous dysplasia is biopsied over a period of years, maturation is still absent. This fundamental histologic abnormality makes it possible to distinguish fibrous dysplasia from other lesions. In some instances, however, particularly in femoral lesions, the differential diagnosis becomes nearly impossible.[757]

Occasionally, lesions of fibrous dysplasia show calcified spherules similar to those seen in cementifying fibromas.[756,762,763a] Other cases show highly cellular areas that may be diagnosed incorrectly as sarcoma. Focal areas of hyaline cartilage and cystic areas may also be present. The former are more common in the polyostotic variety and can dominate the microscopic picture to such a degree that a mistaken diagnosis of a cartilaginous tumor can be made.[755] The transition of normal to abnormal bone is often abrupt. This is helpful in distinguishing it radiographically from osteitis fibrosa cystica resulting from hyperparathyroidism.

It has been suggested that some rib lesions resembling fibrous dysplasia but showing progressive maturation of the bone toward the periphery are secondary to trauma ("post-

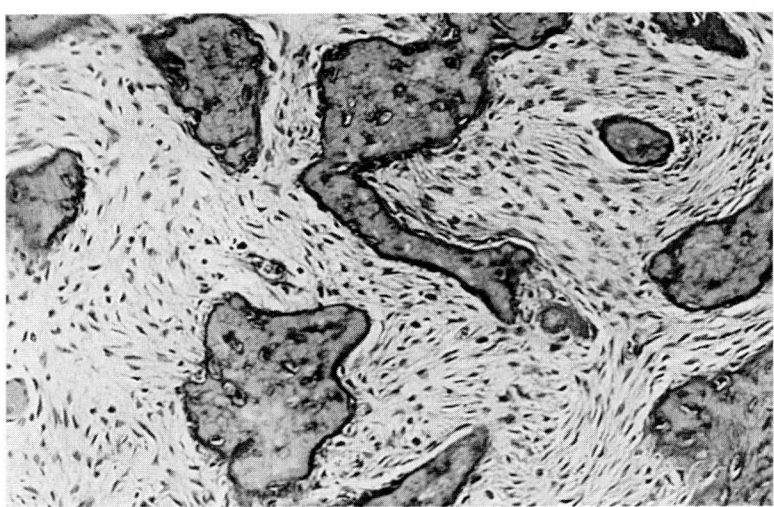

Fig. 24-96 Typical fibrous dysplasia of rib demonstrating spicules of new bone formation with intervening cellular fibrous tissue. Trabeculae are not oriented along lines of stress. They form odd geometric patterns and have no osteoblasts on their surfaces. There is no maturation of this coarse fiber bone.

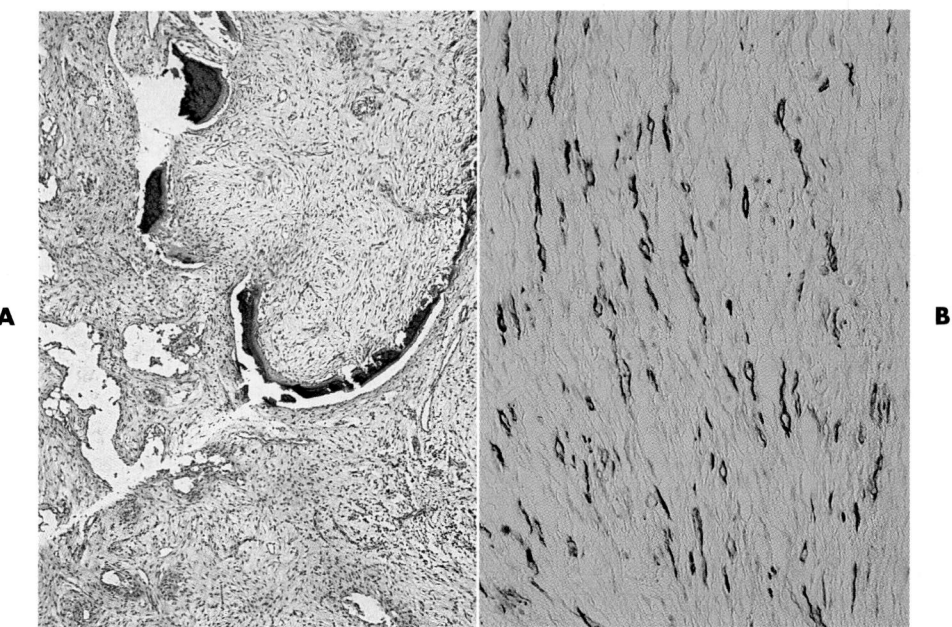

Fig. 24-97 Osteofibrous dysplasia. **A,** The low-power view is similar to that of fibrous dysplasia, but on high power there was osteoblastic rimming of the bone trabeculae. **B,** Immunoreactivity of spindle cells of osteofibrous dysplasia for keratin. This does not occur in fibrous dysplasia.

traumatic dysplasia").[750] Some of these lesions are bilateral and strikingly symmetrical.[745]

Fibrous dysplasia may be accompanied by intramuscular myxoma of the same extremity.[739a] In addition, fibrous dysplasia of either monostotic or polyostotic type can be complicated by the development of a primary bone sarcoma, particularly osteosarcoma[748] but also chondrosarcoma and malignant fibrous histiocytoma.[749,759]

Resection cures fibrous dysplasia in bones such as the rib. Curettement is adequate in long bones such as the tibia. In the maxilla, where some deformity may exist, partial removal of the lesion is all that is necessary.

Osteofibrous dysplasia (fibro-osseous dysplasia, ossifying fibroma) is closely related to fibrous dysplasia.[754] It is distinguished from it microscopically by the osteoblastic rimming of the bone trabeculae and the presence of lamellar bone and radiographically by its cortical rather than medullary location and its greater tendency to recur[741,743,751] (Fig. 24-97, *A*). The tibia and fibula are the bones usually affected, the lesions usually being eccentrically located.[742,753]

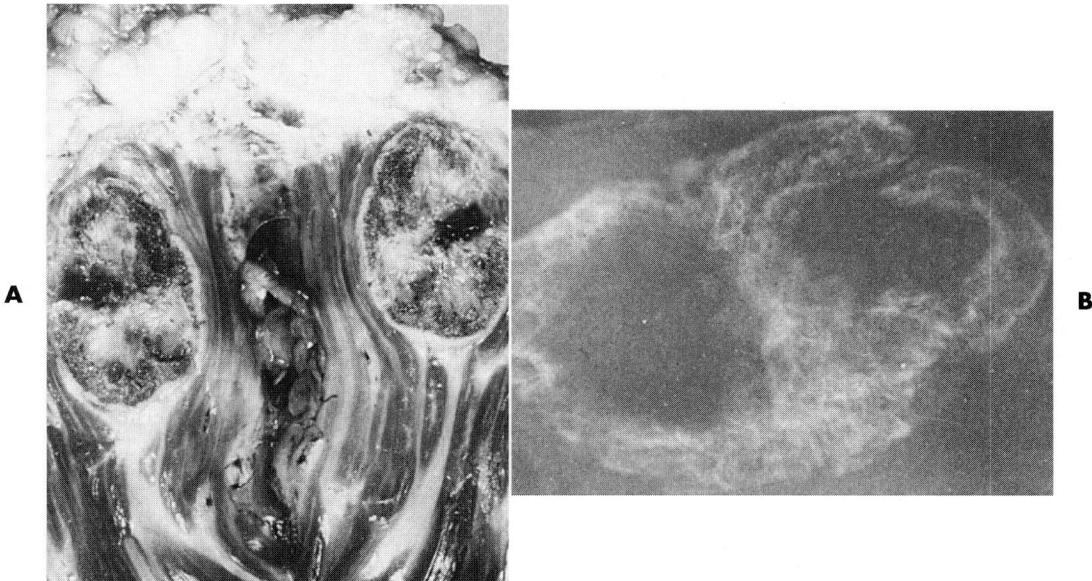

Fig. 24-98 A, Well-defined myositis ossificans occurring in muscle. **B,** Same lesion shown in **A** illustrating bone formation in periphery. (From Ackerman LV: Extraosseous localized nonneoplastic bone and cartilage formation [so-called myositis ossificans]. J Bone Joint Surg **40A:**279-298, 1958.)

Clonal chromosomal abnormalities have been identified in this lesion, suggesting a neoplastic nature.[740] Immunohistochemically, reactivity for keratin can be found in the spindle cells; this has never been the case in lesions of fibrous dysplasia[754,763] (Fig. 24-97, *B*). Furthermore, a peculiar and as yet unexplained relationship exists between osteofibrous dysplasia and adamantinoma of long bones (see p. 1973).

Myositis ossificans

Myositis ossificans is a reactive condition that is sometimes mistaken microscopically for osteosarcoma.[765,769] The term is inaccurate because the muscle may not be involved, and inflammation is virtually absent. A history of trauma is obtained in only half of the patients. The most common locations are the flexor muscles of the upper arm (especially the brachialis anticus), the quadriceps femoris, the adductor muscles of the thigh, the gluteal muscles, and the soft tissues of the hand. Radiographic studies show periosteal reaction and faint soft tissue calcification within 3 to 6 weeks of the injury; these are gradually replaced by mature heterotopic bone by 10 to 12 weeks (Fig. 24-98). Arteriography done during the active stage of the disease shows numerous fine vessels followed by a dense, poorly defined stain in the mass.[770]

Microscopically, there is a highly cellular stroma associated with new bone and, less commonly, cartilage formation. In an early lesion, the centrally placed areas may be very difficult to distinguish from osteosarcoma because of their extreme cellularity. As the process evolves, osteoid appears in an orderly pattern at the periphery of this mass and subsequently matures into well-developed bone. Several microscopic subtypes have been described, which correspond to different stages of the process.[769] The most important diagnostic feature is provided by the maturation pattern ("zonal phenomenon"), characterized by a central cellular

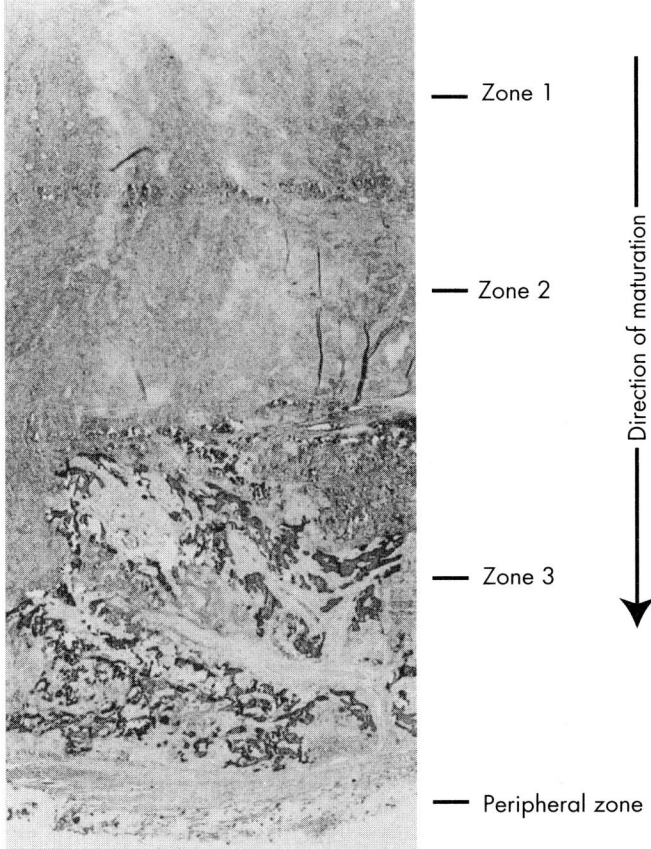

Zone 1

Zone 2

Direction of maturation

Zone 3

Peripheral zone

Fig. 24-99 Schematic representation of zonal phenomenon in myositis ossificans. (From Ackerman LV: Extraosseous localized nonneoplastic bone and cartilage formation [so-called myositis ossificans]. J Bone Joint Surg **40A:**279-298, 1958).

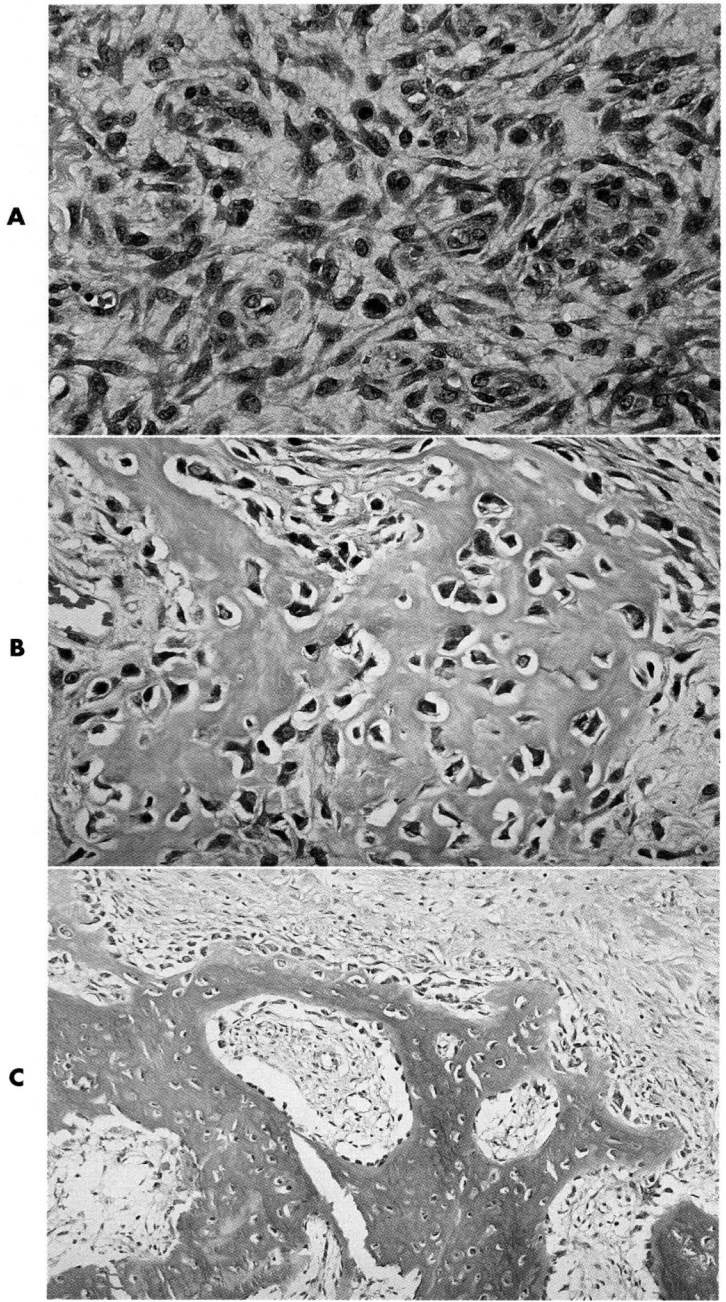

Fig. 24-100 Various appearances of myositis ossificans. **A,** Deep region showing highly cellular appearance that can simulate a soft tissue sarcoma. **B,** Midportion showing osteoid formation by plump osteoblasts. **C,** Peripheral portion showing a shell of well-formed bone.

area, an intermediate zone of osteoid formation, and a peripheral shell of highly organized bone[765] (Figs. 24-99 and 24-100). Ultrastructurally, cells with features of myofibroblasts are prominent, as befits a reactive condition of mesenchymal tissues.[767]

The most important differential diagnosis is with extraosseous osteosarcoma and juxtacortical osteosarcoma. In the former condition, clearly sarcomatous areas are pres-

ent, and the zonal phenomenon does not occur (see Chapter 25). We seriously doubt whether myositis ossificans ever develops into osteosarcoma. We believe that many of the reported cases of this complication actually represent misdiagnosed instances of juxtacortical or extraosseous osteosarcoma.

A reactive lesion histologically and pathogenetically probably related to myositis ossificans has been reported in

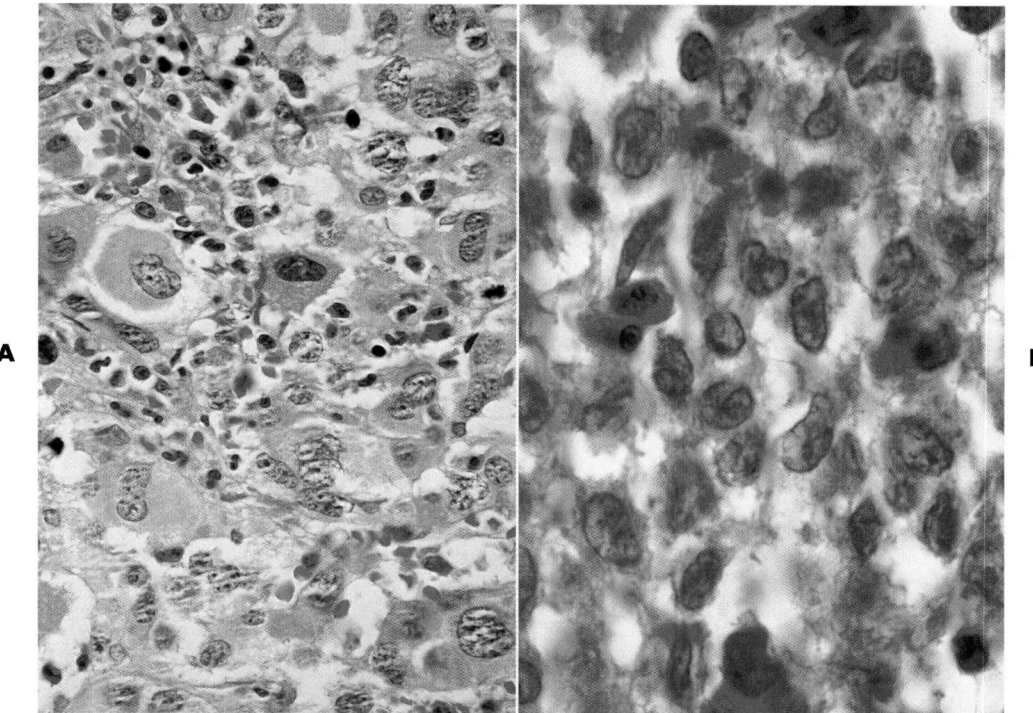

Fig. 24-101 Langerhans' cell granulomatosis. **A,** Polymorphic appearance resulting from admixture of Langerhans' cells, nonspecific histiocytes, lymphocytes, and eosinophils. There is a mild atypia in the Langerhans' cells that can simulate a malignant process. **B,** High-power view showing elongated nuclei with occasional longitudinal grooves in the Langerhans' cells.

the small bones of the hand as *florid reactive periostitis, parosteal fasciitis, fibro-osseous tumor of the digits,* and other descriptive terms.[766,768]

Langerhans' cell granulomatosis

The unifying feature of the group of conditions designated as Langerhans' cell granulomatosis (histiocytosis X, eosinophilic granuloma) is an infiltration by a specific cell of the immune system known as Langerhans' cell. This is accompanied by a variable admixture of eosinophils, giant cells, neutrophils, foamy cells, and areas of fibrosis. Langerhans' cells have a characteristic morphologic appearance[776] (Fig. 24-101). Their nuclei often are lobulated or indented, sometimes with a longitudinal groove; their cytoplasm is, for the most part, distinctly acidophilic. A specific intracytoplasmic organelle, known as Langerhans' or Birbeck's granule, is regularly present on electron microscopic examination (Fig. 24-102, *A*).

Langerhans' cell granulomatosis of bone can be divided into three major categories on the basis of type and extent of the organ involvement:

1 Solitary bone involvement
2 Multiple bone involvement (with or without skin involvement)
3 Multiple organ involvement (bone, liver, spleen, and others)

The cases with solitary bone involvement, which represent the most common variety, have been traditionally referred to as eosinophilic granuloma.[773] Young adults are most commonly affected.[774] Any bone can be involved, with the possible exception of the hands and feet. The most common sites are the cranial vault, jaw, humerus, rib, and femur (Fig. 24-102, *B*). Radiographically, they present as an osteolytic lesion often in the metaphyseal area of long bones, sometimes associated with periosteal bone proliferation. They can be confused radiographically with metastatic carcinoma (Fig. 24-103) or Ewing's sarcoma (Fig. 24-104). After fracture, this process may extend into adjacent soft tissues. Recurrences may develop in soft tissue after surgery. These lesions may spontaneously regress. They are extremely radiosensitive and can be cured with small amounts of radiation. The long-term prognosis is excellent. It is exceptional for these patients to develop other bone lesions or involvement of other organs.

Cases of multiple bone involvement have been traditionally designated as multiple or polyostotic eosinophilic granulomas.[771,772] When strategically located, the bony infiltration may result in proptosis, diabetes insipidus, chronic otitis media, or a combination of these conditions. The eponym of Hand-Schüller-Christian disease has been applied to this variety. Since the circumstances on which this designation is based are fortuitous and erratic, it would probably be better to drop the term entirely. This form is characterized by a prolonged clinical course, often marked by alternating episodes of regressions and recrudescences. The eventual outcome is favorable in most cases.

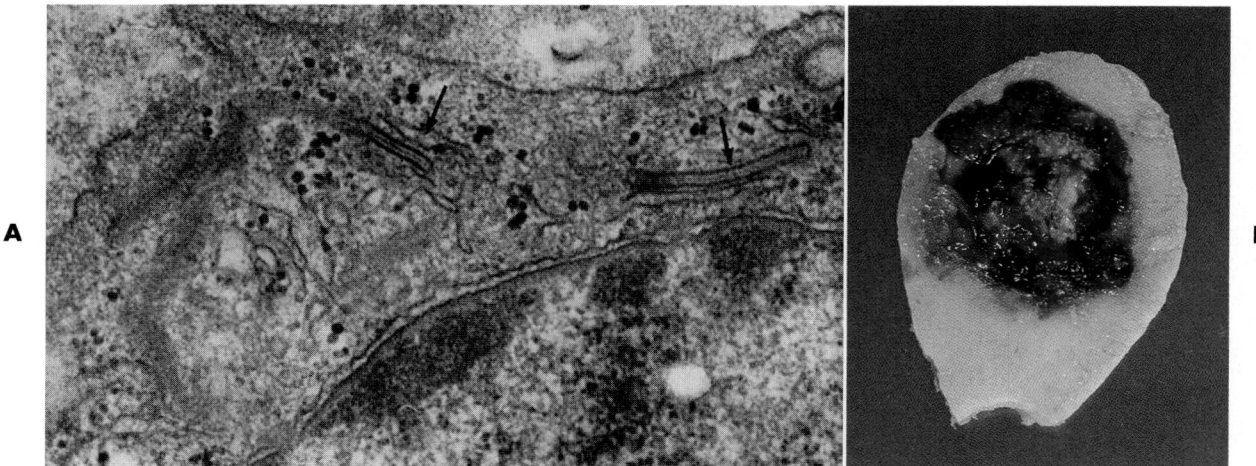

Fig. 24-102 A, This cell from eosinophilic granuloma of bone contains several Langerhans' granules *(arrows).* This is a constant feature of Langerhans' cells in this group of diseases. **B,** Gross appearance of eosinophilic granuloma of skull. Sharply circumscribed, dark brown lesion is seen. (Courtesy Dr. J. Segura, San Jose, Costa Rica.)

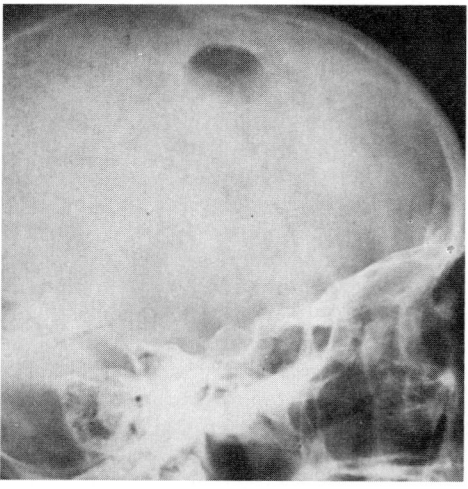

Fig. 24-103 Osteolytic lesion of skull in 25-year-old woman. Radiographically, lesion was thought to be metastatic carcinoma but proved to be solitary lesion of eosinophilic granuloma.

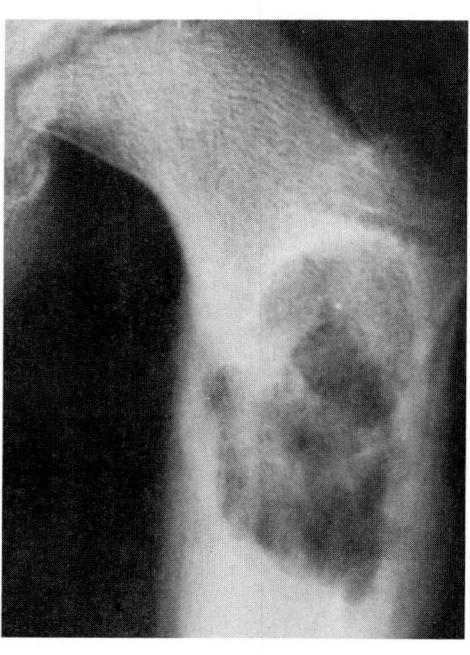

Fig. 24-104 Osteolytic lesion of femur in 12-year-old boy. This was thought to be Ewing's sarcoma but proved microscopically to be eosinophilic granuloma.

This type of Langerhans' cell granulomatosis blends imperceptibly with the form having multiple organ involvement. Following the skeletal system, the skin and the lungs are the two most common sites affected. It is difficult to predict the outcome of the disease in a particular case, but there are several parameters that can be used as guidelines. Poor prognostic factors are young age (under 18 months) at the time of diagnosis, hepatomegaly, anemia and/or thrombocytopenia, bone marrow involvement, and hemorrhagic skin lesions. Features not associated with a poor prognosis are seborrhea-like skin lesions, diabetes insipidus, and pulmonary lesions.[777] Microscopically, it is very difficult to separate the aggressive from the more indolent forms. In a typical case of the former, the infiltrate is more monomor-

phic, with more mitoses and necrosis and fewer giant cells and eosinophils than in a typical case of the latter,[775] but in our experience the overlap has been too great to rely on these features alone.

The differential diagnosis of Langerhans' cell granulomatosis of bone at the microscopic level includes osteomyelitis and the osseous manifestations of sinus histiocytosis with massive lymphadenopathy (Rosai-Dorfman's disease).[778]

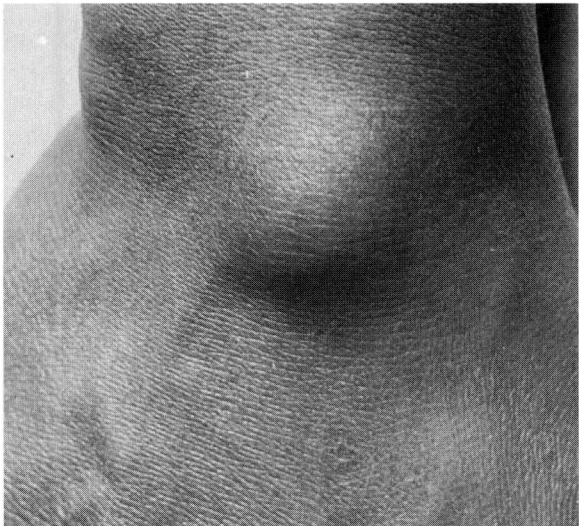

Fig. 24-105 Typical location and appearance of ganglion.

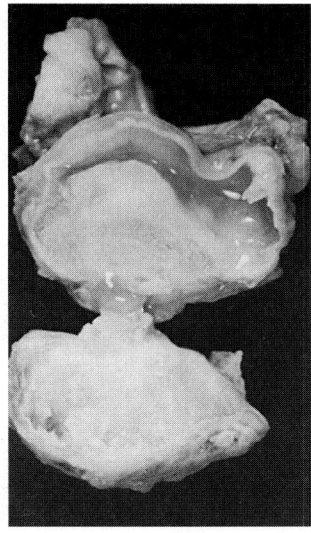

Fig. 24-106 Ganglion illustrating mucoid appearance and poorly defined capsule.

Joints and related structures
NORMAL ANATOMY

Joints that permit free movements of the bone, referred to as *diarthroses,* are covered by hyaline cartilage and enclosed in a joint capsule. This capsule is composed of an outer fibrous layer of dense connective tissues, which is continuous with the periosteum of the bones, and an inner synovial layer. The latter, also referred to as *synovial membrane,* contains fibroblast-like cells (synoviocytes, type B cells)[781] and macrophages of presumed bone marrow derivation (type A cells). Synoviocytes secrete collagen and proteoglycan and have a highly characteristic phenotype that includes the strong expression of vascular cell adhesion molecule-1 (VCAM-1)[780] and of the antigen detected by Mab67,[779] as well as high activity of the enzyme uridine diphosphoglucose dehydrogenase. Synoviocytes are immunoreactive for vimentin but not for keratin or other epithelial markers.

A layer of loose connective tissue or adipose tissue is present in some regions of the joint between the synovial and the fibrous layers, resulting in the formation of folds or "villi," which protrude into the joint cavity. In old age, these villi may contain islands of cartilage.

Tendons are composed of closely packed parallel type I collagen fibers. They are surrounded by a layer of connective tissue known as the *tendon sheath.* In long tendons, this sheath is composed of an inner layer adjacent to the collagen and an outer layer that is loosely bound to the tissues surrounding the tendon. The space between these two layers is somewhat reminiscent of a joint cavity.

NON-NEOPLASTIC DISEASES
Ganglia and cystic meniscus

Ganglia occur around joints and—less commonly—around tendon sheaths. They are annoying deformities that may cause some pain, weakness, partial disability of the joint, and bone changes. Ganglia located in the popliteal space can produce pain or foot drop as result of compression of the common peroneal nerve.[784] Individuals overusing the wrist and fingers (pianists, typists) are prone to this condition. A history of injury preceding ganglion formation may exist.

Ganglia develop by myxoid degeneration and cystic softening of the connective tissue of the joint capsule or tendon sheath.[782,783] The theory of a rent in the synovial membrane of a joint leading to the collection of synovial fluid and the formation of a false capsule can seldom be substantiated.

The most common location of ganglia is on the dorsal carpal area of the hand, where the cystic lesion pushes its way toward the surface between the tendons of the extensor indicis proprius and the extensor carpi radialis (Figs. 24-105 and 24-106). The second most frequent location is the volar surface of the wrist, superficial and medial to the radial artery. Ganglia also arise on the volar surfaces of the fingers just distal to the metacarpophalangeal joints, in the dorsum of the foot, around the ankle and knee, and in the various articular and ligamentous areas of the spine. Intraosseous ganglia are discussed on p. 1979. Ganglia are not lined by synovia and do not communicate with the joint cavity, two features distinguishing them from Baker's cysts (see later section) (Fig. 24-107).

A lesion microscopically similar to soft tissue ganglion may occur in the menisci of the knee and is referred to simply as *cystic meniscus.* The most common site is the peripheral portion of the middle third of the lateral meniscus.[781a,783a] It may remain confined to the meniscus or extend extracapsularly. A traumatic etiology is favored.

Bursae and Baker's cyst

Bursae are found where muscles, tendons, and skin glide over bony prominences. They are subject to all the diseases that occur in large joint spaces. Inflammation may be associated with the formation of cysts, fluid, and loose bodies (Fig. 24-108). The incomplete removal of loose bodies may be followed by the disappearance of the remaining ones from the bursa.

A related lesion is *subdeltoid bursitis* associated with *calcareous tendonitis.* This entity is primarily a degeneration of a tendon or muscle in the rotator cuff of the shoulder followed by deposition of calcium in necrotic collagenous tissue. This calcific material stimulates a secondary inflammatory reaction.[785]

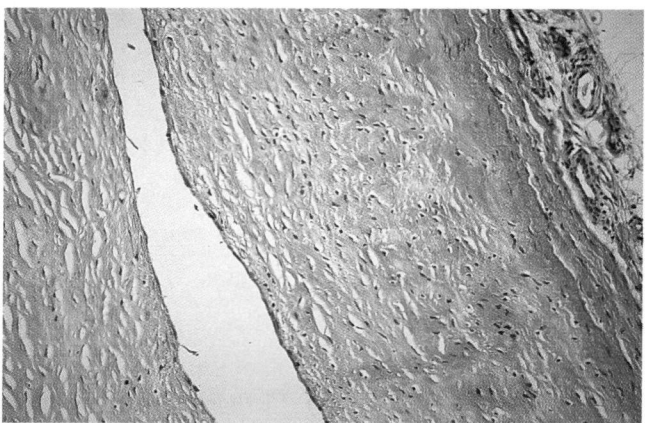

Fig. 24-107 Microscopic appearance of ganglion. The wall is composed of dense fibrous tissue, and there is no synovial lining.

Baker's cyst occurs in the popliteal space from herniation of the synovial membrane through the posterior part of the capsule or from escape of joint fluid through normal anatomic connections of the knee joint with the semimembraneous bursa (Fig. 24-109). The cyst is lined by true synovium and may have cartilage in its wall. Any joint disease leading to increased intra-articular pressure, such as degenerative joint disease, neuropathic arthropathy, and rheumatoid arthritis, may result in the formation of Baker's cyst.[786]

Carpal tunnel syndrome

The carpal tunnel is the space between the flexor retinaculum or transverse carpal ligament and the carpal bones. The medial nerve courses through this tunnel, and its compression in this location by a variety of causes produces the symptoms of carpal tunnel syndrome.[788-790] These include bony deformity following trauma, masses within the canal (i.e., hemangiomas, lipomas, ganglia), rheumatoid arthritis, and amyloidosis.[787] Often, no specific etiology can be demonstrated.

Arthritis

Synovial biopsy

Needle biopsy of the synovium, particularly of the knee joint, is of aid in the assessment of synovial inflammatory conditions[793,797] (Fig. 24-110, *A* and *B*). The procedure is safe, simple, and easily repeated. It is indicated for inflammatory joint diseases when the etiology remains in doubt,

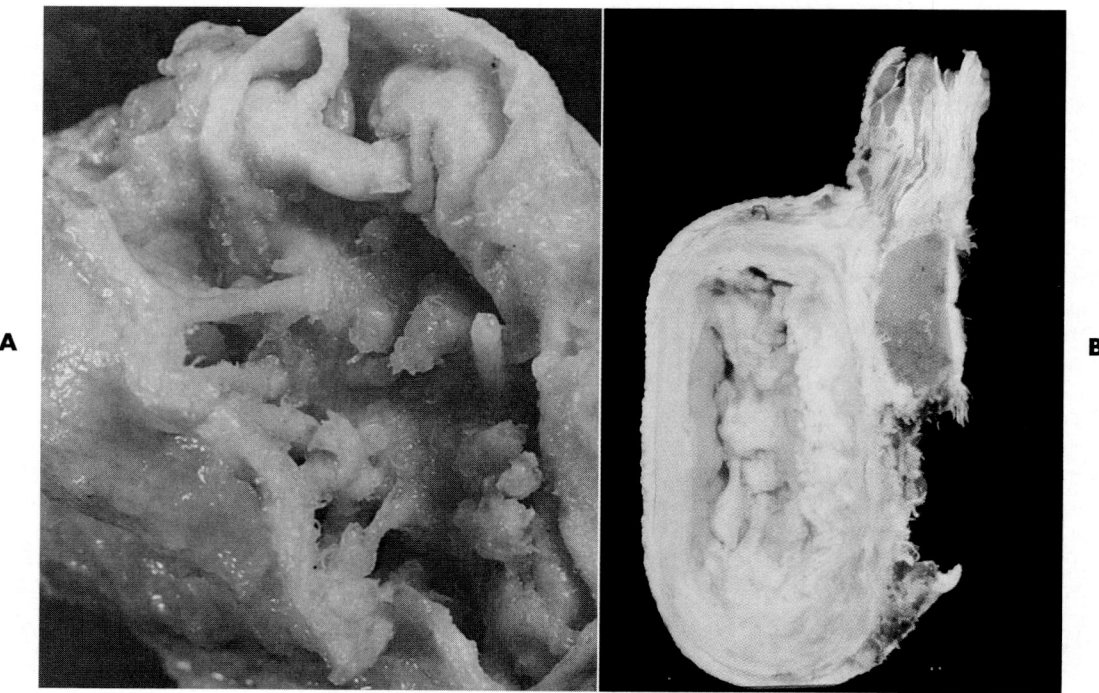

Fig. 24-108 A, Bursal cyst of prepatellar area. Cyst contained fluid. There is extensive proliferation of synovia. **B,** Gross appearance of prepatellar bursa with chronic inflammation.

particularly when only one joint is affected. Examination of the synovial fluid should always be performed before biopsy. It is possible to diagnose tuberculosis and other specific granulomatous lesions by this method.[792-798] Other diagnosable diseases are pigmented villonodular synovitis, amyloidosis, Whipple's disease, hemochromatosis, metastatic disease, and gout. A heavy neutrophilic infiltrate is highly characteristic of infectious arthritis, although it also may be seen in Behçet's disease and familial Mediterranean fever. Unfortunately, the histologic findings in the most common rheumatic diseases are often nonspecific[791]; however, the combination of prominent lymphoid follicles and marked hyperplasia of synovial cells is highly suggestive of rheumatoid arthritis. By the use of a small-caliber synovial biopsy needle (Parker-Pearson technique), Schumacher and Kulka[795] were able to obtain sufficient synovial tissue for diagnosis in 92% of the 109 joint biopsies they performed. Histologic examination proved to be of direct diagnostic value in 38 cases.

Degenerative joint disease (osteoarthritis)

Surgical pathology specimens of legs amputated for traumatic reasons or because of gangrene secondary to vascular disease offer the unique opportunity for study of degenerative joint disease. The term osteoarthritis is inaccurate because this type of joint disease is degenerative and not inflammatory. The pathologic changes are related directly to age and are conditioned by use and occupation of the patient.[815] These morphologic changes have been beautifully

described in the works of Collins,[801,802] Hirsch et al,[806] and Bauer and Bennett.[799,800] The following description is taken from the classic article by Bauer and Bennett[799]:

In degenerative arthritis, the earliest and primary change in the joints is a gradual and uneven degeneration of the hyaline cartilage of the articular surfaces. This is first detected as a fibrillation of the cartilaginous matrix which generally begins near the articular surface and is associated with a disappearance of the spindle-cell perichondrium. As a result of this fibrillation, which takes place usually at right angles to the articular surface, the neighboring carti-

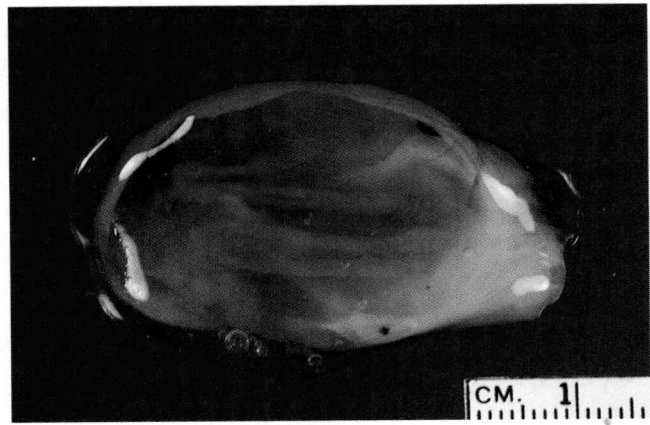

Fig. 24-109 Gross appearance of Baker's cyst.

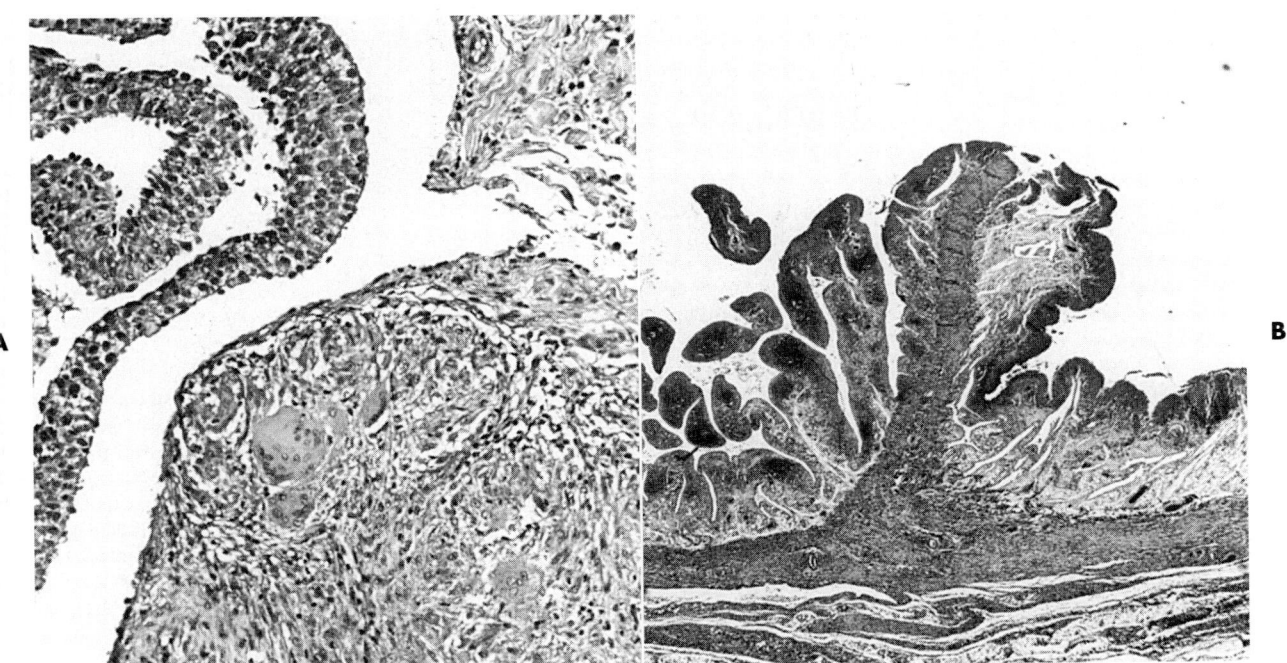

Fig. 24-110 A, Sarcoidosis of joint as seen in synovial biopsy. **B,** Synovium with chronic Lyme arthritis. Hypertrophic synovitis with lymphoplasmacellular aggregates are seen resembling appearance of rheumatoid arthritis. (**B** courtesy Dr. P. Duray, Philadelphia.)

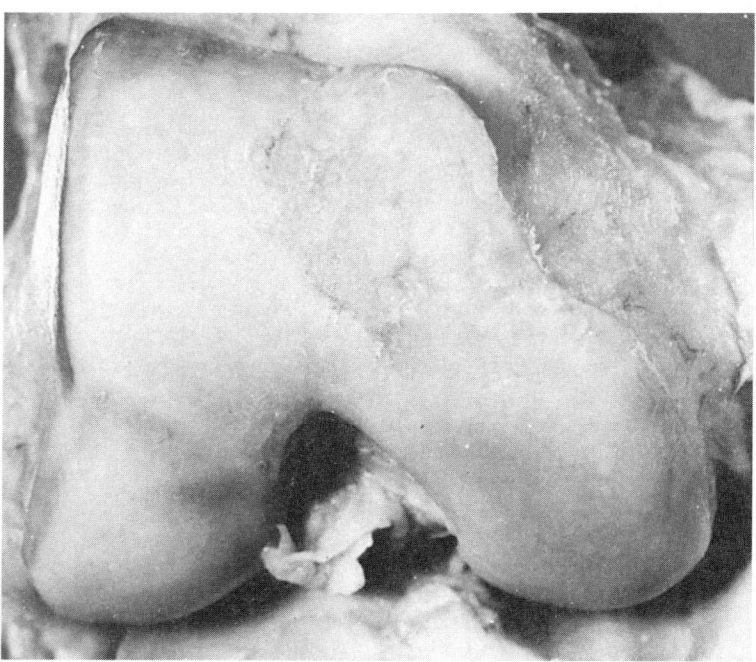

Fig. 24-111 Pronounced degenerative joint disease in 55-year-old man. Note degeneration and destruction of cartilage over wide area.

lage cells are set free and finally disintegrate and disappear. Also, the original smooth articular surface takes on a papillary appearance. At times this fibrillation is responsible for the freeing of minute masses of cartilage and fibrillated matrix. The depth to which this fibrillation extends varies. Sometimes it extends entirely through the cartilage down to the zone of provisional calcification so that masses of cartilage may be peeled away, exposing either the zone of provisional calcification or the underlying bone to the attrition of joint motion [Fig. 24-111]. Occasionally, only a portion of the articular cartilage undergoes degeneration, fibrillation, and destruction [Fig. 24-112]. This leads to thinning of the cartilage over a circumscribed area. To meet this erosion and depression, an overgrowth occurs on the opposite joint surface. This is brought about by increased activity of the perichondrium. As a result, an irregular or somewhat toothed joint line is formed, and finally, with ultimate disappearance of the entire articular cartilage, the two bony surfaces are brought into contact. Since this change takes place gradually and is at first confined only to a portion of the joint, motion is continued with the result that the exposed bone undergoes marked thickening of the trabeculae and narrowing of the marrow spaces until an extremely dense bony structure has been produced. The friction of continued joint motion produces a high degree of polish on the exposed condensed bone which then acquires an appearance closely resembling ivory; hence the term "eburnation of bone."

While this process of fibrillation and destruction of cartilage with erosion is taking place in one portion of the joint and a corresponding overgrowth is occurring on the opposite joint surface, secondary changes in the joint may be produced. Changes in the shape of the joint surface may gradually, over a period of months

or years, lead to more or less extensive subluxations. As a result, the amount of joint motion may be diminished, or, in certain instances, the joint surfaces may become interlocked, producing "ankylosis by deformity." There is no true ankylosis in this type of joint disease. Common among these imperfectly understood secondary changes is an increased activity of the perichondrium at the periphery of the joint where the cartilage and capsule come together. This results in the new formation of cartilage which may be transformed into bone and thus causes an increase in the size of the bone end. As a rule this increase in circumference is not uniform, but is irregular and the contour is nodular, as exemplified by Heberden's node. Since this deposit of new bone is usually within the attachment of the joint capsule, it may in some cases lead to filling up of the original joint cavity, thus producing partial or complete dislocation.

As a rule, no great increase in the thickness of the joint capsules of these joints is observed, and, in many instances, the synovial membrane appears normal. However, in some cases, there is marked thickening of the synovial membrane with the production of papillary or pedunculated masses of connective tissue which may be converted by metaplasia into cartilage or bone or, in some cases, into fat tissue. Detachment of these pedunculated masses may give rise to loose bodies, the so-called joint mice. The breaking off of an osteophyte is another cause of loose-body formation. As a rule, in this type of joint disease there is very little tendency for the synovial membrane to extend over the articular surfaces and in no case does fibrous ankylosis occur.*

---

*From Bauer W, Bennett GA: Experimental and pathologic studies in the degenerative type of arthritis. J Bone Joint Surg **18:**1-18, 1936.

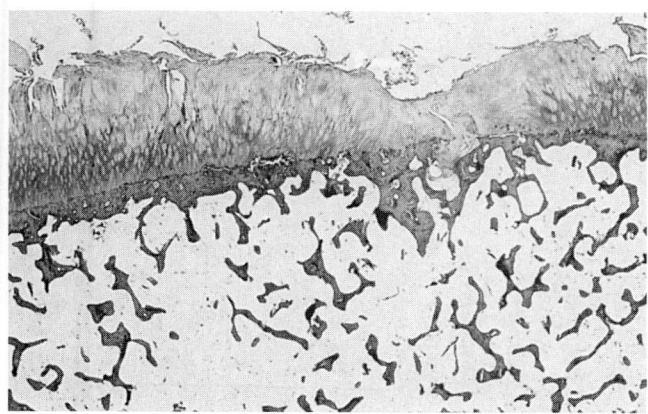

Fig. 24-112 Section taken through zone shown in Fig. 24-111 demonstrating fragmentation and fibrillation of thinned cartilage.

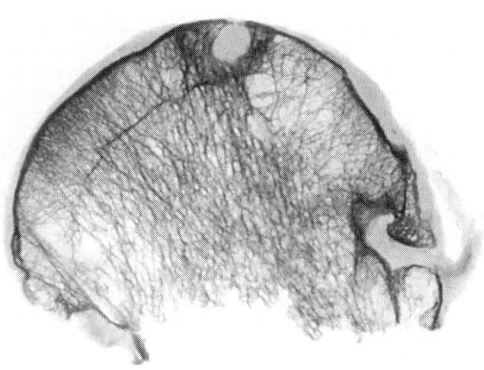

Fig. 24-113 Specimen radiograph of femoral head with osteoarthrosis. Note irregular thinning of articular cartilage and formation of subchondral cyst surrounded by sclerotized bone.

As this lucid description clearly indicates, the changes of degenerative joint disease are centered in the cartilage, a type of tissue notorious for its poor capacity for repair.[804,816] These changes are more prominent on the joint surface exposed to friction, weight bearing, or movement, but they also occur in areas of the joint not subject to these mechanical forces.[805] The mechanical attrition of the cartilage is preceded by a loss of chondroitin sulfate matrix.[810] Loss of cartilage thickness leads to narrowing of the joint space and loss of stability of the chondro-osseous junction. The osteophytes seen at the margins of osteoarthritic joints progress through discrete stages of cartilage differentiation that can be followed with collagen type–specific probes.[798a] The cartilage degradation in osteoarthritis is believed to be mediated by cytokines, in particular IL-1.[814a]

Some degree of synovial hyperplasia with hyperemia and lymphocytic infiltration can be seen in advanced stages of the disease, especially in the hip; these changes should not be confused with rheumatoid arthritis.

A secondary change sometimes seen in the osteoarthritic head of a femur is the presence of cysts located close to the surface. These are surrounded by dense bone and contain fluid or loose connective tissue[805,808,809,814] (Figs. 24-113 to 24-115). Other secondary features of the disease are represented by changes in the capsular and synovial nerves.[802a,813]

Neuropathic arthropathy (Charcot's joint) is a particularly destructive variant of degenerative joint disease (Fig. 24-116). The process is usually slowly progressive, although on rare occasions it may have an extremely rapid evolution.[811] Particles of dead bone and cartilage often are seen in large amounts embedded in the synovial membrane.[807] However, they are not specific for this condition.

Chondromalacia patellae is the name given to a condition of obscure etiology characterized by softening, fibrillation, fissuring, and erosion of the articular cartilage of the patella.[812] Microscopically, the changes are indistinguishable from those of degenerative joint disease.[803]

Rheumatoid arthritis

Rheumatoid arthritis is an immune-complex disease that manifests as a chronic polyarticular arthritis. It is mostly seen in women during the second and third decades of life.[839,840] The joints of the feet and hands are nearly always involved. Other joints frequently affected are the elbows, knees, wrists, ankles, hips, spine, and temporomandibular articulations.

Lysosomes and interleukins are mediators of the inflammatory reaction seen in this disease and in other joint diseases.[826,843,845a] Basic fibroblastic growth factor may play a role in synovial hyperplasia and joint destruction.[831a] The etiology of rheumatoid arthritis is unknown, but viral participation has long been suspected on the basis of epidemiologic, morphologic, and immunohistologic findings.[845] The HLA linkage and the autoantibody production observed in most patients support an autoimmune element in this disease.[844]

The earliest morphologic changes occur in the synovial membrane. Hyperemia of the synovium is followed by proliferation of the synovial lining cells and infiltration by plasma cells and lymphocytes (Fig. 24-117). Lymphoid follicles are often present.[830] The small synovial blood vessels are lined by plump endothelial cells, and fibrin deposits often are seen close to the synovial lining or within the stroma. These changes, although certainly supporting a diagnosis of rheumatoid arthritis in a clinically compatible case, are not pathognomonic of this entity. Two additional microscopic features, which are also nonspecific, include the presence of synovial giant cells and bone and cartilage fragments within the actual synovial membrane. Muirden[835] found synovial giant cells in one third of the 100 biopsies he examined. They need to be distinguished from multinucleated plasma cells, foreign body cells, and Touton giant cells that can also occur in joints with rheumatoid arthritis. Grimley and Sokoloff[824] found them only in patients with active, seropositive disease, although they found no correlation

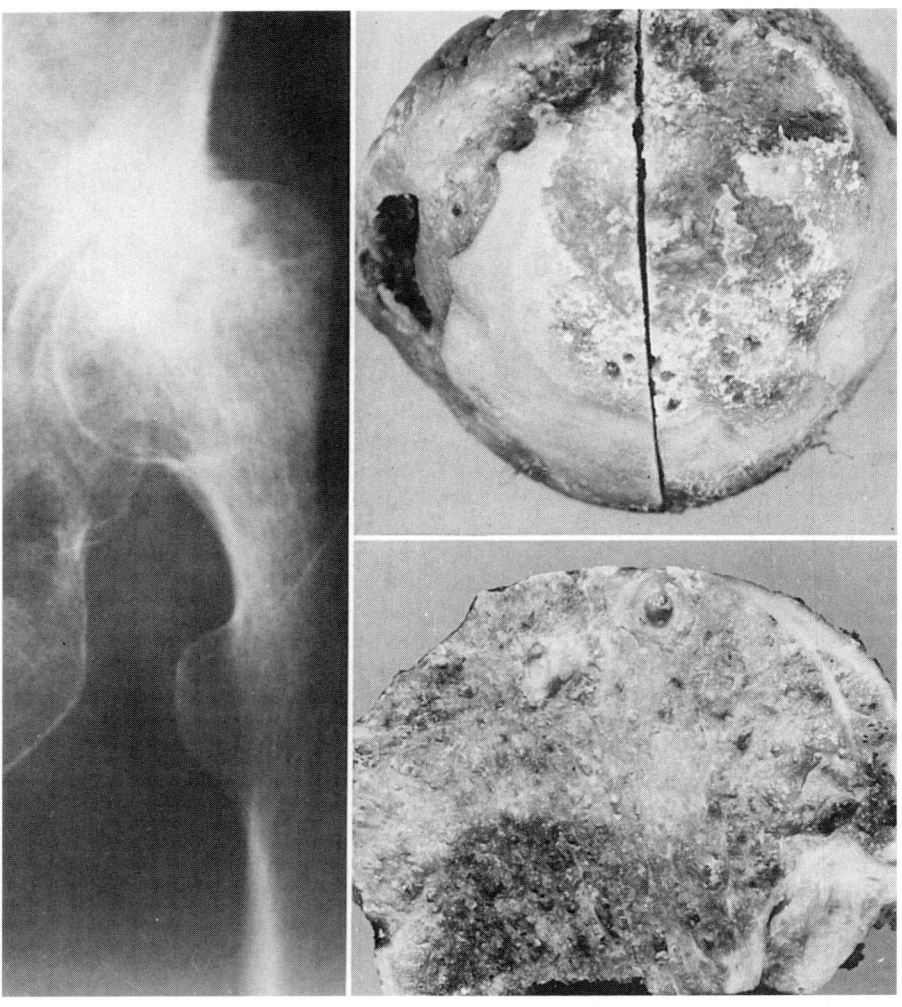

Fig. 24-114 Head of femur demonstrating advanced osteoarthritic changes. There are loss of cartilage and cyst formation.

with the serologic titer. On the other hand, Bhan and Roy[821] found them in seropositive and in seronegative cases, as well as in tuberculosis, traumatic arthritis, and villonodular synovitis. The cartilage and bone fragments tend to occur in joints with advanced disease. They appear to arise as a result of the erosive destructive process of the articular surface and can be distinguished by virtue of their position and clear demarcation from the metaplastic cartilage and bone that sometimes arises from synovial cells. They also have been seen in synovial membranes of osteoarthritis, osteochondritis dissecans, chondromalacia patellae, and particularly in neuropathic joints[829,835] (Fig. 24-118).

In the second phase, granulation tissue grows into the subchondral marrow of the bone.[832] Osteoporosis occurs early and may result in spontaneous fractures of long bones (particularly the femoral neck) and the pelvis.[842] Prominent pannus is formed over the articular cartilage (Fig. 24-119). Cartilage and even bone form in this pannus. The granulation tissue of the subchondral area and the pannus within the joint attack the cartilage.[822] Its destruction may be followed by fibrous ankylosis and eventually bony ankylosis.

Mitchell and Shepard[833] have described the early changes seen by electron microscopy in the articular cartilage. Increased articular pressure may lead to bursting of the joint capsule and acute joint rupture,[823] bone cysts ("rheumatoid geodes"),[836] or herniation of the capsule into the soft tissues.[831] The bone cysts are radiographically similar to those seen in association with degenerative joint disease, but in rheumatoid arthritis they contain granulation tissue instead of fluid or myxoid material.

Rheumatoid arthritis is generally regarded as the expression of a systemic disease.[827,828] Tenosynovitis and "rheumatoid nodules" are the two most common extra-articular manifestations. The latter, which are seen in approximately 20% of the patients, occur most often in tendons and tendon sheaths and periarticular subcutaneous tissue but also have been seen in the heart and large vessels, lung and pleura, kidney, meninges, and synovial membrane itself.[837] In exceptional instances, they have occurred systemically and have been responsible for the patient's death.[820] Microscopically, they are composed of a necrotic center impregnated with fibrin, surrounded by a predominantly histiocytic

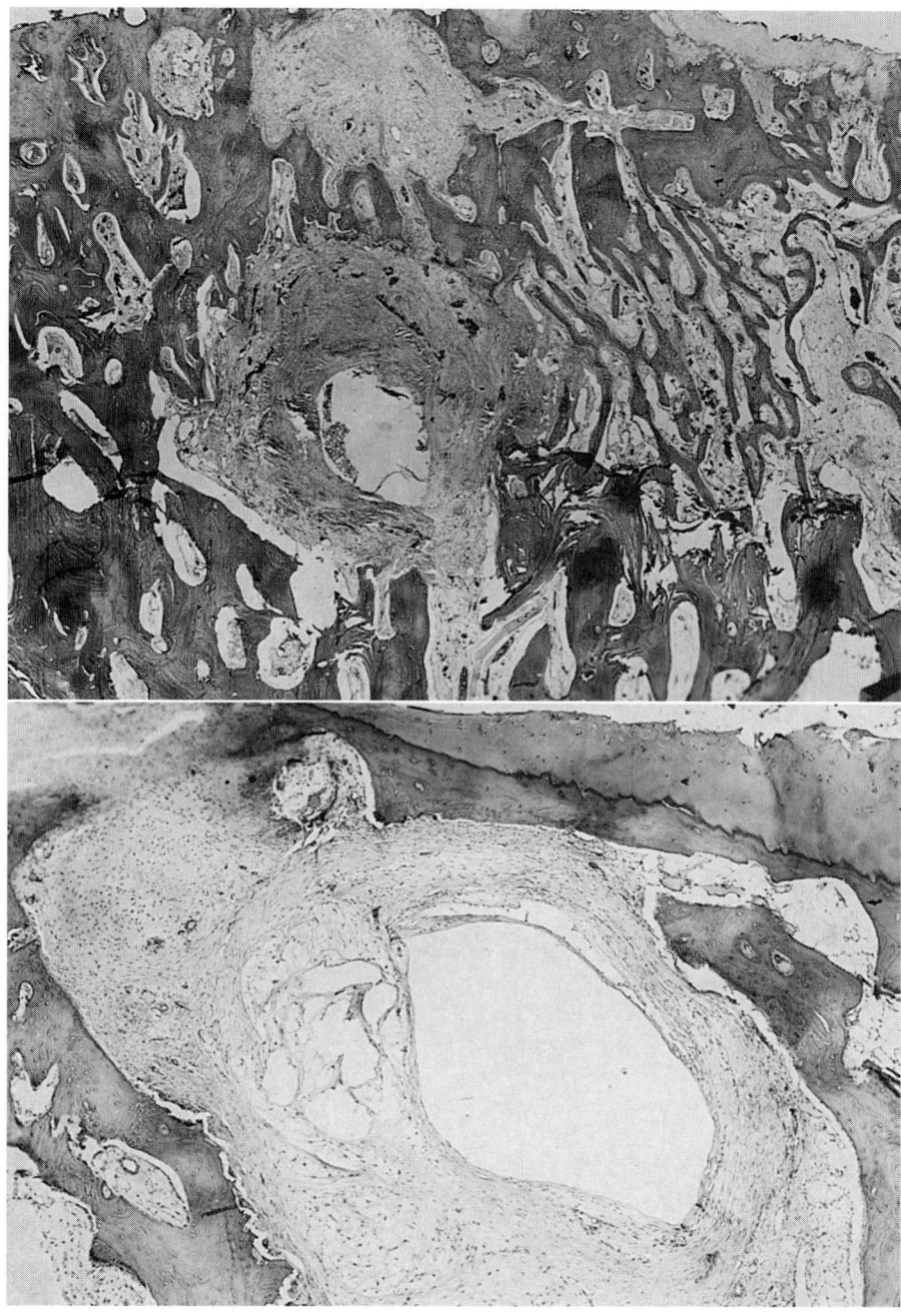

Fig. 24-115 Loss of cartilage, eburnation, and cyst formation in advanced osteoarthritis.

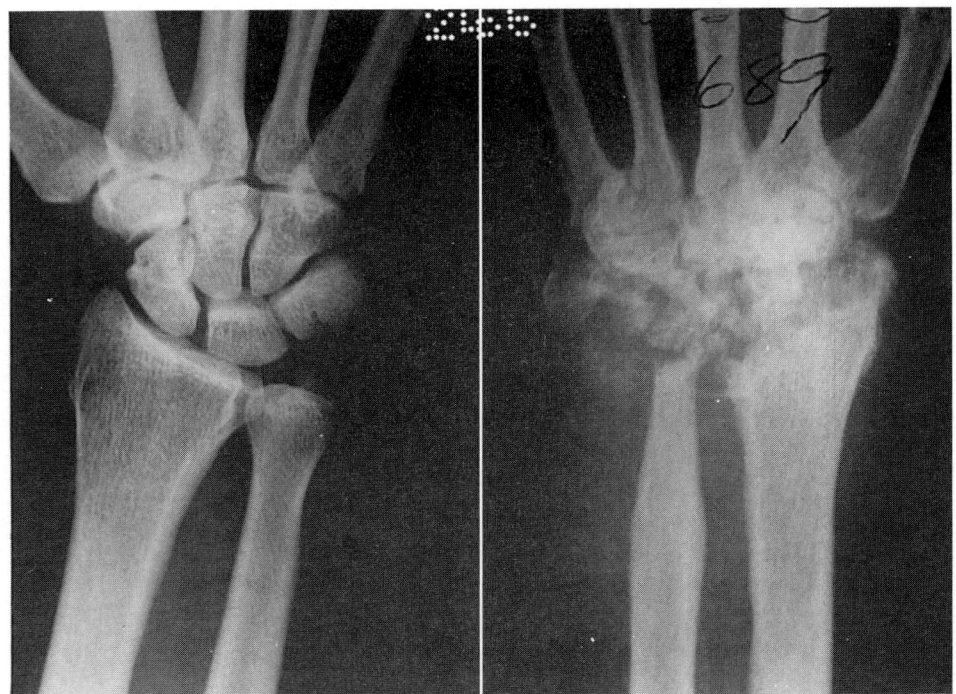

Fig. 24-116 Neuropathic changes in wrist secondary to syringomyelia.

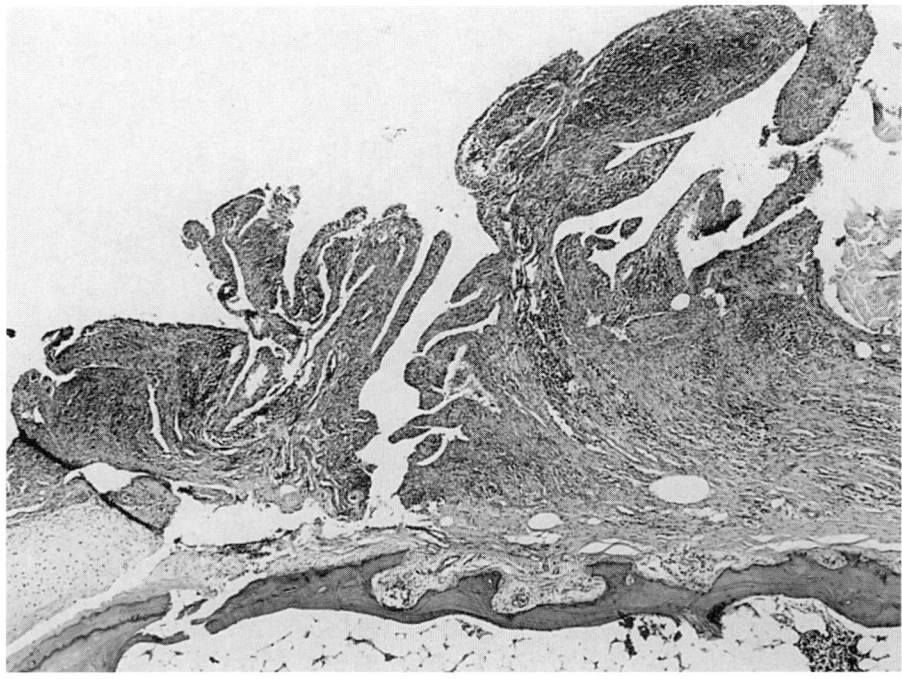

Fig. 24-117 Exuberant papillary projections of inflamed synovium in rheumatoid arthritis involving wrist.

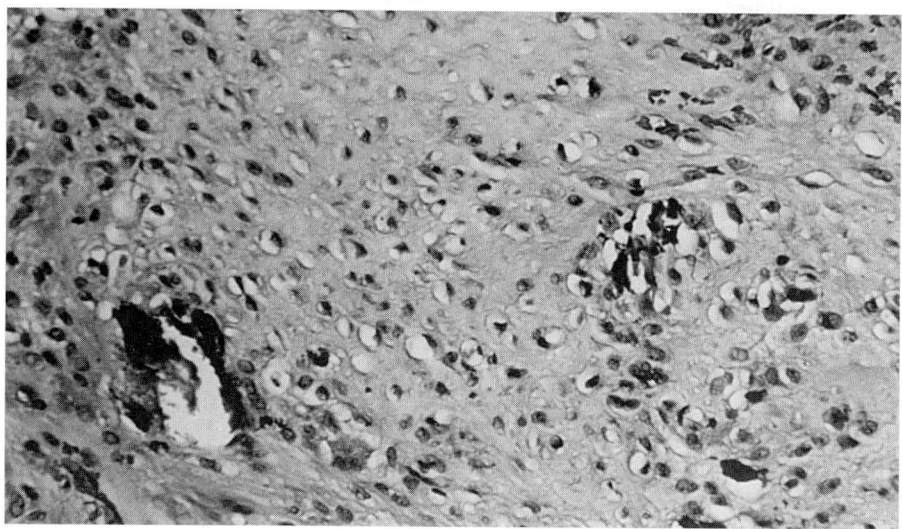

Fig. 24-118 Calcific debris embedded in synovial membrane of Charcot's joint.

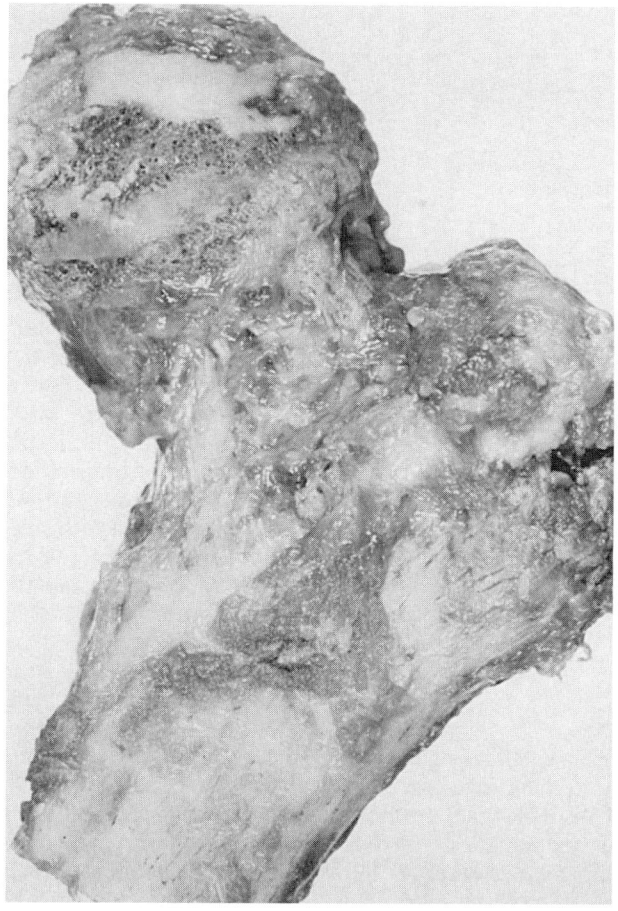

Fig. 24-119 Advanced rheumatoid arthritis involving femur. There is prominent proliferation of synovium and almost complete destruction of overlying articular cartilage.

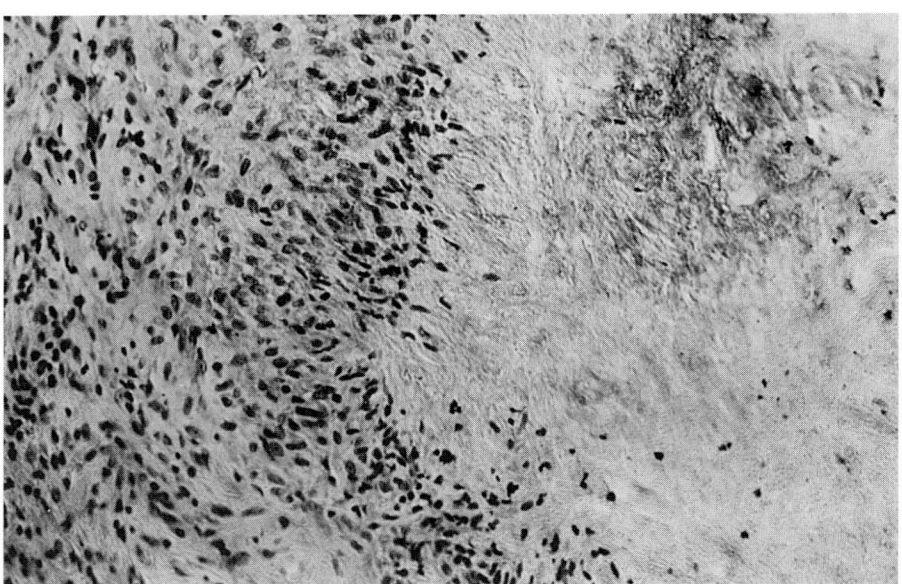

Fig. 24-120 Typical rheumatoid nodule. Note central necrosis, palisading of cells around margin of this area, and chronic inflammatory cells.

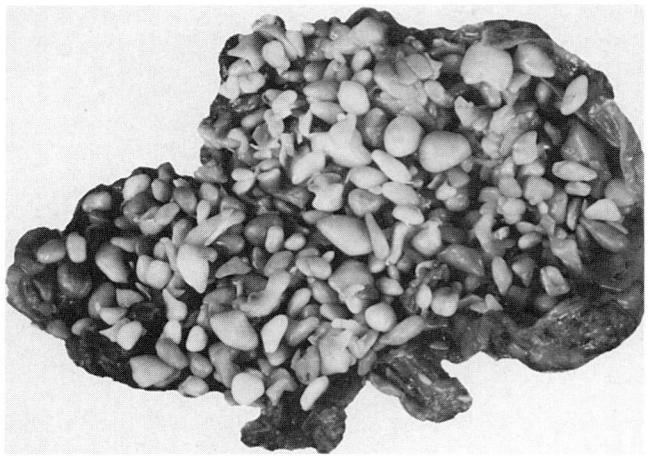

Fig. 24-121 Tuberculous bursitis with innumerable "rice bodies." Latter are mainly composed of fibrin and have no diagnostic significance. (Courtesy Dr. E.F. Lascano, Buenos Aires.)

inflammatory reaction often arranged in a palisading fashion (Fig. 24-120). They are not specific to rheumatoid arthritis. Nodules morphologically indistinguishable can occur in rheumatic fever, in systemic lupus erythematosus, and in children in the absence of any apparent disease.[817,818,825] Berardinelli et al.[819] followed ten cases of the latter and found rheumatoid factor 2 to 16 years after the appearance of the nodules.

Sokoloff et al.[841] found nonnecrotizing arteritis in 10% of patients with rheumatoid arthritis. Necrotizing arteritis has also been described.[834,838] Polyneuritis can be observed.

The pulmonary manifestations of rheumatoid arthritis have been discussed in Chapter 7 and the lymph node changes in Chapter 21.

Amyloidosis is a significant complication of the disease. In the United States, rheumatoid arthritis has displaced tuberculosis as the most common underlying disorder associated with amyloid deposition.

Infectious arthritis

Bacterial, fungal, and parasitic infections can reach the joints either by hematogenous spread or by contiguous extension from a neighboring osteomyelitis (Fig. 24-121). A form of infectious arthritis that has risen dramatically in recognition and frequency in recent years is *Lyme disease,* an arthropod-transmitted spirochetosis that also involves skin, heart, and nervous system.[847,848] The microscopic changes in the synovium are those of a nonspecific chronic synovitis, but the spirochete can occasionally be detected with the Liederle stain[846] (Fig. 24-110, *B*).

Gout

About 2% to 5% of chronic joint disease is caused by gout. The metatarsophalangeal joints are often the first to be involved, but other joints of the hands and feet are also frequently involved. The disease may also involve the joints of the long bones.

Calcification and even ossification of tophi occur frequently.[851] The urate deposits progressively destroy the cartilage and may cause osteolytic, irregular destruction of subchondral bone (Fig. 24-122). These deposits may extend out from a joint into the soft tissue and cause destruction of the ligaments. This destruction eventually leads to subcutaneous deposits that may erode through the skin. The microscopic pattern of gout is unmistakable. Fixation in alcohol is important for the preservation of sodium urate monohydrate

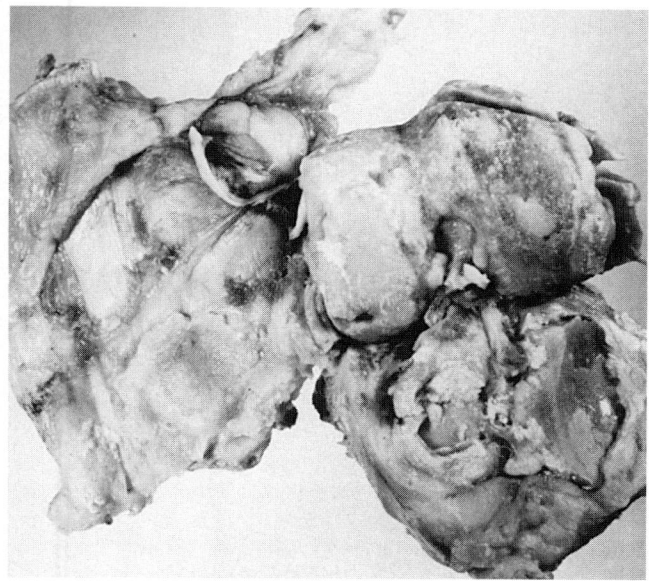

Fig. 24-122 Extensive involvement of knee joint and synovium by gout. In some areas, cartilage of condyles is completely missing and there is involvement of semilunar cartilages as well. Grayish white plaques represent deposits of uric acid and crystals. Patient, 83-year-old woman, had leg amputated because of arterial insufficiency and finding of gout was unexpected.

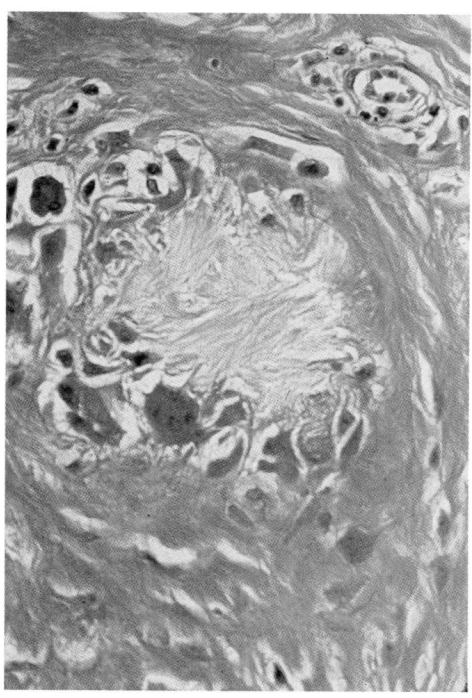

Fig. 24-123 Lesion of periarticular gout showing foreign body–type giant cell reaction to the deposited crystals. The crystalline nature of this material is not obvious in this formalin-fixed specimen.

deposits that appear as needle-shaped, doubly refractile crystals. The deGalantha stain is particularly suited for their demonstration.[850] Even if alcohol fixation is not done, the appearance of tophi is usually diagnostic because of the typical granulomatous response that they elicit (Figs. 24-123 and 24-124). Histiocytes and foreign body giant cells predominate in the infiltrate. Palisading of the histiocytes sometimes occurs and may be a source of confusion with rheumatoid nodules.

Gout should also be differentiated from *chondrocalcinosis* (pseudogout syndrome), a rare condition in which the symptoms result from diffuse deposition of calcium pyrophosphate crystals in the articular cartilage.[849,850a,852]

Intervertebral disk prolapse

Material curetted from an intervertebral disk because of prolapse is a very common surgical specimen. Traditionally, features such as fibrillation, cluttering of chondrocytes, and granular change have been regarded as indicators of degeneration related to prolapse. Weidner et al.[853] found instead that the feature that better correlated with prolapse was neovascularization occurring at the edges of the fibrocartilaginous fragments.

Other articular and periarticular diseases

Scleroderma (progressive systemic sclerosis) is often accompanied by arthralgia or arthritis, and sometimes these dominate the clinical picture. The main microscopic changes in the synovial membrane are superficial deposition of fibrin, mild mononuclear infiltrate, minimal hyperplasia of synovial lining cells, proliferation of collagen fibers, and focal obliteration of small vessels.[861]

In *lupus erythematosus,* the microscopic changes in the synovium can be indistinguishable from those of rheumatoid arthritis. As a rule, however, there is a more intense surface fibrin deposition and a lesser degree of proliferation of synovial cells.[856]

Amyloid can deposit in the synovium, articular cartilage, periarticular tissue, and intervertebral disk in old age, apparently unrelated to osteoarthritis and in the absence of systemic amyloidosis.[854,855,859,860] Heavier amounts can be seen as an expression of primary amyloidosis or multiple myeloma. Amyloidosis is one of the causes of the carpal tunnel syndrome[857,858] (see p. 1988). This amyloid material usually consists of transthyretin (AF/ASCI, prealbumin).[860]

TUMORS AND TUMORLIKE CONDITIONS
Fibrous histiocytoma of tendon sheath (nodular tenosynovitis)

Fibrous histiocytoma of the tendon sheath (also called giant cell tumor of the tendon sheath, xanthogranuloma, and benign synovioma) is a common lesion that occurs more frequently in women than men, usually appearing in young and middle-aged persons. Most cases are distributed between the wrist and fingertips and between the ankle and toe tips. It is more often proximal than distal on both the hands and feet and occurs most frequently on their flexor surfaces.

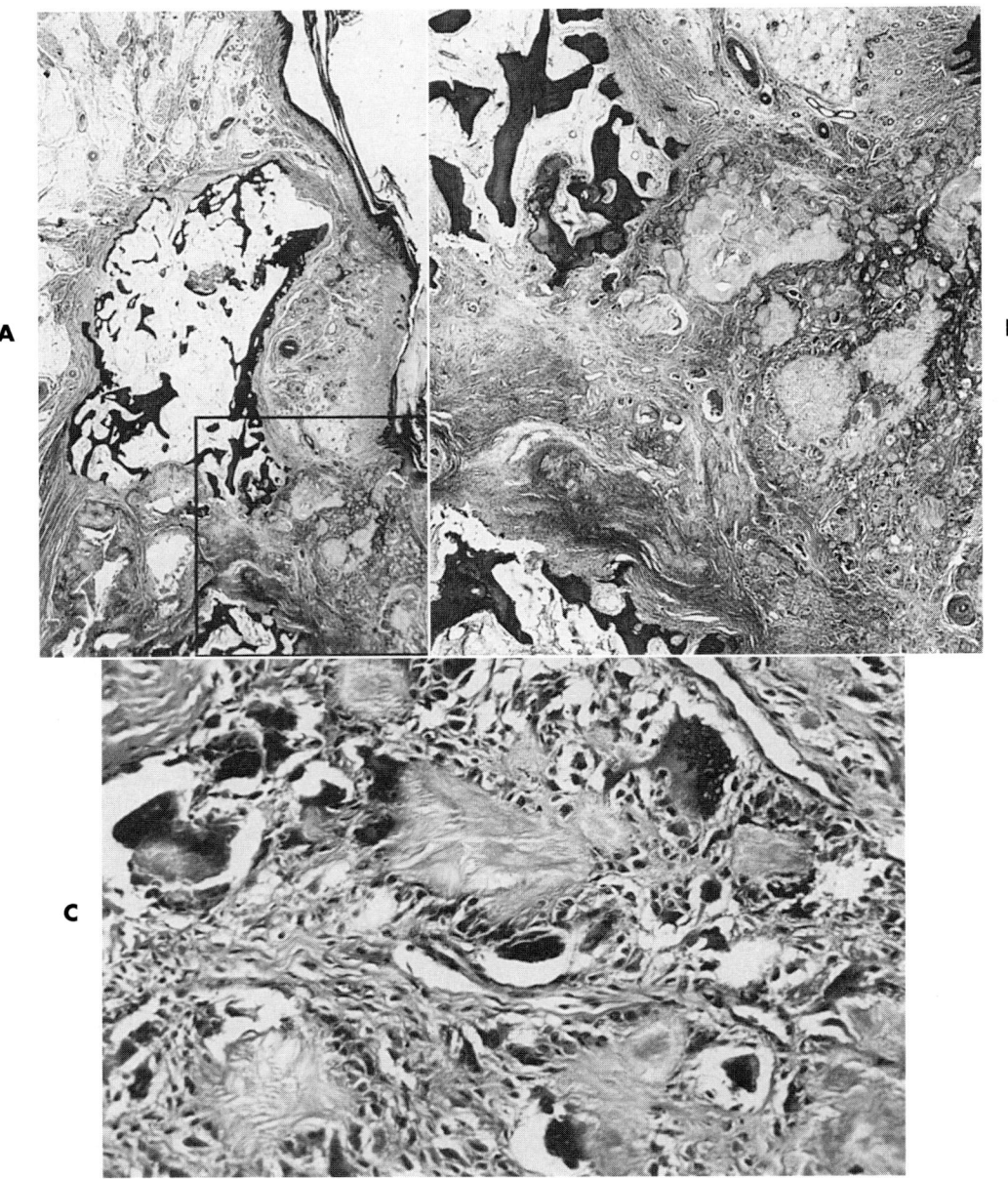

Fig. 24-124 Characteristic lesion of gout. **A** and **B,** Tophaceous deposits that have destroyed joint, with complete destruction of cartilage and extension out into soft tissue and growth just beneath epidermis. **C,** Urate deposits surrounded by characteristic giant cells. Later demonstrates characteristic picture of gout. Patient's trouble began in great toe.

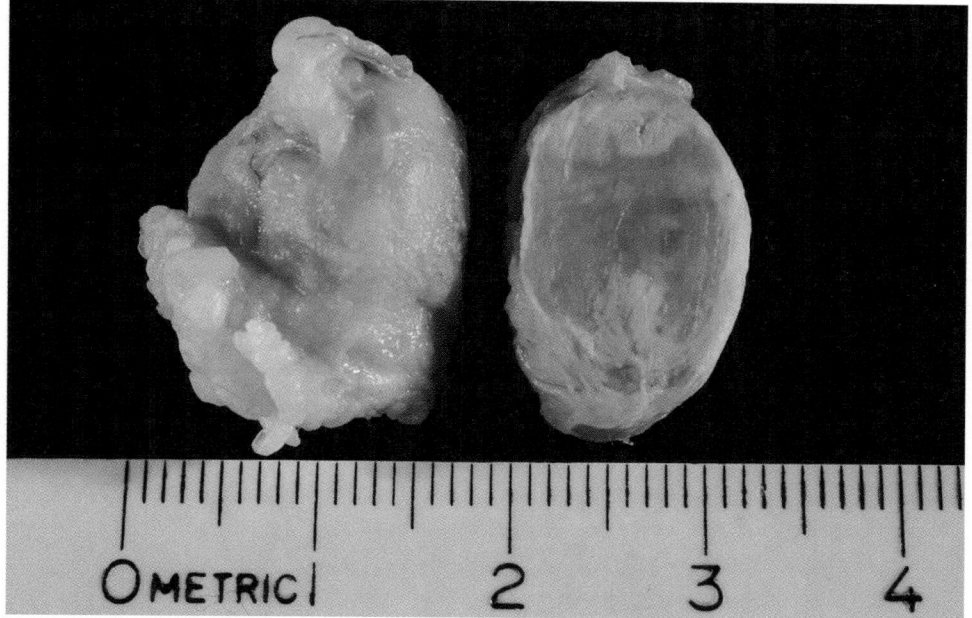

Fig. 24-125 Gross appearance of fibrous histiocytoma of tendon sheath. The lesion is small, well circumscribed, solid, and with a brownish cast.

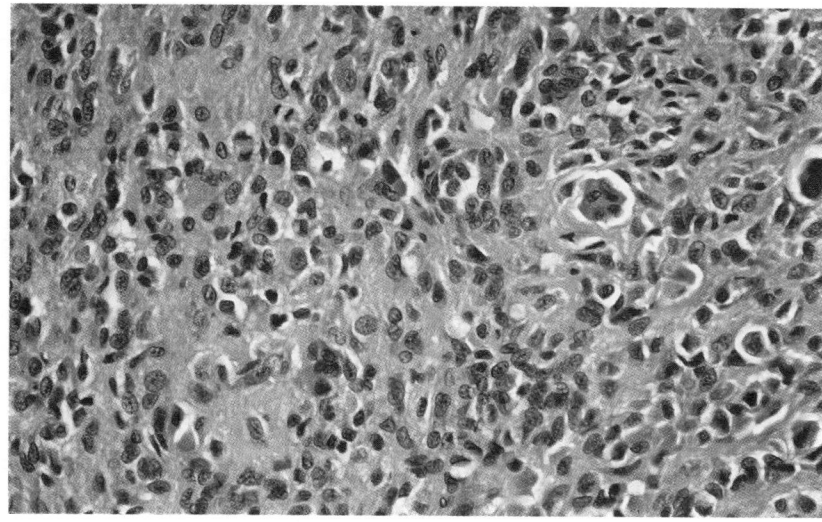

Fig. 24-126 Microscopic appearance of fibrous histiocytoma of tendon sheath. There is a polymorphic infiltrate of small histiocytes and multinucleated giant cells that are embedded in dense fibrous tissue.

Grossly, it presents as a single mass usually measuring 1 to 3 cm in diameter. It has a fairly well-defined capsule, may be somewhat lobulated, and varies in color from whitish gray to yellowish brown (Fig. 24-125).

Microscopically, this lesion contains closely packed medium-sized polyhedral cells with a variable admixture of giant cells containing fat and hemosiderin (Fig. 24-126). Cells in zones of active proliferation may show mitotic figures. Focal zones of hyalinization constitute the more quiescent areas. Sometimes, the whole lesion adopts an hypocellular fibrohyalinized appearance. We suspect that the cases reported as *tendon sheath fibromas* are histogenetically related to fibrous histiocytoma.[863,864a] Their location, clinical presentation, and recurrence rate are certainly comparable. Ultrastructural and immunohistochemical studies of fibrous histiocytomas of tendon sheath have shown cells with the features of synovial cells alternating with fibroblastic elements, histiocytes, and lymphocytes.[862,864b,864c]

The great cellularity of this tumor, its variable pattern, and the presence of mitotic figures may lead to an erroneous diagnosis of sarcoma. However, these tumors are nearly always benign. They may erode contiguous bone by pressure. If incompletely removed, they may recur locally. New lesions also possibly develop after excision.[866]

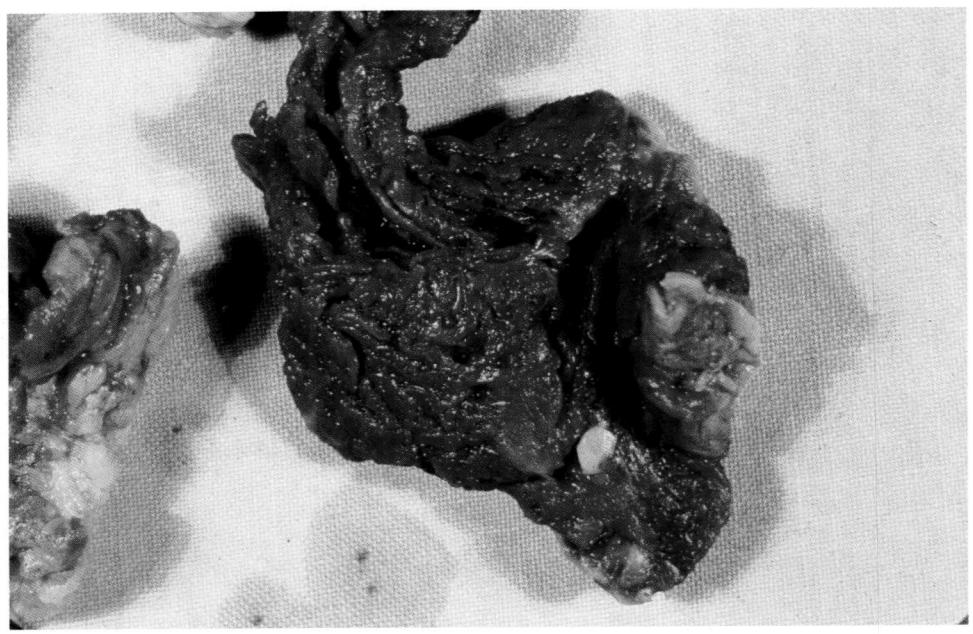

Fig. 24-127 Gross appearance of pigmented villonodular synovitis of knee joint. The lesion has a characteristic dark brown color resulting from extensive hemosiderin deposition. (Courtesy Dr. Jack Uecker, St. Paul, MN.)

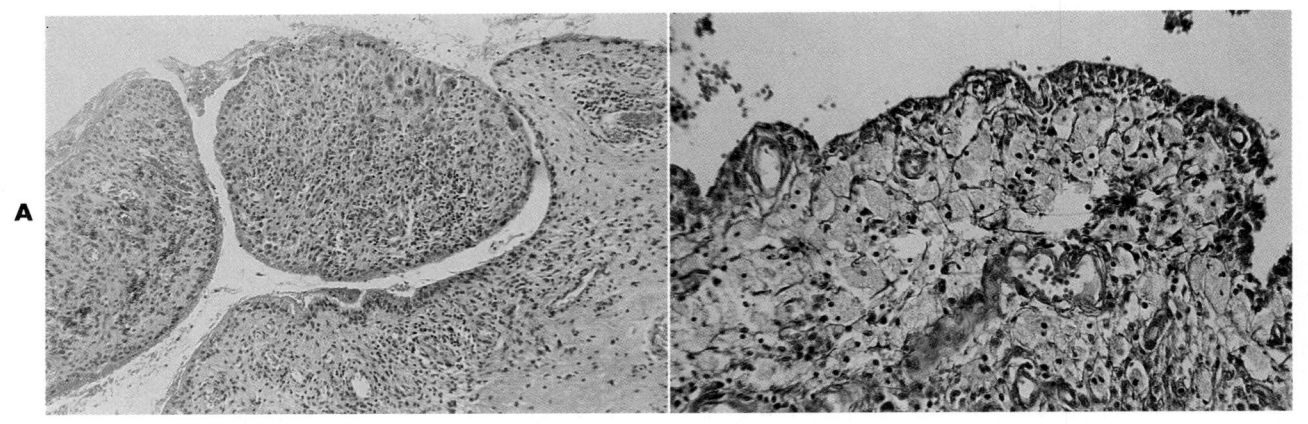

Fig. 24-128 Microscopic appearance of pigmented villonodular synovitis. **A,** Low-power view showing the villous appearance of the proliferation and hyperplastic synovium **B,** High-power view. In this area, foamy cells predominate. In others, there were large collections of hemosiderin-laden macrophages.

The nature of this lesion is still controversial: Jaffe et al.[864] considered it a reactive process—hence the name of nodular tenosynovitis. Most authors currently regard it as neoplastic and as a form of fibrous histiocytoma.

A very rare malignant counterpart of this lesion has been described. Features that should suggest malignancy are a high number of mitotic figures, marked nuclear hyperchromasia, and lack of paucity of multinucleated giant cells.[865] The main differential diagnosis of fibrous histiocytoma of the tendon sheath is epithelioid sarcoma. The presence of granuloma-like formations, necrosis, invasiveness, epithelioid features, and keratin immunoreactivity favors the later.

Pigmented villonodular synovitis and bursitis

Pigmented villonodular synovitis tends to occur in young adults.[870-872] Although the knee joint is the usual site, the process may involve the ankle, hip, shoulder, or even elbow joint.[867,873] Usually only one articulation is affected, instances of bilateral disease being exceptional. Occasionally, the lesion may penetrate within the underlying bone.[875]

The process may be focal or diffuse. When diffuse, it is made up of brownish-yellow spongy tissue. Its appearance depends on the content of hemosiderin pigment. Large amounts of tissue often are present, and complete removal may be impossible (Fig. 24-127). Microscopically, the cel-

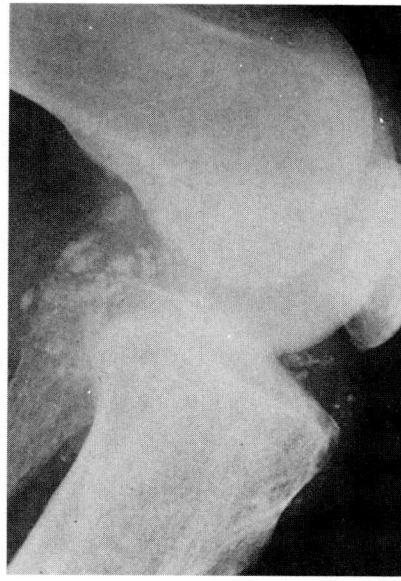

Fig. 24-129 Synovial osteochondromatosis. Nodules can be seen clearly in joint space.

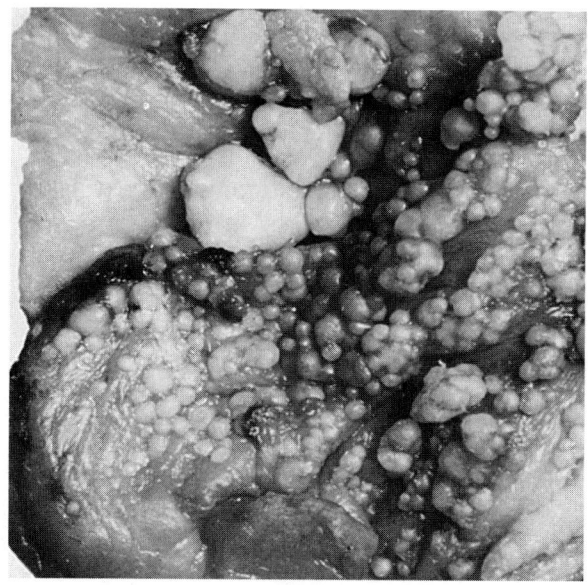

Fig. 24-130 Extensive involvement of synovium of knee joint by osteochondromatosis.

lular component is similar to that of nodular tenosynovitis, but in addition there are papillary projections made up of foamy cells and hemosiderin-containing phagocytes (Fig. 24-128), Large clefts and pseudoglandular or alveolar spaces lined by synovial cells are also present.[876]

The capacity of this lesion to result in bone cyst formation and late cartilage and bone loss has been attributed to the production of metalloproteinases such as collagenase and stromelysin.[869] Trisomy 7 was documented in a case of this disease, suggesting that at least some cases represent clonal, neoplastic proliferations.[874]

This disease can be treated by excision. It may recur locally because complete removal is often impossible.[868] If it recurs locally, radiation therapy may be helpful. In our experience, this lesion has not become malignant. Extensively recurrent lesions, however, have been misdiagnosed as fibrosarcoma and synovial sarcoma.

Synovial osteochondromatosis and chondrosarcoma

Synovial osteochondromatosis (chondrometaplasia) is an infrequent disease of unknown etiology associated with the formation of osteocartilaginous bodies in the synovial membrane.[877] This condition most often is monoarticular, affecting the knee or hip and communicating bursae. It is aggravated by infection and trauma. Sometimes a similar condition is seen in the soft tissue adjacent to but not communicating with the joint.[882a]

Grossly, the osteocartilaginous bodies may remain confined to the synovium or be extruded within the joint cavity. They usually are partially calcified (Fig. 24-129). Innumerable small bodies can be seen grossly in the resected lesion (Figs. 24-130 and 24-131). A single nodule beneath thinned synovium contains hyaline cartilage and at times bone (Fig. 24-132). The disease seems to follow this sequence:

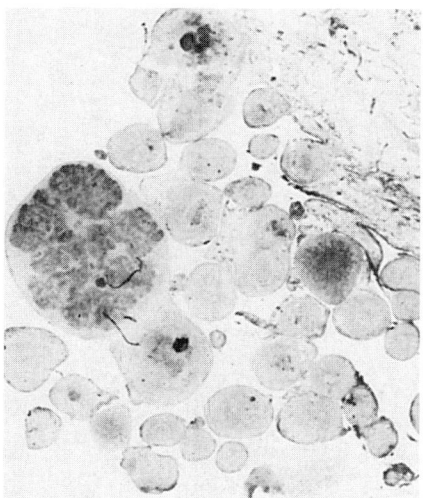

Fig. 24-131 Pattern and formation of synovial osteochondromatosis.

(1) active intrasynovial disease with no loose bodies, (2) intrasynovial proliferation and free loose bodies, and (3) multiple free osteochondral bodies with no demonstrable intrasynovial disease.[881]

To make a diagnosis of synovial osteochondromatosis, one should find cartilaginous or osteocartilaginous bodies attached to the synovial membrane in addition to those free in the joint spaces. The latter also can occur in degenerative joint disease, neuropathic arthropathy, and osteochondritis dissecans, and the process is referred to as *secondary synovial chondrometaplasia*.[883] Microscopically, the cartilage cells of primary synovial osteochondromatosis may show some degree of atypia and even binucleated forms, but this does not necessarily indicate malignancy.[882] Local recrudescence after treatment may supervene.

Synovial chondrosarcoma is an exceptionally rare entity that closely resembles synovial chondromatosis radiographically and grossly[878,879] (Fig. 24-133). The distinction, which may be quite difficult, is made by the presence in the chondrosarcoma of obvious cytologic features of malignancy in the cartilaginous cells.[880]

Other tumors

Most tumors involving the joint space represent direct extension from neoplasms initially located in the adjacent bones.

The only primary tumor of the joints that is seen with any frequency in addition to those already mentioned is ***synovial hemangioma.*** Most patients are young adults, and there is a predominance for the male sex. The knee is the most common site, followed by the elbow and finger. In most cases the tumor is confined to the intra-articular synovium, but sometimes it is located in a bursa adjacent to a joint. The most common microscopic pattern is cavernous hemangioma, followed by lobular capillary hemangioma, arteriovenous hemangioma, and venous hemangioma.[884]

Isolated cases of intra-articular hemangiopericytoma, synovial sarcoma, and epithelioid sarcoma have been observed.[885]

REFERENCES
Bone
NORMAL ANATOMY

1 Anderson HC: Mechanism of mineral formation in bone. Lab Invest **60**:320-330, 1989.
2 Centrella M, McCarthy TL, Canalis E: Skeletal tissue and transforming growth factor beta. FASEB J **2**:3066-3073, 1988.
3 Enneking WF, Kagan A: Transepiphyseal extension of osteosarcoma. Incidence, mechanism, and implications. Cancer **41**:1526-1537, 1978.
4 Fornasier VL: Osteoid. An ultrastructural study. Hum Pathol **8**:243-254, 1977.
5 Glimcher MJ: Mechanism of calcification. Role of collagen fibrils and collagen-phosphoprotein complexes *in vitro* and *in vivo*. Anat Rec **224**:139-153, 1989.
6 Gurley MA, Roth SI: Bone. In Sternberg SS, ed.: Histology for pathologists. New York, 1992, Raven Press, Ltd.
7 Heinegard D, Oldberg A: Structure and biology of cartilage and bone matrix non-collagenous macromolecules. FASEB J **3**:2042-2051, 1989.
8 Huffer WE: Morphology and biochemistry of bone remodeling. Possible control by vitamin D, parathyroid hormone, and other substances. Lab Invest **59**:418-442, 1988.
9 Kukita T, McManus LM, Miller M, Civin C, Roodman GD: Osteoclast-like cells formed in long-term human bone marrow cultures express a similar surface phenotype as authentic osteoclasts. Lab Invest **60**:532-538, 1989.
10 Marks SJ Jr, Popoff SN: Bone cell biology. The regulation of development, structure, and function in the skeleton. Am J Anat **83**:1-44, 1988.

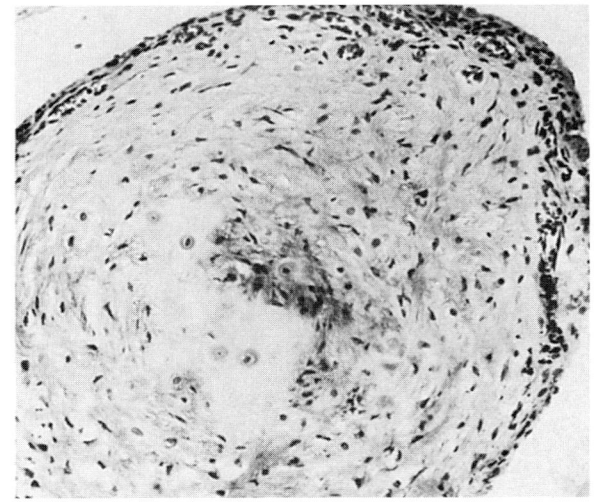

Fig. 24-132 Single nodule of osteochondromatosis forming beneath intact synovium. Note cartilage formation in center of this nodule.

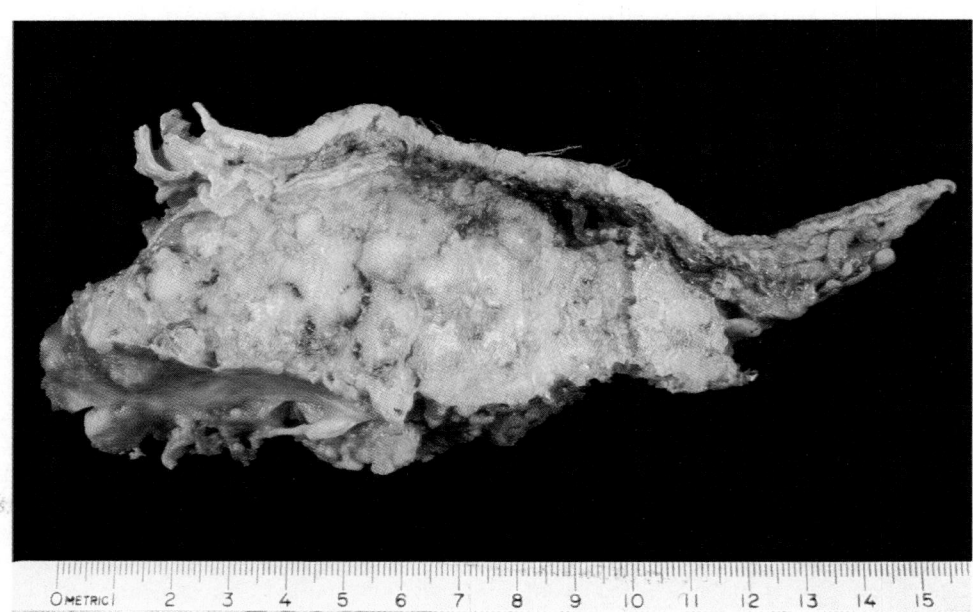

Fig. 24-133 Gross appearance of synovial chondrosarcoma. The lesion has a more expansile quality than the usual synovial osteochondromatosis.

11 Noda M, Vogel RL, Craig AM, Prahl J, De Luca HF, Denhardt DT: Identification of a DNA sequence responsible for binding of the 1,25-dihydroxyvitamin D3 receptor and 1,25-dihydroxyvitamin D3 enhancement of mouse secreted phosphoprotein 1 (SPP-1 or osteopontin) gene expression. Proc Natl Acad Sci USA **87**:9995-9999, 1990.

12 Okada Y, Naka K, Kawamura K, Matsumoto T, Nakanishi I, Fujimoto N, Sato H, Seiki M: Localization of matrix metalloproteinase 9 (92-Kilodalton gelatinase/type IV collagenase = gelatinase B) in osteoclasts. Implications for bone resorption. Lab Invest **72**:311-322, 1995.

13 Owen TA, Bortell R, Yocum SA, Smock SL, Zhang M, Abate C, Shalhoub V, Aronin N, Wright KL, van Wijnen AJ, et al.: Coordinate occupancy of AP-1 sites in the vitamin D-responsive and CCAAT box elements by Fos-Jun in the osteocalcin gene: Model for phenotype suppression of transcription. Proc Natl Acad Sci USA **87**:9990-9994, 1990.

14 Reinholt FP, Hultenby K, Oldberg A, Heinegard D: Osteopontin. A possible anchor of osteoclasts to bone. Proc Natl Acad Sci USA **87**:4473-4475, 1990.

15 Udagawa N, Takahashi N, Akatsu T, Tanaka H, Sasaki T, Nishihara T, Koga T, Martin TJ, Suda T: Origin of osteoclasts. Mature monocytes and macrophages are capable of differentiating into osteoclasts under a suitable microenvironment prepared by bone marrow-derived stromal cells. Proc Natl Acad Sci USA **87**:7260-7264, 1990.

16 Wozney JM, Rosen V, Celeste AJ, Mitsock LM, Whitters MJ, Kriz RW, Hewick RM, Wang EA: Novel regulators of bone formation. Molecular clones and activities. Science **242**:1528-1534, 1988.

17 Zheng MH, Wood DJ, Papadimitriou JM: What's new in the role of cytokines on osteoblast proliferation and differentiation? Pathol Res Pract **188**:1104-1121, 1992.

METABOLIC BONE DISEASES

18 Avioli LV, Krane SM, eds: Metabolic bone disease, vol. I. New York, 1977, Academic Press, Inc.

19 Avioli LV, Teitelbaum SL: The renal osteodystrophies. In Brenner BM, Rector FC, eds: The kidney. Philadelphia, 1976, WB Saunders Co, pp 1542-1591.

20 Becks JS, Nordin BEC: Histological assessment of osteoporosis by iliac crest biopsy. J Pathol Bacteriol **80**:391-397, 1960.

21 Bernstein DS, Sadowsky N, Hegsted DM, Guri CD, Stare FJ: Prevalence of osteoporosis in high- and low-fluoride areas in North Dakota. JAMA **198**:499-504, 1966.

21a Bullough PG: Atlas of orthopedic pathology, ed 2. St. Louis, 1992, Mosby.

22 Caldwell RA: Observations on the incidence, aetiology and pathology of senile osteoporosis. J Clin Pathol **15**:421-431, 1962.

23 Coe FL, Favus MJ, eds: Disorders of bone and mineral metabolism, New York, 1992, Raven Press.

24 Davis ME, Strandjord NM, Lanzl LH: Estrogens and the aging process. JAMA **196**:219-224, 1966.

25 Fallon MD, Teitelbaum SL: The interpretation of fluorescent tetracycline markers in the diagnosis of metabolic bone diseases. Hum Pathol **13**:416-417, 1982.

26 Falvo KA, Bullough PG: Osteogenesis imperfecta. A histometric analysis. J Bone Joint Surg (Am) **55**:275-286, 1973.

27 Fourman P: Calcium metabolism and the bone, ed 2. Philadelphia, 1968, FA Davis Co.

28 Frost HM: Tetracycline-based histological analysis of bone remodeling. Calcif Tissue Res **3**:211-237, 1969.

29 Jowsey J, Kelly PJ, Riggs BL, Bianco AJ Jr, Scholz DA, Gershon-Cohen J: Quantitative microradiographic studies of normal and osteoporotic bone. J Bone Joint Surg (Am) **47**:785-806, 1965.

30 Mankin HJ: Rickets, osteomalacia, and renal osteodystrophy. Part II. J Bone Joint Surg (Am) **56**:352-386, 1974.

31 Raisz LG: Local and systemic factors in the pathogenesis of osteoporosis. N Engl J Med **318**:818-828, 1988.

32 Riggs BL, Melton LJ III: Involutional osteoporosis. N Engl J Med **314**:1676-1686, 1986.

33 Riggs BL, Melton LJ: The prevention and treatment of osteoporosis. N Engl J Med **327**:620-627, 1992.

34 Sillence DO, Horton WA, Rimoin DL: Morphologic studies in the skeletal dysplasias. A review. Am J Pathol **96**:811-870, 1979.

35 Steendijk R: Metabolic bone disease in children. Clin Orthop **77**:247-275, 1971.

36 Stevenson JC, ed: New techniques in metabolic bone diseases. London, 1990, Wright.

37 Teitelbaum SL: Metabolic and other nontumorous disorders of the bone. In Kissane JM, ed: Anderson's pathology, ed 8. St. Louis, 1985, The CV Mosby Co, pp 1705-1777.

38 Teitelbaum SL: Renal osteodystrophy. Hum Pathol **15**:306-323, 1984.

39 Teitelbaum SL, Bullough PG: The pathophysiology of bone and joint disease. Am J Pathol **96**:283-354, 1979.

40 Teitelbaum SL, Hruska KA, Shieber W, Debnam JW, Nichols SH: Tetracycline fluorescence in uremic and primary hyperparathyroid bone. Kidney Int **12**:366-372, 1977.

41 Teitelbaum SL, Nichols SH: Tetracycline-based morphometric analysis of trabecular bone kinetics. In Meunier P, ed: Bone histomorphometry. Second International Workshop on Bone Morphology. Lyon, France, 1976, Armour Co, pp 311-319.

42 Vigorita VJ: The bone biopsy protocol for evaluating osteoporosis and osteomalacia. Am J Surg Pathol **8**:925-930, 1984.

43 Vigorita VJ: Osteoporosis. A diagnosable disorder? Pathol Annu **23**(Pt 2):185-212, 1988.

FRACTURES

44 Collins DH: Structural changes around nails and screws in human bones. J Pathol Bacteriol **65**:109-121, 1953.

45 Collins DH: Tissue changes in human femurs containing plastic appliances. J Bone Joint Surg (Br) **36**:458-563, 1954.

46 Ham AW, Harris WR: Repair and transplantation of bone. In Bourne GH, ed: The biochemistry and physiology of bone, ed 2, vol 3. New York, 1956, Academic Press, Inc, pp 338-379.

47 Mindell ER, Rodbard S, Kwasman BG: Chrondrogenesis in bone repair. A study of the healing fracture callus in the rat. Clin Orthop **79**:187-196, 1971.

48 Odell RT, Leydig SM: The conservative treatment of fractures in children. Surg Gynecol Obstet **92**:69-74, 1951.

49 Schwarz E: Hypercallosis in osteogenesis imperfecta. Am J Roentgenol Radium Ther Nucl Med **85**:645-648, 1961.

OSTEOMYELITIS

50 Berney S, Goldstein M, Bishko F: Clinical and diagnostic features of tuberculous arthritis. Am J Med **53**:36-42, 1972.

51 Bohm E, Josten C: What's new in exogenous osteomyelitis? Pathol Res Pract **188**:254-258, 1992.

52 Cabanela ME, Sim FH, Beabout JW, Dahlin DC: Osteomyelitis appearing as neoplasms. A diagnostic problem. Arch Surg **109**:68-72, 1974.

53 Cozzutto C: Xanthogranulomatous osteomyelitis. Arch Pathol Lab Med **108**:973-976, 1984.

54 Farrow R, Cureton RJR: Carcinomatous invasion of bone in osteomyelitis. Br J Surg **50**:107-109, 1962.

55 Felsberg GJ, Gore RL, Schweitzer ME, Jui V: Sclerosing osteomyelitis of Garre (periostitis ossificans). Oral Surg Oral Med Oral Pathol **70**:117-120, 1990.

56 Garcia A Jr, Grantham SA: Hematogenous pyogenic vertebral osteomyelitis. J Bone Joint Surg (Am) **42**:429-436, 1960.

57 Johnson LL, Kempson RL: Epidermoid carcinoma in chronic osteomyelitis. Diagnostic problems and management. J Bone Joint Surg (Am) **47**:133-145, 1965.

58 Lewis P, Sutter VL, Finegold M: Bone infections involving anaerobic bacteria. Medicine (Baltimore) **57**:279-305, 1978.

59 Moore RM, Green NE: Blastomycosis of bone. A report of six cases. J Bone Joint Surg (Am) **64**:1097-1101, 1982.

60 Schwarz J: What's new in mycotic bone and joint diseases? Pathol Res Pract **178**:617-634, 1984.

61 Silver HK, Simon JL, Clement DH: Salmonella osteomyelitis and abnormal hemoglobin disease. Pediatrics **20**:439-447, 1957.

62 Trueta J: The three types of acute haematogenous osteomyelitis. J Bone Joint Surg (Br) **41**:671-680, 1959.

63 Waldvogel FA, Vasey H: Osteomyelitis. The past decade. N Engl J Med **300**:360-370, 1980.

64 Weisenburger DD, Vinh TN, Levinson B: Malakoplakia of bone. An unusual cause of pathologic fracture in an immunosuppressed patient. Clin Orthop **201**:106-110, 1985.

65 Wu P-C, Khin N-M, Pang S-W: Salmonella osteomyelitis. An important differential diagnosis of granulomatous osteomyelitis. Am J Surg Pathol **9**:531-537, 1985.

66 Yasuma T, Nakajima Y: Clinicopathological study on plasma cell osteomyelitis. Acta Pathol Jpn **31**:835-844, 1981.

BONE NECROSIS
Infarct

67 Galli SJ, Weintraub HP, Proppe KH: Malignant fibrous histiocytoma and pleomorphic sarcoma in association with medullary bone infarcts. Cancer **41**:607-619, 1978.

68 Mirra JM, Bullough PG, Marcove RC, Jacobs B, Huvos AG: Malignant fibrous histiocytoma and osteosarcoma in association with bone infarcts. Report of four cases, two in caisson workers. J Bone Joint Surg (Am) **56:**932-940, 1974.

69 Torres FX, Kyriakos M: Bone infarct-associated osteosarcoma. Cancer **70:**2418-2430, 1992.

Aseptic (avascular) bone necrosis

70 Bohr H, Larsen EJ: On necrosis of the femoral head after fracture of the neck of the femur. J Bone Joint Surg (Br) **47:**330-338, 1965.

71 Golding JSR, Maciver JF, Went LN: The bone changes in sickle-cell anaemia and its genetic variants. J Bone Jont Surg (Br) **41:**711-718, 1959.

72 Mankin HJ: Nontraumatic necrosis of bone (osteonecrosis). N Engl J Med **326:**1473-1479, 1992.

73 Phemister DB: Repair of bone in the presence of aseptic necrosis resulting from fractures, transplantations, and vascular obstruction. J Bone Joint Surg **12:**769-787, 1930.

Osteochondritis dissecans

74 Milgram JW: Radiological and pathological manifestations of osteochondritis of the distal femur. A study of 50 cases. Radiology **126:**305-311, 1978.

Radiation necrosis

75 Sengupta S, Prathap K: Radiation necrosis of the humerus. A report of three cases. Acta Radiol **12:**313-320, 1973.

PAGET'S DISEASE

76 Barry HC: Paget's disease of bone. Edinburgh, 1969, E & S Livingstone, Ltd.

77 Collins DH: Paget's disease of bone. Incidence and subclinical forms. Lancet **2:**51-57, 1956.

78 Collins DH, Winn JM: Focal Paget's disease of the skull (osteoporosis circumscripta). J Pathol Bacteriol **69:**1-9, 1955.

79 Eisman JA, Martin TJ: Osteolytic Paget's disease. Recognition and risks of biopsy. J Bone Joint Surg (Am) **68:**112-117, 1986.

80 Fallon MD, Schwamm HA: Paget's disease of bone. An update on the pathogenesis, pathophysiology, and treatment of osteitis deformans. Pathol Annu **24**(Pt 1):115-159, 1989.

81 Greenspan A, Norman A, Sterling AP: Precocious onset of Paget's disease—a report of three cases and review of the literature. J Can Assoc Radiol **28:**69-72, 1977.

82 Hadjipavlou A, Lander P, Srolovitz H, Enker IP: Malignant transformation in Paget disease of bone. Cancer **70:**2802-2808, 1992.

83 Lake ME: The pathology of fracture in Paget's disease. Aust NZ J Surg **27:**307-312, 1958.

84 Mii Y, Miyauchi Y, Honoki K, Morishita T, Miura S, Aoki M, Tamai S, Tsunoda S, Nishitani M, Sakaki T: Electron microscopic evidence for a viral nature for osteoclast inclusions in Paget's disease of bone. Virchows Arch Pathol **424:**99-104, 1994.

85 Mills BG, Singer FR: Nuclear inclusions in Paget's disease of bone. Science **194:**201-202, 1976.

86 Price CHG, Goldie W: Paget's sarcoma of bone. A study of 80 cases from the Bristol and the Leeds bone tumour registries. J Bone Joint Surg (Br) **51:**205-224, 1969.

87 Reifenstein EC Jr, Albright F: Paget's disease. Its pathologic physiology and the importance of this in the complications arising from fracture and immobilization. N Engl J Med **231:**343-355, 1944.

88 Schmorl G: Ueber Ostitis deformans Paget. Virchows Arch [A] **283:**694-751, 1931.

89 Smith BJ, Eveson JW: Paget's disease of bone with particular reference to dentistry. J Oral Pathol **10:**233-247, 1981.

90 Uehlinger E: Osteofibrosis deformans juvenilis (Polyostotische fibröse Dysplasia Jaffe-Lichtenstein). Virchows Arch [A] **306:**255-299, 1940.

OSTEOPETROSIS

91 Coccia PF, Krivit W, Cervenka J, Clawson C, Kersey JH, Kim TH, Nesbit ME, Ramsay MKC, Warkentin PI, Teitelbaum SL, Kahn AJ, Brown DM: Successful bone marrow transplantation for infantile malignant osteopetrosis. N Engl J Med **302:**701-708, 1980.

91a Key LL Jr, Rodriguiz RM, Willi SM, Wright NM, Hatcher HC, Eyre DR, Cure JK, Griffin PP, Ries WL: Long-term treatment of osteopetrosis with recombinant human interferon gamma. N Engl J Med **332:**1594-1599, 1995.

92 Milgram JW, Murali J: Osteopetrosis. A morphological study of twenty-one cases. J Bone Joint Surg (Am) **64:**912-919, 1982.

TUMORS
Classification and distribution

93 Dorfman HD: Malignant transformation of benign bone lesions. In Proceedings of the Seventh National Cancer Conference, vol 7. Philadelphia, 1973, JB Lippincott Co, pp 901-913.

93a Dorfman HD, Czerniak B: Bone Cancers. Cancer **75:**203-210, 1995.

94 Hudson TM: Radiologic-pathologic correlation of musculoskeletal lesions. Baltimore, 1987, Williams & Wilkins.

95 Schajowicz F, Ackerman LV, Sissons HA: Histologic typing of bone tumours. International Histological Classification of Tumours, No. 6. Geneva, 1972, World Health Organization.

96 Schajowicz F, Sissons HA, Sobin LH: The World Health Organization's histologic classification of bone tumors. A commentary on the second edition. Cancer **75:**1208-1214, 1995.

Bone-forming tumors
Osteoma

96a Bertoni F, Unni KK, Beabout JW, Sim FH: Parosteal osteoma of bones other than of the skull and face. Cancer **75:**2466-2473, 1995.

97 Chang CHJ, Piatt ED, Thomas KE, Watne AL: Bone abnormalities in Gardner's syndrome. Am J Roentgenol Radium Ther Nucl Med **103:**645-652, 1968.

98 Hallberg OE, Begley JW Jr: Origin and treatment of osteomas of the paranasal sinuses. Arch Otolaryngol **51:**750-760, 1950.

Osteoid osteoma and osteoblastoma

99 Ayala AG, Murray JA, Erling MA, Raymond AK: Osteoid-osteoma. Intraoperative tetracycline-fluorescence demonstration of the nidus. J Bone Joint Surg (Am) **68:**747-751, 1986.

100 Bauer TW, Zehr RJ, Belhobek GH, Marks KE: Juxta-articular osteoid osteoma. Am J Surg Pathol **15:**381-387, 1991.

101 Bertoni F, Bacchini P, Donati D, Martini A, Picci P, Campanacci M: Osteoblastoma-like osteosarcoma. The Rizzoli Institute experience. Mod Pathol **6:**707-716, 1993.

102 Bertoni F, Unni KK, Lucas DR, McLeod RA: Osteoblastoma with cartilaginous matrix. An unusual morphologic presentation in 18 cases. Am J Surg Pathol **17:**69-74, 1993.

103 Bertoni F, Unni KK, McLeod RA, Dahlin DC: Osteosarcoma resembling osteoblastoma. Cancer **55:**416-426, 1985.

104 Beyer WF, Kühn H: Can an osteoblastoma become malignant? Virchows Arch [A] **408:**297-305, 1985.

105 Byers PD: Solitary benign osteoblastic lesions of bone—osteoid osteoma and benign osteoblastoma. Cancer **22:**43-57, 1968.

106 Dorfman HD, Weiss SW: Borderline osteoblastic tumors. Problems in the differential diagnosis of aggressive osteoblastoma and low-grade osteosarcoma. Semin Diagn Pathol **1:**215-234, 1984.

107 Hasegawa T, Hirose T, Sakamoto R, Seki K, Ikata T, Hizawa K: Mechanism of pain in osteoid osteomas. An immunohistochemical study. Histopathology **22:**487-491, 1993.

108 Healey JH, Ghalman B: Osteoid osteoma and osteoblastoma. Current concepts and recent advances. Clin Orthop **204:**76-85, 1986.

109 Jaffe HL: Osteoid-osteoma of bone. Radiology **45:**319-334, 1945.

110 Lichtenstein L: Benign osteoblastoma. J Bone Joint Surg (Am) **46:**755-765, 1964.

111 Loizaga JM, Calvo M, Lopez Barea F, Martinez Tello FJ, Perez Villanueva J: Osteoblastoma and osteoid osteoma. Clinical and morphological features of 162 cases. Pathol Res Pract **189:**33-41, 1993.

112 Lucas DR, Unni KK, McLeod RA, O'Connor MI, Sim FH: Osteoblastoma. Clinicopathologic study of 306 cases. Hum Pathol **25:**117-134, 1994.

113 MacLennan DI, Wilson FC Jr: Osteoid osteoma of the spine. A review of the literature and report of six new cases. J Bone Joint Surg (Am) **49:**111-121, 1967.

114 Marcove RC, Heelan RT, Huvos AG, Healey J, Lindeque BG: Osteoid osteoma. Diagnosis, localization, and treatment. Clin Orthop 197-201, 1991.

115 Marsh BW, Bonfiglio M, Brady LP, Enneking WF: Benign osteoblastoma. Range of manifestations. J Bone Joint Surg (Am) **57:**1-9, 1975.

116 McLeod RA, Dahlin DC, Beabout JW: The spectrum of osteoblastoma. Am J Roentgenol **126:**321-335, 1976.

117 Pettine KA, Klassen RA: Osteoid-osteoma and osteoblastoma of the spine. J Bone Joint Surg (Am) **68:**354-361, 1986.

118 Rigault P, Mouterde P, Padovani JP, Jaubert F, Guyonvarch G: Ostéome ostéoïde chez l'enfant. A propos de 29 cas. Rev Chir Orthop **61:**627-646, 1975.

119 Schajowicz F, Lemos C: Osteoid osteoma and osteoblastoma. Acta Orthop Scand **41:**272-291, 1970.

120 Schajowicz F, Lemos C: Malignant osteoblastoma. J Bone Joint Surg (Br) **58:**202-211, 1976.

121 Steiner GC: Ultrastructure of osteoid osteoma. Hum Pathol **7:**309-325, 1976.

122 Wold LE, Pritchard DJ, Bergert J, Wilson DM: Prostaglandin synthesis by osteoid osteoma and osteoblastoma. Mod Pathol **1:**129-131, 1988.

123 Yoshikawa S, Nakamura T, Takagi M, Imamura T, Okano K, Sasaki S: Benign osteoblastoma as a cause of osteomalacia. A report of two cases. J Bone Joint Surg (Br) **59:**279-286, 1977.

Osteosarcoma

124 Ahuja SC, Villacin AB, Smith J, Bullough PG, Huvos AG, Marcove RC: Juxta-cortical (parosteal) osteogenic sarcoma. Histologic grading and prognosis. J Bone Joint Surg (Am) **59:**632-647, 1977.

125 Amstutz HC: Multiple osteogenic sarcomata—metastatic or multicentric? Report of two cases and review of literature. Cancer **24:**923-931, 1969.

126 Arlen M, Higinbotham NL, Huvos AG, Marcove RC, Miller T, Shah IC: Radia-tion-induced sarcoma of bone. Cancer **28:**1087-1099, 1971.

127 Atik OS, Caglar M, Bolukbasi S, Gogus S, Gogus MT: Osteogenic sarcoma of the distal femur in a young child. Hum Pathol **13:**766, 1982.

128 Ayala AG, Raymond AK, Jaffe N: The pathologist's role in the diagnosis and treatment of osteosarcoma in children. Hum Pathol **15:**258-266, 1984.

129 Ayala AG, Raymond AK, Ro JY, Carrasco CH, Fanning CV, Murray JA: Nee-dle biopsy of primary bone lesions. M.D. Anderson experience. Pathol Annu **24**(Pt 1):219-251, 1989.

130 Ayala AG, Ro JY, Raymond AK, Jaffe N, Chawla S, Carrasco H, Link M, Jimenez J, Edeiken J, Wallace S, et al.: Small cell osteosarcoma. A clinico pathologic study of 27 cases. Cancer **64:**2162-2173, 1989.

131 Bacci G, Picci P, Ruggieri P, Mercuri M, Avella M, Capanna R, Brach Del Pre-ver A, Mancini A, Gherlinzoni F, Padovani G, et al.: Primary chemotherapy and delayed surgery (neoadjuvant chemotherapy) for osteosarcoma of the extremi-ties. The Istituto Rizzoli Experience in 127 patients treated preoperatively with intravenous methotrexate (high versus moderate doses) and intraarterial cisplatin. Cancer **65:**2539-2553, 1990.

132 Banta JV, Schreiber RR, Kulik WJ: Hyperplastic callus formation in osteogene-sis imperfecta simulating osteosarcoma. J Bone Joint Surg (Am) **53:**115-122, 1971.

133 Barwick KW, Huvos AG, Smith J: Primary osteogenic sarcoma of the vertebral column. A clinicopathologic correlation of ten patients. Cancer **46:**595-604, 1980.

134 Bauer HC, Kreicbergs A, Silversward C, Tribukait B: DNA analysis in the dif-ferential diagnosis of osteosarcoma. Cancer **61:**2532-2540, 1988.

135 Belli L, Scholl S, Livartowski A, Ashby M, Palangie T, Levasseur P, Pouillart P: Resection of pulmonary metastases in osteosarcoma. A retrospective analysis of 44 patients. Cancer **63:**2546-2550, 1989.

136 Bertoni F, Bacchii P, Fabbri N, Mercuri M, Picci P, Ruggieri P, Campanacci M: Osteosarcoma. Low-grade intraosseous-type osteosarcoma, histologically resem-bling parosteal osteosarcoma, fibrous dysplasia, and desmoplastic fibroma. Cancer **71:**338-345, 1993.

137 Bertoni F, Pignatti G, Bachini P, Picci P, Bacci G, Campanacci M: Telangiectatic or hemorrhagic osteosarcoma of bone. A clinicopathologic study of 41 patients at the Rizzoli Institute. Progr Surg Pathol **10:**63-82, 1989.

138 Bertoni F, Present D, Bacchini P, Pignatti G, Picci P, Campanacci M: The Istituto Rizzoli experience with small cell osteosarcoma. Cancer **64:**2591-2599, 1989.

139 Bjornsson J, Inwards CY, Wold LE, Sim FH, Taylor WF: Prognostic significance of spontaneous tumour necrosis in osteosarcoma. Virchows Arch [A] **423:**195-199, 1993.

140 Bosse A, Vollmer E, Bocker W, Roessner A, Wuisman P, Jones D, Fisher LW: The impact of osteonectin for differential diagnosis of bone tumors. An immuno-histochemical approach. Pathol Res Pract **186:**651-657, 1990.

141 Broström L-A, Harris MA, Simon MA, Cooperman DR, Nilsonne U: The effect of biopsy on survival of patients with osteosarcoma. J Bone Joint Surg (Br) **61:**209-212, 1979.

142 Burgers JM, van Glabbeke M, Busson A, Cohen P, Mazabraud AR, Abbatucci JS, Kalifa C, Tubiana M, Lemerle JS, Voute PA, et al.: Osteosarcoma of the limbs. Report of the EORTC-SIOP 03 trial 20781 investigating the value of adju-vant treatment with chemotherapy and/or prophylactic lung irradiation. Cancer **61:**1024-1031, 1988.

143 Campanacci M, Bacci G, Gertoni F, Picci P, Minutillo A, Franceschi C: The treatment of osteosacoma of the extremities. Twenty years' experience at the Isti-tuto Ortopedico Rizzoli. Cancer **48:**1569-1581, 1981.

144 Campanacci M, Cervellati G: Osteosarcoma. A review of 345 cases. Ital J Orthop Traumatol **1:**5-22, 1975.

145 Campanacci M, Picci P, Gherlinzoni F, Guerra A, Bertoni F, Neff JR: Parosteal osteosarcoma. J Bone Joint Surg (Br) **66:**313-321, 1984.

146 Clark JL, Unni KK, Dahlin DC, Devine KD: Osteosarcoma of the jaw. Cancer **51:**2311-2316, 1983.

147 Dahlin DC, Coventry MB: Osteogenic sarcoma. A study of 600 cases. J Bone Joint Surg (Am) **49:**101-110, 1967.

148 Dahlin DC, Unni KK: Osteosarcoma of bone and its important recognizable vari-eties. Am J Surg Pathol **1:**61-72, 1977.

149 Dardick I, Schatz J, Colgan T: Osteogenic sarcoma with epithelial differentia-tion. Ultrastruct Pathol **16:**463-474, 1992.

150 Davis AM, Bell RS, Goodwin PJ: Prognostic factors in osteosarcoma. A critical review. J Clin Oncol **12:**423-431, 1994.

151 deSantos LA, Murray JA, Ayala AG: The value of percutaneous needle biopsy in the management of primary bone tumors. Cancer **43:**735-744, 1979.

152 deSantos LA, Murray JA, Finklestein JB, Spjut HJ, Ayala AG: The radiographic spectrum of periosteal osteosarcoma. Radiology **127:**123-129, 1978.

153 Devaney K, Vinh TN, Sweet DE: Small cell osteosarcoma of bone. An immuno-histochemical study with differential diagnostic considerations. Hum Pathol **24:** 1211-1225, 1993.

154 Dickersin GR, Rosenberg AE: The ultrastructure of small-cell osteosarcoma, with a review of the light microscopy and differential diagnosis. Hum Pathol **22:**267-275, 1991.

155 Dwinnell LA, Dahlin DC, Ghormley RK: Parosteal (juxtacortical) osteogenic sarcoma. J Bone Joint Surg (Am) **36:**732-744, 1954.

156 Edeiken J, Farrell C, Ackerman LV, Spjut HJ: Parosteal sarcoma. Am J Roentgenol Radium Ther Nucl Med **111:**579-583, 1971.

157 Enneking WF, ed: Osteosarcoma. Symposium. Clin Orthop **111:**1-104, 1975.

158 Enneking WF, Kagan A: "Skip" metastases in osteosarcoma. Cancer **36:**2192-2205, 1975.

159 Farr GH, Huvos AG: Juxtacortical osteogenic sarcoma. J Bone Joint Surg (Am) **51:**1205-1216, 1972.

160 Fechner RE, Huvos AG, Mirra JM, Spjut HJ, Unni KK: A symposium on the pathology of bone tumors. Pathol Annu **19**(Pt 1):125-194, 1984.

161 Frentzel-Beyme R, Wagner G: Malignant bone tumours. Status of aetiological knowledge and needs of epidemiological research. Arch Orthop Trauma Surg **94:**81-89, 1979.

162 Garbe LR, Monges GM, Pellegrin EM, Payan HL: Ultrastructural study of osteosarcomas. Hum Pathol **12:**891-896, 1981.

163 Glasser DB, Lane JM, Huvos AG, Marcove RC, Rosen G: Survival, prognosis, and therapeutic response in osteogenic sarcoma. The Memorial Hospital experi-ence. Cancer **69:**698-708, 1992.

164 Hall RB, Robinson LH, Malawar MM, Dunham WK: Periosteal osteosarcoma. Cancer **55:**165-171, 1985.

165 Harvei S, Solheim O: The prognosis in osteosarcoma. Norwegian national data. Cancer **48:**1719-1723, 1981.

166 Hasegawa T, Hirose T, Kudo E, Hizawa K, Usui M, Ishii S: Immunophenotypic heterogeneity in osteosarcomas. Hum Pathol **22:**583-590, 1991.

167 Hasegawa T, Shibata T, Hirose T, Seki K, Hizawa K: Osteosarcoma with epithe-lioid features. An immunohistochemical study. Arch Pathol Lab Med **117:**295-298, 1993.

168 Hiddemann W, Roessner A, Wörmann B, Mellin W, Klockenkemper B, Bösing T, Büchner T, Grundmann E: Tumor heterogeneity in osteosarcoma as identified by flow cytometry. Cancer **59:**324-328, 1987.

169 Huvos AG: Osteogenic sarcoma of bones and soft tissues in older persons. A clinicopathologic analysis of 117 patients older than 60 years. Cancer **57:**1442-1449, 1986.

170 Huvos AG, Butler A, Bretsky SS: Osteogenic sarcoma associated with Paget's disease of bone. A clinicopathologic study of 65 patients. Cancer **52:**1489-1495, 1983.

171 Huvos AG, Butler A, Bretsky SS: Osteogenic sarcoma in pregnant women. Prog-nosis, therapeutic implications, and literature review. Cancer **56:**2326-2331, 1985.

172 Huvos AG, Rosen G, Bretsky SS, Butler A: Telangiectatic osteogenic sarcoma. A clinicopathologic study of 124 patients. Cancer **49:**1679-1689, 1982.

173 Huvos AG, Sundaresan N, Bretsky SS, Butler A: Osteogenic sarcoma of the skull. A clinicopathologic study of 19 patients. Cancer **56:**1214-1221, 1985.

174 Huvos AG, Woodard HQ, Cahan WG, Higinbotham NL, Stewart FW, Butler A, Bretsky SS: Postradiation osteogenic sarcoma of bone and soft tissues. A clini-copathologic study of 66 patients. Cancer **55:**1244-1255, 1985.

175 Iavarone A, Matthay KK, Steinkirchner TM, Israel MA: Germ-line and somatic p53 gene mutations in multifocal osteogenic sarcoma. Proc Natl Acad Sci USA **89:**4207-4209, 1992.

176 Iwasaki R, Yamamuro T, Kotoura Y, Okumura H, Kasai R, Nakashima Y: Immunohistochemical study of bone GLA protein in primary bone tumors. Cancer 70:619-624, 1992.

177 Jaffe N, Raymond AK, Ayala A, Carrasco CH, Wallace S, Robertson R, Griffiths M, Wang YM: Effect of cumulative courses of intraarterial cisdiamminedichloroplatin-II on the primary tumor in osteosarcoma. Cancer 63:63-67, 1989.

178 Kahn LB, Wood FW, Ackerman LV: Fracture callus associated with benign and malignant bone lesions and mimicking osteosarcoma. Am J Clin Pathol 52:14-24, 1969.

179 Kellie SJ, Pratt CB, Parham DM, Fleming ID, Meyer WH, Rao BN: Sarcomas (other than Ewing's) of flat bones in children and adolescents. A clinicopathologic study. Cancer 65:1011-1016, 1990.

180 Kozakewich H, Perez-Atayde AR, Goorin AM, Wilkinson RH, Gebhardt MC, Vawter GF: Osteosarcoma in young children. Cancer 67:638-642, 1991.

181 Kramer K, Hicks DG, Palis J, Rosier RN, Oppenheimer J, Fallon MD, Cohen HJ: Epithelioid osteosarcoma of bone. Immunocytochemical evidence suggesting divergent epithelial and mesenchymal differentiation in a primary osseous neoplasm. Cancer 71:2977-2982, 1993.

182 Kurt AM, Unni KK, McLeod RA, Pritchard DJ: Low-grade intraosseous osteosarcoma. Cancer 65:1418-1428, 1990.

183 Kyriakos M: Intracortical osteosarcoma. Cancer 56:2525-2533, 1980.

184 Lane JM, Hurson B, Boland PJ, Glasser DB: Osteogenic sarcoma. Clin Orthop 204:93-110, 1986.

185 Lanzer WL, Liotta LA, Yee C, Azar HA, Costa J: Synthesis of pro-collagen type II by a xenotransplanted human chondroblastic osteosarcoma. Am J Pathol 104:217-226, 1981.

186 Levine AM, Resenberg SA: Alkaline phosphatase levels in osteosarcoma tissue are related to prognosis. Cancer 44:2291-2293, 1979.

187 Malawer MM, Dunham WK: Skip metastases in osteosarcoma. Recent experience. J Surg Oncol 22:236-245, 1983.

188 Mankin HJ, Conner JF, Schiller AL, Perlmutter N, Alho A, McGuire M: Grading of bone tumors by analysis of nuclear DNA content using flow cytometry. J Bone Joint Surg (Am) 67:404-413, 1985.

189 Mankin HJ, Lange TA, Spanier SS: The hazards of biopsy in patients with malignant primary bone and soft-tissue tumors. J Bone Joint Surg (Am) 64:1121-1127, 1982.

190 Martin SE, Dwyer A, Kissane JM, Costa J: Small-cell osteosarcoma. Cancer 50:990-996, 1982.

191 Martínez-Tello FJ, Navas-Palacios JJ: The ultrastructure of conventional, parosteal, and periosteal osteosarcomas. Cancer 50:949-961, 1982.

192 Martland HS, Humphries RE: Osteogenic sarcoma in dial painters using luminous paint. Arch Pathol 7:406-417, 1929.

193 Matsuno T, Unni KK, McLeod RA, Dahlin DC: Telangiectatic osteogenic sarcoma. Cancer 38:2538-2547, 1976.

194 Nora FE, Unni KK, Pritchard DJ, Dahlin DC: Osteosarcoma of extragnathic craniofacial bones. Mayo Clin Proc 58:268-272, 1983.

195 O'Hara JM, Hutter RVP, Foote FW Jr, Miller T, Woodward HQ: An analysis of 30 patients surviving longer than ten years after treatment for osteogenic sarcoma. J Bone Joint Surg (Am) 50:335-354, 1968.

196 Okada K, Wold LE, Beabout JW, Shives TC: Osteosarcoma of the hand. A clinicopathologic study of 12 cases. Cancer 72:719-725, 1993.

197 Ottolenghi CE: Diagnosis of orthopaedic lesions by aspiration biopsy. Results of 1,061 punctures. J Bone Joint Surg (Am) 37:443-464, 1955.

198 Ozisik YY, Meloni AM, Peier A, Altungoz O, Spanier SS, Zalupski MM, Leong SP, Sandberg AA: Cytogenetic findings in 19 malignant bone tumors. Cancer 74:2268-2275, 1994.

199 Parham DM, Prat CB, Parvey LS, Webber BL, Champion J: Childhood multifocal osteosarcoma. Clinicopathologic and radiologic correlates. Cancer 55:2653-2658, 1985.

200 Penman HG, Ring PA: Osteosarcoma in association with total hip replacement. J Bone Joint Surg (Br) 66:632-634, 1984.

201 Picci P, Bacci G, Campanacci M, Gasparini M, Pilotti S, Cerasoli S, Bertoni F, Guerra A, Capanna R, Albisinni U, Galletti S, Gherlinzoni F, Calderoni P, Sudanese A, Baldini N, Bernini M, Jaffe N: Histologic evaluation of necrosis in osteosarcoma induced by chemotherapy. Regional mapping of viable and non-viable tumor. Cancer 56:1515-1521, 1985.

202 Polednak AP: Bone cancer among female radium dial workers. Latency periods and incidence rates by time after exposure. Brief communication. J Natl Cancer Inst 60:77-82, 1978.

203 Pritchard DJ, Finkel MP, Reilly CA Jr: The etiology of osteosarcoma. A review of current considerations. Clin Orthop 111:14-22, 1975.

204 Rao BN, Champion JE, Pratt CB, Carnesale P, Dilawari R, Fleming I, Green A, Austin B, Wrenn E, Kumar M: Limb salvage procedures for children with osteosarcoma. An alternative to amputation. J Pediatr Surg 18:901-908, 1983.

205 Raymond AK, Chawla SP, Carrasco CH, Ayala AG, Fanning CV, Grice B, Armen T, Plager C, Papadopoulos NEJ, Edeiken J, Wallace S, Jaffe N, Murray JA, Benjamin RS: Osteosarcoma chemotherapy effect. A prognostic factor. Semin Diagn Pathol 4:212-236, 1987.

206 Reddick RL, Michelitch HJ, Levine AM, Triche TJ: Osteogenic sarcoma. A study of the ultrastructure. Cancer 45:64-71, 1980.

207 Rosen G, Marcove RC, Caparros B, Nirenberg A, Kosloff C, Huvos AG: Primary osteogenic sarcoma. The rationale for preoperative chemotherapy and delayed surgery. Cancer 43:2163-2177, 1979.

208 Scaglietti O, Calandriello B: Ossifying parosteal sarcoma. J Bone Joint Surg (Am) 44:635-647, 1962.

209 Schajowicz F, Derqui JC: Puncture biopsy in lesions of the locomotor system. Review of results in 4,050 cases, including 941 vertebral punctures. Cancer 21:531-548, 1968.

210 Schajowicz F, Santini Araujo E, Berenstein M: Sarcoma complicating Paget's disease of bone. A clinicopathological study of 62 cases. J Bone Joint Surg (Br) 65:299-307, 1983.

211 Schaller RT Jr, Haas J, Schaller J, Morgan A, Bleyer A: Improved survival in children with osteosarcoma following resection of pulmonary metastases. J Pediatr Surg 17:546-550, 1982.

212 Schulz A, Jundt G, Berghäuser K-H, Gehron-Robey P, Termine JD: Immunohistochemical study of osteonectin in various types of osteosarcoma. Am J Pathol 132:233-238, 1988.

212a Sciot R, Samson I, Dal Cin P, Lateur L, Van Damme B, Van Den Berghe H, Desmet V: Giant cell rich parosteal osteosarcoma. Histopathology 27:51-55, 1995.

213 Scranton PE, DeCicco FA, Totten RS, Yunis EJ: Prognostic factors in osteosarcoma. A review of 20 years' experience at the University of Pittsburgh Health Center Hospitals. Cancer 36:2179-2191, 1975.

214 Shapiro F: Ultrastructural observations on osteosarcoma tissue. A study of 10 cases. Ultrastruct Pathol 4:151-161, 1983.

215 Shives TC, Dahlin DC, Sim FH, Pritchard DJ, Earle JD: Osteosarcoma of the spine. J Bone Joint Surg (Am) 68:660-668, 1986.

216 Sim FH, Unni KK, Beabout JW, Dahlin DC: Osteosarcoma with small cells simulating Ewing's tumor. J Bone Joint Surg (Am) 62:207-215, 1979.

217 Simon MA, Bos GD: Epiphyseal extension of metaphyseal osteosarcoma in skeletally immature individuals. J Bone Joint Surg (Am) 62:195-204, 1980.

218 Simon MA, Hecht JD: Invasion of joints by primary bone sarcomas in adults. Cancer 50:1649-1655, 1982.

219 Sindelar WF, Costa J, Ketcham AS: Osteosarcoma associated with Thorotrast administration. Cancer 42:2604-2609, 1978.

220 Smith GD, Chalmers J, McQueen MM: Osteosarcoma arising in relation to an enchondroma. A report of three cases. J Bone Joint Surg (Br) 68:315-319, 1986.

221 Sommer H-J, Knop J, Heise U, Winkler K, Delling G: Histomorphometric changes of osteosarcoma after chemotherapy. Correlation with 99mTC methylene diphosphonate functional imaging. Cancer 59:252-258, 1987.

222 Spjut HJ, Ayala AG, deSantos LA, Murray JA: Periosteal osteosarcoma. In Management of primary bone and soft tissue tumors, M.D. Anderson Hospital and Tumor Institute. Chicago, 1977, Year Book Medical Publishers, Inc, pp 79-95.

223 Stark A, Aparisi T, Ericsson JLE: Human osteogenic sarcoma. Fine structure of the osteoblastic type. Ultrastruct Pathol 4:311-329, 1983.

224 Stark A, Aparisi T, Ericsson JLE: Human osteogenic sarcoma. Fine structure of the chondroblastic type. Ultrastruct Pathol 6:51-67, 1984.

225 Stark A, Aparisi T, Ericsson JLE: Human osteogenic sarcoma. Fine structure of the fibroblastic type. Ultrastruct Pathol 7:301-319, 1984.

226 Stark A, Aparisi T, Ericsson JLE: Human osteogenic sarcoma. Fine structural localization of alkaline phosphatase. Ultrastruct Pathol 8:143-154, 1985.

226a Swanson PE, Dehner LP, Sirgi KE, Wick MR: Cytokeratin immunoreactivity in malignant tumors of bone and soft tissue. A reappraisal of cytokeratin as a reliable marker in diagnostic immunohistochemistry. Appl Immunohistochem 2:103-112, 1994.

227 Tucker MA, DÁngio GJ, Boice JD Jr, Strong LC, Li FP, Stovall M, Stone BJ, Green DM, Lombardi F, Newton W, Hoover RN, Fraumeni JF Jr: Bone sarcomas linked to radiotherapy and chemotherapy in children. N Engl J Med 317:588-593, 1987.

228 Unni KK, Dahlin DC, Beabout JW, Ivins JC: Parosteal osteogenic sarcoma. Cancer 37:2466-2475, 1976.

229 Unni KK, Dahlin DC, Beabout JW: Periosteal osteogenic sarcoma. Cancer 37:2476-2485, 1976.

230 Unni KK, Dahlin DC, McLeod RA, Prtichard DJ: Intraosseous well-differentiated osteosarcoma. Cancer 40:1337-1347, 1977.

231 Uribe-Botero G, Russell WO, Sutow WW, Martin RG: Primary osteosarcoma of bone. A clinicopathologic investigation of 243 cases, with necropsy studies in 54. Am J Clin Pathol **67:**427-435, 1977.

232 Van der Heul RO, Von Ronnen JR: Juxtacortical osteosarcoma. Diagnosis, differential diagnosis, treatment, and an analysis of eighty cases. J Bone Joint Surg (Am) **49:**415-439, 1967.

233 van der Walt JD, Ryan JF: Parosteal osteogenic sarcoma of the hand. Histopathology **16:**75-78, 1990.

234 Varela-Duran J, Dehner LP: Postirradiation osteosarcoma in childhood. A clinicopathologic study of three cases and review of the literature. Am J Pediatr Hematol Oncol **2:**263-271, 1980.

235 Vigorita VJ, Jones JK, Ghelman B, Marcove RC: Intracortical osteosarcoma. Am J Surg Pathol **8:**65-71, 1984.

236 Wakasa K, Sakurai M, Uchida A, Yoshikawa H, Maeda A: Massive pulmonary tumor emboli in osteosarcoma. Occult and fatal complication. Cancer **66:**583-586, 1990.

237 Weatherby RP, Dahlin DC, Ivins JC: Postradiation sarcoma of bone. Review of 78 Mayo Clinic cases. Mayo Clin Proc **56:**294-306, 1981.

238 White VA, Fanning CV, Ayala AG, Raymond AK, Carrasco CH, Murray JA: Osteosarcoma and the role of fine-needle aspiration. A study of 51 cases. Cancer **62:**1238-1246, 1988.

239 Wick MR, Siegal GP, Unni KK, McLeod RA, Greditzer HG III: Sarcomas of bone complicating osteitis deformans (Paget's disease). Fifty years' experience. Am J Surg Pathol **5:**47-59, 1981.

240 Williams AH, Schwinn CP, Parker JW: The ultrastructure of osteosarcoma. A review of twenty cases. Cancer **37:**1293-1301, 1976.

241 Winkler K, Bielack S, Delling G, Salzer-Kuntschik M, Kotz R, Greenshaw C, Jurgens H, Ritter J, Kusnierz-Glaz C, Erttmann R, et al.: Effect of intraarterial versus intravenous cisplatin in addition to systemic doxorubicin, high-dose methotrexate, and ifosfamide on histologic tumor response in osteosarcoma (study COSS-86). Cancer **66:**1703-1710, 1990.

242 Wold LE, Unni KK, Beabout JW, Pritchard DJ: High-grade surface osteosarcomas. Am J Surg Pathol **8:**181-186, 1984.

243 Wold LE, Unni KK, Beabout JW, Sim FH, Dahlin DC: Dedifferentiated parosteal osteosarcoma. J Bone Joint Surg (Am) **66:**53-59, 1984.

244 Yoshida H, Adachi H, Hamada Y, Aki T, Yumoto T, Morimoto K, Orido T: Osteosarcoma. Ultrastructural and immunohistochemical studies on alkaline phosphatase–positive tumor cells constituting a variety of histologic types. Acta Pathol Jpn **38:**325-338, 1988.

245 Yoshida H, Yumoto T, Adachi H, Minamizaki T, Maeda N, Furuse K: Osteosarcoma with prominent epithelioid features. Acta Pathol Jpn **39:**439-445, 1989.

246 Yoshikawa H, Rettig WJ, Takaoka K, Alderman E, Rup B, Rosen V, Wozney JM, Lane JM, Huvos AG, Garin-Chesa P: Expression of bone morphogenetic proteins in human osteosarcoma. Immunohistochemical detection with monoclonal antibody. Cancer **73:**85-91, 1994.

246a Yoshikawa H, Rettig WJ, Lane JM, Takaoka K, Alderman E, Rup B, Rosen V, Healey JH, Huvos AG, Garin-Chesa P: Immunohistochemical detection of bone morphogenetic proteins in bone and soft-tissue sarcomas. Cancer **74:**842-847, 1994.

247 Yunis EJ, Barnes L: The histologic diversity of osteosarcoma. Pathol Annu **21**(Pt 1):121-141, 1986.

Cartilage-forming tumors
Chondroma

248 Boriani S, Bacchini P, Bertoni F, Campanacci M: Periosteal chondroma. A review of twenty cases. J Bone Joint Surg (Am) **65:**205-212, 1983.

249 Brand T, Hatch EI, Schaller RT, Stevenson JK, Arensman Rm, Schwartz MC: Surgical management of the infant with mesenchymal hamartoma of the chest wall. J Pediatr Surg **21:**556-558, 1986.

250 Campbell AN, Wagget J, Mott MG: Benign mesenchymoma of the chest wall in infancy. J Surg Oncol **21:**267-270, 1982.

251 Cannon SR, Sweetnam DR: Multiple chondrosarcomas in dyschondroplasia (Ollier's disease). Cancer **55:**836-840, 1985.

252 Cowan WK: Malignant change and multiple metastases in Ollier's disease. J Clin Pathol **18:**650-653, 1965.

253 Laurence W, Franklin EL: Calcifying enchondroma of long bones. J Bone Joint Surg (Br) **35:**224-228, 1953.

254 Lewis RJ, Ketcham AS: Maffucci's syndrome. Functional and neoplastic significance. Case report and review of the literature. J Bone Joint Surg (Am) **55:**1465-1479, 1973.

255 Lichtenstein L, Hall JE: Periosteal chondroma. A distinctive benign cartilage tumor. J Bone Joint Surg (Am) **34:**691-697, 1952.

256 Liu J, Hudkins PG, Swee RG, Unni KK: Bone sarcomas associated with Ollier's disease. Cancer **59:**1376-1385, 1987.

257 McCarthy EF, Dorfman HD: Vascular and cartilaginous hamartoma of the ribs in infancy with secondary aneurysmal bone cyst formation. Am J Surg Pathol **4:**247-253, 1980.

258 Nojima T, Unni KK, McLeod RA, Pritchard DJ: Periosteal chondroma and periosteal chondrosarcoma. Am J Surg Pathol **9:**666-677, 1985.

259 Nosanchuk JS, Kaufer H: Recurrent periosteal chondroma. Report of two cases and a review of the literature. J Bone Joint Surg (Am) **51:**375-380, 1969.

260 Sun T-C, Swee RG, Shives TC, Unni KK: Chondrosarcoma in Maffucci's syndrome. J Bone Joint Surg (Am) **67:**1214-1215, 1985.

261 Takigawa K: Chondroma of the bones of the hand. J Bone Joint Surg (Am) **53:**1591-1600, 1971.

262 Tamimi HK, Bolen JW: Enchondromatosis (Ollier's disease) and ovarian juvenile granulosa cell tumor. A case report and review of the literature. Cancer **53:**1605-1608, 1984.

Osteochondroma

263 Copeland RL, Meehan PL, Morrissy RT: Spontaneous regression of osteochondromas. Two case reports. J Bone Joint Surg (Am) **67:**971-973, 1985.

264 del Rosario AD, Bui HX, Singh J, Ginsburg R, Ross JS: Intracytoplasmic eosinophilic hyaline globules in cartilaginous neooplasms. A surgical, pathological, ultrastructural, and electron probe x-ray microanalytic study. Hum Pathol **25:**1283-1289, 1994.

265 Fairbank HAT: An atlas of general affections of the skeleton. Edinburgh, 1951, E & S Livingstone, Ltd.

266 Han SK, Henein HG, Novin N, Giargiana FA Jr: An unusual arterial complication seen with a solitary osteochondroma. Am Surg **43:**471-472, 1977.

267 Hwang W-S, McQueen D, Monson RC, Reed MH: The significance of cytoplasmic chondrocyte inclusions in multiple osteochondromatosis, solitary osteochondromas, and chondrodysplasias. Am J Clin Pathol **78:**89-91, 1982.

268 Josefczyk MA, Huvos AG, Smith J, Urmacher C: Bursa formation in secondary chondrosarcoma with intrabursal chondrosarcomatosis. Am J Surg Pathol **9:**309-314, 1985.

269 Landon GC, Johnson KA, Dahlin DC: Subungual exostoses. J Bone Joint Surg (Am) **61:**256-259, 1979.

270 Meneses MF, Unni KK, Swee RG: Bizarre parosteal osteochondromatous proliferation of bone (Nora's lesion). Am J Surg Pathol **17:**691-697, 1993.

271 Miller-Breslow A, Dorfman HD: Dupuytren's (subungual) exostosis. Am J Surg Pathol **12:**368-378, 1988.

272 Nora FE, Dahlin DC, Beaubout JW: Bizarre parosteal osteochondromatous proliferations of the hands and feet. Am J Surg Pathol **7:**245-250, 1983.

273 Ochsner PE: Zum problem der neoplastischen Entartung bei multiplen kartilaginären Exostosen. Z Orthop **116:**369-378, 1978.

274 Unni KK, Dahlin DC: Premalignant tumors and conditions of bone. Am J Surg Pathol **3:**47-60, 1979.

Chondroblastoma

275 Aronsohn RS, Hart WR, Martel W: Metaphyseal chondroblastoma of bone. Am J Roentgenol **127:**686-688, 1976.

276 Birch PJ, Buchanan R, Golding P, Pringle JAS: Chondroblastoma of the rib with widespread bone metastases. Histopathology **25:**583-585, 1994.

277 Brecher ME, Simon MA: Chondroblastoma. An immunohistochemical study. Hum Pathol **19:**1043-1047, 1988.

278 Codman EA: Epiphyseal chondromatous giant cell tumors of the upper end of the humerus. Surg Gynecol Obstet **52:**543-548, 1931.

279 Coleman SS: Benign chondroblastoma with recurrent soft-tissue and intra-articular lesions. J Bone Joint Surg **48:**1554-1560, 1966.

280 Fanning CV, Sneige NS, Carrasco CH, Ayala AG, Murray JA, Raymond AK: Fine needle aspiration cytology of chondroblastoma of bone. Cancer **65:**1847-1863, 1990.

281 Hicks DG, Krasinskas AM, Sickel JZ, Hughes SS, Puzas JE, Moynas R, Rosier RN: Chondroblastoma. In situ hybridization and immunohistochemical evidence supporting a cartilaginous origin. Int J Surg Pathol **1:**155-162, 1994.

282 Huvos AG, Marcove RC, Erlandson RA, Mike V: Chondroblastoma of bone. A clinico-pathologic and electron microscopic study. Cancer **29:**760-771, 1972.

283 Kahn LB, Wood FM, Ackerman LV: Malignant chondroblastoma. Report of two cases and review of the literature. Arch Pathol **88:**371-376, 1969.

284 Kunze E, Graewe TH, Peitsch E: Histology and biology of metastatic chondroblastoma. Report of a case with a review of the literature. Pathol Res Pract **182:**113-120, 1987.

285 Kyriakos M, Land VJ, Penning HL, Parker SG: Metastatic chondroblastoma. Report of a fatal case with a review of the literature on atypical, aggressive, and malignant chondroblastoma. Cancer **55:**1770-1789, 1985.

286 Levine GD, Bensch KG: Chondroblastoma—the nature of the basic cell. A study by means of histochemistry, tissue culture, electron microscopy, and autoradiography. Cancer **29:**1546-1562, 1972.

287 Mii Y, Miyauchi Y, Honoki K, Morishita T, Miura S, Aoki M, Tamai S: Ultra-structural cytochemical demonstration of proteoglycans and calcium in the extracellular matrix of chondroblastomas. Hum Pathol **25:**1290-1294, 1994.

288 Monda L, Wick MR: S-100 protein immunostaining in the differential diagnosis of chondroblastoma. Hum Pathol **16:**287-293, 1985.

289 Nakamura Y, Becker LE, Marks A: S-100 protein in tumors of cartilage and bone. An immunohistochemical study. Cancer **58:**1820-1824, 1983.

290 Reyes CV, Kathuria S: Recurrent and aggressive chondroblastoma of the pelvis with late malignant neoplastic changes. Am J Surg Pathol **3:**449-455, 1979.

291 Schajowicz F, Gallardo H: Epiphysial chondroblastoma of bone. A clinico-pathological study of sixty-nine cases. J Bone Joint Surg (Br) **52:**205-226, 1970.

292 Semmelink HJ, Prusczynski M, Wiersma-van Tilburg A, Smedts F, Ramaekers FC: Cytokeratin expression in chondroblastomas. Histopathology **16:**257-263, 1990.

293 Springfield DS, Capanna R, Gherlinzoni F, Picci P, Campanacci M: Chondro-blastoma. A review of seventy cases. J Bone Joint Surg (Am) **67:**748-754, 1985.

294 Steiner GC: Ultrastructure of benign cartilaginous tumors of intraosseous origin. Hum Pathol **10:**71-86, 1979.

295 Turcotte RE, Kurt AM, Sim FH, Unni KK, McLeod RA: Chondroblastoma. Hum Pathol **24:**944-949, 1993.

296 Valls J, Ottolenghi CE, Schajowicz F: Epiphyseal chondroblastoma of bone. J Bone Joint Surg (Am) **33:**997-1009, 1951.

297 Welsh RA, Meyer AT: A histogenetic study of chondroblastoma. Cancer **17:**578-589, 1964.

Chondromyxoid fibroma and related tumors

298 Bleiweiss IJ, Klein MJ: Chondromyxoid fibroma. Report of six cases with immunohistochemical studies. Mod Pathol **3:**664-666, 1990.

299 Dahlin DC: Chondromyxoid fibroma of bone, with emphasis on its morphological relationship to benign chondroblastoma. Cancer **9:**195-203, 1956.

300 Gherlinzoni F, Rock M. Picci P: Chondromyxoid fibroma. The experience at the Istituto Ortopedico Rizzoli. J Bone Joint Surg (Am) **65:**198-204, 1983.

301 Jaffe HL, Lichtenstein L: Chondromyxoid fibroma of bone. A distinctive benign tumor likely to be mistaken especially for chondrosarcoma. Arch Pathol **45:**541-551, 1948.

302 Kreicbergs A, Lönnquist PA, Willems J: Chondromyxoid fibroma. A review of the literature and a report on our own experience. Acta Pathol Microbiol Immunol Scand (A) **93:**189-197, 1985.

303 Kyriakos M: Soft tissue implantation of chondromyxoid fibroma. Am J Surg Pathol **3:**363-372, 1979.

304 Marcove RC, Kambolis C, Bullough PG, Jaffe HL: Fibromyxoma of bone. Cancer **17:**1209-1213, 1964.

305 Marcove RC, Lindeque BG, Huvos AG: Fibromyxoma of the bone. Surg Gynecol Obstet **169:**115-118, 1989.

306 McClure DK, Dahlin DC: Myxoma of bone. Report of three cases. Mayo Clin Proc **52:**249-253, 1977.

307 Schajowicz F, Gallardo H: Chondromyxoid fibroma (fibromyxoid chondroma) of bone. A clinico-pathological study of thirty-two cases. J Bone Joint Surg (Br) **53:**198-216, 1971.

308 Zillmer DA, Dorfman HD: Chondromyxoid fibroma of bone. Thirty-six cases with clinicopathologic correlation. Hum Pathol **20:**952-964, 1989.

Chondrosarcoma

309 Alho A, Connor JF, Mankin HJ, Schiller AL, Campbell CJ: Assessment of malignancy of cartilage tumors using flow cytometry. A preliminary report. J Bone Joint Surg (Am) **65:**779-785, 1983.

310 Barnes R, Catto M: Chondrosarcoma of bone. J Bone Joint Surg (Br) **48:**729-764, 1966.

311 Bertoni F, Boriani S, Laus M, Campanacci M: Periosteal chondrosarcoma and periosteal osteosarcoma. Two distinct entities. J Bone Joint Surg (Br) **64:**370-376, 1982.

312 Campanacci M, Guernelli N, Leonessa C, Boni A: Chondrosarcoma. A study of 133 cases, 80 with long term follow up. Ital J Orthop Traumatol **1:**387-414, 1975.

313 Castresana J, Barrios C, Gomez L, Kreicbergs A: Amplification of the c-*myc* proto-oncogene in human chondrosarcoma. Diagn Mol Pathol **1:**235-238, 1992.

314 Coltrera MD, Googe PB, Harrist TJ, Hyams VJ, Schiller AL, Goodman ML: Chondrosarcoma of the temporal bone. Diagnosis and treatment of 13 cases and review of the literature. Cancer **58:**2689-2696, 1986.

315 Dahlin DC, Henderson ED: Chondrosarcoma, a surgical and pathological problem. J Bone Joint Surg (Am) **38:**1025-1038, 1956.

316 Dahlin DC, Salvador AH: Chondrosarcomas of bones of the hands and feet. A study of 30 cases. Cancer **34:**755-760, 1974.

317 Dobashi Y, Sugimura H, Sato A, Hirabayashi T, Kanda H, Kitagawa T, Kawaguchi N, Imamura T, Machinami R: Possible association of p53 overexpression and mutation with high-grade chondrosarcoma. Diagn Mol Pathol **2:**257-263, 1993.

318 Erlandson RA, Huvos AG: Chondrosarcoma. A light and electron microscopic study. Cancer **34:**1642-1652, 1974.

319 Evans HL, Ayala AG, Romsdahl MM: Prognostic factors in chondrosarcoma of bone. A clinicopathologic analysis with emphasis on histologic grading. Cancer **40:**818-831, 1977.

320 Garrison RC, Unni KK, McLeod RA, Pritchard DJ, Dahlin DC: Chondrosarcoma arising in osteochondroma. Cancer **49:**1890-1897, 1982.

321 Gitelis S, Bertoni F, Picci P, Campanacci M: Chondrosarcoma of bone. The experience at the Istituto Ortopedico Rizzoli. J Bone Joint Surg (Am) **63:**1248-1257, 1981.

322 Healey JH, Lane JM: Chondrosarcoma. Clin Orthop **204:**119-129, 1986.

323 Huvos AG, Marcove RC: Chondrosarcoma in the young. A clinicopathologic analysis of 790 patients younger than 21 years of age. Am J Surg Pathol **11:**930-942, 1987.

324 Kindblom L, Angervall L: Histochemical characterization of mucosubstances in bone and soft tissue tumors. Cancer **36:**985-994, 1975.

325 Kreicbergs A, Boquist L, Borssén B, Larsson S-E: Prognostic factors in chondrosarcoma. A comparative study of cellular DNA content and clinicopathologic features. Cancer **50:**577-583, 1982.

326 Kreicbergs A, Slezak E, Söderberg G: The prognostic significance of different histomorphologic features in chondrosarcoma. Virchows Arch [A] **390:**1-10, 1981.

327 Kristensen IB, Sunde LM, Jensen OM: Chondrosarcoma. Increasing grade of malignancy in local recurrence. Acta Pathol Microbiol Immunol Scand (A) **94:**73-77, 1986.

328 Lansche WE, Spjut HJ: Chondrosarcoma of the small bones of the hand. J Bone Joint Surg (Am) **40:**1139-1149, 1958.

329 Lichtenstein L, Jaffe HL: Chondrosarcoma of bone. Am J Pathol **19:**553-589, 1943.

330 Mandahl N, Heim S, Arheden K, Rydholm A, Willen H, Mitelman F: Chromosomal rearrangements in chondromatous tumors. Cancer **65:**242-248, 1990.

331 Mankin HJ, Cantley KP, Lippiello L, Schiller AL, Campbell CJ: The biology of human chondrosarcoma. I. Description of the cases, grading, and biochemical analyses. J Bone Joint Surg (Am) **62:**160-176, 1980.

332 Mankin HJ, Cantley KP, Schiller AL, Lippiello L: The biology of human chondrosarcoma. II. Variation in chemical composition among types and subtypes of benign and malignant cartilage tumors. J Bone Joint Surg (Am) **62:**176-188, 1980.

333 Marcove RC, Huvos AG: Cartilaginous tumors of the ribs. Cancer **27:**794-801, 1971.

334 McAfee MK, Pairolero PC, Bergstralh EJ, Piehler JM, Unni KK, McLeod RA, Bernatz PE, Payne WS: Chondrosarcoma of the chest wall. Factors affecting survival. Ann Thorac Surg **40:**535-541, 1985.

335 McKenna RJ, Schwinn CP, Soong KY, Higinbotham NL: Sarcomata of the osteogenic series (osteosarcoma, fibrosarcoma, chondrosarcoma, parosteal osteogenic sarcoma, and sarcomata arising in abnormal bone). J Bone Joint Surg (Am) **48:**1-26, 1966.

336 Mirra JM, Gold R, Downs J, Eckardt JJ: A new histologic approach to the differentiation of enchondroma and chondrosarcoma of the bones. A clinicopathologic analysis of 51 cases. Clin Orthop **201:**214-237, 1985.

337 Nakamura Y, Becker LE, Marks A: S-100 protein in tumors of cartilage and bone. An immunohistochemical study. Cancer **58:**1820-1824, 1983.

338 Okajima K, Honda I, Kitagawa T: Imunohistochemical distribution of S-100 protein in tumors and tumorlike lesions of bone and cartilage. Cancer **61:**792-799, 1988.

339 O'Neal LW, Ackerman LV: Cartilaginous tumors of ribs and sternum. J Thorac Surg **21:**71-108, 1951.

340 O'Neal LW, Ackerman LV: Chondrosarcoma of bone. Cancer **5:**551-577, 1952.

341 Pritchard DJ, Lunke RJ, Taylor WF, Dahlin DC, Medley BE: Chondrosarcoma. A clinicopathologic and statistical analysis. Cancer **45:**149-157, 1980.

342 Sanerkin NG, Gallagher P: A review of the behaviour of chondrosarcoma of bone. J Bone Joint Surg (Br) **61:**395-400, 1979.

343 Schajowicz F: Juxtacortical chondrosarcoma. J Bone Joint Surg (Br) **59:**473-480, 1977.

344 Schiller AL: Diagnosis of borderline cartilage lesions of bone. Semin Diagn Pathol **2:**42-62, 1985.

345 Smith WS, Simon MA: Segmental resection for chondrosarcoma. J Bone Joint Surg (Am) **57:**1097-1103, 1975.

346 Wrba F, Gullick WJ, Fertl H, Amann G, Salzer-Kuntschik M: Immunohistochemical detection of the c-*erb*B-2 proto-oncogene product in normal, benign and malignant cartilage tissues. Histopathology **15**:71-76, 1989.
347 Young CL, Sim FH, Unni KK, McLeod RA: Chondrosarcoma of bone in children. Cancer **66**:1641-1648, 1990.

Clear cell chondrosarcoma

348 Bjornsson J, Unni KK, Dahlin DC, Beabout JW, Sim FH: Clear cell chondrosarcoma of bone. Observations in 47 cases. Am J Surg Pathol **8**:223-230, 1984.
349 Faraggiana T, Sender B, Glicksman P: Light- and electron-microscopic study of clear cell chondrosarcoma. Am J Clin Pathol **75**:117-121, 1981.
350 Unni KK, Dahlin DC, Beabout JW, Sim FH: Chondrosarcoma. Clear-cell variant. A report of sixteen cases. J Bone Joint Surg (Am) **58**:676-683, 1976.
351 Wang LT, Liu TC: Clear cell chondrosarcoma of bone. A report of three cases with immunohistochemical and affinity histochemical observations. Pathol Res Pract **189**:411-415, 1993.
352 Weiss A-PC, Dorfman HD: S-100 protein in human cartilage lesions. J Bone Joint Surg (Am) **68**:521-526, 1986.

Myxoid chondrosarcoma (chordoid sarcoma)

353 Dabska M: Parachordoma. A new clinicopathologic entity. Cancer **40**:1586-1592, 1977.
354 Martin RF, Melnick PJ, Warner NE, Terry R, Bullock WK, Schwinn CP: Chordoid sarcoma. Am J Clin Pathol **59**:623-635, 1972.
355 Miettinen M, Lehto V-P, Dahl D, Virtanen I: Differential diagnosis of chordoma, chondroid, and ependymal tumors as aided by anti-intermediate filament antibodies. Am J Pathol **112**:160-169, 1983.
356 Pardo-Mindan FJ, Guillen FJ, Villas C, Vazquez JJ: A comparative ultrastructural study of chondrosarcoma, chordoid sarcoma, and chordoma. Cancer **47**:2611-2619, 1981.
357 Shin HJ, Mackay B, Ichinose H, Ayala AG, Romsdahl MM: Parachordoma. Ultrastruct Pathol **18**:249-256, 1994.

Dedifferentiated chondrosarcoma

358 Abernoza P, Neumann MP, Manivel JC, Wick MR: Dedifferentiated chondrosarcoma. An ultrastructural study of two cases, with immunocytochemical correlations. Ultrastruct Pathol **10**:529-538, 1986.
359 Bertoni F, Present D, Bacchini P, Picci P, Pignatti G, Gherlinzoni F, Campanacci M: Dedifferentiated peripheral chondrosarcomas. A report of seven cases. Cancer **63**:2054-2059, 1989.
360 Bridge JA, De Boer J, Travis J, Johansson SL, Elmberger G, Noel SM, Neff JR: Simultaneous interphase cytogenetic analysis and fluorescence immunophenotyping of dedifferentiated chondrosarcoma. Implications for histopathogenesis. Am J Pathol **144**:215-220, 1994.
361 Dahlin DC, Beabout JW: Dedifferentiation of low-grade chondrosarcomas. Cancer **28**:461-466, 1971.
362 Dervan PA, O'Loughlin J, Hurson BJ: Dedifferentiated chondrosarcoma with muscle and cytokeratin differentiation in the anaplastic component. Histopathology **12**:517-526, 1988.
363 Jaworski RC: Dedifferentiated chondrosarcoma. An ultrastructural study. Cancer **53**:2674-2678, 1984.
364 Johnson S, Tetu B, Ayala AG, Chawla SP: Chondrosarcoma with additional mesenchymal component (dedifferentiated chondrosarcoma). I. A clinicopathologic study of 26 cases. Cancer **58**:278-286, 1986.
365 McCarthy EF, Dorfman HD: Chondrosarcoma of bone with dedifferentiation. A study of eighteen cases. Hum Pathol **13**:36-40, 1982.
366 McFarland GB, McKinley LM, Reed RJ: Dedifferentiation of low-grade chondrosarcomas. Clin Orthop **122**:157-164, 1977.
367 Meis JM: "Dedifferentiation" in bone and soft-tissue tumors. A histological indicator of tumor progression. Pathol Annu **26**(Pt 1):37-62, 1991.
368 Mirra JM, Marcove RC: Fibrosarcomatous dedifferentiation of primary and secondary chondrosarcoma. Review of five cases. J Bone Joint Surg (Am) **56**:285-296, 1974.
369 Tetu B, Ordóñez NG, Ayala AG, Mackay B: Chondrosarcoma with additional mesenchymal component (dedifferentiated chondrosarcoma). II. An immunohistochemical and electron microscopic study. Cancer **58**:287-298, 1986.

Mesenchymal chondrosarcoma

370 Bertoni F, Picci P, Bacchini P, Capanna R, Innao V, Bacci G, Campanacci M: Mesenchymal chondrosarcoma of bone and soft tissues. Cancer **52**:533-541, 1983.
371 Dabska M, Huvos AG: Mesenchymal chondrosarcoma in the young. A clinicopathologic study of 19 patients with explanation of histogenesis. Virchows Arch [A] **399**:89-104, 1983.

372 Dowlig EA: Mesenchymal chondrosarcoma. J Bone Joint Surg (Am) **46**:747-754, 1964.
373 Frydman CP, Klein MJ, Abdelwahab IF, Zwass A: Primitive multipotential primary sarcoma of bone. A case report and immunohistochemical study. Mod Pathol **4**:768-772, 1991.
374 Goldman RL: "Mesenchymal" chondrosarcoma, a rare malignant chondroid tumor usually primary in bone. Report of a case arising in extraskeletal soft tissue. Cancer **20**:1494-1498, 1967.
375 Guccion JG, Font RL, Enzinger FM, Zimmerman LE: Extraskeletal mesenchymal chondrosarcoma. Arch Pathol **95**:336-340, 1973.
376 Huvos AG, Rosen G, Dabska M, Marcove RC: Mesenchymal chondrosarcoma. A clinicopathologic analysis of 35 patients with emphasis on treatment. Cancer **51**:1230-1237, 1983.
377 Jacobson SA: Polyhistioma. A malignant tumor of bone and extraskeletal tissues. Cancer **40**:2116-2130, 1977.
378 Ling LL-L, Steiner GC: Primary multipotential malignant neoplasm of bone. Chondrosarcoma associated with squamous cell carcinoma. Hum Pathol **17**:317-320, 1986.
379 Nakashima Y, Unni KK, Shives TC, Swee RG, Dahlin DC: Mesenchymal chondrosarcoma of bone and soft tissue. A review of 111 cases. Cancer **57**:2444-2453, 1986.
380 Salvador AH, Beabout JW, Dahlin DC: Mesenchymal chondrosarcoma. Observations on 30 new cases. Cancer **28**:605-615, 1971.
381 Steiner GC, Mirra JM, Bullough PG: Mesenchymal chondrosarcoma. A study of the ultrastructure. Cancer **32**:926-939, 1973.
382 Swanson PE, Lillemoe TJ, Manivel JC, Wick MR: Mesenchymal chondrosarcoma. An immunohistochemical study. Arch Pathol Lab Med **114**:943-948, 1990.

Giant cell tumor

383 Aparisi T: Giant cell tumor of bone. Acta Orthop Scand **173**(Suppl):1-38, 1978.
384 Aparisi T, Arborgh B, Ericsson JLE: Giant cell tumor of bone. Virchows Arch [A] **381**:159-178, 1979.
385 Aqel NM, Pringle JA, Horton MA: Cellular heterogeneity in giant cell tumour of bone (osteoclastoma). An immunohistological study of 16 cases. Histopathology **13**:675-685, 1988.
386 Athanason NA, Bliss E, Gatter KC, Heryet A: An immunohistological study of giant-cell tumour of bone. Evidence for an osteoclast origin of the giant cells. J Pathol **147**:153-158, 1985.
387 Bertoni F, Present D, Enneking WF: Giant-cell tumor of bone with pulmonary metastases. J Bone Joint Surg (Am) **67**:890-900, 1985.
388 Bertoni F, Unni KK, Beabout JW, Ebersold MJ: Giant cell tumor of the skull. Cancer **70**:1124-1132, 1992.
389 Bouropoulou V, Kontogeorgos G, Manika Z: A histological and immunoenzymatic study on the histogenesis of "giant cell tumor of bones." Pathol Res Pract **180**:61-67, 1985.
390 Bridge JA, Neff JR, Bhatia PS, Sanger WG, Murphey MD: Cytogenetic findings and biologic behavior of giant cell tumors of bone. Cancer **65**:2697-2703, 1990.
391 Campanacci M, Giunti A, Olmi R: Giant-cell tumours of bone. A study of 209 cases with long-term follow-up in 130. Ital J Orthop Traumatol **1**:249-277, 1975.
392 Dahlin DC, Cupps RE, Johnson EW Jr: Giant-cell tumor. A study of 195 cases. Cancer **25**:1061-1070, 1970.
393 Eckardt JJ, Grogan TJ: Giant cell tumor of bone. Clin Orthop **204**:45-58, 1986.
394 Emley WE: Giant cell tumor of the sphenoid bone. A case report and review of literature. Arch Otolaryngol **94**:369-374, 1971.
395 Emura I, Inoue Y, Ohnishi Y, Morita T, Saito H, Tajima T: Histochemical, immunohistochemical and ultrastructural investigations of giant cell tumors of bone. Acta Pathol Jpn **36**:691-702, 1986.
396 Fain JS, Unni KK, Beabout JW, Rock MG: Nonepiphyseal giant cell tumor of the long bones. Clinical, radiologic, and pathologic study. Cancer **71**:3514-3519, 1993.
397 Fornasier VL, Flores L, Hastings D, Sharp T: Virus-like filamentous intranuclear inclusions in a giant-cell tumor, not associated with Paget's disease of bone. A case report. J Bone Joint Surg (Am) **67**:333-336, 1985.
398 Fukunaga M, Nikaido T, Shimoda T, Ushigoma S, Nakamori K: A flow cytometric DNA analysis of giant cell tumors of bone including two cases with malignant transformation. Cancer **70**:1886-1894, 1992.
399 Goldring SR, Schiller AL, Mankin HJ, Dayer J-M, Krane SM: Characterization of cells from human giant cell tumors of bone. Clin Orthop **204**:59-75, 1986.
400 Hanaoka H, Friedman B, Mack RP: Ultrastructure and histogenesis of giant-cell tumor of bone. Cancer **25**:1408-1423, 1970.

401 Kasahara K, Yamamuro T, Kasahara A: Giant-cell tumour of bone. Cytological studies. Br J Cancer **40:**201-209, 1979.

402 Ladanyi M, Traganos F, Huvos AG: Benign metastasizing giant cell tumors of bone. A DNA flow cytometric study. Cancer **64:**1521-1526, 1989.

403 Liu TC, Ji ZM, Wang LT: Giant cell tumors of bone. An immunohistochemical study. Pathol Res Pract **185:**448-453, 1989.

404 Mankin HJ, Fogelson FS, Thrasher AZ, Jaffer F: Massive resection and allograft transplantation in the treatment of malignant bone tumors. N Engl J Med **294:**1247-1255, 1976.

405 McDonald DJ, Sim FH, McLeod RA, Dahlin DC: Giant-cell tumor of bone. J Bone Joint Surg (Am) **68:**235-242, 1986.

406 Medeiros J, Beckstead J, Rosenberg A, Warnke R, Wood G: Giant cells and mononuclear cells of giant cell tumor of bone resemble histiocytes. Appl Immunohistochem **1:**115-122, 1993.

407 Meis JM, Dorfman HD, Nathanson SD, Haggar AM, Wu KK: Primary malignant giant cell tumor of bone. "Dedifferentiated" giant cell tumor. Mod Pathol **2:**541-546, 1989.

408 Metze K, Ciplea AG, Hettwer H, Barckhaus RH: Size dependent enzyme activities of multinucleated (osteoclastic) giant cells in bone tumors. Pathol Res Pract **182:**214-221, 1987.

409 Mii Y, Miyauchi Y, Morishita T, Miura S, Honoki K, Aoki M, Tamai S: Osteoclast origin of giant cells in giant cell tumors of bone. Ultrastructural and cytochemical study of six cases. Ultrastruct Pathol **15:**623-629, 1991.

410 Murphy WR, Ackerman LV: Benign and malignant giant-cell tumors of bone. Cancer **9:**317-339, 1956.

411 Nascimento AG, Huvos AG, Marcove RC: Primary malignant giant cell tumor of bone. A study of eight cases and review of the literature. Cancer **44:**1393-1402, 1979.

412 Negoescu A, Mandache E: The ultrastructure of nuclear inclusions in the giant-cell tumor of bone. Pathol Res Pract **184:**410-417, 1989.

413 Parrish FF: Allograft replacement of all or part of the end of a long bone following excision of a tumor. Report of twenty-one cases. J Bone Joint Surg (Am) **55:**1-22, 1973.

414 Peison B, Feigenbaum J: Metaphyseal giant-cell tumor in a girl of 14. Radiology **118:**145-146, 1976.

415 Picci P, Manfrini M, Zucchi V, Gherlinzoni F, Rock M, Bertoni F, Neff JR: Giant-cell tumor of bone in skeletally immature patients. J Bone Joint Surg (Am) **65:**486-490, 1983.

416 Present D, Bertoni F, Hudson T, Enneking WF: The correlation between the radiologic staging studies and histopathologic findings in aggressive stage 3 giant cell tumor of bone. Cancer **57:**237-244, 1986.

417 Regezi JA, Zarbo RJ, Lloyd RV, Unni KK: Muramidase, α-1 antitrypsin, α-1 antichymotrypsin, and S-100 protein immunoreactivity in giant cell lesions. Cancer **59:**64-68, 1987.

418 Rock MG, Pritchard DJ, Unni KK: Metastases from histologically benign giant-cell tumor of bone. J Bone Joint Surg (Am) **66:**269-274, 1984.

419 Roessner A, Bassewitz DBv, Schlake W, Thorwesten G, Grundmann E: Biologic characterization of human bone tumors. III. Giant cell tumor of bone. A combined electron microscopical, histochemical, and autoradiographical study. Pathol Res Pract **178:**431-440, 1984.

420 Sanerkin NG: Malignancy, aggressiveness, and recurrence in giant cell tumor of bone. Cancer **46:**1641-1649, 1980.

421 Sara AS, Ayala AG, el-Naggar A, Ro JY, Raymond AK, Murray JA: Giant cell tumor of bone. A clinicopathologic and DNA flow cytometric analysis. Cancer **66:**2186-2190, 1990.

422 Savini R, Gherlinzoni F, Morandi M, Neff JR, Picci P: Surgical treatment of giant-cell tumor of the spine. Istituto Ortopedico Rizzoli. J Bone Joint Surg (Am) **65:**1283-1290, 1983.

423 Schajowicz F: Giant-cell tumors of bone (osteoclastoma). A pathological and histochemical study. J Bone Joint Surg (Am) **43:**1-29, 1961.

424 Schajowicz F, Ubios AM, Santini Araujo E, Cabrini RL: Virus-like intranuclear inclusions in giant cell tumor of bone. Clin Orthop **201:**247-250, 1985.

425 Steiner GC, Ghosh L, Dorfman HD: Ultrastructure of giant cell tumors of bone. Hum Pathol **3:**569-586, 1972.

426 Sung HW, Kuo DP, Shu WP, Chai YB, Liu CC, Li SM: Giant-cell tumor of bone. Analysis of two hundred and eight cases in Chinese patients. J Bone Joint Surg (Am) **64:**755-761, 1982.

427 Sybrandy S, de la Fuente AA: Multiple giant tumour of bone. Report of a case. J Bone Joint Surg (Br) **55:**350-356, 1973.

428 Wold LE, Swee RG: Giant cell tumor of the small bones of the hands and feet. Semin Diagn Pathol **1:**173-184, 1984.

429 Wolfe JT III, Scheithauer BW, Dahlin DC: Giant-cell tumor of the sphenoid bone. Review of 10 cases. J Neurosurg **59:**322-327, 1983.

430 Yoshida H, Akeho M, Yumoto T: Giant cell tumor of bone. Enzyme histochemical, biochemical and tissue culture studies. Virchows Arch [A] **395:**319-330, 1982.

431 Zheng MH, Fan Y, Wysocki SJ, Lau AT, Robertson T, Beilharz M, Wood DJ, Papadimitriou JM: Gene expression of transforming growth factor-beta 1 and its type II receptor in giant cell tumors of bone. Possible involvement in osteoclast-like cell migration. Am J Pathol **145:**1095-1104, 1994.

Marrow tumors
Ewing's sarcoma

432 Ambros IM, Ambros PF, Strehl S, Kovar H, Gadner H, Salzer-Kuntschik M: MIC2 is a specific marker for Ewing's sarcoma and peripheral primitive neuroectodermal tumors. Evidence for a common histogenesis of Ewing's sarcoma and peripheral primitive neuroectodermal tumors from MIC2 expression and specific chromosome aberration. Cancer **67:**1886-1893, 1991.

433 Bacci G, Toni A, Avella M, Manfrini M, Sudanese A, Ciaroni D, Boriani S, Emiliani E, Campanacci M: Long-term results in 144 localized Ewing's sarcoma patients treated with combined therapy. Cancer **63:**1477-1486, 1989.

434 Bator SM, Bauer TW, Marks KE, Norris DG: Periosteal Ewing's sarcoma. Cancer **58:**1781-1784, 1986.

434a Brinkhuis M, Winjnaendts LC, van der Linden JC, van Unnik AJ, Voute PA, Baak JP, Meijer CJ: Peripheral primitive neuroectodermal tumour and extra-ossseous Ewing's sarcoma; a histological, immunohistochemical and DNA flow cytometric study. Virchows Arch **425:**611-616, 1995.

435 Cangir A, Vietti TJ, Gehan EA, Burgert EO Jr, Thomas P, Tefft M, Nesbit ME, Kissane J, Pritchard D: Ewing's sarcoma metastatic at diagnosis. Results and comparisons of two intergroup Ewing's sarcoma studies. Cancer **66:**887-893, 1990.

436 Carter RL, al-Sams SZ, Corbett RP, Clinton S: A comparative study of immunohistochemical staining for neuron-specific enolase, protein gene product 9.5 and S-100 protein in neuroblastoma, Ewing's sarcoma and other round cell tumours in children. Histopathology **16:**461-467, 1990.

437 Cavazzana AO, Miser JS, Jefferson J, Triche TJ: Experimental evidence for a neural origin of Ewing's sarcoma of bone. Am J Pathol **127:**507-518, 1987.

438 Dehner LP: Primitive neuroectodermal tumor and Ewing's sarcoma. Am J Surg Pathol **17:**1-13, 1993.

439 Delattre O, Zucman J, Melot T, Garau XS, Zucker JM, Lenoir GM, Ambros PF, Sheer D, Turc-Carel C, Triche TJ, et al.: The Ewing family of tumors—a subgroup of small-round-cell tumors defined by specific chimeric transcripts. N Engl J Med **331:**294-299, 1994.

440 Dierick AM, Langlois M, Van Oostveldt P, Roels H: The prognostic significance of the DNA content in Ewing's sarcoma. A retrospective cytophotometric and flow cytometric study. Histopathology **23:**333-339, 1993.

441 Dierick AM, Roels H, Langlois M: The immunophenotype of Ewing's sarcoma. An immunohistochemical analysis. Pathol Res Pract **189:**26-32, 1993.

442 Dockhorn-Dworniczak B, Schafer KL, Dantcheva R, Blasius S, Winkelmann W, Strehl S, Burdach S, van Valen F, Jurgens H, Bocker W: Diagnostic value of the molecular genetic detection of the t(11;22) translocation in Ewing's tumours. Virchows Arch **425:**107-112, 1994.

443 Downing JR, Head DR, Parham DM, Douglass EC, Hulshof MG, Link MP, Motroni TA, Grier HE, Curcio-Brint AM, Shapiro DN: Detection of the (11;22) (q24;q12) translocation of Ewing's sarcoma and peripheral neuroectodermal tumor by reverse transcription polymerase chain reaction. Am J Pathol **143:**1294-1300, 1993.

444 Editorial: Ewing's sarcoma and its congeners. An interim appraisal. Lancet **339:**99-100, 1992.

445 Ehara S, Kattapuram SV, Egglin TK: Ewing's sarcoma. Radiographic pattern of healing and bony complications in patients with long-term survival. Cancer **68:**1531-1535, 1991.

446 Fellinger EJ, Garin-Chesa P, Glasser DB, Huvos AG, Rettig WJ: Comparison of cell surface antigen HBA71 (p30/32MIC2), neuron-specific enolase, and vimentin in the immunohistochemical analysis of Ewing's sarcoma of bone. Am J Surg Pathol **16:**746-755, 1992.

447 Fellinger EJ, Garin-Chesa P, Su SL, De Angelis P, Lane JM, Rettig WJ: Biochemical and genetic characterization of the HBA71 Ewing's sarcoma cell surface antigen. Cancer Res **51:**336-340, 1991.

448 Fellinger EJ, Garin-Chesa P, Triche TJ, Huvos AG, Rettig WJ: Immunohistochemical analysis of Ewing's sarcoma cell surface antigen p30/32MIC2. Am J Pathol **139:**317-325, 1991.

449 Friedman B, Gold H: Ultrastructure of Ewing's sarcoma of bone. Cancer **22:**307-322, 1968.

450 Friedman B, Hanaoka H: Round-cell sarcomas of bone. A light and electron microscopic study. J Bone Joint Surg (Am) **53:**1118-1136, 1971.

451 Friedman JM, Vitale M, Maimon J, Israel MA, Horowitz ME, Schneider BS: Expression of the cholecystokinin gene in pediatric tumors. Proc Natl Acad Sci USA **89:**5819-5823, 1992.

452 Garin-Chesa P, Fellinger EJ, Huvos AG, Beresford HR, Melamed MR, Triche TJ, Rettig WJ: Immunohistochemical analysis of neural cell adhesion molecules. Differential expression in small round cell tumors of childhood and adolescence. Am J Pathol **139:**275-286, 1991.

453 Gasparini M, Barni S, Lattuada A, Musumeci R, Bonadonna G, Fossati-Bellani F: Ten years experience with Ewing's sarcoma. Tumori **63:**77-90, 1977.

454 Hartman KR, Triche TJ, Kinsella TJ, Miser JS: Prognostic value of histopathology in Ewing's sarcoma. Long-term follow-up of distal extremity primary tumors. Cancer **67:**163-171, 1991.

455 Hasegawa T, Hirose T, Kudo E, Hizawa K, Yamawaki S, Ishii S: Atypical primitive neuroectodermal tumors. Comparative light and electron microscopic and immunohistochemical studies on peripheral neuroepitheliomas and Ewing's sarcomas. Acta Pathol Jpn **41:**444-454, 1991.

456 Jaffe R, Santamaria M, Yunis EJ, Tannery NH, Agostini RM Jr, Medina J, Goodman M: The neuroectodermal tumor of bone. Am J Surg Pathol **8:**885-898, 1984.

457 Kaspers GJ, Kamphorst W, van de Graaff M, van Alphen HA, Veerman AJ: Primary spinal epidural extraosseous Ewing's sarcoma. Cancer **68:**648-654, 1991.

458 Kissane JM, Askin FB, Foulkes M, Stratton LB, Shirley SF: Ewing's sarcoma of bone. Clinicopathologic aspects of 303 cases from the Intergroup Ewing's Sarcoma Study. Hum Pathol **14:**773-779, 1983.

459 Kissane JM, Askin FB, Nesbit M, Vietti T, Burgert EO Jr, Cangir A, Gehan EA, Perez CA, Pritchard DJ, Tefft M: Sarcomas of bone in childhood. Pathologic aspects. In Glicksman A, Tefft M, eds: Bone and soft tissue sarcomas. J Natl Cancer Inst Monograph **56:**29-41, 1981.

460 Ladanyi M, Heinemann FS, Huvos AG, Rao PH, Chen QG, Jhanwar SC: Neural differentiation in small round cell tumors of bone and soft tissue with the translocation t(11;22)(q24;q12). An immunohistochemical study of 11 cases. Hum Pathol **21:**1245-1251, 1990.

461 Ladanyi M, Lewis R, Garin-Chesa P, Rettig WJ, Huvos AG, Healey JH, Jhanwar SC: EWS rearrangement in Ewing's sarcoma and peripheral neuroectodermal tumor. Molecular detection and correlation with cytogenetic analysis and MIC2 expression. Diagn Mol Pathol **2:**141-146, 1993.

462 Leong A S-Y, Milios J: Small round cell tumors in childhood. Immunohistochemical studies in rhabdomyosarcoma, neuroblastoma, Ewing's sarcoma, and lymphoblastic lymphoma. Surg Pathol **2:**5-18, 1989.

463 Llombart-Bosch A, Peydro-Olaya A: Scanning and transmission electron microscopy of Ewing's sarcoma of bone (typical and atypical variants). An analysis of nine cases. Virchows Arch [A] **398:**329-346, 1983.

464 Löning TH, Liebsch J, Delling G: Osteosarcomas and Ewing's sarcomas. Comparative immunocytochemical investigation of filamentous proteins and cell membrane determinants. Virchows Arch [A] **407:**323-336, 1985.

465 Mahoney JP, Alexander RW: Ewing's sarcoma. A light and electron microscopic study of 21 cases. Am J Surg Pathol **2:**283-298, 1978.

466 Mawad JK, Mackay B, Raymond AK, Ayala AG: Electron microscopy in the diagnosis of small round cell tumors of bone. Ultrastruct Pathol **18:**263-268, 1994.

467 Maygarden SJ, Askin FB, Siegal GP, Gilula LA, Schoppe J, Foulkes M, Kissane JM, Nesbit M: Ewing sarcoma of bone in infants and toddlers. A clinicopathologic report from the Intergroup Ewing's Study. Cancer **71:**2109-2118, 1993.

468 Mendenhall CM, Marcus RB Jr, Enneking WF, Springfield DS, Thar TL, Million RR: The prognostic significance of soft tissue extension in Ewing's sarcoma. Cancer **51:**913-917, 1983.

469 Miettinen M, Lehto V-P, Virtanen I: Histogenesis of Ewing's sarcoma. An evaluation of intermediate filaments and endothelial cell markers. Virchows Arch [Cell Pathol] **41:**277-284, 1982.

470 Moll R, Lee I, Gould VE, Berndt R, Roessner A, Franke WW: Immunocytochemical analysis of Ewing's tumors. Patterns of expression of intermediate filaments and desmosomal proteins indicate cell type heterogeneity and pluripotential differentiation. Am J Pathol **127:**288-304, 1987.

471 Nascimento AG, Unni KK, Pritchard DJ, Cooper KL, Dahlin DC: A clinicopathologic study of 20 cases of large-cell (atypical) Ewing's sarcoma of bone. Am J Surg Pathol **4:**29-36, 1980.

472 Navarro S, Cavazzana AO, Llombart-Bosch A, Triche TJ: Comparison of Ewing's sarcoma of bone and peripheral neuroepithelioma. An immunocytochemical and ultrastructural analysis of two primitive neuroectodermal neoplasms. Arch Pathol Lab Med **118:**608-615, 1994.

473 Navas-Palacios JJ, Aparicio-Duque R, Valdes MD: On the histogenesis of Ewing's sarcoma. An ultrastructural, immunohistochemical, and cytochemical study. Cancer **53:**1882-1901, 1984.

474 Neff JR: Nonmetastatic Ewing's sarcoma of bone. The role of surgical therapy. Clin Orthop **204:**111-118, 1980.

475 Noguera R, Triche TJ, Navarro S, Tsokos M, Llombart-Bosch A: Dynamic model of differentiation in Ewing's sarcoma cells. Comparative analysis of morphologic, immunocytochemical, and oncogene expression parameters. Lab Invest **66:**143-151, 1992.

476 Pagani A, Fischer-Colbrie R, Sanfilippo B, Winkler H, Cerrato M, Bussolati G: Secretogranin II expression in Ewing's sarcomas and primitive neuroectodermal tumors. Diagn Mol Pathol **1:**165-172, 1992.

477 Perez CA, Razek A, Tefft M, Nesbit M, Burgert EO, Kissane J, Vietti T, Gehan EA: Analysis of local tumor control in Ewing's sarcoma. Cancer **40:**2864-2873, 1977.

478 Perlman EJ, Dickman PS, Askin FB, Grier HE, Miser JS, Link MP: Ewing's sarcoma—routine diagnostic utilization of MIC2 analysis. A Pediatric Oncology Group/Children's Cancer Group Intergroup Study. Hum Pathol **25:**304-307, 1994.

479 Pinto A, Grant LH, Hayes FA, Schell MJ, Parham DM: Immunohistochemical expression of neuron-specific enolase and Leu 7 in Ewing's sarcoma of bone. Cancer **64:**1266-1273, 1989.

480 Ramani P, Rampling D, Link M: Immunocytochemical study of 12E7 in small round-cell tumours of childhood. An assessment of its sensitivity and specificity. Histopathology **23:**557-561, 1993.

481 Razek A, Perez CA, Tefft M, Nesbit M, Vietti T, Burgert EO Jr, Kissane J, Pritchard DJ, Gehan EA: Intergroup Ewing's sarcoma study. Local control related to radiation dose, volume, and site of primary lesion in Ewing's sarcoma. Cancer **46:**516-521, 1980.

482 Rettig WJ, Garin-Chesa P, Huvos AG: Ewing's sarcoma. New approaches to histogenesis and molecular plasticity. Lab Invest **66:**133-137, 1992.

483 Roessner A, Jurgens H: Round cell tumours of bone. Pathol Res Pract **189:**111-136, 1993.

484 Rosen G, Caparros B, Nirenberg A, Marcove RC, Huvos AG, Kosloff C, Lane J, Murphy ML: Ewing's sarcoma. Ten-year experience with adjuvant chemotherapy. Cancer **47:**2204-2213, 1981.

485 Scarpa S, Modesti A, Triche TJ: Extracellular matrix synthesis by undifferentiated childhood tumor cell lines. Am J Pathol **129:**74-85, 1987.

486 Schajowicz F: Ewing's sarcoma and reticulum-cell sarcoma of bone. With special reference to the histochemical demonstration of glycogen as an aid to differential diagnosis. J Bone Joint Surg (Am) **41:**349-356, 1959.

487 Schmidt D, Herrmann C, Jurgens H, Harms D: Malignant peripheral neuroectodermal tumor and its necessary distinction from Ewing's sarcoma. A report from the Kiel Pediatric Tumor Registry. Cancer **68:**2251-2259, 1991.

488 Schmidt D, Mackay B, Ayala AG: Ewing's sarcoma with neuroblastoma-like features. Ultrastruct Pathol **3:**143-151, 1982.

489 Selleri L, Hermanson GG, Eubanks JH, Lewis KA, Evans GA: Molecular localization of the t(11;22)(q24;q12) translocation of Ewing sarcoma by chromosomal in situ suppression hybridization. Proc Natl Acad Sci USA **88:**887-891, 1991.

490 Shishikura A, Ushigome S, Shimoda T: Primitive neuroectodermal tumors of bone and soft tissue. Histological subclassification and clinicopathologic correlations. Acta Pathol Jpn **43:**176-186, 1993.

491 Siegal GP, Oliver WR, Reinus WR, Gilula LA, Foulkes MA, Kissane JM, Askin FB: Primary Ewing's sarcoma involving the bones of the head and neck. Cancer **60:**2829-2840, 1987.

492 Sorensen P, Liu X, Delattre O, Rowland J, Biggs C, Thomas G, Triche T: Reverse transcriptase PCR amplification of EWS/FL-1 fusion transcripts as a diagnostic test for peripheral primitive neuroectodermal tumors of childhood. Diagn Mol Pathol **2:**147-157, 1993.

493 Spjut HJ, Ayala AG: Skeletal tumors in childhood and adolescence. In Finegold M, ed: Pathology of neoplasia in children and adolescents, vol 18, Major Series in Pathology. Philadelphia, 1986, WB Saunders Co.

494 Stephenson CF, Bridge JA, Sandberg AA: Cytogenetic and pathologic aspects of Ewing's sarcoma and neuroectodermal tumors. Hum Pathol **23:**1270-1277, 1992.

495 Stevenson AJ, Chatten J, Bertoni P, Miettinen M: CD99 (p30/32MIC) neuroectodermal/Ewing's sarcoma antigen as an immunohistochemical marker. Review of more than 600 tumors and the literature experience. Appl Immunohistochem **2:**231-240, 1994.

496 Telles NC, Rabson AS, Pomeroy TC: Ewing's sarcoma. An autopsy study. Cancer **41:**2321-2329, 1978.

497 Thomas PRM, Foulkes MA, Gilula LA, Burgert EO, Evans RG, Kissane J, Nesbit ME, Pritchard DJ, Tefft M, Vietti TJ: Primary Ewing's sarcoma of the ribs. A report from the Intergroup Ewing's Sarcoma Study. Cancer **51:**1021-1027, 1983.

498 Triche TJ, Ross WE: Glycogen-containing neuroblastoma with clinical and histopathologic features of Ewing's sarcoma. Cancer **41:**1425-1432, 1978.

499 Tsuneyoshi M, Yokoyama R, Hashimoto H, Enjoji M: Comparative study of neuroectodermal tumor and Ewing's sarcoma of the bone. Histopathologic, immunohistochemical and ultrastructural features. Acta Pathol Jpn **39:**573-581, 1989.

500 Ushigome S, Shimoda T, Takaki K, Nikaido T, Takakuwa T, Ishikawa E, Spjut HJ: Immunocytochemical and ultrastructural studies of the histogenesis of Ewing's sarcoma and putatively related tumors. Cancer **64:**52-62, 1989.

501 Weidner N, Tjoe J: Immunohistochemical profile of monoclonal antibody O13. Antibody that recognizes glycoprotein p30/32MIC2 and is useful in diagnosing Ewing's sarcoma and peripheral neuroepithelioma. Am J Surg Pathol **18:**486-494, 1994.

502 Wilkins RM, Pritchard DJ, Burgert EO Jr, Unni KK: Ewing's sarcoma of bone. Experience with 140 patients. Cancer **58:**2551-2555, 1986.

503 Yunis EJ, Agostini RM Jr, Walpusk JA, Hubbard JD: Glycogen in neuroblastomas. A light- and electron-microscopic study of 40 cases. Am J Surg Pathol **3:**313-323, 1979.

Malignant lymphoma and related lesions

504 Baar J, Burkes RL, Bell R, Blackstein ME, Fernandes B, Langer F: Primary non-Hodgkin's lymphoma of bone. A clinicopathologic study. Cancer **73:**1194-1199, 1994.

505 Bacci G, Jaffe N, Emiliani E, Van Horn J, Manfrini M, Picci P, Bertoni F, Gherlinzoni F, Campanacci M: Therapy for primary non-Hodgkin's lymphoma of bone and a comparison of results with Ewing's sarcoma. Ten years' experience at the Istituto Ortopedico Rizzoli. Cancer **57:**1468-1472, 1986.

506 Boston HC, Dahlin DC, Ivins JC, Cupps RE: Malignant lymphoma (so-called reticulum cell sarcoma) of bone. Cancer **34:**1131-1137, 1974.

507 Chabner BA, Haskell CM, Canellos GP: Destructive bone lesions in chronic granulocytic leukemia. Medicine (Baltimore) **48:**401-410, 1969.

508 Chan JK, Ng CS, Hui PK, Leung WT, Sin VC, Lam TK, Chick KW, Lam WY: Anaplastic large cell Ki-1 lymphoma of bone. Cancer **68:**2186-2191, 1991.

509 Chan K-W, Rosen G, Miller DR, Tan CTC: Hodgkin's disease in adolescents presenting as a primary bone lesion. A report of four cases and review of literature. Am J Pediatr Hematol Oncol **4:**11-17, 1982.

510 Clayton F, Butler JJ, Ayala AG, Ro JY, Zornoza J: Non-Hodgkin's lymphoma in bone. Pathologic and radiologic features with clinical correlates. Cancer **60:**2494-2501, 1987.

511 Dosoretz DE, Raymond AK, Murphy GF, Doppke KP, Schiller AL, Wang CC, Suit HD: Primary lymphoma of bone. The relationship of morphologic diversity to clinical behavior. Cancer **50:**1009-1014, 1982.

512 Falini B, Binazzi R, Pileri S, Mori A, Bertoni F, Canino S, Fagioli M, Minelli O, Ciani C, Pellicioli P: Large cell lymphoma of bone. A report of three cases of B-cell origin. Histopathology **12:**177-190, 1988.

513 Fowles JV, Olweny CLM, Katongole-Mbidde E, Lukanga-Ndawula A, Owor R: Burkitt's lymphoma in the appendicular skeleton. J Bone Joint Surg (Br) **65:**464-471, 1983.

514 Horan FT: Bone involvement in Hodgkin's disease. Br J Surg **56:**277-281, 1969.

515 Howat AJ, Thomas HUW, Waters KD, Campbell PE: Malignant lymphoma of bone in children. Cancer **59:**335-339, 1987.

516 Ivins JC: Reticulum-cell sarcoma of bone. J Bone Joint Surg (Am) **35:**835-842, 1953.

517 Llombart-Bosch A, Blache R, Peydro-Olaya A: Round-cell sarcomas of bone and their differential diagnosis (with particular emphasis on Ewing's sarcoma and reticulosarcoma). A study of 233 tumors with optical and electron microscopic techniques. Pathol Annu **17**(Pt 2):113-145, 1982.

518 Mahoney JP, Alexander RW: Primary histiocytic lymphoma of bone. A light and ultrastructural study of four cases. Am J Surg Pathol **4:**149-161, 1980.

519 Marsh WL Jr, Bylund DJ, Heath VC, Anderson MJ: Osteoarticular and pulmonary manifestations of acute leukemia. Case report and review of the literature. Cancer **57:**385-390, 1986.

520 Ostrowski ML, Unni KK, Banks PM, Shives TC, Evans RG, O'Connell MJ, Taylor WF: Malignant lymphoma of bone. Cancer **58:**2646-2655, 1986.

521 Pettit CK, Zukerberg LR, Gray MH, Ferry JA, Rosenberg AE, Harmon DC, Harris NL: Primary lymphoma of bone. A B-cell neoplasm with a high frequency of multilobated cells. Am J Surg Pathol **14:**329-334, 1990.

522 Radaszkiewicz T, Hansmann ML: Primary high-grade malignant lymphomas of bone. Virchows Arch [A] **413:**269-274, 1988.

523 Reimer RR, Chabner BA, Young RC, Reddick R, Johnson RE: Lymphoma presenting in bone. Results of histopathology, staging, and therapy. Ann Intern Med **87:**50-55, 1977.

524 Rossleigh MA, Smith J, Straus DJ, Engel IA: Osteonecrosis in patients with malignant lymphoma. A review of 31 cases. Cancer **58:**1112-1116, 1986.

525 Shoji H, Miller TR: Primary reticulum cell sarcoma of bone. Significance of clinical features upon the prognosis. Cancer **28:**1234-1244, 1971.

526 Simmons CR, Harle TS, Singleton EB: The osseous manifestations of leukemia in children. Radiol Clin North Am **6:**115-129, 1968.

527 Thomas LB, Forkner CE, Frei E, Besse BE, Stabenau JR: The skeletal lesions of acute leukemia. Cancer **14:**608-621, 1961.

528 Triche TJ, Askin FB, Kissane JM: Neuroblastoma, Ewing's sarcoma, and the differential diagnosis of small-, round-, blue-cell tumors. In Finegold M, ed: Pathology of neoplasia in children and adolescents, vol 18, Major Series in Pathology. Philadelphia, 1986, WB Saunders Co.

529 Vassallo J, Roessner A, Vollmer E, Grundmann E: Malignant lymphomas with primary bone manifestation. Pathol Res Pract **182:**381-389, 1987.

530 Wang CC, Fleischli DJ: Primary reticulum cell sarcoma of bone, with emphasis on radiation therapy. Cancer **22:**994-998, 1968.

Vascular tumors

531 Bollinger BK, Laskin WB, Knight CB: Epithelioid hemangioendothelioma with multiple site involvement. Literature review and observations. Cancer **73:**610-615, 1994.

532 Cai Q, Hodgson SF, Kao PC, Lennon VA, Klee GG, Zinsmiester AR, Kumar R: Brief report. Inhibition of renal phosphate transport by a tumor product in a patient with oncogenic osteomalacia. N Engl J Med **330:**1645-1649, 1994.

533 Campanacci M, Boriani S, Giunti A: Hemangioendothelioma of bone. A study of 29 cases. Cancer **46:**804-814, 1980.

534 Dorfman HD, Steiner GC, Jaffe HL: Vascular tumors of bone. Hum Pathol **2:**349-376, 1971.

535 Goldberg NS, Hebert AA, Esterly NB: Sacral hemangiomas and multiple congenital abnormalities. Arch Dermatol **122:**684-687, 1986.

536 Gorham LW, Stout AP: Massive osteolysis (acute spontaneous absorption of bone, phantom bone, disappearing bone). Its relation to hemangiomatosis. J Bone Joint Surg (Am) **37:**985-1004, 1955.

537 Halliday DR, Dahlin DC, Pugh DG, Young HH: Massive osteolysis and angiomatosis. Radiology **82:**627-644, 1964.

538 Jumbelic M, Feuerstein IM, Dorfman HD: Solitary intraosseous lymphangioma. A case report. J Bone Joint Surg (Am) **66:**1479-1480, 1984.

539 Larsson S-E, Lorentzon R, Boquist L: Malignant hemangioendothelioma of bone. J Bone Joint Surg (Am) **57:**84-89, 1975.

540 Mackenzie DH: Intraosseous glomus tumors. Report of two cases. J Bone Joint Surg (Br) **44:**648-651, 1962.

541 Mirra JM, Kameda N: Myxoid angioblastomatosis of bones. A case report of a rare, multifocal entity with light, ultramicroscopic, and immunopathologic correlation. Am J Surg Pathol **9:**450-458, 1985.

542 Nuovo MA, Dorfman HD, Sun CC, Chalew SA: Tumor-induced osteomalacia and rickets. Am J Surg Pathol **13:**588-599, 1989.

543 O'Connell JX, Kattapuram SV, Mankin HJ, Bhan AK, Rosenberg AE: Epithelioid hemangioma of bone. A tumor often mistaken for low-grade angiosarcoma or malignant hemangioendothelioma. Am J Surg Pathol **17:**610-617, 1993.

544 Ose D, Vollmer R, Shelburne J, McComb R, Harrelson J: Histiocytoid hemangioma of the skin and scapula. A case report with electron microscopy and immunohistochemistry. Cancer **51:**1656-1662, 1983.

545 Otis J, Hutter RVP, Foote FW Jr, Marcove RC, Stewart FW: Hemangioendothelioma of bone. Surg Gynecol Obstet **127:**295-305, 1968.

546 Rosai J, Gold J, Landy R: The histiocytoid hemangiomas. A unifying concept embracing several previously described entities of skin, soft tissue, large vessels, bone, and heart. Hum Pathol **10:**707-730, 1979.

547 Schajowicz F, Aiello CL, Francone MV, Giannini RE: Cystic angiomatosis (hamartomatous haemolymphangiomatosis) of bone. A clinicopathological study of three cases. J Bone Joint Surg (Br) **60:**100-106, 1978.

548 Sellke FW, Laszewski MJ, Robinson RA, Davis R, Rossi NP: Hemangiopericytoma of the sternum. Arch Pathol Lab Med **115:**242-244, 1991.

549 Spjut HJ, Lindbom A: Skeletal angiomatosis. Report of two cases. Acta Pathol Microbiol Scand **55:**49-58, 1962.

550 Steiner GC, Dorfman HD: Ultrastructure of hemangioendothelial sarcoma of bone. Cancer **29:**122-135, 1972.

551 Töpfer DI: Ueber ein infiltrierend wachsendes Hämangiom der Haut und multiple Kapillarektasien der Haut und innergen Organe. II. Zur Kenntnis der Wirbelangiome. Frankfurt Z Pathol **36:**337-345, 1928.

552 Tsuneyoshi M, Dorfman HD, Bauer TW: Epithelioid hemangioendothelioma of bone. A clinicopathologic, ultrastructural, and immunohistochemical study. Am J Surg Pathol **10:**754-764, 1986.

553 Unni KK, Ivins JC, Beabout JW, Dahlin DC: Hemangioma, hemangiopericytoma, and hemangioendothelioma (angiosarcoma) of bone. Cancer **27:**1403-1414, 1971.

554 van Haelst UJ, Pruszczynski M, ten Cate LN, Mravunac M: Ultrastructural and immunohistochemical study of epithelioid hemangioendothelioma of bone. Coexpression of epithelial and endothelial markers. Ultrastruct Pathol **14**:141-149, 1990.

555 Weidner N, Santa Cruz D: Phosphaturic mesenchymal tumors. A polymorphous group causing osteomalacia or rickets. Cancer **59**:1442-1454, 1987.

556 Wold LE, Swee RG, Sim FH: Vascular lesions of bone. Pathol Annu **20**(Pt 2):101-137, 1985.

557 Wold LE, Unni KK, Beabout JW, Ivins JC, Bruckman JE, Dahlin DC: Hemangioendothelial sarcoma of bone. Am J Surg Pathol **6**:59-70, 1982.

558 Wold LE, Unni KK, Cooper KL, Sim FH, Dahlin DC: Hemangiopericytoma of bone. Am J Surg Pathol **6**:53-58, 1982.

Other connective tissue tumors
Desmoplastic fibroma and related lesions

559 Bertoni F, Calderoni P, Bacchini P, Campanacci M: Desmoplastic fibroma of bone. A report of six cases. J Bone Joint Surg (Br) **66**:265-268, 1984.

560 Gebhardt MC, Campbell CJ, Schiller AL, Mankin HJ: Desmoplastic fibroma of bone. A report of eight cases and review of the literature. J Bone Joint Surg (Am) **67**:732-747, 1985.

561 Hasegawa T, Hirose T, Seki K, Hizawa K, Okada J, Nakanishi H: Solitary infantile myofibromatosis of bone. An immunohistochemical and ultrastructural study. Am J Surg Pathol **17**:308-313, 1993.

562 Inwards CY, Unni KK, Beabout JW, Shives TC: Solitary congenital fibromatosis (infantile myofibromatosis) of bone. Am J Surg Pathol **15**:935-941, 1991.

563 Inwards CY, Unni KK, Beabout JW, Sim FH: Desmoplastic fibroma of bone. Cancer **68**:1978-1983, 1991.

564 Lagacé R, Bouchard H-Ls, Delage C, Seemayer TA: Desmoplastic fibroma of bone. An ultrastructural study. Am J Surg Pathol **3**:423-430, 1979.

565 O'Connell JX, Logan PM, Beauchamp CP: Solitary fibrous tumor of the periosteum. Hum Pathol **26**:460-462, 1995.

566 Rabham WN, Rosai J: Desmoplastic fibroma. Report of ten cases and review of the literature. J Bone Joint Surg (Am) **50**:487-502, 1968.

567 Whitesides TE, Ackerman LV: Desmoplastic fibroma. A report of three cases. J Bone Joint Surg (Am) **42**:1143-1150, 1960.

Fibrosarcoma

568 Bertoni F, Capanna R, Calderoni P, Bacchini P, Campanacci M: Primary central (medullary) fibrosarcoma of bone. Semin Diagn Pathol **1**:185-198, 1984.

569 Cunningham MP, Arlen M: Medullary fibrosarcoma of bone. Cancer **21**:31-37, 1968.

570 Dahlin DC, Ivins JC: Fibrosarcoma of bone. A study of 114 cases. Cancer **23**:35-41, 1969.

571 Gilmer WS Jr, MacEwen GD: Central (medullary) fibrosarcoma of bone. J Bone Joint Surg (Am) **40**:121-141, 1958.

572 Hernandez FJ, Fernandez BB: Multiple diffuse fibrosarcoma of bone. Cancer **37**:939-945, 1976.

573 Huvos AG, Higinbotham NL: Primary fibrosarcoma of bone. A clinicopathologic study of 130 patients. Cancer **35**:837-847, 1975.

574 McLeod JJ, Dahlin DC, Ivins JC: Fibrosarcoma of bone. Am J Surg **94**:431-437, 1957.

575 Taconis WK, Van Rijssel ThG: Fibrosarcoma of long bones. A study of the significance of areas of malignant fibrous histiocytoma. J Bone Joint Surg (Br) **67**:111-116, 1985.

Malignant fibrous histiocytoma

576 Abdul-Karim FW, Ayala AG, Chawla SP, Jing B-S, Goepfert H: Malignant fibrous histiocytoma of jaws. A clinicopathologic study of 11 cases. Cancer **56**:1590-1596, 1985.

577 Bagó-Granell J, Aguirre-Canyadell M, Nardi J, Tallada N: Malignant fibrous histiocytoma of bone at the site of a total hip arthroplasty. A case report. J Bone Joint Surg (Br) **66**:38-40, 1984.

578 Belza MG, Urich H: Chordoma and malignant fibrous histiocytoma. Evidence for transformation. Cancer **58**:1082-1087, 1986.

579 Boland PJ, Huvos AG: Malignant fibrous histiocytoma of bone. Clin Orthop **204**:130-134, 1986.

580 Dahlin DC, Unni KK, Matsuno T: Malignant (fibrous) histiocytoma of bone—fact or fancy? Cancer **39**:1508-1516, 1977.

581 Frierson HF Jr, Fechner RE, Stallings RG, Wang G-J: Malignant fibrous histiocytoma in bone infarct. Association with sickle cell trait and alcohol abuse. Cancer **59**:496-500, 1987.

582 Heselson NG, Price SK, Mills EED, Conway SSM, Marks RK: Two malignant fibrous histiocytomas in bone infarcts (case report). J Bone Joint Surg (Am) **65**:1166-1171, 1983.

583 Huvos AG, Heilweil M, Bretsky SS: The pathology of malignant fibrous histiocytoma of bone. A study of 130 patients. Am J Surg Pathol **9**:853-871, 1985.

584 Huvos AG, Woodard HQ, Heilweil M: Postradiation malignant fibrous histiocytoma of bone. A clinicopathologic study of 20 patients. Am J Surg Pathol **10**:9-18, 1986.

585 Kahn LB, Webber B, Mills E, Antsey L, Heleson NG: Malignant fibrous histiocytoma (malignant fibrous xanthoma: xanthosarcoma) of bone. Cancer **42**:640-651, 1978.

586 Katenkamp D, Stiller D: Malignant fibrous histiocytoma of bone. Light microscopic and electron microscopic examination of four cases. Virchows Arch [A] **391**:323-335, 1981.

587 Kristensen IB, Jensen OM: Malignant fibrous histiocytoma of bone. A clinicopathologic study of 9 cases. Acta Pathol Microbiol Immunol Scand (A) **92**:205-210, 1984.

588 Lee Y-S, Pho RWH, Nather A: Malignant fibrous histiocytoma at site of metal implant. Cancer **54**:2286-2289, 1984.

589 Martorell M, Calabuig C, Peydro-Olaya A, Llombart-Bosch A, Terrier-Lacombe MJ, Contesso G: Fibroblast and myofibroblast participation in malignant fibrous histiocytoma (MFH) of bone. Ultrastructural study of eight cases with immunohistochemical support. Pathol Res Pract **184**:582-590, 1989.

590 McCarthy EF, Matsuno T, Dorfman HD: Malignant fibrous histiocytoma of bone. A study of 35 cases. Hum Pathol **10**:57-70, 1979.

591 Miettinen M, Lehto V-P, Virtanen I: Malignant fibrous histiocytoma within a recurrent chordoma. A light microscopic, electron microscopic, and immunohistochemical study. Am J Clin Pathol **82**:738-743, 1984.

592 Nakashima Y, Morishita S, Kotoura Y, Yamamuro T, Tamura K, Onomura T, Sudo Y, Awaya G, Hamashima Y: Malignant fibrous histiocytoma of bone. A review of 13 cases and an ultrastructural study. Cancer **55**:2804-2811, 1985.

593 Spanier SS, Enneking WF, Enriquez P: Primary malignant fibrous histiocytoma of bone. Cancer **36**:2084-2098, 1975.

594 Ushigome S, Shimoda T, Fukunaga M, Takakuwa T, Nakajima H: Immunohistochemical aspects of the differential diagnosis of osteosarcoma and malignant fibrous histiocytoma. Surg Pathol **1**:347-358, 1988.

595 Yokoyama R, Tsuneyoshi M, Enjoji M, Shinohara N, Masuda S: Prognostic factors of malignant fibrous histiocytoma of bone. A clinical and histopathologic analysis of 34 cases. Cancer **72**:1902-1908, 1993.

Muscle tumors

596 Angervall L, Berlin Ö, Kindblom L-G, Stener B: Primary leiomyosarcoma of bone. A study of five cases. Cancer **46**:1270-1279, 1980.

597 Jundt G, Moll C, Nidecker A, Schilt R, Remagen W: Primary leiomyosarcoma of bone. Report of eight cases. Hum Pathol **25**:1205-1212, 1994.

598 Kawai T, Suzuki M, Mukai M, Hiroshima K, Shinmei M: Primary leiomyosarcoma of bone. An immunohistochemical and ultrastructural study. Arch Pathol Lab Med **107**:433-437, 1983.

599 Lamovec J, Zidar A, Bracko M, Golouh R: Primary bone sarcoma with rhabdomyosarcomatous component. Pathol Res Pract **190**:51-60, 1994.

600 Myers JL, Arocho J, Bernreuter W, Dunham W, Mazur MT: Leiomyosarcoma of bone. A clinicopathologic, immunohistochemical, and ultrastructural study of five cases. Cancer **67**:1051-1056, 1991.

601 Oda Y, Tsuneyoshi M, Hashimoto H, Iwashita T, Ushijima M, Masuda S, Iwamoto Y, Sugioka Y: Primary rhabdomyosarcoma of the iliac bone in an adult. A case mimicking fibrosarcoma. Virchows Arch [A] **423**:65-69, 1993.

602 Rashid A, Dickersin GR, Rosenthal DI, Mankin H, Rosenberg AE: Rhabdomyosarcoma of the long bone in an adult. A case report and literature review. Int J Surg Pathol **1**:253-260, 1994.

603 Scheele PM Jr, Von Kuster LC, Krivchenia G: Primary malignant mesenchymoma of bone. Arch Pathol Lab Med **114**:614-617, 1990.

604 von Hochstetter AR, Eberle H, Rüttner JR: Primary leiomyosarcoma of extragnathic bones. Case report and review of literature. Cancer **53**:2194-2200, 1984.

605 Young MP, Freemont AJ: Primary leiomyosarcoma of bone. Histopathology **19**:257-262, 1991.

Adipose tissue tumors

606 Barcelo M, Pathria MN, Abdul-Karim FW: Intraosseous lipoma. A clinicopathologic study of four cases. Arch Pathol Lab Med **116**:947-950, 1992.

607 Chow LT, Lee KC: Intraosseous lipoma. A clinicopathologic study of nine cases. Am J Surg Pathol **16**:401-410, 1992.

608 Mandard JC, Mandard AM, Le Gal Y: Les liposarcomes primitifs de l'os. A propos de 5 cas revue de la littérature. Ann Anat Pathol (Paris) **18**:329-346, 1973.

609 Pardo-Mindan FJ, Ayala H, Joly M, Gimeno E, Vazquez JJ: Primary liposarcoma of bone. Light and electron microscopic study. Cancer **48**:274-280, 1981.

Other primary tumors
Chordoma

610 Abenoza P, Sibley RK: Chordoma. An immunohistologic study. Hum Pathol 17:744-747, 1986.

611 Ariel IM, Verdu C: Chordoma. An analysis of twenty cases treated over a twenty-year span. J Surg Oncol 7:27-44, 1975.

612 Bjornsson J, Wold LE, Ebersold MJ, Laws ER: Chordoma of the mobile spine. A clinicopathologic analysis of 40 patients. Cancer 71:735-740, 1993.

613 Bottles K, Beckstead JH: Enzyme histochemical characterization of chordomas. Am J Surg Pathol 8:443-447, 1984.

614 Campbell WM, McDonald TJ, Unni KK, Laws ER Jr: Nasal and paranasal presentations of chordomas. Laryngoscope 90:612-618, 1980.

615 Chambers PW, Schwinn CP: Chordoma. A clinicopathologic study of metastasis. Am J Clin Pathol 72:765-776, 1979.

616 Chu TA: Chondroid chordoma of the sacrococcygeal region. Arch Pathol Lab Med 111:861-864, 1987.

617 Coffin CM, Swanson PE, Wick MR, Dehner LP: An immunohistochemical comparison of chordoma with renal cell carcinoma, colorectal adenocarcinoma, and myxopapillary ependymoma: A potential diagnostic dilemma in the diminutive biopsy. Mod Pathol 6:531-538, 1993.

618 Coffin CM, Swanson PE, Wick MR, Dehner LP: Chordoma in childhood and adolescence. A clinicopathologic analysis of 12 cases. Arch Pathol Lab Med 117:927-933, 1993.

619 Crawford T: The staining reactions of chordoma. J Clin Pathol 11:110-113, 1958.

620 Erlandson RA, Tandler B, Lieberman PH, Higinbotham NL: Ultrastructure of human chordoma. Cancer Res 28:2115-2125, 1968.

621 Franquemont DW, Katsetos CD, Ross GW: Fatal acute pontocerebellar hemorrhage due to an unsuspected spheno-occipital chordoma. Arch Pathol Lab Med 113:1075-1078, 1989.

622 Gagne EJ, Su WP: Chordoma involving the skin. An immunohistochemical study of 11 cases. J Cutan Pathol 19:469-475, 1992.

623 Heaton JM, Turner DR: Reflections on notochordal differentiation arising from a study of chordomas. Histopathology 9:543-550, 1985.

624 Heffelfinger MJ, Dahlin DC, MacCarty CS, Beabout JW: Chordomas and cartilaginous tumors at the skull base. Cancer 32:410-420, 1973.

625 Higinbotham NL, Phillips RF, Farr HW, Hustu O: Chordoma. Thirty-five-year study at Memorial Hospital. Cancer 20:1841-1850, 1967.

626 Hruban RH, May M, Marcove RC, Huvos AG: Lumbo-sacral chordoma with high-grade malignant cartilaginous and spindle cell components. Am J Surg Pathol 14:384-389, 1990.

627 Jeffrey PB, Biava CG, Davis RL: Chondroid chordoma. A hyalinized chordoma without cartilaginous differentiation. Am J Clin Pathol 103:271-279, 1995.

628 Jeffrey PB, Davis RL, Biava C, Rosenblum M: Microtubule aggregates in a clival chordoma. Arch Pathol Lab Med 117:1055-1057, 1993.

629 Kaiser TE, Pritchard DJ, Unni KK: Clinicopathologic study of sacrococcygeal chordoma. Cancer 54:2574-2578, 1984.

630 Kaneko Y, Iwaki T, Fukui M: Lectin histochemistry of human fetal notochord, ecchordosis physaliphora, and chordomas. Arch Pathol Lab Med 116:60-64, 1992.

631 Lam R: The nature of cytoplasmic vacuoles in chordoma cells. A correlative enzyme and electron microscopic histochemical study. Pathol Res Pract 186:642-650, 1990.

632 Meis JM, Giraldo AA: Chordoma. An immunohistochemical study of 20 cases. Arch Pathol Lab Med 112:553-556, 1988.

633 Meis JM, Raymond AK, Evans HL, Charles RE, Giraldo AA: "Dedifferentiated" chordoma. A clinicopathologic and immunohistochemical study of three cases. Am J Surg Pathol 11:516-525, 1987.

634 Miettinen M: Chordoma. Antibodies to epithelial membrane antigen and carcinoembryonic antigen in differential diagnosis. Arch Pathol Lab Med 108:891-892, 1984.

635 Mindell ER: Current concepts review. Chordoma. J Bone Joint Surg (Am) 63:501-505, 1981.

636 Mitchell A, Scheithauer BW, Unni KK, Forsyth PJ, Wold LE, McGivney DJ: Chordoma and chondroid neoplasms of the spheno-occiput. An immunohistochemical study of 41 cases with prognostic and nosologic implications. Cancer 72:2943-2949, 1993.

637 Nakamura Y, Becker LE, Marks A: S 100 protein in human chordoma and human and rabbit notochord. Arch Pathol Lab Med 107:118-120, 1983.

638 O'Connell JX, Renard LG, Liebsch NJ, Efird JT, Munzrider JE, Rosenberg AE: Base of skull chordoma. A correlative study of histologic and clinical features of 62 cases. Cancer 74:2261-2267, 1994.

639 Pearlman AW, Friedman M: Radical radiation therapy of chordoma. Am J Roentgenol Radium Ther Nucl Med 108:333-341, 1970.

640 Persson S, Kindblom LG, Angervall L: Classical and chondroid chordoma. A light-microscopic, histochemical, ultrastructural and immunohistochemical analysis of the various cell types. Pathol Res Pract 187:828-838, 1991.

641 Rich TA, Schiller A, Suit HD, Mankin HJ: Clinical and pathologic review of 48 cases of chordoma. Cancer 56:182-187, 1985.

642 Richter HJ, Batsakis JG, Boles R: Chordomas. Nasopharyngeal presentation and atypical long survival. Ann Otol Rhinol Laryngol 84:327-332, 1975.

643 Rosenberg AE, Brown GA, Bhan AK, Lee JM: Chondroid chordoma—a variant of chordoma. A morphologic and immunohistochemical study. Am J Clin Pathol 101:36-41, 1994.

644 Rutherfoord GS, Davies AG: Chordomas—ultrastructure and immunohistochemistry. A report based on the examination of six cases. Histopathology 11:775-787, 1987.

645 Salisbury JR, Isaacson PG: Demonstration of cytokeratins and an epithelial membrane antigen in chordomas and human fetal notochord. Am J Surg Pathol 9:791-797, 1985.

646 Sarasa JL, Fortes J: Ecchordosis physaliphora. An immunohistochemical study of two cases. Histopathology 18:273-275, 1991.

647 Sundaresan N: Chordomas. Clin Orthop 204:135-142, 1986.

648 Ueda Y, Nakanishi I, Tsuchiya H, Tomita K: Microtubular aggregates in the rough endoplasmic reticulum of sacrococcygeal chordoma. Ultrastruct Pathol 15:77-82, 1991.

649 Ueda Y, Oda Y, Kawashima A, Tsuchiya H, Tomita K, Nakanishi I: Collagenous and basement membrane proteins of chordoma. Immunohistochemical analysis. Histopathology 21:345-352, 1992.

650 Valderrama E, Kahn LB, Lipper S, Marc J: Chondroid chordoma. Electron-microscopic study of two cases. Am J Surg Pathol 7:625-632, 1983.

651 Volpe R, Mazabraud A: A clinicopathologic review of 25 cases of chordoma (a pleomorphic and metastasizing neoplasm). Am J Surg Pathol 7:161-170, 1983.

652 Walaas L, Kindblom LG: Fine-needle aspiration biopsy in the preoperative diagnosis of chordoma. A study of 17 cases with application of electron microscopic, histochemical, and immunocytochemical examination. Hum Pathol 22:22-28, 1991.

653 Walker WP, Landas SK, Bromley CM, Sturm MT: Immunohistochemical distinction of classic and chondroid chordomas. Mod Pathol 4:661-666, 1991.

654 Wittchow R, Landas SK: Glial fibrillary acidic protein expression in pleomorphic adenoma, chordoma, and astrocytoma. A comparison of three antibodies. Arch Pathol Lab Med 115:1030-1033, 1991.

655 Wojno KJ, Hruban RH, Garin-Chesa P, Huvos AG: Chondroid chordomas and low-grade chondrosarcomas of the craniospinal axis. An immunohistochemical analysis of 17 cases. Am J Surg Pathol 16:1144-1152, 1992.

656 Wold LE, Laws ER Jr: Cranial chordomas in children and young adults. J Neurosurg 59:1043-1047, 1983.

657 Zukerberg LR, Young RH: Chordoma metastatic to the ovary. Arch Pathol Lab Med 114:208-210, 1990.

Adamantinoma of long bones

658 Baker PL, Dockerty MB, Coventry MB: Adamantinoma (so-called) of the long bones. J Bone Joint Surg (Am) 36:704-720, 1954.

659 Benassi MS, Campanacci L, Gamberi G, Ferrari C, Picci P, Sangiorgi L, Campanacci M: Cytokeratin expression and distribution in adamantinoma of the long bones and osteofibrous dysplasia of tibia and fibula. An immunohistochemical study correlated to histogenesis. Histopathology 25:71-76, 1994.

660 Campanacci M, Giunti A, Bertoni F, Laus M, Gitelis S: Adamantinoma of the long bones. The experience at the Istituto Ortopedico Rizzoli. Am J Surg Pathol 5:533-542, 1981.

661 Cohen DM, Dahlin DC, Pugh DG: Fibrous dysplasia associated with adamantinoma of the long bones. Cancer 15:515-521, 1961.

662 Czerniak B, Rojas-Corona RR, Dorfman HD: Morphologic diversity of long bone adamantinoma. The concept of differentiated (regressing) adamantinoma and its relationship to osteofibrous dysplasia. Cancer 64:2319-2334, 1989.

663 Eisenstein W, Pitcock JA: Adamantinoma of the tibia. An eccrine carcinoma. Arch Pathol Lab Med 108:246-250, 1984.

664 Hazelbag HM, Fleuren GJ, v.d.Broek LJ, Taminiau AH, Hogendoorn PC: Adamantinoma of the long bones. Keratin subclass immunoreactivity pattern with reference to its histogenesis. Am J Surg Pathol 17:1225-1233, 1993.

664a Jundt G, Remberger K, Roessner A, Schulz A, Bohndorf K: Adamantinoma of long bones. A histopathological and immunohistochemical study of 23 cases. Pathol Res Pract 191:112-120, 1995.

665 Keeney GL, Unni KK, Beabout JW, Pritchard DJ: Adamantinoma of long bones. A clinicopathologic study of 85 cases. Cancer 64:730-737, 1989.

666 Mills SE, Rosai J: Adamantinoma of the pretibial soft tissue. Clinicopathologic features, differential diagnosis, and possible relationship to intraosseous disease. J Clin Pathol 83:108-114, 1985.

667 Moon NF, Mori H: Adamantinoma of the appendicular skeleton—updated. Clin Orthop **204:**215-237, 1986.

668 Perez-Atayde AR, Kozakewich HPW, Vawter GF: Adamantinoma of the tibia. An ultrastructural and immunohistochemical study. Cancer **55:**1015-1023, 1985.

669 Rosai J: Adamantinoma of the tibia. Electron microscopic evidence of its epithelial origin. Am J Clin Pathol **51:**786-792, 1969.

670 Rosai J, Pinkus GS: Immunohistochemical demonstration of epithelial differentiation in adamantinoma of the tibia. Am J Surg Pathol **6:**427-434, 1982.

671 Schajowicz F, Gallardo H: Adamantinoma de tibia. Revisión bibliográfica y consideración de un nuevo caso. Rev Ortoped Traumatol Lat-Am **12:**105-118, 1967.

672 Ueda Y, Roessner A, Bosse A, Edel G, Bocker W, Wuisman P: Juvenile intracortical adamantinoma of the tibia with predominant osteofibrous dysplasia-like features. Pathol Res Pract **187:**1039-1034, 1991.

673 Unni KK, Dahlin DC, Beabout JW, Ivins JC: Adamantinomas of long bones. Cancer **34:**1796-1805, 1974.

674 Weiss SW, Dorfman HD: Adamantinoma of long bone. An analysis of nine new cases with emphasis on metastasizing lesions and fibrous dysplasia-like changes. Hum Pathol **8:**141-153, 1977.

675 Yoneyama T, Winter WG, Milsow L: Tibial adamantinoma. Its histogenesis from ultrastructural studies. Cancer **40:**1138-1142, 1977.

Peripheral nerve tumors

675a Bullock MJ, Bedard YC, Bell RS, Kandel R: Intraosseous malignant peripheral nerve sheath tumor. Report of a case and review of the literature. Arch Pathol Lab Med **119:**367-370, 1995.

676 De La Monte SM, Dorfman HD, Chandra R, Malawer M: Intraosseous schwannoma. Histologic features, ultrastructure, and review of the literature. Hum Pathol **15:**551-558, 1984.

677 Ducatman BS, Scheithauer BW, Dahlin DC: Malignant bone tumors associated with neurofibromatosis. Mayo Clin Proc **58:**578-582, 1983.

678 Fawcett KJ, Dahlin DC: Neurilemoma of bone. Am J Clin Pathol **47:**759-766, 1967.

679 Hunt JC, Pugh DG: Skeletal lesions in neurofibromatosis. Radiology **76:**1-19, 1961.

680 Myers JL, Bernreuter W, Dunham W: Melanotic schwannoma. Clinicopathologic, immunohistochemical, and ultrastructural features of a rare primary bone tumor. Am J Clin Pathol **93:**424-429, 1990.

681 Turk PS, Peters N, Libbey NP, Wanebo HJ: Diagnosis and management of giant intrasacral schwannoma. Cancer **70:**2650-2657, 1992.

682 Wirth WA, Bray CB: Intra-osseous neurilemoma. Case report and review of thirty-one cases from the literature. J Bone Joint Surg (Am) **59:**252-255, 1977.

Xanthoma

683 Bertoni F, Unni KK, McLeod RA, Sim FH: Xanthoma of bone. Am J Clin Pathol **90:**377-384, 1988.

Fibrocartilaginous mesenchymoma

684 Bulychova IV, Unni KK, Bertoni F, Beabout JW: Fibrocartilaginous mesenchymoma of bone. Am J Surg Pathol **17:**830-836, 1993.

Metastatic tumors

685 Berrettoni BA, Carter JR: Mechanisms of cancer metastasis to bone. J Bone Joint Surg (Am) **68:**308-312, 1986.

686 Caffey J, Andersen DH: Metastatic embryonal rhabdomyosarcoma in the growing skeleton. Clinical, radiographic, and microscopic features. Am J Dis Child **95:**581-600, 1958.

687 Charhon SA, Chapuy MC, Delvin EE, Valentin-Opran A, Edouard CM, Meunier PJ: Histomorphometric analysis of sclerotic bone metastases from prostatic carcinoma with special reference to osteomalacia. Cancer **51:**918-924, 1983.

688 Daroca PJ Jr, Reed RJ, Martin PC: Metastatic amelanotic melanoma simulating giant-cell tumor of bone. Hum Pathol **21:**978-980, 1990.

689 Gurney H, Larcos G, McKay M, Kefford R, Langlands A: Bone metastases in hypernephroma. Frequency of scapular involvement. Cancer **64:**1429-1431, 1989.

690 Healey JH, Turnbull ADM, Miedema B, Lane JM: Acrometastases. A study of twenty-nine patients with osseous involvement of the hands and feet. J Bone Joint Surg (Am) **68:**743-746, 1986.

691 Kahn LB, Wood FW, Ackerman LV: Fracture callus associated with benign and malignant bone lesions and mimicking osteosarcoma. Am J Clin Pathol **52:**14-24, 1969.

692 Morris DM, House HC: The significance of metastasis to the bones and soft tissues of the hand. J Surg Oncol **28:**146-150, 1985.

693 Norman A, Ulin R: A comparative study of periosteal new-bone response in metastatic bone tumors (solitary) and primary bone sarcomas. Radiology **92:**705-708, 1969.

694 Perez CA, Bradfield JS, Morgan HC: Management of pathologic fractures. Cancer **29:**1027-1037, 1972.

695 Quinn JM, Matsumura Y, Tarin D, McGee JO, Athanasou NA: Cellular and hormonal mechanisms associated with malignant bone resorption. Lab Invest **71:**465-471, 1994.

696 Simon MA, Bartucci EJ: The search for the primary tumor in patients with skeletal metastases of unknown origin. Cancer **58:**1088-1095, 1986.

697 Thomas BM: Three unusual carcinoid tumours, with particular reference to osteoblastic bone metastases. Clin Radiol **19:**221-225, 1968.

698 Troncoso A, Ro JY, Grignon DJ, Han WS, Wexler H, von Eschenbach A, Ayala AG: Renal cell carcinoma with acrometastasis. Report of two cases and review of the literature. Mod Pathol **4:**66-69, 1991.

699 Yamashita K, Ueda T, Komatsubara Y, Koyama H, Inaji H, Yonenobu K, Ono K: Breast cancer with bone-only metastases. Visceral metastases-free rate in relation to anatomic distribution of bone metastases. Cancer **68:**634-637, 1991.

TUMORLIKE LESIONS
Solitary bone cyst

699a Amling M, Werner M, Posl M, Maas R, Korn U, Delling G: Calcifying solitary bone cyst. Morphologic aspects and differential diagnosis of sclerotic bone tumours. Virchows Arch **426:**235-242, 1995.

700 Campanacci M, Capanna R, Picci P: Unicameral and aneurysmal bone cysts. Clin Orthop **204:**25-36, 1986.

701 Jaffe HL, Lichtenstein L: Solitary unicameral bone cyst. Arch Surg **44:**1004-1025, 1942.

702 Mirra JM, Bernard GW, Bullough PG, Johnston W, Mink G: Cementum-like bone production in solitary bone cysts (so-called "cementoma" of long bones). Report of three cases. Electron microscopic observations supporting a synovial origin to the simple bone cyst. Clin Orthop **135:**295-307, 1978.

703 Smith RW, Smith CF: Solitary unicameral bone cyst of the calcaneus. A review of twenty cases. J Bone Joint Surg (Am) **56:**49-56, 1974.

704 Stewart MJ, Hamel HA: Solitary bone cyst. South Med J **43:**926-936, 1950.

Aneurysmal bone cyst

705 Aho HJ, Aho AJ, Einola S: Aneurysmal bone cyst. A study of ultrastructure and malignant transformation. Virchows Arch [A] **395:**169-179, 1982.

706 Alles JU, Schulz A: Immunocytochemical markers (endothelial and histiocytic) and ultrastructure of primary aneurysmal bone cysts. Hum Pathol **17:**39-45, 1986.

707 Bertoni F, Bacchini P, Capanna R, Ruggieri P, Biagini R, Ferruzzi A, Bettelli G, Picci P, Campanacci M: Solid variant of aneurysmal bone cyst. Cancer **71:**729-734, 1993.

708 Buraczewski J, Dabska M: Pathogenesis of aneurysmal bone cyst. Relationship between the aneurysmal bone cyst and fibrous dysplasia of bone. Cancer **28:**597-604, 1971.

709 Capanna R, Albisinni U, Picci P, Calderoni P, Campanacci M, Springfield DS: Aneurysmal bone cyst of the spine. J Bone Joint Surg (Am) **67:**527-531, 1985.

710 Clough JR, Price CHG: Aneurysmal bone cyst. Pathogenesis and long term results of treatment. Clin Orthop **97:**52-63, 1973.

711 Dabezies EJ, D'Ambrosia RD, Chuinard RG, Ferguson AB: Aneurysmal bone cyst after fracture. A report of three cases. J Bone Joint Surg (Am) **64:**617-621, 1982.

712 Dabska M, Buraczewski J: Aneurysmal bone cyst. Pathology, clinical course and radiologic appearances. Cancer **23:**371-389, 1969.

713 D'Alonzo RT, Pitcock JA, Milford LW: Giant cell reaction of bone. Report of two cases. J Bone Joint Surg (Am) **54:**1267-1271, 1972.

714 Dehner LP, Risdall RJ, L'Heureux P: Giant cell-containing "fibrous" lesion of the sacrum. Am J Surg Pathol **2:**55-70, 1978.

715 Edling NPG: Is the aneurysmal bone cyst a true entity? Cancer **18:**1127-1130, 1965.

716 Koskinen EVS, Visuri TI, Holmström T, Roukkula MA: Aneurysmal bone cyst. Evaluation of resection and of curettage in 20 cases. Clin Orthop **118:**136-146, 1976.

717 Kyriakos M, Hardy D: Malignant transformation of aneurysmal bone cyst, with an analysis of the literature. Cancer **68:**1770-1780, 1991.

718 Levy WM, Miller AS, Bonakdarpour A, Aegerter E: Aneurysmal bone cyst secondary to other osseous lesions. Report of 57 cases. Am J Clin Pathol **63:**1-8, 1975.

719 Lichtenstein L: Aneurysmal bone cyst. Observations on fifty cases. J Bone Joint Surg (Am) **39:**873-882, 1957.

720 McCarthy EF, Dorfman HD: Vascular and cartilaginous hamartoma of the ribs in infancy with secondary aneurysmal bone cyst formation. Am J Surg Pathol **4:**247-253, 1980.

721 Oda Y, Tsuneyoshi M, Shinohara N: "Solid" variant of aneurysmal bone cyst (extragnathic giant cell reparative granuloma) in the axial skeleton and long bones. A study of its morphologic spectrum and distinction from allied giant cell lesions. Cancer **70:**2642-2649, 1992.

722 Panico L, Passeretti U, De Rosa N, D'Antonio A, De Rosa G: Giant cell reparative granuloma of the distal skeletal bones. A report of five cases with immunohistochemical findings. Virchows Arch **425:**315-320, 1994.

723 Petrik PK, Findlay JM, Sherlock RA: Aneurysmal cyst, bone type, primary in an artery. Am J Surg Pathol **17:**1062-1066, 1993.

724 Rodriguez-Peralto JL, Lopez-Barea F, Sanchez-Herrera S, Atienza M: Primary aneurysmal cyst of soft tissues (extraosseous aneurysmal cyst). Am J Surg Pathol **18:**632-636, 1994.

725 Ruiter DJ, van Rijssel ThG, van der Velde EA: Aneurysmal bone cysts. A clinicopathological study of 105 cases. Cancer **39:**2231-2239, 1977.

726 Sabanathan S, Chen K, Robertson CS, Salama FD: Aneurysmal bone cyst of the rib. Thorax **39:**125-130, 1984.

727 Sanerkin NG, Mott MG, Roylance J: An unusual intraosseous lesion with fibroblastic, osteoclastic, osteoblastic, aneurysmal and fibromyxoid elements. "Solid" variant of aneurysmal bone cyst. Cancer **51:**2278-2286, 1983.

728 Tillman BP, Dahlin DC, Lipscomb PR, Stewart JR: Aneurysmal bone cyst. An analysis of 95 cases. Mayo Clin Proc **43:**478-495, 1968.

729 Vergel De Dios AM, Bond JR, Shives TC, McLeod RA, Unni KK: Aneurysmal bone cyst. A clinicopathologic study of 238 cases. Cancer **69:**2921-2931, 1992.

730 Wold LE, Dobyns JH, Swee RG, Dahlin DC: Giant cell reaction (giant cell reparative granuloma) of the small bones of the hands and feet. Am J Surg Pathol **10:**491-496, 1986.

Ganglion cyst of bone

731 Bauer TW, Dorfman, HD: Intraosseous ganglion. A clinicopathologic study of 11 cases. Am J Surg Pathol **6:**207-213, 1982.

732 Schajowicz F, Sainz MC, Slullitel JA: Juxta-articular bone cysts (intra-osseous ganglia). J Bone Joint Surg (Br) **61:**107-116, 1979.

733 Sim FH, Dahlin DC: Ganglion cysts of bone. Mayo Clin Proc **46:**484-488, 1971.

Metaphyseal fibrous defect (nonossifying fibroma)

734 Arata MA, Peterson HA, Dahlin DC: Pathological fractures through non-ossifying fibromas. Review of the Mayo Clinic experience. J Bone Joint Surg (Am) **63:**980-988, 1981.

735 Clarke BE, Xipell JM, Thomas DP: Benign fibrous histiocytoma of bone. Am J Surg Pathol **9:**806-815, 1985.

736 Cunningham JB, Ackerman LV: Metaphyseal fibrous defects. J Bone Joint Surg (Am) **38:**797-808, 1956.

737 Hatcher CH: Pathogenesis of localized fibrous lesion in the metaphyses of long bones. Ann Surg **122:**1016-1030, 1945.

738 Jaffe HL, Lichtenstein L: Nonosteogenic fibroma of bone. Am J Pathol **18:**205-221, 1942.

Fibrous dysplasia and related lesions

739 Albright F, Butler AM, Hampton AO, Smith P: Syndrome characterized by osteitis fibrosa disseminata, areas of pigmentation and endocrine dysfunction with precocious puberty in females. N Engl J Med **216:**727-746, 1937.

739a Aoki T, Kouho H, Hisaoka M, Hashimoto H, Nakata H, Sakai A: Intramuscular myxoma with fibrous dysplasia. A report of two cases with a review of the literature. Pathol Int **45:**165-171, 1995.

740 Bridge JA, Dembinski A, De Boer J, Travis J, Neff JR: Clonal chromosomal abnormalities in osteofibrous dysplasia. Implications for histopathogenesis and its relationship with adamantinoma. Cancer **73:**1746-1752, 1994.

741 Campanacci M: Osteofibrous dysplasia of long bones. A new clinical entity. Ital J Orthopaed Traumatol **2:**221-237, 1976.

742 Campanacci M, Laus M: Osteofibrous dysplasia of the tibia and fibula. J Bone Joint Surg (Am) **63:**367-375, 1981.

743 Campbell CJ, Hawk T: A variant of fibrous dysplasia (osteofibrous dysplasia). J Bone Joint Surg (Am) **64:**231-236, 1982.

743a Candeliere GA, Glorieux FH, Prud'homme J, St-Arnaud R: Increased expression of the c-*fos* proto-oncogene in bone from patients with fibrous dysplasia. N Engl J Med **332:**1546-1551, 1995.

744 Dorfman HD, Ishida T, Tsuneyoshi M: Exophytic variant of fibrous dysplasia (fibrous dysplasia protuberans). Hum Pathol **25:**1234-1237, 1994.

745 Gouldesbrough DR: Symmetrical fibro-osseous dysplasia of rib—evidence for a traumatic aetiology. Histopathology **17:**267-270, 1990.

746 Greco MA, Steiner GC: Ultrastructure of fibrous dysplasia of bone. A study of its fibrous, osseous, and cartilaginous components. Ultrastruct Pathol **10:**55-66, 1986.

747 Harris WH, Dudley HR, Barry RJ: The natural history of fibrous dysplasia. J Bone Joint Surg (Am) **44:**207-233, 1962.

748 Huvos AG, Higinbotham NL, Miller TR: Bone sarcomas arising in fibrous dysplasia. J Bone Joint Surg (Am) **54:**1047-1056, 1972.

749 Ishida T, Machinami R, Kojima T, Kikuchi F: Malignant fibrous histiocytoma and osteosarcoma in association with fibrous dysplasia of bone. Report of three cases. Pathol Res Pract **188:**757-763, 1992.

750 Kandel RA, Pritzker KPH, Bedard YC: Symmetrical fibro-osseous dysplasia of rib—post-traumatic dysplasia? Histopathology **5:**651-658, 1981.

751 Kempson RL: Ossifying fibroma of the long bones. Arch Pathol **82:**218-233, 1966.

752 Lichtenstein L, Jaffe HL: Fibrous dysplasia of bone. Arch Pathol **33:**777-816, 1942.

753 Nakashima Y, Yamamuro T, Fujiwara Y, Kotoura Y, Mori E, Hamashima Y: Osteofibrous dysplasia (ossifying fibroma of long bones). A study of 12 cases. Cancer **52:**909-914, 1983.

754 Park YK, Unni KK, McLeod RA, Pritchard DJ: Osteofibrous dysplasia. Clinicopathologic study of 80 cases. Hum Pathol **24:**1339-1347, 1993.

755 Pelzmann KS, Nagel DZ, Salyer WR: Polyostotic fibrous dysplasia and fibrochondrodysplasia. Skeletal Radiol **5:**116-118, 1980.

756 Povysil C, Matejovsky Z: Fibro-osseous lesion with calcified spherules (cementifying fibromalike lesion) of the tibia. Ultrastruct Pathol **17:**25-34, 1993.

757 Ragsdale BD: Polymorphic fibro-osseous lesions of bone. An almost site-specific diagnostic problem of the proximal femur. Hum Pathol **24:**505-512, 1993.

758 Reed RJ: Fibrous dysplasia of bone. A review of 25 cases. Arch Pathol **75:**480-495, 1963.

759 Ruggieri P, Sim FH, Bond JR, Unni KK: Malignancies in fibrous dysplasia. Cancer **73:**1411-1424, 1994.

760 Schlumberger HG: Fibrous dysplasia of single bones (monostotic fibrous dysplasia). Milit Surg **99:**504-527, 1946.

761 Schwindinger WF, Francomano CA, Levine MA: Identification of a mutation in the gene encoding the alpha subunit of the stimulatory G protein of adenylyl cyclase in McCune-Albright syndrome. Proc Natl Acad Sci USA **89:**5152-5156, 1992.

762 Sissons HA, Steiner GC, Dorfman HD: Calcified spherules in fibro-osseous lesions of bone. Arch Pathol Lab Med **117:**284-290, 1993.

763 Sweet DE, Vinh TN, Devaney K: Cortical osteofibrous dysplasia of long bone and its relationship to adamantinoma. A clinicopathologic study of 30 cases. Am J Surg Pathol **16:**282-290, 1992.

763a Voytek TM, Ro JY, Edeiken J, Ayala AG: Fibrous dysplasia and cemento-ossifying fibroma. A histologic spectrum. Am J Surg Pathol **19:**775-781, 1995.

Myositis ossificans

765 Ackerman LV: Extraosseous localized nonneoplastic bone and cartilage formation (so-called myositis ossificans). J Bone Joint Surg (Am) **40:**279-298, 1958.

766 Dupree WB, Enzinger FM: Fibro-osseous pseudotumor of the digits. Cancer **58:**2103-2109, 1986.

767 Povýšil C, Matějovský Z: Ultrastructural evidence of myofibroblasts in pseudomalignant myositis ossificans. Virchows Arch [A] **381:**189-203, 1979.

768 Spjut HJ, Dorfman HD: Florid reactive periostitis of the tubular bones of the hands and feet. Am J Surg Pathol **5:**423-433, 1981.

769 Sumiyoshi K, Tsuneyoshi M, Enjoji M: Myositis ossificans. A clinicopathologic study of 21 cases. Acta Pathol Jpn **35:**1109-1122, 1985.

770 Yaghmai I: Myositis ossificans. Diagnostic value of arteriography. AJR **128:**811-816, 1977.

Langerhans' cell granulomatosis

771 Daneshbod K, Kissane JM: Histiocytosis. The prognosis of polyostotic eosinophilic granuloma. Am J Clin Pathol **65:**601-611, 1976.

772 Lieberman PH, Jones CR, Dargeon HWK, Begg CF: A reappraisal of eosinophilic granuloma of bone. Hand-Schüller-Christian syndrome and Letterer-Siwe syndrome. Medicine (Baltimore) **48:**375-400, 1969.

773 Makley JT, Carter JR: Eosinophilic granuloma of bone. Clin Orthop **204:**37-44, 1986.

774 McGavran MH, Spady HA: Eosinophilic granuloma of bone. A study of 28 cases. J Bone Joint Surg (Am) **42:**979-992, 1960.

775 Newton WA, Hamoudi AB: Histiocytosis. A histologic classification with clinical correlation. Perspect Pediatr Pathol **1:**251-283, 1973.

776 Nezelof C, Basset F, Rousseau MF: Histiocytosis X. Histogenetic arguments for a Langerhans cell origin. Biomed **18:**365-371, 1973.

777 Nezelof C, Frileux-Herbet F, Cronier-Sachot J: Disseminated histiocytosis X. Analysis of prognostic factors based on a retrospective study of 50 cases. Cancer **44**:1824-1838, 1979.

778 Walker PD, Rosai J, Dorfman RF: The osseous manifestations of sinus histiocytosis with massive lymphadenopathy. Am J Clin Pathol **75**:131-139, 1981

Joints and related structures
NORMAL ANATOMY

779 Stevens CR, Map PI, Revell PA: A monoclonal antibody (Mab 67) marks type B synoviocytes. Rheumatol Int **10**:103-106, 1990.

780 Wilkinson LS, Edwards JCW, Poston RN, Haskard DO: Expression of vascular cell adhesion molecule-1 in normal and inflamed synovium. Lab Invest **68**:82-88, 1993.

781 Wilkinson LS, Pitsillides AA, Worrall JG, Edwards JCW: Light microscopic characterization of the fibroblast-like synovial intimal cell (synoviocyte). Arthritis Rheum **35**:1179-1184, 1992.

NON-NEOPLASTIC DISEASES
Ganglia and cystic meniscus

781a Glasgow MM, Allen PW, Blakeway C: Arthroscopic treatment of cysts of the lateral meniscus. J Bone Joint Surg Br **75**:299-302, 1993.

782 Lichtenstein L: Tumors of synovial joints, bursae, and tendon sheaths. Cancer **8**:816-830, 1955.

783 McEvedy BV: Simple ganglia. Br J Surg **49**:585-594, 1962.

783a Romanini L, Calvisi V, Collodel M, Masciocchi C: Cystic degeneration of the lateral meniscus. Pathogenesis and diagnostic approach. Ital J Orthop Traumatol **14**:493-500, 1988.

784 Stack RE, Bianco AH Jr, MacCarthy CS: Compression of the common peroneal nerve by ganglion cyst. Report of nine cases. J Bone Joint Surg (Am) **47**:773-778, 1965.

Bursae and Baker's cyst

785 Pederson HE, Key JA: Pathology of calcareous tendinitis and subdeltoid bursitis. Arch Surg **62**:50-63, 1951.

786 Wagner T, Abgarowicz T: Microscopic appearance of Baker's cyst in cases of rheumatoid arthritis. Rheumatologia **8**:21-26, 1970.

Carpal tunnel syndrome

787 Bastian FO: Amyloidosis and the carpal tunnel syndrome. Am J Clin Pathol **61**:711-717, 1974.

788 Entin MA: Carpal tunnel syndrome and its variants. Surg Clin North Am **48**:1097-1112, 1968.

789 Phalen GS: The carpal-tunnel syndrome. Seventeen years' experience in diagnosis and treatment of six hundred and fifty-four hands. J Bone Joint Surg (Am) **48**:211-228, 1966.

790 Spinner RJ, Bachman JW, Amadio PC: The many faces of carpal tunnel syndrome. Mayo Clin Proc **64**:829-836, 1989.

ARTHRITIS
Synovial biopsy

791 Goldenberg DL, Cohen AS: Synovial membrane histopathology in the differential diagnosis of rheumatoid arthritis, gout, pseudogout, systemic lupus erythematosus, infectious arthritis and degenerative joint disease. Medicine **57**:239-252, 1978.

792 Polley HF, Bickel WH: Experiences with an instrument for punch biopsy of synovial membrane. Mayo Clin Proc **26**:273-281, 1951.

793 Revell PA: The synovial biopsy. In Anthony PP, MacSween RNM, eds: Recent advances in histopathology, vol 13. Edinburgh, 1987, Churchill-Livingstone.

794 Rodnan GP, Yunis EJ, Totten RS: Experience with punch biopsy of synovium in the study of joint disease. Ann Intern Med **53**:319-331, 1960.

795 Schumacher HR, Kulka JP: Needle biopsy of the synovial membrane. Experience with the Parker-Pearson technic. N Engl J Med **286**:416-419, 1972.

796 Schwartz S, Cooper N: Synovial membrane punch biopsy. Arch Intern Med **108**:400-406, 1961.

797 Soren A: Histodiagnosis and clinical correlation of rheumatoid and other synovitis. Philadelphia, 1978, JP Lippincott Co.

798 Zevely HA, French AJ, Mikkelsen WM, Duff IF: Synovial specimens obtained by knee joint punch biopsy. Histologic study in joint diseases. Am J Med **20**:510-519, 1956.

Degenerative joint disease (osteoarthritis)

798a Aigner T, Dietz U, Stöss H, Von der Mark K: Differential expression of collagen types I, II, III, and X in human osteophytes. Lab Invest **73**:236-243, 1995.

799 Bauer W, Bennett GA: Experimental and pathological studies in the degenerative type of arthritis. J Bone Joint Surg **18**:1-18, 1936.

800 Bennett GA, Waine H, Bauer W: Changes in the knee joint at various ages. New York, 1942, Commonwealth Fund.

801 Collins DH: The pathology of articular and spinal diseases. London, 1949, Edward Arnold & Co.

802 Collins DH: Recent advances in the pathology of chronic arthritis and rheumatic disorders. Postgrad Med J **31**:602-608, 1955.

802a Di Francesco L, Sokoloff L: Lipochondral degeneration of capsular tissue in osteoarthritic hips. Am J Surg Pathol **19**:278-283, 1995.

803 Haliburton RA, Sullivan CR: The patella in degenerative joint disease. A clinicopathologic study. Arch Surg **77**:677-683, 1958.

804 Hamerman D: The biology of osteoarthritis. N Engl J Med **320**:1322-1330, 1989.

805 Harrison MHM, Schajowicz F, Tureta J: Osteoarthritis of the hip. A study of the nature and evolution of the disease. J Bone Joint Surg (Br) **35**:598-626, 1953.

806 Hirsch C, Schajowicz F, Galante J: Structural changes in the cervical spine. A study on autopsy specimens in different age groups. Acta Orthop Scand (Suppl) **109**:7-77, 1967.

807 Horwitz T: Bone and cartilage debris in the synovial membrane. Its significance in the early diagnosis of neuro-arthropathy. J Bone Joint Surg (Am) **30**:579-588, 1948.

808 Jayson MI, Rubenstein D, Dixon AS: Intra-articular pressure and rheumatoid geodes (bone 'cysts'). Ann Rheum Dis **29**:496-502, 1970.

809 Mankin HJ: The reaction of articular cartilage to injury and osteoarthritis. N Engl J Med **291**:1285-1292, 1335-1340, 1974.

810 Matthews BF: Composition of articular cartilage in osteoarthritis. Changes in collagen/chondroitinsulphate ratio. Br Med J **2**:660-661, 1953.

811 Norman A, Robbins H, Milgram JE: The acute neuropathic arthropathy. A rapid, severely disorganizing form of arthritis. Radiology **90**:1159-1164, 1968.

812 Outerbridge RE: The etiology of chrondromalacia patellae. J Bone Joint Surg (Br) **43**:752-757, 1961.

813 Rabinowicz T, Jacqueline F: Pathology of the capsular and synovial hip nerves in chronic hip diseases. Pathol Res Pract **186**:283-292, 1990.

814 Rhaney K, Lamb DW: The cysts of osteoarthritis of the hip. A radiological and pathological study. J Bone Joint Surg (Br) **37**:663-675, 1955.

814a Sadouk M, Pelletier J-P, Tardif G, Klansa D, Cloutier J-M, Martel-Pelletier J: Human synovial fibroblasts coexpress IL-1 receptor Type I and Type II mRNA. The increased level of the IL-1 receptor in osteoarthritic cells is related to an increased level of the Type I receptor. Lab Invest **74**:347-355, 1995.

815 Silverberg M, Frank EL, Jarrett SR, Silberberg R: Aging and osteoarthritis of the human sternoclavicular joint. Am J Pathol **35**:851-865, 1959.

816 Sokoloff L: Pathology and pathogenesis of osteoarthritis. In McCarty DJ, ed: Arthritis and applied conditions, ed 9. Philadelphia, 1979, Lea & Febiger, pp 1135-1153.

Rheumatoid arthritis

817 Beatty EC Jr: Rheumatic-like nodules occurring in nonrheumatic children. Arch Pathol **68**:154-159, 1959.

818 Bennett GA, Zeller JW, Bauer W: Subcutaneous nodules of rheumatoid arthritis and rheumatic fever. Arch Pathol **30**:70-89, 1940.

819 Berardinelli JL, Hyman CJ, Campbell EE, Fireman P: Presence of rheumatoid factor in ten children with isolated rheumatoid-like nodules. J Pediatr **81**:751-757, 1972.

820 Bevans M, Nadell J, Dmartius F, Ragan C: The systemic lesions of malignant arthritis. Am J Med **16**:197-211, 1954.

821 Bhan AK, Roy S: Synovial giant cells in rheumatoid arthritis and other joint diseases. Ann Rheum Dis **30**:294-298, 1971.

822 Cooper NS: Pathology of rheumatoid arthritis. Med Clin North Am **52**:607-621, 1968.

823 Dixon AStJ, Grant C: Acute synovial rupture in rheumatoid arthritis. Clinical and experimental observations. Lancet **1**:742-745, 1964.

824 Grimley PM, Sokoloff L: Synovial giant cells in rheumatoid arthritis. Am J Pathol **49**:931-954, 1966.

825 Hahn BH, Yardley JH, Stevens MB: "Rheumatoid" nodules in systemic lupus erythematosus. Ann Intern Med **72**:49-58, 1970.

826 Harris ED Jr: Rheumatoid arthritis. Pathophysiology and implications for therapy. N Engl J Med **322**:1277-1289, 1990.

827 Hart FD: Rheumatoid arthritis. Extra-articular manifestations. Br Med J **3**:131-136, 1969.

828 Hart FD: Rheumatoid arthritis. Extra-articular manifestations. Part II. Br Med J **2**:747-752, 1970.

829 Horwitz T: Bone and cartilage debris in the synovial membrane. Its significance in the early diagnosis of neuro-arthropathy. J Bone Joint Surg (Am) **30**:579-588, 1948.

830 Imai Y, Sato T, Yamakawa M, Kasajima T, Suda A, Watanabe Y: A morphological and immunohistochemical study of lymphoid germinal centers in synovial and lymph node tissues from rheumatoid arthritis patients with special reference to complement components and their receptors. Acta Pathol Jpn **39**:127-134, 1989.

831 Jayson MI, Dixon AS, Kates A, Pinder I, Coomes EN: Popliteal and calf cysts in rheumatoid arthritis. Treatment by anterior synovectomy. Ann Rheum Dis **31**:9-15, 1972.

831a Qu Z, Huang X-N, Ahmadi P, Andresevic J, Planck SR, Hart CE, Rosenbaum JT: Expression of basic fibroblast growth factor in synovial tissue from patients with rheumatoid arthritis and degenerative joint disease. Lab Invest **73**:339-346, 1995.

832 Luck JV: Bone and joint diseases. Springfield, Ill, 1950, Charles C Thomas, Publisher.

833 Mitchell N, Shepard N: The ultrastructure of articular cartilage in rheumatoid arthritis. A preliminary report. J Bone Joint Surg (Am) **52**:1405-1423, 1970.

834 Mongan ES, Cass RM, Jacox RF, Vaughan JH: A study of the relation of seronegative and seropositive rheumatoid arthritis to each other and to necrotizing vasculitis. Am J Med **47**:23-25, 1969.

835 Muirden KD: Giant cells, cartilage and bone fragments within rheumatoid synovial membrane. Clinicopathological correlations. Aust Ann Med **2**:105-110, 1970.

836 Palmer DG: Synovial cysts in rheumatoid disease. Ann Intern Med **70**:61-68, 1969.

837 Roberts WC, Kehol JA, Carpenter DF, Golden A: Cardiac valvular lesions in rheumatoid arthritis. Arch Intern Med **122**:141-146, 1968.

838 Schmid FR, Cooper NS, Ziff M, McEwen C: Arteritis in rheumatoid arthritis. Am J Med **30**:56-83, 1961.

839 Sokoloff L: Biopsy in rheumatic diseases. Med Clin North Am **45**:1171-1180, 1961.

840 Sokoloff L: Pathology of rheumatoid arthritis and allied disorders. In McCarty DJ, ed: Arthritis and applied conditions, ed 9. Philadelphia, 1979, Lea & Febiger, pp 429-447.

841 Sokoloff L, Wilens SL, Bunim JJ: Arthritis of striated muscle in rheumatoid arthritis. Am J Pathol **27**:157-173, 1951.

842 Taylor RT, Huskisson EC, Whitehouse GH, Hart FD: Spontaneous fractures of pelvis in rheumatoid arthritis. Br Med J **4**:663-664, 1971.

843 Weissmann G: Lysosomal mechanisms of tissue injury in arthritis. N Engl J Med **286**:141-146, 1972.

844 Winchester R: The molecular basis of susceptibility to rheumatoid arthritis. Adv Immunol **56**:389-466, 1994.

845 Ziegler B, Gay RE, Huang GQ, Fassbender HG, Gay S: Immunohistochemical localization of HTLV-I p19- and p24-related antigens in synovial joints of patients with rheumatoid arthritis. Am J Pathol **135**:1-5, 1989.

845a Zvaifer NJ: Rheumatoid arthritis. The multiple pathways to chronic synovitis (editorial). Lab Invest **73**:307-310, 1995.

Infectious arthritis

846 Johnston YE, Duray PH, Steere AC, Kashgarian M, Buza J, Malawista SE, Askenase PW: Lyme arthritis. Spirochetes found in synovial microangiopathic lesions. Am J Pathol **118**:26-34, 1985.

847 Meyerhoff J: Lyme disease. Am J Med **75**:663-670, 1983.

848 Steere AC: Lyme disease. N Engl J Med **321**:586-596, 1989.

Gout

849 Chaplin AJ: Calcium pyrophosphate. Histological characterization of crystals in pseudogout. Arch Pathol Lab Med **100**:12-15, 1976.

850 deGalantha E: Technic for preservation and microscopic demonstration of nodules in gout. Am J Clin Pathol **5**:165-166, 1935.

850a Ishida T, Dorfman HD, Bullough PG: Tophaceous pseudogout (tumoral calcium pyrophosphate dihydrate crystal deposition disease). Hum Pathol **26**:587-593, 1995.

851 Lichtenstein L, Scott HW, Levin MH: Pathologic changes in gout—survey of eleven necropsied cases. Am J Pathol **32**:871-895, 1956.

852 Moskowitz RW, Katz D: Chondrocalcinosis and chondrocalsynovitis (pseudo-gout syndrome). Analysis of 24 cases. Am J Med **43**:322-334, 1967.

Intervertebral disk prolapse

853 Weidner N, Rice DT: Intervertebral disk material. Criteria for determining probable prolapse. Hum Pathol **19**:406-410, 1988.

Other articular and periarticular diseases

854 Athanasou NA, Sallie B: Localized deposition of amyloid in articular cartilage. Histopathology **20**:41-46, 1992.

855 Cary NRB: Clinicopathological importance of deposits of amyloid in the femoral head. J Clin Pathol **38**:868-872, 1985.

856 Glldenberg DL, Cohen AS: Synovial membrane histopathology in the differential diagnosis of rheumatoid arthritis, gout, pseudogout, systemic lupus erythematosus, infectious arthritis and degenerative joint disease. Medicine (Baltimore) **57**:239-252, 1978.

857 Kyle RA, Eilers SG, Linscheid RL, Gaffey TA: Amyloid localized to tenosynovium at carpal tunnel release. Natural history of 124 cases. Am J Clin Pathol **91**:393-397, 1989.

858 Kyle RA, Gertz MA, Linke RP: Amyloid localized to tenosynovium at carpal tunnel release. Immunohistochemical identification of amyloid type. Am J Clin Pathol **97**:250-253, 1992.

859 Ladefoged C, Merrild U, Jorgensen B: Amyloid deposits in surgically removed articular and periarticular tissue. Histopathology **15**:289-296, 1989.

860 Mihara S, Kawai S, Gondo T, Ishihara T: Intervertebral disc amyloidosis. Histochemical, immunohistochemical and ultrastructural observations. Histopathology **25**:415-420, 1994.

861 Rodnan GP, Medsger TA: The rheumatic manifestations of progressive systemic sclerosis (scleroderma). Clin Orthop **57**:81-93, 1968.

TUMORS AND TUMORLIKE CONDITIONS
Fibrous histiocytoma of tendon sheath (nodular tenosynovitis)

862 Alguacil-Garcia A, Unni KK, Goellner JR: Giant cell tumor of tendon sheath and pigmented villonodular synovitis. An ultrastructural study. Am J Clin Pathol **69**:6-17, 1978.

863 Chung EB, Enzinger FM: Fibroma of tendon sheath. Cancer **44**:1945-1954, 1979.

864 Jaffe HL, Lichtenstein L, Sutro CJ: Pigmented villonodular synovitis, bursitis, and tenosynovitis. Arch Pathol **31**:731-765, 1941.

864a Maluf HM, DeYoung BR, Swanson PE, Wick MR: Fibroma and giant cell tumor of tendon sheath. A comparative histological and immunohistological study. Mod Pathol **8**:155-159, 1995.

864b O'Connell JX, Fanburg JC, Rosenberg AE: Giant cell tumor of tendon sheath and pigmented villonodular synovitis. Immunophenotype suggests a synovial cell origin. Hum Pathol **26**:771-775, 1995.

864c Tashiro H, Iwasaki H, Kikuchi M, Ogata K Okazaki M: Giant cell tumors of tendon sheath. A single and multiple immunostaining analysis. Pathol Int **45**:147-155, 1995.

865 Ushijima M, Hashimoto H, Tsuneyoshi M, Enjoji M, Miyamoto Y, Okue A: Malignant giant cell tumor of tendon sheath. Report of a case. Acta Pathol Jpn **35**:699-709, 1985.

866 Wright CJE: Benign cell synovioma. An investigation of 85 cases. Br J Surg **38**:257-271, 1951.

Pigmented villonodular synovitis and bursitis

867 Atmore WG, Dahlin DC, Ghormley RK: Pigmented villonodular synovitis. A clinical and pathologic study. Minn Med **39**:196-202, 1956.

868 Byers PD, Cotton RE, Deacon OW, Lowy M, Newman PH, Sissons HA, Thomson AD: The diagnosis and treatment of pigmented villonodular synovitis. J Bone Joint Surg (Br) **50**:290-305, 1968.

869 Darling JM, Glimcher LH, Shortkroff S, Albano B, Gravallese EM: Expression of metalloproteinases in pigmented villonodular synovitis. Hum Pathol **25**:825-830, 1994.

870 Greenfield MM, Wallace KM: Pigmented villonodular synovitis. Radiology **54**:350-356, 1950.

871 Myers BW, Masi AT: Pigmented villonodular synovitis and tenosynovitis. A clinical epidemiologic study of 166 cases and literature review. Medicine **59**:223-238, 1980.

872 Nilsonne U, Moberger G: Pigmented villonodular synovitis of joints. Histological and clinical problems in diagnosis. Acta Orthop Scand **40**:448-460, 1969.

873 Rao AS, Vigorita VJ: Pigmented villonodular synovitis (giant-cell tumor of the tendon sheath and synovial membrane). A review of eighty-one cases. J Bone Joint Surg (Am) **66**:76-94, 1984.

874 Ray RA, Morton CC, Lipinski KK, Corson JM, Fletcher JA: Cytogenetic evidence of clonality in a case of pigmented villonodular synovitis. Cancer **67**:121-125, 1991.

875 Scott FM: Bone lesions in pigmented villonodular synovitis. J Bone Joint Surg (Br) **50**:306-311, 1968.

876 Ushijima M, Hashimoto H, Tsuneyoshi M, Enjoji M: Pigmented villonodular synovitis. A clinicopathologic study of 52 cases. Acta Pathol Jpn **36:**317-326, 1986.

Synovial osteochondromatosis and chondrosarcoma

877 Baunsgaard P, Nielsen BB: Primary synovial chondrometaplasia. Histologic variations in the structure of metaplastic nodules. Acta Pathol Microbiol Immunol Scand (A) **92:**455-460, 1984.

878 Bertoni F, Unni KK, Beabout JW, Sim FH: Chondrosarcomas of the synovium. Cancer **67:**155-162, 1991.

879 Goldman RL, Lichtenstein L: Synovial chondrosarcoma. Cancer **12:**1233-1240, 1964.

880 King JW, Spjut HJ, Fechner RE, Vanderpool DW: Synovial chondrosarcoma of the knee joint. J Bone Joint Surg (Am) **49:**1389-1396, 1967.

881 Milgram JW: Synovial osteochondromatosis. A histopathological study of thirty cases. J Bone Joint Surg (Am) **59:**792-801, 1977.

882 Murphy FP, Dahlin DC, Sullivan CR: Articular synovial chondromatosis. J Bone Joint Surg (Am) **44:**77-86, 1962.

882a Sviland L, Malcolm AJ: Synovial chondromatosis presenting as painless soft tissue mass. A report of 19 cases. Histopathology **27:**275-279, 1995.

883 Villacin AB, Brigham LN, Bullough PG: Primary and secondary synovial chondrometaplasia. Histopathologic and clinicoradiologic differences. Hum Pathol **10:**439-451, 1979.

Other tumors

884 Devaney K, Vinh TN, Sweet DE: Synovial hemangioma. A report of 20 cases with differential diagnostic considerations. Hum Pathol **24:**737-745, 1993.

885 Ladefoged C, Jensen NK: Synovial haemangiopericytoma of the knee joint. Histopathology **15:**635-637, 1989.

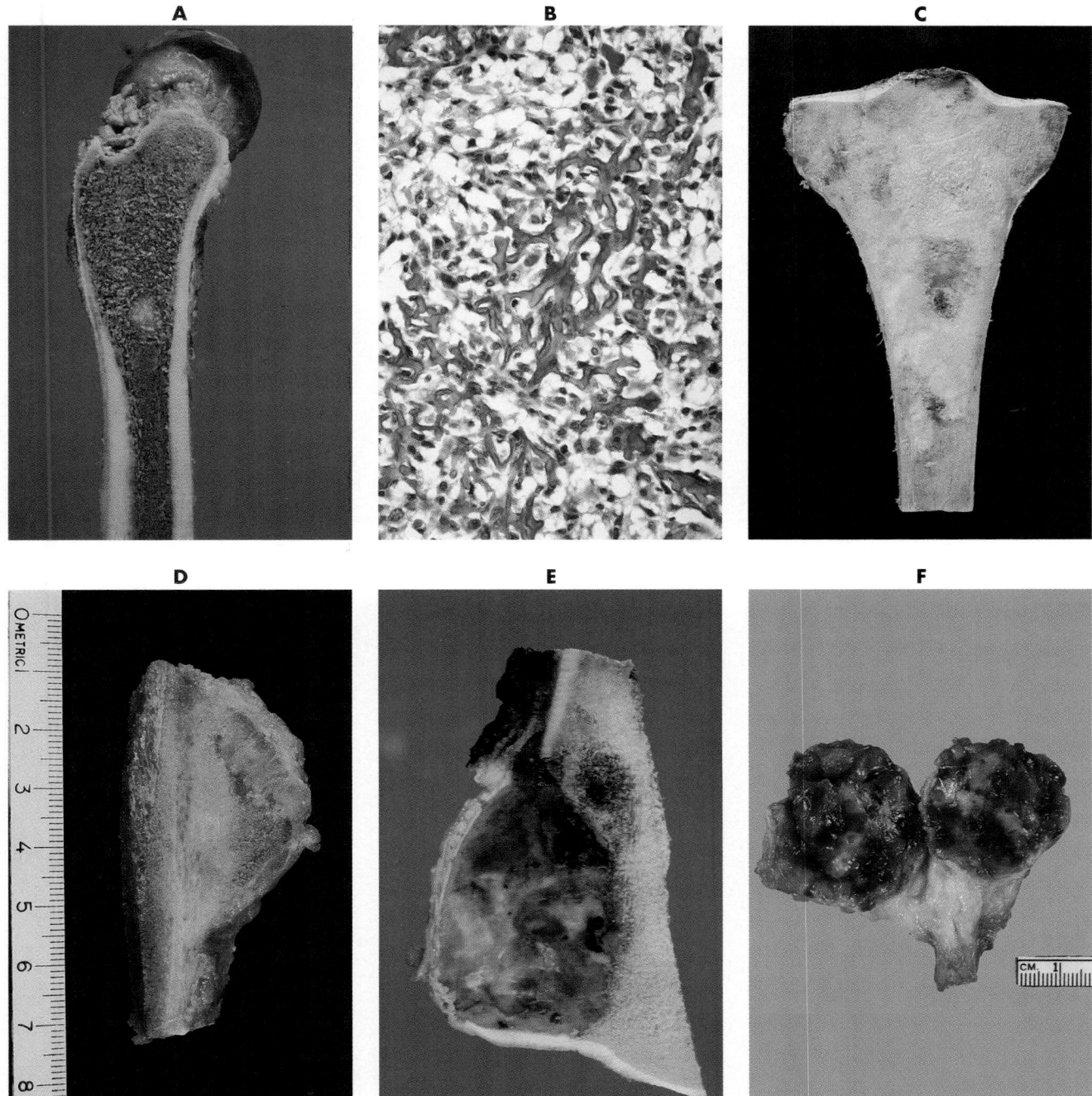

Plate XVII A, So-called skip metastasis located in the upper half of the femur. The primary tumor was located in the lower metaphysis of the same bone. **B,** Microscopic appearance of osteosarcoma showing characteristic basophilic thin trabeculae of neoplastic bone with an appearance that is reminiscent of fungal hyphae. **C,** Gross appearance of intraosseous well-differentiated osteosarcoma of tibia. **D,** Gross appearance of juxtacortical chondroma. The tumor produces a semispherical expansion of the involved bone. **E,** Gross appearance of giant cell tumor of lower end of the femur. Lesion is characteristically peripheral, expansile, well-circumscribed, and hemorrhagic. **F,** Gross appearance of giant cell tumor of ulna. Note well-circumscribed character, expansile quality, and brownish-red discoloration. (**C** courtesy Dr. Juan José Segura, San José, Costa Rica.)

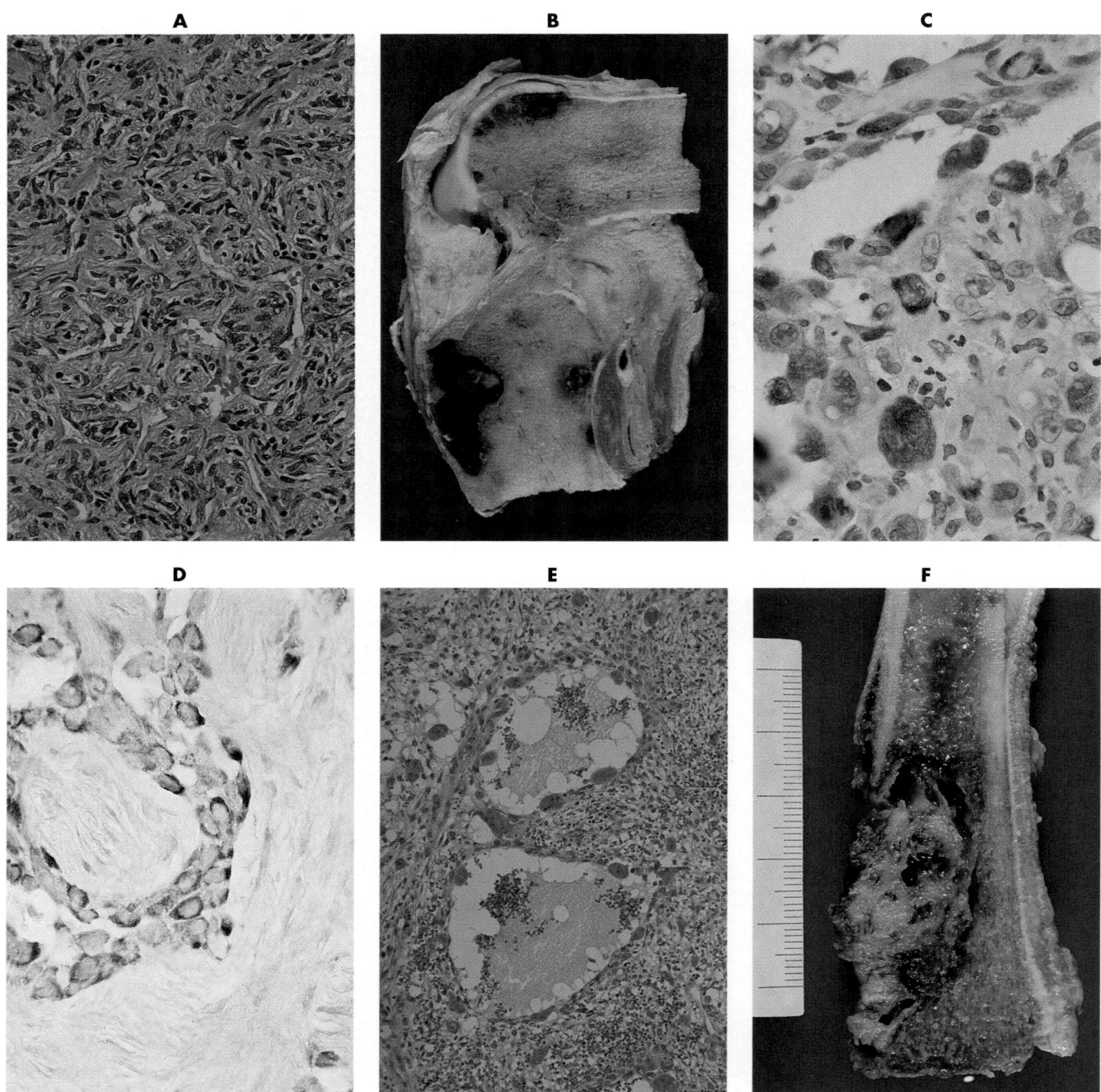

Plate XVIII A, Primary hemangiopericytoma of bone. The appearance is similar to that of the more common soft tissue lesion. **B,** Gross appearance of multicentric epithelioid hemangioendothelioma involving femur and tibia. **C,** Immunoreactivity for factor XVIII in the highly atypical cells of angiosarcoma of bone. **D,** Immunoreactivity for keratin in the tumor cell of adamantinoma of tibia. **E,** Medium-power view of aneurysmal bone cyst. Two large cavities are lined by osteoclast-like multinucleated giant cells. The intervening stroma is rather cellular but contains no malignant osteoid. **F,** Gross appearance of so-called solid variant of aneurysmal bone cyst. A few hemorrhagic cystic areas are present at the periphery.

25 Soft tissues

NORMAL ANATOMY

Soft tissue is loosely defined as the complex of nonepithelial extraskeletal structures of the body exclusive of the supportive tissue of the various organs and the hematopoietic/lymphoid tissue. It is composed of fibrous (connective) tissue, adipose tissue, skeletal muscle, blood and lymph vessels, and peripheral nervous system. Most of the soft tissue is derived embryologically from mesoderm, with a neuroectodermal contribution corresponding to the peripheral nerves.

Fibrous tissue consists primarily of fibroblasts and an extracellular matrix that contains fibrillary structures (collagen and elastin) and nonfibrillary extracellular matrix ("ground substance"). Fibrous tissue is classified according to its texture into loose (most locations) and dense (tendons, aponeuroses, and ligaments). *Fibroblasts* are responsible for the production of the various extracellular material, including the many types of collagen. Their shape varies from spindle (especially when stretched along bundles of collagen fibers) to stellate (in myxoid areas). Immunohistochemically, they are reactive for vimentin and focally for actin. *Fibrocytes* represent the quiescent stage of fibroblasts. *Myofibroblasts* are modified fibroblasts that show features intermediate between fibroblasts and smooth muscle cells.[14]

Adipose tissue is divided into two major types: *white fat,* mainly located in the subcutaneous tissue, mediastinum, abdomen, and retroperitoneum; and *brown fat,* which is restricted to the interscapular region, neck, mediastinum, axillae, and retroperitoneum (especially perirenal region). Brown fat, whose main function is heat production, is much more conspicuous in infants and children. White fat consists of *lipocytes.* These are round or oval cells having most of the cytoplasm occupied by a single large lipid droplet that pushes the crescent-shaped nucleus to the periphery. *Brown fat cells* are smaller, with an acidophilic multivacuolated cytoplasm and a centrally located nucleus showing fine indentations; mitochondria are numerous at the ultrastructural level.

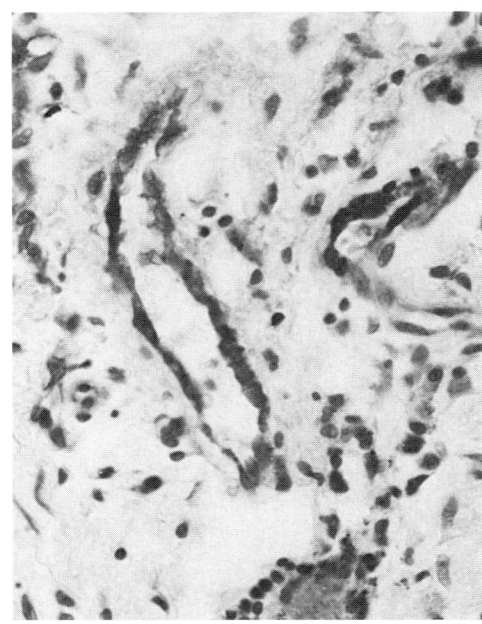

Fig. 25-1 Immunoperoxidase staining of factor VIII–associated protein. Endothelial cells of these proliferating vessels stain intensely. This is used as cytochemical marker for endothelial cells.

Skeletal muscle is mainly derived from within myotomes (but also from mesectoderm in the head and neck region) through the formation of myoblasts and eventually of myotubes (muscle fibers). The most distinguishing feature of these fibers is the presence of myofibrils, which are composed of two types of microfilaments: thin (made of actin) and thick (made of myosin). The periodic arrangement and interdigitation of thin and thick filaments results in the cross-banding seen at a light microscopic level. The I (isotropic) band is made only of thin filaments, the adjacent A (aniso-tropic) band is a zone of overlapping thin and thick filaments, and the H band is made up only of thick myofilaments. The I band is divided in its center by the Z line or disc, which is thought to serve as an attachment site for the *sarcomere* (that is, the repeating individual unit of the muscle fiber).

Blood vessels are divided into arterial and venous compartments joined by a network of capillaries. The several types of cells present in blood vessels are divided into two major types: endothelial cell (located toward the lumen) and a closely related group composed of pericytes, smooth muscle cells, and glomus cells (located toward the outside). Endothelial cells are mainly recognized by their shape and location, but both of these can be greatly altered in neoplastic conditions; therefore one has to rely on the presence of other features to identify them. Ultrastructurally, endothelial cells exhibit numerous pinocytotic vesicles, cytoplasmic microfilaments, specialized cell junctions, microvilli, continuous basal lamina, and—most important—the Weibel-Palade body, a membrane-bound organelle thought to be specific to this cell type[3] and shown to contain the von Willebrand factor.[21]

Immunohistochemically, endothelial cells exhibit reactivity for factor VIII–related antigen (FVIII-RA), vimentin, *Ulex europaeus* I lectin, CD31, CD34, endothelin, and basal lamina components[*] (Fig. 25-1). Of these, the stain for FVIII-RA (see Fig. 25-1) is the most reliable and specific, even if the labile nature of the antigen sometimes results in false-negative results. Use of monoclonal antibodies for other endothelial markers indicates that phenotypic diversity exists among these cells, a fact of potential diagnostic utility.[5,11,19]

Endothelial cells of normal lymph vessels show a much weaker staining for FVIII-RA than endothelial cells from blood vessels, but a similar degree of reactivity for *Ulex*.[2,7]

The cells of the pericyte-smooth muscle-glomus family are characterized ultrastructurally by cytoplasmic microfilaments exhibiting focal condensations, numerous pinocytotic vesicles, and a thick continuous basal lamina. Immunohistochemically, they show reactivity for actin, vimentin, and myosin; positivity for desmin is largely restricted to smooth muscle cells.

Peripheral nerves are formed by axons, Schwann's cells, perineurial cells, and fibroblasts. Most of the fibroblasts are located in the *epineurium,* which is the outer sheath of fully developed nerves. Each nerve fascicle is surrounded by the *perineurium,* a structure continuous with the pia arachnoid of the central nervous system; *perineurial cells* are immuno-reactive for epithelial membrane antigen and negative for S-100 protein. *Schwann's cells* look similar to fibroblasts at the light microscopic level but are easily distinguished from them immunohistochemically because of their strong immunoreactivity for S-100 protein and ultrastructurally by an intimate relationship to axons (with the formation of mesoaxons) and the presence of a continuous basal lamina that coats the surface of the cell facing the endoneurium. Schwann's cells are of neuroectodermal derivation, whereas perineurial cells apparently originate from fibroblasts.[1]

INFECTIONS

Soft tissue involvement by infectious processes usually is the result of direct extension from cutaneous, visceral, or osseous foci or the complication of trauma or surgery. Rarely, the process has a hematogenous source.

The severity of the inflammatory reaction and the type of tissue response observed pathologically depend on the type, dose, and virulence of the infecting organism; the resistance of the host tissues; the presence or absence of necrotic tissue, hematoma, or foreign body; and the anatomic features of the infected area.

Clinical types of infectious processes, such as hemolytic streptococcal gangrene, necrotizing fasciitis, and Meleney's synergistic gangrene, must be diagnosed by clinical appearance and bacteriologic study. In necrotizing fasciitis the process is accompanied by severe systemic toxicity; it is usually caused by group A streptococci, but other bacteria may be involved.[24] All of the pyogenic and necrotizing infections produce acute inflammatory tissue reactions indistinguishable microscopically. Granulomatous inflammations of soft tissue include tuberculosis, atypical mycobacteriosis, actinomycosis, blastomycosis, coccidioidomycosis, sporotrichosis, and dirofilariasis.[21a] A proper search for microorganisms should be made with special stains and cultures.

---

[*]References 2, 4, 4a, 6, 8-10, 12, 13, 15-18, 20.

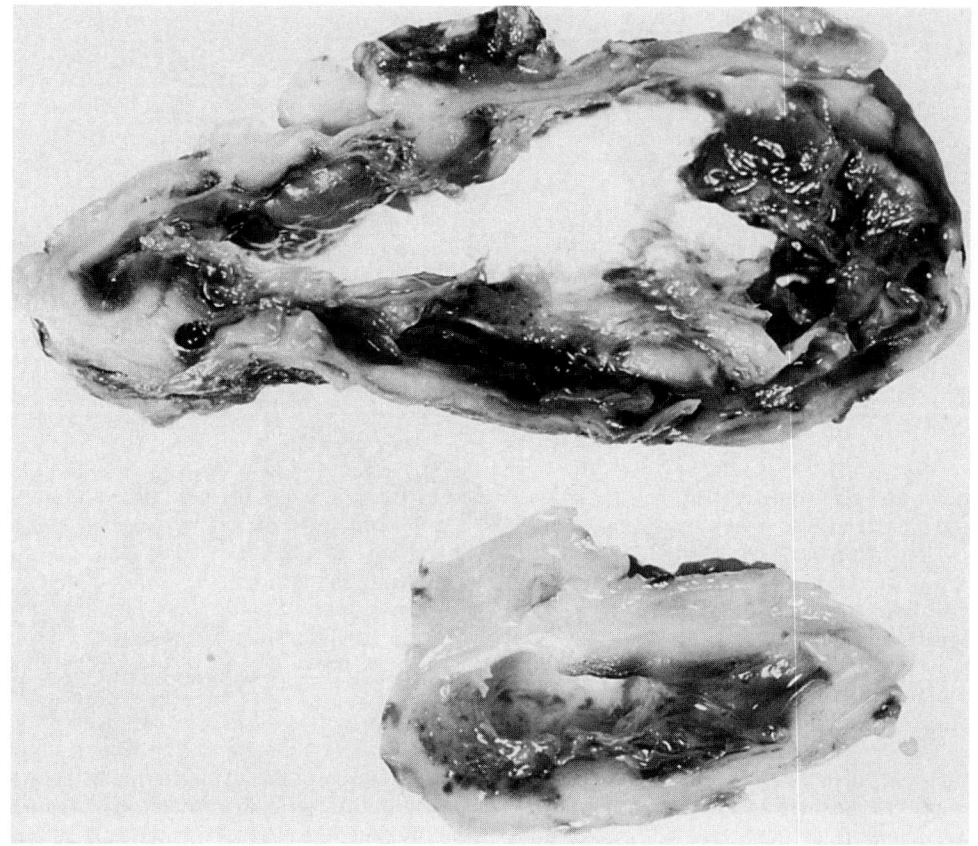

Fig. 25-2 Cystic hematoma of left scapular region excised from 45-year-old woman 2 weeks after injury.

Any chronic pyogenic infection, granulomatous inflammation, or encysted hematoma of soft tissue can mimic clinically a soft tissue tumor[22,23] (Fig. 25-2).

TUMORS
Classification

Soft tissue tumors constitute a large and heterogeneous group of neoplasms. This chapter deals primarily with tumors located in the somatic soft tissues; it excludes those arising from the soft tissues of the mediastinum, retroperitoneum, and visceral organs and those primarily involving the dermis, such as Kaposi's sarcoma.

Traditionally, soft tissue sarcomas have been classified according to a histogenetic concept (e.g., fibrosarcoma as a tumor arising from fibroblasts, osteosarcoma as a tumor arising from osteoblasts, and so on). Morphologic, immunohistochemical, and experimental data instead suggest that most if not all sarcomas arise from primitive multipotential mesenchymal cells, which in the course of neoplastic transformation undergo differentiation along one or more lines.[25] The acceptance of this alternative scheme does not require a change in terminology: A liposarcoma remains such but is now viewed not as a tumor arising from a lipoblast but as a tumor exhibiting lipoblastic differentiation. At a practical level, the importance of this classification based on histogenesis and/or differentiation is that it correlates with a variety of clinical parameters, such as location, pattern of growth,

multiplicity, likelihood of recurrence, incidence and distribution of metastases, prognosis, and patient's age.[26]

Age

A definite relationship exists between soft tissue tumor type and the age of presentation.[28,29] For instance, embryonal rhabdomyosarcoma is typically a tumor of infants and children, synovial sarcoma mainly affects adolescents and young adults, and liposarcomas and malignant fibrous histiocytomas are usually seen in middle-aged and elderly patients. Some of the pediatric cases are congenital. It is interesting that congenital soft tissue tumors rarely behave malignantly, even if an aggressive behavior might have been expected from their microscopic appearance.[27]

Diagnosis and special techniques

For any large soft tissue tumor in which the possibility of malignancy exists, the proper initial diagnostic procedure is to obtain material through incisional biopsy or fine-needle aspiration. The latter technique is being used with increasing frequency in this country, with rates of accuracy equivalent to those obtainable with frozen section.[38] After the tumor has been accurately classified, it can be treated properly. Incisional biopsy has not been shown to result in an increase of recurrence or metastases; on the contrary, when followed by adequate treatment, it is associated with a lower incidence of local recurrence than is primary excision of the

Table 25-1 Major nonrandom chromosomal alterations in soft tissue sarcomas

Tumor Type	Chromosomal alteration	Genes
Ewing's sarcoma/PNET	t(11; 22) (q24; q12)	FLI1, EWS
Clear cell sarcoma	t(12; 22) (q13; q12)	AFT1, EWS
Intra-abdominal desmoplastic cell tumor	t(11; 22) (p13; q12)	WT1, EWS
Myxoid liposarcoma	t(12; 16) (q13; p11)	CHOP, TLS
Atypical lipomatous tumor (well-differentiated liposarcoma)	Marker ring and giant chromosomes	?
Alveolar rhabdomyosarcoma	t(2; 13) (q35; q14)	PAX3, FKHR
Synovial sarcoma	t(x; 18) (p11; q11)	SSX, SYT
Extraskeletal myxoid chondrosarcoma	t(9; 22) (q22; q12)	?

sarcoma performed without prior biopsy.[39] At the time of the definitive surgery the area of the biopsy or aspiration should be excised in continuity with the tumor.

Performance of frozen sections is useful in determining the type of neoplasm, the relative degree of malignancy, and the adequacy of surgical margins.

Light microscopic evaluation of hematoxylin-eosin–stained sections remains the standard technique for the diagnosis of these tumors and is sufficient in the majority of the cases.[33] However, there are special techniques that have been successfully applied to increase diagnostic accuracy; these include conventional special stains, electron microscopy, immunohistochemistry, cytogenetics, and molecular methods. Examples of the first category are reticulin stain for vascular tumors and synovial sarcomas, periodic acid–Schiff for alveolar soft part sarcomas (for the demonstration of intracytoplasmic crystals), phosphotungstic acid–hematoxylin or Masson's trichrome for tumors of striated muscle, and mucin stains for synovial sarcomas and myxoid tumors in general.

Electron microscopy also can be very helpful.[34,45] Smooth and striated muscle cells, Schwann's cells, endothelial cells, glomus cells, and the cells of granular cell tumor and alveolar soft part sarcoma have distinctive ultrastructural features that often provide a specific diagnosis.[32,42] Ultrastructural studies can also be performed on material obtained from fine-needle aspiration.[36]

Enzyme histochemical determinations are of limited use. Alkaline phosphatase is particularly strong in osteosarcoma and vascular endothelial tumors, whereas acid phosphatase and nonspecific esterase are demonstrable in giant cell tumors and malignant fibrous histiocytoma.[31]

Immunohistochemistry for tissue-related markers (such as smooth muscle actin or FVIII-related antigen) has proved of great value and is being extensively used to accurately classify these neoplasms; the specificity, sensitivity, and applicability of this technique to routinely processed material clearly render it the method of choice in most circumstances.[30,40,43] The number of available markers is very large and continues to expand.

The systematic use of cytogenetics has shown the existence of nonrandom chromosomal alterations in association with several types of soft tissue tumors[35,35a,37,41,44] (Table 25-1). Finally, molecular pathology has emerged as a powerful tool for the study of these tumors, particularly those occurring in children.

The specific applications of these various methods are described under the respective tumor types.

Grading and staging

Some degree of microscopic grading of soft tissue is already built into the conventional microscopic classification of these tumors. Thus dermatofibrosarcoma protuberans is by definition a low-grade neoplasm, whereas nearly all malignant fibrous histiocytomas of the storiform-pleomorphic type are high-grade tumors. In addition, several attempts have been made to establish some general guidelines for the grading of soft tissue sarcomas independent of their microscopic type.[46,49,57-59] The number of grades has varied in the different systems: two (low-grade and high-grade), three (I, II, and III, or low-grade, intermediate-grade, and high-grade), and four (I, II, III, and IV) grades have been recognized.

In a two-grade system, tumors are assigned to the low-grade category when their metastasizing potential is low (15% or less).[50,52] Understandably, many clinicians prefer such a system because it makes their therapeutic decision easier. Yet we believe that a three-grade system reflects better the morphologic and behavioral span of these neoplasms.

The criteria used have included degree of cellularity, pleomorphism, mitotic activity, and necrosis, and have been found to be of definite prognostic value for both adult and pediatric soft tissue tumors[48,55,57a]; however, it is misleading to overemphasize grading that is independent of the specific microscopic type of the sarcoma and the circumstances in which it occurs, such as the patient's age or the depth and size of the tumor.[54] For instance, a congenital fibrosarcoma and a superficially located malignant fibrous histiocytoma may both be regarded as grade III tumors, yet their incidence of metastatic spread is extremely low; conversely, a deeply seated malignant peripheral nerve sheath tumor in a patient with Recklinghausen's disease may appear as a grade I tumor because of uniformity of proliferation and low mitotic count, yet it will usually behave in a very aggressive fashion.

ENNEKING STAGING SYSTEM FOR SOFT TISSUE SARCOMA		
Stage I:		
G1	Without metastases	T1
G1	Without metastases	T2
Stage II:		
G2	Without metastases	T1
G2	Without metastases	T2
Stage III:		
G1 or G2	With metastases	T1
G1 or G2	With metastases	T2

A grading system that has proved useful within the constraints just alluded to is that proposed by Costa et al.[51] It is very easy to apply and correlates well with the probability of recurrence or metastasis. Tumors with well-differentiated cytologic features and absence of pleomorphism are classified as grade I. The other tumors are classified as grade II when necrosis is absent or minimal and as grade III when necrosis is moderate or marked. In other words, necrosis governs the grade for tumors other than grade I. The importance of necrosis as an independent prognostic indicator has been confirmed by several independent studies.[56] There is some evidence that microscopic grading can also be used as a predictor of response to systemic chemotherapy.[60]

Two main staging systems for soft tissue sarcoma have been proposed. The one espoused by the American Joint Committee (AJC) is largely based on the TNM system, in that it uses the size of the primary tumor (T), the status of lymph nodes (N), the presence of distant metastases (M), and the tumor's histologic grade (G)[47] (see Appendix G).

In the Enneking system,[53] which is also applied to tumors of bone and which is better suited to lesions in the extremities, soft tissue sarcomas are grouped according to anatomic settings (T1, intracompartmental, or T2, extracompartmental); grades (G1, low, and G2, high) and presence or absence of metastases, giving the scheme shown in the box.

Prognosis

The prognosis of soft tissue tumors depends on a variety of parameters, many of which are interrelated.

1 **Tumor size.** There is a definite relationship between tumor size and outcome. This is true for practically all tumor types in which this parameter has been analyzed.[70,71]

2 **Depth.** Superficially located tumors (dermis and subcutaneous tissue) have a much better prognosis than deep-seated lesions (intermuscular or intramuscular, retroperitoneal) of similar microscopic type. The difference is largely due to the fact that superficial lesions tend to be considerably smaller at the time of excision.

3 **Microscopic type.** Some soft tissue neoplasms (such as atypical lipomatous tumors) are low-grade lesions with no capacity to metastasize, whereas other neo-plasms of similar cell type (such as pleomorphic liposarcoma) are highly aggressive and prone to spread distantly.

4 **Surgical margins.** Not surprisingly, adequacy of surgical margins is statistically associated with local relapse.[62,65,68] Parenthetically, local recurrence is of relatively minor importance in the development of distant metastases.[66,73]

5 **Microscopic grade.** As already indicated, a relationship has been found between various microscopic grading systems and outcome, which at least in some instances has been found to be independent of cell type.

6 **Clinical stage.** As for most other tumors, this determination—which incorporates several of the previously mentioned parameters, as well as the presence or absence of metastases—is the most powerful prognostic determinator.

7 **DNA ploidy.** Several flow cytometric studies performed in soft tissue sarcomas of various microscopic types have shown—as expected—that DNA aneuploidy correlates with a higher microscopic grade, a higher rate of cell proliferation, and decreased survival rates.[61,69] However, it has not yet been determined whether DNA analysis is an independent prognostic factor when applied to soft tissue sarcomas that have been segregated by microscopic type, anatomic site, stage, grade, margin status, and type of therapy.

8 **Cell proliferation.** As already indicated, mitotic activity is incorporated into most grading schemes. Evaluation of proliferation markers such as Ki-67 and p105 has been shown to correlate with prognosis but—as for ploidy values—it remains to be seen whether it qualifies as an independent variable.[72,74]

9 **Oncogene alterations.** It has been shown that soft tissue tumors exhibiting mutations of p53 or altered expression of the retinoblastoma gene behave more aggressively than those lacking these changes,[63,64,67] but similar provisos apply.

Therapy

Soft tissue tumors that are relatively small and/or clearly benign on clinical grounds (such as superficially located lipomas, schwannomas, hemangiomas, and fibrous histiocytomas of the tendon sheath) can be removed directly, but in most others the excision should be preceded by a biopsy. A few tumors (such as schwannomas) can be safely enucleated, but for most others—even if benign—a rim of uninvolved normal tissue should be excised in continuity with the neoplasm to prevent recurrence. Many soft tissue sarcomas, such as fibrosarcoma, myxoid liposarcoma, and leiomyosarcoma, may appear grossly encapsulated, but microscopic examination will often show tumor cells beyond the apparent capsule; therefore enucleation will usually fail. A wide local excision is particularly important for infiltrative lesions such as fibromatosis and dermatofibrosarcoma protuberans.

Full-fledged soft tissue sarcomas in children are currently treated, for the most part, by a combination of surgery, radiation therapy, and multidrug chemotherapy, with results that are vastly superior to those obtained in the prechemotherapy era.[81]

The treatment of high-grade soft tissue sarcomas in adults has undergone radical changes.[76,86] It has been thought for many years that amputation or disarticulation offered the best chances of cure for sarcomas involving an extremity. Contrariwise, many studies done during the past 20 years have shown that for several types of soft tissue sarcomas, a wide local excision offers as good a chance of survival as an amputation, especially if supplemented by other types of therapy.[79,88] Very good results along this line have been obtained by combining limited (even incomplete) surgery with radical-dose radiation therapy (6300 to 7000 rad over $6\frac{1}{2}$ to $7\frac{1}{2}$ weeks).[83,84] Tumor histologic grade correlates well with the incidence of local recurrence and disease-free survival following this therapeutic modality.[83,84,87]

A controversial issue is the usefulness of adjuvant preoperative or postoperative chemotherapy for sarcomas of adult patients.[75,80,85] Results from a randomized study conducted at the National Cancer Institute strongly suggest that chemotherapy diminishes the likelihood of tumor recurrence, at least on a short-term basis, whether the sarcoma is located in the extremities, head and neck region, or trunk.[78,82]

Finally, surgical resection of pulmonary metastases has proved of value in 20% to 25% of the patients who develop this complication.[77]

Pathogenesis

Much has been written in the medical and legal literature on the possible relationship between trauma and soft tissue sarcoma; suffice it to say, no convincing evidence has been provided for a definite cause-to-effect relationship between the two.[96] Individuals subjected to repeated serious trauma (such as football players) do not have an increased incidence of soft tissue tumors. In the overwhelming majority of the cases in which a relation between tumor and trauma seems to exist, careful review of the evidence and doubling rates studies will show that the tumor antedated the trauma and that the latter simply called the attention of the patient to its presence (so-called traumatic determinism).

The large majority of soft tissue sarcomas arise de novo rather than from malignant degeneration of pre-existing benign tumors. Although the latter phenomenon may occur (as in neurofibromas), in most cases in which a given benign tumor is said to have become malignant, review of the original material will show that it was malignant from its inception. Conclusive evidence has accumulated that a variety of soft tissue sarcomas can arise as a complication of radiation therapy.[93,95] Malignant fibrous histiocytomas and soft tissue osteosarcomas are the most common types. The average latent period is about 10 years, and the prognosis is poor. Soft tissue sarcomas have also developed around foreign bodies, such as bullets, shrapnel, and surgically implanted material. The latency period has varied from 2 years to over 50 years, and the most common microscopic types have been malignant fibrous histiocytoma and angiosarcoma.[91]

A possible association between exposure to phenoxy herbicides and development of soft tissue sarcoma has been suggested.[90,94,97] However, several case control studies have failed to show any significant association among the United States soldiers stationed in Vietnam and exposed to Agent Orange, a defoliant that contained dioxin as a contaminant.[89,92]

Tumors and tumorlike conditions of fibrous tissue
Calcifying aponeurotic fibroma

Calcifying aponeurotic fibroma is a distinctive lesion originally described as juvenile aponeurotic fibroma, typically presenting as a soft tissue mass in the hand or wrist of a child or adolescent.[102] At surgery, it may appear as a nodule or as an ill-defined infiltrating mass in the subcutaneous tissue or attached to a tendon. Sometimes, foci of calcification may be detected on gross inspection.[99]

Microscopically, the lesion is characterized by a diffuse fibroblastic growth in which spotty calcification occurs (Fig. 25-3). Infiltration of fat and striated muscle is often seen at the periphery. Mitoses are scarce, and atypical cytologic features are absent. Scattered osteoclast-like giant cells are frequently seen. The cells inside and surrounding the calcified foci have a strong resemblance to chondrocytes. It is this feature that led some authors to postulate that this lesion is basically of cartilaginous origin and represents the cartilaginous analogue of fibromatosis.[100,101,103]

Calcifying aponeurotic fibroma can be confused with rheumatoid nodule, schwannoma, and fibromatosis. Local recurrence is common, especially in young children. However, distant metastases do not occur.[98]

Fibroma of tendon sheath

Fibroma of tendon sheath is a well-circumscribed, often lobulated tumor found attached to tendon or tendon sheath. Microscopically, it is composed of dense fibrous tissue containing spindle and sometimes stellate mesenchymal cells (Fig. 25-4). Frequently, there are dilated or slit-like channels, some of them resembling tenosynovial spaces.[104,106,110] Occasionally, a component of bizarre tumor cells unaccompanied by mitoses is seen.[107] Ultrastructurally, most of the cells have features of myofibroblasts.[105] The behavior is benign. It is not clear whether this is a distinct entity or rather a heterogeneous process representing the end stage of lesions, such as fibrous histiocytoma of tendon sheath or nodular fasciitis.[107a,108,109] We favor the latter interpretation.

Giant cell fibroblastoma

Giant cell fibroblastoma is a mesenchymal neoplasm occurring almost exclusively in children younger than 10 years of age.[113,119] Most of these lesions are located in the superficial soft tissues of back or thigh. Microscopically, an ill-defined proliferation of fibroblasts is seen in a heavily collagenized and focally myxoid stroma. Typical features include the presence of multinucleated cells with a floret-like appearance, other types of atypical tumor cells, and the formation of cystic and sinusoidal structures lined by spindle and floret cells[115,119] (Fig. 25-5). Ultrastructurally and immunohistochemically, the cells have the features of primitive mesenchymal cells.[111] Local recurrence is frequent, but distant metastases do not occur.[114,116]

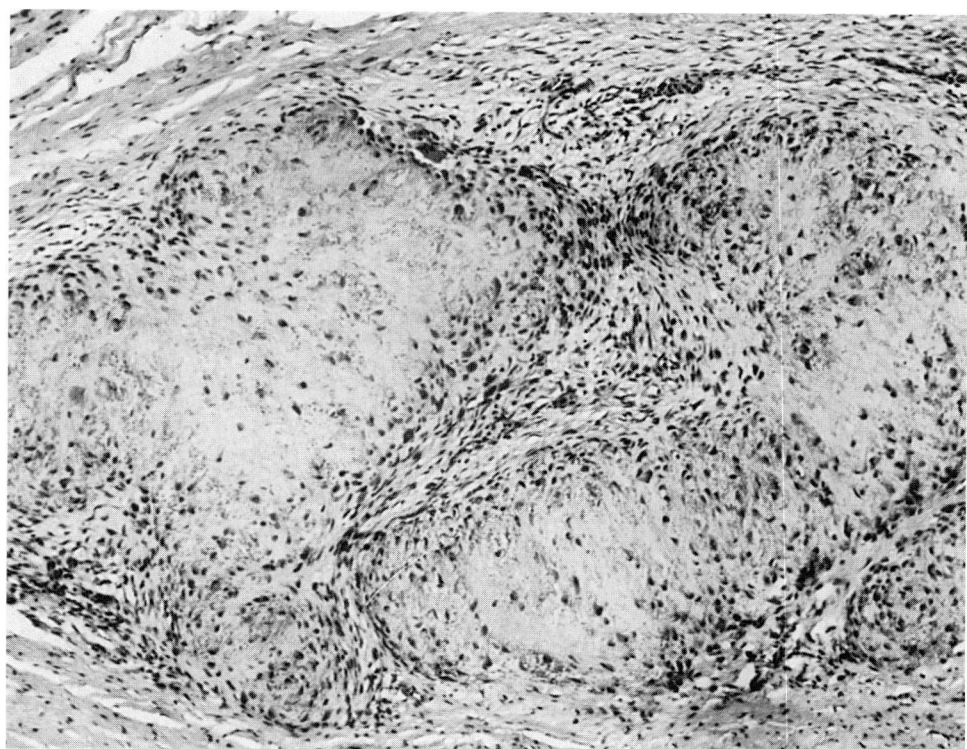

Fig. 25-3 Localized nodular type of calcifying aponeurotic fibroma in 44-year-old man. It appeared as nodule on dorsal surface of wrist. Proliferating cells are cartilaginous in origin. (Slide contributed by Dr. C.P. Schwinn, Los Angeles.)

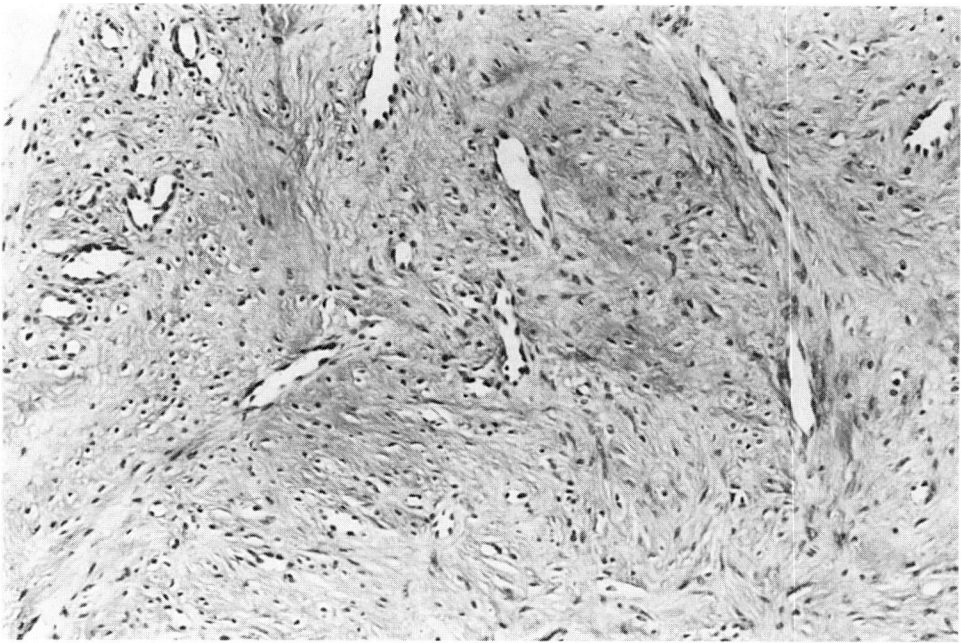

Fig. 25-4 Fibroma of tendon sheath. Nodule is composed of dense fibrous tissue, interspersed with numerous medium-sized vessels.

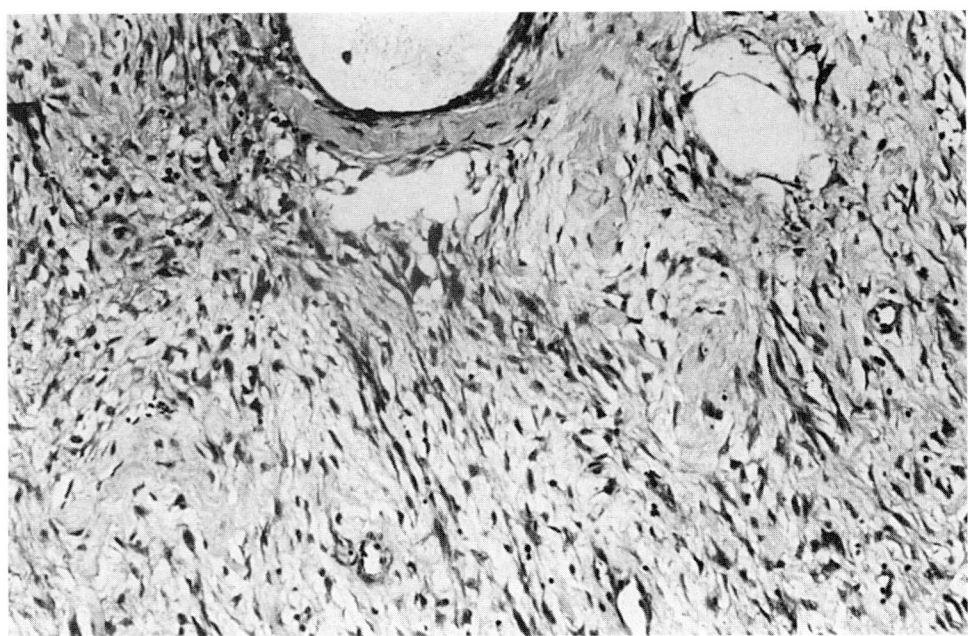

Fig. 25-5 Giant cell fibroblastoma. Vascular-like spaces are present in this fibromyxoid lesion, some multinucleated fibroblasts concentrating beneath them.

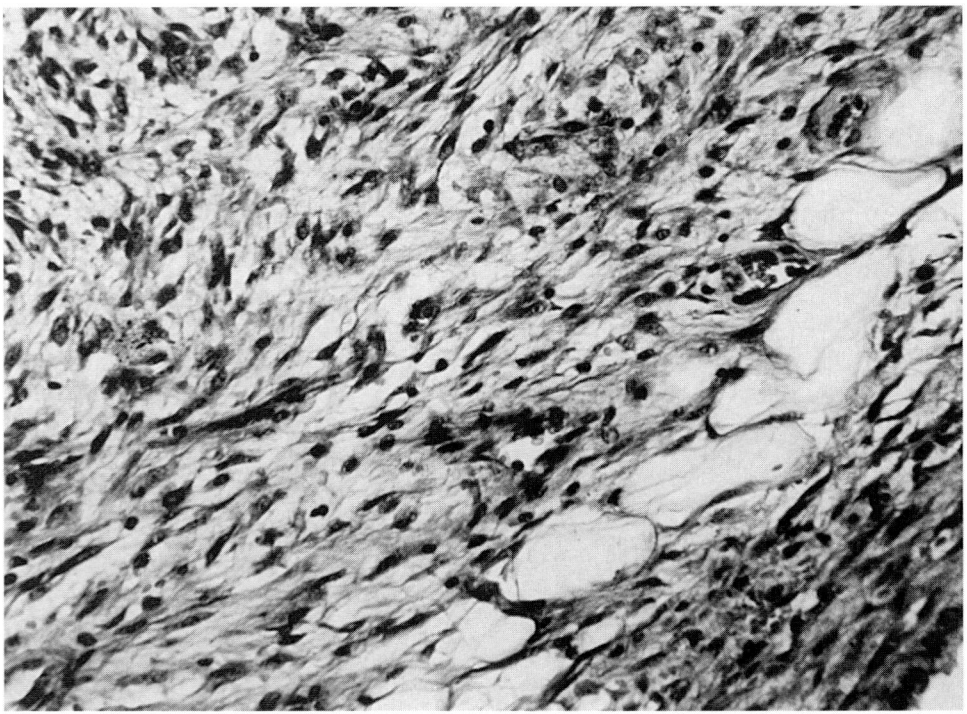

Fig. 25-6 Typical nodular fasciitis in 47-year-old woman who had soft tissue mass just beneath skin in deltopectoral group that measured 3 × 2 × 1 cm and had been present for only 2 weeks. It is highly cellular and vascular and can easily be confused with fibrosarcoma. It infiltrates on its periphery and may show evidence of maturation.

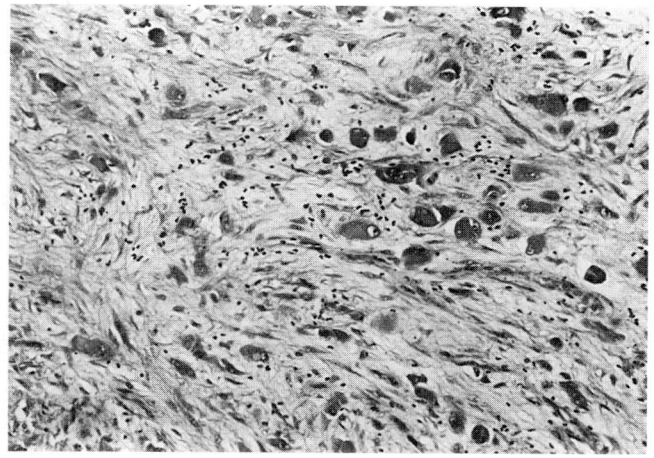

Fig. 25-7 Proliferative fasciitis. Numerous ganglion-like cells are present in fibrous and inflammatory background.

The suggestion that giant cell fibroblastoma is related to dermatofibrosarcoma protuberans and that it may represent its infantile counterpart[119] has received support from the similarities of their ultrastructural and immunohistochemical profiles[116,118] and the description of hybrid and combined cases, whether in the original lesion or in the recurrence.[112,117] In one such case the dermatofibrosarcoma component had pigmented features (Bednar's tumor).[120]

Nodular fasciitis and related lesions

Nodular fasciitis is the preferred designation for the condition originally designated as subcutaneous pseudosarcomatous fibromatosis.[137] It is a distinctive lesion and a very important one because of its ability to simulate a malignant process.[121,122,136,146,148] It can affect patients of all ages but is most prevalent in young adults, the peak age being 40 years.[134,148]

The most common locations are the upper extremities (particularly the flexor aspect of the forearms), trunk, and neck. Two important clinical features of nodular fasciitis are its history of rapid growth (usually a few weeks) and its small size. It usually extends above the fascia into the subcutis, but it may grow beneath it into skeletal muscle, remain within the fascia as a fusiform expansion of this structure, or be centered in the dermis.[130,138,141,147] Like most soft tissue growths of fibrous tissue nature, it has infiltrative margins.

Microscopically, the lesion is characterized by a cellular spindle-cell growth set in a loosely textured mucoid matrix (Fig. 25-6). Vascular proliferation, lymphocytic infiltration, and extravasated red blood cells are also present. A feature of diagnostic significance is the presence of undulating wide bands of collagen lined on the sides by spindle cells, similar to those seen in keloid scars. Storiform areas may be seen focally. Focal metaplastic bone formation may be present, establishing a link between nodular fasciitis and myositis ossificans.[125,126] The high cellularity of the lesion and the presence of mitotic figures are responsible for the frequent

confusion of this lesion with sarcoma, particularly of the malignant fibrous histiocytoid type. Small size, short duration, red blood cell extravasation, keloid-type collagen, and lack of pleomorphic cells are the main features favoring a diagnosis of nodular fasciitis.

Ultrastructurally and immunohistochemically, many of the proliferating spindle cells have features of myofibroblasts.[142,150] The DNA pattern is always diploid.[128] Follow-up studies of this entity have conclusively shown that it is perfectly benign.[134,136,146]

Cranial fasciitis is a distinct variant of nodular fasciitis seen in children and characterized by involvement of the skull with erosion of the underlying cranium.[139]

Intravascular fasciitis is another morphologic variant of fasciitis in which involvement of the wall and lumen of the medium-sized veins and arteries occurs.[144,147]

In *proliferative fasciitis* the location of the lesion, rapidity of growth, and self-limited nature are the same as those of nodular fasciitis, but the presence of large basophilic cells resembling ganglion cells indicates a link with proliferative myositis (see subsequent discussion) (Fig. 25-7). It usually affects adults, although it can also be seen in children.[140] It follows a benign clinical course.[123] As in the other conditions described in this section, myofibroblasts are the cells that predominate ultrastructurally.[124]

Nodular fasciitis and the variants described previously are characteristically located in the somatic soft tissues, but fasciitis-like lesions with a somewhat different morphologic appearance (even more sarcomatoid) can develop from the stromal tissue of a variety of organs, such as the bladder, prostate, vulva, vagina, and cervix (see respective chapters).

Proliferative myositis can be confused with sarcoma not only clinically and at surgery but also microscopically.[135] The skeletal muscles of the shoulder, thorax, and thigh are those most commonly affected. Most patients are over the age of 45 years, but it can also present in children.[140] Grossly, the lesion does not look like a sarcoma but rather like an ill-defined scar-like induration of the muscle. Microscopically, a cellular proliferation rich in fibroblasts is seen surrounding individual fibers. The hallmark of the lesion is the presence of very large basophilic cells with vesicular nuclei and very prominent nucleoli, resembling ganglion cells or rhabdomyoblasts (Fig. 25-8). Their appearance and immunohistochemical profile suggest a myofibroblastic nature.[127] Conservative surgery is curative.[129]

Focal myositis is an altogether different inflammatory condition that affects children and adults. It typically evolves over a period of a few weeks as a localized, painful swelling of the soft tissues.[131,149] Most cases occur in the lower extremities. Both clinically and at surgery, the impression given is often of a neoplasm. Grossly, the lesion is pale and ill-defined. Microscopically, degeneration and regeneration of muscle fibers are seen in association with interstitial inflammation and fibrosis. The lesion is solitary and self-limited and should be distinguished from polymyositis. Enzyme histochemical and electron microscopic studies suggest that the disease may be the result of a denervation process.[132]

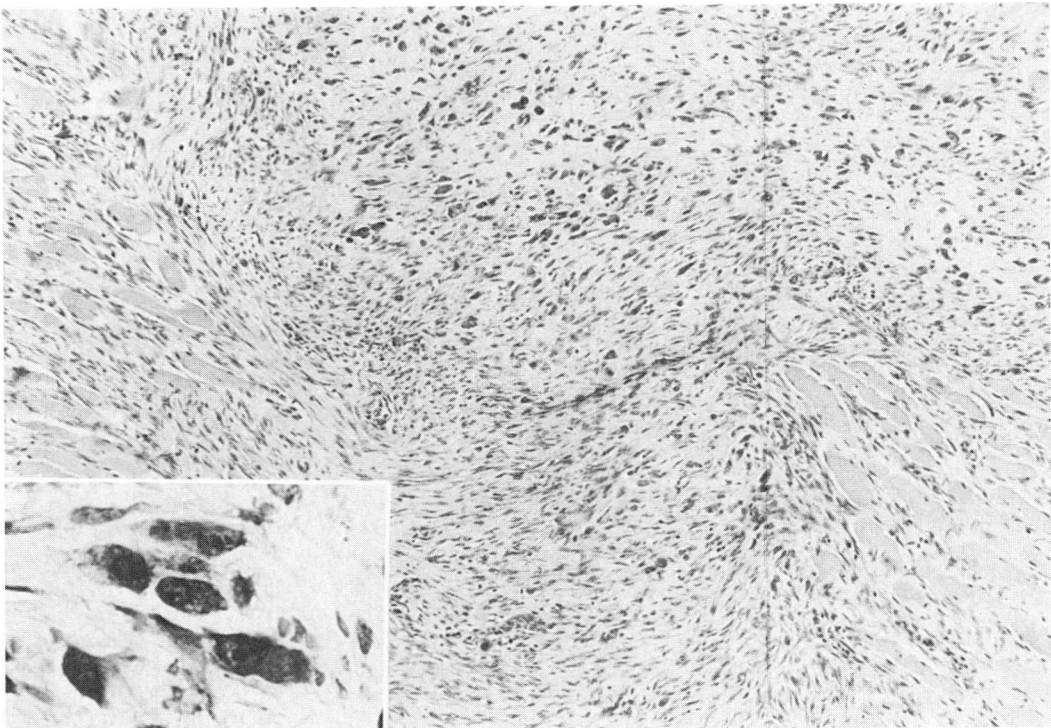

Fig. 25-8 Proliferative myositis. A cellular proliferation accompanied by collagen deposition infiltrates skeletal muscle fibers. **Inset,** Large cells with prominent nuclei and nucleoli are present. Some resemble ganglion cells.

Other pseudoneoplastic myofibroblastic processes pathogenetically related to nodular fasciitis and representing an exaggerated reaction to injury include *proliferative funiculitis* (involving the spermatic cord and probably secondary to ischemia or torsion)[133] and *atypical decubital fibroplasia* (occurring primarily in physically debilitated or immobilized patients).[143] The latter condition merges with *ischemic fasciitis,* in which a central area of necrosis is seen surrounded by a ring of neoformed vessels and proliferating fibroblasts/myofibroblasts.[145]

Nodular fasciitis and the variants described previously are characteristically located in the somatic soft tissues, but fasciitis-like lesions with a somewhat different morphologic appearance (even more sarcomatoid) can develop from the stromal tissue of a variety of organs such as the bladder, prostate, vulva, vagina, and cervix (see respective chapters).

Myositis ossificans

Although myositis ossificans is located in the soft tissue and is pathogenetically and histologically linked to the previous entities, it is discussed in Chapter 24 because of its intimate relation to bone and periosteum.

Elastofibroma

Elastofibroma is a benign, poorly circumscribed tumorlike condition involving almost exclusively the subscapular region of elderly individuals, although isolated cases have been seen in the deltoid muscle, infraolecranon area, hip, thigh, and stomach.[153] Multiple and familial cases have been described, suggesting the existence of a constitutional background.[160] There is often a history of hard manual labor. At surgery, the lesions usually are found at the apex of the scapula, beneath the rhomboid and latissimus dorsi muscles. The right side is affected more commonly than the left. Bilaterality is frequent. A periosteal origin has been suggested.[158]

Microscopically, collagen bundles alternate with numerous acidophilic, refractive cylinders often containing a central dense core, both of which stain strongly with elastic stains (Fig. 25-9). Ultrastructurally, the cylinders are made up of immature amorphous elastic tissue, whereas the central core contains mature fibers.[151,152,155,162] Elastase digestion fully removes this material.[151]

The biochemical composition is that of elastin but with a slightly different amino acid composition than normal elastic tissue.[156a,161] The collagen deposited in the lesion is a mixture of types I, II, and III; the presence of type II collagen is perplexing because this is normally present only in articular cartilage and some ocular structures.[159] This lesion is not a true neoplasm but rather a reactive hyperplasia involving abnormal elastogenesis[154,156]; it would seem that the new material synthesized by the tumor cells is laid down around pre-existing elastic fibers.[157]

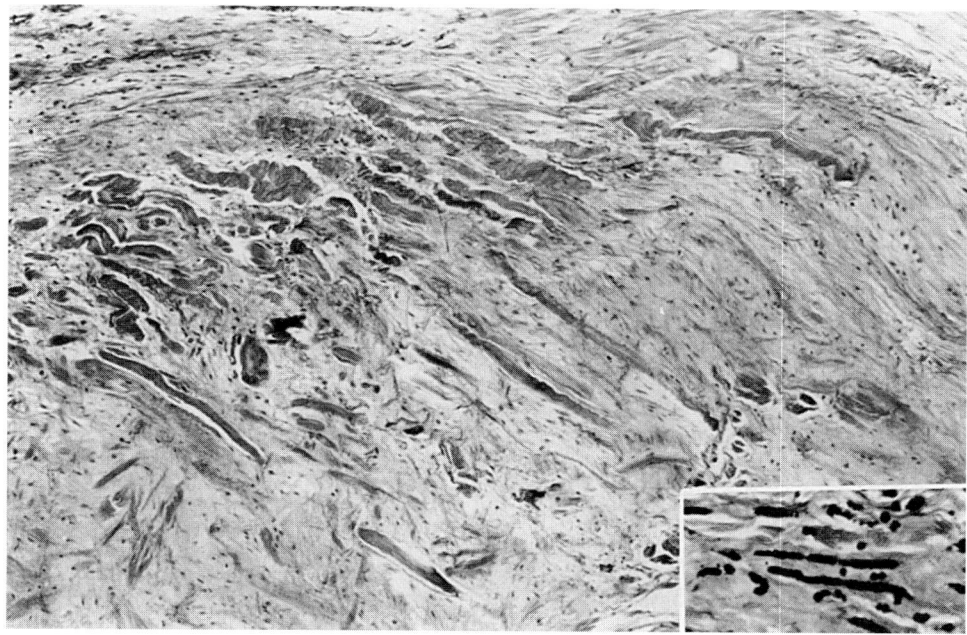

Fig. 25-9 Elastofibroma. **Inset** shows central elastic tissue core demonstrated with Verhoeff–van Gieson stain.

Fibromatosis

The generic term *fibromatosis* was originally proposed by Stout[228] for a group of related conditions having in common the following features:

1 Proliferation of well-differentiated fibroblasts (later shown to be mainly myofibroblasts)
2 Infiltrative pattern of growth
3 Presence of a variable (but usually abundant) amount of collagen between the proliferating cells
4 Lack of cytologic features of malignancy and scanty or absent mitotic activity
5 Aggressive clinical behavior characterized by repeated local recurrences but lack of capacity to metastasize distantly

Grossly, these lesions are often large, firm, and whitish, with ill-defined outlines and an irregularly whorled cut surface[163] (Figs. 25-10 and 25-11). They often arise in a muscular fascia. Microscopically, most of the proliferating cells have features intermediate between those of fibroblasts and smooth muscle cells (i.e., of myofibroblasts). This was first described in a classic ultrastructural study of palmar fibromatosis by Gabbiani and Majno.[192] The authors noted nuclear deformations of the type found in contracted cells (retrospectively identified by light microscopy as cross-banded nuclei) and a cytoplasmic fibrillary system similar to that seen in smooth muscle cells. They suggested that the proliferating fibroblasts had modulated toward a contractile cell—which they proposed to designate the myofibroblast—and that this was responsible for the contracture evident clinically. The myofibroblastic appearance of the cells of fibromatosis has been confirmed by many,[193,206] as has the fact that this cell type is implicated in a large number of reactive conditions as well as neoplasms of soft tissue.[181,183] In an ultrastructural study of fibromatosis, Welsh[234] described intracytoplasmic collagen formation, probably representing a pathologic process in the course of collagen synthesis. This alteration is, however, nonspecific; it has also been detected in a variety of collagen-producing soft tissue sarcomas.[208]

Other light microscopic features commonly encountered in fibromatosis are a perivascular lymphocytic infiltrate located at the advancing edge of the lesion and thick-walled vessels sharply outlined from the surrounding tissue. Dystrophic calcification and metaplastic ossification have also been described.[190]

Some pathologists add the adjective *aggressive* to some forms of fibromatosis to emphasize the biologic behavior. We do not use the term, since we regard it as redundant; most fibromatoses are potentially aggressive. Besides, there is little correlation between the cellularity or other microscopic features of these lesions and their biologic behavior.[237] Other authors have gone even further and have used *differentiated fibrosarcoma* as a synonym for the histologically more cellular or clinically more aggressive types of fibromatosis. We are opposed to this terminology because the designation of sarcoma endows this lesion in the mind of many surgeons with a metastasizing potential that it does not possess. Although we recognize the difficulties involved, we always attempt to make a distinction between fibromatosis and well-differentiated fibrosarcoma, reserving the latter term for tumors showing atypical cytologic features and/or a significant number of mitotic figures (more than one per

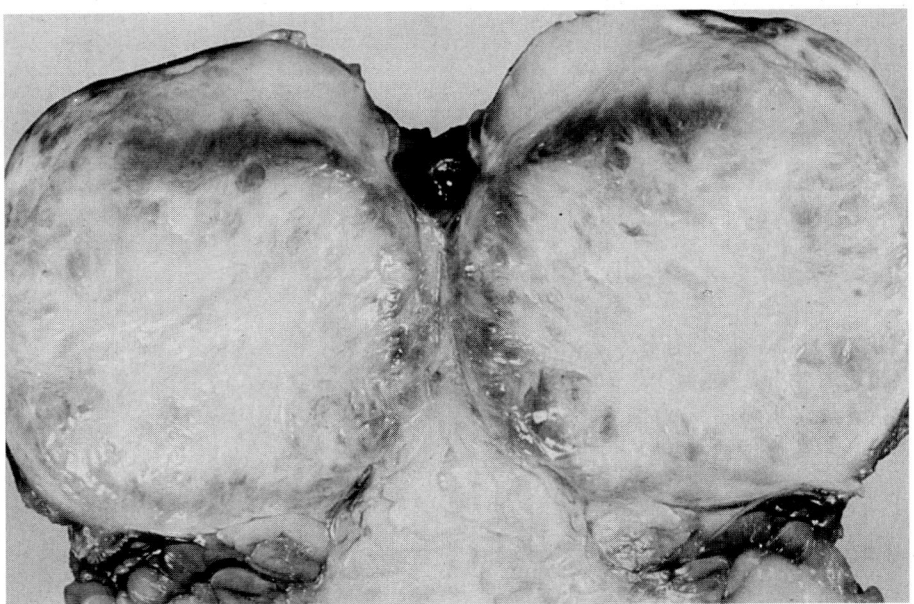

Fig. 25-10 Large fibromatosis of abdominal wall. Note lack of circumscription and almost complete replacement of muscle.

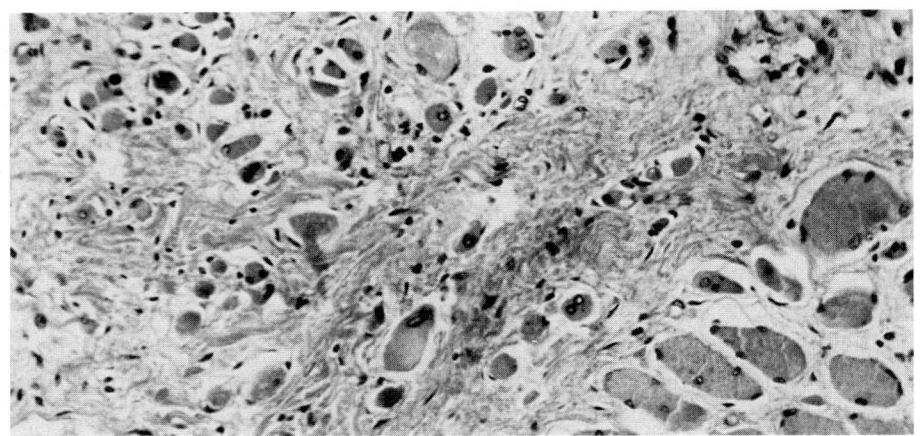

Fig. 25-11 Fibromatosis with adult fibrous tissue growing between muscle bundles.

high-power field). As Enzinger[184] remarked, it is usually not possible on the basis of the histologic examination to predict whether or not a fibromatosis will recur, but it is possible to predict whether a fibrous tumor is or is not capable of metastases.

Most soft tissue fibromatoses are in intimate contact with skeletal muscles—hence their designation as *musculoaponeurotic fibromatosis*.[185] This is preferable to the obsolete term, *desmoid tumor*, traditionally regarded as a neoplasm of the abdominal wall appearing in women during or following pregnancy. In our experience, this lesion is almost as common in men and in other locations, such as the shoulder girdle, head and neck area, and thigh.[198,210,216] It can also

occur in the mediastinum, retroperitoneum, abdominal cavity (see subsequent discussion), and breast.[173,174,221]

The treatment of choice is a prompt radical excision, including a wide margin of involved tissue. Sometimes this requires the removal of the entire muscle involved. The incidence of local recurrence is lower in fibromatoses of the abdominal wall than in those located elsewhere.[198] Some of the latter have recurred as many as five or six times. Only rarely, however, has local aggressiveness forced amputation. Actually, cessation of attempts to excise persistent tissue locally may be followed by failure of the lesion to enlarge further. Because of this observation, some authors have advised against the re-excision of a recurrent lesion that does not appear to be growing.[218] Enzinger and Shiraki[185] analyzed thirty cases located in the shoulder girdle that had been followed for a minimum of 10 years. In 57% of the patients the tumor recurred one or more times. However, at the end of the follow-up period, *all patients* were living without any evidence of continuing tumor growth. A higher incidence of recurrence was seen in young individuals and in those patients with tumors of large size.

Radiation therapy may be effective in achieving local control. It has been used in the form of external radiation following conservative (and sometimes inadequate) surgery[204] and in the form of iridium implantation coupled with surgery for the treatment of recurrences.[239] Some cases of fibromatosis have also been successfully managed with endocrine therapy, such as tamoxifen.[226,235]

Juvenile fibromatosis is a term that has often been applied to examples of fibromatosis occurring in children and adolescents.[165,194,222] Except for their greater frequency in this age group and, in some specific instances, their greater propensity for local recurrence, there is very little either on clinical or microscopic grounds that differentiates fibromatosis in children from that occurring in other age groups.[177] There are, however, three variants of fibromatosis apparently restricted to childhood that present a distinctive clinicopathologic picture: fibromatosis colli (congenital torticollis), infantile digital fibromatosis, and infantile myofibromatosis.

Fibromatosis colli (congenital torticollis) is a type of fibromatosis affecting the lower third of the sternomastoid muscle and appearing at birth or shortly thereafter, sometimes bilaterally.[178] Fibromatosis colli is frequently associated with various congenital anomalies. Thus, Iwahara and Ikeda[200] found congenital (usually ipsilateral) dislocations of the hip in 14% of their patients. An association between complicated deliveries (particularly breech deliveries) and fibromatosis colli has been established. Although some instances of spontaneous disappearance have been recorded, this condition usually necessitates resection of the muscle. Microscopically, the cellularity of the fibrous tissue depends on the age of the process. This condition has been considered to be caused by birth injury, but there is rarely evidence of previous hemorrhage.[172]

Infantile digital fibromatosis is a form of fibromatosis usually restricted to childhood.[217] The typical location is on the exterior surface of the end phalanges of the fingers and toes, but it may also occur outside the digits and at sites such as the oral cavity and breast.[213,215] The lesions are often multiple and either present at birth or appear during the first 2 years of life. However, morphologically identical lesions in adults are on record.[231] The component cells are myofibroblasts.[169] A distinctive microscopic feature, generally not observed in other forms of fibromatosis, is the presence of peculiar eosinophilic cytoplasmic inclusions (Fig. 25-12). These have been examined ultrastructurally and found to be composed of compact masses of granules and filaments without a limiting membrane.[166,175] Their significance is obscure; their similarity with the "virus factories" seen in cells with certain viruses has been commented on, but they are currently thought to derive from cytoplasmic contractile

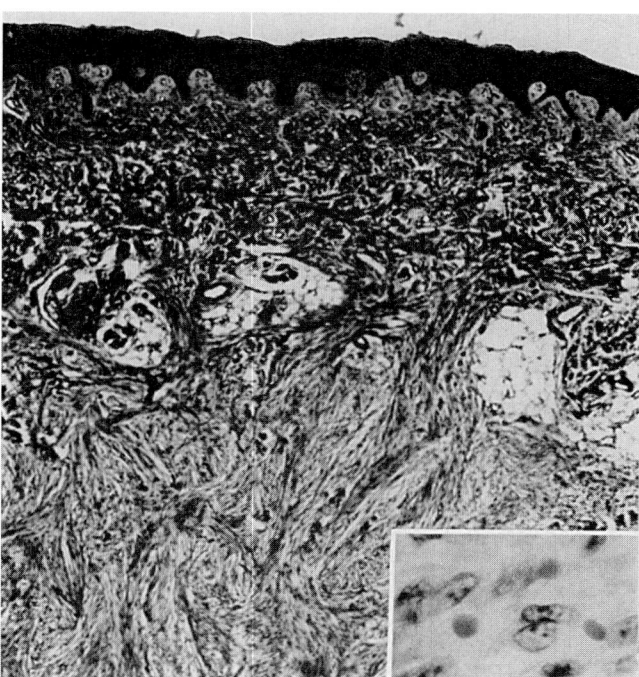

Fig. 25-12 Infantile digital fibromatosis. Involvement is predominantly dermal. **Inset** shows characteristic intracytoplasmic round hyaline inclusions seen in this lesion.

proteins, probably actin.[187,195a,201,211,212,238] This disease has a high tendency for local recurrence.[223]

Infantile myofibromatosis presents as solitary[232] or multiple[171,180,189] nodules in the skin, soft tissues, or bone, either limited to these sites or associated with internal organ involvement.[167,195,220,224,232] A large majority of the cases occur before the age of 2 years, and about 60% are congenital.[176] However, this lesion can also occur in adults, in whom it is also known as *solitary myofibroma*.[168,179,197] Solitary forms are more common in males, and multicentric forms are more common in females.[176] A familial incidence has been detected, and evidence for an autosomal-dominant pattern of transmission has been obtained.[203] Microscopically, peripheral areas that resemble smooth muscle alternate with hemangiopericytoma-like areas and foci having a more typical fibroblastic configuration. Central necrosis and intravascular growth may be present.[176] Ultrastructurally, the lesion is largely composed of myofibroblasts, hence its name[209]; however, a whole range of differentiation exists between fibroblasts and fully developed, desmin-positive smooth muscle cells.[188] Infantile myofibromatosis can undergo spontaneous regression, allegedly through the mechanism of apoptosis.[191] An overlap seems to exist between infantile myofibromatosis and infantile hemangiopericytoma[230] (see p. 2068).

Fibromatosis hyalinica multiplex (multiple juvenile hyaline fibromatosis, systemic hyalinosis) is a morphologically distinctive type of familial multiple fibromatosis affecting children but not present at birth,[199] probably resulting from

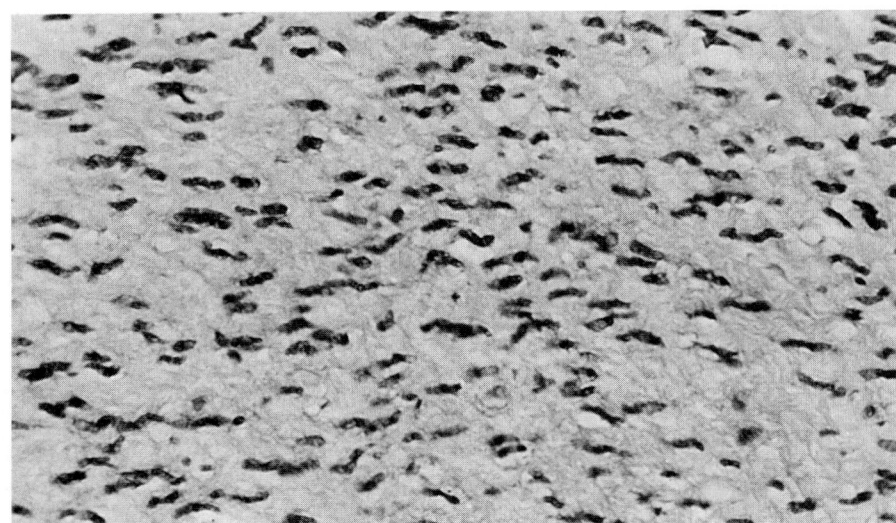

Fig. 25-13 Cellular area in plantar fibromatosis, sometimes incorrectly diagnosed as fibrosarcoma. Note uniformity of nuclei. Mitotic figures are exceptional.

an inborn error of metabolism and characterized microscopically by a conspicuous hyalinization of the connective tissue of the skin, oral cavity, articular capsule, and bone.[182] Ultrastructurally, the cells have the features of fibroblasts; numerous cisternae of endoplasmic reticulum are seen, many of which are dilated ("fibril-filled balls"). Entangled cytoplasmic tubules may also be present.[233,236]

Some forms of fibromatosis derive their names from their particular location.[163] *Penile fibromatosis* (Peyronie's disease) is discussed in Chapter 18. *Palmar fibromatosis* is also known as Dupuytren's contracture and *plantar fibromatosis* as Ledderhose's disease.[202,207,214,225] These conditions occur predominantly in adults. Contracture of the fingers or toes is the leading clinical manifestation. The lesions can be multiple and bilateral and may coexist in the upper and lower extremities. The plantar form tends to be more localized than its palmar counterpart. Microscopically, they have been classified into three phases: proliferative, involutive, and residual.[229] During the proliferative phase, cellularity may be marked (especially for the plantar lesions), and this may lead to a mistaken diagnosis of fibrosarcoma (Fig. 25-13). It is well to remember that fibrosarcoma of the palmar and plantar areas is exceptional[164] and that the differential diagnosis of a cellular spindle-cell tumor of the sole is usually between fibromatosis, synovial sarcoma, malignant melanoma, and Kaposi's sarcoma.

Fibromatoses also have been classified according to the presumed inciting cause, such as *cicatricial fibromatosis* and *postirradiation fibromatosis.* The cicatricial form may follow accidental trauma or arise in the scar of surgical procedures. Postirradiation fibromatosis differs from the other forms by virtue of the common occurrence of bizarre cells with large hyperchromatic nuclei. This feature, which in the absence of radiation exposure would be strong evidence of malignancy, should be interpreted more conservatively under these circumstances.

The association of soft tissue tumors, usually of the fibromatosis type, with multiple colonic polyposis and occasionally multiple osteomas is known as *Gardner's syndrome.*[170,219,227] In this condition, the fibromatosis has a particular tendency to involve intra-abdominal structures, such as the omentum and mesentery,[173,174,205] and to manifest itself following a surgical procedure in the area.

Recently the proposal has been made to designate tumors composed entirely of myofibroblasts as *myofibroblastomas* (or as *myofibrosarcomas* when malignant).[186,196,209a] A closely related lesion has been named *desmoplastic fibroblastoma.*[185a]

Fibrosarcoma

Fibrosarcomas are commonly tumors of adults, although they can occur in any age group and even be present as congenital neoplasms[240,243,246,250,255] (Fig. 25-14). They arise from superficial and deep connective tissues such as fascia, tendon, periosteum, and scar; grow slowly or rapidly; and often appear well circumscribed[251] (Fig. 25-15). They usually are soft and cellular and may contain areas of necrosis and hemorrhage.

Microscopically, the well-differentiated tumors are easily recognized as fibroblastic (Fig. 25-16). The cells are arranged in fascicles that intersect each other at acute angles resulting in a herringbone appearance. The individual cells resemble fibroblasts, and a reticulin stain demonstrates abundant fibers *wrapped around each cell.*[254] Phosphotungstic acid–hematoxylin demonstrates abundant cytoplasmic fibrils. The fibroblastic nature is more difficult to recognize in the undifferentiated tumors. It should be remembered that many other soft tissue tumors, particularly synovial sarcoma, liposarcoma, malignant fibrous histiocytoma, and malignant peripheral nerve sheath tumor, often contain areas closely resembling fibrosarcoma. Only careful examination of different blocks of the tumor will provide the correct diagnosis

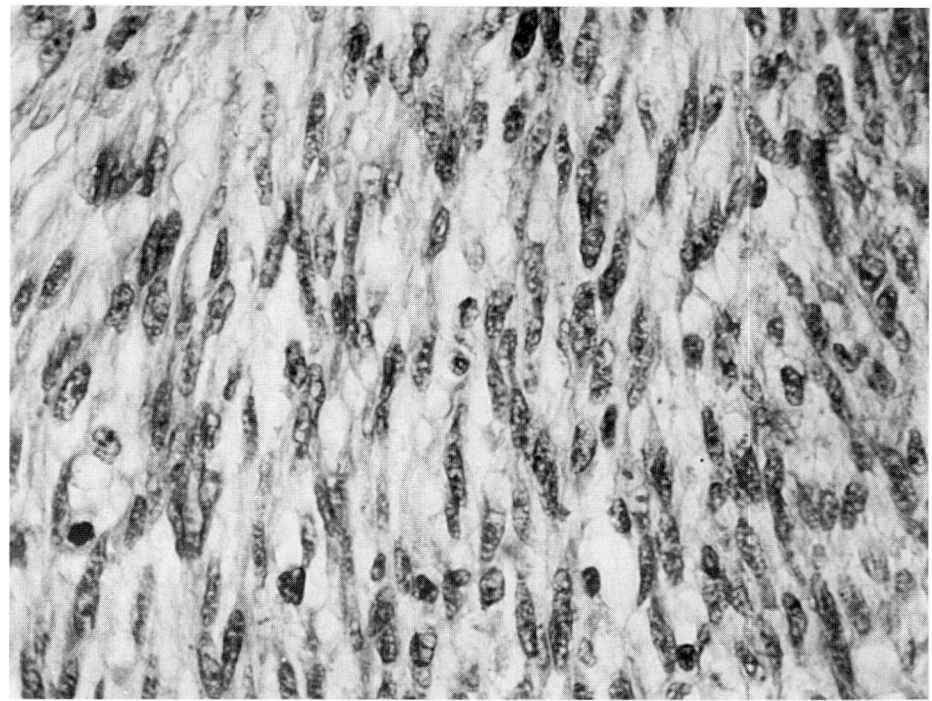

Fig. 25-14 Congenital fibrosarcoma of thigh. Lesion, which was pseudoencapsulated mass, was locally excised, and patient was living 5 years after operation. Patients with such tumor may have an unexpectedly good prognosis.

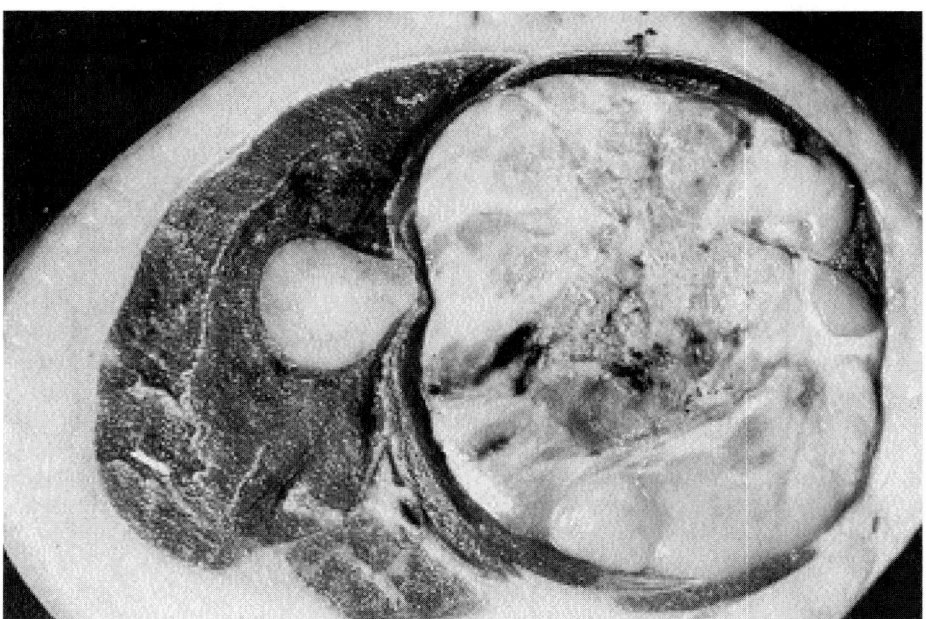

Fig. 25-15 Moderately differentiated fibrosarcoma of thigh. Apparent encapsulation is in contrast to lack of circumscription in fibromatosis.

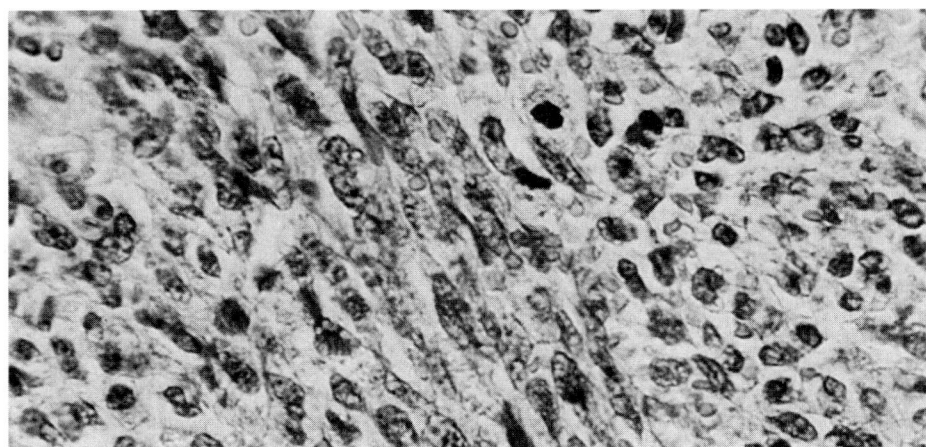

Fig. 25-16 Well-differentiated fibrosarcoma showing fibroblasts with occasional mitotic figures.

in these instances. The presence of giant tumor cells in a soft tissue sarcoma usually means that it is not fibrosarcoma but more probably liposarcoma or malignant fibrous histiocytoma. Ultrastructurally, most of the tumor cells recapitulate the morphology of normal fibroblasts, whereas others have features of myofibroblasts.[241,244,255] Immunohistochemically, there is reactivity for vimentin and type I collagen but not for smooth muscle markers, histiocytic markers, or basal lamina components.[245]

As already indicated, another important differential diagnosis is with fibromatosis. The main light microscopic differences are listed on p. 2032. With special techniques and allowing for some degree of overlap, fibrosarcoma is more likely than fibromatosis to have a high proliferative index, to have an aneuploid DNA pattern, and to exhibit p53 positivity.[248] In contrast to the fibromatoses, fibrosarcomas are capable of distant metastases. The survival rate in a recent large series was 41% at 5 years and 29% at 10 years.[258] Generally, the more superficial and differentiated the tumor, the better the prognosis. Increased mitotic activity and marked cellularity (as expressed by a grading system) are associated with an increased incidence of metastases.[258] In two large series,[249,257] fibrosarcomas in children under 5 years of age at the time of diagnosis were shown to have a high recurrence rate but an incidence of distant metastases of only 7% to 8%. Congenital fibrosarcomas are particularly reluctant to metastasize despite their extreme cellularity, very rapid growth, and extensive local invasion.[242] Conversely, fibrosarcomas occurring in children 10 years old or older have a metastatic rate close to that of adult patients (i.e., 50%).[253] The treatment of choice is radical excision. Postoperative radiation therapy should be considered if microscopic residual or positive margins are encountered. Since subclinical microscopic metastases are presumed to exist in many patients at the time of surgery, adjuvant chemotherapy has been recommended following the surgical excision of the tumor in high-grade lesions.[258]

Inflammatory fibrosarcoma is a controversial entity of the mesentery and retroperitoneum that is seen more commonly in children and adolescents and is often accompanied by anemia and fever.[247] It merges imperceptibly with inflammatory pseu-

dotumor of this region, and it has also been named *inflammatory myofibroblastic tumor*[241a,249a,252] (see Chapter 26).

Epithelioid fibrosarcoma is a recently described peculiar variant of fibrosarcoma that simulates the appearance of infiltrating carcinoma on architectural, cytologic, and immunohistochemical grounds.[273a]

Fibrohistiocytic tumors

This large, complex, and controversial family of tumors is characterized by a dual cellular composition: Cells with a fibroblastic appearance are intimately mixed with others having some of the morphologic and functional attributes of histiocytes.[262,268,274,275] Stout and his colleagues at Columbia Presbyterian Hospital in New York City[273,276] originally proposed that these tumors originate from tissue histiocytes, some of which were said to acquire fibroblastic features; that is, they become "facultative fibroblasts," a property also ascribed to Schwann's cells, smooth muscle cells, and other mesenchymal cells.[279] Another proposed interpretation of these lesions is that they arise from primitive mesenchymal cells and have the capacity for dual differentiation into histiocytes and fibroblasts.[259,267] Both these theories assume the existence of a true neoplastic histiocytic component, in addition to the population of reactive histiocytes that is undoubtedly present. Some of the cells in these tumors do show phagocytic properties, accumulate fat and hemosiderin, exhibit lysosomes ultrastructurally, and manifest immunocytochemical reactivity for hydrolytic enzymes[272,277]; however, the specific cell markers of "true histiocytes" derived from bone marrow have been found to be absent in the tumor cells and present only in the osteoclast-like giant cells occasionally seen in these lesions.[260,278,280] In these and other studies, the tumor cells had a phenotypic appearance resembling that of fibroblasts.[271] Furthermore, the existence of a cell of hematopoietic lineage in a mesenchymal neoplasm would seem highly unlikely on conceptual grounds. There is also the fact that patterns indistinguishable from those of malignant fibrous histiocytoma can be seen in otherwise typical mesenchymal tumors of various well-defined types, particularly liposarcoma and malignant peripheral nerve sheath tumor (PNST).[261,269] Perhaps the tumors in the fibrous histiocytoma group (particularly the malignant ones) do not represent a specific type but rather a common pathway for a variety of other soft tissue sarcomas, including fibrosarcoma, leiomyosarcoma, liposarcoma, and MPNST.[263,271] In any event, these lesions have enough in common to justify discussing them as a distinct group.

Histiocytoma. Pure histiocytoma of skin and soft tissue is probably the only tumor discussed in this section that is composed of true histiocytes. As such, it may be totally unrelated to all the other "fibrohistiocytic" tumors described. Most cases of histiocytoma occur in children. Microscopically, the typical case is made up of closely packed polygonal cells with little or no intervening stroma.[282] The cytoplasm is eosinophilic and may contain lipid droplets. Inflammatory cells are frequently present. Fibrosis, which may be present in the older lesions, should be distinguished from the active fibroblastic proliferation of fibrous histiocytomas. The benign tumors greatly predominate over those exhibiting a malignant behavior, and the differential diagnosis between them may be difficult. Histiocytomas with clinical and/or pathologic features that single them out from the rest are *juvenile xanthogranuloma, reticulohistiocytoma, and generalized eruptive histiocytoma,* all of which are benign. Most of these varieties are discussed in Chapter 4. Although most of these lesions are cutaneous, deep soft tissue examples exist.[281]

Benign fibrous histiocytoma. Well-defined examples of the benign variant of fibrous histiocytoma include *subepidermal nodular fibrosis,* so-called *giant cell tumor of tendon sheath,*[287] and *pigmented villonodular synovitis* (see Chapter 24). The microscopic diagnosis is usually simple. A variable mixture of histiocyte-like cells (some foamy, others multinucleated, still others containing hemosiderin) and fibroblast-like cells is always present.[283,285] Some lesions can be extremely cellular, and some may have large atypical nuclei,[286] but mitotic activity is usually scanty or absent.

Save for the tendosynovial examples previously listed, benign fibrous histiocytoma tends to be a superficial tumor, whereas malignant fibrous histiocytoma is a deep-seated one. However, exceptions exist on both counts.[284]

The distinction between benign and malignant fibrous histiocytoma is not always easy and depends as much on the size and location of the tumor as it does on microscopic features.

Pure *xanthomas* are regarded as the tissue expression of an abnormality of metabolism and not as members of the fibrous histiocytoma group.

Intermediate (borderline) fibrous histiocytoma. This group of tumors is characterized by local aggressiveness (manifested by a high tendency for local occurrence) but is accompanied by an extremely low rate of distant metastasis; the few metastases that develop do so only after repeated failures at local control.[297,314,315] The best example in this category is the tumor traditionally known as *dermatofibrosarcoma protuberans* and also discussed in Chapter 4.[288,291,298] It is typically centered in the dermis, but it can also occur in deeper soft tissues. This lesion is characterized microscopically by lack of circumscription; high cellularity; a relatively monomorphic appearance; nuclear hyperchromasia; high mitotic activity; lack or inconspicuousness of giant, foamy, or hemosiderin-laden cells; and—most of all—

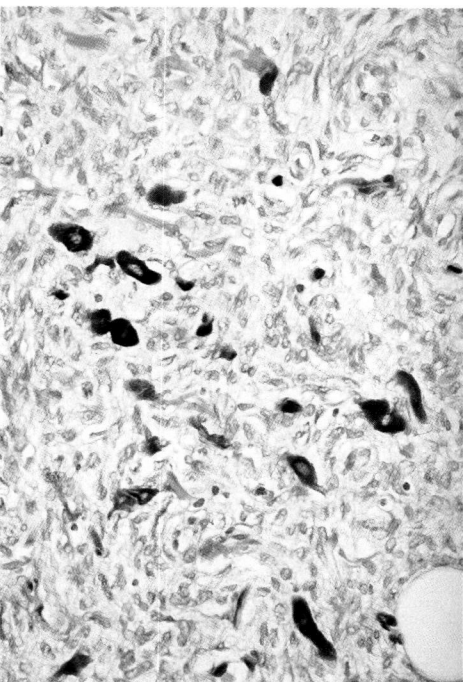

Fig. 25-17 Pigmented dermatofibrosarcoma protuberans (Bednar's tumor). Scattered, heavily pigmented cells are seen among the spindle neoplastic elements.

by the presence of what has been called a *storiform* pattern of growth. This refers to a peculiar arrangement of the tumor cells around a central point, producing radiating "spokes" grouped at right angles to each other. Tridimensional reconstruction studies suggest that this structure develops at the periphery of adjacent proliferating cell groups.[310] This pattern can also be seen in benign fibrous histiocytomas as well as in tumors of totally unrelated types, such as thymoma; however, its most florid manifestation is in the intermediate and malignant forms of fibrous histiocytoma. The collagen deposited in dermatofibrosarcoma appears as nonpolarizable thin strands, in contrast to that present in most dermatofibromas.[289] The histogenesis of this tumor remains controversial; the immunohistochemical profile is more in keeping with a fibroblastic than a fibrohistiocytic or neural derivation,[295a,308] although the existence of a pigmented variant (Bednar's tumor) suggests otherwise (Fig. 25-17).

The main differential diagnosis is with deep-seated benign fibrous histiocytoma[304]; stains for CD34 (positive in dermatofibrosarcoma protuberans) and factor XIIIa (positive in benign fibrous histiocytoma of skin) are helpful in this regard.

As previously noted, a link exists between dermatofibrosarcoma protuberans and giant cell fibroblastoma. Indeed, the latter is regarded by some as the juvenile variant of the former.[290] It should be noted, however, that classical forms of dermatofibrosarcoma can also be seen in the pediatric age group.[309]

Sometimes tumors with the typical appearance of dermatofibrosarcoma protuberans develop foci indistinguishable from fibrosarcoma.[316] Significantly, there is usually a

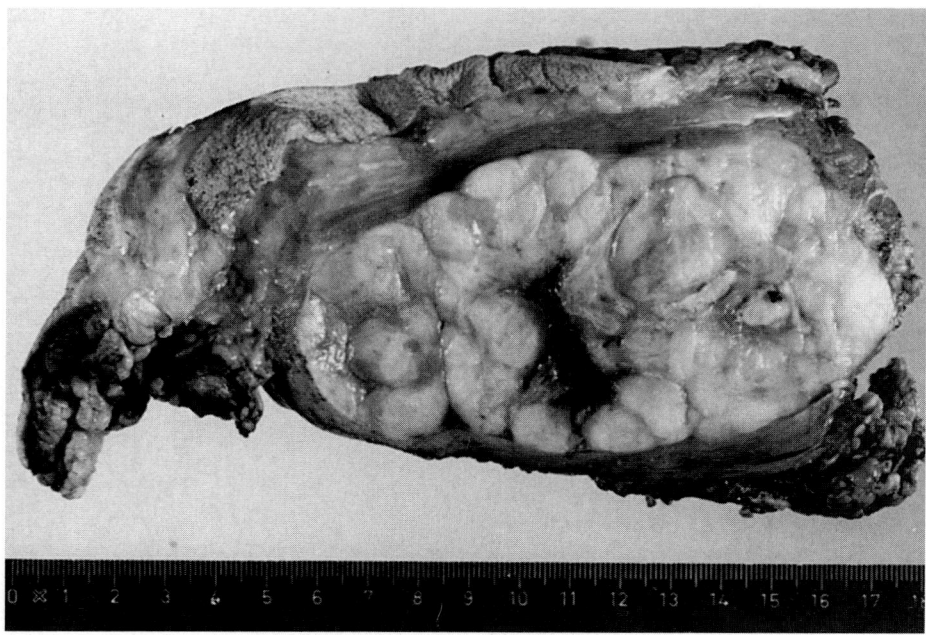

Fig. 25-18 Malignant fibrous histiocytoma. Tumor is located in the deep soft tissues and is surrounded by skeletal muscle. It has multinodular quality and contains hemorrhagic and necrotic areas. (Courtesy Dr. J. Costa, Lausanne, Switzerland.)

loss of CD34 immunoreactivity in these foci.[300a] There is disagreement among the various series as to whether this development is accompanied by a more aggressive clinical course.[292,294] In other instances the tumor progresses to a malignant fibrous histiocytoma pattern.[312]

Pigmented dermatofibrosarcoma (Bednar's tumor) looks like the usual dermatofibrosarcoma protuberans except for the presence of a population of dendritic cells heavily loaded with melanin; the occurrence of this variant is of interest because it raises the possibility of a peripheral nerve origin,[296,311] a possibility that others have also raised for the usual type of dermatofibrosarcoma protuberans.[301] The alternative possibility, that the melanin-containing dendritic cells are not neoplastic but rather represent secondary melanocyte colonization, has been suggested.[295,299] A case with the Bednar's tumor pattern has been seen in the recurrence of a giant cell fibroblastoma, further supporting the relationship between these various neoplasms.[293]

Atypical fibroxanthoma is another tumor that can be placed in an intermediate or borderline category. It typically presents as a small nodule in the sun-exposed skin of elderly individuals.[305,306] Less commonly, it appears as a large mass in the trunk and limbs of younger patients.[300] Some cases develop in parts of the body previously subjected to radiation therapy.[313] The differential diagnosis includes spindle-cell squamous cell carcinoma and spindle-cell (desmoplastic) malignant melanoma. Immunohistochemical stains for S-100 protein and keratin are useful in this differential diagnosis.[307] The large majority of atypical fibroxanthomas are cured by local excision,[300,303] but a few cases accompanied by metastases are on record.[302] This tumor type is also discussed in Chapter 4.

Malignant fibrous histiocytoma (MFH) and related tumors. This tumor, also known as fibroxanthosarcoma and fibrohistiocytic sarcoma, is listed in most recent series as the most common type of soft tissue sarcoma. Many tumors formerly designated pleomorphic rhabdomyosarcoma or pleomorphic liposarcoma are at present diagnosed as MFH. However, as already mentioned, serious doubts have been raised about the existence of MFH as a specific entity.[331] It may well be that this designation embraces sarcomas of various types (particularly fibrosarcomas) having some common morphologic features, such as pleomorphism and a storiform pattern of growth.[352]

Several morphologic variants of MFH have been described. *Storiform-pleomorphic MFH* is the prototypic and most common member of this group.[349,350,368,377] Most cases occur in the deep soft tissues of extremities in adults, with a peak in the seventh decade, but cases have also been recorded in children[359,362,371] (Fig. 25-18). Some develop at the site of previous radiation therapy and actually constitute the most common type of postradiation sarcoma.[358] Still others have appeared around an infarct or a foreign body or at the site of a surgical scar.[336] Nearly half of them involve the deep fascia or the substance of a skeletal muscle.[340,379] Often they are quite large at the time of excision. As the name indicates, the presence of highly pleomorphic tumor cells and a storiform pattern of growth are the two most important microscopic features, even if the latter is not essential for the diagnosis.[348,349] Inflammatory elements, such as lymphocytes, plasma cells, and eosinophils, are usually mixed with the neoplastic cells (Fig. 25-19). Metaplastic bone and cartilage formation may be present focally.[321] Ultrastructurally, MFH consists of a mixture of cells resembling fi-

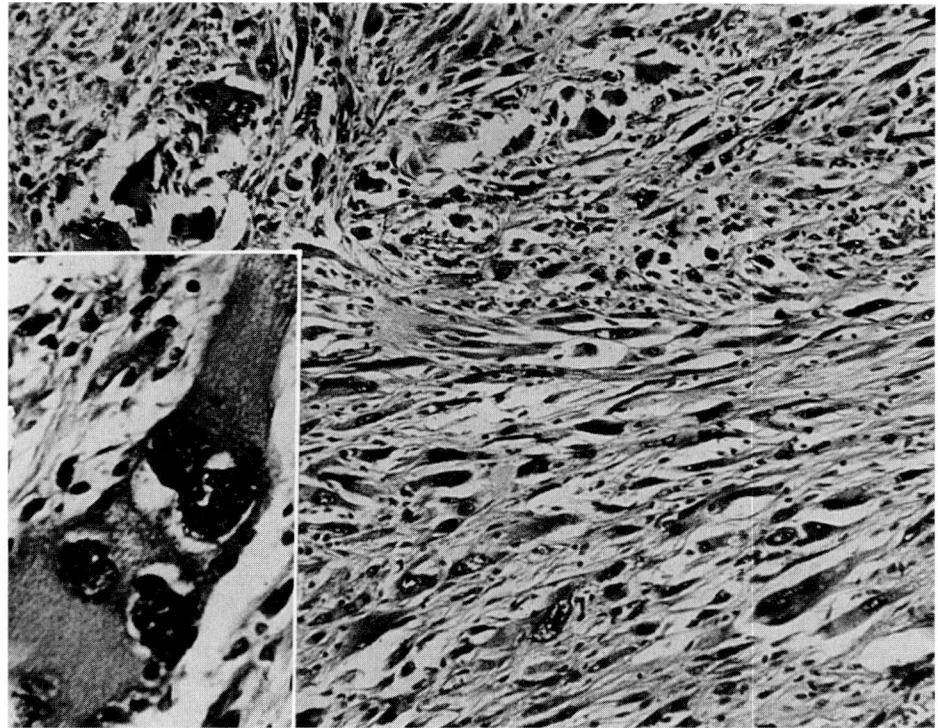

Fig. 25-19 Malignant fibrous histiocytoma of storiform-pleomorphic type. Note bizarre giant cell **(inset)** and characteristic highly malignant spindle-cell stroma.

broblasts, myofibroblasts, histiocytes, and primitive mesenchymal cells.[270,334,344,370,373] Peculiar intranuclear inclusions consisting of closely packed undulating fibrils have been found in some cases.[372] Immunohistochemically, there is usually reactivity for vimentin, alpha-1-antitrypsin, alpha-1-antichymotrypsin, KP1 (CD68), factor XIIIa, ferritin, and the plasma proenzyme factor XIII, and sometimes also for actin, desmin, and lysozyme.* A variety of lysosomal enzymes have also been detected using standard enzyme histochemical techniques.[319,353] It should be remarked that none of these antigens are specific for histiocytes.[366] Some cases of MFH have also shown immunoreactivity for keratin.[333,347,361,363]

This tumor is prone to local recurrence and has the capacity to metastasize to distant sites, especially the lungs and regional lymph nodes.[368] The most important prognostic factors are size and depth of its location, two parameters that are closely related.[320,339,357,362,364] In a series of 200 cases reported by Weiss and Enzinger,[378] tumors that were small, were superficially located, or had a prominent inflammatory component (other than neutrophilic) metastasized only rarely.

Myxoid MFH is probably equivalent to myxofibrosarcoma (a term that we prefer).[317,342] Most of these tumors arise in the extremities of adults, usually are attached to the fascia or within a major muscle, and have a better prognosis than the MFH.[378] Grossly, they are mucoid and resemble myxoid liposarcomas. Microscopically, they also resemble liposarcoma by virtue of an abundant matrix of acid muco-

polysaccharides, high vascularity, and the presence of cells resembling lipoblasts (Fig. 25-20). They are distinguished by the presence elsewhere in the tumor of typical areas of MFH and the absence of true lipoblasts, which should contain neutral fat in the cytoplasmic vacuoles rather than acid mucopolysaccharides. Some electron microscopic differences between the two have also been described.[345,374]

Low-grade fibromyxoid sarcoma is a soft tissue neoplasm characterized by alternating fibrous and myxoid areas, a focally whorled pattern of growth, low cellularity, and a bland appearance of the fibroblastic spindle cells.[328,329] Both local recurrences and distant metastases have been common in the reported cases from a single source.[328,329,331a] The distinction from myxofibrosarcoma is difficult on both conceptual and practical grounds.

Plexiform fibrohistiocytic tumor occurs chiefly in children and young adults. It usually presents as a small, slow-growing dermal or subcutaneous mass, often in an upper extremity. Microscopically, there is a multinodular or plexiform proliferation of fibroblast-like and histiocyte-like cells admixed with osteoclast-like giant cells.[327] The immunohistochemical and ultrastructural features suggest a myofibroblastic derivation.[335] Local recurrence is very common, and a few cases have resulted in regional lymph node metastases.[327]

Inflammatory MFH is a tumor in which the neoplastic cells (some with a bland appearance and others that are bizarre and anaplastic) are mixed with, and even obscured by, an intense inflammatory infiltrate rich in neutrophils[343] (Fig. 25-21). Some of the tumor cells contain phagocytosed

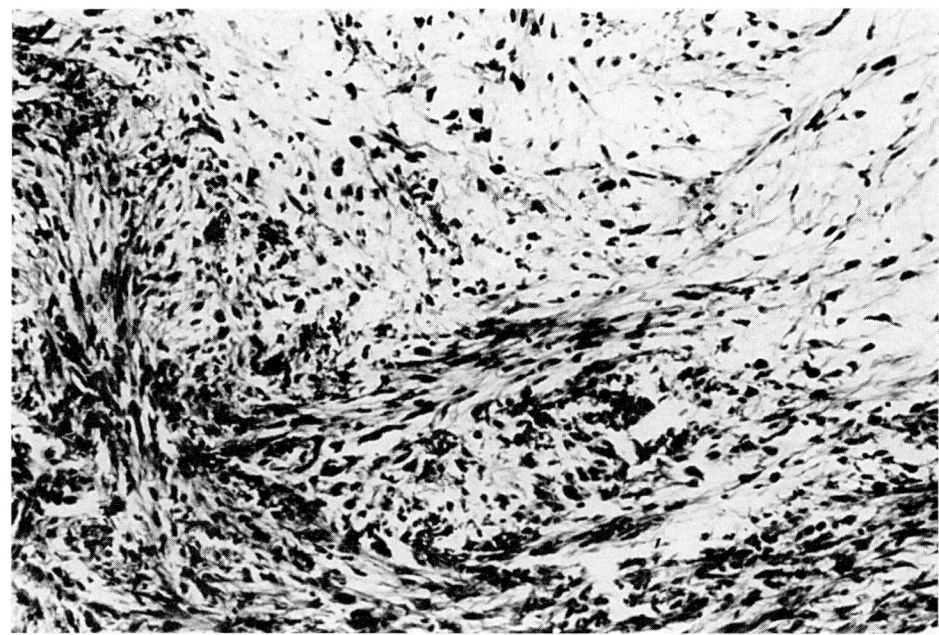

Fig. 25-20 Myxoid variant of MFH. Hypercellular areas with fascicular and vaguely storiform patterns of growth alternate with foci of prominent myxoid change.

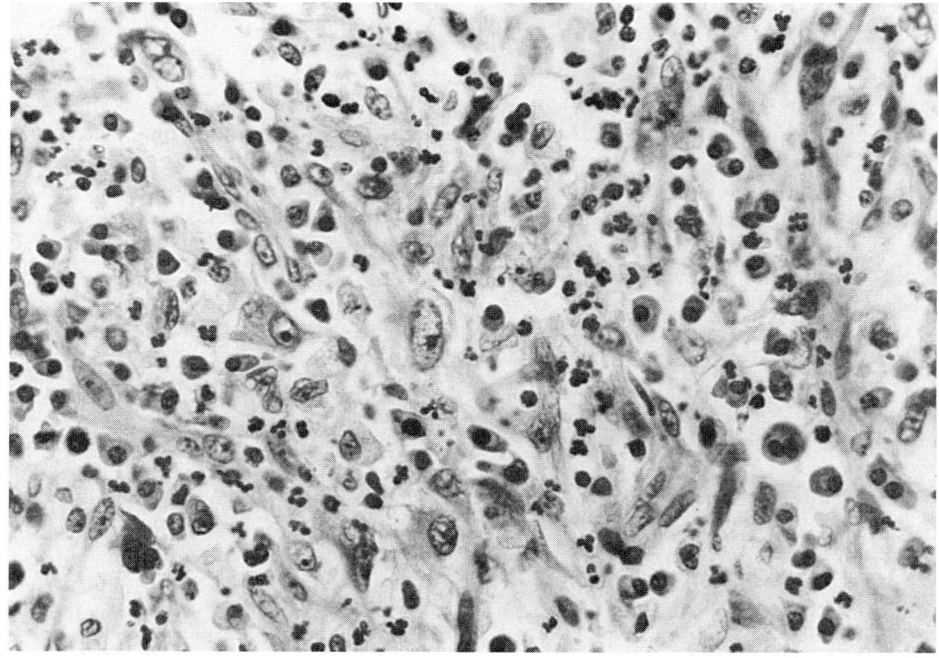

Fig. 25-21 Inflammatory variant of MFH. Atypical cells of histiocytic appearance are seen scattered among dense inflammatory infiltrate rich in neutrophils and plasma cells.

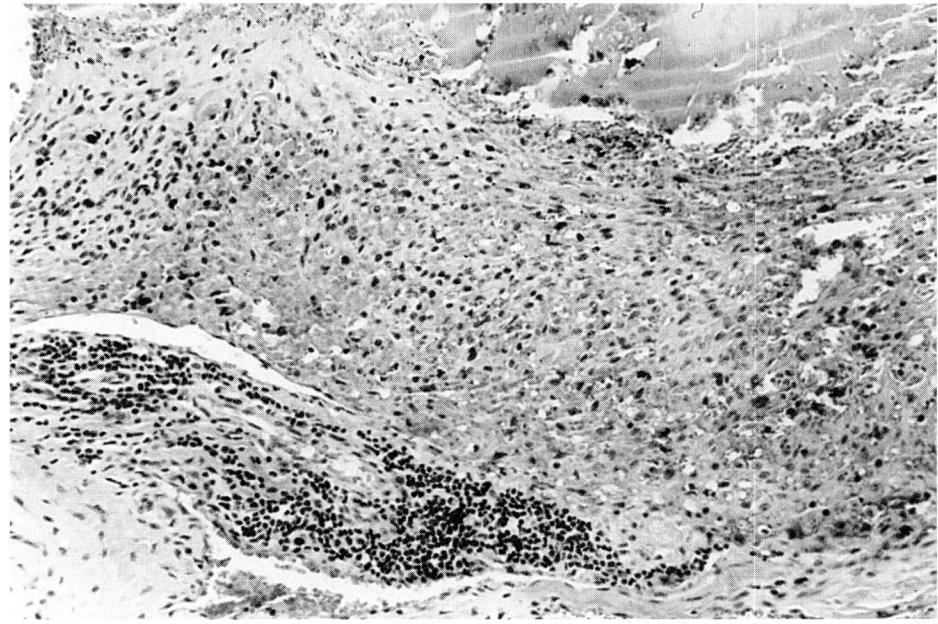

Fig. 25-22 So-called angiomatoid MFH. Lesion is surrounded by heavy perivascular lymphocytic infiltrate and is composed of relatively small and uniform tumor cells arranged in compact fashion around central region of fresh hemorrhage.

neutrophils in their cytoplasm. Storiform pattern, collections of foamy cells, and areas of tissue necrosis are also consistently present. A very similar pattern (i.e., intense neutrophilic infiltration in pleomorphic tumors associated with phagocytosis of neutrophils by the tumor cells) can be seen in otherwise typical myxoid liposarcomas, irradiated osteosarcomas, and metastatic carcinomas from the kidney and adrenal gland. Perhaps the neutrophilic infiltration is simply a tissue response to the production and release of (? biochemically abnormal) lipid by the tumor cells. Sometimes this tissue-inflammatory reaction is accompanied by a peripheral leukemoid reaction and eosinophilia.[375]

Angiomatoid MFH usually appears in the extremities of children and young adults as a circumscribed, multinodular, or multicystic hemorrhagic mass[324,326,356] (Plate XIX-A). Occasional congenital examples have been described.[318] Microscopically, highly cellular foci are mixed with focal areas of hemorrhagic cyst-like spaces and large aggregates of chronic inflammatory cells. The latter are often arranged at the periphery of the tumor in the form of lymphoid follicles and may simulate the appearance of a lymph node (Fig. 25-22). This tumor has been interpreted as a variant of MFH, and some of its immunohistochemical and ultrastructural features support this theory.[376] Other studies have suggested instead that this lesion may be of vascular or myoid nature.[330,338,369] Immunohistochemically, many of the cases show strong reactivity for desmin[330] and for KP1 (CD68).[367] As already stated, the latter marker is not specific for histiocytes.

Angiomatoid MFH is a low-grade malignant tumor that has a tendency for local recurrence and that can also metastasize distantly.[324,326] It is important to recognize that per-

fectly benign dermal fibrous histiocytomas (so-called dermatofibromas) also can be accompanied by hemorrhagic foci and that this does not endow them with any particular aggressive behavior[365] (see Chapter 4).

Most of the retroperitoneal and mediastinal lesions formerly called **xanthogranuloma**[355] are examples of fibrous histiocytomas (usually malignant), whereas others probably represent idiopathic mediastinal or retroperitoneal fibrosis or even malakoplakia[323] (see Chapter 26). We think therefore that the term xanthogranuloma should not be used as a specific diagnosis.

It has been suggested that epithelioid sarcoma and malignant giant cell tumor of soft parts also represent malignant tumors of histiocytes; however, until more definite evidence for this is obtained, it is preferable to categorize them as tumors of uncertain cell type (see pp. 2101 and 2103, respectively).

The microscopic appearance of benign and malignant fibrous histiocytoma can be closely simulated by a number of benign and malignant conditions, including malakoplakia,[323] silica reaction,[380] histioid leprosy, and metastatic carcinoma (particularly from the kidney).

Tumors and tumorlike conditions of peripheral nerves

There are four major lesions in the peripheral nerves: *neuroma,* a benign nonneoplastic overgrowth of nerve fibers and Schwann's cells; *schwannoma (neurilemoma)* and *neurofibroma,* two benign neoplasms; and *malignant peripheral nerve sheath tumor* (MPNST), also designated as *neurofibrosarcoma* or *malignant schwannoma.* Despite the fact that these lesions may overlap and coexist with each other, it is important to make a distinction among them in

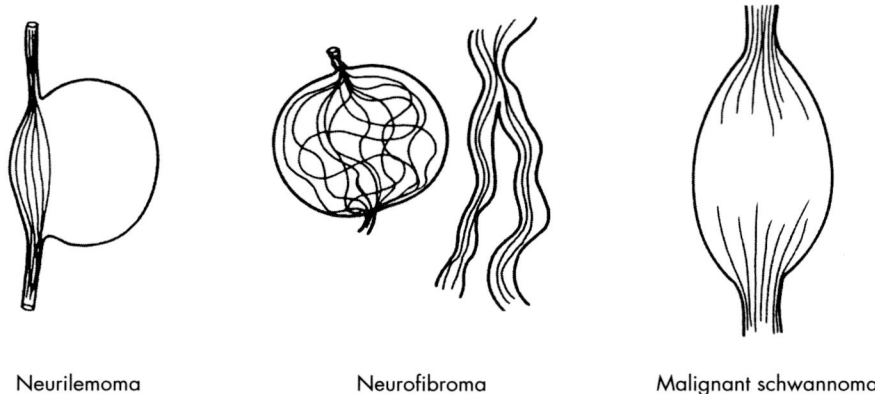

Neurilemoma   Neurofibroma   Malignant schwannoma

Fig. 25-23 Schematic drawing emphasizing main differences between the three major types of peripheral nerve tumors. Note diameter of nerve involved and behavior of neurites (*thin black lines*) in relation to neoplasm.

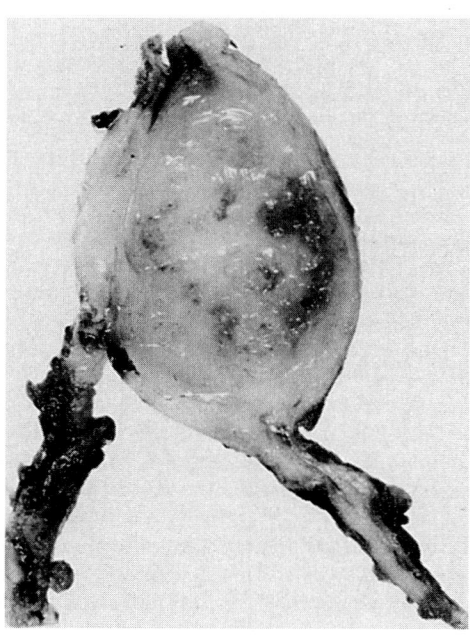

Fig. 25-24 Encapsulated schwannoma with small nerve entering its periphery.

view of their markedly different natural history. For a discussion on the features of schwannoma and neurofibroma in the mediastinum and retroperitoneal area, see Chapters 8 and 26, respectively.

Neuroma

The large majority of neuromas follow trauma—hence their designation as ***traumatic neuromas.*** When a peripheral nerve is severed or crushed, the proximal end regenerates, and if it fails to meet the distal end, a tangled mass of nerve fibers results. Microscopically, all the elements of a nerve can be recognized: axons, Schwann's cells, and perineurial fibroblasts. In addition, scar tissue is often present. Not sur-

prisingly, this lesion is often exquisitely painful. Immunohistochemically, the Schwann's cells of this lesion show aberrant expression of the macrophage-associated antigens CD68 and Ki-M1-P, in keeping with the macrophagic properties that they are known to acquire under these circumstances.[386] ***Amputation neuroma,*** a term made popular during World War I, is merely a type of traumatic neuroma in which the original trauma involves the loss of part or all of an extremity.

Morton's neuroma (Morton's metatarsalgia) can be regarded as a specific variant of traumatic neuroma caused by repeated mild traumas to the region.[385] Its typical location is the interdigital plantar nerve between the third and fourth toes. The lesion is more common in female adults. Microscopically, the affected nerve is markedly distorted. There is extensive perineurial fibrosis often arranged in a concentric fashion. The arterioles are thickened and sometimes occluded by thrombi.[387,388]

Palisaded encapsulated neuroma (solitary circumscribed neuroma) presents as a small, solitary, asymptomatic papule in the skin (see Chapter 4). Its most common location is the face of middle-aged individuals. Microscopically, the lesion is centered in the dermis (in contrast to schwannoma, which is rarely seen in this location) and is characterized by a proliferation of Schwann's cells and numerous axons located within a capsule derived from perineurium.[384] Immunohistochemically, the Schwann's cells are reactive for S-100 protein, the axons for neurofilaments, and the capsule for epithelial membrane antigen.[382,383]

Schwannoma (neurilemoma)

Schwannoma (neurilemoma) is one of the few *truly encapsulated* neoplasms of the human body and is almost always solitary. Its most common locations are the flexor surfaces of the extremities, neck, mediastinum, retroperitoneum, posterior spinal roots, and cerebellopontine angle.[421] The nerve of origin often can be demonstrated in the periphery, flattened along the capsule but not penetrating the substance of the tumor (Figs. 25-23 and 25-24). Since this is a benign neoplasm that only rarely recurs locally, every at-

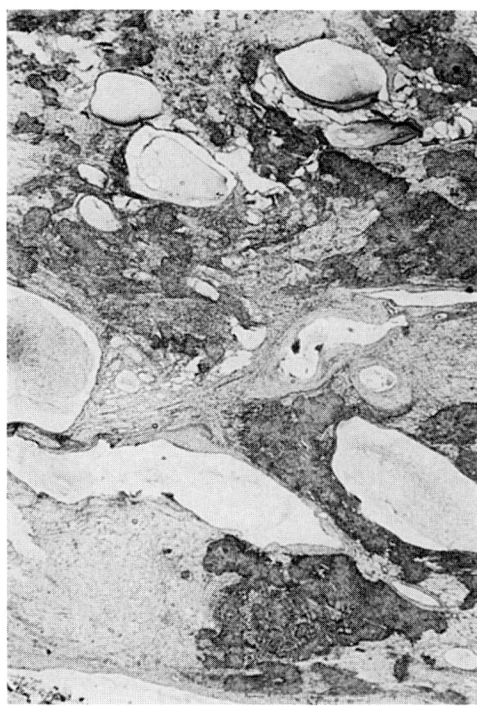

Fig. 25-25 Antoni type A (cellular areas) and Antoni type B (cystic areas) tissue in schwannoma.

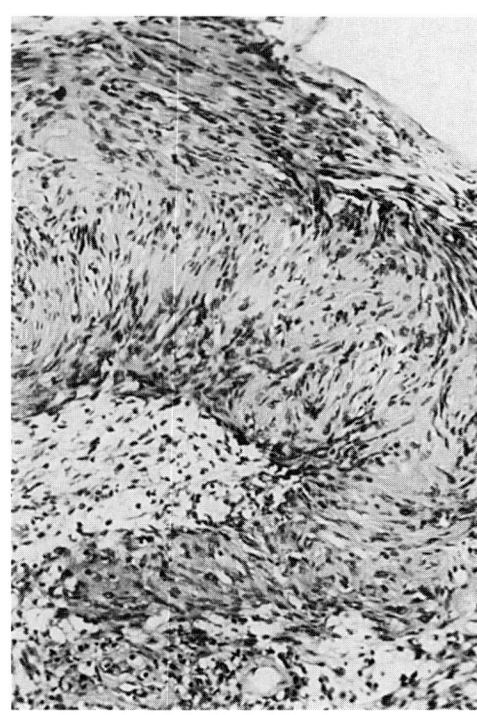

Fig. 25-26 Area of Antoni type A tissue with palisading of cells in schwannoma.

tempt should be made to preserve the nerve, if this is of any clinical significance (e.g., facial nerve or vagus nerve).

Grossly, the larger schwannomas often contain cystic areas (Plate XIX-B). The microscopic appearance is distinctive. Two different patterns usually can be recognized, designated by Antoni as A and B. The type A areas, which in small tumors comprise almost their entirety, are quite cellular, composed of spindle cells often arranged in a palisading fashion or in an organoid arrangement (Verocay bodies) (Figs. 25-25 and 25-26).

In type B areas the tumor cells are separated by abundant edematous fluid that may form cystic spaces (see Fig. 25-25). Occasionally, isolated cells with bizarre hyperchromatic nuclei are observed; they are particularly common in so-called *ancient schwannomas* and are of no particular significance.[394] Mitoses are usually absent or extremely scanty. Blood vessels can be of such prominence as to simulate a vascular neoplasm (Fig. 25-27). By electron microscopy, they have been found to be of the fenestrated type, a rather surprising feature.[409] Thrombosis and hyaline thickening of the adventitia are common. Sometimes, large nodular masses of collagen with radiating edges are seen, a feature sometimes descriptively designated as "amianthoid" fibers or collagenous spherules; we believe that the majority of soft tissue tumors exhibiting these formations are of peripheral nerve sheath derivation.[393,424,425] This does not apply to lesions of lymph nodes containing similar structures (see Chapter 21).

Palisading of nuclei is not unique for schwannoma. It also occurs in leiomyoma, leiomyosarcoma, fibrous histiocytoma, calcifying aponeurotic fibroma, and even in non-neoplastic

smooth muscle of the appendiceal wall. Axons are not present, except in the portion of the capsule where the nerve is attached. Collections of foamy macrophages are sometimes seen, especially in the larger neoplasms. More unusual is the presence of clusters of granular cell similar to those seen in granular cell tumors.[391] The rare occurrence of plexiform areas in schwannoma may cause them to be mistaken for neurofibroma.[399,414] Epithelioid areas can also be present, although much less commonly than in MPNST.[402,427] A few cases containing a glandular component have been described (benign glandular schwannomas)[389,422]; care should be exercised to rule out the possibility of sweat gland entrapment before making this diagnosis.

Rare schwannomas are found to contain melanin pigment.[426] When this feature is prominent and accompanied by psammoma body formation, the possibility of the tumor representing a psammomatous melanotic schwannoma should be considered[390] (see subsequent sections).

Exceptionally, otherwise typical schwannomas or those with epithelioid features have been found to contain foci of small, round hyperchromatic Schwann's cells with scanty cytoplasm, sometimes forming rosettes and simulating neuroblastoma.[396a,404]

It is generally agreed that the neoplasm described in this section originates from Schwann's cells, hence the current preference for the term schwannoma for it.[398] By electron microscopy, the tumor cells have a continuous basal lamina; numerous, extremely thin cytoplasmic processes; aggregates of intracytoplasmic microfibrils; peculiar intracytoplasmic lamellar bodies; and extracellular long-spacing col-

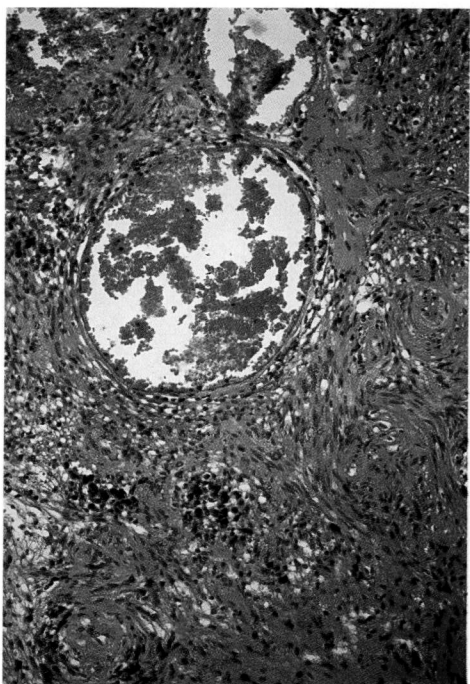

Fig. 25-27 Schwannoma showing large vascular spaces that may lead to confusion with a vascular neoplasm. Hemosiderin-laden macrophages are also present as evidence of previous hemorrhage.

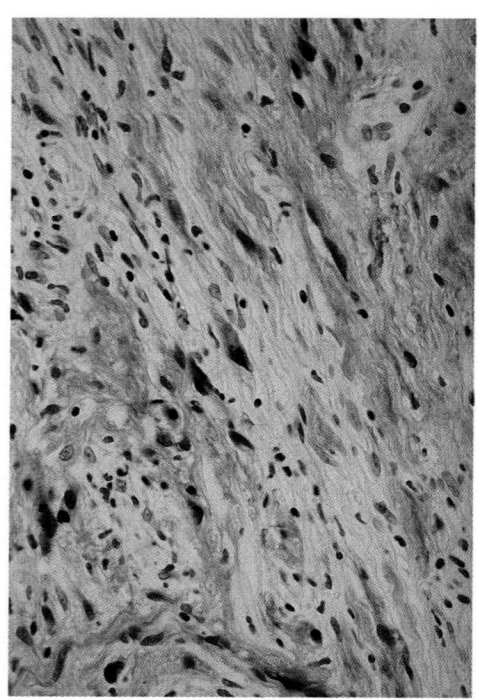

Fig. 25-28 S-100 immunoreactivity in schwannoma.

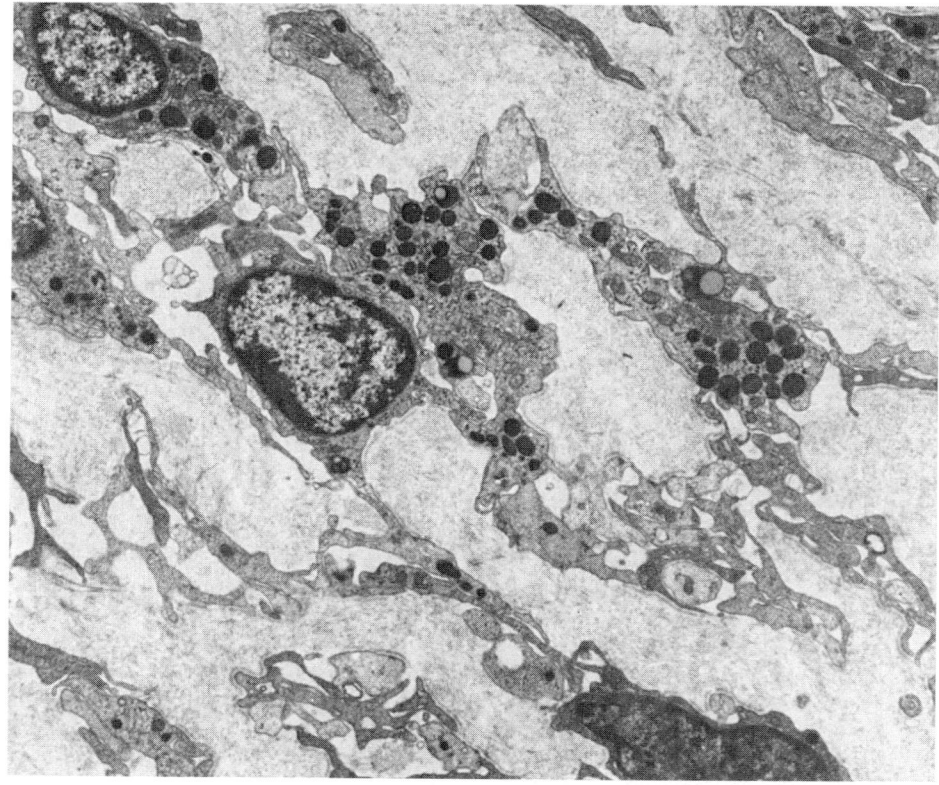

Fig. 25-29 Electron microscopic appearance of schwannoma of retroperitoneum. Elongated cells with narrow processes are partially covered by basal lamina. Cells contain lipid of varied densities.

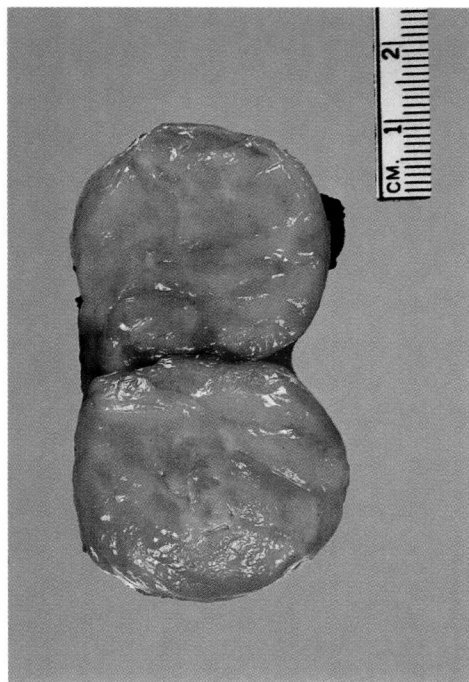

Fig. 25-30 Gross appearance of cellular schwannoma. The tumor is encapsulated and has a golden yellow color.

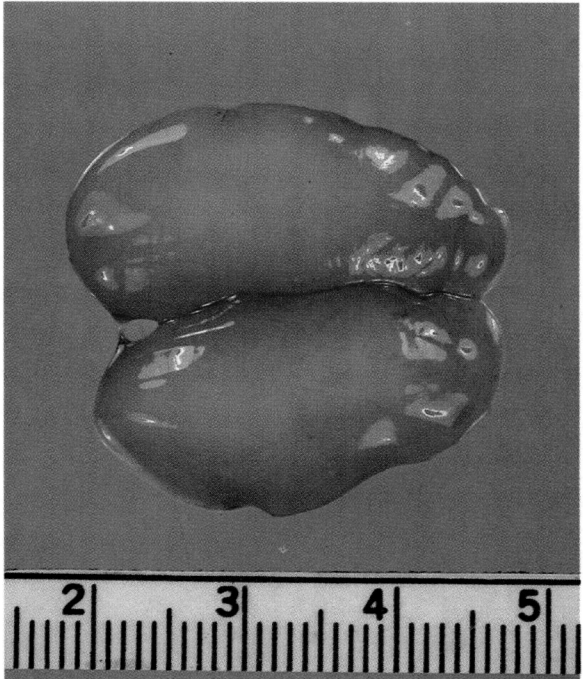

Fig. 25-31 Well-circumscribed neurofibroma of soft tissue. The tumor has a gelatinous appearance.

lagen[396,403,410,428] (Fig. 25-29). Parenthetically, the latter feature is not specific for peripheral nerve cell tumors.[397] Immunohistochemically, the tumor cells show immunoreactivity for S-100 protein, calcinurin, basal lamina components (such as laminin, type IV collagen, and merosin), vimentin, nerve growth factor receptor, lipocortin-1, and sometimes glial fibrillary acidic protein and KP1 (CD68)* (Fig. 25-28). Whether they also exhibit positivity for two markers of myelin—myelin basic protein and P2 protein—remains a disputed issue.[392] Keratin, desmoplakin, neurofilaments, and desmin are not expressed.[406]

Malignant transformation of schwannoma is—in contrast to neurofibroma—an exceptionally rare event. However, several indubitable cases are on record.[408,431] Interestingly, in most of them the malignant component has exhibited an epithelioid morphology.

Cellular schwannoma is the term used for highly cellular schwannomas that are exclusively composed of Antoni A areas but that exhibit no Verocay bodies[400,430] (Fig. 25-30). These changes can be accompanied by nuclear atypia, mitotic activity, and focal necrosis. Most reported cases have been in the retroperitoneum, pelvis, and mediastinum.[391a,429] The differential diagnosis with a low-grade MPNST remains a difficult, somewhat arbitrary, and rather controversial subject.

Psammomatous melanotic schwannoma is a distinctive type of peripheral nerve sheath tumor that occurs as a component of the Carney's syndrome.[390] Most arise from the spinal nerve roots.[401,418] As the name indicates, the tumor is characterized microscopically by the presence of melanin

pigmentation and the deposition of psammoma bodies. In contrast to all other types of schwannoma described in this section, the psammomatous melanotic variety is regarded as a low-grade malignancy because of its tendency for local recurrence and the fact that a few of the reported cases have metastasized.[390]

Neurofibroma

The gross, microscopic, and ultrastructural features of neurofibroma, as well as its natural history, are distinct from those of schwannoma.[473] The fact that in some instances the differential diagnosis may be difficult or that in isolated cases features of both lesions may coexist does not justify lumping them together.

The gross appearance of neurofibroma varies a great deal from lesion to lesion. As a rule, the tumors are not encapsulated and have a softer consistency than schwannoma (Fig. 25-31). The more superficial tumors appear as small, soft, pedunculated nodules protruding from the skin ("molluscum pendulum"). Deeper tumors grow larger. They may result in diffuse tortuous enlargement of peripheral nerves and are then designated as *plexiform neurofibromas* (Fig. 25-32). The diffuse involvement of the nerves may make a complete resection impossible. This particular form of neurofibroma is more commonly seen in the orbit, neck, back, and inguinal region.

Microscopically, neurofibromas are formed by a combined proliferation of all the elements of a peripheral nerve: axons, Schwann's cells, fibroblasts, and (in the plexiform type) perineurial cells. Axons can be demonstrated by silver or acetylcholinesterase stains or by immunostaining for neuron-specific enolase, neurofilaments, or various neu-

*References 395, 403, 405-407, 411-413, 415-417, 419, 420, 423.

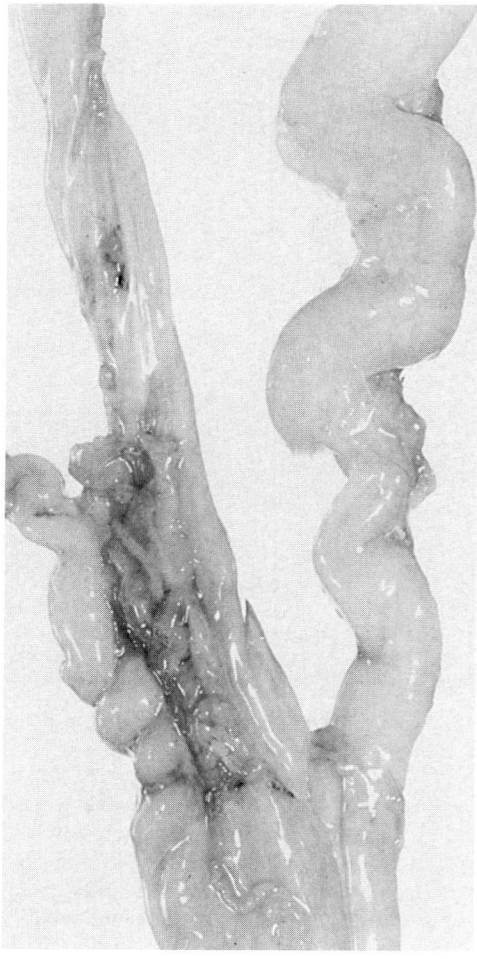

Fig. 25-32 Plexiform neurofibroma involving nerves of lower extremity of young boy. Note enlargement and tortuosity of nerve bundles.

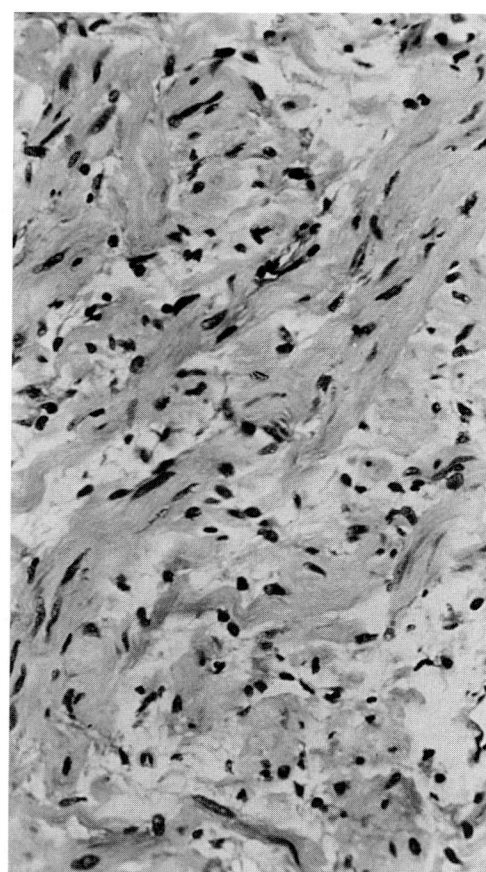

Fig. 25-33 Typical neurofibroma. Note disorderly pattern of fibers.

ropeptides.[456,476] Schwann's cells usually represent the predominant cellular element. Most have markedly elongated nuclei, with a wavy, serpentine configuration and pointed ends (Fig. 25-33). Ultrastructurally, they are seen to enclose axons in plasmalemmal invaginations (mesaxons)[477] (Figs. 25-34 and 25-35). They are immunoreactive for S-100 protein and surrounded by basement membrane components.[440] A population of factor XIIIa–positive and CD34-positive cells is also present; the nature of these cells and their histogenetic relationship with normal nerve constituents is not clear.[474,479] EMA-positive perineurial cells are common in plexiform but not in ordinary neurofibromas.[475] The stroma contains a rich network of collagen fibers, among which almost all major types are represented (I, III, IV, V, and VI).[440,462,463] Mucinous changes in the stroma may be prominent and result in a mistaken diagnosis of myxoma or myxoid liposarcoma.[461] Mitoses are exceptional. Numerous mast cells are present in the stroma.[454,465] Distorted organoid structures resembling Wagner-Meissner or Pacini's corpuscles are sometimes seen. Tumors in which these formations are particularly prominent have sometimes been designated as *tumors of tactile end organs*, and *pacinian neurofibromas*,

respectively.[449,455,457,469] There is some question, however, as to whether the latter lesions are of neoplastic or hyperplastic nature.[444]

In contrast to schwannomas, Verocay's bodies, palisading of nuclei, and hyaline thickening of the vessel wall are almost always absent in neurofibromas. Sometimes, otherwise typical neurofibromas are seen to contain melanin, a feature not unexpected in view of the embryologic relationship between Schwann's cells and melanocytes.[435,437] These *pigmented neurofibromas* should be differentiated from blue nevi and malignant melanomas. Occasionally, an otherwise typical neurofibroma will show foci of skeletal muscle differentiation (neuromuscular hamartomas).[432,459] Some neurofibromas (as well as other types of benign and malignant peripheral nerve tumors) may be partially composed of granular cells, similar in all respects to those of granular cell tumor.[443]

Malignant transformation of neurofibroma should be suspected in the presence of frequent mitoses, overly expressed cell proliferation markers, and the presence of p53 in many tumor cells.[456a]

Neurofibromatosis (Recklinghausen's disease). Multiple neurofibromas represent the most important component of the genetically determined disorder known as neurofibromatosis or Recklinghausen's disease type I.[441,464] This

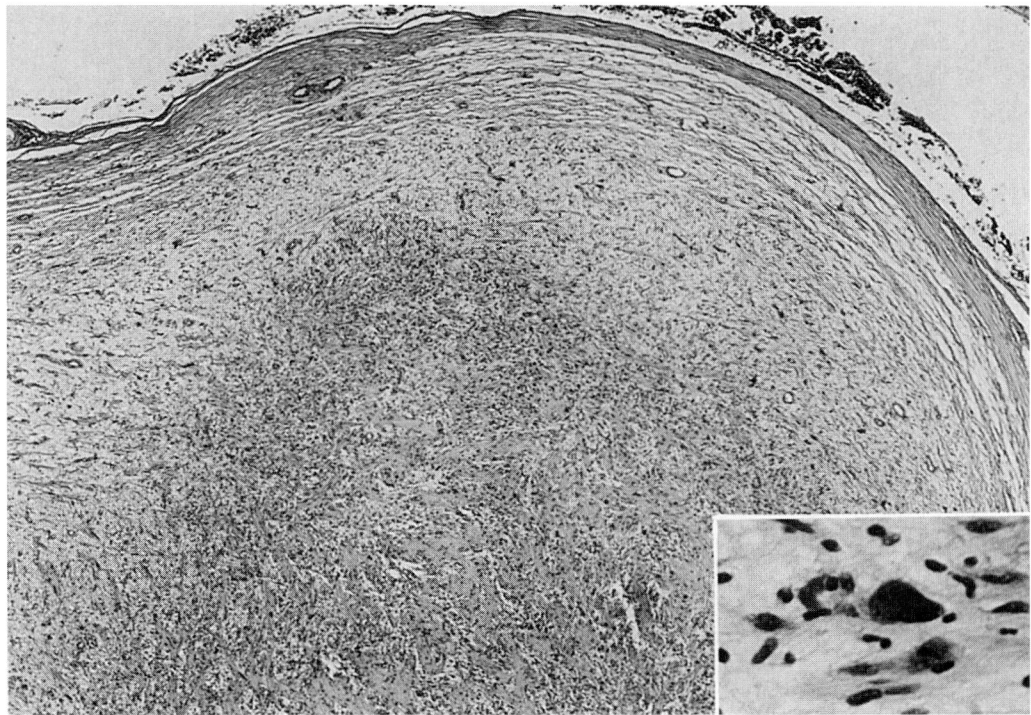

Fig. 25-34 Neurofibroma excised from superficial soft tissues of arm in 36-year-old man. Focus of marked cellularity can be seen in center, surrounded by more typical areas. **Inset,** Cellular center contains scattered giant tumor cells with bizarre hyperchromatic nuclei. This finding per se is not indication of malignant transformation. There were no mitoses.

is one of the most common autosomal-dominant diseases in humans, the prevalence being 1 in 2500 to 3300. The responsible gene (NF1 gene) is located near the centromere of chromosome 17.[433,445,483] This gene encodes a ubiquitous protein known as neurofibromin, which is necessary for correct negative regulation of *ras* proteins.[434,442,448,448a] In this disorder, neurofibromas may occur in every conceivable site: axilla, thigh, buttock, deep-lying soft tissue, orbit, mediastinum, retroperitoneum, tongue, gastrointestinal tract, and many others.[466] Plexiform neurofibromas may result in massive enlargement of a limb or some other part of the body ("elephantiasis neuromatosa") (Fig. 25-36 and Plate XIX-C). In addition to neurofibromas, patients with type I Recklinghausen's disease often have many other associated lesions, the most common being the *café au lait spot.* This consists microscopically of an increase in the amount of melanin in the epidermal basal layer and is sometimes seen overlying a neurofibroma. It can be distinguished from the pigmented spots associated with Albright's syndrome by virtue of its distribution and smooth, delicate margins.[436] Solitary café au lait spots are common in normal individuals. Only when they are present in a number of five or more can a significant association with neurofibromatosis be detected.[481] Other lesions sometimes seen in patients with Recklinghausen's disease include congenital malformations of various types,[450] megacolon, various types of vascular lesions,[458,468] fibrosing alveolitis,[478] schwannoma, lipoma, pheochromocytoma, neuroblastoma,[439,482] ganglioneuroma,[460] carcinoid tumor,[452] gastrointestinal stromal tumor,[446] and

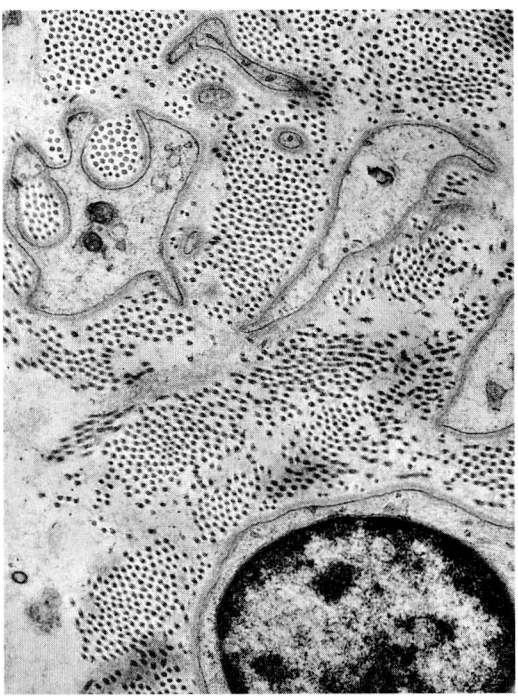

Fig. 25-35 Electron microscopic appearance of plexiform neurofibroma in a patient with Recklinghausen's neurofibromatosis. Schwann cell processes, one of which *(upper left)* is enveloping collagen fibrils. Note the continuous basal lamina. (×14,900.) (Courtesy Dr. Robert A. Erlandson, Memorial Sloan-Kettering Cancer Center.)

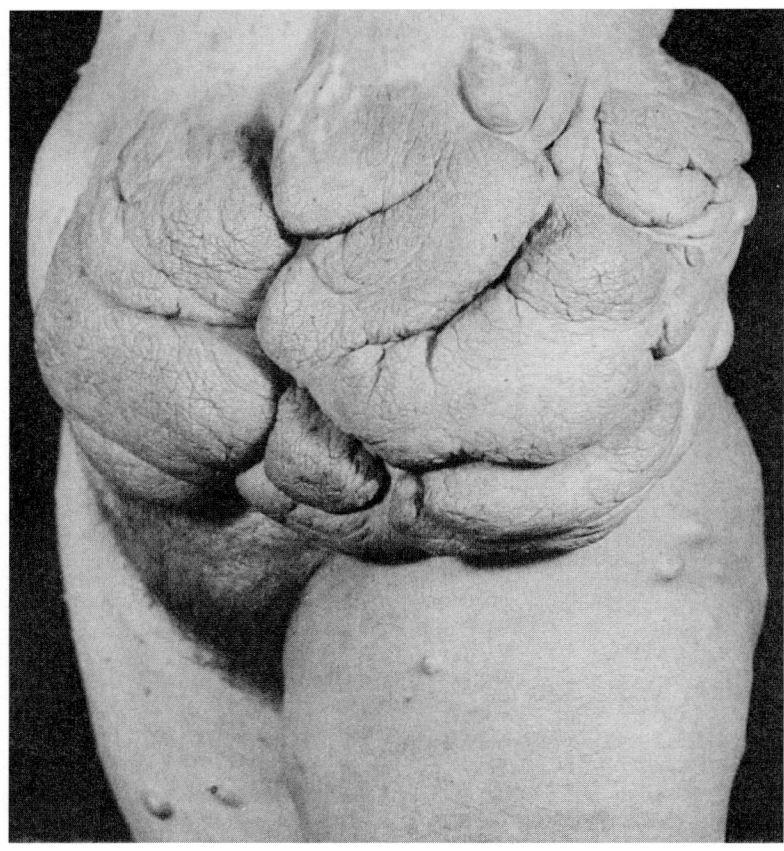

Fig. 25-36 Florid case of Recklinghausen's disease. In addition to typical changes of elephantiasis in lower abdomen, multiple small neurofibromas of chest and extremities are evident.

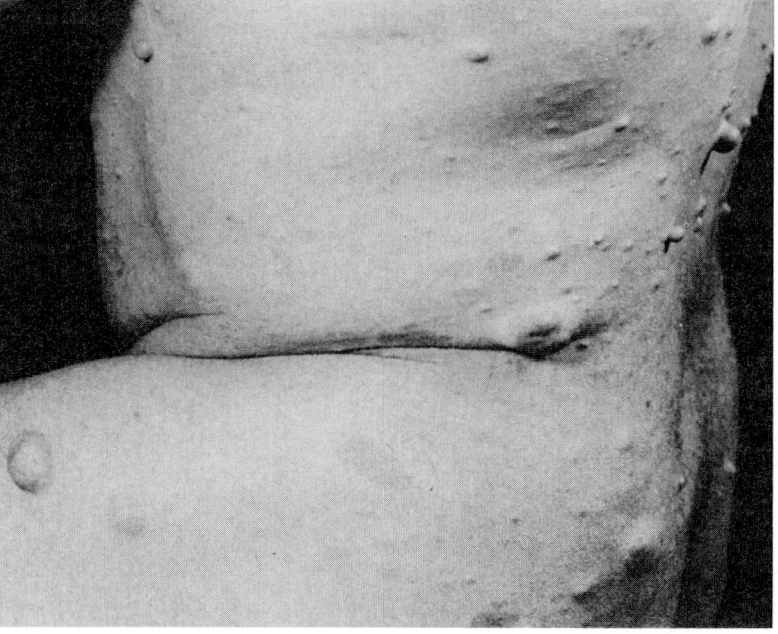

Fig. 25-37 Recklinghausen's disease showing innumerable nodules and café au lait spots.

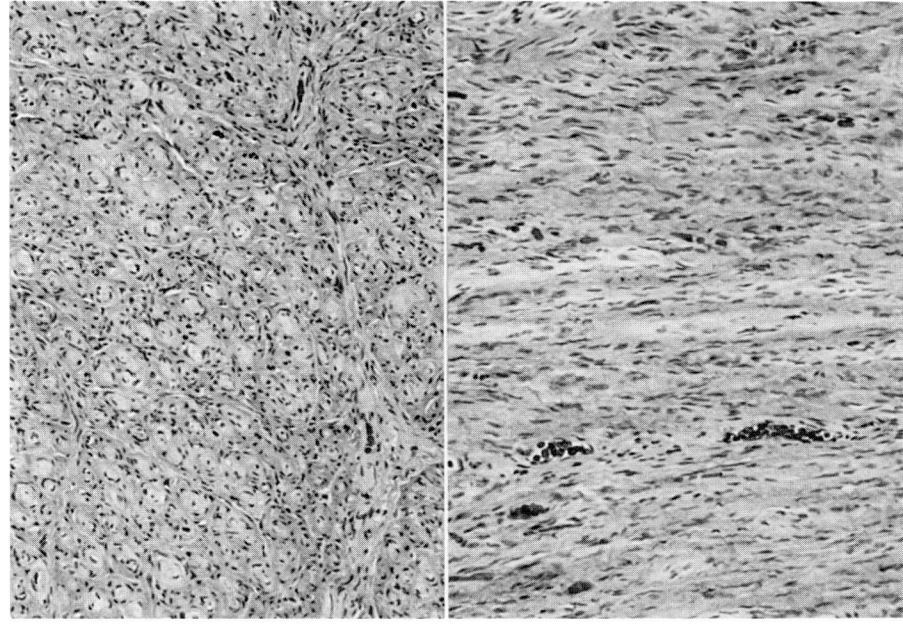

Fig. 25-38 Two different patterns of growth of perineurioma. (Courtesy Dr. J. Bilbao, Toronto.)

Wilms' tumor.[438,472] Increased serum levels of nerve growth factor have been detected in these patients.[470]

Type II (central) Recklinghausen's disease is genetically different from type I, resulting from an alteration of a gene located in chromosome 22.[467,480] It is characterized by the presence of a variety of neoplasms in the central nervous system, the most distinctive of which are bilateral acoustic schwannomas (see Chapter 28). Meningiomas, astrocytomas, and tumors of other types also occur.[453]

A small proportion of patients with type I neurofibromatosis develop MPNST. The incidence quoted ranges between 5% and 13%.[451,471] The malignant tumors arise almost always in *large* nerve trunks of the neck or extremities. For practical purposes, peripheral superficial neurofibromas never become malignant, and the only reasons for surgical removal are size and unsightliness (Fig. 25-37). An increased incidence of nonlymphatic leukemia seems to exist in patients with type I Recklinghausen's disease.[447]

Perineurioma

Benign tumors of the peripheral nerve composed predominantly or exclusively of perineurial cells have been described.[493] Microscopically, they are composed of extremely elongated cells arranged in parallel bundles, the appearance being not too dissimilar from that of neurofibroma or pacinian neurofibroma (Fig. 25-38). Some cases have a storiform pattern of growth and may correspond to the former *storiform perineurial fibromas*.[488] The diagnosis of perineurioma should be suspected in myxoid lesions of soft tissue in which a storiform or fascicular pattern of growth is evident.[489,494] It is unclear whether so-called *localized hypertrophic neuropathy* is a non-neoplastic condition or another morphologic manifestation of perineurioma.[485,492]

Ultrastructurally, perineurioma is characterized by non-branching, thin cytoplasmic processes coated by an external lamina and joined at their ends by a tight junction, few organelles, actin and vimentin filaments, and numerous pinocytotic vesicles[486,487,489] (Fig. 25-39). Immunohistochemically, the tumor cells are positive for epithelial membrane antigen and negative for S-100 protein, recapitulating the profile of normal perineurial cells.[484,490,491] Abnormalities of chromosome 22 have been found in some of the cases.[485a]

Nerve sheath myxoma

This controversial benign tumor of peripheral nerves can occur in the skin, soft tissues, or an intraspinal location.[500] It has a gross and microscopic appearance reminiscent of myxoma, except for the presence of plumper, epithelial-like cells and a distinct fascicular or plexiform arrangement; the latter feature is sometimes so pronounced that some authors have suggested the less committal designation of *plexiform myxoma*[495,501] (Fig. 25-40). It seems likely that nerve sheath myxoma and the cutaneous tumor described as *neurothekeoma*[498] are closely related, if not identical (see Chapter 4). As mentioned in the previous section, the differential diagnosis includes perineurioma (which can show prominent myxoid features and a fascicular or storiform pattern of growth) and myxoid neurofibroma (which is immunoreactive for S-100 protein).[496,497,499]

Malignant peripheral nerve tumor (MPNST)

Malignant peripheral nerve tumor (MPNST) is the currently preferred term for the neoplasm also known as malignant schwannoma, *neurogenic sarcoma*, and *neurofibrosarcoma*.[527] About half of these tumors arise de novo, and the other half from nerves involved by neurofibromas as part of

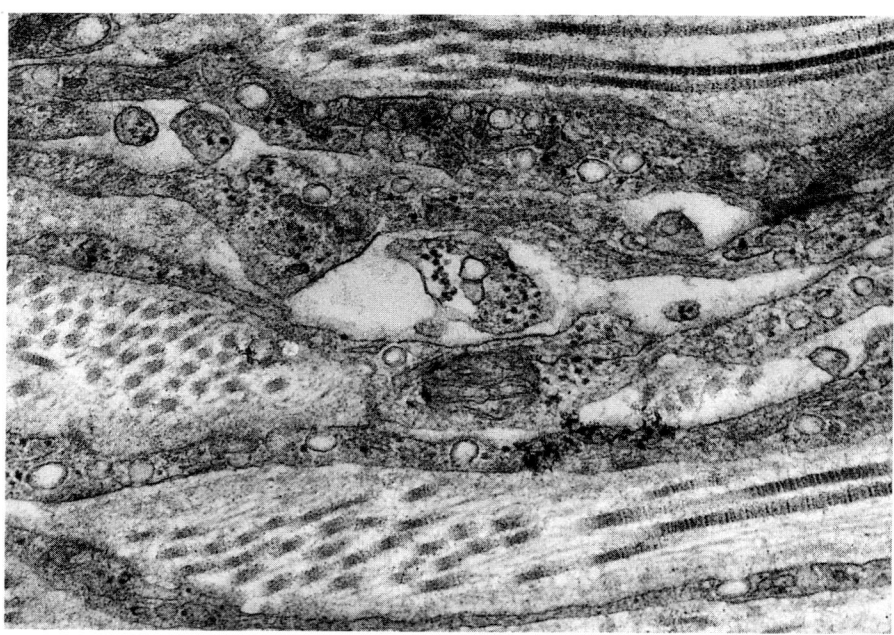

Fig. 25-39 Electron microscopic appearance of perineurioma. Thin perineurial cell cytoplasmic processes with prominent pinocytotic vesicles. The processes are coated by a continuous basal lamina. (×42,000.) (Courtesy Dr. Robert A. Erlandson, Memorial Sloan-Kettering Cancer Center.)

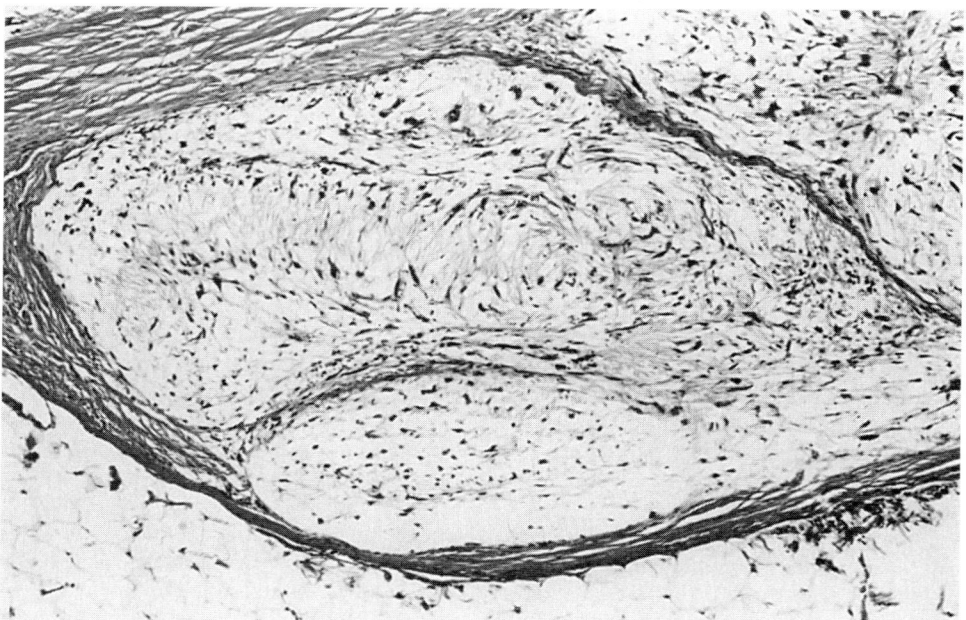

Fig. 25-40 Nerve sheath myxoma. Distinctly fascicular pattern of growth distinguishes this lesion from other myxoid neoplasms.

type I Recklinghausen's disease. Some have occurred in areas of previous irradiation,[520,547] and a few have originated from the Schwann's cell–like (satellite cell) component of ganglioneuroma.[504,524,526,550] The development of MPNST in Recklinghausen's disease has been found to be associated with chromosome 17p deletions and p53 gene mutations.[544]

Because of its difficult microscopic recognition, errors are often made, more often than not by diagnosing MPNST as some other type of soft tissue sarcoma. There are two circumstances in which the diagnosis of MPNST should be the primary consideration in the presence of a malignant tumor of soft tissues composed of spindle cells: (1) when the tumor

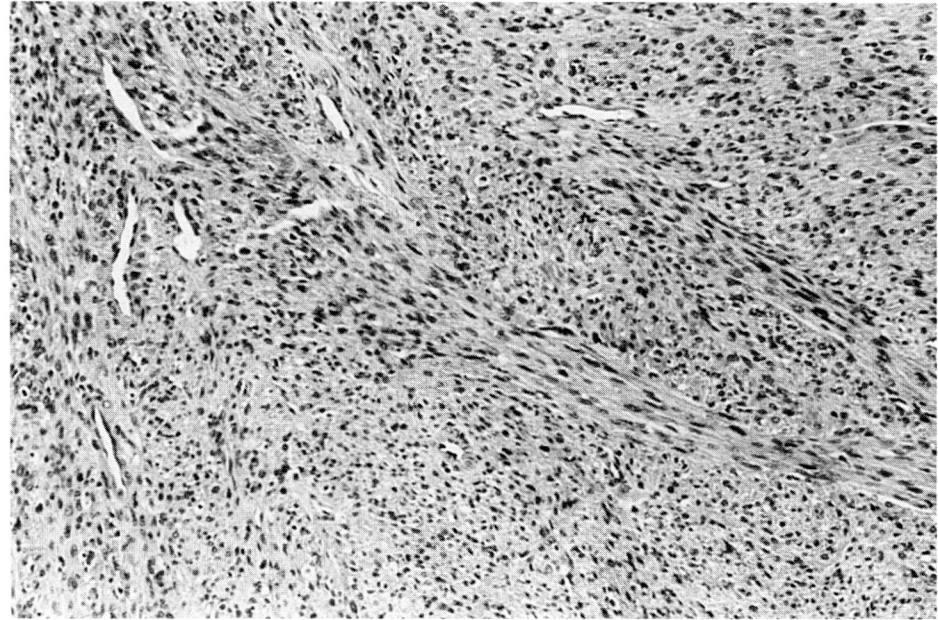

Fig. 25-41 Malignant peripheral nerve tumor (MPNST). Features suggestive of diagnosis are distinctly fascicular arrangement of tumor cells, hypercellular but monomorphic appearance, and focally well-developed vascular pattern.

develops in a patient with type I Recklinghausen's disease or (2) when the tumor is obviously arising within the anatomic compartment of a major nerve or in continuity with a neurofibroma.[513] In the absence of these circumstances the light microscopic diagnosis of MPNST is usually only presumptive and requires corroboration with special techniques. It is true that in some tumors, features suggestive of nerve sheath origin can be identified, such as serpentine cells, arrangement in palisades or whorls, large gaping vascular spaces, perivascular collections of plumper tumor cells and geographic areas of necrosis with tumor palisading at the edges, but none of these features is pathognomonic[530] (Figs. 25-41 to 25-43). In most areas the appearance is that of an extremely cellular spindle-cell neoplasm. Mitoses are usually in abundance. Although most tumors are quite monomorphic, some can be extremely bizarre. At the light microscopic level the latter can simulate the appearance of a pleomorphic liposarcoma or malignant fibrous histiocytoma very closely and may be identified as neural only on ultrastructural examination.[532] Metaplastic tissues such as cartilage, bone, or muscle are present in about 15% of the cases.[521,522] The most spectacular variant is characterized by the presence of well-developed skeletal muscle and has been dignified by the term *malignant triton tumor*.[506,517,567] Areas of recognizable MPNST should be present to make such a diagnosis in these metaplastic tumors; otherwise a diagnosis corresponding to the morphologic appearance of the tumor—such as angiosarcoma of peripheral nerve—is appropriate even if the patient has Recklinghausen's disease.[507,545]

In some MPNST, part or most of the tumor is composed of plump cells with polygonal acidophilic cytoplasm and an

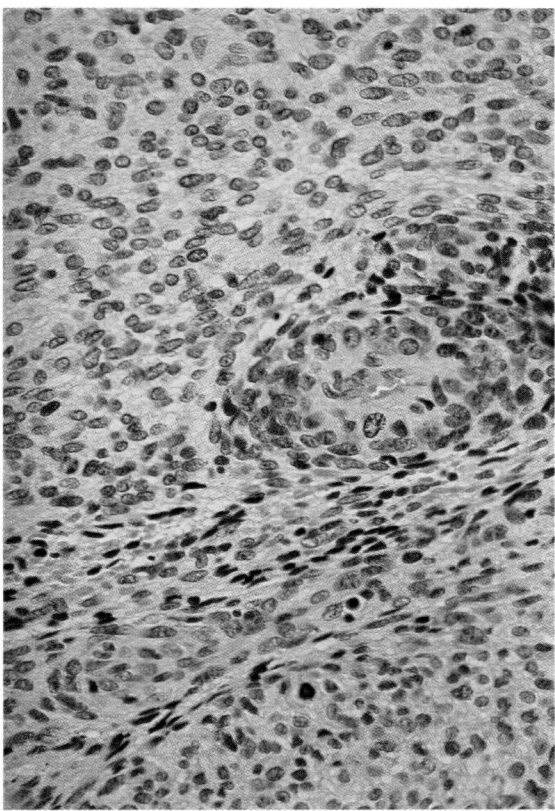

Fig. 25-42 Malignant peripheral nerve sheath tumor. The plump and almost epithelioid appearance of the cells surrounding the vessels is a common feature in this tumor type.

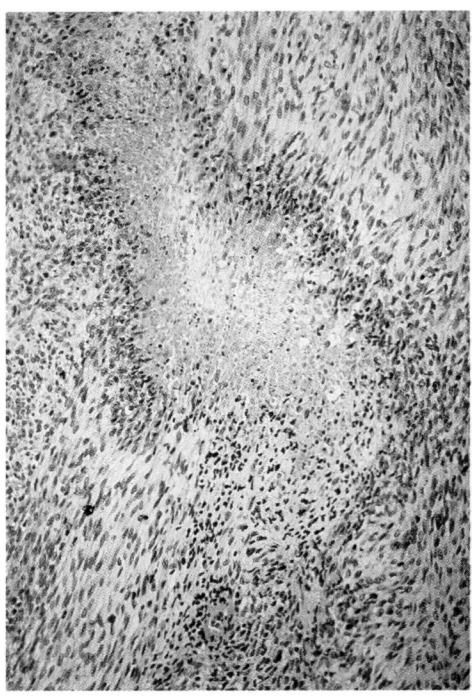

Fig. 25-43 Malignant peripheral nerve sheath tumor. The area of necrosis with irregular borders and palisading at the edges is similar to that seen in glioblastoma multiforme.

epithelioid-like appearance; these are designated as *epithelioid malignant schwannomas*[502,518,538,546] (Figs. 25-45 and 25-46). One such case exhibited squamous differentiation.[503] Epithelioid MPNST of the skin may be associated with HMB-45 immunoreactivity and be indistinguishable from some neurotropic/spindle-cell/desmoplastic forms of malignant melanoma.[553,556] Interestingly, most of the MPNST that have arisen from malignant transformation of schwannomas have been of the epithelioid type.[549,551,569] Occasionally, MPNST show foci of *glandular differentiation,* with or without mucin production and with positivity for keratin, EMA, CEA, chromogranin, somatostatin, serotonin, and some peptide hormones[511,515,566,568]; it has been suggested that these formations represent foci of ependymal or neuroendocrine differentiation, but this view has been contested.[516,561] Glands and skeletal muscle can coexist in the same tumor.[552] In general, any peripheral nerve tumor should be suspected of being malignant if it contains epithelial glandular structures, no matter how well differentiated they are. Melanin can be present in the tumor cells, particularly if the tumor arises from spinal nerve roots; the distinction between melanocytic MPNST and primary malignant melanoma of nerves is difficult to make and has little practical significance.[537]

The belief that these MPNST originate in Schwann's cells is largely based on circumstantial evidence, the reasoning being that if these tumors represent the malignant counterpart of neurofibromas and the latter arise primarily from Schwann's cells, then the former also must have that origin. Some of the microscopic features just mentioned and tissue culture studies[555] favor this hypothesis, which is also supported by the electron microscope description of infoldings

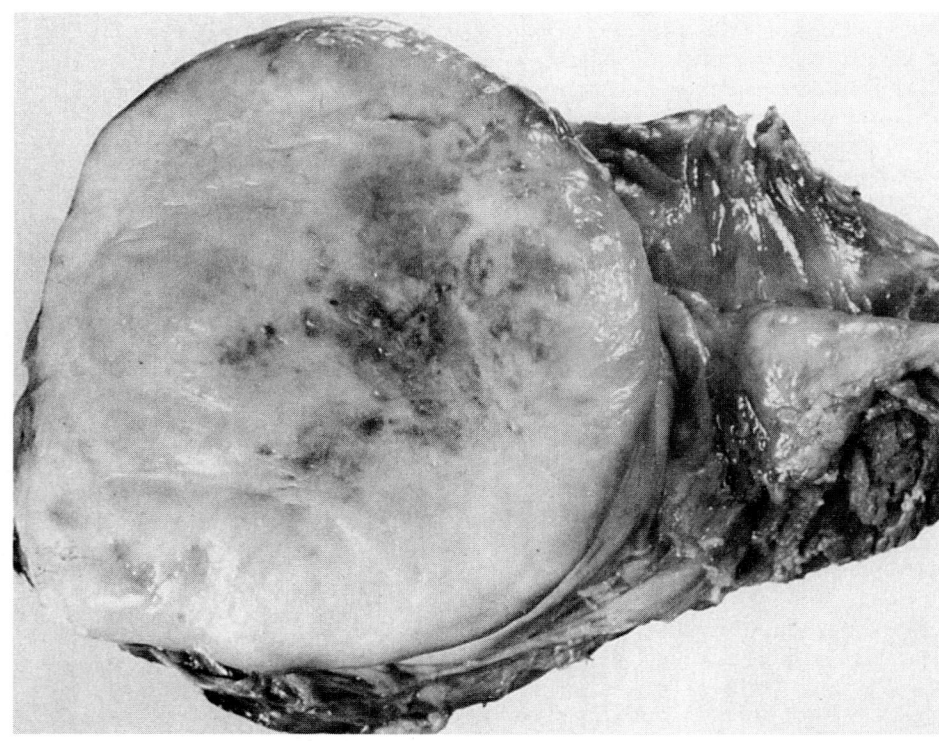

Fig. 25-44 MPNST removed from flank of 16-year-old girl with florid Recklinghausen's disease.

of the cell membrane with lamellar configuration, presence of discontinuous basal lamina material, conspicuous intercellular junctions, and occasional dense-core granules.* Further support comes from the fact that immunohistochemically the tumor cells show reactivity for Schwann's cell markers, such as S-100 protein and Leu7, in about half of the cases,[529,536,563,565] the former being particularly prominent in neurofibroma-like areas and in foci of melanocytic differentiation.[541] However, some MPNST show no discernible schwannian features at any level and may actually exhibit features suggestive of perineurial or fibroblastic nature.[523,533,534] Because of this fact, a histogenetically noncommittal term, such as MPNST, seems preferable to the time-honored malignant schwannoma.

A large majority of MPNST arise in adults, but they have also been recorded in children.[542,543,548] The most common locations are the neck, forearm, lower leg, and buttock.[508,535] Grossly, the finding of a large mass producing fusiform enlargement of a major nerve, such as the sciatic nerve, is characteristic[558] (Fig. 25-44 and Plate XIX-D). Most MPNST are deep-seated, but they can occur in the subcutis or even in the skin.[512,525]

The clinical evolution is that of a highly malignant neoplasm, despite the relatively slow growth rate of some cases.[505,514,528,554,562] Local recurrence (often in the cut nerve ends) and distant metastases are frequent.[514,564] In general, there is little correlation between microscopic grading and prognosis.[522,559] However, a plexiform variant of MPNST occurring in a superficial location in children has been associated with a better prognosis.[543]

———————
*References 509, 510, 519, 531, 555, 557, 560.

Occasionally, malignant tumors are found in major peripheral nerves or elsewhere in the soft tissue, having a light and electron microscopic appearance suggestive of primitive neuroectodermal origin. Sometimes these features are seen together with areas of typical MPNST and sometimes in a pure form.[539,540] The latter form, known as peripheral neuroepithelioma, peripheral or adult neuroblastoma, or primitive neuroectodermal tumor (PNET), is discussed on p. 2105. The rare occurrence of neuroblastoma-like areas in benign schwannoma has already been mentioned (see p. 2043).

Other tumors of peripheral nerves

In addition to benign and malignant tumors composed of the constitutive cells of peripheral nerves, these structures are occasionally involved in a selective fashion by mesenchymal or other neoplasms. Thus isolated cases of hemangioma, lipoma, angiosarcoma, and malignant lymphoma have been described.[570,572] Some of these tumors have occurred in nerves affected by neurofibroma and/or in patients with type I Recklinghausen's disease.[571]

Tumors of adipose tissue
Lipoma

Benign fatty tumors can arise in any location in which fat is normally present. The majority occur in the upper half of the body, particularly the trunk and neck, but they can occur in any other site, including the hand.[593] Most lipomas are subcutaneous, an important point in the differential diagnosis with liposarcomas, which are almost always deep-seated. However, lipomas can also occur in the deep soft tissues; these are subclassified into *intramuscular* (most common in the trunk) and *intermuscular* (most common in the anterior

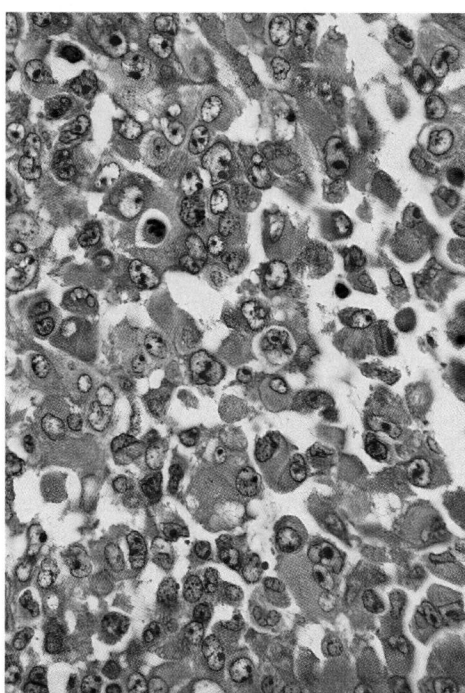

Fig. 25-45 Malignant peripheral nerve sheath tumor of epithelioid type.

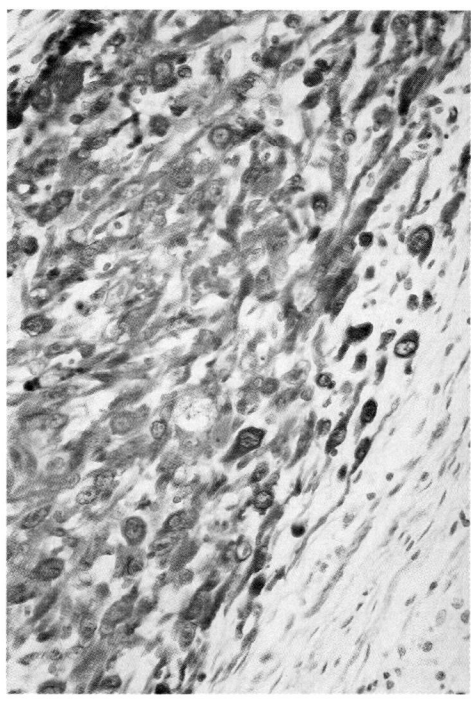

Fig. 25-46 Same case as Fig. 25-45 showing strong immunoreactivity for S-100 protein.

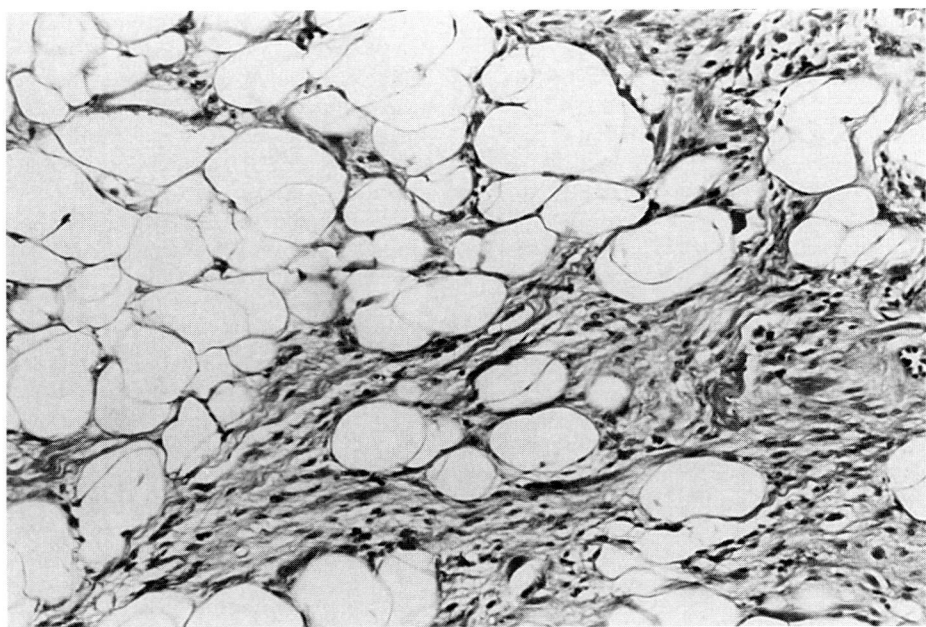

Fig. 25-47 Spindle-cell lipoma. Lobules of mature fat are entrapped by spindle-cell component associated with collagen deposition.

abdominal wall).[581] There are about 120 lipomas for every liposarcoma.[594] Most patients are in the fifth or sixth decade of life. Only rarely are children affected. Lipomas may be single or multiple. Multiple lipomas are more common in women; many are seen in a familial setting, and some occur in patients with neurofibromatosis or multiple endocrine neoplasia. In *diffuse lipomatosis,* massive enlargement of a limb may be seen as a result of diffuse proliferation of mature adipose tissue. In the familial variant of this process, lipomatosis has a symmetric distribution.[576]

Lipomas can grow to a large size; they are usually encapsulated when located in the superficial soft tissues but tend to be poorly circumscribed when arising in deeper structures.[582,589] Grossly, lipomas consist of bright yellow fat separated by fine fibrous trabeculae. Microscopically, lipomas are composed of mature adipose tissue with no cellular atypia.

Areas of fat necrosis, infarct, and calcification may be present. It is important not to confuse the histiocytes associated with fat necrosis with lipoblasts. The fact that they are often seen arranged in a circumferential fashion around a large lipid droplet (as is the case in fat necrosis at other sites) is a helpful diagnostic sign.

Ultrastructurally, only univacuolar mature adipocytes are present in typical lipomas.[588] Although the light microscopic and electron microscopic appearance of a lipoma does not differ significantly from that of normal adult fat, its lipid content as determined by biochemical extraction and the activity of lipoprotein lipase is different.[595,598]

Morphologic variations that lipomas may exhibit include the following:

1 *Fibrolipoma.* This is characterized by the presence of prominent bundles of *mature* fibrous tissue traversing the fatty lobules. It should not be equated with spindle-cell lipoma (see later section).

2 *Myxolipoma.* This tumor features focally well-developed myxoid changes. It should not be overdiagnosed as myxoid liposarcoma.

3 *Chondroid lipoma.* This recently described variant is usually deep-seated. It is characterized by a component of eosinophilic and vacuolated cells containing glycogen and lipid that resembles brown fat cells, lipoblasts, and chondroblasts.[592] These cells are immunoreactive for vimentin, S-100 protein, and CD68; curiously, some are also positive for keratin.[589a,592] Lipomas may also show foci of mature metaplastic cartilage and bone.[587]

4 *Myolipoma.* This tumor is characterized by an admixture in variable proportions of mature adipose tissue and bundles of well-differentiated smooth muscle.[591]

5 *Spindle cell lipoma.* This is a benign fatty tumor characteristically located in the regions of the shoulder and posterior neck of adults, but it has also been found in many other locations, including the limbs, face, oral cavity, trunk, and anus.[580,596] It is composed of an admixture of mature lipocytes and uniform spindle cells set in a mucinous and fibrous background[578] (Fig. 25-47). Features that assist in distinguishing it from myxoid liposarcoma include the absence of lipoblasts and of a prominent plexiform vascular pattern, the presence of thick collagen bundles, and the great uniformity of the proliferating spindle cells. In some instances the appearance of irregular branching spaces with villiform projections results in a pseudoangiomatous appearance.[583] Ultrastructurally, spindle-cell lipomas are composed of a mixture of spindle mesenchymal cells and mature lipocytes.[574]

6 *Pleomorphic lipoma.* This is a lipoma containing hyperchromatic multinucleated ("floret-like") tumor cells

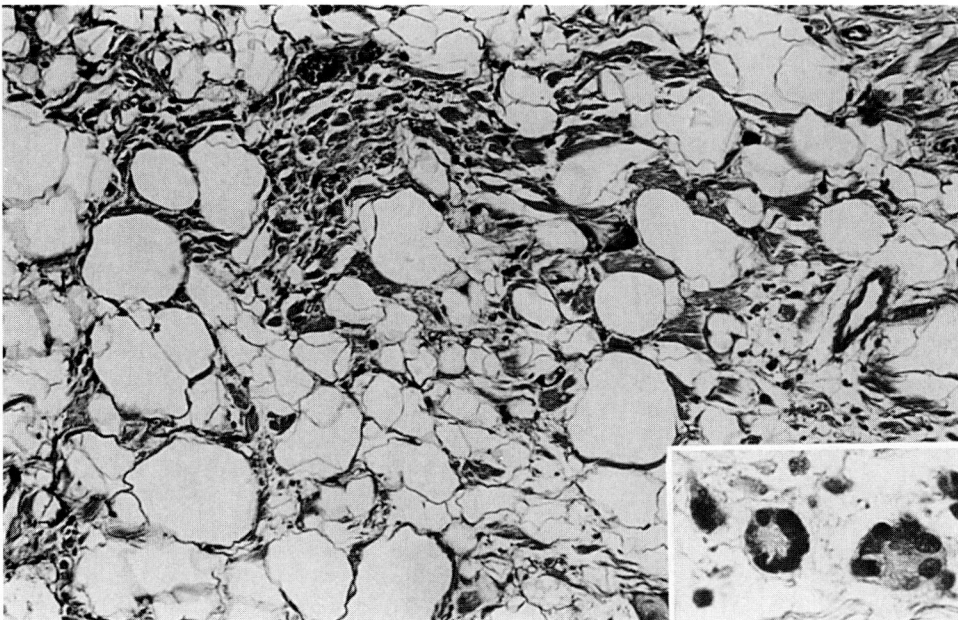

Fig. 25-48 Pleomorphic lipoma. Most of tissue is composed of mature fat, but scattered cells with atypical nuclei are present. **Inset** shows characteristic floret-like cells seen in this lesion.

within the fibrous septa traversing the neoplasm (Fig. 25-48). As for spindle-cell lipoma, its most common location is the shoulder and posterior neck region.[597] We have also seen them in the dermis and beneath mucosal membranes. The most difficult differential diagnosis is with a sclerosing form of well-differentiated liposarcoma (atypical lipomatous tumor); the relative proportion of floret-type giant cells and lipoblasts is the most important distinguishing feature.[573]

7 *Angiolipoma.* These are well-circumscribed small tumors occurring shortly after puberty. They are often painful and characteristically multiple. They are located in the subcutis, most commonly on the trunk or extremities. Vascularity often is limited to a band of tissue on the periphery of the neoplasm. Hyaline thrombi are common and constitute an important diagnostic sign[575] (Fig. 25-49). Angiolipomas in which the vascular component predominates (cellular angiolipomas) can be confused with Kaposi's sarcoma or angiosarcoma.[586] The pain correlates well with the degree of vascularity.[585]

So-called *infiltrating angiolipomas* are unrelated to the lesion just described; Enzinger[577] believes that they probably represent intramuscular large-vessel hemangiomas in which portions of the affected muscle tissue have been replaced by fat.

• • •

Cytogenetically, 80% of solitary lipomas exhibit chromosomal aberrations affecting mainly 12q, 6p, and 13q. In contrast with atypical lipomatous tumors, marker ring or giant chromosomes are extremely rare. Multiple lipomas usually exhibit a normal karyotype. Nearly all spindle-cell and pleomorphic lipomas have aberrations of 16q, this finding sup-

porting the close link between these two tumor types and the fact that they are distinct from atypical lipomatous tumors.[579,584,590]

The gene involved in chromosome region 12q15 of lipoma cells is said to be HMGI-C; this gene encodes an "architectural" transcription factor.[589b]

Lipoblastoma/lipoblastomasis

Lipoblastoma/lipoblastomasis affects infants and young children almost exclusively.[603-605] It commonly involves the proximal portion of the lower and upper extremities. Grossly, the lesion is soft and lobulated. It is subdivided into (benign) lipoblastoma (sometimes also designated as embryonal or fetal lipoma) when well circumscribed and lipoblastomatosis when deep-seated and ill-defined. Microscopically, it closely resembles fetal fat[601] (Fig. 25-50). It has often been confused with myxoid liposarcoma because of the presence of lipoblasts, a plexiform vascular pattern, and an abundant myxoid stroma. Its ultrastructural appearance is also very similar to that of myxoid liposarcoma.[599] It is distinguished from the latter by virtue of the young age of the patient, distinct lobulation, and absence of giant cells or pleomorphic nuclei.[600,604] Cytogenetically, lipoblastoma/lipoblastomasis is often associated with rearrangements of 8q.[602] The clinical course is benign. In the series of Chung and Enzinger,[600] the recurrence rate was 14% and was attributed to incomplete removal of the tumor.

Hibernoma

Hibernoma is a rare benign neoplasm occurring usually in the intercapsular region and in the axilla but also in the mediastinum and retroperitoneum.[611] Its cut surface has a typical brown color, and its microscopic pattern is characteristic—an organoid arrangement of large cells with cen-

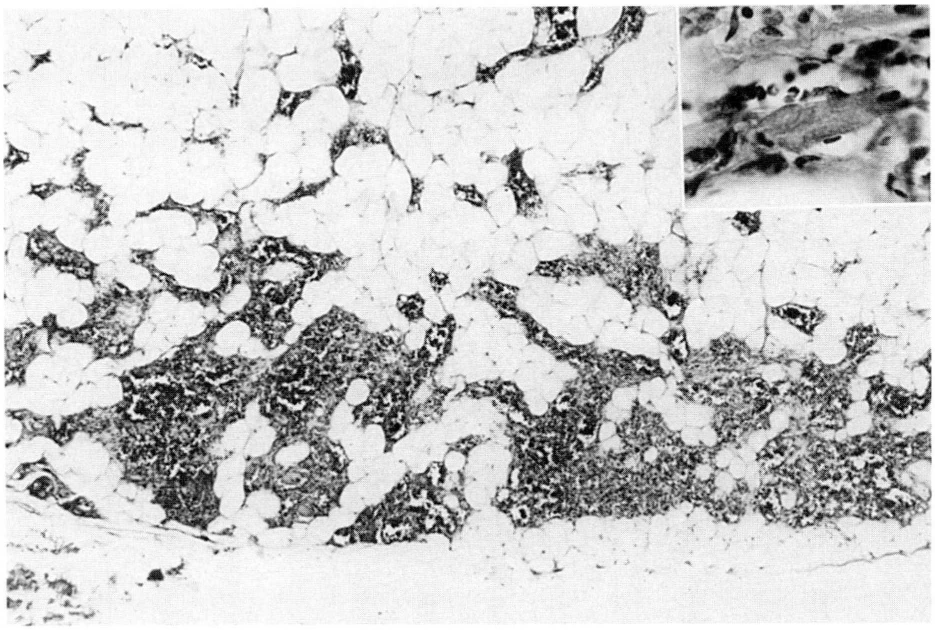

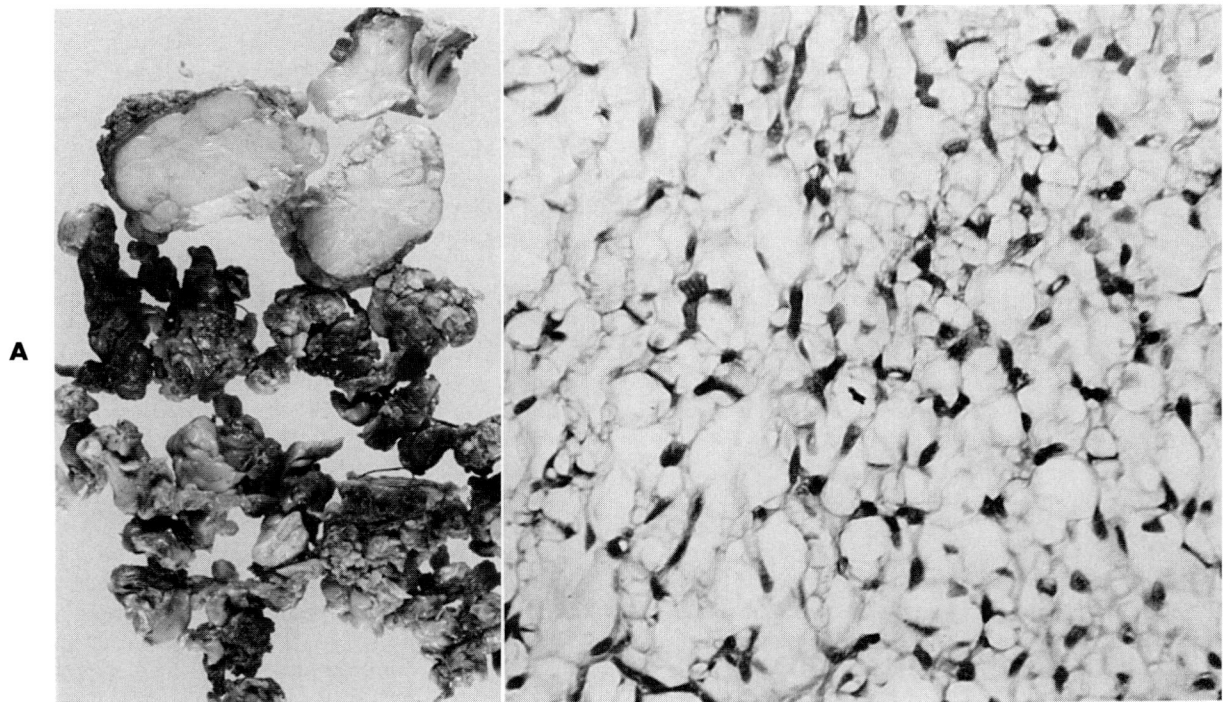

Fig. 25-49 Angiolipoma. Vascular component is particularly prominent at periphery of tumor. **Inset** shows hyaline thrombi that are a constant finding in this lesion.

Fig. 25-50 Lipoblastomatosis. **A,** Gross appearance. Note multinodular and ill-defined appearance. **B,** Microscopic appearance, which closely simulates myxoid liposarcoma. On low power it had distinctly lobular configuration. (**A** Courtesy Dr. J. Costa, Lausanne, Switzerland.)

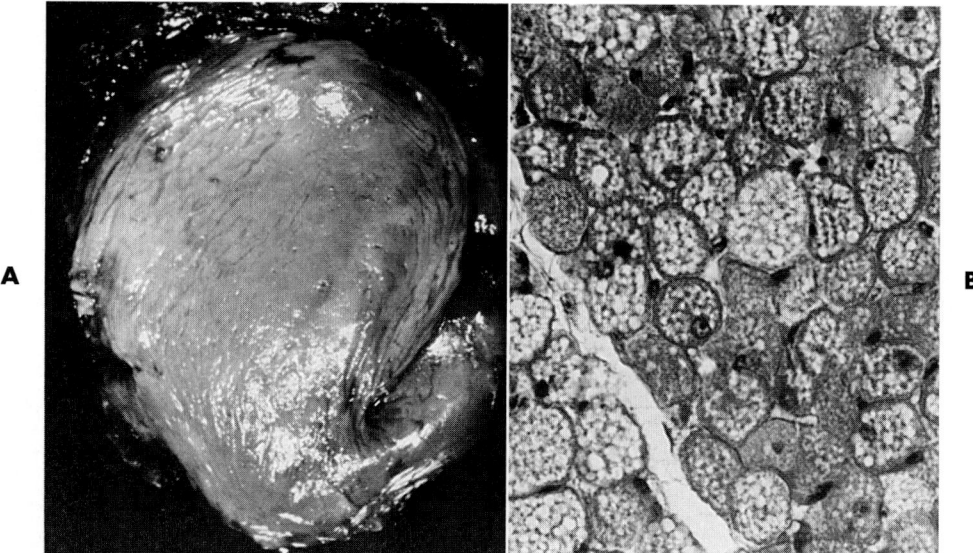

Fig. 25-51 Hibernoma. **A,** Gross appearance. Tumor is well circumscribed and has lobular configuration. In fresh state, it had distinctly brown color. **B,** Microscopic appearance. Cells have abundant, strikingly vacuolated cytoplasm.

trally located nucleus and a cytoplasm filled with many small vacuoles that stain for neutral fat (Fig. 25-51). Cytogenetically, it is often associated with aberrations of 11q.[608]

This tumor has received its name because it resembles the brown fat of the hibernating glands of animals,[607] a similarity that is maintained at the electron microscopic level.[609,610,613] Interestingly, endocrine-like activity resembling that of adrenal cortical tissue has been detected in one case.[606] Sometimes the features of hibernoma are seen mixed with those of ordinary lipoma. Malignant soft tissue tumors in which many of the tumor cells have features of brown fat have been seen; they should be regarded as a morphologic variant of liposarcoma. Interestingly, hibernomas of the interscapular region develop regularly in transgenic mice containing the adipocyte-specific regulatory region from the adipocyte P2 gene linked to the simian virus 40 transforming genes.[612]

Liposarcoma

Liposarcoma is the second most frequent soft tissue sarcoma in adults.[626] Indubitable cases of liposarcoma have also been observed in adolescents and children.[620,639,645,652] However, most cases so diagnosed in this age group (particularly in the past) have been in reality examples of lipoblastomatosis or giant cell fibroblastoma.[622]

Liposarcomas are usually large and occur most frequently in the lower extremities (popliteal fossa and medial thigh); retroperitoneal, perirenal, and mesenteric region; and shoulder area.[649] Grossly, they are well circumscribed but not encapsulated[655] (Fig. 25-52). They may have a mucoid, slimy surface suggestive of myxoma, a bright yellow appearance mimicking lipoma, or a surface resembling cerebral convolutions. Rarely, liposarcomas have multiple foci

of origin[614,634] and/or are associated with independent benign multiple lipomas in the same patient.

In their classic article on the subject, Enzinger and Winslow[627] divided liposarcomas into four types: myxoid, round cell, well differentiated, and pleomorphic, acknowledging the existence of mixed forms. The common morphologic denominator of liposarcoma is the *lipoblast*. This appears as a mononuclear or multinucleated cell with one or more cytoplasmic vacuoles that contain fat. The nucleus may be pushed aside by a single large vacuole, resulting in a signet ring configuration, or it may remain centrally located but exhibit small indentations by multiple small vacuoles, the appearance being similar to that of mature sebaceous cells or spongiocytes of adrenal cortex. This highly characteristic scalloped nuclear appearance can also be appreciated in specimens obtained from fine-needle aspiration.[657]

Myxoid liposarcoma, which is by far the most common type of liposarcoma, shows a marked predilection for the lower extremities, particularly the thigh. Microscopically, it has few or no mitotic figures and features proliferating lipoblasts in different stages of differentiation, a prominent anastomosing capillary network, and a mucoid matrix rich in hyaluronidase-sensitive acid mucopolysaccharides[659] (Fig. 25-53). The presence of a prominent vascular component in myxoid liposarcoma is an important feature in the differential diagnosis with myxoma. The mucoid extracellular material may accumulate in large pools, thus simulating a tumor of lymph vessel origin. Metaplastic cartilage is found in rare instances. Myxoid liposarcomas containing foci of pleomorphic or round cells (designated as "poorly differentiated myxoid type" in Stout's classification) are associated with a decrease in the survival rate.[642] Ultrastructurally, cells varying in appearance from primitive mes-

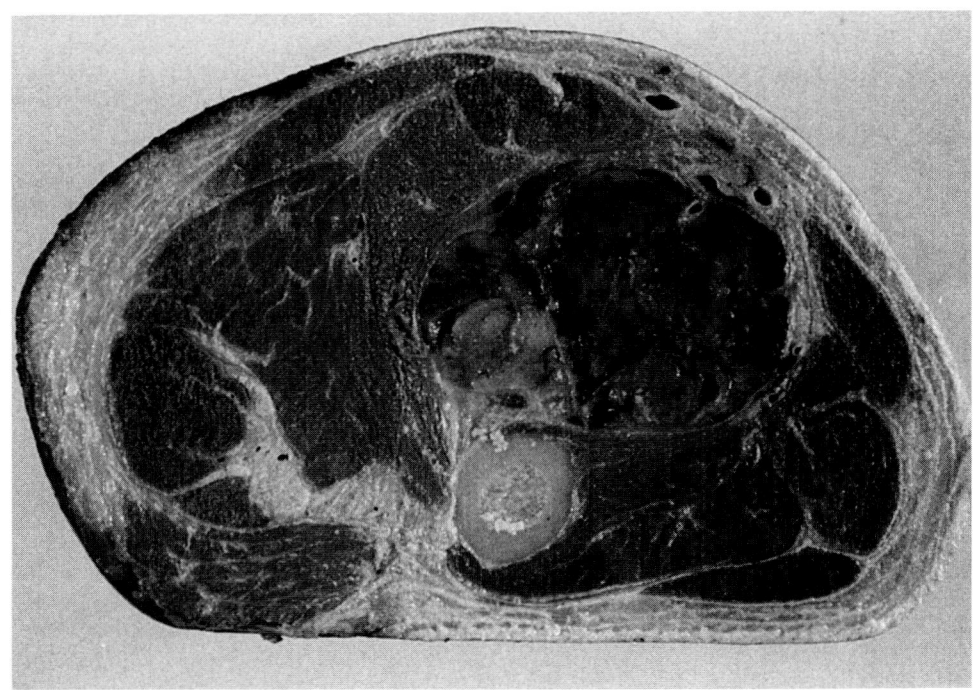

Fig. 25-52 Cross section of thigh with myxoid liposarcoma. Tumor grows in intermuscular planes and has pseudoencapsulated appearance. (Courtesy Dr. J. Costa, Lausanne, Switzerland.)

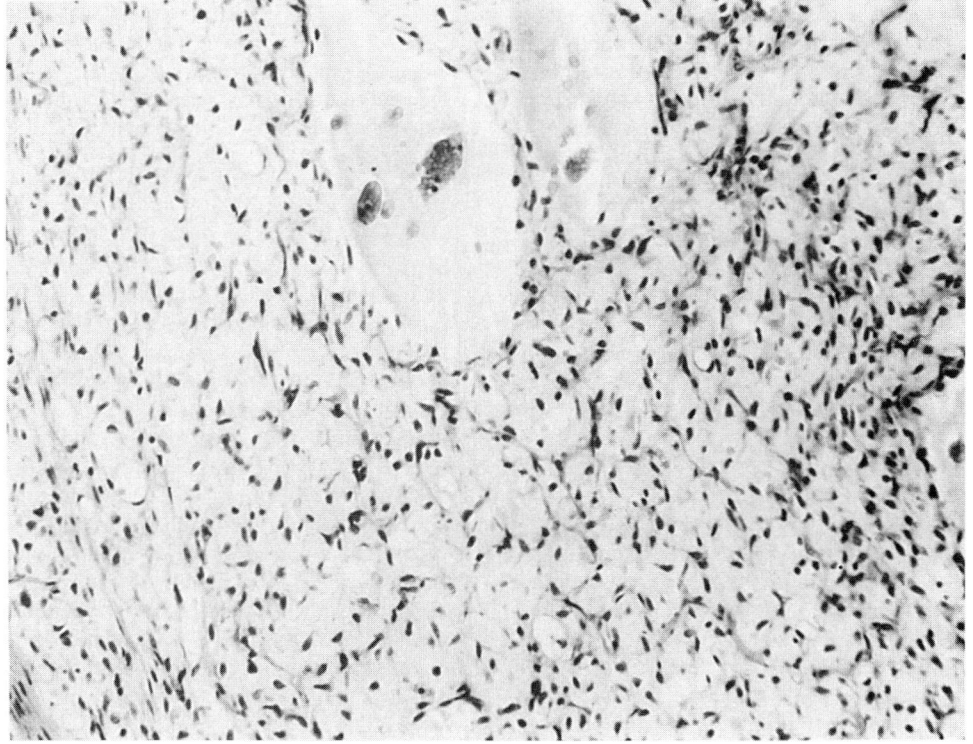

Fig. 25-53 Typical myxoid liposarcoma. Note plexiform vascular pattern and abundant myxoid extracellular material, with formation of large mucoid pools.

enchymal cells to typical multivacuolated and univacuolated lipoblasts are seen.[617,618,650] The abundant capillaries are intimately related to all of these various cell types in a manner analogous to that of developing fetal adipose tissue.[617,643,644]

Cytogenetically, myxoid liposarcoma is characterized by the reciprocal translocation t (12;16) (q 13; p 11), which results in the rearrangement of the transcription factor gene CHOP. The latter is thought to be involved in adipocyte differentiation.[615,624,633,635,654]

In the *round cell type* the tumor cells are small and have a distinctly acidophilic cytoplasm. The presence among them of scattered lipoblasts establishes the diagnosis. Mitoses are more common than in the myxoid form, but the vascular network is less prominent. Pseudoglandular arrangement of the tumor cells is frequent.

It has been pointed out that myxoid liposarcoma can be accompanied by a varying number of round cells and that so-called round cell liposarcoma is the extreme expression of this phenomenon (i.e., a poorly differentiated subtype of myxoid liposarcoma) rather than a specific type of liposarcoma. The commonality of chromosomal aberrations between myxoid and round cell liposarcoma strongly supports this interpretation.[633]

Well-differentiated liposarcoma resembles ordinary lipoma grossly (Plate XIX-E). It also resembles it on low-power examination, but closer inspection shows characteristic tumor cells with large, deep-staining nuclei (Figs. 25-54 and 25-55). The atypical cells may concentrate on the fibrous strands that traverse the adipose tissue lobules (sclerosing subtype) or be scattered among the mature adipocytes (lipoma-like subtype). Since this is nearly always a non-metastasizing neoplasm, there is a question as to whether the designation of *liposarcoma* is justified for it. The alternative terms **atypical lipoma** and **atypical lipomatous tumor**

(which we prefer) have been suggested for this group of tumors.[616,619,629,632,640] The behavior of these atypical lipomatous tumors is substantially different depending on their location.[646] Those situated in the somatic soft tissues may recur, but they practically never result in distant metastases

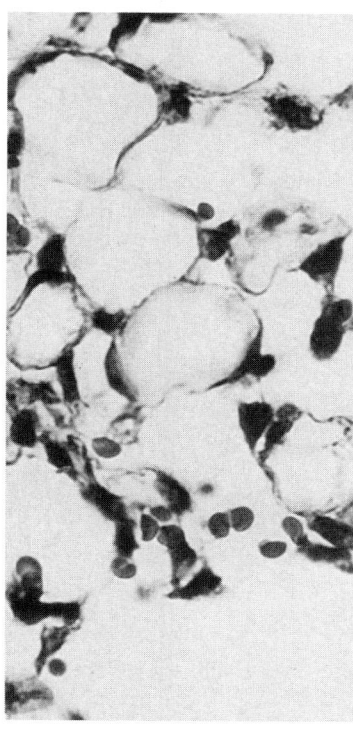

Fig. 25-54 Well-differentiated liposarcoma in which individual nuclei have been compressed to crescentic shape.

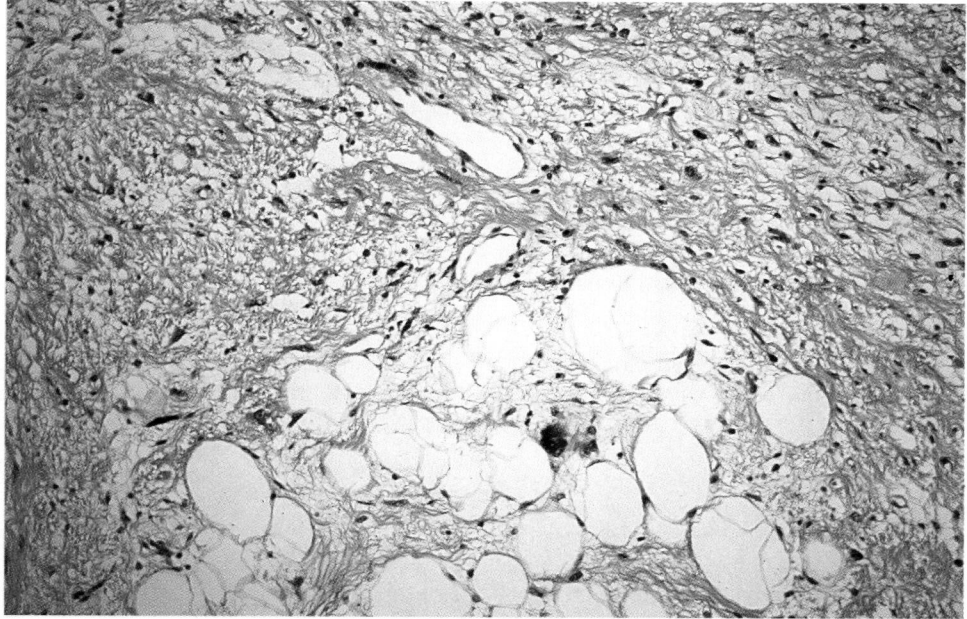

Fig. 25-55 Low-power microscopic view of an atypical lipomatous tumor with prominent sclerosing pattern. This corresponds to the well-differentiated liposarcoma, sclerosing type, of other classification schemes.

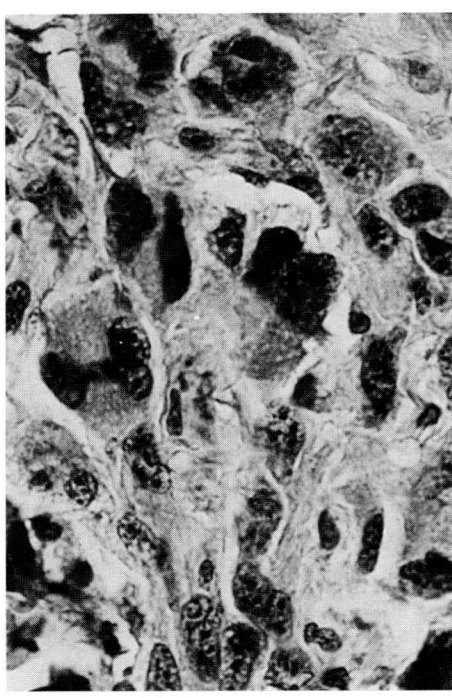

Fig. 25-56 Pleomorphic liposarcoma with innumerable tumor giant cells and great pleomorphism.

or tumor-related deaths; those originating in the retroperitoneum have a very high incidence of recurrence (some of these recurrences having a "dedifferentiated" appearance; see subsequent discussion), and some of the patients die as a result. In view of these findings and based on pragmatic rather than conceptual criteria, Azumi et al.[616] have proposed to use the term *atypical lipoma* for the former and *well-differentiated liposarcoma* for the latter. As already stated, we prefer instead to designate the entire group as **atypical lipomatous tumor,** followed by a statement as to the predicted natural history based on the size and location of the mass.

Occasionally, smooth muscle bundles are seen in these neoplasms, a phenomenon akin to that already mentioned in connection with lipomas.[630] Dei Tos et al.[625] have described a variant of atypical lipomatous tumor characterized by a population of relatively bland spindle cells arrayed in fascicles and whorls, set in a variably myxoid stroma. Most of these tumors (which they named *spindle-cell liposarcomas*) were located in the subcutaneous tissue of the shoulder girdle or upper limbs and therefore appeared different from liposarcomas that had been described as fibroblastic (or even as spindle cell) in the past.

Cytogenetically, close to 80% of the atypical lipomatous tumors (including dedifferentiated examples) show marker ring and giant chromosomes, in stark contrast to lipomas of either ordinary or spindle/pleomorphic type.[633]

The *pleomorphic type* of liposarcoma is highly undifferentiated. It has many tumor giant cells, some of which have the features of lipoblasts (Fig. 25-56). Sometimes a heavy neutrophilic infiltrate is present, some of the neutrophils being located within the cytoplasm of the multinucleated giant cells. Tumors with this appearance have been called *inflammatory liposarcomas*[653] (Fig. 25-58). The differential diagnosis includes malignant fibrous histiocytoma and pleomorphic rhabdomyosarcoma. Fat stains are of little help in the diagnosis of liposarcoma; fat may be totally lacking in some forms of this tumor and may be present in a host of soft tissue neoplasms other than liposarcoma. S-100 protein is focally but consistently found immunohistochemically in the cells of both benign and malignant adipose tissue tumors.[623,636] Benign lesions sometimes confused with liposarcoma are intramuscular myxoma, lipoblastoma/lipoblastosis, spindle-cell and pleomorphic lipoma, inflamed lipoma, localized lipoatrophy (such as that seen at sites of insulin injections), and lipogranuloma (such as the one resulting from injection of liquid silicone). In general, the diagnosis of liposarcoma should be questioned for any tumor seen in the pediatric age group or any tumor that is small, superficial, or embedded within a major muscle. Although true liposarcomas can be found in the neck,[641,651] the diagnostic features of malignancy need to be assessed very critically because of the high frequency with which lesions that simulate liposarcoma occur in this location.

Tumor size and histologic subtype are important prognostic determinators.[648] Both the myxoid and the well-differentiated types tend to recur locally rather than to metastasize.[621] In contrast the round cell and pleomorphic types often give rise to widespread metastases. In the series of Enzinger and Winslow[627] the 5-year survival rate of patients with myxoid and well-differentiated forms exceeded 70%, whereas in the round cell and pleomorphic varieties it was only 18% (Fig. 25-57).

The microscopic appearance of recurrent or metastatic liposarcoma can depart greatly from that of the original tumor; the term **dedifferentiated liposarcoma** has been proposed for the emergence of a nonlipogenic component within an atypical lipomatous tumor (but not in a myxoid liposarcoma). The dedifferentiated component may already be present at the time of the original excision but is much more commonly seen in the recurrent or metastatic foci. It is much more common in retroperitoneal neoplasms, but it has also been documented in tumors of the extremities.[647] Microscopically, the dedifferentiated component is usually high grade, with an appearance reminiscent of fibrosarcoma or malignant fibrous histiocytoma, with or without myxoid features.[628,638,653,656,658] Heterologous elements, such as blood vessels or skeletal muscle, may be present[631]; these are accompanied by their respective immunohistochemical markers.[637] Occasionally, the dedifferentiated component appears in the form of a discontinuous micronodular pattern throughout the tumor.[647] Tumor progression is accompanied by overexpression of p53.[635a]

Tumors and tumorlike conditions of blood and lymph vessels

Hemangioma

Hemangiomas occupy a gray zone between hamartomatous malformations and true neoplasms. They are frequently designated and regarded as tumors because of their usually localized nature and mass effect. Although clearly benign, they can become very large and unsightly and can even be fatal if they affect vital structures. They almost never

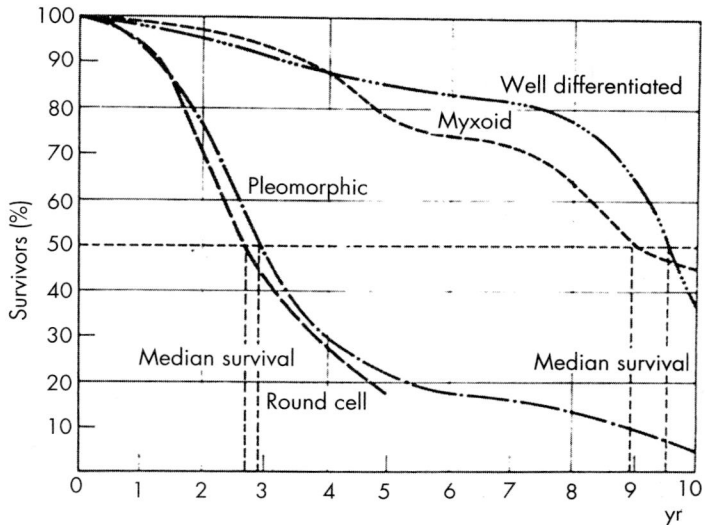

Fig. 25-57 Survival rates according to histologic types in liposarcoma of retroperitoneum and lower extremity. (From Enzinger FM, Winslow DJ: Liposarcoma. A study of 103 cases. Virchows Arch [A] **355:**367-388, 1962.)

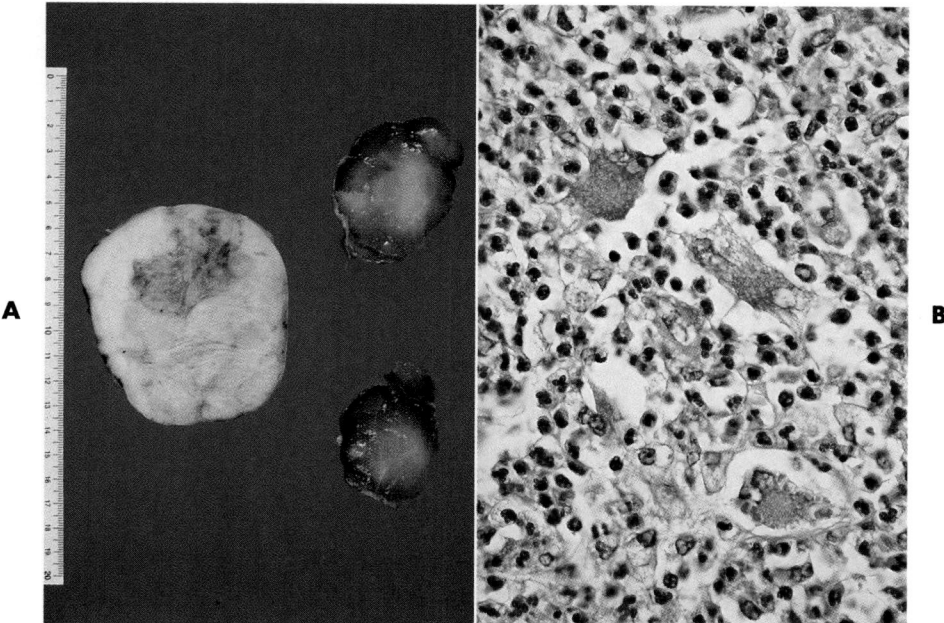

Fig. 25-58 Inflammatory liposarcoma. **A,** Gross appearance. The inflammatory liposarcoma is represented by the larger mass, whereas the others were atypical lipomatous tumors. All three masses were located in the retroperitoneum. **B,** Microscopic appearance showing highly pleomorphic tumor cells surrounded by numerous neutrophils.

become malignant. A high percentage occur in children, and many are already present at birth.[665,679] Over half of the cases are in the head and neck area; they can also occur in the trunk or extremities. Most hemangiomas are solitary; when multiple (with or without associated lesions in internal organs) or affecting a large segment of the body, the condition is known as *(multifocal) angiomatosis.*[671,682]

Hemangiomas have been classified according to their clinical appearance and the caliber of vessel involved. A close correlation exists between these two parameters.

Capillary hemangiomas are made up of small vessels of capillary caliber and can occur in any organ. The most distinctive and common variant of this type is known as *benign hemangioendothelioma* or *juvenile* or *hyperplastic hemangioma.* Its most common location is the skin, where it appears as an elevated nodule with an intense crimson color (Figs. 25-59 and 25-60). Such a hemangioma is traditionally known to dermatologists as a strawberry hemangioma. It is usually present at birth or appears during the first month and enlarges rapidly during the first few months of life, only to

stop growing when the child is about 6 months old. Subsequently, it becomes flaccid, pale blue, and covered with tiny wrinkles, and it eventually disappears completely.[668,677,678]

Other locations for this lesion include the salivary gland and breast. Microscopically, the lesion exhibits a vaguely lobular configuration on low-power examination. Masses of closely packed spindle cells are seen with neoformed spaces that contain little blood (Fig. 25-61). Ultrastructurally and immunohistochemically, most of the cells are endothelial, but there is also a component of pericytes and fibroblasts.[669,672,685,686,690] Mitotic figures are usually present and can be numerous. At the periphery, the tumor may be seen to invade subcutaneous tissue or skeletal muscle. Perineurial involvement has also been observed.[663a,680] Mast cells may be numerous.[667] Some benign hemangioendotheliomas have an appearance that closely simulates Kaposi's sarcoma. These tumors, which have been referred to as *Kaposi-like* or *kaposiform,* are usually located in the retroperitoneum or deep soft tissue of the extremities and are often associated with thrombocytopenia and hemorrhage (Kasabach-Merritt syndrome).[666,687,691]

Cavernous hemangiomas are composed of larger vessels with cystically dilated lumina and thin walls. Those occurring in the skin are traditionally known as *port-wine nevus* or *nevus flammeus.* This lesion, which is present at birth, grows very slowly and in proportion to the growth of the patient; in time, it becomes nodular and soft. In contrast to the strawberry nevus, it does not regress spontaneously.[668] Large, deep cavernous hemangiomas may undergo thrombosis, ulceration, and infection. They can also be associated with thrombocytopenia and with intravascular coagulation, which are corrected by removal of the tumor.[684,688] Cavernous hemangiomas containing dilated, interconnecting, thin-walled channels with occasional pseudopapillary projections have been designated as *sinusoidal hemangiomas.*[663]

Large-vessel hemangiomas may be composed of vessels with the structure of veins (venous hemangiomas) or a combination of veins and arteries (racemose, cirsoid, or arteriovenous hemangiomas).[673] The structure of the vessel wall

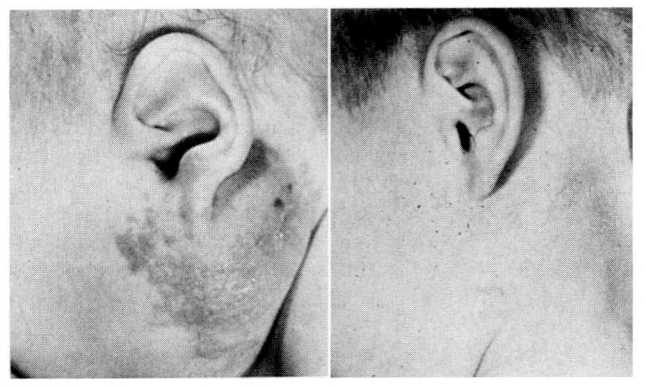

A

B

Fig. 25-59 A, Extensive hemangioma (strawberry nevus) in 3-month-old infant. **B,** Same child 4 years later. Lesion completely disappeared without treatment.

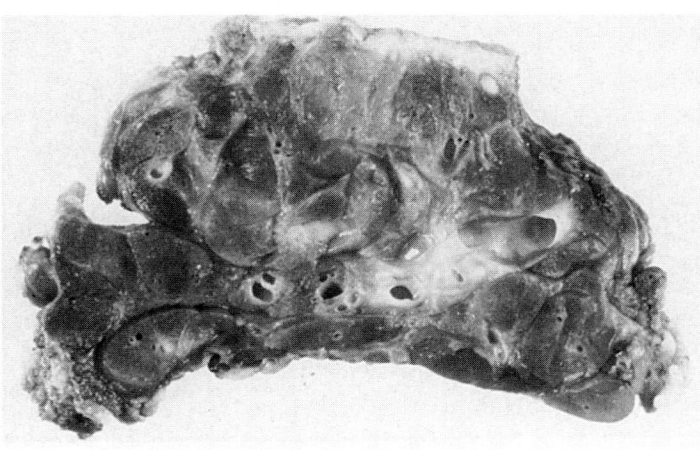

Fig. 25-60 Gross appearance of infantile hemangioendothelioma. Lesion has spongy appearance, dark red color, and lobular configuration. It is centered in subcutaneous tissue, but it extends into both lower dermis and skeletal muscle. (Courtesy Dr. J. Costa, Lausanne, Switzerland.)

is often abnormal and not easily identifiable as arterial or venous. They occur in the back, gluteal region, thigh, and other sites; sometimes an entire extremity is involved. The association of varicose veins, (dysplastic) cutaneous hemangiomas, and soft tissue and bone hypertrophy is known as *Klippel-Trenaunay syndrome.*[675,676] Venous hemangiomas of the feet have been seen in patients with the Turner's syndrome.[689] Thrombosis and calcification are common in large-vessel hemangiomas; the latter can be large enough to be detectable radiographically.

Skeletal muscle (intramuscular) hemangiomas usually have a venous or cavernous microscopic appearance.[662] In

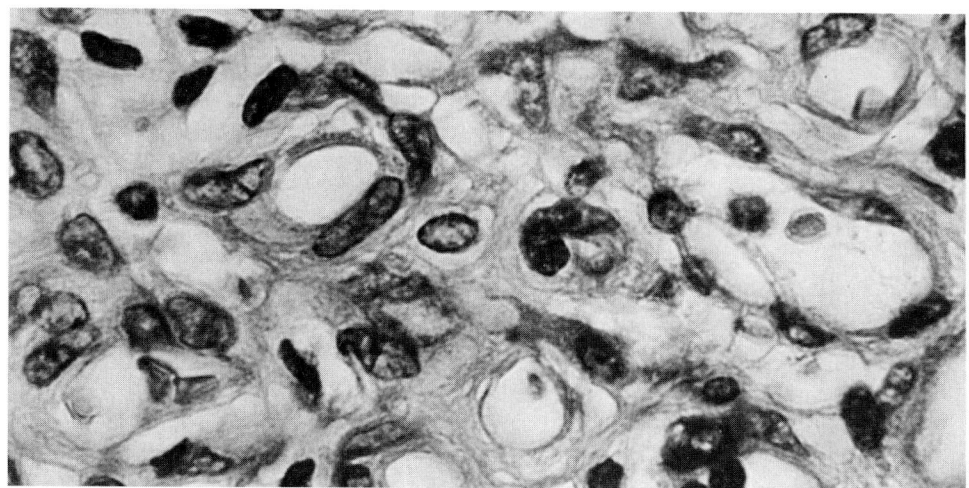

Fig. 25-61 Hemangioma (strawberry nevus) in 1-year-old child. Note vascular channels, decreased cellularity, and increased connective tissue.

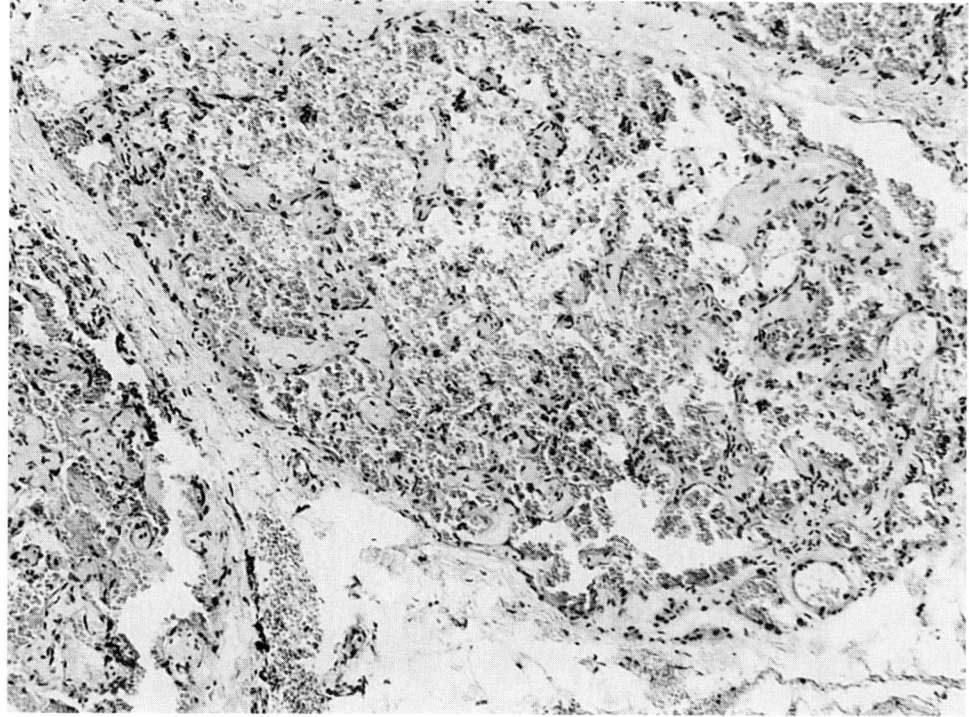

Fig. 25-62 Intravascular papillary endothelial hyperplasia. Large blood vessel shows complex papillary proliferation within lumen, covered by proliferating endothelial cells. There is no atypia or necrosis, and proliferation is confined to vessel lumen. This is not angiosarcoma but rather the result of organizing and recanalizing thrombosis.

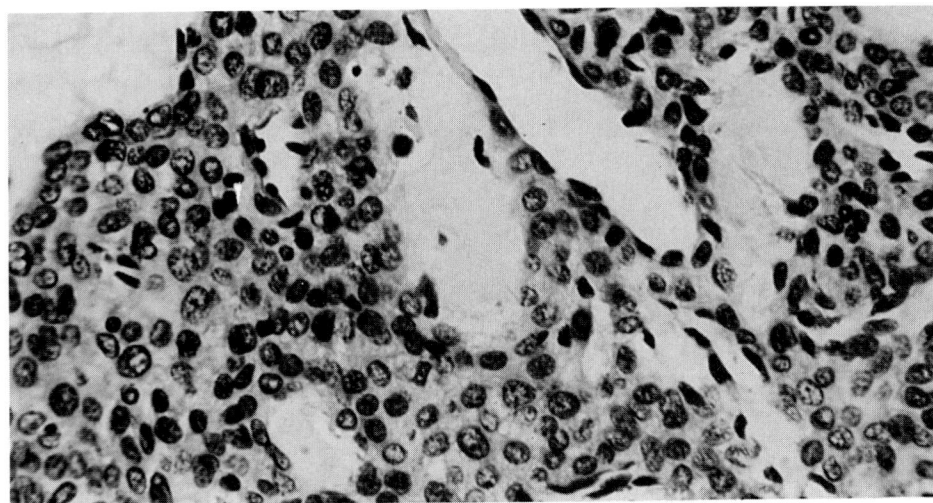

Fig. 25-63 Typical glomus tumor with uniform cells and abundant vessels. It was exquisitely painful and located in subungual area. Cajal stain showed numerous neurites.

other cases, they are very cellular, with plump nuclei, mitotic figures, intraluminal papillary projections, and even infiltration of perineurial spaces.[661] It should be remembered that bona fide angiosarcomas of skeletal muscle are exceptionally rare.

Symplasmic hemangioma is a term we have proposed for a distinctive benign vascular neoplasm featuring bizzare stromal cells. The latter are usually found around the tumor vessels, embedded in a fibrinous material.[687a]

Intravascular papillary endothelial hyperplasia is probably not a true neoplasm but is discussed here because of its capacity to simulate microscopically benign and malignant vascular tumors.[664,674] First described by Masson in hemorrhoidal vessels as "vegetant intravascular hemangioendothelioma,"[664] it is currently thought to represent an exuberant organization and recanalization of a thrombus, an interpretation supported by immunohistochemical studies.[660] It can occur in previously normal vessels or in varices, hemorrhoids, hematomas, pyogenic granulomas, hemangiomas, and angiosarcomas.[674,681,683] The de novo ("pure") form is usually found in the extremities (particularly the fingers) and the head and neck region, whereas the type engrafted on a pre-existing vascular disorder ("mixed") tends to be in the trunk.[670] It simulates angiosarcoma because of the presence of papillary formations, anastomosing vascular channels, and plump endothelial cells. It is identified because of the exclusively intravascular nature of the process; the lack of necrosis, bizarre cells, and atypical mitoses; the characteristically fibrinous and/or hyaline appearance of the papillary stalks; and the frequent finding of residual organizing thrombi (Fig. 25-62).

Glomus tumor

Glomus tumor, also known as *glomangioma,* originates in the neuromyoarterial glomus, a normal arteriovenous shunt abundantly supplied with nerve fibers and fulfilling a temperature-regulating function.[707] The classical location of the glomus tumor is the subungual region, but it can occur elsewhere in the skin, soft tissues (particularly in the flexor surface of the arms and about the knee), nerves, stomach (see

Chapter 11), nasal cavity, and trachea.[694a,695,700,707,711,713] It has also been reported in the sacrococcygeal region, arising from the coccygeal body (glomus coccygeum) and associated with coccydinia,[698] but there is some question as to whether this is a true neoplasm or simply a normal structure of this region.[693,694,710]

Subungual lesions are always supplied by numerous nerve fibers and are exquisitely painful, two features often absent in glomus tumors arising elsewhere. The tumor may erode the terminal phalanx or even present as an intraosseous lesion in this location.[704] Superficial lesions are well circumscribed. Glomus tumors in children tend to be multiple and of an infiltrative nature.[703] They may present clinically as varicosities of the lower extremities.

Microscopically, glomus tumors consist of blood vessels lined by normal endothelial cells and surrounded by a solid proliferation of round or cuboidal "epithelioid" cells with perfectly round nuclei and acidophilic cytoplasm (Figs. 25-63 to 25-65). As seen under an electron microscope, the tumor cells have features of smooth muscle rather than of pericytes.[715] Immunohistochemically, they manifest reactivity for myosin, vimentin, actin, and basal lamina components but not for desmin.[696,697,706,709] Numerous substance P–containing nervefibers have been detected among the glomus cells.[702]

Three microscopic types of glomus tumor have been recognized: solid, angiomatous, and myxoid.[705,714] The solid type can be confused with sweat gland tumor, melanocytic nevus, or metastatic carcinoma[701] (Fig. 25-65). This is particularly the case when the tumor cells are very epithelioid and/or grow in an Indian-file fashion.[710a] An *oncocytic variant* of glomus tumor, in which the cytoplasm of the glomus cells is packed with mitochondria, has also been described.[712] Often the diagnostic relationship between tumor cells and blood vessels can be clearly seen only at the very periphery of the neoplasm. Mast cells are common.

On rare occasions, glomus tumors behave in an aggressive fashion, with local recurrences and invasion of adjacent structures.[699] In other instances, lesions with the typical cyto-

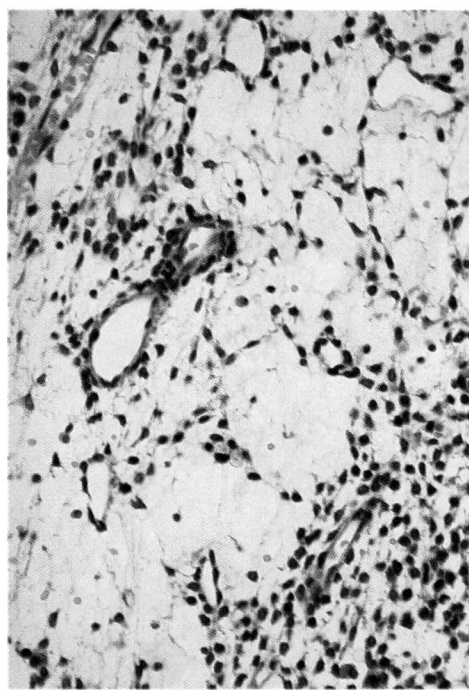

Fig. 25-64 Glomus tumor showing prominent secondary myxoid changes.

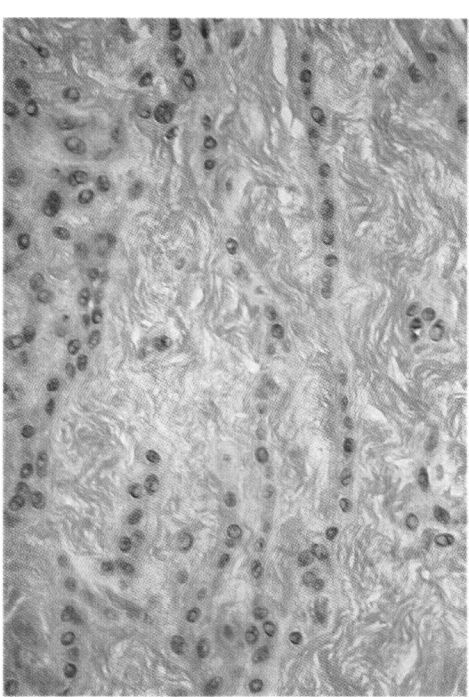

Fig. 25-65 Glomus tumor of finger showing an Indian-file pattern that simulates the appearance of invasive carcinoma.

Table 25-2 Clinical and anatomic features of glomus tumor and hemangiopericytoma

Features	Glomus tumor	Hemangiopericytoma
Pain	Often	Rare
Local invasion	Rare, usually in children	Frequent
Metastases	Never	Sometimes
Location	Skin, superficial soft tissues, stomach	Any tissue
Multiplicity	Sometimes	No
Histology	Organoid cells; round or oval vascular spaces, often dilated; axons are present	Diffuse elongated cells; vascular spaces often collapsed; axons are absent

Modified from Kuhn C III, Rosai J: Tumors arising from pericytes. Ultrastructure and organ culture of a case. Arch Pathol **88**:653-663, 1969.

architectural features of glomus tumor merge with a cytologically malignant tumor; these have been designated *glomangiosarcomas*.[692,699,708] Theoretically, a de novo glomangiosarcoma should also exist, but its morphologic recognition (particularly its distinction from vascular/epithelioid forms of leiomyosarcoma) would be most difficult. No convincing examples of metastasizing glomus tumors have been reported.

Hemangiopericytoma

Stout[737] regarded hemangiopericytoma as a less organoid type of glomus tumor, arising from Zimmerman's pericytes, a theory that he supported with tissue culture studies.[729] The main differences between hemangiopericytoma and glomus tumor are summarized in Table 25-2. The tumor occurs principally in adults and is often deep-seated.[732] In a series of 106 cases reported by Enzinger and Smith,[720]

twenty-seven were in the thigh and twenty-six in the pelvic retroperitoneum. The orbit is another common location. Surgical excision can be difficult because of profuse bleeding.

Grossly, hemangiopericytoma is nearly always solitary and solid, with a smooth surface and a color ranging from grayish white to reddish brown; areas of hemorrhage, necrosis, and cystic degeneration are common (Fig. 25-66). In about three fourths of the cases the tumor is well circumscribed or encapsulated. The marked vascularization of these tumors can be well demonstrated by angiographic and microangiographic studies.[716] Microscopically, the cells are oval to spindle, lack myofibrils with trichrome stains, and have a close relationship with blood vessels; they are separated from the normal-appearing endothelial cells by a layer of silver-staining material composed of basement membrane material mixed with collagen fibers (Fig. 25-67). Many of

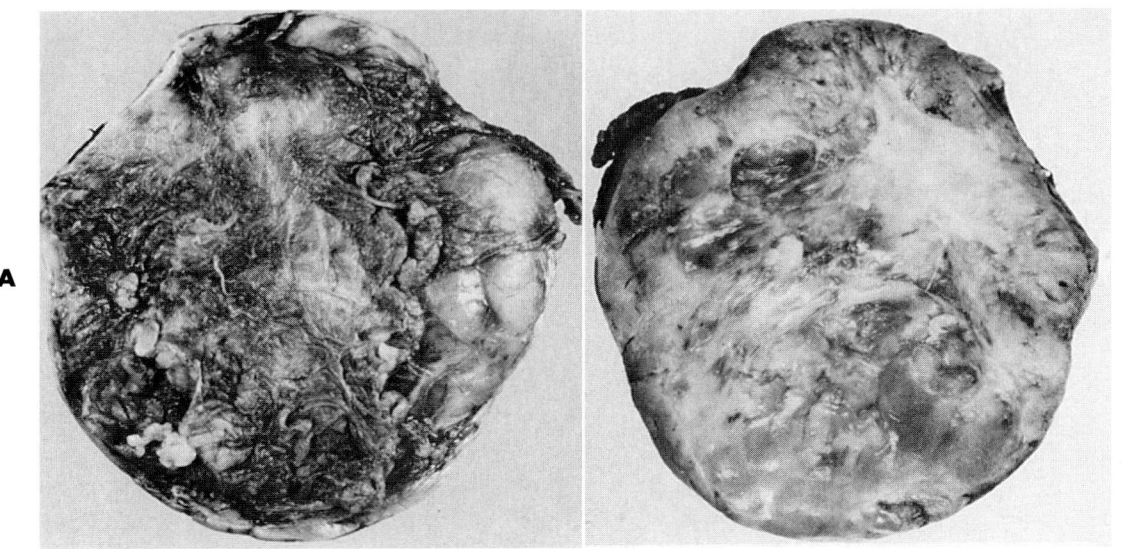

Fig. 25-66 External appearance **(A)** and cross section **(B)** of hemangiopericytoma of soft tissues. Encapsulation is complete, and there are areas of cystic degeneration and fibrosis. Microscopically, mitoses were very scanty.

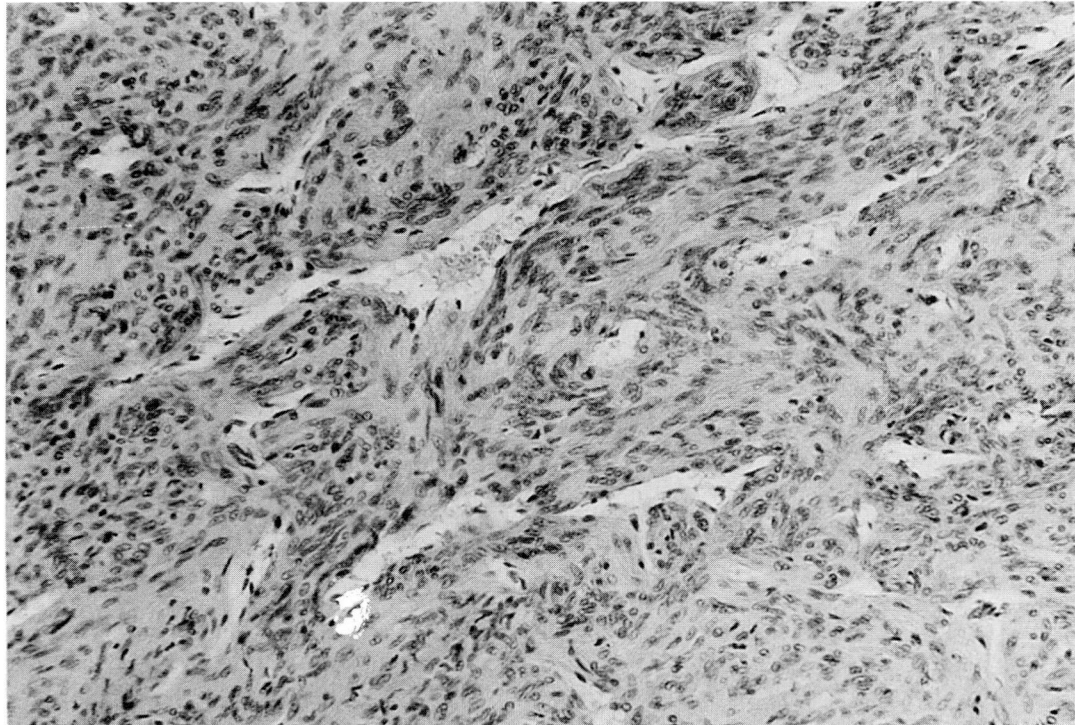

Fig. 25-67 Hemangiopericytoma of soft tissue. Ramifying and somewhat collapsed vascular channels lined by flat endothelial cells show marked proliferation of spindle cells of perithelial appearance.

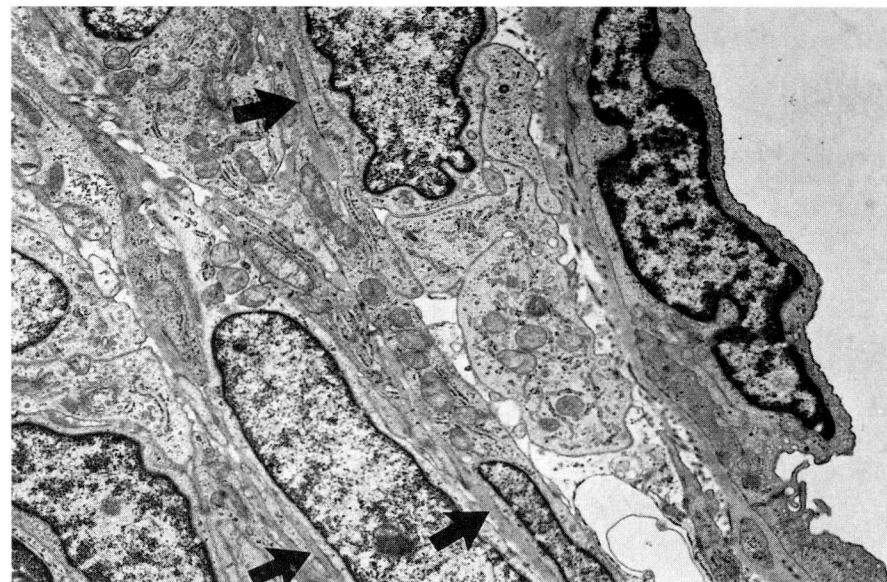

Fig. 25-68 Electron microscopic appearance of hemangiopericytoma of soft tissues. Blood capillary *(right)* surrounded by spindle-shaped tumor cells. Basal lamina *(arrows)* is present between the pericytic tumor cells. (×7900.) (Courtesy Dr. Robert A. Erlandson, Memorial Sloan-Kettering Cancer Center.)

the vessels are branching and exhibit a characteristic "staghorn" configuration. Secondary features that may render the identification difficult include extensive areas of fibrosis and hyalinization (in which the vascular pattern that defines this tumor is lost) and myxoid changes. Immunohistochemically, the tumor cells are invariably positive for vimentin but very rarely and only focally for smooth muscle markers such as actin and desmin.[723,733-735] A subpopulation of tumor cells is also immunoreactive for factor XIIIa and histocompatibility antigen HLA-DR.[730] CD34 usually stains only the endothelial cell component, although sometimes there is a diffusion effect in the immediate vicinity. Stains for basement membrane components, such as type IV collagen and laminin, can be demonstrated between the perithelial and endothelial cells and sometimes surrounding individual perithelial cells.

By electron microscopy, most of the tumor cells have features comparable with those of normal pericytes, whereas others appear as transitional forms with smooth muscle cells and endothelial cells.[717,724,725,731] The most frequently noted features in the tumor cells are cytoplasmic filaments and processes, pinocytotic vesicles, basal lamina, and poorly formed intercellular junctions[719] (Fig. 25-68). Cytogenetically, aberrations of 12q 13-15 have been detected in a subgroup of hemangiopericytomas.[726]

In Stout's series,[736] 11.7% of the cases resulted in distant metastases. He was unable to predict the likelihood of malignant behavior on the basis of the microscopic appearance. In Enzinger and Smith's series,[720] follow-up revealed local recurrence and/or metastases in nineteen of ninety-three patients, the latter being more common in the lung and skeleton. The morphologic features that correlated with aggressive behavior were prominent mitotic activity, necrosis, hemorrhage, and increased cellularity. Local recurrence was an ominous sign, since it often heralded the appearance

of distant metastases. These recurrences can appear 5 or more years after the original excision.[727]

The existence of hemangiopericytoma as a distinct tumor entity represented a controversial concept from its very inception and it remains so at present.[721] We believe that a good point can be made for the theoretical and practical validity of the concept while acknowledging the fact that several other tumors may exhibit a pattern of growth focally indistinguishable from hemangiopericytoma. The most important of these are mesenchymal chondrosarcoma (distinguished by the presence elsewhere in the tumor of islands of mature cartilage), synovial sarcoma, infantile fibrosarcoma, MFH, solitary fibrous tumor, MPNST, and thymoma (which should have more evident epithelial foci elsewhere).[738] The following four other tumors are probably histogenetically related to conventional hemangiopericytoma but have distinctive features of their own:

1 So-called *angioblastic meningioma.* Although originally regarded as a subtype of meningioma, most ultrastructural and immunohistochemical studies have shown the lack of a meningothelial component in this tumor and its close similarities with hemangiopericytoma.[718,730] This low-grade malignant neoplasm, which has a tendency to metastasize to the skeletal system, is further discussed in Chapter 28.

2 *Phosphaturic mesenchymal tumor.* In this neoplasm, hemangiopericytomatous areas are associated with osteoclast-like cells, cartilage, and other patterns (see p. 2107).

3 *Congenital or infantile hemangiopericytoma.* This tumor tends to be more superficially located than its adult counterpart; is often multilobulated; and shows immature cytologic features, increased mitotic activity, and focal necrosis.[733] It also seems to contain a neoplastic component of endothelial cells.[722] The latter feature,

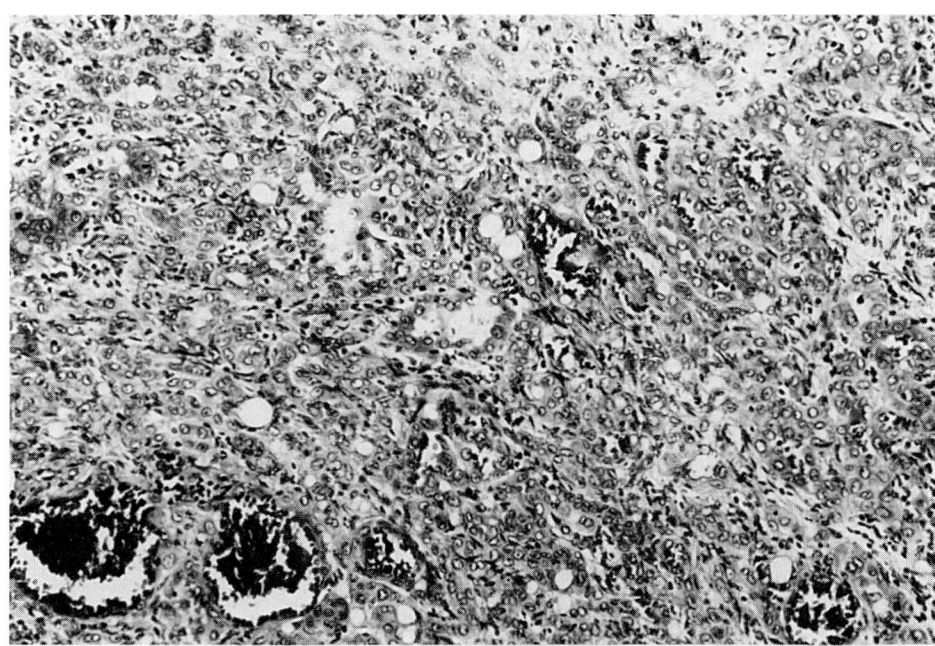

Fig. 25-69 Histiocytoid (epithelioid) hemangioendothelioma. Plump endothelial cells are seen growing in small cords and tubules. Nuclei are vesicular, and cytoplasm contains occasional large vacuoles.

plus its invariably benign behavior despite the alarming microscopic features, suggests a possible relationship with hemangioendothelioma.[720] It has also been pointed out that numerous similarities exist between infantile hemangiopericytoma and infantile myofibromatosis[728] (see p. 2033).

4 *Lipomatous hemangiopericytoma.* We have seen several examples of this peculiar neoplasm, which combines typical hemangiopericytomatous areas with myxoid and sclerosing foci and with islands of mature adipose tissue.[730a]

Hemangioendothelioma

The term *hemangioendothelioma* has been used over the years both for benign and for fully malignant vascular tumors composed of endothelial cells, and therefore it lacks specificity. Currently, its preferred use is for vascular tumors of an endothelial nature that occupy an *intermediate* position between the benign hemangioma and the full-blown angiosarcoma.[740] Because of the possibility of misunderstanding, it is better to always use the term with one of the qualifiers that follow.

Epithelioid (histiocytoid) hemangioendothelioma. This tumor is composed of a distinctive type of endothelial cells having an epithelial-like or histiocyte-like appearance. The cytoplasm is abundant and eosinophilic, often vacuolated. The nucleus is round, vesicular, and occasionally indented. Vascular lumina are present, most of them small; some are located intracellularly and are responsible for the cytoplasmic vacuolation (Fig. 25-69). Mitoses, pleomorphism, and necrosis are variable but usually scanty or absent. An inflammatory infiltrate is often present at the periphery; this may contain well-formed germinal centers and/or a large number of eosinophils. The stroma may be

scanty or have a prominent myxoid appearance. Osteoclast-like multinucleated giant cells may be present.[759] The endothelial nature of the tumor cells has been confirmed ultrastructurally and immunohistochemically.[741] The acidophilic staining quality of the cytoplasm is due to the presence of packed intermediate filaments of vimentin type.

Tumors with this set of morphologic features have been described in a large number of sites, including the skin, bone, lung, pleura, liver, peritoneum, and lymph nodes.[760] Those located in the soft tissue are seen in adults and often arise from the wall of a vein in an extremity.[740,756,758] They also occur in the head and neck area.[744] Most patients are cured by excision, but metastases had developed in one fifth of the cases reported by Weiss et al.[458]

Epithelioid hemangioendothelioma is one of several related proliferative lesions of endothelial cells having as a common denominator an epithelioid or histiocytoid morphology, often accompanied by immunoreactivity for keratin.[747] These were originally embraced under the generic category of *histiocytoid hemangioma,*[739,742,751] but it has become clear that lesions composed of epithelioid (histiocytoid) cells can be present in infectious processes (such as Peruvian verruca and bacillary angiomatosis), in the skin disorder of unknown pathogenesis traditionally known as angiolymphoid hyperplasia with eosinophilia, in the low-grade (borderline) neoplasm described here, and in the fully malignant epithelioid angiosarcoma (see p. 2070).[745,753] Despite early statements to the contrary, Kimura's disease as seen in the Orient does not belong to this group.[755]

Spindle-cell hemangioendothelioma. This vascular tumor of soft tissues may present at any age, has a male predominance, occurs preferentially in the dermis and subcutaneous tissue of the distal extremities, and combines histologically the features of cavernous hemangioma and Kaposi's

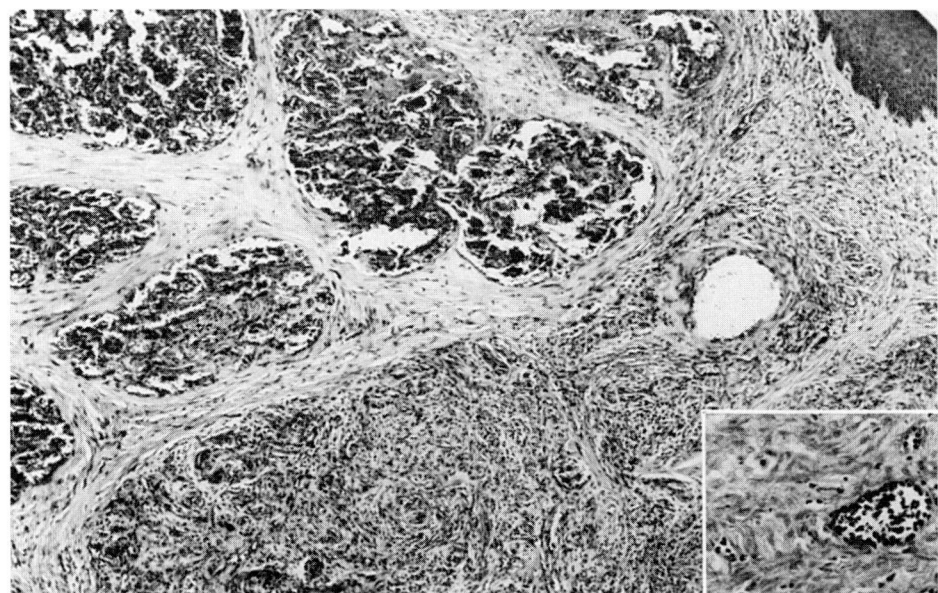

Fig. 25-70 Spindle cell hemangioendothelioma. Areas with appearance of cavernous hemangioma alternate with others reminiscent of Kaposi's sarcoma. **Inset** shows close intermingling of two components.

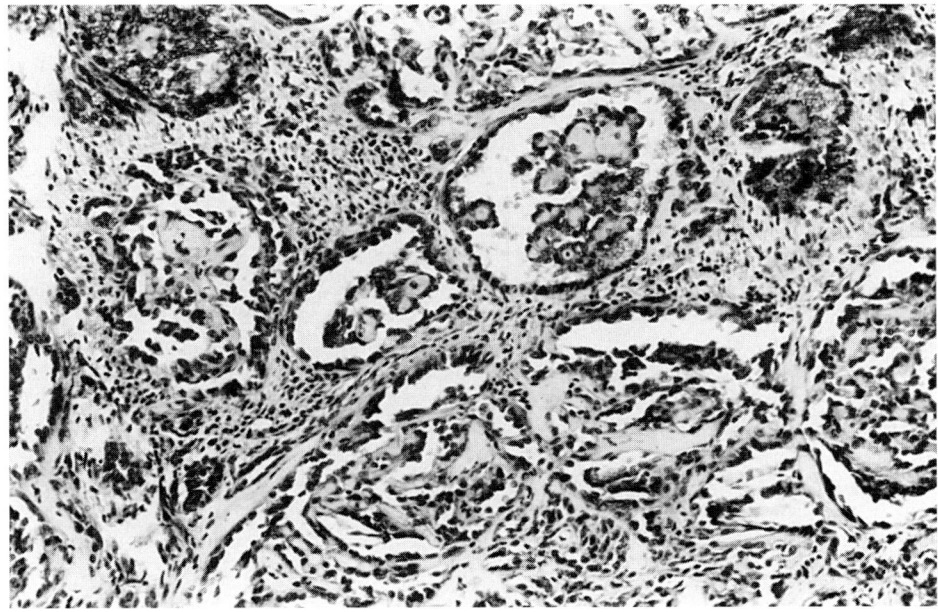

Fig. 25-71 Malignant endovascular papillary angioendothelioma. Papillary projections are formed within neoformed vascular structures, appearance resembling that of immature renal glomeruli.

sarcoma[752,754,757] (Fig. 25-70). The latter areas often have a component of epithelioid (histiocytoid) endothelial cells. The immunohistochemical features are those of endothelial cells.[746a] Development of recurrences or new lesions is common, but metastases have been documented in only one case, following repeated recurrences and radiation therapy.[757] Some cases have occurred in patients with Maffucci's or Klippel-Trenaunay syndrome.[744a,746] Variously interpreted as a low-grade angiosarcoma[757] and a non-neoplastic lesion related to a vascular malformation,[746,748] it probably represents a benign or at most borderline endothelial neoplasm.

Malignant endovascular papillary angioendothelioma (Dabska's tumor). This is an extremely rare but distinctive tumor of childhood, located in the skin or soft tissues and characterized by papillary tufts that are lined by plump endo-

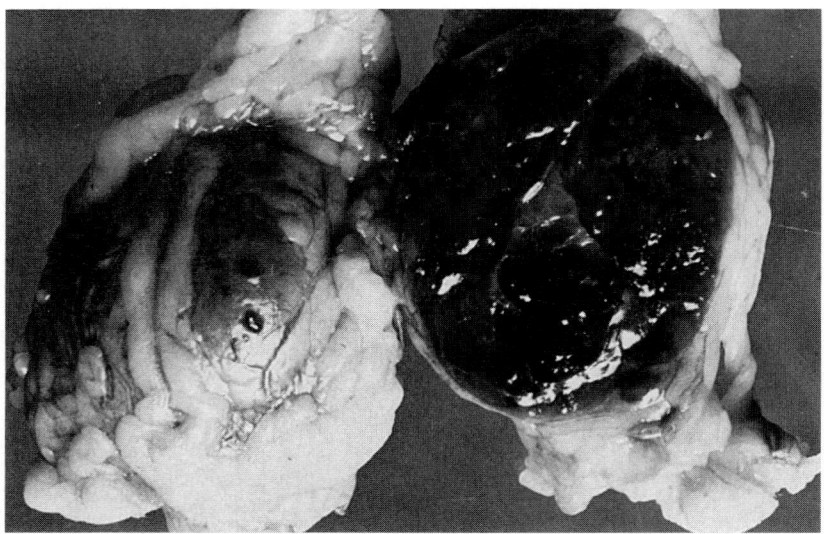

Fig. 25-72 Angiosarcoma of omentum in 41-year-old woman. Tumor nodules also were present in retroperitoneum. On cross section, tumor is dark red, spongy, and of soft consistency. It proved rapidly fatal.

thelial cells located within dilated vascular lumina, some of which have a glomeruloid configuration (Fig. 25-71). Many of the tumor cells have epithelioid or histiocytoid features, including cytoplasmic eosinophilia and vacuolation. The lesion has a uniformly good prognosis, although nodal metastases have occurred in a few instances.[743,749,750]

Retiform hemangioendothelioma. See Chapter 4.

Angiosarcoma

The term *angiosarcoma,* if used without adjectives or prefixes, refers to a malignant neoplasm arising from the *endothelial cells of blood vessels* (i.e., a malignant hemangioendothelioma).[779,782] It is usually seen in adults, the most common sites being the skin, soft tissue, breast, bone, liver, and spleen. Some soft tissue angiosarcomas arise from major vessels, such as the inferior vena cava, pulmonary artery, or aorta.[761,774] These tend to have a very undifferentiated appearance and a solid pattern of growth,[783] to such an extent that they may not be identifiable as being of endothelial nature.[762,763] Accordingly, topographic terms such as intimal sarcoma, luminal sarcoma, and arterial/venous trunk sarcoma have been used for them.[767,774]

Angiosarcomas have been reported in previously irradiated fields,[766,777] around long-standing foreign bodies,[770,771] in arteriovenous fistulas,[764] engrafted on mediastinal or retroperitoneal germ cell tumors,[780] or arising within pre-existing benign tumors, such as hemangioma, neurofibroma, intramuscular lipoma, or leiomyoma.[765,776,784]

Grossly, angiosarcomas tend to be highly hemorrhagic and deeply invasive (Fig. 25-72). Their microscopic appearance ranges from a pattern so well differentiated as to simulate a benign hemangioma to one so undifferentiated and solid as to simulate carcinoma, malignant melanoma, or other types of sarcoma. The diagnostic areas of angiosarcoma are represented by the freely anastomosing vascular channels lined by atypical endothelial cells (Fig. 25-73), a pattern that is accentuated by silver reticulin stains.[778] Lymphoid foci and clumps of hemosiderin are common.

Variations in the appearance of the neoplastic endothelial cells are great. Their shape ranges from very elongated to plump and epithelioid and their size from small to giant, with occasional development of multinucleated forms[768] (Fig. 25-74). The latter are sometimes seen to display prominent hyaline globules containing alpha-1-antitrypsin and alpha-1-antichymotrypsin.[781] In rare cases, foci of granular cells similar to those seen in granular cell tumors are present.[775] The differential diagnosis includes hemangioma for the better differentiated lesions, Kaposi's sarcoma for those with a predominantly spindle component, and carcinoma or amelanotic melanoma for the poorly diferentiated types. Metastatic renal cell carcinoma, because of its high degree of vascularity, is particularly notorious for its ability to simulate angiosarcoma; in this regard, it should be kept in mind that clear tumor cells are not a feature of angiosarcoma.

Immunohistochemically and ultrastructurally, various endothelial markers can be demonstrated depending on the degree of differentiation[772]; in the tumor with epithelioid features, co-expression of keratin is common.[768]

A well-defined clinicopathologic form of angiosarcoma involves the head and neck region (particularly the scalp) of elderly individuals. It begins in the skin but often extends into the subcutis. The clinical course includes repeated local occurrences over a long period of time, followed in some cases by lymph node and pulmonary metastases.[769,773,778]

Neoplastic angioendotheliomatosis, once regarded as a form of multicentric angiosarcoma, is now viewed as a type of malignant lymphoma with a particular tropism for vascular lumina; this entity is discussed in Chapter 4.

Lymphangioma and lymphangiomyoma

Most **lymphangiomas** represent malformations rather than true neoplasms and are thought to result from failure of

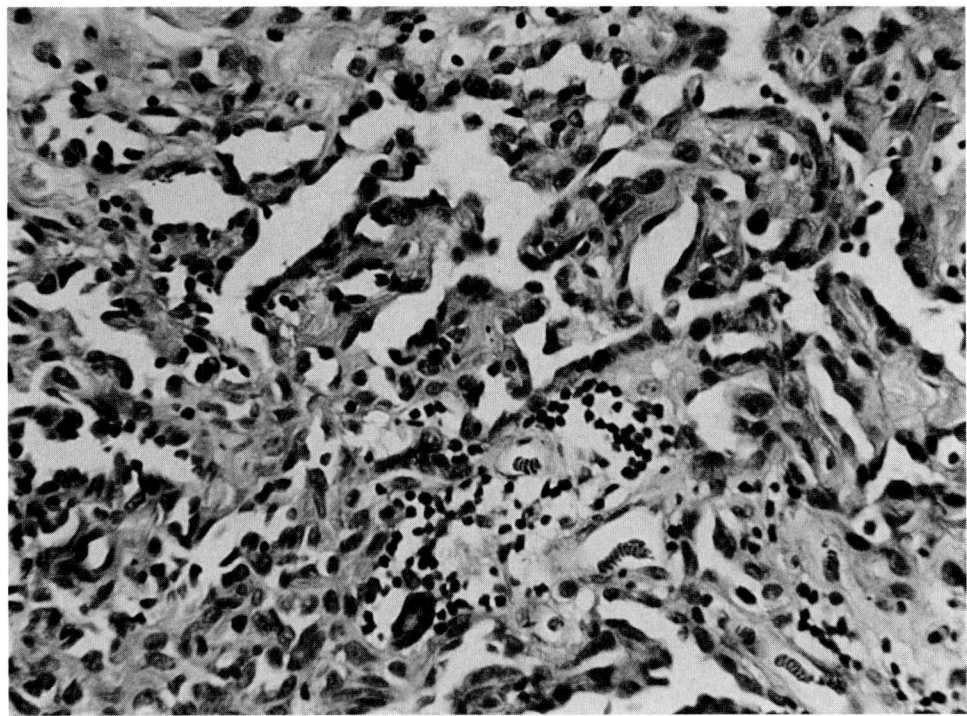

Fig. 25-73 Soft tissue angiosarcoma. Freely anastomosing vascular channels are lined by atypical endothelial cells.

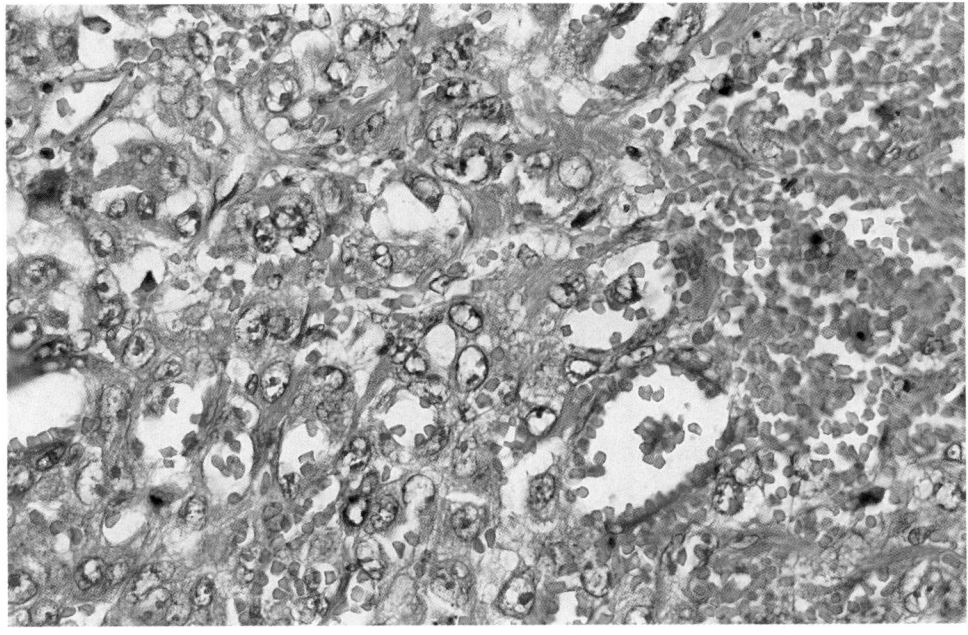

Fig. 25-74 Epithelioid angiosarcoma arising from the region of the seminal vesicle.

the lymphatic system to communicate with the venous system.[789] Three forms exist: capillary, cavernous, and cystic. The capillary form occurs in the skin, whereas the cavernous variety prefers deep soft tissues. Cystic lymphangioma is usually known as *hygroma*. Its most common presentation is in the form of a poorly defined soft tissue mass in the neck

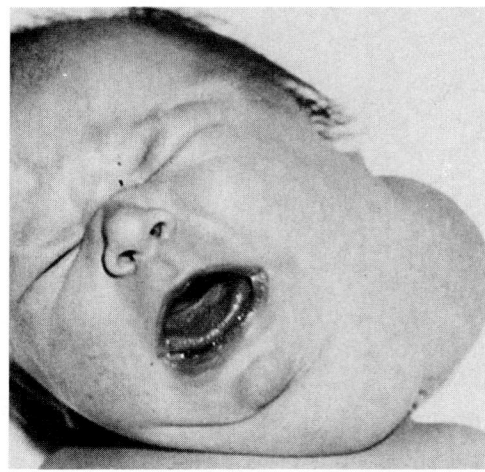

Fig. 25-75 Large cystic hygroma in infant. (From Maxwell JH: Tumors of the face and neck in infancy and childhood. South Med J **45:**292-299,1952.)

of children, usually situated posterior to the sternocleidomastoid muscle and sometimes extending into the mediastinum (Figs. 25-75 and 25-76). Those developing in utero often progress to hydrops and cause fetal death. Many of the fetuses have karyotypes consistent with Turner's syndrome[786,789] or other chromosomal abnormalities. Some lymphangiomas are diffuse and/or multicentric, the condition being designated as *lymphangiomatosis*. These cases may be limited to the soft tissues or be accompanied by osseous and/or visceral manifestations.[799] A preferred location is the thoracic cavity, with resulting chylous pleural effusion and/or chylopericardium.[787] Other cases affect diffusely the extremities.[792]

Microscopically, lymphangioma consists of large lymphatic channels growing in loose connective tissue (Fig. 25-77). A few disorganized bundles of smooth muscle can be present in the wall of the larger channels. Focal areas of papillary endothelial proliferation similar to those described by Masson in blood vessels are sometimes found.[796] Large collections of lymphocytes may be present in the stroma and cause mistakes in interpretation. Lymphangioma does not become malignant and is curable by excision.[794]

Lymphangiomyoma is the preferred term for a benign neoplasm seen exclusively in females and originally described as lymphangiopericytoma.[791,801] The localized form is restricted to the mediastinum and retroperitoneum. It is often seen in close association with the thoracic duct and its tributaries and it often results in chylothorax.[790] Chylous

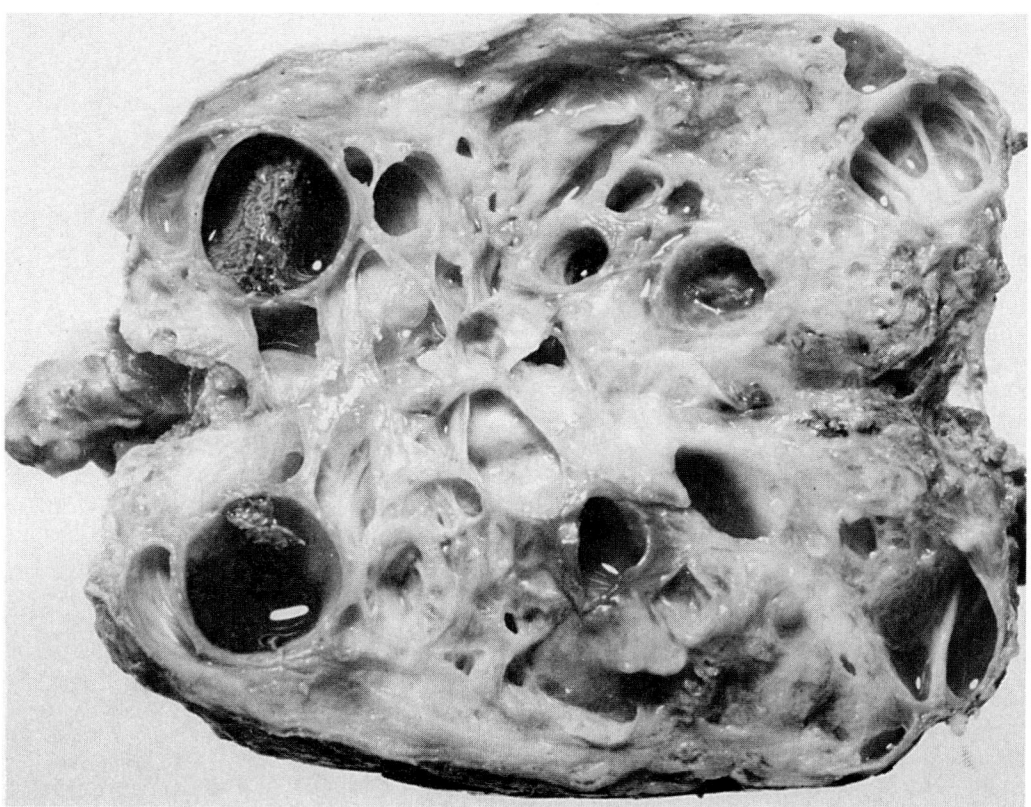

Fig. 25-76 Large cystic hygroma (17 × 15 × 17 cm) in neck of 18-month-old male infant extending into superior portion of mediastinum.

ascites and chyluria (secondary to ureteral wall involvement) may also be present. The diffuse form of the disease, known as lymphangio(leio)myomatosis, typically involves the lung[800] (see Chapter 7). Some cases of lymphangiomyoma/lymphangiomyomatosis are seen in patients with the tuberous sclerosis complex, suggesting a pathogenetic link.[795]

Microscopically, there is a proliferation of intimately mingled lymph vessels and smooth muscle elements (Fig. 25-78). Immunohistochemically, the tumor cells (which are plumper and paler than those of ordinary leiomyomas) are reactive for actin, desmin, and HMB-45.[788] This profile overlaps considerably with that of angiomyolipoma, another neoplasm associated with the tuberous sclerosis complex.

Although immunohistochemical evaluation of hormone receptors in lymphangiomyoma/lymphangiomyomatosis have resulted in conflicting findings,[793,798] good therapeutic results have been reported with progesterone therapy[797] or oophorectomy.[785]

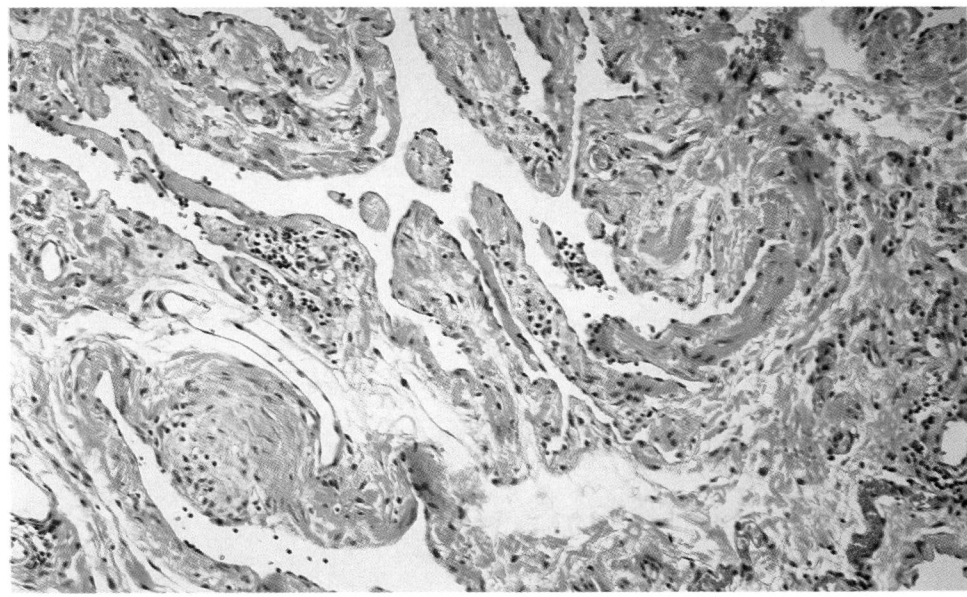

Fig. 25-77 Lymphangioma of soft tissue showing dilated spaces lined by flattened endothelium A scattering of lymphocytes is present in the stroma.

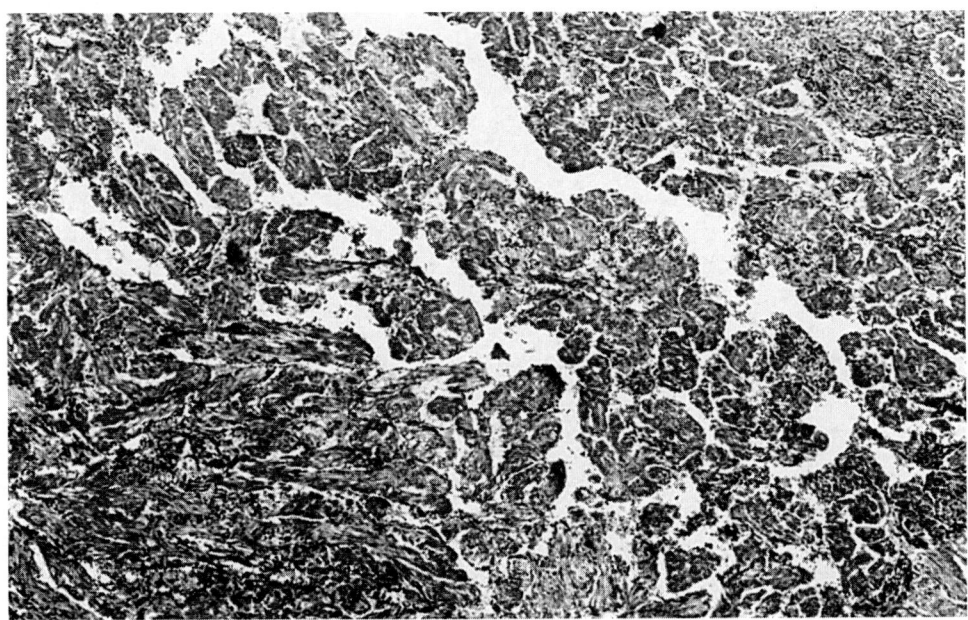

Fig. 25-78 Lymphangioma. Prominent bundles of smooth muscle cells are separated by spaces line by flattened endothelium.

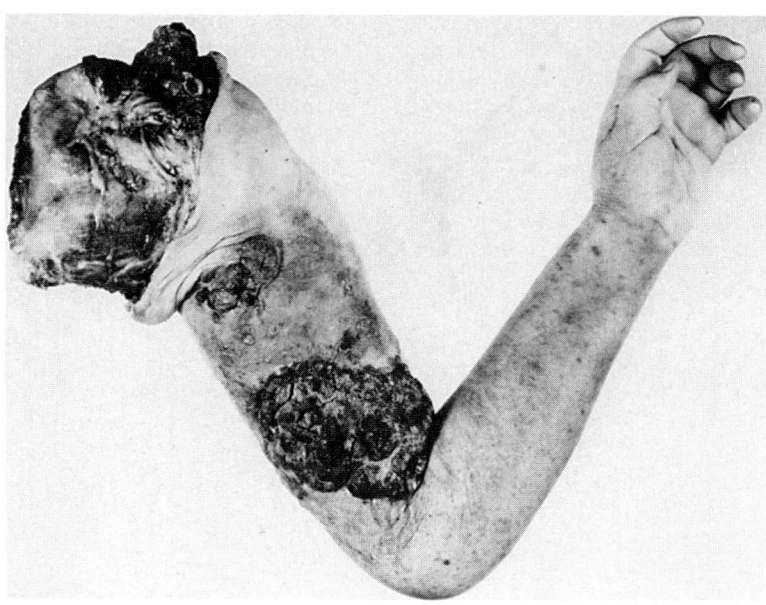

Fig. 25-79 Postmastectomy lymphangiosarcoma treated by disarticulation. Large ulcerated tumor masses are present in background of lymphedema.

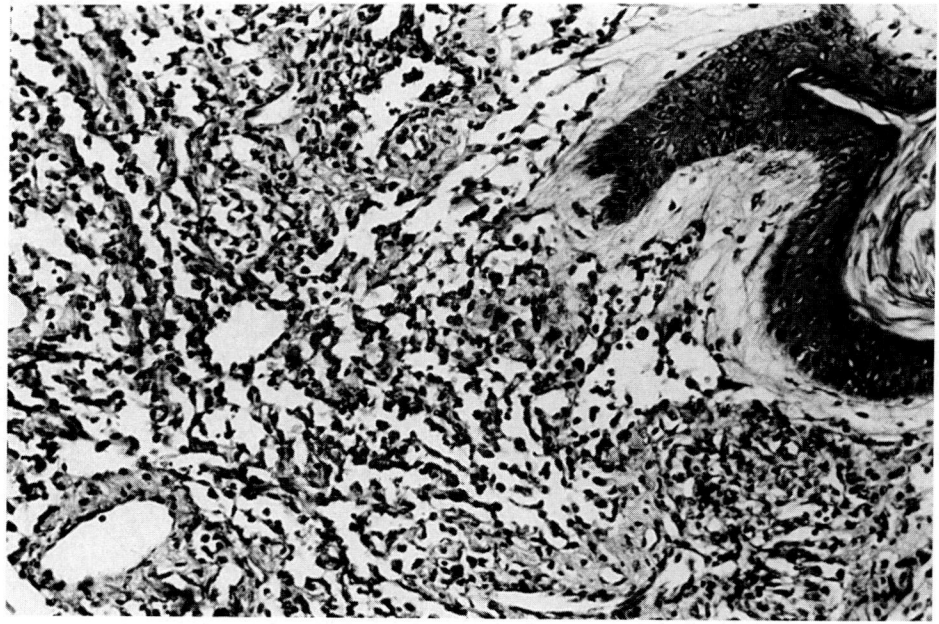

Fig. 25-80 Postmastectomy lymphangiosarcoma. Cellular tumor composed of relatively small cells infiltrates dermis and forms ill-defined anastomosing vascular channels.

Lymphangiosarcoma

Most lymphangiosarcomas arise in patients who have had long-standing massive lymphedema after radical mastectomy, the average interval being approximately 10 years.[804,809,811,812] They also may develop secondarily to chronic lymphedema of the lower leg.[806,810] Sometimes they occur after mastectomy but without being preceded by clinically detectable edema. In other instances, they follow radiation therapy to the area. Clinically, they present as bluish or purple elevations in the edematous skin. They are frequently multiple, although in late stages they coalesce to form a large hemorrhagic mass (Fig. 25-79).

Microscopically, the tumors are composed of areas resembling angiosarcoma and other zones with empty endothe-

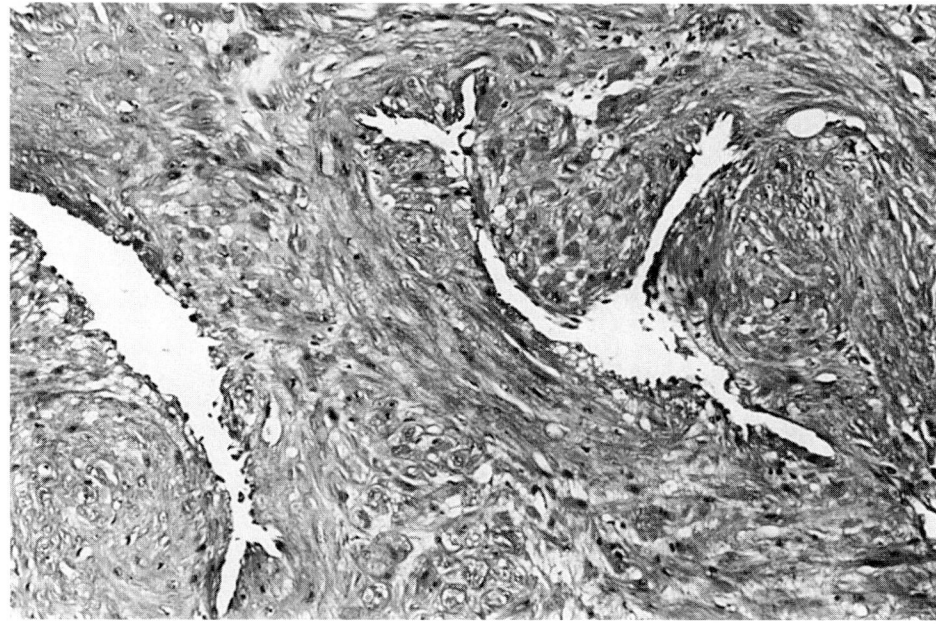

Fig. 25-81 Vascular leiomyoma. Smooth muscle proliferation is clearly related to wall of blood vessels.

lium-lined spaces suggesting lymphatics (Fig. 25-80). The microscopic diagnosis of this lesion may be very difficult in its early phases, for only a small nodule of innocuous-appearing collections of vessels lined by a single layer of endothelium may exist. In some instances the clinical and microscopic features are similar to those of lymphangioma circumscriptum.[803] In such cases, it is wise to use a conservative diagnosis such as "atypical vascular proliferation" and reserve the diagnosis of lymphangiosarcoma for those cases showing clear-cut cytoarchitectural aberrations.

The most typical areas are represented by freely anastomosing vascular channels lined by atypical endothelial cells. These may be accompanied by undifferentiated solid areas that may simulate recurrent breast carcinoma on both microscopic and clinical grounds. Electron microscopy and immunohistochemistry may be needed to make the distinction.[805] Parenthetically, these special techniques reveal that some of these tumors show differentiation toward blood vessels rather than lymph vessels.[802,807,808]

The behavior of Lymphangiosarcoma is extremely malignant. Of 129 patients reviewed by Woodward et al.,[813] only 11 had survived 5 years or more.

Tumors of smooth muscle

Leiomyoma

Several types of leiomyomas exist. ***Cutaneous leiomyomas*** (also discussed in Chapter 4) arise from arrectores pilorum muscles; they are characteristically superficial, small, multiple, and grouped.

Genital leiomyomas are single tumors that arise from smooth muscle bundles located in the superficial subcutaneous tissue of genital areas and structures that are topographically and functionally related to them, such as the nip-

ple, areola, axilla, scrotum, penis, vulvar labia, and anal skin.[823]

Vascular leiomyomas (angioleiomyomas) arise from the smooth muscle of blood vessels (Fig. 25-81). They occur more frequently in females and are usually located in the soft tissues of the lower limbs.[817,822,824] They constitute, together with traumatic neuroma, glomus tumor, eccrine spiradenoma, and angiolipoma, the classic five painful nodules of skin and soft tissues.[821]

Grossly, leiomyomas are yellow or yellowish pink, sharply circumscribed, and fairly firm. Microscopically, they are made up of intersecting fascicles of smooth muscle cells. Mitotic activity is absent, and there is no necrosis or hemorrhage. Foci of cartilaginous metaplasia may be present.[819] Tumors composed of smooth muscle and adipose tissue (myolipomas) are discussed on p. 2054. In vascular leiomyomas the smooth muscle bundles are seen to originate from medium-sized vessels that lack elastic fibers. Islands of mature fat may be present in between. Occasionally, bizarre nuclear forms similar to those seen in uterine symplasmatic leiomyoma are encountered.[814] These tumors have been subdivided into capillary (solid), cavernous, and venous types[817]; transitional forms with glomus tumor and hemangiopericytoma also occur.

The pain often associated with vascular leiomyomas is thought to be mediated by the nerves present within the tumor and in the capsule, whether by mechanical stretching or through mast cell mediation.[815,816,818] Their behavior is benign. Their ultrastructure, immunohistochemistry, and differential diagnosis with leiomyosarcoma are discussed in connection with the latter.

Deep-seated leiomyomas of nonvascular type occur most commonly in the extremities; they may exhibit dystrophic

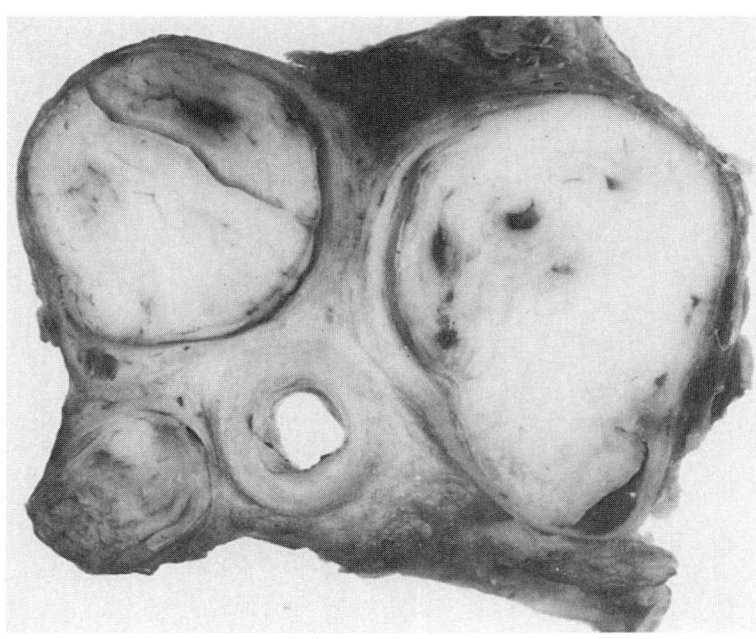

Fig. 25-82 Vascular leiomyosarcoma resulting in occlusive tumor thrombi in three large veins in popliteal region. Artery is uninvolved.

calcification, degenerative nuclear changes, and necrobiotic granuloma-like nodules resembling giant rosettes.[820]

Leiomyosarcoma

Leiomyosarcoma of soft tissue is relatively rare.[829,830,831,834] It is typically a tumor of adults and the elderly, although cases in children are on record.[854,862] The leiomyosarcomas seen with increasing frequency in immunosuppressed patients (HIV-infected individuals and organ transplant recipients) have been found to be associated with the Epstein-Barr virus.[838,841]

Most soft tissue leiomyosarcomas are located in the extremities[834]; many arise from the walls of arteries and veins of widely differing caliber, ranging from large ones (inferior vena cava, saphenous vein, femoral vein, pulmonary artery, femoral artery, and aorta, in that order of frequency) to venules and arterioles* (Fig. 25-82). Those located in the inferior vena cava can result in Budd-Chiari syndrome[836] (see also Chapter 27).

Grossly, leiomyosarcomas can be as well circumscribed as the leiomyomas but are larger and softer and have a tendency for fresh tumor necrosis, hemorrhage, and cystic degeneration. Those arising from major vessels can protrude in a polypoid fashion within the lumen[826] or be predominantly intramural[839] (Plate XIX-F). The intraluminal growth can be demonstrated by phlebography or CT scanning.[826]

Microscopically, the pattern of growth is predominantly fascicular, with the tumor bundles intersecting each other at wide angles. Merging of tumor cells with blood vessel walls is an important diagnostic clue. In some cases the vascular pattern is particularly prominent, resulting in a heman-

giopericytoma-like appearance. We regard these tumors as the malignant counterpart of vascular leiomyoma and designate them as *vascular leiomyosarcomas*[858] (Fig. 25-83). The individual cells have elongated, blunt-ended nuclei and acidophilic fibrillary cytoplasm, features that are also apparent in cytologic preparations.[831] Palisading of nuclei may occur, a feature that may cause confusion with peripheral nerve tumors. The degree of nuclear atypia is highly variable; in extreme cases, it may be reminiscent of malignant fibrous histiocytoma.[835] Cytoplasmic vacuoles located at both ends of the nucleus, sometimes indenting them, represent another diagnostic clue. Focal granular changes can be present in the cytoplasm, approaching those seen in granular cell tumor.[843,845] Myxoid changes[850] and osteoclast-like multinucleated giant cells[842,861] may be prominent.[842,850,861]

Ultrastructurally, the tumor cells exhibit numerous cytoplasmic filaments with focal densities, pinocytotic vesicles, and a thick basal lamina.[840] Myofibrils can be demonstrated in well-differentiated tumors with PTAH. Reticulin stain shows wavy, undulating fibers between long lines of tumor cells, without individual cells being wrapped within. Immunohistochemically, both leiomyomas and well-differentiated leiomyosarcomas show reactivity for vimentin (particularly in those of vascular origin), actin, smooth muscle myosin, desmin, and basal lamina components, including laminin and type IV collagen.* Surprisingly, normal and neoplastic smooth muscle cells have been found also to react strongly with some antikeratin monoclonal antibodies.[828,846,855] Estrogen receptor protein has also been detected in some of these tumors.[859] Cytogenetic analysis has shown

---

*References 825, 826, 833, 837, 848, 849, 856.

*References 827, 832, 844, 847, 851, 857.

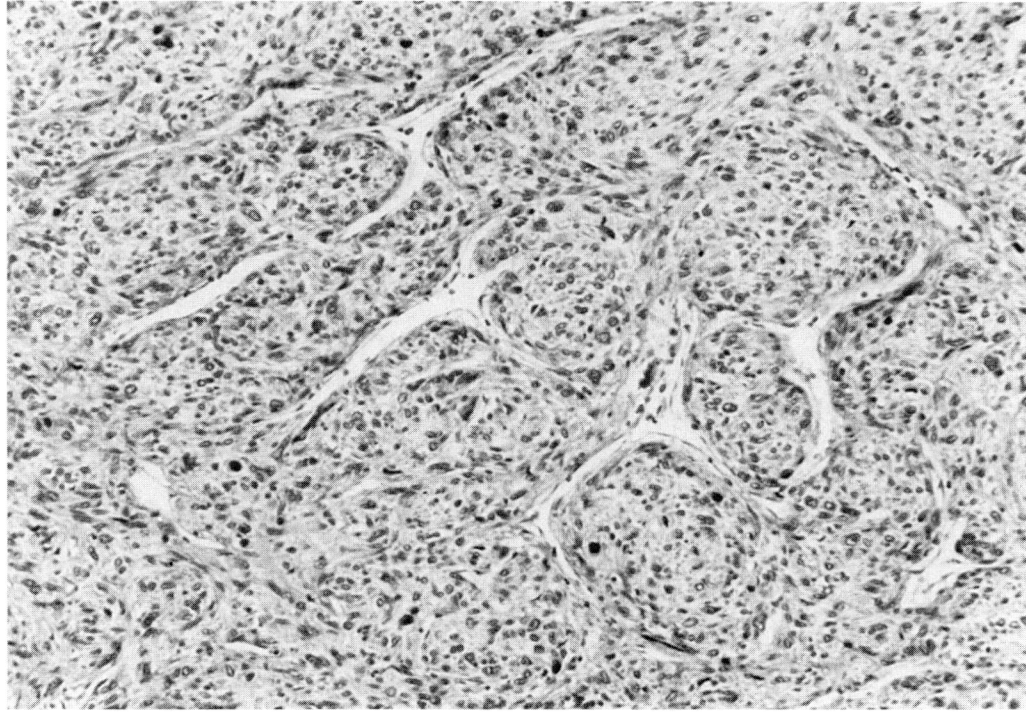

Fig. 25-83 Vascular leiomyosarcoma of soft tissues. In contrast to vascular leiomyoma, mitoses are frequent and cellular atypia is present. Low-power pattern resembles hemangiopericytoma, but tumor cells contain abundant myofibrils.

a variety of chromosomal aberrations but no specific karyotypic marker.[852]

The differential diagnosis between leiomyoma and leiomyosarcoma depends on a combination of gross and microscopic features. High mitotic activity is virtually diagnostic of malignancy. A diagnosis of leiomyosarcoma should also be strongly suspected for smooth muscle tumors of soft tissue that are overly large, necrotic, or hemorrhagic, even if their mitotic count is low[853] (Fig. 25-84). Prognosis in leiomyosarcoma correlates primarily with tumor size and depth, two parameters that are closely related. In one large series, 40% of the cutaneous leiomyosarcomas recurred, but none metastasized; among the subcutaneous tumors, one half recurred, and one third resulted in metastases or tumor-related deaths.[834] Prognosis is even worse for the tumors located intramuscularly. Mitotic activity also correlates with prognosis[860]; however, the fact remains that in many metastasizing leiomyosarcomas of soft tissue, there are less than ten mitoses per high-power field. Simple enucleation of the tumor virtually guarantees local recurrence. The majority of these tumors eventually give rise to distant metastases, sometimes 15 years or more after the original excision.

Clear cell (epithelioid) smooth muscle tumors

Smooth muscle tumors of soft tissues may have a round cell (clear cell, epithelioid) configuration, in whole or in part, similar to that seen more often in smooth muscle tumors of the stomach and other intra-abdominal sites[865] (Fig. 25-85). The term *bizarre leiomyoblastoma* has been used for this tumor type, which has benign and malignant forms. An intravascular variant has also been described.[863] We prefer to designate these tumors as *leiomyomas* or *leiomyosarcomas, clear cell (epithelioid) variant,* and classify them as benign or malignant by using similar criteria to those we apply for smooth muscle tumors in general, although acknowledging the fact that this distinction can be extremely difficult to make in the individual case. Immunohistochemical or ultrastructural markers of smooth muscle differentiation tend to be expressed only focally and imperfectly in these tumors.[864,865]

Tumors of striated muscle
Rhabdomyoma

So-called cardiac rhabdomyomas, seen in association with the tuberous sclerosis complex, are probably not true neoplasms. Bona fide benign tumors of skeletal muscle origin are exceedingly rare.[866,868,877] They can be divided into distinct subtypes, although some overlap exists.[867,875,879,880] Those known as the *adult* type are found almost exclusively in adult patients in the oral cavity and its vicinity. Multifocal and recurrent cases have been described.[871,878] Microscopically, the cells are well differentiated, large, rounded or polygonal, with abundant acidophilic cytoplasm containing variable amounts of lipid and glycogen (Fig. 25-86). Some cells have features of "spider cells." Cross striations and intracytoplasmic rod-like ("jack straw") inclusions are frequent, and intranuclear inclusions may be seen. There is no

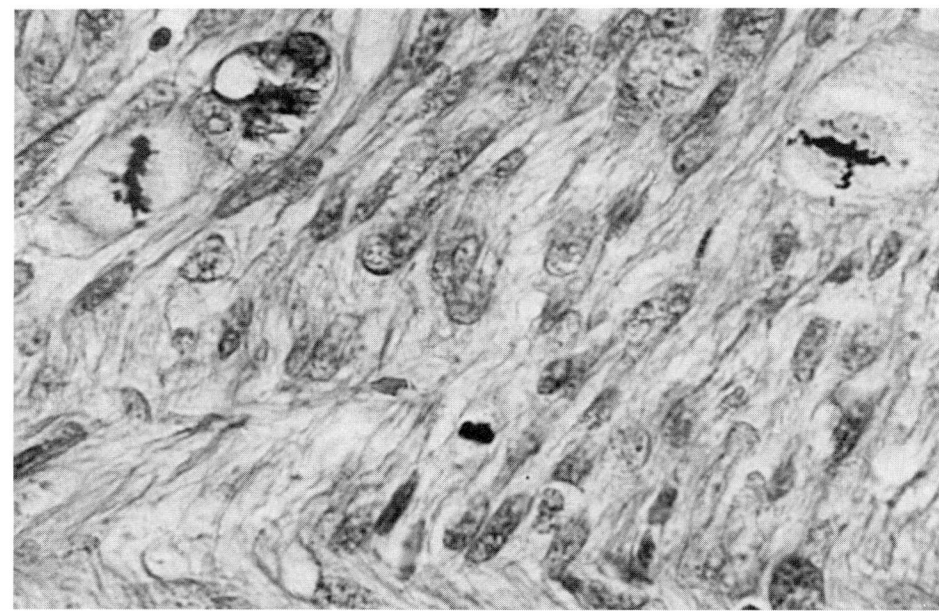

Fig. 25-84 Fairly well-differentiated metastatic leiomyosarcoma. However, it showed numerous mitotic figures, both typical and atypical.

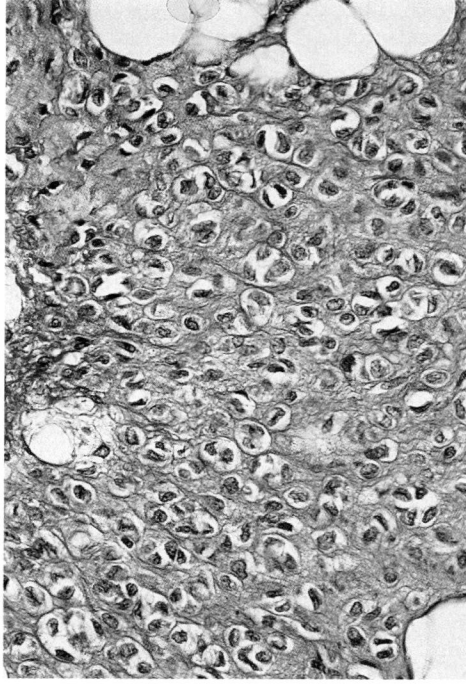

Fig. 25-85 Epithelioid smooth muscle tumor. The PAS stain highlights the thick basement membrane that surrounds individual tumor cells.

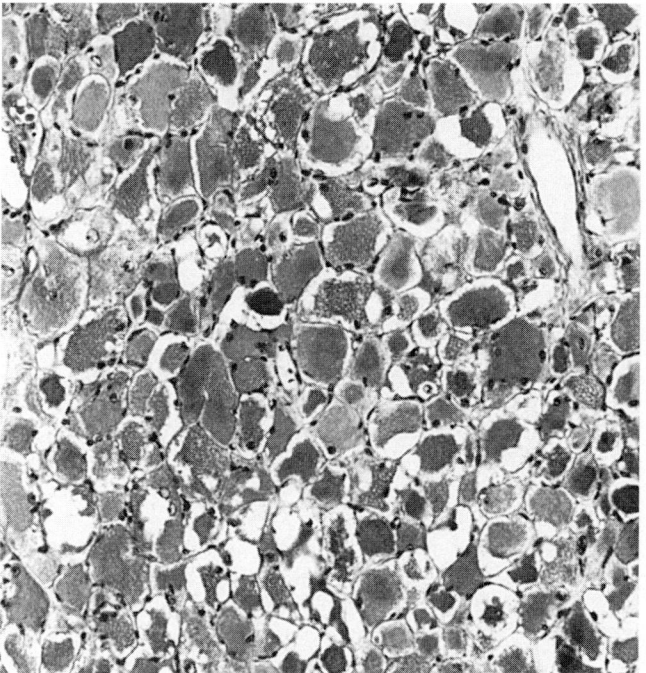

Fig. 25-86 Adult form of rhabdomyoma. Cross striations are identifiable in several of tumor cells.

mitotic activity or nuclear atypia. The differential diagnosis includes granular cell tumor and hibernoma.

The *fetal* form of rhabdomyoma is seen almost exclusively in two locations: the head and neck area (particularly the retroauricular area) in children under 3 years of age and the vulvovaginal region of middle-aged women[869,870,872]

(Fig. 25-87). The latter, also referred to as *genital rhabdomyoma,* is separated by some authors from the other fetal types. Microscopically, both lesions are very cellular, formed by immature skeletal muscle fibers (some containing cross striations) and primitive mesenchymal cells (Fig. 25-88). Their development is equivalent to that of fetal

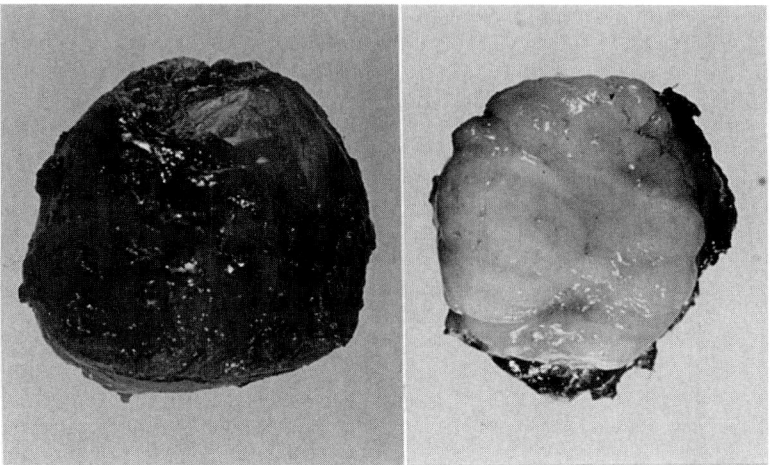

Fig. 25-87 External appearance and cut surface of fetal rhabdomyoma. Tumor is well circumscribed, solid, whitish, and of soft consistency. It was located in parotid soft tissue of a 3-year-old boy. (Courtesy Dr. J. Costa, Lausanne, Switzerland.)

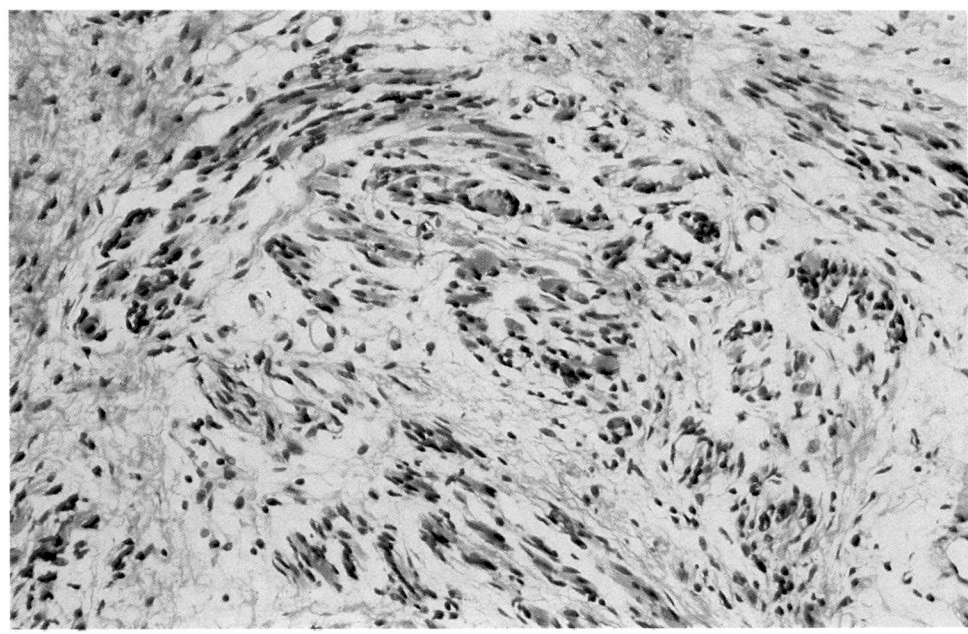

Fig. 25-88 Fetal rhabdomyoma. (Courtesy Dr. Louis Dehner, St. Louis, MO.)

skeletal muscle of 7 to 12 weeks gestation. Nuclear aberrations are absent, and mitoses are generally rare. The vulvovaginal cases tend to have a myxoid quality. Kapadia et al.[872] have divided their cases of fetal rhabdomyoma into "classic" and "intermediate." The latter were characterized by the presence of large, ganglion cell–like rhabdomyoblasts with vesicular nuclei and prominent nucleoli, interlacing ribbon- or strap-like rhabdomyoblasts with deeply acidophilic cytoplasm, fascicles simulating smooth muscle, plexiform patterns with infiltration of fat, and intimate relationship with peripheral nerves.

The main differential diagnosis of fetal rhabdomyoma is with well-differentiated rhabdomyosarcoma. The distinction can be very difficult because of the overlap of many histologic features; nuclear atypia is said to be the most important distinguishing feature.[872,874]

The immunohistochemical features of rhabdomyoma (especially the adult type) recapitulate those of normal skeletal muscle cells[873,876]; the markers that these cells can exhibit are listed in the section on rhabdomyosarcoma. Ultrastructurally, hypertrophied Z-band material, thick and thin filaments, numerous mitochondria (some

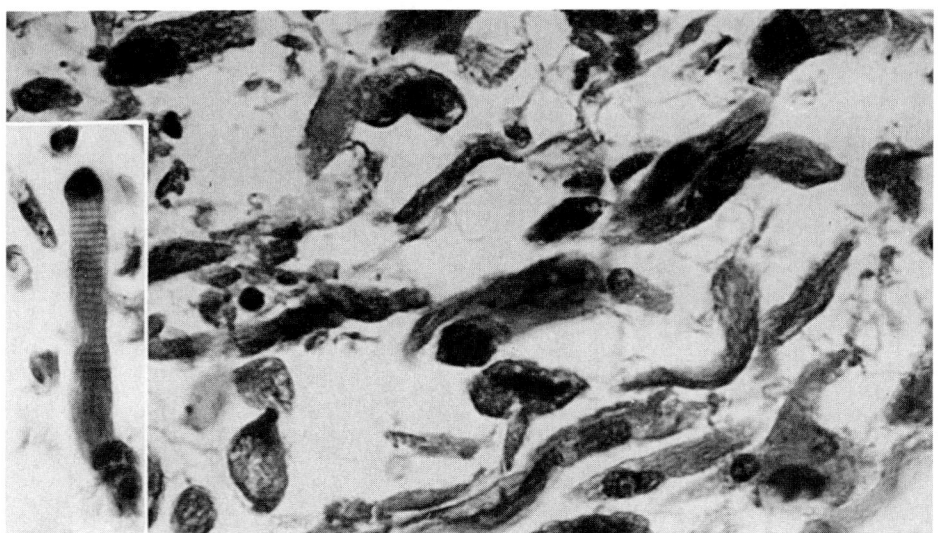

Fig. 25-89 Pleomorphic rhabdomyosarcoma with tumor giant cells and tapering cytoplasmic processes. Cell in **inset** shows well-defined cross striations.

with abnormal configuration or with inclusions), intranuclear bodies, and cytoplasmic bodies have been observed.

Rhabdomyosarcoma

There are three major categories of rhabdomyosarcoma: pleomorphic, embryonal, and alveolar.[881,920]

Pleomorphic rhabdomyosarcoma, which constituted practically all the cases of rhabdomyosarcoma in the older literature, is actually the least common of the three categories. It arises in areas where myotome-derived skeletal muscle occurs and is therefore usually located in an extremity, especially the thigh.[926,935,977] It occurs almost exclusively in adults. Grossly, it may be confined within fascial compartments and have the shape of the muscle from which it arises. Microscopically, the tumor is very pleomorphic, with numerous tumor giant cells. Making a differential diagnosis with liposarcoma and malignant fibrous histiocytoma is so difficult that a diagnosis of pleomorphic rhabdomyosarcoma should not be made unless there is incontrovertible evidence of skeletal muscle differentiation in the form of cross striations (Fig. 25-89) or through the demonstration of specific ultrastructural or immunohistochemical markers (see subsequent discussion). One should be very careful to avoid the following pitfalls: (1) entrapped non-neoplastic skeletal muscle fibers; (2) release of myoglobin from necrotic muscle with subsequent nonspecific absorption by tumor cells, which thus become immunoreactive[909]; and (3) presence of skeletal muscle differentiation in other malignant tumors. In regard to the latter event, it is somewhat ironic that the best evidence of skeletal muscle differentiation in malignant tumors is often found not in rhabdomyosarcoma per se but rather in tumors such as MPNST (see p. 2051), malignant thymoma (see Chapter 8), mixed müllerian tumor of the female genital tract (see Chapter 19), malignant germ cell tumors (particularly extragonadal ones), medulloblastoma (see Chapter 28), and Wilms' tumor (see Chapter 17).

When defined by the restrictive criteria listed previously, pleomorphic rhabdomyosarcoma becomes a very rare neoplasm[946]; however, well-documented cases exist.[898,913] The behavior of pleomorphic rhabdomyosarcoma seems not to be substantially different from that of other pleomorphic sarcomas of soft tissue.

The other two types of rhabdomyosarcomas occur primarily in children and adolescents and actually constitute the most common form of soft tissue sarcoma in this age group.[914,979,981] Sometimes these two types are grouped under the term "juvenile."[953]

Embryonal rhabdomyosarcoma arises from unsegmented and undifferentiated mesoderm and is common in the head and neck region (particularly the orbit, nasopharynx, middle ear, and oral cavity), retroperitoneum, bile ducts, and urogenital tract.[922,939,959] A smaller percentage occur in the extremities, and these are associated with a higher relapse rate and a lower survival rate.[918,976] A few occur initially within the thoracic cavity.[895] Cases with primary presentation in the skin are also on record.[967] The large majority occur in children between the ages of 3 and 12 years, but they can also occur in younger patients[960] and in adults.[919,936] Some cases have been associated with hypercalcemia or with elevated parathormone levels.[905] Grossly, the tumor is poorly circumscribed, white, and soft. When growing beneath a mucosal membrane, such as the vagina, urinary bladder, or nasal cavity, it frequently forms large polypoid masses resembling a bunch of grapes—hence the name *sarcoma botryoides.* The appearance is quite similar to that of an allergic nasal polyp, and, as such, is deceptively benign.

Microscopically, the tumor cells are small and spindle shaped. Some have a deeply acidophilic cytoplasm (Fig. 25-90). A feature of diagnostic value is the presence of highly cellular areas usually surrounding blood vessels, alternating with parvicellular regions that have abundant mucoid intercellular material. A highly characteristic feature of the poly-

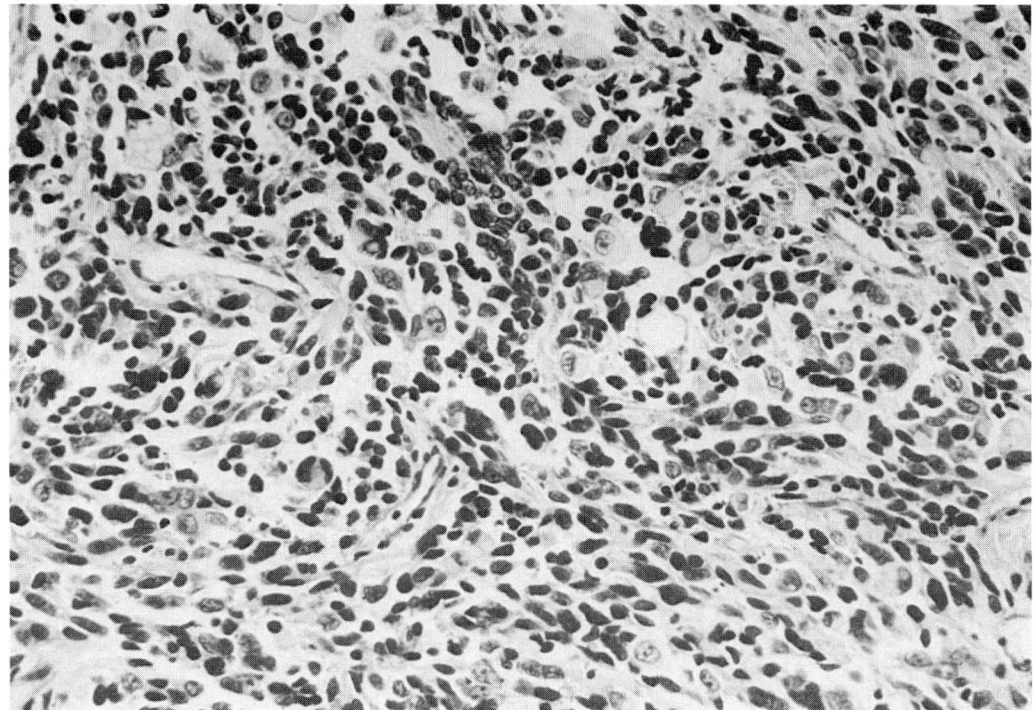

Fig. 25-90 Embryonal rhabdomyosarcoma excised from perineal region of 6-year-old child. Small cells with dark nuclei alternate with larger cells with vesicular nuclei and acidophilic cytoplasm. Cross striations are not seen. (Courtesy Dr. B. Lane, New York.)

poid ("botryoid") tumors is the presence of a dense zone of undifferentiated tumor cells immediately beneath the epithelium, a formation known as *Nicholson's cambium layer* (Fig. 25-91). Cross striations may or may not be present; in contrast to pleomorphic rhabdomyosarcoma in adults, their presence is not indispensable for the light microscopic diagnosis, as long as all the other features are present. Confirmation of the diagnosis, always desirable, can be obtained with ultrastructural and immunohistochemical markers (see the subsequent discussion).

Occasional tumors within the embryonal category usually have focally anaplastic features, with bizarre nuclear forms; these should not be classified as pleomorphic rhabdomyosarcomas but rather as pleomorphic subtypes of embryonal (and rarely alveolar) rhabdomyosarcoma.[930] It has been suggested that they are associated with a more aggressive clinical course, especially when the pleomorphic features are extensive[915,930]; conversely, well-differentiated tumors (with over 50% rhabdomyoblasts) are associated with an excellent response to chemotherapy.[969] Tumors examined following multidrug chemotherapy tend to show a greater degree of differentiation than the pretherapy specimen, suggesting that the drugs have either induced maturation or resulted in a selection of the better differentiated components.[896,947]

The most common sites of metastatic involvement are the soft tissues, serosal surfaces, lung, bone marrow, and lymph nodes.[892,901,961,965] Cases associated with diffuse bone marrow involvement may simulate acute leukemia.[916] Rhabdomyosarcomas arising from genitourinary sites or extrem-

ities are particularly prone to metastasize to lymph nodes,[933] whereas tumors originating in head and neck structures adjacent to meningeal surfaces have a high incidence of direct meningeal extension.

The prognosis of embryonal rhabdomyosarcoma has markedly improved following treatment with excision, radiation therapy, and multidrug chemotherapy.[884,912] Over 80% of children now survive when the disease is localized to the region of origin.[940,941] Age at diagnosis is an independent predictor of outcome.[932]

A prognostically favorable variant of embryonal rhabdomyosarcoma is represented by the *spindle-cell* type, which is composed of elongated spindle cells arranged in a fasciculated or storiform pattern.[890] Most reported cases have been in males, and the most common locations have been the paratesticular area and the head and neck region.[934] This entity bears some resemblance to the tumors described by Lundgren et al.[938] as *infantile rhabdomyofibrosarcomas,* but it is not clear whether the two are identical. The latter microscopically simulated fibrosarcoma and were characterized by an aggressive clinical course.

Very rarely, accumulation of cytoplasmic glycogen or lipids in embryonal rhabdomyosarcoma results in a clear cell appearance that can simulate clear cell carcinoma.[891,987] Another morphologic variation is represented by tumor cells containing cytoplasmic globular inclusions composed of intermediate filaments and resulting in a rhabdoid appearance.[929]

Occasionally, in infants and children, tumors with a location and appearance otherwise characteristic of embryonal

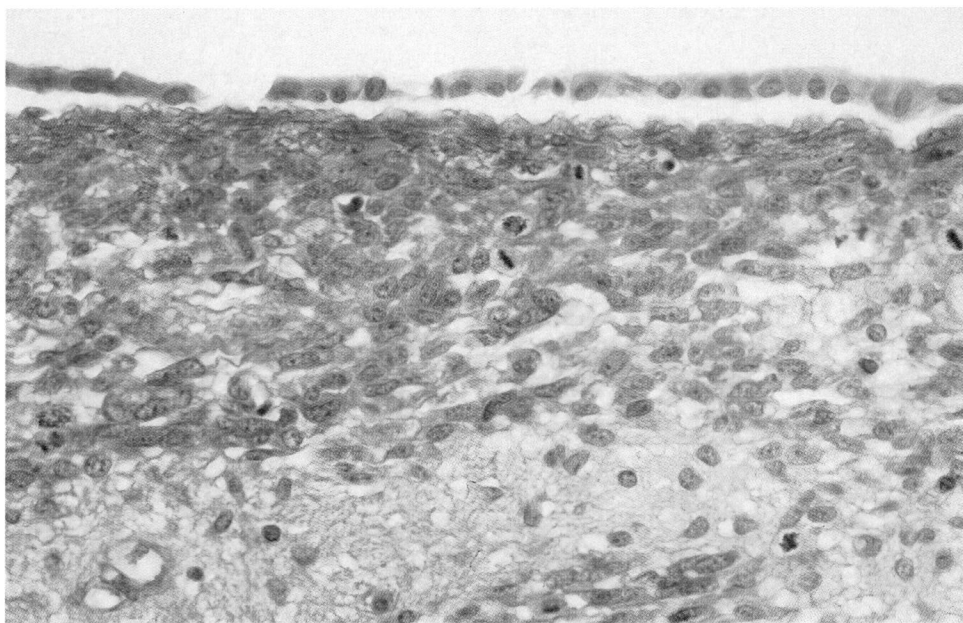

Fig. 25-91 Botryoid rhabdomyosarcoma of bile duct showing a concentration of tumor cells immediately beneath the epithelium ("cambium layer").

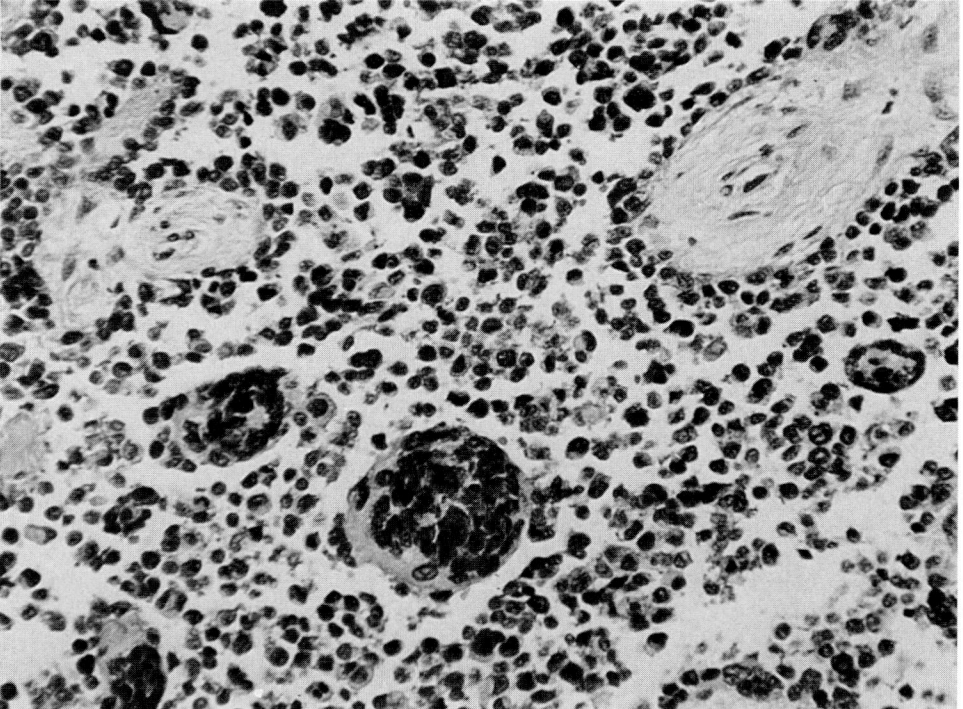

Fig. 25-92 Alveolar rhabdomyosarcoma. Lack of cohesiveness of tumor cells and scattered multinucleated giant tumor cells are characteristic.

rhabdomyosarcoma are seen to contain collections of cells exhibiting neuronal, melanocytic, and/or schwannian differentiation; these have been interpreted by some as originating from the migratory neural crest (ectomesenchyme) and designated as *ectomesenchymomas*.[924,925,968] Others have been given the histogenetically less committal name of *ganglio-rhabdomyosarcoma*.[928] Little is known about their natural history, which does not seem to differ much from that of the ordinary embryonal rhabdomyosarcoma.

Alveolar rhabdomyosarcoma may be related to the embryonal form and occasionally coexists with it; however, it should be regarded as a separate entity because it differs from the latter in several ways. For instance, it predominates in an older age group (10 to 25 years) and occurs more frequently in the extremities. In a series of 110 cases reported by Enzinger,[907] the most common locations were the forearms, arms, and perirectal and perineal regions.

Microscopically, small, round, or oval tumor cells are seen separated in nests by connective tissue septa (Fig. 25-92). The tumor cells in contact with these fibrous strands remain firmly attached to them, but the others tend to detach because of a lack of cohesiveness, which results in a typical alveolar or pseudoglandular appearance. The deep acidophilia of the cytoplasm and the presence of occasional multinucleated giant cells are important diagnostic features.[973] Cases in which the alveolar pattern is poorly developed are referred to as the "solid" variant of alveolar rhabdomyosarcoma and are particularly difficult to diagnose. Before identification of this entity,[906,963] many of these tumors were misdiagnosed as primary malignant lymphoma ("reticulum cell sarcoma") of the soft tissues. The comments made regarding cross striations and special studies for the diagnosis of embryonal rhabdomyosarcomas also apply for the alveolar type.

The prognosis of alveolar rhabdomyosarcoma is distinctly worse than for the embryonal variety, even with the most recent combined modalities of treatment.[917,962,974,984] In the series reported by Enzinger[907] (which antedates current therapeutic regimens), 92% of the patients had died from widespread metastasis within the first 4 years after diagnosis. The lung and regional lymph nodes are the most common metastatic sites. The ovary can also be involved.[985] Peripheral lymph node involvement, sometimes in a multiple fashion, may be the first manifestation of the disease ("lymphadenopathic form"). A common site for occult primary alveolar rhabdomyosarcoma is the perirectal-perineal region.

Electron microscopy. Ultrastructural examination may confirm a diagnosis of rhabdomyosarcoma through the identification of sarcomere-related structures, such as Z bands, thick and thin filaments in a hexagonal array, an A band containing thick filaments, and H and M bands, or leptomeric structures* (Fig. 25-93). Drawbacks of this technique are those related to sampling and the absence of these features in the poorly differentiated cells.[886,894] A good correlation is present between the light and electron microscopic appearance of these tumors.[972]

Immunohistochemistry and other special stains. Conventional special stains such as PTAH, Masson's trichrome, and silver impregnation technique are of only relative use in the diagnosis of rhabdomyosarcoma. They highlight the cross striations when these are already appreciated in a good H & E preparation, but they only rarely detect them if they are not already apparent in the routine preparations.

Immunohistochemistry, on the contrary, has proved of great value. Hardly any other tumor type has been described for which the array of markers is as varied as for rhabdomyosarcoma, and the list continues to grow.* There is a range of specificity and sensitivity among these markers and this translates into their relative practical utility. The most important follow:

1 *Myoglobin.* This protein appears to be specific for striated muscle differentiation, and it would therefore seem well suited for this purpose[885,927,950] (Fig. 25-94). Unfortunately, it is expressed only when the tumor cell has acquired a high degree of differentiation. It is therefore often negative in poorly differentiated tumors.[889] One should also be careful of diffusion from neighboring injured skeletal muscle fibers.[909]

2 *Desmin.* This intermediate filament is a specific indicator for muscle differentiation, but it reacts with both smooth and striated muscle. In general, only tumors with round rhabdomyoblasts or strap cells show positivity for this marker.[948] Nevertheless, in one study, it was found that desmin was the most reliable single marker for the identification of the solid variant of alveolar rhabdomyosarcoma.[978]

3 *Myosin.* This marker has proved very effective.[931,978] Adult sarcomeric and fetal forms of myosin exist; expression of fetal heavy chain skeletal myosin, viewed as the expression of an oncofetal antigen, was found in one series in 81% of rhabdomyosarcomas.[897,898,911]

4 *Tropomyosin alpha-actinin, titin, and Z protein.* These are constituent proteins of sarcomeric muscle and show a high degree of specificity. Unfortunately, most of them stain only well-differentiated cells in a minority of the tumors, a fact that greatly limits their diagnostic application.[952,955]

5 *Actin.* Rhabdomyosarcomas consistently express sarcomeric actin, which represents one of the best markers for this tumor[899,943,951,975] (Fig. 25-95). Schurch et al.[970] made the interesting and surprising observation that the specific sarcomeric actin expressed by these tumors is not of the alpha-skeletal muscle but the alpha-cardiac type.

6 *Vimentin.* This antigen is consistently positive, particularly in the lesser differentiated tumors, but it lacks specificity as a skeletal muscle marker.[948] It is the first marker to appear in the tumor cells, followed sequentially by actin, desmin, fast myosin, and myoglobin.[888,983]

7 *MyoD1.* The MyoD1 gene codes for a nuclear phosphoprotein, which induces skeletal muscle differenti-

---

*References 887, 908, 921, 937, 942, 949.

*References 882, 910, 923, 966, 971, 978, 980.

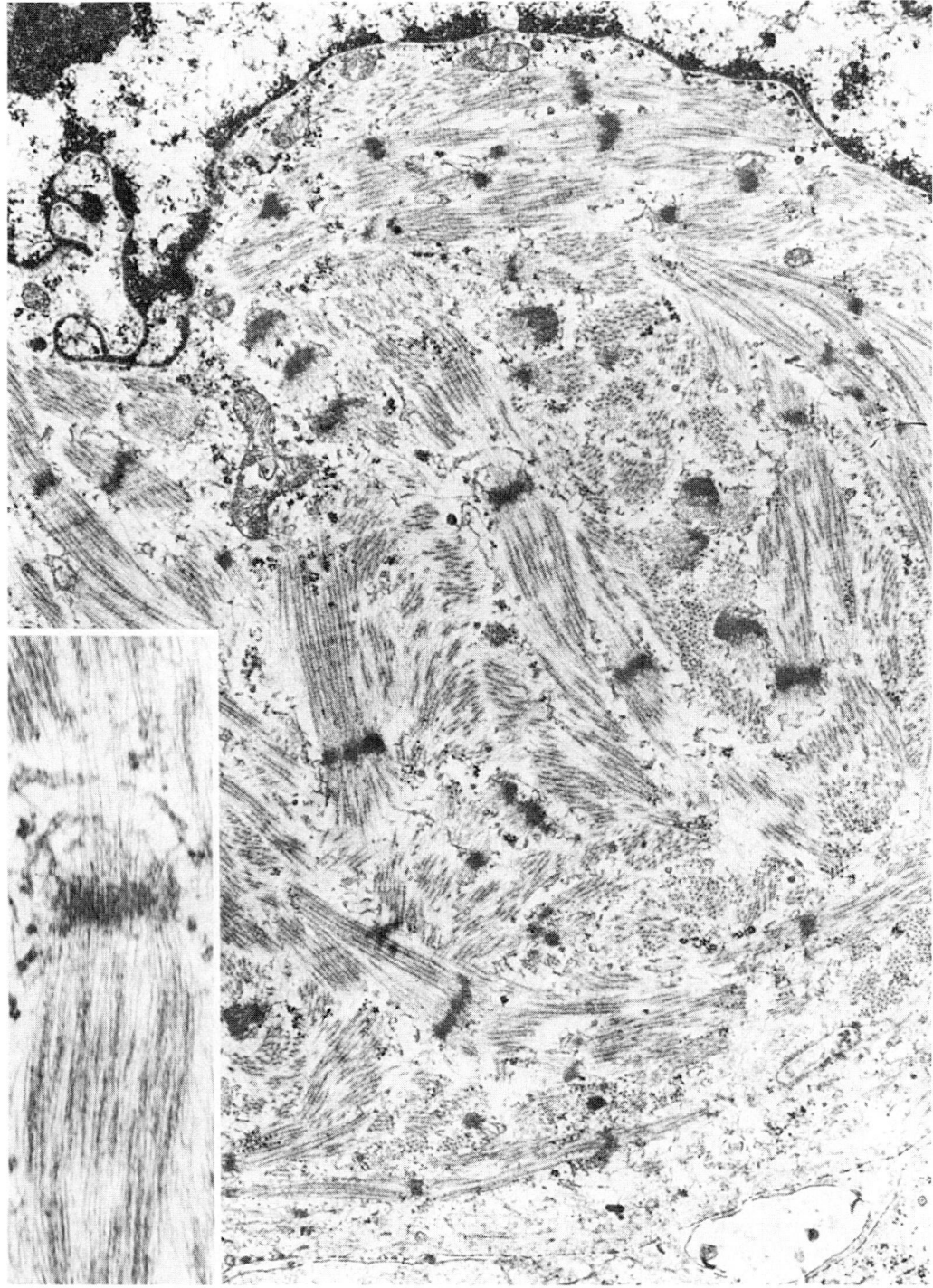

Fig. 25-93 Electron micrograph from same case shown in Fig. 25-92. Cytoplasm of tumor cell contains abortive cross striations, too small and haphazardly oriented to be visible with light microscope. **Inset** shows Z band and clearly visible double set of filaments. (×18,000; **inset** ×45,000.) (Courtesy Dr. B. Lane, New York.)

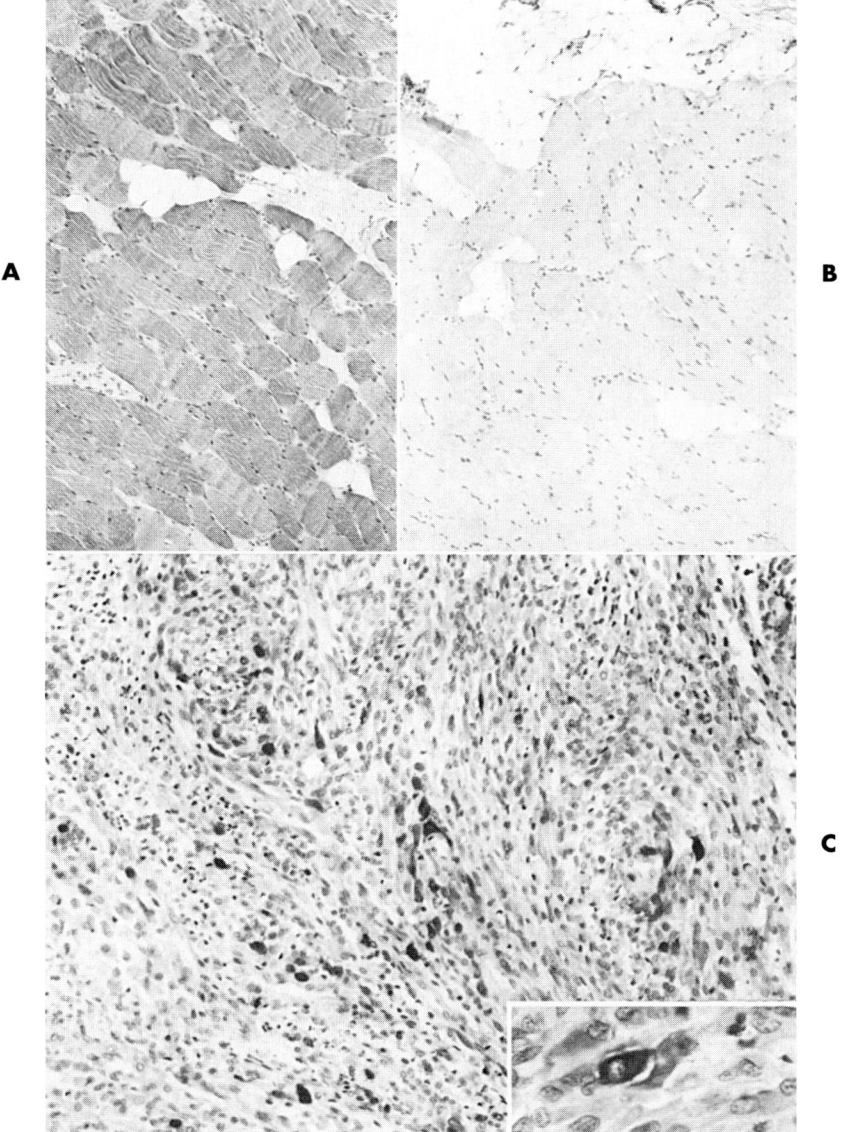

Fig. 25-94 Myoglobin stain with immunoperoxidase technique. **A,** Normal skeletal muscle. Strong diffuse cytoplasmic positivity is evident. **B,** Preabsorption of antiserum with myoglobin abolishes reaction. **C,** Embryonal rhabdomyosarcoma. Cytoplasm of many tumor cells is strongly positive. This is particularly well appreciated in high-power **inset. (A** and **B** from Mukai K, Rosai J, Hallaway BE: Localization of myoglobin in normal and neoplastic human skeletal muscle cells using an immunoperoxidase method. Am J Surg Pathol **3:**373-376, 1979.)

ation in mesenchymal cells.[893,902] This protein product can be consistently detected immunohistochemically in fresh frozen tissue. The results with this marker in paraffin-embedded material are not overly satisfactory and somewhat inferior to those obtained with the related nuclear protein *myogenin*.[903,982b] It has been shown that the MyoD1 protein present in rhabdomyosarcoma cells is capable of binding DNA but is relatively nonfunctional as a transcriptional activator, suggesting the deficiency in these tumors of a factor needed for its activity.[977a]

8 *Enzymes.* These can be demonstrated immunohistochemically or through standard enzymatic histo-
chemical techniques; most of the latter require fresh frozen tissue. They include creatine kinase subunit M (muscle type[900]), myo(pho)sphorilase, acetylcholinesterase, adenosine triphosphatase,[982] and betaenolase.[958,964]

9 *Basal lamina components, such as type IV collagen and laminin.* No specificity can be ascribed to these markers, since they are also present in other types of mesenchymal cells and in epithelial cells.[883]

10 *Antiskeletal muscle antibody from myasthenic patients.* The specific antigen against which this antibody is directed is not known, but it is clearly associated with the skeletal muscle fiber.[954]

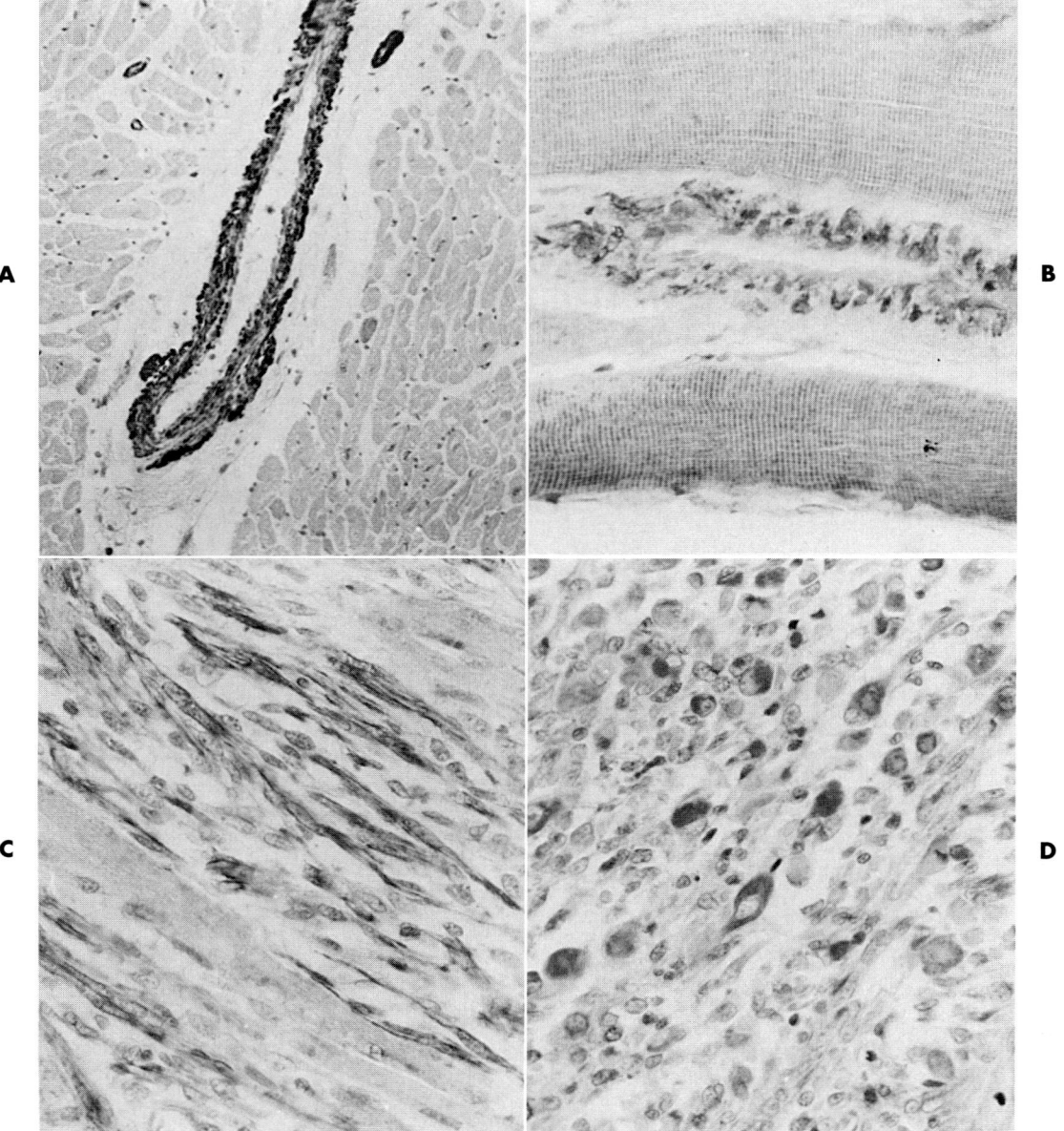

Fig. 25-95 Actin staining of muscle cells whit immunoperoxidase technique. **A,** Normal myocardium. Smooth muscle of vessel wall stains intensely. **B,** Normal skeletal muscle. Cross striations are dramatically demonstrated. Smooth muscle of vessel wall between two skeletal muscle fibers also stains. **C,** Fetal rhabdomyoma. There is marked cytoplasmic positivity in nearly all neoplastic cells. **D,** Embryonal rhabdomyosarcoma. Staining of variable intensity may be seen in tumor cells.

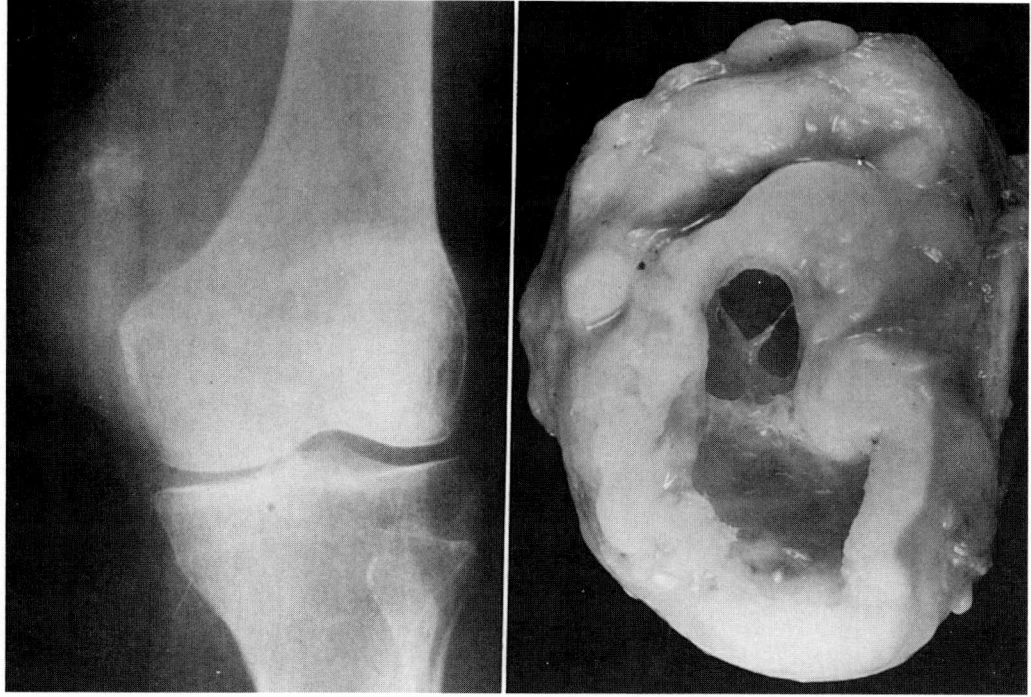

Fig. 25-96 Soft tissue chondroma occurring in knee region of 71-year-old woman. As usual, tumor is partially calcified, lobulated, and focally cystic.

11 **Insulin-like growth factor II.** This has been found to be consistently expressed in rhabdomyosarcomas, in contrast to most other types of childhood malignancy.[986]

12 **Other markers.** Rhabdomyosarcomas have been found to show focal immunoreactivity for keratin, neurofilaments, and S-100 protein.[944]

This is a wide and somewhat confusing choice of options. In our institution, we have chosen the battery of sarcomeric actin, desmin, and myoglobin for the routine investigation of these neoplasms.

Cytogenetics and molecular pathology. Alveolar rhabdomyosarcomas are consistently associated with the translocation t (2;13).[903a,957] This is not present in embryonal rhabdomyosarcomas, which lack a chromosomal marker. MYCN amplification has been detected in close to half of the alveolar tumors but not in the embryonal types.[904]

DNA ploidy. Most rhabdomyosarcomas have been shown to be aneuploid, in contrast to other types of childhood sarcomas.[945] It has been suggested that DNA content is a predictor of outcome in some subsets of embryonal rhabdomyosarcoma.[956]

Tumors of pluripotential mesenchyme

Stout[994] coined the term *mesenchymoma* for tumors consisting of two or more mesenchymal elements in addition to fibrous tissue. Benign and malignant forms exist. The most frequent benign variant is composed of smooth muscle, fat, and blood vessels (angiomyolipoma). Cartilage may also be present, establishing a histogenetic link with the tumors described in the following section.[989-991] It is debatable whether benign mesenchymoma is of a neoplastic or hamartomatous nature.[988] The malignant variant, well described by Stout,[994] contains in the same neoplasm multiple varieties of soft tissue sarcomas, such as chondrosarcoma, liposarcoma, and leiomyosarcoma. Nash and Stout[992] reviewed forty-two cases occurring in children, in nine of which the tumor was present at birth. Most malignant mesenchymomas are high-grade neoplasms, but some cases have been characterized by a low-grade histology and an indolent clinical course.[993]

Tumors of metaplastic mesenchyme

Soft tissue (extraskeletal) chondromas are seen most frequently in the soft tissues of the hands and feet of adults.[1010,1016] Grossly, they are lobulated, have a typical hyaline appearance, and are often calcified (Fig. 25-96). Some nuclear hyperchromasia may be present and should not be interpreted as evidence of malignancy[1010,1024] (Fig. 25-97). Chondrosarcomas of the hands and feet exist, but they are exceptionally rare.[1002] The occasional presence of a cellular fibroblastic growth around the lobules may prompt confusion with calcifying aponeurotic fibroma. Also confusing is the fact that sometimes the cartilaginous cells have an acidophilic cytoplasm simulating that of a histiocyte and sometimes a vacuolated appearance reminiscent of a lipoblast. Histologic variants with proliferation of osteoclast-like giant cells and chrondroblastic activity have been described.[999] Local recurrence is not infrequent.

Soft tissue (extraskeletal) chondrosarcomas exhibit in general a less aggressive behavior than their skeletal coun-

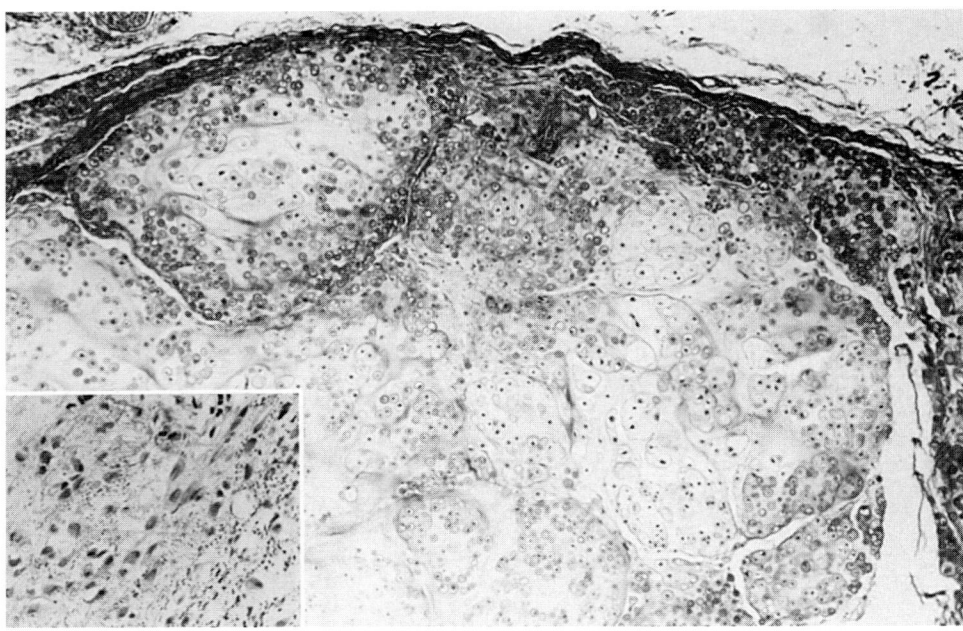

Fig. 25-97 Soft tissue chondroma. Note lobular configuration of lesion. **Inset** shows fine punctate calcification and plump appearance of tumor cells.

terpart.[1029,1034] Most of these tumors fit into the category of *myxoid chondrosarcoma.*[1005] Most occur in the extremities of adult patients, but they have also been reported in the trunk and/or in children.[1009] Microscopically, there are strands and cords of relatively small cells with acidophilic cytoplasm that are occasionally vacuolated, embedded in an abundant myxoid matrix.[1005,1030] Well-differentiated chondrocytes are absent, and this is responsible for the difficulties sometimes encountered in the diagnosis. Glycogen is present in many of the tumor cells. Acid mucopolysaccharides are abundant in the stroma. In contrast with those present in myxoma and myxoid liposarcoma, they are partially resistant to testicular hyaluronidase treatment because they are largely composed of chondroitin-4-sulfate, chondroitin-6-sulfate, and keratan sulfate. The histochemical properties of the mucosubstance formed by most chondrosarcomas (in contrast to those of benign cartilaginous tumors) are those of fetal cartilage.[1015] In some tumors, this myxochondroid stroma is scanty, and the diagnosis may consequently be missed.[1017] Ultrastructurally, the most conspicuous features of the cells of myxoid chondrosarcoma are a well-developed granular endoplasmic reticulum (sometimes containing peculiar parallel microtubules), abundant cytoplasmic filaments, and cytoplasmic glycogen.[1004,1020,1023,1030,1033]

Immunohistochemically, myxoid chondrosarcomas are reactive for S-100 protein, Leu7, and lysozyme but not for keratin (despite their morphologic resemblance to chordoma).[1007] The chromosonal translocation t(9;22) (q22-31;q11-12) has been consistently detected in these tumors.[1026a] Metastases are usually in the lungs[1025]; in some cases, this is the first manifestation of the tumor.[1003] Cases reported as *chordoid sarcoma* or *chordoid tumor*[998a,1019,1031] probably belong to the same category as extraskeletal chon-

drosarcoma, even if some have been found to exhibit epithelial membrane antigen immunoreactivity.[1032] *Parachordoma* is a morphologically somewhat similar neoplasm that typically develops adjacent to tendon, synovium, or osseous structures within extremities. Microscopically, well-circumscribed lobules composed of small cellular aggregates embedded within a hyalinized and chondroid matrix are present.[1001] Some of the tumor cells have the features of physaliphorous cells. Its nature and relationship with soft tissue chondrosarcoma remain unclear.[1013,1026,1027]

Another morphologic variant of chondrosarcoma that can be found in soft tissue and in other extraskeletal sites is *mesenchymal chondrosarcoma.* It has been described in the orbit, dura, trunk, retroperitoneum, extremities, and kidney.* Like its counterpart in the bone, it is characterized microscopically by an alternating pattern of highly cellular undifferentiated small cells (often growing in a hemangiopericytomatous fashion) and islands of well-differentiated cartilage (Fig. 25-98) (see Chapter 24). The prognosis is poor.[1022]

Yet another variant of soft tissue chondrosarcoma is *embryonal chondrosarcoma,* a very rare childhood tumor with a primitive appearance.[1014]

Soft tissue (extraskeletal) osteosarcoma is distinguished from chondrosarcoma by applying the same criteria used for skeletal tumors (i.e., the occurrence of osteoid and bone formation directly produced by the tumor cells, without interposition of cartilage) (Fig. 25-99). It usually occurs in the extremities of adults[995,1006,1011,1028] (Plate XX-A). A small proportion of these tumors arise following exposure to x rays.[1012] As for their most common counterpart in the skeletal system, the predominant histologic pattern may be

*References 997, 1008, 1018, 1022, 1035, 1037.

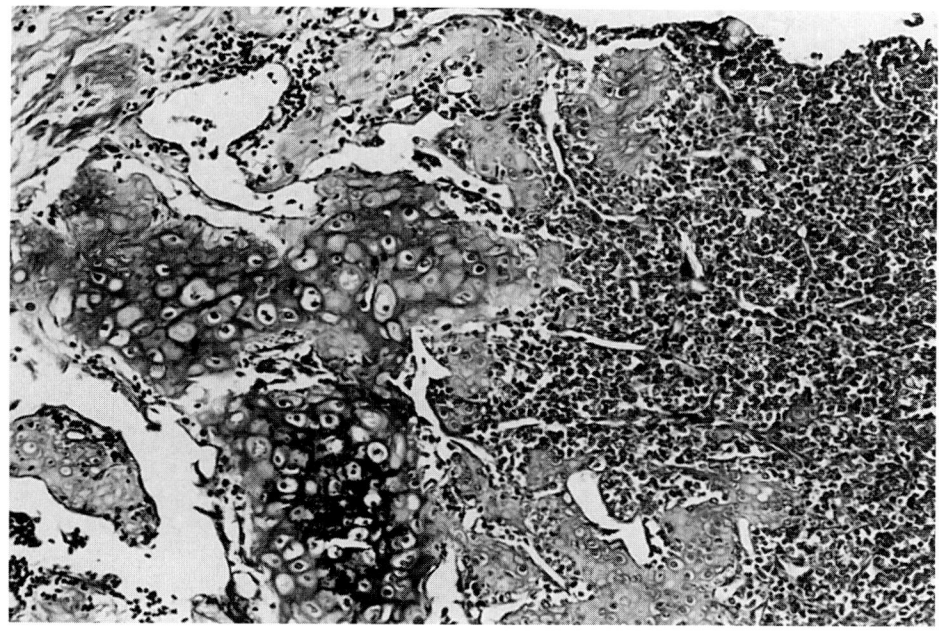

Fig. 25-98 Mesenchymal chondrosarcoma. Areas of highly cellular small round-cell appearance with prominent vascularization alternate with foci of well-differentiated cartilage.

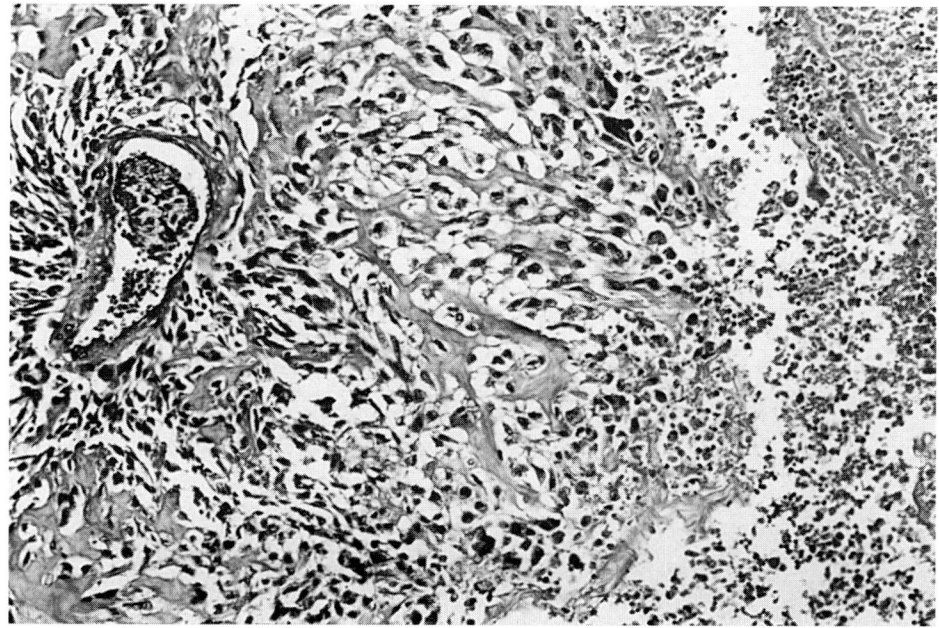

Fig. 25-99 Extraskeletal osteosarcoma. There is extensive osteoid production by tumor cells.

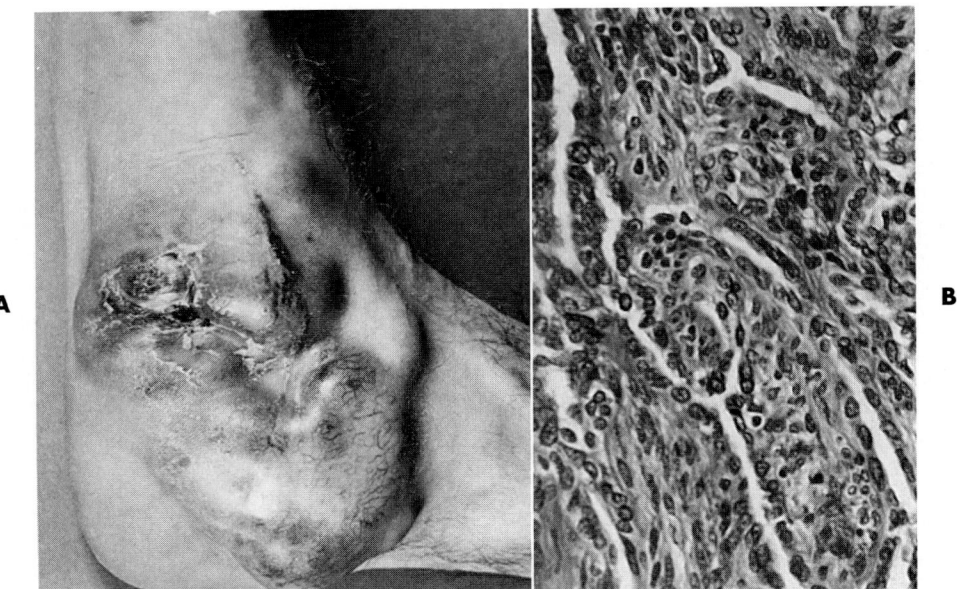

Fig. 25-100 Synovial sarcoma. **A,** Clinical appearance of tumor, which presented as large ulcerated mass in ankle. **B,** Microscopic appearance, showing characteristic biphasic pattern of glands and spindle cells.

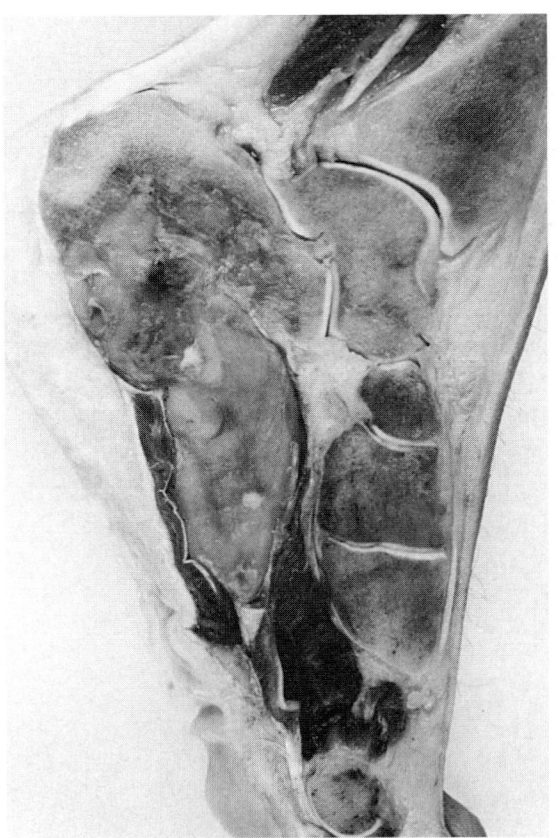

Fig. 25-101 Cut surface of lower extremity amputated for synovial sarcoma of heel. The tumor has solid appearance. It is located in deep soft tissues and is invading the os calcis.

osteoblastic, chondroblastic, fibroblastic, MFH-like, telangiectactic, or well differentiated (the latter being analogous to parosteal osteosarcoma).[996,1021,1036] The prognosis is much worse than for chondrosarcoma, the overall mortality rate being over 60%.[1000] Extraskeletal osteosarcoma should be distinguished from myositis ossificans (see Chapter 24).[1024] The presence of marked nuclear atypia and lack of differentiation ("zone phenomenon") are the most important identifying features. It should also be distinguished from other soft tissue tumors in which metaplastic bone is formed, such as fibrosarcoma, synovial sarcoma, and MFH.[998]

Tumors of synovial tissue

Synovial sarcoma arises in 80% of the cases about the knee and ankle joints of children and young adults[1055,1059,1075,1079,1090] (Figs. 25-100 and 25-101). It also occurs about the shoulder and elbow; in the region of the hip, soft tissues of the neck (particularly the retropharyngeal area),[1039,1082] oral cavity,[1087] anterior abdominal wall,[1049] retroperitoneum,[1086] and mediastinum[1094]; and intravascularly.[1071,1085] This neoplasm often grows close to joints, tendon sheaths, and bursae, but it is very rare for it to involve the synovial membrane.[1067] It is well circumscribed, firm, and grayish pink. Focal calcification is frequent, and it may be detected radiographically.[1092]

Microscopically, the typical example of this tumor has a biphasic pattern resulting from the admixture of gland-like areas and a sarcomatous stroma (Fig. 25-98, *B*). Exceptionally, squamous metaplasia is seen in the epithelial component.[1074] Hyalinization, calcification, osseous metaplasia, or cartilaginous metaplasia can be present in the sarcomatous component; sometimes, the osteoid and bone formation is so extensive as to obscure the true nature of the neoplasm.[1073]

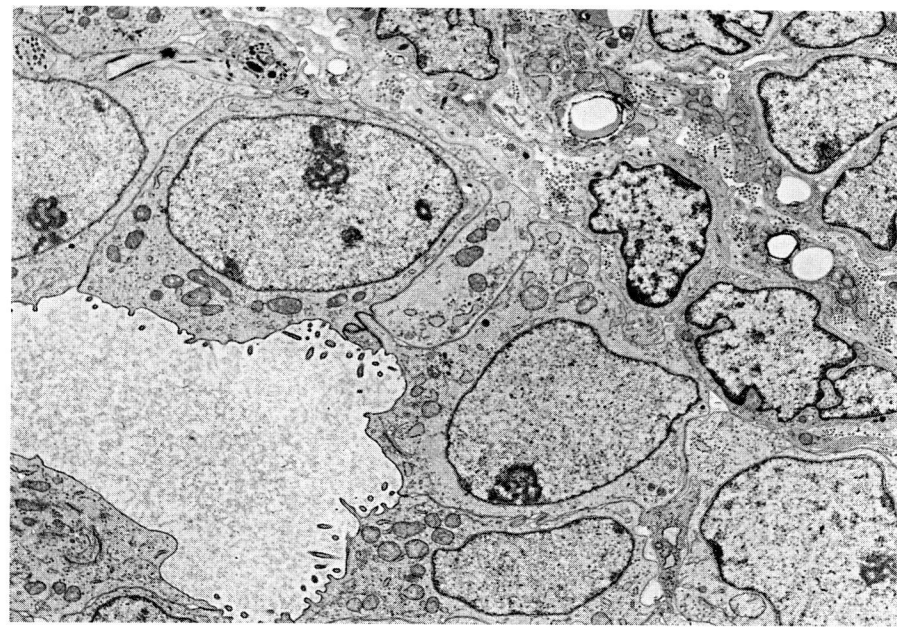

Fig. 25-102 Electron microscopic appearance of biphasic synovial sarcoma. Glandular formation of epithelioid tumor cells with sparse luminal microvilli *(lower left).* (×4300.) (Courtesy Dr. Robert A. Erlandson, Memorial Sloan-Kettering Cancer Center.)

A predominantly epithelial synovial sarcoma may be misdiagnosed as metastatic adenocarcinoma.[1057,1066] Conversely, an incorrect diagnosis of fibrosarcoma may be made when the spindle-cell component predominates. A careful search for an epithelial-like component should be carried out in any tumor with the appearance of fibrosarcoma located in a periarticular area. The possibility of synovial sarcoma should be suspected in the presence of spindle-cell tumors of monotonous appearance having plump-appearing nuclei, scanty mitotic activity, a focally whorled pattern, distinct lobulation, a large number of mast cells, or occasional nests of large, pale cells. It has been proposed that tumors having these features but no clear-cut epithelial foci represent synovial sarcoma with monophasic growth of the fibroblastic component[1065,1070] and that epithelioid sarcoma and other purely epithelial tumors of soft tissue are variants of synovial sarcomas with an almost monophasic growth of the epithelial component.[1048,1056,1093] The occasional coexistence of synovial sarcoma and epithelioid sarcoma[1084] and the ultrastructural similarities between the two tumors[1058,1061] support this contention.

Reticulin stains emphasize the biphasic nature of the tumor. Mucin stains reveal the presence of acid mucopolysaccharides (hyaluronic acid, chondroitin sulfate, heparitin sulfate) in the spindle-cell areas and of PAS-positive, sialic acid–containing glycoproteins in the epithelial foci.[1076]

Ultrastructurally, the epithelial areas have features of true glandular epithelium; subtle features of epithelial differentiation are sometimes also found in the spindle-cell component, such as intercellular spaces within processes and specialized cell junctions* (Figs. 25-102 and 25-103).

Immunohistochemically, there is strong reactivity for keratin in the epithelial areas and often in the spindle cells as well.[1038,1041,1062,1083] Since normal or reactive synovial cells do not express keratin, the possibility has been raised that synovial sarcoma is not differentiating toward synovial structures, as traditionally believed, but toward true epithelium. The corollary of this theory is that tumor should be viewed as a primary carcinoma (or carcinosarcoma) of soft tissue,[1054,1060,1072] whether arising from epithelial rests or— more likely—from mesenchymal tissues that have undergone epithelial metaplasia. Of importance in this regard is the fact that, whereas many types of soft tissue sarcoma (including synovial sarcoma) exhibit immunoreactivity for keratins 8 and 18, only synovial sarcoma shows positivity for keratins 7 and 19, as well as for the desmosome-associated protein desmoplakin.[1069] CEA, epithelial membrane antigen, vimentin and occasionally S-100 protein are also expressed by this tumor.* It has also been found that a significant number of cases of synovial sarcoma are immunoreactive for O13, the marker characteristically associated with Ewing's sarcoma/PNET (see p. 2105).[1044a]

Synovial sarcoma has been found to be associated in about 90% of the cases with the chromosomal translocation t (x;18) (p11.2; q 11.2); this aberration is present in both the biphasic and monophasic types.[1043] The breakpoints have been cloned and shown to involve two novel genes, SSX (in chromosome X) and SYT (in chromosome 18). This results in a chimeric SYT-SSX transcript, of which a minor molecular variant has been described.[1052]

Synovial sarcoma can recur locally and metastasize distantly, particularly to the lung and lymph nodes. The inci-

*References 1044-1046, 1050, 1053, 1058, 1063, 1068, 1090.

*References 1038, 1041, 1051, 1060, 1078, 1080.

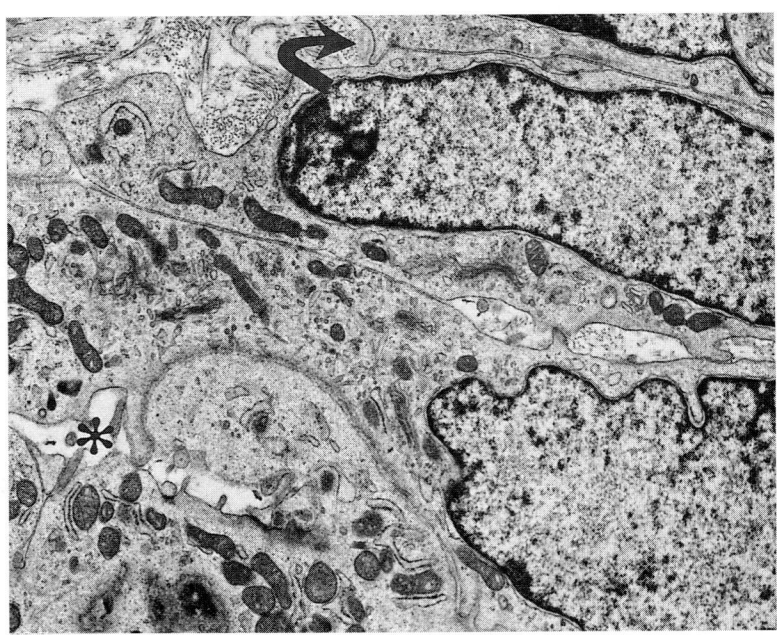

Fig. 25-103 Electron microscopic appearance of monophasic synovial sarcoma. Spindle-shaped tumor cells. Note the rudimentary lumen with microvilli *(asterisk)* and the remnants of basal lamina *(arrow).* (×7700.) (Courtesy Dr. Robert A. Erlandson, Memorial Sloan-Kettering Cancer Center.)

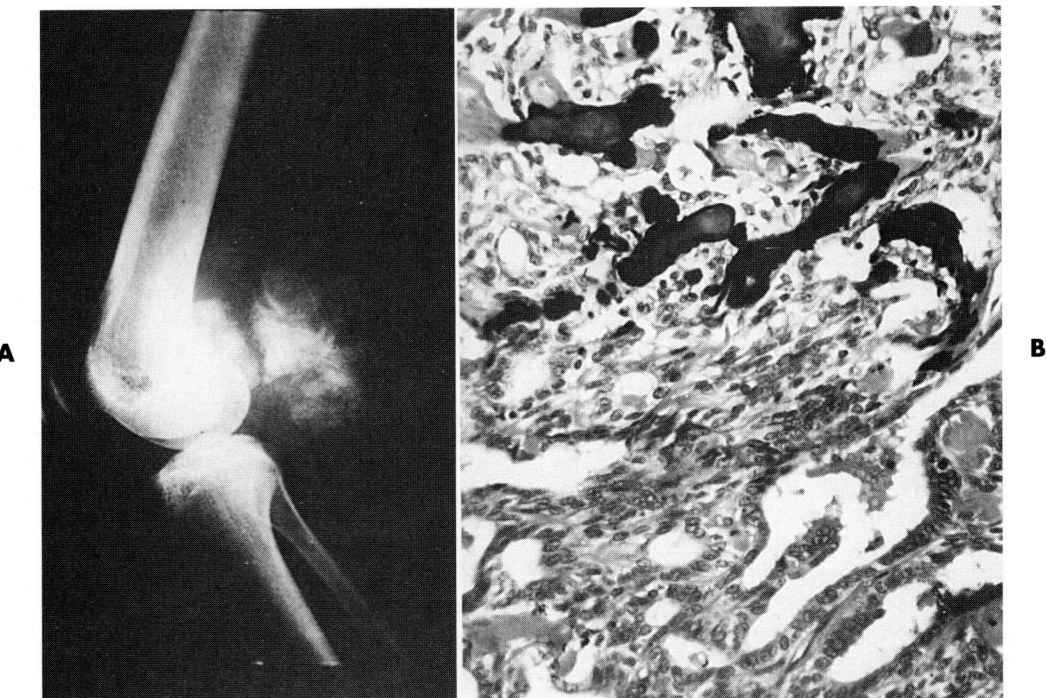

Fig. 25-104 A, Radiograph of large calcifying synovial sarcoma located in popliteal space. **B,** Photomicrograph of same case showing biphasic component and extensive stromal calcification. (From Varela-Duran J, Enzinger FM: Calcifying synovial sarcoma. A clinicopathologic study of 32 cases. Cancer **50:**345-352, 1982.)

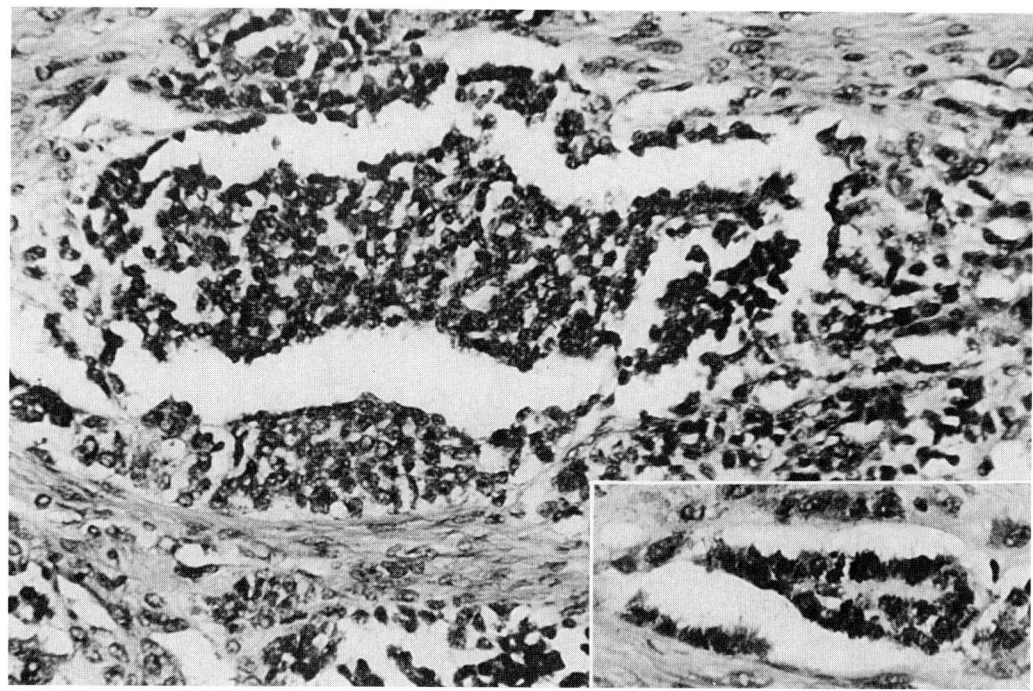

Fig. 25-105 Pigmented neuroectodermal tumor of infancy. Clump of undifferentiated neuroectodermal cells has detached from peripheral portion, resulting in alveolar pattern. **Inset,** Another area of same tumor illustrating melanin-containing elements.

dence of nodal metastases is in the range of 10% to 15% (i.e., much higher than that of most soft tissue sarcomas of adults). The preferred treatment is local excision, with wide margins of normal tissue, supplemented by a high dose of radiation therapy.[1089] Synovial sarcoma has been traditionally regarded as a tumor of ominous prognosis[1055]; in several series, however, the 5-year survival rate has approached 50%.[1042,1064,1091] The prognosis seems to be even better for the synovial sarcomas associated with osseous metaplasia and/or extensive calcification. In a variant characterized by heavy stromal calcification and designated as *calcifying synovial sarcoma* the 5-year survival rate was 84%[1092] (Fig. 25-104). The prognosis is also related to age (better in young patients), site (better for distal lesions), size (better for tumors less than 5 cm in diameter),[1088,1095] mitotic activity (better for tumors having less than fifteen mitoses per ten high-power fields),[1040] necrosis (worse for tumors having tumor necrosis of more than 50%), rhabdoid cells (worse when present), and DNA ploidy pattern (worse for aneuploid tumors).[1047,1077,1081]

Tumors of extragonadal germ cells

Soft tissue teratomas are more frequent in females and are present either at birth or in early childhood.[1096] In some cases, there is an association with twinning or malformations. The most common locations, in descending order of frequency, are the sacrococcygeal area, head and neck, retroperitoneum, mediastinum, and central nervous system.[1097,1101,1104,1105] Taken as a whole, approximately three fourths are benign. However, there are important variations in the incidence of malignancy according to location, age,

and sex.[1099,1100] Nearly all the teratomas presenting in the neck during infancy are benign, usually asymmetric, and massive; the rare teratomas of the neck presenting in adults have a high incidence of malignancy.[1098,1103]

The terminology and diagnostic criteria used in the evaluation of these lesions is the same as for those of gonadal origin (see Chapters 18 and 19). The benign form is often multicystic and contains a variety of well-differentiated tissues. The malignant types may have the appearance of teratocarcinoma, embryonal carcinoma, or yolk sac tumor. Immature neuroectodermal components are common; although they occasionally exhibit metastasizing capacity, their natural tendency is toward spontaneous maturation.[1102]

Tumors of neural tissue (other than peripheral nerves)

Pigmented neuroectodermal tumor of infancy

The neurogenic origin of pigmented neuroectodermal tumor of infancy, also known as melanotic progonoma and retinal anlage tumor, is now established.[1107,1112] The classical location is the maxilla, but it also has been reported in the mandible, skull and other bones, mediastinum, soft tissues (thigh, forearm, cheek), and epididymis.[1108,1110,1111,1115,1117] Microscopically, most tumor cells are small and round, with the appearance of neuroblasts. As a result, this tumor may be misdiagnosed as neuroblastoma. The diagnostic feature is the presence of pseudoglandular or alveolar formations lined by a wall of larger cells containing abundant CNS-type (spiculated) melanin in their cytoplasm (Fig. 25-105). Rarely, a skeletal muscle component is present.[1113] Immunohistochemically, the large

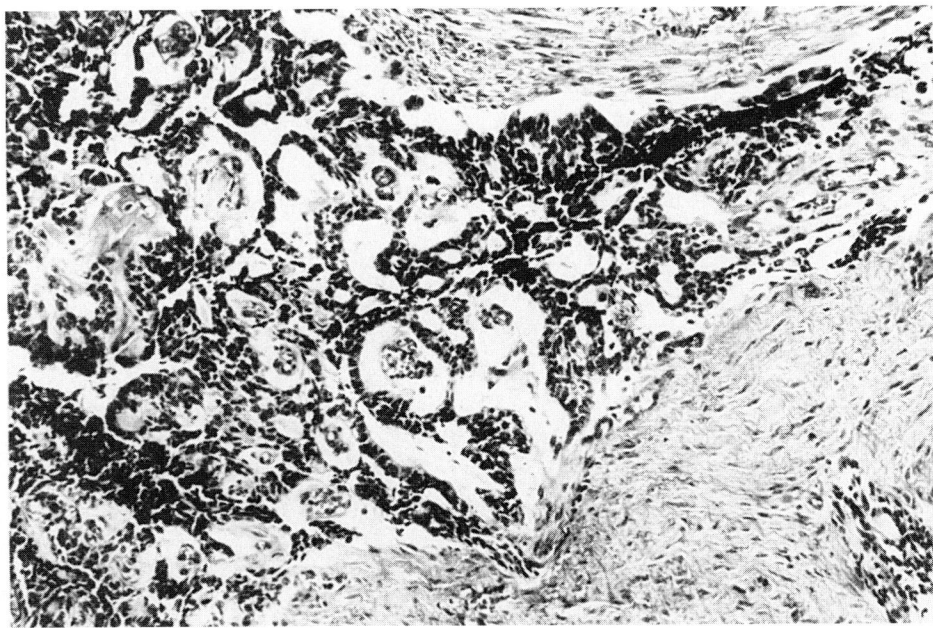

Fig. 25-106 Soft tissue ependymoma located in sacrococcygeal region. Tumor cells form well-defined perivascular structures and are surrounded by dense fibrous tissue.

cells are strongly reactive for keratin and HMB-45 and less so for vimentin and NSE, whereas the small cells show only positivity for NSE. Both cell components are negative for S-100 protein.[1106,1113,1114,1116] Ultrastructurally, there are melanosomes at various stages of maturation in the large cells, and neurosecretory granules and cytoplasmic processes in the small cells.[1113]

The clinical course is usually benign. Most supposedly malignant varieties probably represent malignant teratomas with a pigmented neuroectodermal component. However, unquestionable recurrent and metastatic cases of pigmented neuroectodermal tumor of infancy have been seen.[1109,1110,1117]

Other neural tumors

Meningiomas can present as a soft tissue mass at the base of the nose or scalp[1119] (see Chapters 4 and 7).

Myxopapillary ependymomas can appear as soft tissue masses over the sacrococcygeal area, unconnected with the spine or spinal cord structures[1118,1121] (Plate XX-B). The clinical diagnosis is usually that of pilonidal cyst. Grossly, they are well circumscribed and can be shelled out easily. Their microscopic appearance is homologous to that of their more common counterpart in the filum terminale and cauda equina (see Chapter 28) (Fig. 25-106). Metastases have occurred in approximately one fifth of the cases.[1120]

Myxopapillary ependymomas should be distinguished from sacrococcygeal ependymal rests, which probably represent their precursors. These are small (less than 0.5 cm) nodules that are usually found incidentally in tissue from pilonidal sinuses and that consist of clusters of ependymal cells near the junction of dermis and subcutis.[1122]

Gliomas of soft tissue have been generally located at the root of the nose in infants, but they can occur in other sites;

they are probably not neoplasms but examples of heterotopic glial tissue.[1123]

Primitive neuroectodermal tumors (PNET) are discussed on p. 2105.

Tumors of hematopoietic tissue

Rarely, *malignant lymphomas* first manifest themselves as soft tissue masses, usually located in an extremity.[1129] This occurrence is more common with non-Hodgkin's lymphomas than with Hodgkin's disease. Most cases are of B-cell derivation, but examples of peripheral T-cell lymphoma with primary involvement of soft tissues are on record.[1125,1128] Exceptionally, these lymphomas develop in areas of postmastectomy lymphedema and are confused clinically with angiosarcoma (Stewart-Treves syndrome)[1127]

Most cases of *plasmacytoma* of soft tissue represent direct extension from underlying osseous foci.[1124] However, isolated soft tissue masses also can occur in the absence of bone involvement. They have a tendency to become disseminated.

In rare cases, nodules of *extramedullary hematopoiesis* develop in the mediastinum, retroperitoneum, or other soft tissue areas; they have been described in agnogenic myeloid metaplasia and congenital spherocytosis and in other types of anemia[1126] and should be distinguished from myelolipoma (see Chapter 16).

Tumors of uncertain cell type
Fibrous hamartoma of infancy

Fibrous hamartoma of infancy is a tumorlike condition seen almost exclusively during the first 2 years of life and is sometimes present at birth.[1130,1133] It predominates in boys, and the most common locations are the region of the shoulder, axilla, and upper arm. It is almost always solitary.

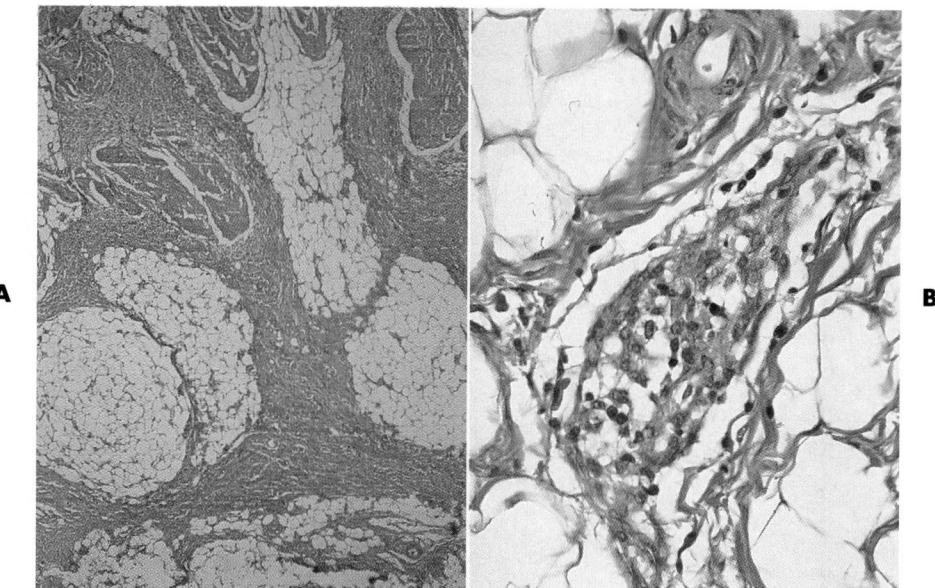

Fig. 25-107 Fibrous hamartoma of infancy. **A,** Low-power microscopic view showing an admixture of islands of mature adipose tissue and cellular fibrous foci. **B,** High-power view showing an oval cluster of plump mesenchymal cells.

Grossly, it is poorly circumscribed and composed of whitish tissue of fibrous appearance intermixed with islands of fat.

Microscopically, the distinctive feature of this lesion is an organoid pattern, three distinct types of tissue being present: (1) well-differentiated spindle cells of fibroblastic/myofibroblastic appearance accompanied by deposition of collagen; (2) mature adipose tissue, and (3) immature, cellular areas arranged in a whorl-like pattern and resembling primitive mesenchyme (Fig. 25-107). Positivity for vimentin occurs in both fibrous and immature areas, whereas reactivity for actin (and sometimes desmin) is found mainly in the spindle-cell areas, suggesting the existence of a myofibroblastic component.[1131,1132,1134] Although there may be local recurrence, the clinical course is basically that of a benign disease.[1130]

Myxoma

Myxomas are rare neoplasms that have a mucoid, slimy gross appearance[1145] (Fig. 25-108, *A*). The majority are poorly circumscribed and may infiltrate neighboring structures. They almost always occur in adults and are more common in females.[1136] The diagnosis of myxoma in a child should be seriously questioned. A high proportion of myxomas arise within skeletal muscle, especially those of the thigh. The prognosis is excellent. In most of the reported series, there was not a single case of local recurrence.[1136,1138] Multiple intramuscular myxomas are nearly always seen in association with fibrous dysplasia of the bones of the same extremity.[1134a,1139,1146] The presence of multiple myxomas in the skin, breast, or other locations should raise the possibility of Carey's syndrome, which also includes spotty cutaneous pigmentation, nodular pigmented adrenal disease, and other endocrine abnormalities.[1135] Another important loca-

tion of myxoma is the juxta-articular region (juxta-articular myxoma), particularly in the knee.[1143]

The differential diagnosis of myxoma should be made with two groups of diseases. The first is a group of neoplasms in which myxomatous change can be a prominent secondary feature, such as liposarcoma, MFH, chondrosarcoma, smooth muscle tumors, embryonal rhabdomyosarcoma, neurofibroma, and aggressive angiomyxoma.[1142] The latter differs from myxoma by its lack of relationship with a skeletal muscle, its great vascularity, and the fact that it is seen almost exclusively in the soft tissues of the female genital region (see Chapter 19).

The second is a variety of non-neoplastic conditions resulting in focal mucinous degeneration of the skin or soft tissues, such as nodular fasciitis, localized myxedema, mucous (myxoid) cyst, ganglion, follicular mucinosis (alopecia mucinosa), papular mucinosis, and cutaneous focal mucinosis.[1140] It should be remembered that in myxoma the cells have a bland and hypocellular appearance throughout, that mitotic activity is practically absent, that lipoblasts are not identified, and, most importantly, that blood vessels are extremely scanty (Fig. 25-108, *B*). The latter feature has been well demonstrated and contrasted with the high vascularity of myxoid liposarcoma in morphologic, angiographic, and microangiographic studies.[1138,1141] Focal aggregates of foamy histiocytes may be present; these are seen to contain neutral fat by oil red O stain and should not be confused with the lipoblasts of myxoid liposarcoma.[1138] The diagnosis of myxoma should be questioned if the lesion is not intramuscular or juxta-articular, if more than occasional vessels are present, and if focal hypercellularity and/or atypia are detected. Admittedly, angiomyxomas of the superficial soft tissue exist.[1134a] However, when hypervascularity is associated in a myxoid tumor with hypercellularity, the alternative

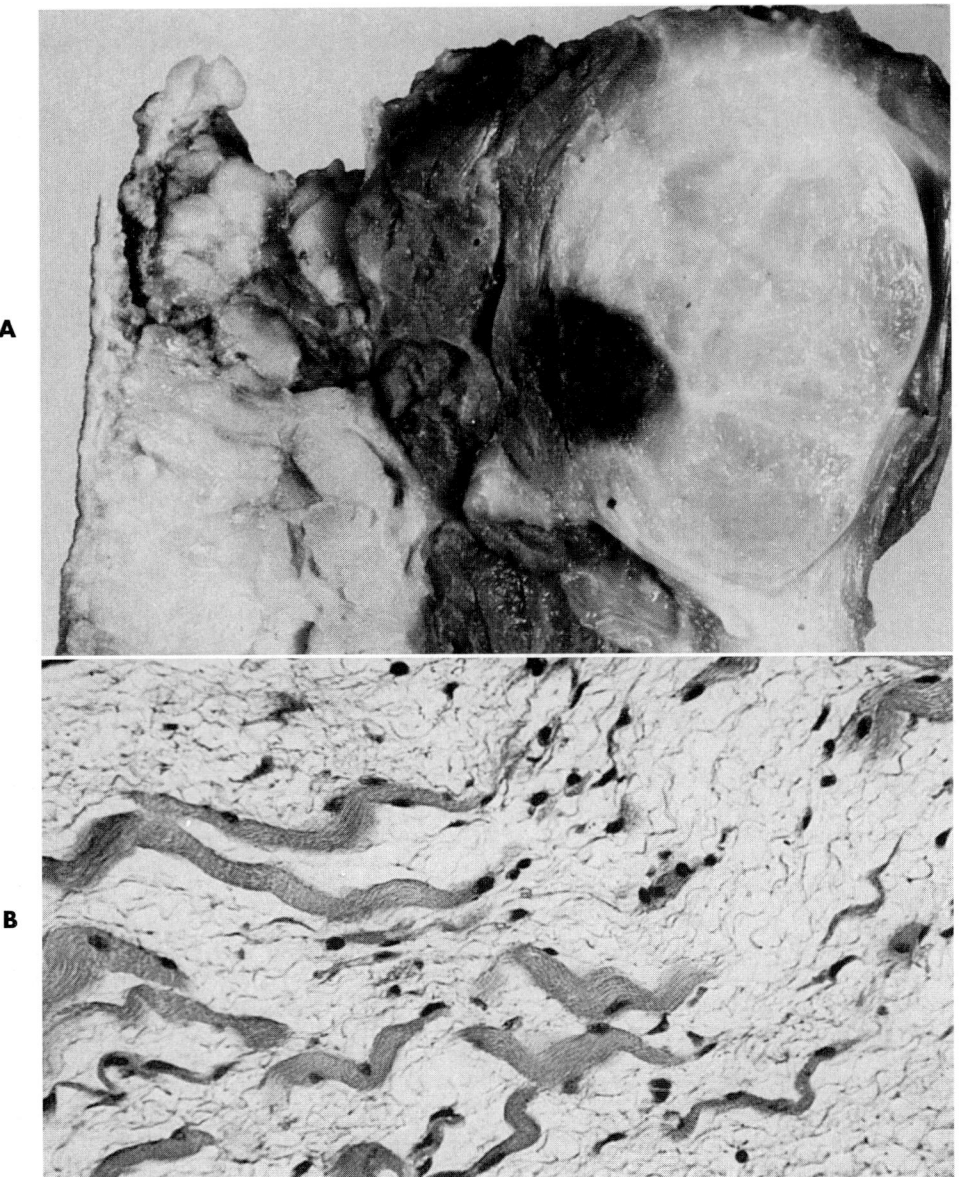

Fig. 25-108 A, Myxoma of vastus lateralis muscle of thigh. **B,** Same tumor shown in **A.** Note myxomatous tissue infiltrating muscle bundles.

possibility of a low-grade form of myxoid MFH (grade I myxofibrosarcoma) or low-grade fibromyxoid sarcoma should be considered. We have seen cases of the latter entity in which multiple local recurrences developed, usually having a similar histology but sometimes acquiring a more pleomorphic appearance.

Ultrastructurally, the principal cell of intramuscular myxoma resembles a fibroblast, with prominent granular endoplasmic reticulum, well-developed Golgi apparatus, and cytoplasmic filaments.[1137] Immunohistochemically, myxoid myxoma shows no reactivity for S-100 protein, this constituting another difference from myxoid liposarcoma.[1138] Desmin is also absent, but vimentin is expressed.[1144] The myxoid material is entirely digestible by hyaluronidase.

Granular cell tumor

The classic location of granular cell tumor, also known as granular cell myoblastoma, is the tongue. It has been seen, however, in many other locations such as the skin, vulva, breast, larynx, bronchus, esophagus, stomach, appendix, rectum, anus, bile ducts, pancreas, urinary bladder, uterus, brain, pituitary gland, and soft tissue.* Multiplicity of lesions can be observed, particularly in black patients.[1173,1185] A few congenital examples have been reported, most of them located in the gingiva,[1155,1163,1165] but some exhibiting systemic involvement.[1180]

*References 1151, 1154, 1156, 1159, 1160, 1162, 1169, 1173, 1184, 1193.

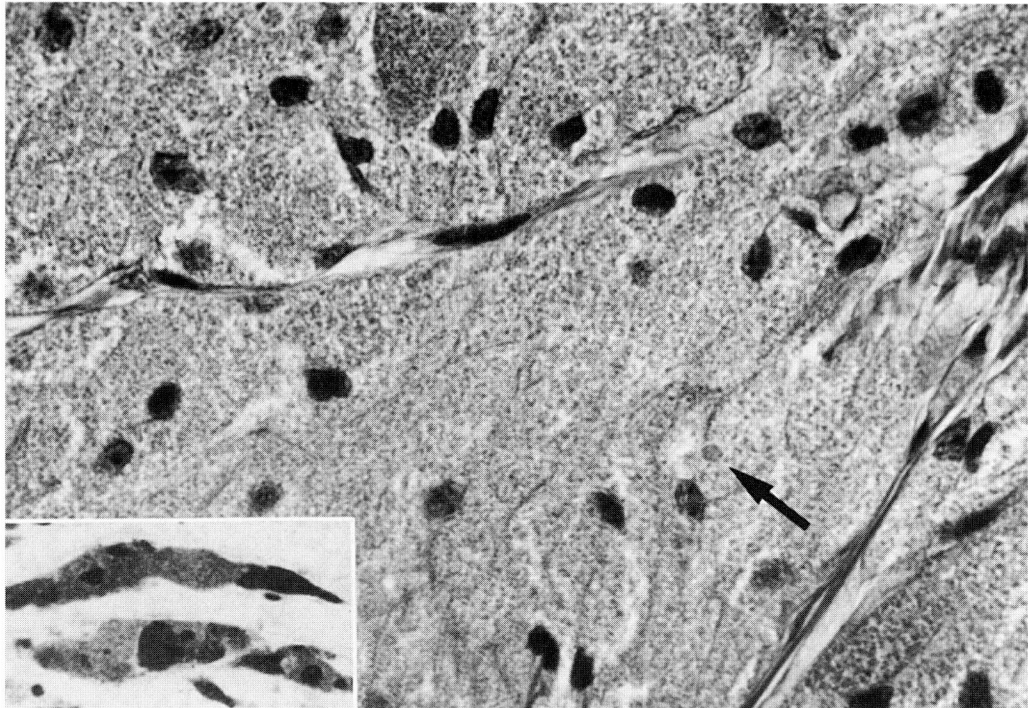

Fig. 25-109 Granular cell tumor. Innumerable small granules are present in cytoplasm of tumor cells, together with occasional larger granules with a droplet-like appearance *(arrow)*. **Inset** shows strong immunoreactivity for S-100 protein in both nucleus and cytoplasm of tumor cells.

These tumors are usually small, although we have seen cases measuring up to 5 cm in diameter. They have a hard consistency and ill-defined margins (Plate XX-C). This, plus the ulceration sometimes complicating the larger cutaneous tumors, explains why they are sometimes confused clinically and on gross inspection with a malignant neoplasm. Rarely, they have a polypoid shape.[1164] The individual cells are large and their cytoplasm highly granular (Fig. 25-109). Most granules are small and regular. They alternate with larger round droplets having a homogeneous eosinophilic appearance and a stronger PAS positivity. If the tumor grows near an epithelial surface, such as the skin, vulva, or larynx, secondary epithelial hyperplasia occurs that may be incorrectly diagnosed as carcinoma[1189] (Fig. 25-110). Elastosis is often present in the stroma.[1168]

Histochemically, the cytoplasmic granules contain large amounts of hydrolytic enzymes (such as acid phosphatase), and they are consistently positive for Luxol fast blue.[1172] Ultrastructurally, they have the appearance of lysosomes. Other interesting electron microscopic findings are the presence of a second cell population with "angulated bodies" resulting in a Gaucher cell–like appearance[1150] and of replicated basal lamina material around the granular cells, the latter suggesting repeated cycles of cellular injury and repair.[1149] Immunohistochemically, positivity has been described (in at least some of the lesions) for S-100 protein, laminin, HLA-DR, myelin basic protein, and CEA.[1167,1174-1176,1181,1188] The presence of the latter two markers remains controversial[1153];

the apparent CEA reactivity may be caused by the presence of a cross-reacting antigen.[1166,1178] The expression of HLA-DR is thought to be related not to the cell of origin but rather to some common immunologic pathogenesis.[1182]

The large majority of the granular cell tumors pursue a benign clinical course. Most cases reported in the old literature as malignant granular cell myoblastomas are in reality examples of alveolar soft part sarcoma. However, there have been several well-documented cases of tumors with a light and electron microscopic appearance comparable with that of granular cell tumor that have resulted in distant metastases.[1147,1161,1183,1190-1192]

The histogenesis of this lesion is still discussed. Most writers on the subject favor a Schwann's cell origin, based on histochemical, immunohistochemical, and ultrastructural findings and on the occurrence of typical lesions, within nerves.[1148,1150,1158,1186] However, in some lesions, there is no evidence of Schwann's cell participation.[1164] Furthermore, changes histochemically and ultrastructurally indistinguishable from those previously discussed have been documented in neoplastic and non-neoplastic smooth muscle cells and in tumoral ameloblasts.[1152,1177,1187] We therefore favor the view that granular cell tumor is not a specific entity but rather the expression of a degenerative change that can occur not only in Schwann's cells but also in a variety of other cell types, whether previously normal or forming part of a benign or a malignant neoplasm, such as MPNST, leiomyosarcoma, or angiosarcoma.[1157,1170,1171,1179] We favor making the diagnosis

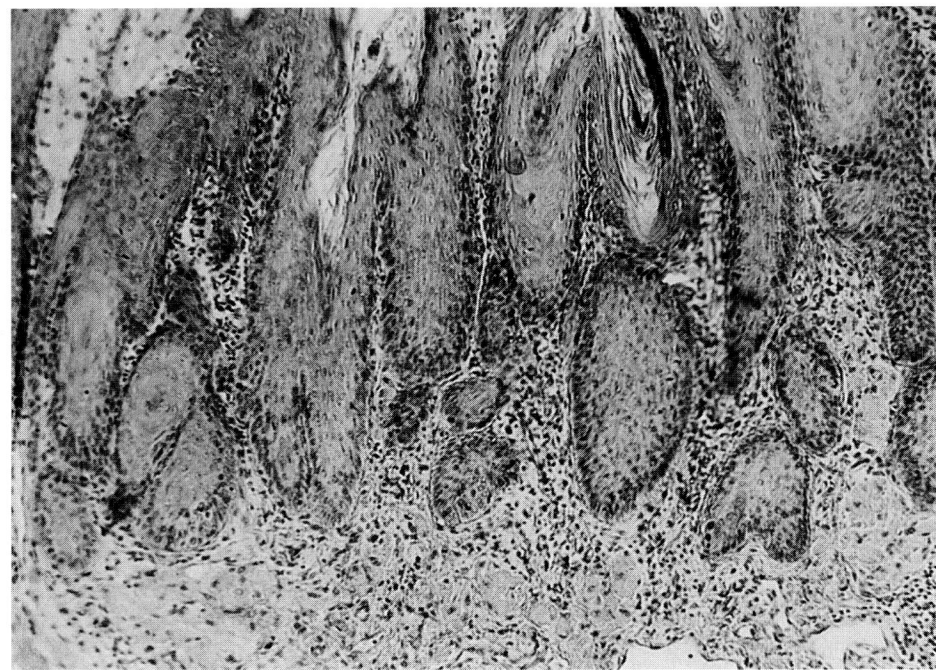

Fig. 25-110 Bizarre epidermal changes overlying granular cell tumor. These changes often lead to incorrect diagnosis of cancer.

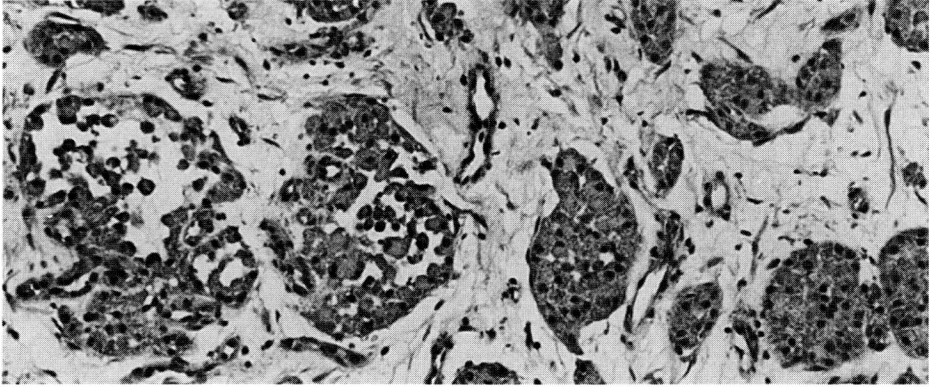

Fig. 25-111 Alveolar soft part sarcoma presenting as mass in oropharyngeal region of young girl. Tumor forms well-defined lobules, some of which show central space simulating alveolus.

of granular cell tumor only when the entire lesion is granular and to designate the other cases according to their basic component, noting that focal granular changes are present.

Alveolar soft part sarcoma

Alveolar soft part sarcoma, a malignant soft tissue tumor designated in the past as malignant organoid granular cell myoblastoma and malignant nonchromaffin paraganglioma, involves most often the deep soft tissues of the thigh and leg.[1204] It has also been seen in the oral cavity and pharynx, mediastinum (sometimes arising from the pul-

monary vein), stomach, retroperitoneum, orbit, uterus, and vagina.[1199,1202,1216,1221,1222] We have also seen it inside the patella. Most patients are young females. Grossly, the tumors are well circumscribed, usually large, moderately firm, and gray or yellowish (Plate XX-D). Areas of necrosis or hemorrhage are common in the larger neoplasms.

Microscopically, the tumor cells are separated by fibrous tissue into well-defined nests. Detachment of the central cells results in a typical alveolar pattern (Fig. 25-111). The individual cells are large and have vesicular nuclei, prominent nucleoli, and a granular cytoplasm (Fig. 25-112). Mito-

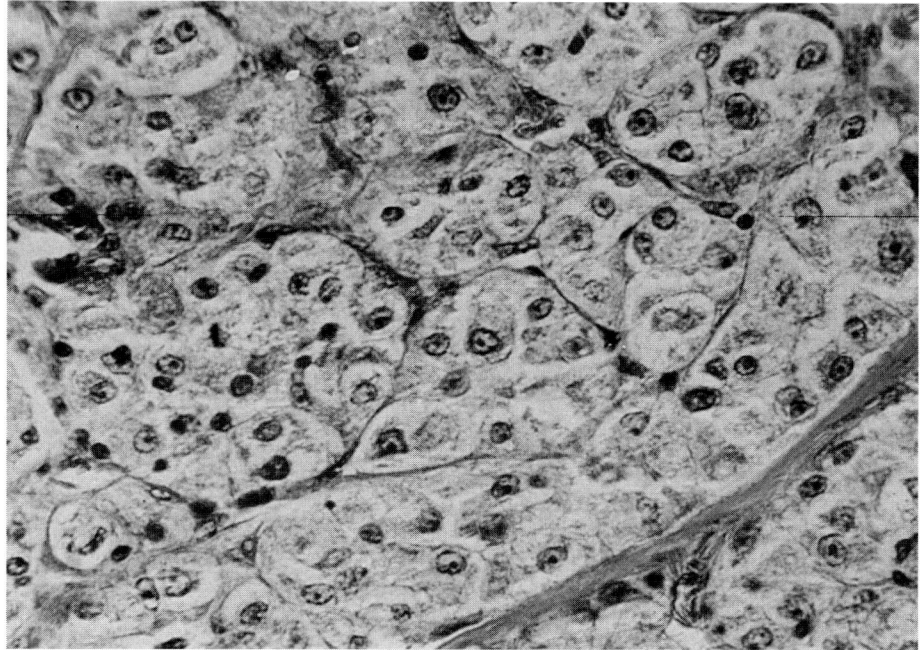

Fig. 25-112 Alveolar soft part sarcoma. Note nesting arrangement of cells, prominent nuclei and nucleoli, and abundant granular cytoplasm.

ses are exceptional. PAS stain sometimes demonstrates the presence of diastase-resistant intracytoplasmic needle-like structures. These are seen by electron microscopy as membrane-bound crystals with a periodicity of 58 to 100 nm, sometimes arranged in a cross-grid pattern[1198] (Fig. 25-113). This feature is of great diagnostic value in lesions of controversial nature.[1220] Other ultrastructural features include numerous vesicles with an electron-dense content in the Golgi region (possibly representing the precursors of the crystals) and smooth tubular aggregates associated with plasmalemmal invaginations.[1213]

The tumor is highly malignant, despite its deceivingly slow and indolent clinical course. Vein invasion is common. Blood-borne metastases appear in the lungs and other organs as long as 30 years or more following excision of the primary tumor.[1205,1206] Not infrequently, a metastasis in the lung or in another organ is the first manifestation of the disease. There is a good correlation between tumor size and survival.[1197]

The histogenesis of this strange neoplasm has not yet been definitely established.[1194,1210] We believe there is no convincing evidence to support the theory that this tumor represents a malignant counterpart of granular cell tumor, that is arises from nonchromaffin paraganglia, or that it is related to renin-producing cells of blood vessel walls.[1196] Instead, a wealth of data has accumulated in recent years supporting the interpretation that alveolar soft part sarcoma is of myogenous derivation and that it represents a distinct variant of rhabdomyosarcoma.[1201] This includes the (admittedly inconsistent) immunohistochemical demonstration of smooth muscle and sarcomeric actin, desmin, Z-protein, fast myosin, beta-enolase, and the MM isozyme of creatine kinase*; the demonstration of ATPase activity in the crystalline inclusions[1207]; the detection of similar membrane-bound cytoplasmic crystals in a normal human muscle spindle[1195]; the presence of T-tubule–like structures at the ultrastructural level[1213]; and the demonstration of MyoD1 protein, a nuclear phosphoprotein that is the product of a regulatory gene that controls the commitment of a cell to a myogenic lineage.[1218] Parenthetically, immunohistochemical staining for this marker in paraffin-embedded material has shown a consistently strong reaction in a *cytoplasmic* location. Whether this represents a cross-reaction or is reflecting the inability of the protein to be transported into the nucleus (thus preventing it from exercising its specific function) remains to be determined.

The few alveolar soft part sarcomas that have been studied cytogenetically have shown an abnormality of 17q25.[1219]

Clear cell sarcoma of tendons and aponeuroses (malignant melanoma of soft parts)

This malignant tumor arises chiefly from large tendons and aponeuroses of the extremities.[1229,1231,1238] The feet are the most common site, but it has been described in several other sites, including the penis.[1240] Most of the patients are young adults.

Grossly, the tumors are firm, well circumscribed, and gray or white and are cut with a gritty sensation. Microscopically, solid nests and fascicles of pale fusiform or cuboidal cells are present (Fig. 25-114). The nucleoli are large and deeply basophilic. Multinucleated giant cells are often seen. Abundant extracellular and intracellular iron is present. In many

---

*References 1200, 1203, 1208, 1209, 1211, 1212, 1214, 1215, 1217.

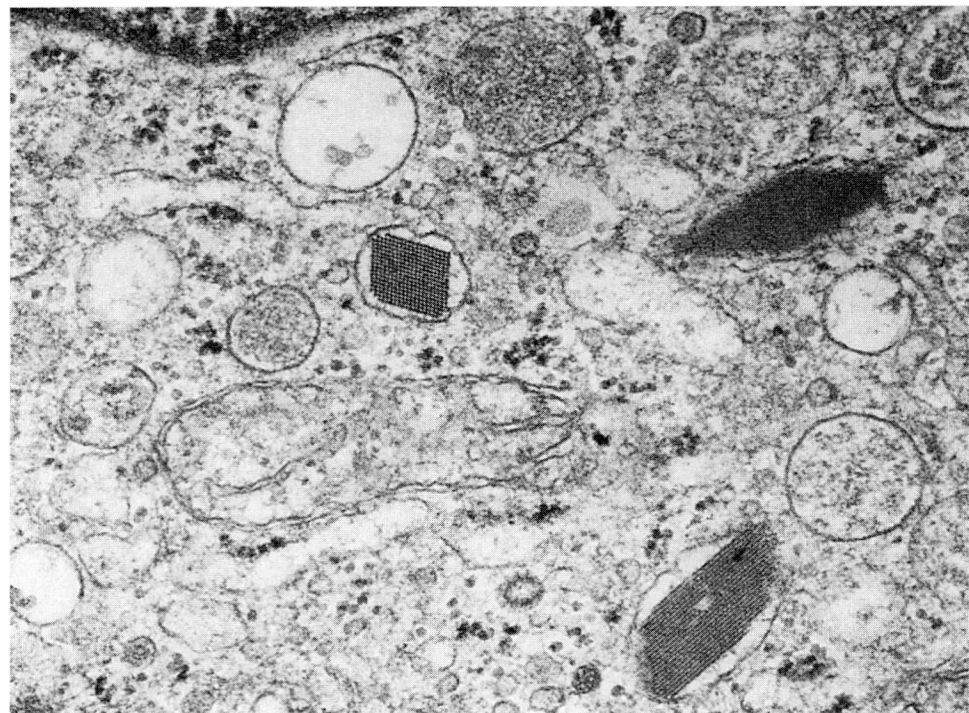

Fig. 25-113 Electron microscopic appearance of alveolar soft part sarcoma. Detailed view of characteristic crystalloid inclusions that demonstrate orderly 70 Å periodicity. Both linear and cross-hatched crystalloid patterns may be noted. (×70,000.) (Courtesy Dr. J. Sciubba, New Hyde Park, NY.)

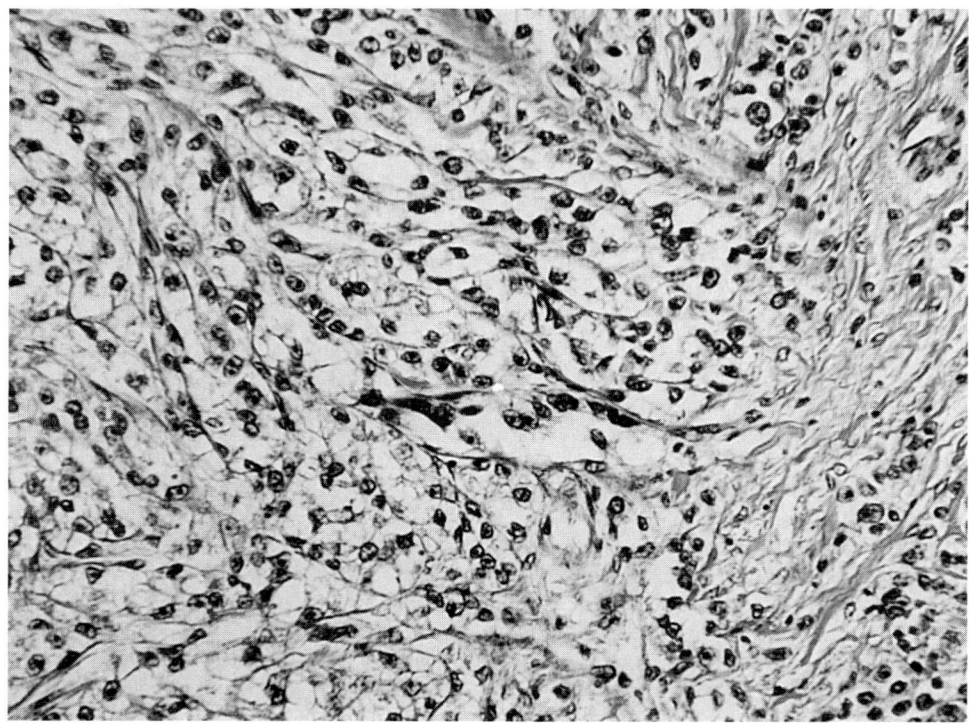

Fig. 25-114 Clear cell sarcoma of soft tissue that occurred in 27-year-old woman and arose from left patellar tendon. (Slide contributed by Dr. F. Enzinger, Bethesda, MD.)

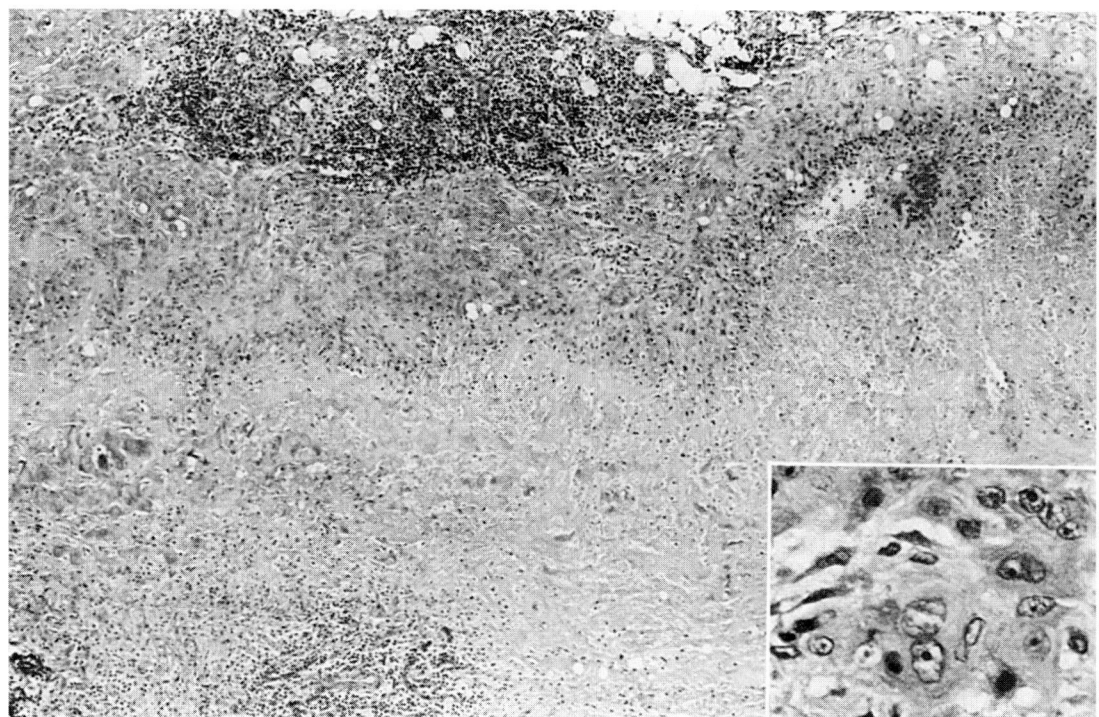

Fig. 25-115 Epithelioid sarcoma. Tumor cells are arranged in granuloma-like fashion around area of necrosis. **Inset** shows plump and epithelioid appearance of tumor cells.

of the cases the tumor cells also contain cytoplasmic melanin,[1225,1228,1242] strongly suggesting that this neoplasm is of neuroectodermal derivation and that it represents a peculiar type of malignant melanoma of soft parts.[1224,1228,1236] In keeping with this interpretation is the fact that the tumor cells consistently exhibit immunoreactivity for S-100 protein, HMB-45, Leu7, NSE, and vimentin[1228,1232,1233,1241] and that ultrastructurally there are melanosomes plus features consistent with a neural derivation.[1226,1237] When compared with conventional melanoma of skin metastatic to soft tissue by DNA ploidy analysis, clear cell sarcoma is more likely to be diploid or to show a lesser degree of aneuploidy.[1230] Like conventional melanoma, the clear cell carcinoma type may exhibit immunoreactivity for keratin.[1235a]

Clear cell sarcoma is associated with the chromosomal translocation t (12;22) (q13; q12).[1227] Of great interest is the fact that the gene involved in 22q12 (EWS) is the same one that is affected in Ewing's sarcoma/PNET and intra-abdominal desmoplastic small cell tumor.

The clinical course of clear cell sarcoma is characterized by slow but relentless progression with frequent local recurrences and eventual nodal and distant metastases.[1223,1231] Large tumor size and necrosis are statistically significant predictors of poor prognosis.[1234,1235,1239]

Epithelioid sarcoma

Epithelioid sarcoma usually affects adolescents and young adults.[1251] A few cases have been reported in patients with neurofibromatosis.[1264] The extremities are the most common location, particularly the hands and fingers. Several instances of vulvar involvement have also been recorded.[1268] The tumors tend to be superficially located and are sometimes centered in the reticular dermis. Others are found in the subcutis or deeper soft tissues, particularly fascial planes, aponeuroses, and tendon sheaths.[1265] The necrosis often seen in the center of the nodules and the epithelioid appearance of the tumor cells often results in a mistaken diagnosis of infectious granuloma or, more frequently, necrobiotic collagen granuloma.[1265]

One of the most characteristic features is the striking acidophilia of the tumor tissue, which is due to the staining characteristics of the cytoplasm and the extensive desmoplasia (Fig. 25-115). Metaplastic elements such as bone and cartilage may be present.[1249] Sometimes, most of the tumor cells have a spindle shape and simulate a fibroma or a dermatofibrosarcoma protuberans.[1258] Sometimes, epithelioid sarcomas of the soft tissue or vulva exhibit rhabdoid features; when these are prominent, it may become difficult to decide whether to diagnose the lesion as an epithelioid sarcoma or as a rhabdoid tumor.[1259,1262]

Ultrastructurally, the tumor cells exhibit abundant intermediate filaments, desmosome-like cell junctions, and small intercellular spaces surrounded by filopodia or microvilli[1244,1254,1256,1260] (Fig. 25-116). Immunohistochemically, there is positivity for keratin, epithelial membrane antigen, vimentin, CD34, tissue polypeptide antigen, and occasion-

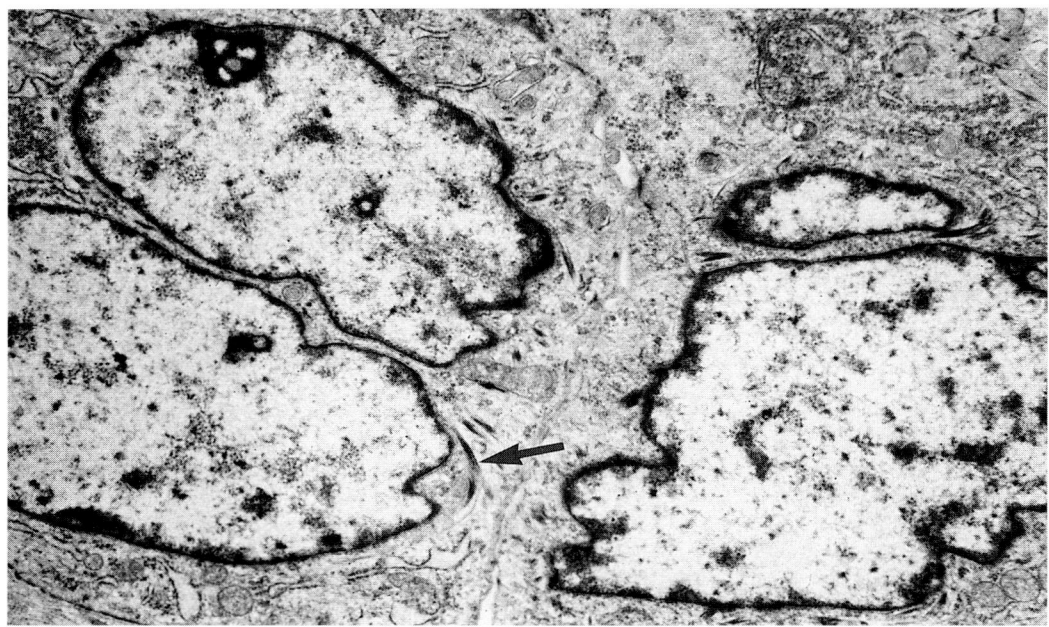

Fig. 25-116 Electron microscopic appearance of epithelioid sarcoma. Small tonofibrils *(arrow)* are present in the epithelioid tumor cells. (×11,100.) (Courtesy Dr. Robert A. Erlandson, Memorial Sloan-Kettering Cancer Center.)

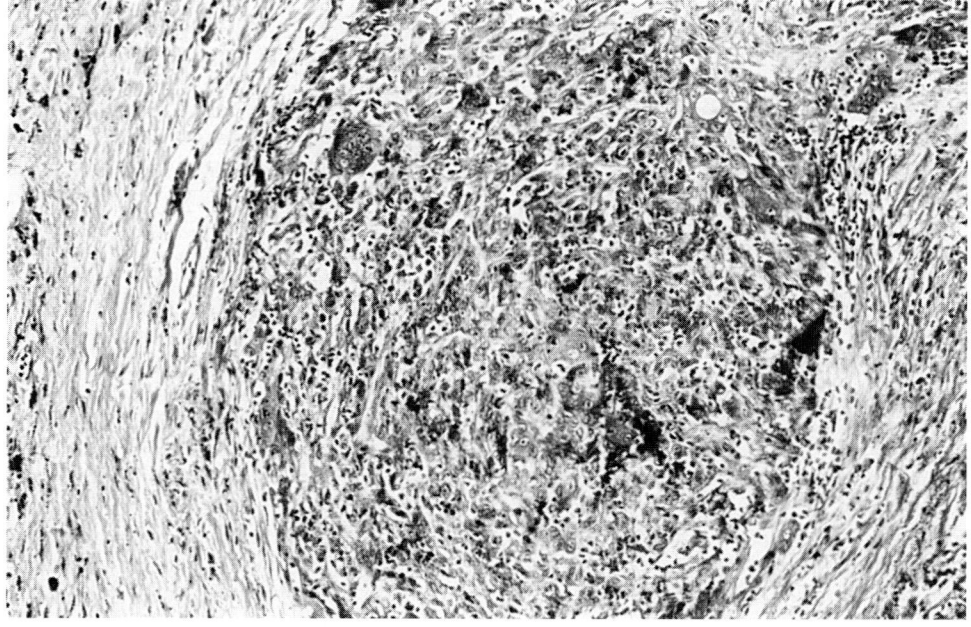

Fig. 25-117 Giant cell tumor of soft parts. Note nodular configuration and large number of osteoclast-like giant cells.

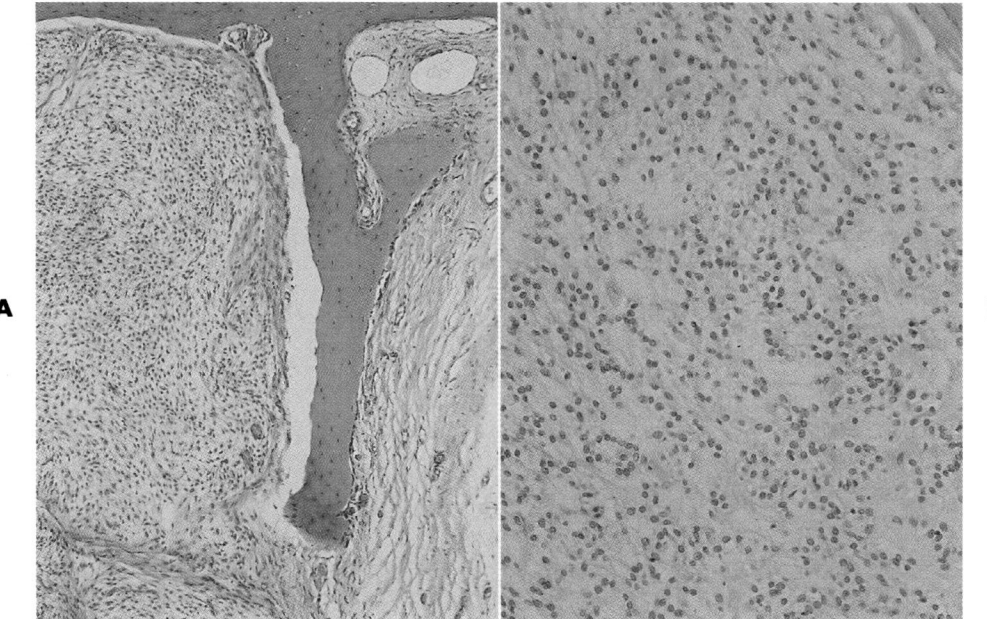

Fig. 25-118 Ossifying fibromyxoid tumor of soft parts. **A,** Low-power microscopic view showing characteristic peripheral rim of mature bone. **B,** Medium-power view showing cords of tumor cells embedded in fibromyxoid stroma. (Courtesy Dr. Christopher D.M. Fletcher, Boston.)

ally CEA.* The coexpression of vimentin and keratin is thought to be characteristic of this tumor; however, vimentin-negative cases that still retain positivity for keratin and CD34 have been reported.[1243]

The histogenesis of this tumor remains obscure. It clearly exhibits features of epithelial differentiation and therefore could be regarded as a form of carcinoma of soft tissue, together with synovial sarcoma and the exceptionally rare adamantinoma of soft tissues.[1257] Whether the epithelial features present in these tumors derive from metaplasia of mesenchymal elements remains to be determined. The tumor spreads to noncontiguous areas of skin, soft tissue, fascia, and bone, as well as by direct extension along fascial planes.[1245,1261] Local recurrence is the rule, although it may take years for this to develop. Lymph node metastases are relatively common and constitute an ominous prognostic sign.[1263] Metastases also occur in the lungs, other organs, and skin; for some peculiar reason, the scalp is a preferred site.[1268] Sometimes a lymph node metastasis is the first clinical manifestation of the disease.[1267] Excision plus radiation therapy achieves a low rate of local recurrence.[1266] A more aggressive clinical course is associated with a proximal or axial tumor location, increased size and depth, hemorrhage, mitotic figures, necrosis, rhabdoid features, and vascular invasion.[1246,1252]

Malignant giant cell tumor of soft parts

Malignant giant cell tumor of soft parts is a rare neoplasm that mainly affects adults and the elderly and is usually located in the extremities. Most cases are located deeply, but a superficial variety in the subcutaneous tissue and fascia has also been described[1271] (Plate XX-E). The tumor is com-

posed of an admixture of osteoclast-like multinucleated giant cells and stromal cells[1269,1272,1274] (Fig. 25-117). The stromal cells are probably the only neoplastic component; some are elongated and fibroblast-like, whereas others are plump, resembling histiocytes. Some of the latter may be multinucleated but different from the osteoclast-like elements. The giant cells resemble osteoclasts not only light microscopically, but also ultrastructurally and in their content of hydrolytic enzymes, such as acid phosphatase. The tumor can occur in the subcutaneous tissues or in deeper structures and has a characteristic multinodular configuration on low-power examination. Vascularity is pronounced, a fact also evident in angiographic studies.[1270] The overall appearance of the tumor is highly reminiscent of giant cell tumor of bones. The histogenesis is unclear, but a relationship with MFH is currently favored.[1269,1272] Indeed, in some classification schemes this tumor is included as one of the histologic types of MFH.[1273]

The behavior directly depends on the depth of the lesion; superficially located tumors are much less likely to recur or metastasize than deeper neoplasms.

Ossifying fibromyxoid tumor

Ossifying fibromyxoid tumor is a newly described soft tissue neoplasm, which usually presents in adult patients as a small, painless, well-circumscribed mass in the subcutaneous tissue or muscle of the extremities.[1276] Microscopically, the tumor cells are typically arranged in a cord- or nest-like pattern within a myxoid matrix that blends with foci of fibrosis and osteoid formation. The low-power appearance is distinctive by virtue of lobulation and an incomplete shell of mature bone in the region corresponding to the tumor capsule[1276] (Fig. 25-118, A). The tumor cells are small and round, with scanty atypia and few mitoses (Fig. 25-118, B).

---

*References 1247, 1248, 1250, 1253, 1255, 1260.

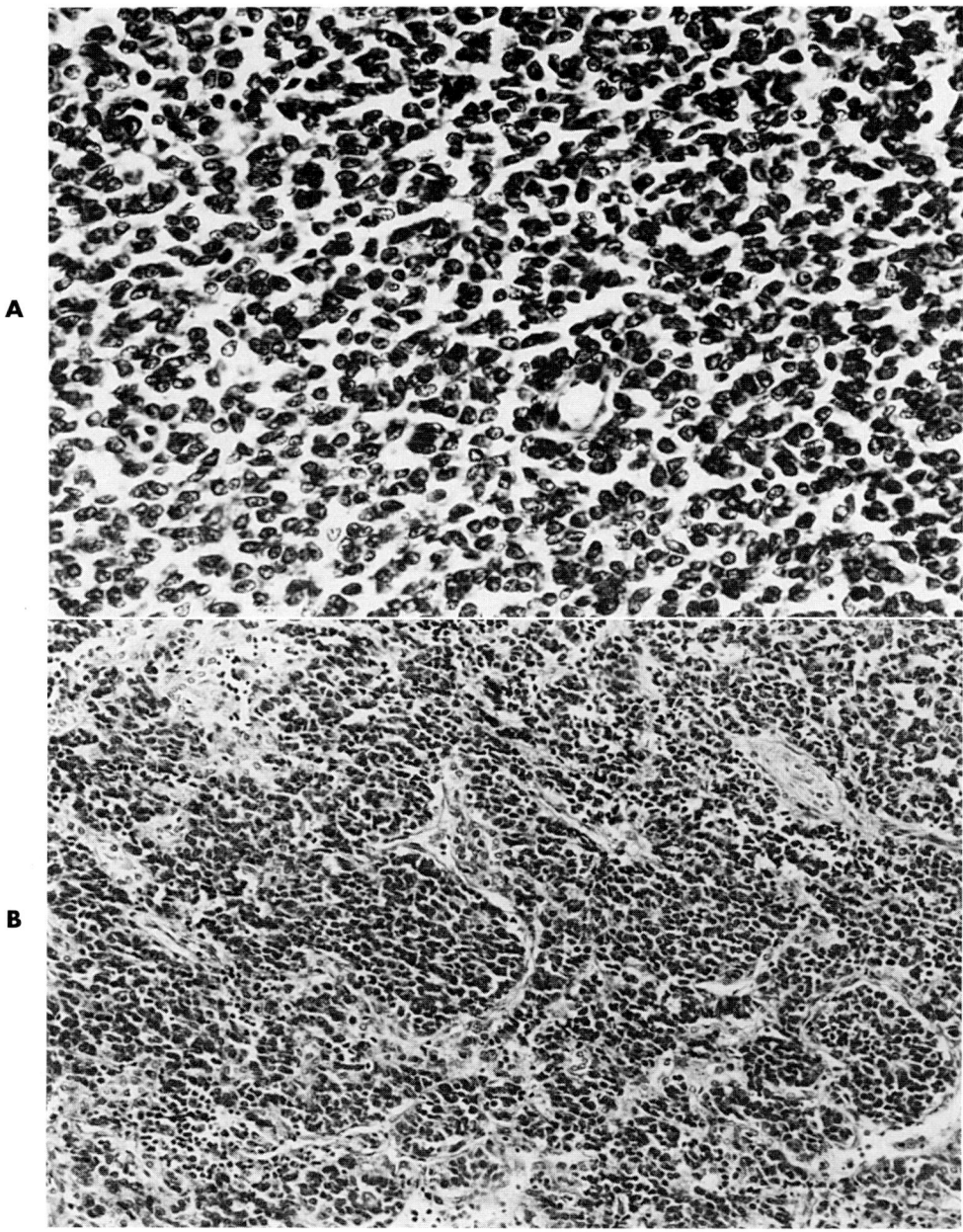

Fig. 25-119 **A,** Extraskeletal Ewing's sarcoma. There is monomorphic proliferation of small round cells with scanty cytoplasm. Some concentration of tumor cells around blood vessels can be appreciated. **B,** Malignant small cell tumor of thoracopulmonary region. Definite nesting is of importance in differential diagnosis with malignant lymphoma.

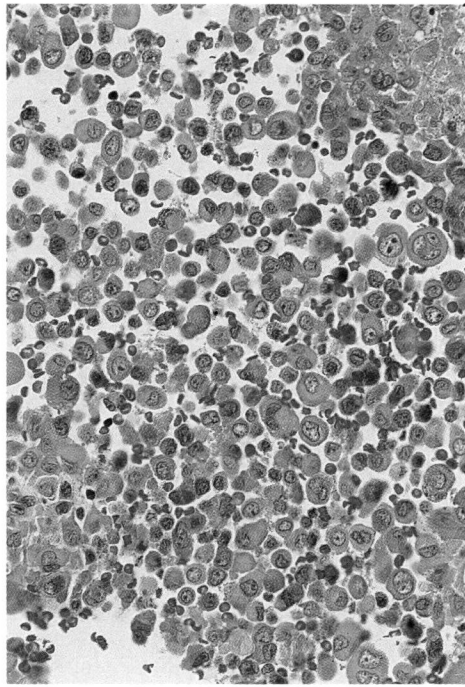

Fig. 25-120 Soft tissue tumor of the vulvar region with rhabdoid features. The tumor cells are small and round to oval, and their nuclei are lateralized.

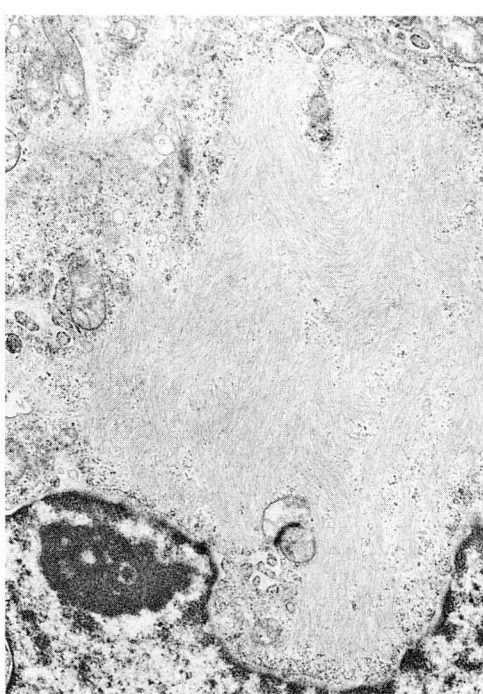

Fig. 25-121 Electron microscopic appearance of rhabdoid tumor of soft tissue. The cytoplasmic organelles of this rhabdoid cell are displaced by a large aggregate of intermediate filaments, immunohistochemically shown to be of vimentin type. (×15,000.) (Courtesy Dr. Robert A. Erlandson, Memorial Sloan-Kettering Cancer Center.)

Immunohistochemically, there is widespread immunoreactivity for S-100 protein and vimentin, associated with focal reactivity for Leu7 and glial fibrillary acidic protein, and negativity for type II collagen. Ultrastructurally, there are complex cell processes and basement membrane deposition. This combination of features is more in keeping with a schwannian than a cartilaginous or other mesenchymal derivation.[1275,1277] However, the detection of desmin and smooth muscle by some authors suggests that a partial differentiation toward a smooth muscle phenotype may be taking place in these tumors.[1278,1279]

The behavior of this tumor is indolent, but local recurrences developed in a quarter of the cases reported by Enzinger et al.[1276] in whom follow-up information was available. Additional atypical and malignant cases have been reported by Kilpatrick et al.[1276a]

Extraskeletal Ewing's sarcoma/PNET

Tumors morphologically indistinguishable from *Ewing's sarcoma* of the skeletal system can present as soft tissue masses. In many cases, they simply represent soft tissue extensions of tumor originating in the underlying bone. In others, bone involvement is absent, and these are regarded as primary Ewing's sarcomas of soft tissues.[1302,1306,1309] Most of the patients are adolescents or young adults, and the usual sites of involvement are the soft tissues of the lower extremity and paravertebral region.[1281] Like their skeletal counterpart, they are composed of uniform small, round, or oval cells containing cytoplasmic glycogen and sometimes arranged in a "peritheliomatous" pattern (Fig. 25-119, *A*).

Ultrastructurally, the cells are rather primitive, with abundant cytoplasmic glycogen, poorly developed cell junctions, and no evidence of neural differentiation.[1290,1294,1316] The course is aggressive and distant metastases are common, particularly to lung and skeleton.

As already discussed in Chapter 24, Ewing's sarcoma of both osseous and extraosseous sites is currently regarded as merging imperceptibly with *primitive neurectodermal tumor* (PNET)[1295,1303,1314] and subsuming the clinicopathologic entity originally described as malignant small cell tumor of the thoracopulmonary region[1282,1284,1291,1299] (Fig. 25-119 and Plate XX-F). The nosologic unity of Ewing's sarcoma/PNET is strongly supported by the existence of numerous intermediate forms,[1296,1306,1307,1317] the strong immunoreactivity for O13 (HBA71;12E7;RFB-1),[1315] and—most important—the presence of a consistent chromosomal translocation (11:22; q24; q12),[1312] which leads to the fusion of Ewing's sarcoma gene (ESG) in chromosome 22 to fli-1 gene in chromosome 11 and the production of a chimeric transcript.[1286] O13 recognizes a cell membrane protein of yet unknown function (p30/32 MIC 2; CD99), which is the product of MIC2, a pseudoautosomal gene located on the short arm of the X and Y chromosomes.[1280,1289,1310] It is not specific for Ewing's sarcoma/PNET (see p. 2091). Other markers that have been detected immunohistochemically in this family of tumors—many of them pointing toward a neuroepithelial line of differentiation—include neuron-specific enolase, synaptophysin, S-100 protein, PGP 9.5, secretogranin II, vimentin, and keratin.[1283,1292,1293,1297,1301] The 11;22 translocation, present in about 90% of the cases, can be detected by Southern blotting reverse transcriptase PCR or chromosomal in situ suppression hybridization.[1288,1298,1305,1308]

The claim has been made that tumors in this family having easily detectable neuroepithelial markers have a more aggressive clinical course than those with a more undifferen-

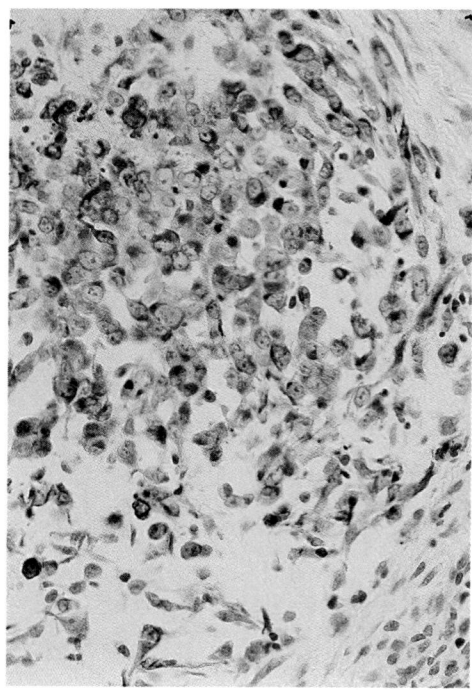

Fig. 25-122 Epithelioid sarcoma immunostained for keratin. The reaction has a characteristic punctate quality (same case as Fig. 25-120).

tiated appearance.[1285,1295,1303,1304] However, most attempts to subdivide them on phenotypic grounds have been unsuccessful.[1300,1308] The fact remains that—statistically speaking—tumors located in bone are more likely to exhibit a more undifferentiated phenotype (in keeping with the original Ewing's sarcoma concept), whereas those located in soft tissues—including most thoracopulmonary examples—tend to display various degrees of neuroepithelial differentiation.[1299]

The differential diagnosis of Ewing's sarcoma/PNET of soft tissues includes embryonal and alveolar rhabdomyosarcoma (especially the solid variant of the latter), malignant lymphoma, and so-called rhabdoid tumor.[1287,1311]

Rhabdoid tumor

Rhabdoid tumor was originally described as a primary renal neoplasm (see Chapter 17), but examples of a morphologically similar neoplasm have now been identified in other sites, particularly soft tissues.[1326] Some of the cases have involved major nerves.[1320] Most patients are infants or children, but it can also occur in adults. Microscopically, solid sheets of cells are present with areas of compartmentalization. The most striking morphologic feature is the deeply and homogeneously acidophilic cytoplasm of the tumor cells (the result of packing by intermediate filaments), with occasional lateral displacement of the nucleus[1318] (Figs. 25-120 and 25-121). Myxoid, pseudoalveolar, and hyalinized areas may be present.[1323] Immunohistochemically, there is positivity for vimentin and often for keratin and EMA but generally not for skeletal muscle markers or S-100 protein[1321] (Fig. 25-122). However, a great deal of phenotypical diversity has been recorded in these lesions.[1322,1325]

Metastases are early (to the lungs, liver, and lymph nodes), response to therapy is poor, and the clinical course is extremely aggressive.[1324,1326] Most evidence suggests that

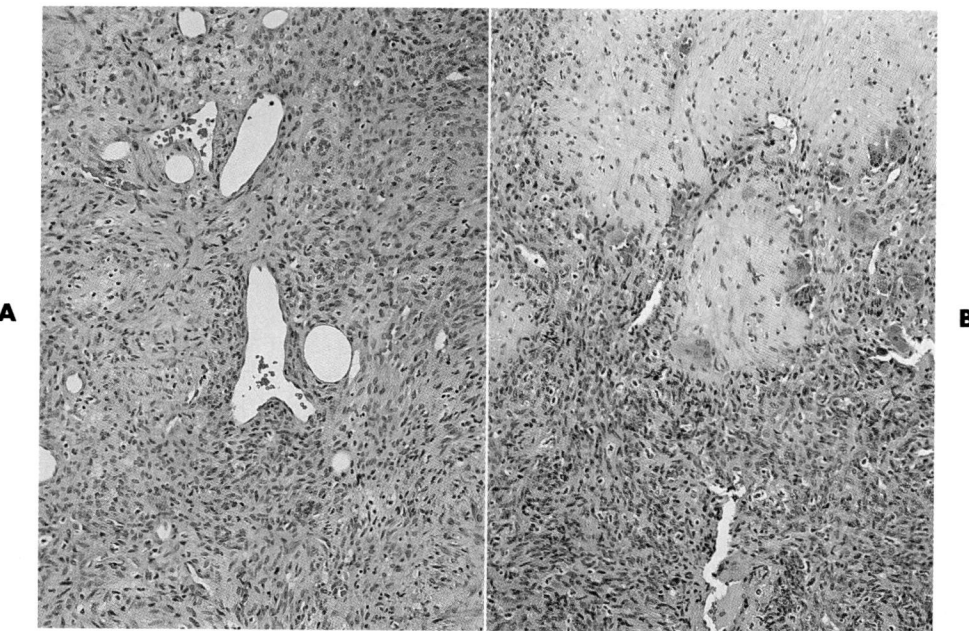

Fig. 25-123 Phosphaturic mesenchymal tumor. **A,** This area has a hemangiopericytoma-like quality. **B,** In this area from the same tumor, there is chondroid differentiation and a scattering of osteoclast-like giant cells.

rhabdoid tumor of soft tissues is not a specific tumor entity but rather that a "rhabdoid" phenotype can develop in a wide variety of tumor types, including epithelioid sarcoma, intra-abdominal desmoplastic small cell tumor, rhabdomyo-sarcoma, malignant melanoma, and various types of carcinoma.[1322,1327,1327a] Of practical importance is the fact that the emergence of the rhabdoid phenotype is invariably associated with an aggressive and almost always lethal clinical course.[1319]

Phosphaturic mesenchymal tumor

An interesting association has been reported between some tumors of soft tissue or bone and osteomalacia or rickets.[1331] The syndrome results from tumor production of a renal phosphaturic substance that depletes total-body phosphates by inhibiting tubular reabsorption of phos-

phate.[1328,1330] It is characterized biochemically by hypophosphatemia, renal phosphate wasting, and decreased serum 1,25-dihydroxyvitamin D3 levels.[1329] The soft tissue tumors associated with this complication have shown an admixture of microscopic features.[1331] In our experience the most characteristic feature has been the association of hemangiopericytoma-like areas and osteoclast-like giant cells, with or without foci of osseous and cartilaginous metaplasia (Fig. 25-123). The behavior has been generally benign.[1329,1331]

Metastatic carcinoma

Skeletal muscle or other deep soft tissue metastases of carcinoma occur, but only rarely do they represent the first clinical manifestation of the disease. Reported cases include metastases from carcinoma of the kidney, lung, and large bowel.[1332]

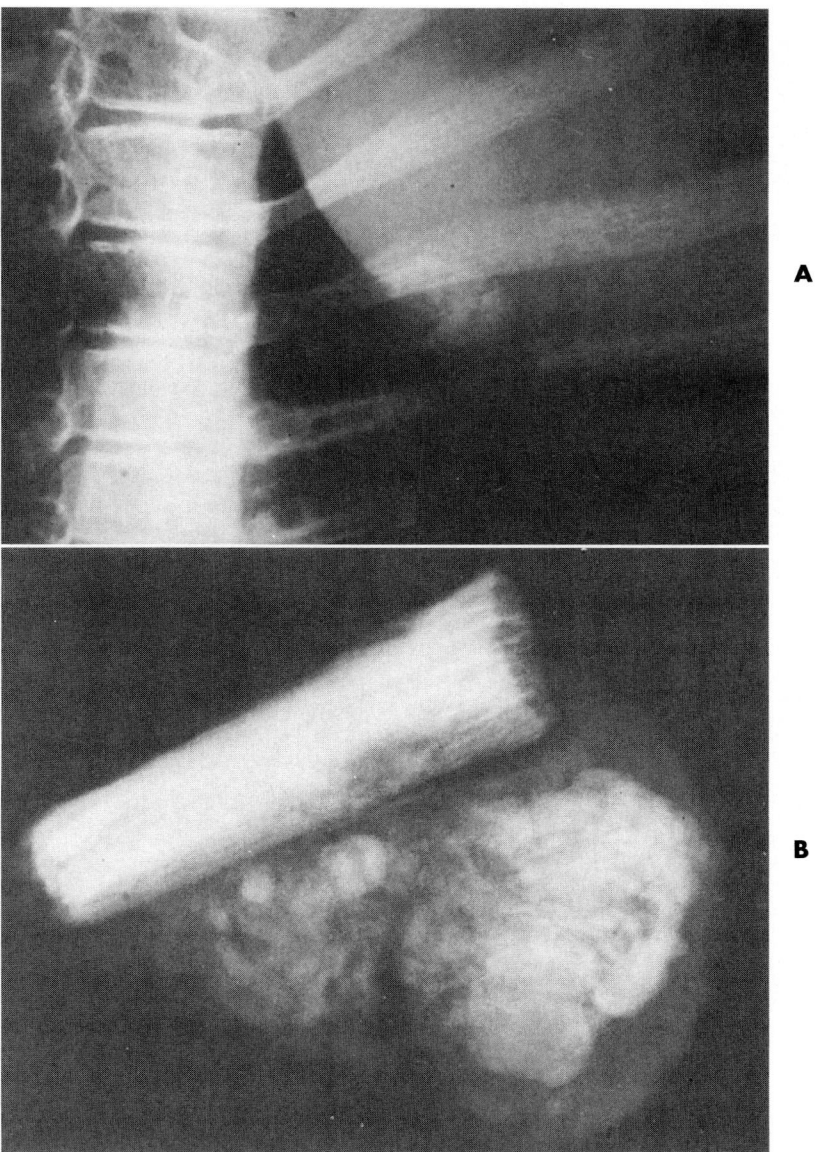

A

B

Fig. 25-124 **A,** Radiograph showing area of tumoral calcinosis adjacent to posterior rib in 9-year-old child. **B,** Radiograph of excised specimen. Calcification is lobulated, splotchy, and independent of eighth rib.

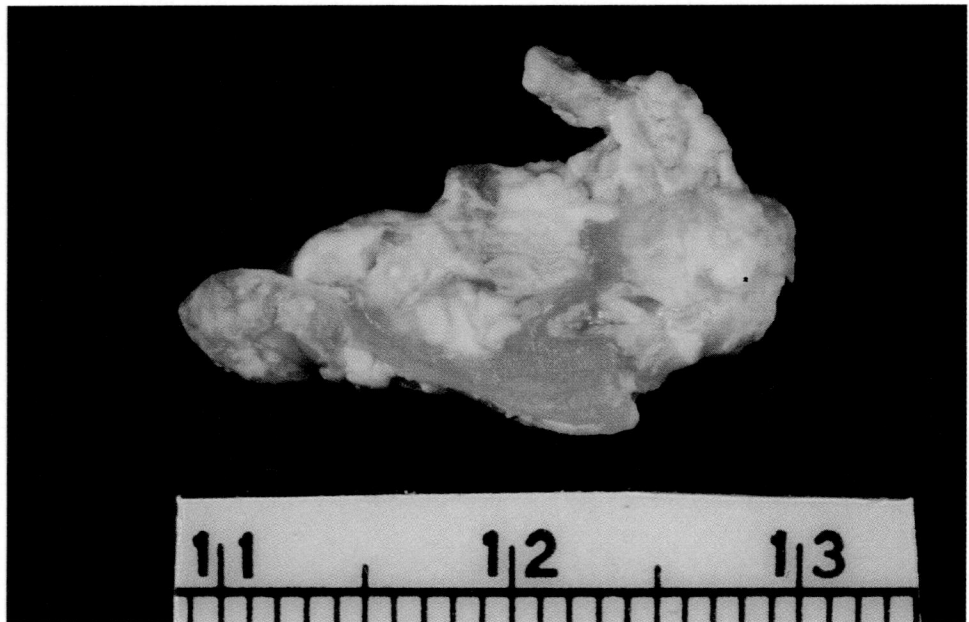

Fig. 25-125 Gross appearance of tumoral carcinosis. The appearance is characteristically multi-nodular, and the material has a chalky quality.

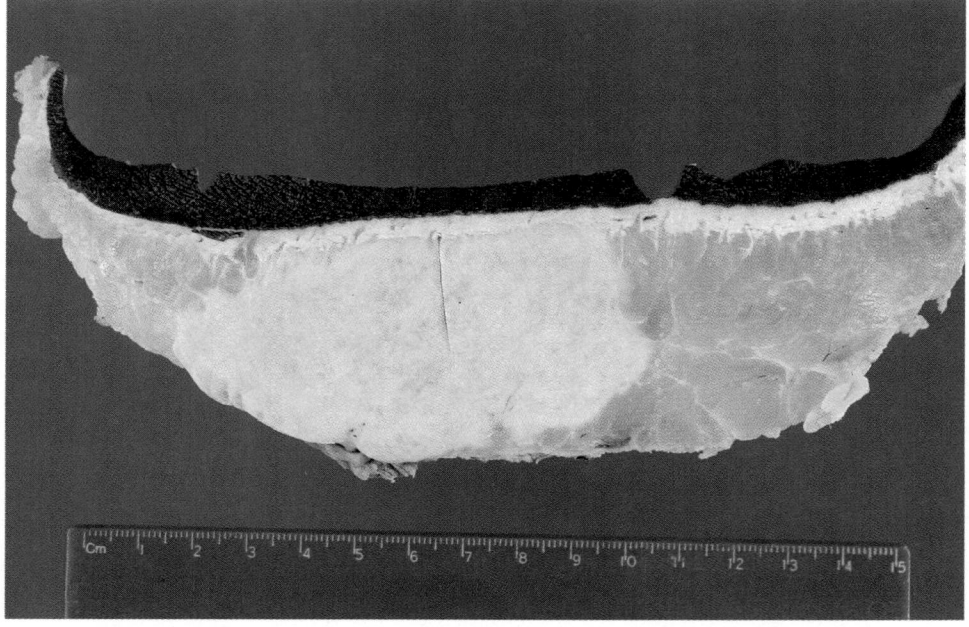

Fig. 25-126 Gross appearance of sinus histiocytosis with massive lymphadenopathy (Rosai-Dorfman disease) involving skin and soft tissues in the buttock region.

Other tumorlike conditions

Tumoral calcinosis is characterized by the formation of large, painless, calcified masses in the periarticular soft tissues, especially along extensor surfaces (Figs. 25-124 and 25-125). The elbows and hips are the most common sites. Curiously, the knee is always spared.

The disease has a genetic basis. It is inherited as an autosomal-dominant trait with variable clinical expressivity. The serum calcium is usually normal, but there is hyperphosphatemia and elevated serum dihydroxyvitamin D levels.[1341] The disease may recur after excision.[1337]

Calcifying fibrous pseudotumor is a benign and probably non-neoplastic fibrous lesion characterized by the presence of abundant hyalinized collagen with psammomatous or dystrophic calcifications and a lymphoplasmacytic infiltrate. Most patients are adolescents and young adults, and the behavior is benign.[1335]

Amyloid tumor (amyloidoma) can present as a localized mass in the soft tissues. The mediastinum and retroperitoneum are the most common locations. The amyloid may be of AL (more frequently) or AA type.[1339]

Aneurysmal cyst morphologically similar to that more commonly seen in the skeletal system can develop in the soft tissues.[1343]

Sinus histiocytosis with massive lymphadenopathy (Rosai-Dorfman disease) may present as a mass in the soft tissue, with or without associated lymph node involvement (Fig. 25-126). It is most commonly located in the extremities, but it can also occur in the trunk and head and neck region. As is also the case in other extranodal sites, emperipolesis is usually inconspicuous, and secondary collagen deposition is prominent.[1342]

Castleman's disease has been described in the form of a subcutaneous mass in a distal extremity.[1345]

Polyvinylpyrrolidone (PVP) granuloma is a tumorlike condition of skin or soft tissue that follows injections of drugs containing PVP.[1333,1338] The prominent myxoid features and focal cellularity may simulate a neoplastic process, particularly myxoid liposarcoma and signet ring carcinoma.[1340] PVP is localized in the cytoplasm of foamy histiocytes and multinucleated giant cells, many of which appear vacuolated. These cells are positive for mucicarmine, colloidal iron, GMS, Congo red, Sudan black B, and argentaffin stains[1340]; the presence of PVP can be detected by infrared spectrophotometry.[1338]

Bronchogenic cysts of skin and soft tissue are usually discovered at or seen after birth in male infants. The most common location is the suprasternal notch and manubrium sterni[1336]; despite their name, they are probably of branchial arch derivation (i.e., *branchiogenic*)[1334,1344] (see Chapter 4).

REFERENCES
NORMAL ANATOMY

1 Bunge MB, Wood PM, Tynan LB, Bates ML, Sanes JR: Perineurium originates from fibroblasts. Demonstration in vitro with a retroviral marker. Science **243**:229-231, 1989.

2 Burgdorf W, Mukai K, Rosai J: Immunohistochemical identification of factor VIII-related antigen in endothelial cells of cutaneous lesions of alleged vascular nature. Am J Clin Pathol **75**:167-171, 1981.

3 Carstens PH: The Weibel-Palade body in the diagnosis of endothelial tumors. Ultrastruct Pathol **2**:315-325, 1981.

4 Cohen PR, Rapini RP, Farhood AI: Expression of the human hematopoietic progenitor cell antigen CD34 in vascular and spindle cell tumors. J Cutan Pathol **20**:15-20, 1993.

4a DeYoung BR, Swanson PE, Argenyi ZB, Ritter JH, Fitsgibbon JF, Stahl DJ, Hoover W, Wick MR: CD31 immunoreactivity in mesenchymal neoplasms of the skin and subcutis. Report of 145 cases and review of putative immunohistologic markers of endothelial differentiation. J Cutan Pathol **22**:215-222, 1995.

5 Fajardo LF: The complexity of endothelial cells. A review. Am J Clin Pathol **92**:241-250, 1989.

6 Gottlieb AI, Langille BL, Wong MK, Kim DW: Structure and function of the endothelial cytoskeleton. Lab Invest **65**:123-137, 1991.

7 Hultberg BM, Svanholm H: Immunohistochemical differentiation between lymphangiographically verified lymphatic vessels and blood vessels. Virchows Arch [A] **414**:209-215, 1989.

8 Miettinen M, Holthofer H, Lehto V-P, Miettinen A, Virtanen I: *Ulex europaeus* I lectin as a marker for tumors derived from endothelial cells. Am J Clin Pathol **79**:32-36, 1983.

9 Miettinen M, Lindenmayer AE, Chaubal A: Endothelial cell markers CD31, CD34, and BNH9 antibody to H- and Y-antigens. Evaluation of their specificity and sensitivity in the diagnosis of vascular tumors and comparison with von Willebrand factor. Mod Pathol **7**:82-90, 1994.

10 Mukai K, Rosai J, Burgdorf W: Localization of factor VIII-related antigen in vascular endothelial cells using an immunoperoxidase method. Am J Surg Pathol **4**:273-276, 1980.

11 Page C, Rose M, Yacoub M, Pigott R: Antigenic heterogeneity of vascular endothelium. Am J Pathol **141**:673-683, 1992.

12 Ramani P, Bradley NJ, Fletcher CD: QBEND/10, a new monoclonal antibody to endothelium. Assessment of its diagnostic utility in paraffin sections. Histopathology **17**:237-242, 1990.

13 Rubanyi GM, Botelho LH: Endothelins. FASEB J **5**:2713-2720, 1991.

14 Schmitt-Graff A, Desmouliere A, Gabbiani G: Heterogeneity of myofibroblast phenotypic features. An example of fibroblastic cell plasticity. Virchows Arch **425**:3-24, 1994.

15 Stephenson TJ, Mills PM: Monoclonal antibodies to blood group isoantigens. An alternative marker to factor VIII-related antigen for benign and malignant vascular endothelial cells. J Pathol **147**:139-148, 1985.

16 Suzuki Y, Hashimoto K, Crissman J, Kanzaki T, Nishiyama S: The value of blood group-specific lectin and endothelial associated antibodies in the diagnosis of vascular proliferations. J Cutan Pathol **13**:408-419, 1986.

17 Tokunaga O, Fan J, Watanabe T, Kobayashi M, Kumazaki T, Mitsui Y: Endothelin. Immunohistologic localization in aorta and biosynthesis by cultured human aortic endothelial cells. Lab Invest **67**:210-217, 1992.

18 Traweek ST, Kandalaft PL, Mehta P, Battifora H: The human hematopoietic progenitor cell antigen (CD34) in vascular neoplasia. Am J Clin Pathol **96**:25-31, 1991.

19 Turner RR, Beckstead JH, Warnke RA, Wood GS: Endothelial cell phenotypic diversity. In situ demonstration of immunologic and enzymatic heterogeneity that correlates with specific morphologic subtypes. Am J Clin Pathol **87**:569-575, 1987.

20 Voigt J, Gorguet B, Szekeres G, Saati T, Delsol G: Comparison of the reactivities of monoclonal antibodies QBEND10 (CD34) and BNH9 in vascular tumors. Appl Immunohistochem **1**:51-57, 1993.

21 Warhol MJ, Sweet JM: The ultrastructural localization of von Willebrand factor in endothelial cells. Am J Pathol **117**:310-315, 1984.

INFECTIONS

21a Herzberg AJ, Boyd PR, Gutierrez Y: Subcutaneous dirofilariasis in Collier County, Florida, USA. Am J Surg Pathol **19**:934-939, 1995.

22 Michelson E: Syndrome of trauma to the psoas muscle. Arch Surg **50**:77-81, 1945.

23 Picket WJ, Friedell MT: Large nonpulsating hematoma (false aneurysm). Surg Clin North Am **27**:153-155, 1947.

24 Woo ML, Patrick WGD, Simon MTP, French GL: Necrotising fasciitis caused by *Vibrio vulnificus*. J Clin Pathol **37**:1301-1304, 1984.

TUMORS
Classification

25 Mills SE: Sometimes we don't look like our parents (editorial). Mod Pathol **8**:347, 1995.

26 Ross J, Hendrickson MR, Kempson RL: The problem of the poorly differentiated sarcoma. Semin Oncol **9**:467-483, 1982.

Age

27 Kauffman SL, Stout AP: Congenital mesenchymal tumors. Cancer **18**:460-476, 1965.

28 Rydholm A, Berg NO, Gullberg B, Thorngren K-G, Persson BM: Epidemiology of soft-tissue sarcoma in the locomotor system. A retrospective population-based study of the inter-relationships between clinical and morphologic variables. Acta Pathol Microbiol Immunol Scand (A) **92**:363-374, 1984.

29 Soule EH, Mahour GH, Mills SD, Lynn HB: Soft-tissue sarcomas of infants and children. A clinicopathologic study of 135 cases. Mayo Clin Proc **43**:313-326, 1968.

Diagnosis and special techniques

30 Altmannsberger M, Dirk T, Osborn M, Weber K: Immunohistochemistry of cytoskeletal filaments in the diagnosis of soft tissue tumors. Semin Diagn Pathol **3**:306-316, 1986.

31 Bendix-Hansen K, Myhre-Jensen O: Enzyme histochemical investigations on bone and soft tissue tumours. Acta Pathol Microbiol Immunol Scand (A) **93**:73-80, 1985.

32 Dickersin GR: Embryonic ultrastructure as a guide in the diagnosis of tumors. Ultrastruct Pathol **11**:609-652, 1987.

33 Enjoji M, Hashimoto H: Diagnosis of soft tissue sarcomas. Pathol Res Pract **178**:215-226, 1984.

34 Fisher C: The value of electronmicroscopy and immunohistochemistry in the diagnosis of soft tissue sarcomas. A study of 200 cases. Histopathology **16**:441-454, 1990.

35 Fletcher JA, Kozakewich HP, Hoffer FA, Lage JM, Weidner N, Tepper R, Pinkus GS, Morton CC, Corson JM: Diagnostic relevance of clonal cytogenetic aberrations in malignant soft-tissue tumors. N Engl J Med **324**:436-442, 1991.

35a Goodlad JR, Fletcher CDM: Recent developments in soft tissue tumours. Histopathology **27**:103-120, 1995.

36 Kindblom L-G, Walaas L, Widehn S: Ultrastructural studies in the preoperative cytologic diagnosis of soft tissue tumors. Semin Diagn Pathol **3**:317-344, 1986.

37 Ladanyi M: The emerging molecular genetics of sarcoma translocations. Diagn Mol Pathol **4**:162-173, 1995.

38 Layfield LJ, Anders KH, Glasgow BJ, Mirra JM: Fine-needle aspiration of primary soft-tissue lesions. Arch Pathol Lab Med **110**:420-424, 1986.

39 Lieberman Z, Ackerman LV: Principles in management of soft tissue sarcomas. Surgery **35**:350-365, 1954.

40 Miettinen M: Immunohistochemistry of soft-tissue tumors. Possibilities and limitations in surgical pathology. Pathol Annu **25**(Pt 1):1-36, 1990.

41 Molenaar WM, De Jong B, Buist J, Idenburg VJ, Seruca R, Vos AM, Hoekstra HJ: Chromosomal analysis and the classification of soft tissue sarcomas. Lab Invest **60**:266-274, 1989.

42 Nakanishi I, Katsuda S, Ooi A, Kajikawa K, Matsubara F: Diagnostic aspect of spindle-cell sarcomas by electron microscopy. Acta Pathol Jpn **33**:425-437, 1983.

43 Parham DM: Immunohistochemistry of childhood sarcomas. Old and new markers. Mod Pathol **6**:133-138, 1993.

44 Sreekantaiah C, Ladanyi M, Rodriguez E, Chaganti RS: Chromosomal aberrations in soft tissue tumors. Relevance to diagnosis, classification, and molecular mechanisms. Am J Pathol **144**:1121-1134, 1994.

45 van Haelst UJGM: General considerations on electron microscopy of tumors of soft tissues. Progr Surg Pathol **2**:225-257, 1980.

Grading and staging

46 Angervall L, Kindblom L-G, Rydholm A, Stener B: The diagnosis and prognosis of soft tissue tumors. Semin Diagn Pathol **3**:240-258, 1986.

47 Beahrs OH, Henson DE, Hutter RVP, Kennedy BJ: Manual for staging of cancer, ed 4. Philadelphia, 1992, JB Lippincott Co.

48 Coindre JM, Nguyen BB, Bonichon F, de Mascarel I, Trojani M: Histopathologic grading in spindle cell soft tissue sarcomas. Cancer **61**:2305-2309, 1988.

49 Coindre JM, Trojani M, Contesso G, David M, Rouesse J, Bui NB, Bodaert A, De Mascarel I, De Mascarel A, Goussot J-F: Reproducibility of a histopathologic grading system for adult soft tissue sarcoma. Cancer **58**:306-309, 1986.

50 Cooper JE, Allen PW: Low-grade sarcomas. Pathol Annu **25**(Pt 2):1-18, 1990.

51 Costa J, Wesley RA, Glatstein E, Rosenberg SA: The grading of soft tissue sarcomas. Results of a clinicohistopathologic correlation in a series of 163 cases. Cancer **53**:530-541, 1984.

52 Donohue JH, Collin C, Friedrich C, Godbold J, Hajdu SI, Brennan MF: Low-grade soft tissue sarcomas of the extremities. Analysis of risk factors for metastasis. Cancer **62**:184-193, 1988.

53 Enneking WF: Musculoskeletal tumor staging: 1988 update. Cancer Treat Res **44**:39-49, 1989.

54 Hashimoto H, Daimaru Y, Takeshita S, Tsuneyoshi M, Enjoji M: Prognostic significance of histologic parameters of soft tissue sarcomas. Cancer **70**:2816-2822, 1992.

55 Heise HW, Myers MH, Russell WO, Suit HD, Enzinger FM, Edmonson JH, Cohen J, Martin RG, Miller WT, Hajdu SI: Recurrence-free survival time for surgically treated soft tissue sarcoma patients. Multivariate analysis of five prognostic factors. Cancer **57**:172-177, 1986.

56 Kulander BG, Polissar L, Yang CY, Woods JS: Grading of soft tissue sarcomas. Necrosis as a determinant of survival. Mod Pathol **2**:205-208, 1989.

57 Myhre-Jensen O, Kaae S, Madsen EH, Sneppen O: Histopathological grading in soft-tissue tumours. Relation to survival in 261 surgically treated patients. Acta Pathol Microbiol Immunol Scand (A) **91**:145-150, 1983.

57a Parham DM, Webber BL, Jenkins JJ III, Cantor AB, Maurer HM: Nonrhabdomyosarcomatous soft tissue sarcomas of childhood. Formulation of a simplified system for grading. Mod Pathol **8**:705-710, 1995.

58 Russell WO, Cohen J, Enzinger F, Hajdu SI, Heise H, Martin RG, Meissner W, Miller WT, Schmidtz RL, Suit HD: A clinical and pathological staging system for soft tissue sarcomas. Cancer **40**:1562-1570, 1977.

59 Trojani M, Contesso G, Coindre JM, Rouesse J, Bui NB, De Mascarel A, Goussot JF, David M, Bonichon F, Lagarde C: Soft-tissue sarcomas of adults. Study of pathological prognostic variables and definition of a histopathological grading system. Int J Cancer **33**:37-42, 1984.

60 van Haelst-Pisani CM, Buckner JC, Reiman HM, Schaid DJ, Edmonson JH, Hahn RG: Does histologic grade in soft tissue sarcoma influence response rate to systemic chemotherapy? Cancer **68**:2354-2358, 1991.

Prognosis

61 Agarwal V, Greenebaum E, Wersto R, Koss LG: DNA ploidy of spindle cell soft-tissue tumors and its relationship to histology and clinical outcome. Arch Pathol Lab Med **115**:558-562, 1991.

62 Bell RS, O'Sullivan B, Liu FF, Powell J, Langer F, Fornasier VL, Cummings B, Miceli PN, Hawkins N, Quirt I, et al.: The surgical margin in soft-tissue sarcoma. J Bone Joint Surg (Am) **71**:370-375, 1989.

63 Cance WG, Brennan MF, Dudas ME, Huang CM, Cordon-Cardo C: Altered expression of the retinoblastoma gene product in human sarcomas. N Engl J Med **323**:1457-1462, 1990.

64 Drobnjak M, Latres E, Pollack D, Karpeh M, Dudas M, Woodruff JM, Brennan MF, Cordon-Cardo C: Prognostic implications of p53 nuclear overexpression and high proliferation index of Ki-67 in adult soft-tissue sarcomas. J Natl Cancer Inst **86**:549-554, 1994.

65 Enneking WF, Maale GE: The effect of inadvertent tumor contamination of wounds during the surgical resection of musculoskeletal neoplasms. Cancer **62**:1251-1256, 1988.

66 Gustafson P, Rooser B, Rydholm A: Is local recurrence of minor importance for metastases in soft tissue sarcoma? Cancer **67**:2083-2086, 1991.

67 Herbert SH, Corn BW, Solin LJ, Lanciano RM, Schultz DJ, McKenna WG, Coia LR: Limb-preserving treatment for soft tissue sarcomas of the extremities. The significance of surgical margins. Cancer **72**:1230-1238, 1993.

68 Kawai A, Noguchi M, Beppu Y, Yokoyama R, Mukai K, Hirohashi S, Inoue H, Fukuma H: Nuclear immunoreaction of p53 protein in soft tissue sarcomas. A possible prognostic factor. Cancer **73**:2499-2505, 1994.

69 Kroese MC, Rutgers DH, Wils IS, van Unnik JA, Roholl PJ: The relevance of the DNA index and proliferation rate in the grading of benign and malignant soft tissue tumors. Cancer **65**:1782-1788, 1990.

70 Rooser B, Attewell R, Berg NO, Rydholm A: Prognostication in soft tissue sarcoma. A model with four risk factors. Cancer **61**:817-823, 1988.

71 Stotter AT, A'Hern RP, Fisher C, Mott AF, Fallowfield ME, Westbury G: The influence of local recurrence of extremity soft tissue sarcoma on metastasis and survival. Cancer **65**:1119-1129, 1990.

72 Swanson SA, Brooks JJ: Proliferation markers Ki-67 and p105 in soft-tissue lesions. Correlation with DNA flow cytometric characteristics. Am J Pathol **137**:1491-1500, 1990.

73 Tanabe KK, Pollock RE, Ellis LM, Murphy A, Sherman N, Romsdahl MM: Influence of surgical margins on outcome in patients with preoperatively irradiated extremity soft tissue sarcomas. Cancer **73**:1652-1659, 1994.

74 Ueda T, Aozasa K, Tsujimoto M, Ohsawa M, Uchida A, Aoki Y, Ono K, Matsumoto K: Prognostic significance of Ki-67 reactivity in soft tissue sarcomas. Cancer **63**:1607-1611, 1989.

Therapy

75 Casper ES, Gaynor JJ, Harrison LB, Panicek DM, Hajdu SI, Brennan MF: Preoperative and postoperative adjuvant combination chemotherapy for adults with high grade soft tissue sarcoma. Cancer **73**:1644-1651, 1994.

76 Editorial: Changes in treating soft-tissue sarcomas. Br Med J **2**:562-563, 1979.

77 Eilber FR, Huth JF, Mirra J, Rosen G: Progress in the recognition and treatment of soft tissue sarcomas. Cancer **65**:660-666, 1990.

78 Glenn J, Kinsella T, Glatstein E, Tepper J, Baker A, Sugarbaker P, Sindelar W, Roth J, Brennan M, Costa J, Seipp C, Wesley R, Young RC, Rosenberg SA: A randomized, prospective trial of adjuvant chemotherapy in adults with soft tissue sarcomas of the head and neck, breast and trunk. Cancer **55**:1206-1214, 1985.

79 Karakousis CP, Emrich LJ, Rao U, Krishnamsetty RM: Feasibility of limb salvage and survival in soft tissue sarcomas. Cancer **57**:484-491, 1986.

80 Mazanet R, Antman KH: Adjuvant therapy for sarcomas. Semin Oncol **18**:603-612, 1991.

81 Nesbit ME Jr: Advances and management of solid tumors in children. Cancer **65**:696-702, 1990.

82 Potter DA, Kinsella T, Glatstein E, Wesley R, White DE, Seipp CA, Chang AE, Lack EE, Costa J, Rosenberg SA: High-grade soft tissue sarcomas of the extremities. Cancer **58**:190-205, 1986.

83 Suit HD, Russell WO, Martin RG: Sarcoma of soft tissue. Clinical and histopathologic parameters and response to treatment. Cancer **35**:1478-1483, 1975.

84 Tepper JE: Role of radiation therapy in the management of patients with bone and soft tissue sarcomas. Semin Oncol **16**:281-288, 1989.

85 Ueda T, Aozasa K, Tsujimoto M, Hamada H, Hayashi H, Ono K, Matsumoto K: Multivariate analysis for clinical prognostic factors in 163 patients with soft tissue sarcoma. Cancer **62**:1444-1450, 1988.

86 Walker MJ, Wood DK, Briele HA, Greager JA, Patel M, Das Gupta TK: Soft tissue sarcomas of the distal extremities. Surgery **99**:392-398, 1986.

87 Willett CG, Schiller AL, Suit HD, Mankin HJ, Rosenberg A: The histologic response of soft tissue sarcoma to radiation therapy. Cancer **60**:1500-1504, 1987.

88 Yang JC, Rosenberg SA: Surgery for adult patients with soft tissue sarcomas. Semin Oncol **16**:289-296, 1989.

Pathogenesis

89 Greenwald P, Kovasznay B, Collins DN et al.: Sarcoma of soft tissues after Vietnam service. J Natl Cancer Inst **73**:1107-1109, 1984.

90 Hardell L, Eriksson M: The association between soft tissue sarcomas and exposure to phenoxyacetic acids. A new case-referent study. Cancer **62**:652-656, 1988.

91 Jennings TA, Peterson L, Axiotis CA, Friedlaender GE, Cooke RA, Rosai J: Angiosarcoma associated with foreign body material. A report of three cases. Cancer **62**:2436-2444, 1988.

92 Kang H, Enzinger FM, Breslin P et al.: Soft tissue sarcoma and military service in Vietnam. A case control study. J Natl Cancer Inst **79**:693-699, 1987.

93 Laskin WB, Silverman TA, Enzinger FM: Postradiation soft tissue sarcomas. An analysis of 53 cases. Cancer **62**:2330-2340, 1988.

94 Lynge E, Storm HH, Jensen OM: The evaluation of trends in soft tissue sarcoma according to diagnostic criteria and consumption of phenoxyherbicides. Cancer **60**:1896-1901, 1987.

95 Mark RJ, Bailet JW, Poen J, Tran LM, Calcaterra TC, Abemayor E, Fu YS, Parker RG: Postirradiation sarcoma of the head and neck. Cancer **72**:887-893, 1993.

96 Monkman GR, Orwoll G, Ivins JC: Trauma and oncogenesis. Mayo Clin Proc **49**:157-163, 1974.

97 Wingren G, Fredrikson M, Brage HN, Nordenskjold B, Axelson O: Soft tissue sarcoma and occupational exposures. Cancer **66**:806-811, 1990.

Tumors and tumorlike conditions of fibrous tissue
Calcifying aponeurotic fibroma

98 Allen PM, Enzinger FM: Juvenile aponeurotic fibroma. Cancer **26**:857-867, 1970.

99 Chung EB: Pitfalls in diagnosing benign soft tissue tumors in infancy and childhood. Pathol Annu **20**(Pt 2):323-386, 1985.

100 Goldman RL: The cartilage analogue of fibromatosis (aponeurotic fibroma). Further observations based on 7 new cases. Cancer **26**:1325-1331, 1970.

101 Iwasaki H, Kikuchi M, Eimoto T, Enjoji M, Yoh S, Sakurai H: Juvenile aponeurotic fibroma. An ultrastructural study. Ultrastruct Pathol **4**:75-83, 1983.

102 Keasbey LE: Juvenile aponeurotic fibroma (calcifying fibroma). Cancer **6**:338-346, 1953.

103 Lichtenstein L, Goldman RL: The cartilage analogue of fibromatosis. Cancer **17**:810-816, 1964.

Fibroma of tendon sheath

104 Chung EB, Enzinger FM: Fibroma of tendon sheath. Cancer **44**:1945-1954, 1979.

105 Hashimoto H, Tsuneyoshi M, Daimaru Y, Ushijima M, Enjoji M: Fibroma of tendon sheath. A tumor of myofibroblasts. A clinicopathologic study of 18 cases. Acta Pathol Jpn **35**:1099-1107, 1985.

106 Humphreys S, McKee PH, Fletcher CDM: Fibroma of tendon sheath. A clinicopathologic study. J Cutan Pathol **13**:331-338, 1986.

107 Lamovec J, Bracko M, Voncina D: Pleomorphic fibroma of tendon sheath. Am J Surg Pathol **15**:1202-1205, 1991.

107a Maluf HM, De Young BR, Swanson PE, Wick MR: Fibroma and giant cell tumor of tendon sheath. A comparative histological and immunohistological study. Mod Pathol **8**:155-159, 1995.

108 Pulitzer DR, Martin PC, Reed RJ: Fibroma of tendon sheath. A clinicopathologic study of 32 cases. Am J Surg Pathol **13**:472-479, 1989.

109 Satti MB: Tendon sheath tumours. A pathological study of the relationship between giant cell tumour and fibroma of tendon sheath. Histopathology **20**:213-220, 1992.

110 Smith PS, Pieterse AS, McClure J: Fibroma of tendon sheath. J Clin Pathol **35**:842-848, 1982.

Giant cell fibroblastoma

111 Abdul-Karim FW, Evans HL, Silva EG: Giant cell fibroblastoma. A report of three cases. Am J Clin Pathol **83**:165-170, 1985.

112 Alguacil-Garcia A: Giant cell fibroblastoma recurring as dermatofibrosarcoma protuberans. Am J Surg Pathol **15**:798-801, 1991.

113 Chou P, Gonzalez-Crussi F, Mangkornkanok M: Giant cell fibroblastoma. Cancer **63**:756-762, 1989.

114 Chung EB: Pitfalls in diagnosing benign soft tissue tumors in infancy and childhood. Pathol Annu **20**(Pt 2):323-386, 1985.

115 Dymock RB, Allen PW, Stirling JW, Gilbert EF, Thornbery JM: Giant cell fibroblastoma. A distinctive, recurrent tumor of childhood. Am J Surg Pathol **11**:263-271, 1987.

116 Fletcher CD: Giant cell fibroblastoma of soft tissue: A clinicopathological and immunohistochemical study. Histopathology **13**:499-508, 1988.

117 Michal M, Zamecnik M: Giant cell fibroblastoma with a dermatofibrosarcoma protuberans component. Am J Dermatopathol **14**:549-552, 1992.

118 Pinto A, Hwang W, Wong A, Seagram C: Giant cell fibroblastoma in childhood. Immunohistochemical and ultrastructural study. Mod Pathol **5**:639-642, 1992.

119 Shmookler BM, Enzinger FM, Weiss SW: Giant cell fibroblastoma. A juvenile form of dermatofibrosarcoma protuberans. Cancer **64**:2154-2161, 1989.

120 Zamecnik M, Michal M: Giant-cell fibroblastoma with pigmented dermatofibrosarcoma protuberans component. Am J Surg Pathol **18**:736-740, 1994.

Nodular fasciitis and related lesions

121 Allen PW: Nodular fasciitis. Pathology **4**:9-26, 1972.

122 Bernstein KE, Lattes R: Nodular (pseudosarcomatous) fasciitis, a nonrecurrent lesion. Cancer **49**:1668-1678, 1982.

123 Chung EB, Enzinger FM: Proliferative fasciitis. Cancer **36**:1450-1458, 1975.

124 Craver JL, McDivitt RW: Proliferative fasciitis. Ultrastructural study of two cases. Arch Pathol Lab Med **105**:542-545, 1981.

125 Dahl I, Angervall L: Pseudosarcomatous proliferative lesions of soft tissue with or without bone formation. Acta Pathol Microbiol Scand (A) **85**:577-589, 1977.

126 Daroca PJ Jr, Pulitzer DR, LoCicero J III: Ossifying fasciitis. Arch Pathol Lab Med **106**:682-685, 1982.

127 el-Jabbour JN, Bennett MH, Burke MM, Lessells A, O'Halloran A: Proliferative myositis. An immunohistochemical and ultrastructural study. Am J Surg Pathol **15**:654-659, 1991.

128 el-Jabbour JN, Wilson GD, Bennett MH, Burke MM, Davey AT, Eames K: Flow cytometric study of nodular fasciitis, proliferative fasciitis, and proliferative myositis. Hum Pathol **22**:1146-1149, 1991.

129 Enzinger FM, Dulcey F: Proliferative myositis. Report of 33 cases. Cancer **20**:2213-2223, 1967.

130 Goodlad JR, Fletcher CD: Intradermal variant of nodular 'fasciitis.' Histopathology **17**:569-571, 1990.

131 Heffner RR Jr, Armbrustmacher VW, Earle KM: Focal myositis. Cancer **40**:301-306, 1977.

132 Heffner RR Jr, Barron SA: Denervating changes in focal myositis, a benign inflammatory pseudotumor. Arch Pathol Lab Med **104**:261-264, 1980.

133 Hollowood K, Fletcher CD: Pseudosarcomatous myofibroblastic proliferations of the spermatic cord ("proliferative funiculitis"). Histologic and immunohistochemical analysis of a distinctive entity. Am J Surg Pathol **16**:448-454, 1992.

134 Hutter RVP, Stewart FW, Foote FW Jr: Fasciitis. A report of 70 cases with follow-up proving the benignity of the lesion. Cancer **15**:992-1003. 1962.

135 Kern WH: Proliferative myositis. A pseudosarcomatous reaction to injury. Arch Pathol **69**:209-216, 1960.

136 Kleinstiver BJ, Rodriguez HA: Nodular fasciitis. A study of 45 cases and review of the literature. J Bone Joint Surg (Am) **50**:1204-1212, 1968.

137 Konwaler BE, Keasbey L, Kaplan L: Subcutaneous pseudosarcomatous fibromatosis (fasciitis). Report of 8 cases. Am J Clin Pathol **25**:241-252, 1955.

138 Lai FM, Lam WY: Nodular fasciitis of the dermis. J Cutan Pathol 20:66-69, 1993.

139 Lauer DH, Enzinger FM: Cranial fasciitis of childhood. Cancer 45:401-406, 1980.

140 Meis JM, Enzinger FM: Proliferative fasciitis and myositis of childhood. Am J Surg Pathol 16:364-372, 1992.

141 Meister P, Bückmann FW, Konrad E: Extent and level of fascial involvement in 100 cases with nodular fasciitis. Virchows Arch [A] 380:177-185, 1978.

142 Montgomery EA, Meis JM: Nodular fasciitis. Its morphologic spectrum and immunohistochemical profile. Am J Surg Pathol 15:942-948, 1991.

143 Montgomery EA, Meis JM, Mitchell MS, Enzinger FM: Atypical decubital fibroplasia. A distinctive fibroblastic pseudotumor occurring in debilitated patients. Am J Surg Pathol 16:708-715, 1992.

144 Patchefsky AS, Enzinger FM: Intravascular fasciitis. A report of 17 cases. Am J Surg Pathol 5:29-36, 1981.

145 Perosio PM, Weiss SW: Ischemic fasciitis. A juxta-skeletal fibroblastic proliferation with a predilection for elderly patients. Mod Pathol 6:69-72, 1993.

146 Price EB Jr, Silliphant WM, Shuman R: Nodular fasciitis. A clinicopathologic analysis of 65 cases. Am J Clin Pathol 35:122-136, 1961.

147 Price SK, Kahn LB, Saxe N: Dermal and intravascular fasciitis. Unusual variants of nodular fasciitis. Am J Dermatopathol 15:539-543, 1993.

148 Shimuzu S, Hashimoto H, Enjoji M: Nodular fasciitis. An analysis of 250 patients. Pathology 16:161-166, 1984.

149 Toti P, Catella AM, Benvenuti A: Focal myositis. A pseudotumoral lesion. Histopathology 24:171-173, 1994.

150 Wirman JA: Nodular fasciitis, a lesion of myofibroblasts. An ultrastructural study. Cancer 38:2378-2389, 1976.

Elastofibroma

151 Banfield WG, Lee CK: Elastofibroma. An electron microscopic study. J Natl Cancer Inst 40:1067-1077, 1968.

152 Dixon AY, Lee SH: An ultrastructural study of elastofibromas. Hum Pathol 11:257-262, 1980.

153 Enjoji M, Sumiyoshi K, Sueyuski K: Elastofibromatous lesion of the stomach in a patient with elastofibroma dorsi. Am J Surg Pathol 9:233-237, 1985.

154 Fukuda Y, Miyake H, Masuda Y, Masugi Y: Histogenesis of unique elastinophilic fibers of elastofibroma. Ultrastructural and immunohistochemical studies. Hum Pathol 18:424-429, 1987.

155 Govoni E, Severi B, Laschi R, Lorenzini P, Ronchetti IP, Baccarani M: Elastofibroma. An in vivo model of abnormal neoelastogenesis. Ultrastruct Pathol 12:327-339, 1988.

156 Järvi OH, Saxén AE, Hopsu-Havu VK, Wartiovaara JJ, Vaissalo VT: Elastofibroma. A degenerative pseudotumor. Cancer 23:42-63, 1969.

156a Kahn HJ, Hanna WM: "Aberrant elastic" in elastofibroma. An immunohistochemical and ultrastructural study. Ultrastruct Pathol 19:45-50, 1995.

157 Kindblom L-G, Spicer SS: Elastofibroma. A correlated light and electron microscopic study. Virchows Arch [A] 396:127-140, 1982.

158 Kumaratilake JS, Krishnan R, Lomax-Smith J, Cleary EG: Elastofibroma. Disturbed elastic fibrillogenesis by periosteal-derived cells? An immunoelectron microscopic and in situ hybridization study. Hum Pathol 22:1017-1029, 1991.

159 Madri JA, Dise CA, LiVolsi VA, Merino MJ, Bibro MC: Elastofibroma dorsi. An immunochemical study of collagen content. Hum Pathol 12:186-190, 1981.

160 Nagamine N, Nohara Y, Ito E: Elastofibroma in Okinawa. A clinicopathologic study of 170 cases. Cancer 50:1794-1805, 1982.

161 Nakamura Y, Okamoto K, Tanimura A, Kato M, Morimatsu M: Elastase digestion and biochemical analysis of the elastin from an elastofibroma. Cancer 58:1070-1075, 1986.

162 Stemmermann GN, Stout AP: Elastofibroma dorsi. Am J Clin Pathol 37:490-506, 1962.

Fibromatosis

163 Allen PW: The fibromatoses. A clinicopathologic classification based on 140 cases. Am J Surg Pathol 1:255-270, 305-321, 1977.

164 Allen RA, Woolner LB, Ghormley RK: Soft-tissue tumors of the sole. With special reference to plantar fibromatosis. J Bone Joint Surg (Am) 37:14-26, 1955.

165 Ayala AG, Ro JY, Goepfert H, Cangir A, Khorsand J, Flake G: Desmoid fibromatosis. A clinicopathologic study of 25 children. Semin Diagn Pathol 3:138-150, 1986.

166 Battifora H, Hines JR: Recurrent digital fibromas of childhood. An electron microscope study. Cancer 27:1530-1536, 1971.

167 Beatty EC Jr: Congenital generalized fibromatosis in infancy. Am J Dis Child 103:620-624, 1962.

168 Beham A, Badve S, Suster S, Fletcher CD: Solitary myofibroma in adults. Clinicopathological analysis of a series. Histopathology 22:335-341, 1993.

169 Bhawan J, Bacchetta C, Joris I, Majno G: A myofibroblastic tumor. Infantile digital fibroma (recurrent digital fibrous tumor of childhood). Am J Pathol 94:19-28, 1979.

170 Bochetto JF, Raycroft JE, Delnnocentes LW: Multiple polyposis, exostosis, and soft tissue tumors. Surg Gynecol Obstet 117:489-494, 1963.

171 Briselli MF, Soule EH, Gilchrist GS: Congenital fibromatosis. Report of 18 cases of solitary and 4 cases of multiple tumors. Mayo Clin Proc 55:554-562, 1980.

172 Brown JB, McDowell F: Wry-neck facial distortion prevented by resection of fibrosed sternomastoid muscle in infancy and childhood. Ann Surg 131:721-733, 1950.

173 Burke AP, Sobin LH, Shekitka KM: Mesenteric fibromatosis. A follow-up study. Arch Pathol Lab Med 114:832-835, 1990.

174 Burke AP, Sobin LH, Shekitka KM, Federspiel BH, Helwig EB: Intraabdominal fibromatosis. A pathologic analysis of 130 tumors with comparison of clinical subgroups. Am J Surg Pathol 14:335-341, 1990.

175 Burry AF, Kerr JFR, Pope JH: Recurring digital fibrous tumour of childhood. An electron microscopic and virological study. Pathology 2:287-291, 1970.

176 Chung EB, Enzinger FM: Infantile myofibromatosis. Cancer 48:1807-1818, 1981.

177 Cooper PH: Fibrous proliferations of infancy and childhood. J Cutan Pathol 19:257-267, 1992.

178 Coventry MB, Harris LE, Bianco AJ, Bulbulian AH: Congenital muscular torticollis (wry neck). Postgrad Med 28:383-392, 1960.

179 Daimaru Y, Hashimoto H, Enjoji M: Myofibromatosis in adults (adult counterpart of infantile myofibromatosis). Am J Surg Pathol 13:859-865, 1989.

180 Dimmick JE, Wood WS: Congenital multiple fibromatosis. Am J Dermatopathol 5:289-295, 1983.

181 Dominguez-Malagon H: Proliferative disorders of myofibroblasts. Ultrastruct Pathol 17:211-220, 1993.

182 Drescher E, Woyke S, Markiewicz C, Tegi J: Juvenile fibromatosis in siblings (fibromatosis hyalinica multiplex juvenilis). J Pediatr Surg 2:427-430, 1967.

183 Editorial: The myofibroblast. Lancet 2:1290-1291, 1978.

184 Enzinger FM: Histological typing of soft tissue tumours. International histological classification of tumours, No 3. Geneva, 1969, World Health Organization.

185 Enzinger FM, Shiraki M: Musculo-aponeurotic fibromatosis of the shoulder girdle (extra-abdominal desmoid). Analysis of 30 cases followed up for ten or more years. Cancer 20:1131-1140, 1967.

185a Evans HL: Desmoplastic fibroblastoma. A report of seven cases. Am J Surg Pathol 19:1077-1081, 1995.

186 Eyden BP, Banerjee SS, Harris M, Mene A: A study of spindle cell sarcomas showing myofibroblastic differentiation. Ultrastruct Pathol 15:367-378, 1991.

187 Faraggiana T, Churg J, Strauss L: Ultrastructural histochemistry of infantile digital fibromatosis. Ultrastruct Pathol 2:241-247, 1981.

188 Fletcher CDM, Achu P, Van Noorden S, McKee PH: Infantile myofibromatosis. A light microscopic, histochemical and immunohistochemical study suggesting true smooth muscle differentiation. Histopathology 11:245-258, 1987.

189 Fletcher CDM, Stirling RW, Smith MA, Pambakian H, McKee PH: Multicentric extra-abdominal "myofibromatosis." Report of a case with ultrastructural findings. Histopathology 10:713-724, 1986.

190 Fromowitz FB, Hurst LC, Nathan J, Badalamente M: Infantile (desmoid type) fibromatosis with extensive ossification. Am J Surg Pathol 11:66-75, 1987.

191 Fukasawa Y, Ishikura H, Takada A, Yokoyama S, Imamura M, Yoshiki T, Sato H: Massive apoptosis in infantile myofibromatosis. A putative mechanism of tumor regression. Am J Pathol 144:480-485, 1994.

192 Gabbiani G, Majno G: Dupuytren's contracture. Fibroblast contraction? An ultrastructural study. Am J Pathol 66:131-138, 1972.

193 Goellner JR, Soule EH: Desmoid tumors. An ultrastructural study of eight cases. Hum Pathol 11:43-50, 1980.

194 Goslee L, Clermont V, Bernstein J, Woolley PW Jr: Superficial connective tissue tumors in early infancy. J Pediatr 65:377-387, 1964.

195 Hasegawa T, Hirose T, Seki K, Hizawa K, Okada J, Nakanishi H: Solitary infantile myofibromatosis of bone. An immunohistochemical and ultrastructural study. Am J Surg Pathol 17:308-313, 1993.

195a Hayashi T, Tsuda N, Chowdhury PR, Anami M, Kishikawa M, Iseki M, Kobayashi K: Infantile digital fibromatosis. A study of the development and regression of cytoplasmic inclusion bodies. Mod Pathol 8:548-552, 1995.

196 Herrera GA, Johnson WW, Lockard VG, Walker BL: Soft tissue myofibroblastomas. Mod Pathol 4:571-577, 1991.

197 Hogan SF, Salassa JR: Recurrent adult myofibromatosis. A case report. Am J Clin Pathol 97:810-814, 1992.

198 Hunt RT, Morgan HC, Ackerman LV: Principles in the management of extra-abdominal desmoids. Cancer 13:825-836, 1960.

199 Ishikawa H, Mori S: Systemic hyalinosis or fibromatosis hyalinica multiplex juvenilis as a congenital syndrome. A new entity based on the inborn error of the acid mucopolysaccharide metabolism in connective tissue cells? Acta Derm Venereol **53:**185-191, 1973.

200 Iwahara T, Ikeda A: On the ipsilateral involvement of congenital muscular torticollis and congenital dislocation of the hip. J Jpn Orthop Assoc **35:**1221-1226, 1962.

201 Iwasaki H, Kikuchi M, Ohtsuki I, Enjoji M, Suenaga N, Mori R: Infantile digital fibromatosis. Identification of actin filaments in cytoplasmic inclusions by heavy meromyosin binding. Cancer **52:**1653-1661, 1983.

202 Iwasaki H, Müller H, Stutte HJ, Brennscheidt U: Palmar fibromatosis (Dupuytren's contracture). Ultrastructural and enzyme histochemical studies of 43 cases. Virchows Arch [A] **405:**41-53, 1984.

203 Jennings TA, Duray PH, Collins FS, Sabetta J, Enzinger FM: Infantile myofibromatosis. Evidence for an autosomal-dominant disorder. Am J Surg Pathol **8:**529-538, 1984.

204 Kiel KD, Suit HD: Radiation therapy in the treatment of aggressive fibromatoses (desmoid tumors). Cancer **54:**2051-2055, 1984.

205 Kim D-H, Goldsmith HS, Quan SH, Huvos AG: Intraabdominal desmoid tumor. Cancer **27:**1041-1043, 1971.

206 Kiryu H, Tsuneyoshi M, Enjoji M: Myofibroblasts in fibromatoses. An electron microscopic study. Acta Pathol Jpn **35:**533-547, 1985.

207 Larsen RD, Posch JL: Dupuytren's contracture. With special reference to pathology. J Bone Joint Surg (Am) **40:**773-792, 1958.

208 Levine AM, Reddick R, Triche T: Intracellular collagen fibrils in human sarcomas. Lab Invest **39:**531-540, 1978.

209 Liew S-H, Haynes M: Localized form of congenital generalized fibromatosis. A report of 3 cases with myofibroblasts. Pathology **13:**257-266, 1981.

209a Mackay B, Ordóñez NG, Salter JE Jr, Pollock RE: Myofibroblastoma of the axilla. Ultrastruct Pathol **19:**265-268, 1995.

210 Masson JK, Soule EH: Desmoid tumors of head and neck. Am J Surg **112:**615-622, 1966.

211 Mortimer G, Gibson AAM: Recurring digital fibroma. J Clin Pathol **35:**849-854, 1982.

212 Mukai M, Torikata C, Iri H, Hata J, Naito M, Shimoda T: Immunohistochemical identification of aggregated actin filaments in formalin-fixed, paraffin-embedded sections. I. A study of infantile digital fibromatosis by a new pretreatment. Am J Surg Pathol **16:**110-115, 1992.

213 Pettinato G, Manivel JC, Gould EW, Albores-Saavedra J: Inclusion body fibromatosis of the breast. Two cases with immunohistochemical and ultrastructural findings. Am J Clin Pathol **101:**714-718, 1994.

214 Pickren JW, Smith AG, Stevenson TW Jr, Stout AP: Fibromatosis of the plantar fascia. Cancer **4:**846-856, 1951.

215 Purdy LJ, Colby TV: Infantile digital fibromatosis occurring outside the digit. Am J Surg Pathol **8:**787-790, 1984.

216 Reitamo JJ, Hayry P, Nykyri E, Saxén AE: The desmoid tumor. Incidence, sex, age, and anatomical distribution in the Finnish population. Am J Clin Pathol **77:**665-684, 1982.

217 Reye RDK: Recurring digital fibrous tumors of childhood. Arch Pathol **80:**228-231, 1965.

218 Rock MG, Pritchard DJ, Reiman HM, Soule EH, Brewster RC: Extra-abdominal desmoid tumors. J Bone Joint Surg (Am) **66:**1369-1374, 1984.

219 Rodriguez-Bigas MA, Mahoney MC, Karakousis CP, Petrelli NJ: Desmoid tumors in patients with familial adenomatous polyposis. Cancer **74:**1270-1274, 1994.

220 Roggli VL, Kim H-S, Hawkins E: Congenital generalized fibromatosis with visceral involvement. A case report. Cancer **45:**954-960, 1980.

221 Rosen PP, Ernsberger D: Mammary fibromatosis. A benign spindle-cell tumor with significant risk for local recurrence. Cancer **63:**1363-1369, 1989.

222 Rosenberg HS, Stenback WA, Spjut HJ: The fibromatoses of infancy and childhood. Perspect Pediatr Pathol **4:**269-348, 1978.

223 Santa Cruz DJ, Reiner CB: Recurrent digital fibroma of childhood. J Cutan Pathol **5:**339-346, 1978.

224 Shnitka TK, Douglas MA, Horner RH: Congenital generalized fibromatosis. Cancer **11:**627-639, 1958.

225 Skoog T: Dupuytren's contracture. Pathogenesis and surgical treatment. Surg Clin North Am **47:**433-444, 1967.

226 Sportiello DJ, Hoogerland DL: A recurrent pelvic desmoid tumor successfully treated with tamoxifen. Cancer **67:**1443-1446, 1991.

227 Staley CJ: Gardner's syndrome. Simultaneous occurrence of polyposis coli, osteomatosis and soft tissue tumors. Arch Surg **82:**420-422, 1961.

228 Stout AP: Juvenile fibromatosis. Cancer **7:**953-978, 1954.

229 Ushijima M, Tsuneyoshi M, Enjoji M: Dupuytren type fibromatoses. A rare cause of neonatal intestinal obstruction. A clinicopathologic study of 62 cases. Acta Pathol Jpn **34:**991-1001, 1984.

230 Variend S, Bax NMA, Van Gorp J: Are infantile myofibromatosis, congenital fibrosarcoma and congenital haemangiopericytoma histogenetically related? Histopathology **26:**57-62, 1995.

231 Viale G, Doglioni C, Iuzzolino P, Bontempini L, Colombi R, Coggi G, Dell'Orto P: Infantile digital fibromatosis-like tumour (inclusion body fibromatosis) of adulthood. Report of two cases with ultrastructural and immunocytochemical findings. Histopathology **12:**415-424, 1988.

232 Walts AF, Asch M, Raj C: Solitary lesion of congenital fibromatosis. Am J Surg Pathol **6:**255-260, 1982.

233 Wang N-S, Knaack J: Fibromatosis hyalinica multiplex juvenilis. Ultrastruct Pathol **3:**153-160, 1982.

234 Welsh RA: Intracytoplasmic collagen formations in desmoid fibromatosis. Am J Pathol **49:**515-535, 1966.

235 Wilcken N, Tattersall MH: Endocrine therapy for desmoid tumors. Cancer **68:**1384-1388, 1991.

236 Woyke S, Domagala W, Olszewski W: Ultrastructure of a fibromatosis hyalinica multiplex juvenilis. Cancer **26:**1157-1168, 1970.

237 Yokoyama R, Tsuneyoshi M, Enjoji M, Shinohara N, Masuda S: Extra-abdominal desmoid tumors. Correlations between histologic features and biologic behavior. Surg Pathol **2:**29-42, 1989.

238 Yun K: Infantile digital fibromatosis. Immunohistochemical and ultrastructural observations of cytoplasmic inclusions. Cancer **61:**500-507, 1988.

239 Zelefsky MJ, Harrison LB, Shiu MH, Armstrong JG, Hajdu SI, Brennan MF: Combined surgical resection and iridium 192 implantation for locally advanced and recurrent desmoid tumors. Cancer **67:**380-384, 1991.

Fibrosarcoma

240 Chung EB, Enzinger FM: Infantile fibrosarcoma. Cancer **38:**729-739, 1976.

241 Churg AM, Kahn LB: Myofibroblasts and related cells in malignant fibrous and fibrohistiocytic tumors. Hum Pathol **8:**205-218, 1977.

241a Coffin CM, Watterson J, Priest JR, Dehner LP: Extrapulmonary inflammatory myofibroblastic tumor (inflammatory pseudotumor). A clinicopathologic and immunohistochemical study of 84 cases. Am J Surg Pathol **19:**859-872, 1995.

242 Dehner LP, Askin FB: Tumors of fibrous tissue origin in childhood. A clinicopathologic study of cutaneous and soft tissue neoplasms in 66 children. Cancer **38:**888-900, 1976.

243 Gonzalez-Crussi F, Wiederhold MD, Sotelo-Avila C: Congenital fibrosarcoma. Presence of a histiocytic component. Cancer **46:**77-86, 1980.

244 Guber S, Rudolph R: The myofibroblast. Surg Gynecol Obstet **146:**641-649, 1978.

245 Hall J, Tseng SCG, Timpl R, Hendrix MJC, Stern R: Collagen types in fibrosarcoma. Absence of type III collagen in reticulin. Hum Pathol **16:**439-446, 1985.

246 Iwasaki H, Enjoji M: Infantile and adult fibrosarcomas of the soft tissues. Acta Pathol Jpn **29:**377-388, 1979.

247 Meis JM, Enzinger FM: Inflammatory fibrosarcoma of the mesentery and retroperitoneum. A tumor closely simulating inflammatory pseudotumor. Am J Surg Pathol **15:**1146-1156, 1991.

248 Oshiro Y, Fukuda T, Tsuneyoshi M: Fibrosarcoma versus fibromatoses and cellular nodular fasciitis. A comparative study of their proliferative activity using proliferating cell nuclear antigen, DNA flow cytometry, and p53. Am J Surg Pathol **18:**712-719, 1994.

249 Pritchard DJ, Soule EH, Taylor WF, Ivins JC: Fibrosarcoma. A clinicopathologic and statistical study of 199 tumors of the soft tissues of the extremities and trunk. Cancer **33:**888-897, 1974.

249a Ramachandra S, Hollowood K, Bisceglia M, Fletcher CDM: Inflammatory pseudotumour of soft tissues. A clinicopathological and immunohistochemical analysis of 18 cases. Histopathology **27:**313-323, 1995.

250 Schofield DE, Fletcher JA, Grier HE, Yunis EJ: Fibrosarcoma in infants and children. Application of new techniques. Am J Surg Pathol **18:**14-24, 1994.

251 Scott SM, Reiman HM, Pritchard DJ, Ilstrup DM: Soft tissue fibrosarcoma. A clinicopathologic study of 132 cases. Cancer **64:**925-931, 1989.

252 Souid AK, Ziemba MC, Dubansky AS, Mazur M, Oliphant M, Thomas FD, Ratner M, Sadowitz PD: Inflammatory myofibroblastic tumor in children. Cancer **72:**2042-2048, 1993.

253 Soule EH, Pritchard DJ: Fibrosarcoma in infants and children. A review of 110 cases. Cancer **40:**1711-1721, 1977.

254 Stout AP: Fibrosarcoma. The malignant tumor of fibroblasts. Cancer **1:**30-63, 1948.

255 Stout AP: Fibrosarcoma in infants and children. Cancer **15:**1028-1040, 1962.

256 Suh CH, Ordonez NG, Mackay B: Fibrosarcoma. Observations on the ultrastructure. Ultrastruct Pathol **17:**221-229, 1993.

257 van der Werf-Messing B, van Unnik JAM: Fibrosarcoma of the soft tissue. A clinicopathologic study. Cancer 18:1113-1123, 1965.
258 Weiss SW: Proliferative fibroblastic lesions. From hyperplasia to neoplasia. Am J Surg Pathol 10(Suppl 1):14-25, 1986.

Fibrohistiocytic tumors

259 Alguacil-Garcia A, Unni KK, Goellner JR: Malignant fibrous histiocytoma. An ultrastructural study of six cases. Am J Clin Pathol 69:121-129, 1978.
260 Brecher ME, Franklin WA: Absence of mononuclear phagocyte antigens in malignant fibrous histiocytoma. Am J Clin Pathol 86:344-348, 1986.
261 Enzinger FM: Malignant fibrous histiocytoma 20 years after Stout. Am J Surg Pathol 10(Suppl 1):43-53, 1986.
262 Fisher ER, Vuzevski VD: Cytogenesis of the schwannoma (neurilemoma), neurofibroma, dermatofibroma, and dermatofibrosarcoma as revealed by electron microscopy. Am J Clin Pathol 49:141-154, 1968.
263 Fletcher CD: Pleomorphic malignant fibrous histiocytoma. Fact or fiction? A critical reappraisal based on 159 tumors diagnosed as pleomorphic sarcoma. Am J Surg Pathol 16:213-228, 1992.
267 Fu Y, Gabbiani G, Kaye GI, Lattes R: Malignant soft tissue tumors of probable histiocytic origin (malignant fibrous histiocytomas). General considerations and electron microscopic and tissue culture studies. Cancer 35:176-198, 1975.
268 Harris M: The ultrastructure of benign and malignant fibrous histiocytomas. Histopathology 4:29-44, 1980.
269 Herrera GA, Reimann BE, Salinas JA: Malignant schwannomas presenting as malignant fibrous histiocytomas. Ultrastruct Pathol 3:253-261, 1982.
270 Iwasaki H, Isayama T, Johnzaki H, Kikuchi M: Malignant fibrous histiocytoma. Evidence of perivascular mesenchymal cell origin. Immunocytochemical studies with monoclonal anti-MFH antibodies. Am J Pathol 128:528-537, 1987.
271 Iwasaki H, Isayama T, Ohjimi Y, Kikuchi M, Yoh S, Shinohara N, Yoshitake K, Ishiguro M, Kamada N, Enjoji M: Malignant fibrous histiocytoma. A tumor of facultative histiocytes showing mesenchymal differentiation in cultured cell lines. Cancer 69:437-447, 1992.
272 Iwasaki H, Kikuchi M, Takii M, Enjoji M: Benign and malignant fibrous histiocytomas of the soft tissues. Functional characterization of the cultured cells. Cancer 50:520-530, 1982.
273 Lattes R: Malignant fibrous histiocytoma. A review article. Am J Surg Pathol 6:761-771, 1982.
273a Meis-Kindblom JM, Kindblom L-G, Enzinger FM: Sclerosing epithelioid fibrosarcoma. A variant of fibrosarcoma simulating carcinoma. Am J Surg Pathol 19:979-993, 1995.
274 O'Brien JE, Stout AP: Malignant fibrous xanthomas. Cancer 17:1445-1455, 1964.
275 Ozzello L, Hamels J: The histiocytic nature of dermatofibrosarcoma protuberans—tissue culture and electron microscopic study. Am J Clin Pathol 65:136-148, 1976.
276 Ozzello L, Stout AP, Murray MR: Cultural characteristics of malignant histiocytoma and fibrous xanthomas. Cancer 16:331-344, 1963.
277 Reed R: Histiocytes, fibrocytes, and facultative transformations. Am J Dermatopathol 4:253-262, 1982.
278 Roholl PJ, Kleyne J, Van Unnik JAM: Characterization of tumor cells in malignant fibrous histiocytomas and other soft-tissue tumors, in comparison with malignant histiocytes. II. Immunoperoxidase study on cryostat sections. Am J Pathol 121:269-274, 1985.
279 Vernon-Roberts B: The macrophage. Cambridge, 1972, Cambridge University Press.
280 Wood GS, Beckstead JH, Turner RR, Hendrickson MR, Kempson RL, Warnke RA: Malignant fibrous histiocytoma tumor cells resemble fibroblasts. Am J Surg Pathol 10:323-335, 1986.

Histiocytoma

281 Janney CG, Hurt MA, Santa Cruz DJ: Deep juvenile xanthogranuloma. Subcutaneous and intramuscular forms. Am J Surg Pathol 15:150-159, 1991.
282 Kauffman SL, Stout AP: Histiocytic tumors (fibrous xanthoma and histiocytoma) in children. Cancer 14:469-482, 1961.

Benign fibrous histiocytoma

283 Black WC, McGavran MH, Graham P: Nodular subepidermal fibrosis. A clinical pathologic study emphasizing the frequency of clinical misdiagnoses. Arch Surg 98:296-300, 1969.
284 Fletcher CDM: Benign fibrous histiocytoma of subcutaneous and deep soft tissue. A clinicopathologic analysis of 21 cases. Am J Surg Pathol 14:801-809, 1990.
285 Niemi KM: The benign fibrohistiocytic tumours of the skin. Acta Derm Venereol (Stockh) 50(Suppl 63):1-66, 1970.

286 Tamada S, Ackerman AB: Dermatofibroma with monster cells. Am J Dermatopathol 9:380-387, 1987.
287 Ushijima M, Hashimoto H, Tsuneyoshi M, Enjoji M: Giant cell tumor of the tendon sheath (nodular tenosynovitis). A study of 207 cases to compare the large joint group with the common digit group. Cancer 57:875-884, 1986.

Intermediate (borderline) fibrous histiocytoma

288 Barnes L, Coleman JA Jr, Johnson JT: Dermatofibrosarcoma protuberans of the head and neck. Arch Otolaryngol 110:398-404, 1984.
289 Barr RJ, Young EM, King DF: Non-polarized collagen in dermatofibrosarcoma protuberans. A useful diagnostic aid. J Cutan Pathol 13:339-346, 1986.
290 Beham A, Fletcher CD: Dermatofibrosarcoma protuberans with areas resembling giant cell fibroblastoma. Report of two cases. Histopathology 17:165-167, 1990.
291 Burkhardt BR, Soule EH, Winkelman RK, Ivins JC: Dermatofibrosarcoma protuberans. Study of 56 cases. Am J Surg 111:638-644, 1966.
292 Connelly JH, Evans HL: Dermatofibrosarcoma protuberans. A clinicopathologic review with emphasis on fibrosarcomatous areas. Am J Surg Pathol 16:921-925, 1992.
293 De Chadarevian JP, Coppola D, Billmire DF: Bednar tumor pattern in recurring giant cell fibroblastoma. Am J Clin Pathol 100:164-166, 1993.
294 Ding J, Hashimoto H, Enjoji M: Dermatofibrosarcoma protuberans with fibrosarcomatous areas. A clinicopathologic study of nine cases and a comparison with allied tumors. Cancer 64:721-729, 1989.
295 Ding JA, Hashimoto H, Sugimoto T, Tsuneyoshi M, Enjoji M: Bednar tumor (pigmented dermatofibrosarcoma protuberans). An analysis of six cases. Acta Pathol Jpn 40:744-754, 1990.
295a Dominguez-Malagon HR, Ordóñez NG, Mackay B: Dermatofibrosarcoma protuberans. Ultrastructural and immunocytochemical observations. Ultrastruct Pathol 19:281-290, 1995.
296 Dupree WB, Langloss JM, Weiss SW: Pigmented dermatofibrosarcoma protuberans (Bednar tumor). A pathologic, ultrastructural, and immunohistochemical study. Am J Surg Pathol 9:630-639, 1985.
297 Fisher ER, Hellstrom HR: Dermatofibrosarcoma with metastases simulating Hodgkin's disease and reticulum cell sarcoma. Cancer 19:1165-1171, 1966.
298 Fletcher CDM, Evans BJ, MacArtney JC, Smith N, Wilson Jones E, McKee PH: Dermatofibrosarcoma protuberans. A clinicopathologic and immunohistochemical study with a review of the literature. Histopathology 9:921-938, 1985.
299 Fletcher CD, Theaker JM, Flanagan A, Krausz T: Pigmented dermatofibrosarcoma protuberans (Bednar tumour). Melanocytic colonization or neuroectodermal differentiation? A clinicopathological and immunohistochemical study. Histopathology 13:631-643, 1988.
300 Fretzin DF, Helwig EB: Atypical fibroxanthoma of the skin. A clinicopathologic study of 140 cases. Cancer 31:1541-1552, 1973.
300a Goldblum JR: CD34 positivity in fibrosarcomas which arise in dermatofibrosarcoma protuberans. Arch Pathol Lab Med 119:238-241, 1995.
301 Hashimoto K, Brownstein MH, Jakobiec FA: Dermatofibrosarcoma protuberans. A tumor with perineural and endoneural features. Arch Dermatol 110:874-885, 1974.
302 Helwig EB, May D: Atypical fibroxanthoma of the skin with metastasis. Cancer 57:368-376, 1986.
303 Hudson AW, Winkelmann RK: Atypical fibroxanthomas of the skin. A reappraisal of 19 cases in which the original diagnosis was spindle-cell squamous carcinoma. Cancer 29:413-422, 1972.
304 Kamino H, Jacobson M: Dermatofibroma extending into the subcutaneous tissue. Differential diagnosis from dermatofibrosarcoma protuberans. Am J Surg Pathol 14:1156-1164, 1990.
305 Kempson RL, McGavran MH: Atypical fibroxanthoma of the skin. Cancer 17:1463-1471, 1964.
306 Kroe DJ, Pitcock JA: Atypical fibroxanthoma of the skin. Report of ten cases. Am J Clin Pathol 51:487-492, 1969.
307 Kuwano H, Hashimoto H, Enjoji M: Atypical fibroxanthoma distinguishable from spindle cell carcinoma in sarcoma-like skin lesions. A clinicopathologic and immunohistochemical study of 21 cases. Cancer 55:172-180, 1985.
308 Lautier R, Wolff HH, Jones RE: An immunohistochemical study of dermatofibrosarcoma protuberans supports its fibroblastic character and contradicts neuroectodermal or histiocytic components. Am J Dermatopathol 12:25-30, 1990.
309 McKee PH, Fletcher CD: Dermatofibrosarcoma protuberans presenting in infancy and childhood. J Cutan Pathol 18:241-246, 1991.
310 Meister P, Höhne N, Konrad E, Eder M: Fibrous histiocytoma. An analysis of the storiform pattern. Virchows Arch [A] 383:31-41, 1979.
311 Nakamura T, Ogata H, Katsuyama T: Pigmented dermatofibrosarcoma protuberans. Report of two cases as a variant of dermatofibrosarcoma protuberans with partial neural differentiation. Am J Dermatopathol 9:18-25, 1987.

312 O'Dowd J, Laidler P: Progression of dermatofibrosarcoma protuberans to malignant fibrous histiocytoma. Report of a case with implications for tumor histogenesis. Hum Pathol **19:**368-370, 1988.

313 Rachmaninoff N, McDonald JR, Cook JC: Sarcoma-like tumors of the skin following irradiation. Am J Clin Pathol **36:**427-437, 1961.

314 Taylor HB, Helwig EB: Dermatofibrosarcoma protuberans. A study of 115 cases. Cancer **15:**717-725, 1962.

315 Volpe E, Carbone A: Dermatofibrosarcoma protuberans metastatic to lymph nodes and showing a dominant histiocytic component. Am J Dermatopathol **5:**327-334, 1983.

316 Wrotnowski U, Cooper PH, Shmookler BM: Fibrosarcomatous change in dermatofibrosarcoma protuberans. Am J Surg Pathol **12:**287-293, 1988.

Malignant fibrous histiocytoma (MFH) and related tumors

317 Angervall L, Kindblom L-G, Merck C: Myxofibrosarcoma. A study of 30 cases. Acta Pathol Microbiol Scand (A) **85:**127-140, 1977.

318 Argenyi ZB, Goodenberger ME, Strauss JS: Congenital neural hamartoma ("fascicular schwannoma"). A light microscopic, immunohistochemical, and ultrastructural study. Am J Dermatopathol **12:**283-293, 1990.

319 Bendix-Hansen K, Myhre-Jensen O: Enzyme histochemical investigations on bone and soft tissue tumours. Acta Pathol Microbiol Immunol Scand (A) **93:**73-80, 1985.

320 Bertoni F, Capanna R, Biagini R, Bacchini P, Guerra A, Ruggieri P, Present D, Campanacci M: Malignant fibrous histiocytoma of soft tissue. An analysis of 78 cases located and deeply seated in the extremities. Cancer **56:**356-367, 1985.

321 Bhagavan BS, Dorfman HD: The significance of bone and cartilage formation in malignant fibrous histiocytoma of soft tissue. Cancer **49:**480-488, 1982.

322 Binder SW, Said JW, Shintaku IP, Pinkus GS: A histiocyte-specific marker in the diagnosis of malignant fibrous histiocytoma. Use of monoclonal antibody KP-1 (CD68). Am J Clin Pathol **97:**759-763, 1992.

323 Colby TV: Malakoplakia. Two unusual cases which presented diagnostic problems. Am J Surg Pathol **2:**377-382, 1978.

324 Costa MJ, Weiss SW: Angiomatoid malignant fibrous histiocytoma. A follow-up study of 108 cases with evaluation of possible histologic predictors of outcome. Am J Surg Pathol **14:**1126-1132, 1990.

325 Du Boulay CE: Demonstration of alpha-1-antitrypsin and alpha-1-antichymotrypsin in fibrous histiocytomas using the immunoperoxidase technique. Am J Surg Pathol **6:**559-564, 1982.

326 Enzinger FM: Angiomatoid malignant fibrous histiocytoma. A distinct fibrohistiocytic tumor of children and young adults simulating a vascular neoplasm. Can-cer **44:**2147-2157, 1979.

327 Enzinger FM, Zhang RY: Plexiform fibrohistiocytic tumor presenting in children and young adults. An analysis of 65 cases. Am J Surg Pathol **12:**818-826, 1988.

328 Evans HL: Low-grade fibromyxoid sarcoma. A report of two metastasizing neoplasms having a deceptively benign appearance. Am J Clin Pathol **88:**615-619, 1987.

329 Evans HL: Low-grade fibromyxoid sarcoma. A report of 12 cases. Am J Surg Pathol **17:**595-600, 1993.

330 Fletcher CD: Angiomatoid "malignant fibrous histiocytoma." An immunohistochemical study indicative of myoid differentiation. Hum Pathol **22:**563-568, 1991.

331 Fletcher CD: Pleomorphic malignant fibrous histiocytoma. Fact or fiction? A critical reappraisal based on 159 tumors diagnosed as pleomorphic sarcoma. Am J Surg Pathol **16:**213-228, 1992.

331a Goodlad JR, Mentzel T, Fletcher CD: Low grade fibromyxoid sarcoma. Clinicopathological analysis of eleven new cases in support of a distinct entity. Histopathology **26:**229-237, 1995.

332 Hirose T, Kudo E, Hasegawa T, Abe J, Hizawa K: Expression of intermediate fil-aments in malignant fibrous histiocytomas. Hum Pathol **20:**871-877, 1989.

333 Hirose T, Sano T, Abe J, Hizawa K, Hatakeyama S, Mori I: Malignant fibrous histiocytoma with epithelial differentiation? Ultrastruct Pathol **12:**529-536, 1988.

334 Hoffman MA, Dickersin GR: Malignant fibrous histiocytoma. An ultrastructural study of 11 cases. Hum Pathol **14:**913-922, 1983.

335 Hollowood K, Holley MP, Fletcher CD: Plexiform fibrohistiocytic tumour. Clinicopathological, immunohistochemical and ultrastructural analysis in favour of a myofibroblastic lesion. Histopathology **19:**503-513, 1991.

336 Inoshita T, Youngberg GA: Malignant fibrous histiocytoma arising in previous surgical sites. Report of two cases. Cancer **53:**176-183, 1984.

337 Inoue A, Aozasa K, Tsujimoto M, Tamai M, Chatani F, Ueno H: Immunohistologic study on malignant fibrous histiocytoma. Acta Pathol Jpn **34:**759-765, 1984.

338 Kay S: Angiomatoid malignant fibrous histiocytoma. Report of two cases with ultrastructural observations of one case. Arch Pathol Lab Med **109:**934-937, 1985.

339 Kearney MM, Soule EH, Ivins JC: Malignant fibrous histiocytoma. A retrospective study of 167 cases. Cancer **45:**167-178, 1980.

340 Kempson RL, Kyriakos M: Fibroxanthosarcoma of the soft tissues. A type of malignant fibrous histiocytoma. Cancer **29:**961-976, 1972.

341 Kindblom L-G, Jacobsen GK, Jacobsen M: Immunohistochemical investigations of tumors of supposed fibroblastic-histiocytic origin. Hum Pathol **13:**834-840, 1982.

342 Kindblom L-G, Merck C, Angervall L: The ultrastructure of myxofibrosarcoma. A study of 11 cases. Virchows Arch [A] **381:**121-139, 1979.

343 Kyriakos M, Kempson RL: Inflammatory fibrous histiocytoma. An aggressive and lethal lesion. Cancer **37:**1584-1606, 1976.

344 Lagacé R: The ultrastructural spectrum of malignant fibrous histiocytoma. Ultrastruct Pathol **11:**153-159, 1987.

345 Lagacé R, Delage C, Seemayer TA: Myxoid variant of malignant fibrous histiocytoma. Ultrastructural observations. Cancer **43:**526-534, 1979.

346 Lawson CW, Fisher C, Gatter KC: An immunohistochemical study of differentiation in malignant fibrous histiocytoma. Histopathology **11:**375-383, 1987.

347 Litzky LA, Brooks JJ: Cytokeratin immunoreactivity in malignant fibrous histiocytoma and spindle cell tumors. Comparison between frozen and paraffin-embedded tissues. Mod Pathol **5:**30-34, 1992.

348 Meister P, Konrad E, Höhne N: Incidence and histological structure of the storiform pattern in benign and malignant fibrous histiocytomas. Virchows Arch [A] **393:**93-101, 1981.

349 Meister P, Konrad E, Krauss F: Fibrous histiocytoma. A histological and statistical analysis of 155 cases. Pathol Res Pract **162:**361-379, 1978.

350 Meister P, Konrad EA, Nothrath W, Eder M: Malignant fibrous histiocytoma. Histological patterns and cell types. Pathol Res Pract **168:**193-212, 1980.

351 Miettinen M, Lehto V-P, Badley RA, Virtanen I: Expression of intermediate filaments in soft tissue sarcomas. Int J Cancer **30:**541-546, 1982.

352 Miettinen M, Soini Y: Malignant fibrous histiocytoma. Heterogeneous patterns of intermediate filament proteins by immunohistochemistry. Arch Pathol Lab Med **113:**1363-1366, 1989.

353 Nakanishi S, Hizawa K: Enzyme histochemical observation of fibrohistiocytic tumors. Acta Pathol Jpn **34:**1003-1016, 1984.

354 Nemes Z, Thomazy V: Factor XIIIa and the classic histiocytic markers in malignant fibrous histiocytoma. A comparative immunohistochemical study. Hum Pathol **19:**822-829, 1988.

355 Oberling C: Retroperitoneal xanthogranuloma. Am J Cancer **23:**477-489, 1935.

356 Pettinato G, Manivel JC, De Rosa G, Petrella G, Jaszcz W: Angiomatoid malignant fibrous histiocytoma. Cytologic, immunohistochemical, ultrastructural, and flow cytometric study of 20 cases. Mod Pathol **3:**479-487, 1990.

357 Pezzi CM, Rawlings MS Jr, Esgro JJ, Pollock RE, Romsdahl MM: Prognostic factors in 227 patients with malignant fibrous histiocytoma. Cancer **69:**2098-2103, 1992.

358 Pinkston JA, Sekine I: Postirradiation sarcoma (malignant fibrous histiocytoma) following cervix cancer. Cancer **49:**434-438, 1982.

359 Raney RB, Allen A, O'Neill J, Handler SD, Uri A, Littman P: Malignant fibrous histiocytoma of soft tissue in childhood. Cancer **57:**2198-2201, 1986.

360 Reid MB, Gray C, Fear JD, Bird CC: Immunohistological demonstration of factors XIIIA and XIIIS in reactive and neoplastic fibroblastic and fibro-histiocytic lesions. Histopathology **10:**1171-1178, 1986.

361 Roholl PJ, Prinsen I, Rademakers LP, Hsu SM, van Unnik JA: Two cell lines with epithelial cell-like characteristics established from malignant fibrous histiocytomas. Cancer **68:**1963-1972, 1991.

362 Rooser B, Willen H, Gustafson P, Alvegard TA, Rydholm A: Malignant fibrous histiocytoma of soft tissue. A population-based epidemiologic and prognostic study of 137 patients. Cancer **67:**499-505, 1991.

363 Rosenberg AE, O'Connell JX, Dickersin GR, Bhan AK: Expression of epithelial markers in malignant fibrous histiocytoma of the musculoskeletal system. An immunohistochemical and electron microscopic study. Hum Pathol **24:**284-293, 1993.

364 Rydholm A, Syk I: Malignant fibrous histiocytoma of soft tissue. Correlation between clinical variables and histologic malignancy grade. Cancer **57:**2323-2324, 1986.

365 Santa Cruz DJ, Kyriakos M: Aneurysmal ("angiomatoid") fibrous histiocytoma of the skin. Cancer **47:**2053-2061, 1981.

366 Smith ME, Costa MJ, Weiss SW: Evaluation of CD68 and other histiocytic antigens in angiomatoid malignant fibrous histiocytoma. Am J Surg Pathol **15:**757-763, 1991.

367 Soini Y, Miettinen M: Alpha-1-antitrypsin and lysozyme. Their limited significance in fibrohistiocytic tumors. Am J Clin Pathol **91:**515-521, 1989.

368 Soule EH, Enriquez P: Atypical fibrous histiocytoma, malignant fibrous histiocytoma, malignant histiocytoma and epithelioid sarcoma. A comparative study of 65 tumors. Cancer **30:**128-143, 1972.

369 Sun C-CJ, Toker C, Breitenecker R: An ultrastructural study of angiomatoid fibrous histiocytoma. Cancer **49:**2103-2111, 1982.

370 Taxy JB, Battifora H: Malignant fibrous histiocytoma. An electron microscopic study. Cancer **40:**254-267, 1977.

371 Tracy T Jr, Neifield JP, DeMay RM, Salzberg AM: Malignant fibrous histiocytomas in children. J Pediatr Surg **19:**81-83, 1984.

372 Tralka TS, Yee C, Triche TJ, Costa J: Unusual intranuclear inclusions in malignant fibrous histiocytoma. Presence in primary tumor, metastases, and xenografts. Ultrastruct Pathol **3:**161-167, 1982.

373 Tsuneyoshi M, Enjoji M, Shinohara N: Malignant fibrous histiocytoma. An electron microscopic study of 17 cases. Virchows Arch [A] **392:**135-145, 1981.

374 Tsuneyoshi M, Hashimoto H, Enjoji M: Myxoid malignant fibrous histiocytoma versus myxoid liposarcoma. A comparative ultrastructural study. Virchows Arch [A] **400:**187-199, 1983.

375 Vilanova JR, Burgos-Bretones J, Simon R, Rivera-Pomar JM: Leukaemoid reaction and eosinophilia in "inflammatory fibrous histiocytoma." Virchows Arch [A] **388:**237-243, 1980.

376 Wegmann W, Heitz PU: Angiomatoid malignant fibrous histiocytoma. Evidence for the histiocytic origin of tumor cells. Virchows Arch [A] **406:**59-66, 1985.

377 Weiss SW: Malignant fibrous histiocytoma. A reaffirmation. Am J Surg Pathol **6:**773-784, 1982.

378 Weiss SW, Enzinger FM: Myxoid variant of malignant fibrous histiocytoma. Cancer **39:**1672-1685, 1977.

379 Weiss SW, Enzinger FM: Malignant fibrous histiocytoma. An analysis of 200 cases. Cancer **41:**2250-2266, 1978.

380 Weiss SW, Enzinger FM, Johnson FB: Silica reaction simulating fibrous histiocytoma. Cancer **42:**2738-2743, 1978.

381 Wood GS, Beckstead JH, Turner RR, Henrickson MR, Kempson RL, Warnke RA: Malignant fibrous histiocytoma tumor cells resemble fibroblasts. Am J Surg Pathol **10:**323-335, 1986.

Tumors and tumorlike conditions of peripheral nerves

Neuroma

382 Albrecht S, Kahn HJ, From L: Palisaded encapsulated neuroma. An immunohistochemical study. Mod Pathol **2:**403-406, 1989.

383 Argenyi ZB: Immunohistochemical characterization of palisaded, encapsulated neuroma. J Cutan Pathol **17:**329-335, 1990.

384 Dakin MC, Leppard B, Theaker JM: The palisaded, encapsulated neuroma (solitary circumscribed neuroma). Histopathology **20:**405-410, 1992.

385 Ha'Eri GB, Fornasier VL, Schatzker J: Morton's neuroma pathogenesis and ultrastructure. Clin Orthop **141:**256-259, 1979.

386 Kaiserling E, Xiao JC, Ruck P, Horny HP: Aberrant expression of macrophage-associated antigens (CD68 and Ki-M1P) by Schwann cells in reactive and neoplastic neural tissue. Light- and electron-microscopic findings. Mod Pathol **6:**463-468, 1993.

387 Reed RJ, Bliss BO: Morton's neuroma. Regressive and productive inter metatarsal elastofibrositis. Arch Pathol **95:**123-129, 1973.

388 Scotti TM: The lesion of Morton's metatarsalgia (Morton's toe). Arch Pathol **63:**91-102, 1957.

Schwannoma (neurilemoma)

389 Brooks JJ, Draffen RM: Benign glandular schwannoma. Arch Pathol Lab Med **116:**192-195, 1992.

390 Carney JA: Psammomatous melanotic schwannoma. A distinctive, heritable tumor with special associatrs, including cardiac myxoma and the Cushing syndrome. Am J Surg Pathol **14:**206-222, 1990.

391 Carpenter PM, Grafe MR, Varki NM: Granular cells in a cellular neurilemoma. Arch Pathol Lab Med **116:**1083-1085, 1992.

391a Casadei GP, Scheithauer BW, Hirose T, Manfrini M, Van Houton C, Wood MB: Cellular schwannoma. A clinicopathologic, DNA flow cytometric, and proliferation marker study of 70 patients. Cancer **75:**1109-1119, 1995.

392 Clark HB, Minesky JJ, Agrawal D, Agrawal HC: Myelin basic protein and P2 protein are not immunohistochemical markers for Schwann cell neoplasms. A comparative study using antisera to S-100, P2, and myelin basic proteins. Am J Pathol **121:**96-101, 1985.

393 Connolly CE: "Crystalline" collagen production by an unusual benign soft tissue tumour ("amianthioma"). Histopathology **5:**11-20, 1981.

394 Dahl I, Hagmar B, Idvall I: Benign solitary neurilemmoma (schwannoma). A correlative cytological and histological study of 28 cases. Acta Pathol Microbiol Immunol Scand (A) **92:**91-101, 1984.

395 Dei Tos AP, Doglioni C, Laurino L, Fletcher CD: KP1 (CD68) expression in benign neural tumours. Further evidence of its low specificity as a histiocytic/myeloid marker. Histopathology **23:**185-187, 1993.

396 Dickersin GR: The electron microscopic spectrum of nerve sheath tumors. Ultrastruct Pathol **11:**103-146, 1987.

396a Fisher C, Chappell ME, Weiss SW: Neuroblastoma-like epithelioid schwannoma. Histopathology **26:**193-194, 1995.

397 Fisher ER, Vuzevski VD: Cytogenesis of schwannoma (neurilemoma), neurofibroma, dermatofibroma and dermatofibrosarcoma as revealed by electron microscopy. Am J Clin Pathol **49:**141-154, 1968.

398 Fletcher CD: Peripheral nerve sheath tumors. A clinicopathologic update. Pathol Annu **25**(Pt 1):53-74, 1990.

399 Fletcher CDM, Davies SE: Benign plexiform (multinodular) schwannoma. A rare tumour unassociated with neurofibromatosis. Histopathology **10:**971-980, 1986.

400 Fletcher CDM, Davies SE, McKee PH: Cellular schwannoma. A distinct pseudosarcomatous entity. Histopathology **11:**21-35, 1987.

401 Font RL, Truong LD: Melanotic schwannoma of soft tissues. Electron-microscopic observations and review of literature. Am J Surg Pathol **8:**129-138, 1984.

402 Franks AJ: Epithelioid neurilemmoma of the trigeminal nerve. An immunohistochemical and ultrastructural study. Histopathology **9:**1339-1350, 1985.

403 Gay RE, Gay S, Jones RE Jr: Histological and immunohistological identification of collagens in basement membranes of Schwann cells of neurofibromas. Am J Dermatopathol **5:**317-325, 1983.

404 Goldblum JR, Beals TF, Weiss SW: Neuroblastoma-like neurilemoma. Am J Surg Pathol **18:**266-273, 1994.

405 Goto S, Matsukado Y, Mihara Y, Inoue N, Miyamoto E: An immunocytochemical demonstration of calcineurin in human nerve cell tumors. A comparison with neuron-specific enolase and glial fibrillary acidic protein. Cancer **60:**2948-2957, 1987.

406 Gould VE, Moll R, Moll I, Lee I, Schwechheimer K, Franke WW: The intermediate filament complement of the spectrum of nerve sheath neoplasms. Lab Invest **55:**463-474, 1986.

407 Gown AM, Thompson SJ, Bothwell M: Monoclonal antibody to nerve growth factor receptor. A new marker for nerve sheath tumors (abstract). Lab Invest **58:**35A, 1988.

408 Hanada M, Tanaka T, Kanayama S, Takami M, Kimura M: Malignant transformation of intrathoracic ancient neurilemoma in a patient without von Recklinghausen's disease. Acta Pathol Jpn **32:**527-536, 1982.

409 Hirano A, Dembitzer HM, Zimmerman HM: Fenestrated blood vessels in neurilemoma. Lab Invest **27:**305-309, 1972.

410 Hwang WS, Benediktsson H: Lamellar bodies in benign and malignant schwannomas. Acta Pathol Microbiol Immunol Scand (A) **90:**89-93, 1982.

411 Johnson MD, Glick AD, Davis BW: Immunohistochemical evaluation of Leu-7, myelin basic protein, S100-protein glial-fibrillary acidic-protein, and LN3 immunoreactivity in nerve sheath tumors and sarcomas. Arch Pathol Lab Med **112:**155-160, 1988.

412 Johnson MD, Kamso-Pratt J, Pepinsky RB, Whetsell WO Jr: Lipocortin-1 immunoreactivity in central and peripheral nervous system glial tumors. Hum Pathol **20:**772-776, 1989.

413 Kahn HJ, Marks A, Thom H, Baumal R: Role of antibody to S 100 protein in diagnostic pathology. Am J Clin Pathol **79:**341-347, 1983.

414 Kao GF, Laskin WB, Olsen TG: Solitary cutaneous plexiform neurilemmoma (schwannoma). A clinicopathologic, immunohistochemical, and ultrastructural study of 11 cases. Mod Pathol **2:**20-26, 1989.

415 Kawahara E, Oda Y, Ooi A, Katsuda S, Nakanishi I, Umeda S: Expression of glial fibrillary acidic protein (GFAP) in peripheral nerve sheath tumors. A comparative study of immunoreactivity of GFAP, vimentin, S-100 protein, and neurofilament in 38 schwannomas and 18 neurofibromas. Am J Surg Pathol **12:**115-120, 1988.

416 Leivo I, Engvall E, Laurila P, Miettinen M: Distribution of merosin, a laminin-related tissue-specific basement membrane protein, in human Schwann cell neoplasms. Lab Invest **61:**426-432, 1989.

417 Memoli VA, Brown EF, Gould VE: Glial fibrillary acidic protein (GFAP). Immunoreactivity in peripheral nerve sheath tumors. Ultrastruct Pathol **7:**269-275, 1984.

418 Mennemeyer RP, Hammar SP, Tytus JS, Hallman KO, Raisis JE, Bockus D: Melanotic schwannoma. Clinical and ultrastructural studies of three cases with evidence of intracellular melanin synthesis. Am J Surg Pathol **3:**3-10, 1979.

419 Miettinen M: Melanotic schwannoma coexpression of vimentin and glial fibrillary acidic protein. Ultrastruct Pathol **11:**39-46, 1987.

420 Miettinen M, Foidart J-M, Ekblom P: Immunohistochemical demonstration of laminin, the major glycoprotein of basement membranes, as an aid in the diagnosis of soft tissue tumors. Am J Clin Pathol **79:**306-311, 1983.

421 Oberman HA, Sullenger G: Neurogenous tumors of the head and neck. Cancer **20:**1992-2001, 1967.

422 Oda Y, Hashimoto H, Tsuneyoshi M, Iwata Y: Benign glandular peripheral nerve sheath tumor. Pathol Res Pract **190:**466-473, 1994.

423 Ogawa K, Oguchi M, Yamabe H, Nakashima Y, Hamashima Y: Distribution of collagen type IV in soft tissue tumors. An immunohistochemical study. Cancer **58:**269-277, 1986.

424 Orenstein JM: Amianthoid fibers in a synovial sarcoma and a malignant schwannoma. Ultrastruct Pathol **4:**163-176, 1983.

425 Skelton HG III, Smith KJ, Lupton GP: Collagenous spherulosis in a schwannoma. Am J Dermatopathol **16:**549-553, 1994.

426 Szpak CA, Shelburne J, Linder J, Klintworth GK: The presence of stage II melanosomes (premelanosomes) in neoplasms other than melanomas. Mod Pathol **1:**35-43, 1988.

427 Taxy JB, Battifora H: Epithelioid schwannoma. Diagnosis by electron microscopy. Ultrastruct Pathol **2:**19-24, 1981.

428 Waggener JD: Ultrastructure of benign peripheral nerve sheath tumors. Cancer **19:**699-709, 1966.

429 White W, Shiu MH, Rosenblum MK, Erlandson RA, Woodruff JM: Cellular schwannoma. A clinicopathologic study of 57 patients and 58 tumors. Cancer **66:**1266-1275, 1990.

430 Woodruff JM, Godwin TA, Erlandson RA, Susin M, Martini N: Cellular schwannoma. A variety of schwannoma sometimes mistaken for a malignant tumor. Am J Surg Pathol **5:**733-744, 1981.

431 Yousem SA, Colby TV, Urich H: Malignant epithelioid schwannoma arising in a benign schwannoma. A case report. Cancer **55:**2799-2803, 1985.

Neurofibroma

432 Azzopardi JG, Eusebi V, Tison V, Betts C: Neurofibroma with rhabdomyomatous differentiation. Benign "triton" tumour of the vagina. Histopathology **7:**561-572, 1983.

433 Barker D, Wright E, Nguyen K, Cannon L, Fain P, Goldgar D, Bishop DT, Carey J, Baty B, Kivlin J, Willard H, Waye JS, Greig G, Leinwand L, Nakamura Y, O'Connell P, Leppert M, Lalouel J-M, White R, Skolnick M: Gene for von Recklinghausen neurofibromatosis is in the pericentromeric region of chromosome 17. Science **236:**1100-1102, 1987.

434 Basu TN, Gutmann DH, Fletcher JA, Glover TW, Collins FS, Downward J: Aberrant regulation of *ras* proteins in malignant tumour cells from type 1 neurofibromatosis patients. Nature **356:**713-715, 1992.

435 Bednár B: Storiform neurofibromas of skin, pigmented and nonpigmented. Cancer **10:**368-376, 1957.

436 Benedict PH, Szabó G, Fitzpatrick TB, Sinesi SJ: Melanotic macules in Albright's syndrome and in neurofibromatosis. JAMA **205:**618-626, 1968.

437 Bird CC, Willis RA: The histogenesis of pigmented neurofibromas. J Pathol **97:**631-637, 1969.

438 Blatt J, Jaffe R, Deutsch M, Adkins JC: Neurofibromatosis and childhood tumors. Cancer **57:**1225-1229, 1986.

439 Bolande RP, Towler WF: A possible relationship of neuroblastoma to von Recklinghausen's disease. Cancer **26:**162-172, 1970.

440 Chanoki M, Ishii M, Fukai K, Kobayashi H, Hamada T, Muragaki Y, Ooshima A: Immunohistochemical localization of type I, III, IV, V, and VI collagens and laminin in neurofibroma and neurofibrosarcoma. Am J Dermatopathol **13:**365-373, 1991.

441 Crowe FW, Schull WJ, Neel JV: Multiple neurofibromatosis. Springfield, Ill, 1956, Charles C Thomas, Publisher.

442 De Clue JE, Cohen BD, Lowy DR: Identification and characterization of the neurofibromatosis type 1 protein product. Proc Natl Acad Sci USA **88:**9914-9918, 1991.

443 Finkel G, Lane B: Granular cell variant of neurofibromatosis. Ultrastructure of benign and malignant tumors. Hum Pathol **13:**959-963, 1982.

444 Fletcher CD, Theaker JM: Digital pacinian neuroma. A distinctive hyperplastic lesion. Histopathology **15:**249-256, 1989.

445 Fountain JW, Wallace MR, Bruce MA, Seizinger BR, Menon AG, Gusella JF, Michels VV, Schmidt MA, Dewald GW, Collins FS: Physical mapping of a translocation breakpoint in neurofibromatosis. Science **244:**1085-1087, 1989.

446 Fuller CE, Williams GT: Gastrointestinal manifestations of type 1 neurofibromatosis (von Recklinghausen's disease). Histopathology **19:**1-11, 1991.

447 Goerg C, Goerg K, Pflueger KH, Havemann K: Neurofibromatosis and acute monocytic leukemia in adults. Cancer **64:**1717-1719, 1989.

448 Gutmann DH, Wood DL, Collins FS: Identification of the neurofibromatosis type 1 gene product. Proc Natl Acad Sci USA **88:**9658-9662, 1991.

448a Hermonen J, Hirvonen O, Ylä-Outinen H, Lakkakorpi J, Björkstrand A-S, Laurikainen L, Kallionen M, Oikarinen A, Peltonen S, Peltonen J: Neurofibromin. Expression by normal human keratinocytes *in vivo* and *in vitro* and in epidermal malignancies. Lab Invest **73:**221-228, 1995.

449 Hill RP: Neuroma of Wagner-Meissner tactile corpuscles. Cancer **4:**879-882, 1951.

450 Holt JF: Neurofibromatosis in children. Am J Roentgenol **130:**651-658, 1978.

451 Hosoi K: Multiple neurofibromatosis (von Recklinghausen's disease), with special reference to malignant transformation. Arch Surg **22:**258-281, 1931.

452 Hough DR, Chan A, Davidson H: Von Recklinghausen's disease associated with gastrointestinal carcinoid tumors. Cancer **51:**2206-2208, 1983.

453 Ilgren EB, Kinnier-Wilson LM, Stiller CA: Gliomas in neurofibromatosis. A series of 89 cases with evidence for enhanced malignancy in associated cerebellar astrocytomas. Pathol Annu **20**(Pt 1):331-358, 1985.

454 Johnson MD, Kamso-Pratt J, Federspiel CF, Whetsell WO Jr: Mast cell and lymphoreticular infiltrates in neurofibromas. Comparison with nerve sheath tumors. Arch Pathol Lab Med **113:**1263-1270, 1989.

455 Kaiserling E, Geerts ML: Tumour of Wagner-Meissner touch corpuscles. Wagner-Meissner neurilemmoma. Virchows Arch [A] **409:**241-250, 1986.

456 Kamata Y: Study on the ultrastructure and acetylcholinesterase activity in von Recklinghausen's neurofibromatosis. Acta Pathol Jpn **28:**393-410, 1978.

456a Kindblom L-G, Ahldén M, Meis-Kindblom JM, Stenman G: Immunohistochemical and molecular analysis of p53, MDM2, proliferating cell nuclear antigen and Ki67 in benign and malignant peripheral nerve sheath tumours. Virchows Arch **427:**19-26, 1995.

457 MacDonald DM, Wilson-Jones E: Pacinian neurofibroma. Histopathology **1:**247-255, 1977.

458 Malecha M, Rubin R: Aneurysms of the carotid arteries associated with von Recklinghausen's neurofibromatosis. Pathol Res Pract **188:**145-147, 1992.

459 Markel SF, Enzinger FM: Neuromuscular hamartoma. A benign "triton tumor" composed of mature neural and striated muscle elements. Cancer **49:**140-144, 1982.

460 McCarroll HR: Clinical manifestations of congenital neurofibromatosis. J Bone Joint Surg (Am) **32:**601-617, 1950.

461 Megahed M: Histopathological variants of neurofibroma. A study of 114 lesions. Am J Dermatopathol **16:**486-495, 1994.

462 Peltonen J, Jaakkola S, Hsiao LL, Timpl R, Chu ML, Uitto J: Type VI collagen. In situ hybridizations and immunohistochemistry reveal abundant mRNA and protein levels in human neurofibroma, schwannoma and normal peripheral nerve tissues. Lab Invest **62:**487-492, 1990.

463 Peltonen J, Jaakkola S, Lebwohl M, Renvall S, Risteli L, Virtanen I, Uitto J: Cellular differentiation and expression of matrix genes in type 1 neurofibromatosis. Lab Invest **59:**760-771, 1988.

464 Piccardi VM: Von Recklinghausen neurofibromatosis. N Engl J Med **305:**1617-1628, 1981.

465 Pineada A: Mast cells. Their presence and ultrastructural characteristics in peripheral nerve tumors. Arch Neurol **13:**372-382, 1965.

466 Raszkowski HJ, Hufner RF: Neurofibromatosis of the colon. A unique manifestation of von Recklinghausen's disease. Cancer **27:**134-142, 1971.

467 Rouleau GA, Merel P, Lutchman M, Sanson M, Zucman J, Marineau C, Hoang-Xuan K, Demczuk S, Desmaze C, Plougastel B, et al.: Alteration in a new gene encoding a putative membrane-organizing protein causes neurofibromatosis type 2. Nature **363:**515-521, 1993.

468 Salyer WR, Salyer DC: The vascular lesions of neurofibromatosis. Angiology **25:**510-519, 1974.

469 Saxén E: Tumours of tactile end-organs. Acta Pathol Microbiol Scand **25:**66-79, 1948.

470 Schenkein I, Beuker ED, Helson L, Axelrod F, Dancis J: Increased nerve-growth-stimulating activity in disseminated neurofibromatosis. N Engl J Med **290:**613-614, 1974.

471 Sorensen SA, Mulvihill JJ, Nielsen A: Long-term follow-up of von Recklinghausen neurofibromatosis. Survival and malignant neoplasms. N Engl J Med **314:**1010-1015, 1986.

472 Stay EJ, Vater G: The relationship between nephroblastoma and neurofibromatosis (von Recklinghausen's disease). Cancer **39:**2550-2555, 1977.

473 Stout AP: Neurofibroma and neurilemoma. Clin Proc **5:**1-12, 1946.

474 Takata M, Imai T, Hirone T: Factor-XIIIa-positive cells in normal peripheral nerves and cutaneous neurofibromas of type-1 neurofibromatosis. Am J Dermatopathol **16:**37-43, 1994.

475 Theaker JM, Fletcher CD: Epithelial membrane antigen expression by the perineurial cell. Further studies of peripheral nerve lesions. Histopathology **14:**581-592, 1989.

476 Vaalasti A, Suomalainen H, Kuokkanen K, Rechardt L: Neuropeptides in cutaneous neurofibromas of von Recklinghausen's disease. J Cutan Pathol **17:**371-373, 1990.

477 Waggener JD: Ultrastructure of benign peripheral nerve sheath tumors. Cancer **19:**699-709, 1966.

478 Webb WR, Goodman PC: Fibrosing alveolitis in patients with neurofibromatosis. Radiology **122:**289-293, 1977.

479 Weiss SW, Nickoloff BJ: CD-34 is expressed by a distinctive cell population in peripheral nerve, nerve sheath tumors, and related lesions. Am J Surg Pathol **17:**1039-1045, 1993.

480 Wertelecki W, Rouleau GA, Superneau DW, Forehand LW, Williams JP, Haines JL, Gusella JF: Neurofibromatosis 2. Clinical and DNA linkage studies of a large kindred. N Engl J Med **319:**278-283, 1988.

481 Whitehouse D: Diagnostic value of the cafe-au-lait spots in children. Arch Dis Child **41:**316-319, 1966.

482 Witzleben CL, Landy RA: Disseminated neuroblastoma in a child with von Recklinghausen's disease. Cancer **34:**786-790, 1974.

483 Yagle MK, Parruti G, Xu W, Ponder BA, Solomon E: Genetic and physical map of the von Recklinghausen neurofibromatosis (NF1) region on chromosome 17. Proc Natl Acad Sci USA **87:**7255-7259, 1990.

Perineurioma

484 Ariza A, Bilbao JM, Rosai J: Immunohistochemical detection of epithelial membrane antigen in normal perineurial cells and perineurioma. Am J Surg Pathol **12:**678-683, 1988.

485 Bilbao JM, Khoury NJS, Hudson AR, Briggs SJ: Perineurioma (localized hypertrophic neuropathy). Arch Pathol Lab Med **108:**557-560, 1984.

485a Emory TS, Scheithauer BW, Hirose T, Wood M, Onofrio BM, Jenkins RB: Intraneural perineurioma. A clonal neoplasm associated with abnormalities of chromosome 22. Am J Clin Pathol **103:**696-704, 1995.

486 Erlandson RA: The enigmatic perineurial cell and its participation in tumors and in tumorlike entities. Ultrastruct Pathol **15:**335-351, 1991.

487 Lazarus SS, Trombetta LD: Ultrastructural identification of a benign perineurial cell tumor. Cancer **41:**1823-1829, 1978.

488 Mentzel T, Dei Tos AP, Fletcher CDM: Perineurioma (storiform perineurial fibroma). Clinico-pathological analysis of four cases. Histopathology **25:**261-268, 1994.

489 Ohno T, Park P, Akai M, Kamura S, Murase K, Kimura H, Kadoya H, Manabe S, Nagao K, Sugano I: Ultrastructural study of a perineurioma. Ultrastruct Pathol **12:**495-504, 1988.

490 Perentes E, Nakagawa Y, Ross GW, Stanton C, Rubinstein LJ: Expression of epithelial membrane antigen in perineurial cells and their derivatives. An immuno histochemical study with multiple markers. Acta Neuropathol **75:**160-165, 1987.

491 Theaker JM, Gatter KC, Puddle J: Epithelial membrane antigen expression by the perineurium of peripheral nerve and in peripheral nerve tumours. Histopathology **13:**171-179, 1988.

492 Tsang W, Chan JKC, Chow L, Tse C: Perineurioma. An uncommon soft tissue neoplasm distinct from localized hypertrophic neuropathy and neurofibroma. Am J Surg Pathol **16:**756-763, 1992.

493 Weidenheim KM, Campbell WG Jr: Perineurial cell tumor. Immunocytochemical and ultrastructural characterization. Relationship to other peripheral nerve tumors with a review of the literature. Virchows Arch [A] **408:**375-383, 1986.

494 Weidner N, Nasr A, Johnston J: Plexiform soft tissue tumor composed predominantly of perineurial fibroblasts (perineurioma). Ultrastruct Pathol **17:**251-262, 1993.

Nerve sheath myxoma

495 Angervall L, Kindblom L-G, Haglid K: Dermal nerve sheath myxoma. A light and electron microscopic, histochemical and immunohistochemical study. Cancer **53:**1752-1759, 1984.

496 Blumberg AK, Kay S, Adelaar RS: Nerve sheath myxoma of digital nerve. Cancer **63:**1215-1218, 1989.

497 Fletcher CDM, Chan JK-C, MacKee PH: Dermal nerve sheath myxoma. A study of three cases. Histopathology **10:**135-145, 1986.

498 Gallager RL, Helwig EB: Neurothekeoma—a benign cutaneous tumor of neural origin. Am J Clin Pathol **74:**759-764, 1980.

499 Goldstein J, Lifshitz T: Myxoma of the nerve sheath. Report of three cases, observations by light and electron microscopy and histochemical analysis. Am J Dermatopathol **7:**423-429, 1985.

500 Paulus W, Jellinger K, Perneczky G: Intraspinal neurothekeoma (nerve sheath myxoma). A report of two cases. Am J Clin Pathol **95:**511-516, 1991.

501 Pulitzer DR, Reed RJ: Nerve-sheath myxoma (perineurial myxoma). Am J Dermatopathol **7:**409-421, 1985.

Malignant peripheral nerve tumor (MPNST)

502 Alvira MM, Mandybur TI, Menefee MG: Light microscopic and ultrastructural observations of a metastasizing malignant epithelioid schwannoma. Cancer **38:**1977-1982, 1976.

503 Axiotis CA, Merino MJ, Tsokos M: Epithelioid malignant peripheral nerve sheath tumor with squamous differentiation. A light microscopic, ultrastructural, and immunohistochemical study. Surg Pathol **3:**301-308, 1990.

504 Banks E, Yum M, Brodhecker C, Goheen M: A malignant peripheral nerve sheath tumor in association with a paratesticular ganglioneuroma. Cancer **64:**1738-1742, 1989.

505 Bojsen-Moller M, Myhre-Jensen O: A consecutive series of 30 malignant schwannomas. Survival in relation to clinico-pathological parameters and treatment. Acta Pathol Microbiol Immunol Scand [A] **92:**147-155, 1984.

506 Brooks JSJ, Freeman M, Enterline HT: Malignant triton tumors. Natural history and immunohistochemistry of nine new cases with literature review. Cancer **55:**2543-2549, 1985.

507 Brown RW, Tornos C, Evans HL: Angiosarcoma arising from malignant schwannoma in a patient with neurofibromatosis. Cancer **70:**1141-1144, 1992.

508 Bruner JM: Peripheral nerve sheath tumors of the head and neck. Semin Diagn Pathol **4:**136-149, 1987.

509 Chen KTK, Latorraca R, Fabich D, Padgug A, Hafez GR, Gilbert EF: Malignant schwannoma. A light microscopic and ultrastructural study. Cancer **45:**1585-1593, 1980.

510 Chitale AR, Dickersin GR: Electron microscopy in the diagnosis of malignant schwannomas. A report of six cases. Cancer **51:**1448-1461, 1983.

511 Christensen WN, Strong EW, Bains MS, Woodruff JM: Neuroendocrine differentiation in the glandular peripheral nerve sheath tumor. Pathologic distinction from the biphasic synovial sarcoma with glands. Am J Surg Pathol **12:**417-426, 1988.

512 Dabski C, Reiman HM Jr, Muller SA: Neurofibrosarcoma of skin and subcutaneous tissues. Mayo Clin Proc **65:**164-172, 1990.

513 D'Agostino AN, Soule EH, Miller RH: Primary malignant neoplasms of nerves (malignant neurilemomas) in patients without manifestations of multiple neurofibromatosis (von Recklinghausen's disease). Cancer **16:**1003-1013, 1963.

514 D'Agostino AN, Soule EH, Miller RH: Sarcomas of the peripheral nerves and somatic soft tissues associated with multiple neurofibromatosis (von Recklinghausen's disease). Cancer **16:**1015-1027, 1963.

515 Daimaru Y, Hashimoto H, Enjoji M: Malignant peripheral nerve-sheath tumors (malignant schwannomas). An immunohistochemical study of 29 cases. Am J Surg Pathol **9:**434-444, 1985.

516 DeSchryver K, Santa Cruz DJ: So-called glandular schwannoma. Ependymal differentiation in a case. Ultrastruct Pathol **6:**167-175, 1984.

517 Dewit L, Albus-Lutter CE, De Jong ASH, Voute PA: Malignant schwannoma with a rhabdomyoblastic component, a so-called triton tumor. A clinicopathologic study. Cancer **58:**1350-1356, 1986.

518 DiCarlo EF, Woodruff JM, Bansal M, Erlandson RA: The purely epithelioid malignant peripheral nerve sheath tumor. Am J Surg Pathol **10:**478-490, 1986.

519 Dickersin GR: The electron microscopic spectrum of nerve sheath tumors. Ultrastruct Pathol **11:**103-146, 1987.

520 Ducatman BS, Scheithauer BW: Postirradiation neurofibrosarcoma. Cancer **51:**1028-1033, 1983.

521 Ducatman BS, Scheithauer BW: Malignant peripheral nerve sheath tumors with divergent differentiation. Cancer **54:**1049-1057, 1984.

522 Ducatman BS, Scheithauer BW, Piepgras DG, Reiman HM, Ilstrup DM: Malignant peripheral nerve sheath tumors. Cancer **57:**2006-2021, 1986.

523 Fisher C, Carter RL, Ramachandra S, Thomas DM: Peripheral nerve sheath differentiation in malignant soft tissue tumours. An ultrastructural and immunohistochemical study. Histopathology **20:**115-125, 1992.

524 Fletcher CD, Fernando IN, Braimbridge MV, McKee PH, Lyall JR: Malignant nerve sheath tumour arising in a ganglioneuroma. Histopathology **12:**445-448, 1988.

525 George E, Swanson PE, Wick MR: Malignant peripheral nerve sheath tumors of the skin. Am J Dermatopathol **11:**213-221, 1989.

526 Ghali VS, Gold JE, Vincent RA, Cosgrove JM: Malignant peripheral nerve sheath tumor arising spontaneously from retroperitoneal ganglioneuroma. A case report, review of the literature, and immunohistochemical study. Hum Pathol **23:**72-75, 1992.

527 Ghosh BC, Ghosh L, Huvos AG, Fortner JG: Malignant schwannoma. A clinicopathologic study. Cancer **31:**184-190, 1973.

528 Gore I: Primary malignant tumors of nerve. A report of eight cases. Cancer **5:**278-296, 1952.

529 Gray MH, Rosenberg AE, Dickersin GR, Bhan AK: Glial fibrillary acidic protein and keratin expression by benign and malignant nerve sheath tumors. Hum Pathol **20:**1089-1096, 1989.

530 Guccion JG, Enzinger FM: Malignant schwannoma associated with von Recklinghausen's neurofibromatosis. Virchows Arch [A] **383:**43-57, 1979.

531 Herrera GA, Pinto de Moraes H: Neurogenic sarcomas in patients with neurofibromatosis (von Recklinghausen's disease). Light, electron microscopy and immunohistochemistry study. Virchows Arch [A] **403**:361-376, 1984.

532 Herrera GA, Reimann BE, Salinas JA: Malignant schwannomas presenting as malignant fibrous histiocytomas. Ultrastruct Pathol **3**:253-261, 1982.

533 Hirose T, Hasegawa T, Kudo E, Seki K, Sano T, Hizawa K: Malignant peripheral nerve sheath tumors. An immunohistochemical study in relation to ultra structural features. Hum Pathol **23**:865-870, 1992.

534 Hirose T, Sano T, Hizawa K: Heterogeneity of malignant schwannomas. Ultrastruct Pathol **12**:107-116, 1988.

535 Hruban RH, Shiu MH, Senie RT, Woodruff JM: Malignant peripheral nerve sheath tumors of the buttock and lower extremity. A study of 43 cases. Cancer **66**:1253-1265, 1990.

536 Johnson TL, Lee MW, Meis JM, Zarbo RJ, Crissman JD: Immunohistochemical characterization of malignant peripheral nerve sheath tumors. Surg Pathol **4**:121-135, 1994.

537 Krausz T, Azzopardi JG, Pearse E: Malignant melanoma of the sympathetic chain. With a consideration of pigmented nerve sheath tumours. Histopathology **8**:881-894, 1984.

538 Laskin WB, Weiss SW, Bratthauer GL: Epithelioid variant of malignant peripheral nerve sheath tumour (malignant epithelioid schwannoma). Am J Surg Pathol **15**:1136-1145, 1991.

539 Lattes R: Peripheral neuroepithelioma. Proceedings of the 39th Annual Anatomic Pathology Slide Seminar of the American Society of Clinical Pathologists. Chicago, 1975, American Society of Clinical Pathology, pp. 49-52.

540 Mackay B, Luna MA, Butler JJ: Adult neuroblastoma. Electron microscopic observations in nine cases. Cancer **37**:1334-1351, 1976.

541 Matsunou H, Shimoda T, Kakimoto S, Yamashita H, Ishikawa E, Mukai M: Histopathologic and immunohistochemical study of malignant tumors of peripheral nerve sheath (malignant schwannoma). Cancer **56**:2269-2279, 1985.

542 Meis JM, Enzinger FM, Martz KL, Neal JA: Malignant peripheral nerve sheath tumors (malignant schwannomas) in children. Am J Surg Pathol **16**:694-707, 1992.

543 Meis-Kindblom JM, Enzinger FM: Plexiform malignant peripheral nerve sheath tumor of infancy and childhood. Am J Surg Pathol **18**:479-485, 1994.

544 Menon AG, Anderson KM, Riccardi VM, Chung RY, Whaley JM, Yandell DW, Farmer GE, Freiman RN, Lee JK, Li FP, et al.: Chromosome 17p deletions and p53 gene mutations associated with the formation of malignant neurofibrosarcomas in von Recklinghausen neurofibromatosis. Proc Natl Acad Sci USA **87**:5435-5439, 1990.

545 Millstein DI, Tang C-K, Campbell EW Jr: Angiosarcoma developing in a patient with neurofibromatosis (von Recklinghausen's disease). Cancer **47**:950-954, 1981.

546 Morgan KG, Gray C: Malignant epithelioid schwannoma of superficial soft tissue? A case report with immunohistology and electron microscopy. Histopathology **9**:765-775, 1985.

547 Newbould MJ, Wilkinson N, Mene A: Post-radiation malignant peripheral nerve sheath tumour: A report of two cases. Histopathology **17**:263-265, 1990.

548 Raney B, Schnaufer L, Ziegler M, Chatten J, Littman P, Jarrett P: Treatment of children with neurogenic sarcoma. Experience at the Children's Hospital of Philadelphia, 1958-1984. Cancer **59**:1-5, 1987.

549 Rasbridge SA, Browse NL, Tighe JR, Fletcher CD: Malignant nerve sheath tumour arising in a benign ancient schwannoma. Histopathology **14**:525-528, 1989.

550 Ricci A Jr, Parham DM, Woodruff JM, Callihan T, Green A, Erlandson RA: Malignant peripheral nerve sheath tumors arising from ganglioneuromas. Am J Surg Pathol **8**:19-29, 1984.

551 Robson DK, Ironside JW: Malignant peripheral nerve sheath tumour arising in a schwannoma. Histopathology **16**:295-297, 1990.

552 Rose DS, Wilkins MJ, Birch R, Evans DJ: Malignant peripheral nerve sheath tumour with rhabdomyoblastic and glandular differentiation. Immunohistochemical features. Histopathology **21**:287-290, 1992.

553 Shimizu S, Teraki Y, Ishiko A, Shimizu H, Harada T, Mukai M, Nishikawa T: Malignant epithelioid schwannoma of the skin showing partial HMB-45 positivity. Am J Dermatopathol **15**:378-384, 1993.

554 Storm FK, Eilber FR, Mirra J, Morton DL: Neurofibrosarcoma. Cancer **45**:126-129, 1980.

555 Stout AP: Discussion of case 5, Seventeenth Seminar of the American Society of Clinical Pathologists, Chicago, Ill, October, 1951.

556 Suster S, Amazon K, Rosen LB, Ollague JM: Malignant epithelioid schwannoma of the skin. A low-grade neurotropic malignant melanoma? Am J Dermatopathol **11**:338-344, 1989.

557 Taxy JB, Battifora H, Trujillo Y, Dorfman HD: Electron microscopy in the diagnosis of malignant schwannoma. Cancer **48**:1381-1391, 1981.

558 Thomas JE, Piepgras DG, Scheithauer B, Onofrio BM, Shives TC: Neurogenic tumors of the sciatic nerve. Mayo Clin Proc **58**:640-647, 1983.

559 Trojanowski JQ, Kleinman GM, Proppe KH: Malignant tumors of nerve sheath origin. Cancer **46**:1202-1212, 1980.

560 Tsuneyoshi M, Enjoji M: Primary malignant peripheral nerve tumors (malignant schwannomas). A clinicopathologic and electron microscopic study. Acta Pathol Jpn **29**:363-375, 1979.

561 Uri AK, Witzelben CL, Raney RB: Electron microscopy of glandular schwannoma. Cancer **53**:493-497, 1984.

562 Wanebo JE, Malik JM, Vanden Berg SR, Wanebo HJ, Driesen N, Persing JA: Malignant peripheral nerve sheath tumors. A clinicopathologic study of 28 cases. Cancer **71**:1247-1253, 1993.

563 Weiss SW, Langloss JM, Enzinger FM: Value of S-100 protein in the diagnosis of soft tissue tumors with particular reference to benign and malignant Schwann cell tumors. Lab Invest **49**:299-308, 1983.

564 White HR Jr: Survival in malignant schwannoma. An 18-year study. Cancer **27**:720-729, 1971.

565 Wick MR, Swanson PE, Scheithauer BW, Manivel JC: Malignant peripheral nerve sheath tumor. An immunohistochemical study of 62 cases. Am J Clin Pathol **87**:425-433, 1987.

566 Woodruff JM: Peripheral nerve tumors showing glandular differentiation (glandular schwannomas). Cancer **37**:2399-2413, 1976.

567 Woodruff JM, Chevnik NL, Smith MC, Millett WB, Foote FW: Peripheral nerve tumors with rhabdomyosarcomatous differentiation (malignant "triton" tumors). Cancer **37**:2426-2439, 1973.

568 Woodruff JM, Christensen WN: Glandular peripheral nerve sheath tumors. Cancer **72**:3618-3628, 1993.

569 Woodruff JM, Selig AM, Crowley K, Allen PW: Schwannoma (neurilemoma) with malignant transformation. A rare, distinctive peripheral nerve tumor. Am J Surg Pathol **18**:882-895, 1994.

Other tumors of peripheral nerves

570 Eusebi V, Bondi A, Cancellieri A, Canedi L, Frizzera G: Primary malignant lymphoma of sciatic nerve. Report of a case. Am J Surg Pathol **14**:881-885, 1990.

571 Radi MJ, Foucar E, Palmer CH, Gooding RA: Malignant lymphoma arising in a large congenital neurofibroma of the head and neck. Report of a case. Cancer **61**:1667-1673, 1988.

572 Vigna PA, Kusior MF, Collins MB, Ross JS: Peripheral nerve hemangioma. Potential for clinical aggressiveness. Arch Pathol Lab Med **118**:1038-1041, 1994.

Tumors of adipose tissue
Lipoma

573 Azzopardi JG, Iocco J, Salm R: Pleomorphic lipoma. A tumour simulating liposarcoma. Histopathology **7**:511-523, 1983.

574 Bolen JW, Thorning D: Spindle-cell lipoma. A clinical, light- and electron-microscopic study. Am J Surg Pathol **5**:435-441, 1981.

575 Dixon AY, McGregor DH, Lee SH: Angiolipomas. An ultrastructural and clinicopathological study. Hum Pathol **12**:739-747, 1981.

576 Enzi G: Multiple symmetric lipomatosis. An updated clinical report. Medicine (Baltimore) **63**:56-64, 1984.

577 Enzinger FM: Benign lipomatous tumors simulating a sarcoma. In M.D. Anderson Tumor Institute. Management of primary bone and soft tissue tumors. Chicago, 1977, Year Book Medical Publishers Inc, pp. 11-24.

578 Enzinger FM, Harvey DA: Spindle cell lipoma. Cancer **36**:1852-1859, 1975.

579 Fletcher CDM, Akerman M, Dal Cin P, De Wever I, Mandahl N, Mertens F, Mitelman F, Rosai J, Rydholm A, Sciot R, Tallini G, Van den Berghe H, Van de Ven W, Vanni R, Willen H: Correlation between clinicopathologic features and karyotype in lipomatous tumors. A report of 178 cases from the chromosomes and morphology (CHAMP) collaborative study group. Am J Pathol (in press).

580 Fletcher CDM, Martin-Bates E: Spindle cell lipoma. A clinicopathological study with some original observations. Histopathology **11**:803-817, 1987.

581 Fletcher CD, Martin-Bates E: Intramuscular and intermuscular lipoma: Neglected diagnoses. Histopathology **12**:275-287, 1988.

582 Greenberg SD, Isensee C, Gonzalez-Angulo A, Wallace SA: Infiltrating lipomas of the thigh. Am J Clin Pathol **39**:66-72, 1963.

583 Hawley IC, Krausz T, Evans DJ, Fletcher CD: Spindle cell lipoma—a pseudoangiomatous variant. Histopathology **24**:565-569, 1994.

584 Heim S, Mandahl N, Rydholm A, Willen H, Mitelman F: Different karyotypic features characterize different clinico-pathologic subgroups of benign lipogenic tumors. Int J Cancer **42**:863-867, 1988.

585 Howard WR, Helwig EB: Angiolipoma. Arch Dermatol **82**:924-931, 1960.

586 Hunt SJ, Santa Cruz DJ, Barr RJ: Cellular angiolipoma. Am J Surg Pathol **14**:75-81, 1990.

587 Katzer B: Histopathology of rare chondroosteoblastic metaplasia in benign lipomas. Pathol Res Pract **184**:437-445, 1989.

588 Kin YH, Reiner L: Ultrastructure of lipoma. Cancer **50**:102-106, 1982.

589 Kindblom L-G, Angervall L, Stener B, Wickbom I: Intermuscular and intramuscular lipomas and hibernomas. A clinical, roentgenologic, histologic, and prognostic study of 46 cases. Cancer **33**:754-762, 1974.

589a Kindblom L-G, Meis-Kindblom JM: Chondroid lipoma. An ultrastructural and immunohistochemical analysis with further observations regarding its differentiation. Hum Pathol **26**:706-715, 1995.

589b Lovell-Badge R: Living with bad architecture. Nature **376**:725-726, 1995.

590 Mandahl N, Heim S, Arheden K, Rydholm A, Willen H, Mitelman F: Three major cytogenetic subgroups can be identified among chromosomally abnormal solitary lipomas. Hum Genet **79**:203-208, 1988.

591 Meis JM, Enzinger FM: Myolipoma of soft tissue. Am J Surg Pathol **15**:121-125, 1991.

592 Meis JM, Enzinger FM: Chondroid lipoma. A unique tumor simulating liposarcoma and myxoid chondrosarcoma. Am J Surg Pathol **17**:1103-1112, 1993.

593 Paarlberg D, Linscheid RL, Soule EH: Lipomas of the hand. Including a case of lipoblastomatosis in a child. Mayo Clin Proc **47**:121-124, 1972.

594 Pack GT, Pierson JC: Liposarcoma. Surgery **36**:687-712, 1954.

595 Popper H, Knipping G: A histochemical and biochemical study of a liposarcoma with several aspects on the development of fat synthesis. Pathol Res Pract **171**:373-380, 1981.

596 Robb JA, Jones RA: Spindle cell lipoma in a perianal location. Hum Pathol **13**:1052, 1982.

597 Shmookler BM, Enzinger FM: Pleomorphic lipoma. A benign tumor simulating liposarcoma. A clinicopathologic analysis of 48 cases. Cancer **47**:126-133, 1981.

598 Solvonuk PF, Taylor GP, Hancock R, Wood WS, Frohlich J: Correlation of morphologic and biochemical observations in human lipomas. Lab Invest **51**:469-474, 1984.

Lipoblastoma/lipoblastomasis

599 Bolen JW, Thorning D: Benign lipoblastoma and myxoid liposarcoma. A comparative light- and electron-microscopic study. Am J Surg Pathol **4**:163-174, 1980.

600 Chung EB, Enzinger FM: Benign lipoblastomatosis. An analysis of 35 cases. Cancer **32**:482-492, 1973.

601 Coffin CM: Lipoblastoma. An embryonal tumor of soft tissue related to organogenesis. Semin Diagn Pathol **11**:98-103, 1994.

602 Fletcher CDM, Akerman M, Dal Cin P, De Wever I, Mandahl N, Mertens F, Mitelman F, Rosai J, Rydholm A, Sciot R, Tallini G, Van den Berghe H, Van de Ven W, Vanni R, Willen H: Correlation between clinicopathologic features and karyotype in lipomatous tumors. A report of 178 cases from the chromosomes and morphology (CHAMP) collaborative study group. Am J Pathol (in press).

603 Greco AMA, Garcia RL, Vuletin JC: Benign lipoblastomatosis. Ultrastructure and histogenesis. Cancer **45**:511-515, 1980.

604 Mentzel T, Calonje E, Fletcher CD: Lipoblastoma and lipoblastomatosis. A clinicopathological study of 14 cases. Histopathology **23**:527-533, 1993.

605 Vellios F, Baez MF, Schumacher HB: Lipoblastomatosis. A tumor of fetal fat different from hibernoma. Am J Pathol **34**:1149-1155, 1958.

Hibernoma

606 Allegra SR, Gmuer C, O'Leary GP Jr: Endocrine activity in a large hibernoma. Hum Pathol **14**:1044-1052, 1983.

607 Brines OA, Johnson MH: Hibernoma, a special fatty tumor. Report of a case. Am J Pathol **25**:467-479, 1949.

608 Fletcher CDM, Akerman M, Dal Cin P, De Wever I, Mandahl N, Mertens F, Mitelman F, Rosai J, Rydholm A, Sciot R, Tallini G, Van den Berghe H, Van deVen W, Vanni R, Willen H: Correlation between clinicopathologic features and karyotype in lipomatous tumors. A report of 178 cases from the chromosomes and morphology (CHAMP) collaborative study group. Am J Pathol (in press).

609 Gaffney EF, Hargreaves HK, Semple E, Vellios F: Hibernoma. Distinctive light and electron microscopic features and relationship to brown adipose tissue. Hum Pathol **14**:677-687, 1983.

610 Levine GD: Hibernoma. An electron microscopic study. Hum Pathol **3**:351-359, 1972.

611 Rigor VU, Goldstone SE, Jones J, Bernstein R, Gold MS, Weiner S: Hibernoma. A case report and discussion of a rare tumor. Cancer **57**:2207-2211, 1986.

612 Ross SR, Choy L, Graves RA, Fox N, Solevjeva V, Klaus S, Ricquier D, Spiegelman BM: Hibernoma formation in transgenic mice and isolation of a brown adipocyte cell line expressing the uncoupling protein gene. Proc Natl Acad Sci USA **89**:7561-7565, 1992.

613 Seemayer TA, Knaack J, Wang N, Ahmed MN: On the ultrastructure of hibernoma. Cancer **36**:1785-1793, 1975.

Liposarcoma

614 Ackerman LV: Multiple primary liposarcomas. Am J Pathol **20**:789-798, 1944.

615 Aman P, Ron D, Mandahl N, Fioretos T, Heim S, Arheden K, Willen H, Rydholm A, Mitelman F: Rearrangement of the transcription factor gene CHOP in myxoid liposarcomas with t(12; 16)(q13; p11). Genes Chromosom Cancer **5**:278-285, 1992.

616 Azumi N, Curtis J, Kempson RL, Hendrickson MR: Atypical and malignant neoplasms showing lipomatous differentiation. A study of 111 cases. Am J Surg Pathol **11**:161-183, 1987.

617 Battifora H, Nunez-Alonso C: Myxoid liposarcoma. Study of 10 cases. Ultrastruct Pathol **1**:157-169, 1980.

618 Bolen JW, Thorning D: Liposarcomas. A histogenetic approach to the classification of adipose tissue neoplasms. Am J Surg Pathol **8**:3-17, 1984.

619 Brooks JJ, Connor AM: Atypical lipoma of the extremities and peripheral soft tissues with dedifferentiation. Implications for management. Surg Pathol **3**:169-178, 1990.

620 Castleberry RP, Kelly DR, Wilson ER, Cain WS, Salter MR: Childhood liposarcoma. Report of a case and review of the literature. Cancer **54**:579-584, 1984.

621 Chang HR, Hajdu SI, Collin C, Brennan MF: The prognostic value of histologic subtypes in primary extremity liposarcoma. Cancer **64**:1514-1520, 1989.

621a Cheng EY, Springfield DS, Mankin HJ: Frequent incidence of extrapulmonary sites of initial metastasis in patients with liposarcoma. Cancer **75**:1120-1127, 1995.

622 Chung EB: Pitfalls in diagnosing benign soft tissue tumors in infancy and childhood. Pathol Annu **20**(Pt 2):323-386, 1985.

623 Cocchia D, Lauriola L, Stolfi VM, Tallini G, Michetti F: S-100 antigen labels neoplastic cells in liposarcoma and cartilaginous tumours. Virchows Arch [A] **402**:139-145, 1983.

624 Crozat A, Aman P, Mandahl N, Ron D: Fusion of CHOP to a novel RNA-binding protein in human myxoid liposarcoma. Nature **363**:640-644, 1993.

625 Dei Tos AP, Mentzel T, Newman PL, Fletcher CD: Spindle cell liposarcoma, a hitherto unrecognized variant of liposarcoma. Analysis of six cases. Am J Surg Pathol **18**:913-921, 1994.

626 Enterline HT, Culberson JD, Rochlin DB, Brady LW: Liposarcoma. A clinical and pathological study of 53 cases. Cancer **13**:932-950, 1960.

627 Enzinger FM, Winslow DJ: Liposarcoma. A study of 103 cases. Virchows Arch [A] **335**:367-388, 1962.

628 Evans HL: Liposarcoma. A study of 55 cases with a reassessment of its classification. Am J Surg Pathol **3**:507-523, 1979.

629 Evans HL: Liposarcomas and atypical lipomatous tumors. A study of 66 cases followed for a minimum of 10 years. Surg Pathol **1**:41-54, 1988.

630 Evans HL: Smooth muscle in atypical lipomatous tumors. A report of three cases. Am J Surg Pathol **14**:714-718, 1990.

631 Evans HL, Khurana KK, Kemp BL, Ayala AG: Heterologous elements in the dedifferentiated component of dedifferentiated liposarcoma. Am J Surg Pathol **18**:1150-1157, 1994.

632 Evans HL, Soule EH, Winkelmann RK: Atypical lipoma, atypical intramuscular lipoma, and well-differentiated retroperitoneal liposarcoma. A reappraisal of 30 cases formerly classified as well differentiated liposarcoma. Cancer **43**:574-584, 1979.

633 Fletcher CDM, Akerman M, Dal Cin P, De Wever I, Mandahl N, Mertens F, Mitelman F, Rosai J, Rydholm A, Sciot R, Tallini G, Van den Berghe H, Van de Ven W, Vanni R, Willen H: Correlation between clinicopathologic features and karyotype in lipomatous tumors. A report of 178 cases from the chromosomes and morphology (CHAMP) collaborative study group. Am J Pathol (in press).

634 Georgiades DE, Alcalais CB, Karabela VG: Multicentric well-differentiated liposarcomas. A case report and a brief review of the literature. Cancer **24**:1091-1097, 1969.

635 Gibas Z, Miettinen M, Limon J, Nedoszytko B, Mrozek K, Roszkiewicz A, Rys J, Niezabitowski A, Debiec-Rychter M: Cytogenetic and immunohistochemical profile of myxoid liposarcoma. Am J Clin Pathol **103**:20-26, 1995.

635a Goldblum JR, Frank TS, Poy EL, Weiss SW: p53 mutations and tumor progression in well-differentiated liposarcoma and dermatofibrosarcoma protuberans. Int J Surg Pathol **3**:35-42, 1995.

636 Hashimoto H, Daimaru Y, Enjoji M: S-100 protein distribution in liposarcoma. An immunoperoxidase study with special reference to the distinction of liposarcoma from myxoid malignant fibrous histiocytoma. Virchows Arch [A] **405**:1-10, 1984.

637 Hashimoto H, Daimaru Y, Tsuneyoshi M, Enjoji M: Soft tissue sarcoma with additional anaplastic components. A clinicopathologic and immunohistochemical study of 27 cases. Cancer **66**:1578-1589, 1990.

638 Hashimoto H, Enjoji M: Liposarcoma. A clinicopathologic subtyping of 52 cases. Acta Pathol Jpn **32**:933-948, 1982.

639 Kauffman SL, Stout AP: Lipoblastic tumors of children. Cancer **12**:912-923, 1959.

640 Kindblom L-G, Angervall L, Fassina AS: Atypical lipoma. Acta Pathol Microbiol Immunol Scand (A) **90**:27-36, 1982.

641 Kindblom L-G, Angervall L, Jarlstedt J: Liposarcoma of the neck. A clinico-pathologic study of 4 cases. Cancer **42**:774-780, 1978.

642 Kindblom L-G, Angervall L, Svendsen P: Liposarcoma. A clinicopathologic, radiographic and prognostic study. Acta Pathol Microbiol Scand **253**(Suppl):1-71, 1975

643 Kindblom L-G, Säve-Söderbergh J: The ultrastructure of liposarcoma. A study of 10 cases. Acta Pathol Microbiol Scand (A) **87**:109-121, 1979.

644 Lagacé R, Jacob S, Seemayer TA: Myxoid liposarcoma. An electron microscopic study. Biological and histogenetic considerations. Virchows Arch [A] **384**:159-172, 1979.

645 La Quaglia MP, Spiro SA, Ghavimi F, Hajdu SI, Meyers P, Exelby PR: Liposarcoma in patients younger than or equal to 22 years of age. Cancer **72**:3114-3119, 1993.

646 Lucas DR, Nascimento AG, Sanjay BK, Rock MG: Well-differentiated liposarcoma. The Mayo Clinic experience with 58 cases. Am J Clin Pathol **102**:677-683, 1994.

647 McCormick D, Mentzel T, Beham A, Fletcher CD: Dedifferentiated liposarcoma. Clinicopathologic analysis of 32 cases suggesting a better prognostic subgroup among pleomorphic sarcomas. Am J Surg Pathol **18**:1213-1223, 1994.

648 Reitan JB, Kaalhus O, Brennhovd IO, Sager EM, Stenwig AE, Talle K: Prognostic factors in liposarcoma. Cancer **55**:2482-2490, 1985.

649 Reszel PA, Soule EH, Coventry MB: Liposarcoma of extremities and limb girdles. Study of 222 cases. J Bone Joint Surg (Am) **48**:229-244, 1966.

650 Rossouw DJ, Cinti S, Dickersin GR: Liposarcoma. An ultrastructural study of 15 cases. Am J Clin Pathol **85**:649-667, 1986.

651 Saunders JR, Jaques DA, Casterline PF, Percarpio B, Goodloe S Jr: Liposarcomas of the head and neck. A review of the literature and addition of four cases. Cancer **43**:162-168, 1979.

652 Schmookler BM, Enzinger FM: Liposarcoma occurring in children. An analysis of 17 cases and review of the literature. Cancer **52**:567-574, 1983.

653 Snover DC, Sumner HW, Dehner LP: Variability of histologic pattern in recurrent soft tissue sarcomas originally diagnosed as liposarcoma. Cancer **49**:1005-1015, 1982.

654 Sreekantaiah C, Karakousis CP, Leong SP, Sandberg AA: Cytogenetic findings in liposarcoma correlate with histopathologic subtypes. Cancer **69**:2484-2495, 1992.

655 Stout AP: Liposarcoma. The malignant tumor of lipoblasts. Ann Surg **119**:86-197, 1944.

656 Tallini G, Erlandson RA, Brennan MF, Woodruff JM: Divergent myosarcomatous differentiation in retroperitoneal liposarcoma. Am J Surg Pathol **17**:546-556, 1993.

657 Walaas L, Kindblom L-G: Lipomatous tumors. A correlative cytologic and histologic study of 27 tumors examined by fine needle aspiration cytology. Hum Pathol **16**:6-18, 1985.

658 Weiss SW, Rao VK: Well-differentiated liposarcoma (atypical lipoma) of deep soft tissue of the extremities, retroperitoneum, and miscellaneous sites. A follow-up study of 92 cases with analysis of the incidence of "dedifferentiation." Am J Surg Pathol **16**:1051-1058, 1992.

659 Winslow DJ, Enzinger FM: Hyaluronidase-sensitive acid mucopolysaccharides in liposarcomas. Am J Pathol **37**:497-505, 1960.

Tumors and tumorlike conditions of blood and lymph vessels
Hemangioma

660 Albrecht S, Kahn HJ: Immunohistochemistry of intravascular papillary endothelial hyperplasia. J Cutan Pathol **17**:16-21, 1990.

661 Allen PW, Enzinger FM: Hemangioma of skeletal muscle. An analysis of 89 cases. Cancer **29**:8-22, 1972.

662 Beham A, Fletcher CD: Intramuscular angioma. A clinicopathological analysis of 74 cases. Histopathology **18**:53-59, 1991.

663 Calonje E, Fletcher CD: Sinusoidal hemangioma. A distinctive benign vascular neoplasm within the group of cavernous hemangiomas. Am J Surg Pathol **15**:1130-1135, 1991.

663a Calonje E, Mentzel T, Fletcher CD: Pseudomalignant perineurial invasion in cellular ('infantile') capillary haemangiomas. Histopathology **26**:159-164, 1995.

664 Clearkin KP, Enzinger FM: Intravascular papillary endothelial hyperplasia. Arch Pathol Lab Med **100**:441-444, 1976.

665 Coffin CM, Dehner LP: Vascular tumors in children and adolescents. A clinicopathologic study of 228 tumors in 222 patients. Pathol Annu **28**(Pt 1):97-120, 1993.

666 Dabashi Y, Eisen RN: Infantile hemangioendothelioma of the pelvis associated with Kasabach-Merritt syndrome. Pediatr Pathol **10**:407-415, 1990.

667 Dethlefsen SM, Mulliken JB, Glowacki J: An ultrastructural study of mast cell interactions in hemangiomas. Ultrastruct Pathol **10**:175-183, 1986.

668 Finn MC, Glowacki J, Mulliken JB: Congenital vascular lesions. Clinical application of a new classification. J Pediatr Surg **18**:894-900, 1983.

669 Gonzalez-Crussi F, Reyes-Mugica M: Cellular hemangiomas ("hemangioendotheliomas") in infants. Light microscopic, immunohistochemical, and ultrastructural observations. Am J Surg Pathol **15**:769-778, 1991.

670 Hashimoto H, Daimaru Y, Enjoji M: Intravascular papillary endothelial hyperplasia. A clinicopathologic study of 91 cases. Am J Dermatopathol **5**:539-546, 1983.

671 Koblenzer PJ, Bukowski MJ: Angiomatosis (hamartomatous hem-lymphangiomatosis). Report of a case with diffuse involvement. Pediatrics **28**:65-76, 1961.

672 Kojimahara M, Baba Y, Nakajima T: Ultrastructural study of hemangiomas. Acta Pathol Jpn **37**:605-609, 1987.

673 Koutlas IG, Jessurun J: Arteriovenous hemangioma. A clinicopathological and immunohistochemical study. J Cutan Pathol **21**:343-349, 1994.

674 Kuo T-T, Sayers CP, Rosai J: Masson's "vegetant intravascular hemangioendothelioma." A lesion often mistaken for angiosarcoma. Study of seventeen cases located in the skin and soft tissues. Cancer **38**:1227-1236, 1976.

675 Lie JT: Pathology of angiodysplasia in Klippel-Trenaunay syndrome. Pathol Res Pract **183**:747-755, 1988.

676 Lindenauer SM: The Klippel-Trenaunay syndrome. Varicosity, hypertrophy and hemangioma with no arteriovenous fistula. Ann Surg **162**:303-314, 1965.

677 Lister WA: The natural history of strawberry nevi. Lancet **1**:1429-1434, 1938.

678 Modlin JJ: Capillary hemangiomas of the skin. Surgery **38**:169-180, 1955.

679 Mulliken JB, Young AE: Vascular birthmarks. Hemangiomas and malformations. Philadelphia, 1988, WB Saunders.

680 Perrone T: Vessel-nerve intermingling in benign infantile hemangioendothelioma. Hum Pathol **16**:198-200, 1985.

681 Pins MR, Rosenthal DI, Springfield DS, Rosenberg AE: Florid extravascular papillary endothelial hyperplasia (Masson's pseudoangiosarcoma) presenting as a soft-tissue sarcoma. Arch Pathol Lab Med **117**:259-263, 1993.

682 Rao VK, Weiss SW: Angiomatosis of soft tissue. An analysis of the histologic features and clinical outcome in 51 cases. Am J Surg Pathol **16**:764-771, 1992.

683 Salyer WR, Salyer DC: Intravascular angiomatosis. Development and distinction from angiosarcoma. Cancer **36**:995-1004, 1975.

684 Shim WKT: Hemangiomas of infancy complicated by thrombocytopenia. Am J Surg **116**:896-906, 1968.

685 Smoller BR, Apfelberg DB: Infantile (juvenile) capillary hemangioma. A tumor of heterogeneous cellular elements. J Cutan Pathol **20**:330-336, 1993.

686 Taxy JB, Gray SR: Cellular angiomas of infancy. An ultrastructural study of two cases. Cancer **43**:2322-2331, 1979.

687 Tsang WY, Chan JK: Kaposi-like infantile hemangioendothelioma. A distinctive vascular neoplasm of the retroperitoneum. Am J Surg Pathol **15**:982-989, 1991

687a Tsang WYW, Chan JKC, Fletcher CDM, Rosai J: Symplastic hamangioma. A distinctive vascular neoplasm featuring bizarre stromal cells (abstract). Int J Surg Pathol **1**:202, 1994.

688 Weinblatt ME, Kahn E, Kochen JA: Hemangioendothelioma with intravascular coagulation and ischemic colitis. Cancer **54**:2300-2304, 1984.

689 Weiss SW: Pedal hemangioma (venous malformation) occurring in Turner's syndrome. An additional manifestation of the syndrome. Hum Pathol **19**:1015-1018, 1988.

690 Yasunaga C, Sueishi K, Ohgami H, Suita S, Kawanami T: Heterogenous expression of endothelial cell markers in infantile hemangioendothelioma. Immunohistochemical study of two solitary cases and one multiple one. Am J Clin Pathol **91**:673-681, 1989.

691 Zukerberg LR, Nickoloff BJ, Weiss SW: Kaposiform hemangioendothelioma of infancy and childhood. An aggressive neoplasm associated with Kasabach-Merritt syndrome and lymphangiomatosis. Am J Surg Pathol **17**:321-328, 1993.

Glomus tumor

692 Aiba M, Hirayama A, Kuramochi S: Glomangiosarcoma in a glomus tumor. An immunohistochemical and ultrastructural study. Cancer **61**:1467-1471, 1988.

693 Albrecht S, Zbieranowski I: Incidental glomus coccygeum. When a normal structure looks like a tumor. Am J Surg Pathol **14**:922-924, 1990.

694 Bell RS, Goodman SB, Fornasier VL: Coccygeal glomus tumors. A case of mistaken identity? J Bone Joint Surg (Am) **64**:595-597, 1982.

694a Calonje E, Fletcher CDM: Cutaneous intraneural glomus tumor. Am J Dermatopathol **17**:395-398, 1995.

695 Carroll RE, Berman AT: Glomus tumors of the hand. Review of the literature and report of 28 cases. J Bone Joint Surg (Am) **54**:691-703, 1972.

696 Dervan PA, Tobbia IN, Casey M, O'Loughlin J, O'Brien M: Glomus tumours. An immunohistochemical profile of 11 cases. Histopathology **14**:483-491, 1989.

697 Di Sant'Agnese PA, De Mesy Jensen KL: Thick (myosin) filaments in a glomus tumor. Am J Clin Pathol **79**:130-134, 1983.

698 Duncan L, Halverson J, De Schryver-Kecskemeti K: Glomus tumor of the coccyx. A curable cause of coccygodynia. Arch Pathol Lab Med **115**:78-80, 1991.

699 Gould EW, Manivel JC, Albores-Saavedra J, Monforte H: Locally infiltrative glomus tumors and glomangiosarcomas. A clinical, ultrastructural, and immunohistochemical study. Cancer **65:**310-318, 1990.

700 Ito H, Motohiro K, Nomura S, Tahara E: Glomus tumor of the trachea. Immunohistochemical and electron microscopic studies. Pathol Res Pract **183:**778-784, 1988.

701 Kaye VM, Dehner LP: Cutaneous glomus tumor. A comparative immunohisto-chemical study with pseudoangiomatous intradermal melanocytic nevi. Am J Dermatopathol **13:**2-6, 1991.

702 Kishimoto S, Nagatani H, Miyashita A, Kobayashi K: Immunohistochemical demonstration of substance P-containing nerve fibers in glomus tumors. Br J Dermatol **113:**213-218, 1985.

703 Kohout E, Stout AR: The glomus tumor in children. Cancer **14:**555-556, 1961.

704 Lattes R, Bull DC: A case of glomus tumor with primary involvement of bone. Ann Surg **127:**187-191, 1948.

705 Masson P: Le glomus neuromyo-artériel des régions tactiles et ses tumeurs. Lyon Chir **21:**259-280, 1924.

706 Miettinen M, Lehto V-P, Virtanen I: Glomus tumor cells. Evaluation of smooth muscle and endothelial cell properties. Virchows Arch [Cell Pathol] **43:**139-149, 1983.

707 Murray MR, Stout AP: The glomus tumor. Investigations of its distribution and behavior, and the identity of its "epithelioid" cell. Am J Pathol **18:**183-203, 1942.

708 Noer H, Krogdahl A: Glomangiosarcoma of the lower extremity. Histopathology **18:**365-366, 1991.

709 Nuovo MA, Grimes MM, Knowles DM: Glomus tumors. A clinicopathologic and immunohistochemical analysis of forty cases. Surg Pathol **3:**31-46, 1990.

710 Pambakian H, Smith MA: Glomus tumours of the coccygeal body associated with coccydynia. A preliminary report. J Bone Joint Surg (Br) **633:**424-426, 1981.

710a Pulitzer DR, Martin PC, Reed RJ: Epithelioid glomus tumor. Hum Pathol **26:**1022-1027, 1995.

711 Shugart RR, Soule EH, Johnson EW: Glomus tumor. Surg Gynecol Obstet **117:**334-340, 1963.

712 Slater DN, Cotton DWK, Azzopardi JG: Oncocytic glomus tumour. A new variant. Histopathology **11:**523-531, 1987.

713 Stout AP: Tumors of the neuromyoarterial glomus. Am J Cancer **24:**255-272, 1935.

714 Tsuneyoshi M, Enjoji M: Glomus tumor. A clinicopathologic and electron microscopic study. Cancer **50:**1601-1607, 1982.

715 Venkatachalam MA, Greally JG: Fine structure of glomus tumor. Similarity of glomus cells to smooth muscle. Cancer **23:**1176-1184, 1969.

Hemangiopericytoma

716 Angervall L, Kindblom L-G, Nielsen JM, Stener B, Svendsen P: Hemangiopericytoma. A clinicopathologic, angiographic and microangiographic study. Cancer **42:**2412-2427, 1978.

717 Battifora H: Hemangiopericytoma. Ultrastructural study of five cases. Cancer **31:**1418-1432, 1973.

718 D'Amore ES, Manivel JC, Sung JH: Soft-tissue and meningeal hemangiopericytomas. An immunohistochemical and ultrastructural study. Hum Pathol **21:**414-423, 1990.

719 Dardick I, Hammar SP, Scheithauer BW: Ultrastructural spectrum of hemangiopericytoma. A comparative study of fetal, adult, and neoplastic pericytes. Ultrastruct Pathol **13:**111-154, 1989.

720 Enzinger FM, Smith BH: Hemangiopericytoma. An analysis of 106 cases. Hum Pathol **7:**61-82, 1976.

721 Fletcher CDM: Haemangiopericytoma—a dying breed? Reappraisal of an 'entity' and its variants. A hypothesis. Curr Diagn Pathol **1:**19-23, 1994.

722 Hayes MMM, Dietrich BE, Uys CJ: Congenital hemangiopericytomas of skin. Am J Dermatopathol **8:**148-153, 1986.

723 Hultberg BM, Daugaard S, Johansen HF, Mouridsen HT, Hou-Jensen K: Malignant haemangiopericytomas and haemangioendotheliosarcomas. An immunohistochemical study. Histopathology **12:**405-414, 1988.

724 Kuhn C III, Rosai J: Tumors arising from pericytes. Ultrastructure and organ culture of a case. Arch Pathol **88:**653-663, 1969.

725 Llombart-Bosch A, Peydro-Olaya A, Pellin A: Ultrastructure of vascular neoplasms. Pathol Res Pract **174:**1-41, 1982.

726 Mandahl N, Orndal C, Heim S, Willen H, Rydholm A, Bauer HC, Mitelman F: Aberrations of chromosome segment 12q13-15 characterize a subgroup of hemangiopericytomas. Cancer **71:**3009-3013, 1993.

727 McMaster MJ, Soule EH, Ivins JC: Hemangiopericytoma. A clinicopathologic study and long-term follow-up of 60 patients. Cancer **36:**2232-2244, 1975.

728 Mentzel T, Calonje E, Nascimento AG, Fletcher CD: Infantile hemangiopericytoma versus infantile myofibromatosis. Study of a series suggesting a continuous spectrum of infantile myofibroblastic lesions. Am J Surg Pathol **18:**922-930, 1994.

729 Murray MR, Stout AP: The glomus tumor. Investigation of its distribution and behavior, and the identity of its "epithelioid" cell. Am J Pathol **18:**183-203, 1942.

730 Nemes Z: Differentiation markers in hemangiopericytoma. Cancer **69:**133-140, 1992.

730a Nielsen GP, Dickersin GR, Provenzal JM, Rosenberg AE: Lipomatous hemangiopericytoma. A histologic, ultrastructural and immunohistochemical study of a unique variant of hemangiopericytoma. Am J Surg Pathol **19:**748-756, 1995.

731 Nunnery EW, Kahn LB, Reddick RL, Lipper S: Hemangiopericytoma. A light microscopic and ultrastructural study. Cancer **47:**906-914, 1981.

732 O'Brien P, Brasfield RD: Hemangiopericytoma. Cancer **14:**249-252, 1965.

733 Ordóñez NG, Mackay B, el-Naggar AK, Byers RM: Congenital hemangiopericytoma. An ultrastructural, immunocytochemical, and flow cytometric study. Arch Pathol Lab Med **117:**934-937, 1993.

734 Porter PL, Bigler SA, McNutt M, Gown AM: The immunophenotype of hemangiopericytomas and glomus tumors, with special reference to muscle protein expression. An immunohistochemical study and review of the literature. Mod Pathol **4:**46-52, 1991.

735 Schurch W, Skalli O, Lagace R, Seemayer TA, Gabbiani G: Intermediate filament proteins and actin isoforms as markers for soft-tissue tumor differentiation and origin. III. Hemangiopericytomas and glomus tumors. Am J Pathol **136:**771-786, 1990.

736 Stout AP: Hemangiopericytoma (a study of 25 new cases). Cancer **2:**1027-1054, 1949.

737 Stout AP: Tumors featuring pericytes. Glomus tumor and hemangiopericytoma. Lab Invest **5:**217-223, 1965.

738 Tsuneyoshi M, Daimaru Y, Enjoji M: Malignant hemangiopericytoma and other sarcomas with hemangiopericytoma-like pattern. Pathol Res Pract **178:**446-453, 1984.

Hemangioendothelioma

739 Allen PW, Ramakrishna B, MacCormac LB: The histiocytoid hemangiomas and other controversies. Pathol Annu **27**(Pt 2):51-87, 1992.

740 Angervall L, Kindblom L-G, Karlsson K, Stener B: Atypical hemangioendothelioma of venous origin. A clinicopathologic, angiographic, immunohistochemical, and ultrastructural study of two endothelial tumors within the concept of histiocytoid hemangioma. Am J Surg Pathol **9:**504-516, 1985.

741 Arnold G, Klein PJ, Fischer R: Epithelioid hemangioendothelioma. Report of a case with immuno-lectin histochemical and ultrastructural demonstration of its vascular nature. Virchows Arch [A] **408:**435-443, 1986.

742 Cooper PH: Is histiocytoid hemangioma a specific pathologic entity? Am J Surg Pathol **12:**815-817, 1988.

743 Dabska M: Malignant endovascular papillary angioendothelioma of the skin in childhood. Clinicopathologic study of six cases. Cancer **24:**503-510, 1969.

744 Ellis GL, Kratochvil FJ III: Epithelioid hemangioendothelioma of the head and neck. A clinicopathologic report of twelve cases. Oral Surg Oral Med Oral Pathol **61:**61-68, 1986.

744a Fanburg JC, Meis-Kindblom JM, Rosenberg AE: Multiple enchondromas associated with spindle-cell hemangioendotheliomas. An overlooked variant of Maffucci's syndrome. Am J Surg Pathol **19:**1029-1038, 1995.

745 Fetsch JF, Weiss SW: Observations concerning the pathogenesis of epithelioid hemangioma (angiolymphoid hyperplasia). Mod Pathol **4:**449-455, 1991.

746 Fletcher CD, Beham A, Schmid C: Spindle cell haemangioendothelioma. A clinicopathological and immunohistochemical study indicative of a non-neoplastic lesion. Histopathology **18:**291-301, 1991.

746a Fukunaga M, Ushigome S, Nikaido T, Ishikawa E, Nakamori K: Spindle cell hemangioendothelioma. An immunohistochemical and flow cytometric study of six cases. Pathol Int **45:**589-595, 1995.

747 Gray MH, Rosenberg AE, Dickersin GR, Bhan AK: Cytokeratin expression in epithelioid vascular neoplasms. Hum Pathol **21:**212-217, 1990.

748 Imayama S, Murakamai Y, Hashimoto H, Hori Y: Spindle cell hemangioendothelioma exhibits the ultrastructural features of reactive vascular proliferation rather than of angiosarcoma. Am J Clin Pathol **97:**279-287, 1992.

749 Morgan J, Robinson MJ, Rosen LB, Unger H, Niven J: Malignant endovascular papillary angioendothelioma (Dabska tumor). A case report and review of the literature. Am J Dermatopathol **11:**64-68, 1989.

750 Patterson K, Chandra RS: Malignant endovascular papillary angioendothelioma. Cutaneous borderline tumor. Arch Pathol Lab Med **109:**671-673, 1985.

751 Rosai J, Gold J, Landy R: The histiocytoid hemangiomas. A unifying concept embracing several previously described entities of skin, soft tissue, large vessels, bone and heart. Hum Pathol **10:**707-730, 1979.

752 Scott GA, Rosai J: Spindle cell hemangioendothelioma. Report of seven additional cases of a recently described vascular neoplasm. Am J Dermatopathol **10**:281-288, 1988.

753 Tsang WY, Chan JK: The family of epithelioid vascular tumors. Histopathology **8**:187-212, 1993.

754 Tsang WY, Chan JK, Fletcher CD: Recently characterized vascular tumours of skin and soft tissues. Histopathology **19**:489-501, 1991.

755 Urabe A, Tsuneyoshi M, Enjoji M: Epithelioid hemangioma versus Kimura's disease. A comparative clinicopathologic study. Am J Surg Pathol **11**:758-766, 1987.

756 Weiss SW, Enzinger FM: Epithelioid hemangioendothelioma. A vascular tumor often mistaken for a carcinoma. Cancer **50**:970-981, 1982.

757 Weiss SW, Enzinger FM: Spindle cell hemangioendothelioma. A low-grade angiosarcoma resembling a cavernous hemangioma and Kaposi's sarcoma. Am J Surg Pathol **10**:521-530, 1986.

758 Weiss SW, Ishak KG, Dail DH, Sweet DE, Enzinger FM: Epithelioid hemangioendothelioma and related lesions. Semin Diagn Pathol **3**:259-287, 1986.

759 Williams SB, Butler BC, Gilkey FW, Kapadia SB, Burton DM: Epithelioid hemangioendothelioma with osteoclastlike giant cells. Arch Pathol Lab Med **117**:315-318, 1993.

760 Yousem SA, Hochholzer L: Unusual thoracic manifestations of epithelioid hemangioendothelioma. Arch Pathol Lab Med **111**:459-463, 1987.

Angiosarcoma

761 Abratt RP, Williams M, Dodd NF, Uys CJ: Angiosarcoma of the superior vena cava. Cancer **52**:740-743, 1983.

762 Baker PB, Goodwin RA: Pulmonary artery sarcomas. A review and report of a case. Arch Pathol Lab Med **109**:35-39, 1985.

763 Burke AP, Virmani R: Sarcomas of the great vessels. A clinicopathologic study. Cancer **71**:1761-1773, 1993.

764 Byers RJ, McMahon RF, Freemont AJ, Parrott NR, Newstead CG: Epithelioid angiosarcoma arising in an arteriovenous fistula. Histopathology **21**:87-89, 1992.

765 Chaudhuri B, Ronan SG, Manaligod JR: Angiosarcoma arising in a plexiform neurofibroma. A case report. Cancer **46**:605-610, 1980.

766 Davies JD, Rees GJG, Mera SL: Angiosarcoma in irradiated post-mastectomy chest wall. Histopathology **7**:947-956, 1983.

767 Fitzmaurice RJ, McClure J: Aortic intimal sarcoma. An unusual case with pulmonary vasculature involvement. Histopathology **17**:457-462, 1990.

768 Fletcher CD, Beham A, Bekir S, Clarke AM, Marley NJ: Epithelioid angiosarcoma of deep soft tissue. A distinctive tumor readily mistaken for an epithelial neoplasm. Am J Surg Pathol **15**:915-924, 1991.

769 Girard C, Johnson WC, Graham JH: Cutaneous angiosarcoma. Cancer **26**:868-883, 1970.

770 Hayman J, Huygens H: Angiosarcoma developing around a foreign body. J Clin Pathol **36**:515-518, 1986.

771 Jennings TA, Peterson L, Friedlaender GE, Cooke RA, Axiotis A, Hayman JA, Rosai J: Angiosarcoma associated with foreign bodies. Report of three cases. Cancer **62**:2436-2444, 1988.

772 Mackay B, Ordóñez NG, Huang WL: Ultrastructural and immunocytochemical observations on angiosarcomas. Ultrastruct Pathol **13**:97-110, 1989.

773 Maddox JC, Evans HL: Angiosarcoma of skin and soft tissue. A study of 44 cases. Cancer **48**:1907-1921, 1981.

774 McGlennen RC, Manivel JC, Stanley SJ, Slater DL, Wick MR, Dehner LP: Pulmonary artery trunk sarcoma. A clinicopathologic, ultrastructural, and immunohistochemical study of four cases. Mod Pathol **2**:486-494, 1989.

775 McWilliam LJ, Harris M: Granular cell angiosarcoma of the skin. Histology, electron microscopy and immunohistochemistry of a newly recognized tumor. Histopathology **9**:1205-1216, 1985.

776 Millstein DI, Tang C-K, Campbell EW Jr: Angiosarcoma developing in a patient with neurofibromatosis (von Recklinghausen's disease). Cancer **47**:950-954, 1981.

777 Nanus DM, Kelsen D, Clark DGC: Radiation-induced angiosarcoma. Cancer **60**:777-779, 1987.

778 Rosai J, Sumner HW, Kostianovsky M, Perez-Mesa C: Angiosarcoma of skin. A clinicopathologic and fine structural study. Hum Pathol **7**:83-109, 1976.

779 Stout AP: Hemangio-endothelioma. A tumor of blood vessels featuring vascular endothelial cells. Ann Surg **118**:445-464, 1943.

780 Ulbright TM, Clark SA, Einhorn LH: Angiosarcoma associated with germ cell tumors. Hum Pathol **16**:268-272, 1985.

781 Vuletin JC, Wajsbort RR, Ghali V: Primary retroperitoneal angiosarcoma with eosinophilic globules. A combined light-microscopic, immunohistochemical, and ultrastructural study. Arch Pathol Lab Med **114**:618-622, 1990.

782 Wilson-Jones E: Malignant vascular tumours. Clin Exp Dermatol **1**:287-312, 1976.

783 Wright EP, Virmani R, Glick AD, Page DL: Aortic intimal sarcoma with embolic metastases. Am J Surg Pathol **9**:890-897, 1985.

784 Zagzag D, Yang G, Seidman I, Lusskin R: Malignant epithelioid hemangioendothelioma arising in an intramuscular lipoma. Cancer **71**:764-768, 1993.

Lymphangioma and lymphangiomyoma

785 Banner A, Carrington C, Emory W, Kittle F, Leonard G, Ringus J, Taylor P, Addington W: Efficacy of oophorectomy in lymphangioleiomyomatosis and benign metastasizing leiomyoma. N Engl J Med **305**:204-210, 1981.

786 Byrne J, Blanc WA, Warburton D, Wigger J: The significance of cystic hygroma in fetuses. Hum Pathol **15**:61-67, 1984.

787 Carlson KC, Parnassus WN, Klatt EC: Thoracic lymphangiomatosis. Arch Pathol Lab Med **111**:475-477, 1987.

788 Chan JK, Tsang WY, Pau MY, Tang MC, Pang SW, Fletcher CD: Lymphangiomyomatosis and angiomyolipoma. Closely related entities characterized by hamartomatous proliferation of HMB-45-positive smooth muscle. Histopathology **22**:445-455, 1993.

789 Chervenak FA, Isaacson G, Blakemore KJ, Breg WR, Hobbins JC, Berkowitz RL, Tortora M, Mayden K, Mahoney MJ: Fetal cystic hygroma. N Engl J Med **309**:822-825, 1983.

790 Cornog JL Jr, Enterline HT: Lymphangiomyoma, a benign lesion of chyliferous lymphatics synonymous with lymphangiopericytoma. Cancer **19**:1909-1930, 1966.

791 Enterline HT, Roberts D: Lymphangiopericytoma. Case report of a previously undescribed tumor type. Cancer **8**:582-587, 1955.

792 Gomez CS, Calonje E, Ferrar DW, Browse NL, Fletcher CDM: Lymphangiomatosis of the limbs; clinicopathologic analysis of a series with a good prognosis. Am J Surg Pathol **19**:125-133, 1995.

793 Graham ML II, Spelsberg TC, Dines DE, Payne WS, Bjornsson J, Lie JT: Pulmonary lymphangiomyomatosis. With particular reference to steroid-receptor assay studies and pathologic correlation. Mayo Clin Proc **59**:3-11, 1984.

794 Gross RE, Hurwitt ES: Cervicomediastinal and mediastinal cystic hygromas. Surg Gynecol Obstet **87**:599-610, 1948.

795 Jao J, Gilbert S, Messer R: Lymphangiomyoma and tuberous sclerosis. Cancer **29**:1188-1192, 1972.

796 Kuo T-T, Gomez LG: Papillary endothelial proliferation in cystic lymphangiomas. Arch Pathol Lab Med **103**:306-308, 1979.

797 McCarty KS Jr, Mossler JA, McLelland R, Sieker HO: Pulmonary lymphangiomyomatosis responsive to progesterone. N Engl J Med **303**:1461-1465, 1980.

798 Ohori NP, Yousem SA, Sonmez-Alpan E, Colby TV: Estrogen and progesterone receptors in lymphangioleiomyomatosis, epithelioid hemangioendothelioma, and sclerosing hemangioma of the lung. Am J Clin Pathol **96**:529-535, 1991.

799 Ramani P, Shah A: Lymphangiomatosis. Histologic and immunohistochemical analysis of four cases. Am J Surg Pathol **17**:329-335, 1993.

800 Taylor JR, Ryu J, Colby TV, Raffin TA: Lymphangioleiomyomatosis. Clinical course in 32 patients. N Engl J Med **323**:1254-1260, 1990.

801 Wolff M: Lymphangiomyoma. Clinicopathologic study and ultrastructural confirmation of its histogenesis. Cancer **31**:988-1007, 1973.

Lymphangiosarcoma

802 Capo V, Ozzello L, Fenoglio CM, Lombardi L, Rilke F: Angiosarcomas arising in edematous extremities. Immunostaining for factor VIII-related antigen and ultrastructural features. Hum Pathol **16**:144-150, 1985.

803 Drachman D, Rosen L, Sharaf D, Weissmann A: Postmastectomy low-grade angiosarcoma. An unusual case clinically resembling a lymphangioma circumscriptum. Am J Dermatopathol **10**:247-251, 1988.

804 Eby CS, Brennan MJ, Fine G: Lymphangiosarcoma. A lethal complication of chronic lymphedema. Arch Surg **94**:223-230, 1967.

805 Hashimoto K, Matsumoto M, Eto H, Lipinski J, LaFond AA: Differentiation of metastatic breast carcinoma from Stewart-Treves angiosarcoma. Use of anti-keratin and anti-desmosome monoclonal antibodies and factor VIII-related antibodies. Arch Dermatol **121**:742-746, 1985.

806 Herman JB: Lymphangiosarcoma of the chronically edematous extremity. Surg Gynecol Obstet **121**:1107-1115, 1965.

807 Lagacé R, Leroy J-P: Comparative electron microscopic study of cutaneous and soft tissue angiosarcomas, post-mastectomy angiosarcoma (Stewart-Treves syndrome) and Kaposi's sarcoma. Ultrastruct Pathol **11**:161-173, 1987.

808 McWilliam LJ, Harris M: Histogenesis of post-mastectomy angiosarcoma. An ultrastructural study. Histopathology **9**:331-343, 1985.

809 Miettinen M, Lehto V-P, Virtanen I: Postmastectomy angiosarcoma (Stewart-Treves syndrome). Light-microscopic, immunohistological, and ultrastructural characteristic of two cases. Am J Surg Pathol **7**:329-339, 1983.

810 Muller R, Hajdu SI, Brennan MF: Lymphangiosarcoma associated with chronic filarial lymphedema. Cancer **59**:179-183, 1987.

811 Sordillo PP, Chapman R, Hajdu SI, Magill GB, Golbey RB: Lymphangiosarcoma. Cancer **48**:1674-1679, 1981.

812 Stewart FW, Treves N: Lymphangiosarcoma in post-mastectomy lymphedema. A report of six cases in elephantiasis chirurgica. Cancer **1**:64-81, 1948.

813 Woodward AH, Ivins JC, Soule EH: Lymphangiosarcoma arising in chronic lymphedematous extremities. Cancer **30**:562-572, 1972.

Tumors of smooth muscle
Leiomyoma

814 Carla TG, Filotico R, Filotico M: Bizarre angiomyomas of superficial soft tissues. Pathologica **83**:237-242, 1991.

815 Fox SB, Heryet A, Khong TY: Angioleiomyomas. An immunohistological study. Histopathology **16**:495-496, 1990.

816 Geddy PM, Gray S, Reid WA: Mast cell density and PGP 9.5-immunostained nerves in angioleiomyoma. Their relationship to painful symptoms. Histopathology **22**:387-390, 1993.

817 Hachisuga T, Hashimoto H, Enjoji M: Angioleiomyoma. A clinicopathologic reappraisal of 562 cases. Cancer **54**:126-130, 1984.

818 Hasegawa T, Seki K, Yang P, Hirose T, Hizawa K: Mechanism of pain and cytoskeletal properties in angioleiomyomas. An immunohistochemical study. Pathol Int **44**:66-72, 1994.

819 Khalluf E, DeYoung BR, Swanson PE: Soft tissue leiomyoma with cartilaginous metaplasia. Report of an unusual phenomenon. Int J Surg Pathol **1**:235-238, 1994.

820 Kilpatrick SE, Mentzel T, Fletcher CD: Leiomyoma of deep soft tissue. Clinicopathologic analysis of a series. Am J Surg Pathol **18**:576-582, 1994.

821 Lendrum AC: Painful tumors of the skin. Ann R Coll Surg Engl **1**:62-67, 1947.

822 MacDonald DM, Sanderson KV: Angioleiomyoma of the skin. Br J Dermatol **91**:161-168, 1974.

823 Stout AP: Solitary cutaneous and subcutaneous leiomyoma. Am J Cancer **29**:435-469, 1937.

824 Yokoyama R, Hashimoto H, Daimaru Y, Enjoji M: Superficial leiomyomas. A clinicopathologic study of 34 cases. Acta Pathol Jpn **37**:1415-1422, 1987.

Leiomyosarcoma

825 Baker PB, Goodwin RA: Pulmonary artery sarcomas. A review and report of a case. Arch Pathol Lab Med **109**:35-39, 1985.

826 Berlin O, Stener B, Kindblom L-G, Angervall L: Leiomyosarcomas of venous origin in the extremities. A correlated clinical, roentgenologic, and morphologic study with diagnostic and surgical implications. Cancer **54**:2147-2159, 1984.

827 Brooks JJ: Immunohistochemistry of soft tissue tumors. Hum Pathol **13**:969-974, 1982.

828 Brown DC, Theaker JM, Banks PM, Gatter KC, Mason DY: Cytokeratin expression in smooth muscle and smooth muscle tumours. Histopathology **11**:477-486, 1987.

829 Bulmer JH: Smooth muscle tumors of limbs. J Bone Joint Surg (Br) **49**:52-58, 1967.

830 Dahl I, Angervall L: Cutaneous and subcutaneous leiomyosarcoma. A clinicopathologic study of 47 patients. Pathol Europ **9**:307-315, 1974.

831 Dahl I, Hagmar B, Angervall L: Leiomyosarcoma of the soft tissue. A correlative cytological and histological study of 11 cases. Acta Pathol Microbiol Immunol Scand (A) **89**:285-291, 1981.

832 Donner L, DeLanerolle P, Costa J: Immunoreactivity of paraffin-embedded normal tissues and mesenchymal tumors for smooth muscle myosin. Am J Clin Pathol **80**:677-681, 1983.

833 Dorfman HD, Fishel ER: Leiomyosarcomas of the greater saphenous vein. Am J Clin Pathol **39**:73-78, 1963.

834 Fields JP, Helwig EB: Leiomyosarcoma of the skin and subcutaneous tissue. Cancer **47**:156-169, 1981.

835 Hashimoto H, Daimaru Y, Tsuneyoshi M, Enjoji M: Leiomyosarcoma of the external soft tissues. A clinicopathologic, immunohistochemical, and electron microscopic study. Cancer **57**:2077-2088, 1986.

836 Imakita M, Yutani C, Ishibashi-Ueda H, Hiraoka H, Naito H: Primary leiomyosarcoma of the inferior vena cava with Budd-Chiari syndrome. Acta Pathol Jpn **39**:73-77, 1989.

837 Kevoskian J, Cento DP: Leiomyosarcoma of large arteries and veins. Surgery **73**:390-400, 1973.

838 Lee ES, Locker J, Nalesnik M, Reyes J, Jaffe R, Alashari M, Nour B, Tzakis A, Dickman PS: The association of Epstein-Barr virus with smooth-muscle tumors occurring after organ transplantation. N Engl J Med **332**:19-25, 1995.

839 Leu HJ, Makek M: Intramural venous leiomyosarcomas. Cancer **57**:1395-1400, 1986.

840 Mackay B, Ro J, Floyd C, Ordóñez NG: Ultrastructural observations on smooth muscle tumors. Ultrastruct Pathol **11**:593-607, 1987.

841 McClain KL, Leach CT, Jenson HB, Joshi VV, Pollock BH, Parmley RT, Di Carlo FJ, Chadwick EG, Murphy SB: Association of Epstein-Barr virus with leiomyosarcomas in children with AIDS. N Engl J Med **332**:12-18, 1995.

842 Mentzel T, Calonje E, Fletcher CD: Leiomyosarcoma with prominent osteoclast-like giant cells. Analysis of eight cases closely mimicking the so-called giant cell variant of malignant fibrous histiocytoma. Am J Surg Pathol **18**:258-265, 1994.

843 Mentzel T, Wadden C, Fletcher CD: Granular cell change in smooth muscle tumours of skin and soft tissue. Histopathology **24**:223-231, 1994.

844 Miettinen M, Lehto V-P, Badley RA, Virtanen I: Expression of intermediate filaments in soft-tissue sarcomas. Int J Cancer **30**:541-546, 1982.

845 Nistal M, Paniagua R, Picazo ML, Cermeño deGiles F, Ramos Guerreira JL: Granular changes in vascular leiomyosarcoma. Virchows Arch [A] **386**:239-248, 1980.

846 Norton AJ, Thomas JA, Isaacson PG: Cytokeratin-specific monoclonal antibodies are reactive with tumours of smooth muscle derivation. An immunocytochemical and biochemical study using antibodies to intermediate filament cytoskeletal proteins. Histopathology **11**:487-499, 1987.

847 Ogawa K, Oguchi M, Yamabe H, Nakashima Y, Hamashima Y: Distribution of collagen type IV in soft tissue tumors. An immunohistochemical study. Cancer **58**:269-277, 1986.

848 Phelan JT, Sherer W, Perez-Mesa C: Malignant smooth-muscle tumors (leiomyosarcomas) of soft-tissue origin. N Engl J Med **266**:1027-1030, 1962.

849 Saku T, Tsuda N, Anami M, Okabe H: Smooth and skeletal muscle myosins in spindle cell tumors of soft tissue. An immunohistochemical study. Acta Pathol Jpn **35**:125-136, 1985.

850 Salm R, Evans DJ: Myxoid leiomyosarcoma. Histopathology **9**:159-169, 1985.

851 Schürch W, Skalli O, Seemayer TA, Gabbiani G: Intermediate filament proteins and actin isoforms as markers for soft tissue tumor differentiation and origin. I. Smooth muscle tumors. Am J Pathol **128**:91-103, 1987.

852 Sreekantaiah C, Davis JR, Sandberg AA: Chromosomal abnormalities in leiomyosarcomas. Am J Pathol **142**:293-305, 1993.

853 Stout AP, Hill WT: Leiomyosarcoma of the superficial soft tissue. Cancer **11**:844-854, 1958.

854 Swanson PE, Wick MR, Dehner LP: Leiomyosarcoma of somatic soft tissues in childhood. An immunohistochemical analysis of six cases with ultrastructural correlation. Hum Pathol **22**:569-577, 1991.

855 Tauchi K, Tsutsumi Y, Yoshimura S, Watanabe K: Immunohistochemical and immunoblotting detection of cytokeratin in smooth muscle tumors. Acta Pathol Jpn **40**:574-580, 1990.

856 Thomas MA, Fine G: Leiomyosarcoma of veins. Report of 2 cases and review of the literature. Cancer **13**:96-101, 1960.

857 Tsukada T, McNutt MA, Ross R, Gown AM: HHF35, a muscle actin-specific monoclonal antibody. II. Reactivity in normal, reactive, and neoplastic human tissues. Am J Pathol **127**:389-402, 1987.

858 Varela-Duran J, Oliva H, Rosai J: Vascular leiomyosarcoma. The malignant counterpart of vascular leiomyoma. Cancer **44**:1684-1691, 1979.

859 Weiss SW, Langloss JM, Shmookler BM, Malawer MM, D'Avis J, Enzinger FM, Stanton R: Estrogen receptor protein in bone and soft tissue tumors. Lab Invest **54**:689-694, 1986.

860 Wile AG, Evans HL, Romsdahl MM: Leiomyosarcoma of soft tissue. A clinicopathologic study. Cancer **48**:1022-1032, 1981.

861 Wilkinson N, Fitzmaurice RJ, Turner PG, Freemont AJ: Leiomyosarcoma with osteoclast-like giant cells. Histopathology **20**:446-449, 1992.

862 Yannopoulos K, Stout AP: Smooth muscle tumors in children. Cancer **15**:958-971, 1962.

Clear cell (epithelioid) smooth muscle tumors

863 Chen KTK, Ma CK: Intravenous leiomyoblastoma. Am J Surg Pathol **7**:591-596, 1983.

864 Evans DJ, Lampert IA, Jacobs M: Intermediate filaments in smooth muscle tumours. J Clin Pathol **36**:57-61, 1983.

865 Suster S: Epithelioid leiomyosarcoma of the skin and subcutaneous tissue. Clinicopathologic, immunohistochemical, and ultrastructural study of five cases. Am J Surg Pathol **18**:232-240, 1994.

Tumors of striated muscle
Rhabdomyoma

866 Agamanolis DP, Dasu S, Krill CE: Tumors of skeletal muscle. Hum Pathol **17**:778-795, 1986.

867 Crotty PL, Nakhleh RE, Dehner LP: Juvenile rhabdomyoma. An intermediate form of skeletal muscle tumor in children. Arch Pathol Lab Med **117**:43-47, 1993.

868 Czernobilsky B, Cornog JL, Enterline HT: Rhabdomyoma. Report of case with ultrastructural and histochemical studies. Am J Clin Pathol 49:782-789, 1968.

869 Dehner LP, Enzinger FM: Fetal rhabdomyoma. An analysis of nine cases. Cancer 30:160-166, 1972.

870 di Sant'Agnese PA, Knowles DM II: Extracardiac rhabdomyoma. A clinicopathologic study and review of the literature. Cancer 46:780-789, 1980.

871 Golz R: Multifocal adult rhabdomyoma. Case report and literature review. Pathol Res Pract 183:512-518, 1988.

872 Kapadia SB, Meis JM, Frisman DM, Ellis GL, Heffner DK: Fetal rhabdomyoma of the head and neck. A clinicopathologic and immunophenotypic study of 24 cases. Hum Pathol 24:754-765, 1993.

873 Kapadia SB, Meis JM, Frisman DM, Ellis GL, Heffner DK, Hyams VJ: Adult rhabdomyoma of the head and neck. A clinicopathologic and immunophenotypic study. Hum Pathol 24:608-617, 1993.

874 Kodet R, Fajstavr J, Kabelka Z, Koutecky J, Eckschlager T, Newton WA Jr: Is fetal cellular rhabdomyoma an entity or a differentiated rhabdomyosarcoma? A study of patients with rhabdomyoma of the tongue and sarcoma of the tongue enrolled in the intergroup rhabdomyosarcoma studies I, II, and III. Cancer 67:2907-2913, 1991.

875 Konrad EA, Meister P, Hübner G: Extracardiac rhabdomyoma. Report of different types with light microscopic and ultrastructural studies. Cancer 49:898-907, 1982.

876 Lehtonen E, Asikainen U, Badley RA: Rhabdomyoma. Ultrastructural features and distribution of desmin, muscle type of intermediate filament protein. Acta Pathol Microbiol Immunol Scand (A) 90:125-129, 1982.

877 Morgan JJ, Enterline HT: Benign rhabdomyoma of the pharynx. A case report, review of the literature, and comparison with cardiac rhabdomyoma. Am J Clin Pathol 42:174-181, 1964.

878 Scrivner D, Meyer JS: Multifocal recurrent adult rhabdomyoma. Cancer 46:790-795, 1980.

879 Whitten RO, Benjamin DR: Rhabdomyoma of the retroperitoneum. A report of a tumor with both adult and fetal characteristics. A study by light and electron microscopy, histochemistry, and immunochemistry. Cancer 59:818-824, 1987.

880 Willis J, Abdul-Karim FW, di Sant'Agnese PA: Extracardiac rhabdomyomas. Semin Diagn Pathol 11:15-25, 1994.

Rhabdomyosarcoma

881 Agamanolis DP, Dasu S, Krill CE: Tumors of skeletal muscle. Hum Pathol 17:778-795, 1986.

882 Altmannsberger M, Dirk T, Osborn M, Weber K: Immunohistochemistry of cytoskeletal filaments in the diagnosis of soft tissue tumors. Semin Diagn Pathol 3:306-316, 1986.

883 Autio-Harmainen H, Apaja-Sarkkinen M, Martikainen J, Taipale A, Rapola J: Production of basement membrane laminin and type IV collagen by tumors of striated muscle. An immunohistochemical study of rhabdomyosarcomas of different histologic types and a benign vaginal rhabdomyoma. Hum Pathol 17:1218-1224, 1986.

884 Bale PM, Parsons RE, Stevens MM: Diagnosis and behavior of juvenile rhabdomyosarcoma. Hum Pathol 14:596-611, 1983.

885 Brooks JJ: Immunohistochemistry of soft tissue tumors. Myoglobin as a tumor marker for rhabdomyosarcoma. Cancer 50:1757-1763, 1982.

886 Bundtzen JL, Norback DH: The ultrastructure of poorly differentiated rhabdomyosarcomas. A case report and literature review. Hum Pathol 13:301-313, 1982.

887 Carstens PHB: Soft tissue tumor with prominent leptomeric fibrils and complexes (rhabdomyosarcoma). Ultrastruct Pathol 10:137-144, 1986.

888 Carter RL, Jameson CF, Philp ER, Pinkerton CR: Comparative phenotypes in rhabdomyosarcomas and developing skeletal muscle. Histopathology 17:301-309, 1990.

889 Carter RL, McCarthy KP, Machin LG, Jameson CF, Philp ER, Pinkerton CR: Expression of desmin and myoglobin in rhabdomyosarcomas and in developing skeletal muscle. Histopathology 15:585-595, 1989.

890 Cavazzana AO, Schmidt D, Ninfo V, Harms D, Tollot M, Carli M, Treuner J, Betto R, Salviati G: Spindle cell rhabdomyosarcoma. A prognostically favorable variant of rhabdomyosarcoma. Am J Surg Pathol 16:229-235, 1992.

891 Chan JK, Ng HK, Wan KY, Tsao SY, Leung TW, Tse KC: Clear cell rhabdomyosarcoma of the nasal cavity and paranasal sinuses. Histopathology 14:391-399, 1989.

892 Cho KR, Olson JL, Epstein JI: Primitive rhabdomyosarcoma presenting with diffuse bone marrow involvement. An immunohistochemical and ultrastructural study. Modern Pathol 1:23-28, 1988.

893 Choi J, Costa ML, Mermelstein CS, Chagas C, Holtzer S, Holtzer H: MyoD converts primary dermal fibroblasts, chondroblasts, smooth muscle, and retinal pigmented epithelial cells into striated mononucleated myoblasts and multinucleated myotubes. Proc Natl Acad Sci USA 87:7988-7992, 1990.

894 Churg A, Ringus J: Ultrastructural observations on the histogenesis of alveolar rhabdomyosarcoma. Cancer 41:1355-1361, 1978.

895 Crist WM, Raney RB Jr, Newton W, Lawrence W Jr, Tefft M, Foulkes MA: Intrathoracic soft tissue sarcomas in children. Cancer 50:598-604, 1982.

896 D'Amore ES, Tollot M, Stracca-Pansa V, Menegon A, Meli S, Carli M, Ninfo V: Therapy associated differentiation in rhabdomyosarcomas. Mod Pathol 7:69-75, 1994.

897 De Jong ASH, Albus-Lutter ChE, van Raamsdonk W, Voûte PA: Myosin and myoglobin as tumor markers in the diagnosis of rhabdomyosarcom. Am J Surg Pathol 8:521-528, 1984.

898 De Jong ASH, van Kessel–van Vark M, Albus-Lutter ChE: Pleomorphic rhabdomyosarcoma in adults. Immunohistochemistry as a tool for its diagnosis. Hum Pathol 18:298-303, 1987.

899 De Jong ASH, van Kessel–van Vark M, Albus-Lutter ChE, van Raamsdonk W, Voûte PA: Skeletal muscle actin as tumor marker in the diagnosis of rhabdomyosarcoma in childhood. Am J Surg Pathol 9:467-474, 1985.

900 De Jong ASH, van Kessel–van Vark M, Albus-Lutter ChE, Voûte PA: Creatine kinase subunits M and B as markers in the diagnosis of poorly differentiated rhabdomyosarcomas in children. Hum Pathol 16:924-928, 1985.

901 de la Monte SM, Hutchins GM, Moore GW: Metastatic behavior of rhabdomyosarcoma. Pathol Res Pract 181:148-152, 1986.

902 Dias P, Dilling M, Houghton P: The molecular basis of skeletal muscle differentiation. Semin Diagn Pathol 11:3-14, 1994.

903 Dias P, Parham DM, Shapiro DN, Webber BL, Houghton PJ: Myogenic regulatory protein (MyoD1) expression in childhood solid tumors. Diagnostic utility in rhabdomyosarcoma. Am J Pathol 137:1283-1291, 1990.

903a Downing JR, Khandekar A, Shurtleff SA, Head DR, Parham DM, Webber BL, Pappo AS, Hulshof MG, Conn WP, Shapiro DN: Multiplex RT-PCR assay for the differential diagnosis of alveolar rhabdomyosarcoma and Ewing's sarcoma. Am J Pathol 146:626-634, 1995.

904 Driman D, Thorner PS, Greenberg ML, Chilton-MacNeill S, Squire J: MYCN gene amplification in rhabdomyosarcoma. Cancer 73:2231-2237, 1994.

905 Elomaa I, Lehto V-P, Selander R-K: Hypercalcemia and elevated serum parathyroid hormone level in association with rhabdomyosarcoma. Arch Pathol Lab Med 108:701-703, 1984.

906 Enterline HT, Horn RC: Alveolar rhabdomyosarcoma. A distinctive tumor type. Am J Clin Pathol 20:356-366, 1958.

907 Enzinger FM: Alveolar rhabdomyosarcoma. An analysis of 110 cases. Cancer 24:18-31, 1969.

908 Erlandson RA: The ultrastructural distinction between rhabdomyosarcoma and other undifferentiated "sarcomas." Ultrastruct Pathol 11:83-101, 1987.

909 Eusebi V, Bondi A, Rosai J: Immunohistochemical localization of myoglobin in nonmuscular cells. Am J Surg Pathol 8:51-55, 1984.

910 Eusebi V, Ceccarelli C, Gorza L, Schiaffino S, Bussolati G: Immunocytochemistry of rhabdomyosarcoma. The use of four different markers. Am J Surg Pathol 10:293-299, 1986.

911 Eusebi V, Rilke F, Ceccarelli C, Fedeli F, Schiaffino S, Bussolati G: Fetal heavy chain skeletal myosin. An oncofetal antigen expressed by rhabdomyosarcoma. Am J Surg Pathol 10:680-686, 1986.

912 Flamant F, Hill C: The improvement in survival associated with combined chemotherapy in childhood rhabdomyosarcoma. Cancer 53:2417-2421, 1984.

913 Gaffney EF, Dervan PA, Fletcher CD: Pleomorphic rhabdomyosarcoma in adulthood. Analysis of 11 cases with definition of diagnostic criteria. Am J Surg Pathol 17:601-609, 1993.

914 Gonzalez-Crussi F, Black-Schaffer S: Rhabdomyosarcoma of infancy and childhood. Problems of morphologic classification. Am J Surg Pathol 3:157-171, 1979.

915 Hawkins HK, Camacho-Velasquez JV: Rhabdomyosarcoma in children. A correlation of form and prognosis in one institution's experience. Am J Surg Pathol 11:531-542, 1987.

916 Hayashi Y, Kikuchi F, Oka T, Itoyama S, Mohri N, Usuki K, Takaku F, Murakami T, Saitoh Y, Urano Y: Rhabdomyosarcoma with bone marrow metastasis simulating acute leukemia. Report of two cases. Acta Pathol Jpn 38:789-798, 1988.

917 Hays DM, Newton W Jr, Soule EH, Foulkes MA, Raney RB, Tefft M, Ragab A, Maurer HM: Mortality among children with rhabdomyosarcomas of the alveolar histologic subtype. J Pediatr Surg 18:412-417, 1983.

918 Hays DM, Soule EH, Lawrence W Jr, Gehan EA, Maurer HM, Donaldson M, Raney RB, Tefft M: Extremity lesions in the Intergroup Rhabdomyosarcoma Study (IRS-I). A preliminary report. Cancer 49:1-8, 1982.

919 Hollowood K, Fletcher CD: Rhabdomyosarcoma in adults. Semin Diagn Pathol 11:47-57, 1994.

920 Horn RC Jr, Enterline HT: Rhabdomyosarcoma. A clinicopathological study and classification of 39 cases. Cancer 11:181-199, 1958.

921 Horvat BI, Caines M, Fisher ER: The ultrastructure of rhabdomyosarcoma. Am J Clin Pathol **53**:555-564, 1970.

922 Jaffe BF, Fox JE, Batsakis JG: Rhabdomyosarcoma of the middle ear and mastoid. Cancer **27**:29-37, 1971.

923 Kahn HJ, Yeger H, Kassim O, Jorgensen AO, MacLennan DH, Baumal R, Smith CR, Phillips MJ: Immunohistochemical and electron microscopic assessment of childhood rhabdomyosarcoma. Increased frequency of diagnosis over routine histologic methods. Cancer **51**:1897-1903, 1983.

924 Karcioglu Z, Someren A, Mathes SJ: Ectomesenchymoma. A malignant tumor of migratory neural crest (ectomesenchyme) remnants showing ganglionic, schwannian, melanocytic and rhabdomyoblastic differentiation. Cancer **39**:2486-2496, 1977.

925 Kawamoto EH, Weidner N, Agostini RM Jr, Jaffe R: Malignant ectomesenchymoma of soft tissue. Report of two cases and review of the literature. Cancer **59**:1791-1802, 1987.

926 Keyhani A, Booher RJ: Pleomorphic rhabdomyosarcoma. Cancer **22**:956-967, 1968.

927 Kindblom L-G, Seidal T, Karlsson K: Immunohistochemical localization of myoglobin in human muscle tissue and embryonal and alveolar rhabdomyosarcoma. Acta Pathol Microbiol Immunol Scand [A] **90**:167-174, 1982.

928 Kodet R, Kasthuri N, Marsden HB, Coad NAG, Raafat F: Gangliorhabdomyosarcoma. A histopathological and immunohistochemical study of three cases. Histopathology **10**:181-193, 1986.

929 Kodet R, Newton WA Jr, Hamoudi AB, Asmar L: Rhabdomyosarcomas with intermediate-filament inclusions and features of rhabdoid tumors. Light microscopic and immunohistochemical study. Am J Surg Pathol **15**:257-267, 1991.

930 Kodet R, Newton WA Jr, Hamoudi AB, Asmar L, Jacobs DL, Maurer HM: Childhood rhabdomyosarcoma with anaplastic (pleomorphic) features. A report of the Intergroup Rhabdomyosarcoma Study. Am J Surg Pathol **17**:443-453, 1993.

931 Koh S-J, Johnson WW: Antimyosin and antirhabdomyo sera. Their use for the diagnosis of childhood rhabdomyosarcoma. Arch Pathol Lab Med **104**:118-122, 1980.

932 La Quaglia MP, Heller G, Ghavimi F, Casper ES, Vlamis V, Hajdu S, Brennan MF: The effect of age at diagnosis on outcome in rhabdomyosarcoma. Cancer **73**:109-117, 1994.

933 Lawrence W, Hays DM, Heyn R, Tefft M, Crist W, Beltangady M, Newton W Jr, Wharam M: Lymphatic metastases with childhood rhabdomyosarcoma. A report from the Intergroup Rhabdomyosarcoma Study. Cancer **60**:910-915, 1987.

934 Leuschner I, Newton WA Jr, Schmidt D, Sachs N, Asmar L, Hamoudi A, Harms D, Maurer HM: Spindle cell variants of embryonal rhabdomyosarcoma in the paratesticular region. A report of the Intergroup Rhabdomyosarcoma Study. Am J Surg Pathol **17**:221-230, 1993.

935 Linscheid RL, Soule EH, Henderson ED: Pleomorphic rhabdomyosarcomata of the extremities and limb girdles. J Bone Joint Surg (Am) **47**:715-726, 1965.

936 Lloyd RV, Hajdu SI, Knapper WH: Embryonal rhabdomyosarcoma in adults. Cancer **51**:557-565, 1983.

937 Lombardi L, Pilotti S: Ultrastructural characterization of poorly differentiated rhabdomyosarcomas. Ultrastruct Pathol **17**:669-680, 1993.

938 Lundgren L, Angervall L, Stenman G, Kindblom LG: Infantile rhabdomyofibrosarcoma. A high-grade sarcoma distinguishable from infantile fibrosarcoma and rhabdomyosarcoma. Hum Pathol **24**:785-795, 1993.

939 Masson JK, Soule EH: Embryonal rhabdomyosarcoma of head and neck. Report of 88 cases. Am J Surg **110**:585-591, 1965.

940 Maurer HM, Beltangady M, Gehan EA, Crist W, Hammond D, Hays DM, Heyn R, Lawrence W, Newton W, Ortega J, Ragab AH, Raney RB, Ruymann FB, Soule E, Tefft M, Webber B, Wharam M, Vietti TJ: The Intergroup Rhabdomyosarcoma Study. I. A final report. Cancer **61**:209-220, 1988.

941 Maurer HM, Gehan EA, Beltangady M, Crist W, Dickman PS, Donaldson SS, Fryer C, Hammond D, Hays DM, Herrmann J, et al.: The Intergroup Rhabdomyosarcoma Study-II. Cancer **71**:1904-1922, 1993.

942 Mierau GW, Favara BE: Rhabdomyosarcoma in children. Ultrastructural study of 31 cases. Cancer **46**:2035-2040, 1980.

943 Miettinen M: Antibody specific to muscle actins in the diagnosis and classification of soft tissue tumors. Am J Pathol **130**:205-215, 1988.

944 Miettinen M, Rapola J: Immunohistochemical spectrum of rhabdomyosarcoma and rhabdomyosarcoma-like tumors. Expression of cytokeratin and the 68-kD neurofilament protein. Am J Surg Pathol **13**:120-132, 1989.

945 Molenaar WM, Dam-Meiring A, Kamps WA, Cornelisse CJ: DNA-aneuploidy in rhabdomyosarcomas as compared with other sarcomas of childhood and adolescence. Hum Pathol **19**:573-579, 1988.

946 Molenaar WM, Oosterhuis AM, Ramaekers FCS: The rarity of rhabdomyosarcomas in the adult. A morphologic and immunohistochemical study. Pathol Res Pract **180**:400-404, 1985.

947 Molenaar WM, Oosterhuis JW, Kamps WA: Cytologic "differentiation" in childhood rhabdomyosarcomas following polychemotherapy. Hum Pathol **15**:973-979, 1984.

948 Molenaar WM, Oosterhuis JW, Oosterhuis AM, Ramaekers FCS: Mesenchymal and muscle-specific intermediate filaments (vimentin and desmin) in relation to differentiation in childhood rhabdomyosarcoma. Hum Pathol **16**:838-843, 1985.

949 Morales AR, Fine G, Horn RC Jr: Rhabdomyosarcoma. An ultrastructural appraisal. Pathol Annu **7**:81-106, 1972.

950 Mukai K, Rosai J, Hallaway BE: Localization of myoglobin in normal and neoplastic human skeletal muscle cells using an immunoperoxidase method. Am J Surg Pathol **3**:373-376, 1979.

951 Mukai K, Schollmeyer JV, Rosai J: Immunohistochemical localization of actin. Its applications in surgical pathology. Am J Surg Pathol **5**:91-97, 1981.

952 Mukai M, Iri H, Torikata C, Kageyama K, Morikawa Y, Shimizu K: Immunoperoxidase demonstration of a new muscle protein (Z-protein) in myogenic tumors as a diagnostic aid. Am J Pathol **114**:164-170, 1984.

953 Nakhleh RE, Swanson PE, Dehner LP: Juvenile (embryonal and alveolar) rhabdomyosarcoma of the head and neck in adults. A clinical, pathologic, and immunohistochemical study of 12 cases. Cancer **67**:1019-1024, 1991.

954 Om A, Ghose T: Use of anti-skeletal muscle antibody from myasthenic patients in the diagnosis of childhood rhabdomyosarcomas. Am J Surg Pathol **11**:272-276, 1987.

955 Osborn M, Hill C, Altmannsberger M, Weber K: Monoclonal antibodies to titin in conjunction with antibodies to desmin separate rhabdomyosarcomas from other tumor types. Lab Invest **55**:101-108, 1986.

956 Pappo AS, Crist WM, Kuttesch J, Rowe S, Ashmun RA, Maurer HM, Newton WA, Asmar L, Luo X, Shapiro DN: Tumor-cell DNA content predicts outcome in children and adolescents with clinical group III embryonal rhabdomyosarcoma. The Intergroup Rhabdomyosarcoma Study Committee of the Children's Cancer Group and the Pediatric Oncology Group. J Clin Oncol **11**:1901-1905, 1993.

957 Parham DM, Shapiro DN, Downing JR, Webber BL, Douglass EC: Solid alveolar rhabdomyosarcomas with the t(2; 13). Report of two cases with diagnostic implications. Am J Surg Pathol **18**:474-478, 1994.

958 Parham DM, Webber B, Holt H, Williams WK, Maurer H: Immunohistochemical study of childhood rhabdomyosarcomas and related neoplasms. Results of an Intergroup Rhabdomyosarcoma study project. Cancer **67**:3072-3080, 1991.

959 Peters E, Cohen M, Altini M, Murray J: Rhabdomyosarcoma of the oral and paraoral region. Cancer **63**:963-966, 1989.

960 Ragab AH, Heyn R, Tefft M, Hays DN, Newton WA Jr, Beltangady M: Infants younger than 1 year of age with rhabdomyosarcoma. Cancer **58**:2606-2610, 1986.

961 Raney RB Jr, Tefft M, Maurer HM, Ragab AH, Hays DM, Soule EH, Foulkes MA, Gehan EA: Disease patterns and survival rate in children with metastatic soft-tissue sarcoma. A report from the Intergroup Rhabdomyosarcoma Study (IRS)-I. Cancer **62**:1257-1266, 1988.

962 Reboul-Marty J, Quintana E, Mosseri V, Flamant F, Asselain B, Rodary C, Zucker JM: Prognostic factors of alveolar rhabdomyosarcoma in childhood. An International Society of Pediatric Oncology study. Cancer **68**:493-498, 1991.

963 Riopelle JL, Thériault JP: Sur une forme méconnue de sarcome des parties molles; le rhabdomyosarcome alvéolaire. Ann Anat Pathol (Paris) **1**:88-111, 1956.

964 Royds JA, Variend S, Timperley WR, Taylor CB: Comparison of ß-enolase and myoglobin as histological markers of rhabdomyosarcoma. J Clin Pathol **38**:1258-1260, 1985.

965 Ruymann FB, Newton WA Jr, Ragab AH, Donaldson MH, Foulkes M: Bone marrow metastases at diagnosis in children and adolescents with rhabdomyosarcoma. A report from the Intergroup Rhabdomyosarcoma Study. Cancer **53**:368-373, 1984.

966 Sarnat HB, de Mello DE, Siddiqui SY: Diagnostic value of histochemistry in embryonal rhabdomyosarcoma. Am J Surg Pathol **3**:177-183, 1979.

967 Schmidt D, Fletcher CD, Harms D: Rhabdomyosarcomas with primary presentation in the skin. Pathol Res Pract **189**:422-427, 1993.

968 Schmidt D, Mackay B, Osborne BM, Jaffe N: Recurring congenital lesion of the cheek. Ultrastruct Pathol **3**:85-90, 1982.

969 Schmidt D, Reimann O, Treuner J, Harms D: Cellular differentiation and prognosis in embryonal rhabdomyosarcoma. A report from the Cooperative Soft Tissue Sarcoma Study 1981 (CWS 81). Virchows Arch [A] **409**:183-194, 1986.

970 Schurch W, Bochaton-Piallat ML, Geinoz A, d'Amore E, Laurini RN, Cintorino M, Begin LR, Boivin Y, Gabbiani G: All histological types of primary human rhabdomyosarcoma express alpha-cardiac and not alpha-skeletal actin messenger RNA. Am J Pathol **144**:836-846, 1994.

971 Scupham R, Gilbert EF, Wilde J, Wiedrich TA: Immunohistochemical studies of rhabdomyosarcoma. Arch Pathol Lab Med **110**:818-821, 1980.

972 Seidal T, Kindblom L-G: The ultrastructure of alveolar and embryonal rhabdomyosarcoma. A correlative light and electron microscopic study of 17 cases.
Acta Pathol Microbiol Immunol Scand (A) **92**:231-248, 1984.

973 Seidal T, Mark J, Hagmar B, Angervall L: Alveolar rhabdomyosarcoma. A
cytogenetic and correlated cytological and histological study. Acta Pathol
Microbiol Immunol Scand (A) **90**:345-354, 1982.

974 Shimada H, Newton WA Jr, Soule EH, Beltangady MS, Maurer HM: Pathology
of fatal rhabdomyosarcoma. Report from Intergroup Rhabdomyosarcoma Study
(IRS-I and IRS-II). Cancer **59**:459-465, 1987.

975 Skalli O, Gabbiani G, Babaï F, Seemayer TA, Pizzolato G, Schürch W: Intermediate filament proteins and actin isoforms as markers for soft tissue tumor differentiation and origin II. Rhabdomyosarcomas. Am J Pathol **130**:515-531, 1988.

976 Soule EH, Geitz M, Henderson ED: Embryonal rhabdomyosarcoma of the
limbs and limb-girdles. A clinicopathologic study of 61 cases. Cancer **23**:1336-
1346, 1969.

977 Stout AP: Rhabdomyosarcoma of the skeletal muscles. Ann Surg **123**:447-
472, 1946.

977a Tapscott SJ, Thayer MJ, Weintraub H: Deficiency in rhabdomyosarcomas of a
factor required for MyoD activity and myogenesis. Science **259**:1450-1453, 1995.

978 Tsokos M: The role of immunocytochemistry in the diagnosis of rhabdomyosarcoma. Arch Pathol Lab Med **110**:776-778, 1986.

979 Tsokos M: The diagnosis and classification of childhood rhabdomyosarcoma.
Semin Diagn Pathol **11**:26-38, 1994.

980 Tsokos M, Howard R, Costa J: Immunohistochemical study of alveolar and
embryonal rhabdomyosarcoma. Lab Invest **48**:148-155, 1983.

981 Tsokos M, Webber BL, Parham DM, Wesley RA, Miser A, Miser JS, Etcubanas
E, Kinsella T, Grayson J, Glatstein E, et al.: Rhabdomyosarcoma. A new classification scheme related to prognosis. Arch Pathol Lab Med **116**:847-855, 1992.

982 Variend S, Loughlin MA: An evaluation of enzyme histochemistry in the diagnosis of childhood rhabdomyosarcoma. Histopathology **9**:389-400, 1985.

982a Wang NP, Marx J, McNutt MA, Rutledge JC, Gown AM: Expression of myogenic regulatory proteins (myogenin and MyoD1) in small blue round cell
tumors of childhood. Am J Pathol (in press).

982b Wesche WA, Fletcher CD, Dias P, Houghton PJ, Parham DM: Immunohistochemistry of MyoD1 in adult pleomorphic soft tissue sarcomas. Am J Surg
Pathol **19**:261-269, 1995.

983 Wijnaendts LC, van der Linden JC, van Unnik AJ, Delemarre JF, Barbet JP,
Butler-Browne GS, Meijer CJ: Expression of developmentally regulated muscle proteins in rhabdomyosarcomas. Am J Pathol **145**:895-901, 1994.

984 Wijnaendts LC, van der Linden JC, van Unnik AJ, Delemarre JF, Voute PA,
Meijer CJ: Histopathological classification of childhood rhabdomyosarcomas.
Relationship with clinical parameters and prognosis. Hum Pathol **25**:900-
907, 1994.

985 Young RH, Scully RE: Alveolar rhabdomyosarcoma metastatic to the ovary. A
report of two cases and a discussion of the differential diagnosis of small cell
malignant tumors of the ovary. Cancer **64**:899-904, 1989.

986 Yun K: A new marker for rhabdomyosarcoma. Insulin-like growth factor II.
Lab Invest **67**:653-664, 1992.

987 Zuppan CW, Mierau GW, Weeks DA: Lipid-rich rhabdomyosarcoma—a
potential source of diagnostic confusion. Ultrastruct Pathol **15**:353-359, 1991.

Tumors of pluripotential mesenchyme

988 Bures C, Barnes L: Benign mesenchymomas of the head and neck. Arch Pathol
Lab Med **102**:237-241, 1978.

989 Dorfman HD, Levin S, Robbins H: Cartilage-containing benign mesenchymomas
of soft tissue. Report of two cases. J Bone Joint Surg (Am) **62**:472-475, 1980.

990 Hollingsworth H, Pogrebniak H, Baker A, Merino M: Unusual mesenchymoma
with prominent chondro-osseous elements. Int J Surg Pathol **1**:129-134, 1993.

991 Milchgrub S, McMurry NK, Vuitch F, Dorfman HD: Chondrolipoangioma. A
cartilage-containing benign mesenchymoma of soft tissue. Cancer **66**:2636-
2641, 1990.

992 Nash A, Stout AP: Malignant mesenchymomas in children. Cancer **14**:524-
533, 1961.

993 Newman PL, Fletcher CD: Malignant mesenchymoma. Clinicopathologic analysis of a series with evidence of low-grade behaviour. Am J Surg Pathol
15:607-614, 1991.

994 Stout AP: Mesenchymoma, the mixed tumor of mesenchymal derivatives. Ann
Surg **127**:278-290, 1948.

Tumors of metaplastic mesenchyme

995 Allan CJ, Soule EH: Osteogenic sarcoma of the somatic soft tissues. Clinicopathologic study of 26 cases and review of literature. Cancer **27**:1121-1133, 1971.

996 Bane BL, Evans HL, Ro JY, Carrasco CH, Grignon DJ, Benjamin RS, Ayala
AG: Extraskeletal osteosarcoma. A clinicopathologic review of 26 cases. Cancer **65**:2762-2770, 1990.

997 Bertoni F, Picci P, Bacchini P, Capanna R, Innao V, Bacci G, Campanacci
M: Mesenchymal chondrosarcoma of bone and soft tissues. Cancer **52**:533-
541, 1983.

998 Bhagavan BS, Dorfman HD: The significance of bone and cartilage formation
in malignant fibrous histiocytoma of soft tissue. Cancer **49**:480-488, 1982.

998a Carstens PHB: Chordoid tumor. A light, electron microscopic, and immunohistochemical study. Ultrastruct Pathol **19**:291-296, 1995.

999 Chung EB, Enzinger FM: Chondroma of soft parts. Cancer **41**:1414-
1424, 1978.

1000 Chung EB, Enzinger FM: Extraskeletal osteosarcoma. Cancer **60**:1132-
1142, 1987.

1001 Dabska M: Parachordoma. A new clinicopathologic entity. Cancer **40**:1586-
1592, 1977.

1002 Dahlin DC, Salvador AH: Cartilaginous tumors of the soft tissues of the hands
and feet. Mayo Clin Proc **49**:721-726, 1974.

1003 D'Ambrosio RG, Shiu MH, Brennan MF: Intrapulmonary presentation of
extraskeletal myxoid chondrosarcoma of the extremity. Report of two cases.
Cancer **58**:1144-1148, 1986.

1004 De Blois G, Wang S, Kay S: Microtubular aggregates within rough endoplasmic reticulum. An unusual ultrastructural feature of extraskeletal myxoid chondrosarcoma. Hum Pathol **17**:469-475, 1986.

1005 Enzinger FM, Shiraki M: Extra-skeletal myxoid chondrosarcoma. An analysis
of 34 cases. Hum Pathol **3**:421-435, 1972.

1006 Fine G, Stout AP: Osteogenic sarcoma of the extraskeletal soft tissues. Cancer
9:1027-1043, 1956.

1007 Fletcher CDM, Powell G, McKee PH: Extraskeletal myxoid chondrosarcoma. A
histochemical and immunohistochemical study. Histopathology **10**:489-499, 1986.

1008 Guccion JG, Font RL, Enzinger FM, Zimmerman LE: Extraskeletal mesenchymal chondrosarcoma. Arch Pathol **95**:336-340, 1973.

1009 Hachitanda Y, Tsuneyoshi M, Daimaru Y, Enjoji M, Nakagawara A, Ikeda K,
Sueishi K: Extraskeletal myxoid chondrosarcoma in young children. Cancer
61:2521-2526, 1988.

1010 Humphreys S, Pambakian H, McKee PH, Fletcher CDM: Soft tissue chondroma. A study of 15 tumours. Histopathology **10**:147-159, 1986.

1011 Huvos AG: Osteogenic sarcoma of bones and szoft tissues in older persons.
A clinicopathologic analysis of 117 patients older than 60 years. Cancer **57**:1442-
1449, 1986.

1012 Huvos AG, Woodard HQ, Cahan WG, Higinbotham NL, Stewart FW, Butler A,
Bretsky SS: Postradiation osteogenic sarcoma of bone and soft tissues. A clinicopathologic study of 66 patients. Cancer **55**:1244-1255, 1985.

1013 Ishida T, Oda H, Oka T, Imamura T, Machinami R: Parachordoma. An ultrastructural and immunohistochemical study. Virchows Arch [A] **422**:239-246, 1993.

1014 Jessurun J, Rojas ME, Albores-Saavedra J: Congenital extraskeletal embryonal
chondrosarcoma. J Bone Joint Surg (Am) **64**:293-296, 1982.

1015 Kindblom L-G, Angervall L: Histochemical characterization of mucosubstances in bone and soft tissue tumors. Cancer **36**:985-994, 1975.

1016 Lichtenstein L, Goldman RL: Cartilage tumors in soft tissues, particularly in the
hand and foot. Cancer **17**:1203-1208, 1964.

1017 Mackenzie DH: The unsuspected soft tissue chondrosarcoma. Histopathology
7:759-766, 1983.

1018 Malhotra CM, Doolittle CH, Rodil JV, Vezeridis MP: Mesenchymal chondrosarcoma of the kidney. Cancer **54**:2495-2499, 1984.

1019 Martin RF, Melnick PJ, Warner NE, Terry R, Bullock WK, Schwinn CP: Chordoid sarcoma. Am J Clin Pathol **59**:623-635, 1973.

1020 Martinez-Tello FJ, Navas-Palacios JJ: Ultrastructural study of conventional
chondrosarcomas and myxoid- and mesenchymal-chondrosarcoma. Virchows
Arch [A] **396**:197-211, 1982.

1021 Mirra JM, Fain JS, Ward WG, Eckardt JJ, Eilber F, Rosen G: Extraskeletal
telangiectatic osteosarcoma. Cancer **71**:3014-3019, 1993.

1022 Nakashima Y, Unni KK, Shives TC, Swee RG, Dahlin DC: Mesenchymal chondrosarcoma of bone and soft tissue. A review of 111 cases. Cancer **57**:2444-
2453, 1986.

1023 Payne C, Dardick I, Mackay B: Extraskeletal myxoid chondrosarcoma with
intracisternal microtubules. Ultrastruct Pathol **18**:257-261, 1994.

1024 Reiman HM, Dahlin DC: Cartilage- and bone-forming tumors of the soft tissues. Semin Diagn Pathol **3**:288-305, 1986.

1025 Saleh G, Evans HL, Ro JY, Ayala AG: Extraskeletal myxoid chondrosarcoma.
A clinicopathologic study of ten patients with long-term follow-up. Cancer
70:2827-2830, 1992.

1026 Sangueza OP, White CR Jr: Parachordoma. Am J Dermatopathol **16**:185-
188, 1994.

1026a Sciot R, Dal Cin P, Fletcher C, Samson I, Smith M, De Vos R, Van Damme
B, Van den Berghe H: t(9;22)(q22-31;q11-12) is a consistent marker of
extraskeletal myxoid chondrosarcoma. Evaluation of three cases. Mod Pathol
8:765-768, 1995.

1027 Shin HJ, Mackay B, Ichinose H, Ayala AG, Romsdahl MM: Parachordoma. Ultrastruct Pathol 18:249-256, 1994.

1028 Sordillo PP, Hajdu SI, Magill GB, Golbey RB: Extraosseous osteogenic sarcoma. A review of 48 patients. Cancer 51:727-734, 1983.

1029 Stout AP, Verner EW: Chondrosarcoma of the extraskeletal soft tissue. Cancer 6:581-590, 1953.

1030 Tsuneyoshi M, Enjoji M, Iwasaki H, Shinohara N: Extraskeletal myxoid chondrosarcoma. A clinicopathologic and electron microscopic study. Acta Pathol Jpn 31:439-447, 1981.

1031 Weiss SW: Ultrastructure of the so-called "chordoid sarcoma." Evidence supporting cartilaginous differentiation. Cancer 37:300-306, 1976.

1032 Wick MR, Burgess JH, Manivel JC: A reassessment of "chordoid sarcoma." Ultrastructural and immunohistochemical comparison with chordoma and skeletal myxoid chondrosarcoma. Mod Pathol 1:433-443, 1988.

1033 Wolford JF, Bedetti CI: Skeletal myxoid chondrosarcoma with microtubular aggregates within rough endoplasmic reticulum. Arch Pathol Lab Med 112:77-81, 1988.

1034 Wu KK, Collon DJ, Guise ER: Extra-osseous chondrosarcoma. Report of five cases and review of the literature. J Bone Joint Surg (Am) 62:189-194, 1980.

1035 Wu WQ, Lapi A: Primary non-skeletal intracranial cartilaginous neoplasm. Report of a chondroma and a mesenchymal chondrosarcoma. J Neurol Neurosurg Psychiatry 33:469-475, 1970.

1036 Yi ES, Shmookler BM, Malawer MM, Sweet DE: Well-differentiated extraskeletal osteosarcoma. A soft-tissue homologue of parosteal osteosarcoma. Arch Pathol Lab Med 115:906-909, 1991.

1037 Zucker DK, Horopian DS: Dural mesenchymal chondrosarcoma. Case report. J Neurosurg 48:829-833, 1978.

Tumors of synovial tissue

1038 Abenoza P, Manivel JC, Swanson PE, Wick MR: Synovial sarcoma. Ultrastructural study and immunohistochemical analysis by a combined peroxidase-antiperoxidase/avidin-biotin-peroxidase complex procedure. Hum Pathol 17:1107-1115, 1986.

1039 Batsakis JG, Nishiyama RH, Sullinger GD: Synovial sarcomas of the neck. Arch Otolaryngol 85:327-331, 1967.

1040 Cagle LA, Mirra JM, Storm FK, Roe DJ, Eilber FR: Histologic features relating to prognosis in synovial sarcoma. Cancer 59:1810-1814, 1987.

1041 Corson JM, Weiss LM, Banks-Schlegel SP, Pinkus GS: Keratin proteins and carcinoembryonic antigen in synovial sarcomas. An immunohistochemical study of 24 cases. Hum Pathol 15:615-621, 1984.

1042 Crocker EW, Stout AP: Synovial sarcoma in children. Cancer 12:1123-1133, 1959.

1043 Dal Cin P, Rao U, Jani-Sait S, Karakousis C, Sandberg AA: Chromosomes in the diagnosis of soft tissue tumors. I. Synovial sarcoma. Mod Pathol 5:357-362, 1992.

1044 Dardick I, Ramjohn S, Thomas MJ, Jeans D, Hammar SP: Synovial sarcoma. Pathol Res Pract 187:871-885, 1991.

1044a Dei Tos AP, Wadden C, Calonje E, Sciot R, Pauwels P, Knight JC, Dal Cin P, Fletcher CDM: Immunohistochemical demonstration of glycoprotein p30/32^{MIC2}(CD99) in synovial sarcoma. A potential cause of diagnostic confusion. Appl Immunohistochem 3:168-173, 1995.

1045 Dickersin GR: Synovial sarcoma. A review and update, with emphasis on the ultrastructural characterization of the nonglandular component. Ultrastruct Pathol 15:379-402, 1991.

1046 Dische FE, Darby AJ, Howard ER: Malignant synovioma. Electron microscopical findings in three patients and review of the literature. J Pathol 124:149-155, 1978.

1047 el-Naggar AK, Ayala AG, Abdul-Karim FW, McLemore D, Ballance WW, Garnsey L, Ro JY, Batsakis JG: Synovial sarcoma. A DNA flow cytometric study. Cancer 65:2295-2300, 1990.

1048 Farris AB, Reed RJ: Monophasic, glandular, synovial sarcomas and carcinomas of the soft tissues. Arch Pathol Lab Med 106:129-132, 1982.

1049 Fetsch JF, Meis JM: Synovial sarcoma of the abdominal wall. Cancer 72:469-477, 1993.

1050 Fisher C: Synovial sarcoma. Ultrastructural and immunohistochemical features of epithelial differentiation in monophasic and biphasic tumors. Hum Pathol 17:996-1008, 1986.

1051 Fisher C, Schofield JB: S-100 protein positive synovial sarcoma. Histopathology 19:375-377, 1991.

1052 Fligman I, Lonardo F, Jhanwar SC, Gerald WL, Woodruff J, Ladanyi M: Molecular diagnosis of synovial sarcoma and character of a novel SYT-SSX fusion transcript. Am J Pathol (in press).

1053 Gabbiani G, Kaye GI, Lattes R, Majno G: Synovial sarcoma. Electron microscopic study of a typical case. Cancer 28:1031-1039, 1971.

1054 Ghadially FN: Is synovial sarcoma a carcinosarcoma of connective tissue? Ultrastruct Pathol 11:147-151, 1987.

1055 Haagensen CD, Stout AP: Synovial sarcoma. Ann Surg 120:826-842, 1944.

1056 Hajdu SI, Shiu MH, Fortner JG: Tendosynovial sarcoma. A clinicopathological study of 136 cases. Cancer 39:1201-1217, 1977.

1057 Ishida T, Kojima T, Iijima T, Oka T, Kuroda M, Horiuchi H, Imamura T, Machinami R: Synovial sarcoma with a predominant epithelial component. Int J Surg Pathol 1:261-268, 1994.

1058 Krall RA, Kostianovsky M, Patchefsky AS: Synovial sarcoma. A clinical, pathological, ultrastructural study of 26 cases supporting the recognition of a monophasic variant. Am J Surg Pathol 5:137-151, 1981.

1059 Ladenstein R, Treuner J, Koscielniak E, d'Oleire F, Keim M, Gadner H, Jurgens H, Niethammer D, Ritter J, Schmidt D: Synovial sarcoma of childhood and adolescence. Report of the German CWS-81 study. Cancer 71:3647-3655, 1993.

1060 Leader M, Patel J, Collins M, Kristin H: Synovial sarcomas. True carcinosarcomas? Cancer 59:2096-2098, 1987.

1061 Lombardi L, Rilke F: Ultrastructural similarities and differences of synovial sarcoma, epithelioid sarcoma, and clear cell sarcoma of the tendons and aponeuroses. Ultrastruct Pathol 6:209-219, 1984.

1062 Lopes JM, Bjerkehagen B, Holm R, Bruland O, Sobrinho-Simoes M, Nesland JM: Immunohistochemical profile of synovial sarcoma with emphasis on the epithelial-type differentiation. A study of 49 primary tumours, recurrences and metastases. Pathol Res Pract 190:168-177, 1994.

1063 Lopes JM, Bjerkehagen B, Sobrinho-Simoes M, Nesland JM: The ultrastructural spectrum of synovial sarcomas. A study of the epithelial type differentiation of primary tumors, recurrences, and metastases. Ultrastruct Pathol 17:137-151, 1993.

1064 Mackenzie DH: Synovial sarcoma. A review of 58 cases. Cancer 19:169-180, 1966.

1065 Mackenzie DH: Monophasic synovial sarcoma—a histological entity? Histopathology 1:151-157, 1977.

1066 Majeste RM, Beckman EN: Synovial sarcoma with an overwhelming epithelial component. Cancer 61:2527-2531, 1988.

1067 McKinney CD, Mills SE, Fechner RE: Intraarticular synovial sarcoma. Am J Surg Pathol 16:1017-1020, 1992.

1068 Mickelson MR, Brown GA, Maynard JA, Cooper RR, Bonfiglio M: Synovial sarcoma. An electron microscopic study of monophasic and biphasic forms. Cancer 45:2109-2118, 1980.

1069 Miettinen M: Keratin subsets in spindle cell sarcomas. Keratins are widespread but synovial sarcoma contains a distinctive keratin polypeptide pattern and desmoplakins. Am J Pathol 138:505-513, 1991.

1070 Miettinen M, Lehto V-P, Virtanen I: Monophasic synovial sarcoma of spindle-cell type. Virchows Arch [A] 44:187-199, 1983.

1071 Miettinen M, Santavirta S, Släts P: Intravascular synovial sarcoma. Hum Pathol 18:1075-1077, 1987.

1072 Miettinen M, Virtanen I: Synovial sarcoma—a misnomer. Am J Pathol 117:18-25, 1984.

1073 Milchgrub S, Ghandur-Mnaymneh L, Dorfman HD, Albores-Saavedra J: Synovial sarcoma with extensive osteoid and bone formation. Am J Surg Pathol 17:357-363, 1993.

1074 Mirra JM, Wang S, Bhuta S: Synovial sarcoma with squamous differentiation of its mesenchymal glandular elements. A case report with light-microscopic, ultramicroscopic, and immunologic correlation. Am J Surg Pathol 8:791-796, 1984.

1075 Moberger G, Nilsonne U, Friberg S Jr: Synovial sarcoma. Histologic features and prognosis. Acta Orthop Scand (Suppl) 3:1-38, 1968.

1076 Nakamura T, Nakata K, Hata S, Ono K, Katsuyama T: Histochemical characterization of mucosubstances in synovial sarcoma. Am J Surg Pathol 8:429-434, 1984.

1077 Oda Y, Hashimoto H, Tsuneyoshi M, Takeshita S: Survival in synovial sarcoma. A multivariate study of prognostic factors with special emphasis on the comparison between early death and long-term survival. Am J Surg Pathol 17:35-44, 1993.

1078 Ordóñez NG, Mahfouz SM, Mackay B: Synovial sarcoma. An immunohistochemical and ultrastructural study. Hum Pathol 21:733-749, 1990.

1079 Pappo AS, Fontanesi J, Luo X, Rao BN, Parham DM, Hurwitz C, Avery L, Pratt CB: Synovial sarcoma in children and adolescents. The St Jude Children's Research Hospital experience. J Clin Oncol 12:2360-2366, 1994.

1080 Pinkus GS, Kurtin PJ: Epithelial membrane antigen—a diagnostic discriminant in surgical pathology. Immunohistochemical profile in epithelial, mesenchymal, and hematopoietic neoplasms using paraffin sections and monoclonal antibodies. Hum Pathol 16:929-940, 1985.

1081 Rooser B, Willen H, Hugoson A, Rydholm A: Prognostic factors in synovial sarcoma. Cancer **63**:2182-2185, 1989.

1082 Roth JA, Enzinger FM, Tannenbaum M: Synovial sarcoma of the neck. A follow-up study of 24 cases. Cancer **35**:1243-1253, 1975.

1083 Salisbury JR, Isaacson PG: Synovial sarcoma. An immunohistochemical study. J Pathol **147**:49-57, 1985.

1084 Schiffman R: Epithelioid sarcoma and synovial sarcoma in the same knee. Cancer **45**:158-166, 1980.

1085 Shaw GR, Lais CJ: Fatal intravascular synovial sarcoma in a 31-year-old woman. Hum Pathol **24**:809-810, 1993.

1086 Shmookler BM: Retroperitoneal synovial sarcoma. Am J Clin Pathol **77**:686-691, 1982.

1087 Shmookler BM, Enzinger FM, Brannon RB: Orofacial synovial sarcoma. A clinicopathologic study of 11 new cases and review of the literature. Cancer **50**:269-272, 1982.

1088 Soule EH: Synovial sarcoma. Am J Surg Pathol **10**(Suppl 1):78-82, 1986.

1089 Suit HD, Russell WO, Martin RG: Management of patients with sarcoma of soft tissue in an extremity. Cancer **31**:1247-1255, 1973.

1090 Tsuneyoshi M, Yokoyama K, Enjoji M: Synovial sarcoma. A clinicopathologic and ultrastructural study of 42 cases. Acta Pathol Jpn **33**:23-36, 1983.

1091 van Andel JG: Synovial sarcoma. A review and analysis of treated cases. Radiol Clin Biol **41**:145-159, 1972.

1092 Varela-Duran J, Enzinger FM: Calcifying synovial sarcoma. A clinicopathologic study of 32 cases. Cancer **50**:345-352, 1982.

1093 Weidner N, Goldman R, Johnston J: Epithelioid monophasic synovial sarcoma. Ultrastruct Pathol **17**:287-294, 1993.

1094 Witkin GB, Rosai J: A biphasic tumor of the mediastinum with features of synovial sarcoma. A report of 4 cases (abstract). Lab Invest **58**:104A, 1988.

1095 Wright PH, Sim EH, Soule EH, Taylor WF: Synovial sarcoma. J Bone Joint Surg (Am) **64**:112-122, 1982.

Tumors of extragonadal germ cells

1096 Berry CL, Keelnig J, Hilton C: Teratoma in infancy and childhood. A review of 91 cases. J Pathol **98**:241-252, 1969.

1097 Billmire DF, Grosfeld JL: Teratomas in childhood. Analysis of 142 cases. J Pediatr Surg **21**:548-551, 1986.

1098 Colton JJ, Batsakis JG, Work WP: Teratomas of the neck in adults. Arch Otolaryngol **104**:271-272, 1978.

1099 Conklin J, Abell MR: Germ cell neoplasms of sacrococcygeal region. Cancer **20**:2105-2117, 1967.

1100 Dehner LP: Intrarenal teratoma occurring in infancy. Report of a case with discussion of extragonadal germ cell tumors in infancy. J Pediatr Surg **8**:369-378, 1973.

1101 Dehner LP, Mills A, Talerman A, Billman GF, Krous HF, Platz CE: Germ cell neoplasms of head and neck soft tissues. A pathologic spectrum of teratomatous and endodermal sinus tumors. Hum Pathol **21**:309-318, 1990.

1102 Gonzalez-Crussi F, Winkler RF, Mirkin DL: Sacrococcygeal teratomas in infants and children. Relationship of histology and prognosis in 40 cases. Arch Pathol Lab Med **102**:420-425, 1978.

1103 Mochizuki Y, Noguchi S, Yokoyama S, Murakami N, Moriuchi A, Aisaka K, Yamashita H, Nakayama I: Cervical teratoma in a fetus and an adult. Two case reports and review of literature. Acta Pathol Jpn **36**:935-943, 1986.

1104 Tapper D, Lack EE: Teratomas in infancy and childhood. A 54-year experience at the Children's Hospital Medical Center. Ann Surg **198**:398-410, 1983.

1105 Willis RA: Pathology of tumors, ed 4. London, 1968, Butterworth.

Tumors of neural tissue (other than peripheral nerves)
Pigmented neuroectodermal tumor of infancy

1106 Argenyi ZB, Schelper RL, Balogh K: Pigmented neuroectodermal tumor of infancy. A light microscopic and immunohistochemical study. J Cutan Pathol **18**:40-45, 1991.

1107 Borello ED, Gorlin RH: Melanotic neuroectodermal tumor of infancy—a neoplasm of neural crest origin. Report of a case associated with high urinary excretion of vanilmandelic acid. Cancer **19**:196-206, 1966.

1108 Clark BE, Parsons H: An embryological tumor of retinal anlage involving the skull. Cancer **4**:78-85, 1951.

1109 Dehner LP, Sibley RK, Sauk JJ Jr, Vickers RA, Nesbit ME, Leonard AS, Waite DE, Neeley JE, Ophoven J: Malignant melanotic neuroectodermal tumor of infancy. A clinical, pathologic, ultrastructural and tissue culture study. Cancer **43**:1389-1410, 1979.

1110 Johnson RE, Scheithauer BW, Dahlin DC: Melanotic neuroectodermal tumor of infancy. A review of seven cases. Cancer **52**:661-666, 1983.

1111 Koudstaal J, Oldhoff J, Panders AK, Hardonk MJ: Melanotic neuroectodermal tumor of infancy. Cancer **22**:151-161, 1968.

1112 Neustein HB: Fine structure of a melanotic progonoma or retinal anlage tumor of the anterior fontanel. Exp Mol Pathol **6**:131-142, 1967.

1113 Pettinato G, Manivel JC, d'Amore ES, Jaszcz W, Gorlin RJ: Melanotic neuroectodermal tumor of infancy. A reexamination of a histogenetic problem based on immunohistochemical, flow cytometric, and ultrastructural study of 10 cases. Am J Surg Pathol **15**:233-245, 1991.

1114 Raju U, Zarbo R, Regezi J, Krutchkoff D, Perrin E: Melanotic, neuroectodermal tumors of infancy. Intermediate filament-, neuroendocrine-, and melanoma-associated antigen profiles. Appl Immunohistochem **1**:69-76, 1993.

1115 Scheck O, Ruck P, Harms D, Kaiserling E: Melanotic neuroectodermal tumor of infancy occurring in the left thigh of a 6-month-old female infant. Ultrastruct Pathol **13**:23-33, 1989.

1116 Stirling RW, Powell G, Fletcher CD: Pigmented neuroectodermal tumour of infancy. An immunohistochemical study. Histopathology **12**:425-435, 1988.

1117 Young S, Gonzalez-Crussi F: Melanocytic neuroectodermal tumor of the foot. Report of a case with multicentric origin. Am J Clin Pathol **84**:371-378, 1985.

Other neural tumors

1118 Anderson MS: Myxopapillary ependymomas presenting in the soft tissue over the sacrococcygeal region. Cancer **19**:585-590, 1966.

1119 Bain GO, Shnitka TK: Cutaneous meningioma (psammoma). Arch Dermatol **74**:590-594, 1956.

1120 Helwig EB, Stern JB: Subcutaneous sacrococcygeal myxopapillary ependymoma. A clinicopathologic study of 32 cases. Am J Clin Pathol **81**:156-161, 1984.

1121 King P, Cooper PN, Malcolm AJ: Soft tissue ependymoma. A report of three cases. Histopathology **22**:394-396, 1993.

1122 Pulitzer DR, Martin PC, Collins PC, Ralph DR: Subcutaneous sacrococcygeal ("myxopapillary") ependymal rests. Am J Surg Pathol **12**:672-677, 1988.

1123 Shepherd NA, Coates PJ, Brown AA: Soft tissue gliomatosis—heterotopic glial tissue in the subcutis. A case report. Histopathology **11**:655-660, 1987.

Tumors of hematopoietic tissue

1124 Akosa AB, Ali MH: Extramedullary plasmacytoma of skeletal muscle. A case report with immunocytochemistry and ultrastructural study. Cancer **64**:1504-1507, 1989.

1125 Axiotis CA, Fuks J, Jennings TA, Kadish AS: Peripheral T-cell lymphoma presenting as a soft-tissue mass of the extremity. Arch Pathol Lab Med **112**:850-851, 1988.

1126 Condon WB, Safarik LR, Elzi EP: Extramedullary hematopoiesis simulating intrathoracic tumor. Arch Surg **90**:643-648, 1965.

1127 D'Amore ES, Wick MR, Geisinger KR, Frizzera G: Primary malignant lymphoma arising in postmastectomy lymphedema. Another facet of the Stewart-Treves syndrome. Am J Surg Pathol **14**:456-463, 1990.

1128 Lanham GR, Weiss SW, Enzinger FM: Malignant lymphoma. A study of 75 cases presenting in soft tissue. Am J Surg Pathol **13**:1-10, 1989.

1129 Travis WD, Banks FM, Reiman HM: Primary extranodal soft tissue lymphoma of the extremities. Am J Surg Pathol **11**:359-366, 1987.

Tumors of uncertain cell type
Fibrous hamartoma of infancy

1130 Enzinger FM: Fibrous hamartoma of infancy. Cancer **18**:241-248, 1965.

1131 Fletcher CDM, Powell G, Van Noorden S, McKee PH: Fibrous hamartoma of infancy. A histochemical and immunohistochemical study. Histopathology **12**:65-74, 1988.

1132 Groisman G, Lichtig C: Fibrous hamartoma of infancy. An immunohistochemical and ultrastructural study. Hum Pathol **22**:914-918, 1991.

1133 Maung R, Lindsay R, Trevenen C, Hwang WS: Fibrous hamartoma of infancy. Hum Pathol **18**:652-653, 1987.

1134 Michal M, Mukensnabl P, Chlumska A, Kodet R: Fibrous hamartoma of infancy. A study of eight cases with immunohistochemical and electron microscopical findings. Pathol Res Pract **188**:1049-1053, 1992.

Myxoma

1134a Allen PW, Dymock RB, MacCormac LB: Superficial angiomyxomas with and without epithelial components. Report of 30 tumors in 28 patients. Am J Surg Pathol **12**:519-530, 1988.

1134b Aoki T, Kouho H, Hisaoka M, Hashimoto H, Nakata H, Sakai A: Intramuscular myxoma with fibrous dysplasia. A report of two cases with a review of the literature. Pathol Int **45**:165-171, 1995.

1135 Carney JA, Gordon H, Carpenter PC, Shenoy BV, Go VLW: The complex of myxomas, spotty pigmentation, and endocrine overactivity. Medicine **64**:270-283, 1985.

1136 Enzinger FM: Intramuscular myxoma. A review and follow-up study of 34 cases. Am J Clin Pathol **43**:104-113, 1965.

1137 Feldman PS: A comparative study including ultrastructure of intramuscular myxoma and myxoid liposarcoma. Cancer **43:**512-525, 1979.

1138 Hashimoto H, Tsuneyoshi M, Daimaru Y, Enjoji M, Shinohara N: Intramuscular myxoma. A clinicopathologic, immunohistochemical, and electron microscopic study. Cancer **58:**740-747, 1986.

1139 Ireland DCR, Soule EH, Ivins JC: Myxoma of somatic soft tissues. A report of 58 patients, 3 with multiple tumors and fibrous dysplasia of bone. Mayo Clin Proc **48:**401-410, 1973.

1140 Johnson WC, Helwig EB: Cutaneous focal mucinosis. A clinicopathological and histochemical study. Arch Dermatol **93:**13-20, 1966.

1141 Kindblom L, Stener B, Angervall L: Intramuscular myxoma. Cancer **34:**1737-1744, 1974.

1142 Mackenzie DH: The myxoid tumors of somatic soft tissues. Am J Surg Pathol **5:**443-458, 1981.

1143 Meis JM, Enzinger FM: Juxta-articular myxoma. A clinical and pathologic study of 65 cases. Hum Pathol **23:**639-646, 1992.

1144 Miettinen M, Hockerstedt K, Reitamo J, Totterman S: Intramuscular myxoma. A clinicopathological study of twenty-three cases. Am J Clin Pathol **84:**265-272, 1985.

1145 Stout AP: Myxoma, the tumor of primitive mesenchyme. Ann Surg **127:**706-719, 1948.

1146 Wirth WA, Leavitt D, Enzinger FM: Multiple intramuscular myxomas. Another extraskeletal manifestation of fibrous dysplasia. Cancer **27:**1167-1173, 1971.

Granular cell tumor

1147 Al-Sarraf M, Loud AV, Vaitkevicius VK: Malignant granular cell tumor. Histochemical and electron microscopic study. Arch Pathol **91:**550-558, 1971.

1148 Bedetti CD, Martinez AJ, Beckford NS, May M: Granular cell tumor arising in myelinated peripheral nerves. Light and electron microscopy and immunoperoxidase study. Virchows Arch [A] **402:**175-183, 1983.

1149 Bhawan J, Malhotra R, Naik DR: Gaucher-like cells in a granular cell tumor. Hum Pathol **14:**730-733, 1983.

1150 Budzilovich GN: Granular cell "myoblastoma" of vagus nerve. Acta Neuropathol **10:**162-169, 1968.

1151 Chandrasoma P, Fitzgibbons P: Granular cell tumor of the intrapancreatic common bile duct. Cancer **53:**2178-2182, 1984.

1152 Christ ML, Ozzello L: Myogenous origin of a granular cell tumor of the urinary bladder. Am J Clin Pathol **56:**736-749, 1971.

1153 Clark HB, Minesky JJ, Agrawal D, Agrawal HC: Myelin basic protein and P2 protein are not immunohistochemical markers for Schwann cell neoplasms. A comparative study using antisera to S-100, P2, and myelin basic proteins. Am J Pathol **121:**96-101, 1985.

1154 Copas P, Dyer M, Hall DJ, Diddle AW: Granular cell myoblastoma of the uterine cervix. Diagn Gynecol Obstet **3:**251-254, 1981.

1155 de la Monte SM, Radowsky M, Hood AF: Congenital granular-cell neoplasms. An unusual case report with ultrastructural findings and a review of the literature. Am J Dermatopathol **8:**57-63, 1986.

1156 Demay RM, Kay S: Granular cell tumor of the breast. Pathol Annu **19**(Pt 2):121-148, 1984.

1157 Finkel G, Lane B: Granular cell variant of neurofibromatosis. Ultrastructure of benign and malignant tumors. Hum Pathol **13:**959-963, 1982.

1158 Fisher ER, Wechsler H: Granular cell myoblastoma—a misnomer. Electron microscopic and histochemical evidence concerning its Schwann cell derivation and nature (granular cell schwannoma). Cancer **15:**936-957, 1962.

1159 Garancis JC, Komorowski RA, Kuzma JF: Granular cell myoblastoma. Cancer **25:**542-550, 1970.

1160 Johnston J, Helwig EB: Granular cell tumours of the gastrointestinal tract and perianal region. A study of 74 cases. Dig Dis Sci **26:**807-816, 1981.

1161 Kindblom L-G, Olsson K-M: Malignant granular cell tumor. A clinicopathologic and ultrastructural study of a case. Pathol Res Pract **172:**384-393, 1981.

1162 Lack EE, Worsham GF, Callihan MD, Crawford BE, Klappenbach S, Rowden G, Chun B: Granular cell tumor. A clinicopathologic study of 110 patients. J Surg Oncol **13:**301-316, 1980.

1163 Lack EE, Worsham GF, Callihan MD, Crawford BE, Vawter GF: Gingival granular cell tumors of the newborn (congenital "epulis"). A clinical and pathologic study of 21 patients. Am J Surg Pathol **5:**37-46, 1981.

1164 Le Boit PE, Barr RJ, Burall S, Metcalf JS, Yen TS, Wick MR: Primitive polypoid granular-cell tumor and other cutaneous granular-cell neoplasms of apparent nonneural origin. Am J Surg Pathol **15:**48-58, 1991.

1165 Lifshitz MS, Flotte TJ, Greco MA: Congenital granular cell epulis. Immunohistochemical and ultrastructural observations. Cancer **53:**1845-1848, 1984.

1166 Matthews JB, Mason GI: Granular cell myoblastoma. An immunoperoxidase study using a variety of antisera to human carcinoembryonic antigen. Histopathology **7:**77-82, 1983.

1167 Mazur MT, Shultz JJ, Myers JL: Granular cell tumor. Immunohistochemical analysis of 21 benign tumors and one malignant tumor. Arch Pathol Lab Med **114:**692-696, 1990.

1168 McMahon JN, Rigby HS, Davies JD: Elastosis in granular cell tumours. Prevalence and distribution. Histopathology **16:**37-41, 1990.

1169 McSwain GR, Colpitts R, Kreutner A, O'Brien PH, Spicer S: Granular cell myoblastoma. Surg Gynecol Obstet **150:**703-710, 1980.

1170 McWilliam LJ, Harris M: Granular cell angiosarcoma of the skin. Histology, electron microscopy and immunohistochemistry of a newly recognized tumor. Histopathology **9:**1205-1216, 1985.

1171 Miettinen M, Lehtonen E, Lehtola H, Ekblom P, Lehto V, Virtanen I: Histogenesis of granular cell tumor. An immunohistochemical and ultrastructural study. J Pathol **142:**221-229, 1984.

1172 Mittal KR, True LD: Origin of granules in granular cell tumor. Intracellular myelin formation with autodigestion. Arch Pathol Lab Med **112:**302-303, 1988.

1173 Moscovic EA, Azar HA: Multiple granular cell tumors ("myoblastomas"). Case report with electron microscopic observations and review of the literature. Cancer **20:**2032-2047, 1967.

1174 Mukai M: Immunohistochemical localization of S-100 protein and peripheral nerve myelin proteins (P2 protein, P0 protein) in granular cell tumors. Am J Pathol **112:**139-146, 1983.

1175 Nakazato Y, Ishizeki J, Takahashi K, Yamaguchi H: Immunohistochemical localization of S-100 protein in granular cell myoblastoma. Cancer **49:**1624-1628, 1982.

1176 Nathrath WBJ, Remberger K: Immunohistochemical study of granular cell tumours. Demonstration of neurone specific enolase, S 100 protein, laminin and alpha-1-antichymotrypsin. Virchows Arch [A] **408:**421-434, 1986.

1177 Navarrette AR, Smith M: Ultrastructure of granular cell ameloblastoma. Cancer **27:**948-955, 1971.

1178 Nielsen K, Paulsen SM, Johansen P: Carcinoembryonic antigen like antigen in granular cell myoblastomas. An immunohistochemical study. Virchows Arch [A] **401:**159-162, 1983.

1179 Nistal M, Paniagua R, Picazo ML, Cermeño deGiles F, Ramos Guerreira L: Granular changes in vascular leiomyosarcoma. Virchows Arch [A] **386:**239-248, 1980.

1180 Park SH, Kim TJ, Chi JG: Congenital granular cell tumor with systemic involvement. Immunohistochemical and ultrastructural study. Arch Pathol Lab Med **115:**934-938, 1991.

1181 Penneys NS, Adachi K, Ziegels-Weissman J, Nadji M: Granular cell tumors of the skin contain myelin basic protein. Arch Pathol Lab Med **107:**302-303, 1983.

1182 Regezi JA, Zarbo RJ, Courtney RM, Crissman JD: Immunoreactivity of granular cell lesions of skin, mucosa, and jaw. Cancer **64:**1455-1460, 1989.

1183 Robertson AJ, McIntosh W, Lamont P, Guthrie W: Malignant granular cell tumour (myoblastoma) of the vulva. Report of a case and review of the literature. Histopathology **5:**69-79, 1981.

1184 Sakurama N, Matsukado Y, Marubayashi T, Kodama T: Granular cell tumour of the brain and its cellular identity. Acta Neurochir (Wien) **56:**81-94, 1981.

1185 Seo IS, Azzarelli B, Warner TF, Goheen MP, Senteney GE: Multiple visceral and cutaneous granular cell tumors. Ultrastructural and immunocytochemical evidence of Schwann cell origin. Cancer **53:**2104-2110, 1984.

1186 Shimamura K, Osamura RY, Ueyama Y, Hata J-I, Tamaoki N, Machida N, Fukuda H, Uemura K: Malignant granular cell tumor of the right sciatic nerve. Report of an autopsy case with electron microscopic, immunohistochemical, and enzyme histochemical studies. Cancer **53:**524-529, 1984.

1187 Sobel JH, Marquet E, Schwarz R: Granular degeneration of appendiceal smooth muscle. Arch Pathol **92:**427-432, 1971.

1188 Stefansson K, Wollmann RL: S-100 protein in granular cell tumors (granular cell myoblastomas). Cancer **49:**1834-1838, 1982.

1189 Strong, EW, McDivitt RW, Brasfield RD: Granular cell myoblastoma. Cancer **25:**415-422, 1970.

1190 Troncoso P, Ordonez NG, Raymond AK, Mackay B: Malignant granular cell tumor. Immunocytochemical and ultrastructural observations. Ultrastruct Pathol **12:**137-144, 1988.

1191 Usui M, Ishii S, Yamawaki S, Sasaki T, Minami A, Hizawa K: Malignant granular cell tumor of the radial nerve. Cancer **39:**1547-1555, 1977.

1192 Uzoaru I, Firfer B, Ray V, Hubbard-Shepard M, Rhee H: Malignant granular cell tumor. Arch Pathol Lab Med **116:**206-208, 1992.

1193 Vance SF III, Hudson RP: Granular cell myoblastoma. Clinicopathologic study of 42 patients. Am J Clin Pathol **52:**208-211, 1969.

Alveolar soft part sarcoma

1194 Auerbach HE, Brooks JJ: Alveolar soft part sarcoma. A clinicopathologic and immunohistochemical study. Cancer **60:**66-73, 1987.

1195 Carstens HB: Membrane-bound cytoplasmic crystals, similar to those in alveolar soft part sarcoma, in a human muscle spindle. Ultrastruct Pathol **14**:423-428, 1990.

1196 DeSchryver-Kecskemeti K, Kraus FT, Engleman W, Lacy PE: Alveolar soft-part sarcoma—a malignant angioreninoma. Histochemical, immunocytochemical, and electron-microscopic study of four cases. Am J Surg Pathol **6**:5-18, 1982.

1197 Evans HL: Alveolar soft-part sarcoma. A study of 13 typical examples and one with a histologically atypical component. Cancer **55**:912-917, 1985.

1198 Fisher ER, Reidford H: Electron microscopic evidence suggesting the myogenous derivation of the so-called alveolar soft part sarcoma. Cancer **27**:150-159, 1971.

1199 Font RL, Jurco S III, Zimmerman LE: Alveolar soft-part sarcoma of the orbit. A clinicopathologic analysis of 17 cases and a review of the literature. Hum Pathol **13**:569-579, 1982.

1200 Foschini MP, Ceccarelli C, Eusebi V, Skalli O, Gabbiani G: Alveolar soft part sarcoma. Immunological evidence of rhabdomyoblastic differentiation. Histopathology **13**:101-108, 1988.

1201 Foschini MP, Eusebi V: Alveolar soft-part sarcoma. A new type of rhabdomyosarcoma? Semin Diagn Pathol **11**:58-68, 1994.

1202 Gray GF Jr, Glick AD, Kurtin PJ, Jones HW III: Alveolar soft part sarcoma of the uterus. Hum Pathol **17**:297-300, 1986.

1203 Hirose T, Kudo E, Hasegawa T, Abe J, Hizawa K: Cytoskeletal properties of alveolar soft part sarcoma. Hum Pathol **21**:204-211, 1990.

1204 Lieberman PH, Brennan MF, Kimmel M, Erlandson RA, Garin-Chesa P, Flehinger BY: Alveolar soft-part sarcoma. A clinico-pathologic study of half a century. Cancer **63**:1-13, 1989.

1205 Lieberman PH, Foote FW, Stewart FW, Berg JW: Alveolar soft-part sarcoma. JAMA **198**:1047-1051, 1966.

1206 Lillehei KO, Kleinschmidt-De Masters B, Mitchell DH, Spector E, Kruse CA: Alveolar soft part sarcoma. An unusually long interval between presentation and brain metastasis. Hum Pathol **24**:1030-1034, 1993.

1207 Machinami R, Kikuchi F: Adenosine triphosphatase activity of crystalline inclusions in alveolar soft part sarcoma. An ultrahistochemical study of a case. Pathol Res Pract **181**:357-361, 1986.

1208 Matsuno Y, Mukai K, Itabashi M, Yamauchi Y, Hirota T, Nakajima T, Shimosato Y: Alveolar soft part sarcoma. A clinicopathologic and immunohistochemical study of 12 cases. Acta Pathol Jpn **40**:199-205, 1990.

1209 Miettinen M, Ekfors T: Alveolar soft part sarcoma. Immunohistochemical evidence for muscle cell differentiation. Am J Clin Pathol **93**:32-38, 1990.

1210 Mukai M, Iri H, Nakajima T, Hirose S, Torikata C, Kageyama K, Ueno N, Murakami K: Alveolar soft-part sarcoma. A review on its histogenesis and further studies based on electron microscopy, immunohistochemistry, and biochemistry. Am J Surg Pathol **7**:679-689, 1983.

1211 Mukai M, Torikata C, Iri H, Mikata A, Hanaoka H, Kato K, Kageyama K: Histogenesis of alveolar soft part sarcoma. An immunohistochemical and biochemical study. Am J Surg Pathol **10**:212-218, 1986.

1212 Ogawa K, Nakashima Y, Yamabe H, Hamashima Y: Alveolar soft part sarcoma, granular cell tumor, and paraganglioma. An immunohistochemical comparative study. Acta Pathol Jpn **36**:895-904, 1986.

1213 Ohno T, Park P, Higaki S, Miki H, Kamura S, Unno K: Smooth tubular aggregates associated with plasmalemmal invagination in alveolar soft part sarcoma. Ultrastruct Pathol **18**:383-388, 1994.

1214 Ordóñez NG, Hickey RC, Brooks TE: Alveolar soft part sarcoma. A cytologic and immunohistochemical study. Cancer **61**:525-531, 1988.

1215 Ordóñez NG, Ro JY, Mackay B: Alveolar soft part sarcoma. An ultrastructural and immunocytochemical investigation of its histogenesis. Cancer **63**:1721-1736, 1989.

1216 O'Toole RV, Tuttle SE, Lucas JG, Sharma HM: Alveolar soft part sarcoma of the vagina. An immunohistochemical and electron microscopic study. Int J Gynecol Pathol **4**:258-265, 1985.

1217 Persson S, Willems JS, Kindblom LG, Angervall L: Alveolar soft part sarcoma. An immunohistochemical, cytologic and electron-microscopic study and a quantitative DNA analysis. Virchows Arch [A] **412**:499-513, 1988.

1218 Rosai J, Dias P, Parham DM, Shapiro DN, Houghton P: MyoD1 protein expression in alveolar soft part sarcoma as confirmatory evidence of its skeletal muscle nature. Am J Surg Pathol **15**:974-981, 1991.

1219 Sciot R, Dal Cin P, De Vos R, Van Damme B, De Wever I, Van den Berghe H, Desmet VJ: Alveolar soft-part sarcoma. Evidence for its myogenic origin and for the involvement of 17q25. Histopathology **23**:439-444, 1993.

1220 Shipkey IH, Lieberman PH, Foote FW Jr, Stewart FW: Ultrastructure of alveolar soft part sarcoma. Cancer **17**:821-830, 1964.

1221 Tsutsumi Y, Deng YL: Alveolar soft part sarcoma of the pulmonary vein. Acta Pathol Jpn **41**:771-777, 1991.

1222 Yagihashi S, Yagihashi N, Hase Y, Nagai K, Alguacil-Garcia A: Primary alveolar soft-part sarcoma of stomach. Am J Surg Pathol **15**:399-406, 1991.

Clear cell sarcoma of tendons and aponeuroses (malignant melanoma of soft parts)

1223 Angervall L, Stener B: Clear-cell sarcoma of tendons. A study of 4 cases. Acta Pathol Microbiol Scand **77**:589-597, 1969.

1224 Azumi N, Turner RR: Clear cell sarcoma of tendons and aponeuroses. Electron microscopic findings suggesting Schwann cell differentiation. Hum Pathol **14**:1084-1089, 1983.

1225 Bearman RM, Noe J, Kempson RL: Clear cell sarcoma with melanin pigment. Cancer **36**:977-984, 1975.

1226 Benson JD, Kraemer BB, Mackay B: Malignant melanoma of soft parts. An ultrastructural study of four cases. Ultrastruct Pathol **8**:57-70, 1985.

1227 Bridge JA, Borek DA, Neff JR, Huntrakoon M: Chromosomal abnormalities in clear cell sarcoma. Implications for histogenesis. Am J Clin Pathol **93**:26-31, 1990.

1228 Chung EB, Enzinger FM: Malignant melanoma of soft parts. A reassessment of clear cell sarcoma. Am J Surg Pathol **7**:405-413, 1983.

1229 Eckardt JJ, Pritchard DJ, Soule EH: Clear cell sarcoma. A clinicopathologic study of 27 cases. Cancer **52**:1482-1488, 1983.

1230 el-Naggar AK, Ordonez NG, Sara A, McLemore D, Batsakis JG: Clear cell sarcomas and metastatic soft tissue melanomas. A flow cytometric comparison and prognostic implications. Cancer **67**:2173-2179, 1991.

1231 Enzinger FM: Clear-cell sarcoma of tendons and aponeuroses. An analysis of 21 cases. Cancer **18**:1163-1174, 1965.

1232 Hasegawa T, Hirose T, Kudo E, Hizawa K: Clear cell sarcoma. An immunohistochemical and ultrastructural study. Acta Pathol Jpn **39**:321-327, 1989.

1233 Kindblom L-G, Lodding P, Angervall L: Clear-cell sarcoma of tendons and aponeuroses. An immunohistochemical and electron microscopic analysis indicating neural crest origin. Virchows Arch [A] **401**:109-128, 1983.

1234 Lucas DR, Nascimento AG, Sim FH: Clear cell sarcoma of soft tissues. Mayo Clinic experience with 35 cases. Am J Surg Pathol **16**:1197-1204, 1992.

1235 Montgomery E, Meis J, Ramos A, Frisman D, Mertz K: Clear cell sarcoma of tendons and aponeuroses. A clinicopathologic study of 58 cases with analysis of prognostic factors. Am J Surg Pathol **1**:89-100, 1993.

1235a Mooi WJ, Deenik W, Peterse JL, Hogendoorn PCW: Keratin immunoreactivity in melanoma of soft parts (clear cell sarcoma). Histopathology **27**:61-65, 1995.

1236 Mukai M, Torikata C, Iri H, Mikata A, Kawai T, Hanaoka H, Yakumaru K, Kageyama K: Histogenesis of clear cell sarcoma of tendons and aponeuroses. Am J Pathol **114**:264-272, 1984.

1237 Ohno T, Park P, Utsunomiya Y, Hirahata H, Inoue K: Ultrastructural study of a clear cell sarcoma suggesting Schwannian differentiation. Ultrastruct Pathol **10**:39-48, 1986.

1238 Pavlidis NA, Fisher C, Wiltshaw E: Clear-cell sarcoma of tendons and aponeuroses. A clinicopathologic study. Presentation of six additional cases with review of the literature. Cancer **54**:1412-1417, 1984.

1239 Sara AS, Evans HL, Benjamin RS: Malignant melanoma of soft parts (clear cell sarcoma). A study of 17 cases, with emphasis on prognostic factors. Cancer **65**:367-374, 1990.

1240 Saw D, Tse CH, Chan J, Watt CY, Ng CS, Poon YF: Clear cell sarcoma of the penis. Hum Pathol **17**:423-425, 1986.

1241 Swanson PE, Wick MR: Clear cell sarcoma. An immunohistochemical analysis of six cases and comparison with other epithelioid neoplasms of soft tissue. Arch Pathol Lab Med **113**:55-60, 1989.

1242 Tsuneyoshi M, Enjoji M, Kubo T: Clear cell sarcoma of tendons and aponeuroses. A comparative study of 13 cases with a provisional subgrouping into the melanotic and synovial types. Cancer **42**:243-252, 1978.

Epithelioid sarcoma

1243 Arber DA, Kandalaft PL, Mehta P, Battifora H: Vimentin-negative epithelioid sarcoma. The value of an immunohistochemical panel that includes CD34. Am J Surg Pathol **17**:302-307, 1993.

1244 Bloustein PA, Silverberg SG, Waddell WR: Epithelioid sarcoma. Case report with ultrastructural review, histogenetic discussion, and chemotherapeutic data. Cancer **38**:2390-2400, 1976.

1245 Bryan RS, Soule EH, Dobyns JH, Pritchard DJ, Linscheid RL: Primary epithelioid sarcoma of the hand and forearm. J Bone Joint Surg (Am) **56**:458-465, 1974.

1246 Chase DR, Enzinger FM: Epithelioid sarcoma. Diagnosis, prognostic indicators, and treatment. Am J Surg Pathol **9**:241-263, 1985.

1247 Chase DR, Enzinger FM, Weiss SW, Langloss JM: Keratin in epithelioid sarcoma. An immunohistochemical study. Am J Surg Pathol **8**:435-441, 1984.

1248 Chase DR, Enzinger FM, Weiss SW, Langloss JM: Coexpression of keratin and vimentin in epithelioid sarcoma. Am J Surg Pathol **9:**460-463, 1985.

1249 Chetty R, Slavin JL: Epithelioid sarcoma with extensive chondroid differentiation. Histopathology **24:**400-401, 1994.

1250 Daimaru Y, Hashimoto H, Tsuneyoshi M, Enjoji M: Epithelial profile of epithelioid sarcoma. An immunohistochemical analysis of eight cases. Cancer **59:**134-141, 1987.

1251 Enzinger FM: Epithelioid sarcoma. A sarcoma simulating a granuloma or a carcinoma. Cancer **25:**1029-1041, 1970.

1252 Evans HL, Baer SC: Epithelioid sarcoma. A clinicopathologic and prognostic study of 26 cases. Semin Diagn Pathol **10:**286-291, 1993.

1253 Fisher C: Epithelioid sarcoma. The spectrum of ultrastructural differentiation in seven immunohistochemically defined cases. Hum Pathol **19:**265-275, 1988.

1254 Gabbiani G, Fu Y-S, Kaye GI, Lattes R, Majno G: Epithelioid sarcoma. A light and electron microscopic study suggesting a synovial origin. Cancer **30:**486-499, 1972.

1255 Manivel JC, Wick MR, Dehner LP, Sibley RK: Epithelioid sarcoma. An immunohistochemical study. Am J Clin Pathol **87:**319-326, 1987.

1256 Miettinen M, Lehto V-P, Vartio T, Virtanen I: Epithelioid sarcoma. Ultrastructural and immunohistologic features suggesting a synovial origin. Arch Pathol Lab Med **106:**620-623, 1982.

1257 Mills SE, Rosai J: Adamantinoma of the pretibial soft tissue. Clinicopathologic features, differential diagnosis, and possible relationship to intraosseous disease. Am J Clin Pathol **83:**108-114, 1985.

1258 Mirra JM, Kessler S, Bhuta S, Eckardt J: The fibroma-like variant of epithelioid sarcoma. A fibrohistiocytic/myoid cell lesion often confused with benign and malignant spindle cell tumors. Cancer **69:**1382-1395, 1992.

1259 Molenaar WM, De Jong B, Dam-Meiring A, Postma A, De Vries J, Hoekstra HJ: Epithelioid sarcoma or malignant rhabdoid tumor of soft tissue? Epithelioid immunophenotype and rhabdoid karyotype. Hum Pathol **20:**347-351, 1989.

1260 Mukai M, Torikata C, Iri H, Hanaoka H, Kawai T, Yakumaru K, Shimoda T, Mikata A, Kageyama K: Cellular differentiation of epithelioid sarcoma—electron-microscopic, enzyme-histochemical, and immunohistochemical study. Am J Pathol **119:**44-56, 1985.

1261 Peimer CA, Smith RJ, Sirota RL, Cohen BE: Epithelioid sarcoma of the hand and wrist. Patterns of extension. J Hand Surg **2:**275-282, 1977.

1262 Perrone T, Swanson PE, Twiggs L, Ulbright TM, Dehner LP: Malignant rhabdoid tumor of the vulva. Is distinction from epithelioid sarcoma possible? A pathologic and immunohistochemical study. Am J Surg Pathol **13:**848-858, 1989.

1263 Prat J, Woodruff JM, Marcove RC: Epithelioid sarcoma. An analysis of 22 cases indicating the prognostic significance of vascular invasion and regional lymph node metastasis. Cancer **41:**1472-1487, 1978.

1264 Rose DSC, Fisher C, Smith MEF: Epithelioid sarcoma arising in a patient with neurofibromatosis type 2. Histopathology **25:**379-380, 1994.

1265 Santiago H, Feinerman LK, Lattes R: Epithelioid sarcoma. A clinical and pathologic study of nine cases. Hum Pathol **3:**133-147, 1972.

1266 Shimm DS, Suit HD: Radiation therapy of epithelioid sarcoma. Cancer **52:**1022-1025, 1983.

1267 Sugarbaker PH, Auda S, Webber BL, Triche TJ, Shapiro E, Cook WJ: Early distant metastases from epithelioid sarcoma of the hand. Cancer **48:**852-855, 1981.

1268 Weissmann D, Amenta PS, Kantor GR: Vulvar epithelioid sarcoma metastatic to the scalp. A case report and review of the literature. Am J Dermatopathol **12:**462-468, 1990.

Malignant giant cell tumor of soft parts

1269 Alguacil-Garcia A, Unni KK, Goellner JR: Malignant giant cell tumor of soft parts. An ultrastructural study of four cases. Cancer **40:**244-253, 1977.

1270 Angervall L, Hagmar B, Kindblom L-G, Merck C: Malignant giant cell tumor of soft tissues. A clinicopathologic, cytologic, ultrastructural, angiographic, and microangiographic study. Cancer **47:**736-747, 1981.

1271 Gould E, Albores-Saavedra J, Rothe M, Mnaymneh W, Menendez-Aponte S: Malignant giant cell tumor of soft parts presenting as a skin tumor. Am J Dermatopathol **11:**197-201, 1989.

1272 Guccion JG, Enzinger FM: Malignant giant cell tumor of soft parts. An analysis of 32 cases. Cancer **29:**1518-1529, 1972.

1273 Kearney MM, Soule EH, Ivins JC: Malignant fibrous histiocytoma. A retrospective study of 167 cases. Cancer **45:**167-178, 1980.

1274 Salm R, Sissons HA: Giant-cell tumours of soft tissues. J Pathol **107:**27-39, 1972.

Ossifying fibromyxoid tumor

1275 Donner LR: Ossifying fibromyxoid tumor of soft parts. Evidence supporting Schwann cell origin. Hum Pathol **23:**200-202, 1992.

1276 Enzinger FM, Weiss SW, Liang CY: Ossifying fibromyxoid tumor of soft parts. A clinicopathological analysis of 59 cases. Am J Surg Pathol **13:**817-827, 1989.

1276a Kilpatrick SE, Ward WG, Mozes M, Miettinen M, Fukunaga M, Fletcher CDM: Atypical and malignant variants of ossifying fibromyxoid tumor. Clinicopathologic analysis of six cases. Am J Surg Pathol **19:**1039-1046, 1995.

1277 Miettinen M: Ossifying fibromyxoid tumor of soft parts. Additional observations of a distinctive soft tissue tumor. Am J Clin Pathol **95:**142-149, 1991.

1278 Schofield JB, Krausz T, Stamp GW, Fletcher CD, Fisher C, Azzopardi JG: Ossifying fibromyxoid tumour of soft parts. Immunohistochemical and ultrastructural analysis. Histopathology **22:**101-112, 1993.

1279 Yang P, Hirose T, Hasegawa T, Gao Z, Hizawa K: Ossifying fibromyxoid tumor of soft parts. A morphological and immunohistochemical study. Pathol Int **44:**448-453, 1994.

Extraskeletal Ewing's sarcoma/PNET

1280 Ambros IM, Ambros PF, Strehl S, Kovar H, Gadner H, Salzer-Kuntschik M: MIC2 is a specific marker for Ewing's sarcoma and peripheral primitive neuroectodermal tumors. Evidence for a common histogenesis of Ewing's sarcoma and peripheral primitive neuroectodermal tumors from MIC2 expression and specific chromosome aberration. Cancer **67:**1886-1893, 1991.

1281 Angervall L, Enzinger FM: Extraskeletal neoplasm resembling Ewing's sarcoma. Cancer **36:**240-251, 1975.

1282 Askin FB, Rosai J, Sibley RK, Dehner LP, McAlister WH: Malignant small cell tumor of the thoracopulmonary region in childhood. A distinctive clinicopathologic entity of uncertain histogenesis. Cancer **43:**2438-2451, 1979.

1283 Cavazzana AO, Ninfo V, Roberts J, Triche TJ: Peripheral neuroepithelioma. A light microscopic, immunocytochemical, and ultrastructural study. Mod Pathol **5:**71-78, 1992.

1284 Contesso G, Llombart-Bosch A, Terrier P, Peydro-Olaya A, Henry-Amar M, Oberlin O, Habrand JL, Dubousset J, Tursz T, Spielmann M, et al.: Does malignant small round cell tumor of the thoracopulmonary region (Askin tumor) constitute a clinicopathologic entity? An analysis of 30 cases with immunohistochemical and electron-microscopic support treated at the Institute Gustave Roussy. Cancer **69:**1012-1020, 1992.

1285 Dehner LP: Primitive neuroectodermal tumor and Ewing's sarcoma. Am J Surg Pathol **17:**1-13, 1993.

1286 Delattre O, Zucman J, Melot T, Garau XS, Zucker JM, Lenoir GM, Ambros PF, Sheer D, Turc-Carel C, Triche TJ, et al.: The Ewing family of tumors—a sub group of small-round-cell tumors defined by specific chimeric transcripts. N Engl J Med **331:**294-299, 1994.

1287 Dickman PS, Triche TJ: Extraosseous Ewing's sarcoma versus primitive rhabdomyosarcoma. Diagnostic criteria and clinical correlation. Hum Pathol **17:**881-893, 1986.

1288 Downing JR, Head DR, Parham DM, Douglass EC, Hulshof MG, Link MP, Motroni TA, Grier HE, Curcio-Brint AM, Shapiro DN: Detection of the (11; 22)(q24; q12) translocation of Ewing's sarcoma and peripheral neuroectodermal tumor by reverse transcription polymerase chain reaction. Am J Pathol **143:**1294-1300, 1993.

1289 Fellinger EJ, Garin-Chesa P, Triche TJ, Huvos AG, Rettig WJ: Immunohistochemical analysis of Ewing's sarcoma cell surface antigen p30/32MIC2. Am J Pathol **139:**317-325, 1991.

1290 Gillespie JJ, Roth LM, Wills ER, Einhorn LH, Willman J: Extraskeletal Ewing's sarcoma. Histologic and ultrastructural observations in three cases. Am J Surg Pathol **3:**99-108, 1979.

1291 Gonzalez-Crussi F, Wolfson SL, Misugi K, Nakajima T: Peripheral neuroectodermal tumors of the chest wall in childhood. Cancer **54:**2519-2527, 1984.

1292 Gould VE, Moll R, Berndt R, Roessner A, Franke WW, Lee I: Immunohistochemical analysis of Ewing's tumors (abstract). Lab Invest **56:**28A, 1987.

1293 Harris MD, Moore IE, Steart PV, Weller RO: Protein gene product (PGP) 9.5 as a reliable marker in primitive neuroectodermal tumours—an immunohistochemical study of 21 childhood cases. Histopathology **16:**271-277, 1990.

1294 Hashimoto H, Tsuneyoshi M, Daimaru Y, Enjoji M: Extraskeletal Ewing's sarcoma. A clinicopathologic and electron microscopic analysis of 8 cases. Acta Pathol Jpn **35:**1087-1098, 1985.

1295 Jürgens H, Bier V, Harms D, Beck J, Brandeis W, Etspüler G, Gadner H, Schmidt D, Treuner J, Winkler K, Göbel U: Malignant peripheral neuroectodermal tumors. A retrospective analysis of 42 patients. Cancer **61:**349-357, 1988.

1296 Kawaguchi K, Koike M: Neuron-specific enolase and leu-7 immunoreactive small round-cell neoplasm. The relationship to Ewing's sarcoma in bone and soft tissue. Am J Clin Pathol **86:**79-83, 1986.

1297 Ladanyi M, Heinemann FS, Huvos AG, Rao PH, Chen QG, Jhanwar SC: Neural differentiation in small round cell tumors of bone and soft tissue with the translocation t(11; 22)(q24; q12). An immunohistochemical study of 11 cases. Hum Pathol **21:**1245-1251, 1990.

1298 Ladanyi M, Lewis R, Garin-Chesa P, Rettig WJ, Huvos AG, Healey JH, Jhanwar SC: EWS rearrangement in Ewing's sarcoma and peripheral neuroectodermal tumor. Molecular detection and correlation with cytogenetic analysis and MIC2 expression. Diagn Mol Pathol 2:141-146, 1993.

1299 Linnoila RI, Tsokos M, Triche TJ, Marangos PJ, Chandra RS: Evidence for neural origin and PAS-positive variants of the malignant small cell tumor of thoracopulmonary region ("Askin tumor"). Am J Surg Pathol 10:124-133, 1986.

1300 Navarro S, Cavazzana AO, Llombart-Bosch A, Triche TJ: Comparison of Ewing's sarcoma of bone and peripheral neuroepithelioma. An immunocytochemical and ultrastructural analysis of two primitive neuroectodermal neoplasms. Arch Pathol Lab Med 118:608-615, 1994.

1301 Pagani A, Fischer-Colbrie R, Sanfilippo B, Winkler H, Cerrato M, Bussolati G: Secretogranin II expression in Ewing's sarcomas and primitive neuroectodermal tumors. Diagn Mol Pathol 1:165-172, 1992.

1302 Rud NP, Reiman HM, Pritchard DJ, Frassica FJ, Smithson WA: Extraosseous Ewing's sarcoma. A study of 42 cases. Cancer 64:1548-1553, 1989.

1303 Schmidt D, Harms D, Burdach S: Malignant peripheral neuroectodermal tumours of childhood and adolescence. Virchows Arch [A] 406:351-365, 1985.

1304 Schmidt D, Herrmann C, Jurgens H, Harms D: Malignant peripheral neuroectodermal tumor and its necessary distinction from Ewing's sarcoma. A report from the Kiel Pediatric Tumor Registry. Cancer 68:2251-2259, 1991.

1305 Selleri L, Hermanson GG, Eubanks JH, Lewis KA, Evans GA: Molecular localization of the t(11; 22)(q24; q12) translocation of Ewing sarcoma by chromosomal in situ suppression hybridization. Proc Natl Acad Sci USA 88:887-891, 1991.

1306 Shimada H, Newton WA Jr, Soule EH, Qualman SJ, Aoyama C, Maurer HM: Pathologic features of extraosseous Ewing's sarcoma. A report from the Intergroup Rhabdomyosarcoma Study. Hum Pathol 19:442-453, 1988.

1307 Shishikura A, Ushigome S, Shimoda T: Primitive neuroectodermal tumors of bone and soft tissue. Histological subclassification and clinicopathologic correlations. Acta Pathol Jpn 43:176-186, 1993.

1308 Sorensen P, Liu X, Delattre O, Rowland J, Biggs C, Thomas G, Triche T: Reverse transcriptase PCR amplification of EWS/FLI-1 fusion transcripts as a diagnostic test for peripheral primitive neuroectodermal tumors of childhood. Diagn Mol Pathol 2:147-157, 1993.

1309 Soule EH, Newton W Jr, Moon TE, Tefft M: Extraskeletal Ewing's sarcoma—a preliminary review of 26 cases encountered in the intergroup rhabdomyosarcoma study. Cancer 42:259-264, 1978.

1310 Stevenson AJ, Chatten J, Bertoni F, Miettinen M: CD99 (p30/32MIC2) neuroectodermal/Ewing's sarcoma antigen as an immunohistochemical marker. Review of more than 600 tumors and the literature experience. Appl Immunohistochem 2:231-240, 1994.

1311 Triche TJ, Askin FB, Kissane JM: Neuroblastoma, Ewing's sarcoma, and the differential diagnosis of small-, round-, blue-cell tumors. In Finegold M, ed: Pathology of neoplasia in children and adolescents, vol 18. Philadelphia, 1986, WB Saunders, p. 145.

1312 Turc-Carel C, Philip I, Berger MP, Philip T, Lenoir GM: Chromosome study of Ewing's sarcoma (ES) cell lines. Consistency of a reciprocal translocation t(11;22)(q24;=-q12). Cancer Genet Cytogenet 12:1-12, 1984.

1313 Ushigome S, Shimoda T, Nikaido T, Nakamori K, Miyazawa Y, Shishikura A, Takakuwa T, Ubayama Y, Spjut HJ: Primitive neuroectodermal tumors of bone and soft tissue. With reference to histologic differentiation in primary or metastatic foci. Acta Pathol Jpn 42:483-493, 1992.

1314 Variend S: Small cell tumours in childhood. A review. J Pathol 145:1-25, 1985.

1315 Weidner N, Tjoe J: Immunohistochemical profile of monoclonal antibody O13. Antibody that recognizes glycoprotein p30/32MIC2 and is useful in diagnosing Ewing's sarcoma and peripheral neuroepithelioma. Am J Surg Pathol 18:486-494, 1994.

1316 Wigger HJ, Salazar GH, Blane WA: Extraskeletal Ewing sarcoma. An ultrastructural study. Arch Pathol Lab Med 101:446-449, 1977.

1317 Yunis EJ: Ewing's sarcoma and related small round cell neoplasms in children. Am J Surg Pathol 10(Suppl 1):54-62, 1986.

Rhabdoid tumor

1318 Frierson HF, Mills SE, Innes DJ Jr: Malignant rhabdoid tumor of the pelvis. Cancer 55:1963-1967, 1985.

1319 Gururangan S, Bowman LC, Parham DM, Wilimas JA, Rao B, Pratt CB, Douglass EC: Primary extracranial rhabdoid tumors. Clinicopathologic features and response to ifosfamide. Cancer 71:2653-2659, 1993.

1320 Kent AL, Mahoney DH Jr, Gresik MV, Steuber CP, Fernbach DJ: Malignant rhabdoid tumor of the extremity. Cancer 60:1056-1059, 1987.

1321 Kodet R, Newton WA Jr, Sachs N, Hamoudi AB, Raney RB, Asmar L, Gehan EA: Rhabdoid tumors of soft tissues. A clinicopathologic study of 26 cases enrolled on the Intergroup Rhabdomyosarcoma Study. Hum Pathol 22:674-684, 1991.

1322 Parham DM, Weeks DA, Beckwith JB: The clinicopathologic spectrum of putative extrarenal rhabdoid tumors. An analysis of 42 cases studied with immunohistochemistry or electron microscopy. Am J Surg Pathol 18:1010-1029, 1994.

1323 Schmidt D, Leuschner I, Harms D, Sprenger E, Schafer HJ: Malignant rhabdoid tumor. A morphological and flow cytometric study. Pathol Res Pract 184:202-210, 1989.

1324 Sotelo-Avila C, Gonzalez-Crussi F, De Mello D, Vogler C, Gooch WM, Gale G, Pena R: Renal and extrarenal rhabdoid tumors in children. A clinicopathologic study of 14 patients. Semin Diagn Pathol 3:151-163, 1986.

1325 Tsokos M, Kouraklis G, Chandra RS, Bhagavan BS, Triche TJ: Malignant rhabdoid tumor of the kidney and soft tissues. Evidence for a diverse morphological and immunocytochemical phenotype. Arch Pathol Lab Med 113:115-120, 1989.

1326 Tsuneyoshi M, Daimaru Y, Hashimoto H, Enjoji M: Malignant soft tissue neoplasms with the histologic features of renal rhabdoid tumors. An ultrastructural and immunohistochemical study. Hum Pathol 16:1235-1242, 1985.

1327 Weeks DA, Beckwith JB, Mierau GW: Rhabdoid tumor. An entity or a phenotype? Arch Pathol Lab Med 113:113-114, 1989.

1327a Wick MR, Ritter JH, Dehner LP: Malignant rhabdoid tumors. A clinicopathologic review and conceptual discussion. Semin Diagn Pathol 12:233-248, 1995.

Phosphaturic mesenchymal tumor

1328 Cai Q, Hodgson SF, Kao PC, Lennon VA, Klee GG, Zinsmeister AR, Kumar R: Brief report. Inhibition of renal phosphate transport by a tumor product in a patient with oncogenic osteomalacia. N Engl J Med 330:1645-1649, 1994.

1329 Weidner N: Review and update. Oncogenic osteomalacia-rickets. Ultrastruct Pathol 15:317-333, 1991.

1330 Weidner N, Bar RS, Weiss D, Strottmann MP: Neoplastic pathology of oncogenic osteomalacia/rickets. Cancer 55:1691-1705, 1985.

1331 Weidner N, Santa Cruz D: Phosphaturic mesenchymal tumors. A polymorphous group causing osteomalacia or rickets. Cancer 59:1442-1454, 1987.

Metastatic carcinoma

1332 Alexiou G, Papadopoulou-Alexiou M, Karakousis CP: Renal cell carcinoma presenting as skeletal muscle mass. J Surg Oncol 27:23-25, 1984.

Other tumorlike conditions

1333 Cabanne F, Chapuis JL, Duperrat B, Putelat R: L'infiltration cutanée par la polyvinylpyrrolidone. Ann Anat Pathol 11:385-396, 1966.

1334 Coleman WR, Homer RS, Kaplan RP: Branchial cleft heterotopia of the lower neck. J Cutan Pathol 16:353-358, 1989.

1335 Fetsch JF, Montgomery EA, Meis JM: Calcifying fibrous pseudotumor. Am J Surg Pathol 17:502-508, 1993.

1336 Fraga S, Helwig EB, Rosen SM: Bronchogenic cysts in the skin and subcutaneous tissue. Am J Clin Pathol 56:230-238, 1971.

1337 Harkness JW, Peters HJ: Tumoral calcinosis, a report of six cases. J Bone Joint Surg (Am) 49:721-731, 1967.

1338 Hizawa K, Inaba H, Nakanishi S, Otsuka H, Izumi K: Subcutaneous pseudosarcomatous polyvinylpyrrolidone granuloma. Am J Surg Pathol 8:393-398, 1984.

1339 Krishnan J, Chu WS, Elrod JP, Frizzera G: Tumoral presentation of amyloidosis (amyloidomas) in soft tissues. A report of 14 cases. Am J Clin Pathol 100:135-144, 1993.

1340 Kuo T-T, Hsueh S: Mucicarminophilic histiocytosis. A polyvinylpyrrolidone (PVP) storage disease simulating signet-ring cell carcinoma. Am J Surg Pathol 8:419-428, 1984.

1341 Lyles KW, Burkes EJ, Ellis GJ, Lucas EJ, Dolan EA, Drezner MK: Genetic transmission of tumoral calcinosis. Autosomal dominant with variable clinical expressivity. J Clin Endocrinol Metab 60:1093-1096, 1985.

1342 Montgomery E, Meis J, Ramos A, Frisman D, Mertz K: Clear cell sarcoma of tendons and aponeuroses. A clinicopathologic study of 58 cases with analysis of prognostic factors. Int J Surg Pathol 1:89-100, 1993.

1343 Rodriguez-Peralto JL, Lopez-Barea F, Sanchez-Herrera S, Atienza M: Primary aneurysmal cyst of soft tissues (extraosseous aneurysmal cyst). Am J Surg Pathol 18:632-636, 1994.

1344 Shareef DS, Salm R: Ectopic vestigial lesions of the neck and shoulders. J Clin Pathol 34:1155-1162, 1981.

1345 Sleater J, Mullins D: Subcutaneous Castleman's disease of the wrist. Am J Dermatopathol 17:174-178, 1995.

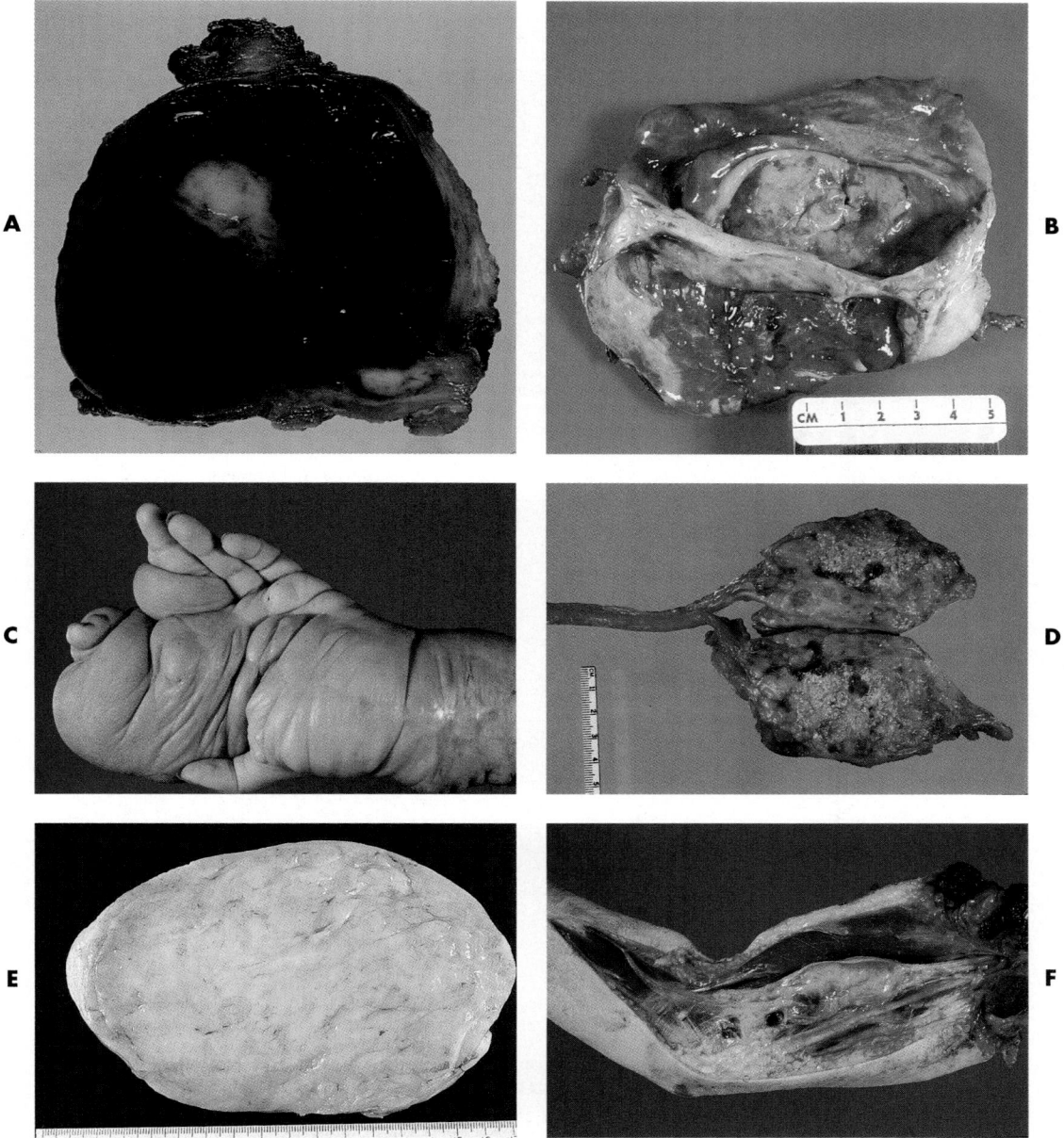

Plate XIX A, Angiomatoid malignant fibrous histiocytoma. A small solid focus of white tumor is seen within a large hemorrhage cyst. B, Schwannoma of the mediastinum that has undergone marked cystic degeneration (so-called ancient
schwannoma). C, Marked deformation of distal upper extremity by diffuse neurofibromatosis. This patient developed a
malignant peripheral nerve sheath tumor. D, Malignant peripheral nerve sheath tumor producing a characteristic fusiform
expansion of the sciatic nerve. Foci of necrosis and hemorrhage are present. E, Atypical lipomatous tumor. The neoplasm
is well circumscribed and not very different from an ordinary lipoma. F, Leiomyosarcoma of soft tissues of arm. The fusiform
shape of the tumor cell is due to the fact that the tumor is following the course of the large blood vessels from which it arose.
(A courtesy Dr. Hector Rodriguez-Martinez, Mexico City.)

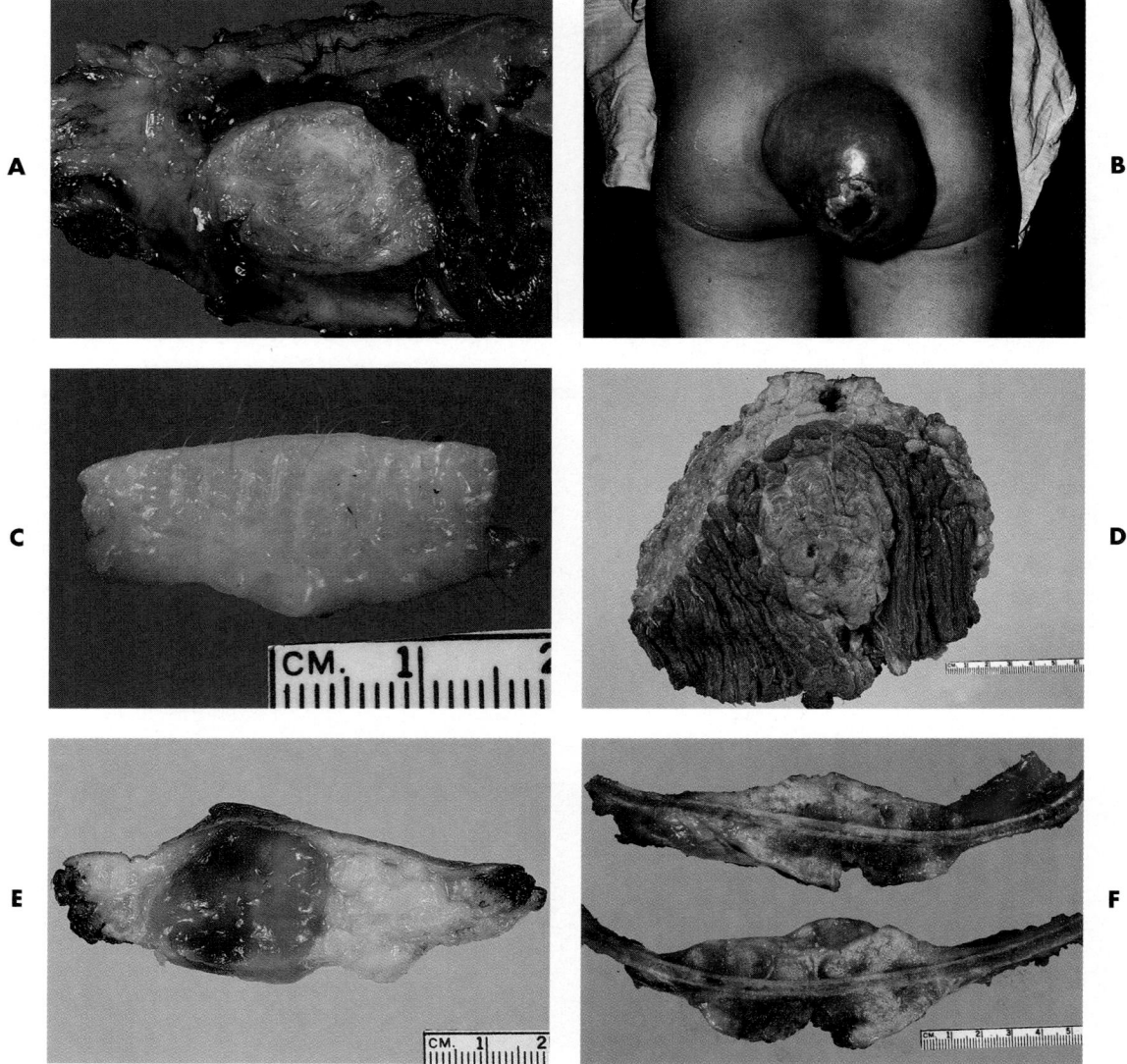

Plate XX **A,** Extraskeletal osteosarcoma. Neoplasm is embedded within skeletal muscle and is relatively well circumscribed. **B,** Myxopapillary ependymoma of the sacrococcygeal region resulting in a huge protruding mass that is focally ulcerated. **C,** Granular cell tumor of skin. There is an ill-defined permeation of the dermis by whitish tissue. **D,** Alveolar soft-part sarcoma. The tumor is multinodular, relatively well circumscribed, and embedded within skeletal muscle. **E,** Malignant giant cell tumor of soft parts. The tumor is relatively well circumscribed, bulges on the cut surface, and is focally hemorrhagic. **F,** Ewing's sarcoma/PNET of thoracopulmonary region. The tumor is present on both sides of the rib, but the bone was only minimally involved. (**B** courtesy Dr. Juan Josè Segura, San Josè, Costa Rica.)

26 Peritoneum, retroperitoneum, and related structures

Peritoneum
NORMAL ANATOMY

The peritoneal cavity is lined by mesodermally derived tissues consisting of a layer of surface mesothelium resting on vascularized subserosal tissue and separated from it by a continuous basal lamina. It is characterized ultrastructurally by the presence of apical tight junctions, desmosomes, surface microvilli, and tonofilaments. Immunohistochemically, it exhibits strong reactivity to cytokeratin, epithelial membrane antigen (EMA), and basal lamina components. It is negative for CEA, Leu-M1, and B72.3. The surprising fact that normal mesothelium expresses parathyroid hormone–like peptide activity has been recently reported.[2] Just as interesting is the fact that developing mesothelium in the embryo exhibits transient immunoreactivity for desmin before switching to its adult keratin-based intermediate filament profile.

The resting subserosal cells have the overall structure of fibroblasts, are negative for keratin, and express vimentin.[1] These cells are sometimes referred to as "multipotential subserosal cells" because they are thought to have the capacity to serve as replicative cells that can differentiate into surface mesothelium. In females, these subserosal cells can be conspicuous, especially in the pelvic parietal peritoneum and on the bladder dome. They are sensitive to sex hormones and are probably the progenitors of lesions such as endometriosis, endosalpingiosis, ectopic decidual reaction, leiomyomatosis peritonealis disseminata, and tumors of ovarian or uterine type[3] (see p. 2146). This large group of peritoneal disorders related to the female genital tract is also discussed in Chapter 19, Ovary and Uterine corpus.

Structures or regions topographically related to the peritoneum and retroperitoneum are the omentum, mesentery, hernia sacs, umbilicus, and sacrococcygeal region. Since an overlapping of pathologic processes exists among all of them, they are discussed in this chapter, with appropriate references to other sections of the text when indicated.

INFLAMMATION

Chemical peritonitis can be caused by bile, pancreatic juice, gastric juice, meconium, and barium sulfate.[11] Barium peritonitis has been seen following perforation of large bowel occurring during the course of radiographic examinations performed because of obstruction[14]; it is the result of the bacteria that accompany the contrast material.

Extravasation of *bile* as a result of trauma or disease of the gallbladder, bile ducts, or duodenum causes an acute or subacute peritonitis that is initially limited to the upper quadrant of the abdomen.[7] *Gastric juice* produces a severe peritoneal reaction because of its hydrochloric acid content, although it may be bacteriologically sterile. The release of *pancreatic juice* causes fat necrosis. The formation of calcium salts in large areas of fat necrosis may cause hypocalcemia.

Bacterial peritonitis may be either primary or secondary. The *primary* form usually is caused by streptococci and is seen more commonly in children (particularly in those affected by the nephrotic syndrome). Adult patients with ascites secondary to liver disease are also susceptible. This form of peritonitis tends to produce marked constitutional symptoms with minimal localizing findings. Aspiration of intra-abdominal fluid discloses an inflammatory exudate containing only a single type of organism. Large amounts of extracellular fluid are lost into the exudate, equivalent to those of a burn covering one half to three fourths of the cutaneous surface.[6]

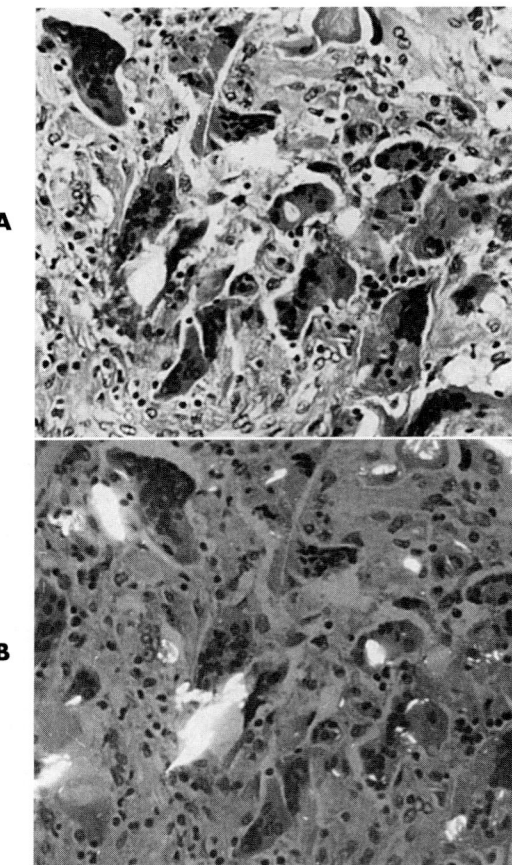

Fig. 26-1 Histologic appearance of talc granuloma without **(A)** and with **(B)** polarized light. With latter, talc crystals can be seen vividly.

Perforation of a viscus such as the colon produces *secondary* peritonitis. If the fluid is aspirated, a mixture of bacterial flora rather than a single organism is found. *Tuberculous peritonitis* may occur with few constitutional symptoms, despite extensive involvement of the peritoneum.[4,9,10,17] In a review of forty-seven cases, Singh et al.[16] found radiographic evidence of pulmonary parenchymal lesions in only 6% of the cases. The search for acid-fast organisms on a direct smear of ascitic fluid is often unrewarding. The best diagnostic methods are culture of the fluid and percutaneous biopsy of the peritoneum.[12,13] Singh et al.[16] found the latter to be useful in 64% of their cases. Chemotherapy is the treatment of choice; surgery is reserved for those cases associated with enteritis leading to bowel obstruction, perforation, fistula, or a mass that does not resolve with drug therapy.[15] Other specific forms of peritonitis are *coccidioidomycosis* and *actinomycosis*.[5] Exceptionally, *Oxyuris vermicularis* may escape from the appendix or other portions of the gastrointestinal tract into the peritoneal cavity and elicit the formation of granulomas.[18]

Meconium peritonitis is the result of perforation of the small bowel during intrauterine life. It may present in infants as intestinal obstruction requiring surgical intervention. With healing, only scattered calcific foci remain. These can be located in the main peritoneal cavity, inguinal region, or scrotum; the latter can simulate clinically a testicular tumor.[8]

Vernix caseosa peritonitis represents a rare complication of Cesarean section, and it has distinctive microscopic features.[8a]

ADHESIONS

Adhesions, with the possibility of subsequent intestinal obstruction, follow all intra-abdominal operations. They can be minimized by careful handling of tissues, reperitonealization where feasible, and removal of intraperitoneal blood clots. Ryan et al.[24] showed in an experimental model that drying of the serosa plus bleeding consistently resulted in the formation of adhesions. There is good experimental evidence to suggest that formation of peritoneal adhesions is related to a local depression of peritoneal plasminogen activator, which is the principal peritoneal fibrin-clearing system known.[20]

Innumerable agents, including sodium citrate, heparin, olive oil, liquid paraffin, ACTH, cortisone, pepsin, fibrinolysin, and amniotic fluid, have been used to prevent adhesions, but none has accomplished this goal. Adhesions become collagenous and strong as the cellularity of their fibrous tissue decreases with maturation. Postoperative adhesions are the most frequent cause of intestinal obstruction today.

Extensive peritoneal fibrosis *(sclerosing* or *fibrosing peritonitis)* also has been described as a reaction to asbestos, to silica in drug abusers,[22] in patients with the carcinoid syndrome, in women with luteinized thecomas and related proliferative stromal lesions of the ovary,[23] and as a complication of the administration of beta-adrenergic–blocking drugs.[21] In many instances, the etiologic agent cannot be identified; some of these "idiopathic" cases are probably pathogenetically related to mesenteric panniculitis and—as such—are examples of the inflammatory fibrosclerosis group of diseases[19] (see p. 2155).

REACTION TO FOREIGN MATERIALS

The peritoneum reacts briskly to foreign substances. One of the better known peritoneal reactions to foreign material is "talc powder granuloma," which is secondary to the talc (hydrated magnesium silicate) used in the past on surgical gloves. Spillage of this material into the peritoneal cavity at surgery results in nodules that can be mistaken grossly for tuberculosis or metastatic carcinoma.[33] Microscopically, they are formed by foreign body granulomas containing birefringent crystals. The latter are made apparent with polarizing lenses or simply by lowering the condenser of the microscope (Fig. 26-1).

Talc used for surgical gloves has long been recognized as a hazard and has been replaced by other substances, such as modified starch. Although these materials elicit a lesser degree of reaction, intraperitoneal granulomas may still develop,[34,39] usually between 10 days and 4 weeks after a laparotomy. These usually have the appearance of foreign-body granulomas but sometimes exhibit tuberculoid features with caseum-like necrosis.[38] At reoperation, the findings are ascites, miliary peritoneal nodules, serosal inflammation, and adhesions. The gross appearance can closely simulate metastatic carcinoma, tuberculosis, or Crohn's disease. The nature of the granulomas can be identified by the presence of granules that are PAS-positive and birefringent (with a

Maltese cross pattern) within the cytoplasm of histiocytes and foreign body giant cells.[30,32] Levison et al.[36] have pointed out that the Maltese cross pattern is characteristic of corn starch, whereas other types of starch particles may have different shapes, sizes, and surface markings.[36] The diagnosis may be suspected through the finding of starch granules in the aspirated peritoneal fluid. Fortunately, the disease is usually self-limited.

Another source of surgical contamination is the cellulose fibers derived from disposable surgical gowns and drapes.[40] Sometimes the starch found in peritoneal granulomas does not originate in surgical gloves but from food starch that has gained its access to the peritoneal cavity through perforation of the bowel[31] or from starch contained in contraceptive devices.[36]

Mineral oil or paraffin placed in the peritoneal cavity years ago to prevent adhesions was responsible for the formation of nodules that could be grossly mistaken for metastatic carcinoma.[37] Microscopically, these nodules exhibit foreign body giant cells, chronic inflammation, and foamy macrophages. Similar changes follow rupture of a cystic teratoma of the ovary, in which large amounts of oily material cause a profound nodular peritoneal reaction.[25]

Keratin from endometrioid adenocarcinomas with squamous differentiation (adenoacanthomas) of the endometrium, ovary, or both can detach from the main tumor, reach the peritoneal cavity (through the fallopian tube in the case of uterine tumors), and elicit a brisk foreign body–type granulomatous reaction. The presence of these keratin granulomas has no prognostic significance and should not be equated with the presence of viable tumor implants.[27,35]

Peritoneal endometriosis may result in the formation of *necrotic pseudoxanthomatous nodules*; this may follow diathermy ablation of the lesion, but it may also be seen spontaneously.[28,29]

Although not a foreign body, one could mention here the curious phenomenon of implantation of normal splenic tissue in the peritoneal cavity following traumatic rupture of the spleen, a process known as *splenosis*[26] (see Chapter 22).

CYSTS AND LOOSE BODIES

Pseudocysts of the peritoneal cavity (lacking a mesothelial or epithelial lining) may follow inflammatory processes such as perforated ulcerative colitis or perforated appendicitis.

Solitary cysts varying in size from 1 to 6 cm can be found incidentally within the peritoneal cavity, either attached to the wall or lying loose in the lower pelvis. They have a translucent wall, watery fluid in the lumen, and a lining composed of one or more layers of mesothelial cells[45] (Fig. 26-2). They probably represent acquired inclusion cysts related to chronic inflammation. A case of multilocular *melanotic* peritoneal cyst has been described.[42]

A probably related condition has been designated *cystic* or *multicystic benign mesothelioma*.[44,47,48,53] This process nearly always occurs in the pelvis of adult females, the average age at diagnosis being around 35 years. It has also been described involving most of the peritoneum, and a few cases have been seen in males. Often there is a history of previous pelvic surgery, endometriosis, or pelvic inflammatory disease. This entity may result in pelvic pain, present clinically

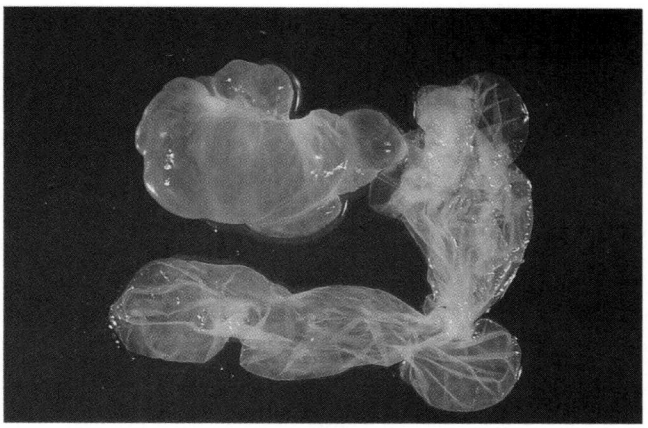

Fig. 26-2 Gross appearance of peritoneal cysts. They have a thin, translucent wall and contain a clear fluid. (Courtesy Dr. Juan Jose Segura, San Jose, Costa Rica.)

as a mass, or be found incidentally at laparotomy (often at the time of a tubal ligation) or within a hernia sac. Grossly, multiple cysts are present, measuring up to 15 cm or more in diameter, attached to or engulfing pelvic organs (Fig. 26-4, *A*). Microscopically, the cysts are lined by flattened or cuboidal mesothelial cells (Fig. 26-4, *B*). When flat, the cells closely simulate the appearance of endothelial cells. They react immunohistochemically for keratin; are negative for FVIII-related antigen and other endothelial markers; and exhibit desmosomes, tonofibrils, and slender microvilli on ultrastructural examination.[48,52] The wall, which is devoid of smooth muscle, usually shows foci of chronic inflammation, hemorrhage, and fibrin deposition. Sometimes the reactive mesothelial proliferation in the wall of these cysts is prominent enough to simulate a malignancy.[46]

The natural history of this disorder is characterized by a great tendency to local recurrence. This fact, plus the tumor-like appearance that these lesions exhibit grossly, is responsible for the assumption that they represent benign mesotheliomas. We agree with Ross et al.[50] that they probably are instead *multiple peritoneal inclusion cysts* forming as a result of peritoneal reactive proliferation. Their tendency for recurrence can be explained by persistence of the original inciting factor. The main differential diagnosis is with cystic lymphangioma[41] (see pp. 2152, 2153, and 2159).

Cysts of müllerian origin can occur between the bladder and rectum in the true pelvis of males.[43] They result from persistence of müllerian duct derivatives and are usually lined by fallopian tube–type epithelium.[51] They have also been described in the mesentery (see p. 2153). Occasionally, they may be the site of malignant transformation.[49]

Appendix epiploica may twist, undergo massive fat necrosis, and present as a sclerocalcified nodule either attached to its original site or free-floating in the abdominal cavity[54] (Fig. 26-3, *A* and *B*).

HYPERPLASIA AND METAPLASIA

The mesothelial lining surface has a great capacity to undergo florid hyperplastic changes when irritated. This

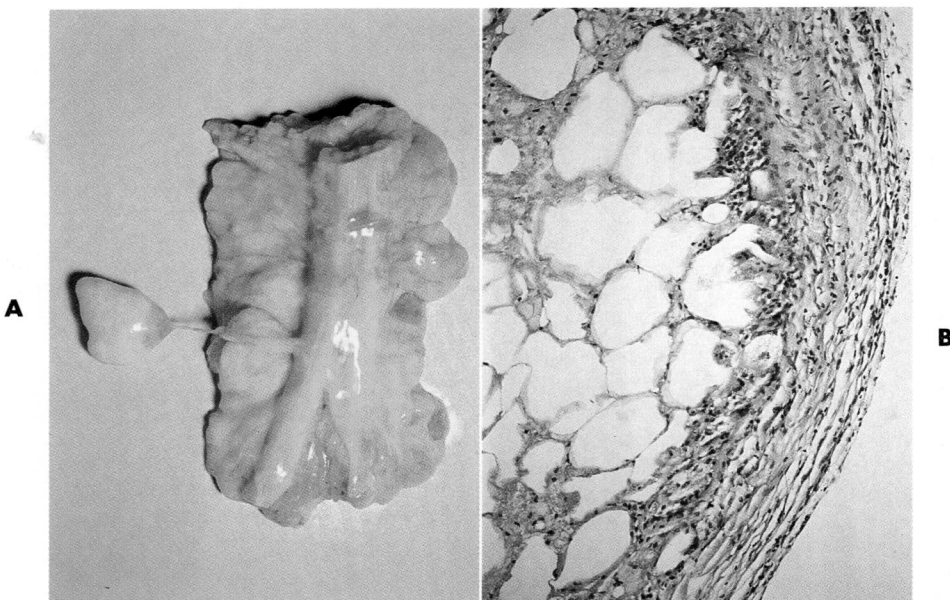

Fig. 26-3 Twisted appendix epiploica. **A,** Gross appearance. **B,** Microscopic appearance, showing inflammatory reaction to fat necrosis.

hyperplasia can occur in a diffuse fashion throughout the peritoneal cavity in cases of liver cirrhosis, collagen vascular diseases (such as lupus erythematosus), and viral infections. Actually, mesothelial hyperplasia may supervene in any long-standing effusion regardless of its cause. It can also occur in a localized fashion as a response to injury. Hernia sacs can exhibit florid foci of *nodular mesothelial hyperplasia* following incarceration or some other mechanical insult; this is particularly common in children and may simulate malignancy.[60] A similar change may occur in the serosa of an acutely inflamed appendix or a fallopian tube following rupture of an ectopic pregnancy, simulating implants from a serous papillary tumor of the ovary. The danger of misinterpreting these reactive mesothelial changes as neoplastic is even greater when they develop in association with ovarian neoplasms, sometimes in intimate closeness to them.[56]

Microscopically, these mesothelial hyperplastic changes may appear as papillary projections, solid nests, or tubular structures. They may project on the surface or interact in a complex fashion with the underlying stroma, simulating invasion.[59] Psammoma bodies may be present in the stroma of the papillary formations[60] (Figs. 26-4 and 26-5). The cells may be vacuolated or have an entirely clear cytoplasm[59]; these vacuoles do not stain for mucin or fat.

The differential diagnosis between reactive mesothelial hyperplasia and mesothelioma can be very difficult. Features favoring malignancy are the presence of *grossly visible* nodular or papillary foci, marked nuclear atypia, increase in nucleo-cytoplasmic ratio, and presence of necrosis in the desmoplastic areas.[59] The latter finding is one of the most useful signs, since it is extremely unusual in the reactive processes.

Immunohistochemically, reactive mesothelial cells stain strongly for keratin of various molecular weights; reactive subserosal connective tissue cells retain their expression of vimentin but also acquire immunoreactivity for low-molecular-weight keratin and develop the ultrastructural features of myofibroblasts.[55] Unfortunately, these features are of little practical use in the differential diagnosis with mesothelioma. Instead, immunohistochemistry can be of value in the differential diagnosis between reactive mesothelial hyperplasia and epithelial tumor implants in patients with borderline or malignant ovarian serous neoplasms (see Chapter 19). It has been claimed that morphometric analysis can also aid in this distinction.[58]

Mesothelial cells can also undergo metaplastic changes, the most important being *squamous metaplasia*[57,61] and *müllerian metaplasia*. The latter change is seen almost exclusively in females; predominates in the pelvic region; and is mainly represented by endometriosis, endosalpingiosis, and ectopic decidual reaction.[62] (This is further discussed on p. 2146 and in Chapter 19, Ovary.) Focal *cartilaginous metaplasia* also occurs, but this probably originates from the submesothelial mesenchymal elements rather than the mesothelium itself (Fig. 26-6).

TUMORS
Mesothelioma

The mesotheliomas seen in the peritoneum are qualitatively similar to those occurring in the pleural cavity (see Chapter 7), but the relative proportions among the various types and the criteria used for the differential diagnosis with metastatic carcinoma (ovary and lung, respectively) are somewhat different. Traditionally, peritoneal mesotheliomas

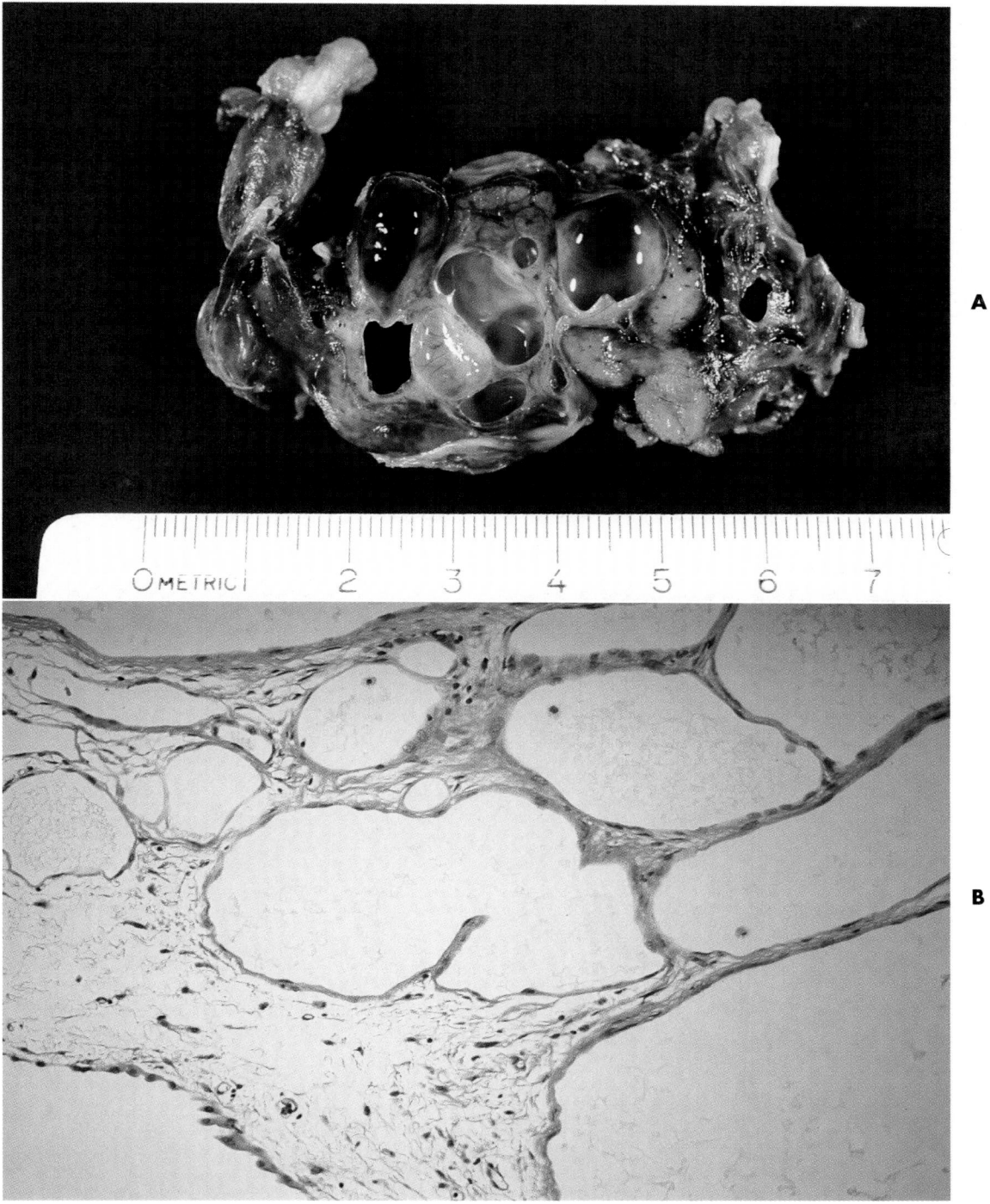

Fig. 26-4 So-called benign multicystic mesothelioma. **A,** Gross appearance. **B,** Microscopic appearance. The flat shape of the mesothelium lining the cyst simulates the appearance of a lymphangioma.

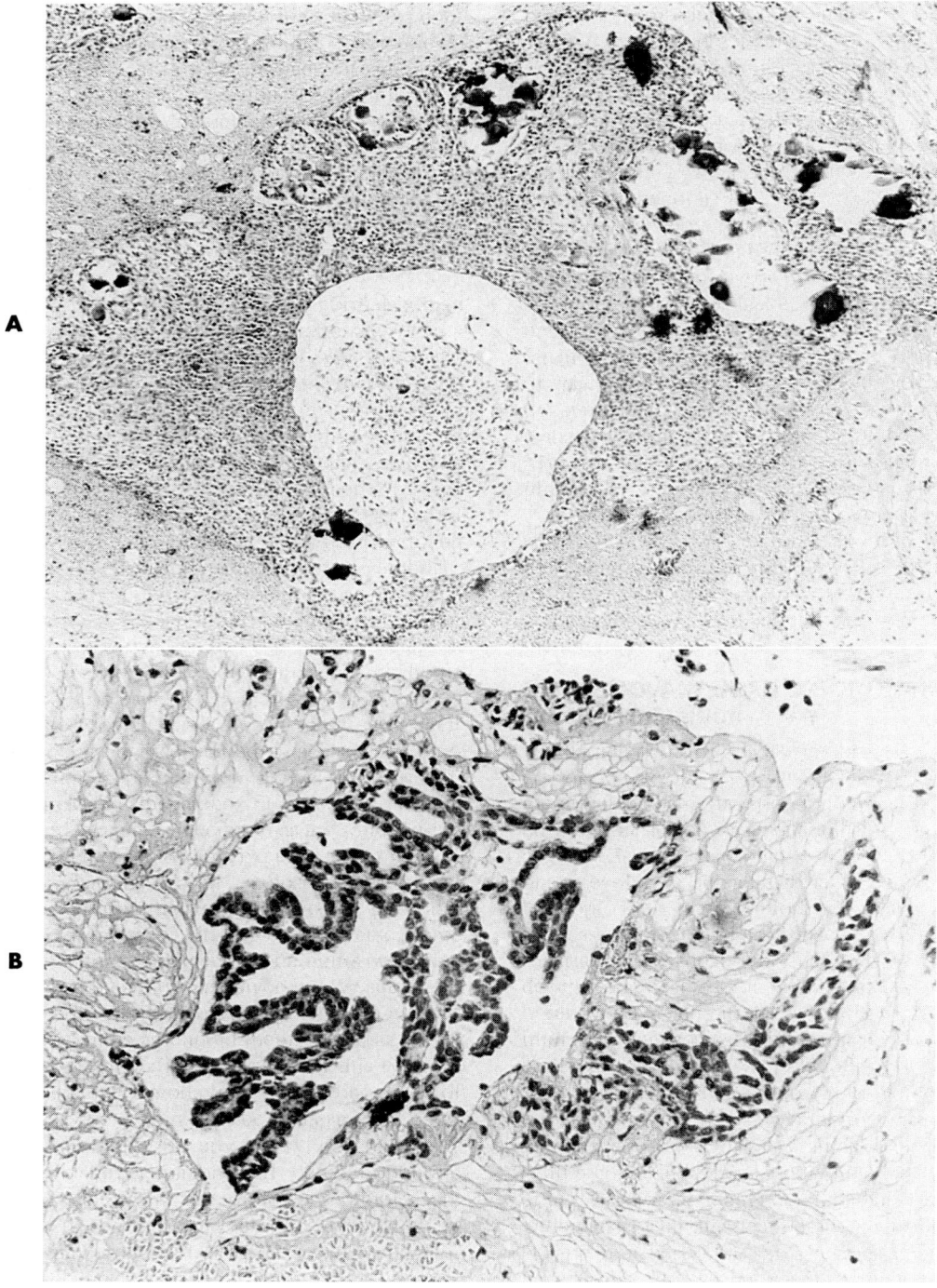

Fig. 26-5 Nodular mesothelial hyperplasia in hernia sac. **A,** Predominantly solid nodule of hyperplastic mesothelial cells lines sac and obliterates lumen. Numerous psammoma bodies are present. **B,** This focus of mesothelial proliferation within sac shows papillary arrangement that may simulate mesothelioma or metastatic ovarian carcinoma.

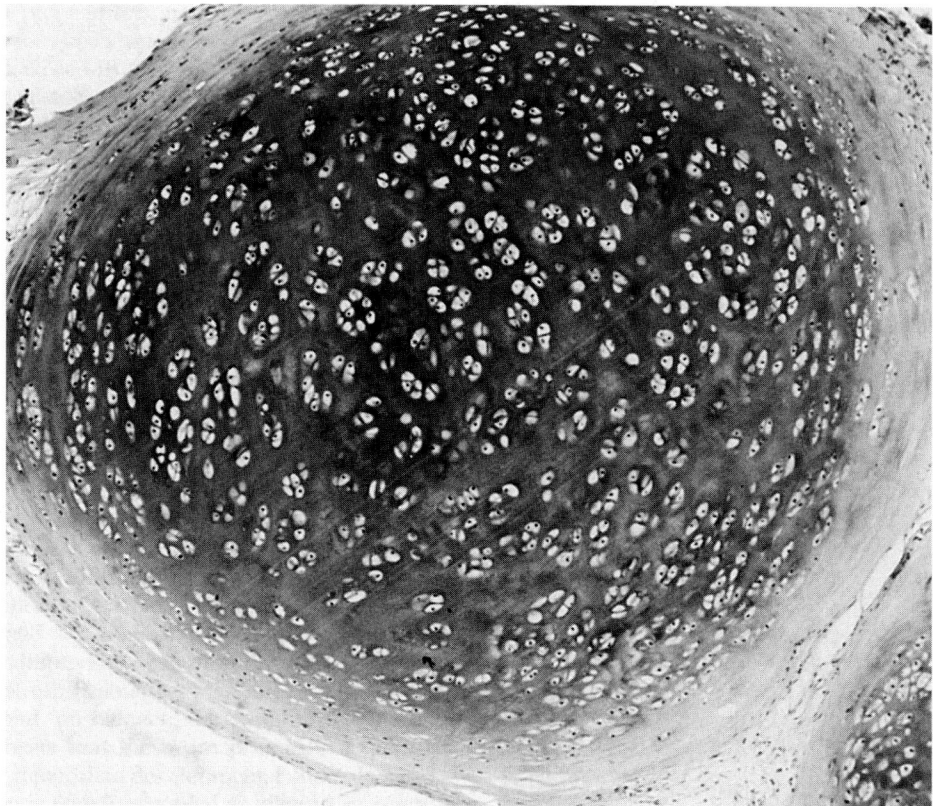

Fig. 26-6 Peritoneal cartilaginous metaplasia. (Slide contributed by Dr. J. Bauer, St. Louis.)

have been divided into epithelial and fibrous, but the latter tumor is no longer considered a type of mesothelioma and is discussed separately (see p. 2146). The majority of true mesotheliomas are either solitary and benign or diffuse and malignant, but exceptions occur in both directions.

Benign mesothelioma

The benign form of mesothelioma usually presents as a solitary small papillary structure resembling grossly and microscopically the appearance of choroid plexus[77] (Fig. 26-7). Most examples are incidental findings at the time of laparotomy. A few are pedunculated and may undergo torsion. We suspect that many of these lesions are reactive (i.e., examples of focal papillary mesothelial hyperplasia) rather than true neoplasms. There is no evidence that they undergo malignant transformation, and they are not related to asbestos exposure.

Daya et al.[75,76] have described a type of *well-differentiated papillary mesothelioma* of the peritoneum that shows a great predilection for females and that is usually multifocal. They pointed out that most of these tumors appeared to be indolent or inactive and recommended a conservative therapeutic approach to them.[75]

Malignant mesothelioma

Most cases of peritoneal malignant mesothelioma occur in individuals past 40 years of age, but they have been described in young adults,[79] children,[65,82,100] and neonates.[94] A definite male predominance has been noted. Their frequency is on the increase.[64] About half of the cases are associated with asbestos exposure[95]; interestingly, peritoneal mesotheliomas are common in patients with heavy asbestos exposure, whereas pleural mesotheliomas predominate in the larger population of transiently exposed individuals. The latency period is 15 years and over.[98] Major asbestos usage in the United States began around 1950 and continued through the 1960s, and therefore it is not unreasonable to expect a further increase in the incidence of this neoplasm. Some peritoneal mesotheliomas have occurred after exposure to Thorotrast[89] and others following repeated mesothelial irritation.[70,92] In some instances, they have been found to coexist with pleural mesotheliomas.

The usual clinical presentation is in the form of recurrent ascites, which may be associated with abdominal cramps and increased abdominal girth. Intermittent partial bowel obstruction is common. Occasionally, the disease may first be manifested in a hernia sac or in the umbilicus.[71,86] In other instances, inguinal or cervical lymphadenopathy resulting from metastatic disease is the first sign of the tumor.[97]

Grossly, peritoneal mesothelioma usually appears as multiple plaques or nodules scattered over the visceral and parietal peritoneum[80,104] (Fig. 26-8). It may be accompanied by dense intraperitoneal adhesions and shortening of the mesentery (Fig. 26-9, *A*). Ascites is almost universally pre-

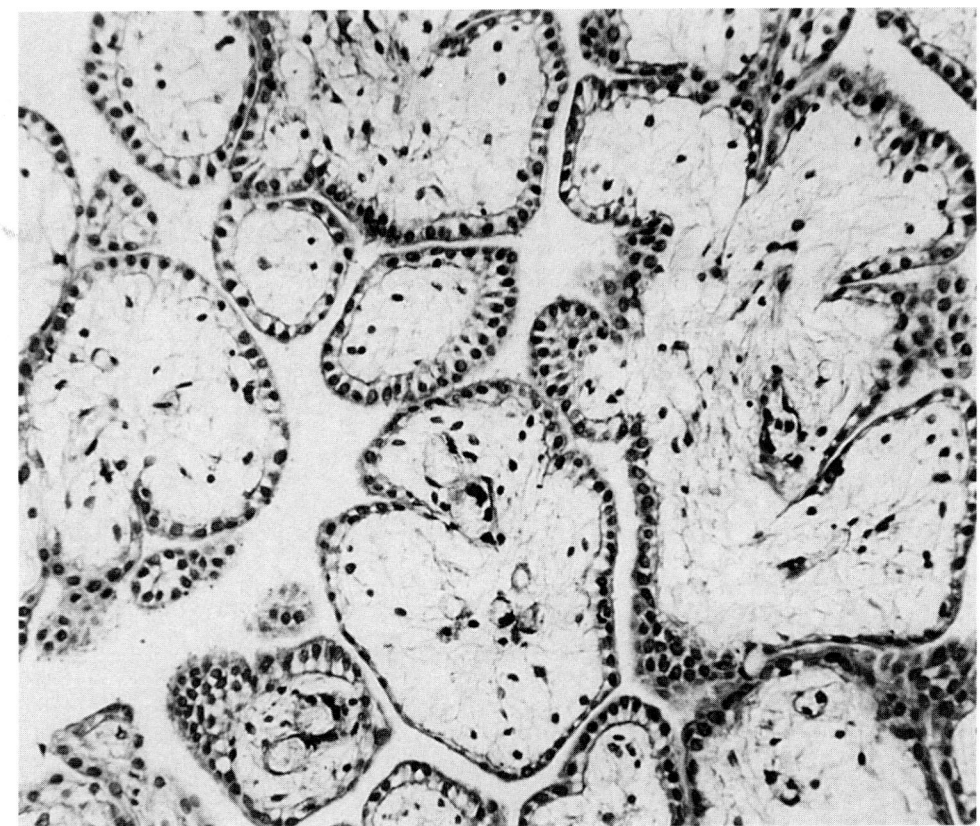

Fig. 26-7 Benign papillary mesothelioma occurring in 41-year-old man. Lesion had been present for at least 3 years. (Slide contributed by Dr. M.J. Zbar, Miami.)

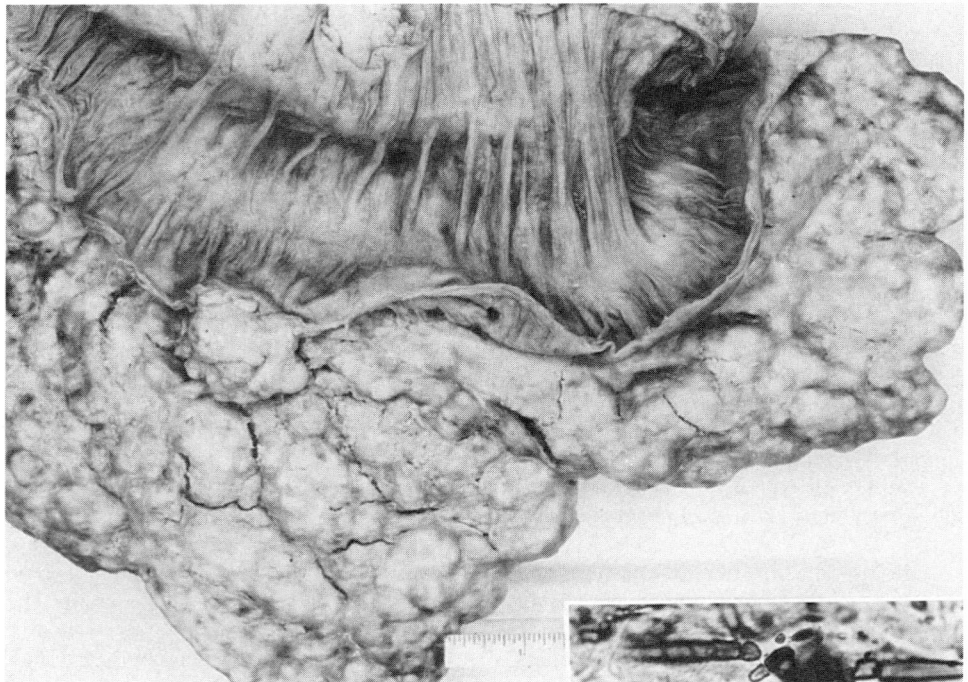

Fig. 26-8 Portion of malignant mesothelioma overlying dilated transverse colon. Lesion occurred in 65-year-old male with no history of industrial exposure to asbestos. In three sections of lower lobe of lung, foci of asbestosis were present with asbestos bodies, fibrosis, and occasional giant cells. There were no asbestos bodies found in upper lobes. **Inset,** Classic asbestos body in lower lobe. Note chair rung appearance. (Courtesy Dr. J.G. Thomson, Cape Town, South Africa.)

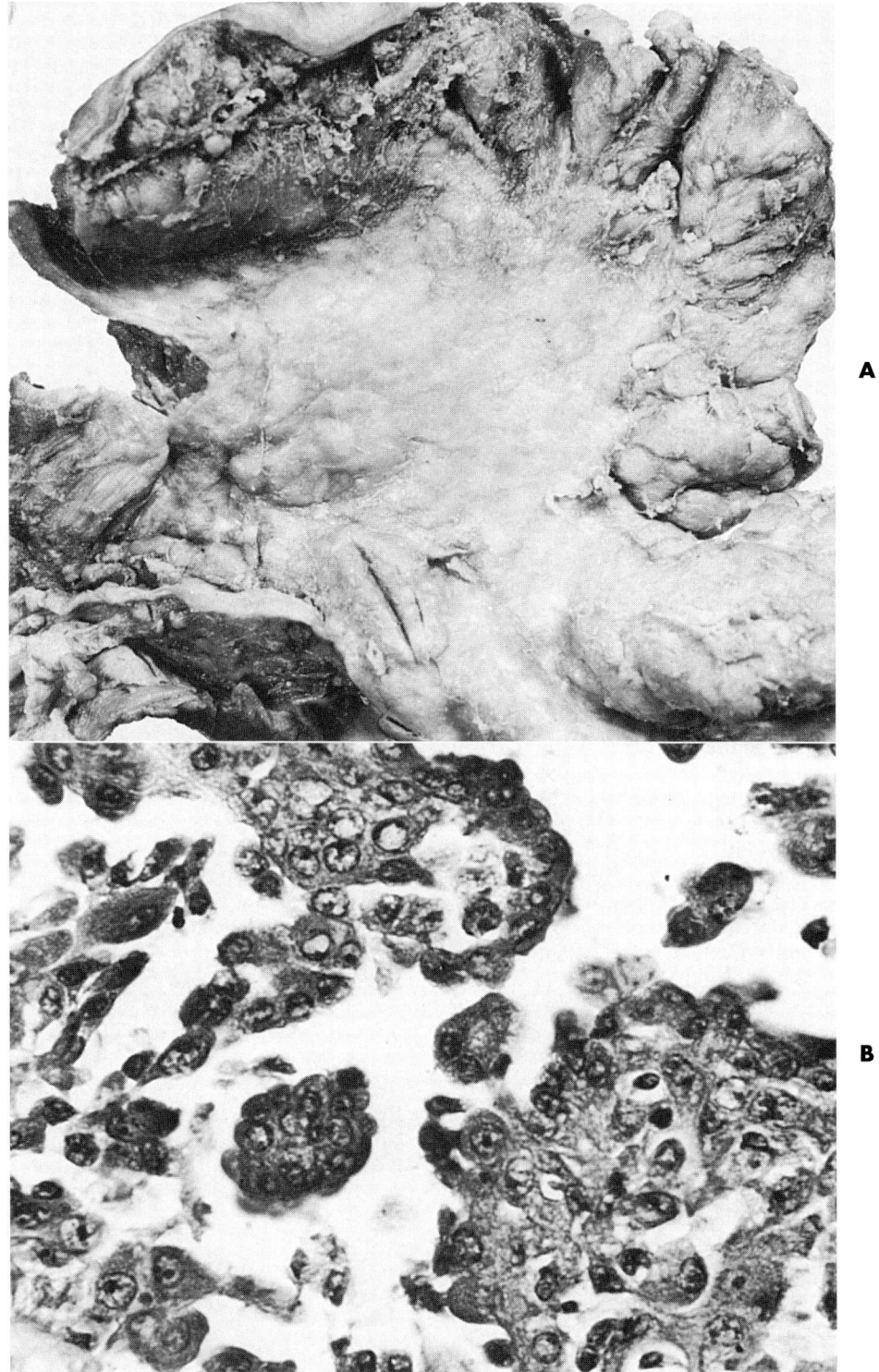

Fig. 26-9 **A,** Malignant mesothelioma that diffusely involved peritoneal cavity. Fibrosis and shortening of mesentery are prominent. **B,** Microscopic appearance of same lesion. Papillary projections are prominent.

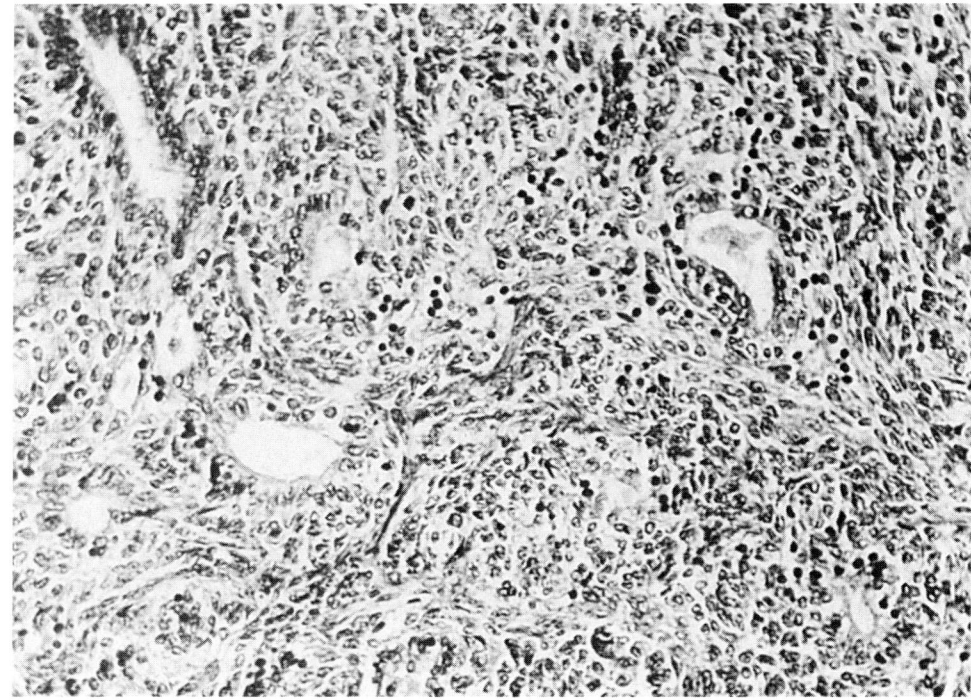

Fig. 26-10 Malignant mesothelioma assuming pattern reminiscent of synovial sarcoma. Note intimate admixture of stromal and glandular components.

sent. Coexisting fibrous pleural plaques are common, more so than with pleural mesotheliomas; sometimes fibrous plaques are also present within the abdominal cavity.[63] Complete obliteration of the peritoneal cavity by tumor may develop. In advanced stages, the tumor may locally invade the intestinal wall, hilum of the spleen and liver, gastric wall, pancreas, bladder, anterior abdominal wall, and retroperitoneum. Metastases to retroperitoneal or pelvic lymph nodes may develop, but metastases to lung or other distant sites are relatively rare. On rare occasions, the tumor presents as an isolated mass; such a lesion is distinguished from benign mesothelioma by virtue of its more solid appearance and the presence of atypia.[74]

The microscopic pattern of malignant mesothelioma is highly variable. The most common arrangement is that of papillae or tubules lined by atypical mesothelial cells, the former having vascularized fibrous cores that may contain psammoma bodies (Fig. 26-9, *B*). In other instances, the mesothelial-like cells alternate with sarcomatoid spindle cells in a biphasic fashion (Fig. 26-10). The individual cells are, in general, fairly uniform, with acidophilic or vacuolated cytoplasm and large vesicular or hyperchromatic nuclei.[68] Sometimes the abundant ground glass cytoplasm and the sharply outlined polygonal shape give the cells a hepatoid or deciduoid appearance; such tumors are more common in young females and are apparently unrelated to asbestos.[91] In some cases, the tumor cells show prominent vacuoles or are entirely clear, as a result of hydropic changes. In other instances, the cells may appear foamy as a result of lipid accumulation; some of these are multinucleated and resem-

ble Touton's giant cells.[84] Mitoses may be difficult to find. Exceptionally, the tumor may exhibit foci of cartilaginous or other types of mesenchymal metaplasia.[101]

Extracellular mucosubstances are often present. These represent acid mucopolysaccharides, since they stain with colloidal iron and Alcian blue, are removed at least partially by hyaluronidase digestion, and are PAS negative. According to Kannerstein et al.,[81] a *definitely positive* diastase-resistant PAS reaction in a poorly differentiated peritoneal malignancy rules out mesothelioma and establishes the diagnosis of metastatic carcinoma.[78] The latter tumor also may contain colloidal iron–positive material, but hyaluronidase digestion would have little effect on the reaction. The detection of high levels of hyaluronic acid by histochemistry or biochemical extraction favors a diagnosis of mesothelioma, but it is not a specific finding.[72] Immunocytochemically, the cells of malignant mesotheliomas are strongly positive for keratin, epithelial membrane antigen, and basement membrane–related proteins (type IV collagen, laminin, and laminin receptors) and are generally negative for CEA, B72.3, and Leu-M1 (and related "myelomonocytic" antigens).[78,79a,96,103] The tumor cells may also exhibit positivity for vimentin[66,73] and occasionally also for actin and desmin;[85] when the latter is the case, the tumors have been referred to as *leiomyoid* mesotheliomas.[90] Some malignant mesotheliomas also express bcl-2 protein.[93]

By electron microscopy, the cells of a well-differentiated mesothelioma exhibit polarity, abundant microvilli covered with fuzzy material, extracellular and intracellular neolumina formation, glycogen granules, junctional structures,

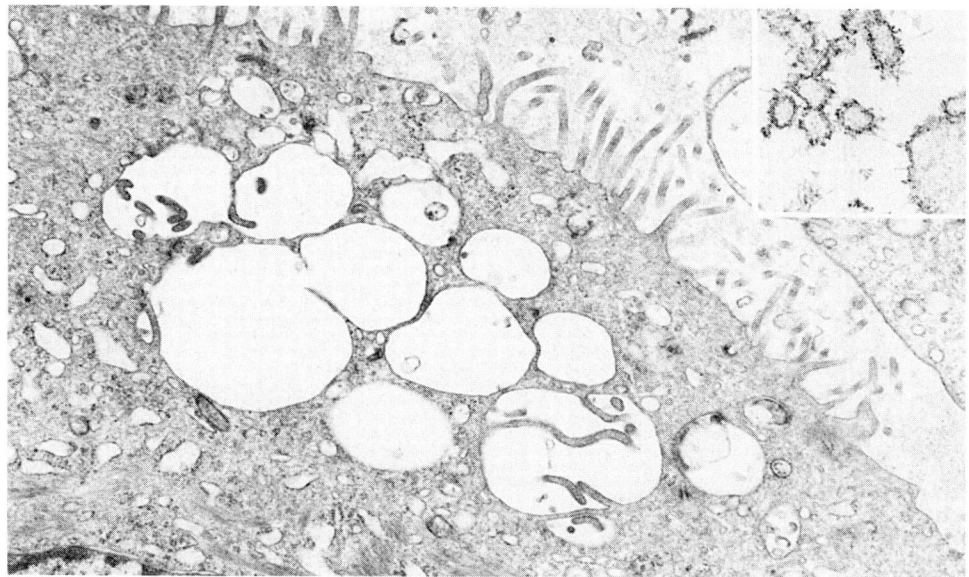

Fig. 26-11 Electron microscopic appearance of cell from malignant mesothelioma demonstrating numerous microvilli in luminal surface and intracellular vacuoles also equipped with microvilli. **Inset** shows microvilli coated with acid mucopolysaccharides. (×8000; **inset** Hale's colloidal iron; ×45,000; from Suzuki Y, Churg J, Kannerstein M: Ultrastructure of human malignant diffuse mesothelioma. Am J Pathol **85:**241-262, 1976.)

tonofilaments, and basal lamina[99] (Fig. 26-11). Transitions are found between typical mesothelial cells and cells with a mesenchymal, fibroblast-like appearance.[67]

The main differential diagnoses of malignant mesothelioma are reactive mesothelial hyperplasia and metastatic carcinoma, particularly of the serous papillary type. The latter usually originates in the ovary, but it can also present as an extra-ovarian mass in the peritoneal cavity of females. This group of müllerian-related tumors is further discussed in Chapter 19. Suffice it to say here that immunohistochemically these serous neoplasms are more likely to be reactive for CEA, Leu-M1, B72.3, CA-125, S-100 protein, placental alkaline phosphatase, and amylase than the mesotheliomas.[69,83] Of these, CEA, Leu-M1, and B72.3 have the most discriminatory value.[83]

The prognosis for malignant mesothelioma is extremely poor. Most patients die of the disease within 2 years of the diagnosis.[88,102] Some encouraging results have been obtained with a combination of surgical debulking, combination chemotherapy, and whole-abdomen irradiation.[87]

Intra-abdominal desmoplastic small cell tumor

Intra-abdominal desmoplastic small cell tumor (IADSCT) is a highly malignant neoplasm that characteristically presents as a single mass or multiple nodules within the abdominal cavity in adolescents and young adults, usually of the male sex.[108,111,113,116] One case has been reported in a patient with Peutz-Jeghers syndrome.[117] There is a definite predilection for the pelvic region, but sometimes there is extension to the entire peritoneal cavity, scrotum, and/or retroperitoneum. Accompanying ascites is the rule. Grossly, the tumor nodules are firm to hard, variously sized, and ranging

in shape from plaque-like to spherical (Fig. 26-12). Invasion of intra-abdominal organs (such as the gastrointestinal tract) is usually restricted to the serosa. However, cases with prominent involvement of sites such as liver, pancreas, and ovary have been observed.[120]

Microscopically, there are sharply outlined islands of tumor cells separated by a generally abundant stroma that tends to be very cellular ("desmoplastic") (Fig. 26-13, *A*). The tumor cells are usually small, round, and monotonous, with hyperchromatic nuclei, high mitotic activity, and very scanty cytoplasm. Some of these cells may have a rhabdoid appearance. The stroma is largely made up of fibroblasts and myofibroblasts, but it also contains proliferating vessels sometimes exhibiting a lobular configuration. These structures are similar to those seen in other malignant tumors composed of primitive neuroepithelial/neuroendocrine cells and perhaps resulting from the secretion of angiogenic factor by the tumor cells.[107] Morphologic variations include tumors with very scanty stroma, presence of tubular or glandular formations, and clusters of pleomorphic large tumor cells.

The immunohistochemical profile of this neoplasm is distinctive in the sense that it displays simultaneous expression of epithelial (keratin, epithelial membrane antigen), muscular (desmin), and neural (neuron-specific enolase) markers (Figs. 26-13, *B*, and 26-14, *A* and *B*). The keratin reactivity has a diffuse cytoplasmic quality, whereas that for desmin tends to have a localized, dot-like ("globoid") quality. Vimentin is also strongly expressed, but stains for actin are characteristically negative. O13 (an antigen associated with Ewing's sarcoma) is usually negative, although focal cytoplasmic stain may be observed. Occasional reactivity for chromogranin has also been described. At the ultrastructural

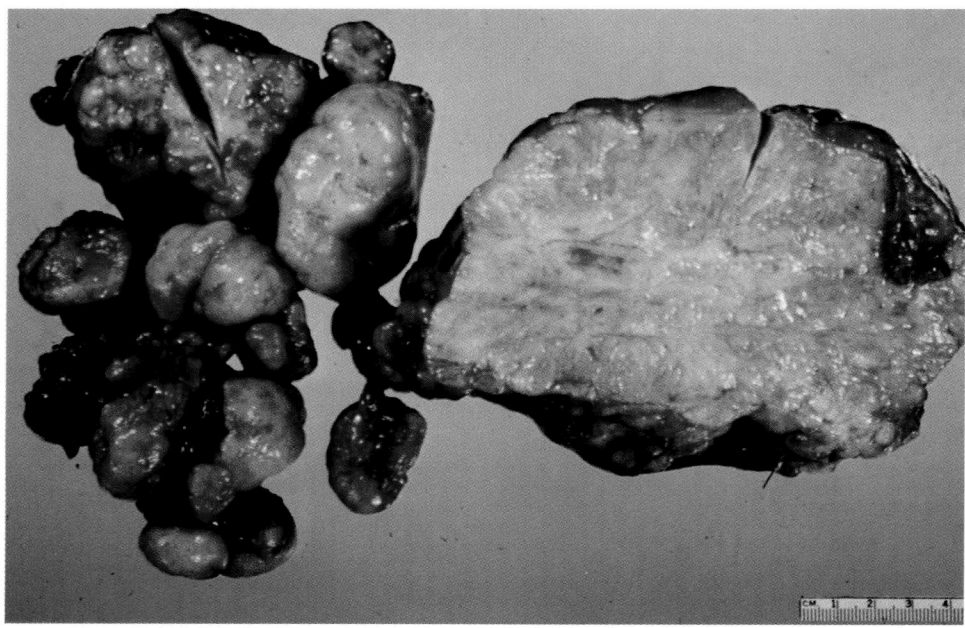

Fig. 26-12 Gross appearance of desmoplastic small cell tumor. There are multiple nodules, one of them of considerable size. Note the large areas of fibrosis.

level the cells have a rather primitive appearance with a few specialized junctions, scattered membrane-bound dense core cytoplasmic granules, and a variable amount of intermediate filaments that tend to cluster in a paranuclear location.

IADSCT is associated with a unique karyotypic aberration involving the reciprocal translocation t (11;22) (p13; q24).[115] The genes involved are EWS (Ewing's sarcoma gene) in 22q24 and the WT1 (Wilms' tumor gene 1) in 11p13.[110,112] This remarkable finding is of practical importance in the differential diagnosis with other small round cell tumors of childhood.[106] It may also explain why the phenotypical features of this neoplasm overlap somewhat with those of Ewing's sarcoma/PNET and Wilms' tumor. The peculiar topographic distribution of IADSCT also suggests a relationship with the mesothelial lining and the possibility that it may represent a "mesothelioblastoma."[108] The transient expression of desmin by the normal developing mesothelium (see p. 2135), the selective expression of WT1 gene products in malignant mesothelioma,[105] and the description of three cases of desmoplastic small cell tumor in the pleural cavity[114] support this contention. On the other hand, the identification of a typical case of this entity in the cerebellum suggests a link with the family of primitive neuroepithelial neoplasms.[118]

The behavior of IADSCT is extremely aggressive, perhaps more than that of any other malignant small round cell tumor of infancy.[109,113,119] Most patients are dead of disease within 2 years of initial diagnosis.

Other primary tumors

Primary peritoneal tumors, other than mesotheliomas, not connected with either the omentum or the mesentery are extremely rare.

Solitary fibrous tumor (formerly known as solitary fibrous mesothelioma) is much less common in the peritoneal than in the pleural cavity, but its morphologic features are identical (see Chapter 7).[124] It presents in adulthood and —like its pleural counterpart—may be accompanied by hypoglycemia. Most cases have followed a benign clinical course.[122,125] The phenotype of the tumor cell is the same as that of the normal submesothelial mesenchyme.

Angiosarcomas have been described following administration of radiation therapy.[123] ***Epithelioid hemangioendothelioma*** can coat the peritoneal cavity in a diffuse fashion, simulating the pattern of growth of malignant mesothelioma; similar cases have been described in the pleural cavity.[126]

Gonzalez-Crussi et al.[121] have described several ***undifferentiated sarcomas*** of undetermined histogenesis involving the peritoneal cavity of children.

Lesions of the secondary müllerian system

The term "secondary müllerian system" has been applied to the pelvic and lower abdominal mesothelium and the subjacent mesenchyme of females, on the basis of its close embryologic relationship with the primary müllerian system (i.e., the müllerian ducts).[136] The potentiality of this tissue is manifested by the existence in the peritoneal cavity (most often in the pelvic region) of a large variety of metaplastic and neoplastic lesions that are analogous in all regards to those more commonly found in the ovary, uterus, or other organs of the female genital tract.[140]

1 ***Endosalpingiosis***. This is discussed in Chapter 19.
2 ***Endometriosis***. This is discussed in Chapter 19 (see also p. 2137).
3 ***Ectopic decidual reaction***. It is most commonly seen in the pelvis and omentum, where it appears as tiny,

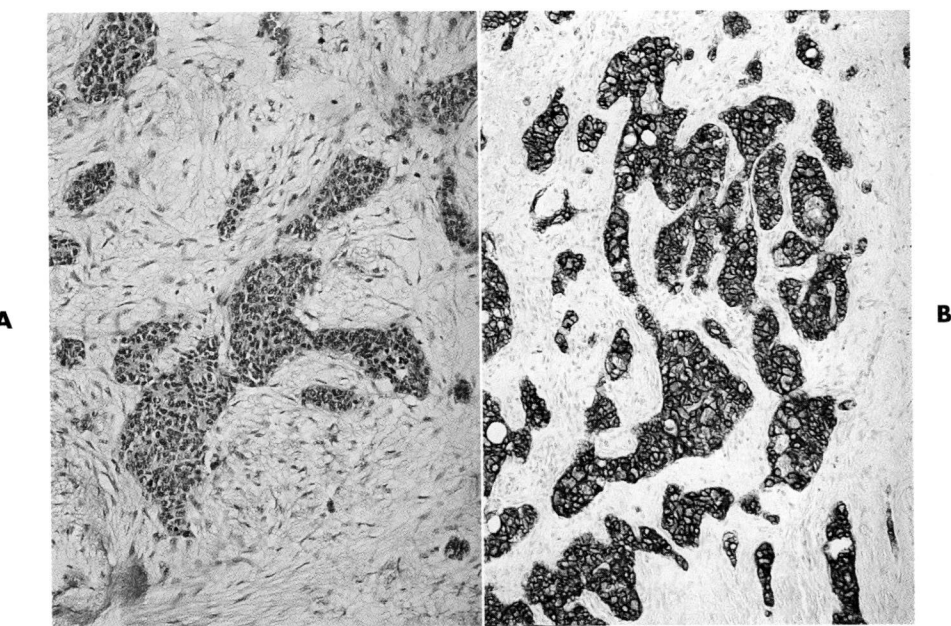

Fig. 26-13 Microscopic appearance of intra-abdominal desmoplastic small cell tumor. **A,** Low-power view of a routinely stained section showing well-defined tumor nests surrounded by cellular stroma. **B,** Immunostain for keratin.

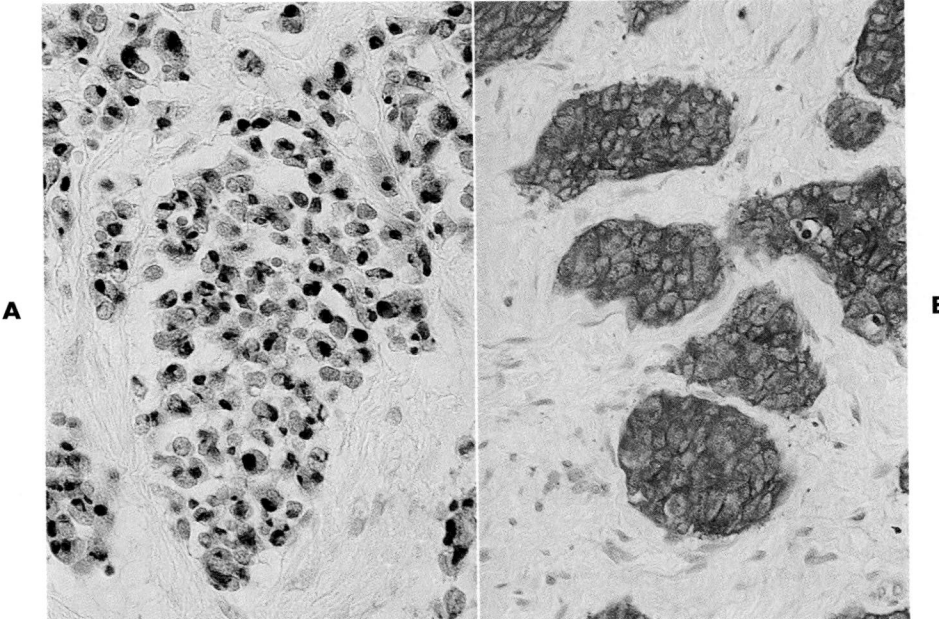

Fig. 26-14 Microscopic appearance of intra-abdominal desmoplastic small cell tumor. **A,** Immunostain for desmin. Note the punctate (globoid) quality of the reaction. **B,** Immunostain for neuron specific enolase.

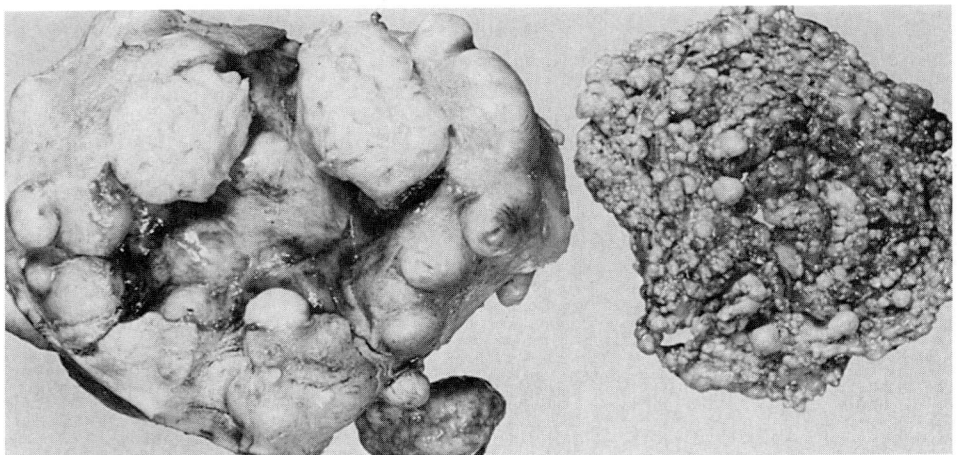

Fig. 26-15 Multiple leiomyomas of uterus associated with innumerable nodules composed of smooth muscle in omentum. This is an example of leiomyomatosis peritonealis disseminata. Patient was 45 years old at time of operation. She remained well 20 years later. (Specimen contributed by Dr. J. Hobbs, St. Louis.)

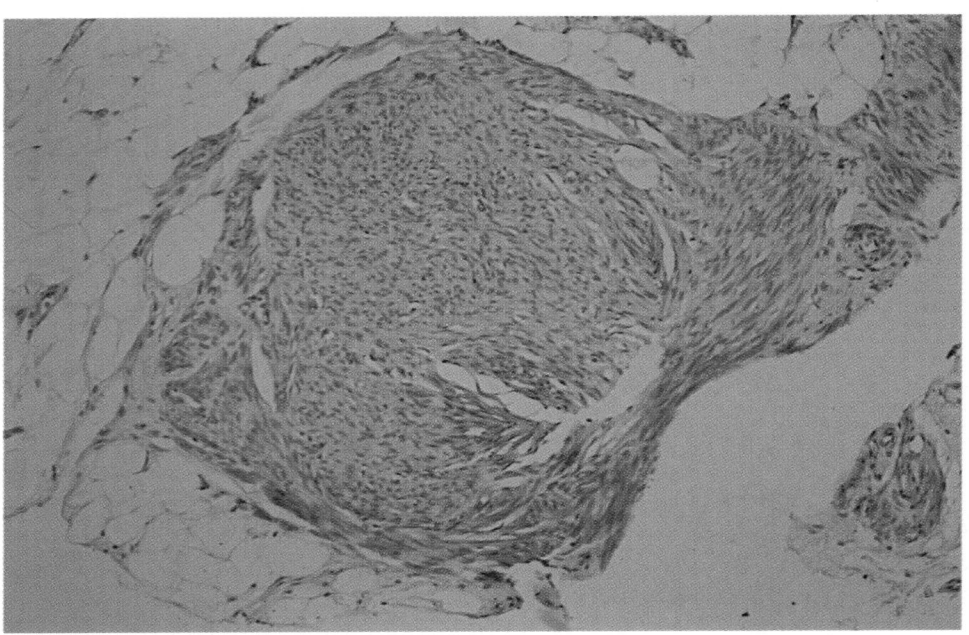

Fig. 26-16 Low-power view of leiomyomatosis peritonealis disseminata.

gray submesothelial nodules.[128,130] Microscopically, the decidual cells may exhibit bizarre hyperchromatic nuclei and be confused with metastatic squamous cell carcinoma. Vascular changes may occur as an expression of regression.[128]

4 *Leiomyomatosis peritonealis disseminata.* This is a rare benign condition in which typical uterine leiomyomas are associated with multiple small nodules of mature smooth muscle distributed throughout the omentum and both visceral and parietal layers of the peritoneum (Figs. 26-15 and 26-16). A mistaken diagnosis of metastatic leiomyosarcoma may result. Rarely, the disease coexists with endometriosis. Exceptionally, a sex-cord–like pattern is observed.[137] A strong association with pregnancy exists.[139] Steroid hormone receptors have been detected in the proliferating cells.[132,138] In most instances, spontaneous regression of the nodules occurs.

5 *(Papillary) serous tumors of the peritoneum.* They include peritoneal serous micropapillomatosis of low malignant potential, serous psammocarcinoma, and (extraovarian) serous carcinoma.[127,131,133,134] They are discussed in Chapter 19.

6 *Endometrial stromal sarcoma and malignant mixed müllerian tumor.*[129,135] These are discussed in Chapter 19.

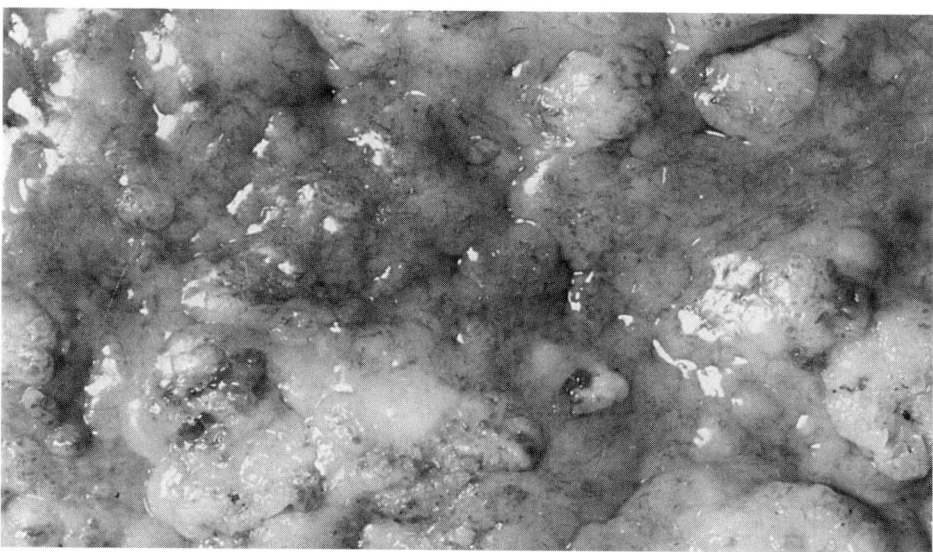

Fig. 26-17 Diffuse involvement of peritoneum by metastatic squamous cell carcinoma simulating primary malignant mesothelioma.

Metastatic tumors

All types of metastatic tumors may involve the peritoneal cavity. The most common sites of the primary tumors are the female genital tract (particularly ovary), followed by large bowel and pancreas.[143] The gross pattern varies from single, well-defined nodules to a diffuse peritoneal thickening. Variations in consistency depend on cellularity, amount of fibrous tissue, and mucin content. Metastatic carcinoma may simulate closely the gross and microscopic appearance of malignant mesothelioma (Fig. 26-17). This is particularly the case with papillary serous carcinoma of the ovary (Fig. 26-18).

Pseudomyxoma peritonei is a distinctive form of tumor implant in which the peritoneal cavity contains large amounts of mucinous material[145,149,151,161] (Fig. 26-19). The primary tumor is usually a borderline or malignant mucinous neoplasm of the appendix, ovary, or pancreas (see Chapters 11, 15, and 19). Several studies done recently on the subject have led to the conclusion that the appendix is the primary site of origin of pseudomyxoma in the vast majority of the cases in both men and women.[156,159,164] The further suggestion has been made that the associated mucinous ovarian tumors—when present—are most likely additional implants from the appendiceal lesions rather than independent synchronous neoplasms.[156,159,164] The subject is further discussed in Chapter 19.

Microscopically, large pools of mucus are seen accompanied by hyperemic vessels and chronic inflammatory cells. *Viable epithelial glandular cells must be identified within the mucus to diagnose pseudomyxoma peritonei* (Fig. 26-20). These cells usually have a deceivingly bland appearance. The disease is characterized by a slow but relentless clinical course, with recurrent ascites that eventually reaches massive proportions ("jelly-belly syndrome"). Aggressive surgical resection is the standard treatment, with most patients requiring multiple laparotomies.[152] It should be noted that mucinous cystadenomas of the ovary and appendix can rupture and pour their content into the peritoneal cavity; the resulting condition, which is self-limited and microscopically lacks tumor cells, should not be designated as pseudomyxoma peritonei.[142,147]

Another very distinctive form of tumor implantation is the *gliomatosis peritonei* resulting from the selective growth of glial tissue from ovarian teratoma[146]; this is discussed in Chapter 19.

Metastatic carcinoma in the peritoneal cavity is often accompanied by recurrent ascites. This is sometimes treated by peritoneovenous shunting, by which the effusion is returned to the general circulation; amazingly, this technique has not resulted in an increase in the number of extra-abdominal metastases.[163]

Cytology

The diagnosis of metastatic carcinoma in the peritoneal cavity is possible in about 75% of the cases on the basis of cytologic examination of ascitic fluid[141,157] (Figs. 26-21 and 26-22). With malignant lymphoma and leukemia, the overall yield is approximately 60%, these figures being slightly higher for large cell lymphoma.[153,157]

The two most difficult problems in cytology of ascitic fluid are the distinction between reactive and neoplastic mesothelium and that between malignant mesothelioma and metastatic carcinoma. False-positive diagnoses have been caused by liver cirrhosis and other disorders associated with mesothelial hyperplasia; confusion occurs because the reactive cells may form pseudoacini closely resembling the true acini of adenocarcinoma, have multiple nuclei or a signet ring appearance, or undergo mitotic division.[148,162] Evaluation of the nucleo-cytoplasmic ratio and of nuclear features are essential in this differential diagnosis.

Malignant mesothelioma often grows in papillary clusters.[155,158] It differs from metastatic adenocarcinoma by the

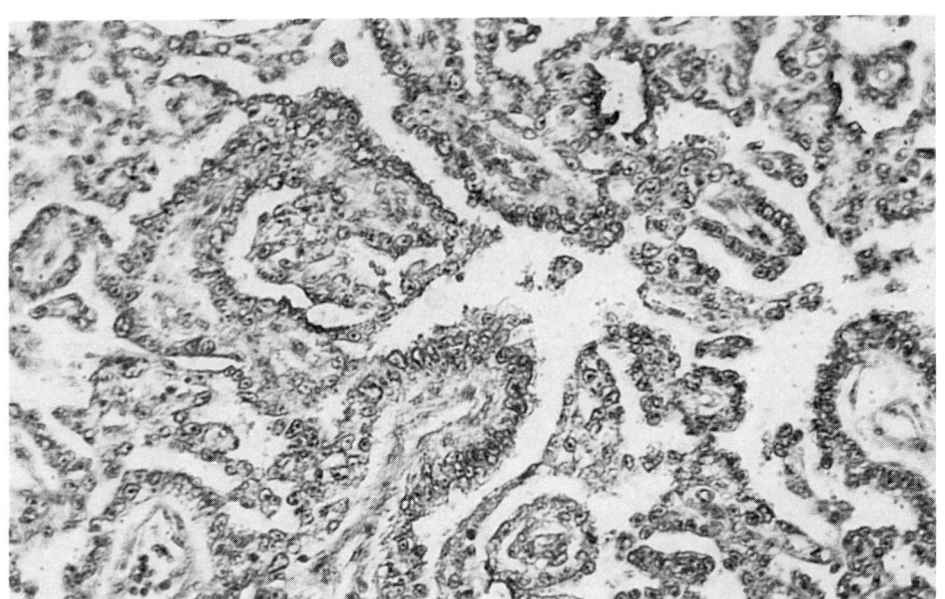

Fig. 26-18 Metastatic ovarian cancer of papillary serous type closely resembling primary malignant mesothelioma.

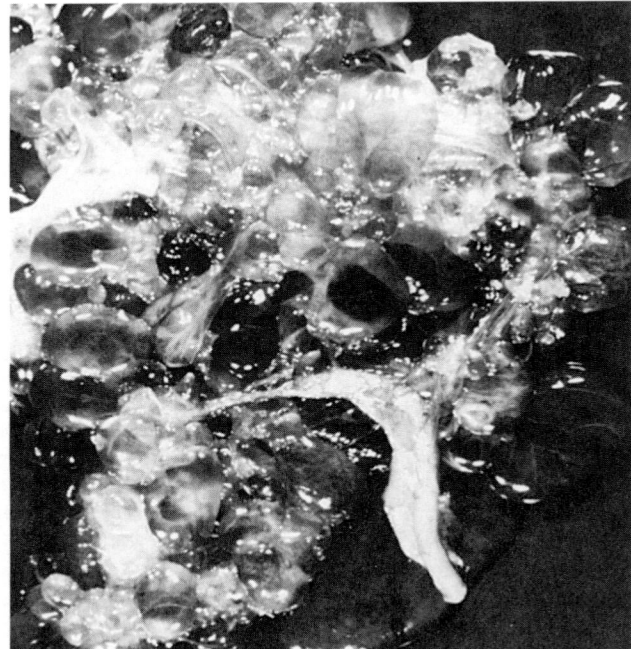

Fig. 26-19 Pseudomyxoma peritonei. Large cystic formations containing mucus surround an uninvolved appendix. Primary lesion was ovarian mucinous cystadenocarcinoma.

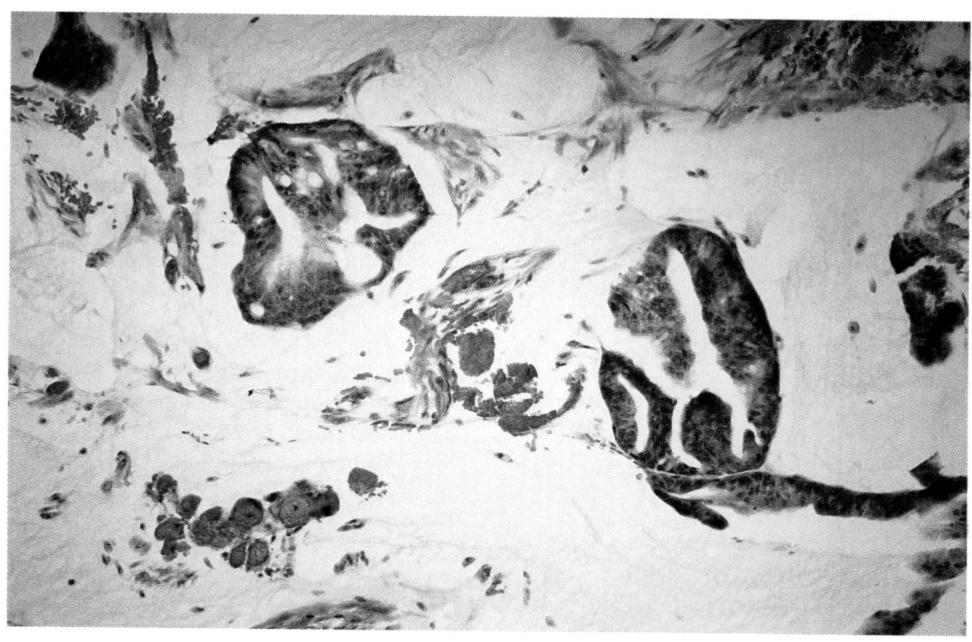

Fig. 26-20 Microscopic appearance of pseudomyxoma peritonei. Clusters of well-differentiated mucin-producing glandular cells are seen floating in a sea of mucin.

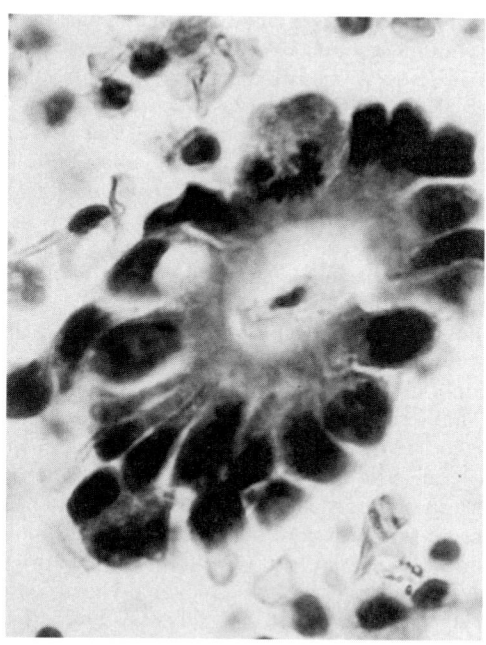

Fig. 26-21 Easily identified metastatic adenocarcinoma in ascitic fluid. Note large, dense nuclei and atypical mitotic figure in acinus.

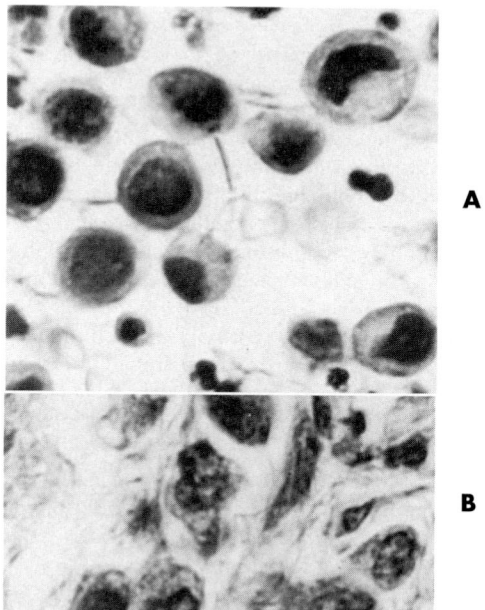

Fig. 26-22 A, Ascitic fluid sediment with numerous tumor cells identified by their dense, large atypical appearance. **B,** Same tumor shown in **A,** which was primary in stomach.

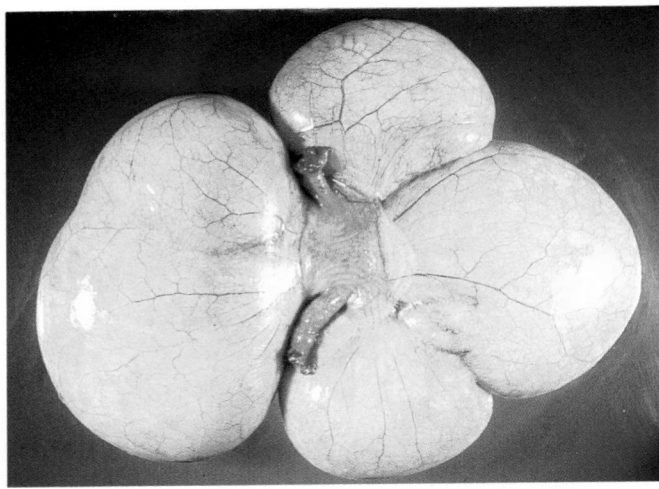

Fig. 26-23 Outer aspect of a mesenteric chylous cyst.

absence of true acini, a more frequent bi-nucleation and multinucleation, and the presence of a range of differentiation among the mesothelial cells.[150] Electron microscopic and immunohistochemical techniques have been successfully applied to cytologic preparations in an effort to increase the diagnostic accuracy.[144,154,160]

Omentum

Hemorrhagic infarct of the omentum may result from torsion or strangulation in a hernia sac. *Primary idiopathic segmental infarction* of the greater omentum is an acute abdominal lesion of obscure etiology usually mistaken clinically for acute appendicitis or cholecystitis. Characteristically, the infarcted segment of omentum is on the right side adherent to the cecum, ascending colon, and anterior parietal peritoneum.[167]

The large majority of the omental neoplasms in adults are *metastatic carcinomas* from the ovary, gastrointestinal tract, pancreas, or other intra-abdominal sites. The omentum is also consistently involved by *diffuse malignant mesothelioma* of the peritoneum.

Cystic lymphangioma represents the single most frequent tumor of the omentum in children[170]; its gross and microscopic appearance is analogous to that of the more common "cystic hygroma" of the neck.[168]

Primary solid tumors of the omentum are exceptionally rare. Smooth muscle tumors predominate among both the benign and malignant categories.[166,172] A high percentage of these tumors are of the epithelioid (clear cell or leiomyoblastoma) type.[172]

A peculiar lesion characterized by the formation of multiple nodules in the omentum and mesentery of children has been described as *myxoid* or *multicentric hamartoma*[169,170]; microscopically, plump mesenchymal cells are seen in a background with prominent myxoid and inflammatory

changes. Whatever the nature of this lesion may ultimately prove to be, its behavior so far has been benign.

Other reported omental lesions include *teratoma* (usually mature),[171] *elastofibroma*,[173] and *cryptococcosis,* resulting in a tumorlike mass ("cryptococcoma").[165]

Mesentery

Mesenteric panniculitis (also called *isolated lipodystrophy of the mesentery, retractile mesenteritis,* and *sclerosing mesenteritis*) is a rare disorder grossly appearing as a diffuse, localized, or multinodular thickening of the mesentery of the small and/or large bowel.[188,201,204] The process may lead to retraction and distortion of the intestinal loops and formation of adhesions between them. Microscopically, there is an infiltration by inflammatory cells, myofibroblasts, and foamy macrophages, the latter probably representing a reaction to fat necrosis[182,196] (Fig. 26-24). The vessels traversing the lesion are often inflamed and sometimes thrombosed. The differential diagnosis includes Weber-Christian disease and Whipple's disease. In eight of the fifty-three patients reported by Kipfer et al.,[189] a malignant lymphoma ultimately developed; other series did not show such an association. Retrospectively, some of these cases might have been malignant lymphoma with a prominent degree of sclerosis, simulating an inflammatory condition. It is likely that at least some examples of mesenteric panniculitis represent a mesenteric extension of idiopathic retroperitoneal fibrosis and, as such, members of the family of disorders collectively known as *inflammatory fibrosclerosis.*[200]

Inflammatory pseudotumor (plasma cell granuloma) presents as an intra-abdominal mass in children and adolescents. It is often associated with fever, weight loss, and anemia, manifestations that often regress following excision of the mass.[181,199,207] Microscopically there is a polymorphic infiltrate composed of plump myofibroblasts arranged in a vaguely fascicular fashion, plasma cells, lymphocytes, and other inflammatory elements. It was originally reported as a pseudoneoplastic inflammatory process because of the rich inflammatory component and the generally favorable outcome following surgical excision. However, further experience has shown that these cases blend imperceptibly with others showing a more neoplastic appearance of the fibroblastic/myofibroblastic component and/or running an aggressive clinical course, including the development of metastases. The term *inflammatory fibrosarcoma*[192] has been proposed for the more neoplastic-appearing members of this group. There is also cytogenetic and molecular evidence that even some of the more inflammatory-appearing lesions may be neoplastic.[205] Because of these facts, we prefer the recently proposed term *inflammatory myofibroblastic tumor*[181,198] for this process.

Mesenteric cysts are usually incidental findings, but they may be large enough to produce symptoms.[190,206] Some are seen as a component of the basal cell–nevus syndrome.[183] They are round and smooth, with a thin wall and a content that may be a serous fluid resembling plasma or a white milky fluid, particularly if located near the jejunum. In the latter instance, they are referred to as *chylous cysts* (Fig. 26-23). Most of these cysts arise from lymph vessels and are lined by endothelium.[176] When they are large and multiloc-

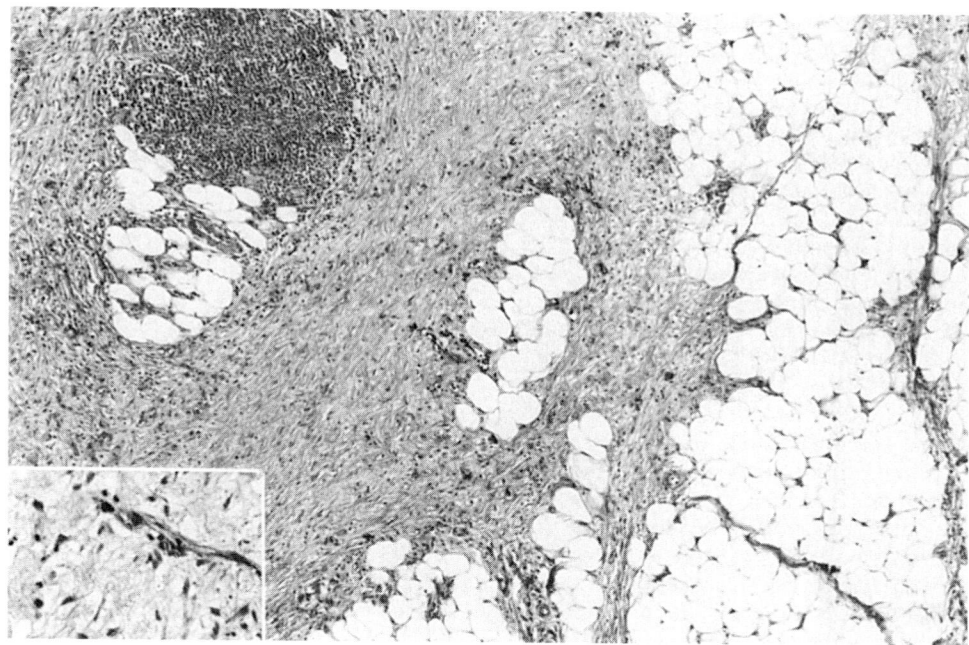

Fig. 26-24 Mesenteric panniculitis. Ill-defined inflammatory and fibrosing process surrounds adipose tissue and accentuates its lobular quality. Prominent vascularity and proliferation of mesenchymal cells as seen in **inset** may simulate appearance of mesenchymal neoplasm.

ular and/or have smooth muscle in their walls, we prefer to regard them as *cystic lymphangiomas*.[180,202]

Other types of mesenteric cysts occur. One is *bowel duplication,* in which the cyst is lined by intestinal mucosa, there is a layer of smooth muscle, and there is an anatomic connection with the bowel by way of an interlacing muscular wall and blood supply; over half of these are diagnosed before 6 months of age.[202] Other mesenteric cysts are lined by mesothelium and are examples of so-called *benign cystic (or multicystic) mesothelioma* (see p. 2137). Others are lined by *müllerian (fallopian tube–like) epithelium,* similar to those more commonly seen in the true pelvis[185] (see Chapter 19). Still others, seen in females who have had previous pelvic surgery, are lined by luteinized cells and have ovarian stroma in their wall; these are referred to as *ovarian remnant syndrome*[203] or *mesenteric cyst–ovarian implant syndrome*.[197]

Cystic mucinous tumors of benign and borderline type have been described in the mesentery and retroperitoneum of females.[174] They are analogous in all regards to the homonymous tumors in the ovary, of which they can be regarded as the peritoneal counterparts.[174]

Most solid tumors involving the mesentery in adults are *metastatic carcinomas.* Yannopoulos and Stout[208] studied forty-four *primary solid tumors* of the mesentery. Two thirds were benign. There were twelve cases of fibromatosis, seven tumors of smooth muscle origin, six tumors of adipose tissue origin, six "xanthogranulomas" (most of which today would probably be regarded to as "fibrous histiocytomas"), five vascular neoplasms, three neurofibromas, and five miscellaneous tumors (Fig. 26-25). Adipose tissue tumors can be benign or malignant.[194] The smooth muscle tumors,

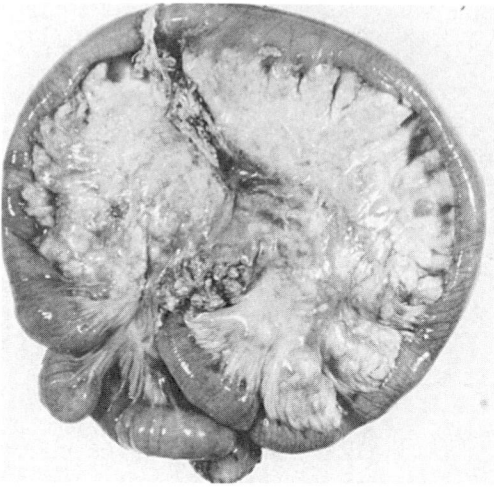

Fig. 26-25 Extremely large plexiform neurofibroma involving mesentery of small bowel. It was necessary to remove 140 cm of ileum to obtain this mass, which measured 24 cm × 11 cm. Six years following operation, 22-year-old male patient was well. (From Leach WB: Giant neurofibroma of mesentery. Arch Surg **74:**438-441, 1957.)

when large, usually behave in a malignant fashion even if their mitotic count is low[186]; a third of these tumors show an epithelioid (clear cell) appearance, and a similar proportion exhibit pleomorphic areas reminiscent of malignant fibrous histiocytoma.[186] Infantile mesenteric hemangioendotheliomas can be associated with thrombocytopenia.[184] In the presence of *fibromatosis* of the mesentery, the possibility of

Gardner's syndrome should always be investigated, particularly if it develops following a surgical procedure.[178,179,191] Some of these cases have shown immunoreactivity for CD34.[193]

Castleman's disease (giant lymph node hyperplasia) may present as a mesenteric mass associated with hematologic disturbances.[195] Some cases are accompanied by heavy calcification.

Other reported mesenteric tumors include an allegedly primary *carcinoid tumor*[175] and several examples of *germ cell tumor,* including yolk sac tumor[187] and a mature cystic teratoma (dermoid cyst) associated with autoimmune hemolytic anemia.[177]

Hernia sacs

This rather mundane specimen is one of the most common to be received in the surgical pathology laboratory. In most instances, there is not much of interest microscopically: an attenuated lining of mesothelial cells resting on a thin layer of connective tissue (corresponding to the processus vaginalis in indirect inguinal hernias), adipose tissue, dense fibrous tissue belonging to fascia and/or aponeurosis, and sometimes fascicles of skeletal muscle (from the transversus abdominis in the inguinal hernias). The preperitoneal fat that covers the sac may be abundant and be designated as "lipoma" by the surgeon, but it does not represent a neoplasm. Once in a while, however, the hernial sac will show one or more startling pathologic changes. *Mesothelial hyperplasia* resulting from trauma or another injury can be so extreme as to simulate a malignancy (see p. 2137); the

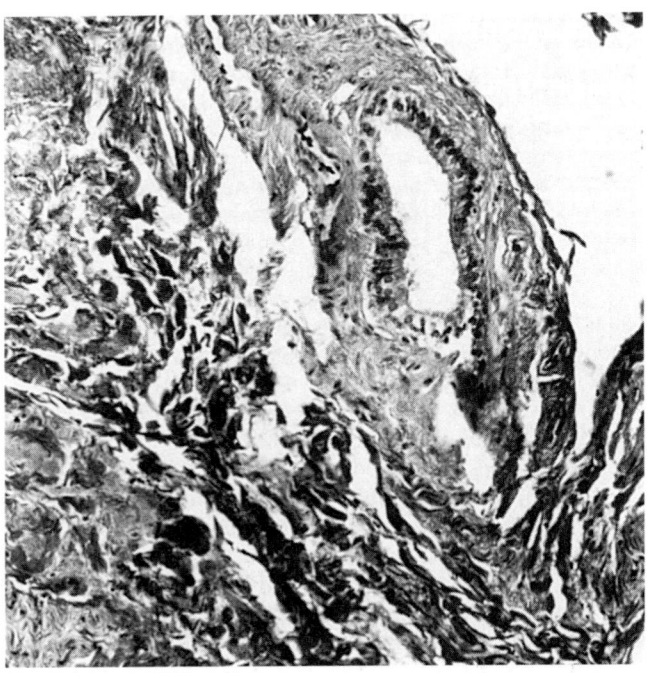

Fig. 26-26 Tubular structure lined by ciliated columnar epithelium found incidentally in hernia sac. This finding is of no clinical significance.

accompanying inflammation, hyperemia, and fibrin deposition will point toward its reactive nature. Sometimes a *mesothelioma* or a *metastatic carcinoma* will first become evident from the study of a herniorrhaphy specimen. The most common sources for the primary are the gastrointestinal tract, ovary, prostate, and appendix.[210,212] The pseudomyxoma peritonei that sometimes accompanies appendiceal mucinous tumors may result in filling of the hernia sac by viscid mucin (see p. 2149). A particularly exotic tumor reported within an umbilical hernia sac is an *extragonadal sex-cord tumor with annular tubules*.[209] Parenthetically, the other reported case of extragonadal tumor of this type was located in the fallopian tube and associated with endometriosis.[211]

Other changes one may encounter in a hernia sac are *endometriosis* in females and *glandular inclusions* from müllerian remnants in prepuberal males. The latter are lined by ciliated epithelium and surrounded by a mantle of fibrous tissue; they should not be misinterpreted as portions of the vas deferens or epididymis[213,215] (Fig. 26-26).

Crystalline foreign particulate material largely composed of talc was consistently detected in hernia sacs by polarized microscopy and X-diffraction studies by Pratt et al.[214] They suggest that the source of this talc was ingestion with food or medication, but it seems to us that they did not satisfactorily rule out the alternative possibility that the source was the surgical procedure or the processing of the specimen.

Umbilicus

The umbilicus is subject to a variety of diseases resulting from its unique anatomy and the important structures with which it is connected during development. Excluding conditions such as hernias, omphaloceles, neonatal infections, and extensive fetal malformations, the group of disorders of importance to the surgical pathologist that can affect this structure are those that follow.

Urachal remnant anomalies may present as a patent sinus between the umbilicus and the bladder, as blind sinuses at any level between these two structures, and as a closed but persistently attached urachus. Steck and Helwig[222] have suggested that most cases of granulomatous omphalitis, umbilical granuloma, and pilonidal sinus of the umbilicus are related to urachal anomalies because of the fact that an attached urachus is found in nearly half of these cases (see Chapter 17, Urinary bladder).

Omphalomesenteric duct remnant anomalies include patency of the duct, "umbilical polyp," sinus tract, attachment of Meckel's diverticulum to the umbilicus by an incompletely obliterated duct, and formation of a cyst in the umbilicus or along the course of the incompletely obliterated duct[219] (see Chapter 11, Small bowel).

Endometriosis of the umbilicus is the most common form of cutaneous endometriosis, except for those occurring in surgical scars[220] (see Chapter 19, Uterine corpus).

Keratinous cysts of epidermal type are relatively common.[221]

Benign tumors of the umbilical region can be of various types; most of them belong to the category of benign melanocytic nevus and fibroepithelial polyp (papilloma).[220,223]

Malignant tumors involving the umbilicus can be primary or metastatic. The most common primary malignant tumor is malignant melanoma, followed by basal cell carcinoma and adenocarcinoma.[218,221] Metastatic tumors are much more common. Most of them originate in the stomach, pancreas, large bowel, or ovary.[221] The colloquial term "Sister Joseph's nodule" refers to umbilical metastases from malignancies of the female genital tract, usually ovarian carcinoma.[216] Several cases have been described of rapid development of umbilical metastases after laparoscopic cholecystectomy for unsuspected gallbladder carcinoma.[217]

Retroperitoneum
NORMAL ANATOMY

The retroperitoneal space is the portion of the lumboiliac region limited anteriorly by the peritoneal covering, posteriorly by the posterior abdominal wall, superiorly by the twelfth rib and vertebra, inferiorly by the base of the sacrum and iliac crest, and laterally by the side borders of the quadratus lumbora muscles. It contains, embedded in a meshwork of loose connective tissue, the adrenal glands, kidneys and ureters, aorta and its branches, inferior vena cava and its tributaries, and numerous lymph nodes.

This potentially large space allows both primary and metastatic tumors to grow silently before clinical signs and symptoms appear.

NON-NEOPLASTIC CONDITIONS

Inflammatory processes from the kidney (pyelonephritis), large bowel (diverticulitis), appendix, and pancreas may result in a retroperitoneal abscess, usually resulting from coliform bacteria. In children, nontuberculous psoas abscesses are, in most cases, due to gram-positive cocci originating from a focus of tonsillitis, otitis media, or cutaneous furuncle. Perforation of the biliary system may occur within the retroperitoneum, with formation of a bile-containing cystic mass. Infection from a tuberculous vertebra may form a retroperitoneal cold abscess, which is often confined to the psoas muscle. *Malakoplakia* can involve the retroperitoneum and be confused with malignant fibrous histiocytoma.[247] Massive retroperitoneal *hemorrhage* in the adult is most often the result of a ruptured aortic aneurysm, trauma, hemorrhagic diathesis, or anticoagulant drug therapy.[238] Less commonly, it is of renal or adrenal origin. Lawson et al.[237] reviewed ten cases of the latter phenomenon. In five instances the adrenal gland was the site of a pheochromocytoma, but in the other five, there was no demonstrable abnormality. We have also seen massive retroperitoneal hemorrhage as a complication of adrenal metastases of malignant melanoma. Perirenal hemorrhagic cysts sometimes contain equally spaced radial striations that are probably the expression of the Liesegang phenomenon and that should not be mistaken for parasites.[246]

Benign retroperitoneal cysts may occur not connected with the adrenal gland or kidney. Their inner lining is usually compatible with either a mesothelial or mesonephric origin.[236] In some instances, the lining is instead of müllerian type, with either a serous or a mucinous appearance.[227] Upper retroperitoneal cysts of bronchogenic type presenting as an adrenal mass have also been described.[228]

Idiopathic retroperitoneal fibrosis (Ormond's disease, sclerosing fibrosis, sclerosing retroperitonitis) is a rare disease of obscure etiology that results in progressive renal failure by producing constriction and final obliteration of the ureters.[239] Grossly, an ill-defined fibrous mass occupies the retroperitoneal midline, encircles the lower abdominal aorta, and displaces the ureters medially. The latter feature is of value to the radiologist in the differential diagnosis, since most retroperitoneal neoplasms displace the ureter laterally. More localized forms exist, in which the process is sharply circumscribed in the periureteral or renal pelvic region (Fig. 26-27), around one kidney, or around the bladder.[230] Microscopically, a prominent inflammatory infiltrate composed of lymphocytes, plasma cells, histiocytes, and eosinophils, often containing germinal centers, is seen accompanied by foci of fat necrosis, fibroblastic proliferation, and collagen deposition.[241] Cell marker studies have shown that a high percentage of the spindle cells present in this lesion express the immunophenotype of tissue macrophages.[232] The plasma cells, which can be very numerous, show a polyclonal immunoglobulin staining pattern[245]; a significant proportion of the immunoglobulin produced is of the IgA type, a finding of potential diagnostic significance.[243] The fibrous tissue in the midline tends to be more mature than that of the periphery.[224] The wall of veins is often involved by the inflammation.[233,240] Mitchinson[241] also found aortic involvement in three of his cases.

Idiopathic retroperitoneal fibrosis may be associated with a similar process in the mediastinum, sclerosing cholangitis, Riedel's thyroiditis, pseudotumor of the orbit, or generalized vasculitis. Any possible combination among these various processes has been encountered and is generally referred to as *multifocal fibrosclerosis*.[225,231] Several cases of retroperitoneal fibrosis have been reported secondary to the administration of methysergide and other drugs[229]; in many cases, cessation of therapy resulted in dramatic regression of the lesion. The available evidence strongly suggests that idiopathic retroperitoneal fibrosis represents an immunologic hypersensitivity disorder. Surgical ureterolysis is the treatment of choice[226,244]; sometimes corticosteroid therapy has resulted in dramatic improvement.[242]

Occasionally the clinical and pathologic features of idiopathic retroperitoneal fibrosis can be simulated by malignant neoplasms accompanied by chronic inflammation and fibrosis, notably malignant lymphoma and signet ring cell carcinoma of the stomach.[234,235,248]

TUMORS

Primary tumors of the retroperitoneal area can be of many types.[270,278,289,292,300] In a generic sense, neoplasms arising in the kidney, adrenal gland, and retroperitoneal lymph nodes qualify in the category and are actually the most common. The large majority of the retroperitoneal *malignant lymphomas* are of non-Hodgkin's type and B-cell derivation. Most are follicular center cell lymphomas; many of these are associated with extensive fibrosis, which can simulate the pattern of idiopathic retroperitoneal fibrosis.[324] Others are of B-immunoblastic type and run a very aggressive clinical course.[323] These tumors can be diagnosed by fine-needle aspiration, supplemented if necessary by immunostains.[257]

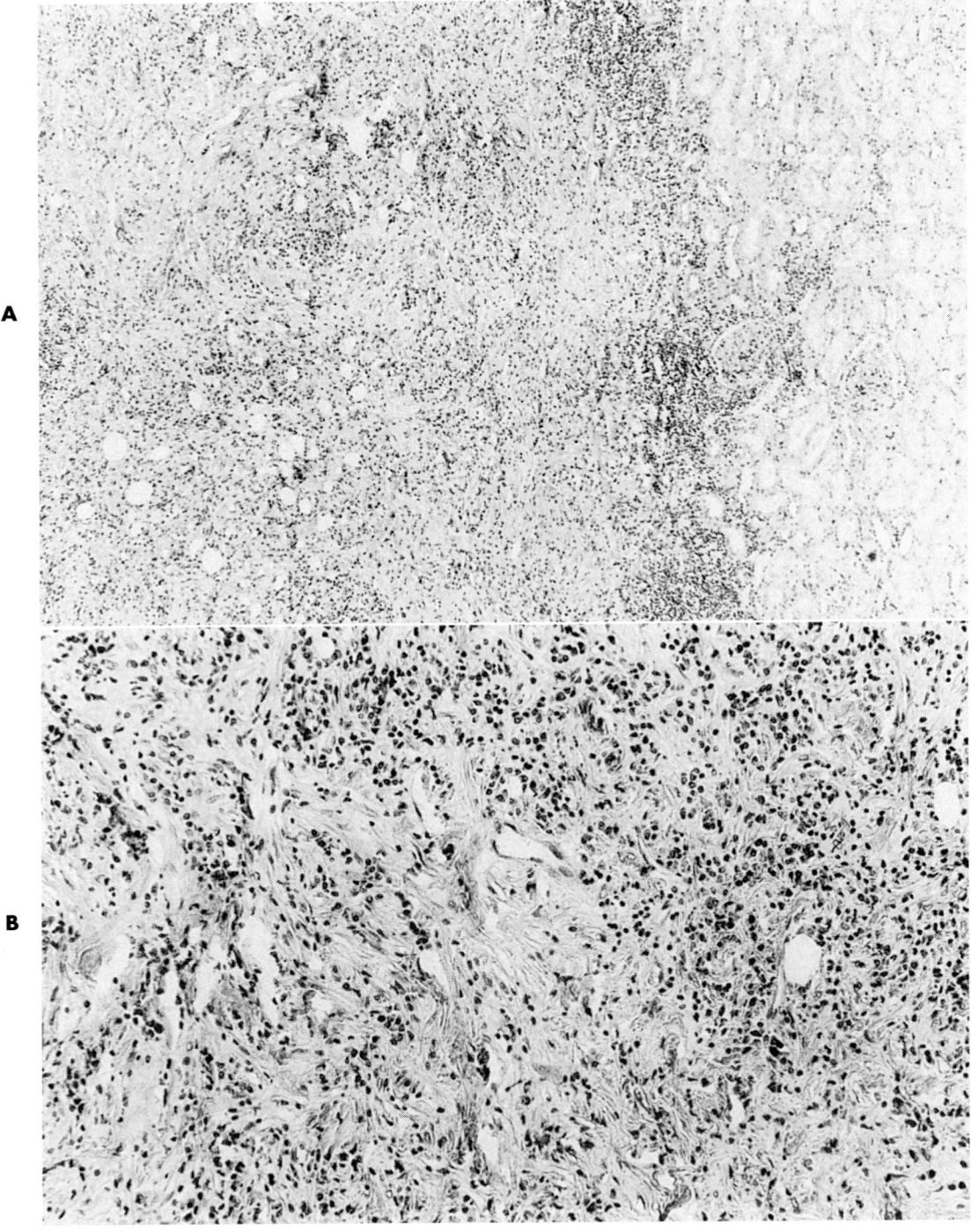

Fig. 26-27 A, Idiopathic retroperitoneal fibrosis involving region of renal pelvis and extending into renal parenchyma. **B,** At higher magnification, fibrosing nature of process and heavy inflammatory component are evident. This should not be confused with fibromatosis or with malignant fibrous histiocytoma.

By convention, the designation of primary retroperitoneal tumors has been reserved for tumors in this area arising outside of the previously discussed structures. Most of them have been already discussed elsewhere, particularly in Chapter 25. Here, only the frequency and peculiarities of these neoplasms as they pertain to their retroperitoneal location will be considered.

Symptoms secondary to retroperitoneal neoplasms are vague and appear late in the course of the disease. They are related to displacements of organs and obstructive phenomena[302] (Fig. 26-28).

The classic radiologic methods for the evaluation of retroperitoneal tumors have been plain roentgenograms, barium studies of the gastrointestinal tract, and intravenous/retrograde pyelograms. These were later supplemented by selective arteriography and inferior cavography, but these techniques in turn have been largely superseded by ultrasonography, CT scanning, and nuclear magnetic resonance imaging[271,312] (Fig. 26-29).

Soft tissue tumors

As a group, retroperitoneal soft tissue sarcomas are associated with a very poor long-term survival rate, the main reason being the extreme difficulty encountered in performing a complete surgical removal with a rim of normal tissue around the tumor.[261,280,319]

Liposarcoma is the most frequent retroperitoneal sarcoma. It is particularly prone to arise and grow in the perirenal region (Figs. 26-30 and 26-31). At the time of excision, it is usually extremely large. Some cases present as multiple independent tumor nodules. Liposarcomas in this location have a worse prognosis than those located in the extremities (39% versus 71% survival rate in the series of Enzinger and Winslow,[265] the former figure falling to 4% at 10 years). Total or near-total excision followed by radiation therapy offers the best chances of cure.[282] The large majority of retroperitoneal liposarcomas are of well-differentiated type (also known as atypical lipomatous tumors) or of pleomorphic type. Myxoid liposarcomas are very unusual at this site.

Lipoma is much less common than its malignant counterpart. As the latter, it is usually very large at the time of diagnosis and can be multiple. Any adipose tissue tumor of the retroperitoneum with atypical features should be designated as well-differentiated liposarcoma or atypical lipomatous tumor, no matter how focal these features are, in view of its marked tendency for recurrence and poor long-term prognosis.[252] Many cases reported in the literature as retroperitoneal lipomas are actually examples of atypical lipomatous tumors, particularly those in which a malignant transformation is said to have occurred.

Both atypical lipomatous tumors and lipomas may contain bundles of well-differentiated smooth muscle; when benign, these tumors are referred to as *myolipomas*[293]; angiomyolipoma is the obvious differential diagnosis (see later section).

Malignant fibrous histiocytoma is the second most common retroperitoneal sarcoma. All variants of this tumor entity have been described in this location, including the inflammatory type.[279] The latter may be associated with

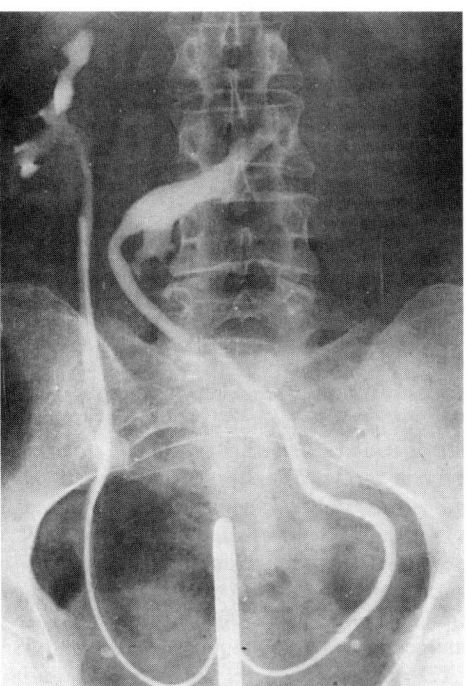

Fig. 26-28 Extreme displacement of kidney and ureter in patient with large retroperitoneal tumor.

marked peripheral leukocytosis.[320] It is inadvisable to classify these deep-seated lesions as benign no matter how bland their microscopic appearance may be, in view of the fact that some of them will result in repeated recurrences and even metastases. Along these lines, it should be mentioned that the majority of the cases reported in the past as retroperitoneal xanthogranulomas probably represent examples of MFH with a prominent component of foamy macrophages.[297] This is not to say that true inflammatory processes having a prominent histiocytic component cannot occur in this region. They certainly can, specific examples being sinus histiocytosis with massive lymphadenopathy (Rosai-Dorfman's disease), Langerhans' cell granulomatosis, the nebulous entity known as Erdheim-Chester disease, and malakoplakia.[264] The differential diagnosis of MFH in this region also includes other types of sarcomas and sarcomatoid renal carcinoma.

Leiomyosarcoma is the third most common sarcoma in this area.[272,273] This tumor has a particular tendency to undergo massive cystic degeneration when occurring in this region.[290] Retroperitoneal smooth muscle tumors containing five or more mitoses per high-power field should be classified as leiomyosarcomas. Tumor cell necrosis or a tumor size greater than 10 cm is strongly suggestive of malignancy, even in the presence of a low mitotic count. When these criteria are applied to retroperitoneal tumors, it will be found that nearly all of them qualify as leiomyosarcomas. The prognosis has been extremely poor in all the reported series; over 85% of the patients have died of tumor, usually within 2 years of diagnosis.[273,281,305,311]

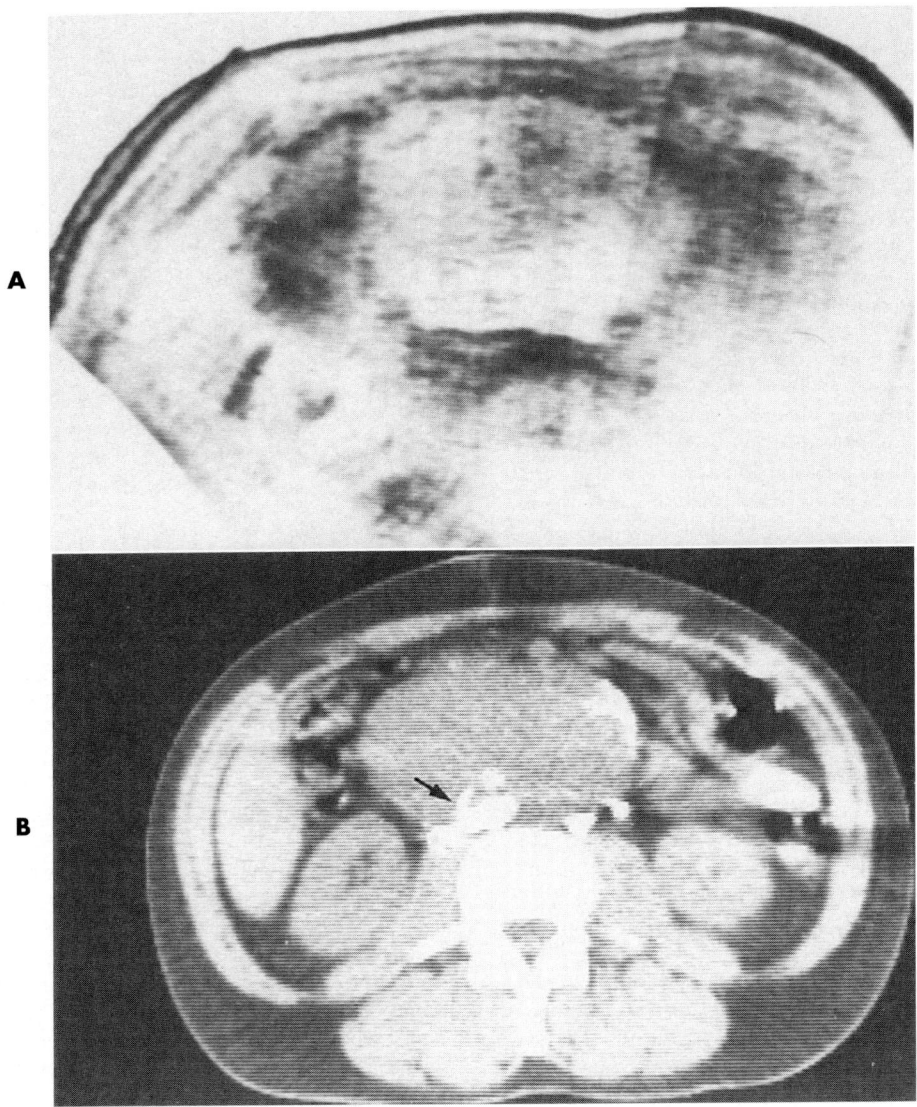

Fig. 26-29 **A,** Transverse ultrasonography in patient with retroperitoneal metastases from testicular germ cell tumor. Echo demonstrates massive retroperitoneal tumor lying against spine and protruding into abdominal cavity. Complex echo pattern within tumor indicates areas of fibrosis, probably secondary to necrosis. **B,** Transverse computed tomography in same patient whose sonogram is shown in **A.** Mass is again clearly shown. Its borders are better demarcated than in sonogram, but internal architecture is less distinct. Darker areas at periphery of mass *(arrow)* represent iodide material from previous lymphangiogram. (Courtesy Dr. S. Feinberg, Minneapolis.)

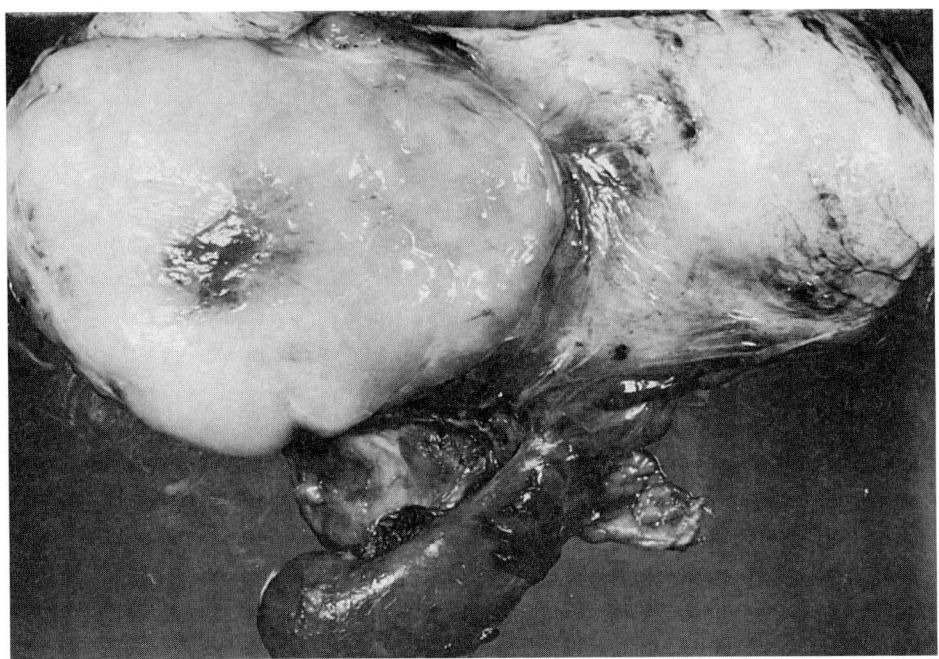

Fig. 26-30 Large slimy retroperitoneal liposarcoma growing in perirenal region.

Some of the malignant stromal neoplasms of this region have shown an epithelioid (clear cell) morphology, and a subset of them have exhibited focal granular cell changes.[304] Others have shown ultrastructural features suggestive of neural differentiation (so-called gastrointestinal autonomic nerve tumors).[286]

Renal angiomyolipoma is a benign retroperitoneal tumor that can be easily confused with leiomyosarcoma in a biopsy specimen because of the atypia commonly seen in the smooth muscle elements (see Chapter 17). The primarily intrarenal location, the admixture with mature fat and thick-walled blood vessels, and the immunoreactivity for HMB-45 should allow the recognition of this entity. It should also be noted that primary extrarenal examples of this tumor exist.

Leiomyoma is exceptionally rare and perhaps even non-existent as a primary retroperitoneal neoplasm. When encountering a tumor in this region with a leiomyomatous appearance, one should consider the possibilities of a uterine leiomyoma extending posteriorly, a well-differentiated leiomyosarcoma, lymphangiomyoma, and the previously discussed angiomyolipoma[254] (see Fig. 17-108).

Rhabdomyosarcoma of retroperitoneum is usually of the embryonal type (including its botryoid variety) and rarely of the alveolar type and is limited for all practical purposes to infants and children.[262,306] Multimodality treatment has resulted in greater than 50% tumor response, but the long-term prognosis remains poor.[262,306] The differential diagnosis of retroperitoneal rhabdomyosarcoma in children includes malignant lymphoma, Ewing's sarcoma/PNET in all its manifestations (including so-called paravertebral round cell tumor),[315,328] and (intra-abdominal) desmoplastic small cell

tumor (i.e., the whole gamut of small cell tumors of childhood). The distinction between these various entities is often very difficult to make, to say the least, and it may be impossible in the individual case, even after performing ultrastructural and immunohistochemical studies.[263,266,316] This fact was clearly shown in a study from the Intergroup Rhabdomyosarcoma Study Committee,[262] in which almost 30% of 101 retroperitoneal soft tissue sarcomas were classified as undifferentiated or unspecified. The situation has greatly improved following the systematic evaluation of these tumors with cytogenetic and molecular techniques (see Chapter 25).

Rhabdomyoma is practically nonexistent in the retroperitoneum; however, a convincing case combining features of the fetal and adult types of this tumor has been reported in a neonate.[326]

Fibromatosis may occur, sometimes in association with mediastinal involvement. In contrast to idiopathic retroperitoneal fibrosis (a disorder with which it is often confused), it lacks a prominent inflammatory component, except for perivascular lymphocytic cuffing at the growing edge.

Fibrosarcoma is one of the rarest retroperitoneal tumors in our experience. We believe that most cases so designated in the literature would today be labeled liposarcomas, leiomyosarcomas, or malignant fibrous histiocytomas.[250]

Solitary fibrous tumor can present as a primary retroperitoneal mass, sometimes accompanied by hypoglycemia. Some of the reported cases were associated with independent pleural tumors of similar appearance.[277]

Vascular tumors of several types have been described, including hemangioma, hemangiopericytoma, lymphangioma, lymphangiomyoma, and angiosarcoma.[288] Some of the angiosarcomas are of the epithelioid variety; prominent

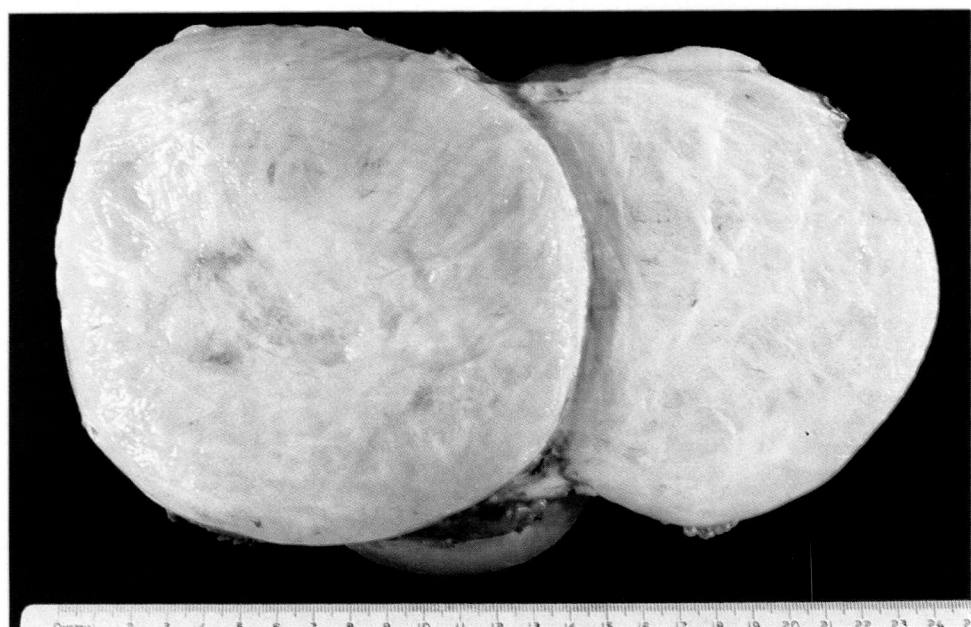

Fig. 26-31 Cut surface of liposarcoma of the well-differentiated sclerosing type.

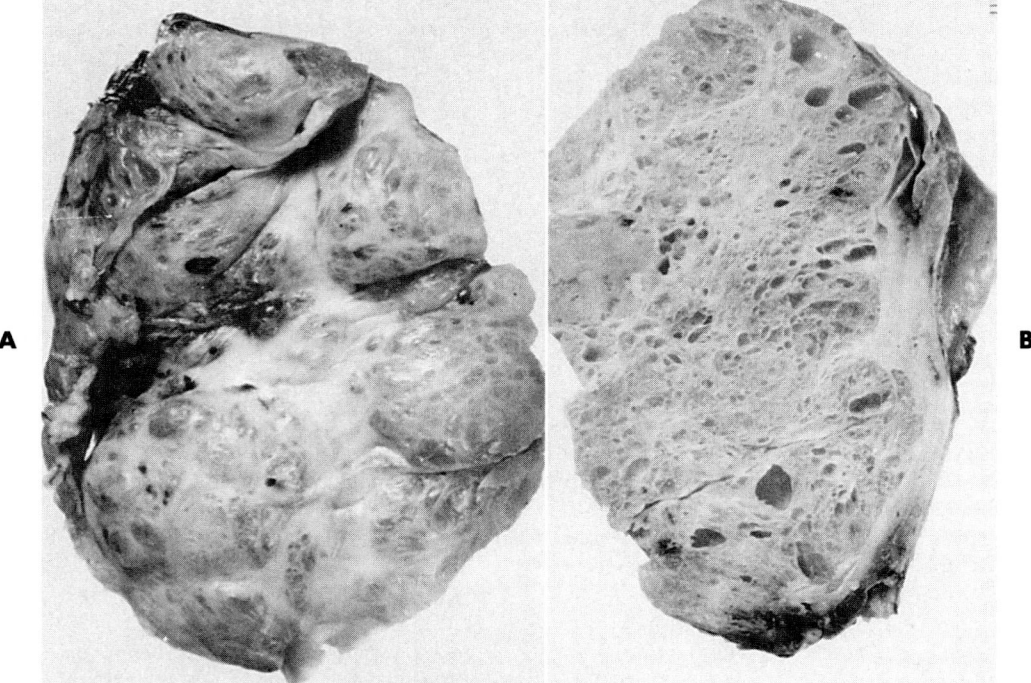

Fig. 26-32 External appearance **(A)** and cross section **(B)** of benign cystic lymphangioma that was present in retroperitoneum and mesentery of 77-year-old woman who had progressive abdominal enlargement of number of years. It weighed 900 g. Note honeycombing of specimen. Patient has remained well for over 2 years.

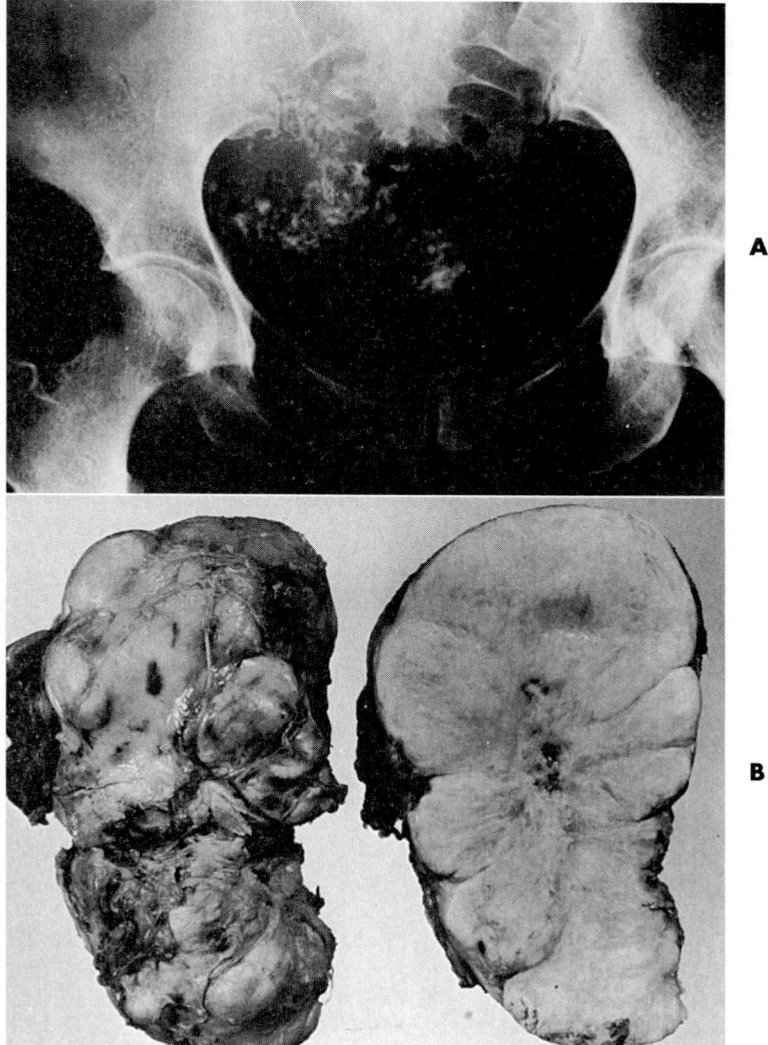

Fig. 26-33 A, Partially calcified retroperitoneal malignant peripheral nerve sheath tumor. **B,** Gross appearance of same lesion. It was firm and grayish white and directly invaded vertebra, metastasized distantly, and caused death.

eosinophilic globules may be present in the cytoplasm of the tumor cells.[321] A peculiar variant of infantile hemangioendothelioma mimicking Kaposi's sarcoma and often accompanied by thrombocytopenia and hemorrhage (Kasabach-Merritt syndrome) has a special tendency for a retroperitoneal location.[317]

Peripheral nerve tumors (Fig. 26-32) of benign type are not as common as in the mediastinum. Both schwannomas and neurofibromas have been described.[313] Malignant peripheral nerve tumors are proportionally more frequent in this location; they may involve the bone directly, and they metastasize widely[294] (Fig. 26-33). Some of the cases have arisen from retroperitoneal ganglioneuromas.[269]

Synovial sarcoma, alveolar soft part sarcoma,[309] and *extraskeletal osteosarcoma* can present as primary retroperitoneal neoplasms[260]; all of the few reported cases of the former have shown a characteristic biphasic pattern.[310] There has also been a report of a *dendritic follicular tumor* arising extranodally from periduodenal retroperitoneal soft tissue.[275]

Germ cell tumors

Retroperitoneal germ cell tumors in children are represented by mature and immature teratoma, embryonal carcinoma, and yolk sac tumor.[251,253,274,285] Their features merge with those of sacrococcygeal teratomas, which are discussed in more detail on p. 2163.

Retroperitoneal germ cell tumors in adults can arise in this location or represent metastases from primaries in the gonads.[249,256,295] Both types are much more common in males. The entire microscopic gamut is represented, including seminoma (germinoma), embryonal carcinoma, teratocarcinoma, mature and immature teratoma, mature teratoma with malignant transformation, yolk sac tumor, and choriocarcinoma[296,329] (Fig. 26-34). The chances of a retroperitoneal germ cell tumor in a male being metastatic from a

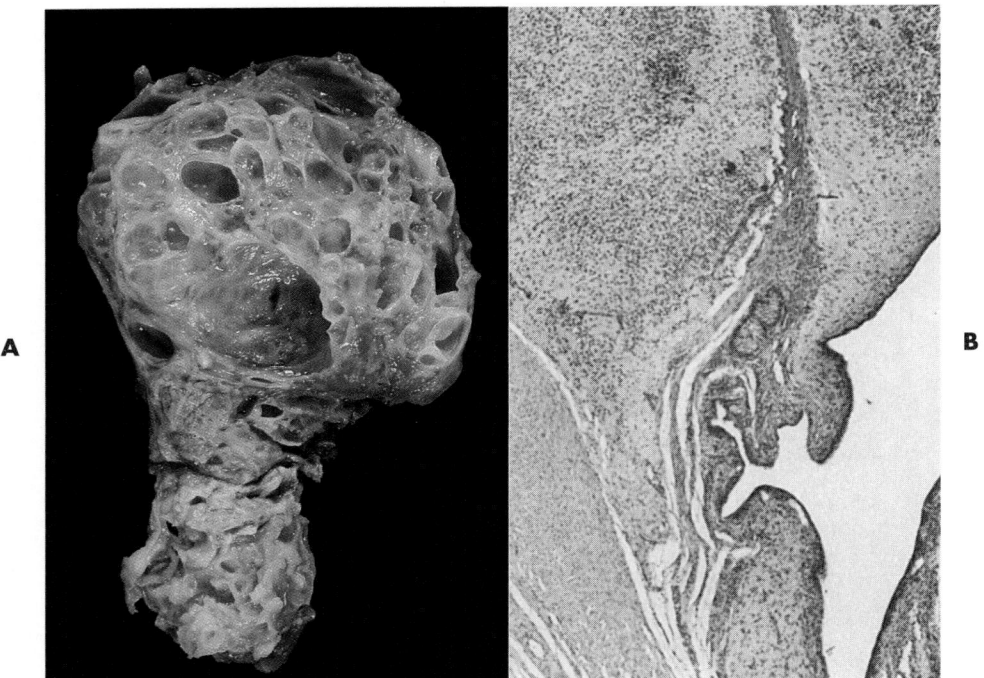

Fig. 26-34 Mature retroperitoneal teratoma. **A,** Gross appearance, showing multiple cystic spaces. **B,** Microscopic appearance from a different case. The tumor is made up of a large variety of tissues from all three layers, including prominent neural component.

small testicular primary tumor are much higher than for a mediastinal tumor of the same type. The gross appearance of the tumor may give a clue in this regard: in general, primary retroperitoneal neoplasms are formed by a single mass, whereas those metastatic from the testis tend to involve several nodes, often on both sides of the peritoneum.[325] Also, seminomas are more likely to be primary than nonseminomatous germ cell tumors. The testicular primary tumor, when present, may be clinically apparent, may be occult, or may have been excised many years previously.[291] In some cases, only intratubular germ cell neoplasia is found in the testicle, suggesting the possibility of independent neoplastic events.[258] Careful palpation, roentgenograms, sonography, and scrotal thermography have been employed to detect occult testicular tumors; of these, sonography has proved to be the most useful.[287]

Other primary tumors and tumorlike conditions

Tumors of sympathetic nervous tissue of the type more commonly seen in the adrenal gland can also be present in the retroperitoneum outside this gland, as indicated in Chapter 16. This includes neuroblastoma, ganglioneuroblastoma, ganglioneuroma, and their variants (Fig. 26-35).

Paragangliomas arise outside the adrenal gland in approximately 10% of the cases. They may occur anywhere along the midline of the retroperitoneum, the best known location being the Zuckerkandl's body (at the origin of the inferior mesenteric artery).[284,298,299] Tumors arising in *heterotopic adrenal cortex* have also been reported.

Myelolipomas similar to those of the adrenal glands can be encountered in the presacral area. They are well-circum-

scribed, can attain a huge size, and are composed of a mixture of fat cells and normal marrow hematopoietic elements.[255] These are usually asymptomatic, whereas mass-forming foci of extramedullary hematopoiesis (which lack fat and are ill defined) are associated with myeloproliferative diseases, hemolytic anemia, or severe skeletal diseases.[259,267]

Carcinoid tumor has been described as a primary retroperitoneal neoplasm; whether it represents a metastasis from an undetected primary tumor, the expression of a monodermal teratoma, or a neoplasm from endocrine cells normally present in this location remains to be determined.[327]

Tumors of müllerian type are occasionally seen as primary retroperitoneal masses in the pelvis or rectovaginal septum (see Chapter 19, Ovary). They can be of serous, mucinous, or endometrioid type, benign or malignant. They arise either from heterotopic ovarian tissue or, more likely, from invaginations of the peritoneal mesothelial layer with concurrent or subsequent metaplasia.[257a,276,301,303,307,318] Some mucinous retroperitoneal tumors have shown evidence of gastric mucosal differentiation, suggesting a totally different histogenesis.[308]

Wilms' tumor has been reported in the retroperitoneum outside the kidney in the absence of teratomatous elements.[283,314,322] Some of these lesions may represent teratomas predominantly or exclusively composed of nephrogenic elements. Most of these cases have occurred in children, but they have also been recorded in adults.[268]

Myoepithelioma has been described, simulating microscopically the appearance of a schwannoma.[255a]

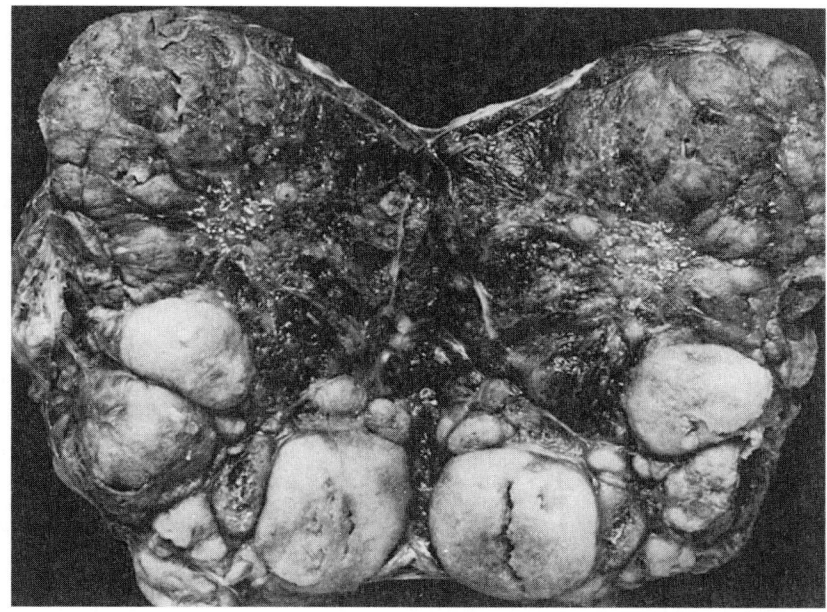

Fig. 26-35 Hemorrhagic nodular ganglioneuroblastoma. (Courtesy Dr. M. Dockerty, Rochester, MN.)

Metastatic tumors

Secondary neoplasms may appear in the retroperitoneal space as a result of local extension or because of lymph node involvement. The former is mainly represented by pancreatic carcinoma and primary bone neoplasms, notably sacrococcygeal chordoma.

The carcinomas most commonly giving rise to retroperitoneal lymph node metastases are those originating in the testis, prostate, pancreas, uterine cervix, endometrium, and kidney.

Sacrococcygeal region
DEVELOPMENTAL ANOMALIES

A large and complex number of malformations can occur in the sacrococcygeal region, the most common being meningocele and spina bifida.[333,342] Some of these are discussed in Chapter 28. *Tailgut cyst (retrorectal cystic hamartoma)* presents in the presacrococcygeal area, usually in adult patients but sometimes in children, as a multiloculated cyst lined by squamous, transitional, or glandular epithelium[334,335,345,346,355,357] (Fig. 26-36). Disorganized fascicles of smooth muscle may be seen in the wall. Prominent glomus bodies may also be present.[356] This benign malformative lesion should be distinguished from teratoma, epidermal cyst, rectal or anal duplication, and anal gland cyst.[354,365] In rare cases, adenocarcinoma and carcinoid tumors arise within tailgut cysts.[353]

GERM CELL TUMORS

Sacrococcygeal germ cell tumors in neonates and infants are nearly always primary.[332] From 75% to 90% of the cases occur in females. They can arise in the retroperitoneum proper, arise in the sacrococcygeal region, or involve both compartments.[340,343,360] Chromosomal analysis of these extragonadal teratomas suggests that they have arisen from

postmitotic, premeiotic cells.[347] The most common type is the *mature teratoma* presenting at birth in the sacrococcygeal region (Fig. 26-37) or protruding through the abdominal cavity (Fig. 26-38).[334,339] It may be very large, is usually cystic and multilocular, and may appear malignant to the surgeon because of its stubborn adherence to neighboring structures. This fixation is of an inflammatory nature, caused by reaction to extravasated material. Total excision is curative; the tip of the coccyx should be removed as part of the operation to prevent recurrence.[367] Microscopically, this tumor is composed of mature tissues throughout. Hepatic tissue is present in one quarter of the cases.[358] The presence of immature elements in regard to amount and microscopic type should be evaluated with care.[366] If this immaturity is restricted to neuroectodermal components (which is often the case), the tendency is toward spontaneous differentiation. As a result, the behavior of this type of immature teratoma is usually benign, although occasional cases will recur or metastasize.[341,366]

Most of the clearly malignant teratomas in this age group have the appearance of *yolk sac (endodermal sinus) tumor,* either pure or associated with other germ cell components, and are accompanied by the production of oncofetal antigens.[340,348,362] They often contain immature hepatic tissue.[358] These tumors run an extremely aggressive clinical course.[336,341,350] A component of Wilms' tumor can sometimes be found within these teratomas.

An interesting clinical observation is that the large majority of sacrococcygeal teratomas present at birth are benign, whereas tumors in the same general location discovered after the age of 2 months are often malignant.[339] This has been taken by some to indicate that a malignant transformation has supervened in that short period. We doubt that this is the case. It seems to us that this clinical observation can better be explained by postulating the existence of two

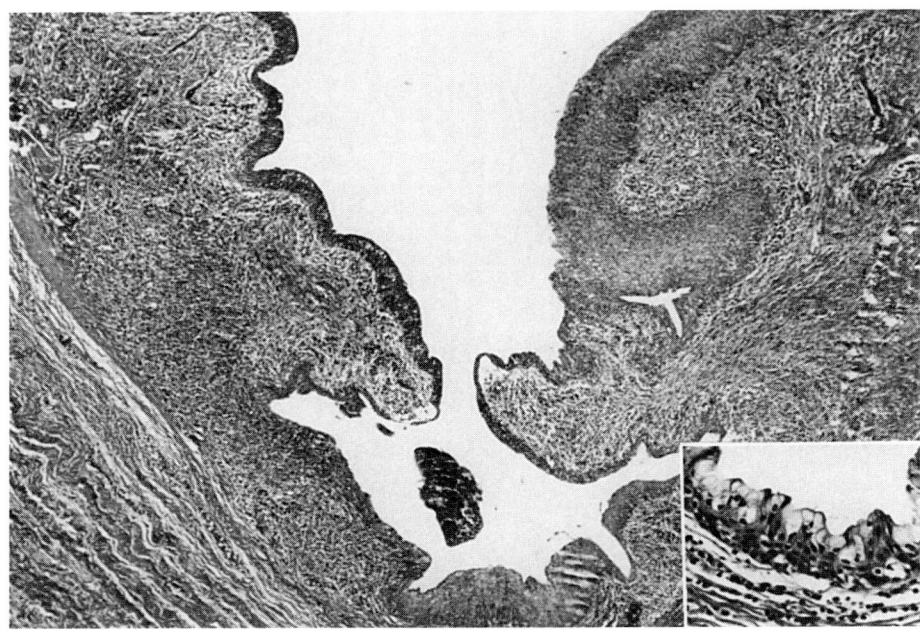

Fig. 26-36 So-called tailgut cyst. Epithelium is squamous in some areas and of glandular type in others. Wall is thick and chronically inflamed. **Inset** shows stratified and partially mucinous nature of epithelium lining a portion of the cyst.

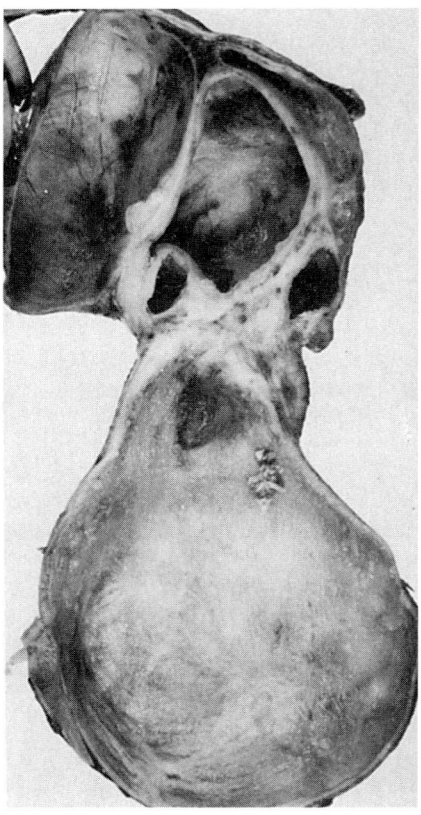

Fig. 26-37 Benign multicystic teratoma of sacrococcygeal region present at birth. It was mainly composed of adult skin and neural tissue.

groups of teratomas. One arises in the very distal portion of the sacrococcygeal region, is therefore clinically obvious at the time of birth, and is nearly always mature. The other arises more proximally, in the retrorectal or adjacent retroperitoneal region, is malignant from the start, and grows into the sacrococcygeal area to become clinically evident only some time after birth. It also grows within the abdominal cavity, this being responsible for the clinical observation that teratomas associated with marked bowel or bladder dysfunction are often malignant. Exceptions in both directions certainly occur, but the large majority of teratomas in this region fit into this scheme.

A sacrococcygeal presentation of teratoma in adults is exceptional. Most are benign and probably have been there since birth. A few show malignant foci, either in the form of germ cell (trophoblastic, yolk sac) components or of adult-type carcinomatous tissues.[331,367] Mature teratomas excised in early life may recur in adulthood in the form of a microscopically similar neoplasm,[351] as a malignant germ cell tumor (such as yolk sac tumor),[363] or as a somatic-type malignant tumor, such as adenocarcinoma.[349]

The differential diagnosis of benign sacrococcygeal teratoma includes the already mentioned developmental abnormalities of this region, a discussion of which is beyond the scope of this book. A comprehensive review of these anomalies can be found in an article by Bale.[333]

PILONIDAL DISEASE

Pilonidal sinuses appear as small openings in the intergluteal fold about 3.5 to 5 cm posterior to the anal orifice. Hairs are sometimes seen protruding from them. The opening is continued by a sinus tract, which is directed upward in

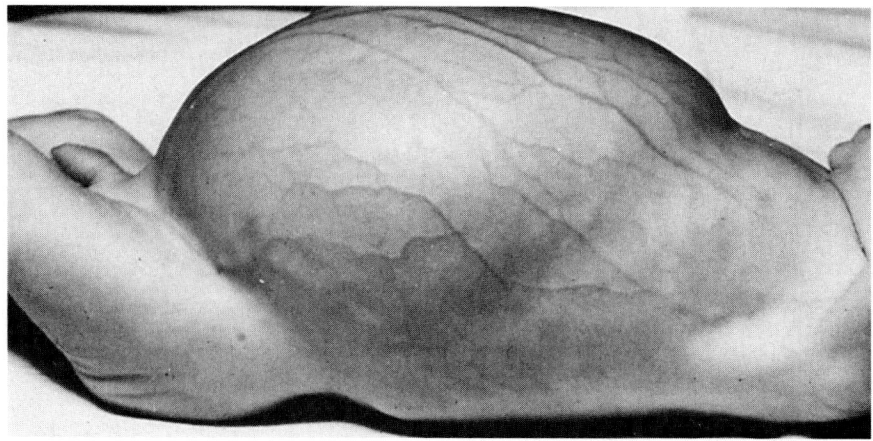

Fig. 26-38 Huge benign cystic retroperitoneal teratoma in infant. Teratoma was removed successfully and child is well.

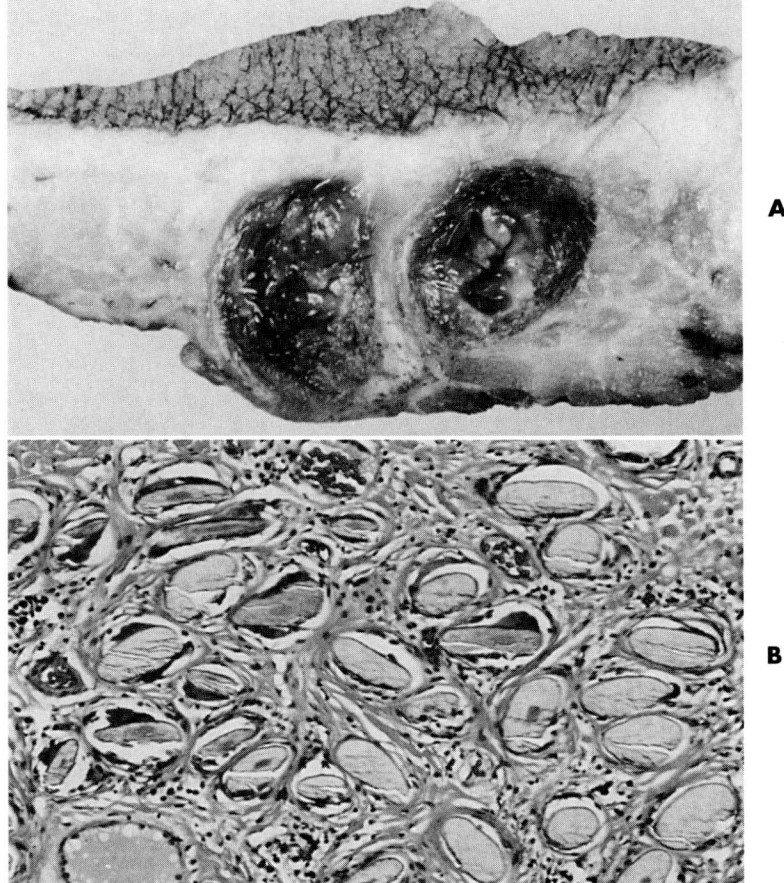

Fig. 26-39 **A,** Pilonidal sinus removed from sacrococcygeal area of 19-year-old youth. Hair-containing cystic structures in dermis are characteristic. They communicated with each other in another plane of section. **B,** Microscopic appearance of pilonidal sinus. Numerous hair shafts penetrate into dermis and elicit foreign body giant cell reaction.

93% of the cases.[361] The disease is most often seen in young white males with dark, straight hair. Although congenital anomalies related to the closure of the neural canal can certainly occur in this area, it is now believed that the large majority of pilonidal sinuses have an acquired pathogenesis.[338] Hairs penetrate areas of inflammation from without, lodge in the dermis, and elicit a foreign body type of reaction (Fig. 26-39). The sinus is lined by granulation tissue. In approximately 25% of the cases, hairs are not found within the lesion.

Pilonidal sinuses also have been described in other areas where skin folds are prominent, such as the umbilicus, clitoris, and axilla.[337] A further observation favoring the theory of the acquired origin is the fact that barbers and hairdressers occasionally develop a disease equivalent to pilonidal sinus between their fingers, the sinuses containing somebody else's hairs!

Cases of *squamous cell carcinoma*[353,364] and *verrucous carcinoma* (giant condyloma acuminatum)[359] developing within pilonidal sinuses have been described.

OTHER TUMORS

Neoplasms other than germ cell tumors can involve the sacrococcygeal region primarily or as an extension from adjacent sites. Most cases of *cellular blue nevus* involve this area (see Chapter 4). Cases of coccydynia have been reported secondarily to *tumors of the coccygeal glomus,* although the neoplastic nature of this process has been questioned (see Chapter 25). *Myxopapillary ependymoma* can involve the soft tissues of the buttock, unconnected with the spine[344,352] (see Chapter 28).

Carcinoid tumor has been seen in a presacral location, presumably primary at this site.[330]

Chordoma arising in the sacrum can produce a large retrorectal or sacrococcygeal mass (see Chapter 24). Finally, *carcinomas* of the anus or rectum (particularly those of the mucinous adenocarcinoma type) can spread to this region by direct extension (see Chapter 11).

REFERENCES
Peritoneum
NORMAL ANATOMY

1 Bolen JLW, Hammar SP, McNutt MA: Reactive and neoplastic serosal tissue. A light-microscopic, ultrastructural, and immunocytochemical study. Am J Surg Pathol **10**:34-47, 1986.
2 McAuley P, Asa SL, Chiu B, Henderson J, Goltzman D, Drucker DJ: Parathyroid hormone-like peptide in normal and neoplastic mesothelial cells. Cancer **66**:1975-1979, 1990.
3 Ober WB, Black MB: Neoplasms of the subcoelomic mesenchyme. Arch Pathol **59**:698-705, 1955.

INFLAMMATION

4 Bastani B, Shariatzadeh MR, Dehdashti F: Tuberculous peritonitis. Report of 30 cases and review of the literature. Q J Med **56**:549-557, 1985.
5 Chen KTK: Coccidioidal peritonitis. Am J Clin Pathol **80**:514-516, 1983.
6 Davis JH: Current concepts of peritonitis. Am Surg **33**:673-681, 1967.
7 Ellis H, Adair HM: Bile peritonitis. A report of fifteen patients. Postgrad Med J **50**:713-717, 1974.
8 Forouhar F: Meconium peritonitis. Pathology, evolution, and diagnosis. Am J Clin Pathol **78**:208-213, 1982.
8a George E, Leyser S, Zimmer HL, Simonowitz DA, Agress RL, Nordin DD: Vernix caseosa peritonitis. An infrequent complication of Cesarean section with distinctive histopathologic features. Am J Clin Pathol **103**:681-684, 1995.
9 Gilinsky NH, Marks IN, Kottler RE, Price SK: Abdominal tuberculosis. A 10-year review. S Afr Med J **64**:849-857, 1983.
10 Gonnella JS, Hudson EK: Clinical patterns of tuberculous peritonitis. Arch Intern Med **117**:164-169, 1966.
11 Kay S: Tissue reaction to barium sulfate contrast medium. Histopathologic study. Arch Pathol **57**:279-284, 1954.
12 Levine H: Needle biopsy of peritoneum in exudative ascites. Arch Intern Med **120**:542-545, 1967.
13 Levine H: Needle biopsy diagnosis of tuberculous peritonitis. Am Rev Respir Dis **97**:889-894, 1968.
14 Seaman WB, Wells J: Complications of the barium enema. Gastroenterology **48**:728-737, 1965.
15 Sherman S, Rohwedder JJ, Ravikrishnan KP, Weg JLG: Tuberculous enteritis and peritonitis. Report of 36 general hospital cases. Arch Intern Med **140**:506-507, 1980.
16 Singh MM, Bhargava AN, Jain KP: Tuberculous peritonitis. An evaluation of pathogenetic mechanisms, diagnostic procedures and therapeutic measures. N Engl J Med **281**:1091-1094, 1969.
17 Sochocky S: Tuberculous peritonitis. A review of 100 cases. Am Rev Respir Dis **95**:398-401, 1967.
18 Vinuela A, Fernandez-Rojo F, Martinez-Merino A: Oxyuris granulomas of pelvic peritoneum and appendicular wall. Histopathology **3**:69-77, 1979.

ADHESIONS

19 Black W, Nelson D, Walker W: Multifocal subperitoneal sclerosis. Surgery **63**:706-710, 1968.
20 Bockman RF, Woods M, Sargent L, Gervin AS: A unifying pathogenetic mechanism in the etiology of intraperitoneal adhesions. J Surg Res **20**:1-5, 1976.
21 Brown P, Baddeley H, Read AE, Davies JD, McGarry JMc: Sclerosing peritonitis. An unusual reaction to a ß-adrenergic-blocking drug (Practolol). Lancet **2**:1477-1481, 1974.
22 Castelli MJ, Armin A-R, Husain A, Orfei E: Fibrosing peritonitis in a drug abuser. Arch Pathol Lab Med **109**:767-769, 1985.
23 Clement PB, Young RH, Hanna W, Scully RE: Sclerosing peritonitis associated with luteinized thecomas of the ovary. A clinicopathological analysis of six cases. Am J Surg Pathol **18**:1-13, 1994.
24 Ryan GB, Grobety J, Majno G: Postoperative peritoneal adhesions. A study of the mechanisms. Am J Pathol **65**:117-140, 1971.

REACTION TO FOREIGN MATERIALS

25 Auer EA, Dockerty MB, Mayo CW: Reaction to foreign material. Ruptured dermoid cyst of the ovary simulating abdominal carcinomatosis. Mayo Clin Proc **26**:489-497, 1951.
26 Carr N, Turk E: The histological features of splenosis. Histopathology **21**:549-554, 1992.
27 Chen KTK, Kostich ND, Rosai J: Peritoneal foreign body granulomas to keratin in uterine adenoacanthoma. Arch Pathol Lab Med **102**:174-177, 1978.
28 Clarke TJ, Simpson RH: Necrotizing granuloma of peritoneum following diathermy ablation of endometriosis. Histopathology **16**:400-402, 1990.
29 Clement PB, Young RH, Scully RE: Necrotic pseudoxanthomatous nodules of ovary and peritoneum in endometriosis. Am J Surg Pathol **12**:330-397, 1988.
30 Coder DM, Olander GA: Granulomatous peritonitis caused by starch glove powder. Arch Surg **105**:83-86, 1972.
31 Davies JD, Ansell ID: Food-starch granulomatous peritonitis. J Clin Pathol **36**:435-438, 1983.
32 Davies JD, Neely J: The histopathology of peritoneal starch granulomas. J Pathol **107**:265-278, 1972.
33 Eiseman B, Seelig MG, Womack NA: Talcum powder granuloma. Frequent and serious postoperative complication. Ann Surg **126**:820-832, 1947.
34 Holmes EC, Eggleston JC: Starch granulomatous peritonitis. Surgery **71**:85-90, 1972.
35 Kim KR, Scully RE: Peritoneal keratin granulomas with carcinomas of endometrium and ovary and atypical polypoid adenomyoma of endometrium. A clinicopathological analysis of 22 cases. Am J Surg Pathol **14**:925-932, 1990.
36 Levison DA, Crocker PR, Jones S, Owen RA, Barnard NJ: The varied appearances of starch particles in smears and paraffin sections. Histopathology **13**:667-674, 1988.
37 Marshall SF, Rorse RA: Peritoneal adhesions. Report of a case of paraffinoma. Surg Clin North Am **32**:903-908, 1952.
38 Nissim F, Ashkenazy M, Borenstein R, Czernobilsky B: Tuberculoid cornstarch granulomas with caseous necrosis. A diagnostic challenge. Arch Pathol Lab Med **105**:86-88, 1981.
39 Saxen L, Saxen E: Starch granulomas as a problem in surgical pathology. Acta Pathol Microbiol Scand **64**:55-70, 1965.

40 Tinker MA, Burdman D, Deysine M, Teicher I, Platt N, Aufses AH Jr: Granulomatous peritonitis due to cellulose fibers from disposable surgical fabrics. Laboratory investigations and clinical implications. Ann Surg 180:831-835, 1974.

CYSTS AND LOOSE BODIES

41 Carpenter HA, Lancaster JR, Lee RA: Multilocular cysts of the peritoneum. Mayo Clin Proc 57:634-638, 1982.
42 Drachenberg CB, Papadimitriou JC: Melanotic peritoneal cyst. Light-microscopic and ultrastructural studies. Arch Pathol Lab Med 114:463-467, 1990.
43 Eickhoff JH: Müllerian duct cyst. Report of a case and review of the literature. Scand J Urol Nephrol 12:89-92, 1978.
44 Katsube Y, Mukai K, Silverberg SG: Cystic mesothelioma of the peritoneum. Cancer 50:1615-1622, 1982.
45 Lascano EF, Villamayor RD, Llauro JL: Loose cysts of the peritoneal cavity. Ann Surg 152:836-844, 1960.
46 McFadden DE, Clement PB: Peritoneal inclusion cysts with mural mesothelial proliferation. A clinicopathological analysis of six cases. Am J Surg Pathol 10:844-854, 1986.
47 Mennemeyer R, Smith M: Multicystic, peritoneal mesothelioma. A report with electron microscopy of a case mimicking intraabdominal cystic hygroma (lymphangioma). Cancer 44:692-698, 1979.
48 Moore JH Jr, Crum CP, Chandler JG, Feldman PS: Benign cystic mesothelioma. Cancer 45:2395-2399, 1980.
49 Novak RW, Raines RB, Sollee AN: Clear cell carcinoma in a müllerian duct cyst. Am J Clin Pathol 76:339-341, 1981.
50 Ross MJ, Welch WR, Scully RE: Multilocular peritoneal inclusion cysts (so-called cystic mesotheliomas). Cancer 64:1336-1346, 1989.
51 Sarto GE, Simpson JL: Abnormalities of the müllerian and wolffian duct systems. Birth Defects 14:37-55, 1978.
52 Schneider V, Partridge JR, Gutierrez F, Hurt WG, Maizels MS, Demay RM: Benign cystic mesothelioma involving the female genital tract. Report of four cases. Am J Obstet Gynecol 145:355-359, 1983.
53 Villaschi S, Autelitano F, Santeusanio G, Balistreri P: Cystic mesothelioma of the peritoneum. A report of three cases. Am J Clin Pathol 94:758-761, 1990.
54 Vuong PN, Guyot H, Moulin G, Houissa-Vuong S, Berrod JL: Pseudotumoral organization of a twisted epiploic fringe or 'hard-boiled egg' in the peritoneal cavity. Arch Pathol Lab Med 114:531-533, 1990.

HYPERPLASIA AND METAPLASIA

55 Bolen JW, Hammar SP, McNutt MA: Reactive and neoplastic serosal tissue. A light-microscopic, ultrastructural, and immunocytochemical study. Am J Surg Pathol 10:34-47, 1986.
56 Clement PB, Young RH: Florid mesothelial hyperplasia associated with ovarian tumors. A potential source of error in tumor diagnosis and staging. Int J Gynecol Pathol 12:51-58, 1993.
57 Crone L: Squamous metaplasia of the peritoneum. J Pathol Bacteriol 62:61-68, 1950.
58 Deligdisch L, Kerner H, Cohen CJ, Dargent D, Gil J: Morphometric differentiation between responsive tumor cells and mesothelial hyperplasia in second-look operations for ovarian cancer. Hum Pathol 24:143-147, 1993.
59 McCaughey WTE, Al-Jabi M: Differentiation of serosal hyperplasia and neoplasia in biopsies. Pathol Annu 21(Pt 1):271-293, 1986.
60 Rosai J, Dehner LP: Nodular mesothelial hyperplasia in hernia sacs. A benign reactive condition simulating a neoplastic process. Cancer 35:165-175, 1975.
61 Schatz JE, Colgan TJ: Squamous metaplasia of the peritoneum. Arch Pathol Lab Med 115:397-398, 1991.
62 Zaytsev P, Taxy JB: Pregnancy-associated ectopic decidua. Am J Surg Pathol 11:526-530, 1987.

TUMORS
Mesothelioma

63 Andrion A, Pira E, Mollo F: Peritoneal plaques and asbestos exposure. Arch Pathol Lab Med 107:609-610, 1983.
64 Antman KH: Malignant mesothelioma. N Engl J Med 303:200-202, 1980.
65 Armstrong GR, Raafat F, Ingram L, Mann JR: Malignant peritoneal mesothelioma in childhood. Arch Pathol Lab Med 112:1159-1162, 1988.
66 Bolen JW, Hammar SP, McNutt MA: Reactive and neoplastic serosal tissue. A light-microscopic, ultrastructural, and immunocytochemical study. Am J Surg Pathol 10:34-47, 1986.
67 Bolen JW, Thorning D: Mesotheliomas. A light-and electron-microscopical study concerning histogenetic relationships between the epithelial and the mesenchymal variants. Am J Surg Pathol 4:451-464, 1980.

68 Bolio-Cicero A, Aguirre J, Perez-Tamayo R: Malignant peritoneal mesothelioma. Am J Clin Pathol 36:417-426, 1961.
69 Bollinger DJ, Wick MR, Dehner LP, Mills SE, Swanson PE, Clarke RE: Peritoneal malignant mesothelioma versus serous papillary adenocarcinoma. A histochemical and immunohistochemical comparison. Am J Surg Pathol 13:659-670, 1989.
70 Brown JW, Kristensen KAB, Monroe LS: Peritoneal mesothelioma following pneumoperitoneum maintained for 12 years. Report of a case. Am J Dig Dis 13:830-835, 1968.
71 Chen KT: Malignant mesothelioma presenting as Sister Joseph's nodule. Am J Dermatopathol 13:300-303, 1991.
72 Chiu B, Churg A, Tengblad A, Pearce R, McCaughey WTE: Analysis of hyaluronic acid in the diagnosis of malignant mesothelioma. Cancer 54:2195-2199, 1984.
73 Churg A: Immunohistochemical staining for vimentin and keratin in malignant mesothelioma. Am J Surg Pathol 9:360-365, 1985.
74 Crotty TB, Myers JL, Katzenstein A-LA, Tazelaar HD, Swensen SJ, Churg A: Localized malignant mesothelioma. A clinicopathologic and flow cytometric study. Am J Surg Pathol 18:357-363, 1994.
75 Daya D, McCaughey WT: Well-differentiated papillary mesothelioma of the peritoneum. A clinicopathologic study of 22 cases. Cancer 65:292-296, 1990.
76 Daya D, McCaughey WT: Pathology of the peritoneum. A review of selected topics. Semin Diagn Pathol 8:277-289, 1991.
77 Goepel JR: Benign papillary mesothelioma of peritoneum. A histological, histochemical and ultrastructural study of six cases. Histopathology 5:21-30, 1981.
78 Gosh AK, Butler EB: Immunocytological staining reactions of anticarcinoembryonic antigen, CA and antihuman milk fat globule monoclonal antibodies on benign and malignant exfoliated mesothelial cells. J Clin Pathol 40:1424-1427, 1987.
79 Kane MJ, Chahinian AP, Holland JF: Malignant mesothelioma in young adults. Cancer 65:1449-1455, 1990.
79a Kallianpur AR, Carstens PH, Liotta LA, Frey KP, Siegal GP: Immunoreactivity in malignant mesotheliomas with antibodies to basement membrane components and their receptors. Mod Pathol 3:11-18, 1990.
80 Kannerstein M, Churg J: Peritoneal mesothelioma. Hum Pathol 8:83-94, 1977.
81 Kannerstein M, Churg J, Magner D: Histochemistry in the diagnosis of malignant mesothelioma. Ann Clin Lab Sci 3:207-211, 1973.
82 Kauffman SL, Stout AP: Mesothelioma in children. Cancer 17:539-544, 1964.
83 Khoury N, Raju U, Crissman JD, Zarbo RJ, Greenawald KA: A comparative immunohistochemical study of peritoneal and ovarian serous tumors, and mesotheliomas. Hum Pathol 21:811-819, 1990.
84 Kitazawa M, Kaneko H, Toshima M, Ishikawa H, Kobayashi H, Sekiya M: Malignant peritoneal mesothelioma with massive foamy cells. Codfish roe-like mesothelioma. Acta Pathol Jpn 34:687-692, 1984.
85 Kung ITM, Thallas V, Spencer EJ, Wilson SM: Expression of muscle actin in diffuse mesotheliomas. Hum Pathol 26:565-570, 1995.
86 Kwee WS, Veldhuizen RW, Vermorken JB, Golding RP, Donner R: Peritoneal mesothelioma presenting as umbilical tumor. Pathol Res Pract 174:159-165, 1982.
87 Lederman GS, Recht A, Herman T, Osteen R, Corson J, Antman KH: Long-term survival in peritoneal mesothelioma. The role of radiotherapy and combined modality treatment. Cancer 59:1882-1886, 1987.
88 Lerner HJ, Schoenfeld DA, Martin A, Falkson G, Borden E: Malignant mesothelioma. The Eastern Cooperative Oncology Group (ECOG) experience. Cancer 52:1981-1985, 1983.
89 Maurer R, Egloff B: Malignant peritoneal mesothelioma after cholangiography with Thorotrast. Cancer 36:1381-1385, 1975.
90 Mayall FG, Goddard H, Gibbs AR: Intermediate filament expression in mesotheliomas. Leiomyoid mesotheliomas are not uncommon. Histopathology 21:453-457, 1992.
91 Nascimento AG, Keeney GL, Fletcher CD: Deciduoid peritoneal mesothelioma. An unusual phenotype affecting young females. Am J Surg Pathol 18:439-445, 1994.
92 Riddell RH, Goodman MJ, Moossa AR: Peritoneal malignant mesothelioma in a patient with recurrent peritonitis. Cancer 48:134-139, 1981.
93 Segers K, Ramael M, Singh SK, Weyler J, Van Meerbeeck J, Vermeire P, Van Marck E: Immunoreactivity for bcl-2 protein in malignant mesothelioma and non-neoplastic mesothelium. Virchows Arch 424:631-634, 1994.
94 Silberstein MJ, Lewis JE, Blair JD, Graviss ER, Brodeur AE: Congenital peritoneal mesothelioma. J Pediatr Surg 18:243-246, 1983.
95 Smither WJ: Asbestos and mesothelioma of the pleura. Proc R Soc Med 59:57-61, 1966.

96 Strickler JG, Herndier BG, Rouse RV: Immunohistochemical staining in malignant mesotheliomas. Am J Clin Pathol **88:**610-614, 1987.

97 Sussman J, Rosai J: Lymph node metastasis as the initial manifestation of malignant mesothelioma. Report of six cases. Am J Surg Pathol **14:**819-828, 1990.

98 Suzuki Y: Diagnostic criteria for human diffuse malignant mesothelioma. Acta Pathol Jpn **42:**767-786, 1992.

99 Suzuki Y, Churg J, Kannerstein M: Ultrastructure of human malignant diffuse mesothelioma. Am J Pathol **85:**241-251, 1976.

100 Talerman A, Montero JR, Chilcote RR, Okagaki T: Diffuse malignant peritoneal mesothelioma in a 13-year-old girl. Report of a case and review of the literature. Am J Surg Pathol **9:**73-80, 1985.

101 Trotter BB, Palmer WS: Mesenchymomatous mesothelioma. Report of a case with unusual histological features. Cancer **12:**884-888, 1959.

102 Vogelzang NJ, Schultz SM, Iannucci AM, Kennedy BJ: Malignant mesothelioma. The University of Minnesota experience. Cancer **53:**377-383, 1984.

103 Wick MR, Mills SE, Swanson PE: Expression of "myelomonocytic" antigens in mesotheliomas and adenocarcinomas involving the serosal surfaces. Am J Clin Pathol **94:**18-26, 1990.

104 Winslow DJ, Taylor HB: Malignant peritoneal mesotheliomas. Cancer **13:**127-136, 1960.

Intra-abdominal desmoplastic small cell tumor

105 Amin KM, Litzky LA, Smythe WR, Mooney AM, Morris JM, Mews DJY, Pass HI, Kari C, Rodeck U, Rauscher III FJ, Kaiser LR, Albelda SM: Wilms' tumor 1 susceptibility (WT1) gene products are selectively expressed in malignant mesothelioma. Am J Pathol **146:**344-356, 1995.

106 de Alava E, Ladanyi M, Rosai J, Gerald WL: Detection of chimeric transcripts in desmoplastic small round cell tumor and related developmental tumors by RT-PCR. A specific diagnostic assay. Am J Pathol 1995 (in press).

107 Gaudin PB, Rosai J: Florid vascular proliferation associated with neural and neuroendocrine neoplasms. A diagnostic clue and potential pitfall. Am J Surg Pathol **19:**642-652, 1995.

108 Gerald WL, Miller HK, Battifora H, Miettinen M, Silva EG, Rosai J: Intra-abdominal desmoplastic small round-cell tumor. Report of 19 cases of a distinctive type of high-grade polyphenotypic malignancy affecting young individuals. Am J Surg Pathol **15:**499-513, 1991.

109 Gerald WL, Rosai J: Desmoplastic small cell tumor with multi-phenotypic differentiation. Zentralbl Pathol **139:**141-151, 1993.

110 Gerald WL, Rosai J, Ladanyi M: Characterization of the genomic breakpoint and chimeric transcripts in the EWS-WT1 gene fusion of desmoplastic small round cell tumor. Proc Natl Acad Sci USA **92:**1028-1032, 1995.

111 Gonzalez-Crussi F, Crawford SE, Sun CC: Intraabdominal desmoplastic small-cell tumors with divergent differentiation. Observations on three cases of childhood. Am J Surg Pathol **14:**633-642, 1990.

112 Ladanyi M, Gerald W: Fusion of the EWS and WT1 genes in the desmoplastic small round cell tumor. Cancer Res **54:**2837-2840, 1994.

113 Ordóñez NG, el-Naggar AK, Ro JY, Silva EG, Mackay B: Intra-abdominal desmoplastic small cell tumor. A light microscopic, immunocytochemical, ultrastructural, and flow cytometric study. Hum Pathol **24:**850-865, 1993.

114 Parkash V, Gerald WL, Parma A, Miettinen M, Rosai J: Desmoplastic small round cell tumor of the pleura. Am J Surg Pathol **19:**659-665, 1995.

115 Rodriguez E, Sreekantaiah C, Gerald W, Reuter VE, Motzer RJ, Chaganti RS: A recurring translocation, t(11; 22)(p13; q11.2), characterizes intra-abdominal desmoplastic small round-cell tumors. Cancer Genet Cytogenet **69:**17-21, 1993.

116 Schmidt D, Koster E, Harms D: Intraabdominal desmoplastic small-cell tumor with divergent differentiation. Clinicopathological findings and DNA ploidy. Med Pediatr Oncol **22:**97-102, 1994.

117 Shintaku M, Baba Y, Fujiwara T: Intra-abdominal desmoplastic small cell tumour in a patient with Peutz-Jeghers syndrome. Virchows Arch **425:**211-215, 1994.

118 Tison V, Cerasoli S, Morigi F, Ladanyi M, Gerald WL, Rosai J: Intracranial desmoplastic small-cell tumor. Report of a case. Am J Surg Pathol (in press).

119 Wills EJ: Peritoneal desmoplastic small round cell tumors with divergent differentiation. A review. Ultrastruct Pathol **17:**295-306, 1993.

120 Young RH, Eichhorn JH, Dickersin GR, Scully RE: Ovarian involvement by the intra-abdominal desmoplastic small round cell tumor with divergent differentiation. A report of three cases. Hum Pathol **23:**454-464, 1992.

Other primary tumors

121 Gonzalez-Crussi F, Sotelo-Avila C, de Mello DE: Primary peritoneal, omental, and mesenteric tumors in childhood. Semin Diagn Pathol **3:**122-137, 1986.

122 Goodlad JR, Fletcher CD: Solitary fibrous tumour arising at unusual sites. Analysis of a series. Histopathology **19:**515-522, 1991.

123 McCaughey WTE, Dardick I, Barr JR: Angiosarcoma of serous membranes. Arch Pathol Lab Med **107:**304-307, 1983.

124 Stout AP: Solitary fibrous mesothelioma of the peritoneum. Cancer **3:**820-825, 1950.

125 Young RH, Clement PB, McCaughey WT: Solitary fibrous tumors ('fibrous mesotheliomas') of the peritoneum. A report of three cases and a review of the literature. Arch Pathol Lab Med **114:**493-495, 1990.

126 Yousem SA, Hochholzer L: Unusual thoracic manifestations of epithelioid hemangioendothelioma. Arch Pathol Lab Med **111:**459-463, 1987.

Lesions of the secondary müllerian system

127 Bell DA, Scully RE: Benign and borderline serous lesions of the peritoneum in women. Pathol Annu **24**(Pt 2):1-21, 1989.

128 Buttner A, Bassler R, Theele C: Pregnancy-associated ectopic decidua (deciduosis) of the greater omentum. An analysis of 60 biopsies with cases of fibrosing deciduosis and leiomyomatosis peritonealis disseminata. Pathol Res Pract **189:**352-359, 1993.

129 Chang KL, Crabtree GS, Lim-Tan SK, Kempson RL, Hendrickson MR: Primary extrauterine endometrial stromal neoplasms. A clinicopathologic study of 20 cases and a review of the literature. Int J Gynecol Pathol **12:**282-296, 1993.

130 Clement PB, Young RH, Scully RE: Nontrophoblastic pathology of the female genital tract and peritoneum associated with pregnancy. Semin Diagn Pathol **6:**372-406, 1989.

131 Dalrymple JC, Bannatyne P, Russell P, Solomon HJ, Tattersall MH, Atkinson K, Carter J, Duval P, Elliott P, Friedlander M, et al.: Extraovarian peritoneal serous papillary carcinoma. A clinicopathologic study of 31 cases. Cancer **64:**110-115, 1989.

132 Due W, Pickartz H: Immunohistologic detection of estrogen and progesterone receptors in disseminated peritoneal leiomyomatosis. Int J Gynecol Pathol **8:**46-53, 1989.

133 Fox H: Primary neoplasia of the female peritoneum. Histopathology **23:**103-110, 1993.

134 Fromm GL, Gershenson DM, Silva EG: Papillary serous carcinoma of the peritoneum. Obstet Gynecol **75:**89-95, 1990.

135 Garamvoelgyi E, Guillou L, Gebhard S, Salmeron M, Seematter RJ, Hadji MH: Primary malignant mixed Müllerian tumor (metaplastic carcinoma) of the female peritoneum. A clinical, pathologic, and immunohistochemical study of three cases and a review of the literature. Cancer **74:**854-863, 1994.

136 Lauchlan SC: The secondary müllerian system revisited. Int J Gynecol Pathol **13:**73-79, 1994.

137 Ma KF, Chow LT: Sex cord–like pattern leiomyomatosis peritonealis disseminata. A hitherto undescribed feature. Histopathology **21:**389-391, 1992.

138 Sutherland JA, Wilson EA, Edger DE, Powell D: Ultrastructure and steroid-binding studies in leiomyomatosis peritonealis disseminata. Am J Obstet Gynecol **136:**992-996, 1980.

139 Tauber H-D, Wissner SE, Haskins AL: Leiomyomatosis peritonealis disseminata. An unusual complication of genital leiomyomata. Obstet Gynecol **25:**561-574, 1965.

140 Thor AD, Young RH, Clement PB: Pathology of the fallopian tube, broad ligament, peritoneum, and pelvic soft tissues. Hum Pathol **22:**856-867, 1991.

Metastatic tumors; Cytology

141 Cardozo PL: A critical evaluation of 3,000 cytologic analyses of pleural fluid, ascitic fluid and pericardial fluid. Acta Cytol (Baltimore) **10:**455-460, 1966.

142 Cariker M, Dockerty M: Mucinous cystadenomas and mucinous cystadenocarcinomas of the ovary. A clinical and pathorical study of 355 cases. Cancer **7:**302-310, 1954.

143 Chu DZ, Lang NP, Thompson C, Osteen PK, Westbrook KC: Peritoneal carcinomatosis in nongynecologic malignancy. A prospective study of prognostic factors. Cancer **63:**364-367, 1989.

144 Esteban JM, Yokota S, Husain S, Battifora H: Immunocytochemical profile of benign and carcinomatous effusions. A practical approach to difficult diagnosis. Am J Clin Pathol **94:**698-705, 1990.

145 Fernandez RN, Daly JM: Pseudomyxoma peritonei. Arch Surg **115:**409-414, 1980.

146 Harms D, Janig U, Gobel U: Gliomatosis peritonei in childhood and adolescence. Pathol Res Pract **184:**422-430, 1989.

147 Higa E, Rosai J, Pizzimbono CA, Wise L: Mucosal hyperplasia, mucinous cystadenoma and mucinous cystadenocarcinoma of appendix. A re-evaluation of appendiceal "mucocele." Cancer **32:**1325-1341, 1973.

148 Johnson WD: The cytological diagnosis of cancer in serous effusion. Acta Cytol (Baltimore) **10:**161-172, 1966.

149 Kahn MA, Demopoulos RI: Mucinous ovarian tumors with pseudomyxoma peritonei. A clinicopathological study. Int J Gynecol Pathol **11:**15-23, 1992.

150 Klempman S: The exfoliative cytology of diffuse pleural mesothelioma. Cancer **15:**691-704, 1962.

151 Long RTL, Spratt JS, Dowling E: Pseudomyxoma peritonei. New concepts in management with a report of 17 patients. Am J Surg **117:**162-168, 1969.

152 Mann WJ, Jr, Wagner J, Chumas J, Chalas E: The management of pseudomyxoma peritonei. Cancer **66:**1636-1640, 1990.

153 Melamed MR: The cytological presentation of malignant lymphomas and related diseases in effusions. Cancer **16:**413-431, 1963.

154 Nance KV, Silverman JF: Immunocytochemical panel for the identification of malignant cells in serous effusions. Am J Clin Pathol **95:**867-874, 1991.

155 Naylor B: The exfoliative cytology of diffuse malignant mesothelioma. J Pathol Bacteriol **86:**293-298, 1963.

156 Prayson RA, Hart WR, Petras RE: Pseudomyxoma peritonei. A clinicopathologic study of 19 cases with emphasis on site of origin and nature of associated ovarian tumors. Am J Surg Pathol **18:**591-603, 1994.

157 Reagan JW: Exfoliative cytology of pleural, peritoneal and pericardial fluids. CA **10:**153-159, 1960.

158 Roberts HG, Campbell GM: Exfoliative cytology of diffuse mesothelioma. J Clin Pathol **23:**577-582, 1972.

159 Ronnett BM, Kurman RJ, Zahn CM, Schmookler BM, Jablonski KA, Kass ME, Sugarbaker PH: Pseudomyxoma peritoneum in women. A clinicopathologic analysis of 30 cases with emphasis on site of origin, prognosis, and relationship to ovarian mucinous tumors of low malignant potential. Hum Pathol **26:**509-524, 1995.

160 Ruitenbeek T, Gouw AS, Poppema S: Immunocytology of body cavity fluids. MOC-31, a monoclonal antibody discriminating between mesothelial and epithelial cells. Arch Pathol Lab Med **118:**265-269, 1994.

161 Smith JW, Kemeny N, Caldwell C, Banner P, Sigurdson E, Huvos A: Pseudomyxoma peritonei of appendiceal origin. The Memorial Sloan-Kettering Cancer Center experience. Cancer **70:**396-401, 1992.

162 Takagi F: Studies on tumor cells in serous effusion. Am J Clin Pathol **24:**663-675, 1954.

163 Tarin D, Price JE, Kettlewell MGW, Souter RG, Vass ACR, Crossley B: Mechanisms of human tumor metastasis studied in patients with peritoneovenous shunts. Cancer Res **44:**3584-3592, 1984.

164 Young RH, Gilks CB, Scully RE: Mucinous tumors of the appendix associated with mucinous tumors of the ovary and pseudomyxoma peritonei. A clinicopathological analysis of 22 cases supporting an origin in the appendix. Am J Surg Pathol **15:**415-429, 1991.

Omentum

165 Chong PY, Panabokke RG, Chew KH: Omental cryptococcoma. An unusual presentation of cryptococcosis. Arch Pathol Lab Med **110:**239-241, 1986.

166 Dixon AY, Reed JS, Dow N, Lee SH: Primary omental leiomyosarcoma masquerading as hemorrhagic ascites. Hum Pathol **15:**233-237, 1984.

167 Epstein LI, Lempke RE: Primary idiopathic segmental infarction of the greater omentum. Case report and collective review of the literature. Ann Surg **167:**437-443, 1968.

168 Galifer RB, Pous JG, Juskiewenski S, Pasquie M, Gaubert J: Intra-abdominal cystic lymphangiomas in childhood. Prog Pediatr Surg **11:**173-239, 1978.

169 Gonzalez-Crussi F, de Mello DE, Sotelo-Avila C: Omental-mesenteric myxoid hamartomas. Infantile lesions simulating malignant tumors. Am J Surg Pathol **7:**567-578, 1983.

170 Gonzalez-Crussi F, Sotelo-Avila C, de Mello DE: Primary peritoneal, omental, and mesenteric tumors in childhood. Semin Diagn Pathol **3:**122-137, 1986.

171 Ordóñez NG, Manning JT Jr, Ayala AG: Teratoma of the omentum. Cancer **51:**955-958, 1983.

172 Stout AP, Hendry J, Purdie FJ: Primary solid tumors of the great omentum. Cancer **16:**231-243, 1963.

173 Tsutsumi A, Kawabata K, Taguchi K, Doi K: Elastofibroma of the greater omentum. Acta Pathol Jpn **35:**233-241, 1985.

Mesentery

174 Banerjee R, Gough J: Cystic mucinous tumours of the mesentery and retroperitoneum. Report of three cases. Histopathology **12:**527-532, 1988.

175 Barnardo DE, Stavrou M, Bourne R, Bogomoletz W: Primary carcinoid tumor of the mesentery. Hum Pathol **15:**796-798, 1984.

176 Barr WB, Yamashita T: Mesenteric cysts. Review of the literature and report of a case. Am J Gastroenterol **41:**53-57, 1964.

177 Buonanno G, Gonella F, Pettinato G, Castaldo C: Autoimmune hemolytic anemia and dermoid cyst of the mesentery. A case report. Cancer **54:**2533-2536, 1984.

178 Burke AP, Sobin LH, Shekitka KM: Mesenteric fibromatosis. A follow-up study. Arch Pathol Lab Med **114:**832-835, 1990.

179 Burke AP, Sobin LH, Shekitka KM, Federspiel BH, Helwig EB: Intra-abdominal fibromatosis. A pathologic analysis of 130 tumors with comparison of clinical subgroups. Am J Surg Pathol **14:**335-341, 1990.

180 Carpenter HA, Lancaster JR, Lee RA: Multilocular cysts of the peritoneum. Mayo Clin Proc **57:**634-638, 1982.

181 Coffin CM, Watterson J, Priest JR, Dehner LP: Extrapulmonary inflammatory myofibroblastic tumor (inflammatory pseudotumor). A clinicopathologic and immunohistochemical study of 84 cases. Am J Surg Pathol **19:**859-872, 1995.

182 Crane JT, Aguilar MJ, Grimes OR: Isolated lipodystrophy. A form of mesenteric tumor. Am J Surg **90:**169-179, 1955.

183 Gorlin RJ, Sedano HO: The multiple nevoid basal cell carcinoma syndrome revisited. Birth Defects **7:**140-148, 1971.

184 Hansen RC, Castelino RA, Lazerson J, Probert J: Mesenteric hemangioendothelioma with thrombocytopenia. Cancer **32:**136-141, 1973.

185 Harpaz N, Gellman E: Urogenital mesenteric cyst with fallopian tubal features. Arch Pathol Lab Med **111:**78-80, 1987.

186 Hashimoto H, Tsuneyoshi M, Enjoji M: Malignant smooth muscle tumors of the retroperitoneum and mesentery. A clinicopathologic analysis of 44 cases. J Surg Oncol **28:**177-186, 1985.

187 Jones MA, Clement PB, Young RH: Primary yolk sac tumors of the mesentery. A report of two cases. Am J Clin Pathol **101:**42-47, 1994.

188 Kelly JK, Hwang WS: Idiopathic retractile (sclerosing) mesenteritis and its differential diagnosis. Am J Surg Pathol **13:**513-521, 1989.

189 Kipfer RE, Moertel CG, Dahlin DC: Mesenteric lipodystrophy. Ann Intern Med **80:**582-588, 1974.

190 Kurtz RJ, Heimann TM, Holt J, Beck AR: Mesenteric and retroperitoneal cysts. Ann Surg **203:**109-112, 1986.

191 Magid D, Fishman EK, Jones B, Hoover HC, Feinstein R, Siegelman SS: Desmoid tumors in Gardner syndrome. Use of computed tomography. AJR **142:**1141-1145, 1984.

192 Meis JM, Enzinger FM: Inflammatory fibrosarcoma of the mesentery and retroperitoneum. A tumor closely simulating inflammatory pseudotumor. Am J Surg Pathol **15:**1146-1156, 1991.

193 Monihan JM, Carr NJ, Sobin LH: CD34 immunoexpression in stromal tumours of the gastrointestinal tract and in mesenteric fibromatoses. Histopathology **25:**469-474, 1994.

194 Moyana TN: Primary mesenteric liposarcoma. Am J Gastroenterol **83:**89-92, 1988.

195 Neerhout RC, Larson W, Mansur P: Mesenteric lymphoid hamartoma associated with chronic hypoferremia, anemia, growth failure and hypoglobulinemia. N Engl J Med **280:**922-925, 1969.

196 Ogden WM, Bradburn DM, Rives JD: Mesenteric panniculitis. Review of 27 cases. Ann Surg **161:**864-875, 1965.

197 Payan HM, Gilbert EF: Mesenteric cyst-ovarian implant syndrome. Arch Pathol Lab Med **111:**282-284, 1987.

198 Pettinato G, Manivel JC, De Rosa N, Dehner LP: Inflammatory myofibroblastic tumor (plasma cell granuloma). Am J Clin Pathol **94:**538-546, 1990.

199 Pisciotto PT, Gray GF Jr, Miller DR: Abdominal plasma cell pseudotumor. J Pediatr **93:**628-630, 1978.

200 Remmele W, Muller-Lobeck H, Paulus W: Primary mesenteritis, mesenteric fibrosis and mesenteric fibromatosis. Pathol Res Pract **184:**77-85, 1988.

201 Reske M, Namiki H: Sclerosing mesenteritis. Report of two cases. Am J Clin Pathol **64:**661-667, 1975.

202 Ros PR, Olmstead WW, Moser RP Jr, Dachman AH, Hjermstad BH, Sobin LH: Mesenteric and omental cysts. Histologic classification with imaging correlation. Radiology **164:**327-332, 1987.

203 Shemwell RE, Weed JC: Ovarian remnant syndrome. Obstet Gynecol **36:**299-303, 1970.

204 Tedeschi CG, Botta GC: Retractile mesenteritis. N Engl J Med **266:**1035-1040, 1962.

205 Treissman SP, Gillis DA, Lee CL, Giacomantonio M, Resch L: Omental-mesenteric inflammatory pseudotumor. Cytogenetic demonstration of genetic changes and monoclonality in one tumor. Cancer **73:**1433-1437, 1994.

206 Vanek VW, Phillips AK: Retroperitoneal, mesenteric, and omental cysts. Arch Surg **119:**838-842, 1984.

207 Wu JP, Yunis EJ, Fetterman G, Jaeschke WF, Gilbert EF: Inflammatory pseudotumors of the abdomen. Plasma cell granulomas. J Clin Pathol **26:**943-948, 1973.

208 Yannopoulos K, Stout AP: Primary solid tumors of the mesentery. Cancer **16:**914-927, 1963.

Hernia sacs

209 Baron BW, Schraut WH, Azizi F, Talerman A: Extragonadal sex cord tumor with annular tubules in an umbilical hernia sac. A unique presentation with implications for histogenesis. Gynecol Oncol **30:**71-75, 1988.

210 Bostwick D, Eble J: Prostatic adenocarcinoma metastatic to inguinal hernia sac. J Urol Pathol **1**:193-200, 1993.

211 Griffith LM, Carcangiu ML: Sex cord tumor with annular tubules associated with endometriosis of the fallopian tube. Am J Clin Pathol **96**:259-262, 1991.

212 Nicholson CP, Donohue JH, Thompson GB, Lewis JE: A study of metastatic cancer found during inguinal hernia repair. Cancer **69**:3008-3011, 1992.

213 Popek EJ: Embryonal remnants in inguinal hernia sacs. Hum Pathol **21**:339-349, 1990.

214 Pratt PC, George MH, Mastin JP, Roggli VL: Crystalline foreign particulate material in hernia sacs. Hum Pathol **16**:1141-1146, 1985.

215 Walker AN, Mills SE: Glandular inclusions in inguinal hernial sacs and spermatic cords. Müllerian-like remnants confused with functional reproductive structures. Am J Clin Pathol **82**:85-89, 1984.

Umbilicus

216 Brustman L, Seltzer V: Sister Joseph's nodule. Seven cases of umbilical metastases from gynecologic malignancies. Gynecol Oncol **19**:155-162, 1984.

217 Clair DG, Lautz DB, Brooks DC: Rapid development of umbilical metastases after laparoscopic cholecystectomy for unsuspected gallbladder carcinoma. Surgery **113**:355-358, 1993.

218 Ross JE, Hill RB Jr: Primary umbilical adenocarcinoma. A case report and review of literature. Arch Pathol **99**:327-329, 1975.

219 Steck WD, Helwig EB: Cutaneous remnants of the omphalomesenteric duct. Arch Dermatol **90**:463-470, 1964.

220 Steck WD, Helwig EB: Cutaneous endometriosis. JAMA **191**:101-104, 1965.

221 Steck WD, Helwig EB: Tumors of the umbilicus. Cancer **18**:907-915, 1965.

222 Steck WD, Helwig EB: Umbilical granulomas, pilonidal disease, and the urachus. Surg Gynecol Obstet **120**:1043-1057, 1965.

223 Vicente J, Vazquez-Doval J, Quintanilla E: Fibroepithelial papilloma of the umbilicus. Int J Dermatol **33**:791-792, 1994.

Retroperitoneum
NON-NEOPLASTIC CONDITIONS

224 Catino D, Torack RM, Hagstrom JWC: Idiopathic retroperitoneal fibrosis. Histochemical evidence for lateral spread of the process from the midline. J Urol **98**:191-194, 1967.

225 Comings DE, Skubi KB, van Eyes J, Motulsky AG: Familial multifocal fibrosclerosis. Findings suggesting that retroperitoneal fibrosis, mediastinal fibrosis, sclerosing cholangitis, Riedel's thyroiditis, and pseudo-tumor of the orbit may be different manifestations of a single disease. Ann Intern Med **66**:884-892, 1967.

226 Cooksey G, Powell PH, Singh M, Yeates WK: Idiopathic retroperitoneal fibrosis. A long-term review after surgical treatment. Br J Urol **54**:628-631, 1982.

227 de Peralta MN, Delahoussaye PM, Tornos CS, Silva EG: Benign retroperitoneal cysts of mullerian type. A clinicopathologic study of three cases and review of the literature. Int J Gynecol Pathol **13**:273-278, 1994.

228 Foerster HM, Sengupta EE, Montag AG, Kaplan EL: Retroperitoneal bronchogenic cyst presenting as an adrenal mass. Arch Pathol Lab Med **115**:1057-1059, 1991.

229 Graham JR, Suby HI, LeCompte PR, Sadowsky NL: Fibrotic disorders associated with methysergide therapy for headache. N Engl J Med **274**:359-368, 1966.

230 Harbrecht PJ: Variants of retroperitoneal fibrosis. Ann Surg **165**:388-401, 1967.

231 Hellstrom HR, Perez-Stable ED: Retroperitoneal fibrosis with disseminated vasculitis and intrahepatic sclerosing cholangitis. Am J Med **40**:184-187, 1966.

232 Hughes D, Buckley PJ: Idiopathic retroperitoneal fibrosis is a macrophage-rich process. Implications for its pathogenesis and treatment. Am J Surg Pathol **17**:482-490, 1993.

233 Jones JH, Ross EJ, Matz LR, Edwards D, Davies DR: Retroperitoneal fibrosis. Am J Med **48**:203-208, 1970.

234 Jonsson G, Lindstedt E, Rubin S-O: Two cases of metastasizing scirrhous gastric carcinoma simulating idiopathic retroperitoneal fibrosis. Scand J Urol Nephrol **1**:299-302, 1967.

235 Kendall AR, Lakey WH: Sclerosing Hodgkin's disease vs. idiopathic retroperitoneal fibrosis. J Urol **35**:284-291, 1961.

236 Kurtz RJ, Heiman TM, Holt J, Beck AR: Mesenteric and retroperitoneal cysts. Arch Surg **203**:109-112, 1986.

237 Lawson DW, Corry RJ, Patton AS, Austen WG: Massive retroperitoneal adrenal hemorrhage. Surg Gynecol Obstet **129**:989-994, 1969.

238 Leake R, Wayman TB: Retroperitoneal encysted hematomas. J Urol **68**:69-73, 1952.

239 Lepor H, Walsh PC: Idiopathic retroperitoneal fibrosis. J Urol **122**:1-6, 1979.

240 Meyer S, Hausman R: Occlusive phlebitis in multifocal fibrosclerosis. Am J Clin Pathol **65**:274-283, 1976.

241 Mitchinson MJ: The pathology of idiopathic retroperitoneal fibrosis. J Clin Pathol **23**:681-689, 1970.

242 Mitchinson MJ: Retroperitoneal fibrosis revisited. Arch Pathol Lab Med **110**:784 786, 1986.

243 Munro JM, van der Walt JD, Cox EL: A comparison of cytoplasmic immunoglobulins in retroperitoneal fibrosis and abdominal aortic aneurysms. Histopathology **10**:1163-1169, 1986.

244 Osborn DE, Rao PN, Barnard RJ, Ackrill P, Ralston AJ, Best JJK: Surgical management of idiopathic retroperitoneal fibrosis. Br J Urol **53**:292-296, 1981.

245 Osborne BM, Butler JJ, Bloustein P, Sumner G: Idiopathic retroperitoneal fibrosis (sclerosing retroperitonitis). Hum Pathol **18**:735-739, 1987.

246 Sneige N, Dekmezian RH, Silva EG, Cartwright J Jr, Ayala AG: Pseudoparasitic Liesegang structures in perirenal hemorrhagic cysts. Am J Clin Pathol **89**:148-153, 1988.

247 Terner JY, Lattes R: Malakoplakia of colon and retroperitoneum. Report of a case with a histochemical study of the Michaelis-Gutmann inclusion bodies. Am J Clin Pathol **44**:20-31, 1965.

248 Thomas MH, Chisholm GD: Retroperitoneal fibrosis associated with malignant disease. Br J Cancer **28**:453-458, 1973.

TUMORS

249 Abell MR, Fayos JV, Lampe I: Retroperitoneal germinomas (seminomas) without evidence of testicular involvement. Cancer **18**:273-290, 1965.

250 Ackerman LV: Tumors of the peritoneum and retroperitoneum. In Atlas of tumor pathology, 1st Series, Fasc. 23 and Fasc. 24. Washington, DC, 1953, Armed Forces Institute of Pathology.

251 Arnheim EE: Retroperitoneal teratomas in infancy and childhood. Pediatrics **8**:309-327, 1951.

252 Azumi N, Curtis J, Kempson RL, Hendrickson MR: Atypical and malignant neoplasms showing lipomatous differentiation. A study of 111 cases. Am J Surg Pathol **11**:161-183, 1987.

253 Berry CL, Keelnig J, Hilton C: Teratoma in infancy and childhood. A review of 91 cases. J Pathol **98**:241-252, 1969.

254 Bhattacharyya AK, Balogh K: Retroperitoneal lymphangioleiomyomatosis. A 36-year benign course in a postmenopausal woman. Cancer **56**:1144-1146, 1985.

255 Brietta LK, Watkins D: Giant extra-adrenal myelolipoma. Arch Pathol Lab Med **118**:188-190, 1994.

255a Burke T, Sahin A, Johnson DE, Ordóñez NG, Mackay B: Myoepithelioma of the retroperitoneum. Ultrastruct Pathol **19**:269-274, 1995.

256 Buskirk SJ, Evans RG, Farrow GM, Earle JD: Primary retroperitoneal seminoma. Cancer **49**:1934-1936, 1982.

257 Cafferty LL, Katz RL, Ordóñez NG, Carrasco CH, Cabanillas FR: Fine needle aspiration diagnosis of intraabdominal and retroperitoneal lymphomas by a morphologic and immunocytochemical approach. Cancer **65**:72-77, 1990.

257a Carabias E, Garcia Muñoz H, Dihmes FP, López Pino MA, Ballestín C: Primary mucinous cystadenocarcinoma of the retroperitoneum. Report of a case and literature review. Virchows Archiv **426**:641-645, 1995.

258 Chen KT, Cheng AC: Retroperitoneal seminoma and intratubular germ cell neoplasia. Hum Pathol **20**:493-495, 1989.

259 Chen KTK, Felix EL, Flam MS: Extraadrenal myelolipoma. Am J Clin Pathol **78**:386-389, 1982.

260 Chung EB, Enzinger FM: Extraskeletal osteosarcoma. Cancer **60**:1132-1142, 1987.

261 Cody HS III, Turnbull AD, Fortner JG, Hajdu SI: The continuing challenge of retroperitoneal sarcomas. Cancer **47**:2147-2152, 1981.

262 Crist WM, Raney RB, Tefft M, Heyn R, Hays DM, Newton W, Beltangady M, Maurer HM: Soft tissue sarcomas arising in the retroperitoneal space in children. A report from the Intergroup Rhabdomyosarcoma Study (IRS) Committee. Cancer **56**:2125-2132, 1985.

263 Dickman PS, Triche TJ: Extraosseous Ewing's sarcoma versus primitive rhabdomyosarcoma. Diagnostic criteria and clinical correlation. Hum Pathol **17**:881-893, 1986.

264 Eble JN, Rosenberg AE, Young RH: Retroperitoneal xanthogranuloma in a patient with Erdheim-Chester disease. Am J Surg Pathol **18**:843-848, 1994.

265 Enzinger FM, Winslow DJ: Liposarcoma. A study of 103 cases. Virchows Arch [A] **335**:367-388, 1962.

266 Erlandson RA: The ultrastructural distinction between rhabdomyosarcoma and other undifferentiated "sarcomas." Ultrastruct Pathol **11**:83-101, 1987.

267 Fowler MR, Williams GB, Alba JM, Byrd CR: Extra-adrenal myelolipomas compared with extra medullary hematopoietic tumors. A case of presacral myelolipoma. Am J Surg Pathol **6:**363-374, 1982.

268 Fukutomi Y, Shibuya C, Yamamoto S, Okuno F, Nishiwaki S, Kashiki Y, Muto Y: Extrarenal Wilms' tumor in the adult patient. A case report and review of the world literature. Am J Clin Pathol **90:**618-622, 1988.

269 Ghali VS, Gold JE, Vincent RA, Cosgrove JM: Malignant peripheral nerve sheath tumor arising spontaneously from retroperitoneal ganglioneuroma. A case report, review of the literature, and immunohistochemical study. Hum Pathol **23:**72-75, 1992.

270 Gill W, Carter DC, Durie B: Retroperitoneal tumors. A review of 134 cases. J R Coll Surg Edinb **15:**213-221, 1970.

271 Goldberg BB, ed: Abdominal gray scale ultrasonography. New York, 1977, John Wiley & Sons, Inc.

272 Golden T, Stout AP: Smooth muscle tumors of the gastrointestinal tract and retroperitoneal tissues. Surg Gynecol Obstet **73:**784-810, 1941.

273 Hashimoto H, Tsuneyoshi M, Enjoji M: Malignant smooth muscle tumors of the retroperitoneum and mesentery. A clinicopathologic analysis of 44 cases. J Surg Oncol **28:**177-186, 1985.

274 Hawkins EP, Finegold MJ, Hawkins HK, Krischer JP, Starling KA, Weinberg A: Nongerminomatous malignant germ cell tumors in children. A review of 89 cases from the pediatric oncology group, 1971-1984. Cancer **58:**2579-2584, 1986.

275 Hollowood K, Stamp G, Zouvani J, Fletcher CDM: Extranodal follicular dendritic cell sarcoma of the gastrointestinal tract. Morphologic, immunohistochemical and ultrastructural analysis of two cases. Am J Clin Pathol **103:**90-97, 1995.

276 Hyman MP: Extraovarian endometrioid carcinoma. Review of the literature and report of two cases with unusual features. Am J Clin Pathol **68:**522-528, 1977.

277 Ibrahim NB, Briggs JC, Corrin B: Double primary localized fibrous tumours of the pleura and retroperitoneum. Histopathology **22:**282-284, 1993.

278 Jacobsen S, Juul-Jorgensen S: Primary retroperitoneal tumors. A review of 26 cases. Acta Chir Scand **140:**498-500, 1974.

279 Kahn LB: Retroperitoneal xanthogranuloma and xanthosarcoma (malignant fibrous xanthoma). Cancer **31:**411-422, 1973.

280 Karakousis CP, Velez AF, Emrich LJ: Management of retroperitoneal sarcomas and patient survival. Am J Surg **150:**376-380, 1985.

281 Kay S, McNeill DD: Leiomyosarcoma of retroperitoneum. Surg Gynecol Obstet **129:**285-288, 1969.

282 Kinne DW, Chu FCH, Huvos AG, Yagoda A, Fortner JG: Treatment of primary and recurrent retroperitoneal liposarcoma. Twenty-five-year experience at Memorial Hospital. Cancer **31:**53-64, 1973.

283 Koretz MJ, Wang S, Klein FA, Lawrence W Jr: Extrarenal adult Wilms' tumor. Cancer **60:**2484-2488, 1987.

284 Kryger-Baggesen N, Kjaergaard J, Sehested M: Nonchromaffin paraganglioma of the retroperitoneum. J Urol **134:**536-538, 1985.

285 Lack EE, Travis WD, Welch KJ: Retroperitoneal germ cell tumors in childhood. A clinical and pathologic study of 11 cases. Cancer **56:**602-608, 1985.

286 Lauwers GY, Erlandson RA, Casper ES, Brennan MF, Woodruff JM: Gastrointestinal autonomic nerve tumors. A clinicopathological, immunohistochemical, and ultrastructural study of 12 cases. Am J Surg Pathol **17:**887-897, 1993.

287 Lee Y-TN, Gold RH: Localization of occult testicular tumor with scrotal thermography. JAMA **236:**1975-1976, 1976.

288 Leonidas JC, Brill PW, Bhan I, Smith TH: Cystic retroperitoneal lymphangioma in infants and children. Radiology **127:**203-208, 1978.

289 Lofgren L: Primary retroperitoneal tumors. A histopathological, clinical and follow-up study supplemented by follow-up study of a series from the Finnish Cancer Register. Ann Acad Sci Fenn (Med) **129:**5-86, 1967.

290 Lumb G: Smooth-muscle tumours of the gastrointestinal tract and retroperitoneal tissues presenting as large cystic masses. J Pathol Bacteriol **63:**139-147, 1951.

291 Maatman T, Bukowski RM, Montie JE: Retroperitoneal malignancies several years after initial treatment of germ cell cancer of the testis. Cancer **54:**1962-1965, 1984.

292 Melicow MM: Primary tumors of the retroperitoneum. A clinico-pathologic analysis of 162 cases. Review of the literature and tables of classification. J Int Coll Surg **19:**401-449, 1953.

293 Michal M: Retroperitoneal myolipoma. A tumour mimicking retroperitoneal angiomyolipoma and liposarcoma with myosarcomatous differentiation. Histopathology **25:**86-88, 1994.

294 Moazam F, Rogers BM, Talbert JL: Retroperitoneal malignant schwannoma. A case report. J Pediatr Surg **18:**189-192, 1983.

295 Montague DK: Retroperitoneal germ cell tumors with no apparent testicular involvement. J Urol **113:**505-508, 1975.

296 Moss JF, Slayton RE, Economou SG: Primary retroperitoneal pure choriocarcinoma. Two long-term complete responders from a rare fatal disease. Cancer **62:**1053-1054, 1988.

297 Oberling C: Retroperitoneal xanthogranuloma. Am J Cancer **23:**477-489, 1935.

298 Oguma S, Okazaki H, Nakamichi G, Endo Y: A case of nonfunctioning paraganglioma arising from the retroperitoneum. Angiographic and scintigraphic features. J Urol **133:**73-76, 1985.

299 Olson JR, Abell MR: Nonfunctional nonchromaffin paragangliomas of the retroperitoneum. Cancer **23:**1358-1367, 1969.

300 Pack GT, Tabah EJ: Primary retroperitoneal tumors. A study of 120 cases. Surg Gynecol Obstet **90(Suppl):**209-231, 313-341, 1954.

301 Park U, Han KC, Chang HK, Huh MH: A primary mucinous cystoadenocarcinoma of the retroperitoneum. Gynecol Oncol **42:**64-67, 1991.

302 Parkinson MC, Chabrel CM: Clinicopathological features of retroperitoneal tumours. Br J Urol **56:**17-23, 1984.

303 Pennell TC, Gusdon JP: Retroperitoneal mucinous cystadenoma. Am J Obstet Gynecol **160:**1229-1231, 1990.

304 Piana S, Roncaroli F: Epithelioid leiomyosarcoma of retroperitoneum with granular cell change. Histopathology **25:**90-93, 1994.

305 Ranchod M, Kempson RC: Smooth muscle tumors of the gastrointestinal tract and retroperitoneum. A pathologic analysis of 100 cases. Cancer **39:**255-262, 1977.

306 Ransom JL, Pratt CB, Hustu O, Kumar APM, Howarth CB, Bowles D: Retroperitoneal rhabdomyosarcoma in children. Results of multimodality therapy. Cancer **45:**845-850, 1980.

307 Roth LM, Ehrlich CE: Mucinous cystadenocarcinoma of the retroperitoneum. Obstet Gynecol **49:**486-488, 1977.

308 Rothacker D, Knolle J, Stiller D, Borchard F: Primary retroperitoneal mucinous cystadenomas with gastric epithelial differentiation. Pathol Res Pract **189:**1195-1204, 1993.

309 Schmidt D, Mackay B, Sinkovics JG: Retroperitoneal tumor with vertebral metastasis in a 25-year-old female. Ultrastruct Pathol **2:**383-388, 1981.

310 Shmookler BM: Retroperitoneal synovial sarcoma. A report of four cases. Am J Clin Pathol **77:**686-691, 1982.

311 Shmookler BM, Lauer DH: Retroperitoneal leiomyosarcoma. A clinicopathologic analysis of 36 cases. Am J Surg Pathol **7:**269-280, 1983.

312 Stanley P: Computed tomographic evaluation of the retroperitoneum in infants and children. J Comput Tomogr **7:**63-75, 1983.

313 Steers WD, Hodge GB, Johnson DE, Chaitin BA, Charnsangavej C: Benign retroperitoneal neurilemoma without von Recklinghausen's disease. A rare occurrence. J Urol **133:**846-848, 1985.

314 Tang C-K, Toker C, Wybel RE, Desai RG: An unusual pelvic tumor with benign glandular, sarcomatous, and Wilms' tumor-like components. Hum Pathol **12:**940-944, 1981.

315 Tefft M, Vawter GF, Mitus A: Paravertebral "round cell" tumors in children. Radiology **92:**1501-1509, 1969.

316 Triche RJ, Askin FB, Kissane JM: Neuroblastoma, Ewing's sarcoma, and the differential diagnosis of small-, round-, blue-cell tumors. In Finegold M, ed: Pathology of neoplasia in children and adolescents, vol 18 of Major problems in pathology. Philadelphia, 1986, WB Saunders Co.

317 Tsang WY, Chan JK: Kaposi-like infantile hemangioendothelioma. A distinctive vascular neoplasm of the retroperitoneum. Am J Surg Pathol **15:**982-989, 1991.

318 Ulbright TM, Morley DJ, Roth LM, Berkow RL: Papillary serous carcinoma of the retroperitoneum. Am J Clin Pathol **79:**633-637, 1983.

319 van Doorn RC, Gallee MP, Hart AA, Gortzak E, Rutgers EJ, van Coevorden F, Keus RB, Zoetmulder FA: Resectable retroperitoneal soft tissue sarcomas. The effect of extent of resection and postoperative radiation therapy on local tumor control. Cancer **73:**637-642, 1994.

320 Vilanova JR, Burgos-Bretones J, Simon R, Rivera-Pomar JM: Leukaemoid reaction and eosinophilia in "inflammatory fibrous histiocytoma." Virchows Arch [A] **388:**237-243, 1980.

321 Vuletin JC, Wajsbort RR, Ghali V: Primary retroperitoneal angiosarcoma with eosinophilic globules. A combined light-microscopic, immunohistochemical, and ultrastructural study. Arch Pathol Lab Med **114:**618-622, 1990.

322 Wakely PE, Jr, Sprague RI, Kornstein MJ: Extrarenal Wilms' tumor. An analysis of four cases. Hum Pathol **20:**691-695, 1989.

323 Waldron JA, Magnifico M, Duray PH, Cadman EC: Retroperitoneal mass presentations of B-immunoblastic sarcoma. Cancer **56:**1733-1741, 1985.

324 Waldron JA, Newcomer LN, Katz ME, Cadman E: Sclerosing variants of follicular center cell lymphomas presenting in the retroperitoneum. Cancer **52:**712-720, 1983.

325 Weissbach L, Boedefeld EA: Localization of solitary and multiple metastases in stage II nonseminomatous testis tumor as basis for a modified staging lymph node dissection in stage I. J Urol **138:**77-82, 1987.

326 Whitten RO, Benjamin DR: Rhabdomyoma of the retroperitoneum. A report of a tumor with both adult and fetal characteristics. A study by light and electron microscopy, histochemistry, and immunochemistry. Cancer **59:**818-824, 1987.

327 Yajima A, Toki T, Morinaga S, Sasano H, Sasano N: A retroperitoneal endocrine carcinoma. Cancer **54:**2040-2042, 1984.

328 Yunis EJ: Ewing's sarcoma and related small round cell neoplasms in children. Am J Surg Pathol **10:**S54-S62, 1986.

329 Zaino RJ: Paget's disease in a retroperitoneal teratoma. Hum Pathol **15:**622-624, 1984.

Sacrococcygeal region

330 Addis BJ, Rao SG, Finnis D, Carvell JE: Pre-sacral carcinoid tumour. Histopathology **18:**563-565, 1991.

331 Ahmed HA, Pollock DJ: Malignant sacrococcygeal teratoma in the adult. Histopathology **9:**359-363, 1985.

332 Arnheim EE: Retroperitoneal teratomas in the infancy and childhood. Pediatrics **8:**309-327, 1951.

333 Bale PM: Sacrococcygeal developmental abnormalities and tumors in children. Perspect Pediatr Pathol **1:**9-56, 1984.

334 Berry CL, Keelnig J, Hilton C: Teratoma in infancy and childhood. A review of 91 cases. J Pathol **98:**241-252, 1969.

335 Caropreso PR, Wengert PA Jr, Milford HE: Tailgut cyst. A rare retrorectal tumor. Report of a case and review. Dis Colon Rectum **18:**597-600, 1975.

336 Chretien PB, Milam JD, Foote FW, Miller TR: Embryonal adenocarcinomas (a type of malignant teratoma) of the sacrococcygeal region. Clinical and pathologic aspects of 21 cases. Cancer **26:**522-535, 1970.

337 Culp CE: Pilonidal disease and its treatment. Surg Clin North Am **47:**1007-1014, 1967.

338 Davage ON: The origin of sacrococcygeal pilonidal sinuses based on an analysis of four hundred and sixty-three cases. Am J Pathol **30:**1191-1205, 1954.

339 Donnellan WA, Swenson O: Benign and malignant sacrococcygeal teratomas. Surgery **64:**834-846, 1968.

340 Ein SH, Mancer K, Adeyemi SD: Malignant sacrococcygeal teratoma—endodermal sinus, yolk sac tumor—in infants and children. A 32-year review. J Pediatr Surg **20:**473-477, 1985.

341 Gonzalez-Crussi F, Winkler RF, Mirkin DL: Sacrococcygeal teratomas in infants and children. Relationship of histology and prognosis in 40 cases. Arch Pathol Lab Med **102:**420-425, 1978.

342 Harrist TY, Gang DL, Kleinman GM, Mihm MC Jr, Hendren WH: Unusual sacrococcygeal embryologic malformations with cutaneous manifestations. Arch Dermatol **118:**643-648, 1982.

343 Hawkins EP, Finegold MJ, Hawkins HK, Krischer JP, Starling KA, Weinberg A: Nongerminomatous malignant germ cell tumors in children. A review of 89 cases from the pediatric oncology group, 1971-1984. Cancer **58:**2579-2584, 1986.

344 Helwig EB, Stern JB: Subcutaneous sacrococcygeal myxopapillary ependymoma. A clinicopathologic study of 32 cases. Am J Clin Pathol **81:**156-161, 1984.

345 Hjernstad BM, Helwig EB: Tailgut cysts. Report of 53 cases. Am J Clin Pathol **89:**139-147, 1988.

346 Hood DL, Petras RE, Grundfest-Broniatowski S, Jagelman DG: Retrorectal cystic hamartoma. Report of five cases with carcinoid tumor arising in two (abstract). Am J Clin Pathol **89:**433, 1988.

347 Kaplan CG, Askin FB, Benirschke K: Cytogenetics of extragonadal tumors. Teratology **19:**261-266, 1979.

348 Kuhajda FP, Taxy JB: Oncofetal antigens in sacrococcygeal teratomas. Arch Pathol Lab Med **107:**239-242, 1983.

349 Lack EE, Glaun RS, Hefter LG, Seneca RP, Steigman C, Athari F: Late occurrence of malignancy following resection of a histologically mature sacrococcygeal teratoma. Report of a case and literature review. Arch Pathol Lab Med **117:**724-728, 1993.

350 Lack EE, Travis WE, Welch KJ: Retroperitoneal germ cell tumors in childhood. A clinical and pathologic study of 11 cases. Cancer **56:**602-608, 1985.

351 Lahdenne P, Heikinheimo M, Nikkanen V, Klemi P, Siimes MA, Rapola J: Neonatal benign sacrococcygeal teratoma may recur in adulthood and give rise to malignancy. Cancer **72:**3727-3731, 1993.

352 Lemberger A, Stein M, Doron J, Fried G, Goldsher D, Feinsod M: Sacrococcygeal extradural ependymoma. Cancer **64:**1156-1159, 1989.

353 Lineaweaver WC, Brunson MB, Smith JF, Franzini DA, Rumley TO: Squamous carcinoma arising in a pilonidal sinus. J Surg Oncol **27:**239-242, 1984.

354 MacLeod JH, Purves JKB: Duplications of the rectum. Dis Colon Rectum **13:**133-137, 1970.

355 Marco V, Autonell J, Farre J, et al.: Retrorectal cyst-hamartoma. Report of two cases with adenocarcinoma developing in one. Am J Surg Pathol **6:**707-714, 1982.

356 McDermott NC, Newman J: Tailgut cyst (retrorectal cystic hamartoma) with prominent glomus bodies. Histopathology **18:**265-266, 1991.

357 Mills SE, Walker AN, Stallings RG, Allen MS: Retrorectal cystic hamartoma. Report of three cases, including one with a perirenal component. Arch Pathol Lab Med **108:**737-740, 1984.

358 Nakashima N, Fukatsu T, Nagasaka T, Sobue M, Takeuchi J: The frequency and histology of hepatic tissue in germ cell tumors. Am J Surg Pathol **11:**682-692, 1987.

359 Norris CS: Giant condyloma acuminatum (Buschke-Lowenstein tumor) involving a pilonidal sinus. A case report and review of the literature. J Surg Oncol **22:**47-50, 1981.

360 Noseworthy J, Lack EE, Kozakewich HPW, Vawter GF, Welch KJ: Sacrococcygeal germ cell tumors in childhood. An updated experience with 118 patients. J Pediatr Surg **16:**358-364, 1981.

361 Notaras MJ: A review of three popular methods of treatment of postanal (pilonidal) sinus disease. Br J Surg **57:**886-890, 1970.

362 Olsen MM, Raffensperger JG, Gonzalez-Crussi F, Luck SR, Kaplan WE, Morgan ER: Endodermal sinus tumor. A clinical and pathological correlation. J Pediatr Surg **17:**832-840, 1982.

363 Oosterhuis J, van Berlo R, de Jong B, Dam A, Buist J, Tamminga R, Zwierstra R: Sacral teratoma with late recurrence of yolk sac tumor. J Urol Pathol **1:**257-268, 1993.

364 Pilipshen SJ, Gray G, Goldsmith E, Dineen P: Carcinoma arising in pilonidal sinuses. Ann Surg **193:**506-512, 1981.

365 Tagart REB: Congenital anal duplication. A cause of para-anal sinus. Br J Surg **64:**525-528, 1977.

366 Valdiserri RO, Yunis EJ: Sacrococcygeal teratomas. A review of 68 cases. Cancer **48:**217-221, 1981.

367 Whalen TV Jr, Mahour GH, Landing BH, Woolley MM: Sacrococcygeal teratomas in infants and children. Am J Surg **150:**373-375, 1985.

27 Cardiovascular system

Heart
Arteries
Veins
Lymph vessels

Heart

INTRODUCTION

Most operations for congenital cardiovascular malformations are directed toward improvement in the flow of oxygenated blood by such procedures as ligation or division of a patent ductus or the closure of interatrial and interventricular septal defects.[1] Methods have been devised to relieve pulmonary, aortic, and mitral valvular stenosis. Coronary artery bypass graft surgery has become a widely used and effective procedure for the symptomatic treatment of ischemic heart disease.[2] These various cardiac abnormalities and their methods of treatment will not be presented in detail.

Another cardiac operation that has become almost routine in some medical centers is cardiac transplantation; here the pathologist plays a very important role in monitoring the possibility of rejection.

NORMAL ANATOMY

The major histologic components of the heart are pericardium, myocardium, endocardium, and valves. The *pericardium* is divided into fibrous (parietal) and serous (visceral, epicardium) portions. It is lined by a single layer of mesothelial cells resting on a basement membrane. The *myocardium* consists of bundles of cardiac muscle fibers (myocytes) separated by fibrous bands. These fibers form a syncytium with end-to-end junctions, called intercalated discs, and sometimes side-to-side junctions. The nuclei of myocytes are centrally located, in contrast to those of skeletal muscle fibers. The *endocardium* consists of a single layer of endothelial cells that are continuous with those of the major blood vessels. The *semilunar (pulmonary and aortic) valves* are composed of three layers: fibrosa (made of dense collagen), spongiosa (containing large amounts of proteoglycans, loosely arranged collagen fibers, and scattered fibroblasts), and ventricularis (identified by its profusion of elastic fibers). The *atrioventricular (mitral and tricuspid) valves* are composed of the annulus (a ring of circumferentially oriented collagen and elastic fibers), leaflets, chordae tendineae, and papillary muscles. The leaflets, like those of the semilunar valves, are composed of three layers: fibrosa, ventricularis (on the ventricular side, rich in elastic fibers), and the spongiosa (on the atrial side, rich in proteoglycans).

The morphologic features of blood and lymph vessels are discussed in Chapter 25.

MYOCARDIAL BIOPSY

The performance of myocardial or endomyocardial biopsies has become a common procedure.[17,24,33,34] These biopsies can be obtained through a catheter inserted in a systemic vein through a transthoracic route or at the time of surgery for congenital or acquired heart disease.[24,34] Examination of multiple levels increases the sensitivity of the procedure, particularly in cases of myocarditis.[10,27] Ultrastructural examination can be of importance, especially for the evaluation of drug toxicity.[26]

The current complication rate with the intravascular procedure at specialized centers is less than 1%; the most common complication is hemopericardium (which rarely requires thoracotomy), and the most serious is cardiac perforation. The two most important indications of myocardial biopsy are monitoring of heart transplant recipients and grading of Adriamycin toxicity.[46] These and other diseases in which myocardial biopsy has provided useful information are discussed in the following paragraphs.[31,48]

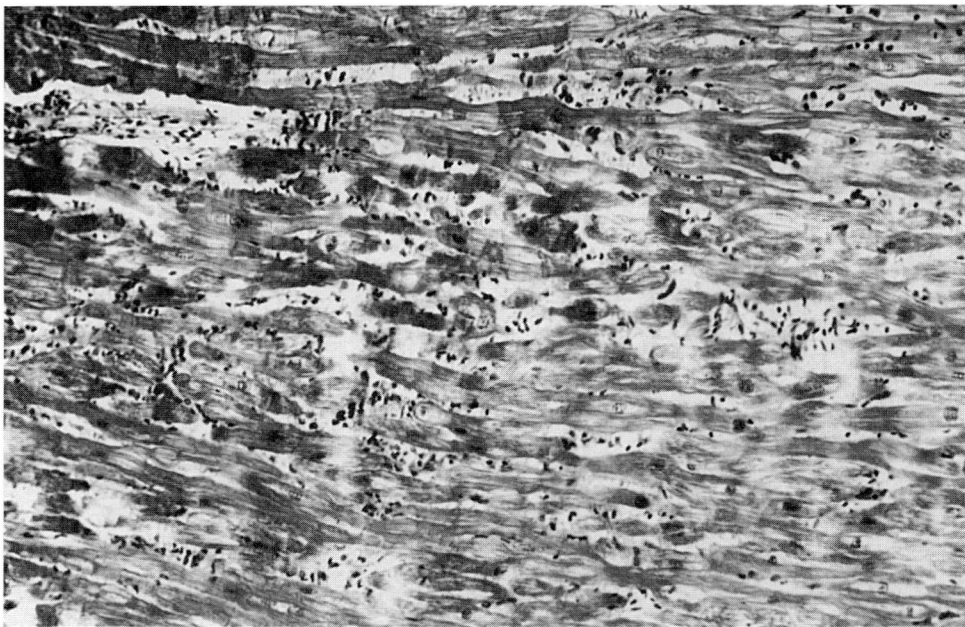

Fig. 27-1 Myocardial biopsy showing active pericarditis. Mononuclear infiltrate is present in interstitium, associated with degenerative changes in some of myocardial fibers.

Idiopathic hypertrophic cardiomyopathy. The main microscopic changes in this condition,[13a,41] as seen in whole hearts, septal myomectomy specimens, or biopsies obtained at thoracotomy, are myofiber disarray and hypertrophy and interstitial fibrosis.[21,43] Transvascular biopsy specimens are less informative, but they still show disarray of myofibrils and myofilaments within individual myocytes by ultrastructural examination. Unfortunately, these changes are not specific for this condition.[32,43] Another nonspecific change that is commonly found in idiopathic hypertrophic myocardiopathy is *basophilic degeneration* of myocardium. This appears as basophilic, finely granular material in the cytoplasm of isolated myocardial fibers and consists of polyglucosan deposits.[37a,41a]

Idiopathic dilated cardiomyopathy. Abnormalities in the myocardial biopsy are consistently present but, again, are of a nonspecific nature. They consist mainly of hypertrophy and degenerative changes of the myocardial fibers.[20,25,39]

A good correlation has been found between the severity of the condition clinically and the extent and degree of microscopic abnormalities,[20] although the sometimes focal nature of the changes may be misleading. Leukocytic infiltrates are present in about one half of the myocardial biopsies in this condition, a fact to remember in the differential diagnosis with myocarditis.[42]

Restrictive (restrictive/obliterative) myocardiopathy. In the *eosinophilic* form of this disease in its active stage, a myocarditis with a heavy component of eosinophils is present; in the inactive stage of this form and in the *noneosinophilic* form (the most common in the United States), the biopsy findings are nonspecific.[15]

Infiltrative myocardiopathies. This is the group of cardiac diseases in which endomyocardial biopsy can be par-

ticularly rewarding. This includes amyloidosis,[35] hemosiderosis,[9] hemochromatosis, and glycogenosis. However, as Ferrans and Roberts[22] have aptly pointed out, the diagnosis of most of these conditions can be made more readily by biopsy of another, more readily accessible organ.

Other myocardiopathies. *Ischemic myocardiopathy* is secondary to severe coronary artery disease with myocardial infarct and is characterized by congestive heart failure and cardiac dilatation. Cases with similar features occurring in the absence of a myocardial infarct have been described.[6]

Right ventricular dysplasia is a strongly familial idiopathic cardiomyopathy that mainly involves the right ventricle. The anatomic substrate is variable infiltration of the right ventricular myocardium by adipose and fibrous tissue.[30]

Myocarditis. It is agreed that the diagnosis of myocarditis requires the presence of an inflammatory infiltrate *and* myocyte necrosis or degeneration ("Dallas criteria")[4] (Fig. 27-1). The infiltrate is usually of lymphocytic nature, easily identifiable, often admixed with histiocytes, and amenable to semiquantification in routine sections.[16] Most of these lymphocytes are of T-cell type.[12] Some authors have suggested the use of leukocyte common antigen in immunohistochemical preparations to quantify the number of lymphocytes, but this seems hardly necessary.[40] In *hypersensitivity myocarditis,* the infiltrate is rich in eosinophils, is predominantly perivascular, and is accompanied by a lesser degree of necrotizing changes.[11,13,18]

The myocyte alterations can take the form of frank necrosis, vacuolization, or disruption and are better appreciated in longitudinal sections. The presence of edema should not be used as a criterion for myocarditis. Fibrosis, if present, should be quantified (mild, moderate, or severe) and qualified (interstitial, endocardial, or replacement).

Diagnostic terms to be used in subsequent biopsies, using the first specimen as a reference point, are *ongoing* or *persistent myocarditis* when both the myocyte damage and the inflammation persist, *resolving* or *healing myocarditis* when these changes are substantially reduced, and *resolved* or *healed myocarditis* when these changes are no longer present.[4] Fenoglio et al.[19] divided their cases of myocarditis into *acute, rapidly progressive,* and *chronic;* they found a good correlation between these types and the clinical course.

The etiology of myocarditis can be viral, bacterial, fungal, parasitic (particularly Chagas' disease and toxoplasmosis, the latter often seen in AIDS patients), caused by a collagen-vascular disease (especially rheumatic fever), drug-induced, radiation-induced, or an expression of transplant rejection.[3,5,37,45,47] Rare forms of granulomatous myocarditis include tuberculosis and sarcoidosis.[36,38] In many cases of myocarditis, the condition remains idiopathic. In the form known as *giant cell myocarditis,* the giant cells exhibit the immunophenotype of histiocytes rather than cardiac muscle fibers.[44]

Drug-induced cardiomyopathy. The myocardial changes resulting from *Adriamycin* toxicity have been well documented.[28,29] Vacuolization of cardiac myocytes, resulting from dilatation of the sarcotubular system, is the earliest change. This is followed by the appearance of the so-called "adria cell," characterized light microscopically by loss of cross striations and myofilamentous bundles and accompanied by a homogeneous basophilic staining ("myocytolysis"). Ultrastructurally, there is dissociation of sarcomeres and fragmentation and loss of myofilaments. Immunohistochemically, cells with myocytolysis retain reactivity for myoglobin and various enzymes, suggesting that the myocyte is viable and that the change may be reversible.[14] This alteration is in no way specific for Adriamycin toxicity but can be seen in a large variety of diseases.[14] Inflammation is nil or absent, and this constitutes an important differential feature with other myocardial lesions (Figs. 27-2 and 27-3).

The changes are rather diffuse but seem to predominate in the subendocardial region. They are dose dependent and are enhanced if radiation therapy has also been used. In the latter instance, the changes just described will be in addition to those resulting from the radiation, which are mainly located in the capillaries.[8]

Cyclophosphamide may produce hemorrhagic necrosis, extensive capillary thrombosis, interstitial hemorrhage and fibrin deposition, and necrosis of myocardial fibers.[7]

Tumors. Primary and metastatic tumors of the heart have been diagnosed with endomyocardial biopsy.[23]

HEART TRANSPLANT

Myocardial biopsy is the most sensitive indicator of rejection.* The criteria used for the diagnosis depend on the immunosuppressive regimen used (i.e., cyclosporine-based or azathioprine-based).[54] The main microscopic sign of rejection is a perivascular and interstitial inflammatory infiltrate, predominantly lymphocytic, accompanied by focal necrosis of myocytes and edema. Clusters of neutrophils may be present around the necrotic myocytes.

One should be careful not to misinterpret a previous biopsy site as indicative of rejection; it appears as a sharply outlined area of necrotic myocytes, sometimes associated with a thrombus and granulation tissue (Fig. 27-4, *A*). Rejection should also be distinguished from ischemic changes (Fig. 27-5, *A*) and from *drug-induced hypersensitivity myocarditis,* a self-limited condition that does not cause heart failure and usually resolves without residual injury.[56]

The most widely used grading system of acute rejection episodes is that proposed by Billingham[51]:

Early rejection (reversible) (Figs. 27-4, *B,* and 27-5, *B*)
  Endocardial and interstitial edema
  Scanty perivascular and endocardial infiltrate of pyroninophilic lymphocytes with prominent nucleoli
  Pyroninophilia of endocardial and endothelial cells
Moderate rejection (reversible) (Figs. 27-4, *C,* and 27-5, *C*)
  Interstitial, perivascular, and endocardial infiltrate of pyroninophilic lymphocytes with prominent nucleoli
  Early focal myocytolysis
Severe rejection (irreversible or very difficult to reverse) (Fig. 27-4, *D*)
  Interstitial hemorrhage and infiltrate of pyroninophilic lymphocytes and polymorphonuclear leukocytes, vascular and myocyte necrosis
Resolving rejection (Fig. 27-5, *D*)
  Active fibrosis, residual small lymphocytes (nonpyroninophilic), plasma cells, and hemosiderin deposits

Some modifications to this scheme have been proposed,[58,61,68] but it remains to be seen whether they represent an improvement over the original scheme.[60] Perhaps the most important of these additions is that of ***vascular rejection,*** a process that injures the endothelium in the absence of significant intramyocardial lymphocytic infiltration[62a] (Fig. 27-5, *E*).

The long-term successfully transplanted heart characteristically shows some degree of hypertrophy and fibrosis of muscle fibers.[65,66] Accelerated arteriosclerosis is now the major long-term complication of heart transplantation. Gaudin et al.[55] have shown that ischemic injury to the heart during the peritransplant period—as detected in endomyocardial biopsies—contributes to the development of this complication (Fig. 27-5, *F*).

In about 10% of heart transplant cases, endocardial lymphoid collections develop in which the presence of the Epstein-Barr virus genome can be demonstrated. When intense, this change has been referred to as *EBV-associated post-transplant lymphoproliferative disorder.*[49,59] In addition to the heart, the infiltrate may involve the lung, gastrointestinal tract, lymph nodes, and other sites.[52,62] The proliferating cells are B-lymphocytes of host origin, and the process ranges from atypical lymphoid hyperplasia to malignant lymphoma.[52,57,67a] Some of these cases (particularly when located in the lung and gastrointestinal tract) respond to a reduction in immunosuppression.[52]

Cytomegalovirus infection can be diagnosed through the demonstration of viral inclusion bodies, with immunohistochemical or in situ hybridization techniques, or by PCR. The

---

*References 51, 53, 55a, 58, 63, 64, 67.

Text continued on p. 2180

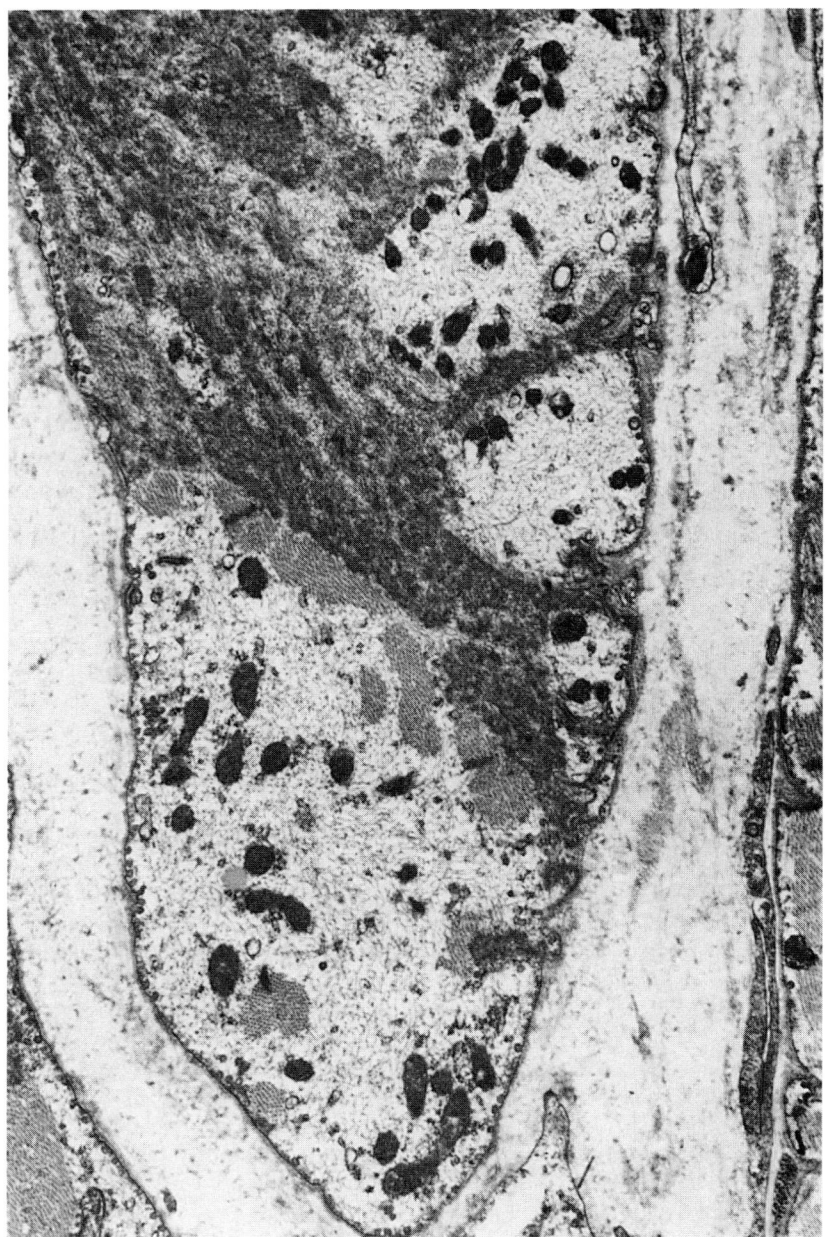

Fig. 27-2 Adriamycin cardiotoxicity. Myocyte in center ("adria cell") shows extensive pale areas of loss of myofibrils and fragmentation of myofilaments. Mitochondria (dark oval structures in same areas) are not qualitatively altered. Remnants of Z bands form diagonal dense area in center. Note intact myofibril in adjacent myocyte (right edge). (×5600; courtesy Dr. L.F. Fajardo, Stanford, CA.)

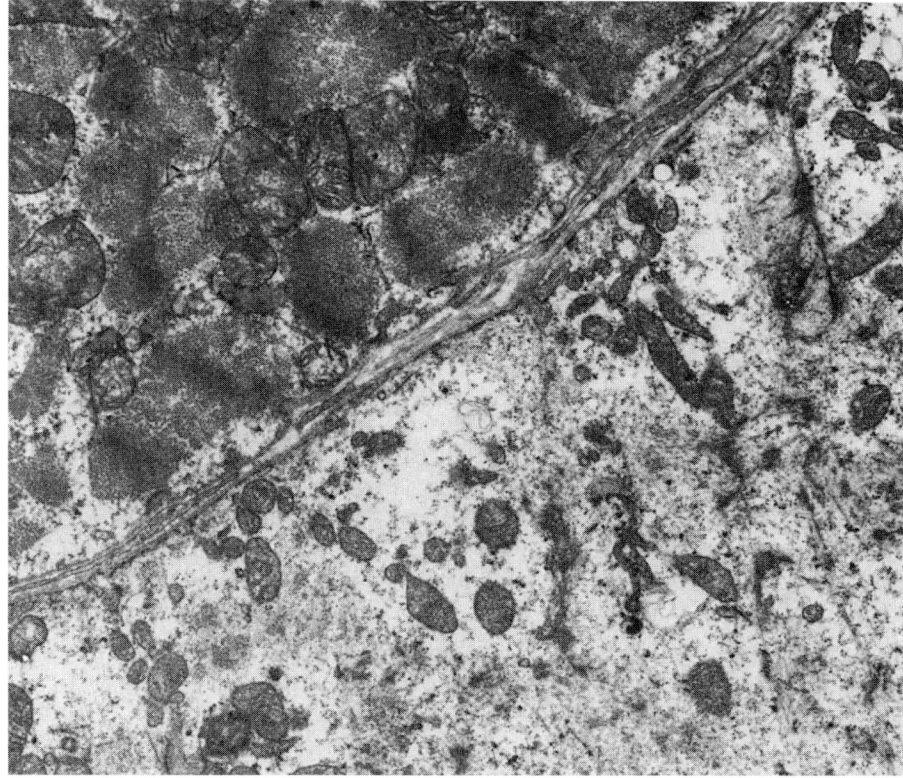

Fig. 27-3 Compare transverse section of normal cardiac myocyte (*upper left*) with myocyte severely affected by Adriamycin (*lower right*). There is complete disorganization of sarcomeres and extensive fragmentation of myofilaments. Mitochondria are small (compare with *top*). Remnants of Z bands are present near right edge. This complete loss of contractile elements in one myocyte, with preservation of adjacent cell, creates sharply defined amphophilic or basophilic areas that characterize "adria cells" in paraffin sections. (×8200; courtesy Dr. L.F. Fajardo, Stanford, CA.)

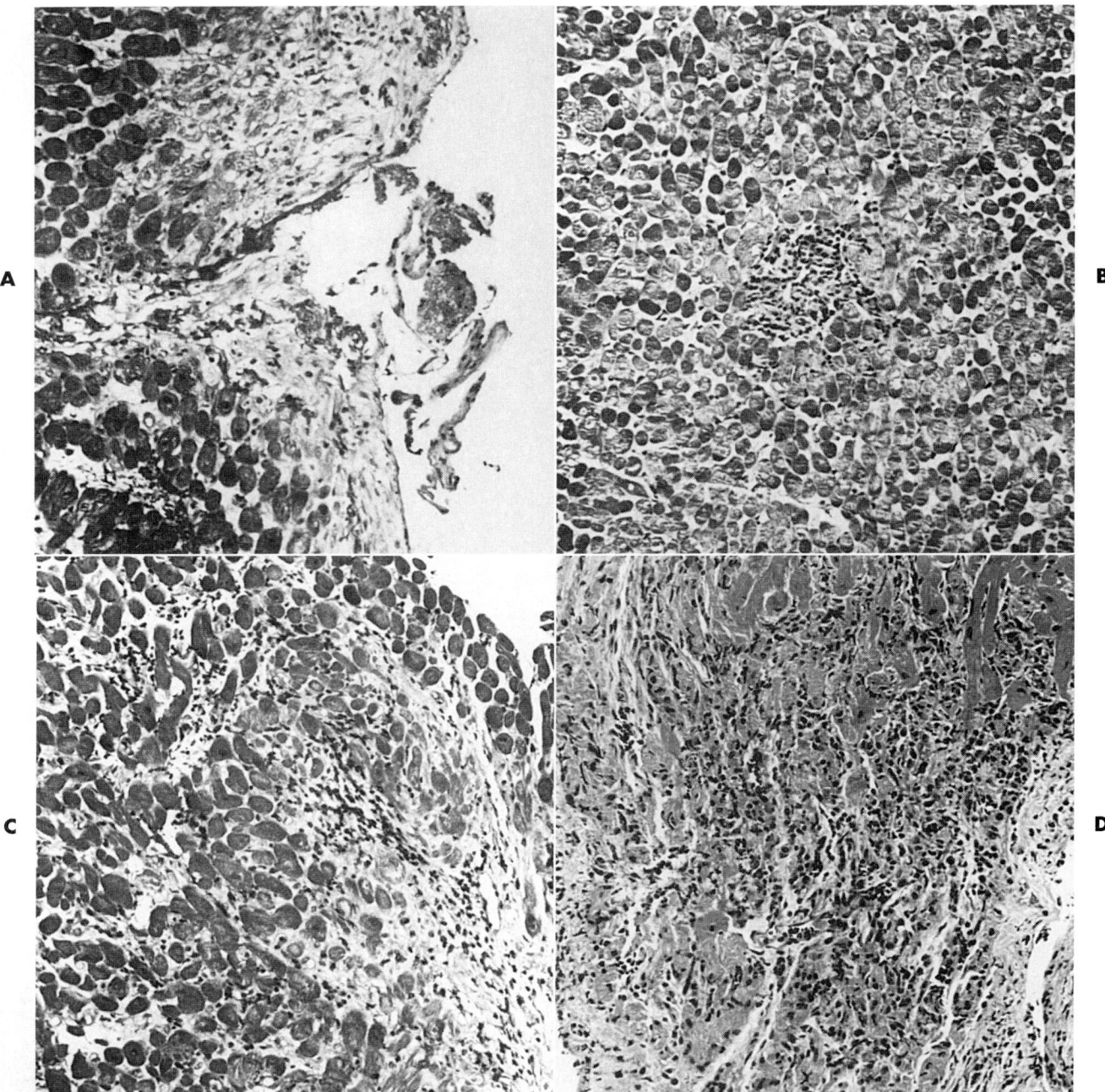

Fig. 27-4 Endomyocardial biopsy in transplanted hearts. **A,** Site of previous biopsy. Sharply circumscribed area of necrosis of myocardial fibers is seen immediately beneath endocardium, covered by organizing mural thrombus. This physiologic repair should not be misinterpreted as evidence of rejection. **B,** Mild rejection. Isolated collection of perivascular lymphocytes is only abnormality present. **C,** Moderate rejection. Lymphocytic infiltrate is of greater intensity and accompanied by some deposition of collagen. **D,** Severe rejection. Inflammatory infiltrate is extensive and accompanied by marked degenerative changes in myocardial fibers.

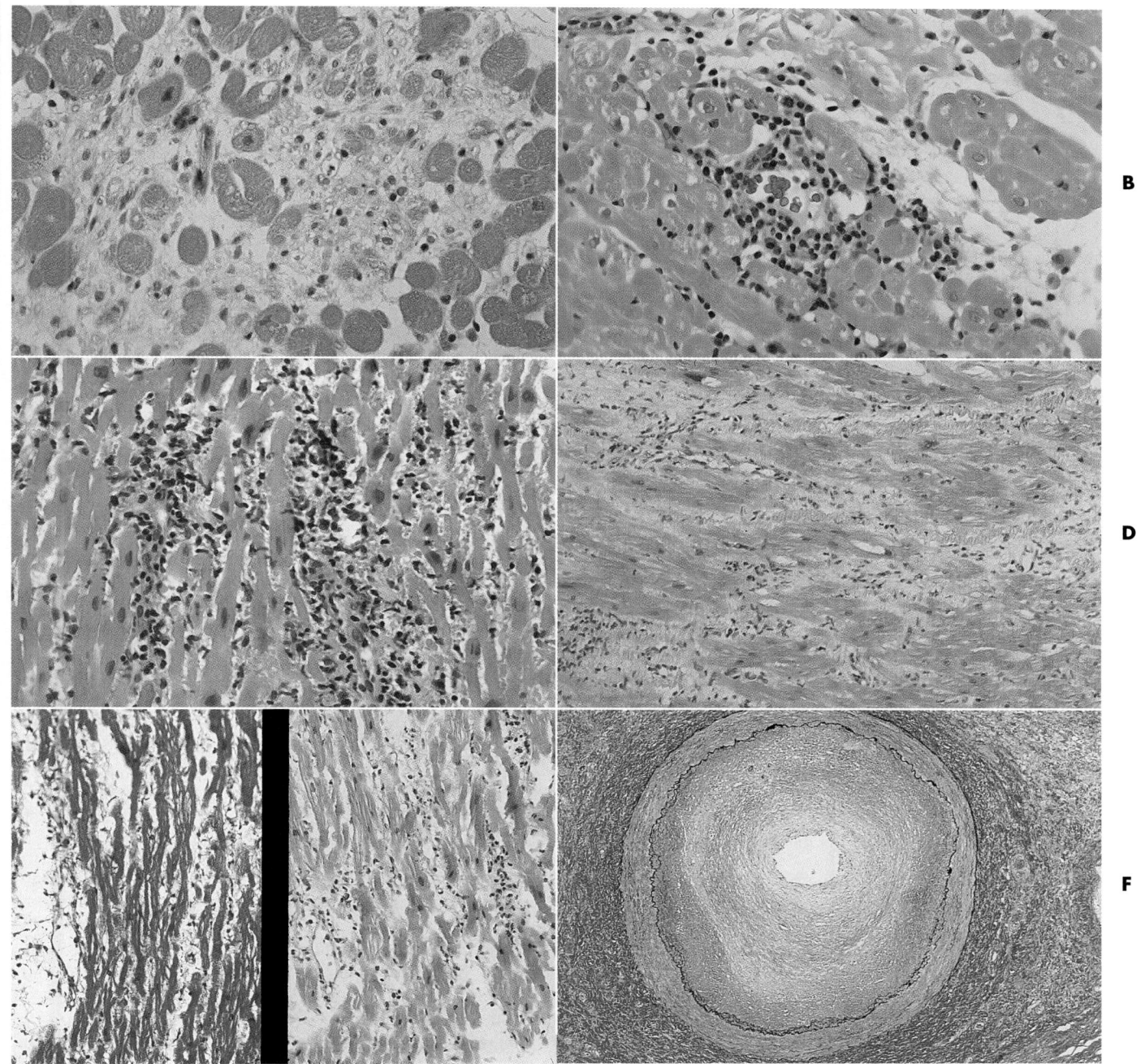

Fig. 27-5 Various microscopic appearance of heart transplant. **A,** Endomyocardial biopsy with healing ischemic changes. There is focal dropout of myofibers with sparse infiltrate of mononuclear cells, including pigment-laden histiocytes. **B,** Mild acute cellular rejection. There is patchy perivascular lymphocytic infiltrate with no myocyte injury. **C,** Moderate acute rejection showing myocyte injury or damage. **D,** Resolving rejection. There is a diminished inflammatory infiltrate with interstitial fibrosis after treatment for moderate acute rejection. **E,** Acute vascular rejection. There is a sparse inflammatory infiltrate with dilated small vessels and edema, shown with H&E *(left)* and trichrome *(right).* **F,** Chronic rejection (transplant vasculopathy). There is concentric narrowing of epicardial coronary artery by fibromuscular intimal proliferation. Note the preservation of internal elastic lamina (EVG). (Courtesy Dr. Richard N. Eisen, Greenwich, CT.)

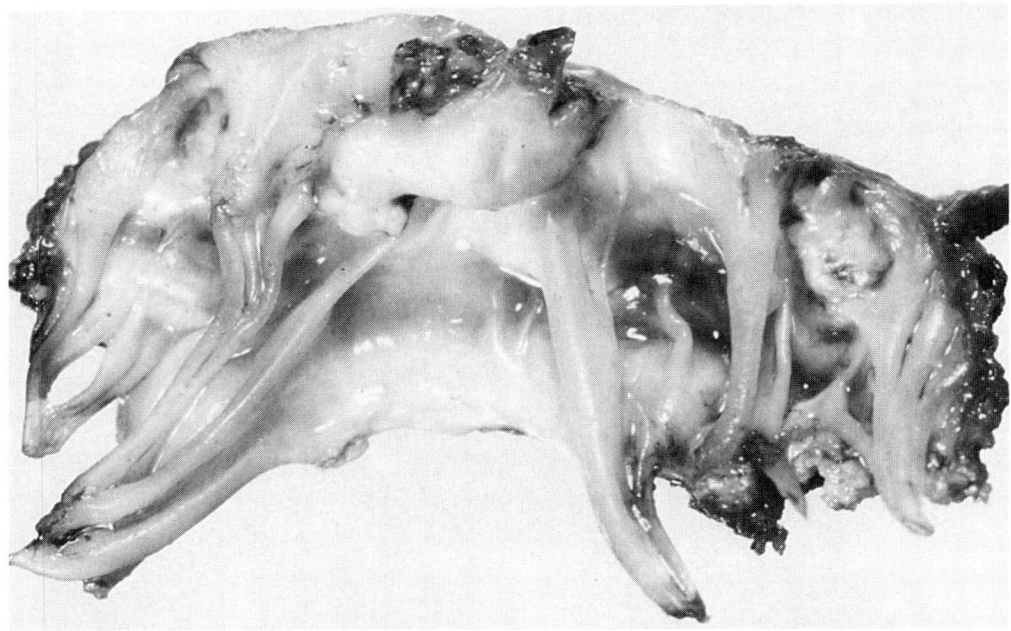

Fig. 27-6 Surgical specimen of mitral valve distorted by rheumatic heart disease in 40-year-old man who had disease for over 10 years. Valve was resected and replaced by prosthesis. Unfortunately, it failed.

Table 27-1 Gross morphologic assessment of abnormal cardiac valvular function

Pathologic feature	Stenotic valve	Purely regurgitant valve
For all valves		
Valve weight	Increased	Normal or slightly increased or decreased
Fibrous thickening	Diffuse	Diffuse, focal, or none
Calcific deposits	None to heavy	Minimal (if any)
Tissue loss (perforation, indentation)	None	May be present
Vegetations	Minimal	May be present
Commissural fusion	May be present	Minimal (if any)
Annular circumference	Normal	Normal or increased
For aortic valves		
Number of cusps	One to three	Two or three
For mitral (or tricuspid) valves		
Abnormal papillary muscles	No	May be present
Chordae tendineae		
Fusion	Usually present	Absent
Elongation	Absent	May be present
Shortening	Usually present	May be present
Rupture	Absent	May be present

latter method is the most sensitive; however, PCR demonstration of HCMV DNA in otherwise negative endomyocardial specimens is of questionable significance.[50]

CARDIAC VALVES

Surgery to correct major defects of the valves by resection and prosthetic replacement is frequently performed (Fig. 27-6). It should be emphasized that the most precise diagnosis will be made from the gross appearance of the valve and that usually the microscopic examination is of little value.[75,88,93,100] Photographic and radiographic examination of the specimen is also indicated. Careful examination of the gross specimen with knowledge of the clinical history often allows a distinction to be made between a rheumatic or congenital origin for a chronic valvulopathy.[89] Microscopically, both show fibrosis, calcification, occasional inflammatory cells, and sometimes foci of dystrophic amyloid deposition.[72]

The major etiologies of valvular disease, the gross morphologic assessment, and the etiologic assessment are shown in the box and Tables 27-2 to 27-3.[90]

Nearly all cases of *mitral valve* stenosis (with or without mitral insufficiency) are acquired and postinflammatory.[73] Among the cases of mitral insufficiency, Olson et al.[84] found that 38% were caused by a floppy valve (myxoid heart disease) and 31% by postinflammatory disease. They observed a floppy valve in 73% of the cases of chordal rupture and in 38% of the cases of infective endocarditis. They further noted that the relative frequency of floppy mitral valve as a cause of insufficiency has increased in recent years. Grossly, the floppy valve shows leaflet thickening and redundancy, leading to the formation of dome-like deformities reaching above the level of the annulus, which appears dilated. The

Table 27-2 Etiologic assessment of valvular heart disease

	Senile degeneration	Myxomatous degeneration	Rheumatic	Infective	Secondary
Gross features					
Leaflet/cuspal thickening	0	0/1	1	0	0
Calcification	1	0	0/1	0	0
Commissural chordal fusion	0	0	1	0	0
Leaflet cuspal redundancy	0	1	0	0	0
Leaflet cuspal defects	0	0	0	1	0
Chordal rupture	0	0/1	0	0/1	0
Histologic features					
Preservation of layered architecture	1	1	0	0/1	1
GAG accumulation in spongiosa	0	1	0	0	0/1
Thinned fibrosa	0	1	0	0	0
Neovascularization	0	0	0/1	0/1	0
Superficial fibrosis only	0/1	0/1	0	0/1	0/1

Abbreviations and symbols: 0, absent; 1, present; 0/1, present in some cases; GAG, glycosaminoglycan.
From Schoen FJ: Surgical pathology of removed natural and prosthetic heart valves. Hum Pathol **18**:558-567, 1987.

chordae are often thin and attenuated, with fibrosis or fusion at the anchoring sites.[84,100,101] Chordal rupture is seen in over one half of the cases.[79] Microscopically, stromal accumulation of glycosaminoglycans is the distinguishing feature, leading to the appearance of "myxoid degeneration." A lesser degree of accumulation of this material is seen in the neural and conduction system of these patients, pointing to a more general myxoid alteration.[82] Whether this alteration is the result of a genetically determined disease or a degenerative process of nonspecific nature remains controversial. The existence of familial forms of this disorder points toward the former.[77]

Specimens of *aortic valves* removed because of stenosis may show calcification of congenitally bicuspid valves (48%), calcification of a normally tricuspid valve without commissural fusion (so-called senile type) (28%), calcification of an acquired bicuspid valve (13%), a fibrous (rheumatic) type valve (10%), or calcification of congenitally unicuspid valves (1%).[85,86,98] Exceptionally, cartilaginous metaplasia is encountered.[78] In combined aortic stenosis and insufficiency, the most common changes are those of postinflammatory disease (69%) or calcification of congenitally bicuspid (19%) and unicommissural (6%) valves.[99] Pure aortic insufficiency is not related to calcification but to causes such as aortic root dilatation, bicuspid valve, and others.[74]

Specimens of *pulmonary valve* may be received in the surgical pathology laboratory because of pure pulmonary stenosis (the majority as a component of tetralogy of Fallot), pure pulmonary insufficiency, or combined stenosis and insufficiency. Congenital heart disease accounts for 95% of the cases, and tetralogy of Fallot is the most common form. Bicuspid pulmonary valve is the most common anomaly.[69]

Specimens of *tricuspid valve* can be the result of operations for pure insufficiency (by far the most common), combined stenosis and insufficiency, and pure stenosis (very rare). The most common causes of insufficiency are postinflammatory diseases, congenital disorders, pulmonary venous hypertension, and infective endocarditis.[80]

MAJOR ETIOLOGIES OF ACQUIRED MITRAL AND AORTIC VALVE DISEASE

Mitral valve disease
Mitral stenosis
 Post-inflammatory scarring(rheumatic)
 Calcification of mitral annulus
Mitral regurgitation
 Abnormalities of leaflets and commissures
 Post-inflammatory scarring (rheumatic)
 Infective endocarditis
 Floppy mitral valve
 Abnormalities of mitral apparatus
 Rupture of papillary muscle
 Papillary muscle dysfunction (fibrosis or ischemia)
 Rupture of chordae tendineae
 Left ventricular enlargement (e.g., congestive cardiomyopathy)
 Calcification of mitral annulus
Aortic valve disease
Aortic stenosis
 Calcification of congenitally deformed valve
 Senile calcific aortic stenosis
 Post-inflammatory scarring (rheumatic)
Aortic regurgitation
 Abnormalities of cusps and commissures
 Post-inflammatory scarring (rheumatic)
 Infective endocarditis
Aortic disease
 Syphilitic aortitis
 Ankylosing spondylitis
 Rheumatoid arthritis
 Marfan's syndrome
 Aortic dissection
 Trauma

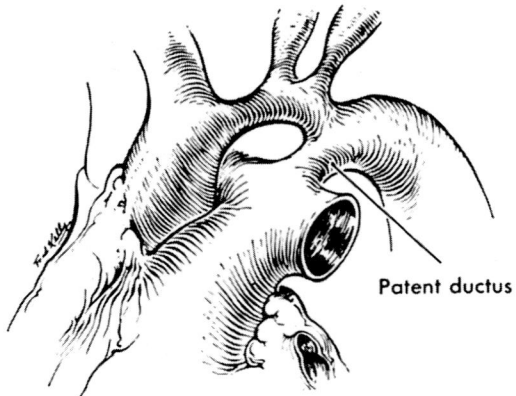

Fig. 27-7 Infantile (diffuse) type of coarctation of aorta. (From Burford TH: Symposium on clinical surgery. Coarctation of aorta and its treatment. Surg Clin North Am **30**:1249-1258, 1950.)

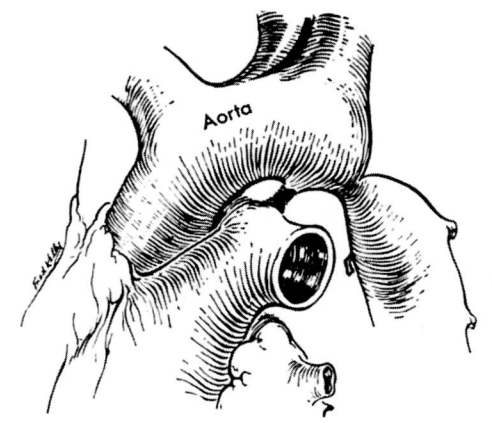

Fig. 27-8 Adult (localized) type of coarctation of aorta. (From Burford TH: Symposium on clinical surgery. Coarctation of aorta and its treatment. Surg Clin North Am **30**:1249-1258, 1950.)

An easy system for the identification of the many different types of *artificial heart valve prostheses* by the pathologist has been developed.[97] Microscopic study of these prosthetic valves has shown that, following insertion, a neo-endocardium develops at the junction with the heart wall, and from there it grows centripetally over the sewing cloth toward the valve lumen.

The pathologic changes that may be found in removed bioprosthetic heart valves include thrombosis, infection, cuspal tears and perforations, fibrous sheathing, calcification, intracuspal hematomas, and several others.* Mechanical valves may show thrombosis, infection, and various alterations associated with the valve design and the composition of the various elements.[91,96] Cuspal retraction without stenosis can also occur, leading to wide-open regurgitation.[83]

At the time of the correction of a mitral stenosis, the surgeon may perform a biopsy of the *atrial appendage*. These appendages are always abnormal, showing hypertrophy of the muscle and various other alterations. About one half of them show Aschoff nodules.[71] These are formed by collections of plump cells arranged in a granuloma-like fashion. The cells are positive for vimentin and negative for actin and desmin, suggesting a mesenchymal but not myocardial derivation.[81] The presence of these nodules does not correlate with the postoperative course or with clinical evidence of activity of the rheumatic process.

CORONARY ARTERY BYPASS

A vast number of coronary artery bypass operations have been done during the past 20 years using a segment of saphenous vein to join the aorta to a segment of the coronary artery distal to the obstruction. The patency rate of these grafts is over 80% after 5 years. Graft failure necessitating reoperation may result from the intimal fibrous hyperplasia that develops after the first month in all grafts becoming occlusive or from atherosclerosis in older grafts.[105] This

*References 70, 76, 87, 92, 94, 95.

atherosclerosis is typically concentric, diffuse, without a fibrous cap, with numerous foamy and inflammatory cells (including multinucleated giant forms), and associated with erosion of the media.[103] Secondary thrombosis is common.[102,104]

COARCTATION OF AORTA

Coarctation of aorta is divided into infantile (diffuse, preductal) and adult (localized, postductal) types (Figs. 27-7 and 27-8).

In the first type, the coarctated segment lies proximal to the ductus arteriosus. In the second type, which is by far the most common, the short, narrowed segment of the aorta is at the level of the aortic insertion of the ductus or just distal to it. If resection is not done, about 60% of patients die before 40 years of age of aortic rupture, endocarditis, hypertension, or congestive failure.[107] With present techniques, the operative risk is small, and the long-term results are excellent. The operation, which consists in the removal of the coarctation with end-to-end anastomosis, is best done when the patient is between 5 and 7 years of age.[106,108]

Grossly, the vessel is narrowed at the point of insertion of the ligamentum arteriosum. On opening the aorta, a diaphragm-like structure lies across the lumen, through which there is an aperture usually 1 mm or less in diameter (Fig. 27-9). Often there is localized subintimal thickening, and beneath this the media is distorted and thickened (Fig. 27-10).

Operations for coarctation of the aorta are more difficult in older patients because of advanced arteriosclerotic changes in the aorta.

CARDIAC TUMORS
Myxoma

Myxomas constitute approximately 50% of primary tumors of the heart. They occur in two settings: sporadic and familial.[111] The sporadic tumor occurs in middle-aged women (76%), usually in the left atrium (86%), nearly always as a single tumor, and without associated conditions. The famil-

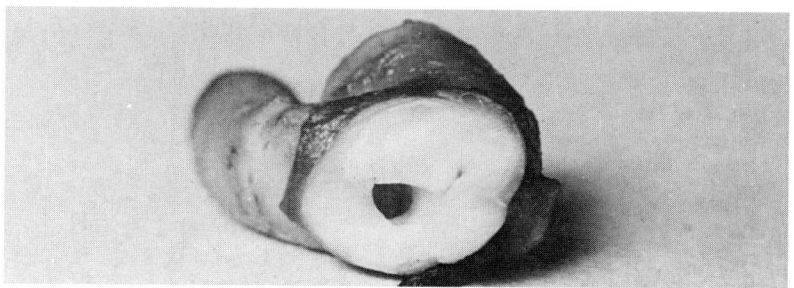

Fig. 27-9 Coarctation of aorta, adult type, showing greatly narrowed lumen.

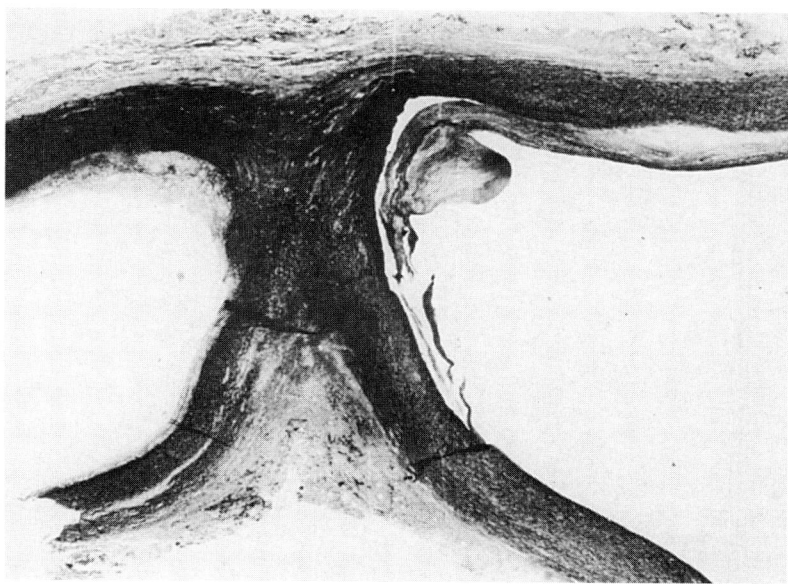

Fig. 27-10 Coarctation of aorta at point of constriction showing subintimal thickening and medial distortion.

ial variety is a disorder of young people, slightly more frequent in men, less commonly located in the left atrium (62%), multicentric in one third of the cases, and associated in 20% of the patients with extracardiac abnormalities. These include cutaneous and labial lentiginosis, eyelid and cutaneous myxomas, myxoid mammary fibroadenomas (often multiple and bilateral), adrenocortical nodular dysplasia associated with Cushing's syndrome, and large cell calcifying Sertoli cell tumor of the testis.[111] This genetically determined complex is known as *Carney's syndrome.*

Left-sided cardiac myxomas may present with signs of mitral stenosis or insufficiency, and right-sided tumors with dyspnea, syncope, distention of neck veins, and other symptoms. They may also lead to multiple emboli in the systemic or pulmonary circulation, depending on their location[127] (Fig. 27-11). Myocardial, pulmonary, or cerebral infarcts may thus supervene. Some cases have resulted in polycythemia or hypergammaglobulinemia.[118,136] A heart murmur that changes with time and position is a typical sign but is found in less than one half of the patients. The diagnosis can be established by echocardiography, gated radionuclide blood-pool scan, or cardiac catheterization.[125,137] Occasionally, the diagnosis is made by histologic examination of an embolus removed at operation (Fig. 27-10).

Grossly, myxomas are soft, polypoid, pale, lobulated masses often attached by a stalk to the septum near the foramen ovale. A papillary configuration may be apparent, especially if the specimen is examined under water. Calcification may occur, and this seems to be more common in those located in the right atrium. Microscopically, round, polygonal, or stellate cells are seen surrounded by abundant loose stroma rich in acid mucopolysaccharides. Some of these cells form solid cords and vascular channels, sometimes continuous with the endocardial lining.[115] Mitoses, pleomorphism, or necrosis is absent or minimal. Other microscopic variations include surface thrombosis, Gamna-Gandy bodies, ossification ("petrified" myxoma), occurrence of cartilaginous tissue, extramedullary hematopoiesis, and presence of thymic and foregut remnants.[110,119,122,139] The latter may be somehow related to the most peculiar change that cardiac myxoma can exhibit (i.e., the presence of well-developed mucin-producing glands)[116] (Fig. 27-12, *A* and

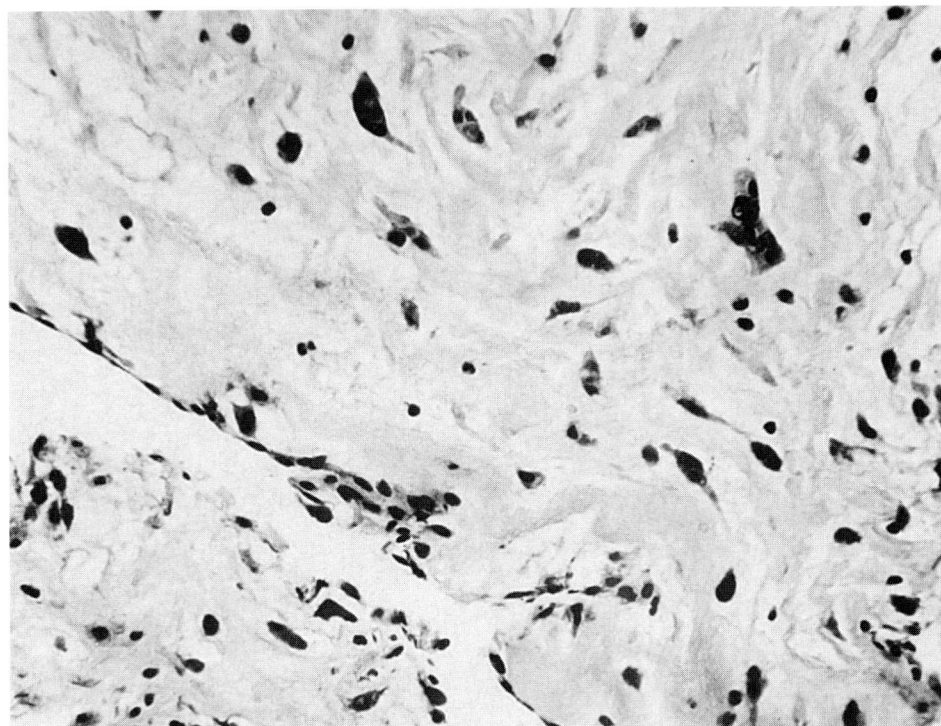

Fig. 27-11 Patient (33-year-old woman), who was thought to have rheumatic heart disease, developed signs of embolism to one of large arteries of leg. Artery was opened, and peculiar jelly-like clot was found. It was thought by surgeon to be extremely atypical. Microscopically, it showed cells with bizarre nuclei against mucoid background. This pattern was thought to be typical of myxoma, and it was predicted that patient had myxoma of left side of heart. Appropriate studies were made, and thoracic surgeon removed myxoma found in left atrium. Patient had uneventful postoperative recovery. She did not have rheumatic heart disease.

B). This phenomenon, which has been referred to as *glandular myxoma,* should not be confused with metastatic adenocarcinoma.

The controversy that existed as to whether cardiac myxoma is a true neoplasm or an expression of exuberant thrombus formation[130] has been laid to rest. Convincing evidence in favor of a neoplastic nature is provided by the existence of (1) occasional aggressive examples with invasion of the chest wall or distant metastases[126,129,131,135]; (2) cases with malignant transformation at the morphologic level[120]; (3) cases with aneuploid DNA levels[134]; and (4) cases with chromosomal aberrations.[112]

The cell of origin has also been in dispute. Ultrastructural examinations have suggested that myxomas arise from multipotential mesenchymal cells.[113,114] Immunohistochemically, some authors have found strong positivity for factor VIII–related antigen in all cases and have used this as an argument in favor of the endothelial (endocardial) origin of this tumor.[124] Most others, including ourselves, have found that reactivity for factor VIII, although usually present, is focal and often restricted to the cells lining invaginations rather than to those embedded in the stroma.[109,119,121,123,133] Positive staining has also been reported for vimentin, actin, desmin, smooth muscle myosin, alpha-1-antitrypsin, and alpha-1-antichymotrypsin.[109,117,121,138] The areas of glandular differ-

entiation are positive for CEA, EMA, and keratin.[116,119,132] This combination of findings is also in keeping with the interpretation that myxomas arise from mesenchymal cells with the capacity for multidirectional differentiation.[117,138]

Surgical excision of the ordinary myxoma is often curative. Several instances of local recurrence have been reported in the past; with the routine performance of partial atrial septectomy, together with the excision of the tumor, they have become very rare.[128]

Other benign tumors and tumorlike conditions

Rhabdomyoma and *rhabdomyomatosis* are mostly seen during the first decade of life, and many are congenital.[144,166] Some of the patients have tuberous sclerosis, and others suffer from congenital heart disease.[143] Grossly, rhabdomyomas present as one or more firm, white, well-circumscribed nodules. Microscopically, the most distinctive feature is the presence of "spider cells," so named because of their radial cytoplasmic extensions. Immunohistochemically, they show reactivity for myoglobin, actin, desmin, vimentin, and sometimes HMB-45.[143,171] The latter is of interest because of the link of rhabdomyoma with tuberous sclerosis and the morphologic similarities with angiomyolipoma, another HMB-45–positive lesion.[171] Rarely, cardiac rhabdomyomas

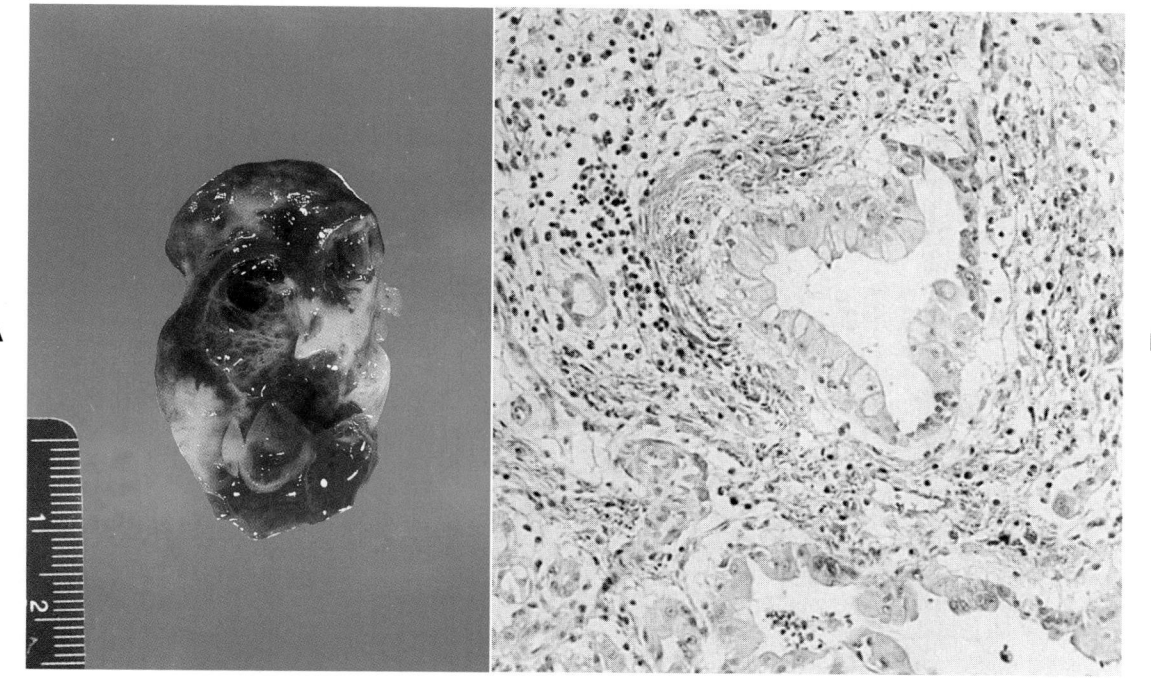

Fig. 27-12 Glandular myxoma. **A,** Gross appearance. Note the myxoid quality and extensive hemorrhage. **B,** Microscopic appearance. The epithelium is tall columnar and contains intracytoplasmic mucin. This rare type of myxoma should not be confused with metastatic adenocarcinoma.

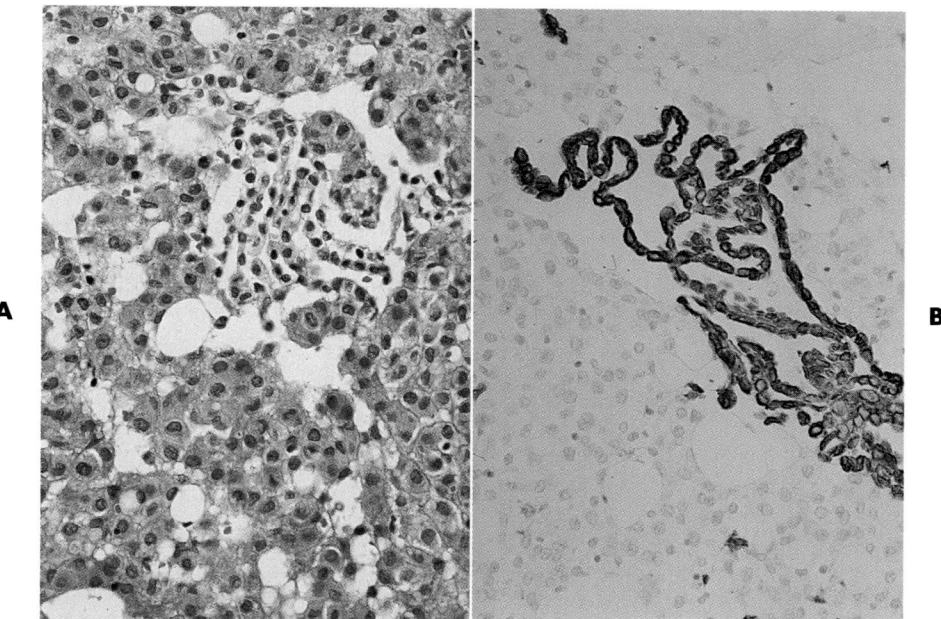

Fig. 27-13 So-called cardiac MICE. **A,** This process is composed of an admixture of plump histiocytes and ribbons of small cuboidal mesothelial cells. **B,** The immunostain for keratin highlights the mesothelial cell component, which is surrounded by the negative histiocytes and other mononuclear cells.

in adults have a morphologic appearance similar to that of the extracardiac type of this tumor.[172]

Mesothelial/monocytic incidental cardiac excrescenses ("cardiac MICE") are incidental microscopic findings at the time of cardiac surgery (usually for valvular disease) or in an endomyocardial biopsy. They may be found attached to the endocardium, free-floating in the pericardial cavity, or even inside an aortic dissecting aneurysm.[161,170] Although some of its morphologic features originally suggested a histiocytoid endothelial nature,[165] ultrastructural and immunohistochemical studies have shown that the lesion is composed of an admixture of keratin-positive mesothelial cells and KP-1–positive histiocytes[161] (Fig. 27-13, *A* and *B*). Microscopically, the mesothelial cells form strips, tubular and micropapillary formations surrounded by the smaller histiocytes. Huge round vacuoles are often present. Except for the latter, the appearance is very similar to that of nodular mesothelial hyperplasia as seen in hernia sacs.[164]

The process is clearly benign, non-neoplastic, and clinically of no significance. The pathogenesis remains unclear. Ingrowth of pericardial cells along a perforation tract has been suggested.[161,170] Others have postulated an artefact produced by suctioning of the pericardial cavity during cardiac surgery.[146] Their main practical importance resides in the fact that a pathologist unaware of their existence may mistake them for a metastatic carcinoma or some other neoplasm. Parenthetically, thoroughly convincing cases of histiocytoid (epithelioid) hemangioma of the heart are on record.[159]

Cystic tumor of the atrioventricular nodal region was regarded as a mesothelioma for many years, but there is now conclusive evidence that it represents a developmental abnormality of epithelial nature and endodermal origin.[141,147,153] It may be associated with other congenital anomalies.[142] Because of its crucial location, it may result in complete heart block. All reported cases have been found at autopsy.

Microscopically, the lesion consists of ductular structures, cysts, and solid nests of epithelial-like cells, which on electron microscopy show desmosomes and microvilli.[142,151] Immunohistochemically, the cells are reactive for keratin, CEA, and B72.3 but not for factor VIII.[142,147,160] It should be pointed out that not all nodular lesions of the atrioventricular node are examples of this entity; some are of vascular or neural nature.[154,155]

Papillary fibroelastoma (fibroelastic hamartoma, fibroma, papilloma, papillary fibroblastoma) is a small papillary growth that usually occurs on the surface of the valves but may also be seen in other endocardial locations[140] (Fig. 27-14, *A*). It is nearly always an incidental finding and is formed microscopically by a lining of hyperplastic endocardial cells covering a core of hyalinized hypocellular stroma[149,165a] (Fig. 27-14, *B*). It probably represents the end stage of the organization of a mural thrombus rather than a true neoplasm.[148]

Paraganglioma (extra-adrenal pheochromocytoma) can present as a primary intracardiac neoplasm. The left atrium is the most common location; hypertension and elevated urine catecholamine levels are often present. In general, the microscopic, ultrastructural, and immunohistochemical features are those of paraganglioma[156] (see Chapter 16).

Other primary tumors of the heart include *granular cell tumor* (not to be mistaken for rhabdomyoma),[150] *heman-*

gioma,[168] *lymphangioma, lipoma*,[169] *angiolipoma*,[158] *schwannoma*,[162] *ganglioneuroma*,[152,163] and *benign teratoma*.[167] A few cases of intracardiac *ectopic thyroid* have also been observed,[157] and a case of *plasma cell granuloma* of the heart has been seen in a 10-month-old female infant.[145]

Primary malignant tumors

Sarcomas of the heart are exceptionally rare.[174,180,188,190] Some of them are highly pleomorphic and unclassifiable even with the help of ultrastructural and immunohistochemical techniques (Fig. 27-15). Of those that can be placed into a specific category, *angiosarcoma* is probably the most common.[183,185,193] It is typically located in the atrium, where it presents as a large mass (Fig. 27-16, *A*). Its microscopic appearance may be similar to that of angiosarcoma elsewhere (see Chapter 25), but the majority are poorly differentiated. Ultrastructural and immunohistochemical features of endothelial differentiation can usually be demonstrated.[197] *Kaposi's sarcoma* can involve the heart in its generalized form, an event that seems to be more common in the AIDS setting. The second most common category of sarcoma is that of *myosarcoma*, either *leiomyosarcoma* or *rhabdomyosarcoma* (particularly the latter).[173] Other types described include *malignant fibrous histiocytoma*,[189,192] *osteosarcoma*,[175] *fibrosarcoma, liposarcoma, synovial sarcoma*,[186,194] and *malignant peripheral nerve tumor*.[196] It is possible that some of the sarcomas with prominent myxoid features represent the malignant counterpart of cardiac myxoma.[187] All of these tumor types occur almost always in adults, but a handful of pediatric cases are on record, including examples of *rhabdoid tumor*.[195]

Most patients with primary heart sarcomas present with intractable congestive heart failure, arrhythmias, or signs of superior vena cava obstruction. In rare cases, a metastatic lesion is the first manifestation of the disease.[182] It has been pointed out that malignant tumors are more frequently found in the right side of the heart and that benign neoplasms are more common on the left side.[173]

Malignant lymphoma presenting as a primary heart tumor is very rare.[176,177,179] Most of the reported cases have been of diffuse large cell type. AIDS patients are at an increased risk.[178,181,184] Secondary cardiac involvement by advanced malignant lymphoma or leukemia is a relatively common event, although it is rarely detected antemortem; in a few instances, it constitutes the immediate cause of death.[191] The lymphoproliferative lesion associated with EBV seen in cardiac transplant recipients is discussed on p. 2175.

Metastatic tumors

Involvement of the heart by metastatic carcinoma or by generalized malignant lymphoma is a more common event than primary malignancy of this organ, by a factor of 30 to 1[199,204]; however, it is rarely seen as a biopsy or surgical specimen unless the disease affects the pericardium preferentially.[198,203]

In the majority of the carcinomas metastatic to the heart, the primary tumor is in the thoracic cavity or contiguous areas, and the tumor reaches the heart by metastasizing to the mediastinal lymph nodes and from there extending in a retrograde fashion to the cardiac lymph vessels.[200] Malig-

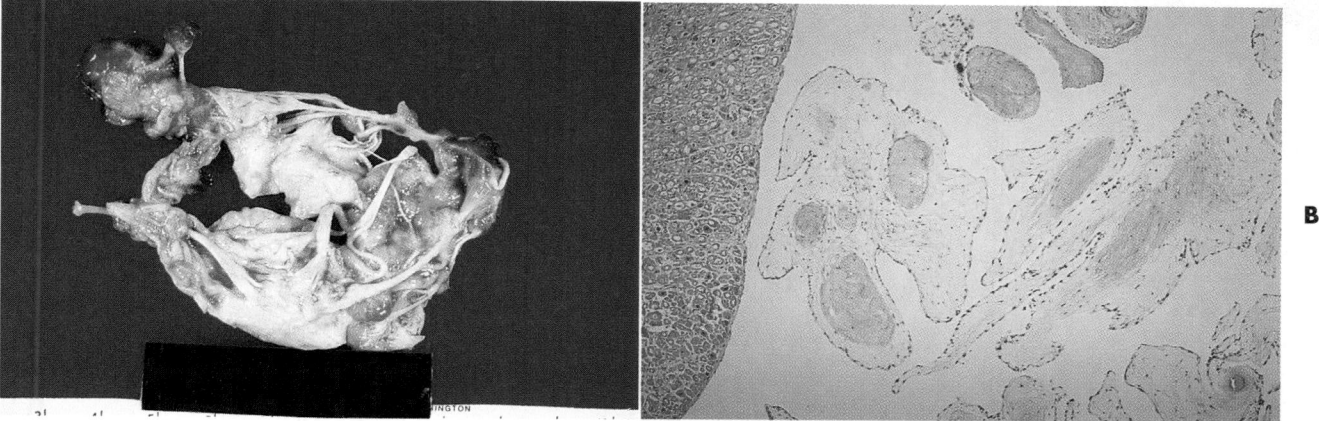

Fig. 27-14 So-called papillary elastofibroma. **A,** Gross appearance. **B,** Low-power microscopic appearance. Notice the densely hyalinized central core and the flat endocardial lining.

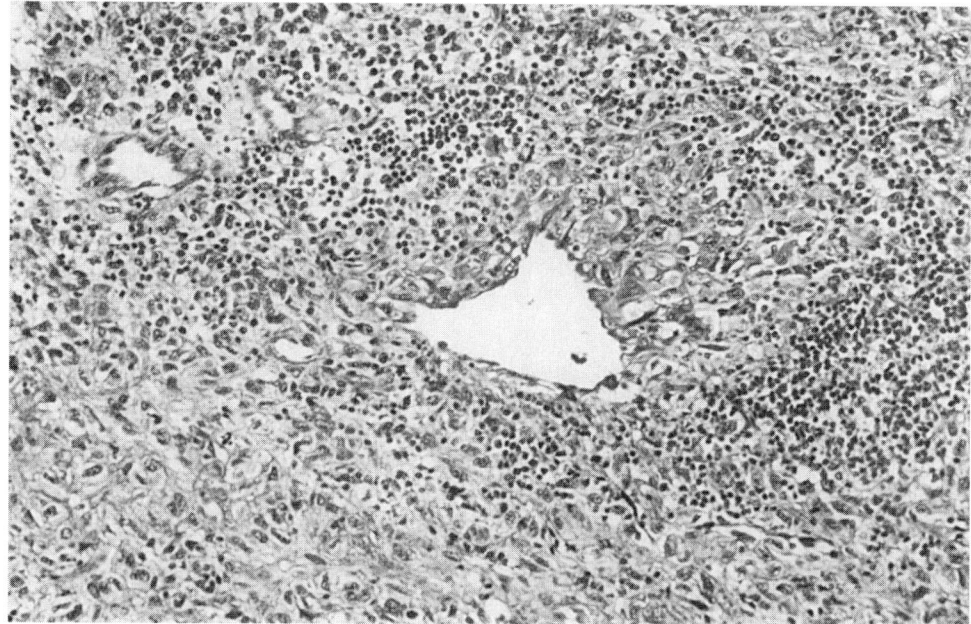

Fig. 27-15 Sarcoma of heart accompanied by marked inflammatory infiltration. It was not possible to classify this tumor into one of major categories of soft tissue sarcoma. Concentric arrangement of tumor cells around large vessel is common feature in heart sarcomas.

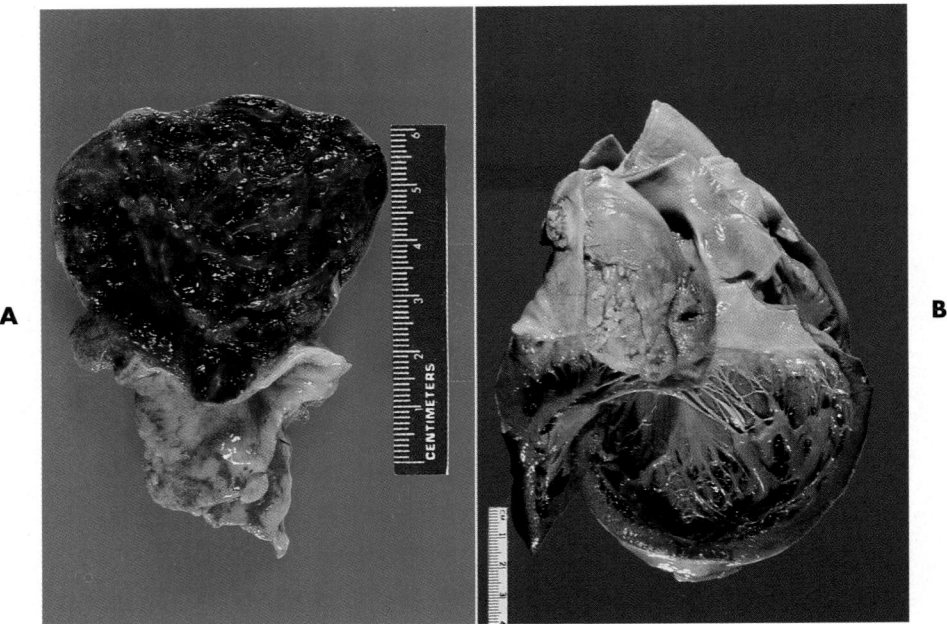

Fig. 27-16 A, Gross appearance of a large angiosarcoma of the heart. **B,** Large metastatic carcinoma in left atrium that was continuous with tumor in left pulmonary vein. This mass simulated an atrial myxoma by echocardiography. The primary tumor was a mucoepidermoid carcinoma of left submaxillary gland.

nant tumors with a marked tendency to spread to the heart by the hematogenous route are malignant melanoma; carcinomas of kidney, lung, and breast; choriocarcinomas; and childhood rhabdomyosarcoma[202] (Fig. 27-16, *B*). Exceptionally, the metastatic heart lesion presents as an isolated nodule, amenable to surgical therapy.[201]

PERICARDIUM

Pericardial (coelomic) cysts are discussed together with all other mediastinal cysts in Chapter 9.

Pericarditis is of importance to the surgical pathologist for several reasons. A diagnosis of tuberculous pericarditis or sarcoidosis can be made from a pericardial open biopsy.[216] Acute nonspecific pericarditis[212] and purulent pericarditis[210] are rarely biopsied, but the former may be troublesome because of the sometimes extreme degree of mesothelial hyperplasia that accompanies it and that can simulate malignancy (Fig. 27-17). Chronic pericarditis is often accompanied by fibrosis and calcification, which may lead to constriction (so-called constrictive pericarditis). This may result from tuberculosis and other infections, collagen-vascular diseases, malignant tumors, trauma, surgery, radiation therapy, or chemotherapy.[217,219] Chronic pericarditis and pericardial constriction are the most common manifestations of radiation damage to the heart.[209,219] The interval between the radiation and the onset of the disease is usually between 50 and 125 months. Pathologic examination usually shows only dense fibrosis with deposits of calcium and a scanty inflammatory infiltrate. Residual granulomas may be found in the cases of tuberculous etiology, and atypical fibroblasts in those related to radiation.

Castleman's disease located within the pericardial sac has been described.[220]

Mesotheliomas of the pericardium occur, but their frequency is much less than that for similar tumors in the pleura or peritoneum. They have been reported in the setting of tuberous sclerosis[213] and may present as a single well-circumscribed mass, as multiple tumors, or as a diffuse growth encasing the heart. Sometimes, they coexist with a pleural mesothelioma. Microscopically, the appearance varies from epithelial to spindle shaped, with a frequent admixture of these elements. Pure spindle-cell (sarcomatoid) mesotheliomas are particularly unusual.[208] As in the pleura, acid mucopolysaccharides are often produced by the tumor cells. The differential diagnosis is with mesothelial hyperplasia and metastatic carcinoma. Demonstration of a continuity between the tumor and the mesothelial lining cells favors a mesothelial nature for the proliferation. Because of the extreme rarity of pericardial mesotheliomas and the fact that reactive mesothelial proliferation can be particularly florid in the pericardium, one should be very cautious in making a diagnosis of malignancy under these circumstances.

Most mesotheliomas of the pericardium occur in adults and are diffuse and malignant. They may locally infiltrate the superficial myocardium and even metastasize to the mediastinal lymph nodes and lungs.[207] Localized mesotheliomas are amenable to surgical excision.[215]

Other primary tumors of the pericardium are exceptionally rare. One such group is represented by germ cell tumors; both mature teratoma and yolk sac tumor (endodermal sac tumor) have been reported in this location.[206,214] Angiosar-

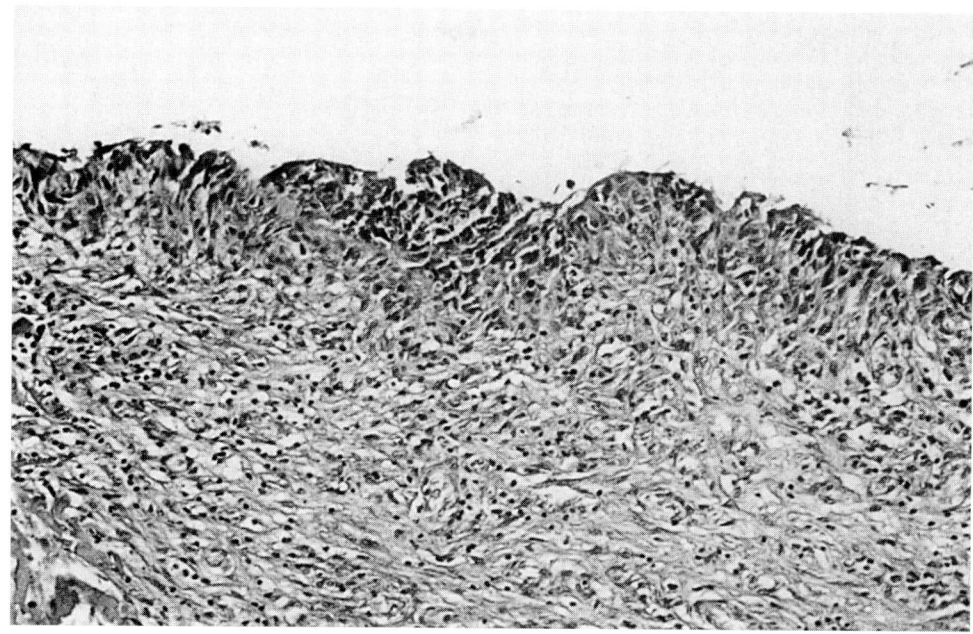

Fig. 27-17 Intense mesothelial proliferation in chronic pericarditis. It is accompanied by fibrosis, inflammation, and fibrin deposition. This type of mesothelial hyperplasia can be misinterpreted as malignant both on cytologic examination and on pericardial biopsy.

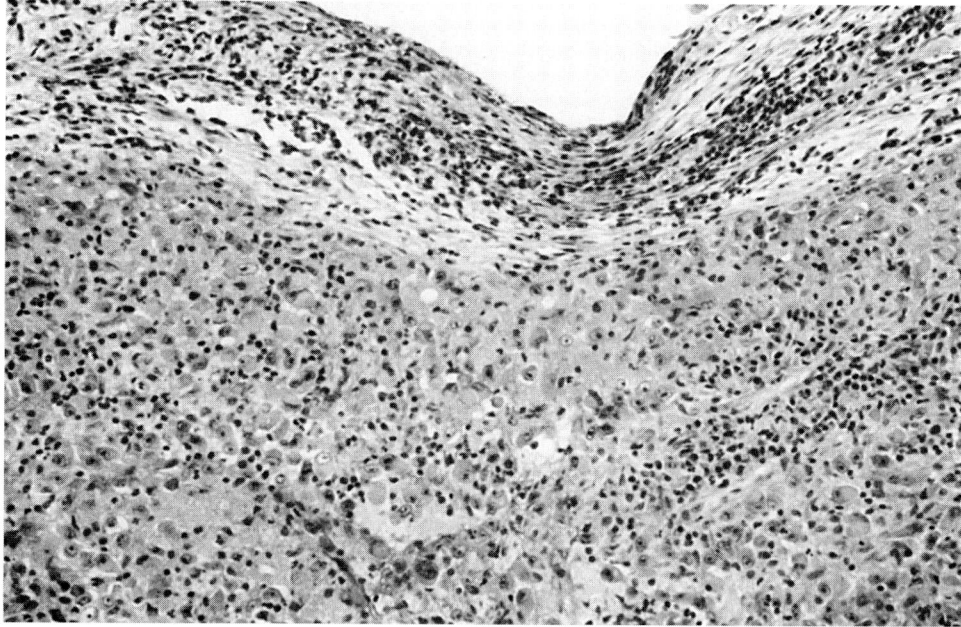

Fig. 27-18 Malignant melanoma metastatic to pericardium. Tumor is covered by thick and inflamed serosa.

coma of pericardium may coat the pericardium in a diffuse fashion, thus simulating the pattern of growth of mesothelioma.[218]

Metastatic carcinoma to the pericardium usually originates in the lung in the form of direct extension or lymphatic permeation. It may result in constrictive "pericarditis" as a result of the associated intense desmoplastic reaction (see p. 2188). Other tumors that commonly give rise to pericardial metastases are breast carcinoma, malignant melanoma, and malignant lymphoma[205,211] (Fig. 27-18).

REFERENCES

INTRODUCTION

1 Castaneda AR: Cardiac surgery of the neonate and infant. Philadelphia, 1994, W.B. Saunders.

2 Marks C: Fundamentals of cardiac surgery. London, 1993, Chapman & Hall.

MYOCARDIAL BIOPSY

3 Anderson DW, Virmani R: Emerging patterns of heart disease in human immunodeficiency virus infection. Hum Pathol 21:253-259, 1990.

4 Aretz HT: Myocarditis. The Dallas criteria. Hum Pathol 18:619-624, 1987.

5 Atkinson JB, Connor DH, Robinowitz M, McAllister HA, Virmani R: Cardiac fungal infections. Review of autopsy finding in 60 patients. Hum Pathol 15:935-942, 1984.

6 Atkinson JB, Virmani R: Congestive heart failure due to coronary artery disease without myocardial infarction. Clinicopathologic description of an unusual cardiomyopathy. Hum Pathol 20:1155-1162, 1989.

7 Billingham ME: Some recent advances in cardiac pathology. Hum Pathol 10:367-386, 1979.

8 Billingham ME, Bristow MR, Glatstein E, Mason JW, Masek MA, Daniels JR: Adriamycin cardiotoxicity. Endomyocardial biopsy evidence of enhancement by irradiation. Am J Surg Pathol 1:17-23, 1977.

9 Buja LM, Roberts WC: Iron in the heart, etiology and clinical significance. Am J Med 51:209-221, 1971.

10 Burke AP, Farb A, Robinowitz M, Virmani R: Serial sectioning and multiple level examination of endomyocardial biopsies for the diagnosis of myocarditis. Mod Pathol 4:690-693, 1991.

11 Burke AP, Saenger J, Mullick F, Virmani R: Hypersensitivity myocarditis. Arch Pathol Lab Med 115:764-769, 1991.

12 Chow LH, Ye Y, Linder J, McManus BM: Phenotypic analysis of infiltrating cells in human myocarditis. An immunohistochemical study in paraffin-embedded tissue. Arch Pathol Lab Med 113:1357-1362, 1989.

13 Darcy T, Mullick F, Schell L, Virmani R: Distinguishing features of myocarditis. Hypersensitivity vs. idiopathic myocarditis (abstract). Lab Invest 58:21A, 1988.

13a Davies MJ, McKernna WJ: Hypertrophic cardiomyopathy. Pathology and pathogenesis. Histopathology 26:493-500, 1995.

14 Edwalds GM, Said JW, Block MI, Herscher LL, Siegel RJ, Fishbein MC: Myocytolysis (vacuolar degeneration) of myocardium. Immunohistochemical evidence of viability. Hum Pathol 15:753-756, 1984.

15 Edwards WD: Cardiomyopathies. Hum Pathol 18:625-635, 1987.

16 Edwards WD, Holmes DR Jr, Reeder GS: Diagnosis of active lymphocytic myocarditis by endomyocardial biopsy. Quantitative criteria for light microscopy. Mayo Clin Proc 57:419-425, 1982.

17 Fenoglio JJ, Marboe CC: Endomyocardial biopsy. An overview. Hum Pathol 18:609-612, 1987.

18 Fenoglio JJ Jr, McAllister HA Jr, Mullick FG: Drug related myocarditis. I. Hypersensitivity myocarditis. Hum Pathol 12:900-907, 1981.

19 Fenoglio JJ Jr, Ursell PC, Kellogg CF, Drusin RE, Weiss MB: Diagnosis and classification of myocarditis by endomyocardial biopsy. N Engl J Med 308:12-18, 1983.

20 Ferrans VJ, Massumi RA, Shugoll GL, Ali N, Roberts WC: Ultrastructural studies of myocardial biopsies in 45 patients with obstructive or congestive cardiomyopathy. In Bajusz E, Rona G, Brink AJ, Lochner A, eds: Recent advances in studies on cardiac structure and metabolism, vol 2. The cardio-myopathies. Baltimore, 1973, University Park Press, pp 231-272.

21 Ferrans VJ, Morrow AG, Roberts WC: Myocardial ultrastructure in idiopathic hypertrophic subaortic stenosis. A study of operatively excised left ventricular outflow tract muscle in 14 patients. Circulation 45:769-792, 1972.

22 Ferrans VJ, Roberts WC: Myocardial biopsy. A useful diagnostic procedure or only a research tool? Am J Cardiol 41:965-967, 1978.

23 Flipse TR, Tazelaar HD, Holmes DR Jr: Diagnosis of malignant cardiac disease by endomyocardial biopsy. Mayo Clin Proc 65:1415-1422, 1990.

24 Fujita M, Neustein HB, Lurie PR: Transvascular endomyocardial biopsy in infants and small children. Myocardial findings in 10 cases of cardiomyopathy. Hum Pathol 10:15-30, 1979.

25 Gravanis MB, Ansari AA: Idiopathic cardiomyopathies. A review of pathologic studies and mechanism of pathogenesis. Arch Pathol Lab Med 111:915-929, 1987.

26 Hammond EH: Utility of ultrastructural studies of cardiac biopsy specimens. Ultrastruct Pathol 18:201-202, 1994.

27 Hauck AJ, Kearney DL, Edwards WD: Evaluation of postmortem endomyocardial biopsy specimens from 38 patients with lymphocytic myocarditis. Implications for role of sampling error. Mayo Clin Proc 64:1235-1245, 1989.

28 Henderson IC, Frei E III: Adriamycin and the heart (editorial). N Engl J Med 300:310-311, 1979.

29 Jaenke RS, Fajardo LF: Adriamycin-induced myocardial lesions. Report of a workshop. Am J Surg Pathol 1:55-60, 1977.

30 Kollo IJ, Edwards WD, Seward JB: Right ventricular dysplasia. The Mayo Clinic experience. Mayo Clin Proc 70:541-548, 1995.

31 Lie JT: Diagnostic histology of myocardial disease in endomyocardial biopsies and at autopsy. Pathol Annu 24(Pt 2):255-293, 1989.

32 Maron BJ, Bonow RO, Cannon RO III, Leon MB, Epstein SE: Hypertrophic cardiomyopathy. Interrelations of clinical manifestations, pathophysiology, and therapy. N Engl J Med 316:780-789; 844-852, 1987.

33 Nippoldt TB, Edwards WD, Holmes DR Jr, Reeder GS, Hartzler GO, Smith HC: Right ventricular endomyocardial biopsy. Clinicopathologic correlates in 100 consecutive patients. Mayo Clin Proc 57:407-418, 1982.

34 Olsen EGJ: Endomyocardial biopsy. Invest Cell Pathol 1:139-157, 1978.

35 Olson LJ, Gertz MA, Edwards WD, Li C-Y, Pellikka PA, Holmes DR Jr, Tajik AJ, Kyle RA: Senile cardiac amyloidosis with myocardial dysfunction. Diagnosis by endomyocardial biopsy and immunohistochemistry. N Engl J Med 317:738-742, 1987.

36 Roberts WC, McAllister HA Jr, Ferrans VJ: Sarcoidosis of the heart. A clinicopathologic study of 35 necropsy patients (group I) and review of 78 previously reported necropsy patients (group II). Am J Med 63:86-108, 1977.

37 Roldan EO, Moskowitz L, Hensley GT: Pathology of the heart in acquired immunodeficiency syndrome. Arch Pathol Lab Med 111:943-946, 1987.

37a Rosai J, Lascano EF: Basophilic (mucoid) degeneration of myocardium. A disorder of glycogen metabolism. Am J Pathol 61:99-116, 1970.

38 Rose AG: Cardiac tuberculosis. A study of 19 patients. Arch Pathol Lab Med 111:422-426, 1987.

39 Rose AG, Beck W: Dilated (congestive) cardiomyopathy. A syndrome of severe cardiac dysfunction with remarkably few morphological features of myocardial damage. Histopathology 9:367-379, 1985.

40 Schnitt SJ, Ciano PS, Schoen FJ: Quantitation of lymphocytes in endomyocardial biopsies. Use and limitations of antibodies to leukocyte common antigen. Hum Pathol 18:796-800, 1987.

41 Spirito P, Chiarella F, Carratino L, Berisso MZ, Bellotti P, Vecchio C: Clinical course and prognosis of hypertrophic cardiomyopathy in an outpatient population. N Engl J Med 320:749-755, 1989.

41a Tamura S, Takahashi M, Kawamura S, Ishihara T: Basophilic degeneration of the myocardium. Histological, immunohistochemical and immunoelectronmicroscopic studies. Histopathology 26:501-508, 1995.

42 Tazelaar HD, Billingham ME: Leukocytic infiltrates in idiopathic dilated cardiomyopathy. A source of confusion with active myocarditis. Am J Surg Pathol 10:405-412, 1986.

43 Tazelaar HD, Billingham ME: The surgical pathology of hypertrophic cardiomyopathy. Arch Pathol Lab Med 111:257-260, 1987.

44 Theaker JM, Gatter KC, Brown DC, Heryet A, Davies MJ: An investigation into the nature of giant cells in cardiac and skeletal muscle. Hum Pathol 19:974-979, 1988.

45 Ursell PC, Albala A, Fenoglio JJ Jr: Diagnosis of acute rheumatic carditis by endomyocardial biopsy. Hum Pathol 13:677-679, 1982.

46 Ursell PC, Fenoglio JJ: Spectrum of cardiac disease diagnosed by endomyocardial biopsy. Pathol Annu 19(Pt 2):197-219, 1984.

47 Weinstein C, Fenoglio JJ: Myocarditis. Hum Pathol 18:613-618, 1987.

48 Winters GL, Costanzo-Nordin MR: Pathological findings in 2300 consecutive endomyocardial biopsies. Mod Pathol 4:441-448, 1991.

HEART TRANSPLANT

49 Abu-Farsakh H, Cagle PT, Buffone GJ, Bruner JM, Weilbaecher D, Greenberg SD: Heart allograft involvement with Epstein-Barr virus-associated posttransplant lymphoproliferative disorder. Arch Pathol Lab Med 116:93-95, 1992.

50 Arbustini E, Grasso M, Diegoli M, Percivalle E, Grossi P, Bramerio M, Campana C, Goggi C, Gavazzi A, Vigano M: Histopathologic and molecular profile of human cytomegalovirus infections in patients with heart transplants. Am J Clin Pathol **98**:205-213, 1992.

51 Billingham ME: Some recent advances in cardiac pathology. Hum Pathol **10**:367-386, 1979.

52 Chen JM, Barr ML, Chadburn A, Frizzera G, Schenkel FA, Sciacca RR, Reison DS, Addonizio LJ, Rose EA, Knowles DM, et al: Management of lymphoproliferative disorders after cardiac transplantation. Ann Thorac Surg **56**:527-538, 1993.

53 Chomette G, Auriol M, Delcourt A, Karkouche B, Cabrol A, Cabrol C: Human cardiac transplants. Diagnosis of rejection by endomyocardial biopsy. Causes of death (about 30 autopsies). Virchows Arch [A] **407**:295-307, 1985.

54 Forbes RD, Rowan RA, Billingham ME: Endocardial infiltrates in human heart transplants. A serial biopsy analysis comparing four immunosuppression protocols. Hum Pathol **21**:850-855, 1990.

55 Gaudin PB, Rayburn BK, Hutchins GM, Kasper EK, Baughman KL, Goodman SN, Lecks LE, Baumgartner WA, Hruban RH: Peritransplant injury to the myocardium associated with the development of accelerated arteriosclerosis in heart transplant recipients. Am J Surg Pathol **18**:338-346, 1994.

55a Hammond EH: Solid organ transplantation pathology. Major problems in pathology, vol 30. Philadelphia, 1994, W.B. Saunders.

56 Hawkins ET, Levine TB, Goss SJ, Moosvi A, Levine AB: Hypersensitivity myocarditis in the explanted hearts of transplant recipients. Reappraisal of pathologic criteria and their clinical implications. Pathol Annu **30**(Pt 1):287-304, 1995.

57 Kemnitz J, Cohnert TR: Lymphoma like lesion in human orthotopic cardiac allografts (abstract). Am J Clin Pathol **89**:430, 1988.

58 Kemnitz J, Cohnert T, Schnäfers H-J, Helmke M, Wahlers T, Herrmann G, Schmidt RM, Haverich A: A classification of cardiac allograft rejection. A modification of the classification by Billingham. Am J Surg Pathol **11**:503-515, 1987.

59 Kottke-Marchant K, Ratliff NB: Endomyocardial lymphocytic infiltrates in cardiac transplant recipients. Incidence and characterization. Arch Pathol Lab Med **113**:690-698, 1989.

60 Kottke-Marchant K, Ratliff NB: Endomyocardial biopsy. Pathologic findings in cardiac transplant recipients. Pathol Annu **25**(Pt 1):211-244, 1990.

61 McAllister HA, Schnee MJ, Radiovancevic B, Frazier H: A system for grading cardiac allograft rejections. Tex Heart Inst J **13**:1-2, 1986.

62 Morrison VA, Dunn DL, Manivel JC, Gajl-Peczalska KJ, Peterson BA: Clinical characteristics of post-transplant lymphoproliferative disorders. Am J Med **97**:14-24, 1994.

62a Olsen SL, Wagoner LE, Hammond EH, Taylor DO, Yowell RL, Ensley RD, Bristow MR, O'Connell JB, Renlund DG: Vascular rejection in heart transplantation. Clinical correlation, treatment options, and future considerations. J Heart Lung Transplant **12**:S135-142, 1993.

63 Pardo-Mindan FJ, Lozano MD, Contreras-Mejuto F, de Alava E: Pathology of heart transplant through endomyocardial biopsy. Semin Diagn Pathol **9**:238-248, 1992.

64 Pomerance A, Stovin P: Heart transplant pathology. The British experience. J Clin Pathol **38**:146-159, 1985.

65 Rowan RA, Billingham ME: Pathologic changes in the long-term transplanted heart. A morphometric study of myocardial hypertrophy, vascularity, and fibrosis. Hum Pathol **21**:767-772, 1990.

66 Tazelaar HD, Gay RE, Rowan RA, Billingham ME, Gay S: Collagen profile in the transplanted heart. Hum Pathol **21**:424-428, 1990.

67 Uys CJ, Rose AG: Cardiac transplantation. Aspects of the pathology. Pathol Annu **17**(Pt 2):147-178, 1982.

67a Weissman DJ, Ferry JA, Harris NL, Louis DN, Delmonico F, Spiro I: Posttransplantation lymphoproliferative disorders in solid organ recipients are predominantly aggressive tumors of host origin. Am J Clin Pathol **103**:748-755, 1995.

68 Zerbe TR, Arena V: Diagnostic reliability of endomyocardial biopsy for assessment of cardiac allograft rejection. Hum Pathol **19**:1307-1314, 1988.

CARDIAC VALVES

69 Altrichter PM, Olson LJ, Edwards WD, Puga FJ, Danielson GK: Surgical pathology of the pulmonary valve. A study of 116 cases spanning 15 years. Mayo Clin Proc **64**:1352-1360, 1989.

70 Billingham ME: Some recent advances in cardiac pathology. Hum Pathol **10**:367-386, 1979.

71 Clark RM, Anderson W: Rheumatic activity in auricular appendages removed at mitral valvoplasty. Am J Pathol **31**:809-819, 1955.

72 Cooper JH: Localized dystrophic amyloidosis of heart valves. Hum Pathol **14**:649-653, 1983.

73 Dare AJ, Harrity PJ, Tazelaar HD, Edwards WD, Mullany CJ: Evaluation of surgically excised mitral valves. Revised recommendations based on changing operative procedures in the 1990s. Hum Pathol **24**:1286-1293, 1993.

74 Dare AJ, Veinot JP, Edwards WD, Tazelaar HD, Schaff HV: New observations on the etiology of aortic valve disease. A surgical pathologic study of 236 cases from 1990. Hum Pathol **24**:1330-1338, 1993.

75 Davies MJ: Pathology of cardiac valves. London, 1980, Butterworth & Co, Ltd.

76 Ferrans VJ, Tomita Y, Hilbert SL, Jones M, Roberts WC: Pathology of bioprosthetic cardiac valves. Hum Pathol **18**:586-595, 1987.

77 Gravanis MB, Campbell WG Jr: The syndrome of prolapse of the mitral valve. Arch Pathol Lab Med **106**:369-374, 1982.

78 Groom DA, Starke WR: Cartilaginous metaplasia in calcific aortic valve disease. Am J Clin Pathol **93**:809-812, 1990.

79 Hanson TP, Edwards BS, Edwards JE: Pathology of surgically excised mitral valves. One hundred consecutive cases. Arch Pathol Lab Med **109**:823-828, 1985.

80 Hauck AJ, Freeman DP, Ackermann DM, Danielson GK, Edwards WD: Surgical pathology of the tricuspid valve. A study of 363 cases spanning 25 years. Mayo Clin Proc **63**:851-863, 1988.

81 Love GL, Restrepo C: Aschoff bodies of rheumatic carditis are granulomatous lesions of histiocytic origin. Mod Pathol **1**:256-261, 1988.

82 Morales AR, Romanelli R, Boucek RJ, Tate LG, Alvarez RT, Davis JT: Myxoid heart disease. An assessment of extravalvular cardiac pathology in severe mitral valve prolapse. Hum Pathol **23**:129-137, 1992.

83 Murphy SK, Rogler WC, Fleming WH, McManus BM: Retraction of bioprosthetic heart valve cusps. A cause of wide-open regurgitation in right-sided heart valves. Hum Pathol **19**:140-147, 1988.

84 Olson LJ, Subramanian R, Ackermann DM, Orszulak TA, Edwards WD: Surgical pathology of the mitral valve. A study of 712 cases spanning 21 years. Mayo Clin Proc **62**:22-34, 1987.

85 Passik CS, Ackermann DM, Pluth JR, Edwards WD: Temporal changes in the causes of aortic stenosis. A surgical pathologic study of 646 cases. Mayo Clin Proc **62**:119-123, 1987.

86 Peterson MD, Roach RM, Edwards JE: Types of aortic stenosis in surgically removed valves. Arch Pathol Lab Med **109**:829-832, 1985.

87 Robboy SJ, Kaiser J: Pathogenesis of fungal infection on heart valve prostheses. Hum Pathol **6**:711-715, 1975.

88 Roberts WC, Morrow AG: Cardiac valves and the surgical pathologist. Arch Pathol **82**:309-313, 1966.

89 Rose AG: Etiology of acquired valvular heart disease in adults. A survey of 18,132 autopsies and 100 consecutive valve-replacement operations. Arch Pathol Lab Med **110**:385-388, 1986.

90 Schoen FJ: Surgical pathology of removed natural and prosthetic heart valves. Hum Pathol **18**:558-567, 1987.

91 Schoen FJ, Hobson CE: Anatomic analysis of removed prosthetic heart valves. Causes of failure of 33 mechanical valves and 58 bioprostheses, 1980 to 1983. Hum Pathol **16**:549-559, 1985.

92 Schoen FJ, Levy RJ, Piehler HR: Pathological considerations in replacement cardiac valves. Cardiovasc Pathol **1**:29-52, 1992.

93 Schoen FJ, Sutton MSJ: Contemporary issues in the pathology of valvular heart disease. Hum Pathol **18**:568-576, 1987.

94 Silver MD: Cardiac pathology. A look at the last five years. II. The pathology of cardiovascular prostheses. Hum Pathol **5**:127-138, 1974.

95 Silver MD: Late complications of prosthetic heart valves. Arch Pathol Lab Med **102**:281-284, 1978.

96 Silver MD, Butany J: Mechanical heart valves. Methods of examination, complications, and modes of failure. Hum Pathol **18**:577-585, 1987.

97 Silver MD, Datta BN, Bowes VF: A key to identify heart valve prostheses. Arch Pathol **99**:132-138, 1975.

98 Subramanian R, Olson LJ, Edwards WD: Surgical pathology of pure aortic stenosis. A study of 374 cases. Mayo Clin Proc **59**:683-690, 1984.

99 Subramanian R, Olson LJ, Edwards WD: Surgical pathology of combined aortic stenosis and insufficiency. A study of 213 cases. Mayo Clin Proc **60**:247-254, 1985.

100 van der Bel-Kahn J, Becker AE: The surgical pathology of rheumatic and floppy mitral valves. Distinctive morphologic features upon gross examination. Am J Surg Pathol **10**:282-292, 1986.

101 Virmani R, Atkinson JB, Forman MB, Robinowitz M: Mitral valve prolapse. Hum Pathol **18**:596-602, 1987.

CORONARY ARTERY BYPASS

102 Kern WH, Wells WJ, Meyer BW: The pathology of surgically excised aortocoronary saphenous vein bypass grafts. Am J Surg Pathol **5**:491-496, 1981.

103 Ratliff NB, Myles JL: Rapidly progressive atherosclerosis in aortocoronary saphenous vein grafts. Possible immune-mediated disease. Arch Pathol Lab Med 113:772-776, 1989.

104 Smith SH, Geer JC: Morphology of saphenous vein-coronary artery bypass grafts. Seven to 116 months after surgery. Arch Pathol Lab Med 107:13-18, 1983.

105 Yutani C, Imakita M, Ishibashi-Ueda H: Histopathological study of aorto-coronary bypass grafts with special reference to fibrin deposits on grafted saphenous veins. Acta Pathol Jpn 39:425-432, 1989.

COARCTATION OF AORTA

106 Bergdahl L, Bjork VO, Jonasson R: Surgical correction of coarctation of the aorta. Influence of age on late results. J Thorac Cardiovasc Surg 85:532-536, 1983.

107 Campbell M: Natural history of coarctation of the aorta. Br Heart J 32:633-640, 1970.

108 Lerberg DB, Hardesty RL, Siewers RD, Zuberbuhler JR, Bahnson HT: Coarctation of the aorta in infants and children. 25 years experience. Ann Thorac Surg 33:159-170, 1982.

CARDIAC TUMORS
Myxoma

109 Boxer ME: Cardiac myxoma. An immunoperoxidase study of histogenesis. Histopathology 8:861-872, 1984.

110 Burke AP, Virmani R: Cardiac myxoma. A clinicopathologic study. Am J Clin Pathol 100:671-680, 1993.

111 Carney JA: Differences between nonfamilial and familial cardiac myxoma. Am J Surg Pathol 9:53-55, 1985.

112 Dewald GW, Dahl RJ, Spurbeck JL, Carney JA, Gordon H: Chromosomally abnormal clones and nonrandom telomeric translocations in cardiac myxomas. Mayo Clin Proc 62:558-567, 1987.

113 Feldman PS, Horvath E, Kovacs K: An ultrastructural study of seven cardiac myxomas. Cancer 40:2216-2232, 1977.

114 Ferrans VJ, Roberts WC: Structural features of cardiac myxomas. Histology, histochemistry and electron microscopy. Hum Pathol 4:111-146, 1973.

115 Fine G, Morales A, Horn RC Jr: Cardiac myxoma. A morphologic and histogenetic appraisal. Cancer 22:1156-1162, 1968.

116 Goldman BI, Frydman C, Harpaz N, Ryan SF, Loiterman D: Glandular cardiac myxomas. Histologic, immunohistochemical, and ultrastructural evidence of epithelial differentiation. Cancer 59:1767-1775, 1987.

117 Govoni E, Severi B, Cenacchi G, Laschi R, Pileri S, Rivano MT, Alampi G, Branzi A: Ultrastructural and immunohistochemical contribution to the histogenesis of human cardiac myxoma. Ultrastruct Pathol 12:221-233, 1988.

118 Heath D: Pathology of cardiac tumors. Am J Cardiol 21:315-327, 1968.

119 Johansson L: Histogenesis of cardiac myxomas. An immunohistochemical study of 19 cases, including one with glandular structures, and review of the literature. Arch Pathol Lab Med 113:735-741, 1989.

120 Kasugai T, Sakurai M, Yutani C, Hirota S, Waki N, Adachi S, Kitamura Y: Sequential malignant transformation of cardiac myxoma. Acta Pathol Jpn 40:687-692, 1990.

121 Landon G, Ordòñez NG, Guarda LA: Cardiac myxomas. An immunohistochemical study using endothelial, histiocytic, and smooth-muscle cell markers. Arch Pathol Lab Med 110:116-120, 1986.

122 Lie JT: Petrified cardiac myxoma masquerading as organized atrial mural thrombus. Arch Pathol Lab Med 113:742-745, 1989.

123 McComb RD: Heterogeneous expression of factor VIII/von Willebrand factor by cardiac myxoma cells. Am J Surg Pathol 8:539-544, 1984.

124 Morales AR, Fine G, Castro A, Nadji M: Cardiac myxoma (endocardioma). An immunocytochemical assessment of histogenesis. Hum Pathol 12:896-899, 1981.

125 Pohost GM, Pastore JO, McKusick KA, Chiotellis PN, Kapellakis GZ, Meyers GS, Dinsmore RE, Block PC: Detection of left atrial myxoma by gated radionuclide cardiac imaging. Circulation 55:88-92, 1977.

126 Read RC, White HJ, Murphy ML, Williams D, Sun CN, Flanagan WH: The malignant potentiality of left atrial myxoma. J Thorac Cardiovasc Surg 68:857-868, 1974.

127 Reed RJ, Utz MP, Terezakis N: Embolic and metastatic cardiac myxoma. Am J Dermatopathol 11:157-165, 1989.

128 Richardson JV, Brandt B III, Doty DB, Ehrenhaft JL: Surgical treatment of atrial myxomas. Early and late results of 111 operations and review of the literature. Ann Thorac Surg 28:354-358, 1979.

129 Rupp GM, Heyman RA, Martinez AJ, Sekhar LN, Jungreis CA: The pathology of metastatic cardiac myxoma. Am J Clin Pathol 91:221-227, 1989.

130 Salyer WR, Page DL, Hutchins GM: The development of cardiac myxomas and papillary endocardial lesions from mural thrombus. Am Heart J 89:14-17, 1975.

131 Samaratunga H, Searle J, Cominos D, Le Fevre I: Cerebral metastasis of an atrial myxoma mimicking an epithelioid hemangioendothelioma. Am J Surg Pathol 18:107-111, 1994.

132 Schmitt-Graff A, Borchard F: Cardiac myxoma with a cytokeratin-immunoreactive glandular component. Pathol Res Pract 188:217-215, 1992.

133 Schuger L, Ron N, Rosenmann E: Cardiac myxoma. A retrospective immunohistochemical study. Pathol Res Pract 182:63-66, 1987.

134 Seidman JD, Berman JJ, Hitchcock CL, Becker RL Jr, Mergner W, Moore GW, Virmani R, Yetter RA: DNA analysis of cardiac myxomas. Flow cytometry and image analysis. Hum Pathol 22:494-500, 1991.

135 Seo IS, Warner TFCS, Colyer RA, Winkler RF: Metastasizing atrial myxoma. Am J Surg Pathol 4:391-399, 1980.

136 Silverman J, Olwin JS, Graettinger JS: Cardiac myxomas with systemic embolization. Review of the literature and report of a case. Circulation 26:99-103, 1962.

137 Silverman NA: Primary cardiac tumors. Ann Surg 191:127-138, 1980.

138 Tanimura A, Kitazono M, Nagayama K, Tanaka S, Kosuga K: Cardiac myxoma. Morphologic, histochemical, and tissue culture studies. Hum Pathol 19:316-322, 1988.

139 Trotter SE, Shore DF, Olsen EG: Gamna-Gandy nodules in a cardiac myxoma. Histopathology 17:270-272, 1990.

Other benign tumors and tumorlike conditions

140 Almagro UA, Perry LS, Choi H, Pintar K: Papillary fibroelastoma of the heart. Report of six cases. Arch Pathol Lab Med 206:318-321, 1982.

141 Aqel NM, Shousha S: Glandular inclusions in fetal myocardium. Histopathology 24:85-87, 1994.

142 Burke AP, Anderson PG, Virmani R, James TN, Herrera GA, Ceballos R: Tumor of the atrioventricular nodal region. A clinical and immunohistochemical study. Arch Pathol Lab Med 114:1057-1062, 1990.

143 Burke AP, Virmani R: Cardiac rhabdomyoma. A clinicopathologic study. Mod Pathol 4:70-74, 1991.

144 Chan HSL, Sonley MJ, Möes CAF, Daneman A, Smith CR, Martin DJ: Primary and secondary tumors of childhood involving the heart, pericardium, and great vessels. A report of 75 cases and review of the literature. Cancer 56:825-836, 1985.

145 Chou P, Gonzalez-Crussi F, Cole R, Reddy VB: Plasma cell granuloma of the heart. Cancer 62:1409-1413, 1988.

146 Courtice RW, Stinson WA, Walley VM: Tissue fragments recovered at cardiac surgery masquerading as tumoral proliferations. Evidence suggesting iatrogenic or artefactual origin and common occurrence. Am J Surg Pathol 18:167-174, 1994.

147 Duray PH, Mark EJ, Barwick KW, Madri JA, Strom RL: Congenital polycystic tumor of the atrioventricular node. Arch Pathol Lab Med 109:30-34, 1985.

148 Fekete PS, Nassar VH, Talley JD, Boedecker EA: Cardiac papilloma. Arch Pathol Lab Med 107:246-248, 1983.

149 Feldman PS, Meyer MW: Fibroelastic hamartoma (fibroma) of the heart. Cancer 38:314-323, 1976.

150 Fenoglio JJ, McAllister HA: Granular cell tumors of the heart. Arch Pathol Lab Med 100:276-278, 1976.

151 Fenoglio JJ Jr, Jacobs DW, McAllister HA Jr: Ultrastructure of the mesothelioma of the atrioventricular node. Cancer 40:721-727, 1977.

152 Fine G: Primary tumors of the pericardium and heart. In Edwards JE, et al, eds: The heart. Baltimore, 1974, The Williams & Wilkins Co, pp 189-210.

153 Fine G, Raju U: Congenital polycystic tumor of the atrioventricular node (endodermal heterotopia, mesothelioma). A histogenetic appraisal with evidence for its endodermal origin. Hum Pathol 18:791-795, 1987.

154 Hoyt JC, Hutchins GM: Angiomatous variants of so-called mesothelioma of the atrioventricular node. Arch Pathol Lab Med 110:851-852, 1986.

155 Jaffe R: Neuroma in the region of the atrioventricular node. Hum Pathol 12:375-376, 1981.

156 Johnson TL, Shapiro B, Beierwaltes WH, Orringer MB, Lloyd RV, Sisson JC, Thompson NW: Cardiac paragangliomas. A clinicopathologic and immunohistochemical study of four cases. Am J Surg Pathol 9:827-834, 1985.

157 Kantelip B, Lusson JR, De Riberolles C, Lamaison D, Bailly P: Intracardiac ectopic thyroid. Hum Pathol 17:1293-1296, 1986.

158 Kiaer HW: Myocardial angiolipoma. Acta Pathol Microbiol Immunol Scand (A) 92:291-292, 1984.

159 Kuo T-T, Hsueh S, Su I-J, Gonzalez-Crussi F, Chen J-S: Histiocytoid hemangioma of the heart with peripheral eosinophilia. Cancer 55:2854-2861, 1985.

160 Linder J, Shelburne JD, Sorge JP, Whalen RE, Hackel DB: Congenital endodermal heterotopia of the atrioventricular node. Evidence for the endodermal origin of so-called mesotheliomas of the atrioventricular node. Hum Pathol 15:1093-1098, 1984.

161 Luthringer DJ, Virmani R, Weiss SW, Rosai J: A distinctive cardiovascular lesion resembling histiocytoid (epithelioid) hemangioma. Evidence suggesting mesothelial participation. Am J Surg Pathol 14:993-1000, 1990.

162 Monroe B, Federman M, Balogh K: Cardiac neurilemoma. Report of a case with electron microscopic examination. Arch Pathol Lab Med **108:**300-304, 1984.

163 Prichard RW: Tumors of the heart. Review of the subject and report of one hundred and fifty cases. Arch Pathol **51:**98-128, 1951.

164 Rosai J, Dehner LP: Nodular mesothelial hyperplasia in hernia sacs. A benign reactive condition simulating a neoplastic process. Cancer **35:**165-175, 1975.

165 Rosai J, Gold J, Landy R: The histiocytoid hemangiomas. A unifying concept embracing several previously described entities of skin, soft tissue, large vessels, bone and heart. Hum Pathol **10:**707-730, 1979.

165a Rubin MA, Snell JA, Tazelaar HD, Lack EE, Austenfeld JL, Azumi N: Cardiac papillary fibroelastoma. An immunohistochemical investigation and unusual clinical manifestations. Mod Pathol **8:**402-407, 1995.

166 Silverman JF, Kay S, McCue M, Lower RR, Brough AJ, Chang CH: Rhabdomyoma of the heart. Ultrastructural study of three cases. Lab Invest **35:**596-606, 1976.

167 Swalwell CI: Benign intracardiac teratoma. A case of sudden death. Arch Pathol Lab Med **117:**739-742, 1993.

168 Tabry IF, Nassar VH, Rizk G, Touma A, Dagher IK: Cavernous hemangioma of the heart. Case report and review of the literature. J Thorac Cardiovasc Surg **69:**415-420, 1975.

169 Tazelaar HD, Locke TJ, McGregor CG: Pathology of surgically excised primary cardiac tumors. Mayo Clin Proc **67:**957-965, 1992.

170 Veinot JP, Tazelaar HD, Edwards WD, Colby TV: Mesothelial/monocytic incidental cardiac excrescences. Cardiac MICE. Mod Pathol **7:**9-16, 1994.

171 Weeks DA, Chase DR, Malott RL, Chase RL, Zuppan CW, Bekwith JB, Mierau GW: HMB-45 staining in angiomyolipoma, cardiac rhabdomyoma, other mesenchymal processes, and tuberous sclerosis-associated brain lesions. Int J Surg Pathol **1:**191-198, 1994.

172 Yu GH, Kussmaul WG, Di Sesa VJ, Lodato RF, Brooks JS: Adult intracardiac rhabdomyoma resembling the extracardiac variant. Hum Pathol **24:**448-451, 1993.

Primary malignant tumors

173 Bearman RM: Primary leiomyosarcoma of the heart. Report of a case and review of the literature. Arch Pathol **98:**62-65, 1974.

174 Burke AP, Cowan D, Virmani R: Primary sarcomas of the heart. Cancer **69:**387-395, 1992.

175 Burke AP, Virmani R: Osteosarcomas of the heart. Am J Surg Pathol **15:**289-295, 1991.

176 Cairns P, Butany J, Fulop J, Rakowski H, Hassaram S: Cardiac presentation of non-Hodgkin's lymphoma. Arch Pathol Lab Med **111:**80-83, 1987.

177 Chou S-T, Arkles LB, Gill GD, Pinkus N, Parkin A, Hicks JD: Primary lymphoma of the heart. A case report. Cancer **52:**744-747, 1983.

178 Constantino A, West TE, Gupta M, Loghmanee F: Primary cardiac lymphoma in a patient with acquired immune deficiency syndrome. Cancer **60:**2801-2805, 1987.

179 Curtsinger CR, Wilson MJ, Yoneda K: Primary cardiac lymphoma. Cancer **64:**521-525, 1989.

180 Fabian JT, Rose AG: Tumours of the heart. A study of 89 cases. S Afr Med J **61:**71-77, 1982.

181 Guarner J, Brynes RK, Chan WC, Birdsong G, Hertzler G: Primary non-Hodgkin's lymphoma of the heart in two patients with the acquired immunodeficiency syndrome. Arch Pathol Lab Med **111:**254-256, 1987.

182 Herhusky MJ, Gregg SB, Virmani R, Chun PKC, Bender H, Gray GF Jr: Cardiac sarcomas presenting as metastatic disease. Arch Pathol Lab Med **109:**943-945, 1985.

183 Herrmann MA, Shankerman RA, Edwards WD, Shub C, Schaff HV: Primary cardiac angiosarcoma. A clinicopathologic study of six cases. J Thorac Cardiovasc Surg **103:**655-664, 1992.

184 Holladay AO, Siegel RJ, Schwartz DA: Cardiac malignant lymphoma in acquired immune deficiency syndrome. Cancer **70:**2203-2207, 1992.

185 Janigan DT, Husain A, Robinson NA: Cardiac angiosarcomas. A review and a case report. Cancer **57:**852-859, 1986.

186 Karn CM, Socinski MA, Fletcher JA, Corson JM, Craighead JE: Cardiac synovial sarcoma with translocation (X; 18) associated with asbestos exposure. Cancer **73:**74-78, 1994.

187 Klima T, Milam JD, Bossart MI, Cooley DA: Rare primary sarcomas of the heart. Arch Pathol Lab Med **110:**1155-1159, 1986.

188 Lam KY, Dickens P, Chan AC: Tumors of the heart. A 20-year experience with a review of 12,485 consecutive autopsies. Arch Pathol Lab Med **117:**1027-1031, 1993.

189 Laya MB, Mailliard JA, Bewtra C, Levin HS: Malignant fibrous histiocytoma of the heart. A case report and review of the literature. Cancer **59:**1026-1031, 1987.

190 McAllister HA Jr, Fenoglio JJ: Tumors of the cardiovascular system. In Atlas of tumor pathology, Second Series, Fasc. 15. Washington, DC, 1978, Armed Forces Institute of Pathology.

191 McDonnell PJ, Mann RB, Bulkley BH: Involvement of the heart by malignant lymphoma. A clinicopathologic study. Cancer **49:**944-951, 1982.

192 Ovcak Z, Masera A, Lamovec J: Malignant fibrous histiocytoma of the heart. Arch Pathol Lab Med **116:**872-874, 1992.

193 Rossi NP, Kioschos JM, Aschenbrener CA, Ehrenhaft JL: Primary angiosarcoma of the heart. Cancer **37:**891-894, 1976.

194 Sheffield EA, Corrin B, Addis BJ, Gelder C: Synovial sarcoma of the heart arising from so-called mesothelioma of the atrio-ventricular node. Histopathology **12:**191-202, 1988.

195 Small EJ, Gordon GJ, Dahms BB: Malignant rhabdoid tumor of the heart in an infant. Cancer **55:**2850-2853, 1985.

196 Ursell PC, Albala A, Fenoglio JJ Jr: Malignant neurogenic tumor of the heart. Hum Pathol **13:**640-645, 1982.

197 Yang H-Y, Wasielewski JF, Lee W, Lee E, Paik YK: Angiosarcoma of the heart. Ultrastructural study. Cancer **47:**72-80, 1981.

Metastatic tumors

198 Hanfling SM: Metastatic cancer to the heart. Circulation **22:**474-483, 1960.

199 Klatt EC, Heitz DR: Cardiac metastases. Cancer **65:**1456-1459, 1990.

200 Kline IK: Cardiac lymphatic involvement by metastatic tumor. Cancer **29:**799-808, 1972.

201 Lagrange J-L, Despins P, Spielman M, Le Chevalier T, De Lajartre A-Y, Fontaine F, Sarrazin D, Contesso G, Génin J, Rouesse J, Grossetête R: Cardiac metastases. Case report on an isolated cardiac metastasis of a myxoid liposarcoma. Cancer **58:**2333-2337, 1986.

202 Pratt CB, Dugger DL, Johnson WW, Ainger LE: Metastatic involvement of the heart in childhood rhabdomyosarcoma. Cancer **31:**1492-1497, 1973.

203 Roberts WC, Glancy DL, DeVita VT Jr: Heart in malignant lymphoma (Hodgkin's disease, lymphosarcoma, reticulum cell sarcoma and mycosis fungoides). Study of 196 autopsy cases. Am J Cardiol **22:**85-107, 1968.

204 Smith C: Tumors of the heart. Arch Pathol Lab Med **110:**371-374, 1986.

PERICARDIUM

205 Adenle AD, Edwards JE: Clinical and pathologic features of metastatic neoplasms of the pericardium. Chest **81:**166-169, 1982.

206 Cox JN, Friedli B, Mechmeche R, Ben Ismail M, Oberhaensli I, Faidutti B: Teratoma of the heart. A case report and review of the literature. Virchows Arch [A] **402:**163-174, 1983.

207 Fine G: Primary tumors of the pericardium and heart. In Edwards JE et al, eds: The heart. Baltimore, 1974, The Williams & Wilkins Co, pp 189-210.

208 Fukuda T, Ishikawa H, Ohnishi Y, Tachikawa S, Oguma F, Kasuya S, Sakashita I: Malignant spindle cell tumor of the pericardium. Evidence of sarcomatous mesothelioma with aberrant antigen expression. Acta Pathol Jpn **39:**750-754, 1989.

209 Hancock EW: Heart disease after radiation (editorial). N Engl J Med **308:**588, 1983.

210 Klacsmann PG, Bulkley BH, Hutchins GM: The changed spectrum of purulent pericarditis. An 86 year autopsy experience in 200 patients. Am J Med **63:**666-673, 1977.

211 Mambo NC: Diseases of the pericardium. Morphologic study of surgical specimens from 35 patients. Hum Pathol **12:**978-987, 1981.

212 Martin A: Acute non-specific pericarditis. A description of nineteen cases. Br Med J **2:**279-281, 1966.

213 Naramoto A, Itoh N, Nakano M, Shigematsu H: An autopsy case of tuberous sclerosis associated with primary pericardial mesothelioma. Acta Pathol Jpn **39:**400-406, 1989.

214 Nelson E, Stenzel P: Intrapericardial yolk sac tumor in an infant girl. Cancer **60:**1567-1569, 1987.

215 Sane AC, Roggli VL: Curative resection of a well-differentiated papillary mesothelioma of the pericardium. Arch Pathol Lab Med **119:**266-267, 1995.

216 Shiff AD, Blatt CJ, Kolp C: Recurrent pericardial effusion secondary to sarcoidosis of the pericardium. A biopsy-proved case. N Engl J Med **281:**141-143, 1967.

217 Stewart JR, Fajardo LF: Radiation-induced heart disease. An update. Prog Cardiovasc Dis **27:**173-194, 1984.

218 Terada T, Nakanuma Y, Matsubara T, Suematsu T: An autopsy case of primary angiosarcoma of the pericardium mimicking malignant mesothelioma. Acta Pathol Jpn **38:**1345-1351, 1988.

219 Tötterman KJ, Pesonen E, Siltanen P: Radiation-related chronic heart disease. Chest **83:**875-878, 1983.

220 Virmani R, Bewtra C, McAllister HA, Schulte RD: Intrapericardial giant lymph node hyperplasia. Am J Surg Pathol **6:**475-481, 1982.

Arteries

ARTERIOSCLEROSIS

Arteriosclerosis is a generalized progressive arterial disease associated with localized arterial occlusions and aneurysms. It is the principal cause of heart attack, stroke, and gangrene of the extremities and is responsible for about 50% of all deaths in the United State, Europe, and Japan. The lesions result from an excessive inflammatory and proliferative response to various forms of injury to the endothelium and smooth muscle of the arterial wall. Numerous growth factors, cytokines, and vasoregulatory molecules participate in the process.[7-9] The pathology of arteriosclerosis has gained greater surgical significance with the development of direct operative therapy for lesions of major arteries.

The pathology of arteriosclerosis primarily consists of the following:

1 Formation of intimal *plaques,* composed of lipid deposits and proliferated spindle cells. The latter seem to be of heterogenous nature, fibroblasts and smooth muscle cells predominating.[6,10]

2 Reduplication and fragmentation of the internal elastic lamina.

3 Degeneration of the media indicated by fragmentation of elastic tissue network; by hyaline, mucinoid, and collagenous degeneration of the smooth muscle; and by medial calcification.

4 Adventitial fibrosis and chronic inflammatory cellular infiltration

Arteriosclerosis may present as an occlusive process when the disease attacks the intima more rapidly than the media and adventitia, but may present as an aneurysm when the reverse is true. Occlusive disease and aneurysm may co-exist in the same arterial system.[5]

The pathogenesis of arteriosclerosis is probably multifactorial.[8] Factors thought important in its pathogenesis include changes in lipid metabolism, increased endothelial permeability to serum lipoprotein complexes, susceptibility of the intima to mechanical injury from flow turbulence at major bifurcations, and in the presence of hypertension, elastic tissue fragmentation and thrombosis or disruption of vasa vasorum.

The areas of the arterial tree involved by arteriosclerosis that are successfully treated surgically have rapidly increased so that only occlusions of the smaller peripheral arteries of the extremities remain outside the realm of operative attack.

Surgical therapy for occlusive disease of the coronary, carotid, and mesenteric arteries is now frequently undertaken. The principal manifestations of arteriosclerosis that at present are treated surgically with some success are fusiform and saccular aneurysms of the aorta or other major arteries; dissecting aneurysm; and occlusive disease of the abdominal aorta, the iliofemoral arterial system, and less often, the popliteal, subclavian, brachial, renal, and carotid arterial systems.[1-3,11]

Aneurysms
Aortic aneurysms

Aneurysms secondary to arteriosclerosis occur most frequently in the abdominal aorta, but the mechanism of development and the pathologic changes are similar in other arteries.[13]

Arterial dilatation is likely initiated by a loss of elasticity or weakening of the recoil strength in the arterial wall, which results in elongation and tortuosity, as well as dilatation. Initially, this dilatation is most often fusiform. At the same intraluminal pressure, the larger the diameter of the artery the greater the tension in the arterial wall. The tendency for dilatation thus increases rapidly after it has begun.[21] The progressive dilatation often results in a break in the arterial wall and the development of sacculation of the aneurysm.[32] The sacculations nearly always are partially filled with laminated clot, which may be the source of emboli into the arteries peripheral to the aneurysm (Fig. 27-19).

Microscopically, there are medial fibrosis and calcification, atherosclerosis, periaortic fibrosis, and thickening of the vasa vasorum. Those located in the ascending aorta have a high incidence of fragmentation of elastic fibers and cystic medial change.[30] A mild to moderate lymphoplasmacytic infiltrate may be seen in the adventitia; this is still consistent with an arteriosclerotic pathogenesis and is not necessarily indicative of a primary vasculitis (see p. 2209).[22,26,37] The pattern of expression of the adhesion molecules suggests that they may play a role in the initiation and progression of the chronic inflammatory changes associated with advanced atherosclerosis.[35]

Superimposed bacterial infection may complicate an aortic aneurysm of arteriosclerotic origin.[23] *Salmonella* is the predominant organism, followed by *Staphylococcus.*[14,34]

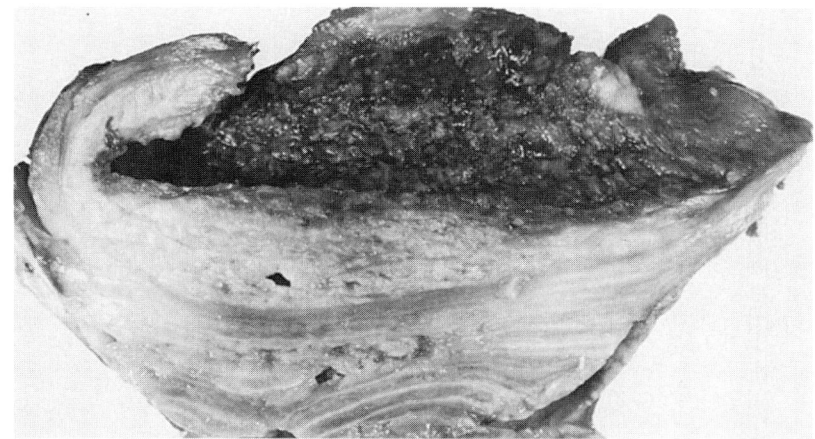

Fig. 27-19 Resected abdominal aortic aneurysm that has been transected to show lamination of clot.

Cases of aortic aneurysm have also been reported secondary to lupus erythematosus.[39]

The patient with an abdominal aneurysm may be asymptomatic and without clinical findings except for prominent abdominal aortic pulsations. The majority, however, seek treatment because of dull midabdominal or back pain associated with a pulsating, tender epigastric or retroumbilical mass that has enlarged rapidly or has been noted only recently. Painful and rapidly enlarging aneurysms will soon rupture if operative therapy is not undertaken. Retroperitoneal hemorrhages from small aneurysms may produce severe back pain with few abdominal symptoms or signs. Fistulas may develop from these aneurysms; there may be leakage into the vena cava or the duodenum or other portions of small bowel.[36] Significantly, aortoenteric fistulas also may occur as a late complication of reconstructive aortic surgery.[29] Aneurysms of the hepatic artery may rupture into the common bile duct; those of the splenic artery into the stomach, colon, or pancreatic duct; and those of the internal iliac artery into the rectosigmoid.[12,16,25]

Patients with aneurysms of the thoracic aorta survive but a short time without surgical correction.[15] Kampmeir[27] showed the average life expectancy after onset of symptoms to be 6 to 8 months. The prognosis in abdominal aneurysm appears better than that in aneurysm of the thoracic aorta.[24,28,33]

Schatz et al.[38] reviewed 141 untreated cases of abdominal aortic aneurysms at the Mayo Clinic. The prognosis was poor when the aneurysms were accompanied by symptomatic heart disease, when they were symptomatic, and when they exceeded 7.5 cm in diameter. Only 20% of the patients with aneurysm associated with symptomatic heart disease survived 5 years. Of those in whom the cause of death was known, 44% died of ruptured aneurysm.

Klippel and Butcher[31] reported thirty patients with abdominal aortic aneurysms not treated operatively. Only two died of rupture. Szilagyi et al.[40] compared 223 untreated abdominal aortic aneurysms with a group of 480 treated surgically. They were able to show that modern operative mortality was significantly less than the likelihood of rupture without operation.

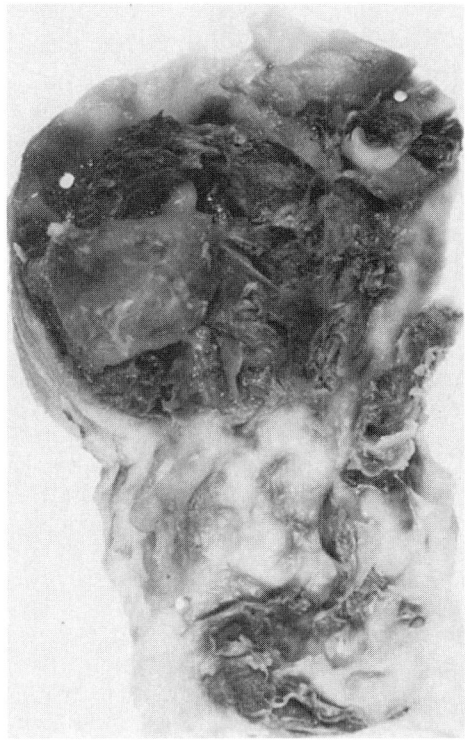

Fig. 27-20 Popliteal artery aneurysm, partially thrombosed.

It may be concluded that once an aneurysm of the aortic system is of significant size, its excision and aortic reconstitution are mandatory.[17-20]

Popliteal artery aneurysms

Arteriosclerotic aneurysms of arteries in the extremities are rare except for the popliteal and femoral arteries[43] (Fig. 27-20). The pathologic changes and the progressive enlargement of these aneurysms are similar to those in larger arteries, although the rate of progressive dilatation usually is less.

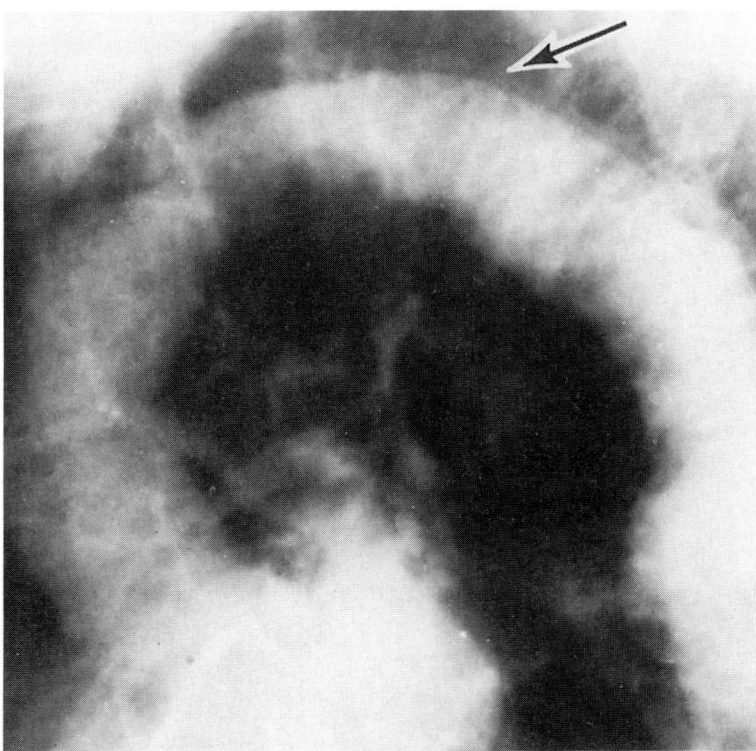

Fig. 27-21 Dissecting aneurysm in 68-year-old man who died of rupture into pericardium on way to operating room. Double aortic shadow characteristic of dissecting aneurysm is indicated *(arrow).*

Their treatment is essential to avoid acute thrombosis, embolic phenomena, or rupture as causes of severe peripheral flow deficiency and gangrene.[44] Most patients with popliteal aneurysms are first seen because of these complications. Occasionally, such patients seek medical aid because of anterior tibial muscular necrosis. The popliteal arterial elongation associated with aneurysm formation may kink and occlude the anterior tibial artery as it passes through the interosseous membrane.[42]

Patients with popliteal aneurysms frequently have multiple aneurysms. In 69 patients having 100 popliteal aneurysms, hypertension and occlusive arterial disease were frequent.[41] Only 3 of these patients were women.

Ninety-two of the aneurysms were considered purely arteriosclerotic. Syphilis, mycotic infections, and trauma entered into the diagnosis of the remaining ones. In the absence of extensive gangrene, popliteal aneurysms with or without the presence of complications are best treated by excision of the aneurysm and insertion of autologous vein grafts.

Dissecting aneurysms

Dissecting aneurysms of the aorta, if untreated, are associated with a rapidly fatal course in 75% to 90% of the patients. Their etiology is related to an underlying degeneration of the elements of the media. Factors associated with dissection are hypertension, Marfan's syndrome, pregnancy, bicuspid aortic valve, and traumatic, atherosclerotic, or inflammatory injuries of the aortic media.[45,52] This includes recently introduced procedures such as insertion of an intra-aortic balloon pump and aortic cannulation during cardiopulmonary bypass operation.

The process of dissection most commonly begins in a transverse intimal tear associated with an intimal plaque located either in the ascending aorta or in the upper descending thoracic aorta near the origin of the left subclavian artery.[48] Once this tear develops, the intramural layers of the aorta are rapidly separated by the force of the blood entering the wall. The dissection usually involves the entire circumference of the aorta as it progresses distally. Perforation often occurs through the adventitia, resulting in early death from hemorrhage into the pericardium or pleural cavity. Lower extremity symptoms and signs of acute occlusion of the abdominal aorta may be prominent because of distal aortic or iliac luminal occlusion by the leading point of the dissection. Diagnostic imaging is essential in the evaluation of suspected aortic dissection.[46]

Three major types of dissection are recognized depending on the location and extent.[48,49] Type I begins in the ascending aorta and extends beyond; type II is confined to the ascending aorta; type IIIA begins in the descending aorta and stops above the diaphragm; type IIIB also begins in the descending aorta but extends below it. Dissecting aneurysms can also be classified according to their duration as acute, subacute, and chronic. The subacute type characteristically begins abruptly and then progresses gradually for several days before rupture and death (Fig. 27-21). The chronic form occurs in a few patients who develop a re-entry site from the dissected passage back into the lumen of the aorta. The occasional long-term survivor of dissecting aneurysm is encountered among these patients.

The objective of surgical treatment is to excise the intimal tear, obliterate entry into the false channel proximally and distally, and reconstitute the aorta, usually with the interposition of a synthetic sleeve graft; aortic valve repair or replacement may be also necessary in proximal dissections.[47,48] Medical therapy consists in lowering the arterial blood pressure and diminishing the velocity of ventricular contraction.[50,51]

There is a need for proper selection in deciding surgical versus medical therapy. There is now general agreement that acute proximal dissections should be treated surgically whenever possible, whereas the treatment of distal dissections is more controversial.

Wheat et al.[51] reported the successful treatment of patients with acute dissecting aortic aneurysm by the use of antihypertensive agents. In a series of thirty-three patients so treated, McFarland et al.[50] reported that the survival rate was 52%, the mean follow-up period being more than 3 years. These authors emphasized the need for proper selection in deciding a surgical versus a medical therapy.

Exceptionally, dissecting aneurysms can occur in arteries other than the aorta, such as the renal, coronary, pulmonary, and carotid vessels.[53]

Diffuse arterial tortuosity and dilatation

Occasionally, a more or less generalized arterial dilatation and extreme tortuosity are seen in patients suffering from generalized arteriosclerosis (Figs. 27-22 and 27-23). Leriche[54] reported such instances as *dolicho et mega arteria*. The mechanism of the tortuosity and generalized dilatation is thought to relate to weakening of the arterial wall, but the cause for its generalized nature is not clearly understood.

One needs to know that such arterial dilatation and tortuosity may be mistaken for intra-abdominal aneurysm, since surgical attack on such generalized tortuosity is probably not warranted in the absence of complications.

Arterial substitution

Arteriosclerotic aneurysms of the abdominal aorta and the iliac arteries are best treated by excision and replacement of the involved arterial segment by synthetic prostheses.[56] Aneurysms of the popliteal arteries are probably best replaced by venous autografts. Arterial homografts are no longer used to replace diseased arterial segments because of the superiority of synthetic arterial prostheses.[55]

After implantation, homografts are partially replaced or encased by host collagenous tissue (Fig. 27-24). In a few months, they lose much of their elasticity, although fragmented elastic tissue is still demonstrable histologically over a year after implantation. The evolution of the intimal surface of both homografts and synthetic cloth prostheses after implantation consists of the organization of the fibrin layer initially deposited and the development of a lining of flattened cells, which by special staining techniques, appears nearly like normal vascular endothelium.[57] True endothelial ingrowth from the host artery occurs across the suture line for a variable distance.

Szilagyi et al.[58] reported late aneurysm formation in two of fifty-five aortic homografts and tortuous dilatation in twelve of sixty-six femoral homografts within 3 years after insertion. Calcification may appear in the wall of homografts after long implantation. Implantation of synthetic cloth prostheses is followed by their encasement with collagen and a decline in tensile strength of some of them.

Arterial occlusive disease

Thrombotic occlusions of the major arteries are often associated with arteriosclerotic changes such as calcification, atheromatosis, and ulceration of the intima.[69] The occlusive process is often insidious, although final thrombotic obliteration of the lumen is occasionally quite rapid and may be clinically indistinguishable from embolization. Indeed, the differentiation of the two pathologically and at surgery is quite difficult in older individuals in whom arteriosclerosis of the abdominal aorta is nearly universal. The process of occlusion probably begins in the iliac arteries near the aortic bifurcation from which thrombus formation propagates cephalad in the aorta, occasionally to the level of the renal arteries. Thrombi and emboli can become secondarily infected by fungi, particularly *Aspergillus* and *Mucor* (Fig. 27-25).

The syndrome of distal aortic thrombosis (Leriche's syndrome) manifests itself with an insidious onset and gradual progression of symptoms of pain and easy fatigability in the legs, hips, and back; intermittent claudication; and sexual impotence (Fig. 27-26).[73] In this condition, arterial insufficiency in the lower extremities usually is manifested clinically by the absence of pulses below the umbilicus. If the process is partial, weak pulsations may be felt or a characteristic systolic murmur heard over the abdominal aorta and the femoral arteries.

Despite the presence of intermittent claudication and the absence of pulses, many patients are found by arteriography to have near-normal distal arteries.[64] This patency of the peripheral arteries is probably responsible for the relative absence of muscular atrophy or of atrophy of skin appendages in the legs and feet of many of the patients despite their symptoms of peripheral blood flow insufficiency and lack of pulses.

Arteriosclerotic occlusive disease also frequently involves other major arterial bifurcations in the lower extremity such as those of the common iliac and common femoral arteries. In the latter instance, the intimal disease and thrombosis occur frequently in the external femoral artery just distal to the bifurcation. Other arterial segments in the lower extremity prone to early thrombotic occlusion are those associated with some degree of fascial fixation. Such areas exist (1) in the external iliac artery behind the inguinal ligament, (2) in the superficial femoral artery as it passes through the fascial ring beneath the adductor longus tendon, and (3) in the anterior tibial artery where it passes through the interosseous membrane.[65]

Although arteriosclerosis is a generalized arterial disease, the tendency for occlusive complications to develop early in its evolution at the sites just noted makes possible the suc-

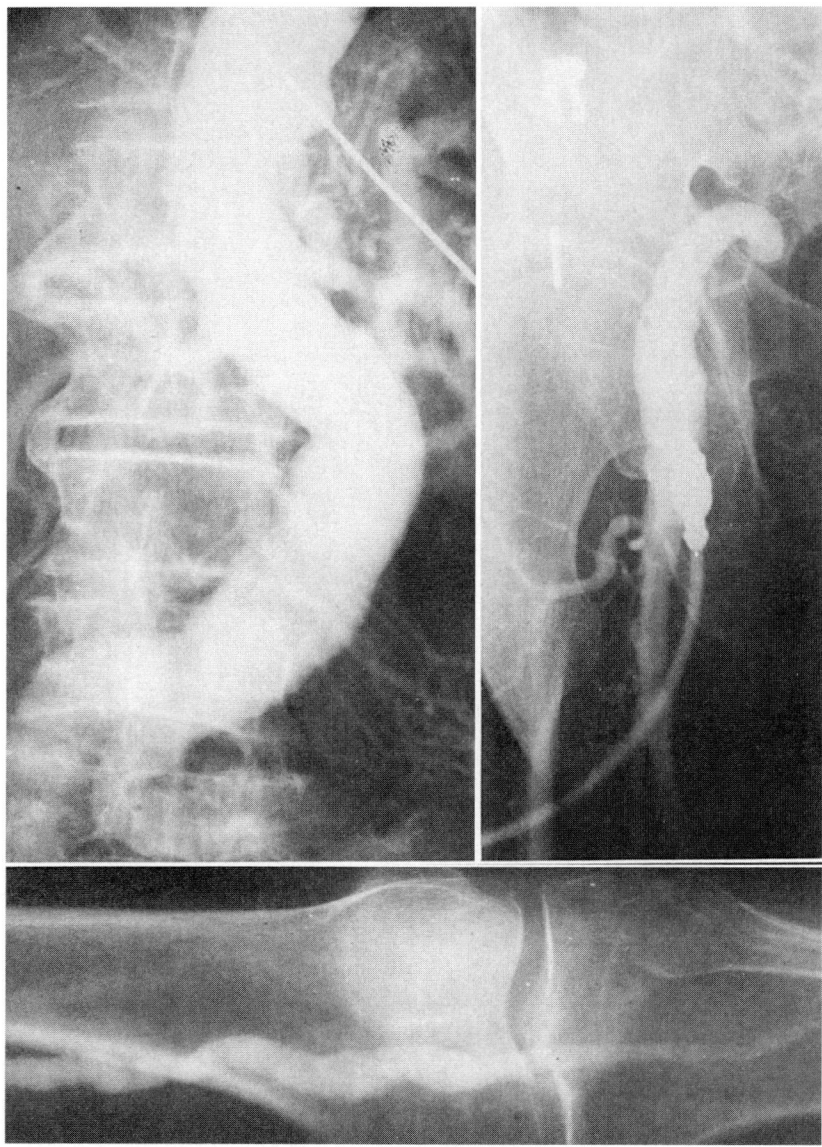

Fig. 27-22 Arteriograms of abdominal aorta and femoral and popliteal arteries illustrating generalized arterial dilatation and tortuosity in patient who had pulsating intra-abdominal mass initially diagnosed as aneurysm.

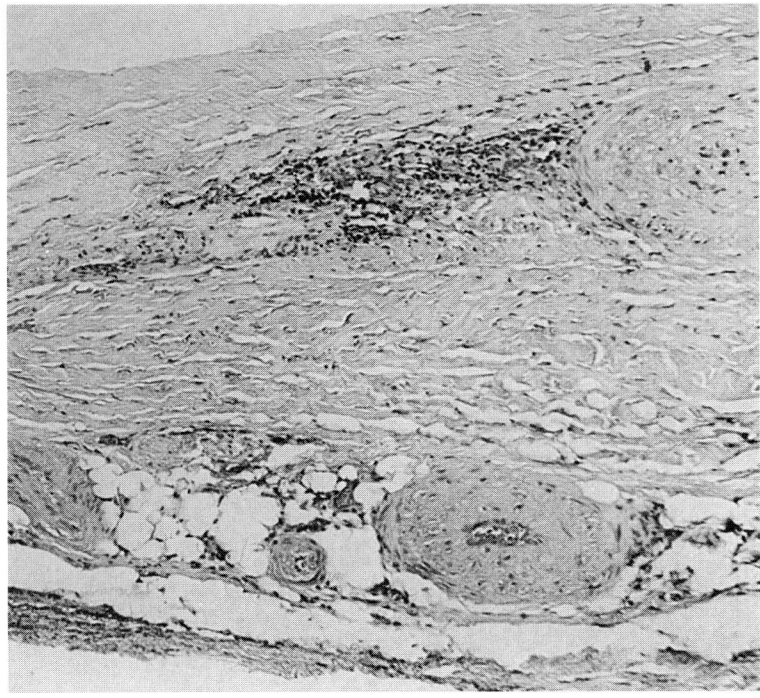

Fig. 27-23 Appearance of arterial wall after amputation for gangrene secondary to embolization from mural thrombi in dilated and tortuous femoral artery.

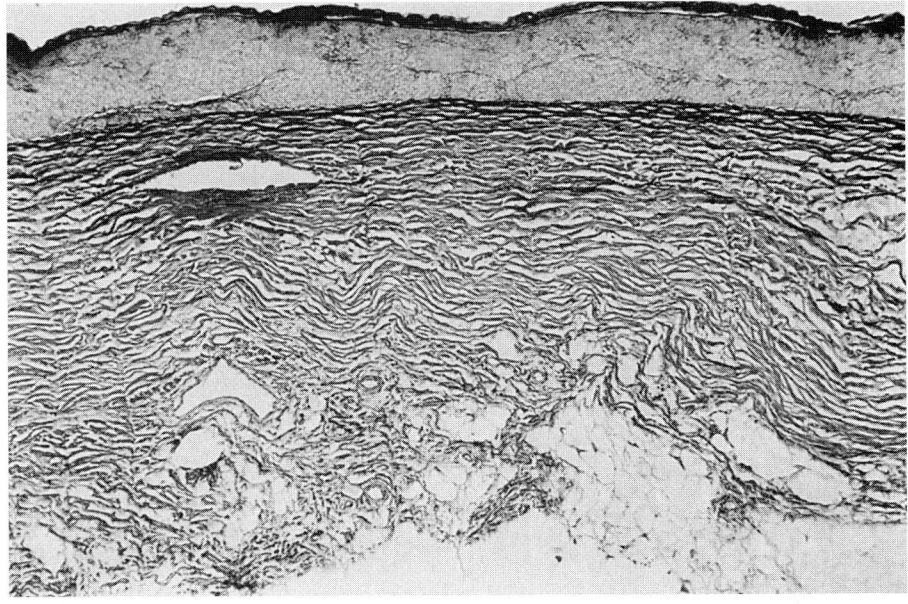

Fig. 27-24 Collagenous encasement of iliac homograft 18 months after implantation.

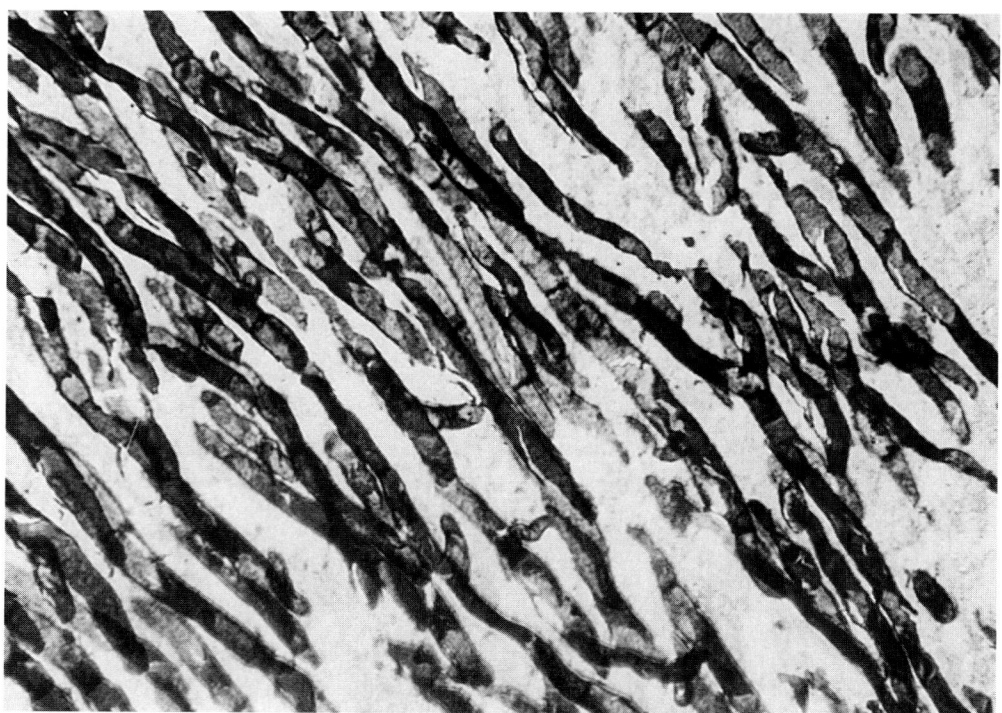

Fig. 27-25 Infection of femoral artery embolus by *Aspergillus*. Hyphae are thick and septate. Patient, 59-year-old woman, had cold, pulseless lower extremity 10 weeks following initial valve replacement. (Gomori's methenamine silver.)

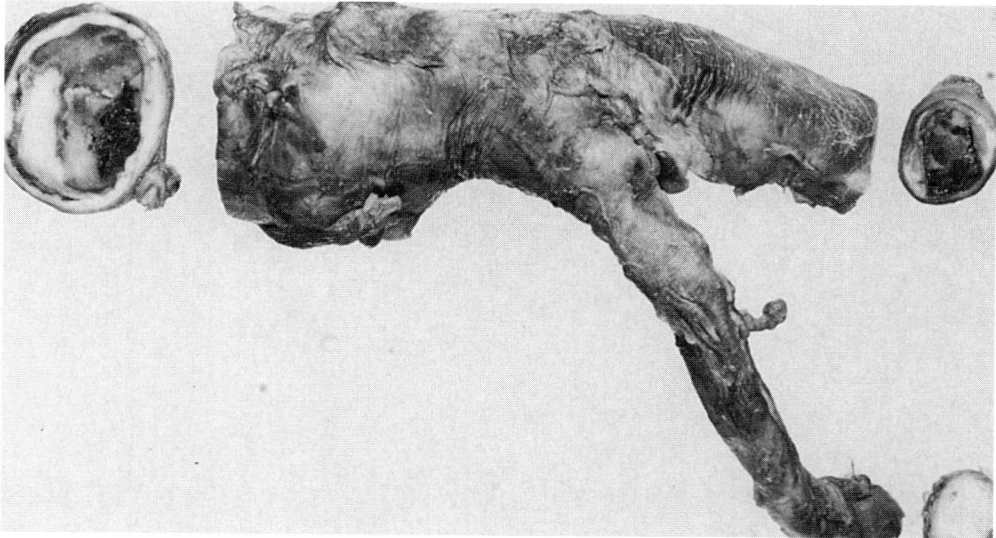

Fig. 27-26 Thrombotic occlusion of distal abdominal aorta and common iliac arteries (Leriche's syndrome).

cessful treatment of patients with marked peripheral blood flow deficiency. Surgical correction of the obstructive disease, however, often only temporarily improves the peripheral blood flow because of the progressive nature of generalized arteriosclerosis.[77] Successful operative therapy of arterial occlusive disease relieves symptoms of ischemia but actually prevents amputation of but a few extremities. However, aggressive operative therapy in properly selected patients with limited gangrene of the extremities may permit healing after amputation of only the gangrenous part.[74]

The surgical treatment of major arterial occlusive disease is performed by using two general methods: arterial substitutes and thromboendarterectomy (intimectomy).

Thromboendarterectomy is superior to arterial replacement early after treatment of arterial occlusive disease of the aorta and iliac arteries.[62] Autogenous venous bypass for femoral arterial occlusive disease appears to be associated with patency rates superior to those following endarterectomy and synthetic bypass grafts.[63,72]

Successful results in 85% to 95% of patients with occlusions of the aortic and iliac arteries have been reported with both methods of treatment. Postoperative aneurysm formation and vascular thrombosis have also been reported following the use of both methods. The correction of femoral occlusive disease by endarterectomy or by the bypass arterial substitution technique has proved less beneficial than for larger arteries. Approximately 70% of the patients with femoral grafts develop late thrombosis.

The incidence of late failure of both endarterectomy and arterial grafting procedures will likely always be higher in the smaller femoral artery than in the aorta and iliac arteries.

Thromboendarterectomy of major arteries is a technique in which the diseased intima and thrombotic material filling the lumen are dissected from the inner portion of the media in a smooth and uniform manner so that the remaining adventitia and media of the artery can continue to conduct blood (Figs. 27-27 and 27-28). The remaining arterial tube is lined rapidly by a fibrinoid layer that develops a pseudoendothelial surface similar to that lining an implanted arterial substitute. Likewise, early thrombosis does not occur in these segments if the transit time of the blood through them is rapid. Endarterectomized arterial segments, examined months after the operative procedure, show a fibrous type of intima with an endothelium-like covering and preservation of the remaining media and elastic tissue.[60]

Extensive medial calcification of the Mönckeberg type may occasionally be a contraindication to endarterectomy.

Studies of the elastic properties of normal human arteries and of arteriosclerotic arteries obtained at autopsy from patients of the same age have shown insignificant variations of elasticity coefficients between the two. The progressive encasement of synthetic prostheses with collagen and the similar encasement and invasion of fibrous tissue into the wall of homografts are associated with a reduction in the elastic properties of the implants. Their distensibility becomes much less after implantation.[61] Studies of both cloth prostheses and homografts at varying times after implantation indicate that the result is a collagen-like tube through which the blood flows. The response of the wall of the graft to distention is no longer that of the adjacent host vessels.

Arterial embolism of atheromatous origin is an important complication of arterial occlusive disease. It may occur spontaneously or following aortic surgery or angiographic procedures.[66,67,76] The complications vary according to the vessels affected and include livedo reticularis and gangrene of the lower extremities, ocular symptoms, cerebral infarct, gastrointestinal bleeding, renal hypertension, and renal failure.[59,68,70,71] The frequency of atheromatous embolism correlates with the severity of ulcerative atheromatous changes in the aorta. Simultaneous embolism to various organs may lead to a mistaken clinical diagnosis of polyarteritis nodosa.[75] Random biopsies of skeletal muscle may be diagnostic in these cases.[59]

CYSTIC ADVENTITIAL DEGENERATION

Cystic adventitial degeneration, a rare condition almost always affecting the popliteal artery, may cause luminal obstruction.[79,80] A collection of jelly-like material distends the wall and bulges into the lumen[82] (Fig. 27-29). Most cases occur in young men without a history of trauma and without general arterial change. The microscopic appearance of the involved arterial segments is that of mucinous degeneration. The pathogenesis is probably related to that of soft tissue ganglion.[81] Other arteries may exceptionally be affected by this condition.[78]

FIBROMUSCULAR DYSPLASIA

Fibromuscular dysplasia is a nonarteriosclerotic, noninflammatory vascular disease of unknown pathogenesis.[88] Humoral, mechanical, and genetic factors may play a role. It usually becomes manifest during the third or fourth decades of life, although it also can be seen in children.[90] It involves large and medium-sized muscular arteries, such as the renal, carotid, axillary, and mesenteric arteries, sometimes in a multicentric fashion.[86] Imaging techniques useful for the evaluation of this disease include CT scans, MRI, and angiography.[85] Morphologically, it is characterized by a disorderly arrangement and proliferation of the cellular and extracellular elements of the wall, particularly the media, with the resulting distortion of the vessel lumen.[83] The absence of necrosis, calcification, inflammation, and fibrinoid necrosis are important negative diagnostic features. Morphologic varieties with predominant intimal or adventitial involvement have been described.[84,87] Surgical techniques for this condition include graduated or balloon intraluminal dilatation (either isolated or associated with resection-anastomosis), saphenous graft, and reconstructive aneurysmorrhaphy.[89]

MESENTERIC VASCULAR OCCLUSION

Mesenteric vascular occlusion may originate in veins or arteries. Rarely, occlusion of both occurs simultaneously. Arterial occlusion is the more frequent of the two[93,103] (62% of cases). After the initiation of arterial or venous thrombosis, hemorrhagic infarction of the intestine and its mesentery develops if the process is rapid in onset and extensive.

Venous mesenteric thrombosis often is associated with infection and cancer.[95,96] However, infection and cancer per se are not directly related to the mesenteric venous thrombosis.

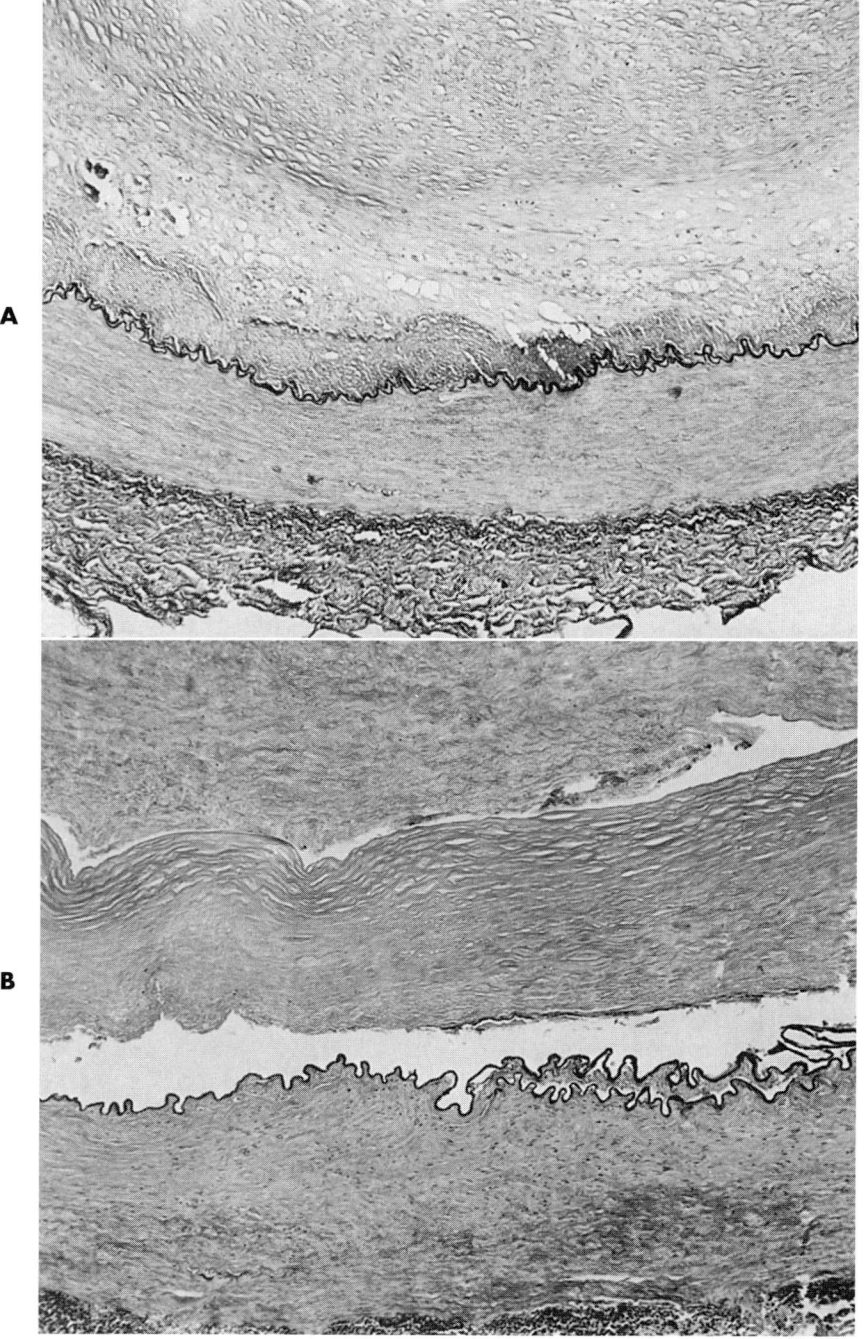

Fig. 27-27 Result of endarterectomy performed on occluded femoral artery removed at autopsy. **A,** Vessel was transected and section made from one of cut ends. **B,** Tissue section made from other cut end after simple wire loop endarterectomy. Freed intimal core was left in situ to demonstrate plane of cleavage developed.

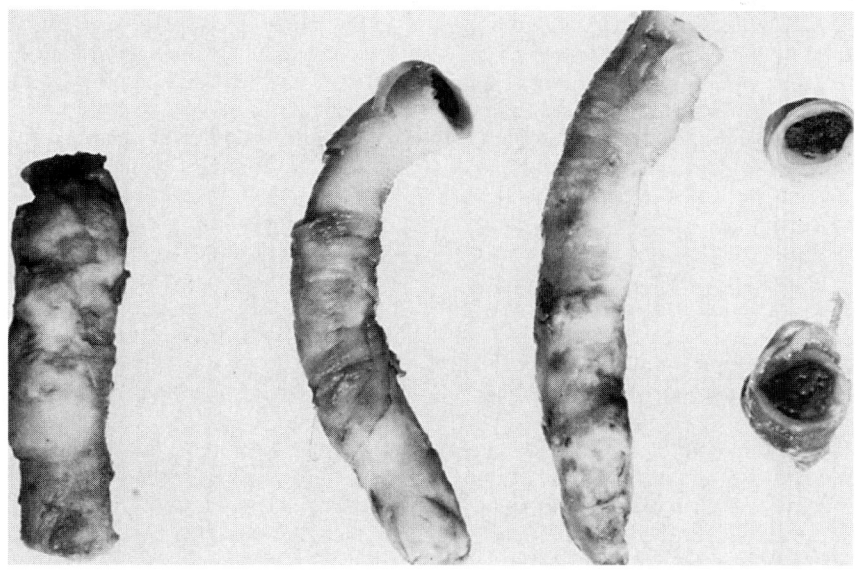

Fig. 27-28 Operative specimen from femoral endarterectomy removed in cleavage plane similar to that shown in Fig. 27-27.

A

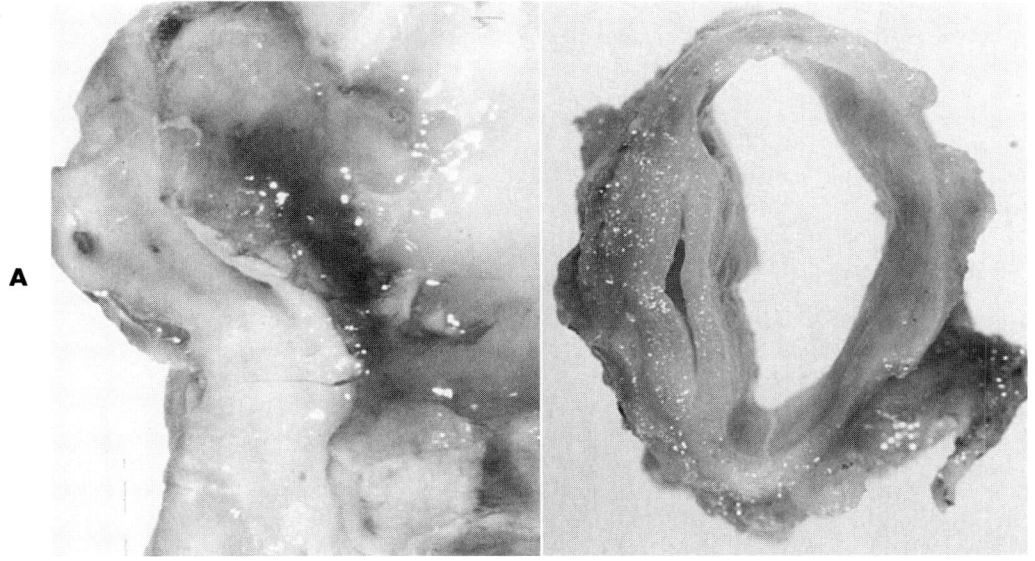

B

Fig. 27-29 Cystic adventitial degeneration of popliteal artery. **A,** Mucoid mass is present in adventitia of artery, resulting in marked distortion of vessel. **B,** Cross section of another case showing large cystic mass in adventitial region of popliteal artery. Collapsed arterial lumen is seen on left. (**B** Courtesy Dr. J. Costa, Lausanne, Switzerland.)

The relative reduction in the frequency of mesenteric venous occlusion is probably due to antibiotic control of many intra-abdominal infections.

Occlusion of the mesenteric arterial system may be caused by emboli from thrombi in an arteriosclerotic aorta, from a fibrillating atrium, or from a mural thrombus secondary to myocardial infarction.[100] Mesenteric arterial occlusion also may follow arteriosclerotic change in the superior mesenteric artery with local thrombosis and such rare conditions as polyarteritis, septic arteritis, and thromboangiitis obliterans.[97] Mesenteric arteries can be involved in rheumatoid disease and cause infarction.[92] Arterial and venous thrombosis, followed by ulceration and necrosis of the bowel, has been described following surgical repair of aortic coarctation.[94] The pathogenesis of this condition, which has been erroneously designated as "mesenteric arteritis," is probably related to the occurrence of hypertension during the first 2 postoperative days.

The technique of color-flow Duplex imaging can detect the presence of significant arterial stenosis in over 80% of the cases.[101]

Infarction of the small intestine or colon, perforation, and peritonitis do not always follow mesenteric vascular occlusion, either arterial or venous. As a matter of fact, many patients with significant disease of the celiac and superior mesenteric arteries as detected by Doppler sonography are asymptomatic.[99] Johnson and Baggenstoss[95] reported the presence of infarction in only fifty-two of ninety-nine patients found to have mesenteric vascular occlusions postmortem. Conversely, mesenteric infarct can be seen in the absence of arterial or venous occlusion.[98,102]

Infarction of the bowel depends on the location, extent of occlusion, rapidity of its onset, and state of the collateral circulation, as well as the general physical condition of the patient. Patients with cirrhosis of the liver and portal hypertension often have episodes of cramping abdominal pain associated with low-grade fever and moderate leukocytosis that gradually recede. Several such episodes may take place before a sufficient amount of the portal venous system is occluded to cause the clinical picture of intra-abdominal catastrophe.

The clinical diagnosis of mesenteric vascular thrombosis is difficult at times because the patient does not have the classic severe abdominal pain, distention, nausea, vomiting, leukocytosis, and shock. Such a picture depends on a massive sudden occlusion of the superior mesenteric artery or vein.

Acute occlusion of mesenteric arteries produces bowel necrosis without the early marked hypovolemic disturbances seen with extensive venous thrombosis. Bloody diarrhea is less common in arterial than in venous occlusions, but abdominal pain is generally more prominent in arterial occlusions. If the occlusion is sufficiently extensive to cause gangrene of the bowel, death from peritonitis follows if the bowel is not resected. A hypovolemic death in less than 24 hours, however, is often the outcome in the presence of massive venous occlusion.

Of the two types of occlusion, arterial embolic occlusion is more likely to be amenable to successful treatment than is venous thrombosis. The treatment of both conditions consists primarily of early abdominal exploration and resection of nonviable bowel. The determination of viability of laparotomy may be quite difficult. The extent of small bowel resection compatible with survival has been shown to be as much as three fourths of the organ.

To date, embolectomy has but rarely remedied occlusion of the superior mesenteric artery. However, because of the serious prognosis associated with extensive small intestinal and colonic resection, this procedure should probably be attempted more often.

Chronic intestinal ischemia produces the syndrome of abdominal angina. Segmental intestinal infarction may be incident to disease of small mesenteric arteries without involvement of the proximal superior mesenteric artery. So-called nonocclusive intestinal infarction is probably related to disease in these vessels in most instances[91] (Fig. 27-30).

Renal artery disease and its relationship to hypertension are discussed in Chapter 17.

TRAUMATIC AND IATROGENIC INJURIES
Rupture

Rupture of a major vessel in the absence of an aneurysm may follow open or blunt trauma; may exceptionally occur in a spontaneous fashion through an atheromatous plaque or an area destroyed by degeneration (as in Ehlers-Danlos syndrome) or inflammation[106-108]; or may be seen as a major complication of balloon dilatation, surgery, or radiation therapy.[104] Fajardo and Lee[105] reviewed eleven vascular ruptures in patients who had had previous treatment for carcinoma. The vessels involved were the aorta and the carotid and femoral arteries. Most patients were men who had been subjected to surgery and radiation therapy for epidermoid carcinomas of the oropharynx, esophagus, or genitalia. In most cases, the rupture was due to surgical rather than radiotherapeutic complications, such as necrosis of skin flaps, infections, and fistulas.

Thrombosis

Nonpenetrating trauma may result in occlusive thrombosis of a major artery such as the carotid artery following blunt trauma to the paratonsillar area.[110,112] In children, trauma and arteritis constitute the two most common causes of acquired occlusions of major arteries.[109,114] Organizing and recanalizing thrombi can exhibit a papillary pattern of anastomosing channels reminiscent of angiosarcoma[111] or else acquire a myxomatous appearance with primitive mesenchymal cells, similar to that of cardiac myxoma.[113]

Pulsating hematoma

Pulsating hematoma or false aneurysm usually results from a small perforation in the artery usually produced by a sharp instrument or a small missile.[117] Traumatic aneurysms may also follow injury to an artery by blunt trauma[115] (Fig. 27-31). The defect is only a few millimeters in diameter but is sufficiently large to allow the escape of blood into the immediately surrounding tissues.

Cohen[116] emphasized the role of the adventitial layer in the development of the aneurysmal sac because of its tendency to seal off the defect in the arterial wall. Of equal importance is the nature of the surrounding tissue and the

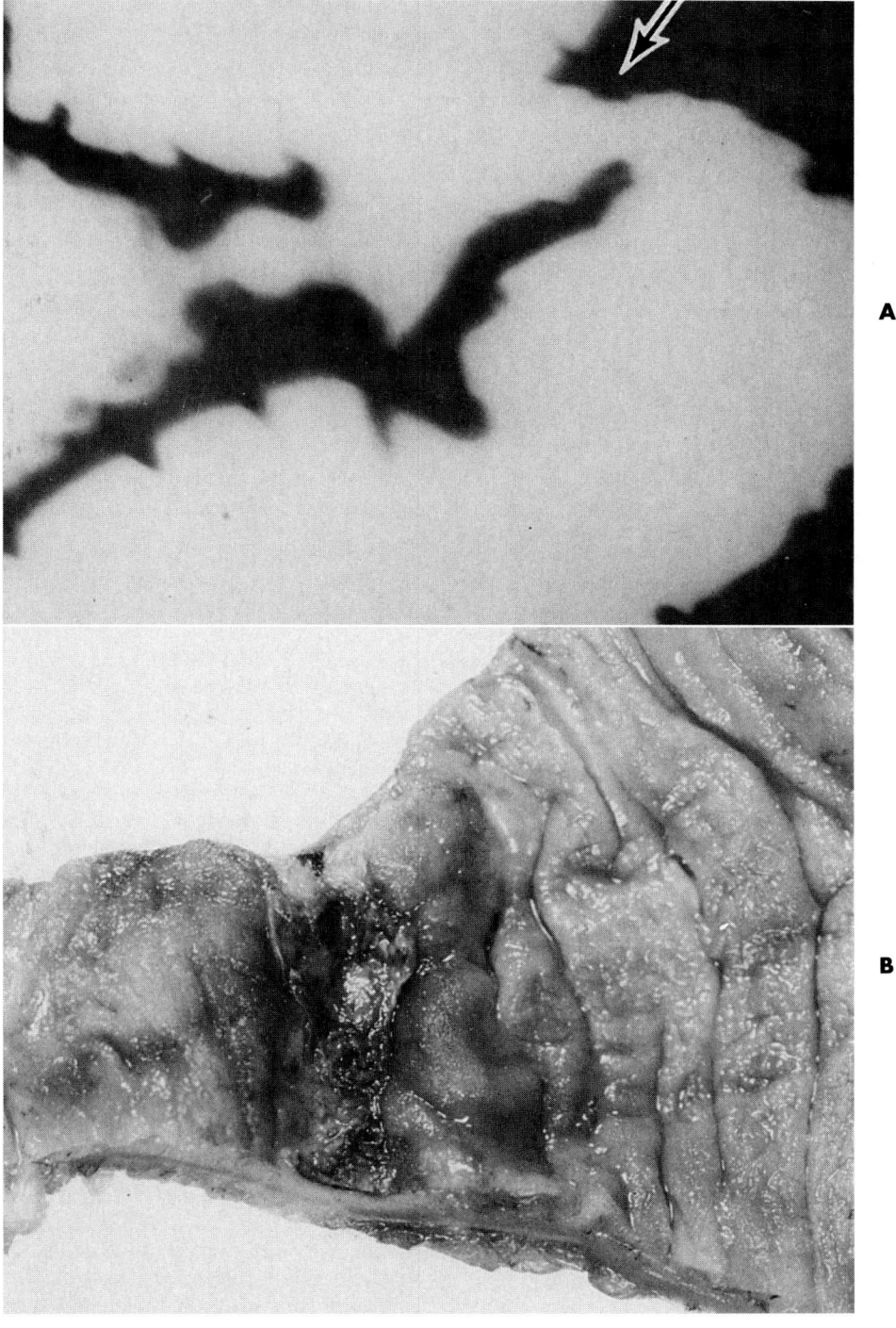

Fig. 27-30 A, Segmented area of constriction *(arrow)* in small bowel interpreted as possible malignant neoplasm. **B,** Excised segment of lesion shown in **A** revealing well-delimited ulcer. Small segment of attached mesentery showed organized thrombi. Ulcer was on basis of vascular insufficiency.

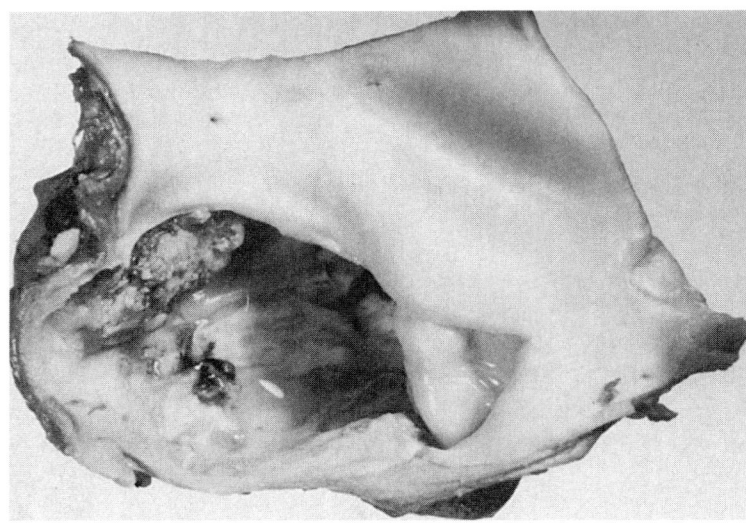

Fig. 27-31 Traumatic aneurysm of thoracic aorta in 23-year-old man caused by automobile accident 5 years before operation. Note sharp line of demarcation between normal aorta and aneurysm. Aneurysm was excised, and defect was replaced with synthetic graft.

strength of its fascial structures. When strong fascial surroundings are absent, the rate of aneurysmal enlargement is quite rapid. It is slower when the area of injury is within a circumscribed fascial channel such as Hunter's canal. The blood collects about the defect in the artery until the pressure within the hematoma approaches the mean blood pressure. Enlargement of the hematoma then slows because blood returns to the arterial lumen during diastole. It is this situation that produces the characteristic to-and-fro murmur heard over the pulsating hematoma. This murmur has a rather harsh systolic component and a softer diastolic component. The murmur is not constant as is the murmur of arteriovenous fistula. The walls of the pulsating hematoma contain varying amounts of laminated clot, which in turn is surrounded by a rather dense fibrous tissue reaction.

The operative treatment of pulsating hematoma is often not difficult. Usually the arterial wall defect can be closed by simple suture after evacuation of the hematoma and excision of the fibrotic aneurysmal sac. Occasionally, however, arterial substitution is required.

These lesions should be treated immediately on diagnosis to prevent continued enlargement, pain on compression of adjacent nerves and other structures, and ischemia of the tissues peripheral to them. Since ligation of the afflicted artery (if it is a major one) is no longer the treatment of choice, waiting for collateral vessels to develop is not indicated.

Acquired arteriovenous fistula

Acquired arteriovenous fistulas are seen most frequently during times of war and are produced in a manner quite similar to that of traumatic aneurysm. However, in this instance, the perforating injury involves both the artery and the adjacent vein. Such an injury usually results in a pulsating hematoma that communicates with both the arterial and venous lumina.[118]

Following trauma, the fistula may be established almost immediately. However, the communication between the arterial and venous systems is frequently delayed until the wound is partially organized and the thrombus in the hematoma surrounding the artery and vein is partially absorbed. Most patients present with a pulsating mass in the region of injury that can be differentiated from simple pulsating hematoma in several ways. The murmur over the pulsating region is usually continuous because of a continuous flow of arterial blood into the vein. In other words, during diastole the pressure in the pulsating hematoma about the arteriovenous communication is never sufficient to produce reversal of blood flow. In some slowly developing, long-standing arteriovenous communications in the absence of a pulsating hematoma, a massive sacculation of the adjacent vein may slowly develop.

Patients with an arteriovenous fistula usually show venous dilatation about and peripheral to the fistula, as well as increased skin temperature in the area of the fistula. Despite increased temperature near the lesion, the extremity peripheral to it is usually cooler than normal, since the actual peripheral blood flow is less.

When arteriovenous fistulas develop between smaller arteries and veins, the sac may be excised and the vessels ligated without difficulty. Those involving the larger arteries, such as the femoral, axillary, or popliteal artery, require the maintenance of arterial continuity. Some type of arterial substitution may be necessary occasionally in larger arteriovenous aneurysms, although transvenous closure of the defect in the arterial wall usually can be accomplished satisfactorily.

The dilatation of the major artery entering an arteriovenous fistula of long standing may be marked, and the degenerative changes in the arterial wall may be extensive. These changes consist of atherosclerosis, calcification, disruption of the elastic tissue network, and fibrosis. If the degenera-

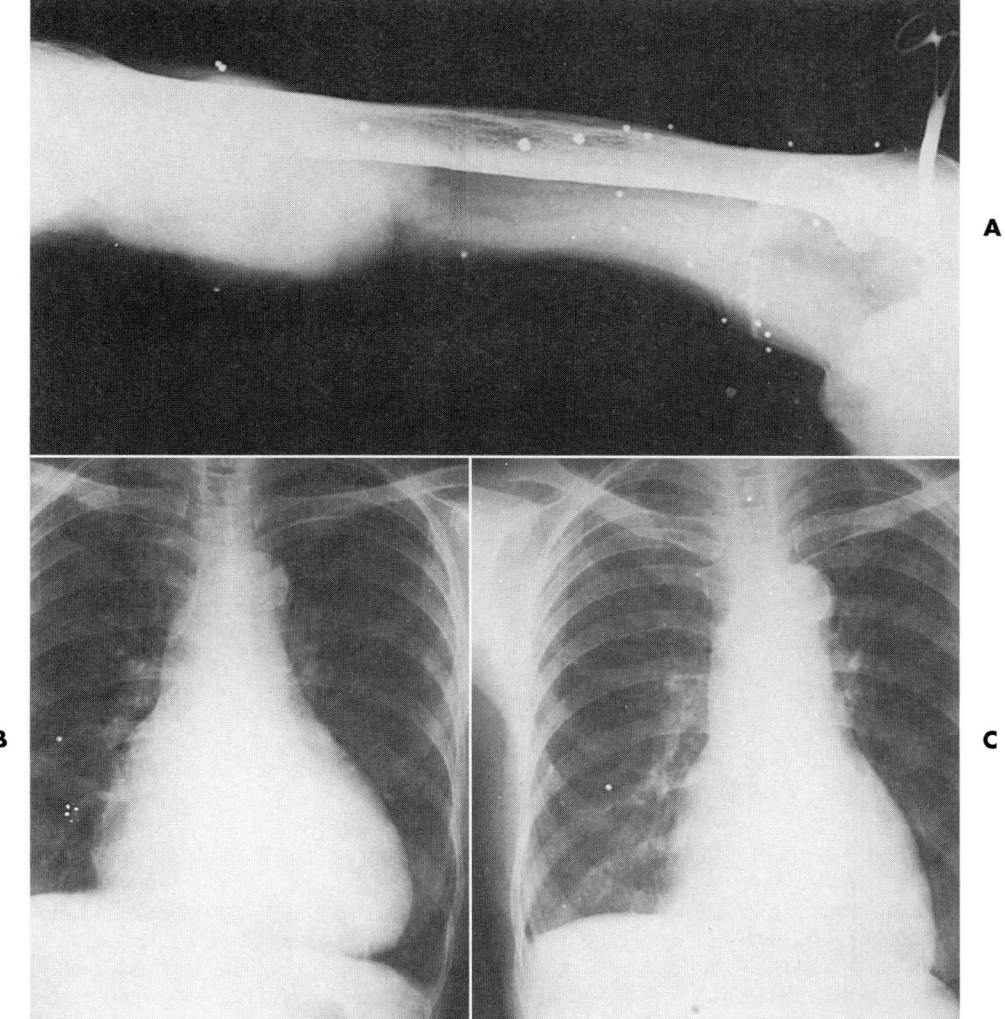

Fig. 27-32 Arteriovenous fistula in 68-year-old woman. **A,** Arteriogram showing markedly enlarged femoral artery entering region of arteriovenous fistula. Pellets from original shotgun wound 30 years previously are visible. **B,** Radiograph before correction of arteriovenous fistula. **C,** Radiograph 5 days after operation.

tion is sufficiently advanced, it is irreversible. In such arteries, aneurysms may develop despite the cure of the arteriovenous fistula. The dilatation of the artery entering the arteriovenous fistula is thought to result from the increased flow of blood through it.

Arteriovenous fistulas are associated with increase in cardiac output, pulse rate, and blood volume, which may lead to congestive heart failure (Fig. 27-32). Such systemic results rarely, if ever, develop from a single congenital arteriovenous fistula with the exception of those that appear in the pulmonary tree. Congenital arteriovenous fistulas usually present as tumefactions containing many relatively small arteries and veins surrounded by moderately large amounts of fibrous tissue. Their treatment is primarily excisional.

THROMBOANGIITIS OBLITERANS

Thromboangiitis obliterans (Buerger's disease) is a rare thrombotic and inflammatory disease of the arteries and veins of unknown etiology that has no single diagnostic, clinical, or pathologic sign.[119] Its inflammatory component may involve entire neurovascular bundles. Although it is a generalized vascular disease, the involvement of the arteries of the lower extremities is usually most advanced, and the resultant flow deficiency is the usual reason for the patient to seek therapy. A form preferentially involving mesenteric vessels has also been described.[128] The onset of the condition occurs most often in men between 20 and 35 years of age and may be heralded by superficial migratory acute thrombophlebitis that is precipitated by undue exertion or

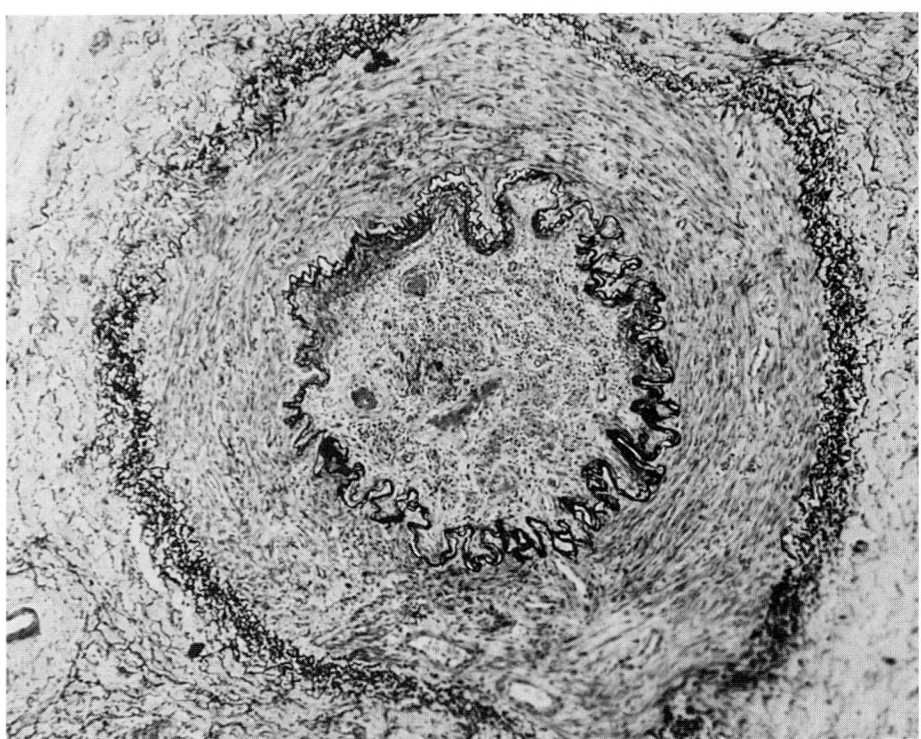

Fig. 27-33 Cellular organization of occluding thrombus with small recanalizing channels thought to be compatible with Buerger's disease. Note absence of calcification.

exposure to cold. Study of biopsies of such involved veins shows the histologic changes associated with acute intravascular thrombosis. Pathologic involvement in the arterial tree is segmental and is usually present primarily in the smaller arteries. There is a paucity of collateral flow.[121] This process has a widespread geographic distribution[125] but has been reported with increased frequency in Korea and Japan.[124]

Microscopic examination of early arterial lesions shows panarteritis often associated with thrombosis. Endothelial proliferation and periarterial fibrosis soon become prominent. The inflammatory process attacks the entire thickness of the vessel wall and perivascular tissues. Where nerves are in close proximity to the vascular tree, it involves the perineural stroma. Extension of the inflammatory process about peripheral sensory nerves may be responsible in part for the severe pain so common in afflicted extremities. Calcification in the arterial wall is absent. Arterial calcification on x-ray examination indicates arteriosclerosis rather than Buerger's disease.

The arterial and venous thrombosis associated with the angiitic process becomes partially recanalized. Cellularity of the organizing fibrous tissue replacing the thrombus is often prominent. Recanalization of thrombi is incomplete and is characterized by numerous small vascular channels passing through the remaining fibrous tissue (Fig. 27-33).

The pathologic process ascribed to Buerger's disease may be difficult to distinguish microscopically from inflammatory and fibrotic changes that may accompany arteriosclerotic thromboses.[120,123]

The vascular process tends generally to be progressive, but in some instances the acute manifestation seems to subside, partially in patients who cease using tobacco.

Treatment is largely symptomatic and includes the control of pain, the avoidance of tobacco, and cleanliness of the extremity. Late in the disease, amputations may be necessary. Sympathectomy may benefit patients with cold, temperature-sensitive feet or hands and those with peripheral gangrenous ulcers.

The death of patients with Buerger's disease may follow complications attending gangrene of the extremities. However, many patients with this affliction die of myocardial infarction, renal insufficiency, occlusions of mesenteric vessels, and strokes.

With the use of arteriography and careful pathologic examination, a high proportion of cases of alledged Buerger's disease have actually been shown to be arteriosclerosis. This pathologic process can be mimicked with considerable exactitude by the development of embolism and thrombosis.[130] This has led some investigators to postulate that Buerger's disease is not a distinct entity but rather a peculiar manifestation of arteriosclerosis.[131] Although we agree that many cases originally diagnosed as Buerger's disease are indeed examples of arteriosclerosis, we believe that the entity thromboangiitis obliterans exists.[122,126,127,129,132]

ARTERITIS

Inflammatory diseases of the arteries have been classified on the basis of the etiologic agent involved, the caliber and

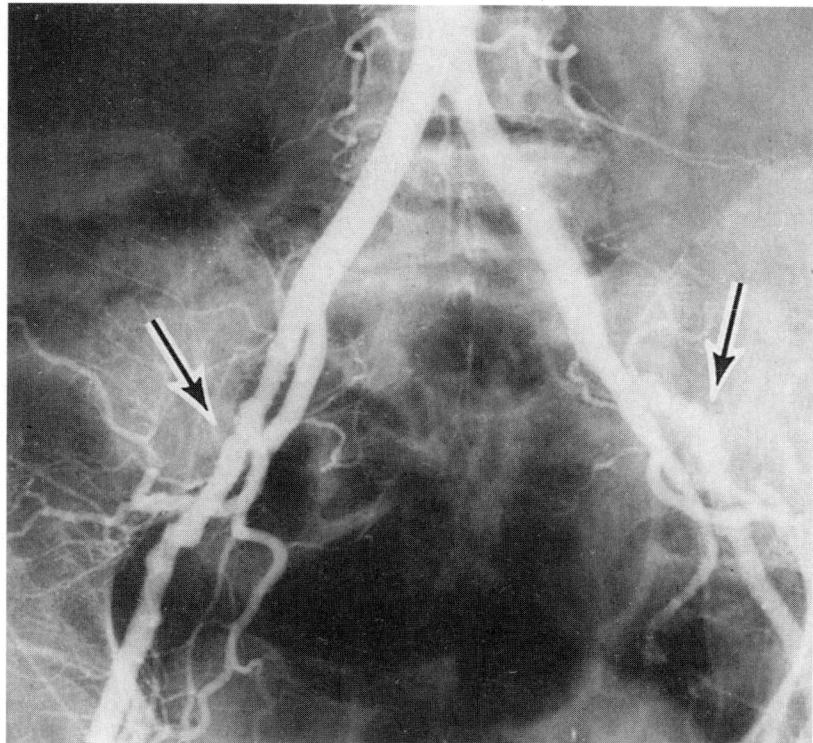

Fig. 27-34 Vasculitis in 52-year-old woman showing scalloped irregularities limited to external iliac arteries.

location of the vessel affected, and the type of microscopic change observed. The former is obviously the most desirable but, at present, impractical, since a specific etiologic agent can be detected for only a minority of the cases, such as in pneumococcal, syphilitic, mycotic, or tuberculous arteritis.[133,135] Imperfect as it is, a division based on the vessel caliber is quite useful. Within each group, the arteritides can be further subdivided into more or less specific types on the basis of the associated condition and/or pathologic appearance.[134]

Large vessel arteritis

There is a group of related nonsyphilitic diseases primarily affecting the aorta and its main branches and characterized by chronic inflammation and patchy destruction of the elements of the media.[138,153,157] They may result in aortic insufficiency, diffuse aortic tortuosity and elongation, the aortic arch syndrome, aneurysm formation, and dissection of the vessel (Fig. 27-34). They are more common in adults but have also been described in children.[141]

In some aortic aneurysms, there is a thick outer wall composed of fibroblasts and collagen that entrap fat, nerves, and lymph nodes and that are accompanied by a heavy lymphoplasmatic infiltrate.[137] These have been referred to as *inflammatory aneurysms,*[139] but it is not clear whether they represent a distinct entity or simply a variant of atherosclerotic aneurysm, perhaps induced by antigens in the atheromatous plaque, and/or mediated by adhesion molecules (see p. 2194); the latter possibility seems the most likely.[148,154]

In the variety of arteritis known as ***Takayasu's disease,*** there is chronic inflammation and fibrosis of the arterial wall, which has a predilection for the aortic arch branches and results in the absence of pulses in the upper extremities, ocular changes, and neurologic symptoms.[142,144,150] In later stages, superimposed changes of arteriosclerosis may obscure the diagnosis.[143] In general, the possibility of an underlying arteritis should always be considered when arteriosclerotic changes in the aorta are seen in young or middle-aged individuals and when these changes are either segmental or occur at an unusual site. Most patients with Takayasu's disease are young, Asian, and female. The disease is rare in the United States, but it has been well documented.[145] In a series of sixteen autopsy cases reported from South Africa,[155] there was segmental coronary arteritis in three patients, with development of coronary aneurysms in two. There was co-existent tuberculosis in 37.5% of the patients, but this might well have been coincidental.

In Kawasaki's disease of infants, arterial changes are prominent and may result in sudden death from acute myocardial ischemia. Microscopically, the coronary and other arteries show reactive proliferative changes in the media, panarteritis, and frequent aneurysmal dilatation.[147] Marked fibrosis is present in the healed stage.[140] The etiology is unknown, but the pathologic changes are thought to be immune-mediated.[136,146] Specifically, it has been suggested that the disease may be caused by a toxin that acts as a "superantigen."[149,152]

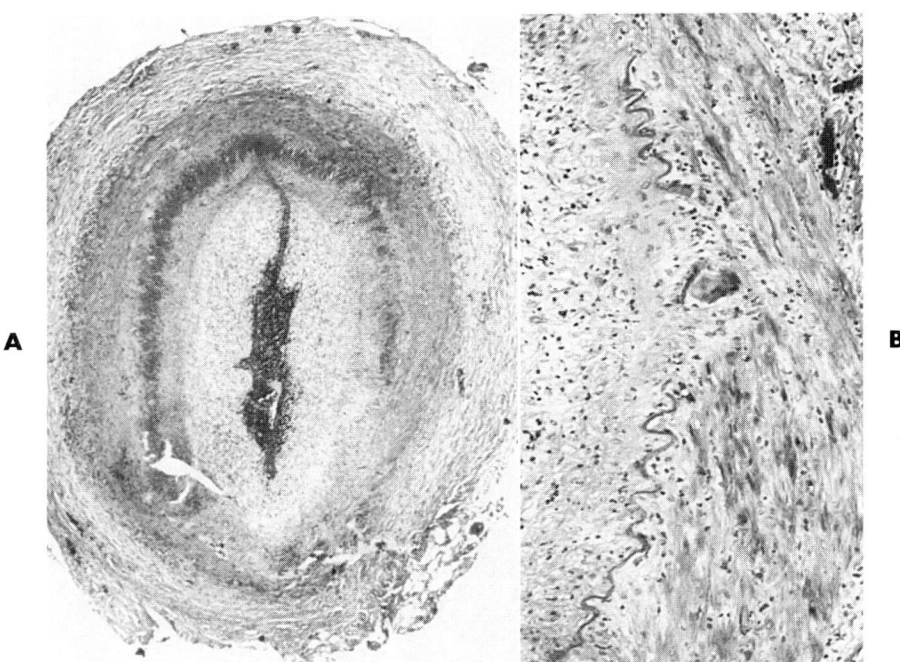

Fig. 27-35 Temporal arteritis. **A,** Low-power view of involved artery showing marked subintimal fibrosis accompanied by partial destruction of muscle layer. **B,** Internal elastic layer is interrupted. Foreign body type giant cells are seen in process of phagocytosing fragments of elastic tissue.

Aortic arteritis can be seen associated with rheumatoid arthritis, ankylosing spondylitis, and scleroderma.[156,158] There is a definite relationship between the type and location of the vessel and the frequency and etiology of the inflammatory diseases it may be affected by. Tuberculosis characteristically involves small vessels; rarely, it may be seen in larger vessels and results in stenosis or aneurysms.[151]

Most of the reported cases of aneurysms of the superior mesenteric artery have been either syphilitic or mycotic; the majority of the latter were associated with bacterial endocarditis.

Medium-sized vessel arteritis

The classic example of medium-sized vessel arteritis is *polyarteritis nodosa,* classically described at autopsy as visible nodular lesions at the points of arterial branchings. This condition should be suspected clinically if there is a history suggesting hypersensitivity, with fever, eosinophilia, and involvement of many organ systems. Infrequently, there are skin manifestations. A muscle or peripheral nerve biopsy may be diagnostic.[168] A biopsy is most rewarding in the presence of a nodule. Rarely, organs such as the gallbladder, appendix, or colon may show unsuspected lesions typical of polyarteritis (see respective chapters).

In *Wegener's granulomatosis,* the arteritis is accompanied by necrosis and granulomatous reaction. The organs most commonly involved are the upper respiratory tract, lung, and kidney (see respective chapters).

Temporal arteritis (cranial arteritis, giant cell arteritis, Horton's disease) was originally thought to be restricted to the temporal, cerebral, and retinal arteries. However, many cases with generalized arterial involvement have been described, indicating that it is a systemic disease.[167,172] This condition, which is most common in the older age group, is characterized by pain in the distribution of the temporal artery and localized tenderness. In other patients, central nervous system manifestations predominate.[166] Sometimes, nodulations can be palpated along the course of the artery. Microscopically, partial destruction of the wall by an inflammatory infiltrate containing multinucleated giant cells is present. Some of the multinucleated giant cells are of Langhans' type, and others are of foreign body type. Many of them are intimately associated with the internal elastic lamina, and some may even contain fragments of phagocytosed elastica in their cytoplasm (Fig. 27-35). The pathogenesis of this disease remains unknown, but immune factors are thought to play an important role.[164]

Ultrastructurally, there is an accumulation of histiocytes, epithelioid cells, and giant cells at the intimal-medial junction, followed by fragmentation, degeneration, and dissolution of the internal elastic lamina.[171] Immunohistochemical deposition of immunoglobulins and fibrinogen occurs in the vessel wall, but this is probably the result of diffusion from the lumen rather than a primary deposit of immune complexes.[160] It is important to emphasize that the changes are often segmental and that a negative biopsy does not rule out the diagnosis. In one series, only 60% of patients with clinical evidence of temporal arteritis had positive biopsies but the other 40% (showing arteriosclerosis or atherosclerosis) also responded to steroid therapy.[159]

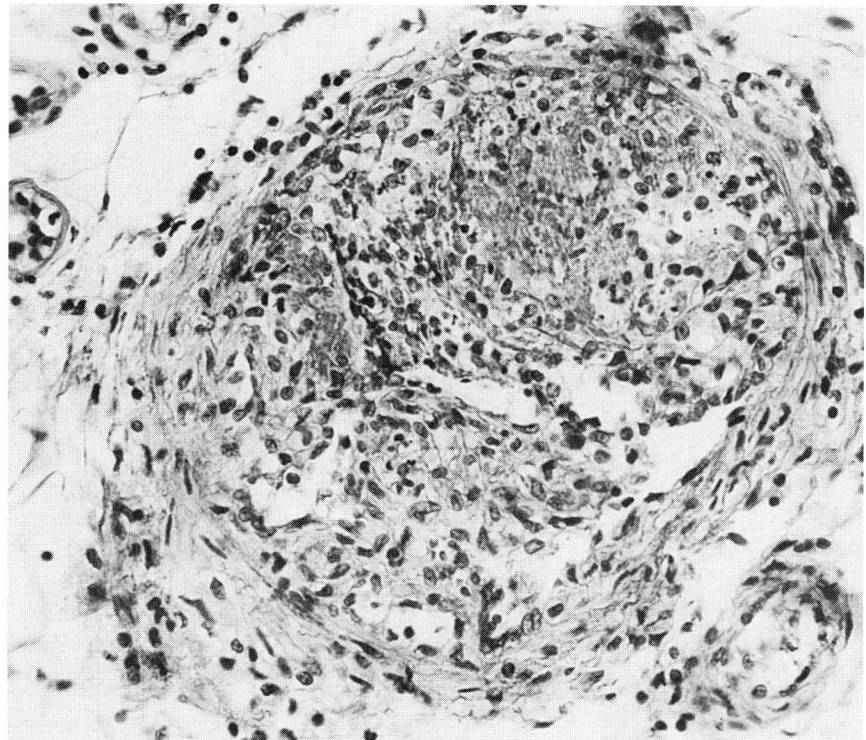

Fig. 27-36 Vasculitis involving small vessel of subcutaneous tissue. Note thrombosis, inflammation, and eccentric involvement.

Serial sections should always be performed[165] and contralateral biopsies should be considered in selected cases.[162] Angiography can be useful by guiding the surgeon to biopsy the diseased area.[161]

It should also be remembered that not all cases of arteritis involving the temporal artery represent examples of the entity temporal arteritis.[169,170]

The syndrome of *polymyalgia rheumatica,* characterized by muscle pain and tenderness involving mainly the muscles of the neck, shoulder, and pelvic girdle and accompanied by elevated erythrosedimentation rate, is often a manifestation of generalized giant cell arteritis.[163,173]

Degos' disease, a progressive subendothelial fibrous thickening of the wall of medium-sized arteries and arterioles, leads to vascular occlusions in many organs, particularly the skin and the digestive system, where ischemic infarcts result.[174]

Small vessel arteritis (arteriolitis)

Small vessel arteritis is the most common variety of arterial inflammation. Most examples are secondary to hypersensitivity to drugs or bacterial antigens or appear as a component of one of the collagen-vascular diseases. The two most important morphologic features to be determined are the nature of the inflammatory infiltrate (whether lymphocytic or neutrophilic) and the presence or absence of necrosis of the vessel wall. In a large majority of the cases, skin manifestations are prominent (see Chapter 4) (Fig. 27-36).

Sneddon's syndrome is an inflammatory syndrome of small arteries of unknown pathogenesis that is characteristically followed by smooth muscle proliferation.[175,176] The diagnosis can be suggested by skin biopsy.

TUMORS

The general subject of vascular tumors is dealt with in Chapter 25. Only those neoplasms involving major vessels are discussed here.

Primary tumors of the *aorta* or *pulmonary artery* are almost invariably malignant and represent various types of sarcoma. Cases have been reported with names such as fibrosarcoma, leiomyosarcoma, rhabdomyosarcoma, fibromyxosarcoma, malignant fibrous histiocytoma, and malignant histiocytoma.* In some instances, abundant metaplastic cartilage and bone formation have been present.[177,186]

Some sarcomas are thought to originate from the intima and to represent a type of *angiosarcoma* (malignant hemangioendothelioma or intimal sarcoma). In contrast to those arising in smaller vessels, these tumors tend to have a predominantly solid pattern of growth, making the diagnosis very difficult.[191,193] Because of these interpretative problems and the fact that the clinical presentation correlates better with the location of the tumor than its microscopic type, it has been suggested that these sarcomas be simply classified as *intimal* (obstructive or nonobstructive)

---

*References 178, 180, 181, 183, 184, 190, 194.

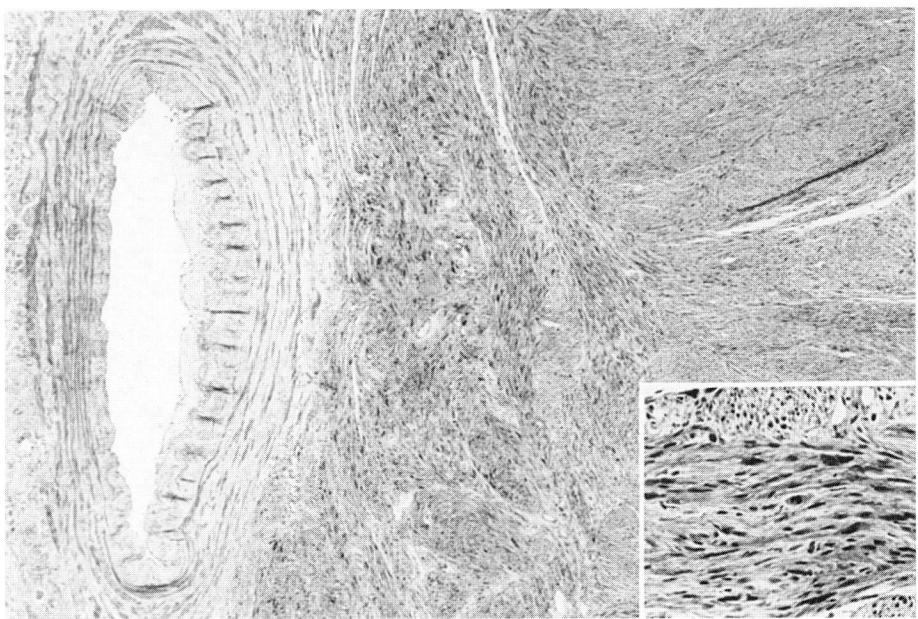

Fig. 27-37 Leiomyosarcoma of posterior tibial vein. Adjacent artery is uninvolved. **Inset** shows typical fascicular arrangement of tumor cells. There is hypercellularity, nuclear atypia, and mitotic figures.

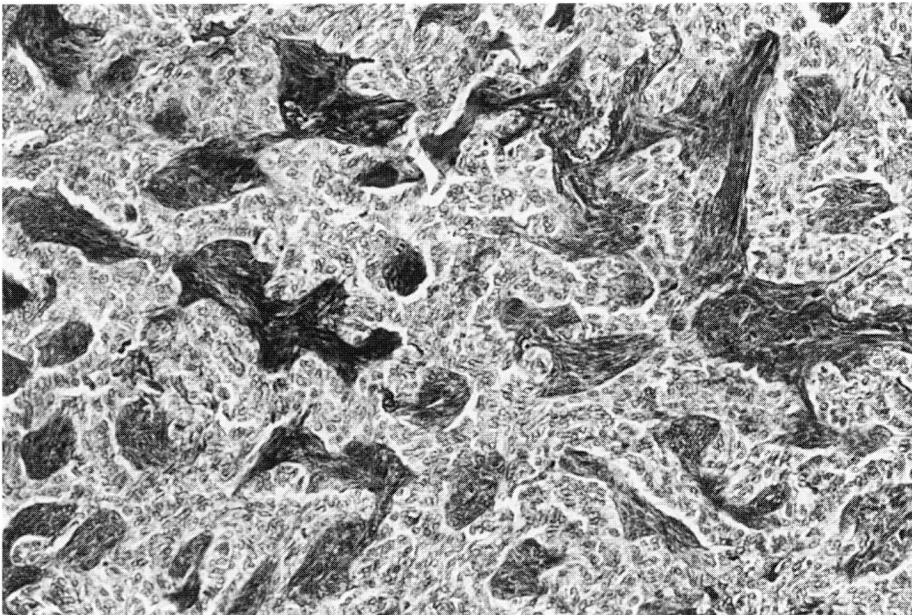

Fig. 27-38 Synovial sarcoma presenting as intraluminal mass within femoral artery. (Courtesy Dr. M. Miettinen, Philadelphia.)

or *mural.*[179,192,196] Some of these tumors have arisen at the site of a vascular prosthesis.[182,195] Embolic metastases are common.

Most tumors arising in large veins are malignant and are largely represented by *leiomyosarcoma*[185] (see Chapter 25) (Fig. 27-37).

Additional primary tumors and tumorlike conditions that may exhibit a predominant or exclusive intravascular location are epithelioid hemangioendothelioma,[189] pyogenic granuloma, intravascular papillary endothelial hyperplasia, nodular fasciitis, so-called systemic or malignant angioendotheliomatosis (which in reality is an angiotropic malignant lymphoma), and synovial sarcoma (Fig. 27-38). These entities are discussed in Chapters 4 and 25. We have also seen a case of entirely intravascular Kaposi's sarcoma. Arterial masses having a morphologic appearance similar to that of aneurysmal bone cyst have been recorded.[187]

Metastatic tumors can lodge in large vessels and produce occlusion. Cases of major arterial occlusion from lung carcinoma have been well documented.[188]

REFERENCES
ARTERIOSCLEROSIS

1 DeBakey ME, Crawford ES, Cooley DA, Morris GC Jr: Surgical considerations of occlusive disease of the abdominal aorta and iliac and femoral arteries. Analysis of 803 cases. Ann Surg **148**:306-324, 1958.

2 DeBakey ME, Crawford ES, Cooley DA, Morris GC Jr, Garrett HE, Fields WS: Cerebral arterial insufficiency. One to 11-year results following arterial reconstructive operation. Ann Surg **161**:921-945, 1965.

3 DeBakey ME, Crawford ES, Morris GC Jr, Cooley DA: Surgical considerations of occlusive disease of the innominate, carotid, subclavian, and vertebral arteries. Ann Surg **154**:698-725, 1961.

4 Hort W: Arteriosclerosis. Its morphology in the past and today. Basic Res Cardiol **89**:1-15, 1994.

5 Kannel WB, Shurtleff D: The natural history of arteriosclerosis obliterans. Cardiovasc Clin **3**:37-52, 1971.

6 Raines EW, Ross R: Smooth muscle cells and the pathogenesis of the lesions of atherosclerosis. Br Heart J **69**:S30-S37, 1993.

7 Ross R: Atherosclerosis. Current understanding of mechanisms and future strategies in therapy. Transplant Proc **25**:2041-2043, 1993.

8 Ross R: The pathogenesis of atherosclerosis. A perspective for the 1990s. Nature **362**:801-809, 1993.

9 Ross R: Rous-Whipple Award Lecture. Atherosclerosis. A defense mechanism gone awry. Am J Pathol **143**:987-1002, 1993.

10 Stary HC, Chandler AB, Glagov S, Guyton JR, Insull W Jr, Rosenfeld ME, Schaffer SA, Schwartz CJ, Wagner WD, Wissler RW: A definition of initial, fatty streak, and intermediate lesions of atherosclerosis. A report from the Committee on Vascular Lesions of the Council on Arteriosclerosis, American Heart Association. Arterioscler Thromb **14**:840-856, 1994.

11 Thompson JE, Kartchner MM, Austin DJ, Wheeler CG, Patman RD: Carotid endarterectomy for cerebrovascular insufficiency (stroke). Follow-up of 359 cases. Ann Surg **163**:751-763, 1966.

Aneurysms
Aortic aneurysms

12 Ariyan S, Cahow CE, Greene FL, Stansel HC: Successful treatment of hepatic artery aneurysm with erosion into the common duct. Ann Surg **182**:169-172, 1975.

13 Belkin M, Donaldson MC, Whittemore AD: Abdominal aortic aneurysms. Curr Opin Cardiol **9**:581-590, 1994.

14 Bennett DE, Cherry JK: Bacterial infection of aortic aneurysms. A clinicopathological study. Am J Surg **113**:321-326, 1967.

15 Borst HG, Laas J: Surgical treatment of thoracic aortic aneurysms. Adv Card Surg **4**:47-87, 1993.

16 Bowers J, Koehler PR, Hammar SP, Nelson JA, Tolman KG: Rupture of a splenic artery aneurysm into the pancreatic duct. Gastroenterology **70**:1152-1155, 1976.

17 Darling RC, Messina CR, Brewster DC, Ottinger LW: Autopsy study of unoperated abdominal aortic aneurysms. The case for early resection. Circulation **56**(Suppl):161-164, 1977.

18 DeBakey ME, Cooley DA, Creech O Jr: Resection of aneurysms of thoracic aorta. Surg Clin North Am **36**:969-982, 1956.

19 DeBakey ME, Crawford ES, Cooley DA, Morris GC Jr, Royster TS, Abbott WP: Aneurysm of abdominal aorta. Analysis of results of graft replacement therapy one to eleven years after operation. Ann Surg **160**:622-639, 1964.

20 DeBakey ME, Creech O Jr, Morris GC Jr: Aneurysm of thoracoabdominal aorta involving the celiac, superior mesenteric, and renal arteries. Report of 4 cases treated by resection and homograft replacement. Ann Surg **144**:549-573, 1956.

21 de Takats G, Pirani CL: Aneurysms. General considerations. Angiology **5**:173-208, 1954.

22 De Vries DP, Van Schil PE, Vanmaele RG, Schoofs EL: Inflammatory aneurysms of the abdominal aorta. A five years experience. Acta Chir Belg **94**:7-11, 1994.

23 Farkas JC, Fichelle JM, Laurian C, Jean-Baptiste A, Gigou F, Marzelle J, Goldstein FW, Cormier JM: Long-term follow-up of positive cultures in 500 abdominal aortic aneurysms. Arch Surg **128**:284-288, 1993.

24 Hatswell EM: Abdominal aortic aneurysm surgery. I. An overview and discussion of immediate perioperative complications. Heart Lung **23**:228-241, 1994.

25 Hirst AE Jr, Affeidt JE: Abdominal aortic aneurysm with rupture into the duodenum. A report of eight cases. Gastroenterology **17**:504-514, 1951.

26 Imakita M, Yutani C, Ishibashi-Ueda H, Nakajima N: Atherosclerotic abdominal aneurysms. Comparative data of different types based on the degree of inflammatory reaction. Cardiovasc Pathol **1**:65-73, 1992.

27 Kampmeir RH: Saccular aneurysm of the thoracic aorta. A clinical study of 633 cases. Ann Intern Med **12**:624-651, 1938.

28 Kiell CS, Ernst CB: Advances in management of abdominal aortic aneurysm. Adv Surg **26**:73-98, 1993.

29 Kiernan PD, Pairolero PC, Hubert JP Jr, Mucha P Jr, Wallace RB: Aortic graft-enteric fistula. Mayo Clin Proc **55**:731-738, 1980.

30 Klima T, Spjut HJ, Coelho A, Gray AG, Wukasch DC, Reul GJ Jr, Cooley DA: The morphology of ascending aortic aneurysms. Hum Pathol **14**:810-817, 1983.

31 Klippel AP, Butcher HR Jr: The unoperated abdominal aortic aneurysm. Am J Surg **111**:629-631, 1966.

32 MacSweeney ST, Powell JT, Greenhalgh RM: Pathogenesis of abdominal aortic aneurysm. Br J Surg **81**:935-941, 1994.

33 Money SR, Hollier LH: The management of thoracoabdominal aneurysms. Adv Surg **27**:285-294, 1994.

34 Oskoui R, Davis WA, Gomes MN: Salmonella aortitis. A report of a successfully treated case with a comprehensive review of the literature. Arch Intern Med **153**:517-525, 1993.

35 Ramshaw AL, Parums DV: The distribution of adhesion molecules in chronic periaortitis. Histopathology **24**:23-32, 1994.

36 Reckless JPD, McColl I, Taylor GW: Aorto-enteric fistulae. An uncommon complication of abdominal aneurysms. Br J Surg **59**:458-460, 1972.

37 Rose AG, Dent DM: Inflammatory variant of abdominal atherosclerotic aneurysm. Arch Pathol Lab Med **105**:409-413, 1981.

38 Schatz IJ, Fairbairn JF II, Juergens JL: Abdominal aortic aneurysms. A reappraisal. Circulation **26**:200-205, 1962.

39 Stehbens WE, Delahunt B, Shirer WC, Naik DK: Aortic aneurysm in systemic lupus erythematosus. Histopathology **22**:275-277, 1993.

40 Szilagyi DE, Smith RF, DeRusso FJ, Elliott JP, Sherrin FW: Contribution of abdominal aortic aneurysmectomy to prolongation of life. Ann Surg **164**:678-699, 1966.

Popliteal artery aneurysms

41 Gifford RW Jr, Hines EA Jr, Janes JM: An analysis and follow-up study of 100 popliteal aneurysms. Surgery **33**:284-293, 1953.

42 Julian OC, Dye WS, Javid H: The use of vessel grafts in the treatment of popliteal aneurysms. Surgery **38**:970-980, 1955.

43 Pappas G, Janes JM, Bernatz PE, Schirger A: Femoral aneurysms. Review of surgical management. JAMA **190**:489-493, 1964.

44 Roggo A, Brunner U, Ottinger LW, Largiader F: The continuing challenge of aneurysms of the popliteal artery. Surg Gynecol Obstet **177**:565-572, 1993.

Dissecting aneurysms

45 Cavanzo FJ, Taylor HB: Effect of pregnancy on the human aorta and its relationship to dissecting aneurysms. Am J Obstet Gynecol **105**:567-568, 1969.

46 Cigarroa JE, Isselbacher EM, De Sanctis RW, Eagle KA: Diagnostic imaging in the evaluation of suspected aortic dissection. Old standards and new directions. N Engl J Med **328**:35-43, 1993.

47 DeBakey ME, McCollum CH, Crawford ES, Morris GC Jr, Howell J, Noon GP, Lawrie G: Dissection and dissecting aneurysms of the aorta. Twenty-year follow-up of five hundred twenty-seven patients treated surgically. Surgery **92**:1118-1134, 1982.

48 DeSanctis RW, Doroghazi RM, Austen WG, Buckley MJ: Aortic dissection. N Engl J Med **317:**1060-1067, 1987.

49 Guilmet D, Bachet J, Goudot B, Dreyfus G, Martinelli GL: Aortic dissection. Anatomic types and surgical approaches. J Cardiovasc Surg (Torino) **34:**23-32, 1993.

50 McFarland J, Willerson JT, Dinsmore RE, Austen WG, Buckley MJ, Sanders CA, DeSanctis RW: The medical treatment of dissecting aortic aneurysms. N Engl J Med **286:**115-155, 1972.

51 Wheat MW Jr, Harris PD, Malm JR, Kaiser G, Bowman FO Jr, Palmer RF: Acute dissecting aneurysms of the aorta. Treatment and results in 64 patients. J Thorac Cardiovasc Surg **58:**344-351, 1969.

52 Wilson SK, Hutchins GM: Aortic dissecting aneurysms. Causative factors in 204 subjects. Arch Pathol Lab Med **106:**175-180, 1982.

53 Wychulis AR, Kincaid OW, Wallace RB: Primary dissecting aneurysms of peripheral arteries. Mayo Clin Proc **44:**804-810, 1969.

Diffuse arterial tortuosity and dilatation

54 Leriche R: Physiologie, pathologique et traitement chirurgical des maladies artérielles de la vasomotricité. Paris, 1945, Masson et Cie.

Arterial substitution

55 Meade JW, Linton RR, Darling RC, Menendez CV: Arterial homografts. A long-term clinical follow-up. Arch Surg **93:**392-399, 1966.

56 Stanley JC, ed: Biologic and synthetic vascular prostheses. New York, 1982, Grune & Stratton.

57 Stump MM, Jordan GL Jr, DeBakey ME, Halpert B: The endothelial lining of homografts and Dacron prostheses in the canine aorta. Am J Pathol **40:**487-491, 1962.

58 Szilagyi DE, McDonald RT, Smith RF, Whitcomb JG: Biologic fate of human arterial homografts. Arch Surg **75:**506-529, 1957.

Arterial occlusive disease

59 Anderson WR, Richards AM, Weiss L: Hemorrhage and necrosis of stomach and small bowel due to atheroembolism. Am J Clin Pathol **48:**30-38, 1967.

60 Barker WJ, Cannon JA, Zeldis LJ, Perry A: Anatomical results of endarterectomy. Surg Forum **6:**266-269, 1955.

61 Bennett DE, Cherry JK: Bacterial infection of aortic aneurysms. A clinicopathological study. Am J Surg **113:**321-326, 1967.

62 Darling RC, Linton RR: Aortoiliofemoral endarterectomy for atherosclerotic occlusive disease. Surgery **55:**184-194, 1964.

63 DeWeese JA, Barner HB, Mahoney EB, Rob CG: Autogenous venous by-pass grafts and thromboendarterectomies for atherosclerotic lesions of the femoropopliteal arteries. Ann Surg **163:**205-214, 1966.

64 DeWolfe VG, Beven EG: Arteriosclerosis obliterans in the lower extremities. Correlation of clinical and angiographic findings. Cardiovasc Clin **3:**65-92, 1971.

65 Dible JH: The pathology of limb ischaemia. St. Louis, 1966, Warren H. Green, Inc.

66 Drost H, Buis B, Haan D, Hillers JA: Cholesterol embolism as a complication of left heart catheterization. Report of seven cases. Br Heart J **52:**339-342, 1984.

67 Harrington JT, Sommers SC, Kassirer JP: Atheromatous emboli with progressive renal failure. Renal arteriography as the probable inciting factor. Ann Intern Med **68:**152-160, 1968.

68 Hollenhorst RW: Vascular status of patients who have cholesterol emboli in the retina. Am J Ophthalmol **61:**1159-1165, 1966.

69 Jorgensen L: Mechanisms of thrombosis. Pathobiology **2:**139-204, 1972.

70 Kalter DC, Rudolph A, McGavran M: Livedo reticularis due to multiple cholesterol emboli. J Am Acad Dermatol **13:**235-242, 1985.

71 Kassirer JP: Atheroembolic renal disease. N Engl J Med **280:**812-818, 1969.

72 Kouchoukos NT, Levy JF, Balfour JF, Butcher HR Jr: Operative therapy for femoral-popliteal arterial occlusive disease. A comparison of therapeutic methods. Circulation **35**(Suppl 1):174-182, 1967.

73 Krotovsky GS, Turpitko SA, Gerasimov VB, Zabelskaya TF, Mamedov DM, Klokov KI, Uchkin IG, Papandopoulos E: Surgical treatment and prevention of vasculopathic impotence in conjunction with revascularisation of the lower extremities in Leriche's syndrome. J Cardiovasc Surg **32:**340-343, 1991.

74 Morris GC Jr, Wheeler CG, Crawford ES, Cooley DA, DeBakey ME: Restorative vascular surgery in the presence of impending and overt gangrene of the extremities. Surgery **51:**50-57, 1962.

75 Richards AM, Eliot RS, Kanjuh VI, Bloemendaal RD, Edwards JE: Cholesterol embolism. A multiple system disease masquerading as polyarteritis nodosa. Am J Cardiol **15:**696-707, 1965.

76 Stout C, Hartsuck JM, Howe J, Richardson JL: Atheromatous embolism after aortofemoral bypass and aortic ligation. Arch Pathol **93:**271-275, 1972.

77 Warren R, Gomez RL, Marston JAP, Cox JST: Femoropopliteal arteriosclerosis obliterans. Arteriographic patterns and rates of progression. Surgery **55:**135-143, 1964.

CYSTIC ADVENTITIAL DEGENERATION

78 Blackstrom CG, Linell F, Ostberg G: Cystic myxomatous adventitial degeneration of the radial artery with development of ganglion in the connective tissue. Acta Chir Scand **129:**447-451, 1965.

79 Flanigan DP, Burnham SJ, Goodreau JJ, Bergan JJ: Summary of cases of adventitial cystic disease of the popliteal artery. Ann Surg **189:**165-175, 1979.

80 Haid SP, Conn I Jr, Bergan JJ: Cystic adventitial disease of the popliteal artery. Arch Surg **101:**765-770, 1970.

81 Lewis GJT, Douglas DM, Reid W, Watt JK: Cystic adventitial disease of the popliteal artery. Br Med J **3:**411-415, 1967.

82 Terry JD, Schenken JR, Lohff MR, Neis DD: Cystic adventitial disease. Hum Pathol **23:**639-643, 1981.

FIBROMUSCULAR DYSPLASIA

83 Claiborne TS: Fibromuscular hyperplasia. Report of a case with involvement of multiple arteries. Am J Med **49:**103-105, 1970.

84 Crocker DW: Fibromuscular dysplasias of renal artery. Arch Pathol **85:**602-613, 1968.

85 Furie DM, Tien RD: Fibromuscular dysplasia of arteries of the head and neck. Imaging findings. AJR Am J Roentgenol **162:**1205-1209, 1994.

86 Harrison EG, Hung JC, Bernatz PE: Morphology of fibromuscular dysplasia of the renal artery in renovascular hypertension. Am J Med **43:**97-112, 1967.

87 Hunt JC, Harrison EG Jr, Kincaid OW, Bernatz PE, Davis GP: Idiopathic fibrous and fibromuscular stenoses of the renal arteries associated with hypertension. Mayo Clin Proc **37:**181-216, 1962.

88 Lüscher TF, Lie JT, Stanson AW, Houser OW, Hollier LH, Sheps SG: Arterial fibromuscular dysplasia. Mayo Clin Proc **62:**931-952, 1987.

89 Moreau P, Albat B, Thevenet A: Fibromuscular dysplasia of the internal carotid artery. Long-term surgical results. J Cardiovasc Surg **34:**466-472, 1993.

90 Price RA, Vawter GF: Arterial fibromuscular dysplasia in infancy and childhood. Arch Pathol **93:**419-426, 1972.

MESENTERIC VASCULAR OCCLUSION

91 Arosemena E, Edwards JE: Lesions of the small mesenteric arteries underlying intestinal infarction. Geriatrics **22:**122-138, 1967.

92 Bienenstock H, Minick R, Rogoff B: Mesenteric arteritis and intestinal infarction in rheumatoid disease. Arch Intern Med **119:**359-364, 1967.

93 Flaherty MJ, Lie JT, Haggitt RC: Mesenteric inflammatory veno-occlusive disease. A seldom recognized cause of intestinal ischemia. Am J Surg Pathol **18:**779-784, 1994.

94 Ho ECK, Moss AJ: The syndrome of "mesenteric arteritis" following surgical repair of aortic coarctation. Report of 9 cases and review of literature. Pediatrics **49:**40-45, 1972.

95 Johnson CC, Baggenstoss AH: Mesenteric vascular occlusion. I. Study of 99 cases of occlusion of veins. Mayo Clin Proc **24:**628-636, 1949.

96 Johnson CC, Baggenstoss AH: Mesenteric vascular occlusion. II. Study of 60 cases of occlusion of arteries and of 12 cases of occlusion of both arteries and veins. Mayo Clin Proc **24:**649-665, 1949.

97 Kempczinski RF, Clark SM, Blebea J, Koelliker DD, Fenoglio-Preiser C: Intestinal ischemia secondary to thromboangiitis obliterans. Ann Vasc Surg **7:**354-358, 1993.

98 Ottinger LW, Austen WG: A study of 136 patients with mesenteric infarction. Surg Gynecol Obstet **124:**251-261, 1967.

99 Roobottom CA, Dubbins PA: Significant disease of the celiac and superior mesenteric arteries in asymptomatic patients. Predictive value of Doppler sonography. AJR Am J Roentgenol **161:**985-988, 1993.

100 Schneider TA, Longo WE, Ure T, Vernava AM: Mesenteric ischemia. Acute arterial syndromes. Dis Colon Rectum **37:**1163-1174, 1994.

101 Volteas N, Labropoulos N, Leon M, Kalodiki E, Chan P, Nicolaides AN: Detection of superior mesenteric and coeliac artery stenosis with colour flow Duplex imaging. Eur J Vasc Surg **7:**616-620, 1993.

102 Williams LF, Anastasia LF, Hasiotis CA, Bosniak MA, Byrne JJ: Nonocclusive mesenteric infarction. Am J Surg **114**:376-381, 1967.

103 Wilson GSM, Block J: Mesenteric vascular occlusion. Arch Surg **73**:330-345, 1956.

TRAUMATIC AND IATROGENIC INJURIES
Rupture

104 Eeckhout E, Beuret P, Lobrinus A, Genton CY, Goy JJ: Coronary artery rupture during transluminal coronary recanalization and angioplasty in a case of acute myocardial infarction and shock. Clin Cardiol **16**:355-356, 1993.

105 Fajardo LF, Lee A: Rupture of major vessels after radiation. Cancer **36**:904-913, 1975.

106 Hasan RI, Krysiak P, Deiranyia AK, Hooper T: Spontaneous rupture of the internal mammary artery in Ehlers-Danlos syndrome (letter). J Thorac Cardiovasc Surg **106**:184-185, 1993.

107 Rodriguez HF, Rivera E: Spontaneous rupture of the thoracic aorta through an atheromatous plaque. Ann Intern Med **54**:307-313, 1961.

108 Worrell JT, Buja LM, Reynolds RC: Pneumococcal aortitis with rupture of the aorta. Report of a case and review of the literature. Am J Clin Pathol **89**:565-568, 1988.

Thrombosis

109 Bickerstaff ER: Aetiology of acute hemiplegia in childhood. J Neurosurg **2**:82-87, 1964.

110 Houck WS, Jackson JR, Odom GL, Young WG: Occlusion of internal carotid artery in neck secondary to closed trauma to head and neck. Report of two cases. Ann Surg **159**:219-221, 1964.

111 Kuo T, Sayers CP, Rosai J: Masson's "vegetant intravascular hemangioendothelioma." A lesion often mistaken for angiosarcoma. Study of seventeen cases located in the skin and soft tissues. Cancer **38**:1227-1236, 1976.

112 Pitner SE: Carotid thrombosis due to intraoral trauma. An unusual complication of a common childhood accident. N Engl J Med **274**:764-767, 1966.

113 Salyer WR, Salyer DC: Myxoma-like features of organizing thrombi in arteries and veins. Arch Pathol **99**:307-311, 1975.

114 Shillito J Jr: Carotid arteritis. Cause of hemiplegia in childhood. J Neurosurg **21**:540-551, 1964.

Pulsating hematoma

115 Bennett DE, Cherry JK: The natural history of traumatic aneurysms of the aorta. Surgery **61**:516-523, 1967.

116 Cohen SM: Peripheral aneurysm and arteriovenous fistula. Ann R Coll Surg Engl **11**:1-30, 1952.

117 Gallen J, Wiss DA, Cantelmo N, Menzoin JO: Traumatic pseudoaneurysm of the axillary artery. Report of three cases and literature review. J Trauma **24**:350-354, 1984.

Acquired arteriovenous fistula

118 Gomes MMR, Bernatz PE: Arteriovenous fistulas. A review of ten-year experience at the Mayo Clinic. Mayo Clin Proc **45**:81-102, 1970.

THROMBOANGIITIS OBLITERANS

119 Colburn MD, Moore WS: Buerger's disease. Heart Dis Stroke **2**:424-432, 1993.

120 Gore I, Burrows S: A reconsideration of the pathogenesis of Buerger's disease. Am J Clin Pathol **29**:319-330, 1958.

121 Hershey FB, Pareira MD, Ahlvin RC: Quadrilateral peripheral vascular disease in the young adult. Circulation **26**:1261-1269, 1962.

122 Ishikawa K, Kawase S, Mishima Y: Occlusive arterial disease in extremities, with special reference to Buerger's disease. Angiology **13**:398-411, 1962.

123 Kelly PJ, Dahlin DJ, Janes JM: Clinicopathological study of ninety-four limbs amputated for occlusive vascular disease. J Bone Joint Surg **40**:72-78, 1958.

124 McKusick VA, Harris WS: The Buerger syndrome in the Orient. Bull Johns Hopkins Hosp **109**:241-291, 1961.

125 McKusick VA, Harris WS, Ottesen OE, Goodman RM: The Buerger syndrome in the United States. Bull Johns Hopkins Hosp **110**:145-176, 1962.

126 McKusick VA, Harris WS, Ottesen OE, Shelley WM, Bloodwell DB: Buerger's disease. A distinct clinical and pathologic entity. JAMA **181**:93-100, 1962.

127 Mills JL, Porter JM: Buerger's disease. A review and update. Semin Vasc Surg **6**:14-23, 1993.

128 Schellong SM, Bernhards J, Ensslen F, Schafers HJ, Alexander K: Intestinal type of thromboangiitis obliterans (Buerger's disease). J Intern Med **235**:69-73, 1994.

129 Shionoya S: Buerger's disease. Diagnosis and management. Cardiovasc Surg **1**:207-214, 1993.

130 Theis FV: Thromboangiitis obliterans. A 30-year study. J Am Geriatr Soc **6**:106-117, 1958.

131 Wessler S, Ming S-C, Guerwich V, Greiman DG: A critical evaluation of thromboangiitis obliterans. The case against Buerger's disease. N Engl J Med **262**:1149-1160, 1960.

132 Williams G: Recent views on Buerger's disease. J Clin Pathol **22**:573-577, 1969.

ARTERITIS

133 Manion WC: Infectious angiitis. In Orbison JL, Smith DE, eds: The peripheral blood vessels. Baltimore, 1963, The Williams & Wilkins Co, pp 221-231.

134 Parums DV: The arteritides. Histopathology **25**:1-20, 1994.

135 Worrell JT, Buja LM, Reynolds RC: Pneumococcal aortitis with rupture of the aorta. Report of a case and review of the literature. Am J Clin Pathol **89**:565-568, 1988.

Large vessel arteritis

136 Arav-Boger R, Assia A, Jurgenson U, Spirer Z: The immunology of Kawasaki disease. Adv Pediatr **41**:359-367, 1994.

137 Beckman EN: Plasma cell infiltrates in atherosclerotic abdominal aortic aneurysms. Am J Clin Pathol **85**:21-24, 1986.

138 Domingo RT, Maramba MD, Torres LF, Wesolowski SA: Acquired aortoarteritis. A worldwide vascular entity. Arch Surg **95**:780-790, 1967.

139 Feiner HD, Raghavendra BN, Phelps R, Rooney L: Inflammatory abdominal aortic aneurysm. Report of six cases. Hum Pathol **15**:454-459, 1984.

140 Fujiwara H, Fujiwara T, Kao T-C, Ohshio G, Hamashima Y: Pathology of Kawasaki disease in the healed stage. Relationships between typical and atypical cases of Kawasaki disease. Acta Pathol Jpn **36**:857-867, 1986.

141 Gonzalez-Cerna JL, Villavicencio L, Molina B, Bessudo L: Nonspecific obliterative aortitis in children. Ann Thorac Surg **4**:193-204, 1967.

142 Hall S, Barr W, Lie JT, Stanson AW, Kazmier FJ, Hunder GG: Takayasu arteritis. A study of 32 North American patients. Medicine **64**:89-99, 1985.

143 Ishikawa K, Maetani S: Long-term outcome for 120 Japanese patients with Takayasu's disease. Clinical and statistical analyses of related prognostic factors. Circulation **90**:1855-1860, 1994.

144 Judge RD, Currier RD, Gracie WA, Figley MM: Takayasu arteritis and the aortic arch syndrome. Am J Med **32**:379-392, 1962.

145 Kerr GS, Hallahan CW, Giordano J, Leavitt RY, Fauci AS, Rottem M, Hoffman GS: Takayasu arteritis. Ann Intern Med **120**:919-929, 1994.

146 Leung DY: Kawasaki disease. Curr Opin Rheumatol **5**:41-50, 1993.

147 Masuda H, Shozawa T, Naoe S, Tanaka N: The intercostal artery in Kawasaki disease. A pathologic study of 17 autopsy cases. Arch Pathol Lab Med **110**:1136-1142, 1986.

148 Mitchinson MJ: Chronic periaortitis and periarteritis. Histopathology **8**:589-600, 1984.

149 Nadel S, Levin M: Kawasaki disease. Curr Opin Pediatr **5**:29-34, 1993.

150 Nasu T: Pathology of pulseless disease. A systematic study and critical review of 21 autopsy cases reported in Japan. Angiology **14**:225-242, 1963.

151 O'Leary M, Nollet DJ, Blomberg DJ: Rupture of a tuberculous pseudoaneurysm of the innominate artery into the trachea and esophagus. Report of a case and review of the literature. Hum Pathol **8**:458-467, 1977.

152 Pariser KM: Takayasu's arteritis. Curr Opin Cardiol **9**:575-580, 1994.

153 Restrepo C, Tejeda C, Correa P: Nonsyphilitic aortitis. Arch Pathol **87**:1-12, 1969.

154 Rose AG, Dent DM: Inflammatory variant of abdominal atherosclerotic aneurysm. Arch Pathol Lab Med **105**:409-413, 1981.

155 Rose AG, Sinclair-Smith CC: Takayasu's arteritis. A study of 16 autopsy cases. Arch Pathol Lab Med **104**:231-237, 1980.

156 Roth LM, Kissane JM: Panaortitis and aortic valvulitis in progressive systemic sclerosis (scleroderma). Report of case with perforation of an aortic cusp. Am J Clin Pathol **41**:287-296, 1964.

157 Schrire V, Asherson RA: Arteritis of the aorta and its major branches. Q J Med **33**:439-463, 1964.

158 Valaitis J, Pilz CG, Montgomery MM: Aortitis with aortic valve insufficiency in rheumatoid arthritis. Arch Pathol **63**:207-212, 1957.

Medium-sized vessel arteritis

159 Allsop CJ, Gallagher PJ: Temporal artery biopsy in giant-cell arteritis. A reappraisal. Am J Surg Pathol **5**:317-323, 1981.

160 Banks PM, Cohen MD, Ginsburg WW, Hunder GG: Immunohistologic and cyto-chemical studies of temporal arteritis. Arthritis Rheum **26**:1201-1207, 1983.

161 Elliott PD, Baker HL Jr, Brown AL Jr: The superficial temporal artery angiogram. Radiology **102**:635-638, 1972.

162 Goodman BW Jr: Temporal arteritis. Am J Med **67**:839-852, 1979.

163 Hamilton CR Jr, Shelley WM, Tumulty PA: Giant cell arteritis including tempo-ral arteritis and polymyalgia rheumatica. Medicine (Baltimore) **50**:1-27, 1971.

164 Hunder GG, Lie JT, Goronzy JJ, Weyand CM: Pathogenesis of giant cell arteri-tis. Arthritis Rheum **36**:757-761, 1993.

165 Klein RG, Campbell RJ, Hunder GG, Carney JA: Skip lesions in temporal arteri-tis. Mayo Clin Proc **51**:504-510, 1976.

166 Kolodny EH, Rebeiz JJ, Caviness VS, Richardson EP: Granulomatous angiitis of the central nervous system. Arch Neurol **19**:510-524, 1968.

167 Lie JT, Failoni DD, Davis DC Jr: Temporal arteritis with giant cell aortitis, coro-nary arteritis, and myocardial infarction. Arch Pathol Lab Med **110**:857-860, 1986.

168 Maxeiner SR, McDonald JR, Kirklin JW: Muscle biopsy in the diagnosis of peri-arteritis nodosa. Surg Clin North Am **32**:1225-1233, 1952.

169 Morgan GJ Jr, Harris ED Jr: Non-giant cell temporal arteritis. Arthritis Rheum **21**:362-366, 1978.

170 O'Brien JP: A concept of diffuse actinic arteritis. Br J Dermatol **98**:1-13, 1978.

171 Parker F, Healey LA, Wilske KR, Odland GF: Light and electron microscopic studies on human temporal arteries with special reference to alterations related to senescence, atherosclerosis and giant cell arteritis. Am J Pathol **79**:57-80, 1975.

172 Parums DV: The arteritides. Histopathology **25**:1-20, 1994.

173 Royster TS, DiRe JJ: Polymyalgia rheumatica and giant cell arteritis with bilat-eral axillary artery occlusion. Am Surg **37**:421-426, 1971.

174 Strole WE Jr, Clark WH, Isselbacher KJ: Progressive arterial occlusive disease (Kohlmeier-Degos). A frequently fatal cutaneosystemic disorder. N Engl J Med **276**:195-201, 1967.

Small vessel arteritis (arteriolitis)

175 Sepp N, Zelger B, Schuler G, Romani N, Fritsch P: Sneddon's syndrome. An inflammatory disorder of small arteries followed by smooth muscle proliferation. Immunohistochemical and ultrastructural evidence. Am J Surg Pathol **19**:448-453, 1995.

176 Zelger B, Sepp N, Stockhammer G, Dosch E, Hilty E, Ofner D, Aichner F, Fritsch PO: Sneddon's syndrome. A long-term follow-up of 21 patients. Arch Dermatol **129**:437-447, 1993.

TUMORS

177 Baker PB, Goodwin RA: Pulmonary artery sarcomas. A review and report of a case. Arch Pathol Lab Med **109**:35-39, 1985.

178 Bleisch VR, Kraus FT: Polypoid sarcoma of the pulmonary trunk. Analysis of the literature and report of a case with leptomeric organelles and ultrastructural fea-tures of rhabdomyosarcoma. Cancer **46**:314-324, 1980.

179 Burke AP, Virmani R: Sarcomas of the great vessels. A clinicopathologic study. Cancer **71**:1761-1773, 1993.

180 Chen KTK: Primary malignant fibrous histiocytoma of the aorta. Cancer **48**:840-844, 1981.

181 Emmert-Buck MR, Stay EJ, Tsokos M, Travis WD: Pleomorphic rhab-domyosarcoma arising in association with the right pulmonary artery. Arch Pathol Lab Med **118**:1220-1222, 1994.

182 Fehrenbacher JW, Bowers W, Strate R, Pittman J: Angiosarcoma of the aorta associated with a Dacron graft. Ann Thorac Surg **32**:297-301, 1981.

183 Iwasaki I, Iwase H, Horie H, Ide G, Saito T, Furukawa Y: Leiomyosarcoma of pulmonary truncus. Acta Pathol Jpn **34**:863-867, 1984.

184 Johansson L, Carlen B: Sarcoma of the pulmonary artery. Report of four cases with electron microscopic and immunohistochemical examinations, and review of the literature. Virchows Arch **424**:217-224, 1994.

185 Kaiser LR, Urmacher C: Primary sarcoma of the superior pulmonary vein. Cancer **66**:789-795, 1990.

186 Murthy MSN, Meckstroth CV, Merkle BH, Huston JT, Cattaneo SM: Primary intimal sarcoma of pulmonary valve and trunk with osteogenic sarcomatous ele-ments. Report of a case considered to be pulmonary embolus. Arch Pathol Lab Med **100**:649-651, 1976.

187 Petrik PK, Findlay JM, Sherlock RA: Aneurysmal cyst, bone type, primary in an artery. Am J Surg Pathol **17**:1062-1066, 1993.

188 Prioleau PG, Katzenstein AA: Major peripheral arterial occlusion due to malig-nant tumor embolism. Cancer **42**:2009-2014, 1978.

189 Rosai J, Gold J, Landy R: The histiocytoid hemangiomas. A unifying concept embracing several previously described entities of skin, soft tissue, large vessels, bone and heart. Hum Pathol **10**:707-730, 1979.

190 Salm R: Primary fibrosarcoma of aorta. Cancer **29**:73-83, 1972.

191 Schmid E, Port J, Carroll RM, Freidman NB: Primary metastasizing aortic endothelioma. Cancer **54**:1407-1411, 1984.

192 Sladden RA: Neoplasia of aortic intima. J Clin Pathol **17**:602-607, 1964.

193 Steffelaar JW, van der Heul RO, Blackstone E, Vos A: Primary sarcoma of the aorta. Arch Pathol **99**:139-142, 1975.

194 Stevenson JE, Burkhead H, Trueheart RE, McLaren J: Primary malignant tumor of the aorta. Am J Med **51**:553-559, 1971.

195 Weinberg DS, Maini BS: Primary sarcoma of the aorta associated with a vascu-lar prosthesis. A case report. Cancer **46**:398-402, 1980.

196 Wright EP, Virmani R, Glick AD, Page DL: Aortic intimal sarcoma with embolic metastases. Am J Surg Pathol **9**:890-897, 1985.

Veins

THROMBOPHLEBITIS AND THROMBOEMBOLISM

Thrombophlebitis is a thrombotic disease of veins accompanied by varying degrees of inflammation. The venous wall is edematous, the intima irregularly ulcerated, and the media infiltrated with chronic inflammatory cells (Fig. 27-39). As the acute inflammatory phase of the disease subsides, varying amounts of fibrous tissue are deposited in the adventitia and in the media. During the acute phase, the thrombus becomes attached more or less firmly to the denuded intima.

The process of thrombophlebitis is associated with edema of the extremity, which may be minimal or marked. When there is but little edema and few or no clinical signs of acute inflammation in the extremity, the venous thrombosis has been termed *phlebothrombosis* or bland noninflammatory venous thrombosis.[10] The noninflammatory type of thrombophlebitis is probably more frequently associated with pulmonary emboli than is thrombophlebitis with more marked signs of inflammation. However, the rigid separation of phlebothrombosis from thrombophlebitis is not pathologically possible or clinically practical. In most instances, these two conditions are merely different degrees of the same process.

Thrombophlebitis may involve only the superficial veins such as the saphenous vein. The vein is acutely inflamed and tender, and the overlying skin is usually red. When such thrombosis of the superficial veins occurs, there is usually little edema. However, thrombophlebitic edema may develop with marked rapidity and may be of great volume if the process extends into the deep venous system. Rapid shifts of extracellular fluid into the leg may be sufficiently massive to cause shock. In such instances, the extremity may become so swollen that cutaneous blebs develop, followed by cutaneous necrosis (phlegmasia ceruleadolens).[14] Thrombophlebitis of this severity, however, is rare. The usual postoperative or post-traumatic acute thrombophlebitis initially causes painful, tender, swollen, cool, and mottled or grayish white extremity. Clinical examination is notoriously inaccurate in the diagnosis of deep vein thrombosis. Useful diagnostic tests are ascending contrast venography, radiolabeled fibrinogen leg scanning, and impedance plethysmography.[9]

Purulent or septic thrombophlebitis is occasionally seen in association with abscess or other infection usually occurring in the peritoneal cavity or pelvis. Stein and Pruitt[15] found this complication in 4.6% of 521 burned patients who had been treated by venous catheterization. Purulent thrombophlebitis at any location is associated with marked chills and high temperature because of the bacteremia arising from the infected intravascular thrombus.

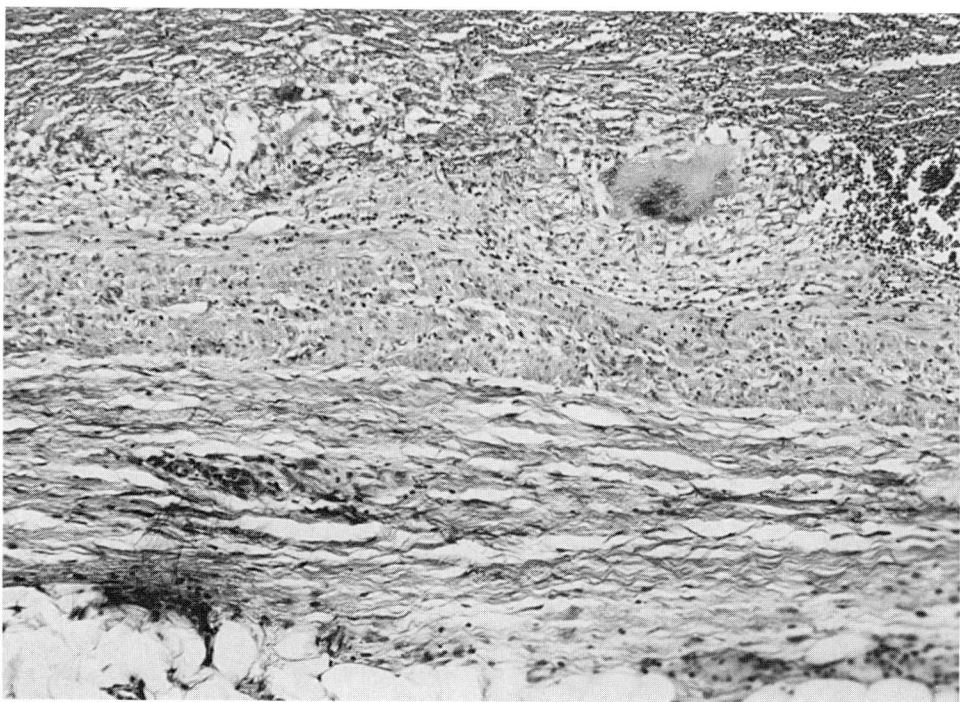

Fig. 27-39 Acute venous thrombosis accompanied by inflammatory cellular infiltration containing giant cells.

There is a statistically significant association between deep vein thrombosis and the subsequent development of cancer (Trousseau's syndrome).[11] Many of the tumors have been mucin-producing adenocarcinomas, and most of them have arisen from the pancreas.

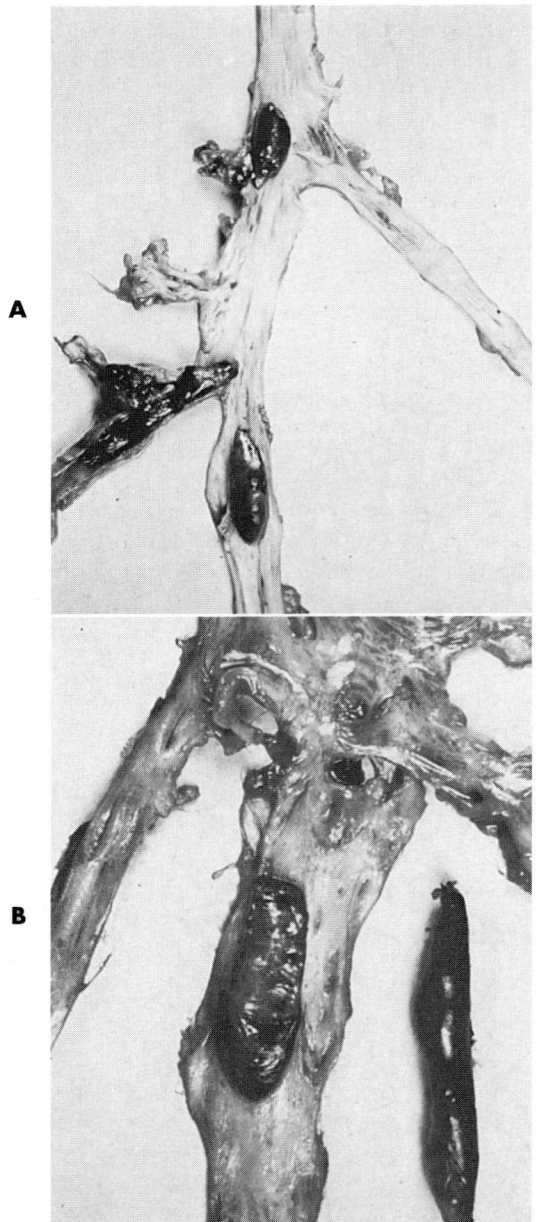

Fig. 27-40 **A,** Multiple venous thrombi. Lower thrombus is lying in valve pocket at upper end of superficial femoral vein. Middle one on left is lying in proximal end of profunda femoris vein, whereas upper thrombus is lying in common femoral vein at junction of long saphenous vein. **B,** Thrombus arising in valve pocket at upper end of superficial femoral vein. Lines of Zahn can be clearly seen. Postmortem clot is shown for comparison. (From McLachlin J, Paterson JC: Some basic observations on venous thrombosis and pulmonary embolism. Surg Gynecol Obstet **93:**1-8, 1951.)

Pulmonary embolism is often thought to be primarily a complication of some surgical procedure or trauma such as fracture, particularly of the lower extremity, but the incidence of this complication is as high on medical as on surgical services.[7] Some of the factors thought to favor intravenous thrombosis and subsequent pulmonary embolism are neoplasms, cardiac disease, venous stasis from any cause, infection in the immediate area of veins, trauma, spasm of vessels, intimal injury, increased coagulability, and immobilization of the limbs.[3] The use of oral contraceptives with early regimens was found to be causally related to the presence of thromboembolic phenomena.[5,13,16] Irey et al.[6] described distinctive vascular lesions in association with thrombosis in arteries and veins of twenty young women receiving oral contraceptives. The incidence of this complication has greatly diminished with modifications in the type and dosage of contraceptive drugs.

Pulmonary embolism is seen in all forms of thrombophlebitis. Sudden massive pulmonary emboli frequently occur in patients without antecedent symptoms or signs of peripheral thrombophlebitis.

The greatest percentage of thrombi resulting in pulmonary embolization are thought to originate in the veins of the lower extremity. In a classic study, Rössle[12] found that 27% of patients over 20 years of age harbored thrombi in the veins of the calf at autopsy. The study of Hunter et al.[4] confirmed these observations and indicated that the thrombosis occurred in over 50% of middle-aged or older persons confined to bed.

McLachlin and Paterson[8] stressed the finding of intravascular thromboses arising in relationship to the valve pockets. In 100 complete dissections of the veins of the pelvis and lower extremities, they showed gross venous thrombi in 34%, and in over one half of these there were pulmonary emboli (Fig. 27-40). In their series, the thrombi found in 34 patients totaled 76—6 in the pelvic veins, 49 in the thigh veins, and 21 in the leg veins. They found that 75% of the venous thrombi arose in the veins of the thigh and pelvis and 25% in the smaller veins of the calf and feet, with 92% arising in the lower extremities. Similar findings were reported by Beckering and Titus.[1]

Crane[2] concluded that approximately 85% of fatal pulmonary emboli arise in the legs (90% in postsurgical patients and 80% in cardiac or medical patients).

STASIS ULCERS

The chief immediate complication of thrombophlebitis is pulmonary embolus, and the principal long-term complication is stasis ulceration.

The treatment of acute thrombophlebitis attempts to limit the extension of the process and to prevent pulmonary embolization. Elevation, rest with the maintenance of good hydration, elastic support, and possibly anticoagulant therapy are the initial measures. The effectiveness of anticoagulant therapy as usually administered for thromboembolic disease has been questioned.[17] Ligation of the venous system above the area of intravascular clotting is occasionally indicated when lesser measures fail to prevent pulmonary embolus.

As the acute phase of the disease subsides, measures must be taken to avoid later stasis disease in the lower extremity.

The use of elastic supports to help control any dependent edema in the extremity is imperative and may be required for many months or years. With the passage of time, collateral venous channels may develop and communicate with the superficial venous systems, resulting in secondary superficial varicosities. Recanalization of the major deep veins is usually associated with the process. Any significant varicosities in the postphlebitic extremity should be removed.

For reasons not clearly understood, the prevention and control of stasis ulceration are quite difficult in the presence of subcutaneous varicosities. The preventive measures directed toward control of dependent edema are not often carried out by patients suffering from thrombophlebitis, so after several years, cutaneous pigmentation, brawny edema, dermal and subcutaneous fibrosis, extensive secondary varicosities, and ulceration of the skin in the lower one third of

the leg develop. Although stasis ulcers are seen in patients who have a history of past thrombophlebitis, such a history is commonly absent. Even in patients having thrombophlebitis, the exact pathogenesis of the process leading to ulceration is unknown.

The diagnosis of stasis disease is not usually difficult. Only occasionally are ulceration, pigmentation, and surrounding fibrosis confused with other forms of ulceration. Before extensive treatment of a patient with advanced chronic leg ulcer, careful evaluation of the arterial blood supply should be made. Any significant arterial flow deficiency will likely result in failure of surgical therapy for ulceration. Correction of major arterial occlusion should be made when possible, before treatment of the stasis ulcer in those patients in whom both are present. Obviously, the other rare causes of ulceration such as specific infections and neoplasms must

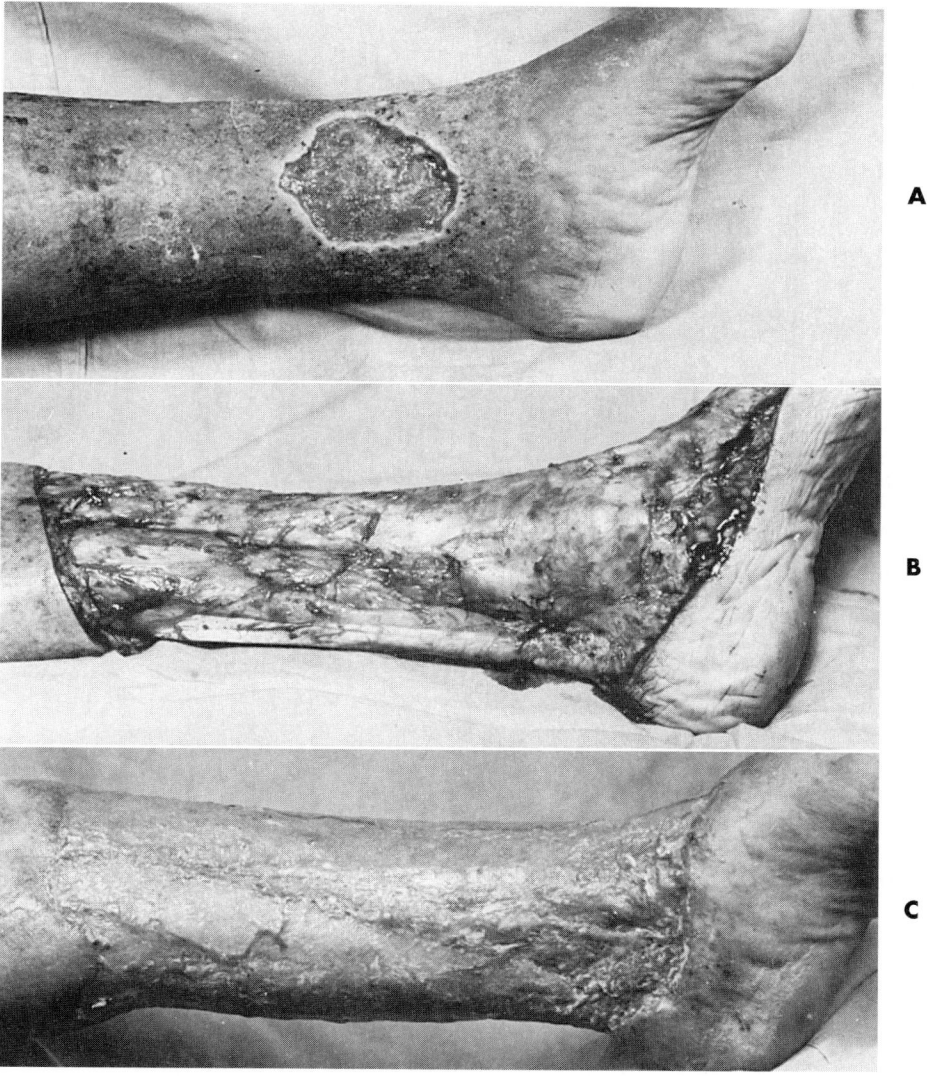

Fig. 27-41 A, Long-standing chronic stasis ulcer refractory to nonoperative therapy. **B,** Fibrotic skin, subcutaneous tissue, and fascia have been widely excised. Periosteum and peritendineum were not removed. **C,** Extremity 2 years after operation.

be excluded. All ulcers should be cultured and any unusual-appearing ones biopsied before excisional therapy is undertaken.

If ulceration has not yet appeared or is not extensive or chronic in nature, the total removal of the varicose veins with ligation of perforating veins may control the process. If stasis ulceration is extensive, chronic, and long standing, it is best treated by excision and stripping of all superficial varicosities of the extremity after high ligation and division of the saphena magna and its tributaries at the saphenous-femoral junction. The ulcer and its base should be excised down to normal tissue, with removal of all the inelastic thickened skin and fascia about it. The cutaneous-fascial defect should then be covered with a partial thickness cutaneous autograft.

The extent of excision often required for advanced stasis ulceration is shown in Fig. 27-41. In most instances, the depth of the excision should include the fascia overlying the muscle, for in the presence of long-standing stasis ulcers, the fascial fibrosis and thickening are quite extensive. This also facilitates ligation of the perforating veins that are invariably present beneath the area of stasis fibrosis.

VARICOSE VEINS

Varicose veins occur more frequently in women than in men. Their incidence is much higher in obese women, particularly those who have had several pregnancies. Varicosities developing in women after pregnancy may be secondary to deep venous thrombosis.

Larson and Smith[19] reported that 213 of 491 patients (43%) had a definite family history of varicose veins, indicating some hereditary disposition. The superficial veins of the leg become dilated and tortuous and lose valvular function. Microscopically, there is fibrosis beneath the endothelium and in the wall, with secondary elastosis and loss of muscle. Calcification may occur.

Primary or simple varicosities often develop in the second and third decades of life and may be present for many years without causing symptoms or complications. The likelihood of thrombosis with propagation into the deep venous system and the likelihood of the development of the postphlebitic syndrome are sufficiently great to warrant the removal of varicose veins. The use of sclerosing agents is contraindicated because of the danger of deep venous thrombosis, as well as the temporary nature of the superficial venous occlusion obtained. The surgical removal of varicosities is best performed by venous stripping techniques and excisions.[18,20]

REFERENCES
THROMBOPHLEBITIS AND THROMBOEMBOLISM

1 Beckering RE Jr, Titus JL: Femoral-popliteal venous thrombosis and pulmonary embolism. Am J Clin Pathol **52**:530-537, 1969.
2 Crane C: Deep venous thrombosis and pulmonary embolism. N Engl J Med **257**:147-157, 1957.
3 DeBakey ME: Critical evaluation of problem of thromboembolism. Int Abstr Surg **98**:1-27, 1954.
4 Hunter WC, Krygier JJ, Kennedy JC, Sneedend VD: Etiology and prevention of thrombosis of the deep leg veins. Surgery **17**:178-190, 1945.
5 Inman WHW, Vessey MP: Investigation of deaths from pulmonary coronary and cerebral thrombosis and embolism in women in childbearing age. Br Med J **2**:193-199, 1968.
6 Irey NS, Manion WC, Taylor HB: Vascular lesions in women taking oral contraceptives. Arch Pathol **89**:1-8, 1970.
7 McCartney JS: Postoperative pulmonary embolism. N Engl J Med **257**:147-157, 1957.
8 McLachlin J, Paterson JC: Some basic observations on venous thrombosis and pulmonary embolism. Surg Gynecol Obstet **93**:1-8, 1951.
9 Mohr DN, Ryu JH, Litin SC, Rosenow EC III: Recent advances in the management of venous thromboembolism. Mayo Clin Proc **63**:281-290, 1988.
10 Ochsner A, DeBakey ME, DeCamp PT: Venous thrombosis, analysis of 580 cases. Surgery **29**:1-20, 1951.
11 Prandoni P, Lensing AW, Buller HR, Cogo A, Prins MH, Cattelan AM, Cuppini S, Noventa F, ten Cate JW: Deep-vein thrombosis and the incidence of subsequent symptomatic cancer. N Engl J Med **327**:1128-1133, 1992.
12 Rössle R: Ueber die Bedeutung und die Entstehung der Wadenvenenthrombosen. Virchows Arch [A] **300**:180-189, 1937.
13 Sartwell PE, Masi AT, Arthes FG, Greene GR, Smith HE: Thromboembolism and oral contraceptives. An epidemiological case-control study. Am J Epidemiol **90**:365-380, 1969.
14 Stallworth JM, Bradham GB, Kletke RR, Price RG Jr: Phlegmasia cerulea dolens. A 10-year review. Ann Surg **161**:802-811, 1965.
15 Stein JM, Pruitt BA Jr: Suppurative thrombophlebitis. A lethal iatrogenic disease. N Engl J Med **282**:1452-1455, 1970.
16 Vessey MP, Doll R: Investigation of relation between use of oral contraceptives and thromboembolic disease. A further report. Br Med J **2**:651-657, 1969.

STASIS ULCERS

17 Butcher HR Jr: Anticoagulant drug therapy for thrombophlebitis in the lower extremities. An evaluation. Arch Surg **80**:864-875, 1960.

VARICOSE VEINS

18 Agrifoglio G, Edwards EA: Results of surgical treatment of varicose veins. JAMA **178**:906-911, 1961.
19 Larson RA, Smith FS: Varicose veins. Evaluation of observations in 491 cases. Mayo Clin Proc **18**:400-408, 1943.
20 Myers TT: Results of the stripping operation in the treatment of varicose veins. Mayo Clin Proc **29**:583-590, 1954.

Lymph vessels

With the exception of tumors of lymph vessels, such as lymphangioma and lymphangiosarcoma (see Chapter 25), the only primary lymphatic disease encountered clinically with some frequency is lymphedema. Chylothorax and chyloascites also occur, but in nearly all instances these processes are secondary to trauma, neoplastic disease, or some infectious process.

LYMPHEDEMA

Lymphedema may be classified as postinfectious, posttraumatic, obstructive, and idiopathic. In some parts of the world, lymphedema resulting from *Schistosoma (Filaria)* is very common.[1] Obstructive lymphedema is most often seen following obstruction of regional lymph nodes by malignant tumor or following node removal, as in radical mastectomy or in radical groin dissection. The development of lymphedema of the arm after radical mastectomy is more common in patients in whom postoperative infection has produced fibrosis in the axilla or in patients having persistent cancer in the axilla. However, lymphedema can also be seen in patients who give a history of as little trauma as a severely sprained ankle or following such infections as a furuncle.

Many patients give no history of trauma or infection associated with the onset of their lymphedema. In such instances, the lymphedema is usually termed idiopathic.[3] This type is further subdivided into *lymphedema congenita, praecox* (beginning before the age of 35 years), and *tarda*.[2,4] Congenital idiopathic lymphedema, also known as Milroy's disease, is inherited as an autosomal dominant trait.

Postmastectomy lymphedema and, to a lesser degree, Milroy's disease can be complicated by the development of lymphangiosarcoma (see Chapter 25). Curiously, this complication is extremely rare in the cases of lymphedema resulting from schistosomiasis, although cases have been described.

Pathology

The obstructive pathogenesis of neoplastic involvement of regional lymph nodes is obvious. Injection techniques combined with magnification radiography have served to delineate accurately normal fine lymphatic channels, as well as tumor involvement[8,9,11] (Fig. 27-42).

The swelling of lymphedema is usually slowly progressive. There is dilatation of the dermal lymphatics, as well as the deeper fascial lymphatics[5] (Fig. 27-43). When the degree of swelling is advanced, there is a depression of hair follicles and gross dermal edema. In such cases, the cutaneous lymphatics may be sufficiently dilated to be associated with lymphorrhea following minor cutaneous abrasions or needle punctures (Fig. 27-44). Tissue sections of such skin usually show markedly dilated dermal lymphatics.

All forms of lymphedema are probably in some way associated with inadequate lymphatic drainage. Drinker and Yaffey[6] postulated that the increased protein content of the lymph present in chronic lymphatic stasis stimulates the deposition of fibrous tissue in the skin, subcutaneous tissue, and fascia. Such fibrosis aggravates the degree of inadequate lymphatic drainage and makes the disease slowly progressive.

Whatever the mechanism, the slowly progressive nature of lymphedema in many patients is associated with dermal thickening and collagenous deposition in the subcutaneous tissues and fascia. Bouts of superficial cellulitis and lymphangitis often become superimposed on the lymphedema in an extremity. In some patients, recurrent bouts of such infections are completely incapacitating. The presence of recurrent infection in such an extremity appears to hasten the deposition of collagen and may result in such a large amount of fibrotic replacement of subcutaneous fat and normal dermal structures as to make demonstration of dermal lymphatics impossible.

Kinmonth et al.[7] reported the presence of dilated, valveless, deep lymphatic channels in idiopathic lymphedema. These were visualized at operation after the injection of patent blue dye and by roentgenologic lymphangiography. Although many varicose-like lymphatic trunks were found in their patients, in none was a definite proximal site of lymphatic channel obstruction discovered.

In a few patients with idiopathic lymphedema having no clinical evidence or history of lymphangitis or cellulitis in the extremity, enlarged regional lymph nodes have been removed. Microscopically, they contain a mild chronic inflammatory response, sinusoidal fibrosis, and markedly dilated lymphatic channels (Fig. 27-45). Direct communication between lymph nodes and veins has been demonstrated.[10]

Treatment

Treatment of lymphedema consists primarily of elevation of the extremity, compression, and massage, which must be maintained during many years of supervision. Recurrent bouts of streptococcal lymphangitis may be prevented by daily administration of antibiotics orally. Such conservative measures will control the lymphedema sufficiently to avoid operation in many patients.[12,13] Operative therapy is indicated only in about 15% of the cases when the extent of subcutaneous fibrosis, infection, and massive swelling is sufficient to markedly handicap the patient.[17,19]

The operation most commonly performed is the excision of the thickened fibrotic skin, the edematous subcutaneous tissue, and the thickened fascia overlying the muscles, followed by the immediate application of split-thickness cutaneous autografts[16,18] (Fig. 27-46). The technique most frequently used is the Kinmonth's modification of Homans' procedure.[15] A second group of operations, referred to as physiologic, aim to provide or enhance lymph drainage[14]; these procedures are controversial and have not met with widespread acceptance.

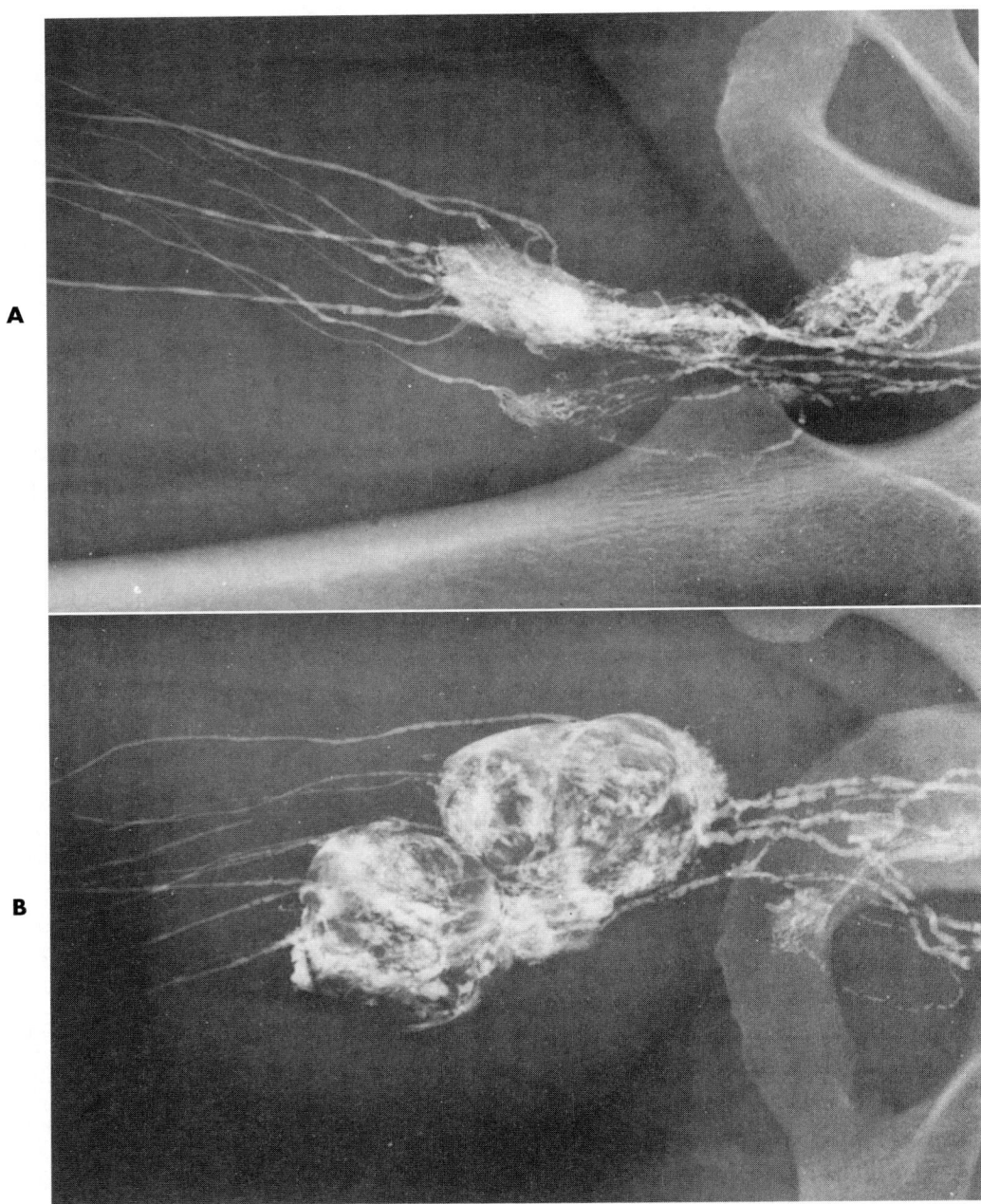

Fig. 27-42 **A,** Magnification radiograph of normal left superficial subinguinal lymph node with afferent and efferent lymphatic channels in 40-year-old woman. **B,** Magnification radiograph of enlarged right superficial subinguinal lymph node with malignant infiltration secondary to primary melanoma of skin of heel. Same patient as shown in **A.** (From Isard HJ, Ostrum BJ, Cullinan JE: Magnification roentgenography. A "spot-film" technic. Med Radiogr Photogr **38:**92-109, 1962.)

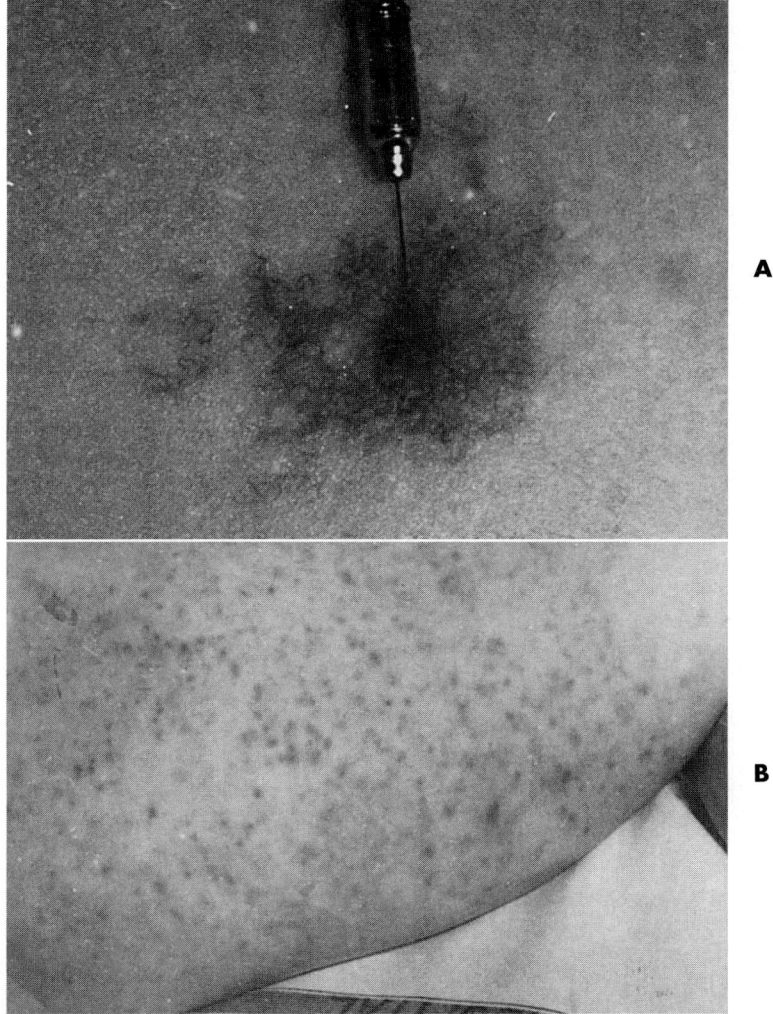

Fig. 27-43 Injection of enlarged cutaneous lymphatics with 4% sky blue dye. Patient had obstructive lymphedema in inguinal region caused by Hodgkin's disease. **A,** Initial injection was made on lateral aspect of thigh. **B,** Four hours after injection, extensive retrograde filling of cutaneous lymphatics on skin of medial thigh had occurred. (From Butcher HR Jr, Hoover AL: Abnormalities of human superficial cutaneous lymphatic cannulation. Ann Surg **142:**633-753, 1955.)

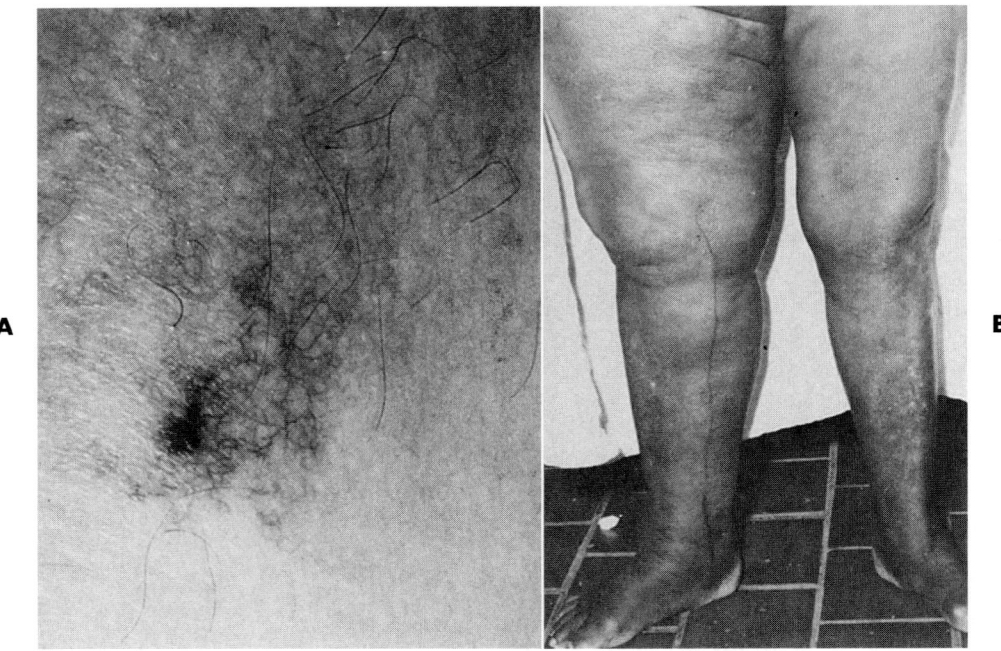

Fig. 27-44 **A,** Dye-filled skin lymphatics in leg of patient with obstructive lymphedema. **B,** Following cutaneous puncture for injection of lymphatics, dye-containing lymph flowed from site. (From Butcher HR Jr, Hoover AL: Abnormalities of human superficial cutaneous lymphatic cannulation. Ann Surg **142:**633-653, 1955.)

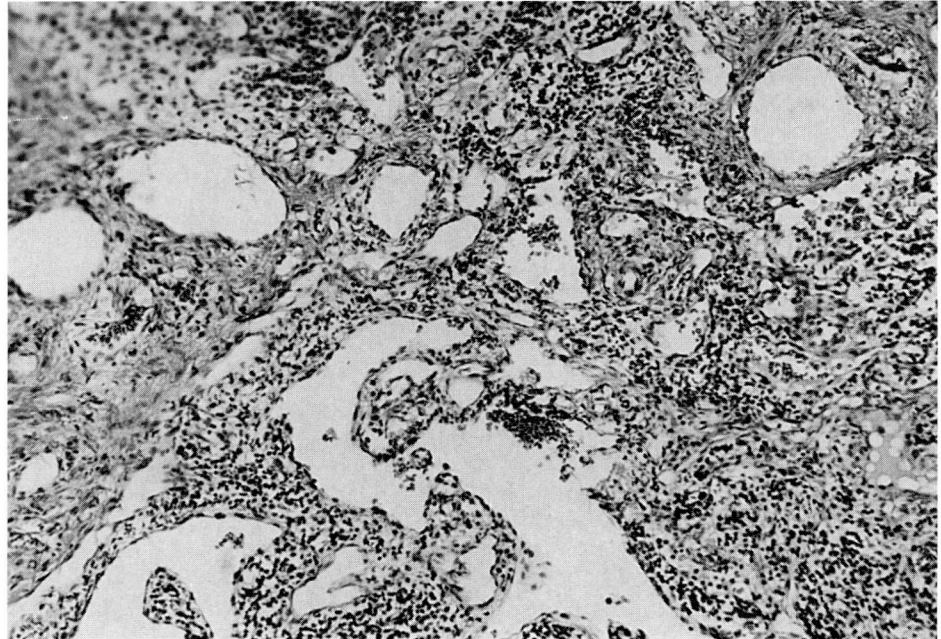

Fig. 27-45 Markedly dilated lymph channels in enlarged lymph node removed from groin of patient with idiopathic lymphedema of obstructive type.

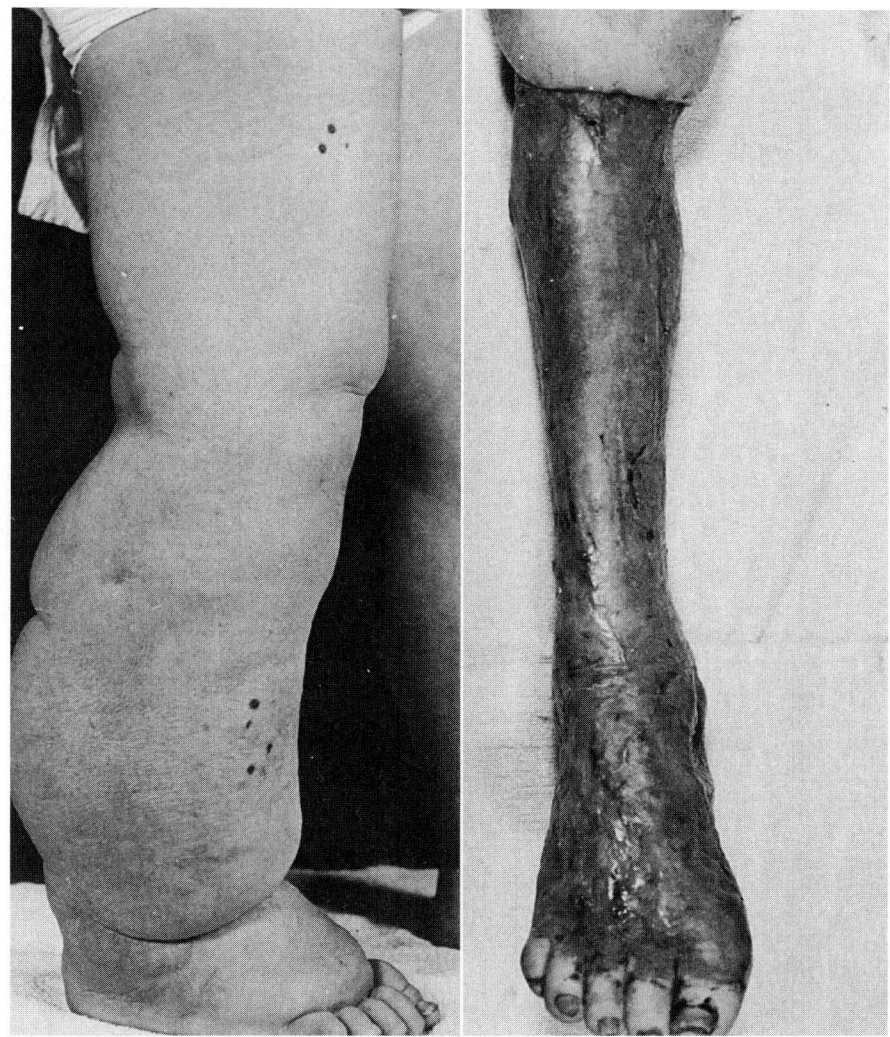

Fig. 27-46 Preoperative and postoperative photographs of patient with long-standing infectious lymphedema. All fibrotic skin, subcutaneous tissue, and fascia were removed, and defect was covered with split-thickness cutaneous autografts. (From Butcher HR Jr, Hoover AL: Abnormalities of human superficial cutaneous lymphatic cannulation. Ann Surg **142:**633-653, 1955.)

In patients with sufficiently severe lymphedema to require excision of the skin, subcutaneous tissue, and fascia of the extremity, gross examination of the excised portions shows dense fibrotic bands and sheets extending through the markedly swollen subcutaneous tissue. Pockets of fluid may be found in the intervening tissue spaces at operation. The skin over the fibrotic dermis may be atrophic in some areas and hyperplastic and keratotic in others. The collagenous thickening of the dermis is usually extreme. Lymphatic channels as such are not often seen histologically in such skin and subcutaneous tissue. This is particularly true if the process has been associated with multiple episodes of dermal infection. Dilated dermal lymphatics may be demonstrated histologically and by dye injection techniques in the skin of a lymphedematous extremity unassociated with long-standing episodes of infection (Fig. 27-47).

The dermal and subcutaneous fibrosis similar to that seen in advanced forms of lymphedema also occurs about long-standing chronic stasis ulcers. The obliteration of dermal lymphatics, however, cannot be related primarily to the etiology of stasis ulcers since similar obliteration occurs in the fibrotic skin of long-standing lymphedema, a condition rarely associated with chronic ulceration of the lower extremity.

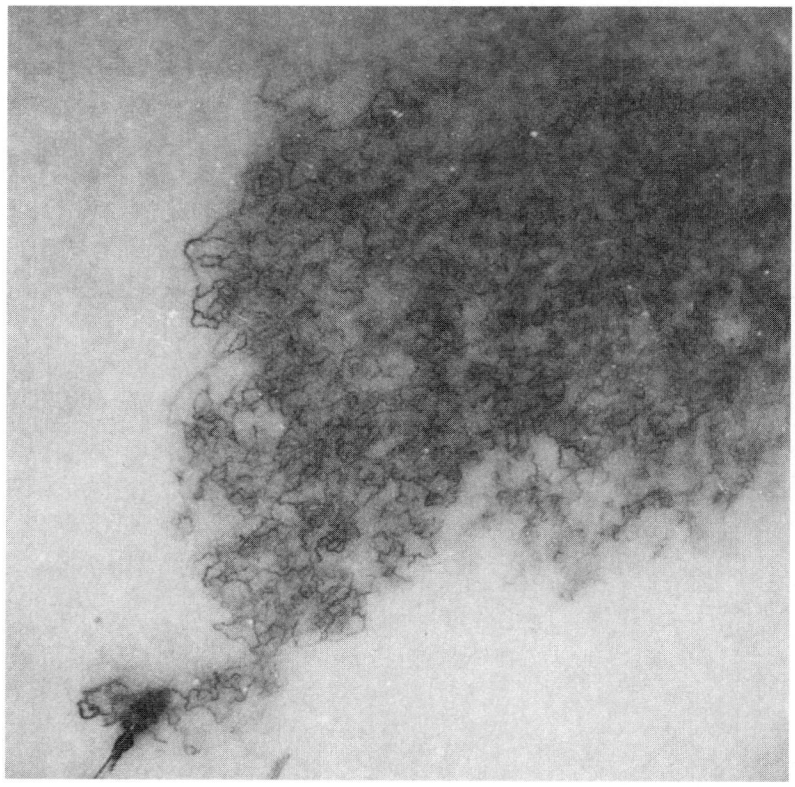

Fig. 27-47 Unusually dilated superficial cutaneous lymphatics in skin of patient with idiopathic lymphedema. (From Butcher HR Jr, Hoover AL: Abnormalities of human superficial cutaneous lymphatic cannulation. Ann Surg **142:**633-653, 1955.)

REFERENCES

LYMPHEDEMA

1 Dandapat MC, Mohapatro SK, Mohanty SS: Filarial lymphoedema and elephantiasis of lower limb. A review of 44 cases. Br J Surg **73:**451-453, 1986.
2 Lewis JM, Wald ER: Lymphedema praecox. J Pediatr **104:**641-648, 1984.
3 Schirger A, Harrison EG Jr, Janes JM: Idiopathic lymphedema. JAMA **182:**124-132, 1962.
4 Smeltzer DM, Stickler GB, Schirger A: Primary lymphedema in children and adolescents. A follow-up study and review. Pediatrics **76:**206-218, 1985.

Pathology

5 Butcher HR Jr, Hoover AL: Abnormalities of human superficial cutaneous lymphatics associated with stasis ulcers, lymphedema, scars and cutaneous autografts. Ann Surg **142:**633-653, 1955.
6 Drinker CK, Yaffey JM: Lymphatics, lymph and lymphoid tissue. Their physiological and clinical significance. Cambridge, Mass, 1941, Harvard University Press.
7 Kinmonth JB, Taylor GW, Tracy GD, Marsh JD: Primary lymphoedema. Clinical and lymphangiographic studies of a series of 107 patients in which the lower limbs were affected. Br J Surg **95:**1-10, 1957.
8 McPeak CJ, Constantinides SG: Lymphangiography in malignant melanoma. A comparison of clinicopathologic and lymphangiographic findings in 21 cases. Cancer **17:**1586-1594, 1964.

9 Pomerantz M, Ketcham AS: Lymphangiography and its surgical applications. Surgery **53:**589-597, 1963.
10 Pressman JJ, Simon MB: Experimental evidence of direct communications between lymph nodes and veins. Surgery **113:**537-541, 1961.
11 Wallace S: Dynamics of normal and abnormal lymphatic systems as studied with contrast media. Cancer Chemother Rep **52:**31-58, 1968.

Treatment

12 Browse NL: The diagnosis and management of primary lymphedema. J Vasc Surg **3:**181-184, 1986.
13 Foldi E, Foldi M, Weissleder H: Conservative treatment of lymphoedema of the limbs. Angiology **36:**171-180, 1985.
14 Huang GK, Hu RQ, Liu ZZ, Shen YL, Lan TD, Pan GP: Microlymphaticovenous anastomosis in the treatment of lower limb obstructive lymphedema. Analysis of 91 cases. Plast Reconstr Surg **76:**671-685, 1985.
15 Kinmonth JB: The lymphatics. Surgery, lymphography and disease of the chyle and lymph systems, ed 2. London, 1982, Edward Arnold Ltd.
16 Savage RC: The surgical management of lymphedema. Surg Gynecol Obstet **160:**283-290, 1985.
17 Schirger A, Harrison EG Jr, Janes JM: Idiopathic lymphedema. JAMA **182:**124-132, 1962.
18 Servelle M: Surgical treatment of lymphedema. A report of 652 cases. Surgery **101:**485-495, 1987.
19 Thompson N: Surgical treatment of chronic lymphedema of extremities. Surg Clin North Am **47:**445-503, 1967.

28 Neuromuscular system

Marc K. Rosenblum, Juan M. Bilbao, and L.C. Ang

Central nervous system
Peripheral nerves
Skeletal muscle

Central nervous system

Marc K. Rosenblum, M.D.

ACKNOWLEDGMENTS: To Joy Ivry, who uncomplainingly prepared the manuscript and even encouraged all along the way; Kin Kong, expert (and patient) medical photographer principally responsible for the illustrations used in this chapter; Dr. Robert Erlandson, kind purveyor of the included electron photomicrographs (unless otherwise stated in the accompanying legends); Dr. Rosemary Purrazzella, my wife, and our children, Julia and Michael, who forbore—for whatever satisfaction they may bring, the author's thanks and apologies.

NORMAL ANATOMY

Dauntingly complex and characterized by extraordinary variation in regional architecture, the gross and microscopic anatomy of the human central nervous system (CNS) cannot be surveyed here in any methodic fashion. We preface this account of neurosurgical pathology with a brief review of those anatomic landmarks and topographic relationships that bear particularly on issues of differential diagnosis. The cellular composition of the brain, the spinal cord, and their coverings are addressed only insofar as these topics are relevant to the current nosology of primary neoplasms arising in these locations, whereas considerations of traditional neurohistochemistry and immunohistology are deferred to those sections of this chapter dealing with specific tumor types and non-neoplastic conditions (e.g., demyelinating disease) that require application of such techniques for definitive classification.

Confined within the cranium and vertebral canal, the CNS is sheathed by connective tissue membranes that include a densely collagenous outer covering termed the pachymeninx or, more familiarly, dura mater and delicate inner investments known as the leptomeninges or pia-arachnoid. Under normal circumstances, these are closely apposed and loosely joined by a layer of dural border cells that are easily disrupted (artefactually or by expanding lesions such as hematomas) to yield a "subdural" space that is, in fact, only a potential tissue compartment. A sagittal dural fold referred to as the *falx cerebri* lies between the cerebral hemispheres, a second such fold—the *tentorium cerebelli*—separating the superior cerebellar surfaces from the cerebrum's overlying temporal lobes. Enclosed within the cranial dura, in addition to meningeal artery branches, are venous sinuses that serve both to drain the cerebral veins and to carry away cerebrospinal fluid (CSF) transported from the subarachnoid space by arachnoid villi that project into these conduits. Termed *pacchionian granulations* as they achieve grossly visible proportions with normal aging, these villi are draped by specialized arachnoidal cells of interest to surgical pathologists as the likely progenitors of the meningioma, a relatively common, dural-based neoplasm. Whereas the dura adheres tightly to the endosteal surfaces of the skull, at the spinal levels, it is attached only anteriorly to the vertebral bodies and is surrounded on its lateral and posterior aspects by a true compartment—the *epidural space*—which contains segments of the spinal nerve roots, blood vessels, and a very modest amount of adipose tissue.

We introduce at this juncture several localizing terms current in clinical parlance that encode information of potential utility to the pathologist and that may be encountered in neuroimaging reports and on specimen requisitions. Because the substance of the brain and spinal cord constitute the central "neuraxis," lesions localized to the neuroparenchyma proper are often described as *intra-axial,* whereas those that simply abut the CNS from a meningeal or juxtameningeal site are said to be *extra-axial.* The qualifiers *intramedullary* or *extramedullary* may be further invoked for masses lying within or adjacent to the spinal cord, respectively. The brain itself may be broadly but usefully parcelled into *supratentorial* versus *infratentorial* components, the former situated above and the latter below the tentorium cerebelli. The cerebellum and most of the brainstem, including the pons and medulla in their entirely, are infratentorial structures that may be collectively designated the posterior fossa contents.

The supratentorial CNS consists of the cerebrum (subdivided into frontal, parietal, temporal, and occipital lobes) and deep nuclei of the basal ganglia, thalamus, and hypothalamus.

Within the CNS, connective tissue is scant and essentially restricted to the adventitia of blood vessels. There are no resident lymphoid elements. The parenchyma of the brain and spinal cord is composed principally of the bodies and cytoplasmic processes of neuroepithelial cell types, including neurons and the various classes of glia. Subsumed under the latter designation are the nervous system's supporting astrocytes, its myelinating oligodendrocytes, and the ependymal cells that line ventricular surfaces. These all have their neoplastic counterparts, classified generically as gliomas and subclassified as astrocytomas, oligodendrogliomas, and ependymomas, respectively. Close kin of the ependyma are the specialized epithelial elements of the choroid plexus, which are responsible for the production of CSF and are represented among brain tumors by papillomas and carcinomas. The neurosecretory parenchymal cells of the pineal gland, situated posterior to the midbrain's tectal plate, may also be the targets of transformative events—thus the pineoblastoma and pineocytoma.

We close this necessarily truncated summary on a practical note. There can be no gainsaying the importance of lesion location in the formulation of differential clinical and histologic diagnoses, particularly when tumors are at issue. Meningioma, for example, should be a remote consideration for the pathologist confronted by neurosurgical material from an intra-axial mass but looms large if the lesion in question is dural based or fills the cerebellopontine angle (where schwannoma might also be reasonably suspected). By contrast, astrocytomas of diffuse fibrillary type, oligodendrogliomas, and metastatic carcinoma account for most cerebral hemispheric tumors (particularly in adulthood). Pilocytic astrocytomas, which mainly affect young persons, exhibit a decided predilection for the cerebellum and third ventricular/hypothalamic region, whereas ependymomas frequent the fourth ventricles of children and the spinal cords of adults (where they constitute the most common intramedullary tumors). Primary CNS lymphomas are most often situated within deep, periventricular white matter structures or the basal ganglia, whereas germ cell tumors only exceptionally arise outside of a midline, pineal region–suprasellar axis and central neurocytomas are typically confined within the lateral ventricles. In a similar vein, the distal spinal cord's tapering conus medullaris and filum terminale are the nearly exclusive hosts of myxopapillary ependymomas and CNS paragangliomas. Many other examples of regional CNS vulnerability to particular tumor types and non-neoplastic lesions are to be found in the rest of this chapter. The foregoing should serve to underscore the potential benefits of a dialog among pathologists, neuroradiologists, and neurosurgeons.

CONGENITAL ABNORMALITIES
Craniospinal dysraphism

Defective midline closure of the embryonic neural tube or its mesodermally derived coverings accounts for the varied malformations collectively referred to as *dysraphic states.* Expressions of craniospinal dysraphism range from trivial skeletal abnormalities that pass undetected through life to lethal anomalies of the nervous system proper that result in intrauterine fetal demise. Considered here are those representatives of this complex group most likely to be approached by the neurosurgeon.

The large majority of dysraphic malformations occur along the spinal axis, where they are chiefly localized, although by no means restricted, to the lumbosacral region.[1,7] The minimal lesion—simple agenesis of the posterior vertebral arches—ranks among the most prevalent of congenital anomalies and is termed *spina bifida occulta.* Its presence may be suggested in otherwise asymptomatic cases by the finding of an overlying skin dimple or sinus tract, hyperpigmented patch, hairy tuft, angioma, or lipoma. Spina bifida cystica or aperta refers to the less common situation in which meningeal or neural tissues protrude through the osseous defect. The resulting lesion, generically designated a "cystocele," typically bulges from the posterior midline in saccular fashion and is subclassified according to the nature of its herniated elements, the major variants being meningocele and meningomyelocele. The latter, by definition, contains elements derived from the spinal cord, as well as its ensheathing meninges, and accounts for 80% to 90% of dysraphic cystoceles complicating spina bifida.[1,7] Cystoceles may also present as ventrally positioned, pelvic, or laterally situated, paravertebral masses. The former are associated with sacral defects, the latter with hemivertebrae. It should be noted, however, that most "lateral meningoceles" are not true dysraphic lesions; instead they represent arachnoidal diverticula that exit the spinal canal via widened neural foramina. These are most common at the thoracic levels and are often encountered in the setting of type 1 neurofibromatosis.[6] Rarely, meningomyeloceles present as tail-like appendages in the low sacral region.[3]

The resected *meningocele* is a discoid mass covered on its external aspect by skin that may be attenuated but that is not usually ulcerated or otherwise disrupted. A narrow pedicle representing the cystocele's attachment to the spinal canal may hang from its smooth, membranous inner surface. The sac proper is composed of collagenous tissue containing meningothelial cells disposed along irregular clefts, around alveolar spaces, in nests and long cords. Distinct dural and arachnoid membranes are not formed. Some examples are associated with tumorous accumulations of mature adipose tissue ("lipomeningocele"), and the sac wall may also exhibit a disorganized proliferation of nerve twigs, smooth muscle bundles, and blood vessels. Displaced but otherwise normal spinal nerve roots may lie within the meningocele cavity but can often be successfully repositioned and thus do not usually appear in surgical specimens. The finding of neuroglial tissue in any form mandates a diagnosis of *meningomyelocele.*[1] This ranges in volume and organization from microscopic nests of glia embedded in the cystocele's wall to recognizable, albeit deformed, spinal cord. Variants include the lipomeningomyelocele and the syringomyelocele (or myelocystocele), the latter characterized by gross distention of its included spinal cord's central canal. Rarely, meningomyeloceles are encountered in complex with intraspinal cysts lined by enteric epithelium—the so-called split notochord syndrome[5]—or with bona fide teratomas.[10] In any of these guises, the meningomyelocele is often covered by little more than a translucent membrane that represents atretic cutis and may contain plaques of ependymoglial tissue. This is prone to ulceration and predisposes to bacterial invasion of the CSF with ascending meningoventricular infection.

The outcome for infants afflicted by spina bifida cystica depends on the size and complexity of the malformation, particularly on the extent to which spinal cord elements participate in its genesis, and is frequently influenced by the presence of associated anomalies involving the spinal cord rostral to the cystocele, the cranium, and brain.[1,7] Simple meningoceles are often unassociated with neurologic debility or attended by relatively mild paraparesis, are generally closed without incident, and only exceptionally prove fatal. Unfortunately, the far more common meningomyelocele is usually complicated by significant and irreversible impairment of lower extremity and bladder function. Furthermore, nearly all affected children also suffer an associated Arnold-Chiari malformation with hydrocephalus, the main structural features of this second anomaly being caudal displacement of the medulla and cerebellar vermis, kinking of the cervicomedullary junction, widening and shallowing of the posterior fossa, and in many instances, deformation of the midbrain and aqueductal stenosis. Untreated, few patients survive childhood, and even with aggressive surgical intervention the mortality rate ranges from 30% to 60%. The leading immediate causes of death are meningitis, pyelonephritis, pneumonia, and progressive hydrocephalus. Rarely, squamous carcinomas arise from the chronically irritated epidermis overlying unattended cystoceles.[2]

To the externally evident malformations just described should be added various intraspinal and juxtaspinal anomalies, often referred to as occult or "closed" dysraphisms, that similarly occur in complex with spina bifida and its cutaneous stigmata but are imperceptible on physical examination because of their deep location. These, too, exhibit a decided predilection for the lumbosacral region, where they are typically discovered on neuroradiologic evaluation for myelopathy. It is fixation of the filum terminale or spinal roots to these abnormal structures, with resulting traction on the cord (as evidenced by displacement of the conus medullaris below the level of the L2 vertebral body), that is often responsible for their principal neurologic manifestations—disturbed gait, bladder spasticity or hypotonia, and anococcygeal and perineal pain. Maldevelopmental lesions that may present as this *"tethered cord" syndrome*[1,4] include intraspinal lipomas; dermoid, epidermoid, or hindgut cysts; intrasacral meningeal diverticula ("occult meningoceles"); and cystic intradural masses composed of neuroglial tissue ("occult meningomyeloceles"). The dividing collagenous or chondro-osseous septum characteristically present in cases of congenitally split spinal cord (diastematomyelia) is yet another potentially tethering anomaly, whereas the offending lesion in some instances is simply a short filum (typically thickened owing to fatty infiltration) or a fibrous band extending into the exposed spinal canal from the sacral subcutis. The latter is often associated with a telltale skin dimple or dermal sinus and may rarely exhibit a hamartomatous proliferation of included pacinian corpuscles.[1] Fortunately, many of the tethered cord's associated malformations are amenable to surgical correction, division of the immobilized

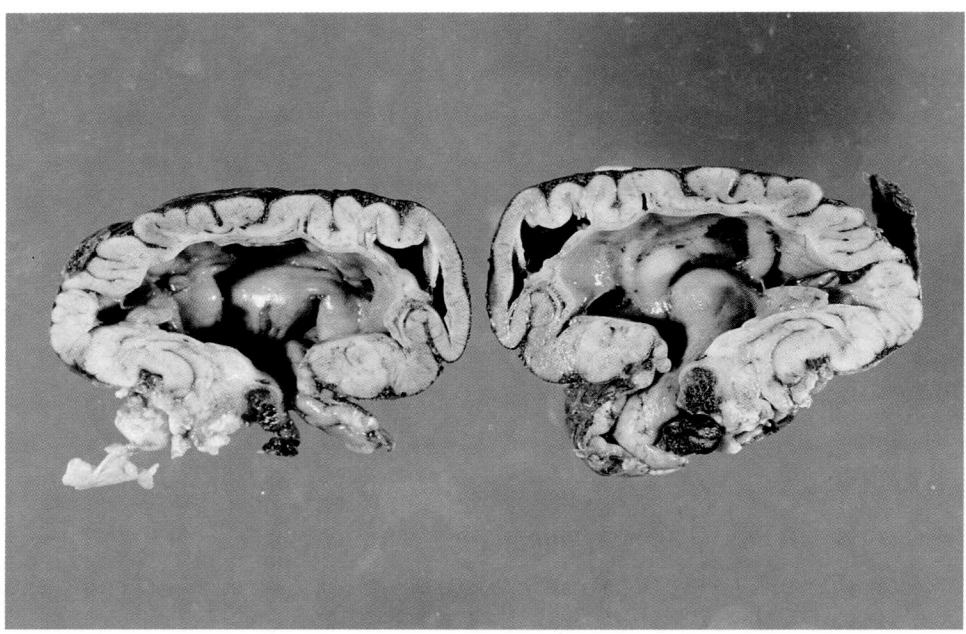

Fig. 28-1 Encephalocele. A well-developed, gyriform cortical mantle characterizes this neurosurgical specimen from the occipital region of a newborn. (Courtesy Dr. Humberto Cravioto, New York.)

filum frequently resulting in substantial neurologic improvement and relief of pain.[4]

A distant second in incidence to the dysraphic cystoceles of the lumbosacral region are those involving the cranium. These, too, hug the midline and, like their spinal counterparts, may contain meningeal derivatives alone or associated neural tissues. The latter, termed *encephaloceles*, vastly predominate. Approximately 80% of encephaloceles exit the cranial cavity in the region of the occiput via defects in the posterior wall of the foramen magnum or occipital bone.[7,9] These are generally covered by intact scalp, subjacent to which are recognizable dural and leptomeningeal membranes, and may contain choroid plexus, cerebellar, and brainstem elements in addition to substantial volumes of cerebral hemispheric tissue (Fig. 28-1). The extruded brain, which encloses a central CSF-filled chamber that may communicate freely with the ventricular system, can appear remarkably well formed but commonly exhibits microscopic abnormalities of cortical architecture, if not grossly anomalous gyration, and its covering leptomeninges frequently contain islands of heterotopic neuroglial tissue. Vascular compression at the level of the encephalocele's narrow intraosseous neck may result in secondary alterations such as hemorrhage and infarction. Excision and closure can often be effected without complication, but a regrettably large percentage of occipital encephaloceles are attended by malformations of the intracranial contents, microcephaly, and mental retardation.

Extraoccipital encephaloceles may protrude through defects in other portions of the cranial vault or bulge into the anterior or posterior fontanels but are more commonly of the sincipital or basilar types.[7,9] Sincipital encephaloceles present as visible facial swellings in the region of the forehead, nasal bridge, or orbit, whereas basal variants are situated in the nasal cavity, sphenoid sinus, nasopharynx, or pterygopalatine fossa and therefore are not externally evident. The latter group includes the transethmoidal encephaloceles that herniate through defects in the cribriform plate and constitute the most common polypoid intranasal masses encountered in the newborn. Prior to biopsy or resection, a subcutaneous or submucosal mass in any of these locations must be carefully evaluated for evidence of extension into the cranial cavity. Inasmuch as the encephalocele communicates with the subarachnoid space via its associated osseous defect, intracranial repair with dural closure is required if CSF leakage and meningitis are to be avoided. Simple neuroglial heterotopias occurring in these same regions, by contrast, are defined as maintaining no open connection to the intracranial compartment and thus may be safely approached transnasally or transorally, depending on their precise situation. These are addressed separately later in this chapter. Suffice it to say that the results of neuroimaging study are often decisive in the classification of a given lesion because both the heterotopia and true encephalocele often consist solely of aggregated astroglia embedded in fibrous tissue. Either may contain admixed neurons. Heterotopias of the nasal region rarely if ever harbor ependymal elements, a feature of some encephaloceles, but these may be encountered in examples situated in other sincipital or basilar locations. Included meninges are an inconstant feature of specimens derived from extraoccipital encephaloceles, but, when identified, exclude heterotopia from further consideration.

Although this discussion is restricted to congenital anomalies, it should be noted that meningoceles and encephaloceles may be the acquired consequences of trauma or preceding neurosurgical procedures. "Endaural" examples may complicate chronic otitis media or mastoiditis and have recently been described as a late effect of cranial irradiation in childhood.[8]

Neuroglial and meningeal heterotopias

The *neuroglial heterotopia,* introduced in the preceding discussion of cranial dysraphism, is a displaced mass of mature central neuroepithelial tissue unconnected to the brain proper. Leptomeningeal examples constitute occasional incidental findings on postmortem examination and are frequently noted in association with major structural anomalies of the underlying nervous system (e.g., craniospinal cystoceles).[15] These are of little clinical import save for their hypothesized role as progenitors of the odd primary leptomeningeal glioma. Similarly, intrapulmonary neuroglial rests are an autopsy curiosity virtually restricted to fetuses and neonates harboring severe neural tube defects such as anencephaly.[17] The heterotopias most likely to engage the surgical pathologist frequent the same locations favored by sincipital and basal encephaloceles—the bridge of the nose and nasal cavity, paranasal sinuses, palatal region, and nasopharynx—and are probably best regarded as "sequestered" variants of their obviously dysraphic counterparts.[19] By far the most common of these maldevelopmental lesions is the so-called nasal glioma, addressed in Chapter 7. Neuroglial heterotopias may also present in the cranial bones, scalp, orbit, and submandibular region.[19] Their structure varies. Most consist solely of solid glial nests embedded in fibrous tissues, only about 10% containing neurons and these rarely in abundance. Astrocytes usually predominate and are often the only neuroepithelial elements present in nasal examples. Pharyngeal lesions are typically more complex, often containing ependyma-lined clefts and choroid plexus–like formations. Pigmented neuroepithelial structures suggesting retinal differentiation may also be encountered in the latter. An intraorbital heterotopia composed of cerebellar tissue is on record.[13]

The neuroglial nature of the lesions under discussion is usually obvious in routinely prepared histologic sections but may be confirmed in a questionable case by immunolabeling of the heterotopia's matrix and included astrocytic elements with antibodies to glial fibrillary acidic protein (GFAP).[19] The distinction of these rests from encephaloceles, a matter of considerable clinical significance, has already been addressed in the discussion of craniospinal dysraphism. It should be noted that neuroglial heterotopias occasionally exhibit worrisome cytologic abnormalities and troubling hypercellularity but are generally cured by simple excision. Even the small percentage that have reportedly recurred have been controlled with conservative local reoperation. Rare heterotopias interpreted as having undergone focal neoplastic transformation are to be found in the literature. The diminutive neoplasms purported to arise in this setting have included an oligodendroglioma,[12] a mixed glioma composed of oligodendroglial and astrocytic elements,[16] and a melanotic neuroectodermal tumor of infancy.[18] A probable instance of frontal lobe astrocytoma penetrating the cribriform plate to masquerade as a nasal glial heterotopia has also been depicted.[14]

In contrast to some sincipital and basal encephaloceles, neuroglial heterotopias do not contain elements derived from the meninges. Displaced meningothelium, however, may be encountered in curious lesions of the scalp variously interpreted as hamartomas or as meningeal dysraphias that have lost their connection to the intracranial compartment in the course of development ("sequestered meningoceles").[11,20] These *extracranial meningeal heterotopias* are often noted at birth but may not come to surgical attention until adulthood. They are situated most often in the dermis or subcutis of the midline occipital region, at the vertex, in the posterior fontanel, or overlying the lambdoid suture. Regional alopecia is a common associated finding. The lesion consists of collagenous tissue containing irregular slit-like spaces lined by flattened meningothelial cells. These may also form solid cords or, rarely, small nests. Central neuroepithelial derivatives are not present, but islands of necrotic cellular material that could conceivably represent degenerated neuroglial components have been described in some cases. Extracranial meningeal heterotopias may be misconstrued as melanocytic lesions, lymphangiomas, or even angiosarcomas but can be distinguished in problematic cases by their expression of epithelial membrane antigen on immunocytochemical assay. Although neoplastic transformation has not been described, these maldevelopmental lesions could theoretically serve as precursors to the rare bona fide meningiomas arising in the scalp. These are addressed along with other ectopic meningiomas in the discussion of meningothelial tumors.

The reader is referred to the section dealing with ependymal neoplasms for comment on myxopapillary ependymal rests of the sacrococcygeal region and their relationship to extramedullary ependymomas.

Choristomas

Maldevelopmental rests composed of tissues foreign to the nervous system—**"choristomas"**—are only rarely encountered within the confines of the dura mater. *Ecchordosis physaliphora* is the term used to describe an intracranial heterotopia exhibiting the histologic and ultrastructural features characteristic of the notochord and its neoplastic offspring, the chordoma.[23] Ecchordoses are typically situated just ventral to the belly of the pons, are frequently connected to notochordal remnants in the adjacent clivus via attenuated transdural stalks, and usually take the form of bosselated, gelatinous nodules loosely adherent to the basilar artery. They generally measure no more than 1 to 2 cm in greatest dimension and, for the most part, are autopsy curiosities. Whether some larger, symptomatic examples are best regarded as "giant" ecchordoses or as bona fide intradural chordomas is controversial (see the section on chordoma). *Leptomeningeal rhabdomyomatosis* refers to microscopic aggregates of mature striated myofibers characteristically located in the prepontine region or cerebellopontine angles.[22] These may, in addition, harbor well-differentiated adipocytes, displaced neuroglial tissue, and aberrant peripheral nerve fibers and are usually detected in complex with major developmental anomalies of the CNS. Rarely, choristomatous nodules composed of striated[28] or smooth muscle[24] are encountered in cranial nerve divisions. Also on record are

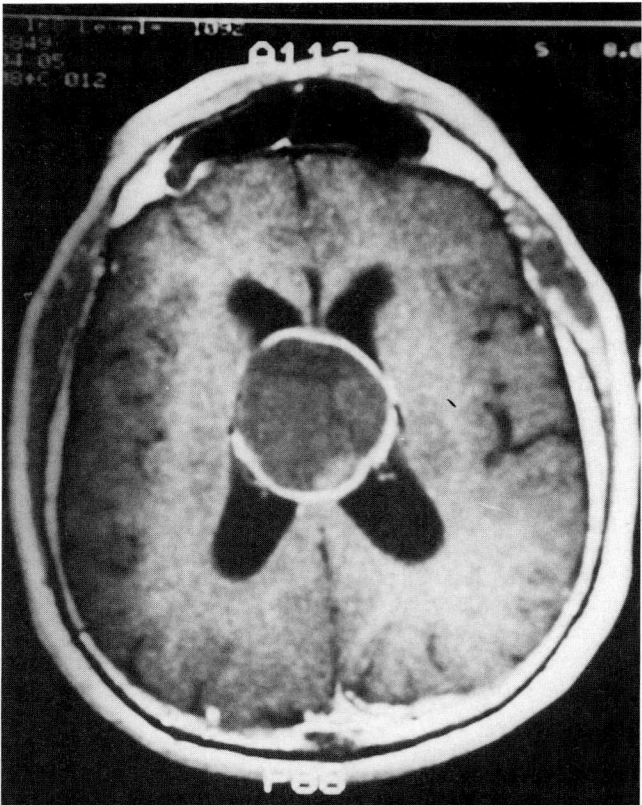

Fig. 28-2 Colloid cyst. The obstructive ventricular dilatation (hydrocephalus) associated with this large example is characteristic of these lesions. Note the well-delineated cyst wall, bright in this contrast-enhanced magnetic resonance image.

several müllerian choristomas of the lumbosacral region associated with spina bifida, one intradural example containing endometrium, endocervical glands, and smooth muscle bundles.[26] We mention here isolated depictions of intracerebral[27] and intraspinal[25] endometriosis, although these are properly regarded as acquired, rather than developmental, lesions. Finally, there is the bizarre account of a minute adenoid cystic carcinoma arising in a cerebellopontine angle mass otherwise composed of mature salivary gland tissue.[21]

Cysts of the central neuraxis

This section considers various non-neoplastic lesions, maldevelopmental or secondarily acquired, only some of which qualify as "true" (i.e., epithelium-lined) cysts. Chief among the latter are the *colloid cysts* of the anterosuperior third ventricle.[40] These generally present in the third through fifth decades of life with manifestations of ventricular outflow obstruction, a consequence of their intimate relation to the foramen of Monro (Fig. 28-2). Thin-walled and often draped by adherent choroid plexus, colloid cysts are filled with a viscous, mucoid material that rapidly congeals on fixation (Fig. 28-3). Their lining epithelium is prone to a low cuboidal attenuation resulting from pressure exerted by the cyst contents but when well preserved is found to be of columnar type and is frequently populated by ciliated and

goblet cell elements (Fig. 28-4). Only a basement membrane, inapparent at the light microscopic level, separates these from a delicate, fibrous capsule. The cyst contents are PAS positive and commonly include the hyphae-like aggregates of degenerate nucleoproteins so characteristic of this entity as to be diagnostic in the absence of identifiable epithelium[41] (Fig. 28-5). An inflammatory reaction to the contents of ruptured colloid cysts is responsible for most, if not all, cases of so-called xanthogranuloma situated in the third ventricle.[39]

Ultrastructural[32] and immunocytochemical[35,37,42] investigations of the colloid cyst have rendered untenable its traditional classification as a neuroepithelial derivative, suggesting instead an origin from misplaced endodermal tissues. Its constituent epithelial cell types correspond closely to those typical of respiratory mucosae, sport an apical glycocalyx coating particularly characteristic of endodermally derived epithelia, and express cytokeratin, epithelial membrane antigen, and carcinoembryonic antigen but not GFAP or the choroid plexus–associated transthyretin (prealbumin). Their occasional designation as "neuroepithelial" notwithstanding, similar histogenetic considerations apply to rare cysts of comparable structure situated within the posterior fossa,[30,31] cerebral hemispheres or interhemispheric fissure,[36] and optic nerve.[34] Although properly treated in the context of pituitary disorders (see Chapter 29), the Rathke cleft cyst,[43] a lesion having its origin in remnants of the stomodeum, is briefly noted here for the striking resemblance of its lining epithelium to that of the colloid cyst. Curiously, however, the latter rarely contains the metaplastic squamous elements common to Rathke cleft cysts and other cystic intracranial lesions putatively of endodermal lineage.

Intraspinal cysts resulting, in all likelihood, from the incomplete separation of developing endodermal and notochordal tissues in early embryonic life have been variously designated as "neurenteric," "foregut," "enterogenous," and "teratomatous."[29] These intradural extramedullary lesions are typically situated anterior to the spinal cord, are often associated with local vertebral abnormalities, and may be encountered in complex with other evidences of faulty development such as intestinal reduplication and dermal sinuses.[38] Most exhibit a simple mural structure and columnar epithelial lining similar to that of the colloid cyst, but occasional examples are endowed with a specialized respiratory or gastroenteric-type "mucosa" and the organized supporting elements (e.g., seromucinous glands, muscularis, cartilaginous rings, ganglion cells) of the developed alimentary tract or tracheobronchial tree.[33]

Two major variants of ectodermally derived neuraxis cyst are recognized, both lined by keratinizing squamous epithelium. The *epidermoid cyst,* by definition, is devoid of cutaneous-type adnexal structures and filled by friable, often lamellated keratinous debris that radiates a pearly sheen when viewed through the lesion's thin fibrous capsule. *Dermoid cysts,* by contrast, are endowed with skin appendages, including pilosebaceous units, eccrine and, occasionally, apocrine glands, as well as mural adipose tissue foreign to their epidermoid counterparts. They may contain a greasy, yellowish-gray material admixed with hairs or just friable, keratin-rich debris similar to that of their epidermoid counterparts (Fig. 28-6). Cysts of both types are, for the most part, maldevelopmental in origin, presumably arising from sur-

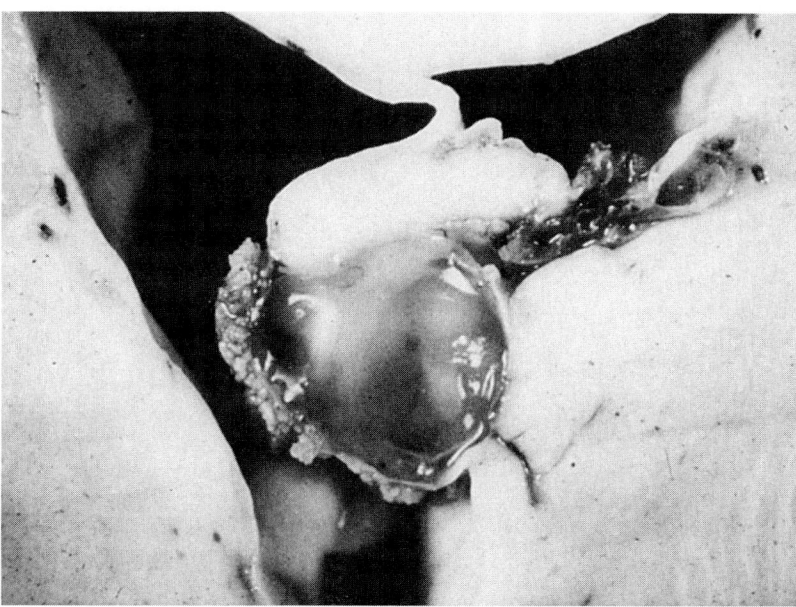

Fig. 28-3 Colloid cyst. Demonstrated here is the colloid cyst's typical location in the anterosuperior third ventricle at the level of the interventricular foramina of Monro. Note the draping choroid plexus. (Courtesy Dr. J.E. Olvera-Rabiela, Mexico City.)

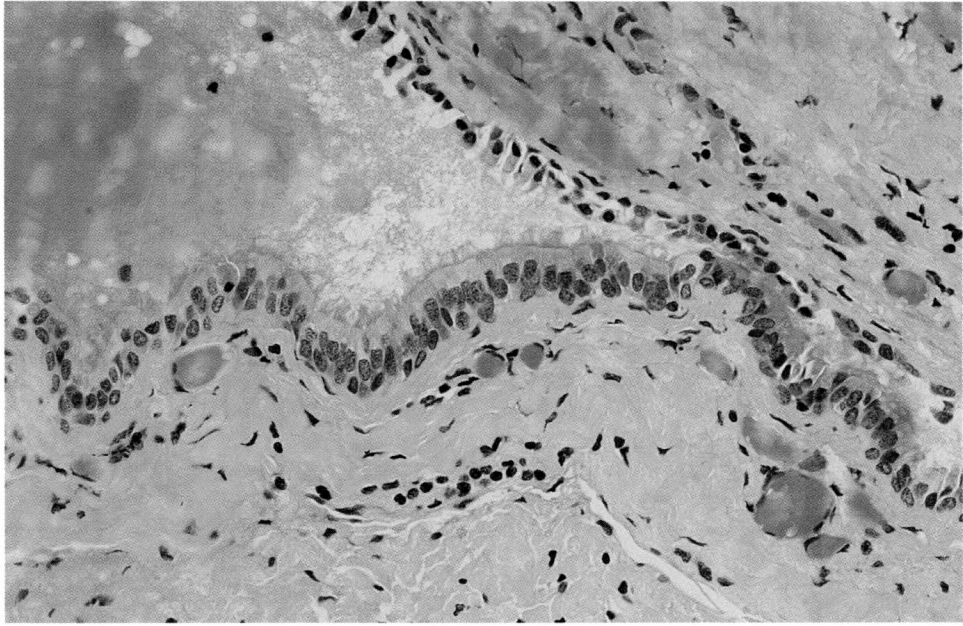

Fig. 28-4 Colloid cyst. A pseudostratified and ciliated columnar epithelium lines well-preserved colloid cysts. Note the supporting collagenous tissue of the cyst wall, yellow in this hematoxylin-phloxine-saffronin preparation.

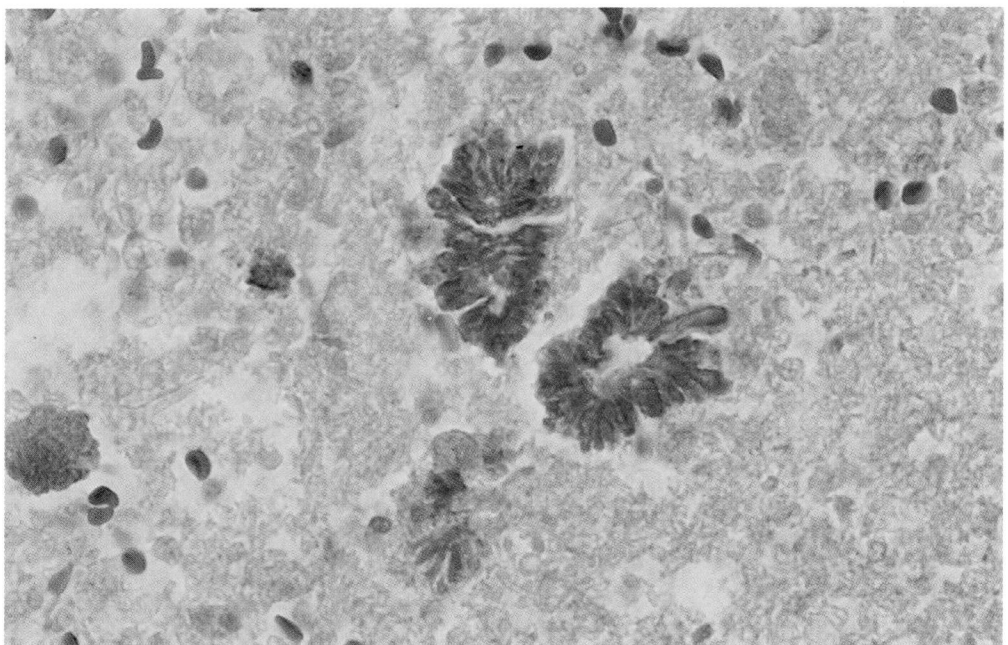

Fig. 28-5 Colloid cyst. The radiate, hyphae-like structures shown here are often found admixed with the liquid contents of colloid cysts and, for practical purposes, are diagnostic of this entity.

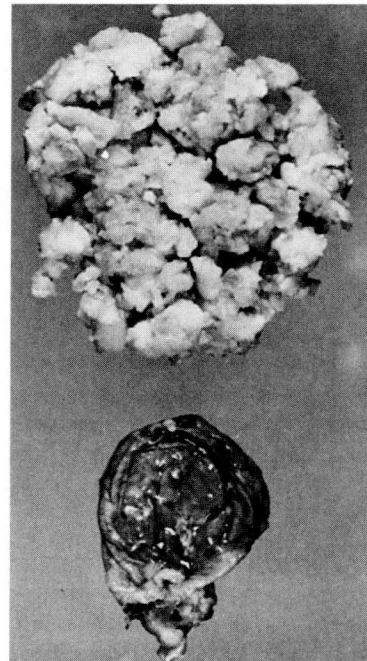

Fig. 28-6 Dermoid cyst. The contents of this lesion, removed from the frontal region of a 15-year-old boy, consist of granular, white, keratinous debris shown at top. The cyst wall, below, was lined by mature squamous epithelium and contained skin adnexae on histologic study.

face ectodermal elements trapped in association with the developing central nervous system on closure of the neural groove or formation of the secondary cerebral vesicles. The occurrence of some examples, particularly dermoids, in complex with craniovertebral anomalies (e.g., spina bifida), malformations of the spinal cord, and dermal sinuses attests to their dysembryogenetic basis. Well documented, however, are acquired variants, most of them epidermoid, resulting from the traumatic[53] or iatrogenic[46] implantation of cutaneous tissues in the cranial or spinal subdural space.

Epidermoid and dermoid cysts are characterized by distinctive clinical as well as histologic features. The former affect subjects of all ages, most coming to attention in young adulthood or middle age, whereas the latter usually present in childhood or adolescence. Cysts of epidermoid type are widely distributed along the neuraxis, but the great majority are positioned intracranially, the cerebellopontine angle being their single most common location.[54] Rarely, posterior fossa examples conspicuously erode into or lie embedded within the cerebellum or brainstem.[51] Supratentorial representatives exhibit a predilection for the parasellar region, but may also be situated within the ventricular system, in the cerebral hemispheres, suprasellar, or pineal regions.[54] Intraspinal epidermoid cysts are typically intradural and extramedullary in location but may on rare occasion lie entirely within the substance of the cord.[52]

Compared with its epidermoid counterpart, the dermoid cyst clings tightly to the midline. It, too, favors the posterior fossa but in this location characteristically occupies the cerebellar vermis or fourth ventricle.[49] When situated above the tentorium, the dermoid cyst tends to a frontal, paramedian position on the skull base.[48] An infantile, subgaleal variant typically resides in the anterior fontanel. Although generally outnumbered by epidermoid cysts, dermoids actually predominate at spinal levels. These exhibit a decided predilection for the lumbosacral region, where they constitute a manifestation of spinal dysraphism.

Although the clinical manifestations of dermoid and epidermoid cysts are principally referable to their local mass effects, either may present with signs and symptoms of "chemical" or infectious meningitis. The former results from cyst rupture and the spillage of irritating keratinous and lipid-rich debris into the ventricular system and subarachnoid space.[50] Repeated episodes of bacterial meningitis are a recognized complication of cysts associated with dermal sinuses offering access to the nervous system. Patients harboring posterior fossa dermoids and occipital sinuses may also suffer cerebellar abscesses. Neoplastic transformation is a well-documented but, fortunately, rare occurrence. In most cases, the underlying lesion is a cyst of epidermoid type and the secondary cancer a squamous carcinoma.[45] Isolated dermoid cysts have given rise to tumors described as anaplastic sebaceous carcinoma[44] or atypical hidradenoma.[47] Even histologically conventional cysts can recur following incomplete resection of their walls.[54]

Inasmuch as epidermoid cysts may arise, albeit rarely, in the suprasellar region, their differential diagnosis includes **Rathke cleft cysts** with extensive squamous metaplasia and **craniopharyngiomas**. The former will usually harbor scattered mucicarminophilic cells of cuboidal or low columnar

configuration atop their squamous elements and do not evidence the advanced keratinization typical of the epidermoid cyst. The formation of cytoplasmic keratohyaline granules, typical of the epidermoid cyst's maturing squames, is foreign to the craniopharyngioma. Furthermore, epidermoid cysts lack the latter's islands of "ghost cell" keratinocytes and its "machinery oil"–like contents and do not exhibit the basaloid elements and stellate reticulum of the adamantinomatous craniopharyngioma or the filiform architecture of its papillary variant (see Chapter 29 for details). The exceptional dermoid cyst presenting in the pineal or suprasellar region should be separable from the mature cystic teratoma by its lack of glandular components (indicative of endodermal differentiation), muscle, or cartilage.

Glioependymal cysts are most commonly situated in the paraventricular white matter of the frontal and parietal lobes but may also lie within the cerebellum, brainstem, or spinal cord.[55-57,59] A derivation from ventricular lining elements displaced in the course of neuroembryogenesis seems most plausible for these intraparenchymal examples, rare variants positioned in the cerebellopontine angle and other extra-axial sites conceivably originating from subarachnoid neuroglial heterotopias.[58] As their name implies, glioependymal cysts are lined by cells resembling mature ependymocytes. Like the cells lining the more common cysts of endodermal type, these may be ciliated but differ in that they do not exhibit goblet cell differentiation, are not coated by an apical glycocalyx, and do not rest on a basal lamina, being directly apposed to fibrillary neuroglial tissue. Representatives presenting in the subarachnoid space may, however, contain "supporting" astrocytic elements that fashion a continuous basement membrane separating them from a delicate fibrous capsule, much as the normal glia limitans are delimited from the connective tissues of the pia-arachnoid by a basal lamina.[55,58]

The limited immunocytochemical studies reported to date suggest that the cells lining glioependymal cysts can express GFAP, S-100 protein, and, possibly, cytokeratin.[55,58,59] Failure to elaborate carcinoembryonic antigen or transthyretin (prealbumin) may serve to distinguish these lesions from cysts of endodermal or choroid plexus type, respectively. By definition, the latter are lined by cells having the immunohistochemical and fine structural attributes of the native plexus epithelium,[61,62] considered in the discussion of this structure's epithelial neoplasms. We mention only for completeness sake cystic alterations that are a transient feature of some fetal choroid plexi.[60] These are of no consequence to the surgical pathologist.

Rarely, intraparenchymal brain cysts exhibit no specialized lining elements and are not associated with historical or tissue evidence of underlying trauma, hemorrhage, infarction, neoplasia, demyelinating disease, or infection that might account for their genesis.[63-66] Most numerous are examples termed "simple" or "gliotic" cysts, presenting in the cerebellar hemispheric white matter of middle-aged or elderly adults.[64,65] That at least some of these clinically benign lesions are not congenital anomalies but represent instead "burntout" pilocytic astrocytomas has been suggested in view of the latter tumor's proneness to macrocystic alterations and the presence around many simple cerebellar cysts of a dense mesh of glial processes rich in Rosenthal fibers and containing scattered atypical astrocytes.[64] Inasmuch as the neoplastic components of cerebellar cysts associated with pilocytic astrocytomas and hemangioblastomas may be confined to diminutive mural nodules, careful inspection of cystic lesions in this location following drainage at surgery is mandatory, and biopsy of various portions of their linings is prudent. Exceptional cysts arising outside the cerebellum are lined only by normal or mildly reactive neuroglial tissue, are juxtaventricular in location, and contain a fluid similar in its composition to CSF.[63,66] These likely derive from ventricular diverticula or represent collections of CSF that have dissected into the neuropil via congenital or acquired breaches in the ependyma.

Particularly prone to cystic change is the normal human pineal gland, but only rarely does this alteration result in a lesion of symptomatic proportions.[67] *Pineal cysts* that come to neurosurgical attention generally do so in the third through fifth decades of life, their presenting manifestations being indistinguishable from those of neoplasms in this region and including evidences of obstructive hydrocephalus, as well as disturbances of ocular motility. Like the cerebellar lesions previously described, these are lined by a dense weave of piloid astroglial processes containing Rosenthal fibers and granular bodies but do not exhibit the microcystic architecture characteristic of the pilocytic astrocytoma or approach the latter in cellularity. A second differential diagnostic consideration is the *pineocytoma,* as the cysts under discussion regularly contain elements of residual pineal parenchyma within their walls. These usually retain the organoid appearances typical of the normal gland, but in some cases their uniform, telltale lobularity is obscured as a result of longstanding compression. Appreciation of a given lesion's neuroradiologic features and appearance at operation is quite helpful in this regard, because pineocytomas are solid masses rather than thin-walled cysts. Simple excision is curative.

Loculated accumulations of CSF enclosed by fibroconnective tissues derived from the leptomeninges are generally referred to as *arachnoid cysts.* Etiologically diverse, some arachnoid cysts develop as sequelae of meningitis or trauma and are circumscribed by adhesions traversing the subarachnoid space. Most, however, are considered to begin as maldevelopmental clefts in the arachnoid membrane that subsequently undergo cystic dilatation.[72] Lesions of this type are lined by an attenuated meningothelium resting on a layer of supporting fibrous tissue so thin as to be transparent at operation. They most commonly occupy the sylvian fissures,[70] followed by the cisterna magna and cerebellopontine angles,[73] but suprasellar[71] and intradiploic[76] examples are also well recognized. By virtue of their very gradual inflation, these lesions may produce striking deformities in neighboring neural tissues that are often unaccompanied by mass effects such as midline shifts or internal herniae and thus have a malformation–like appearance. In fact, examples of so-called temporal lobe agenesis likely represent the protracted compressive effects of long-standing arachnoid cysts situated about the sylvian fissures.[75]

Most arachnoid "cysts" presenting at spinal levels are actually meningeal diverticula that can be shown to communicate with the subarachnoid space.[69] These may lie within or outside the dural sleeve, are often multifocal, and can be lined by meningothelial cells or composed solely of membranous fibrous tissue. Only a minority achieve symptomatic proportions, producing myelopathy or radicular syndromes, at times associated with erosion of adjacent vertebral bodies or the sacrum. Extradural variants arising in association with the posterior spinal roots, typically at lumbosacral levels, are often eponymously designated as *Tarlov's perineurial cysts.* Only exceptionally do these prompt neurosurgical intervention by causing perineal pain, sciatica, or bladder or bowel dysfunction. Rarely, cystically dilated or otherwise enlarged arachnoid granulations masquerade as dermoid (or other true) cysts[68] or produce sizable lytic skull defects that arouse suspicion of neoplastic disease.[74]

Yet another cystic lesion that may impinge on the spinal neuraxis is the *synovial ("ganglion") cyst,* a mass of acellular myxoid material bound within a fibrous capsule devoid of specialized lining elements. A degenerative abnormality, the synovial cyst typically presents at lumbar levels in association with osteoarthritic changes of the vertebral column.[77,78] Myeloradiculopathy and bony erosion are its principal complications.

Finally, we mention the intracranial extension of sinonasal mucoceles[79] and report of a multiloculated, cystic frontal lobe mass having the appearance of allergic nasal polyposis,[80] the latter associated with a bony abnormality of the anterior fossa floor and complicated by CSF rhinorrhea and meningitis.

CEREBROVASCULAR DISORDERS
Cerebral infarction

Characterized by an abrupt loss of neurologic function ("stroke") referable to a circumscribed arterial territory within the affected brain, the common variety of cerebral infarct is an ischemic lesion of later adult life confidently diagnosed at the bedside. Occasional examples, however, are silent at onset, evolve in subacute fashion as expansile intracranial "tumors" indistinguishable from neoplasms on neuroradiologic assessment, and are consequently sampled by the neurosurgeon. Obviously, the histology of a given infarct will depend on the stage at which the dynamic cytologic and organizational alterations that follow irreversible ischemic injury are iatrogenically interrupted.[81] Biopsied tissues generally exhibit a spongy rarefaction reflective of the edematous transudation that is largely to blame for these lesions' associated mass effects, commonly evidence intense vascular congestion, and may be frankly hemorrhagic. Neurons, if at all recognizable, persist only in faded, "ghost"-like profile or appear shrunken, angulated, and abnormally eosinophilic with a loss of intranuclear detail. Neutrophilic exudates may be apparent early, but most lesions approached surgically have evolved to the point where mononuclear phagocytes, including lipid-laden foam cells, constitute their principal reactive elements. These lend to organizing infarcts a potentially alarming hypercellularity all the more misleading when accompanied, as is often the case, by capillary proliferation and endothelial hypertrophy resembling glioma-associated vascular hyperplasia. Inasmuch as the cytologic features by which macrophages are recognized tend to be obscured in conventional frozen sections but are immediately apparent in squash and smear preparations, routine use of the latter is justly urged for purposes of intraoperative consultation. Once a lesion has been identified as being rich in phagocytes, the major differential consideration is demyelinating disease, given detailed consideration elsewhere in this chapter. Suffice it to say that demyelinating pseudotumors only exceptionally progress to tissue necrosis, are usually characterized by perivascular lymphoid cuffing and a relative preservation of axons foreign to brain infarcts, and generally afflict patients younger than those at risk of ischemic cerebral events.

Intracranial aneurysms

The *saccular* or *"berry" aneurysm* (Fig. 28-7) ranks chief among surgically correctable cerebrovascular abnormalities and is unrivaled as a cause of massive subarachnoid hemorrhage in adults. These common lesions (their prevalence in the general population falls in the neighborhood of 5%) are somewhat more frequent in women and are encountered at all ages beyond puberty, although symptomatic examples cluster in the fifth through seventh decades of life.[86-88,91] Exceptional cases occur on a familial basis. The factors critical in initiating the formation of saccular intracranial aneurysms remain undefined, and the majority are unassociated with local or systemic conditions known to promote vascular injury, but hemodynamic stress probably plays the major role in their development and, on balance, the weight of evidence supports the hypothesis that these are primarily acquired, degenerative lesions rather than developmental anomalies.[87,91] Arterial hypertension is widely regarded as playing an aggravating role in their evolution and may underlie their association with the adult form of aortic coarctation and type III polycystic kidney disease.[91] Connective tissue disorders that result in increased vascular fragility also predispose to the development of saccular aneurysms, these having been described in the settings of type III collagen deficiency (Ehlers-Danlos syndrome type IV), pseudoxanthoma elasticum, and Marfan's syndrome.[91] Aneurysms of the saccular variety occasionally occur in complex with fibromuscular dysplasia of the renal arteries, intracranial arteriovenous malformations or fistulae, and persistent primitive carotid-basilar anastomoses or other anomalies of the circle of Willis.[87] The latter observations notwithstanding, the localization of most saccular aneurysms (discussed later) is at odds with the theory that they commonly originate in vestigial remnants of the embryonic cerebral vasculature.

Frequently multifocal, saccular intracranial aneurysms usually lie within 3 cm of the internal carotid artery termini at the circle of Willis, and 80% involve divisions of the cerebral vasculature ventral to the posterior communicating arteries.[87,88] It is clear from autopsy studies that the middle cerebral arteries are most commonly affected, but most clinical series are dominated by anterior communicating and internal carotid artery examples because these are more prone to rupture.[85-88] That saccular aneurysms almost invariably bulge from points of acute-angle vascular bifurcation has been interpreted by some observers as the natural consequence of increased hemodynamic impact or turbulence at these points and by others as reflecting an inherent local weakness of the vessel wall secondary to focal gaps in the arterial media known to occur near circulatory forks.[87,91]

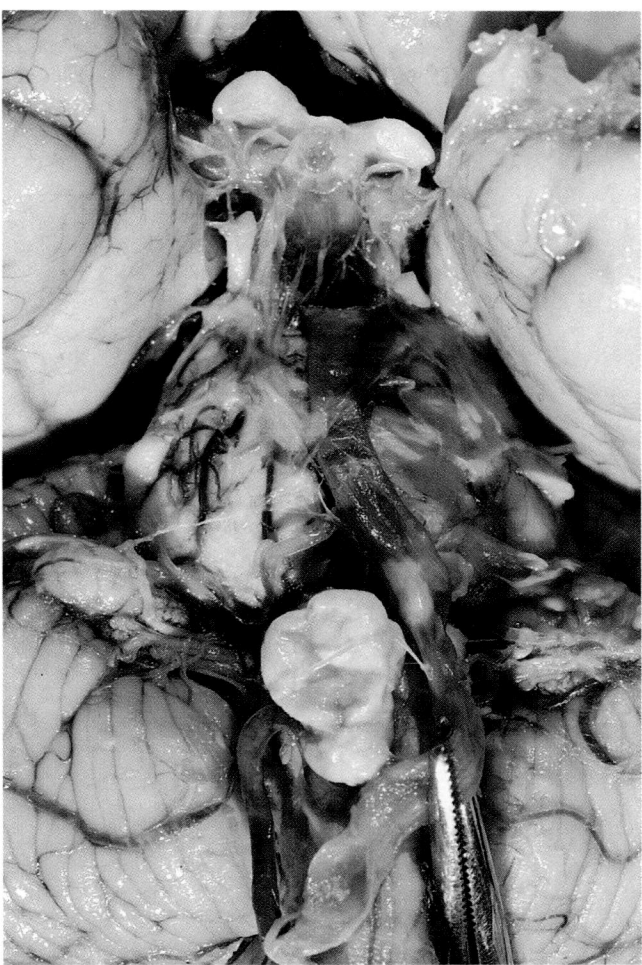

Fig. 28-7 Saccular aneurysm. Depicted is an intact example incidentally discovered at autopsy. In contrast to most saccular aneurysms, this arises from the posterior cerebral vasculature.

Although such "defects" could theoretically influence the localization of some lesions, there actually appears to be little topographic concordance between their major distribution in the human cerebrovascular tree and that of saccular aneurysms.[91]

On histologic examination, the walls of saccular intracranial aneurysms are composed principally of fibrous tissue, their parent vessels' muscular coats and elastic laminae typically terminating abruptly at the points of aneurysmal outpouching.[87,88] Atheromatous changes are common and may be florid but are characteristically confined to the aneurysmal sac and thus probably represent superimposed alterations of little direct etiologic significance. Much the same can be said of chronic inflammatory mural infiltration. Other secondary phenomena include partial or, in select instances, complete thrombotic occlusion, the latter presumably accounting for the occasional "disappearance" of untreated aneurysms assessed by periodic angiographic study.

Most saccular aneurysms remain asymptomatic, and even frank rupture may be followed by spontaneous thrombotic closure of the aneurysmal sac and clinical resolution, but this is not to trivialize the associated risk of catastrophic intracranial hemorrhage. Long-term follow-up studies of patients with angiographically proven saccular aneurysms suggest a 1% to 2% annual incidence of rupture; approximately half of these bleeding episodes prove fatal.[86] Although subarachnoid hemorrhage alone may be lethal, it is the dissection of blood into the brain itself or ventricular system that kills in many cases. Massive intraparenchymal hematomas are most often a consequence of middle cerebral artery aneurysms, whereas anterior communicating examples are generally responsible for most episodes of fatal intraventricular hemorrhage (blood usually entering the anterior horn of the lateral ventricle after dissecting through the inferomedial frontal lobe).[85] Another grave complication is cerebral infarction related to postrupture vasospasm, again encountered most commonly in patients harboring aneurysms of the anterior communicating arteries.

Although most observers have concluded that considerable risk of rupture is attached to saccular aneurysms exceeding 1 cm in diameter and relatively little to examples measuring 5 mm or less,[87] none of these lesions can be regarded as entirely innocent. In fact, nearly 70% of saccular aneurysms that ruptured in the course of a recently reported long-term follow-up study measured 6 mm or less in diameter on angiographic assessment.[86] Aneurysms that achieve "giant" proportions (usually defined as having diameters of at least 3 cm) typically present with cranial neuropathies, evidence of ventricular outflow obstruction, or other mass effects, rather than hemorrhage. Rarely, the surgical management of saccular aneurysms is complicated by a local granulomatous response to shredded gauze employed as reinforcement following aneurysmal clipping.[83] These "gauzomas" can achieve considerable size, presenting as contrast-enhancing masses with significant accompanying edema, and may produce headache, fever, obstructive hydrocephalus, cranial nerve palsies, and endocrinopathy.

Although the designation of *mycotic aneurysm* would seem to connote an infectious process specifically of fungal etiology, this term has been applied in practice to focal arteritides of diverse cause having in common only an element of vascular dilatation. Most mycotic intracranial aneurysms are, in fact, bacterial in nature and evolve as complications of endocarditis or, less frequently, suppurating pulmonary infection.[82] Streptococci and staphylococcal species are the usual offenders. Experimental observations suggest that aneurysms of this type are produced by septic embolization to the vasa vasorum, organisms secondarily infiltrating the affected vessel from its adventitial aspect.[89] The resulting lesions, often multifocal, tend to be situated on distal branches of the cerebral vasculature, are more often fusiform or irregular than berry-like in configuration, and are frequently of diminutive proportions. Fungal aneurysms are specifically addressed in the discussion of CNS mycoses. In brief, these are most often caused by *Aspergillus* and *Candida* species, generally involve the large cerebral arteries at the base of the brain, and tend to have greater diameters on presentation than their bacterial counterparts.

Atherosclerotic intracranial aneurysms generally afflict older adults, usually arise in the setting of advanced and generalized cerebrovascular atheromatosis, typically involve supraclinoid portions of the internal carotid arteries or the basilar artery, and may assume saccular, fusiform, cylindrical, or conical configurations.[87] Fusiform lesions of the vertebrobasilar trunk are the single most common variant.[87,90] Atherosclerotic aneurysms are generally of large size and frequently achieve giant proportions. Their presenting manifestations are more often related to compression of neighboring CNS structures or ischemic complications of progressive thrombosis than to hemorrhage, although some observers assert that the associated risk of rupture is underestimated.[90] Far more common than discrete aneurysm formation is atherosclerotic "dolichoectasia"—diffuse dilatation and tortuous elongation of the basilar or internal carotid arteries—and the two processes may coexist.

Dissecting aneurysms of the intracranial vasculature are rarities.[87] Most documented cases are without satisfactory etiologic explanation, although some have been attributed to trauma, syphilis, cystic medionecrosis, arteriosclerosis, fibromuscular dysplasia, or other local abnormalities of vascular structure. Stenosis of the involved vessel's lumen secondary to the intramural accumulation of blood may result in bulbar or cerebral infarction; rupture typically produces catastrophic subarachnoid hemorrhage. Symptoms referable to mass effect constitute the least frequent manifestation of intracranial arterial dissection.

Exceptionally, tumors metastatic to the CNS present as "spontaneous" intracerebral or subarachnoid hemorrhages that ultimately prove the consequences of neoplastic aneurysm formation. Most **neoplastic intracranial aneurysms** result from the embolization of cardiac myxomas to the cerebral vasculature, but examples caused by ovarian choriocarcinoma and non–small cell carcinoma of the lung are also on record.[84]

Charcot-Bouchard microaneurysms are saccular or fusiform lesions most commonly found on lenticulostriate, perforating pontine, and corticomedullary junction arteries measuring 40 to 200 μm in diameter.[87] These are particularly prevalent in hypertensive subjects, and their rupture is widely regarded as a major cause of basal ganglionic, bulbar, and cerebellar hemorrhage in this patient cohort. That aneurysms of Charcot-Bouchard type have received little attention in the surgical pathology literature may simply reflect the specialized tissue handling requisite to their identification. Studies in which surgically evacuated hematomas have been subjected to meticulous examination under the dissecting microscope (and serial thin-sectioning of suspect lesions) suggest that microaneurysms are under-appreciated as a factor predisposing to atraumatic lobar cerebral hemorrhage in both hypertensive and normotensive individuals.[92,93]

Vascular malformations

Generically designated as vascular malformations are various non-neoplastic lesions resulting from focal anomalies in the development of the cerebrospinal circulation. These are usefully divided into four relatively discrete morphologic categories, namely, capillary telangiectases, angiomas of venous or cavernous type, and arteriovenous malformations.[94,95] Also considered in this section are arteriovenous fistulas, since these are, strictly speaking, malformations,

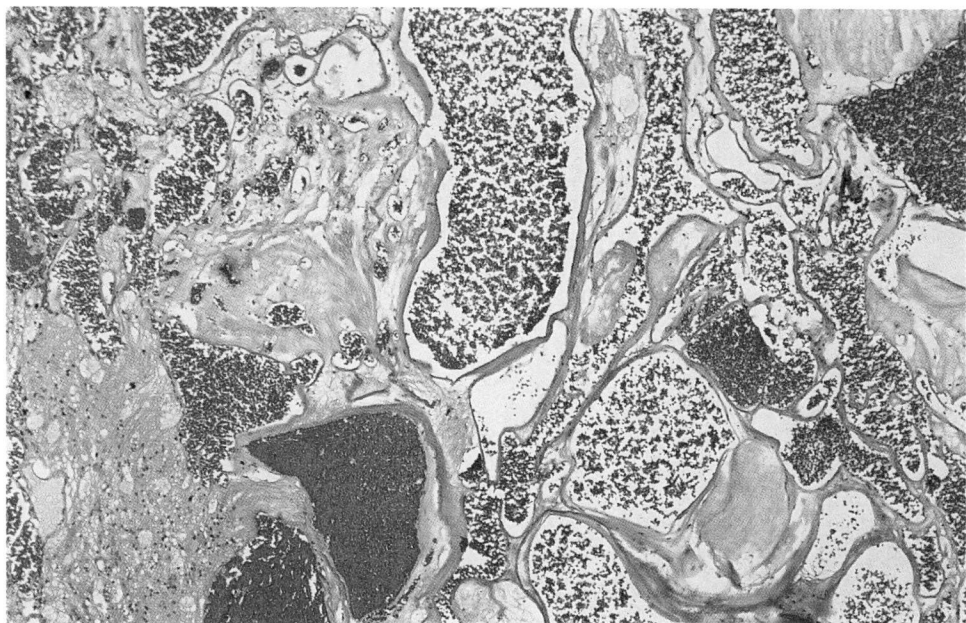

Fig. 28-8 Cavernous angioma. As illustrated, the cavernous angioma consists of ectatic and fibrous-walled vascular channels devoid of intervening neuroglial tissue. Neighboring brain parenchyma is present at lower left.

although they are generally regarded as acquired, rather than developmental, abnormalities.

Capillary telangiectases exhibit a curious predilection for the basis pontis (particularly the region of the median raphe), but are occasionally found to involve the cerebral hemispheres and spinal cord.[94,95] They usually constitute only incidental findings at autopsy, but isolated examples complicated by symptomatic hemorrhage are on record,[95] as is a massive pontomedullary case associated with a protracted history of bulbar dysfunction.[96] The lesion consists of loosely aggregated and variably ectatic capillary-type vessels (i.e., devoid of elastic or muscular mural elements) separated by normal or only mildly gliotic neuropil. A densely mineralized variant—the "calcified telangiectatic hamartoma" or "haemangioma calcificans"—is a recognized, albeit rare, cause of epilepsy, particularly of temporal lobe type.[97]

The *venous angioma* is a loose collection of dilated veins found typically in the digitate or deep white matter of the cerebral or cerebellar hemispheres.[94,95,98,99] The radial convergence of their ectatic vessels on a central draining varix lends to many of these lesions a diagnostic "caput medusae"—like profile on angiographic study. Although venous angiomas are the most common vascular malformations of the human central nervous system, it is the exceptional example that is responsible for intracranial hemorrhage or is otherwise symptomatic.

The *cavernous angioma* differs from all other vascular malformations in that its constituent vessels are fashioned into a compact, globose mass devoid of intervening neural elements.[94,95] On gross inspection, a spongy core of blood-filled channels is encircled by a thin rind of indurated

(because gliotic) and rusted-appearing (because hemosiderin-laden) neural parenchyma. Histologic study will reveal closely apposed, engorged vessels composed solely of fibrous tissue (Fig. 28-8). Secondary alterations such as thrombosis and dystrophic calcification are common, some lesions undergoing extensive metaplastic ossification as well. The existence of hybrid variants exhibiting in part the structure of capillary telangiectases has fueled speculation that cavernous angiomas may evolve from malformations of the former type,[106] but the fact remains that "mixed" lesions are exceptional. Cavernous angiomas may be situated anywhere along the neuraxis. Most examples lie above the tentorium,[94,95,109] often in cerebral white matter subjacent to the motor strip, but the cerebellum and brainstem,[109] spinal cord,[100] cauda equina,[105] and cranial nerves[103] may also be involved. Multifocal examples are by no means rare. The designation of cavernous angioma has also been extended to certain extra-axial vascular malformations affecting dural venous sinuses, but these depart structurally from their counterparts positioned in the CNS proper in that they contain, in addition to compact cavernous elements, capillaries and muscular vessels of both arterial and venous type.[104] These distinctive lesions, which usually present as a consequence of cranial nerve compression and are generally mistaken for meningiomas on preoperative neuroimaging study, are not given further consideration here.

Cavernous angiomas may become manifest in childhood,[108] but most symptomatic lesions are encountered in the third and fourth decades of life.[109] Familial cases transmitted in autosomal dominant fashion have been well delineated, an apparent excess involving Mexican-American kindreds,[111]

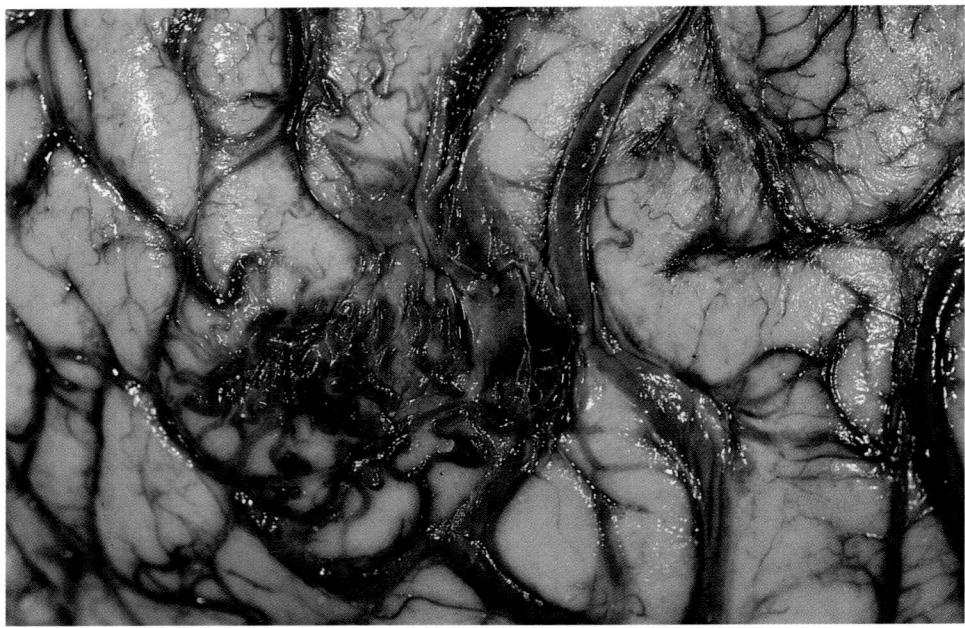

Fig. 28-9 Arteriovenous malformation. This variety of vascular anomaly often involves the leptomeninges (as well as underlying brain) and may be apparent on inspection of the cortical surface as a tangle of vascular channels and ectatic, draining veins.

and include variants occurring in complex with cavernous angiomas of the retina and skin.[102] That seizures are their dominant clinical manifestation reflects the proximity of most such lesions to epileptogenic cerebrocortical tissues. Less frequent complaints include focal neurologic deficits and headache. Although catastrophic hemorrhage is decidedly rare, cavernous angiomas are a recognized cause of intracranial hematomas, including both acutely symptomatic[110] and "encapsulated" lobar types,[107] the latter resulting in all likelihood from repeated subclinical episodes of bleeding and subsequent organization. A confident preoperative diagnosis of cavernous angioma may be established by neuroradiologic means. The typical lesion, although "angiographically occult" (i.e., not apparent on arteriographic study), appears in T2-weighted magnetic resonance images as an irregularly hyperdense nodule unassociated with significant edema or mass effect but surrounded by a hypodense penumbra resulting from the accumulation of hemosiderin in adjoining neural tissues.[101]

The most threatening of the congenital cerebrovascular anomalies under discussion is the ***arteriovenous malformation*** (AVM), a tangle of deformed arterial afferents and draining veins devoid of an interposed capillary bed.[94,95,117] AVMs may be situated in any region of the brain or spinal cord and can be restricted to the dura or choroid plexus,[113] but most lie within the distribution of the middle cerebral arteries and involve the hemispheric convexities in contiguity with their covering leptomeninges (Fig. 28-9). A majority present in early and mid-adulthood as a consequence of intracranial hemorrhage, other common manifestations including seizures, focal sensorimotor deficits, and headaches not clearly referable to episodes of bleeding.[112,119] Familial cases have been

described.[121] The turbulent shunting of blood through AVMs of the brain is sometimes audible as a cranial or orbital bruit, can often be demonstrated to diagnostic advantage on angiographic study, and may precipitate high-output cardiac failure in afflicted infants and children, particularly those harboring extensive lesions drained by aneurysmally dilated galenic veins. Unfortunately, AVMs are complicated by fatal rupture with distressing frequency. Long-term observations suggest that symptomatic examples carry a 2% to 4% risk of clinically significant hemorrhage per year and, left untreated, will eventuate in the deaths of at least one fourth of affected patients as a direct result of rupture.[112,119] Feeding arteries are prone to develop saccular aneurysms, and it is occasionally one of these, rather than the malformation itself, that is responsible for the lethal hemorrhagic ictus.

AVMs vary in size from cryptic lesions not demonstrable by angiographic means and discovered only on sampling of surgically evacuated hematomas[115] to enormous lobar examples that may focally span the full thickness of a cerebral hemisphere. As their tortuous, cirsoid vascular components form a complex network of blood-filled channels, the nature of these lesions is often apparent on casual gross inspection. Intervening neural tissues are typically attenuated, and there is evidence of rust-brown discoloration attesting to prior hemorrhage. Involved leptomeninges are thickened, opacified, and frequently siderotic as well. On histologic study, the lesion is composed of variably ectatic and hyalinized veins, abnormally muscularized arteries, and structurally ambiguous vessels formed solely of fibrous tissue or displaying both arterial and venous characteristics.[94,95,117] Critical to the distinction of the true AVM from normal leptomeningeal vessels that may assume a malformative appearance in neurosurgical material as a result of artefac-tual compaction are the former's conspicuous mural anoma-lies. Chief among these are striking fluctuations in medial thickness, architectural disarray or focal disappearance of the media altogether, or its separation into inner and outer coats by a seemingly aberrant elastic lamina.[117] Cushions of fibromuscular tissue may also appear to project in polypoid fashion into the lumens of these abnormal vessels, and focal duplications and disruptions of the internal elastic lamina are common. Superimposed alterations include mural fibro-plasia and atheromatosis, aneurysmal dilatation, calcifica-tion, and thrombosis, which, if extensive, may preclude the visualization of even sizable malformations by angiographic methods.[115] Lesions subjected to preoperative embolization with bucrylate[120] or polyvinyl alcohol[114] in an attempt to minimize blood loss during resection exhibit a foreign body response to the occluding material and may undergo focal necrosis. Entrapped neuropil usually manifests dense astrogliosis, neuronal depopulation, and ferruginous encrus-tation of included neuroglial elements. The reader's atten-tion is also called to the presence, in the interstices of select AVMs, of oligodendroglioma-like regions that may be intrinsic to the underlying maldevelopmental process or the result of abnormal oligodendroglial aggregation caused by the ischemic contraction of entrapped white matter.[116,118] The association of AVMs and bona fide gliomas is discussed under the heading of "Gliomesenchymal Tumors," as are malformation-like alterations occurring in the vascular stroma of neuroepithelial tumors.

To the sporadic and familial malformations mentioned in preceding paragraphs can be added a host of vascular anoma-lies constituting manifestations of certain neurocutaneous syndromes ("phakomatoses"), some clearly heritable and others the apparent result of spontaneous mutation. The most widely recognized of these disorders is *encephalo-trigeminal angiomatosis,* known by the eponym of *Sturge-Weber syndrome* and defined as a florid venocapillary pro-liferation involving the leptomeninges and cortical mantle of one cerebral hemisphere in complex with a cutaneous hemangioma ("port-wine stain") lying at least in part in the ophthalmic distribution of the ipsilateral trigeminal nerve.[123,124] Progressive mineralization of the involved cor-tex, centered initially on its abnormal perforating vessels, results in a gyriform, "tram-track" profile of radiologically demonstrable intracranial calcifications characteristic of the disease. Atrophy of the affected cerebral hemisphere is the rule, and patients typically suffer contralateral hemiparesis, often attended by motor seizures and mental retardation. The association of unilateral retinal angiomatosis and a cutaneous hemangioma in an ipsilateral trigeminal distribu-tion with an AVM of the midbrain is referred to as *mesen-cephalo-oculo-facial angiomatosis* (also termed neuroreti-nal angiomatosis, Bonnet-Dechaume-Blanc syndrome, or Wyburn-Mason syndrome).[123] Capillary telangiectases and AVMs are also recognized, albeit rare, CNS manifestations of hereditary hemorrhagic telangiectasia (Osler-Weber-Rendu disease).[122]

Arteriovenous fistulas of the craniospinal vasculature are accorded only passing consideration here because their cur-rent management—surgical clipping or selective embolic occlusion of the offending communication—does not usu-ally yield specimens for anatomic study. It is the absence of a plexiform, angiomatous nidus interposed between its feed-ing arteries and venous efferents that serves to distinguish the simple fistula from the AVM on angiographic and mor-phologic evaluation, although the latter's participating ves-sels may develop fistulous connections.[129] Trauma clearly figures in the genesis of some examples (particularly carotid-cavernous sinus and vertebrovertebral types) as does neuro-surgical injury, but many arteriovenous fistulas present in a spontaneous fashion. Those involving the cerebral arteries proper typically come to attention in childhood or early adult life, their clinical manifestations including headache, seizures, focal sensorimotor deficits, cardiac decompensation, and intracranial hemorrhage. Catastrophic rupture, however, appears to be exceptional. Fistulas developing below the tentorium are often localized to the dural sheaths of spinal nerve roots in the low thoracic region.[125,128] Lesions of this sort afflict men far more commonly than women, usually become symptomatic in or beyond middle age, and result in an ischemic myelopathy characterized by progressive para-paresis, paresthesias of the lower extremities, and sphincter disturbances. Known eponymously as *Foix-Alajouanine syn-drome* or *angiodysgenetic myelomalacia,* this disorder is typified by serpentine elongation and distention of veins coursing over the dorsal surface of the thoracic spinal cord and is likely the result of protracted local venous hyperten-sion caused by an overlap in the vascular drainage of the adjacent dural fistula and the cord itself. Fistulas involving the perimedullary vascular plexus[129] or distantly situated in the cranial or sacral dura [127] may eventuate in a similar pic-ture. Dural-based arteriovenous fistulas have also been implicated in the pathogenesis of vascular malformations occupying the sigmoid and transverse sinuses.[126]

Primary angiitis

Among the less common forms of cerebrovascular disease is the idiopathic disorder variously described as "isolated," "granulomatous," or "primary" angiitis of the CNS.[131,132] Inasmuch as many histopathologically con-firmed cases have not evidenced overtly granulomatous fea-tures and as autopsy studies have disclosed exceptional instances of extraneural vascular involvement, the last of these designations would seem the most accurate and is adopted here.

Primary angiitis of the CNS can occur at any age but usu-ally afflicts young or middle-aged adults, its principal clini-cal manifestations including headache, mental status changes, and focal neurologic deficits (particularly hemiparesis) that may evolve in progressive fashion or present abruptly as "stroke." Signs and symptoms of myelopathy occasionally dominate the clinical picture, but only rarely is morphologic evidence of vascular injury accentuated at, or confined to, spinal levels.[130,133] If not promptly diagnosed and managed, the disorder generally progresses to tetraparesis, coma, and death.

Short of biopsy for tissue confirmation, angiography is the most useful investigative procedure and findings typical of vasculitis—particularly multifocal, segmental stenosis, dilatation, or "beading" of small- to medium-caliber lep-tomeningeal arteries—are considered by some to constitute sufficient grounds for the institution of corticosteroid or

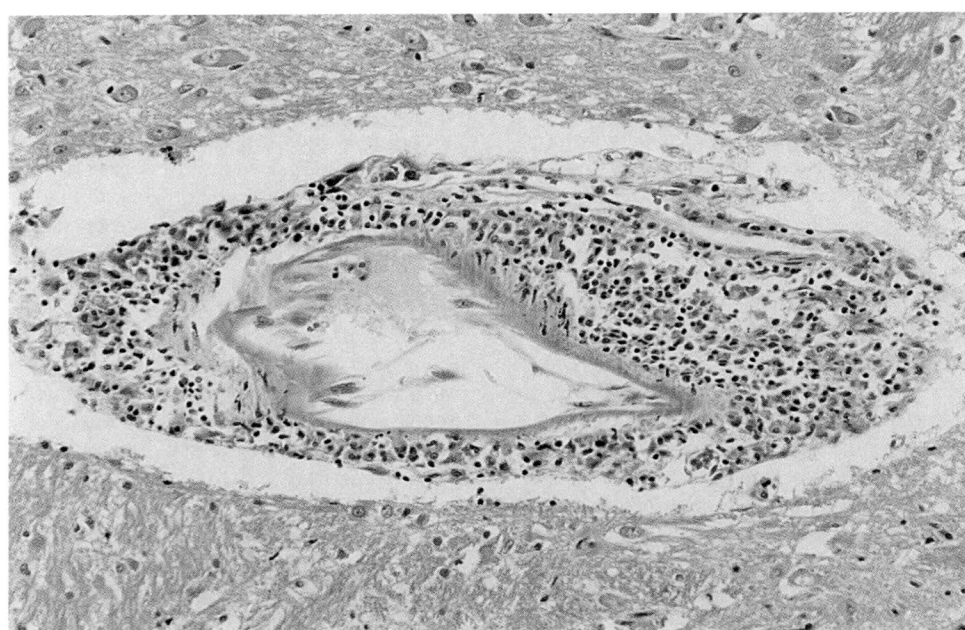

Fig. 28-10 Primary angiitis of the CNS. A lymphohistiocytic infiltrate is centered on the wall of this small perforating artery, found in biopsy material from a young woman with headache and progressive confusion.

cytotoxic therapy in the appropriate setting (i.e., when underlying infection and other systemic processes associated with secondary CNS angiitis have been excluded from further diagnostic consideration). However, arteriograms may be unrevealing even in the face of florid vascular disease.[131] Less commonly encountered neuroradiologic abnormalities include aneurysm formation and focal "mass" lesions secondary to infarction, often hemorrhagic.

Most observers regard biopsy as the sole means of confirming a presumptive clinical diagnosis of primary CNS angiitis, although false-negative samplings are a common consequence of the disorder's segmental distribution. Small and midsized leptomeningeal arteries usually bear the brunt of the injury, but neighboring veins are often involved in concert, and the process may affect the large vessels at the base of the brain as well. Rarely, however, are inflammatory alterations confined to the latter. That the histologic presentation of primary CNS angiitis is subject to considerable variation merits emphasis.[131] Most frequently encountered are necrotizing, polyarteritis-like, or non-necrotizing lymphoplasmacytic variants. Mural infiltration by histiocytes, including epithelioid forms, and multinucleated giant cells of foreign body and Langhans' type characterize granulomatous examples, but, again, this is an inconstant feature (Fig. 28-10). When present, giant cells are not strictly associated with the elastic lamina and may lie in any part of the vessel wall. Secondary changes include thrombosis and, in long-standing cases, mural scarring and exuberant fibrointimal hyperplasia.

Notwithstanding the fact that its histologic features are shared by cerebral vasculitides complicating a variety of systemic disorders,[131] primary angiitis of the CNS would seem to merit its distinct nosologic status on clinical grounds. This is not to deny the possibility that this curious process might be triggered by diverse offenses to the cerebrospinal circulation. Although long suspected, an infectious etiology remains unproved. Noteworthy in this regard, however, is the epidemiologic association of primary CNS angiitis with cutaneous herpes zoster infection and with underlying conditions, chiefly hematolymphoid neoplasia, predisposing to this and other viral opportunists. In fact, most patients with leukemia or lymphoma reportedly complicated by primary angiitis of the nervous system have suffered from prior or synchronous zoster.[131] These observations are especially intriguing in view of the undisputed role of the varicella-zoster virus as agent of a large-vessel cerebral arteritis, potentially indistinguishable from primary CNS angiitis, addressed in our discussion of viral disorders (see p. 2263).

Cerebral amyloid angiopathy

The deposition of amyloid in the walls of cerebral blood vessels is a fact of aging and a conspicuous accompanying feature of varied disorders, including Alzheimer's disease, Down's syndrome, dementia pugilistica, and certain types of spongiform encephalopathy.[139] It is the association of this process—cerebral amyloid angiopathy—with intracranial hemorrhage that compels the attention of the neurosurgeon and surgical pathologist. *Cerebral amyloid angiopathy* may well be the most common nontraumatic cause of lobar cerebral hematoma in elderly subjects (the cohort at greatest risk) and has been estimated to account for some 5% to 10% of all primary, atraumatic brain hemorrhages.[139] The disorder is not a manifestation of systemic amyloidosis in any of its guises and typically presents in sporadic fashion, although Dutch and Icelandic kindreds afflicted by a heritable (autosomal-dominant) syndrome of florid cerebrovascular amyloidosis and early death as a result of recurrent intracerebral hemorrhages have been delineated. Beta-protein, found also in the infiltrated vessels and neuritic plaques characteristic of asymptomatic senescence and Alzheimer's disease, constitutes the amyloid responsible for both the common sporadic and familial Netherlandish variants, whereas cystatin C, an inhibitor of cysteine proteases normally present in various body fluids, is the offending amyloidogenic protein implicated in the heritable Icelandic form.[134] Although a substantial proportion of affected patients suffer also from senile dementia of the Alzheimer's type, cerebral amyloid angiopathy, even when severe, is not necessarily associated with cognitive impairment or with the characteristic cortical alterations of Alzheimer's disease.

The peripheral, lobar location of amyloid-associated cerebral hematomas contrasts sharply with the basal ganglionic or bulbar situation typical of hypertensive hemorrhages and reflects the particular susceptibility of superficial cortical and leptomeningeal vessels to amyloidotic infiltration.[138,139] Chiefly affected are small-caliber arteries and arterioles, but veins may be involved as well. These exhibit mural expansion and, in advanced cases, effacement by acellular, eosinophilic material deposited in the adventitia and media. By definition, this possesses the histochemical properties (Fig. 28-11) and fine structural attributes common to all amyloids. Its definitive identification is most readily accomplished by demonstration of a dichroic, bluish-green birefringence in Congo red–stained sections viewed under polarized light. Other defining characteristics include thioflavin S or T fluorescence under ultraviolet light. Ultrastructural study should reveal randomly arrayed, nonbranching extracellular fibrils averaging 9 nm in diameter but is not requisite to the diagnosis if the appropriate reactions are obtained on Congo red or thioflavin assay. Amyloid-laden cerebral vessels generally maintain their patency but are subject to a variety of "vasculopathic" alterations. These include "double-barreling" (a targetoid, vessel-within-vessel configuration produced by what would appear to be a circumferential cleft in the media), glomeruloid arteriolar changes, obliterative fibrointimal proliferation, perivascular or intramural lymphocytic infiltration, the development of microaneurysms, and finally, fibrinoid necrosis.[138,140] Restricted to vessels bearing a heavy amyloid burden, this last abnormality appears to play a particularly significant role in the pathogenesis of vascular rupture.[140]

As is often the case in extracranial locations, amyloid deposited in the cerebral vasculature occasionally elicits a foreign body–type response replete with multinucleated giant cells that surround affected vessels and attempt to phagocytize the offending material. Much rarer are examples of cerebral amyloid angiopathy associated with a true vasculitis of necrotizing and granulomatous type.[135,136] Most reported cases probably represent idiosyncratic host reactions to the offending protein, but it is conceivable that primary cerebral vasculitides could aggravate, if not trigger, local amyloidogenic processes. Instances of cerebral amyloid angiopathy

and vasculitis occurring in patients with rheumatoid arthritis are noteworthy in this regard.[137] Interestingly, the few examples of "angiitic" cerebrovascular amyloidosis that we have encountered presented not with hemorrhage but as pseudoneoplastic, infiltrative masses associated with seizures and focal neurologic deficits of a subacutely progressive nature. Much the same can be said of cases reported under the rubric of combined granulomatous angiitis and cerebral amyloid angiopathy.[135,136]

Epidural hematoma

The great majority of ***epidural hematomas*** follow cranial trauma complicated by temporal bone fracture and result from laceration of middle meningeal artery branches that penetrate the skull in the region of the pterion.[141] The accumulation of blood between the calvarium and endosteal surface of the dura mater is typically rapid, associated with acute deterioration of consciousness, and soon eventuates in death as a result of transtentorial herniation with brainstem compression if not promptly evacuated. Uncommon variants become symptomatic only long after their initiating injuries. Delimited by encapsulating neomembranes formed of vascularized fibrous tissue, chronic epidural hematomas of this sort are usually of venous origin.

Subdural hematoma

Subdural hematomas result from the dissection of blood into the potential space separating the arachnoid and dura mater, closely apposed under normal circumstances.[146] Most overlie the cerebral convexities in the frontoparietal region (Fig. 28-12) and are thought to follow rupture of delicate bridging veins that traverse the arachnoid-dura interface enroute to the superior sagittal sinus.[143] These vessels are particularly susceptible to shearing forces generated by sudden angular acceleration of the head, as commonly occurs in the setting of trauma, and many subdural hematomas are clearly associated with cranial injury. Most "spontaneous" examples occur in the elderly, possibly because cerebral atrophy and resultant traction on these bridging vessels reduce their capacity to withstand otherwise trivial stresses. A similar phenomenon may promote the development of subdural hematomas following ventricular decompression for hydrocephalus. Patients who have received anticoagulants, who are thrombocytopenic, or who have been treated with long-term hemodialysis are also at increased risk of subdural hemorrhage.[143,147] A small subset of subdural hematomas result from arterial injury.[145] These are usually associated with major craniocerebral trauma.

The pathology of the subdural hematoma is a function of its age. If evacuated within days of onset, it consists simply of clotted blood. Often, however, the original bleeding episode passes unnoticed, and the hematoma becomes symptomatic only after it has elicited an organizational response resulting in its enclosure within a discoid sac fashioned of grayish brown, collagenous neomembranes that adhere to the dura but develop no attachments to the underlying arachnoid. The latter feature reflects the fact that the mesenchymal elements responsible for the hematoma's encapsulation derive entirely from the dura, the leptomeninges remaining curiously unmoved by the presence of blood in the subdural space and

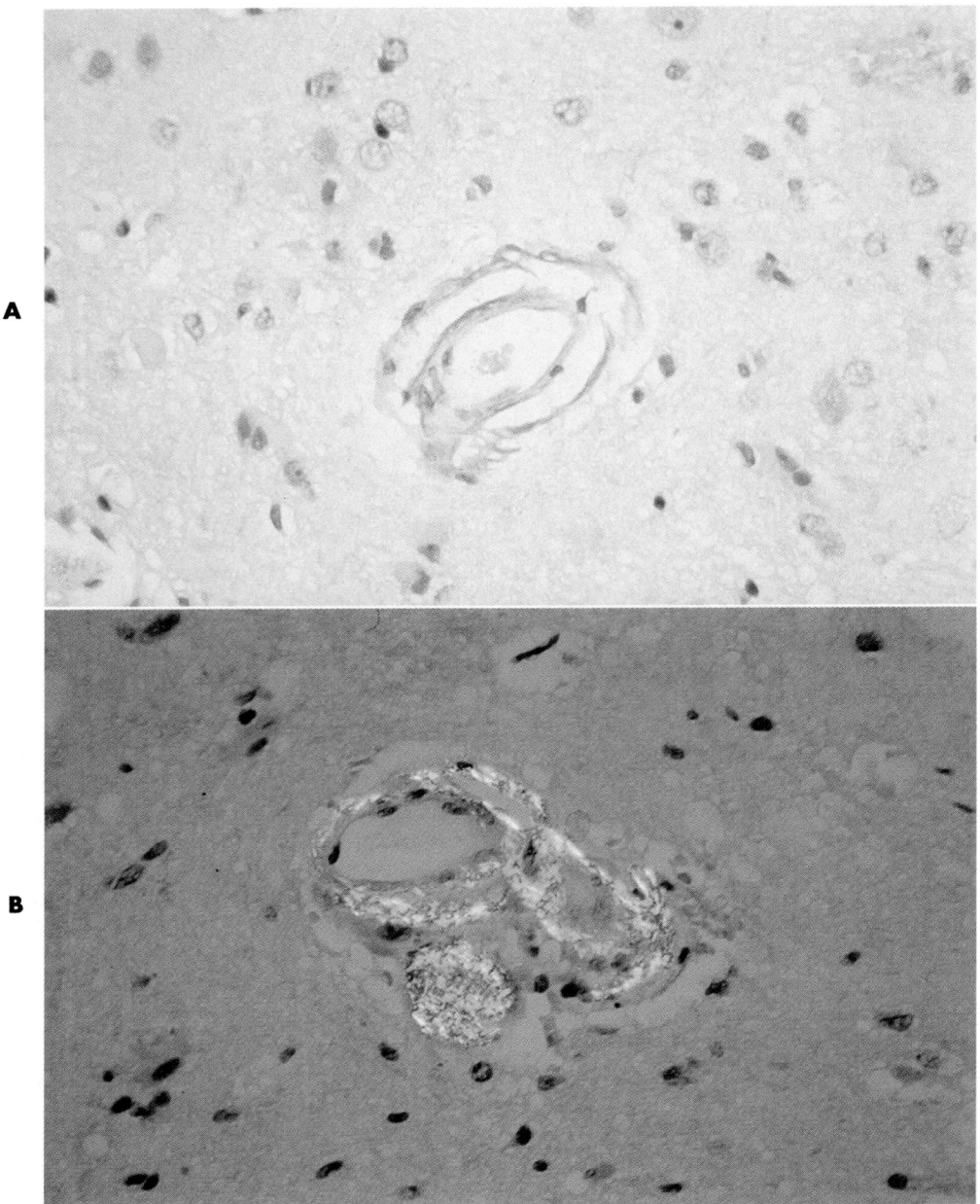

Fig. 28-11 Cerebral amyloid ("congophilic") angiopathy. As in extraneural locations, amyloid in the walls of cerebral vessels takes the Congo red stain **(A)** and exhibits an "apple green" birefringence when sections thus prepared are viewed under polarized light **(B)**. The apparent "double-barrel" lumen evident in **A** is a common feature of amyloid-laden cerebral vessels.

playing no part in its organization. Inasmuch as the histologic maturation of these limiting membranes proceeds in temporally predictable fashion, the chronicity of a given lesion may be estimated by thorough assessment of the membranes.[143] Surgical pathologists, however, are generally spared this exercise because current management of the chronic subdural hematoma is usually restricted to evacua-

tion of its sac's clotted and liquefied contents. Suffice it to say that the outer (juxtadural) membrane, which may attain a thickness of several millimeters, consists in the early stages of proliferating spindle cells and budding capillaries that penetrate the hematoma's superficial aspect and come to lie in a loose connective tissue matrix containing admixed siderophages, scattered lymphocytes, and in some cases,

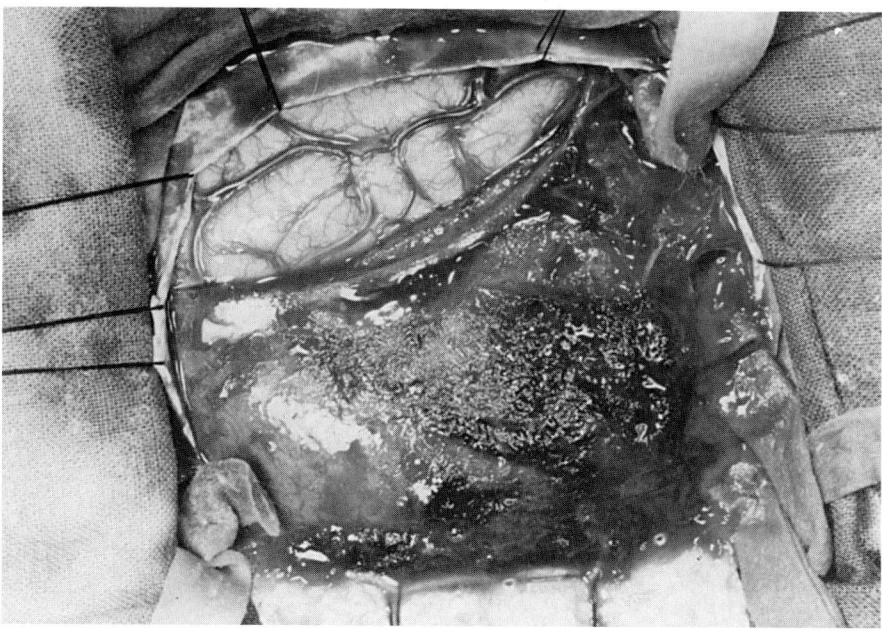

Fig. 28-12 Subdural hematoma. The dura has been reflected, exposing the neomembrane and organizing hematoma. Note, in upper portion of field, how the latter peel freely from the leptomeningeal surface. (Courtesy Dr. H.G. Schwartz, St. Louis.)

hematopoietic elements. The inner membrane, by contrast, has a simpler structure and is thinner and relatively avascular. The precise cytogenesis of the spindly, fibroblastic elements populating these neomembranes and responsible for their ensuing collagenization remains a matter of speculation, but an origin from "dural border" cells that normally form a complex lamina apposed to the arachnoid has been suggested on the strength of fine structural observations.[142,146,148] In any event, both membranes undergo progressive hyalinization and, with complete resorption of the hematoma, fuse to form a thin fibrous rind closely resembling the adjacent dura mater on microscopic study. In exceptional instances, the hematoma sac is transformed into a calcific, even ossified, shell.[144]

The chronic subdural hematoma's capacity to present in clinically delayed fashion as an expanding intracranial mass would seem a paradox. Once completed, the enclosing hematoma sac could conceivably function as a semipermeable membrane and permit the ingress of fluid drawn by osmotic forces from the CSF compartment or the capillary network in its outer lamina. A prosaic (but, perhaps, more likely) explanation would incriminate these delicate vessels in episodes of rebleeding. Not infrequently, subdural hematomas that first come to attention in their chronic, encapsulated phases disclose evidence of recent, superimposed hemorrhage in the form of fresh blood layered subjacent to their vascularized outer membranes.

INFLAMMATORY DISEASES
Demyelinating diseases

The idiopathic demyelinating diseases of the CNS, of which multiple sclerosis is by far the most common, are usu-

ally regarded as "medical" disorders diagnosed on clinical grounds or at autopsy. In fact, a number of reports have called attention to the fact that demyelinating lesions of the cerebral hemispheric white matter and spinal cord may present as space-occupying "tumors" associated with considerable mass effect, edema, and disruption of the blood-brain barrier evidenced, on CT or MR study, by diffuse or ring-like enhancement following administration of contrast media[152,153,156,157] (Fig. 28-13). Few patients harboring such lesions carry a diagnosis of multiple sclerosis when they present with symptoms and signs referable to an expanding intracranial mass. Solitary examples, not surprisingly, prompt consideration of aggressive glial neoplasia or abscess formation, whereas multifocal variants suggest metastatic disease or even cerebral parasitosis when lesions exhibit cystic characteristics on scan. Such demyelinating "pseudotumors" understandably occasion neurosurgical intervention for purposes of definitive diagnosis and thus enter the domain of the surgical pathologist.

The *tumefactive demyelinating lesion* shares with the active "plaque" typical of subacute multiple sclerosis[155] a sharp delineation from adjacent, uninvolved white matter evident in biopsy samples that include its perimeter. Affected tissues exhibit diffuse infiltration by foamy, lipid-laden macrophages; reactive astrocytosis of variable intensity; and perivascular aggregates of small (mostly T) lymphocytes and occasional plasma cells[152,153,155,157] (Fig. 28-14). The definitive characterization of the process as a demyelinating one ultimately requires the demonstration of relative axonal preservation in foci devoid of stainable myelin. This is readily accomplished by comparing serial sections assessed for myelin and axons by traditional neurohistochemical methods (Fig. 28-15) or

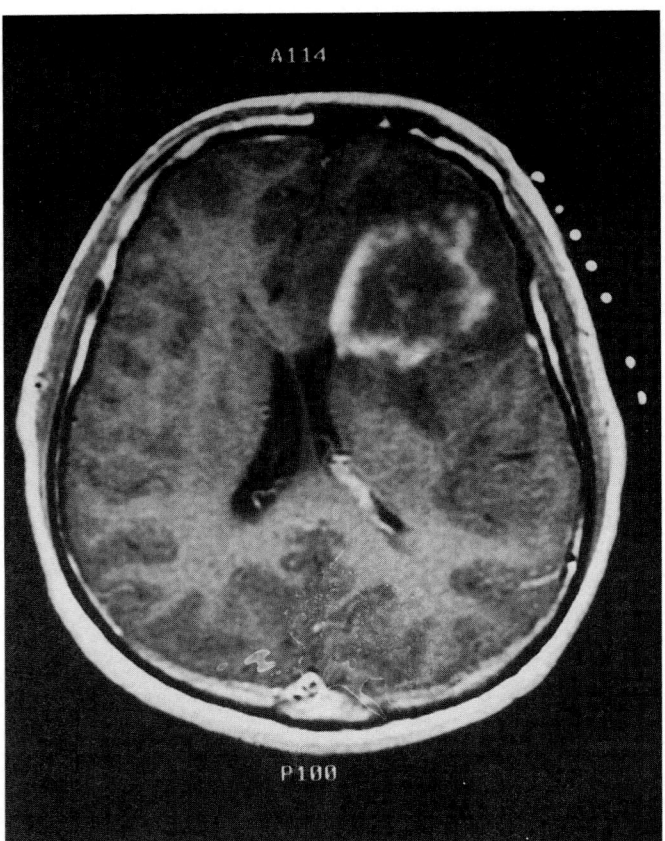

Fig. 28-13 Demyelinating pseudotumor. Taken following administration of a "contrast" agent that serves to delineate foci of blood-brain barrier breakdown as regions of bright signal, this magnetic resonance image demonstrates a lesion characterized by "ring" enhancement, conspicuous hypodensity of the surrounding white matter (indicative of edema), and "mass effect" evidenced by obliteration of the ipsilateral ventricular angle and shift of the neighboring cingulate gyrus across the midline. The neuroradiologic diagnosis was "probably glioblastoma, abscess also a possibility." The patient, a 32-year-old man with subacutely progressive hemiparesis and somnolence, recovered completely following limited biopsy and a short course of corticosteroids. He remains asymptomatic 3 years after diagnosis.

assayed for components of the myelin sheath and axon using commercially available antibodies to myelin basic protein and neurofilaments, respectively. In the typical case, large numbers of axons will course uninterrupted through regions in which myelin, if at all demonstrable, persists only as phagocytized debris in the cytoplasm of macrophages. It should be pointed out, however, that a variable element of axonal depopulation is the rule, some particularly destructive examples progressing to cavitation.

In our experience, demyelinating pseudotumors are the non-neoplastic lesions most often misinterpreted on biopsy as gliomas, specifically as diffuse fibrillary astrocytomas or, rarely, as oligodendrogliomas. The consequences to patients subjected to cerebral irradiation may be devastating.[156] The potential causes for error are many.[152,153,156,157] A diagnosis of glioma may be prompted by the florid and cytologically atypical astrogliosis that characterizes some examples—an impression likely to be reinforced by the finding of scattered

mitotic figures, as well as astrocytes that appear to be in atypical mitosis by virtue of a peculiar parcellation of their nuclear material (Fig. 28-16). Perivascular lymphoid infiltrates are an inconstant feature of demyelinating lesions sampled at craniotomy and even when conspicuous are no guarantee that a glial proliferation is not neoplastic. Even in their absence, however, the orderly spacing of gemistocytic astrocytes typical of hyperplastic states—a "logic" maintained in these lesions—should suggest a reactive process.

Especially confounding is failure to appreciate the high content of macrophages that lend to tissues undergoing demyelination their alarmingly hypercellular appearance. The voluminous foamy or granular cytoplasm typical of these cells when engaged in the digestion of phagocytized myelin and useful in their distinction from glia may be obscured in suboptimally procured or processed samples. As this is particularly true of frozen sections, the use of cytologic preparations wherein these features are likely to be

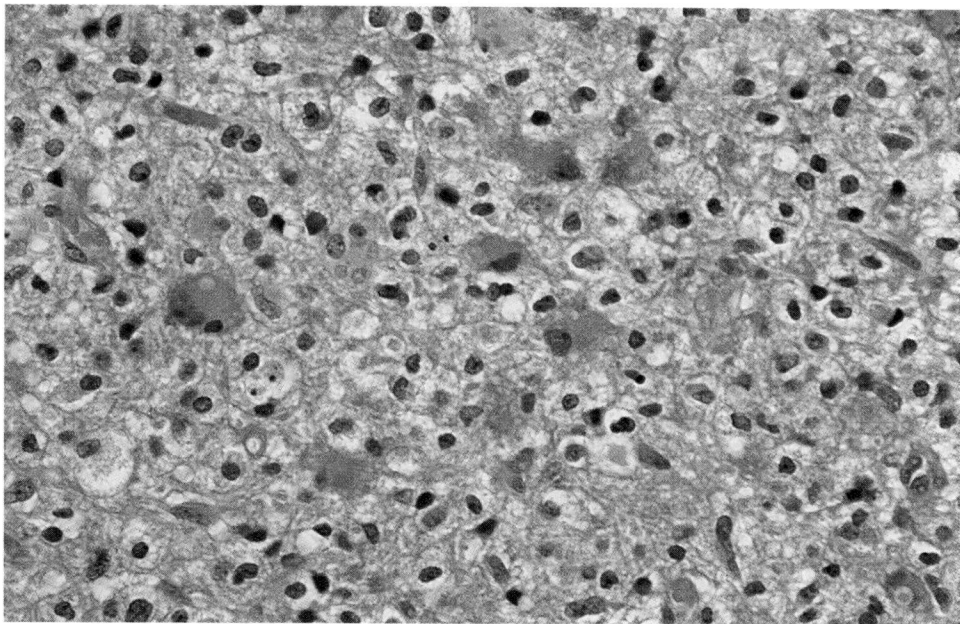

Fig. 28-14 Demyelinating pseudotumor. The hypercellularity of this lesion reflects infiltration by macrophages in large number, recognizable on careful study by their granular or foamy cytoplasm. Also apparent are several hyperplastic astrocytes.

preserved is strongly advocated for purposes of intraoperative consultation (Fig. 28-17). Lectin or immunocytochemical assay for monocyte/macrophage markers such as HAM-56 (Fig. 28-18) may also aid in circumventing problems of cell identification,[151] particularly as applied to neurosurgical specimens exhibiting artefactual distortion or dominated by newly arrived mononuclear cells interrupted in their labors and thus not evidencing the cytoplasmic characteristics of fully developed, lipid-engorged phagocytes (Fig. 28-16). Diffuse infiltration by macrophages is so rarely a feature of the untreated glioma as to virtually exclude this diagnosis. The ready identification of such cells in smears, crush preparations, or tissue sections should instead suggest a non-neoplastic, necrotizing process (such as organizing infarction) or a selectively demyelinating disorder. Primary CNS lymphomas inadvertently treated by the preoperative administration of corticosteroids may vanish on neuroradiologic scan and can further simulate demyelinating disease by leaving behind only reactive lymphohistiocytic infiltrates but do not cause selective, regionally circumscribed myelin loss (see discussion of lymphoproliferative and myeloproliferative disorders for references). Patients suffering from multiple sclerosis on occasion do develop glial neoplasms,[149,154] but there is no compelling evidence that the incidence of the latter is increased in this population.

As mentioned, only exceptionally do tumefactive demyelinating lesions complicate the course of established multiple sclerosis. Interestingly, only three of thirty-one patients presenting with solitary or multifocal demyelinating pseudotumors in the series of Kepes,[153] the largest reported

to date, developed additional cerebral lesions during follow-up periods ranging from 9 months to 12 years. This intriguing observation suggests that the biology of tumefactive demyelinating disease differs significantly from that of classic multiple sclerosis and is perhaps more akin to that of the monophasic "allergic" encephalomyelitides triggered by viral infection or vaccination. Last, mention is made of a *multifocal inflammatory leukoencephalopathy* described as complicating the chemotherapy of colorectal adenocarcinoma with 5-fluorouracil and levamisole.[150] The lesions in question are demyelinative and morphologically indistinguishable from active multiple sclerosis plaques. Whether one or both of these agents are directly responsible for this condition or somehow precipitate attacks of multiple sclerosis in patients predisposed to the disorder is unclear.

Idiopathic inflammatory and reactive disorders, xanthomatous lesions, and "histiocytoses"

This section discusses various oddities that have little in common beyond their etiologic obscurity and inflammatory or otherwise "reactive" histologic appearances. Most are better known for their systemic manifestations and are given detailed consideration elsewhere in these volumes. Specific description is here accorded only those entities unique to the nervous system.

Idiopathic hypertrophic cranial pachymeningitis is, as its name implies, a chronic inflammatory and fibrosing disorder of unknown cause.[159,160] The examples reported to date, all of adult onset, have been characterized chiefly by headache, progressive cranial neuropathies, and cerebellar

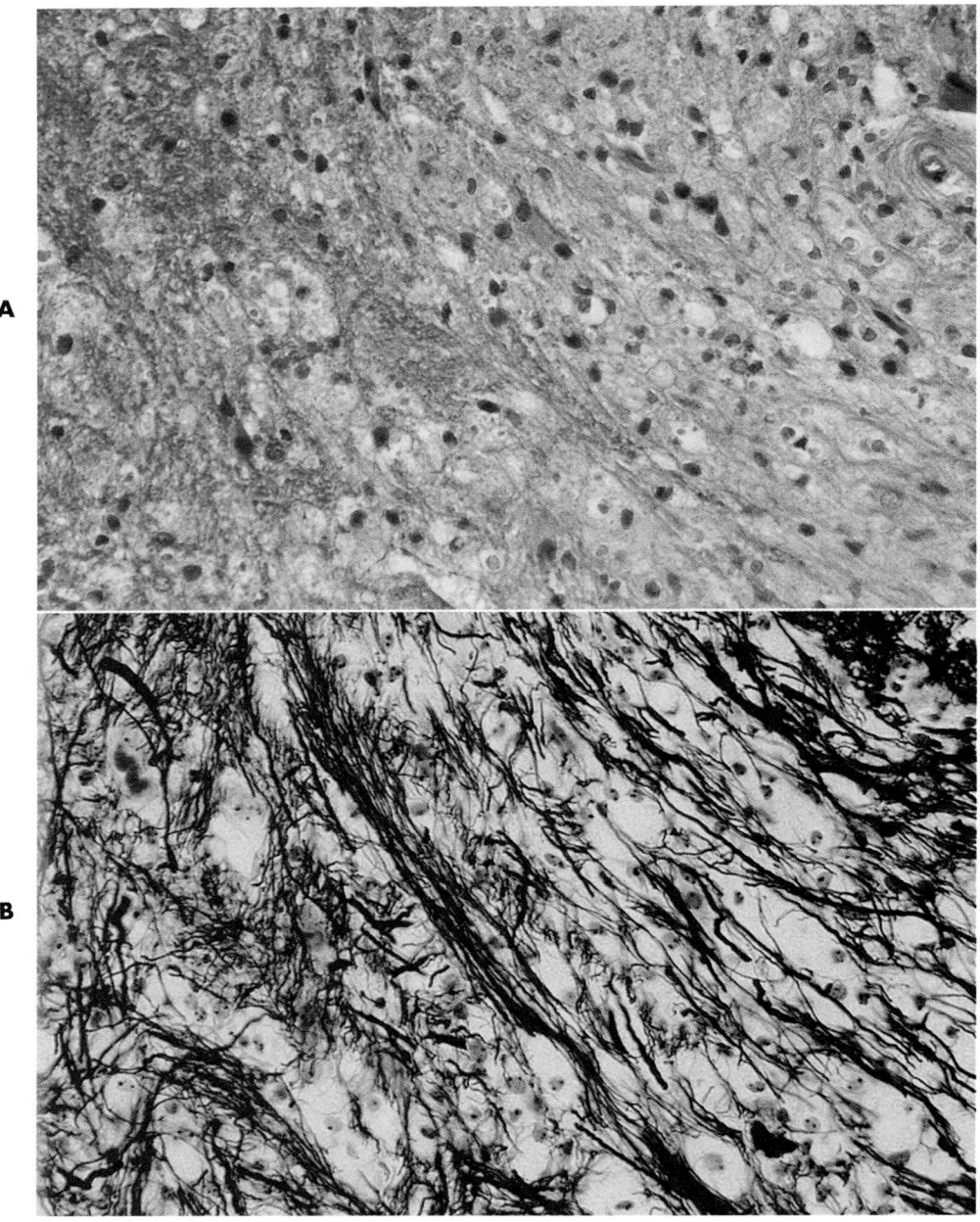

Fig. 28-15 Demyelinating pseudotumor. The interface of a demyelinated plaque *(right)* and normal white matter *(left)* is shown here in serial sections stained for myelin **(A)** and axons **(B)** by the Luxol fast blue and Bielschowsky methods, respectively. Myelin, blue in **A,** persists in the plaque only as globules present in the cytoplasm of macrophages. Axons, stained black in **B,** course uninterrupted into the region of demyelination.

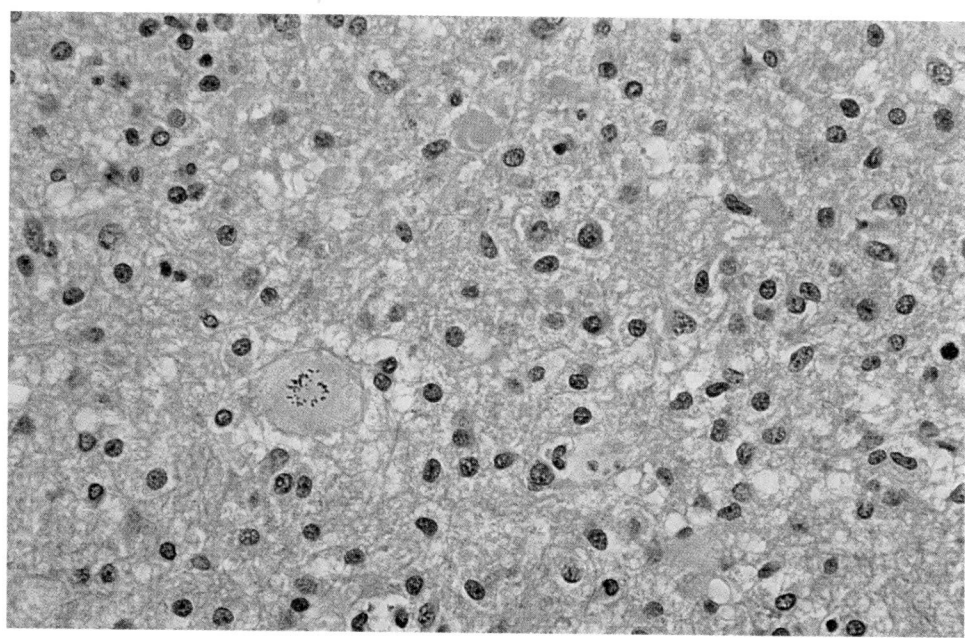

Fig. 28-16 Demyelinating pseudotumor. An apparently atypical mitotic figure and diffuse infiltrate of mononuclear cells lacking the cytoplasmic features of fully developed macrophages may lead to the incorrect diagnosis of glioma.

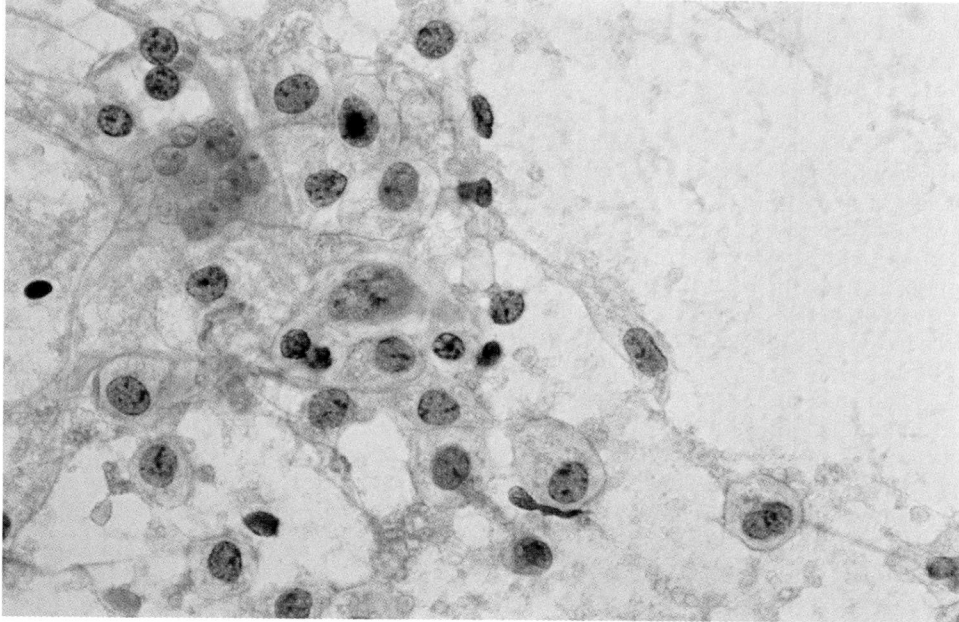

Fig. 28-17 Demyelinating pseudotumor. The presence of foamy macrophages in cytologic preparations argues strongly against a diagnosis of glioma at the time of intraoperative consultation. As shown here, somewhat atypical-appearing, multinucleate astrocytes are not uncommonly encountered in such specimens.

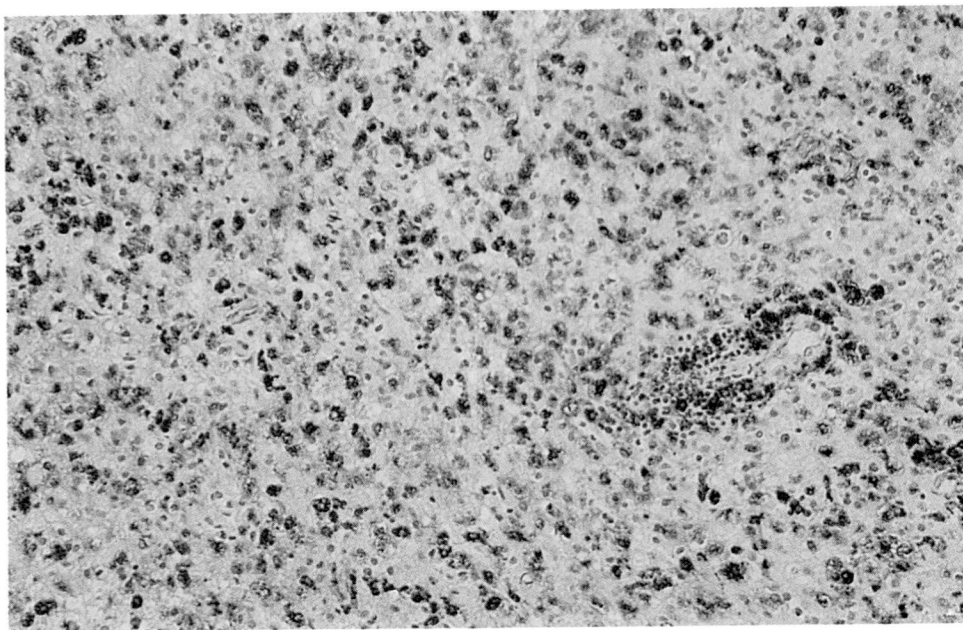

Fig. 28-18 Demyelinating pseudotumor. The density of infiltrating macrophages characteristic of demyelinating lesions is demonstrated in this immunoperoxidase assay for HAM-56.

ataxia occurring in association with radiographically demonstrable thickening and abnormal contrast enhancement of the peribulbar meninges, tentorium, and falx. The process may involve the dura over the cerebral convexities or extend into the orbit and cause painful ophthalmoplegia as a result of mural inflammation of the cavernous sinus. Idiopathic hypertrophic spinal pachymeningitis, a disease of the cervical and upper thoracic region typified by symptoms and signs of compressive radiculopathy, may represent a variant of the same basic disorder.[158] Meningeal biopsies disclose dispersed lymphoplasmacytic infiltrates, exuberant fibroplasia, and in some instances, necrotizing granulomas. Obviously, a confident diagnosis can only be rendered following exclusion of tuberculosis, syphilis, mycotic infections, sarcoidosis, Wegener's granulomatosis, rheumatoid disease, and other defined causes of chronic fibrosing meningitis.[159,160]

Noteworthy is the occasional association of these craniospinal pachymeningitides with extracranial disorders collected under the rubric of *multifocal fibrosclerosis*.[159,160] The latter include inflammatory orbital pseudotumor, idiopathic mediastinal and retroperitoneal fibrosis, sclerosing cholangitis, Riedel's struma, Peyronie's disease, Dupuytren's contracture, fibrosing orchitis, systemic vasculitis, and fibroinflammatory lesions of the subcutaneous tissues and lungs. Secondary extension to the cavernous sinus and neighboring intracranial meninges of inflammatory pseudotumors confined initially to the orbit is also a recognized, albeit uncommon, phenomenon.[161] Unfortunately, the idiopathic craniospinal meningitides are often inexorably progressive disorders, although neurologic deterioration may be delayed by

corticosteroid administration and the resection of compressing fibroinflammatory meningeal masses.

Turning from the meninges to the brain proper, we briefly mention a form of chronic encephalitis, known eponymously as *Rasmussen's syndrome,* long suspected to represent a persistent viral infection but provisionally cataloged here under idiopathic disorders pending convincing demonstration of its infectious basis.[162-164] Afflicted patients suffer intractable unilateral focal seizures or epilepsia partialis continua of childhood onset and often develop progressive hemiparesis and cognitive impairment over the protracted course of the disease. The syndrome's neuropathologic substrate is a nonspecific, chronic encephalitis characterized by lymphoid infiltration of the cerebrocortical perivascular compartment and neuropil, microglial nodule formation, astrogliosis, and variable neuronal loss. There is no reproducibly effective treatment for this curious disorder, but some patients have reportedly benefited from limited resection of localized epileptogenic foci, lobectomy, or extended hemispherectomy.

Limbic encephalitis is a subacutely evolving amnestic syndrome of adulthood that usually represents a paraneoplastic complication of pulmonary small cell carcinoma, although the disorder has also been reported in association with other tumor types (e.g., Hodgkin's disease and nonseminomatous testicular germ cell tumors) and, rarely, in the absence of demonstrable cancer.[165,166] Clinical manifestations consist principally of short-term memory loss (sufficiently profound as to occasionally mimic Korsakoff's psychosis), confusion, disordered affect, and evidences of complex partial seizure activity, including olfactory and visual hallucinations. Many examples present or evolve as one facet of a complex paraneoplastic neurologic disorder that may involve the dorsal root ganglia, brainstem, cerebellum, spinal cord, autonomic ganglia, and myenteric plexi.[167,168]

Neuroimaging studies in cases of limbic encephalitis often disclose focal abnormalities of the medial temporal regions that may prompt considerations of herpes simplex encephalitis or an infiltrative neoplastic process and precipitate biopsy for definitive diagnosis. The brunt of the injury falls on the amygdaloid nuclei, hippocampi, and entorhinal cortices, consisting of florid reactive astrocytosis, perivascular lymphoid cuffing, microglial or "neuronophagic" nodule formation, and in some cases, conspicuous neuronal depopulation. In contrast to herpes simplex encephalitis, the process is never overtly necrotizing, hemorrhagic, or attended by nuclear alterations suggestive of viral infection. Especially useful in the clinical evaluation of suspected limbic encephalitis (which characteristically presents in patients harboring otherwise silent tumors of diminutive proportions) is assay of serum or CSF for a specific autoantibody, designated anti-Hu, directed against neuronal nucleoproteins in the 35 to 40 kd size range and strongly associated with small cell carcinomas of the lung.[167,168] Demonstration of this autoantibody constitutes compelling evidence for the paraneoplastic etiology of a patient's neurologic complaints and mandates a careful evaluation for underlying cancer, beginning with targeted investigation of the chest. Anti-Hu IgG appears to be elaborated in response to aberrant tumoral expression of this neuron-specific protein, prompting articulation of the concept that an immunologic response directed initially against an inciting neoplasm comes ultimately to involve the nervous system in a cross-reaction having devastating neurologic consequences.[168]

Reported as **calcifying pseudoneoplasms of the neural axis**[169] or **unusual fibro-osseous lesions**[170] are histologically distinctive masses composed centrally of an amorphous, hyaline, and vaguely chondroid matrix material exhibiting plate-like or dusty mineralization and rimmed by palisading histiocytes and foreign body–type giant cells. Some examples contain, or are surrounded in part by, spicules of metaplastic bone. These peculiar lesions favor the cranial floor and spinal epidural space but may present within the substance of the brain itself. Although properly regarded as non-neoplastic, they can progress to extensive destruction of the skull base complicated by considerable neurologic morbidity if inadequately treated. Simple excision appears to suffice in this regard. Mineralizing deposits indistinguishable from these fibro-osseous lesions may be found in association with foci of cortical meningioangiomatosis, discussed in the section on meningothelial tumors. Ossified intracranial nodules lacking the calcifying pseudoneoplasm's defining matrix may be formed in non-specific response to trauma, infection, or hemorrhage, and are termed cerebral calculi or simply "brain stones."

Of those principally extraneural disorders occasionally engaging the talents of the neurosurgeon, most deserving of mention are Langerhans' cell granulomatosis (eosinophilic granuloma or histiocytosis X), sarcoidosis, and sinus histiocytosis with massive lymphadenopathy (Rosai-Dorfman dis-

ease). *Langerhans' cell granulomatosis* of the CNS typically follows infiltration of the calvarial floor and exhibits a striking tropism for the region of the hypothalamus and infundibulum, the eponym Hand-Schüller-Christian disease being applied to the classic clinical triad of diabetes insipidus, proptosis, and defects of the skull base on roentgenographic study. A similar topography is characteristic of those exceptional examples restricted (on presentation, at least) to the nervous system,[171] but rare unifocal lesions situated entirely within the cerebral hemispheres are on record,[172] as are isolated instances of brain invasion from contiguous primary foci in the cranial vault.[173]

Neurosarcoidosis most commonly assumes the form of a granulomatous basilar meningitis (Fig. 28-19) complicated by cranial neuropathies or, with extension of the process to the hypothalamic region, diabetes insipidus and other diencephalic syndromes.[176] Although the overwhelming majority of patients have established systemic disease, primary CNS presentations have been described, including tumoral involvement of the meninges,[175] brain,[174] and spinal cord.[177] A granulomatous vasculitis may accompany meningeal disease.

Dural-based masses clinically indistinguishable from meningiomas constitute the pattern of intracranial and intraspinal disease characteristic of *extranodal sinus histiocytosis with massive lymphadenopathy*.[178,179] These lesions can represent the sole manifestations of the disorder and may be solitary or multifocal. A similar predilection for the dura characterizes inflammatory pseudotumors of the neuraxis that have been dubbed *plasma cell granulomas*,[180] although isolated cerebral[181] and intraventricular[183] examples have been depicted. A unique variant possibly analogous to the hyalinizing plasmacytic granuloma of pulmonary origin contains "raft-like" islands of acellular, hyaline connective tissue associated with a foreign body–type giant cell response.[182]

Collectively designated as "xanthomatous" are diverse lesions sharing only a conspicuous complement of foamy, lipid-laden macrophages. Mention has already been made of so-called xanthogranulomas forming in relation to colloid cysts of the third ventricle. Lesions similarly composed of foamy macrophages, foreign body–type giant cells, cholesterol clefts, and reactive lymphoid infiltrates commonly occur in the glomus of the choroid plexus but only rarely attain symptomatic proportions.[184] Dural-based masses described as xanthomas or xanthogranulomas, some of immense proportions, have been encountered in otherwise healthy subjects,[189,194] in association with abnormalities of lipid metabolism such as familial hypercholesterolemia and phytosterolemia,[190,191,195] and in the setting of systemic Weber-Christian disease (relapsing nodular nonsuppurative panniculitis).[193] Some reported examples have complicated a disorder having the clinical features of Hand-Schüller-Christian disease.[185] Whereas the foregoing are clearly non-neoplastic, the nature of some benign xanthomatous lesions containing fibroblasts in storiform array and termed *intracranial fibroxanthomas* is questionable.[186] The literature also contains accounts of solitary masses involving the region of the Gasserian ganglion (Meckel's cave), one a xanthoma of probably traumatic origin[187] and the other a histiocytic proliferation indistinguishable from cutaneous juvenile xan-

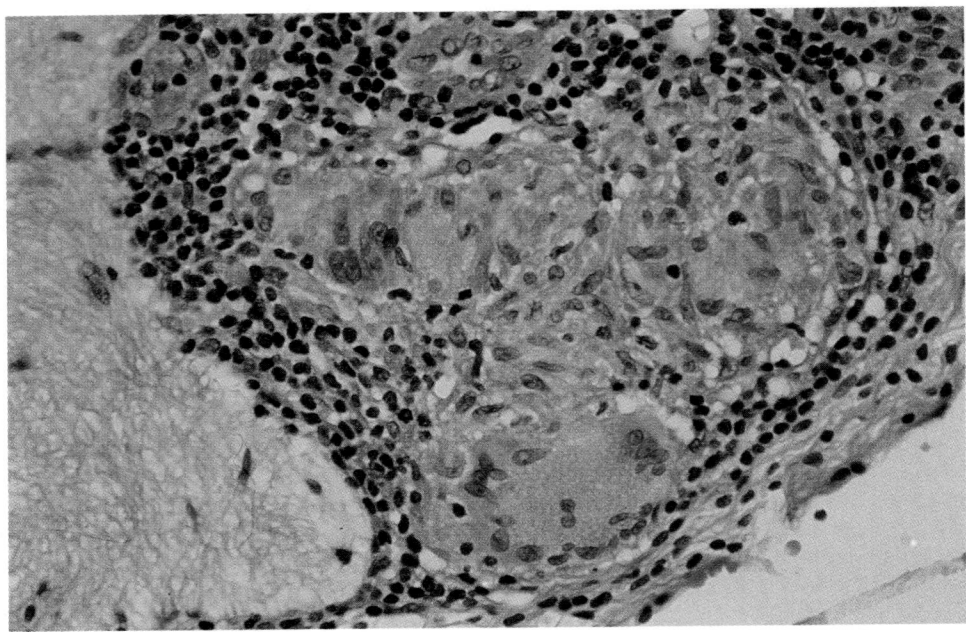

Fig. 28-19 Neurosarcoidosis. A non-necrotizing, granulomatous leptomeningitis replete with multinucleated giant cells of monocytic derivation characterizes this inflammatory disorder in its usual CNS presentation.

thogranuloma ("nevoxanthoendothelioma").[192] CNS infiltration is, in addition, a recognized complication of "xanthoma disseminatum," a systemic syndrome characterized by the widespread eruption of juvenile xanthogranuloma–like lesions.[188]

Other odd processes that have been documented in neurosurgical material include cerebral malakoplakia,[198,199] the pseudoparasitic red blood cell alteration known as myospherulosis,[201] and a bizarre, likely reactive lesion reported as "inflammatory myofibrohistiocytic proliferation simulating sarcoma in children," one multifocal example of which presented with synchronous pulmonary and cerebral masses.[204] An isolated account depicts tumorous cerebellar infiltration by cytologically atypical histiocytes exhibiting immunoreactivity for S-100 protein and conspicuous emperipolesis (lymphophagocytosis),[197] this possibly representing an unusual variant of extranodal sinus histiocytosis with massive lymphadenopathy (Rosai-Dorfman disease). Finally, we mention several described CNS complications of systemic autoimmunologic (collagen vascular) disorders, including rheumatoid nodules of the meninges,[200,203] intracranial extension of sinonasal Wegener's granulomatosis,[202] and a low-grade, corticosteroid-responsive meningoencephalitis associated with cognitive decline in the setting of Sjögren's syndrome.[196]

Infectious diseases
Bacterial infections

Bacteria are responsible for the overwhelming majority of suppurative infections involving the CNS and its coverings. Of particular concern to surgical pathologists are the common forms of localized suppuration: abscesses of the brain and spinal epidural space.

Approximately 20% of brain abscesses are not associated with conditions predisposing to bacterial invasion of the nervous system, the remainder arising in patients with established pyogenic infections at extraneural sites, facilitating anatomic anomalies or histories of penetrating cranial trauma or prior neurosurgery.[210,224] Obviously, their demographic features, localization, number, and microbiologic characteristics will vary with the risk factors in individual cases.

The extraneural bacterial infections predisposing to brain abscess are usefully divided into those involving contiguous meningeal or parameningeal sites versus those more distantly placed. Curious is the fact that cerebral abscesses rarely complicate bacterial meningitis, a notable exception to this rule being their significant association with neonatal leptomeningitides caused by Proteus mirabilis and Citrobacter diversus.[215,217] More frequently implicated among local sources of bacillary invasion are infected paranasal sinuses, middle ear cavities, and mastoids.[210,224] Although their pathogenesis remains imprecisely defined, abscesses associated with these various infections are commonly held to result from the retrograde thrombophlebitic carriage of organisms into the cranial cavity via emissary veins. Typically solitary, these tend to stereotyped topographic presentations. Thus cerebral abscesses related to frontoethmoid sinusitis characteristically settle in the anterobasal frontal lobes, whereas "otitic" examples (including those associated with chronic mastoiditis) are usually encountered in the temporal lobes or cerebellar hemispheres. Lesions complicating sphenoid sinusitis frequent both the frontal and temporal regions. The organisms most often isolated from brain abscesses in these clinical circumstances include aerobic or microaerophilic streptococci (especially members of the *S. milleri* group), aerobic gram-negative bacilli *(Proteus, Escherichia coli, Klebsiella-Enterobacter,* and *Haemophilus* species), and *Bacteroides* species; mixed infections are common. Other local suppurative processes associated with the subsequent development of brain abscess include dental sepsis and pyogenic infections of the face and scalp. Usually frontal in location, "odontogenic" abscesses typically follow tooth extraction or other dental manipulation and harbor mixed aerobic and anaerobic populations dominated by *Fusobacterium, Bacteroides,* and *Streptococcus* species. *Staphylococcus aureus* is the main offender when facial or scalp infections are incriminated; cerebral abscesses in this setting usually occur in cases complicated by cavernous sinus thrombosis. Mandibulofacial actinomycosis may also eventuate in brain abscess.[220]

Hematogenous seeding of the CNS from distant foci of infection usually results in a multiplicity of abscesses that commonly lie within the territories subtended by the middle cerebral arteries. Most germinate at the junction of the cortical mantle and underlying white matter, but the cerebellum, basal ganglia, thalami, and brainstem may also be involved. "Metastatic" lesions of this sort most often have their origin in the thorax, chronic suppurating pulmonary disorders such as lung abscess and bronchiectasis leading the list of conditions predisposing to their development.[210,224] Much less common among underlying "donors" are bacterial endocarditis (characteristically acute), empyema, osteomyelitis, and infections of deep pelvic organs or abdominal viscera. Additional risk factors of note include various conditions in which the filtering function of the lung's capillary bed is abrogated (e.g., pulmonary arteriovenous fistulae) and cyanotic congenital heart diseases when complicated by right-to-left shunts (as encountered in tetralogy of Fallot, patent foramen ovale, ventricular septal defect, and transposition of the great vessels). The secondary polycythemia that regularly attends these anomalies may further promote the genesis of abscesses from infective emboli by causing microcirculatory sludging and regional brain hypoxia. Similar mechanisms may account for the significant risk of cerebral abscess in hereditary hemorrhagic telangiectasia (Osler-Weber-Rendu disease); most patients with this complication harbor pulmonary AVMs and exhibit hypoxemia with resultant cyanosis, clubbing, and polycythemia.[213] Among iatrogenic causes of metastatic brain abscess, instrumentation of the esophagus in attempts to relieve caustic strictures or treat varices by the endoscopic injection of sclerosing agents merits citation.[218]

The microbiology of the foregoing lesions is complex, but a few generalizations are possible. *Fusobacterium, Bacteroides,* and streptococci are the organisms most commonly recovered from brain abscesses associated with pulmonary sepsis, actinomycotic[220] and nocardial[209] lesions (the latter often encountered in debilitated and immunosuppressed subjects) also representing secondary deposits from foci of established lung infection in a majority of cases. Streptococci and *Haemophilus* species are the typical offenders in cases related to congenital heart disease, whereas *S. aureus*

dominates isolates from examples complicating acute bacterial endocarditis.

With regard to the direct inoculation of bacteria into CNS tissues, abscess formation is probably the least frequent cerebral consequence of either penetrating cranial trauma or neurosurgery.[221,224] *S. aureus* is the organism most often recovered from lesions arising in these circumstances, followed by *Streptococcus, Enterobacter,* and *Clostridium* species. *Propionibacterium acnes,* a gram-positive, anaerobic rod that causes a syndrome of shunt malfunction and immune-complex nephritis in patients with intraventricular catheters, is also emerging as an increasingly common agent of traumatically and surgically acquired brain abscesses.[205,224] Trauma and intracranial hematoma accumulation, in addition, predispose to cerebral *Salmonella* abscess.[224]

Brain abscesses remain a diagnostic challenge to the clinician because their presenting manifestations and neuroradiologic appearances are nonspecific. Noteworthy is the fact that only 40% to 50% of patients are febrile on evaluation. The more common signs and symptoms are those of any expanding intracranial mass: headache, altered mental status, focal sensorimotor deficits, seizure, nausea, and vomiting.[210,224] Although central hypodensity, "ring" enhancement, and surrounding edema are characteristic on CT or MRI studies (Fig. 28-20), these appearances may be shared by malignant neoplasms and, on occasion, demyelinating disease.

Experimental, clinical, and histopathologic observations suggest that abscesses of the human brain begin as ill-defined zones of bacterial multiplication and polymorphonuclear leukocytic infiltration (cerebritis) most commonly situated in white matter immediately subjacent to the cortical ribbon or at the gray-white junction.[207] With time, proliferating fibroblasts come to surround a central mass of fibrinopurulent debris and fashion a collagenous capsule resembling the pyogenic membranes formed in response to suppurative infections outside the nervous system (Fig. 28-21). This, in turn, is bordered by edematous, chronically inflamed, and gliotic brain tissue that may evidence foci of acute cerebritis attesting to the host's failure to entirely wall off the primary locus of infection.

The rate at which encapsulation proceeds and its completeness vary considerably. Hematogenous bacterial seeding of the brain from distant sites of suppuration generally results in abscesses with capsules less developed than those that surround examples arising secondary to contiguous pyogenic processes. Especially notorious for their poor encapsulation are nocardial lesions. That capsular organization is typically most advanced along the superficial, juxtacortical perimeter of brain abscesses is reflected in the tendency of "daughter" lesions to bud from their deep aspects and in their tendency to rupture into the ventricular system rather than subarachnoid space. Because the mesenchymal elements responsible for capsule formation presumably derive from the adventitia of regional blood vessels and require oxygen for collagen fibrillogenesis, the relatively retarded organizational responses of paraventricular, as compared with cortical and paracortical, tissues may be a consequence of their less extensive vasculature. The intraventricular discharge of purulent material is among the most feared of

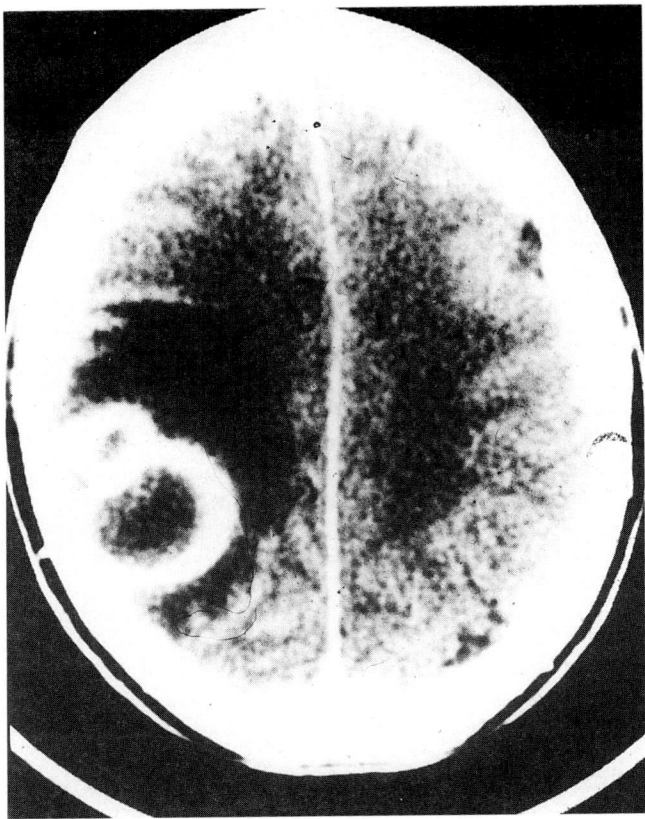

Fig. 28-20 Cerebral abscess. Ring enhancement of their developing pseudocapsules, budding of "daughter" lesions, and marked hypodensity of adjacent white matter reflecting severe edema are all characteristic of cerebral abscesses on CT or MR study. This example complicated mandibulofacial actinomycosis.

all abscess-related complications, almost invariably proving fatal.

In contrast to the largely intracranial localization of bacterial abscesses involving the CNS proper, 90% of epidural examples are situated at spinal levels.[211,212] Here a "true" (as opposed to potential) space, containing adipose tissue, nutrient arteries, and an elaborate venous plexus, expands posterior and lateral to the dura mater, whereas above the foramen magnum this fibrous sheath adheres tightly to the inner aspect of the skull. Anterior tethering of the dura to adjacent vertebral bodies presumably accounts for the fact that most epidural abscesses evolving along the length of the spinal cord are posteriorly or posterolaterally positioned. Approximately half of these settle in the thoracic region and one third in the lumbar region. Less accommodating is the epidural space at cervical levels, where the spinal canal is nearly filled by the cord itself, and sacral lesions are rare.

Roughly 40% of spinal epidural abscesses arise "spontaneously," the remainder (like their neuroparenchymal counterparts) secondarily complicating infections established at contiguous or distant sites, trauma, intravenous drug abuse, spinal surgery, or other invasive procedures, including epidural catheterization and lumbar puncture. Of particular impor-

tance among predisposing infections are contiguous foci of vertebral osteomyelitis, psoas and perinephric abscesses, decubitus ulcers, and other cutaneous and soft tissue suppurations. Diabetes mellitus, alcoholism, and renal failure are also recognized as significant risk factors. Presenting clinical manifestations typically include fever, malaise, and backache. If antimicrobial therapy and neurosurgical decompression are delayed, these early symptoms may progress in stepwise fashion to radiculopathy, sensorimotor and sphincter disturbances indicative of spinal cord dysfunction, and finally, paralysis. *S. aureus* remains the most common culprit, distantly trailed by gram-negative aerobes such as *E. coli* and *Pseudomonas aeruginosa,* streptococci, and various anaerobes.

Although *Mycobacterium tuberculosis* is among the more common agents of spinal epidural abscess,[211,212,225] especially among intravenous drug abusers, the lesions it produces are typically granulomatous and caseating rather than suppurative. These usually arise in the low thoracic or lumbar region by extension from contiguous foci of tuberculous vertebral osteomyelitis or disk infection, but "primary" examples not associated with osseous, pulmonary, or extraosseous disease may be encountered. Diagnosis is complicated by the fact that patients often present with back pain of insidious onset and chronic evolution unattended by fever, leukocytosis, or evidence of tuberculosis on chest film. As with nontuberculous epidural abscesses, the consequence of delayed intervention is progressive neurologic dysfunction culminating in myelopathy or "Pott's paraplegia." Other localized forms of mycobacterial CNS infection include tuberculoma,[219,225] focal tuberculous meningoencephalitis,[222] and the rare tuberculous abscess.[223] Tuberculoma, defined as an encapsulated, granulomatous, and centrally caseating inflammatory mass, is by far the most common variant of neuroparenchymal tuberculosis, is usually unaccompanied by evidence of co-extant meningeal infection, and may settle anywhere along the neuraxis but favors the intracranial contents. An excess of pediatric examples present in the cerebellum, constituting the posterior fossa "tumors" encountered most frequently in some countries (e.g., India), where tuberculosis is rampant. At substantially increased risk of developing both tuberculous meningitis and neuroparenchymal tuberculomas are HIV-1–seropositive subjects,[206,225] instances of CNS infection by atypical mycobacteria of the avium-intracellulare complex having also been documented in this setting.[214]

Other distinctive bacterial infections of the nervous system proper include a bulbar encephalitis ("rhombencephalitis") caused by *Listeria monocytogenes*[216] and cerebral Whipple's disease, resulting from invasion of the neuropil by *Tropheryma whippelii.*[208] The latter process is characterized in the brain, as elsewhere, by infiltrates of foamy macrophages exhibiting an intense, granular PAS positivity of their cytoplasm and containing numerous rod-shaped bacillary forms on ultrastructural study. A florid reactive astrogliosis is the rule.

Mycoses

The incidence of CNS mycosis has risen dramatically over the past several decades, reflecting the expanded population of immunocompromised patients susceptible to microbial

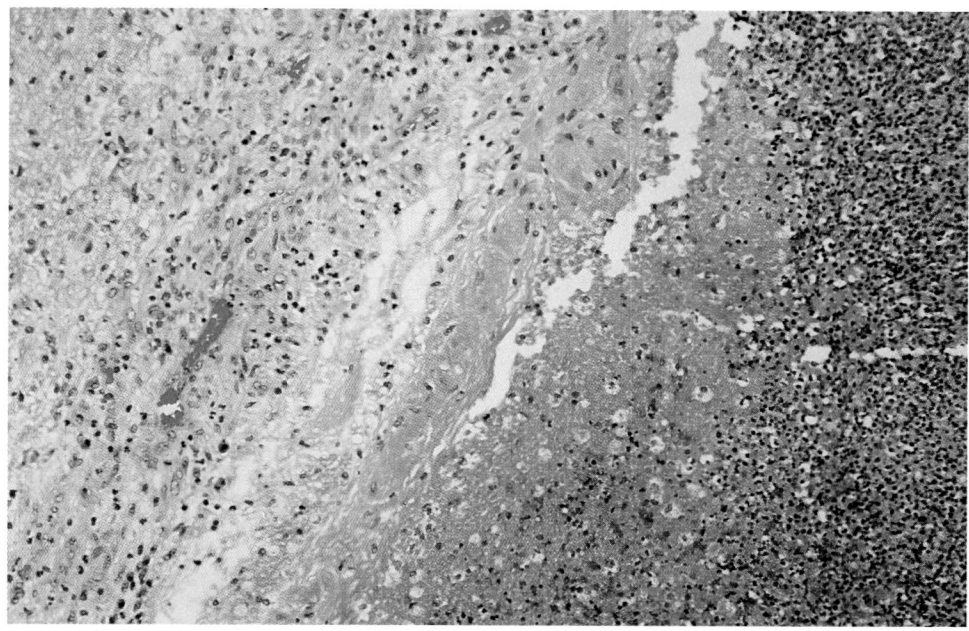

Fig. 28-21 Cerebral abscess. The lesion's purulent contents are separated from neighboring white matter by a granulation tissue-like zone of angioblastic and fibroblastic activity.

opportunists. Still, neuroinvasive fungal infection only exceptionally occasions diagnostic operative intervention and thus remains a curiosity to the surgical pathologist. Most space-occupying intracranial and intraspinal lesions of mycotic etiology develop in association with diffuse meningeal or disseminated systemic infection and, consequently, are diagnosed by study of the CSF or, in the latter scenario, are treated empirically without recourse to tissue examination. Many are discovered only at autopsy. *Cryptococcus neoformans,* pathogenic molds, *Candida* species, and the dimorphic and dematiaceous fungi collectively account for the vast majority of lesions encountered in neurosurgical practice.[240]

C. neoformans, the agent of a diffuse leptomeningitis that is the single most common CNS mycosis, occasionally proliferates in localized neuroparenchymal or choroid plexus–based, intraventricular masses known as ***cryptococcomas.***[229,238,240] Noteworthy is the fact that fewer than 5% of these unusual lesions arise in association with systemic disorders predisposing to opportunistic infection. Cryptococcal meningitis, by contrast, often afflicts immunosuppressed patients (e.g., HIV-1–seropositive adults, diabetics, organ transplant recipients, and patients being treated for hematologic or lymphoid neoplasia). The appearance of the cryptococcoma varies with the host's reaction, which may range from inertia to necrotizing granuloma formation and pronounced desmoplasia. When cryptococci hold the advantage, the lesion consists mainly of mucoid or gelatinous material that reflects the conspicuous elaboration of capsular mucopolysaccharides characteristic of these organisms. This is often traversed in honeycomb-like fashion by fibrous connective tissue septa. At the other extreme are sclerotic, granulomatous masses containing only rare yeast forms. Exceptional examples mimic bacterial abscesses, containing

purulent debris bound by a well-developed pyogenic membrane. *Cryptococcus* is typically ovoid or spheric in profile, measures 2 to 15 μm in diameter, replicates by budding from a narrow base, and is reliably distinguished from other yeast by demonstration of its mucicarminophilic capsule.

Fungi existing in pure hyphal form at both room temperature and 37° C are termed molds. The major CNS pathogens in this group include *Aspergillus* species, the Mucoraceae, and *Pseudallescheria boydii. Fusarium, Paecilomyces,* and *Penicillium* species, *Streptomyces griseus,* and *Acremonium alabamensis* have also proved neuroinvasive on occasion.[240] Opportunists all, these ubiquitous organisms only rarely attack otherwise healthy individuals and share a particular predilection for patients receiving maintenance doses of broad-spectrum antibiotics through protracted periods of neutropenia, as commonly occurs in the management of leukemias and lymphomas. CNS infections that occur in such settings result from fungemia, are primarily intraparenchymal (as opposed to meningeal), are usually multifocal, and typically accompanied by evidence of systemic mycosis. The development of cerebral aspergillosis in patients treated for hematologic neoplasms, for example, is almost invariably preceded by symptomatic fungal infection of the lungs. Also at risk of blood-borne CNS seeding by pathogenic molds are patients taking corticosteroids, intravenous drug abusers, and, in the case of *P. boydii,*[234] victims of near drowning. Alcoholic liver disease and Cushing's syndrome have also been associated with CNS aspergillosis.[240,244] A second important form of meningeal and neuroparenchymal mycosis caused by these agents follows their direct intracranial spread from foci of orbital or paranasal sinus infection. This pattern of disease is typified by rhinocerebral mucormycosis, a disorder classically associated with diabetic ketoacidosis but also complicating other acidemic states (e.g., sepsis, profound dehydration, uremia), renal transplantation, and desferoxamine therapy.[240] Prior to the application of immunosuppressive chemotherapeutic regimens to the treatment of cancer, *Aspergillus* generally invaded the CNS from primary foci of ocular, sinonasal or middle ear infection. In addition, skull fracture, penetrating trauma, and craniotomy may set the stage for neural infection by molds.

The neurologic manifestations, distribution, and morphology of CNS lesions caused by these agents vary with the clinical circumstances surrounding infection and the immune status of the host. Particularly characteristic of cerebral disease evolving in the setting of disseminated systemic mycosis is a syndrome of multifocal stroke that reflects the shared tendency of pathogenic molds to occlude, invade, and trigger thrombosis of the leptomeningeal and perforating cerebral vasculature. The resulting lesions are basically infarcts, often hemorrhagic, that are secondarily colonized by fungi migrating through damaged blood vessel walls and that frequently exhibit little inflammatory reaction or limited superimposed suppuration. These are typically scattered in both cerebral hemispheres and often involve the deep nuclei, cerebellum, and brainstem. Contiguous fungal infiltration of the leptomeninges is common, but infection limited to these tissues is rare. Solitary lesions are exceptional, but examples produced by *Aspergillus* species,[230,246] *P. boydii*,[234] and other molds[240] are on record. These present with symptoms referable to an expanding intracranial mass, tend to occur in patients whose immune reflexes are relatively preserved, and may assume an abscess-like or even granulomatous character. Of particular note is a distinctive form of localized CNS mucormycosis characterized by a remarkably stereotypic predilection for the basal ganglia of intravenous drug abusers.[227,241] The more common rhino-cerebral infections caused by advancing Mucoraceae are manifest as poorly delimited, necrotizing lesions again evidencing the ischemic and hemorrhagic qualities typical of these angioinvasive organisms. True mycotic aneurysm has also been described as a consequence of cerebral aspergillosis.[237]

The definitive taxonomic classification of molds requires their isolation in culture and cannot be accomplished on the basis of their morphology in tissue sections. Of the major CNS pathogens, both *Aspergillus* species and *P. boydii* appear in biopsy material as septate hyphae. *Aspergillus* species are usually somewhat stouter and branch (at acute angles) more frequently, but these are not reliably distinguishing features. By contrast, the Mucoraceae are broad, ribbon-like hyphal organisms that are nonseptate and branch at right angles.

Blastomyces dermatitidis, Histoplasma capsulatum, Coccidioides immitis, and *Paracoccidioides brasiliensis* are traditionally grouped as "dimorphic" fungi because of their growth as filamentous mycelia at room temperature and yeast at 37° C. All are capable of infecting the CNS, usually in the form of a chronic granulomatous meningitis in patients with co-extant, active systemic mycoses. Limited extension to the cerebral cortex from contiguous foci of leptomeningeal infection is common but typically of no clinical consequence. Only rarely do neuroparenchymal lesions attain symptomatic proportions. Again, these unusual fungal masses are generally, although not invariably, associated with evident infection of extraneural tissues. Examples have been described

both in the obviously immunodeficient and in patients with no clear risk factors for opportunistic disease.* Worth noting are observations that roughly half of the intracranial blastomycomas and a majority of the histoplasmomas reported to date presented as solitary lesions. Brain invasion by *C. immitis* and *P. brasiliensis* is, by contrast, infrequently unifocal. The interested reader is referred to the cited literature for details regarding the pathogenesis and morphology of these curious lesions and the appearances of their causative agents. Suffice it to say that these organisms as a rule evoke a necrotizing, granulomatous tissue response replete with multinucleated giant cells and, in cases of blastomycoma and histoplasmoma, foci of caseation that may prompt considerations of tuberculous infection. A suppurative infiltrate of polymorphonuclear leukocytes is also commonly observed in otherwise granulomatous masses caused by *B. dermatitidis*. Mycotic intracranial aneurysm caused by *C. immitis* infection has been described.[231]

The dematiaceous fungi are a group of pigmented hyphal yeasts best known as the agents of chronic skin and subcutaneous infections such as Madura foot and tinea capitis. Extracutaneous disease is exceptional, but the brain is a common target in disseminated mycoses caused by these organisms. One member of the group, *Xylohypha bantiana (Cladosporium trichoides)*, appears to be specifically neurotropic and is responsible for most CNS infections,[228,240] which are often classed with other deep mycoses caused by pigmented fungi under the rubric of **phaeohyphomycosis.** This organism is fully capable of invading the nervous systems of apparently immunocompetent hosts and, in many cases, does so in the absence of demonstrable foci of extraneural infection. Isolated patients have suffered immunosuppressive underlying conditions; exhibited pre-existent phaeohyphomycotic infections of the paranasal sinuses, ear, or lungs; or have apparently acquired the infection through traumatic intracerebral implantation or intravenous drug abuse.[233] Neuroparenchymal lesions consist of necrotizing granulomas, multifocal in about 50% of cases. A similar fraction are attended by fungal meningitis. In tissue sections, the agent appears as branching, septate hyphal, and yeast-like structures with a brown or olive-green hue. Isolation in culture is required for definitive classification. Other pigmented fungi that have been reported to cause CNS disease include *Drechslera-Bipolaris-Exserohilum* and *Curvularia* species, *Fonsecaea pedrosoi, Wangiella dermatitidis, Dactylaria constricta,* and *Ramichloridium oboroideum*.[240]

If *Candida* species appear to receive short shrift in these pages, it is not because the threat they pose to the nervous system is trivial in epidemiologic terms. Actually, cerebral candidiasis has emerged in recent years as one of the most common CNS mycoses encountered in immunosuppressed patients.[235,240] The fact remains, however, that the great majority of cerebral *Candida* infections are discovered only at autopsy, resulting from fungemia in debilitated, moribund patients. The typical lesions are diminutive foci of suppuration scattered widely in the neuropil and associated in some cases with fungal meningitis. The formation of granulomas or macroabscesses, disease limited to the meninges, and vas-

---

*References 226, 236, 239, 240, 242, 243, 245.

culitis, with resultant infarction or the development of mycotic aneurysms,[237,240] have also been described, as has the extraordinary presentation of CNS candidiasis as a localized fungal mass.[232]

Viral infections

Herpes simplex encephalitis Herpes viruses are responsible for a wide variety of neurologic infections, our concern here being with a distinctive form of focal, necrotizing, and hemorrhagic encephalitis caused principally by herpes simplex virus type 1 (HSV-1).[254] *Herpes simplex encephalitis* (HSE) afflicts only 2 to 4 persons per 1,000,000 inhabitants a year but leads the list of potentially fatal, nonepidemic cerebral infections of viral etiology. Individuals of any age may be affected. The disease is often fulminant in its evolution and is characterized by fever, disordered affect, dysphasia, seizure activity, and deterioration of consciousness. CSF pleocytosis is the rule and may be accompanied by xanthochromia, whereas abnormalities are usually localized to one or both frontotemporal regions on electroencephalographic study, CT scan, or MRI (Fig. 28-22). Isolation of the agent from neurosurgical material remains the most sensitive and specific means of diagnosis in general use at this time, though the need for brain biopsy in the management of suspected HSE has become a matter of some controversy with the advent of efficacious antiviral therapy in the form of acyclovir.[254] Among the more compelling arguments in favor of biopsy is that many diseases, including neoplasms and infections of nonviral etiology, can masquerade as HSE. Assays of CSF for HSV-specific antigens[254] and genomic sequences[247] hold great promise as noninvasive methods of rapid and definitive diagnosis.

A remarkably stereotypic predilection for the anteromedial temporal lobes, orbitofrontal cortex, insulae, and cingulate gyri typifies HSE.[249,250,254] Experimental observations support the hypothesis that this "limbic" distribution reflects transolfactory spread of the agent to the CNS and suggest that at least some cases of HSE follow activation of virus residing latently in cerebral tissues.[254] The histologic appearances of the disorder vary considerably with the duration of the clinical illness.[249,250] The earliest appreciable changes, evident prior to the arrival of inflammatory infiltrates, include neuronal shrinkage and eosinophilia accompanied by vascular congestion, spongy cortical rarefaction, and pallor. We have seen this picture, which closely mimics that of hypoxic-ischemic brain injury, misdiagnosed as acute cerebral infarction, although close scrutiny of these degenerating neurons often reveals a ground-glass alteration of their nucleoplasm that should suggest a viral cytopathic effect. It is during this early phase of symptomatic disease that careful search for the eosinophilic intranuclear inclusion bodies typical of herpetic infection is most likely to be rewarded (Fig. 28-23). These may be identified in the nuclei of cortical astrocytes and satellite oligodendroglia, as well as neurons, but are an inconstant feature of the disorder.

The pronounced inflammatory reaction characteristic of fully developed HSE is usually in evidence by the second week of clinical disease. Lymphocytes and plasma cells colonize the meninges, cuff penetrating blood vessels, and migrate into the devastated cortex. Mononuclear cells may

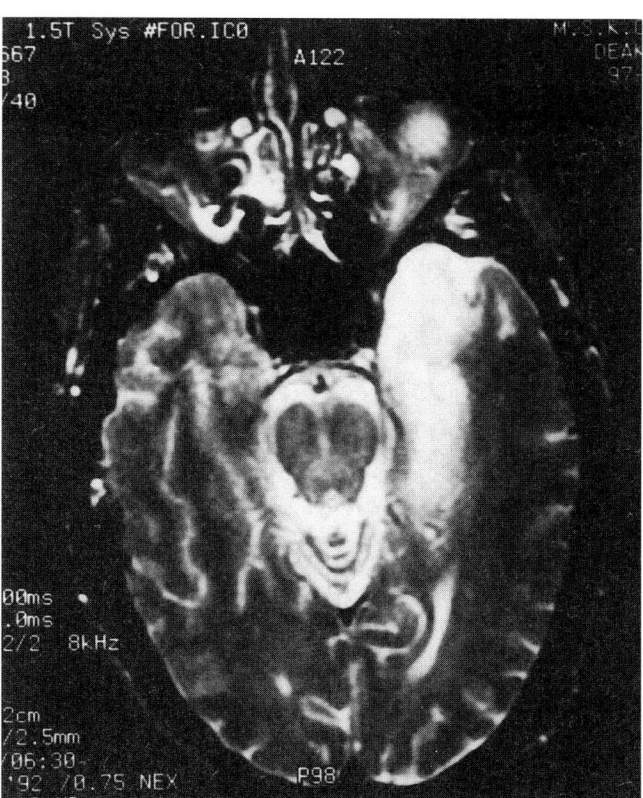

Fig. 28-22 HSE. This MRI, from a middle-aged man with headache, fever, and disordered affect, demonstrates the anteromedial temporal lobe localization of signal abnormalities ("bright" in this study) typical of HSE on neuroradiologic assessment.

converge on infected neurons to form neuronophagic or so-called microglial nodules. These changes are often accompanied by hemorrhage and, in some cases, thrombosis and even fibrinoid necrosis of the cerebral vasculature. Foamy macrophages eventually come to dominate the invading cellular elements and ultimately clear the necrotic debris, only cavitated and gliotic remnants persisting at sites of prior infection.

Electron microscopy,[253] immunocytochemistry[249,253] and in situ hybridization techniques[248] may all be profitably applied to the diagnosis of HSE and may in select cases provide evidence of HSV infection in biopsy material exhibiting little alteration at the light microscopic level. Ultrastructural study is the most laborious and least sensitive of these methods but is the only one to afford direct visualization of the agent in infected cells. Assembled in the nucleus, the mature HSV particle is an icosahedral nucleocapsid averaging 100 to 120 nm in diameter and containing a central density representing the agent's genomic DNA (Fig. 28-24). Virions typically acquire a lipid envelope derived from the host nuclear membrane on transport into the cytoplasm. Inasmuch as similar appearances are shared by other encephalitogenic herpes viruses, electron microscopy is of limited utility in specifically identifying the offender as HSV. Commercially available antibodies to this agent are now routinely employed for this purpose, and immunohistochem-

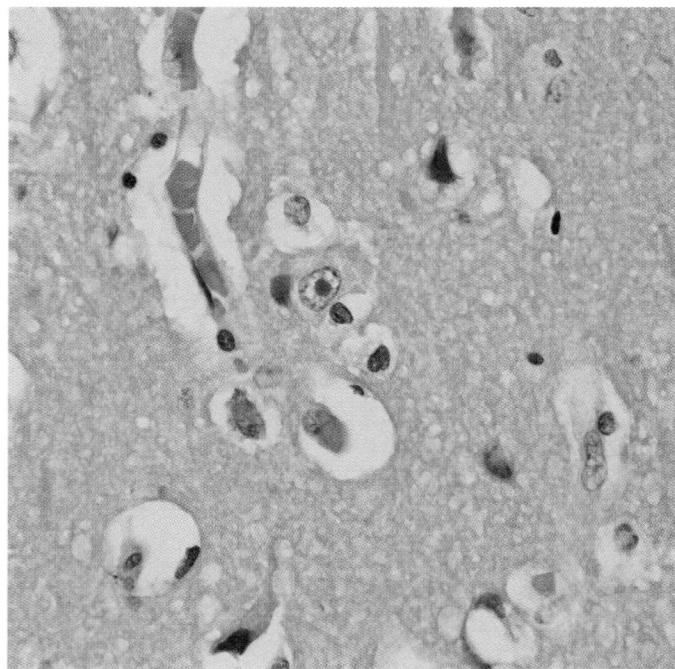

Fig. 28-23. HSE. As shown here, herpes simplex encephalitis may masquerade as a noninfectious, ischemic process (particularly if biopsied early in its clinical evolution). Note the noninflammatory appearance, neuronal shrinkage, pyknosis, and dissolution. The nucleus of an astrocyte in the center of this field contains a well-defined inclusion body.

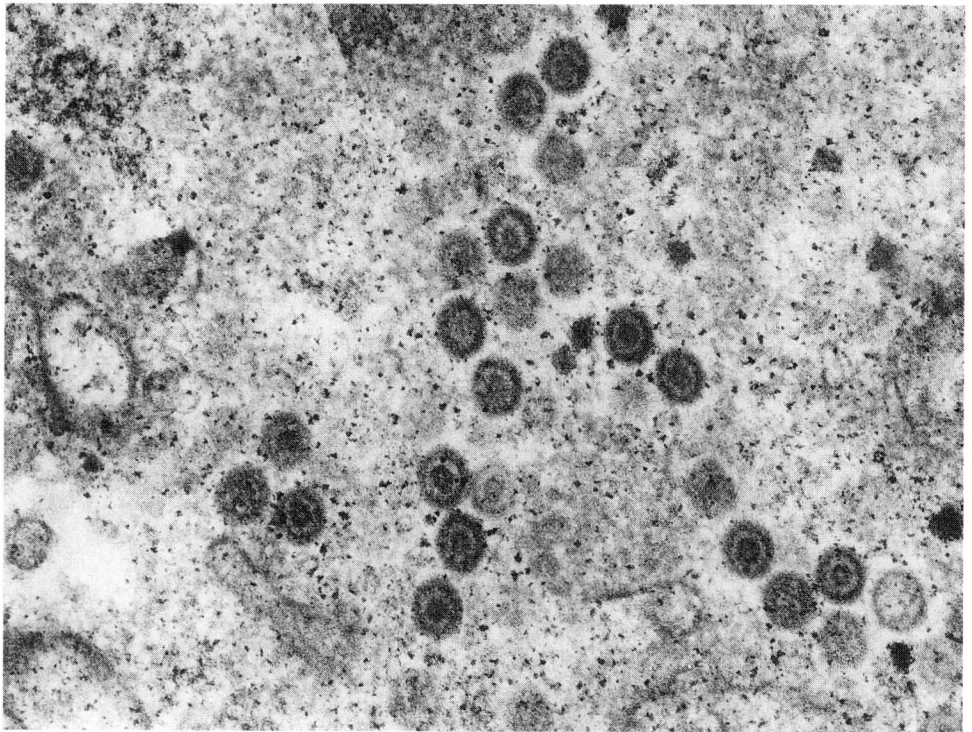

Fig. 28-24 HSE. This transmission electron photomicrograph reveals enveloped nucleocapsids with an average diameter of 100 nm in the cytoplasm of an infected cell. (×62,000.)

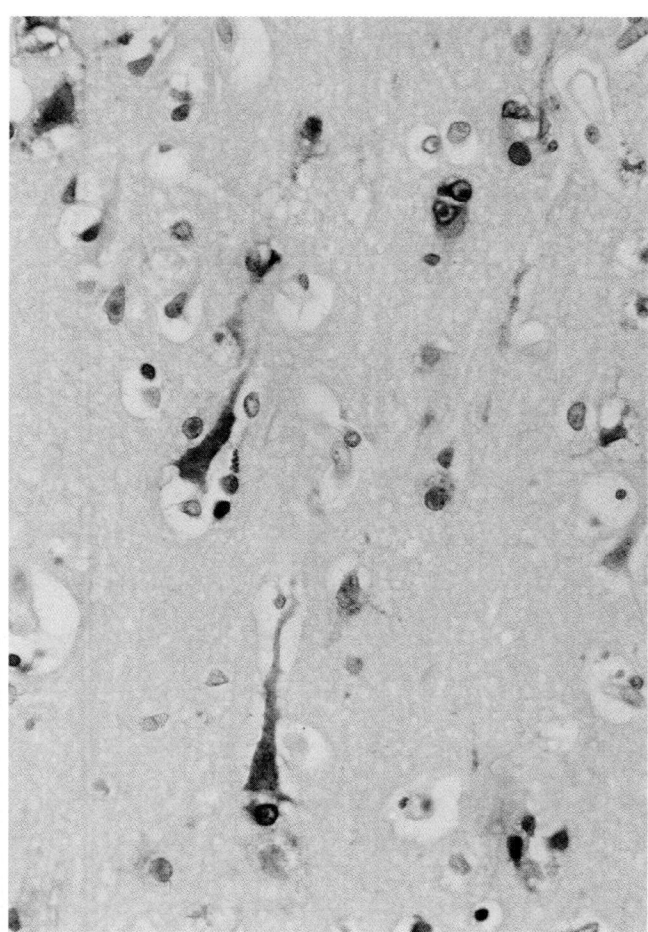

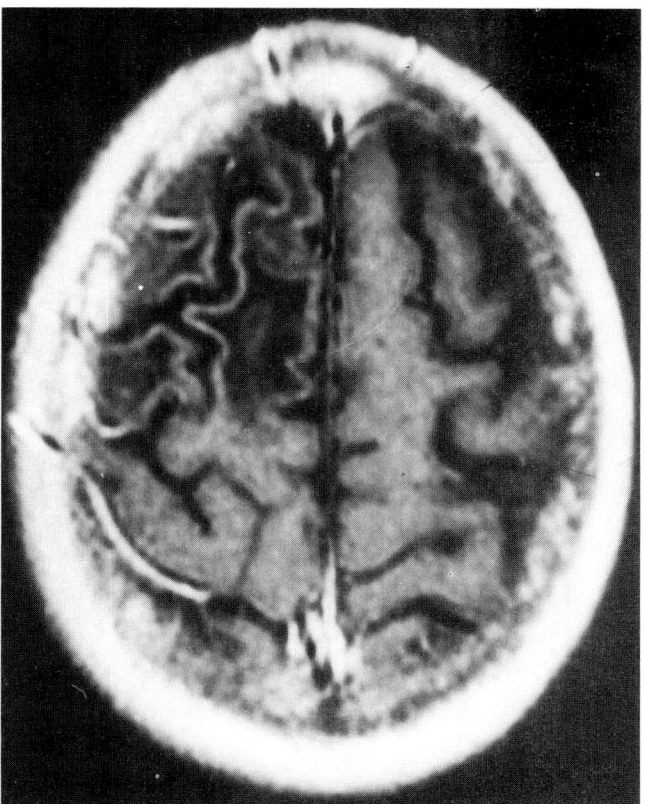

Fig. 28-26 Progressive multifocal leukoencephalopathy. A postcontrast injection MRI demonstrates the regional white matter hypodensity, absence of mass effect or abnormal enhancement, and cortical preservation that typify this demyelinating infection.

Fig. 28-25 HSE. In this immunoperoxidase preparation, the cytoplasm of neurons and inclusion bodies within the nuclei of satellite glia are labeled by antibodies to herpes simplex type 1.

ical assay, although not supplanting viral isolation procedures, is a technique strongly recommended in all cases of clinically suspected HSE, regardless of whether inspection of biopsy material reveals evidence of an inflammatory process (Fig. 28-25). In fact, Esiri's elegant correlative studies[249] indicate that attempts at HSV antigen detection are most likely to succeed during the first week of encephalitic symptoms. Coincident with a mounting inflammatory reaction, antigen expression declines steadily through the second and third weeks of the clinical illness and is not usually demonstrable thereafter. We have noted, however, the unusual persistence of viral antigens beyond this period in cases of HSE involving immunocompromised hosts. These appeared to be arrested at the noninflammatory, pseudoischemic phase characteristic of early HSE in otherwise normal individuals. A similarly inert histologic picture characterized an example of protracted HSE involving an anergic patient with Hodgkin's disease.[251] Viral persistence and a paucity of reactive lymphoid elements have been documented in the setting of acquired immune deficiency syndrome (AIDS).[252]

Progressive multifocal leukoencephalopathy *Progressive multifocal leukoencephalopathy* (PML) is an oppor-

tunistic demyelinating disease of the CNS caused by DNA viruses of the polyoma group.[266] Nearly all clinical isolates responsible for the disorder have been strains of the ubiquitous *JC virus* (so designated for the initials of the first afflicted patient from whose brain the agent was recovered), with only exceptional cases linked to the related SV-40. Originally delineated as a paraneoplastic complication of Hodgkin's disease and chronic lymphocytic leukemia,[255] PML is almost always associated with defective cell-mediated immunity, is currently encountered most frequently in the setting of underlying human immunodeficiency virus type 1 (HIV-1) infection, and may be the presenting manifestation of AIDS.[256] An estimated 0.5% to 1.0% of HIV-1–infected individuals develop this disorder, PML having become the viral infection most likely to prompt diagnostic brain biopsy in hospitals serving large HIV-1–seropositive populations. The disease is characterized by subacutely evolving neurologic symptoms indicative of a multifocal process. Chief among these are motor deficits, cognitive decline, and visual loss. Although tumefactive variants have been described,[259,264] neuroimaging studies usually provide a clue to the nature of the process by demonstrating scattered foci

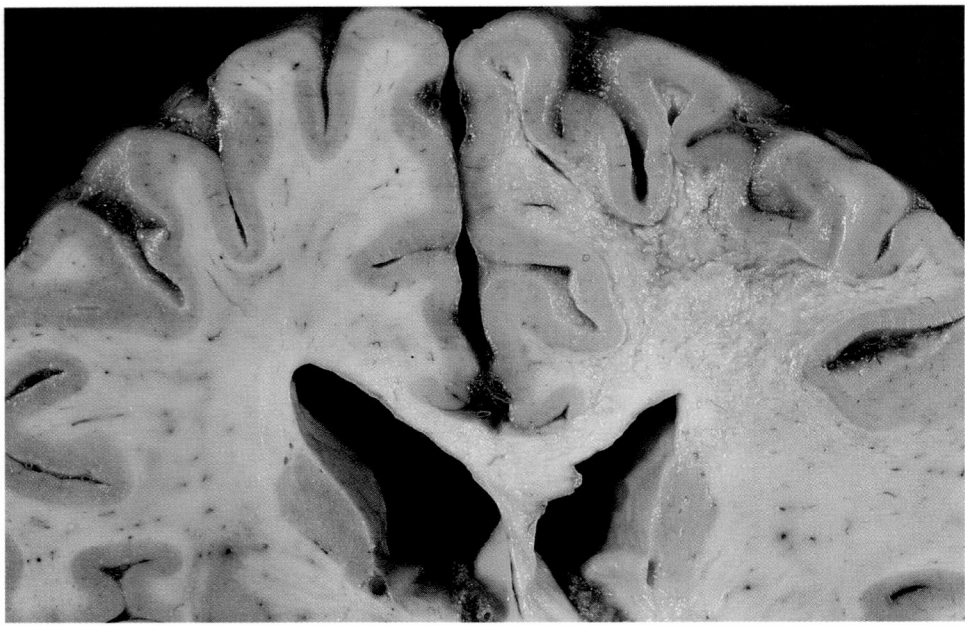

Fig. 28-27 Progressive multifocal leukoencephalopathy. Note an intact cortical ribbon overlying devastated white matter of the right frontal lobe.

of white matter hypodensity not associated with mass effect or contrast enhancement (Fig. 28-26). At present, brain biopsy remains the usual method of definitive diagnosis, but the selective amplification of JC virus–specific DNA sequences from the CSF of afflicted patients can be accomplished.[258]

Any level of the central neuraxis may be affected in PML, but the cerebral hemispheric white matter generally bears the brunt of the injury (Fig. 28-27). Cerebellar and bulbar localizations are less common, and the spinal cord is usually spared. It is the remarkable tropism of the JC virus for, and its replication within, oligodendroglia that are responsible for the alterations pathognomonic of PML. Productive infection of these cells results in progressive enlargement of their nuclei, dissolution of their compacted chromatin, and its replacement by homogeneously dense and basophilic or "ground-glass," amphophilic material (Fig. 28-28). Considerably less common than this transformation of the entire nucleoplasm are demarcated eosinophilic inclusions of the sort that typify herpes virus infections. At the fine structural level, the oligodendrocytopathy characteristic of PML corresponds to a distention of the nucleus by nonenveloped, spheric, or icosahedral particles measuring 33 to 45 nm in diameter. These are frequently aggregated in paracrystalline arrays and may be admixed with filamentous viral strands 15 to 25 nm in diameter (Fig. 28-29). Although immunocytochemical assay,[260] in situ hybridization,[260] and gene amplification techniques[263] may also be used to demonstrate JC virus infection, the highly specific nature of the oligodendroglial karyomegaly and nucleoplasmic alterations typical of PML cannot be overemphasized. A confident (and eco-

nomic) diagnosis requires only their recognition in routinely processed and stained tissue sections examined by conventional light microscopy.

With the ongoing infection and lysis of target cells, PML evolves as centrifugally expanding zones of oligodendroglial depletion and subsequent infiltration by foamy macrophages engaged in the scavenging and digestion of degenerating myelin sheaths. Early on, small plaques tend to a miliary clustering at the gray-white junction that probably reflects hematogenous seeding of the CNS following reactivation of the agent in sites of systemic latency.[262] Geographic zones of demyelination, resulting from the coalescence of these small lesions, become grossly evident as regions of white matter retraction, granularity, and yellowish-gray discoloration (Fig. 28-27). In most cases, a relatively undisturbed cortical ribbon will span these devastated areas. This, and the characteristic persistence of axons in the face of total demyelination, reflect the resistance of neurons (cerebellar granule cells excepted) to JC virus infection. Some thinning of the axonal population, however, is the rule, and PML can progress to extensive white matter cavitation. Particularly widespread and destructive examples have been described in the setting of co-infection by HIV-1.[260,265]

A histologic feature of PML meriting further comment is atypical astrocytic hyperplasia (Fig. 28-30). In addition to florid astrogliosis—a constant finding—the demyelinating lesions of PML often contain greatly enlarged astrocytes exhibiting bizarre nuclear abnormalities indistinguishable from those usually associated with neoplasia. These changes, often seen in concert with atypical mitotic figures, are

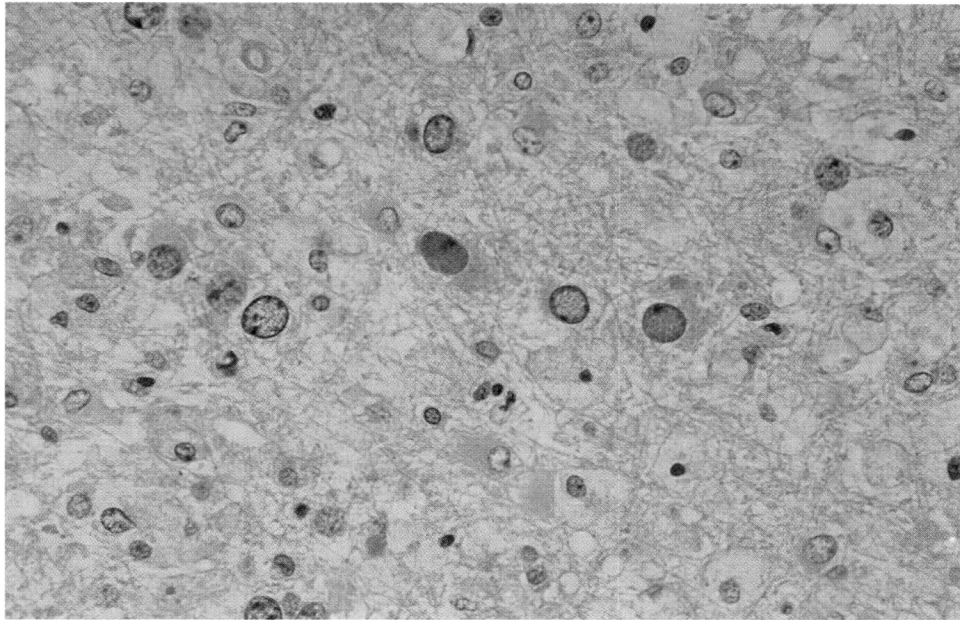

Fig. 28-28 Progressive multifocal leukoencephalopathy. JC virus–infected oligodendrocytes in the center of this field exhibit the nuclear swelling, chromatin dissolution, and replacement by amphophilic, "ground-glass" inclusion material that are peculiar to this disorder. Note presence of scattered hyperplastic astrocytes and admixed foamy macrophages.

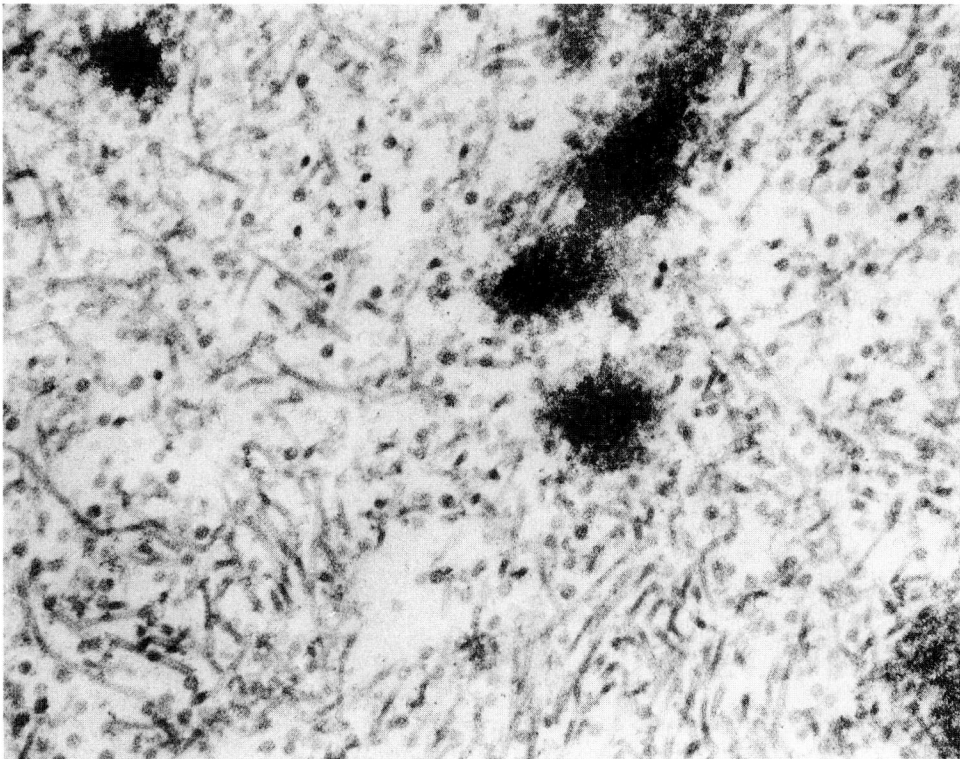

Fig. 28-29 Progressive multifocal leukoencephalopathy. This transmission electron micrograph of an oligodendrocyte's nucleus depicts nonenveloped virions of 37-nm diameter lying singly and in the filamentous arrays that are a common feature of JC infection. (×45,150.)

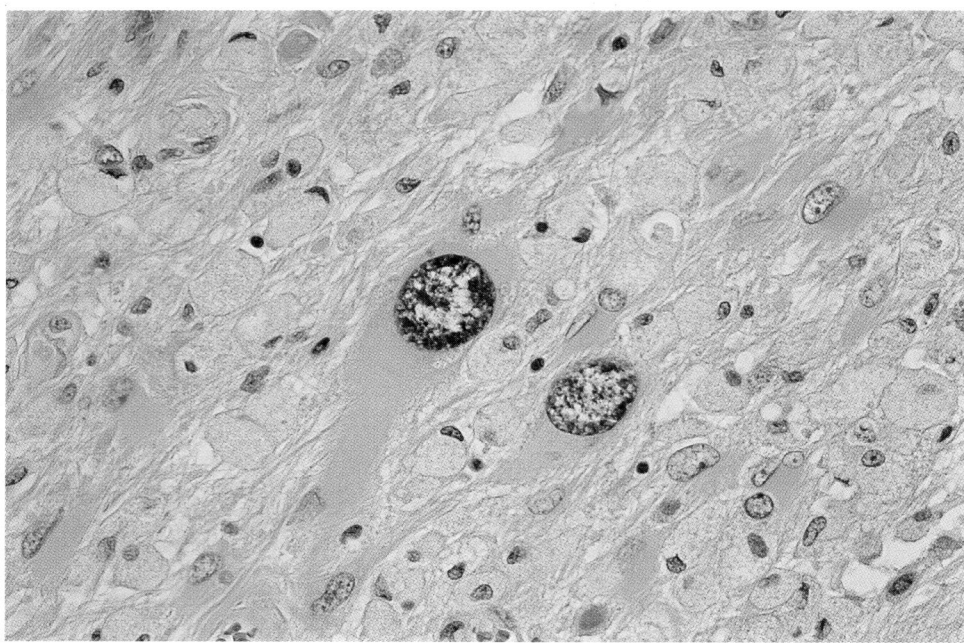

Fig. 28-30 Progressive multifocal leukoencephalopathy. Grotesque cytologic alterations may result from infection of astrocytes by the JC virus. An accompanying infiltrate of foamy macrophages should militate strongly against the diagnosis of neoplasia, despite the worrisome appearances of these bizarre cells.

believed to reflect a form of nonpermissive infection in which the agent's genome is spliced into that of the host cell, a process integral to the recognized capacity of polyomaviruses, including JC virus isolates from patients with PML, to induce central neuroepithelial tumors in the experimental situation. The precise role, if any, of these viruses in the pathogenesis of human brain tumors remains to be clarified, but it is noteworthy that the association of PML with multifocal astrocytomas has been documented, albeit rarely.[261]

PML is usually characterized by minimal inflammatory response to the agent; however, some variants evidence intense perivascular and interstitial lymphoid infiltration.[257] The latter often contain very few oligodendrocytes manifesting the nuclear cytopathic effects pathognomonic of JC virus infection and may prompt considerations of primary cerebral lymphoma, another recognized complication of the immunosuppressed state occurring with particular frequency in HIV-1–seropositive patients. It is this unusual form of PML that is most likely to present as a space-occupying, contrast-enhancing mass on CT or MRI study, further complicating the clinical delineation of these entities. A conspicuous inflammatory response typifies biopsy material from a small subset of AIDS patients surviving for considerably longer than the 3- to 6-month interval in which most cases of PML progress ineluctably to death.[257] The rare examples of spontaneously remitting PML that we have seen have been of this unusually inflammatory type and presumably reflect elimination or immunologic containment of the JC virus following a transitory abrogation of its enforced dormancy.

Varicella-zoster virus encephalitis and cerebral vasculitis. The varicella-zoster virus (VZV), agent of chickenpox and shingles, causes a rare form of encephalitis sharing certain clinical and histologic features with PML.[270,271] The condition has to date been described exclusively in immunocompromised hosts (including patients treated for Hodgkin's disease, other cancers, and AIDS) and may present months following resolution of cutaneous zoster or in the absence of a preceding exanthem. Described by some authors as a "leukoencephalitis," this chronic infection can settle anywhere along the central neuraxis, but exhibits a striking predilection for the cerebral hemispheric white matter. It is characterized by multifocal, centrifugally expanding, and coalescent foci of demyelination and frank necrosis with little inflammatory reaction. The nuclei of oligodendrocytes situated on the periphery of these lesions exhibit a ground-glass transformation or homogeneous filling by basophilic material superficially similar to the cytopathy induced in such cells by the JC virus but differ in not being conspicuously enlarged. Furthermore, neighboring astrocytes (and, in some cases, neurons and ependymal cells) infected by the VZV contain well-demarcated Cowdry A–type intranuclear inclusions of the sort that typify herpes virus replication and are not driven to the atypical hyperplasia characteristic of PML. Fine structural study will disclose herpes-type nucleocapsids averaging approximately 100 nm in diameter within the nuclei of infected cells. These differ slightly from herpes simplex–type virions in that their core densities tend to be eccentrically positioned, but definitive

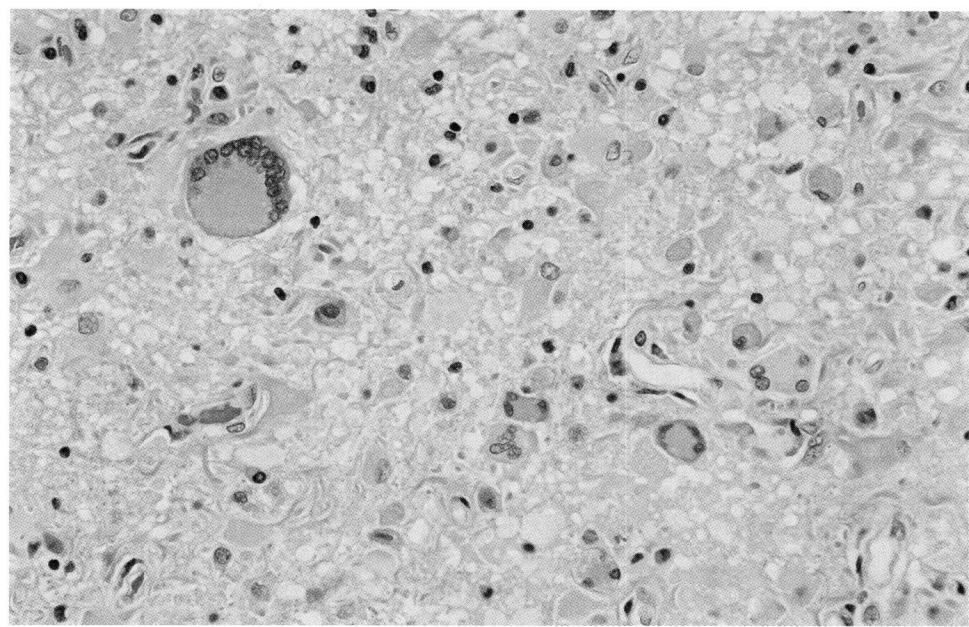

Fig. 28-31 HIV encephalitis. Nongranulomatous infiltrates centered loosely about blood vessels in the cerebral white matter (shown here) or basal ganglia and dominated by macrophages, including multinucleated forms resulting from retrovirally mediated cell fusion, characterize infection of the CNS by this agent. The associated astrogliosis and spongy rarefaction are common accompanying features.

identification of the agent requires immunocytochemical assay, molecular hybridization studies, or culture.

In addition to being an encephalitogen, the VZV is recognized as a rare cause of cerebral vasculitis. This involves predominantly the large arteries at the base of the brain and their major branches. Like the encephalitis associated with this agent, vasculitic complications of zoster typically follow resolution of the cutaneous exanthem. Two major variants have been described. One, a noninflammatory "angiopathy" afflicting immunocompromised hosts, is characterized by striking fibrointimal proliferation, thrombosis, and in some cases, disruption of the elastica and thinning of the media without evident necrosis of mural elements.[268,271] The other is an overtly inflammatory and necrotizing angiitis designated by some observers as "granulomatous" because of the presence of multinucleated histiocytes within damaged vessel walls. This often presents as hemiplegic stroke weeks after an episode of contralateral zoster ophthalmicus in a patient with no major evidences of defective immunity.[267] In fact, we have seen several examples—all in patients seropositive for HIV-1—displaying both angiopathic and angiitic features, depending on the portion of vessel sampled, and suspect that the former simply represent the chronic sequelae of what is primarily an inflammatory process. In addition to thrombosis with consequent cerebral infarction, VZV angiitis may result in fusiform aneurysmal dilatation, mural rupture, and subarachnoid hemorrhage.[269] Definitive diagnosis requires localization of the agent by immunocytochemical assay or ultrastructural study to elements of the vessel

wall, typically smooth muscle cells in the media or intimal (myo)fibroblasts. See p. 2263 for further consideration of VZV as a cerebrovascular pathogen.

HIV-1 encephalomyelitis. HIV-1 encephalomyelitis is not a disorder likely to engage the surgical pathologist but demands, nevertheless, some consideration in view of the current AIDS epidemic and the unique nature of the neuropathologic alterations associated with this retroviral infection.[273,274] HIV-1 is alone among viral encephalitogens in exhibiting no particular tropism for neuroectodermal cell types, its replication in the nervous system taking place largely within marrow-derived phagocytes and microglia. CNS infection is characterized by loosely arrayed, vasocentric, or paravascular inflammatory infiltrates concentrated in the cerebral hemispheric white matter, basal ganglia, and rostral brainstem (Fig. 28-31). These are dominated by mononucleated and multinucleated macrophages, the latter reflecting a process of virally mediated cell fusion that is the characteristic cytopathic effect of this and other members of the lentivirus subfamily of retroviruses. These cells, and their mononuclear precursors, harbor and release fully formed virions, which may be found budding from their plasmalemma, aggregated in membrane-delimited intracytoplasmic vacuoles, or lying free in the cytoplasm (Fig. 28-32). The mature particle is spherical, averages 100 to 120 mm in diameter, and possesses a cylindrical or bar-shaped nucleoid usually positioned eccentrically and enclosed by a limiting membrane.[272] Attendant changes include diffuse astrogliosis and microglial activation, generalized pallor of the cerebral

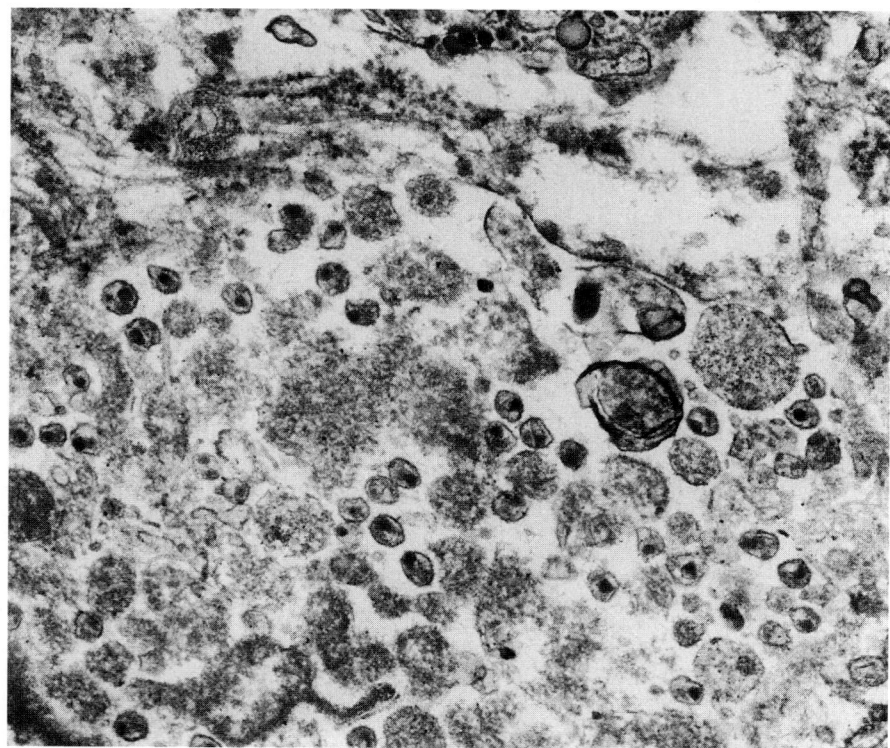

Fig. 28-32 HIV encephalitis. This transmission electron micrograph shows intracytoplasmic HIV particles measuring 110 to 120 nm in diameter. Note the well-defined envelopes and eccentrically positioned core densities. (×40,000.) (Courtesy Dr. Leroy Sharer, Newark, NJ.)

white matter, and brain atrophy. The precise relationship of local HIV-1 replication to these indices of widespread CNS injury remains to be clarified.

Parasitoses

The CNS parasitoses include a great variety of protozoal and helminthic infections given comprehensive consideration elsewhere.[275-278] This discussion is limited to two representatives of particular importance to the surgical pathologist—neurocysticercosis and toxoplasmosis.

Neurocysticercosis, caused by larvae of the pork tapeworm, *Taenia solium,* is the most common parasitic cerebral infection encountered in worldwide neurosurgical practice.[278] Endemic to nearly all continents, the disease is particularly prevalent in Mexico (where it is the leading cause of space-occupying intracranial lesions), Central and South America, India, Africa, and China. An increasing incidence in the United States is largely attributable to cases occurring in immigrants from these regions.[279] Infection is acquired by ingestion of food or water contaminated by feces containing the cestode's ova. These are partially digested in the host's stomach, evolving to oncospheres and subsequently penetrating the small intestinal mucosa to disseminate throughout the body, preferentially encysting in ocular tissues, striated muscle, and brain. The ensuing clinical disorder is named for the designation given the organism at this larval stage, *Cysticercus cellulosae.*

Cysticerci actually persist in parasitized tissues for long periods without eliciting symptoms of any kind. The active clinical phase of neurocysticercosis is triggered by the host's inflammatory response to the larva's death (approximately 18 months following primary infection). The high incidence of focal or generalized seizures associated with the disorder reflects the fact that oncospheres reaching the CNS settle mainly in the epileptogenic cerebral cortex, but they may also colonize the ventricular system and basal cisterns in a distinctive pattern of infestation ("racemose" cysticercosis), resulting in obstructive hydrocephalus and consequent manifestations of elevated intracranial pressure. The presence of multifocal, rim-enhancing cerebral cysts on neuroimaging study suffices in many cases to prompt a diagnostic as well as therapeutic course of antihelminthic chemotherapy, but a substantial proportion of patients present with solitary lesions, and the host's reaction to the decaying parasite may convert the cyst to a deceptively solid inflammatory pseudotumor. Neurosurgical intervention may be obviated by a positive immunoelectrotransfer blot serologic assay, but false-negative results have been reported, especially in subjects with unifocal disease.[282]

When not completely obscured by secondary inflammatory changes, the gross appearance of cysticerci excised in toto is virtually pathognomonic (Fig. 28-33). Individual cysts are of small diameter, are circumscribed by a rubbery fibrous pseudocapsule, and contain a single larval scolex repre-

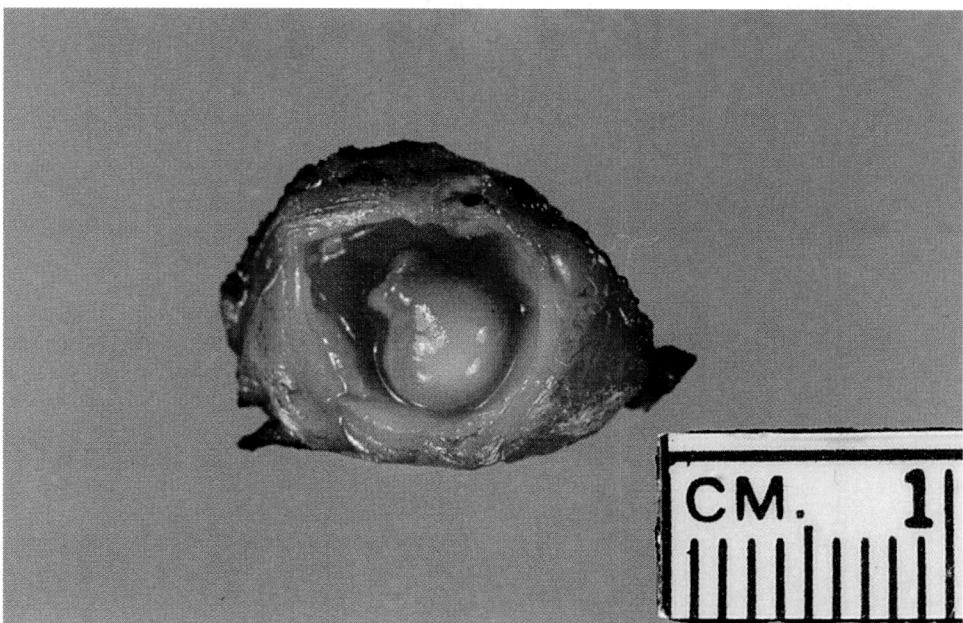

Fig. 28-33 Neurocysticercosis. Typical of cerebral *Taenia solium* infestation is the solitary, encysted scolex demonstrated in this neurosurgical specimen from the left frontal cortex of a 32-year-old Haitian man with a history of seizures.

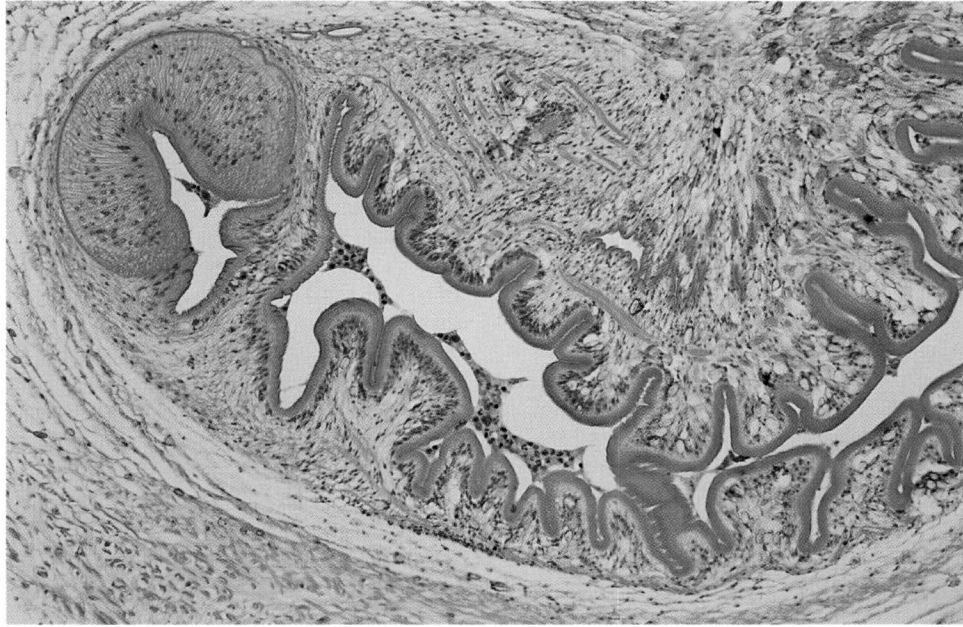

Fig. 28-34 Neurocysticercosis. The parasite's main structural features include a prominent investing tegument or "cuticle," aggregated subcuticular cells, smooth muscle fibers, and four suckers, one of which is depicted at upper left.

sented by a spheric or ovoid grayish-white nodule measuring no more than 3 to 4 mm in greatest dimension. By contrast, cestode larval cysts produced by the morphologically similar *Multiceps multiceps* contain numerous scolices and those caused by *Echinococcus granulosus* are considerably larger and endowed with a characteristically laminated wall. On histologic examination, the fibrous pseudocapsule is typically infiltrated by lymphocytes and plasma cells in large numbers, may contain eosinophils in abundance, and in some cases, is the site of an active granulomatous reaction. The mummified remains of the degenerate scolex are covered by a wavy, somewhat refractile cuticle and consist largely of loose, reticular tissue containing numerous calcospherites. Relatively intact scolices possess a discernible subcuticular "pseudoepithelial" layer, small myofiber bundles, and four suckers armed with birefringent hooklets (Fig. 28-34). Racemose cysticerci evacuated from the ventricles or subarachnoid space present as grape-like clusters of interconnected larval "bladders" lacking organized scolices.

Toxoplasmosis is the generic designation applied to localized or systemic infections caused by the obligate intracellular protozoan *Toxoplasma gondii.* CNS involvement may assume a number of distinctive clinicomorphologic guises,[275,278] this discussion focusing on a "tumefactive" variant largely confined to immunocompromised hosts and typically unassociated with clinical manifestations of extraneural parasitosis. Once regarded as rare and encountered principally among patients treated for hematolymphoid neoplasms (Hodgkin's disease, particularly), this form of toxoplasmosis is now known to physicians the world over as a common AIDS-defining disorder and is in fact the leading cause of space-occupying intracranial lesions in the HIV-1 seropositive.[280,281] Bone marrow transplant recipients have also emerged in recent years as a population prone to CNS infections of this type. Common to the afflicted is a breakdown of cell-mediated immune surveillance thought, in most cases, to permit recrudescence of the agent in dormantly parasitized neural tissues. *T. gondii* is noted for its silent persistence in the brain following primary infection, which is usually asymptomatic and acquired by the consumption of inadequately cooked red meats containing encysted organisms or by the inadvertent ingestion of foodstuffs, soil, or other materials contaminated by protozoal oocytes shed in the feces of domestic cats.

The clinical and neuroradiologic features of CNS toxoplasmosis are quite variable, are nonspecific, and do not suffice for definitive diagnosis. Because *Toxoplasma* "abscesses" favor neuron-rich gray matter structures such as the cerebral cortex, basal ganglia, and brainstem, it should come as no surprise that seizures, progressive hemipareses, and cranial nerve deficits figure prominently among their initial manifestations. Many patients, however, present without localizing complaints, evidencing instead fever, headache, lethargy, and diffuse encephalopathy, subacute in its evolution. Cranial MR imaging typically discloses multifocal, nodular lesions characterized by ring-like peripheral enhancement, surrounding edema, and mass effect, but exceptional examples are nonenhancing or diffusely so, and solitary abscesses at presentation are not rare. Studies in the HIV-1 seropositive have demonstrated that, in this population at least, cere-

bral toxoplasmosis only occasionally develops in patients with no serologic evidence of contact with the organism.[281] A negative serum anti-*Toxoplasma* IgG titer militates against, but does not exclude, the diagnosis in this setting. Although an etiologically specific diagnosis requires the demonstration of the protozoan in biopsy material, it has become common practice to institute antimicrobial therapy on empiric grounds in suspect cases and to reserve neurosurgical intervention for the patient who does not respond satisfactorily to such management. Most HIV-1–seropositive individuals whose intracranial masses fail to resolve on anti-*Toxoplasma* chemotherapy prove to harbor primary CNS lymphomas.

The *Toxoplasma* "abscess," as it is commonly called, consists of a central mass of necrotic cellular debris surrounded by edematous and inflamed brain tissue typically exhibiting conspicuous vascular abnormalities. The latter include perivascular and intramural lymphoid infiltration, endothelial swelling, thrombosis, fibrinoid necrosis, and in long-standing lesions, fibrous obliteration. It is within this perimeter zone that *Toxoplasma* are most numerous, the necrotic core often being devoid of identifiable organisms. Two protozoal forms are evident in active lesions. Responsible for tissue injury is the rapidly proliferating tachyzoite. This is faintly basophilic, measures approximately 2×6 μm, and typically exhibits a slightly crescentic or lunate profile (the Greek *toxon* means bow or arc). Because it is often difficult to visualize tachyzoites in routine histologic preparations and to confidently distinguish them from cellular detritus, the screening of suspect biopsy material with *Toxoplasma*-specific antibodies is strongly advised. More readily apparent, although present in lesser numbers, are intracellular pseudocysts and "true" (i.e., membrane-delimited) cysts that may attain diameters of up to 200 μm (Fig. 28-35). These are filled with minute, PAS-positive bradyzoites (named for their slow replicative cycles); are immunologically inert; and represent the form in which *Toxoplasma* chronically persist in brain and other tissues. Within the CNS, bradyzoites appear to collect preferentially within neurons and perivascular macrophages. Again, it is immune failure that is believed to somehow trigger their metamorphosis to tachyzoites and subsequent destructive invasion of neural tissues. Careful inspection of active lesions often reveals ruptured cysts that appear to be disgorging their content of protozoa into the neuropil. Like tachyzoites, bradyzoites are labeled by commercially available *Toxoplasma*-specific antibodies.

Spirochetal infections

The two major CNS spirochetoses are neurosyphilis,[283,284] caused by *Treponema pallidum,* and neuroborreliosis complicating infection by the agent of Lyme arthritis, *Borrelia burgdorferi.*[285,286] No attempt is made here to discuss the pathogenesis and varied clinical expressions of these complex syndromes, matters largely irrelevant to the surgical pathologist. Suffice it to say that intracerebral inflammatory pseudotumors (known as "gummas" in the case of treponemal disease and accompanied by necrosis and fibroplasia in this setting) are restricted to the late stages of systemic infection by these organisms, constitute their least common manifestations, and are usually approached surgically only

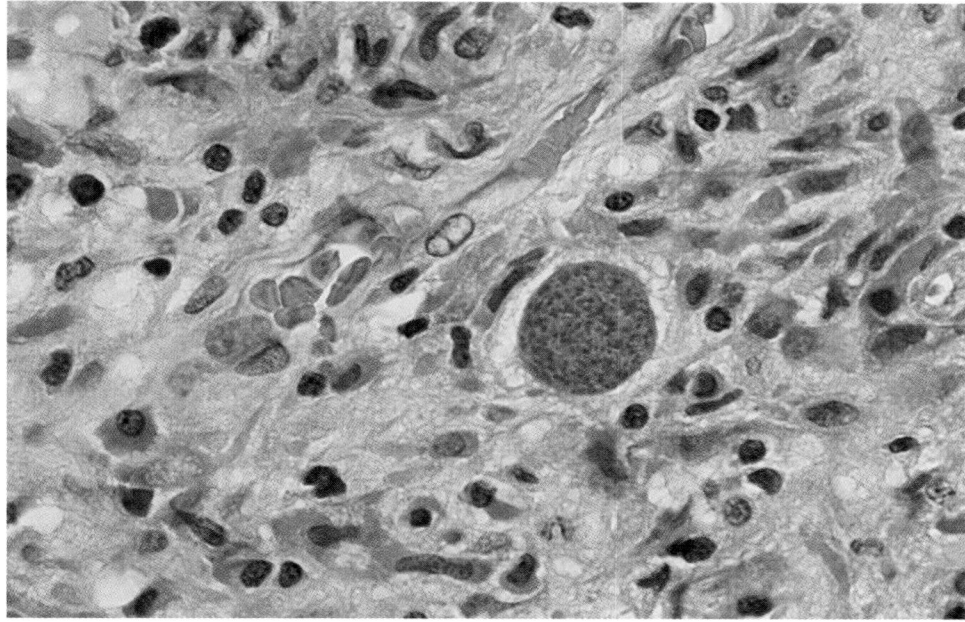

Fig. 28-35 Toxoplasmosis. Minute, basophilic structures representing bradyzoites fill a protozoal pseudocyst lying among infiltrating lymphocytes, plasma cells, and macrophages.

when the diagnosis is unsuspected on clinical grounds and so not established by the appropriate serologic methods. The reader is referred to the cited literature for further details.

Prion-associated diseases

Although often classed among viral disorders of the nervous system, the rare diseases traditionally designated as *subacute spongiform encephalopathies* are caused by transmissible agents that have resisted placement in the conventional taxonomy of infectious pathogens. Concerted efforts to isolate nonhuman genomic material from the tissues of affected patients have proved uniformly unsuccessful to date. By contrast, such tissues are characterized by the accumulation of amyloidogenic proteins or *prions* that may be host derived and somehow capable of engineering their own replication and acting as the "infectious" moieties of these transmissible illnesses.[291] The biology, molecular cytogenetics, and expanding clinical spectrum of prion-associated disorders are complex subjects beyond the scope of this discussion, which is limited to practical considerations in the diagnosis of *Creutzfeldt-Jakob disease* (CJD), the variant most commonly encountered in neurologic practice and most likely to prompt brain biopsy.

The iatrogenic transmission of CJD via contaminated neurosurgical instruments and a variety of transplanted human tissues has been recorded,[291] but most examples involve middle-aged or older adults having no evident exposure to potentially contaminated materials or other individuals suffering the disorder. A heredofamilial variant associated with mutations in the gene encoding the prion protein precursor accounts for approximately 10% to 15% of cases.[291] Although there is some variation in the early manifestations and tem-

poral evolution of the disorder, the course of most patients is dominated by cognitive decline that progresses relentlessly and in subacute fashion to profound dementia, often attended by generalized myoclonus. Electroencephalographic studies are almost invariably abnormal, often demonstrating a "burst-suppression" pattern of periodic spike and wave complexes considered particularly characteristic of CJD. The afflicted are typically left vegetative within 6 to 8 months of symptom onset and rarely survive longer than a year after diagnosis.

The appearance of biopsy material, usually secured from the nondominant frontal lobe, depends on disease duration.[291,293,295] The earliest perceptible change consists of a spongy vacuolization of the cortex most pronounced in its deeper laminae (Fig. 28-36). At the light microscopic level, rare vacuoles may be localizable to neuronal perikarya, but most appear randomly scattered in the neuropil. The latter are situated principally within neuronal processes on fine structural study, are often traversed by membrane-derived septa, and may contain granular or curled membranous profiles. With disease progression, spongiform change becomes increasingly florid and is attended by conspicuous astrogliosis, neuronal shrinkage, and depopulation. The end-stage cortex may be left virtually devoid of recognizable neurons and largely replaced by the tangled processes of hyperplastic astrocytes. At no stage of the disorder is there evidence of an inflammatory response, and white matter abnormalities, typically restricted to long-standing examples, are limited to secondary axonal loss save for rare variants exhibiting spongy leukoencephalopathy.[290] An arresting feature of CJD, but one evident in only a minority of cases, is the deposition in the cerebellar (and, to a lesser extent, cerebral) cor-

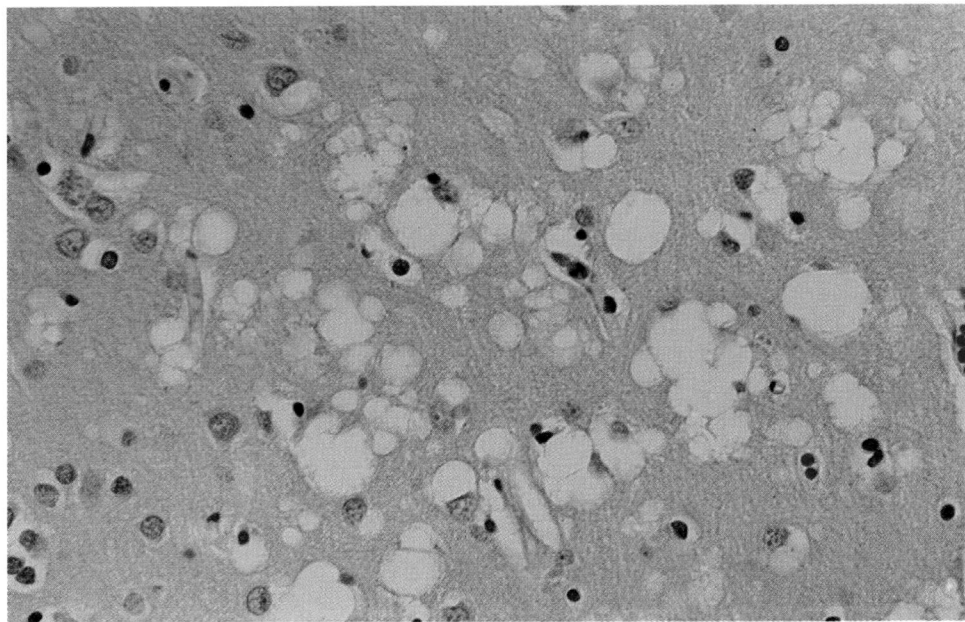

Fig. 28-36 Spongiform encephalopathy (Jakob-Creutzfeldt disease). Noninflammatory vacuolization of the cerebral cortex is the dominant alteration evident in this biopsy specimen from an elderly man with progressive dementia and myoclonus. This change typically precedes conspicuous neuronal dropout and astrogliosis, the other dominant findings in this prion-related disorder.

tex of amyloid plaques that often display radiate, spicular contours and are specifically recognized by antibodies to prion proteins.[291,293,294,298] These tend to be particularly numerous in familial examples and are a defining histopathologic feature of the dominantly inherited variant known as Gerstmann-Straussler syndrome,[291,294,297] also associated with mutations of the prion-encoding gene and characterized by progressive cerebellar ataxia.

Biopsy material from cases of suspected CJD requires special handling. The agent is clearly resistant to the fixation and sterilization procedures in routine use, even formalinized and paraffin-embedded archival specimens retaining the capacity to transmit the disease. Although there are no documented instances of CJD involving general pathologists, neuropathologists, or autopsy technicians, isolated examples occurring in histotechnologists are on record, including the autopsy-proven case of an individual known to have processed contaminated brain tissues.[296] The simplest method of inactivating the agent in small biopsy specimens would appear to be 48-hour fixation in formalin, followed by immersion in 50 to 100 ml of pure formic acid for 1 hour and subsequent transfer to fresh formalin for an additional 48-hour period.[287] Continuous gentle agitation is employed throughout processing. This protocol yields histologic sections of excellent quality, preserves the antigenic integrity of the tissues, and may actually enhance their immunoreactivity with prion-specific antibodies. Consult Brown and colleagues for additional details.[287] Neutral buffered formalin to which phenol has been added (15 g/dl) can also be recommended for use, particularly with whole brain specimens.[288] These should remain immersed for at

least 4 weeks prior to sectioning. Other methods of proven efficacy for the decontamination of suspect tissues and instruments are outlined in a report of the American Neurological Association's Committee on Health Care Issues.[289]

We would close this abbreviated discussion of prion-associated disorders by reminding the reader that the histopathologic alterations typical of CJD are not uniformly distributed in the involved brain. Consequently, a negative biopsy should not reassure hospital staff handling tissues and fluids from suspect patients. We would also caution against the diagnosis of spongiform encephalopathy on minimal histologic criteria because scattered intracortical vacuoles and shrunken-appearing neurons commonly represent artefacts of surgical manipulation. Finally, pathologists should be aware that spongy changes indistinguishable on histologic grounds from those of CJD may, on occasion, be encountered in otherwise typical examples of Alzheimer's disease, in cerebrocortical Lewy body disease, and in a dementing disorder combining the morphologic features of both these entities.[292] Spongiform vacuolization in these circumstances is typically restricted to the temporal cortex, insula, or amygdala and is unattended by the deposition of prion antibody-positive amyloid. To date, animal inoculation studies have not shown such hybrid cases to be transmissible.

PRIMARY TUMORS
Glial tumors
Astrocytic neoplasms
Fibrillary astrocytomas. Named for their permeative growth patterns and the filamentous cytoplasmic processes that lend to their constituent cells a resemblance, however

distorted, to the "fibrous" astrocytes populating the normal brain and spinal cord, ***astrocytomas of diffuse fibrillary type*** collectively constitute the most common primary neoplasms of the human CNS.[301] Although most are unassociated with obvious predisposing factors, radiation-related cases are well documented,[335,338] and occasional examples complicate type 1 neurofibromatosis[312] or define Turcot's syndrome,[323] the heritable complex of adenomatous colonic polyposis, colorectal adenocarcinoma, and central neuroepithelial neoplasia. HIV-1–seropositive patients appear also to be at increased risk of developing CNS tumors, including neoplasms of the astrocytic series.[329]

Diffuse fibrillary astrocytomas afflict subjects of all ages and may arise at any level of the central neuraxis, but there can be no doubt of their predilection for the cerebral hemispheres of adults. Here they are characteristically centered in white matter, a minority originating in deep gray structures such as the basal ganglia and thalami. Headaches, seizures, focal sensorimotor deficits, and alterations of affect are the principal clinical manifestations of these supratentorial lesions. The common variety of brainstem glioma, encountered in childhood or adolescence as progressive cranial nerve and long tract dysfunction associated with "pseudohypertrophic" enlargement of the pons on neuroradiologic investigation, is also an astrocytoma of diffuse fibrillary type.[299,301,337] Intraspinal examples figure prominently among primary tumors of the cervical and upper thoracic cord,[304,307] but are vastly outnumbered by ependymomas at more caudal levels. Exceptional variants are situated entirely within the leptomeninges and subarachnoid space, where they may derive from heterotopic neuroglial rests.[313,332]

Neuro-oncologic practice demands that the diffuse fibrillary astrocytomas be subclassified according to their perceived biologic potential. Despite general agreement among observers as to the histologic features of greatest predictive value in this regard, a uniform system of grading and reporting has not been adopted to date, and various schemae for the subcategorization of these neoplasms are currently in use.[301] The diagnostic terminology and criteria employed here conform, except where indicated, to those recommended in the revised classification of CNS tumors issued by the World Health Organization (WHO) in 1993.[318]

In this three-tiered system, astroglial neoplasms of the diffuse fibrillary variety are designated as astrocytoma (without other specification), anaplastic astrocytoma, or glioblastoma multiforme, according to histologic indices presently outlined. The reader will note that the diagnosis of glioblastoma is reserved for astrocytic tumors of the highest grade and is not applied to poorly differentiated gliomas that clearly exhibit oligodendroglial or ependymal differentiation. We would emphasize from the outset the disheartening tendency of the diffuse fibrillary astrocytoma, however differentiated and indolent at inception, to grow increasingly alarming to the morphologist and clinically aggressive with the passage of time. A consequence of this inherent instability that bears on practical issues of diagnosis and management is the resulting regional heterogeneity for which this neoplasm is notorious. Zonal variations in histologic appearance, ploidy, proliferative activity, karyotype, and molecular cytogenetic profile potentially confound the interpretation of observations based on limited tissue samples, a particu-

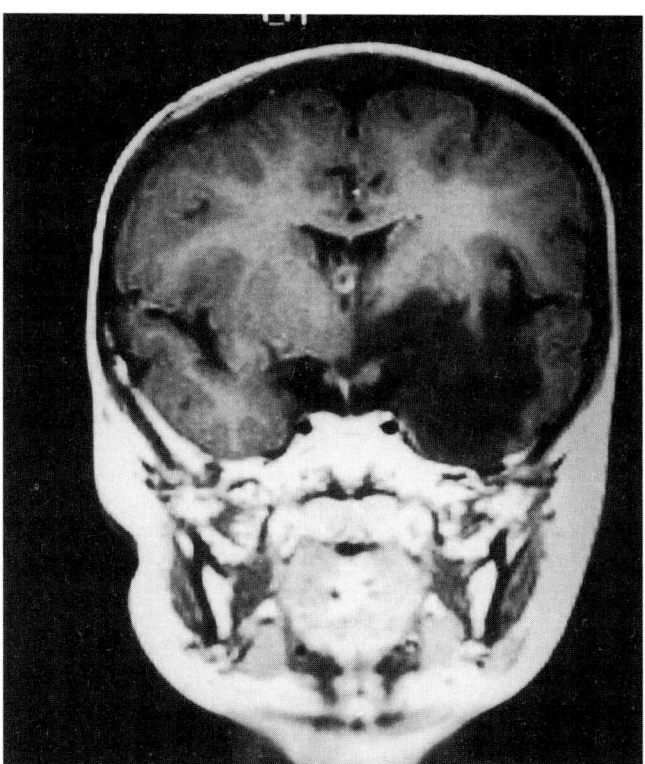

Fig. 28-37 Diffuse fibrillary astrocytoma. Neuroradiologic features common to the low-grade fibrillary astrocytoma in postcontrast MRIs, such as this temporal example, include generalized expansion and hypodensity of infiltrated regions with only modest mass effect and no foci of bright signal enhancement that would indicate blood-brain barrier disruption (see Fig. 28-45 for comparison).

larly vexing problem in the era of stereotactic biopsy. The biology of astrocytoma progression is a complex topic beyond the scope of this survey, but we would be remiss not to cite evidence that this phenomenon may be driven by mutations or allelic loss involving the tumor-suppressing p53[321] and retinoblastoma[310] genes.

Well-differentiated or low-grade fibrillary astrocytic neoplasms, hereafter referred to simply as astrocytomas, typically present in the third or fourth decade of life and are decidedly uncommon after age 40. Beyond this, the overwhelming majority of fibrillary astrocytic tumors exhibit anaplastic histologic features or are frank glioblastomas. Particularly suggestive of a slowly evolving supratentorial astrocytoma (or other low-grade neoplasm) is a protracted preoperative course characterized by intermittent seizures or headache unassociated with focal neurologic deficits. Complaints referable to such lesions may be present for years prior to their discovery, although the advent of sophisticated neuroradiologic techniques has considerably shortened the average predetection interval.[324] Because astrocytomas do not usually provoke significant neovascularization of the infiltrated neural parenchyma, they appear in CT scans and MR images as regions of diminished density that are not delineated ("enhanced") by contrast media employed to define foci of blood-brain barrier disruption (Fig. 28-37).

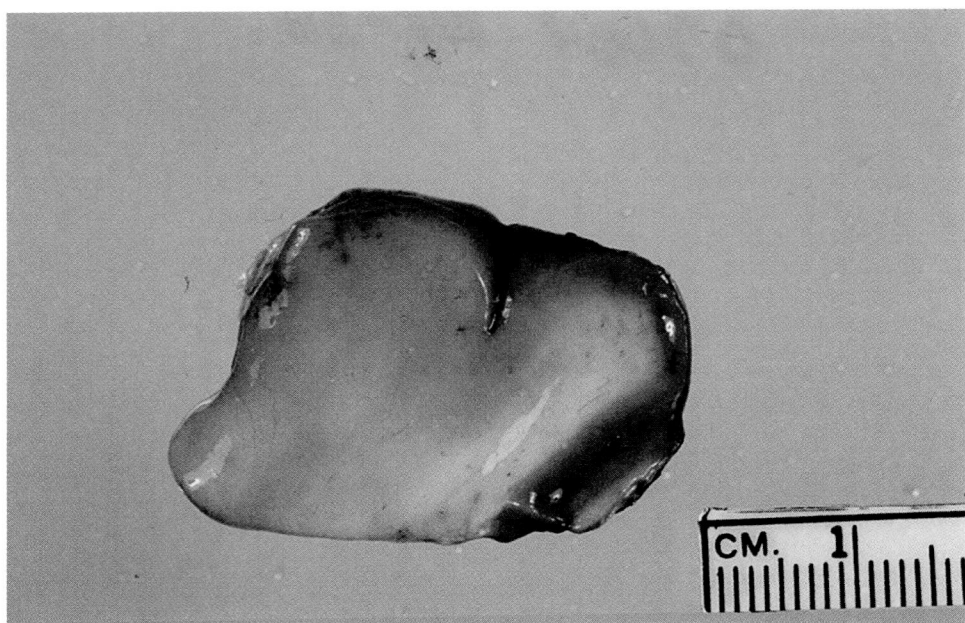

Fig. 28-38 Diffuse fibrillary astrocytoma. The insidious permeation typical of the fibrillary astrocytoma is illustrated in this anterior temporal lobectomy specimen. The gyrus at right maintains a clearly demarcated cortical ribbon over its digitate white matter. Moving to the left, there is diffuse gyral expansion and effacement of these landmarks, reflecting tumoral infiltration. No discrete mass is formed, and as is characteristic of low-grade examples, there is no evident hemorrhage or necrosis (see Fig. 28-46 for comparison).

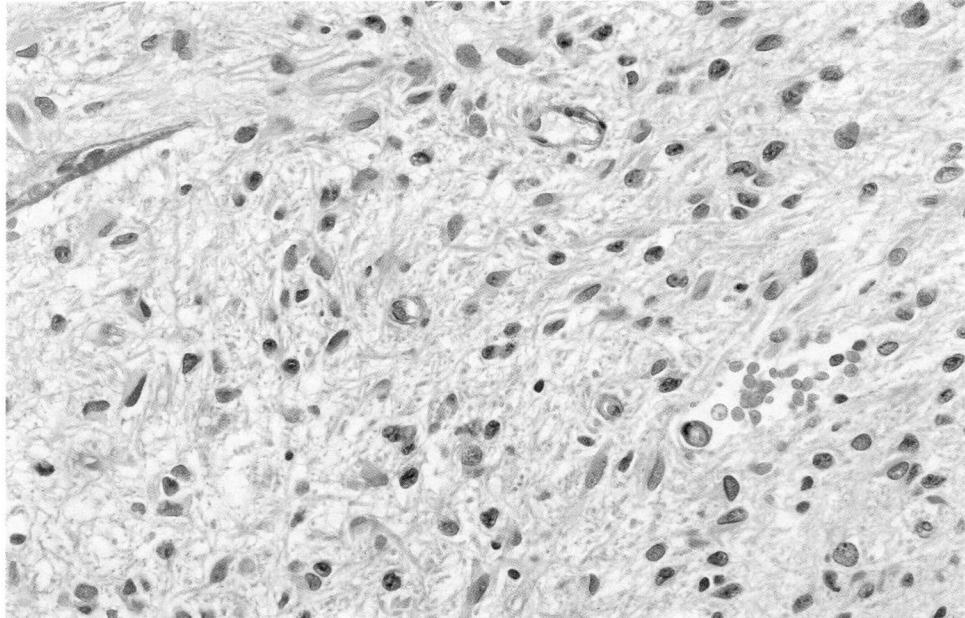

Fig. 28-39 Diffuse fibrillary astrocytoma. Conspicuous cytoplasmic processes, mild nuclear pleomorphism, and only modest hyperchromasia are evidenced by the cells of this well-differentiated astrocytoma. The absence of mitotic activity supports its classification as a low-grade lesion. Note the dyscohesive growth pattern.

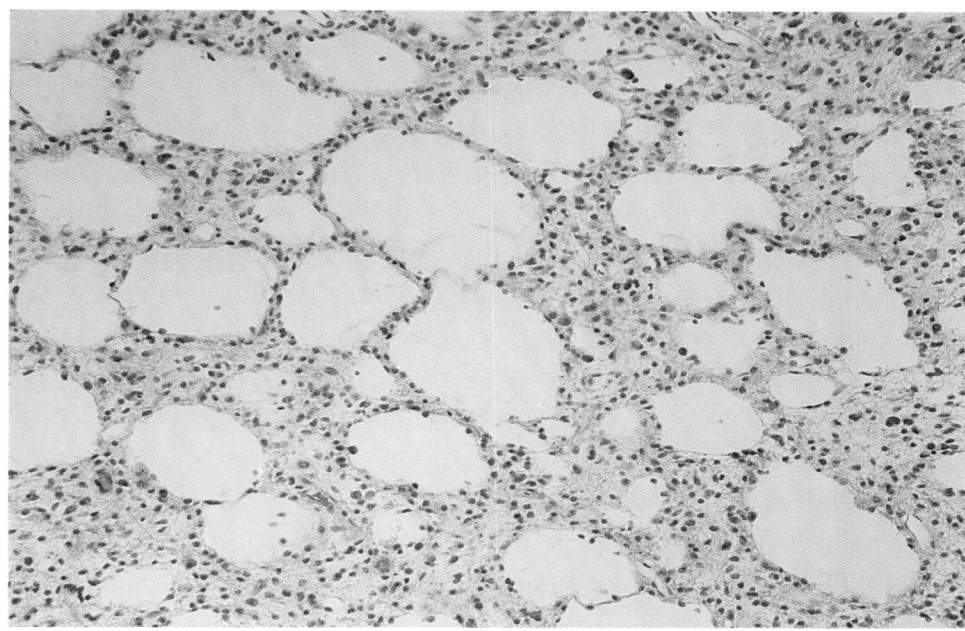

Fig. 28-40 Diffuse fibrillary astrocytoma. Foreign to reactive astroglial proliferations, microcystic change is a particularly conspicuous feature of low-grade astrocytomas and other glial neoplasms.

The presence of such enhancement suggests that a lesion shown by biopsy to be an astrocytoma has undergone focal anaplastic progression and should prompt careful review of postoperative neuroradiologic studies to ascertain the region of tumor sampled.

At operation, astrocytomas are spatially indistinct, producing a diffuse expansion and induration of permeated CNS structures along with a highly characteristic blurring or effacement of gray-white landmarks (Fig. 28-38). They may acquire a somewhat mucoid consistency as a result of myxoid change but are not prone to spontaneous hemorrhage or necrosis. Histologic study typically discloses a dyscohesive cellular infiltrate percolating through recognizable neuropil in a patternless array that stands in sharp contrast to the even distribution of hyperplastic astrocytes characteristic of reactive glial proliferations (Fig. 28-39). Samples of invaded cortex often disclose striking aggregation of tumor cells beneath the pia and about neurons, the latter phenomenon known as *satellitosis,* but it should be pointed out that these formations are shared by tumors of oligodendroglial lineage. A common architectural feature of immeasurable utility in establishing the neoplastic nature of the process in question is microcystic change (Fig. 28-40), an alteration to which a variety of glial neoplasms (generally low-grade) are prone but rarely, if ever, encountered in a reactive setting. A similar significance attaches to the finding of scattered calcospherites in biopsy material. Admixed foamy macrophages, on the other hand, militate strongly against the diagnosis of astrocytoma in the absence of prior therapy and should instead prompt considerations of demyelinating disease and infarction.

Conspicuous lymphocytic cuffing of regional blood vessels, the hallmark of inflammatory CNS disorders, occasionally attends astrocytic neoplasms of the "garden variety" but among neuroepithelial tumors is far more often a feature of the gemistocytic astrocytoma, pleomorphic xanthoastrocytoma, and ganglioglioma. Finally, survey of a candidate for the diagnosis of low-grade astrocytoma should not reveal foci of dense cellularity, proliferation of vascular elements, mitotic activity, or zones of necrosis.

At the cytologic level, astrocytomas are composed, at least in part, of cells invested with delicate processes that taper from a modest perinuclear expanse of eosinophilic cytoplasm or are represented only as a background fibrillar meshwork in which "naked" nuclei appear to lie embedded (Fig. 28-39). Particularly arresting in smear or crush preparations (Fig. 28-41), which are indispensable adjuncts (and expedient alternatives) to frozen section for purposes of intraoperative consultation, these may be unipolar or multipolar but, in contrast to the cytoplasmic extensions characteristic of hyperplastic astroglia, do not sprout from the cell body in the radial, stellate array for which the astrocyte is named.[301,302] On ultrastructural study,[336] these processes contain bundles of 7- to 11-nm ("intermediate") filaments composed of GFAP (Fig. 28-42), the principal cytoskeletal constituent elaborated by human astrocytes, and vimentin.[305] Nuclei are typically oval in configuration with smooth contours, do not contain conspicuous nucleoli, often have a vesicular quality, but may be somewhat hyperchromatic. Mild variation in size and shape is to be expected, but conspicuous nuclear pleomorphism calls the diagnosis of astrocytoma into serious question.

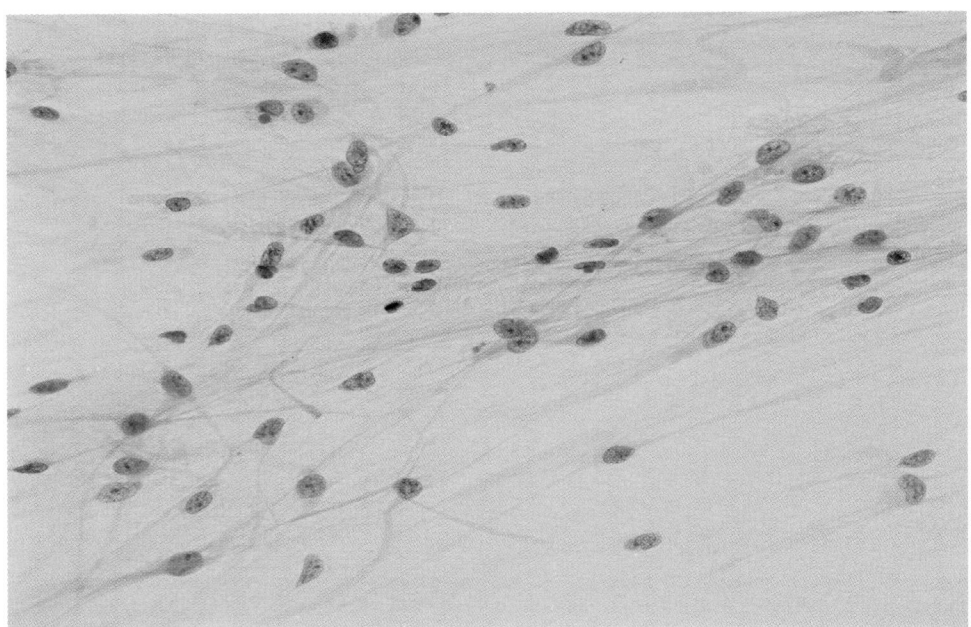

Fig. 28-41 Diffuse fibrillary astrocytoma. A lack of cellular cohesion, delicate oval nuclei without nucleoli, and conspicuous cytoplasmic processes—features that collectively serve to distinguish astrocytomas from metastatic carcinomas, lymphomas, and other neoplasms—are all apparent in this intraoperative squash preparation.

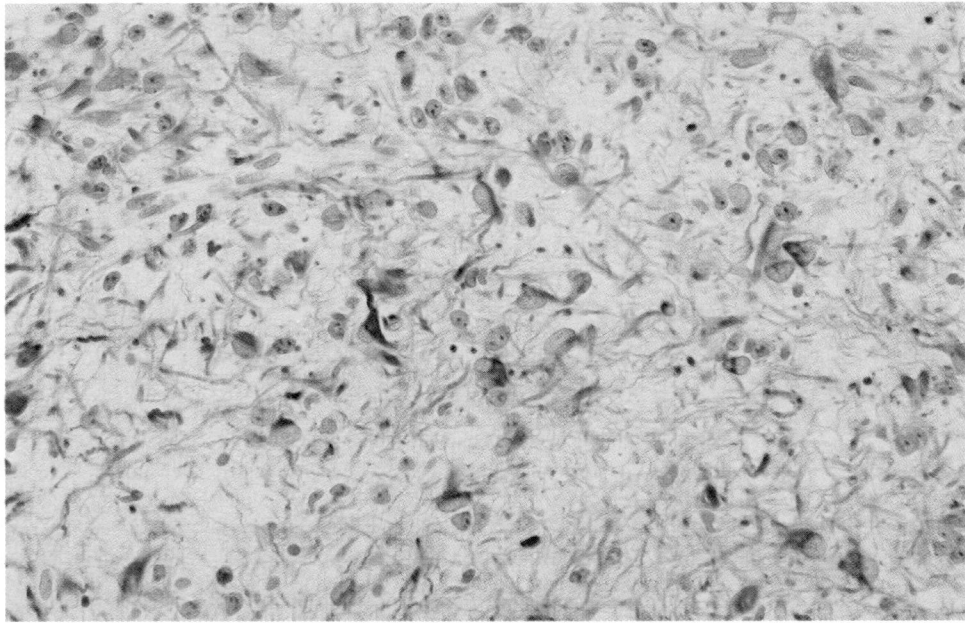

Fig. 28-42 Diffuse fibrillary astrocytoma. An immunoperoxidase preparation demonstrates labeling of tumor cell bodies and processes by a monoclonal antibody to glial fibrillary acidic protein.

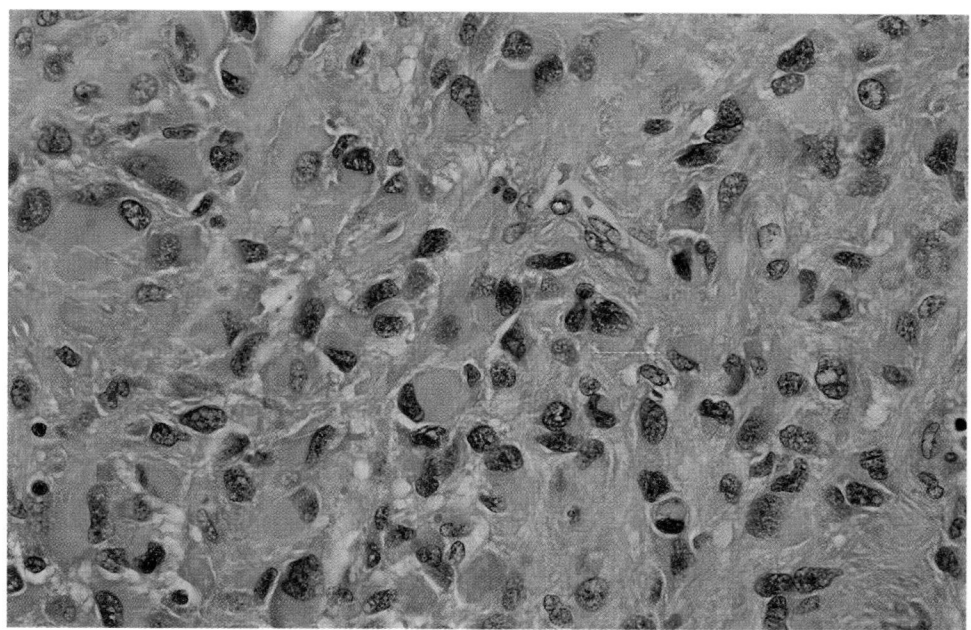

Fig. 28-43 Anaplastic astrocytoma. Compared with its low-grade counterpart (see Fig. 28-39), this lesion exhibits increased cellularity and the cytologic features of a fully malignant neoplasm, including conspicuous nuclear pleomorphism and dense hyperchromasia. Mitotic figures, foreign to the low-grade astrocytoma, were also found (not shown).

The **anaplastic astrocytoma** often evolves from a well-differentiated precursor lesion of the type described. Accordingly, morphologic evidence of tumor progression may constitute a focal finding in what would otherwise qualify as a histologically favorable lesion.[301] Microscopic examination of the prototypical case reveals an infiltrate that is at a glance more alarmingly cellular and pleomorphic than that of the low-grade astrocytoma (Fig. 28-43), although biopsies derived from the tumor-CNS interface may contain only scattered neoplastic elements. Nuclear alterations commonly include angulation, dense hyperchromasia, and considerable variation in contour and dimension. The diagnosis rests on particularly firm ground if mitotic figures can be demonstrated, because these are foreign to the low-grade astrocytoma. An increase in regional blood vessels is permissible, as is hypertrophy of their lining endothelium, but disorderly endothelial proliferation or zones of coagulative tumor necrosis in the setting of a cytologically malignant fibrillary astrocytic neoplasm mandate classification of the lesion as a glioblastoma (see the following sections).

In light of their predictably aggressive clinical evolution,[319] we also regard as anaplastic those astrocytomas richly endowed with gemistocytic elements (Fig. 28-44). The latter possess a globose paranuclear mass of dense, eosinophilic cytoplasm from which one or more short, stout processes may radiate, often terminating on a nearby blood vessel. Pure gemistocytic astrocytomas are exceptionally uncommon. In fact, most tumors possessed of a prominent gemistocytic component also harbor a subpopulation of small, poorly differentiated neoplastic cells that are thought to represent their actively proliferative compartment. As noted,

perivascular lymphoid infiltrates are a striking feature of many gemistocytic astrocytomas but do not augur well for afflicted patients, the majority of these lesions degenerating into glioblastomas in relatively short order. Care must be taken lest this designation be extended to oligodendrogliomas composed of diminutive or "mini"-gemistocytes (discussed in the section on oligodendroglioma). These do not manifest the perivascular lymphocytic cuffing or dense fibrillary matrix of the gemistocytic astrocytoma; often exhibit a cohesive, lobular, or pavement-like architecture; and almost invariably harbor telltale oligodendroglial elements of classic clear-cell type.

Although its unfortunate title would imply a derivation from embryonal or stem cell elements, the **glioblastoma multiforme** is now widely regarded as arising principally via the neoplastic transformation of mature astrocytes. "Primary" and "secondary" variants are recognized, the former occurring de novo (i.e., unassociated with demonstrable precursor lesions), the latter resulting from the successful expansion of particularly anaplastic and aggressive clones generated within pre-existent, differentiated astrocytic neoplasms.[301] Noteworthy is the observation that the glioblastoma associated with historical or histologic evidence of a progenitory low-grade astrocytoma may present at a younger age and evolve in a somewhat less menacing fashion than the common variety encountered in older adults.[341] That this clinicopathologic duality reflects divergent molecular oncogenetic mechanisms has been suggested, mutations or deletions of the tumor-suppressing p53 allele being specifically implicated in the "secondary" pathway.[321,340] Loss of heterozygosity involving chromosome 10 and asso-

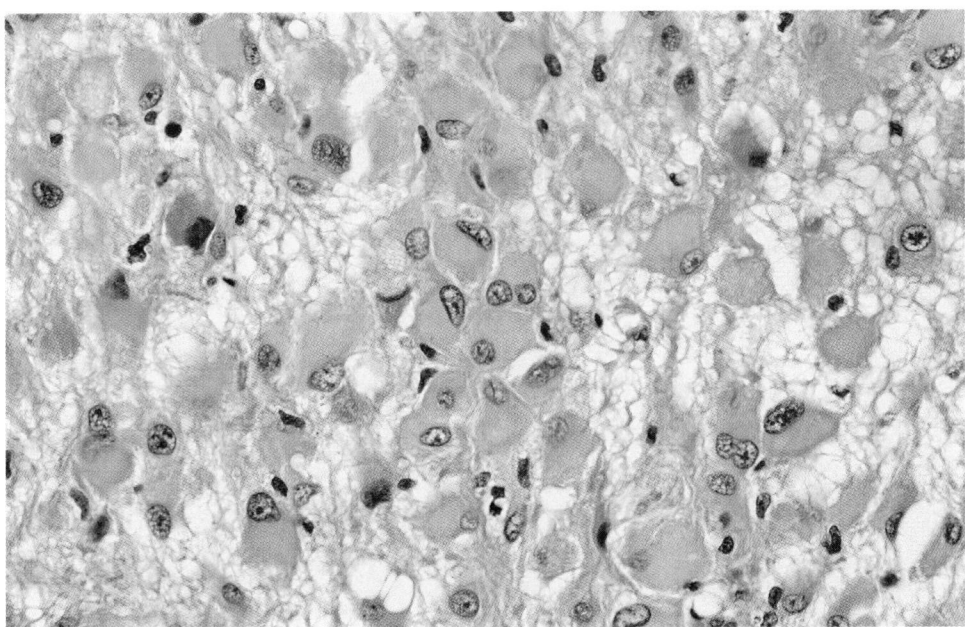

Fig. 28-44 Gemistocytic astrocytoma. Heavily dominated on initial resection by the large gemistocytes shown here, this example recurred 11 months after radiotherapy and chemotherapy. Re-resection demonstrated progression to glioblastoma. Note that these cells retain the oval and somewhat vesicular nuclei of astrocytes. For a comparison with the "minigemistocytic" variant of oligodendroglioma, see Fig. 28-63, *B*.

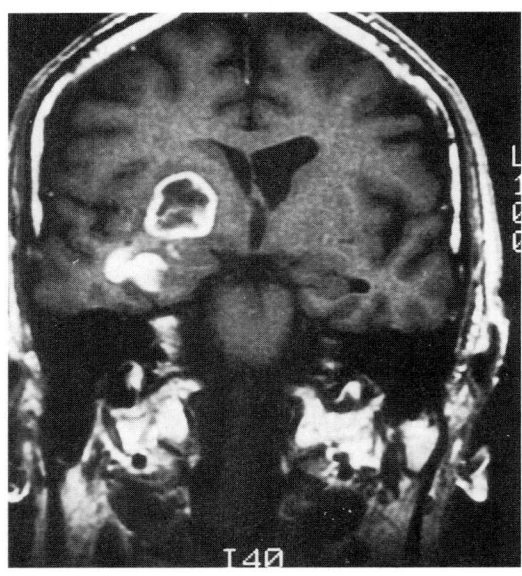

Fig. 28-45 Glioblastoma multiforme. In postcontrast injection CT or (shown here) MR studies, many glioblastomas are characterized by a bright ("enhancing") ring (representing intact, abnormally vascularized tumor tissue in which the blood-brain barrier is disrupted) that surrounds a region of hypodensity (central necrosis). The gyriform temporal lobe enhancement below this basal ganglionic example attests to neoplastic infiltration beyond the deceptively well-delimited ring margin.

ciated amplification of the locus on chromosome 7 encoding the epidermal growth factor receptor may, on the other hand, underlie the genesis of de novo examples.[340] These latter molecular cytogenetic phenomena are restricted to astrocytic neoplasms exhibiting the morphologic features of glioblastoma, whereas p53 abnormalities are also observed in fibrillary astrocytomas of well-differentiated and anaplastic type.[321]

Like astrocytomas of lower grade, glioblastomas may be discovered on evaluation for seizures or headache but are often attended by subacutely evolving neurologic deficits indicative of their more rapid growth and destructive invasion. A subset present in sudden, stroke-like fashion as a consequence of intratumoral hemorrhage, and occasional examples mimic metastatic disease by virtue of their multifocality.[300,301] Especially characteristic on CT or MR evaluation is a pattern of ring-like contrast enhancement that reflects their abnormal vascularization and tendency to spontaneous central necrosis (Fig. 28-45). On gross inspection, these aggressive lesions may seem relatively circumscribed and often appear to be more clearly demarcated from neighboring tissues than their better-differentiated counterparts—deceptively so, inasmuch as neoplastic cells regularly invade neuropil well beyond a given tumor's apparent perimeter.[301,314] Hemorrhagic discoloration and foci of yellow softening indicative of coagulative necrosis impart a variegated appearance to most examples that should immediately suggest their virulent nature (Fig. 28-46).

On histologic study, the glioblastoma is a highly cellular, pleomorphic, and mitotically active neoplasm. Its cytologic

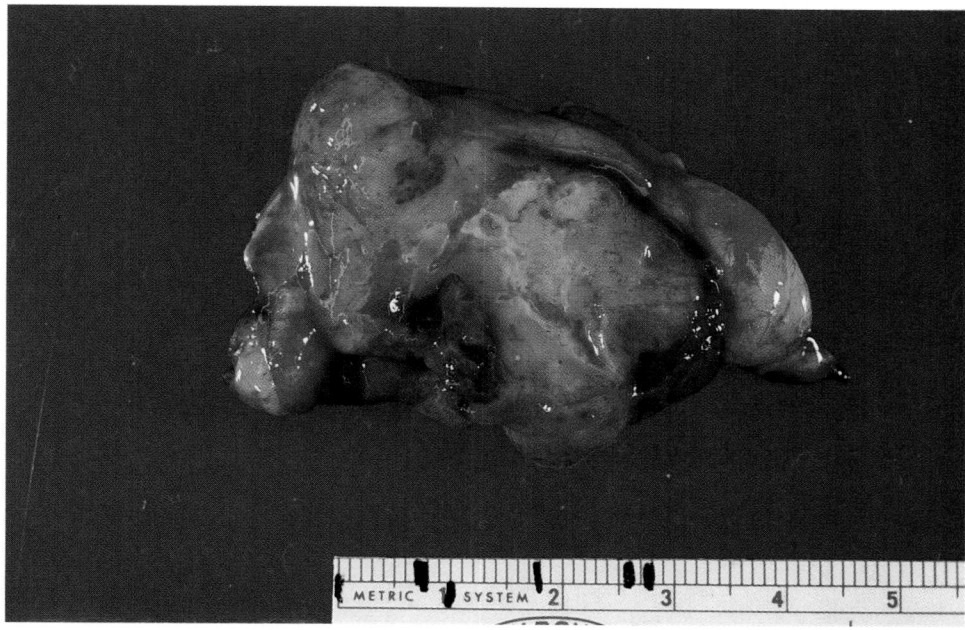

Fig. 28-46 Glioblastoma multiforme. Foci of hemorrhage and geographic yellow discoloration indicative of necrosis impart a variegated appearance to this example.

makeup is subject to extreme variation.[301] Differentiated elements may be intermingled with bizarre multinucleated tumor giant cells or small anaplastic forms altogether devoid of identifying astrocytic features (Fig. 28-47). The latter often come to dominate the histologic picture at recurrence, selectively repopulating tumors subjected to therapy, but may also constitute the nearly exclusive elements of select small-cell glioblastomas at presentation.

An arresting phenomenon common to many glioblastomas is a complex form of microvascular hyperplasia, likely driven by tumor-derived mitogens (e.g., platelet-derived growth factor, epidermal growth factor, transforming growth factor beta), in which proliferating blood vessels come to be lined by cells heaped up in disorderly fashion and are ultimately transformed into glomeruloid or solid tufts (Fig. 28-48). Although often referred to simply as "endothelial" hyperplasia, this process involves a number of vessel-associated cell types, prominent among which are pericytic/myoid elements expressing smooth muscle–related antigens.[309,340a] Its identification in neurosurgical material from patients not previously subjected to radiation therapy suffices for a diagnosis of glioblastoma multiforme by WHO criteria, as does the finding of focal coagulative tumor necrosis, regardless of whether neoplastic cells align themselves about such zones in the prototypical palisades that are a "textbook" feature of this lesion[301,318] (Fig. 28-47). We should point out, however, that many neuropathologists are reluctant to accept a high-grade fibrillary astrocytic neoplasm as a glioblastoma in the absence of tumor necrosis, because this finding has emerged from several clinical series as being especially predictive of an accelerated clinical course and short survival.[301]

Irradiation induces in the glioblastoma a variety of morphologic alterations,[301] the most predictable being widespread necrosis, unrelated to regional tumor cell density (usually much reduced) and vasculopathic changes that include ectasia, fibrinoid necrosis, and obliterative mural fibroplasia (Fig. 28-49). Florid astrogliosis and infiltration by macrophages, the latter identifiable by their immunoreactivity for HAM-56 and other histiocytic "markers," may complicate the recognition of neoplastic elements. Some reresection specimens, in fact, consist solely of necrotic debris or contain only scattered suspect cells exhibiting cytopathic alterations, presumably treatment-related, such as grotesque karyomegaly and dense hyperchromasia with chromatin smudging and nuclear vacuolization. Although we favor the view that these cells are neoplastic, albeit damaged, it is conceivable that they represent in some cases hyperplastic astrocytes displaying radiation atypia. Whatever their origin, these elements do not imply disease progression, and we report such specimens as exhibiting treatment effect with only minimal evidence of persistent, injured tumor. The diagnosis of recurrence rests on firmest grounds when aggregates of cytologically unaltered and mitotically active tumor cells can be demonstrated, cellular palisading about foci of necrosis also constituting unimpeachable testimony to treatment failure. In some instances, the necrotizing and vasculopathic changes described here will be found to involve brain tissue (typically white matter, which is particularly susceptible to ionizing irradiation) manifesting no tumoral infiltration. This toxic process *cerebral radionecrosis* characteristically interrupts a period of apparent remission and neurologic recovery measured in months (or, in

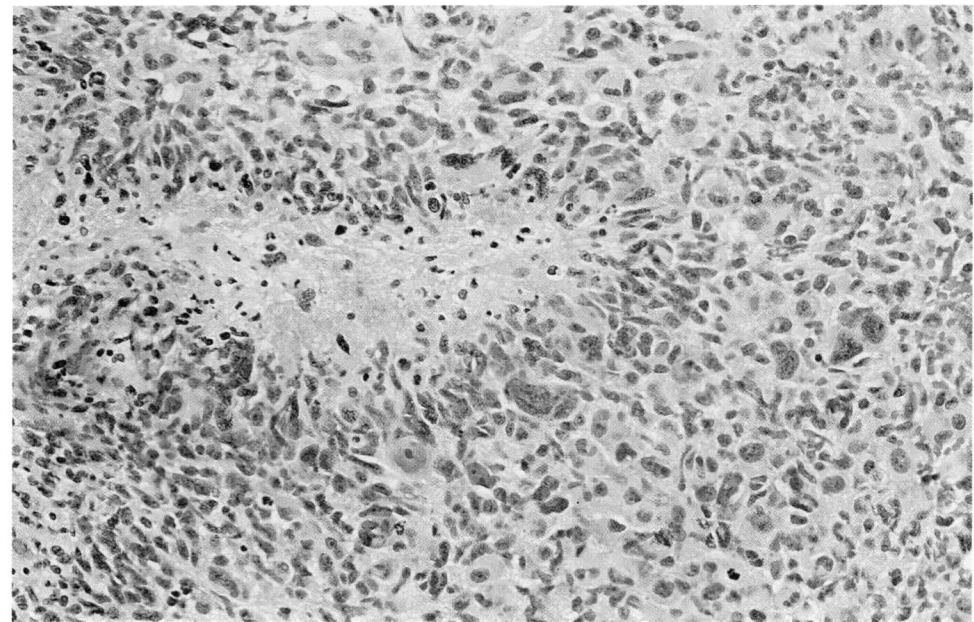

Fig. 28-47 Glioblastoma multiforme. Dense cellularity, striking pleomorphism, and zones of coagulative necrosis lined by "palisading" tumor cells characterize the prototypical glioblastoma.

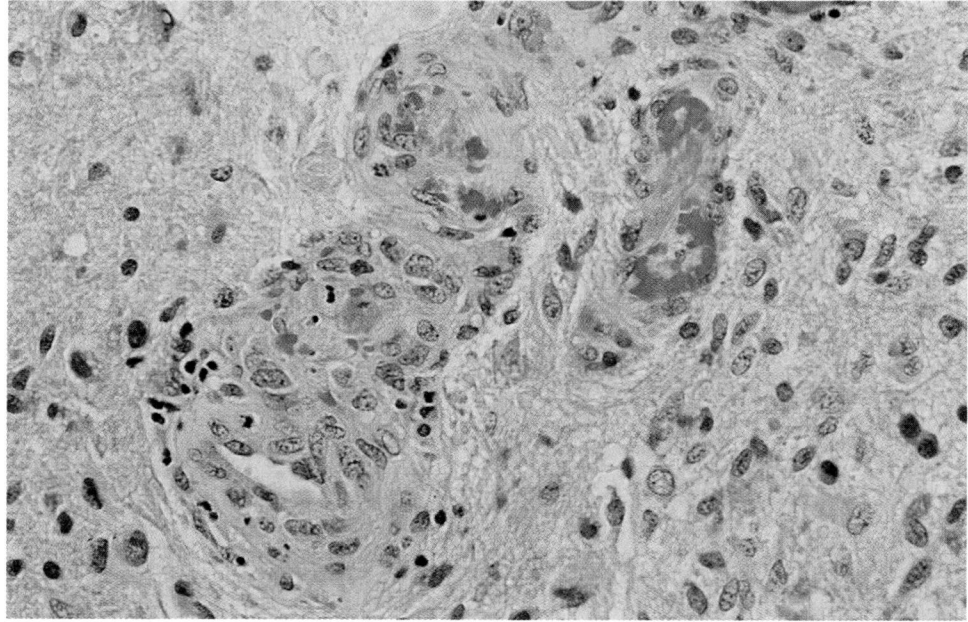

Fig. 28-48 Glioblastoma multiforme. Small blood vessels exhibiting a disorderly proliferation of their mural elements ("microvascular hyperplasia") are a feature of many high-grade fibrillary astrocytomas and, along with necrosis, constitute a defining characteristic of the glioblastoma by WHO criteria.

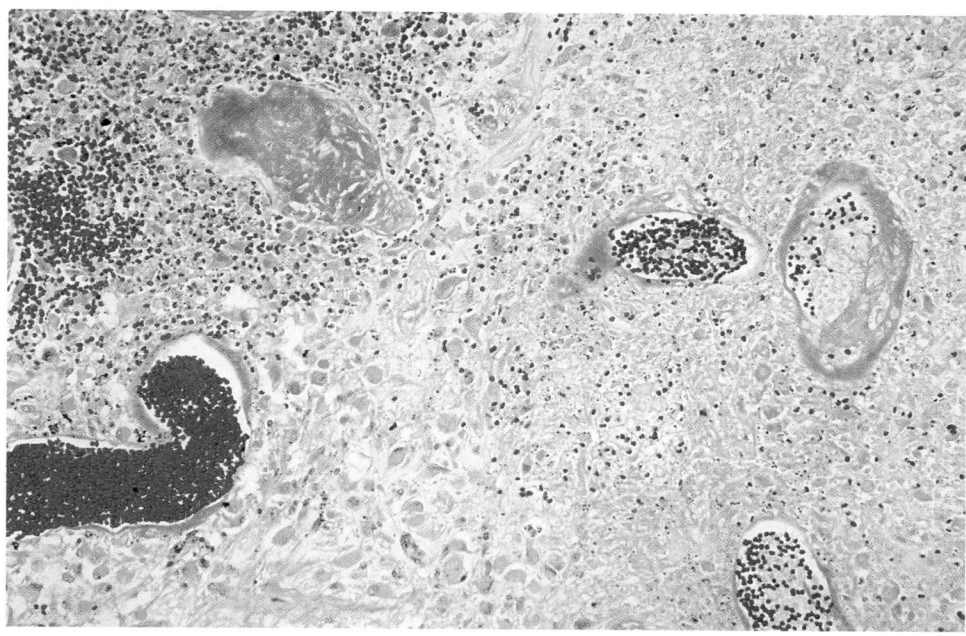

Fig. 28-49 Radiation effect. A marked reduction in cellularity, extensive necrosis, and necrotizing fibrinoid vasculopathy with vascular thrombosis and ectasia typify astrocytic neoplasms injured by irradiation.

some cases, years) and may mimic post-therapy relapse to clinical and neuroradiologic perfection.

Although most of the astrocytic neoplasms under discussion are confidently distinguished from primary cerebral sarcomas and tumors metastatic to the CNS by virtue of their characteristic cytologic features and typically dyscohesive patterns of infiltration, select variants of anaplastic astrocytoma and glioblastoma may occasion considerable confusion in this regard. A case in point is the *giant cell glioblastoma,* a tumor noted for its unusual circumscription, sarcomatoid cytologic features, and reticulin-rich matrix.[322] Although long regarded by some observers as a "monstrocellular" sarcoma, the glial nature of this neoplasm can be demonstrated by positive immunocytochemical assay for GFAP. The same can be said for spindle cell and "xanthosarcomatous," lipid-rich variants of glioblastoma.[316,333] We have seen a number of high-grade astrocytic neoplasms misclassified as fibrosarcomas or malignant fibrous histiocytomas because immunohistochemical studies demonstrated cytoplasmic labeling for vimentin, alpha$_1$-antitrypsin, or antichymotrypsin, but failed to include examination for GFAP expression. Still other aggressive and poorly differentiated astrocytic tumors contain gland-like ("adenoid") formations,[315] undergo squamous metaplasia,[328] or assume clear cell cytologic features (owing to cytoplasmic lipidization) and a cohesive disposition in nests and sheets that bring "balloon cell" melanoma and carcinomas of renal or adrenocortical origin to mind.[333] Immunolabeling for cytokeratin[305,330] and epithelial membrane antigen (EMA)[311] may further conspire to obscure the glial lineage of these and other astrocytic neoplasms. Again, assay for GFAP expres-

sion may be decisive in their unmasking, although the literature—analyzed elsewhere[333]—contains isolated depictions of carcinomas (mainly renal) that were decorated by antisera to this marker protein (see section on secondary tumors). Glioblastomas may also harbor primitive-appearing papillary structures that invite confusion with the medulloepithelioma.[327] Lastly, we call the reader's attention to the existence of astrocytic tumors that undergo a striking granular cell metamorphosis resulting from the intracytoplasmic accumulation of engorged secondary lysosomes.[325] Although their granular cell components exhibit remarkably benign cytologic features, these peculiar neoplasms are characterized by an aggressive clinical evolution.

The four-tiered Daumas-Duport scheme for the grading of diffuse fibrillary astrocytomas, also known as the St. Anne–Mayo system, merits comment as an attractive alternative to the WHO classification in that it requires of the pathologist only binary decisions regarding clearly defined and easily identified histologic variables.[306] Specimens are assessed for the presence of nuclear atypia (i.e., hyperchromasia or obvious variation in size or shape), mitotic figures, endothelial proliferation (defined as vascular lumina lined by at least two layers of piled-up or haphazardly arrayed endothelial cells), and foci of coagulative necrosis. Variables are simply scored as present or absent and astrocytomas assigned to grade 1 if none, grade 2 if any one, grade 3 if any two, and grade 4 if three or all of these features are identified. Although the equal weighting of such findings as nuclear atypism and necrosis would seem inappropriate in theory, this method succeeds in stratifying lesions in a hierarchy of escalating biologic potential because the evaluated indices of anaplasia accrue to evolving astrocytic tumors in a predictable sequence. Thus it is nuclear atypism alone that comes in practice to distinguish the grade 2 from the grade 1 astrocytoma, the additional presence of mitoses that defines the grade 3 lesion, and the superimposed appearance of endothelial proliferation or necrosis that characterizes tumors of grade 4. The last three Daumas-Duport grades generally correspond, then, to the tripartite astrocytoma–anaplastic astrocytoma–glioblastoma construct of the WHO classification, the former system also identifying a small subset of patients with particularly indolent (grade 1) lesions and favorable outcomes. The latter, unfortunately, are exceedingly rare. The results of randomized, prospective clinical trials employing the Daumas-Duport model have yet to be reported, but the interobserver reproducibility of this method and its ability to generate four distinct survival curves have been confirmed in large studies of archival material from multiple institutions,[306,317] as has a strong correlation of its ascending grades with increasing proliferative index as assessed by bromodeoxyuridine labeling methods.[320]

The prognosis of a given fibrillary astrocytic neoplasm is a complex function of both clinical and morphologic variables. Patient age, functional status on presentation, tumor location, and histology all affect the outcome of supratentorial examples.[301] Faring best are young subjects harboring low-grade lesions that are unassociated with focal neurologic deficits and that are situated in the cerebral hemispheres (as opposed to corpus callosum, basal ganglia, or thalami). Follow-up studies of patients identified and managed since the advent of CT imaging (i.e., in the era of "early" detection) suggest median survivals in the 7- to 10-year range under such relatively favorable circumstances, death typically following tumor "dedifferentiation".[301,321a,324] Whether attempted resection or radiotherapy prolongs the lives of patients with low-grade cerebral hemispheric astrocytomas is a contentious matter; some neuro-oncologists elect to simply follow affected individuals until there is clear clinical or neuroradiologic evidence of tumor progression. Comparably situated anaplastic astrocytomas and glioblastomas, by contrast, are unarguably aggressive neoplasms associated with median postoperative survival periods of 24 to 36 and 12 months, respectively, despite irradiation and adjuvant chemotherapy.[301] Again, young patients tend to live longer than middle-aged or elderly adults, as do some individuals with evidence of a pre-existing astrocytoma of low grade.[341] There is also evidence, admittedly controversial, to suggest that gross total excision lengthens survival.[341] Ultimately, however, the insidious manner in which these lesions permeate brain tissues beyond their neuroradiologically defined and grossly apparent confines frustrates operative attempts at local disease control and sets the stage for progressive infiltration of neighboring cerebral parenchyma by chemoresistant clones. This, the primary pattern of treatment failure, is occasionally complicated by the development of CSF-borne neuraxial metastases and, rarely, by spread to somatic sites, such as bone, lung, liver, or lymph node.[301] Most unusual, but well documented, are cases in which systemic metastases have been apparent on initial patient presentation,[308] and the bizarre phenomenon of inadvertent tumor transplantation via hepatic and renal allografts has also been the subject of isolated reports.[339]

Similarly dismal is the prognosis attached to diffusely invasive astrocytic neoplasms of the brainstem, most of which are histologically anaplastic, if not obvious glioblastomas at diagnosis.[299,301,337] It is the exceptional patient who remains alive more than 2 years from symptom onset. These lesions may mimic pilocytic astrocytomas in the generally limited biopsies secured from the bulbar region by virtue of a certain spindling imposed on their constituent cells as these infiltrate the compact fiber traits of the pontine base. Dense hyperchromasia and conspicuous nuclear pleomorphism usually serve to distinguish these cells from well-differentiated piloid astrocytes, but in questionable cases, their elongate nuclei can be shown by the appropriate histochemical methods to lie among myelinated axons rather than in a meshwork of bipolar, GFAP-immunoreactive cytoplasmic processes. It should also be pointed out that pilocytic astrocytomas (discussed later) tend at bulbar levels to a sharp circumscription and exophytic growth from the dorsal pontomedullary junction generally foreign to fibrillary astrocytic neoplasms of the brainstem. Not surprisingly, patients with high-grade astrocytomas of the cerebellum[303] and spinal cord[304,307] do very poorly, whereas a subset of indolent, well-differentiated lesions occurring in the latter location appear amenable to radical resection and are compatible with long-term survival.[307]

Although conventional histologic examination remains the only technique routinely applied to the prognostic assessment of fibrillary astrocytomas, we would call the reader's attention to quantifiable methods for the determination of these tumors' proliferative capacities as adjuncts to traditional morphologic classification.[301,320,326,331] These may, in fact, prove more accurate than histopathologic grading in the prediction of a given lesion's clinical evolution. Technical details may be found in the cited literature. Of the varied published methods, immunocytochemical assays for a cell cycle–associated, nonhistone nucleoprotein recognized by the commercially available Ki-67[326] and MIB-1[331] monoclonal antibodies are most easily performed and interpreted (Fig. 28-50). Whereas Ki-67 studies require frozen sections (reactivity is rapidly lost on routine tissue processing), MIB-1 is applicable to formalin-fixed, paraffin-embedded material. Ki-67 labeling indices (i.e., fraction of decorated tumor cell nuclei) in excess of 3% have been associated with a potential for aggressive growth in supratentorial fibrillary astrocytomas.[326] Flow cytometry has also been applied to this problem, one study suggesting that patients with anaplastic astrocytomas characterized by an aneuploid histogram fare somewhat better than individuals whose morphologically comparable tumors are demonstrably diploid.[334]

Protoplasmic astrocytoma. In contrast to the fibrous astrocyte, assumed progenitor of the fibrillary astrocytoma, the protoplasmic astrocyte normally resides in gray, rather than white, matter (e.g., cerebral cortex, deep nuclei) and fashions elongated, GFAP-rich cytoplasmic processes only in pathologic circumstances. Tumor cells resembling protoplasmic astrocytes (i.e., poorly fibrillated) are often apparent in foci of cortical invasion by conventional fibrillary astrocytomas and populate the microcystic regions common to astrocytomas of juvenile pilocytic type (discussed later). Uncommon neoplasms traditionally dubbed *protoplasmic astrocytomas* are composed predominantly or exclusively of

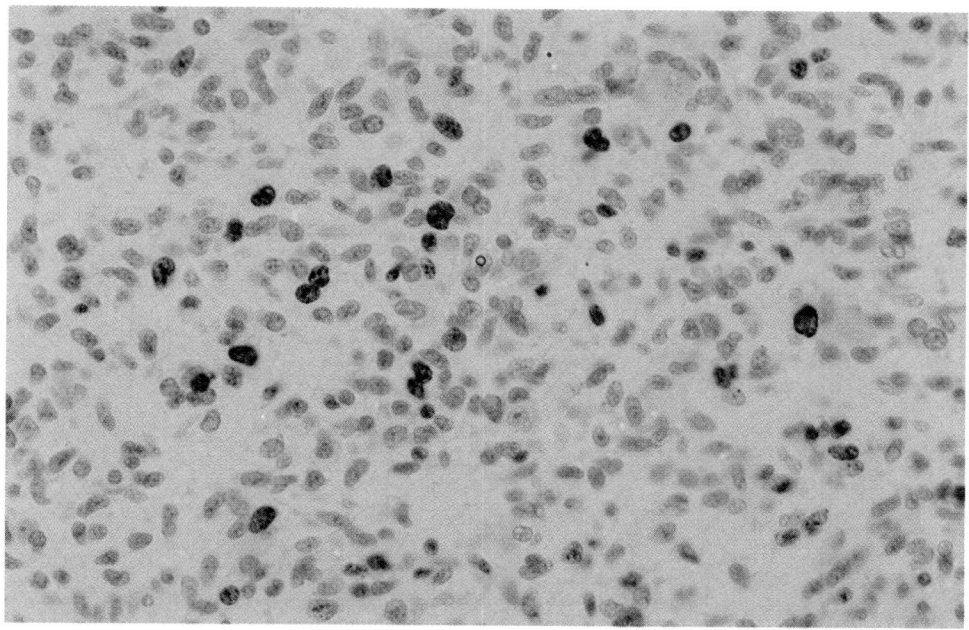

Fig. 28-50 Markers of cellular proliferation. Actively cycling tumor cells within a glioblastoma are identified in this immunoperoxidase preparation by their nuclear labeling with the MIB-1 monoclonal antibody.

such cells.[343] These generally arise in the cerebral cortices of children and young adults, presenting as superficially situated masses of somewhat gelatinous gray tissue. Histologic study reveals cytologically uniform cells evenly suspended in a cobweb-like matrix of short cytoplasmic fibrils and myxoid material that tends to accumulate in microcysts of varying diameter. Nuclei are generally round or slightly oval, showing little variation in size, and the overall appearance is typically that of a low-grade neoplasm. Mitotic activity is exceptional and constitutes evidence of increased biologic potential. Recent immunocytochemical studies demonstrating that these cortically based tumors may harbor only a minor subset of cells exhibiting the cytoplasmic GFAP expression and surface ganglioside profile characteristic of fibrillary astroglia have been taken as evidence of their derivation from protoplasmic astrocytes.[342] In practice, we find that distinction of these lesions from microcystic oligodendrogliomas is problematic.

Pilocytic astrocytomas. *Pilocytic astrocytomas* typically present in childhood, adolescence, or early adult life, hence their common designation by the prefacing term *juvenile,* and exhibit a decided predilection for the cerebellum,[348,360] third ventricular (hypothalamic) region,[358] optic nerves, and chiasm.[344,363] They constitute the great majority of tumors collected under the traditional appellations of "cerebellar astrocytoma" and "optic nerve glioma," including those examples of the latter, often bilateral, complicating type 1 neurofibromatosis (von Recklinghausen's disease). Noteworthy in this regard is the recent demonstration that some pilocytic astrocytomas harbor deletions of the long arm of chromosome 17 that include the locus (17q11.2) to which

the type 1 neurofibromatosis gene has been mapped.[362] A significant percentage of pediatric astrocytomas arising at spinal levels appear to be of juvenile pilocytic type[359]; the same can be said of a clinically distinctive subset of bulbar neoplasms that deviate from the diffuse fibrillary astrocytomas typical of the brainstem by virtue of their circumscription, by their tendency to bulge into the fourth ventricle in "dorsally exophytic" fashion and their relatively favorable prognosis.[352] Pilocytic astrocytomas may also be situated in the cerebral hemispheres,[347] basal ganglia, and thalami.[354]

Save for those tumors positioned in the anterior visual pathway, which produce a fusiform, "pseudohypertrophic" expansion of the optic nerve, and a subset of cerebellar examples having diffusely invasive components,[348] pilocytic astrocytomas tend to be sharply demarcated, tend to be nodular in contour, and frequently project into sizable cysts that may account for most of their mass effect and associated neurologic symptoms (Fig. 28-51). Homogeneous contrast enhancement typifies the solid elements of the pilocytic astrocytoma, a feature serving, along with the neoplasm's tendency to cystic change and the high signal intensity displayed by many examples on both T1- and T2-weighted MRI study, to distinguish this lesion from the diffuse fibrillary astrocytoma on neuroradiologic examination (Fig. 28-52).

The prototypical pilocytic astrocytoma is an architecturally and cytologically biphasic neoplasm composed of tumor cells in both fascicular and microcystic array (Fig. 28-53). The former component is fashioned of elements bearing the delicate, bipolar cytoplasmic processes for which the tumor is named, the adjectival *pilocytic* deriving from the

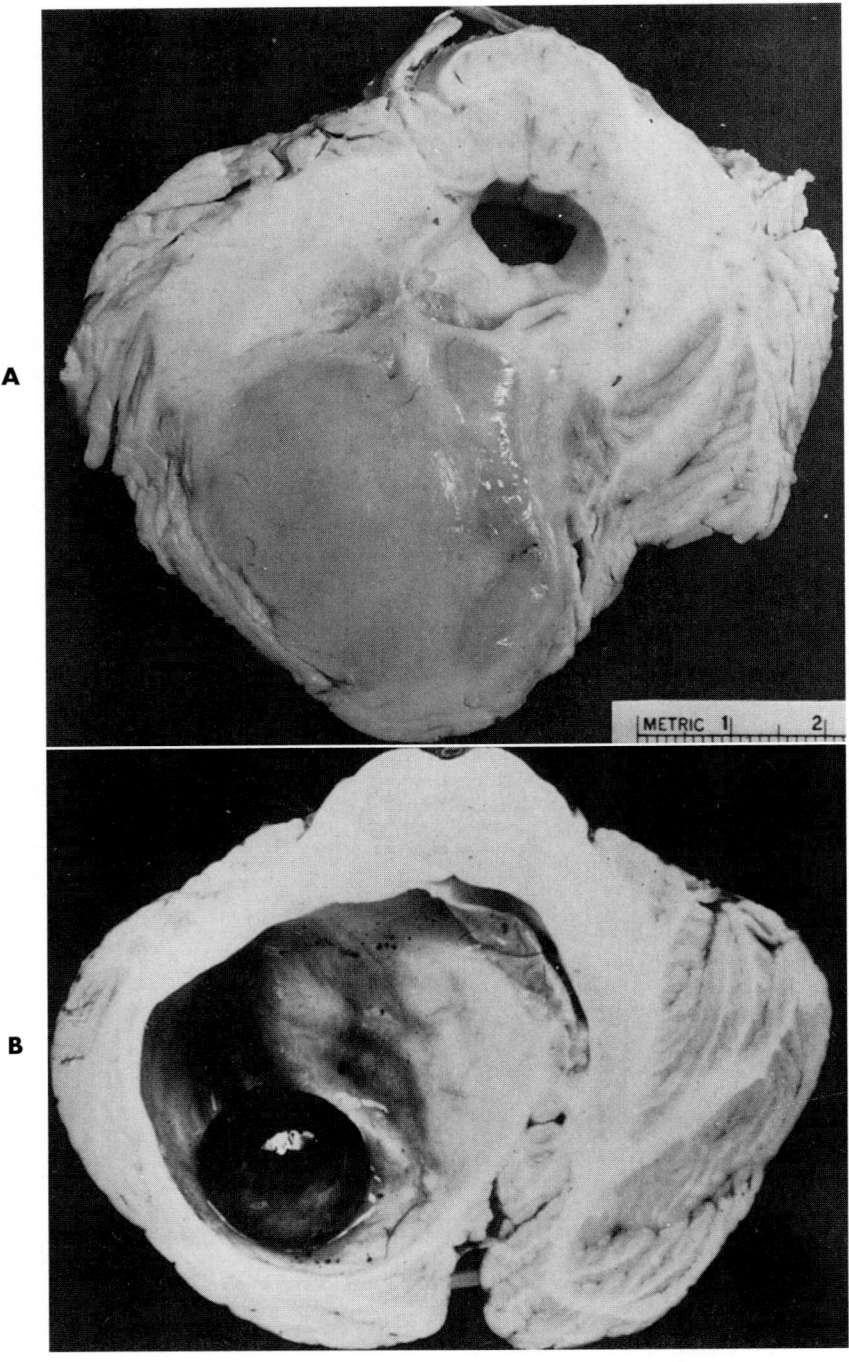

Fig. 28-51 Pilocytic astrocytoma. Two childhood cerebellar examples illustrate macroscopic variants of the pilocytic astrocytoma. The neoplasm is well delimited in both cases, forming a solid gray mass **(A)** or constituting a somewhat hemorrhagic, discrete mural nodule projecting from the wall of a cyst **(B)**. (**B** from Rubinstein LJ: Seminario de Neuropatología, Mérida, Yucatán. Bol Asoc Mex Patol AC **7**:13-59, 1969; courtesy Dr. J.E. Olvera-Rabiela, Mexico City.)

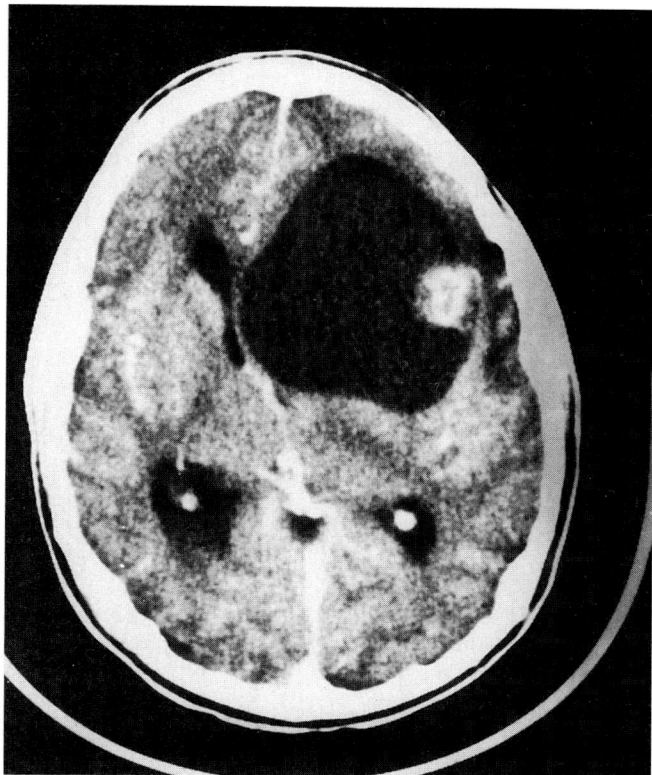

Fig. 28-52 Pilocytic astrocytoma. This postcontrast injection CT study of a frontal lobe example emphasizes that pilocytic astrocytomas may be localized to the cerebral hemispheres, where they commonly maintain the cyst/mural nodule configuration assumed by many of their more prevalent cerebellar counterparts. Diffuse contrast enhancement of the lesion's solid, nodular component *(right)* is the rule. A similar neuroradiologic presentation is manifested by many gangliogliomas and pleomorphic xanthoastrocytomas, as discussed in the text.

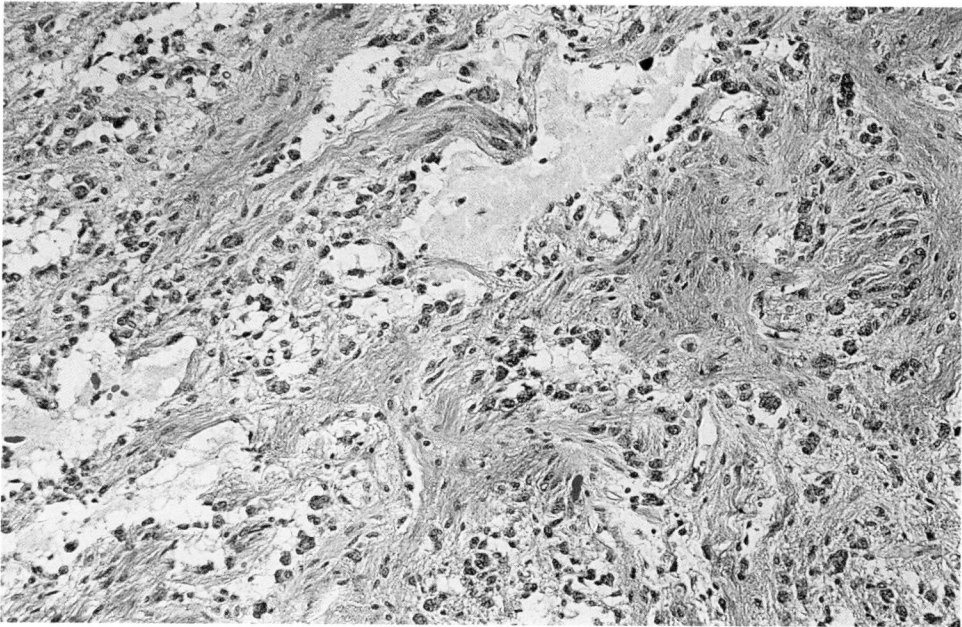

Fig. 28-53 Pilocytic astrocytoma. The biphasic cellular populations and architecture of the classic pilocytic astrocytoma are in evidence. The lesion's process-bearing spindle-cell ("piloid") constituents fashion a densely fibrillar matrix, whereas its process-poor ("protoplasmic") elements aggregate in regions of myxoid change that often progress to microcyst formation.

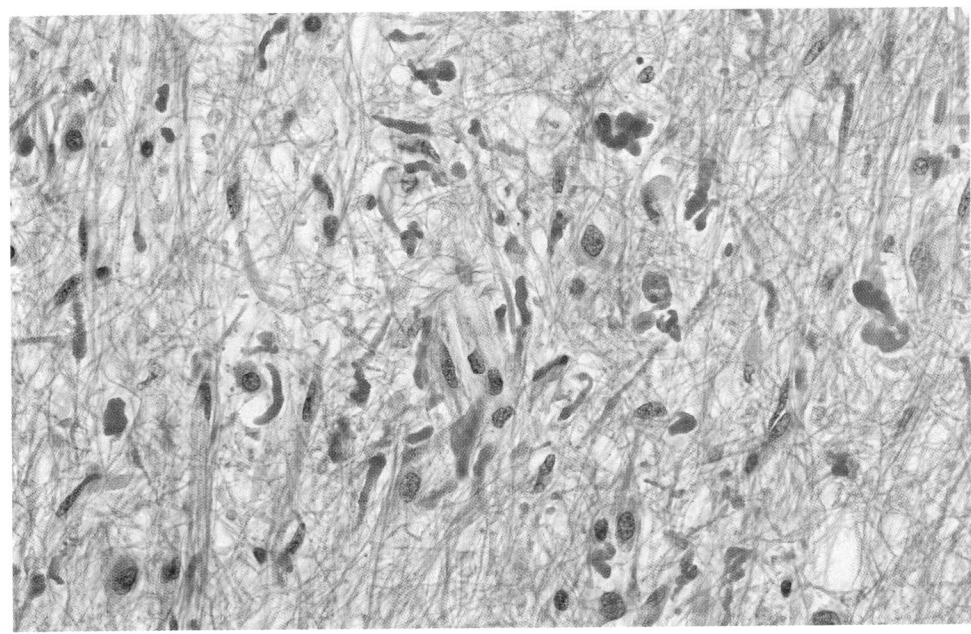

Fig. 28-54 Pilocytic astrocytoma. Varicose Rosenthal fibers lie among the otherwise delicate and hair-like cytoplasmic processes for which the pilocytic astrocytoma is named.

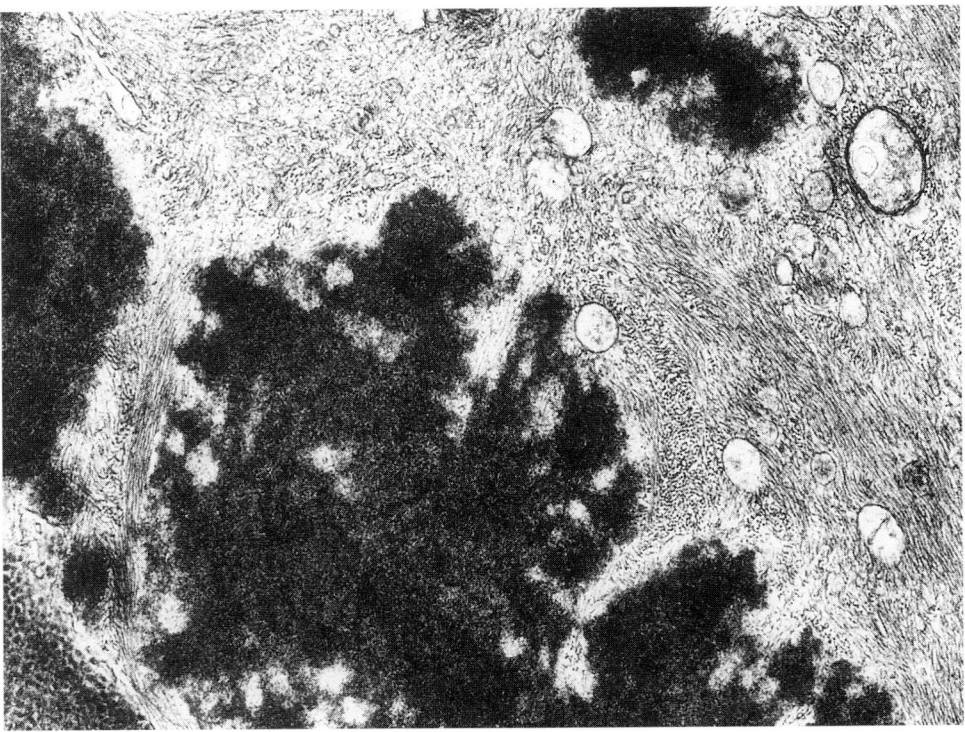

Fig. 28-55 Pilocytic astrocytoma. On transmission electron microscopic study, Rosenthal fibers are intracytoplasmic aggregates of granular, electron-dense material intimately associated with intermediate filaments, the latter composed principally of glial fibrillary acidic protein. (×25,350.)

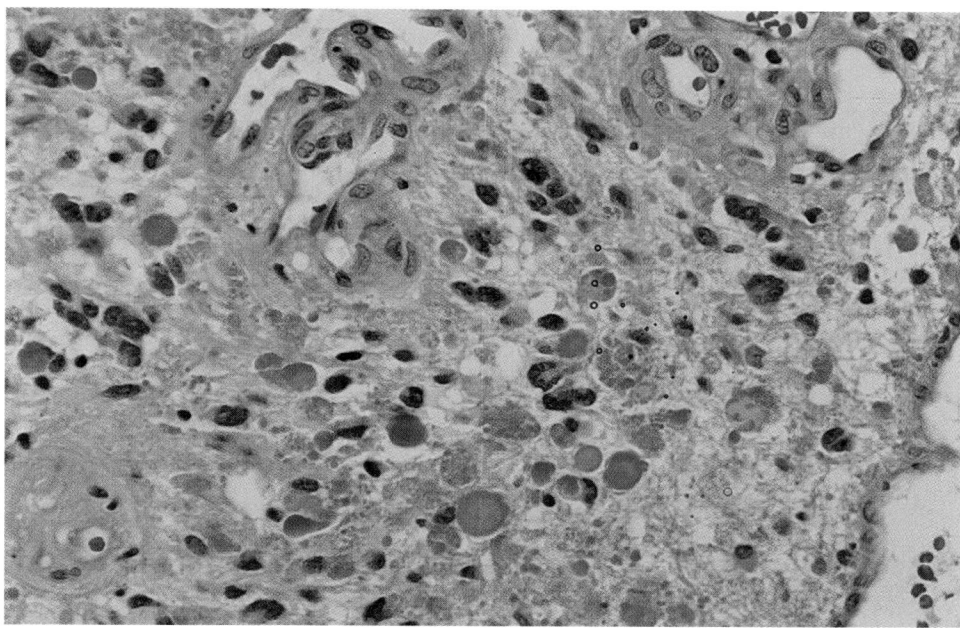

Fig. 28-56 Pilocytic astrocytoma. Eosinophilic, hyaline globular bodies are typically associated with, although not restricted to, three indolent neuroepithelial tumors: the pilocytic astrocytoma, pleomorphic xanthoastrocytoma, and ganglioglioma.

Greek root for hair. These are typically woven in a dense fibrillar matrix in which oval or spindly tumor cell nuclei appear to lie embedded, a given cell's slender and remarkably elongated processes being optimally visualized in cytologic preparations that are useful adjuncts to the study of frozen sections during intraoperative consultation. In microcystic regions, neoplastic cells are arranged about, or float suspended in, pools of basophilic, myxoid material. Here a "protoplasmic" cytology is assumed, tumor cells exhibiting rounded nuclear contours and manifesting little tendency to elaborate cytoplasmic extensions. It should be noted that the relative admixture of piloid and microcystic elements varies greatly from case to case. The latter are particularly likely to dominate cerebellar examples in children. Other common histologic features include oligodendroglioma-like clear cell foci and an angiomatoid vasculature characterized by complex arborization, hyaline mural fibroplasia, and ectasia.

Classically associated with the juvenile pilocytic astrocytoma are the cytoplasmic structures known as Rosenthal fibers and eosinophilic granular bodies. Vermiform acidophilic densities typically restricted to the tumor's richly fibrillated regions (Fig. 28-54), *Rosenthal fibers* represent masses of granular, electron-dense material surrounded by glial filaments (Fig. 28-55). They may be labeled by antisera to alpha B-crystallin and a related 27-kd heat shock protein but are not immunoreactive in GFAP preparations.[350,353] *Eosinophilic granular bodies* are clustered acidophilic globules (Fig. 28-56) that probably derive from lysosomes and are immunoreactive for alpha$_1$-antitrypsin, alpha$_1$-antichymotrypsin, ubiquitin, and alpha B-crystallin.[351,355] At the

ultrastructural level, granular bodies represent membrane-bound collections of amorphous osmiophilic material and myelin-like figures lying within the cytoplasm of tumor cells[351,355] (Fig. 28-57). It is important to note that neither of these cytoplasmic alterations is constant to, or pathognomic of, the pilocytic astrocytoma. Rosenthal fibers, for example, typically abound in the gliotic tissues adjacent to hemangioblastomas and craniopharyngiomas, whereas eosinophilic granular bodies are a conspicuous feature of many gangliogliomas and pleomorphic xanthoastrocytomas, as discussed in the sections dealing with these entities.

The exacting histologic indices by which the diffuse fibrillary astrocytoma's biologic potential is gauged simply cannot be applied to the juvenile pilocytic variant, a neoplasm that is among the most indolent of all central neuroepithelial tumors. Isolated mitotic figures, glomeruloid vascular proliferation, multinucleated giant cell formation, and nuclear atypism (at times alarming, particularly in the tumor's microcystic regions) are divorced, in this setting, from any sinister prognostic import, as is the rather common finding of extension into the subarachnoid space. This is not to deny the existence of lesions meriting the designation of "anaplastic" pilocytic astrocytoma by virtue of their conspicuous mitotic activity, dense cellularity, and foci of coagulative necrosis, but such cases are rare and, in fact, do not necessarily evolve in a clinically malignant manner.[347,348] In a similar vein, an elevated bromodeoxyuridine labeling (proliferative) index—a feature more commonly encountered in pilocytic astrocytomas derived from children—does not appear to be predictive of a poor outcome, the suggestion

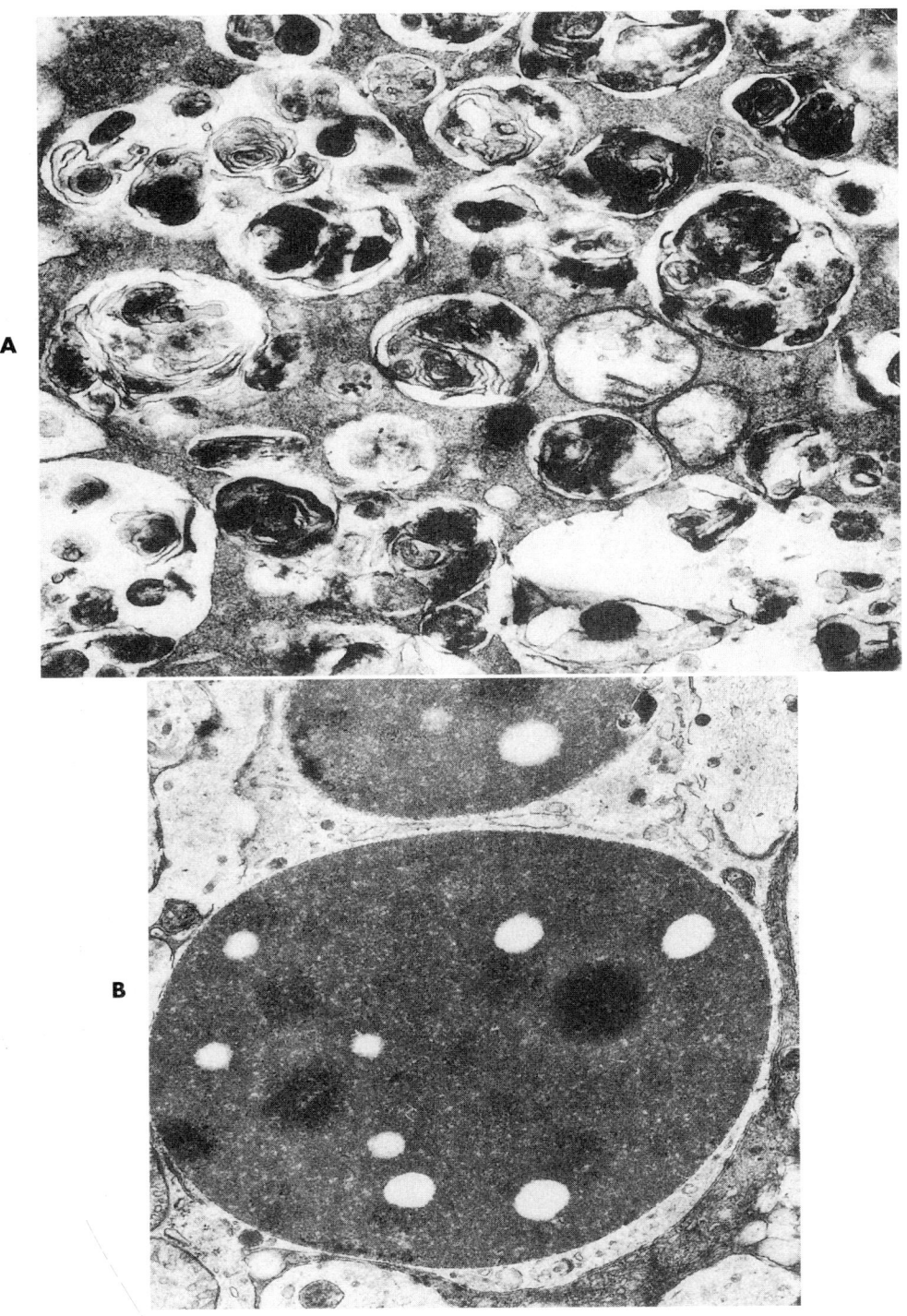

Fig. 28-57 Pilocytic astrocytoma. At the ultrastructural level, eosinophilic globular bodies appear to represent engorged lysosomes containing **(A)** membranous debris ("myelin figures") or amorphous, variably electron-dense material **(B)**. (**A** ×26,500; **B** ×14,200.)

having been offered that the growth rate of these tumors may actually decelerate over time.[349]

Pilocytic astrocytomas confined to the optic nerve and cerebellum lend themselves to curative neurosurgical resection, as do those arising in accessible cerebral hemispheric sites. Well documented is the phenomenon of cure following less-than-total operative ablation of cerebellar examples, but instances of late recurrence (even decades) after their radical removal are also on record.[345,348,356] A less favorable prognosis attaches, understandably, to lesions involving the optic chiasm, hypothalamus, and other regions that preclude concerted neurosurgical attack, but even in these loci the clinical evolution of pilocytic astrocytomas that ultimately prove fatal may be protracted. Irradiation and chemotherapy are reserved for such inaccessible lesions and for the occasional tumor that behaves in an unexpectedly aggressive fashion.[346] Dissemination via the CSF is exceptional[357] despite the fact that pilocytic astrocytomas frequently infiltrate the adjacent subarachnoid space and leptomeninges extensively, and "malignant degeneration" remains the stuff of which case reports are made.[361] Radiotherapy may play a role in promoting the latter development, because nearly all tumors evidencing this biologic progression were subjected to such treatment years prior to recurring in anaplastic and aggressive form. In fact, some of these may have represented independent, radiation-induced glioblastomas. Extracranial spread of opticohypothalamic pilocytic astrocytoma to the abdominal cavity via a ventriculoperitoneal shunt has been described,[357] but is a clinical and pathologic curiosity.

We close this discussion of the pilocytic astrocytoma by emphasizing the importance of segregating this surgically curable neoplasm from the diffuse fibrillary astrocytoma, which may arise in the cerebellum. The latter is typically resistant to all forms of therapy and, with rare exception, progresses inexorably to death within 12 to 18 months of diagnosis. Pilocytic astrocytomas of the cerebellum occasionally consist in part of diffusely permeative elements, but these are noteworthy for their remarkable cytologic uniformity and lack of atypism.[348] The finding of such components, particularly in a pediatric case, should prompt a careful search for piloid or microcystic foci and a review of preoperative neuroimaging studies. The sharp demarcation, largely cystic configuration, and homogeneously contrast-enhancing solid components often evidenced by the pilocytic astrocytoma are generally foreign to astrocytic neoplasms of the diffuse fibrillary variety. Similar neuroradiologic considerations apply above the tentorium (i.e., to cerebral hemispheric lesions), as discussed previously.

Pleomorphic xanthoastrocytoma. The *pleomorphic xanthoastrocytoma*[367] is a histologically alarming, yet relatively indolent, neoplasm that typically presents in adolescence or early adult life as a well-demarcated, superficially positioned, and partially cystic mass situated in the temporal or, less commonly, parieto-occipital region (Fig. 28-58). Infratentorial variants have been described but are clearly exceptional.[364,368] At operation, the lesion may appear to lie largely above the cortical mantle. Evaluation of surgical specimens that permit assessment of the tumor-brain interface generally confirms that much of the xanthoastrocytoma occupies the leptomeninges and subarachnoid space but invariably discloses foci of parenchymal invasion in which neoplastic cells permeate Virchow-Robin spaces and the neuropil proper.

The tumor is named for its often bizarre cytologic characteristics and the tendency of its constituent cells to intracytoplasmic lipid accumulation, although the latter is not a uniformly conspicuous feature. Most examples are composed of spindle-shaped elements in loose fascicular array admixed with tumor giant cells displaying worrisome, even grotesque nuclear abnormalities (Fig. 28-59). Their abundant cytoplasm may appear foamy or coarsely vacuolated—attesting to advanced lipidization—but more commonly assumes a ground-glass or finely granular quality. Reactive lymphoid infiltrates, at times extensive, and aggregated eosinophilic globular bodies representing lysosomes distended by autophagic debris or imbibed proteinaceous material round out the histologic picture. The latter phenomenon is shared by certain other slow-growing neuroepithelial neoplasms, notably the juvenile pilocytic astrocytoma and ganglioglioma, and thus likely reflects a process of gradual cellular degeneration (i.e., senescence). In fact, isolated gangliogliomas composed in part of xanthoastrocytomatous elements have been reported (see section on ganglion cell tumors), and we have encountered cerebral hemispheric astrocytomas of juvenile pilocytic type exhibiting foci of leptomeningeal spread conforming in all respects to the histology of the pleomorphic xanthoastrocytoma in its unalloyed form. Additional features described in select cases have included a cohesive, nesting, or alveolar growth pattern[365] and a hyalinizing, angiomatoid stromal vascular response.[370]

The pathologist unacquainted with the pleomorphic xanthoastrocytoma is likely to mistakenly classify it as an atypical, if not frankly malignant, "fibrohistiocytic" tumor. The sarcomatoid histologic presentation of the lesion is rendered all the more misleading by an intricate pericellular pattern of reticulin deposition in flagrant violation of the neurohistochemical principle that such staining in glial, as opposed to mesodermally derived, neoplasms typically remains confined to the stromal vasculature. This feature actually reflects the elaboration by tumor cells of encircling basal lamina material, demonstrable at the ultrastructural level or by recourse to antisera directed against type IV collagen or laminin,[365] and has been taken, along with the characteristically superficial location of the xanthoastrocytoma, as evidence of its derivation from a class of astrocytes normally situated just beneath the pia-arachnoid and invested by basement membranes that envelop their radially oriented cytoplasmic processes.[367] GFAP expression, a feature mandatory for definitive diagnosis, allies this curious tumor with other astrocytic neoplasms and effectively segregates it from lesions of mesenchymal lineage,[367,368] but otherwise typical examples may contain few immunolabeled cells. Diffuse cytoplasmic immunoreactivity for S-100 protein is the rule and tumor cells may be labeled by antisera to alpha$_1$-antitrypsin, antichymotrypsin, and other "histiocytic" antigens.[368] The latter finding has prompted some to question the existence of the pleomorphic xanthoastrocytoma as an entity distinct from the leptomeningeal fibrous histiocytoma, but such

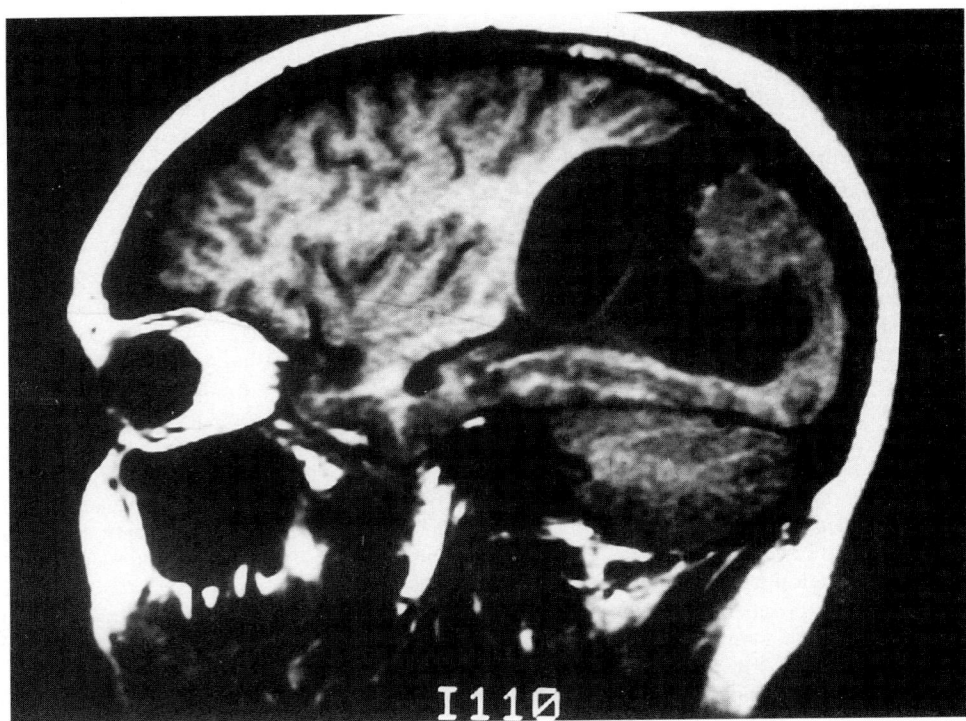

Fig. 28-58 Pleomorphic xanthoastrocytoma. This nonenhanced, parasagittal MRI shows the tendency of this tumor's nodular or plaque-like solid components to be superficially positioned and associated with sizable subjacent cysts.

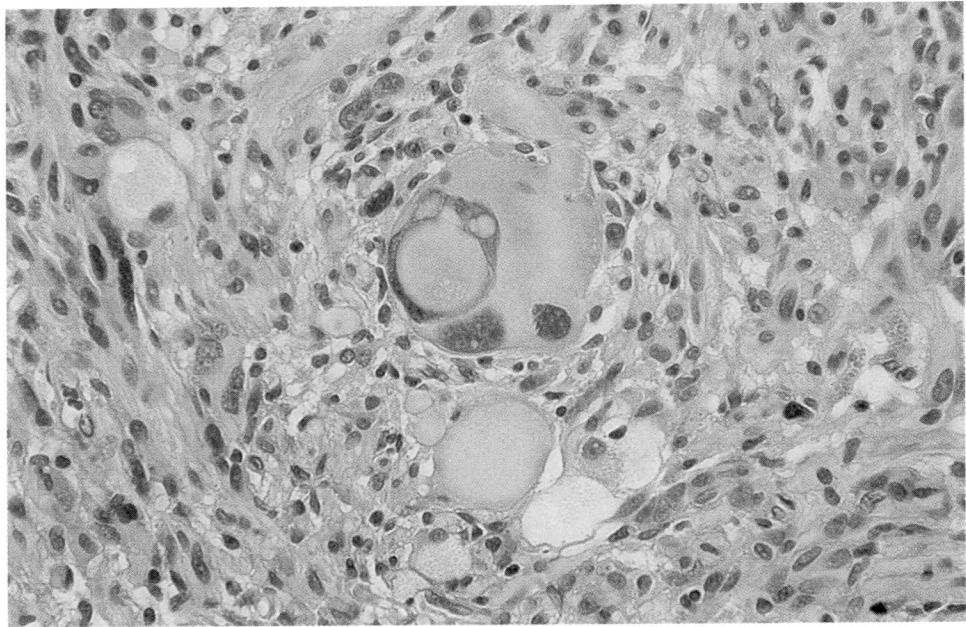

Fig. 28-59 Pleomorphic xanthoastrocytoma. Spindle and giant cells, including bizarre multinucleated forms, combine to give this relatively indolent neoplasm a most disturbing appearance. Note hyaline, granular, and vacuolar cytoplasmic alterations, the last attesting to lipid accumulation.

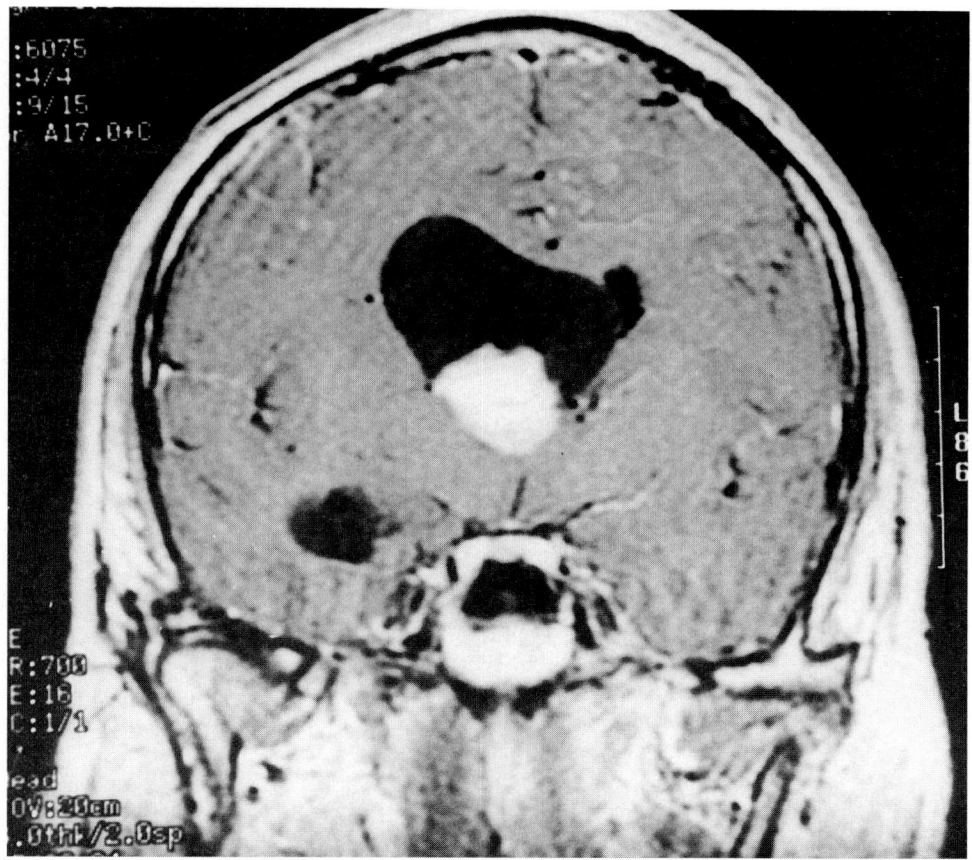

Fig. 28-60 Subependymal giant cell astrocytoma. This postcontrast injection MRI demonstrates the subependymal giant cell astrocytoma's typically intraventricular location near the foramen of Monro (with resulting obstructive hydrocephalus), as well as its characteristic circumscription. This example was not associated with tuberous sclerosis.

reagents decorate a variety of neoplastic (including glial) cell types and thus are of notoriously little discriminatory value in the classification and differential diagnosis of CNS tumors.

Despite their disturbing morphology, most of the pleomorphic xanthoastrocytomas reported to date have exhibited a remarkably benign clinical evolution. Gross total excision is usually feasible and is the treatment of choice. These tumors may recur following resection and can degenerate into full-blown glioblastomas,[366] but this appears to be exceptional. The presence of scattered mitotic figures does not seem to constitute an ominous prognostic sign in this setting, whereas conspicuous proliferative activity, the emergence of an anaplastic small cell component, and foci of coagulative necrosis have been associated with fatal outcomes and imply malignant transformation.[366,369]

Subependymal giant cell astrocytoma (tuberous sclerosis). The *subependymal giant cell astrocytoma* typically presents in the first or second decade of life as an intraventricular mass associated with obstructive hydrocephalus, a consequence of its practically unvarying situation near the foramen of Monro[377] (Fig. 28-60). Although by no means restricted to this setting, it is the intracranial tumor classi-

cally associated with tuberous sclerosis (Bourneville's disease), a disorder transmissible via loci on chromosomes 9 and 16[373] but more often encountered in a nonfamilial form that presumably results from spontaneous mutation. Traditionally defined by the triad of mental retardation, epilepsy, and midfacial angiofibromatosis ("adenoma sebaceum"), this phakomatosis is named for distinctive foci of gyral expansion ("tubers") populated by enlarged, dysmorphic neurons and astrocytes in obvious disarray and possessed of an unusual firmness as a result of extensive glial overgrowth ("sclerosis"). Also characteristic are periventricular "candle gutterings," essentially miniature versions of the tumors under discussion, composed of outsized astrocytes aggregated in a fibrillary matrix prone to calcification. The dominant extracranial manifestations of the tuberous sclerosis complex include renal angiomyolipomas, cardiac rhabdomyomas, pulmonary lymphangioleiomyomatosis, fibrous dysplasia of bone, and various cutaneous lesions (hypopigmented macules, subungual fibromas, and shagreen patches).[374] Some afflicted patients also harbor retinal hamartomas similar to the subependymal nodules just described.

A sharply delineated, spherical, or multinodular mass of fleshy, grayish-pink tissue, the subependymal giant cell astro-

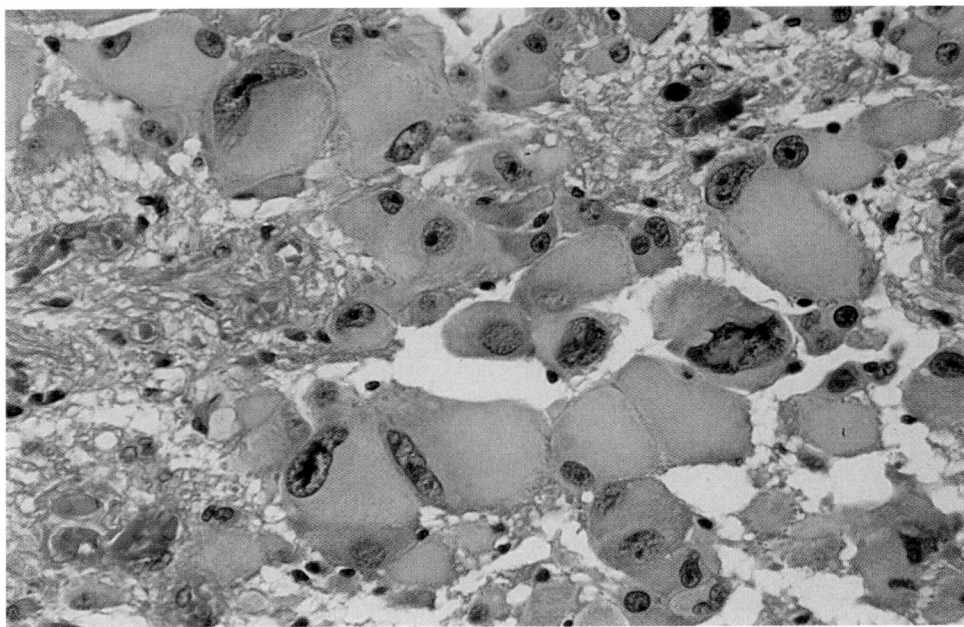

Fig. 28-61 Subependymal giant cell astrocytoma. Tumor cells that achieve truly giant proportions, often polygonal in contour and closely apposed in lobular array, are responsible for this neoplasm's name (but not evident in all cases).

cytoma is typically anchored to the ventricular wall over a broad front. Calcifications are a common feature, and some cases exhibit foci of cystic change. The tumor's constituent cells are large, closely apposed, and characterized by rounded (gemistocyte-like), polygonal (ganglion cell–like), or in some instances, spindly profiles (Fig. 28-61). Only rarely do these actually attain the monstrous proportions of the giant cells observed in high-grade astrocytic neoplasms such as the giant cell glioblastoma. Their eosinophilic cytoplasm often has a glassy or hyaline appearance, and their eccentrically positioned, vesicular nuclei and conspicuous nucleoli distinctly resemble those of large neurons or ganglion cells. An intersecting fibrovascular stroma lends a lobular architecture to many examples, and tumor cell processes often condense about adjacent blood vessels in an ependymoma-like fashion. A curious feature of the lesion is its tendency to contain infiltrating mast cells, often in large numbers. Results of immunocytochemical studies may be disappointing, even misleading, as the subependymal giant cell astrocytoma, its name and suggestive cytology notwithstanding, often contains few GFAP-reactive cells.[371] Furthermore, elements labeled by antibodies to neurofilament proteins may be demonstrated in some cases,[371] and cells harboring dense-core vesicles and forming synapse-like structures have been encountered in isolated examples.[375] These ambiguous features are particularly characteristic of tumors associated with the tuberous sclerosis complex.

Subependymal giant cell astrocytomas enlarge at a remarkably slow rate, are reluctant to invade adjacent cerebral structures, and do not exploit the CSF as a means of escaping their ventricular confines. Cure is often effected by gross total removal, and prolonged survival usually follows

such seemingly inadequate procedures as subtotal resection and ventriculoperitoneal shunting for relief of obstructive hydrocephalus. Although reported cases are few, tumors evidencing mitotic activity and foci of necrosis do not appear to behave in a particularly sinister manner.[372,377] Neoplasms interpreted as overtly malignant giant cell astrocytomas or glioblastomas have been described in the setting of tuberous sclerosis but are clearly exceptional.[376]

Desmoplastic cerebral astrocytoma of infancy. The rare *desmoplastic cerebral astrocytoma of infancy*[378-380] presents in the first year of life with manifestations of increased intracranial pressure that usually include irritability, vomiting, macrocephaly, bulging fontanels, and forced downward deviation of the eyes (the so-called sunset sign). The lesion characteristically possesses a superficially situated and contrast-enhancing nodular or plaque-like frontoparietal component that adheres to the dura mater and is associated with a large, subjacent cyst. The bulk of the tumor is heavily collagenized and dominated by spindle cells in sweeping fascicular, whorled, or storiform arrays that invite its confusion with meningeal fibrous histiocytoma, intracranial fibromatosis, or fibroblastic meningioma (Fig. 28-62). Most examples also contain miniature gemistocyte-like elements and small, embryonal-appearing cells, often mitotically active, arranged about microcystic spaces, or aggregated in densely populous nests (Fig. 28-62). Definitive diagnosis requires the demonstration of GFAP expression, diffuse cytoplasmic reactivity for S-100 protein also being the rule.

At the ultrastructural level, the desmoplastic cerebral astrocytoma's constituent cells, like those of the pleomorphic xanthoastrocytoma, are invested by basal lamina material, a

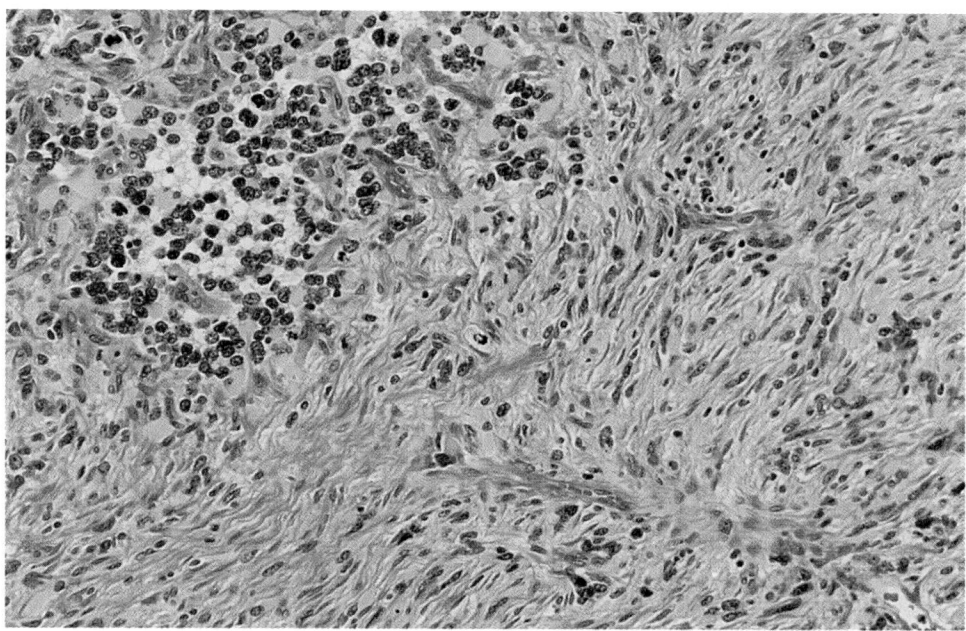

Fig. 28-62 Desmoplastic cerebral astrocytoma of infancy. This distinctive, variably collagenized neoplasm is dominated by spindly astrocytes in fascicular or storiform array but often harbors, as shown here, small, primitive-appearing cells aggregated in micronodules.

finding that has prompted some observers to postulate that it, too, is of subpial astrocytic lineage and possibly a "prelipidized," infantile variant of the latter. By definition this variant is devoid of identifiable neuronal elements, but this peculiar neoplasm bears a striking clinicobiologic and morphologic resemblance to the desmoplastic infantile ganglioglioma (discussed later). The two may be close histogenetic kin or a unified entity. The favorable outcomes of the few cases reported to date suggest that desmoplastic cerebral astrocytomas, whatever their derivation, are indolent tumors despite their disturbingly dense cellularity and evident proliferative activity.

Oligodendroglioma

The oligodendroglioma typically presents in the cerebral hemisphere of a young or middle-aged adult. Characteristic clinical features include a protracted history of intermittent seizures or headache, a frontotemporal or parietal lobe location, and partial calcification on neuroradiologic study.[381,392,397] A minority of oligodendrogliomas afflict children; some observers assert that an excess of pediatric examples arise in the posterior fossa.[396] Only rarely is the spinal cord involved.[386] Cases restricted to leptomeninges have been described.[383a]

On gross inspection, oligodendrogliomas may appear as well-demarcated masses of soft, grayish-pink tissue situated largely in the subcortical white matter, but extension to the overlying cortical ribbon is frequently noted at operation. Cystic changes are common, and the accumulation of a myxoid interstitial matrix lends to many a gelatinous consistency. A vulnerability to artefactual cytoplasmic dissolution accounts for the "classic" oligodendroglioma's histo-

logic presentation as a sheet-like or permeative proliferation of uniform, round nuclei surrounded by optically clear halos (Fig. 28-63, *A*). In select cases, a fusiform spindling of tumor cells may be apparent. A majority of oligodendrogliomas contain scattered calcospherites, and many are subtended by a plexiform, "chicken wire"–like network of thin-walled blood vessels. An additional feature of diagnostic utility is a tendency to pronounced perineuronal aggregation ("satellitosis") on the part of tumor cells infiltrating cortical tissues. Typical of well-differentiated variants is microcystic change, believed by some investigators to connote a favorable prognosis.[381,394] In exceptional instances, tumor cells are segregated into prominent lobules by their fibrovascular stroma or stagger across the microscopic field in rhythmic palisades.

Oligodendrogliomas may contain cells distended by an intracytoplasmic, PAS-positive mucosubstance, "mini-gemistocytes" harboring inclusion-like whorls of GFAP-positive fibrillar material[382,388] (Fig. 28-63, *B*) or eosinophilic granular cells stuffed with autophagic vacuoles[399] or miniature Rosenthal fibers.[390,393] GFAP expression has occasionally been documented in neoplastic oligodendrocytes of clear cell type,[384,388] again evidencing the close cytogenetic kinship between oligodendroglia and astroglia. Some neuropathologists have suggested that the emergence of minigemistocytic elements is a harbinger of biologic aggression in the setting of oligodendroglial neoplasia,[382] but others have been able to demonstrate a particularly poor outcome only for patients whose oligodendrogliomas harbor large gemistocytes of the type found in fibrillary astrocytomas.[391] Neoplastic transformation of a glial progenitor normally programmed to bidirectional maturation along

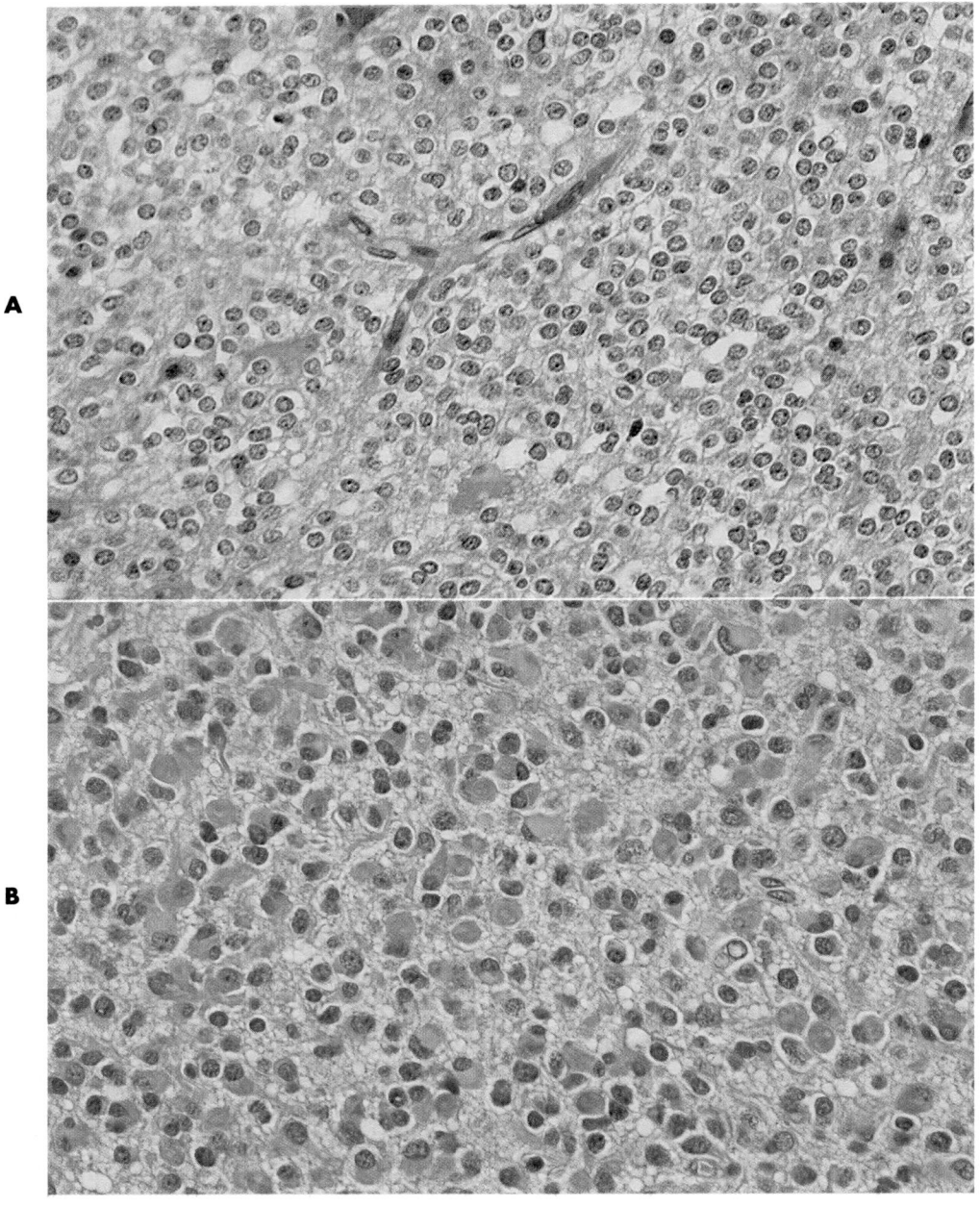

Fig. 28-63 Oligodendroglioma. Uniform, round nuclei and clear perinuclear halos (artefacts of delayed fixation) typify well-differentiated oligodendrogliomas (A). "Minigemistocytic" variants (B) maintain oligodendroglial nuclear features while amassing globose paranuclear expanses of eosinophilic, hyaline or whorling fibrillar cytoplasm. Compare the size of these cells and their nuclear features with those of the gemistocytic astrocytoma depicted at identical magnification in Fig. 28-44.

oligodendrocytic and astrocytic lines may explain the frequency with which oligodendrogliomas evidence astroglial differentiation,[385,389a] as well as the fact that, of all mixed gliomas, those composed exclusively of these two cell types are by far the most common. Noteworthy in this regard is the recent demonstration that oligodendrogliomas and mixed "oligo-astrocytomas" may share allelic losses involving chromosomes 1p and 19q.[389a]

Unfortunately, there exists at present no immunocytochemical reagent that consistently and specifically identifies neoplastic cells as oligodendroglial.[384,395] Membranous Leu7 reactivity is characteristic but not specific.[395] Cytoplasmic galactocerebroside labeling may be of diagnostic utility,[385] but is inconstant. Only rarely do neoplastic oligodendroglia, even when highly differentiated, express carbonic anhydrase C, myelin-associated glycoprotein, or myelin basic protein.[395] Definitive ultrastructural markers are similarly lacking in most instances. Oligodendrogliomas may elaborate cytoplasmic processes arranged in a complex, lamellar fashion reminiscent of myelin sheath formation, but this would appear to be exceptional.[393] Promptly fixed examples usually contain abundant microtubules, free ribosomes, and mitochondria, but no truly unique organellar structures or distinctive inclusions. It is thus what the oligodendroglioma fails to accomplish that is often most useful in its distinction from potential mimickers. Save for the transitional variants alluded to previously, it does not fashion compact intermediate filament bundles as do neoplasms of the astrocytic series, or the zonulae adherentes, microvilli, and cilia of clear cell ependymomas. The central neurocytoma, a neoplasm that may be indistinguishable from the oligodendroglioma at the light microscopic level, is unmasked in like fashion by its synaptic arrays, clear and dense-core vesicles, and frequent expression of synaptophysin. This entity is further considered below along with another lesion that often contains oligodendroglioma-like tissues, the dysembryoplastic neuroepithelial tumor. Proliferations resembling oligodendroglioma have also been described in association with AVMs (see section on cerebrovascular disorders).[116,118]

Numerous studies have addressed the relation of histology to outcome in cases of oligodendroglioma and a variety of schema proposed for their grading.[381,392,394,397] Well-differentiated examples that do not exhibit mitotic activity, nuclear pleomorphism, vascular hyperplasia, or necrosis tend to behave in a relatively indolent fashion. Rarely, however, do these lend themselves to complete excision, and most patients progress inexorably to death following local recurrence, although their course may extend over many years. Conspicuous mitotic activity and foci of coagulative necrosis appear to be especially unfavorable histologic findings predictive of an accelerated clinical course. Tumors exhibiting these features—often accompanied by dense cellularity, nuclear atypism and endothelial hyperplasia—are appropriately designated as **anaplastic oligodendrogliomas.**

Noteworthy is mounting clinical evidence that oligodendroglial neoplasms and mixed oligodendrogliomas-astrocytomas are chemosensitive tumors.[383,387] Whereas irradiation remains the cornerstone of treatment for the patient harboring fibrillary astrocytoma, neuro-oncologists in growing numbers are turning to chemotherapy as the initial approach to aggressive oligodendrogliomas and mixed gliomas composed partly of oligodendroglial elements. Although this does not appear to be as frequent an event in the context of oligodendroglial neoplasia, malignant degeneration of the sort regularly observed in cases of diffuse fibrillary astrocytoma may occur in the initially well-differentiated oligodendroglioma. Recurrent lesions may maintain some cytologic fidelity to their oligodendrocytic lineage or, progressively overgrown by anaplastic astroglial elements, result in a histologic picture indistinguishable from that of the glioblastoma. Gliosarcomatous transformation has also been reported to complicate the evolution of oligodendroglial tumors (see section on gliomesenchymal tumors). Like their fibrillary astrocytic counterparts, oligodendrogliomas kill by virtue of progressive cerebral infiltration following local recurrence. Only a small minority seed the craniospinal leptomeninges after gaining access to the ventricles or subarachnoid space, and extracranial metastasis is vanishingly rare.[389,398]

Ependymal tumors

Ependymomas constitute no more than 5% to 7% of all primary CNS neoplasms, but their prevalence relative to other tumor types varies considerably with patient age and presenting location.[427,433] A majority of intracranial examples arise in childhood, whereas intramedullary lesions usually afflict adults. The incidence of the former peaks in the first decade of life, ependymomas comprising approximately 10% of intracranial neoplasms in the pediatric population and up to 30% of those encountered in children under 3 years of age. At least two thirds of these childhood tumors are situated within the fourth ventricle and consequently present with evidence of increased intracranial pressure secondary to obstructive hydrocephalus.[421,429] Supratentorial lesions are more evenly distributed among children and adults and more likely to be associated with seizure activity and focal motor deficits.[400,410]

Ependymomas of the spinal cord exhibit a decided predilection for the fourth and fifth decades of life, constituting the most common intramedullary neoplasms of adulthood and some 60% to 70% of tumors so situated.[409] Roughly half of all ependymomas originating at spinal levels involve the conus medullaris, filum terminale, or cauda equina.[427] These are typically of myxopapillary type and are considered separately. The principal clinical manifestations of those arising at cervicothoracic levels are pain localized to the neck or back, numbness and paresthesias of the distal extremities, atrophy of the hands, and gait disturbances. An intraspinal location typifies ependymomas complicating "central" von Recklinghausen's disease (type 2 neurofibromatosis). These tend to be multifocal and may be associated with intramedullary ependymal ectopias.[436] Ependymomas may very rarely be confined to cranial nerves.[419] A recent report suggesting that childhood ependymomas and choroid plexus tumors harbor DNA sequences closely related, if not identical, to those of the simian virus 40 (SV-40) is particularly intriguing given the recognized ability of this and other polyoma viruses to induce a similar spectrum of neoplasms in animal hosts.[403]

Wherever situated, ependymomas are characterized by grayish-white coloration, a granular texture and friable con-

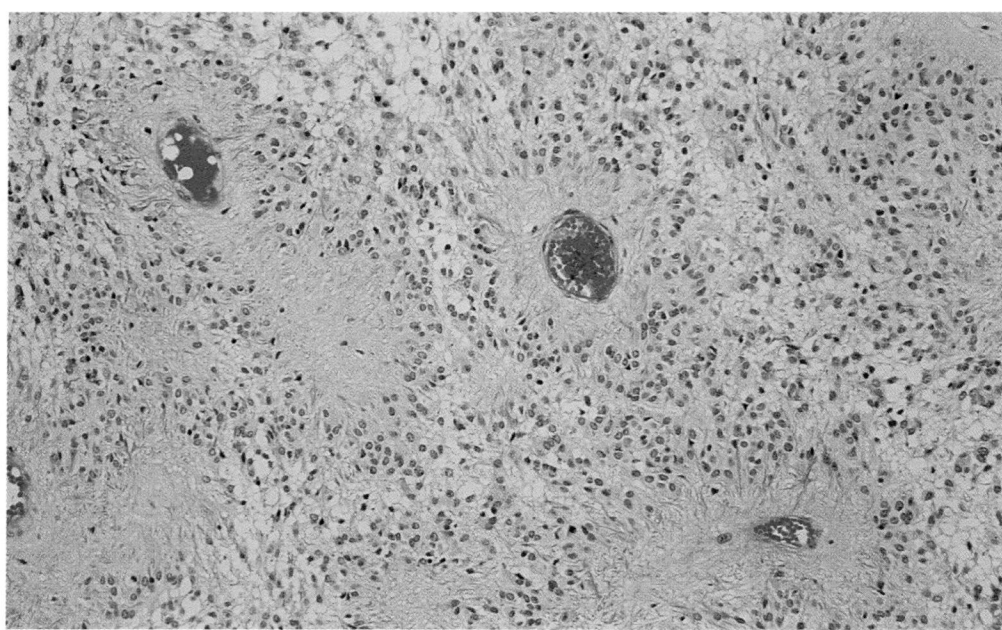

Fig. 28-64 Ependymoma. The cytoplasmic processes of ependymal tumor cells condense about blood vessels to form pseudorosettes.

sistency, lobulated contours, and a remarkable circumscription. Supratentorial examples are often, although not invariably, found to communicate with the ventricular system, lobar types frequently exhibiting cystic change and foci of dense calcification.[400] The latter is also a common feature of posterior fossa lesions evident on neuroradiologic study and useful in their distinction from medulloblastomas, tumors that only exceptionally undergo any appreciable mineralization. Posterior fossa ependymomas tend, furthermore, to be anchored to the floor of the fourth ventricle, whereas medulloblastomas that come to fill this chamber hang from its roof. Designated as "plastic" ependymomas are those examples that exploit CSF exit foramina to escape the restrictive confines of the fourth ventricle and, in so doing, encircle the medulla and rostral cervical spinal cord. Intramedullary variants typically produce a fusiform widening of involved segments and are not uncommonly associated with syrinx formation, cystic dissection of the cord usually progressing rostrally from the tumor's superior pole.[409]

Specific adjectival designations have been extended to the varied histologic presentations of the ependymoma.[412] Most common by far are *cellular* variants typified by the dense meshwork of fibrillary cytoplasmic processes that condense, collar-like, about their stromal blood vessels in formations known as perivascular pseudorosettes (Fig. 28-64). These are accompanied in a minority of cases by canals, tubules, or actual rosettes lined by cells closely resembling normal ependymocytes (Fig. 28-65). Longitudinal nuclear grooving has been emphasized by some observers as a consistent cytologic feature of ependymomas, optimally visualized in touch or crush preparations, that facilitates identification of these tumors at the time of surgery.[405] Dystrophic calcification is a common finding, and some examples undergo

osseous or chondroid metaplasia.[424] Rare melanotic variants have also been depicted.[434]

At the ultrastructural level, cellular ependymomas exhibit a number of specialized cytoplasmic features characteristic of non-neoplastic ependyma.[438] Elaborate, zipper-like junctional complexes (zonulae adherentes) bind their constituent cells and are likely responsible in some measure for the cohesive growth pattern and "pushing" margins typical of such tumors. Prominent arrays of slender, curving microvilli and cilia sprout into the lumina of rosettes or intercellular clefts, again framed by membrane junctions of zonula adherens type (Fig. 28-66). Cilia usually evidence a normal 9 + 2 arrangement of axial doublet complexes but may deviate from this. Their anchoring basal bodies can at times be visualized by light microscopy as abluminal or juxtanuclear cytoplasmic granules and rod-shaped structures ("blepharoplasts") evident in phosphotungstic acid–hematoxylin (PTAH) preparations. Intermediate filaments composed principally of vimentin and GFAP[413,417,425] are additional cytoskeletal elements conspicuous in the cellular processes of ependymal neoplasms.

Although maintaining their ultrastructural fidelity to the ependymal line, a subset of ependymomas exhibit confounding histologic features. ***"Tanycytic" ependymomas*** may be confused with highly fibrillated astrocytomas by virtue of their spindly cytologic features; fascicular growth patterns; and poorly developed, inconspicuous pseudorosettes.[412] Ependymomas commonly contain, in addition to admixed astrocytic elements, cells characterized by perinuclear cytoplasmic clearing. Variants dominated by the latter, ***"clear cell" ependymomas,*** are often misconstrued as oligodendroglial, particularly those containing scattered calcospherules and manifesting a plexiform vascular network.[418] Because

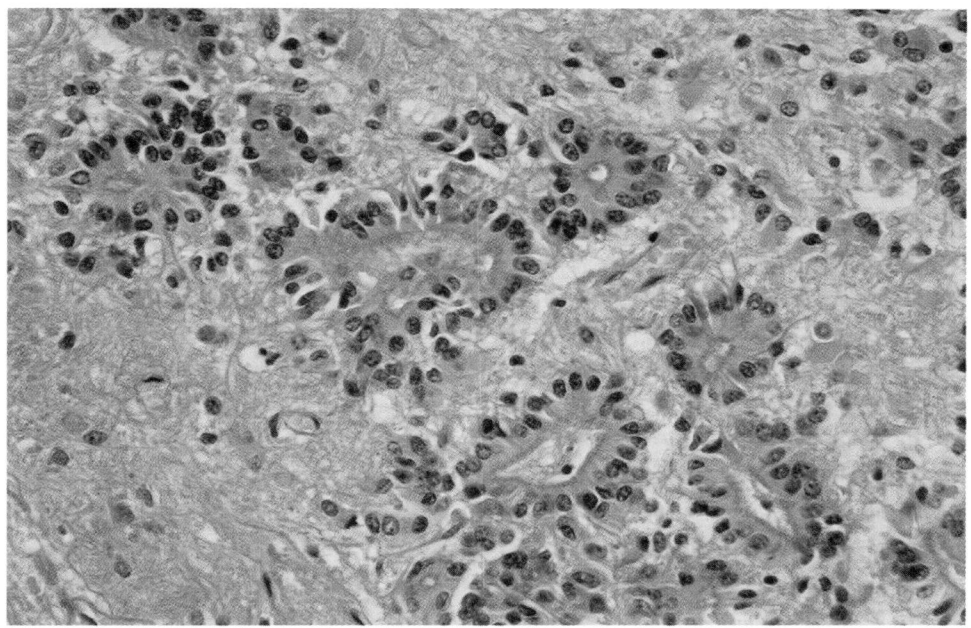

Fig. 28-65 Ependymoma. The true ependymal rosette contains a well-defined central lumen. Clustered ciliary basal bodies ("blepharoplasts") are responsible for the enhanced, granular staining of tumor cell apices.

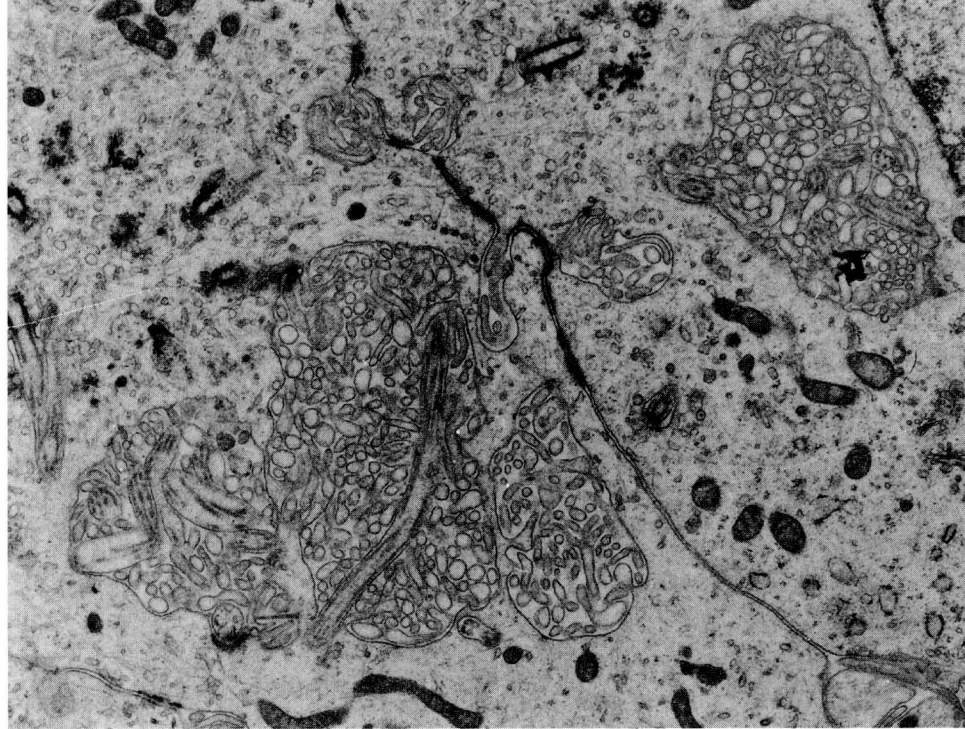

Fig. 28-66 Ependymoma. Features indicative of ependymal differentiation at the ultrastructural level include the joining of tumor cells by grouped junctional complexes and the formation of lumens filled with microvilli and, in lesser number, cilia. (×8800.)

such tumors retain their identifying ependymal features at the electron microscopic level, they are readily segregated from the oligodendroglioma and the central neurocytoma, another neoplasm figuring prominently in the differential diagnosis of supratentorial clear cell tumors, especially those presenting as intraventricular growths (see later discussion). The formation of intracytoplasmic lumina is responsible for signet–ring cell variants of ependymoma.[440]

Finally, rare ependymomas are largely *papillary* in configuration. The distinction of such neoplasms from choroid plexus tumors and metastatic papillary carcinomas has traditionally rested on the fact that their columnar lining elements are supported by a fibrillary glial "stroma" rather than vascularized connective tissue cores. In recent years, immunocytochemical techniques have been applied to this problem.[401,413,417,422,425] Like other ependymomas, papillary variants typically express both vimentin and GFAP, may exhibit labeling for EMA along the apices of their villous and tubular structures, but only exceptionally display cytokeratin reactivity, a consistent feature of choroid plexus neoplasms and metastatic carcinomas. If present at all, cytokeratin-positive cells are typically few in number. Occasional choroid plexus tumors manifest immunoreactivity for GFAP (generally interpreted as evidence of ependymal differentiation), but such foci are usually minor components of these transitional cases. Furthermore, differentiated papillary tumors of the choroid plexus elaborate basement membranes that can be demonstrated by immunocytochemical assay for laminin, a feature generally foreign to intracranial ependymomas.[413] The distinguishing features of the astroblastoma, a papillary tumor closely related to the ependymal series, are discussed later.

That most ependymomas grow slowly is evidenced by their relatively protracted clinical evolution and low proliferative indices in assays employing the in situ bromodeoxyuridine method.[428] Numerous studies, only a representative sample of which are cited here, have sought to define those clinicopathologic variables bearing on the prognosis of patients harboring such tumors.* Location weighs heavily on outcome. Refinements of microsurgical technique, coupled with the accessibility of many intramedullary ependymomas and their clear demarcation from neighboring neural tissues, have rendered feasible the curative resection of these tumors.[409] By contrast, few intracranial ependymomas lend themselves to complete excision, and their long-term prognosis is consequently poor. Whether specific histologic features have an impact on survival separable from considerations of tumor site, extent of resection, and patient age at diagnosis remains controversial. Poorly differentiated tumors exhibiting dense cellularity and conspicuous mitotic activity certainly merit the designation of **anaplastic ependymoma** on morphologic grounds and have proved more aggressive than their low-grade counterparts in some studies, but these histologic findings are not consistently predictive of an accelerated clinical course.[435] Necrosis is a common finding in cellular ependymomas, particularly in those occupying the fourth ventricle, and alone does not brand a lesion as anaplastic. Suffice it to say that the large majority of intracranial

*References 400, 410, 411, 421, 427, 429, 433.

ependymomas ultimately prove fatal, regardless of histologic grade, because of uncontrolled progression at the primary site. Despite their preferential distribution in and around the ventricular system, only a small minority give rise to symptomatic CSF-borne metastases; the utility of histologic assessment in predicting this complication is, again, open to question.[433] Occasional examples infiltrate contiguous cranial and paraspinal tissues, some traveling to distant extraneural sites such as the lymph node, lung, or (via ventriculoperitoneal shunts) abdominal cavity.

The ***myxopapillary ependymoma*** is a morphologically distinctive variant virtually restricted to the region of the conus medullaris and filum terminale, a structure to which it bears certain resemblances at both the light and electron microscopic levels.[439] An origin in cervicothoracic segments of the spinal cord is exceptional and an intracranial presentation exceedingly rare.[423] Typically of myxopapillary type are those unusual extradural ependymomas that arise principally in the subcutaneous tissues overlying the sacrococcyx,[414] less often in the presacral region or sacrum itself.[426] These curious lesions probably originate from extramedullary ependymal rests representing remnants of the extradural filum terminale or coccygeal medullary vestige, a derivative of the caudal neural tube persisting beneath the skin of the postanal pit as an ependyma-lined cleft. Such rests can exhibit myxopapillary features and should not be construed as neoplastic by sole virtue of this growth pattern.[432] We mention here the occurrence of extramedullary ependymomas in the female pelvis[408] and mediastinum,[430] although these are suspected by many observers to represent particularly "lopsided" variants of monodermal teratoma. A primary pulmonary example is also on record.[406]

Myxopapillary lesions share with other intramedullary ependymomas a predilection for the third, fourth, and fifth decades of life, though nearly one fifth of those in the large Mayo Clinic series reported by Sonneland et al.[439] involved patients younger than 20 years of age, some of them children. Nearly all produce low back pain; other common manifestations include sciatica, sensorimotor deficits, urinary and/or fecal incontinence, and impotence. Neuroimaging studies usually demonstrate a sharply delimited lesion of the conus or filum associated with complete blockage to CSF flow on myelography. Surgical exploration typically discloses a highly vascularized, ovoid or sausage-shaped mass that may be invested by a fibrous pseudocapsule derived from the stroma of the filum terminale. Advanced examples can envelop the cauda equina, erode into neighboring bony structures, and infiltrate paraspinal soft tissues. A gelatinous appearance is characteristic on sectioning, and many tumors exhibit hemorrhagic discoloration.

The myxopapillary ependymoma is named for the manner in which its cuboidal cells drape themselves about a basophilic, mucinous material that in turn collars stromal blood vessels and collects in microcystic spaces (Fig. 28-67). Many examples contain, in addition, spindly elements that may engage in the formation of gliovascular pseudorosettes. Present in select cases are eosinophilic spherules ("balloons") possibly representing amalgamated collagen fibrils, myxoid matrix, and basal lamina materials.[439] Degenerative alterations are common and include progres-

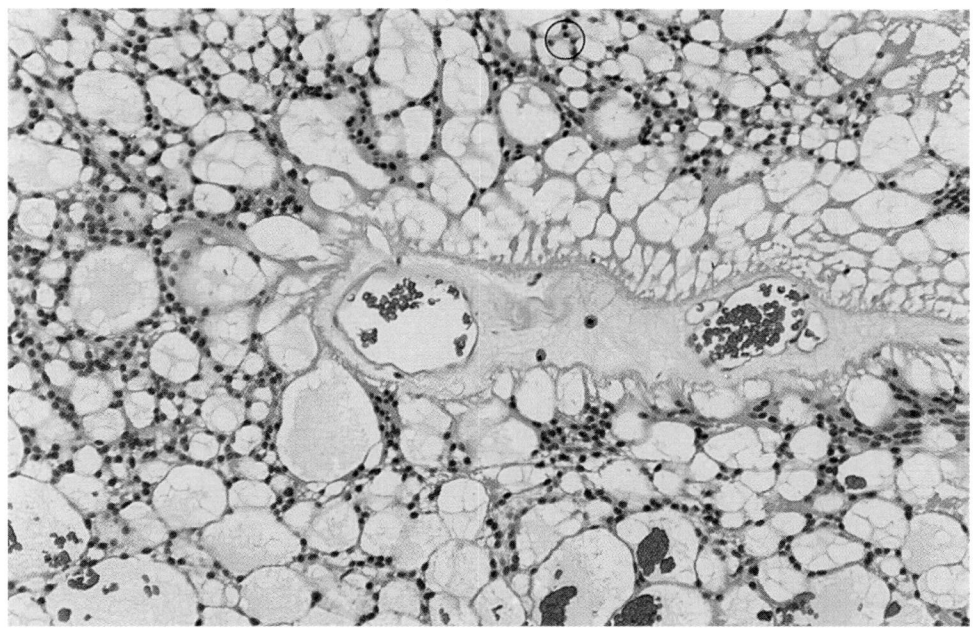

Fig. 28-67 Myxopapillary ependymoma. Note the manner in which mucinous material separates draping tumor cells from a hyalinized vascular core and accumulates in rounded microcysts.

sive collagenization, vascular sclerosis, thrombosis, hemorrhage, and hemosiderin deposition. Long-standing cases are at times characterized by extensive fibrous tissue overgrowth and virtual obliteration of their cellular elements.

The histologic presentation of the myxopapillary ependymoma is in most cases sufficiently distinctive as to render it instantly recognizable to the pathologist familiar with this entity. Particularly myxomatous variants may assume a chordoma-like appearance, whereas examples dominated by spindle-cell elements may be mistaken for schwannomas of spinal nerve root origin. A characteristic immunophenotype and ultrastructure distinguish the myxopapillary ependymoma from these tumors and the rare paragangliomas of the cauda equina region.[404,439] Like other ependymomas, myxopapillary types consistently co-express vimentin and GFAP. They may be labeled by antisera to S-100 protein but do not elaborate cytokeratins, EMA, chromogranin, or carcinoembryonic antigen (CEA).

At the ultrastructural level,[438,439] these tumors possess intermediate filament-laden cytoplasmic processes that interdigitate in complex fashion and are joined by the elaborate junctional complexes typical of ependymal neoplasms in general. Cilia and microvilli further attest to their ependymal lineage, although these are not displayed as conspicuously by myxopapillary ependymomas compared with cellular ependymomas. The consistent elaboration of basal lamina material, often investing cells as a continuous basement membrane, generally distinguishes myxopapillary lesions from other ependymomas, whereas the presence of microtubular aggregates within cisternae of the rough endoplasmic reticulum has been proposed as an ultrastructural

marker shared by no other primary neoplasms of the spinal cord or brain.[416]

The myxopapillary ependymoma is an indolent tumor amenable in many cases to surgical cure. Five of seventy-seven (6.5%) afflicted patients described in the Mayo Clinic series[439] ultimately died of their disease but only following repeated local recurrences over periods ranging from 12 to 15 years. The presence of cytologic atypism and modest mitotic activity did not alter the prognosis in this study, but lesions whose gross features permitted only subtotal resection clearly recurred and progressed more frequently than tumors lending themselves to complete removal. The need for prolonged postoperative surveillance is underscored by the fact that 15% of patients experienced late recurrences that became manifest an average of 5.8 years following gross total resection. Myxopapillary ependymomas occasionally spread to higher levels of the central neuraxis via the CSF, and isolated examples metastasize to the lung, liver, bone, and lymph node.[407] The latter phenomenon typically complicates stubbornly recurring tumors that have gained access to extravertebral soft tissues. Extradural primary tumors presenting in the sacrococcygeal region are associated with a substantially increased risk of such dissemination.[414,426]

While recognizing its commitment to an ependymal phenotype and proper position among tumors of this series, we defer consideration of the ependymoblastoma to our discussion of primitive neuroepithelial neoplasms and conclude this section with a brief account of the *subependymoma,* a distinctive lesion named for the resemblance of its constituent cells to, and proposed origin from, the subepend-

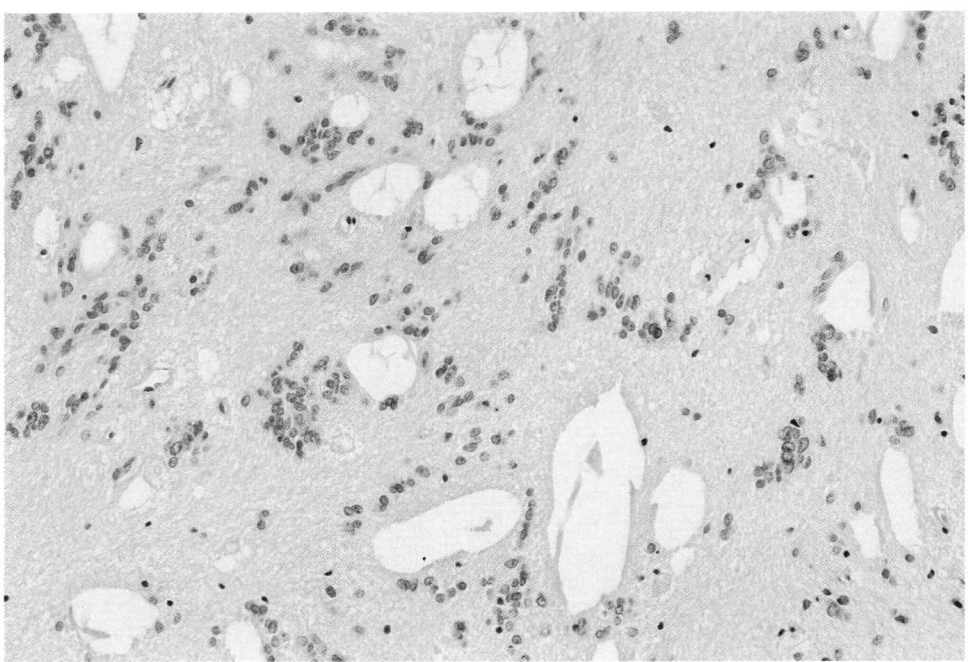

Fig. 28-68 Subependymoma. Characteristic of this entity is the huddling of small tumor cells in an expansive fibrillar meshwork. Microcystic changes commonly round out the histologic picture.

mal neuroglia distributed along the ventricular system. The large majority of these tumors are confined to the fourth ventricle, typically arising from its floor, and are diminutive lesions incidentally discovered at autopsy of older men, but occasional examples attain obstructing proportions.[420] More likely to achieve symptomatic size are subependymomas situated in the lateral ventricles, particularly those originating about the foramen of Monro or from the septum pellucidum. Only rarely do subependymomas present in the third ventricle or cerebral aqueduct. Similarly exceptional are extraventricular examples arising at spinal cord levels.[431] Multifocal variants may arise in association with conditions producing long-standing obstructive hydrocephalus. This, and the histologic resemblance of subependymomas to the ependymal granulations characteristic of processes associated with protracted irritation of the ventricular surfaces, have been taken as evidence that these tumors may have a reactive etiology. Noteworthy in this regard is the report of a third ventricular example developing adjacent to a craniopharyngioma, a tumor that consistently provokes an intense proliferative glial reaction.[415] As pointed out by the authors, local irradiation may also have played a critical role in the genesis of this unique lesion. Rare cases of familial subependymoma are found in the literature.[437]

Although some symptomatic examples have been described as infiltrating adjacent neural parenchyma, subependymomas are typically noninvasive and characterized by well-defined, lobulated contours. Those encountered at autopsy are solid nodules composed of tough white tissue, whereas larger lesions often exhibit cystic change and foci of hemorrhagic discoloration. Many cases display calcification, at times extensive. Histologic examination characteristically

discloses small aggregates of tumor cells haphazardly disposed in a hypovascular fibrillary meshwork that may be densely compacted or evidence spongy rarefaction (Fig. 28-68). Their uniform nuclei tend to have delicate oval contours and a punctate chromatin distribution reminiscent of the cellular ependymoma. These cells may contain blepharoplasts, may occasionally fashion small rosettes, and can be shown to elaborate the zonulae adherentes, ciliary, and microvillous arrays typical of ependymal neoplasms.[402] That they are allied with this series is further suggested by the occurrence of hybrid or transitional variants composed in part of conventional ependymoma.[420] These evidences of ependymal differentiation notwithstanding, many subependymomas contain recognizably astrocytic elements of fibrillary or even gemistocytic type (as well as transitional forms exhibiting features of both cell lines) that have fueled the controversy surrounding their precise cytogenesis. We would emphasize the fact that some of these benign neoplasms exhibit potentially alarming nuclear atypism, modest mitotic activity, and small foci of coagulative necrosis devoid of marginal palisading.[420] These findings are not predictive of an aggressive course. A melanotic example has been depicted,[434] as has a case containing sarcomatous elements interpreted as deriving from the tumor's stromal vasculature (see section on gliomesenchymal tumors).

Astroblastoma

The rare glial neoplasm known as ***astroblastoma*** usually presents as a well-demarcated, cerebral hemispheric mass in a child, adolescent, or young adult.[441] The frontoparietal region is favored. The lesion is characterized by a papilliform architecture, its radially arranged cellular elements

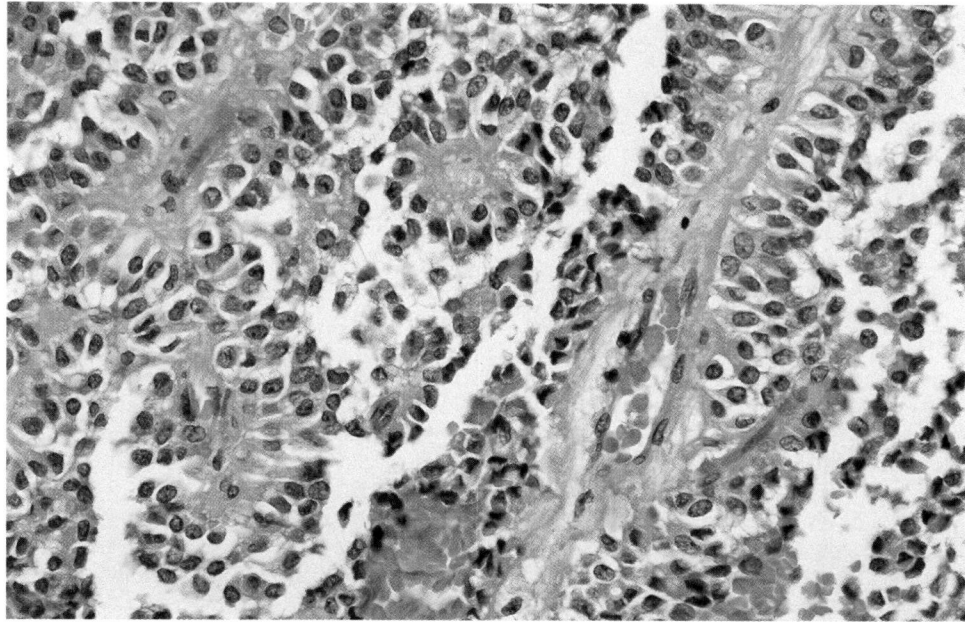

Fig. 28-69 Astroblastoma. The stout cytoplasmic processes of this papillary neoplasm's constituent cells taper rapidly toward supporting vascular cores.

directing unipolar cytoplasmic processes in "cartwheel" fashion toward centrally placed stromal blood vessels (Fig. 28-69). The latter are prone to progressive collagenous thickening and hyalinization, a striking feature of most cases that may advance, in long-standing examples, to partial fibrous obliteration of the neoplastic tissue. In contrast to the ependymoma's perivascular pseudorosettes, which generally lie embedded in a dense fibrillar matrix, the astroblastoma's gliovascular structures are only tenuously supported by an intervening population of astrocytic-appearing tumor cells and often appear to float unanchored in tissue sections.

Astroblastomatous cell processes are shorter and stouter than those of ependymocytes and differ further in terminating on their target vessels as expanded footplates. The lesion's more constant ultrastructural attributes include a rich cytoplasmic complement of intermediate filaments and glycogen, intercellular junctional complexes (these may be well developed but usually fall short of the ependymoma's elaborate zonulae adherentes), and an investing basal lamina separating polar processes from adjoining stroma vessels.[442-444] Noteworthy in regard to the astroblastoma's cytogenesis is the observation that its component cells may display certain ultrastructural features characteristic of tanycytes, ependymal-lining elements that normally extend basal cytoplasmic processes toward regional capillaries.[444] These include, in addition to the basal lamina deposition just mentioned, "purse-string" microvillous arrays atop tumor cells and lamellar cytoplasmic interdigitations ("pleats") along their lateral edges. On immunohistochemical assay, cytoplasmic vimentin reactivity is the rule, whereas GFAP expression, apparently subject to considerable variation, may be faint, only focally evident, or not demonstrable.[441-444] Cyto-

plasmic labeling for S-100 protein, cytokeratins, and EMA has also been depicted.[443]

Inasmuch as diffuse fibrillary astrocytomas, particularly those of the gemistocytic variety, may focally evidence gliovascular formations comparable to those of the astroblastoma, the latter designation should be reserved for tumors with a pure, or at least dominant, papillary architecture of the type described. These may be further divided into prognostically favorable and unfavorable variants, although the correlation of histology and outcome is, admittedly, imperfect.[441] Tumors characterized by an orderly growth pattern and little in the way of mitotic activity have been associated with protracted disease-free survival following resection and varied forms of irradiation and chemotherapy. Examples manifesting conspicuous mitotic activity, vascular hyperplasia, and large zones of coagulative necrosis ("anaplastic astroblastomas") often evidence histologic transition to infiltrating, high-grade astrocytoma of conventional type and can rapidly eventuate in the picture of glioblastoma. That this aggressive-looking variant may yet retain the circumscription typical of its well-differentiated counterpart, rendering operative extirpation feasible, probably accounts for instances of long-term survival in this setting.[441]

Mixed gliomas

Although there can be no disclaiming the presence within many gliomas of elements suggesting differentiation along more than a single cell line, the point at which this phenomenon merits recognition in the reporting of neurosurgical specimens remains very much a matter of subjective interpretation and personal prejudice. Some observers insist that a candidate's constituent populations be regionally segregated, as well as cytologically distinct, or that dissimilar cell types, when closely intermingled, be represented in roughly equivalent proportion if the status of mixed glioma is to be granted. The most common variant, in either guise, is the *mixed oligodendroglioma-astrocytoma* or *"oligoastrocytoma."*[301,445,446] That this tumor is closely allied to the pure oligodendroglioma is suggested by recent observations that it shares with the latter allelic losses involving chromosomes 1p and 19q.[389a] We agree that this diagnosis should be reserved for the tumor harboring neoplastic astrocytes that exhibit the cytologic features expected of the conventional fibrillary astrocytoma. Oligodendrogliomas composed in part of GFAP-positive, "minigemistocytic" elements retaining the oligodendrocyte's rounded nuclear profile and compacted chromatin do not qualify.[301,446] In a similar vein, oligodendroglioma-like regions are not infrequently encountered in pilocytic astrocytomas but, in this setting, are considered part of the diagnosis.

Oligoastrocytomas are largely supratentorial tumors of adulthood that favor the frontoparietal and temporal regions. They may be divided into low-grade (i.e., well-differentiated) and anaplastic variants, the latter characterized by dense cellularity, conspicuous pleomorphism, mitotic activity, and in some cases, vascular hyperplasia and coagulative necrosis. In light of recent observations suggesting that at least some of these mixed neoplasms share the chemosensitivity of the pure oligodendroglioma,[387] we think it important that the presence of even a minor oligodendroglial component within an otherwise astrocytic tumor be "captured" in the surgical pathology report and so apply the label oligoastrocytoma rather liberally. More common, in fact, than clearly biphasic lesions are hybrids populated by elements that resist rigid classification as either oligodendrocytes or astroglia. The optimal approach to these transitional neoplasms, which we descriptively term *gliomas with astrocytic and oligodendroglial features,* remains to be clarified.

As previously discussed, clear cell components histologically identical to oligodendroglioma may be found within otherwise conventional ependymomas, particularly supratentorial examples. The demonstration that these elements retain ependymocytic features at the ultrastructural level calls into question descriptions of mixed oligodendroglial and ependymal tumors.[445] In fact, we have not encountered a glioma that could be proved to differentiate along divergent, oligoependymal lines. With regard to other forms of mixed glial neoplasia, we have, on rare occasion, resorted halfheartedly to the diagnosis of ependymoastrocytoma for tumors of predominantly astrocytic character exhibiting foci of conspicuous pseudorosette formation. The neoplastic cells forming such gliovascular structures, however, typically retain astrocytic nuclear features and elaborate cytoplasmic processes considerably coarser than those of the classic cellular ependymoma. These invasive lesions are probably best approached as variants of diffuse fibrillary astrocytoma. The diagnosis of ependymoastrocytoma should not be extended to the common fourth ventricular ependymoma harboring a minor astrocytic component.

Gliomatosis cerebri

The brain of a patient treated for an aggressive fibrillary astrocytoma will commonly exhibit, at autopsy, diffuse invasion of structures adjoining the primary tumor bed, as well as subtle infiltration of neuropil at a considerable distance from what is grossly evident recurrent disease.

Gliomatosis cerebri, by contrast, is a rare condition in which large portions of the brain are found to be diffusely permeated by tumor cells in such a manner as to suggest a neoplastic "field effect," rather than centrifugal expansion of a pre-existent glioblastoma or another anaplastic glioma.[447-449] Affected regions are typically expanded in "pseudohypertrophic" fashion, their internal architectural markings obscured without formation of recognizable tumor nodules. The process may be remarkably diffuse, involving, ab initio, both cerebral hemispheres, deep gray matter, the brainstem, and even the spinal cord. The diagnosis was at one time restricted to cases examined at autopsy, but is now rendered clinically when biopsy material from a patient with widespread neuroradiologic abnormalities discloses a diffusely infiltrating glioma, usually a fibrillary astrocytoma.

It should be stressed that gliomatosis cerebri is neither a unified cytogenetic entity nor a condition that can be diagnosed on cytologic or histologic grounds alone. Whereas most examples exhibit astrocytic features, neoplastic oligodendroglia may participate in this process, and pure oligodendrogliomatosis has been described.[448] Although unusually elongated nuclear profiles and a tendency to pronounced subpial, perivascular, and circumneuronal cellular aggregation are often emphasized as especially characteristic, these are by no means specific or even constant morphologic features. Gliomatosis cerebri may pursue a protracted clinical course, particularly if the neoplastic infiltrate is of low histologic grade, but is a uniformly fatal disease. Focal or multicentric progression to anaplastic astrocytoma or glioblastoma is encountered in the evolution of some examples.

Gliomesenchymal tumors

This section discusses a variety of unusual tumors characterized by their "mixed" neuroepithelial (specifically glial) and mesenchymal features. The most common of these peculiar neoplasms is the *gliosarcoma,* widely regarded as a variant of glioblastoma multiforme in which mesodermal elements associated with the latter's hyperplastic vasculature secondarily undergo neoplastic transformation.[453] Sarcomatous change has been estimated to occur in some 2%[462] to 8%[464] of glioblastomas. The designation of *sarcoglioma* has been extended to exceedingly rare malignant gliomesenchymal tumors for which the reverse of the foregoing scenario is postulated (i.e., intracranial sarcomas and meningiomas complicated by the progression to neoplasia of commingled, reactive astrocytic elements).[460,463]

The clinical profile of the gliosarcoma is essentially that of the pure glioblastoma, although some observers have noted a distinct predilection for the temporal lobe and a higher incidence of extracranial dissemination on the part of the former.[464] Most tumors arise in the absence of recognized predisposing factors, but isolated examples have been associated with the intracranial instillation of Thorotrast.[467,471] At operation, many are initially mistaken for cerebral metastases or, when attached to the dura, are mistaken for meningiomas, the errors resulting from their characteristic circumscription and firm textures. These attributes in turn reflect the high content of connective tissue fibers typical of the

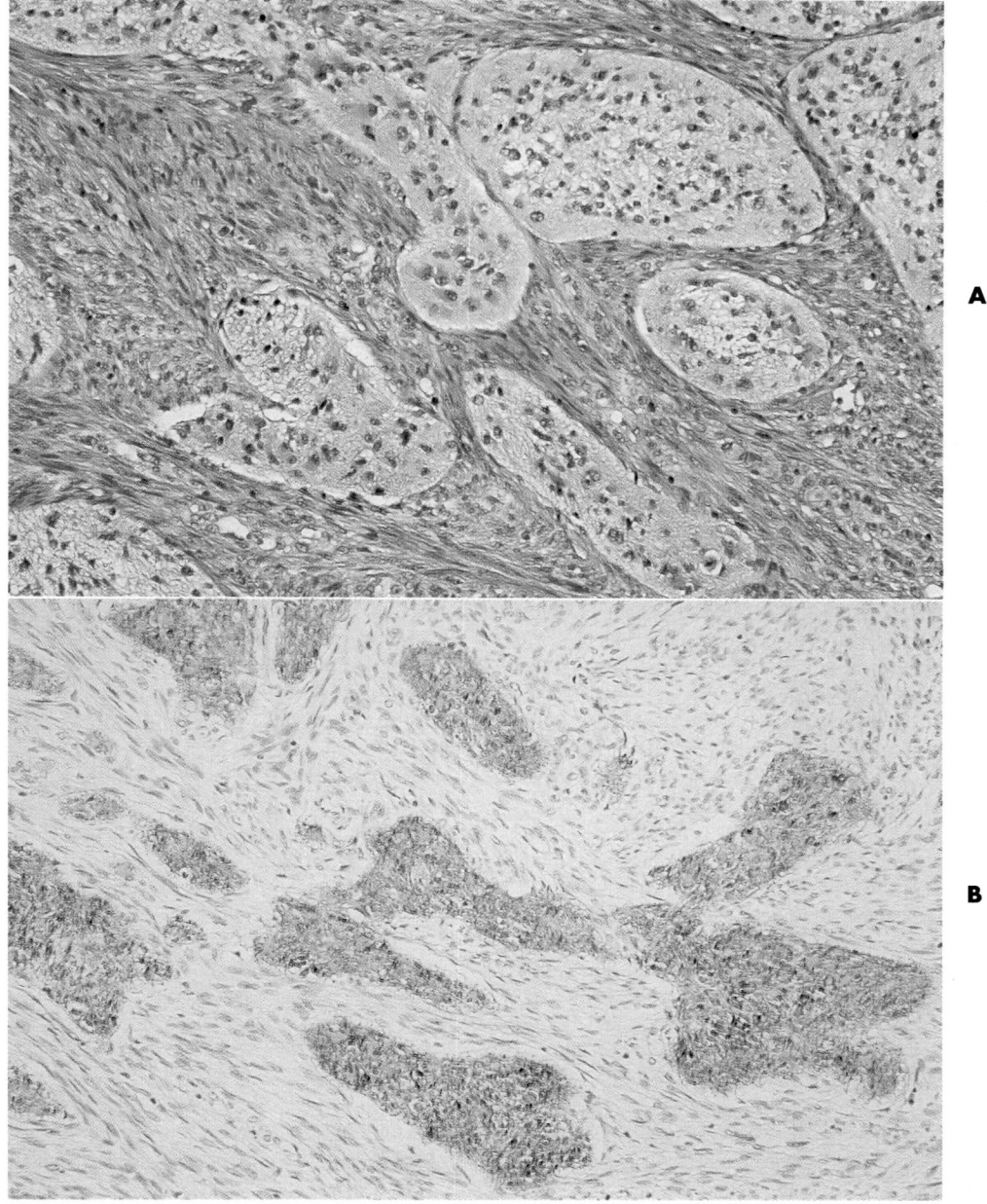

Fig. 28-70 Gliosarcoma. Islands of astrocytic tumor tissue lie embedded in what otherwise appears to be a spindle-cell sarcoma (A). On immunoperoxidase assay (B), only astrocytic elements are labeled for glial fibrillary acidic protein.

gliosarcoma but foreign to most other neuroepithelial neoplasms. A marmoreal admixture of gliomatous and sarcomatous tissues lends to these tumors a strikingly biphasic architecture on histologic study (Fig. 28-70, A). The former are nearly always astrocytic and overtly high grade, most exhibiting the features of full-blown glioblastoma, although examples derived from oligodendrogliomas[465] and subependymomas[461] are on record. Gland-like or "adenoid" formations and squamous metaplasia may be observed in the glial por-

tions of select cases.[315,328] The tumor's mesenchymal components usually evidence appearances that would prompt the diagnosis of fibrosarcoma or malignant fibrous histiocytoma in a soft tissue setting. A subset contain chondro-osseous,[457] muscle,[450,456] or mixed mesenchymal[466] elements and differentiation along endothelial lines has also been described.[469] A unique example of multifocal intramedullary "astrolipoma" composed of low-grade astroglial and well-differentiated adipocytic elements has also been recorded.[467a]

Distinction of the gliosarcoma's neuroepithelial and mesenchymal constituents can be accomplished using a combination of traditional histochemical and immunocytochemical techniques.[453,455,462,464,469] The latter are richly invested with connective tissue fibers demonstrable by reticulin impregnation methods and preparations for collagen, such as the Mallory trichrome stain, but do not express GFAP, the reverse being true of the tumor's glial component (Fig. 28-70, B). The identification of an architecturally and cytologically distinct, GFAP-negative component is requisite to the segregation of the true gliosarcoma from collagenized, sarcomatous-appearing glioblastomas and gliomas associated with a florid fibroblastic reaction by virtue of meningeal invasion. We agree that "desmoplastic" or "metaplastic" glioblastomas—tumors in which glial cells appear responsible for connective tissue formation[452]—should also be separated from the ranks of the gliosarcomas.[453] Similar considerations apply to rare variants of astrocytoma and ependymoma that give rise to GFAP-immunoreactive, cartilaginous elements.[459]

As previously discussed in the context of fibrillary astrocytic neoplasms, the florid vascular hyperplasia characteristic of glioblastomas is a process driven by the tumoral elaboration of mitogens that act not only on endothelium, but also on pericytes, smooth muscle cells, and fibroblasts. The "glomeruloid" stromal formations typical of such tumors appear, in fact, to be dominated by pericytic/myoid elements that express alpha-smooth muscle actin.[309,340a] That this phenomenon eventuates in the sarcomatous components of these tumors—a notion based on perceived histologic transitions from the hyperplastic to the unarguably malignant—has recently received support from the demonstration that neoplastic cells with a comparable immunophenotype populate some gliosarcomas.[456] Like others,[455] we have been largely unable to reproduce reports that the latter harbor tumor cells labeling with antisera to factor VIII R-Ag and the lectin UEA-1 or containing Weibel-Palade bodies on ultrastructural study,[469] but the possibility that at least some of these neoplasms are composed of "dedifferentiated" endothelial elements is obviously impossible to exclude. Also championed as progenitors of the gliosarcoma's mesenchymal compartment are perivascular histiocytes, fibroblasts, myofibroblasts, or other, uncommitted stromal cells in the vascular adventitia.[453] Some observers have taken the position that gliosarcomas are simply "metaplastic" glioblastomas (i.e., derived solely from glial cell types that secondarily adopt mesodermal profiles).[458] We are not inclined to this reductive view.

The designation *"gliofibroma"* has been extended to a somewhat heterogeneous group of neoplasms encountered for the most part in childhood and having in common a population of astrocytes invested by basal lamina material and embedded in a variably collagenized matrix.[453] Some appear to represent desmoplastic astrocytomas in which neoplastic glia, unaided by mesenchymal derivatives, are directly responsible for the elaboration of connective tissues, whereas other examples contain a second cellular population variously interpreted as fibroblastic or schwannian.[468,470] The rarity and disparate morphologic features of the tumors reported under this rubric obviously preclude useful generalizations

regarding their histogenesis and clinical biology. A number of recorded cases have evidenced conspicuous cytologic atypism and mitotic activity, pursuing an aggressive course (with CSF-borne metastasis) and ending fatally, the benign connotations of the term gliofibroma notwithstanding.[453] A more favorable outcome seems to be attached to those lacking features of histologic anaplasia.

This discussion of gliomesenchymal tumors is concluded with passing reference to the various uses of the term *"angioglioma."* Originally applied to what would now be classified as the cellular variant of cerebellar hemangioblastoma, this designation has been most frequently invoked in reference to gliomas exhibiting degenerative alterations of their vasculature resembling AVMs or cavernous angiomas.[116] Slow-growing lesions such as pilocytic astrocytomas and oligodendrogliomas seem especially prone to such changes. These lesions may appear hypervascular on angiographic study, exhibiting a tumoral "blush," but as a rule do not evidence the shunting characteristic of true AVMs. Only exceptionally are the latter found in contiguity with glial neoplasms. Most such lesions are regarded as "collision" tumors in which gliomatous and malformative tissues are fortuitously associated, but isolated reports of glial neoplasms secondarily arising at the sites of pre-existent AVMs and angiomas suggest that the gliotic reaction typical of tissues surrounding such long-standing vascular anomalies may rarely progress to neoplasia.[454] A strikingly increased concentration of oligodendrocytes in and around some AVMs appears to result from "collapse" of chronically edematous and ischemic white matter or to represent part of the malformation process and should not prompt a diagnosis of oligodendroglioma.[116,118] Finally, we call attention to a group of exceedingly uncommon "mixed" tumors composed of gliomatous and hemangioblastomatous elements.[451] These, too, have been described as a form of "angioglioma," a nonspecific and potentially misleading term that is probably best abandoned.

Choroid plexus tumors

A secretory organ responsible for the production of CSF, the choroid plexus consists of a richly vascularized fibrous stroma draped by an epithelium that derives from neuroectodermal cells abutting the embryonic ventricular system. Only rarely do its specialized epithelial elements give rise to neoplasms. Most of these uncommon tumors present sporadically and affect otherwise healthy subjects, particularly children, but examples have been reported in siblings[477] and as components of the Li-Fraumeni[481] and Aicardi[494] syndromes. *Li-Fraumeni syndrome,* transmitted in autosomal dominant fashion and linked to germ line mutations of the p53 tumor suppressor gene, is a complex of multiple familial cancers, chief among which are carcinomas of the breast and adrenal cortex, sarcomas of bone and soft tissue, leukemias, and various central neuroepithelial neoplasms. Major manifestations of the *Aicardi syndrome* include infantile flexor spasms, agenesis of the corpus callosum, and chorioretinal anomalies. Noteworthy is the recent demonstration that human choroid plexus tumors, like ependymomas, may harbor DNA sequences similar to those of SV-40,[403] since expression of this agent's T antigen in transgenic mice is

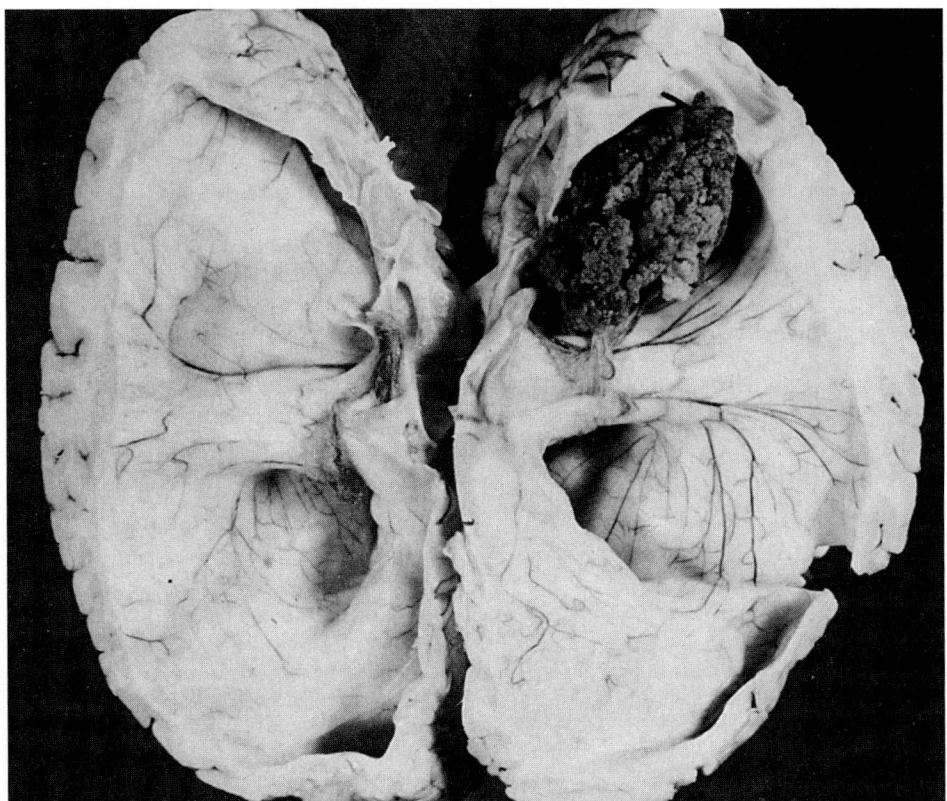

Fig. 28-71 Choroid plexus papilloma. Advanced hydrocephalus is associated with this typically bosselated example lying in the lateral ventricle of an infant.

specifically associated with the induction of choroid plexus neoplasms.

Tumors derived from the epithelium of the choroid plexus exhibit considerable morphologic and biologic diversity. The great majority, however, are benign neoplasms that replicate the parent organ's villous architecture and are consequently termed *choroid plexus papillomas.* Most of the latter come to attention during early childhood, displaying a predilection for the lateral ventricles of young boys.[480,490] Adult cases, by contrast, are situated more often in the fourth ventricle or its lateral recesses, some presenting as tumors of the cerebellopontine angle.[490] Associated clinical manifestations are largely those of hydrocephalus resulting from ventricular outflow obstruction or the excessive production of CSF by these highly differentiated neoplasms. Rarely, congenital plexus–related hydrocephalus is caused by villous hypertrophy of this organ.[486]

On gross inspection, the choroid plexus papilloma is a globose mass of friable reddish-brown tissue having a bosselated surface often likened to that of a cauliflower (Fig. 28-71). Calcification, common to these tumors, imparts to some a gritty consistency or, when extensive, stony hardness that may hinder sectioning in the undecalcified state. Histologic examination typically discloses a complex array of branching fibrovascular fronds covered by a monolayer of uniform cuboidal or columnar epithelial cells exhibiting minimal nuclear atypism or mitotic activity (Fig. 28-72). On ultrastructural study these cells rest on an uninterrupted basement membrane, are joined at their apices by elaborate junctional complexes, are crowned by microvilli, and occasionally, are ciliated.[488] The tumoral stroma, like that of the normal choroid plexus, may be conspicuously infiltrated by foamy macrophages and is, in select cases, the site of metaplastic bone or cartilage formation.[495] The epithelial elements of some tumors undergo oncocytic change,[475,478] and a rare melanotic variant of the choroid plexus papilloma has also been reported.[493] These neoplasms may, in addition, evidence limited ependymal differentiation, signaled by foci in which tumor cells extend tapering, GFAP-immunoreactive cytoplasmic processes toward their fibrovascular cores.[475] This finding presumably reflects the ontogeny of the plexus epithelium as a form of specialized ependyma, but choroid plexus papillomas do not elaborate the fibrillary glial "stroma" characteristic of ependymomas, including those of papillary type, an important differential diagnostic feature. Exceptional cases exhibit a glandular, rather than papillary, growth pattern—an arrangement for which the designations of acinar or tubular choroid plexus adenoma have been invoked.[473,479,487] Several of these curious variants have been mucin-producing.

The well-differentiated choroid plexus papilloma is a noninvasive growth that is often amenable to curative resec-

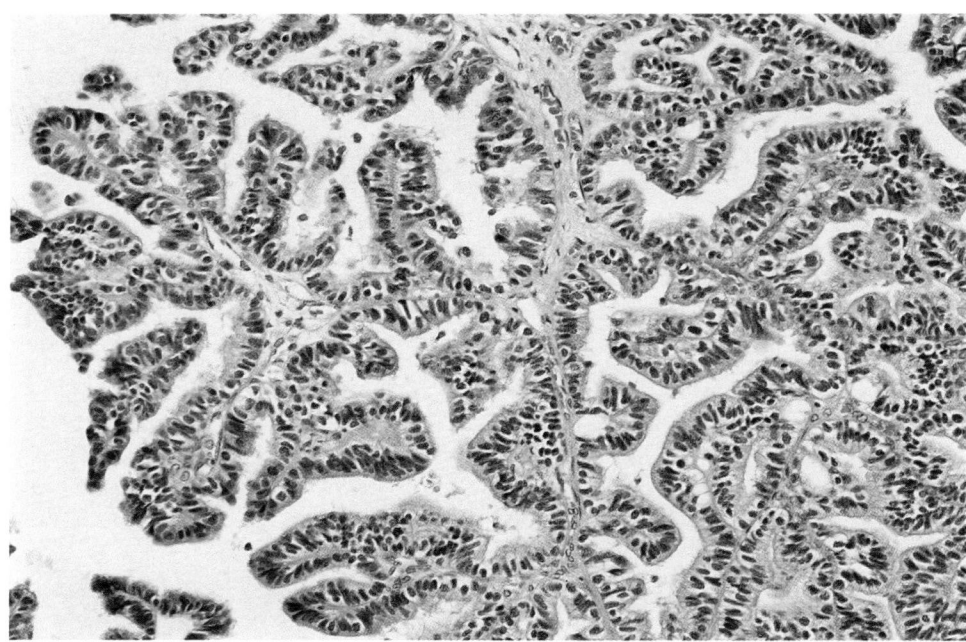

Fig. 28-72 Choroid plexus papilloma. This example's delicate fibrovascular fronds are covered by an orderly, low columnar epithelium.

tion.[490] The capacity of otherwise conventional examples to seed the CSF and metastasize along the central neuraxis is a well-recognized but, fortunately, uncommon phenomenon.[496] More problematic is a subset of tumors, often dubbed atypical choroid plexus papillomas, that fall short of overt histologic malignancy while evidencing an unexpectedly complex architecture, cytologic atypism, mitotic activity, or penetration of juxtatumoral brain tissue.[492] Some have noted an increased likelihood of recurrence and progression to histologic anaplasia on the part of tumors exhibiting worrisome morphologic traits of this sort,[492] but such has not been the experience of all observers.[490]

Choroid plexus carcinoma is the appropriate designation for frankly malignant epithelial neoplasms of plexus origin. The overwhelming majority of these rare tumors present in infancy or childhood and are situated in a lateral ventricle,[480,491] but third[483] and fourth[484] ventricular examples are also on record. In contrast to their benign counterparts, choroid plexus carcinomas are invasive, destructive, and typified by geographic foci of necrosis and hemorrhage. Many, while focally maintaining a half-hearted fidelity to the villiform architecture of the native plexus, contain foci in which their papillary structure breaks down and is replaced by nests and patternless sheets of anaplastic cells exhibiting alarming pleomorphism and mitotic activity. Isolated cases have been described as containing melanotic cytoplasmic pigments[474] or eosinophilic, PAS-positive, and diastase-resistant globules.[489] These aggressive neoplasms usually prove fatal, frequently escaping the confines of the ventricular system and seeding the subarachnoid space.

A few useful generalizations can be offered regarding the feasibility of distinguishing choroid plexus tumors from other neoplasms by immunocytochemical means, a problem addressed in numerous studies.[401,476,482] The epithelium of the native plexus rests on a basement membrane demonstrable by immunohistochemical assay for laminin, its constituent cells typically exhibiting diffuse cytoplasmic labeling by antibodies to vimentin, cytokeratins, and S-100 protein (expressed in nuclei as well).[425,476] Choroid plexus tumors generally remain faithful to the parental immunophenotype,* although some observers have found muted S-100 protein expression to be a common feature of malignant variants.[476,492] Plexus neoplasms may facilitate recognition of their neuroepithelial lineage by expressing GFAP, but this is the exception rather than the rule and is usually restricted to a very small subset of cells populating any given tumor.[422,425,475,476,492] As discussed (on p. 2294), intracranial ependymomas (including those of papillary type) often exhibit widespread GFAP reactivity and contain few if any cytokeratin-positive elements. There is, unfortunately, no antigenic profile that altogether segregates metastatic carcinomas from GFAP-negative plexus primaries, but the former are far more likely to exhibit immunoreactivity for the surface epithelial antigens identified by monoclonal antibodies HEA125 and Ber EP4,[482] as well as for CEA,[401,492] and are less often S-100 protein positive.[401] Cytoplasmic labeling with antibodies to transthyretin (prealbumin) has been identified as an attribute of normal choroid plexus epithelium and proposed as a marker of its associated neoplasms,[485] but the diagnostic utility of this approach is somewhat compromised by the fact that expression of the antigen, as immunocytochemically defined, is an inconstant

---

*References 401, 413, 422, 425, 476, 482, 492.

feature of the latter and has been noted on the part of select carcinomas metastatic to brain.[472] The diagnosis of choroid plexus carcinoma in an adult must be regarded with considerable skepticism (regardless of a tumor's location, morphology, or antigenic characteristics) because these are vanishingly rare beyond childhood and the overwhelming majority of older patients presenting with intracranial carcinomas, including well-differentiated lesions of papillary configuration, are ultimately found to harbor systemic primaries. With regard to the prognostic implications of immunophenotype in the setting of choroid plexus neoplasia, we would emphasize that the benign and malignant cannot be reliably distinguished on the basis of antigenic profile, although dampened expression of transthyretin and S-100 protein seem to be more characteristic of the latter and of papillomas that recur following resection.[476,492] CEA expression, generally foreign to epithelial tumors of the plexus,[492] may be somewhat more common among malignant variants.[476]

Neuronal and glioneuronal tumors, hamartomas, and related lesions

Ganglion cell tumors

The uncommon neoplasms collectively designated as **ganglion cell tumors** are composed, in part or exclusively, of large, mature neurons assumed, like their extracranial counterparts in lesions such as the peripheral ganglioneuroma, to represent the terminally differentiated progeny of neuroblastic precursors. By definition, the appellation is reserved for tumors devoid of distinct embryonal elements, although a variety of primitive neuroepithelial neoplasms are capable of neuronal differentiation and may exhibit ganglion cell maturation. A majority of ganglion cell tumors come to neurosurgical intervention within the first three decades of life. By most accounts,[498,501,505] these favor the supratentorial compartments, but examples have been described at all levels of the central neuraxis, and some observers regard the brainstem and spinal cord as relatively common sites of origin.[510] Even optic nerve cases have been depicted.[508] A predilection for the frontotemporal regions accounts for the discovery of many ganglion cell tumors in the course of evaluation for epilepsy, often of protracted duration. Albeit nonspecific, neuroradiologic presentation as a well-demarcated, partially cystic mass evidencing contrast enhancement of its solid components and foci of calcification is particularly characteristic (Fig. 28-73). In our experience, the cerebral hemispheric lesion presenting as a mural nodule within a cyst usually proves to be a ganglion cell tumor, pilocytic astrocytoma, or pleomorphic xanthoastrocytoma.

Although defined by their neuronal component, most ganglion cell tumors contain admixed glial elements and are consequently termed **gangliogliomas.** Those exceptional lesions composed solely of differentiated neurons merit designation as **gangliocytomas.**[499] Common to both is the irregular distribution of variably sized neurons, including large forms resembling mature ganglion cells, in a delicate fibrillary matrix that often contains scattered calcospherules and exhibits a proneness to spongy rarefaction (Fig. 28-74). Microcystic changes are common in regions dominated by

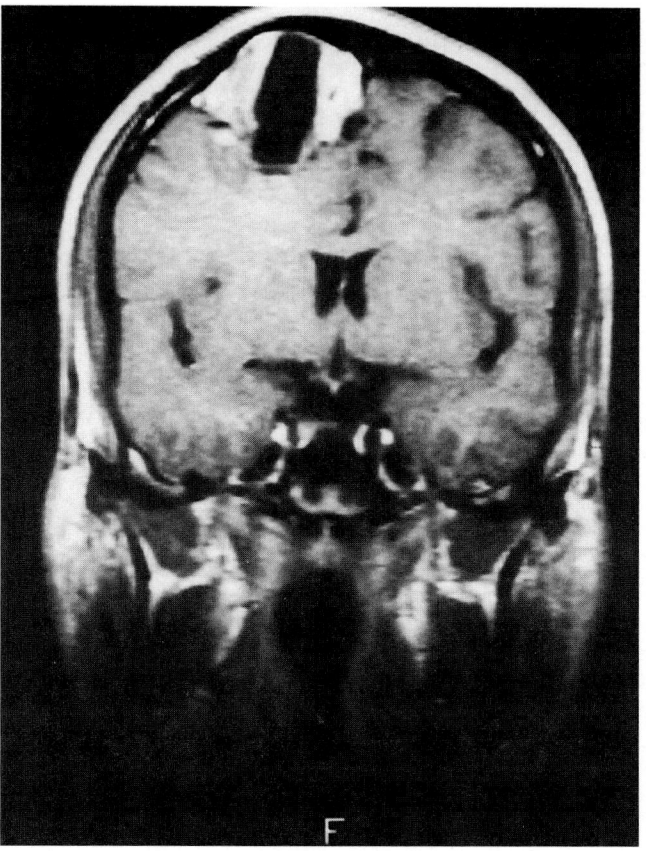

Fig. 28-73 Ganglioglioma. As demonstrated in this postcontrast injection MRI, the ganglioglioma frequently presents as a cystic cerebral hemispheric mass with brightly enhancing solid components. The absence of mass effect or hypodensity of the adjoining white matter (indicative of edema) are particularly suggestive of a slow-growing lesion.

neoplastic glia. Whereas native neurons trapped in an advancing glial neoplasm generally manifest little cytologic alteration and tend to an even distribution and orderly polarity, the ganglion cell tumor's neuronal elements often display, in addition to obvious architectural disarray and anomalous clustering, conspicuous morphologic alterations, chief among which are pleomorphism, multinucleation, cytoplasmic vacuolation and, in some cases, gigantism. Rare examples have been reported to contain Alzheimer disease–type neurofibrillary tangles and other cytoplasmic inclusions seen in neurodegenerative and neuronal storage disorders.[503] A melanotic variant has also been described,[512] as have ganglion cell tumors associated with (possibly progenitory) glioneuronal hamartomas,[517] discussed later.

Lymphoid infiltration merits emphasis as being of some diagnostic utility to the pathologist not distracted by this common, "pseudoencephalitic" presentation of the ganglion cell tumor. In fact, a florid inflammatory reaction extending into the substance of the lesion (i.e., not simply confined to the perivascular compartment) is characteristic among central neuroepithelial tumors only of this entity and the pleo-

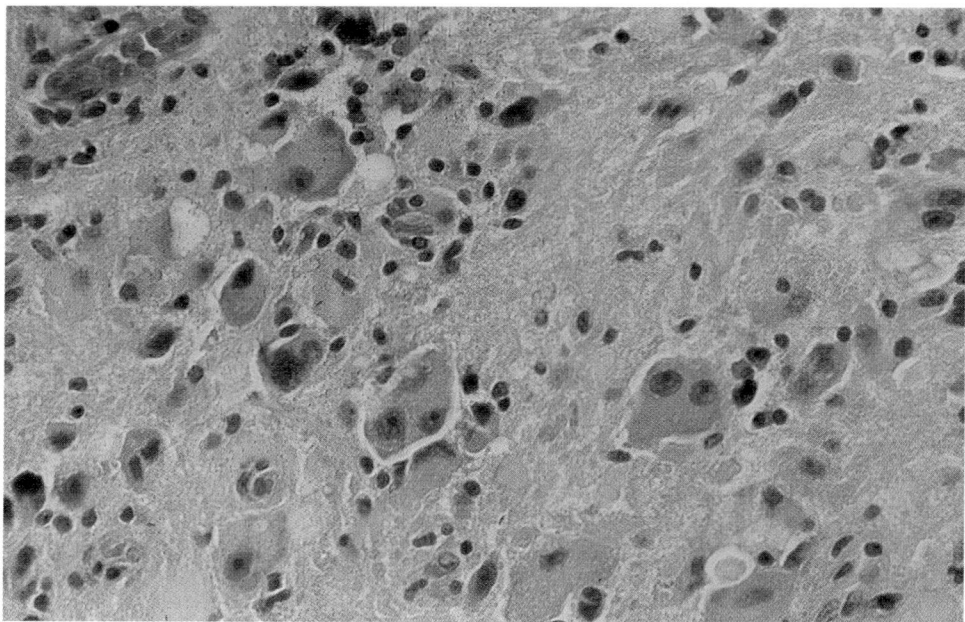

Fig. 28-74 Ganglioglioma. The neoplastic nature of the ganglion cell tumor's large neurons is readily apparent when abnormal clustering and cytologic abnormalities such as multinucleation are in evidence. Note admixed small lymphocytes, a common feature. Elsewhere this example harbored astrocytic elements.

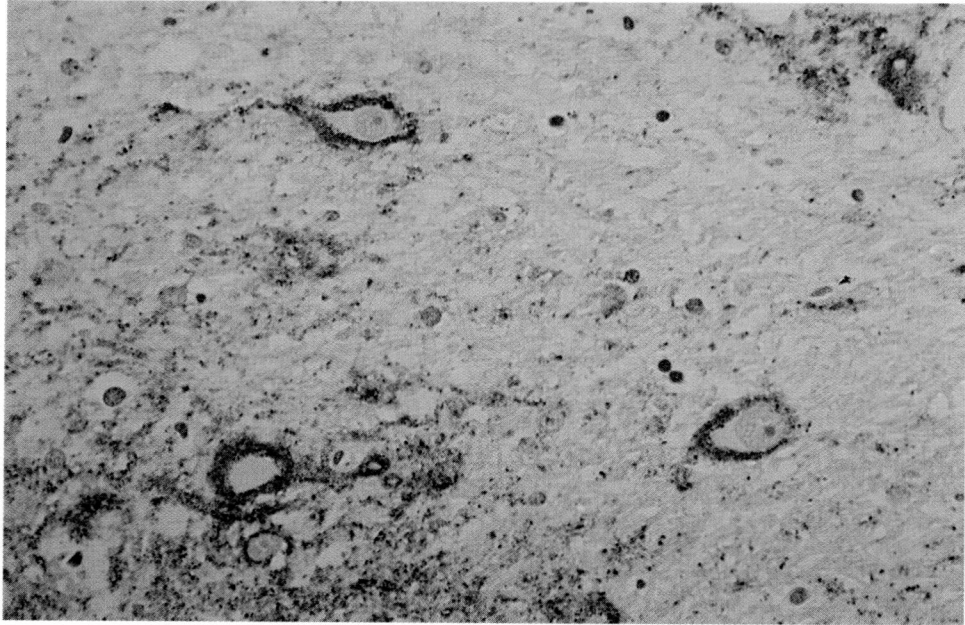

Fig. 28-75 Ganglioglioma. Surface perikaryal labeling for synaptophysin characterizes the neuronal elements of some ganglion cell tumors on immunohistochemical assay.

morphic xanthoastrocytoma, the more so if plasma cells are found to participate. Also noteworthy is desmoplasia, another phenomenon uncommonly associated with neoplasms of neuroepithelial derivation but one that lends to some ganglion cell tumors a fascicular or vaguely storiform architecture, imposing a disfiguring and deceptive spindling on their constituent neuronal elements. Eosinophilic globules of lysosomal derivation that aggregate in the matrices of many ganglion cell tumors are yet another clue to the diagnosis, because only the pilocytic astrocytoma and pleomorphic xanthoastrocytoma exhibit this presumably degenerative alteration with comparable frequency (see Fig. 28-56 for an illustration of such structures). Stromal blood vessels are often prominent and frequently undergo sclerosis, select ganglion cell tumors masquerading as vascular malformations on angiographic and gross neurosurgical assessment.

Given their differentiated cytologic appearances, it should come as no surprise that the ganglion cell tumor's neuronal populace elaborates cytoplasmic processes demonstrating the argyrophilia typical of axons on neurohistochemical study and containing parallel microtubular arrays and clear, presynaptic-type vesicles on ultrastructural examination.[510] These processes may also harbor membrane-bound, dense-core ("neurosecretory") granules—rarely found in native CNS neurons—and can terminate in synaptic complexes. Although tumors of astrocytic lineage may occasionally assume ganglion cell–like cytologic appearances, they manifest none of these specialized features and in most instances are readily unmasked by their expression of GFAP.

The formation of aberrant synapses of axosomatic type may be responsible for the presence in many ganglion cell tumors of large neurons exhibiting a coarsely granular or linear deposition of reaction product about their perikarya on immunocytochemical assay for synaptophysin (Fig. 28-75), a glycoprotein component of the presynaptic vesicle membrane.[498,509-511] A similar phenomenon has been reproduced utilizing antibodies to synapsin I, a phosphoprotein normally localized to the synaptic vesicle's cytoplasmic surface.[511] Whether this circumperikaryal labeling pattern is restricted to neoplastic neurons, as has been claimed,[509,511] is open to question. An identical immunocytochemical phenomenon has been depicted in an account of postradiation neuronal gigantism involving the cerebral cortex.[497] Certainly we have not observed (and know of no reports describing) a similar reaction on anti-synaptophysin assay of normal cerebrocortical tissues, but have encountered comparable labeling about native neurons in the striatum, deep cerebellar nuclei, brainstem, and (especially) spinal cord.[517a] The last observation could explain the unusually large percentage of intramedullary "gangliogliomas" reported in one recent series,[510] as well as the "paradoxical" tendency of the tumors so diagnosed to recur following apparently complete resection,[506] behavior at odds with that of intracranial ganglion cell tumors (see later discussion). We suspect that at least some of these lesions, classified as gangliogliomas on the basis of their synaptophysin immunoreactivity, instead represented low-grade astrocytomas containing entrapped spinal neurons. Neoplastic ganglion cells may also exhibit immunoreactivity for neurofilament proteins, a variety of neuropeptides, enzymes integral to catecholamine meta-

bolism and chromogranin A.[498,499,502,513,517] Conspicuous perikaryal labeling for the last of these antigens, presumably a reflection of dense-core granule formation, may, like circumneuronal synaptophysin expression, be of some diagnostic utility inasmuch as native CNS neurons outside the hypothalamus and brainstem react only weakly, if at all, with commercially available antibodies to chromogranin A.

The ganglioglioma's glial component is typically astrocytic and GFAP positive and may exhibit fibrillary, gemistocytic, piloid, or even pleomorphic xanthoastrocytomatous features.[500,507] Although some contain bona fide oligodendroglial elements, the oligodendrocyte-like clear cells present in select gangliogliomas may alternatively represent diminutive neurons ("neurocytes").[510] Most gangliogliomas evidence no overtly anaplastic histologic characteristics, are remarkably indolent, and if accessible, are cured by resection alone.[498,501,505,506] Malignant degeneration appears to be most uncommon and is almost invariably restricted to the ganglion cell tumor's glial components, which may on occasion assume the appearances of frank glioblastoma. Noteworthy, however, is the observation that the presence of high-grade glial elements does not necessarily augur poorly in this setting,[505,506] a happy discrepancy likely resulting from the fact that gangliogliomas tend to expand in a compact, relatively noninvasive fashion that lends itself to the purposes of the neurosurgeon. Although the appropriate management of the histologically anaplastic ganglioglioma will remain in doubt pending the documentation of outcome in additional examples, a number of authors have concluded that observation alone is reasonable following gross total resection.[505,506] Whether irradiation or chemotherapy is of benefit to patients with residual or recurrent disease is unclear. That gangliogliomas only exceptionally kill is apparent from the recently reported experience of several major referral centers[498,501,505,506] and the critical analysis of Wacker et al.[516] As noted by the latter authors, their remarkable case of diffuse leptomeningeal gangliogliomatosis may actually have represented advanced glioneuronal maturation of a metastasizing cerebellar medulloblastoma. We note, in passing, the recent description of a unique ganglioglioma that recurred (3 years after subtotal resection and irradiation) as a high-grade neoplasm populated by cells exhibiting a hybrid neuronal and astrocytic phenotype on immunocytochemical and ultrastructural study.[504]

Included among the mixed glioneuronal neoplasms are the unusual tumors described as ***desmoplastic infantile gangliogliomas.***[514,515] Complex admixtures of fibroblastic and neuroepithelial components, the latter evidencing divergent astrocytic and neuronal differentiation, these are typified by a frontoparietal location and presentation as large, cystic meningocerebral masses in patients younger than 2 years of age. Despite their often considerable size at diagnosis, cellular pleomorphism, and content of embryonal-appearing, mitotically active small-cell elements, a favorable outcome following resection is the rule. Of interest is the fact that basal lamina material often invests this lesion's neoplastic glia. This finding is characteristic of what would appear to be a closely allied neoplasm, the desmoplastic cerebral astrocytoma of infancy, as well as the pleomorphic xanthoastrocytoma, and as discussed previously in reference to

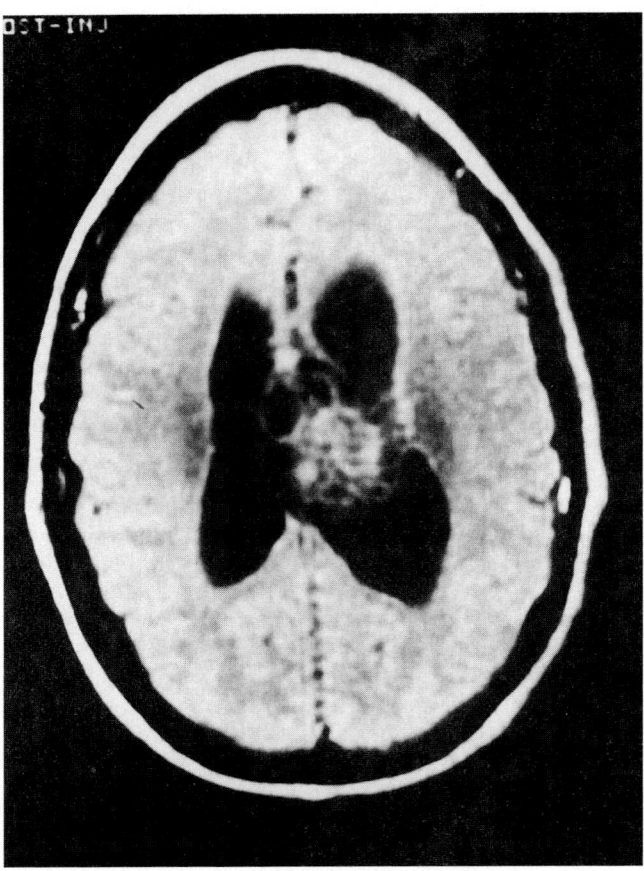

Fig. 28-76 Central neurocytoma. This postcontrast injection MRI shows the neurocytoma's predilection for the lateral ventricles, its tendency to be centered about the septum pellucidum, its often multicystic structure, regions of bright enhancement, and associated ventriculomegaly indicative of obstructive hydrocephalus.

these tumor types, is generally taken as evidence of differentiation along subpial astrocytic lines. In fact, the desmoplastic infantile ganglioglioma and cerebral astrocytoma differ only in the former's content of neuronal elements, their otherwise comparable morphologic and biologic features suggesting that these may represent a unified pathologic entity.

Central neurocytoma

Noted for its largely intraventricular situation and oligodendroglioma-like histology, the **central neurocytoma** is a neoplasm composed of essentially mature, albeit diminutive, neurons.[519,520,522,529] The tumor typically produces symptoms and signs of increased intracranial pressure in young adulthood, its peak incidence spanning the third and fourth decades of life. There is no gender predilection. A consequence of obstructive hydrocephalus, the lesion's presenting manifestations are typically found on neuroimaging study to reflect blockade of the foramen of Monro by a sizable mass occupying the anterior aspect of the lateral ventricles and extending, in some cases, to the third ventricle as well. On occasion, the lesion is confined to the latter chamber. Attach-

ment to the septum pellucidum is particularly characteristic, but the central neurocytoma may be anchored anywhere along the wall of the lateral ventricles, a feature suggesting its origin from remnants of the subependymal germinal matrix that retain postnatal proliferative capabilities.[520] MR images generally reveal the lesion to contain a heterogeneous admixture of tissues isodense and hypodense relative to normal cerebral cortex, contrast enhancement on gadolinium administration being the rule (Fig. 28-76). Foci of conspicuous calcification are common, as is cystic change, and approximately half of these richly vascularized neoplasms exhibit a tumoral "blush" on angiographic assessment.

The central neurocytoma is a neoplasm remarkable for the cytologic conformity of its constituent cells (Fig. 28-77). These possess nuclei of uniformly small diameter and rounded contour whose granular chromatin is distributed in a diffuse, peppery fashion. A striking tendency to perinuclear cytoplasmic clearing further contributes to the lesion's oligodendroglioma-like appearance, a mimicry abetted in many instances by admixed calcospherules and a plexiform capillary arcade. The tumor deviates from the oligodendroglioma, however, in its elaboration of a fibrillary, neuropil-like matrix that may separate streams or regimented columns of neoplastic cells, appear as circumscribed, acellular islands embedded in foci of sheet-like tumor growth, or collar stromal vessels in the manner of the ependymoma—another lesion that can exhibit clear cell features and that figures prominently in the differential diagnosis. Although it may attain dense cellularity, the usual neurocytoma is virtually devoid of mitotic activity and does not exhibit vascular hyperplasia or undergo necrosis. Only isolated cases have been reported to manifest worrisome features of this sort.[529] The formation of Homer Wright rosettes and admixed ganglion cell forms—findings more typical of the differentiating cerebral neuroblastoma—likewise appears to have characterized only exceptional examples.[520,529]

The neurocytoma's stereotypic clinical presentation and neuroradiologic and histologic features should prompt ultrastructural or immunocytochemical investigations that are required to confirm the diagnosis. Electron microscopy will reveal its fibrillar matrix to be composed of entwined cytoplasmic processes replete with microtubules in parallel array; membrane-bound, dense-core granules; and clear vesicles (Fig. 28-78).[519,522] Synapses, typical or abortive, further attest in some cases to this neoplasm's advanced neuronal maturation. As expected given its fine structure, the neurocytoma has been shown to be capable of expressing a variety of antigens restricted in the normal CNS to cells of neuronal lineage. These include synaptophysin, synapsin, neurofilament proteins, class III beta tubulin, microtubule-associated proteins, the L1 adhesion molecule, and 180-kd neural cell adhesion molecule isoform.[511,519-521,528] A hormonally active hypothalamic neurocytoma exhibiting vasopressin immunoreactivity has also been reported.[523] That the vast majority of central neurocytomas studied to date have demonstrated labeling of their fibrillar matrices by monoclonal antibodies to synaptophysin merits particular emphasis, as a positive assay utilizing these commercially available reagents obviates the need for time-consuming ultrastructural examination.[519,520] Although rare variants have been described as

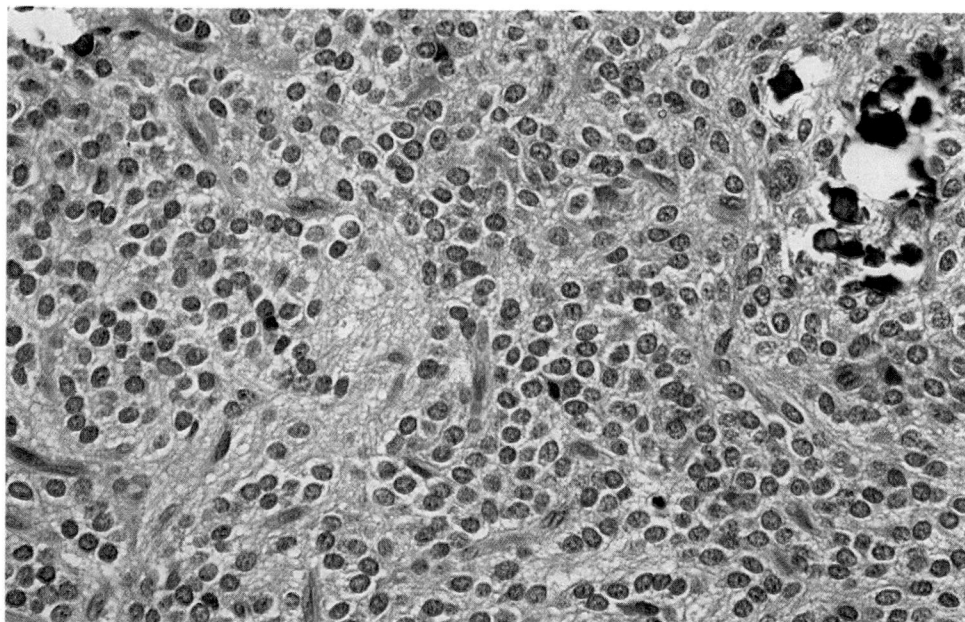

Fig. 28-77 Central neurocytoma. The typical neurocytoma is rather densely populated by small, monomorphous cells embedded in a variably abundant, delicate fibrillar matrix. Rounded nuclear contours, perinuclear clearing, a plexiform capillary arcade, and associated microcalcifications (the basophilic structures present at upper right) impart an oligodendroglioma-like appearance to this small cell neuronal neoplasm.

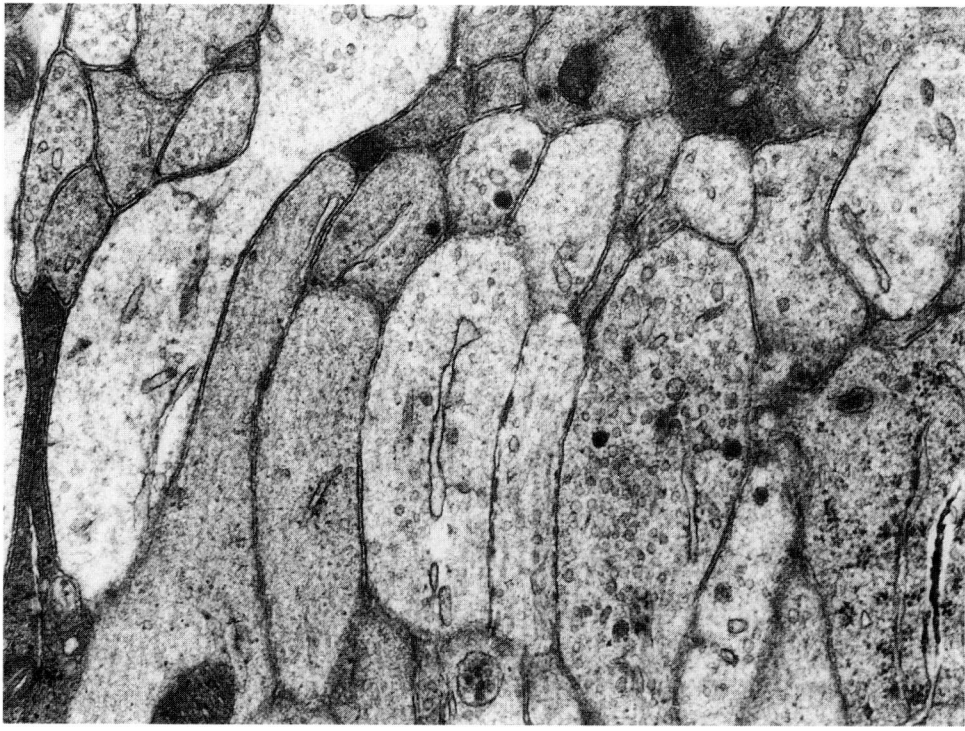

Fig. 28-78 Central neurocytoma. This transmission electron micrographic study readily discloses the neuronal nature of this neoplasm, demonstrating arrays of "neuritic" processes replete with microtubules, clear synaptic-type vesicles, and dense-core neurosecretory granules. (×27,000.)

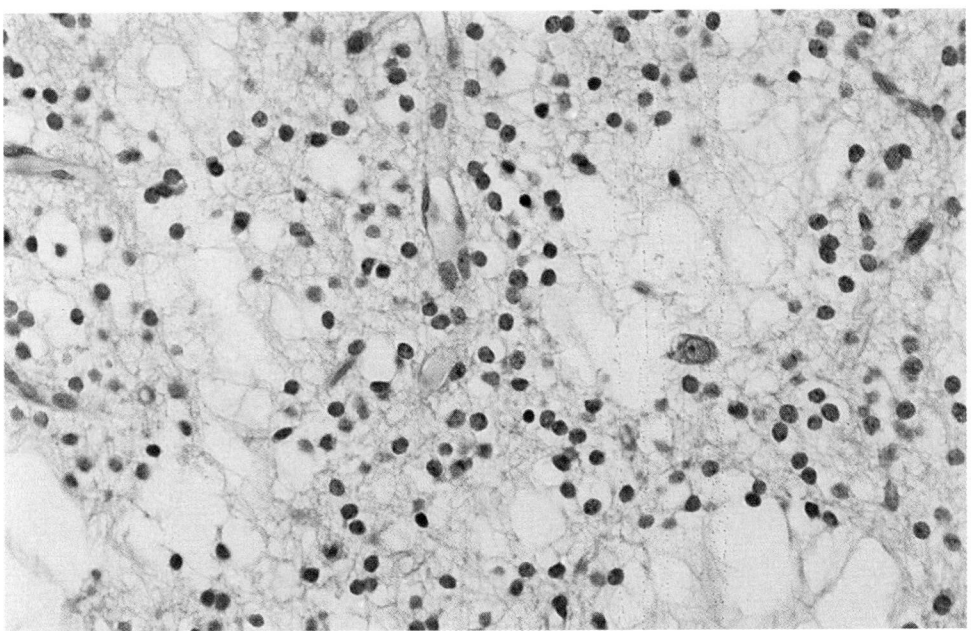

Fig. 28-79 Dysembryoplastic neuroepithelial tumor. The diagnostic features of this lesion include a dominant population of oligodendrocyte-like cells disposed about small capillaries and the formation of myxoid microcysts that contain "floating" neurons (such as the one present to right of center).

containing GFAP-reactive glial elements,[528] most investigators have been unable to reproduce this finding and regard these tumors as committed to a neuronal phenotype.[519,520]

Follow-up data indicate that the prognosis for patients with central neurocytomas is favorable,[519,520,522,529] these tumors growing slowly and remaining confined to the ventricles. Infiltration of periventricular tissues is clearly exceptional, and dissemination via the CSF has not been documented. Cure may be effected by excision, the treatment of choice, and some patients have remained stable for protracted periods following ventriculoperitoneal shunting alone. At least some lesions have proved radiosensitive.

We briefly note descriptions of neurocytomas, mixed "glioneurocytomas," or "ganglioneurocytomas" (i.e., differentiated neuronal neoplasms composed of both small neurons and mature ganglion cells) presenting as extraventricular, cerebral hemispheric,[510,525,526] or intramedullary[527] growths. Also on record is a cerebellar neoplasm composed of neurocytic and adipocytic elements (neurolipocytoma), possibly a mature variant of the lipidized medulloblastoma (see p. 2313). Obviously, the spectrum of differentiated, small cell neuronal tumors remains to be delineated. An overtly malignant, pleomorphic neuronal neoplasm that may masquerade as small cell glioblastoma has been described[524] and may represent the anaplastic counterpart of the central neurocytoma.

Dysembryoplastic neuroepithelial tumor

Usually discovered in childhood, adolescence, or early adult life, the dysembryoplastic neuroepithelial tumor is typically associated with a protracted history of partial complex seizures refractory to conventional pharmacologic manage-

ment—a consequence of its tendency to lie, at least in part, within epileptogenic temporal cortex.[530,531] Extratemporal examples favor the frontal lobes. Subcortical cases, including apparently multifocal variants, have been described and may involve deep gray nuclei and posterior fossa contents.[533] Characteristic is a lobular growth pattern in which multiple tumor nodules are separated by limited expanses of cerebral cortex exhibiting cytoarchitectural disorganization (dysplasia). Individual nodules are populated by oligodendrocyte-like cells that often manifest striking perinuclear clearing and by larger, mature-appearing neurons that seem to float in a basophilic, myxoid matrix (Fig. 28-79). The former constitute the dominant cellular component and tend to a linear alignment in close proximity to traversing capillaries arrayed in parallel fashion, some possessing short cytoplasmic processes and forming perivascular pseudorosettes. "Oligodendrocytic" rosettes containing a central core of fibrillary eosinophilic material are also encountered in some cases. GFAP-reactive astroglial elements are only sparsely represented in simple variants of the dysembryoplastic neuroepithelial tumor, but complex examples harboring foci with the appearance of pilocytic astrocytoma have been delineated.[530,531,533]

The frequent association of the dysembryoplastic neuroepithelial tumor with cortical dysplasia and its clinical biology suggest that this may represent a hamartomatous, rather than neoplastic, lesion. In fact, no tumor-related deaths have been recorded to date, and no published example has exhibited clinical evidence of rapid growth or other aggressive behavior. Surgical extirpation renders patients seizure-free and suffices for cure.[530,531] Although the cytogenesis of this peculiar entity's oligodendrocyte-like elements is not entirely clear, recent immunocytochemical and ultrastructural studies suggest that at least a subset are diminutive neurons ("neurocytes") rather than oligodendroglia.[532] An origin from remnants of the embryonic subpial granular layer that have been found to persist in the frontotemporal regions of normal infants could explain the dysembryoplastic neuroepithelial tumor's characteristic topography and largely intracortical presentation.[530]

Hypothalamic neuronal hamartoma and choristoma

The *hypothalamic neuronal hamartoma* typically presents as a rubbery grayish-white nodule no more than 1 or 2 cm in diameter that bulges into the suprasellar cistern from a broad-based stalk anchoring it to the tuber cinereum or mammillary body.[538] The lesion is usually discovered on evaluation of a boy for precocious puberty, but young females and older individuals may be affected, and an association with other endocrinologic syndromes, principally acromegaly, is recognized. The hamartoma consists of large, mature neurons that may closely resemble those populating the principal hypothalamic nuclei. The former are embedded in a matrix of myelinated and nonmyelinated axons. Some examples have a gliotic appearance, but astrocytes and oligodendroglia are only minor cellular elements. That their misplaced neurons retain hypothalamic hormonal activity is currently the most attractive hypothesis regarding the functional manifestations of these unusual lesions. Immunohistochemical assay of select examples, among them cases associated with sexual precocity, has revealed reactivity of their neuronal elements for gonadotropin-releasing hormones, including luteinizing hormone–releasing factor.[536,540] Hamartomas (described as hypothalamic "gangliocytomas") harbored by acromegalic patients have been reported to elaborate growth hormone–releasing factor[534] and, in so doing, may drive the adenohypophysis to neoplasia, as evidenced by their association with growth hormone–producing pituitary adenomas.[541] Neurons of hypothalamic type displaced to the anterior pituitary gland, referred to as *intrasellar gangliocytomas* or *adenohypophyseal neuronal choristomas,* may promote the development of adenomas by a similar mechanism.[537,541] Rarely, a congenital hypothalamic hamartoma is found as part of a complex malformative process that includes imperforate anus, cryptorchidism, polydactyly, pituitary aplasia, hypoplasia of the adrenal and thyroid glands, and various cardiac and renal anomalies.[535,539] This infantile variant, composed of small, immature-appearing neuronal elements, is designated as **hypothalamic hamartoblastoma,** and its associated malformations are often referred to as the *Hall-Pallister syndrome.*

Glioneuronal hamartomas, cortical dysplasias, and other epileptogenic lesions

A spate of recent publications attest to an ongoing interest in the neurosurgical management of refractory seizure disorders and in the delineation of their anatomic substrates.[542-546] Inasmuch as operative approaches to this problem are practiced largely in specialized referral centers and so do not engage the general surgical pathologist, we specifically consider here only one of the more commonly encountered lesions not addressed elsewhere in this text, the glioneuronal hamartoma.

Although by no means restricted to this site, *glioneuronal hamartomas* are often found in and about the amygdala, figuring prominently among seizure-associated lesions in series detailing the surgical treatment of chronic temporal lobe epilepsy.[544,545] Ranging from the microscopic to expansile gray nodules that may be grossly evident on evaluation of lobectomy specimens and visualized by neuroradiographic means, these lesions are sometimes found to be multifocal, are often associated with other evidences of faulty development (such as patchy cortical dysgenesis and neuronal ectopias in the temporal white matter), and may occur in complex with low-grade neuroepithelial neoplasms of varied type. Whether they serve as the progenitors of select gliomas, gangliogliomas, or dysembryoplastic neuroepithelial tumors (the more commonly associated lesions) is open to question. Populated, in most cases rather sparsely, by neurons of medium to large size and admixed astrocytes that may exhibit hyperplastic features, glioneuronal hamartomas do not evidence the cellularity, pleomorphism, or conspicuous inflammatory infiltration of the bona fide ganglioglioma, nor do they manifest microcystic change or the myxoid alterations characteristic of the dysembryoplastic neuroepithelial tumor. Some, like the latter, harbor aggregated oligodendrocyte-like clear cell elements, but these are a minor component and further deviate in evidencing no special relationship to the stromal vasculature. Spongiform change may be apparent within the lesion and can involve associated cortex in patchy fashion, this possibly representing a seizure-induced tissue disturbance. Finally, select variants contain scattered bizarre cells of neuronal, astrocytic, or indeterminate lineage resembling those of the cortical tuber (the tuberous sclerosis complex is discussed in relation to subependymal giant cell astrocytomas) or neurons with a chromatolytic, "ballooned" appearance.[542-546]

Lhermitte-Duclos disease

The curious condition known as *Lhermitte-Duclos disease* consists of a grossly evident, regional thickening of the cerebellar folia that, in turn, reflects replacement of their granule and Purkinje cell layers by an array of large, abnormal neurons with attendant expansion and abnormal myelination of the overlying molecular layer.[547] The subjacent folial white matter, by contrast, is typically attenuated or undergoes complete degeneration. The disorder's principal clinical manifestations are those of any posterior fossa mass (e.g., headache, nausea, vomiting, visual disturbances, and ataxia). Most patients present in the third or fourth decades of life.[550]

It is particularly noteworthy that Ambler and colleagues,[547] reporting the first familial examples of this condition and noting its frequent association with megalencephaly and other malformations, should have inclined to the prescient classification of Lhermitte-Duclos disease "with tuberous sclerosis, von Recklinghausen's neurofibromatosis, and Sturge-Weber disease as a developmental disorder of cell growth." In fact, several independent studies have recently underscored the association of this cerebellar lesion with Cowden's syndrome, the autosomal dominant complex of oral papillomatosis, acral keratoses, multiple cutaneous tricholemmomas, macrocephaly, gastrointestinal polyposis, and an increased risk of malignant neoplasms, particularly mammary carcinoma.[551,553,554] Neuroimaging studies[550,554] usually reveal a non enhancing cerebellar hemispheric mass, may demonstrate the calcification to which the abnormal molecular layer is prone, and can suggest the specific diagnosis by delineating the folial expansion characteristic of the disease. Surgical debulking is the treatment of choice, although the condition may occasionally recur following resection.[550,554]

The nature and pathogenesis of Lhermitte-Duclos disease have resisted satisfactory explication. On neurohistochemical and ultrastructural study, the abnormal neurons typical of the disorder seem to represent outsized caricatures of the granule cells that they appear to replace, elaborating axons that course, as expected, toward the pial surface while undergoing myelination foreign to the normal molecular layer.[548] Most observers believe that these neuronal elements are, in fact, native granule cells stimulated to hypertrophy, possibly in compensatory response to faulty development of the fetal external granular layer, but a subset may be rimmed by axosomatic complexes in the manner of normal Purkinje cells and express select antigens characteristic of the latter.[549,552]

Embryonal neuroepithelial tumors

Collectively described as "embryonal" are diverse neoplasms sharing, in addition to a postulated derivation from primitive neuroepithelial precursors, a peak incidence in the early years of life and an aggressive clinical biology. Most such tumors are dominated by small, anaplastic cells apparently uncommitted to any particular cytogenetic pathway on conventional histologic assessment, but the capacity of these lesions to differentiate along neuronal, glial, and on occasion, mesenchymal lines has long been recognized and is manifest in their bewildering morphologic and immunophenotypic heterogeneity.[557-560]

Few subjects in surgical neuropathology have occasioned controversy as heated as that surrounding the nomenclature appropriate to these complex neoplasms. Their original designations were predicated on the theory that the histologic appearances of CNS tumors reflect the neoplastic transformation of specific cell types at recognizable stages of neuroembryogenesis.[562] Thus *medulloepithelioma* was the name given to a tumor harboring structures resembling, and so presumed to originate from, the neural tube's primitive medullary epithelium, whereas *ependymoblastoma* was used for an embryonal neoplasm seemingly committed to differentiation along ependymal lines alone, and so forth. The theoretical underpinnings of this scheme have been justly questioned and an alternative, operational approach suggested in which the generic *primitive neuroectodermal tumor* (PNET) is accorded all such neoplasms and then qualified to indicate a lesion's site and differentiating characteristics.[561] Implied is the common origin of embryonal tumors from indifferent stem cells that either remain undifferentiated or exercise any of a number of maturational options following their neoplastic transformation. Specifically, targeting of undifferentiated neuroepithelial cells known to persist in the subependymal plate and pineal anlage is hypothesized to account for the occurrence of histologically similar neoplasms of primitive character at various sites along the neuraxis.

Simply stated, the cytogenesis of these embryonal tumors remains, at present, wholly speculative. It is our practice to employ the time-honored designations first applied to these neoplasms, flawed as they may be; this traditional terminology is retained in the newly revised classification of CNS tumors issued by the WHO.[560] The pineoblastoma is treated under pineal parenchymal neoplasms. We call the reader's attention to the association of embryonal neoplasms arising in the brain and kidney, specifically to the occurrence of renal rhabdoid tumors in complex with medulloblastoma, pineoblastoma, and cerebral neuroblastoma.[555] Examples of Wilms' tumor associated with medulloblastoma,[560a] glioblastoma,[560a] and cerebellar medulloepithelioma[555] are also on record (the first two cited cases involving siblings). This curious phenomenon remains unexplained. Embryonal neuroepithelial tumors capable of neuronal or mixed neuronoglial differentiation have also been described following prophylactic cranial irradiation for childhood leukemia and lymphoma.[556]

Medulloblastoma

The cerebellar tumors traditionally designated as ***medulloblastomas*** are the most common of the primitive neuroepithelial neoplasms.[557,573] Noted for a peak incidence in the latter half of life's first decade, these embryonal lesions account for 20% to 25% of all intracranial tumors arising in childhood and for some 40% of those situated in the posterior fossa. Roughly one fourth of afflicted patients are beyond their teenage years[575] and approximately 65% are male. Although most medulloblastomas present in sporadic fashion, they may complicate a variety of heritable multisystem disorders. Chief among the latter is the *nevoid basal cell carcinoma*—or *"Gorlin"—syndrome,* an autosomal dominant disorder characterized principally by skeletal anomalies (including craniomegaly), lamellar calcium deposition in the falx cerebri and diaphragma sellae, cutaneous epidermoid cysts and pits on the palms and soles, odontogenic keratocysts, calcifying ovarian fibromas, and multifocal basal cell carcinomas noted for their early age at presentation, involvement of hidden, as well as sun-exposed, skin, melanotic pigmentation, associated calcifications and clinical indolence.[581] Medulloblastomas may also constitute a defining feature of Turcot's syndrome, previously mentioned in relation to diffuse fibrillary astrocytomas and characterized by the occurrence of central neuroepithelial neoplasms in complex with polyposis coli.[323]

The cellular origins of the medulloblastoma are unclear. Certainly, the human cerebellum has not been shown to harbor a cell type having the properties ascribed to the putative "medulloblast" (i.e., the capacity to spawn successive generations of uncommitted offspring able, in turn, to differentiate along both neuronal and glial lines). Enthusiastically championed in this regard are remnants of the fetal external granular cell layer, known to persist after birth, as well as elements of the posterior medullary velum and hypothesized stem cells in the subependymal matrix.[557,561] Given the morphologic and immunophenotypic heterogeneity of neoplasms to which the designation of medulloblastoma is currently extended, a nonuniform cytogenesis would not be surprising.

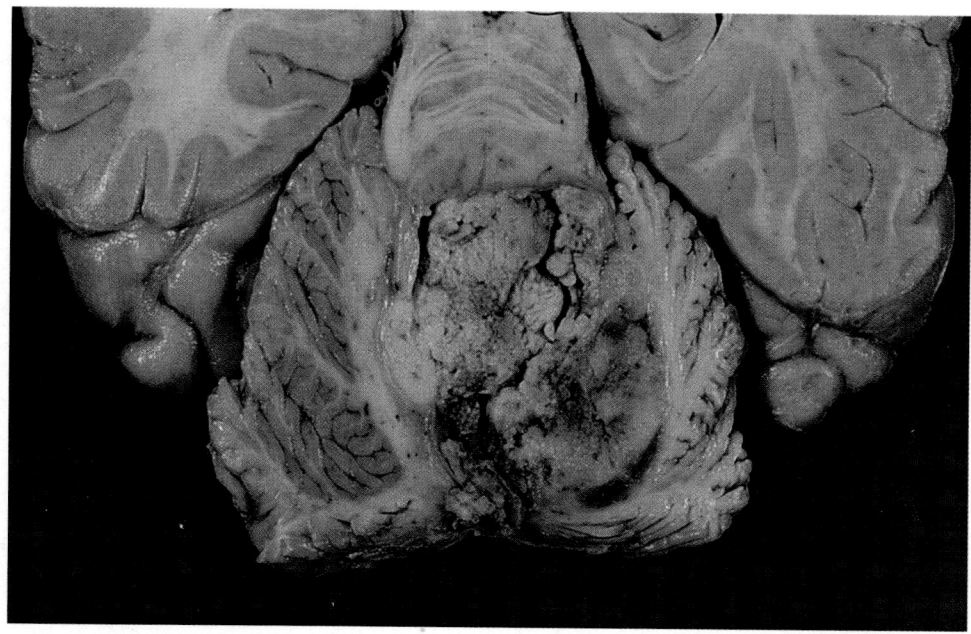

Fig. 28-80 Medulloblastoma. As shown, examples arising in the cerebellar vermis commonly come to fill the fourth ventricle.

At least 75% of childhood medulloblastomas arise in the midline, occupying the cerebellar vermis and expanding to fill the fourth ventricle (Fig. 28-80). Consequently, their presenting manifestations usually reflect intracranial hypertension secondary to CSF blockade and consist most commonly of lethargy, headache, and morning emesis. These are frequently accompanied by truncal ataxia and disturbed gait. The relative proportion of laterally positioned, hemispheric lesions increases with age. In either location, medulloblastomas appear as solid, intensely and homogeneously contrast-enhancing masses on CT or MR imaging. Unlike ependymomas, the major differential diagnostic consideration in the region of the fourth ventricle, they are not prone to conspicuous calcification and hang from the ventricle's roof rather than bulge upward from its floor. Not infrequently, brainstem invasion is apparent on neuroradiologic assessment at diagnosis, and CSF-borne metastases, also common, may be visualized as foci of nodular or diffuse contrast enhancement in the subarachnoid space.

Medulloblastomas have long been separated into "classical" and "desmoplastic" variants, although there would now appear to be no compelling clinical reason to do so. *Classical medulloblastomas,* at their most primitive, are solid masses of friable, grayish-white tissue composed of diminutive, undifferentiated-appearing cells closely arrayed in packed sheets (Fig. 28-81). Nuclei are often densely hyperchromatic, round or angulated, and invested with little or no definable cytoplasm and are thus prone to deformation or "molding" by their neighbors. A tendency to swirling or a fascicular architecture and fusiform cellular profiles may be encountered, as may nuclei disposed in perivascular pseu-

dorosettes or regimented in compact, rhythmic palisades. Stromal elements are typically scanty, consisting of scattered small blood vessels that only exceptionally exhibit hyperplastic changes and these rarely comparable to the glomeruloid microvascular alterations characteristic of high-grade gliomas. Mitotic figures and the karyorrhectic remains of singly degenerate cells usually abound, but most medulloblastomas exhibit little evidence of zonal coagulative necrosis—a phenomenon seemingly at odds with their high cellular density and proliferative activity. When present, however, such foci may be bordered by tumor cells in a palisading array. Patterns of local spread commonly encountered in neurosurgical material include diffuse permeation of adjoining neural parenchyma along the lesion's perimeter, arresting subpial accumulations of neoplastic cells that invite comparison to a persistent fetal external granular layer, and extension into the subarachnoid compartment with reinvasion of the underlying cerebellar cortex along a broad front or via penetrating perivascular spaces.

The *desmoplastic medulloblastoma* may occupy a midline, vermal position and present in childhood but is clearly over-represented among laterally situated tumors of adult onset, characteristically lying in the superior aspect of the affected cerebellar hemisphere. Here it may appear at operation as a leptomeningeal-based, lobulated, and sharply delimited mass. A firm consistency reflects the collagenization for which the lesion is named, a process that forces tumor cells into regimented Indian-file and trabecular arrangements, vague whorls, or even storiform arrays. Because a fibroplastic reaction selectively characterizes foci of subarachnoid space invasion by otherwise classic medulloblas-

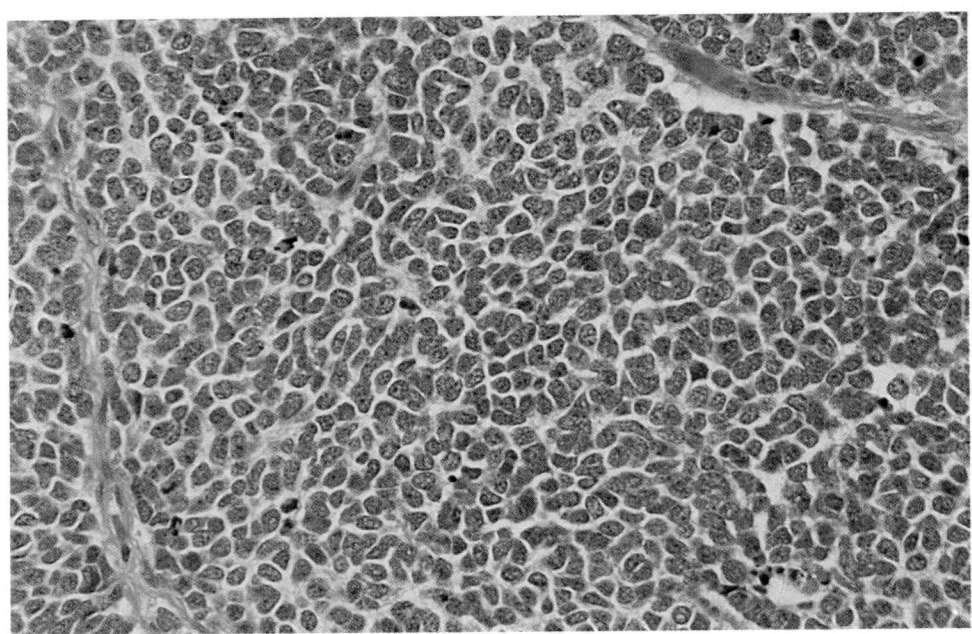

Fig. 28-81 Medulloblastoma. The classic medulloblastoma is a highly cellular neoplasm composed of diminutive, undifferentiated-looking elements possessed of little definable cytoplasm and prone to nuclear molding.

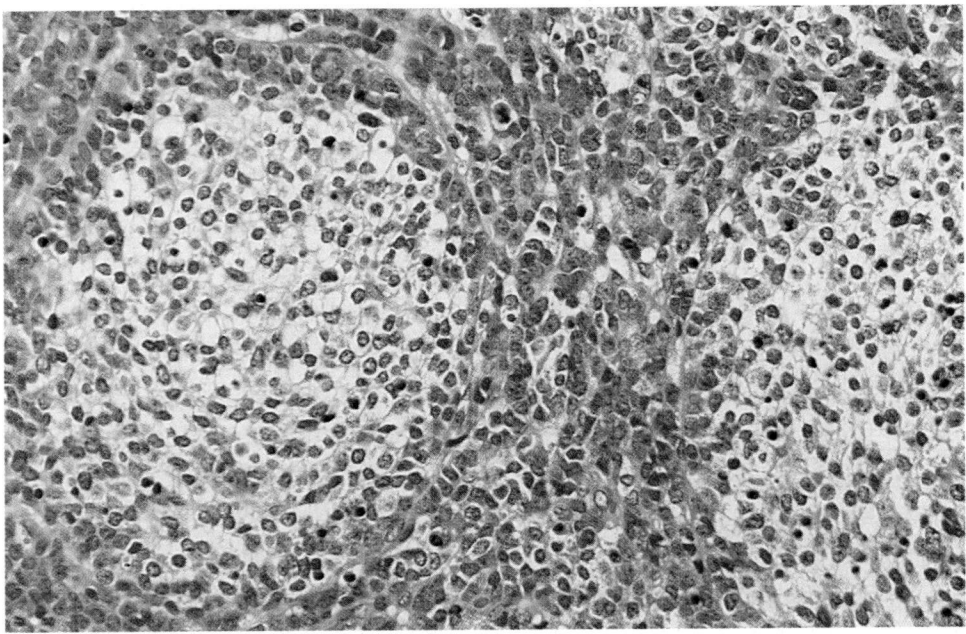

Fig. 28-82 Desmoplastic medulloblastoma. Micronodular zones of somewhat reduced cellularity ("pale islands") are a striking feature of this medulloblastoma variant.

tomas, the desmoplastic variant's histology has been interpreted as resulting simply from the reaction of mesenchymal leptomeningeal elements to tumoral permeation. Noteworthy, however, is this lesion's tendency to harbor micronodular, reticulin-free zones ("pale islands") that lend to some examples an appearance likened to that of lymph nodes exhibiting follicular hyperplasia (Fig. 28-82). Characterized by reduced cellularity, a rarefied fibrillary matrix, and the frequent emergence of an oligodendroglial-like populace, the pseudofollicle is not merely free of connective tissues but appears, as presently discussed, to represent a locus of progressive neuronal and, possibly, astrocytic differentiation.[577,578]

Select neoplasms depicted as variants of medulloblastoma merit additional comment. An especially aggressive subtype is a tumor composed wholly, or in part, of large cells possessing vesicular nuclei, prominent nucleoli, and variably abundant eosinophilic cytoplasm.[574] These bring to mind the primary CNS rhabdoid tumors of the cerebellar region discussed later, but their cytoplasm lacks globular hyaline inclusions and is reactive for neuron-specific enolase and synaptophysin, rather than EMA, on immunocytochemical assay. One of four reported cases contained admixed small cell elements typical of conventional medulloblastoma, whereas another was found on cytogenetic analysis to harbor the latter's most common karyotypic abnormality, isochromosome 17q.[573] The *melanotic medulloblastoma* is defined by its content of pigmented cells disposed in clusters, tubules, and papillae.[564,576] These are appropriately stained by conventional histochemical methods for the demonstration of melanin and can be shown to contain melanosomes in varying stages of maturation. Although this lesion bears a certain histologic resemblance to the indolent melanotic neuroectodermal tumors of infancy that arise in the maxillary and epididymal regions, it is a virulent neoplasm prone to early and widespread neuraxis dissemination along CSF pathways.

The *medullomyoblastoma* is a small cell neuroepithelial neoplasm containing heterologous rhabdomyoblastic elements.[557,584] This curious neoplasm has been variously interpreted as a medulloblastoma evidencing the extreme plasticity of its multipotential neuroepithelial progenitors; as a tumor of neural crest (ectomesenchymal) derivation; as a composite lesion whose myoblastic constituents arise via the secondary neoplastic induction of vessel-associated, or leptomeningeal, stromal elements; and finally, as a bidermal teratoma. Although otherwise typical medulloblastomas have been reported to contain scattered desmin-immunoreactive tumor cells,[559] supporting their capacity for divergent differentiation along mesenchymal lines, noteworthy is an account of a cystic, tridermal cerebellar teratoma harboring solid regions evidencing medullomyoblastomatous features.[567] Tumors containing both muscular and melanotic elements have been described,[572] as have medulloblastomas exhibiting chondroid differentiation[563] and lipoblastic and adipocytic features.[566,570]

Although controversy still surrounds the conventional medulloblastoma's cellular origins, most observers grant its capacity to differentiate along both neuronal and glial lines.[557] It is the former option that is exercised most frequently, although maturation to recognizable neurons (ganglion cells) is exceptional. Reliable indices of neuronal differentiation that can be apprehended at the light microscopic level include the radial arrangement of tumor cell nuclei about small tangles of fibrillar material to form Homer Wright rosettes (Fig. 28-83) and the emergence of "pale islands," previously described as a particularly arresting feature of some desmoplastic medulloblastomas but occasionally encountered in classical variants. Ultrastructural studies have confirmed that the cells participating in these distinctive formations elaborate neurite-like cytoplasmic processes joined by specialized adhesion plaques and laden with microtubules in parallel, longitudinal array—features restricted in combination to embryonal neurons.[578] Furthermore, both the Homer Wright rosette and pale island constitute loci of concentrated immunoreactivity for neuron-specific enolase and various cytoplasmic antigens of a more restricted neuronal distribution (e.g., the class III beta-tubulin isotype, microtubule-associated protein 2, and synaptophysin).[577,578] The latter's oligodendroglia-like constituents are actually neuroblastic in nature.

Ultrastructural evidences of more advanced neuronal maturation that include the presence of clear and dense-core secretory vesicles and, in some cases, synapse formation characterize select *neuroblastic medulloblastomas* that have also been termed *cerebellar neuroblastomas*.[557,583] These tumors often contain elements of conventional desmoplastic medulloblastoma but exhibit a more strikingly lobular microarchitecture, their reticulin-free zones having unusually elongated profiles, being particularly rich in fibrillary matrix material and populated by cells arrayed in linear streams (Fig. 28-84). Neoplasms of this sort have been shown to occasionally undergo sequential maturation to highly differentiated ganglion cell tumors.[571] It has been suggested that they constitute a subset of medulloblastomas carrying an especially favorable prognosis.[585]

Only rarely is glial differentiation sufficiently advanced as to be obvious on routine histologic assessment of a medulloblastoma. Immunocytochemical screening for GFAP expression, however, may disclose included astrocytic elements of an unquestionably neoplastic nature, these varying greatly in number and distribution.[557,568,580] Noteworthy is the observation that the desmoplastic medulloblastoma often harbors within its pale islands a conspicuous network of GFAP-reactive cells, suggesting that these micronodular zones are organized loci of divergent astroglial, as well as neuronal, outgrowth.[577,578] The possibility, however, that such cells are reactive astrocytes recruited to these foci is not easily dismissed. It should be pointed out that many medulloblastomas contain scattered GFAP-positive elements that tend to lie near stromal blood vessels and that display the stellate cytoplasmic configurations typical of non-neoplastic astroglia. Their presence should not be construed as evidence of a tumor's ability to differentiate along astrocytic lines. We mention in passing immunocytochemical studies suggesting that medulloblastomas share with retinoblastomas and pineoblastomas the capacity to express photoreceptor-associated proteins such as opsin and the S-antigen.[569,580] Although interpreted as supporting the unified cytogenesis of these embryonal neuroepithelial neoplasms,

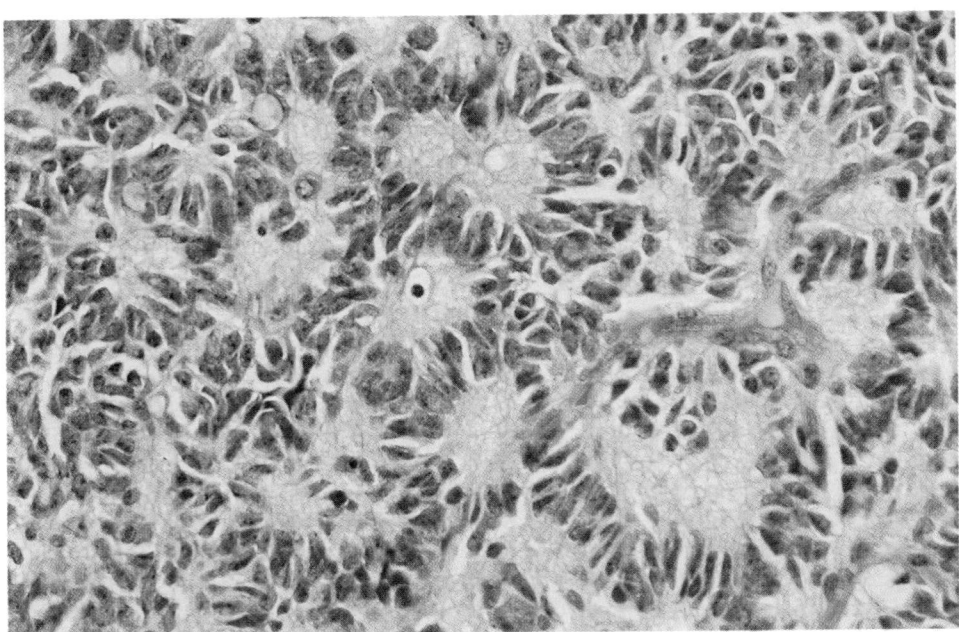

Fig. 28-83 Medulloblastoma. Homer Wright rosettes consist of tumor cell nuclei disposed in circular fashion about tangled cytoplasmic processes. These structures are indicative of differentiation along neuronal lines.

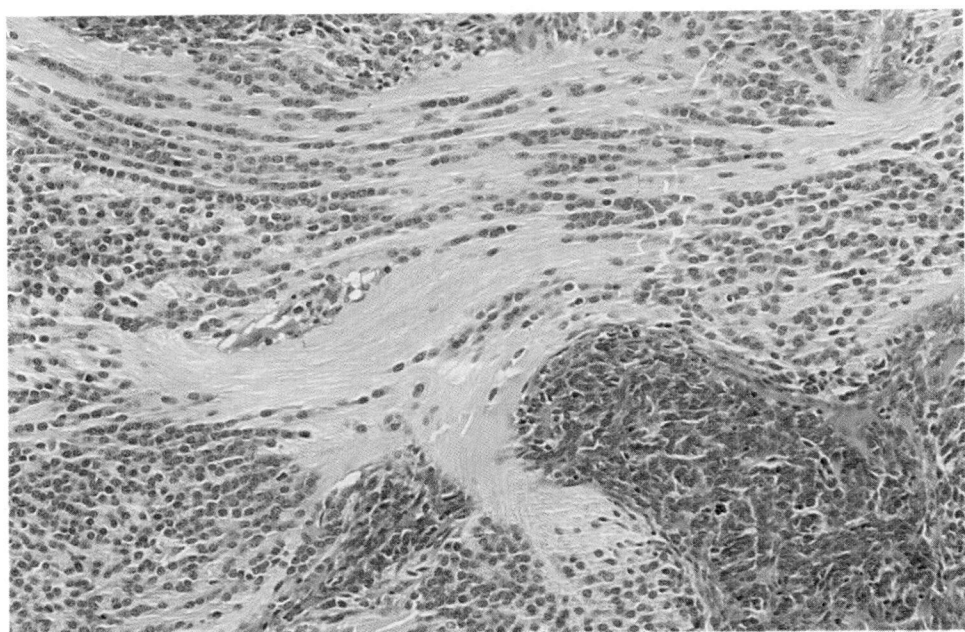

Fig. 28-84 "Neuroblastic" medulloblastoma. This variant of medulloblastoma is typified by the linear streaming of rounded, "neurocytic" tumor cell nuclei within amassed cytoplasmic processes.

the biologic significance of this phenomenon is far from clear.

The reader should note that we have elected to cite only a small sample of the more recent studies detailing the medulloblastoma's immunohistochemical profile and make no attempt to analyze the conflicting data that have emerged from repeated efforts to correlate the expression of neuronal, glial, or photoreceptor-associated antigens with this tumor's clinical behavior. Simply put, neither immunophenotype nor conventional light microscopic evidences of differentiation along specific cell lines have been shown to influence outcome in a consistently predictable fashion,[557,575,580] although the neuroblastic medulloblastoma ("cerebellar neuroblastoma") may well emerge as a relatively indolent variant.[585] Features associated with decreased survival rates include conspicuous mitotic activity, necrosis, a diploid DNA histogram, a high proliferative index, and amplification of the c-*myc* gene,[565,573,579,585] but none of these are widely applied to management planning, and all medulloblastomas are currently approached as potentially aggressive neoplasms. Among clinical variables, only disseminated disease at diagnosis (i.e., cytologic or neuroradiologic evidence of CSF seeding) has clearly emerged as being of independent (and understandably ominous) prognostic import.[573,582] The excess mortality noted in infants and very young children may simply reflect the particularly high incidence of neuraxis metastasis at diagnosis in this cohort and the reluctance of treating physicians to expose the immature nervous system to the tumoricidal, but ultimately toxic, doses of radiation required to control this disease. Whether less than total resection prejudices matters against afflicted patients remains uncertain, but most neuro-oncologists and neurosurgeons believe that operative extirpation of all visible tumor should be the immediate goal of therapy if technically feasible.

The prognosis for patients with medulloblastomas has improved dramatically over the last several decades, largely because of recognition that disease control requires, in addition to high-dose irradiation of the posterior fossa contents, inclusion of the entire craniospinal subarachnoid space in the treatment field to address the tendency of these aggressive neoplasms to disseminate via CSF pathways. Five-year survival rates of 70% or better have been achieved by irradiation alone in patients with tumors confined at diagnosis to the posterior fossa and free of the brainstem.[573] The addition of chemotherapy has succeeded in increasing the 5-year actuarial survival of patients with locally advanced disease (including bulbar infiltration) to better than 80%.[582] Unfortunately, however, many children evidence leptomeningeal metastasis on initial evaluation, and the outlook for such patients is not nearly so favorable. Although late relapses are well documented,[586] the great majority of pediatric medulloblastomas conform to Collins' law, which defines the risk period for recurrence of an embryonal childhood neoplasm as equal to the patient's age at diagnosis plus 9 months. Most deaths occur within 2 to 3 years of presentation.

Local (i.e., posterior fossa) recurrence has been the major pattern of treatment failure in the era of whole neuraxis irradiation, but the incidence of systemic metastases may well be on the rise with increasingly effective control of CNS disease.[586] In fact, no neuroepithelial tumor rivals the medulloblastoma in its proclivity for extraneural spread,[557,573] a complication that may ultimately supervene in more than 10% to 15% of conventionally treated patients.[586] Inasmuch as skeletal deposits, often widespread, account for more than 90% of systemic metastases and occasionally develop early in the medulloblastoma's clinical evolution, neuro-oncologists now routinely include bone marrow examination in the staging evaluation of afflicted patients. Lymph nodes and lungs may also be involved and ventriculoperitoneal shunts inserted to relieve persistent hydrocephalus can grant tumors access to the abdominal cavity. The addition of chemotherapy to the initial treatment regimen may exert some protective effect against distant metastasis[586] and is also being explored as a means of lowering the radiation doses required to effect cure. Disheartening is the price exacted of many survivors by childhood irradiation for this tumor, its complications including growth failure, serious intellectual impairment, behavioral disturbances, and the induction of secondary neoplasms.[573] References to radiation-associated meningiomas, sarcomas, and glioblastomas arising in this setting are provided in the sections dealing with these specific tumor types.

Regarding matters of differential diagnosis, it is the neuronal immunophenotype of many medulloblastomas that merits emphasis. Although relatively few can be shown to elaborate neurofilament protein on assay with commercially available reagents, the large majority at least focally express synaptophysin. In problematic cases, this property may be exploited to exclude from further consideration such potentially confounding lesions as the poorly differentiated fourth ventricular ependymoma, other anaplastic gliomas, and primary cerebellar lymphomas (typified by a B-cell immunoprofile). We have not encountered a solitary cerebellar metastasis as the presenting manifestation of an otherwise occult small cell carcinoma, but this diagnosis may be entertained by the pathologist confronted with an adult-onset medulloblastoma. Although synaptophysin reactivity may be shared by both neoplasms, it has been our experience that the expression of EMA, a conspicuous feature of anaplastic small cell carcinomas, is generally foreign to the medulloblastoma. The latter, it should be noted, may contain cytokeratin-positive elements,[559] although these are usually few and far between.

Medulloepithelioma

The *medulloepithelioma* is a highly aggressive, embryonal neoplasm that typically arises in the cerebrum of an infant or child younger than 5 years of age.[590] The tumor's frequent association with a lateral ventricle has been cited in support of its postulated origin from the lining germinal matrix of the developing forebrain, although lesions situated in the cerebellum, brainstem, and cauda equina have also been accorded this designation.[590] Often attaining enormous proportions, medulloepitheliomas are usually well circumscribed and composed of friable, grayish-pink tissue evidencing hemorrhage, necrosis, and in some cases, cystic degeneration. Their defining feature is the formation of tubules, ribbons, or papillae resembling, and believed to rep-

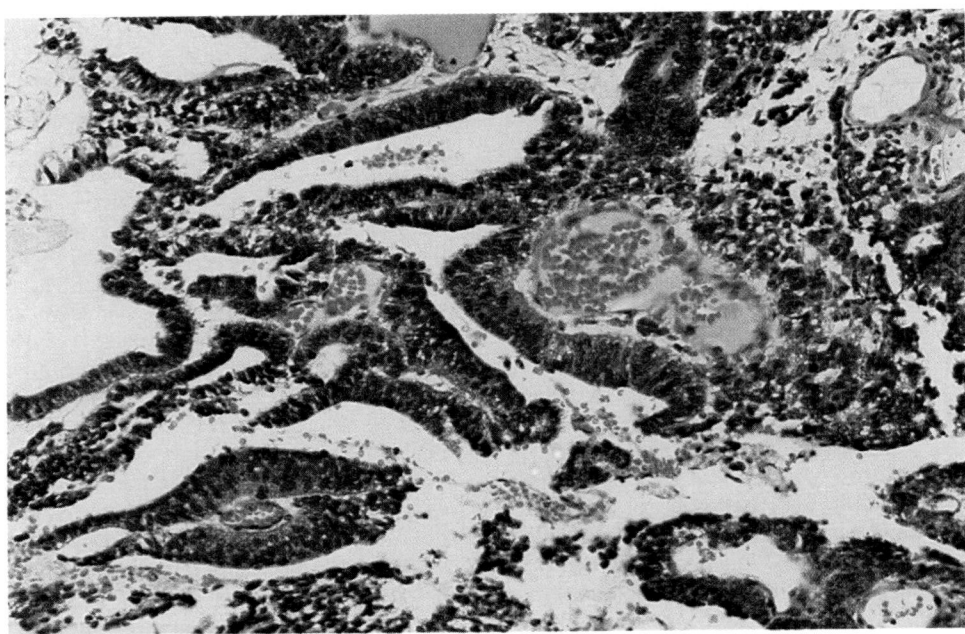

Fig. 28-85 Medulloepithelioma. A tubulopapillary disposition of its columnar elements characterizes this primitive neuroepithelial neoplasm.

resent, a recapitulation of the neural tube's primitive medullary epithelium (Fig. 28-85). These are fashioned of pseudostratified columnar cells that rest on a continuous, PAS-positive basement membrane and are sometimes capped by apical cytoplasmic protrusions ("blebs"). PAS-positive material may also coat these cells' luminal surfaces in limiting membrane–like fashion. Mitotic figures are readily identified and are generally abluminal in location, a pattern reminiscent of the juxtaventricular proliferative activity that characterizes early neurocytogenesis. Medullary epithelial structuring varies widely in extent and may constitute only a focal finding in an otherwise patternless, small cell malignant neoplasm.

In keeping with their proposed stem cell derivation, these tumors are clearly capable of, and often manifest, divergent differentiation and maturation, at times advanced, along astrocytic, ependymal, neuronal, and possibly, oligodendroglial lines.[589,590] An example containing chondroid, osseous, and skeletal muscle elements has also been depicted,[587] although the exact nosologic position of this lesion in relation to the immature teratoma, which may also harbor medullary-type neuroepithelial formations, is problematic. Obviously, the presence of admixed nonteratomatous germ cell components and evidence of endodermal or somatic ectodermal differentiation should be sought and excluded before a diagnosis of medulloepithelioma is rendered, particularly if neoplastic mesenchymal tissues are identified.

Given its tubulopapillary growth pattern, the differential diagnosis of the medulloepithelioma must also include the high-grade ependymoma, ependymoblastoma, and choroid plexus carcinoma. The few ultrastructural studies recorded to date indicate that the cells composing medullary epithelial structures are neither crowned by the microvilli and cilia nor joined by the complex zonulae adherentes–type junctions typical of ependymal derivatives.[590,591] Their elaboration of both a basal lamina and internal limiting membrane is yet another feature distinguishing medulloepithelioma from these other tumor types. Because immunocytochemical investigation has been limited to isolated cases,[558,587,588,591] it is impossible to generalize regarding the antigenic phenotype of this embryonal neoplasm. If its reported cytokeratin and S-100 negativity prove a consistent finding, this might serve as a further point of distinction from malignant epithelial tumors of choroid plexus origin. The latter, it should be noted, tend to a more obviously papilliform architecture than is exhibited by most medulloepitheliomas and are incapable of neuronal or astrocytic differentiation. Last, we mention the existence of glioblastomas containing medulloepithelioma-like structures, cited in our discussion of the diffuse fibrillary astrocytomas. The fact that bona fide medulloepitheliomas may contain regions exhibiting the features of ependymoma, ependymoblastoma, and glioblastoma clearly complicates matters.

Clinical experience with the medulloepithelioma, although limited, has served to sufficiently characterize its biology.[590] The large majority of affected patients have succumbed within 1 year of diagnosis, their courses frequently complicated by widespread leptomeningeal metastasis.

Neuroblastoma

The diagnosis of **neuroblastoma** is probably best reserved for extracerebellar neoplasms of embryonal character that can be shown to differentiate along neuronal, but not glial, lines. We concur with the view that the cerebellar "neuroblastoma" represents a variant of medulloblastoma and label as "primitive neuroectodermal tumor" the unusual extracerebellar neoplasm of embryonal type that evidences bidirectional, glioneuronal maturation. Also to be segregated from the tumors under discussion are the largely intraventricular central neurocytoma and superficially positioned desmoplastic infantile ganglioglioma, previously given separate consideration. Delimited in this fashion, neuroblastomas of the CNS are typified by a deep cerebral hemispheric localization and a presentation in the first decade of life, most recorded cases having been discovered in children younger than 5 years of age.[593,596]

Consisting of friable gray tissue prone to necrosis and cystic change, neuroblastomas are often quite large by the time patients come to surgery but usually appear to be sharply demarcated. Induction of a collagenous stroma lends to some examples a firm consistency and unusually lobulated contours. Although the division seems to be of no practical biologic significance, several subtypes can be distinguished on histologic grounds. The "classic" neuroblastoma is composed of small, mitotically active cells possessed of densely hyperchromatic nuclei and disposed in highly populous sheets variably punctuated by a delicate, fibrillary matrix material representing their tangled cytoplasmic processes. It is this variant that is most likely to contain diagnostic Homer Wright rosettes and large, differentiated neurons ("ganglion" cells). The "desmoplastic" neuroblastoma is defined by a fibrous stroma, most developed in regions where tumor contacts the leptomeninges, that imposes a lobular, trabecular, or Indian-file arrangement on its constituent cells. Larger than classic neuroblasts, the latter are characterized by vesicular nuclei and often prominent nucleoli and may possess a more clearly defined, albeit modest, expanse of hematoxyphylic or plum-colored cytoplasm. *Transitional neuroblastomas,* as their name implies, combine features of both the classical and desmoplastic variants. Still other neuroblastomas exhibit a compact nuclear palisading that imparts a polar spongioblastoma-like appearance.[597] It should be pointed out that central neuroblastic tumors only rarely evidence the graded, maturational nuclear and cytoplasmic alterations so often displayed by their retroperitoneal and posterior mediastinal counterparts.[592,595,598] Exceptional neoplasms of this sort merit designation as **ganglioneuroblastomas.**

In the absence of Homer Wright rosettes or included neurons that are clearly intrinsic to the neoplasm rather than entrapped, the diagnosis of neuroblastoma requires ultrastructural or immunocytochemical confirmation. On electron microscopic study, tumor cell processes can be shown to contain microtubules (often in parallel array) and dense-core or clear secretory vesicles. Attempts at synapse formation, usually abortive, are apparent in only a small minority of cases.

Immunohistochemical assay may supplant ultrastructural examination if cytoplasmic synaptophysin or neurofilament protein expression can be documented. Synaptophysin labeling, in our experience, is the far more sensitive index and is typically concentrated in the tumor's fibrillar matrix. Cell bodies and cytoplasmic processes are also characteristically reactive with antibodies to neuron-specific enolase, but such labeling is by no means restricted to central neuroepithelial tumors of neuronal type. The capacity of central ganglioneuroblastomas to differentiate along Schwann cell lines, sup-

ported by ultrastructural studies, may account for the presence of GFAP-positive elements in select tumors of this type,[595] but expression of this antigen should otherwise be limited to the processes of cells reasonably interpreted as reactive astrocytes. These are most numerous at the tumor-brain interface, but may also lie embedded deep within the lesion's substance, usually lying near penetrating blood vessels.

The interpretation of survival data reported for patients with cerebral neuroblastomas is complicated by the inclusion in some clinical series of cases that would now be reclassified as examples of central neurocytoma or desmoplastic infantile ganglioglioma, both associated with a favorable prognosis, as well as anaplastic small cell tumors exhibiting no convincing evidence of neuronal differentiation. Still, neuroblastomas seem more amenable to surgical and radiotherapeutic management than other primitive extracerebral neoplasms,[593] and a particularly gratifying outcome following resection of largely cystic lesions has been reported.[594] Unfortunately, the risks of local regrowth and CSF-borne metastasis are high, occasional examples spreading to extraneural sites.[593,596] Noteworthy are isolated cases of late local recurrence in which reoperation has demonstrated maturation of cerebral neuroblastomas to fully differentiated ganglion cell tumors.[592,598]

Ependymoblastoma

The *ependymoblastoma* is a rare neuroepithelial neoplasm of infancy and early childhood that is usually cerebral in location but that may also present in the posterior fossa.[599,601] A minority arise in contact with the ventricular system. The tumor is densely populated by small, monomorphic cells disposed in anastomosing cords and sheets punctuated by "ependymoblastic" rosettes. These are distinguished from rosettes of mature ependymal type by a multilayered stratification of their encircling nuclei and by their manifest proliferative activity, mitotic figures often lying in a juxtaluminal position.[601] As such, these structures more closely resemble the retinoblastoma's Flexner-Wintersteiner rosettes. Although tubules and canals lined by a monolayer of well-differentiated ependymal cells may be present, the perivascular pseudorosettes characteristic of the ependymoma are not formed. Foci of necrosis are common but not surrounded by tumor cells in palisaded array, and there is generally no evidence of vascular ("endothelial") proliferation—additional features segregating this embryonal neoplasm from conventional ependymomas that have undergone anaplastic change. Ultrastructural studies have confirmed the lesion's capacity for advanced maturation along ependymal lines, demonstrating that its rosette-forming elements are joined at their apices by elaborate junctional complexes and richly endowed with microvilli and cilia,[600] but the few examples subjected to immunocytochemical assay have not shared the ependymoma's expression of GFAP.[599] We have already alluded to regional ependymoblastic differentiation on the part of medulloepitheliomas. Ependymoblastomas, by definition, are devoid of medullary epithelial formations and their primitive small cell elements exhibit no differentiation along neuronal lines. Local leptomeningeal invasion is the rule and may be complicated by disseminated, CSF-borne neuraxial metastases. Survival is usually measured in months.

Polar spongioblastoma

The *polar spongioblastoma* is composed of spindled cells whose fusiform nuclei appear suspended in compact palisades between delicate unipolar or bipolar cytoplasmic processes arrayed in close parallel fashion. This arresting histologic presentation has been likened to the radial arrangement of migrating glia ("spongioblasts") that characterizes the 16- to 18-week stage of human neuroembryogenesis.[604]

It is in deference to the view that the polar spongioblastoma represents a primitive neuroepithelial neoplasm that we briefly address it here, but there is, in fact, considerable controversy as to whether the peculiar tumors awarded this designation constitute a unified pathologic entity.[604,605] Skeptics point to the fact that a rhythmic, palisading architecture may be encountered in neoplasms that otherwise qualify as classic oligodendrogliomas, pilocytic astrocytomas, glioblastomas, ependymomas, cerebral neuroblastomas, or medulloblastomas.[605] To believers, however, the frequent admixture of identifiably oligodendroglial and astrocytic elements is simply evidence of the polar spongioblastoma's derivation from embryonic forebears largely committed to differentiation along glial lines.[604] Other than a predilection for children, no distinctive topographic or biologic features serve to ally the lesions reported under this rubric, further complicating their uncritical acceptance as representatives of a defined neoplastic process. Neither has a diagnostic immunocytochemical or ultrastructural profile emerged from the handful of cases studied to date. The tumor's constituent "spongioblasts" are said to be nonreactive for GFAP, a finding interpreted as consonant with their primitive nature.[603,604] Whether examples reported to contain intracytoplasmic dense-core granules and microtubules[602] are not better regarded as variants of neuroblastoma is open to question.

It is our view that the diagnosis of polar spongioblastoma, if resorted to at all, should be reserved for neoplasms that exhibit a compact, palisaded growth pattern throughout. Careful search should be made for telltale foci exhibiting the features of any of the conventional tumors listed and classification based on the histology of such areas, however limited in volume. Ultrastructural examination is required to exclude the alternative diagnosis of palisaded cerebral neuroblastoma.

Primitive neuroectodermal tumor

The term *primitive neuroectodermal tumor (PNET)* was originally coined not as a generic alternative to "embryonal neuroepithelial neoplasm," which it has become, but to designate a cerebral tumor of infancy and childhood characterized by a medulloblastoma-like histologic presentation and propensity for widespread dissemination along CSF pathways.[608] As originally defined, at least 90% of the lesion's constituent cells were altogether devoid of differentiated features, uniformly small, densely hyperchromatic, and disposed in patternless sheets. Desmoplastic mesenchymal components were a conspicuous feature of many cases, additional findings including sharp tumor circumscription, high mitotic rates, necrosis, and cystic change. Histologic appearances suggestive of limited glial, neuronal, or bidirectional differentiation were often noted.[608,610]

The problems inherent in defining a tumor largely on the basis of its undifferentiated, primitive appearance should be obvious. The diagnosis of PNET would seem to rest on firmest grounds in the presence of divergent neuronoglial differentiation. The demonstration of a polymorphous immunophenotype may prove especially useful in this regard, because some PNETs have been shown to co-express synaptophysin and multiple intermediate filament proteins (usually the complex of vimentin-GFAP-neurofilament protein but, occasionally, cytokeratin and desmin as well).[559] The nosologic status in relation to cerebral neuroblastomas of PNETs containing isolated Homer Wright rosettes or evidencing neuronal characteristics on immunocytochemical or ultrastructural study is problematic in the absence of attendant glial differentiation. Similarly murky is the distinction of the PNET exhibiting glial differentiation alone from a highly anaplastic glioma. In practice, we find ourselves applying the former label to largely monomorphic, small cell neoplasms of childhood composed, in part, of GFAP-reactive elements but exhibiting neither the glomeruloid vascular hyperplasia nor the tendency for tumor cells to palisade about foci of necrosis that typify high-grade gliomas (particularly astrocytomas) of conventional type. Immunolabeled cells often huddle in small clusters or aggregate about stromal blood vessels, are poorly fibrillated, and may assume a microgemistocytic or even rhabdoid appearance. We would caution the reader against the "low percentage" diagnosis of PNET in the adult because the patient so labeled almost invariably proves to harbor a glioblastoma with small cell features at reoperation or autopsy. Again, convincing ultrastructural and immunocytochemical evidence of divergent glioneuronal differentiation should be sought to substantiate the diagnosis in this setting.

The spectrum of primitive neuroepithelial neoplasia occurring outside the confines of the cerebellum includes embryonal tumors evidencing choroid plexus[609] and smooth[612] and striated muscle[606] differentiation. A lesion harboring ganglioneuroblastomatous and schwannian elements but otherwise bearing a close clinical and morphologic resemblance to the desmoplastic infantile ganglioglioma has been depicted,[607] as has a "mixed" tumor composed of neuroblasts and astrocytes unaccompanied by a demonstrable "stem cell" (i.e., undifferentiated) population.[611] Also noteworthy are neoplasms interpreted as intracranial examples of the melanotic neuroectodermal tumor of infancy[614] and PNETs that occur following prophylactic cranial irradiation for childhood leukemia and lymphoma.[556] Last, there is report of a unique, desmoplastic embryonal neoplasm arising in the cerebellum but conforming to no recognized variant of medulloblastoma.[613] The described case was characterized by a cellular, immature-appearing "stroma," populated by desmin-immunoreactive elements, embedded within which were nests and cords of small neuroepithelial cells variably labeled by antisera to synaptophysin, neurofilament protein, GFAP, and cytokeratin. At recurrence, this peculiar lesion exhibited strikingly epithelioid features and overt neuronal (ganglion cell) differentiation.

Pineal parenchymal tumors

Tumors of specialized pineal parenchymal lineage include an embryonal variant designated as pineoblastoma, a differentiated subtype termed the pineocytoma, and lesions manifesting transitional or mixed features.[623a,627]

The *pineoblastoma* is largely, although not exclusively, a pediatric entity, most cases presenting in the first decade of life with signs and symptoms of intracranial hypertension secondary to ventricular outflow obstruction at the level of the cerebral aqueduct. Pressure exerted on the mesencephalic tectum may also result in disturbances of ocular motility. Primitive and medulloblastoma-like in appearance, this densely populated neoplasm is composed of diminutive, hyperchromatic, and mitotically active cells disposed in patternless sheets or lobules that are often punctuated by zones of coagulative necrosis and dystrophic calcification.[621,623a,627] The monotony may be relieved by the formation of Homer Wright rosettes, identical to those of the medulloblastoma and neuroblastoma, that attest to this embryonal tumor's shared capacity to differentiate along neuronal lines. Rare variants contain mature ganglion cells or glial elements,[621,629] whereas occasional examples evince an atavistic potential for photosensory differentiation that recapitulates the parent organ's phylogenesis as the primary photoreceptor of low vertebrates and "third eye" of some mammalian species. The pineoblastoma may thus fashion Flexner-Wintersteiner rosettes and fleurettes a la the retinoblastoma,[621] elaborate club-shaped cilia having the 9 + 0 axonemal array characteristic of photosensory cells,[624] and express rhodopsin, the rhodopsin-binding S-antigen (normally involved in visual signal transduction), and a retinoid-binding glycolipoprotein that appears early in retinal genesis.[623,623a,625]

The pineal gland's vestigial photosensory attributes are also obliquely evidenced by the documented occurrence of pineoblastomas, some exhibiting photoreceptor-associated features, in complex with retinoblastomas.[618,622] The ocular neoplasms in such cases are typically of the heritable, bilateral variety—prompting designation of this curious phenomenon as the syndrome of "trilateral retinoblastoma." Mention should also be made in this regard of rare pineoblastomas harboring melanotic elements that have been likened to pigmented ciliary or retinal-type epithelium,[626,628] similar cellular components transiently populating the fetal pineal gland and, parenthetically, typifying the melanotic neuroectodermal ("retinal anlage") tumor of infancy.[619] Such lesions may manifest, in addition to melanotic tubules, evidence of neuronal, ependymal, retinoblastomatous, and rhabdomyoblastic differentiation. The similarity of complex tumors of this type to neoplasms derived from the primitive medullary epithelium of the optic vesicle (teratoid ocular medulloepitheliomas or "diktyomas") has been noted.[626]

A highly aggressive lesion, the pineoblastoma cannot be controlled by surgical means. Local irradiation may result in apparent clinical and radiologic remission but is almost invariably followed in short order by recurrence at the primary site and widespread dissemination within the ventricular system and subarachnoid space. Patients treated in this fashion usually succumb to their disease within 2 years of diagnosis, but there is evidence to suggest that inclusion of the entire craniospinal axis in the radiation port substantially improves the outlook for afflicted individuals and that adjuvant or "salvage" chemotherapy may be of some benefit.[627]

In contrast to the pineoblastoma, the *pineocytoma* generally presents in young or middle-aged adults. Several histologic variants have been depicted,* although whether all merit such classification is open to question,[615,627] as discussed. A major subtype is the tumor in which anastomosing cords of neoplastic cells are arrayed in a conspicuous meshwork of delicate, synaptophysin-immunoreactive[616,623a] cytoplasmic processes, aggregating about this anuclear fibrillary matrix to form structures dubbed *pineocytomatous rosettes.*[615,627] Resembling outsized versions of the Homer Wright rosette (Fig. 28-86), these are unique to the pineocytoma and are composed at the ultrastructural level of neurite-like cytoplasmic extensions laden with microtubules and dense-core vesicles and joined by occasional synaptic complexes.[624] These features have prompted some observers to label tumors of this type as *pineocytomas with neuronal differentiation.*[621] Such lesions frequently harbor admixed multinucleated tumor giant cells[615] but are dominated by monomorphous, cytologically benign-appearing elements largely devoid of mitotic activity. Other examples lack pineocytomatous rosettes but rather closely mimic the microscopic architecture of the pineal gland in their organoid division, by a delicate fibrovascular stroma, into well-demarcated lobules. The latter display a greater variation in size and configuration than those constituting the pineal parenchyma and further deviate therefrom in not being separated by intervening astroglial elements.

Either variant may contain, as may the exceptional pineoblastoma, cells resembling non-neoplastic pinealocytes by virtue of their elaboration of unipolar cytoplasmic processes terminating in rounded varicosities,[621] although these do not maintain the strict juxtavascular polarity characteristic of their normal counterparts. Considered a specific indication of pinealocytic differentiation, such processes can be visualized by silver carbonate impregnation methods applicable to formalin-fixed, paraffin-embedded material.[617,621] Ultrastructural study will disclose their content of microtubules, "neurosecretory" granules, clear vesicles, and, in some cases, symmetric membrane thickenings or vesicle-crowned rodlets (also known as synaptic ribbons, a feature of mammalian pinealocytes).[624] Also shared with the cells of the normal pineal parenchyma are paired intracytoplasmic filaments, 8 nm in diameter, arrayed in helices exhibiting a 26 to 30 nm periodicity.[620] Like the pineoblastoma, these more mature pineal parenchymal tumors have been reported to exhibit divergent gangliogliomatous differentiation[621] and can express rhodopsin and the retinal S-antigen.[623a,625]

Survey of the literature shows that tumors of widely disparate biologic potential have been grouped under the appellation of pineocytoma.[627] There is general agreement that neoplasms characterized by pineocytomatous rosette formation ("pineocytomas with neuronal differentiation") grow slowly and tend not to invade neighboring tissues or to disseminate via CSF pathways.[615,623a,627] It is to these tumors that we restrict the designation of pineocytoma, after the suggestion of Borit et al.[615] Such lesions may ultimately kill by compressing adjacent bulbar structures but usually run a course considerably more protracted than that of the pineoblastoma. By contrast, the potential for both locally

---

*References 615, 621, 623a, 627, 630, 631.

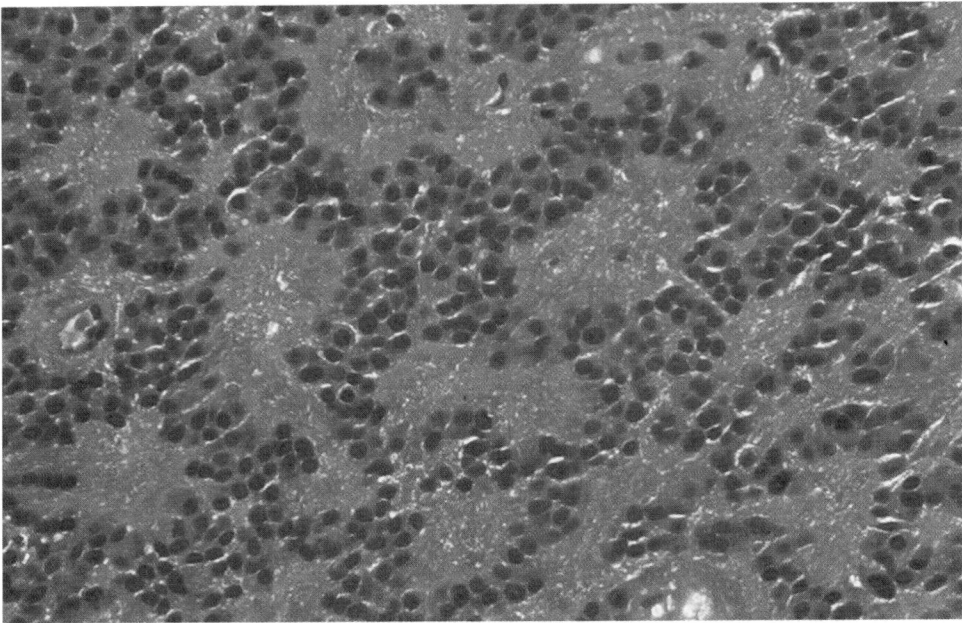

Fig. 28-86 Pineocytoma. Shown here are the conspicuous rosettes that constitute a defining feature of this neoplasm. Note the benign nuclear features, monomorphism, and absence of mitotic activity.

aggressive behavior and CSF-borne spread has been attached to lobular examples that fail to fashion rosettes of pineocytomatous type. Noteworthy is the fact that a subset of these metastasizing "pineocytomas" evidenced dense cellularity, conspicuous mitotic activity, necrosis, and pineoblastoma-like appearances in their secondary deposits.[621] Arguably, at least some represented unusually organoid variants of pineoblastoma from the outset or merited placement in a category of "**transitional pineal parenchymal neoplasm**" or "**pineal parenchymal tumor of intermediate differentiation**" reserved for the lesion seeming to occupy a position somewhere between the embryonal and mature extremes.[627] Similar nosologic considerations apply to rare tumors described as **papillary pineocytomas,**[630,631] one of which progressed rapidly.[630] Although appearing to exhibit advanced pinealocytic differentiation, this particular example manifested foci of sheet-like growth, necrosis, and the formation of fleurettes and rosettes of Flexner-Wintersteiner but not pineocytomatous type. Certainly, composite or "mixed" neoplasms harboring discrete pineocytomatous and pineoblastomatous elements have been depicted.[623a,627] These should be approached as potentially aggressive lesions.

Meningothelial tumors and related lesions

The designation of *meningioma* has been extended through the years to diverse neoplasms sharing only a tendency to arise within the histogenetically complex tissues of the leptomeninges or dura mater. Thus such dissimilar entities as the meningeal hemangiopericytoma and hemangioblastoma—currently accorded separate nosologic status among tumors of the CNS and its coverings—were once yoked under the regrettable rubric of "angioblastic" meningioma

and widely assumed to derive from a common progenitor. Most neuropathologists now label as meningiomas only those neoplasms exhibiting morphologic or immunophenotypic evidence of an origin from meningothelial cells, specialized elements that populate the arachnoid membranes and cap the arachnoidal villi associated with intradural venous sinuses and their tributaries.

Meningiomas may make their appearance in childhood or adolescence,[637,640] but most are encountered in middle adult life.[647,652] Females are afflicted far more commonly than males, and some studies suggest a particularly increased incidence in women with mammary carcinomas,[652] rare meningiomas actually harboring metastatic deposits derived from breast primaries.[675] Coupled with their frequent expression of progesterone (as well as androgen) receptors[657] and the rapid enlargement of some examples during pregnancy or the luteal phase of the menstrual cycle, these observations indicate that the growth of meningiomas is subject to hormonal influence. Noteworthy is the association of multifocal meningiomas with type 2 ("central") neurofibromatosis (NF-2),[647] the genetic locus for which resides on chromosome 22. Allelic loss involving this chromosome is a regular feature of meningiomas, whether they are sporadic or NF-2 related,[650a,671] suggesting that inactivation of a tumor-suppressing gene figures in their genesis. Familial examples occurring outside the setting of classic NF-2 have also been described.[647] Ionizing cranial irradiation has emerged from a number of epidemiologic studies as conferring significant risk for subsequent meningioma development,[652] radiation-related lesions being more often multiple, histologically atypical, and clinically aggressive than those arising in sporadic fashion.[642] Less clear is the etiologic role of craniocerebral

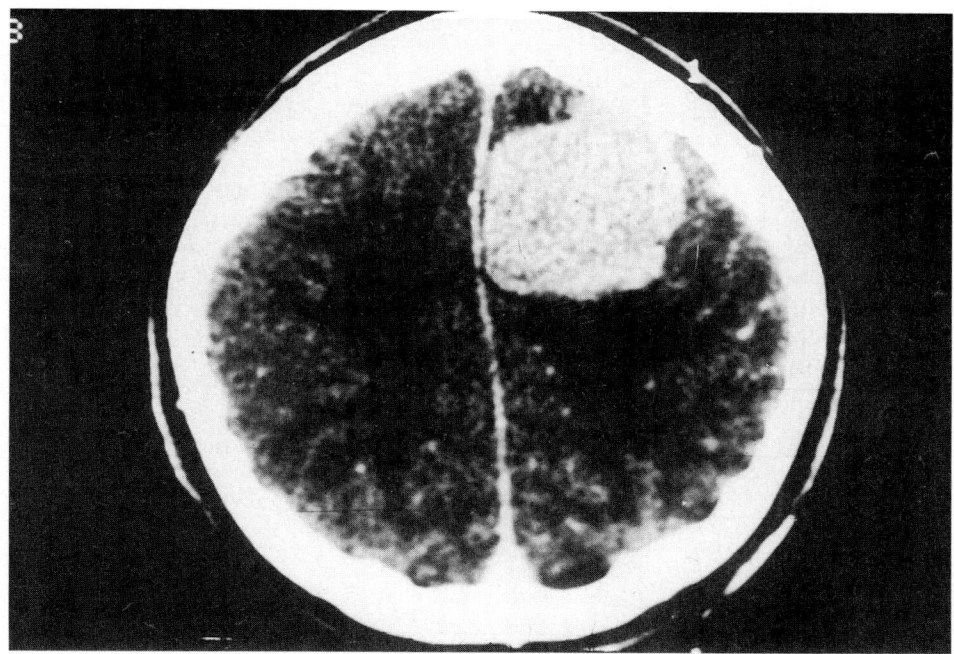

Fig. 28-87 Meningioma. Sharp circumscription, homogeneous enhancement, and broad anchorage to the dura (demonstrated at upper right of this CT scan) are hallmarks of the meningioma on postcontrast injection neuroimaging study.

trauma,[652] but the presentation of select meningiomas in the immediate vicinity of a prior skull fracture or in close physical association with traumatically implanted foreign bodies has been convincingly documented.[633,668] Also on record are meningiomas found to lie just over a glioblastoma or other glioma.[647,656a,672] Most "collision" tumors of this sort are undoubtedly fortuitous lesions, but it is conceivable that the occasional meningioma evokes a hyperplastic glial reaction that subsequently progresses to neoplasia.[656a] As noted in our discussion of gliomesenchymal neoplasms, the term *sarcoglioma* has been extended to some mixed tumors postulated to have arisen in this fashion.[460]

Most meningiomas arise within the cranial cavity, are dural based, and are found in the vicinity of the superior sagittal sinus, over the cerebral convexities or in contact with the falx cerebri. Basally positioned examples favor the sphenoid ridge, olfactory grooves, tuberculum sellae, and parasellar region. Still others are anchored to the petrous ridge, presenting as cerebellopontine angle tumors when posteriorly situated. Intracranial meningiomas may also originate within the tela choroidea or stroma of the choroid plexus and rest entirely within the ventricular system. At spinal levels, meningiomas clearly favor the thoracic region, cervical examples being uncommon and lumbar lesions rare. Also recognized are epidural (intradiploic), calvarial, and intrapetrous meningiomas as well as variants located entirely outside the craniospinal confines.[647] The latter are usually encountered in the head and neck region and include orbital (i.e., optic sheath), glabellar, sinonasal, oropharyngeal, subgaleal, juxtaparotid, and cutaneous examples.[647,653] Rarely, ectopic meningiomas are situated at even greater removes from the central neuraxis (e.g., in the medi-

astinum,[673] lung,[666] or brachial plexus[636]). As discussed elsewhere in these volumes, the so-called minute pulmonary chemodectoma is actually composed of cells having the ultrastructure and immunophenotype of meningothelium.

On neuroradiologic (Fig. 28-87) and gross assessment (Fig. 28-88), the typical meningioma is a solid, lobulated, or globose mass broadly anchored to the dura mater. Cystic variants, although uncommon, are well recognized,[663] and the term *meningioma en plaque* may be invoked for the occasional lesion that presents (usually over the sphenoid ridge) as a poorly delimited, blanket-like growth. Adjoining neural tissues are generally deflected at the neoplasm's "pushing" perimeter, but grossly evident dural infiltration or invasion of nearby venous sinuses is not uncommon. Some examples insidiously permeate the neighboring skull, provoking a highly characteristic form of osteoplastic expansion and bony remodeling known as hyperostosis or, neglected, come to attention as visible masses in the scalp. None of these findings brand a meningioma as malignant (a determination to be made on a given tumor's histologic appearance), although involvement of the cranial floor greatly prejudices matters against the neurosurgeon and so predisposes to tumor recurrence and progression following attempted resection. Highly suspect, however, is the lesion that cannot be easily separated from the adjacent brain or spinal cord because this implies transgression of the pia-arachnoid and invasion of the neuroparenchyma proper— traditionally regarded as prima facie evidence of malignancy in the setting of meningothelial neoplasia.

On sectioning, most meningiomas are grayish-tan and soft, but collagenized examples have a rubbery texture and a whorled or trabeculated cut surface (resembling that of the leiomyoma), whereas variants rich in stromal mucopolysac-charides acquire a somewhat gelatinous consistency. Calci-fication is often readily apparent and infiltration by foamy macrophages at times results in foci of yellow discoloration, a phenomenon that may also reflect the accumulation of lipids within tumor cells.

Meningiomas are notorious for the variety of their cyto-logic and histologic presentations, but most assume one of several prototypical guises.[647] "Meningotheliomatous" vari-ants are characterized by a lobular microarchitecture and are populated by cells having delicate round or oval nuclei, inconspicuous nucleoli, lightly eosinophilic cytoplasm, and indistinct cytoplasmic borders (thus their alternative desig-

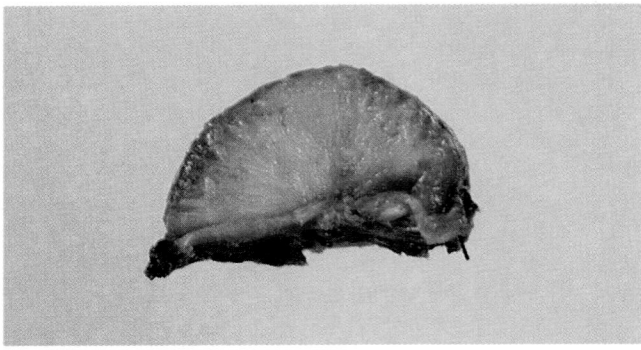

Fig. 28-88 Meningioma. The broad dural base depicted here is char-acteristic.

nation as *syncytial meningiomas*). Common to these (and other subtypes) are tumor cells concentrically wrapped in tight whorls, pale nuclear "pseudoinclusions" consisting of invaginated cytoplasm, and the lamellated calcospherules known as psammoma bodies (Fig. 28-89). While none of these features are pathognomonic of meningioma, their demonstration in the setting of an extra-axial, dural-based mass carries considerable diagnostic weight. In contrast to the epithelioid appearances of meningotheliomatous vari-ants, *fibroblastic* or *fibrous meningiomas* adopt a mesenchy-mal profile, being variably collagenized and consisting of spindly tumor cells in fascicular or storiform array (Fig. 28-90). *Transitional meningiomas,* as their name implies, are hybrids, maintaining a lobular arrangement but evidencing a tendency to cellular elongation and streaming. These are often particularly rich in compact cellular whorls and endowed with psammoma bodies in conspicuous numbers. When the latter are present in profusion, the term *psammo-matous meningioma* may be applied. Such tumors exhibit a particular predilection for the intraspinal compartment. It should be noted that none of the foregoing growth patterns is of any special biologic significance, most neuropatholo-gists dispensing with these qualifying adjectives in their reporting of surgical material.

To these classic subtypes of meningioma can be added histologic variants too numerous to be accorded (and too uncommon to merit) detailed discussion or depiction here. Only the more distinctive are acknowledged. Unless other-wise stated, these depart in no way from the benign course pursued by meningiomas of more conventional appearance.

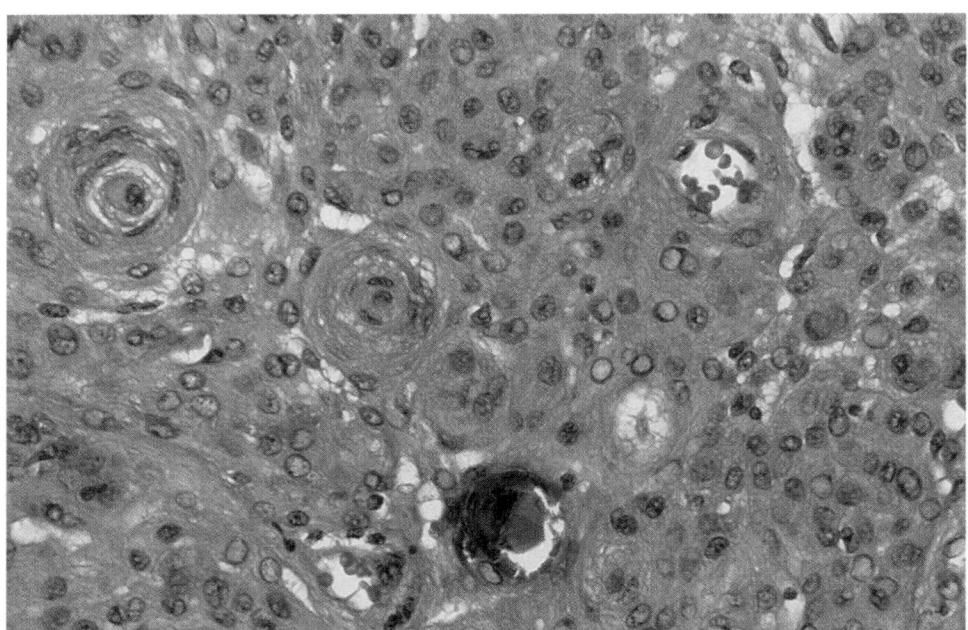

Fig. 28-89 Meningioma. Indistinct cytoplasmic boundaries, nuclear clearing ("pseudoinclusions"), cel-lular whorls, and a psammoma body are all apparent in this view of a meningotheliomatous (syncytial) meningioma.

The *microcystic meningioma*[658,662] is named for its content of variably sized intercellular vacuoles, these often appearing empty but in some instances containing a lightly PAS-positive fluid derived in all likelihood via the transudation of plasma across the neoplasm's characteristically rich, and frequently hyalinized, stromal vasculature. Some examples actually progress to the formation of macrocysts and harbor only minor solid components. The tumor's constituent cells may exhibit cytoplasmic clearing because of glycogen or lipid accumulation and often assume spindly or stellate profiles that, along with their tendency to disaggregation, can prompt consideration of a low-grade, microcystic astrocytoma in the differential diagnosis. Nuclear pleomorphism, karyomegaly, and a smudgy hyperchromasia may be in evidence but are unattended by mitotic activity and are divorced from any sinister prognostic import.

The *secretory meningioma*,[632] a variant of the meningotheliomatous subtype, is distinguished by its content of "pseudopsammoma bodies"—globular hyaline inclusions that are eosinophilic, intensely PAS positive, and diastase resistant (Fig. 28-91, *A*). On ultrastructural study, these can be shown to lie within microvillus-lined intracellular lumina and may be immunolabeled for human secretory component, IgM, IgA, and CEA (Fig. 28-91, *B*). Although entirely benign, the secretory meningioma may masquerade as a malignant neoplasm by virtue of its occasional association with elevated serum CEA levels,[654] an especially confounding phenomenon in the patient with a prior history of systemic cancer, and with subacutely progressive neurologic deficits referable to severe edema of juxtatumoral cerebral tissues. The latter,

generally foreign to conventional meningiomas and usually encountered as a complication of malignant meningeal neoplasms (primary or metastatic), may be related to a curious pericytic proliferation occurring in the vascular bed of select examples.[632,660]

The "inflammatory" meningioma is a tumor infiltrated by lymphoid and plasmacellular elements, at times so heavily as to obscure its meningothelial (and neoplastic) nature.[641,643] There can be no doubt that at least some reported cases would be better classified as dural-based examples of inflammatory pseudotumor ("plasma cell granuloma") or sinus histiocytosis with massive lymphadenopathy (Rosai-Dorfman disease). Peritumoral lymphoplasmacytic infiltrates with germinal center formation are also conspicuous features of a peculiar meningeal tumor noteworthy for its chordoid histology and presentation in childhood or adolescence with manifestations of the Castleman syndrome—polyclonal dysgammaglobulinemia, iron-refractory anemia, hepatosplenomegaly, and retarded growth and sexual maturation.[648] Resection typically effects a remission of the systemic disorder, but this obscure neoplasm may recur and behave in locally aggressive fashion.

Metaplastic meningiomas can contain bone, cartilage, or adipocytic elements.[647,669] We would call particular attention to a rare variant that may be misconstrued as sarcoma because of its lipoblastic cytologic features and the occurrence in some examples of troubling nuclear abnormalities that are probably degenerative in nature.[650] Meningiomas can also masquerade as chordomas or metastatic colloid carcinomas as a result of pronounced myxoid alterations[634,677] and may

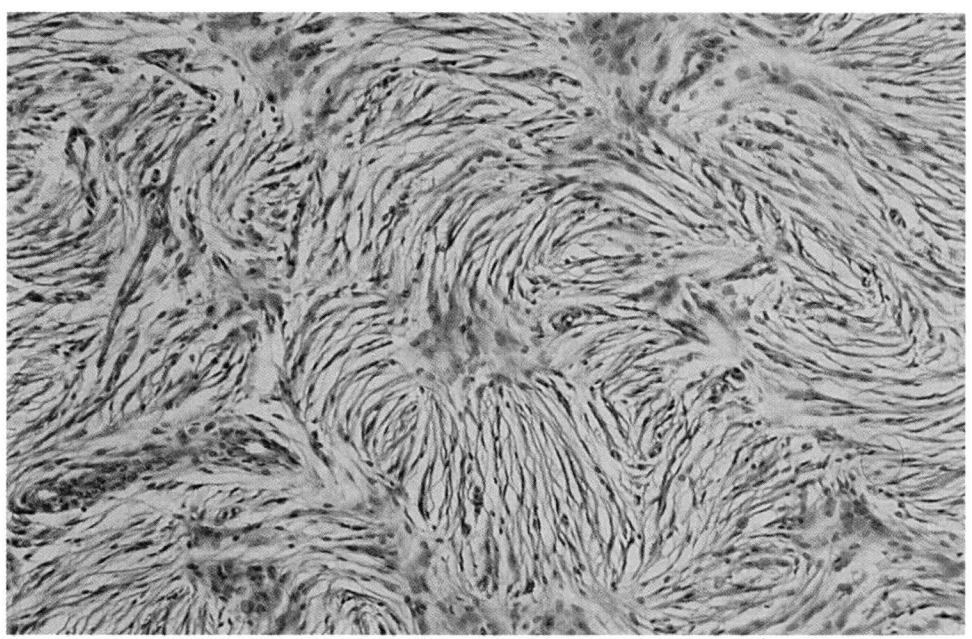

Fig. 28-90 Meningioma. Cellular spindling and a fascicular or storiform architecture are evidenced by meningiomas of "fibroblastic" type.

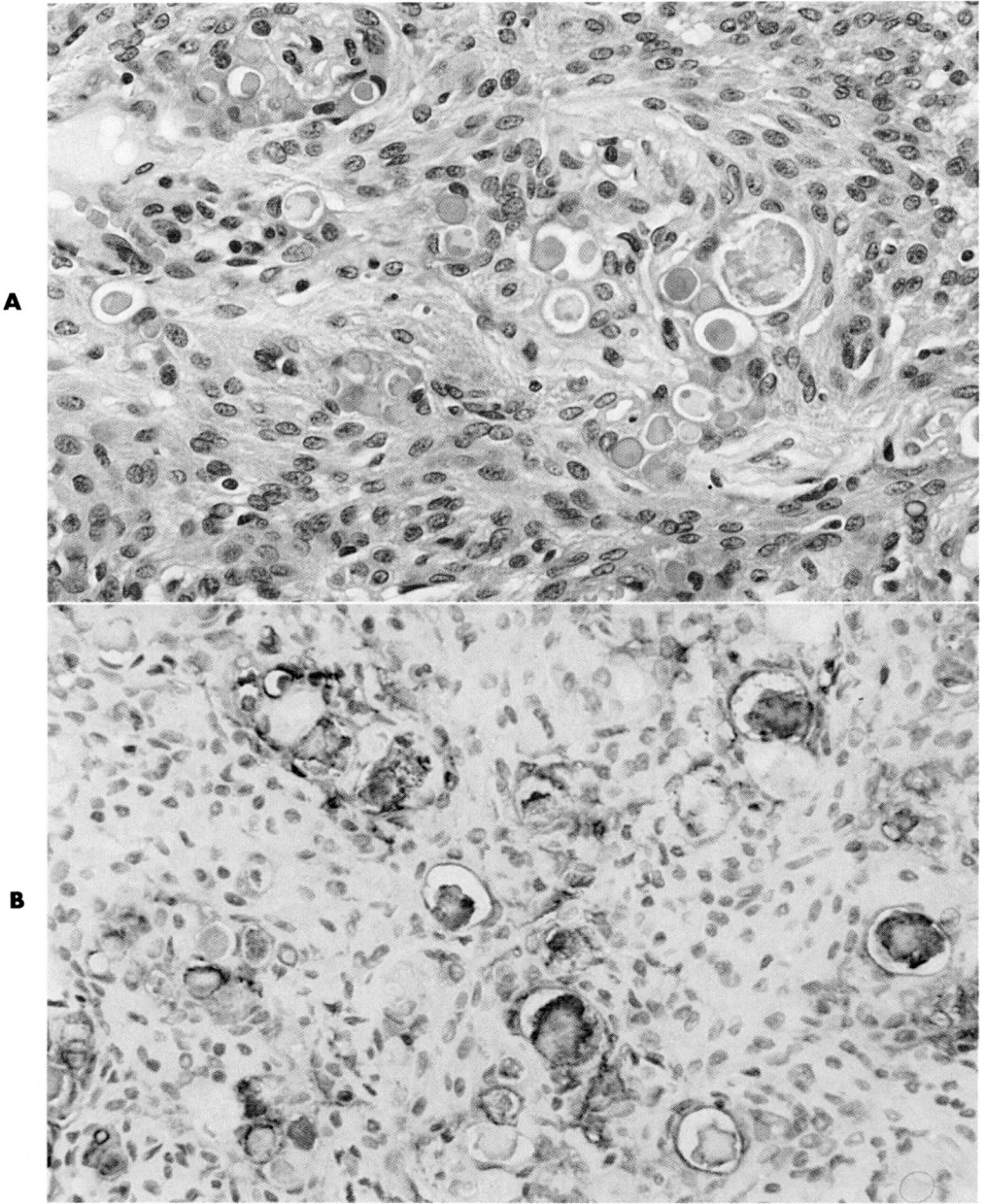

Fig. 28-91 Secretory meningioma. This variant of meningotheliomatous meningioma harbors eosinophilic globules **(A)** that label with antibodies to carcinoembryonic antigen **(B)**.

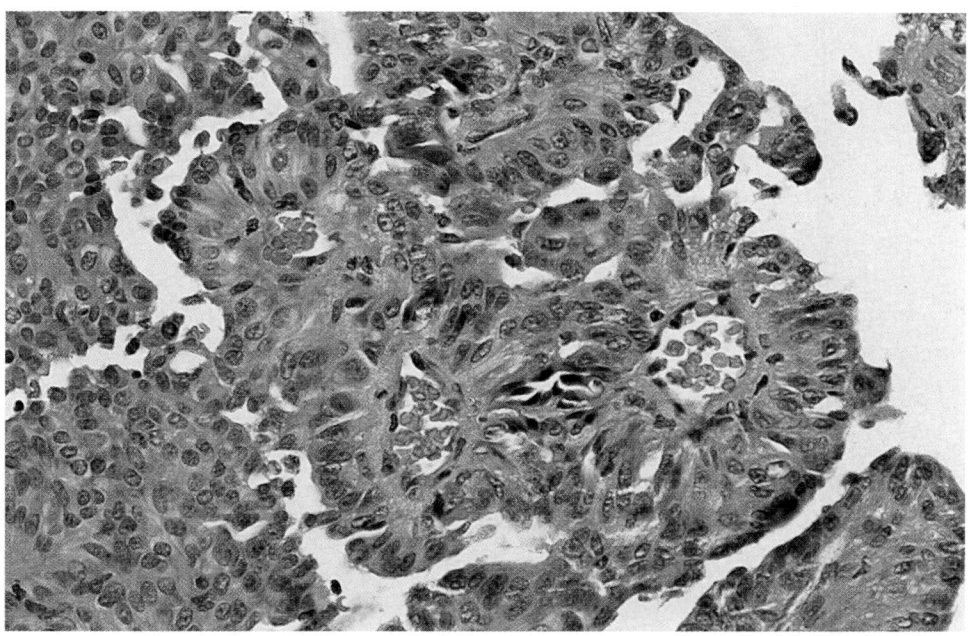

Fig. 28-92 Papillary meningioma. This intraspinal example, which elsewhere exhibited the histology of an atypical meningotheliomatous meningioma with increased mitotic activity and foci of necrosis, metastasized to lung, lymph node, and bone.

exhibit hyaline, granular, or clear cell features, the last potentially mimicking oligodendrogliomas and being prone to aggressive recurrence.[676] Still others evidence foci of schwannoma-like nuclear palisading; pseudoglandular structures[649]; a nesting arrangement reminiscent of paraganglioma; or a hyalinized stromal vasculature so exuberant and domineering as to suggest an angiomatous malformation.[647] A variety of eosinophilic cytoplasmic inclusions have also been described in the cells of meningiomas.[646,647] A sclerosing subtype that appears to undergo progressive fibrous obliteration is noteworthy for its presentation in the pediatric group and favorable outcome despite a tendency to foci of disturbing hypercellularity, pleomorphism, and cerebrocortical invasion.[637] As noted later, some observers have suggested a possible origin for this variant in the hamartomatous lesion known as meningioangiomatosis.

A final variant meriting specific comment in view of its distinctive histology and clinical biology is the *papillary meningioma,* a tumor characterized by the ependymoma-like perivascular structuring of its constituent cells.[655,664] The latter can be seen to extend variably elongated cytoplasmic processes toward vessel walls, fashioning pseudorosettes that frequently appear to float unanchored in tissue sections (Fig. 28-92). Regions exhibiting a more conventional meningothelial appearance are invariably identifiable but usually depart from the typical in evidencing worrisome hypercellularity, brisk mitotic activity, and in some cases, foci of coagulative necrosis. As these features would suggest, papillary meningiomas are potentially aggressive neoplasms noted for their tendency for stubborn local recurrence, their capacity for extraneural metastasis, and their

often fatal outcome. An excess of reported cases have presented in childhood or adolescence.

Distinction of the meningioma from potential counterfeits occasionally requires the use of the electron microscope or immunocytochemical assay. The former's most constant and distinctive ultrastructural feature is the complex interdigitation of tumor cell processes without intervening basal lamina material (elaborated by both the meningeal hemangiopericytoma and schwannoma), although fibroblastic variants tend to a more parallel alignment. Intercellular junctional complexes are frequent and include well-developed desmosomes, a conspicuous cytoplasmic complement of intermediate filaments rounding out the ultrastructural picture (Fig. 28-93). The latter consist of vimentin, regularly demonstrable by immunohistochemical methods regardless of a given meningioma's histologic pattern.[674] Of particular diagnostic utility is the observation that a large majority of meningiomas exhibit membranous, as well as diffuse, cytoplasmic immunolabeling for EMA[674] (Fig. 28-94), a feature foreign to tumors of pericytic, schwannian, or fibrocytic derivation. Reactivity for S-100 protein, if present, is generally weak and is limited to the cytoplasm of only a minor subset of neoplastic cells. Also exceptional is cytokeratin expression, though some investigators have noted focal immunoreactivity in up to 30% of routinely processed (i.e., formalin-fixed) cases.[665] The elaboration of cytokeratin proteins by cells of meningothelial lineage would appear to be correlated with ultrastructural evidences of epithelial differentiation such as intracellular tonofilament bundle accumulation and lumen formation, being characteristic among meningiomas only of the inclusion-bearing elements found

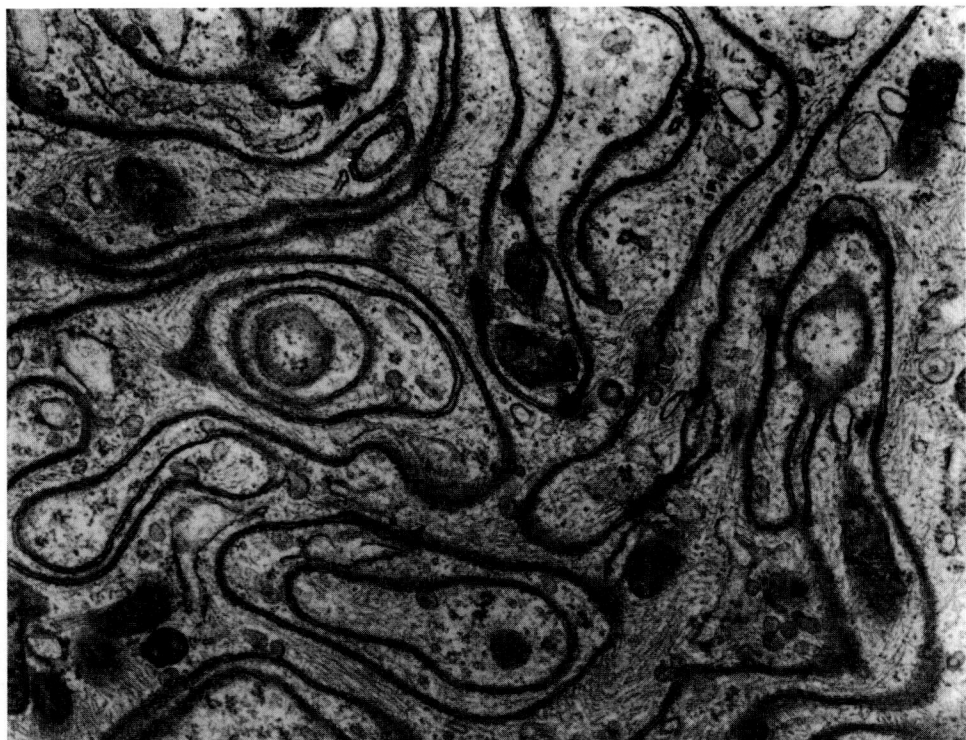

Fig. 28-93 Meningioma. Ultrastructural examination of meningiomas will often disclose complex, jig-saw puzzle–like arrays of interdigitated cytoplasmic processes laden with intermediate filaments and joined by desmosomes. As demonstrated here, neoplastic meningothelial cells are not typically coated by basement membranes (a feature of Schwann cells), nor does basal lamina material accumulate in their matrices (a characteristic of the hemangiopericytoma illustrated in Fig. 28-97). (×18,000.)

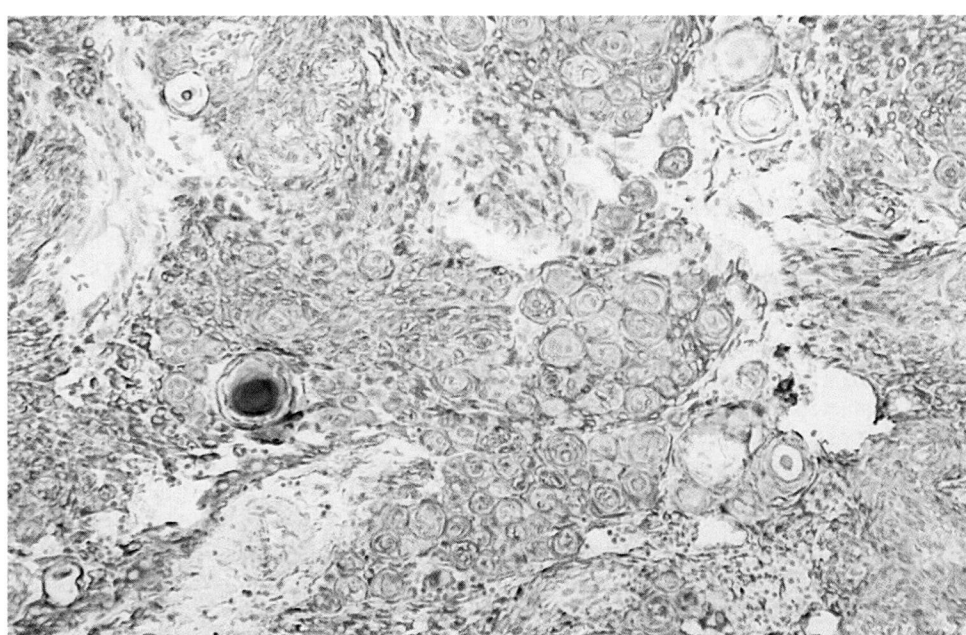

Fig. 28-94 Meningioma. Cytoplasmic labeling for epithelial membrane antigen on immunoperoxidase assay, depicted here, characterizes the overwhelming majority of meningiomas, regardless of their histologic subtype.

in the secretory subtype.[665,674] The presence of widespread cytokeratin reactivity militates strongly against the diagnosis of meningioma and suggests instead that a dural-based mass represents metastatic carcinoma. A GFAP-reactive neoplasm interpreted as a papillary meningioma has been described[635] but would appear to be unique. We know of no other depictions of meningiomas expressing GFAP and have not succeeded in reproducing this observation.

Meningiomas are amenable to cure by surgical methods alone when complete excision can be effected, as is usually the case for examples arising over the cerebral convexity or along the spinal axis. Even tumors so favorably situated, however, may recur following apparently total resection, the magnitude of this risk emerging only on long-term observation of patients treated for these slow-growing neoplasms. Mirimanoff and colleagues,[659] for example, found that the respective local relapse rates for intraspinal and convexity tumors (0% and 3% at 5 years) rose to 13% and 25% by the end of the first postoperative decade.[659] By all accounts, the likelihood of regrowth is substantially higher for olfactory groove and sphenoid wing meningiomas (41% and 54% at 10 years, respectively, in the study just quoted); en plaque examples and lesions invasive of the cranial floor prove particularly troublesome.[645]

Although there can be no gainsaying the influence of tumor location (i.e., surgical accessibility) on outcome in cases of meningioma, the fact remains that certain morphologic features serve to define a subset of neoplasms far more likely to behave in locally aggressive fashion than their histologically benign counterparts. Findings correlated with an increased postoperative failure rate (and shortened time to tumor regrowth) include the proliferation of tumor cells in patternless sheets rather than lobules, nucleolar prominence, mitotic figures (these are generally absent or identified only on patient search in cases of conventional meningioma), single cell or regional necrosis, and brain invasion.[638,644,656] Accounting for some 5% to 10% of meningothelial neoplasms, lesions exhibiting such worrisome characteristics span a histologic spectrum extending from the "borderline" to the overtly high grade. In practice, most fall far short of frank anaplasia and merit designation as "atypical meningiomas," mainly because of their modest mitotic activity and tendency to undergo coagulative necrosis limited to small, punched-out zones at the centers of their abnormally populous lobules. These tumors may burrow into adjacent cortex via penetrating Virchow-Robin spaces, but their advancing elements retain cohesive and "pushing" contours, remaining sharply delimited from the neuropil proper and typically eliciting little by way of a cellular response. Fully malignant ("anaplastic") meningiomas, by contrast, usually exhibit advanced architectural disarray and cytologic atypism (some assuming carcinoma-like or fibrosarcomatous appearances), are typified by florid proliferative activity, often undergo extensive geographic necrosis, and may send irregular cords or tongues of tumor cells dissecting into the substance of the neighboring brain, trapping bits of neuropil in their wake and provoking a conspicuous glial reaction. It should be pointed out that features suggesting an aggressive potential may constitute only focal findings in what is an otherwise benign-appearing tumor; some initially differentiated menin-

giomas undergo histologic and biologic progression with repeated recurrence. The emergence of rhabdomyosarcomatous elements has been reported in this setting.[639]

The identification of potentially aggressive meningiomas cannot be reliably accomplished solely on clinical grounds, although neuroimaging findings that should prompt concern include indistinct tumoral margins, a "mushrooming" growth pattern characterized by multinodular projections from the main mass, foci that fail to enhance on administration of contrast media (these representing regions of necrosis), and edema of the neighboring brain.[644,656] That the pathologist's recognition of these lesions has definite prognostic implications is underscored by observation of patients undergoing seemingly total surgical extirpation of their tumors. Jääskeläinen et al. recorded 5-, 10-, and 15-year recurrence rates of 38%, 49%, 54%, respectively, for atypical meningiomas following ostensibly complete resection.[644] Fully 78% of anaplastic (i.e., overly malignant) examples encountered in this study had recurred by the fifth postoperative year, whereas respective 5-, 15-, and 25-year relapse rates for histologically benign meningiomas were 3%, 15%, and 21%. In a similar vein, Mahmood and colleagues noted respective 5-, 10-, and 15-year recurrence rates of 50%, 67%, and 67% for atypical meningiomas following gross total resection.[656] At these same follow-up intervals, respectively, 33%, 66%, and 100% of completely excised tumors judged to be histologically malignant had recurred. Clinically aggressive meningiomas tend to an elevated fraction of cycling tumor cells when compared with their benign counterparts,[651,663a,667,670] but whether quantitative determinations of proliferative activity (or ploidy analysis) are of prognostic value independent of histology and extent of resection is unclear.

Although local regrowth is the major pattern of treatment failure, malignant meningiomas can spread via the CSF and, on occasion, travel to extraneural sites such as the lung, liver, bone, and lymph node.[647] We would point out, however, that an excess of distant metastases recorded in the literature have derived from "angioblastic" variants that would now be classified as meningeal hemangiopericytomas (see p. 2230). Examples of "benign metastasizing meningioma" have been well documented but remain curiosities.[661] As noted, venous sinus invasion is a feature of many meningiomas and is not predictive of hematogenous dissemination or germane to the designation of a given lesion as atypical or malignant. In a similar vein, little significance attaches to foci of pronounced nuclear pleomorphism, provided that nucleolar enlargement, mitotic activity, or other atypical features are not in evidence. Pathologists should also bear in mind that foci of necrosis may result from radiotherapy or attempts to reduce a lesion's vascularity (and thus facilitate its removal) by preoperative embolization, cases of the latter type often manifesting an intravascular foreign body–type giant cell reaction.

Meningioangiomatosis is the designation traditionally applied to an epileptogenic hamartoma often, although by no means invariably, occurring in association with NF-2.[680] The lesion consists of a circumscribed, en plaque proliferation of blood vessels and accompanying spindle cells—the latter occasionally in whorled array—that dissects the subjacent cerebral cortex. Extensive calcification, including the presence of numerous psammoma bodies, is common as are fibrous tissue overgrowth and vascular hyalinization. A curious feature is the tendency of entrapped neurons to contain Alzheimer-type neurofibrillary tangles. The term *meningioangiomatosis* notwithstanding, the lesion's perivascular, spindle-cell component may not exhibit EMA immunoreactivity or a meningothelial fine structure and has been interpreted by some observers as predominantly fibroblastic.[679] Rare examples of bona fide meningioma interpreted as originating in foci of meningioangiomatosis are on record,[678] reference having already been made to the suggestion that the sclerosing meningothelial tumors of childhood may arise in this setting. We have recently encountered a leptomeningeal hemangiopericytoma overlying a focus of cortical meningioangiomatosis replete with tangle-bearing neurons. In exceptional cases, subcortical structures play host to this peculiar hamartomatous process. A possible example of bulbar meningioangiomatosis has recently been reported.[681] Simple excision is the treatment of choice, often resulting in long-term seizure control.

Nonmeningothelial, mesenchymal tumors

Excepting the obscure process known as primary meningeal sarcomatosis and the congenital lipomatous tumors of the lumbosacral spinal canal and cranial cavity, the varied lesions surveyed in this section represent the homologs of neoplasms encountered far more frequently in the somatic soft tissues and bones than along the central neuraxis.[682] Accordingly, little attempt is made to describe or depict their histopathologic, ultrastructural, and immunophenotypic profiles, all of which are given detailed attention elsewhere in these volumes. However, we would emphasize the hazards in diagnosis occasioned by the existence of both neuroepithelial and meningothelial tumors that pretend to inclusion among the select company under discussion. Whereas CNS neoplasms exhibiting spindly or bizarre, "monstrocellular" cytologic features were once presumed to be mesodermal in derivation if they could be shown to elaborate an intercellular reticulin network, it is now clear that candidates fulfilling this criterion also must be subjected to immunohistochemical assay for evidence of cytoplasmic GFAP expression if entities such as the sarcomatoid or "giant cell" glioblastoma, desmoplastic cerebral astrocytoma, and pleomorphic xanthoastrocytoma are to be unmasked. In addition, the possibility has always to be borne in mind, particularly in adult cases, that the biopsy demonstrating bona fide sarcoma derives, in fact, from a malignant mixed gliomesenchymal tumor (i.e., a gliosarcoma). Especially suspect in this regard are limited specimens evidencing the features of fibrosarcoma or malignant fibrous histiocytoma, but the gliosarcoma, as already indicated, may also contain angiosarcomatous, osteosarcomatous, chondrosarcomatous, and myosarcomatous tissues. Inasmuch as primitive neuroepithelial neoplasms such as the medullomyoblastoma and certain variants of pineoblastoma contain striated muscle elements, putative embryonal rhabdomyosarcomas of the CNS must be screened for telltale evidence of neuroglial differentiation at the ultrastructural level or for the expression of GFAP, synaptophysin, neurofilament proteins, and other

neuroepithelial antigens. Finally, electron microscopic study and immunocytochemical assay for EMA labeling may serve to distinguish the fibrosarcoma- or hemangiopericytoma-like meningioma from the genuine article. These guidelines are offered, of course, with the full realization that malignant neoplasms readily forego such luxury functions as the manufacture of marker proteins convenient to the surgical pathologist.

Lipoma and liposarcoma

Intradural tumors composed of mature adipose tissue may be encountered anywhere along the neuraxis but are most common at spinal levels, where they can be divided into a congenital, maldevelopmental group situated principally in the lumbosacral region and a smaller, arguably neoplastic subset tending to a thoracic location.[685] The former have already been discussed as manifestations of spinal dysraphism. Commonly occurring in complex with spina bifida and its cutaneous stigmata, "lipomas" of this type figure prominently among intraspinal anomalies complicated by fixation of the filum terminale, caudal displacement of the conus medullaris, and the traction-induced myelopathy known as the "tethered cord" syndrome (see p. 2229). These malformative lesions not infrequently contain heterotopic components such as smooth and striated muscle, aberrant peripheral nerve fibers, meningothelial derivatives ("occult" lipomeningocele), ependyma, and other neuroglial elements ("occult" lipomeningomyelocele).[695] We have encountered an example that harbored mesonephroid tubules and glomeruloid structures lined by an orderly cuboidal epithelium. Although entrapment of the cauda equina and permeation of the conus usually preclude thorough resection of these intraspinal masses, dramatic neurologic improvement can often be effected by debulking, division of the tethered filum, and dural reconstruction.[4]

In contrast to the congenital lipomatous tumors of the lumbosacral canal, **lipomas** occurring at higher levels of the spinal axis are typically unassociated with regional anomalies of the vertebrae or intraspinal contents and consist solely of mature fat.[685,686] Only rarely are these entirely intramedullary.[686a] Much more common are *leptomyelolipomas,*[685,686] which present as subpial masses plastered over a highly variable length of the spinal cord, incorporating its roots and blending into its parenchyma proper. These features frustrate attempts at complete excision, but again, long-term symptomatic relief is often achieved by simple debulking. Uncommon examples contain conspicuous vascular elements and are dubbed angiolipomas or angiomyolipomas, but such lesions are more often epidural in location.[688] Symptomatic accumulation of adipose tissue in this compartment is also a recognized, albeit rare, complication of corticosteroid administration known as **spinal epidural lipomatosis,**[689] one example of which consisted of brown fat ("hibernoma").[687]

Intracranial lipomas are usefully segregated into a midline group (Fig. 28-95) and a laterally situated variant involving the eighth cranial nerve. The former exhibit a decided predilection for the region of the corpus callosum but may also settle along the tuber cinereum, above the quadrigeminal plate, in the ambient cisterns, and in the third ventricle.[683]

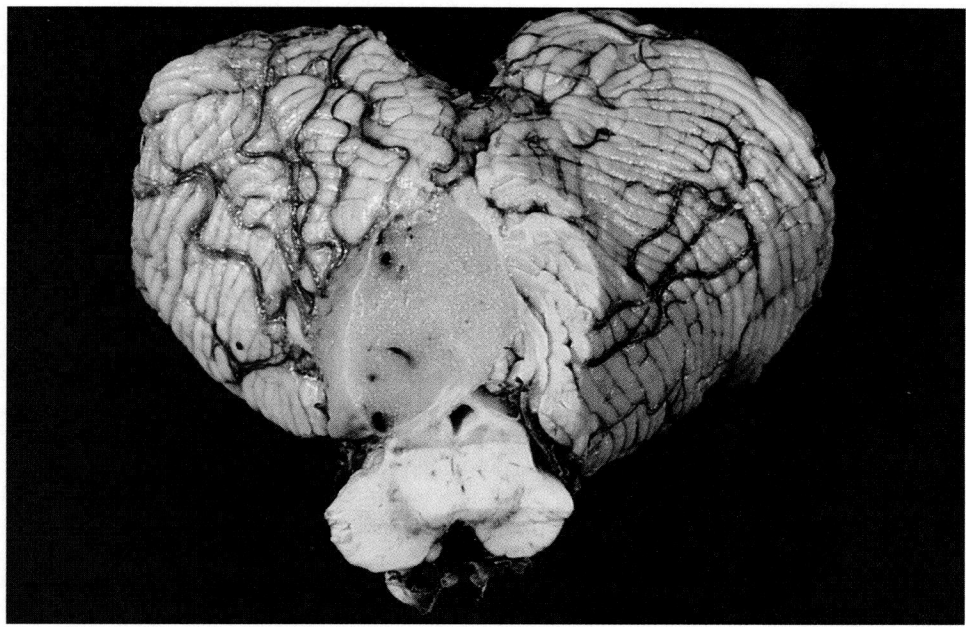

Fig. 28-95 Lipoma. Intracranial lipomas often present in a midline or paramedian position, as illustrated by this example—a mass of bright yellow adipose tissue occupying the cerebellar vermis and impinging on the tectum.

Most are incidentally discovered at autopsy, but epileptogenic callosal examples are well recognized, tuberal variants may eventuate in hypothalamic dysfunction, and lesions impinging on the third ventricle or aqueduct of Sylvius may be complicated by progressive hydrocephalus. Sleep apnea has exceptionally been recorded in association with lipomas involving the mesencephalic tectum and rostral pons.[691] In any of these locations, the midline lipoma is clearly maldevelopmental, being frequently associated with structural anomalies of neighboring neural tissues (e.g., agenesis of the corpus callosum) and occasionally occurring in complex with cranial defects or congenital intracranial cysts of the colloid or epidermoid type. The added presence, in some instances, of cartilage, bone, smooth or striated muscle, heterotopic peripheral nerves, ganglion cells, neuroglia, and choroid plexus further attests to their malformative basis, although some observers have speculated that these more complex lesions may represent teratomas or teratoid neoplasms.[694] Exceptional variants merit designation as angiolipomas.[692]

Intracranial lipomas situated off the midline tend to present in the cerebellopontine angle[684] or internal auditory canal[690] and are usually mistaken for acoustic schwannomas on clinical evaluation. The eighth cranial nerve is typically permeated in diffuse fashion, its fibers divided into small fascicles embedded in mature adipose tissue, and other cranial nerves may be engulfed in like manner by large lesions lying adjacent to the brainstem. Because attempts at en bloc resection may result in severe neurologic deficits, some observers have suggested that cerebellopontine angle examples be subjected to the minimum debulking required to relieve local mass effects.[684] The intrinsically high signal

characteristic of fat on T_1-weighted MR study may facilitate the accurate preoperative identification of these (and other) neuraxial masses as lipomas.

Liposarcomas are among the least common of all malignant mesenchymal tumors reported to involve the CNS or its coverings. Only isolated meningeal examples are on record.[693] The reader is reminded that cells resembling bizarre lipoblasts may be encountered in "lipidized" neoplasms of meningothelial and astrocytic lineage.

Osseous and cartilaginous tumors

Osseous plaques adherent to the falx cerebri and undersurface of the dura in the region of the superior sagittal sinus are common incidental findings at autopsy, are asymptomatic, and are of no clinical significance. Although termed *osteomas,* these almost certainly represent reactive, metaplastic lesions and may occur with increased frequency in the setting of chronic renal failure.[700] Only isolated examples of bona fide **osteogenic sarcoma** arising from the dura[702] or brain[706] have been depicted. Bosselated masses of mature hyaline cartilage known as *chondromas* (or osteochondromas when they contain bony elements) may bulge into the cranial cavity from its floor or, less commonly, are found attached to the inner aspect of the dura.[703,707] Cystic variants have been described,[701] as have examples complicating the generalized skeletal chondromatoses designated as Maffucci's syndrome[698] and Ollier's disease.[710]

Intracranial *chondrosarcomas* of conventional type usually originate in the skull base, but meningeal and neuroparenchymal primaries are recognized,[682,696,699] including radiation-associated variants.[697] Curiously, the **mesenchymal chondrosarcoma** seems to have a special predilection for the dura among extraosseous sites.[709] Cases arising in the spinal pia[705] and brain[704] are also on record. Rarest of all cartilaginous intracranial neoplasms is the **extraskeletal myxoid chondrosarcoma.**[708]

Fibroblastic and "fibrohistiocytic" tumors

Unfortunately, it is the *fibrosarcoma,* an aggressive neoplasm, that dominates the family of fibroblastic and "fibrohistiocytic" tumors arising within the craniospinal confines. Sporadic,[713] familial,[712] and radiation-associated[718,720,724] variants are all recognized, the last typically complicating treatment of pituitary adenomas and originating in the region of the sella turcica. Attachment to the dura or leptomeninges is common, but some examples are situated entirely within the substance of the cerebrum. Symptomatic local recurrence is the rule even after gross total resection of circumscribed, superficially positioned lesions, and most patients succumb to their disease within 1 year of diagnosis, often after developing leptomeningeal and distant, extracranial metastases. Similarly lethal is the intracranial *malignant fibrous histiocytoma* (a dubious entity from the histogenetic perspective and probably better regarded as a pleomorphic variant of fibrosarcoma).[682,723] This tumor, too, may be radiation induced.[714] The spectrum of malignant fibroblastic tumors encountered along the neuraxis includes an example of **low-grade fibromyxoid sarcoma** histologically similar to its soft tissue counterpart.[682]

Benign neuraxial tumors composed of fibroblasts or related cell types, all exceedingly rare, include the **fibroma** (sometimes referred to as fibromyxoma or, simply, myxoma owing to mucoid alterations of its stroma),[715,719,722] **angiofibroma,**[716] and **myofibroblastoma.**[721] Several examples of dural fibromatosis have also been described, some following neurosurgical procedures.[711,717] Fibroblasts additionally participate in the formation of intracranial masses known as fibroxanthomas, but these, dominated by foam cells, are probably reactive in nature and are considered under the rubric of *xanthomatous lesions* (see p. 2251).

To our opening caveats regarding neuroglial tumors that may masquerade as neoplasms of fibroblastic or fibrohistiocytic lineage, we would add the warning that astrocytic lesions routinely exhibit immunolabeling with antisera to vimentin and may also be positive on assay for alpha$_1$-antitrypsin and antichymotrypsin. No differential diagnostic significance should be attached to these findings.

Endothelial tumors

The overwhelming majority of vasoformative tumors involving the CNS are maldevelopmental anomalies (see p. 2238). Endothelial neoplasms of the neuraxis include *epithelioid hemangioendotheliomas,*[726] probably best regarded as tumors of relatively low malignant potential ("borderline" lesions), and aggressive **angiosarcomas** of conventional type that usually are fatal.[727,728] We have not encountered an example of cutaneous or visceral angiosarcoma presenting as a neuraxial mass, but an account of metastatic atrial myxoma masquerading as intracranial epithelioid hemangioendothelioma has been published.[731]

Noteworthy is the fact that most endothelial tumors of the CNS arise in the cerebral hemispheres proper rather than in the meninges; mesenchymal tumors of nonendothelial lineage that present in the intracranial or spinal compartments usually originate from the dura mater. The designation of hemangioendothelioma has also been extended to vasogenic meningocerebral lesions that structurally resemble the cellular ("juvenile") capillary hemangiomas encountered as cutaneous "nevi" in infancy.[729,730] We have also had the opportunity to study an epileptogenic frontal lobe mass, associated with a history of antecedent cranial trauma, which exhibited the features of lobular capillary hemangioma (or so-called pyogenic granuloma) and are familiar with a case in which morphologically similar, but multifocal cerebral hemispheric lesions regressed after corticosteroid administration.[725] Diffuse involvement of the spinal cord by a lesion having capillary hemangiomatous features has also been described.[726a]

Finally, the spectrum of primary endothelial proliferations potentially involving the nervous system includes the process known as **intravascular papillary endothelial hyperplasia** or **Masson's vegetant intravascular hemangioendothelioma.**[732,733] Intracerebral variants, which may evolve from pre-existing vascular malformations, can achieve enormous proportions and have occasionally proved fatal as a result of associated mass effects. Manifestations of intracranial hypertension secondary to impaired cerebral venous outflow led to the discovery of a dural sinus example situated at the torcular Herophili.[733]

Meningeal hemangiopericytoma

Although their cytogenesis remains a contentious issue, recent studies have clearly shown that select dural-based tumors long regarded as "angioblastic" variants of meningioma are immunophenotypically, as well as morphologically, indistinguishable from hemangiopericytomas arising in the somatic soft tissues[674,734-738] (Fig. 28-96). That these are now widely accepted as the latter's neuraxial homologs is reflected in their recent reclassification as nonmeningothelial, mesenchymal neoplasms by the WHO.[736]

Meningeal hemangiopericytomas are largely tumors of adulthood that do not exhibit the distinct predilection for women characteristic of meningiomas and that strongly favor the intracranial compartment. Their distinction from meningiomas evidencing potentially misleading pericytomatous growth patterns is usually straightforward because the latter often contain psammomatous calcospherites and tumor cells concentrically arrayed in tight whorl formations—both foreign to the hemangiopericytoma, as are the intranuclear pseudoinclusions typical of meningothelial elements and their neoplastic derivatives. Also alien to the meningioma, but a feature of many hemangiopericytomas, is a network of "reticulin" investing individual tumor cells. This appears to represent basal lamina material at the ultrastructural level[734,737,738] (Fig. 28-97). The hemangiopericytoma further departs from the meningioma on electron microscopic study in that the cytoplasmic processes elaborated by its consistent cells, although joined by rudimentary junctions, are neither bound by well-developed desmosomes nor intertwined in complex fashion. Serving also to segregate these lesions from neoplasms of meningothelial lineage is their failure to express EMA on immunocytochemical assay.[674,734,737,738] Mesenchymal chondrosarcomas of dural

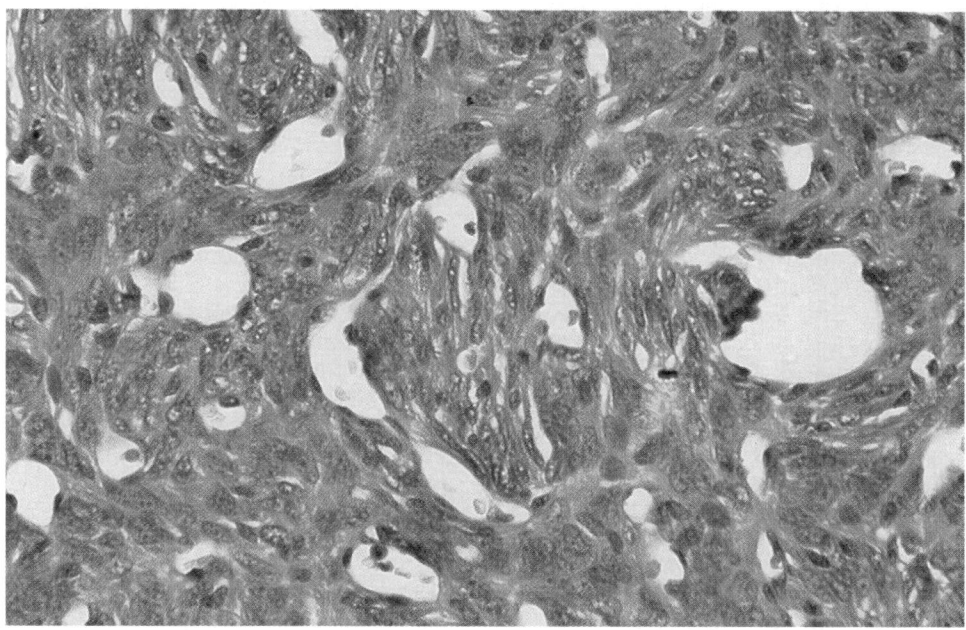

Fig. 28-96 Meningeal hemangiopericytoma. Long regarded as a form of "angioblastic" meningioma, this lesion is now widely accepted as the homolog of its extraneural soft tissue counterpart.

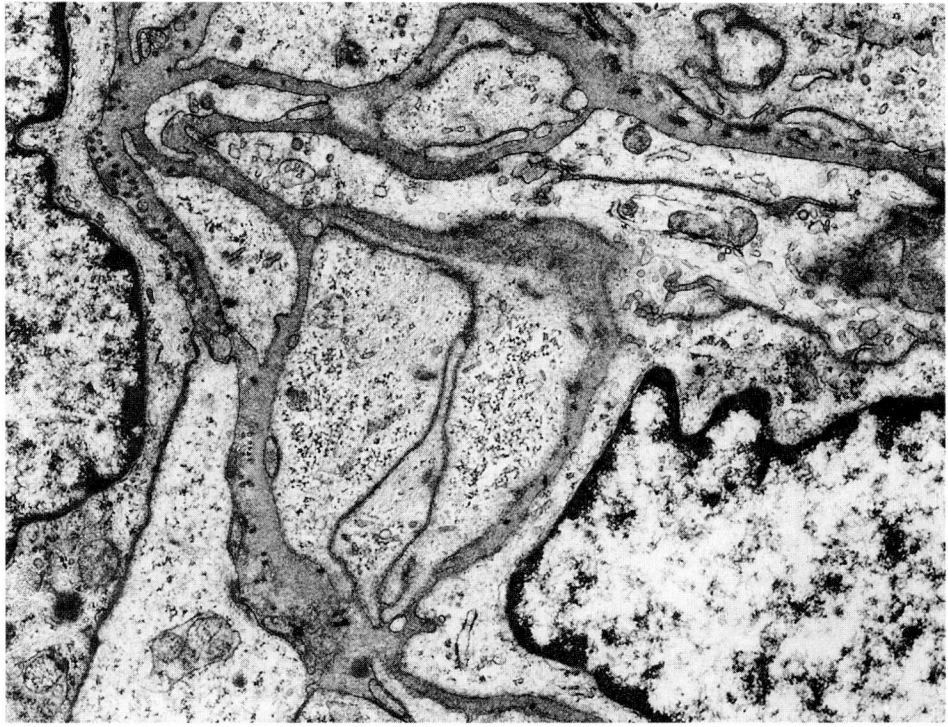

Fig. 28-97 Meningeal hemangiopericytoma. Unlike the cytoplasmic processes of meningothelial tumor cells (compare Fig. 28-93), those of the hemangiopericytoma's constituent neoplastic elements are separated by basal lamina material demonstrable on ultrastructural examination. (×11,360.)

origin routinely harbor anaplastic small cell elements in pericytomatous architectural array and thus enter the differential diagnosis, but the meningeal hemangiopericytoma lacks these tumors' distinctive chondroid components.

Regrowth at the primary site despite seemingly complete initial resection is typical of the meningeal hemangiopericytoma, although this may take years to become clinically apparent. Even with the addition of postoperative radiotherapy, most afflicted patients die as a direct result of intracranial tumor progression, often after a protracted course characterized by repeated local recurrence.[735,737] Extracranial metastasis, usually a late complication, occurs with surprising frequency. Most often seeded are the lungs, bones, and liver, but retroperitoneal organs, such as kidney and pancreas, may also be involved.[735,737] Some observers have found such features as conspicuous mitotic activity and foci of necrosis to be of ominous prognostic import,[737] whereas others have been unable to correlate outcome with histology.[735] In our view, all meningeal hemangiopericytomas are best regarded as potentially aggressive sarcomas.

Myogenous tumors

Embryonal rhabdomyosarcomas account for nearly all primary myogenous neoplasms of the CNS reported to date.[740,745,748] These tend to segregate into a posterior fossa subset, characterized by a presentation in childhood and a predilection for the cerebellum, and a supratentorial group of adult onset typified by a cerebral hemispheric localization. The midline, vermal position of many intracranial rhabdomyosarcomas arising in the pediatric population and the recognized capacity of the cerebellar medulloblastoma to differentiate along skeletal muscle lines ("medullomyoblastoma") have prompted speculation that both tumor types might originate from a common, primordial progenitor in the rhombic roof.[745] Whatever their histogenesis, primary rhabdomyosarcomas of the CNS are high-grade neoplasms; few patients live 2 years after diagnosis despite aggressive irradiation and chemotherapy. Neuraxis dissemination and extracranial metastasis may complicate local tumor progression. Mention should be made of a diffuse leptomeningeal variant unassociated with a demonstrable neuroparenchymal component,[746] but this diagnosis requires rigorous exclusion of an occult primary focus in the orbit, paranasal sinuses, nasopharynx, or middle ear because rhabdomyosarcomas originating in these parameningeal regions frequently seed the subarachnoid space (see p. 2344).

Primary smooth muscle tumors of the CNS are vanishingly rare, but intrasellar[742] and suprasellar[749] **leiomyomas** are on record, as are isolated intracranial and intraspinal **leiomyosarcomas**.[739,741,744] The recent account of a thoracic epidural leiomyoma occurring in an HIV-1–seropositive man is particularly noteworthy in view of the emerging association of this retroviral infection with benign and malignant smooth muscle tumors occurring at unusual sites.[747] A single report describes the intracranial occurrence of a neoplasm interpreted as a **pleomorphic angioleiomyoma**.[743]

Other primary CNS sarcomas

In addition to the varied forms of CNS neoplasia exhibiting differentiation along specific mesenchymal lines, there is a disparate collection of anaplastic tumors to which only descriptive appellations such as "spindle cell" or "polymorphic cell" sarcoma have been given.[751] These are presumed to derive from mesodermal precursors, but their histogenesis, in fact, is totally obscure. Children are more often affected than adults, and most cases appear to originate from the dura or pia arachnoid. Reported cases have been composed of spindled, polygonal, or round cells said to be without further identifying characteristics, but inasmuch as no systematic investigation of the tumors' fine structure or immunophenotype has been undertaken, it is impossible to conclude (and there is much reason to doubt) that this is a unified pathologic entity. Reported under the rubric of **primary leptomeningeal sarcomatosis** are variants characterized by diffuse tumoral proliferation restricted to the subarachnoid space and unaccompanied by dominant foci of bulky disease.[750-752] These may present with signs and symptoms of polyradiculopathy, spinal cord compression, or intracranial mass effect and are often misdiagnosed initially as chronic meningitides of infectious etiology or as manifestations of neurosarcoidosis or other inflammatory disorders. The differential diagnosis includes leptomeningeal carcinomatosis, gliomatosis, lymphomatosis, and medulloblastomatosis. Last, we call attention to rare mention in the literature of poorly characterized meningeal tumors classified as primary intracranial examples of **Ewing's sarcoma**.[682]

Nerve sheath tumors of the craniospinal axis

Inasmuch as nerve sheath tumors arising within the cranial cavity and spinal canal are the morphologic and biologic homologs of their more common, peripherally situated counterparts, the reader is referred to Chapter 25 of this text for a detailed treatment of their diagnostic structural and immunophenotypic features.

Schwannomas are the most frequent variant to abut the central neuraxis, usually presenting in adulthood as tumors of the cerebellopontine angle or lumbosacral spinal extramedullary space.[763,775] Only exceptionally do these benign neoplasms afflict children.[753] Nearly all cerebellopontine angle tumors originate in the vestibular branch of cranial nerve VIII (*acoustic schwannoma or neuroma*) and produce hearing loss. Schwannomas arising at spinal levels exhibit a similar predilection for sensory divisions of the neuraxis, typically involving the posterior roots. These often assume a "dumbbell" configuration as they squeeze through adjacent intervertebral foramina and expand into the paravertebral soft tissues. Schwannomas rarely lie within the substance of the brain,[756] can be embedded within the spinal cord proper, and may involve cranial nerves other than the acoustic.[775] Bilateral eighth nerve examples are a defining feature of NF-2, an autosomal dominant disorder transmitted by allelic loss involving chromosome 22.[770] Affected kindreds are prone to an assortment of neoplasms, all typified in this setting by multiplicity, that includes craniospinal schwannomas, meningiomas, and intramedullary ependymomas. Loss of heterozygosity involving chromosome 22 is also a feature of acoustic schwannomas occurring in sporadic fashion.[776]

The schwannoma's characteristic Antoni A and B structure, nuclear palisading (Verocay bodies), infiltration by

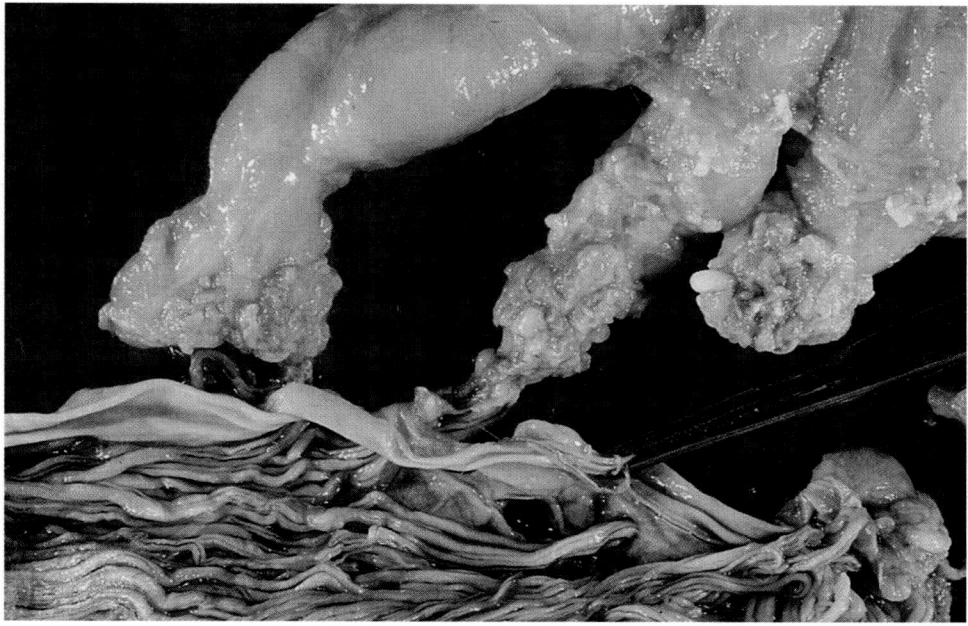

Fig. 28-98 Neurofibromatosis. Neurofibromas of the spinal nerve roots are principally encountered in the setting of type 1 neurofibromatosis (classic von Recklinghausen disease). Multiple spinal roots of this afflicted patient exhibit plexiform neurofibromatous expansion. Normal cauda equina are present at bottom.

foamy macrophages, and vascular hyalinization usually suffice for its recognition, but meningiomas on occasion exhibit similar features and are the former's most frequent counterfeit. Immunocytochemical techniques and electron microscopic study may both be usefully applied to this problem. Schwannomas are characterized by diffuse cytoplasmic S-100 protein expression and pericellular immunolabeling for laminin and type IV collagen, the latter reflecting investment of their elongated cellular processes by a continuous basal lamina foreign to the typical meningioma. Our experience, consonant with that of Perentes et al.,[774] is that cytoplasmic expression of EMA—a regular feature of meningothelial tumors—is absent from the schwannoma or restricted to normal perineurial cells incorporated into the latter's capsule and thus limited to its periphery. Admittedly, however, other researchers have described EMA-reactive neoplastic elements in the substance of some schwannomas.[674] These are said to exhibit diffuse cytoplasmic reactivity without the cell membrane accentuation characteristic of meningothelial tumors. It is worth remembering that meningiomas only rarely present in the lumbosacral regions favored by schwannomas of the spinal roots.[775]

A variant of schwannoma recognized for its elaboration of melanosomal melanin exhibits a decided predilection for the spinal nerve roots.[765] An intramedullary example has also been recorded.[769] Most of the ***melanotic schwannomas*** reported to date have evolved in a benign fashion. The risk of local recurrence following incomplete resection, however, is substantial,[765] and an aggressive course characterized by visceral and cerebral metastases has been documented.[758] A subset of melanotic schwannomas containing

psammomatous concretions constitutes part of a heritable complex that includes cardiac, cutaneous, and mammary myxomas; spotty pigmentation; Sertoli cell tumors of the testis; and evidence of endocrine hyperfunction (principally Cushing's syndrome and acromegaly).[754]

A small minority of intracranial and intraspinal schwannomas are of the "cellular" type.[756a,759,777] In contrast to its histologically conventional counterpart, the ***cellular schwannoma*** is a densely populated spindle-cell tumor, typically devoid of Antoni B areas and Verocay bodies, that may contain foci of mitotic activity and is likely to be misconstrued as a sarcoma. The lesion shares with the classical schwannoma foci of vascular hyalinization, infiltration by lymphocytes and foamy macrophages, diffuse S-100 protein immunoreactivity, and highly differentiated Schwann cell features at the ultrastructural level. Such tumors may recur locally following excision, but a metastasizing example has never been described. Finally, **granular cell tumors** of schwannian lineage have been noted to involve the trigeminal nerve and to present as intracranial masses.[755]

Most craniospinal **neurofibromas** represent manifestations of NF-1 ("peripheral" or classic von Recklinghausen's disease), transmitted in autosomal dominant fashion by a locus on chromosome 17.[763,767,775] This complex disorder includes, in addition to multifocal cutaneous and more deeply situated plexiform neurofibromas, dermatologic abnormalities (café au lait spots and axillary freckling), pigmented hamartomas of the iris (Lisch nodules), various skeletal defects, and glial neoplasms, chief among which are pilocytic astrocytomas of the anterior optic pathways. Spinal neurofibromas arising in this setting typically do so at multiple levels (Fig. 28-98). Only rarely are cranial nerves involved.

Well documented, but exceedingly uncommon, are *malignant nerve sheath tumors* originating in cranial or spinal nerve roots. The former are said to arise most commonly within the trigeminal nerve[768] or gasserian ganglion.[766] Several "acoustic" examples are also on record,[771,772] including a so-called Triton tumor (i.e., a variant exhibiting rhabdomyoblastic differentiation).[764] Also noteworthy is a report of a malignant nerve sheath tumor arising in a lateral ventricle.[764a] Malignant nerve sheath tumors often originate in neurofibromas, particularly those of plexiform type, and so are strongly associated with NF-1.[761,762] Isolated craniospinal examples have also followed local irradiation.[760]

Other reported lesions relevant to the present discussion include an intracranial **nerve sheath "myxoma" or "neurothekeoma"** that involved the gasserian ganglion[773] and examples of **localized hypertrophic mononeuropathy** affecting cranial nerves[757] or cauda equina.[778] The latter exhibited segmental expansion of the involved nerves secondary to "onion bulb," periaxonal Schwann cell proliferations.

Lymphoproliferative and myeloproliferative disorders

Because secondary spread of systemic lymphoproliferative and myeloproliferative disorders to the CNS does not often occasion neurosurgical intervention for diagnostic purposes, only a few general observations on this problem are offered. At greatest risk of such dissemination are patients suffering from acute leukemias,[782] particularly of lymphoblastic type; diffuse leptomeningeal infiltration is the dominant pattern of CNS involvement encountered in this setting. In some cases, extensive permeation of cranial and spinal nerve roots accompanies the unrestrained proliferation of leukemic cells in the subarachnoid compartment. Circumscribed, dural-based, or (rarely) intracerebral masses composed of leukemic cells principally complicate the acute myelogenous leukemias but have virtually disappeared from clinical practice because of modern cytoreductive therapy. Variously designated as **chloromas, granulocytic sarcomas,** or **myeloblastomas,** these tumors usually develop in subjects who are demonstrably leukemic but exceptionally constitute the initial manifestation of relapse following apparently successful treatment, or they present in otherwise normal individuals as harbingers of subsequent bone marrow and peripheral blood involvement.[820,825] Parameningeal **masses of extramedullary hematopoietic tissue** have been reported to produce neurologic dysfunction, mainly as a result of spinal cord compression, in patients with thalassemia or myelofibrosis.[787,806]

Involvement of the CNS in the course of node-based **non-Hodgkin's lymphoma** is uncommon and usually limited to permeation of the leptomeninges ("lymphomatous meningitis") or, less often, infiltration of the spinal epidural space.[801] Cerebral infiltrates are decidedly unusual in this setting and typically complicate advanced (stage IV) disease, an excess of cases occurring in patients with diffuse large cell or lymphoblastic subtypes and involvement of other extranodal sites, chief among which is the bone marrow.[801] By contrast, patients presenting with non-Hodgkin's lymphoma of the

eye—an extension of the CNS—frequently develop lymphomatous lesions of the brain proper.[815] A subset of malignant lymphomas, principally non-Hodgkin's variants, are confined at diagnosis to paraspinal tissues, usually arising in the midthoracic region and prompting evaluation for epidural compressive myelopathy.[797,799] Only exceptionally are the meninges colonized or the neural parenchyma penetrated in the course of systemic **Hodgkin's disease,**[817] **plasma cell myeloma,**[808,821] **Waldenström's macroglobulinemia,**[793] or **mycosis fungoides.**[781]

The designation of *primary central nervous system lymphoma* (PCNSL) is reserved for malignant lymphoid neoplasms of non-Hodgkin's type restricted at presentation to the brain, spinal cord, or meninges.[783,802,811] Although the association of PCNSL with states of diminished immune responsiveness has long been appreciated and its particular predilection for victims of AIDS documented in numerous studies,[780,802,810,811] most afflicted patients suffer no predisposing illness, and epidemiologic data suggest a dramatic increase in the general incidence of PCNSL that is not attributable to advances in diagnosis or the epidemic spread of HIV-1.[792] Sporadic cases most often present in the sixth or seventh decades of life and manifest a 1.5:1 to 2:1 male/female ratio, whereas AIDS-related examples are characterized by a younger age at onset and an overwhelming predominance in men, reflecting the demography of HIV-1 infection. Most patients suffer the usual symptoms of an expanding intracranial mass, although PCNSLs tend to arise in the deep cerebral hemispheric white matter, corpus callosum, and basal ganglia and thus are not as prone to produce seizures as gliomas or metastatic deposits that involve epileptogenic cortical tissues. Frontocallosal and periventricular examples may prompt evaluation for personality change, depression, progressive psychomotor retardation, or frank psychosis. Some tumors are discovered in the course of workup for persistent uveocyclitides unresponsive to conventional ophthalmologic treatment, a manifestation of ocular involvement that often occurs in complex with cerebral infiltration.[815]

Neuroradiologic features (Fig. 28-99) that suggest the diagnosis of PCNSL on CT or MR study include tumoral hyperdensity in precontrast images, diffuse (as opposed to rim) enhancement on administration of contrast media, evidence of widespread subependymal infiltration, and multifocality.[802] The last is apparent in some 30% to 40% of sporadic, and the great majority of HIV-1–associated, cases. Especially suspect are masses that regress substantially with corticosteroid administration alone prior to biopsy; occasional lymphomas disappear (transiently) with such treatment and masquerade as multiple sclerosis.[795,802,804] Inasmuch as extensive central necrosis lends to many HIV-1–associated PCNSLs a "ring"-enhancing radiologic appearance indistinguishable from *Toxoplasma* abscesses,[780] it has become common practice in this setting to offer patients what amounts to a diagnostic as well as therapeutic trial of antimicrobial therapy. Lesions that do not respond promptly must be regarded as lymphomas until proved otherwise. A definitive diagnosis of PCNSL usually requires biopsy, but may be accomplished by demonstration of malignant lymphoid cells in CSF.

PCNSLs may arise anywhere along the neuraxis. Roughly 75% are situated in the supratentorial compartment, these favoring the deep structures enumerated.[783,802,811] Most of the remainder involve the cerebellum or brainstem, only rare examples being isolated to the spinal cord.[802,822] Approximately 5% present as diffuse leptomeningeal infiltrates in the absence of demonstrable intraparenchymal disease.[798,805] Lesions are poorly defined in most instances and composed of dry, granular tan-white or grayish-pink tissue that may evidence small foci of necrotic softening or hemorrhagic discoloration. Extensive necrosis and conspicuous hemorrhage are most commonly encountered in AIDS-related cases, which may closely mimic *Toxoplasma* abscesses on gross examination (particularly after irradiation). Some examples diffusely permeate the neuropil, producing little distortion of the brain's architecture save for a slight pallor of gray matter landmarks and expansion of involved structures ("lymphomatosis cerebri"). A striking histologic feature of many cases is the tendency for tumor cells to aggregate in Virchow-Robin spaces and to infiltrate the walls of cerebral vessels (Fig. 28-100). Most PCNSLs are high-grade lesions of large cell type,[783,802,811,818] although all major cytologic variants have been reported in this location, including such oddities as signet-ring cell[813] and anaplastic, Ki-1[814] lymphoma. Follicular (nodular) lesions, however, have yet to be described in this setting. Some observers have noted an overrepresentation of immunoblastic and small noncleaved cell types among PCNSLs, particularly those involving AIDS patients and other immunosuppressed hosts, compared with node-based or other extranodal primary tumors.[783,802,811] Regardless of the cytologic variety, touch preparations are useful in establishing the lymphoid nature of a given tumor at the time of intraoperative consultation (Fig. 28-101).

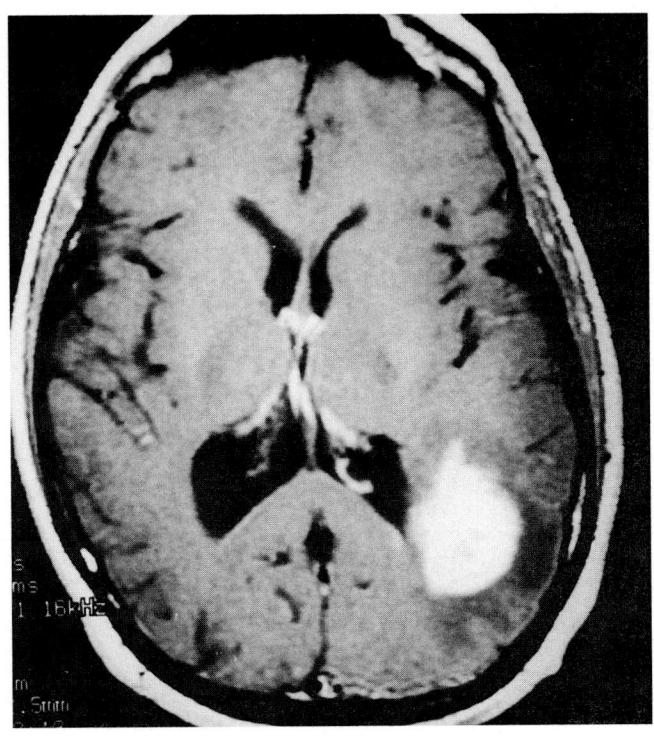

Fig. 28-99 Primary CNS lymphoma. As demonstrated in this postcontrast injection MRI, primary cerebral lymphomas exhibit a predilection for the deep, paraventricular white matter and tend to striking and fairly homogeneous enhancement in "sporadic" (as opposed to AIDS-related) cases.

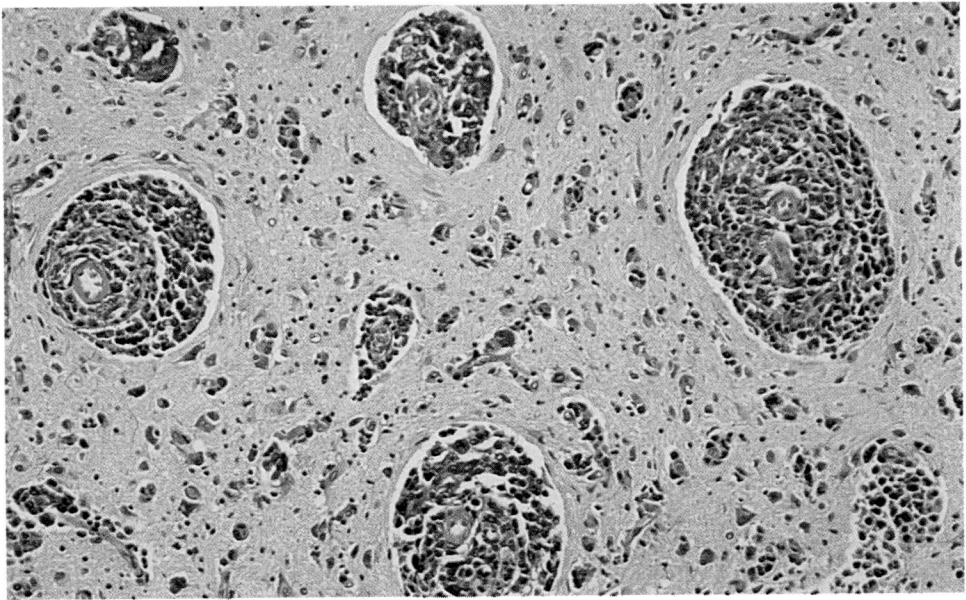

Fig. 28-100 Primary CNS lymphoma. Although not apparent in all cases, a vasocentric growth pattern with tumoral infiltration of blood vessel walls and Virchow-Robin spaces is common to primary CNS lymphomas. Systemic lymphomas secondarily involving the neuroparenchyma may also preferentially grow in this fashion.

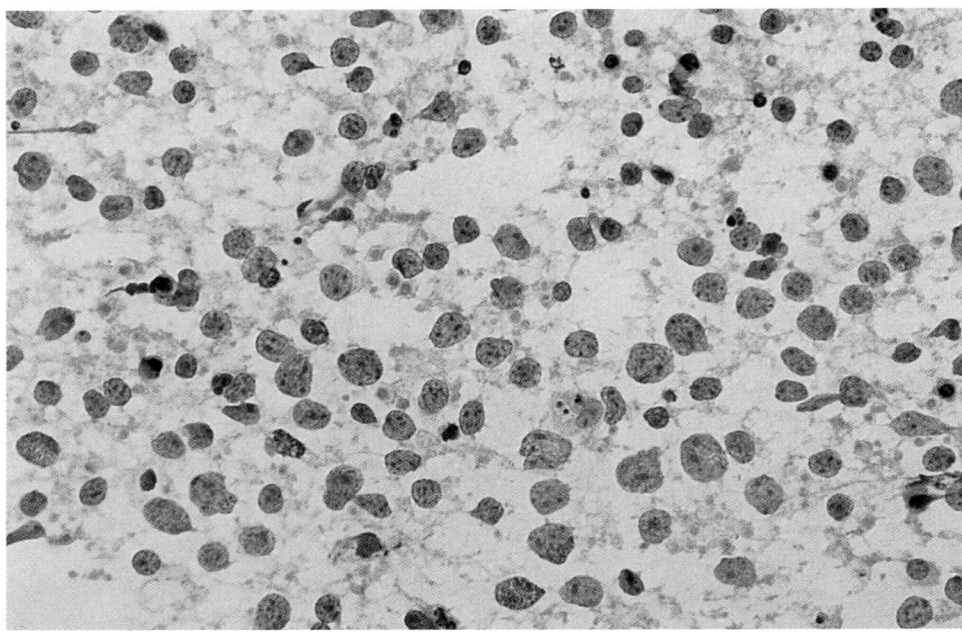

Fig. 28-101 Primary CNS lymphoma. An intraoperative smear preparation demonstrates the large cell cytology and nuclear features characteristic of CNS lymphoma. The lack of cellular cohesion or cytoplasmic processes, respectively, is useful in discriminating this tumor from metastatic carcinoma and glioblastoma multiforme, two neoplasms that commonly enter the clinical differential diagnosis.

By all accounts, the overwhelming majority of PCNSLs exhibit a B-cell immunophenotype[783,802,810,811,818] (Fig. 28-102). Molecular hybridization methods have also been successfully applied to the demonstration of their B-lymphocytic lineage and clonal nature.[803,804] These lesions often harbor a conspicuous complement of admixed T cells that can confound interpretation of the histologic and immunohistochemical picture, but these reactive elements usually appear as small, well-differentiated lymphocytes that are readily distinguished from the large, atypical B cells on which the diagnosis rests. Particularly deceptive are biopsies deriving from the perimeter of PCNSLs, where reactive T lymphocytes often constitute a dominant and obscuring population, or from lesions evidencing marked shrinkage on preoperative corticosteroid administration. These may be selectively relieved of their neoplastic B-cell components and heavily infiltrated by foamy macrophages, a phenomenon that may prompt, along with their radiologic and clinical resolution, acceptance of multiple sclerosis as the primary disease process.[795,804,818] It is worth remembering that multiple sclerosis is, for the most part, a disorder of the young. Furthermore, it has been our experience that inadvertently "treated" lymphomas do not leave behind the sharply demarcated foci of selective myelin loss and relative axonal preservation typical of garden-variety multiple sclerosis or demyelinating pseudotumors. T-cell lymphomas of the brain and leptomeninges have been described[798,809,811a,814] but are clearly exceptional.

The detection of Epstein-Barr viral (EBV) nucleic acid sequences in PCNSLs, including a large percentage of those derived from the immunocompromised, is deserving of mention in view of this agent's recognized ability to immortalize B cells in vitro and to drive a polyclonal, systemic lymphoproliferation that may evolve to lymphoma in the immunodeficient host.[786,816] EBV has also been incriminated in the case of a cerebellar lymphoproliferative lesion, initially polyclonal, that progressed to lymphoma in an apparently immunocompetent adult.[788]

Although limited clinical evidence suggests that small cleaved and noncleaved subtypes fare somewhat better than large cell variants,[802] all PCNSLs are currently approached as high-grade neoplasms. AIDS patients with PCNSL usually die within 2 to 3 months of diagnosis and cerebral irradiation but often succumb to opportunistic infections rather than their intracranial tumors.[780] Tumors occurring in otherwise healthy individuals typically regress following similar treatment but almost invariably recur, often at CNS sites remote from the initial focus, and generally kill within 18 months of discovery.[783,802] Recent studies indicate that the addition of chemotherapy substantially lengthens survival.[796] The usual pattern of treatment failure is progressive and frequently multifocal infiltration of the CNS proper attended, in some cases, by leptomeningeal dissemination. Ocular involvement is experienced by many patients as the disease evolves,[815] but systemic lymphomatous infiltrates develop in no more than 10% of cases.

Primary lymphoproliferative disorders of the CNS other than non-Hodgkin's lymphoma merit little discussion. Only rarely is **Hodgkin's disease** confined, on presentation, to the CNS.[784] Histologic and immunocytochemical reassessment[823]

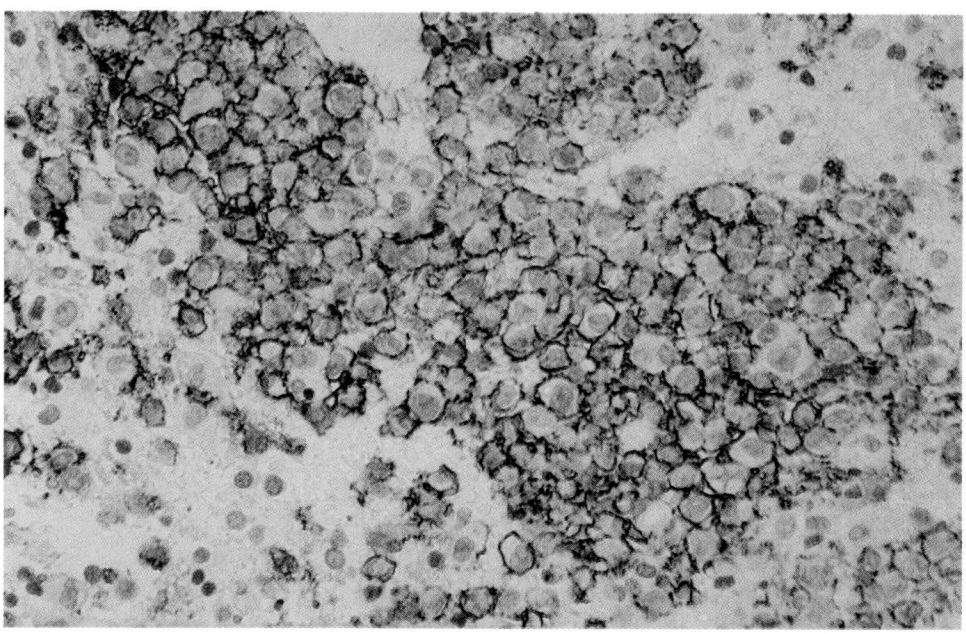

Fig. 28-102 Primary CNS lymphoma. The great majority of lymphomas arising in the CNS are of B-cell type and, as shown here, label for CD20 on immunoperoxidase (L-26) assay.

of the sole series in which cases of Hodgkin's disease reportedly constituted a significant percentage of primary cerebral lymphomas revealed that the tumors so diagnosed were, in fact, B-cell neoplasms with somewhat pleomorphic features. The peculiar disorder described as *neoplastic angioendotheliomatosis,* formerly regarded as an intravascular variant of angiosarcoma, is now known to be an unusual form of malignant lymphoma, usually of large B-cell type, exhibiting a remarkable tropism for blood vessels in the skin, adrenal glands, and CNS.[789,794] A more accurate designation for this process is **intravascular malignant lymphomatosis.** Patients often present with neurologic dysfunction—progressive encephalopathy, dementia, or stroke—that reflects multifocal cerebral infarction resulting from occlusion of vascular lumina by malignant lymphoid cells (Fig. 28-103). Rare cases have been described as limited to the brain or spinal cord,[791] one of which occurred in a child with AIDS.[790]

Other oddities include **Castleman's disease** confined to the leptomeninges,[819] primary dural or intracerebral **plasmacytomas,**[807,826] and **amyloidomas,**[785,812,824] neither of the latter appearing to herald systemic myeloma. Finally, there is so-called **lymphomatoid granulomatosis,** an angiocentric and necrotizing lymphoproliferative disorder usually described as involving the CNS in association with pulmonary disease but occasionally reported to localize in brain alone.[779,800] Several of these isolated cerebral variants involved patients with AIDS[779] and a number eventuated in recognizable lymphoma. Whether such cases represent, ab initio, an angiocentric form of malignant lymphoma is open to question, as is the existence of lymphomatoid granulomatosis as a unified pathologic entity. At least some cases would appear to be EBV driven.[800]

Germ cell tumors

The neoplastic transformation of primordial germ cells that wander into the region of the developing CNS from the fetal yolk sac is presumed to account for the intracranial presentation of a diverse group of tumors morphologically identical to germ cell neoplasms occurring in the gonads, sacrococcygeum, retroperitoneum, and mediastinum.[833,837,838,848] In Western series, these constitute no more than 0.5% of all intracranial tumors and approximately 3% of those encountered in children, but their incidence is greatly increased among the Japanese and in Taiwan.[838] *Intracranial germ cell tumors* share with other extragonadal primaries a predilection for the midline, 95% arising along an axis extending from the suprasellar cistern to, and including, the pineal gland. They are, in fact, the most common neoplasms presenting in the latter location. A small subset involves the suprasellar and pineal regions simultaneously, exceptional examples lying in the basal ganglia, thalami, cerebral hemispheres,[839,842,849] sella turcica,[842] spinal cord,[836,846] and lateral or fourth ventricles.[827,842] Congenital lesions, typically teratomas, may attain virtually holocranial proportions.[843]

The vast majority of intracranial germ cell tumors are diagnosed during the first three decades of life, their peak incidence corresponding to the onset of puberty. This observation, coupled with their stereotypic proximity to the dien-

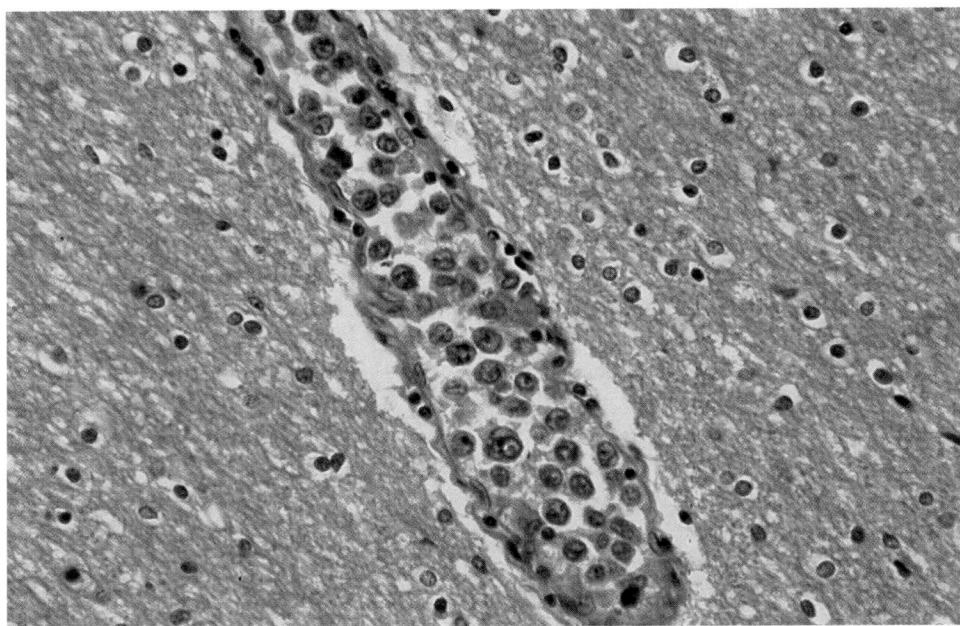

Fig. 28-103 Intravascular malignant lymphomatosis. Large, highly atypical cells fill a small blood vessel in the white matter of a 63-year-old woman subjected to brain biopsy for progressive cognitive impairment. Positive immunoassays for leukocyte common antigen and CD20 confirmed their lymphoid nature and B-cell phenotype, respectively.

cephalic centers that regulate gonadotrophic activity, has occasioned speculation that the neuroendocrine events surrounding puberty facilitate the escape of dormant germ cells from normal proliferative controls.[838] Males are afflicted more than twice as frequently as females. Suprasellar examples produce visual field defects, diabetes insipidus, and hypothalamopituitary failure, whereas pineal region tumors compress the tectal plate and obstruct the aqueduct, presenting with symptoms and signs of hydrocephalus often accompanied by a vertical gaze paresis eponymously designated as Parinaud's syndrome. Intracranial (as well as other extragonadal) germ cell tumors are a recognized, albeit infrequent, complication of Klinefelter's syndrome.[829]

The macroscopic features and histologic criteria governing the subclassification of intracranial germ cell tumors differ in no way from those discussed elsewhere in relation to their gonadal homologs (see Chapter 18). Exceeding in incidence all other tumor types combined is the neoplasm now termed *germinoma* but formerly designated as a variant of "pinealoma" because of its frequent location in the pineal region and fancied structural resemblance to that of the embryonic gland.[833,837,838,848] Morphologically identical to the seminoma, germinomas in pure form constituted 65% of 389 histologically verified intracranial germ cell tumors culled from the English language literature published between 1950 and 1981.[838] The correct diagnosis may be suggested by isolated elevation of placental alkaline phosphatase (PLAP) activity in the serum or CSF, because immunohistochemical studies have confirmed that pure germinomas, like their seminomatous counterparts, elaborate cytoplasmic PLAP but not alpha-fetoprotein (AFP) or beta-human chorionic gonadotropin (beta-HCG).[833,837,848] Bifocal tumors involving the pineal and suprasellar regions are nearly always germinomas.[838]

Although the histologic diagnosis is usually straightforward, a germinoma that has elicited a florid lymphocytic and granulomatous reaction may masquerade as tuberculosis, sarcoidosis, or another inflammatory process.[840] The neoplastic nature of this lesion can be especially difficult to appreciate in the limited neurosurgical material obtained by stereotactic techniques. Immunocytochemical assay for PLAP may aid in the detection of tumor cells obscured by an overwhelming granulomatous infiltrate, but the potential for sampling error and the apparent failure of some germinomas to express the antigen should be borne in mind. Mention should also be made of germinomas containing admixed syncytiotrophoblastic giant cells that can be shown to elaborate beta-HCG.[833,837,848] These tumors may prompt preoperative considerations of choriocarcinoma by producing elevated levels of beta-HCG in the serum and CSF.

The prognostic significance of included syncytiotrophoblastic elements in germinomas is unclear. It has been suggested that such tumors are more likely to recur after treatment than germinomas devoid of syncytiotrophoblastic cells,[850] but the identification and follow-up of many more patients harboring this variant will be required to settle the issue. Certainly, these neoplasms do not behave in the highly aggressive fashion of choriocarcinomas and should be clearly delineated from the latter. The elaboration of beta-HCG may be responsible for the association of CNS germ cell tumors (principally germinomas) containing syncytiotrophoblastic giant cells with precocious puberty or isosexual pseudoprecocity.[828,836,841]

The nongerminomatous CNS germ cell tumors include **teratomas,**[837,843,846] **embryonal carcinomas,**[839,844] **endodermal sinus ("yolk sac") tumors,**[831,837] **choriocarcinomas,**[832,845] and all mixtures thereof.[833,837,838,848] The teratoma group encompasses mature and immature types, the extraordinarily organized variant known as intracranial fetus in fetu,[827,849a] and rare examples exhibiting rhabdomyosarcomatous transformation.[847] We have also studied two cases in which elements of mucin-producing adenocarcinoma, derived from teratomatous glands or foci of enteric differentiation in included yolk sac tumor components, came to dominate pineal germ cell tumors.[834] Elevated levels of AFP in the serum or CSF are justly considered prima facie evidence of a nongerminomatous germ cell tumor inasmuch as this antigen, characteristic of the endodermal sinus tumor and expressed by some examples of embryonal carcinoma and teratoma, is not elaborated by the pure germinoma.[833,837,848]

The clinical management of intracranial germ cell neoplasms has been governed largely by their division into germinoma in unalloyed form versus tumors composed, in part or wholly, of nongerminomatous elements. Most patients with localized intracranial germinoma can be cured by external beam irradiation, a gratifying testament to these lesions' exquisite radiosensitivity.[830] Although a few patients harboring mature teratomas are candidates for curative resection, patients whose neoplasms contain elements of embryonal carcinoma, choriocarcinoma, or endodermal sinus tumor usually succumb to progressive disease despite irradiation and conventional chemotherapy.[833,838,848] It is hoped that high-dose chemotherapeutic regimens currently under trial will alter the outlook for afflicted patients. Given their proximity to CSF pathways, it should come as no surprise that intracranial germ cell tumors (including the germinoma) often seed the ventricular surfaces and subarachnoid space.[838] Cytologic examination of the CSF is thus critical in the preoperative evaluation and follow-up monitoring of affected individuals. Extraneural (i.e., systemic) spread is a rare complication that includes "spontaneous" metastasis to sites outside the neuraxis, as well as seeding of the peritoneal cavity via ventriculoperitoneal shunts placed for relief of obstructive hydrocephalus.[831,835]

Melanocytic tumors

Mention has already been made of melanogenesis as a function occasionally exercised by nerve sheath tumors and central neuroepithelial neoplasms such as the ependymoma, subependymoma, choroid plexus papilloma or carcinoma, ganglioglioma, pineoblastoma, and medulloblastoma. The CNS and its coverings may also host neoplasms posited to derive from melanocytes of neural crest origin that normally populate the pia arachnoid.[862] Cells of this type are especially numerous over the ventral aspects of the caudal medulla and high cervical spinal cord, regions that often evidence a peppery discoloration on gross inspection, but the growths for which they are held accountable exhibit no predilection for these areas and, although largely leptomeningeal-based, may be anchored to the dura mater or buried in the substance

of the brain or spinal cord proper. Although these diverse lesions are often collectively discussed (particularly in the older literature) under inclusive designations such as melanoma, melanoblastoma, or melanoblastomatosis, it would appear that most examples of clinical importance fall into one of several fairly homogeneous diagnostic categories. Addressed in greater detail later, these include relatively indolent tumors termed melanocytomas, as well as frankly malignant melanomas occurring in either localized or diffuse leptomeningeal form. Neoplasms of this sort in some instances constitute manifestations of a generalized neurocristopathy. The syndrome of **neurocutaneous melanosis,** for example, is defined by the association of giant or multifocal nevi of congenital type with discrete meningeal melanomas or, more commonly, an unrestrained (and ultimately fatal) proliferation of melanocytic elements, often deceptively benign in appearance, throughout the subarachnoid space and within craniospinal perivascular compartments.[855,860] In addition, both meningeal melanocytomas and melanomas have been reported to arise in complex with Ota's nevus, characterized by congenital cutaneous, ocular, and retrobulbar soft tissue hyperpigmentation in a maxillo ophthalmic, trigeminal nerve distribution.[852,863] Intracranial melanoma has also been described as a complication of NF-1.[854]

Melanocytomas usually present in middle age or later adult life as circumscribed, extra-axial masses attached to the leptomeninges or dura mater. Most arise in association with spinal nerve roots, intracranial examples exhibiting a curious predilection for the trigeminal nerve and typically lying adjacent to the pons or within Meckel's cave.[856,858,858a,864,865] Consisting of grossly pigmented, tan-brown to coal-black tissue, melanocytomas are composed of variably admixed spindle and epithelioid cells, the former disposed in interlacing fascicles, broad streams, or whorls that have prompted misclassification of some reported examples as melanotic meningiomas[858] (Fig. 28-104). Nucleoli may be prominent, but candidates for this diagnosis should not evidence conspicuous mitotic activity, nuclear pleomorphism, or foci of necrosis. Cytoplasmic melanization is usually advanced, at least focally, and can obscure all cytologic detail. Ultrastructural study will confirm the presence of melanosomes in varying stages of maturation. Basement membrane material may invest some cells and occasional junctional complexes may be apparent, but the extensive basal lamina deposition and complex cytoplasmic interdigitation characteristic of the melanotic schwannoma are foreign to the melanocytoma.[856,858,858a] Tumor cells are reactive for S-100 protein, vimentin, and HMB-45 on immunocytochemical assay but do not express epithelial membrane antigen.[856,858a,864] Gross total excision should be the immediate goal of therapy and may prove curative, although local recurrence is common.[865]

Aggressive neuroparenchymal invasion and CSF seeding are not usual features of the melanocytoma, although we have recently encountered a histologically typical example that arose in the cervical spinal meninges and was complicated by multiple subarachnoid deposits, including "drop" metastases that filled the thecal sac. Given its dendritic cellular profiles and relatively indolent clinical biology, it should come as no surprise that this tumor has been likened

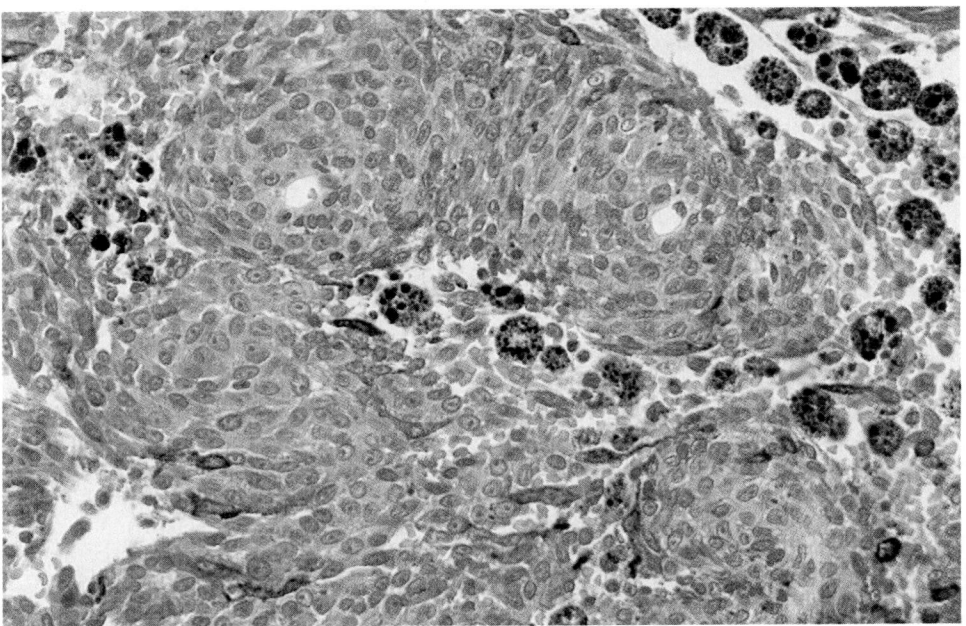

Fig. 28-104 Meningeal melanocytoma. The tendency to cellular whorling manifested by this example, resected from the cervical region of a 34-year-old man with a protracted history of neck pain and gait disturbance, accounts for the classification of many melanocytomas as melanotic meningiomas. Note finely divided brown pigment in the cytoplasm of some tumor cells (as opposed to coarse pigment granules in melanophages), delicate and monomorphous nuclear features, lack of mitotic activity, and absence of necrosis.

to both the ocular melanomas of spindle A and B types and the cellular blue nevus.[856,858]

A *malignant melanoma* is diagnosed as indigenous to the CNS only after meticulous search for a cutaneous, mucosal, or ocular primary proves unrewarding. Because malignant melanomas arising along the central neuraxis are the morphologic and immunophenotypic homologs of their peripherally situated counterparts, they are not described separately here other than to emphasize their ability to present, ab initio, as diffuse leptomeningeal growths[853,862] or as discrete masses[861] that carry a substantial risk of subsequent CSF dissemination. Proliferations of the former sort are particularly characteristic of childhood examples occurring as part of the neurocutaneous melanosis complex[855,860] but may be encountered at any age and in the absence of unusual dermal nevi. Signs and symptoms of intracranial hypertension, cranial nerve deficits, and a meningitic or subarachnoid hemorrhage–like picture are typical of primary leptomeningeal melanomatosis, which can be diagnosed by the demonstration of malignant cells in the CSF. Solitary variants, which mainly arise in adulthood, become symptomatic by virtue of their compression or invasion of neural parenchyma from sites of origin in the pia arachnoid or, less commonly, the dura.[859] In either form, CNS melanomas are aggressive neoplasms that often prove fatal within months of diagnosis, although a small subset arising within the spinal cord have been reported to evolve in a considerably more protracted fashion,[857] being amenable to resection and local irradiation.

Conceivably, at least some of the latter represented melanocytomas. We note recent description of an intracerebral **balloon cell melanoma** that may have arisen from a meningocortical melanocytic "nevus."[851]

Paraganglioma

Primary *paragangliomas* of the craniospinal axis are virtually restricted to the region of the cauda equina, where they present as delicately encapsulated intradural masses attached to the filum terminale or, less commonly, spinal roots.[869,870] Afflicted patients are typically in their fifth or sixth decade of life, present with low back pain and sciatica (occasionally accompanied by sensorimotor deficits and incontinence), and are found on myelography to have subarachnoid block. Clinically and radiographically indistinguishable from other neoplasms arising in this location (notably myxopapillary ependymomas and tumors of nerve sheath origin), these functionally silent lesions are histologically, ultrastructurally, and immunophenotypically similar to their extraspinal counterparts and so are not separately described here. They do, however, manifest a greater tendency to ganglion cell and schwannian differentiation. The designation *gangliocytic paraganglioma* is sometimes extended to tumors evidencing such features, but these do not constitute a clinically distinctive subset.[870] Occasional variants are characterized by radial perivascular arrays and pseudopapillary structures superficially similar to those of the myxopapillary ependymoma but do not generally elaborate any mucoid matrix and are readily unmasked by their argyrophilia, content of intra-cytoplasmic dense-core granules, and labeling with antisera to neurofilament proteins, chromogranin, and synaptophysin.[868-870] Some examples can, in addition, be shown to contain serotonin, somatostatin, and other neuropeptides.[868,870] A tumor of the cauda equina exhibiting both paraganglionic and ependymal differentiation has been recently described[866] but is clearly exceptional.

With regard to outcome, paragangliomas of the cauda equina are usually amenable to curative resection but may recur and, rarely, kill if inadequately excised.[870] Intraoperative manipulation of such tumors may be complicated by significant elevations of blood pressure and tachycardia,[871] presumably resulting from the release of biogenic amines. One locally aggressive case was reported to exhibit unusual oncocytic features.[867]

Chordoma

Chordomas are familiar to all pathologists as destructive tumors of the clivus and sacrococcygeum generally thought to originate from remnants of the primitive notochord persisting at these sites. Attention is called to entirely extra-osseous, intradural variants that typically lie ventral to the brainstem and that present in adulthood by reason of progressive hydrocephalus or bulbar or intratumoral hemorrhage.[876] Isolated examples have also been described as occupying the anterior third ventricle,[872] spinal epidural space,[874] or foramen magnum[873] or as arising from the tentorium.[875] The relationship of the intradural chordoma to the ecchordosis physaliphora, a notochordal heterotopia of comparable morphology that also favors the prepontine regions, remains a subject of debate.[876] Although some lesions designated as intradural chordomas are clearly neoplasms and are likely derived from displaced notochordal remnants, others may simply represent outsized, symptomatic ecchordoses. The differential diagnosis necessarily includes the rare intracranial myxoid chondrosarcoma. Intradural chordomas share with their osseous counterparts expression of cytokeratins and EMA, both alien to the chondrosarcoma, and so are readily distinguished by immunocytochemical assay. The number of reported cases is small; gross total excision of these circumscribed masses seems to hold the promise of cure, and no instances of neuraxial or extraneural dissemination have been described.

Hemangioblastoma (von Hippel–Lindau disease)

The great majority of **hemangioblastomas** present in young adulthood or middle age as cerebellar tumors associated with headache, nausea and vomiting, ataxia, and other evidences of an expanding posterior fossa mass.[892,894] Favored extracerebellar sites include the spinal cord and medulla, odd examples arising in the optic nerves,[893] spinal roots (including cauda equina), cerebral hemispheres,[892a] craniospinal meninges, and retina.[892,894] In any of these locations, familial hemangioblastomas are the hallmark of von Hippel–Lindau disease, a complex, autosomal dominant syndrome that commonly includes retinal angiomatosis, cysts and carcinomas of renocortical and pancreatic origin, adrenal pheochromocytomas, and papillary cystadenomas of the epididymis.[888] Affected kindreds are also reportedly at risk

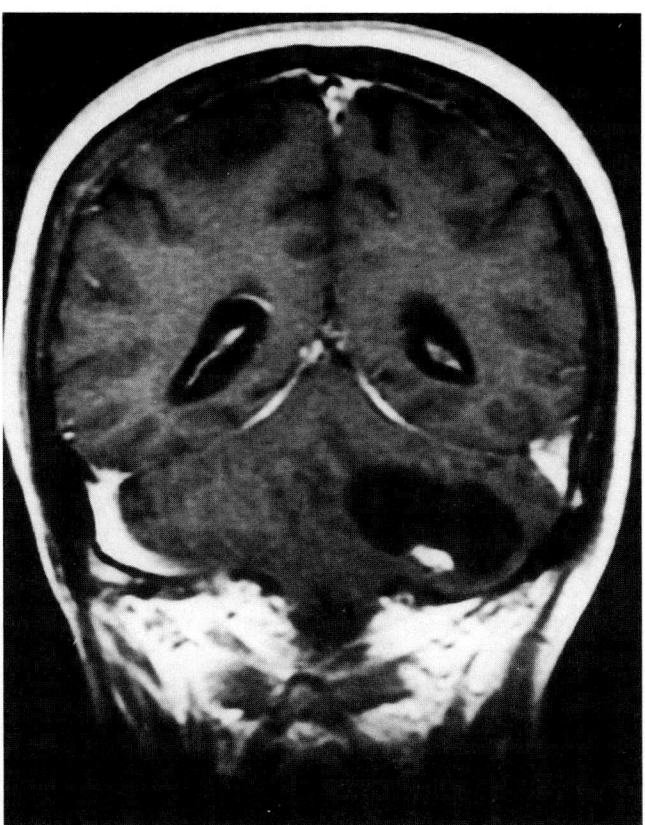

Fig. 28-105 Hemangioblastoma. Most hemangioblastomas arise in the cerebellar hemispheres, where, as emphasized in this postcontrast injection MRI, they present as diminutive, brightly enhancing, and sharply delimited mural nodules projecting into sizable cysts.

for angiomas and cysts of the liver, spleen, or lung; hepatocellular adenomas and carcinomas; paragangliomas; endocrine tumors of the thyroid gland, pancreas, and gastrointestinal tract; a variety of central neuroepithelial neoplasms; syringomyelia; and recently, aggressive papillary tumors of the middle ear and papillary cystadenomas of probable mesonephric origin arising in the female genital adnexae.[882] Noteworthy is the demonstration that even sporadic hemangioblastomas, which constitute some 75% to 80% of examples encountered in clinical practice, may harbor mutations of a tumor-suppressor gene incriminated in the pathogenesis of von Hippel–Lindau disease and mapped to chromosome 3.[887] A minority of hemangioblastomas present with erythrocytosis, a consequence of tumoral erythropoietin production,[883,895] and some contain foci of extramedullary hematopoiesis.[894]

The hemangioblastoma often constitutes a sharply circumscribed mural nodule, at times diminutive, in what is otherwise a smooth-walled cyst or, at spinal levels, syrinx (Fig. 28-105). The tumor tends to be clearly demarcated from adjacent non-neoplastic tissues (Fig. 28-106). Its characteristic reddish-brown and yellow coloration reflects a rich vasculature and high lipid content, respectively. The former, an anastomosing network of delicate, capillary-like channels

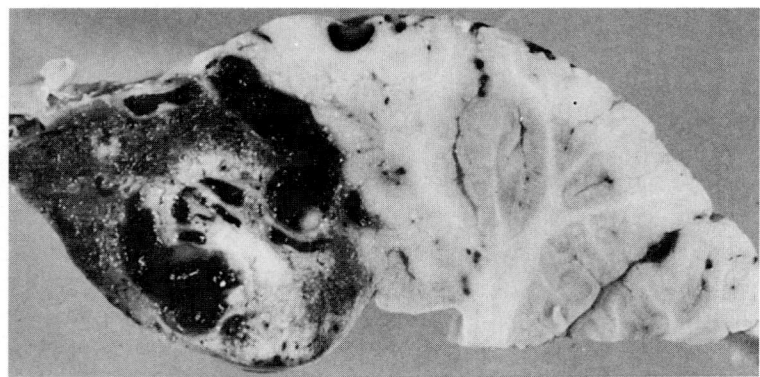

Fig. 28-106 Hemangioblastoma. Another cerebellar example is illustrated to underscore this benign neoplasm's circumscription and conspicuous vascularization. (Courtesy Dr. J.E. Olvera-Rabiela, Mexico City.)

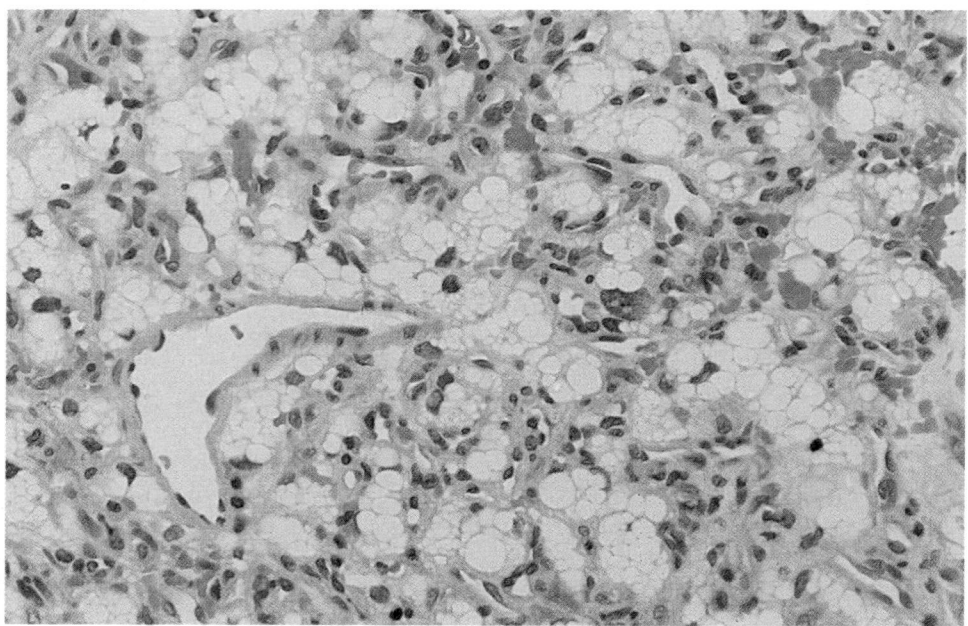

Fig. 28-107 Hemangioblastoma. The neoplasm's defining "stromal" cells are most readily visualized when lipid accumulation imparts a foamy or vacuolated quality to the pale cytoplasm.

supplied by feeding vessels of larger caliber, is responsible for the lesion's name and traditional classification as a primary vascular neoplasm. In fact, the sole neoplastic element of the hemangioblastoma is probably its so-called "stromal cell," which inhabits the interstices between the tumor's ramifying vascular arcade and is recognized by a pale cytoplasm often rich in neutral fats and, as a consequence, finely vacuolated or foamy in appearance (Fig. 28-107). Aggregation of stromal cells in cohesive nests and lobules lends to "cellular" hemangioblastomas an epithelioid histologic presentation that invites confusion with metastatic renocortical carcinoma of clear cell type, whereas their paucity in "reticular" variants results in a picture that may be mis-construed as simply angiomatous. Potentially misleading as well is the tendency for some stromal cells to exhibit conspicuous nuclear abnormalities, presumably degenerative, reminiscent of those encountered in neoplasms of endocrine type. These changes, which include alarming karyomegaly, pleomorphism, and chromatin smudging, are unaccompanied by mitotic activity and are of no prognostic import. A regular feature of the tumor-brain interface is a florid piloid astrogliosis replete with Rosenthal fibers but lacking the microcystic elements typical of the juvenile pilocytic astrocytoma. The designation *angioglioma* has been extended to rare tumors interpreted as containing a mixture of hemangioblastomatous and neoplastic glial tissues (see p. 2300).

Examples of hemangioblastoma arising in association with AVM have also been reported.[889]

Despite repeated investigations into its ultrastructure and antigenic profile,[877,880,881,884,891] the cytogenesis of the stromal cell remains an enigma and there is no compelling evidence that would support its widely assumed derivation from vasoformative elements such as endothelium or pericytes. Suffice it to say that this cell remains unlabeled by endothelial "markers" such as antisera to factor VIII–related antigen and the lectin *Ulex europaeus* agglutinin-I; its ultrastructure—an electron-lucent cytoplasm possessed of lipid droplets, microfilaments, and profiles of smooth and rough endoplasmic reticulum—does not conform to that of any cell type normally associated with blood vessels or, for that matter, other human tissues[885,886] (Fig. 28-108). GFAP immunoreactivity is typically restricted to entrapped astrocytes or a subset of stromal cells situated along the periphery of the tumor, a phenomenon reasonably interpreted as reflecting phagocytosis or nonspecific adsorption of antigen produced in neighboring gliotic parenchyma.

That stromal cells may be capable of neuroendocrine differentiation is suggested by positive immunoassays for S-100 protein, neuron-specific enolase, and a variety of neuropeptides.[877,880] Select cases have also exhibited intracytoplasmic dense-core granules on ultrastructural analysis.[886] Others have concluded that these are undifferentiated mesenchymal cells,[881] or mesodermally derived elements capable of differentiating along "fibrohistiocytic" lines.[891] On a practical note, we would point out that the hemangioblastoma may exceptionally contain cytokeratin-reactive elements, but the stromal cell's consistent failure to express epithelial membrane antigen readily distinguishes this tumor from metastatic renocortical carcinoma and the occasional meningioma characterized by an unusually rich vasculature and tumor cell lipidization.[884]

Their histogenesis notwithstanding, hemangioblastomas are benign neoplasms that usually lend themselves to curative resection. Excised examples can recur, however, and patients (particularly those afflicted with von Hippel–Lindau disease) may develop additional, multifocal primary tumors.[878,879,892] Some observers have noted a solid gross configuration and paucity of stromal cells to be correlated with symptomatic tumor regrowth.[878] Dissemination of histologically conventional hemangioblastomas by the CSF has been reported[890] but is exceedingly rare.

Rhabdoid and atypical teratoid tumors

Although few acceptable cases have been reported to date, **primary rhabdoid tumors of the CNS** appear to be highly aggressive neoplasms characterized by a peak incidence in early childhood and infancy and a capacity for early neuraxis dissemination by the CSF.[897,898,900,900a] Although their histologic, ultrastructural, and immunophenotypic features conform, by definition, to those of rhabdoid tumors arising in the kidney, addressed elsewhere in this text, the question of a more fundamental homology will remain unanswered until the cytogenesis of both entities is clarified. Noteworthy in this regard are examples described as simultaneously involving kidney and brain,[899] although these, admittedly, could be dismissed as instances of metastasis

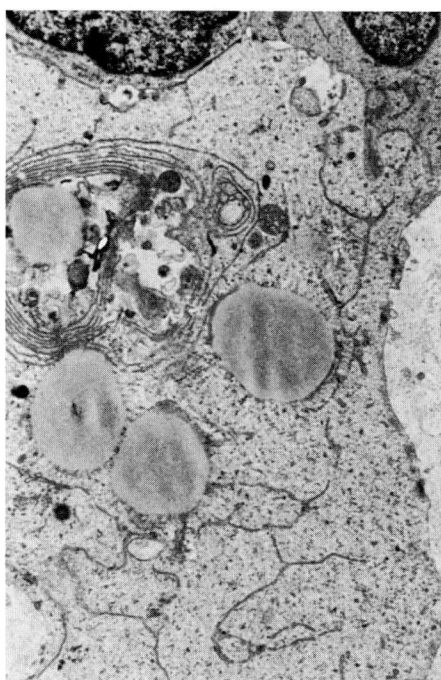

Fig. 28-108 Hemangioblastoma. Lipid droplets and membranous profiles, some in concentric array, are demonstrated in this transmission electron photomicrograph of a "stromal" cell. (3 8,400.)

rather than multifocal neoplastic transformation of a shared progenitor. As noted in the discussion of embryonal neoplasms, renal rhabdoid tumors may occur together with primitive neuroepithelial neoplasms arising in the brain.[555]

Because cells exhibiting rhabdoid cytologic features may be encountered in a variety of intracranial neoplasms, notably primitive neuroepithelial tumors exhibiting glial differentiation[901] and bona fide rhabdomyosarcomas, immunoassays for the expression of GFAP and muscle-associated antigens, respectively, are critical in the exclusion of these alternative diagnoses. The large cell medulloblastoma is another consideration but lacks the hyaline perinuclear inclusions typical of the rhabdoid tumor, does not express EMA, and is further distinguished by its labeling with antibodies to synaptophysin.[574] An obscure posterior fossa neoplasm, the *atypical teratoid tumor,* has been described as containing a rhabdoid component admixed with spindly neuroepithelial and mesenchymal elements.[896] The relationship, if any, of this poorly characterized lesion to the pure CNS rhabdoid tumor is unclear, but select examples of each have been characterized by monosomy 22 on cytogenetic analysis.[896]

Other primary tumors

The list of neoplastic oddities that have been encountered along the central neuraxis includes a single intraspinal mass interpreted as an **adrenocortical adenoma,**[902] a lesion of the sellar region described as a **heterotopic follicular carcinoma of thyroid gland type,**[905] and a number of ectopic, suprasellar **pituitary adenomas** situated in the third ventricle/hypothalamic region.[903,904] A survey of intracranial sarcomas previously cited in the discussion of nonmeningothelial, mesenchymal neoplasms includes an example of **cerebral ectomesenchymoma**—a tumor composed of ganglion cell and rhabdomyosarcomatous elements.[682]

SECONDARY TUMORS

Secondary involvement of the CNS by direct extension or hematogenous metastasis is a common complication of systemic cancer and a phenomenon that frequently prompts diagnostic, as well as palliative, neurosurgical intervention. Because we have already touched on this subject in reference to lymphoproliferative and myeloproliferative disorders, this discussion is concerned only with invasion of the central neuraxis by solid tumors.

That neoplasms arising in and around the skeletal confines of the brain and spinal cord often come to impinge on these structures should come as no surprise. Examples include the pituitary adenoma with suprasellar or retrosellar expansion, the glomus jugulare tumor (paraganglioma) that exploits neighboring foramina of the calvarial floor to present as a mass in the pontocerebellar angle, and sacrococcygeal chordomas that engulf the roots of the cauda equina.[928] Ceruminous gland carcinomas of the ear may occasionally billow into the middle cranial fossa.[912] A substantial risk of local skull base destruction and invasion of contiguous meninges, potentially complicated by dissemination in the subarachnoid space, is seen in embryonal rhabdomyosarcomas originating in head and neck sites, particularly the nasopharynx, paranasal sinuses, and middle ear.[908] Similarly situated carcinomas of mucosal or minor salivary gland derivation may behave in like fashion, but some of the latter instead track insidiously along regional nerve fiber bundles to achieve radiologically detectable proportions only within the cranial compartment.[915,926] Neglected, basal cell or squamous carcinomas of the face and scalp may also reach the CNS by permeating the calvarium or by propagation within perineural spaces. Cancers arising in more distant sites may secondarily infiltrate the nervous system after first metastasizing to juxtaneural structures, the vertebral column apparently serving as an especially important way station in this regard. Epidural spinal cord compression by malignant tumors, for example, is most frequently caused by carcinomas of pulmonary, prostatic, or mammary origin that have spread to the vertebrae, neoplastic cells commonly entering the spinal canal via the bony foramina traversed by the vertebral veins.[910] A similar sequence of events is postulated to account for the high incidence of vertebral and paravertebral metastases in cancer patients developing diffuse leptomeningeal carcinomatosis, principally a complication of adenocarcinomas derived from the lung and breast.[918] This diagnosis is usually established by the demonstration of malignant cells on cytologic inspection of the CSF.[909]

More common than instances of secondary CNS infiltration by contiguous malignant tumors are blood-borne neuraxial metastases. The principal offenders in this regard are carcinomas of the lung and breast, followed by malignant melanomas, renocortical carcinomas, and adenocarcinomas of colorectal origin.[928] Carcinomas of the lung are the systemic cancers most likely to present initially as intracerebral tumors, accounting for roughly half of all such cases[919] and up to 85% of lesions exhibiting adenocarcinomatous histol-

ogy.[922] Increasingly effective management of systemic disease may account for the rising incidence of intracranial deposits from ovarian carcinomas[920] and osseous or soft tissue sarcomas,[921] but the latter remain rare as neurosurgical specimens. Sarcomas typically spread to the lungs en route to the brain but may give rise to isolated cerebral or dural-based metastases that, in exceptional instances, herald discovery of the primary tumor.[925] Noteworthy is the prominence of alveolar soft part sarcoma, one of the rarest tumor types, among mesenchymal neoplasms giving rise to intracranial metastases.[921,925] Mention should also be made of HIV-1–associated Kaposi's sarcoma traveling to the cranial compartment,[907] but this remains a curiosity even in the presence of widespread cutaneous and visceral involvement.

Although blood-borne tumor emboli may lodge at any level of the central neuraxis, a few useful generalizations can be made regarding the topography of metastatic lesions. Intramedullary metastases (i.e., those involving the spinal cord parenchyma) are rare,[913] the great majority of metastatic deposits coming to lie in the supratentorial or infratentorial compartments. In general, the distribution of metastases within the latter conforms to their relative volumes and blood supply.[914] Thus most lesions settle within frontoparietal cerebral tissues subtended by the middle cerebral artery (the dominant tributary of the circle of Willis); tumor emboli often lodge within the "watershed" zone representing the terminus of this vessel's territory. For reasons that are not clear, colorectal, uterine, and renocortical carcinomas are overrepresented among cancers seeding the cerebellum.[914] Prostatic adenocarcinomas also exhibit a curious predilection for this structure when they metastasize to the brain, but their deposits are typically dural based and only exceptionally involve the neural parenchyma proper.[911] Dural metastases in women usually derive from mammary primary tumors.[930] As a rule, those tumors that frequently travel to the CNS (e.g., malignant melanoma and carcinomas of the lung) tend to produce multiple metastases, whereas cancers that only occasionally involve the brain (e.g., gastrointestinal adenocarcinomas) are often represented by solitary deposits. Noteworthy is a clinical study in which nearly one half of cancer patients with brain metastases were found to have unifocal lesions on neuroradiologic assessment.[914] A particularly compelling case for neurosurgical intervention can be made in this setting because metastatic lesions are usually compact in their growth patterns and thus lend themselves to excision. Patients who undergo surgical extirpation of single metastases (usually followed by whole brain radiotherapy) may be restored to many months, or even years, of useful function; live longer; and enjoy a better quality of life than those whose tumors are simply irradiated.[924] It is to be hoped that the advent of refined stereotactic and radiosurgical techniques will improve the outlook for patients with deep-seated or multifocal lesions.

In contrast to the common glial neoplasms of adulthood, metastatic nodules tend to be sharply circumscribed and possessed of "pushing" margins (Fig. 28-109). Much of their mass effect may be derived from edematous expansion of neighboring white matter, often disproportionate to the small size of the offending deposits and usually more pronounced than the edema accompanying primary brain tumors. Most

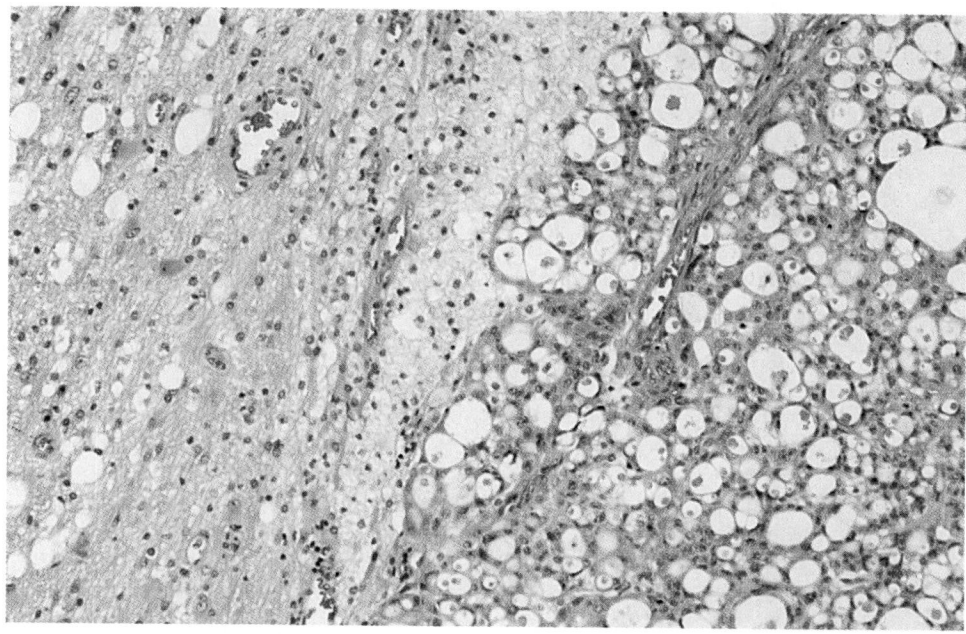

Fig. 28-109 Metastatic carcinoma. A cohesive growth pattern and clearly delimited tumor-CNS interface are hallmarks of neoplasms metastatic to the brain. The adenocarcinoma *(right),* derived from a primary in the left lung, "pushes" against adjacent cerebral white matter.

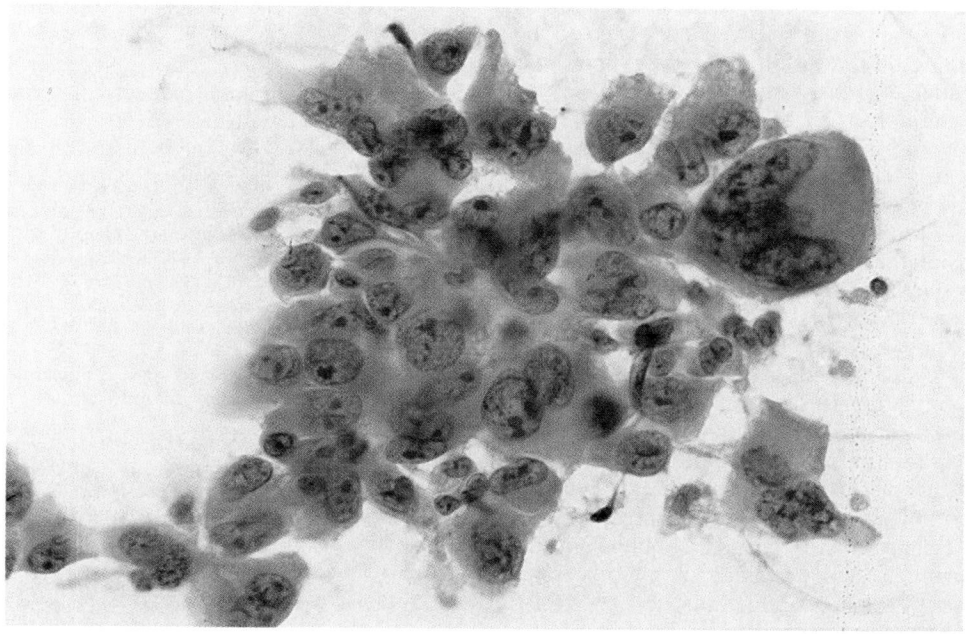

Fig. 28-110 Metastatic carcinoma. The cellular cohesion characteristic of most epithelial neoplasms and foreign to gliomas and lymphomas is generally maintained in cytology preparations, facilitating rapid intraoperative diagnosis. Note also the absence of cytoplasmic processes and presence of conspicuous nucleoli, the latter also alien to most neuroepithelial tumors, in this smear preparation of a poorly differentiated pulmonary adenocarcinoma that presented as a solitary, right frontal lobe brain mass.

metastases are relatively superficial in location, straddling the gray-white junction to involve both cerebral cortex (thus the high incidence of associated seizures) and digitate white matter. Intralesional hemorrhage occasionally brings brain metastases to light and is especially common in examples of melanoma[927] and in germ cell tumors (particularly chorio-carcinoma).[928]

On histologic examination, most secondary cancers conform to the histology of their donor tumors and are readily distinguished from primary neoplasms of the brain or meninges on casual inspection. Features that aid in the segregation of poorly differentiated carcinomas from anaplastic gliomas include a cohesive architecture, abrupt interface with adjacent neural tissue, "peritheliomatous" pattern of tumor cell preservation about stromal blood vessels in cases evidencing coagulative necrosis, and absence of complex microvascular hyperplasia. The last, however, is an arresting feature of some metastatic small cell carcinomas derived from the lung and has even been reported to undergo sarcomatous transformation in isolated instances.[916] A confident diagnosis of metastatic carcinoma can often be made at the time of surgery by examination of smear or crush preparations in which the cellular cohesion of most epithelial neoplasms is preserved (Fig. 28-110). The reader is reminded that glial neoplasms of varied type, including fibrillary astrocytomas, may be labeled by antibodies to cytokeratins[305,330] and, on occasion, EMA.[311] Assay for GFAP should thus be performed before one concludes that a poorly differentiated tumor expressing these markers is, in fact, a carcinoma. We have not succeeded in duplicating reports of GFAP expression on the part of select renocortical carcinomas.[635,884] Depending on the histologic findings in a given case, the differential diagnosis of a suspected metastasis may include, in addition to an epithelioid or sarcomatous glioblastoma, the capillary hemangioblastoma, papillary ependymoma, choroid plexus tumor, and meningioma. Each of these is considered separately elsewhere in this chapter. We refer the reader to the foregoing discussion of fibrillary astrocytic neoplasms for a brief account of lipid-rich, adenoid or partially squamous glioblastomas and gliosarcomas that may masquerade as cerebral metastases.

In closing, mention is made of certain unusual forms or presentations of secondary CNS involvement by malignant neoplasms. These include diffuse seeding of the periventricular tissues by metastatic small cell carcinomas of the lung[931] (a pattern of spread mimicking the topography of some primary CNS lymphomas), miliary or "encephalitic" cerebral carcinomatosis or melanomatosis with widespread vascular cuffing by tumor cells on microscopic study but no conspicuous mass lesions,[917,929] and occlusion of major cerebral vessels by neoplastic emboli resulting in ischemic stroke.[923] Intracardiac tumors such as myxomas are the lesions most often implicated in cerebral infarction secondary to neoplastic embolization, but this phenomenon has also been recorded in association with carcinomas arising in the head and neck, lungs, colon, and other visceral sites. As mentioned in the discussion of primary mesenchymal tumors of the CNS, deposits derived from occult atrial myxomas may be misconstrued as cerebral epithelioid hemangioendotheliomas.[731] Neoplastic aneurysms are discussed in the section

dealing with cerebrovascular disorders. Yet another vascular complication of intracranial metastasis is subdural hemorrhage secondary to dural-based lesions.[906]

REFERENCES
CONGENITAL ABNORMALITIES
Craniospinal dysraphism

1 Bale PM: Sacrococcygeal developmental abnormalities and tumors in children. Perspect Pediatr Pathol 1:9-56, 1984.
2 Chadduck WM, Uthman EL: Squamous cell carcinoma and meningomyelocele. Neurosurgery 14:601-603, 1984.
3 Chakrabortty S, Oi S, Yoshida Y, Yamada H, Yamaguchi M, Tamaki N, Matsumoto S: Myelomeningocele and thick filum terminale with tethered cord appearing as a human tail. J Neurosurg 78:966-969, 1993.
4 Chapman PH, Beyerl B: The tethered spinal cord, with particular reference to spinal lipoma and diastematomyelia. In Hoffman HJ, Epstein F, eds: Disorders of the developing nervous system. Diagnosis and treatment. Boston, 1986, Blackwell Scientific, pp 109-131.
5 Ebisu T, Odake G, Fujimoto M, Ueda S, Tsujii H, Morimoto M, Sawada T: Neurenteric cysts with meningomyelocele or meningocele. Split notochord syndrome. Childs Nerv Syst 6:465-467, 1990.
6 Erkulvrawtr S, Gammal TE, Hawkins J, Green JB, Srinivasan G: Intrathoracic meningoceles and neurofibromatosis. Arch Neurol 36:557-559, 1979.
7 Fisher RG, Uihlein A, Keith HM: Spina bifida and cranium bifidum. Study of 530 cases. Proc Staff Meet Mayo Clin 27:33-38, 1952.
8 Lalwani AK, Jackler RK, Harsh IV GR, Butt F Y-S: Bilateral temporal bone encephaloceles after cranial irradiation. Case report. J Neurosurg 79:596-599, 1993.
9 McLaurin RL: Encephalocele and related anomalies. In Hoffman HJ, Epstein F, eds: Disorders of the developing nervous system. Diagnosis and treatment. Boston, 1986, Blackwell Scientific, pp 153-171.
10 Mitang RN: Teratoma occurring within a myelomeningocele. J Neurosurg 37:448-451, 1972.

Neuroglial and meningeal heterotopias

11 Bale PM, Hughes L, de Silva M: Sequestered meningoceles of scalp. Extracranial meningeal heterotopia. Hum Pathol 21:1156-1163, 1990.
12 Boessen EH, Hudson WR: Oligodendroglioma arising in heterotopic brain tissue of the soft palate and nasopharynx. Am J Surg Pathol 11:571-574, 1987.
13 Call NB, Baylis HI: Cerebellar heterotopia in the orbit. Arch Ophthalmol 98:717-719, 1980.
14 Chan JKC, Lau W: Nasal astrocytoma or nasal glial heterotopia? Arch Pathol Lab Med 113:943-945, 1989.
15 Cooper JS, Kernohan JW: Heterotopic glial nests in the subarachnoid space. Histopathologic characteristics, mode of origin and relation to meningeal gliomas. J Neuropathol Exp Neurol 10:16-29, 1951.
16 Gold AH, Sharer LR, Walden RH: Central nervous system heterotopia in association with cleft palate. Plast Reconstr Surg 66:434-441, 1980.
17 Kershisnik MM, Kaplan C, Craven CM, Carey JC, Townsend JJ, Knisely AS: Intrapulmonary neuroglial heterotopia. Arch Pathol Lab Med 116:1043-1046, 1992.
18 Lee SC, Henry MM, Gonzalez-Crussi F: Simultaneous occurrence of melanotic neuroectodermal tumor and brain heterotopia in the oropharynx. Cancer 38:249-253, 1976.
19 Patterson K, Kapur S, Chandra RS: "Nasal gliomas" and related brain heterotopias. A pathologist's perspective. Pediatr Pathol 5:353-362, 1986.
20 Suster S, Rosai J: Hamartoma of scalp with ectopic meningothelial elements. A distinctive benign soft tissue lesion that may simulate angiosarcoma. Am J Surg Pathol 14:1-11, 1990.

Choristomas

21 Curry B, Taylor CW, Fisher AWF: Salivary gland heterotopia. A unique cerebellopontine angle tumor. Arch Pathol Lab Med 106:35-38, 1982.
22 Fix SE, Nelson J, Schochet SS Jr: Focal leptomeningeal rhabdomyomatosis of the posterior fossa. Arch Pathol Lab Med 113:872-873, 1989.
23 Ho KL: Ecchordosis physaliphora and chordoma. A comparative ultrastructural study. Clin Neuropathol 4:77-86, 1985.
24 Lena G, Dufour T, Gambarelli D, Chabrol B, Mancini J: Choristoma of the intracranial maxillary nerve in a child. Case report. J Neurosurg 81:788-791, 1994.
25 Lombardo L, Mateos JH, Barroeta FF: Subarachnoid hemorrhage due to endometriosis of the spinal canal. Neurology 18:423-426, 1968.
26 Molleston MC, Roth KA, Wipold II FJ, Grubb RL Jr: Tethered cord syndrome from a choristoma of müllerian origin. Case report. J Neurosurg 74:497-500, 1991.

27 Thibodeau LL, Prioleau GR, Manuelidis EE, Merino MJ, Heafner MD: Cerebral endometriosis—case report. J Neurosurg **66**:609-610, 1987.

28 Zwick DL, Livingston K, Clapp L, Kosnik E, Yates A: Intracranial trigeminal nerve rhabdomyoma/choristoma in a child. A case report and discussion of possible histogenesis. Hum Pathol **20**:390-392, 1989.

Cysts of the central neuraxis

29 Agnoli A, Laun A, Schonmayr R: Enterogenous intraspinal cysts. J Neurosurg **61**:834-840, 1984.

30 Del Bigio M, Jay V, Drake JM: Prepontine cyst lined by respiratory epithelium with squamous metaplasia. Immunohistochemical and ultrastructural study. Acta Neuropathol **83**:564-568, 1992.

31 Harris CP, Dias MS, Brockmeyer DL, Townsend JJ, Willis BK, Apfelbaum RI: Neurenteric cysts of the posterior fossa. Recognition, management and embryogenesis. Neurosurgery **29**:893-897, 1991.

32 Ho K-L, Garcia JH: Colloid cysts of the third ventricle. Ultrastructural features are compatible with endodermal differentiation. Acta Neuropathol **83**:605-612, 1992.

33 Ho K-L, Tiel R: Intraspinal bronchogenic cyst. Ultrastructural study of the lining epithelium. Acta Neuropathol **78**:513-520, 1989.

34 Isla A, Palacios J, Roda J, Gutierrez M, Gonzalez C, Blazquez M: Neuroepithelial cyst in the optic nerve. Case report. J Neurosurg **67**:137-139, 1987.

35 Lach B, Scheithauer BW, Gregor A, Wick MR: Colloid cyst of the third ventricle. A comparative immunohistochemical study of neuraxis cysts and choroid plexus epithelium. J Neurosurg **78**:101-111, 1993.

36 List CF, Williams JR: Subdural epithelial cyst in the interhemispheral fissure. Report of a case with some remarks concerning the classification of intracranial epithelial cysts. J Neurosurg **18**:690-693, 1961.

37 Mackenzie IRA, Gilbert JJ: Cysts of the neuraxis of endodermal origin. J Neurol Neurosurg Psychiatry **54**:572-575, 1991.

38 Millis RR, Holmes AE: Enterogenous cyst of the spinal cord with associated intestinal reduplication, vertebral anomalies, and a dorsal dermal sinus. Case report. J Neurosurg **38**:73-77, 1973.

39 Montaldi S, Deruaz J-P, Cai Z-T, de Tribolet N: Symptomatic xanthogranuloma of the third ventricle. Report of two cases and review of the literature. Surg Neurol **32**:200-205, 1989.

40 Nitta M, Symon L: Colloid cysts of the third ventricle. A review of 36 cases. Acta Neurochir **75**:136-146, 1985.

41 Powers J, Dodds H: Primary actinomycoma of the third ventricle—the colloid cyst. A histochemical and ultrastructural study. Acta Neuropathol **37**:21-26, 1977.

42 Tsuchida T, Hruban RH, Carson B, Phillips P: Colloid cysts of the third ventricle. Immunohistochemical evidence for nonneuroepithelial differentiation. Hum Pathol **23**:811-816, 1992.

43 Voelker JL, Campbell RL, Muller J: Clinical, radiographic, and pathological features of symptomatic Rathke's cleft cysts. J Neurosurg **74**:535-544, 1991.

44 Gluszcz A: A cancer arising in a dermoid of the brain. A case report. J Neuropathol Exp Neurol **21**:383-387, 1962.

45 Goldman SA, Gandy SE: Squamous cell carcinoma as a late complication of intracerebroventricular epidermoid cyst. Case report. J Neurosurg **66**:618-620, 1987.

46 Halcrow SJ, Crawford PJ, Craft AW: Epidermoid spinal cord tumour after lumbar puncture. Arch Dis Child **60**:978-979, 1985.

47 Keogh AJ, Timperley WR: Atypical hidradenoma arising in a dermoid cyst of the spinal canal. J Pathol **117**:207-209, 1975.

48 Lunardi P, Missori P: Supratentorial dermoid cysts. J Neurosurg **75**:262-266, 1991.

49 Lunardi P, Missori P, Gagliardi F, Fortuna A: Dermoid cysts of the posterior cranial fossa in children. Report of nine cases and review of the literature. Surg Neurol **34**:39-42, 1990.

50 Lunardi P, Missori P, Rizzo A, Gagliardi F: Chemical meningitis in ruptured intracranial dermoid. Case report and review of the literature. Surg Neurol **32**:449-452, 1989.

51 Obana WG, Wilson CB: Epidermoid cysts of the brain stem. Report of three cases. J Neurosurg **74**:123-128, 1991.

52 Roux A, Mercier C, Larbrisseau A, Dube L-J, Dupuis C, Del Carpio R: Intramedullary epidermoid cysts of the spinal cord. Case report. J Neurosurg **76**:528-533, 1992.

53 Smith C, Timperley WR: Multiple intraspinal and intracranial epidermoids and lipomata following gunshot injury. Neuropathol Appl Neurobiol **10**:235-239, 1984.

54 Yamakawa K, Shitara N, Genka S, Manaka S, Takakura K: Clinical course and surgical prognosis of 33 cases of intracranial epidermoid tumors. Neurosurgery **24**:568-573, 1989.

55 Ciricillo SF, Davis RL, Wilson CB: Neuroepithelial cysts of the posterior fossa. Case report. J Neurosurg **72**:302-305, 1990.

56 Friede RL, Yasargil MG: Supratentorial intracerebral epithelial (ependymal) cysts. review, case reports, and fine structure. J Neurol Neurosurg Psychiatry **40**:127-137, 1977.

57 Gherardi R, Lacombe M, Poirier J, Roucayrol A, Wechsler J: Asymptomatic encephalic intraparenchymatous neuroepithelial cysts. Acta Neuropathol **63**:264-268, 1984.

58 Ho K-L, Chason JL: A glioependymal cyst of the cerebellopontine angle. Immunohistochemical and ultrastructural studies. Acta Neuropathol **74**:382-388, 1987.

59 Robertson D, Kirkpatrick JB, Harper RL, Mawad ME: Spinal intramedullary ependymal cyst. Report of three cases. J Neurosurg **75**:312-316, 1991.

60 Chitkara U, Cogswell C, Norton K, Wilkins I, Mehalek K, Berkowitz R: Choroid plexus cysts in the fetus. A benign anatomic variant or pathologic entity? Report of 41 cases and review of the literature. Obstet Gynecol **72**:185-189, 1988.

61 Inoue T, Matsushima T, Fukui M, Matsubara T, Kitamoto T: Choroidal epithelial cyst of the cerebral hemisphere. An immunohistochemical study. Surg Neurol **28**:119-122, 1987.

62 Odake G, Tenjin H, Murakami N: Cyst of the choroid plexus in the lateral ventricle. case report and review of the literature. Neurosurgery **27**:470-476, 1990.

63 Nakasu Y, Hanada J, Watanabe K: Progressive neurological deficits with benign intracerebral cysts. Report of two cases. J Neurosurg **65**:706-709, 1986.

64 Silverberg GD: Simple cysts of the cerebellum. J Neurosurg **35**:320-327, 1971.

65 Weisberg LA: Non-neoplastic gliotic cerebellar cysts. Clinical and computed tomography correlations. Neuroradiology **24**:53-57, 1982.

66 Wilkins RH, Burger PC: Benign intraparenchymal brain cysts without an epithelial lining. J Neurosurg **68**:378-382, 1988.

67 Fain JS, Tomlinson FH, Scheithauer BW, Parisi JE, Fletcher GP, Kelly PJ, Miller GM: Symptomatic glial cysts of the pineal gland. J Neurosurg **80**:454-460, 1994.

68 Beatty R, Hornig G, Hanson EJ: Protruding arachnoid granulations mimicking dermoid cysts. J Pediatr Surg **24**:411-413, 1989.

69 Nabors MW, Pait TG, Byrd EB, Karim NO, Davis DO, Kobrine AI, Rizzoli HV: Updated assessment and current classification of spinal meningeal cysts. J Neurosurg **68**:366-377, 1988.

70 Passero S, Filosomi G, Cioni R, Venturi C, Volpini B: Arachnoid cysts of the middle cranial fossa. A clinical, radiological and follow-up study. Acta Neurol Scand **82**:94-100, 1990.

71 Pierre-Kahn A, Capelle L, Brauner R, Sainte-Rose C, Renier D, Rappaport R, Hirsch J-F: Presentation and management of suprasellar arachnoid cysts. Review of 20 cases. J Neurosurg **73**:355-359, 1990.

72 Rengachary SS, Watanabe I: Ultrastructure and pathogenesis of intracranial arachnoid cysts. J Neuropathol Exp Neurol **40**:61-83, 1981.

73 Rock J, Zimmerman R, Bell W, Fraser R: Arachnoid cysts of the posterior fossa. Neurosurgery **18**:176-179, 1986.

74 Rosenberg AE, O'Connell J, Ojemann R, Plata M: Giant cystic arachnoid granulations. A rare cause of lytic skull lesions. Hum Pathol **24**:438-441, 1993.

75 Shaw C-M: "Arachnoid cysts" of the Sylvian fissure versus "temporal lobe agenesis" syndrome. Ann Neurol **5**:483-485, 1979.

76 Weinand M, Rengachary SS, McGregor D, Watanabe I: Intradiploic arachnoid cysts. Report of two cases. J Neurosurg **70**:954-958, 1989.

77 Gorey MT, Hyman RA, Black KS, Scuderi DM, Cinnamon J, Kim KS: Lumbar synovial cyst eroding bone. Am J Neuroradiol **13**:161-163, 1992.

78 Hemminghytt S, Daniles D, Williams A, Haughton V: Intraspinal synovial cysts. Natural history and diagnosis by CT. Radiology **145**:375-376, 1982.

79 Close LG, O'Connor WE: Sphenoethmoidal mucoceles with intracranial extension. Otolaryngol Head Neck Surg **91**:350-357, 1983.

80 Reddy PK, Rao GP, Prakasham A, Purnand A, Sulochana C, Kumar RSA, Reddy YR, Chandramala MS, Indumathi D: Intracerebral polyposis. Case report. J Neurosurg **78**:294-296, 1993.

CEREBROVASCULAR DISORDERS
Cerebral infarction

81 Chuaqui R, Tapia J: Histologic assessment of the age of recent brain infarcts in man. J Neuropathol Exp Neurol **52**:481-489, 1993.

Intracranial aneurysms

82 Bohmfalk GL, Story JL, Wissinger JP, Brown WE Jr: Bacterial intracranial aneurysm. J Neurosurg **48**:369-382, 1978.

83 Chambi I, Tasker RR, Gentili F, Lougheed WM, Smyth HS, Marshall J, Young I, Deck J, Shrubb J: Gauze-induced granuloma ("gauzoma"). An uncommon complication of gauze reinforcement of berry aneurysms. J Neurosurg **72**:163-170, 1990.

84 Ho K-L: Neoplastic aneurysm and intracranial hemorrhage. Cancer **50**:2935-2940, 1982.

85 Inagawa T, Hirano A: Ruptured intracranial aneurysms. An autopsy study of 133 patients. Surg Neurol **33**:117-123, 1990.

86 Juvela S, Porras M, Heiskanen O: Natural history of unruptured intracranial aneurysms. A long-term follow-up study. J Neurosurg **79**:174-182, 1993.

87 McCormick WF: Vascular diseases. In Rosenberg RN, ed: The clinical neurosciences. Neuropathology, vol 3. New York, 1983, Churchill Livingstone, pp 35-47.

88 McCormick WF, Nofzinger JD: Saccular intracranial aneurysms. An autopsy study. J Neurosurg 22:155-159, 1965.

89 Molinari GF, Smith L, Goldstein MN, Satran R: Pathogenesis of cerebral mycotic aneurysms. Neurology 23:325-332, 1972.

90 Shokunbi MT, Vinters HV, Kaufmann JCE: Fusiform intracranial aneurysms. Clinicopathologic features. Surg Neurol 29:263-270, 1988.

91 Stehbens WE: Etiology of intracranial berry aneurysms. J Neurosurg 70:823-831, 1989.

92 Wakai S, Kumakura N, Nagai M: Lobar intracerebral hemorrhage—a clinical, radiographic and pathological study of 29 consecutive cases with negative angiography. J Neurosurg 76:231-238, 1992.

93 Wakai S, Nagai M: Histological verification of microaneurysms as a cause of cerebral haemorrhage in surgical specimens. J Neurol Neurosurg Psychiatry 52:595-599, 1989.

Vascular malformations

94 Jellinger K: Vascular malformations of the central nervous system. A morphological overview. Neurosurg Rev 9:177-216, 1986.

95 Russell DS, Rubinstein LJ: Pathology of tumours of the nervous system, ed 5. Baltimore, 1989, Williams & Wilkins, pp 727-746.

96 Farrell DF, Forno LS: Symptomatic capillary telangiectasis of the brainstem without hemorrhage. Report of an unusual case. Neurology 20:341-346, 1970.

97 Vaquero J, Manrique M, Oya S, Cabezudo JM, Bravo G: Calcified telangiectatic hamartomas of the brain. Surg Neurol 13:453-457, 1980.

98 Garner TB, Del Curling O, Kelly Jr DL, Laster DW: The natural history of intracranial venous angiomas. J Neurosurg 75:715-722, 1991.

99 Rigamonti D, Spetzler RF, Medina M, Rigamonti K, Geckle DS, Pappas C: Cerebral venous malformations. J Neurosurg 773:560-564, 1990.

100 Anson JA, Spetzler RF: Surgical resection of intramedullary spinal cord cavernous malformations. J Neurosurg 78:446-451, 1993.

101 Del Curling Jr O, Kelly Jr DL, Elster AD, Craven TE: An analysis of the natural history of cavernous angiomas. J Neurosurg 75:702-708, 1991.

102 Dobyns WB, Michels VV, Groover RV, Mokri B, Trautmann JC, Forbes GS, Laws ER Jr: Familial cavernous malformations of the central nervous system and retina. Ann Neurol 21:578-583, 1987.

103 Matias-Guiu X, Alejo M, Sole T, Ferrer I, Noboa R, Bertumeus F: Cavernous angiomas of the cranial nerves. Report of two cases. J Neurosurg 73:620-622, 1990.

104 Meyer FB, Lombardi D, Scheithauer B, Nichols DA: Extra-axial cavernous hemangiomas involving the dural sinuses. J Neurosurg 73:187-192, 1990.

105 Pagni CA, Canavero S, Forni M: Report of a cavernoma of the cauda equina and review of the literature. Surg Neurol 30:124-131, 1990.

106 Rigamonti D, Johnson PC, Spetzler RF, Hadley MN, Drayer BP: Cavernous malformations and capillary telangiectasia. A spectrum within a single pathological entity. Neurosurgery 28:60-64, 1991.

107 Roda JM, Carceller F, Pérez-Higueras A, Morales C: Encapsulated intracerebral hematomas. A defined entity. J Neurosurg 78:829-833, 1993.

108 Scott RM, Barnes P, Kupsky W, Adelman LS: Cavernous angiomas of the central nervous system in children. J Neurosurg 76:38-46, 1992.

109 Simard JM, Garcia-Bengochea F, Ballinger WE Jr, Mickle JP, Quisling RG: Cavernous angioma. A review of 126 collected and 12 new clinical cases. Neurosurgery 18:162-172, 1986.

110 Tung H, Giannotta SL, Chandrasoma PT, Zee C-S: Recurrent intraparenchymal hemorrhages from angiographically occult vascular malformations. J Neurosurg 73:174-180, 1990.

111 Zabramski JM, Wascher TM, Spetzler RF, Johnson B, Golfinos J, Drayer BP, Brown B, Rigamonti D, Brown G: The natural history of familial cavernous malformations. Results of an ongoing study. J Neurosurg 80:422-432, 1994.

112 Brown RD Jr, Wiebers DO, Forbes G, O'Fallon WM, Piepgras DG, Marsh WR, Maciunas RJ: The natural history of unruptured intracranial arteriovenous malformations. J Neurosurg 68:352-357, 1988.

113 Carleton CC, Cauthen JC: Vascular ("arteriovenous") malformations of the choroid plexus. Arch Pathol 99:286-288, 1975.

114 Germano IM, Davis RL, Wilson CB, Hieshima GB: Histopathological follow-up study of 66 cerebral arteriovenous malformations after therapeutic embolization with polyvinyl alcohol. J Neurosurg 76:607-614, 1992.

115 Lobato RD, Perez C, Rivas JJ, Cordobes F: Clinical, radiological, and pathological spectrum of angiographically occult intracranial vascular malformations. Analysis of 21 cases and review of the literature. J Neurosurg 68:518-531, 1988.

116 Lombardi D, Scheithauer BW, Piepgras D, Meyer FB, Forbes GS: "Angioglioma" and the arteriovenous malformation-glioma association. J Neurosurg 75:589-596, 1991.

117 Mandybur TI, Nazek M: Cerebral arteriovenous malformations. A detailed morphological and immunohistochemical study using actin. Arch Pathol Lab Med 114:970-973, 1990.

118 Nazek M, Mandybur TI, Kashiwagi S: Oligodendroglial proliferative abnormality associated with arteriovenous malformation. Report of three cases with review of the literature. Neurosurgery 23:781-785, 1988.

119 Ondra SL, Troupp H, George ED, Schwab K: The natural history of symptomatic arteriovenous malformations of the brain. A 24-year follow-up assessment. J Neurosurg 73:387-391, 1990.

120 Vinters HV, Lundie MJ, Kaufman JCE: Long-term pathological follow-up of cerebral arteriovenous malformations treated by embolization with bucrylate. N Engl J Med 314:477-483, 1986.

121 Yokoyama K, Asano Y, Murakawa T, Takada M, Ando T, Sakai N, Yamada H, Iwata H: Familial occurrence of arteriovenous malformation of the brain. J Neurosurg 74:585-589, 1991.

122 Román G, Fisher M, Perl DP, Poser CM: Neurological manifestations of hereditary hemorrhagic telangiectasia (Rendu-Osler-Weber disease). Report of 2 cases and review of the literature. Ann Neurol 4:130-144, 1978.

123 Russell DS, Rubinstein LJ: Pathology of tumours of the nervous system, ed 5. Baltimore, 1989, Williams & Wilkins, pp 766-808.

124 Wohlwill FJ, Yakovlev PI: Histopathology of meningofacial angiomatosis (Sturge-Weber's disease). Report of four cases. J Neuropathol Exp Neurol 16:341-364, 1957.

125 Benhaiem N, Poirier J, Hurth M: Arteriovenous fistulae of the meninges draining into the spinal veins. A histological study of 28 cases. Acta Neuropathol 62:103-111, 1983.

126 Nishijima M, Takaku A, Endo S, Kuwayama N, Koizumi F, Sato H, Owada K: Etiological evaluation of dural arteriovenous malformation of the lateral and sigmoid sinuses based on histopathological examinations. J Neurosurg 76:600-606, 1992.

127 Partington MD, Rüfenacht DA, Marsh WR, Piepgras DG: Cranial and sacral dural arteriovenous fistulas as a cause of myelopathy. J Neurosurg 76:615-622, 1992.

128 Rosenblum B, Oldfield EH, Doppman JL, DiChiro G: Spinal arteriovenous malformations. A comparison of dural arteriovenous fistulas and intradural AVMs in 81 patients. J Neurosurg 67:795-802, 1987.

129 Tomlinson FH, Rüfenacht DA, Sundt Jr TM, Nichols DA, Fode NC: Arteriovenous fistulas of the brain and spinal cord. J Neurosurg 79:16-27, 1992.

Primary angiitis

130 Caccamo DV, Garcia JH, Ho K-L: Isolated granulomatous angiitis of the spinal cord. Ann Neurol 32:580-582, 1992.

131 Lie JT: Primary (granulomatous) angiitis of the central nervous system. A clinicopathologic analysis of 15 new cases and review of the literature. Hum Pathol 23:164-171, 1992.

132 Rhodes RH, Madelaire NC, Petrelli M, Cole M, Karaman BA: Primary angiitis and angiopathy of the central nervous system and their relationship to systemic giant cell arteritis. Arch Pathol Lab Med 119:334-349, 1995.

133 Yoong MF, Blumberg PC, North JB: Primary (granulomatous) angiitis of the central nervous system with multiple aneurysms of spinal arteries—case report. J Neurosurg 79:603-607, 1993.

Cerebral amyloid angiopathy

134 Castaño EM, Frangione B: Human amyloidosis, Alzheimer disease and related disorders. Lab Invest 58:122-132, 1988.

135 Gray F, Vinters HV, LeNoan H, Salama J, Delaporte P, Poirier J: Cerebral amyloid angiopathy and granulomatous angiitis. Immunohistochemical study using antibodies to the Alzheimer A4 peptide. Hum Pathol 21:1290-1293, 1990.

136 LeCoz P, Mikol J, Ferrand J, Woimant F, Masters C, Beyreuther K, Haguenau M, Cophignon J, Pepin B: Granulomatous angiitis and cerebral amyloid angiopathy presenting as a mass lesion. Neuropathol Appl Neurobiol 17:149-155, 1991.

137 Mandybur TI: Cerebral amyloid angiopathy. Possible relationship to rheumatoid vasculitis. Neurology 29:1336-1340, 1979.

138 Mandybur TI: Cerebral amyloid angiopathy. The vascular pathology and complications. J Neuropathol Exp Neurol 45:79-90, 1986.

139 Vinters HV: Cerebral amyloid angiopathy—a critical review. Stroke 18:311-324, 1987.

140 Vonsattel JPG, Myers RH, Hedley-White ET, Ropper AH, Bird ED, Richardson Jr EP: Cerebral amyloid angiopathy without and with cerebral hemorrhages. A comparative histological study. Ann Neurol 30:637-649, 1991.

Epidural hematoma

141 Hardman JM: Cerebrospinal trauma. In Davis RL, Robertson DM, eds: Textbook of neuropathology, ed 2. Baltimore, 1991, Williams & Wilkins, pp 973-974.

Subdural hematoma

142 Friede RL, Schachenmayr W: The origin of subdural neomembranes. II. Fine structure of neomembranes. Am J Pathol **92**:69-84, 1978.

143 Hardman JM: Cerebrospinal trauma. In Davis RL, Robertson DM, eds: Textbook of neuropathology, ed 2. Baltimore, 1991, Williams & Wilkins, pp 974-979.

144 Niwa J, Nakamura T, Fujishige M, Hashi K: Removal of a large asymptomatic calcified chronic subdural hematoma. Surg Neurol **30**:135-139, 1988.

145 Rengachary SS, Szymanski DC: Subdural hematomas of arterial origin. Neurosurgery **8**:166-172, 1981.

146 Schachenmayr W, Friede RL: The origin of subdural neomembranes. I. Fine structure of the dura-arachnoid interface in man. Am J Pathol **92**:53-68, 1978.

147 Wintzen AR: The clinical course of subdural haematoma. A retrospective study of aetiological, chronological, and pathological features in 212 patients and a proposed classification. Brain **103**:855-867, 1980.

148 Yamashima T, Yamamoto S: The origin of inner membranes in chronic subdural hematomas. Acta Neuropathol **67**:219-225, 1985.

INFLAMMATORY DISEASES
Demyelinating diseases

149 Aarli JA, Mork SJ, Myrseth E, Larsen J: Glioblastoma associated with multiple sclerosis. Coincidence or induction? Eur Neurol **29**:312-316, 1989.

150 Hook CC, Kimmel DW, Kvols LK, Scheithauer BW, Forsyth P, Rubin J, Moertel C, Rodriguez M: Multifocal inflammatory leukoencephalopathy with 5-fluorouracil and levamisole. Ann Neurol **31**:262-267, 1992.

151 Hulette CM, Downey BT, Burger PC: Macrophage markers in diagnostic neuropathology. Am J Surg Pathol **16**:493-499, 1992.

152 Hunter SB, Ballinger WE, Rubin JJ: Multiple sclerosis mimicking primary brain tumor. Arch Pathol Lab Med **111**:464-468, 1987.

153 Kepes JJ: Large focal tumor-like demyelinating lesions of the brain. Intermediate entity between multiple sclerosis and acute disseminated encephalomyelitis? A study of 31 cases. Ann Neurol **33**:18-27, 1993.

154 Nahser HC, Vieregge P, Nau HE, Reinhardt V: Coincidence of multiple sclerosis and glioma. Clinical and radiological remarks on two cases. Surg Neurol **26**:45-51, 1986.

155 Nesbit G, Forbes G, Scheithauer BW, Okazaki H, Rodriguez M: Multiple sclerosis. Histopathologic and MR and/or CT correlation in 37 cases at biopsy and three cases at autopsy. Radiology **180**:467-474, 1991.

156 Peterson K. Rosenblum MK, Powers JM, Alvord E, Walker RW, Posner JB: Effect of brain irradiation on demyelinating lesions. Neurology **43**:2105-2112, 1993.

157 Zagzag D, Miller D, Kleinman G, Abati A, Donnenfeld H, Budzilovich G: Demyelinating disease versus tumor in surgical neuropathology—clues to a correct pathological diagnosis. Am J Surg Pathol **17**:537-545, 1993.

Idiopathic inflammatory and reactive disorders, xanthomatous lesions, and "histiocytoses"

158 Ashkenazi E, Constantini S, Pappo O, Gomori M, Averbuch-Heller L, Umansky F: Hypertrophic spinal pachymeningitis. Report of two cases and review of the literature. Neurosurgery **28**:730-732, 1991.

159 Mamelak AN, Kelly WM, Davis RL, Rosenblum ML: Idiopathic hypertrophic cranial pachymeningitis—report of three cases. J Neurosurg **79**:270-276, 1993.

160 Masson C, Henin D, Hauw JJ, Rey A, Raverdy P, Masson M: Cranial pachymeningitis of unknown origin. A study of seven cases. Neurology **43**:1329-1334, 1993.

161 Noble SC, Chandler WF, Lloyd RV: Intracranial extension of orbital pseudotumor. A case report. Neurosurgery **18**:798-801, 1986.

162 Farrell MA, DeRosa MJ, Curran JG, Secor DL, Cornford ME, Comair YG, Peacock WJ, Shields WD, Vinters HV: Neuropathologic findings in cortical resections (including hemispherectomies) performed for the treatment of childhood epilepsy. Acta Neuropathol **83**:246-259, 1992.

163 Piatt Jr. JH, Hwang PA, Armstrong DC, Becker LE, Hoffman HJ: Chronic focal encephalitis (Rasmussen syndrome). Six cases. Epilepsia **29**:268-279, 1988.

164 Vinters, HV, Wang R, Wiley CA: Herpesviruses in chronic encephalitis associated with intractable childhood epilepsy. Hum Pathol **24**:871-879, 1993.

165 Burton GV, Bullard DE, Walther PJ, Burger PC: Paraneoplastic limbic encephalopathy with testicular carcinoma. A reversible neurologic syndrome. Cancer **62**:2248-2251, 1988.

166 Corsellis JAN, Goldberg GJ, Norton AR: "Limbic encephalitis" and its association with carcinoma. Brain **91**:481-496, 1968.

167 Dalmau J, Graus F, Rosenblum MK, Posner JB: Anti-Hu-associated paraneoplastic encephalomyelitis/sensory neuronopathy. A clinical study of 71 patients. Medicine **71**:59-72, 1992.

168 Rosenblum MK: Paraneoplasia and autoimmunologic injury of the nervous system. The anti-Hu syndrome. Brain Pathol **3**:199-212, 1993.

169 Bertoni F, Unni KK, Dahlin DC, Beabout JW, Onofrio BM: Calcifying pseudoneoplasms of the neural axis. J Neurosurg **72**:42-48, 1990.

170 Smith DM, Berry III AD: Unusual fibro-osseous lesion of the spinal cord with positive staining for glial fibrillary acidic protein and radiological progression. A case report. Hum Pathol **25**:835-838, 1994.

171 Kepes JJ, Kepes M: Predominantly cerebral forms of histiocytosis-X. A reappraisal of "Gagel's hypothalamic granuloma," "granuloma infiltrans of the hypothalamus" and "Ayala's disease" with a report of four cases. Acta Neuropathol **14**:77-98, 1969.

172 Montine TJ, Hollensead SC, Ellis WG, Martin JS, Moffat EJ, Burger PC: Solitary eosinophilic granuloma of the temporal lobe. A case report and long-term follow-up of previously reported cases. Clin Neuropathol **13**:225-228, 1994.

173 Reznik M, Stevenaert A, Bex V, Kratzenberg E: Focal brain invasion as the first manifestation of Langerhans cell granulomatosis in an adult. Clin Neuropathol **12**:179-183, 1993.

174 Powers WJ, Miller EM: Sarcoidosis mimicking glioma. Case report and review of intracranial sarcoid mass lesions. Neurology **31**:907-910, 1981.

175 Ranoux D, Devaux B, Lamy C, Mear JY, Roux FX, Mas JL: Meningeal sarcoidosis, pseudo-meningioma, and pachymeningitis of the convexity. J Neurol Neurosurg Psychiatry **55**:300-303, 1992.

176 Stern BJ, Krumholz A, Johns C, Scott P, Nissim J: Sarcoidosis and its neurological manifestations. Arch Neurol **42**:909-917, 1985.

177 Terunuma H, Konno H, Iizuka H, Yamamoto T, Yoshimoto T: Sarcoidosis presenting as progressive myelopathy. Clin Neuropathol **7**:77-80, 1988.

178 Foucar E, Rosai J, Dorfman R: Sinus histiocytosis with massive lymphadenopathy (Rosai-Dorfman disease). Review of the entity. Semin Diagn Pathol **7**:19-73, 1990.

179 Shaver EG, Rebsamen SL, Yachnis AT, Sutton LN: Isolated extranodal sinus histiocytosis in a 5-year old boy. Case report. J Neurosurg **79**:769-773, 1993.

180 Cannella DM, Prezyna AP, Kapp JP: Primary intracranial plasma cell granuloma. J Neurosurg **69**:785-788, 1988.

181 Gochman GA, Kuffy K, Crandall PH, Vinters HV: Plasma cell granuloma of the brain. Surg Neurol **33**:347-352, 1990.

182 Nazek M, Mandybur TI, Sawaya R: Hyalinizing plasmacytic granulomatosis of the falx. Am J Surg Pathol **12**:308-313, 1988.

183 Pimentel J, Costa A, Tavora L: Inflammatory pseudotumor of the choroid plexus. Case report. J Neurosurg **79**:939-942, 1993.

184 Brück W, Sander U, Blanckenberg P, Friede RL: Symptomatic xanthogranuloma of choroid plexus with unilateral hydrocephalus. J Neurosurg **75**:324-327, 1991.

185 Jamjoon ZAB, Raina V, Al-Jamali A, Jamjoom AB, Yacub B, Sharif HS: Intracranial xanthogranuloma of the dura in Hand-Schüller-Christian disease. J Neurosurg **78**:297-300, 1993.

186 Kamiryo T, Abiko S, Orita T, Aoki H, Watanabe Y, Hiraoka K: Bilateral intracranial fibrous xanthoma. Surg Neurol **29**:27-31, 1988.

187 Kimura H, Oka K, Nakayama Y, Tomonaga M: Xanthoma in Meckel's cave. A case report. Surg Neurol **35**:317-320, 1991.

188 Knobler RM, Neumann RA, Gebhart W, Radaskiewicz T, Perenci P, Widhalm K: Xanthoma disseminatum with progressive involvement of the central nervous and hepatobiliary systems. J Am Acad Dermatol **23**:341-344, 1990.

189 Koyama S, Tsubokawa T, Katayama Y, Hirota H: A huge intracranial xanthogranuloma in the middle cranial fossa. Case report. Neurosurgery **28**:436-439, 1991.

190 Miyachi S, Kobayashi T, Takahashi T, Saito K, Hashizume Y, Sugita K: An intracranial mass lesion in systemic xanthogranulomatosis. Case report. Neurosurgery **27**:822-826, 1990.

191 Okabe H, Ishizawa M, Matsumoto K, Ogata M, Nishioka J, Hukuda S, Hidaka H, Yosuda H, Ochi Y: Immunohistochemical analysis of spinal intradural xanthomatosis developed in a patient with phytosterolemia. Acta Neuropathol **83**:554-558, 1992.

192 Paulus W, Kirchner T, Ott MM, Kühl J, Warmuth-Metz M, Sörensen N, Müller-Hermelink HK, Roggendorf W: Histiocytic tumor of Meckel's cave—an intracranial equivalent of juvenile xanthogranuloma of the skin. Am J Surg Pathol **16**:76-83, 1992.

193 Pick P, Jean E, Horoupian D, Factor S: Xanthogranuloma of the dura in systemic Weber-Christian disease. Neurology **33:**1067-1070, 1983.

194 Vaquero J, Leunda G, Cabezudo JM, de Juan M, Herrero J, Bravo G: Posterior fossa xanthogranuloma. Case report. J Neurosurg **51:**718-722, 1979.

195 Yamada H, Kurata H, Nomura K, Utsunomiya K, Shimizu M, Isogai Y: Adult xanthogranulomatous lesion involving familial hypercholesterolemia. Jpn J Med **28:**757-761, 1989.

196 Caselli RJ, Scheithauer BW, Bowles CA, Trenerry MR, Meyer FB, Smigielski JS, Rodriguez M: The treatable dementia of Sjögren's syndrome. Ann Neurol **30:**98-101, 1991.

197 Figarella-Branger D, Gambarelli D, Perez-Castillo M, Regis J, Peragut JC, Pellissier JF: Atypical inflammatory histiocytic tumor of the cerebellum. A histological, immunohistochemical, and ultrastructural study. Am J Surg Pathol **14:**778-783, 1990.

198 Gal R, Gukovsky-Oren S, Sandbank U, Baharav E, Kessler E: Michaelis-Gutmann bodies in a healing brain infarct. Stroke **18:**947-950, 1987.

199 Ho K-L: Morphogenesis of Michaelis-Gutmann bodies in cerebral malacoplakia. An ultrastructural study. Arch Pathol Lab Med **113:**874-879, 1989.

200 Kim RC, Collins GH: The neuropathology of rheumatoid disease. Hum Pathol **12:**5-15, 1981.

201 Mills SE, Lininger JR: Intracranial myospherulosis. Hum Pathol **13:**596-597, 1982.

202 Nishino H, Rubino FA, DeRemee RA, Swanson JW, Parisi JE: Neurological involvement in Wegener's granulomatosis. An analysis of 324 consecutive patients at the Mayo Clinic. Ann Neurol **33:**4-9, 1993.

203 Spurlock RG, Richman AV: Rheumatoid meningitis. a case report and review of the literature. Arch Pathol Lab Med **107:**129-131, 1983.

204 Tang TT, Segura AD, Oechler HW, Harb JM, Adair SE, Gregg DC, Camitta BM, Franciosi RA: Inflammatory myofibroblastic proliferation simulating sarcoma in children. Cancer **65:**1626-1634, 1990.

Infectious diseases
Bacterial infections

205 Berensen CS, Bia FJ: *Propionobacterium acnes* causes postoperative brain abscesses unassociated with foreign bodies. Case reports. Neurosurgery **25:**130-134, 1989.

206 Bishburg E, Sunderam G, Reichman LB, Kapila R: Central nervous system tuberculosis with the acquired immunodeficiency syndrome and its related complex. Ann Intern Med **105:**210-213, 1986.

207 Britt RH, Enzmann DR: Clinical stages of human brain abscesses on serial CT scans after contrast infusion. Computerized tomographic, neuropathological, and clinical correlations. J Neurosurg **59:**972-989, 1983.

208 Brown AP, Lane JC, Murayama S, Vollmer DG: Whipple's disease presenting with isolated neurological symptoms. Case report. J Neurosurg **73:**623-627, 1990.

209 Byrne E, Brophy BP, Perrett LV: Nocardial cerebral abscess. New concepts in diagnosis, management and prognosis. J Neurol Neurosurg Psychiatry **42:**1038-1045, 1979.

210 Chun CH, Johnson JD, Hofstetter M, Raff MJ: Brain abscess. A study of 45 consecutive cases. Medicine **65:**415-431, 1986.

211 Del Curling O, Gower DJ, McWhorter JM: Changing concepts in spinal epidural abscess. A report of 29 cases. Neurosurgery **27:**185-192, 1990.

212 Gellin BG, Weingarten K, Gamache Jr. FW, Hartman BJ: Epidural abscess. In Scheld WM, Whitley RJ, Durack DT, eds: Infections of the central nervous system. New York, 1991, Raven Press, pp 499-514.

213 Hall WA: Hereditary hemorrhagic telangiectasia (Rendu-Osler-Weber disease) presenting with polymicrobial brain abscess. Case report. J Neurosurg **81:**294-296, 1994.

214 Hawkins CC, Gold JWM, Whimbey E, Kiehn TE, Brannon P, Cammarata R, Brown AE, Armstrong D: *Mycobacterium avium* complex infections in patients with the acquired immunodeficiency syndrome. Ann Intern Med **105:**184-188, 1986.

215 Kline MW: *Citrobacter* meningitis and brain abscess in infancy. Epidemiology, pathogenesis and treatment. J Pediatr **113:**430-433, 1988.

216 Pollock SS, Pollock TM, Harrison MJ: Infection of the central nervous system by *Listeria monocytogenes*. A review of 54 adult and juvenile cases. Q J Med **53:**331-340, 1984.

217 Renier D, Flaudin C, Hirsch E, Hirsch J-F: Brain abscess in neonates. A study of 30 cases. J Neurosurg **69:**877-882, 1988.

218 Schlitt M, Mitchem L, Zorn G, Dismukes W, Morawetz RB: Brain abscess after esophageal dilation for caustic stricture. Report of three cases. Neurosurgery **17:**947-951, 1985.

219 Sinh G, Pandya SK, Dastur DK: Pathogenesis of unusual intracranial tuberculomas and tuberculous space-occupying lesions. J Neurosurg **29:**149-159, 1968.

220 Smego Jr. RA: Actinomycosis of the central nervous system. Rev Infect Dis **9:**855-865, 1987.

221 Tenney JH: Bacterial infections of the central nervous system in neurosurgery. Neurol Clin **4:**91-114, 1986.

222 Trautmann M, Lindner O, Haase C, Bruckner O: Focal tuberculous meningoencephalitis. Eur Neurol **22:**417-420, 1983.

223 Whitener DR: Tuberculous brain abscess. Report of a case and review of the literature. Arch Neurol **35:**148-155, 1978.

224 Wispelwey B, Dacey Jr. RG, Scheld WM: Brain abscess. In Scheld WM, Whitley RJ, Durack DT, eds: Infections of the central nervous system. New York, 1991, Raven Press, pp 457-486.

225 Zuger A, Lowy FD: Tuberculosis of the central nervous system. In Scheld WM, Whitley RJ, Durack DT, eds: Infections of the central nervous system. New York, 1991, Raven Press, pp 425-456.

Mycoses

226 Araujo JC, Werneck L, Cravo MA: South American blastomycosis presenting as a posterior fossa tumor. J Neurosurg **49:**425-428, 1978.

227 Cuadrado LM, Guerrero A, Lopez Garcia Asenjo JA, Martin F, Palau E, Urra DG: Cerebral mucormycosis in two cases of acquired immunodeficiency syndrome. Arch Neurol **45:**109-111, 1988.

228 Dixon DM, Walsh TJ, Merz WG, McGinnis MR: Infections due to *Xylohypha bantiana (Cladosporium trichoides)*. Rev Infect Dis **11:**515-525, 1989.

229 Fujita NK, Reynard M, Sapico FL, Guze LB, Edwards JE: Cryptococcal intracerebral mass lesions. Ann Intern Med **94:**382-388, 1981.

230 Goodman ML, Coffey RJ: Stereotactic drainage of *Aspergillus* brain abscess with long-term survival. Case report and review. Neurosurgery **24:**96-99, 1989.

231 Hadley MN, Martin NA, Spetzler RF, Johnson PC: Multiple intracranial aneurysms due to *Coccidioides immitis* infection. J Neurosurg **66:**453-456, 1987.

232 Ilgren EB, Westmorland D, Adams CBT, Mitchell RG: Cerebellar mass caused by *Candida* species. J Neurosurg **60:**428-430, 1984.

233 Kasantikul V, Shuangshoti S, Sampatanukul P: Primary chromoblastomycosis of the medulla oblongata. Complication of heroin addiction. Surg Neurol **29:**319-321, 1988.

234 Kershaw P, Freeman R, Templeton D, DeGirolami PC, DeGirolami U, Tarsy D, Hoffman S, Eliopoulos G, Karchmer AW: *Pseudallescheria boydii* infection of the central nervous system. Arch Neurol **47:**468-472, 1990.

235 Lipton SA, Hickey WF, Morris JH, Loscalzo J: Candidal infection in the central nervous system. Am J Med **76:**101-108, 1984.

236 Mendel E, Milefchik EN, Amadi J, Gruen P: Coccidioidomycosis brain abscess. Case report. J Neurosurg **81:**614-616, 1994.

237 Mielke B, Weir B, Oldring D, von Westarp C: Fungal aneurysm. Case report and review of the literature. Neurosurgery **9:**578-581, 1981.

238 Penar PL, Kim J, Chyatte D, Sabshin JK: Intraventricular cryptococcal granuloma. J Neurosurg **68:**145-148, 1988.

239 Roos KL, Bryan JP, Maggio WM, Jane JA, Scheld WM: Intracranial blastomycoma. Medicine **66:**224-235, 1987.

240 Sepkowitz K, Armstrong D: Space-occupying fungal lesions of the central nervous system. In Scheld WM, Whitley RJ, Durack DT, eds: Infections of the central nervous system. New York, 1991, Raven Press, pp 741-764.

241 Stave GM, Heimberger T, Kerkering TM: Zygomycosis of the basal ganglia in intravenous drug abusers. Am J Med **86:**115-117, 1989.

242 Venger BH, Landon G, Rose JE: Solitary histoplasmoma of the thalamus. Case report and literature review. Neurosurgery **20:**784-787, 1987.

243 Voelker JL, Muller J, Worth RM: Intramedullary spinal histoplasma granuloma—case report. J Neurosurg **70:**959-961, 1989.

244 Walsh TJ, Hier DB, Caplan LR: Aspergillosis of the central nervous system. Clinicopathological analysis of 17 patients. Ann Neurol **18:**574-582, 1985.

245 Wheat LJ, Batteiger BE, Sathapatayavongs B: *Histoplasma capsulatum* infections of the central nervous system—a clinical review. Medicine **69:**244-260, 1990.

246 Yanai Y, Wakao T, Fukamachi A, Kunimine H: Intracranial granuloma caused by *Aspergillus fumigatus*. Surg Neurol **23:**597-604, 1985.

Viral infections
Herpes simplex encephalitis

247 Aurelius E, Johansson B, Sköldenberg B, Staland A, Forsgren M: Rapid diagnosis of herpes simplex encephalitis by nested polymerase chain reaction assay of cerebrospinal fluid. Lancet **337:**189-192, 1991.

248 Bruner JM: Oligonucleotide probe for herpes virus. Use in paraffin sections. Mod Pathol **3:**635-638, 1990.

249 Esiri MM: Herpes simplex encephalitis—an immunohistologic study of the distribution of viral antigen within the brain. J Neurol Sci **54:**209-226, 1982.

250 Kennedy PGE, Adams JH, Graham DI, Clements GB: A clinicopathological study of herpes simplex encephalitis. Neuropathol Appl Neurobiol **14:**395-415, 1988.

251 Price RW, Chernik NL, Horta-Barbosa L, Posner JB: Herpes simplex encephalitis in an anergic patient. Am J Med **54:**222-228, 1973.

252 Tan SV, Guiloff RJ, Scaravilli F, Klapper PE, Cleator GM, Gazzard BG: Herpes simplex type 1 encephalitis in acquired immune deficiency syndrome. Ann Neurol **34**:619-622, 1993.

253 White CL III, Taxy JB: Early morphologic diagnosis of herpes simplex virus encephalitis. Advantages of electron microscopy and immunoperoxidase staining. Hum Pathol **14**:135-139, 1983.

254 Whitley RJ, Schlitt M: Encephalitis caused by herpes viruses, including B virus. In Scheld WM, Whitley RJ, Durack DT, eds: Infections of the central nervous system. New York, 1991, Raven Press, pp 41-86.

Progressive multifocal leukoencephalopathy

255 Astrom K-E, Mancall EL, Richardson EP Jr: Progressive multifocal leukoencephalopathy—a hitherto unrecognized complication of chronic lymphatic leukaemia and Hodgkin's disease. Brain **81**:93-111, 1958.

256 Berger JR, Kaszovitz B, Post MJ, Dickinson G: Progressive multifocal leukoencephalopathy associated with human immunodeficiency virus infection. A review of the literature with a report of sixteen cases. Ann Intern Med **107**:78-87, 1987.

257 Hair LS, Nuovo G, Powers JM, Sisti MB, Britton CB, Miller JR: Progressive multifocal leukoencephalopathy in patients with human immunodeficiency virus. Hum Pathol **23**:663-667, 1992.

258 McGuire D, Barhite S, Hollander H, Miles M: JC virus DNA in cerebrospinal fluid of human immunodeficiency virus–infected patients. Predictive value for progressive multifocal leukoencephalopathy. Ann Neurol **37**:395-399, 1995.

259 Preskorn SH, Watanabe I: Progressive multifocal leukoencephalopathy-cerebral mass lesions. Surg Neurol **12**:231-234, 1979.

260 Schmidbauer M, Budka H, Shah KV: Progressive multifocal leukoencephalopathy (PML) in AIDS and in the pre-AIDS era. A neuropathological comparison using immunocytochemistry and in situ DNA hybridization for virus detection. Acta Neuropathol **80**:375-380, 1990.

261 Sima AAF, Finkelstein SD, McLachlan DR: Multiple malignant astrocytomas in a patient with spontaneous progressive multifocal leukoencephalopathy. Ann Neurol **14**:183-188, 1983.

262 Tornatore C, Berger JR, Houff SA, Curfman B, Meyers K, Winfield D, Major EO: Detection of JC virus DNA in peripheral lymphocytes from patients with and without progressive multifocal leukoencephalopathy. Ann Neurol **31**:454-462, 1992.

263 Ueki K, Richardson EP Jr, Henson JW, Louis DN: In situ polymerase chain reaction demonstration of JC virus in progressive multifocal leukoencephalopathy, including an index case. Ann Neurol **36**:670-673, 1994.

264 Vanneste JAL, Bellott SM, Stam FC: Progressive multifocal leukoencephalopathy presenting as a single mass lesion. Eur Neurol **23**:113-118, 1984.

265 Vazeux R, Cumont M, Girard PM, Nassif X, Trotot P, Marche C, Mathiessen L, Vedrenne C, Mikol J, Henin D, Katlama C, Bolgert F, Montagnier L: Severe encephalitis resulting from coinfections with HIV and JC virus. Neurology **40**:944-948, 1990.

266 Walker DL: Progressive multifocal leukoencephalopathy. In Vinken PJ, Bruyn GW, Klawans HL, eds: Handbook of clinical neurology (revised series), vol 47. Amsterdam, 1985, North Holland, pp 503-524.

Varicella-zoster virus encephalitis and cerebral vasculitis

267 Doyle PW, Gibson G, Dolman CL: Herpes zoster ophthalmicus with contralateral hemiplegia. Identification of cause. Ann Neurol **14**:84-85, 1983.

268 Eidelberg D, Sotrel A, Horoupian DS, Neumann PE, Pumarola-Sune T, Price RW: Thrombotic cerebral vasculopathy associated with herpes zoster. Ann Neurol **19**:7-14, 1986.

269 Fukumoto S, Kinjo M, Hokamura K, Tanaka K: Subarachnoid hemorrhage and granulomatous angiitis of the basilar artery. Demonstration of the varicella-zoster virus in the basilar artery lesions. Stroke **17**:1024-1028, 1986.

270 Horten BC, Price RW, Jimenez D: Multifocal varicella-zoster virus leukoencephalitis temporally remote from herpes zoster. Ann Neurol **9**:251-266, 1981.

271 Morgello S, Block GA, Price RW, Petito CK: Varicella-zoster virus leukoencephalitis and cerebral vasculopathy. Arch Pathol Lab Med **112**:173-177, 1988.

HIV-1 encephalomyelitis

272 Meyenhofer MF, Epstein LG, Cho E-S, Sharer LR: Ultrastructural morphology and intracellular production of human immunodeficiency virus (HIV) in brain. J Neuropathol Exp Neurol **46**:474-484, 1987.

273 Rosenblum MK: Infection of the central nervous system by the human immunodeficiency virus type 1. Morphology and relation to syndromes of progressive encephalopathy and myelopathy in patients with AIDS. Pathol Annu **25**(Pt1):117-169, 1990.

274 Sharer LR: Pathology of HIV-1 infection of the central nervous system. A review. J Neuropathol Exp Neurol **51**:3-11, 1992.

Parasitoses

275 Brown WJ, Voge M: Neuropathology of parasitic infections. Oxford, 1982, Oxford University Press.

276 Cameron ML, Durack DT: Helminthic infections of the central nervous system. In Scheld W, Whitley R, Durack D, eds: Infections of the central nervous system. New York, 1991, Raven Press, pp 825-858.

277 Cegielski JP, Durack DT: Protozoal infections of the central nervous system. In Scheld W, Whitley R, Durack D, eds: Infections of the central nervous system. New York, 1991, Raven Press, pp 767-800.

278 Dukes CS, Luft BJ, Durack DT: Toxoplasmosis of the central nervous system. In Scheld WM, Whitley RJ, Durack DT, eds: Infections of the central nervous system. New York, 1991, Raven Press, pp 801-824.

279 Earnest MP, Reller LB, Filley CM, Grek AJ: Neurocysticercosis in the United States. 35 cases and a review. Rev Infect Dis **9**:961-979, 1987.

280 Navia BA, Petito C, Gold J, Cho E, Jordan B, Price R: Cerebral toxoplasmosis complicating the acquired immune deficiency syndrome. Clinical and neuropathological findings in 27 patients. Ann Neurol **19**:224-238, 1986.

281 Porter SB, Sande MA: Toxoplasmosis of the central nervous system in the acquired immunodeficiency syndrome. N Engl J Med **327**:1643-1648, 1992.

282 Wilson M, Bryan RT, Fried JA, Ware DA, Schantz PM, Pilcher JB, Tsang VCW: Clinical evaluation of the cysticercosis enzyme-linked immunoelectrotransfer blot in patients with neurocysticercosis. J Infect Dis **164**:1007-1009, 1991.

Spirochetal infections

283 Hook III EW: Central nervous system syphilis. In Scheld W, Whitley R, Durack D, eds: Infections of the central nervous system. New York, 1991, Raven Press, pp 639-656.

284 Horowitz HW, Valsamis MP, Wicher V, Abbruscato F, Larsen SA, Wormser GP, Wicker K: Brief report. Cerebral syphilitic gumma confirmed by the polymerase chain reaction in a man with human immunodeficiency virus infection. N Engl J Med **331**:1488-1491, 1994.

285 Murray R, Morawetz R, Kepes J, El Gammal T, Le Doux M: Lyme neuroborreliosis manifesting as an intracranial mass lesion. Neurosurgery **30**:769-773, 1992.

286 Reik L Jr: Lyme disease. In Scheld W, Whitley R, Durack D, eds: Infections of the central nervous system. New York, 1991, Raven Press, pp 657-689.

Prion-associated diseases

287 Brown P, Wolff A, Gajdusek DC: A simple and effective method for inactivating virus infectivity in formalin-fixed tissue samples from patients with Creutzfeldt-Jakob disease. Neurology **40**:887-890, 1990.

288 Brumback RA: Routine use of phenolized formalin in fixation of autopsy brain tissue to reduce risk of inadvertent transmission of Creutzfeldt-Jakob disease. N Engl J Med **319**:654, 1988.

289 Committee on Health Care Issues, American Neurological Association: Precautions in handling tissues, fluids and other contaminated materials from patients with documented or suspected Creutzfeldt-Jakob disease. Ann Neurol **19**:75-77, 1986.

290 Cruz-Sanchez F, Lafuente J, Gertz H-J, Stoltenburg-Didinger G: Spongiform encephalopathy with extensive involvement of white matter. J Neurol Sci **82**:81-87, 1987.

291 DeArmond SJ, Prusiner SB: Etiology and pathogenesis of prion diseases. Am J Pathol **146**:785-811, 1995.

292 Hansen LA, Masliah E, Terry RD, Mirra SS: A neuropathological subset of Alzheimer's disease with concomitant Lewy body disease and spongiform change. Acta Neuropathol **78**:194-201, 1989.

293 Leestma JE: Viral infections of the nervous system. In Davis RL, Robertson DM, eds: Textbook of neuropathology, 2nd ed. Baltimore, 1991, Williams & Wilkins, pp 879-889.

294 Masters CL, Gajdusek DC, Gibbs Jr CJ: Creutzfeldt-Jakob disease virus isolations from the Gerstmann-Sträussler syndrome—with an analysis of the various forms of amyloid plaque deposition in the virus-induced spongiform encephalopathies. Brain **104**:559-588, 1981.

295 Masters CL, Richardson Jr EP: Subacute spongiform encephalopathy (Creutzfeldt-Jakob disease)—the nature and progression of spongiform change. Brain **101**:333-344, 1978.

296 Miller DC: Creutzfeldt-Jakob disease in histopathology technicians. N Engl J Med **318**:853-854, 1988.

297 Nochlin D, Sumi SM, Bird T, Snow A, Leventhal C, Beyreuther K, Masters CL: Familial dementia with PrP-positive amyloid plaques. A variant of Gerstmann-Sträussler syndrome. Neurology **39**:910-918, 1989.

298 Piccardo P, Safar J, Ceroni M, Gajdusek DC, Gibbs CJ: Immunohistochemical localization of prion protein in spongiform encephalopathies and normal tissue. Neurology **40**:518-522, 1990.

PRIMARY TUMORS
Glial tumors
Astrocytic neoplasms
Fibrillary astrocytomas

299 Albright AL, Guthkelch AN, Packer RJ, Price RA, Rourke LB: Prognostic factors in pediatric brain-stem gliomas. J Neurosurg 65:751-755, 1986.

300 Barnard RO, Geddes JF: The incidence of multifocal cerebral gliomas. A histologic study of large hemisphere sections. Cancer 60:1519-1531, 1987.

301 Burger PC, Scheithauer BW: Tumors of the central nervous system. Atlas of Tumor Pathology, third series. Fascicle 10. Washington, DC, 1994, Armed Forces Institute of Pathology, pp 25-161.

302 Burger PC, Vogel FS: Frozen section interpretation in surgical neuropathology. I. Intracranial lesions. Am J Surg Pathol 1:323-347, 1977.

303 Chamberlain MC, Silver P, Levin VA: Poorly differentiated gliomas of the cerebellum. A study of 18 patients. Cancer 65:337-340, 1990.

304 Cohen AR, Wisoff JH, Allen JC, Epstein F: Malignant astrocytomas of the spinal cord. J Neurosurg 70:50-54, 1989.

305 Cosgrove M, Fitzgibbons PL, Sherrod A, Chandrasoma PT, Martin SE: Intermediate filament expression in astrocytic neoplasms. Am J Surg Pathol 13:141-145, 1989.

306 Daumas-Duport C, Scheithauer B, O'Fallon J, Kelly P: Grading of astrocytomas. A simple and reproducible method. Cancer 62:2152-2165, 1988.

307 Epstein FJ, Farmer J-P, Freed D: Adult intramedullary astrocytomas of the spinal cord. J Neurosurg 77:355-359, 1992.

308 Gamis AS, Egelhoff J, Roloson G, Young J, Woods GM, Newman R, Freeman AI: Diffuse bony metastases at presentation in a child with glioblastoma multiforme. A case report. Cancer 66:180-184, 1990.

309 Haddad SF, Moore SA, Schelper RL, Goeken J: Vascular smooth muscle hyperplasia underlies the formation of glomeruloid vascular structures of glioblastoma multiforme. J Neuropathol Exp Neurol 51:488-492, 1992.

310 Henson JW, Schnitker BL, Correa KM, von Deimling A, Fassbender F, Xu H-J, Benedict WF, Yandell DW, Louis DN: The retinoblastoma gene is involved in malignant progression of astrocytomas. Ann Neurol 36:714-721, 1994.

311 Hitchcock E, Morris CS: Cross reactivity of anti-epithelial membrane antigen monoclonal for reactive and neoplastic glial cells. J Neurooncol 4:345-352, 1987.

312 Ilgren EB, Kinnier-Wilson LM, Stiller CA: Gliomas in neurofibromatosis. A series of 89 cases with evidence of enhanced malignancy in associated cerebellar astrocytomas. In Sommers SC, Rosen PP, Fechner RE, eds: Pathology annual, vol. 20 (1), Norwalk, Conn, 1985, Appleton-Century-Crofts, pp 331-358.

313 Kakita A, Wakabayashi K, Takahashi H, Ohama E, Ikuta F, Tokiguchi S: Primary leptomeningeal glioma. Ultrastructural and laminin immunohistochemical studies. Acta Neuropathol 83:538-542, 1992.

314 Kelly PJ, Daumas-Duport C, Kispert DB, Kall BA, Scheithauer BW, Illig JJ: Imaging-based stereotaxic serial biopsies in untreated glial neoplasms. J Neurosurg 66:865-874, 1987.

315 Kepes JJ, Fulling KH, Garcia JH: The clinical significance of "adenoid" formations of neoplastic astrocytes imitating metastatic carcinoma in gliosarcomas. A review of five cases. Clin Neuropathol 1:139-150, 1982.

316 Kepes JJ, Rubinstein LJ: Malignant gliomas with heavily lipidized (foamy) tumor cells. A report of three cases with immunoperoxidase study. Cancer 47:2451-2459, 1981.

317 Kim TS, Halliday AL, Hedley-Whyte ET, Convery K: Correlates of survival and the Daumas-Duport grading system for astrocytomas. J Neurosurg 74:27-37, 1991.

318 Kleihues P, Burger PC, Scheithauer BW: Histological typing of tumours of the central nervous system. 2nd ed. Berlin, 1993, Springer-Verlag, pp 11-14.

319 Krouwer HGJ, Davis RL, Silver P, Prados M: Gemistocytic astrocytomas. A reappraisal. J Neurosurg 74:399-406, 1991.

320 Labrousse F, Daumas-Duport C, Batorski L, Hoshino T: Histological grading and bromodeoxyuridine labeling index of astrocytomas. J Neurosurg 75:202-205, 1991.

321 Louis DN: The p53 gene and protein in human brain tumors. J Neuropathol Exp Neurol 53:11-21, 1994.

321a Lunsford LD, Somaza S, Kondziolka D, Flickinger JC: Survival after stereotactic biopsy and irradiation of cerebral nonanaplastic, nonpilocytic astrocytoma. J Neurosurg 82:523-529, 1995.

322 Margetts JC, Kalyan-Raman UP: Giant-celled glioblastoma of brain. A clinicopathological and radiological study of ten cases (including immunohistochemistry and ultrastructure). Cancer 63:524-531, 1989.

323 Mastronardi L, Ferrante L, Lunardi P, Cervoni L, Fortuna A: Association between neuroepithelial tumor and multiple intestinal polyposis (Turcot's syndrome). Report of a case and critical analysis of the literature. Neurosurgery 28:449-452, 1991.

324 McCormack BM, Miller DC, Budzilovich GN, Voorhees GJ, Ransohoff J: Treatment and survival of low-grade astrocytoma in adults—1977-1988. Neurosurgery 31:636-642, 1992.

325 Melaragno MJ, Prayson RA, Murphy MA, Hassenbusch SJ, Estes ML: Anaplastic astrocytoma with granular cell differentiation. Case report and review of the literature. Hum Pathol 24:805-808, 1993.

326 Montine TJ, Vandersteenhoven JJ, Aguzzi A, Boyko OB, Dodge RK, Kerns B-J, Burger PC: Prognostic significance of Ki-67 proliferation index in supratentorial fibrillary astrocytic neoplasms. Neurosurgery 34:674-679, 1994.

327 Mørk SJ, Rubinstein LJ, Kepes JJ: Patterns of epithelial metaplasia in malignant gliomas. I. Papillary formations mimicking medulloepithelioma. J Neuropathol Exp Neurol 47:93-100, 1988.

328 Mørk SJ, Rubinstein LJ, Kepes JJ, Perentes E, Uphoff DF: Patterns of epithelial metaplasia in malignant gliomas. II. Squamous differentiation of epithelial-like formations in gliosarcomas and glioblastomas. J Neuropathol Exp Neurol 47:101-118, 1988.

329 Moulignier A, Mikol J, Pialoux G, Eliaszewicz M, Thurel C, Thiebaut J-B: Cerebral glial tumors and human immunodeficiency virus-1 infection. More than a coincidental association. Cancer 74:686-692, 1994.

330 Ng H-K, Lo STH: Cytokeratin immunoreactivity in gliomas. Histopathology 14:359-368, 1989.

331 Onda K, Davis RL, Shibuya M, Wilson CB, Hoshino T: Correlation between the bromodeoxyuridine labeling index and the MIB-1 and Ki-67 proliferating cell indices in cerebral gliomas. Cancer 74:1921-1926, 1994.

332 Ramsay DA, Goshko V, Nag S: Primary spinal leptomeningeal astrocytoma. Acta Neuropathol 80:338-341, 1990.

333 Rosenblum MK, Erlandson RA, Budzilovich GN: The lipid-rich epithelioid glioblastoma. Am J Surg Pathol 15:925-934, 1991.

334 Salmon I, Kiss R, Dewitte O, Gras T, Pasteels J-L, Brotchi J, Flament-Durand J: Histopathologic grading and DNA ploidy in relation to survival among 206 adult astrocytic tumor patients. Cancer 70:538-546, 1992.

335 Salvati M, Artico M, Caruso R, Rocchi G, Ramundo Orlando E, Nucci F: A report on radiation-induced gliomas. Cancer 67:392-397, 1991.

336 Scheithauer BW, Bruner JM: The ultrastructural spectrum of astrocytic neoplasms. Ultrastruct Pathol 11:535-581, 1987.

337 Stroink AR, Hoffman HJ, Hendrick EB, Humphreys RP: Diagnosis and management of pediatric brain-stem gliomas. J Neurosurg 65:745-750, 1986.

338 Tsang RW, Laperriere NJ, Simpson WJ, Brierley J, Panzarella T, Smyth HS: Glioma arising after radiation therapy for pituitary adenoma. A report of four patients and estimation of risk. Cancer 72:2227-2233, 1993.

339 Val-Bernal F, Ruiz JC, Cotorruelo JG, Arias M: Glioblastoma multiforme of donor origin after renal transplantation. Report of a case. Hum Pathol 24:1256-1259, 1993.

340 von Deilming A, von Ammon K, Schoenfeld D, Wiestler OD, Seizinger BR, Louis DN: Subsets of glioblastoma multiforme defined by molecular genetic analysis. Brain Pathol 3:19-26, 1993.

340a Wesseling P, Schlingemann RO, Rietveld FJR, Link M, Burger PC, Ruiter DJ: Early and extensive contribution of pericytes/vascular smooth muscle cells to microvascular proliferation in glioblastoma multiforme. An immuno-light and immuno-electron microscopic study. J Neuropathol Exp Neurol 54:304-310, 1995.

341 Winger MJ, Macdonald DR, Cairncross JG: Supratentorial anaplastic gliomas in adults. The prognostic importance of extent of resection and prior low-grade glioma. J Neurosurg 71:487-493, 1989.

Protoplasmic astrocytoma

342 Piepmeier JM, Fried I, Makuch R: Low-grade astrocytomas may arise from different astrocyte lineages. Neurosurgery 33:627-632, 1993.

343 Russell DS, Rubinstein LJ: Pathology of tumours of the nervous system, 5th ed. Baltimore, 1989, Williams & Wilkins, pp 100-101.

Pilocytic astrocytoma

344 Alvord EC Jr, Lofton S: Gliomas of the optic nerve or chiasm—outcome by patients' age, tumor site, and treatment. J Neurosurg 68:85-98, 1988.

345 Austin EJ, Alvord EC Jr: Recurrences of cerebellar astrocytomas. A violation of Collins' law. J Neurosurg 68:41-47, 1988.

346 Brown MT, Friedman HS, Oakes WJ, Boyko OB, Hockenberger B, Schold SC Jr: Chemotherapy for pilocytic astrocytomas. Cancer 71:3165-3172, 1993.

347 Forsyth PA, Shaw EG, Scheithauer BW, O'Fallon JR, Layton DD Jr, Katzmann JA: Supratentorial pilocytic astrocytomas. A clinicopathologic, prognostic, and flow cytometric study of 51 patients. Cancer 72:1335-1342, 1993.

348 Hayostek CJ, Shaw EG, Scheithauer BW, O'Fallon JR, Weiland TL, Schomberg PJ, Kelly PJ, Hu TC: Astrocytomas of the cerebellum. A comparative clinicopathologic study of pilocytic and diffuse astrocytomas. Cancer **72**:856-869, 1993.

349 Ito S, Hoshino T, Shibuya M, Prados M, Edwards M, Davis R: Proliferative characteristics of juvenile pilocytic astrocytomas determined by bromodeoxyuridine labeling. Neurosurgery **31**:414-419, 1992.

350 Iwaki T, Iwaki A, Tateishi J, Sakaki Y, Goldman JE: α B-crystallin and 27-kd heat shock protein are regulated by stress conditions in the central nervous system and accumulate in Rosenthal fibers. Am J Pathol **143**:487-495, 1993.

351 Katsetos CD, Krishna L, Friedberg E, Reidy J, Karkavelas G, Savory J: Lobar pilocytic astrocytomas of the cerebral hemispheres: II. Pathobiology—morphogenesis of the eosinophilic granular bodies. Clin Neuropathol **13**:306-314, 1994.

352 Khatib Z, Heidemann R, Kovnar E, Sanford R, Fairclough D, Langston J, Douglass E, Ochs J, Jenkins J, Ogle L, Kun L: Pilocytic dorsally exophytic brainstem gliomas. A distinct clinicopathologic entity. Ann Neurol **32**:458-459, 1992.

353 Lach B, Sikorska M, Rippstein P, Gregor A, Staines W, Davie TR: Immunoelectron microscopy of Rosenthal fibers. Acta Neuropathol **81**:503-509, 1991.

354 McGirr SJ, Kelly PJ, Scheithauer BW: Stereotactic resection of juvenile pilocytic astrocytomas of the thalamus and basal ganglia. Neurosurgery **20**:447-452, 1987.

355 Murayama S, Bouldin T, Suzuki K: Immunocytochemical and ultrastructural studies of eosinophilic granular bodies in astrocytic tumors. Acta Neuropathol **83**:408-414, 1992.

356 Pagni CA, Giordana MT, Canavero S: Benign recurrence of a pilocytic cerebellar astrocytoma 36 years after radical removal. Case report. Neurosurgery **28**:606-609, 1991.

357 Pollack IF, Hurtt M, Pang D, Albright AL: Dissemination of low grade intracranial astrocytomas in children. Cancer **73**:2869-2878, 1994.

358 Rodriguez LA, Edwards MSB, Levin VA: Management of hypothalamic gliomas in children. An analysis of 33 cases. Neurosurgery **26**:242-247, 1990.

359 Rossitch E Jr, Zeidman SM, Burger PC, Curnes JT, Harsh C, Anscher M, Oakes WJ: Clinical and pathological analysis of spinal cord astrocytomas in children. Neurosurgery **27**:193-196, 1990.

360 Schneider JH Jr, Raffel C, McComb JG: Benign cerebellar astrocytomas of childhood. Neurosurgery **30**:58-63, 1992.

361 Schwartz AM, Ghatak NR: Malignant transformation of benign cerebellar astrocytoma. Cancer **65**:333-336, 1990.

362 von Deimling A, Louis DN, Menon AG, von Ammon K, Petersen I, Ellison D, Wiestler OD, Seizinger BR: Deletions on the long arm of chromosome 17 in pilocytic astrocytoma. Acta Neuropathol **86**:81-85, 1993.

363 Wong JYC, Uhl V, Wara WM, Sheline GE: Optic gliomas—a reanalysis of the University of California, San Francisco experience. Cancer **60**:1847-1855, 1987.

Pleomorphic xanthoastrocytoma

364 Herpers MJHM, Freling G, Beuls EAM: Pleomorphic xanthoastrocytoma in the spinal cord. Case report. J Neurosurg **80**:564-569, 1994.

365 Iwaki T, Fukui M, Kondo A, Matsushima T, Takeshita I: Epithelial properties of pleomorphic xanthoastrocytomas determined in ultrastructural and immunohistochemical studies. Acta Neuropathol **74**:142-150, 1987.

366 Kepes JJ, Rubinstein LJ, Ansbacher L, Schreiber DJ: Histopathological features of recurrent pleomorphic xanthoastrocytomas. Further corroboration of the glial nature of this neoplasm. A study of three cases. Acta Neuropathol **78**:585-593, 1989.

367 Kepes JJ, Rubinstein LJ, Eng LF: Pleomorphic xanthoastrocytoma. A distinctive meningocerebral glioma of young subjects with relatively favorable prognosis. A study of 12 cases. Cancer **44**:1839-1852, 1979.

368 Kros JM, Vecht CJ, Stefanko SZ: The pleomorphic xanthoastrocytoma and its differential diagnosis—a study of five cases. Hum Pathol **22**:1128-1135, 1991.

369 Macaulay RJB, Jay V, Hoffman HJ, Becker LE: Increased mitotic activity as a negative prognostic indicator in pleomorphic xanthoastrocytoma. J Neurosurg **79**:761-768, 1993.

370 Sugita Y, Kepes JJ, Shigemori M, Kuramoto S, Reifenberger G, Kiwit JCW, Wechsler W: Pleomorphic xanthoastrocytoma with desmoplastic reaction. Angiomatous variant. Report of two cases. Clin Neuropathol **9**:271-278, 1990.

Subependymal giant cell astrocytoma (tuberous sclerosis)

371 Bonnin JM, Rubinstein LJ, Papasozomenos SC, Marangos PJ: Subependymal giant cell astrocytoma. Significance and possible cytogenetic implications of an immunohistochemical study. Acta Neuropathol **62**:185-193, 1984.

372 Chow CW, Klug GL, Lewis EA: Subependymal giant cell astrocytoma in children. An unusual discrepancy between histological and clinical features. J Neurosurg **68**:880-883, 1988.

373 European Chromosome 16 Tuberous Sclerosis Consortium: Identification and characterization of the tuberous sclerosis gene on chromosome 16. Cell **75**:1305-1315, 1993.

374 Gomez MR: Tuberous sclerosis, 2nd ed. New York, 1988, Raven Press.

375 Nakamura Y, Becker LE: Subependymal giant-cell tumor. Astrocytic or neuronal? Acta Neuropathol **60**:271-277, 1983.

376 Padmalatha C, Harruff RC, Ganick D, Hafez G-R: Glioblastoma multiforme with tuberous sclerosis. Report of a case. Arch Pathol Lab Med **104**:649-650, 1980.

377 Shepherd CW, Scheithauer BW, Gomez MR, Altermatt HJ, Katzmann JA: Subependymal giant cell astrocytoma. A clinical, pathological and flow cytometric study. Neurosurgery **28**:864-868, 1991.

Desmoplastic cerebral astrocytoma of Infancy

378 Aydin F, Ghatak NR, Salvant J, Muizelaar P: Desmoplastic cerebral astrocytoma of infancy. A case report with immunohistochemical, ultrastructural and proliferation studies. Acta Neuropathol **86**:666-670, 1993.

379 Louis DN, von Deimling A, Dickersin GR, Dooling EC, Seizinger BR: Desmoplastic cerebral astrocytomas of infancy. A histopathologic, immunohistochemical, ultrastructural, and molecular genetic study. Hum Pathol **23**:1402-1409, 1992.

380 Taratuto AL, Monges J, Lylyk P, Leiguarda R: Superficial cerebral astrocytoma attached to dura. Report of six cases in infants. Cancer **54**:2505-2512, 1984.

Oligodendroglioma

381 Burger PC, Rawlings CE, Cox EB, McLendon RE, Schold SC Jr, Bullard DE: Clinicopathologic correlations in the oligodendroglioma. Cancer **59**:1345-1352, 1987.

382 Burger PC, Scheithauer BW, Vogel FS: Surgical pathology of the nervous system and its coverings, ed 3. New York, Churchill Livingstone, 1991, pp 306-324.

383 Cairncross JG, Macdonald DR, Ramsay DA: Aggressive oligodendroglioma. A chemosensitive tumor. Neurosurgery **81**:78-82, 1992.

383a Chen R, Macdonald DR, Ramsay DA: Primary diffuse leptomeningeal oligodendroglioma. Case report. J Neurosurg **83**:724-728, 1995.

384 Cruz-Sanchez FF, Rossi ML, Buller JR, Carboni P Jr, Fineron PW, Coakham HB: Oligodendrogliomas. A clinical, histological, immunocytochemical and lectin-binding study. Histopathology **19**:361-367, 1991.

385 de la Monte SM: Uniform lineage of oligodendrogliomas. Am J Pathol **135**:529-540, 1989.

386 Fortuna A, Celli P, Palma L: Oligodendrogliomas of the spinal cord. Acta Neurochir **52**:305-329, 1980.

387 Glass J, Hochberg FH, Gruber ML, Louis DN, Smith D, Rattner B: The treatment of oligodendrogliomas and mixed oligodendrogliomas-astrocytomas with PCV chemotherapy. J Neurosurg **76**:741-745, 1992.

388 Herpers M, Budka H: Glial fibrillary acidic protein (GFAP) in oligodendroglial tumors. Gliofibrillary oligodendroglioma and transitional oligoastrocytoma as subtypes of oligodendroglioma. Acta Neuropathol **64**:265-272, 1984.

389 Jellinger K. Minauf M, Salzer-Kuntschik M: Oligodendroglioma with extraneural metastases. J Neurol Neurosurg Psychiatry **32**:249-253, 1969.

389a Kraus JA, Koopmann J, Kaskel P, Maintz D, Brandner S, Schramm J, Louis DN, Wiestler OD, von Deimling A: Shared allelic losses on chromosome 1p and 19q suggest a common origin of oligodendroglioma and oligoastrocytoma. J Neuropathol Exp Neurol **54**:91-95, 1995.

390 Kros JM, de Jong AAW, van der Kwast TH: Ultrastructural characterization of transitional cells in oligodendrogliomas. J Neuropathol Exp Neurol **51**:186-193, 1992.

391 Kros JM, Van Eden CG, Stefanko SZ, Waayer-Van Batenburg M, van der Kwast TH: Prognostic implications of glial fibrillary acidic protein containing cell types in oligodendrogliomas. Cancer **66**:1204-1212, 1990.

392 Ludwig C, Smith M, Godfrey A, Armbrustmacher V: A clinicopathologic study of 323 patients with oligodendrogliomas. Ann Neurol **19**:15-21, 1986.

393 Min K-W, Scheithauer BW: Oligodendroglioma. The ultrastructural spectrum. Ultrastruct Pathol **18**:47-60, 1994.

394 Mørk SJ, Halvorsen TB, Lindegaard K-F, Eide GE: Oligodendroglioma. Histologic evaluation and prognosis. J Neuropathol Exp Neurol **45**:65-78, 1986.

395 Nakagawa Y, Parentes E, Rubinstein LJ: Immunohistochemical characterization of oligodendrogliomas. An analysis of multiple markers. Acta Neuropathol **72**:15-22, 1986.

396 Packer RJ, Sutton LN, Rorke LB, Zimmerman RA, Littman P, Bruce DA, Schut L: Oligodendroglioma of the posterior fossa in childhood. Cancer **56**:195-199, 1985.

397 Shaw E, Scheithauer B, O'Fallon J, Tazelaar H, Davis D: Oligodendrogliomas. The Mayo Clinic experience. J Neurosurg **76**:428-434, 1992.

398 Spataro J, Sacks O: Oligodendroglioma with remote metastases. Case report. J Neurosurg **28**:373-379, 1968.

399 Takei Y, Mirra SS, Miles ML: Eosinophilic granular cells in oligodendrogliomas. An ultrastructural study. Cancer **38**:1968-1976, 1976.

Ependymal tumors

400 Afra D, Muller W, Slowik F, Wilcke O, Budka H, Turoczy L: Supratentorial lobar ependymomas. Reports on the grading and survival periods in 80 cases, including 46 recurrences. Acta Neurochir **69**:243-251, 1983.

401 Ang LC, Taylor AR, Bergin D, Kaufmann JCE: An immunohistochemical study of papillary tumors in the central nervous system. Cancer **65**:2712-2719, 1990.

402 Azzarelli B, Rekate HL, Roessmann U: Subependymoma. A case report with ultrastructural study. Acta Neuropathol **40**:279-282, 1977.

403 Bergsagel DJ, Finegold MJ, Butel JS, Kupsky WJ, Garcea RL: DNA sequences similar to those of simian virus 40 in ependymomas and choroid plexus tumors of childhood. N Engl J Med **326**:988-993, 1992.

404 Coffin CM, Swanson PE, Wick MR, Dehner LP: An immunohistochemical comparison of chordoma with renal cell carcinoma, colorectal adenocarcinoma, and myxopapillary ependymoma. A potential diagnostic dilemma in the diminutive biopsy. Mod Pathol **6**:531-538, 1993.

405 Craver RD, McGarry P: Delicate longitudinal nuclear grooves in childhood ependymomas. Arch Pathol Lab Med **118**:919-921, 1994.

406 Crotty TB, Hooker RP, Swensen SJ, Scheithauer BW, Myers JL: Primary malignant ependymoma of the lung. Mayo Clin Proc **67**:373-378, 1992.

407 Davis C, Barnard RO: Malignant behavior of myxopapillary ependymoma. Report of three cases. J Neurosurg **62**:925-929, 1985.

408 Duggan MA, Hugh J, Nation JG, Robertson DI, Stuart GCE: Ependymoma of the uterosacral ligament. Cancer **64**:2565-2571, 1989.

409 Epstein FJ, Farmer J-P, Freed D: Adult intramedullary spinal cord ependymomas. The result of surgery in 38 patients. J Neurosurg **79**:204-209, 1993.

410 Ernestus RI, Wilcke O, Schröder R: Supratentorial ependymomas in childhood. Clinicopathological findings and prognosis. Acta Neurochir **111**:96-102, 1991.

411 Figarella-Branger D, Gambarelli D, Dollo C, Devictor B, Perez-Castillo AM, Genitori L, Lena G, Choux M, Pellissier JF: Infratentorial ependymomas of childhood. Correlation between histological features, immunohistological phenotype, silver nucleolar organizer region staining values and post-operative survival in 16 cases. Acta Neuropathol **82**:208-216, 1991.

412 Friede RL, Pollack A: The cytogenetic basis for classifying ependymomas. J Neuropathol Exp Neurol **37**:103-118, 1978.

413 Furness PN, Lowe J, Tarrant GS: Subepithelial basement membrane deposition and intermediate filament expression in choroid plexus neoplasms and ependymomas. Histopathology **16**:251-255, 1990.

414 Helwig EB, Stern JB: Subcutaneous sacrococcygeal myxopapillary ependymoma. A clinicopathologic study of 32 cases. Am J Clin Pathol **81**:156-161, 1984.

415 Ho K-C, Meyer J, Caya J, Tieu TM, Prentiss A: Craniopharyngioma and "reactive" subependymoma of the third ventricle. Clin Neuropathol **6**:12-15, 1987.

416 Ho K-L: Microtubular aggregates within rough endoplasmic reticulum in myxopapillary ependymoma of the filum terminale. Arch Pathol Lab Med **114**:956-960, 1990.

417 Kaneko Y, Takeshita I, Matsushima T, Iwaki T, Tashima T, Fukui M: Immunohistochemical study of ependymal neoplasms. Histological subtypes and glial and epithelial characteristics. Virchows Arch [A] **417**:97-103, 1990.

418 Kawano N, Yada K, Yagishita S: Clear cell ependymoma. A histological variant with diagnostic implications. Virchows Arch [A] **415**:467-472, 1989.

419 Little NS, Morgan MK, Eckstein RP: Primary ependymoma of a cranial nerve. Case report. J Neurosurg **81**:792-794, 1994.

420 Lombardi D, Scheithauer BW, Meyer FB, Forbes GS, Shaw EG, Gibney DJ, Katzmann JA: Symptomatic subependymoma. A clinicopathological and flow cytometric study. J Neurosurg **75**:583-588, 1991.

421 Lyons MK, Kelly PJ: Posterior fossa ependymomas. Report of 30 cases and review of the literature. Neurosurgery **28**:659-665, 1991.

422 Mannoji H, Becker LE: Ependymal and choroid plexus tumors—cytokeratin and GFAP expression. Cancer **61**:1377-1385, 1988.

423 Maruyama R, Koga K, Nakahara T, Kishida K, Nabeshima K: Cerebral myxopapillary ependymoma. Hum Pathol **23**:960-962, 1992.

424 Mathews T, Moossy J: Gliomas containing bone and cartilage. J Neuropathol Exp Neurol **33**:456-471, 1974.

425 Miettinen M, Clark R, Virtanen I: Intermediate filament proteins in choroid plexus and ependyma and their tumors. Am J Pathol **123**:231-240, 1986.

426 Miralbell R, Louis DN, O'Keeffe D, Rosenberg AE, Suit HD: Metastatic ependymoma of the sacrum. Cancer **65**:2353-2355, 1990.

427 Mørk SJ, Løken AC: Ependymoma. A follow-up study of 101 cases. Cancer **40**:907-915, 1977.

428 Nagashima T, Hoshino T, Cho KG, Edwards MSB, Hudgins RJ, Davis RL: The proliferative potential of human ependymomas measured by in situ bromodeoxyuridine labeling. Cancer **61**:2433-2438, 1988.

429 Nazar GB, Hoffman HJ, Becker LE, Jenkin D, Humphreys RP, Hendrick EB: Infratentorial ependymomas in childhood. Prognostic factors and treatment. J Neurosurg **72**:408-417, 1990.

430 Nobles E, Lee R, Kircher T: Mediastinal ependymoma. Hum Pathol **22**:94-96, 1991.

431 Pagni CA, Canavero S, Giordana MT, Mascalchi M, Arnetoli G: Spinal intramedullary subependymomas. Case report and review of the literature. Neurosurgery **30**:115-117, 1992.

432 Pulitzer DR, Martin PC, Collins PC, Ralph DR: Subcutaneous sacrococcygeal ("myxopapillary") ependymal rests. Am J Surg Pathol **12**:672-677, 1988.

433 Rawlings III CE, Giangaspero F, Burger PC, Bullard DE: Ependymomas. A clinicopathologic study. Surg Neurol **29**:271-281, 1988.

434 Rosenblum MK, Erlandson RA, Aleksic SN, Budzilovich GN: Melanotic ependymoma and subependymoma. Am J Surg Pathol **14**:729-736, 1990.

435 Ross GW, Rubinstein LJ: Lack of histopathological correlation of malignant ependymomas with postoperative survival. J Neurosurg **70**:31-36, 1989.

436 Russell DS, Rubinstein LJ: Pathology of tumours of the nervous system, ed 5. Baltimore, 1989, Williams & Wilkins, pp 769-784.

437 Ryken TC, Robinson RA, Van Gilder JC: Familial occurrence of subependymoma. J Neurosurg **80**:1108-1111, 1994.

438 Sara A, Bruner JM, Mackay B: Ultrastructure of ependymoma. Ultrastruct Pathol **18**:33-42, 1994.

439 Sonneland PRL, Scheithauer BW, Onofrio BM: Myxopapillary ependymoma. A clinicopathologic and immunocytochemical study of 77 cases. Cancer **56**:883-893, 1985.

440 Zuppan CW, Mierau GW, Weeks DA: Ependymoma with signet-ring cells. Ultrastruct Pathol **18**:43-46, 1994.

Astroblastoma

441 Bonnin JM, Rubinstein LJ: Astroblastomas. A pathological study of 23 tumors, with a postoperative follow-up in 13 patients. Neurosurgery **25**:6-13, 1989.

442 Cabello A, Madero S, Castresana A, Diaz-Lobato R: Astroblastoma. Electron microscopy and immunohistochemical findings. Case report. Surg Neurol **35**:116-121, 1991.

443 Jay V, Rutka J: Astroblastoma. Report of a case with ultrastructural, cell kinetic, and cytogenetic analysis. Pediatr Pathol **13**:323-332, 1993.

444 Rubinstein LJ, Herman MM: The astroblastoma and its possible cytogenetic relationship to the tanycyte. An electron microscopic, immunohistochemical, tissue—and organ—culture study. Acta Neuropathol **78**:472-483, 1989.

Mixed gliomas

445 Hart MN, Petito CK, Earle KM: Mixed gliomas. Cancer **33**:134-140, 1974.

446 Kleihues P, Burger PC, Scheithauer BW: Histological typing of tumours of the central nervous system, ed 2. Berlin, 1993, Springer-Verlag, pp 19-20.

Gliomatosis cerebri

447 Artigas J, Cervos-Navarro J, Iglesias JR, Eberhardt G: Gliomatosis cerebri. Clinical and histological findings. Clin Neuropathol **4**:135-148, 1985.

448 Balko MG, Blisard KS, Samaha FJ: Oligodendroglial gliomatosis cerebri. Hum Pathol **23**:706-707, 1992.

449 Kandler RH, Smith CML, Broome JC, Davies-Jones GAB: Gliomatosis cerebri. A clinical, radiological and pathological report of four cases. Br J Neurosurg **5**:187-193, 1991.

Gliomesenchymal tumors

450 Barnard RO, Bradford R, Scott T, Thomas D: Gliomyosarcoma—report of a case of rhabdomyosarcoma arising in a malignant glioma. Acta Neuropathol **69**:23-27, 1986.

451 Bonnin JM, Peña CE, Rubinstein LJ: Mixed capillary hemangioblastoma and glioma. A redefinition of the "angioglioma." J Neuropathol Exp Neurol **42**:504-516, 1983.

452 Bozóky B, Kemény E, Krenacs T, Razga T, Barzó P: Gliosarcomas as a result of sarcomatous differentiation of glial tumor cells. Brain Tumor Pathol **8**:45-49, 1991.

453 Cerda-Nicolas M, Kepes JJ: Gliofibromas (including malignant forms) and gliosarcomas. A comparative study and review of the literature. Acta Neuropathol **85**:349-361, 1993.

454 Goodkin R, Zaias B, Michelsen WJ: Arteriovenous malformation and glioma. Coexistent or sequential? J Neurosurg **72**:798-805, 1990.

455 Grant JW, Steart PV, Aguzzi A, Jones DB, Gallagher PJ: Gliosarcoma. An immunohistochemical study. Acta Neuropathol **79**:305-309, 1989.

456 Haddad SF, Moore SA, Schelper RL, Goeken J: Smooth muscle cells can comprise the sarcomatous component of gliosarcomas. J Neuropathol Exp Neurol **51**:493-498, 1992.

457 Hayashi K, Ohara N, Jeon HJ, Akagi S, Takahashi K, Akagi T, Namba S: Gliosarcoma with features of chondroblastic osteosarcoma. Cancer **72**:850-855, 1993.

458 Jones H, Steart PV, Weller RO: Spindle cell glioblastoma or gliosarcoma? Neuropathol Appl Neurobiol **17**:177-187, 1991.

459 Kepes JJ, Rubinstein LJ, Chiang H: The role of astrocytes in the formation of cartilage in gliomas. An immunohistochemical study of four cases. Am J Pathol **117**:471-483, 1984.

460 Lalitha VS, Rubinstein LJ: Reactive glioma in intracranial sarcoma. A form of mixed sarcoma and glioma ("sarcoglioma"). Report of eight cases. Cancer **43**:246-257, 1979.

461 Louis DN, Hedley-Whyte ET, Martuza RL: Sarcomatous proliferation of the vasculature in a subependymoma. Acta Neuropathol **78**:332-335, 1989.

462 Meis JM, Martz KL, Nelson JS: Mixed glioblastoma multiforme and sarcoma. A clinicopathologic study of 26 Radiation Therapy Oncology Group cases. Cancer **67**:2342-2349, 1991.

463 Montpetit VJ, Pokrupa R, Richard MT, Clapin DF: Myofibroblastic differentiation of a primary intracerebral sarcoma with gliomatous reaction. Clin Neuropathol **7**:1-9, 1988.

464 Morantz RA, Feigin I, Ransohoff J: Clinical and pathological study of 24 cases of gliosarcoma. J Neurosurg **45**:398-408, 1976.

465 Pasquier B, Couderc P, Pasquier D, Panh M, N'Golet A: Sarcoma arising in oligodendroglioma of the brain. A case with intramedullary and subarachnoid spinal metastases. Cancer **42**:2753-2758, 1978.

466 Paulus W, Jellinger K: Mixed glioblastoma and malignant mesenchymoma, a variety of gliosarcoma. Histopathology **22**:277-279, 1993.

467 Reid PM, Barber PC: Gliosarcoma developing in close relationship to an abscess cavity injected with thorotrast. Surg Neurol **29**:67-72, 1988.

467a Roda JM, Gutierrez-Molina M: Multiple intraspinal low-grade astrocytomas mixed with lipoma (astrolipoma). Case report. J Neurosurg **82**:891-894, 1995.

468 Schober R, Bayindir C, Canbolat A, Urich H, Wechsler W: Gliofibroma. Immunohistochemical analysis. Acta Neuropathol **83**:207-210, 1992.

469 Slowik F, Jellinger K, Gazso L, Fisher J: Gliosarcomas. Histological, immunohistochemical, ultrastructural and tissue culture studies. Acta Neuropathol **67**:201-210, 1985.

470 Vazquez M, Miller DC, Epstein F, Allen JC, Budzilovich GN: Glioneurofibroma. Renaming the pediatric "gliofibroma." A neoplasm composed of Schwann cells and astrocytes. Mod Pathol **4**:519-523, 1991.

471 Wargotz ES, Sidawy MK, Jannotta FS: Thorotrast-associated gliosarcoma— including comments on Thorotrast use and review of sequelae with particular reference to lesions of the central nervous system. Cancer **62**:58-66, 1988.

Choroid plexus tumors

472 Albrecht S, Rouah E, Becker L, Bruner J: Transthyretin immunoreactivity in choroid plexus neoplasms and brain metastases. Mod Pathol **4**:610-614, 1991.

473 Andreini L, Doglioni C, Giangaspero F: Tubular adenoma of choroid plexus. A case report. Clin Neuropathol **10**:137-140, 1991.

474 Boesel CP, Suhan JP: A pigmented choroid plexus carcinoma. Histochemical and ultrastructural studies. J Neuropathol Exp Neurol **38**:177-186, 1979.

475 Bonnin JM, Colon LE, Morawetz RB: Focal glial differentiation and oncocytic transformation in choroid plexus papilloma. Acta Neuropathol **72**:277-280, 1987.

476 Coffin CM, Wick MR, Braun J, Dehner LP: Choroid plexus neoplasms. Clinicopathologic and immunohistochemical studies. Am J Surg Pathol **10**:394-404, 1986.

477 Coons S, Johnson PC, Dickman CA, Rekate H: Choroid plexus carcinoma in siblings. A study in light and electron microscopy with Ki-67 immunocytochemistry. J Neuropathol Exp Neurol **48**:483-493, 1989.

478 Diengdoh JV, Shaw MDD: Oncocytic variant of choroid plexus papilloma. Evolution from benign to malignant "oncocytoma." Cancer **71**:855-858, 1993.

479 Duckett S, Osterholm J, Schaefer D, Gonzales C, Schwartzman RJ: Ossified mucin-secreting choroid plexus adenoma. Case report. Neurosurgery **29**:130-132, 1991.

480 Ellenbogen RG, Winston KR, Kupsky WJ: Tumors of the choroid plexus in children. Neurosurgery **25**:327-335, 1989.

481 Garber JE, Burke EM, Lavally BL, Billett AL, Sallan SE, Scott RM, Kupsky W, Li FP: Choroid plexus tumors in the breast cancer-sarcoma syndrome. Cancer **66**:2658-2660, 1990.

482 Gottschalk J, Jautzke G, Paulus W, Goebel S, Cervos-Navarro J: The use of immunomorphology to differentiate choroid plexus tumors from metastatic carcinomas. Cancer **72**:1343-1349, 1993.

483 Gradin WC, Taylon C, Fruin AH: Choroid plexus carcinoma of the third ventricle. Case report and review of the literature. Neurosurgery **12**:217-220, 1983.

484 Griffin BR, Stewart GR, Berger MS, Geyer JR, O'Dell M, Rostad S: Choroid plexus carcinoma of the fourth ventricle. Pediatr Neurosci **14**:134-139, 1988.

485 Herbert J, Cavallaro T, Dwork AJ: A marker for primary choroid plexus neoplasms. Am J Pathol **136**:1317-1325, 1990.

486 Hirano H, Hirahara K, Asakura T, Shimozuru T, Kadota K, Kasamo S, Shimohonji M, Kimotsuki K, Goto M: Hydrocephalus due to villous hypertrophy of the choroid plexus in the lateral ventricles. Case report. J Neurosurg **80**:321-323, 1994.

487 Hoenig EM, Ghatak N, Hirano A, Zimmerman H: Multiloculated cystic tumor of the choroid plexus of the fourth ventricle. Case report. J Neurosurg **27**:574-579, 1967.

488 Matsushima T: Choroid plexus papillomas and human choroid plexus. A light and electron microscopic study. J Neurosurg **59**:1054-1062, 1983.

489 McComb RD, Burger PC: Choroid plexus carcinoma—report of a case with immunohistochemical and ultrastructural observations. Cancer **51**:470-475, 1983.

490 McGirr SJ, Ebersold M, Scheithauer BW, Quast LM, Shaw EG: Choroid plexus papillomas. Long-term follow-up results in a surgically treated series. J Neurosurg **69**:843-849, 1988.

491 Packer RJ, Perilongo G, Johnson D, Sutton L, Vezina G, Zimmerman R, Ryan J, Reaman G, Schut L: Choroid plexus carcinoma of childhood. Cancer **69**:580-585, 1992.

492 Paulus W, Jänisch W: Clinicopathologic correlations in epithelial choroid plexus neoplasms. A study of 52 cases. Acta Neuropathol **80**:635-641, 1990.

493 Reimund EL, Sitton JE, Harkin JC: Pigmented choroid plexus papilloma. Arch Pathol Lab Med **114**:902-905, 1990.

494 Robinow M, Johnson GF, Minella PA: Aicardi syndrome, papilloma of the choroid plexus, cleft lip, and cleft of the posterior palate. J Pediatr **104**:404-405, 1984.

495 Salazar J, Vaquero J, Aranda I, Menendez J, Jimenez J, Bravo G: Choroid plexus papilloma with chondroma. Case report. Neurosurgery **18**:781-783, 1986.

496 Wolfson WL, Brown WJ: Disseminated choroid plexus papilloma. An ultrastructural study. Arch Pathol Lab Med **101**:366-368, 1977.

Neuronal and glioneural tumors, hamartomas, and related lesions
Ganglion cell tumors

497 Caccamo D, Herman MM, Urich H, Rubinstein LJ: Focal neuronal gigantism and cerebral cortical thickening after therapeutic irradiation of the central nervous system. Arch Pathol Lab Med **113**:880-885, 1989.

498 Diepholder HM, Schwechheimer K, Mohadjer M, Knoth R, Volk B: A clinicopathologic and immunomorphologic study of 13 cases of ganglioglioma. Cancer **68**:2192-2201, 1991.

499 Felix I, Bilbao JM, Asa SL, Tyndel F, Kovacs K, Becker LE: Cerebral and cerebellar gangliocytomas. A morphological study of nine cases. Acta Neuropathol **88**:246-251, 1994.

500 Furuta A, Takahashi H, Ikuta F, Onda K, Takeda N, Tanaka R: Temporal lobe tumor demonstrating ganglioglioma and pleomorphic xanthoastrocytoma. J Neurosurg **77**:143-147, 1992.

501 Haddad SF, Moore SA, Menezes AH, Van Gilder JC: Ganglioglioma. 13 years of experience. Neurosurgery **31**:171-178, 1992.

502 Hirose T, Kannuki S, Nishida K, Matsumoto K, Sano T, Hizawa K: Anaplastic ganglioglioma of the brain stem demonstrating active neurosecretory features of neoplastic neuronal cells. Acta Neuropathol **83**:365-370, 1992.

503 Hori A, Weiss R, Schaake T: Ganglioglioma containing osseous tissue and neurofibrillary tangles. Arch Pathol Lab Med **112**:653-655, 1988.

504 Jay V, Squire J, Becker LE, Humphreys R: Malignant transformation in a ganglioglioma with anaplastic neuronal and astrocytic components. Report of a case with flow cytometric and cytogenetic analysis. Cancer **73**:2862-2868, 1994.

505 Krouwer HGJ, Davis RL, McDermott MW, Hoshino T, Prados MD: Gangliogliomas. A clinicopathological study of 25 cases and review of the literature. J Neurooncol 17:139-154, 1993.

506 Lang FF, Epstein FJ, Ransohoff J, Allen JC, Wisoff J, Abbott IR, Miller DC: Central nervous system gangliogliomas. Part 2. Clinical outcome. J Neurosurg 79:867-873, 1993.

507 Lindboe CF, Cappelen J, Kepes JJ: Pleomorphic xanthoastrocytoma as a component of cerebellar ganglioglioma. Case report. Neurosurgery 31:353-355, 1992.

508 Lu WY, Goldman M, Young B, Davis DG: Optic nerve ganglioglioma. Case report. J Neurosurg 78:979-982, 1993.

509 Miller DC, Koslow M, Budzilovich G, Burstein DE: Synaptophysin. A sensitive and specific marker for ganglion cells in central nervous system neoplasms. Hum Pathol 21:271-276, 1990.

510 Miller DC, Lang FF, Epstein FJ: Central nervous system gangliogliomas. Part I. Pathology. J Neurosurg 79:859-866, 1993.

511 Smith TW, Nikulasson S, De Girolami U, De Gennaro LJ: Immunohistochemistry of synapsin I and synaptophysin in human nervous system and neuroendocrine tumors. Applications in diagnostic neuro-oncology. Clin Neuropathol 12:335-342, 1993.

512 Soffer D, Lach B, Constantini S: Melanotic cerebral ganglioglioma. Evidence for melanogenesis in neoplastic astrocytes. Acta Neuropathol 83:315-323, 1992.

513 Takahashi H, Wakabayashi K, Kawai K, Ikuta F, Tanaka R, Takeda N, Washiyama K: Neuroendocrine markers in central nervous system neuronal tumors (gangliocytoma and ganglioglioma). Acta Neuropathol 77:237-243, 1989.

514 VandenBerg SR: Desmoplastic infantile ganglioglioma and desmoplastic cerebral astrocytoma of infancy. Brain Pathol 3:275-281, 1993.

515 VandenBerg SR, May EE, Rubinstein LJ, Herman MM, Parentes E, Vinores SA, Collins VP, Park TS: Desmoplastic supratentorial neuroepithelial tumors of infancy with divergent differentiation potential ("desmoplastic infantile gangliogliomas"). Report on 11 cases of a distinctive embryonal tumor with favorable prognosis. J Neurosurg 66:58-71, 1987.

516 Wacker MR, Cogen PH, Etzell JE, Daneshvar L, Davis RL, Prados MD: Diffuse leptomeningeal involvement by ganglioglioma in a child. J Neurosurg 77:302-306, 1992.

517 Wolf HK, Müller MB, Spänle M, Zentner J, Schramm J, Wiestler OD: Ganglioglioma. A detailed histopathological and immunohistochemical analysis of 61 cases. Acta Neuropathol 88:166-173, 1994.

517a Zhang P, Rosenblum M: Synaptophysin expression in the human spinal cord. Diagnostic implications of an immunohistochemical study. Am J Surg Pathol (in press).

Central neurocytoma

518 Ellison DW, Zygmunt SC, Weller RO: Neurocytoma/lipoma (neurolipocytoma) of the cerebellum. Neuropathol Appl Neurobiol 19:95-98, 1993.

519 Figarella-Branger D, Pellissier JF, Daumas-Duport C, Delisle MB, Pasquier B, Parent M, Gambarelli D, Rougon G, Hassoun J: Central neurocytomas. Critical evaluation of a small-cell neuronal tumor. Am J Surg Pathol 16:97-109, 1992.

520 Hassoun J, Söylemezoglu F, Gambarelli D, Figarella-Branger D, von Ammon K, Kleihues P: Central neurocytoma. A synopsis of clinical and histological features. Brain Pathol 3:297-306, 1993.

521 Hessler RB, Lopes MBS, Frankfurter A, Reidy J, VandenBerg SR: Cytoskeletal immunohistochemistry of central neurocytomas. Am J Surg Pathol 16:1031-1038, 1992.

522 Kim DG, Chi JG, Park SH, Chang KH, Lee SH, Jung H-W, Kim HJ, Cho B-K, Choi KS, Han DH: Intraventricular neurocytoma—clinicopathological analysis of seven cases. J Neurosurg 76:759-765, 1992.

523 Maguire JA, Bilbao JM, Kovacs K, Resch L: Hypothalamic neurocytoma with vasopressin immunoreactivity. Immunohistochemical and ultrastructural observations. Endocr Pathol 3:99-104, 1992.

524 Mrak RE: Malignant neurocytic tumor. Hum Pathol 25:747-752, 1994.

525 Nishio S, Takeshita I, Fukui M: Primary cerebral ganglioneurocytoma in an adult. Cancer 66:358-362, 1990.

526 Nishio S, Takeshita I, Kaneko Y, Fukui M: Cerebral neurocytoma. A new subset of benign neuronal tumors of the cerebrum. Cancer 70:529-537, 1992.

527 Tatter SB, Borges LF, Louis DN: Central neurocytomas of the cervical spinal cord. Report of two cases. J Neurosurg 81:288-293, 1994.

528 Von Deimling A, Kleihues P, Saremaslani P, Yasargil MG, Spoerri O, Sudhof TC, Wiestler OD: Histogenesis and differentiation potential of central neurocytomas. Lab Invest 64:585-591, 1991.

529 Yasargil MG, von Ammon K, von Deimling A, Valavanis A, Wichmann W, Wiestler OD: Central neurocytoma—histopathological variants and therapeutic approaches. J Neurosurg 76:32-37, 1992.

Dysembryoplastic neuroepithelial tumor

530 Daumas-Duport C: Dysembryoplastic neuroepithelial tumors. Brain Pathol 3:283-295, 1993.

531 Daumas-Duport C, Scheithauer BW, Chodkiewicz J-P, Laws ER, Vedrenne C: Dysembryoplastic neuroepithelial tumor. A surgically curable tumor of young patients with intractable partial seizures. Report of thirty-nine cases. Neurosurgery 23:545-556, 1988.

532 Hirose T, Scheithauer BW, Lopes BS, VandenBerg S: Dysembryoplastic neuroepithelial tumor (DNT). An immunohistochemical and ultrastructural study. J Neuropathol Exp Neurol 53:184-195, 1994.

533 Leung SY, Gwi E, Ng HK, Fung CF, Yam KY: Dysembryoplastic neuroepithelial tumor. A tumor with small neuronal cells resembling oligodendroglioma. Am J Surg Pathol 18:604-614, 1994.

Hypothalamic neuronal hamartoma and choristoma

534 Asa SL, Scheithauer BW, Bilbao JM, Horvath E, Ryan N, Kovacs K, Randall RV, Laws ER, Singer W, Linfoot JA, Thorner MO, Vale W: A case for hypothalamic acromegaly. A clinicopathological study of six patients with hypothalamic gangliocytomas producing growth hormone-releasing factor. J Clin Endocrinol Metab 58:796-803, 1984.

535 Clarren SK, Alvord EC Jr, Hall JG: Congenital hypothalamic hamartoblastoma, hypopituitarism, imperforate anus, and postaxial polydactyly—a new syndrome? Part II. Neuropathological considerations. Am J Med Genet 7:75-83, 1980.

536 Culler FL, James HE, Simon ML, Jones KL: Identification of gonadotropin-releasing hormone in neurons of a hypothalamic hamartoma in a boy with precocious puberty. Neurosurgery 17:408-412, 1985.

537 Li JY, Racadot O, Kujas M, Kouadri M, Peillon F, Racadot J: Immunocytochemistry of four mixed pituitary adenomas and intrasellar gangliocytomas associated with different clinical syndromes. Acromegaly, amenorrhea—galactorrhea, Cushing's disease and isolated tumoral syndrome. Acta Neuropathol 77:320-328, 1989.

538 Nishio S, Fujiwara S, Aiko Y, Takeshita I, Fukui M: Hypothalamic hamartoma—report of two cases. J Neurosurg 70:640-645, 1989.

539 Nurbhai MA, Tomlinson BE, Lorigan-Forsythe B: Infantile hypothalamic hamartoma with multiple congenital abnormalities. Neuropathol Appl Neurobiol 11:61-70, 1985.

540 Price RA, Lee PA, Albright AL, Ronnekleiv OK, Gutai JP: Treatment of sexual precocity by removal of a luteinizing hormone–releasing hormone secreting hamartoma. JAMA 251:2247-2249, 1984.

541 Scheithauer BW, Kovacs K, Randall RV, Horvath E, Okazaki H, Laws ER Jr: Hypothalamic neuronal hamartoma and adenohypophyseal neuronal choristoma. Their association with growth hormone adenoma of the pituitary gland. J Neuropathol Exp Neurol 42:648-663, 1983.

Glioneuronal hamartomas, cortical dysplasias, and other epileptogenic lesions

542 Armstrong DD: The neuropathology of temporal lobe epilepsy. J Neuropathol Exp Neurol 52:433-443, 1993.

543 Mischel PS, Nguyen LP, Vinters HV: Cerebral cortical dysplasia associated with pediatric epilepsy. Review of neuropathologic features and proposal of a grading system. J Neuropathol Exp Neurol 54:137-153, 1995.

544 Plate KH, Wieser H-G, Yasargil MG, Wiestler OD: Neuropathological findings in 224 patients with temporal lobe epilepsy. Acta Neuropathol 86:433-438, 1993.

544a Prayson RA, Estes ML: Cortical dysplasia. A histopathologic study of 52 cases of partial lobectomy in patients with epilepsy. Hum Pathol 26:493-500, 1995.

545 Wolf HK, Campos MG, Zentner J, Hufnagel A, Schramm J, Elger CE, Wiestler OD: Surgical pathology of temporal lobe epilepsy. Experience with 216 cases. J Neuropathol Exp Neurol 52:499-506, 1993.

546 Wolf HK, Zentner J, Hufnagel A, Campos MG, Schramm J, Elger CE, Wiestler OD: Surgical pathology of chronic epileptic seizure disorders. Experience with 63 specimens from extratemporal corticectomies, lobectomies, and functional hemispherectomies. Acta Neuropathol 86:466-472, 1993.

Lhermitte-Duclos disease

547 Ambler M, Pogacar S, Sidman R: Lhermitte-Duclos disease (granule cell hypertrophy of the cerebellum). Pathological analysis of the first familial cases. J Neuropathol Exp Neurol 28:622-647, 1969.

548 Ferrer I, Isamat F, Acebes J: A Golgi and electron microscopic study of a dysplastic gangliocytoma of the cerebellum. Acta Neuropathol **47:**163-165, 1979.

549 Hair LS, Symmans F, Powers JM, Carmel P: Immunohistochemistry and proliferative activity in Lhermitte-Duclos disease. Acta Neuropathol **84:**570-573, 1992.

550 Milbouw G, Born JD, Martin D, Collignon F, Hans P, Reznick M, Bonnal J: Clinical and radiological aspects of dysplastic gangliocytoma (Lhermitte-Duclos disease). A report of two cases with review of the literature. Neurosurgery **22:**124-128, 1988.

551 Padberg GW, Schot JDL, Vielvoye GJ, Bots GTAM, de Beer FC: Lhermitte-Duclos disease and Cowden disease. A single phakomatosis. Ann Neurol **29:**517-523, 1991.

552 Shiurba RA, Gessaga EC, Eng LF, Sternberger LA, Sternberger NH, Urich H: Lhermitte-Duclos disease. An immunohistochemical study of the cerebellar cortex. Acta Neuropathol **75:**474-480, 1988.

553 Wells GB, Lasner TM, Yousem DM, Zager EL: Lhermitte-Duclos disease and Cowden's syndrome in an adolescent patient. Case report. J Neurosurg **81:**133-136, 1994.

554 Williams III DW, Elster AD, Ginsberg LE, Stanton C: Recurrent Lhermitte-Duclos disease. Report of two cases and association with Cowden's disease. Am J Neuroradiol **13:**287-290, 1992.

Embryonal neuroepithelial tumors

555 Bonnin JM, Rubinstein LJ, Palmer NF, Beckwith JB: The association of embryonal tumors originating in the kidney and in the brain. A report of seven cases. Cancer **54:**2137-2146, 1984.

556 Brüstle O, Ohgaki H, Schmitt HP, Walter GF, Ostertag H, Kleihues P: Primitive neuroectodermal tumors after prophylactic central nervous system irradiation in children. Association with an activated K-*ras* gene. Cancer **69:**2385-2392, 1992.

557 Burger PC, Scheithauer BW: Tumors of the central nervous system. Atlas of tumor pathology, 3rd series. Fascicle 10. Washington, DC, 1994, Armed Forces Institute of Pathology, pp 193-225.

558 Cruz-Sanchez FF, Rossi ML, Hughes JT, Moss TH: Differentiation in embryonal neuroepithelial tumors of the central nervous system. Cancer **67:**965-971, 1991.

559 Gould VE, Jansson DS, Molenaar WM, Rorke LB, Trojanowski JQ, Lee VMY, Packer RJ, Franke WW: Primitive neuroectodermal tumors of the central nervous system. Patterns of expression of neuroendocrine markers and all classes of intermediate filament proteins. Lab Invest **62:**498-509, 1990.

560 Kleihues P, Burger PC, Scheithauer BW: Histological typing of tumours of the central nervous system, ed 2. Berlin, 1993, Springer-Verlag, pp 27-30.

560a Rainov NG, Lübbe J, Renshaw J, Pritchard-Jones K, Lüthy AR, Aguzzi A: Association of Wilms' tumor with primary brain tumor in siblings. J Neuropathol Exp Neurol **54:**214-223, 1995.

561 Rorke LB: The cerebellar medulloblastoma and its relationship to primitive neuroectodermal tumors. J Neuropathol Exp Neurol **42:**1-15, 1983.

562 Rubinstein LJ: Embryonal central neuroepithelial tumors and their differentiating potential. A cytogenetic view of a complex neuro-oncological problem. J Neurosurg **62:**795-805, 1985.

Medulloblastoma

563 Anwer UE, Smith TW, De Girolami U, Wilkinson HA: Medulloblastoma with cartilaginous differentiation. Arch Pathol Lab Med **113:**84-88, 1989.

564 Boesel CP, Suhan JP, Sayers MP: Melanotic medulloblastoma. Report of a case with ultrastructural findings. J Neuropathol Exp Neurol **37:**531-543, 1978.

565 Chatty EM, Earle KM: Medulloblastoma. A report of 201 cases with emphasis on the relationship of histologic variants to survival. Cancer **28:**977-983, 1971.

566 Chimelli L, Hahn MD, Budka H: Lipomatous differentiation in medulloblastoma. Acta Neuropathol **81:**471-473, 1991.

567 Chowdhury C, Roy S, Mahapatra AK, Bhatia R: Medullomyoblastoma. A teratoma. Cancer **55:**1495-1500, 1985.

568 Coffin CM, Braun JT, Wick MR, Dehner LP: A clinicopathologic and immunohistochemical analysis of 53 cases of medulloblastoma with emphasis on synaptophysin expression. Mod Pathol **3:**164-170, 1990.

569 Czerwionka M, Korf HW, Hoffman O, Busch H, Schachenmayr W: Differentiation in medulloblastomas. Correlation between the immunocytochemical demonstration of photoreceptor markers (S-antigen, rod-opsin) and the survival rate in 66 patients. Acta Neuropathol **78:**629-636, 1989.

570 Davis DG, Wilson D, Schmitz M, Markesbery WR: Lipidized medulloblastoma in adults. Hum Pathol **24:**990-995, 1993.

571 de Chadarevian J-P, Montes JL, O'Gorman AM, Freeman CR: Maturation of cerebellar neuroblastoma into ganglioneuroma with melanosis. A histologic, immunocytochemical, and ultrastructural study. Cancer **59:**69-76, 1987.

572 Dúinkerke SJ, Slooff JL, Gabrëëls FLM, Renier WO, Thijssen HOM, Biesta JH: Melanotic rhabdomyomedulloblastoma or teratoid tumor of cerebellar vermis. Clin Neurol Neurosurg **83:**29-33, 1981.

573 Friedman HS, Oakes WJ, Bigner SH, Wilkstrand CJ, Bigner DD: Medulloblastoma. Tumor biological and clinical perspectives. J Neurooncol **11:**1-15, 1991.

574 Giangaspero F, Rigobello L, Badiali M, Loda M, Andreini L, Basso G, Zorzi F, Montaldi A: Large-cell medulloblastomas. A distinct variant with highly aggressive behavior. Am J Surg Pathol **16:**687-693, 1992.

575 Hubbard JL, Scheithauer BW, Kispert DB, Carpenter SM, Wick MR, Laws ER: Adult cerebellar medulloblastomas. The pathological, radiographic and clinical disease spectrum. J Neurosurg **70:**536-544, 1989.

576 Jimenez CL, Carpenter BF, Robb IA: Melanotic cerebellar tumor. Ultrastruct Pathol **11:**751-759, 1987.

577 Katsetos CD, Herman MM, Frankfurter A, Gass P, Collins P, Walker CC, Rosemberg S, Barnard RO, Rubinstein LJ: Cerebellar desmoplastic medulloblastomas—a further immunohistochemical characterization of the reticulin-free pale islands. Arch Pathol Lab Med **113:**1019-1029, 1989.

578 Katsetos CD, Liu HM, Zacks SI: Immunohistochemical and ultrastructural observations on Homer Wright (neuroblastic) rosettes and the "pale islands" of human cerebellar medulloblastomas. Hum Pathol **19:**1219-1227, 1988.

579 Kopelson G, Linggood RM, Kleinman GM: Medulloblastoma. The identification of prognostic subgroups and implications for multimodality management. Cancer **51:**312-319, 1983.

580 Maraziotis T, Perentes E, Karamitopoulou E, Nakagawa Y, Gessage EC, Probst A, Frankfurter A: Neuron-associated class III β-tubulin isotype, retinal S-antigen, synaptophysin, and glial fibrillary acidic protein in human medulloblastomas. A clinicopathological analysis of 36 cases. Acta Neuropathol **84:**355-363, 1992.

581 Naguib MG, Sung JH, Erickson DL, Gold LHA, Seljeskog EL: Central nervous system involvement in the nevoid basal cell carcinoma syndrome. Case report and review of the literature. Neurosurgery **11:**52-56, 1982.

582 Packer RJ, Sutton LN, Elterman R, Lange B, Goldwein J, Nicholson S, Mulne L, Boyett J, D'Angio G, Wechsler-Jentzsch K, Reaman G, Cohen BH, Bruce DA, Rorke LB, Molloy P, Ryan J, La Fond D, Evans AE, Schut L: Outcome for children with medulloblastoma treated with radiation and cisplatin, CCNU, and vincristine chemotherapy. J Neurosurg **81:**690-698, 1994.

583 Pearl GS, Takei Y: Cerebellar "neuroblastoma." Nosology as it relates to medulloblastoma. Cancer **47:**772-779, 1981.

584 Rao C, Friedlander ME, Klein E, Anzil AP, Sher JH: Medullomyoblastoma in an adult. Cancer **65:**157-163, 1990.

585 Schofield DE, Yunis EJ, Geyer JR, Albright AL, Berger MS, Taylor SR: DNA content and other prognostic features in childhood medulloblastoma. Proposal of a scoring system. Cancer **69:**1307-1314, 1992.

586 Tarbell NJ, Loeffler JS, Silver B, Lynch E, Lavally BL, Kupsky W, Scott M, Sallan SE: The change in patterns of relapse in medulloblastoma. Cancer **68:**1600-1604, 1991.

Medulloepithelioma

587 Auer RN, Becker LE: Cerebral medulloepithelioma with bone, cartilage, and striated muscle. Light microscopic and immunohistochemical study. J Neuropathol **42:**256-267, 1983.

588 Caccamo DV, Herman MM, Rubinstein LJ: An immunohistochemical study of the primitive and maturing elements of human cerebral medulloepitheliomas. Acta Neuropathol **79:**248-254, 1989.

589 Deck JHN: Cerebral medulloepithelioma with maturation into ependymal cells and ganglion cells. J Neuropathol Exp Neurol **28:**442-454, 1989.

590 Russell DS, Rubinstein LJ: Pathology of tumours of the nervous system, ed 5. Baltimore, 1989, Williams & Wilkins, pp 247-251.

591 Troost D, Jansen GH, Dingemans KP: Cerebral medulloepithelioma—electron microscopy and immunohistochemistry. Acta Neuropathol **80:**103-107, 1990.

Neuroblastoma

592 Ahdevaara P, Kalimo H, Törmä T, Haltia M: Differentiating intracerebral neuroblastoma. Report of a case and review of the literature. Cancer **40:**784-788, 1977.

593 Bennett JP Jr., Rubinstein LJ: The biological behavior of primary cerebral neuroblastomas. A reappraisal of the clinical course in a series of 70 cases. Ann Neurol **16:**21-27, 1984.

594 Berger MS, Edwards MSB, Wara WM, Levin VA, Wilson CB: Primary cerebral neuroblastoma. Long-term follow-up review and therapeutic guidelines. J Neurosurg **59**:418-423, 1983.

595 Dehner LP, Abenoza P, Sibley RK: Primary cerebral neuroectodermal tumors. Neuroblastoma, differentiated neuroblastoma, and composite neuroectodermal tumor. Ultrastruct Pathol **12**:479-494, 1988.

596 Horten BC, Rubinstein LJ: Primary cerebral neuroblastoma. A clinicopathological study of 35 cases. Brain **99**:735-756, 1976.

597 Ojeda VJ, Spagnolo DV, Vaughan RJ: Palisades in primary neuroblastoma simulating so-called polar spongioblastoma. A light and electron microscopical study of an adult case. Am J Surg Pathol **11**:316-322, 1989.

598 Torres LF, Grant N, Harding BN, Scaravilli F: Intracerebral neuroblastoma. Report of a case with neuronal maturation and long survival. Acta Neuropathol **68**:110-114, 1985.

Ependymoblastoma

599 Cruz-Sanchez FF, Haustein J, Rossi ML, Cervos Navarro J, Hughes JT: Ependymoblastoma. A histological, immunohistological and ultrastructural study of five cases. Histopathology **12**:17-27, 1988.

600 Langford LA: The ultrastructure of the ependymoblastoma. Acta Neuropathol **71**:136-141, 1988.

601 Mørk SJ, Rubinstein LJ: Ependymoblastoma—a reappraisal of a rare embryonal tumor. Cancer **55**:1536-1542, 1985.

Polar spongioblastoma

602 de Chadarévian JP, Guyda HJ, Hollenberg RD: Hypothalamic polar spongioblastoma associated with the diencephalic syndrome. Ultrastructural demonstration of a neuroendocrine organization. Virchows Arch [A] **402**:465-474, 1984.

603 Jansen GH, Troost D, Dingemans KP: Polar spongioblastoma. An immunohistochemical and electron microscopical study. Acta Neuropathol **81**:228-232, 1990.

604 Russell DS, Rubinstein LJ: Pathology of tumours of the nervous system, ed 5. Baltimore, 1989, Williams & Wilkins, pp 169-172.

605 Schiffer D, Cravioto H, Giordana MT, Migheli A, Pezzullo T, Vigliani MC: Is polar spongioblastoma a tumor entity? J Neurosurg **78**:587-591, 1993.

Primitive neuroectodermal tumor

606 Abenoza P, Wick MR: Primitive cerebral neuroectodermal tumor with rhabdomyoblastic differentiation. Ultrastruct Pathol **10**:347-354, 1986.

607 Gambarelli D, Hassoun J, Choux M, Toga M: Complex cerebral tumor with evidence of neuronal, glial and Schwann cell differentiation. A histologic, immunocytochemical and ultrastructural study. Cancer **49**:1420-1428, 1982.

608 Hart MN, Earle KM: Primitive neuroectodermal tumors of the brain in children. Cancer **32**:890-897, 1973.

609 Janzer RC, Kleihues P: Primitive neuroectodermal tumor with choroid plexus differentiation. Clin Neuropathol **4**:93-98, 1985.

610 Kosnik EJ, Boesel CP, Bay J, Sayers MP: Primitive neuroectodermal tumors of the central nervous system in children. J Neurosurg **48**:741-746, 1978.

611 Tang TT, Harb JM, Mørk SJ, Sty JR: Composite cerebral neuroblastoma and astrocytoma. A mixed central neuroepithelial tumor. Cancer **56**:1404-1412, 1985.

612 Vuia O, Hager H: Central neuroblastic tumour associated with smooth muscle fibers. Eur Neurol **13**:258-272, 1975.

613 Yachnis AT, Rorke LB, Biegal JA, Perilongo G, Zimmerman RA, Sutton LN: Desmoplastic primitive neuroectodermal tumor with divergent differentiation. Broadening the spectrum of desmoplastic infantile neuroepithelial tumors. Am J Surg Pathol **16**:998-1006, 1992.

614 Yu JS, Moore MR, Kupsky WJ, Scott RM: Intracranial melanotic neuroectodermal tumor of infancy. Two case reports. Surg Neurol **37**:123-129, 1992.

Pineal parenchymal tumors

615 Borit A, Blackwood W, Mair WGP: The separation of pineocytoma from pineoblastoma. Cancer **45**:1408-1418, 1980.

616 Coca S, Vaquero J, Escandon J, Moreno M, Peralba J, Rodriguez J: Immunohistochemical characterization of pineocytomas. Clin Neuropathol **11**:298-303, 1992.

617 De Girolami U, Zvaigzne O: Modification of the Achúcarro-Hortega pineal stain for paraffin-embedded formalin-fixed tissue. Stain Technol **48**:48-50, 1973.

618 Donoso LA, Rorke LB, Shields JA, Augsburger JJ, Brownstein S, Lahoud S: S-antigen immunoreactivity in trilateral retinoblastoma. Am J Ophthalmol **103**:57-62, 1987.

619 Dooling EC, Chi JG, Gilles FH: Melanotic neuroectodermal tumor of infancy. Its histological similarities to fetal pineal gland. Cancer **39**:1535-1541, 1977.

620 Hassoun J, Devictor B, Gambarelli D, Peragut JC, Toga M: Paired twisted filaments. A new ultrastructural marker of human pinealomas? Acta Neuropathol **65**:163-165, 1984.

621 Herrick MK, Rubinstein LJ: The cytological differentiating potential of pineal parenchymal neoplasms (true pinealomas). A clinicopathologic study of 28 tumours. Brain **102**:298-320, 1979.

622 Holladay DA, Holladay A, Montebello JF, Redmond KP: Clinical presentation, treatment, and outcome of trilateral retinoblastoma. Cancer **67**:710-715, 1991.

623 Lopes MBS, Gonzalez-Fernandez F, Scheithauer BW, VandenBerg SR: Differential expression of retinal proteins in a pineal parenchymal tumor. J Neuropathol Exp Neurol **52**:516-524, 1993.

623a Mena H, Rushing EJ, Ribas JL, Delahunt B, McCarthy WF: Tumors of pineal parenchymal cells. A correlation of histological features, including nucleolar organizer regions, with survival in 35 cases. Hum Pathol **28**:20-30, 1995.

624 Min K-W, Scheithauer BW, Bauserman SC: Pineal parenchymal tumors. An ultrastructural study with prognostic implications. Ultrastruct Pathol **18**:69-85, 1994.

625 Perentes E, Rubinstein LJ, Herman MM, Donoso LA: S-antigen immunoreactivity in human pineal glands and pineal parenchymal tumors. A monoclonal antibody study. Acta Neuropathol **71**:224-227, 1986.

626 Raisanen J, Vogel H, Horoupian DS: Primitive pineal tumor with retinoblastomatous and retinal/ciliary epithelial differentiation. An immunohistochemical study. J Neurooncol **9**:165-170, 1990.

627 Schild SE, Scheithauer BW, Schomberg PJ, Hook CC, Kelly PJ, Frick L, Robinow JS, Buskirk SJ: Pineal parenchymal tumors. Clinical, pathologic and therapeutic aspects. Cancer **72**:870-880, 1993.

628 Schmidbauer M, Budka H, Pilz P: Neuroepithelial and ectomesenchymal differentiation in a primitive pineal tumor ("pineal anlage tumor"). Clin Neuropathol **8**:7-10, 1989.

629 Sobel RA, Trice JE, Nielsen SL, Ellis WG: Pineoblastoma with ganglionic and glial differentiation. Report of two cases. Acta Neuropathol **55**:243-246, 1981.

630 Trojanowski JQ, Tascos NA, Rorke LB: Malignant pineocytoma with papillary features. Cancer **50**:1789-1793, 1982.

631 Vaquero J, Coca S, Martinez R, Escandon J: Papillary pineocytoma. J Neurosurg **73**:135-137, 1990.

Meningothelial tumors and related lesions

632 Alguacil-Garcia A, Pettigrew NM, Sima AAF: Secretory meningioma. A distinct subtype of meningioma. Am J Surg Pathol **10**:102-111, 1986.

633 Barnett GH, Chou SM, Bay JW: Post traumatic intracranial meningioma. A case report and review of the literature. Neurosurgery **18**:75-78, 1986.

634 Berho M, Suster S: Mucinous meningioma. Report of an unusual variant of meningioma that may mimic metastatic mucin-producing carcinoma. Am J Surg Pathol **18**:100-106, 1994.

635 Budka H: Non-glial specificities of immunocytochemistry for glial fibrillary acidic protein (GFAP). Triple expression of GFAP, vimentin and cytokeratins in papillary meningioma and metastasizing renal carcinoma. Acta Neuropathol **72**:43-54, 1986.

636 Coons SW, Johnson PC: Brachial plexus meningioma. Report of a case with immunohistochemical and ultrastructural examination. Acta Neuropathol **77**:445-448, 1989.

637 Davidson GS, Hope JK: Meningeal tumors of childhood. Cancer **63**:1205-1210, 1989.

638 de la Monte SM, Flickinger J, Linggood RM: Histopathologic features predicting recurrence of meningiomas following subtotal resection. Am J Surg Pathol **10**:836-843, 1986.

639 Ferracini R, Poggi S, Frank G, Azzolini U, Sabattini E, Spagnotti F, Cenacchi G, Pileri S: Meningeal sarcoma with rhabdomyoblastic differentiation. Case report. Neurosurgery **30**:782-785, 1992.

640 Germano IM, Edwards MSB, Davis RL, Schiffer D: Intracranial meningiomas of the first two decades of life. J Neurosurg **80**:447-453, 1994.

641 Gi H, Nagao S, Yoshizumi H, Nishioka T, Uno J, Shingu T, Fujita Y: Meningioma with hypergammaglobulinemia. Case report. J Neurosurg **73**:628-629, 1990.

642 Harrison MJ, Wolfe DE, Lau T-S, Mitnick RJ, Sachdev VP: Radiation-induced meningiomas. Experience at the Mount Sinai Hospital and review of the literature. J Neurosurg **75**:564-574, 1991.

643 Horten BC, Urich H, Stefoski D: Meningiomas with conspicuous plasma cell-lymphocytic components. A report of five cases. Cancer **43**:258-264, 1979.

644 Jääskeläinen J, Haltia M, Servo A: Atypical and anaplastic meningiomas. Radiology, surgery, radiotherapy, and outcome. Surg Neurol **25**:233-242, 1986.

645 Kallio M, Sankila R, Hakulinen T, Jääskeläinen J: Factors affecting operative and excess long-term mortality in 935 patients with intracranial meningiomas. Neurosurgery **31:**2-12, 1992.

646 Kawasaki K, Takahashi H, Kaneko H, Sato H, Fusahiro I: Novel eosinophilic intracytoplasmic inclusions in a meningioma. Cancer **72:**2675-2679, 1993.

647 Kepes JJ: Meningiomas. Biology, pathology and differential diagnosis. New York, 1982, Masson.

648 Kepes JJ, Chen W Y-K, Connors MH, Vogel FS: "Chordoid" meningeal tumors in young individuals with peritumoral lymphoplasmacellular infiltrates causing systemic manifestations of the Castleman syndrome. Cancer **62:**391-406, 1988.

649 Kepes JJ, Goldware S, Leoni R: Meningioma with pseudoglandular pattern. A case report. J Neuropathol Exp Neurol **42:**61-68, 1983.

650 Lattes R, Bigotti G: Lipoblastic meningioma. "Vacuolated meningioma." Hum Pathol **22:**164-171, 1991.

650a Lekanne Deprez RH, Riegman PH, van Drunen E, Warringa UL, Groen NA, Stefanko SZ, Koper JW, Avezaat CJJ, Mulder PGH, Zwarthoff EC, Hagemeijer A: Cytogenetic, molecular genetic and pathological analyses in 126 meningiomas. J Neuropathol Exp Neurol **54:**224-235, 1995.

651 Lee KS, Hoshino T, Rodriguez LA, Bederson J, Davis RL, Wilson CB: Bromodeoxyuridine labeling study of intracranial meningiomas. Proliferative potential and recurrence. Acta Neuropathol **80:**311-317, 1990.

652 Longstreth WT Jr, Dennis LK, McGuire VM, Drangsholt MT, Koepsell TD: Epidemiology of intracranial meningioma. Cancer **72:**639-648, 1993.

653 Lopez DA, Silvers DN, Helwig EB: Cutaneous meningiomas. A clinicopathologic study. Cancer **34:**728-744, 1974.

654 Louis DN, Hamilton AJ, Sobel RA, Ojemann RG: Pseudopsammomatous meningioma with elevated serum carcinoembryonic antigen. A true secretory meningioma. Case report. J Neurosurg **74:**129-132, 1991.

655 Ludwin SK, Rubinstein LJ, Russell DS: Papillary meningioma. A malignant variant of meningioma. Cancer **36:**1363-1373, 1975.

656 Mahmood A, Caccamo DV, Tomecek FJ, Malik GM: Atypical and malignant meningiomas. A clinicopathological review. Neurosurgery **33:**955-963, 1993.

656a Matyja E, Kuchna I, Kroh H, Mazurowski W, Zabek M: Meningiomas and gliomas in juxtaposition. Casual or causal coexistence? Report of two cases. Am J Surg Pathol **19:**37-41, 1995.

657 Maxwell M, Galanopoulos T, Neville-Golden J, Antoniades HN: Expression of androgen and progesterone receptors in primary human meningiomas. J Neurosurg **78:**456-462, 1993.

658 Michaud J, Gagne F: Microcystic meningioma. Clinicopathologic report of eight cases. Arch Pathol Lab Med **107:**75-80, 1983.

659 Mirimanoff RO, Dosoretz DE, Linggood RM, Ojemann RG, Martuza RL: Meningioma. Analysis of recurrence and progression following neurosurgical resection. J Neurosurg **62:**18-24, 1985.

660 Mirra SS, Miles ML: Unusual pericytic proliferation in a meningotheliomatous meningioma. An ultrastructural study. Am J Surg Pathol **6:**573-580, 1982.

661 Ng HK, Wong MP, Chan KW: Benign metastasizing meningioma. Clin Neurol Neurosurg **92:**152-154, 1990.

662 Ng H-K, Tse CCH, Lo STH: Microcystic meningiomas—an unusual morphologic variant of meningiomas. Histopathology **14:**1-9, 1989.

663 Odake G: Cystic meningioma. Report of three patients. Neurosurgery **30:**935-940, 1992.

663a Ohta M, Iwaki T, Kitamoto T, Takeshita I, Tateishi J, Fukui M: MIB-1 staining index and scoring of histologic features in meningioma. Indicators for the prediction of biologic potential and postoperative management. Cancer **74:**3176-3189, 1994.

664 Pasquier B, Gasnier F, Pasquier D, Keddari E, Morens A, Couderc P: Papillary meningioma. Clinicopathologic study of seven cases and review of the literature. Cancer **58:**299-305, 1986.

665 Radley MG, di Sant'Agnese PA, Eskin TA, Wilbur DC: Epithelial differentiation in meningiomas. An immunohistochemical, histochemical, and ultrastructural study—with review of the literature. Am J Clin Pathol **92:**266-272, 1989.

666 Robinson PG: Pulmonary meningioma. Report of a case with electron microscopic and immunohistochemical findings. Am J Clin Pathol **97:**814-817, 1992.

667 Roggendorf W, Schuster T, Peiffer J: Proliferative potential of meningiomas determined with the monoclonal antibody Ki-67. Acta Neuropathol **73:**361-364, 1987.

668 Saleh J, Silberstein HJ, Salner AL, Uphoff DF: Meningioma. The role of a foreign body and irradiation in tumor formation. Neurosurgery **29:**113-119, 1991.

669 Salibi SS, Nauta HJ, Brem H, Epstein JI, Cho KR: Lipomeningioma. Report of three cases and review of the literature. Neurosurgery **25:**122-126, 1989.

670 Salmon I, Kiss R, Levivier M, Remmelink M, Pasteels J-L, Brotchi J, Flament-Durand J: Characterization of nuclear DNA content, proliferation index, and nuclear size in a series of 181 meningiomas, including benign primary, recurrent and malignant tumors. Am J Surg Pathol **17:**239-247, 1993.

671 Vagner-Capodano AM, Grisoli F, Gambarelli D, Sedan R, Pellet W, DeVictor B: Correlation between cytogenetic and histopathological findings in 75 human meningiomas. Neurosurgery **32:**892-900, 1993.

672 Vaquero J, Coca S, Martínez R, Jiménez C: Convexity meningioma and glioblastoma in collision. Surg Neurol **33:**139-141, 1990.

673 Wilson AJ, Ratliff JL, Lagios MD, Aguilar MJ: Mediastinal meningioma. Am J Surg Pathol **3:**557-562, 1979.

674 Winek RR, Scheithauer BW, Wick MR: Meningioma, meningeal hemangiopericytoma (angioblastic meningioma), peripheral hemangiopericytoma, and acoustic schwannoma. A comparative immunohistochemical study. Am J Surg Pathol **13:**251-261, 1989.

675 Zon LI, Johns WD, Stomper PC, Kaplan WD, Connolly JL, Morris JH, Harris JR, Henderson IC, Skarin AT: Breast carcinoma metastatic to a meningioma. Case report and review of the literature. Arch Intern Med **149:**959-962, 1989.

676 Zorludemir S, Scheithauer BW, Hirose T, Van Houten C, Miller G, Meyer FB: Clear cell meningioma. A clinicopathologic study of a potentially aggressive variant of meningioma. Am J Surg Pathol **19:**493-505, 1995.

677 Zuppan CW, Liwnicz BH, Weeks DA: Meningioma with chordoid features. Ultrastruct Pathol **18:**29-32, 1994.

678 Blumenthal D, Berho M, Bloomfield S, Schochet SS, Kaufman HH: Childhood meningioma associated with meningioangiomatosis. Case report. J Neurosurg **78:**287-289, 1993.

679 Goates JJ, Dickson DW, Horoupian DS: Meningioangiomatosis. An immunocytochemical study. Acta Neuropathol **82:**527-532, 1991.

680 Halper J, Scheithauer BW, Okazaki H, Laws Jr ER: Meningioangiomatosis. A report of six cases with special reference to the occurrence of neurofibrillary tangles. J Neuropathol Exp Neurol **45:**426-446, 1986.

681 Kollias SS, Crone KR, Ball Jr WS, Prenger EC, Ballard ET: Meningioangiomatosis of the brain stem. J Neurosurg **80:**732-735, 1994.

Nonmeningothelial, mesenchymal tumors

682 Paulus W, Slowik F, Jellinger K: Primary intracranial sarcomas. Histopathological features of 19 cases. Histopathology **18:**395-402, 1991.

Lipoma and liposarcoma

683 Budka H: Intracranial lipomatous hamartomas (intracranial "lipomas"). A study of 13 cases including combinations with medulloblastoma, colloid and epidermoid cysts, angiomatosis and other malformations. Acta Neuropathol **28:**205-222, 1974.

684 Christensen WN, Long DM, Epstein JI: Cerebellopontine angle lipoma. Hum Pathol **17:**739-743, 1986.

685 Giuffre R: Intradural spinal lipomas. Review of literature (99 cases) and report of an additional case. Acta Neurochir **14:**69-95, 1966.

686 Harrison MJ, Mitnick RJ, Rosenblum BR, Rothman AS: Leptomyelolipoma. Analysis of 20 cases. J Neurosurg **73:**360-367, 1990.

686a Lee M, Rezai AR, Abbott R, Coelho DH, Epstein FJ: Intramedullary spinal cord lipomas. J Neurosurg **82:**394-400, 1995.

687 Perling LH, Laurent JP, Cheek WR: Epidural hibernoma as a complication of corticosteroid treatment. Case report. J Neurosurg **69:**613-616, 1988.

688 Preul MC, Leblanc R, Tampieri D, Robitaille Y, Pokrupa R: Spinal angiolipomas. Report of three cases. J Neurosurg **78:**280-286, 1993.

689 Quint DJ, Boulos RS, Sanders WP, Mehta BA, Patel SC, Tiel RL: Epidural lipomatosis. Radiology **169:**485-490, 1988.

690 Saunders JE, Kwartler JA, Wolf HK, Brackmann DE, McElveen JT Jr: Lipomas of the internal auditory canal. Laryngoscope **101:**1031-1036, 1991.

691 Sheridan F, Scharf D, Henderson VW, Miller CA: Lipomas of the mesencephalic tectum and rostral pons associated with sleep apnea syndrome. Clin Neuropathol **9:**152-156, 1990.

692 Shuangshoti S, Vajragupta L: Angiolipoma of thalamus presenting with abrupt onset suggestive of cerebrovascular disease. Clin Neuropathol **14:**82-85, 1995.

693 Sima A, Kindblom LG, Pellettieri L: Liposarcoma of the meninges. Acta Pathol Microbiol Scand (A) **84:**306-310, 1976.

694 Tresser N, Parveen T, Roessmann U: Intracranial lipomas with teratomatous elements. Arch Pathol Lab Med **117:**918-920, 1993.

695 Walsh JW, Markesbery WR: Histological features of congenital lipomas of the lower spinal canal. J Neurosurg **52:**564-569, 1980.

Osseous and cartilaginous tumors

696 Adegbite ABO, McQueen JD, Paine KWE, Rozdilsky B: Primary intracranial chondrosarcoma. A report of two cases. Neurosurgery 17:490-494, 1985.

697 Bernstein M, Perrin RG, Platts ME, Simpson WJ: Radiation-induced cerebellar chondrosarcoma. Case report. J Neurosurg 61:174-177, 1984.

698 Chakrabortty S, Tamaki N, Kondoh T, Kojima N, Kamikawa H, Matsumoto S: Maffucci's syndrome associated with intracranial enchondroma and aneurysm. Case report. Surg Neurol 36:216-220, 1991.

699 Cybulski GR, Russel EJ, D'Angelo CM, Bailey OT: Falcine chondrosarcoma. Case report and literature review. Neurosurgery 16:412-415, 1985.

700 Fallon MD, Ellerbrake D, Teitelbaum SL: Meningeal osteomas and chronic renal failure. Hum Pathol 13:449-453, 1982.

701 Hadadian K, Abtahiih H, Asil ZT, Rakhshan M, Vessal P: Cystic falcine chondroma. Case report and review of the literature. Neurosurgery 29:909-912, 1991.

702 Lam RMY, Malik GM, Chason JL: Osteosarcoma of meninges. Clinical, light, and ultrastructural observations of a case. Am J Surg Pathol 5:203-208, 1981.

703 Mapstone TB, Wongmongkolrit T, Roessman U, Ratcheson RA: Intradural chondroma. A case report and review of the literature. Neurosurgery 12:111-114, 1983.

704 Parker JR, Zarabi MC, Parker JC: Intracerebral mesenchymal chondrosarcoma. Ann Clin Lab Sci 19:401-407, 1989.

705 Ranjan A, Chacko G, Joseph T, Chandi SM: Intraspinal mesenchymal chondrosarcoma. Case report. J Neurosurg 80:928-930, 1994.

706 Reznik M, Lenelle J: Primary intracerebral osteosarcoma. Cancer 68:793-797, 1991.

707 Salazar-Calderon Perriggo VH, Oommen KJ, Sobonya RE: Silent right parietal chondroma resulting in secondary mania. Clin Neuropathol 12:325-329, 1993.

708 Sato K, Kubota T, Yoshida K, Murata H: Intracranial extraskeletal myxoid chondrosarcoma with special reference to lamellar inclusions in the rough endoplasmic reticulum. Acta Neuropathol 86:525-528, 1993.

709 Scheithauer BW, Rubinstein LJ: Meningeal mesenchymal chondrosarcoma. Report of 8 cases with review of the literature. Cancer 42:2744-2752, 1978.

710 Traflet RF, Babaria AR, Barolat G, Doan HT, Gonzalez C, Mishkin MM: Intracranial chondroma in a patient with Ollier's disease. Case report. J Neurosurg 70:274-276, 1989.

Fibroblastic and "fibrohistiocytic" tumors

711 Friede RL, Pollack A: Neurosurgical desmoid tumors. Presentation of four cases with a review of the differential diagnoses. J Neurosurg 50:725-732, 1979.

712 Gainer JV, Chou SM, Chadduck WM: Familial cerebral sarcomas. Arch Neurol 32:665-668, 1975.

713 Gaspar LE, Mackenzie IRA, Gilbert JJ, Kaufmann JCE, Fisher BF, Macdonald DR, Cairncross JG: Primary cerebral fibrosarcomas. Clinicopathologic study and review of the literature. Cancer 72:3277-3281, 1993.

714 Gonzalez-Vitale JC, Slavin RE, McQueen JD: Radiation-induced intracranial malignant fibrous histiocytoma. Cancer 37:2960-2963, 1976.

715 Hisaoka M, Furuta A, Rikimaru S: Sclerosing fibrous tumor of the cauda equina. A fibroblastic variant of peripheral nerve tumor? Acta Neuropathol 86:193-197, 1993.

716 Iyer GV, Vaishya ND, Bhaktaviziam A, Taori G, Abraham J: Angiofibroma of the middle cranial fossa. J Neurosurg 35:90-94, 1971.

717 Mitchell A, Scheithauer BW, Ebersold MJ, Forbes GS: Intracranial fibromatosis. Neurosurgery 29:123-126, 1991.

718 Pagès A, Pagès M, Ramos J, Bénézech J: Radiation-induced intracranial fibrochondrosarcoma. J Neurol 233:309-310, 1986.

719 Palma L, Spagnoli LG, Yusuf MA: Intracerebral fibroma. Light and electron microscopic study. Acta Neurochir 77:152-156, 1985.

720 Pieterse S, Dinning TAR, Blumbergs PC: Postirradiation sarcomatous transformation of a pituitary adenoma. A combined pituitary tumor. J Neurosurg 56:283-286, 1982.

721 Prayson RA, Estes ML, McMahon JT, Kalfas I, Sebek BA: Meningeal myofibroblastoma. Am J Surg Pathol 17:931-936, 1993.

722 Reyes-Mugica M, Chou P, Gonzalez-Crussi F, Tomita T: Fibroma of the meninges in a child. Immunohistological and ultrastructural study. J Neurosurg 76:143-147, 1992.

723 Roosen N, Cras P, Pasquier P, Martin JJ: Primary thalamic malignant fibrous histiocytoma of the dominant hemisphere causing severe neuropsychological symptoms. Clin Neuropathol 8:16-21, 1989.

724 Waltz TA, Brownell B: Sarcoma. A possible late result of effective radiation therapy for pituitary adenoma. Report of two cases. J Neurosurg 24:901-907, 1966.

Endothelial tumors

725 Abe M, Tabuchi K, Takagi M, Matsumoto S, Shimokama T, Kishikawa T: Spontaneous resolution of multiple hemangiomas of the brain. Case report. J Neurosurg 73:448-452, 1990.

726 Chow LT, Chow W, Dawson TF: Epithelioid hemangioendothelioma of the brain. Am J Surg Pathol 16:619-625, 1992.

726a Hida K, Tada M, Iwasaki Y, Abe H: Intramedullary disseminated capillary hemangioma with localized spinal cord swelling. Case report. Neurosurgery 33:1099-1101, 1993.

727 Kuratsu J, Seto H, Kochi M, Itoyama Y, Uemura S, Ushio Y: Metastatic angiosarcoma of the brain. Surg Neurol 35:305-309, 1991.

728 Mena H, Ribas JL, Enzinger FM, Parisi JE: Primary angiosarcoma of the nervous system. Study of eight cases and review of the literature. J Neurosurg 75:73-76, 1991.

729 Pearl GS, Takei Y: Hemangioendothelioma of the neuraxis. An ultrastructural study. Neurosurgery 11:486-490, 1982.

730 Pearl GS, Takei Y, Tindall GT, O'Brien MS, Payne NS, Hoffman JC: Benign hemangioendothelioma involving the central nervous system. "Strawberry nevus" of the neuraxis. Neurosurgery 7:249-256, 1980.

731 Samaratunga H, Searle J, Cominos D, Le Fevre I: Cerebral metastasis of an atrial myxoma mimicking an epithelioid hemangioendothelioma. Am J Surg Pathol 18:107-111, 1994.

732 Sickler GK, Langford LA: Intracranial tumor-forming papillary endothelial hyperplasia—a case report. Clin Neuropathol 9:125-128, 1990.

733 Wen DY, Hardten DR, Wirtschafter JD, Sung JH, Haines SJ: Elevated intracranial pressure from cerebral venous obstruction by Masson's vegetant intravascular hemangioendothelioma. J Neurosurg 75:787-790, 1991.

Meningeal hemangiopericytoma

734 d'Amore ES, Manivel JC, Sung JH: Soft-tissue and meningeal hemangiopericytomas. An immunohistochemical and ultrastructural study. Hum Pathol 21:414-423, 1990.

735 Guthrie BL, Ebersold MJ, Scheithauer BW, Shaw EG: Meningeal hemangiopericytoma. Histopathologic features, treatment, and long-term follow-up of 44 cases. Neurosurgery 25:514-522, 1989.

736 Kleihues P, Burger PC, Scheithauer BW: Histological typing of tumours of the central nervous system. Berlin, 1993, Springer-Verlag, pp 38-39.

737 Mena H, Ribas JL, Pezeshkpour GH, Cowan DN, Parisi JE: Hemangiopericytoma of the central nervous system. A review of 94 cases. Hum Pathol 22:84-91, 1991.

738 Nakamura M, Inoue HK, Ono N, Kunimine H, Tamada J: Analysis of hemangiopericytic meningiomas by immunohistochemistry, electron microscopy and cell culture. J Neuropathol Exp Neurol 46:57-71, 1987.

Myogenous tumors

739 Asai A, Yamada H, Murata S, Matsuno A, Tsutsumi K, Takemura T, Matsutani M, Takakura K: Primary leiomyosarcoma of dura. Case report. J Neurosurg 68:308-311, 1988.

740 Dropcho EJ, Allen JC: Primary intracranial rhabdomyosarcoma. Case report and literature review. J Neurooncol 5:139-150, 1987.

741 Kidooka M, Okada T, Takayama S, Nakasu S, Handa J: Primary leiomyosarcoma of the spinal dura mater. Neuroradiology 33:173-174, 1991.

742 Kroe DJ, Hudgins WR, Simmons JCH, Blackwell CF: Primary intrasellar leiomyoma. Case report. J Neurosurg 29:189-191, 1968.

743 Lach B, Duncan E, Rippstein P, Benoit BG: Primary intracranial pleomorphic angioleiomyoma—a new morphologic variant. An immunohistochemical and electron microscopic study. Cancer 74:1915-1920, 1994.

744 Louis DN, Richardson Jr. EP, Dickersin GR, Petrucci DA, Rosenberg AE, Ojeman RG: Primary intracranial leiomyosarcoma. Case report. J Neurosurg 71:279-282, 1989.

745 Russell DS, Rubinstein LJ: Pathology of tumours of the nervous system, ed 5. Baltimore, 1989, Williams & Wilkins, p 689.

746 Smith MT, Armbrustmacher VW, Violett TW: Diffuse meningeal rhabdomyosarcoma. Cancer 47:2081-2086, 1981.

747 Steel TR, Pell MF, Turner JJ, Lim GHK: Spinal epidural leiomyoma occurring in an HIV-infected man. Case report. J Neurosurg 79:442-445, 1993.

748 Taratuto AL, Molina HA, Diez B, Zúccaro G, Monges J: Primary rhabdomyosarcoma of brain and cerebellum. Report of four cases in infants. An immunohistochemical study. Acta Neuropathol 66:98-104, 1985.

749 Thieruf P, Weiland H: Uber ein intrakranielles Leiomyom. Med Welt 29:1280-1282, 1978.

Other primary CNS sarcomas

750 Budka H, Pilz P, Guseo A: Primary leptomeningeal sarcomatosis. Clinico-pathological report of six cases. J Neurol **211**:77-93, 1975.

751 Russell DS, Rubinstein LJ: Pathology of tumours of the nervous system, ed 5. Baltimore, 1989, Williams & Wilkins, pp 507-514.

752 Thibodeau LL, Ariza A, Piepmeier JM: Primary leptomeningeal sarcomatosis. J Neurosurg **68**:802-805, 1988.

Nerve sheath tumors of the craniospinal axis

753 Allcutt DA, Hoffman HJ, Isla A, Becker LE, Humphreys RP: Acoustic schwannomas in children. Neurosurgery **29**:14-18, 1991.

754 Carney JA: Psammomatous melanotic schwannoma. A distinctive, heritable tumor with special associations, including cardiac myxoma and the Cushing syndrome. Am J Surg Pathol **14**:206-222, 1990.

755 Carvalho GA, Lindeke A, Tatagiba M, Ostertag H, Samii M: Cranial granular-cell tumor of the trigeminal nerve. Case report. J Neurosurg **81**:795-798, 1994.

756 Casadei GP, Komori T, Scheithauer BW, Miller GM, Parisi JE, Kelly PJ: Intracranial parenchymal schwannoma. A clinicopathological and neuroimaging study of nine cases. J Neurosurg **79**:217-222, 1993.

756a Casadei GP, Scheithauer BW, Hirose T, Manfrini M, Van Houton C, Wood MB: Cellular schwannoma. A clinicopathologic, DNA flow cytometric, and proliferation marker study of 70 patients. Cancer **75**:1109-1119, 1995.

757 Chang Y, Horoupian D, Jordan J, Steinberg G: Localized hypertrophic mono-neuropathy of the trigeminal nerve. Arch Pathol Lab Med **117**:170-176, 1993.

758 Cras P, De Groote CC, Van Vyve M, Vercruyssen A, Martin JJ: Malignant pigmented spinal nerve root schwannoma metastasizing in the brain and viscera. Clin Neuropathol **9**:290-294, 1990.

759 Deruaz JP, Janzer RC, Costa J: Cellular schwannomas of the intracranial and intraspinal compartment. Morphological and immunological characteristics compared with classical benign schwannomas. J Neuropathol Exp Neurol **52**:114-118, 1993.

760 Ducatman BS, Scheithauer BW: Postirradiation neurofibrosarcoma. Cancer **51**:1028-1033, 1983.

761 Ducatman BS, Scheithauer BW, Peipgras DG, Reiman HM, Illstrup DM: Malignant peripheral nerve sheath tumors. A clinicopathologic study of 120 cases. Cancer **57**:2006-2021, 1986.

762 Graccion JG, Enzinger FM: Malignant schwannoma associated with von Recklinghausen's neurofibromatosis. Virchows Arch [A] **383**:43-57, 1979.

763 Halliday AL, Sobel RA, Martuza RL: Benign spinal nerve sheath tumors. Their occurrence sporadically and in neurofibromatosis types 1 and 2. J Neurosurg **74**:248-253, 1991.

764 Han DH, Kim DG, Chi JG, Park SH, Jung H-W, Kim YG: Malignant Triton tumor of the acoustic nerve—case report. J Neurosurg **76**:874-877, 1992.

764a Jung J-M, Shin H-J, Chi JG, Park IS, Kim ES, Han JW: Malignant intraventricular schwannoma. Case report. J Neurosurg **82**:121-124, 1995.

765 Killeen RM, Davy CL, Bauserman SC: Melanocytic schwannoma. Cancer **62**:174-183, 1988.

766 Levy WJ, Ansbacher L, Byer J, Nutkiewicz A, Fratkin J: Primary malignant nerve sheath tumor of the gasserian ganglion. A report of two cases. Neurosurgery **13**:572-576, 1983.

767 Levy WJ, Latchow J, Hahn JF, Sawhny B, Bay J, Dohn DF: Spinal neurofibromas. A report of 66 cases and a comparison with meningiomas. Neurosurgery **18**:331-334, 1986.

768 Liwnicz BH: Bilateral trigeminal neurofibrosarcoma. Case report. J Neurosurg **50**:253-256, 1979.

769 Marchese MJ, McDonald JV: Intramedullary melanotic schwannoma of the cervical spinal cord. Report of a case. Surg Neurol **33**:353-355, 1990.

770 Martuza RL, Eldridge R: Neurofibromatosis 2 (bilateral acoustic neurofibromatosis). N Engl J Med **318**:684-688, 1988.

771 McLean CA, Laidlaw JD, Brownbill DSB, Gonzales MF: Recurrence of acoustic neurilemoma as a malignant spindle cell neoplasm. Case report. J Neurosurg **73**:946-950, 1990.

772 Mrak RE, Flanigan S, Collins CL: Malignant acoustic schwannoma. Arch Pathol Lab Med **118**:557-561, 1994.

773 Paulus W, Warmuth-Metz M, Sörensen N: Intracranial neurothekeoma (nerve-sheath myxoma). J Neurosurg **79**:280-282, 1993.

774 Perentes E, Nakagawa Y, Ross GW, Stanton C, Rubinstein LJ: Expression of epithelial membrane antigen in perineurial cells and their derivatives. An immunohistochemical study with multiple markers. Acta Neuropathol **75**:160-165, 1987.

775 Russell DS, Rubinstein LJ: Pathology of tumours of the nervous system, ed 5. Baltimore, 1989, Williams & Wilkins, pp 533-589.

776 Seizinger BR, Martuza RL, Gusella JF: Loss of genes on chromosome 22 in tumorigenesis of human acoustic neuroma. Nature **322**:644-647, 1986.

777 Seppälä MT, Haltia MJJ: Spinal malignant nerve-sheath tumor or cellular schwannoma. A striking difference in prognosis. J Neurosurg **79**:528-532, 1993.

778 Yassini PR, Sauter K, Schochet SS, Kaufman HH, Bloomfield SM: Localized hypertrophic mononeuropathy involving spinal roots and associated with sacral meningocele. Case report. J Neurosurg **79**:774-778, 1993.

Lymphoproliferative and myeloproliferative disorders

779 Anders KH, Latta H, Chang BS, Tomiyasu U, Quddusi AS, Vinters HV: Lymphomatoid granulomatosis and malignant lymphoma of the central nervous system in the acquired immunodeficiency syndrome. Hum Pathol **20**:326-334, 1989.

780 Baumgartner JE, Rachlin JR, Beckstead JH, Meeker TC, Levy RM, Wara WM, Rosenblum ML: Primary central nervous system lymphomas. Natural history and response to radiation therapy in 55 patients with acquired immunodeficiency syndrome. J Neurosurg **73**:206-211, 1990.

781 Bodensteiner DC, Skikne B: Central nervous system involvement in mycosis fungoides. Diagnosis, treatment and literature review. Cancer **50**:1181-1184, 1982.

782 Bojsen-Møller M, Nielsen JL: CNS involvement in leukaemia. An autopsy study of 100 consecutive patients. Acta Pathol Microbiol Scand (A) **91**:209-216, 1983.

783 Bonnin JM, Garcia JH: Primary malignant non-Hodgkin's lymphoma of the central nervous system. Pathol Annu **22**(Pt1):353-375, 1987.

784 Clark WC, Callihan T, Schwartzberg L, Fontanesi J: Primary intracranial Hodgkin's lymphoma without dural attachment. Case report. J Neurosurg **76**:692-695, 1992.

785 Cohen M, Lanska D, Roessmann U, Karaman B, Ganz E, Whitehouse P, Gambetti P: Amyloidoma of the CNS. I. Clinical and pathologic study. Neurology **42**:2019-2023, 1992.

786 DeAngelis LM, Wong E, Rosenblum M, Furneaux H: Epstein-Barr virus in acquired immune deficiency syndrome (AIDS) and non-AIDS primary central nervous system lymphoma. Cancer **70**:1607-1611, 1992.

787 De Klippel N, Dehou MF, Bourgain C, Schots R, De Keyser J, Ebinger G: Progressive paraparesis due to thoracic extramedullary hematopoiesis in myelofibrosis. Case report. J Neurosurg **79**:125-127, 1993.

788 Demetrick DJ, Hamilton MG, Curry B, Tranmer BI: Epstein-Barr virus-associated primary lymphoproliferative disorder of the cerebellum in an immune competent man. Cancer **70**:519-528, 1992.

789 Demirer T, Dail DH, Aboulafia DM: Four varied cases of intravascular lymphomatosis and a literature review. Cancer **73**:1738-1745, 1994.

790 Dozic S, Suvakovic V, Cvetkovic D, Jevtovic DJ, Skender M: Neoplastic angioendotheliomatosis (NAE) of the CNS in a patient with AIDS subacute encephalitis, diffuse leukoencephalopathy and meningo-cerebral cryptococcosis. Clin Neuropathol **9**:284-289, 1990.

791 Dubas F, Saint-Andre JP, Pouplard-Barthelaix A, Delestre F, Emile J: Intravascular malignant lymphomatosis (so-called malignant angioendotheliomatosis)—a case confined to the lumbosacral spinal cord and nerve roots. Clin Neuropathol **9**:115-120, 1990.

792 Eby NL, Grufferman S, Flannelly CM, Schold SC Jr, Vogel FS, Burger PC: Increasing incidence of primary brain lymphoma in the US. Cancer **62**:2461-2465, 1988.

793 Edgar R, Dutcher TF: Histopathology of the Bing-Neel syndrome. Neurology **11**:239-245, 1961.

794 Ferry JA, Harris NL, Picker LJ, Weinberg DS, Rosales RK, Tapia J, Richardson EP Jr.: Intravascular lymphomatosis (malignant angioendotheliomatosis)—a B-cell neoplasm expressing surface homing receptors. Mod Pathol **1**:444-452, 1988.

795 Geppert M, Ostertag CB, Seitz G, Kiessling M: Glucocorticoid therapy obscures the diagnosis of cerebral lymphoma. Acta Neuropathol **80**:629-634, 1990.

796 Glass J, Gruber ML, Cher L, Hochberg FH: Preirradiation methotrexate chemotherapy of primary central nervous system lymphoma. Long-term outcome. J Neurosurg **81**:188-195, 1994.

797 Grant JW, Kaech D, Jones DB: Spinal cord compression as the first presentation of lymphoma. A review of 15 cases. Histopathology **10**:1191-1202, 1986.

798 Grove A, Vyberg M: Primary leptomeningeal T-cell lymphoma. A case and review of primary T-cell lymphoma of the central nervous system. Clin Neuropathol **12**:7-12, 1993.

799 Haddad P, Thaell JF, Kiely JM, Harrison EG, Miller RH: Lymphoma of the spinal extradural space. Cancer **38**:1862-1866, 1976.

800 Hamilton MG, Demetrick DJ, Tranmer BI, Curry B: Isolated cerebellar lymphomatoid granulomatosis progressing to malignant lymphoma. Case report. J Neurosurg **80**:314-320, 1994.

801 Herman TS, Hammond N, Jones SE, Butler JJ, Byrne GE Jr, McKelvey EM: Involvement of the central nervous system by non-Hodgkin's lymphoma. The Southwest Oncology Group Experience. Cancer 43:390-397, 1979.

802 Hochberg FH, Miller DC: Primary central nervous system lymphoma. J Neurosurg 68:835-853, 1988.

803 Kumanishi T, Washiyama K, Nishiyama A, Abe S, Saito T, Ichikawa T: Primary malignant lymphoma of the brain. Demonstration of immunoglobulin gene rearrangements in four cases by the Southern blot hybridization technique. Acta Neuropathol 79:23-26, 1989.

804 Kuroda Y, Kawasaki T, Haraoka S, Fujiyama F, Kakigi R, Abe M, Tabuchi K, Kuroiwa T, Kishikawa T, Sugihara H: Autopsy report of primary CNS B-cell lymphoma indistinguishable from multiple sclerosis. Diagnosis with the immunoglobulin gene rearrangements analysis. J Neurol Sci 111:173-179, 1992.

805 Lachance DH, O'Neill BP, Macdonald DR, Jaeckle KA, Witzig TE, Li C-Y, Posner JB: Primary leptomeningeal lymphoma. Report of 9 cases, diagnosis with immunocytochemical analysis, and review of the literature. Neurology 41:95-100, 1991.

806 Landolfi R, Colosimo C Jr, De Candia E, Castellana MA, De Cristofaro R, Trodella L, Leone G: Meningeal hematopoiesis causing exophthalmus and hemiparesis in myelofibrosis. A case report. Cancer 62:2346-2349, 1988.

807 Mancardi GL, Mandybur TI: Solitary intracranial plasmacytoma. Cancer 51:2226-2233, 1983.

808 McCarthy J, Proctor SJ: Cerebral involvement in multiple myeloma. Case report. J Clin Pathol 31:259-264, 1978.

809 McCue MP, Sandrock AW, Lee JM, Harris NL, Hedley-Whyte ET: Primary T-cell lymphoma of the brainstem. Neurology 43:377-381, 1993.

810 Morgello S, Petito CK, Mouradian JA: Central nervous system lymphoma in the acquired immune deficiency syndrome. Clin Neuropathol 9:205-215, 1990.

811 Nakleh RE, Manivel JC, Hurd D, Sung JH: Central nervous system lymphomas—immunohistochemical and clinicopathologic study of 26 autopsy cases. Arch Pathol Lab Med 113:1050-1056, 1989.

811a Novak JA, Katzin WE: Primary central nervous system T-cell lymphoma with a predominant CD8 immunophenotype. Cancer 75:2180-2185, 1995.

812 O'Brien TJ, McKelvie PA, Vrodos N: Bilateral trigeminal amyloidoma. An unusual case of trigeminal neuropathy with a review of the literature. Case report. J Neurosurg 81:780-783, 1994.

813 Pappas CTE, Johnson PC, Sonntag VKH: Signet-ring cell lymphoma of the central nervous system. Case report. J Neurosurg 69:789-792, 1988.

814 Paulus W, Ott MM, Strik H, Keil V, Müller-Hermelink HK: Large cell anaplastic (Ki-1) brain lymphoma of T-cell genotype. Hum Pathol 25:1253-1256, 1994.

815 Peterson K, Gordon KB, Heinemann M-H, DeAngelis LM: The clinical spectrum of ocular lymphoma. Cancer 72:843-849, 1993.

816 Rouah E, Rogers BB, Wilson DR, Kirkpatrick JB, Buffone GJ: Demonstration of Epstein-Barr virus in primary central nervous system lymphomas by the polymerase chain reaction and in situ hybridization. Hum Pathol 21:545-550, 1990.

817 Sapozink MD, Kaplan HS: Intracranial Hodgkin's disease. A report of 12 cases and review of the literature. Cancer 52:1301-1307, 1983.

818 Schwechheimer K, Braus DF, Schwarzkopf G, Feller AC, Volk B, Müller-Hermelink HK: Polymorphous high-grade B cell lymphoma is the predominant type of spontaneous primary cerebral malignant lymphomas. Histological and immunomorphological evaluation of computed tomography-guided stereotactic brain biopsies. Am J Surg Pathol 18:931-937, 1994.

819 Severson GS, Harrington DS, Weisenburger DD, McComb RD, Casey JH, Gelber BR, Varet B, Abelanet R, Rappaport HH: Castleman's disease of the leptomeninges. Report of three cases. J Neurosurg 69:283-286, 1988.

820 Simpson TA, Anderson ML, Garcia JH, Barton JC: Myeloblastoma of the brain. Acta Neuropathol 78:444-447, 1989.

821 Slager UT, Taylor WF, Opfell RW, Myers A: Leptomeningeal myeloma. Arch Pathol Lab Med 103:680-682, 1979.

822 Slowik F, Mayer A, Afra D, Deak G, Havel J: Primary spinal intramedullary lymphoma. A case report. Surg Neurol 33:132-138, 1990.

823 Taylor CR, Russell R, Lukes RJ, Davis RL: An immunohistological study of immunoglobulin content of primary central nervous system lymphomas. Cancer 41:2197-2205, 1978.

824 Vidal RG, Ghiso J, Gallo G, Cohen M, Gambetti P-L, Frangione B: Amyloidoma of the CNS. II. Immunohistochemical and biochemical study. Neurology 42:2024-2028, 1992.

825 Voessing R, Berthold F, Richard K-E, Thun F, Schroeder R, Krueger GRF: Primary myeloblastoma of the pineal region. Clin Neuropathol 11:11-15, 1992.

826 Wisniewski T, Sisti M, Inhirami G, Knowles DM, Powers JM: Intracerebral solitary plasmacytoma. Neurosurgery 27:826-829, 1990.

Germ cell tumors

827 Afshar F, King TT, Berry CL: Intraventricular fetus-in-fetu. Case report. J Neurosurg 56:845-849, 1982.

828 Aguzzi A, Hedinger CE, Kleihues P, Yasargil MG: Intracranial mixed germ cell tumor with syncytiotrophoblastic giant cells and precocious puberty. Acta Neuropathol 75:427-431, 1988.

829 Arens R, Marcus D, Engelberg S, Findler G, Goodman RM, Passwell JH: Cerebral germinomas and Klinefelter syndrome. A review. Cancer 61:1228-1231, 1988.

830 Aydin F, Ghatak NR, Radie-Keane K, Kinard J, Land SD: The short-term effect of low-dose radiation on intracranial germinoma—a pathologic study. Cancer 69:2322-2326, 1992.

831 Bamberg M, Metz K, Alberti W, Heckemann R, Schulz U: Endodermal sinus tumor of the pineal region—metastasis through a ventriculoperitoneal shunt. Cancer 54:903-906, 1984.

832 Bjornsson J, Scheithauer BW, Leech RW: Primary intracranial choriocarcinoma. A case report. Clin Neuropathol 5:242-245, 1986.

833 Bjornsson J, Scheithauer BW, Okazaki H, Leech RW: Intracranial germ cell tumors. Pathobiological and immunohistochemical aspects of 70 cases. J Neuropathol Exp Neurol 44:32-46, 1985.

834 Freilich RJ, Thompson SJ, Walker RW, Rosenblum MK: Adenocarcinomatous transformation of intracranial germ cell tumors. Am J Surg Pathol 19:537-544, 1995.

835 Gay JC, Janco RL, Lukens JN: Systemic metastases in primary intracranial germinoma. Case report and literature review. Cancer 55:2688-2690, 1985.

836 Hisa S, Morinaga S, Kobayashi Y, Ojima M, Chikaoka H, Sasano N: Intramedullary spinal cord germinoma producing HCG and precocious puberty in a boy. Cancer 55:2845-2849, 1985.

837 Ho DM, Liu H-C: Primary intracranial germ cell tumor—pathologic study of 51 patients. Cancer 70:1577-1584, 1992.

838 Jennings MT, Gelman R, Hochberg F: Intracranial germ cell tumors. Natural history and pathogenesis. J Neurosurg 63:155-167, 1985.

839 Koeleveld RF, Cohen AR: Primary embryonal cell carcinoma of the parietal lobe. J Neurosurg 75:468-471, 1991.

840 Kraichoke S, Cosgrove M, Chandrasoma PT: Granulomatous inflammation in pineal germinoma—a cause of diagnostic failure at stereotaxic brain biopsy. Am J Surg Pathol 12:655-660, 1988.

841 Laidler P, Pounder DJ: Pineal germinoma with syncytiotrophoblastic giant cells. A case with panhypopituitarism and isosexual pseudopuberty. Hum Pathol 15:285-287, 1984.

842 Masuzawa T, Shimabukuro H, Nakahara N, Iwasa H, Sato F: Germ cell tumors (germinoma and yolk sac tumor) in unusual sites in the brain. Clin Neuropathol 5:190-202, 1986.

843 Oi S, Tamaki N, Kondo T, Nakamura H, Kudo H, Suzuki H, Sasaki M, Matsumoto S, Ueda Y, Katayama K, Mochizuki M: Massive congenital intracranial teratoma diagnosed in utero. Childs Nerv Syst 6:459-461, 1990.

844 Packer RJ, Sutton LN, Rorke LB, Rosenstock JG, Zimmerman RA, Littman P, Bilaniuk LT, Bruce DA, Schut L: Intracranial embryonal cell carcinoma. Cancer 54:520-524, 1984.

845 Page R, Doshi B, Sharr MM: Primary intracranial choriocarcinoma. J Neurol Neurosurg Psychiatry 49:93-95, 1986.

846 Pickens JM, Wilson J, Myers GG, Grunnet ML: Teratoma of the spinal cord. Report of a case and review of the literature. Arch Pathol 99:446-448, 1975.

847 Preissig SH, Smith MT, Huntington HW: Rhabdomyosarcoma arising in a pineal teratoma. Cancer 44:281-284, 1979.

848 Rueda-Pedraza ME, Heigetz SA, Sesterhan IA, Clark GB: Primary intracranial germ cell tumors in the first two decades of life. A clinical, light-microscopic and immunohistochemical analysis of 54 cases. Perspect Pediatr Pathol 10:160-207, 1987.

849 Tamaki N, Lin T, Shirataki K, Hosada K, Kurata H, Matsumoto S, Ito H: Germ cell tumors of the thalamus and basal ganglia. Childs Nerv Syst 6:3-7, 1990.

849a ten Cate LN, Vermeij-Keers C, Smit DA, Cohen-Overbeek TE, Gerssen-Schoorl BJG, Dijkhuizen T: Intracranial teratoma with multiple fetuses. Pre- and post-natal appearance. Hum Pathol 26:804-807, 1995.

850 Uematsu T, Tsuura Y, Miyamoto K, Itakura T, Hayashi S, Komai N: The recurrence of primary intracranial germinomas. Special reference to germinoma with syncytiotrophoblastic giant cells. J Neurooncol **13**:247-256, 1992.

Melanocytic tumors

851 Adamek D, Kaluza J, Stachura K: Primary balloon cell malignant melanoma of the right temporo-parietal region arising from meningeal naevus. Clin Neuropathol **14**:29-32, 1995.

852 Balmaceda CM, Fetell MR, Powers J, O'Brien JL, Housepian EH: Nevus of Ota and leptomeningeal melanocytic lesions. Neurology **43**:381-386, 1993.

853 Bamborschke S, Ebhardt G, Szelies-Stock B, Dreesbach HA, Heiss WD: Review and case report. Primary melanoblastosis of the leptomeninges. Clin Neuropathol **4**:47-55, 1985.

854 Haddad FS, Jamali AF, Rebeiz JJ, Fahl M, Haddad GF: Primary malignant melanoma of the gasserian ganglion associated with neurofibromatosis. Surg Neurol **35**:310-316, 1991.

855 Kadonaga JN, Frieden IJ: Neurocutaneous melanosis. Definition and review of the literature. J Am Acad Dermatol **24**:747-755, 1991.

856 Lach B, Russell N, Benoit B, Atack D: Cellular blue nevus ("melanocytoma") of the spinal meninges. Electron microscopic and immunohistochemical features. Neurosurgery **22**:773-780, 1988.

857 Larson III TC, Houser OW, Onofrio BM, Piepgras DG: Primary spinal melanoma. J Neurosurg **66**:47-49, 1987.

858 Limas C, Tio FO: Meningeal melanocytoma ("melanotic meningioma"). Its melanocytic origin as revealed by electron microscopy. Cancer **30**:1286-1294, 1972.

858a O'Brien TF, Moran M, Miller JH, Hensley SD: Meningeal melanocytoma. An uncommon diagnostic pitfall in surgical neuropathology. Arch Pathol Lab Med **119**:542-546, 1995.

859 Özden B, Barlas O, Hacihanefioglu U: Primary dural melanomas. Report of two cases and review of the literature. Neurosurgery **15**:104-107, 1984.

860 Reyes-Mugica M, Chou P, Byrd S, Ray V, Castelli M, Gattuso P, Gonzalez-Crussi F: Nevomelanocytic proliferations in the central nervous system of children. Cancer **72**:2277-2285, 1993.

861 Rodriguez y Baena R, Gaetani P, Danova M, Bosi F, Zappoli F: Primary solitary intracranial melanoma. Case report and review of the literature. Surg Neurol **38**:26-37, 1992.

862 Russell DS, Rubinstein LJ: Pathology of tumours of the nervous system, ed 5. Baltimore, 1989, Williams & Wilkins, pp 792-797.

863 Theunissen P, Spincemaille G, Pannebakker M, Lambers J: Meningeal melanoma associated with nevus of Ota. Case report and review. Clin Neuropathol **12**:125-129, 1993.

864 Uematsu Y, Yukawa S, Yokote H, Itakura T, Hayashi S, Komai N: Meningeal melanocytoma. Magnetic resonance imaging characteristics and pathological features. Case report. J Neurosurg **76**:705-709, 1992.

865 Winston KR, Sotrel A, Schnitt S: Meningeal melanocytoma. Case report and review of the clinical and histological features. J Neurosurg **66**:50-57, 1987.

Paraganglioma

866 Caccamo DV, Ho K-L, Garcia JH: Cauda equina tumor with ependymal and paraganglionic differentiation. Hum Pathol **23**:835-838, 1992.

867 Gaffney EF, Doorly T, Dinn JJ: Aggressive oncocytic neuroendocrine tumour ("oncocytic paraganglioma") of the cauda equina. Histopathology **10**:311-319, 1986.

868 Hirose T, Sano T, Mori K, Kagawa N, Sakaki A, Kuwamura Y, Hizawa K: Paraganglioma of the cauda equina. An ultrastructural and immunohistochemical study of two cases. Ultrastruct Pathol **12**:235-243, 1988.

869 Pigott TJD, Lowe JS, Morrell K, Kerslake RW: Paraganglioma of the cauda equina—report of three cases. J Neurosurg **73**:455-458, 1990.

870 Sonneland PRL, Scheithauer BW, LeChago J, Crawford BG, Onofrio BM: Paraganglioma of the cauda equina region. Clinicopathologic study of 31 cases with special reference to immunocytology and ultrastructure. Cancer **58**:1720-1735, 1986.

871 Toyota B, Barr HWK, Ramsay D: Hemodynamic activity associated with a paraganglioma of the cauda equina. Case report. J Neurosurg **79**:451-455, 1993.

Chordoma

872 Commins D, Baran GA, Molleston M, Vollmer D: Hypothalamic chordoma. Case report. J Neurosurg **81**:130-132, 1994.

873 Katayama Y, Tsubokawa T, Hirasawa T, Takahata T, Nemoto N: Intradural extraosseous chordoma in the foramen magnum region. Case report. J Neurosurg **75**:976-979, 1991.

874 Tomlinson FH, Scheithauer BW, Miller GM, Onofrio BM: Extraosseous spinal chordoma. Case report. J Neurosurg **75**:980-984, 1991.

875 Warnick RE, Raisanen J, Kaczmar Jr T, Davis RL, Prados MD: Intradural chordoma of the tentorium cerebelli. Case report. J Neurosurg **74**:508-511, 1991.

876 Wolfe III JT, Scheithauer BW: "Intradural chordoma" or "giant ecchordosis physaliphora"? Report of two cases. Clin Neuropathol **6**:98-103, 1987.

Hemangioblastoma (von Hippel–Lindau disease)

877 Becker I, Paulus W, Roggendorf W: Histogenesis of stromal cells in cerebellar hemangioblastomas. An immunohistochemical study. Am J Pathol **134**:271-275, 1989.

878 de la Monte SM, Horowitz SA: Hemangioblastomas. Clinical and histopathological factors correlated with recurrence. Neurosurgery **25**:695-698, 1989.

879 Faiss J, Wild G, Schroth G, Heiss E, Melms A: Multiple supratentorial hemangioblastomas following primary infratentorial manifestation. Clin Neuropathol **10**:21-25, 1991.

880 Feldenzer JA, McKeever PE: Selective localization of g-enolase in stromal cells of cerebellar hemangioblastoma. Acta Neuropathol **72**:281-285, 1987.

881 Frank TS, Trojanowski JQ, Roberts SA, Brooks JJ: A detailed immunohistochemical analysis of cerebellar hemangioblastoma. An undifferentiated mesenchymal tumor. Mod Pathol **2**:638-651, 1989.

882 Gaffey MJ, Mills SE, Boyd JC: Aggressive papillary tumor of middle ear/temporal bone and adnexal papillary cystadenoma. Manifestations of von Hippel–Lindau disease. Am J Surg Pathol **18**:1254-1260, 1994.

883 Horton JC, Harsh GR, Fisher JW, Hoyt WF: von Hoppel–Lindau disease and erythrocytosis. Radioimmunoassay of erythropoietin in cyst fluid from a brainstem hemangioblastoma. Neurology **41**:753-754, 1991.

884 Hufnagel TJ, Kim JH, True LD, Manuelidis EE: Immunohistochemistry of capillary hemangioblastoma. Immunoperoxidase-labeled antibody staining resolves the differential diagnosis with metastatic renal cell carcinoma, but does not explain the histogenesis of the capillary hemangioblastoma. Am J Surg Pathol **13**:207-216, 1989.

885 Ishwar S, Taniguiche RM, Vogel FS: Multiple supratentorial hemangioblastomas. Case study and ultrastructural characteristics. J Neurosurg **35**:396-405, 1971.

886 Ismail SM, Jasani B, Cole G: Histogenesis of hemangioblastomas. An immunocytochemical and ultrastructural study in a case of von Hippel–Lindau syndrome. J Clin Pathol **38**:417-421, 1985.

887 Kanno H, Kondo K, Ito S, Yamamoto I, Fujii S, Torigoe S, Sakai N, Hosaka M, Shuin T, Yao M: Somatic mutations of the von Hippel–Lindau tumor suppressor gene in sporadic central nervous system hemangioblastomas. Cancer Res **54**:4845-4847, 1994.

888 Lamiell JM, Salazar FG, Hsia YE: von Hippel–Lindau disease affecting 43 members of a single kindred. Medicine **68**:1-29, 1989.

889 Medvedev YA, Matsko DE, Zubkov YN, Pak VA, Alexander LF: Coexistent hemangioblastoma and arteriovenous malformation of the cerebellum. J Neurosurg **75**:121-125, 1991.

890 Mohan J, Brownell B, Oppenheimer DR: Malignant spread of hemangioblastoma. Report on two cases. J Neurol Neurosurg Psychiatry **39**:515-525, 1976.

891 Nemes Z: Fibrohistiocytic differentiation in capillary hemangioblastoma. Hum Pathol **23**:805-810, 1992.

892 Neumann HPH, Eggert HR, Weigel K, Friedburg H, Wiestler OD, Schollmeyer P: Hemangioblastomas of the central nervous system. J Neurosurg **70**:24-30, 1989.

892a Richmond BK, Schmidt III JH: Congenital cystic supratentorial hemangioblastoma. Case report. J Neurosurg **82**:113-115, 1995.

893 Rubio A, Meyers SP, Powers JM, Nelson CN, de Papp EW: Hemangioblastoma of the optic nerve. Hum Pathol **25**:1249-1251, 1994.

894 Russell DS, Rubinstein LJ: Pathology of tumours of the nervous system, ed 5. Baltimore, 1989, Williams & Wilkins, pp 639-657.

895 Tachibana O, Yamashima T, Yamashita J: Immunohistochemical study of erythropoietin in cerebellar hemangioblastomas associated with secondary polycythemia. Neurosurgery **28**:24-26, 1991.

Rhabdoid and atypical teratoid tumors

896 Biegel JA, Rorke LB, Packer RJ, Emanuel BS: Monosomy 22 in rhabdoid or atypical tumors of the brain. J Neurosurg **73**:710-714, 1990.

897 Biggs PJ, Garen PD, Powers JM, Garvin AJ: Malignant rhabdoid tumor of the central nervous system. Hum Pathol **18**:332-337, 1987.

898 Chou SM, Anderson JS: Primary CNS malignant rhabdoid tumor (MRT). Report of two cases and review of the literature. Clin Neuropathol **10:**1-10, 1991.

899 de Chadarévian J-P, Russo P: Central nervous system-renal neoplasia. A puzzling emerging association in young children (abstract). Lab Invest **50:**2, 1984.

900 Horn M, Schlote W, Lerch KD, Steudel WI, Harms D, Thomas E: Malignant rhabdoid tumor. Primary intracranial manifestation in an adult. Acta Neuropathol **83:**445-448, 1992.

900a Olson TA, Bayar E, Kosnik E, Hamoudi AB, Klopfenstein KJ, Pieters RS, Ruymann FB: Successful treatment of disseminated central nervous system malignant rhabdoid tumor. J Pediatr Hematol Oncol **17:**71-75, 1995.

901 Weeks DA, Malott RL, Zuppan CW, Liwnicz BH, Beckwith JB: Primitive cerebral tumor with rhabdoid features. A case of phenotypic rhabdoid tumor of the central nervous system. Ultrastruct Pathol **18:**23-28, 1994.

Other primary tumors

902 Kepes JJ, O'Boynick P, Jones S, Baum D, McMillan J, Adams ME: Adrenal cortical adenoma in the spinal canal of an 8-year old girl. Am J Surg Pathol **14:**481-484, 1990.

903 Kleinschmidt-DeMasters BK, Winston KR, Rubinstein D, Samuels MH: Ectopic pituitary adenoma of the third ventricle. Case report. J Neurosurg **72:**139-142, 1990.

904 Lindboe CF, Unsgard G, Myhr G, Scott H: ACTH and TSH producing ectopic suprasellar pituitary adenoma of the hypothalamic region. Case report. Clin Neuropathol **12:**138-141, 1993.

905 Ruchti C, Balli-Antunes M, Gerber HA: Follicular tumor in the sellar region without primary cancer of the thyroid. Heterotopic carcinoma? Am J Clin Pathol **87:**776-780, 1987.

SECONDARY TUMORS

906 Ambiavagar P-C, Sher J: Subdural hematoma secondary to metastatic neoplasm. Report of two cases and a review of the literature. Cancer **42:**2015-2018, 1978.

907 Ariza A, Kim JH: Kaposi's sarcoma of the dura mater. Hum Pathol **19:**1461-1463, 1988.

908 Berry MP, Jenkin RDT: Parameningeal rhabdomyosarcoma in the young. Cancer **48:**281-288, 1981.

909 Bigner SH, Schold SC: The diagnosis of metastases to the central nervous system. Pathol Annu **19**(Pt 2):89-119, 1984.

910 Byrne TN: Spinal cord compression from epidural metastases. N Engl J Med **327:**614-619, 1992.

911 Castaldo JE, Bernat JL, Meier FA, Schned AR: Intracranial metastases due to prostatic carcinoma. Cancer **52:**1739-1747, 1983.

912 Cilluffo JM, Harner SG, Miller RH: Intracranial ceruminous gland adenocarcinoma. J Neurosurg **55:**952-956, 1981.

913 Costigan DA, Winkelman MD: Intramedullary spinal cord metastasis. A clinicopathological study of 13 cases. J Neurosurg **62:**227-233, 1985.

914 Delattre J-Y, Krol G, Thaler HT, Posner JB: Distribution of brain metastases. Arch Neurol **45:**741-744, 1988.

915 Dolan EJ, Schwartz ML, Lewis AJ, Kassel EE, Cooper PW: Adenoid cystic carcinoma. An unusual neurosurgical entity. Can J Neurol Sci **12:**65-68, 1985.

916 Feigin I, Budzilovich GN: Sarcoma arising in metastatic carcinoma in the brain. A second instance. Cancer **54:**2047-2050, 1984.

917 Floeter MK, So YT, Ross DA, Greenberg D: Miliary metastasis to the brain. Clinical and radiologic features. Neurology **37:**1817-1818, 1987.

918 Kokkoris CP: Leptomeningeal carcinomatosis. How does cancer reach the piaarachnoid? Cancer **51:**154-160, 1983.

919 Le Chevalier T, Smith FP, Caille P, Constans JP, Rouesse JG: Sites of primary malignancies in patients presenting with cerebral metastases. A review of 120 cases. Cancer **56:**880-882, 1985.

920 LeRoux PD, Berger MS, Elliott JP, Tamimi HK: Cerebral metastases from ovarian carcinoma. Cancer **67:**2194-2199, 1991.

921 Lewis AJ: Sarcoma metastatic to the brain. Cancer **61:**593-601, 1988.

922 Mrak RE: Origins of adenocarcinomas presenting as intracranial metastases. An ultrastructural study. Arch Pathol Lab Med **117:**1165-1169, 1993.

923 O'Neill BP, Dinapoli RP, Okazaki H: Cerebral infarction as a result of tumor emboli. Cancer **60:**90-95, 1987.

924 Patchell RA, Tibbs PA, Walsh JW, Dempsey RJ, Maruyama Y, Kryscio RJ, Markesberry WR, MacDonald JS, Young B: A randomized trial of surgery in the treatment of single metastases in the brain. N Engl J Med **322:**494-500, 1990.

925 Perry JR, Bilbao JM: Metastatic alveolar soft part sarcoma presenting as a dural-based cerebral mass. Neurosurgery **34:**168-170, 1994.

926 Piepmeier JM, Virapongse C, Kier EL, Kim J, Greenberg A: Intracranial adenocystic carcinoma presenting as a primary brain tumor. Neurosurgery **12:**348-352, 1983.

927 Retsas S, Gershuny AR: Central nervous system involvement in malignant melanoma. Cancer **61:**1926-1934, 1988.

928 Russell DS, Rubinstein LJ: Pathology of tumours of the nervous system, ed 5. Baltimore, 1989, Williams & Wilkins, pp 809-854.

929 Scully RE, ed: Case records of the Massachusetts General Hospital, Case 28—1992. N Engl J Med **327:**107-116, 1992.

930 Tsukada Y, Fouad A, Pickren JW, Lane WW: Central nervous system metastasis from breast carcinoma. Autopsy study. Cancer **52:**2349-2354, 1983.

931 Vannier A, Gray F, Gherardi R, Marsault C, Degos JD, Poirier J: Diffuse subependymal periventricular metastases. Report of three cases. Cancer **58:**2720-2725, 1986.

Peripheral Nerves

Juan M. Bilbao, M.D.

NORMAL ANATOMY
BASIC PATHOLOGIC MECHANISMS
NEUROPATHIES
    Inherited neuropathy
    Inflammatory neuropathy
    Leprous neuritis
    Vasculitis
    Amyloidosis
    Neuropathy of dysproteinemia
    Toxic-metabolic neuropathy
    Other neuropathies

The peripheral nervous system may be affected by a variety of multifocal and systemic disorders, and in selected patients, the **biopsy of a peripheral nerve** is a valuable method for the evaluation of peripheral neuropathy. The mere demonstration of peripheral nerve dysfunction is not an indication for nerve biopsy. The latter is more informative in patients in whom a proper clinical history, thorough physical examination, evaluation of kindred (even of patients without a phenotype suggestive of inherited neuropathy), examination of CSF, and electrophysiologic and immunologic studies have failed to determine the cause of nerve disorder. Conditions masquerading as a cryptogenic neuropathy, such as chronic inflammatory neuropathy, amyloidosis, and vasculitis, are occasionally revealed only at biopsy. In many of the metabolic and toxic neuropathies, history and biochemical analysis alone are sufficient to make a diagnosis. Included in these are the neuropathies of chronic alcoholism and malnutrition, porphyria, renal failure, toxic agents and pharmaceuticals, and diabetes mellitus. Some of the inherited metabolic diseases (such as Fabry's disease, Krabbe's disease, and metachromatic leukodystrophy) that produce pathognomonic morphologic and histochemical changes in nerves are now readily identified by biochemical analysis of tissue samples.[1] Furthermore, neuropathies caused by amyloidosis or vasculitis can be diagnosed by biopsy of other tissues (see later discussion).

The diagnostic usefulness of the peripheral nerve biopsy varies considerably. It is important to recognize that in many specimens the histologic changes will be nonspecific, without providing clues as to a definite etiology. Over a 23-year-period (1972 to 1995) 683 consecutive subcutaneous nerve biopsies were performed in adult patients at St. Michael's Hospital, University of Toronto. The sural nerve was selected in 668 patients, a branch of the radial nerve in 9, a branch of the ulnar nerve in 3 and the lateral peroneal nerve in 3. Four additional specimens showed no nerve. A specific diagnosis was made in 28% of cases (Table 28-1). Specimens were either normal or showed minimal change in 12.9% of biopsies. Cases with normal histology included nerve biopsies in patients suspected of having vasculitis but with no clinical evidence of peripheral neuropathy; other patients with symp-toms thought to represent neuropathy were found to have disorders of the spinal cord or muscle. Of the remaining 58.4% of cases the histologic abnormalities, although significant, were considered to be nonspecific (Table 28-2). Many of the patients in the latter group had a distal symmetric neuropathy of the type associated with most nutritional or metabolic-toxic conditions. In these cases, interaction between physician and pathologist is essential in reaching a final diagnosis.[2,3,5]

Removal of a segment of peripheral nerve for diagnostic purposes should result in only a minimal morbidity. Because of the muscular deficit that its resection induces, biopsy of a terminal motor nerve should be reserved for very special cases.[4] The site of biopsy should avoid areas where local trauma to nerve may produce changes or artefacts that may be confused with a polyneuropathy. A distal nerve is favored because in most neuropathies the longest fibers are more often affected. The selected nerve should be accessible to conduction studies and have a constant anatomic course and fascicular composition. The **sural nerve,** a purely sensory subcutaneous nerve, combines all of these requirements and is therefore the most common biopsy site. Alternatively, the saphenous nerve, the superficial peroneal nerve, or a cutaneous branch of the radial nerve at the wrist is sometimes used. The sural nerve (a branch of the tibial nerve) is composed of six to sixteen fascicles. It lies superficial to deep fascia, in the lateral retromalleolar region adjacent to the lesser saphenous vein, between the Achilles tendon and the tendon of the peroneus longus muscle. Although a technique for fascicular biopsy of the sural nerve has been described,

Table 28-1 Specific diagnoses among 683 nerve biopsies*

Diagnosis	No.
Guillain-Barré, CIDP	66
Vasculitis	49
HMSN	25
Leprosy	10
Diabetic neuropathy—angiopathy	10
Amyloid	7
Tomaculous neuropathy	6
Paraprotein neuropathy	6
Granulomatous (non-leprosy)	4
Amiodarone neuropathy	3
Niemann-Pick disease	3
Filamentous axonopathy (disulfiram)	2
Sensory perineuritis	1
Fabry's disease	1
Fungal neuritis	1
Lymphoma	1
Chloroquine neuropathy	1

*196 cases = 28.7% (St. Michael's Hospital).
CIPD, Chronic inflammatory demyelinating polyneuropathy; *HMSN,* hereditary motor and sensory neuropathy.

Table 28-2 Diagnostic sensitivity of sural nerve biopsy (N = 683 cases)

	No. of cases	Percentage
Specific diagnosis	196	28.7
Axonal degeneration	297	43.5
Mixed axonal degeneration—demyelination	59	8.6
Focal chronic inflammation and axonal degeneration	43	6.3
Normal or minimal change	88	12.9

removal of a 5- to 7-cm long segment of the entire nerve is preferable. Four types of preparations should be made for a proper evaluation of a nerve specimen: paraffin embedding after B5 fixation, teased nerve fibers, cryostat sections after "quench" freezing in isopentane-liquid nitrogen, and plastic resin embedding for light and electron microscopy. Because large fibers are greatly susceptible to artefacts, indelicate handling and the use of hyperosmolar fixatives should be avoided. The segment of nerve selected for electron microscopy should be received slightly stretched on a wooden stick and immediately immersed in chilled 2.5% glutaraldehyde in 0.05-M cacodylate buffer at pH 7.4 with an osmolarity of 340 mOs, where it should be left undisturbed for at least 2 hours before trimming. In the paraffin-embedded tissue, we routinely use hematoxylin-eosin–Luxol fast-blue, LCA immunostain, PAS, and Congo red. Of the plastic blocks four contain segments of nerve that comprise the entire cross-sectional area, and four represent fascicles in longitudinal orientation; the remaining blocks include one to three fascicles in transverse section. Examination of plas

tic-embedded (20 to 30 blocks), semithin sections counterstained with toluidine blue is essential in assessing a nerve specimen. Few structural changes will be found by electron microscopy if they were not first appreciated in semithin sections, particularly if viewing was done under oil immersion. Although examination of "teased" nerve fiber preparation may unveil unique morphologic features in some cases, the method is laborious and not cost efficient. We recommend postfixation in osmium tetroxide of a 12-mm segment of nerve, followed by maceration in glycerine for 48 hours before dissection. However gentle, the separation of single nerve fibers from their fascicular bundles with forceps may produce artefacts. An experienced dissector is needed for this time-consuming technique because at least 100 fibers of ten internodes in length (about 1 cm) should be examined to obtain meaningful data.

NORMAL ANATOMY

Three areas can be defined in peripheral nerves[22] (Fig. 28-111). The ***intrafascicular compartment*** contains myelinated and unmyelinated nerve fibers (Fig. 28-112; see also Figs. 28-114, *B*; 28-119, *A*; and 28-143, *A*), Schwann cells, microvessels and venules, fibroblasts, mast cells, macrophages,[14] collagen, oxytalan filaments (Fig. 28-113), and endoneurial fluid. The presence of more than three to four endoneurial cells (per fascicle on cross section) labeled with LCA is an abnormal finding. Endoneurial capillaries differ from their counterpart in muscle in that they invariably have a pericytic complement and that their endothelium is non-fenestrated and displays tight junctions. Like the endothelium of brain, it is impermeable to the transport of protein tracers.[19] An exception is the spinal ganglia, where there is always leakage to most substances. Poorly visualized in

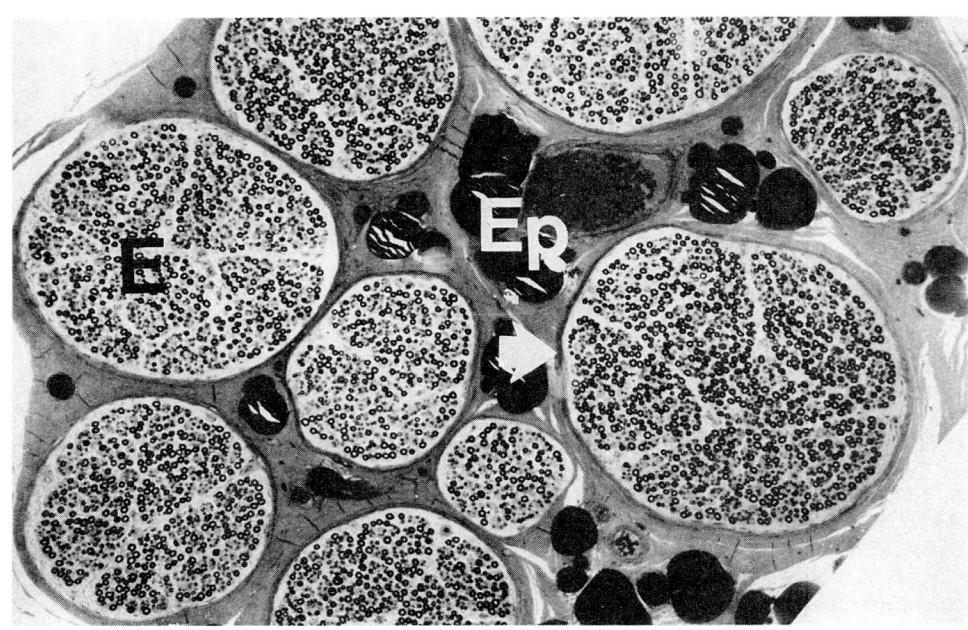

Fig. 28-111 Cross section of normal sural nerve: epineurium *(Ep)*, perineurium *(arrow)*, and endoneurium *(E)*. (Plastic.)

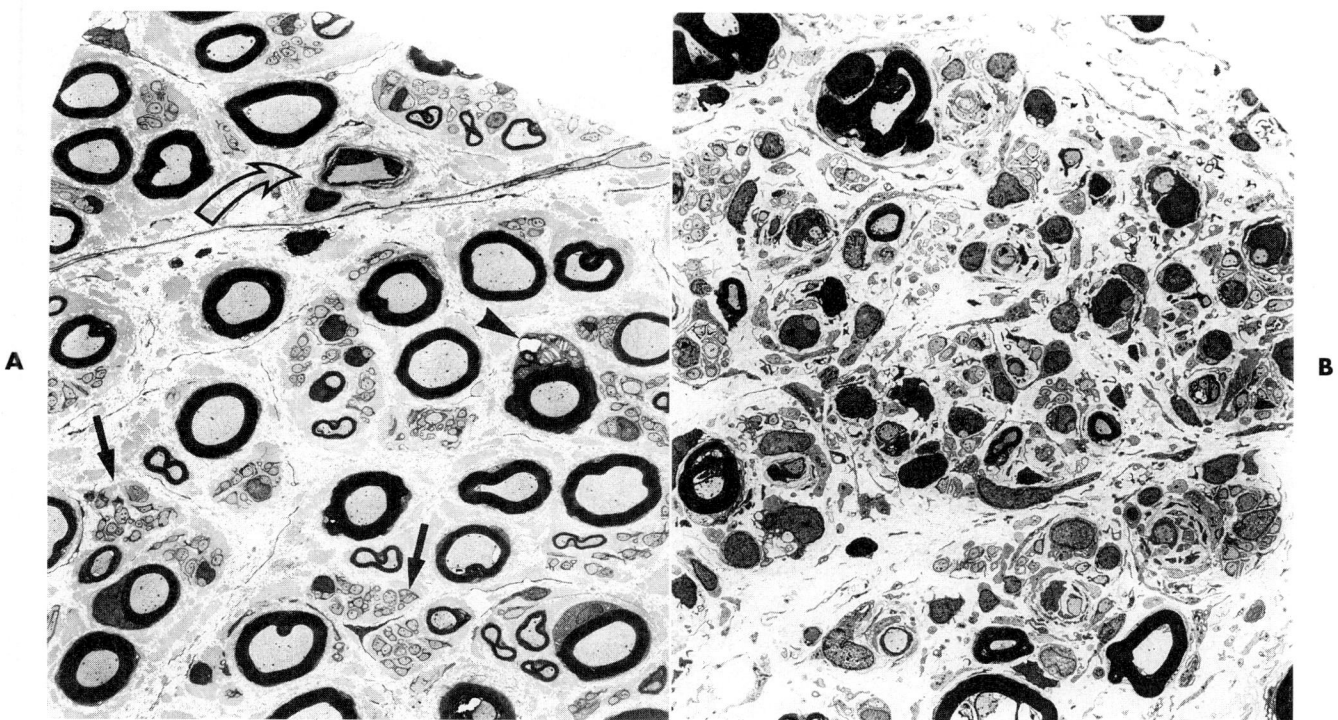

Fig. 28-112 Sural nerve. **A,** Normal. Note the unmyelinated fibers *(arrow),* Reich's pi granule *(arrowhead),* a macrophage, and a mast cell adjacent to microvessel *(open arrow).* (×990.) **B,** Dropout of fibers and hypercellularity in CIDP. (×990.)

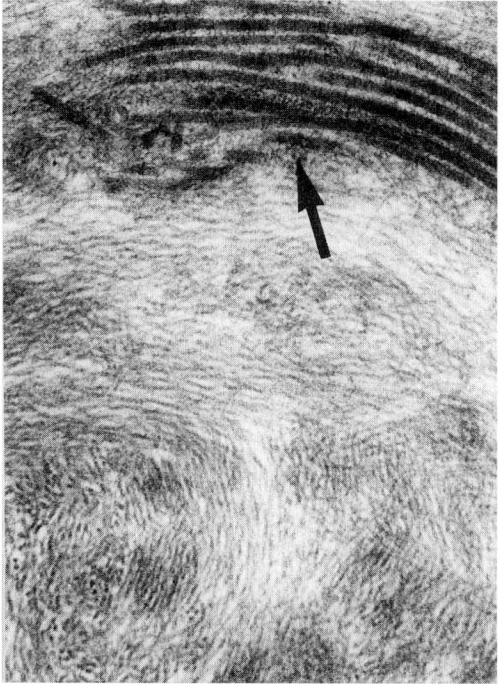

Fig. 28-113 Bundles of oxytalan filaments in endoneurium should not be confused with amyloid deposits. Compare size of oxytalan with collagen *(arrow).* (×21,000.)

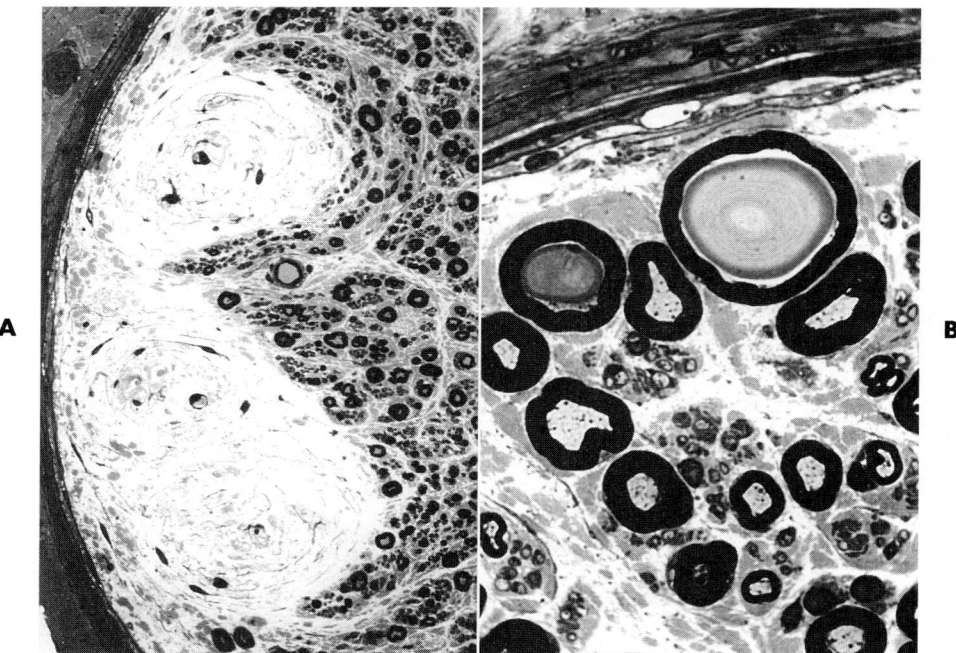

Fig. 28-114 Normal sural nerves. **A,** Renaut body. **B,** Intra-axonal polyglucosan bodies. (Plastic.)

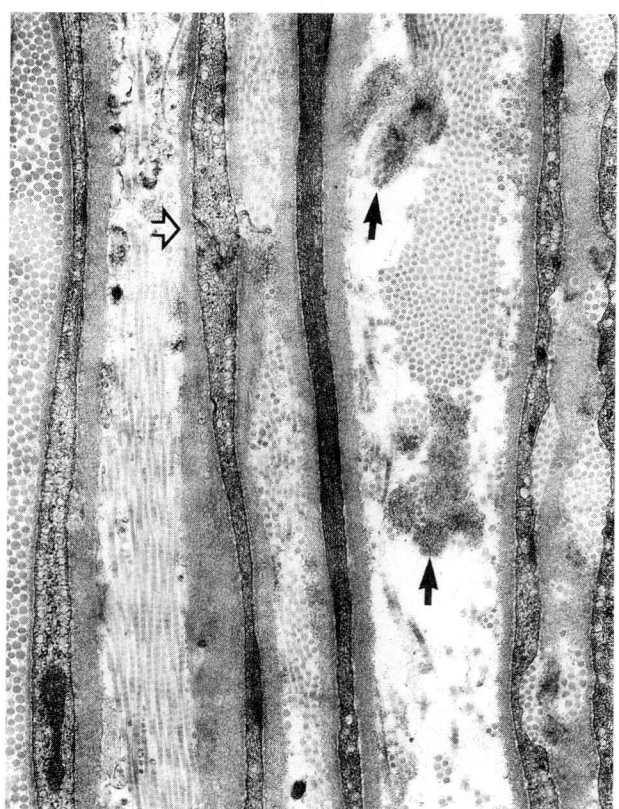

Fig. 28-115 Cross section of perineurium. Perineurial cells are linked by tight junctions *(open arrow)*. Note intervening elaunin *(arrows)* and collagen fibers oriented longitudinally and circumferentially. Cell membrane shows pinocytotic vesicles. (×12,800.)

paraffin sections, ***Renaut bodies*** are enigmatic structures that insinuate into the endoneurium. In semithin sections, they appear as whorled "cushions" adjacent to inner perineurium and are composed of ground substance, randomly oriented fibrils, and fibroblasts with slender processes[7] (Fig.28-114, *A*). In transverse sections, Renaut's bodies may be seen to involve several fascicles; in some they extend for the entire circumference of subperineurium. Ultrastructurally, Renaut bodies contain abundant extracellular filaments of 8 to 14 nm in diameter corresponding in size to the microfibrils described by Haust[15] and to the oxytalan filament of elastic fibers[25] (see Fig. 28-113). Renaut bodies are not seen during fetal life and seem to increase in number during age, particularly near or at entrapment sites, suggesting that chronic trauma may play a role in their pathogenesis.

Each nerve fascicle is ensheathed by the ***perineurium,*** which consists of overlapping layers of flattened cells with interleaved collagen and elastin[21] (Fig. 28-115). Ultrastructurally, the perineurial cell features prominent pinocytotic vesicles, bundles of cytoplasmic filaments, and a continuous basal lamina on the free surface that allows extensive ***zonulae occludentes*** at points of contact between cells,[11] thus conferring on the perineurium the characteristics of a bidirectional diffusion barrier.[19] At the neuromuscular junction, the perineurial sleeve terminates before it reaches the endplate.[11] At this point the perineurium is open ended, and the endoneurium and epineurium are continuous, without an intervening structural barrier. Perineurial cell lineage studies using a recombinant retroviral vector in tissue cultures have elucidated the embryogenesis of this structure. Fibroblasts infected with a recombinant retrovirus (having an *E. coli* Lac z gene that encodes beta-galactosidase) give rise to Lac Z–positive perineurial cells, whereas Schwann cells do

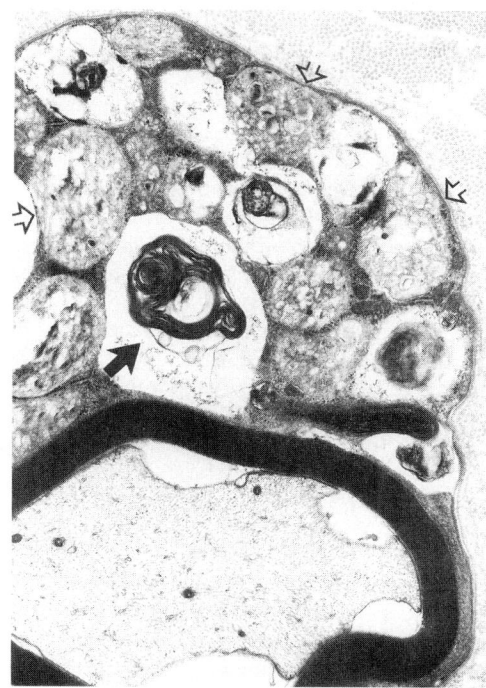

Fig. 28-116 Metachromatic leukodystrophy. Schwann cell cytoplasm is distended with "Tuffstone" bodies *(open arrows)* and a myeloid body *(arrow)*. (×8800.)

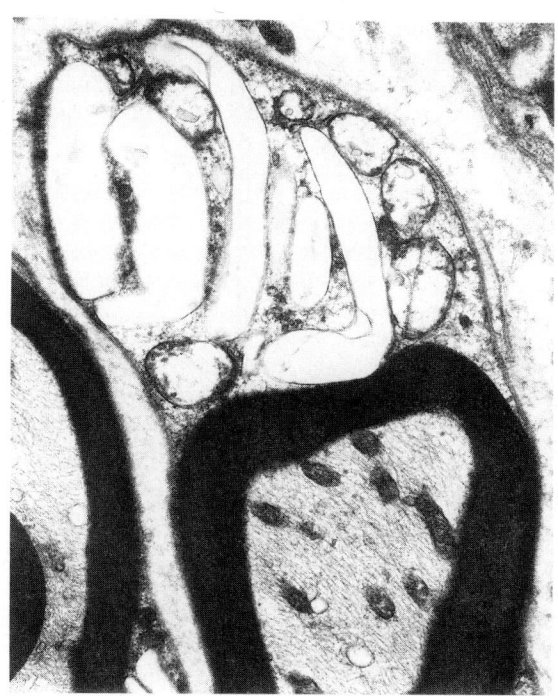

Fig. 28-117 Sural nerve. Farber disease. Typical "banana" bodies in cytoplasm of Schwann cell. (×13,490.)

not.[20] Immunopositivity for epithelial membrane antigen and lack of immunoreaction for S-100 protein are characteristics that distinguish the perineurial cell from the Schwann cell.[6] The *epineurium* is the outermost covering of the peripheral nerves and is composed of loose connective tissue, fat cells, and rare elastic fibers. Nerves are richly vascularized structures. Branches from the nearest limb artery bifurcate into ascending and descending rami that give off vasa nervorum that connect with longitudinal epineurial plexuses. The veins follow a similar course. A lymphatic system in the epineurium has been described.

Schwann cells originate from the neural crest and migrate into the peripheral nervous system to ensheath every myelinated and unmyelinated nerve fiber (see Fig. 28-112, *A*) from the roots to the axonal termination. These cells display a continuous basal lamina,[10,12] and their nucleus lies lengthwise on the nerve fiber. The perinuclear cytoplasm accumulates lysosomal metachromatic lipid inclusions (pi-granule of Reich)[24] and Marchi-positive globules (Elzholz body) during aging, and abnormal deposits in many lipid storage diseases (Figs. 28-116 and 28-117). Lipofuscin is seen in the Schwann cell cytoplasm of unmyelinated fibers. Schwann cells readily proliferate in response to axonal damage and myelin disintegration. They exhibit a passive response to invasion by *Mycobacterium leprae,* with long-term bacterial survival and proliferation (see Fig. 28-135, *B*).

Myelin is a proteophospholipid spiral formed by the invagination of the apposed and compacted Schwann cell membrane. The major protein components of peripheral myelin are protein 0, myelin-associated glycoprotein (anti-

bodies against this protein cause demyelinating neuropathy in some IgM paraproteinemias) (see Fig. 28-141), P1 protein (myelin basic protein), P2 glycoprotein (the major antigen in the production of experimental allergic neuritis), and peripheral myelin protein 22. Compact myelin corresponds to a sequence to two layers of fused Schwann cell membrane without intervening cytoplasm, which during formation is extruded to a paranodal and perinuclear position and to the intramyelinic incisures (or cytoplasmic pockets) of Schmidt-Lanterman.[16] The repetitive structures or periodicity of compact myelin comprises the major dense line (derived from the opposed cytoplasmic aspect of each pair of membranes) and the intraperiod line (formed by the opposed outer surface of each pair of membranes). The thickness of the myelin sheath and internodal length is proportional to axonal diameter. The basic myelinating unit of the peripheral nervous system is the internodal segment, which is delineated by the node of Ranvier, the latter defined as the point of separation of two contiguous Schwann cell territories.

Myelinated nerve fibers vary in outside diameter from 2 to 18 μm (see Fig. 28-112, *A*). Intra-axonal structures analogous to corpora amylacea are incidentally found within myelinated fibers in peripheral nerves of older individuals (see Fig. 28-114, *B*). These polyglucosan bodies are composed partly of glucose polymers and an unidentified protein; they stain strongly with PAS and variably with silver protargol. In a sural nerve biopsy the demonstration of large numbers of polyglucosan bodies is diagnostic of a rare neurodegenerative disease.[13] Nerve fibers of less than 2 μm in diameter are unmyelinated (see Fig. 28-112, *A*) and lie incorporated within a simple invagination of the Schwann cell membrane called mesaxon. The study of pathologic changes in unmyelinated fibers requires silver impregnation and electron microscopy, because they are barely discernible under the light microscope with routine stains. By quantitative morphologic techniques the density of myelinated fibers is calculated to be about 7000 and that of unmyelinated fibers about 30,000 per sural nerve.[8,17] The surface area of endoneurium in the sural nerve is estimated at 0.60 to 1.20 mm[2], excluding Renaut bodies, vessels, and subperineurial space.[9] These measurements have been taken after fixation and dehydration, which produces a shrinkage of the endoneurial area of between 10% and 24%. Age changes in peripheral nerves include a slight dropout of myelinated and unmyelinated fibers. This may explain the common occurrence of mild distal neuropathy in elderly individuals.[18,23]

BASIC PATHOLOGIC MECHANISMS

Peripheral nerve fibers respond to injury in a stereotyped fashion.[26] In *wallerian degeneration,* the cardinal feature is the degeneration of axon and disintegration of myelin that occurs throughout the distal segment of nerve after transection.[31] It usually follows trauma and affects the whole nerve trunk or several fascicles. The degeneration of the distal segment of nerve is absolute,[32] and in the case of motor nerves the muscle undergoes denervation atrophy. The earliest axoplasmic changes are triggered by an increase in axoplasmic calcium concentration and include the accumulation of mitochondria and osmiophilic bodies, followed by disintegration and dissolution of microtubules and neurofilaments (Fig. 28-118, *C*). The myelin breakdown that follows is initiated in the Schwann cell cytoplasm (Fig. 28-118, *D*) and then processed in macrophages, most of which are blood borne.[27] Nerve regeneration from the proximal sement begins almost immediately. Nerve growth factor released by fibroblasts in the extracellular matrix of the distal stump and the expression of nerve growth factor receptors by denervated Schwann cells create a favorable environment for the regrowth of axons.[29,30] If there is proper alignment and approximation of the severed ends, the influx of regenerating axons will reestablish connections through preserved perineurial tubes and columns of Schwann cells (known as bands of Büngner). When the separation is too wide to bridge, a *traumatic neuroma* results from an exuberant and disorganized proliferation of nerve fibers and accompanying Schwann cells and perineurium, which form tangled miniature fascicles embedded in fibrovascular stroma.

Axonal degeneration results either from a metabolic disturbance of the neuron (neuronopathy) leading to a retrograde atrophy and degeneration of the axon ("dying-back" phenomenon),[28] or from a direct injury to the axon (axonopathy).[33] This pattern of degeneration will usually affect large and long fibers early (Fig. 28-118, *A*), but if the metabolic insult is severe, fibers of smaller caliber will also be involved. The myelin sheath breaks down concomitantly with the axon (Fig. 28-118, *A* and *B*). Eventually, columns of empty Schwann cells and basal lamina remain. Nerve conduction velocity in nerves undergoing mild to moderate axonal degeneration is either normal or slightly reduced. Selective depletion of small myelinated and unmyelinated fiber has

been observed in amyloidosis, diabetes, Fabry's disease, Tangier disease, chronic idiopathic anhydrosis, and hereditary sensory and autonomic neuropathies.

Axonal regeneration is slow and variable. It is better appreciated on transverse sections in chronic neuropathies, in which over a background of myelinated fiber loss, "clusters" or "units" of three to seven myelinated fibers of complementary shapes stand out (see Fig. 28-145) These are indicative of sprouting of previously degenerated axons. A small number of regenerating "clusters" are seen in "normal" nerves, particularly in aging.

Primary segmental demyelination is an alteration of the Schwann cell resulting in the destruction of its myelin, with the initial changes observed at the paranodal region at multiple sites in nerve[34] (see Fig. 28-146, *B*). Subsequently, the process extends to the whole internode, leaving the axon denuded and surrounded by myelin debris within Schwann cell processes. In the Guillain-Barré syndrome, a unique mechanism of demyelination is the stripping of myelin off the axon by invading macrophages (see Fig. 28-127, *B*). *Secondary segmental demyelination* is a process of myelin breakdown and remodeling triggered by axonal atrophy; thus it is always encountered over a background of axonal degeneration and is not associated with prominent onion bulb formation. Segmental demyelination can best be demonstrated in teased nerve fiber preparations. In semithin sections, segmental myelin alteration can also be inferred by the loss of myelin about large axons and by disproportionately thin myelin sheaths with respect to axonal diameter. Remyelination from migrating Schwann cells from neighboring areas usually follows. Nerve conduction studies in demyelinating neuropathies typically demonstrate marked slowing.

NEUROPATHIES
Inherited neuropathy

Repeated episodes of primary segmental demyelination and remyelination lead to the formation of "onion bulbs," a term that refers to imbricated layers of supernumerary Schwann cell processes (and intervening collagen) arranged in rings around longitudinally oriented nerve fibers. Onion bulbs, the pathologic hallmark of *hypertrophic neuropathy,* can only be detected in cross sections (Figs. 28-119, *B*, through 28-121). In advanced cases the added accumulation of extracellular matrix and collagen in the endoneurium results in distention of the fascicles caused by expansion of the intrafascicular area, which is easily recognizable on low-power examination. Hypertrophic neuropathy is a prominent feature of several of the genetically determined neuropathies; onion bulbs are also encountered in chronic inflammatory and demyelinating polyneuropathy (see Fig. 28-128, *B* and *C*) and to a lesser extent in diabetic neuropathy.

Dejerine-Sottas disease (hereditary motor-sensory neuropathology type III) appears in childhood and is autosomal-recessive. The clinical features include sensory motor neuropathy, skeletal abnormalities, and markedly enlarged nerves. The CSF protein content is elevated, presumably because spinal roots are involved. A progressive and debilitating clinical course is the rule. Nerve biopsy shows large numbers of onion bulbs, endoneurial fibrosis, loss of axons, and

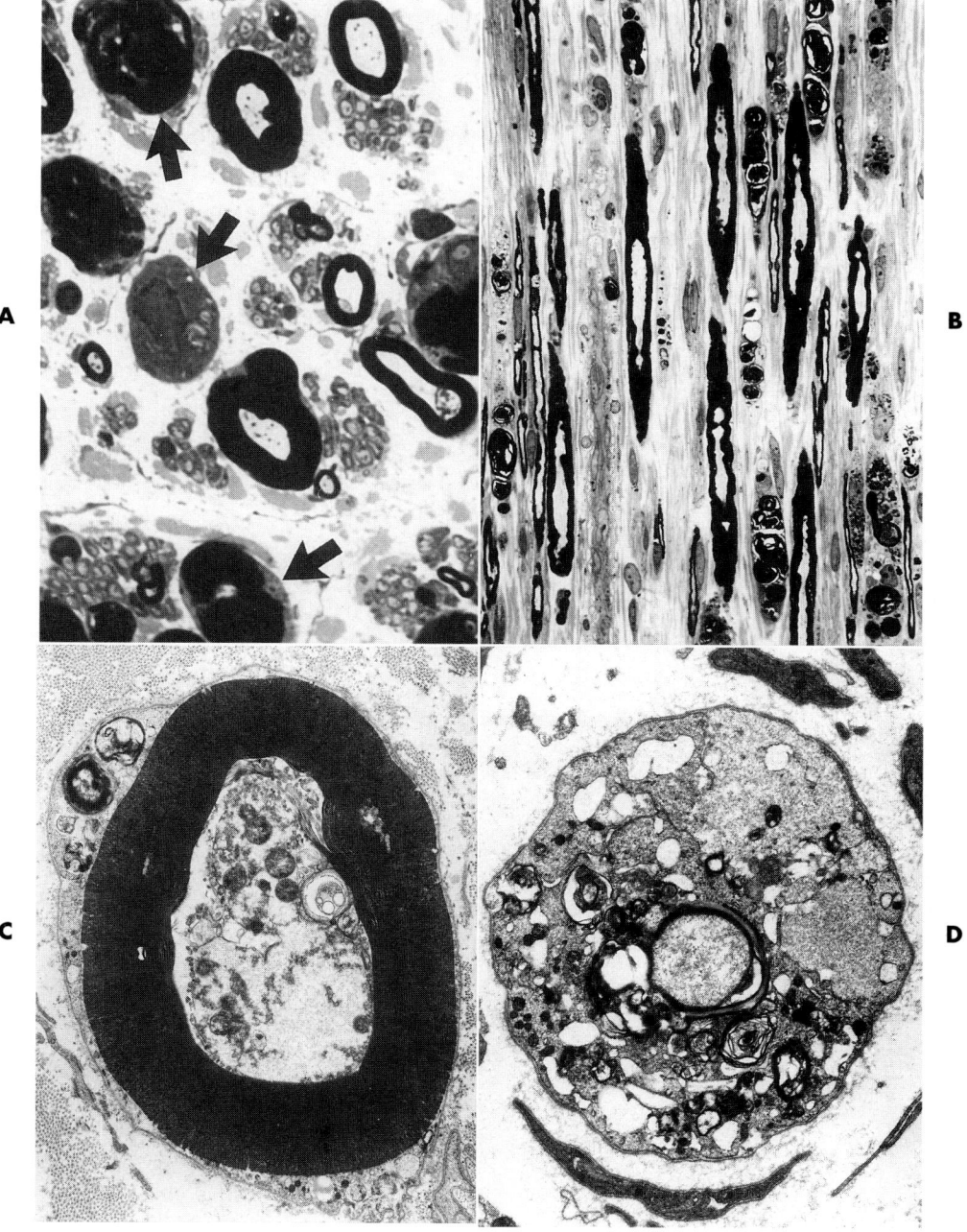

Fig. 28-118 Sural nerve. Severe, subacute, and sensory polyneuropathy in a 66-year-old woman with adenosquamous carcinoma of cervix treated with radiotherapy and 800 mg of misonidazole per day for a total dose of 17.6 mg. Note degeneration of large myelinated fibers *(arrows)* and myelin ovoids (**A** and **B**). (Plastic.) Electron microscopy shows the range of axonal degeneration with granular disintegration of axoplasm **(C)** and fragmentation of myelin within S.C. tube **(D)**. (**C** ×7360; **D** ×7360.)

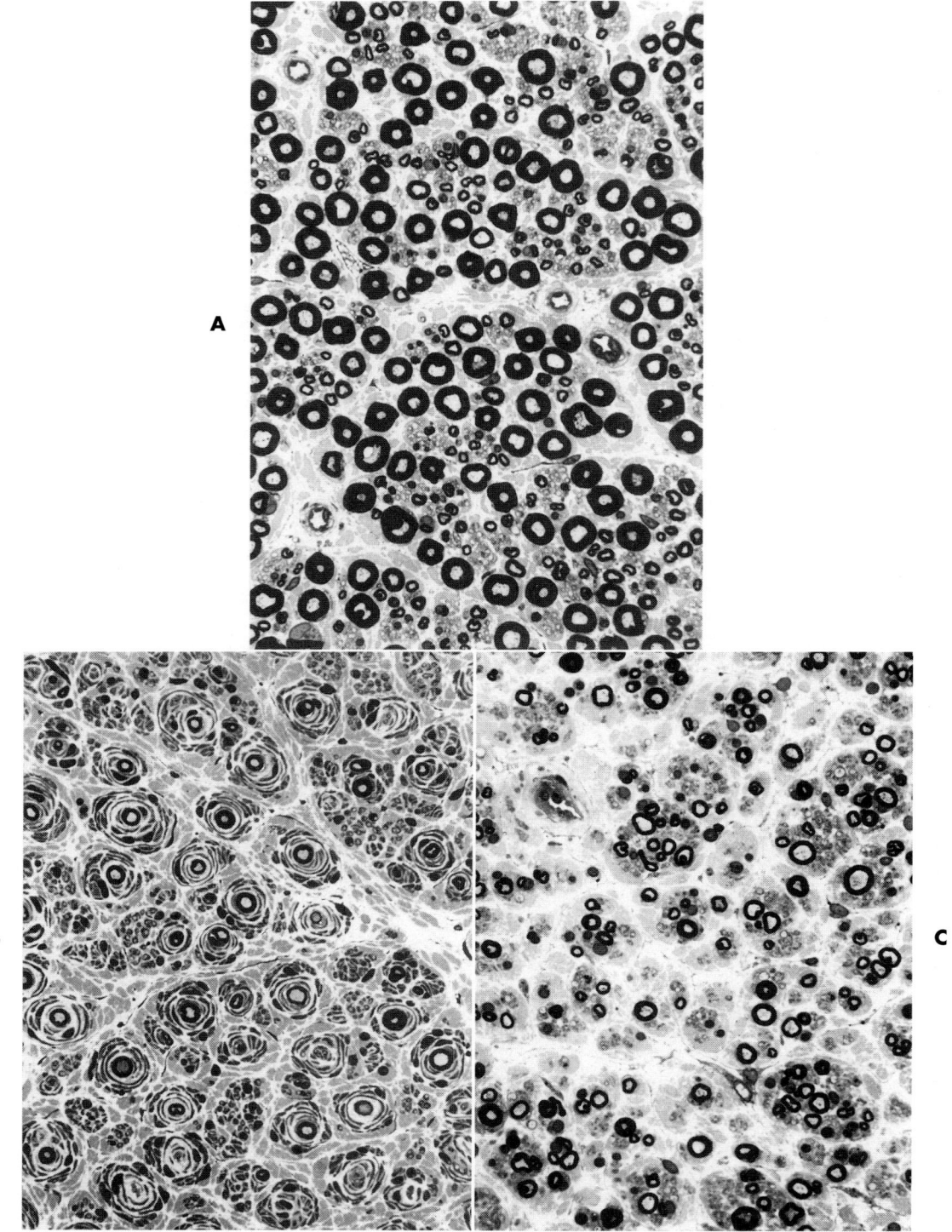

Fig. 28-119 Transverse sections of sural nerves. **A,** Normal. **B,** Hereditary motor sensory neuropathy type I. **C,** Hereditary motor sensory neuropathy type II. (Plastic.)

hypomyelination. The latter is manifested by the fact that many fibers that for axon diameter should be myelinated are amyelinate or show disproportionately thin myelin sheaths[42] (see Fig. 28-120). Nerve pathology in a group of patients with this condition shows onion bulbs formed mostly by basal lamina.

Hereditary motor and sensory neuropathy type I (HMSN-I), the most common variant of *Charcot-Marie-Tooth* disease, is most often an autosomal dominant peroneal muscular atrophy disorder (types Ia and Ib).[41,44] Rare autosomal recessive and X-linked forms have been described. The onset is during the first to fourth decade of life, and the clinical course is more indolent. Patients develop weakness and wasting distally in lower extremities, associated with areflexia and sensory loss. The upper extremities are involved at a later stage. Pes cavus and scoliosis may supervene. Marked slowness of nerve conduction is always present. The histology is similar to that of Dejerine-Sottas disease, except that many fibers exhibit full myelination[46,47,50] (Figs. 28-119, *B,* through 28-121). Variable amounts of chronic inflammation can be found in some cases (see later text). It has been proposed that the primary defect in HMSN-I originates in the Schwann cell, specifically in the expression of the Schwann cell protein peripheral myelin protein 22 (PMP 22). In most families a duplicated gene has been located on chromosome 17.[52] Messenger RNA for PMP 22 is significantly elevated in nerve biopsies of patients with HMSN-Ia.[54] In contrast, a clinically related disorder, ***hereditary motor sensory neuropathy type II*** (also known as Charcot-Marie-Tooth disease, neuronal type) displays mostly chronic axonal degeneration without hypertrophy[37,43,48] (Fig. 28-119, *C*) and only a moderate slowing of motor and sensory nerve conduction velocities.

It is of interest that an abnormality in chromosome 17 (ap 11.2 deletion that includes the gene for PMP 22) has also been documented in a rare polyneuropathy called *hereditary neuropathy with liability to pressure palsies,* also known as *"tomaculous neuropathy."*[35,39] Typically the patients experience recurrent episodes of paralytic mononeuropathy often precipitated by trivial trauma to the nerve, usually lasting days to weeks. Nerve biopsy shows segmental demyelination, rare onion bulbs, and most characteristically segmental thickening of myelin with a "jelly roll" appearance that on electron microscopy corresponds to the wrapping of redundant loops of myelin around the axon[45] (Fig. 28-122).

Because of the increasing reliance on biochemical determination for diagnosis of inherited lysosomal enzyme deficiency, tissue biopsy for histologic diagnosis is now an exception. Nonetheless, three of the **sphingolipidoses** will be briefly discussed because the microscopic changes are so characteristic that a specific pathologic diagnosis is possible even when clinically the condition was not suspected.

Peripheral nerves are often involved in ***Krabbe's globoid-cell leukodystrophy***.[38] This autosomal recessive disease is caused by a deficiency of galactocerebroside beta-galactosidase, which results in the accumulation of psichosine in oligodendrocytes and Schwann cells. Of histiocytic origin, multinucleated "globoid" cells in the cerebral white matter constitute the morphologic basis for diagnosis. Although nerves show histiocytic infiltration, typical globoid cells are

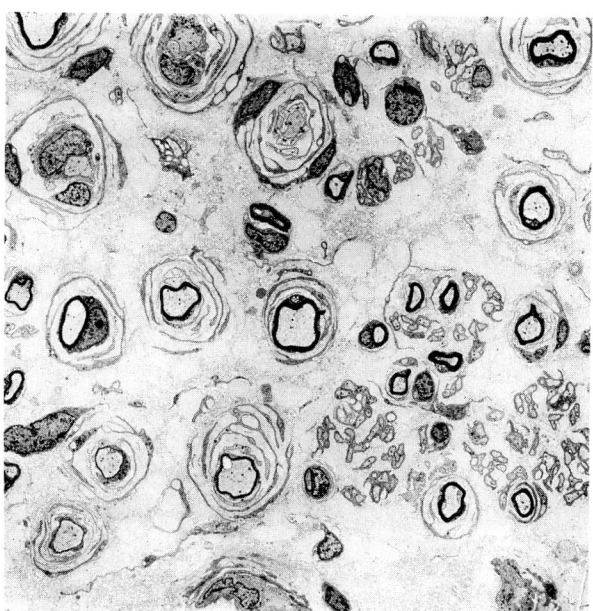

Fig. 28-120 Sural nerve. Universal hypomyelination is characteristic of Dejerine-Sottas disease. (×1170.)

not found. Peripheral nerve lesions include axonal degeneration and segmental demyelination-remyelination with hypertrophic features. Ultrastructurally, pathognomonic inclusions in Schwann cell cytoplasm and macrophages consist of straight or curved prismatic or tubular inclusions[51] (Fig. 28-123). Depending on the plane of section they may appear as empty clefts or hollow, needle-like structures.

Metachromatic leukodystrophy is transmitted as an autosomal recessive trait and is characterized by the accumulation of galactosyl sulfatide in the white matter of brain and in peripheral nerves. Most cases are due to a deficiency of arylsulfatase A. Regardless of age of onset, most patients show evidence of demyelinating polyneuropathy, with onion bulb formation being more obvious in older individuals. The salient feature of the neuropathy is the accumulation of granules in Schwann cells and endoneurial macrophages. Such lipid deposits give a brown metachromasia when frozen section is treated with a solution of acidified cresyl violet or when stained with toluidine blue or thionine; with pseudo-isocyanine the stored material develops a red-violet metachromasia.[36] Pretreatment of section with lipid solvents abolishes the metachromatic reaction. By electron microscopy, many lysosomal lamellated inclusions can be seen, the most characteristic being the **"tuffstone bodies"**[53] (see Fig. 28-116).

Fabry's disease is a sex-linked inborn error of glycosphingolipid catabolism resulting from the deficiency of the lysosomal hydrolase alphagalactosidase in tissues. Affected males have extensive deposition of globotriaosylceramide (Gb Ose3 Cer) in the lysosomes of endothelium, pericytes, and smooth muscle cells of blood vessels. There is also deposition in the ganglion cells, heart, kidneys, cornea, and

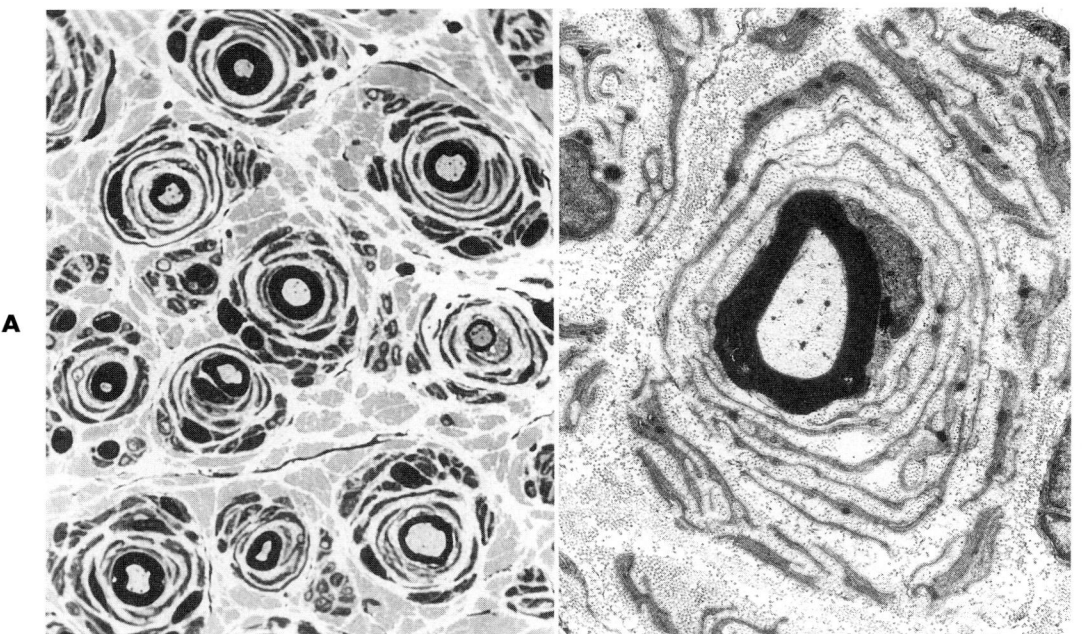

Fig. 28-121 Hereditary motor and sensory neuropathy type I. **A,** Semithin sections show numerous "onion bulbs" surrounding myelinated fibers. (Plastic.) **B,** Electron micrograph shows the typical configuration of an "onion bulb": rings of Schwann cell processes around a myelinated nerve fiber. (×5000.)

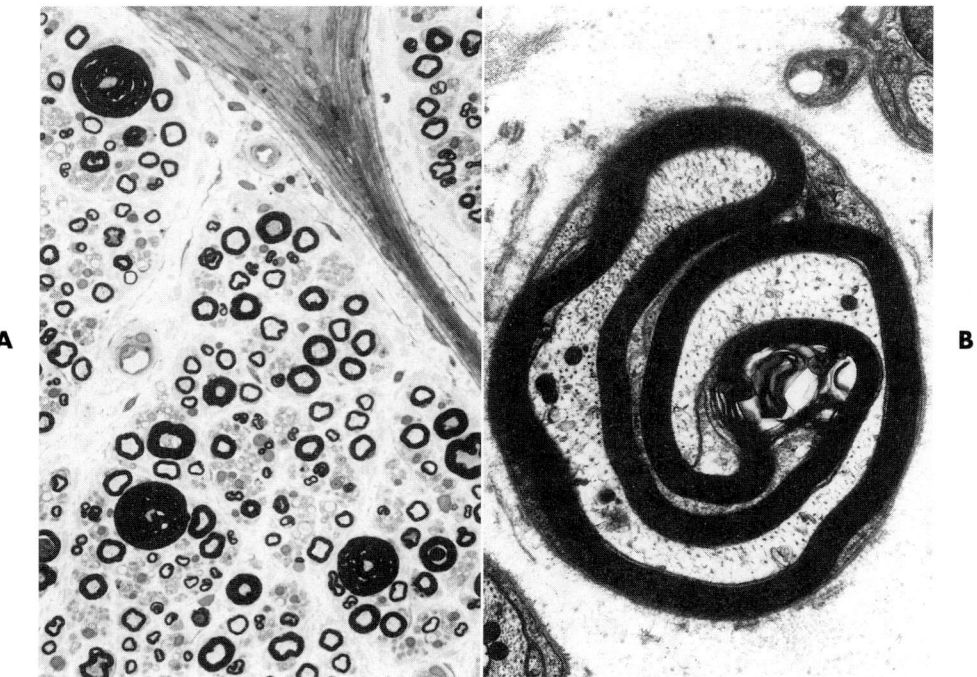

Fig. 28-122 Since the age of 12, this 42-year-old man has had recurrent episodes of peripheral nerve dysfunction considered typical of inherited liability to pressure palsies. Two sons are clinically normal but have slow nerve conduction velocities. **A,** Transverse sections showing typical "jelly rolls." **B,** Internalized redundant loops of myelin, characteristic of tomaculous neuropathy, are shown in this electron micrograph. (×14,200.)

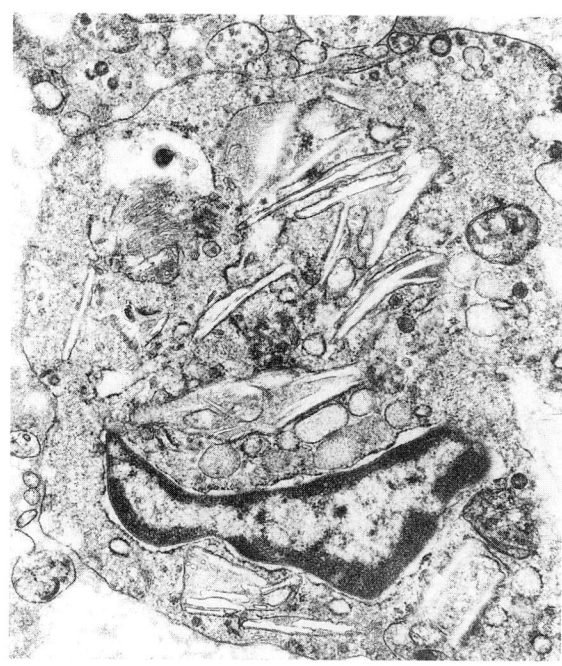

Fig. 28-123 Krabbe's disease. Characteristic inclusions in endoneurial macrophage. (×17,680.)

most other tissues. Clinical manifestations include painful neuropathy, corneal whorl dystrophy, renal failure, and cutaneous angiokeratomata. In nerve biopsies, massive accumulation of glycosphingolipids occurs in perineurium, endothelial cells, and smooth muscle cells but not in Schwann cells[49] (Figs. 28-124, *A*, and 28-125). Frozen sections examined under polarized light disclose birefringent "Maltese crosses" (see Fig. 28-124, *B*). In frozen section, the material stains with lipid-soluble dyes, and in paraffin section, it stains with PAS and Luxol fast blue. Treatment of formalin-fixed tissue with 3% potassium chromate helps preserve the lipid. Ultrastructurally the lipid inclusions display a typical pattern of concentric lamellar inclusions with alternating light- and dark-staining bands having a periodicity of 6.3 nm (see Fig. 28-125, *B*). In some areas the deposit has a spiral configuration[40] (see Fig. 28-125, *B*).

Inflammatory neuropathy

Guillain-Barré syndrome (GBS) is an acute or subacute paralytic illness caused by an autoimmune disorder of T-cell lymphocyte activation as an aberrant response to a precipitating trivial viral infection or another immunologic stimulus such as immunization. The syndrome characteristically has a monophasic course; it begins with paresthesias in toes or fingertips, followed by weakness that usually ascends from the legs to the arms in a matter of days, associated with loss of reflexes. The typical patient becomes bedridden, and in severe cases difficulties in swallowing and respiratory failure ensue. Conduction block is demonstrated in the motor nerves, and the CSF shows few lymphocytes and usually a high protein concentration.

Although this syndrome is well defined clinically, nerve biopsy is sometimes indicated.[66,67] The salient pathologic feature is a widespread focal and perivascular lymphohistiocytic infiltration in the endoneurium (Fig. 28-126, *A*). In many cases, only macrophages seem to permeate into the fascicles. The changes are more pronounced in the proximal segments of the peripheral nervous system, such as the spinal roots and plexuses; however, the sural nerve may show a subtle mononuclear cell infiltration.[55] In semithin sections, the endoneurium appears hypercellular because of the presence of numerous debris-laden macrophages that surround denuded axons (Figs. 28-126, *B*, through 28-127, *A*). Other nerve fibers exhibit disproportionately thin myelin sheaths[74] (see Fig. 28-126, *B* and *C*). In patients with no clinical or electrophysiologic evidence of sensory nerve involvement, examination of a terminal motor nerve may be more informative albeit rarely indicated.[63]

Ultrastructural studies reveal a cell-mediated demyelination; macrophage tongues disrupt and penetrate the Schwann cell basal lamina and displace Schwann cell cytoplasm (see Fig. 28-127, *B*). Macrophage processes, now intratubal (i.e., within the perimeter of Schwann cell basal lamina), begin to dissect along the intraperiod line and strip and engulf the normal myelin with the axon usually being unaffected[74] (see Fig. 28-127, *B*). Recovery, which is common, is associated with remyelination. When inflammation is particularly severe, axonal damage occurs as a bystander effect.[60,66] Treatment in the early stages with plasmapheresis and, more recently, intravenous immune globulin has been shown to improve outcome.[69]

A clinical variant of the GBS is ***chronic inflammatory demyelinating polyneuropathy*** (CIDP) with its more gradual onset and progressive or relapsing course. Nerve biopsy shows axonal degeneration, hypercellularity (see Fig. 28-112, *B*), fenestration of endothelium in intrafascicular microvessels resulting in endoneurial edema, widespread macrophage-mediated segmental demyelination, and occasionally prominent hypertrophic changes[75] (Fig. 28-128, *B* and *C*). Nerve involvement in CIDP lacks uniformity. Although some fascicles are relatively spared, others show changes of varying severity[58,68] (see Fig. 28-128, *C*). Chronic inflammation in the form of perivascular collars varies considerably from case to case (see Fig. 28-128, *A*). The use of serial sections and immunohistochemical markers may help detect inconspicuous lymphocytic infiltrates, typically located in the endoneurium. Not uncommonly, however, perivascular lymphocytes may be confined to the epineurium with no inflammation demonstrable in the endoneurium. In the absence of clear-cut signs of segmental demyelination, the demonstration of occasional mononuclear cells in a nerve biopsy should not be taken as evidence for CIDP. A small number of perivascular lymphocytes in epineurium is considered a normal finding. Some patients with CIDP improve in response to steroid treatment, plasmapheresis, or immunoglobulin. A false-positive diagnosis of CIDP is possible in patients with inherited neuropathy because of the demonstration of focal lymphocytic infiltrates in up to 12% of sural nerve specimens of patients with HMSN-1.[61] Whereas CSF protein is consistently elevated in CIPD, a normal value is the rule in HMSN-1.

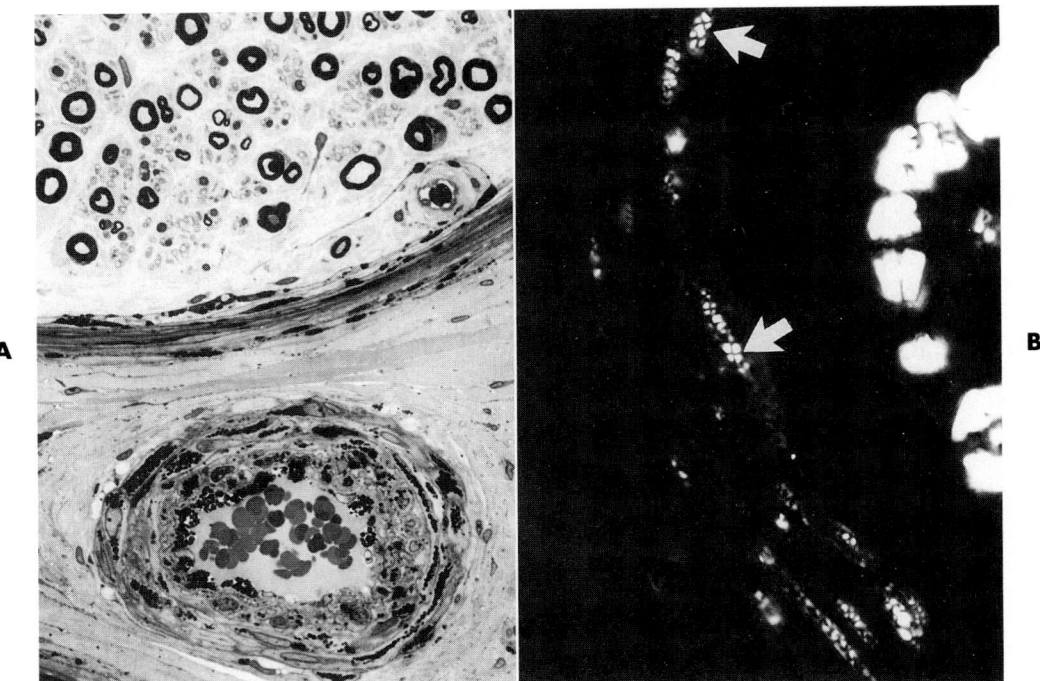

Fig. 28-124 Sural nerve Fabry's disease. **A,** Cross section shows numerous lipid deposits in perineurium and epineurial vessel. (Plastic.) **B,** Unstained frozen section photographed under polarized light. Numerous maltese crosses are demonstrated along perineurium *(white arrows).*

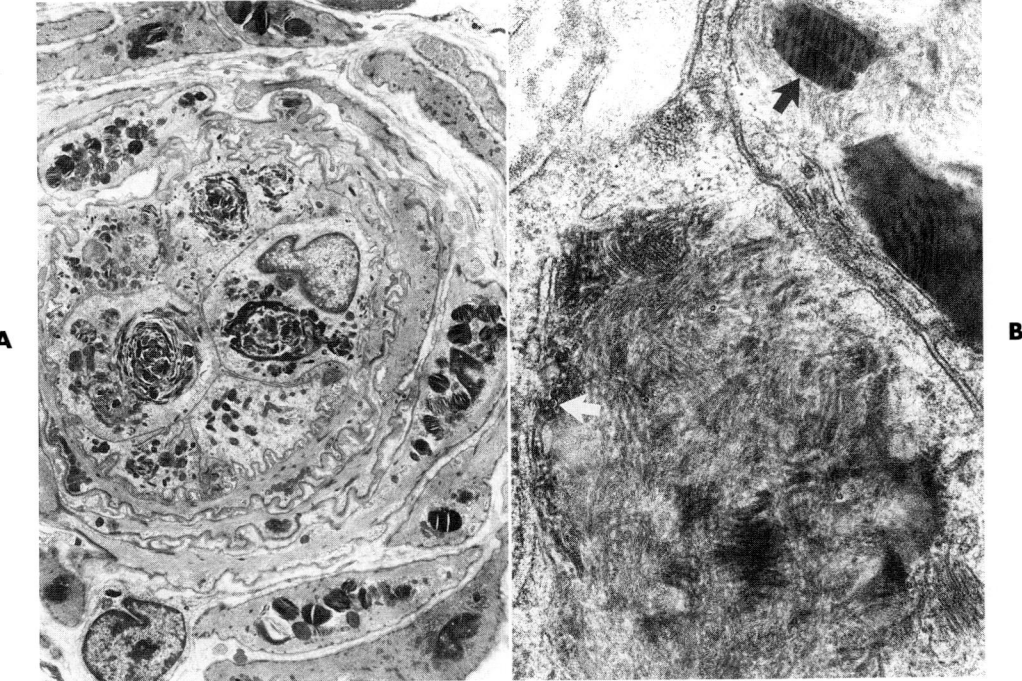

Fig. 28-125 Fabry's disease. **A,** Lipid inclusions in the endothelial cells and pericytes. (×4800.) **B,** Inclusions with alternating bands *(solid arrow)* and curvilinear profiles *(white arrow)* in endothelial cells. (×59,100.)

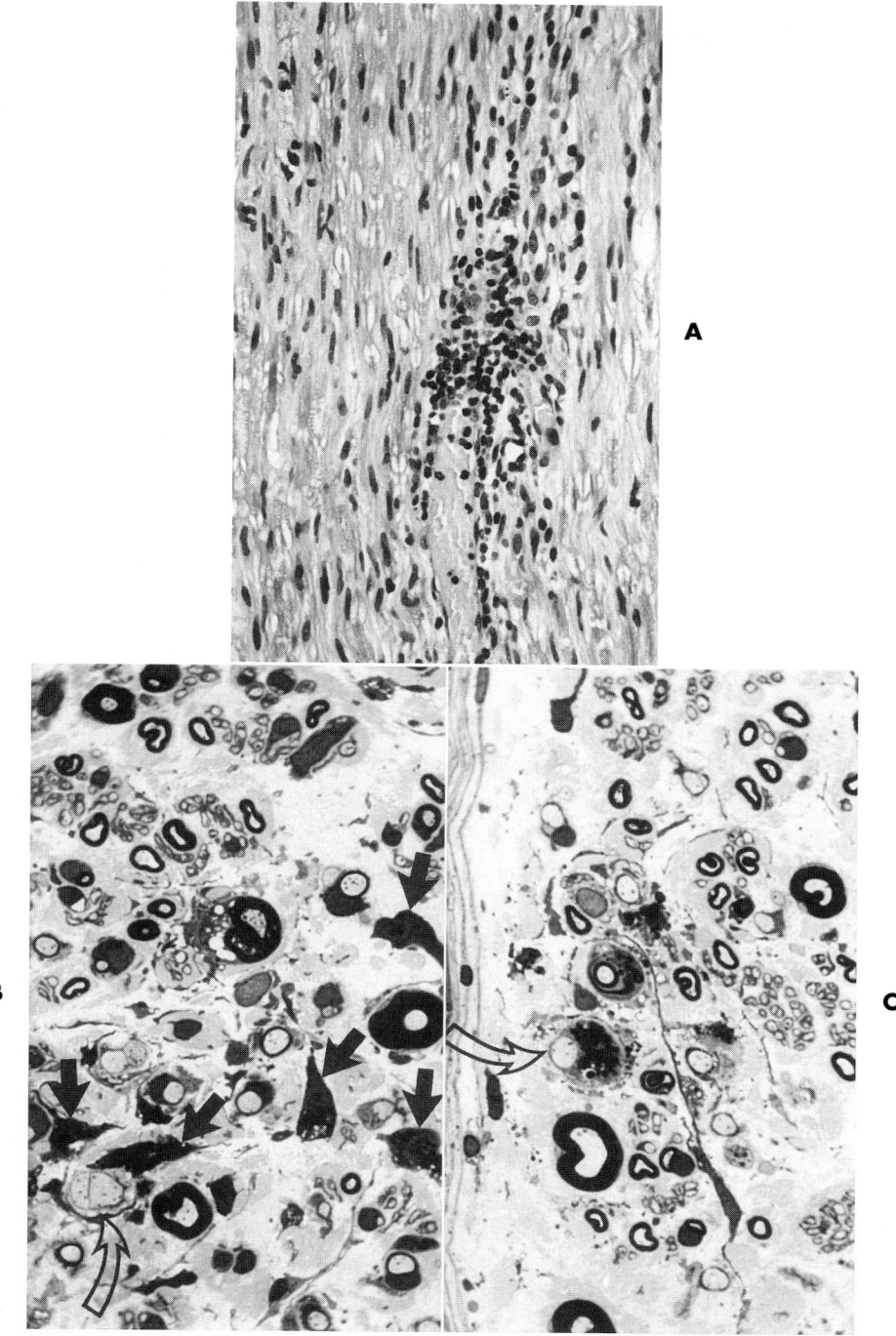

Fig. 28-126 Fourteen-year-old boy with Guillain-Barré syndrome. Sural nerve biopsy performed 5 weeks after onset of symptoms. **A,** Perivascular lymphocytic infiltrate in endoneurium. **B** and **C**, Endoneurial area shows infiltrates by macrophages *(solid arrows)*, segmental demyelination *(open arrows)*, and dropout of myelinated fibers. Compare with normal nerve in Fig. 28-119, *A*. (Plastic.)

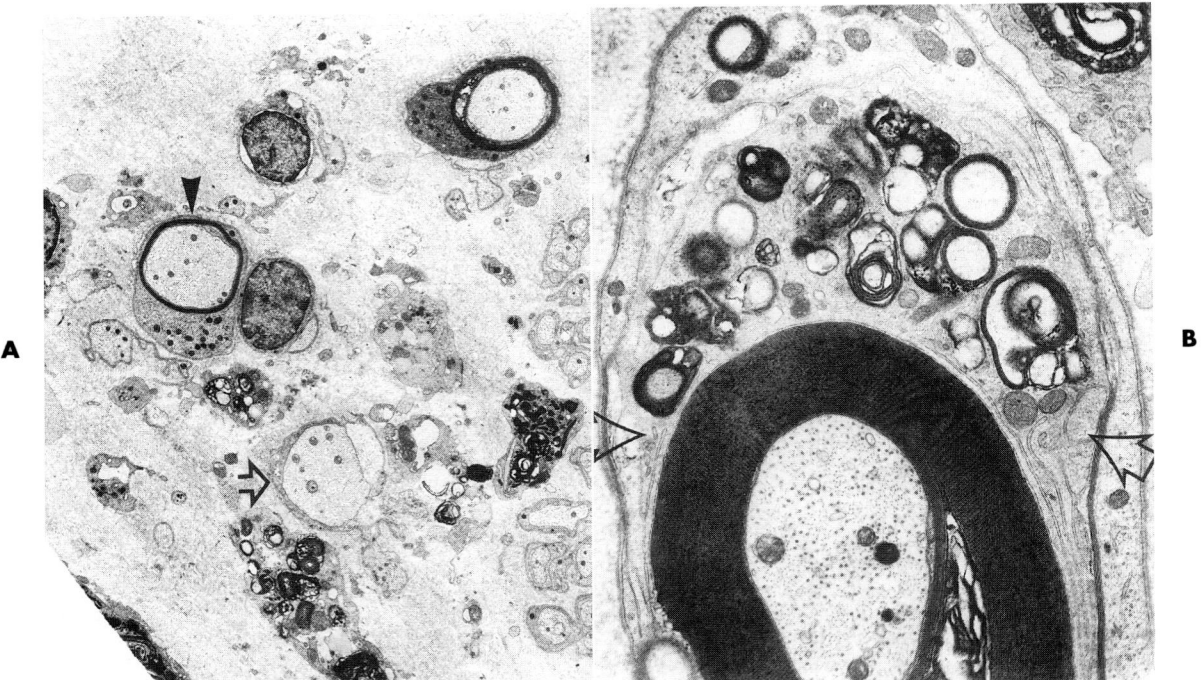

Fig. 28-127 Ultrastructural features of the Guillain-Barré syndrome. **A,** Low-power view of endoneurium shows macrophage processes laden with myelin debris and axons that are demyelinated *(open arrow)* and remyelinating *(arrowhead).* (×4500.) **B,** Macrophagic processes penetrate Schwann cell tube and separate and strip myelin *(open arrows)* off nerve fiber. The axon is spared. (×5700.)

Acute and chronic inflammatory demyelinating polyneuropathies are not uncommon complications during the early stages of infection with the human immunodeficiency virus. Except for pleocytosis in CSF, these cases are clinically indistinguishable from GBS and CIDP. Histologically, the chronic inflammation in subcutaneous nerves is much more intense.[57] A more common neuropathy in *AIDS* appears late in the disease and is characterized by painful dysesthesias, symmetric distal sensory loss, and areflexia.[57,59] Peripheral nerves show axonal degeneration, demyelination, sparse chronic inflammation, and occasionally necrotizing vasculitis[78] (Fig. 28-129, *A*), which is associated with distinctive tubuloreticular inclusions in the endothelium (Fig. 28-129, *B*). A multifocal, necrotizing, inflammatory neuropathy with associated endoneurial cytomegalovirus cytopathy has also been reported in patients with AIDS.[79] The inflammatory infiltrate is composed of mononuclear and polymorphonuclear leukocytes. The diagnosis of CMV-mediated neuropathy is important because its treatment may be lifesaving[73] (Fig. 28-130).

Nerve biopsies in patients with *Lyme borreliosis* and neuropathy have shown nonspecific perivascular (endoneurial, perineurial, and epineurial) lymphoplasmacytic cuffings and endarteritis obliterans.[70] Although spirochetes have never been observed in nerve tissue of patients infected with *Borrelia burgdorferi,* relief of signs and symptoms of neuropathy follows antibiotic therapy.

Sural nerve biopsies of patients affected by the toxic syndrome produced by ingestion of *adulterated rapeseed oil* have shown prominent perineurial mononuclear cell infiltrates, as well as perivenular and pericapillary lymphocytic cuffings mostly in epineurium, in the absence of vasculitis.[77]

About 5% of the patients with *sarcoidosis* develop symptoms of neurologic involvement. The most salient clinical feature of sarcoidosis of the peripheral nervous system is the occurrence of a fluctuating cranial polyneuritis, the facial nerve being most often involved. A symmetric peripheral neuropathy has also been described.[81] Sural nerve biopsy in at least five such cases has shown epithelioid cell granulomata in epineurium and endoneurium[56,71,72,83] (Fig. 28-131); multinucleated giant cells are uncommon in nerve lesions. A granulomatous angiitis and periangiitis have been proposed as a mechanism for nerve damage.[72,76] Nerve biopsy alone is not advisable for the diagnosis of sarcoidosis. Granulomata are more likely to be found in muscle than in peripheral nerves in patients with active disease.[80]

Focal perivascular collections of lymphocytes have been shown in peripheral nerves in patients with the *eosinophilia-myalgia syndrome.*[65]

Patients suffering from carcinomas of various sites may develop neuropathies not related to direct invasion by neoplastic cells. In *paraneoplastic subacute sensory neuropathy,* there are neuronal cell loss and perivascular lymphocytic infiltrates in spinal ganglia. In other patients, a *nonmetastatic carcinomatous sensory motor polyneuropathy* may develop. In these cases the sural nerve shows axonal degeneration and rarely sparse chronic inflammation.

Although benign lymphocytic aggregates are relatively common in nerve biopsies, pathologists should be aware that selective and extensive lymphocytic infiltration of periph-

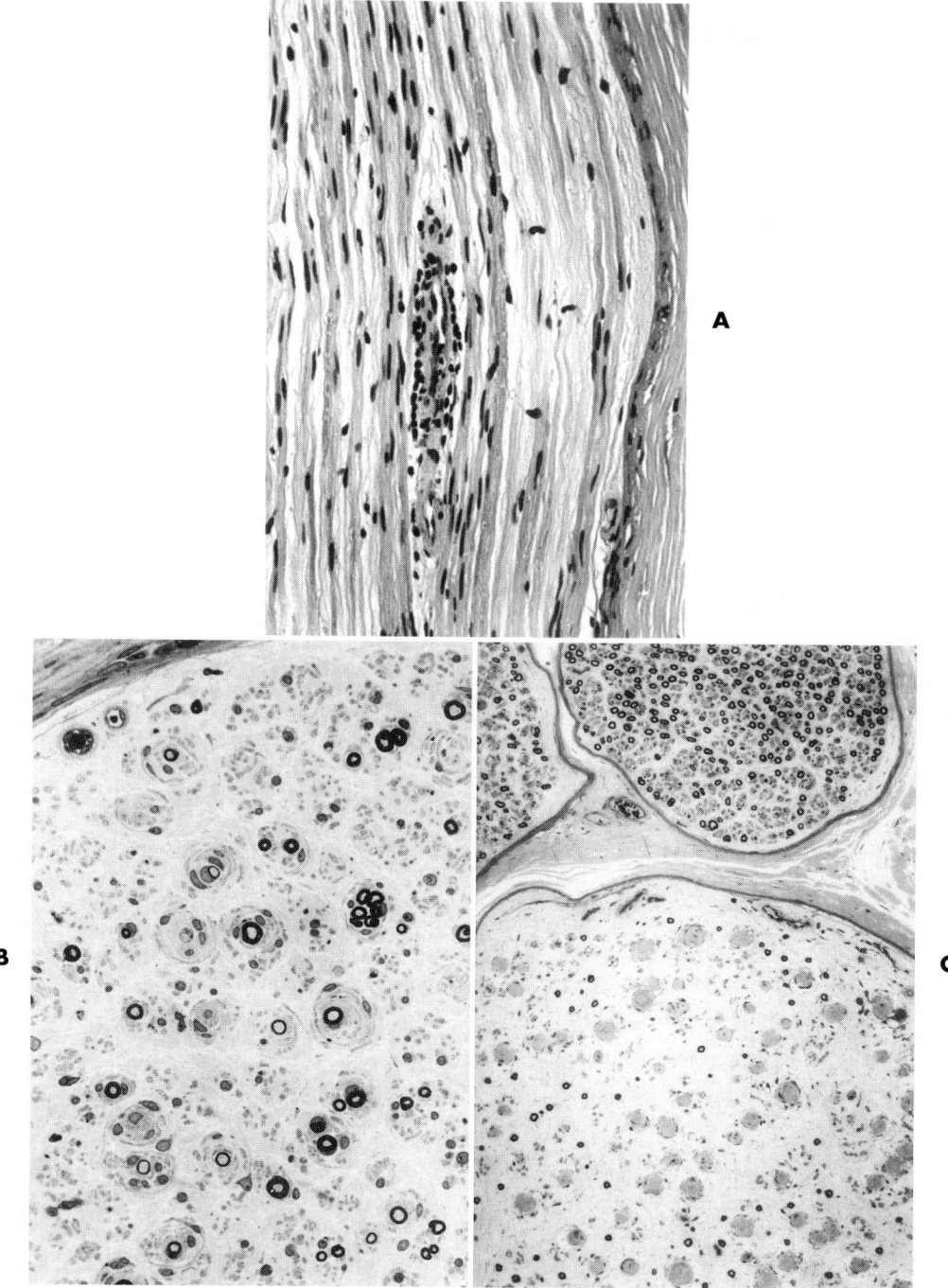

Fig. 28-128 Sural nerve in chronic inflammatory demyelinating polyneuropathy. **A,** Perivascular lymphocytic cuffing in endoneurium. **B,** Myelinated nerve fiber loss, onion bulb formation, and regenerating clusters in a transverse section. **C,** Nonuniform involvement of fascicles. (**B** and **C** Plastic.)

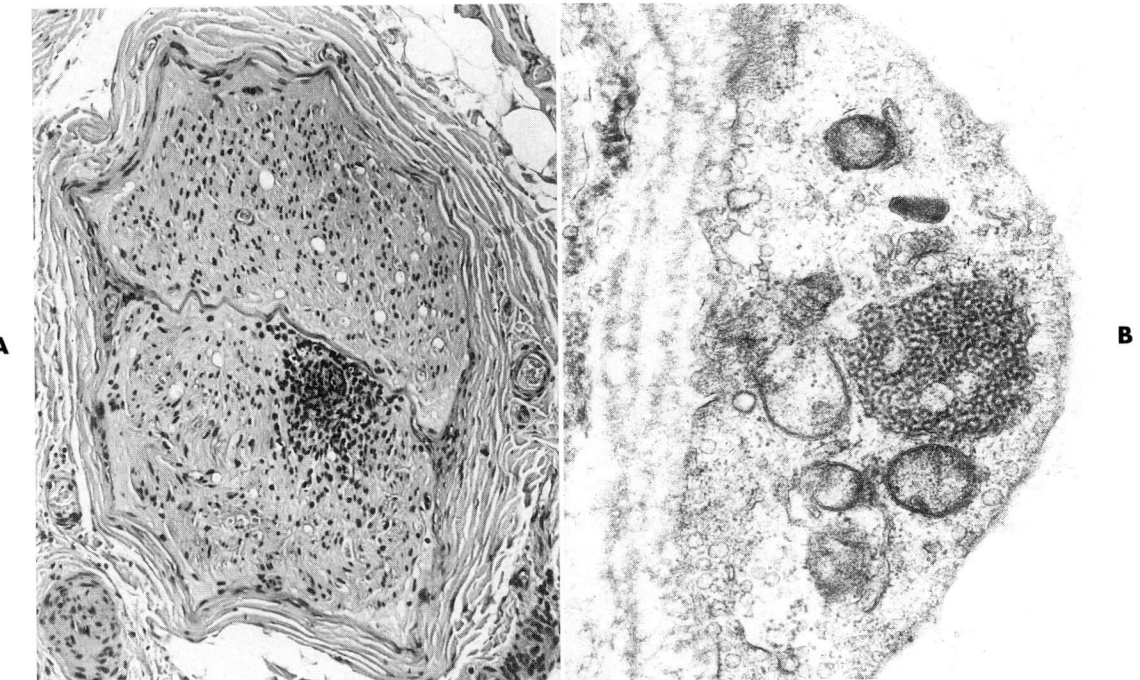

Fig. 28-129 Sural nerve. Endoneurial microvasculitis in a patient with AIDS. Tubuloreticular inclusions in endothelium. (×33,516.)

eral nerves may be the initial manifestation of *malignant lymphoma*. The patients may present with a progressive or relapsing subacute and asymmetric painful neuropathy. Pathologically this *neurolymphomatosis* is widespread and involves nerves, roots, and plexuses. The diagnosis lies in the recognition of the atypical features and the immunophenotype of the mononuclear cell infiltrate.[62,82] Peripheral nerves can be involved in *malignant angioendotheliomatosis (angiotropic large cell lymphoma)*[64] and in lymphomatoid granulomatosis (Fig. 28-132).

Leprous neuritis

Mycobacterium leprae has an unexplained affinity for peripheral nerves that are affected in all forms and stages of leprosy[89,92] (Fig. 28-133). In a patient with leprosy, biopsy of a subcutaneous nerve may reveal pathologic changes that are greater than (or at variance with) those suggested by skin biopsy or clinical examination.[85,95] The tissue response to *M. leprae* infection is largely determined by the natural resistance of the host, the bacillus itself being of low pathogenicity.[94] A two-stage model for genetic control of innate susceptibility to leprosy has been proposed. The expression of a single recessive autosomal gene may determine the susceptibility to disease per se,[96] whereas the progression of the disease and the histologic reaction ultimately developed are associated with genes of the major histocompatibility complex.[91]

The histologic lesions of leprosy are classified within the spectrum of the pure tuberculoid and the pure lepromatous poles. The true borderline form is most unstable, with downgrading (toward lepromatous form) in the absence of treatment, or upgrading (toward tuberculoid form) with treatment. In *tuberculoid leprosy* there is an exuberant inflammatory response; lesions occur early during the disease and may be confined to a single nerve trunk near the portal of entry of the bacillus. The subcutaneous nerve is thickened, with obliteration of the fascicular anatomy by confluent granulomata composed of epithelioid histiocytes, multinucleated giant cells, and lymphocytes (Fig. 28-133, *A*). This may affect the whole cross section of nerve, to the point that the structure becomes unrecognizable. In this instance, immunohistochemical studies for EMA and S-100 protein may help detect residual perineurium and Schwann cells. Caseation necrosis centered in nerves may occur (see Fig. 28-133, *A*). The finding of normal or marginally affected nerve bundles within a granuloma almost excludes the possibility of leprosy. In tuberculoid leprosy, bacilli are very rarely demonstrable with conventional stains. A specific DNA probe and polymerase chain reaction for the detection of picogram quantities of *M. leprae* in tissues has been developed.[90,97]

Lepromatous leprosy is characterized by a selective anergy to *M. leprae* and its antigens.[88] A defect in cell-mediated immunity associated with decreased interferon-gamma production leads to unchecked bacillary proliferation in dermal macrophages, hematogenous spread, and eventually colonization of subcutaneous nerves. A symmetric polyneuropathy develops late in the disease with a peculiar pattern of sensory loss involving the legs (sparing the soles of the feet), dorsal aspect of the forearms, pinnae of the ears, nose, and supraorbital regions. This distribution depends on temperature gradients—*M. leprae* proliferates more freely in cooler

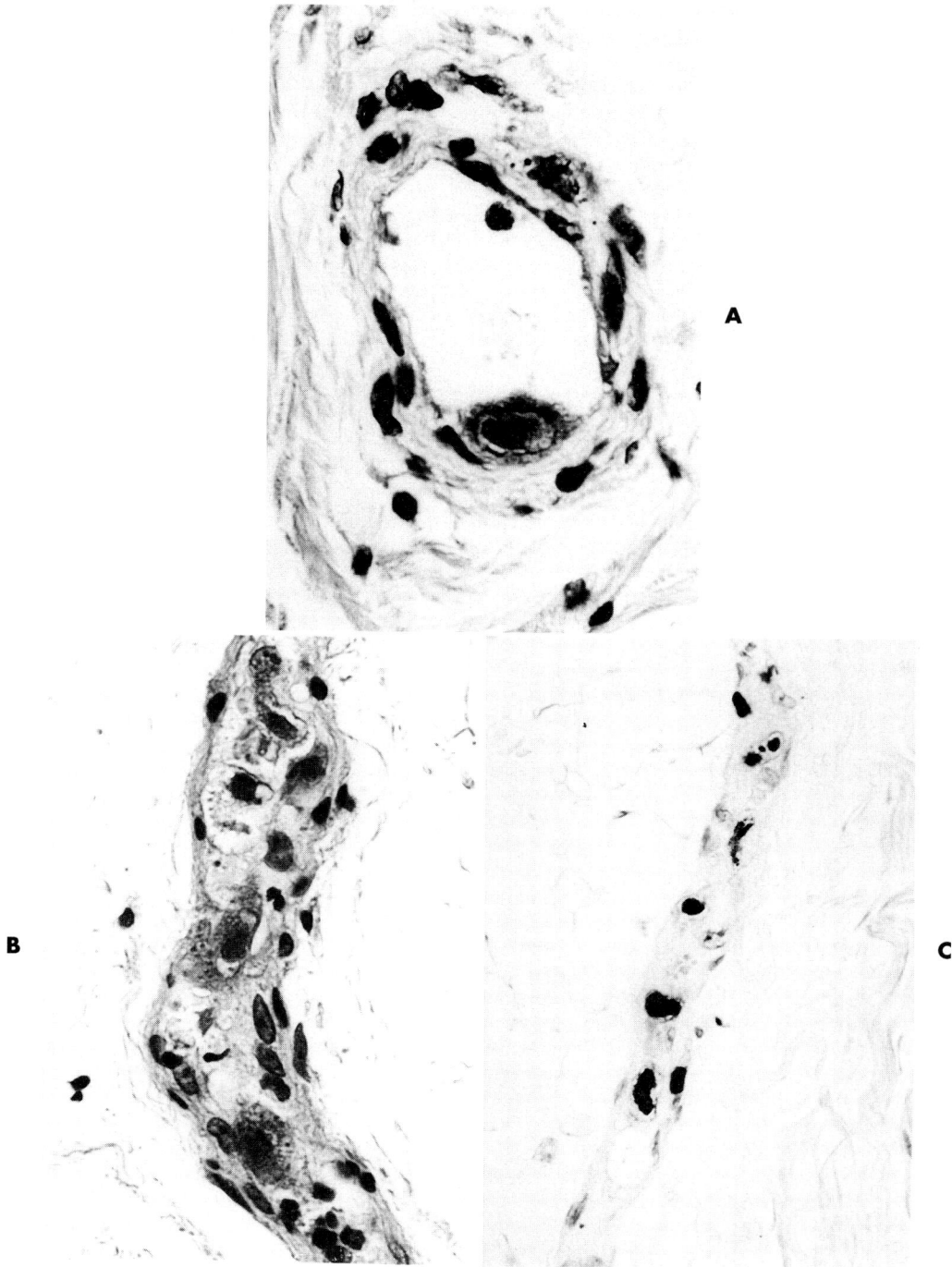

Fig. 28-130 Sural nerve. CMV neuropathy in immunosuppressed patient. Endothelial cells of epineural vessels show diagnostic intranuclear inclusions. Specific immunostaining shown in **C.** (ABC method.)

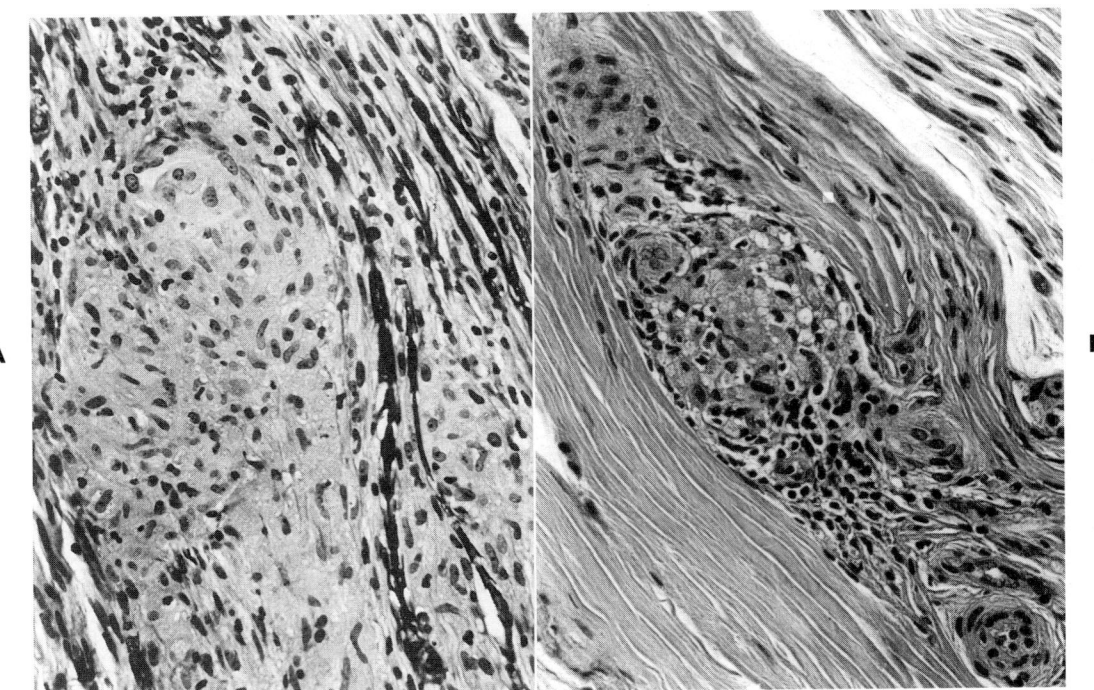

Fig. 28-131 Sarcoid neuropathy shows a "naked" epithelioid histiocytic granuloma in the endoneurium **(A)** and epineurium **(B)**.

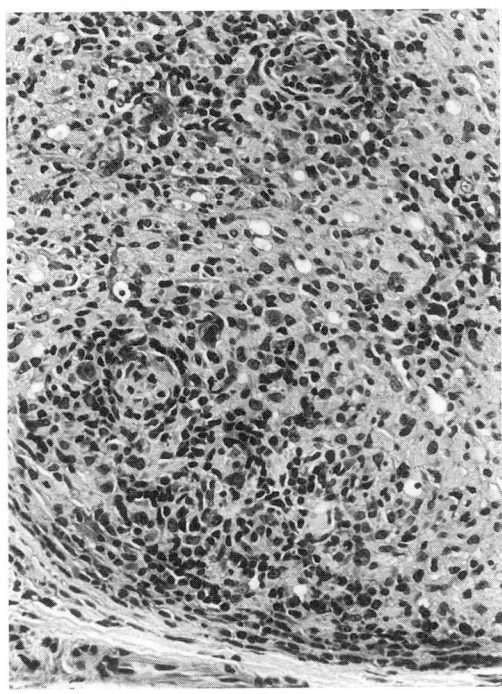

Fig. 28-132 Polyneuropathy was the initial clinical manifestation of lymphomatoid granulomatosis in this 30-year-old miner. The sural nerve disclosed a multifocal and angiocentric pleomorphic mononuclear cell infiltrate in all fascicles. Most cells stain with CD43 and UCHL-1. No progression toward lymphoma has been noted after 10-year follow-up. (Case courtesy Dr. John Deck, Toronto.)

areas. Superficial nerves are enlarged, often with an abrupt transition with normal deeper segments. In transverse sections, there appears an uneven involvement of fascicles, with some being heavily infiltrated by foamy histiocytes and a variable number of plasma cells.[87] Lymphocytes may increase after treatment. Large numbers of bacilli are demonstrable in macrophages, Schwann cells, perineurial cells, endothelium (Fig. 28-134), and perhaps axons (Fig. 28-135). The bacilli are mainly found in "globi" that contain dozens and even hundreds of organisms (see Figs. 28-134, *A*, and 28-135, *B*). The widespread bacillary multiplication may change to fibrosis and atrophy of nerve bundles. Bacilli may persist in nerves even after years of apparently successful treatment.[85] Regressive changes include large vacuolated cells that contain much lipid and sometimes remnants of bacilli (Fig. 28-136, *B*). Both axonal loss and demyelination are prominent in lepromatous leprosy, but the mechanism of damage is not well understood. The perineurium is often greatly involved with lamination by foamy macrophages and separation of the perineurial leaves (see Fig. 28-133, *C*).

Vasculitic lesions may occur within cutaneous nerves in *erythema nodosum leprosum.* Typically, arterioles in the vicinity of perineurium are involved; they show fibrinoid necrosis and acute inflammation indistinguishable from those of hypersensitivity vasculitis. In *borderline leprosy,* where the immunologic polarity is only partially expressed, the lesions are often early, widespread, and severe. The histologic features of this form of leprous neuropathy may have an incongruous appearance, with both lepromatous and tuberculoid patterns being present in the same specimen[93] (see Fig. 28-136, *A*). Lymphocytes are most abundant in

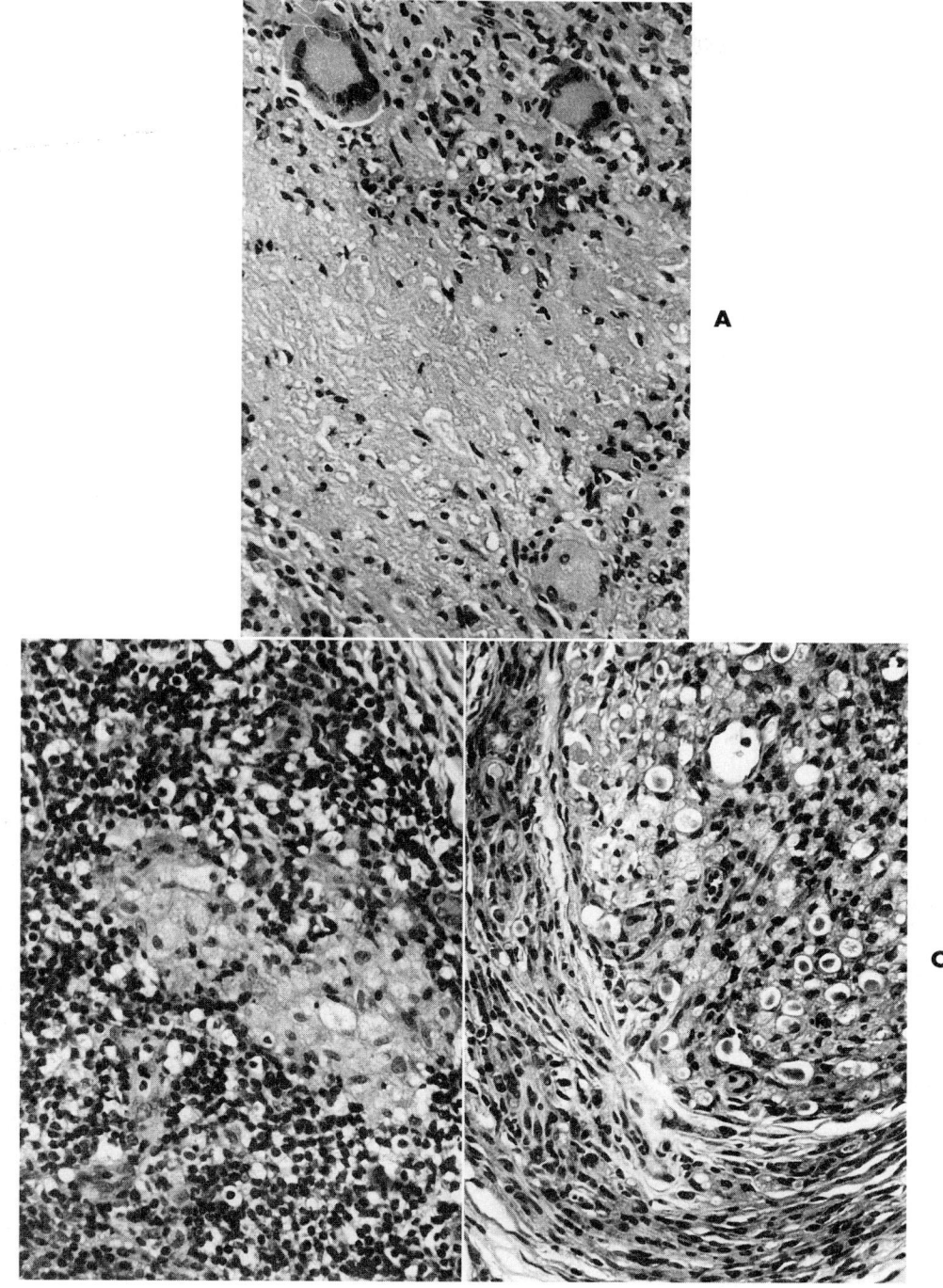

Fig. 28-133 Sural nerve biopsies in leprous neuropathy. **A,** Multinucleated giant cell granuloma about caseation necrosis in the endoneurium in tuberculoid leprosy. **B,** Nerve bundle heavily infiltrated with lymphocytes around a cluster of epithelioid cells in borderline tuberculous leprosy. **C,** Nerve fascicles infiltrated by lepra cells in lepromatous leprosy. Note infiltration of perineurium and paucity of lymphocytes. (**A** from Midroni G, Bilbao JM: Biopsy diagnosis of peripheral neuropathy. Newton, Mass, 1995, Butterworth-Heinemann.)

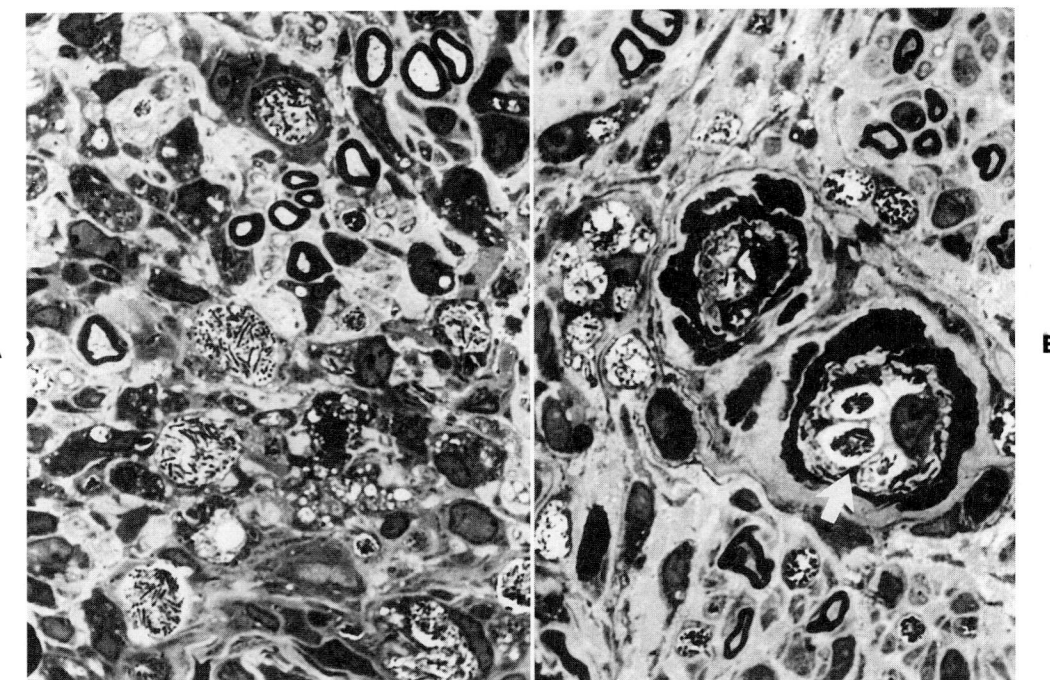

Fig. 28-134 Lepromatous neuropathy. Cross section of sural nerve shows globi in endoneurium. Clusters of bacilli are seen in endothelial cells as well *(white arrow)*. (Plastic.)

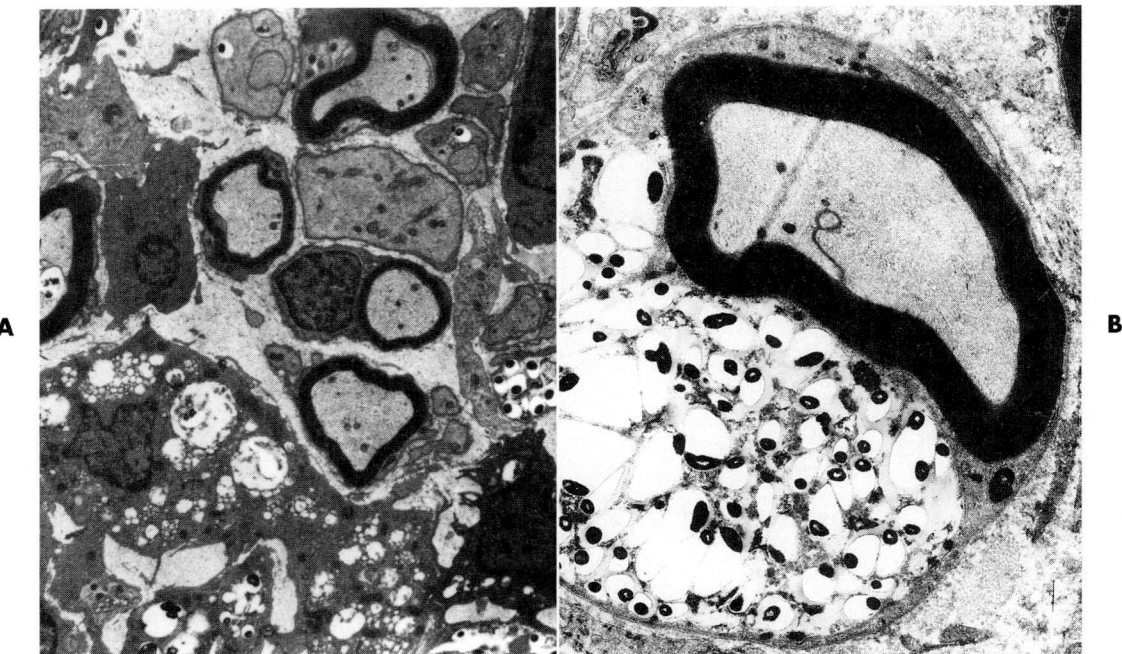

Fig. 28-135 Same patient as in Fig. 28-134. Electron micrographs. **A,** Low-power view of endoneurium shows *M. leprae* in macrophages, Schwann cells, and axon *(arrow)*. (×3960.) **B,** This picture illustrates tolerance of Schwann cells to *M. leprae*. Numerous organisms are seen within a single viable cell. (×6200.)

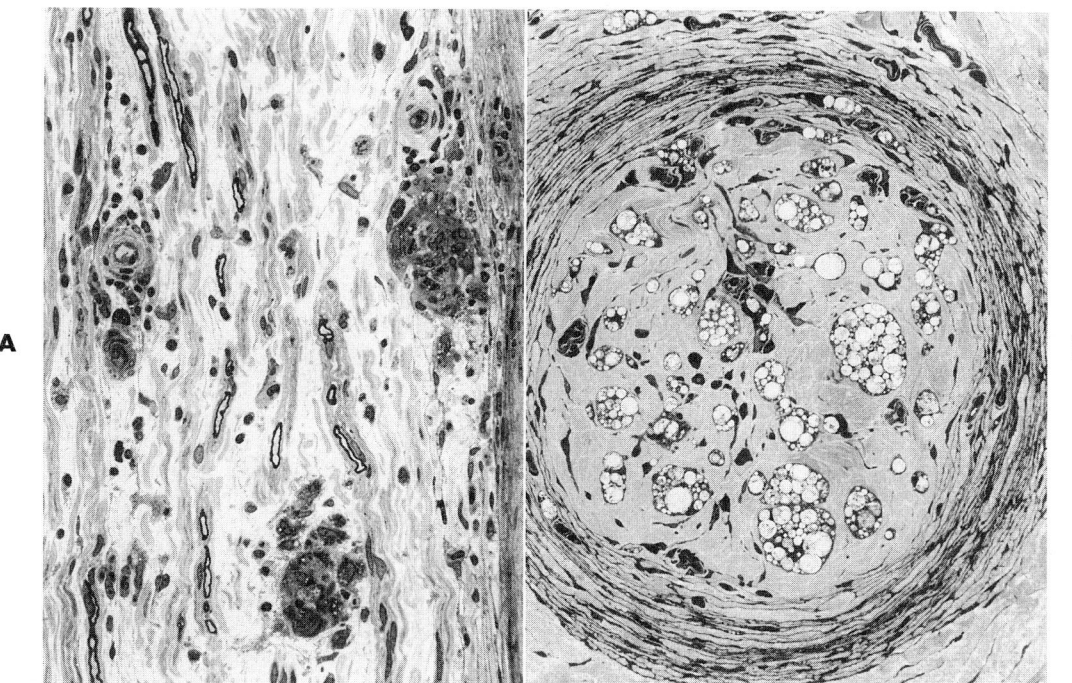

Fig. 28-136 Sural nerve biopsy specimens in leprous neuropathy. **A,** Miniature epithelioid granulomata in endoneurium in dimorphous leprosy. (Plastic.) **B,** Atrophic fascicle displaying no residual nerve fibers. Foamy cells stand out in a hyalinized endoneurium. Fite stain demonstrates rare fragmented bacilli (not shown). Treated lepromatous lesion. (Plastic.) (**A** from Midroni G, Bilbao JM: Biopsy diagnosis of peripheral neuropathy. Newton, Mass, 1995, Butterworth-Heinemann.)

borderline leprosy (see Fig. 28-133, *B*). They may appear densely packed in the epineurium or in the endoneurium adjacent to granulomas or may infiltrate the perineurium. Bacilli are almost always found in borderline lesions.[84]

Patients with *pure neuritic leprosy* display no skin lesions and are skin smear negative for acid-fast bacilli. The diagnosis of this imperfectly known form of leprosy depends exclusively on nerve biopsy,[86] in which the entire spectrum of leprosy lesions can be observed. In a nerve biopsy study of thirty-nine such patients, a significant proportion showed lepromatous histology and nearly two thirds had a moderate to heavy bacterial load within the nerves.[89]

Vasculitis

Although peripheral nerves are resistant to the development of infarcts because of large vessel occlusive disease, sensory motor polyneuropathy is not an uncommon syndrome either in established systemic vasculitis or as the first manifestation of the disease. In most cases, nerve biopsy alone cannot distinguish the *necrotizing vasculitis* of polyarteritis nodosa, rheumatoid arthritis, and most other systemic vasculitis because they are morphologically, immunohistochemically, and probably pathogenetically similar.[103,107] The necrotizing angiitis involves arterioles (up to 300 μm in diameter) and occasionally veins of the epineurial compartment. In *isolated peripheral nerve vasculitis,* the process seems to affect smaller epineurial arterioles.[100] Capillaries and venules are as a rule spared. Acute lesions display segmental fibrinoid necrosis of the vessel and transmural infil-

tration of polymorphonuclear leukocytes and mononuclear cells (Fig. 28-137, *B*). In some cases, the only evidence of necrosis is karyorrhexis within the vascular inflammatory infiltrate. The observation of necrotizing vasculitis with numerous eosinophils and perivascular collections of plasma cells and monocytes argues for the *Churg-Strauss syndrome*.[98,104]

Step sections are essential in the search for vasculitis when the original sample shows perivascular mononuclear cell infiltration without destruction of arterial wall. We have obtained good results by cutting serial sections through the block and staining them in succession with H&E, elastica, Perl's prussian blue, Martius scarlet blue, and leukocyte common antigen. Perivascular aggregates of mononuclear cells without transmural inflammation and necrosis are not diagnostic of vasculitis because similar changes are demonstrable in inflammatory neuropathies. However, studies on simultaneous muscle and nerve biopsies have indicated that in the proper clinical setting the diagnosis of probable vasculitis can be made when massive wallerian degeneration is associated with perivascular cuffing of mononuclear cells, whereas in inflammatory neuropathy endoneurial subtle inflammatory infiltrates and segmental demyelination are seen. Older vasculitic lesions are sometimes shown by recanalized vessels with fragmentation of internal elastica (Fig. 28-137, *A*). Hemosiderin-laden macrophages may be found around these older lesions. In acute cases there is obvious wallerian degeneration, predominantly in central fascicular areas, but clear-cut infarction is exceptional. Vas-

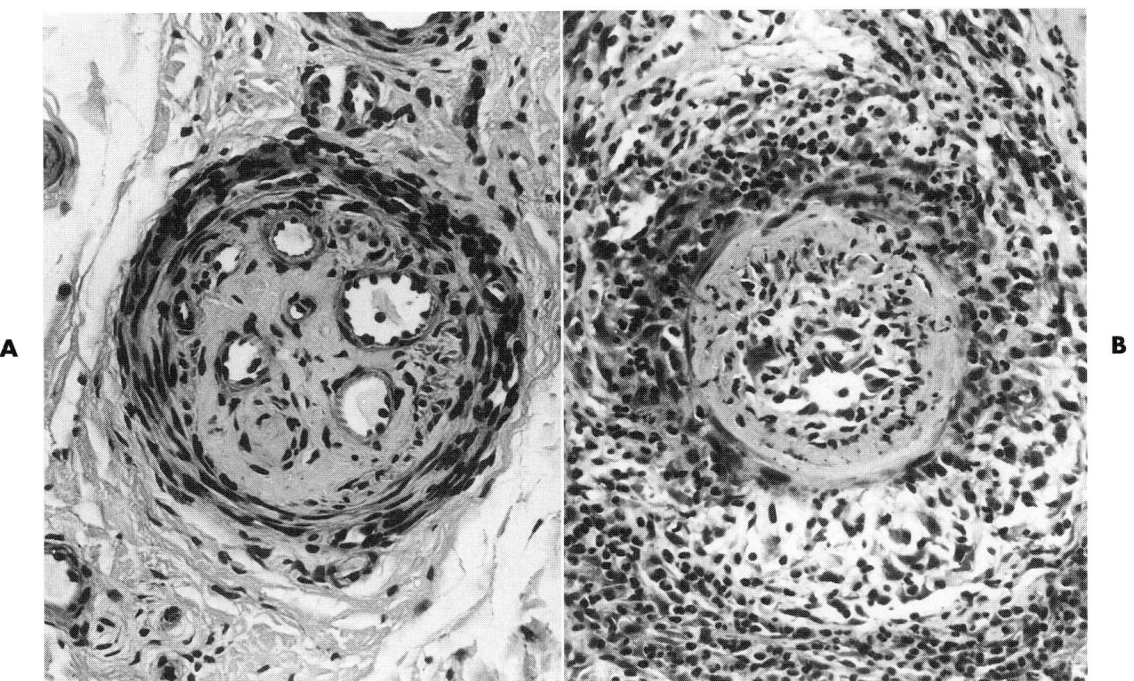

Fig. 28-137 Healed and necrotizing vasculitis in sural nerve is suggestive of the polyphasic course of PAN. (From Midroni G, Bilbao JM: Biopsy diagnosis of peripheral neuropathy. Newton, Mass, 1995, Butterworth-Heinemann.)

culitic neuropathy may be an early manifestation of poly-arteritis nodosa, whereas in rheumatoid arthritis necrotizing vasculitis is a late development; most cases occur after many years of chronic arthritis.

The classical clinical feature of vasculitis is that of *mononeuritis multiplex,* a term that indicates focal and painful involvement of several nerves.[101] Although most often the neurologic deficit is asymmetric, the lesions may summate to produce a symmetric picture. The value of nerve biopsy for the diagnosis of vasculitis depends on (1) clinical evidence of neuropathy, (2) electrodiagnostic studies to demonstrate the extent and distribution of nerve involvement and to help in the selection of nerve for biopsy, and (3) the amount of tissue removed.[102,106] We favor a combination biopsy, through a single incision, of the sural nerve and the gastrocnemius muscle. For this procedure the nerve is found as it courses in the midline of dorsal calf between the two heads of the muscle. Delay in wound healing at the biopsy site may be seen in some patients as the result of corticosteroid therapy. Although good functional recovery follows vasculitic neuropathy, long-term survival is poor.[99]

About 15% of patients with systemic lupus erythematosus develop peripheral neuropathy, some of which is due to *microvasculitis* affecting the endoneurial capillaries. We have seen prominent tubuloreticular inclusions in endoneurial endothelium in a case of lupus vasculitis. A microvasculitis causing neuropathy as a remote effect of cancer has recently emerged.[105] Elsewhere in this chapter reference is made to the peripheral nerve vasculitis of mixed cryoglobulinemia, leprous neuritis, AIDS, Lyme borreliosis, and sarcoidosis.

Amyloidosis

Involvement of the peripheral nerve is found in primary amyloidosis, in amyloidosis secondary to plasma cell dyscrasias, and in the hereditary forms of amyloidosis. The precursor protein of most types of *familial amyloidotic polyneuropathy* (FAP) has been identified as variant types of transthyretin (TTR; originally called prealbumin), an acronym for a serum transport protein that binds thyroxin and vitamin A (retinoic acid).[108] Mutations of a single copy gene on chromosome 18 are associated with most of the autosomal dominant hereditary amyloidosis. Each mutation in the transthyretin protein is the result of a single nucleotide change. Thus far, 26 different point mutations in the TTR gene have been associated with the deposition of TTR as the amyloid major protein. The substitution of methionine for valine at position 30 of the prealbumin molecule is the most common form of FAP (type I) resulting in a peripheral neuropathy (Portuguese, Swedish, and Japanese types).[114,118] Carriers of variant TTR can be detected by Southern blot analysis of isolate DNA from peripheral blood leukocytes.[116] Endoneurial deposits of amyloid in secondary (reactive) amyloidosis have not been properly documented.

The clinical picture of the neuropathy of light chain amyloidosis and of the FAP type I is similar. It consists of slowly progressive distal symmetric sensory polyneuropathy affecting primarily the lower limbs. Spontaneous pain occurs, and there are associated autonomic features. Motor involvement is late. Smaller fibers, both unmyelinated and myelinated, are affected initially, with loss of sensation to pain and temperature (Fig. 28-138). In the peripheral nerve the amyloid

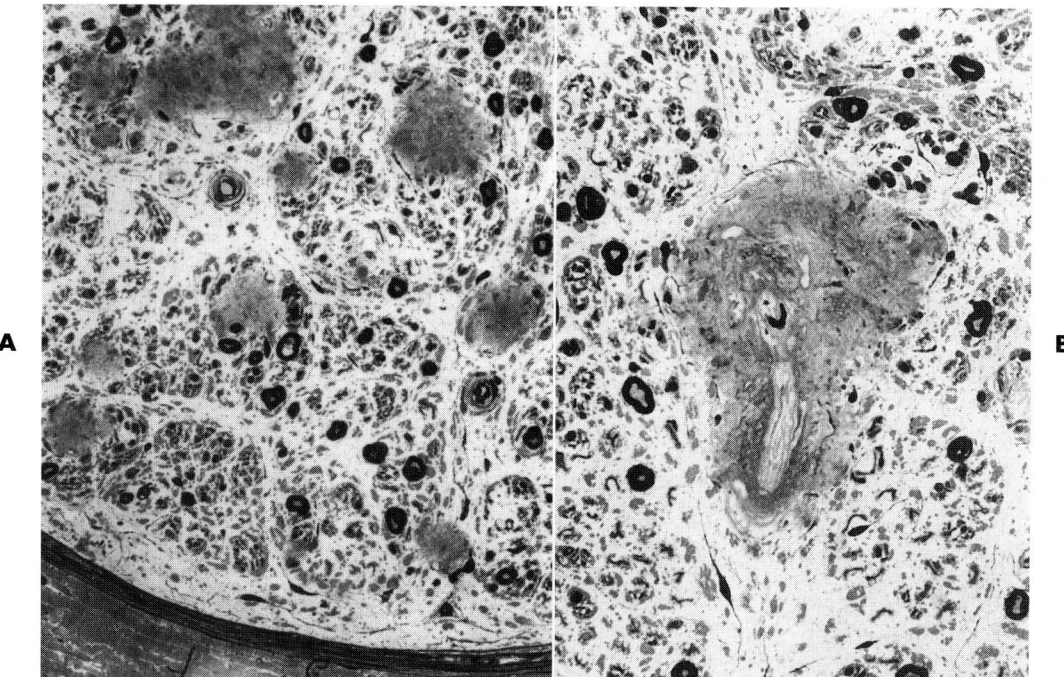

Fig. 28-138 A 48-year-old man with FAP. During a 4-year-period the patient developed a severe distal polyneuropathy with muscle atrophy, impotence, and stocking and glove loss of pain and temperature sensation. Position sense was minimally affected. **A,** Transverse section from sural nerve biopsy specimen shows patchy amyloid deposits, loss of axons, and partial preservation of large myelinated fibers. **B,** Endoneurial capillary with a thick collar of amyloid. (Plastic.) (From Midroni G, Bilbao JM: Biopsy diagnosis of peripheral neuropathy. Newton, Mass, 1995, Butterworth-Heinemann.)

deposits of light chain protein and TTR are indistinguishable without immunohistochemistry.[115] They are extremely variable in amount and may be present in the vessel wall and perivascular spaces of the epineurium and endoneurium, along the perineurium (Figs. 28-138 and 28-139), and as masses of amyloid in the endoneurium, presumably an extension of perivascular deposits[113] (see Fig. 28-139).

Although the sensitivity of sural nerve biopsy for the diagnosis of amyloidosis with peripheral neuropathy is high, we have seen three patients in whom no amyloid was detected in sural nerves, and yet amyloidosis was diagnosed in concomitant muscle biopsy in two and by autopsy a year later in another. Some authors claim a higher yield of positive diagnosis with biopsy of either muscle or abdominal fat pad. The binding capacity of Congo red for amyloid (which results in the typical apple green–yellow birefringence) is best demonstrated on fresh frozen sections, whereas prolonged formalin fixation interferes with this reaction. The use of fluorochromic dyes is also a reliable method for the screening of amyloid in paraffin and frozen sections.[119] In both **light chain amyloid** and **TTR amyloid,** affinity for Congo red stain is preserved after treatment with potassium permanganate.

Nerve deposits in FAP show positive immunostaining with antihuman TTR antiserum1[116] (Fig. 28-140). The majority of light chain amyloid-containing biopsies can be characterized as to light chain type by using anti–light chain antisera. The use of commercially available antibodies is valuable in the categorization of sporadic amyloidotic neuropathy because light chain amyloid may be detected in patients without biochemical evidence of light chain disease, and TTR amyloid may be demonstrable in the nerve of patients without history of an inherited disorder. Dalakas and Cunningham[110] characterized the deposits in 15 cases of *"sporadic"* (nonfamilial or plasma cell dyscrasia) *amyloidotic neuropathy.* Eleven had antigenic determinants for light chain and three for prealbumin. They concluded that characterization of amyloid protein in tissues is useful in sporadic cases because those who were shown to have TTR could receive genetic counseling and those who had light chain amyloid might receive chemotherapy.

In amyloidotic neuropathy, the degree of fiber loss as seen on histologic sections depends largely on the evolution of the disease. In severe cases, no myelinated or unmyelinated fibers may be detectable, whereas in the early stage, there is preservation of fibers of larger diameter. This pattern of predominantly small fiber vulnerability is so characteristic of amyloid neuropathy that notwithstanding negative staining (and this must comprise step sections of the entire block) the diagnosis of amyloidosis is likely to be made with biopsy of other sites. Ultrastructurally the deposits consist of 10-nm unbranched "rigid" or straight fibrils in irregular arrangement or forming fan-shaped clusters. In the intercellular matrix of endoneurium, perivascular spaces, and perineurium, oxytalan filaments of 8 to 14 nm in diameter may simulate amyloid fibrils (see Fig. 28-113). They are dis-

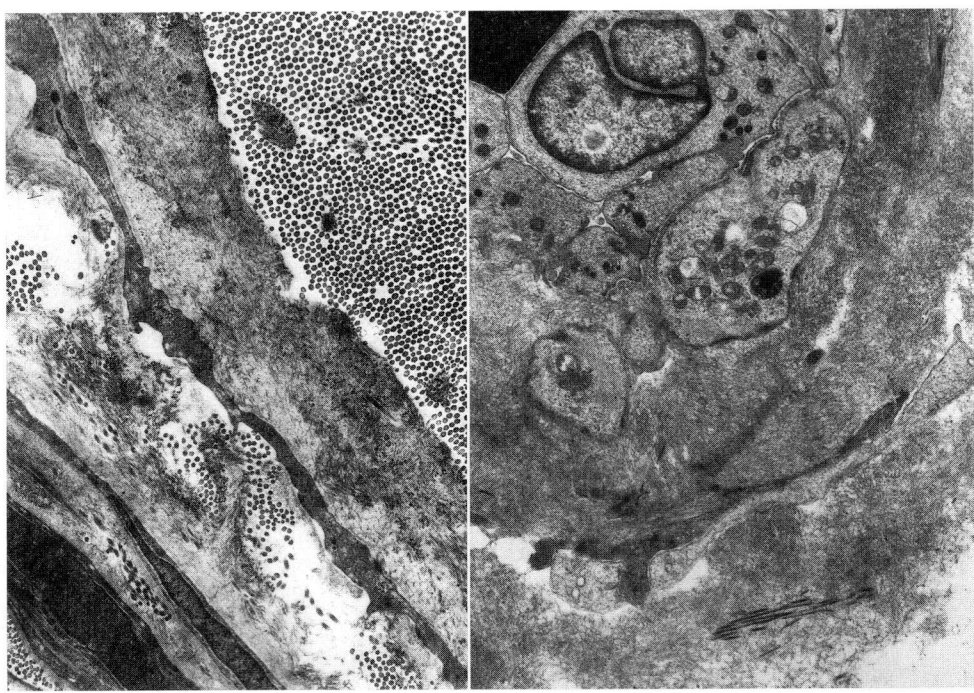

Fig. 28-139 FAP. Electron micrographs show amyloid fibrils in perineurium and perivascular spaces. Basal lamina of perineural and endothelial cells is focally effaced at points of contact with amyloid. Note intervening collagen fibers. (*Left* ×9000; *right* ×6800.)

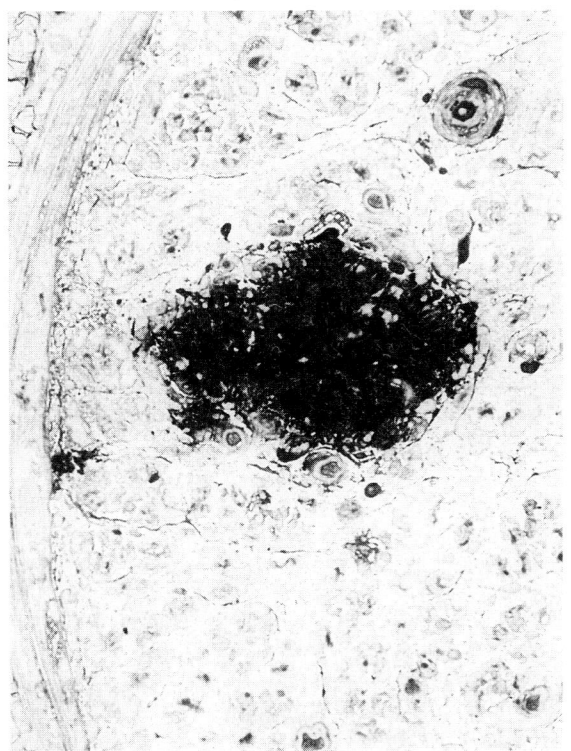

Fig. 28-140 Same patient as in Fig. 28-138. Positive immunostaining for transthyretin in sural nerve deposits. (ABC method.)

tinguished by their wavy or curved shape and by a slightly larger size. In the pathogenesis of amyloid neuropathy, ischemia ascribed to vascular involvement and mechanical damage of nerve fibers resulting from the accumulation of large endoneurial deposits have been proposed. However, autopsy studies have shown massive deposition of amyloid in spinal and autonomic ganglia, which may account for neuronal death and secondary axonal degeneration.

Another type of familial amyloidotic polyneuropathy (type II, ***Rukayina or Indiana form***) presents with carpal tunnel syndrome related to deposits (TTR mutation: serine 84) in the flexor retinaculum, causing compression of the median nerve. The carpal tenosynovium is also the site of localized amyloid deposits in patients on long-term hemodialysis. Beta$_2$-microglobulin has been identified by immunoperoxidase as the main protein of this peculiar form of amyloid.[109,111,112] Transthyretin is not involved in the FAP type III (*Van Allen* or *Iowa form*), which presents as a symmetric polyneuropathy, duodenal ulceration, and renal failure. The amyloid deposits here are derived from a variant of **apolipoprotein Al.** Regardless of ethnic background the amyloid protein in FAP type IV is related to a mutation of **gelsolin,** an actin-modulating protein encoded in a single copy gene located on the long arm of chromosome 9. The amyloid protein deposited in the tissues is an abnormal degradation product of the mutant gelsolin. Although amyloid deposits may be detected throughout the peripheral nervous system, FAP IV (Finnish and Japanese types) is clinically characterized by progressive cranial neuropathy and corneal lattice dystrophy.[117]

Neuropathy of dysproteinemia

Polyneuropathy is not an uncommon development in patients suffering from **monoclonal gammopathy**.[122] The neuropathy may be the presenting feature before an underlying plasma cell dyscrasia becomes detectable, or it may develop during established multiple myeloma, solitary plasmacytoma, or Waldenström's macroglobulinemia. The polyneuropathy is more often seen in patients with **benign monoclonal gammopathy** (i.e., in persons without evidence of plasma cell proliferation or other related diseases). The peripheral nerve deficit may be sensory, motor, or mixed sensory motor. The mechanism of nerve damage in the setting of monoclonal gammopathy is not invariably caused by amyloidosis (see previous text); lymphocytic infiltration of nerve and damage on an immunologic basis are also important.

The incidence of neuropathy associated with *IgM monoclonal proteins* is much higher than that associated with IgG or IgA.[124,125] Studies have demonstrated binding to normal peripheral nerve structures of paraproteins from the patient's serum. The most prevalent antibody activity among these IgM proteins is directed against myelin-associated glycoprotein (MAG).[126] The patients whose IgM binds to MAG form a major and well-characterized subgroup, associated with a distinct clinical picture. Elderly individuals are usually affected; the onset of the neuropathy is insidious, with predominantly demyelinating features. CSF levels are commonly elevated. Pathologically, both axonal degeneration and segmental demyelination with occasional hypertrophic changes have been documented in nerve biopsies. By immunofluorescence, anti-MAG antibody can be localized to areas of myelin splitting.[126] Ultrastructurally, this is termed *widely spaced myelin* (Fig. 28-141) and represents focal separation of the intraperiod line; it is considered to be a unique feature of dysglobulinemic neuropathy.[127] By contrast, a similar abnormality—uncompacted myelin—consists of widening of the major dense line and is a common finding in diverse neuropathies.

Nonamyloid light chain deposition may occur against a background of myeloma, Waldenström's macroglobulinemia, and monoclonal gammopathy of undetermined significance. The deposits appear as coalescent amorphous eosinophilic pools within the endoneurium associated with blood vessels and appear as hyaline bluish deposits in the toluidine blue semithin plastic sections[123] (Fig. 28-142, *A*). This material is PAS positive, resistant to diastase digestion, and Congo red negative. Most of the cases exhibit positive immunoreactivity for kappa light chain (Fig. 28-142, *B*). Ultrastructurally, nonamyloid deposits are amorphous granular or finely reticulated.

Curved tubular structures arranged in a fingerprint pattern may be seen in the endoneurium adjacent to Schwann cells and in the cytoplasm of endothelial cells and pericytes in cases of IgG myeloma with **cryoglobulinemia**.[128,129] A vasculitis involving peripheral nerves resulting in ischemic neuropathy has been described in mixed cryoglobulinemia.[130] Ischemia of nerve may also be caused by intravascular cryoglobulin deposition in the absence of inflammation.[121]

A chronic demyelinating polyneuropathy with predominant and severe motor dysfunction is the salient clinical feature in *osteosclerotic myeloma* and the *POEMS syndrome* (polyneuropathy, organomegaly, endocrinopathy, M-protein, and skin changes).[120] The M protein in these rare variants of multiple myeloma is usually of the IgG or IgA heavy chain class; most are lambda light chain type.

Toxic-metabolic neuropathy

Axonal degeneration of varying severity is the usual pathologic finding in the neuropathy caused by systemic metabolic disorders (vitamin deficiency, uremia, porphyria),[138] exogenous toxins and pharmaceuticals such as alcohol,[136,139] isoniazid, metronidazole, misonidazole[133] (see Fig. 28-118), *cis*-platinum, taxol,[131] thalidomide, heavy metals (arsenic, thallium, mercury), and chemical agents.[137] In the sural nerve, chronic axonal degeneration is manifested by loss of myelinated fibers. Fibers of larger diameter are always more severely affected. In the acute stage, ongoing degeneration may affect a few fibers or the vast majority of them. The breakdown of myelin is best seen on longitudinal sections as rows of osmiophilic debris. Later, fat-laden macrophages appear. In long-standing neuropathy the salient features are fiber loss, denervated Schwann cells, and clusters of myelinated fibers of complementary shapes indicative of regeneration.

Only in rare instances does a toxin induce tissue changes that may be pathognomonic or highly suggestive of a particular compound. *Hexacarbons and glue-sniffing neuropathy* (and rarely disulfiram) will produce characteristic segmental distention of axons as a result of the accumulation of neurofilaments[131] (Fig. 28-143, *C*). The di-iodinated benzofuran derivative *amiodarone*, used in the treatment of cardiac rhythm abnormalities, occasionally gives rise to a sensory motor neuropathy[132]; this typically occurs in a patient who

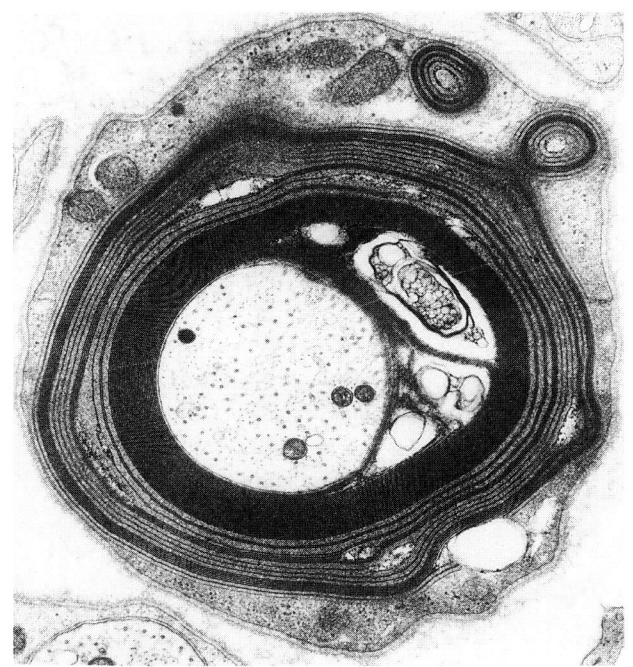

Fig. 28-141 Sural nerve. Widely spaced myelin is typical of the neuropathy associated with IgM paraproteinemia. (×19,600.)

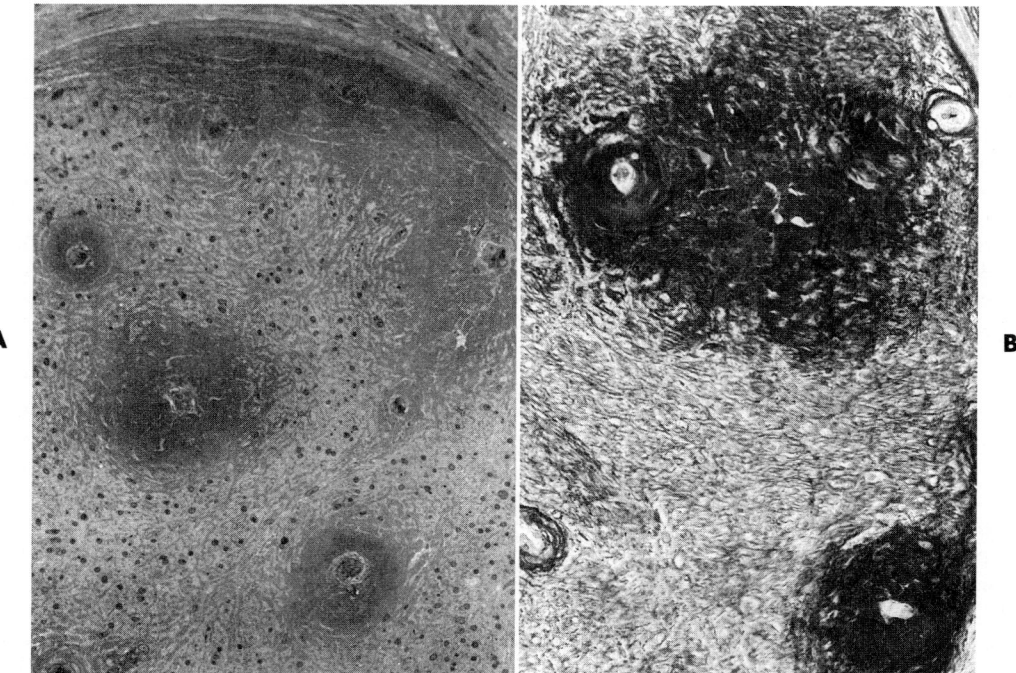

Fig. 28-142 Sural nerve biopsy of a 70-year-old woman with monoclonal gammopathy (IgM, 6.62 g/L) and severe chronic polyneuropathy. **A,** Loss of the entire population of myelinated fibers. Note confluent pools of amorphous material in perivascular spaces and subperineurially. (Plastic.) **B,** Intense immunostaining for IgM kappa is demonstrated in this Congo red–negative perivascular material. (ABC method.)

has been taking the drug for several months at a dosage of 200 to 600 mg per day. Sural nerve biopsy discloses, in addition to axonal degeneration and rare segmental demyelination, phospholipid-containing cytosomes in Schwann cells, perineurium, vascular endothelial cells, and nerve fibers[134] (Fig. 28-143, *B*). Amiodarone and its metabolite desethylamiodarone pass readily into human nerves, either directly or following endothelial injury. The drug inhibits lysosomal phospholipases leading to the formation of typical whorled, lamellar, and paracrystalline inclusions (Fig. 28-144). *Diphtheria toxin* and *perhexilene maleate* induce a primary demyelination,[135] an unusual feature in toxic neuropathy.

Other neuropathies

The most common known cause of peripheral neuropathy in North America is *diabetes mellitus*. Two types of neuropathies have been described in long-standing diabetes: (1) a focal and multifocal neuropathy affecting proximal nerves and (2) more commonly, a symmetric distal polyneuropathy[144] in which the sural nerve biopsy displays a mixture of axonal degeneration, segmental demyelination (see Fig. 28-146, *B*) and hypertrophy, and regeneration clusters (Fig. 28-145) suggesting a dying-back process.[155,167,168] Electron microscopy has revealed thickening of the basal lamina of Schwann cells and perineurium[155] and—more importantly—thickening of the walls of endoneurial capillaries by layers

of duplicated basal lamina (Fig. 28-146, *A*). Autopsy studies in diabetics with neuropathy have shown focal areas of myelinated fiber loss, perineurial damage, miniature neuroma formation (Fig. 28-147), and microangiopathy in the sciatic nerve suggesting a vascular lesion. It is postulated that in some cases the accumulation of many proximal insults causes a severe and diffuse fiber loss distally to produce a symmetric neuropathy. It seems likely, however, that both metabolic and ischemic factors are involved in the pathogenesis of diabetic neuropathy. We have occasionally observed perivascular lymphocytic cuffing in sural nerves from patients with diabetic polyneuropathy.[166]

Nerve biopsy may yield clues to a specific diagnosis or show significant abnormality in the following conditions: *adrenoleukodystrophy* (lamellar inclusions consisting of two parallel electron-dense 2- to 5-nm leaflets separated by a clear space varying from 2 to 7 nm in width in Schwann cells),[163,164] *cerebrotendinous xanthomatosis*,[161] *ceroid lipofuscinosis* (curvilinear bodies and fingerprint structures),[149,156] *Chediak-Higashi disease* (giant lysosomes in Schwann cells),[159,160] *chloroquine neuropathy*,[169] Farber disease[173] (see Fig. 28-117), *gangliosidosis*,[158] *Gaucher's disease*,[1] *giant axonal neuropathy*[148,150] (Fig. 28-148), *leukemic infiltrate*,[172] *neurofibromatous neuropathy*,[170] *Niemann-Pick disease*,[140,154] *polyglucosan body disease* (hyaline concentrically laminated PAS-positive intra-axonal bodies)[145,147,154] (see Fig.

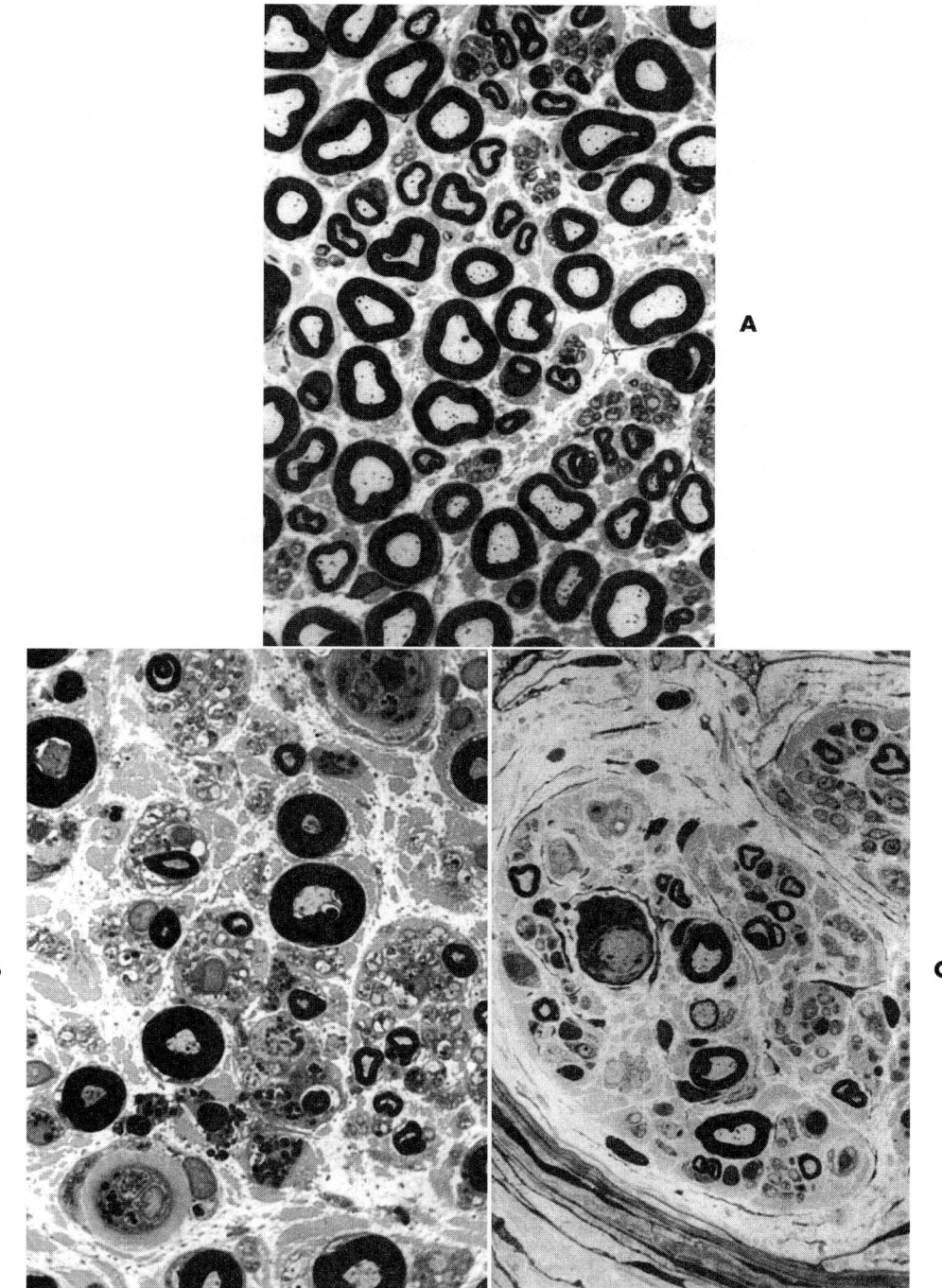

Fig. 28-143 Sural nerve biopsies. **A,** Normal. (Plastic.) **B,** Amiodarone neuropathy shows lipid inclusions in endothelium and Schwann cells and marked dropout of fibers. (Plastic.) **C,** Axonal swelling in disulfiram neuropathy. Axonal loss is severe. (Plastic.)

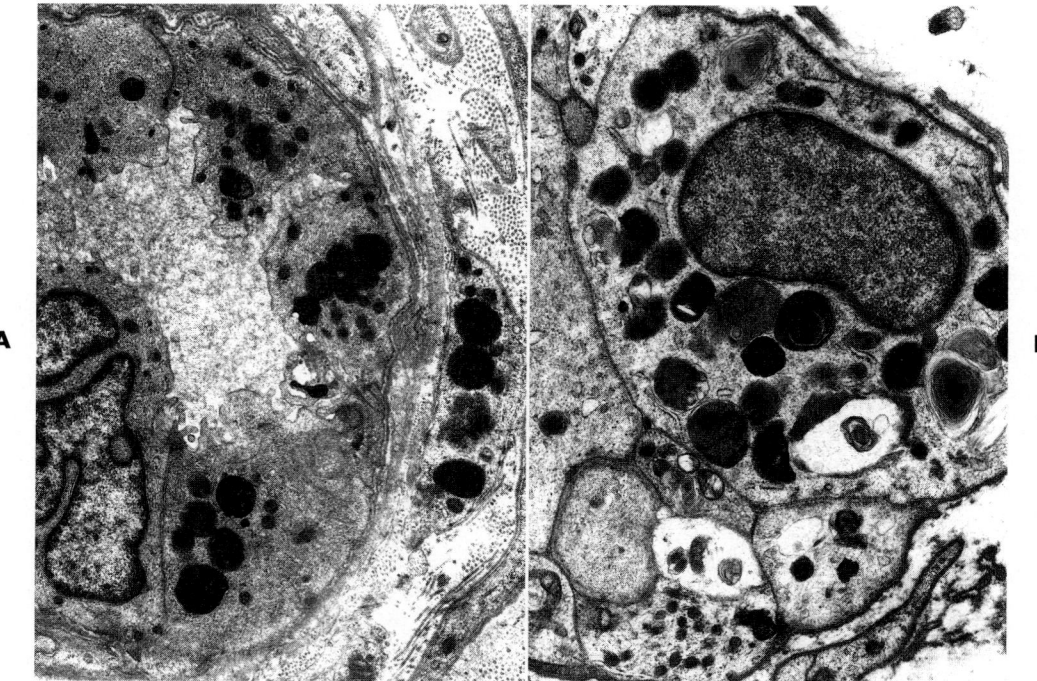

Fig. 28-144 Amiodarone neuropathy. Viewed under the electron microscope this sural nerve reveals lysosomal inclusions in the form of osmiophilic bodies and lamellar and paracrystalline structures in endothelium, pericytes **(A)**, and Schwann cells **(B)**. (**A** ×12,100; **B** ×12,100.)

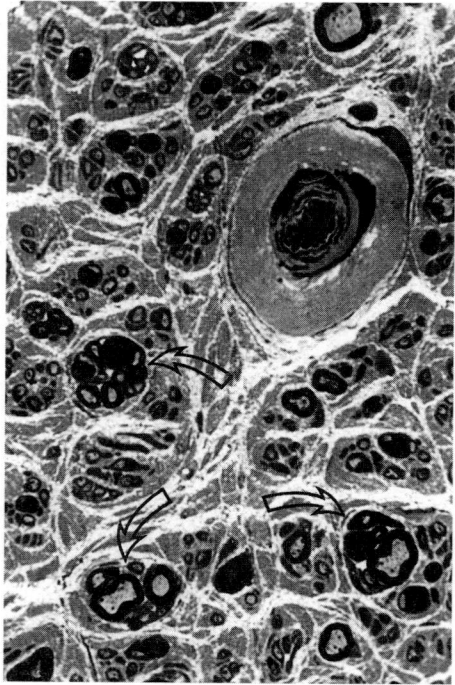

Fig. 28-145 Diabetic neuropathy. Transverse section of sural nerve shows dropout of fibers, regenerating clusters *(arrows),* and thickening of basal lamina of endoneurial capillaries. (Plastic.)

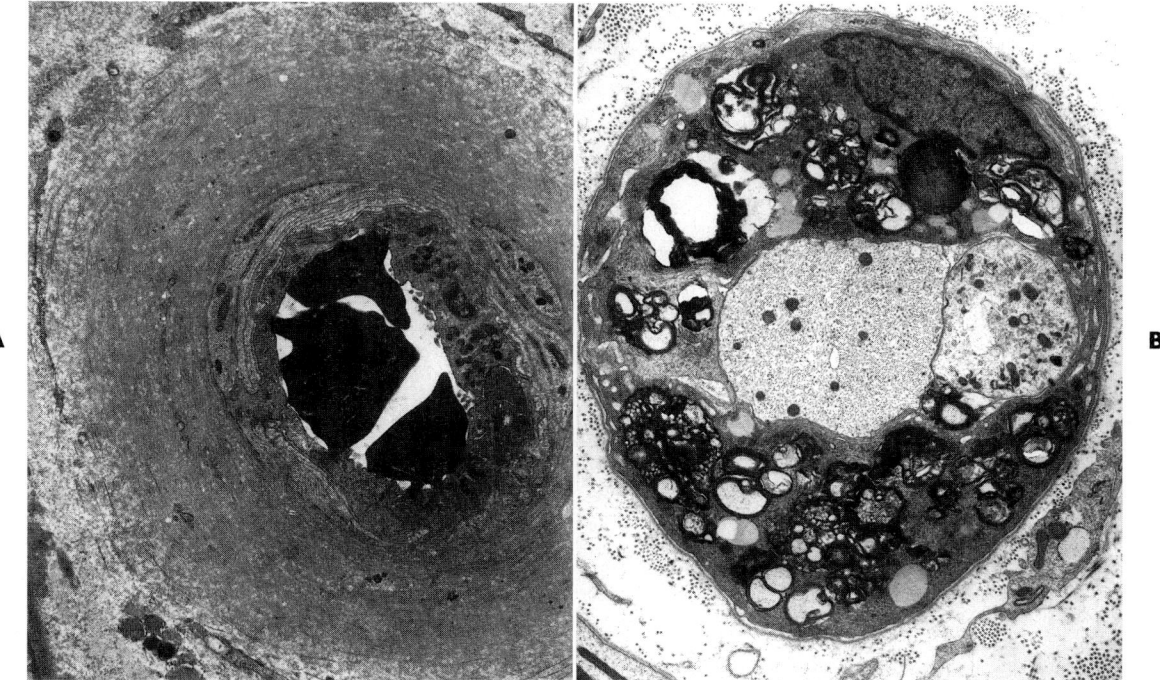

Fig. 28-146 Diabetic neuropathy. Electron micrographs of endoneurium show reduplication of basal lamina about capillary **(A)**; segmental demyelination **(B)**. Axon at center is unaffected while myelin is breaking down. (**A** ×7370; **B** ×9300.)

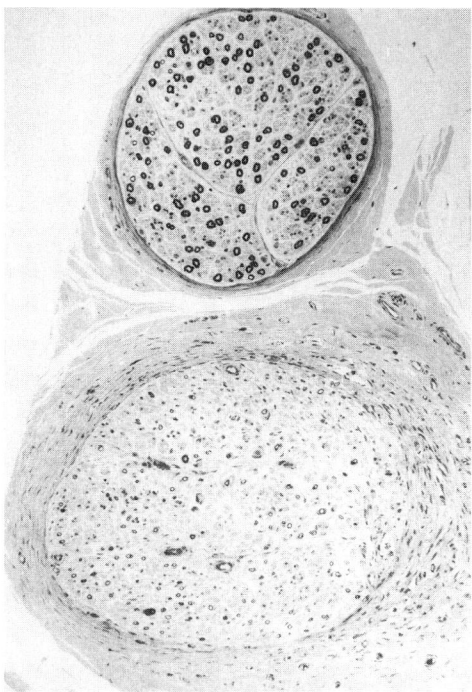

Fig. 28-147 Sural nerve. Diabetic neuropathy. Minineuroma resulting from focal ischemic damage to nerve fascicle. (Plastic.)

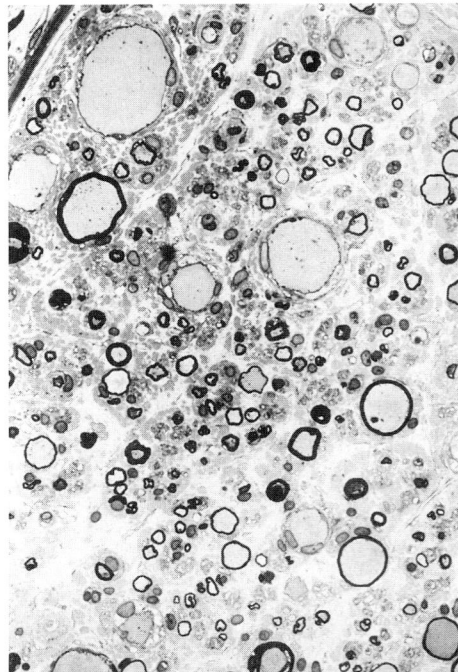

Fig. 28-148 Sural nerve. Giant axonal neuropathy. Numerous enlarged axons are surrounded by attenuated myelin sheaths or are devoid of myelin. (Plastic.)

28-114, *B*), *Pompe's disease,*[141,153] *primary hyperoxaluria,*[142] *Refsum's disease* (abundant though nonspecific paracrystalline inclusions in Schwann cells),[152] *Tangier disease* (lipid droplets and pleomorphic inclusions in the cytoplasm of Schwann cells),[151,157,162] *vincristine toxicity,*[143,165] *Wolman's disease,*[146] and *xanthomatous neuropathy in primary biliary cirrhosis.*[171]

REFERENCES

1 Bischoff A: The peripheral nerves. In Johannessen JV, ed: Electron microscopy in human medicine, vol 6, Nervous system, sensory organs, and respiratory tract. New York, 1979, McGraw-Hill.
2 Dyck PJ, Oviatt KF, Lambert EH: Intensive evaluation of referred unclassified neuropathies yields improved diagnosis. Ann Neurol 10:222-226, 1981.
3 Fagius J: Chronic cryptogenic polyneuropathy. The search for a cause. Acta Neurol Scand 67:173-180, 1983.
4 Hall SM, Hughes RA, Atkinson PF, McColl I, Gale A: Motor nerve biopsy in severe Guillain-Barré syndrome. Ann Neurol 31:441-444, 1992.
5 McLeod JG, Pollard JD, Cameron J, Walsh JC: Chronic polyneuropathy of undetermined cause. J Neurol Neurosurg Psychiatry 47:530-535, 1984.

NORMAL ANATOMY

6 Ariza A, Bilbao JM, Rosai J: Immunohistochemical detection of epithelial membrane antigen in normal perineurial cells and perineurioma. Am J Surg Pathol 12:678-683, 1988.
7 Asbury AK, Johnson PC: Pathology of peripheral nerve. In Bennington JL, ed: Major problems in pathology, vol 9. Philadelphia, 1978, WB Saunders.
8 Behse F: Morphometric studies on the human sural nerve. Acta Neurol Scand Suppl 132:1-38, 1990.
9 Behse F, Buchtal F, Carlsen F, Knappeis GG: Endoneurial space and its constituents in the sural nerve of patients with neuropathy. Brain 97:773-784, 1974.
10 Bunge MB, Bunge RP. Linkage between Schwann cell extracellular matrix production and ensheathment function. Ann NY Acad Sci 486:241-247, 1986.
11 Burkel WE: The histological fine structure of perineurium. Anat Rec 158:177-189, 1967.

12 Dziadek M, Edgar D, Paulsson M, Timpl R, Fleischmajer R: Basement membrane proteins produced by Schwann cells and in neurofibromatosis. Ann NY Acad Sci 486:248-259, 1986.
13 Gray F, Gherardi R, Marshall A, Janota I, Poirier J: Adult polyglucosan body disease (APBD). J Neuropathol Exp Neurol 47:459-474, 1988.
14 Griffin JW, George R, Ho T: Macrophage systems in peripheral nerves. A review. J Neuropathol Exp Neurol 52:553-560, 1993.
15 Haust Daria M: Fine fibrils of extracellular space (microfibrils), their structure and role in connective tissue organization. Am J Pathol 47:1113-1136, 1965.
16 Mugnaini E, Osen KK, Schnapp B, Friedrich VL Jr: Distribution of Schwann cell cytoplasm and plasmalemmal vesicles (caveolae) in peripheral myelin sheaths. An electron microscopic study with thin sections and freeze fracturing. J Neurocytol 6:647-648, 1977.
17 Ochoa J, Mair WG: The normal sural nerve in man. I. Ultrastructure and numbers of fibres and cells. Acta Neuropathol 13:197-216, 1969.
18 Ochoa J, Mair WG: The normal sural nerve in man. II.- Changes in the axons and Schwann cells due to aging. Acta Neuropathol 13:217-239, 1969.
19 Olsson Y, Reese TS: Permeability of vasa nervorum and perineurium in mouse sciatic nerve studied by fluorescence and electron microscopy. J Neuropathol Exp Neurol 30:105-119, 1971.
20 Sanes JR: Analyzing cell lineage with a recombinant retrovirus. Trends Neurosci 12:21-28, 1989.
21 Shanta TR, Bourne GH: The perineurial epithelium — a new concept. In Bourne GH, ed: The structure and function of nervous tissue. Structure I. New York, 1968, Academic Press.
22 Sunderland S: Nerve and nerve injuries, ed 2. New York, 1978, Churchill Livingstone.
23 Tohgi H, Tsukagoshi H, Toyokura Y: Quantitative changes with age in normal sural nerves. Acta Neuropathol 38:213-220, 1977.
24 Tomonaga M, Sluga E: Zur ultrastruktur der pi-granula. Acta Neuropathol 15:56-69, 1970.
25 Weis J, Alexianu ME, Heide G, Schroder JM: Renaut bodies contain elastic fiber components. J Neuropathol Exp Neurol 52:444-451, 1993.

BASIC PATHOLOGIC MECHANISMS

26 Asbury AK, Johnson PC: Pathology of peripheral nerve. In Bennington JL, ed: Major problems in pathology, vol 9. Philadelphia, 1978, W.B. Saunders.
27 Beuche W, Friede RL: The role of non-resident cells in Wallerian degeneration. J Neurocytol 13:767-796, 1984.
28 Cavanagh JB: The "dying-back" process. A common denominator in many naturally occurring and toxic neuropathies. Arch Pathol Lab Med 103:659-664, 1979.
29 Heumann R, Lindholm D, Bandtlow C, et al: Differential regulation of MRNA encoding nerve growth factor and its receptor in rat sciatic nerve during development, degeneration, and regeneration. Role of macrophages. Proc Natl Acad Sci USA 84:8735-8739, 1987.
30 Johnson FM Jr, Taniuchi M, DiStefano PS: Expression and possible function of nerve growth factor receptors on Schwann cells. Trends Neurosci 11:299-304, 1988.
31 Lubinska L: Patterns of wallerian degeneration of myelinated fibres in short and long peripheral stumps and in isolated segments of rat phrenic nerve. Interpretation of the role of axoplasmic flow of the trophic factor. Brain Res 233:227-240, 1982.
32 Malbouisson AM, Ghabriel MN, Allt G: The non-directional pattern of axonal changes in wallerian degeneration. A computer-aided morphometric analysis. J Anat 139:159-174, 1984.
33 Spencer PS, Schaumburg HH: Central-peripheral distal axonopathy. The pathology of dying-back polyneuropathies. Prog Neuropathol 3:253-295, 1976.
34 Weller RO: Diphtheritic neuropathy in the chicken, an electron microscopic study. J Pathol Bacteriol 89:591-598, 1965.

NEUROPATHIES
Inherited neuropathy

35 Behse F, Buchthal F, Carlsen F, Knappeis GG: Hereditary neuropathy with liability to pressure palsies. Electrophysiological and histopathological aspects. Brain 95:777-794, 1972.
36 Benz HU, Harzer K. Metachromatic reaction of pseudoisocyanine with sulfatides in metachromatic leukodystrophy. I. Technical and histochemical staining. Acta Neuropathol 27:177-180, 1974.
37 Berciano J, Combarros O, Figols J, Calleja J, Cabello A, Silos I, Coria F: Hereditary motor and sensory neuropathy type II. Clinicopathological study of a family. Brain 109:897-914, 1986.
38 Bischoff A, Ulrich J: Peripheral neuropathy in globoid cell leukodystrophy (Krabbe's disease). Ultrastructural and histochemical findings. Brain 92:861-870, 1969.

39 Chance PF, Alderson MK, Leppig KA, Lensch MW, Matsunami N, Smith B, Swanson PD, Odelberg SJ, Disteche CM, Bird TD: DNA deletion associated with hereditary neuropathy with liability to pressure palsies. Cell **72:**143-151, 1993.

40 Desnick RJ, Bishop DF: Fabry disease. Alpha galactosidase deficiency. Schindler disease. Alpha-*N*-acetyl galactosaminidase deficiency. In Scriver CR, Beaudet AL, Sly WS, Valle D, eds: The metabolic basis of inherited disease. New York, 1989, McGraw-Hill.

41 Gabreels-Festen A, Gabreels F: Hereditary demyelinating motor and sensory neuropathy. Brain Pathol **3:**135-146, 1993.

42 Guzzetta F, Ferriere G, Lyon G: Congenital hypomyelination polyneuropathy. Pathological findings compared with polyneuropathies starting later in life. Brain **105:**395-416, 1982.

43 Hahn AF: Hereditary motor and sensory neuropathy. HMSN type 11 (neuronal type and X-linked HMSN. Brain Pathol **3:**147-155, 1993.

44 Hoogendijk JE, De Visser M, Bolhuis PA, Hart AAM, Ongerboer De Visser BM: Hereditary motor and sensory neuropathy type I. Clinical and neurographical features of the 17 p duplication subtype. Muscle Nerve **17:**85-90, 1994.

45 Madrid R, Bradley WG: The pathology of neuropathies with focal thickening of the myelin sheath (tomaculous neuropathy). J Neurol Sci **25:**415-448, 1975.

46 Madrid R, Bradley WG, Davis CJ: The peroneal muscular atrophy syndrome. Clinical, genetic, electrophysiological and nerve biopsy studies. Part 2. Observations on pathological changes in sural nerve biopsies. J Neurol Sci **32:**91-122, 1977.

47 Ouvrier RA, McLeod JG, Conchin TE: The hypertrophic forms of hereditary motor and sensory neuropathy. A study of hypertrophic Charcot-Marie-Tooth disease (HMSN type I) and Dejerine-Sottas disease (HMSN type III) in childhood. Brain **110 :**121-148, 1987.

48 Ouvrier RA, McLeod JG, Morgan GJ, Wise GA, Conchin TE: Hereditary motor and sensory neuropathy of neuronal type with onset in early childhood. J Neurol Sci **51:**181-197, 1981.

49 Pellissier JF, Van Hoof F, Bourdet-Bonerandi D, Monier-Faugere MC, Toga M: Morphological and biochemical changes in muscle and peripheral nerve in Fabry's disease. Muscle Nerve **4:**381-387, 1981.

50 Smith TW, Bhawan J, Keller RB, DeGirolami U: Charcot-Marie-Tooth disease associated with hypertrophic neuropathy. A neuropathologic study of two cases. J Neuropathol Exp Neurol **39:**420-440, 1980.

51 Suzuki K, Suzuki Y: Galactosylceramide lipidosis. Globoid-cell leukodystrophy (Krabbe disease). In Scriver CR, Beaudet AL, Sly WS, Valle D, eds: The metabolic basis of inherited disease. New York, 1989, McGraw-Hill.

52 Suter U, Welcher AA, Snipes GJ: Progress in the molecular understanding of hereditary peripheral neuropathies reveals new insights into the biology of the peripheral nervous system. Trends Neurosci **16:**50-56, 1993.

53 Thomas PK, King RH, Kocen RS, Brett EM: Comparative ultrastructural observations on peripheral nerve abnormalities in the late infantile, juvenile and late onset forms of metachromatic leukodystrophy. Acta Neuropathol **39:**237-245, 1977.

54 Yoshikawa 11, Nishimura T, Nakatsuji Y, Fujimura H, Himoro M, Hayasaka K, Sakoda S, Yanagihara T: Elevated expression of messenger RNA for peripheral myelin protein 22 in biopsied peripheral nerves of patients with Chacot-Marie-Tooth disease type 1A. Ann Neurol **35:**445-450, 1994.

Inflammatory neuropathy

55 Asbury AK, Arnason BG, Adams RD: The inflammatory lesion in idiopathic polyneuritis. Its role in pathogenesis. Medicine **48:**173-215, 1969.

56 Brochet B, Louiset P, Lagueny A, Coquet M, Vital C, Loiseau P: Neuropathie peripherique revelatrice d'une sarcoidose. Rev Neurol **144:**590-595, 1988.

57 Cornblath D. McArthur JC, Kennedy PG, Witte AS, Griffin JW: Inflammatory demyelinating peripheral neuropathies associated with human T-cell lymphotropic virus type III infection. Ann Neurol **21:**32-40, 1987.

58 Cusimano MD, Bilbao JM, Cohen SM: Hypertrophic brachial plexus neuritis. A pathological study of two cases. Ann Neurol **24:**615-622, 1988.

59 Dalakas MC, Pezeshkpour GH: Neuromuscular diseases associated with human immunodeficiency virus infection. Ann Neurol **23** (Suppl):S38-S48, 1988.

60 Dyck PJ: Is there an axonal variety of GBS? Neurology **43:**1277-1280, 1993.

61 Gabreels-Festen AAWM, Gabreels FJM, Hoogendijk DA, Bolhuis PA, Jongen PJH, Vingerhoets HM: Chronic inflammatory demyelinating polyneuropathy or hereditary motor and sensory neuropathy? Diagnostic value of morphological criteria. Acta Neuropathol **86:**630-635, 1993.

62 Guberman A, Rosenbaum H, Braciale T, Schlaepfer WW: Human neurolymphomatosis. J Neurol Sci **36:**1-12, 1978.

63 Hall SM, Hughes RA, Atkinson PF, McColl I, Gale A: Motor nerve biopsy in severe Guillain-Barré syndrome. Ann Neurol **31:**441-444, 1992.

64 Harris CP, Sigman JD, Jaeckle KA: Intravascular malignant lymphomatosis. Amelioration of neurological symptoms with plasmapheresis. Ann Neurol **35:**357-359, 1994.

65 Heiman-Patterson TD, Bird SJ, Parry Gi, Varga J, Shy ME, Culligan NW, Edelsohn L, Tatarian GT, Heyes MP, Garcia CA, Tahmoush AJ: Peripheral neuropathy associated with eosinophilia-myalgia syndrome. Ann Neurol **28:**522-528, 1990.

66 Hughes R, Atkinson P, Coates P, Hall S, Leibowitz S: Sural nerve biopsies in Guillain-Barré syndrome. Axonal degeneration and macrophage-associated demyelination and absence of cytomegalovirus genome. Muscle Nerve **15:**568-575, 1992.

67 Krendel DA, Parks HP, Anthony DC, St. Clair MB, Graham DG: Sural nerve biopsy in chronic inflammatory demyelinating polyradiculoneuropathy. Muscle Nerve **12:**257-264, 1989.

68 Lewis RA, Sumner AJ, Brown MJ, Asbury AK: Multifocal demyelinating neuropathy with persistent conduction block. Neurology **32:**958-964, 1982.

69 van der Meche, FG, Schmitz PI, and the Dutch Guillain-Barré Study Group: A randomized trial comparing intravenous immune globulin and plasma exchange in Guillain-Barré syndrome. N Eng J Med **326:**1123-1129, 1992.

70 Meier C, Grahmann F, Engelhardt A, Dumas M: Peripheral nerve disorders in Lyme-borreliosis. Nerve biopsy studies from eight cases. Acta Neuropathol **79:**271-278, 1989.

71 Nemni R, Galassi G, Cohen M, Hays AP, Gould R, Singh N, Bressman S, Gamboa ET: Symmetric sarcoid polyneuropathy. Analysis of a sural nerve biopsy. Neurology **31:**1217-1223, 1981.

72 Oh SJ: Sarcoid polyneuropathy. A histologically proved case. Ann Neurol **7:**178-181, 1980.

73 Lange DJ: Neuromuscular diseases associated with HIV-1 infection. Muscle Nerve **17:**16-30, 1994.

74 Prineas JW: Pathology of the Guillain-Barré syndrome. Ann Neurol **9**(Suppl):6-19, 1981.

75 Prineas JW, McLeod JG: Chronic relapsing polyneuritis. J Neurol Sci **27:**427-458, 1976.

76 Reske-Nielsen E, Harmsen A: Periangiitis and panangiitis as a manifestation of sarcoidosis of the brain. Report of a case. J Nerve Ment Dis **135:**399-412, 1962.

77 Ricoy JR, Cabello A, Rodriguez J, Tellez I: Neuropathological studies on the toxic syndrome related to adulterated rapeseed oil in Spain. Brain **106:**817-835, 1983.

78 Said G, Lacroix C, Andrieu JM, Leibowitch J: Necrotizing arteritis in patients with inflammatory neuropathy and immunodeficiency virus (HIV-III) infection. Neurology **37**(Suppl I):176, 1987.

79 Said G, Lacroix C, Chemouilli P, Goulon-Goeau C, Roullet E, Penaud D, de Broucker T, Meduri G, Vincent D, Torchet M, Vittcoq D, Leport C, Vilde JL: Cytomegalovirus neuropathy in acquired immunodeficiency syndrome. A clinical and pathological study. Ann Neurol **29:**139-146, 1991.

80 Silverstein A, Siltzbach LE, et al: Muscle involvement in sarcoidosis. Asymptomatic, myositis, and myopathy. Arch Neurol **21:**235-241, 1969.

81 Stern BJ, Krumholz A, John C, Scott P, Nissim J: Sarcoidosis and its neurological manifestations. Arch Neurol **42:**909-917, 1985.

82 Thomas FP, Vallejos U, Foitl DR: B cell small lymphocytic lymphoma and chronic lymphocytic leukemia with peripheral neuropathy. Two cases with neuropathological findings and lymphocyte marker analysis. Acta Neuropathol **80:**198-203, 1990.

83 Vital C, Aubertin J, Ragnault JM, Amigues H, Mouton L, Bellance R: Sarcoidosis of the peripheral nerve. A histological and ultrastructural study of two cases. Acta Neuropathol **58:**111-114, 1982.

Leprous neuritis

84 Finlayson MH, Bilbao JM, Lough JO: The pathogenesis of the neuropathy in dimorphous leprosy. Electron microscopic and cytochemical studies. J Neuropathol Exp Neurol **33:**446-455, 1974.

85 Haimanot RT, Mshana RN, McDougall AC, Andersen JO: Sural nerve biopsy in leprosy patients after varying periods of treatment. Histopathological and bacteriological findings on light microscopy. Int J Lepr **52:**163-170, 1984.

86 Jacob M, Mathai R: Diagnostic efficacy of cutaneous nerve biopsy in primary neuritic leprosy. Int J Lepr Other Myobact Dis **56:**56-60, 1988.

87 Job CK, Desikan KV: Pathologic changes and their distribution in peripheral nerves in lepromatous leprosy. Int J Lepr **36:**257-270, 1968.

88 Kaplan G: Recent advances in cytokine therapy in leprosy. J Infect Dis **167** (Suppl 1):S18-22, 1993.

89 Kaur G. Girdhar BK, Girdhar A, Malaviya ON, Mukherjee A, Sengupta V, Desikan KV: A clinical, immunological, and histological study of neuritic leprosy patients. Int J Lepr Other Mycobact Dis **59:**385-391, 1991.

90 Nishimura M, Kwon KS, Shibuta K, Yoshikawa Y, Oh CK, Suzuki T, Chung TA, Hori Y: An improved method for DNA diagnosis of leprosy using formaldehyde-fixed, paraffin embedded skin biopsies. Mod Pathol 7:253-256, 1994.

91 Ohenhoff TH, DeVrieS RR: HLA class II immune response and supression genes in leprosy. Int J Lepr Other Mycobact Dis 55:521-534, 1987.

92 Pearson JM, Ross WF: Nerve involvement in leprosy: Pathology, differential diagnosis and principles of management. Lepr Rev 46:199-212, 1975.

93 Ridley DS: Skin biopsy in leprosy. Histological interpretation and clinical application. Basel, 1977, Ciba-Geigy Limited.

94 Ridley DS: Pathogenesis of leprosy and related diseases. London, 1988, Wright.

95 Ridley DS, Ridley MJ: Classification of nerves is modified by the delayed recognition of Mycobacterium leprae. Int J Lepr 54:596-606, 1986.

96 Shields ED, Russell DA, Pericak-Vance MA: Genetic epidemiology of the susceptibility to leprosy. J Clin Invest 79:1139-1143, 1987.

97 Williams DL, Gillis TP, Booth RJ, Looker D, Watson JD: The use of a specific DNA probe and polymerase chain reaction for the detection of Mycobacterium leprae. J Infect Dis 162:193-200, 1990.

Vasculitis

98 Churg J, Strauss L: Allergic granulomatosis, allergic angitis, and periarteritis nodosa. Am J Pathol 27:277-301, 1951

99 Cohen RD, Conn DL, Ilstrup DM: Clinical features, prognosis, and response to treatment in polyarteritis. Mayo Clin Proc 55:146-155, 1980.

100 Dyck PJ, Benstead TJ, Conn DL, et al: Nonsystemic vasculitic neuropathy. Brain 110:843-854, 1987.

101 Hawke SH, Davies L, Pamphlett R, Guo YD, Pollard JD, McLeod JG: Vasculitic neuropathy. A clinical and pathological study. Brain 114:2175-2190, 1991.

102 Kissel JT, Mendell JR: Vasculitic neuropathy. In Dyck PJ, ed: Peripheral neuropathy. New concepts and treatments. Neurol Clin 10:761-781, 1992.

103 Kissel TJ, Riethman JL, Omerza J, Rammohan KW, Mendell JR: Peripheral nerve vasculitis. Immune characterization of the vascular lesions. Ann Neurol 25:291-297, 1989.

104 Lanham JG, Churg J: Churg-Strauss syndrome. In Churg A, Churg J, eds: Systemic vasculitides. New York, 1991, Igaku-Shoin Medical.

105 Oh SJ, Slaughter R, Harrell L: Paraneoplastic vasculitic neuropathy. A treatable neuropathy. Muscle Nerve 14:152-156, 1991.

106 Said G, Lacroix-Ciaudo C, Fujimura H, Blas C, Faux N: The peripheral neuropathy of necrotizing arteritis. A clinicopathological study. Ann Neurol 23:461-465, 1988.

107 Wees SJ, Sunwoo IN, Oh SJ: Sural nerve biopsy in systemic necrotizing vasculitis. Am J Med 71:525-532, 1981.

Amyloidosis

108 Benson MD: Familial amyloidotic polyneuropathy. Trends Neurosci 12:88-92, 1989.

109 Clanet M, Mansat M, Durroux R, Testut MF, Guiraud B, Rascol A, Conte J: Syndrome du canal carpien, tenosynovite amyloide et hemodialyse periodique. Rev Neurol 137:613-624, 1981.

110 Dalakas M, Cunningham G: Characterization of amyloid deposits in biopsies of 15 patients with "sporadic" (non-familial or plasma cell dyscrasia) amyloid polyneuropathy. Acta Neuropathol 69:66-72, 1986.

111 Gagnon RF, Lough JO, Bourgouin PA: Carpal tunnel syndrome and amyloidosis associated with continuous ambulatory peritoneal dialysis. Can Med Assoc J 139:753-755, 1988.

112 Gorevic PD, Munoz PC, Casey TT, DiRaimondo CR, Stone WJ, Prelli FC, et al: Polymerization of intact beta 2-microglobulin in tissue causes amyloidosis in patients on chronic hemodialysis. Proc Natl Acad Sci USA 83:7908-7912, 1986.

113 Hanyu N, Ikeda S, Nakadai A, Yanagisawa N, Powell HC: Peripheral nerve pathological findings in familial amyloid polyneuropathy. A correlative study of proximal sciatic nerve and sural nerve lesions. Ann Neurol 25:340-350, 1989.

114 Ikeda S, Hanyu N, Hongo M, Yoshioka J, Oguchi H, et al: Hereditary generalized amyloidosis with polyneuropathy. A clinicopathological study of 65 Japanese patients. Brain 110:315-337, 1987.

115 Li K, Kyle RA, Dyck PJ: Immunohistochemical characterization of amyloid proteins in sural nerves and clinical associations in amyloid neuropathy. Am J Pathol 141:217-226, 1992.

116 Murakami T, Yi S, Yamamoto K, Maruyama S, Araki S: Familial amyloidotic polyneuropathy. Report of patients heterozygous for the transthyretin Gly42 gene. Ann Neurol 31:340-342, 1992.

117 Sunada Y, Shimizu T, Nakase H, Shigeo O, Asaoka T, Amano S, Sawa M, Kagawa Y, Karasawa I, Mannen T: Inherited amyloid polyneuropathy type IV (Gelsolin variant) in a Japanese family. Ann Neurol 33:57-62, 1993.

118 Takahashi K, Yi S, Kimura Y, Araki S: Familial amyloidotic polyneuropathy type I in Kumamoto, Japan. A clinicopathologic, histochemical, immunohistochemical, and ultrastructural study. Hum Pathol 22:519-527, 1991.

119 Waldrop FS, Puchtler H, Valentine LS: Fluorescent microscopy of amyloid. Arch Pathol 95:37-44, 1973.

Neuropathy of dysproteinemia

120 Scully RE, ed: Case records of the Massachussetts General Hospital #21-1993. N Engl J Med 328:l550-1558, 1993.

121 Chad D, Pariser K, Bradley WG, Adelman LS, Pinn VW: The pathogenesis of cryoglobulinemic neuropathy. Neurology 32:725-729, 1982.

122 Feiner HD: Pathology of dysproteinemia. Light chain amyloidosis, nonamyloid immunoglobulin deposition disease, cryoglobulinemia syndromes, and macroglobulinemia of Waldenström. Hum Pathol 19:1255-1272, 1988.

123 Jay V, Bilbao JM: Peripheral neuropathy associated with monoclonal gammopathy. Anatomic Pathology II, APII 91-6 (APII-174), 15, 1991.

124 Kelly JJ, Kyle RA, Latov N: Polyneuropathies associated with plasma cell dyscrasia. Boston, 1987, Martinus Nijhoff.

125 Meier C, Vandevelde M, Steck A. Zurbriggen A: Demyelinating polyneuropathy associated with monoclonal IgM-paraproteinaemia. J Neurol Sci 63:353-367, 1983.

126 Mendell JR, Sahenk Z, Whitaker JN, Trapp BD, Yates AJ, Griggs RC, Quarles RH: Polyneuropathy and IgM monoclonal gammopathy. Studies on the pathogenetic role of anti-myelin-associated glycoprotein antibody. Ann Neurol 17:243-254, 1985.

127 Smith IS, Kahn SM, Lacey BW: Chronic demyelinating neuropathy associated with benign IgM paraproteinemia. Brain 106:169-195, 1983

128 Vallat JM, Desproges-Gotteron R, Leboutet MJ, Loubet A, Gualde N, Treves R: Cryoglobulinemic neuropathy. A pathological study. Ann Neurol 8:179-185, 1980.

129 Vital A, Vital C, Ragnaud JM, Baquey A, Aubertin J: IgM cryoglobulin deposits in the peripheral nerve. Virchows Arch [A] 418:83-85, 1991.

130 Vital C, Vallat JM, Deminiere C, Loubet A, Leboutet MJ: Peripheral nerve damage during multiple myeloma and Waldenström's macroglobulinemia. An ultrastructural and immunopathologic study. Cancer 50:1491-1497. 1982.

Toxic-metabolic neuropathy

131 Bilbao JM, Briggs SJ, Gray TA: Filamentous axonopathy in disulfiram neuropathy. Ultrastruct Pathol 7:295-300, 1984.

131a Chaudhry V, Rowinsky EK, Sartorius SE, Donehower R, Cornblath DR: Peripheral neuropathy from taxol and cisplatin combination chemotherapy. Clinical and electrophysiological studies. Ann Neurol 35:304-311, 1994.

132 Jacobs JM, Costa-Jussa FR: The pathology of amiodarone neurotoxicity. II. Peripheral neuropathy in man. Brain 108:753-769, 1985.

133 Melgaard B, Hansen HS, Kamieniecka Z, Paulson OB, Pedersen AG, Tang X, Trojaborg W: Misonidazole neuropathy. A clinical, electrophysiological, and histological study. Ann Neurol 12:10-17, 1982.

134 Pellissier JF, Pouget J, Cros D, De Victor B, Serratrice G, Toga M: Peripheral neuropathy induced by amiodarone chlorhydrate. A clinicopathological study. J Neurosci 63:251-266, 1984.

135 Said G: Perhexiline neuropathy. A clinicopathological study. Ann Neurol 3:259-266, 1978.

136 Shields RW Jr: Alcoholic polyneuropathy. Muscle Nerve 8:l83-187, 1985.

137 Spencer PS, Schaumburg HH, eds: Experimental and clinical neurotoxicology. Baltimore, 1980, Williams & Wilkins.

138 Thorner PS, Bilbao JM, Sima AA, Briggs S: Porphyric neuropathy. An ultrastructural and quantitative case study. Can J Neurol Sci 8:281-287, 1981.

139 Tredici G, Minazzi M: Alcoholic neuropathy. An electron-microscopic study. J Neurol Sci 25:333-346, 1975.

Other neuropathies

140 Anzil AP, Blinzinger K, Mehraein P, Dozic S: Niemann-Pick case report with ultrastructural findings. Neuropaediatrie 4:207-225, 1973.

141 Araoz C, Sun CN, Shenefelt R. White HJ: Glycogenosis type II (Pompe's disease). Ultrastructure of peripheral nerves. Neurology 24:739-742, 1974.

142 Bilbao JM, Berry H, Marotta J, Ross RC: Peripheral neuropathy in oxalosis. A case report with electron microscopic observations. Can J Neurol Sci 3:63-67, 1976.

143 Bradley WG, Lassman LP, Pearce GW, Walton JN: The neuromyopathy of vincristine in man. Clinical, electrophysiological and pathological studies. J Neurol Sci 10:107-131, 1970.

144 Brown MJ, Asbury AK: Diabetic neuropathy. Ann Neurol 15:2-12, 1984.

145 Busard HL, Gabreels-Festen AA, van't Hof MA, Renier WO, Gabreels FJ: Polyglucosan bodies in sural nerve biopsies. Acta Neuropathol **80**:554-557, 1990.

146 Byrd JC, Powers JM: Wolman's disease. Ultrastructural evidence of lipid accumulation in central and peripheral nervous system. Acta Neuropathol **45**:37-42, 1979.

147 Cafferty MS, Lovelace RE, Hays AP, Servidei S, Dimauro S, Rowland LP: Polyglucosan body disease. Muscle Nerve **14**:102-107, 1991.

148 Carpenter S, Karpati G, Andermann F, Gold R: Giant axonal neuropathy. A clinically and morphologically distinct neurological disease. Arch Neurol **31**:312-316, 1974.

149 Carpenter S, Karpati G, Andermann F, Jacob JC, Andermann E: The ultrastructural characteristics of the abnormal cytosomes in Batten-Kuf's disease. Brain **100**:137-156, 1977.

150 Donaghy M, King RH, Thomas PK, Workman JM: Abnormalities of the axonal cytoskeleton in giant axonal neuropathy. J Neurocytol **17**:197-208, 1988.

151 Dyck PJ, Ellefson RD, Yao JK, Herbert PN: Adult-onset Tangier disease. Morphometric and pathologic studies suggesting delayed degradation of neutral lipids after fiber degeneration. J Neuropathol Exp Neurol **37**:119-137, 1978.

152 Fardeau M, Abelanet R, Laudat P, Bonduelle M: Maladie de Refsum. Etude histologique, ultrastructurale et biochimique d'une biopsie de nerf peripherique. Rev Neurol **122**:185-196, 1970.

153 Gambetti P, DiMauro S, Baker L: Nervous system in Pompe's disease. Ultrastructure and biochemistry. J Neuropathol Exp Neurol **30**:412-430, 1971.

154 Gumbinas M, Larsen M, Mei Liu H: Peripheral neuropathy in classic Niemann-Pick disease. Ultrastructure of nerves and skeletal muscles. Neurology **25**:107-113, 1975.

155 Johnson PC: Diabetic neuropathy. In Adachi M, Hirano A, Aronson SM, eds: The pathology of the myelinated axon. New York, 1985, Igaku-Shoin.

156 Joosten E, Gabreels F, Stadhouders A, Bolmers D, Gabreels-Festen A: Involvement of sural nerve in neuronal ceroid-lipofuscinoses. Report of two cases. Neuropaediatrie **4**:98-110, 1973.

157 Kocen RS, King RH, Thomas PK, Haas LF: Nerve biopsy findings in two cases of Tangier disease. Acta Neuropathol **26**:317-327, 1973.

158 Kristensson K, Olsson Y, Sourander P: Peripheral nerve changes in Tay-Sachs and Batten-Spielmeyer-Vogt disease. Acta Pathol Microbiol Scand **70**:630-632, 1967.

159 Lockman LA, Kennedy WR, White JG: The Chediak-Higashi syndrome. Electrophysiological and electron microscopic observations on the peripheral neuropathy. J Pediatr **70**:942-951, 1967.

160 Misra VP, King RH, Harding AE, Muddle JR, Thomas PK: Peripheral neuropathy in the Chediak-Higashi syndrome. Acta Neuropathol **81**:354-358, 1991.

161 Ohnishi A, Yamashita Y, Goto I, Kuriowa Y, Murakami S, Ikeda M: De- and remyelination and onion bulb in cerebrotendinous xanthomatosis. Acta Neuropathol **45**:43-45, 1979.

162 Pollock M, Nukada H, Frith RW, Simcock JP, Allpress S: Peripheral neuropathy in Tangier disease. Brain **106**:911-928, 1983.

163 Powers JM, Schaumburg HH: Adreno-leukodystrophy. Similar ultrastructural changes in adrenal cortical and Schwann cells. Arch Neurol **302**:406-408, 1974.

164 Probst A, Ulrich J, Heitz PU, Herschkowitz N: Adrenomyeloneuropathy. A protracted pseudosystematic variant of adrenoleukodystrophy. Acta Neuropathol **49**:105-115, 1980.

165 Sahenk Z, Brady ST, Mendell JR: Studies on the pathogenesis of vincristine-induced neuropathy. Muscle Nerve **10**:80-84, 1987.

166 Said G, Goulon-Goeau C, Lacroix C, Moulonguet A: Nerve biopsy findings in different patterns of proximal diabetic neuropathy. Ann Neurol **35**:559-569, 1994.

167 Said G, Goulon-Goeau C, Slama G, Tchobroutsky G: Severe early-onset polyneuropathy in insulin-dependent diabetes mellitus. A clinical and pathological study. N Engl J Med **326**:1257-1263, 1992.

168 Sugimura K, Dyck PJ: Multifocal fiber loss in proximal sciatic nerve in symmetric distal diabetic neuropathy. J Neurol Sci **53**:501-509, 1982.

169 Tegner R, Tome FM, Godeau P, Lhermitte F, Fardeau M: Morphological study of peripheral nerve changes induced by chloroquine treatment. Acta Neuropathol **75**:253-260, 1988.

170 Thomas PK, King RH, Chiang TR, Scaravilli F, Sharma AK, Downie AW: Neurofibromatous neuropathy. Muscle Nerve **13**:93-101, 1990.

171 Thomas PK, Walker JG: Xanthomatous neuropathy in primary biliary cirrhosis. Brain **88**:1079-1088, 1965.

172 Vital A, Vital C, Ellie E, Ferrer X, Lagueny A, Ferrer AM, Broustet A, Gbikpi-Benissan G: Malignant infiltration of peripheral nerves in the course of acute myelomonoblastic leukemia—neuropathological study of two cases. Neuropathol Appl Neurobiol **19**:159-163, 1993.

173 Vital C, Battin J, Rivel J, Hehunstre JP: Aspects ultrastructuraux des lesions du nerf peripherique dans un cas de malade de Farber. Rev Neurol **132**:419-423, 1976.

174 Vos AJ, Joosten EM, Gabreels-Festen AA: Adult polyglucosan body disease. Clinical and nerve biopsy findings in two cases. Ann Neurol **13**:440-444, 1983.

Skeletal muscle

L.C. Ang, M.B.

J.M. Bilbao, M.D.

Skeletal muscle biopsy is essential for the diagnosis of diseases of the motor unit and for some systemic conditions such as polyarteritis nodosa and amyloidosis (see peripheral nerve section of this chapter). When interpreting a muscle biopsy, the pathologist must have knowledge of the patient's clinical history, physical examination findings, and results of salient laboratory tests such as EMG, nerve conduction, and serum creatinine phosphokinase. The biopsy site should be selected from a muscle that is moderately involved by the disease and not from a muscle that is so severely affected that all that is left is fat and fibrous tissue with only a few scattered atrophic myofibers.[2] Conversely, a biopsy specimen from a muscle that is minimally involved will show hardly any diagnostic changes. Preferably, the physician ordering the biopsy should indicate a site for the procedure on the request form. A muscle that has been previously traumatized, for instance by EMG needles, should be avoided. Interpretation is easier if biopsies are taken consistently from the same muscles (e.g., from the biceps brachialis in the upper limbs and the quadriceps brachialis in the lower limbs). Equally important is that the biopsy be taken from the belly of the muscle and not at the tendon insertion where there are features that simulate myopathic changes, such as increased number of internal nuclei, variability of myofiber size, and endomysial fibrosis.

The biopsy has to be performed with great care and the least amount of trauma, and the size of tissue sample must be sufficient for cryostat sectioning and resin and paraffin embedding. The specimen (about $1 \times 0.5 \times 0.5$ cm in size) selected for cyrostat preparation should be oriented for transverse sectioning and is "quench" frozen in liquid nitrogen–isopentane. Ice crystal growth with vacuolation of sarcoplasm is a common artefact in muscle biopsy and is due to improper freezing technique.[1] Serial cryostat sections are prepared routinely for the following stains: hematoxylin-eosin, Congo red, modified Gomori trichrome,[3] NADH-TR, PAS, Oil red O, and ATPase preincubated at pH 9.4, 4.6, and 4.3. Transverse and longitudinal sections of muscle are obtained from both paraffin and plastic resin blocks.

NORMAL ANATOMY

The transverse sections of muscle fascicle show polygonal myofibers fitting snugly against each other with little endomysial connective tissue in between. The *myocyte* is a syncytial element with the nuclei located subsarcolemally. Up to 7% of muscle fibers in the adult muscle may show internalization of the nuclei. Satellite cells display scanty cytoplasm and are seen closely applied to the periphery of the myofibers.[6] Ultrastructurally, these reserve cells lie between the plasma membrane and the basal lamina of the myofiber. The diameter of individual fibers can vary from 20 to 50 µm. The larger fibers are found in adult males in proximal muscles and in muscles subjected to prolonged exercise. The fascicle is wrapped by a layer of collagen tissue known as a *perimysium* where the arterioles, venules, and nerve bundles are located. Muscle spindles consisting of smaller-diameter striated myofibers covered with fibrous capsule are occasionally seen in the perimysium. A number of fascicles are in turn bound by the epimysium in which the larger vessels and nerves are present. Capillaries in the endomysial connective tissue average one to two per muscle fiber. In the longitudinal section, the fascicular arrangement of the myofiber is not apparent, but the cross striations of the fibers are well visualized.

Ultrastructurally, the *myofibril*, a major component of each individual fiber, is made up of repeating units of regularly aligned sarcomeres. The *sarcomere* is regarded as the functional unit of muscle and can be defined as the myofibrillary element between two consecutive Z lines.[4] It consists of alternating light (I) and dark (A) bands (Fig. 28-149). In the middle of the A band is the M line, which is flanked by the narrower and lighter H zone. In the middle of the I band is the dense Z line, where the thin actin filaments are anchored. The lighter I band has only the actin filaments traversing it, whereas the darker A band consists of the interdigitation of both the actin and myosin filaments. The H zone is where the actin filaments end, and the M line is where the thickening of myosin filaments occurs. When the muscle contracts, the actin filaments slide past the myosin filaments leading to the shortening of the sarcomeres.

In addition to the myofibrils, the muscle fiber contains mitochondria; sarcoplasmic reticulum; transverse tubular system (T-system) which is an extension of the extracellular space[5] (Fig. 28-149); glycogen granules; lipid inclusions; and lysosomes.

HISTOCHEMISTRY

To interpret a muscle biopsy, the pathologist must be acquainted with the changes that are seen in the histochemical stains. The ATPase reaction is very useful for distinguishing fiber types[8] (Fig. 28-150.) *Type I* (slow twitch or red) fibers, which contain more mitochondria and myo-

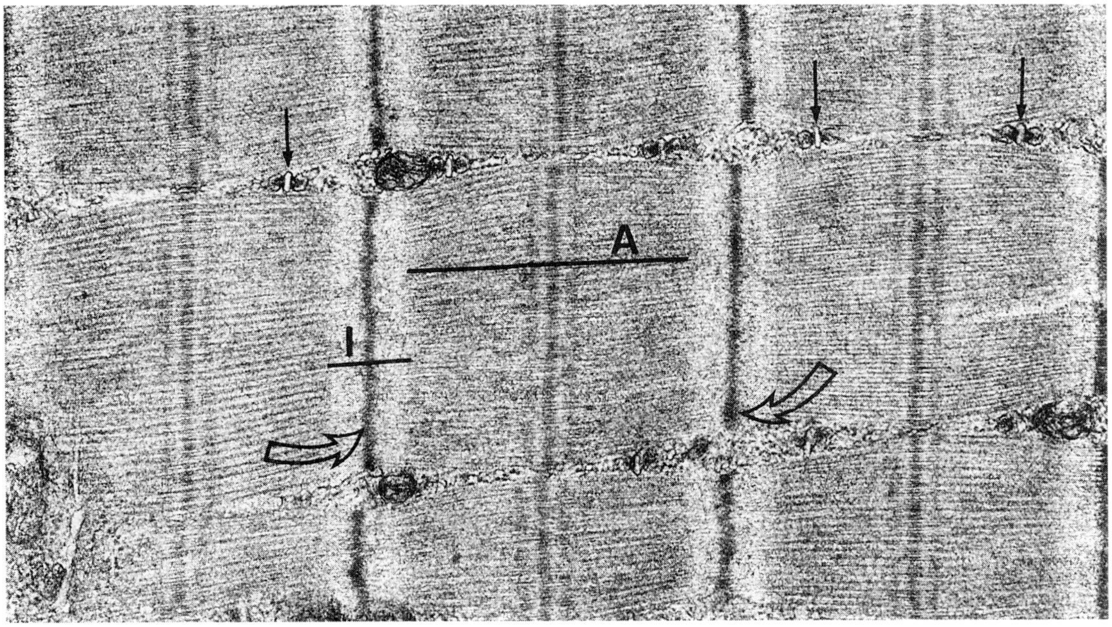

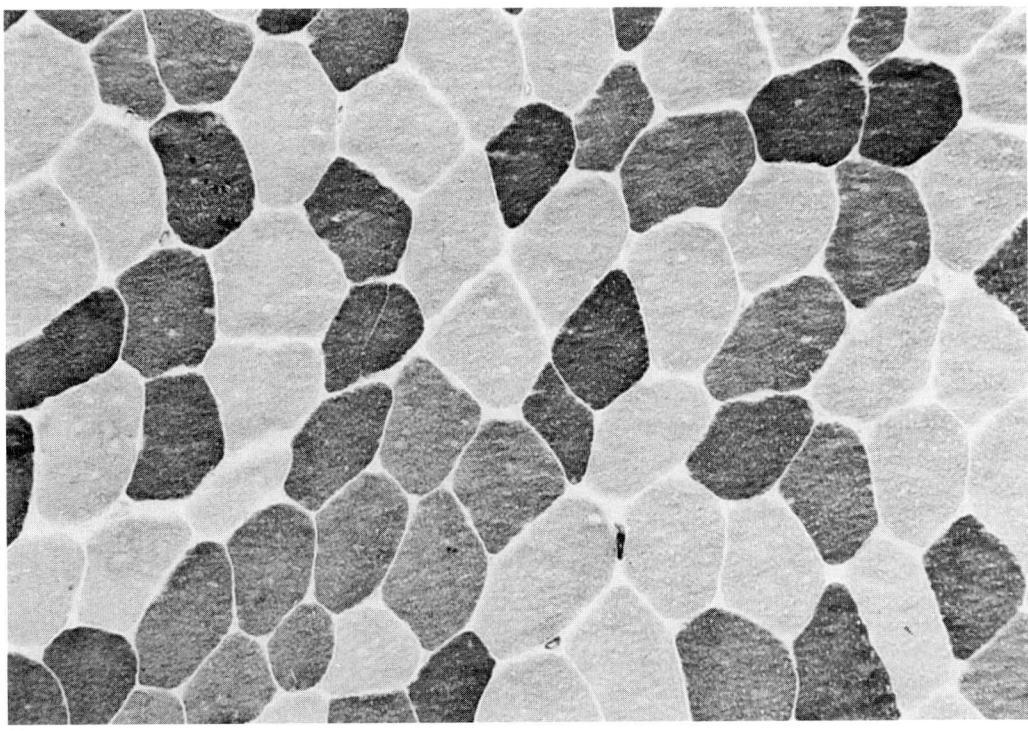

Fig. 28-149 Longitudinal section of normal rat skeletal muscle. The I band is centered by the Z line *(open arrows).* The A band is bisected by the M Line. The T tubules forming triads are shown *(arrows).* (×33,858.)

Fig. 28-150 Normal muscle. In routine ATPase reaction (pH 9.4), type I fibers are light and type II fibers are dark.

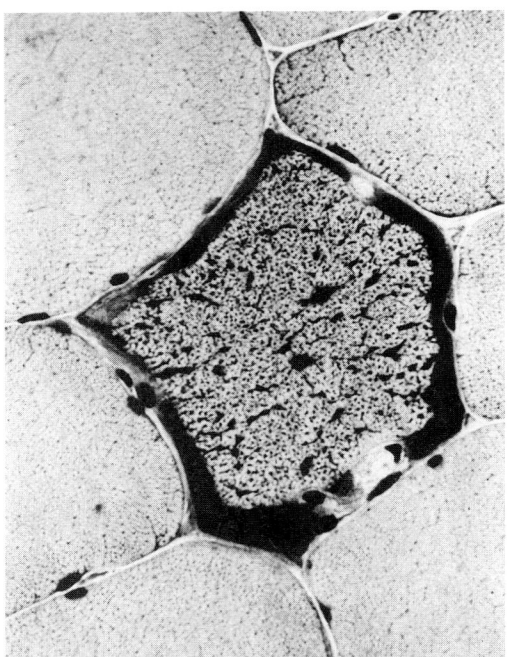

Fig. 28-151 On cryosections, ragged red fibers appear hematoxyphilic with H&E and red with Gomori trichrome and display intense reaction with oxidative enzymes.

globin, utilize aerobic oxidation for their energy requirement. *Type II* (fast twitch or white) fibers, which contain more glycogen, produce energy through the anaerobic glycolysis pathway. With the ATPase reaction at pH 9.4, the type I fibers are pale, and type II fibers are dark. At pH 4.3, this reaction is reversed, with type I fibers appearing dark and the type II fibers pale. ATPase reaction at pH 4.6 highlights the type I and type IIb fibers as darkly stained and the IIa as lightly stained. In the normal muscle, the type I and II fibers are well intermixed in a "checkerboard" pattern (see Fig. 28-150).

In most muscles such as the quadriceps, the proportion of the different types is roughly divided into thirds—one third type I, one third type IIA, and one third type IIB.[7] However, the proportion of type I fibers is higher in muscles that could sustain long contractions such as postural muscles and the proportion of type II is higher in muscles that require fast, powerful, and short contractions. In reinnervation, there is loss of the "checkerboard" pattern with an excessive grouping of one type of fiber, the so-called *fiber type grouping*.

The NADH-TR also identifies the fiber type by virtue of the fact that it reflects the oxidative enzyme activities, although it is less specific than ATPase. Thus the type I fibers appear very dark regardless of the original fiber type. Because it also highlights the distribution of subcellular organelles such as mitochondria and sarcoplasmic reticulum (which are heavily stained), it is a useful stain in the diagnosis of mitochondrial myopathy and structural myopathy such as central core disease. In denervation, target fibers are also best demonstrated by the NADH-TR.

The modified Gomori trichrome stain is useful for showing *ragged red fibers,* which are most frequently associated with mitochondrial myopathy (Fig. 28-151). The inclusions in rod (nemaline) myopathy appear dark red to purple in this stain. PAS and Oil red O stains are used to demonstrate increase of glycogen and lipid stores, respectively.

WORKING CLASSIFICATION

A simple approach to the diagnosis of nonneoplastic skeletal muscle diseases is to divide them into three broad categories: neurogenic atrophy, neuromuscular junction disorders, and primary myopathic diseases.[10] Because muscle biopsies are rarely performed for neuromuscular junction diseases such as myasthenia gravis, the first step in diagnosis is usually to differentiate between neurogenic atrophy and primary myopathic changes.[9] In general, primary myopathic changes are characterized by marked variation of individual fiber size, endomysial fibrosis, and scattered necrotic and regenerative fibers.[9] Often the myopathic changes in a biopsy may be so minimal that it is difficult to distinguish a myopathy from denervation. In such circumstances, access to clinical information, EMG findings, and serum creatine phosphokinase levels is essential before the final interpretation of the biopsy.

The primary myopathic group can be further subdivided into the ***inflammatory myopathy*** and ***noninflammatory myopathy***. Polymyositis, dermatomyositis, and inclusion body myositis are the more common forms of inflammatory myopathy. There are many more diseases in the noninflammatory group, which can be roughly subdivided into four categories: muscular dystrophy, congenital myopathy, metabolic myopathy, and drug-induced myopathy.

Neurogenic atrophy (denervation)

Neurogenic atrophy can be seen in diseases affecting the lower motor neuron such as poliomyelitis, amyotrophic lateral sclerosis, spinal muscular atrophy (Werdnig-Hoffmann and Kugelberg-Welander disease), and predominantly in peripheral neuropathy.[11]

Early denervation changes in a muscle are characterized by random atrophy of type II fibers that are angulated on transverse sections. With progressive denervation, the ATPase reaction shows a mixture of both type I and type II angulated fibers. With the NADH-TR, however, all these atrophied fibers, regardless of the types, are stained darkly. Denervated fibers have little PAS-stainable glycogen.

A more specific change of denervation is the formation of small and later large groups of atrophied fibers. In Werdnig-Hoffmann disease the markedly atrophic fibers have a rounded contour (Fig. 28-152). In about 20% to 30% of cases of denervation atrophy, the NADH-TR reaction may show ***target fibers,*** which have central pallor surrounded by very darkly stained rim that in turn is surrounded by normal-staining sarcoplasm (Fig. 28-153). Target fibers are more common in chronic polyneuropathies than in amyotrophic lateral sclerosis (Fig. 28-154). As a consequence of denervation and reinnervation from collateral sprouting of surviving axons, the typical "checkerboard" pattern is lost. As the motor unit territory enlarges, the newly recruited fibers are converted to single histochemical type, thus forming fiber

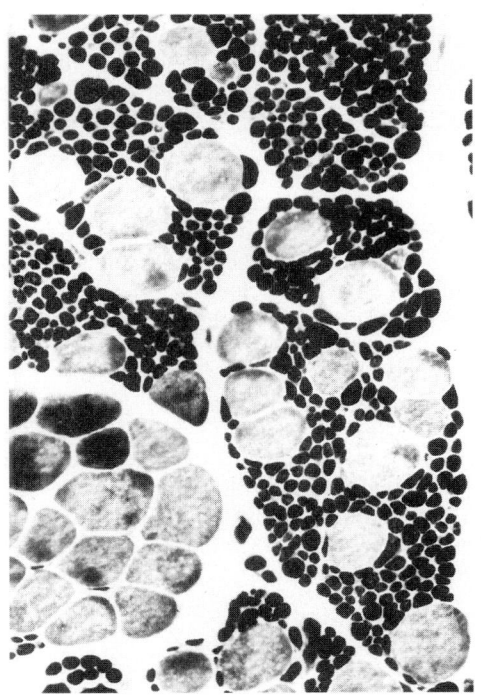

Fig. 28-152 Werdnig-Hoffman Disease. Large group atrophy. Unlike other forms of neurogenic atrophy the small fibers are only occasionally angulated. (Routine ATPase.)

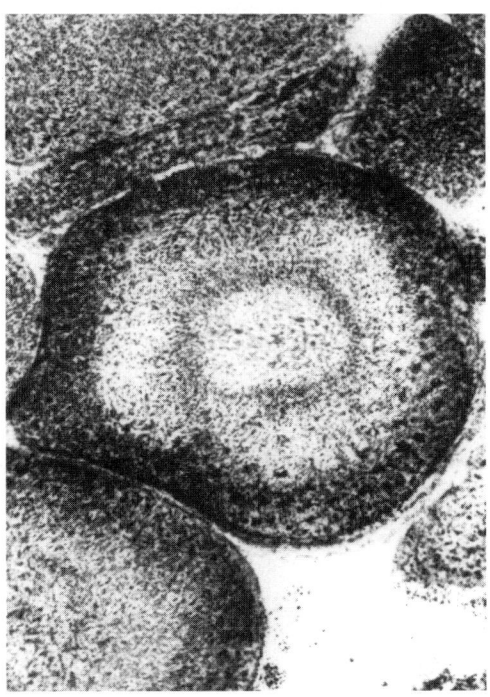

Fig. 28-153 "Target" fiber. Oxidative enzyme reveals the typical pattern (SDH).

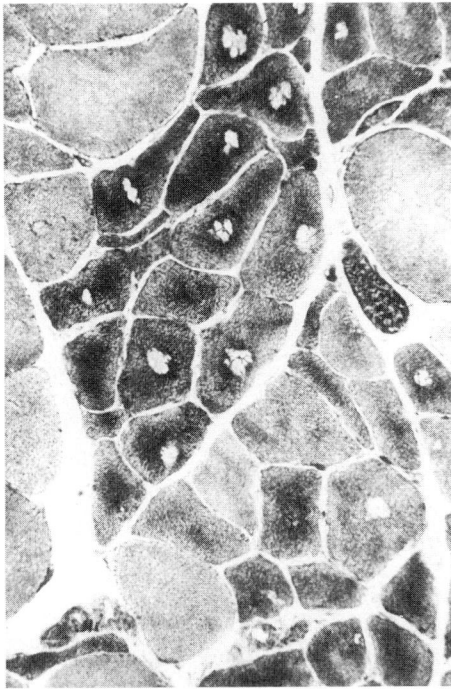

Fig. 28-154 Neurogenic atrophy with reinnervation. Fiber type grouping and "targets" in most type I are shown (SDH).

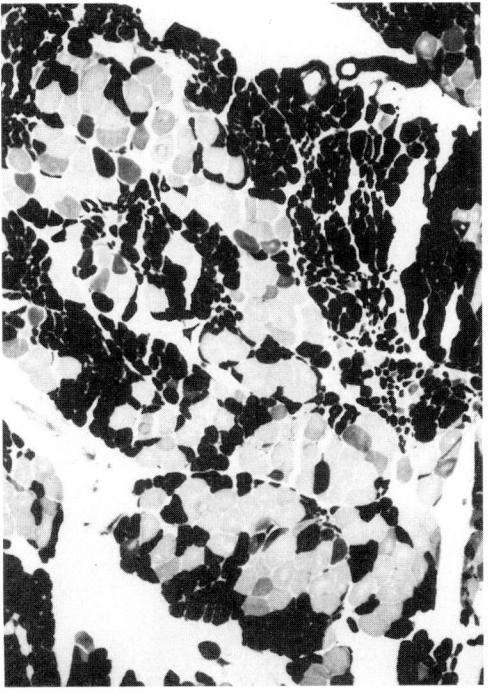

Fig. 28-155 Chronic neurogenic atrophy with reinnervation. The checkerboard staining pattern is altered by fiber type grouping. (ATPase, pH 9.4.)

type grouping (Fig. 28-155). After long-standing denervation, muscle may show hypertrophic fibers, fiber splitting, and even necrotic fibers giving rise to a pseudomyopathic picture.[12] In very advanced neurogenic atrophy, very little muscle may be visualized in a biopsy. Small, inconspicuous bundles of atrophic fibers may be found mingled with adipose tissue.

Inflammatory myopathy

Inflammatory myopathy is an heterogenous group of acquired muscle diseases among which three should be emphasized.[16] *Polymyositis* has an insidious onset without a precipitating event and a subacute or chronic course. The patient complains of symmetric weakness involving the proximal muscles; dysphagia develops later. The histologic appearance is nonspecific; thus polymyositis is a diagnosis of exclusion. The mononuclear cell infiltrate that consists mostly of T cells, particularly activated CD8+ cells and few or no B cells, is intrafascicular (endomysial) surrounding or invading individual non-necrotic muscle fibers.[16,17] Necrotic and regenerating fibers are scattered within the fascicle. In the early phase, the sarcoplasm of the necrotic fibers appears hypereosinophilic and granular with nuclear pyknosis and karyorrhexis. Later, the fibers become pale and vacuolated and undergo phagocytosis. The regenerating fibers are characterized by large vesicular nuclei with prominent nucleoli and basophilia of sarcoplasm. *HIV-associated polymyositis* has a similar histologic picture.

Dermatomyositis is a distinct clinical entity characterized by skin rash heralding the onset of muscle weakness. This myositis may occur alone or can be associated with mixed connective tissue diseases or malignant conditions. The inflammatory infiltrate consists of lymphocytes and plasma cells, and the immunophenotype discloses a higher percentage of B cells and CD4+ T cells. The inflammation is predominantly perivascular, focally in the perimysium and less commonly in the endomysial compartment. Transmural vascular inflammation is not uncommon, and vasculitic changes are prominent in the childhood variant of dermatomyositis.[17] The intramuscular blood vessels show endothelial hyperplasia with obliteration (Fig. 28-156) of capillaries resulting from fibrin thrombi, giving rise to large

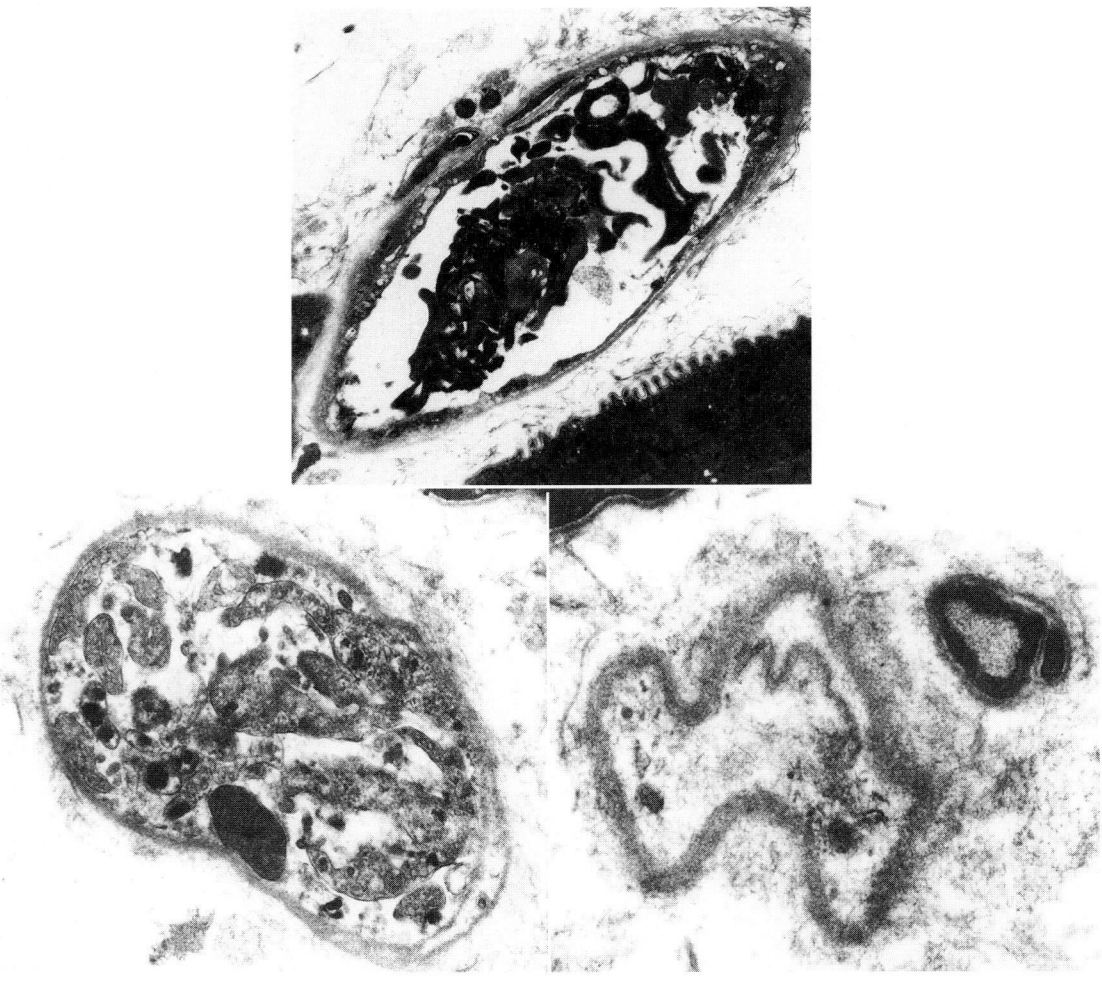

Fig. 28-156 Dermatomyositis. These three microvessels display the spectrum of vasculopathy. (*Top* ×3900; *bottom left* ×10,400; *bottom right* ×15,210.)

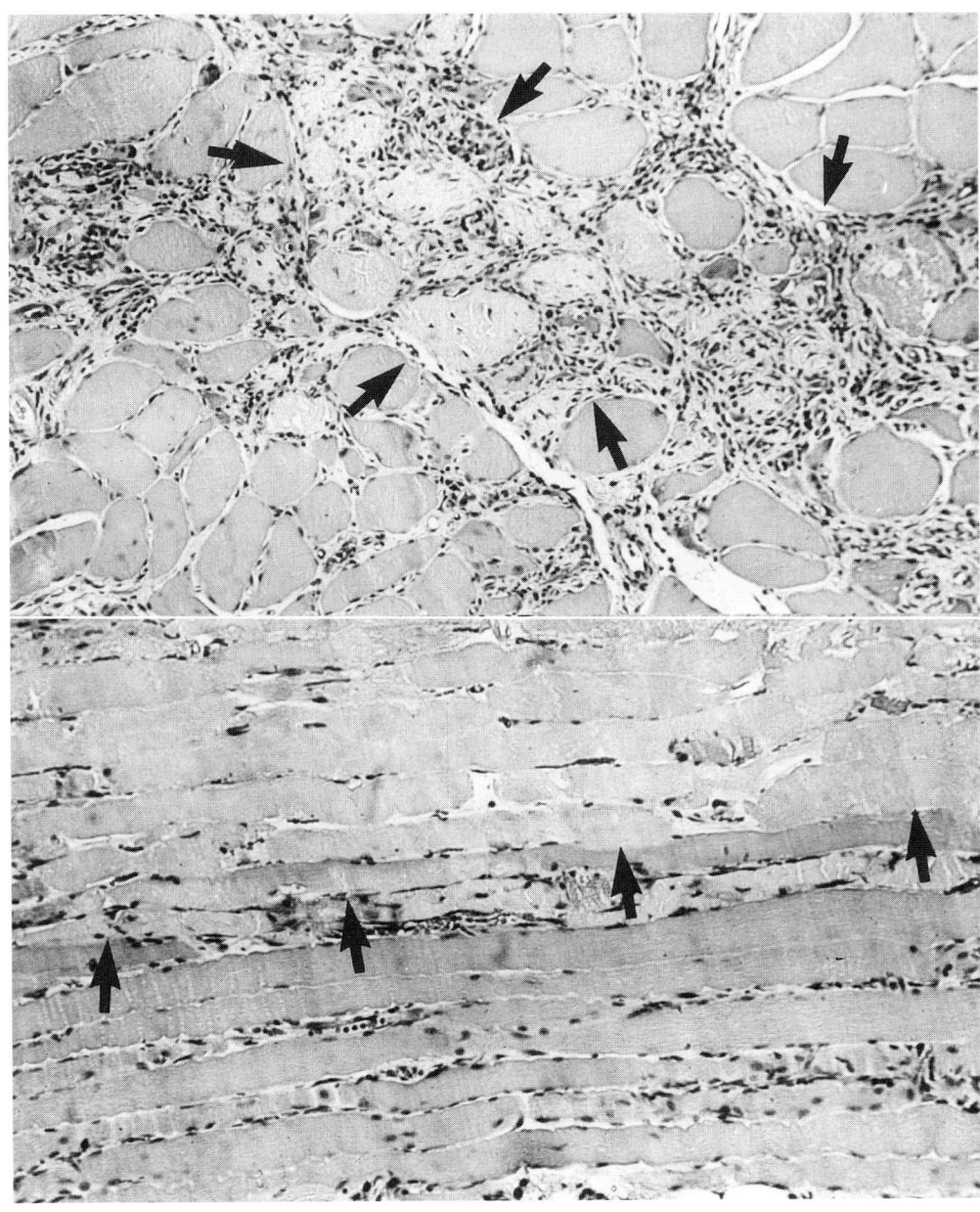

Fig. 28-157 Infarct-like areas *(arrows)* of necrosis are characteristic of dermatomyositis.

areas of necrosis associated with group of regenerating fibers (Fig. 28-157). Atrophic fibers at the periphery of fascicles, known as *perifascicular atrophy*, are highly suggestive of dermatomyositis (Fig. 28-158). These changes are not present in polymyositis or inclusion body myositis. Electron microscopic examination consistently shows tubuloreticular inclusions in the endothelium, a feature not seen in either polymyositis or inclusion body myositis.

The pathologist should suspect *inclusion body myositis* (IBM) when a muscle specimen arrives from a patient with polymyositis that has been unresponsive to therapy. This condition is more frequent in men than in women and affects clinical diagnosis of persons over the age of 50 years. Muscle involvement is asymmetric; weakness of foot and hand muscles is not uncommon. The endomysial inflammation is much like that in polymyositis, most being T cells. Small group atrophy of fibers mimics neurogenic atrophy, and fiber hypertrophy is common. The diagnostic features of inclusion body myositis are slit-like vacuoles in the sarcoplasm surrounded by hematoxyphilic granules called *rimmed vacuoles*[15] (Figs. 28-159 and 28-160) that sometimes contain eosinophilic inclusions. The inclusions of IBM are congophilic, and some of the material associated with them are immunoreactive for beta-amyloid protein[14] and ubiquitin.[13] The intranuclear filamentous inclusions are more easily detected by electron microscopy. The cytoplasmic and intranuclear filaments are similar in size and are rectilinear (Fig. 28-161). In some cases, there are twisted tubulofilaments that resemble the paired helical filaments in brain of Alzheimer's disease.[14]

Pyomyositis refers to localized areas of suppuration within striated muscle. It has been observed in tropical countries,[20]

in addicted patients following contaminated injections, and in immunosuppressed individuals. Other inflammatory myopathies include parasites (e.g., *Trichinella spiralis*[18]) (Fig. 28-162) and *cysticercosis*.[19] Non-necrotizing granulomata suggestive of sarcoidosis can be found in a muscle biopsy.

Muscular dystrophies

This is a group of hereditary primary myopathies with a chronic and progressive course. Within the group the individual entities are sorted by the different mode of inheritance, muscle groups affected, age of onset, clinical course, and severity. With recent advances in molecular genetics, the pathogenesis of some of these conditions has become better understood.

Duchenne muscular dystrophy is an X-linked recessive disease and one of the more common forms of muscular dystrophies with a uniformly poor outcome. The genetic defect is localized to the short arm of the X chromosome and involves a large gene that encodes the protein named *dystrophin*.[28,30] This protein forms an integral part of the skeletal muscle cell membrane, and its deficiency results in an influx of extracellular Ca^{++} and ultimate destruction of the cell.[24,27] The patients experience weakness of the pelvic and shoulder girdles before 5 years of age, and the disease progresses until most patients become nonambulatory by their teens. Death usually occurs at about 20 years of age as a result of respiratory failure and bronchopneumonia. The serum creatine phosphokinase is markedly raised in patients and also moderately increased in about 75% of the carriers. The muscle biopsy features necrotic fibers with myophagocytosis, fiber regeneration (Fig. 28-163), and endomysial fibrosis.[23] Scattered large hyalinized dark fibers are hyper-

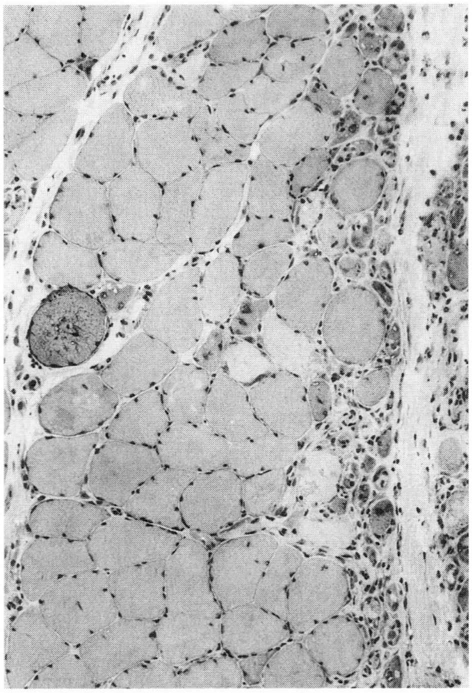

Fig. 28-158 Perifascicular fiber atrophy is typical of dermatomyositis.

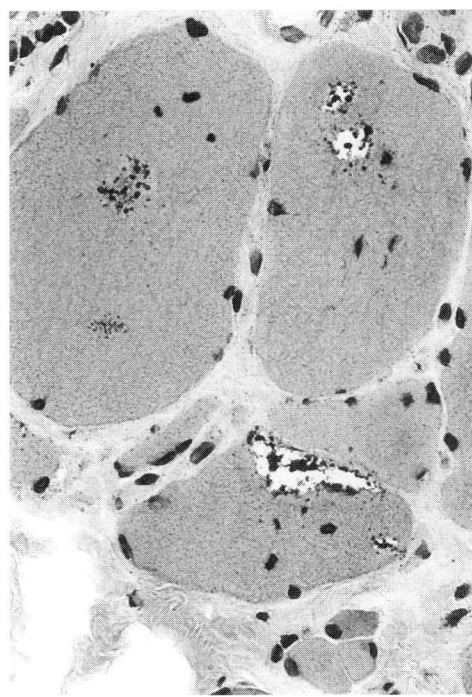

Fig. 28-159 IBM. Sarcoplasmic vacuoles are decorated by hematoxyphilic granules. (Cryosection, H&E.)

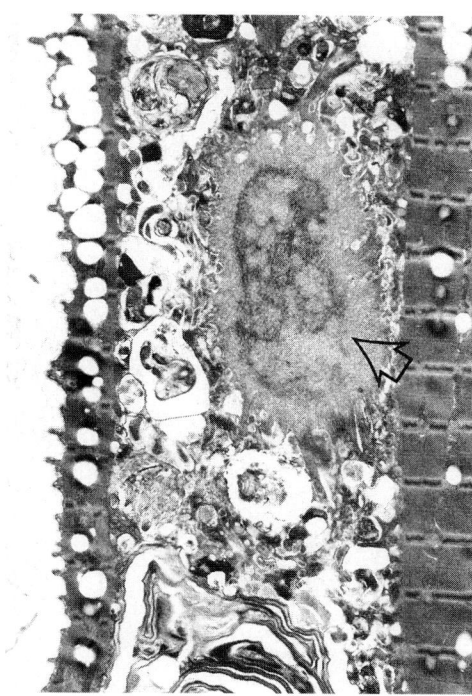

Fig. 28-160 IBM. Myelin-like cytomembranes surround a tangle of abnormal sarcoplasmic filaments *(arrow).* (×4800.)

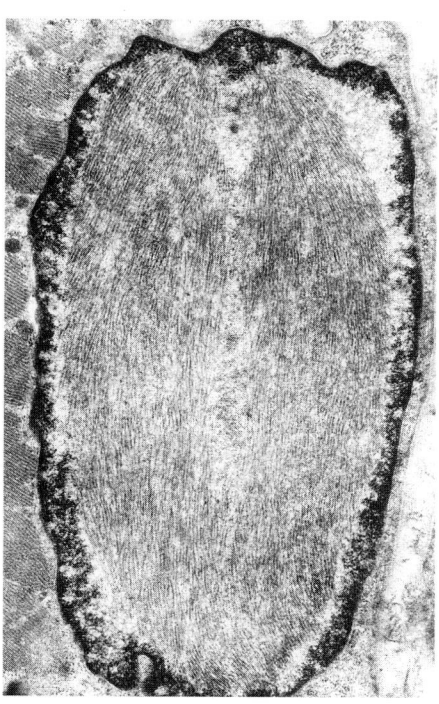

Fig. 28-161 Inclusion body myositis. The intranuclear inclusion is composed of linear filaments. (×1490.)

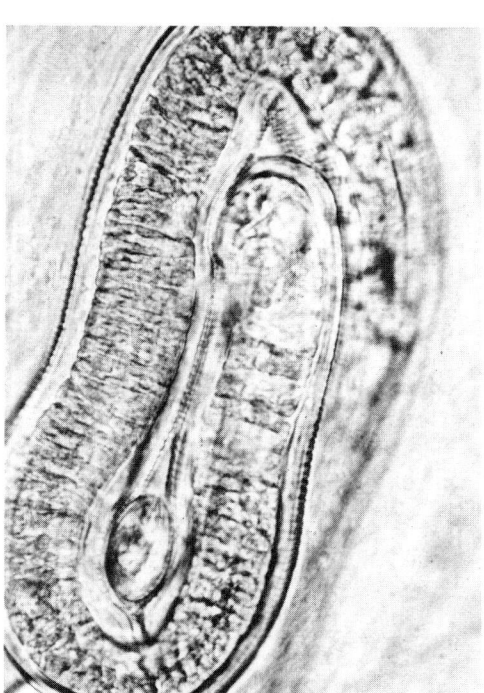

Fig. 28-162 Trichinosis (compression test). The viable worm can be visualized by compressing a piece of fresh muscle between glass slide and coverslip. (Bright field optics.)

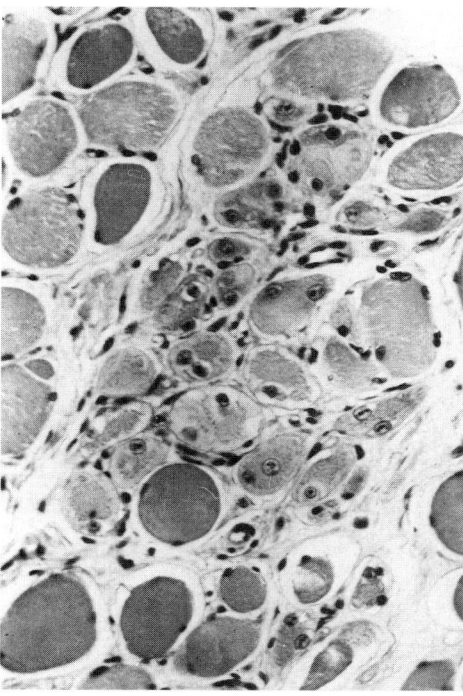

Fig. 28-163 Duchenne dystrophy. Group of regenerating fibers is a common finding.

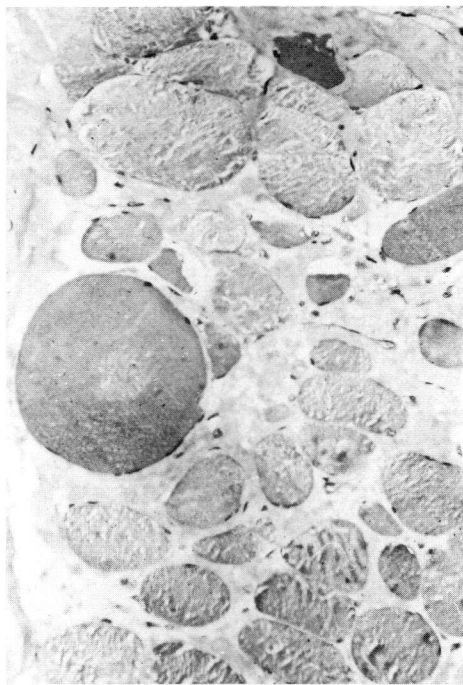

Fig. 28-164 Duchenne dystrophy. Hypercontracted fibers are due to a plasma membrane defect that allows the influx of calcium.

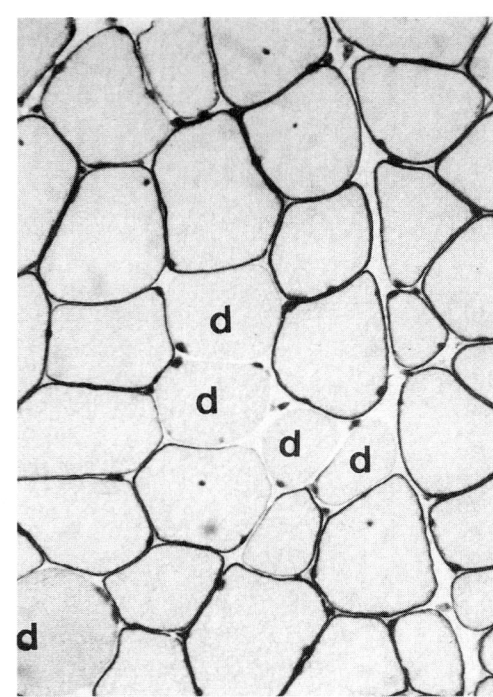

Fig. 28-165 Duchenne dystrophy carrier. A small number of non-necrotic fibers show attenuation or no reaction for dystrophin *(d)* (immunostaining on frozen section).

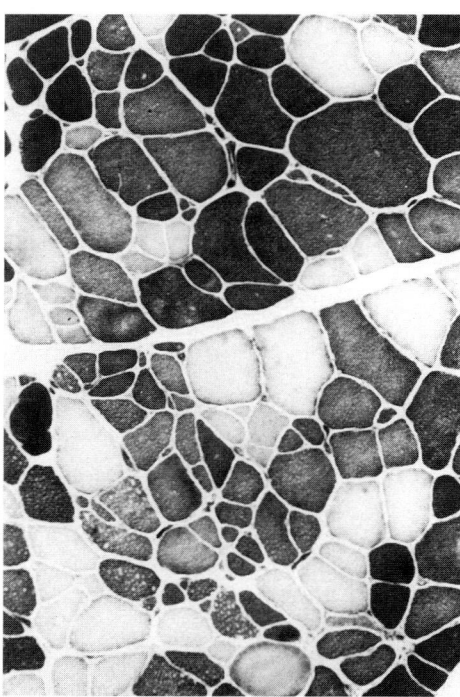

Fig. 28-166 Becker dystrophy. The myopathic changes overlap with those of Duchenne dystrophy.

contracted fibers (Fig. 28-164). Inflammatory reaction is lacking. The dystrophin immunohistochemistry in both patients and carriers reveals defective staining of the protein in the sarcolemmal membrane[21,29] (Fig. 28-165).

Becker dystrophy is an X-linked recessive condition with the defect in the dystrophin gene, but instead of the lack of gene product, there is a structural alteration or decrease in size of the molecule.[29] The onset is later in life than in Duchenne and the clinical course is less severe. The muscle shows endomysial fibrosis, scattered large hypercontracted fibers, and variability of fiber size, but the degenerative and regenerative changes are much less conspicuous than Duchenne (Fig. 28-166). Although attenuated, the sarcolemmal dystrophin immunoreaction is preserved.[26]

Patients suffering from ***facioscapulohumeral dystrophy*** present with progressive weakness involving the muscles of the face, shoulders, and upper arms. The inheritance is autosomal dominant, and the course is slow. The serum creatine phosphokinase can range from normal to five times normal. The changes in the muscle biopsy are nonspecific and include variability in fiber size, fiber splitting, and increase in internal nuclei. A lymphocytic infiltrate is usually slight, but when this is marked, it has to be distinguished from polymyositis.[22,25,32]

Limb girdle dystrophy is an umbrella name for a group of diseases, some with well-characterized chromosomal abnormalities. Patients exhibit proximal weakness of the shoulder and pelvic girdles.[35] The course is slowly progressive. The classical form is autosomal recessive; another variant, of sporadic occurrence, is autosomal dominant. Muscle pathol-

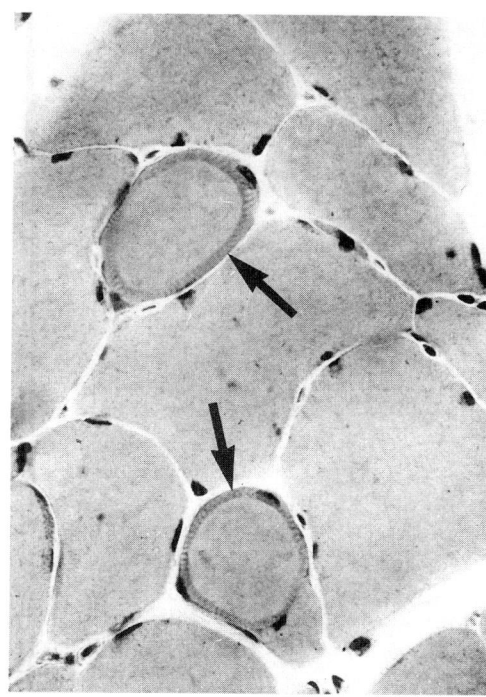

Fig. 28-167 Ring fibers. Circumferentially oriented myofibers are seen at the periphery of two transversely sectioned fibers *(arrows).*

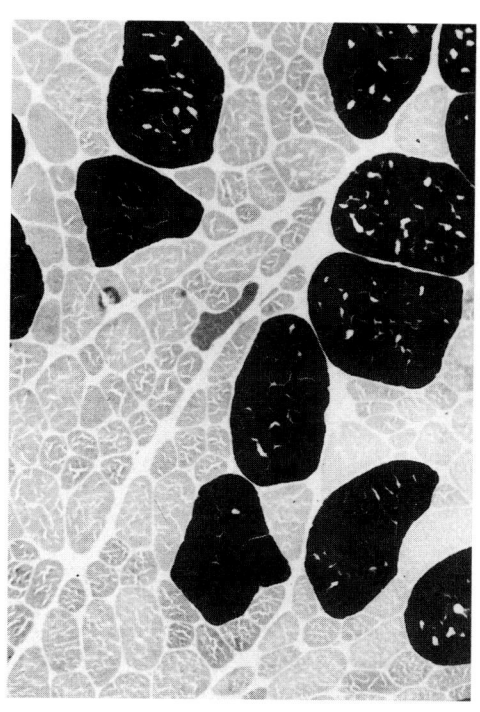

Fig. 28-168 Congenital fiber type disproportion. Hypertrophy of type II fibers and atrophy of type I fibers are shown. (Routine ATPase.)

ogy is rather nonspecific with variability of fiber size and increased internal nuclei. Fiber splitting is prominent.

Myotonic dystrophy is an autosomal dominant disease with the genetic defect being an unstable segment of increased CTG trinucleotide repeats of the gene at chromosome 19 (19q13.3).[31] With successive generations the number of trinucleotide repeats increases, and the gene becomes more unstable, resulting in more severe disease (the phenomenon of anticipation). Clinically, two forms can be distinguished, the congenital and the adult myotonic dystrophy. The *congenital form* is seen in infants presenting with hypotonia and myotonia, although sometimes symptoms may not be noticeable until later in life. In the *adult form* the onset is slow with progressive weakness and stiffness of the distal limbs. The muscles of the face, jaw, and eyelids are most frequently involved, giving rise to a rather characteristic facies. Myotonia typically results in marked delay in grip release, although this may not be always present. Male pattern baldness, cataracts, testicular atrophy, mental subnormality, and cardiac arrhythmias and cardiomyopathy are some of the extramuscular manifestations. Changes in the muscle are variable, but an increase in internal nuclei with type I fiber atrophy and type II hypertrophy is frequent. Ring fibers and sarcoplasmic masses are other significant findings[34] (Fig. 28-167).

Other recognized varieties of muscular dystrophy include **Emery-Dreifuss dystrophy, X-linked myopathy** with **excessive autophagy, distal myopathy, ocular myopathies,** and **oculopharyngeal dystrophy.**[33]

Congenital myopathies

Most patients present as floppy infants with delayed motor development. The course of these myopathies is variable but mostly nonprogressive, and some patients have a normal life expectancy.[37,43] There is, however, some persistent proximal muscle atrophy with weakness throughout life. In this group characteristic structural changes are seen in the light and ultrastructural level, which makes muscle biopsy essential for diagnosis. The three better characterized myopathies in this group are the central core disease, central nuclear myopathy, and rod (nemaline) myopathy. In addition to the structural changes described later, all these conditions exhibit some degree of predominance and hypotrophy in the type I fibers. Sometimes congenital hypotonia is caused by hypotrophy of type I fiber with or without type I fiber predominance in the absence of structural changes. This condition, named ***congenital fiber type disproportion,*** usually has a nonprogressive course (Fig. 28-168).

The change that characterizes ***central core myopathy*** is the central clearing seen in mostly the type I muscle fibers with the NADH-TR[45] (Fig. 28-169). This represents the loss of mitochondria, sarcoplasmic reticulum, glycogen, and lipid demonstrated at the ultrastructural level.[45,47,54] The myofibrillary elements may or may not be disrupted. The difference between the central cores and the targets seen in neurogenic atrophy is that the cores run throughout the whole length of the fibers. The cores are eccentric and smaller or multiple in another type of congenital myopathy known as ***multicore*** or ***minicore disease***[41] (Fig. 28-170). The gene for central core

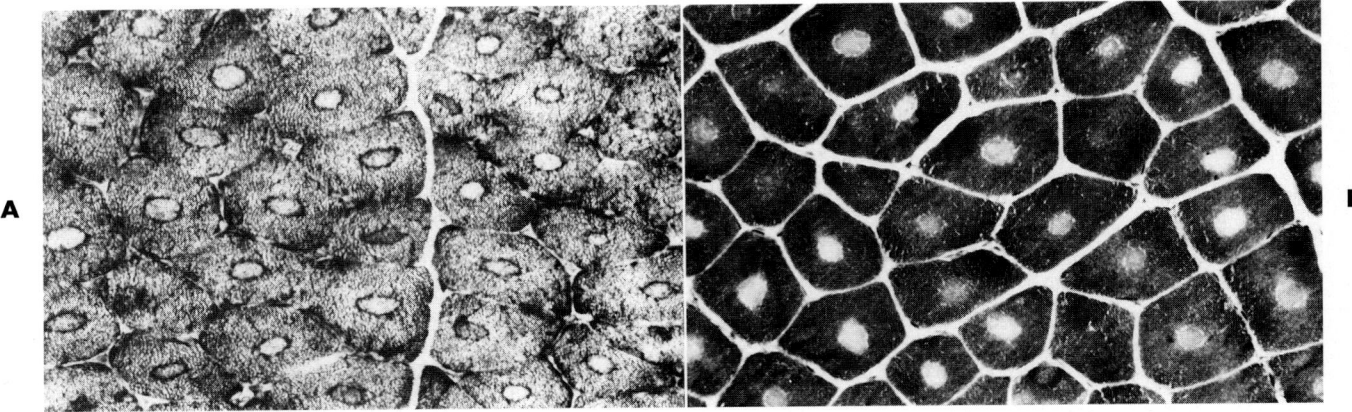

Fig. 28-169 Central core disease. Central areas of reduced activity are seen in all fibers. All fibers react as type 1. (**A** NADH-TR; **B** reverse ATPase.)

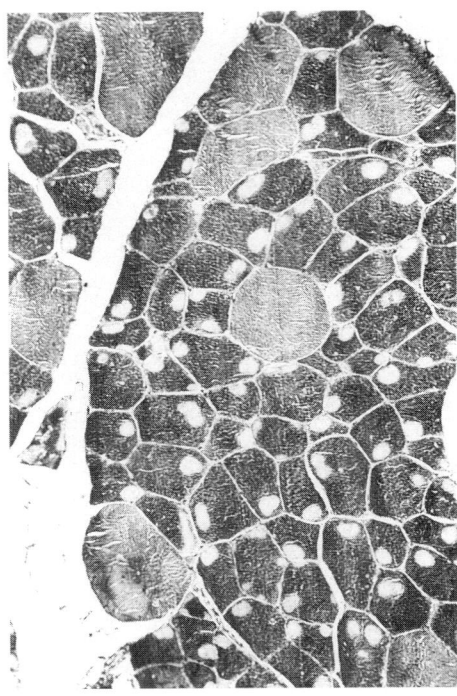

Fig. 28-170 Multicore disease. Spherical zones of reduced enzyme activity are present in type I fibers. Larger type II fibers are unaffected. (PTAH.)

disease is localized to a locus (chromosome 19q13.1) that is closely linked to the gene implicated in malignant hyperthermia.[49,52] Thus molecular genetics has provided an explanation for the known predisposition of central core disease patients to malignant hyperthermia.

In the biopsy of *central nuclear myopathy,* there are at least 25% of the fibers with centrally placed nuclei.[50] In the X-linked recessive type, most fibers with the central nuclei appear small and rounded, similar to the myotubes seen in fetal muscles[36] (Fig. 28-171). Patients from this group usu-

ally present in the prenatal or perinatal period with respiratory failure resulting in high mortality. In those with early and late onset, the clinical course is slower and the fibers appear more matured. In both the early and late onset, both fiber types are involved. Electron microscopy reveals myofibrillary disorganization with accumulation of mitochondria and other membranous organelles around the central nuclei.[48]

In *rod (nemaline) myopathy* the inclusions are inapparent in hematoxylin-eosin and are best seen with modified Gomori trichrome as brilliant red to black granular deposits beneath the sarcolemma (Fig. 28-172). They appear rod shaped on longitudinal semithin sections.[55] These inclusions are not noticeable with ATPase and NADH-TR. Ultrastructurally the rod inclusions that appear elongated or rectangular in the longitudinal sections and polygonal in transverse sections have a similar density to the Z lines [40,46,51] (Fig. 28-173).

Other congenital myopathies that have been described are **fingerprint body myopathy,**[39] **reducing body myopathy,**[38] **spheroid body myopathy,**[44] **trilaminar muscle fiber disease**[53] and **congenital muscular dystrophy**.[42] In one subtype of the congenital muscular dystrophy, **Fukuyama disease,** the associated CNS malformations are thought to be the result of neuronal migration defect.[42]

Metabolic myopathies

This category consists of many different conditions. Only the myopathies associated with periodic paralysis, glycogen storage, lipid storage, and mitochondrial diseases will be discussed here.

Periodic paralysis may be familial (autosomal dominant) or associated with thyrotoxicosis. The periodicity of the paralysis is related to abnormalities in influx and efflux of potassium ions in the muscle fibers, leading to failure in propagation of the action potential. Familial forms are subdivided according to the serum potassium level during the attack into hypokalemic, hyperkalemic, and normokalemic periodic paralysis. The abnormal membrane excitability in skeletal muscle could be attributed to genetic alteration affect-

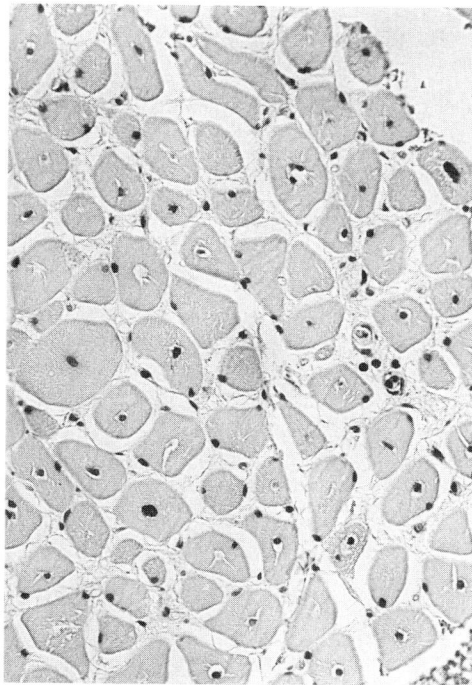

Fig. 28-171 Centronuclear myopathy. Most fibers display central nucleus. Note a perinuclear halo of abnormality of myofibrils.

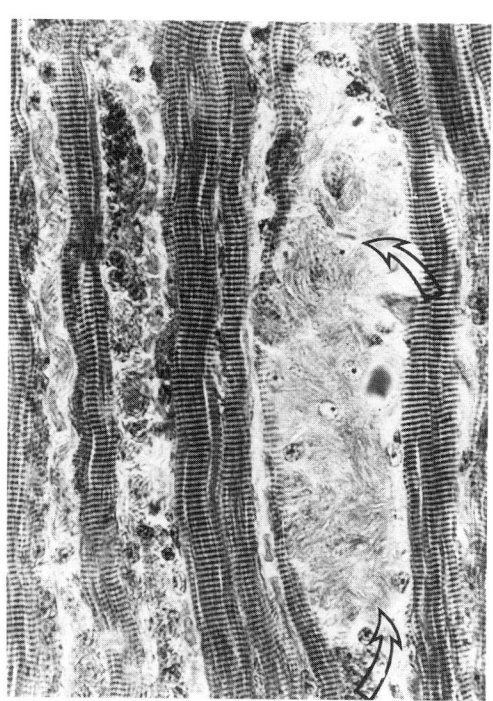

Fig. 28-172 Nemaline myopathy. Thread-like subsarcolemmal aggregates are shown on longitudinal sections *(arrows)*. (PTAH.)

ing the functions in sodium ion channels (hyperkalemic and normokalemic periodic paralysis)[69] and dihydropyridine receptor, a voltage-gated calcium channel (hypokalemic periodic paralysis).[67] In the *hypokalemic form,* the attack of paralysis occurs after a long period of rest such as after a good night's sleep with the patient unable to move on awakening. These attacks usually last from a few hours to 1 day. In the *hyperkalemic form* attacks occur about a half hour's rest after exercise, and each one lasts approximately a few hours. The normokalemic attacks of paralysis are similar to the hyperkalemic but are more severe and can last for days or weeks. The thyrotoxic periodic paralysis may be sporadic or has HLA antigenic association. Biopsy specimens taken during or shortly after periodic paralysis show vacuolar changes in the fibers (Fig. 28-174). Other changes such as variability in fiber size, endomysial fibrosis, fiber degeneration, and regeneration can accompany the vacuolar myopathy. Ultrastructural examination reveals membrane-bound vacuoles that either can be empty or can contain granular material. These vacuoles are the dilated sacs of the sarcoplasmic reticulum. Occasionally there are ultrastructural tubular aggregates that are dense collections of tubules arranged in hexagonal array thought to be derived from the sarcoplamic reticulum.

Glycogen storage diseases (glycogenoses) are a group of inherited (autosomal recessive) diseases characterized by deficiencies of enzymes that degrade glycogen, thus leading to accumulation of glycogen in different organs, such as the liver and heart, and skeletal muscle. The skeletal muscle is affected in at least four types of glycogenoses—namely, acid maltase deficiency, amylo-1,6-glucosidase (debranching

enzyme) deficiency, myophosphorylase deficiency, and phosphofructokinase deficiency.[59,63] In all cases, the ultimate diagnosis can only be confirmed by biochemical assay of the enzyme involved.

Acid maltase deficiency, also known as type II glycogenosis or Pompe's disease, can present at the early infantile, late infantile, juvenile, or adult period. The early infantile form is most severe with involvement of the cardiac muscle, usually leading to cardiac failure and death within the first 2 years of life. The other forms are less severe, and patients survive to adulthood with a progressive myopathy. Vacuolar change is present in all forms, but vacuoles have a tendency to coalesce in the early infantile form, leading to larger vacuoles in most fibers, whereas in the late-onset forms, vacuoles are less conspicuous and may affect selectively type I fibers. In the adult form the biopsy may appear normal. PAS stain is useful in demonstrating glycogen in the vacuoles. Because acid maltase is a lysosomal enzyme, the acid phosphatase is also reactive, even in the absence of obvious glycogen storage. Electron microscopy distinguishes this type of glycogenosis from the other types in that the glycogen granules in maltase deficiency are bound within lysosomal membranes.

In *debranching deficiency* **(type III glycogenosis)** the skeletal muscle is mildly affected although the patient may have growth retardation, hepatomegaly, and hypoglycemia. Vacuolar myopathy is noted in the biopsy, and the vacuoles contain glycogen. Ultrastructural studies reveal storage of free glycogen not bound by any membrane.

Myophosphorylase deficiency **(type IV glycogenosis)** causes a mild myopathy; the patients' main complaints are

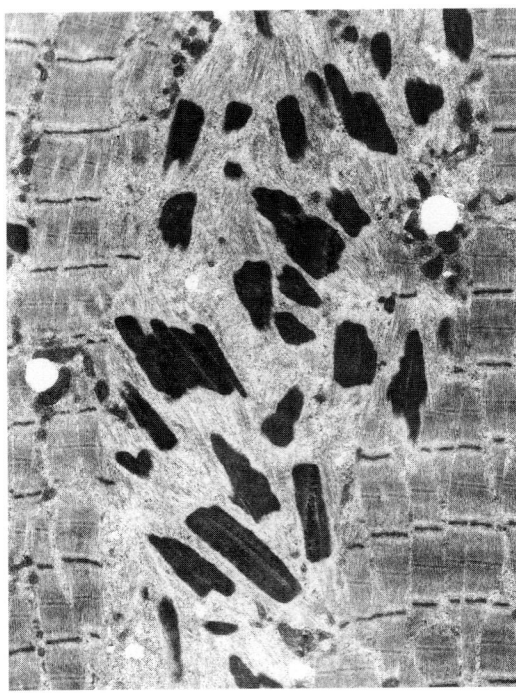

Fig. 28-173 Nemaline myopathy. Rods appear to originate from the Z disks. (×6160.)

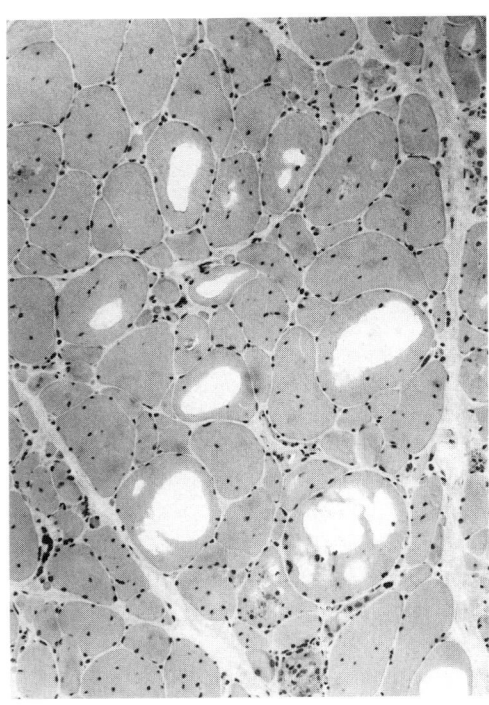

Fig. 28-174 Hypokalemic periodic paralysis. Many fibers display large, optically empty vacuoles.

related to cramps and pains in their muscles, especially those of the calf, during exercise. Myophosphorylase deficiency prevents the muscle from utilizing glycogen during exercise; thus in severe cases, prolonged exercise may lead to rhabdomyolysis. The muscle biopsy usually is normal except that there may be some increase in subsarcolemmal accumulation of glycogen, which is better demonstrated ultrastructurally. The demonstration of the myophosphorylase in the muscle by histochemistry is essential for diagnosis of this condition. The genetic alteration for this disease has been identified in chromosome 11q13.[72]

Clinically, *phosphofructokinase deficiency* (**type VII glycogenosis**) has the same presentation as type IV glycogenosis, and the muscle alterations are very similar except that histochemically there is an absence of phosphofructokinase instead of myophosphorylase.

An increased number and size of lipid droplets can be best demonstrated in *lipid myopathies* with the use of Oil red O preparation on cryostat sections. Although an increase in lipid storage in the skeletal muscle is seen secondarily in steroid myopathy and acute alcoholic myopathy, there are conditions in which the myopathies are the direct result of abnormalities in the lipid metabolic pathway, namely carnitine deficiency and carnitine palmitoyl transferase deficiency.[60] A number of mitochondrial myopathies can also secondarily lead to increased sarcoplasmic lipid deposition.

Carnitine deficiency affects the skeletal muscle primarily, causing weakness or systemically giving rise to hypoglycemia, cardiomyopathy, bowel dysfunctions, hypochromic anemia, seizures, psychomotor retardation, and failure to thrive. Carnitine is essential for the transport of long chain fatty acids across the inner membrane of the mitochondria; when it is deficient, lipid accumulates in the sarcoplasm. This deficiency could occur as a primary defect in the carrier-mediated carnitine or secondary to disorders of betaoxidation and defects in the respiratory chain. The muscle biopsy shows excessive lipid droplets, but the definitive diagnosis is based on assay of the muscle carnitine.

Carnitine palmitoyl transferase deficiency will affect the transfer of long chain fatty acids into the mitochondria and the beta-oxidation pathway. Mutations on chromosome 1p11-13 are found to be responsible for the deficiency in one of the isoforms of this enzyme.[71] Some patients have exercise intolerance and exercise-induced muscle pain. In severe cases, this may be followed by rhabdomyolysis and myoglobinuria. The muscle usually appears normal with light and electron microscopy, and therefore the diagnosis is dependent on the biochemical assay.

Mitochondrial myopathy is a large and heterogeneous group of diseases characterized by abnormal sarcoplasmic accumulation of mitochondria, most of which are ultrastructurally abnormal. The modified Gomori trichrome stain identifies this abnormal accumulation in affected myofibers as intense red granular staining of the sarcoplasm. When the intermyofibrillary deposits are very numerous, the fiber will have a fragmented appearance; hence the name *ragged red fiber*[57,65] (see Fig. 28-151). These fibers also display intense reaction with the NADH-TR and succinate dehydrogenase. Ultrastructurally, not only is there an increase in the number of mitochondria, but also there are an abnormal configuration, paracrystalline intermembranous inclusions, and abnormal

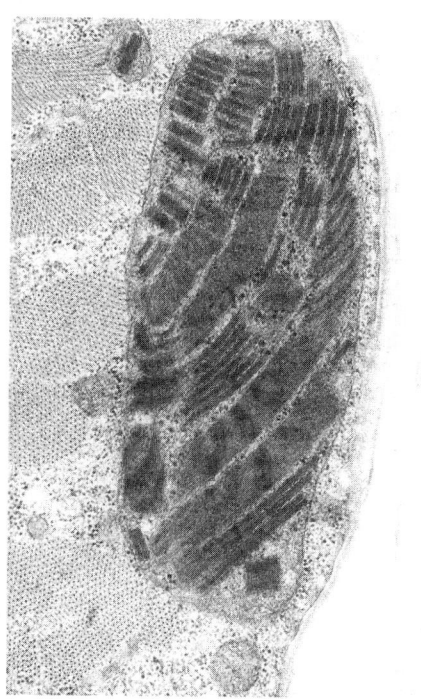

Fig. 28-175 Mitochondrial myopathy. This giant mitochondrion contains paracrystalline arrays. (×19,426.)

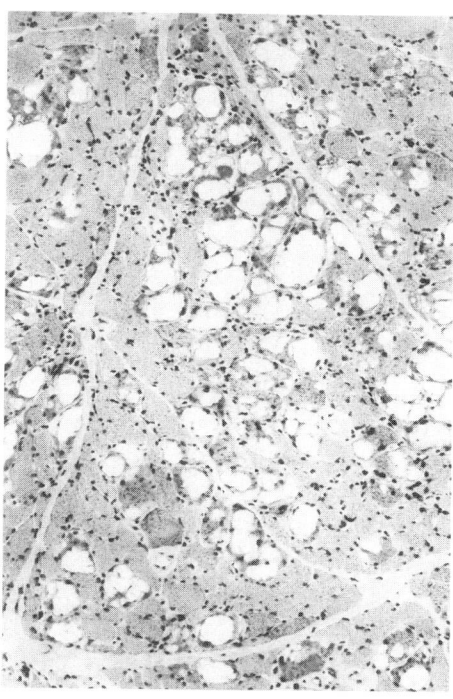

Fig. 28-176 Chloroquine myopathy. Severe vacuolization of myofibers is seen; with ATPase, most of the affected fibers are type I.

cristae with excessive branching[70] (Fig. 28-175). Most of the mitochondrial diseases with known genetic defects involve either the mitochondral genes[56,62] or nuclear genes encoding the respiratory chain polypeptides and Krebs' cycle enzymes.[64] Those with mitochondrial gene mutations are maternally inherited.[56] Even though identification of the genetic defects, deficient enzymes, or polypeptides will provide the final diagnosis, the muscle biopsy very often provides the first clue. The pathologist should also be beware of the fact that a negative biopsy may not exclude a mitochondrial disease.

With the increased understanding of the metabolic pathways in the mitochondria, this group of diseases can be classified according to the types of metabolic defect[64]; for instance, there are derangements in energy transduction[58] (e.g., Luft's disease), substrate utilization[61] (e.g., Leigh's disease) and mitochondrial respiratory chain[66] (e.g., MELAS, MERRF,[57] and Kearns-Sayre syndromes[68]). Some of these diseases, in addition to myopathy, involve other organs such as the heart and brain, resulting in cardiomyopathy, stroke-like syndromes, encephalopathies, seizures, ophthalmoplegia, and deafness.[64,66,73]

Drug-induced myopathy

Rhabdomyolysis is one of the most serious toxic effects of alcohol, amphetamine, heroin, barbiturate, methadone, clofibrate, and amphotericin B.[77,78] It is also a manifestation of malignant hyperthermia, which could be precipitated by general anesthetic agents such as halothane or succinylcholine. Snake, wasp, and spider venoms introduced into the body can also lead to rhabdomyolysis, which appears as

massive acute necrosis of the myofibers with scattered fiber regeneration. The inflammmatory changes seen are only a reaction to the necrosis. Other drugs such as azidothymidine (AZT), emetine, clofibrate, epsilon-aminocaproic acid, and alcohol can cause ***subacute necrotizing myopathy***.[77] In the case of AZT, there are changes in the mitochondria such as ragged red fibers accompanied by ultrastructural abnormalities.[81] Toxic reaction to ***chloroquine*** results in a vacuolar myopathy associated with proximal weakness. These vacuoles are present mainly in type I fibers and contain PAS-positive and acid phosphatase–positive lysosomal inclusions (Fig. 28-176). Ultrastructurally, these lysosomal inclusions can be membranous bodies, myelin figures, or curvilinear inclusions.[76] Vacuolar change and lysosomal inclusions have also been described in ***colchicine-induced myopathy***[79] (Figs. 28-177 and 28-178). Agents such as procainamide, emetine, and D-penicillamine are linked to a form of ***inflammatory myopathy***.[77] In eosinophilia-myalgia syndrome associated with L-tryptophan ingestion, the inflammatory infiltrate consists of lymphocytes, histiocytes, and eosinophils involving mainly the fascia and interstitium.[82]

Although ***type II fiber atrophy*** is very nonspecific, it is a relatively common finding in a muscle biopsy. The most common causes are related to prolonged steriod therapy and disuse related to prolonged bed rest or joint diseases (Fig. 28-179). The other conditions associated with type II atrophy are collagen vascular diseases, polymyalgia rheumatica, and myasthenia gravis.[75] ATPase is essential for the diagnosis and identifies the type II fibers that are angular and only about half the diameter of the normal-looking type I fibers. Patients who receive a combination of high-dose cortico-

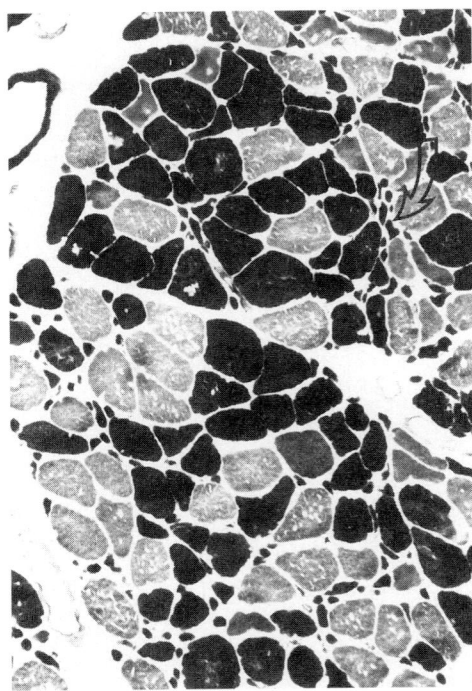

Fig. 28-177 Colchicine neuromyopathy. Type I fibers show vacuolation. Group atrophy of fibers indicates a neurogenic component *(arrow)*. (Routine ATPase.)

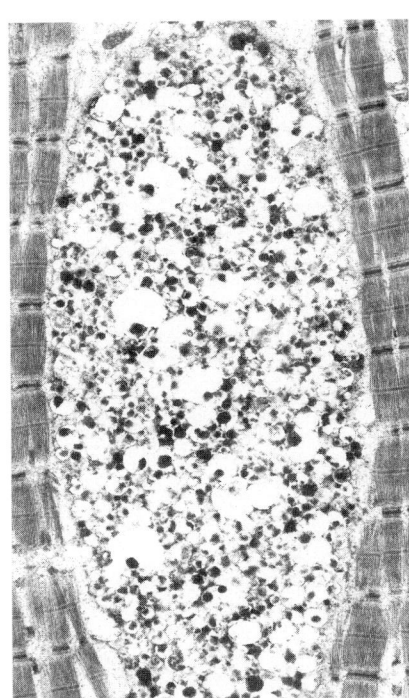

Fig. 28-178 Colchicine myopathy. Vacuoles are formed by aggregates of secondary lysosomes. (×8800.)

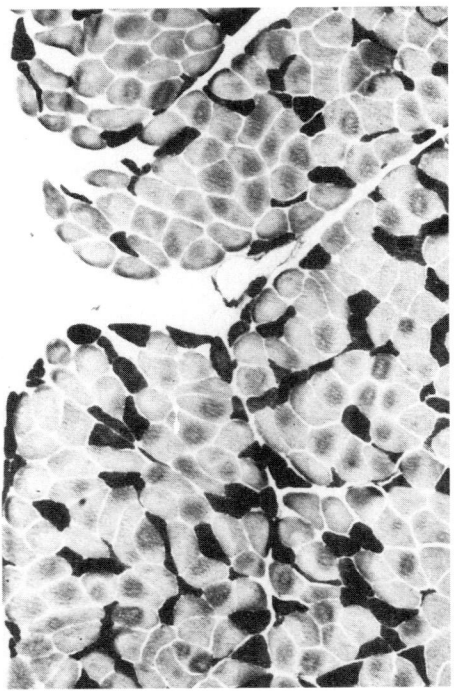

Fig. 28-179 Type II atrophy. This is a consistent finding in steroid-induced myopathy. (Routine ATPase.)

steroids and nondepolarizing neuromuscular blocking agents may develop an acute flaccid quadriparesis and muscle wasting with an elevated CPK level. Muscle biopsy has shown a non-necrotizing noninflammatory myopathy with patchy loss of myofibrillar ATPase staining and selective loss of myosin filaments.[74,80] Slow recovery follows pharmacologic paralysis.

Neuromuscular junction disorders

Myasthenia gravis is an autoimmune disease resulting from autoantibodies produced against the acetylcholine receptors at the motor endplate, causing a defect in neuromuscular transmission.[84] Patients usually suffer from a relapsing and remitting disease with muscle weakness and fatigue. Considerable difference exists in the severity and in the groups of muscles affected. The extraocular muscles are most commonly involved, producing ptosis and diplopia. Depending on the different muscles affected, patients may have dysphagia or even respiratory insufficiency. Typically, the patient is a young female, but when the patient is an elderly male, the presence of a thymoma should be suspected. Muscle biopsy is usually nondiagnostic, although findings such as type II fiber atrophy[75] and scattered collections of lymphocytes without evidence of fiber necrosis have been described.[85] Changes in the neuromuscular junctions such as loss of secondary sarcolemmal folds and widening of the clefts are apparent only on electron microscopy.[86] Unfortunately, in most routine muscle biopsies the neuromuscular junctions are rarely sampled, rendering muscle biopsy unsuitable as a means for the diagnosis of myasthenia gravis.

Similarly in *Eaton-Lambert syndrome,* a paraneoplastic syndrome associated with a defect in the release of acetylcholine from the nerve terminals at the neuromuscular junctions, the muscle biopsy is generally unhelpful and at most demonstrates nonspecific changes such as type II fiber atrophy.[83] The pathogenesis of this disease has been attributed to autoantibodies against the presynaptic voltage-gated calcium channels.[87]

REFERENCES

1 Carpenter S, Karpati G: Methods of tissue removal and preparation. Pathology of skeletal muscle. New York, 1984, Churchill Livingstone, pp 39-61.

2 Dubowitz V: Procedure of muscle biopsy. A practical approach, ed 2. London, 1985, Bailliere Tindall, pp 3-40.

3 Engel WK, Cunningham GG: Rapid examination of muscle tissue. An improved trichrome method for fresh-frozen biopsy sections. Neurology 13:919-923, 1963.

NORMAL ANATOMY

4 Craig R: The structure of the contractile filaments. In Engel AG, Franzini-Armstrong C, eds: Myology, ed. 2. New York, 1994, McGraw-Hill, pp 134-175.

5 Franzini-Armstrong C: The sarcoplasmic reticulum and the transverse tubules. In Engel AG, Franzini-Armstrong C, eds: Myology, ed 2. New York, 1994, McGraw-Hill, pp 176-222.

6 Schmalbruch H, Hellhammer U: The number of satellite cells in normal human muscle. Anat Rec 185:279-287, 1976.

HISTOCHEMISTRY

7 Johnson MA, Polgar J, Weightman D, Appelton D: Data on the distribution of fiber types in thirty-six human muscles. An autopsy study. J Neurol Sci 18:111-129, 1973.

8 Round JM, Matthews Y, Jones DA: A quick, simple and reliable histochemical method for ATPase in human muscle preparations. Histochem J 12:707-709, 1980.

WORKING CLASSIFICATION

9 Dubowitz V: Muscle biopsy. A practical approach, ed 2. London, 1985, Bailliere Tindall, pp 208-219.

10 Weller RO: Muscle biopsy and diagnosis of muscle disease. In Anthony PP, MacSween RNM, eds: Recent advances in pathology, vol 12. Edinburgh, 1984, Churchill Livingstone, pp 259-288.

Neurogenic atrophy (denervation)

11 Brooke MH, Engel WK: The histographic analysis of human muscle biopsies with regard to fiber types. 2. Diseases of the upper and lower motor neuron. Neurology 19:378-393, 1969.

12 Drachman DB, Murphy SR, Nigam MP, Hills JR: "Myopathic" changes in chronically denervated muscle. Arch Neurol 16:14-24, 1967.

Inflammatory myopathy

13 Albrecht S, Bilbao JM: Ubiquitin expression in inclusion-body myositis. Arch Pathol Lab Med 117:789-793, 1993.

14 Askanas V, Engel WK, Mirabella M: Idiopathic inflammatory myopathies. Inclusion-body myositis, polymyositis and dermatomyositis. Curr Opin Neurol 7:448-456, 1994.

15 Chou SM: Inclusion body myositis. A chronic persistent mumps myositis? Hum Pathol 17:765-777, 1986.

16 Dalakas MC: Polymyositis, dermatomyositis and inclusion-body myositis. N Engl J Med 325:1487-1498, 1991.

17 Engel AG, Hohlfeld R, Banker BQ: The polymyositis and dermatomyositis syndromes. In Engel AG, Franzini-Armstrong C, eds: Myology, ed 2. New York, 1994, McGraw-Hill, pp 1335-1383.

18 Gross B, Ochoa J: Trichinosis. Clinical report and histochemistry of muscle. Muscle Nerve 2:394-398, 1979.

19 Jacob JC, Mathew NT: Pseudohypertrophic myopathy in cysticercosis. Neurology 18:767-771, 1968.

20 Levin MJ, Gardner P, Waldvogel FA: Tropical pyomyositis. An unusual infection due to *Staphylococcus aureus*. N Engl J Med 284:196-198, 1971.

Muscular dystrophies

21 Arahata K, Ishihara T, Kamakura K, et al: Mosaic expression of dystrophin in symptomatic carriers of Duchenne's muscular dystrophy. N Engl J Med 320:138-142, 1989.

22 Bates D, Stevens JC, Hudgeon P: "Polymyositis" with involvement of facial and distal musculature. One form of the facio-scapulohumeral syndrome. J Neurol Sci 19:105-108, 1973.

23 Bell CD, Conen PE: Histopathological changes in Duchenne muscular dystrophy. J Neurol Sci 7:529-544, 1968.

24 Carpenter S, Karpati G: Duchenne muscular dystrophy. Plasma membrane loss initiates muscle cell necrosis unless it is repaired. Brain 102:147-161, 1979.

25 Dowben RM, Vawter GF, Bradfonbrenner A, Sniderman P, Kaegy RD: Polymyositis and other diseases resembling muscular dystrophy. Arch Intern Med 115:584-594, 1965.

26 Engel AG, Yamamoto M, Fischbeck KH. Dystrophinopathies. In Engel A, Franzini-Armstrong C, eds: Myology, ed 2. New York, 1994, McGraw-Hill, pp 1133-1187.

27 Fong P, Turner PR, Denetclaw WF, et al: Increased activity of calcium leak channels in myotubes of Duchenne human and mdx mouse origin. Science 250:673-676, 1990.

28 Hoffman EP, Brown RH, Kundel LM: Dystrophin. The product of the Duchenne muscular dystrophy locus. Cell 51:919-928, 1987.

29 Hoffman EP, Fischbeck KH, Brown RH, et al: Characterization of dystrophin in muscle-biopsy specimens from patients with Duchenne's or Becker's muscular dystrophy. N Engl J Med 318:1363-1368, 1988.

30 Koenig M, Monaco AP, Kundel LM: The complete sequence of dystrophin predicts a rod-shaped cytoskeletal protein. Cell 53:219-228, 1988.

31 Mahadevan M, Tsilfidis C, Sabourin L, Shutter G, Amemiya C, Jansen G, Melville C, Narang M, Barcelo J, O'Hoy K, Leblond S, Earle-MacDonald J, deJong P, Wieringa B, Korneluk PG: Myotonic dystrophy mutation. An unstable CTG repeats in the 3 untranslated region of a candidate gene. Science 255:1253-1255, 1992.

32 Munsat TL, Piper D, Cancilla P, Mednick J: Inflammatory myopathy with facioscapulohumeral distribution. Neurology 22:335-347, 1972.

33 Schmalbruch H: The muscular dystrophies. In Mastaglia FL, Walton JN, eds: Skeletal muscle pathology. London, 1992, Churchill Livingstone, pp 283-318.

34 Schroder JM, Adams RD: The ultrastructural morphology of the muscle fiber in myotonic dystrophy. Acta Neuropathol 10:218-241, 1968.

35 Shields RW Jr: Limb girdle syndrome. In Engel A, Franzini-Armstrong C, eds: Myology. New York, 1994, McGraw-Hill, pp 1258-1274.

Congenital myopathies

36 Barth PG, van Wijnbaarten GK, Bethlem J: X-linked myotubular myopathy with fatal neonatal asphyxia. Neurology 25:531-536, 1975.

37 Bodensteiner JB: Congenital myopathies. Muscle Nerve 17:131-144, 1994.

38 Brooke MG, Neville HE: Reducing body myopathy. Neurology 22:829-840, 1972.

39 Engel AG, Angelini C, Gomez MR: Fingerprint body myopathy. A newly recognized congenital muscle disease. Mayo Clin Proc 47:377-388, 1972.

40 Engel AG, Gomez MR: Nemaline (Z disk) myopathy. Observations on the origin, structure, and solubility properties of the nemaline structures. J Neuropathol Exp Neurol 26:601-619, 1967.

41 Engel AG, Gomez MR, Groover RV: Multicore disease. A recently recognized congenital myopathy associated with multifocal degeneration of muscle fibers. Mayo Clin Proc 46:666-681, 1971.

42 Fukayama Y, Kawazura M, Haruna H: A peculiar form of congenital progressive muscular dystrophy report of fifteen cases. Pediatric Universitatis Tokyo 4:5-8, 1960.

43 Goebel HH, Lenard HG: Congenital myopathies. In Rowland LP, DiMauro S, eds: Handbook of clinical neurology, myopathies, vol 28. Amsterdam, 1992, Elsevier, pp 331-367.

44 Goebel HH, Muller J, Gillen HW, Meritt AD: Autosomal dominant "spheroid body myopathy." Muscle Nerve 1:14-26, 1978.

45 Gonatas NK, Perez MC, Shy GM, Evangelista I: Central core disease of skeletal muscle. Ultrastructural and cytochemical observations in 2 cases. Am J Pathol 47:503-524, 1965.

46 Gonatas NK, Shy GM, Godfrey EH: Nemaline myopathy. The origin of nemaline structures. N Engl J Med 274:535-539, 1966.

47 Hayashi K, Miller RG, Brownell AKW: Central core disease. Ultrastructural of the sarcoplasmic reticulum and T-tubules. Muscle Nerve 12:95-102, 1989.

48 Headington JT, McNamara JO, Brownell AK: Centronuclear myopathy. Histochemistry and electron microscopy. Report of two cases. Arch Pathol 99:16-24, 1975.

49 Kausch K, Lehman-Horn F, Janka M, et al: Evidence for linkage of central core disease locus to the proximal long arm of human chromosome 19. Genomics **10**:765-769, 1991.

50 Munsat TL, Thompson LR, Coleman RF: Centronuclear ("myotubular") myopathy. Arch Neurol **20**:120-131, 1969.

51 Price HM, Gordon GB, Pearson CM, Munsat TL, Blumberg JM: New evidence for excessive accumulation of Z band material in nemaline myopathy. Proc Natl Acad Sci USA **54**:1398-1406, 1965.

52 Quene KA, Healy JMS, Keating KZ, et al: Mutations in ryanodine receptor gene in central core disease and malignant hyperthermia. Nature Genet **5**:51-55, 1993.

53 Ringel SP, Neville HE, Duster MC, Carroll JE: A new congenital neuromuscular disease with trilaminar muscle fibers. Neurology **28**:282-289, 1978.

54 Seitelberger F, Wanko T, Gavin MA: The muscle fiber in central core disease. Histochemical and electron microscopic observations. Acta Neuropathol **1**:223-237, 1961.

55 Shy GM, Engel WK, Somers JE, Wanko T: Nemaline myopathy. A new congenital myopathy. Brain **86**:793-810, 1963.

Metabolic myopathies

56 Attardi G, Schatz G: Biogenesis of mitochondria. Annu Rev Cell Biol **4**:290-333, 1988.

57 Berkovic SF, Carpenter S, Evans A, et al: Myoclonus epilepsy and ragged red fibers (MERRF). I. A clinical, pathological, biochemical, magnetic resonance spectrographic and position emission tomographic study. Brain **112**:1231-1260, 1989.

58 DiMauro S, Bonilla E, Lee CP, Schotland D, Scarpa A, Conn H, Chance B: Luft's disease. Further biochemical and ultrastructural studies of skeletal muscle in the second case. J Neurol Sci **27**:217-232, 1976.

59 DiMauro S, Bresolin E, Hays AP: Disorders of glycogen metabolism of muscle. Crit Rev Clin Neurobiol **1**:83-116, 1984.

60 DiMauro S, Trevisan C, Hays A: Disorders of lipid metabolism in muscle. Muscle Nerve **3**:369-388, 1980.

61 DiMauro S, Servidei S, Zeviani M, et al: Cytochrome c oxidase deficiency in Leigh syndrome. Ann Neurol **22**:498-506, 1987.

62 Holt IJ, Harding AE, Morgan-Hughes JA: Deletions of mitochondrial DNA in patients with mitochondrial myopathies. Nature **331**:717-719, 1988.

63 Hug G, Garancis JC, Schubert WK, Kaplan S: Glycogen storage disease, types II, III, VIII, and IX. Am J Dis Child **111**:457-474, 1966.

64 Morgan-Hughes JA: Mitochondrial disease. In Engel AG, Franzini-Armstrong C, eds: Myology, ed 2. New York, 1994, McGraw-Hill, pp 1610-1660.

65 Olson W, Engel WK, Walsh GO, Einaugler R: Oculo-craniosomatic neuromuscular disease with 'ragged-red' fibers. Histochemical and ultrastructural changes in limb muscles of a group of patients with idiopathic progressive external ophthalmophagia. Arch Neurol **26**:193-211, 1972.

66 Pavlakis SG, Phillips PC, DiMauro S, et al: Mitochondrial myopathy encephalopathy, lactic acidosis and stroke-like episodes. A distinctive clinical syndrome. Ann Neurol **16**:481-488, 1984.

67 Ptacek LJ, Tawil R, Griggs RC, Engel AG, Layzer RB, Kwiecinski H, McManis PG, Santiago L, Moore M, Fouad G, Bradley P, Leppert MF: Dihydropyridine receptor mutation causes hypokalamic periodic paralysis. Cell **77**:863-868, 1994.

68 Rivner MH, Shamsnia M, Swift TR, et al: Kearns-Sayne syndrome and complex II deficiency. Neurology **39**:693, 1988.

69 Rudel R, Richer K, Lehman-Hu F: Genotype-phenotype in human skeletal muscle channel diseases. Arch Neurol **50**:1241-1248, 1993.

70 Shy GM, Gonatas NK, Perez M: Two childhood myopathies with abnormal mitochondria. I. Megaconial myopathy. II. Pleconial myopathy. Brain **89**:133-158, 1966.

71 Taroni F, Verderio D, Fiorucci S, Cavadini P, Finocchiaro G, Uziel G, Lamantea E, Gellera C, DiDonato S: Molecular characterization of inherited carnitine palmitoyl transferase II deficiency. Proc Natl Acad Sci USA **89**:8429-8433, 1992.

72 Tsujino S, Shanske S, DiMauro S: Molecular genetic heterogeneity of myophosphorylase deficiency (McArdle's diseases). N Engl J Med **329**:241-245, 1993.

73 Zeviani M, Bonilla E, DeVivo DC, et al: Mitochondrial disease. Neurol Clin **7**:123-155, 1989.

Drug-induced myopathy

74 Dalakas M: Inflammatory and toxic myopathies. Curr Opin Neurol Neurosurg **5**:645-654, 1992.

75 Dubowitz V: Muscle biopsy. A practical approach, ed 2. London, Bailliere Tindall, 1985, pp 82-128.

76 Estes ML, Ewing-Wilson D, Chou SM, et al: Chloroquine neuromyotoxicity. Clinical and pathologic perspective. Am J Med **82**:447-455, 1987.

77 Kakulas BA, Mastaglia FL: Drug-induced, toxic and nutritional myopathies. In Mastaglia FL, Walton JN, eds. Skeletal muscle pathology. London, 1992, Churchill Livingstone, pp 511-540.

78 Klinkerfuss G, Bleisch V, Dioso MM, Perkoff GT: A spectrum of myopathy associated with alcoholism. II. Light and electron microscopic observations. Ann Intern Med **67**:493-510, 1967.

79 Kuncl RW, Duncan G, Watson D, Alderson K, Rogawski IA, Peper M: Colchicine myopathy and neuropathy. N Engl J Med **316**:1562-1568, 1987.

80 Kuncl RW, George EB. Toxic neuropathies and myopathies. Curr Opin Neurol **6**:695-704, 1993.

81 Mhiri C, Baudrimont M, Bonne G, et al: Zidovudine myopathy. A distinctive disorder associated with mitochondrial dysfunction. Ann Neurol **29**:606-614, 1991.

82 Silver RM, Heyes MP, Maize JC, Quearry B, Vionnet-Fausset M, Sternberg EM: Scleroderma, fasciitis, and eosinophilia associated with the ingestion of tryptophan. N Engl J Med **332**:874-881, 1990.

NEUROMUSCULAR JUNCTION DISORDERS

83 Eaton LM, Lambert EH: Electromyography and electrical stimulation of nerves in diseases of the motor units. Observations on a myasthenic syndrome associated with malignant tumours. JAMA **163**:1117-1124, 1957.

84 Lindstrom JM, Seybold ME, Lennon VA, Whittingham S, Duane DD: Antibody to acetylcholine receptor in myasthenia gravis. Neurology **26**:1054-1059, 1976.

85 Russell DS: Histological changes in the striped muscle in myasthenia gravis. J Pathol Bacteriol **65**:279-289, 1953.

86 Santa T, Engel AG, Lambert EH: Histometric study of neuromuscular junction ultrastructure. I. Myasthenia gravis. Neurology **22**:71-82, 1972.

87 Vincent A, Lang B, Newson-Davis J: Autoimmunity to the voltage-gated calcium channel underlies the Lambert-Eaton myasthenic syndrome, a paraneoplastic disorder. Trends Neurosci **12**:496-502, 1989.

29 Pituitary gland

Juan M. Bilbao, M.D.

NORMAL ANATOMY

The pituitary gland consists of the anterior lobe (adenohypophysis), the posterior lobe (neurohypophysis), and the intermediate zone. The adenohypophysis originates from a small ectodermal diverticulum of the stomodeum that extends toward the diencephalic portion of the neural plate. By the sixth week of gestation, the stalk that connects the pouch to the stomodeum disappears, and an infundibular process (the future neurohypophysis) originating in the diencephalon grows to come in contact with the "pinched off" portion of Rathke's pouch.

Grossly, the pituitary gland in the adult is a tan, bean-shaped structure weighing about 600 mg and measuring 13 × 10 × 6 mm. The adenohypophysis (anterior lobe) occupies 80% of the gland and comprises the pars distalis, intermedia, and tuberalis, whereas the neurohypophysis consists of the infundibulum, the pituitary stalk, and the posterior lobe.

Histologically adenohypophysial cells are arranged in intermingling columns and nests demarcated by basal lamina, surrounding reticulin, and a capillary network. In H&E-stained sections, three cell types are recognized in the adenohypophysis: acidophils (40%), basophils (10%), and chromophobes (50%). The pars tuberalis consists of FSH-, LH-,

and less frequently, ACTH-containing cells around the pituitary stalk. These cells may exhibit squamous metaplasia during aging[1,6] (Fig. 29-1). The presence of corticotropic cells in the pars nervosa of the pituitary has been shown often in specimens obtained at autopsy.[4] Immunohistochemistry delineates the five principal cell types and the six hormones that they produce. The ultrastructural features of the five hormone-producing adenohypophysial cells are shown in Figs. 29-2 to 29-6.[2,3,8] Somatotrophs (GH cells) account for 50% of all adenohypophyial cells; lactotrophs (prolactin [PRL]-secreting cells) constitute 20%; corticotrophs (ACTH cells) represent 15% to 20%; thyrotrophs (TSH cells) constitute 5%; and gonadotrophs (FSH and LH cells) account for 10%.[2,3] Histologic and immunohistologic evidence indicates that FSH and LH are produced by the same cell, but these two hormones may also be produced in isolation.

The folliculostellate cell is an element of indeterminate nature found scattered throughout the anterior lobe. Immunohistochemical studies reveal that these cells react strongly for S-100 protein and variably for GFAP, keratin, and vimentin.[7] The functional role of folliculostellate cells has yet to be elucidated.

Cystic structures of variable dimensions lined by cuboidal ciliated epithelium are often found interposed between neurohypophysis and the pars distalis. These are thought to be remnants of Rathke's pouch. Surgical pathologists should be aware of salivary gland rests[9] and nests of granular cells[5] that can rarely be found in the neurohypophysis.

PITUITARY ADENOMA
General and clinical features

Pituitary neoplasms have traditionally made up 10% of the intracranial tumors, but their relative incidence has risen to almost 25% in some institutions as a result of refinement in radioimmunoassay, imaging techniques, and transsphenoidal microsurgery.[15a,22,22a] They arise from the cells of the adenohypophysis and are designated as *pituitary adenomas.* Most examples are found within the confines of the sella turcica. However, since aberrant adenohypophysial cells are known to occur in the diencephalic infundibulum, pituitary stalk,[12] and sphenoid bone between the nasopharynx and pituitary fossa, the appearance of pituitary adenomas in one of these locations (including the root of the nasal cavity) is not unexpected, even if exceptional.[16,17]

Although pituitary adenomas are usually benign lesions, their growth rate is highly variable and unpredictable. Whereas some microadenomas may exhibit little or no detectable change in size over time, others show rapid expansion and invasion of adjacent meninges, bone, sinuses, and brain. Pituitary adenomas may synthesize and release hormones, and in about 70% of cases, there is clinical and/or

The author is indebted to Dr. Kalman Kovacs (Toronto) for his invaluable contribution to this chapter.

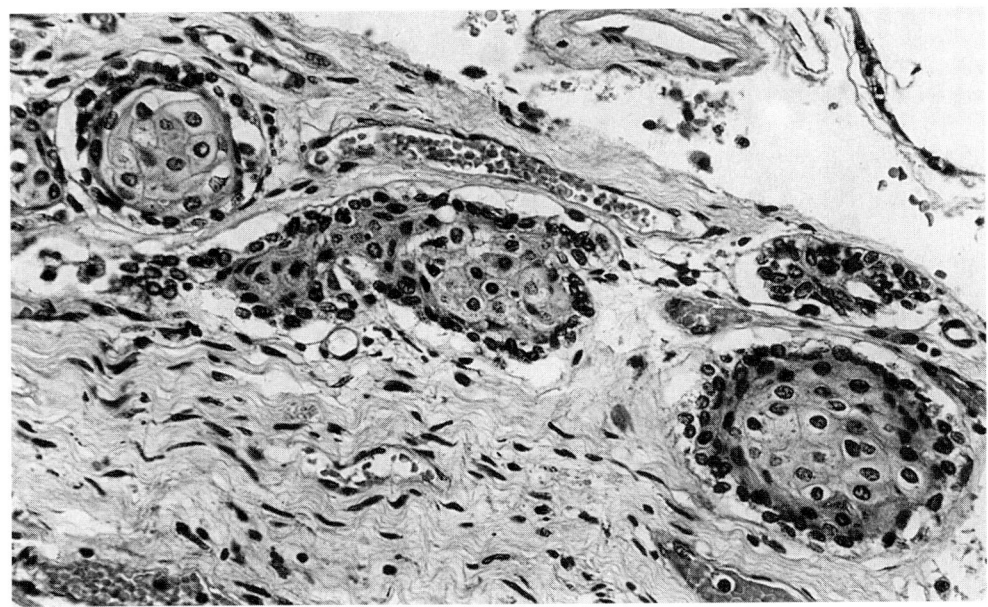

Fig. 29-1 Squamous metaplasia of adenohypophysial cells in pars tuberalis.

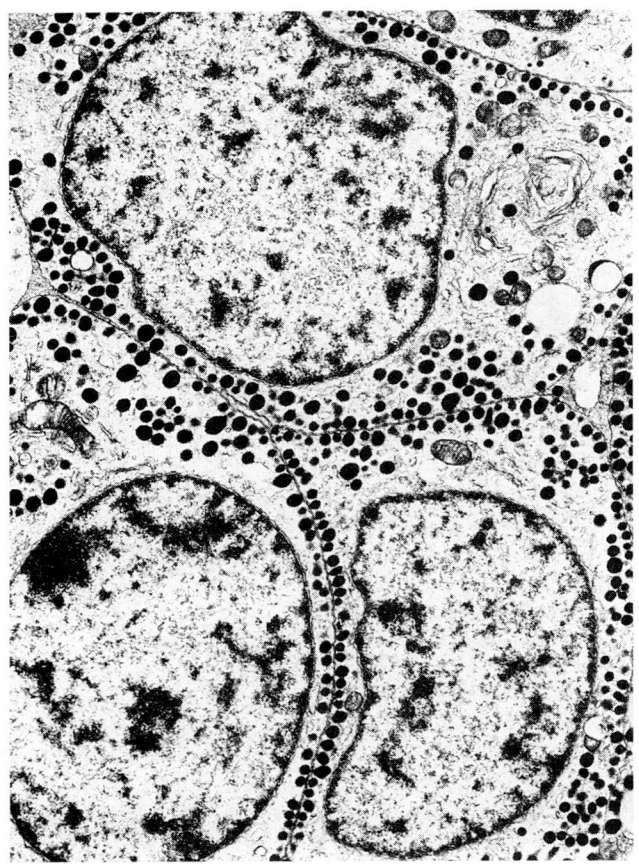

Fig. 29-2 Growth hormone cells have well-developed Golgi complexes and are densely granulated with evenly electron-dense spherical secretory granules measuring 350 to 500 nm in diameter. (Electron micrograph, ×6150; courtesy Dr. E. Horvath, Toronto.)

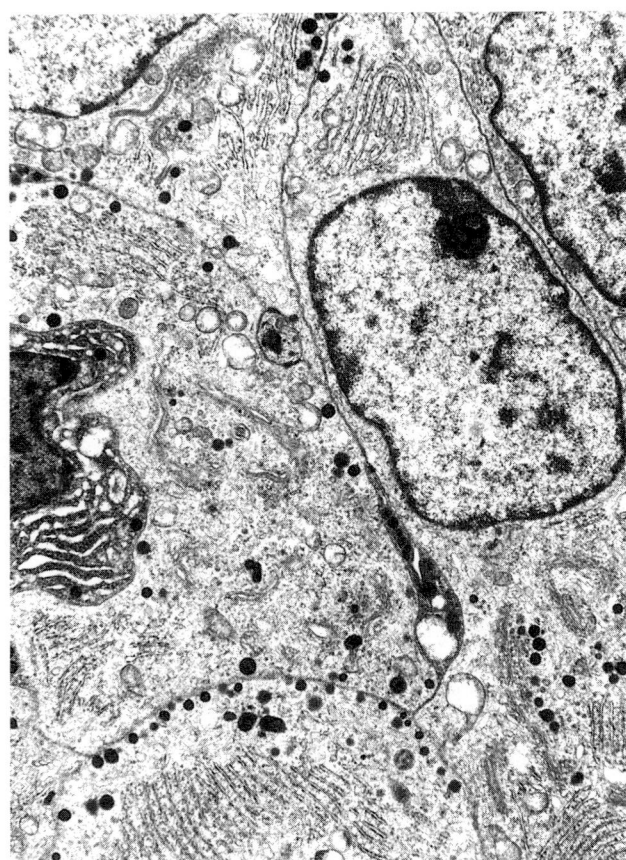

Fig. 29-3 Cytoplasm of prolactin cells displays stacks of well-developed RER and sparse secretory granules measure up to 300 nm. (Electron micrograph, ×5896; courtesy Dr. E. Horvath, Toronto.)

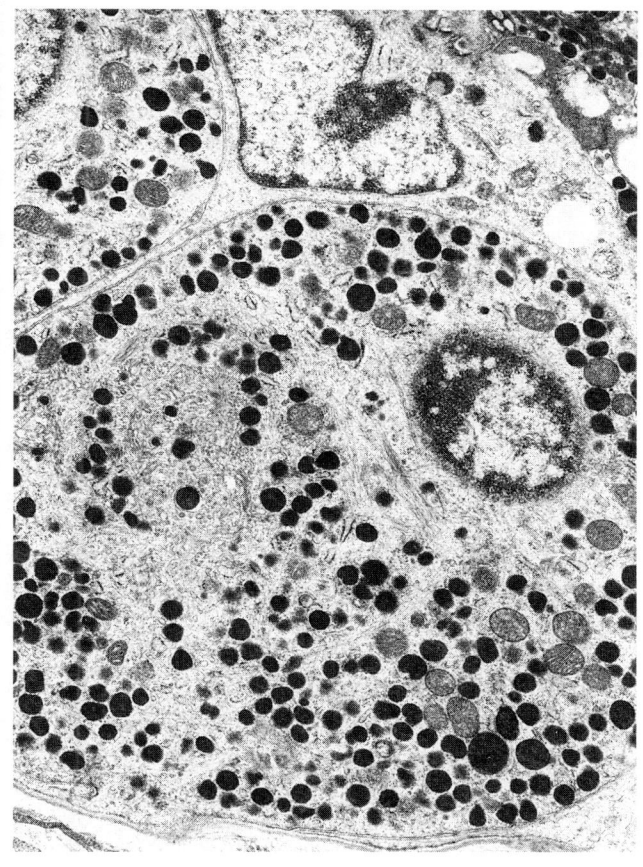

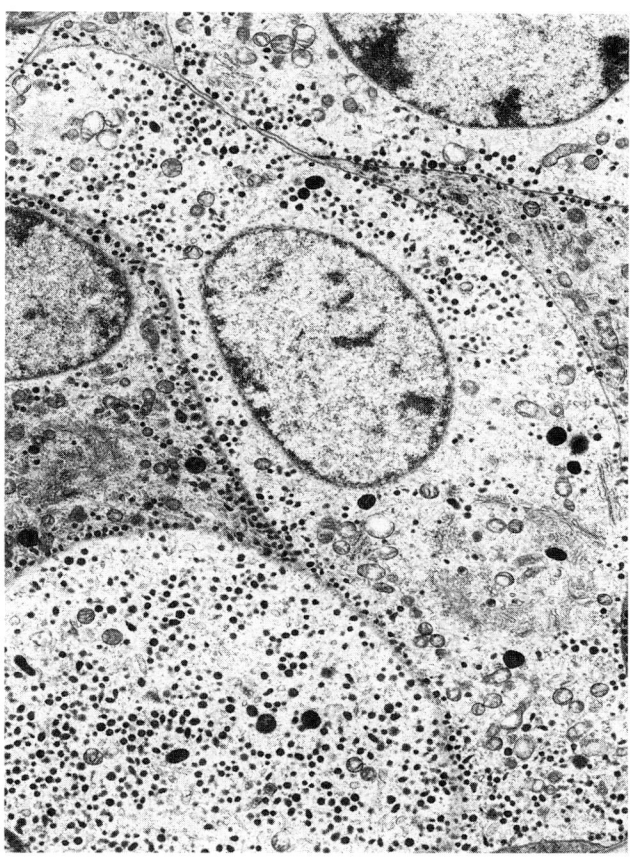

Fig. 29-4 Corticotroph cells show widely distributed RER membranes and prominent Golgi complex displays dilated saccule-containing developing secretory granules. Secretory granules are irregular in shape and measure between 300 to 350 nm. Bundles of filaments are present in perinuclear cytoplasm. (Electron micrograph, ×7480; courtesy Dr. E. Horvath, Toronto.)

Fig. 29-5 Thyrotroph cells are of medium to large size with angular shape and long processes. Secretory granules measure 150 to 200 nm. (Electron micrograph, ×4500; courtesy Dr. E. Horvath, Toronto.)

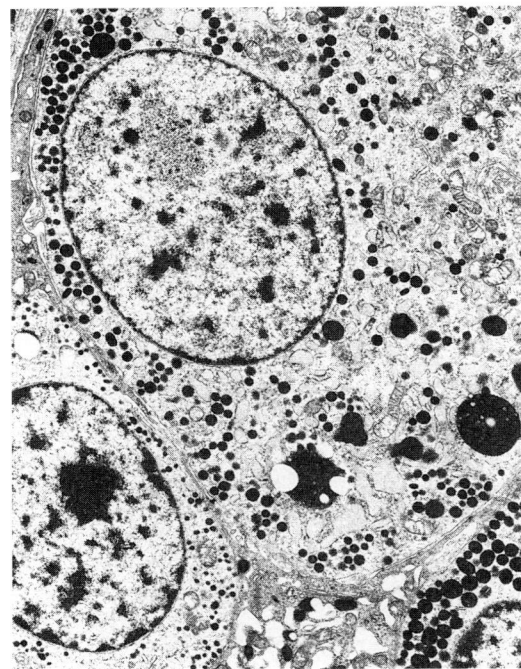

Fig. 29-6 Gonadotroph cells exhibit network of dilated RER and secretory granules whose number, size, electron density, and morphology vary considerably. (Electron micrograph, ×5700; courtesy Dr. E. Horvath, Toronto.)

biochemical evidence of a characteric **hypersecretory syndrome.**[22] Some patients harboring pituitary adenomas may present to the clinician with insidious symptoms of hypopituitarism (secondary to destruction of the normal gland or interference with the delivery of hypothalamic hormones) affecting one or more pituitary hormones.

Pituitary adenomas with suprasellar extension occur in about 10% to 20% of cases. This may give rise to a constellation of neurologic signs and symptoms, not uncommonly as the first manifestation of the disease, related to compression of optic nerves, chiasm, cavernous sinus, and oculomotor nerves. The term **pituitary appoplexy** is reserved for those cases with the abrupt onset of headache, ocular deficits, and altered consciousness. This uncommon but well-known neurosurgical emergency results from hemorrhage and necrosis in an adenoma.[10]

Pituitary adenomas as a group are more frequent in adults and show no major gender difference. Adenomas in younger patients are uncommon.[15,19] Microadenomas are detected in about one fourth of autopsies.[11,20] In a small percentage of patients, the pituitary tumor is one of the components of the multiple endocrine neoplasia syndrome type I.[21] Endocrinologically silent (clinically and biochemically nonfunctional) adenomas tend to be large and constitute about one third of surgically removed pituitary tumors. By contrast, the vast majority of pituitary adenomas in childhood and adolescence are functional.[14]

Enlargement and erosion of the floor of the sella turcica are common findings and important radiologic signs. Currently, magnetic resonance imaging is regarded as the method of choice for the imaging diagnosis of pituitary lesions because of its sensitivity and high resolution[23] (Fig. 29-7).

On the basis of these newer imaging techniques, an anatomic classification of pituitary tumors has been devised.[13,18] Accordingly, microadenomas are intrasellar tumors less than 10 mm in diameter. Macroadenomas with suprasellar extension (SSE) include the following subtypes: grade A (moderate SSE within 10 mm above the jugum sphenoidale, filling the chiasmatic cistern), grade B (large SSE, up to 20 mm, elevating the anterior recess of the third ventricle), grade C (very large SSE, up to 30 mm, filling the anterior third ventricle), and grade D (huge SSE, in excess of 30 mm, above the level of the foramen of Monro, or grade C with asymmetric lateral or multiple expansion).

Gross features

Grossly, pituitary adenomas are usually solid and soft. Their color varies from gray to red according to the degree of vascularity. Cystic, hemorrhagic, and necrotic changes may occur. A characteristic gross appearance is that of a tumor occupying both the intrasellar and suprasellar areas (Fig. 29-8), with a central constriction produced by the diaphragm and the circle of Willis.

Terms that are sometimes used for pituitary adenomas are *enclosed* (when encased within the dural covering of the sella), *invasive* (when infiltrating the dura, the floor of the sella, nasal sinuses, or other structures), and *giant* (when the superior growing edge of the tumor is 20 mm above the jugum sphenoidale)[25] (Fig. 29-9). The most common pattern of gross local invasion is lateral extension and penetration of the cavernous sinus.[24] Even invasive adenomas tend to displace rather than infiltrate the brain. The invasive tendencies of the adenoma can be identified by neuroimaging, by direct inspection at the time of surgery, or by histologic examination if the tissue sample is adequate (Fig. 29-10). Some of the larger adenomas may undergo suprasellar extension, with intrusion into brain mimicking a primary intraventricular tumor if the brain specimen is viewed in isolation (see Fig. 29-9). When massive parasellar extension occurs the tumor may grow intradurally into all the compartments of the base of the brain.

Microscopic features

The microscopic pattern in H&E sections varies from case to case, the differences being based on the relative degrees of cellularity and vascularity. The pattern of growth may be diffuse (solid) (Fig. 29-11, *A*), sinusoidal (trabecular), or papillary (pseudopapillary) (Fig. 29-11, *B*). Glandular arrangement of cells is unusual and suggestive of gonadotroph adenoma (Fig. 29-12, *A*). Some lesions are hypocellular with marked sclerohyalinization of the stroma. The use of reticulin stains facilitates the identification of the tumor-gland interface, with no fibrous capsule in between. The pituitary tissue at the periphery of the adenoma is compressed with condensation of the reticulin network, which is disrupted in the tumor (Fig. 29-13).

The tumor cells are generally round or polygonal and less commonly elongated (Fig. 29-12, *B*). They have a round or oval nucleus and a variable amount of cytoplasm, which may be basophilic, acidophilic, amphophilic, or chromo-

Text continued on p. 2424.

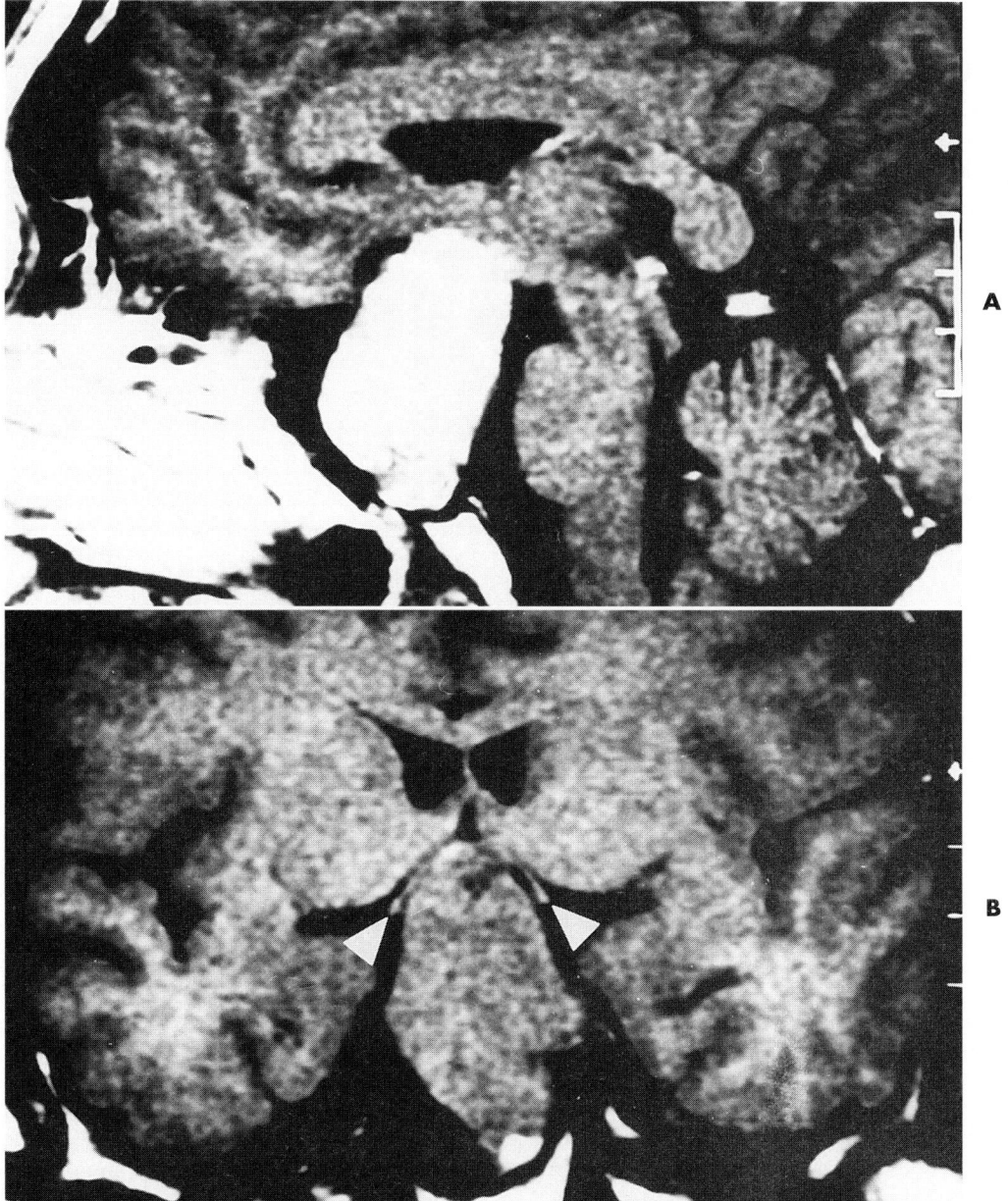

Fig. 29-7 Nuclear magnetic resonance imaging of giant prolactinoma in 50-year-old male. Sagittal view (T$_1$ weighted with gadolinium) shows enhancing sellar and suprasellar mass **(A)**. Coronal image (T1 weighted) discloses isodense mass compressing optic chiasma and nerves *(arrows)* **(B).**

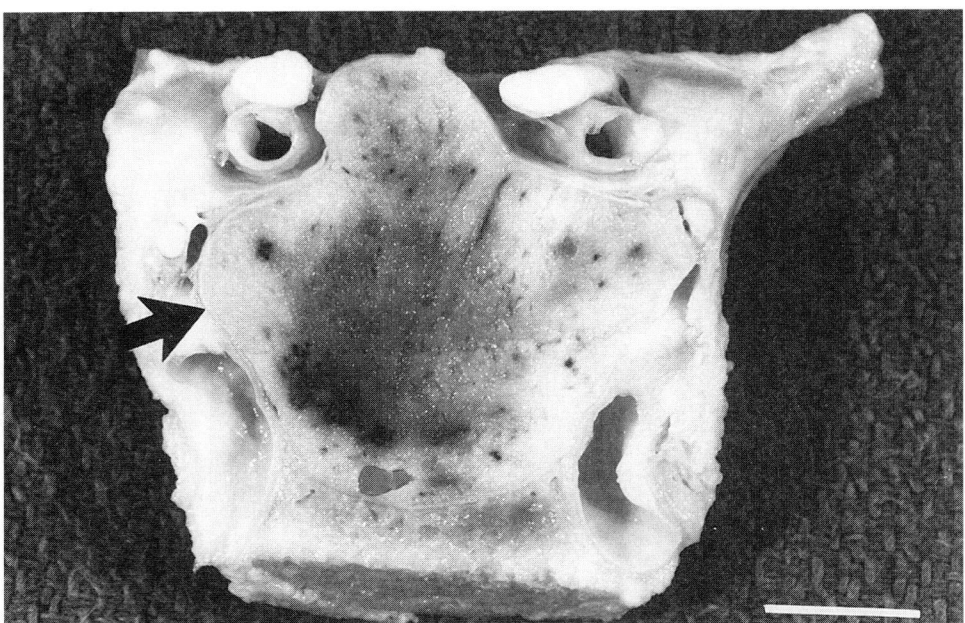

Fig. 29-8 Incidental finding at autopsy of null cell adenoma in a 78-year-old woman. Dorsal view and coronal section of sella showing diffuse tumor that fills sella and compresses residual pituitary tissue into thin peripheral rim (*arrow;* see also Fig. 29-13). Note moderate suprasellar extension. (Bar = 1 cm; specimen courtesy Dr. William Halliday, Winnipeg.)

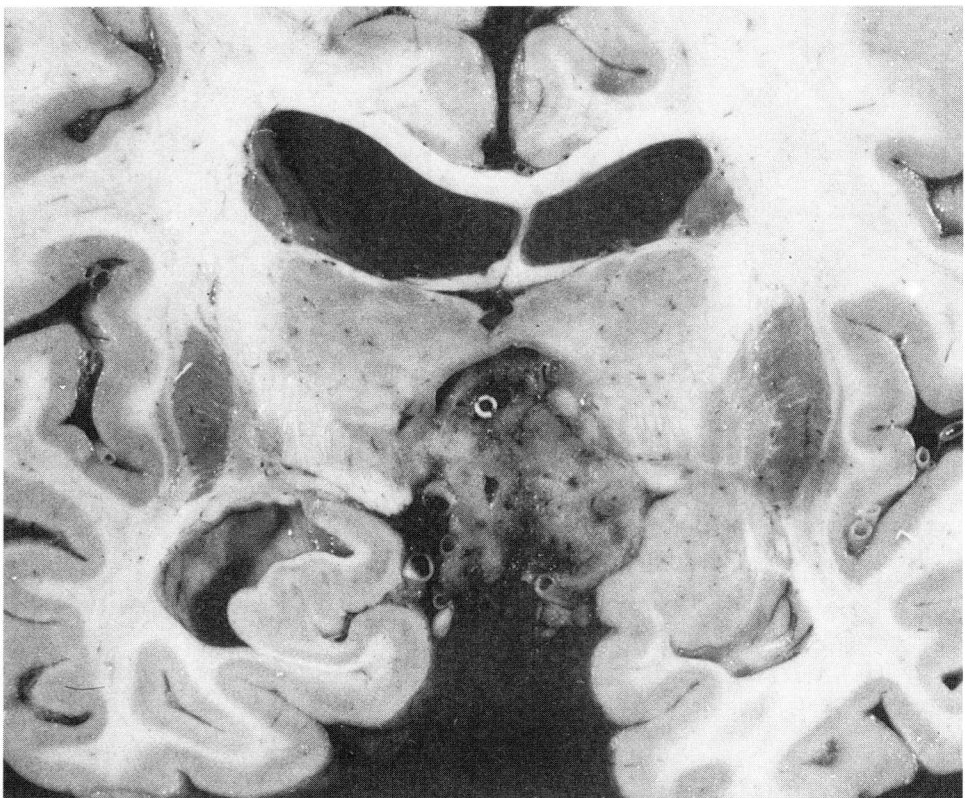

Fig. 29-9 Giant mixed PRL and GH cell adenoma intruding into brain in 74-year-old female with 2-year history of dementia and visual impairment.

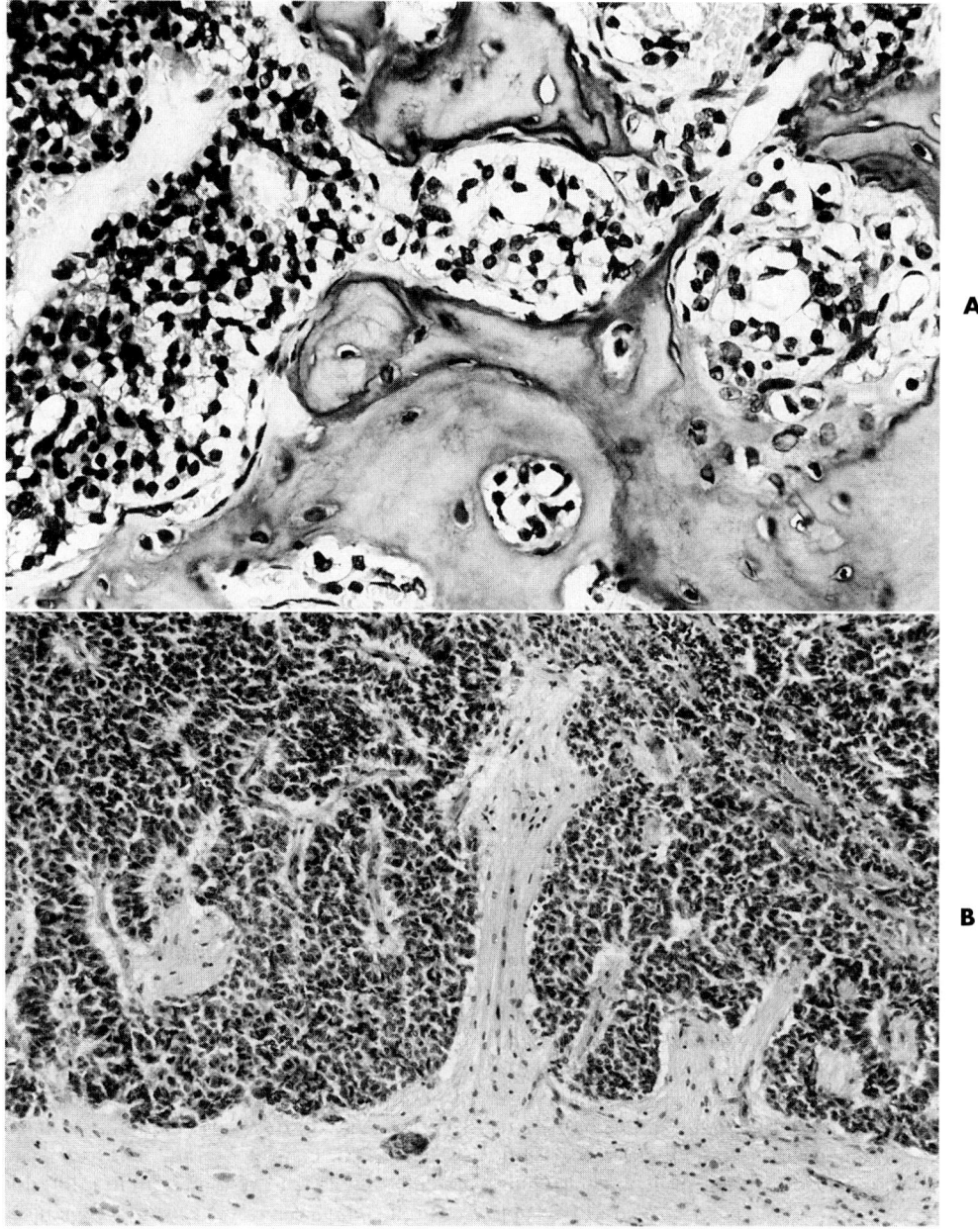

Fig. 29-10 Pituitary adenoma invasive to bone **(A)** and brain **(B)** (same case as in Fig. 30-9).

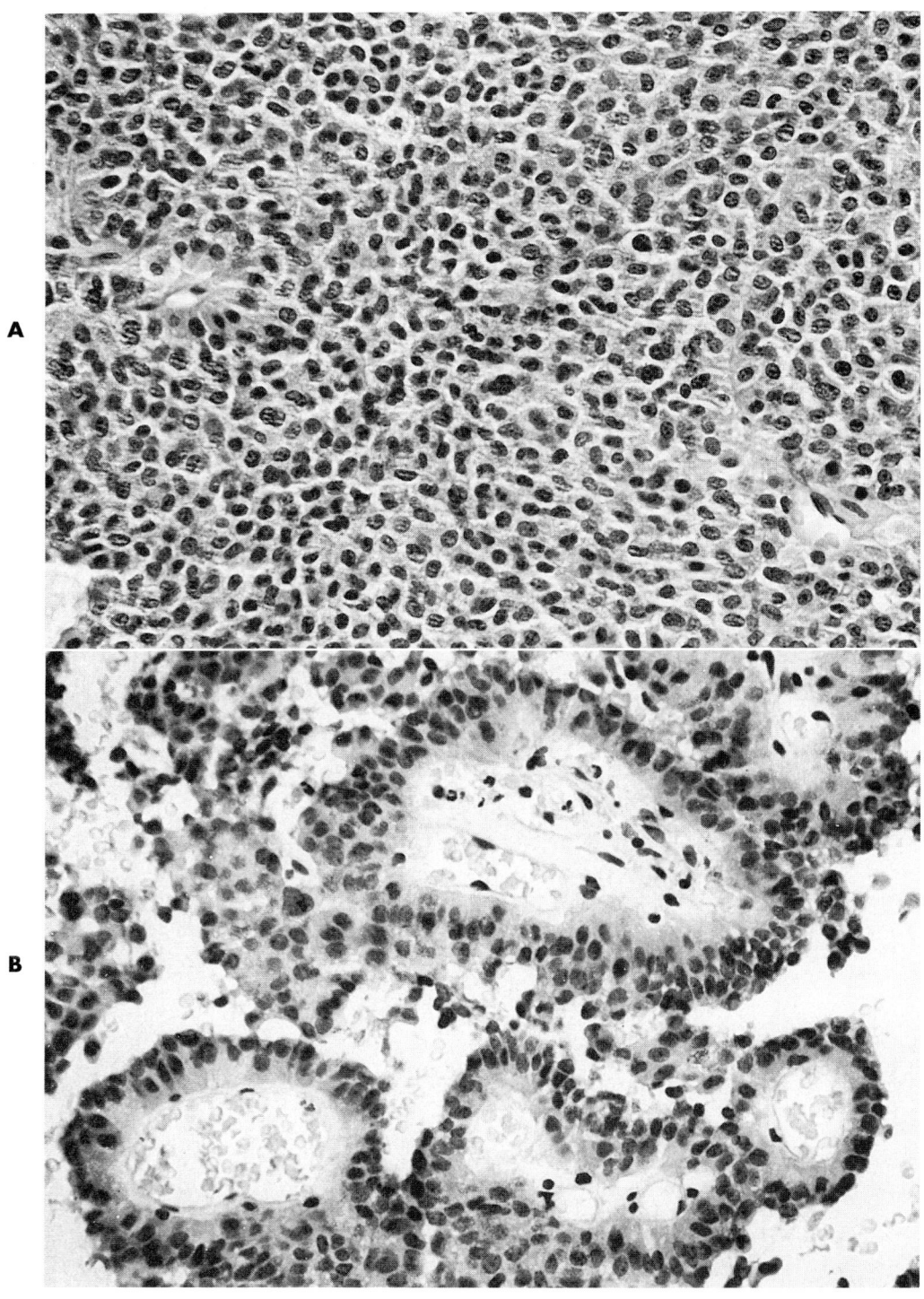

Fig. 29-11 Pituitary adenoma. **A,** Diffuse type. **B,** Papillary type.

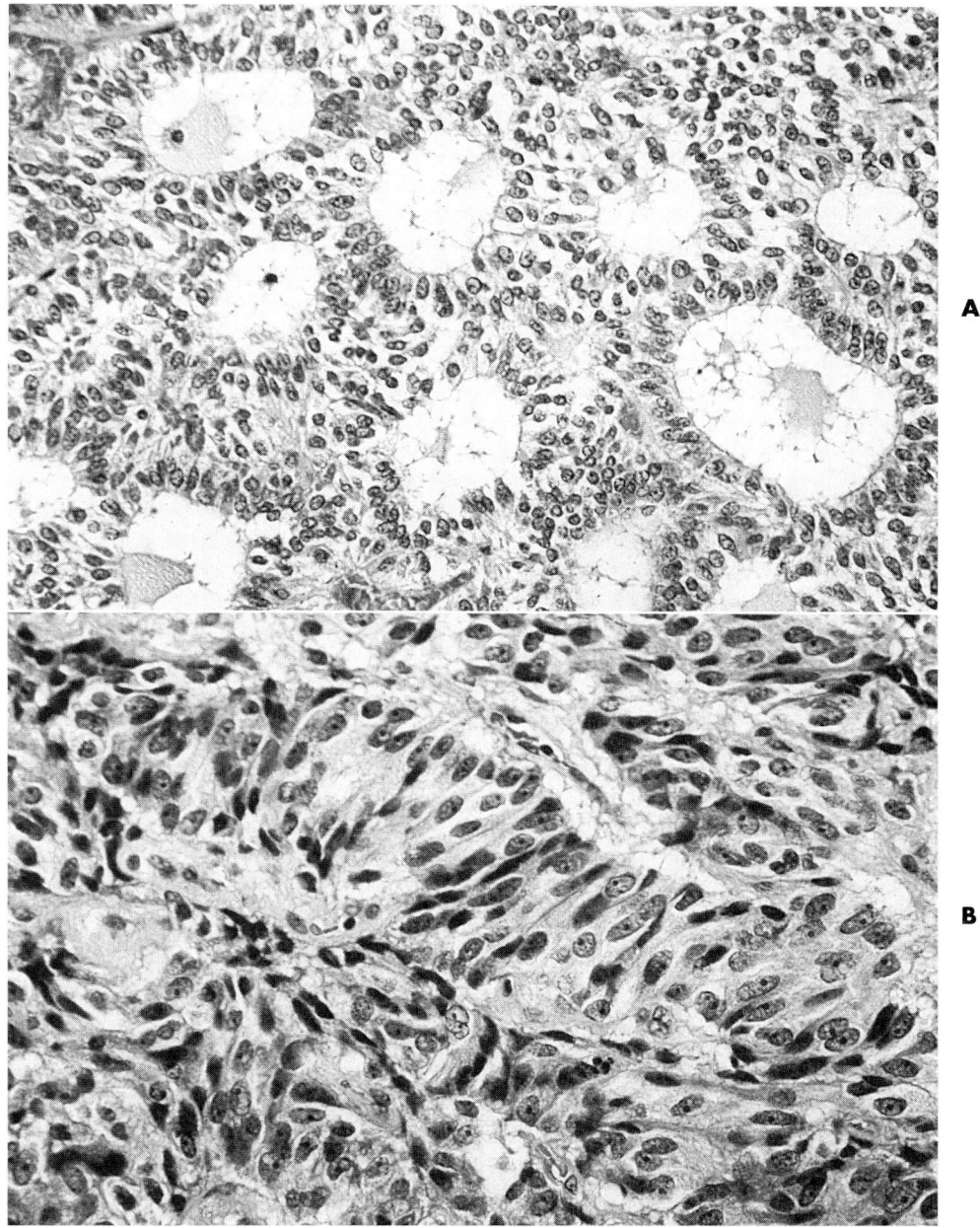

Fig. 29-12 Pituitary adenoma. **A,** Glandular pattern. **B,** Short spindle cells.

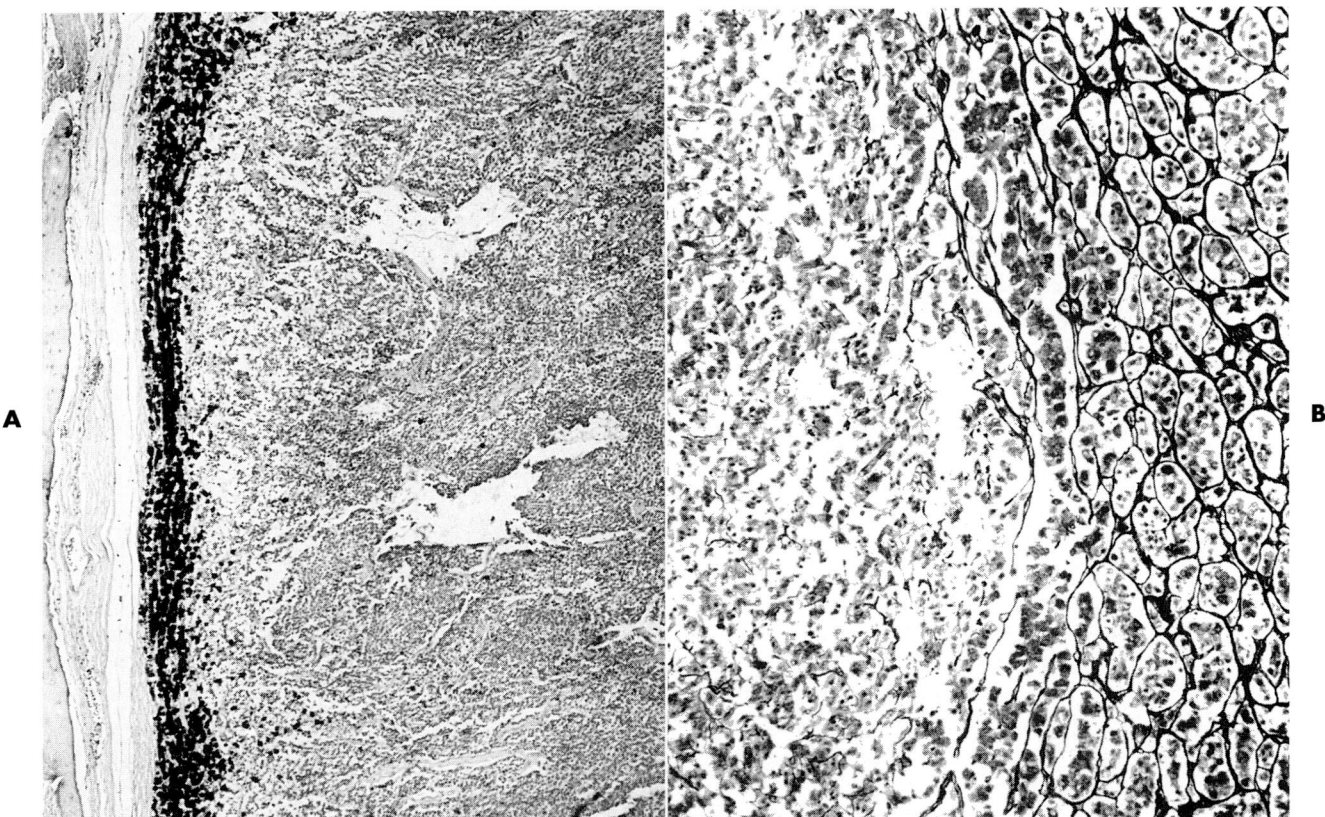

Fig. 29-13 Pituitary adenoma. **A,** Immunostaining of GH highlights residual adenohypophysis at the periphery of enlarged sella (Same case as in Fig. 29-8). **B,** Gordon and Sweet preparation shows dissolution of reticulin network in tumor.

phobic. In intraoperative touch and smear preparations, nuclear pleomorphism and multinucleated cells are readily detected (Fig. 29-14). Mitoses are scanty or absent. Occasional bizarre hyperchromatic nuclei may occur, including giant and ring forms with prominent nucleoli (Fig. 29-14, *C*). Poor correlation exists between histopathologic findings and the aggressiveness of pituitary adenomas. In a study including nonrecurrent and recurrent tumors, the proliferating cell nuclear antigen index was found to be highest among recurrent tumors and in macroadenomas.[27] In some cases, the tumor cells have the morphologic appearance of oncocytes. Calcification occurs in about 7% of pituitary adenomas (Fig. 29-15, *B*), primarily in PRL-secreting neoplasms.[29] The deposition of endocrine amyloid has also been documented in some of these tumors; such deposits are seen mainly in PRL cell adenomas[26,28] (see Fig. 29-15, *A*). In tumors that have undergone hemorrhage and necrosis, the specimen may have the appearance of altered blood, making identification of the adenoma difficult.

Pituitary adenomas composed of uniform cells of clear cytoplasm may be confused with oligodendrogliomas, whereas those consisting of oval cells with acidophilic cytoplasm and eccentric nucleus may be mistaken for plasma cell myeloma. The most common error, however, is the misinterpretation of a papillary type of pituitary adenoma as an ependymoma.

Classification

The traditional classification of pituitary adenomas into chromophobe, acidophil, and basophil variants correlates so poorly with the specific cell types and the corresponding patterns of hormone secretion that there is little use in maintaining it. It has become evident that most normal "chromophobe" cells simply represent specific cells of one kind or another in which the granules are not numerous enough to be obvious at the light microscopic level. The same is true of the so-called chromophobe adenomas. Ultrastructural studies have demonstrated that truly agranular adenomas do not exist.[32-34] Acidophilic pituitary tumors also have been shown to be highly heterogenous. Immunohistochemical studies have demonstrated no detectable hormones in some tumors, whereas others display immunopositivity for GH, PRL, or both.

There is now general agreement that the hormones of the nontumorous adenohypophysis are secreted by a single cell type. The identification of these cells and the correlation with a given hormone have been achieved by careful immunohistochemical and electron microscopic studies under normal and abnormal conditions. The same approach should be followed in the case of neoplasms.[32,37] H&E stains should be routinely supplemented by PAS stain, immunohistochemical (Fig. 29-16), and electron microscopic examination. The contribution of these techniques to the characterization of non-

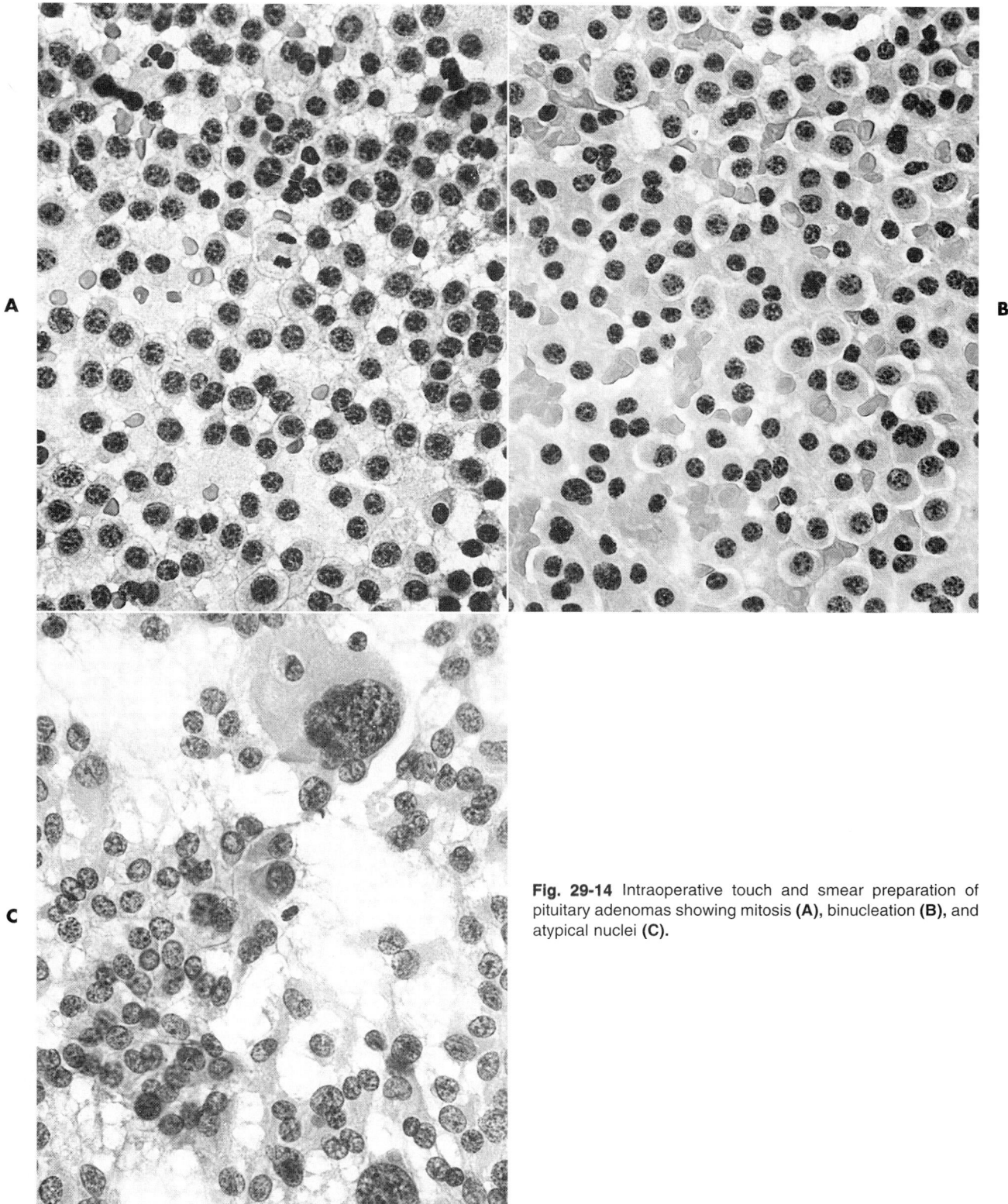

Fig. 29-14 Intraoperative touch and smear preparation of pituitary adenomas showing mitosis **(A),** binucleation **(B),** and atypical nuclei **(C).**

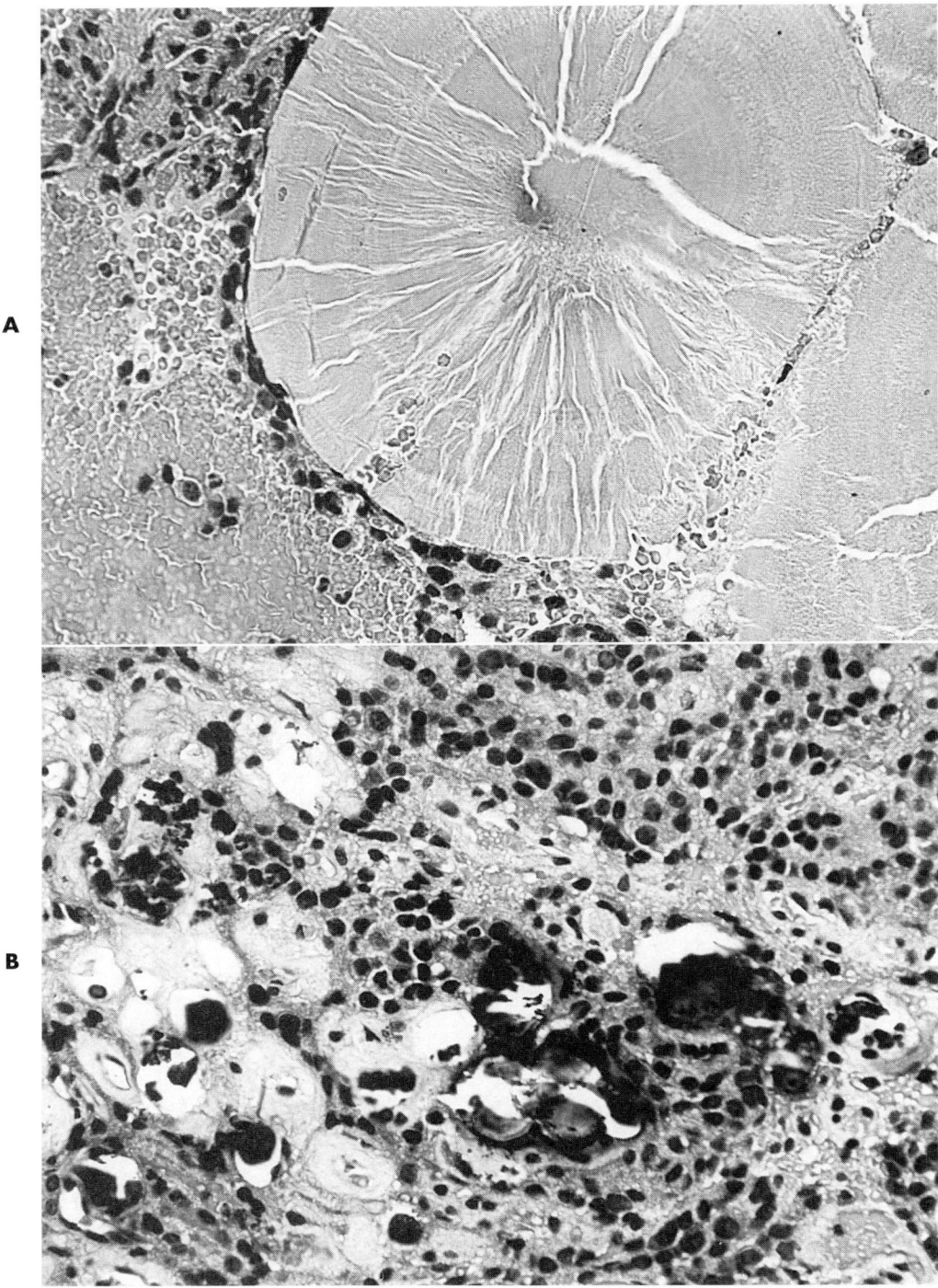

Fig. 29-15 Prolactinomas with amyloid deposition in the form of large spheroids **(A)** and scattered cal-cospherites **(B)**.

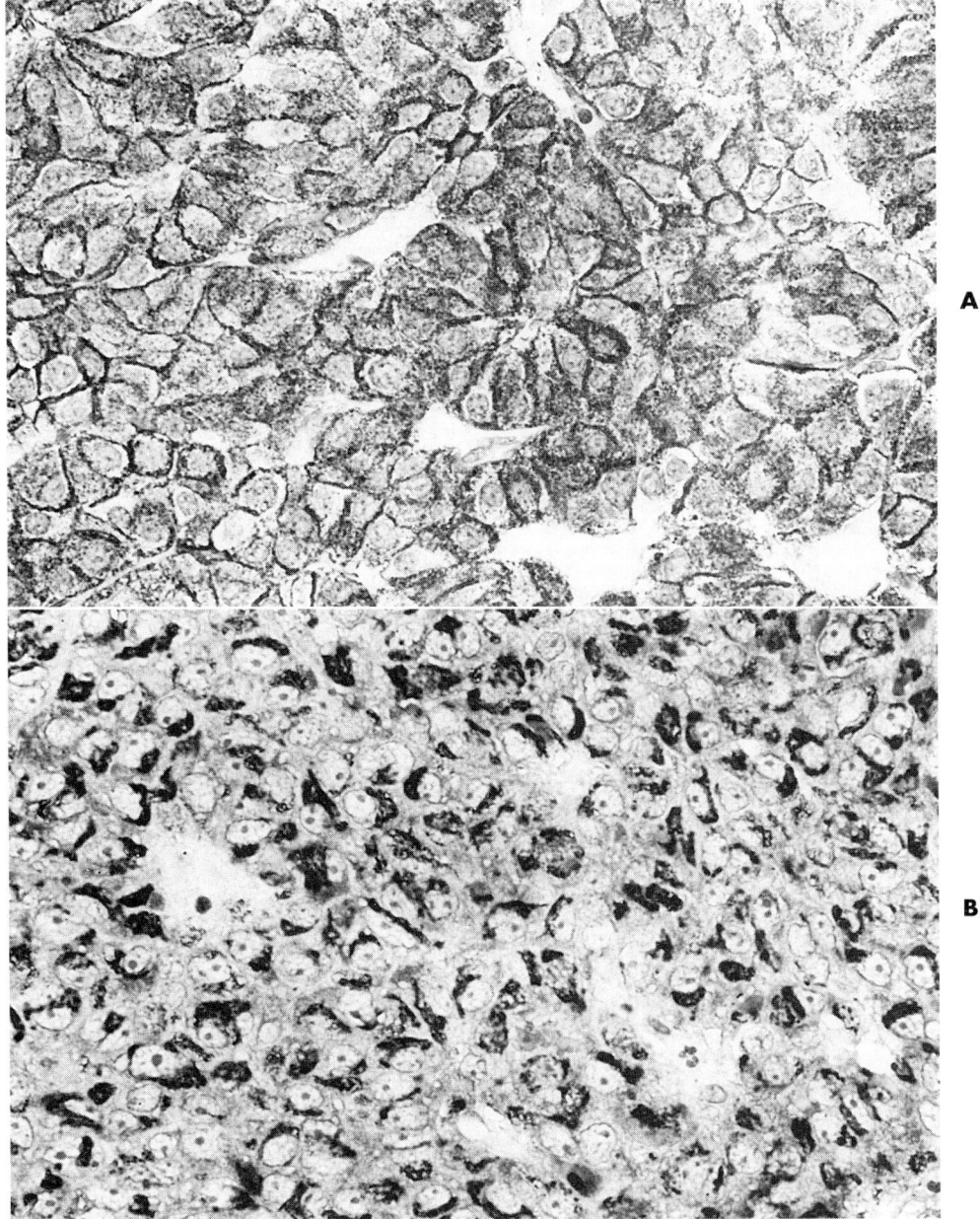

Fig. 29-16 Note different patterns of immunoreactivity of secretory granules, which are restricted to peripheral parts of cytoplasm in ACTH adenoma **(A)** and form typical perinuclear crescents in prolactinoma **(B).**

functioning or "silent" pituitary adenomas is essential.[30,31,38] The substantial majority of clinically nonsecreting adenomas are found to correspond to null cell adenomas, oncocytomas, or gonadotroph adenomas.[35]

The current classification of pituitary adenomas is based on cell type, largely ascertained by immunohistochemical reactions against the specific hormones and by electron microscopy[33,34,37] (Table 29-1). Some pituitary adenomas are also immunoreactive for alpha-subunit, neuron-specific enolase, chromogranin, synaptophysin, and estrogen receptor.[39] Most pituitary adenomas, even those with a plurihormonal phenotype, are considered to be distinct and uniform neoplasms. The occurrence of **double adenomas,** that is, two morphologically and/or imunocytologically distinct patterns in the same surgical specimen, is infrequent.[36]

PRL cell adenoma

PRL cell adenoma is the most common neoplasm arising in the adenohypophysis, accounting for 50% of tumors found incidentally at autopsy[41] and for about 30% of those encountered by the neurosurgeon.[45] The latter group is composed mostly of women of child-bearing age who present with the galactorrhea-amenorrhea syndrome (**Chiari-Frommel syndrome** or **Forbes-Albright syndrome**). The implementation of dopamine agonists as a proven nonsurgical therapeutic alternative for many prolactinomas may explain a decline in their numbers in current surgical series.

Serum level values of PRL above 200 ng/ml are considered diagnostic of PRL-secreting adenomas. Elevation of PRL serum levels up to 150 ng/ml may be the result of a "stalk effect."[46]

In women of child-bearing age, prolactinomas are usually encountered in the microadenoma stage, whereas in males (see Fig. 29-7) and elderly females prolactinomas may acquire large sizes, have a higher incidence of dural invasion, and have usually transgressed the confines of the sella turcica at presentation.

Histologically, these neoplasms are chromophobic or slightly acidophilic, are PAS negative, and exhibit a diffuse or, less commonly, papillary pattern. Some tumors possess a prominent hyalinized stroma, and microcalcification is shown in about one fifth of cases (see Fig. 29-15, *B*). Coarse mineral deposition and ossification with the development of "pituitary stones" rarely occur.[47,48] Endocrine amyloid is not

Table 29-1 Classification of pituitary adenomas*

Cell type	Incidence
Sparsely granulated PRL cell adenoma	26%
Densely granulated PRL cell adenoma	1%
Sparsely granulated GH cell adenoma	7%
Densely granulated GH cell adenoma	7%
Mixed PRL and GH synthesizing adenomas	6%
Acidophil stem cell adenoma	2%
Functioning corticotroph cell adenoma	8%
Silent "corticotroph" cell adenomas	6%
Gonadotroph adenoma	6%
Thyrotroph adenoma	1%
Null cell adenoma (oncocytoma)	26%
Unclassified plurihormonal adenomas	4%

*Relative frequency of each tumor subtype in a series of over 3000 surgically removed pituitary adenomas.
Data from Dr. K. Kovacs and Dr. E. Horvath, St. Michael's Hospital, Toronto, 1994.

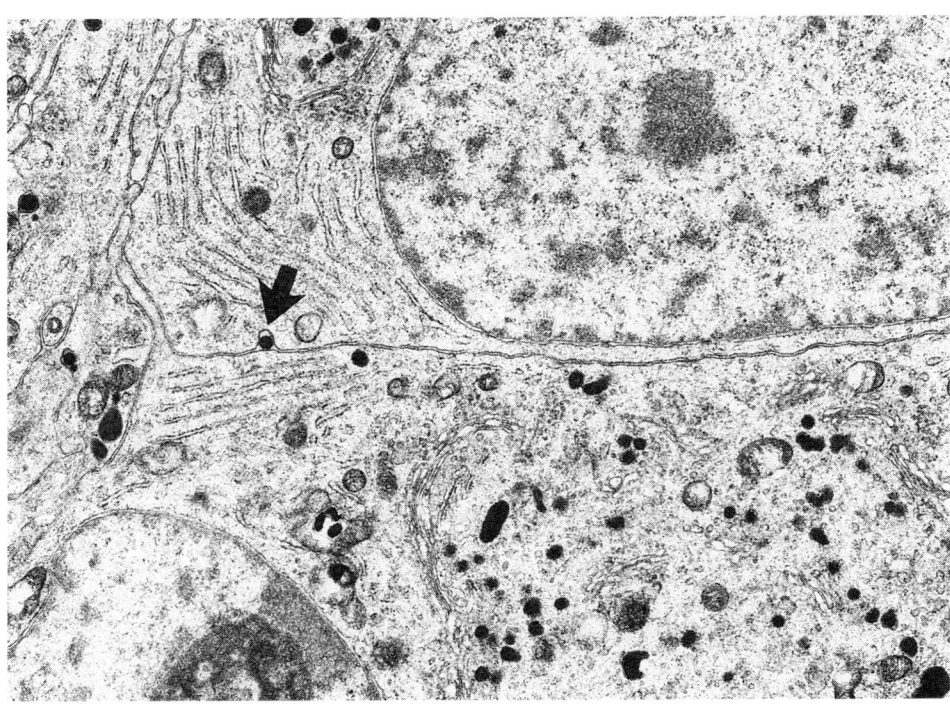

Fig. 29-17 Sparsely granulated PRL cell adenoma showing misplaced exocytosis and pleomorphic granules within the Golgi sacculi. (Electron micrograph, ×4400; courtesy Dr. E. Horvath, Toronto.)

an uncommon feature of PRL-producing adenomas. Amyloid may be present in "wisps" detectable only by electron microscopy both intracellularly and extracellularly[40] or seen in the formation of large extracellular spherules that are pathognomic for this type of neoplasm (see Fig. 29-15, *A*). Prolactin immunopositivity is demonstrated in perinuclear areas corresponding to the prominent Golgi complex, resulting in a crescent-shaped pattern[42] (see Fig. 29-16, *B*).

Ultrastructurally, the cells are irregular and form intricate processes that interdigitate.[44,49] The RER is abundant and consists of parallel arrays of delicate cisternae. A whorl arrangement of RER (nebenkern) is typical of this tumor. In keeping with the chromophobic appearance on H&E stain, the secretory granules are sparse in the range of 150 to 300 nm in diameter. Some of these granules are extruded in the extracellular space between two cells, a phenomenon known as "misplaced exocytosis," and not in the perivascular spaces[43] (Fig. 29-17). A rare variant of PRL adenoma shows marked acidophilia of cytoplasmic granules and, on electron microscopy, densely granulated cells.[43] The sparsely granulated PRL adenoma may occur in the form of a microadenoma typically located laterally in the gland. The macroadenomas may simply expand the sella, whereas others have a predilection of growth downward through sphenoid bone and into the nasopharynx. Dopamine agonists used for the control of hyperprolactinemic states lead to reduction of serum levels of PRL and of the tumor mass. Histologically, such tumors appear to be more cellular because of the involution of the cytoplasm, particularly the RER and Golgi membranes. Tumor fibrosis has been described in long-term treatment with bromocriptine.

GH cell adenoma

Pure adenomas of GH cell type are the densely granulated and sparsely granulated variants. They account for about 14% of all surgically resected pituitary adenomas and may result in gigantism or acromegaly if functioning at a clinical level or, less commonly, unaccompanied by clinical signs of hyperfunction.[50,54,55] Other GH-secreting tumors are bihormonal or plurihormonal and cosecrete PRL, TSH, alpha-subunit, and sometimes other hormones.[52,53,63] These will be discussed elsewhere. Notwithstanding, in situ hybridization studies of mRNA have shown that tumors causing acromegaly not expressing PRL are rare.[51]

The ***densely granulated*** somatotroph adenoma corresponds to the classic acidophilic adenoma of acromegaly. Cytoplasmic granules are plentiful and stain strongly with eosin. By immunostaining they display a diffuse pattern much like normal somatotrophs. No definite correlation exists between serum levels of GH and the intensity of staining for this hormone in the tumor cells. The significant ultrastructural feature is the abundance of large spherical secretory granules measuring 300 to 600 nm.[56,60,61]

The ***sparsely granulated*** GH cell adenoma is chromophobic when stained with H&E,[62] and immunopositivity for GH is meager. When viewed under the electron microscope, scanty secretory granules measure 100 to 300 nm. The area normally occupied by the Golgi region displays a skein of intermediate filaments that immunoreact for keratin[58] and ubiquitin. These fibrous bodies (Fig. 29-18) and multiple centrioles are the distinguishing features of the sparsely granulated variant of GH adenoma.

In both types of GH cell adenomas, tubuloreticular inclusions within capillary endothelium and the accumulation of

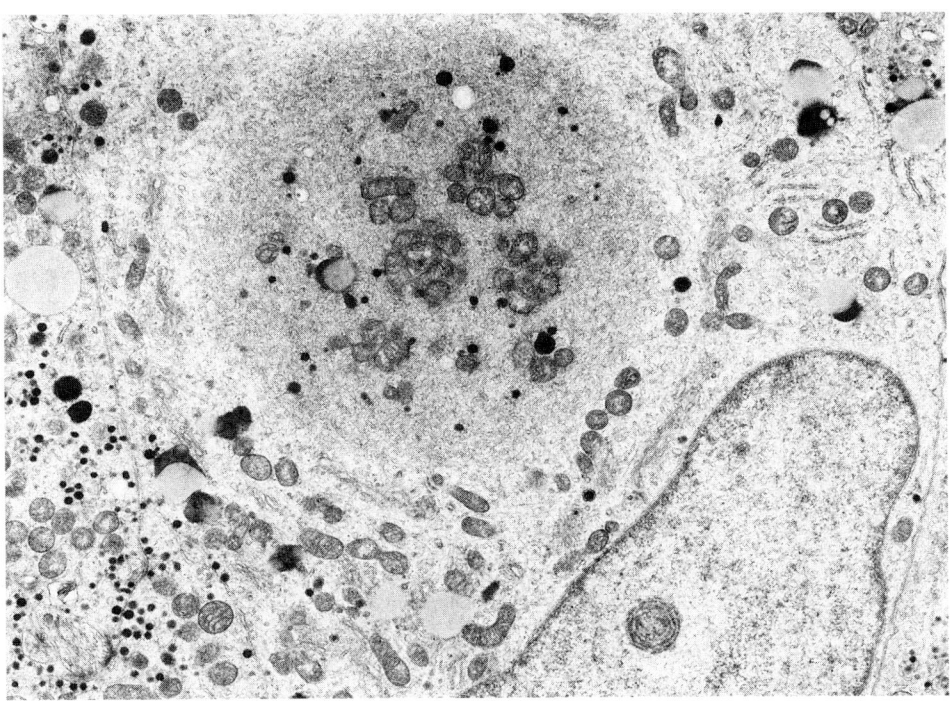

Fig. 29-18 Characteristic appearance of sparsely granulated GH cell adenoma. Note fibrous body. (Electron micrograph, ×7200; courtesy Dr. E. Horvath, Toronto.)

endocrine amyloid may occur, although these changes are poorly understood.[57] Both types of GH cell adenomas are considered variants of the same tumor.[56] From the clinical standpoint, however, the separation of these two types is important because of a difference in prognosis.[63] The densely granulated GH cell adenoma is a slow-growing, well-differentiated tumor that presents in older patients; after surgery it recurs less frequently. By contrast, the sparsely granulated type is larger at presentation, occurs in younger patients, is more aggressive, and is more likely to show invasive tendencies and recurrence.[59]

Mixed PRL- and GH-producing adenomas

Acromegaly is the clinical feature of a heterogeneous group of pituitary adenomas producing GH and PRL.[64,68] It has been postulated that an adenoma arising in a cell committed to GH production can transform toward mammosomatotroph and further to a lactotroph line. The results of a study on GH and PRL gene expression and immunoreactivity in pituitary adenomas producing GH and PRL suggest that somatotroph, mammosomatotroph, and mixed adenomas are closely related neoplasms.[70] They all may be derived from a precursor cell that has the capacity to differentiate to the somatotroph or lactotroph line by the intermediate bihormonal phase—the mammosomatotroph.[66] The exact characterization of these tumors requires immunohistochemistry with double labeling, electron microscopy, and even in situ hybridization.

The *mixed GH cell–PRL cell adenoma* displays a more aggressive course than pure GH cell adenomas (see Fig. 29-9 and 29-10). The patients have elevated levels of serum GH and varying degrees of hyperprolactinemia. Immunohistochemically this is a bimorphous tumor in which GH and PRL are detected in different cell populations randomly arranged. However, bihormonal cells producing both hormones can be demonstrated using the immunogold technique with double labeling. The most common combination is densely granulated GH cells and sparsely granulated PRL cells.

The *mammosomatotroph adenoma* is a slow-growing tumor associated with acromegaly and slight hyperprolactinemia.[65,69] These intensely acidophilic adenomas immunoreact strongly for GH and variably for PRL. With double-labeling immunoelectron microscopy, a mammosomatotroph cell contains both GH and PRL in secretory granules.[67] The distinctive ultrastructural features include very large pleomorphic secretory granules and extruded secretory material that seems to retain its electron density.

Acidophilic stem cell adenoma

Horvath et al.[71] have described under the term *acidophilic stem cell adenoma* neoplasms that share ultrastructural features of GH- and PRL-producing cells. Ultrastructural study is essential for the diagnosis of this fast-growing, invasive macroadenoma that shows an unusual form of mitochondrial gigantism, fibrous bodies, poorly organized rough endoplasmic reticulum, secretory granule extrusion, primitive Golgi apparatus, and oncocytic transformation. Endocrinologically, these tumors are nonfunctioning or cause hyperprolactinemia. Rarely they may also produce GH.[73] The finding

that most of these tumors contain PRL mRNA and PRL immunoreactivity suggests that this adenoma is an offshoot of an immature cell closer to the lactotroph line.[72]

ACTH cell adenoma

Corticotroph adenomas are clinically and biologically a heterogeneous group and constitute approximately between 7% and 14% of all pituitary adenomas.[82] In a retrospective study of 338 consecutive patients with corticotroph adenomas by Thapar et al.,[84] 260 patients were found to have Cushing's disease, 47 presented with Nelson's syndrome, and 31 had hormonally silent masses. In the majority of cases a basophilic microadenoma is responsible for pituitary-dependent Cushing's disease. The size of the neoplasms ranges from 3 to 10 mm in diameter, and most of them are located within the anterior lobe, mainly centrally, and rarely in the lateral lobes. The very small size and fragmentation of a surgical sample may render the diagnosis difficult or even impossible. Immunohistochemical staining for ACTH and endorphin is very helpful in this regard by demonstrating that in one or more of the fragments *all* of the cells are positive for this hormone.

Removal of the hyperplastic adrenal glands in patients with Cushing's disease may result in rapid enlargement of the pituitary neoplasm. Nelson et al.[80] reported that some patients with Cushing's disease and adrenocortical hyperplasia who undergo adrenalectomy later develop clinical signs of a pituitary neoplasm (in the absence of cortisol excess) that is notorious for its invasive tendencies. The condition now known as *Nelson's syndrome* is caused by the loss of the negative corticosteroid feedback mechanism, resulting in the rapid growth of a pre-existing microadenoma.[76]

By light microscopy, the tumor cells are arranged in a distinctive trabecular or sinusoidal pattern (Fig. 29-19) and appear basophil and, less commonly, "chromophobe." However, many adenomas display strong PAS positivity that is ascribed to a carbohydrate moiety contained in proopiomelanocortin, the precursor molecule of ACTH.[77]

Ultrastructurally, the secretory granules may concentrate along the cell membrane or be found scattered throughout the cytoplasm.[77] Their diameters show considerable variations, ranging from 200 to 700 nm. Perinuclear microfilaments, 70 nm in diameter, are usually present and constitute an important diagnostic feature of ACTH-producing tumors (Fig. 29-20). In extreme cases, almost the entire cytoplasm is occupied by Crooke's hyalinization; they are equivalent to the Crooke's hyaline material (keratin and ubiquitin positive, ACTH negative) seen in non-neoplastic ACTH cells in cases of Cushing's disease and ectopic ACTH syndrome (Fig. 29-21). The deposition of microfilaments is dependent on sustained hypercortisolism[81] and glucocorticoid treatment. By contrast, cytoplasmic filaments are not found in tumor cells of Nelson's syndrome because levels of circulating glucocorticoids decline after adrenalectomy. Corticotroph adenomas are usually monohormonal, and immunohistochemically, there is positivity for ACTH (see Fig. 30-16, *A*) and for beta-lipotropic hormone, melanocyte-stimulating hormone, and beta-endorphin in the cytoplasm of adenoma cells.[75,77,78,85]

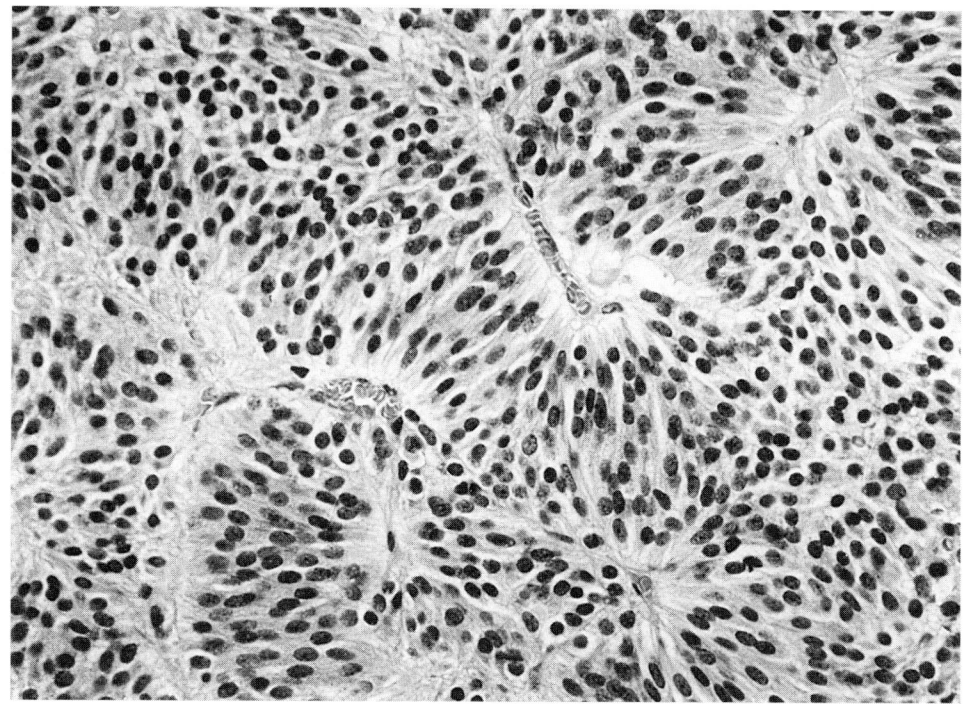

Fig. 29-19 Functioning corticotroph adenoma showing sinusoidal pattern.

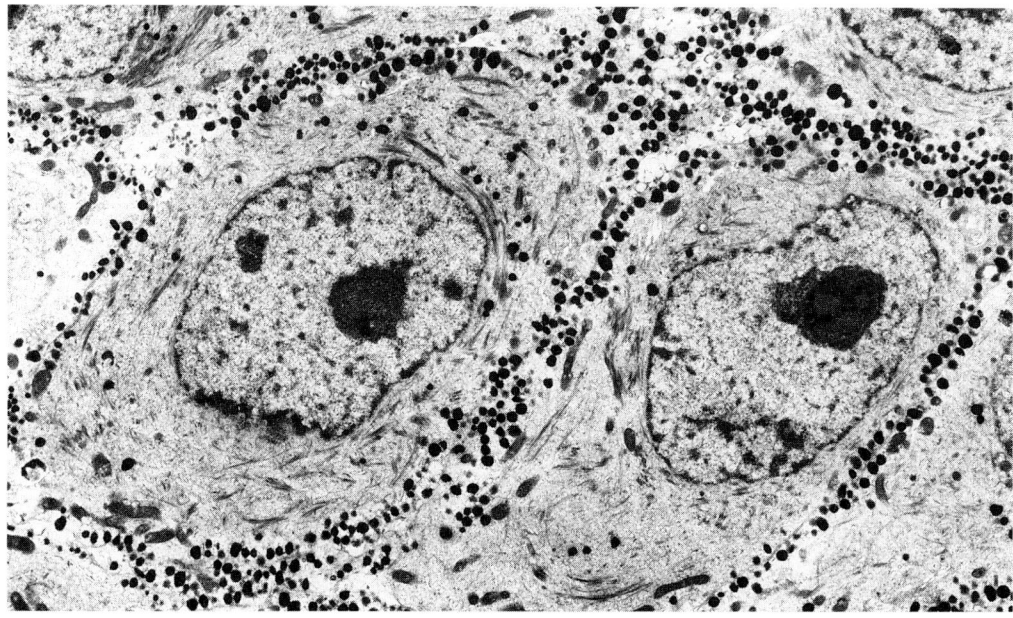

Fig. 29-20 Cells of ACTH-producing adenoma show perinuclear concentric deposits of filaments that are characteristic of Crooke's hyalinization. (Electron micrograph, ×3600; courtesy Dr. E. Horvath, Toronto.)

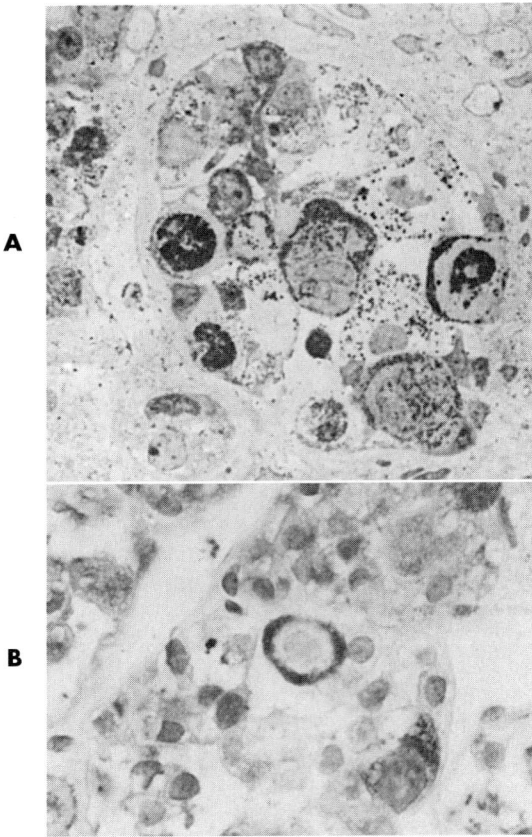

Fig. 29-21 Crooke's change in pituitary cells in patients with Cushing's disease. **A,** Toluidine blue stain of epoxy-embedded section. **B,** ACTH stain (Immunoperoxidase).

About 6% of basophil, densely granulated adenomas that are immunoreactive for ACTH are endocrinologically silent; the reason for this lack of function or hormone release is not known.[77] Some of these **silent ACTH adenomas** have a proclivity to hemorrhage with sudden tumor expansion, leading to the known clinical presentation of pituitary apoplexy. Hyperplasia of corticotroph cells as a cause of Cushing's disease poses a most difficult problem for both neurosurgeons and pathologists.[79,83] Corticotroph hyperplasia is assumed to be the result of hypothalamic dysregulation but may also be secondary to ectopic production of corticotropin-releasing hormone.[74] Ectopic production of ACTH by a neuroendocrine tumor elsewhere in the body may result in Cushing's disease with a pituitary gland of normal size.

Glycoprotein hormone–producing adenoma

The glycoprotein hormone–producing cells of the pituitary gland are gonadotrophs and thyrotrophs. These cells normally synthesize the hormones in a heterodimeric configuration, consisting of an "alpha" subunit common to all members of the class and a "beta" subunit that lends biochemical, immunologic, and functional specificity to the molecule.[87] Abnormal hormone synthesis in gonadotroph and thyrotroph adenomas results in excess production of the alpha-subunit, which can be measured as a diagnostic marker for glycoprotein-producing adenomas[91] and to monitor follow-up after treatment.

The presence of **adenomas of TSH cell type** had been proved by the reports of pituitary adenomas associated with hyperthyroidism and confirmed by Hamilton et al.[89] by the finding of elevated serum TSH levels on radioimmunoassay. However, several of these adenomas arise in patients with long-standing hypothyroidism.[96,99] They are the least common pituitary tumor type, representing only 1% of all neoplasms, with about 100 cases reported so far.[86,88,93,95] Tumors are usually large but may also present as microadenomas. By light microscopy they display a sinusoidal growth pattern. Immunohistochemical reactivity for TSH is essential for diagnosis (Fig. 29-22). The alpha-subunit of the pituitary glycoprotein hormones (TSH, FSH, and LH) can be labeled with immunoreagents in many of the glycoprotein-producing pituitary adenomas. Ultrastructurally, most thyrotroph tumors are well differentiated, the cells resembling nonadenomatous TSH elements[88] with minute secretory granules.

Adenomas of FSH/LH cell type, **gonadotroph adenomas,** represent about 6% of all pituitary adenomas.[94,97,98] These tumors are slow growing, show no evidence of gross invasion, tend to be large at presentation, and rarely are associated with high serum gonadotropin levels. Neoplastic gonadotroph cells have few secretory granules and are therefore rendered chromophobic by conventional stains. Ultrastructurally, the secretory granules have a mean diameter of 150 nm. Immunohistochemically, Trouillas et al.[98] found reactivity for both FSH and LH in fourteen cases, for FSH in seven, and for alpha-subunit in five. The existence of pure alpha-subunit–secreting adenomas has also been documented by other groups.[90,92] Pure LH-producing adenomas are rare. Horvath et al.[91a] found, ultrastructurally, a distinctive vesicular dilatation of the Golgi complex ("honeycomb Golgi") in gonadotropin adenomas occurring in women. Other tumors are less differentiated and resemble null cell adenomas.

Plurihormonal adenoma

Pituitary tumors that produce two or more hormones are designated **plurihormonal adenomas.** The hormones produced may be demonstrated within the same tumor cell, or the tumor may be composed of multiple cell clones, each engaged in the processing of a different hormone.[100,101,103] Most of the plurihormonal adenomas are found in patients with **acromegaly.** These tumors usually co-express GH and PRL[102] and have already been discussed. Not regarded as plurihormonal are adenomas containing ACTH and related proopiomelanocortin peptides because such substances are normally produced in the same cell. In the assessment of the plurihormonality of an adenoma, stringent laboratory methods are essential to avoid spurious labeling caused by cross-reactivity. Nonetheless, there remains a small group of adenomas that cosecrete GH, TSH,[104] alpha-subunit, and any combination of LH, FSH, alpha-subunit, TSH, GH, and PRL. The hormones produced by these tumors are not always accompanied by corresponding elevation in serum hormone levels. Plurihormonal adenomas tend to be large at presentation and have a more aggressive clinical course.

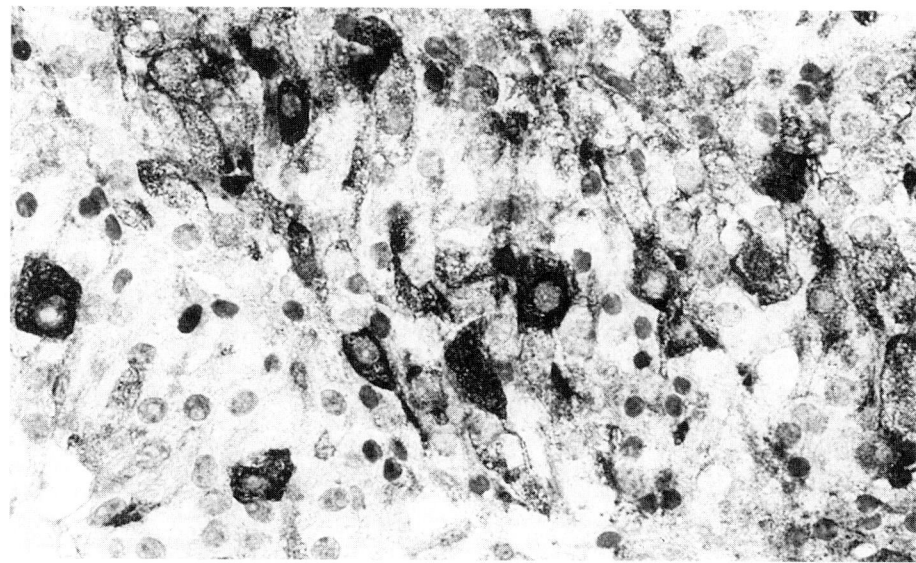

Fig. 29-22 Thyrotroph adenoma. Immunoreaction for TSH is of variable intensity.

Null cell adenoma and oncocytoma

These tumors are pituitary adenomas that manifest no clinical or biochemical evidence of hormone production, show no or faint hormonal immunoreactivity, and when examined under the electron microscope, lack features indicative of any of the five known pituitary cells, showing instead a rudimentary Golgi apparatus and rare secretory granules. Most of such tumors are designated ***null cell adenomas***[108] and are found often as slow-growing sellar and parasellar neoplasms affecting elderly individuals (see Fig. 29-8) who seek medical attention because of progressive loss of vision and hypopituitarism.

These chromophobe tumors are often focally immunoreactive for FSH, LH, TSH, and alpha-subunit[106] and have been found to contain dopamine receptors[110] and estrogen receptors; ultrastructurally they are nononcocytic (Fig. 29-23). The demonstration of gonadotropin release by null cell adenomas maintained in tissue culture has strengthened the hypothesis that null cell adenomas may have a gonadotrophic lineage.[105]

Adenomas having the same morphologic and immunohistochemical attributes as null cell adenomas with added oncocytic change affecting more than 50% of cells have been designated ***pituitary oncocytomas.***[107] When viewed under the electron microscope, mitochondria are found to occupy up to 50% of the cytoplasmic area[109] (Fig. 29-24). These adenomas most likely represent a heterogeneous group, but many, if not most, are transformed null cell adenomas.

Natural history, spread, and metastases

Pituitary apoplexy is a rare complication of adenomas.[111] It represents a spontaneous massive hemorrhagic infarct within a large tumor and is most often seen in nonfunctioning adenomas and in tumors producing ACTH. Pituitary apoplexy often presents as a neurosurgical emergency because of the rapid expansion of the mass upward with compression of anterior hypothalamic area (Fig. 29-25). Bromocriptine treatment may induce the development of pituitary apoplexy in some patients.[115]

In many pituitary tumors, actual invasion of neighboring structures is encountered; these structures may include the brain; anterior, middle, or posterior fossa; cavernous sinus and dura mater; optic nerve; chiasm; sphenoid bone; nasopharynx; and nasal cavity. These tumors should be designated as ***invasive adenomas*** and not as carcinomas. Exceptionally, pituitary neoplasms are found to implant along the subarachnoid space[112,114] and even to metastasize distantly, to the liver, bone, or other organs. In the case of hematogenous metastasis, tumor permeation into the cavernous sinus provides a venous access to the internal jugular vein via the petrosal system.[116] This phenomenon has been reported with nonfunctioning tumors, as well as with neoplasms associated with Nelson's syndrome, acromegaly, and hyperprolactinemia. The behavior of pituitary carcinomas suggests that some tumors result from malignant transformation in a pre-existing benign tumor, whereas others represent de novo malignancy.[113] As in most other endocrine tumors, the correlation between microscopic appearance and biologic behavior is poor. Some of the invasive or metastasizing neoplasms have an obviously malignant cytologic appearance, but the majority do not appreciably differ from the ordinary pituitary adenoma. Evaluation of cell-proliferation markers such as MIB-1 or immunoreactivity for p53, the mutated form of a tumor-suppressor gene product, may provide useful information in the assessment of biologic behavior of adenomas.[116a] Death from pituitary carcinoma is usually caused by extensive intracranial disease.

Treatment

The therapeutic approach to pituitary adenomas varies in different clinics. Both surgical excision and radiation therapy can be used. The choice of therapy sometimes depends on the patient's age, on clinical circumstances, and on the

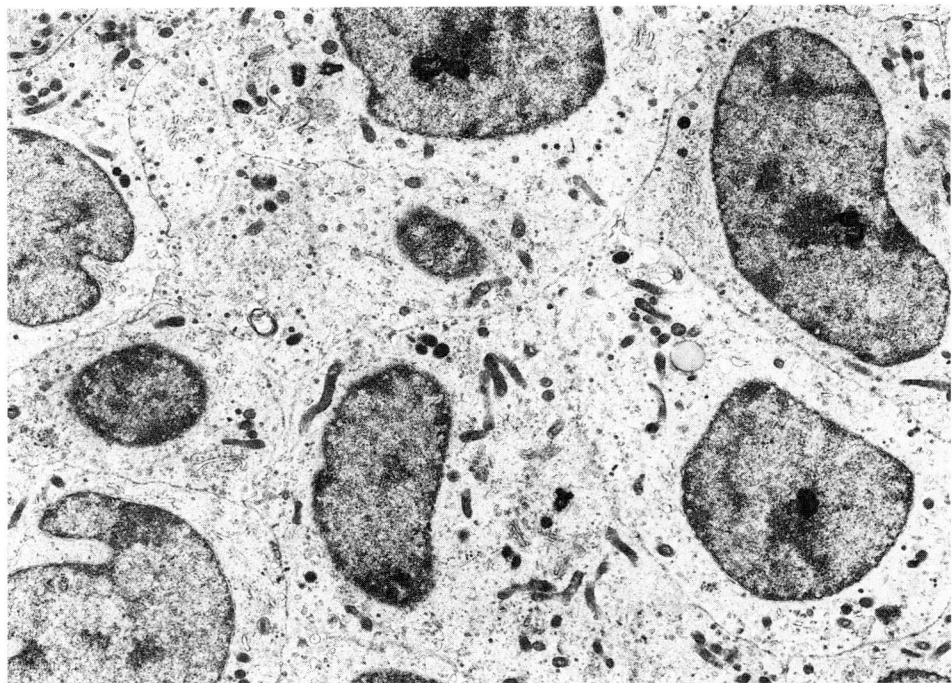

Fig. 29-23 Cytoplasm of null cell adenoma cells contains scanty organelles and small secretory granules. (Electron micrograph, ×5400; courtesy Dr. E. Horvath, Toronto.)

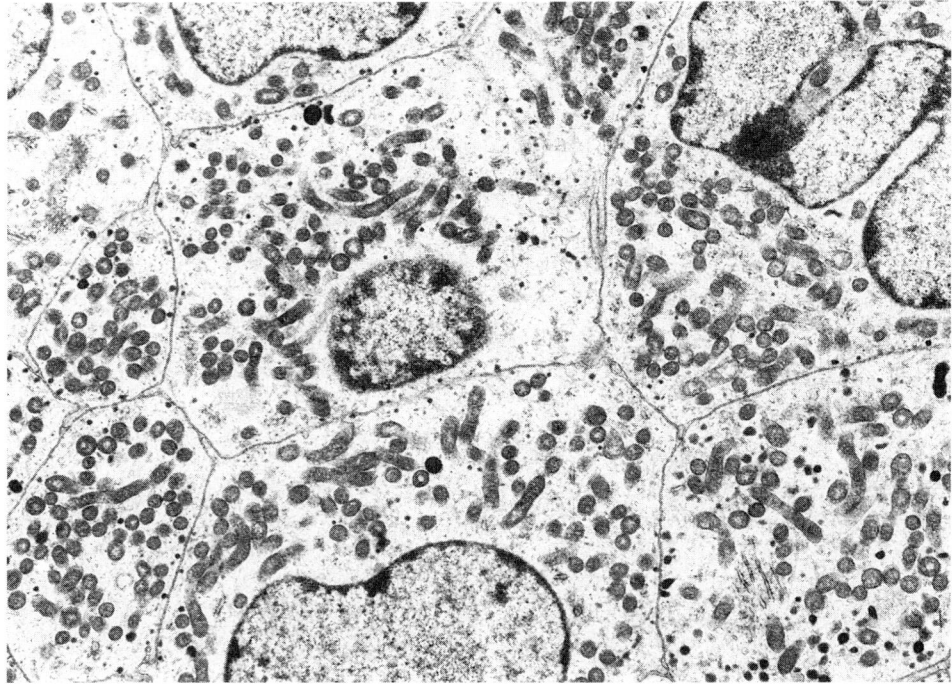

Fig. 29-24 Large numbers of mitochondria and paucity of secretory granules are typical of oncocytoma. (Electron micrograph, ×6000; courtesy Dr. E. Horvath, Toronto.)

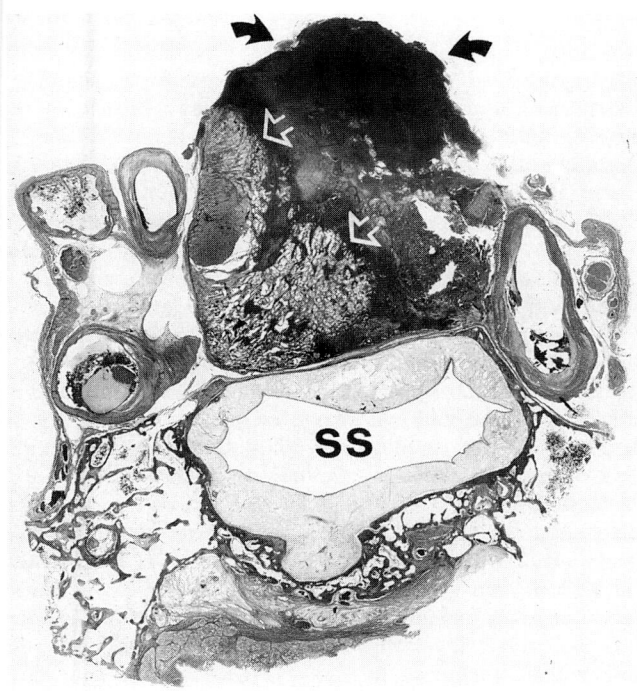

Fig. 29-25 Pituitary apoplexy in 76-year-old man with null cell adenoma. Coronal section of sella and cavernous sinuses showing large intratumoral hemorrage and necrosis with suprasellar extension. Whole mount preparation. *SS,* Sphenoid sinus; *open arrows,* residual tumor; *black arrows,* suprasellar hematoma.

evaluation of postradiation risk of development of malignant bony tumors and hypopituitarism. Radiation results in fibrosis and sometimes cavitation of the adenoma. Transsphenoidal surgery is established as a procedure of low morbidity and mortality.[119,120] A valuable form of therapy, used successfully in cases of adenomas of PRL type, consists of the administration of bromocriptine, a dopamine agonist.[118,122] This results in shrinkage and fibrosis of the mass, recovery of visual field defect, and normalization of the PRL blood level. Clinical symptoms disappear with fertility being restored; this is a reversible effect.

Although no significant shrinkage of the mass has been shown to occur, the long-acting somatostatin analog octreotide has been used with good results in the treatment of patients with acromegaly and pituitary adenomas.[117,118] It is not, however, currently viewed as an alternative to surgery in most patients, but rather as adjuvant therapy.[120] Preoperative treatment with octreotide may prove to be useful in facilitating tumor removal. Refractory acromegaly after surgery can be effectively treated with radiotherapy.[121]

OTHER LESIONS
Gangliocytoma

Gangliocytomas are rare hypothalamic and/or intrasellar tumors composed of large mature nerve cells with a glial stroma.[124,127,129] These lesions exhibit progressive growth, and a number of them are part of a *mixed adenoma-gangliocytoma* (Fig. 29-26) causing acromegaly[125,130] and less often Cushing's disease.[123,131,136] The nerve cells that have morphologic characteristics of hypothalamic elements have been shown to contain not only pituitary hormones and other peptides, but also releasing factors such as GHRH and GnRH.[137] Two theories have been suggested concerning the pathogenesis of adenoma-gangliocytoma: (1) Neurons having a hypothalamic phenotype stimulate GH cells, resulting in adenoma formation; and (2) neuron-like cells may represent transformed adenoma cells.

Gangliocytoma should be differentiated from the *neuronal hypothalamic hamartoma,*[132,133] usually seen in children with the syndrome of precocious puberty[128] and gelastic seizures.[126,135] Histologically, this lesion is composed of a mixture of mature neurons, astrocytes, and oligodendrocytes arranged with a varying degree of organization.

Hypothalamic tumors containing immature neurons are designated *hamartoblastomas.* The constellation of hypothalamic hamartoblastoma with craniofacial anomalies, limb anomalies, and imperforate anus along with hypopituitarism secondary to pituitary dysplasia constitutes the *Pallister-Hall syndrome.*[134]

Lymphocytic hypophysitis

Lymphocytic adenohypophysitis is a rare autoimmune endocrine disease[146] with only about 50 reported cases.[140,141,147] Women in late pregnancy or the immediate postpartum period are primarily affected. The occurrence of this syndrome is rare in males.[142] Patients may present with symptoms of an expanding pituitary mass[144] and/or varying degrees of pituitary dysfunction. Regardless of the form of presentation, most patients will have evidence of partial hypopituitarism or panhypopituitarism at some time during the course of the disease before surgical intervention. About one third of patients develop visual field defects.

Magnetic resonance imaging discloses enlargement of the pituitary fossa with suprasellar extension in most cases.[145] In the initial stages, the pituitary has a firm, tough appearance, very different from that of an adenoma. The salient histologic picture is a polymorphic lymphoplasmacytic infiltration associated with destruction of the anterior pituitary cells[138] (Fig. 29-27). In rare instances, lymphoid follicles with germinal centers are formed.[140] Later stages of the disease are characterized by fibrosis, parenchymal atrophy, and residual lymphocytic aggregates. Electron microscopy has shown interdigitation of mononuclear cells with adenohypophysial cells.[138] Antibodies to pituitary cell have been detected in some cases, and about one third of the patients had other endocrine or immune diseases or chronic lymphocytic infiltration of other endocrine organs at autopsy.

Corticosteroid therapy may be beneficial, with full endocrinologic recovery well documented in one patient.[140,143] Some cases may require surgical decompression and replacement therapy for residual hypopituitarism.[138,139] Indirect evidence suggests spontaneous resolution in some cases.

Rathke's cleft cyst

Cysts of the hypophysial cleft, arising from the remnants of Rathke's pouch, are usually incidental postmortem findings within the pituitary gland.[151,155] On occasion they reach a large size and may exhibit suprasellar extension. Thus they become clinically apparent with compression of the hy-

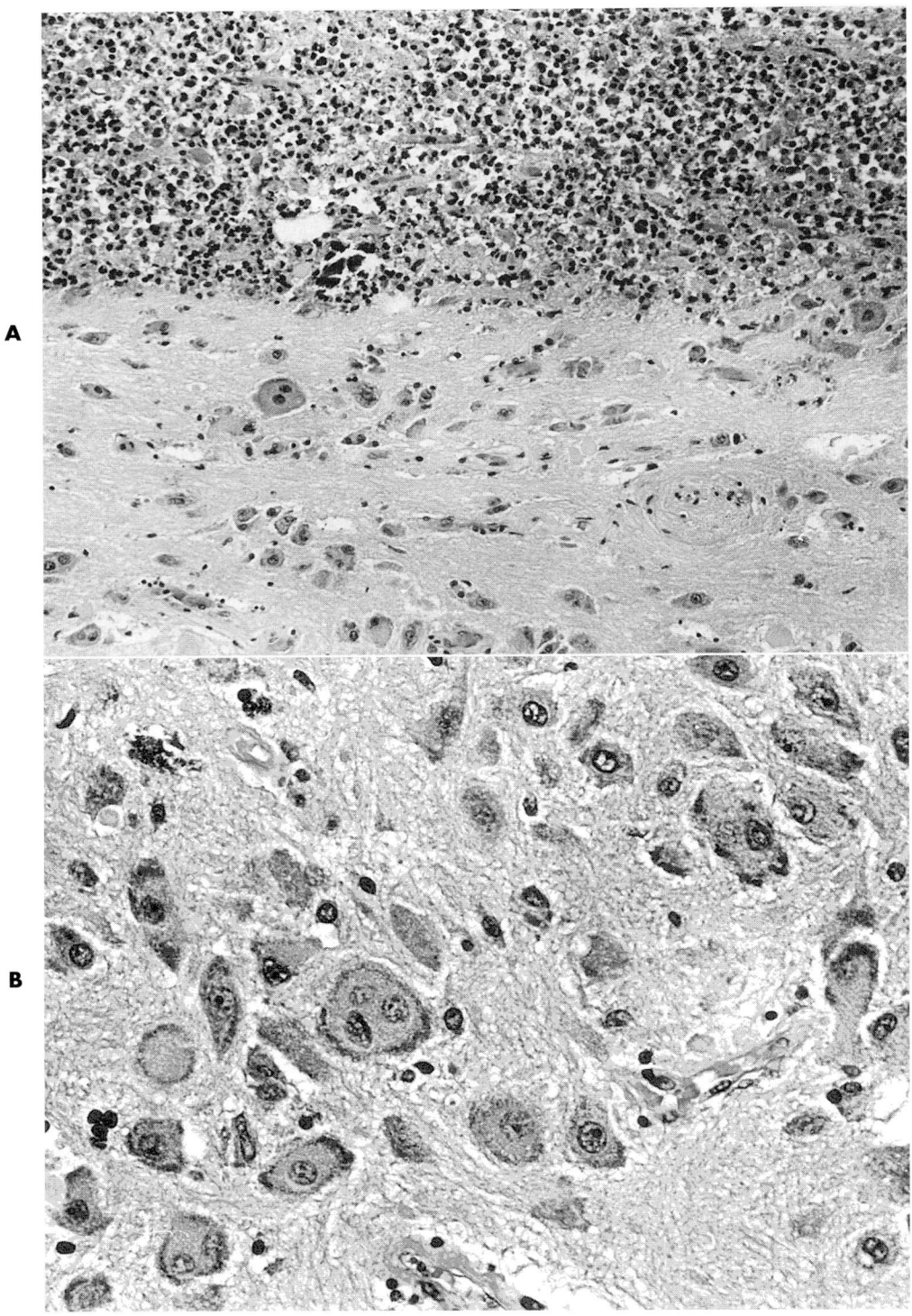

Fig. 29-26 Intrasellar mixed gangliocytoma-adenoma. **A,** Interface between gangliocytoma and adenoma is shown. Multinucleated neurons and glial stroma are illustrated in **B.**

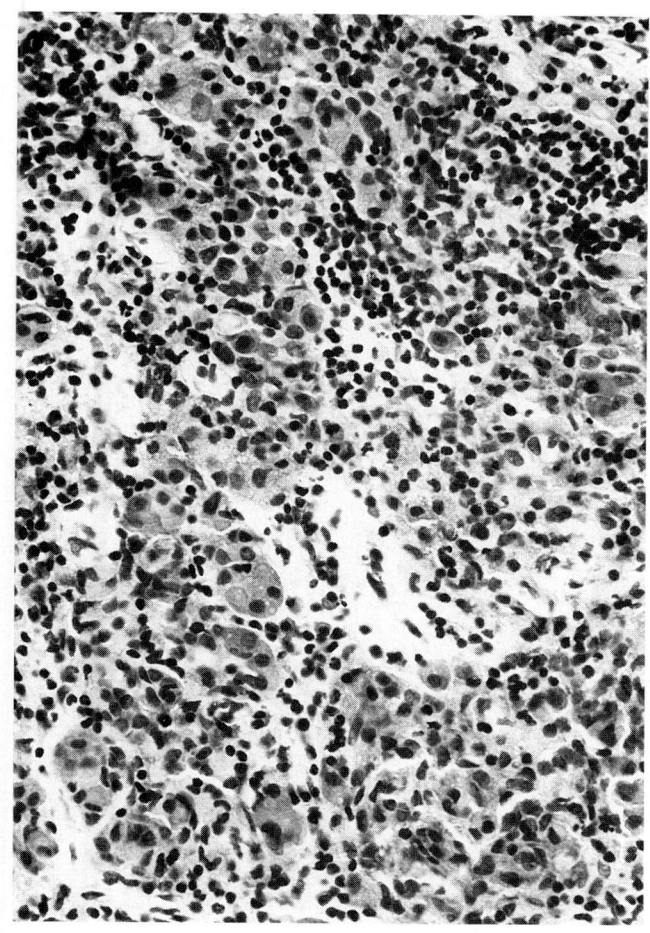

Fig. 29-27 Lymphocytic hypophysitis. Note disorganization of normal histology caused by infiltration of lymphocytes and plasma cells.

pothalamus and optic chiasm.[152] Some purely suprasellar cases have been described.[148] In a review of symptomatic cases, the presenting symptoms included visual disturbances, diabetes insipidus, hypopituitarism, and hydrocephalus.[156,157] Some cases are associated with septic meningitis.[154] The smaller cyst can be found in up to 20% of pituitaries obtained at autopsy. They usually measure less that 5 mm in diameter.

Histologically, the cysts are lined by predominantly columnar ciliated cells (Fig. 29-28), rare goblet cells, and adenohypophysial cells. Foci of squamous differentiation are also demonstrable. Lining cells exhibit strong immunopositivity for low-molecular-weight keratin and focal immunoreaction for S-100 protein. Rare cells may immunoreact for GFAP and vimentin. Evidence of old hemorrhage may be seen in up to 40% of cases.[152] Confusion with craniopharyngioma is possible because of a calcified rim in some Rathke's pouch cysts. Magnetic resonance imaging has a high sensitivity in disclosing the lesion.[152] The cyst content has a high T1- and T2-weighted image on magnetic resonance imaging.[150,158] Association with pituitary adenoma has been reported.[153] Surgical drainage and excision is the treatment of choice; recurrence is unusual.[149,152]

Craniopharyngioma

Most patients with **craniopharyngioma** are in the first or second decades of life,[168] although some are in their 70s and 80s.[171] The tumor has also been reported in fetuses and newborns.[160,169] Its location is usually suprasellar, although it may occupy the sella as well (Fig. 29-29, *A*). It may develop dorsal or ventral to the optic chiasm and, in rare cases, within the chiasm itself.[163,164] Occasional cases located within the third ventricle have been reported.[170] The tumor may achieve giant proportions, growing in the parasellar region and into brain.[180] Craniopharyngiomas can be implanted in other areas of the brain by repeated needle aspiration.[161] Craniopharyngioma constitutes about 3% of all brain tumors.[174]

Cystic degeneration is an extremely common finding, the content of the cyst being a viscous fluid resembling "machinery oil" sparkling with cholesterol crystals. Focal calcification is almost invariably present. In about 75% of the cases, it is prominent enough to be detectable by x-ray studies. The microscopic appearance resembles that of ameloblastoma of the jaws. Anastomosing epithelial islands with a palisaded layer of cells and a center of stellate cells are characteristic (Fig. 29-29, *B*). Foci of squamous metaplasia with solid nests of keratinization, degenerative changes, calcification, and a mixed inflammatory reaction that may be granulomatous are often found.

Gliosis with Rosenthal fiber formation in the adjacent brain may be so intense as to be mistaken for a pilocytic astrocytoma. Small epithelial strands trapped in the peripheral reactive glial tissue may result in a mistaken diagnosis of carcinoma. Cystic craniopharyngiomas should also be distinguished from epidermoid and other cysts occurring in this region, although this may prove difficult in a small sample. The most important features that favor a diagnosis of craniopharyngioma are the basal palisading, the absence of keratohyaline granules, the stratified masses of keratin, and the stellate reticulum. Cavitation may develop from dissociation of the stellate cells, from degeneration of the stromal elements, and from accumulation of desquamated debris. The electron microscopic appearance of craniopharyngioma has been described by Ghatak et al.[166]

In about 10% of cases, seen only in adults, the tumor has a macroscopic papillary appearance (Fig. 29-30), lacks calcification and nodules of keratin, and is composed microscopically of solid, well-differentiated pseudopapillary squamous epithelium with keratinization of individual cells[167] (Fig. 29-31). Malignant transformation in craniopharyngiomas is a rarity.[173]

Although some microscopic differences exist between craniopharyngioma and ameloblastoma of the jaws, the striking morphologic similarity of craniopharyngioma to another odontogenic lesion, the "calcifying odontogenic cyst of Gorlin,"[162,165] and the finding in several cases of craniopharyngioma of undeniable tooth structures[176] is supportive evidence of a related embryologic origin, the intracranial tumor probably arising from a buccal equivalent of the embryonic enamel organ present in Rathke's pouch. **Squamous cell nests** found in the pars tuberalis in about 24% of autopsy cases, once thought to be precursors of craniopharyngiomas, are now considered to be unrelated (see Fig. 29-1). The simul-

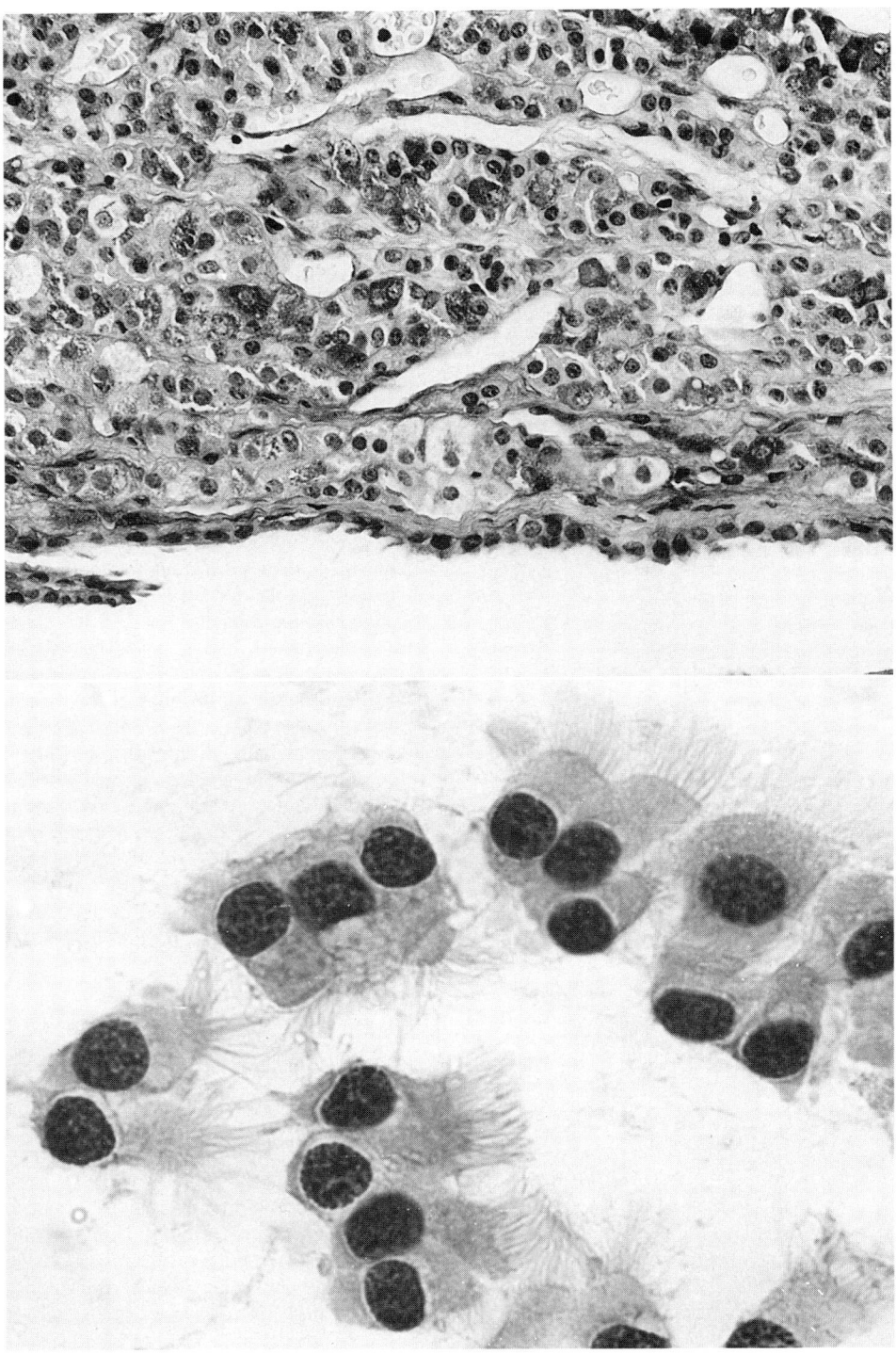

Fig. 29-28 Intrasellar Rathke's cleft cyst within the pituitary gland. The unilocular lesion is lined by columnar epithelium. Ciliated cells are readily demonstrable on a needle aspirate.

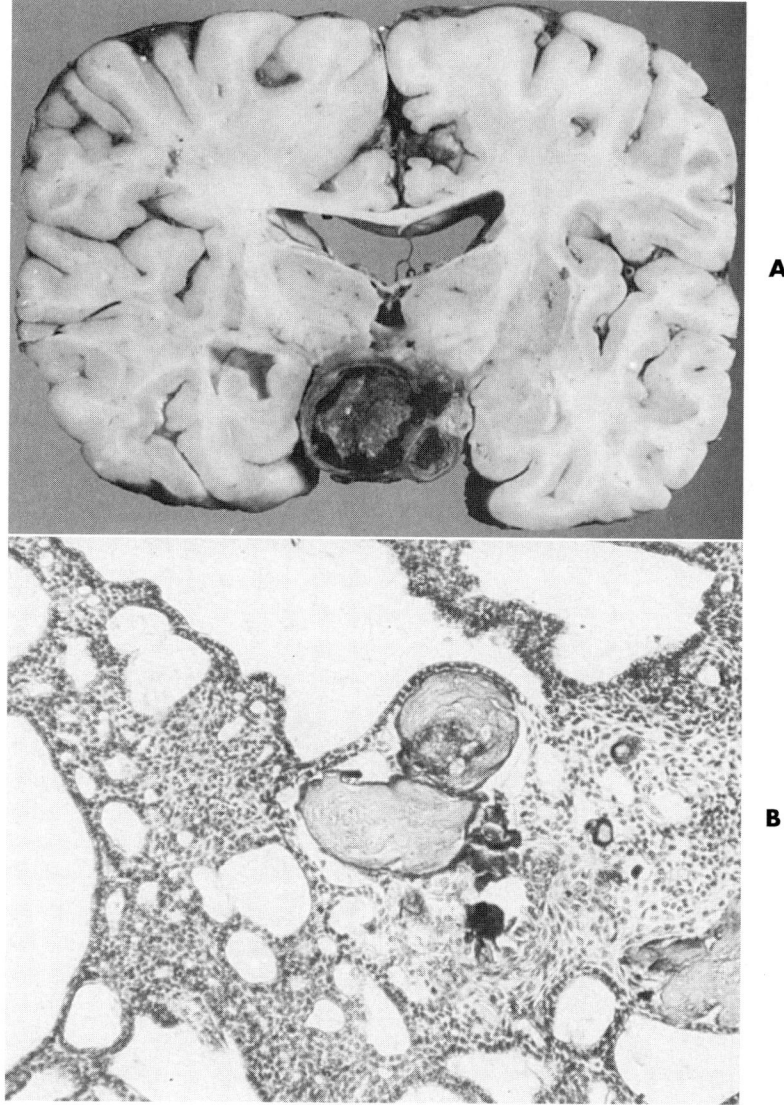

Fig. 29-29 A, Suprasellar craniopharyngioma in 47-year-old man who had surgery 15 years previously, but tumor could not be excised because of its size. Despite subsequent radiation therapy, progressive tumor growth led to compression of optic chiasm, pituitary gland, and cerebral peduncles. Note good circumscription of tumor and its variegated appearance. **B,** Microscopic appearance of craniopharyngioma of suprasellar region. Solid epithelial nests with calcification, collections of "shadow cells," and peripheral palisading alternate with cystic areas.

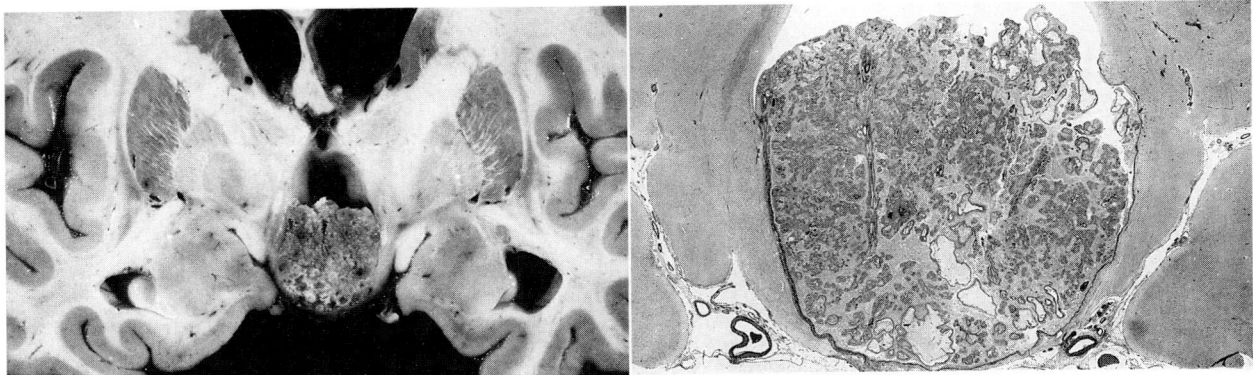

Fig. 29-30 Intraventricular craniopharyngioma of papillary type. This is well-demarcated solid lesion showing no calcification.

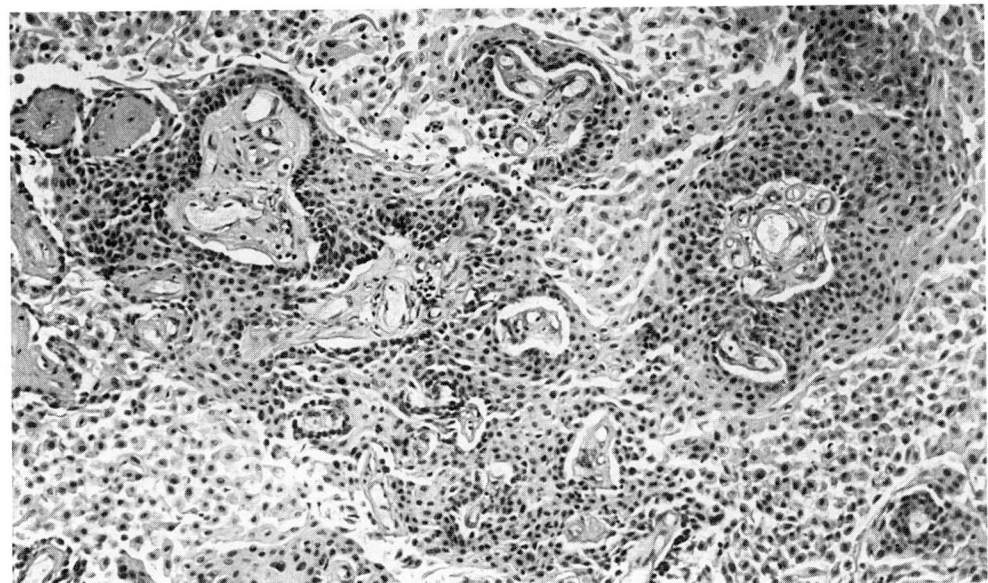

Fig. 29-31 Separation and desquamation of the epithelium along artefactual fissures results in pseudopapillary formation in this craniopharyngioma. Note absence of keratin nodules.

taneous immunohistochemical demonstration of keratin and pituitary hormones in these squamous cells indicates a metaplastic derivation from adenohypophysial cells.[177]

Symptoms are dominated by those of hydrocephalus, especially in the younger patients, and of pressure on the chiasm and optic tracts. *Craniopharyngiomas* can also present with signs of dwarfism, hypogonadism, panhypopituitarism, diabetes insipidus, and hyperprolactinemia caused by a compression of the pituitary stalk. The diagnosis is often delayed until visual disturbances occur. Magnetic resonance imaging is thought to be superior to CT scan in outlining the lesion and in distinguishing scarring from recurrent tumor.[175]

Total or subtotal surgical excision, in some cases followed by radiation therapy, is the treatment of choice.[178,179] In one series, most postoperative morbidity and all postop-

erative mortality occurred after the second and third operations for recurrent tumor. Some authors also achieved good results with stereotactic endocavitary irradiation.[172] Depending on the therapy instituted, recurrence takes place in 20% to 30% of patients. Better results have been reported for the papillary variant of craniopharyngioma.[159] Severe mental retardation may follow radiotherapy in children.

Granular cell tumor

Granular cell tumors (also known as choristoma of neurohypophysis or granular cell pituicytoma) arising from the stalk or posterior lobe of the pituitary usually represent incidental autopsy findings in adults,[184] but in a few cases they have attained sufficient size to produce symptoms of visual impairment requiring surgical intervention.[191,192] Diabetes insipidus was the initial manifestation in one case.[186] Shank-

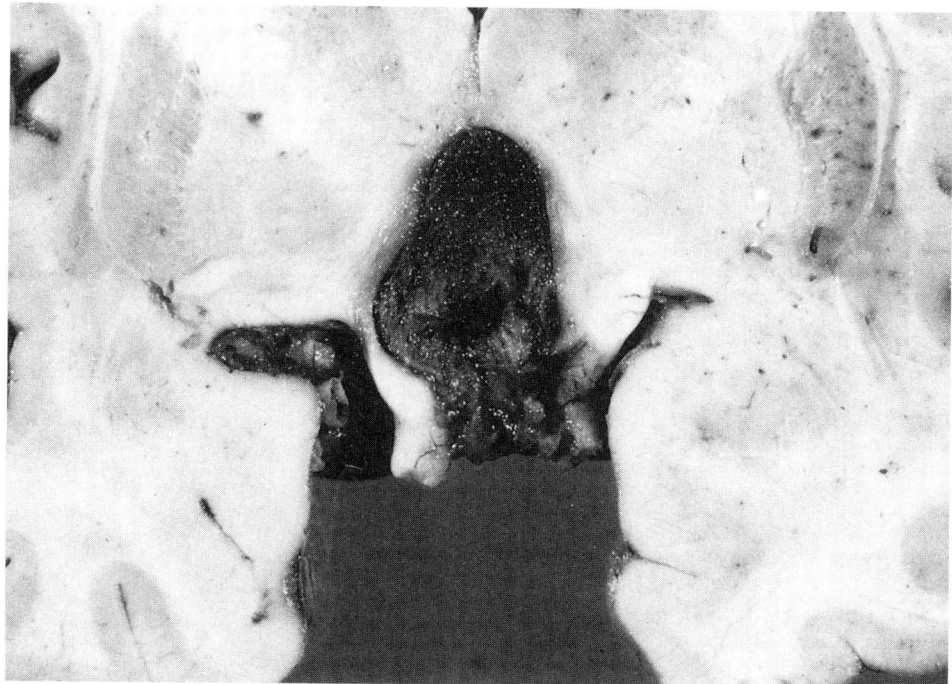

Fig. 29-32 Metastatic malignant carcinoid to posterior pituitary gland extending into hypothalamus.

lin,[187] in a detailed study of pituitaries obtained post mortem, demonstrated small clusters of granular cells that he designated "tumorettes" in up to 17% of unselected specimens; they were found within the posterior pituitary or in the infundibulum. The absence of these nodules in the first and second decades of life suggests that they are acquired rather than congenital.

The histologic and ultrastructural appearance and histochemical reactions of granular cell tumors of neurohypophysis are similar to those of their more common peripheral counterpart: namely, tightly packed polyhedral cells arranged in sheets or ill-defined lobules. They display an abundant granular cytoplasm that is PAS positive–diastase resistant. For some authors the immunophenotype seems to be consistent with Schwannian differentiation.[181] Others have not been able to confirm this finding.[190] Although this lesion is consistently negative when stained for GFAP,[185,190] Nishioka[185] has provided immunohistochemical evidence in support of the hypothesis that granular cell tumors of neurohypophysis may originate from granular pituicytes, a modified glial cell.

The association of granular cell tumors of the pituitary with pituitary adenomas[188] and multiple endocrine neoplasia[189] must be interpreted as fortuitous rather than evidence for a common precursor cell. Hypothalamic granular cell tumors should be differentiated from similar tumors in the cerebral hemispheres where an astrocytic differentiation can be demonstrated by immunohistochemistry.[182] Of the symptomatic cases reported in the literature, most present in the fifth decade and affect females predominantly.[183,191]

Postradiation tumors

Malignant gliomas in the parasellar area have been reported following radiotherapy for pituitary adenoma, craniopharyngioma, suprasellar germinoma, and acute lymphoblastic leukemia.[195,197-205,209,210] Except for a single oligodendroglioma, most cases described are astrocytomas.[196] The latency period ranges from 5 to 25 years, and the radiation doses ranges from 42.5 to 66 Gy. Osteosarcoma and fibrosarcoma of the sphenoid bone and skull have been described following radiotherapy for pituitary adenoma and craniopharyngioma.[193,194,202,208] Postirradiation malignant gliomas are aggressive, with most patients dying within a few months after histologic diagnosis. Meningiomas have rarely been reported following irradiation for pituitary adenoma and craniopharyngioma.[206,207]

Metastatic tumors

Autopsy data indicate that metastasis to the pituitary is not rare; the prevalence is 3% to 5%.[214,216,217] Metastatic carcinoma is more common in the neurohypophysis[212] (Fig. 29-32), with many patients displaying diabetes insipidus.[215] Carcinoma of the breast, lung, or GI tract is the most frequent primary lesion.[211,213,220] Occasionally, no primary tumor can be identified, even at autopsy.

Most pituitary metastases are asymptomatic and constitute incidental findings at autopsy in patients with widespread cancer.[219] However, nine of fourteen patients in one series presented with symptomatic pituitary metastasis with no prior history of malignancy.[211] Metastatic carcinoma to pituitary adenoma has also been reported.[218]

Miscellaneous lesions

Although involvement of the hypothalamic pituitary axis in disseminated *Langerhans cell histiocytosis* is not uncommon,[233,251] isolated lesions are extremely rare and probably analogous to *Gagel's hypothalamic granuloma* and *Ayala's disease*.[240,250]

In about half the cases of adult *acute lymphoblastic leukemia,* periglandular (subcapsular) pituitary infiltration is demonstrable.[243] However, true intraparenchymal deposits are a rarity. Massive leukemic infiltrate of the sella mimicking pituitary adenoma has been reported in *chronic lymphocytic leukemia*.[249] When primary CNS *lymphoma* involves the anterior hypothalamus and pituitary stalk, evidence of hypopituitarism and chiasmal syndrome may develop.[232,245]

Plasmacytoma may develop in the area of the sphenoid bone and thus mimic pituitary adenoma.[231] Most of the patients reported eventually developed multiple myeloma. Ultrastructural and immunohistochemical studies are essential in differentiating plasmacytoma from *plasma cell granuloma* (inflammatory pseudotumor),[235] which is assumed to be a reactive lesion composed of a mixed inflammatory infiltrate.

Other tumors of bone that may arise at the base of the skull involving the sellar and parasellar region are *giant cell tumors,*[271] *chondromyxoid fibroma,*[268] *chordoma,*[224,244] *(en)chondroma,*[221,246] and *chondrosarcoma*.[265] Even a *bony spur* may become significant when located in the sella.[254]

Schwannomas have been reported in both the intrasellar compartment and the parasellar region.[238,253,269] Most uncommon are *hemangioblastoma,*[229] *hemangiopericytoma,*[242] *hemangioma (cavernous),*[227,260] *glomangioma,*[222] *paraganglioma,*[225,266] *neurocytoma,*[241] *primary melanoma,*[228,248,263] *ectopic salivary gland tissue* in the pituitary gland,[262] *primary sellar thyroid follicular tumor,*[258] and *sphenoid sinus mucocele* presenting as pituitary adenoma.[236]

Purely *intrasellar meningiomas* are a rarity[239]; more often the pituitary gland is involved by extension of a *suprasellar meningioma*.[240a,256] Also uncommon are *gliomas* infiltrating the pituitary gland or the sella turcica.[270] Radiologically and clinically they mimic adenomas.[257]

Germ cell tumors account for 0.3% to 0.7% of intracranial tumors,[259] and the most commonly involved sites are the epithalamus and the parasellar area. Three reports describe the distinctly uncommon situation of a germ cell tumor limited to the pituitary fossa.[234,237,255] Morphologically, these neoplasms are indistinguishable from their gonadal and extragonadal counterparts, with *germinomas* predominating.

Sarcoidosis may involve the cranial and spinal leptomeninges throughout and the parasellar area affecting the anterior hypothalamus, resulting in hypopituitarism.[226,247,264,267] Furthermore, both the anterior and posterior lobes of the pituitary may be affected in this condition, leading to a complex pattern of endocrine disturbance.

In some patients well-formed non-necrotizing granulomas without a lymphocytic component remain confined to the region. *Giant cell granulomatous hypophysitis* is considered by some to be a distinct clinicopathologic entity.[223,261,272] Isolated reports document intrasellar *cysticercosis*[230] and *hydatid cyst*.[252]

REFERENCES
NORMAL ANATOMY

1 Asa SL, Kovacs K, Bilbao JM: Pars tuberalis of the human pituitary. A histologic, immunohistochemical, ultrastructural, and immunoelectron microscopic analysis. Virchows Arch [A] **49:**399, 1983.

2 Horvath E, Kovacs K: Fine structural cytology of the adenohypophysis in rat and man. J Electron Microsc Technol **8:**401-432, 1988.

3 Horvath E, Kovacs K: The adenohypophysis. In Functional endocrine pathology. Boston, 1991, Blackwell, pp. 245-281.

4 Lloyd RV, D'Amato CJ, Thiny MT, Jin L, Hicks SP, Chandler WF: Corticotroph (basophil) invasion of the pars nervosa in the human pituitary. Localization of proopiomelanocortin peptides, galanin, and peptidylglycine alpha-amidating monoxygenase-like immunoreactivities. Endocr Pathol **4:**86-94, 1993.

5 Luse SA, Kernohan JW: Granular-cell tumors of the stalk and posterior lobe of the pituitary gland. Cancer **8:**616-622, 1955.

6 Luse SA, Kernohan JW: Squamous nests of the pituitary gland. Cancer **8:**623-628, 1955.

7 Nishioka H, Llena JF, Hirano A: Immunohistochemical study of folliculo-stellate cells in pituitary lesions. Endocr Pathol **2:**155-160, 1991.

8 Pelletier G, Robert F, Hardy J: Identification of human anterior pituitary cells by immunoelectron microscopy. J Clin Endocrinol Metab **46:**534-542, 1978.

9 Schochet SS, McCormick WF, Halmi NS: Salivary gland rests in the human pituitary. Arch Pathol **98:**193-200, 1974.

PITUITARY ADENOMA
General and clinical features

10 Bills DC, Meyer FB, Laws ER Jr, Davis DH, Ebersold MJ, Scheithauer BW, Ilstrup DM, Abboud CF: A retrospective analysis of pituitary apoplexy. Neurosurgery **33:**602-609, 1993.

11 Burrow G, Wortzman G, Rewcastle B, Holgate RC, Kovacs K: Microadenomas of the pituitary and abnormal sellar tomograms in an unselected autopsy series. N Engl J Med **304:**156-158, 1981.

12 Colohan ART, Grady MS, Bonnin JM, Thorner MO, Kovacs K, Jane JA: Ectopic pituitary gland simulating a suprasellar tumor. Neurosurgery **20:**43-48, 1987.

13 Hardy J, Vezina JL: Transsphenoidal neurosurgery of intracranial neoplasms. In Thompson RA, Green JR, eds: Advances in neurology. New York, 1976, Raven Press, pp. 261-274.

14 Kane LA, Leinung MC, Scheithauer BW, Groover RV, Rini JN, Bergstralh EJ, Laws ER Jr, Kovacs K, Horvath E, Zimmerman D: Pituitary adenomas in childhood and adolescence. A clinicopathologic study of the Mayo Clinic experience. Endocr Pathol **3:**517-518, 1992.

15 Kanter SL, Mickle P, Hunter SB, et al: Pituitary adenomas in pediatric patients. Are they more invasive? Pediatr Neurosci **12:**202-204, 1985-86.

15a Klibanski A, Zernas N: Diagnosis and management of hormone-secreting pituitary adenomas. New Engl J Med **324:**822-831, 1991.

16 Lloyd RV, Chandler WF, Kovacs K, et al.: Ectopic pituitary adenomas with normal anterior pituitary glands. Am J Surg Pathol **10:**546-552, 1986.

17 McGrath P: Volume and histology of the human pharyngeal hypophysis. Anat N Z J Surg **37:**16-27, 1967.

18 Mohr G, Hardy J, Comtois R, Beauregard H: Surgical management of giant pituitary adenomas. Can Neurol Sci **17:**62-66, 1990.

19 Mukai K, Seljeskog L, Dehner LP: Pituitary adenomas in patients under 20 years old. A clinicopathological study of 12 cases. J Neurooncol **4:**79-89, 1986.

20 Parent AD, Brown B, Smith EE: Incidental pituitary adenomas. A retrospective study. Surgery **92:**880-883, 1982.

21 Scheithauer BW, Laws ER, Kovacs K: Pituitary adenomas of the multiple endocrine neoplasia type I syndrome. Semin Diagn Pathol **4:**405-411, 1987.

22 Thapar K, Kovacs K, Laws ER, Muller P: Pituitary adenomas. Current concepts in classification, histopathology and molecular biology. Endocrinologist **3:**39-57, 1993.

22a Thapar K, Kovacs K, Muller PJ: Clinical-pathological correlations of pituitary tumours. Bailliere's Clin Endocrin Metab **9:**243-270, 1995.

23 Zimmerman RA: Imaging of intrasellar, suprasellar and parasellar tumors. Semin Roentgenol **25:**174-197, 1990.

Gross features

24 Knosp E, Steiner E, Kitz K, Matula C: Pituitary adenomas with invasion of the cavernous sinus space. A magnetic resonance imaging classification compared with surgical findings. Neurosurgery **33:**610-618, 1993.

25 Kovacs K, Horvath E: Tumors of the pituitary gland. In Atlas of tumor pathology, Series 2, vol 21. Washington, D.C.: 1986, Armed Forces Institute of Pathology.

Microscopic features

26 Bilbao JM, Horvath E, Hudson AR, Kovacs K: Pituitary adenomas producing amyloid-like substance. Arch Pathol **99:**411-415, 1975.

27 Hsu DW, Hakim F, Biller BMK, de La Monte S, Zervas NT, Klibanski A, Hedley-White ET: Significance of proliferating cell nuclear antigen index in predicting pituitary adenoma recurrence. J Neurosurg **78:**753-761, 1993.

28 Landolt AM, Kleihues P, Heitz PU: Amyloid deposits in pituitary adenomas. Arch Pathol Lab Med **111:**453-458, 1987.

29 Landolt AM, Rothenbuhler V: Pituitary adenoma calcification. Arch Pathol Lab Med **101:**22-27, 1977.

Classification

30 Black PM, Hsu DW, Klibanski A, et al: Hormone production in clinically nonfunctioning pituitary adenomas. J Neurosurg **66:**244-250, 1987.

31 Croue A, Beldent V, Rousselet MC, Guy G, Rohmer V, Bigorgne JC, Saint-Andre JP: Contribution of immunohistochemistry, electron microscopy, and cell culture to the characterization of nonfunctioning pituitary adenomas. A study of 40 cases. Hum Pathol **23:**1332-1339, 1992.

32 Girod C, Mazzuca M, Trouillas J, et al: Light microscopy, fine structure and immunohistochemistry studies of 278 pituitary adenomas. In Derome PJ, Gedynak CP, Peillon F, eds: Pituitary adenomas. Paris, 1980, Esdefrios Publishing.

33 Heitz PU, Landolt AM, Zenklusen HR, Kasper M, Reubi JC, Oberholzer M, et al: Immunocytochemistry of pituitary tumors. J Histochem Cytochem **35:**1005-1011, 1987.

34 Horvath E, Kovacs K: The adenohypophysis. In Kovacs K, Asa SL, eds: Functional endocrine pathology. Boston, 1991, Blackwell, pp. 245-281.

35 Kontogeorgos G, Kovacs K, Horvath E, Scheithauer BW: Null cell adenomas, oncocytomas, and gonadotroph adenomas of the human pituitary. An immunocytochemical and ultrastructural analysis of 300 cases. Endocr Pathol **4:**20-27, 1993.

36 Kontogeorgos G, Scheithauer BW, Horvath E, Kovacs K, Lloyd RV, Smyth HS, Rologis D: Double adenomas of the pituitary. A clinicopathological study of 11 tumors. Neurosurgery **31:**840-849, 1992.

37 Mukai K: Pituitary adenomas. Immunocytochemical study of 150 tumors with clinicopathologic correlations. Cancer **52:**648-653, 1983.

38 Saeger W, Gunzl H, Meyer M, et al: Immunohistological studies on clinically silent pituitary adenomas. Endocr Pathol **1:**37-44, 1990.

39 Stefaneanu L, Kovacs K, Horvath E, Lloyd RV, Buchfelder M, Fahlbusch R, Smyth H: In situ hybridization study of estrogen receptor messenger ribonucleic acid in human adenohypophysial cells and pituitary adenomas. J Clin Endocrinol Metab **78:**83-88, 1994.

PRL cell adenoma

40 Bilbao JM II, Horvath E, Hudson AR, Kovacs K: Pituitary adenomas producing amyloid-like substance. Arch Pathol **99:**411-415, 1975.

41 Burrow GN, Wortzman G, Rewcastle NB, Holgate RC, Kovacs K: Microadenomas of the pituitary and abnormal sellar tomograms in an unselected autopsy series. N Engl J Med **304:**156-158, 1981.

42 Esiri MM, Adams CBT, Burke C, Underdown R: Pituitary adenomas. Immunohistology and ultrastructural analysis of 118 tumors. Acta Neuropathol (Berl) **62:**1-14, 1983.

43 Horvath E, Kovacs K: The adenohypophysis. In Functional endocrine pathology. Boston, 1991, Blackwell, pp. 245-281.

44 Kameya T, Tsumuraya M, Adachi I, et al: Ultrastructure, immunohistochemistry and hormone release of pituitary adenomas in relation to prolactin production. Virchows Arch [A] **387:**31-46, 1980.

45 Kovacs K, Horvath E: Tumors of the pituitary gland. In Hartmann WH, ed: Atlas of tumor pathology, Series 2, fasc. XXI. Washington, D.C., 1986, Armed Forces Institute of Pathology, pp. 1-264.

46 Lees PD, Pickard JD, Chir M: Hyperprolactinemia, intrasellar pituitary tissue pressure, and the pituitary stalk compression syndrome. J Neurosurg **67:**192-196, 1987.

47 Mukada K, Ohta M, Uozumi T, Arita K, Kurisu K, Inai K: Ossified prolactinoma. Case report. Neurosurgery **20:**473-475, 1987.

48 Rasmussen C, Larsson SG, Bergh T: The occurrence of macroscopical pituitary calcifications in prolactinomas. Neuroradiology **31:**507-511, 1990.

49 Saeger W, Mohr K, Caselitz J, et al: Light and electron microscopical morphometry of pituitary adenomas in hyperprolactinemia. Pathol Res Pract **181:**544-550, 1986.

GH cell adenoma

50 Asa SL, Kovacs K: Pituitary pathology in acromegaly. Endocrinol Metab Clin North Am **21:**553-574, 1992.

51 Furuhata S, Kameya T, Otani M, Toya S: Prolactin presents in all pituitary tumours of acromegalic patients. Hum Pathol **24:**10-15, 1993.

52 Halmi NS: Occurrence of both growth hormone- and prolactin-immunoreactive material in the cells of human somatotropic pituitary adenomas containing mammotropic elements. Virchows Arch [A] **398:**19-31, 1982.

53 Kanie N, Kageyama N, Kuwayama A, Nakane T, Watanabe M, Kawea A: Pituitary adenomas in acromegalic patients. An immunohistochemical and endocrinological study with special reference to prolactin-secreting adenoma. J Clin Endocrinol Metab **57:**1093-1101, 1983.

54 Klibanski A, Zeras NT, Kovacs K, Ridgway EC: Clinically silent hypersecretion of growth hormone in patients with pituitary tumors. J Neurosurg **66:**806-811, 1987.

55 Kovacs K: Pathology of growth hormone excess. Pathol Res Pract **183:**565-568, 1988.

56 Kovacs K, Horvath E: Pathology of growth hormone-producing tumors of the human pituitary. Semin Diagn Pathol **3:**18-33, 1986.

57 Mori H, Mori S, Saitoh Y, Moriwaki K, Iida S, Matsumoto K: Growth hormone-producing pituitary adenoma with crystal-like amyloid immunohistochemically positive for growth hormone. Cancer **55:**96-102, 1985.

58 Neumann PE, Goldman JE, Horoupian DS, Hess MA: Fibrous bodies in growth hormone-secreting adenomas contain cytokeratin filaments. Arch Pathol Lab Med **109:**505-508, 1985.

59 Robert F: Electron microscopy of pituitary tumors. In Tindall GT, Collins WF, eds: Clinical management of pituitary disorders. New York, 1979, Raven Press, pp. 113-131.

60 Saeger W: Pathology of the pituitary gand. In Belchetz PE, ed: Management of pituitary disease. London, 1984, Chapman & Hall, pp. 253-289.

61 Saeger W, Rubenach-Gerz K, Caselitz J, Ludecke DK: Electron microscopical morphometry of GH-producing pituitary adenomas in comparison with normal GH cells. Virchows Arch [A] **411:**467-472, 1987.

62 Trouillas J, Girod C, Lheritier M, Claustrat B, Dubois MP: Morphological and biochemical relationships in 31 human pituitary adenomas with acromegaly. Virchows Arch [A] **389:**127-142, 1980.

63 Yamada S, Aiba T, Sano T, Kovacs K, Shishiba Y, Sawano S, Takada K: Growth hormone-producing pituitary adenomas. Correlations between clinical characteristics and morphology. Neurosurgery **33:**20-27, 1993.

Mixed PRL- and GH-producing adenomas

64 Bassetti M, Spada A, Arosio M, Vallar L, Brina M, Giannattasio G: Morphologic studies on mixed growth hormone (GH) and prolactin (PRL) secreting human pituitary adenomas. Coexistence of GH and PRL in the same secretory granule. J Clin Endocrinol Metab **62:**1093-1100, 1986.

65 Felix IA, Horvath E, Kovacs K, Smyth HS, Killinger DW, Vale J: Mammosomatotroph adenoma of the pituitary associated with gigantism and hyperprolactinemia. A morphological study including immunoelectron microscopy. Acta Neuropathol (Berl) **71:**76-82, 1986.

66 Frawley LS, Boockfor FR: Mammosomatotropes. Presence and functions in normal and neoplastic pituitary tissue. Endocr Rev **12:**337-355, 1991.

67 Furuhata S, Kameya T: Subdivisions of 26 mixed growth hormone and prolactin-producing pituitary adenomas. Endocr Pathol **3:**812-813, 1992.

68 Halmi NS: Occurrence of both growth hormone- and prolactin-immunoreactive material in the cells of human somatotropic pituitary adenomas containing mammotropic elements. Virchows Arch [A] **398:**19-31, 1982.

69 Horvath E, Kovacs K, Killinger DW, Smyth HS, Weiss MH, Ezrin C: Mammosomatotroph cell adenoma of the human pituitary. A morphologic entity. Virchows Arch [A] **398:**277-289, 1983.

70 Li J, Stefaneanu L, Kovacs K, Horvath E, Smyth H: Growth hormone (GH) and prolactin (PRL) gene expression and immunoreactivity in GH- and PRL-producing human pituitary adenomas. Virchows Archive [A] **422:**193-201, 1993.

Acidophilic stem cell adenoma

71 Horvath E, Kovacs K, Singer W, Smyth HS, Killinger DW, Ezriin C, et al: Acidophil stem cell adenoma of the human pituitary. Clinico-pathological analysis of 15 cases. Cancer **47:**761-771, 1981.

72 Li J, Stefaneanu L, Kovacs K, Horvath E, Smyth H: Growth hormone (GH) and prolactin (PRL) gene expression and immunoreactivity in GH- and PRL-producing human pituitary adenomas. Virchows Archiv [A] **422:**193-201, 1993.

73 McNicol AM, Walker E, Farguharson MA, Teasdale GM: Pituitary macroadenomas associated with hyperprolactinaemia. Immunocytochemical and in situ
hybridization studies. Clin Endocrinol 35:239-244, 1991.

ACTH cell adenoma

74 Belsky JL, Cuello B, Swanson LW, Simmons DM, Jarrett RM, Braza F: Cushing's syndrome due to ectopic production of corticotropin-releasing factor. J Clin
Endocrinol Metab 60:496-500, 1985.

75 Charpin C, Hassoun J, Oliver C, Jacquet P, Argemi B, Grisoli F, et al: Immunohistochemical and immunoelectron-microscopic study of pituitary adenomas
associated with Cushing's disease. A report of 13 cases. Am J Pathol 109:1-
7, 1982.

76 Findling JW, Aron DC, Tyrrell JB: Cushing's disease. In Imura H, ed: The pituitary gland. New York, 1985, Raven Press, pp. 441-466.

77 Kovacs K: The pathology of Cushing's disease. J Steroid Biochem Mol Biol
45:179-182, 1993.

78 Lloyd RV, Chandler WF, McKeever PE, et al: The spectrum of ACTH-producing pituitary lesions. Am J Surg Pathol 10:618-626, 1986.

79 McKeever PE, Koppelman MCS, Metcalf D, Quindler E, Kornblith PL, Strott
CA, et al: Refractory Cushing's disease caused by multinodular ACTH-cell
hyperplasia. J Neuropathol Exp Neurol 41:490-499, 1982.

80 Nelson DH, Meakin JW, Thorn GW: ACTH-producing pituitary tumors following adrenalectomy for Cushing's syndrome. Ann Intern Med 52:560-569, 1960.

81 Neumann PE, Horoupian DS, Goldman JE, Hess MA: Cytoplasmic filaments of
Crooke's hyaline change belong to the cytokeratin class. An immunocytochemical and ultrastructural study. Am J Pathol 116:214-222, 1984.

82 Robert F, Hardy J: Human corticotroph cell adenomas. Semin Diagn Pathol 3:34-
41, 1986.

83 Schnall AM, Kovacs K, Brodkey JS, Pearson OH: Pituitary Cushing's disease
without adenoma. Acta Endocrinol (Copenh) 94:297-303, 1980.

84 Thapar K, Smith MV, Elliot E, Kovacs K, Laws E: Corticotroph adenomas of the
pituitary. Long term results of operative treatment. Endocr Pathol 3:S51-
S53, 1992.

85 Wowra B, Peiffer J: An immunoperoxidase study of a human pituitary adenoma
associated with Cushing's syndrome. Pathol Res Pract 178:349-354, 1984.

Glycoprotein hormone producing adenomas

86 Gesundheit N, Petrick PA, Nissim M, Dahlberg PA, Doppman JL, Emerson GH,
Braverman LF, Oldfield: Thyrotropin-secreting pituitary adenomas. Clinical and
biochemical heterogeneity. Case reports and follow-up of nine patients. Ann
Intern Med 111:827-835, 1989.

87 Gharib SD, Weirman MF, Shupnik MA, Chin WW: Molecular biology of pituitary gonadotropins. Endocr Rev 11:177-199, 1990.

88 Girod C, Trouillas J, Claustrat B: The human thyrotropic adenoma. Pathologic
diagnosis in five cases and critical review of the literature. Semin Diagn Pathol
3:58-68, 1986.

89 Hamilton CRJ, Adams LC, Maloof F: Hyperthyroidism due to thyrotropin-pro-
ducing pituitary chromophobe adenoma. N Engl J Med 283:1077-1080, 1970.

90 Klibanski A, Ridgway EC, Zervas NT: Pure alpha subunit-secreting pituitary
tumors. J Neurosurg 59:585-589, 1983.

91 Klibanski A, Zervas N: Diagnosis and management of hormone-secreting pituitary adenomas. N Engl J Med 324:822-831, 1991.

91a Kovacs K, Asa SL, eds: The adenohypophysis. Functional endocrine pathology,
Boston, 1991, Blackwell, pp. 245-281.

92 Landolt AM, Heitz PU: Alpha-subunit-producing pituitary adenomas. Immunocytochemical and ultrastructural studies. Virchows Arch [A] 409:417-
431, 1986.

93a McCutcheon IA, Weitraub BE, Oldfield EH: Surgical treatment of thyrotropin-
secreting pituitary adenomas. J Neurosurg 73:674-683, 1990.

94 Miura M, Matsukado Y, Kodama T, Mihara Y: Clinical and histopathological
characteristics of gonadotropin-producing pituitary adenomas. J Neurosurg
62:376-382, 1985.

95 Saeger W, Ludecke DK: Pituitary adenomas with hyperfunction of TSH. Frequency, histological classification, immunocytochemistry and ultrastructure.
Virchows Arch [A] 394:255-267, 1982.

96 Samaan NA, Osborne BM, Mackay B, Leavens ME, Duello T, Halmi NS:
Endocrine and morphologic studies of pituitary adenomas secondary to primary
hypothyroidism. J Clin Endocrinol Metab 45:903-911, 1977.

97 Snyder PJ: Gonadotroph cell adenomas of the pituitary. Endocr Rev 6:552-
563, 1985.

98 Trouillas J, Girod C, Sassolas G, Claustrat B: The human gonadotropic adenoma. Pathologic diagnosis and hormonal correlations in 26 tumors. Semin
Diagn Pathol 3:42-57, 1986.

99 Wajchenberg BL, Tsanaclis AMC, Marino R Jr: TSH-containing pituitary adenoma associated with primary hypothyroidism manifested by amenorrhoea and
galactorrhoea. Acta Endocrinol (Copenh) 106:61-66, 1984.

Plurihormonal adenoma

100 Giannattasio G, Bassetti M: Human pituitary adenomas. Recent advances in
morphological studies. J Endocrinol Invest 13:435-454, 1990.

101 Kovacs K, Horvath E, Asa SL, et al: Pituitary cells producing more than one
hormone. Human pituitary adenomas. TEM 1:104-107, 1989.

102 Lloyd RV, Cano M, Chandler WF: Human growth hormone and prolactin
secreting pituitary adenomas analyzed by in situ hybridization. Am J Pathol
134:605-613, 1989.

103 Thapar K, Stefaneanu L, Kovacs K, Horvath E, Asa SL: Plurihormonal pituitary
tumors. Beyond the one cell-one hormone theory. Endocr Pathol 4:1-3, 1993.

104 Yamada S, Aiba T, Sano T, Kovacs K, Shishiba Y, Sawano S, Takada K:
Growth hormone-producing pituitary adenomas. Correlations between clinical
characteristics and morphology. Neurosurgery 33:20-27, 1993.

Null cell adenoma and oncocytoma

105 Asa SL, Cheng Z, Ranyar L, Singer W, Kovacs K, Smyth HS, Muller P: Human
pituitary null cell adenomas and oncocytomas in vitro. Effects of adenohy-
pophysiotropic hormone and gonadal steroids on hormone secretion and tumor
cell morphology. J Clin Endocrinol Metab 74:1128-1134, 1992.

106 Kontogeorgos G, Kovacs K, Horvath E, Scheithauer B: Null cell adenomas,
oncocytomas and gonadotroph cell adenomas of the human pituitary. An
immunocytochemical and ultrastructural analysis of 300 cases. Endocr Pathol
4:20-27, 1993.

107 Kovacs K, Horvath E: Pituitary "chromophobe" adenoma composed of oncocytes. A light and electron microscopic study. Arch Pathol 95:235-239, 1973.

108 Kovacs K, Horvath E, Ryan N, Ezrin C: Null cell adenoma of the human pituitary. Virchows Arch [A] 387:165-174, 1980.

109 Landolt AM, Oswald UW: Histology and ultrastructure of an oncocytic adenoma of the human pituitary. Cancer 31:1099-1105, 1973.

110 Lloyd RV, Anagnostou D, Chandler WF: Dopamine receptors in immunohistochemically characterized null cell adenomas and normal human pituitaries. Mod
Pathol 1:51-56, 1988.

Natural history, spread, and metastases

111 Ahmed M, Rifai A, Al-Jurf M, et al: Classical pituitary apoplexy. Presentation
and follow-up of 13 patients. Horm Res 31:125-132, 1989.

112 Hashimoto N. Handa H, Nishi S: Intracranial and intraspinal dissemination from
a growth hormone-secreting pituitary tumor. J Neurosurg 64:140-144, 1986.

113 Mountcastle RB, Roof BS, Mayfield RK, et al: Case report. Pituitary adenocarcinoma in an acromegalic patient. Response to bromocriptine and pituitary testing. A review of the literature on 36 cases of pituitary carcinoma. Am J Med Sci
298:109-118, 1989.

114 Plangger CA, Twerdy K, Grunert V, et al: Subarachnoid metastases from a prolactinoma. Neurochirurgia 28:235-237, 1985.

115 Shirataki K, Chihara K, Shibata Y, Tamaki N, Matsumoto S, Fujita T: Pituitary
apoplexy manifested during a bromocriptine test in a patient with a growth
hormone and prolactine producing pituitary adenoma. Neurosurgery 23:395-
398, 1988.

116 Thapar K, Kovacs K, Laws ER: The classification and molecular biology of
pituitary adenomas. Advances and technical standards in neurosurgery. Wein-
Vienna, 1995, Springer-Verlag.

116a Thapar K, Kovacs K, Scheithauer BW, et al: Proliferative activity and invasiveness among pituitary adenomas and carcinomas. An analysis using the MIB-
1 antibody. Neurosurgery 1995 (in press).

Treatment

117 Beckers A, Kovacs K, Horvath E, Abs R, Reznik M, Stevenaert A: Effect of
treatment with octreotide on the morphology of growth hormone-secreting pituitary adenomas. Study of 24 cases. Endocr Pathol 2:123-131, 1991.

118 Bevan JS, Adams CBT, Burke CW, Morton KE, Molyneux AJ, Moore RA, et
al: Factors in the outcome of transsphenoidal surgery for prolactinoma and nonfunctioning pituitary tumor, including pre-operative bromocriptine therapy. Clin
Endocrinol 26:541-556, 1987.

119 Black PM, Zervas NT, Candia GL: Incidence and management of complications of transsphenoidal operation for pituitary adenomas. Neurosurgery **20**:920-924, 1987.

120 Davis DH, Laws ER Jr, Ilstrup DM, Speed JK, Caruso M, Shaw EG, Abboud CF, Scheithauer BW, Rott LY, Schleck C: Results of surgical treatment for growth hormone-secreting pituitary adenomas. J Neurosurg **79**:70-75, 1993.

121 Goffman TE, Dewan R, Arakaki R, et al: Persistent or recurrent acromegaly. Long-term endocrinologic efficacy and neurologic safety of postsurgical radiation therapy. Cancer **69**:271-275, 1992.

122 Schettini G, Lombardi G, Merola B, Colao A, Miletto P, Caruso E, Lancranjan I: Rapid and longlasting suppression of prolactin secretion and shrinkage of prolactinomas after infection of long-acting repeatable form of bromocriptine (Parlodel Lar). Clin Endocrinol **33**:161-169, 1990.

OTHER LESIONS
Gangliocytoma

123 Asa SL, Kovacs K, Tindall GT, Barrow DL, Horvath E, Vecsei P: Cushing's disease associated with an intrasellar gangliocytoma producing corticotrophin-releasing factor. Ann Intern Med **101**:789-793, 1984.

124 Asa SL, Scheithauer BW, Bilbao JM, et al: A case for hypothalamic acromegaly. A clinicopathological study of six patients with hypothalamic gangliocytomas producing growth hormone-releasing factor. J Clin Endocrinol Metab **58**:796-803, 1984.

125 Bevan JS, Asa SL, Rossi ML, Esiri MM, Adams CBT, Burke CW: Intrasellar gangliocytoma containing gastrin and growth hormone-releasing hormone associated with a growth hormone-secreting pituitary adenoma. Clin Endocrinol **30**:213-224, 1989.

126 Curatolo P, Cusmai R, Finocchi G, Boscherini B: Gelastic epilepsy and true precocious puberty due to hypothalamic hamartoma. Dev Med Child Neurol **26**:509-514, 1984.

127 Fischer EG, Morris JH, Kettyle WM: Intrasellar gangliocytoma and syndromes of pituitary hypersecretion. Case report. J Neurosurg **59**:1071-1075, 1983.

128 Hirsch-Pescovitz O, Comite F, Hench K, et al: The NIH experience with precocious puberty. Diagnostic subgroups and response to short-term luteinizing hormone releasing hormone analogue therapy. J Pediatr **108**:47-54, 1986.

129 Jakumeit HD, Zimmerman V, Guiot G: Intrasellar gangliocytomas. Report of four cases. J Neurosurg **40**:626-630, 1974.

130 Kamel OW, Horoupian DS, Silverberg GD: Mixed gangliocytoma-adenoma. A distinct neuroendocrine tumor of the pituitary fossa. Hum Pathol **20**:1198-1203, 1989.

131 Li JY, Racadot O, Kujas M, Kouadri M, Peillon F, Racadot J: Immunocytochemistry of four mixed pituitary adenomas and intrasellar gangliocytomas associated with different clinical syndromes. Acromegaly, amenorrhea-galactorrhea, Cushing's disease and isolated tumoral syndrome. Acta Neuropathol **77**:320-328, 1989.

132 Markin RS, Leibrock LG, Huseman CA, McComb RD: Hypothalamic harmartoma. A report of two cases. Pediatr Neurosci **13**:19-26, 1987.

133 Nishio S, Fujiwara S, Aiko Y, Takeshita I, Fukui M: Hypothalamic hamartoma. Report of two cases. J Neurosurg **70**:640-645, 1989.

134 Pallister PD, Hecht F, Herrman J: Three additional cases of the congenital hypothalamic "hamartoblastoma" (Pallister-Hall) syndrome (letter). Am J Med Genet **33**:500-501, 1989.

135 Ponsot G, Diebler C, Plouin P, et al: Hamartomes hypothalamiques et crises de rire. A propos de 7 observations. Arch Fr Pediatr **40**:757-761, 1983.

136 Puchner MJA, Ludecke DK, Valdueza JM, Saeger W, Willig RP, Stalla GK, Odink RJ: Cushing's disease in a child caused by a corticotropin releasing hormone–secreting intrasellar gangliocytoma associated with an adrenocorticotropic hormone–secreting pituitary adenoma. Neurosurgery **33**:920-925, 1993.

137 Yamada S, Stefaneanu L, Kovacs K, Aiba T, Shishiba Y, Hara M: Intrasellar gangliocytoma with multiple immunoreactives. Endocr Pathol **1**:58-63, 1990.

Lymphocytic hypophysitis

138 Asa SL, Bilbao JM, Kovacs K, et al: Lymphocytic hypophysis in pregnancy resulting in hypopituitarism. A distinct clinicopathologic entity. Ann Intern Med **95**:166, 1981.

139 Bitton RN, Slavin M, Decker RE, Zito J, Schneider BS: The course of lymphocytic hypophysitis. Surg Neurol **36**:40-43, 1991.

140 Cosman F, Post KD, Holub DA, Wardlaw SL: Lymphocytic hypophysitis. Report of three new cases and review of the literature. Medicine **68**:240-256, 1989.

141 Feigenbaum SL, Martin MC, Wilson Ch B, Jaffe RB: Lymphocytic adenohypophysitis. A pituitary mass lesion occurring in pregnancy. Am J Obstet Gynecol **164**:1549-1555, 1991.

142 Lee JH, Laws ER, Guthrie BL, Dina TS, Nochomovitz LE: Lymphocytic hypophysitis. Occurrence in two men. Neurosurgery **34**:159-163, 1994.

143 Megrail KM, Beyerl BD, Black PM, Klibanski A, Zervas NT: Lymphocytic adenohypophysitis of pregnancy with complete recovery. Neurosurgery **20**:791-793, 1987.

144 Meichner RH, Riggio S, Manz HJ, Earll JM: Lymphocytic adenohypophysitis causing pituitary mass. Neurology **37**:158-161, 1987.

145 Nussbaum CE, Okawara SH, Jacobs LS: Lymphocytic hypophysitis with involvement of the cavernous sinus and hypothalamus. Neurosurgery **28**:440-444, 1991.

146 Pestell RG, Best JD, Alford FP: Lymphocytic hypophysitis. The clinical spectrum of the disorder and evidence for an autoimmune pathogenesis. Clin Endocrinol **33**:457-466, 1990.

147 Reuch JEB, Kleinschmidt-DeMasters BK, Lillehei KO, Rappe D: Preoperative diagnosis of lymphocytic hypophysitis (adenohypophysitis) unresponsive to short course dexamethasone. Case report. Neurosurgery **30**:268-272, 1992.

Rathke's cleft cyst

148 Barrow DL, Spector RH, Takei Y, Tindall GT: Symptomatic Rathke's cleft cysts located entirely in the suprasellar region. Review of diagnosis, management and pathogenesis. Neurosurgery **16**:766-772, 1985.

149 Baskin DS, Wilson CB: Transsphenoidal treatment of non-neoplastic intrasellar cysts. Report of 38 cases. J Neurosurg **60**:8-13, 1984.

150 Kucharczyk W, Peck WW, Kelly WM, Norman D, Newton TH: Rathke cleft cysts. CT, MR imaging, and pathologic features. Radiology **165**:491-495, 1987.

151 McGrath P: Cysts of sellar and pharyngeal hypophyses. Pathology **3**:123-131, 1971.

152 Midha R, Jay V, Smyth HS: Transsphenoidal management of Rathke's cleft cysts. A clinicopathological review of 10 cases. Surg Neurol **35**:446-454, 1991.

153 Nishio S, Mizuno J, Barrow DL, Takei Y, Tindall GT: Pituitary tumors composed of adenohypophysial adenoma and Rathke's cleft cyst elements. A clinicopathological study. Neurosurgery **21**:371-377, 1987.

154 Obenchain TG, Becker DP: Abscess formation in a Rathke's cleft cyst. Case report. J Neurosurg **36**:359-362, 1972.

155 Shuangshoti S, Netsky MG, Nashold BS: Epithelial cysts related to sella turcica. Proposed origin from neuroepithelium. Arch Pathol **90**:444-450, 1970.

156 Steinberg GK, Koenig GH, Golden JB: Symptomatic Rathke's cleft cysts. Report of two cases. J Neurosurg **56**:290-295, 1982.

157 Yoshida J, Kobayashi T, Kageyama N, Kanzaki M: Symptomatic Rathke's cleft cyst. Morphological study with light and electron microscopy and tissue culture. J Neurosurg **47**:451-458, 1977.

158 Zimmerman RA: Imaging of intrasellar, suprasellar and parasellar tumors. Semin Roentgenol **25**:174-197, 1990.

Craniopharyngioma

159 Adamson TE, Wiestler OD, Kleihues P, Yasargil MG: Correlation of clinical and pathological features in surgically treated craniopharyngiomas. J Neurosurg **73**:12-17, 1990.

160 Azar-Kia B, Krishnan UR, Schechter MM: Neonatal craniopharyngioma. Case report. J Neurosurg **42**:91-93, 1975.

161 Barloon TJ, Yuh WTC, Sato Y, Sickels WJ: Frontal lobe implantation of craniopharyngioma by repeated needle aspirations. Am J Neuroradiol **9**:406-407, 1988.

162 Berstein ML, Buchino JJ: The histologic similarity between craniopharyngioma and odontogenic lesions. A reappraisal. Oral Surg **56**:502-511, 1983.

163 Brodsky MC, Hoyt WF, Barnwell SL, Wilson CB: Intrachiasmatic craniopharyngioma. A rare cause of chiasmal thickening. Case report. J Neurosurg **68**:300-302, 1988.

164 Duff TA, Levine R: Intrachiasmatic craniopharyngioma. Case report. J Neurosurg **59**:176-178, 1983.

165 Freedman PD, Lumerman H, Gee JK: Calcifying odontogenic cyst. Oral Surg **40**:93-106, 1975.

166 Ghatak NY, Hirano A, Zimmerman HM: Ultrastructure of a craniopharyngioma. Cancer **27**:1467-1475, 1971.

167 Giangaspero F, Burger PC, Osborne DR, Stein RB: Suprasellar papillary squamous epithelium ("papillary craniopharyngioma"). Am J Surg Pathol **8**:57-64, 1984.

168 Hoffman HJ: Craniopharyngiomas. Can J Neurol Sci **12**:348-352, 1985.

169 Janish W, Flegel HG: Kranipharingiom bei einem Feten. Zentralbl Allg Pathol **135**:65-69, 1989.

170 Kunishio K, Yamamoto Y, Sunami N, Asari S, Akagi T, Ohtsuki Y: Craniopharyngioma in the third ventricle. Necropsy findings and histogenesis. J Neurol Neurosurg Psychiatry **50**:1053-1056, 1987.

171 Lederman GS, Recht A, Loeffler JS, Dubuisson D, Kleefield J, Schnitt SJ: Craniopharyngioma in an elderly patient. Cancer **60:**1077-1080, 1987.

172 Munari C, Landre E, Musolino A, Terak B, Habert MO, Chodkiewicz JP: Long term results of stereotactic endocavitary beta irradiation of craniopharyngioma. J Neurosurg Sci **33:**99-105, 1989.

173 Nelson GA, Bastian FO, Schlitt M, White RL: Malignant transformation in craniopharyngioma. Neurosurgery **22:**427-429, 1988.

174 Petito CK, DeGirolami U, Earle KM: Craniopharyngiomas. A clinical and pathological review. Cancer **37:**1944-1952, 1976.

175 Pigeau I, Sigal R, Halimi P, Comoy J, Doyon D: MRI features of craniopharyngiomas at 1.5 tesla. J Neuroradiol **15:**276-287, 1988.

176 Seemayer TA, Blundell JS, Wiglesworth FW: Pituitary craniopharyngioma with tooth formation. Cancer **29:**423-430, 1972.

177 Sumi T, Stefaneanu L, Kovacs K: Squamous-cell nests in the pars tuberalis of the human pituitary. Immunocytochemical and in situ hybridization studies. Endocr Pathol **4:**155-161, 1993.

178 Weiss M, Sutton L, Marcial V, et al: The role of radiation therapy in the management of childhood craniopharyngioma. Int J Radiat Oncol Biol Phys **17:**1313-1321, 1989.

179 Yasargil MG, Curcic M, Kis M, Siegenthaler G, Teddy PJ, Roth P: Total removal of craniopharyngiomas. Approaches and long-term results in 144 patients. J Neurosurg **73:**3-11, 1990.

180 Young SC, Zimmerman RA, Nowell MA, et al: Giant cystic craniopharyngiomas. Neuroradiology **29:**468-473, 1987.

Granular cell tumor

181 Buley ID, Gatter KC, Kelly PMA, Heryet A, Millard PR: Granular cell tumors revisited. An immunohistochemical and ultrastructural study. Histopathology **12:**263-274, 1988.

182 Dickson DW, Suzuki KI, Kanner R, Weitz S, Horoupian DS: Cerebral granular cell tumor. Immunohistochemical and electron microscopic study. J Neuropathol Exp Neurol **45:**304-314, 1986.

183 Landolt A: Granular cell tumors of the neurohypophysis. Acta Neurochir (Wien) **22**(Suppl):120-128, 1975.

184 Luse SA, Kernohan JW: Granular cell tumors of the stalk and posterior lobe of the pituitary gland. Cancer **8:**616-622, 1955.

185 Nishioka H: Immunohistochemical study of granular cell tumors and granular pituicytes of the neurohypophysis. Endocr Pathol **4:**140-145, 1993.

186 Schlachter LB, Tindall GT, Pearl GS: Granular cell tumor of the pituitary gland associated with diabetes insipidus. Neurosurgery **6:**418-421, 1980.

187 Shanklin WM: The origin, histology and senescence of tumorettes in the human neurohypophysis. Acta Anat **18:**1-20, 1953.

188 Tomita T, Kuziez M, Watanabe I: Double tumors of anterior and posterior pituitary gland. Acta Neuropathol (Berl) **54:**161-164, 1981.

189 Tuch BE, Carter JN, Armellin GM, Newland RC: The association of a tumor of the posterior pituitary gland with multiple endocrine neoplasia type 1. Aust N Z J Med **12:**179-181, 1982.

190 Ulrich J, Heitz PU, Fischer T, Obrist E, Gullotta F: Granular cell tumors. Evidence for heterogeneous tumor cell differentiation. An immunocytochemical study. Virchows Arch [Cell Pathol] **53:**52-57, 1987.

191 Vaquero J, Leunda G, Cabezudo JM, Solazar AR, Miguel J: Granular pituicytomas of the pituitary stalk. Acta Neurochir (Wien) **59:**209-215, 1981.

192 Waller RR, Riley FC, Sundt TM: A rare cause of the chiasmal syndrome. Arch Ophthalmol **88:**269-272, 1972.

Postradiation tumors

193 Ahmad K, Fayos JV: Pituitary fibrosarcoma secondary to radiation therapy. Cancer **42:**107-110, 1978.

194 Amine ARC, Sugar O: Suprasellar osteogenic sarcoma following radiation for pituitary adenoma. Case report. J Neurosurg **44:**88-91, 1976.

195 Fontana M, Stanton C, Pompili A, et al: Late multifocal gliomas in adolescents previously treated for acute lymphoblastic leukemia. Cancer **60:**1510-1518, 1987.

196 Huang CI, Chiou WH, Ho DM: Oligodendroglioma occurring after radiation therapy for pituitary adenoma. J Neurol Neurosurg Psychiatry **50:**1619-1624, 1987.

197 Hufnagel TJ, Kim JH, Lesser R, et al: Malignant glioma of the optic chiasm eight years after radiotherapy for prolactinoma. Arch Ophthalmol **106:**1701-1705, 1988.

198 Kitanaka C, Shitara N, Nakagomi T, et al: Postradiation astrocytoma. Report of two cases. J Neurosurg **70:**469-474, 1989.

199 Liwnicz BH, Berger TS, Liwnicz RG, Aron BS: Radiation-associated gliomas. A report of four cases and analysis of postradiation tumors of the central nervous system. Neurosurgery **17:**436-445, 1985.

200 Maat-Schieman MLC, Bots GTAM, Thomeer RTWM, Vielvoye GJ: Malignant astrocytoma following radiotherapy for craniopharyngioma. Br J Radiol **58:**480-482, 1985.

201 Marus G, Levin CV, Rutherfoord GS: Malignant glioma following radiotherapy for unrelated primary tumors. Cancer **58:**886-894, 1986.

202 Meredith JM, Mandeville FB, Kay S: Osteogenic sarcoma of the skull following roentgen-ray therapy for benign pituitary tumor. J Neurosurg **17:**792-799, 1960.

203 Piatt JH, Blue JM, Schold SC, Burger PC: Glioblastoma multiforme after radiotherapy for acromegaly. Neurosurgery **13:**85-89, 1983.

204 Ron E, Modan B, Boice JD, et al: Tumors of the brain and nervous system after radiotherapy in childhood. N Engl J Med **319:**1033-1039, 1988.

205 Sogg RL, Donaldson SS, Yorke CH: Malignant astrocytoma following radiotherapy of a craniopharyngioma. J Neurosurg **48:**622-627, 1978.

206 Spallone A: Meningioma as a sequel to radiotherapy for pituitary adenoma. Neurochirurgia (Stuttg) **25:**68-72, 1982.

207 Sridhar K, Ramamurthi B: Intracranial meningioma subsequent to radiation for a pituitary tumor. Case report. Neurosurgery **25:**643-645, 1989.

208 Tanaka S, Nishio S, Morioka T, Fukui M, Kitamura K, Hikita K: Radiation-induced osteosarcoma of the sphenoid bone. Neurosurgery **25:**640-643, 1989.

209 Ushio Y, Arita N, Yoshimine T, Nagatani M, Mogami H: Glioblastoma after radiotherapy for craniopharyngioma: Case report. Neurosurgery **21:**33-38, 1987.

210 Zampieri P, Zorat PL, Migrino S, Soattin GB: Radiation-associated cerebral gliomas. A report of two cases and review of the literature. J Neurosurg Sci **33:**271-279, 1989.

Metastatic tumors

211 Branch CL, Laws ER: Metastatic tumors of the sella turcica masquerading as primary pituitary tumors. J Clin Endocrinol Metab **65:**469-474, 1987.

212 Felix IA: Pathology of the neurohypophysis. Pathol Res Pract **183:**535-537, 1988.

213 Gurling KJ, Scott GBD, Baron DN: Metastasis in pituitary tissue removed at hypophysectomy in women with mammary carcinoma. Br J Cancer **11:**519-523, 1957.

214 Kattah JC, Silgals RM, Manz H, Toro JG, Dritschilo A, Smith FP: Presentation and management of parasellar and suprasellar metastatic mass lesions. J Neurol Neurosurg Psychiatry **48:**44-49, 1985.

215 Kimmel DW, O'Neill BP: Systemic cancer presenting as diabetes insipidus. Clinical and radiographic features of 11 patients with a review of metastatic-induced diabetes insipidus. Cancer **52:**2355-2358, 1983.

216 Max MB, Deck MDF, Rottenberg DA: Pituitary metastasis. Incidence in cancer patients and clinical differentiation from pituitary adenoma. Neurology **31:**998-1002, 1981.

217 McCormick PC, Post KD, Kandji AD, Hays AP: Metastatic carcinoma to the pituitary gland. Br J Neurosurg **3:**71-79, 1989.

218 Post KD, McCormick PC, Hays AP, Kandji AD: Metastatic carcinoma to pituitary adenoma. Report of two cases. Surg Neurol **30:**286-292, 1988.

219 Roessmann U, Kaufman B, Friede RL: Metastatic lesions in the sella turcica and pituitary gland. Cancer **25:**478-480, 1970.

220 Teears RJ, Silverman EM: Clinicopathologic review of 88 cases of carcinoma metastatic to the pituitary gland. Cancer **36:**216-220, 1975.

Miscellaneous lesions

221 Angiari P, Torcia E, Botticelli RA, Villani M, Merli GA, Crisi G: Ossifying parasellar chondroma. Case report. J Neurosurg Sci **31:**59-63, 1987.

222 Asa SL, Kovacs K, Horvath E, Ezrin C, Weiss MH: Sellar glomangioma. Ultrastruct Pathol **7:**49-54, 1984.

223 Bachour E, Perrin G, Ciriano P, Trouillas J, Sassolas G, Tommasi M, Goutelle A: Les granulomes idiopathiques a cellules geantes de l'hypophyse. Neurochirurgie **37:**253-257, 1991.

224 Belza J: Double midline intracranial tumors of vestigial origin. Contiguous intrasellar chordoma and suprasellar craniopharyngioma. Case report. J Neurosurg **25:**199, 1966.

225 Bilbao JM, Horvath E, Kovacs K, Singer W, Hudson AR: Intrasellar paraganglioma associated with hypopituitarism. Arch Pathol Lab Med **102:**95-98, 1978.

226 Capellan JIL, Olmedo LC, Martin JM, et al: Intrasellar mass with hypopituitarism as a manifestation of sarcoidosis. Case report. J Neurosurg **73:**283-286, 1990.

227 Castel JP, Delorge-Kerdiles C, Rivel J: Angiome caverneux du chiasma optique. Neurochirurgie **35:**252-256, 1989.

228 Copeland DD, Sink JD, Seigler HF: Primary intracranial melanoma presenting as a suprasellar tumor. Neurosurgery 6:542-545, 1980.

229 Dan NG, Smith DE: Pituitary hemangioblastoma in a patient with von Hippel-Lindau disease. J Neurosurg 42:232-235, 1975.

230 Del Brutto OH, Guevara J, Sotelo J: Intrasellar cysticercosis. J Neurosurg 69:58-60, 1988.

231 Dhanani AN, Bilbao JM, Kovacs K: Multiple myeloma presenting as a sellar plasmacytomas mimicking a pituitary tumor. Report of a case and review of the literature. Endocr Pathol 1:245-248, 1990.

232 Duchen LW, Treip CS: Microgliomatosis presenting with dementia and hypopituitarism. J Pathol 98:143-146, 1969.

233 Favara BE, Jaffe R: Pathology of Langerhans cell histiocytosis. Hematol Oncol Clin North Am 1:75-97, 1987.

234 Furukawa F, Haebara H, Hamashima Y: Primary intracranial choriocarcinoma arising from the pituitary fossa. Report of an autopsy case with literature review. Acta Pathol Jpn 36:773-781, 1986.

235 Gartman JJ, Powers SK, Fortune M: Pseudotumor of the sellar and parasellar areas. Neurosurgery 24:896-901, 1989.

236 Gerlings PG: Sphenoid sinus mucocele presenting as hypophyseal tumor. Acta Neurochir 61:167-171, 1982.

237 Ghatak NR, Hirano A, Zimmerman HM: Intrasellar germinomas. A form of ectopic pinealoma. J Neurosurg 31:670-675, 1969.

238 Goebel HH, Shimokawa K, Schaake T, Kremp A: Schwannoma of the sellar region. Acta Neurochir (Wien) 48:191-198, 1979.

239 Grisoli F, Vincentelli F, Raybaud C, Harter M, Guibout M, Baldini M: Intrasellar meningioma. Surg Neurol 20:36-41, 1983.

240 Kepes JJ, Kepes M: Predominantly cerebral forms of histiocytosis-X. A reappraisal of "Gagel's hypothalamic granuloma," "granuloma infiltrans of the hypothalamus," and "Ayala's disease" with a report of four cases. Acta Neuropathol (Berl) 14:77-98, 1969.

240a Kinjo T, al-Mefty O, Ciric I: Diaphragma sella meningiomas. Neurosurgery 36:1082-1092, 1995.

241 Maguire JA, Bilbao JM, Kovacs K, Resch L: Hypothalamic neurocytoma with vasopressin immunoreactivity. Immunohistochemical and ultrastructural observations. Endocr Pathol 3:93-96, 1992.

242 Mangiardi JR, Flamm ES, Cravioto H, et al: Hemangiopericytoma of the pituitary fossa. Case report. Neurosurgery 13:58-61, 1983.

243 Masse SR, Wolk RW, Conklin RH: Peripituitary gland involvement in acute leukemia in adults. Arch Pathol 96:141-142, 1973.

244 Mathews W, Wilson CB: Ectopic intrasellar chordoma. Case report. J Neurosurg 40:260, 1974.

245 Miauri F: Primary cerebral lymphoma presenting as steroid-responsive chiasmal syndrome. Br J Neurosurg 1:499-502, 1987.

246 Miki K, Kawamoto K, Kawamura Y, Matsumura H, Asada Y, Hamada A: A rare case of Maffucci's syndrome combined with tuberculum sellae enchondroma, pituitary adenoma and thyroid adenoma. Acta Neurochir (Wien) 87:79-85, 1987.

247 Missler U, Mack M, Nowak G, et al: Pituitary sarcoidosis. Klin Wochenschr 68:342-345, 1990.

248 Neilson JM, Moffat AD: Hypopituitarism caused by a melanoma of the pituitary gland. J Clin Pathol 16:144-149, 1963.

249 Nemato K, Ohnishi Y, Tsukada T: Chronic lymphocytic leukemia showing pituitary tumor with massive leukemic cell infiltration, and special reference to clinicopathological findings of CLL. Acta Pathol Jpn 28:797-805, 1978.

250 Nishio S, Mizuno J, Barrow DL, Takei Y, Tindall GT: Isolated histocytosis X of the pituitary gland. Case report. Neurosurgery 21:718-721, 1987.

251 Ober KP, Alexander E, Challa VR, Ferree C, Elster A: Histiocytosis X of the hypothalamus. Neurosurgery 24:93-95, 1989.

252 Osgen T, Bertan V, Kansu T, et al: Intrasellar hydatid cyst. Case report. J Neurosurg 60:647-648, 1984.

253 Perone TP, Robinson B, Holmes SM: Intrasellar schwannoma. Case report. Neurosurgery 14:71-73, 1984.

254 Petrus M, Mignonat M, Netter JC, Bat P, Chateaneuf R, Bildstein G: Association epine intrasellaire et hyperprolactinemie. Ann Pediatr (Paris) 35:201-203, 1988.

255 Poon W, Ng HK, Wong K, South JR: Primary intrasellar germinoma presenting with cavernous sinus syndrome. Surg Neurol 30:402-405, 1988.

256 Rohringer M, Sutherland GR, Louw DF, Sima AAF: Incidence and clinicopathological features of meningioma. J Neurosurg 71:665-672, 1989.

257 Rossi ML, Bevan JS, Esiri MM, Hughes JT, Adams CBT: Pituicytoma (pilocytic astrocytoma). Case report. J Neurosurg 67:768-772, 1987.

258 Ruchti C, Balli-Antunes M, Gerber HA: Follicular tumor in the sellar region without primary cancer of the thyroid. Heterotopic carcinoma? Am J Clin Pathol 87:776-780, 1987.

259 Rueda-Pedraza ME, Heifetz SA, Sesterhenn IA, Clark GB: Primary intracranial germ cell tumors in the first two decades of life. Perspect Pediatr Pathol 10:160-207, 1987.

260 Sansone ME, Liwnicz BH, Mandybur TI: Giant pituitary cavernous hemangioma. Case report. J Neurosurg 53:124-126, 1980.

261 Scanarini M, D'Avella D, Rotilio A, Kitromilis N, Mingrino S: Giant cell granulomatous hypophysitis. A distinct clinicopathological entity. J Neurosurg 71:681-686, 1989.

262 Schochet SS, McCormick WF, Halmi NS: Salivary gland rests in the human pituitary. Light and electron microscopical study. Arch Pathol 98:193-200, 1974.

263 Scholtz CL, Siu K: Melanoma of the pituitary. Case report. J Neurosurg 45:101-103, 1976.

264 Scott IA, Stocks AE, Saines N: Hypothalamic/pituitary sarcoidosis. Aust N Z J Med 17:243-245, 1987.

265 Sindou M, Daher A, Vighetto A, Goutelle A: Chondrosarcome parasellaire rapport d'un cas opere par voie pterionotemporale et reuve de la litterature. Neurochirurgie 35:186-190, 1989.

266 Steel TR, Dailey AT, Born D, Berger MS, Mayberg MR: Paragangliomas of the sellar region. Report of two cases. Neurosurgery 32:844-847, 1993.

267 Vesley DL: Hypothalamic sarcoidosis. A new cause of morbid obesity. South Med J 82:758-761, 1989.

268 Viswanathan R, Jegathraman AR, Ganapathy K, Bharati AS, Govindan R: Parasellar chondromyxoid fibroma with ipsilateral total internal carotid artery occlusion. Surg Neurol 28:141-144, 1987.

269 Wilberger JE: Primary intrasellar schwannoma. Case report. Surg Neurol 32:156-158, 1989.

270 Winer JB, Lidov H, Scaravilli F: An ependymoma involving the pituitary fossa. J Neurol Neurosurg Psychiatry 52:1443-1444, 1989.

271 Wolfe JT, Scheithauer BW, Dahlin DC: Giant cell tumor of the sphenoid bone. Review of ten cases. J Neurosurg 20:329-331, 1987.

272 Yamada S, Sawano S, Aiba T, Shishiba Y, Sano T, Takahashi S, Takebe K, Yanagiya S: Idiopathic giant-cell granuloma of the pituitary with unusual clinical and histologic features. Endocrine Pathol 4:169-173, 1993.

30 Eye and ocular adnexa

This chapter will cover primarily those entities that come to the attention of the surgical pathologist; therefore entities seen most often at postmortem examination will be excluded. For a more detailed description of these and other entities, the reader is referred to one of the many specialized textbooks available.[1-14] As with all surgical specimens, a complete description of the lesion and a meaningful clinical history are invaluable. Clinical photographs are especially helpful in ophthalmic pathology.

NORMAL ANATOMY

The *eyelids* are divided into a cutaneous and a conjunctival portion. The former is composed of stratified squamous epithelium and the latter of a much thinner conjunctival epithelium. Skin appendages of eyelids include the sebaceous glands (glands of Zeis and meibomian glands), apocrine glands (glands of Moll), and eccrine sweat glands.

The *lacrimal gland* is largely of serous type, with a minor mucinous component in the ductal portion and a layer of myoepithelial cells in the larger peripheral ducts.

The *orbit* contains, in addition to the ocular globe and the lacrimal gland, the following structures: optic nerve and its meningeal covering, Tenon's capsule, the extraocular muscles, blood vessels, and a delicate framework of fibroadipose connective tissue.

The *conjunctiva* is a thin mucous membrane, which lines the inner surface of the eyelids and most of the anterior surface of the ocular globe. The conjunctival epithelium is composed of two to five layers of columnar cells that rest on a continuous basal lamina. This epithelium contains mucin--secreting goblet cells and melanocytes.

The *cornea* consists of six distinct layers: epithelium, epithelial basal lamina, Bowman's layer (an acellular structure made up of collagen fibers), stroma, Descemet's membrane (a true basal lamina produced by the underlying corneal endothelial cells), and a single layer of very flat cells traditionally known as "endothelium."

The *sclera* is mainly composed of a dense collagenous stroma admixed with occasional elastic fibers and scattered fibroblasts.

The *intraocular tissues* comprise the uveal tract (iris, ciliary body, and choroid), the retina, the crystalline lens, and the various intraocular compartments. A detailed description of these structures is beyond the scope of this book.

EYELIDS

Most of the pathologic processes that involve the eyelids are those that involve the skin in general and are considered in detail in Chapter 4. Some consideration, however, is given in this chapter to those lesions that either are peculiar to the lids or present particular problems in this location.

Developmental anomalies

Dermoid cysts typically involve the upper eyelid along the brow margin and may represent forward extension of a mass primarily intraorbital (Fig. 30-1). These lesions rest on and are often firmly attached to the periosteum of the bony orbital rim. They are soft, nontender, oval or round, and usually about 1 cm in diameter.

Microscopically the cysts are lined by well-differentiated epidermal and dermal tissues containing all of the usual skin appendages (Fig. 30-2). The lumen is filled with keratinous debris, sebum, and hairs. In places where these contents have been extruded into the surrounding tissues, a severe foreign body inflammatory reaction may be observed.

Inflammation

Inflammation of the eyelids may be the result of viral, rickettsial, bacterial, mycotic, or parasitic infections; chemical or physical irritants; hypersensitivity states; or systemic dermatologic disorders. These inflammatory processes are rarely biopsied and are of relatively little practical significance to pathologists.

Pseudorheumatoid nodules (deep granuloma annulare) can involve the eyelid and eyebrow and rarely the episcleral and orbital tissues.[17]

Necrobiotic xanthogranuloma with paraproteinemia is characterized by multiple nodules or plaques that involve

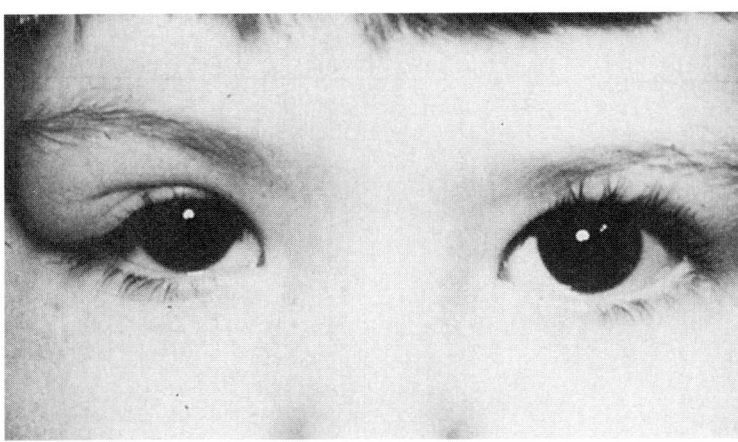

Fig. 30-1 Dermoid cyst of right upper eyelid.

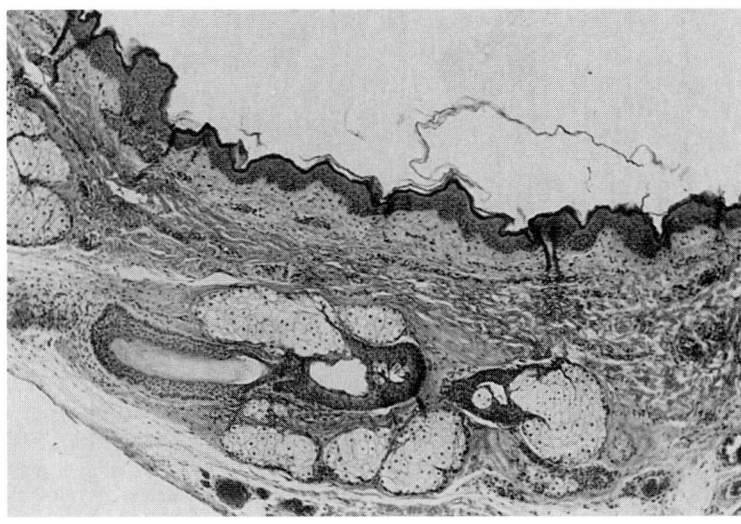

Fig. 30-2 Dermoid cyst of eyelid and brow. Cyst lumen is located in upper right corner.

the periorbital areas (including eyelids) along with other parts of the body. A dysproteinemia caused by an IgG paraprotein is consistently present. Microscopically the granulomas are characterized by collagen "necrobiosis" together with foamy macrophages and Touton giant cells.[15]

Silica granulomas are of noncaseating type and composed of epithelioid cells and multinucleated giant cells and birefringent crystals. They are surrounded by areas of fibrosis.[16]

Chalazion

Chalazion is an extremely common lesion. It represents a lipogranuloma that develops in and about a meibomian gland, presumably as a consequence of the combined effects of obstruction and nonspecific infection of the excretory passages of the gland. The sebaceous material discharged into the tarsus provokes an intense granulomatous inflammatory reaction (Fig. 30-3).

Although chalazion begins as a deep-seated process, not infrequently it erupts through the conjunctival surface of the eyelid. Ordinarily, this lesion is readily recognized and treated, but if, after curettage, one or more recurrences develop, the clinician should be alert to the possibility of a meibomian gland tumor that has previously escaped recognition. In such cases, excision and histopathologic study are indicated.

Microscopically the typical chalazion reveals multiple foci of granulomatous inflammation (Fig. 30-4). In the center of many of the focal granulomas there is a small globule of fat, which in paraffin sections presents as an empty round to ovoid space (Fig. 30-5).

Cysts

Benign cysts of the skin of the eyelids and along the lid margins are relatively common, comprising about one third of lesions removed from the lids. The most common of these are the *keratinous* cysts discussed in Chapter 4. Another relatively frequent lesion is the *cyst of Moll's glands*, often referred to as sudoriferous cyst or simply ductal cyst. These present as thin-walled transparent vesicles at the lid margin. Microscopically they are simple cysts lined by atrophic cuboidal or flattened epithelial cells with an empty lumen (Fig. 30-6).

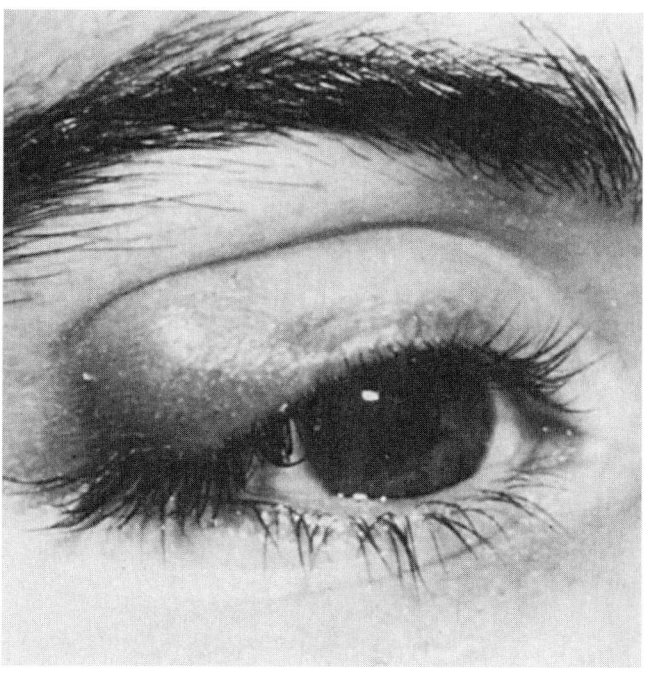

Fig. 30-3 Chalazion of right upper eyelid.

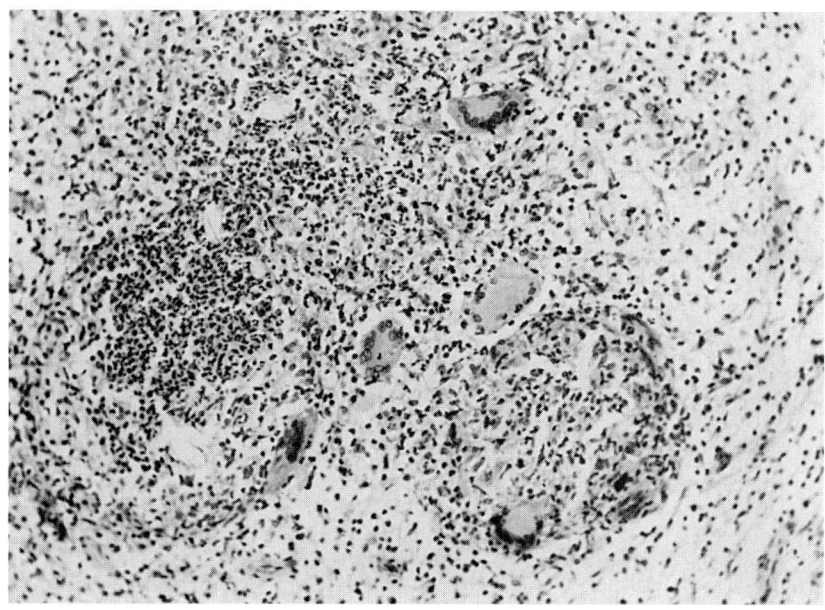

Fig. 30-4 Multiple foci of granulomatous inflammation with microabscesses and Langhans' giant cells in chalazion.

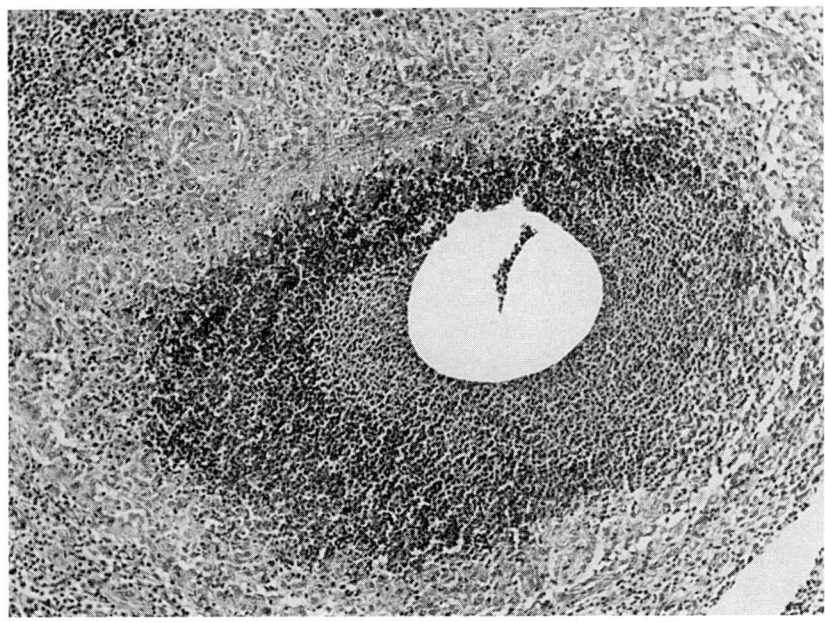

Fig. 30-5 Presence of pools of fat in center of many of granulomas is characteristic of chalazion.

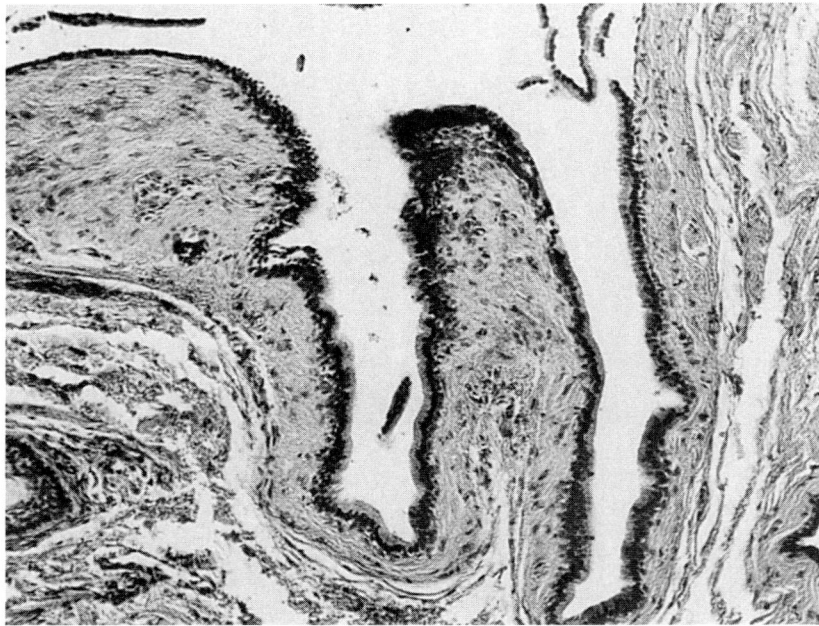

Fig. 30-6 Simple cyst of eyelid margin believed to be secondary to obstruction of duct of Moll's gland (sudoriferous cyst).

Tumors and tumorlike lesions
Tumors and tumorlike lesions of surface epithelium

Basal cell carcinoma is by far the most frequent neoplasm arising in any of the palpebral tissues.[18,19] The overwhelming majority are easily excised without sequelae. On rare occasion, they may invade the orbit, nose, or both, and exenteration of the orbit may become necessary. Microscopic examination of the margins by frozen section at the time of surgery is a useful technique for ensuring that total removal of the tumor has been achieved.[23]

Basal cell carcinomas arise from the cutaneous surface of the eyelids and rarely, if ever, from the conjunctiva. This point is of some diagnostic significance, for a *papilloma* of the palpebral conjunctiva may resemble basal cell carcinoma. When such a lesion is excised and sectioned in such a way that its topographic orientation in relation to the conjunctival surface of the lid is not apparent and if the pathologist is not informed of the clinical appearance of the tumor, an erroneous diagnosis of basal cell carcinoma can result (Fig. 30-7).

Squamous cell carcinoma is cited in most series as responsible for about 10% to 20% of all malignant epithelial tumors of the eyelid. In our experience, it is much less frequent than that, accounting for less than 3% of malignant tumors of the eyelids.[24] A small percentage of these tumors are of the adenoid (pseudoglandular) type.[22]

Merkel cell carcinoma can occur in the eyelid, its morphologic appearance being the same as elsewhere in the skin. Most reported cases have been located in the upper eyelid, where they have presented as large, nontender, red, or violaceous masses.[25]

Non-neoplastic keratotic lesions may resemble squamous cell carcinomas so closely that even experienced clinicians and pathologists have difficulty in differential diagnosis.

The lesions include such entities as papilloma, pseudoepitheliomatous hyperplasia, keratoacanthoma, inverted follicular keratosis, seborrheic keratosis, actinic keratosis, and cutaneous horns.[20,21] The histopathologic features of these lesions are described in Chapter 4.

Adnexal tumors

Sebaceous gland adenomas and adenocarcinomas may arise from the cutaneous sebaceous glands, the glands of Zeis, or the meibomian glands (Fig. 30-8).

Solitary adenomas of the meibomian and Zeis glands are rarely seen in the laboratory, although they may be more common than is generally believed. The meibomian gland tumors, for example, may simulate a chalazion and be removed by curettage. Such curettings are rarely submitted for microscopic examination. Hence, one does not know how often such tumors are missed. In the case of malignant

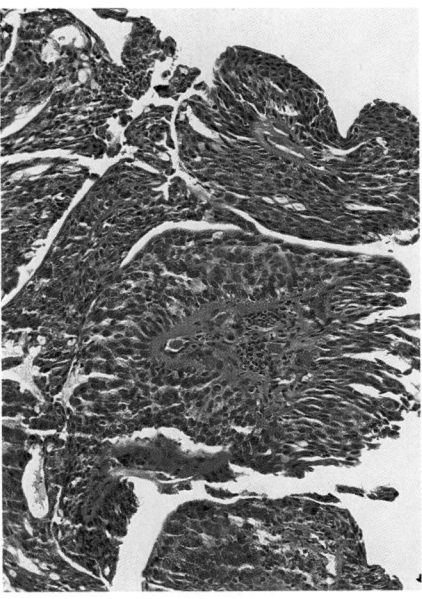

Fig. 30-7 Papilloma of conjunctiva. A papillomatous growth of well-differentiated epithelial cells is supported by a prominent central fibrovascular core.

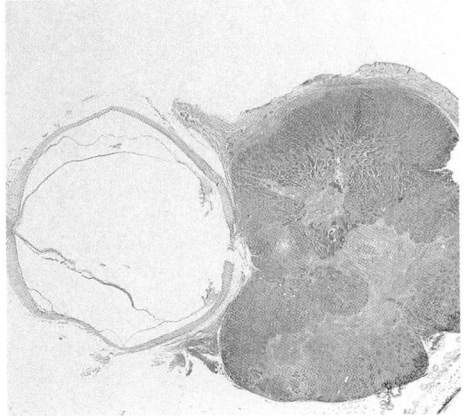

Fig. 30-8 Whole mount of sebaceous gland carcinoma compressing but not infiltrating the ocular globe. The tumor is sharply circumscribed and very cellular and has areas of necrosis.

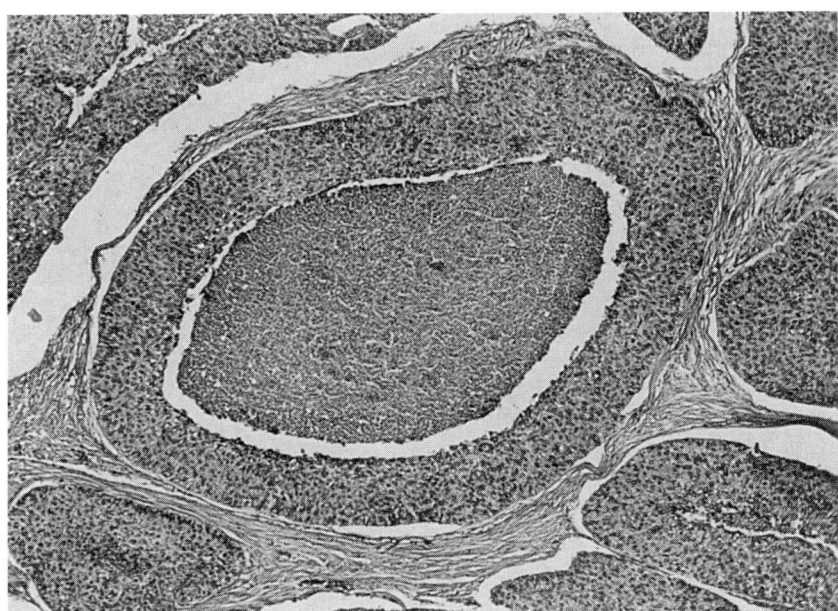

Fig. 30-9 Adenocarcinoma of meibomian gland. Plugs of necrotic tumor fill central portions of duct-like tubular masses of neoplastic tissue.

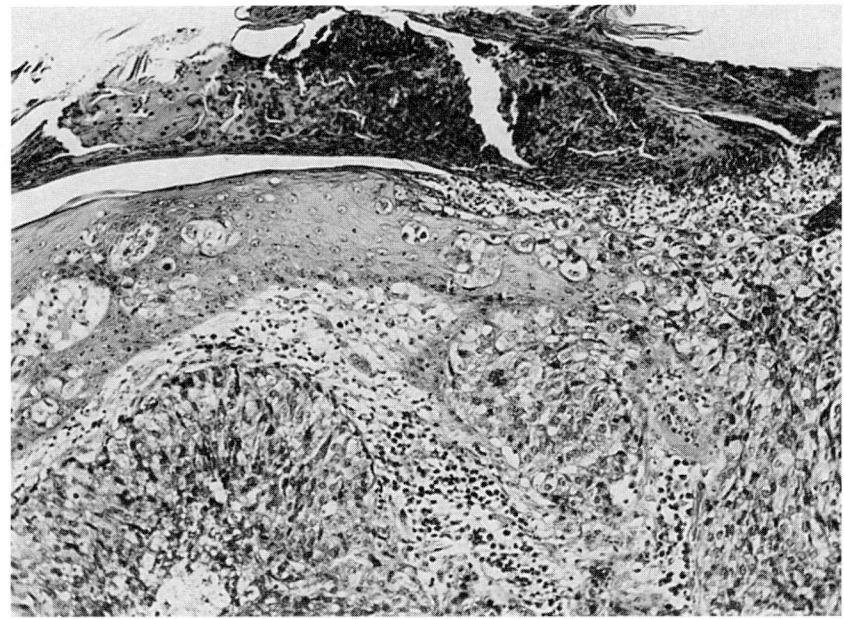

Fig. 30-10 Pagetoid involvement of skin of eyelid in patient with carcinoma of meibomian gland.

tumors, however, recurrence is likely. It is for this reason that recurrent chalazia are often excised and sent to the pathology laboratory. In reviewing the histories of patients with meibomian gland carcinomas, it is impressive that the usual story is one of repeated curettages for chalazia before a neoplasm is suspected and a biopsy obtained.[33]

Malignant meibomian gland tumors show considerable histologic and cytologic variation, merging with adenomas on the one hand and with very anaplastic epithelial tumors of uncertain histogenesis on the other. The former are easily recognized, first by their position within the tarsus and their obvious anatomic relation to the meibomian gland and second by their cytologic characteristics. In such tumors the cells continue to exhibit sebaceous differentiation, which is very dramatically brought out by frozen sections stained for fat. More rapidly growing tumors may be characterized by

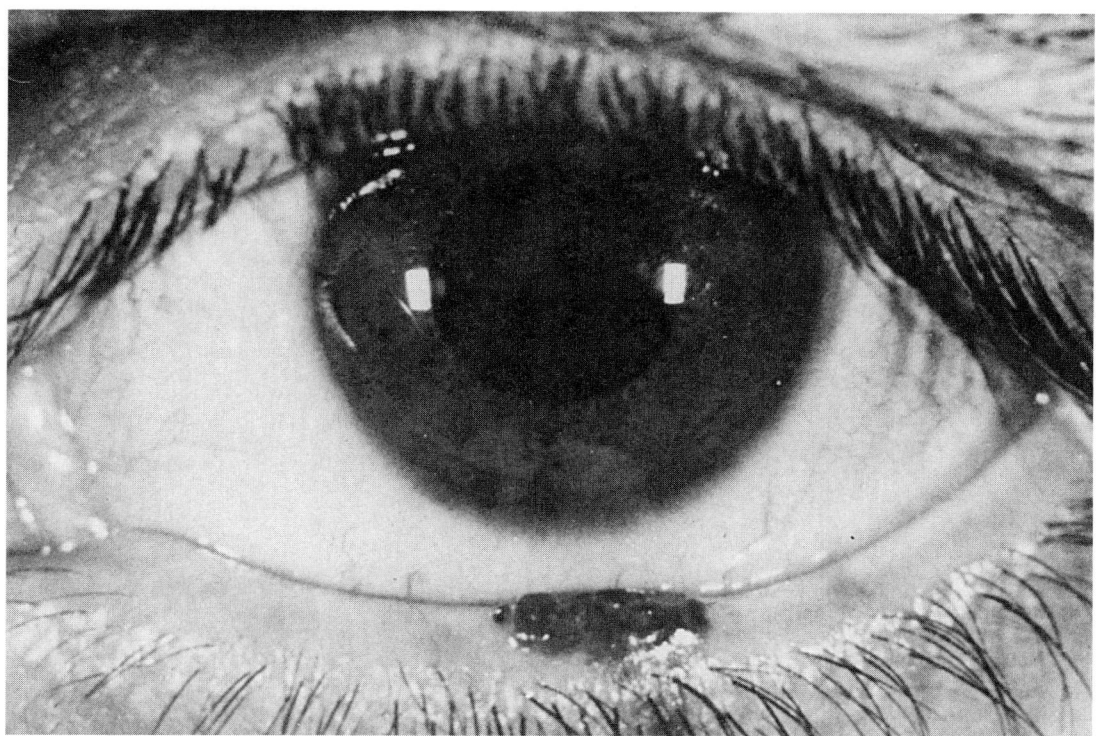

Fig. 30-11 Nevus of margin of lower eyelid.

extensive necrosis of the central areas of neoplastic lobules, giving rise to a comedocarcinoma pattern (Fig. 30-9). Pagetoid involvement of the overlying skin can occur, resulting in a clinical picture of chronic blepharoconjunctivitis[26,31] (Fig. 30-10).

In the series of Rao et al.,[27] 23 out of 104 patients died from metastatic disease, confirming the fact that sebaceous carcinoma is a more aggressive neoplasm when located in the ocular adnexae. Features indicative of a poor prognosis were orbital or vascular invasion, involvement of both eyelids, poor differentiation, multicentric origin, large size, a highly infiltrative pattern, and pagetoid spread.[29]

Trichilemmoma, a benign adnexal tumor believed to originate from the outer hair sheath (trichilemma) and mostly composed of glycogen-rich clear cells, can involve the eyelid and eyebrow[27] (see Chapter 4).

Benign sweat gland tumors of the region include apocrine hidrocystoma[28] and papillary oncocytoma.[30]

Mucinous sweat gland adenocarcinoma of the eyelid is a tumor homologous to the adenocystic carcinoma of the skin seen in other locations[32,34] (see Chapter 4). Local recurrence is common, but distant metastases occurred in only one of the twenty-one cases reported by Wright and Font.[34]

Melanocytic tumors

Melanocytic nevi may be observed in either the cutaneous or the conjunctival surface of the eyelids. The lid margin is a particularly common site (Fig. 30-11). Most are of the junctional or compound type. Like those in other areas, they may give rise to malignant melanoma. Fortunately, this is a very rare event.

A more diffuse and deeply situated melanotic lesion of the lids is the *nevus of Ota* (congenital oculodermal melanosis). This is a form of extrasacral mongolian spot involving the face in areas supplied by the first and second branches of the trigeminal nerve. This type of nevus occurs more frequently in Orientals and blacks than in whites. The latter have an increased incidence of ocular and orbital melanomas.[35]

Melanosis oculi (ocular melanocytosis) is an uncommon congenital anomaly characterized by variable hyperpigmentation of the conjunctiva, episclera, sclera, uveal tract, and occasionally, the optic nerve. It is generally regarded as a variant of nevus of Ota. Patients with this disorder also have an increased incidence of ocular malignant melanoma.[36]

So-called *acquired melanosis* is a disorder that may involve either surface or both surfaces of the eyelid in association with the conjunctiva and is described in the section on conjunctiva (p. 2471).

Malignant melanoma of the eyelid is rare. It may originate from a nevus that has been present for many years, from an acquired melanosis of variable duration, or de novo.

In general, malignant melanomas of the lid carry a grave prognosis, because they tend to metastasize early by the lymphatics and bloodstream. This is in contrast to malignant melanomas of the bulbar conjunctiva (p. 2471) and of the uvea (p. 2489), which have a more favorable prognosis.

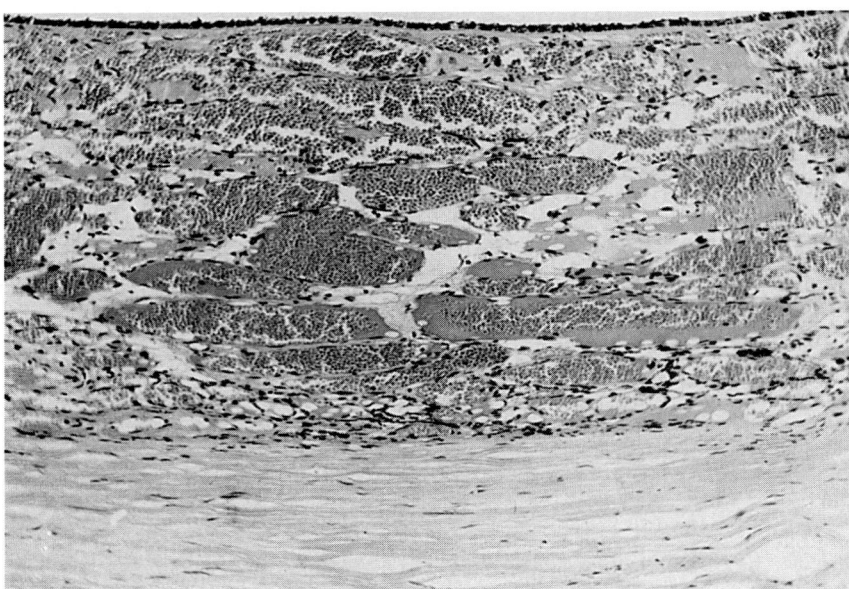

Fig. 30-12 Hemangioma of choroid in eye enucleated from 42-year-old woman who had had a port-wine facial hemangioma since birth and ipsilateral glaucoma since early childhood.

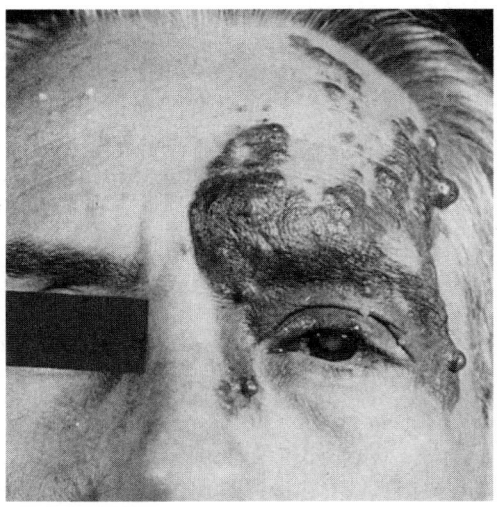

Fig. 30-13 Sturge-Weber syndrome. Patient, 42-year-old man, had had facial hemangioma all his life and was blind in ipsilateral eye because of retinal degeneration, glaucoma, and cataract. Choroidal hemangioma was found in enucleated eye, but clinical study failed to disclose evidence of intracranial lesion. (Courtesy Veterans Administration Hospital, Hines, IL.)

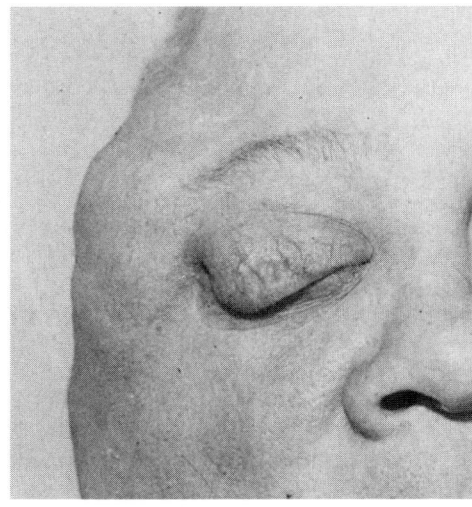

Fig. 30-14 Severe unilateral deformity of face in patient with Recklinghausen's neurofibromatosis. (Courtesy Dr. L.L. Calkins, Kansas City, KS.)

Lymphoid tumors and tumorlike conditions

The morphologic appearances and diagnostic problems presented by these lesions when located in the eyelid are largely similar to those of analogous lesions of the conjunctiva and orbit and are fully discussed on p. 2464. The only difference of note is that the percentage of malignant tumors seems to be higher for lymphoid masses in the eyelid than for those in the other sites.

Eyelid involvement is not an uncommon finding in late cases of *mycosis fungoides*.[37]

Mesenchymal tumors and tumorlike conditions

Angiomas may present as small lesions confined to the eyelid or may extend deep into the orbit. Hemangiomas are more common than lymphangiomas. Their histopathologic characteristics are described in Chapter 4.

The so-called *port-wine stain* (nevus flammeus) is of special interest not only because of its great cosmetic effect, but also because it may be associated with malformations in other tissues (Fig. 30-12). In the *Sturge-Weber syndrome,* the facial hemangioma may be associated with a choroidal hemangioma, glaucoma, and a meningeal hemangioma, all on the ipsilateral side (Fig. 30-13).

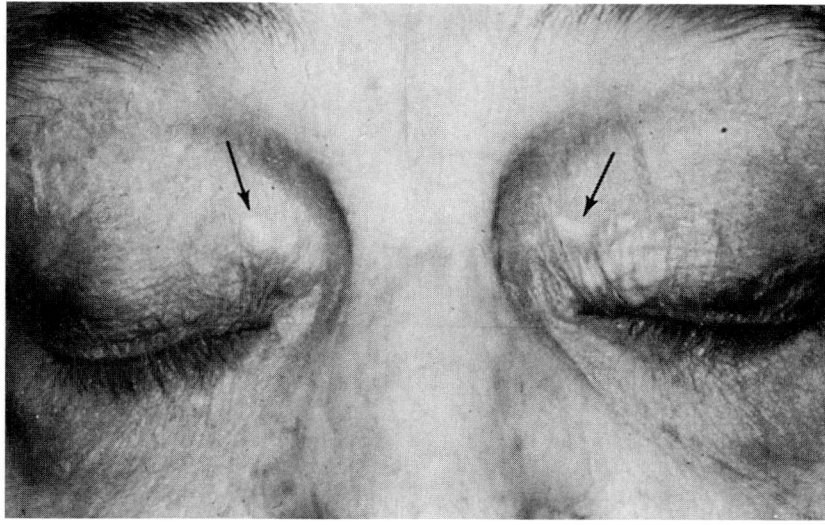

Fig. 30-15 Xanthelasma of upper eyelids in patient who had no other systemic findings.

Masson's hemangioma (intravascular papillary endothelial hyperplasia) can develop in the eyelid, either de novo or engrafted on a pre-existing vascular lesion.[40]

Neurofibromas can present as isolated lesions or as a component of Recklinghausen's disease. Although believed to be present from birth, these tumors frequently show accelerated growth during childhood or later. When associated with Recklinghausen's disease, there may be marked asymmetry of the face caused by diffuse hypertrophy and pendulousness of all of the facial tissues on one side (Fig. 30-14).

Xanthelasmas are slightly elevated yellow plaques located on the medial aspect of the upper and lower eyelids (Fig. 30-15). They are rarely indicative of any serious systemic disturbance and are usually removed for cosmetic reasons. Most of the patients are in the fifth or sixth decade of life. Patients with familial hypercholesterolemia may develop these lesions at a younger age.

Microscopically these lesions show large, pale-staining, fat-laden histiocytes throughout the subepithelial tissues.

Amyloidosis can occur in the eyelid and conjunctiva as a localized mass. It presents as a chronic painless tumefaction usually not associated with any systemic disease.[38,39]

LACRIMAL PASSAGES

Diseases of the lacrimal passages that are of importance to the surgical pathologist are characterized by epiphora (the imperfect drainage of tears so that they flow over the lid margin onto the cheek) and by varying degrees of swelling, induration, and inflammation of the lower eyelid at its nasal end. Although inflammatory obstructions of these passages are common, neoplastic lesions are rare.

Canaliculitis and dacryocystitis

Canaliculitis and dacryocystitis may be the result of direct spread of inflammatory processes in neighboring structures such as the conjunctiva or nose, but more often their pathogenesis is obscure. Acute and chronic types are recognized, and the inflammatory reaction may be suppurative, granulo-matous, or necrotizing, with the formation of fistulous tracts to the skin surface below the eyelid near the base of the nose.

The lacrimal passages become filled with purulent exudate in the acute suppurative types, whereas in the chronic forms the passages are narrowed by the inflammatory thickening of the walls of the lacrimal canal or sac. Frequently there are also hyperplasia of the lining epithelium and hypersecretion of mucus. At times the degree of papillomatous or adenomatous hyperplasia of the sac may give rise to difficulties in differential diagnosis.

Sarcoidosis may involve the lacrimal sac as an extension of upper respiratory tract disease.[41]

Mucocele

Lacrimal mucocele is another complication of chronic inflammation of the lacrimal sac. A low-grade obstructive lesion with a relatively intact and possibly hypersecreting mucosa may lead to great distention of the sac by accumulated secretions.

The contents of the cyst may be clear or milky, fluid or gelatinous, fibrinous or flocculent, sterile or infected. Microscopically the cyst wall reveals varying degrees of atrophy, degeneration, hyperplasia, hypersecretion of the mucosa, and chronic inflammation of the subepithelial tissues.

Dacryolithiasis

Dacryolithiasis and concretions in the lacrimal canaliculus ("tear stones") are of uncertain pathogenesis, but they are generally believed to be the result of low-grade inflammatory processes, including mycoses. If such concretions are crushed and examined microscopically, they will be seen to contain myriad mycelial elements embedded in a relatively acellular matrix. Others, however, are laminated, mineralized stones with recognizable fungous or bacterial forms.

Tumors

Neoplasms of the lacrimal passages are rare. *Papillomas* similar to those arising in the conjunctival surface of the

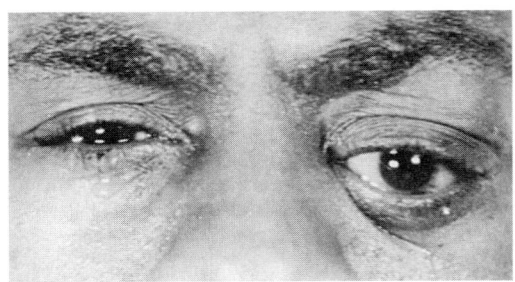

Fig. 30-16 Benign mixed tumor of left lacrimal gland in 38-year-old man. Proptosis was accompanied by severe visual loss. (Courtesy Veterans Administration Hospital, Jefferson Barracks, MO.)

eyelid (p. 2453) may form in the punctum, within the canaliculus, or in the sac. Inflammatory pseudoepitheliomatous hyperplasia, however, is seen more often.

From the clinical point of view, it is usually not possible to distinguish malignant tumors of the lacrimal passages from benign neoplasms and pseudotumors. Dacryocystography has become an important part of the clinical evaluation of lacrimal sac tumors.

Oncocytomas (oxyphil cell adenomas) may occur in the lacrimal sac or in the caruncle. Most of the cases have been seen in elderly women, and local excision has been curative.[42]

All malignant tumors of the lacrimal passages except carcinoma are exceedingly rare, and even carcinoma is distinctly uncommon. These tumors are usually moderately well-differentiated *squamous cell carcinomas,* similar in appearance to those arising from the mucosa of the nose or in the conjunctiva. They tend to form papillary projections into the lumen and spread along natural surfaces, but they also infiltrate directly into adjacent tissues.[45]

Other reported malignancies of the lacrimal sac include *mucoepidermoid carcinoma*[44] and *malignant melanoma.*[43]

LACRIMAL GLAND

Lacrimal gland lesions are divided into nonepithelial and epithelial. The nonepithelial lesions, which make up about 65% of lacrimal gland lesions, include inflammatory pseudotumor, lymphoid hyperplasia, nonspecific dacryoadenitis, Sjögren's syndrome, sarcoidosis, malignant lymphoma, and leukemia. Of the epithelial tumors, benign mixed cell tumor (pleomorphic adenoma) is the most common.

Mikulicz's disease

When chronic dacryoadenitis is associated with enlargement of the parotid or other salivary glands, it has been referred to as *Mikulicz's syndrome.* This may be the result of Mikulicz's disease or a variety of other specific diseases, including sarcoidosis, tuberculosis, syphilis, mumps, Graves' disease, malignant lymphoma, and leukemia.

Mikulicz's disease (benign lymphoepithelial lesion) is the most common cause of Mikulicz's syndrome.[46-48] Microscopically the two essential features are lymphocytic infiltration and formation of "epimyoepithelial islands." The appearance is thus similar to that seen in a more exuberant

form in the salivary glands (see Chapter 12). Sometimes these changes affect only one lacrimal gland, with no salivary gland involvement or systemic manifestations. In fact, this is the type of dacryoadenitis the pathologist sees most frequently.

When Mikulicz's disease is accompanied by failure of lacrimal and conjunctival secretions and consequent keratoconjunctivitis sicca, the term *Sjögren's syndrome* is used. Most of the cases are seen in postmenopausal women.

Tumors

Most neoplasms of the lacrimal gland arise in the orbital lobe where the gland is firmly attached to the orbital rim about the lacrimal fossa. The bone tends to restrict growth in its direction. Hence the enlarging tumor characteristically displaces the eye downward and nasally (Fig. 30-16).

The histopathologic, ultrastructural, and immunohistochemical characteristics of lacrimal gland tumors are similar to those of the salivary glands[52] (see Chapter 12). *Benign mixed tumors* account for about 50% to 60%, *malignant mixed tumors* for 5% to 10%, *adenoid cystic carcinomas* for 20% to 30%, and other carcinomas for 5% to 10%.[49,53,54] Gamel and Font[51] found that adenoid cystic carcinomas with a basaloid pattern of growth had a decidedly worse prognosis than the nonbasaloid type. Because so many of these lacrimal gland tumors have not been completely and adequately removed at the initial operation, there has been an excessively high recurrence rate.[55] It is even more difficult to treat the recurrences, for they are often multiple. The carcinomas have a very poor prognosis.[50,56]

In addition to the epithelial tumors of the lacrimal gland, *malignant lymphomas, lymphoid pseudotumors,* and *chronic inflammatory processes* are important causes of enlargement of the gland. In a patient who is in good general health and who presents no evidence of a systemic disease, the discovery of a lymphoid mass in the lacrimal fossa rarely heralds the development of malignant lymphoma or leukemia. In fact, in the majority of cases there is a polymorphism suggestive of a reactive inflammatory process, although in other cases the rather pure proliferation of lymphocytes makes it quite impossible to rule out a lymphocytic lymphoma or leukemia. The lacrimal glands may, of course, become involved along with other tissues in a leukemia or malignant lymphoma.

ORBIT

The clinical hallmark of disease of the orbit is exophthalmos. This may not necessarily be caused by a true neoplasm, and therefore the surgical pathologist may never see any specimen from many patients who present with this finding. For example, the most common cause for exophthalmos is dysthyroid ophthalmopathy, and rarely is a biopsy taken in these cases.

As for the relative frequency of lesions that cause exophthalmos, many of the statistics that have been reported merely reflect the bias of the specialist involved. For example, to the radiologist one of the most common orbital lesions producing displacement of the eye is a mucocele arising from a paranasal sinus. The ophthalmologist, however, would place mucocele far below such entities as dysthyroid ophthalmopathy, hemangioma, and inflammatory pseudotumor.[58] Procedures useful for the diagnostic evaluation of orbital masses include CT scan, MRI, and fine-needle aspiration.[57,59]

Dysthyroid ophthalmopathy

The most common cause of orbital disease and of exophthalmos is dysthyroid ophthalmopathy in which there is some dysfunction of the pituitary-thyroid axis.[60] When seen with ocular problems, the patient may be hyperthyroid, hypothyroid, or euthyroid. Often there is a history of hyperthyroidism or some form of treatment.

Unilateral orbital involvement occurs with sufficient frequency in both forms of dysthyroid ophthalmopathy to warrant this condition always being considered in the differential diagnosis of orbital tumors (Fig. 30-17).

Histopathologic changes observed in severe cases, which are most likely to come to the attention of surgical pathologists, include widespread edema and chronic inflammation of all the orbital tissues. The most striking gross alterations are observed in the extraocular muscles, which may be massively enlarged (see Fig. 30-17). Muscle fibers degenerate and become hyalinized. A great increase in the interstitial connective tissue, including both cellular elements and ground substance, is observed particularly in the muscles but also in the other orbital tissues.

Inflammatory processes

The orbit may become secondarily inflamed by lesions arising in the face, eyes, nose, sinuses, orbital bones, blood vessels, brain, and meninges.[67] Generally, it is only when such inflammations simulate neoplasms that orbital exploration is undertaken and tissue is obtained for histopathologic diagnosis.

Specific granulomas, including those of tuberculosis, mycosis, and sarcoidosis, are rare.

Mucocele is the result of chronic inflammatory disease of the frontal or ethmoid sinuses. The lesion erodes through the wall of the sinus to produce an inferolateral displacement of the globe. The onset is usually insidious, and the enlargement is symptomless and slow (Fig. 30-18).

Histopathologically, this cystic mass is lined by mucus-secreting sinus mucosa with variable degrees of inflammation and scarring.

Inflammatory pseudotumors of the orbit are much more frequent than the specific infectious granulomas. Undoubtedly these pseudotumors represent an etiologically and pathogenetically heterogeneous group.[61] In some instances, they have been found associated with involvement of paranasal sinuses.[62] In others, they have been the orbital manifestation of sinus histiocytosis with massive lymphadenopathy (SHML, Rosai-Dorfman's disease).[63] Still others represent the orbital manifestation of inflammatory fibrosclerosis (idiopathic sclerosing inflammation), a process that may also involve the retroperitoneum, mediastinum, extrahepatic bile ducts, and thyroid.[68] The pathologic features they share include the following:

1 The formation of an indurated orbital mass often surrounding the optic nerve and incorporating one or more of the extraocular muscles (Fig. 30-19)

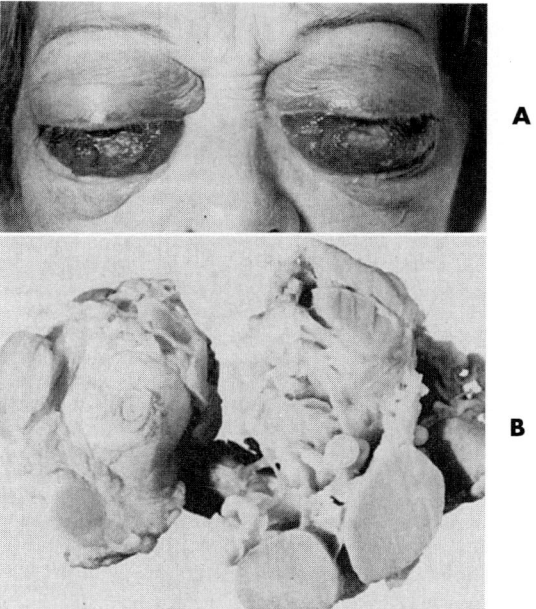

Fig. 30-17 A, Malignant exophthalmos of about 10-month duration in 65-year-old woman who finally died of congestive heart failure. **B,** At autopsy, extraocular muscles were found to be massively thickened.

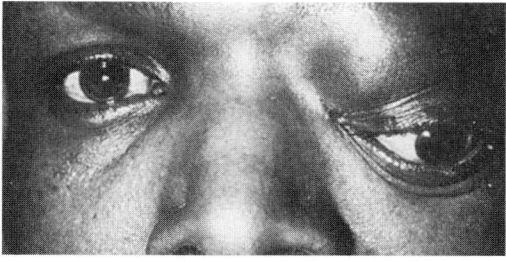

Fig. 30-18 Mucocele producing downward and lateral displacement of left eye. (From del Regato JA, Spjut HJ: Ackerman and del Regato's cancer, ed. 6. St. Louis, 1985, Mosby.)

2 A tissue reaction that includes exudation of fluid, excessive production of ground substance, mobilization of chronic inflammatory cells, vascular proliferation, and hyperplasia of connective tissue (Fig. 30-20)

3 The absence of demonstrable etiologic agents or of otherwise diagnostic histopathologic alterations indicative of specific disease entities such as Hodgkin's disease, temporal arteritis, or lupus erythematosus[66]

This is not to say, however, that the microscopic features are uniform from case to case. In some instances the proliferation of blood vessels and ground substance resembles that of exuberant granulation tissue.[65] At times, there is lymphoid hyperplasia with follicle formation (p. 2464). Other cases with prominent involvement of extraocular muscles suggest the possibility of dysthyroid ophthalmopathy. In cases that are caused by SHML the infiltrate is composed of

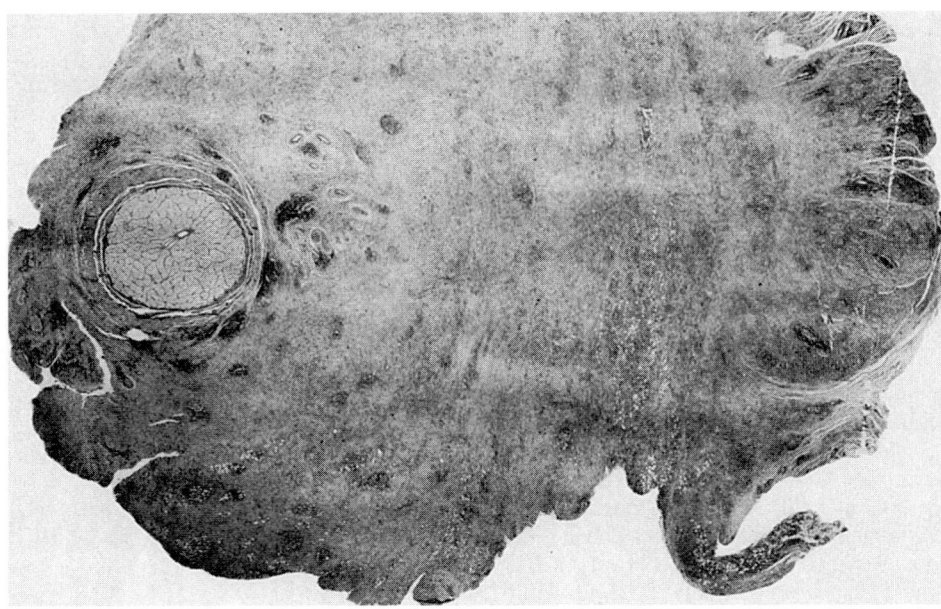

Fig. 30-19 Inflammatory pseudotumor of orbit. Optic nerve and other orbital tissues are "frozen" in dense mass of nonspecific chronic inflammatory tissue.

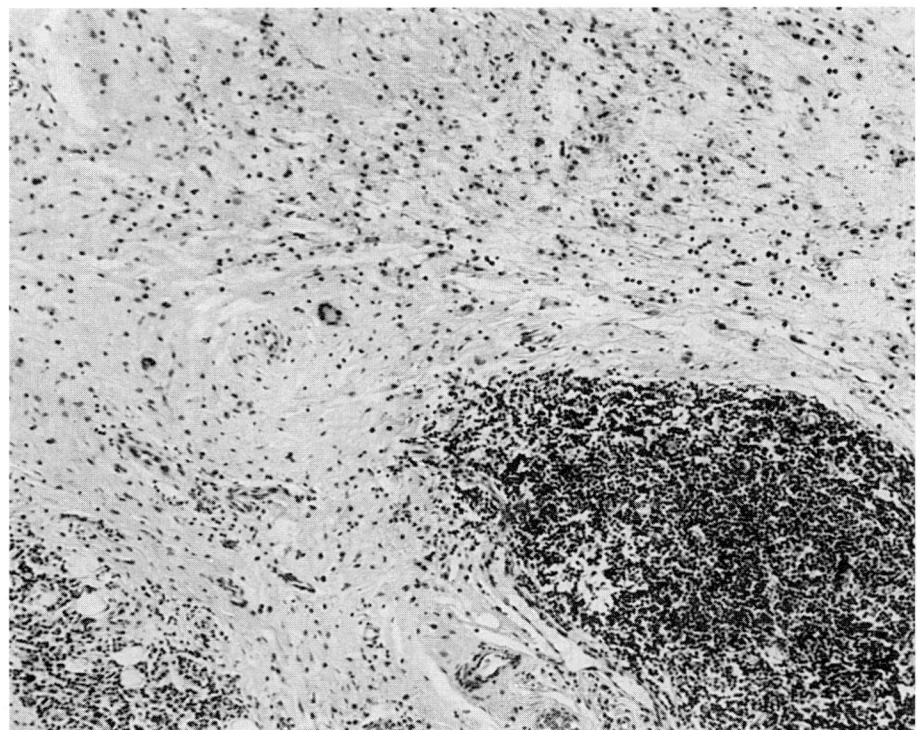

Fig. 30-20 Inflammatory pseudotumor of orbit showing infiltration by chronic inflammatory cells, giant cells, and generalized fibrosis.

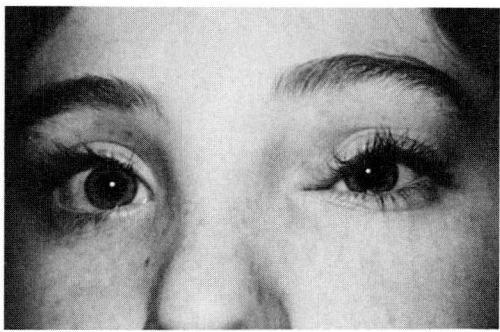

Fig. 30-21 Rhabdomyosarcoma presenting as palpable mass in upper medial quadrant of left orbit with only minimal downward and lateral displacement of eye. (From Smith ME: The differential diagnosis of unilateral exophthalmos. In Gay AJ, Burde RM, eds: Clinical concepts in neuro-ophthalmology. International Ophthalmology Clinics, vol 7, no 4, Boston, 1967, Little, Brown & Co.)

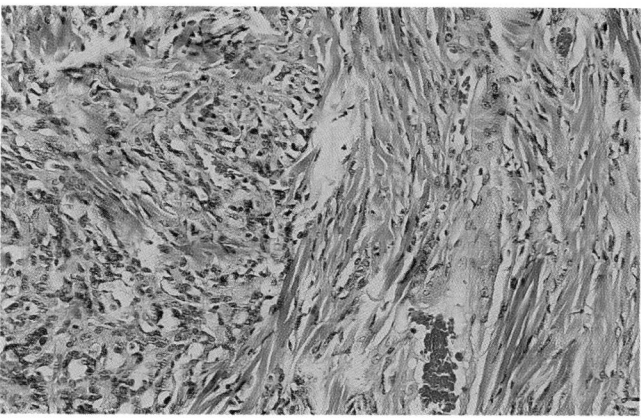

Fig. 30-22 Solitary fibrous tumor of orbit. The alternation of hypercellular and hypocellular areas is characteristic. The collagen has a keloid-type quality. This tumor was strongly immunoreactive for CD34.

large histiocytes (some exhibiting lymphocytophagocytosis), lymphocytes, and plasma cells; fibrosis can be very prominent.[63] Other types of inflammatory pseudotumors are composed of cholesterol granulomas or accumulation of keratin ("epidermoid cholesteatomas").[69]

A well-developed granulomatous reaction about small pools of fat is observed in certain cases. Such lesions may suggest traumatic fat necrosis. Others containing large numbers of cholesterol clefts and many foamy macrophages and giant cells suggest an area of old suppuration or hemorrhage. Periphlebitis is prominent in certain cases, and some of these may present a significant eosinophilia, suggesting the possibility of a hypersensitivity angiitis.

Patients with pseudotumors are usually in the third to fifth decade and in good health. The exophthalmos is of relatively sudden onset and in at least one half of the patients is associated with moderate to severe orbital pain and with lid and conjunctival edema. Diplopia is often present secondary to limitation of ocular motility in one or more fields of gaze, but visual acuity is usually unimpaired. Intracranial extension can occur.[64]

The lesion often can be palpated through the eyelids; if so, the surgeon may be able to reach it easily for a biopsy. Deeper lesions are not so readily accessible for biopsy, and if the clinical signs and symptoms are characteristic for inflammatory pseudotumor, steroids are often given without a biopsy, especially since systemic steroids often produce dramatic alleviation of signs and symptoms. The CT scan can be helpful in localizing the lesion.

Primary tumors

Mesenchymal tumors and tumorlike conditions

Rhabdomyosarcoma is the most common soft tissue sarcoma of the orbit in childhood[80] (Fig. 30-21). The types seen in this age group are embryonal and alveolar, the latter being associated with a more aggressive clinical course.

Fibrous histiocytoma is the most common primary mesenchymal orbital tumor in adults.[72] The upper and nasal portions of the orbit are the most common sites. Font and Hidayat[72] divided their cases into benign, locally aggressive, and malignant; the 10-year survival rate was 100%, 92%, and 23%, respectively.

Hemangiopericytoma is another mesenchymal tumor seen with a relatively high frequency in the orbit.[77] In the series of Croxatto and Font,[70] the recurrence rate was 30%, and the metastatic rate was 15%. The metastases usually developed late in the course of the disease.

Solitary fibrous tumor having an appearance identical to that of the homonymous pleural lesion can occur in the orbit (Fig. 30-22). Immunohistochemically, it is characterized by a strong and widespread reactivity for vimentin and CD34.[71,84] It is likely that cases previously diagnosed as hemangiopericytoma would be reclassified today as solitary fibrous tumor. A close histogenetic relationship seems to exist between these two neoplasms.

Alveolar soft-part sarcoma can present as a primary orbital tumor.[73] The age of occurrence, microscopic appearance, and evolution are similar to those seen in the other location of this tumor (see Chapter 25). The clinical course is indolent, distant metastases sometimes occurring 10 years or more after initial therapy.[73]

Osteosarcoma has been reported most often as a late complication of radiation therapy to the area.[76]

Other malignant mesenchymal tumors, all extremely rare, include **leiomyosarcoma,**[86] **fibrosarcoma,**[83] **mesenchymal chondrosarcoma,**[79] **angiosarcoma,**[78] and **Ewing's sarcoma/ PNET.**[85]

Angiomas are relatively common orbital tumors, with hemangiomas occurring much more commonly than lymphangiomas.[87]

In the infant, these soft, blue, compressible tumors are diffuse throughout the orbit and often extend forward into

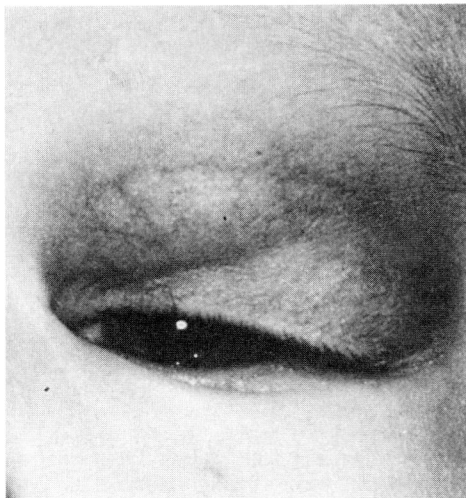

Fig. 30-23 Capillary hemangioma of left orbit and eyelid.

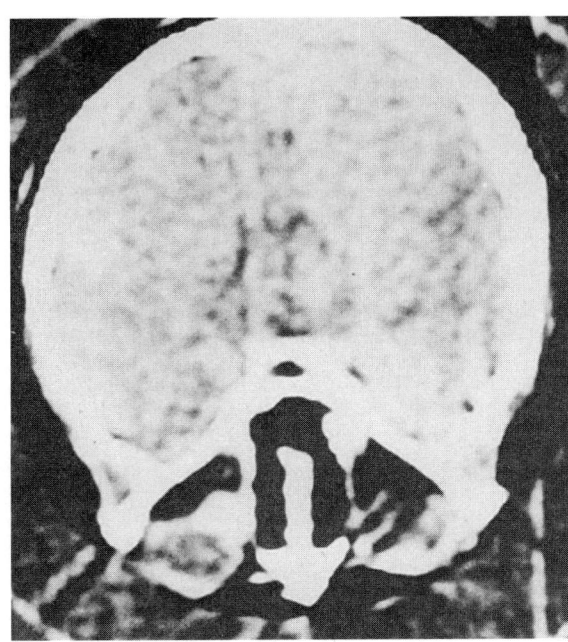

Fig. 30-24 CT scan showing hemangioma of right orbit.

the eyelids (Fig. 30-23). Surgical removal is difficult; fortunately, however, most of these lesions spontaneously regress by 4 years of age. If the tumor is so large that the visual axis of the eye is covered and the eye is at risk for the development of deprivation amblyopia, such lesions can often be reduced in size following a short course of systemic steroids or small doses of radiotherapy.

In the adult, these tumors are usually encapsulated, are situated close to the back of the eye, and can be surgically "shelled" out. The CT scan reveals a discrete round mass that is enhanced by contrast dye (Fig. 30-24).

These tumors rarely present difficulties in histopathologic diagnosis, for they are not significantly dissimilar from angiomas elsewhere. In the infant the lesion is usually of capillary type and in the adult of cavernous type.

Schwannoma and *neurofibroma* represent a small percentage of orbital tumors. Almost all orbital schwannomas are benign, well-encapsulated tumors, which can be completely removed surgically by orbitotomy.[82] Orbital neurofibromas are usually but not always an expression of Recklinghausen's disease.[81] There may be a gross deformity of the orbit and eyelid (see Fig. 30-14) and, on palpation, the lid has been referred to as "a bag of worms."

Other benign mesenchymal tumors that have been observed at this site are *lipoma, chondroma,* and *osteoma*.

Tumorlike proliferations also occur within the orbit, including *nodular fasciitis*[75] and *Masson's hemangioma* (intravascular papillary endothelial hyperplasia).[74]

Langerhans' cell granulomatosis (histiocytosis X) can involve the orbit and result in prominent exophthalmos.

Glioma of optic nerve

Gliomas of the optic nerve are relatively rare, slow-growing tumors that usually arise within the orbital segment of the nerve.

Considerable cytologic variation exists among the gliomas, not only from case to case but also in different portions of a given tumor. Varying degrees of cellularity are observed, but generally these neoplasms are characterized by a low order of anaplasia. This is especially true about the margins of the tumor, where it is often impossible to be certain where reactive gliosis ends and neoplasia begins. Typically there are areas of intense mucinous degeneration within the tumor. Frequently in such areas the tumor cells appear to be virtually lost in the abundant hyaluronidase-sensitive mucoid accumulations.

Small tumors limited to the optic nerve can be adequately managed by resection alone; for the more extensive lesions, biopsy followed by definitive irradiation is recommended.[89,91]

As these gliomas increase in size, they tend to form a bulbous enlargement of the nerve (Fig. 30-25). They also extend along the nerve peripherally toward the eye and centrally toward the brain. In so doing, they often produce great enlargement of the optic canal, an important diagnostic sign for the radiologist. In such cases the optic nerve fibers are likely to be completely destroyed, and the optic disc typically presents the ophthalmoscopic characteristics of primary optic atrophy.

Another growth pattern exhibited by a majority of optic nerve gliomas is infiltration through the pia. This leads to great thickening of the arachnoid (Fig. 30-26). This is partly the result of more exuberant growth of the tumor cells once they have reached the arachnoid, but equally important is the reactive proliferation of arachnoidal cells. At times, this has created difficulties in differential diagnosis between glioma and meningioma.

Microscopically, almost all optic gliomas are low-grade pilocytic astrocytomas, similar to those occurring in the

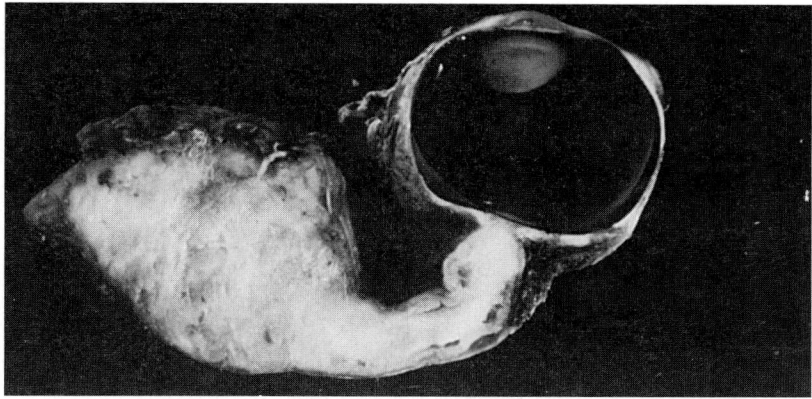

Fig. 30-25 Glioma that has produced massive enlargement of orbital segment of optic nerve. Tumor has completely effaced characteristic architectural features of nerve and its meninges.

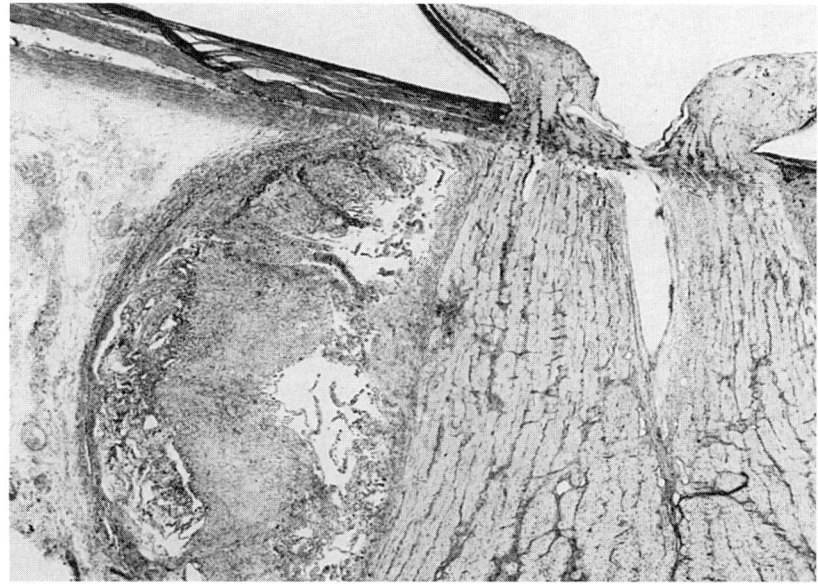

Fig. 30-26 Section through optic nerve just anterior to main mass of this glioma reveals minimal alteration of parenchyma of nerve but greatly thickened meninges. Combination of infiltrating tumor and arachnoidal proliferation is responsible for this meningeal thickening.

cerebellum and in the region of the third ventricle.[88,90] Rarely, malignant tumors characterized by dense cellularity, high mitotic index, marked pleomorphism, necrosis, and vascular proliferation are encountered.[90]

Gliomas of the optic nerve typically make their presence known during the first decade of life with minimal exophthalmos, optic nerve atrophy, or papilledema and with a characteristic thickening of the nerve on CT scan. There is a distinct association of these tumors and Recklinghausen's disease. The majority of optic nerve gliomas are so slow growing that surgical intervention is seldom warranted.

Meningioma

Meningiomas of the orbit arising from the meninges of the optic nerve (Fig. 30-27) are felt to be more aggressive tumors than the meningiomas of the sphenoidal ridge.[92] However, some authors feel that they need not be operated on unless severe proptosis or proof of posterior extension occurs.

Those tumors arising from the orbital meninges generally produce some visual loss, optic atrophy, and exophthalmos. Those arising from the inner portion of the sphenoidal ridge produce more severe compression of the optic nerve within the optic canal, resulting in papilledema or optic atrophy before proptosis. The CT scan has facilitated the diagnosis and localization of these tumors (Fig. 30-28). Microscopically, most orbital meningiomas are of the meningothelial variety. The differential diagnosis includes exuberant arachnoidal hyperplasia, fibrous histiocytoma, hemangiopericytoma, and metastatic carcinoma.[93]

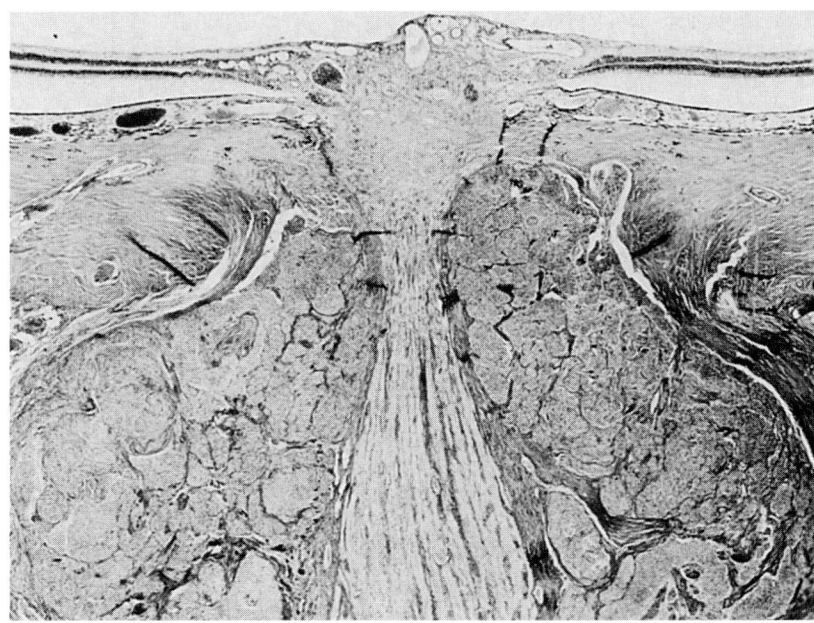

Fig. 30-27 Meningioma of optic nerve Meninges are greatly thickened, and optic nerve reveals severe compression atrophy.

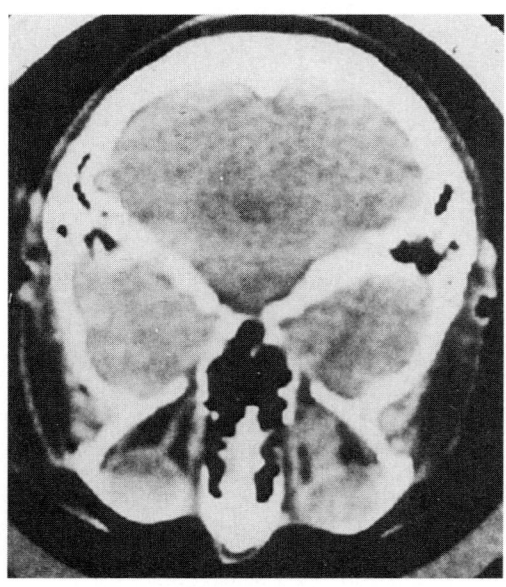

Fig. 30-28 CT scan showing perioptic meningioma of left orbit.

Lymphoid tumors and tumorlike conditions

Lymphoid lesions of the orbit and other ocular sites may present great difficulties in histopathologic diagnoses. Some of these lesions develop in the course of a previously recognized malignant lymphoma or leukemia.[108] Others present initially in the orbit, but thorough clinical and laboratory examination reveals the presence of systemic involvement.[95,101] Still others, perhaps the majority, show involvement of the orbit, conjunctiva, or eyelid not accompanied by any clinical or hematologic evidence of systemic disease.[107]

Microscopically the latter lesions fall into three groups:
1. Those lesions that are quite obviously of malignant nature, usually non-Hodgkin's lymphomas.[109]
2. Those lesions that are fairly obvious examples of reactive hyperplasia. There are considerable polymorphism, a variety of cell types, vascular proliferation, and prominent follicles with germinal centers.
3. Those lesions that are characterized by a rather uniform and monotonous but widespread proliferation of lymphocytes (small lymphocytic proliferations), frequently associated with involvement of orbital fat, blood vessels, and nerves (Figs. 30-29 to 30-31). It is this group that presents the most difficult problems in differential diagnosis.[94,98,105] Some of these lesions are accompanied by plasmacytoid differentiation, Dutcher bodies, and an associated serum paraproteinemia.[96]

Most studies that have been carried out with the third group of lesions have shown that it is very difficult to predict which of them will develop into systemic lymphomas, whether one evaluates them by standard morphologic criteria, by cell marker analysis, or by gene rearrangement techniques.[97,99,106,110] Other studies have shown a better correlation between immunohistochemical features and outcome,[103,104] but perhaps the most important conclusion of all these studies is that the majority of patients with small lymphocytic proliferations localized to the ocular tissues enjoy a relatively benign clinical course and long survival with only minimal therapeutic intervention whether they are of polyclonal or monoclonal nature.[99,102] Some interesting clinicopathologic correlations have also emerged from these studies: Lymphoid infiltrates of the conjunctiva are associated with a lower incidence of extraocular lymphoma (20%) than those of the orbit (35%) or eyelid (67%); and small lymphocytic and intermediate lymphocytic lymphomas are

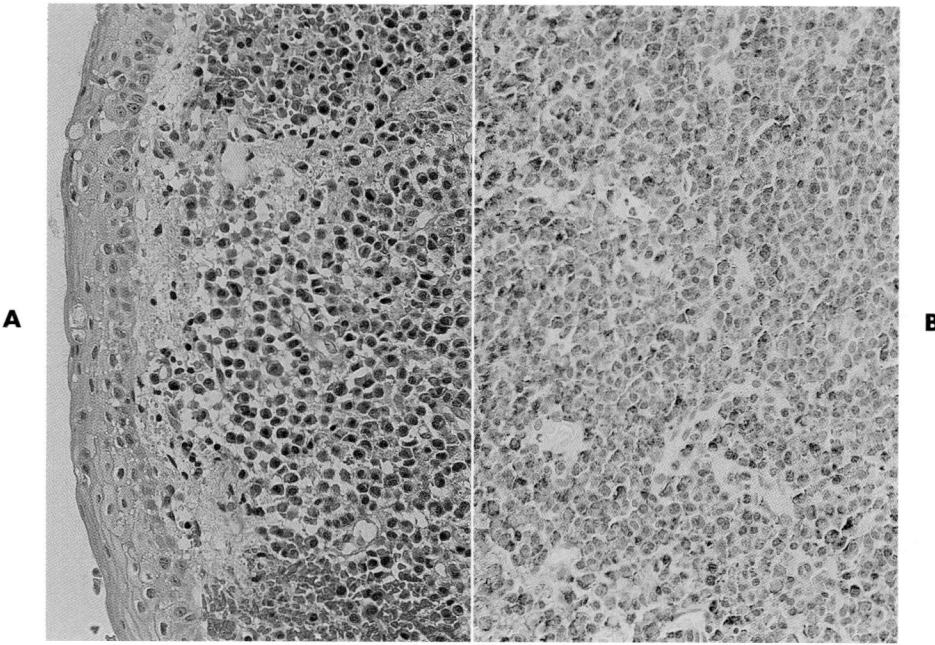

Fig. 30-29 **A** and **B,** Malignant lymphoid proliferation of conjunctiva composed of small tumor cells with prominent plasmacytoid features. **B** shows strong immunoreactivity for kappa light chain.

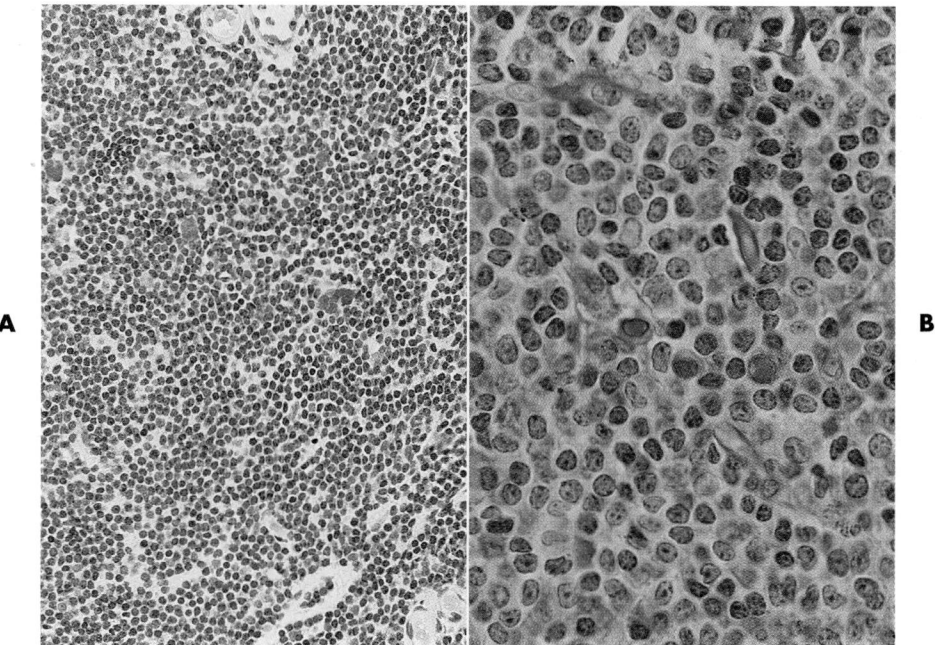

Fig. 30-30 Small lymphocytic proliferation of orbit. **A,** Low-power appearance showing monotonous infiltrate of small lymphoid cells. **B,** PAS stain on another case, showing PAS-positive intranuclear inclusions composed of inspissated immunoglobulin (Dutcher body). The occurrence of these formations is strong evidence in favor of a neoplastic nature for the proliferation.

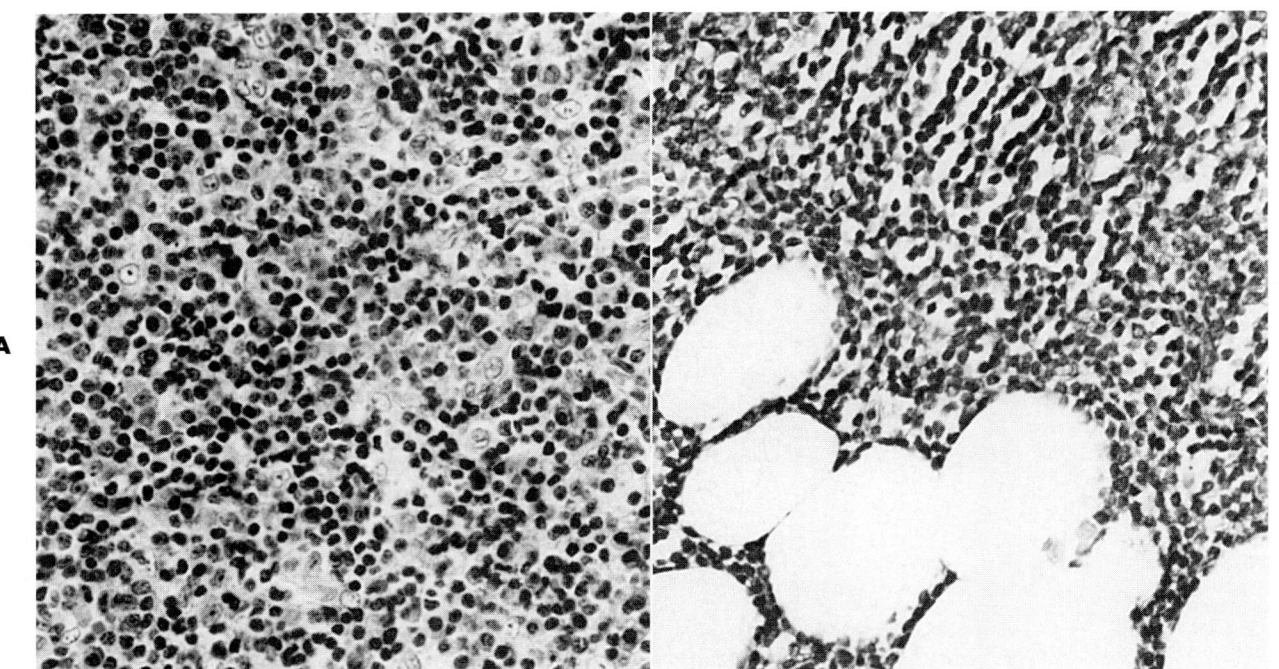

A   B

Fig. 30-31 Small lymphocytic infiltrations of orbit. **A,** Predominantly small lymphocytic proliferation accompanied by occasional histiocytes. This infiltrate was found to be polyclonal on immunohistochemical evaluation, but patient developed similar lesion in breast 1 year later. **B,** Small lymphocytic proliferation infiltrating adipose tissue of orbit. Infiltrate has very monomorphic appearance, but patient remains alive and well 4 years later.

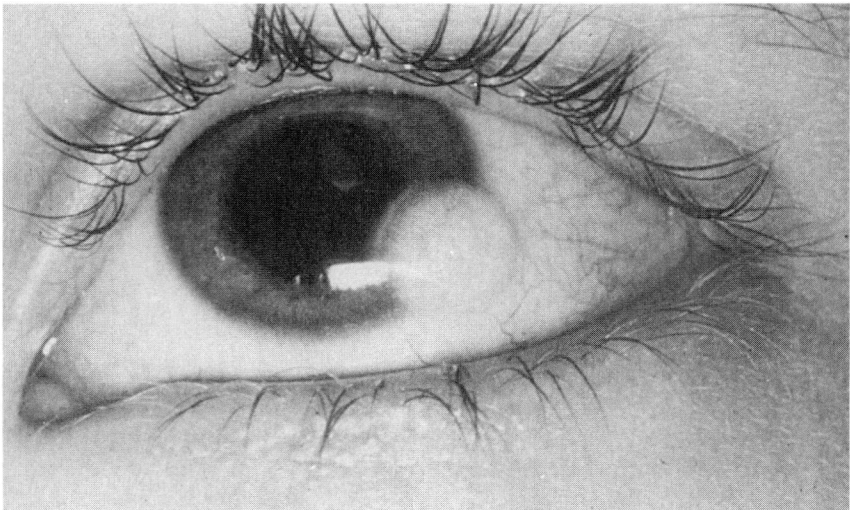

Fig. 30-32 Limbal dermoid in child.

less often associated with extraocular lymphoma (27%) than lymphomas of all other histologic types (46%).[100] The most important prognostic factor is the extent of the disease at the time of presentation.[100] It has been postulated that most conjunctival lymphomas of small lymphocytic type belong to the MALT type, and that this fact is responsible for their generally favorable prognosis.[111]

Metastatic tumors

Direct spread from adjacent structures can occur with primary intraocular tumors such as retinoblastoma or uveal malignant melanomas. Carcinomas of the paranasal sinuses may also fail to produce diagnostic symptoms until orbital extension has occurred.

Hematogenous metastases to the orbit may be seen, on occasion, with many different tumors, but rarely are these initial manifestations of a carcinoma. Even neuroblastoma, which has a notorious reputation for orbital metastases, rarely does so before other diagnostic signs appear.

Most important in this regard is the distinct possibility that a primary embryonal rhabdomyosarcoma might be misinterpreted as a metastatic tumor. Another important possibility to be considered when an undifferentiated "round cell sarcoma" is found in a child's orbital tissues is acute leukemia. Such orbital lesions may make their appearance before peripheral blood studies are diagnostic, but bone marrow aspirates will usually furnish a conclusive answer. In the case of adults an orbital metastasis may, on rare occasions, be the initial manifestation of carcinoma of the breast, bronchus, kidney, or prostate[112]; the latter can be identified by immunoperoxidase techniques.[113]

Carcinoid tumors of the lung or small bowel can also metastasize to the orbit or ocular globe; occasionally an orbital carcinoid tumor is found in the absence of any other disease, suggesting the possibility that it may be primary at this site.[114,115]

CONJUNCTIVA

Lesions of the conjunctiva are thin and tend to fold into distorted patterns when placed into fixative. To prepare the tissue so that the pathologist can orient it properly, the surgeon should spread the lesion onto a small piece of filter paper and allow it to dry for a few seconds before gently placing the filter paper with the adherent specimen into the jar of fixation. Specimens should never be put onto sponges of any kind since these will expand when placed into the fixative, thus distorting the specimen.

Developmental anomalies

Dermoid tumors of the bulbar conjunctiva are firm, localized, elevated opaque masses that typically occur at the limbus, often encroaching on the cornea (Fig. 30-32). These are solid choristomatous masses, not to be confused with dermoid cysts of the orbit.

Over the lesion, the surface epithelium and the subepithelial connective tissue present the histologic features characteristic of epidermis and dermis, respectively. Typically a few hairs project from the tumor. The bulk of the mass is composed of thick bundles of collagen. In some lesions, skin appendages are few, and adipose tissue is abundant. These are known as *dermolipomas,* and they are usually situated in the upper outer fornix. Ocular dermoids may be part of *Goldenhar's syndrome* in which there are extra-auricular appendages and vertebral abnormalities.

Cysts

Benign epithelial-lined inclusion cysts of the conjunctiva usually arise after accidental or surgical trauma or, rarely, de novo.

Degeneration

Pinguecula is a very common degenerative process affecting primarily the subepithelial connective tissues of the bulbar conjunctiva in the interpalpebral region. This gives rise to an elevated yellowish lesion over which the epithelium may become atrophic or thickened. Since these lesions are not progressive, they are seldom excised.

Histologically the most characteristic feature is actinic elastosis affecting a band-like zone beneath the epithelium. Secondary hyalinization and calcareous degeneration also may be observed. Typically the epithelium over pingueculae becomes atrophic, but at times it becomes so acanthotic and dyskeratotic that the erroneous diagnosis of carcinoma may be made.

Pterygium extends into the cornea and is therefore a more important lesion than the pinguecula (Fig. 30-33). Microscopically there is usually some actinic elastosis but also a variable amount of acute and chronic inflammation and congestion of blood vessels.

A morphologically somewhat similar lesion of the conjunctiva has been interpreted as the ocular equivalent of *elastofibroma*.[116]

Graft-versus-host disease

The major histopathologic changes seen in the eyes of patients undergoing bone marrow transplantation involve the conjunctiva, cornea, choroid, and lacrimal gland. The major change in the cornea is keratinization, as appreciated in biopsy specimens.[117]

Inflammation

Inflammatory lesions of the conjunctiva do not often give rise to the type of diagnostic or therapeutic problem that requires excision and histopathologic study. One lesion that deserves mention is the noncaseating granulomatous inflammation found in about one fourth of patients with ***sarcoidosis***[118] (Fig. 30-34). ***Ligneous conjunctivitis*** is a peculiar form of chronic pseudomembranous conjunctivitis that presents as a woody induration of the eyelids plus the formation of a pseudomembrane on the tarsal conjunctiva. The cardinal feature histologically is the presence of large hyaline masses that may simulate amyloid.[119,120]

Inclusion conjunctivitis is seen in adults as an acute or chronic infection. It is produced by *Chlamydia,* and it shows the microscopic appearance of follicular conjunctivitis indistinguishable from viral infection. The diagnosis is based on the finding of so-called Halberstaedter-Prowazek inclusions on conjunctival scrapings.[123]

Actinic granuloma can develop in the conjunctiva, its microscopic appearance being equivalent to that of its more common cutaneous counterpart.[122]

Sjögren's syndrome manifests itself in the conjunctiva by metaplasia of the epithelium, associated with a decreased number of goblet cells and a polymorphic inflammatory infiltrate in the stroma.[121]

Tumors and tumorlike conditions
Tumors of surface epithelium

Papillomas are relatively common lesions of the conjunctiva with a tendency for recurrence after apparent complete excision. In children the papillomas are often multiple. The lesions have a typical papillomatous or "mulberry" surface appearance with small vessels coming up to the surface (Fig. 30-35).

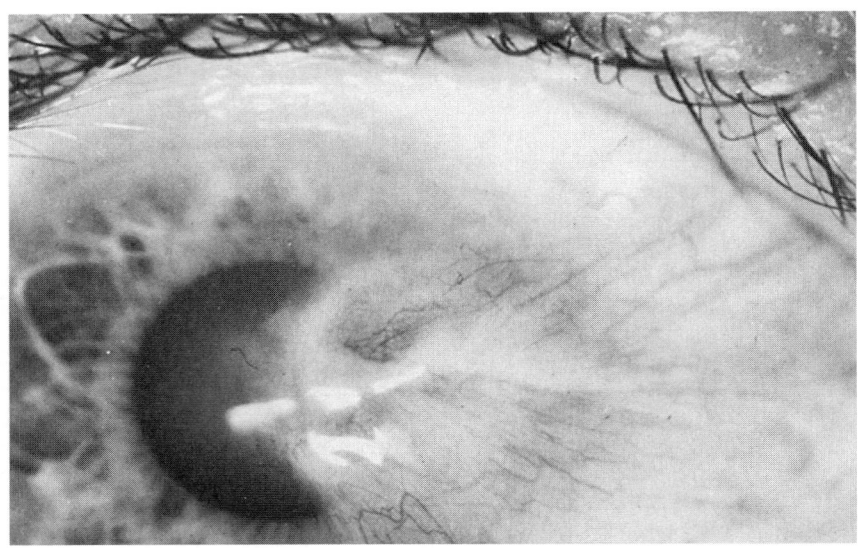

Fig. 30-33 Pterygium that has grown over pupillary axis and has interfered with vision.

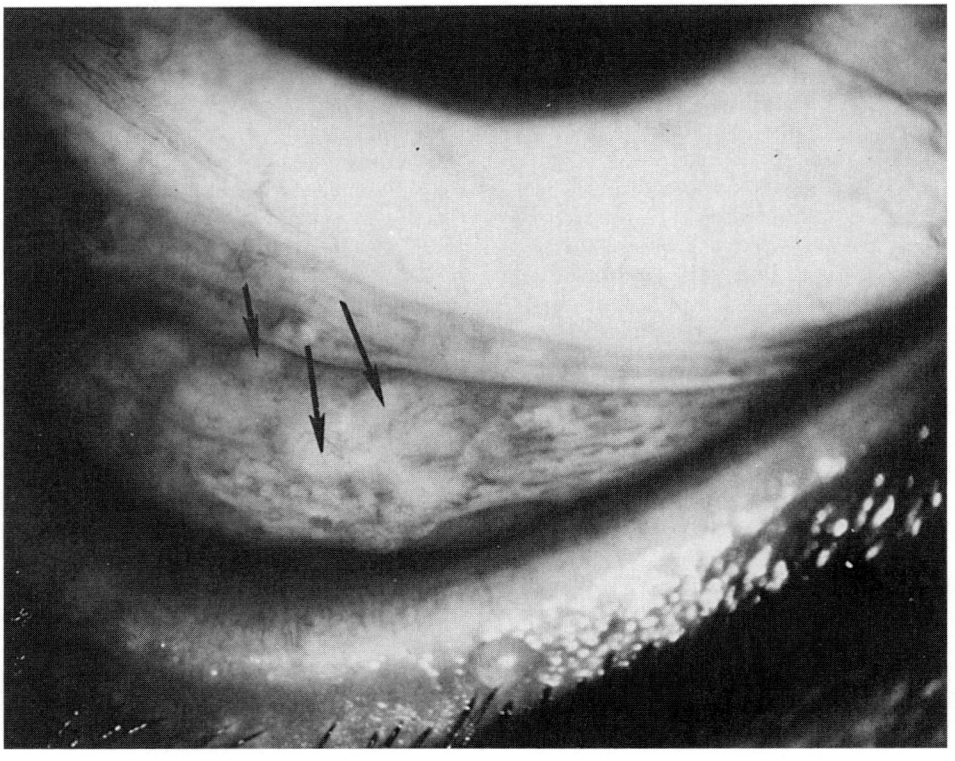

Fig. 30-34 Conjunctival granulomas in sarcoidosis.

Microscopically the typical papilloma reveals pronounced acanthosis and varying degrees of keratinization, koilocytosis, and nonspecific inflammation (see Fig. 30-7). Human papillomavirus type 6/11 has been found in these lesions by in situ hybridization techniques.[128]

Carcinoma in situ of the bulbar conjunctiva varies considerably in its clinical appearance. It may present as an area of leukoplakia, as a papilloma, or as a complication of pterygium or pinguecula (Fig. 30-36).

The histopathologic characteristics of carcinoma in situ of the conjunctiva and cornea are similar to those observed elsewhere in the mucous membranes (Fig. 30-37), or the lesion may mimic Bowen's disease of the skin.[126]

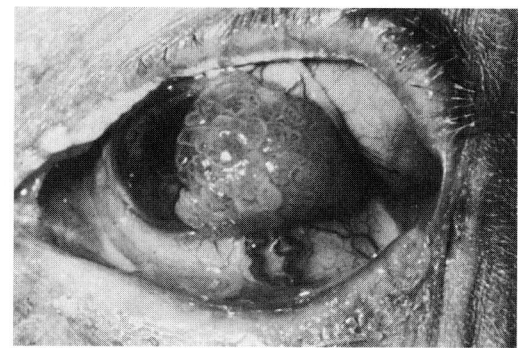

Fig. 30-35 Extensive papilloma of bulbar conjunctiva.

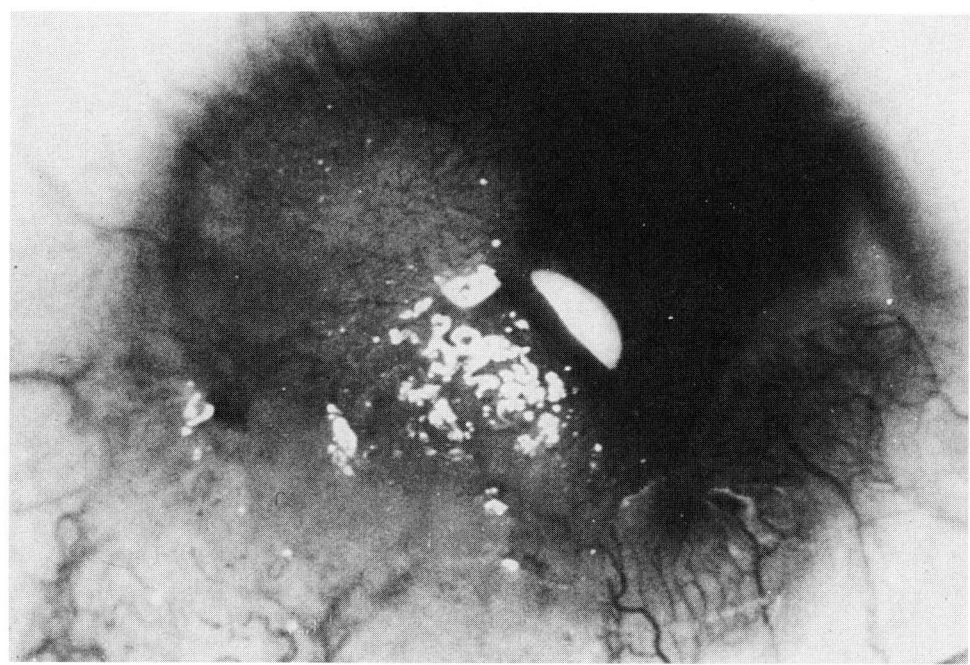

Fig. 30-36 Carcinoma in situ of conjunctiva and cornea.

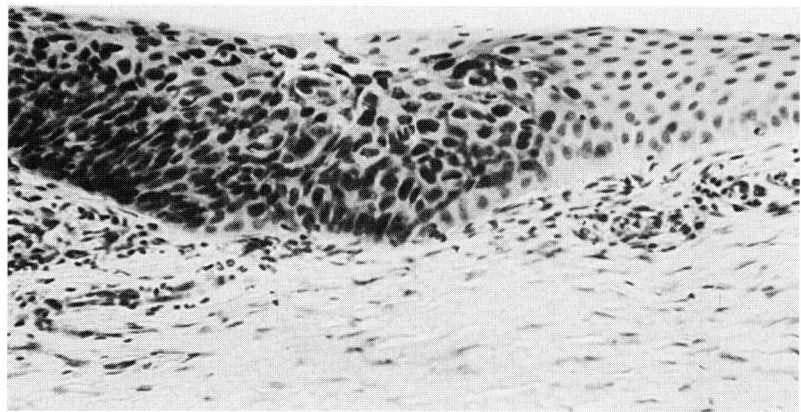

Fig. 30-37 Carcinoma in situ in which there is abrupt transition from essentially normal conjunctival epithelium to intraepithelial neoplasm.

There are many lesions removed from the conjunctiva that do not fall clearly into either of the categories of papilloma or carcinoma in situ. They are often not quite so benign as to be called papilloma, yet there are not enough changes to warrant a classification of carcinoma in situ. These are referred to as *dysplasia* of the conjunctiva; the suggestion has been made of placing these lesions within a spectrum of *conjunctival (or corneal) intraepithelial neoplasia*.[130] The dysplastic lesions have been found to contain HPV type 16 in a substantial number of cases.[127]

Invasive squamous cell carcinoma of the conjunctiva is rare but is still more common than basal cell carcinoma at this site.[124] Clinically, carcinomas of the conjunctiva with significant infiltration (Fig. 30-38) are seldom observed in the United States, probably because it is a common practice

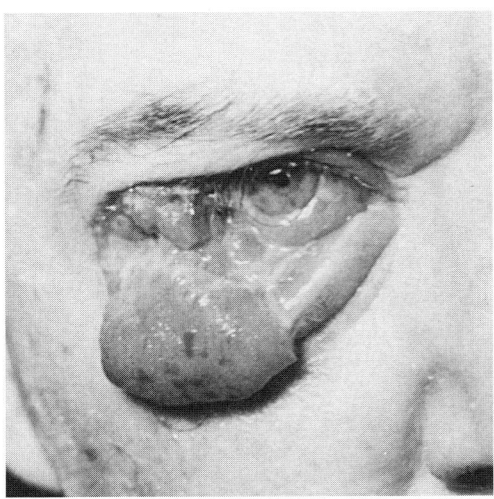

Fig. 30-38 Squamous cell carcinoma of conjunctiva. Tumor grew rapidly over 4-month period.

to excise early "precancerous" or "in situ cancerous" lesions long before this stage occurs. Such lesions, as well as the majority of early invasive carcinomas of the limbal area, can be adequately controlled by excisional therapy. If untreated, these tumors will invade the anterior chamber and other portions of the ocular globe. A high proportion of the deeply invasive conjunctival carcinomas have *adenosquamous* ("mucoepidermoid") features.[125,129] Radical surgery is necessary in these cases[126] (Fig. 30-39).

Melanocytic tumors and tumorlike conditions

Nevi. Nevi of the bulbar conjunctiva, like those of the skin, may be observed from birth, or they may become noticeable at any time during childhood, adolescence, or later.[140] At times a nevus known to have been present since infancy appears to become much larger and more pigmented at puberty (Fig. 30-40).

Characteristically, conjunctival nevi are discrete, flat, or slightly elevated lesions located on the globe in the interpalpebral zone near the limbus, but they vary greatly in size, shape, and position. They also exhibit much variation in degree of pigmentation, about one third being essentially amelanotic.

Microscopically, conjunctival nevi are almost always of the junctional (Fig. 30-41) or compound variety. Counterparts of the common dermal nevus of the skin are rarely observed. A few of the conjunctival nevi are of the epithelioid or spindle-cell type.[138] Frequently, there are numerous solid and cystic inclusions of conjunctival epithelium intimately incorporated into the subepithelial component of these nevi. At times the epithelial inclusions may so dominate the clinical and histopathologic picture that the nevoid nature of the lesion is overlooked (Fig. 30-42). The presence of the epithelial inclusions is supportive evidence for benignity, since they are rare in melanomas.

Malignant melanoma. Malignant melanoma of the conjunctiva, a very rare lesion, may arise without an apparent pre-

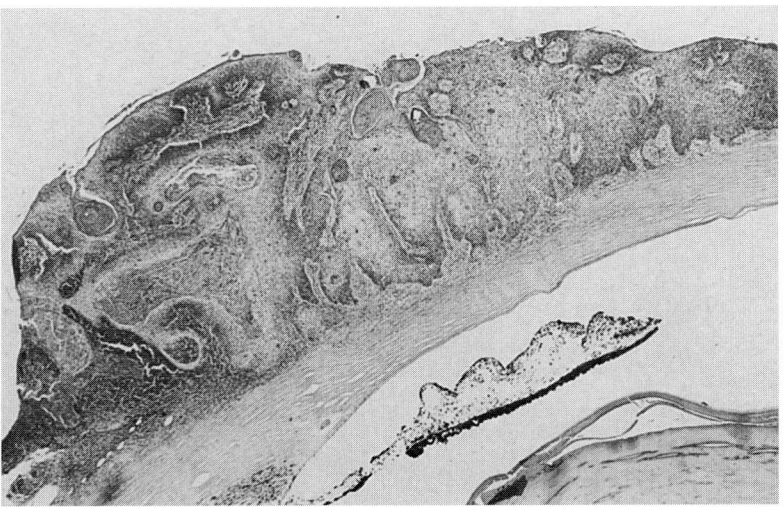

Fig. 30-39 Carcinoma of limbus. Exophytic growth pattern with formation of papillomatous mass is typical of more advanced limbal carcinomas. Even in such large tumors, corneoscleral stroma tends to prevent neoplasm from invading intraocular tissues.

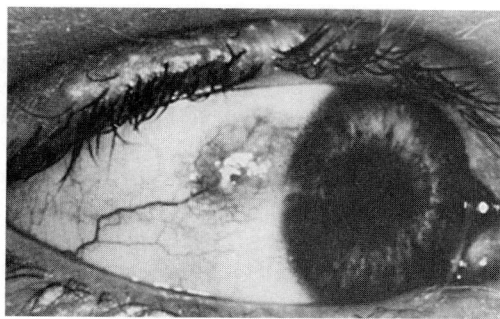

Fig. 30-40 Pigmented lesion at limbus that proved to be benign nevus. (From Regato JA, Spjut HJ: Ackerman and del Regato's Cancer, ed. 5. St. Louis, 1977, Mosby; courtesy Registry of Ophthalmic Pathology, Armed Forces Institute of Pathology, Washington, DC).

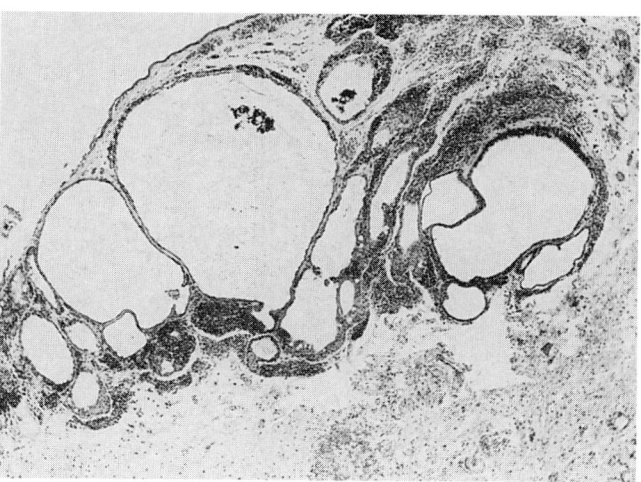

Fig. 30-42 Conjunctival nervus with many associated cystic epithelial inclusions. Small round cells about large cysts are not inflammatory cells but nevus cells. This epibulbar lesion may be analogous to hair dermal nevus of skin.

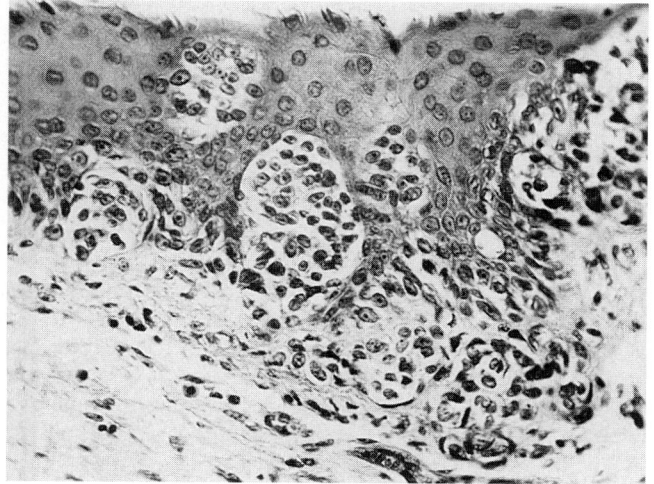

Fig. 30-41 Junctional nevus of bulbar conjunctiva.

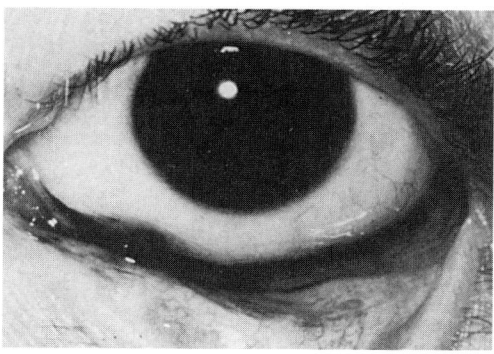

Fig. 30-43 Malignant melanoma of conjunctiva in lower cul-de-sac arising from lesion of acquired melanosis. (From Zimmerman LE: Discussion of pigmented tumors of the conjunctiva. In Boniuk M, ed: Ocular and adnexal tumors. St. Louis, 1964, Mosby; courtesy Registry of Ophthalmic Pathology, Armed Forces Institute of Pathology, Washington, DC.)

cursor lesion, or it may be the sequela of a nevus or of so-called acquired melanosis (see later discussions)[139-141] (Figs. 30-43 and 30-44). The microscopic appearance is similar to that of its cutaneous counterpart. The prognosis is closely related to the subsite and size of the primary tumor. Small localized bulbar tumors have an excellent prognosis, diffuse bulbar melanomas have an intermediate prognosis, and melanomas of the fornix and caruncle have a poor prognosis.[140] Metastatic spread is very uncommon with melanomas less than 1.5 cm in maximum thickness. In the series of 131 cases reported by Folberg et al.[135] the overall mortality was 26%; no prognostic differences were found among the melanomas arising de novo, those with an accompanying nevus, and those associated with so-called acquired melanosis.

The treatment varies from local excision to exenteration of the eye, depending on the extent of the disease.

So-called acquired melanosis. Acquired melanosis is the term most commonly used among ophthalmologists and ophthalmic pathologists for a melanocytic proliferative lesion of the conjunctiva that has also been referred to as pri-

mary acquired melanosis, precancerous melanosis, atypical melanocytic hyperplasia, and malignant melanoma in situ.[131,133,143] Most cases are seen in the fifth decade of life or later, and the typical presentation is that of a diffuse nonelevated granular pigmentation of the conjunctiva. The most common site of involvement is the bulbar conjunctiva, but it can also be present in the cornea, palpebral conjunctiva, or skin of the eyelid. The extent of the lesion and the degree of pigmentation may fluctuate during the course of the years.

Microscopically an increase in the number of melanocytes is seen along the basal layer, individually or in clusters, associated with various degrees of atypicality[136] (Fig. 30-45).

The nature and significance of this lesion have been controversial. Considerations that have been made are similar to

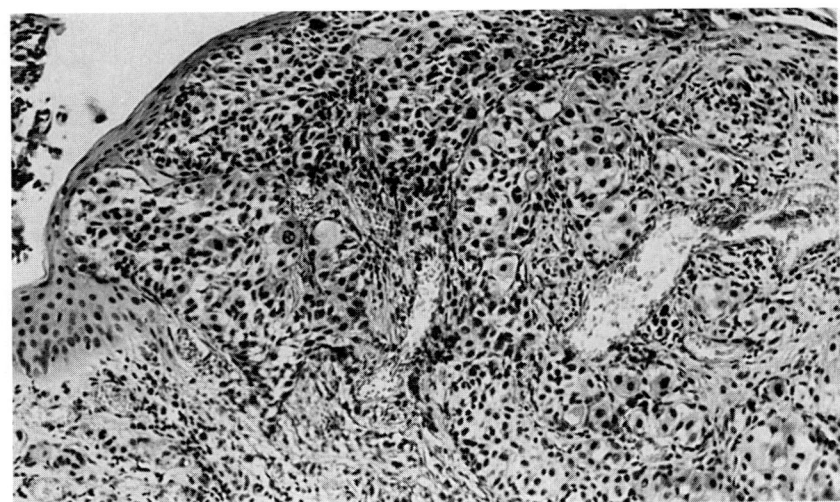

Fig. 30-44 Malignant melanoma arising in nevus known to have been present since childhood. Patient, 59-year-old woman, stated that lesion suddenly became quite large several months before it was excised.

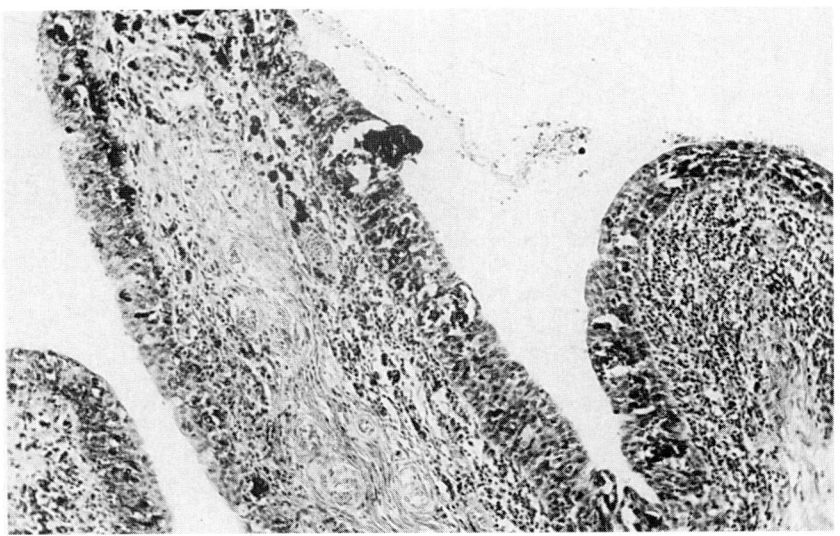

Fig. 30-45 Widespread acquired melanosis of conjunctiva.

those expressed for other acquired melanocytic proliferations of the skin, notably Hutchinson's freckle. Specifically it has been postulated that all cases of acquired melanosis (at least those exhibiting atypia) are malignant melanomas in situ.[131] Guillén and co-workers[137,142] have divided these conjunctival lesions into three groups: (1) conjunctival hypermelanosis (with or without melanocytic hyperplasia but lacking atypia), (2) atypical melanocytic hyperplasia, and (3) malignant melanoma. We believe that the latter term should be reserved for the rare intraepithelial lesions in which the cytoarchitectural features are clearly indicative of a malignant process, fully realizing the subjective nature of this evaluation. From a practical standpoint, the important fact to remember is that the propensity for the development of invasive melanoma is directly related to the presence and degree of atypia.[134,136] In the series of Folberg et al.,[136] none of the lesions without atypia progressed to invasive melanoma, whereas 40% of those with atypia did. Accordingly, the recommendation has been made to extirpate by excision or cryotherapy all of these lesions.[132,136]

Lymphoid tumors and tumorlike conditions

The morphologic appearances and diagnostic problems posed by these lesions when they present in the conjunctiva are similar to those of analogous lesions of the eyelid and orbit and are discussed on p. 2464. The clinical appearance of the conjunctival lesions is that of salmon-colored, smooth masses[144] (Fig. 30-46).

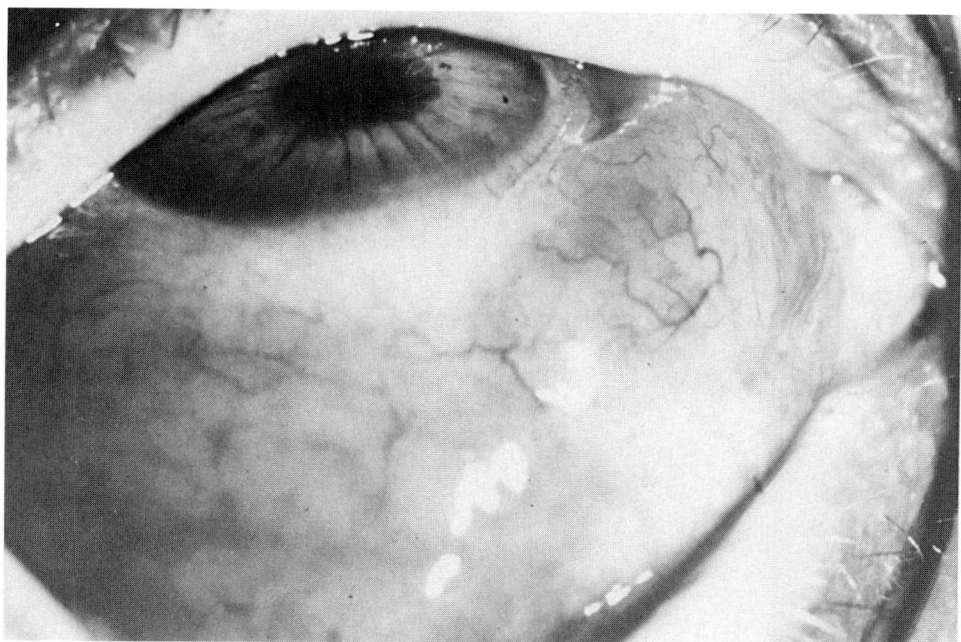

Fig. 30-46 Lymphoid infiltration of conjunctiva.

Other tumors

Myxoma has been reported as a primary tumor in the conjunctiva, cornea, eyelid, and orbit. Grossly, the conjunctival lesions have a smooth, fleshy, gelatinous appearance. Local excision is curative.[147]

Intravenous pyogenic granuloma has been observed in the region of the canthus and in the lacrimal sac.[148]

Vascular tumors of various types can also involve the conjunctiva. They include hemangioma, Kaposi's sarcoma,[146] and angiosarcoma.[145]

CORNEA

A major source of knowledge about corneal pathology comes from the study of corneal "buttons" submitted to the laboratory after corneal transplantation (keratoplasty). The most common diseases that account for keratoplasties are primary and secondary endothelial decompensation, fibrosis and vascularization (such as herpes simplex keratitis), keratoconus, and failed previous grafts.

Other entities for which keratoplasties are sometimes done include interstitial keratitis and the various hereditary dystrophies.

Endothelial decompensation

When the endothelium of the cornea decompensates, it leads to chronic edema of the stroma and epithelium. Bullae of the epithelium break down, causing severe pain, and eventually there is diffuse scarring with reduced vision. When the process is primary (i.e., with no apparent antecedent factors), it is referred to as *Fuchs' dystrophy* and occurs most frequently in females past 50 years of age. It is a bilateral process, although often asymmetric.

When the endothelial decompensation occurs some time after intraocular surgery, especially after cataract extraction, it is often clinically referred to as *aphakic bullous keratopathy.* The clinical appearance and the histopathologic appearance of these buttons are similar in both situations.

Microscopically there are a paucity of endothelial cells, a thickening of Descemet's membrane, and the formation of excrescences of Descemet's membrane, clinically referred to as guttata (Fig. 30-47). If the process has been severe, changes in the epithelium occur, including edema of the basal cells, bullae formation, and pannus formation. A pannus is a fibrovascular ingrowth between the epithelium and Bowman's membrane.[149]

Fibrosis and vascularization

Many buttons from keratoplasty procedures will show a diffuse, nonspecific fibrosis and vascularization throughout the corneal stroma. Such a histopathologic picture can be seen with traumatic scars, chemical burns, or healed ulcerative keratitis secondary to infections. One particular infection that is common is *herpes simplex keratitis* in which the histopathology is characterized by irregularity of the epithelium, patchy loss of Bowman's membrane, infiltration of the anterior stroma by lymphocytes and plasma cells, and diffuse fibrosis and vascularization of the stroma (Fig. 30-48). In severe cases, there is often a granulomatous reaction surrounding Descemet's membrane.[150] Inclusion bodies are only occasionally seen.

Keratoconus

Keratoconus is a congenital ectasia of the central cornea usually becoming manifest in the first decade of life. It tends

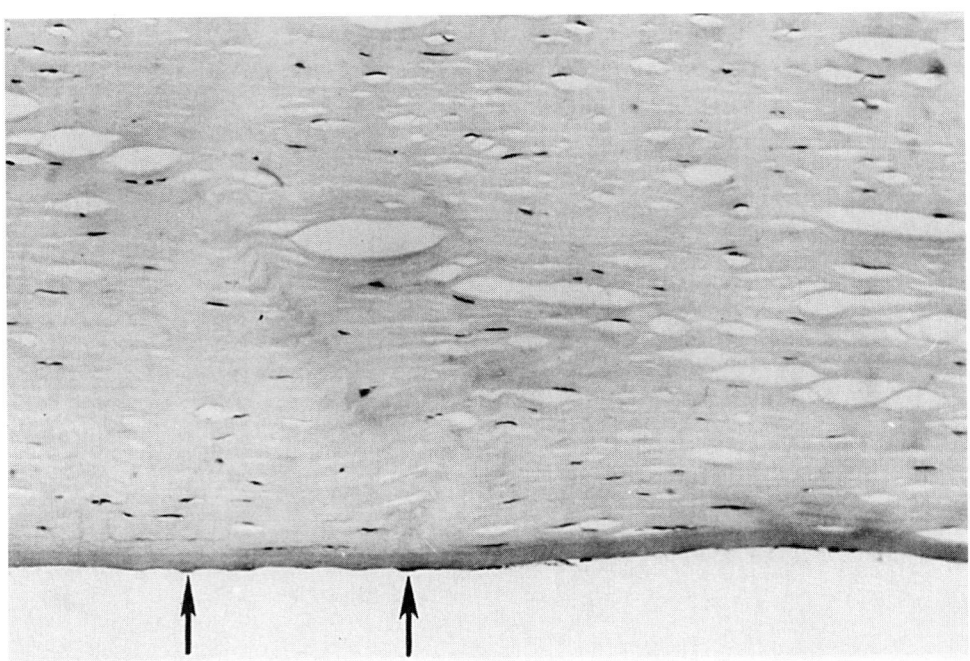

Fig. 30-47 Endothelial decompensation. There is paucity of endothelial cells. Descemet's membrane is thickened, and there are excrescences along its posterior edge *(arrows)*.

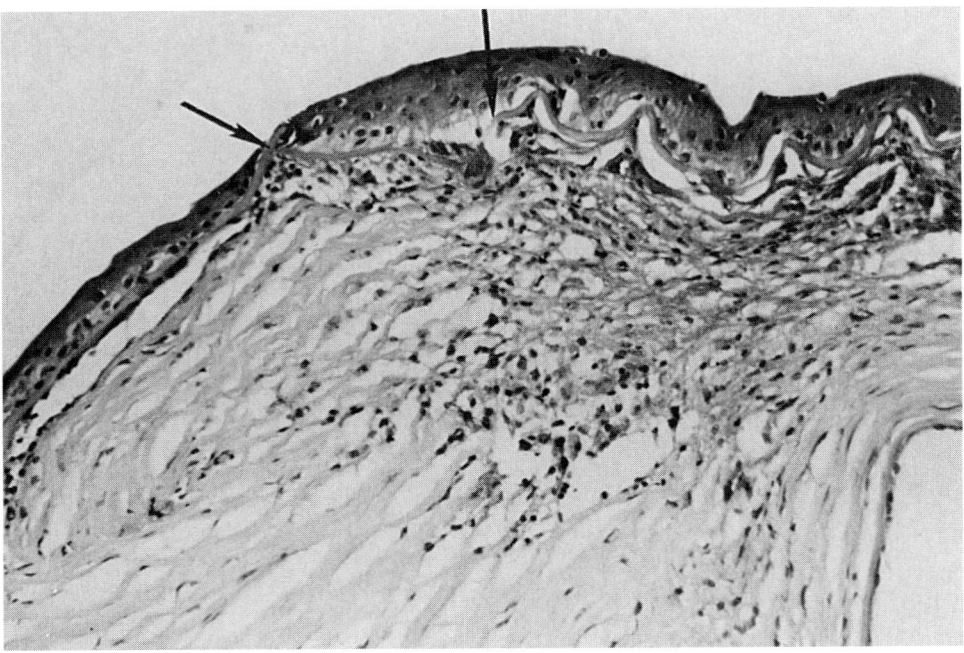

Fig. 30-48 Herpes simplex keratitis. Epithelium is irregular, and there is fragmentation of Bowman's membrane *(arrows)*. Chronic inflammatory cells infiltrate anterior stroma.

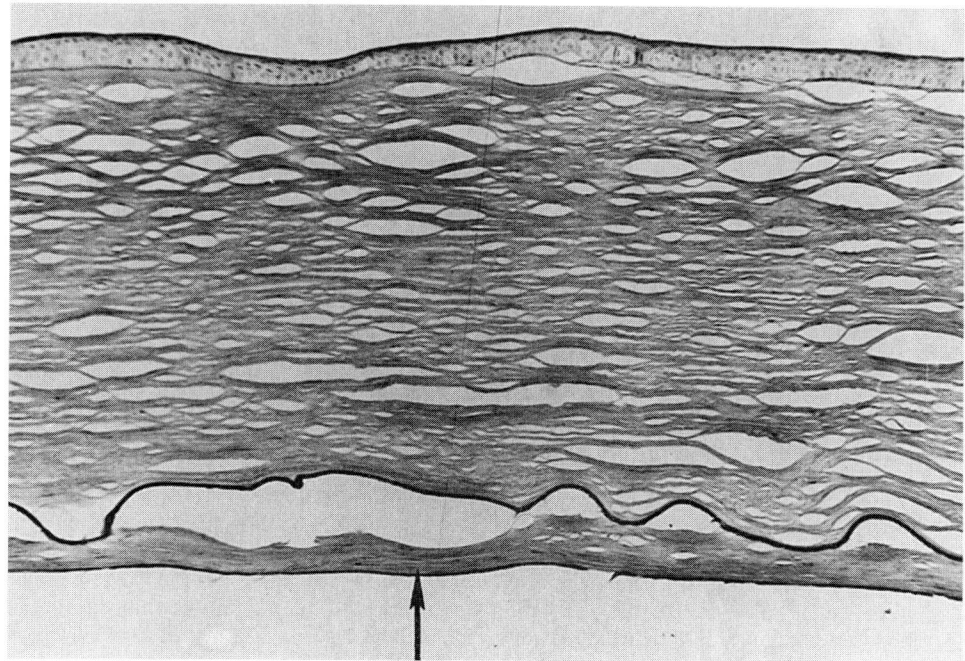

Fig. 30-49 Regraft of corneal button. Note fibrous retrocorneal membrane posterior to Descemet's membrane *(arrow).*

to progress until fibrosis decreases the vision and necessitates corneal transplantation. Histopathologically, there are central thinning and fibrosis. Often the "button" will appear wrinkled on the slide, and this artifact is an instant clue to the diagnosis.

Failed previous grafts

For a variety of reasons, corneal grafts may become opaque, and a second graft is done. The button from the second procedure will often show nonspecific changes such as fibrosis, vascularization, and inflammatory cell infiltration throughout the stroma. At the peripheral edges of the button, there are the full-thickness scars of the previous procedure. A fibrous retrocorneal membrane is present in about one half the cases (Fig. 30-49).

INTRAOCULAR TISSUES

Surgical pathology of the eye itself differs from most of the rest of surgical pathology for several important reasons.

In the first place, biopsies of intraocular tissues are rarely feasible. The important exceptions are the iris and the ciliary body. Lesions of the iris and ciliary body can be removed by iridectomy or iridocyclectomy. This is especially true for melanomas confined to these structures.

In the second place, most of the eyes reaching the surgical pathology laboratory are obtained as a result of enucleation. Usually the globe is intact but free of such accessory tissues as the extraocular muscles and orbital fat. Much less often the eye is eviscerated, and only fragments of the intraocular tissues are submitted for microscopic study. In such cases it is rarely possible to arrive at a satisfactory diagnosis and clinicopathologic correlation. Eyes that are enucleated or eviscerated usually have been diseased for a long time and have become blind. Severe pain and unsightliness are the common immediate reasons for removing the eye. In these cases it is the responsibility of the pathologist not to merely arrive at a definitive diagnosis but to also reconstruct the sequence of events that took place from the onset of ocular disease to the final stages that led to enucleation.

This brings us to another distinctive characteristic of ophthalmic pathology. Frequently the initial pathologic process becomes completely obscured by the subsequent series of events. For example, the patient may first complain of visual disturbance produced by a cataract. The lens opacification progresses, and cataract extraction is performed. Defective wound healing follows, and surface epithelium grows down into the anterior chamber. This leads to secondary glaucoma for which one or more additional surgical procedures are performed. These, in turn, may be complicated by hemorrhage, infection, or retinal detachment. Finally, the eye may become shrunken (phthisic) and disfiguring. A period of several years to a decade or more is usually required for such a series of events to take place.

Intraocular neoplasms represent an exception to the generalization just given. Since only in the case of iris and small ciliary body tumors is it ordinarily possible to excise the neoplasm, the procedure usually followed is to recommend enucleation for other uveal and retinal neoplasms. The aim here is to arrive at a correct clinical diagnosis early, long before such secondary pathologic processes as cataract formation, massive retinal detachment, glaucoma, uveitis, or phthisis complicate the picture. Therefore the pathologist often observes a much less confusing array of pathologic changes and has less difficulty making a diagnosis in eyes

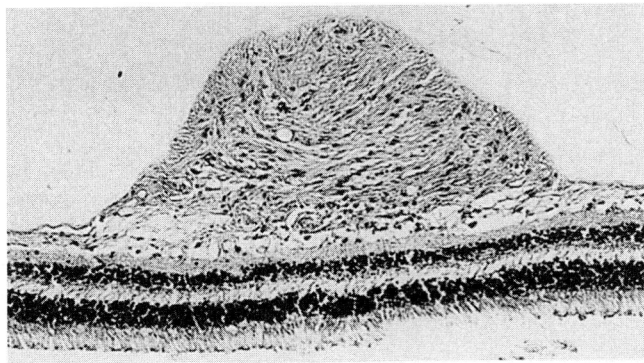

Fig. 30-50 Tuberous sclerosis showing glial nodule or hamartoma projecting against vitreous body from nerve fiber layer of retina.

removed because of intraocular neoplasms rather than in other enucleated eyes. This, however, is not invariably the case, for if the tumor has been present and growing for a long time, it, too, may lead to a wide assortment of secondary processes that sometimes confuse the pathologist as well as the clinician.

Developmental anomalies

Most congenital and developmental malformations of the eye are not seen by the surgical pathologist but only at postmortem examination.[151] Congenital abnormalities typify the point made earlier—that is, the initial pathologic process becomes completely obscured by the subsequent series of events occurring in that eye.

Congenital glaucoma

Congenital glaucoma is characterized by an elevation in the intraocular pressure caused by a malformation of the tissues in the region of the anterior chamber angle. The precise nature of this malformation is still not clear, but there seems to be either an incomplete separation of the iris root from the trabeculae or the retention of an embryonic membrane, or both.

The increased intraocular pressure leads to retinal and optic nerve degeneration, corneal edema and scarring, and global enlargement (buphthalmos). Unilateral congenital glaucoma may occur in Recklinghausen's disease or in the Sturge-Weber syndrome.

When there is a more obvious architectural distortion of the iris and angle of the anterior chamber, it is referred to as the anterior chamber cleavage syndrome[152] or iridogoniodysgenesis. Depending on the degree of angle malformation, other various designations are used (e.g., Rieger's syndrome and Axenfeld's syndrome). This group of malformations is also often associated with a developmental glaucoma.

Retrolental fibroplasia

Retrolental fibroplasia, also called the retinopathy of prematurity, is an acquired form of developmental disorder resulting from the unique sensitivity of retinal blood vessels of the premature retina to oxygen.[153]

Much of the retinal periphery of a baby born after only 6 or 7 months of gestation is completely avascular. If such a premature infant is given high concentrations of oxygen, normal vascularization of the retinal periphery may be inhibited. Vasoconstriction and actual obliteration of the terminal vessels may follow prolonged oxygen therapy. Later, on withdrawal of oxygen, pathologic neovascularization occurs. These newly formed vessels frequently invade the vitreous, leak serum or blood, and eventually lead to organization of the vitreous, retinal detachment, and blindness.

Phakoma

Phakomas are hamartomatous malformations often associated with extraocular lesions as a part of well-defined clinicopathologic syndromes.[154] These include tuberous sclerosis (Bourneville's syndrome), Recklinghausen's disease (neurofibromatosis), Sturge-Weber syndrome (encephalotrigeminal angiomatosis), von Hippel–Lindau disease (angiogliomatosis), ataxia-telangiectasia, and Wyburn-Mason syndrome.

In tuberous sclerosis the most characteristic intraocular lesions are glial plaques and nodules in the nerve fiber layer of the retina, which clinically may simulate a retinoblastoma (Fig. 30-50). Neurofibromas (including the plexiform variety) of the eyelid and orbit and gliomas of the optic nerve are the usual lesions observed in neurofibromatosis.

Hemangioma of the choroid (see Fig. 30-12) is the most common intraocular lesion of the Sturge-Weber syndrome. Ipsilateral glaucoma is often associated with the Sturge-Weber syndrome or Recklinghausen's disease. Abnormally large tortuous arteries and veins leading to a retinal nodule composed of vascular, endothelial, and glial tissues are characteristic of von Hippel–Lindau disease. Vitreous disturbance and retinal detachment are common complications. In ataxia-telangiectasia there are telangiectatic conjunctival vessels, and in the Wyburn-Mason syndrome there are arteriovenous shunts of the retinal vessels.

Persistent hyperplastic primary vitreous

A congenital condition, persistent hyperplastic primary vitreous refers to the persistence and hyperplasia of the fibrovascular tunic of the lens and part of the hyaloid vascular system.[155] It is usually unilateral and occurs in a microphthalmic eye. Clinically this anomaly is manifested by a white reflex behind the pupil (leukokoria). Varying degrees of fibrous tissue are seen behind the lens, and often there is a cataract. Distinction from retinoblastoma is not so great a problem as in the past, but occasionally these eyes are enucleated because retinoblastoma cannot be ruled out.

Histologically there is a dense fibrovascular retrolental mass, and the elongated ciliary processes are enmeshed in this tissue. Remnants of the hyaloid artery system are present, and the retina may appear normal or show evidence of retinal dysplasia (Figs. 30-51 and 30-52).

Retinal dysplasia

Retinal dysplasia is a congenital anomaly that may occur as part of the 13-15 trisomy syndrome or merely in a unilateral malformed eye not associated with other systemic anoma-

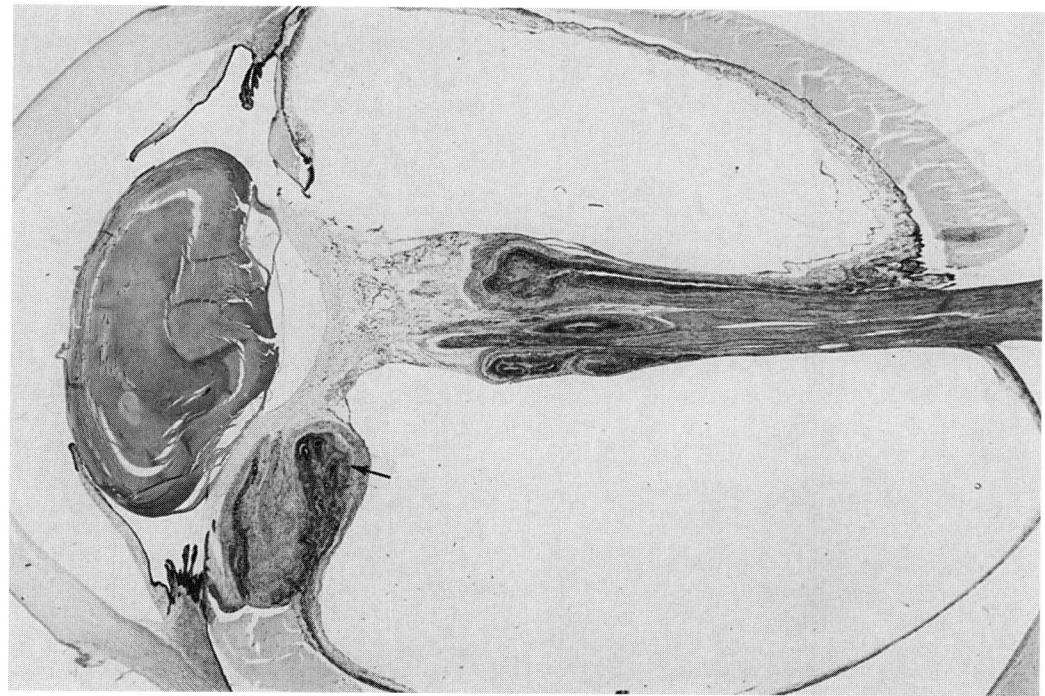

Fig. 30-51 Persistent hyperplastic primary vitreous. Behind lens lies fibrovascular mass to which remnant of hyaloid system attaches. In some cases of persistent hyperplastic primary vitreous, there may be areas of retinal dysplasia *(arrow)*.

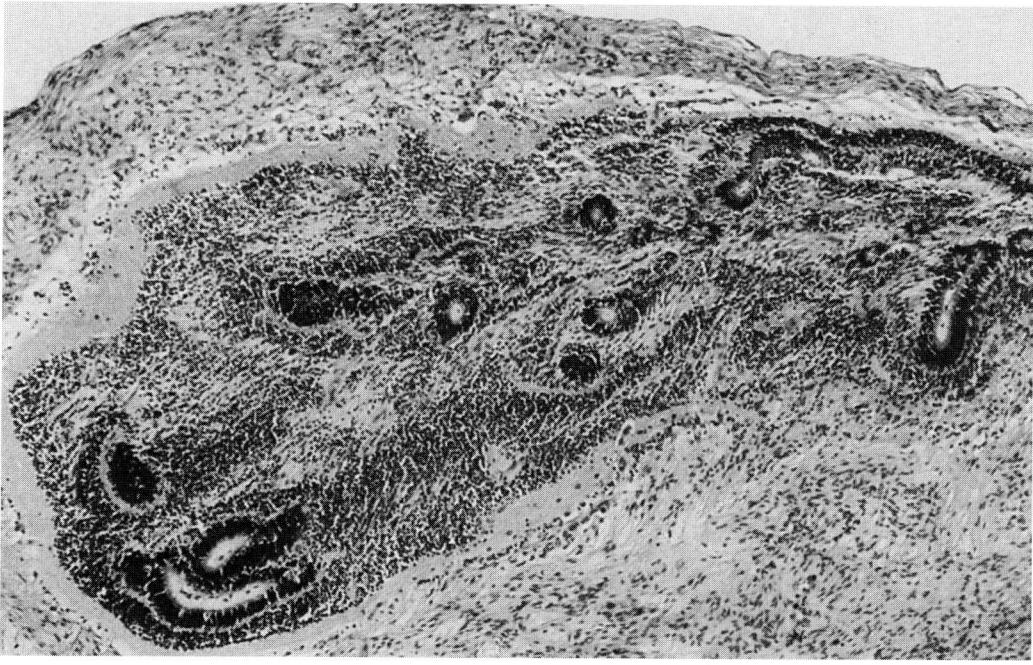

Fig. 30-52 Retinal dysplasia. Within retina are branching tubes composed of abortive elements of rod and cone layer.

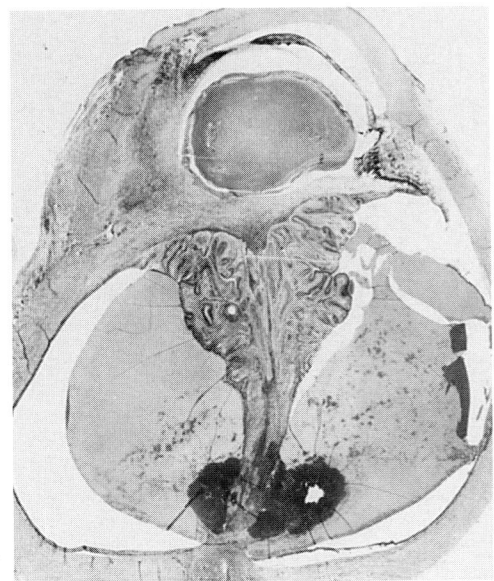

Fig. 30-53 Penetrating wound of eye and multiple minute intraocular foreign bodies (palm splinters) led to formation of dense mass of inflammatory tissue in anterior segment on one side. Organization of vitreous has been complicated by retinal detachment. Blood clots are attached to stalk of detached retina near optic disc.

lies.[156,157] An example of the latter situation would be in the case of persistent hyperplastic primary vitreous, as previously mentioned.

Dysplastic retina is characterized histologically by a series of straight branching tubes composed of abortive elements of the rod and cone layers (see Fig. 30-52). It is believed that this represents disturbed differentiation of neural ectoderm.

Other developmental anomalies

Other congenital entities that are only rarely seen by the surgical pathologist include the rubella syndrome,[158,161] Lowe's syndrome, Fabry's syndrome,[159] and aniridia, in which the nonfamilial case may be associated with Wilms' tumor.[160]

Trauma

Trauma to the globe can be accidental or surgical. The complications that may ensue after severe trauma may eventually lead to blindness and pain, necessitating enucleation. In fact, ocular trauma is the most common reason for eyes reaching the ophthalmic pathology laboratory of a general hospital. Often there are instances in which the surgical pathologist will be expected to identify tissue that has been removed from an eye that is being sutured following a severe laceration. What the ophthalmic surgeon wants to

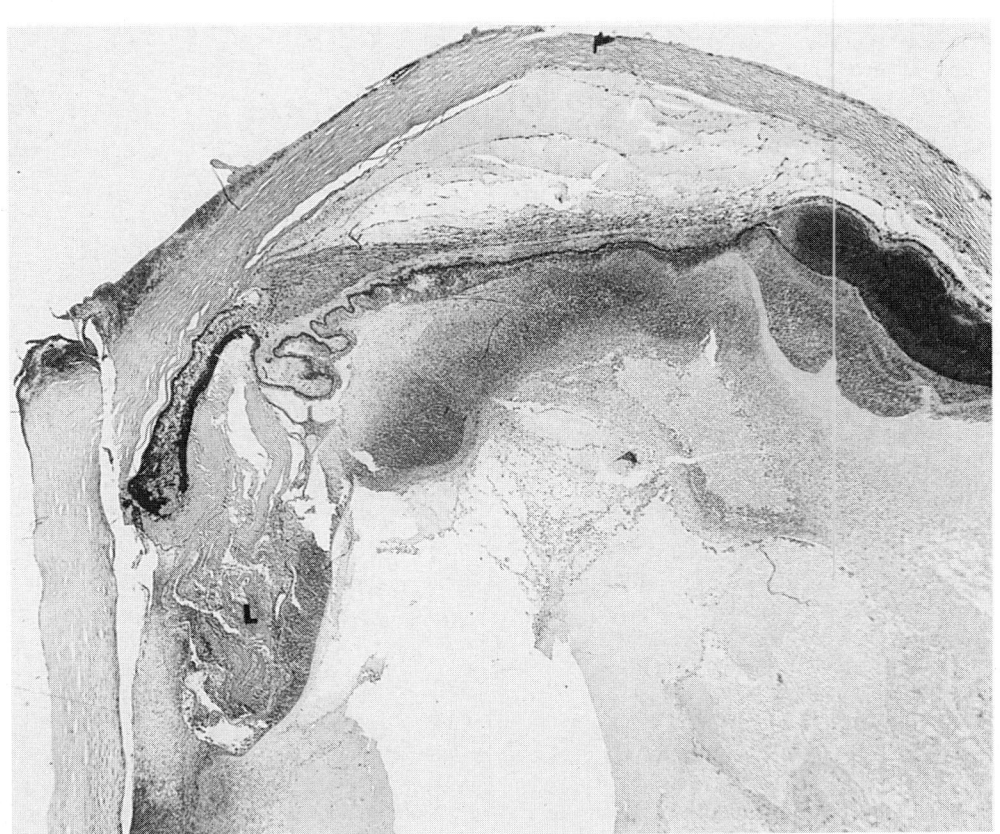

Fig. 30-54 Endophthalmitis showing infiltration of all intraocular structures by acute inflammatory cells. Lens L is necrotic. Organism presumably gained entrance through corneal wound.

know is whether any retina is extruded through the wound. If so, this information may influence further management of the case.

Although some eyes are so extensively damaged that immediate removal is necessary, most of the injured eyes are removed at varying intervals because of secondary changes such as organization of hemorrhage, glaucoma, retinal detachment, infections, inflammation, or complete atrophy (phthisis bulbi) (Fig. 30-53).

Histopathologic diagnosis is not usually a problem, but a search should be made for retained intraocular foreign bodies such as metal, vegetation, and cilia. Retained intraocular iron and copper may produce siderosis and chalcosis, respectively.

Beside the aforementioned secondary changes (e.g., diffuse fibrosis, secondary glaucoma, inflammation), certain specific complications associated with trauma include sympathetic ophthalmia, phacoanaphylactic endophthalmitis, postcontusion angle deformity, fibrous downgrowth, and epithelial downgrowth. These are considered subsequently under other headings.

Inflammation

Inflammation of the eye, as elsewhere, may be acute or chronic, granulomatous or nongranulomatous.

Acute inflammation

Acute intraocular inflammation is often infectious in origin. The causative organism is usually a bacterium or fungus and is generally introduced through a perforating wound (Fig. 30-54). Occasionally, however, the infection is hematogenous. There have been reports of endogenous fungous endophthalmitis,[162,164] and metastatic endophthalmitis also has been reported after injection of addictive drugs.[165]

Initially there is a massive purulent reaction in the anterior and vitreous chambers, and the process is called endophthalmitis. As the infection spreads, other intraocular tissues, such as the retina, uvea, and eventually the cornea and sclera, may become involved. At this stage the term *panophthalmitis* is applicable. Before the advent of antibiotic therapy, eyes affected by severe panophthalmitis were frequently eviscerated or enucleated early. Today the infection can often be controlled, but subsequent organization of the exudate leads to *phthisis bulbi* (see p. 2484). A common cause of noninfectious endophthalmitis or panophthalmitis is massive necrosis of a uveal malignant melanoma or a metastatic carcinoma.[163]

Chronic nongranulomatous inflammation

In chronic nongranulomatous inflammation of the eye, the uveal tract is primarily involved. In *anterior uveitis (iridocyclitis),* the tissues are typically infiltrated by plasma cells in a rather diffuse fashion (Fig. 30-55, *A*), but occasionally the inflammation is in the form of nodular lymphocytic infiltrates. In *posterior uveitis (choroiditis)* the round cell infiltration may also be diffuse, but frequently it is focal or scattered as multiple discrete lesions. In *choroiditis* the overlying retina is usually involved by spread of the inflammatory reaction—hence the alternative term *chorioretinitis.* A complication of inflammatory diseases of the uveal tract is the formation of a *cyclitic membrane* that can contract and lead to detachment of the retina and ciliary body.[166]

In choroiditis, even if prolonged, enucleation is not often necessary, for the eyes do not become painful. However, with recurrent iridocyclitis the inflammatory reaction often produces adhesions between the iris and the cornea (anterior synechiae) (Fig. 30-55, *B*) or between the iris and the lens (posterior synechiae) (Fig. 30-56), and secondary glaucoma results. If this condition is intractable, enucleation is almost inevitable. Often the process is of such a long-term nature that when the eye is enucleated, all that is recognized is the massive scarring that is found in phthisis bulbi, which is due to any cause.

The etiology and pathogenesis of nongranulomatous uveitis can rarely be ascertained clinically or pathologically. Occasionally an entity presents a characteristic picture such as is seen in *herpes zoster ophthalmicus* in which there is a chronic inflammatory cell infiltration around the posterior ciliary nerves and vessels.[167] *Behçet's disease* produces an obliterative vasculitis of the retinal vessels.

Granulomatous inflammation

Granulomatous inflammation may be the result of a specific infection such as toxoplasmosis, tuberculosis, syphilis, nematodiasis, and cytomegalic inclusion disease. Also associated with granulomatous reactions are entities such as sarcoidosis and the collagen diseases. It should be kept in mind, however, that as with the nongranulomatous cases, the etiology cannot often be ascertained. This is the case with the entity designated as *idiopathic solitary granuloma* of the uveal tract.[169] This disorder is unilateral, accompanied by uveal effusion and total retinal detachment, and typically located between the pars plana ciliaris and the equator.[169]

The inflammatory process in granulomatous uveitis may be diffuse, or there is a more localized area of destruction in which the causative agent or otherwise diagnostic lesion will be found.

The term granulomatous uveitis is misleading, for often the most diagnostic lesions are not found in the iris, ciliary body, or choroid but rather in the retina, vitreous, or sclera. The diagnostic lesions of toxoplasmosis are found in the retina, those of nematodiasis in the vitreous or retina, and those of the rheumatoid group in the sclera between the limbus and the equator.

Toxoplasmosis. Although ocular toxoplasmosis is an important entity, it is actually quite rare to receive such globes in the pathology laboratory. The histopathology is characterized by a focal area of coagulative necrosis of the retina surrounded by a granulomatous inflammation in the adjacent choroid and sclera. Within the area of necrotic retina, cysts of *Toxoplasma gondii* can be found[172] (Fig. 30-57). Cases of toxoplasmosis resulting in diffuse retinal necrosis have been observed in patients with AIDS.[170]

Nematodiasis. Nematodiasis is a broad term encompassing a variety of parasitic diseases. The one form of ocular nematodiasis that has been found with considerable frequency in the United States and Great Britain is a type of visceral larva migrans, probably produced in most cases by wandering larvae of *Toxocara canis.*[168] This is principally an infection of children between the ages of 3 and 14 years.[173]

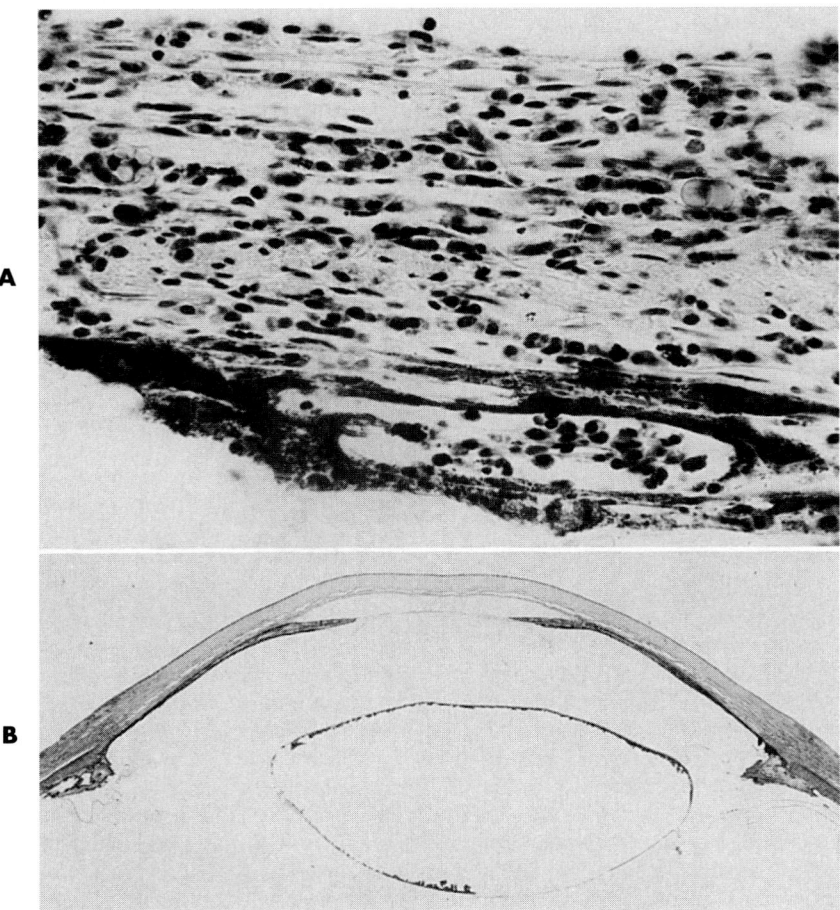

Fig. 30-55 **A,** Nongranulomatous iritis in which atrophic iris is diffusely infiltrated by plasma cells and several Russell bodies are present. Irregular degenerative and proliferative changes may be observed in pigment epithelium. **B,** Same lesion illustrated in **A** showing chronically inflamed iris almost completely adherent to cornea and anterior chamber virtually obliterated.

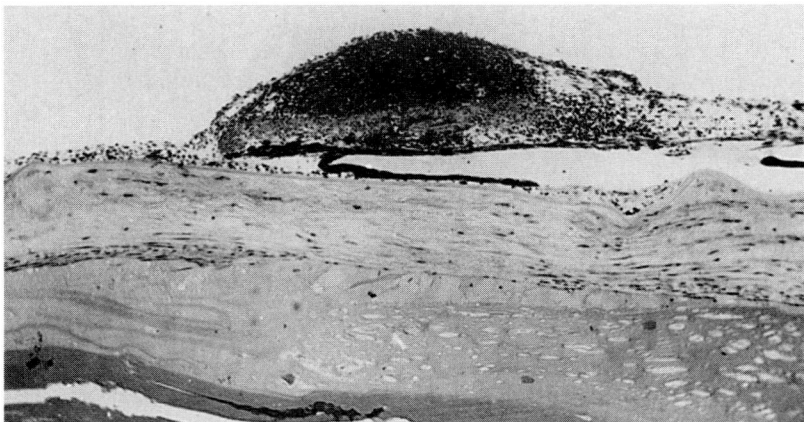

Fig. 30-56 Nongranulomatous iritis with posterior synechiae. Iris is firmly attached to lens, which reveals widespread degeneration of its cortex and fibrous metaplasia of its subcapsular epithelium.

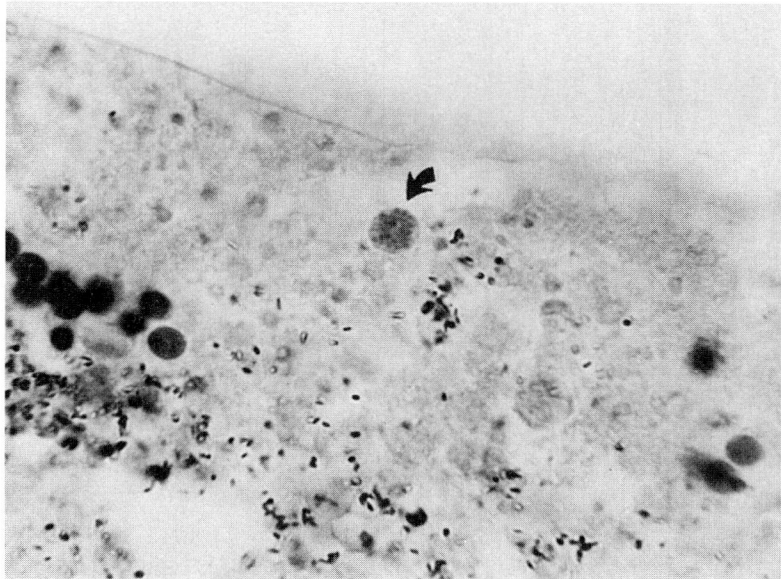

Fig. 30-57 Encysting proliferative forms *(arrow)* of *Toxoplasma gondii* found in necrotic retina. Small particles are pigment granules from necrotic retinal pigment epithelium, whereas larger round structures represent pyknotic retinal nuclei.

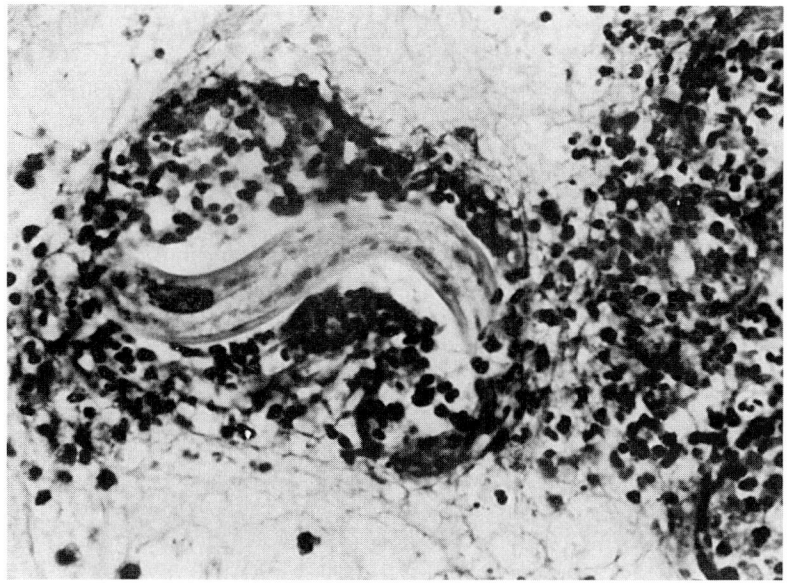

Fig. 30-58 Nematode larva, probably *Toxocara canis,* surrounded by inflammatory cells in vitreous body.

Almost without exception, those children who have had ocular infection have not had clinical evidence of systemic visceral larva migrans, and those who have had the systemic form have not had ocular lesions. Typically a single migrating larva finds its way, hematogenously, into the eye and comes to rest in the vitreous or on the inner surface of the retina (Fig. 30-58).

A pronounced infiltration by acute and chronic inflammatory cells, often with intense eosinophilia, is observed in these tissues.

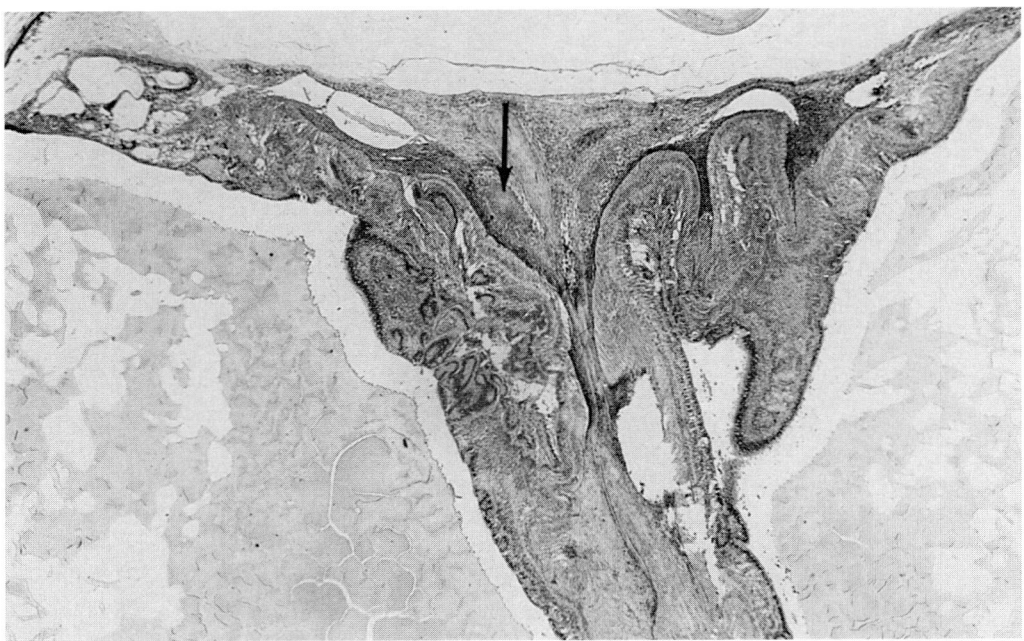

Fig. 30-59 Nematode endophthalmitis in which inflammatory reaction in vitreous has led to retinal detachment. Parasite was found in area of necrosis *(arrow).*

Eventually the inflammatory reaction in the vitreous leads to organization and contracture of this structure with consequent detachment of the retina (Fig. 30-59). This leads to leukokoria, and the eye is enucleated because retinoblastoma cannot be ruled out.

As the nematode larvae die, they often stimulate the formation of a typical granulomatous inflammatory reaction about them. It is usually necessary to make serial sections to find these minute granulomas. The typical inflammatory reaction with intense eosinophilia observed in the vitreous is presumptive evidence of nematodiasis.[171]

Post-traumatic uveitis

Following penetrating injury of the eye, the development of a granulomatous uveitis always causes great concern because of the possibility of *sympathetic uveitis,* a dreaded disease in which injury to one eye gives rise to severe inflammation that sometimes progresses to blindness in the uninjured eye as well as in the injured eye. Fortunately, sympathetic uveitis is extremely rare today. Other causes of post-traumatic granulomatous inflammation are lens-induced endophthalmitis (phacoanaphylaxis), foreign bodies, and blood in the vitreous.

Sympathetic uveitis. Sympathetic uveitis is probably the best example of a pure granulomatous uveitis, for the significant lesion in this disease is confined to the uveal tissues. Typically the process involves the entire uveal tract. There may, of course, be associated inflammatory lesions in other tissues attributable to the original trauma or to the presence of foreign bodies, but the reaction of sympathetic uveitis itself is purely uveal.

There is a dense, diffuse infiltration of the choroid by lymphocytes (Fig. 30-60), and often the ciliary body and iris are similarly involved. Superimposed on this lymphocytic infiltrate are small, irregular, patchy accumulations of large, pale-staining epithelioid cells, which on high magnification, will often be found to contain finely dispersed melanin granules (Fig. 30-61). Polymorphonuclear leukocytes are characteristically lacking, plasma cells are rare, but eosinophils are often included in moderate numbers.

The reaction involves the outer and middle coats of the choroid, extending into the scleral canals along ciliary vessels and nerves, sometimes to the episcleral surface. The choriocapillaris, on the other hand, is typically uninvolved. Clusters of epithelioid cells between Bruch's membrane and the retinal pigment epithelium, referred to as Dalen-Fuchs nodules, are often seen.

Phacoanaphylaxis. Phacoanaphylactic endophthalmitis usually follows penetrating injury to the lens, but a few cases have been observed following spontaneous rupture of a swollen cataractous lens. It is characterized by a granulomatous inflammatory reaction centered about an area of lens perforation. The process is believed to be the result of acquired hypersensitivity to lens protein.

A typical zonal pattern of inflammatory reaction is observed in most cases (Fig. 30-62, *A*). In the area in which the lens capsule is broken, there is a massive invasion of the lens by inflammatory cells. Centrally and immediately surrounding individual lens fibers are polymorphonuclear leukocytes. Peripheral to this is a wall of epithelioid and giant cells about which is a broader, more diffuse zone of granulation tissue and round cell infiltration (Fig. 30-62, *B*).

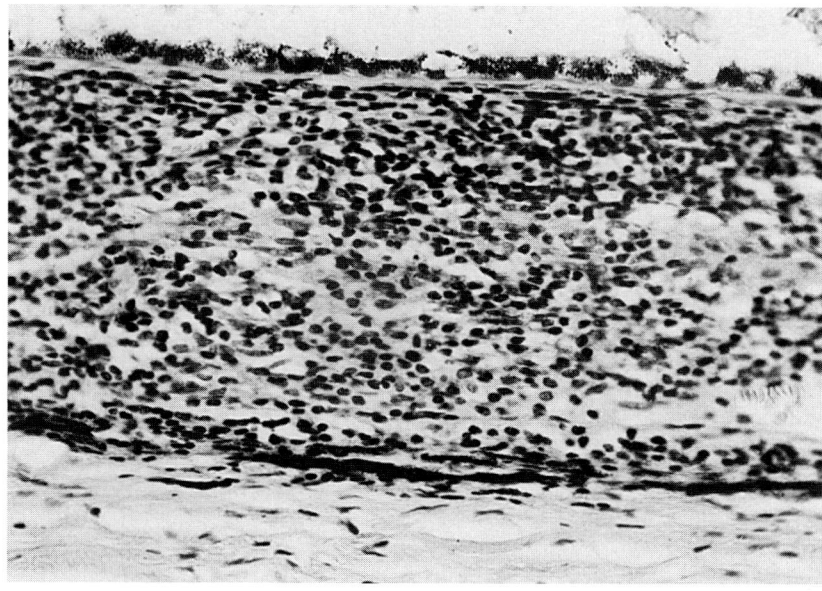

Fig. 30-60 Sympathetic uveitis. Uveal tissues are diffusely infiltrated by lymphocytes, and there are small, irregular collections of pale-staining epithelioid cells.

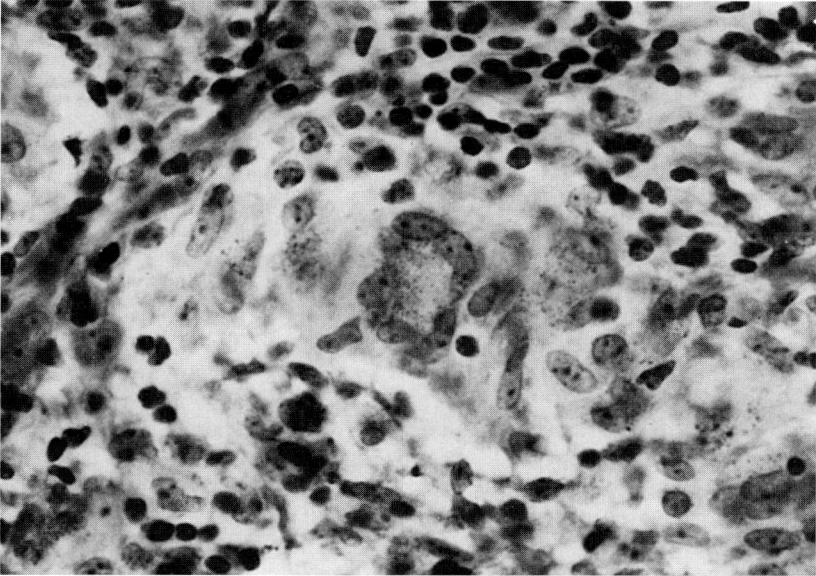

Fig. 30-61 Epithelioid cells and giant cells containing finely dispersed uveal pigment granules that are characteristically present in sympathetic uveitis. (From Friedenwald JS, Wilder HC, Maumenee AE, Sanders TE, Keyes JEL, Hogan MJ, Owens WC, Owens EU: Ophthalmic pathology. An atlas and textbook. Philadelphia, 1952, W.B. Saunders Co.)

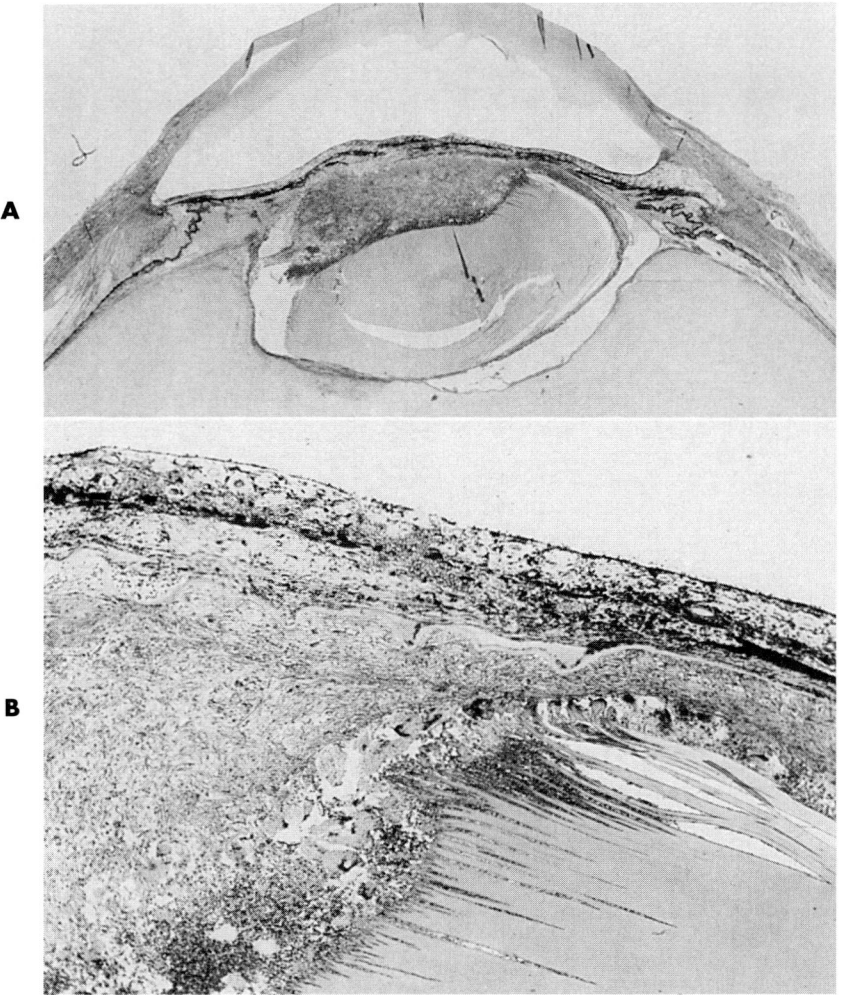

Fig. 30-62 A, Phacoanaphylactic endophthalmitis resulting from penetrating wound that ruptured capsule of anterior lens. Dense infiltrate of acute and chronic inflammatory cells is present in area of lens damage. **B,** Higher magnification of lesion illustrated in **A**. Polymorphonuclear leukocytes are present in and about disintegrating lens fibers. Peripheral to them is wall of macrophages, epithelioid cells, and giant cells, and there is broad zone of granulation tissue about entire lesion.

The iris reveals a variable degree of plasma cell infiltration, and posterior synechiae are commonly formed.

Ordinarily the posterior uveal tract is not inflamed, but characteristically there is a perivasculitis of the retinal vessels. In a considerable number of cases, however, phacoanaphylactic endophthalmitis and sympathetic uveitis are co-existent.[174]

Degeneration

Degenerative changes are usually the result of other primary processes such as trauma or inflammation. The most advanced stage of ocular degeneration in which all tissues are involved is called phthisis bulbi.

Phthisis bulbi

Phthisis bulbi represents the final stage of ocular degeneration in which the production of aqueous humor is so markedly reduced that the intraocular pressure falls (hypotony) and the globe shrinks (Fig. 30-63).

The causes of phthisis bulbi are myriad, but most phthisic eyes reaching the surgical pathology laboratory have been injured, either accidentally or as a result of surgical procedures.

Phthisic eyes are enucleated for several reasons. Many are enucleated because they are disfiguring and others because they become irritated as a result of periodic hemorrhages or bouts of uveitis. Some are enucleated for prophylactic reasons—the fear of sympathetic uveitis or malignant melanoma, either of which may develop long after the eye has become blind and phthisic.

All tissues are affected to varying degrees in phthisis bulbi, and the degree of shrinkage is also variable. The eye may be soft and spongy or stony hard because of calcification and ossification. Typically the media are opaque.

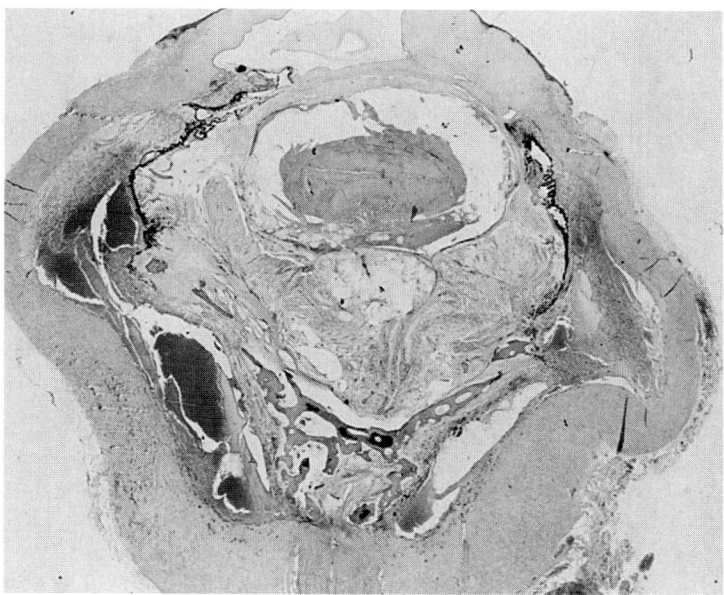

Fig. 30-63 Phthisis bulbi in which globe is markedly shrunken, sclera is wrinkled, and all intraocular tissues reveal severe degenerative changes, including foci of ossification.

Corneal scars, exudates in the anterior and posterior chambers, and advanced cataract formation prevent visualization of the inner eye. The vitreous is usually destroyed, and the retina is completely detached. Extensive areas of osseous metaplasia are frequently observed along the inner surface of the choroid posteriorly. The uvea is often edematous, and pools of serous exudate may separate it from the wrinkled sclera.

In phthisis bulbi that has followed extensive endophthalmitis or panophthalmitis, the various intraocular tissues are often so necrotic and replaced by scar tissue that most of the internal architecture of the eye is effaced.

Glaucoma

Glaucoma is conveniently placed here, since it represents another condition of diverse etiology characterized by widespread degeneration of ocular tissues. The essential feature of the glaucomas is an unphysiologic state of increased intraocular pressure, caused in almost all cases by impaired outflow of aqueous humor. Aqueous humor is produced by the ciliary processes and discharged into the posterior chamber. It flows forward between the lens and the iris, through the pupil, and into the anterior chamber. Aqueous humor leaves the anterior chamber via the trabecular meshwork, which is present in the deep layers of the peripheral cornea, just in front of the anterior chamber angle (Fig. 30-64). After passing through the trabecula, aqueous humor enters Schlemm's canal and leaves the eye via the plexus of intrascleral and episcleral veins along the corneoscleral limbus. When the impaired aqueous drainage follows some known or suspected antecedent disease, the condition is known as secondary glaucoma. Here the surgical pathologist may play an important role in determining the antecedent disease.

Primary glaucoma. The primary glaucomas are not associated with antecedent disease but are either the "chronic simple" type or the "angle-closure" type. In the former, there are certain degenerative changes in the trabecular meshwork and the connective tissues about Schlemm's canal. The exact nature of these changes remains obscure. These eyes seldom reach the pathology laboratory, since the process is usually insidious and often does not cause enough pain to necessitate enucleation.

Acute and chronic angle-closure glaucoma is caused by anatomic and physiologic peculiarities of the tissues and the spaces of the anterior chamber that predispose to blockage of the outflow channels by the iris root. Chronic attacks of angle-closure glaucoma may lead to extensive adhesions of the iris root to the trabecular meshwork (peripheral anterior synechia, Fig. 30-65), and if this glaucoma becomes intractable, it may necessitate enucleation because of pain.[177]

Secondary glaucoma. Secondary glaucoma may be a complication of numerous primary processes, including trauma, inflammation, neoplasia, and malformation. The sites of obstruction to the outflow of aqueous humor are numerous, but the most vulnerable areas are the pupil and the angle of the anterior chamber. Formation of pupillary membranes as a result of organization of hemorrhages and exudates or the development of extensive adhesions between the iris and the lens (posterior synechiae) as a consequence of iritis (see Fig. 30-56) are the usual mechanisms leading to pupillary obstruction.

The outflow channels in the anterior chamber angle may become obstructed by particulate matter or by the formation of extensive adhesions between the root of the iris and the peripheral cornea (peripheral anterior synechiae) (see Fig. 30-65). Particulate matter clogging the passages between the anterior chamber and Schlemm's canal is usually cellular—

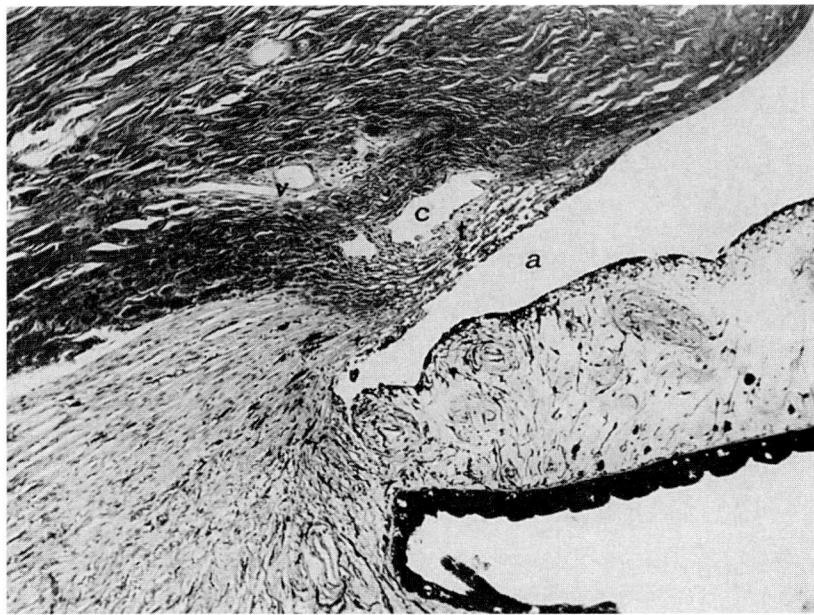

Fig. 30-64 Normal outflow channels for passage of aqueous humor from anterior chamber angle *(a)* include corneoscleral trabecula *(t)*, Schlemm's canal *(c)*, and intrascleral plexus of veins *(v)*. (Verhoeff–van Gieson.)

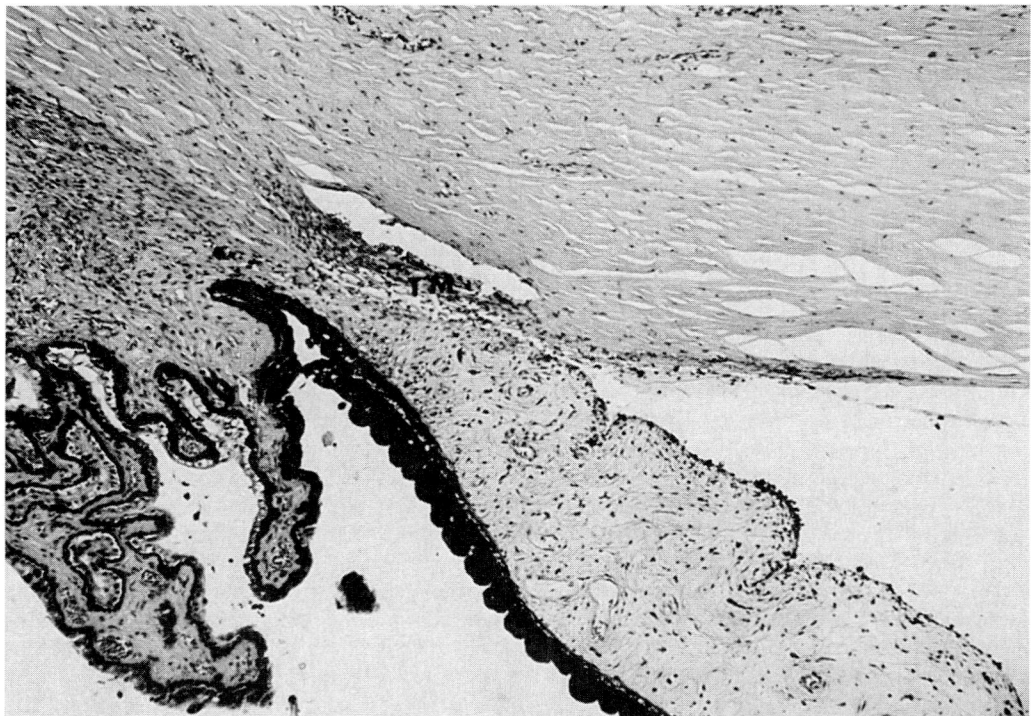

Fig. 30-65 Peripheral aspect of iris lying against trabecular meshwork *(TM)* producing peripheral anterior synechia and blocking outflow of aqueous.

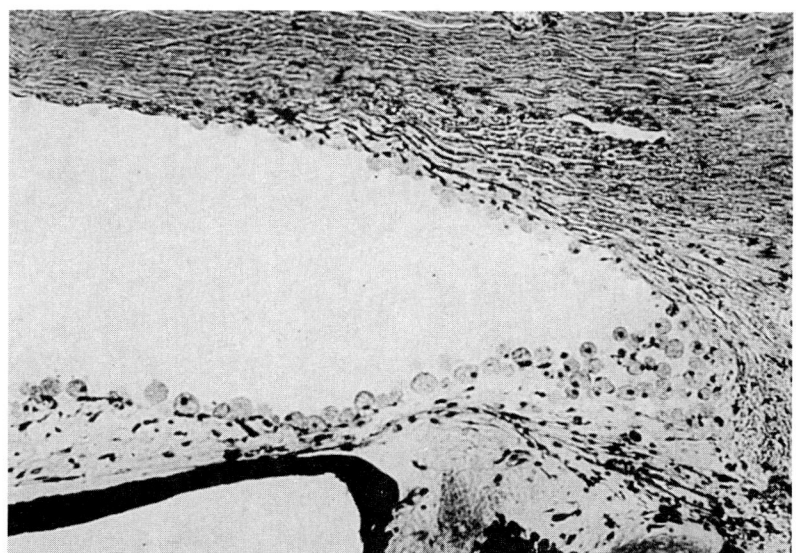

Fig. 30-66 Outflow channels blocked by macrophages in anterior chamber in phacolytic glaucoma (glaucoma secondary to lysis and escape of lens protein into aqueous humor). (From Flocks M, Littwin CS, Zimmerman LE: Phacolytic glaucoma. Clinicopathologic study of 138 cases of glaucoma associated with hypermature cataract. Arch Ophthalomol **54**:37-45, 1955.)

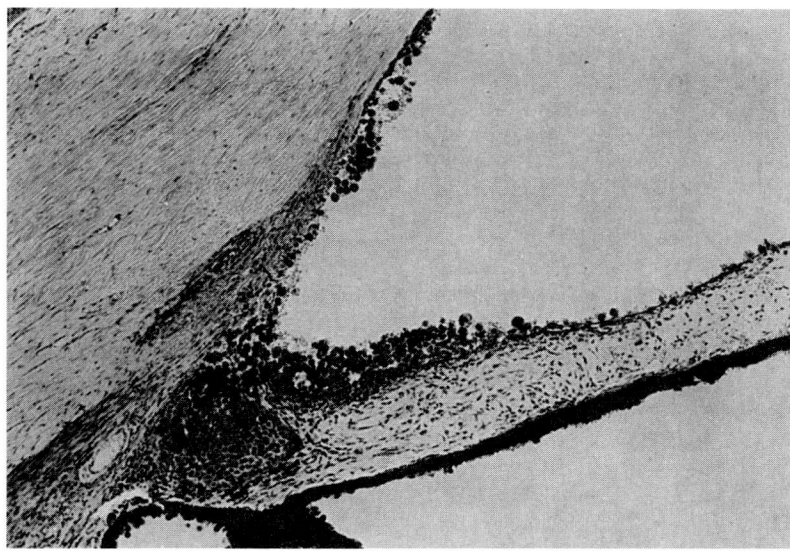

Fig. 30-67 Anterior chamber angle and outflow channels filled with deeply pigmented cells dispersed into aqueous humor from malignant melanoma of iris.

red blood cells after massive hemorrhage into the anterior chamber,[175] leukocytes in certain types of uveitis[176] (Fig. 30-66), or tumor cells, particularly with diffuse melanomas of the iris (Fig. 30-67). Following accidental trauma or surgery, conjunctival and/or corneal epithelium may grow between the wound edges and eventually line the anterior chamber and iris, thus blocking the outflow of aqueous (clinically referred to as "epithelial downgrowth") (Fig. 30-68). Fibrous downgrowth is the extension of dense fibrous tissue from the cornea into the anterior chamber through a gap in the posterior aspect of a corneal wound.

One of the common causes of secondary glaucoma encountered by the ophthalmic pathologist is the development of a neovascular membrane on the surface of the iris. This membrane, known as *rubeosis iridis,* is eventually associated with some degree of peripheral anterior synechia, thus causing blockage of the outflow channels (Fig. 30-69).

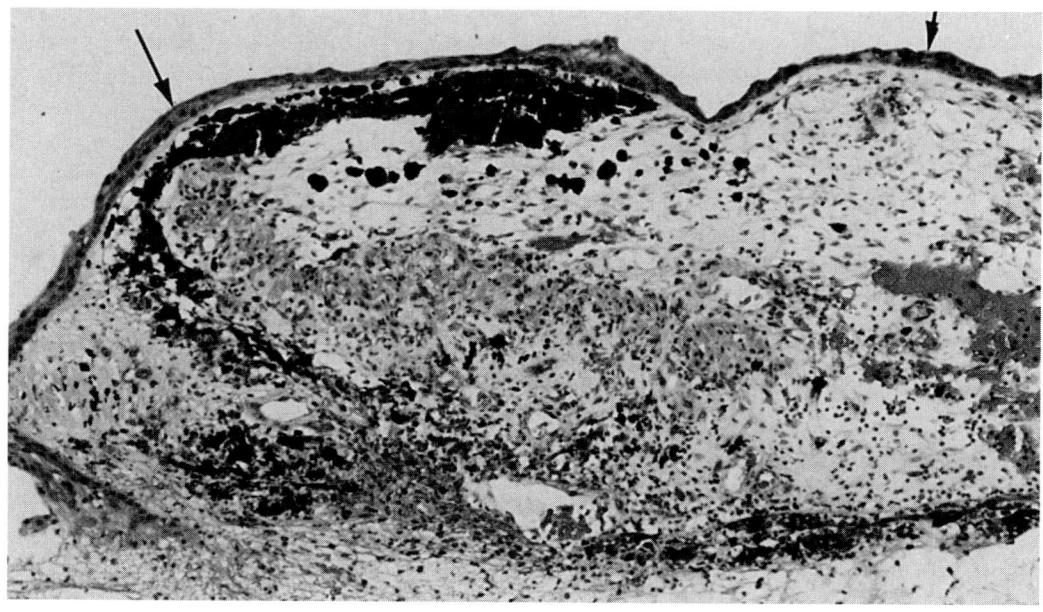

Fig. 30-68 In this case of postcataract extraction, layer of epithelium has grown down wound into anterior chamber to lie on surface of iris *(arrows).*

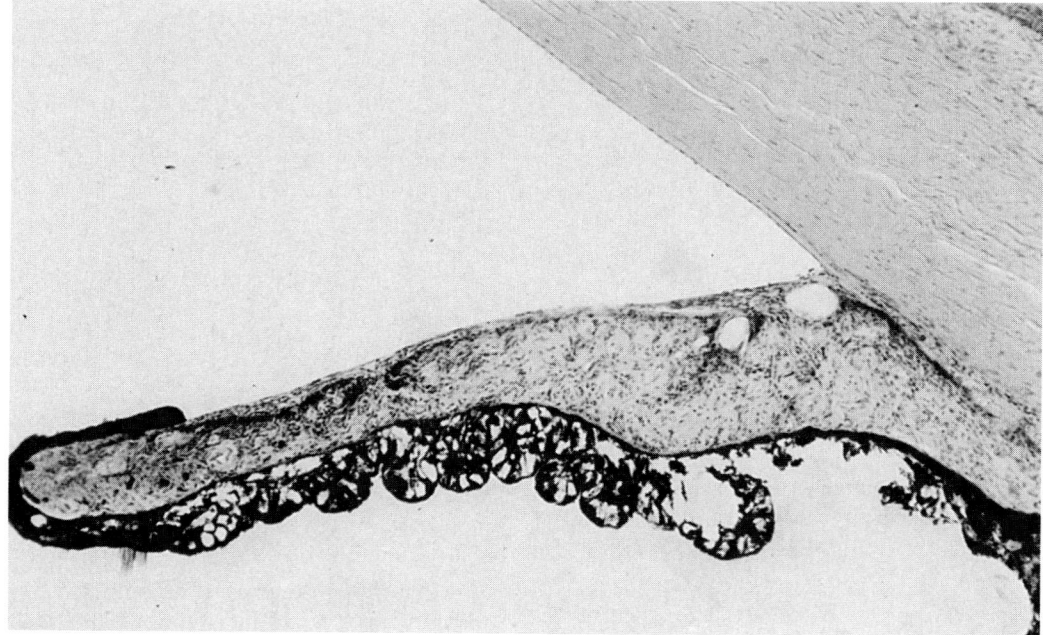

Fig. 30-69 Rubeosis iridis in diabetes. Angle of anterior chamber is occluded by peripheral anterior synechia, and fibrovascular membrane (rubeosis iridis) covers anterior surface of iris. Contraction of this membrane has pulled pigment epithelium anteriorly to produce "ectropion uvea." There is marked diabetic vacuolization of pigment epithelial cells.

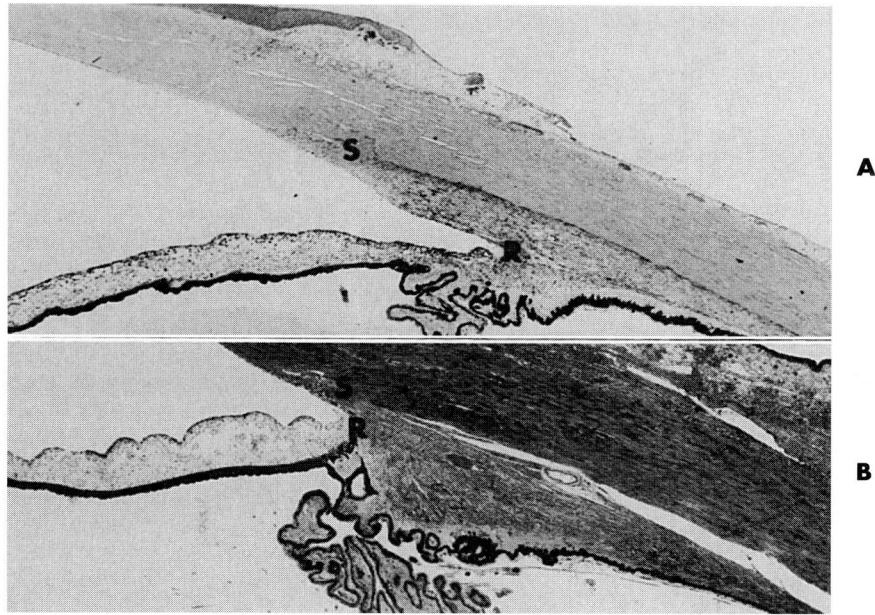

Fig. 30-70 A, Recession of angle of anterior chamber. **B,** Normal angle. In **A,** iris root *(R)* is retrodisplaced with reference to scleral spur *(S),* and contour of atrophic ciliary body is fusiform instead of normal wedge shape.

Rubeosis iridis can occur following several different conditions. It occurs most commonly in diabetes or following occlusion of the central retinal artery or vein. Other conditions associated with rubeosis include carotid artery occlusion, long-standing retinal detachment, chronic uveitis, and intraocular neoplasms.

Damage to the outflow channels may occur as a result of blunt trauma to the eye and give rise to a chronic glaucoma. This situation is often associated with a recession of the anterior chamber angle. Histologically the iris root insertion appears retrodisplaced, and there is atrophy of the ciliary body (Fig. 30-70).

Regardless of the type and cause of glaucoma, certain degenerative changes are typically produced after periods of variable duration. When glaucoma begins in childhood, the tissues tend to stretch, and the globe may become greatly enlarged (buphthalmos). When its onset is in adult life, however, the tissues tend to resist stretching, and normal ocular dimensions are maintained.

The elevated intraocular pressure typically affects the inner retinal layers to a more pronounced degree than it does the outer layers. A common observation is the presence of rather well-preserved rods and cones and an intact outer nuclear layer when virtually all ganglion cells have disappeared and the nerve fiber and inner nuclear layers have become reduced to one half or one third their normal thickness (Fig. 30-71).

Degeneration of nerve fibers is especially noteworthy in the region of the optic disc. This leads to excavation or cupping of the nerve head, posterior bowing of the lamina cribrosa, and severe atrophy of the optic nerve (Fig. 30-72). Often, discrete areas of scleral ectasia are observed, particu-

larly in the equatorial regions. These are lined by uveal tissue and therefore have a bluish color—hence the name *staphyloma* (grape-like swelling).

Diabetes

Ocular diabetes has become one of the most common causes of blindness in Western society. Diabetes can cause a variety of pathologic conditions within the eye. These conditions may lead to complete blindness and if associated with pain, the eyes often reach the pathology laboratory.[179]

The retina often shows scattered hemorrhages and exudates, and there may be the development of neovascular tissue that grows from the inner surface of the retina into the vitreous (Fig. 30-73, *A*). This condition, known as proliferative retinopathy, can cause a retinal detachment that usually does not respond well to surgical treatment (Fig. 30-73, *B*).

As previously mentioned, secondary glaucoma may result from the development of diabetic rubeosis iridis with peripheral anterior synechia (see Fig. 30-69). Many eyes from diabetic patients will also manifest vacuolization of the iris pigment epithelium. These vacuoles have been demonstrated to contain glycogen (see Fig. 30-69) and are related to the level of the blood glucose at the time of enucleation, similarly to Armanni-Ebstein nephropathy.[178]

Tumors and tumorlike conditions

Malignant melanoma

General and clinical features. Melanomas arising from the pigmented or potentially pigment-producing cells of the uvea are the most frequent primary intraocular neoplasms in adults, although they can also occur in adolescents, children, and even neonates.[181,183] It has been suggested that most of

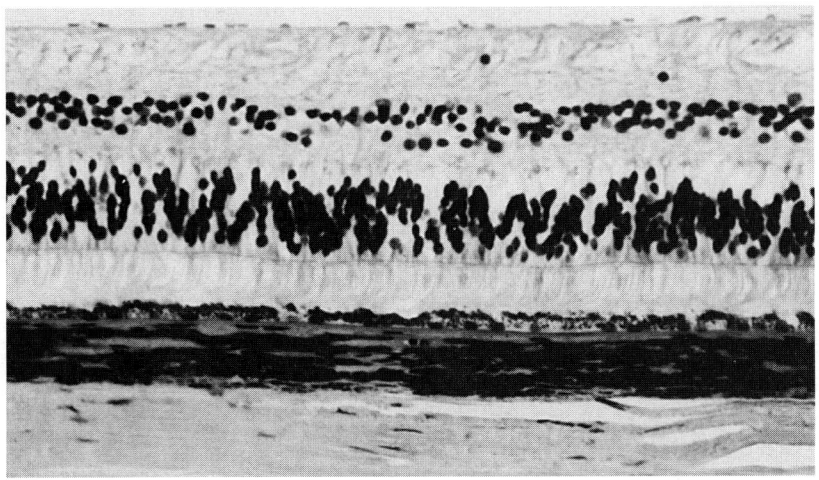

Fig. 30-71 Retina in chronic glaucoma revealing widespread loss of ganglion cells and nerve fibers and reduction of cells in inner nuclear layer but relatively well-preserved visual cells. (From Friedenwald JS, Wilder HC, Maumenee AE, Sanders TE, Keyes JEL, Hogan MJ, Owens WC, Owens EU: Ophthalmic pathology. An atlas and textbook. Philadelphia, 1952, W.B. Saunders Co.)

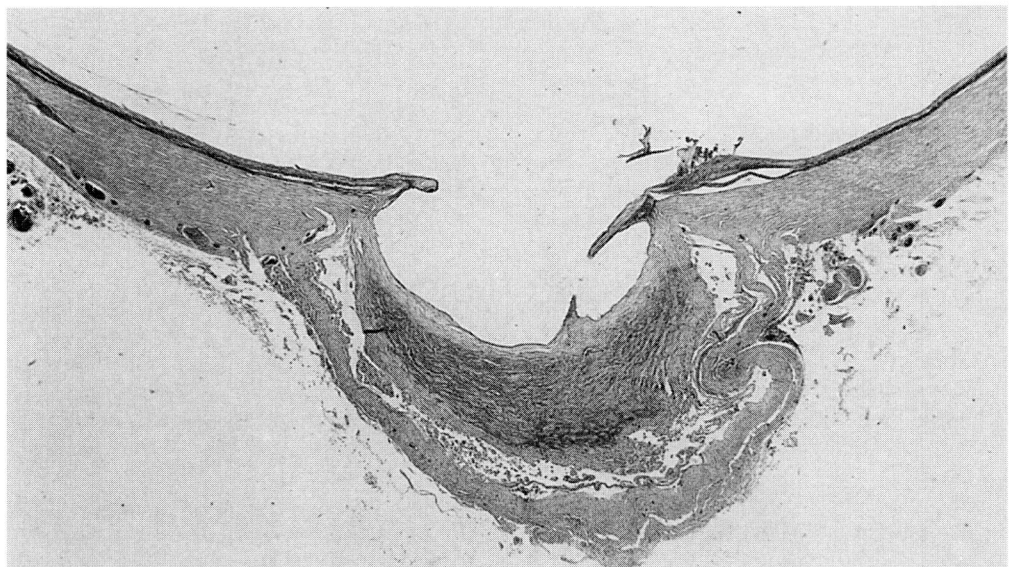

Fig. 30-72 Deep excavation *(cupping)* of optic disc and severe atrophy of optic nerve, which are important complications of chronic glaucoma.

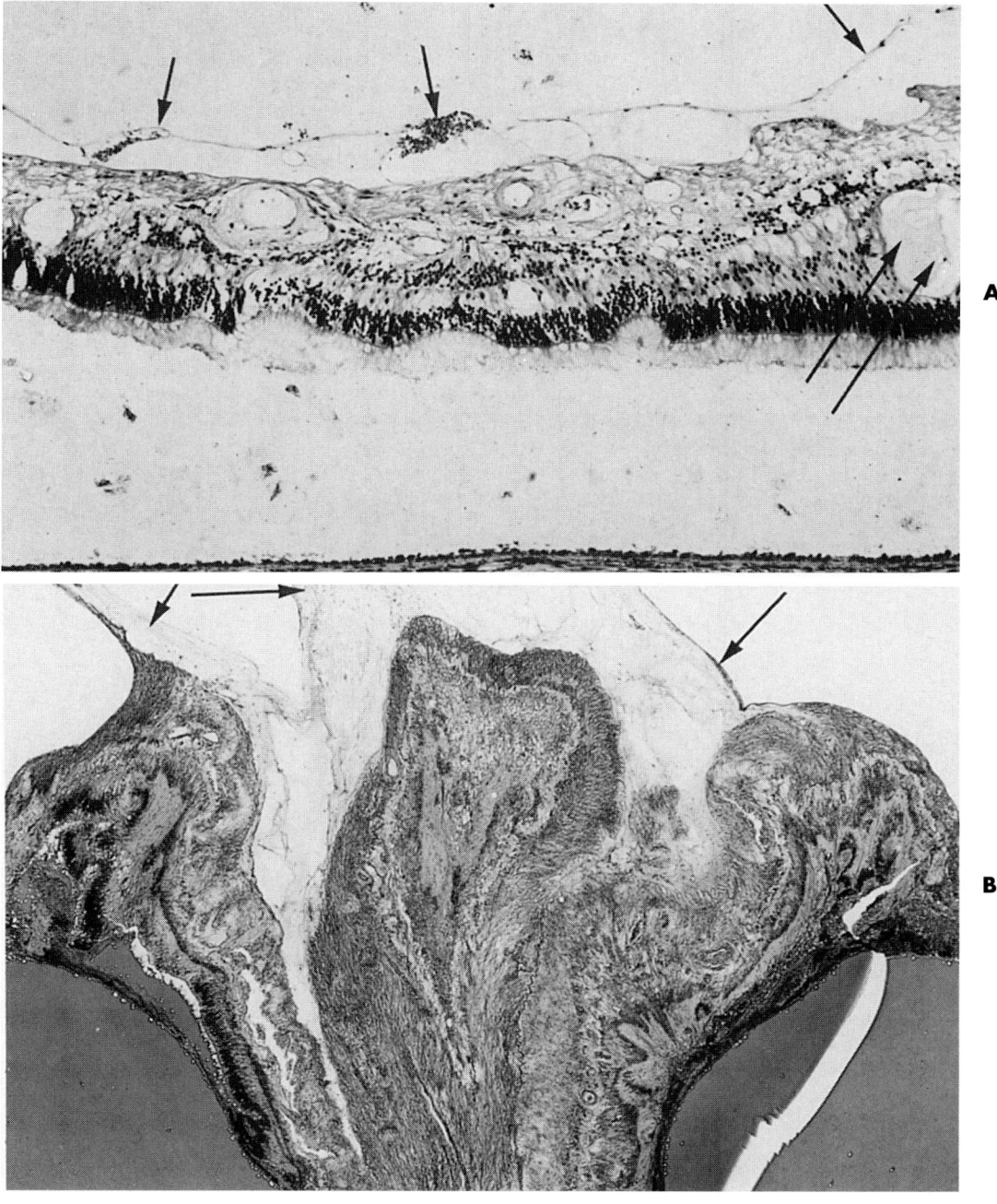

Fig. 30-73 A, Diabetic retinopathy with scattered exudates in deep retinal layers *(double arrows)* and early neovascularization extending from inner surface of retina into vitreous *(single arrows).* **B,** Diabetic proliferative retinopathy *(arrows)* has caused complete retinal detachment.

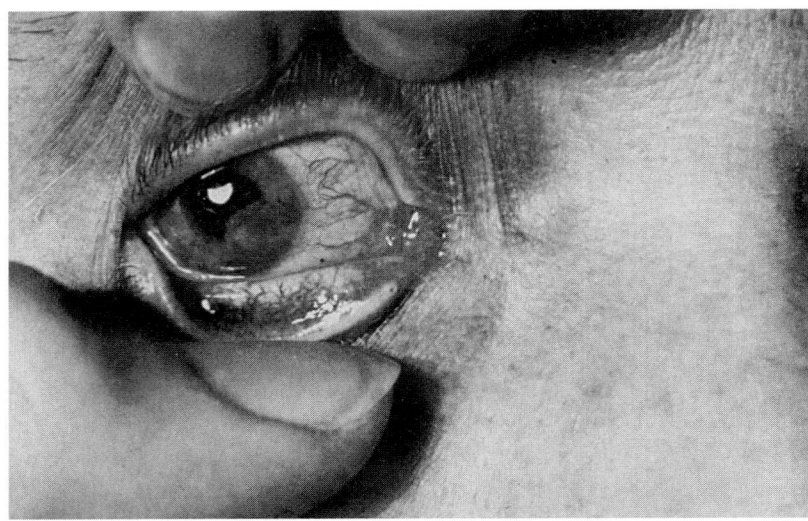

Fig. 30-74 Tumor of iris that had been observed over period of 10 years, during which time it became progressively larger and encroached on pupil. Iridectomy revealed it to be of spindle A cell type. Tumor recurred and necessitated enucleation for secondary glaucoma 15 years after iridectomy. (Courtesy Dr. M.E. Nugent, Bismarck, ND.)

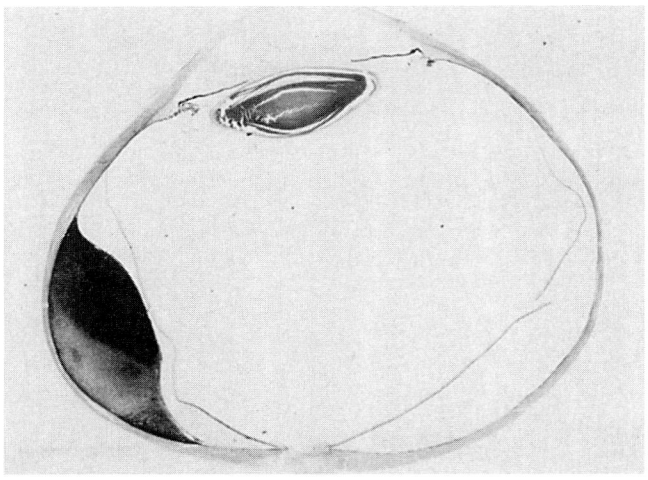

Fig. 30-75 Malignant melanoma of choroid that has not broken through Bruch's membrane but has elevated retina. Most of retinal separation observed in this section is artifactitious. (From Friedenwald JS, Wilder HC, Maumenee AE, Sanders TE, Keyes JEL, Hogan MJ, Owens WC, Owens EU: Ophthalmic pathology. An atlas and textbook. Philadelphia, 1952, W.B. Saunders Co.)

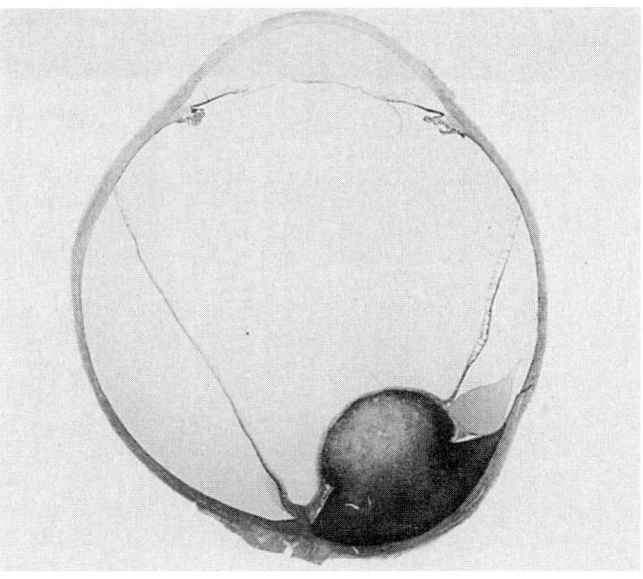

Fig. 30-76 Malignant melanoma of choroid that, by erupting through Bruch's membrane, has formed mushroom-shaped subretinal mass.

them arise on the basis of pre-existing benign nevi.[219-221] A syndrome has been described in which bilateral diffuse melanocytic uveal tumors are seen in association with systemic malignant neoplasms.[182]

Malignant melanoma may be located at any point in the uveal tract, with the choroid and ciliary body being more frequent locations than the iris. Melanoma of the iris presents as an elevated mass with varying degrees of pigmentation and often with distortion of the pupil and the presence of prominent vessels on the tumor (Fig. 30-74). Choroidal melanoma also may vary in pigmentation but characteristically is an irregular, slate-gray, solid, subretinal tumor producing an overlying retinal detachment and decreased vision (Figs. 30-75 and 30-76). It may appear as a discoid, globular, or mushroom-shaped mass. Less commonly, it spreads diffusely and extends out along scleral canals into the orbit[195,212] (Figs. 30-77 to 30-79).

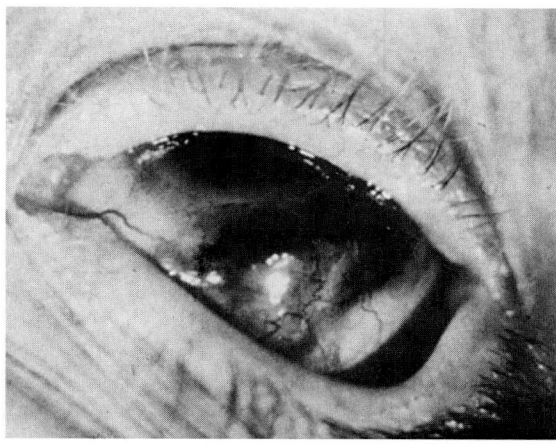

Fig. 30-77 Malignant melanoma of choroid breaking through sclera and presenting under conjunctiva. (From del Regato JA, Spjut HJ: Ackerman and del Regato's cancer, ed. 5. St. Louis, 1977, Mosby; courtesy Registry of Ophthalmic Pathology, Armed Forces Institute of Pathology, Washington, DC.)

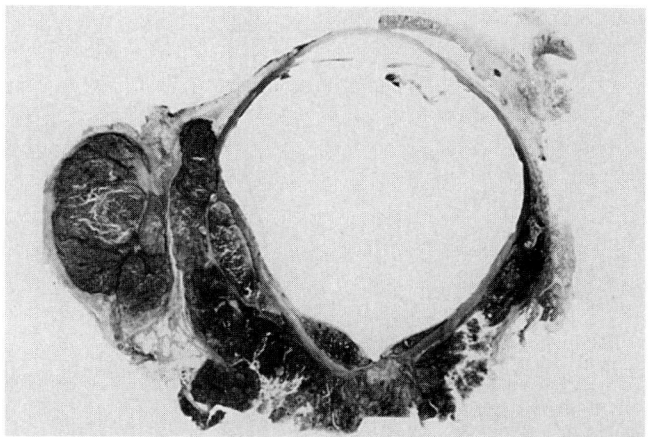

Fig. 30-78 Massive orbital extension from small choroid melanoma that has occurred as result of diffuse spread along natural passages through sclera and optic nerve. (From Friedenwald JS, Wilder HC, Maumenee AE, Sanders TE, Keyes JEL, Hogan MJ, Owens WC, Owens EU: Ophthalmic pathology. An atlas and textbook. Philadelphia, 1952, W.B. Saunders Co.)

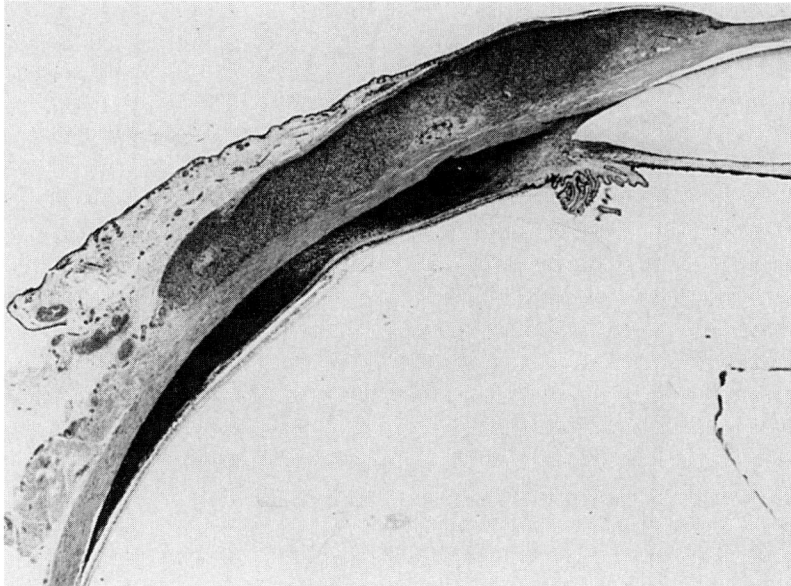

Fig. 30-79 Diffuse malignant melanoma of ciliary body and choroid that extended forward through scleral canals to form large subconjunctival mass that enroached on cornea.

Visual disturbance caused by retinal detachment is a much more frequent presenting complaint than the formation of an orbital tumor. Not infrequently the patient remains asymptomatic until the tumor has grown sufficiently to become necrotic and produce complications such as endophthalmitis, massive intraocular hemorrhage, and/or secondary glaucoma.

At times, malignant melanomas of the posterior uvea are not discovered until the enucleated eye is examined in the laboratory. Iris tumors are more often recognized early, for they can be seen by the patient and family long before other symptoms appear (Figs. 30-74 and 30-80).

Clinically, there are many lesions that simulate uveal malignant melanoma.[185,191,192,200] The most important are metastatic carcinoma, localized hemorrhage beneath the retina or between the pigment epithelium and choroid (Fig. 30-81), focal areas of proliferation of the retinal pigment epithelium (Fig. 30-82), posterior scleritis, and benign tumors such as nevi and hemangiomas.

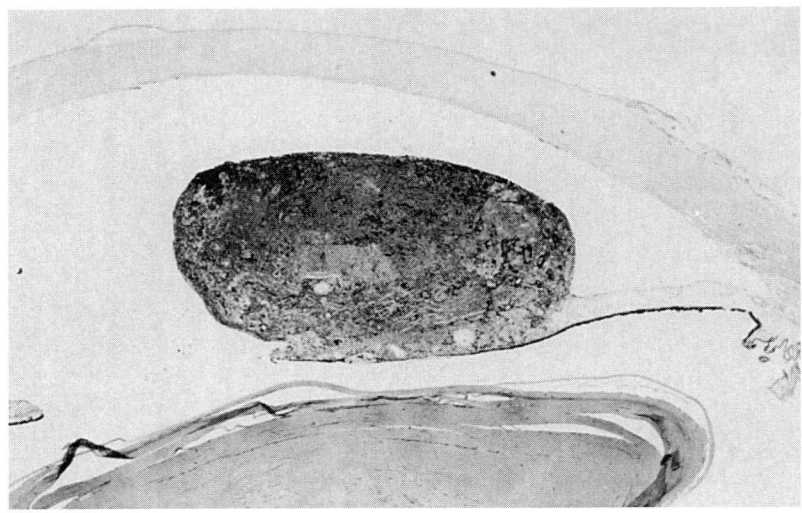

Fig. 30-80 Melanomas of iris are frequently visible through cornea. Hence their duration and rate of growth are often known by patient or family long before other subjective or objective manifestations appear.

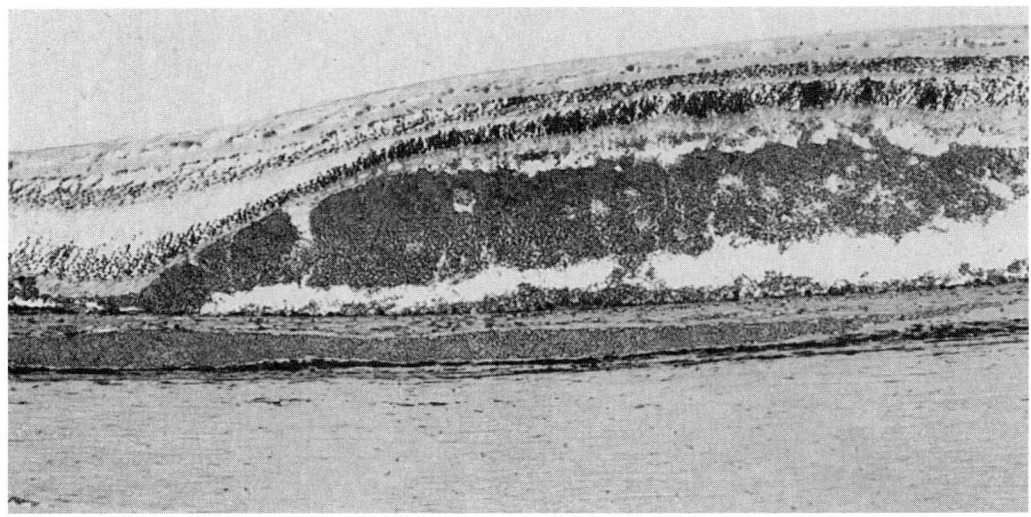

Fig. 30-81 Focal hemorrhage under retina was clinically mistaken for melanoma.

Microscopic features. Microscopically, uveal melanomas have been traditionally divided into three types: spindle A, spindle B, and epithelioid, which may occur singly or in combination.[184,209] Spindle A cells are slender, benign-appearing spindle-shaped cells that have relatively small fusiform nuclei and no nucleoli (Fig. 30-83). Frequently the chromatin is arranged in a linear fashion along the central axis of the nucleus.

Spindle B cells are larger and more pleomorphic, merging on the one hand with spindle A cells and on the other with epithelioid cells. Typically they possess large ovoid nuclei containing prominent nucleoli (Fig. 30-84). Mitotic activity may be more marked. Both spindle A and spindle B tumors tend to be quite cohesive. Some of these tumors have a distinctly fascicular pattern of growth (Figs. 30-85 and 30-86).

Epithelioid cells are still larger and more irregular (Fig. 30-87). They have an abundance of cytoplasm and may be truly gigantic. Multinucleated forms are not unusual. The nuclei are large, and their nucleoli are often strikingly prominent. In some tumors, many bizarre nuclei may be seen. Epithelioid cells are characteristically less cohesive than the spindle cells.

It is rather unusual for these tumors to be composed of a single cell type. Mixtures of spindle A and B cells or mixtures of spindle and epithelioid cells are common.

The microscopic differential diagnosis of primary uveal melanoma includes benign pigmented nevi[202,215] and intraocular metastases of cutaneous malignant melanoma.[187,189,205] In addition, amelanotic melanomas raise the differential diagnosis with metastatic carcinoma, and spin-

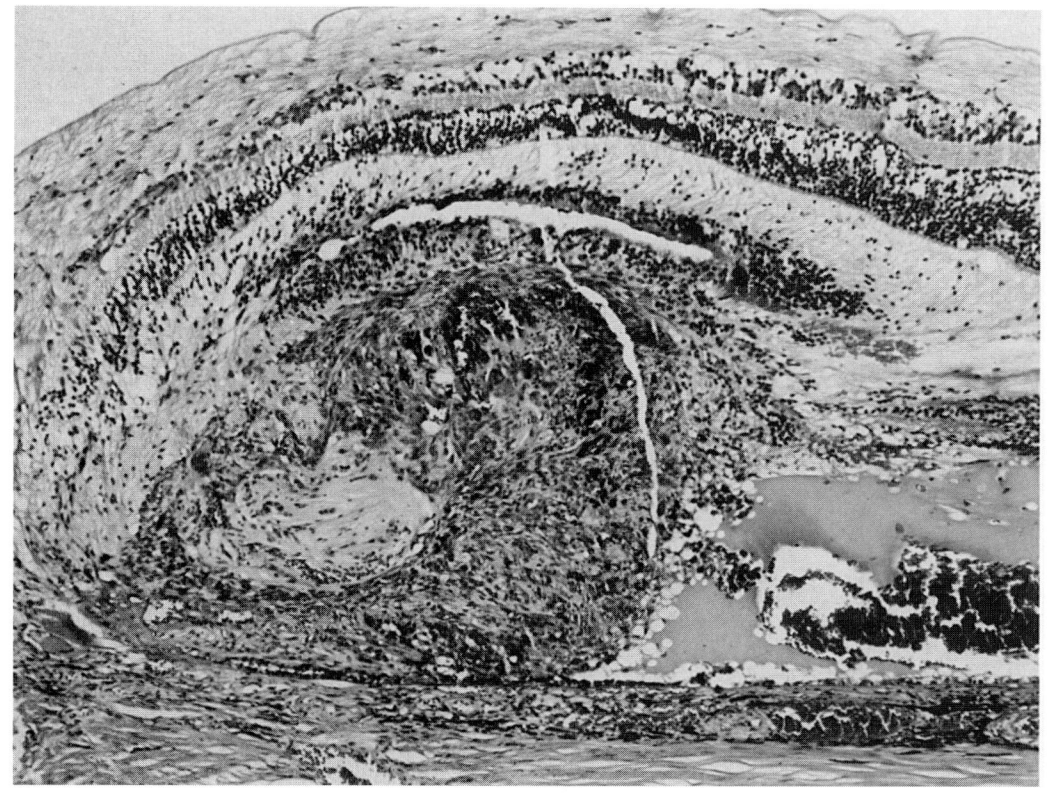

Fig. 30-82 Focal area of proliferation of retinal pigment epithelium that has elevated retina to simulate melanoma.

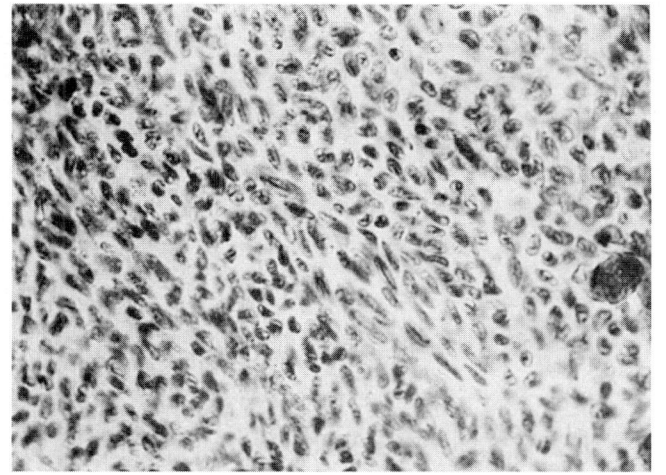

Fig. 30-83 Spindle A type of melanocytic cells.

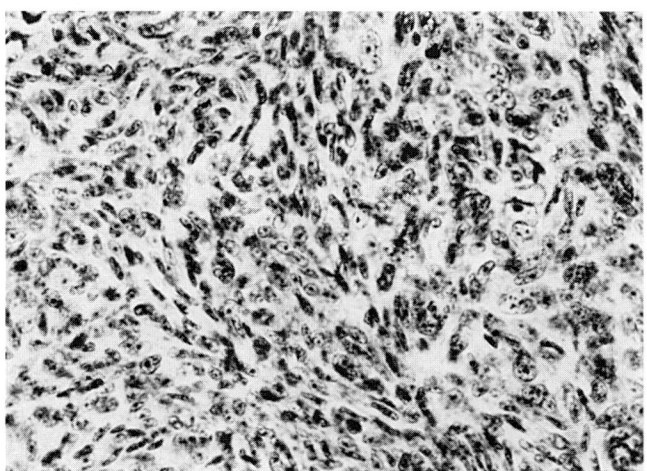

Fig. 30-84 Spindle B type of melanocytic cells, which are larger and more pleomorphic than spindle A cells. Most of nuclei contain prominent nucleoli.

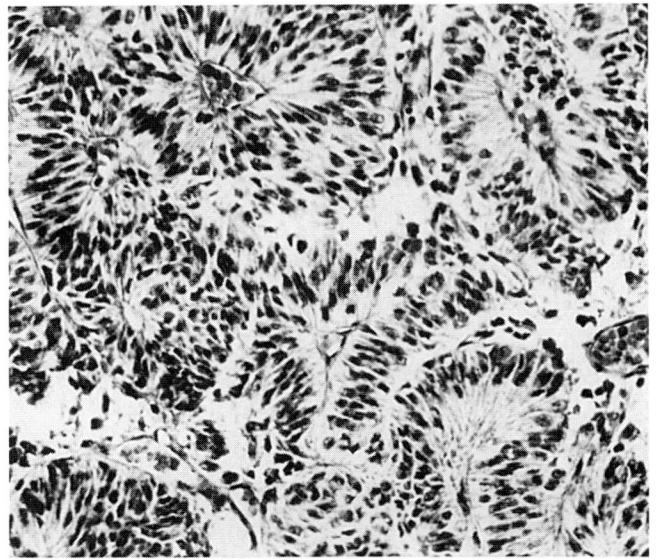

Fig. 30-85 Fascicular type of melanoma composed of spindle cells arranged about dilated capillaries.

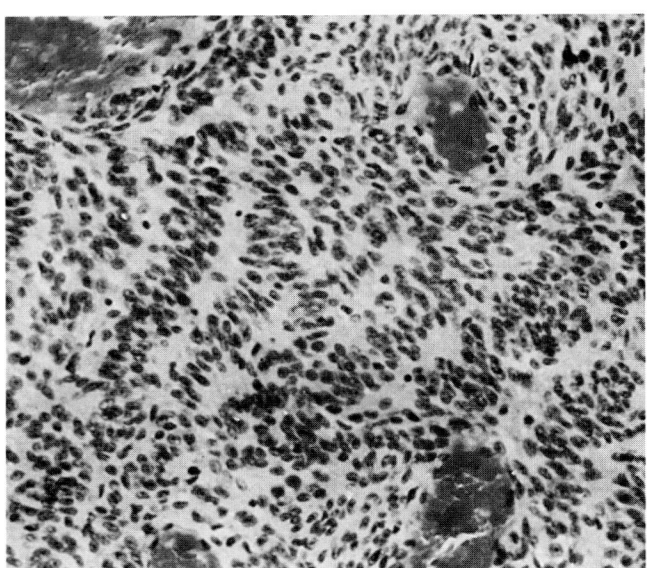

Fig. 30-86 Fascicular type of melanoma in which spindle-shaped cells are arranged with their nuclei in parallel rows.

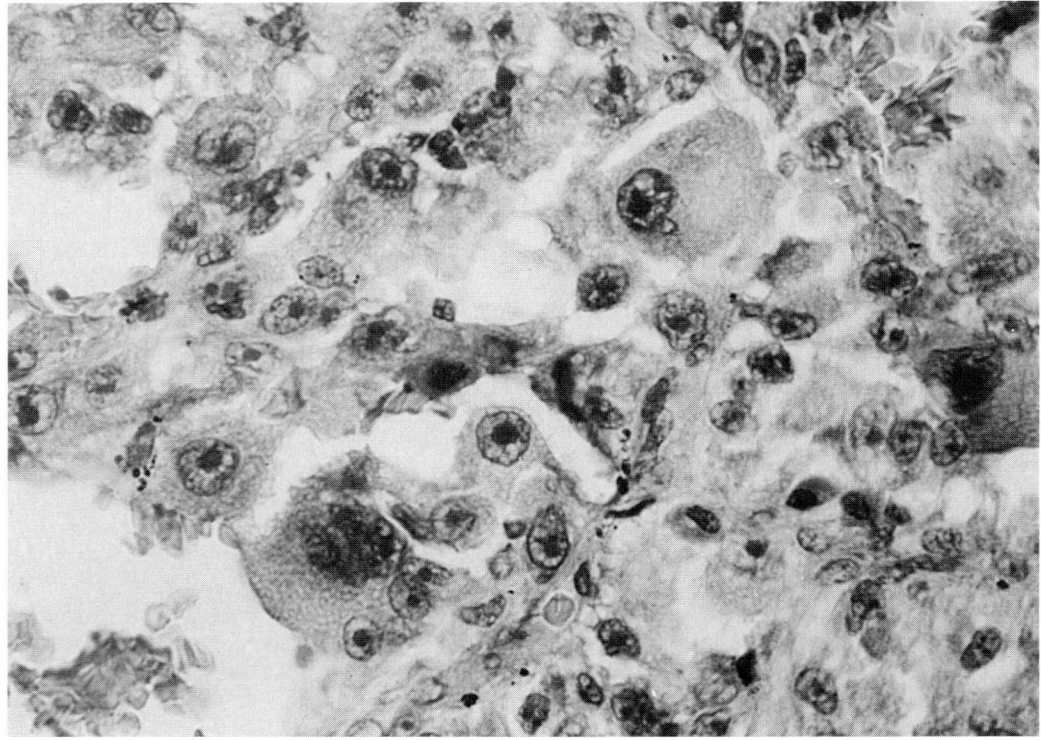

Fig. 30-87 Epithelioid cells with abundant cytoplasm, large nuclei, and extremely prominent nucleoli. (From del Regato JA, Spjut HJ: Ackerman and del Regato's cancer, ed. 6. St. Louis, 1985, Mosby.)

dle cell melanomas with a fascicular pattern of growth may resemble neurofibromas, schwannomas, or leiomyomas. The latter consideration applies particularly to tumors of the ciliary body.

Special techniques. Immunohistochemically, malignant melanomas are reactive for S-100 protein and HMB-45. They are also positive for vimentin and often for low-molecular-weight keratins, such as those demonstrated with Cam 5.2.[197]

Cytogenetically the consistent occurrence of monosomy 3 and trisomy 8q has been documented.[201]

DNA ploidy studies have shown that all spindle A melanomas are diploid, whereas a varying number of spindle B and epithelioid melanomas are aneuploid.[188]

Spread and metastases. The great tendency of uveal melanoma to spread along the course of the optic nerve has already been mentioned. The most common sites of distant metastatic involvement are the liver, lung, bone, and skin.[204]

Therapy. The standard treatment of melanoma of the choroid is removal of the eye. Small melanomas of the iris can be treated by iridectomy or iridocyclectomy.[196] The suggestion has been made that enucleation may stimulate the development of metastatic disease,[206,222,223] but this has not been confirmed in other studies.[206,214] It is not clear whether the use of adjunctive radiation therapy improves prognosis.[186]

Prognosis. The overall mortality from metastasis of melanoma of the uveal tract 15 years after enucleation is close to 50%.[208] The prognosis of this tumor depends on several factors:

1 *Cell type.* This is an extremely important parameter. There are no deaths with pure spindle A tumors, the proposal having therefore been made for these neoplasms to be regarded as spindle-cell nevi rather than melanomas.[209] The 5-year survival rate is 66% to 75% for spindle B melanomas, 50% for mixed (spindle B and epithelioid) melanomas, and 25% to 33% for pure epithelioid melanomas.

2 *Tumor size.* Larger tumors have a worse prognosis than smaller ones.[193,199,208,210] It has been shown that tumor dimension is a better predictor of prognosis than height or volume.[213]

3 *Location.* Tumors located in the iris have an excellent prognosis. This is in part related to their smaller size at the time of diagnosis and also to their less malignant cytologic features.[180,208] As a matter of fact, it has been suggested that most pigmented lesions of the iris traditionally designated as spindle A melanomas are benign nevi, as indicated previously.[203]

4 *Extension into the optic nerve.* This is said to be associated with a decreased survival, but there are conflicting data in this regard. A juxtapapillary location for the tumor does not result in significantly different survival rates if the optic nerve is not involved.[218]

5 *Extension into the sclera.* Extrascleral extension occurs in 10% to 28% of patients with choroidal melanoma.[210,211] In one series the 5-year mortality was 66% for patients with extrascleral extension and 33% for those with no extension.[217]

6 *Necrosis.* This is a sign of poor prognosis; it is usually associated with epithelioid type tumors.

7 *Lymphocytic infiltration.* The presence of a large number of lymphocytes in the tumor stroma has been found to be significantly associated with decreased survival.[190]

8 *Neovascularization.* Melanomas with "closed vascular loops" behave more aggressively than others, but this morphologic feature is associated with other unfavorable morphologic indicators, such as epithelioid cells.[194]

9 *Nucleolar prominence.* Nucleolar large size and pleomorphism are associated with aggressive behavior in uveal melanoma. Various methods have been devised to quantify this determination, which is still unlikely to be widely used.[198,207,216]

10 *Amount of pigmentation.* This feature does not have independent prognostic significance.

11 *DNA ploidy.* Most studies have found no significant correlations between DNA ploidy status and prognosis once the melanomas have been stratified into the major morphologic subtypes.[188]

Retinoblastoma and related lesions

General features. Retinoblastoma is the most common intraocular neoplasm of children. Generally believed to be congenital and derived from primitive neuroectodermal cells exhibiting retinal differentiation,[244,250,251] they nevertheless are seldom recognized until considerable growth has taken place.[229] They are usually diagnosed between the ages of 16 months and 2 years. About 60% of the cases are sporadic, and the other 40% are familial, with the predisposition to tumor development transmitted in an autosomal dominant pattern. Retinoblastoma will develop in 80% to 90% of persons who carry any one of a variety of mutant alleles associated with a predisposition to the tumor.[261]

The responsible gene has been located in chromosome 13q14 and designated the retinoblastoma (Rb) gene.[234,252] Mutations of this tumor-suppressing gene are known to cause both the hereditary and sporadic forms of retinoblastoma and have been implicated in the development of several other malignant tumors. Sporadic retinoblastoma is caused by a somatic mutation, whereas hereditary retinoblastoma is caused by a germ-cell mutation (most often a new one).[235,263] These mutations result in inactivation of the Rb protein, which is believed to function as a negative regulator of cell growth.[239,262,264] These findings have fully confirmed the brilliant "two-hit" hypothesis advanced by Knudson, which has become a paradigm of tumor development.

Clinical features. Retinoblastomas characteristically present as a leukocoria (white pupillary reflex) (Fig. 30-88) or less often as a strabismus when the tumor is in the macula. Rarely, extraocular extension with the formation of an orbital mass is the presenting manifestation.

Retinoblastomas may be flat and diffuse or elevated and may show multicentric foci of origin, especially in the hereditary type. They may protrude into the vitreous (endophytic type) (Fig. 30-89) often with vitreous seeding, or they may grow between the retina and the pigment epithelium

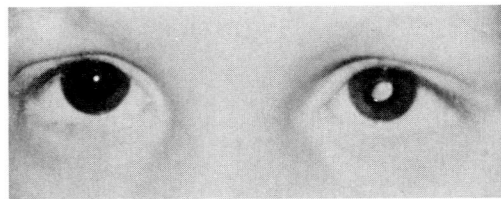

Fig. 30-88 Prominent white reflex attributed to retinoblastoma present in dilated pupil of left eye.

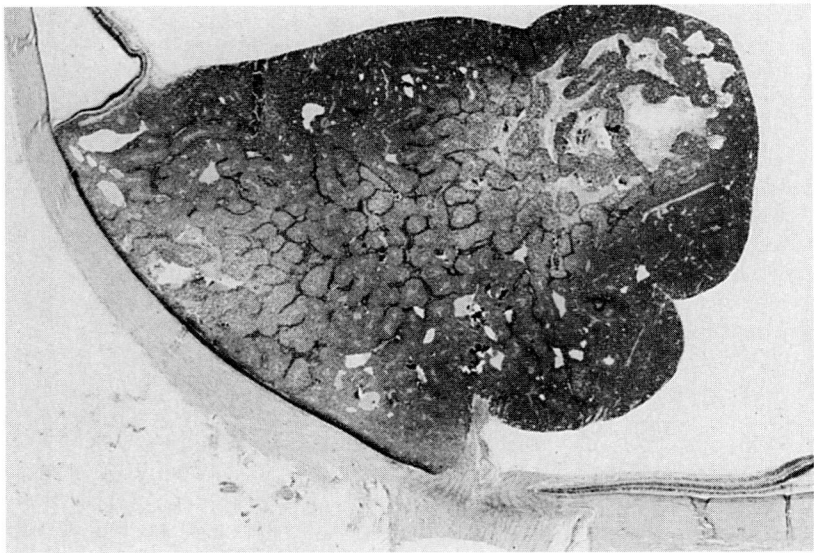

Fig. 30-89 Retinoblastoma presenting as highly cellular neoplasm with scanty stroma. Tumor tends to outgrow its blood supply, and irregular areas of necrosis are commonly observed.

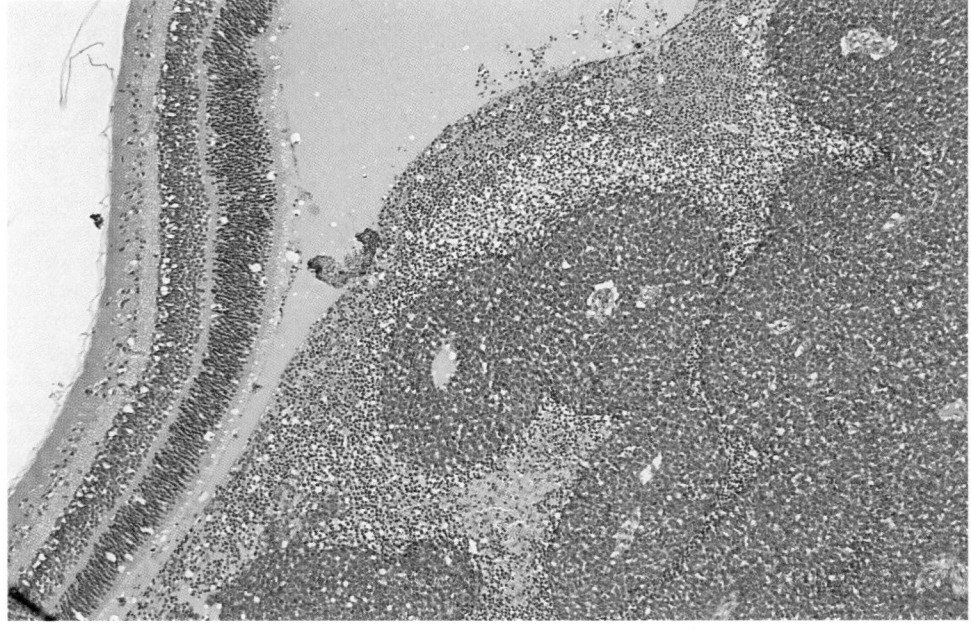

Fig. 30-90 Low-power view of retinoblastoma. There is a collar of viable cell about new nutrient vessels. The normal retina is seen on the left.

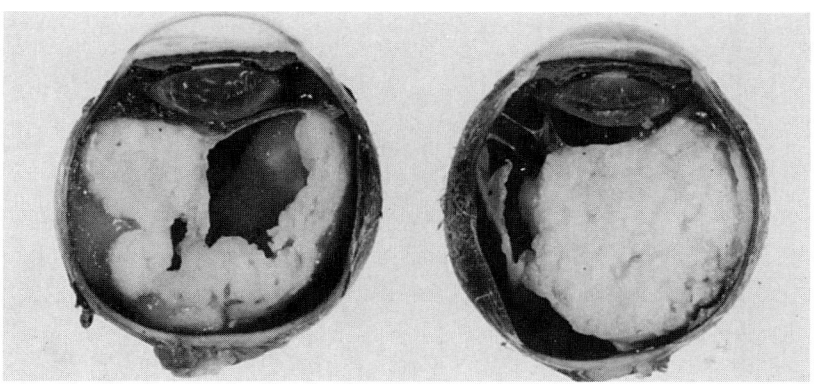

Fig. 30-91 Bilateral retinoblastoma showing presence of white mass consisting of detached retina and neoplastic tissue immediately behind lens in each eye.

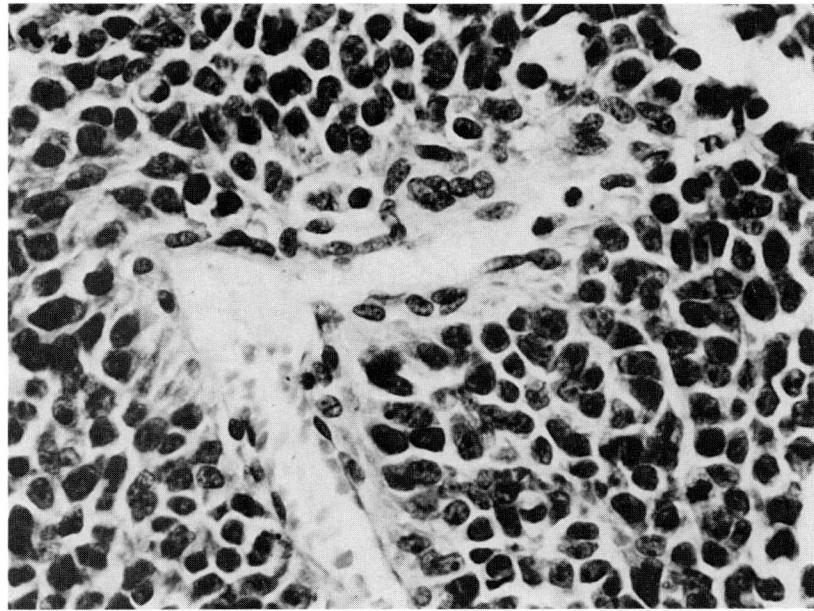

Fig. 30-92 Undifferentiated retinoblastomas composed of relatively large anaplastic cells have less favorable prognosis than those that contain highly differentiated rosettes. (From Friedenwald JS, Wilder HC, Maumenee AE, Sanders TE, Keyes JEL, Hogan MJ, Owens WC, Owens EU: Ophthalmic pathology. An atlas and textbook. Philadelphia, 1952, W.B. Saunders Co.)

(exophytic type). Since the tumors tend to outgrow their blood supply, necrosis is often extensive, and many minute foci of calcification are often present in these areas of necrosis (Fig. 30-90). In fact, these areas of calcification may be appreciated by x-ray examination prior to enucleation.

Bilaterality is present in 30% of all cases and in over 90% of the familial cases (Fig. 30-91). Some patients have presented with bilateral retinoblastoma and a morphologically similar intracranial neoplasm localized in the region of the pineal gland, in keeping with the "third eye" nature of the latter structure.[241] These are referred as *trilateral retinoblastomas*.[230,238]

The clinical differential diagnosis of retinoblastoma includes any disease process that leads to retinal detachment or a retrolental mass in a child under 6 years of age.[240,242] Lesions in this category include traumatic or idiopathic retinal detachments, retrolental fibroplasia, persistent hyperplastic primary vitreous, massive retinal gliosis, Coats' disease, nematodiasis, astrocytomas of tuberous sclerosis, and medulloepitheliomas. Some of these disorders are discussed elsewhere in this chapter.

Microscopic features. Microscopically the tumors are composed of dense masses of small round cells with hyperchromatic nuclei and scanty cytoplasm[245] (Fig. 30-92). Trabecular and nesting formations are common.[255] Hematoxyphilic deposits in and around blood vessel walls are often seen in necrotic areas, similar to those found in pulmonary small cell carcinomas.[231] A sign of differentiation

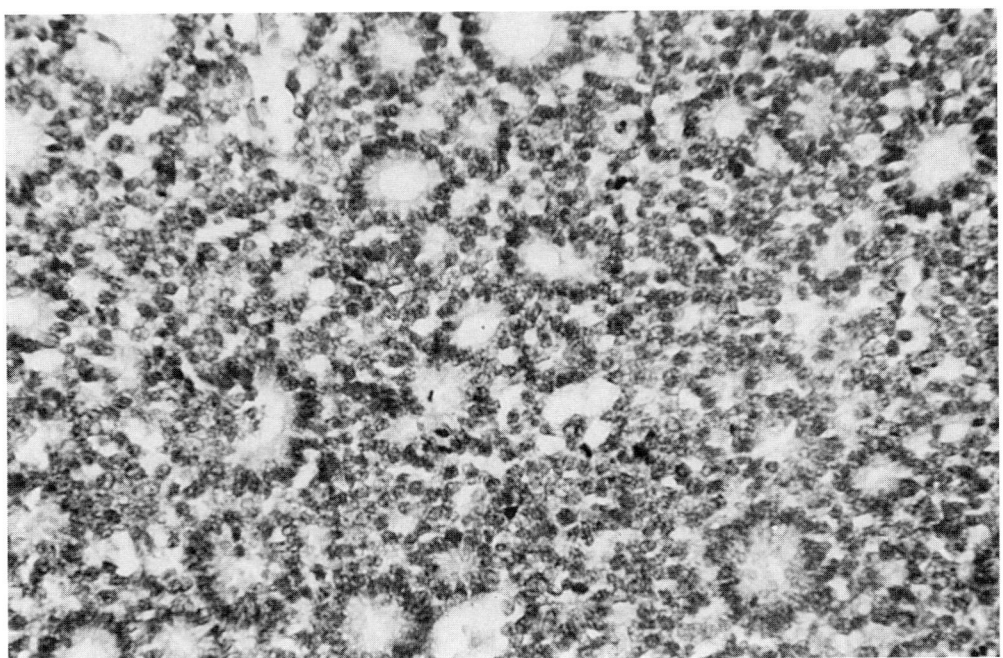

Fig. 30-93 Retinoblastoma with typical rosettes. (From Ackerman LV, del Regato JA: Cancer, ed. 6. St. Louis, 1985, Mosby.)

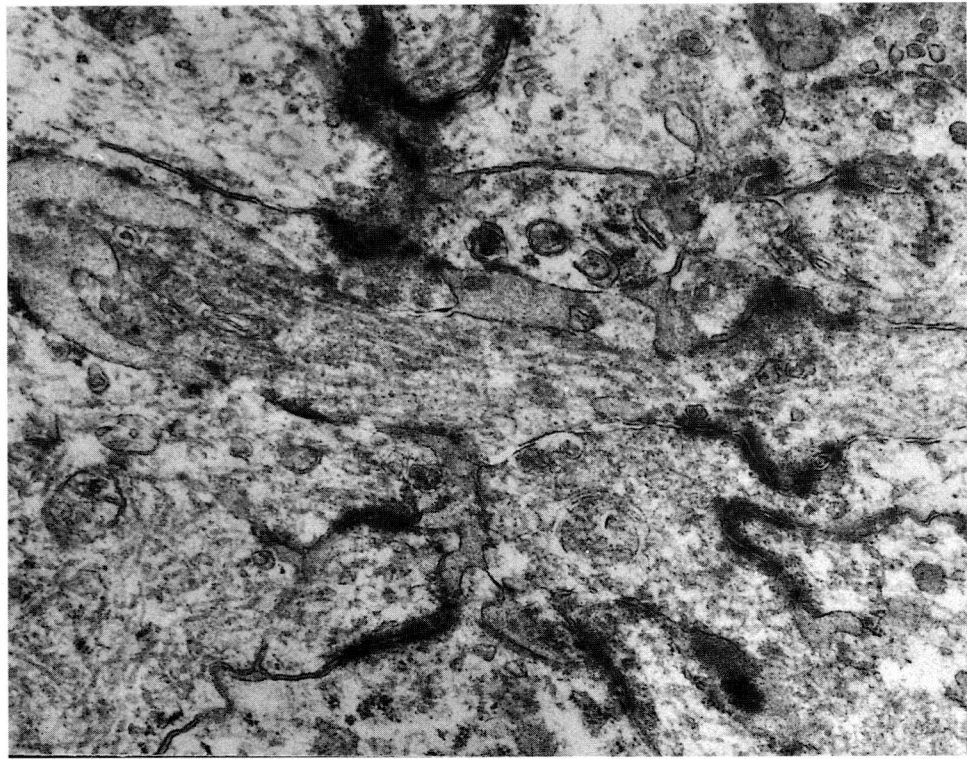

Fig. 30-94 Electron micrograph of retinoblastoma. Portion of the center of a rudimentary Flexner-Wintersteiner rosette illustrating a bulbous apical microtubule-containing cytoplasmic process and numerous cell junctions. (×20,800.) (Courtesy Dr. Robert A. Erlandson, Memorial Sloan-Kettering Cancer Center.)

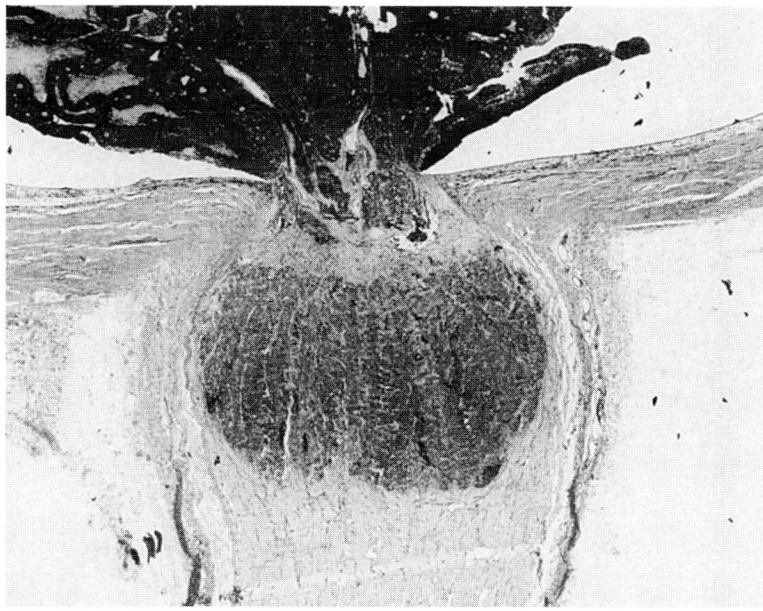

Fig. 30-95 Retinoblastomas exhibit definite tendency to spread out of globe by way of optic nerve. It is therefore of utmost importance for surgical pathologist to determine whether such optic nerve extension has occurred and, if it has, to what extent.

toward retinal structures is provided by the presence of so-called Flexner-Wintersteiner rosettes and fleurettes (Fig. 30-93). *Differentiated neuroblastoma* is characterized by the presence of a bipolar-like cell element.[237] Tumors showing an extreme degree of differentiation are designated as *retinocytomas* and regarded as benign.[248] These lesions carry the same genetic implications as conventional neuroblastomas; they present as small placoid, noninvasive lesions composed entirely of benign-appearing cells with numerous fleurettes, lacking necrosis or mitotic activity.[248]

Ultrastructural and other special techniques. Ultrastructurally, evidence of photodifferentiation has been found in the tumor cells of retinoblastoma[257,258] (Fig. 30-94). Immunohistochemically, there is reactivity for neuron-specific enolase, synaptophysin, S-100 protein, GFAP, myelin basic protein, and Leu7, in keeping with an origin from a pluripotential neuroectodermal cell that retains neuronal and glial features.[247,255,256,263a] In addition, allegedly specific markers of retinal differentiation such as retinal-binding protein, retinal S-antigen, interphotoreceptor retinal-binding protein, cone opsin, and rod opsin have been found in these tumors.[233,236,247,249] Interestingly, retinal S-antigen has also been detected in tumors of the pineal gland and in cerebellar medulloblastomas.[243,249] Further evidence of the retinal nature of this tumor has been obtained in vitro, where differentiation toward photoreceptors has been observed spontaneously or after the addition of differentiating agents.[259]

Spread and metastases. Retinoblastoma has a tendency to invade the optic nerve from which it can extend to the brain or be carried there by the subarachnoid fluid.[254] Large exophytic tumors with secondary glaucoma are at highest risk for optic nerve invasion.[254] Retinoblastoma can also invade the uveal tract. Distant metastases can be limited to the cranial vault or involve distant sites, particularly the skeletal system.[246]

Treatment. The treatment depends on the extent of the disease.[253] Early cases can be managed with conservative measures aimed at preserving the vision, such as unilateral radiation, cryopexy, or xenon arc photocoagulation.[227] When the tumor is so large that the eye is no longer salvageable, enucleation should be performed.[266] If tumor has extended to the surgically cut end of the nerve, irradiation of the orbit and systemic chemotherapy are performed. In patients with bilateral retinoblastoma, the less affected eye is treated with radiotherapy, at times in combination with chemotherapy. Other bilateral cases have been treated with simultaneous bilateral irradiation.[224,225,228] The success rate for life of the patient and for preservation of vision is quite good. If tumor recurrences develop, these are treated with photocoagulation, cryotherapy, and cobalt disks.

Prognosis. The 5-year survival of unilateral retinoblastoma following adequate treatment is over 90% and slightly less for the bilateral cases.[265,266] Two morphologic features indicative of a less favorable prognosis are (1) invasion of optic nerve (Fig. 30-95) and (2) massive invasion of the uveal tract. Ordinarily the ophthalmic surgeon who suspects a retinoblastoma will try to obtain a long segment of optic nerve attached to the globe. Transverse sections of the nerve should be examined microscopically at the level of surgical transection and at various levels along the nerve. The prognosis is poor in tumors that have invaded the nerve and extended to the plane of transection or into the meninges.[251]

Long-term survivors have a greater incidence of development of malignant tumors. The incidence has ranged from 6% to 20% after 10 years and in one series has reached 90% at 30 years. The most common types have been osteosar-

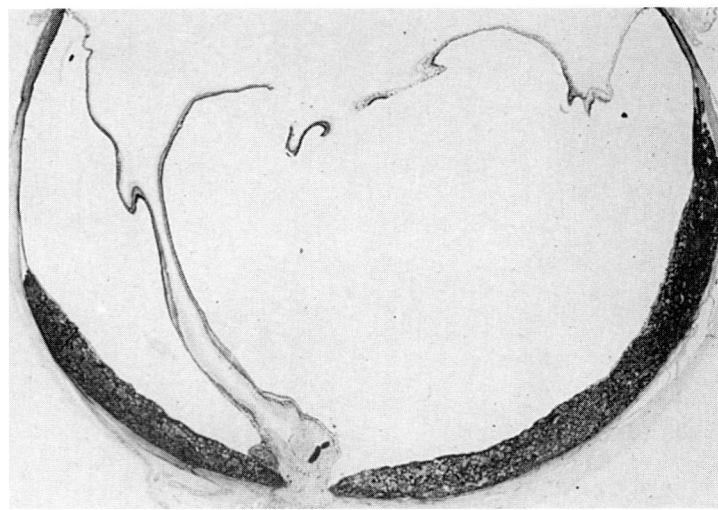

Fig. 30-96 Metastatic carcinoma from breast producing diffuse thickening of choroid posteriorly.

coma and rhabdomyosarcoma, but several other types have been encountered, including rhabdoid tumors.[226,260] This predisposition for a second malignancy is seen almost exclusively with the hereditary form of the disease.[232]

Massive retinal gliosis. Massive retinal gliosis is a relatively uncommon condition in which a large elevated scar develops near the disc and posterior pole following hemorrhage (e.g., in newborn) or inflammation.

Coats' disease. Coats' disease is an exudative retinopathy associated with retinal detachment and foci of telangiectatic retinal vessels. It is usually unilateral and occurs in young children, more often in males.

Lymphoid tumors and tumorlike conditions

Abnormalities of intraocular tissues are present in about 50% of patients with leukemia at autopsy.[267] This is in the form of leukemic infiltrates and hemorrhages, particularly in the choroid and retina.[267,272]

Intraocular *malignant lymphoma* is a rare disease. In over 90% of the cases the eye lesion heralds the presence or development of extraocular lymphoma, which is located in the central nervous system in one half or more of the cases.[269] Sometimes the lymphomatous process involves preferentially the optic nerve.[268]

Reactive lymphoid hyperplasia can also occur within the ocular globe[270,271]; the criteria for distinguishing it from lymphoma are similar to those applied elsewhere.

Other primary tumors

Fuchs' adenoma (benign ciliary epithelioma, Fuchs' epithelioma, coronal adenoma) is a benign tumor of the ciliary body usually found incidentally in a surgically enucleated eye or on postmortem examination. Microscopically it is formed by interlacing trabeculae of uniform, nonpigmented ciliary epithelial cells surrounded by an amorphous hyaline PAS-positive material.[278]

Medulloepithelioma, also known as diktyoma, is a rare tumor that histologically resembles the embryonal retina;

most cases arise from the ciliary epithelium, but a few have been found in the optic nerve or retina.

Leiomyomas can develop in the ciliary body or the iris. *Hemangiomas, hemangioblastomas* (as a component of von Hippel–Lindau disease), *neurofibromas,* and *astrocytomas* are sometimes found in the retina.[275-277]

Juvenile xanthogranuloma can occur in the iris and result in spontaneous hyphema and/or secondary glaucoma.[274] It occurs almost exclusively in young children and is associated with skin lesions of similar microscopic appearance.[279]

Glioneuroma has been described in the iris and ciliary body,[273] and *malignant lymphoma* has been reported involving the entire uveal tract.[276a]

Metastatic tumors

The intraocular tissues can be involved by metastatic carcinoma and, less commonly, by metastatic cutaneous melanoma and metastatic sarcoma. In fact, if one were to routinely do serial sections on all autopsy eyes, cases of metastatic carcinoma would outnumber the primary tumors. The difference, of course, is that most of the patients were asymptomatic for ocular symptoms while alive. The most common primary lesions involved are in the breast in the female and in the lung in the male, with the gastrointestinal tract next in frequency.[280-284] Occasionally the ocular metastasis may be the initial manifestation of the disease, and the primary lesion is discovered only after the eye has been enucleated.

The posterior choroid is the most common site for these metastases (Fig. 30-96). Anterior uveal involvement is much less common, and retinal metastases are rare. Diffuse thickening of the choroid along both sides of the optic nerve is the most common presentation, but bulky tumor masses resembling malignant melanomas also may be observed.

Cytology

In certain cases the pathologist may be called on to examine material that has been aspirated from either the aqueous or the vitreous and has been passed through a Millipore filter. Cases in which this has proved useful include large cell lymphoma,[285] retinoblastoma,[287] and phacolytic glaucoma.[286]

REFERENCES
NORMAL ANATOMY

1 Apple D, Rabb M: Clinicopathologic correlation of ocular disease. A text and stereoscopic atlas, ed 2. St. Louis, 1978, Mosby.

2 Beck K, Jensen OA: External ocular tumors. Textbook and atlas. Philadelphia, 1978, W.B. Saunders Co.

3 Duane T, ed: Clinical ophthalmology, rev ed. New York, 1988, Harper & Row, Publishers, Inc.

4 Ferry AP, ed: Ocular and adnexal tumors. Int Ophthalmol Clin **12:**1-269, 1972.

5 Fine B, Yanoff M: Ocular histology. A text and atlas, ed 2. New York, 1979, Harper & Row, Publishers, Inc.

6 Henderson JW: Orbital tumors. Philadelphia, 1973, W.B. Saunders Co.

7 Hogan MJ, Alvarado JA, Weddell JE: Histology of the human eye. An atlas and textbook. Philadelphia, 1971, W.B. Saunders Co.

8 Hogan MJ, Zimmerman LE: Ophthalmic pathology. An atlas and textbook. ed 2. Philadelphia, 1962, W.B. Saunders Co.

9 Jakobiec FA: Ocular and adnexal tumors. Birmingham, AL, 1978, Aesculapius Publishing Co.

10 Mclean IW, Burnier MN, Zimmerman LE, Jakobiec FA: Atlas of tumor pathology. Tumors of the eye and ocular adnexa, third series. Fascicle 12, Bethesda, 1994, Armed Forces Institute of Pathology.

11 Peyman G, Apple D, Sanders D: Intraocular tumors. New York, 1977, Appleton-Century-Crofts.

12 Reese AB: Tumors of the eye, ed 3. New York, 1976, Harper & Row, Publishers, Inc.

13 Spencer WH, Font RL, Green WR, Homes EL Jr, Jakobiec FA, Zimmerman LE: Ophthalmic pathology. An atlas and textbook, ed 3, 6 vols. Philadelphia, 1985-1986, W.B. Saunders Co.

14 Yanoff M, Fine B: Ocular pathology. A text and atlas. Philadelphia, 1989, Lippincott.

EYELIDS
Inflammation

15 Codère F, Lee RD, Anderson RL: Necrobiotic xanthogranuloma of the eyelid. Arch Ophthalmol **101:**60-63, 1983.

16 Riddle PJ, Font RL, Johnson FB, McLean IW: Silica granuloma of eyelid and ocular adnexa. Arch Ophthalmol **99:**683-689, 1981.

17 Ross MJ, Cohen KL, Peiffer RL Jr, Grimson BS: Episcleral and orbital pseudorheumatoid nodules. Arch Ophthalmol **101:**418-421, 1983.

Tumors and tumorlike lesions
Tumors and tumorlike lesions of surface epithelium

18 Aurora AL, Blodi FC: Lesions of the eyelids. A clinicopathologic study. Surv Ophthalmol **15:**94-104, 1970.

19 Boniuk M: Tumors of the eyelids. Int Ophthalmol Clin **2:**239-317, 1962.

20 Boniuk M, Zimmerman LE: Eyelid tumors with reference to lesions confused with squamous cell carcinoma. II. Inverted follicular keratosis. Arch Ophthalmol **69:**698-707, 1963.

21 Boniuk M, Zimmerman LE: Eyelid tumors with reference to lesions confused with squamous cell carcinoma. III. Keratoacanthoma. Arch Ophthalmol **77:**29-40, 1967.

22 Caya JG, Hidayat AA, Weiner JM: A clinicopathologic study of 21 cases of adenoid squamous cell carcinoma of the eyelid and periorbital region. Am J Ophthalmol **99:**291-297, 1985.

23 Chaflin J, Putterman AM: Frozen section control in the surgery of basal cell carcinoma of the eyelid. Am J Ophthalmol **87:**802-809, 1979.

24 Kwitko ML, Boniuk M, Zimmerman LE: Eyelid tumors with reference to lesions confused with squamous cell carcinoma. I. Incidence and errors in diagnosis. Arch Ophthalmol **69:**693-697, 1963.

25 Searl SS, Boynton JR, Markowitch W, di Sant'Agnese PA: Malignant Merkel cell neoplasm of the eyelid. Arch Ophthalmol **102:**907-911, 1984.

Adnexal tumors

26 Doxanas MT, Green WR: Sebaceous gland carcinoma. Review of 40 cases. Arch Ophthalmol **102:**245-249, 1984.

27 Hidayat AA, Font RL: Trichilemmoma of eyelid and eyebrow. A clinicopathologic study of 31 cases. Arch Ophthalmol **98:**844-847, 1980.

28 Langer K, Konrad K, Smolle J: Multiple apocrine hidrocystomas on the eyelids. Am J Dermatopathol **11:**570-573, 1989.

29 Rao NA, Hidayat AA, McLean IW, Zimmerman LE: Sebaceous carcinomas of the ocular adnexa. A clinicopathologic study of 104 cases, with five-year follow-up data. Hum Pathol **13:**113-122, 1982.

30 Rodgers IR, Jakobiec FA, Krebs W, Hornblass A, Gingold MP: Papillary oncocytoma of the eyelid. A previously undescribed tumor of apocrine gland origin. Ophthalmology **95:**1071-1076, 1988.

31 Russel WG, Page DL, Hough AJ, Rogers LW: Sebaceous carcinoma of meibomian gland origin. The diagnostic importance of pagetoid spread of neoplastic cells. Am J Clin Pathol **73:**504-511, 1980.

32 Snow SN, Reizner GT: Mucinous eccrine carcinoma of the eyelid. Cancer **70:**2099-2104, 1992.

33 Wolfe JT III, Yeatts RP, Wick MR, Campbell RJ, Waller RR: Sebaceous carcinoma of the eyelid. Errors in clinical and pathologic diagnosis. Am J Surg Pathol **8:**597-606, 1984.

34 Wright JD, Font RL: Mucinous sweat gland adenocarcinoma of eyelid. A clinicopathologic study of 21 cases with histochemical and electron microscopic observations. Cancer **44:**1757-1768, 1979.

Melanocytic tumors

35 Henkind P, Friedman A: External ocular pigmentation. Int Ophthalmol Clin **11:**87-111, 1971.

36 Pomeranz GA, Bunt AH, Kalina RE: Multifocal choroidal melanoma in ocular melanocytosis. Arch Ophthalmol **99:**857-863, 1981.

Lymphoid tumors and tumorlike conditions

37 Stenson S, Ramsay DL: Ocular findings in mycosis fungoides. Arch Ophthalmol **99:**272-277, 1981.

Mesenchymal tumors and tumorlike conditions

38 Fett DR, Putterman AM: Primary localized amyloidosis presenting as an eyelid margin tumor. Arch Ophthalmol **104:**584-585, 1986.

39 Smith ME, Zimmerman LE: Amyloidosis of the eyelid and conjunctiva. Arch Ophthalmol **75:**42-56, 1966.

40 Sorenson RL, Spencer WH, Stewart WB, Miller WW, Kleinhenz RJ: Intravascular papillary endothelial hyperplasia of the eyelid. Arch Ophthalmol **101:**1728-1730, 1983.

LACRIMAL PASSAGES
Canaliculitis and dacryocystitis

41 Harris GJ, Williams GA, Clarke GP: Sarcoidosis of the lacrimal sac. Arch Ophthalmol **99:**1198-1201, 1981.

Tumors

42 Lamping KA, Albert DM, Ni C, Fournier G: Oxyphil cell adenomas. Three case reports. Arch Ophthalmol **102:**263-265, 1984.

43 Lloyd WC III, Leone CR Jr: Malignant melanoma of the lacrimal sac. Arch Ophthalmol **102:**104-107, 1984.

44 Ni C, Wagoner MD, Wang W-J, Albert DM, Fan CO, Robinson N: Mucoepidermoid carcinomas of the lacrimal sac. Arch Ophthalmol **101:**1572-1574, 1983.

45 Ryan SJ, Font RL: Primary epithelial neoplasms of the lacrimal sac. Am J Ophthalmol **76:**73-88, 1973.

LACRIMAL GLAND
Mikulicz's disease

46 Font RL, Yanoff M, Zimmerman LE: Benign lymphoepithelial lesion of the lacrimal gland and its relationship to Sjögren's syndrome. Am J Clin Pathol **48:**365-376, 1967.

47 Godwin JT: Benign lymphoepithelial lesion of the parotid gland (adenolymphoma, chronic inflammation, lymphoepithelioma, lymphocytic tumor, Mikulicz's disease). Cancer **5:**1089-1103, 1952.

48 Meyer D, Yanoff M, Hanno H: Differential diagnosis in Mikulicz syndrome, Mikulicz's disease, and similar disease entities. Am J Ophthalmol **70:**516-524, 1971.

Tumors

49 DeRosa G, Zeppa P, Tranfa F, Bonavolontà G: Acinic cell carcinoma arising in a lacrimal gland. First case report. Cancer **57:**1988-1991, 1986.

50 Forrest AW: Pathologic criteria for effective management of epithelial lacrimal gland tumors. Am J Ophthalmol **71:**178-192, 1971.

51 Gamel JW, Font RL: Adenoid cystic carcinoma of the lacrimal gland. The clinical significance of a basaloid histologic pattern. Hum Pathol **13:**219-225, 1982.

52 Iwamoto T, Jakobiec FA: A comparative ultrastructural study of the normal lacrimal gland and its epithelial tumors. Hum Pathol **13:**236-262, 1982.

53 Ludwig ME, LiVolsi VA, McMahon RT: Malignant mixed tumor of the lacrimal gland. Am J Surg Pathol **3:**457-462, 1979.

54 Perzin KH, Jakobiec FA, LiVolsi VA, Desjardins L: Lacrimal gland malignant mixed tumors (carcinomas arising in benign mixed tumors). A clinico-pathologic study. Cancer **45:**2593-2606, 1980.

55 Sanders TE, Ackerman LV, Zimmerman LE: Epithelial tumors of the lacrimal gland. A comparison of the pathologic and clinical behavior with those of the salivary glands. Am J Surg **104:**657-665, 1962.

56 Zimmerman LE, Sanders TE, Ackerman LV: Epithelial tumors of the lacrimal gland. Prognostic and therapeutic significance of histologic types. Int Ophthalmol Clin **2:**337-367, 1962.

ORBIT

57 Char DH: Management of orbital tumors. Mayo Clin Proc **68:**1081-1096, 1993.

58 Shields JA, Bakewell B, Augsburger JJ, Flanagan JC: Classification and incidence of space-occupying lesions of the orbit. A survey of 645 biopsies. Arch Ophthalmol **102:**1606-1611, 1984.

59 Zajdela A, Vielh P, Schlienger P, Haye C: Fine-needle cytology of 292 palpable orbital and eyelid tumors. Am J Clin Pathol **93:**100-104, 1990.

Dysthyroid ophthalmopathy

60 Bahn RS, Heufelder AE: Pathogenesis of Graves' ophthalmopathy. N Engl J Med **329:**1468-1475, 1993.

Inflammatory processes

61 Blodi F, Gass D: Inflammatory pseudotumor of the orbit. Trans Am Acad Ophthalmol Otolaryngol **71:**303-323, 1967.

62 Eshaghian J, Anderson RL: Sinus involvement in inflammatory orbital pseudotumor. Arch Ophthalmol **99:**627-630, 1981.

63 Foucar E, Rosai J, Dorfman RF: The ophthalmologic manifestations of sinus histiocytosis with massive lymphadenopathy. Am J Ophthalmol **87:**354-367, 1979.

64 Frohman LP, Kupersmith MJ, Lang J, Reede D, Bergeron RT, Aleksic S, Trasi S: Intracranial extension and bone destruction in orbital pseudotumor. Arch Ophthalmol **104:**380-384, 1986.

65 Garner A: Pathology of "pseudotumors" of the orbit. A review. J Clin Pathol **26:**639-648, 1973.

66 Grimson BS, Simons KB: Orbital inflammation, myositis, and systemic lupus erythematosus. Arch Ophthalmol **101:**736-738, 1983.

67 Harris GJ: Subperiosteal abscess of the orbit. Arch Ophthalmol **101:**751-757, 1983.

68 McCarthy JM, White VA, Harris G, Simons KB, Kennerdell J, Rootman J: Idiopathic sclerosing inflammation of the orbit. Immunohistologic analysis and comparison with retroperitoneal fibrosis. Mod Pathol **6:**581-587, 1993.

69 Parke DW II, Font RL, Boniuk M, McCrary JA III: "Cholesteatoma" of the orbit. Arch Ophthalmol **100:**612-616, 1982.

Primary tumors
Mesenchymal tumors and tumorlike conditions

70 Croxatto JO, Font RL: Hemangiopericytoma of the orbit. A clinicopathologic study of 30 cases. Hum Pathol **13:**210-218, 1982.

71 Dorfman DM, To K, Dickersin GR, Rosenberg AE, Pilch BZ: Solitary fibrous tumor of the orbit. Am J Surg Pathol **18:**281-287, 1994.

72 Font RL, Hidayat AA: Fibrous histiocytoma of the orbit. A clinicopathologic study of 150 cases. Hum Pathol **13:**199-209, 1982.

73 Font RL, Jurco S III, Zimmerman LE: Alveolar soft-part sarcoma of the orbit. A clinicopathologic analysis of seventeen cases and a review of the literature. Hum Pathol **13:**569-579, 1982.

74 Font RL, Wheeler TM, Boniuk M: Intravascular papillary endothelial hyperplasia of the orbit and ocular adnexa. A report of five cases. Arch Ophthalmol **101:**1731-1736, 1983.

75 Font RL, Zimmerman LE: Nodular fasciitis of the eye and adnexa. A report of ten cases. Arch Ophthalmol **75:**475-481, 1966.

76 Forrest AW: Tumors following radiation about the eye. Int Ophthalmol Clin **2:**543-553, 1962.

77 Henderson JW, Farrow GM: Primary orbital hemangiopericytoma. An aggressive and potentially malignant neoplasm. Arch Ophthalmol **96:**666-673, 1978.

78 Hufnagel T, Ma L, Kuo T-T: Orbital angiosarcoma with subconjunctival presentation. Report of a case and literature review. Ophthalmology **94:**72-77, 1987.

79 Jacobs JL, Merriam JC, Chadburn A, Garvin J, Housepian E, Hilal SK: Mesenchymal chondrosarcoma of the orbit. Report of three new cases and review of the literature. Cancer **73:**399-405, 1994.

80 Knowles D, Jakobiec F, Potter G, Jones IS: Ophthalmic striated muscle neoplasms. Surv Ophthalmol **21:**219-261, 1976.

81 Krohel GB, Rosenberg PN, Wright JE, Smith RS: Localized orbital neurofibromas. Am J Ophthalmol **100:**458-464, 1985.

82 Shields JA, Kapustiak J, Arbizo V, Augsburger JJ, Schnitzer RE: Orbital neurilemoma with extension through the superior orbital fissure. Arch Ophthalmol **104:**871-873, 1986.

83 Weiner JM, Hidayat AA: Juvenile fibrosarcoma of the orbit and eyelid. A study of five cases. Arch Ophthalmol **101:**253-259, 1983.

84 Westra WH, Gerald WL, Rosai J: Solitary fibrous tumor. Consistent CD34 immunoreactivity and occurrence in the orbit. Am J Surg Pathol **18:**992-998, 1994.

85 Wilson WB, Roloff J, Wilson HL: Primary peripheral neuroepithelioma of the orbit with intracranial extension. Cancer **62:**2595-2601, 1988.

86 Wojno T, Tenzel RR, Nadji M: Orbital leiomyosarcoma. Arch Ophthalmol **101:**1566-1568, 1983.

87 Yamasaki T, Handa H, Yamashita J, Paine JT, Tashiro Y, Uno A, Ishikawa M, Asato R: Intracranial and orbital cavernous angiomas. A review of 30 cases. J Neurosurg **64:**197-208, 1986.

Glioma of optic nerve

88 Borit A, Richardson EP Jr: The biological and clinical behaviour of pilocytic astrocytomas of the optic pathways. Brain **105:**161-187, 1982.

89 Dosoretz DE, Blitzer PH, Wang CC, Linggood RM: Management of glioma of the optic nerve and/or chiasm. An analysis of 20 cases. Cancer **45:**1467-1471, 1980.

90 Marquardt MD, Zimmerman LE: Histopathology of meningiomas and gliomas of the optic nerve. Hum Pathol **13:**226-235, 1982.

91 Pierce SM, Barnes PD, Loeffler JS, McGinn C, Tarbell NJ: Definitive radiation therapy in the management of symptomatic patients with optic glioma. Survival and long-term effects. Cancer **65:**45-52, 1990.

Meningioma

92 Karp L, Zimmerman LE, Borit A, Spencer W: Primary intraorbital meningiomas. Arch Ophthalmol **91:**24-28, 1974.

93 Marquardt MD, Zimmerman LE: Histopathology of meningiomas and gliomas of the optic nerve. Hum Pathol **13:**226-235, 1982.

Lymphoid tumors and tumorlike conditions

94 Astarita RW, Minckler D, Taylor CR, Levine A, Lukes RJ: Orbital and adnexal lymphomas. A multiparameter approach. Am J Clin Pathol **73:**615-621, 1980.

95 Bennett CL, Putterman A, Bitran JD, Recant W, Shapiro CM, Karesh J, Kalokhe U: Staging and therapy of orbital lymphomas. Cancer **57:**1204-1208, 1986.

96 Brisbane JU, Lessell S, Finkel HE, Neiman RS: Malignant lymphoma presenting in the orbit. A clinicopathologic study of a rare immunoglobulin-producing variant. Cancer **47:**548-553, 1981.

97 Evans HL: Extranodal small lymphocytic proliferation. A clinicopathologic and immunocytochemical study. Cancer **49:**84-96, 1982.

98 Knowles DM II, Jakobiec FA: Orbital lymphoid neoplasms. A clinicopathologic study of 60 patients. Cancer **46:**576-589, 1980.

99 Knowles DM II, Jakobiec FA: Cell marker analysis of extranodal lymphoid infiltrates. To what extent does the determination of mono- or polyclonality resolve the diagnostic dilemma of malignant lymphoma *v* pseudolymphoma in an extranodal site? Semin Diagn Pathol **2:**163-168, 1985.

100 Knowles DM, Jakobiec FA, McNally L, Burke JS: Lymphoid hyperplasia and malignant lymphoma occurring in the ocular adnexa (orbit, conjunctiva, and eyelids). A prospective multiparametric analysis of 108 cases during 1977 to 1987. Hum Pathol **21:**959-973, 1990.

101 Lazzarino M, Morra E, Rosso R, Brusamolino E, Pagnucco G, Castello A, Ghisolfi A, Tafi A, Zennaro G, Bernasconi C: Clinicopathologic and immunologic characteristics of non-Hodgkin's lymphomas presenting in the orbit. A report of eight cases. Cancer **55:**1907-1912, 1985.

102 McNally L, Jakobiec FA, Knowles DM II: Clinical, morphologic, immunophenotypic, and molecular genetic analysis of bilateral ocular adnexal lymphoid neoplasms in 17 patients. Am J Ophthalmol **103:**555-568, 1987.

103 Medeiros LJ, Harris NL: Lymphoid infiltrates of the orbit and conjunctiva. A morphologic and immunophenotypic study of 99 cases. Am J Surg Pathol **13:**459-471, 1989.

104 Medeiros LJ, Harris NL: Immunohistologic analysis of small lymphocytic infiltrates of the orbit and conjunctiva. Hum Pathol **21:**1126-1131, 1990.

105 Morgan G, Harry J: Lymphocytic tumours of indeterminate nature. A 5-year follow-up of 98 conjunctival and orbital lesions. Br J Ophthalmol **62:**381-383, 1978.

106 Neri A, Jakobiec FA, Pelicci P-G, Dalla-Favera R, Knowles DM II: Immunoglobulin and T cell receptor β chain gene rearrangement analysis of ocular adnexal lymphoid neoplasms. Clinical and biologic implications. Blood **70:**1519-1529, 1987.

107 Peterson K, Gordon KB, Heinemann MH, De Angelis LM: The clinical spectrum of ocular lymphoma. Cancer **72:**843-849, 1993.

108 Shome DK, Gupta NK, Prajapati NC, Raju GM, Choudhury P, Dubey AP: Orbital granulocytic sarcomas (myeloid sarcomas) in acute nonlymphocytic leukemia. Cancer **70:**2298-2301, 1992.

109 Tewfik HH, Platz CE, Corder MP, Panther SK, Blodi FC: A clinicopathologic study of orbital and adnexal non-Hodgkin's lymphomas. Cancer **44:**1022-1028, 1979.

110 Turner RR, Egbert P, Warnke RA: Lymphocytic infiltrates of the conjunctiva and orbit. Immunohistochemical staining of 16 cases. Am J Clin Pathol **81:**447-452, 1984.

111 Wotherspoon AC, Diss TC, Pan LX, Schmid C, Kerr-Muir MG, Lea SH, Isaacson PG: Primary low-grade B-cell lymphoma of the conjunctiva. A mucosa-associated lymphoid tissue type lymphoma. Histopathology **23:**417-424, 1993.

Metastatic tumors

112 Freedman MI, Folk JC: Metastatic tumors to the eye and orbit. Patient survival and clinical characteristics. Arch Ophthalmol **105:**1215-1219, 1987.

113 Reifler DM, Kini SR, Liu D, Littleton RH: Orbital metastasis from prostatic carcinoma. Identification by immunocytology. Arch Ophthalmol **102:**292-295, 1984.

114 Riddle PJ, Font RL, Zimmerman LE: Carcinoid tumors of the eye and orbit. A clinicopathologic study of 15 cases, with histochemical and electron microscopic observations. Hum Pathol **13:**459-469, 1982.

115 Zimmerman LE, Stangl R, Riddle PJ: Primary carcinoid tumor of the orbit. A clinicopathologic study with histochemical and electron microscopic observations. Arch Ophthalmol **101:**1395-1398, 1983.

CONJUNCTIVA
Degeneration

116 Austin P, Jakobiec FA, Iwamoto T, Hornblass A: Elastofibroma oculi. Arch Ophthalmol **101:**1575-1579, 1983.

Graft-versus-host disease

117 Jabs DA, Hirst LW, Green WR, Tutschka PJ, Santos GW, Beschorner WE: The eye in bone marrow transplantation. II. Histopathology. Arch Ophthalmol **101:**585-590, 1983.

Inflammation

118 Bornstein J, Frank M, Radnec D: Conjunctival biopsy in the diagnosis of sarcoidosis. N Engl J Med **267:**60-64, 1962.

119 Chambers J, Blodi F, Golden B, McKee A: Ligneous conjunctivitis. Trans Am Acad Ophthalmol Otolaryngol **73:**996-1004, 1969.

120 Hidayat AA, Riddle PJ: Ligneous conjunctivitis. A clinicopathologic study of 17 cases. Ophthalmology **94:**949-959, 1987.

121 Raphael M, Bellefqih S, Piette JC, Le Hoang P, Debre P, Chomette G: Conjunctival biopsy in Sjögren's syndrome. Correlations between histological and immunohistochemical features. Histopathology **13:**191-202, 1988.

122 Steffen C: Actinic granuloma of the conjunctiva. Am J Dermatopathol **14:**253-254, 1992.

123 Stenson S: Adult inclusion conjunctivitis. Clinical characteristics and corneal changes. Arch Ophthalmol **99:**605-608, 1981.

Tumors and tumorlike conditions
Tumors of surface epithelium

124 Blodi FC: Squamous cell carcinoma of the conjunctiva. Doc Ophthalmol **34:**93--108, 1973.

125 Gamel JW, Eiferman RA, Guibor P: Mucoepidermoid carcinoma of the conjunctiva. Arch Ophthalmol **102:**730-731, 1984.

126 Irvine AR Jr: Epibulbar squamous cell carcinoma and related lesions. In Ferry AP, ed: Ocular and adnexal tumors. Int Ophthalmol Clin **12:**71-83, 1972.

127 McDonnell JM, Mayr AJ, Martin WJ: DNA of human papillomavirus type 16 in dysplastic and malignant lesions of the conjunctiva and cornea. N Engl J Med **320:**1442-1446, 1989.

128 McDonnell PJ, McDonnell JM, Kessis T, Green WR, Shah KV: Detection of human papillomavirus type 6/11 DNA in conjunctival papillomas by in situ hybridization with radioactive probes. Hum Pathol **18:**1115-1119, 1987.

129 Searl SS, Krigstein HJ, Albert DM, Grove AS Jr: Invasive squamous cell carcinoma with intraocular mucoepidermoid features. Conjunctival carcinoma with intraocular invasion and diphasic morphology. Arch Ophthalmol **100:**109-111, 1982.

130 Waring GO III, Roth AM, Ekins MB: Clinical and pathologic description of 17 cases of corneal intraepithelial neoplasia. Am J Ophthalmol **97:**547-559, 1984.

Melanocytic tumors and tumorlike conditions

131 Ackerman AB, Sood R, Koenig M: Primary acquired melanosis of the conjunctiva is melanoma in situ. Mod Pathol **4:**253-263, 1991.

132 Brownstein S, Jakobiec FA, Wilkinson RD, Lombardo J, Jackson WB: Cryotherapy for precancerous melanosis (atypical melanocytic hyperplasia) of the conjunctiva. Arch Ophthalmol **99:**1224-1231, 1981.

133 Folberg R, Jakobiec FA, McLean IW, Zimmerman LE: Is primary acquired melanosis of the conjunctiva equivalent to melanoma in situ? Mod Pathol **5:**2-8, 1992.

134 Folberg R, McLean IW: Primary acquired melanosis and melanoma of the conjunctiva. Terminology, classification, and biologic behavior. Hum Pathol **17:**652-654, 1986.

135 Folberg R, McLean IW, Zimmerman LE: Malignant melanoma of the conjunctiva. Hum Pathol **16:**136-143, 1985.

136 Folberg R, McLean IW, Zimmerman LE: Primary acquired melanosis of the conjunctiva. Hum Pathol **16:**129-135, 1985.

137 Guillén FJ, Albert DM, Mihm MC Jr: Pigmented melanocytic lesions of the conjunctiva. A new approach to their classification. Pathology **17:**275-280, 1985.

138 Jakobiec FA, Zuckerman BD, Berlin AJ, Odell P, MacRae DW, Tuthill RJ: Unusual melanocytic nevi of the conjunctiva. Am J Ophthalmol **100:**100-113, 1985.

139 Jay B: Naevi and melanomata of the conjunctiva. Br J Ophthalmol **49:**169-204, 1965.

140 Jeffrey IJM, Lucas DR, McEwan C, Lee WR: Malignant melanoma of the conjunctiva. Histopathology **10:**363-378, 1986.

141 Liesegang TJ: Pigmented conjunctival and scleral lesions. Mayo Clin Proc **69:**151-161, 1994.

142 Mihm MC Jr, Guillén FJ: Classification of non-nevoid pigmented lesions of the conjunctiva (letter to the editor). Hum Pathol **16:**1078, 1985.

143 Reese AB: Precancerous and cancerous melanosis. Am J Ophthalmol **61:**1272-1277, 1966.

Lymphoid tumors and tumorlike conditions

144 Morgan G: Lymphocytic tumours of the conjunctiva. J Clin Pathol **24:**585-595, 1971.

Other tumors

145 Hufnagel T, Ma L, Kuo T-T: Orbital angiosarcoma with subconjunctival presentation. Report of a case and literature review. Ophthalmology **94:**72-77, 1987.

146 Jaimovich L, Calb I, Kaminsky A: Kaposi's sarcoma of the conjunctiva. J Am Acad Dermatol **14:**589-592, 1986.

147 Patrinely JR, Green WR: Conjunctival myxoma. A clinicopathologic study of four cases and a review of the literature. Arch Ophthalmol **101:**1416-1420, 1983.

148 Truong L, Font RL: Intravenous pyogenic granuloma of the ocular adnexa. Report of two cases and review of the literature. Arch Ophthalmol **103:**1364-1367, 1985.

CORNEA
Endothelial decompensation

149 Waring C, Rodrigues M, Laibson P: Corneal dystrophies. II. Endothelial dystrophies. Surv Ophthalmol **23:**147-168, 1978.

Fibrosis and vascularization

150 Green WR, Zimmerman LE: Granulomatous reaction to Descemet's membrane. Am J Ophthalmol **64:**555-558, 1967.

INTRAOCULAR TISSUES
Developmental anomalies

151 Zimmerman LE, Font RL: Some recent advances in the pathogenesis and histopathology of congenital malformations of the eye. JAMA **196:**684-696, 1966.

Congenital glaucoma

152 Reese AB, Ellsworth RM: The anterior chamber cleavage syndrome. Arch Ophthalmol **75:**307-318, 1968.

Retrolental fibroplasia

153 Reese AB (moderator): Symposium on retrolental fibroplasia. Trans Am Acad Ophthalmol Otolaryngol **59:**7-41, 1955.

Phakoma

154 Font RL, Ferry AP: The phakomatoses. In Ferry AP, ed: Ocular and adnexal tumors. Int Ophthalmol Clin **12:**1-50, 1972.

Persistent hyperplastic primary vitreous

155 Jensen OA: Persistent hyperplastic primary vitreous. Acta Ophthalmol **46**:418-429, 1968.

Retinal dysplasia

156 Cogan DG, Kuwabara T: Ocular pathology of the 13-15 trisomy syndrome. Arch Ophthalmol **72**:246-247, 1964.

157 Hunter WS, Zimmerman LE: Unilateral retinal dysplasia. Arch Ophthalmol **74**:23-30, 1965.

Other developmental anomalies

158 Boniuk M, Zimmerman LE: Ocular pathology in the rubella syndrome. Arch Ophthalmol **77**:455-473, 1967.

159 Font RL, Fine BS: Ocular pathology in Fabry's disease. Histochemical and electron microscopic observations. Am J Ophthalmol **73**:419-430, 1972.

160 Miller RW, Fraumeni JF Jr, Manning MD: Association of Wilms' tumor with aniridia, hemihypertrophy, and other congenital malformations. N Engl J Med **270**:922-927, 1964.

161 Zimmerman LE: The histopathologic basis for ocular manifestations of the congenital rubella syndrome. Am J Ophthalmol **65**:837-862, 1968.

Inflammation
Acute inflammation

162 Fishman LS, Griffin JR, Sapico FL, Hecht R: Hematogenous *Candida* endophthalmitis. N Engl J Med **286**:675-681, 1972.

163 Levine R, Williamson DE: Metastatic carcinoma simulating a postoperative endophthalmitis. Arch Ophthalmol **83**:59-60, 1970.

164 Michelson PE, Stark W, Reeser F, Green WR: Endogenous *Candida* endophthalmitis. Report of 13 cases and 16 from the literature. Int Ophthalmol Clin **11**:125-147, 1971.

165 Sugar S, Mandell G, Shaler J: Metastatic endophthalmitis associated with injection of addictive drugs. Am J Ophthalmol **71**:1055-1058, 1971.

Chronic nongranulomatous inflammation

166 Chan C-C, Fujikawa LS, Rodrigues MM, Stevens G Jr, Nussenblatt RB: Immunohistochemistry and electron microscopy of cyclitic membrane. Report of a case. Arch Ophthalmol **104**:1040-1045, 1986.

167 Naumann G, Gass D, Font R: Histopathology of herpes zoster ophthalmicus. Am J Ophthalmol **65**:533-541, 1968.

Granulomatous inflammation

168 Beaver PC: Larva migrans. Exp Parasitol **5**:587-621, 1956.

169 Margo C, Zimmerman LE: Idiopathic solitary granuloma of the uveal tract. Arch Ophthalmol **102**:732-735, 1984.

170 Parke DW II, Font RL: Diffuse toxoplasmic retinochoroiditis in a patient with AIDS. Arch Ophthalmol **104**:571-575, 1986.

171 Wilder HC: Nematode endophthalmitis. Trans Am Acad Ophthalmol Otolaryngol **54**:99-109, 1950.

172 Wilder HC: Toxoplasma chorioretinitis in adults. Arch Ophthalmol **48**:127-136, 1952.

173 Wilkinson C, Welch R: Intraocular *Toxocara*. Am J Ophthalmol **71**:921-930, 1971.

Post-traumatic uveitis

174 Easom H, Zimmerman LE: Sympathetic ophthalmia and bilateral phacoanaphylaxis. Arch Ophthalmol **72**:9-15, 1964.

Degeneration
Glaucoma

175 Fenton R, Zimmerman LE: Hemolytic glaucoma. Arch Ophthalmol **70**:236-239, 1963.

176 Flocks M, Littwin CS, Zimmerman LE: Phacolytic glaucoma. Arch Ophthalmol **54**:37-45, 1955.

177 Kolker AE, Hetherington J Jr: Becker-Shaffer's diagnosis and therapy of the glaucomas, ed 4. St. Louis, 1976, The C.V. Mosby Co.

Diabetes

178 Smith ME, Glickman P: Diabetic vacuolation of the iris pigment epithelium. Am J Ophthalmol **79**:875-877, 1975.

179 Yanoff M: Ocular pathology in diabetes mellitus. Am J Ophthalmol **67**:21-38, 1969.

Tumors and tumorlike conditions
Malignant melanoma

180 Ashton N, Wybar K: Primary tumours of the iris. Ophthalmologica **151**:97-113, 1966.

181 Barr CC, McLean IW, Zimmerman LE: Uveal melanoma in children and adolescents. Arch Ophthalmol **99**:2133-2136, 1981.

182 Barr CC, Zimmerman LE, Curtin VT, Font RL: Bilateral diffuse melanocytic uveal tumors associated with systemic malignant neoplasms. A recently recognized syndrome. Arch Ophthalmol **100**:249-255, 1982.

183 Broadway D, Lang S, Harper J, Madanat F, Pritchard J, Tarawneh M, Taylor D: Congenital malignant melanoma of the eye. Cancer **67**:2642-2652, 1991.

184 Callender GR: Malignant melanotic tumors of the eye. A study of histologic types in 111 cases. Trans Am Acad Ophthalmol Otolaryngol **36**:131-142, 1931.

185 Chang M, Zimmerman LE, McLean I: The persisting pseudomelanoma problem. Arch Ophthalmol **102**:726-727, 1984.

186 Char DH, Phillips TL: The potential for adjuvant radiotherapy in choroidal melanoma. Arch Ophthalmol **100**:247-248, 1982.

187 Cole EL, Zakov ZN, Meisler DM, Tuthill RJ, McMahon JT: Cutaneous malignant melanoma metastatic to the vitreous. Arch Ophthalmol **104**:98-101, 1986.

188 Coleman K, Baak JPA, van Diest PJ, Curran B, Mullaney J, Fenton M, Leader M: DNA ploidy status in 84 ocular melanomas. A study of DNA quantitation in ocular melanomas by flow cytometry and automatic and interactive static image analysis. Hum Pathol **26**:99-105, 1995.

189 de Bustros S, Augsburger JJ, Shields JA, Shakin EP, Pryor CC II: Intraocular metastases from cutaneous malignant melanoma. Arch Ophthalmol **103**:937-940, 1985.

190 de la Cruz PO Jr, Specht CS, McLean IW: Lymphocytic infiltration in uveal malignant melanoma. Cancer **65**:112-115, 1990.

191 Ferry AP: Lesions mistaken for malignant melanoma of posterior uvea. Arch Ophthalmol **72**:463-469, 1964.

192 Ferry AP: Lesions mistaken for malignant melanoma of iris. Arch Ophthalmol **74**:9-18, 1965.

193 Flocks M, Gerende JH, Zimmerman LE: The size and shape of malignant melanomas of the choroid and ciliary body in relation to prognosis and histologic characteristics. A statistical study of 210 tumors. Trans Am Acad Ophthalmol Otolaryngol **59**:740-758, 1955.

194 Folberg R, Pe'er J, Gruman LM, Woolson RF, Jeng G, Montague PR, Moninger TO, Yi H, Moore KC: The morphologic characteristics of tumor blood vessels as a marker of tumor progression in primary human uveal melanoma. A matched case-control study. Hum Pathol **23**:1298-1305, 1992.

195 Font RL, Spaulding A, Zimmerman LE: Diffuse malignant melanoma of the uveal tract. A clinicopathologic report of 54 cases. Trans Am Acad Ophthalmol Otolaryngol **72**:877-895, 1968.

196 Forrest A, Keeper R, Spencer W: Iridocyclectomy for melanomas of the ciliary body. A follow-up study of pathology and surgical morbidity. Am J Ophthalmol **85**:1237-1249, 1978.

197 Fuchs U, Kivela T, Summanen P, Immonen I, Tarkkanen A: An immunohistochemical and prognostic analysis of cytokeratin expression in malignant uveal melanoma. Am J Pathol **141**:169-181, 1992.

198 Gamel JW, McLean I, Greenberg RA, Naids RM, Folberg R, Donoso LA, Seddon JM, Albert DM: Objective assessment of the malignant potential of intraocular melanomas with standard microslides stained with hematoxylin-eosin. Hum Pathol **16**:689-692, 1985.

199 Gamel JW, McLean IW, McCurdy JB: Biologic distinctions between cure and time to death in 2892 patients with intraocular melanoma. Cancer **71**:2299-2305, 1993.

200 Gass JMD: Differential diagnosis of intraocular tumors. St. Louis, 1974, The C.V. Mosby Co.

201 Horsman DE, White VA: Cytogenetic analysis of uveal melanoma. Consistent occurrence of monosomy 3 and trisomy 8q. Cancer **71**:811-819, 1993.

202 Howard GM, Forrest AW: Incidence and location of melanocytomas. Arch Ophthalmol **77**:61-66, 1967.

203 Jakobiec FA, Silbert G: Are most iris 'melanomas' really nevi? A clinicopathologic study of 189 lesions. Arch Ophthalmol **99**:2117-2132, 1981.

204 Kath R, Hayungs J, Bornfeld N, Sauerwein W, Hoffken K, Seeber S: Prognosis and treatment of disseminated uveal melanoma. Cancer **72**:2219-2223, 1993.

205 Letson AD, Davidorf FH: Bilateral retinal metastases from cutaneous malignant melanoma. Arch Ophthalmol **100**:605-607, 1982.

206 Manschot WA, Van Peperzeel HA: Uveal melanoma. Location, size, cell type, and enucleation as risk factors in metastasis (letter to the editor). Hum Pathol **13**:1147-1148, 1982.

207 McCurdy J, Gamel J, McLean I: A simple, efficient, and reproducible method for estimating the malignant potential of uveal melanoma from routine H & E slides. Pathol Res Pract **187:**1025-1027, 1991.

208 McLean IW, Foster WD, Zimmerman LE: Uveal melanoma. Location, size, cell type, and enucleation as risk factors in metastasis. Hum Pathol **13:**123-132, 1982.

209 McLean IW, Zimmerman LE, Evans R: Reappraisal of Callender's spindle A type of malignant melanoma of choroid and ciliary body. Am J Ophthalmol **86:**557-564, 1978.

210 Miller MV, Herdson PB, Hitchcock GC: Malignant melanoma of the uveal tract. A review of the Auckland experience. Pathology **17:**281-284, 1985.

211 Pach JM, Robertson DM, Taney BS, Martin JA, Campbell RJ, O'Brien PC: Prognostic factors in choroidal and ciliary body melanomas with extrascleral extension. Am J Ophthalmol **101:**325-331, 1986.

212 Sassani JW, Weinstein JM, Graham WP: Massively invasive diffuse choroidal melanoma. Arch Ophthalmol **103:**945-948, 1985.

213 Seddon JM, Albert DM, Lavin DT, Robinson N: A prognostic factor study of disease-free interval and survival following enucleation for uveal melanoma. Arch Ophthalmol **101:**1894-1899, 1983.

214 Seigel D, Myers M, Ferris F III, Steinhorn SC: Survival rates after enucleation of eyes with malignant melanoma. Am J Ophthalmol **87:**761-765, 1979.

215 Shields JA, Karan DS, Perry HD, Donoso LA: Epithelioid cell nevus of the iris. Arch Ophthalmol **103:**235-237, 1985.

216 Sorensen FB, Gamel JW, McCurdy J: Stereologic estimation of nucleolar volume in ocular melanoma. A comparative study of size estimators with prognostic impact. Hum Pathol **24:**513-518, 1993.

217 Starr HJ, Zimmerman LE: Extrascleral extension and orbital recurrence of malignant melanomas of the choroid and ciliary body. Int Ophthalmol Clin **2:**369-385, 1962.

218 Weinhaus RS, Seddon JM, Albert DM, Gragoudas ES, Robinson N: Prognostic factor study of survival after enucleation for juxtapapillary melanomas. Arch Ophthalmol **103:**1673-1677, 1985.

219 Yanoff M, Zimmerman LE: Histogenesis of malignant melanomas of the uvea. I. Nevi of choroid and ciliary body. Arch Ophthalmol **76:**784-796, 1966.

220 Yanoff M, Zimmerman LE: Histogenesis of malignant melanomas of the uvea. II. The relationship of uveal nevi to malignant melanomas. Cancer **20:**493-507, 1967.

221 Yanoff M, Zimmerman LE: Histogenesis of malignant melanomas of the uvea. III. The relationship of congenital ocular melanocytosis and neurofibromatosis to uveal melanomas. Arch Ophthalmol **77:**331-336, 1967.

222 Zimmerman LE, McLean IW: An evaluation of enucleation in the management of uveal melanomas. Am J Ophthalmol **87:**741-760, 1979.

223 Zimmerman LE, McLean IW, Foster W: Does enucleation of the eye containing a malignant melanoma prevent or accelerate the dissemination of tumor cells? Br J Ophthalmol **62:**420-425, 1978.

Retinoblastoma and related lesions

224 Abramson DH, Ellsworth RM, Tretter P, Adams K, Kitchin FD: Simultaneous bilateral radiation for advanced bilateral retinoblastoma. Arch Ophthalmol **99:**1763-1766, 1981.

225 Abramson DH, Ellsworth RM, Tretter P, Javitt J, Kitchin FD: Treatment of bilateral groups I through III retinoblastoma with bilateral radiation. Arch Ophthalmol **99:**1761-1762, 1981.

226 Abramson DH, Ellsworth R, Zimmerman L: Nonocular cancer in retinoblastoma survivors. Trans Am Acad Ophthalmol Otolaryngol **81:**454-457, 1976.

227 Abramson DH, Marks RF, Ellsworth RM, Tretter P, Kitchin FD: The management of unilateral retinoblastoma without primary enucleation. Arch Ophthalmol **100:**1249-1252, 1982.

228 Amendola BE, Lamm FR, Markoe AM, Karlsson UL, Shields J, Shields CL, Augsburger J, Brady LW, Woodleigh R, Miller C: Radiotherapy of retinoblastoma. A review of 63 children treated with different irradiation techniques. Cancer **66:**21-26, 1990.

229 Bishop J, Madson E: Retinoblastoma. Review of the current status. Surv Ophthalmol **19:**342-366, 1975.

230 Brownstein S, de Chaderèvian J-P, Little JM: Trilateral retinoblastoma. Report of two cases. Arch Ophthalmol **102:**257-262, 1984.

231 Bunt AH, Tso MOM: Feulgen-positive deposits in retinoblastoma. Incidence, composition, and ultrastructure. Arch Ophthalmol **99:**144-150, 1981.

232 DerKinderen DJ, Koten JW, Nagelkerke NJD, Tan KEWP, Beemer FA, Den Otter W: Nonocular cancer in patients with hereditary retinoblastoma and their relatives. Int J Cancer **41:**499-504, 1988.

233 Donoso LA, Hamm H, Dietzschold B, Augsburger JJ, Shields JA, Arbizo V: Rhodopsin and retinoblastoma. A monoclonal antibody histopathologic study. Arch Ophthalmol **104:**111-113, 1986.

234 Eng C, Ponder BA: The role of gene mutations in the genesis of familial cancers. FASEB J **7:**910-919, 1993.

235 Gallie BL, Squire JA, Goddard A, Dunn JM, Canton M, Hinton D, Zhu XP, Phillips RA: Mechanism of oncogenesis in retinoblastoma. Lab Invest **62:**394-408, 1990.

236 Gonzalez-Fernandez F, Lopes MB, Garcia-Fernandez JM, Foster RG, De Grip WJ, Rosemberg S, Newman SA, Vanden Berg SR: Expression of developmentally defined retinal phenotypes in the histogenesis of retinoblastoma. Am J Pathol **141:**363-375, 1992.

237 He W, Hashimoto H, Tsuneyoshi M, Enjoji M, Inomata H: A reassessment of histologic classification and an immunohistochemical study of 88 retinoblastomas. A special reference to the advent of bipolar-like cells. Cancer **70:**2901-2908, 1992.

238 Holladay DA, Holladay A, Montebello JF, Redmond KP: Clinical presentation, treatment, and outcome of trilateral retinoblastoma. Cancer **67:**710-715, 1991.

239 Horowitz JM, Park SH, Bogenmann E, Cheng JC, Yandell DW, Kaye FJ, Minna JD, Dryja TP, Weinberg RA: Frequent inactivation of the retinoblastoma anti-oncogene is restricted to a subset of human tumor cells. Proc Natl Acad Sci U S A **87:**2775-2779, 1990.

240 Howard GM, Ellsworth RM: Differential diagnosis of retinoblastoma. A statistical survey of 500 children. Am J Ophthalmol **60:**610-612, 1965.

241 Johnson DL, Chandra R, Fisher WS, Hammock MK, McKeown CA: Trilateral retinoblastoma. Ocular and pineal retinoblastomas. J Neurosurg **63:**367-370, 1985.

242 Kogan L, Boniuk M: Causes for enucleation in childhood with special reference to pseudogliomas and retinoblastomas. Int Ophthalmol Clin **2:**507-524, 1962.

243 Korf H-W, Czerwionka M, Reiner J, Schachenmayr W, Schalken JJ, de Grip W, Gery I: Immunocytochemical evidence of molecular photoreceptor markers in cerebellar medulloblastomas. Cancer **60:**1763-1766, 1987.

244 Kyritsis AP, Tsokos M, Triche TJ, Chader GJ: Retinoblastoma. Origin from a primitive neuroectodermal cell? Nature **307:**471-473, 1984.

245 Lueder GT, Smith ME: Retinoblastoma. Semin Diagn Pathol **11:**104-106, 1994.

246 MacKay CJ, Abramson DH, Ellsworth RM: Metastatic patterns of retinoblastoma. Arch Ophthalmol **102:**391-396, 1984.

247 Manivel JC, Asaikar S, Cameron JD, Wick MR: Retinoblastoma. An immunohistochemical study (abstract). Lab Invest **58:**60A, 1988.

248 Margo C, Hidayat A, Kopelman J, Zimmerman LE: Retinocytoma. A benign variant of retinoblastoma. Arch Ophthalmol **101:**1519-1531, 1983.

249 Perentes E, Rubinstein LJ: Recent applications of immunoperoxidase histochemistry in human neuro-oncology. An update. Arch Pathol Lab Med **111:**796-812, 1987.

250 Rubinstein LJ: Embryonal central neuroepithelial tumors and their differentiating potential. A cytogenetic view of a complex neuro-oncological problem. J Neurosurg **62:**795-805, 1985.

251 Sang DN, Albert DM: Retinoblastoma. Clinical and histopathologic features. Hum Pathol **13:**133-147, 1982.

252 Schubert EL, Hansen MF, Strong LC: The retinoblastoma gene and its significance. Ann Med **26:**177-184, 1994.

253 Shields CL, Shields JA, Baez K, Cater JR, De Potter P: Optic nerve invasion of retinoblastoma. Metastatic potential and clinical risk factors. Cancer **73:**692-698, 1994.

254 Shields JA, Shields CL: Current management of retinoblastoma. Mayo Clin Proc **69:**50-56, 1994.

255 Shuangshoti S, Chaiwun B, Kasantikul V: A study of 39 retinoblastomas with particular reference to morphology, cellular differentiation and tumour origin. Histopathology **15:**113-124, 1989.

256 Terenghi G, Polak JM, Ballesta J, Cocchia D, Michetti F, Dahl D, Marangos PJ, Garner A: Immunocytochemistry of neuronal and glial markers in retinoblastoma. Virchows Arch [A] **404:**61-73, 1984.

257 Ts'o MO, Fine BS, Zimmerman LE: The nature of retinoblastoma. II. Photoreceptor differentiation. An electron microscopic study. Am J Ophthalmol **69:**350-359, 1970.

258 Ts'o MO, Zimmerman LE, Fine BS: The nature of retinoblastoma. I. Photoreceptor differentiation. A clinical and histopathologic study. Am J Ophthalmol **69:**339-349, 1970.

259 Tsokos M, Kyritsis AP, Chader GJ, Triche TJ: Differentiation of human retinoblastoma in vitro into cell types with characteristics observed in embryonal or mature retina. Am J Pathol **123:**542-552, 1986.

260 Walford N, Deferrai R, Slater RM, Delemarre JF, Dingemans KP, Van den Bergh Weerman MA, Voute PA: Intraorbital rhabdoid tumour following bilateral retinoblastoma. Histopathology **20:**170-173, 1992.

261 Wiggs J, Nordenskjöld M, Yandell D, Rapaport J, Grondin V, Janson M, Werelius B, Petersen R, Craft A, Riedel K, Liberfarb R, Walton D, Wilson W, Dryja TP: Prediction of the risk of hereditary retinoblastoma, using DNA polymorphisms within the retinoblastoma gene. N Engl J Med **318:**151-157, 1988.

262 Wiman KG: The retinoblastoma gene. Role in cell cycle control and cell differentiation. FASEB J **7:**841-845, 1993.

263 Yandell DW, Campbell TA, Dayton SH, Petersen R, Walton D, Little JB, McConkie-Rosell A, Buckley EG, Dryja TP: Oncogenic point mutations in the human retinoblastoma gene. Their application to genetic counseling. N Engl J Med **321:**1689-1695, 1989.

263a Yuge K, Nakajima M, Uemura Y, Miki H, Uyama M, Tsubura A: Immunohistochemical features of the human retina and retinoblastoma. Virchows Arch **426:**571-575, 1995.

264 Zacksenhaus E, Bremner R, Jiang Z, Gill RM, Muncaster M, Sopta M, Phillips RA, Gallie BL: Unravelling the function of the retinoblastoma gene. Adv Cancer Res **61:**115-141, 1993.

265 Zelter M, Damel A, Gonzalez G, Schwartz L: A prospective study on the treatment of retinoblastoma in 72 patients. Cancer **68:**1685-1690, 1991.

266 Zelter M, Gonzalez G, Schwartz L, Gallo G, Schvartzman E, Damel A, Muriel FS: Treatment of retinoblastoma. Results obtained from a prospective study of 51 patients. Cancer **61:**153-160, 1988.

Lymphoid tumors and tumorlike conditions

267 Allen R, Straatsma B: Ocular involvement in leukemia and allied disorders. Arch Ophthalmol **66:**490-508, 1961.

268 Kline LB, Garcia JH, Harsh GR III: Lymphomatous optic neuropathy. Arch Ophthalmol **102:**1655-1657, 1984.

269 Qualman SJ, Mendelsohn G, Mann RB, Green WR: Intraocular lymphomas. Natural history based on a clinicopathologic study of eight cases and review of theliterature. Cancer **52:**878-886, 1983.

270 Ryan S, Zimmerman LE, King FM: Reactive lymphoid hyperplasia. An unusual form of intraocular pseudotumor. Trans Am Acad Ophthalmol Otolaryngol **76:**652-671, 1972.

271 Shields JA, Augsburger JJ, Gonder JR, MacLeod D: Localized benign lymphoidtumor of the iris. Arch Ophthalmol **99:**2147-2148, 1981.

272 Vogel M, Font RL, Zimmerman LE, Levine R: Reticulum cell sarcoma of the retina and uvea. Am J Ophthalmol **66:**205-215, 1968.

Other primary tumors

273 Addison DJ, Font RL: Glioneuroma of iris and ciliary body. Arch Ophthalmol **102:**419-421, 1984.

274 Bruner WE, Stark WJ, Green WR: Presumed juvenile xanthogranuloma of the iris and ciliary body in an adult. Arch Ophthalmol **100:**457-459, 1982.

275 Ehlers N, Jensen OA: Juxtapapillary retinal hemangioblastoma (angiomatosis retinae) in an infant. Light microscopical and ultrastructural examination. Ultrastruct Pathol **3:**325-333, 1982.

276 Messmer E, Font RL, Laqua H, Höpping W, Naumann GOH: Cavernous hemangioma of the retina. Immunohistochemical and ultrastructural observations. Arch Ophthalmol **102:**413-418, 1984.

276a Pe'er J, Neudorfer M, Ron N, Anteby I, Lazar M, Rosenmann E: Panuveal malignant mesenchymoma. Arch Pathol Lab Med **118:**844-847, 1995.

277 Ulbright TM, Fulling KH, Helveston EM: Astrocytic tumors of the retina. Differentiation of sporadic tumors from phakomatosis-associated tumors. Arch Pathol Lab Med **108:**160-163, 1984.

278 Zaidman GW, Johnson BL, Salamon SM, Mondino BJ: Fuchs' adenoma affecting the peripheral iris. Arch Ophthalmol **101:**771-773, 1983.

279 Zimmerman LE: Ocular lesions of juvenile xanthogranuloma. Nevoxanthoendothelioma. Trans Am Acad Ophthalmol Otolaryngol **69:**412-442, 1965.

Metastatic tumors

280 Albert DM, Rubenstein R, Scheie H: Tumor metastasis to the eye. Part I. Incidence in 213 adult patients with generalized malignancy. Am J Ophthalmol **63**(Pt1):724-726, 1967.

281 Ferry AP: Metastatic carcinoma of the eye and ocular adnexa. Int Ophthalmol Clin **7:**615-658, 1967.

282 Ferry A, Font R: Carcinoma metastatic to the eye and orbit. Arch Ophthalmol **92:**276-286, 1974.

283 Freedman MI, Folk JC: Metastatic tumors to the eye and orbit. Patient survival and clinical characteristics. Arch Ophthalmol **105:**1215-1219, 1987.

284 Merrill CF, Kaufman DI, Dimitrov NV: Breast cancer metastatic to the eye is a common entity. Cancer **68:**623-627, 1991.

Cytology

285 Barr CC, Green WR, Payne JW, Knox DI, Jensen AD, Thompson RL: Intraocular reticulum-cell sarcoma. Clinicopathologic study of four cases and review of the literature. Surv Ophthalmol **19:**224-239, 1975.

286 Goldberg MF: Cytological diagnosis of phacolytic glaucoma utilizing Millepore filtration of the aqueous. Br J Ophthalmol **51:**847-853, 1967.

287 Wolter JR, Naylor B: A membrane filter method used to diagnose intraocular tumor. J Pediatr Ophthalmol **5:**36-38, 1968.

31 Ear

INTRODUCTION

Nearly all the diseases that can involve the ear also occur in other sites of the body. However, some of these diseases either have a predilection for the ear or pose special problems when occurring at this site. Only the features of these lesions as they pertain to their location in the ear will be discussed here. The general features of the respective entities are dealt with in the respective chapters.

The reader is referred to the specialized books on the subjet for an authoritative discussion of the specific diseases of this structure.[1a,1b,1c]

NORMAL ANATOMY

The ear is divided into the external, middle, and inner segments. The external ear consists of the auricle (pinna) and the external auditory canal, which is further divided into an outer (cartilaginous) portion and an inner (osseous) portion. Microscopically, both the auricle and the canal are covered by skin that differs little from that of the skin elsewhere, except for the fact that in the inner half of the canal the epidermis is very thin and lacks rete pegs. Adnexal structures are present in both areas; they are represented by hair follicles, sebaceous glands, and eccrine sweat glands in the auricle and by hair follicles, sebaceous glands, and a special type of apocrine sweat gland (known as ceruminous glands) in the canal, most of which are located in the outer third of this structure.

The inner portion of the canal is separated from the middle ear by the *tympanic membrane,* a thin fibrous structure lined by an attenuated layer of keratinizing squamous epithelium on the outer surface and by a single layer of cuboidal cells on the inner surface.

The middle ear (tympanic cavity) contains the three auditory ossicles (malleus, incus, and stapes); it connects with the pharynx through the eustachian tube and with the mastoid cavity and its contiguous pneumatic spaces. The middle ear proper and the mastoid are lined by a layer of flat epithelium; the eustachian tube is covered by tall ciliated epithelium, with smooth transitions between the two types.[1d]

The inner ear, which is located in the medial portion of the temporal bone, contains the cochlea and the *vestibular labyrinth.* These structures are supplied by the eighth cranial nerve, which enters the region through the internal auditory canal together with the seventh nerve. The vestibular labyrinth includes the blind *endolymphatic sac,* which is located in the middle of the posteromedial plate of the petrous bone. It has an intraosseous *rugose* portion and a *distal* portion that lies within the dura. It is lined by a flat to low columnar epithelium resting on a well-vascularized stroma.[2] The sac is connected to the *utricle* and *saccule* (the two main membranous structures of the vestibule) by the *endolymphatic duct,* which passes across the petrous bone.

DISEASES OF EXTERNAL EAR
Non-neoplastic disorders

Congenital abnormalities of this region are common. *Preauricular sinuses, cysts,* and *fistulae* are derived from the first or second branchial clefts.[14,18,21] They are lined by squamous or respiratory epithelium and often contain lymphoid tissue in the wall. Cartilage and skin adnexae may also be present. Secondary inflammatory features are common.[14,21] *Accessory tragi* are unilateral or bilateral nodules present at birth, located anteriorly to the auricle in the pretragal area.[3] Like the previous lesions, they are the expression of a branchial cleft anomaly. Microscopically they are composed of a covering of skin; numerous tiny, mature hair follicles, and a core of fibrofatty tissue that may contain cartilage.[17] Depending on the relative amounts of these components, these lesions can be variously misdiagnosed as papillomas, fibromas, or soft tissue chondromas. *Ectopic salivary gland tissue* is not uncommon in the region of the middle ear; it can also be found in the external auditory canal.

Keratinous cysts are common in and around the ear. Some are probably development anomalies related to the branchial cleft (see preceding discussion), and others are equivalent to those seen elsewhere in the skin and, as such, are either of infundibular hair follicle derivation or of epidermal inclusion type. They are all lined by keratinized squamous epithelium and filled by keratin of epidermal type (Fig. 31-1). Ker-

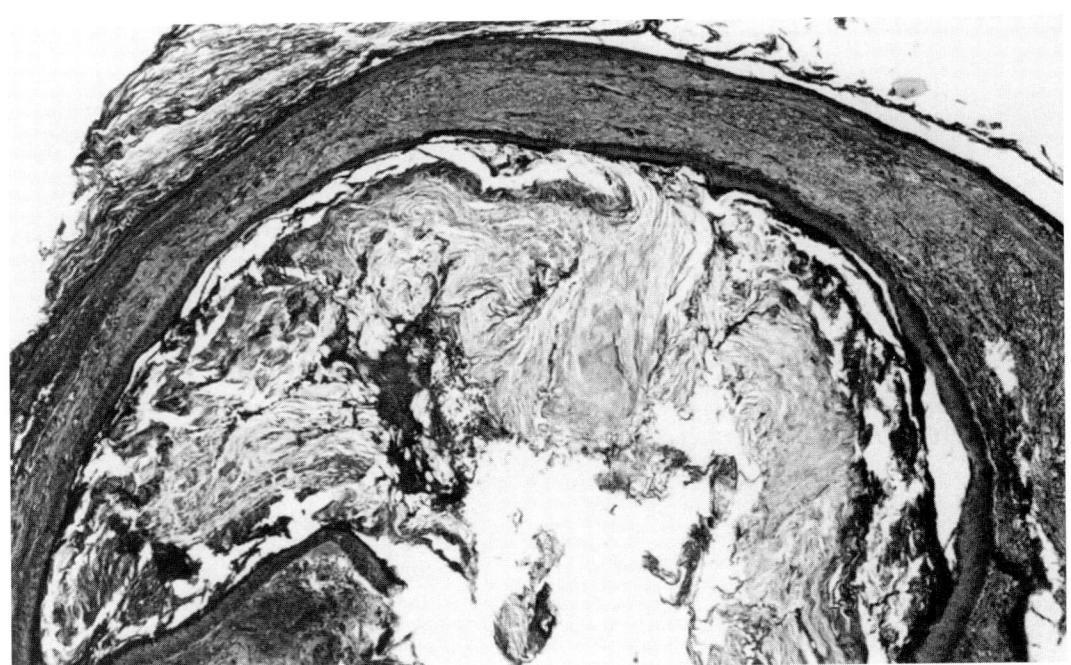

Fig. 31-1 Keratinous cyst of epidermal type involving external ear. Lining of cyst is made up of squamous epithelium and lacks skin adnexae.

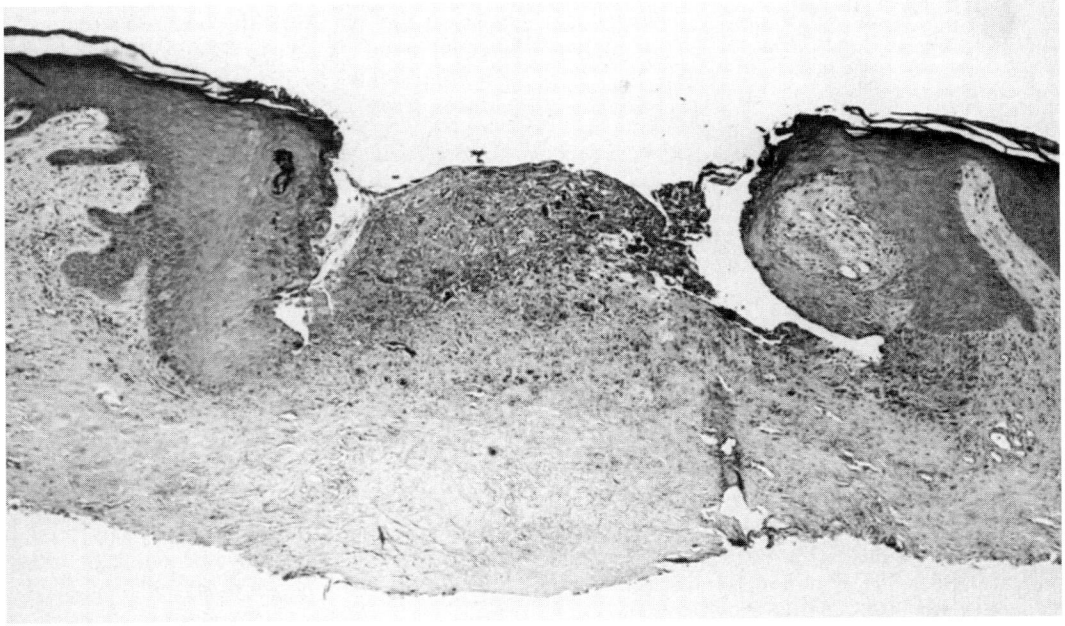

Fig. 31-2 Chondrodermatitis nodularis helicis. Central area of ulceration covered by granulation tissue is surrounded by hyperplastic and keratotic epithelium. Underlying stroma shows chronic inflammation and fibrosis.

atinous cysts of pilar type are common in the periauricular area but not in the ear itself.

Cholesteatoma of the external auditory canal is composed of a cystic mass of keratinized squamous epithelium overlying an area of bone sequestration in the inner half of the canal.[15] This rare condition should not be confused with cholesteatoma of the middle ear spaces (see p. 2513) or with *keratosis obturans,* a disorder characterized by a diffuse acanthosis and hyperkeratosis of the skin of the canal associated with underlying chronic inflammation.[13,15]

Epithelioid (histiocytoid hemangioma (also known as angiolymphoid hyperplasia with eosinophilia) has a

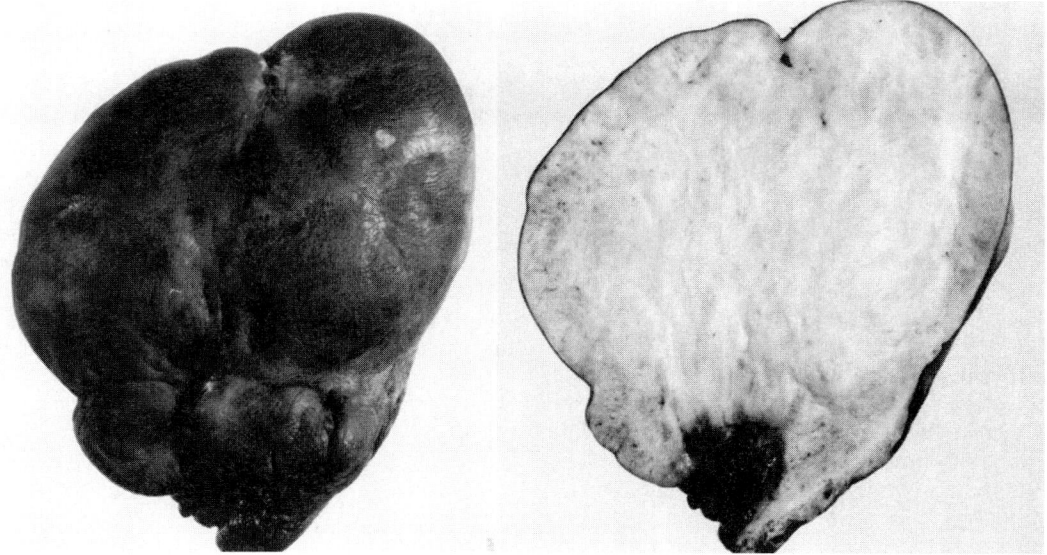

Fig. 31-3 Outer aspect and cut surface of keloid involving earlobe. This is one of most common locations for this lesion. (Courtesy Dr. J. Costa, Lausanne, Switzerland.)

predilection for the skin of the ear, external auditory canal, and periauricular region[19] (see Chapter 4).

Malignant external otitis, also known as necrotizing granulomatous otitis, is caused by *Pseudomonas aeruginosa* and affects mainly elderly patients who have diabetes. Microscopically, it is characterized by a necrotizing inflammatory reaction involving skin, soft tissue, cartilage, and bone.[22]

Chondrodermatitis nodularis chronica helicis (Winkler's disease) usually involves the upper portion of the helix in older patients, but it can also occur in the antihelix and in younger individuals. Clinically, it presents as a painful, small, round nodule often covered by a crust.[10] It is often thought clinically to be squamous cell carcinoma or actinic keratosis. Microscopically, there is marked hyperkeratosis and parakeratosis, acanthosis, and hyperplasia of the epidermis, which can reach pseudoepitheliomatous degrees. The center is usually ulcerated and covered by granulation tissue (Fig. 31-2). The underlying inflammation reaches the perichondrium and is characterized by a mononuclear infiltrate and vascular proliferation. The latter may be so pronounced as to simulate a vascular neoplasm, particularly glomus tumor.[4]

Idiopathic cystic chondromalacia (pseudocyst) results from degeneration of the auricular cartilage and is more commonly seen as a painless localized ear enlargement (sometimes bilaterally) in young males. Grossly, there is a cystic formation within the external auricular cartilage, which is filled by a watery fluid. Microscopically, the cyst has no lining, and there is no associated inflammation.[6]

Relapsing polychondritis is characterized by episodic painful inflammation of cartilage, most commonly in the outer and inner ear, nose, costochondral junctions, a variety of joints, and sometimes the cartilage of the respiratory tract. Aortic insufficiency is a life-threatening complication. The external ear is affected in almost 90% of the patients, and it represents the initial site of involvement in one third of the cases.[8,12]

Microscopically, there are degenerative changes in the cartilage (decrease in basophilic staining, loss of lacunae, and eventual replacement of collagen) and an inflammatory infiltrate, which is neutrophilic initially and mononuclear in the late stages.[8] The etiology is unknown, but the detection in these patients of antibodies to type II collagen suggests an autoimmune mechanism.[7,9]

Localized disorders of the external ear formed by the accumulation of extracellular material include *keloid* (see Chapter 4), localized *amyloidosis,* the uric acid tophi of *gout, elastotic nodules,* and *collagenous papules* (Fig. 31-3). Elastotic nodules are small papules and nodules most commonly noted on the antihelix as a result of actinic damage. Microscopically, they are composed of dermal clumps of elastic tissue.[5,20] Collagenous papules are smooth, firm, small papules, located bilaterally on the inner aspects of the aural pinnae and in rare cases, in the external auditory canal. Microscopically, there is a dense collagenous mass in which dilated vessels and scattered fibroblasts are identified.[16] It has been suggested that auricular lesions with the microscopic features of *granuloma annulare* may be a consequence of trauma.[11]

Tumors and tumorlike conditions
Keratotic lesions

The external ear is a common site for *seborrheic keratosis* and *actinic keratosis* (see Chapter 4). Some ear lesions designated as fibroepithelial papillomas or squamous papillomas are probably variants of seborrheic keratosis. Other *squamous papillomas* present as branching complex polypoid structures in the external auditory canal. Additional types of keratotic lesions that can occur at this site are *keratoacanthoma, inverted follicular keratosis, verruca vulgaris,* and *molluscum contagiosum.* It has been estimated that 8.5% of all keratoacanthomas involve the skin of the external ear.[23] All of these entities are discussed in Chapter 4.

Basal cell carcinoma

Basal cell carcinoma is a common tumor of the auricle and external auditory canal, the ratio between the two sites being 5:1. In the auricle, basal cell carcinoma predominates over squamous cell carcinoma, the ratio being reversed in the external auditory canal. The microscopic features and behavior of this lesion are described in Chapter 4. If un treated, basal cell carcinomas of the canal may extend into the middle ear, mastoid, or even the cranial cavity.[25] These tumors may be treated with surgery or radiation therapy, the choice depending on the size and location.[24]

Squamous cell carcinoma

Squamous cell carcinoma of the external ear comprises one fourth of all squamous cell cutaneous carcinomas of the head and neck region.[26] Most patients are elderly. The tumors are more common in the auricle (particularly the helix) than in the canal.[28,34,37] Many of the latter present clinically with symptoms of otitis.[35] Grossly and microscopically, they do not differ significantly from those seen elsewhere in sun-exposed skin. Some are of the adenoid (pseudoglandular) variety; a few others belong to the *verrucous* type[32,36] (see Chapter 4). The pattern of local spread varies depending on the initial location of the tumor, a finding that also applies to basal cell carcinomas. Tumors of the helix spread initially along the helix and then anteriorly to the antihelix and posteriorly to the posterior surface of the ear; tumors of the antihelix spread concentrically; tumors of the posterior surface of the ear spread to the helix and along that structure.[27] Tumors of the canal tend to invade bone and often destroy the tympanic membrane to penetrate into the middle ear. Like their basal cell counterparts, squamous cell carcinomas can be treated by either surgery or radiation therapy, the choice being determined by the size, location, and degree of invasiveness of the lesion.[32,33]

The prognosis is much better for tumors of the auricle than for those in the canal, a fact that is at least partially related to the earlier diagnosis of the former type of tumor.[27,31] In one series, tumor-related deaths occurred in only one of seventeen patients with tumors of the auricle but in eleven of twenty-one patients with tumors of the canal.[29] The prognosis is particularly ominous for tumors of the inner portion of the canal exhibiting deep involvement of the temporal bone.[30,38]

Adnexal tumors

Almost any type of adnexal tumor can involve the skin of the external ear.[48] One of the most common is *pilomatrixoma,* often seen in children and sometimes confused microscopically with basal cell carcinoma. Other reported cases of - adnexal tumors of this region include other types of *hair-follicle neoplasms*[41] and *sebaceous adenoma.*[47]

Adnexal tumors of the external auditory canal are generally assumed to be of ceruminous gland origin, and the generic term "ceruminoma" has been used for them.[39] The clinical presentation is similar, although the malignant tumors are more often painful and ulcerated.[43] Four major categories are recognized[50]:

Adenoma is sharply demarcated but not encapsulated. Variously sized glandular formations lined by apocrine cells are seen microscopically.[40] A myoepithelial layer can be discerned at the base. Mitotic figures, pleomorphism, necrosis, and invasiveness are lacking.

Benign mixed tumor (pleomorphic adenoma) has an appearance similar to that of its cutaneous or salivary gland counterpart.[42] In some cases, the epithelial component exhibits apocrine features similar to those of adenoma.[49]

Syringocystadenoma papilliferum is morphologically equivalent to the tumor occurring elsewhere in the skin, particularly in the scalp (see Chapter 4). Connection with the surface of the canal is characteristic.

Adenocarcinoma may be well differentiated and therefore difficult to distinguish from adenoma. The presence of more than occasional mitotic activity, pleomorphism, the absence of myoepithelial layer, necrosis, and invasiveness are the main identifying features[44] (Fig. 31-4). The main problem with this tumor is local recurrence; nodal or distant metastases are exceedingly rare.[46]

Adenoid cystic carcinoma has an appearance similar to that of its more common equivalent in the salivary glands (see Chapter 12). Like the latter, it has a great tendency for local (including perineural) invasion and distant (rather than nodal) metastases, particularly to the lungs.[45] The death rate is approximately 50%.

The differential diagnosis of these tumors includes direct invasion from so-called adenomas and paragangliomas of the middle ear and adnexal tumors of the auricle. It is particularly important to distinguish the benign eccrine dermal cylindroma arising from the conchal portion of the auricle from adenoid cystic carcinoma arising from the canal.

Melanocytic tumors

Nevi of any of the known microscopic types can occur in the auricle or, less commonly, in the canal.

Malignant melanomas of the external ear comprise about 10% of all melanomas of the head and neck region.[51] Nearly all are located in the auricle rather than in the canal.[52] The most common type is superficially spreading. Nodal metastases are to the upper cervical, intraparotid, or occipital groups, depending on the exact location of the tumor in the auricle.

Other tumors

Osteoma of the external auditory canal presents as a solitary pedunculated osseous mass attached by a narrow pedicle to the tympanosquamous or tympanomastoid suture line. Microscopically, it is formed by mature lamellar bone containing bone marrow and covered by keratinized squamous epithelium.[54]

Exostoses are sessile, often multiple and bilateral masses that seem to be particularly common in swimmers. Microscopically, the appearance is similar to that of osteoma except for the absence of bone marrow spaces.[54]

Myxomas of the external ear occur in patients with Carney's syndrome, sometimes bilaterally. Microscopically, they are nonencapsulated circumscribed nodules composed of scattered stellate and spindle cells set in a myxoid, capillary-rich matrix.[53]

Other primary tumors of the external ear include various types of soft tissue neoplasms, including those of peripheral

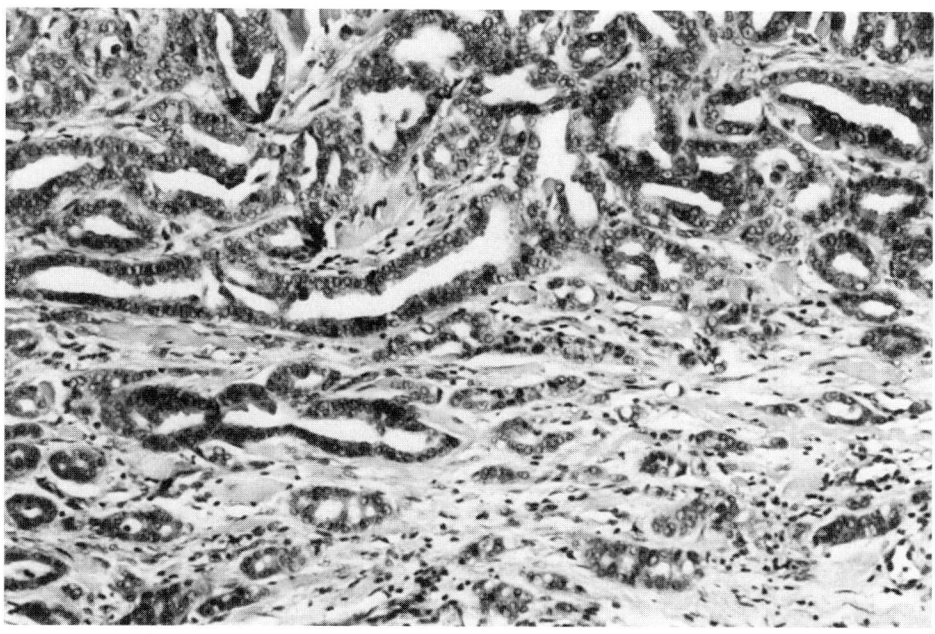

Fig. 31-4 Adenocarcinoma of external ear. Irregularities in gland formations and stromal invasion distinguish this lesion from adenoma.

nerve origin.[55] As already mentioned, the canal can be secondarily involved by tumors of the middle ear or salivary gland.

DISEASES OF MIDDLE AND INNER EAR
Non-neoplastic disorders

Developmental anomalies of the middle ear include encephalocele[64,74] and ectopic salivary gland tissue (sometimes designated as choristoma).[71]

Inflammatory polyp ("otic polyp") arises in the middle ear on the basis of a chronic otitis but often presents in the external auditory canal following perforation of the tympanic membrane. Microscopically, the appearance is that of chronically inflamed stroma, sometimes with the features of granulation tissue. The overlying mucosa may be of columnar ciliated type (consistent with its middle ear origin) or squamous (as a result of metaplasia). Cystically dilated glands may be seen embedded in the stroma.

Inflammations of the middle ear are usually of a nonspecific nature microscopically.[61,62,72] This structure can also be involved by specific conditions such as tuberculosis, aspergillosis, malacoplakia, and Wegener's granulomatosis.[57,58,60,63,69]

Cholesteatoma usually presents during the third or fourth decade, but it may appear at any age. It is the result of chronic otitis media and may involve the middle ear, peritympanic space, mastoid cavities, and petrous portion of the temporal bone. In rare cases, it has been found to extend into the soft tissues of the neck or the intracranial region.[56,65] Grossly, the appearance is that of a cyst filled with a granular waxy material. Microscopically, the membrane that bounds the lesion peripherally is made up of keratinizing squamous epithe-

lium, and the content is composed of keratin squames.[67] Chronic inflammatory cells, cholesterol clefts, and foreign body–type giant cell granulomas are common. It should be noted that although *cholesterol granulomas* are often seen in the middle ear as a consequence of cholesteatoma, they may also occur independently from it as a result of hemorrhage or otitis media.

The pathogenesis of cholesteatoma is controversial; origin of the squamous epithelium from metaplasia of middle ear mucosa, migration from the external auditory canal, migration from the external surface of the tympanic membrane following a perforation, or retraction of the tympanic membrane into the middle ear have all been considered.[66,70,73] In the congenital form, the disease is thought to be the result of inclusions of squamous epithelium in the temporal bone.

The treatment is surgical and aimed at removal of the entire lesion, including the limiting membrane.[68]

Otosclerosis is a disorder of abnormal bone remodeling of unknown etiology involving the otic capsule of the temporal bone. It is characterized by a combination of bone resorption (otospongiosis) and bone production (otosclerosis).[67] This results in the formation of Paget's disease–like woven bone with prominent cement lines.[59] The disease causes hearing loss because of fixation of the stapes footplate in the oval window. Usually, the only specimens received in the pathology laboratory are portions of the stapes head and crura, which are almost always unaffected by the disease.[59]

Presbycusis (hearing loss) is a very common condition but certainly not one likely to generate a surgical specimen. In any event, the morphologic changes described by

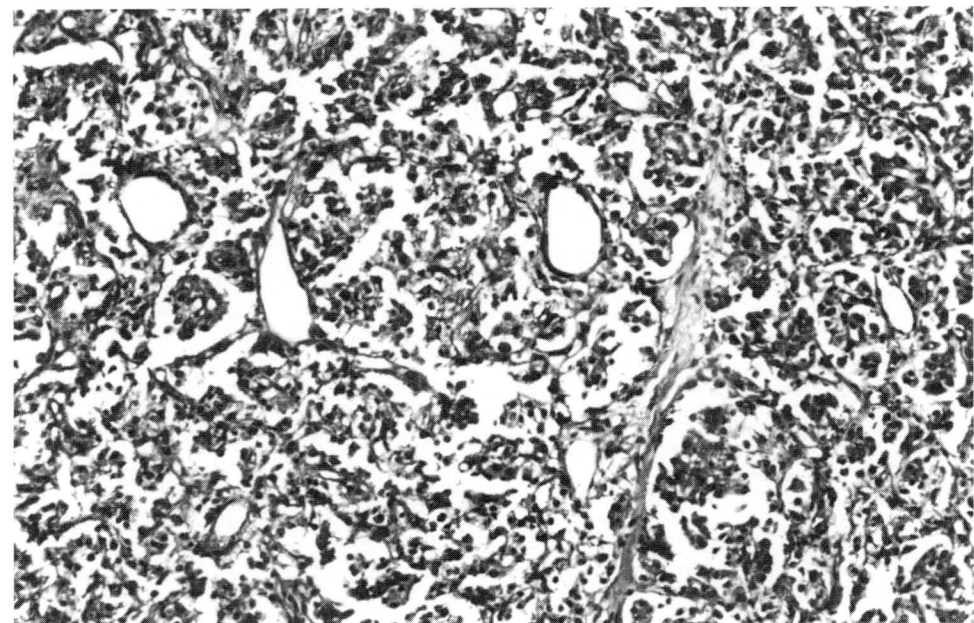

Fig. 31-5 Paraganglioma of middle ear arising from glomus jugulare. Tumor is very well vascularized and is divided in nests by connective tissue septa.

Michaels[67] in this disorder are hair cell degeneration of the cochlea and a process that he calls giant stereociliary degeneration.

Tumors and tumorlike conditions

Paraganglioma

Paraganglioma of the glomus jugulare or glomus tympanicum is the most common neoplasm of the middle ear[75] (Fig. 31-5). The general features of this tumor are discussed in Chapter 16. It can be found in the jugular bulb area, within the middle ear, in the external auditory canal, or around the eustachian tube.[77] In contrast to paragangliomas of other sites, those of the middle ear region have a marked predilection for females.[78] They can be familial, bilateral, or associated with paragangliomas elsewhere. Clinically, the typical presentation is that of a red mass protruding behind the tympanic membrane or extending in the canal. Profuse bleeding may be encountered at the time of biopsy. This tumor has a tendency to infiltrate adjacent bone; a few cases associated with distant metastases are on record. The initial treatment is usually in the form of local excision, but the incidence of local recurrence is over 50%.[78] Radiation therapy has also been used as an adjunct to surgery or as the primary treatment.[76]

Meningioma

About 6% of all meningiomas arise from the surface of the petrous bone, from which they may invade this structure and reach the middle ear.[79] In addition, meningiomas seemingly localized to the middle ear have been described.[80] The tumor may involve the external ear canal, mastoid cavity, or jugular fossa. The microscopic appearance is described in Chapter 28. The treatment is surgical. The prognosis is sub-stantially better for meningiomas limited to the middle ear than for those reaching this site through invasion of the petrous bone.

Schwannoma (acoustic neuroma)

The tumor traditionally known as acoustic neuroma is simply a type of schwannoma arising from the eighth (or sometimes the seventh) nerve, which grows within the internal auditory canal and can reach the middle ear. Its features are described in Chapters 25 and 28. These tumors are bilateral in 8% of the cases and associated with type II Recklinghausen's disease in 16%.[81] The treatment is surgical.

So-called middle ear adenoma and carcinoid tumor

Middle ear adenoma is the term that has been traditionally used for a distinctive tumor of the middle ear mostly seen in patients between 20 and 40 years of age. Grossly, the lesion is grayish white and firm, not as vascular as paragangliomas, and relatively well circumscribed. Microscopically, the pattern of growth may be solid, glandular, or trabecular.[86,91] The tumor cells are uniform, cuboidal or cylindric, with a moderately abundant acidophilic cytoplasm. Mitoses are exceedingly rare, pleomorphism is minimal, and necrosis is absent.

Histochemically, there may be intraluminal positivity for mucin and intracytoplasmic argyrophilia. Ultrastructurally, the tumor cells exhibit desmosomes and microvilli; in addition, membrane-bound dense-core granules are present in many of the tumor cells.[82] Immunohistochemically, positivity for keratin and lysozyme has been described.[88,89]

The histogenetic problem posed by middle ear adenoma mainly concerns its possible neuroendocrine nature and rela-

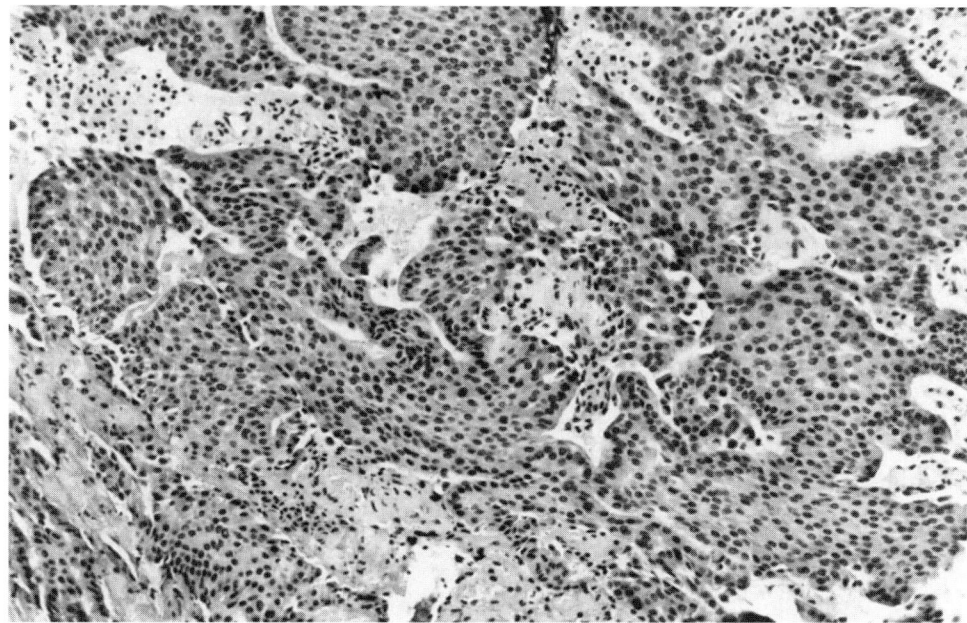

Fig. 31-6 Carcinoid tumor of middle ear. Nesting appearance, artifactual retraction from stroma, and granular cytoplasm are similar to those of carcinoid tumor in other locations. This neoplasm was positive immunohistochemically for chromogranin and exhibited neurosecretory granules on electron microscopic examination.

tionship with the reported cases of **carcinoid tumors** of the middle ear[90,94] (Fig. 31-6). The latter tumors have many cytoarchitectural features in common with middle ear adenoma but also exhibit undeniable evidence of neuroendocrine differentiation.[87] Some authors like to view middle ear adenomas and carcinoid tumors as separate entities and regard the former as tumors of the middle ear mucosa.[89,90] However, a large number of studies performed in recent years have convincingly shown that these two tumors merge imperceptibly, in the sense of showing various portions of exocrine and neuroendocrine differentiation.[83,85,92,93,95] As such, they could be regarded as analogous to adenocarcinoids or amphicrine neoplasms of other sites.[84] The presence of a neuroendocrine component is supported by the previously mentioned argyrophilia, presence of dense core granules ultrastructurally, and reported immunoreactivity for neuron-specific enolase, chromogranin, serotonin, and numerous peptide hormones (such as pancreatic polypeptide, glucagon, cholecystokinin, and leucine-enkephalin).[85,94] Cases associated with systemic manifestations are also on record.[87]

The treatment of choice of middle ear adenoma/carcinoid tumor is surgical excision. The prognosis is excellent, with only an occasional example of local recurrence.[85,93,95]

Adenocarcinoma

Adenocarcinoma of the middle and inner ear is a somewhat confusing and controversial entity.[99,101-103] The term has sometimes been used for adenocarcinomas of the external auditory canal secondarily invading the ear and for so-called middle ear adenoma.[96] However, there is a distinct form of primary adenocarcinoma of this site that is different from

the entities previously mentioned. This is a *papillary adenocarcinoma* composed of uniform cuboidal cells with clear to acidophilic cytoplasm forming papillary structures that rest on a vascular stroma. Cystic dilatation of the glands often occurs, leading to a follicle-like appearance that is very reminiscent of that seen in thyroid tumors.[102,104,105] Tumors with prominent cytoplasmic clearing simulate metastatic renal cell carcinoma. Gaffey et al., who refer to this neoplasm as *aggressive papillary middle-ear tumor* (APMET), favor an origin from middle ear/mastoid epithelium.[98] In a subsequent article, they have shown that this lesion can occur in the setting of von Hippel–Lindau disease, sometimes in association with a microscopically similar tumor in the broad ligament of presumed wolffian (mesonephric) origin.[97] APMET is closely related if not identical to the *low-grade adenocarcinoma of probably endolymphatic sac origin* reported by Heffner.[100] As the name indicates, the author favors an origin from endolymphatic sac epithelium. Regarding the differential diagnosis, it is well to remember that so-called middle ear adenoma does not exhibit papillary formations.

Papillary adenocarcinoma has a tendency to invade bone, from which it may spread to the cranial cavity. The treatment is surgical, but achievement of local control is difficult.[98,99]

Squamous cell carcinoma

Squamous cell carcinoma of the middle ear typically presents in older patients with a history of long-standing ear discharge, which may be hemorrhagic and usually associated with pain and hearing loss.[106,108,110] Rarely, the process is bilateral.[109] An etiologic role for chronic otitis media has

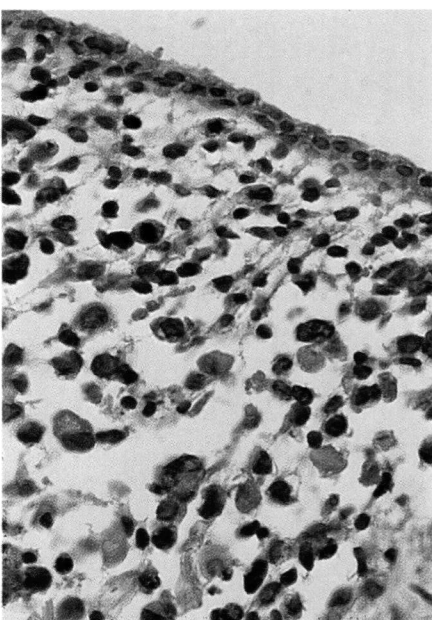

Fig. 31-7 Embryonal rhabdomyosarcoma of the middle ear. Neoplastic tumor cells are seen growing beneath a flattened epithelium. Most of the cell population is small, but there are larger elements with a more abundant fibrillary acidophilic cytoplasm.

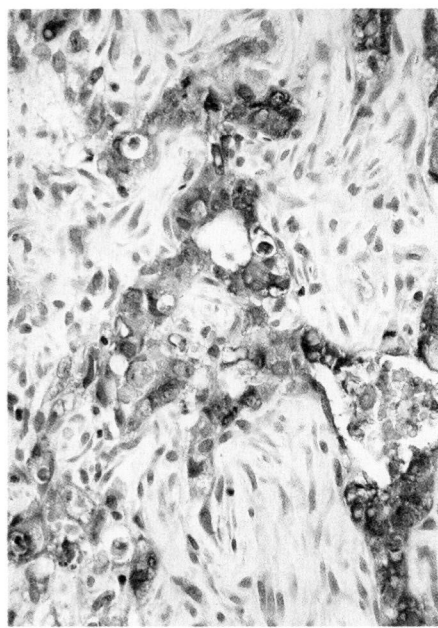

Fig. 31-8 Yolk sac tumor of the middle ear, immunostained for alphafeto protein.

long been suspected.[107] Grossly, the tumor fills the middle ear spaces, from where it may invade the bony walls of the mastoid ear cells, the bone septum that separates the ear from the carotid canal, the internal auditory meatus, the eustachian tube, and the external auditory canal. Eventually, it may reach the intracranial cavity and the soft tissues of the neck.[108] Microscopically, the tumor is an ordinary squamous cell carcinoma of various degrees of differentiation; in rare cases, it may be of *verrucous* type.[111] The differential diagnosis includes secondary invasion of the middle ear by squamous cell carcinomas of the external auditory canal and the eustachian tube. The preferred form of treatment is a combination of surgery and radiation therapy. In the series by Michael and Wells,[108] the 5-year survival rate was 39%.

Rhabdomyosarcoma

Rhabdomyosarcoma of the middle ear occurs almost exclusively in children. At the time of diagnosis, the tumor has often invaded the external canal, mastoid, and meninges.[115] CT scan is the best method to delineate the tumor and to detect intracranial spread. Microscopically, the neoplasms can be of embryonal or botryoid type.[113,114] The microscopic features are described in Chapter 25 (Fig. 31-7). The treatment is a combination of surgery, radiation therapy, and multidrug chemotherapy.[114]

A few cases of rhabdomyosarcoma apparently localized to the external auditory canal have been reported.[112,114]

Other primary tumors

Rare benign primary tumors of the middle ear region include *lipoma, hemangioma, osteoma, ossifying fibroma,*

and *"glioma."*[116,118] The middle ear can also be secondarily involved in cases of *Langerhans' cell granulomatosis (histiocytosis X)*. A middle ear tumor with the histologic and immunohistochemical features of *yolk sac (endodermal sinus) tumor* has been recently reported[117] (Fig. 31-8).

Metastatic tumors

The temporal bone can be involved by malignant tumors arising elsewhere. This involvement can be in the form of direct extension from tumors of the pharynx, salivary glands, or central nervous system or as blood-borne distant metastases. In the latter instance, the most common sites of the primary are the breast, lung, and kidney.[119,120]

REFERENCES
NORMAL ANATOMY
INTRODUCTION

1a Friedmann I: Pathology of the ear. Edinburgh, 1993, Churchill Livingstone.
1b Nager GT: Pathology of the ear and temporal bone. Baltimore, 1993, Williams & Wilkins.
1c Schuknecht HF: Pathology of the ear. Philadelphia, 1993, Lea & Febiger.
1d Lim DJ: Functional morphology of the mucosa of the middle ear and eustachian tube. Ann Otol Rhinol Laryngol **85:**36-43, 1976.
 2 Schindler RA: The ultrastructure of the endolymphatic sac in man. Laryngoscope **21:**1-39, 1980.

DISEASES OF THE EXTERNAL EAR
Non-neoplastic disorders

 3 Brownstein MH, Wanger N, Helwig EB: Accessory tragi. Arch Dermatol **104:**625-631, 1971.
 4 Calnan J, Rossatti B: On the histopathology of chondrodermatitis nodularis helicis chronica. J Clin Pathol **12:**179-182, 1959.
 5 Carter VH, Constantine VS, Poole WL: Elastotic nodules of the antihelix. Arch Dermatol **100:**282-285, 1969.

6 Heffner DK, Hyams VJ: Cystic chondromalacia (endochondral pseudocyst) of the auricle. Arch Pathol Lab Med **110**:740-743, 1986.

7 Herman JH, Dennis MV: Immunopathologic studies in relapsing polychondritis. J Clin Invest **52**:549-558, 1973.

8 Hughes RAC, Berry CL, Siefert M, Lessof MH: Relapsing polychondritis. Three cases with a clinico-pathological study and literature review. Q J Med **41**:363-380, 1972.

9 McCune. WJ, Schiller AL, Dynesius-Trentham RA, Trentham DE: Type II collagen-induced auricular chondritis. Arthritis Rheum **25**:266-273, 1982.

10 Metzger SA, Goodman ML: Chondrodermatitis helicis. A clinical re-evaluation and pathological review. Laryngoscope **86**:1402-1412, 1976.

11 Mills A, Chetty R: Auricular granuloma annulare. A consequence of trauma? Am J Dermatopathol **14**:431-433, 1992.

12 Moloney JR: Relapsing polychondritis. Its otolaryngological manifestations. J Laryngol Otol **92**:9-15, 1978.

13 Naiberg J, Berger G, Hawke M: The pathologic features of keratosis obturans and cholesteatoma of the external auditory canal. Arch Otolaryngol **110**:690-693, 1984.

14 Olsen KD, Maragos NE, Weiland LH: First branchial cleft anomalies. Laryngoscope **90**:423-436, 1980.

15 Piepergerdes JC, Kramer BM, Behnke EE: Keratosis obturans and external auditory canal cholesteatoma. Laryngoscope **90**:383-391, 1980.

16 Sanchez JL: Collagenous papules on the aural conchae. Am J Dermatopathol **5**:231-233, 1983.

17 Satoh T, Tokura Y, Katsumata M, Sonoda T, Takigawa M: Histological diagnostic criteria for accessory tragi. J Cutan Pathol **17**:206-210, 1990.

18 Skau NK, Eriksen KD: Pre-auricular fistula communicating with the external auditory meatus, combined with second branchial cleft anomalies. J Laryngol Otol **100**:203-206, 1986.

19 Thompson JW, Colman M, Williamson C, Ward PH: Angiolymphoid hyperplasia with eosinophilia of the external ear canal. Treatment with laser excision. Arch Otolaryngol **107**:316-319, 1981.

20 Weedon D: Elastotic nodules of the ear. J Cutan Pathol **8**:429-433, 1981.

21 Work WP: Newer concepts of first branchial cleft defects. Laryngoscope **82**:1581-1593, 1972.

22 Zaky DA, Bentley DW, Lowy K, Betts RF, Douglas RG Jr: Malignant external otitis. A severe form of otitis in diabetic patients. Am J Med **61**:298-302, 1976.

Tumors and tumorlike conditions
Keratotic lesions

23 Patterson HC: Facial keratoacanthoma. Otolaryngol Head Neck Surg **91**:263-270, 1983.

Basal cell carcinoma

24 Avila J, Bosch A, Aristizabal S, Frias Z, Marcial V: Carcinoma of the pinna. Cancer **40**:2891-2895, 1977.

25 Goodwin WJ, Jesse RH: Malignant neoplasms of the external auditory canal and temporal bone. Arch Otolaryngol **106**:675-679, 1980.

Squamous cell carcinoma

26 Avila J, Bosch A, Aristizábal S, Frías Z, Marcial V: Carcinoma of the pinna. Cancer **40**:2891-2895, 1977.

27 Bailin PL, Levine HL, Wood BG, Tucker HM: Cutaneous carcinoma of the auricular and periauricular region. Arch Otolaryngol **106**:692-696, 1980.

28 Barnes L, Johnson JT: Clinical and pathological considerations in the evaluation of major head and neck specimens resected for cancer. Part II. Pathol Annu **21**(Pt 2):83-110, 1986.

29 Chen KTK, Dehner LP: Primary tumors of the external and middle ear. Arch Otolaryngol **104**:247-252, 1978.

30 Goodwin WJ, Jesse RH: Malignant neoplasms of the external auditory canal and temporal bone. Arch Otolaryngol **106**:675-679, 1980.

31 Johns ME, Headington JT: Squamous cell carcinoma of the external auditory canal. A clinicopathologic study of 20 cases. Arch Otolaryngol **100**:45-49, 1974.

32 Johnson WC, Helwig EB: Adenoid squamous cell carcinoma (adenoacanthoma). Cancer **19**:1639-1650, 1966.

33 Kinney SE, Wood BG: Malignancies of the external ear canal and temporal bone. Surgical techniques and results. Laryngoscope **97**:158-164, 1987.

34 Lewis JS: Cancer of the ear. CA **37**:78-87, 1987.

35 Paaske PB, Witten J, Schwer S, Hansen HS: Results in treatment of carcinoma of the external auditory canal and middle ear. Cancer **59**:156-160, 1987.

36 Proops DW, Hawke WM, van Nostrand AW, Harwood AR, Lunan M: Verrucous carcinoma of the ear. Case report. Ann Otol Rhinol Laryngol **93**:385-388, 1984.

37 Shiffman NJ: Squamous cell carcinomas of the skin of the pinna. Can J Surg **18**:279-283, 1975.

38 Stell PM, McCormick MS: Carcinoma of the external auditory meatus and middle ear. Prognostic factors and a suggested staging system. J Laryngol Otol **99**:847-850, 1985.

Adnexal tumors

39 Batsakis JG, Hardy GC, Hishivama RH: Ceruminous gland tumors. Arch Otolaryngol **86**:66-69, 1967.

40 Cankar V, Crowley H: Tumors of ceruminous glands. A clinicopathological study of 7 cases. Cancer **17**:67-75, 1964.

41 Cohen C, Davis TS: Multiple trichogenic adnexal tumors. Am J Dermatopathol **8**:241-246, 1986.

42 Collins RJ, Yu HC: Pleomorphic adenoma of the external auditory canal. An immunohistochemical and ultrastructural study. Cancer **64**:870-875, 1989.

43 Lynde CW, McLean DI, Wood WS: Tumors of ceruminous glands. J Am Acad Dermatol **11**:841-847, 1984.

44 Michel RG, Woodard BH, Shelburne JD, Bossen EH: Ceruminous gland adenocarcinoma. A light and electron microscopic study. Cancer **41**:545-553, 1978.

45 Perzin KH, Gullane P, Conley J: Adenoid cystic carcinoma involving the external auditory canal. A clinicopathologic study of 16 cases. Cancer **50**:2873-2883, 1982.

46 Pulec JL: Glandular tumors of the external auditory canal. Laryngoscope **87**:1601-1612, 1977.

47 Raizada RM, Khan NU: Aural sebaceous adenomas. J Laryngol Otol **100**:1413-1416, 1986.

48 Senturia BH, Marcus MD, Lucente SE: Disease of the external ear, ed 2. New York, 1980, Grune & Stratton.

49 Tang X, Tamura Y, Tsutsumi Y: Mixed tumor of the external auditory canal. Pathol Int **44**:80-83, 1994.

50 Wetli CV, Pardo V, Millard M, Gerston K: Tumors of ceruminous glands. Cancer **29**:1169-1178, 1972.

Melanocytic tumors

51 Byers RM, Smith JL, Russell N, Rosenberg V: Malignant melanoma of the external ear. Review of 102 cases. Am J Surg **140**:518-521, 1980.

52 Pack GT, Conley J, Oropeza R: Melanoma of the external ear. Arch Otolaryngol **92**:106-113, 1970.

Other tumors

53 Ferreiro JA, Carney JA: Myxomas of the external ear and their significance. Am J Surg Pathol **18**:274-280, 1994.

54 Graham MD: Osteomas and exostoses of the external auditory canal. Ann Otol Rhinol Laryngol **88**:566-572, 1979.

55 Tran Ba Huy P, Hassan JM, Wassef M, Mikol J, Thurel O: Acoustic schwannoma presenting as a tumor of the external auditory canal. Case report. Ann Otol Rhinol Laryngol **96**:415-418, 1987.

DISEASES OF MIDDLE AND INNER EAR
Non-neoplastic disorders

56 Arkin CF, Millard M, Medeiros LJ: Giant invasive cholesteatoma. Report of a case with cerebellar invasion. Arch Pathol Lab Med **109**:960-961, 1985.

57 Azadeh B, Dabiri S, Moshfegh I: Malakoplakia of the middle ear. Histopathology **19**:276-278, 1991.

58 Barnes L, Beel PL: Diseases of the external auditory canal, middle ear and temporal bone. In Barnes L, ed: Surgical pathology of the head and neck, vol 1. New York, 1985, Marcel Dekker, Inc.

59 Davis GL: Pathology of otosclerosis. A review. Am J Otolaryngol **8**:273-281, 1987.

60 Davis GL: Tumorous and inflammatory conditions of the ear. In Gnepp DR, ed: Pathology of the head and neck, vol 10. Contemporary issues in surgical pathology, New York, 1988, Churchill Livingstone.

61 Friedmann I: Pathology of the ear. London, 1974, Blackwell Scientific Publishers Inc.

62 Friedmann I: Pathology of the ear. Selected topics. Pathol Annu **13**(Pt 1):363-410, 1978.

63 Friedman I: Nose, throat and ears. In Symmers W St C, ed: Systemic pathology, ed 3, vol 1. New York, 1986, Churchill-Livingstone.

64 Kamerer DB, Caparosa RJ: Temporal bone encephalocele. Diagnosis and treatment. Laryngoscope **92**:878-882, 1982.

65 Kreutzer EW, DeBlanc GB: Extra aural spread of acquired cholesteatoma. Arch Otolaryngol **108**:320-323, 1982.

66 Linde RE: Cholesterol granuloma. Ear Nose Throat J **61**:186-189, 1982.

67 Michaels L: The temporal bone. An organ in search of a histopathology. Histopathology **18**:391-394, 1991.

68 Palva T: Surgical treatment of cholesteatomatous ear disease. J Laryngol Otol **99:**539-544, 1985.

69 Ramages LJ, Gertler R: Aural tuberculosis. A series of 25 patients. J Laryngol Otol **99:**1073-1080, 1985.

70 Sade J: Pathogenesis of attic cholesteatomas. J R Soc Med **71:**716-732, 1978.

71 Saeger KL, Gruskin P, Carberry JN: Salivary gland choristoma of the middle ear. Arch Pathol Lab Med **106:**39-40, 1982.

72 Schuknecht HF: Pathology of the ear. Cambridge, Mass., 1974, Harvard University Press.

73 Swartz JD: Cholesteatomas of the middle ear. Diagnosis, etiology, and complications. Radiol Clin North Am **22:**15-35, 1985.

74 Williams DC: Encephalocele of the middle ear. J Laryngol Otol **100:**471-473, 1986.

Tumors and tumorlike conditions
Paraganglioma

75 Alford BR, Guilford FR: A comprehensive study of tumors of the glomus jugulare. Laryngoscope **72:**765-787, 1962.

76 Konefal JB, Pilepich MV, Spector GJ, Perez CA: Radiation therapy in the treatment of chemodectomas. Laryngoscope **97:**1331-1335, 1987.

77 Larson TC III, Reese DF, Baker HL Jr, McDonald TJ: Glomus tympanicum chemodectomas. Radiographic and clinical characteristics. Radiology **163:**801-806, 1987.

78 Reddy EK, Mansfield CM, Hartman GV: Chemodectoma of glomus jugulare. Cancer **52:**337-340, 1983.

Meningioma

79 Nager GT: Meningiomas involving the temporal bone. Springfield, Ill., Charles C Thomas, Publisher.

80 Salama N, Stafford N: Meningiomas presenting in the middle ear. Laryngoscope **92:**92-97, 1982.

Schwannoma (acoustic neuroma)

81 Erickson LS, Sorenson GD, McGavran MH: A review of 140 acoustic neurinomas (neurilemmoma). Laryngoscope **75:**601-626, 1965.

So-called middle ear adenoma and carcinoid tumor

82 Bailey QR, Weiner JM: Middle ear adenoma. A case report with ultrastructural findings. J Laryngol Otol **100:**467-470, 1986.

83 Davies JE, Semeraro D, Knight LC, Griffiths GJ: Middle ear neoplasms showing adenomatous and neuroendocrine components. J Laryngol Otol **103:**404-407, 1989.

84 Faverly DR, Manni JJ, Smedts F, Verhofstad AA, van Haelst UJ: Adeno-carcinoid or amphicrine tumors of the middle ear. A new entity? Pathol Res Pract **188:**162-171, 1992.

85 Hosoda S, Tateno H, Inoue HK, Isojima G, Kondo S, Konishi T: Carcinoid tumor of the middle ear containing serotonin and multiple peptide hormones. A case report and review of the pathology literature. Acta Pathol Jpn **42:**614-620, 1992.

86 Hyams VJ, Michaels L: Benign adenomatous neoplasm (adenoma) of the middle ear. Clin Otolaryngol **1:**17-26, 1976.

87 Latif MA, Madders DJ, Barton RP, Shaw PA: Carcinoid tumour of the middle ear associated with systemic symptoms. J Laryngol Otol **101:**480-486, 1987.

88 McNutt MA, Bolen JW: Adenomatous tumor of the middle ear. An ultrastructural and immunocytochemical study. Am J Clin Pathol **84:**541-547, 1985.

89 Mills SE, Fechner RE: Middle ear adenoma. A cytologically uniform neoplasm displaying a variety of architectural patterns. Am J Surg Pathol **8:**677-685, 1984.

90 Murphy GF, Pilch BZ, Dickersin GR, Goodman ML, Nadol JB Jr: Carcinoid tumor of the middle ear. Am J Clin Pathol **73:**816-823, 1980.

91 Riches WG, Johnston WH: Primary adenomatous neoplasms of the middle ear. Light and electron microscopic features of a group distinct from the ceruminomas. Am J Clin Pathol **77:**153-161, 1982.

92 Ruck P, Pfisterer EM, Kaiserling E: Carcinoid tumour of the middle ear. A morphological and immunohistochemical study with comments on histogenesis and differential diagnosis. Pathol Res Pract **185:**496-503, 1989.

93 Sakurai M, Mori N, Horiuchi O, Matsuura N, Kobayashi Y: Carcinoid tumor of the middle ear. An immunohistochemical and electron microscopic study. Report of a case. Acta Pathol Jpn **38:**1453-1460, 1988.

94 Stanley MW, Horwitz CA, Levinson RM, Sibley RK: Carcinoid tumors of the middle ear. Am J Clin Pathol **87:**592-600, 1987.

95 Wassef M, Kanavaros P, Polivka M, Nemeth J, Monteil JP, Frachet B, Tran Ba Huy P: Middle ear adenoma. A tumor displaying mucinous and neuroendocrine differentiation. Am J Surg Pathol **13:**838-847, 1989.

Adenocarcinoma

96 Fayemi AO, Toker C: Primary adenocarcinoma of the middle ear. Arch Otolaryngol **101:**449-452, 1975.

97 Gaffey MJ, Mills SE, Boyd JC: Aggressive papillary tumor of middle ear/temporal bone and adnexal papillary cystadenoma. Manifestations of von Hippel-Lindau disease. Am J Surg Pathol **18:**1254-1260, 1994.

98 Gaffey MJ, Mills SE, Fechner RE, Intemann SR, Wick MR: Aggressive papillary middle-ear tumor. A clinicopathologic entity distinct from middle-ear adenoma. Am J Surg Pathol **12:**790-797, 1988.

99 Glasscock ME III, McKennan KX, Levine SC, Jackson CG: Primary adenocarcinoma of the middle ear and temporal bone. Arch Otolaryngol Head Neck Surg **113:**822-824, 1987.

100 Heffner DK: Low-grade adenocarcinoma of probable endolymphatic sac origin A clinicopathologic study of 20 cases. Cancer **64:**2292-2302, 1989.

101 Hyans VJ, Batsakis JG, Michaels L: Tumors of the upper respiratory tract and ear. Atlas of tumor pathology, Series 2, Fasc 25, Washington, DC, AFIP, 1988.

102 Pallanch JF, Weiland LH, McDonald TJ, Facer GW, Harner SG: Adenocarcinoma and adenoma of the middle ear, Laryngoscope **92:**47-54, 1982.

103 Schuller DE, Conley JJ, Goodman JH, Clausen KP, Miller WJ: Primary adenocarcinoma of the middle ear. Otolaryngol Head Neck Surg **91:**280-283, 1983.

104 Siedentop KH, Jeantet C: Primary adenocarcinoma of the middle ear. Report of three cases. Ann Otol Rhinol Laryngol **70:**719-733, 1961.

105 Stone HE, Lipa M, Bell RD: Primary adenocarcinoma of the middle ear. Arch Otolaryngol **101:**702-705, 1975.

Squamous cell carcinoma

106 Barnes L, Johnson JT: Clinical and pathological considerations in the evaluation of major head and neck specimens resected for cancer. Part II. Pathol Annu **21**(Pt 2):83-110, 1986.

107 Kenyon GS, Marks PV, Scholtz CL, Dhillon R: Squamous cell carcinoma of the middle ear. A 25-year retrospective study. Ann Otol Rhinol Laryngol **94:**273--277, 1985.

108 Michaels L, Wells M: Squamous cell carcinoma of the middle ear. Clin Otolaryngol **5:**235-248, 1980.

109 Milford CA, Violaris N: Bilateral carcinoma of the middle ear. J Laryngol Otol **101:**711-713, 1987.

110 Morton RP, Stell PM, Derrick PP: Epidemiology of cancer of the middle ear cleft. Cancer **53:**1612-1617, 1984.

111 Woodson GE, Jurco S III, Alford BR, McGavran MH: Verrucous carcinoma of the middle ear. Arch Otolaryngol **107:**63-65, 1981.

Rhabdomyosarcoma

112 Angervall L, Dahl I, Ekedahl C: Embryonal rhabdomyosarcoma in the external ear. Acta Otolaryngol **73:**513-520, 1972.

113 Jaffe BF, Fox JE, Batsakis JG: Rhabdomyosarcoma of the middle ear and mastoid. Cancer **27:**29-37, 1971.

114 Raney RB Jr, Lawrence W Jr, Maurer HM, Lindberg RD, Newton WA Jr, Ragab AH, Tefft M, Foulkes MA: Rhabdomyosarcoma of the ear in childhood. A report from the Intergroup Rhabdomyosarcoma Study—I. Cancer **51:**2356-2361, 1983.

115 Tefft M, Fernandez C, Donaldson M, Newton W, Moon TE: Incidence of meningeal involvement by rhabdomyosarcoma of the head and neck in children. A report of the Intergroup Rhabdomyosarcoma Study (IRS). Cancer **42:**253-258, 1978.

Other primary tumors

116 Cremers CW: Osteoma of the middle ear. J Laryngol Otol **99:**383-386, 1985.

117 Stanley RJ, Scheithauer BW, Thompson EI, Kispert DB, Weiland LH, Pearson BW: Endodermal sinus tumor (yolk sac tumor) of the ear. Arch Otolaryngol Head Neck Surg **112:**200-203, 1987.

118 Stegehuis HR, Guy AM, Anderson KR: Middle-ear lipoma presenting as airways obstruction. Case report and review of literature. J Laryngol Otol **99:**589-591, 1985.

Metastatic tumors

119 Hill BA, Kohut RI: Metastatic adenocarcinoma of the temporal bone. Arch Otolaryngol **102:**568-571, 1976.

120 Schuknecht HF, Allam AF, Murakami Y: Pathology of secondary malignant tumors of the temporal bone. Ann Otol Rhinol Laryngol **77:**5-22, 1968.

Appendix A
Standardization of the surgical pathology report

(This document was prepared by an ad hoc committee of the Association of Directors of Anatomic and Surgical Pathology chaired by Dr. Richard L. Kempson. From Am J Surg Pathol **16:**84-86, 1992.)

Association of Directors of Anatomic and Surgical Pathology

The Association of Directors of Anatomic and Surgical Pathology ("the Association") has concluded that a more standardized surgical pathology report may contribute positively to patient care. As the first step toward achieving this goal, the Association has prepared the following recommendations and urges pathologists to consider seriously adopting these for their own surgical pathology reports. The recommendations concern not only the format of the report but also provide suggestions for information to be included in the report. Widespread adoption of these recommendations should make information transfer from surgical pathology laboratories to clinicians more efficient and complete and also improve communication among surgical pathology laboratories when histologic sections are sent from one institution to another.

Demographic and specimen information

The Association recommends the following:
1 Placing all demographic information in the top portion of the report.
2 Including in the demographic information the patient's name, location, gender, age and/or date of birth, and race, as well as the requesting physician's name, the attending physician's name (if different from the requesting physician), and the medical record or unit number.
3 Printing the name, address, telephone number, and FAX number of the laboratory at the top of the surgical pathology report.
4 Placing the surgical pathology number in the top portion of the report on every page, set off from other information so that it can be easily and quickly identified.
5 Including a summary of the pertinent clinical history as part of every surgical pathology report.
6 Including a separate "specimens submitted" section in every report in which each separately identified tissue submitted for individual examination and diagnosis is clearly identified and listed as a separate specimen.

Gross description

The Association recommends the following:
1 Including an adequate gross description as part of every surgical pathology report. Prerecorded gross descriptions are satisfactory, provided they include specific information about the particular specimen. Each separately identified tissue specimen submitted for individual examination and diagnosis should have its own gross description. Whether "part" or "all" of the specimen has been submitted for microscopic examination should always be recorded in the gross description.
2 Identifying each block with a unique number or letter. Giving multiple blocks the same identification number or letter is discouraged. A summary listing the sites from which each identified block is taken should be placed at the end of the gross description.
3 Augmenting the identification of block selections of complex specimens, when appropriate, by drawings, photographs, xerographs, etc.; but these pictorial records should *not* replace the printed block

identification summary recommended in no. 2 above. Ideally, the pictorial record should accompany the chart copy, the physician copy, and the surgical pathology laboratory copy of the report.

4 Recording in the gross description the fact that margins are inked.

5 Recording the distribution of tissue for special studies in the gross description.

6 Including in the pathology report, when slides or blocks or tissues are received from another laboratory, the numbers of the slides and blocks, the referring hospital's identification numbers or letters, and the referring hospital's demographic data.

Microscopic description and comment section

For purposes of these recommendations, a microscopic description is defined as a description of the cytologic features and the architectural arrangement of the cells in a histologic section. A comment refers to all other pertinent information.

The Association recommends the following:

1 Recording microscopic features whenever the responsible pathologist deems it appropriate, but a microscopic description need not be a part of every report.

2 Placing comments into the report whenever the responsible pathologist considers they are indicated, but a comment need not be written for every case.

3 Making it optional to place microscopic descriptions and comments in separate sections or to combine them.

4 Designating that "special" stains have been performed, listing each stain and the results of the staining in the microscopic or comment section.

5 Listing, when immunohistochemical stains have been performed, each antibody tested and the results of the staining in the microscopic or comment section of the surgical pathology report, in a separate immunohistochemical report, or both.

6 Grading all tumors for which grading has been shown to be a significant prognostic variable. When a grade is given, the grading criteria or scheme should be recorded in a comment or in the diagnosis line unless the grading scheme is standard and well understood by all clinicians.

7 Using a "checklist" approach for recording information needed for patient treatment and prognosis. A statement relating whether each item on the checklist is positive or negative should be made. The checklist is used to ensure that all pertinent information has been included in the pathology report. Such information includes but is not limited to grade, depth of invasion, presence or absence of vascular invasion, size of the tumor, type of tumor, etc., and it is often different for different types of resection specimens. The condition of resection margins should be recorded here if clinically indicated. These checklists may be in manuals, on separate sheets, in computers, etc. It is also recommended that there be routine periodic checks of pathology reports to ensure that this information is present and summarized in an easy-to-find area of the comment or in the diagnosis section.

8 All information needed to formulate the pathologic state of a cancer be present in the report, but this information need not be recorded by a number or letter per se. If a stage number or letter is recorded, then the system used should be specified.

Intraoperative consultation

The Association recommends that the intraoperative consultation report be incorporated verbatim into the final report. The persons responsible for the intraoperative report should be identified. If there is a discrepancy between the intraoperative diagnosis and the final diagnosis, this discrepancy should be recorded and discussed in a comment.

Final diagnosis

The Association recommends the following:

1 Specifying the organ, site, and procedure as well as the diagnosis in the diagnosis section. These can be set off from the diagnosis by a dash or a colon.

2 Standardizing the format of diagnoses within each pathology department.

3 Setting off anatomic diagnoses so that they can be quickly and easily identified.

4 Listing each separately identified tissue submitted for individual examination and diagnosis in the diagnosis section along with the anatomic diagnosis for that specimen.

General considerations

The Association recommends the following:

1 Clearly separating and identifying specimen(s) submitted, clinical information, clinical diagnosis, intraoperative diagnosis, gross description, microscopic description, comments (when they are not combined with the microscopic description), and anatomic diagnoses in such a way as to be found readily and easily in the report. Printing should be of sufficient quality to be read easily.

2 Doing a search for prior histologic and cytologic accession numbers for each case and recording pertinent prior specimen numbers in the current surgical pathology report.

3 Incorporating the results of special studies such as electron microscopy, immunohistochemistry, flow cytometry, receptor status, data, etc., into the surgical pathology report whenever possible. If this information is not a part of the surgical pathology report, the fact that tissue has been sent for the study should be recorded in the surgical pathology report.

4 Recording in the pathology report any information regarding procedures other than routine handling of tissue, such as gross photography, decalcification, specimen x-ray, freezing of samples, and placing specimens in a tissue bank.

5 Documenting intradepartmental consultations in the surgical pathology report, either by identifying the consultant in the comment section or at the end of the surgical pathology report or by having the consultant cosign the report.

6 Noting when external consultation is initiated by the pathologist in the pathology report. When the consultant's report is received, a supplemental report containing the consultant's interpretation and opinions should be issued.

7 Conveying to clinicians any clinically significant unexpected findings and documenting immediately in the surgical pathology report the fact that a call was made.

8 Citing references in the surgical pathology report when pertinent.

9 It is acceptable for the responsible pathologist to make suggestions for additional studies or procedures in the surgical pathology report if the pathologist thinks they will contribute to the case. Such information can be incorporated in the surgical pathology report as long as it is emphasized that they are only suggestions.

10 Note clearly and prominently when an amended report is issued. Changes that have been made in the report should be specified if the new report is a complete one; if only changes are recorded in the amended report, that fact should be specified.

11 Including the date the specimen was received and the date of the final report in all surgical pathology reports.

Appendix B
Incorporation of immunostaining data in anatomic pathology reports

(This document was prepared by an ad-hoc committee of the Association of Directors of Anatomic and Surgical Pathology chaired by Dr. Peter M. Banks. From Am J Surg Pathol **16**:808, 1992.)

The Council of the Association of Directors of Anatomic and Surgical Pathology has reviewed issues in the application of immunostains to diagnostic anatomic pathology. In selected cases this means adding the specificity of immune mechanisms to visual microscopic appearances has become an essential adjunctive method for accurate diagnosis. It has also become evident that no immunologically defined marker is entirely specific for a disease entity. Rather, immunologically defined cellular constituents provide a dimension of resolution regarding cellular differentiation that is additive to that deriving from morphologic observations. As is the case with other ancillary methods, such as special histochemical stains or electron microscopy, immunostaining results must be integrated into a diverse mixture of data, including clinical information, gross and conventional microscopic pathologic findings and, in some cases, other types of ancillary study. It is the responsibility of the pathologist to select appropriate immunostain reagents and to render an informed interpretation of the results of these studies, based on the supplier's description of the reagents' activities, on personal experience, and on reported observations and cumulative experience in the professional literature.

For the purposes of the clarity and exchange of information among pathology laboratories and physicians, the following recommendations are offered for reporting immunostain results.

1 Immunostaining results should always be reported, regardless of perceived significance. Ideally such information should be included in the original main report (surgical, cytology, or autopsy); however, because of time constraints, it may be necessary to report immunostaining separately. When the latter method of reporting is used, it is essential that the initial report state that such studies are pending, and likewise, it is essential that the separate report refer to or even include the original report.

2 A differential diagnosis justifying immunostaining methods should be provided in the report. Reference to differential diagnosis may be very brief or general, for example, "anaplastic large-cell neoplasm of uncertain differentiation" or "epithelial versus lymphoid nature."

3 In the report, or portion of the report, dealing with immunostains the following should be included:

    a. The nature of the studied sample—paraffin sections, frozen sections, aspiration biopsy smears, cellular imprints, cytocentrifuge preparations, etc.

    b The immunoreagents used. These should be specifically described—"HMB-45" rather than simply "melanoma-related antigen." It may be desirable with less commonly encountered reagents to provide a generic designation as well as the specific designation—muscles-specific actin ("HHF-35").

    c Results of the staining for each antibody should be reported in detail sufficient to justify the interpretation—in some cases simply *positive* or *negative*, but in others, cellular patterns of staining or localization of some stain reactivity to certain cellular compartments.

4 Detailed technical information regarding the immunostaining procedures, including fixation, enhancing methods such as enzyme predigestion, and so on, need not be included in the diagnostic report but should be available in permanent laboratory records.

Appendix C
Standardized surgical pathology reports for major tumor types

(Prepared by members of the Department of Pathology, Memorial Sloan-Kettering Cancer Center, New York, NY. From Am J Clin Pathol **100:**240-255, 1993, with additions.)

INDEX FOR STANDARDIZED SURGICAL PATHOLOGY REPORTS

A. Bladder—Biopsy or TUR for carcinoma
B. Bladder—Partial or radical cystectomy for carcinoma
C. Breast—Excision in which only benign disease is present
D. Breast—Excision in which only in situ carcinoma is present
E. Breast—Excision in which only invasive carcinoma is present
F. Breast—Excision in which both in situ and invasive carcinoma are present
G. Esophagus and GE junction—Resection for carcinoma
H. Kidney—Partial or radical nephrectomy for carcinoma
I. Large bowel—Colectomy for carcinoma
J. Larynx—Partial or total laryngectomy for carcinoma
K. Lip, oral cavity, or oropharynx—Resection for carcinoma

L. Liver—Hepatectomy for carcinoma
M. Lung—Pneumonectomy or lobectomy for carcinoma
N. Ovary—Salpingo-oophorectomy for carcinoma
O. Penis and distal urethra—Penectomy for carcinoma
P. Prostate—Radical prostatectomy for carcinoma
Q. Skin—Resection for melanoma
R. Stomach—Partial or total gastrectomy for carcinoma
S. Testis—Orchiectomy for germ cell tumor
T. Thyroid—Resection for carcinoma
U. Uterine cervix—Hysterectomy for cervical carcinoma
V. Uterine corpus—Hysterectomy for endometrial carcinoma
W. Vulva—Vulvectomy for carcinoma
X. Whipple resection for pancreatic, biliary, or ampullary carcinoma

Bladder—biopsy or TUR for carcinoma

Specimen:

Bladder, _____[part #]

_____[procedure]

SP # _____

Pt. Name _____

Fellow/Att _____

Date _____

Diagnosis:

Tumor Type
A1   In situ transitional cell carcinoma
A2   Transitional cell carcinoma
A3   With focal glandular metaplasia
A4   With focal squamous metaplasia
A5   Papilloma
A6   With focal transitional cell carcinoma
A7   Squamous cell carcinoma
A8   Adenocarcinoma
A9   Small cell carcinoma
A10 Mixed carcinoma composed of the following types:
(-)   _____

Histologic Grade
A11 Well differentiated
A12 Moderately differentiated
A13 Poorly differentiated/undifferentiated
(-)   _____

Pattern of Growth
A14 The pattern of growth is papillary
A15 The pattern of growth is flat
A16 The pattern of growth is papillary and flat
A17 The pattern of growth is nodular
A18 The pattern of growth is papillary and nodular
(-)   _____

Local Invasion
A19 The tumor in noninvasive
A20 The tumor invades into the lamina propria
A21 The tumor invades into the muscularis propria
A22 Presence of muscle invasion cannot be evaluated
A23 The tumor extends into periurethral prostatic ducts
A24 The tumor infiltrates the prostatic stroma
(-)   _____

Vascular Invasion
A25 No vascular invasion is identified
A26 Vascular invasion is present
(-)   _____

In Situ Carcinoma (for cases also having an invasive component)
A27 No in situ carcinoma is identified
A28 In situ carcinoma is also present
(-)   _____

Non-Neoplastic Mucosa
A29 The non-neoplastic mucosa is unremarkable
A30 The non-neoplastic mucosa shows the following abnormality(ies):
A31   Chronic cystitis
A32   Granulomatous cystitis
A33   Ulceration
A34   Foreign body reaction
A35   Proliferative cystitis (Brunn's nests, cystitis cystica, cystitis glandularis)

(-)   _____

Bladder—partial or radical cystectomy for carcinoma

Specimen:

Bladder, _____ [part #]

_____ [procedure]

SP # _____

Pt. Name _____

Fellow/Att _____

Date _____

Diagnosis:

B1 No residual carcinoma

B2 No residual invasive carcinoma

Tumor Type

B3 In situ transitional cell carcinoma (pTis) [Use only if there is *NOT* an invasive component]

B4 Transitional cell carcinoma

B5 With focal glandular metaplasia

B6 With focal squamous metaplasia

B7 Papilloma

B8 With focal transitional cell carcinoma

B9 Squamous cell carcinoma

B10 Adenocarcinoma

B11 Small cell carcinoma

B12 Mixed carcinoma composed of the following types:

(-) _____

Histologic Grade

B13 Well differentiated

B14 Moderately differentiated

B15 Poorly differentiated/undifferentiated

(-) _____

Pattern of Growth

B16 The pattern of growth is papillary

B17 The pattern of growth is flat

B18 The pattern of growth is papillary and flat

B19 The pattern of growth is nodular

B20 The pattern of growth is papillary and nodular

(-) _____

Tumor Multicentricity

B21 No evidence of tumor multicentricity is identified

B22 Multicentric foci of invasive carcinoma are present

(-) _____

In Situ Carcinoma (for cases also having an invasive component)

B23 No in situ carcinoma is identified

B24 In situ carcinoma is also present

(-) _____

Local Invasion

B25 The tumor in noninvasive (pTa)

B26 The tumor invades into the lamina propria (pT1)

B27 The tumor invades into the superficial half of the muscularis propria (pT2)

B28 The tumor invades into the deep half of the muscularis propria (pT3a)

B29 The tumor invades into the perivesical soft tissues (pT3b)

(-) _____

Tumor Extension

B30 The tumor does not extend beyond the bladder

B31 The tumor extends beyond the bladder into the following structure(s):

B32 Right ureter

B33 Left ureter

B34 Urethra

B35 Periurethral prostatic ducts

B36 Prostatic stroma

B37 Vagina

(-) _____

Vascular Invasion

B38 No vascular invasion is identified

B39 Vascular invasion is present

(-) _____

Perineurial Invasion

B40 No perineurial invasion is identified

B41 Perineurial invasion is present

(-) _____

Surgical Margins

B42 All surgical margins are free from tumor

B43 The following surgical margin(s) is (are) involved by tumor:

B44 Right ureteral margin

B45 Left ureteral margin

B46 Urethral margin

B47 Perivesical soft tissue margin _____

B48 Bladder mucosal margin _____ [for partial cystectomy]

(-) _____

Non-Neoplastic Mucosa

B49 The non-neoplastic mucosa is unremarkable

B50 The non-neoplastic mucosa shows the following abnormality(ies):

B51 Chronic cystitis

B52 Granulomatous cystitis

B53 Ulceration

B54 Foreign body reaction

B55 Proliferative cystitis (Brunn's nests, cystitis cystica, cystitis glandularis)

(-) _____

NOTE: IF the prostate shows an independent prostatic adenocarcinoma, stop here and continue with the "Prostate" form

Prostate

B56 The prostate is unremarkable

B57 The prostate shows nodular hyperplasia

B58 The prostate shows _____

(-) _____

Bladder—partial or radical cystectomy for carcinoma—cont'd

Seminal Vesicles

B59 The seminal vesicles are unremarkable

B60 The seminal vesicles show _____

(-) _____

Female Genital Organs

B61 All the female genital organs are unremarkable

B62 The vagina shows _____

B63 The cervix shows _____

B64 The endometrium shows _____

B65 The myometrium shows _____

B66 The right fallopian tube shows _____

B67 The left fallopian tube shows _____

B68 The right ovary shows _____

B69 The left ovary shows _____

B70 All other female genital organs are unremarkable

(-) _____

Lymph Nodes

B71 The lymph node status is as follows (expressed as the number of metastatic nodes in relation to the total number of nodes examined):

B72 Right iliac: _____

B73 Right internal iliac: _____

B74 Right external iliac: _____

B75 Left iliac: _____

B76 Left internal iliac: _____

B77 Left external iliac: _____

(-) _____

(-) _____

(-) _____

Breast—excision in which only benign disease is present

Specimen:

Breast, _____[side]

_____[procedure]

SP # _____

Pt. Name _____

Fellow/Att _____

Date _____

Diagnosis:

Breast

C1 No residual in situ or invasive carcinoma

_____

C2 Ductal hyperplasia of mild degree without atypia
C3 Ductal hyperplasia of moderate to florid degree without atypia
C4 Atypical ductal hyperplasia
C5 Lobular hyperplasia without atypia
C6 Atypical lobular hyperplasia
C7 Intraductal papilloma
C8 Sclerosing adenosis
C9 Florid adenosis
C10 Radial scar
C11 Cyst(s)
C12 Apocrine metaplasia
C13 Fibrosis
C14 Calcification
C15 Atrophy
C16 Duct ectasia
C17 Mastitis
C18 Fibroadenoma _____
C19 Fibroadenomatoid hyperplasia
C20 Reactive changes at the biopsy site
C21 Radiation changes
(-) _____

_____

_____

_____

Lymph Nodes

C22 The lymph node status is as follows (expressed as the number of metastatic nodes in relation to the total number of nodes examined):
C23 Level I: _____
C24 Level II: _____
C25 Level III: _____
(-) _____
(-) _____
(-) _____

Breast—excision in which only in situ carcinoma is present

Specimen:

Breast, _____ [side]

_____ [procedure]

SP # _____

Pt. Name _____

Fellow/Att _____

Date _____

Diagnosis:

D1   No residual invasive carcinoma

Tumor Type

D2   Intraductal carcinoma (IDC)

D3   Cribriform type

D4   Solid type

D5   Cribriform and solid type

D6   Papillary type

D7   Micropapillary type

D8   Comedo carcinoma type

D9   With extension into lobules ("lobular cancerization")

(-) _____

Distribution

D10   The IDC is present as a single tumor focus

D11   The IDC is focal with peripheral extension

D12   The IDC is dispersed

(-)

Tumor Size

D13   The estimated diameter for the entire IDC is _____ _____ *mm*

D14   The estimated diameter for the entire IDC is _____ *mm*

D15   The estimated diameter of the IDC cannot be determined because _____

(-) _____

Calcification

D16   No calcification in the IDC is identified

D17   Calcification in the IDC is minimal

D18   Calcification in the IDC is extensive

(-)

For Mastectomy Only

D19   **Tumor Location**
The IDC is located at the following site(s):
Central / UOQ / UIQ / LOQ / LIQ
[circle appropriate one(s)]

(-)

Tumor Multicentricity

D20   No multicentric foci of IDC are identified

D21   Multicentric foci of IDC are present at the following site(s):
Central / UOQ / UIQ / LOQ / LIQ
[circle appropriate one(s)]

(-)

Nipple

D22   No nipple involvement by IDC is identified

D23   The IDC involves the large lactiferous ducts

D24   The IDC involves the nipple (Paget disease)

(-) _____

Surgical Margins

D25   All surgical margins are free from IDC

D26   The IDC is close (within one 40× field) to the following margin(s): _____

D27   The IDC is present at the following margin(s):

(-) _____

Tumor Type

D28   Lobular carcinoma in situ (LCIS)

D29   Classic type (type A)

D30   Large cell type (type B)

D31   With extension into ducts ("pagetoid spread")

(-)

Distribution

D32   The LCIS is present as a single tumor focus

D33   The LCIS is focal with peripheral extension

D34   The LCIS is dispersed

(-)

Calcification

D35   No calcification in the LCIS is identified

D36   Calcification in the LCIS is minimal

D37   Calcification in the LCIS is extensive

(-)

For Mastectomy Only

D38   **Tumor Location**
The IDC is located at the following site(s):
Central / UOQ / UIQ / LOQ / LIQ
[circle appropriate one(s)]

(-)

Tumor Multicentricity

D39   No multicentric foci of IDC are identified

D40   Multicentric foci of IDC are present at the following site(s):
Central / UOQ / UIQ / LOQ / LIQ
[circle appropriate one(s)]

(-)

Surgical Margins

D41   All surgical margins are free from LCIS

D42   The LCIS is close (within one 40× field) to the following margin(s): _____

D43   The LCIS is present at the following margin(s):

_____

_____

(-) _____

Breast—excision in which only in situ carcinoma is present—cont'd

Non-Neoplastic Breast

D44 The non-neoplastic breast is unremarkable
D45 The non-neoplastic breast shows the following abnormality(ies):
D46   Ductal hyperplasia of mild degree without atypia
D47   Ductal hyperplasia of moderate to florid degree without atypia
D48   Atypical ductal hyperplasia
D49   Lobular hyperplasia
D50   Atypical lobular hyperplasia
D51   Intraductal papilloma
D52   Sclerosing adenosis
D53   Radial scar
D54   Apocrine metaplasia
D55   Fibrosis
D56   Calcification
D57   Duct ectasia
D58   Mastitis
D59   Fibroadenoma _____
D60   Fibroadenomatoid hyperplasia
D61   Reactive changes at the biopsy site
D62   Radiation changes
(-)   _____

Lymph Nodes

D63 The lymph node status is as follows (expressed as the number of metastatic nodes in relation to the total number of nodes examined):
D64   Level I: _____
D65   Level II: _____
D66   Level III: _____
(-)   _____
(-)   _____
(-)   _____

Breast—excision in which only invasive carcinoma is present

Specimen:

Breast, _____[side]

_____[procedure]

SP # _____

Pt. Name _____

Fellow/Att _____

Date _____

Diagnosis:

Tumor Type
E1   Invasive ductal carcinoma
E2   NOS type
E3   Tubular type
E4   Cribriform type
E5   Pure mucinous type
E6   Mixed mucinous (mucinous and NOS) type
E7   Papillary type
E8   Medullary type
(-)   _____
E9   Invasive lobular carcinoma
E10   Classic type
E11   Solid type
E12   Trabecular type
E13   Alveolar type
E14   Signet ring type
E15   Tubulo-alveolar type
(-)   _____
E16 Invasive mixed carcinoma:
E17   Ductal _____*type*
E18   Lobular _____*type*
(-)   _____
E19 Invasive carcinoma, type undetermined
(-)   _____

Histologic Grade (for invasive ductal component only)
E20 Histologic Grade I/III (well-developed tubules)
E21 Histologic Grade II/III (moderate tubule formation)
E22 Histologic Grade III/III (slight or no tubule formation)
(-)   _____

Nuclear Grade (for invasive ductal component only)
E23 Nuclear Grade I/III (slight or no variation in size and shape)
E24 Nuclear Grade II/III (moderate variation in size and shape)
E25 Nuclear Grade III/III (marked variation in size and shape)
(-)   _____

Tumor Size
E26 The largest diameter of the tumor, as measured grossly, is _____*cm*
E27 The largest diameter of the tumor, as measured microscopically, is_____*mm*
     [use for tumors ≤ 1.0 cm]
E28 The largest diameter of the tumor cannot be determined because_____
(-)   _____

Tumor Necrosis
E29 No tumor necrosis is identified
E30 Tumor necrosis is minimal
E31 Tumor necrosis is extensive
E32 Tumor necrosis cannot be evaluated because
(-)   _____

Tumor Calcification
E33 No tumor calcification is identified
E34 Tumor calcification is minimal
E35 Tumor calcification is extensive
(-)   _____

Vascular Invasion
E36 No vascular invasion is identified
E37 Vascular invasion is present
E38 Vascular invasion cannot be evaluated because
(-)   _____

Perineurial Invasion
E39 No perineurial invasion is identified
E40 Perineurial invasion is present
(-)   _____

For Mastectomy Only

E41 **Tumor Location**
     The tumor is located at the following site(s):
     Central / UOQ / UIQ / LOQ / LIQ
     [circle appropriate one(s)]
(-)   _____

Tumor Multicentricity
E42 No multicentric tumor foci are identified
E43 Multicentric foci of invasive tumor are present at the following site(s):
     Central / UOQ / UIQ / LOQ / LIQ
     [circle appropriate one(s)]
E44 Number:_____
E45 Type(s)_____
(-)   _____

Nipple
E46 No nipple involvement by invasive carcinoma is identified
E47 The nipple is involved by invasive carcinoma
E48 The nipple is involved by Paget disease
(-)   _____

Skin
E49 No skin involvement by carcinoma is identified
E50 The skin is involved by tumor by direct extension
E51 The skin shows tumor emboli in dermal lymph vessels
E52 The skin shows _____
(-)   _____

Breast—excision in which only invasive carcinoma is present—cont'd

Surgical Margins

E53 All surgical margins are free from tumor

E54 Invasive carcinoma is close (within one 40× field) to the following surgical margin(s):_____

_____

E55 Invasive carcinoma is present at the following surgical margin(s): _____

_____

E56 Involvement of surgical margins by invasive carcinoma cannot be determined because _____

_____

Carcinoma In Situ

E57 No evidence of either ductal or lobular carcinoma in situ is identified

[If there were, you should not have used this form!]

Non-Neoplastic Breast

E58 The non-neoplastic breast is unremarkable

E59 The non-neoplastic breast shows the following abnormality(ies):

E60   Ductal hyperplasia of mild degree without atypia

E61   Ductal hyperplasia of moderate to florid degree without atypia

E62   Atypical ductal hyperplasia

E63   Lobular hyperplasia

E64   Atypical lobular hyperplasia

E65   Intraductal papilloma

E66   Sclerosing adenosis

E67   Radial scar

E68   Apocrine metaplasia

E69   Fibrosis

E70   Calcification

E71   Duct ectasia

E72   Mastitis

E73   Fibroadenoma

E74   Fibroadenomatoid hyperplasia

E75   Reactive changes at the biopsy site

E76   Radiation changes

(-)   _____

Lymph Nodes

E77 The lymph node status is as follows (expressed as the number of metastatic nodes in relation to the total number of nodes examined):

E78   Level I: _____

E79   Level II: _____

E80   Level III: _____

(-)   _____

(-)   _____

(-)   _____

Breast—excision in which both in situ and invasive carcinoma are present

Specimen:

Breast, _____[side]

_____[procedure]

SP # _____

Pt. Name _____

Fellow/Att _____

Date _____

Diagnosis:

Tumor Type
F1 IN SITU AND INVASIVE DUCTAL CARCINOMA
F2   The invasive component is:
F3   NOS type
F4   Tubular type
F5   Cribriform type
F6   Pure mucinous type
F7   Mixed mucinous (mucinous and NOS) type
F8   Papillary type
F9   Medullary type
(-) _____
F10 The in situ component is:
F11   Cribriform type
F12   Solid type
F13   Cribriform and solid type
F14   Papillary type
F15   Micropapillary type
F16   Comedo carcinoma type
F17   with extension into lobules ("lobular canceriza-tion")
(-) _____
F18 IN SITU AND INVASIVE LOBULAR CARCINOMA
F19   The invasive component is:
F20   Classical type
F21   Solid type
F22   Trabecular type
F23   Alveolar type
F24   Signet ring type
F25   Tubulo-alveolar type
(-) _____
F26 The in situ component is:
F27   Classic type (type A)
F28   Large cell type (type B)
(-) _____
F29 IN SITU LOBULAR AND INVASIVE DUCTAL CARCINOMA
F30   The in situ lobular component is *of* _____*type*
F31   The invasive ductal component is *of*_____*type*
F32 IN SITU DUCTAL AND INVASIVE DUCTAL CARCINOMA
F33   The in situ ductal component is *of* _____*type*
F34   The invasive ductal component is *of*_____*type*

Histologic Grade (for invasive ductal component only)
F35 Histologic Grade I/III (well-developed tubules)
F36 Histologic Grade II/III (moderate tubule formation)
F37 Histologic Grade III/III (slight or no tubule formation)
(-) _____

Nuclear Grade (for invasive ductal component only)
F38 Nuclear Grade I/III (slight or no variation in size and shape)
F39 Nuclear Grade II/III (moderate variation in size and shape)
F40 Nuclear Grade III/III (marked variation in size and shape)
(-) _____

Percentage of in situ ductal component
F41 The in situ carcinoma constitutes ≤ 25% of the total tumor mass
F42 The in situ carcinoma constitutes > 25% of the total tumor mass
(-) _____

Tumor Size
F43 The largest diameter of the tumor, as measured grossly, is _____*cm*
F44 The largest diameter of the tumor, as measured micro-scopically, is _____*mm* [use for tumors ≤ 1.0 cm]
F45 The largest diameter of the tumor cannot be determined because_____
(-) _____

Tumor Necrosis in Invasive Component
F46 No tumor necrosis is identified in the invasive component
F47 Tumor necrosis in the invasive component is minimal
F48 Tumor necrosis in the invasive component is extensive
F49 Tumor necrosis in the invasive component cannot be evaluated because_____
(-) _____

Tumor Calcification
F50 No tumor calcification is identified in either the in situ or invasive component
F51 No tumor calcification is identified in the in situ component
F52 Tumor calcification in the in situ component is minimal
F53 Tumor calcification in the in situ component is extensive
F54 No tumor calcification is identified in the invasive component
F55 Tumor calcification in the invasive component is minimal
F56 Tumor calcification in the invasive component is extensive
(-) _____

Breast—excision in which both in situ and invasive carcinoma are present—cont'd

Vascular Invasion
F57 No vascular invasion is identified
F58 Vascular invasion is present
F59 Vascular invasion cannot be evaluated because

(-) _____

_____

Perineurial Invasion
F60 No perineurial invasion is identified
F61 Perineurial invasion is present
(-) _____

For Mastectomy Only

F62 **Tumor Location**
The tumor is located at the following site(s):
Central / UOQ / UIQ / LOQ / LIQ
[circle appropriate one(s)]
(-) _____

Tumor Multicentricity
F63 No multicentric tumor foci are identified
F64 Multicentric foci of invasive tumor are present at
the following site(s):
Central / UOQ / UIQ / LOQ / LIQ
[circle appropriate one(s)]
F65 Number:_____
F66 Type(s)_____
(-) _____
F67 Multicentric foci of in situ carcinoma are present
at the following location(s):
Central / UOQ / UIQ / LOQ / LIQ
[circle appropriate one(s)]
F68 Number:_____
F69 Type(s)_____
(-) _____
F70 Multicentric foci of in situ and invasive carcinoma
are present at the following location(s):
Central / UOQ / UIQ / LOQ / LIQ
[circle appropriate one(s)]
F71 Number:_____
F72 Type(s)_____
(-) _____

Nipple
F73 No involvement of the nipple by either in situ or
invasive carcinoma is identified
F74 The nipple is involved by invasive carcinoma
F75 The IDC involves the large lactiferous ducts
F76 The nipple is involved by IDC (Paget disease)
(-) _____

Skin
F77 No skin involvement by carcinoma is identified
F78 The skin is involved by tumor by direct extension
F79 The skin shows tumor emboli in dermal lymph vessels
F80 The skin shows _____
(-) _____

Surgical Margins
F81 No involvement of the surgical margins by either in
situ or invasive carcinoma is identified
F82 Invasive carcinoma is close (within one 40× field)
to the following surgical margin(s): _____

_____
F83 Invasive carcinoma is present at the following surgical margin(s): _____

_____
F84 Involvement of surgical margins by invasive carcinoma cannot be determined because _____

_____
F85 The in situ carcinoma is close (within one 40× field)
to the following margin(s):_____
F86 The in situ carcinoma is present at the following
margin(s): _____
F87 Involvement of surgical margins by in situ carcinoma cannot be determined because _____

(-) _____
F88 No involvement of the surgical margins by in situ
carcinoma is identified
F89 No involvement of the surgical margins by invasive
carcinoma is identified

Non-Neoplastic Breast
F90 The non-neoplastic breast is unremarkable
F91 The non-neoplastic breast shows the following abnormality(ies):
F92 Ductal hyperplasia of mild degree without atypia
F93 Ductal hyperplasia of moderate to florid degree
without atypia
F94 Atypical ductal hyperplasia
F95 Lobular hyperplasia
F96 Atypical lobular hyperplasia
F97 Intraductal papilloma
F98 Sclerosing adenosis
F99 Radial scar
F100 Apocrine metaplasia
F101 Fibrosis
F102 Calcification
F103 Duct ectasia
F104 Mastitis
F105 Fibroadenoma_____
F106 Fibroadenomatoid hyperplasia
F107 Reactive changes at the biopsy site
F108 Radiation changes
(-) _____

Lymph Nodes
F109 The lymph node status is as follows (expressed as
the number of metastatic nodes in relation to the
total number of nodes examined):
F110 Level I: _____
F111 Level II: _____
F112 Level III:_____
(-) _____
(-) _____
(-) _____

Esophagus and GE junction—resection for carcinoma

Specimen:

Esophagus, _____

_____[procedure]

SP # _____

Pt. Name _____

Fellow/Att _____

Date _____

Diagnosis:

G1 No residual carcinoma
G2 No residual invasive carcinoma
Tumor Type
G3 In situ squamous cell carcinoma
[Use only if there is *NOT* an invasive component]
G4 Invasive squamous cell carcinoma
G5 In situ adenocarcinoma [Use only if there is *NOT* an associated component]
G6 Invasive adenocarcinoma
G7 Invasive basaloid squamous cell carcinoma
(-) _____

Histologic Grade (for invasive tumors only)
G8 Well differentiated
G9 Moderately differentiated
G10 Poorly differentiated/undifferentiated
(-) _____

Tumor Location
G11 Of upper third of esophagus
G12 Of middle third of esophagus
G13 Of lower third of esophagus
G14 Of gastro-esophageal junction
(-) _____

Tumor Size
G15 The tumor length is _____ *cm*
G16 The tumor width is _____ *cm*
G17 The tumor maximal thickness is _____ *cm*
(-) _____

Staging
G18 The tumor does not invade the stroma (Tis)
G19 The tumor invades into the submucosa (T1)
G20 The tumor invades into the muscularis propria (T2)
G21 The tumor invades into the adventitia (T3)
(-) _____
G22 The tumor extends into the following adjacent structure(s) (T4):
_____
(-) _____

Vascular Invasion
G23 No vascular invasion is identified
G24 Vascular invasion is present
(-) _____

Perineurial Invasion
G25 No perineurial invasion is identified
G26 Perineurial invasion is present
(-) _____

Tumor Multicentricity
G27 No evidence of tumor multicentricity is identified
G28 Multicentric foci of invasive carcinoma are present
(-) _____

In Situ Carcinoma
(for cases also having an invasive component)
G29 No in situ carcinoma is identified
G30 In situ carcinoma is also present
(-) _____

Non-Neoplastic Mucosa
G31 The non-neoplastic mucosa is unremarkable
G32 The non-neoplastic mucosa shows chronic inflammation of_____*degree*
G33 The non-neoplastic mucosa shows dysplasia *of* ____ _____*degree*
G34 The adjacent mucosa shows Barrett's esophagus *of* _____*type*
G35 without evidence of dysplasia
G36 with dysplasia *of* _____*degree*
(-) _____

Proximal Margin
G37 The proximal margin is separated from the carcinoma by a distance of _____*cm*
G38 The proximal margin is involved by in situ carcinoma
G39 The proximal margin is involved by invasive carcinoma
(-) _____

Distal Margin
G40 The distal margin is separated from the carcinoma by a distance of_____*cm*
G41 The distal margin is involved by in situ carcinoma
G42 The distal margin is involved by invasive carcinoma
(-) _____

Deep Margin
G43 The deep margin is free from carcinoma
G44 The deep margin is involved by carcinoma
(-) _____

Lymph Nodes
G45 The lymph node status is as follows (expressed as the number of metastatic nodes in relation to the total number of nodes examined):
(-) _____
(-) _____
(-) _____

[For cases with metastatic lymph nodes, regardless of number or site]:
G46 The size of the largest involved node is_____
G47 No perinodal (extracapsular) extension is identified
G48 Perinodal (extracapsular) extension is present
(-) _____

Kidney—partial or radical nephrectomy for carcinoma

Specimen:

*Kidney,*_____

_____[procedure]

SP #_____

Pt. Name _____

Fellow/Att _____

Date _____

Diagnosis:

Tumor Type

H1   Renal cell carcioma
H2   Clear cell type
H3   Granular cell type
H4   Clear and granular cell type
H5   Spindle cell (sarcomatoid) type
H6   Chromophobe cell type
H7   Oncocytoma
H8   Transitional cell carcinoma of renal pelvis
H9   with focal glandular metaplasia
H10   with focal squamous metaplasia
(-)   _____

Nuclear Grade (for renal cell carcinoma only)

H11   Nuclear grade I/IV
H12   Nuclear grade II/IV
H13   Nuclear grade III/IV
H14   Nuclear grade IV/IV
(-)   _____

Histologic Grade (for renal pelvic tumors only)

H15   Well differentiated
H16   Moderately differentiated
H17   Poorly differentiated/undifferentiated
(-)   _____

Pattern of Growth (for renal cell carcinoma only)

H18   The pattern of growth is acinar
H19   The pattern of growth is papillary
H20   The pattern of growth is papillary and acinar
H21   The pattern of growth is papillary and tubular
H22   The pattern of growth is solid
(-)   _____

Tumor Size

H23   The tumor greatest diameter is _____*cm*
(-)   _____

Local Invasion

H24   The tumor is confined within the renal capsule
H25   The tumor extends through the renal capsule but is confined within Gerota's fascia
H26   The tumor extends into the renal pelvis [for renal cell carcinoma only]
(-)   _____

Renal Vein Invasion

H27   No invasion of the renal vein is identified
H28   Invasion of the renal vein is present
(-)   _____

Surgical Margins

H29   All surgical margins are free from tumor
H30   The tumor involves the following surgical margin(s):
H31   Ureteral margin
H32   Renal vein
H33   Soft tissue
H34   Renal parenchymal [for partial nephrectomy specimens only]
(-)   _____

Non-Neoplastic Kidney

H35   The non-neoplastic kidney is unremarkable
H36   The non-neoplastic kidney shows _____
(-)   _____

Adrenal Gland

H37   The adrenal gland is not submitted/not identified
H38   The adrenal gland is unremarkable
H39   The adrenal gland is involved by tumor by direct extension
H40   The adrenal gland is involved by metastatic carcinoma
H41   The adrenal gland shows _____
(-)   _____

Lymph Nodes

H42   The lymph node status is as follows (expressed as the number of metastatic nodes in relation to the total number of nodes examined):
H43   Renal hilar:_____
H44   Right retroperitoneal:_____
H45   Left retroperitoneal: _____
(-)   _____
(-)   _____
(-)   _____

Large bowel—colectomy for carcinoma

Specimen:

Large bowel, _____ [specific site]

_____ [procedure]

SP # _____

Pt. Name _____

Fellow/Att _____

Date _____

Diagnosis:

I1   No residual carcinoma

Tumor Type

I2   Adenocarcinoma

I3   NOS without mucinous component

I4   NOS with mucinous component representing ≤50% of the tumor

I5   With >50% mucinous component (so-called mucinous carcinoma)

I6   Signet ring carcinoma

I7   Adenosquamous carcinoma

I8   Small cell undifferentiated carcinoma

(-) _____

Histologic Grade

I9   Well differentiated

I10 Moderately differentiated

I11 Poorly differentiated/undifferentiated

(-) _____

Tumor Location

I12 Of cecum

I13 Of ascending colon

I14 Of hepatic flexure

I15 Of transverse colon

I16 Of splenic flexure

I17 Of descending colon

I18 Of sigmoid colon

I19 Of rectosigmoid

I20 Of rectum

(-) _____

Gross Configuration

I21 The gross configuration is polypoid

I22 The gross configuration is fungating

I23 The gross configuration is plaque-like

I24 The gross configuration is annular (constrictive)

I25 The gross configuration is ulcerating infiltrative

I26 The gross configuration is diffuse (linitis plastica type)

I27 The gross configuration is _____

(-)

Pre-existing Polyp (At the site of the carcinoma)

I28 No evidence of a pre-existing polyp is identified

I29 There is evidence of a pre-existing polyp *of* _____ _____ *type*

(-) _____

Tumor Size

I30 The tumor length is _____ *cm*

I31 The tumor width is _____ *cm*

I32 The tumor maximal thickness is _____ *cm*

(-) _____

Local Invasion

I33 The tumor is noninvasive (pTis)

I34 The tumor invades into the lamina propria (pTis)

I35 The tumor invades into the submucosa (pT1)

I36 The tumor invades into the muscularis propria (pT2)

I37 The tumor invades into the subserosa or into the non-peritonealized pericolic or perirectal tissue (pT3)

I38 The tumor invades into the following adjacent structure(s) (pT4): _____

(-) _____

Tumor Perforation

I39 No gross tumor perforation is identified

I40 There is gross tumor perforation

(-) _____

Free Serosal Surface (for colonic tumors only)

I41 The free serosal surface is not involved by tumor

I42 The free serosal surface is involved by tumor

(-) _____

Vascular Invasion

I43 No vascular invasion is identified

I44 Vascular invasion is present

(-) _____

Perineurial Invasion

I45 No perineurial invasion is identified

I46 Perineurial invasion is present

(-) _____

Surgical Margins

I47 All surgical margins are free from tumor

I48 Tumor is present at the following surgical margin(s): _____

(-) _____

Distance from Pectinate Line (for rectal tumors only)

I49 The distance between the tumor and the pectinate line is _____ *cm*

(-) _____

Polyps (away from the carcinoma)

I50 No separate polyps are identified

I51 Separate polyp(s) is (are) present

I52   *Type:* _____

I53   *Number:* _____

(-) _____

Non-Neoplastic Bowel

I54 The non-neoplastic bowel is unremarkable

I55 The non-neoplastic bowel shows the following abnormality(ies):

I56   Ulcerative colitis with dysplasia

I57   Ulcerative colitis without dysplasia

I58   Diverticula

(-) _____

Large bowel—colectomy for carcinoma—cont'd

Lymph Nodes

I59 The lymph node status is as follows (expressed as the number of metastatic nodes in relation to the total number of nodes examined):

I60   Pericolic or perirectal_____

I61   Along the course of a named vascular trunk

_____

(-)   _____

Lymph Node Staging

I62 No regional lymph node metastases are identified (pNO)

I63 There are metastases in 1 to 3 pericolic or perirectal lymph nodes (pN1)

I64 There are metastases in 4 or more colic or perirectal lymph nodes (pN2)

I65 There are metastases in 1 or more lymph nodes along course of a major named vascular trunk (pN3)

(-)   _____

Larynx—partial or total laryngectomy for carcinoma

Specimen:

Larynx, _____

_____[procedure]

SP # _____

Pt. Name _____

Fellow/Att _____

Date _____

Diagnosis:

J1 No residual carcinoma
J2 No residual invasive carcinoma

Tumor Type
J3 In situ squamous cell carcinoma [Use only if there is *NOT* an invasive component]
J4 Invasive squamous cell carcinoma
J5 Verrucous carcinoma
J6 Basaloid squamous cell carcinoma
J7 Spindle cell (sarcomatoid) carcinoma
J8 Adenocarcinoma of minor salivary gland origin, _____*type*
J9 Neuroendocrine carcinoma, small cell type
J10 Neuroendocrine carcinoma, large cell type
(-) _____

Histologic Grade
J11 Well differentiated
J12 Moderately differentiated
J13 Poorly differentiated/undifferentiated
(-) _____

Tumor Size
J14 The tumor greatest diameter is _____
J15 The tumor maximal thickness is _____
(-) _____

Tumor Location
J16 The primary tumor location is the supraglottis (_____ _____) [specify site]
J17 The primary tumor location is the glottis (_____ _____) [specify site]
J18 The primary tumor location is the infraglottis (_____ _____) [specify site]
(-) _____

Local Extension
J19 No local extension is identified
J20 There is local extension into the following site(s):
J21   Commissure
J22   Ventricle
J23   Right false vocal cord
J24   Left false vocal cord
J25   Subglottis
(-) _____

Stromal Invasion
J26 No evidence of stromal invasion is identified (Tis)
J27 There is stromal invasion into the following structure(s):
J28   Lamina propria
J29   Muscle
J30   Cartilage (_____) [specify]
J31   Perilaryngeal soft tissues
(-) _____

Vascular Invasion
J32 No vascular invasion is identified
J33 Vascular invasion is present
(-) _____

Perineurial Invasion
J34 No perineurial invasion is identified
J35 Perineurial invasion is present
(-) _____

Tumor Multricentricity
J36 No evidence of tumor multicentricity is identified
J37 Multicentric foci of invasive carcinoma are present
(-) _____

In Situ Carcinoma (for cases also having an invasive component)
J38 No in situ carcinoma is identified
J39 In situ carcinoma is also present
(-) _____

Non-Neoplastic Mucosa
J40 The non-neoplastic mucosa is unremarkable
J41 The non-neoplastic mucosa shows keratosis without dysplasia
J42 The non-neoplastic mucosa shows dysplasia *of* _____ _____*degree*
(-) _____

Surgical Margins
J43 All surgical margins are free from tumor
J44 The tumor involves the following surgical margin(s):
_____
_____
(-) _____

Larynx—partial or total laryngectomy for carcinoma—cont'd

Lymph Nodes

J45 The lymph node status is as follows (expressed as the number of metastatic nodes in relation to the total number of nodes examined):

J46   Right submandibular (level I): _____

J47   Right upper jugular (level II): _____

J48   Right midjugular (level III): _____

J49   Right lower jugular (level IV): _____

J50   Right posterior cervical (level V): _____

J51   Right juxtathyroid (level VI): _____

J52   Right paratracheal and para-esophageal (level VII):

    _____

J53   Left submandibular (level I): _____

J54   Left upper jugular (level II): _____

J55   Left midjugular (level III):_____

J56   Left lower jugular (level IV):_____

J57   Left posterior cervical (level V): _____

J58   Left juxtathyroid (level VI):_____

J59   Left paratracheal and para-esophageal (level VII):

    _____

(-) _____

(-) _____

(-) _____

[For cases with metastatic lymph nodes, regardless of number or site]:

J60 The size of the largest involved node is_____

J61 No perinodal (extracapsular) extension is identified

J62 Perinodal (extracapsular) extension is present

(-) _____

Lip, oral cavity or oropharynx—resection for carcinoma

Specimen:

Oral cavity, _____

_____[procedure]

SP # _____

Pt. Name _____

Fellow/Att _____

Date _____

Diagnosis:

K1 No residual carcinoma
K2 No residual invasive carcinoma

Tumor Type
K3 In situ squamous cell carcinoma [use only if there is *NOT* an invasive component]
K4 Invasive squamous cell carcinoma
K5 Verrucous carcinoma
K6 Spindle cell (sarcomatoid) carcinoma
K7 Adenosquamous carcinoma
K8 Basaloid squamous cell carcinoma
K9 Small cell carcinoma
K10 Adenocarcinoma of minor salivary gland origin, _____type
(-)

Histologic Grade
K11 Well differentiated
K12 Moderately differentiated
K13 Poorly differentiated/undifferentiated
(-)

Tumor Size
K14 The tumor greatest diameter is _____*cm*
K15 The tumor maximal thickness is _____*cm*
(-)

Tumor Location
K16 The tumor location is:
K17   Lower lip
K18   Upper lip
K19   Floor of mouth
K20   Oral tongue
K21   Base of the tongue
K22   Upper gingiva
K23   Lower gingiva
K24   Buccal mucosa (inner surface of cheek)
K25   Hard palate
K26   Soft palate
K27   Retromolar trigone (_____*side*)
K28   Anterior tonsillar pillar (_____*side*)
K29   Tonsillar fossa (_____*side*)
K30   Posterior tonsillar pillar (_____*side*)
K31   Pyriform sinus (_____*side*)
K32   Pharyngeal wall
(-)   _____

Midline Extension
K33 No extension across the midline is identified
K34 The tumor extends across the midline
(-)   _____

Tumor Invasion Within the Oral Cavity
K35 No stromal invasion is present (Tis)
K36 The tumor invades the following structure(s):
K37   Lamina propria
K38   Superficial muscle of tongue
K39   Skeletal muscle [do *NOT* use for tongue tumors]
(-)

Tumor Invasion of Adjacent Structures
K40 The tumor does not invade adjacent structures
K41 The tumor invades the following adjacent structure(s):
K42   Deep muscle of tongue
K43   Periosteum
K44   Cortical bone
K45   Maxillary sinus
K46   Skin
K47   Larynx _____[specify site]
(-)

Tumor Necrosis
K48 No tumor necrosis is identified
K49 Tumor necrosis is minimal
K50 Tumor necrosis is extensive
(-)

Vascular Invasion
K51 No vascular invasion is identified
K52 Vascular invasion is present
(-)

Perineurial Invasion
K53 No perineurial invasion is identified
K54 Perineurial invasion is present
(-)

Tumor Multicentricity
K55 No evidence of tumor multicentricity is identified
K56 Multicentric foci of invasive carcinoma are present
(-)

In Situ Carcinoma
(for cases also having an invasive component)
K57 No in situ carcinoma is identified
K58 In situ carcinoma is also present
(-)

Non-Neoplastic Mucosa
K59 The non-neoplastic mucosa shows no significant abnormalities
K60 The non-neoplastic mucosa shows the following abnormality(ies)
K61   Dysplasia *of*_____*degree*
K62   Keratosis without dysplasia
K63   Atypia, consistent with radiation changes
K64   Chronic inflammation
(-)   _____

Lip, oral cavity or oropharynx—resection for carcinoma—cont'd

Surgical Margins

K65 All surgical margins are free from invasive or in situ carcinoma

K66 All surgical margins are free from invasive carcinoma

K67 Invasive tumor is present at the following margin(s): _____

K68 Invasive tumor is close (40× objective) to the following margin(s): _____

K69 In situ carcinoma is present at the following margin(s): _____

K70 In situ carcinoma is close (40× objective) to the following margin(s): _____

(-) _____

Lymph Nodes

K71 The lymph node status is as follows (expressed as the number of metastatic nodes in relation to the total number of nodes examined):

K72 Right submental (level I): _____

K73 Right submandibular (level I): _____

K74 Right upper jugular (level II): _____

K75 Right midjugular (level III): _____

K76 Right lower jugular (level IV): _____

K77 Right posterior cervical (level V): _____

K78 Right juxtathyroid (level VI): _____

K79 Right paratracheal and para-esophageal (level VII): _____

K80 Left submental (level I): _____

K81 Left submandibular (level I): _____

K82 Left upper jugular (level II): _____

K83 Left midjugular (level III): _____

K84 Left lower jugular (level IV): _____

K85 Left posterior cervical (level V): _____

K86 Left juxtathyroid (level VI): _____

K87 Left paratracheal and para-esophageal (level VII): _____

K88 Pretracheal: _____

(-) _____

(-) _____

[For cases with metastatic lymph nodes, regardless of number or site]:

K89 The size of the largest involved node is _____

K90 No perinodal (extracapsular) extension is identified

K91 Perinodal (extracapsular) extension is present

(-) _____

Liver—hepatectomy for carcinoma

Specimen:

Liver, _____ [laterality and lobe(s)]

_____ [procedure]

SP # _____

Pt. Name _____

Fellow/Att _____

Date _____

Diagnosis:

Tumor Type
L1 Hepatocellular carcinoma, _____ *type*
L2 Cholangiocarcinoma
L3   Of extrahepatic bile ducts
L4   Of intrahepatic bile ducts
L5 Mixed hepatocellular carcinoma/cholangiocarcinoma
L6 Hepatoblastoma
L7   Epithelial type (embryonal subtype)
L8   Epithelial type (fetal subtype)
L9   Epithelial type (embryonal and fetal subtypes)
L10   Epithelial and mesenchymal type (mixed)
L11 Metastatic tumor, adenocarcinoma type
L12 Metastatic tumor, _____ *type*
L13   The tumor is consistent with colorectal origin
L14   The tumor is consistent with _____ *origin*
L15   The number of metastases is _____
(-) _____

Histologic Grade
L16 Well differentiated
L17 Moderately differentiated
L18 Poorly differentiated/undifferentiated
(-) _____

Tumor Size
L19 The greatest tumor diameter is _____ *cm*
L20 The greatest diameter of the largest tumor is _____
_____ *cm*
(-) _____

Tumor Capsule
L21 The tumor is not encapsulated
L22 The tumor is partially surrounded by a fibrous capsule
L23 The tumor is completely surrounded by a fibrous capsule
(-) _____

Tumor Necrosis
L24 The approximate amount of tumor necrosis is _____
(-) _____

Vascular Invasion
L25 No vascular invasion is identified
L26 Vascular invasion is present in the following form(s):
L27   As involvement of the portal vein
L28   As involvement of branches of the portal vein
L29   As tumor thrombi in small vessels
(-) _____

Perineurial Invasion
L30 No perineurial invasion is identified
L31 Perineurial invasion is present
(-) _____

Multifocality (for primary tumors only)
L32 No satellites or multiple tumor foci are identified
L33 Satellite tumor nodules are present
L34 The tumor is multifocal
(-) _____

Hepatic Capsule
L35 The hepatic capsule is free from tumor
L36 The tumor is present beneath the hepatic capsule but not on the surface
L37 The tumor is present on the hepatic capsular surface
(-) _____

Local Extension (for liver tumors only)
L38 The tumor is confined to the liver
L39 The tumor invades the following extrahepatic structure(s): _____
(-) _____

Local Extension (for tumors of extrahepatic bile ducts only)
L40 The tumor is confined to the bile duct wall
L41 The tumor extends into periductal soft tissues
(-) _____

Hepatic Surgical Margins
L42 The surgical margins are free from tumor
L43 The tumor gross clearance is _____ *cm*
L44 The tumor microscopic clearance is _____ *cm*
L45 The surgical margins are involved by tumor
(-) _____

Distal Bile Duct Margin
L46 The distal bile duct margin is free from tumor
L47 The distal bile duct margin is involved by tumor
(-) _____

Non-Neoplastic Liver
L48 The non-neoplastic liver is unremarkable
L49 The non-neoplastic liver shows the following abnormality(ies):
L50   Peritumoral fibrosis
L51   Cirrhosis *of* _____ *type*
L52   Hepatitis *of* _____ *type*
L53   Steatosis *of* _____ *degree*
L54   Hepatocytic dysplasia _____
(-) _____

Lymph Nodes
L55 The lymph node status is as follows (expressed as the number of metastatic nodes in relation to the total number of nodes examined):
(-) _____
(-) _____
(-) _____

Lung—pneumonectomy or lobectomy for carcinoma

Specimen:

Lung, _____[side and lobe]

_____[procedure]

SP # _____

Pt. Name _____

Fellow/Att _____

Date _____

Diagnosis:

M1 No residual carcinoma
M2 No residual invasive carcinoma
Tumor Type
M3 In situ squamous cell carcinoma [use only if there is *NOT* an invasive component]
M4 Squamous cell carcinoma
M5 Spindle cell (sarcomatoid) carcinoma
M6 Adenocarcinoma
M7 N.O.S.
M8 Acinar type
M9 Papillary type
M10 Solid type
M11 Adenosquamous carcinoma
M12 Bronchiolo-alveolar carcinoma
M13 Giant cell carcinoma
M14 Large cell undifferentiated carcinoma
M15 Large cell neuroendocrine carcinoma
M16 Large cell carcinoma with neuroendocrine features
M17 Small cell undifferentiated carcinoma
M18 Oat cell type
M19 Intermediate cell type
M20 Atypical carcinoid tumor
M21 Carcinoid tumor
M22 Metastatic tumor,_____*type*
M23 The tumor is consistent with colorectal origin
M24 The tumor is consistent with _____*origin*
M25 The number of metastases is _____
(-) _____

Histologic Grade
M26 Well differentiated
M27 Moderately differentiated
M28 Poorly differentiated/undifferentiated
(-) _____

Tumor Location
M29 Of right upper lobe
M30 Of right middle lobe
M31 Of right lower lobe
M32 Of left upper lobe
M33 Of left lower lobe
(-) _____

Tumor Size
M34 The tumor greatest diameter is ≤ 3 cm
M35 The tumor greatest diameter is >3 cm
(-) _____

Vascular Invasion
M36 No vascular invasion is identified
M37 Vascular invasion is present
(-) _____

Perineurial Invasion
M38 No perineurial invasion is identified
M39 Perineurial invasion is present
(-) _____

Mainstem Bronchus
M40 The mainstem bronchus is not involved by tumor
M41 The mainstem bronchus is involved by in situ carcinoma
M42 The mainstem bronchus is involved by invasive carcinoma
(-) _____

Bronchial Margin
M43 The bronchial margin is free from tumor
M44 The bronchial margin is involved by in situ carcinoma
M45 The bronchial margin is involved by invasive carcinoma
(-) _____

Pleura
M46 The pleura is free from tumor
M47 The tumor extends subpleurally but not to the pleural surface
M48 The tumor involves the surface of the visceral pleura
M49 The tumor involves the chest wall
(-) _____

In Situ Carcinoma (for cases also having an invasive component)
M50 No in situ carcinoma is identified
M51 In situ carcinoma is also present
(-) _____

Non-Neoplastic Lung
M52 The non-neoplastic lung is unremarkable
M53 The non-neoplastic lung shows the following abnormality(ies):
M54 Focal obstructive pneumonitis
M55 Extensive obstructive pneumonitis
M56 Focal atelectasis
M57 Extensive stelectasis
M58 Emphysematous changes
M59 Interstitial fibrosis

(-) _____
_____

Lung—pneumonectomy or lobectomy for carcinoma—cont'd

Lymph Nodes

M60 The lymph node status is as follows (expressed as the number of metastatic nodes in relation to the total number of nodes examined):

M61   Peribronchial: _____

M62   Hilar: _____

(-)   _____

(-)   _____

(-)   _____

(-)   _____

(-)   _____

(-)   _____

(-)   _____

(-)   _____

(-)   _____

(-)   _____

M63 No direct tumor extension into lymph nodes is identified

M64 Direct tumor extension into lymph nodes is present

(-)   _____

Ovary—salpingo-oophorectomy for carcinoma

Specimen:

_____

_____[procedure]

SP # _____

Pt. Name _____

Fellow/Att _____

Date _____

Diagnosis:

Tumor Type
N1 Papillary serous tumor, borderline (low malignant potential)
N2 Papillary serous carcinoma
N3 Mucinous tumor, borderline (low malignant potential)
N4   Intestinal subtype
N5   Endocervical subtype
N6 Mucinous carcinoma
N7 Endometrioid tumor, borderline (low malignant potential)
N8 Endometrioid carcinoma
N9   With squamous metaplasia
N10 Clear cell tumor, borderline (low malignant potential)
N11 Clear cell carcinoma
N12 Undifferentiated carcinoma
N13 Malignant mullerian mixed tumor
N14   with heterologous elements
N15   without heterologous elements
N16 Mixed carcinoma, composed of the following components: _____
N17 Metastatic carcinoma *of* _____*type*
N18   Consistent with_____*origin*
(-) _____

Histologic Grade
N19 Well differentiated
N20 Moderately differentiated
N21 Poorly differentiated/undifferentiated
(-) _____

Tumor Location
N22 The tumor is unilateral (right ovary)
N23 The tumor is unilateral (left ovary)
N24 The tumor is bilateral
(-) _____

For Unilateral Tumors

Ovarian Surface
N25 The tumor does not involve the ovarian surface
N26 The tumor involves the ovarian surface
Residual Ovary
N27 There is no recognizable residual ovary
N28 The residual ovary shows no significant abnormalities
N29 The residual ovary shows the following abnormality(ies)
N30   Inclusion cyst(s)
N31   Endometriosis
N32   Treatment-related changes
(-) _____

Contralateral Ovary
N33 The contralateral ovary is not present
N34 The contralateral ovary shows no significant abnormalities
N35 The contralateral ovary shows the following abnormality(ies):
N36   Inclusion cyst(s)
N37   Endometriosis
N38   Treatment-related changes
(-) _____

Ovary—salpingo-oophorectomy for carcinoma—cont'd

For Bilateral Tumors

Ovarian Surface

N39   The tumor does not involve the ovarian surface on either side

N40   The tumor involves the ovarian surface on the right side

N41   The tumor involves the ovarian surface on the left side

N42   The tumor involves the ovarian surface on the both sides

Residual Right Ovary

N43   There is no recognizable residual ovary on the right side

N44   The residual ovary on the right side shows no significant abnormalities

N45   The residual ovary on the right side shows the following abnormality(ies)

N46   Inclusion cyst(s)

N47   Endometriosis

N48   Treatment-related changes

(-)   _____

Residual Left Ovary

N49   There is no recognizable residual ovary on the left side

N50   The residual ovary on the left side shows no significant abnormalities

N51   The residual ovary on the left side shows the following abnormality(ies)

N52   Inclusion cyst(s)

N53   Endometriosis

N54   Treatment-related changes

(-)   _____

Right Fallopian Tube

N55   The right fallopian tube is unremarkable

N56   The right fallopian tube is involved by tumor

N57   The right fallopian tube shows _____

(-)   _____

Left Fallopian Tube

N58   The left fallopian tube is unremarkable

N59   The left fallopian tube is involved by tumor

N60   The left fallopian tube shows_____

(-)   _____

NOTE: If carcinoma is present in endometrium, stop here and continue with "Uterine Corpus" form

Endometrium

N61   The endometrium is unremarkable

N62   The endometrium shows the following abnormality(ies):

N63   Atrophy

N64   Simple hyperplasia without atypia

N65   Simple hyperplasia with atypia

N66   Complex hyperplasia without atypia

N67   Complex hyperplasia with atypia

N68   Polyp(s)

N69   Radiation changes

(-)   _____

Myometrium

N70   The myometrium is unremarkable

N71   The myometrium shows the following abnormality(ies):

N72   Adenomyosis

N73   Leiomyoma(s)

(-)   _____

Uterine Serosa

N74   The uterine serosa is unremarkable

N75   The uterine serosa is involved by the ovarian tumor

N76   The uterine serosa shows_____

(-)   _____

Cervix

N77   The cervix is unremarkable

N78   The cervix shows chronic inflammation

N79   The cervix shows _____

(-)   _____

Lymph Nodes

N80   The lymph node status is as follows (expressed as the number of metastatic nodes in relation to the total number of nodes examined):

N81   Right obturator: _____

N82   Right pelvic:_____

N83   Right external iliac: _____

N84   Right internal iliac: _____

N85   Right periaortic: _____

N86   Left obturator: _____

N87   Left pelvic:_____

N88   Left external iliac: _____

N89   Left internal iliac:_____

N90   Left periaortic: _____

(-)   _____

Penis and distal urethra—penectomy for carcinoma

Specimen:

*Penis,*_____

_____[procedure]

SP #_____

Pt. Name _____

Fellow/Att _____

Date _____

Diagnosis:

Tumor Type
O1 Invasive squamous cell carcinoma
O2 Verrucous carcinoma
O3 Spindle cell (sarcomatoid) carcinoma
O4 Spindle and giant cell carcinoma
O5 Mucoepidermoid carcinoma
O6 Adenocarcinoma
O7 Transitional cell carcinoma
(-) _____

Pattern of Growth
O8 The pattern of growth is superficially spreading
O9 The pattern of growth is vertical
O10 The pattern of growth is papillary
O11 The pattern of growth is multicentric
(-) _____

Histologic Grade
O12 Well differentiated
O13 Moderately differentiated
O14 Poorly differentiated/undifferentiated
(-) _____

Tumor Location
O15 The tumor involves the following anatomic site(s):
O16   Glans
O17   Foreskin
O18   Coronal sulcus
O19   Distal urethra
O20   Skin of shaft [Use if this is the *only* area of involvement]
(-) _____

Level of Invasion
O21 The tumor invades to the following level(s):
O22   Lamina propria
O23   Corpus spongiosum
O24   Corpora cavernosa
O25   Buck's fascia
O26   Preputial dartos
O27   Skin
(-) _____

Depth of Invasion
O28 The depth of invasion is_____*mm*
(-)

Vascular Invasion
O29 No vascular invasion is identified
O30 Vascular invasion is present
(-) _____

Perineurial Invasion
O31 No perineurial invasion is identified
O32 Perineurial invasion is present
(-) _____

Tumor Satellitosis
O33 No evidence of tumor satellitosis is present
O34 Tumor satellitosis is present
(-) _____

Extrapenile Extension
O35 The tumor does not extend outside the penis
O36 The tumor extends to the following extrapenile site(s):
O37   Scrotum
O38   Testis
O39   Pubic skin
O40   Abdominal skin
O41   Skin of groin
(-) _____

Surgical Margins
O42 All surgical margins are free from either in situ or invasive carcinoma
O43 The following surgical margin(s) is (are) involved by invasive carcinoma:
O44   Urethra
O45   Skin of shaft
O46   Corpora cavernosa
O47   Foreskin
(-) _____
O48 All surgical margins are free from invasive carcinoma, but the following margin(s) is (are) involved by in situ carcinoma:
O49   Urethra
O50   Foreskin mucosa
O51   Skin of shaft
(-) _____

Tumor Multicentricity
O52 No evidence of tumor multicentricity is identified
O53 Multicentric foci of invasive carcinoma are present
(-) _____

In Situ Carcinoma (for cases also having an invasive component)
O54 No in situ carcinoma is identified
O55 In situ carcinoma is also present
(-) _____

Penis and distal urethra—penectomy for carcinoma—cont'd

Non-Neoplastic Mucosa

O56 The non-neoplastic mucosa is unremarkable

O57 The non-neoplastic mucosa shows the following abnormality(ies):

O58   Chronic inflammation

O59   Fibrosis

O60   Balanitis xerotica obliterans

O61   Epithelial hyperplasia without dysplasia

O62   Dysplasia *of*_____*degree*

O63   Condyloma

O64   Koilocytotic atypia

(-)   _____

Lymph Nodes

O65 The lymph node status is as follows (expressed as the number of metastatic nodes in relation to the total number of nodes examined):

O66   Right sentinel: _____

O67   Right inguinal: _____

O68   Right superficial inguinal: _____

O69   Right deep inguinal:_____

O70   Right pelvic:_____

O71   Left sentinel: _____

O72   Left inguinal: _____

O73   Left superficial inguinal: _____

O74   Left deep inguinal:_____

O75   Left pelvic:_____

(-)   _____

[For cases with metastatic lymph nodes, regardless of number or site]:

O76 The size of the largest involved node is_____

O77 No perinodal (extracapsular) extension is identified

O78 Perinodal (extracapsular) extension is present

(-)   _____

Prostate—radical prostatectomy for carcinoma

Specimen:

Prostate, _____

_____ [procedure]

SP # _____

Pt. Name _____

Fellow/Att _____

Date _____

Diagnosis:

P1 No residual carcinoma

Tumor Type

P2 Adenocarcinoma of prostate

(-) _____

Histologic Grade

P3 Well differentiated
P4 Moderately differentiated
P5 Poorly differentiated/undifferentiated

(-) _____

Gleason's Grade

P6 Gleason's grade is _____ + _____ = _____ /10

(-) _____

Tumor Location

P7 The tumor involves the following quadrant(s):
P8   Right posterior
P9   Right anterior
P10   Left posterior
P11   Left anterior

(-) _____

Vascular Invasion

P12 No vascular invasion is identified
P13 Vascular invasion is present

(-) _____

Perineurial Invasion

P14 No perineurial invasion is identified
P15 Vascular invasion is present

(-) _____

Tumor Multicentricity

P16 No evidence of tumor multicentricity is identified
P17 Multicentric foci of invasive carcinoma are present

(-) _____

Staging

P18 The tumor is confined to the prostate and involves half of a lobe or less (stage pT2a)
P19 The tumor is confined to the prostate and involves more than half a lobe but not both lobes (stage pT2b)
P20 The tumor is confined to the prostate and involves both lobes (stage pT2c)

(-) _____

P21 The tumor invades into the prostatic apex
P22 The tumor invades into the prostatic capsule but not beyond _____
P23 The tumor exhibits unilateral extracapsular extension (stage pT3a)
P24 The tumor exhibits bilateral extracapsular extension (stage pT3b)
P25 The tumor invades into the right seminal vesicle (stage pT3c)
P26 The tumor invades into the left seminal vesicle (stage pT3c)
P27 The tumor invades into both seminal vesicles (stage pT3c)
P28 The tumor invades into bladder neck (stage pT4a)

(-) _____

Surgical Margins

P29 All surgical margins are free from tumor
P30 Tumor is present at the following surgical margin(s):
P31   Apical (urethral)
P32   Soft tissue _____ [specify site]
P33   Bladder neck

(-) _____

Presence of PIN

P34 No evidence of PIN is identified
P35 There is focal PIN ($\leq$ 2 foci)
P36 There is multifocal PIN (> 3 foci)

(-) _____

Location of PIN

P37 The PIN is adjacent to the adenocarcinoma
P38 The PIN is both adjacent and away from the adenocarcinoma
P39 The PIN is away from the adenocarcinoma

(-) _____

Non-Neoplastic Prostate

P40 The non-neoplastic prostate is unremarkable
P41 The non-neoplastic prostate shows the following abnormality(ies):
P42   Nodular hyperplasia
P43   Chronic prostatitis
P44   Infarct
P45   Basal cell hyperplasia

(-) _____

Prostate—radical prostatectomy for carcinoma—cont'd

Lymph Nodes

P46 The lymph node status is as follows (expressed as the number of metastatic nodes in relation to the total number of nodes examined):

P47   Right pelvic:_____

P48   Right internal iliac: _____

P49   Right external iliac: _____

P50   Right periaortic: _____

P51   Left pelvic:_____

P52   Left internal iliac:_____

P53   Left external iliac: _____

P54   Left periaortic: _____

(-)   _____

Lymph Node Staging

P55 No regional lymph node metastases are identified (pNO)

P56 There is metastasis in a single lymph node, 2 cm or less in greatest dimension (pN1)

P57 There is metastasis in a single lymph node, more than 2 cm but no more than 5 cm in greatest dimension, or in multiple lymph nodes, none more than 5 cm in greatest dimension (pN2)

P58 There is metastasis in one or more lymph nodes, more than 5 cm in greatest dimension (pN3)

(-) _____

Skin—resection for melanoma

Specimen:

Skin, _____ [site]

_____ [procedure]

SP # _____

Pt. Name _____

Fellow/Att _____

Date _____

Diagnosis:

Q1 No residual malignant melanoma

Tumor Type

Q2 Malignant melanoma
(-)

Level and Depth

Q3 Clark's level _____

Q4 Depth of invasion _____ *mm*
(-) _____

Radial Growth Phase

Q5 No radial growth phase is identified

Q6 Radial growth phase is present, superficial spreading type

Q7 Radial growth phase is present, lentigo maligna type

Q8 Radial growth phase is present, acral lentiginous type

Q9 Radial growth phase is present, undetermined type

Q10 Radial growth phase cannot be evaluated
(-) _____

Vertical Growth Phase

Q11 No vertical growth phase is identified

Q12 Vertical growth phase is present, epithelioid type

Q13 Vertical growth phase is present, spindle cell type

Q14 Vertical growth phase is present, mixed cell type

Q15 Vertical growth phase cannot be evaluated
(-) _____

Ulceration

Q16 No ulceration is identified

Q17 Ulceration is present, _____ *mm wide*

Q18 Ulceration cannot be evaluated
(-) _____

Pigmentation

Q19 No pigmentation is identified

Q20 Pigmentation is mild to moderate

Q21 Pigmentation is marked
(-) _____

Lymphoid Response at Base (TIL)

Q22 No lymphoid response at base (TIL) is identified

Q23 Lymphoid response at base (TIL) is mild (nonbrisk)

Q24 Lymphoid response at base (TIL) is marked (brisk)

Q25 Lymphoid response at base (TIL) cannot be evaluated
(-) _____

Signs of Regression

Q26 No signs of regression are identified

Q27 Signs of regression are present

Q28 Signs of regression cannot be evaluated
(-) _____

Associated Melanocytic Nevus

Q29 No evidence of an associated melanocytic nevus is identified

Q30 There is an associated melanocytic nevus, _____
_____ *type*
(-) _____

Vascular Invasion

Q31 No vascular invasion is identified

Q32 Vascular invasion is present

Q33 Vascular invasion cannot be evaluated
(-) _____

Microscopic Satellitosis

Q34 No microscopic satellitosis is identified

Q35 Microscopic satellitosis is present

Q36 Microscopic satellitosis cannot be evaluated
(-) _____

Lateral Margins of Excision

Q37 The lateral margins of excision are free from tumor

Q38 The lateral margins of excision are involved by tumor

Q39 The lateral margins of excision cannot be evaluated
(-) _____

Deep Margins of Excision

Q40 The deep margins of excision are free from tumor

Q41 The deep margins of excision are involved by tumor

Q42 The deep margins of excision cannot be evaluated
(-) _____

Non-Neoplastic Skin

Q43 The non-neoplastic skin is unremarkable

Q44 The non-neoplastic skin shows the following abnormality(ies):

Q45   Actinic keratosis

Q46   Melanocytic hyperplasia

Q47   Anatomically separate melanocytic nevus(i) *of*
_____ *type*
(-) _____

Lymph Nodes

Q48 The lymph node status is as follows (expressed as the number of metastatic nodes in relation to the total number of nodes examined):
(-) _____
(-) _____
(-) _____

[For cases with metastatic lymph nodes, regardless of number or site]:

Q49 The size of the largest involved node is _____

Q50 No perinodal (extracapsular) extension is identified

Q51 Perinodal (extracapsular) extension is present
(-) _____

Stomach—partial or total gastrectomy for carcinoma

Specimen:

Stomach, _____

_____[procedure]

SP # _____

Pt. Name _____
Fellow/Att _____
Date _____

Diagnosis:

R1   No residual carcinoma
R2   No residual invasive adenocarcinoma
        Tumor Type
R3   In situ carcinoma [use only if there is *NOT* an invasive component]
R4   Invasive adenocarcinoma
R5   Tubular (intestinal)
R6   Papillary
R7   Signet ring
R8   Mucinous (non–signet ring)
R9   With neuroendocrine features
R10   With squamous metaplasia (adenosquamous carcinoma)
(-)   _____

Histologic Grade
R11   Well differentiated
R12   Moderately differentiated
R13   Poorly differentiated/undifferentiated
(-)   _____

Location
R14   Of upper third (cardiac area/fundus)
R15   Of middle third (corpus)
R16   Of lower third (antral area/pylorus)
(-)   _____

Tumor Size
R17   The tumor length is _____ *cm*
R18   The tumor width is _____ *cm*
R19   The tumor maximal thickness is _____ *cm*
(-)   _____

Pre-existing Polyp (at the site of the carcinoma)
R20   No evidence of a pre-existent polyp is identified
R21   There is evidence of a pre-existing polyp *of* _____
        _____ *type*
(-)   _____

Local Invasion
R22   The tumor in noninvasive (pTis)
R23   The tumor invades into the lamina propria (pT1)
R24   The tumor invades into the submucosa (pT1)
R25   The tumor invades into the muscularis propria (pT2)
R26   The tumor invades into the subserosa (pT2)
R27   The tumor invades at the serosal surface (pT3)
R28   The tumor invades into the following adjacent structure(s) (pT4): _____
(-)   _____

Vascular Invasion
R29   No vascular invasion is identified
R30   Vascular invasion is present
(-)   _____

Perineurial Invasion
R31   No perineurial invasion is identified
R32   Perineurial invasion is present
(-)   _____

Spleen
R33   The spleen was not resected
R34   The spleen is not involved by tumor
R35   The spleen shows direct invasion by tumor
R36   The spleen shows metastatic tumor
(-)   _____

Pancreas
R37   The pancreas was not resected
R38   The pancreas is not involved by tumor
R39   The pancreas shows direct invasion by tumor
R40   The pancreas shows metastatic tumor
(-)   _____

Peritoneum
R41   No peritoneal tumor implants are identified
R42   There are peritoneal tumor implants
(-)   _____

Surgical Margins
R43   All surgical margins are free from tumor
R44   Tumor is present at the following surgical margin(s):
(-)   _____

In Situ Carcinoma (for cases also having an invasive component)
R45   No in situ carcinoma is identified
R46   In situ carcinoma is also present
(-)   _____

Polyps (away from the carcinoma)
R47   No separate polyps are identified
R48   Separate polyp(s) is(are) present:
R49   Type: _____
R50   Number: _____
(-)   _____

Non-Neoplastic Stomach
R51   The non-neoplastic stomach is unremarkable
R52   The non-neoplastic stomach shows the following abnormality(ies):
R53   Dysplasia *of* _____ *degree*
R54   Chronic atrophic gastritis *of* _____ *degree*
R55   without intestinal metaplasia
R56   with intestinal metaplasia
R57   Superficial gastritis
(-)   _____

Stomach—partial or total gastrectomy for carcinoma—cont'd

Lymph Nodes

R58   The lymph node status is as follows (expressed as the number of metastatic nodes in relation to the total number of nodes examined):

R59   Cardiac: _____

R60   Right cardiac: _____

R61   Left cardiac: _____

R62   Lesser curvature: _____

R63   Greater curvature: _____

R64   Suprapyloric: _____

R65   Left gastric artery: _____

R66   Hepatic artery: _____

R67   Celiac: _____

R68   Splenic hilar: _____

R69   Splenic artery: _____

R70   Hepatic hilar: _____

R71   Retropancreatic: _____

R72   Mesenteric:_____

R73   Para-esophageal: _____

(-)   _____

(-)   _____

Testis—orchectomy for germ cell tumor

Specimen:

*Testis,*_____

_____[procedure]

SP #_____

Pt. Name _____

Fellow/Att _____

Date _____

Diagnosis:

Tumor Type

S1   Seminoma
S2   Classic
S3   Spermatocytic
S4   Anaplastic
S5   With trophoblastic giant cells
S6   Embryonal carcinoma
S7   Yolk sac tumor
S8   Mature teratoma
S9   Immature teratoma
S10   Embryonal carcinoma and teratoma (teratocarcinoma)
S11   Teratoma with malignant transformation
S12   Choriocarcinoma
S13   Mixed germ cell tumor composed of the following type(s): _____

(-) _____

Tumor Size

S14   The tumor greatest diameter is _____*cm*
(-) _____

Intratubular Germ Cell Neoplasia (ITGCN)

S15   No ITGCN is identified
S16   ITGCN is present
(-) _____

Vascular Invasion

S17   No vascular invasion is identified
S18   Vascular invasion is present
(-) _____

Tunica Albuginea

S19   The tunica albuginea is free from tumor
S20   The tumor penetrates the tunica albuginea but does not perforate it
S21   The tumor perforates the tunica albuginea
(-) _____

Rete Testis

S22   The rete testis is free from tumor
S23   The rete testis is involved by tumor
(-) _____

Epididymis

S24   The epididymis is free from tumor
S25   The epididymis is involved by tumor
(-) _____

Spermatic Cord and Surgical Margins

S26   The spermatic cord (including its surgical margin) is free from tumor
S27   The spermatic cord if involved by tumor but its surgical margin is free
S28   The surgical margin of the spermatic cord is involved by tumor
(-) _____

Non-Neoplastic Testis

S29   The non-neoplastic testis shows no significant abnormalities
S30   The non-neoplastic testis shows the following abnormality(ies):
S31   Atrophy
S32   Fibrosis
S33   Chronic inflammation
(-) _____

Lymph Nodes

S34   The lymph node status is as follows (expressed as the number of metastatic nodes in relation to the total number of nodes examined):
S35   Right pelvic _____
S36   Right external iliac_____
S37   Right internal iliac _____
S38   Right periaortic _____
S39   Left pelvic _____
S40   Left external iliac_____
S41   Left internal iliac _____
S42   Left periaortic_____
(-) _____

Thyroid—resection for carcinoma

Specimen:

Thyroid, _____

_____[procedure]

SP # _____

Pt. Name _____

Fellow/Att _____

Date _____

Diagnosis:

Tumor Type

T1 Papillary carcinoma
T2   Classic type
T3   Follicular variant
T4   Solid/trabecular variant
T5   Microcarcinoma (occult sclerosing) variant
T6   Diffuse sclerosing variant
T7   Oncocytic (Hurthe cell) variant
T8   Tall cell variant
T9   Columnar cell variant
T10 Follicular carcinoma
T11 Hurthle cell carcinoma
T12 Poorly differentiated carcinoma, insular type
T13 Poorly differentiated carcinoma, _____ _____*type*
T14 Undifferentiated (anaplastic) carcinoma
T15   Without residual well-differentiated component
T16   With residual well-differentiated component *of* _____*type*
T17 Medullary carcinoma
T18   Classic type _____*type*
T19 Mixed medullary-follicular carcinoma
(-) _____

Histologic Grade (for papillary, follicular, or Hurthle cell carcinoma only)
T20 Well differentiated
T21 Moderately differentiated
T22 Poorly differentiated
(-) _____

Mitotic Activity
T23 Mitotic activity is nil
T24 Mitotis activity is mild to moderate
T25 Mitotic activity is marked
(-) _____

Tumor Necrosis
T26 No tumor necrosis is identified
T27 Tumor necrosis is focal
T28 Tumor necrosis is extensive
(-) _____

Other Tumor Features
T29 The tumor also exhibits the following feature(s):
T30   Squamous metaplasia
T31   Cytoplasmic clear cell changes
T32   Focal mucinous features
T33   Psammoma bodies
T34   Calcification of nonpsammoma type
T35   Marked stromal reaction
T36   Necrotic and/or reactive changes probably induced by the fine needle procedure
T37   Amyloid deposition
(-) _____

Tumor Location
T38 The tumor involves the right lobe
T39 The tumor involves the left lobe
T40 The tumor involves the isthmus
T41 The tumor involves the right lobe and isthmus
T42 The tumor involves the left lobe and isthmus
T43 The tumor involves both lobes and isthmus
(-) _____

Tumor Size
T44 The tumor greatest diameter is _____*cm*
(-) _____

Encapsulation
T45 The tumor is totally surrounded by a fibrous capsule
T46 The tumor is partially surrounded by a fibrous capsule
T47 The tumor is not encapsulated
(-) _____

Capsular Invasion
T48 No evidence of capsular invasion is identified
T49 There is focal capsular invasion by tumor
T50 There is extensive capsular invasion by tumor
(-) _____

Blood Vessel Invasion
T51 No evidence of blood vessel invasion is identified
T52 Areas suggestive but not diagnostic of blood vessel invasion are present
T53 Focal vascular invasion is present
T54 Extensive vascular invasion is present
(-) _____

Extrathyroid Extension
T55 No evidence of extrathyroid extension is identified
T56 There is extrathyroid extension into _____
(-) _____

Thyroid—resection for carcinoma—cont'd

Surgical Margins

T57 All surgical margins are free from tumor

T58 The tumor is close (40× objective) to the following surgical margin(s): _____

_____

T59 The tumor is present at the following surgical margin(s) _____

_____

_____

(-) _____

Tumor Multicentricity

T60 No evidence of tumor multicentricity is identified

T61 Gross multicentric foci of carcinoma are present

T62 Microscopic multicentric foci of carcinoma are present

(-) _____

C-Cell Hyperplasia (for medullary carcinoma cases only)

T63 No evidence of C-cell hyperplasia is present

T64 There is C-cell hyperplasia of mild to moderate degree

T65 There is C-cell hyperplasia of marked degree

T66 Presence of C-cell hyperplasia cannot be evaluated

(-) _____

Adenoma(s) (away from the carcinoma)

T67 No separate adenomas are identified

T68 Separate adenoma(s) is (are) identified

T69 *Type:* _____

T70 *Number:* _____

(-) _____

Non-Neoplastic Thyroid

T71 The non-neoplastic thyroid shows no abnormalities

T72 The non-neoplastic thyroid shows the following abnormality(ies):

T73 Nodular hyperplasia

T74 Lymphocytic thyroiditis

T75 Hashimoto's thyroiditis

T76 So-called palpation thyroiditis

T77 Atrophy

T78 Fibrosis

(-) _____

Parathyroid

T79 No parathyroid glands are identified

T80 The following parathyroid glands were identified:

_____

[Specify number and, if possible, the site in parentheses]

T81 These parathyroid glands are not involved by carcinoma

T82 These parathyroid glands are involved by carcinoma

(-)

Lymph Nodes

T83 The lymph node status is as follows (expressed as the number of metastatic nodes in relation to the total number of nodes examined):

T84 Right submandibular (level I): _____

T85 Right upper jugular (level II): _____

T86 Right midjugular (level III): _____

T87 Right lower jugular (level IV): _____

T88 Right posterior cervical (level V): _____

T89 Right juxtathyroid (level VI): _____

T90 Right paratracheal and para-esophageal (level VII): _____

T91 Left submandibular (level I): _____

T92 Left upper jugular (level II): _____

T93 Left midjugular (level III): _____

T94 Left lower jugular (level IV): _____

T95 Left posterior cervical (level V): _____

T96 Left juxtathyroid (level VI): _____

T97 Left paratracheal and para-esophageal (level VII): _____

T98 Superior mediastinal: _____

T99 Pretracheal: _____

(-) _____

(-) _____

[For cases with metastatic lymph nodes, regardless of number or site]

T100 The size of the largest involved node is _____

T101 No perinodal (extracapsular) extension is identified

T102 Perinodal (extracapsular) extension is present

(-) _____

Uterine cervix—hysterectomy for cervical carcinoma

Specimen:

_____

_____[procedure]

SP # _____

Pt. Name _____

Fellow/Att _____

Date _____

Diagnosis:

U1 No residual carcinoma
U2 No residual invasive carcinoma
 Tumor Type
U3 In situ squamous cell carcinoma of uterine cervix [Use only if there is *NOT* an invasive component]
U4 Superficially invasive squamous cell carcinoma of uterine cervix
U5 Large cell keratinizing
U6 Large cell nonkeratinizing
U7 Small cell
U8 Invasive squamous cell carcinoma of uterine cervix
U9 Large cell keratinizing
U10 Large cell nonkeratinizing
U11 Small cell
U12 In situ adenocarcinoma of uterine cervix [Use only if there is *NO* invasive component present]
U13 Invasive adenocarcinoma of uterine cervix
U14 NOS
U15 Mucinous
U16 Endometrioid
U17 Clear cell
U18 Mixed, composed of the following patterns: _____

(-) _____
U19 Invasive adenosquamous carcinoma of uterine cervix
U20 Invasive neuroendocrine carcinoma of uterine cervix
(-) _____

 Histologic Grade
U21 Well differentiated
U22 Moderately differentiated
U23 Poorly differentiated/undifferentiated
(-) _____

 Depth of Invasion
U24 The maximal thickness of the cervical stromal invasion is _____ *mm*
U25 The thickness of the cervix in the area of maximal tumor invasion is _____ *mm*
U26 The maximal superficial spread of the tumor is _____ _____ *mm*
 [For superficially invasive squamous cell carcinoma only]
(-) _____

 Tumor Multicentricity
U27 No evidence of tumor multicentricity is identified
U28 Multicentric foci of invasive carcinoma are present
(-) _____

 In Situ Carcinoma (for cases also having an invasive component)
U29 No in situ carcinoma is identified
U30 In situ carcinoma is also present
(-) _____

 Vascular Invasion
U31 No vascular invasion is identified
U32 Vascular invasion is present
(-) _____

 Perineurial Invasion
U33 No perineurial invasion is identified
U34 Perineurial invasion is present
(-) _____

 Vaginal Extension
U35 No vaginal extension is identified
U36 Vaginal extension is present
(-) _____

 Uterine Corpus Extension
U37 The tumor does not extend into uterine corpus
U38 The tumor extends into the lower uterine segment (mucosa only)
U39 The tumor extends into the lower uterine segment (stroma only)
U40 The tumor extends into the lower uterine segment (mucosa and stroma)
U41 The tumor extends into the uterine fundus (endometrium only)
U42 The tumor extends into the uterine fundus (myometrium only)
U43 The tumor extends into the uterine fundus (endometrium and myometrium)
(-) _____

 Parametrial Involvement
U44 No parametrial involvement is identified
U45 Parametrial involvement is present on the right side only
U46 Parametrial involvement is present on the left side only
U47 Parametrial involvement is present bilaterally
(-) _____

Bladder—biopsy or TUR for carcinoma—cont'd

Surgical Margins
U48 All surgical margins are free from tumor
U49 The following surgical margin(s) are involved by tumor:
U50 Deep cervical *at*_____
U51 Right parametrial
U52 Left parametrial
U53 Right and left parametrial
U54 Anterior vaginal
U55 Posterior vaginal
U56 Anterior and posterior vaginal
(-) _____

Endometrium
U57 The endometrium is unremarkable
U58 The endometrium shows the following abnormality(ies):
U59 Atrophy
U60 Simple hyperplasia without atypia
U61 Simple hyperplasia with atypia
U62 Complex hyperplasia without atypia
U63 Complex hyperplasia with atypia
U64 Polyp(s)
U65 Radiation changes
(-) _____

Myometrium
U66 The myometrium is unremarkable
U67 The myometrium shows the following abnormality(ies):
U68 Adenomyosis
U69 Leiomyoma(s)
(-) _____

Adnexae
U70 All adnexae are unremarkable
U71 The right fallopian tube shows _____
U72 The right ovary shows _____
U73 The left fallopian tube shows_____
U74 The left ovary shows _____
U75 All other adnexae are unremarkable
(-) _____

Lymph Nodes
U76 The lymph node status is as follows (expressed as the number of metastatic nodes in relation to the total number of nodes examined):
U77 Right obturator: _____
U78 Right pelvic:_____
U79 Right external iliac: _____
U80 Right internal iliac: _____
U81 Right periaortic: _____
U82 Left obturator: _____
U83 Left pelvic:_____
U84 Left external iliac: _____
U85 Left internal iliac:_____
U86 Left periaortic: _____
(-) _____

Uterine corpus—hysterectomy for endometrial carcinoma

Specimen:

_____

_____[procedure]

SP #_____

Pt. Name _____

Fellow/Att _____

Date_____

Diagnosis:

V1 No residual endometrial carcinoma

Tumor Type

V2 Adenocarcinoma of endometrium

V3   Endometrioid type, NOS

V4   Endometrioid with squamous metaplasia (adeno-acanthoma)

V5   Endometrioid, adenosquamous subtype

V6   Endometrioid, villoglandular subtype

V7   Clear cell type

V8   Papillary serous type

V9   Mixed type, composed of the following patterns:

_____

(-) _____

V10 Malignant mixed mullerian tumor of endometrium

V11   With heterologous elements

V12   Without heterologous elements

(-) _____

Histologic Grade (for endometrioid types only)

V13 FIGO grade I (≤ 6% solid growth)

V14 FIGO grade II (6%-50% solid growth)

V15 FIGO grade III (> 50% solid growth)

V16 FIGO grade not applicable

(-) _____

Nuclear Grade (for endometrioid types only)

V17 Nuclear grade 1

V18 Nuclear grade 2

V19 Nuclear grade 3

(-) _____

Depth of Invasion

V20 The tumor is limited to the endometrium

V21 The tumor invades to ≤ half of myometrium

V22 The tumor invades to > half of myometrium

V23 The maximal thickness of myometrial invasion is
_____mm [Important!]

V24 The thickness of the myometrium in the area of max-imal tumor invasion is _____mm
[Important!]

(-) _____

Endocervical Invasion

V25 No endocervical invasion is identified

V26 Endocervical invasion is present in the mucosa only

V27 Endocervical invasion is present in the stroma only

V28 Endocervical invasion is present both in the mucosa and the stroma

(-) _____

Vascular Invasion

V29 No vascular invasion is identified

V30 Vascular invasion is present

(-) _____

Endometrium

V31 The endometrium is unremarkable

V32 The endometrium shows the following abnormal-ity(ies):

V33   Atrophy

V34   Simple hyperplasia without atypia

V35   Simple hyperplasia with atypia

V36   Complex hyperplasia without atypia

V37   Complex hyperplasia with atypia

V38   Polyp(s)

V39   Radiation changes

(-) _____

Myometrium

V40 The myometrium is unremarkable

V41 The myometrium shows the following abnormal-ity(ies):

V42   Adenomyosis

V43   Leiomyoma(s)

(-) _____

Adnexae

V44 All adnexae are unremarkable

V45 The right fallopian tube shows _____

V46 The right ovary shows _____

V47 The left fallopian tube shows_____

V48 The left ovary shows _____

V49 All other adnexae are unremarkable

(-) _____

Lymph Nodes

V50 The lymph node status is as follows (expressed as the number of metastatic nodes in relation to the total number of nodes examined):

V51   Right obturator: _____

V52   Right pelvic:_____

V53   Right external iliac: _____

V54   Right internal iliac: _____

V55   Right periaortic: _____

V56   Left obturator: _____

V57   Left pelvic:_____

V58   Left external iliac: _____

V59   Left internal iliac:_____

V60   Left periaortic: _____

(-) _____

For Synchronous Ovarian and Endometrial Car-cinomas of Similar Histology (if applicable):

V61 **Note:** the superficial character of the endometrial carcinoma suggests that it represents an indepen-dent primary rather than a metastasis from the ovarian carcinoma

Vulva—vulvectomy for carcinoma

Specimen:

Vulva, _____

_____ [procedure]

SP # _____

Pt. Name _____

Fellow/Att _____

Date _____

Diagnosis:

W1 No residual carcinoma
W2 No residual invasive carcinoma
Tumor Type
W3 In situ squamous cell carcinoma [Use only if there is *NOT* an invasive component]
W4 Invasive squamous cell carcinoma
W5 Paget's disease
W6   Without invasive adenocarcinoma
W7   With invasive adenocarcinoma
(-) _____

Histologic Grade
W8 Well differentiated
W9 Moderately differentiated
W10 Poorly differentiated/undifferentiated
(-) _____

Tumor Size
W11 The tumor length is _____ *cm*
W12 The tumor width is _____ *cm*
W13 The tumor maximal thickness is _____ *cm*
(-) _____

Tumor Location
W14 The tumor involves the following area(s):
W15   Right labius majus
W16   Left labius majus
W17   Right labius minus
W18   Left labius minus
W19   Clitoris
(-) _____

Vascular Invasion
W20 No vascular invasion is identified
W21 Vascular invasion is present
(-) _____

Perineural Invasion
W22 No perineurial invasion is identified
W23 Perineurial invasion is present
(-) _____

Local Extension
W24 The tumor is limited to the vulva
W25 The tumor extends to the following adjacent area(s):
W26   Vagina
W27   Urethra
W28   Perineum
W29   Anus
(-) _____

Tumor Multicentricity
W30 No evidence of tumor multicentricity is identified
W31 Multicentric foci of invasive carcinoma are present
(-) _____

In Situ Carcinoma (for cases also having an invasive component)
W32 No in situ carcinoma is identified
W33 In situ carcinoma is also present
(-) _____

Surgical Margins
W34 All cutaneous, mucosal, and soft tissue margins are free from tumor
W35 The tumor involves the following surgical margin(s):
W36   Right cutaneous _____
W37   Left cutaneous _____
W38   Superior cutaneous_____
W39   Inferior cutaneous _____
W40   Perineal
W41   Anal
W42   Vaginal
W43   Urethral
W44   Soft tissue at_____
(-) _____
W45 All other margins are free from tumor
(-) _____

Non-Neoplastic Vulva
W46 The non-neoplastic vulva is unremarkable
W47 The non-neoplastic vulva shows the following abnormality(ies):
W48   Lichen sclerosus et atrophicus
W49   Keratosis without dysplasia
W50   Dysplasia *of*_____*degree*
W51   Melanocytic nevus *of* _____*type*
(-) _____

Lymph Nodes
W52 The lymph node status is as follows (expressed as the number of metastatic nodes in relation to the total number of nodes examined):
W53   Right inguinal: _____
W54   Right superficial inguinal: _____
W55   Right deep inguinal:_____
W56   Left inguinal: _____
W57   Left superficial inguinal: _____
W58   Left deep inguinal:_____
(-) _____
(-) _____
(-) _____

Whipple resection for pancreatic, biliary, or ampullary carcinoma

Specimen:

_____

_____[procedure]

SP # _____

Pt. Name _____

Fellow/Att _____

Date _____

Diagnosis:

X1 No residual carcinoma

Tumor Type
X2 Adenocarcinoma
X3 Mucinous adenocarcinoma
X4 Mucinous cystadenocarcinoma
X5 Adenosquamous carcinoma
X6 Sarcomatoid carcinoma
X7 Acinar cell carcinoma
X8 Intraductal papillary carcinoma
X9 Intraductal papillary carcinoma with invasion
(-) _____

Tumor Location
X10 Of pancreas (head)
X11 Of pancreas (body)
X12 Of pancreas (tail)
X13 Of pancreas (_____)
X14 Of common bile duct
X15 Of ampulla
X16 Of nonampullary duodenal mucosa
X17 Of ampullary region, precise site of origin undetermined
(-) _____

Tumor Subtype (for tumors of ampulla only)
X18 Intestinal type
X19 Pancreatobiliary type
X20 Mixed intestinal and pancreatobiliary type
(-) _____

Histologic Grade
X21 Well differentiated
X22 Moderately differentiated
X23 Poorly differentiated/undifferentiated
(-) _____

In Situ Carcinoma (for cases also having an invasive component)
X24 No in situ carcinoma is identified
X25 In situ carcinoma is also present
(-) _____

Residual Benign Lesion (for tumors of ampulla only)
X26 No evidence of a preexisting benign lesion is identified
X27 There is a preexisting benign lesion _of_ _____
_____ _type_
(-) _____

Tumor Size
X28 The tumor greatest diameter is ≤ 2 cm
X29 The tumor greatest diameter is > 2 cm
(-) _____

Direct Extension
X30 The tumor does not extend into the adjacent structures
X31 The tumor extends into the following adjacent structure(s):
X32 Pancreas
X33 Duodenal wall
X34 Duodenal mucosa
X35 Common bile duct
(-) _____

Vascular Invasion
X36 No vascular invasion is identified
X37 Vascular invasion is present
(-) _____

Perineurial Invasion
X38 No perineurial invasion is identified
X39 Perineurial invasion is present
(-) _____

Extrapancreatic Extension (for tumors of pancreas only)
X40 No extrapancreatic extension is identified
X41 Extrapancreatic extension is present
(-) _____

Surgical Margins
X42 All surgical margins are free from tumor
X43 The tumor involves the following surgical margin(s):
X44 Distal pancreatic
X45 Deep pancreatic
X46 Duodenal
X47 Gastric
X48 Bile duct
X49 All other margins are free from tumor
(-) _____

Non-Neoplastic Pancreas
X50 The non-neoplastic pancreas is unremarkable
X51 The non-neoplastic pancreas shows the following abnormality(ies):
X52 Focal chronic pancreatitis
X53 Extensive chronic pancreatitis
X54 Fibrosis
X55 Acute pancreatitis
X56 Islet cell hyperplasia
(-) _____

Whipple resection for pancreatic, biliary, or ampullary carcinoma—cont'd

Lymph Nodes

X57 The lymph node status is as follows (expressed as the number of metastatic nodes in relation to the total number of nodes examined):

X58   Superior pancreatic: _____

X59   Anterior pancreaticoduodenal:

X60   Posterior pancreaticoduodenal:

X61   Posterior pancreatic:

X62   Inferior pancreatic:

X63   Bile duct region:

X64   Splenic hilar: _____

(-)   _____

(-)   _____

(-)   _____

X65   No direct tumor extension into lymph nodes is identified

X66   Direct tumor extension into lymph nodes is noted

(-)   _____

Appendix D
Consultations in surgical pathology

(This document was prepared by an ad-hoc committee of the Association of Directors of Anatomic and Surgical Pathology chaired by Dr. Stephen G. Silverberg. From Am J Surg Pathol **17**:743-745, 1993.)

Consultations are easier to obtain in pathology than in most other medical specialties because of the ability to cut duplicate histologic slides and forward them to any destination. Although this process has been taking place—usually with satisfactory results—for decades, there are numerous steps in the consultation process at which problems can and frequently do arise. Accordingly, the Association of Directors of Anatomic and Surgical Pathology has developed recommendations for consultations in anatomic pathology. Consultations may be generated for many reasons, including (but not limited to) the following:

1 Uncertainty of the referring pathologist about the diagnosis
2 An internal disagreement between two or more pathologists in a group about the diagnosis
3 The patient's request for a second opinion
4 A clinician's request for a second opinion
5 Quality assurance documentation
6 Transfer of the patient to a different hospital or clinic, with a need for diagnosis by a pathologist at the new institution

This appendix consists of two parts: The first considers *personal consultations,* defined as consultations sent to a specific pathologist, usually for one of the first four reasons listed above. The second part deals with *institutional consultations,* in which the sixth reason is generally operative. Specifically excluded are consultations for legal purposes. The Association recommends that the reason for the consultation be specified in the accompanying letter to the consultant.

Personal Consultations

The ideal pathologic consultation proceeds from one pathologist to another; however, consultant pathologists also receive cases for consultation from clinicians, patients, patients' families, and others. The Association makes the following recommendations:

1 The pathologist whose opinion is being solicited has the right to refuse to accept a case for consultation, if he or she believes that the interests of the patient will not be served by its acceptance.
2 The consultant who accepts a case and renders an opinion should always transmit the report to the pathologist in whose laboratory the initial diagnosis was made.

The pathologist sending a case for consultation has certain responsibilities to the consultant, and ultimately to the patient. The Association makes the following recommendations:

1 An accompanying letter should provide the reason for the consultation, specific questions to be answered, the referring pathologist's working diagnosis or differential diagnosis, and appropriate billing information.
2 A copy of the surgical pathology report (or as much of it as has been completed) should accompany the letter and the slides; this should include pertinent demographic and clinical data and a gross description, as well as identification of the exact site of origin of each slide submitted.
3 Adequate material to solve the diagnostic problem should be submitted; in some instances, this material may consist of a single hematoxylin and eosin–stained slide, whereas in others all material available in the case—including special stains, electron micrographs, flow cytometric data, x-ray films, paraffin blocks, frozen or fixed tissue, or other special material or information—may be required. If it is anticipated that immunohistochemical stains or other additional procedures will be needed, the pertinent blocks or appropriately prepared unstained slides should be sent. Previous pathology specimens

and reports from the same patient, if pertinent, should be included. If the referring pathologist has a question about a particular area on one or more slides, this question should be clearly indicated in the consultation letter and marked on the slide. The decision as to what to send should be made initially by the referring pathologist, but the consultant may request more material before making a diagnosis.

The referring pathologist should personally assure that the material sent to the consultant is adequate to demonstrate the lesion in question and that this material is packaged to avoid breakage (Rosen PP, Am J Clin Pathol 1989; 91:348-354). In particular, recut slides should be inspected to ensure that they are representative. If paraffin blocks and glass slides are sent in the same container, a duplicate set of slides should be retained by the referring pathologist.

4 The referring pathologist may state the time frame in which a diagnosis is requested and in this situation attempt to determine that this schedule can be met. This may require telephoning in advance to ensure that the consultant is available, sending the consultation by an express delivery service, providing a telephone or fax number for rapid transmission of the consultant's report, and providing names and contact numbers for other physicians familiar with the case, should the referring pathologist not be available.

5 If the case is sent to more than one consultant, each should be informed of that fact, as well as of the other consultants' diagnoses.

6 If original material must be sent because no duplicates are available (for example, in the case of paraffin blocks or cytologic material), their return should be requested in the consultation letter. Whenever recut slides will suffice, they should be used and the consultant allowed to retain the slides.

7 The opinion of the consultant should be made part of the referring pathologist's report. The referring pathologist has the responsibility of making the final diagnosis and may agree or disagree with the consultant.

The consultant pathologist also has responsibilities to fulfill to optimize the consultation process. The Association recommends the following:

1 If a case is accepted for consultation, a written report providing a diagnostic impression should be issued to identify the exact source of all material reviewed. This policy ultimately protects everyone involved in the process, including the patient.

2 Reports should be issued as expeditiously as possible. If the consultant cannot provide at least a preliminary opinion within 1 week of receipt, arrangements should be made to notify the referring pathologist.

3 When the consultant pathologist's diagnosis may alter immediate patient management, this fact should be communicated to the referring pathologist in a timely fashion.

4 If the consultant cannot make a diagnosis on the basis of the material submitted, he or she may either issue a provisional report on the basis of what is available, with suggestions for further studies to be performed by the referring pathologist, or request more or better material to perform the additional studies in the consultant's laboratory. Such a request is best made by telephone. Occasionally, the consultant may recommend a second consultant who might be more appropriate or, with permission of the referring pathologist, send the case directly to the second consultant.

5 If doing additional studies in the consultant's laboratory would generate additional charges, these charges should be authorized by the referring pathologist before the studies are undertaken.

6 Although the consultant may be asked to make recommendations for therapy and may choose to do so, it should be understood by all concerned that therapeutic recommendations made on the basis of a brief clinical summary and pathologic material alone may not always be applicable to the clinical situation.

7 The consultant should return to its source material that cannot be duplicated (e.g., paraffin blocks, cytologic slides, histologic slides showing lesions that do not persist on other cuts, original x-ray films) and otherwise should be allowed to retain and file all consultation material. The retained slides, whether placed in an institutional or a personal file, should be clearly identified and kept available for subsequent review, as should all written records related to the consultation.

8 It should be assumed that a case sent to a consultant may be published as part of a series by the consultant and that the referring pathologist can be acknowledged if permitted by the journal in which the

report is published. We further recommend that publication of individual case reports by a consultant should be undertaken only with the express approval of the referring pathologist. In either of these situations, the referring pathologist may be asked by the consultant or a collaborator to contribute additional information, including follow-up, on the contributed case.

Institutional Consultations

Many pathologic consultations are transmitted from one laboratory or hospital to another because the patient has been transferred to, or is seeking a second clinical opinion at, a second institution. In most such cases, the clinical consultant or the second institution (or both) will request that pertinent pathology reports and slides be reviewed by the local pathologist. Indeed, the Association recommends that such review be standard institutional policy.

Most of the above recommendations for personal consultations also apply to institutional consultations. In the latter situation, it is even more important that the referred material be retained whenever possible in the second institution, particularly if the patient undergoes treatment there. It is also important that reports be sent directly to the patient's chart and the second institution's clinician(s) (who are more likely to be the official generators of the consultation), as well as to the referring pathologist. In the event of significant disagreement, the case should be promptly discussed with the referring pathologist. In the institutional consultation situation, institutional or departmental rules regarding turnaround time, record-keeping, quality assurance, and so on, take precedence over any mentioned above.

Appendix E
Recommendations on quality control and quality assurance in anatomic pathology

(This document was prepared by the ad-hoc Committee of the Association of Directors of Anatomic and Surgical Pathology chaired by Dr. Juan Rosai. From Am J Surg Pathol **15**:1007-1009, 1991.)

The Association of Directors of Anatomic and Surgical Pathology ("the Association") has prepared the following recommendations regarding Quality Control and Quality Assurance (QC/QA) in surgical pathology and autopsy pathology. This document does not include QC/QA issues as they apply to cytopathology and to specialized anatomic pathology laboratories such as immunohistochemistry or electron microscopy.

The Association wishes to emphasize that the recommendations contained in this document were made taking into consideration the structure, responsibilities, and needs of academic anatomic pathology laboratories that have an active pathology residency or fellowship program. It also wishes to point out that they are to be viewed as being of a generic nature and suitable for modification depending on the specific circumstances of the individual laboratories and the regulations of the respective institutions.

I It is recommended that each Department of Pathology prepare a written QC/QA plan for surgical pathology and autopsy pathology specifically devised for that Department and the respective institution. This document should be updated on a yearly basis. It should be part of the Departmental QC/QA program and, as such, should be structured along the lines of the JCAHO ten-step monitoring process as detailed in The Accreditation Manual for Hospitals.

II It is recommended that each Department establish a QC/QA Committee. The Committee should be appointed by the Chairman on a yearly basis. It should meet monthly, be chaired by a senior pathologist, and have as members representatives from the principal sections or divisions of the Department.

III It is recommended that the QC/QA plan for surgical pathology and autopsy pathology include the components ("indicators") listed below. The first of these indicators is of a prospective nature—i.e., to be carried out before the final report is issued. All others are of a retrospective nature—i.e., to be carried out in a regular fashion independently from the timing of the final report and usually after this has taken place.

Intradepartmental consultation

This function is to be carried out through one or both of the following mechanisms:

1 Review of selected cases by the diagnostic staff as a group, either through a periodic session ("consensus conference") or a written consultation form. The fact that this exercise has taken place should be indicated in the pathology report.

2 Review of selected cases by a second staff pathologist ("consultant"). For those cases in which the entire case is evaluated by the consultant, it is recommended that both pathologists sign the report; for cases in which only a portion of the cases has been reviewed, it is recommended that a note to that effect be added to the report.

Intraoperative consultation

It is recommended that all cases in which an intraoperative consultation has been carried out be reviewed on a regular (i.e., weekly) basis and be placed according to their final disposition in one of the following categories:

1 Agreement
2 Deferral—Appropriate
3 Deferral—Inappropriate
4 Disagreement—Minor
5 Disagreement—Major

For all cases in the "Disagreement—Major" and "Deferral—Inappropriate" categories, it is recommended that the reason for this occurrence be categorized as one of the following:

1 Interpretation
2 Block sampling
3 Specimen sampling
4 Technical inadequacy
5 Lack of essential clinical or pathologic data
6 Other (indicate)

It is further recommended that the medical consequence of the cases included in the "Disagreement—Major" or "Deferral—Inappropriate" categories be listed as one of the following:

1 None
2 Minor/questionable
3 Major

The Association estimates that an acceptable accuracy threshold for intraoperative consultations (as measured by the number of "Disagreement—Major" cases and determined per case) is 3%; an acceptable threshold for "Deferred—Inappropriate" cases is 10%.

The Association believes that it is important for each laboratory to establish its own time thresholds for intraoperative consultation, using as a standard unit the time threshold for the performance of a "basic" frozen section, as defined by a case with a single block, with no other cases being performed by the intraoperative consultation team at the same time.

Random case review

It is recommended that the following cases be reviewed on a random basis:

1 Surgical pathology: 1% or 25/month, whichever is larger
2 Autopsy: 10% or two/month, whichever is larger

The review on the randomly selected cases should include all material related to them, including final report, microscopic slides, turnaround time, and special procedures, if any.

Clinical indicators

It is recommended that a Clinical Indicator be selected on a regular basis on the basis of organ/lesion (i.e., carcinoma of endometrium) or procedure (i.e., TUR), and that *all* cases belonging to that indicator in a given period be evaluated by checking them against a list of predetermined criteria. This activity should be rotated among surgical pathology and autopsy cases.

Intradepartmental and interdepartmental conferences

For all cases presented at intradepartmental and interdepartmental conferences, it is recommended that the diagnosis as listed in the final report be compared with that made by the presenter when reviewing the case for the conference.

Interinstitutional review

For cases in which an outside review has been carried out at the request of the patient, the clinician or other institution, or as part of a cooperative study, it is recommended that the diagnosis as listed in the final report be compared with that made at the outside institution. The Association estimates that an acceptable threshold for clinically significant disagreement following arbitration is 2%, as applied to those cases in which it is decided that the correct interpretation is that from the outside institution.

Surgical pathology turnaround times

The Association believes that the following are acceptable turnaround times for surgical pathology reports, as measured in working days from the time the specimen is accessioned in the laboratory to the time the verbal report is available or the final report is signed.

Type of specimen	Verbal report	Written report
Rushes	1	2
Biopsies	2	3
Surgicals	2	3

Extra time should be allowed for the following procedures, to be measured in days from the time the procedure is initiated or ordered and independently from each other:

1 Overnight fixation, 1
2 Decalcification, 1
3 Resubmission, 1-2
4 Recuts, 1
5 Immunocytochemistry, 1-2
6 Electron microscopy, 2-3
7 Intradepartmental consultation, 1

The Association estimates that an acceptable threshold for these turnaround times is 80%.

Autopsy turnaround time

The Association believes that the following are acceptable turnaround times for autopsy reports, as measured in working days:

1 Provisional report: 1
2 Final report: 30

The Association estimates that an acceptable threshold for the provisional report is 90%; acceptable threshold for the final report is 80%.

Specimen adequacy

It is recommended that the adequacy of submission of specimens to the laboratory be monitored in terms of fixation, safety requirements, and proper identification.

Lost specimen

This is defined as the irretrievable loss of a surgical pathology specimen that has occurred after the case has been accessioned in the laboratory and that prevents an adequate pathologic examination of that specimen. The Association estimates that an acceptable threshold for lost specimens is one in 3,000 cases.

Histology QC

It is recommended that the QC related to the histology lab include:
1 Record of time of delivery of slides
2 Evaluation of slide quality as performed by the pathologist
3 Evaluation of tissue adequacy as performed by the histotechnologist

Isolated event report

It is recommended that isolated events not contemplated in any of the foregoing categories be documented through the issuing of an "Isolated Event Report." All such reports should be kept in a permanent log.

Appendix F
Quality control and quality assurance program for anatomic pathology

The goals of the Anatomic Pathology Departmental Quality Assurance (DQA) program are to ensure (1) accuracy, (2) completeness, and (3) timeliness of all the reports generated by the Division of Anatomic Pathology. These goals are achieved by the continuous monitoring of the following indicators:

Prospective:

1 Intradepartmental consultation (IDC)

Retrospective:

2 Frozen section review (FSR)

3 SP cases random review (SPRR)

4 Autopsy cases random review (ARR)

5 AP clinical indicators (CI)

6 Intradepartmental and interdepartmental conferences (CONF)

7 Interinstitutional review (IIR)

8 Specimen adequacy record (SAR)

9 Lost specimen record (LSR)

10 Single event report (SER)

11 Histology slides delivery (SD)

12 Quality control to histology (TO-H)

13 Quality control from histology (FROM-H)

14 AP turnaround times (TAT)

The meetings of the committee are divided in two portions: (1) one primarily concerned with QC issues, in which all committee members participate, (2) one primarily concerned with QA issues, in which only the attendings participate.

The collection and some of the analysis of the data, organization of the monthly meetings, and all correspondence related to the DQA committee are carried out by a QA assistant working under the supervision of the QA committee chairman.

NOTE: This program does not include cytopathology or specialized tests (such as electron microscopy or immunohistochemistry).

INTRADEPARTMENTAL CONSULTATION (IDC)

Purpose

To provide a prospective system by which all difficult, controversial, and otherwise problematic cases can be presented by any attending for review and discussion before they are signed out.

Frequency

This conference is held daily using a multiheaded microscope. The conference is run by the director of anatomic or surgical pathology. The other participants are the anatomic pathology attendings, particularly those on service rotations. Residents, students, and visitors do not participate.

Procedure

1 The date of the conference and the names of all the attendings present should be recorded.

2 The attendings participating at the conference present for discussion cases of their choice. These cases may be selected on the basis of any of the following criteria:

    a Diagnostic difficulty

    b Controversy in interpretation among attendings and/or residents

    c Discrepancy between frozen section diagnosis and intended final diagnosis

    d Discrepancy between provisional diagnosis and intended final diagnosis

    e Management purposes, such as performance of additional biopsies, special studies, or therapeutic recommendations

    f Request on the part of the clinician or patient

    g Interesting or unusual nature of the case

3 The material presented should include all pertinent microscopic slides, a summary of the clinical data, and when indicated, gross specimens or gross photographs, x rays, and electron micrographs.

4 The individual presenting the case should state his diagnostic impression and reason for presentation.

5 The case is examined simultaneously by all participants, the director of anatomic or surgical pathology leading the discussion.

6 Upon completion of the presentation and discussion of each case, the director of anatomic or surgical pathology will enter in the corresponding form the following information:

    a Pathology number

    b Name of presenter

    c Diagnosis of presenter and reason for presentation

    d Consensus reached

7 If indicated, the nature of the discussion having taken place and the recommendations made.

8 All cases presented at these conferences should be so identified by entering "Conference Case" in the final report, immediately following the diagnosis.

FROZEN SECTION REVIEW (FSR)

Purpose

To monitor the adequacy in the performance of frozen sections in surgical pathology in terms of diagnostic accuracy, timing of the procedure, and consequences of the diagnosis rendered.

Frequency

Weekly.

Procedure

1 The copy of the frozen section forms filed in surgical pathology should include the following information: time at which the specimen was received, time at which the frozen section diagnosis was given, frozen section diagnosis, and final diagnosis.

2 The DQA manager should collect the above forms weekly and evaluate them in regard to time employed to perform the procedure and concordance between frozen section and final diagnosis. In cases in which a discordance exists (including deferred cases) the following information should be entered:

   a Pathology number

   b Frozen section diagnosis

   c Initials of resident(s) and attending(s) who performed the frozen section

   d Final diagnosis, including initials of attending

   e Final disposition, according to the following categories:

      1 Agreement

      2 Deferment— Appropriate

      3 Deferment—Inappropriate

      4 Disagreement—Minor

      5 Disagreement—Major

   f For categories 3 to 5, explanation for the lack of agreement according to the following categories:

      1 Interpretation

      2 Block sampling

      3 Tissue sampling

      4 Technical inadequacy

      5 Lack of important clinical or previous pathologic information

   g For categories 3 to 5, consequence to the patient according to the following categories:

      1 None

      2 Minor/questionable

      3 Major

   h Notes, if indicated

   i Action taken

Steps (e) through (i) of this procedure should be completed by the DQA committee chairman. When indicated, the FS and permanent slides should be reviewed. In addition, the DQA manager should record the above information in a separate form, divided according to the attending who performed the procedure.

Review

1 All FS forms from the preceding month should be presented and discussed at the monthly DQA meeting.

2 A formal review of the FS forms should be carried out by the DQA committee chairman on a quarterly basis, according to the general QA review procedure. The results of the review are to be presented at the monthly DQA meeting.

SP CASES RANDOM REVIEW (SPRR)

Purpose

To monitor on a random basis the adequacy of the surgical pathology report in all of its aspects.

Frequency

Weekly.

Procedure

1 The DQA manager should collect on a random basis one of every fiftieth surgical pathology case for the purposes of this review. The material collected should consist of:
   a Copy of requisition form
   b Copy of final surgical pathology report
   c All microscopic slides
   d All material from special studies (immunohistochemistry, electron microscopy, etc.), if any
   e All gross photographs and specimen x rays, if any
2 This material will be given to the DQA committee chairman, who will evaluate it for the following criteria:
   a Clinical history
   b Gross description
   c Gross photographs, if any
   d Sampling for histology
   e Quality of slides
   f Diagnosis
   g Note, if any
   h SNOMED (topography and morphology) coding
   i Special studies, if any
   j Turnaround time
   k Other

If indicated, assistance for the evaluation should be requested from other members of the pathology department or from outside consultants. Cases in which an important deficiency is detected, especially regarded the diagnosis, should be immediately brought to the attention of the director of anatomic pathology.

Review

1 All SP forms in which deficiencies have been entered should be presented and discussed at the monthly DQA meeting.
2 A formal review of the SP forms should be carried out by the DQA chairman quarterly, according to the general QA review procedure. The results of the review are to be presented at the monthly DQA meeting.

AUTOPSY CASES RANDOM REVIEW (ARR)

Purpose

To monitor on a random basis the adequacy of the autopsy report in all of its aspects.

Frequency

Monthly.

Procedure

1 The DQA manager should collect on a random basis one of every tenth autopsy pathology case for the purposes of this review. The material collected should consist of:

  a Copy of autopsy requisition
  b Copy of final autopsy report
  c All microscopic slides
  d All material from special studies (immunohistochemistry, electron microscopy, etc.), if any
  e All gross photographs and specimen x-rays, if any

2 This material will be given to the DQA Committee chairman, who will evaluate it for the following criteria:

  a Patient identification and history
  b Gross description
  c Gross photographs, if any
  d Sampling for histology
  e Quality of slides
  f Diagnosis
  g Clinicopathologic correlation and bibliography
  h SNOMED (topography & morphology) coding
  i Special studies, if any
  j Turn-around time
  k Other

If indicated, assistance for the evaluation should be requested from other members of the pathology department or from outside consultants. Cases in which an an important deficiency is detected, especially regarding the diagnosis, should be immediately brought to the attention of the director of anatomic pathology.

Review

1 All AUT forms in which deficiencies have been entered should be presented and discussed at the monthly DQA meeting.

2 A formal review of the AUT forms should be carried out by the DQA chairman on a quarterly basis, according to the general QA review procedure. The results of the review are to be presented at the monthly DQA meeting.

AP CLINICAL INDICATORS (CI)

Purpose

To monitor the completeness and consistency of the information provided in the pathology report (surgical, cytology, or autopsy) for specific specimens or diseases, and to correct any deficiencies encountered.

Frequency

Monthly.

Procedure

1 The DQA committee chairman should identify on a monthly basis a specimen or disease to be evaluated. The selection can be made on the basis of tissue received regardless of the pathology present in it (e.g., transurethral prostatectomy) or on the basis of a specific disease entity (e.g., carcinoma of large bowel). It should include, on a rotational basis, cases from surgical pathology, diagnostic cytology, and autopsy pathology.

2 The DQA manager should retrieve all consecutive reports from cases corresponding to the selected specimen/disease that had been accessioned for a predetermined period, which may vary from 2 to 12 months depending on the frequency of the selected item.

3 The reports should be given to the attending designated by the DQA committee chairman for this purpose, who will review them for completeness, accuracy, and consistency by cross-checking them with a predetermined list of required items. The result of the review should be tabulated, and the information obtained should be submitted to the DQA manager.

Review

1 The results of the review should be presented at the monthly DQA meeting.

2 If significant deficiencies are encountered in the review, a follow-up study should be carried out in 3 to 12 months depending on the nature of the material.

INTRADEPARTMENTAL AND INTERDEPARTMENTAL CONFERENCES (CONF)

Purpose

To monitor the degree of agreement between the final diagnosis as expressed in the pathology report (surgical, cytology, or autopsy) and the consensus reached at the intradepartmental or interdepartmental conference(s) in which the case is presented.

Frequency

Monthly.

Procedure

Attendings who present and/or discuss anatomic pathology cases at intradepartmental or interdepartmental conferences should review the diagnostic material on those cases and compare their diagnostic impression and the consensus reached at the conference with the diagnosis as stated in the official report. This information should be entered in the CONF form. In any case in which a discrepancy exists, the nature and importance of the problem should be stated, and the case should be discussed with the attending who signed the pathology report.

Review

1 All CONF forms should be presented and reviewed at the monthly DQA meeting.
2 A formal review of the CONF forms should be carried out by the DQA chairman quarterly, according to the general QA review procedure. The results of the review are to be presented at the monthly DQA meeting.

INTERINSTITUTIONAL REVIEW (IIR)

Purpose

To monitor the degree of diagnostic agreement rate among YNHH cases that have been sent to other institutions for one of the following reasons:
1 At the clinician's or patient's request
2 Because the patient is being treated elsewhere
3 Because the case has been entered in a cooperative study

If a significant discrepancy between the two diagnoses exists, the director of anatomic or surgical pathology should resolve it by subjecting the case to inside or outside arbitration and submit an addendum report with the final resolution.

Procedure

The DQC manager should collect and record the diagnoses made at other institutions and compare those diagnoses with those made on the same cases at our institution. All the cases in which a major discrepancy exists should be recorded, including the arbitration outcome.

Review

1 All ICC from the preceding period should be presented at the monthly DQA meeting.
2 A formal review of the ICC forms should be carried out by the DQA committee chairman bi-annually, according to the general QA review procedure. The results of the review should be presented at the monthly DQA meeting.

SPECIMEN ADEQUACY RECORD (SAR)

Purpose

To monitor the adequacy of submission of specimens to the pathology laboratory in terms of fixation, safety requirements, and proper identification and to correct any deficiencies encountered.

Frequency

Daily.

Procedure

1 The SP accessioner should examine all material received in the laboratory for the deficiencies listed below and record them in the SAR form if present:

   a Specimen not bagged or bagged inadequately

   b Requisition placed inside bag

   c Staples in bag

   d Lid not sealed properly and/or fluid spill contamination

   e Inadequate amount of fixative fluid

   f No clinical history

   g Requisition form missing

   h No physician name

   i No physician signature

   j No specimen

   k Discordant information between requisition form and container

   l Radioactivity detected in specimen

If deficiencies g to l were encountered, the specimen should not be accessioned. The SP assistant or an SP chief resident should be contacted to resolve the matter.

2 The SP assistant should review the SAR form weekly and contact the appropriate services.

Review

1 The completed SAR forms should be filed in the SP office.

2 The SP assistant should review the SAR forms quarterly, tabulate the findings according to type of problem and service, and present the results at the monthly DQA meeting.

LOST SPECIMEN RECORD (LSR)

Purpose

To document all incidents in which a specimen is lost, destroyed, misidentified, or otherwise mishandled so as to make impossible its pathologic interpretation, to determine their cause, and to prevent their further occurrence.

Frequency

Monthly.

Procedure

All "lost specimen" incidents should be recorded in the LSR form should be sent to the DQA files.

Review

The review of the LSR forms should be carried out by the DQA chairman monthly, according to the general QA review procedure. The results of the review are to be presented at the monthly DQA meeting.

SINGLE EVENT REPORT (SER)

Purpose

1 To document the occurrence of single events that could reflect on the delivery of care by the division of anatomic pathology and that are brought to the attention of the DQA chairman through a notification by any member of the medical or technical hospital staff, either within or outside the department.

2 To evaluate the event, and to take a corrective measure if indicated.

Frequency

Monthly.

Review

The review of the SER form should be carried out monthly, and the results of the review should be presented at the monthly DQA meeting.

HISTOLOGY SLIDES DELIVERY (SD)

Purpose

To monitor the time of delivery of microscopic slides by the histology laboratory to surgical pathology, and to correct any deficiencies encountered.

Frequency

Daily.

Procedure

1 A pathology attending or resident should record the time at which the microscopic slides from biopsies and surgical cases are delivered from the histology laboratory. If there is more than one delivery of any of the categories, each should be recorded. Comments regarding any departures from the norm should be made, such as explanations for undue delays.

2 At the end of each month, the completed form should be given to the DQA manager, who will send copies to the director of anatomic or surgical pathology and to the histology manager. The original should be kept in the DQA files.

Review

1 All SD forms from the preceding month should be presented and discussed at the monthly meeting held between the histology laboratory personnel and the director of anatomic or surgical pathology. Minutes from this meeting should be sent to the DQA manager.

2 A formal review of the SD forms should be carried out by the DQA committee chairman on a monthly basis, according to the general QA review procedure. The results of the review are to be presented at the monthly DQA meeting.

QUALITY CONTROL TO HISTOLOGY (TO-H)

Purpose

To monitor the quality of microscopic slides produced by the histology laboratory for surgical pathology, autopsy pathology, and diagnostic cytology (cell blocks), and to correct any deficiencies encountered.

Frequency

Daily.

Procedure

1 Attendings signing out surgical pathology, autopsy pathology, and diagnostic cytology (cell block) material should fill out one TO-H form per diagnostic session regardless of the number of cases examined. The form should be completed even if the technical quality of all the material examined is deemed to be satisfactory. In the cases thought to be of inadequate quality, the following information should be entered: pathology number, block identification, and type of problem. An attempt should be made to be as specific as possible about the nature of technical deficiency and the time of the preliminary slide. Each attending should complete a separate form.

2 Depending on the nature of the problem, the attending may elect to submit the problem slide(s) or a photocopy of the slide(s) to the histology laboratory in conjunction with the TO-H form.

3 Once completed, the forms (and any accompanying material) should be placed by the attending or resident in the histology mailbox in order for them to be hand delivered daily to the histology manager in the histology laboratory.

4 The histology manager should review the submitted forms within 48 hours of reception, evaluate independently the problem, identify the cutter if indicated, and record in the form any comments and corrective action taken. If necessary, the histology manager should examine personally the microscopic slides and discuss the problem with the corresponding attending. The form should be signed, dated, and filed in the histology office. A copy should be sent to the DQA manager.

Review

1 All TO-H forms from the preceding period should be presented and discussed at the monthly meeting held between the histology laboratory personnel and the director of anatomic pathology. Minutes from this meeting should be sent to the DQA manager.

2 A formal review of the TO-H forms should be carried out by the DQA committee chairman on a monthly basis, according to the general QA review procedure. The results of the review should be presented at the monthly DQA meeting.

QUALITY CONTROL FROM HISTOLOGY (FROM-H)

Purpose

1 To monitor the appropriateness of the material and information supplied by the pathologists to the histology laboratory (e.g., case and block identification, size and thickness of samples, decalcification, special fixation, procedures).

2 To monitor the appropriateness of the requests made to the histology laboratory (e.g., recuts, special stains, re-embedding).

3 To correct any deficiencies encountered.

Procedure

The histology manager should send memos through the electronic mail to the individuals involved. A copy should be sent to the director of anatomic pathology or SP team leader, and another copy should be filed in the office of the histology manager.

Review

1 All FROM-H forms from the preceding period should be discussed at the monthly meeting held between the histology laboratory personnel and the director of anatomic or surgical pathology. Minutes from this meeting should be sent to the DQA manager.

2 A formal review of the FROM-H forms should be carried out by the DQA committee chairman monthly, according to the general QA review procedure. The results of this review should be presented at the monthly DQA meeting.

ANATOMIC PATHOLOGY TURNAROUND TIMES (TAT)

Purpose

To monitor the timely reporting of surgical pathology specimens (surgical, cytology, and autopsy) and to correct any deficiencies encountered.

Frequency

Daily.

Procedure

1 A computer printout should be obtained daily listing overdue cases, according to the following criteria:
   a Cytologies not finalized within 2 days of receipt
   b Biopsies not finalized within 2 days of receipt
   c Surgical specimens (routines) not finalized with 3 days of receipt
   d Autopsies in which a provisional diagnosis has not been sent out in 2 days
   e Autopsies not finalized within 30 days of receipt
2 Additional time will be allowed for special procedures according to the schedule recommended by the Association of Directors of Anatomic and Surgical Pathology (see Appendix C). These extra times will be calculated by the computer in a noncumulative fashion and taking into account the day in which those special procedures were ordered.
3 The SP manager, cytology manager, or autopsy PA should determine and record in each case the reason for the delay by checking the corresponding record as entered in the departmental computer and, if necessary, by communicating with the resident and/or attending assigned to the case.
4 Once the information has been collected on all cases, the completed form should be given to the SP team leader, cytology director, or autopsy director, and a copy should be filed in the DQA office.
5 The surgical pathology director, cytology director, or autopsy director, depending on the type of case, will take remedial action on the overdue cases for which no justifiable delay (i.e., waiting for a special study) has been identified.

Review

The formal review of the TAT forms should be carried out by the DQA chairman monthly, according to the general QA review procedure. The results of the review are to be presented at the monthly DQA meeting.

Appendix G
Staging of cancer

(Adapted from Beahrs OH, Henson DE, Hutter RVP, Kennedy BJ, eds: Manual for staging of cancer, 4th Ed. American Joint Committee on Cancer. Philadelphia, 1992, J. B. Lippincott.)

General rules of the TNM system

The TNM system for describing the anatomic extent of disease is based on the assessment of three components:

- T   The extent of the primary tumor
- N   The absence or presence and extent of regional lymph node metastasis
- M   The absence or presence of distant metastasis

TNM clinical classification

The following general definitions are used throughout:

Primary tumor (T)

TX	Primary tumor cannot be assessed
T0	No evidence of primary tumor
Tis	Carcinoma in situ
T1, T2, T3, T4	Increasing size and/or local extent of the primary tumor

Regional lymph nodes (N)

NX	Regional lymph nodes cannot be assessed
N0	No regional lymph node metastasis
N1, N2, N3	Increasing involvement of regional lymph nodes

Note: Direct extension of the primary tumor into lymph nodes is classified as lymph node metastasis.

Note: Metastasis in any lymph node other than regional is classified as a distant metastasis.

A grossly recognizable metastatic nodule in the connective tissue of a lymph drainage area without histologic evidence of residual lymph node is classified in the N category as a regional lymph node metastasis.

A microscopic deposit, up to 2 or 3 mm, is classified in the T category, that is, as discontinuous extension.

Distant metastasis (M)

MX	Presence of distant metastasis cannot be assessed
M0	No distant metastasis
M1	Distant metastasis

Stage grouping

For purposes of tabulation and analysis, the categories resulting from the combination of the above designations are condensed into a convenient number of TNM stage-groupings. In this system, carcinoma in situ is always categorized as Stage 0, and cases with distant metastases are always categorized as Stage IV.

Carcinoma of the skin (excluding eyelid, vulva, and penis)

Primary tumor (T)

TX	Primary tumor cannot be assessed
T0	No evidence of primary tumor
Tis	Carcinoma in situ

T1	Tumor 2 cm or less in greatest dimension
T2	Tumor more than 2 cm but not more than 5 cm in greatest dimension
T3	Tumor more than 5 cm in greatest dimension
T4	Tumor invades deep extradermal structures, i.e., cartilage, skeletal muscle or bone

Lymph node (N)

NX	Regional lymph nodes cannot be assessed
N0	No regional lymph node metastasis
N1	Regional lymph node metastasis

Distant metastasis (M)

MX	Presence of distant metastasis cannot be assessed
M0	No distant metastasis
M1	Distant metastasis

Stage grouping

0	Tis	N0	M0
I	T1	N0	M0
II	T2	N0	M0
	T3	N0	M0
III	T4	N0	M0
	Any T	N1	M0
IV	Any T	Any N	M1

Malignant melanoma of the skin (excluding eyelid)

Primary tumor (pT)

pTX	Primary tumor cannot be assessed
pT0	No evidence of primary tumor
pTis	Melanoma in situ (atypical melanocytic hyperplasia, severe melanocytic dysplasia, not an invasive lesion) (Clark's level I)
pT1	Tumor 0.75 mm or less in thickness and invades the papillary dermis (Clark's level II)
pT2	Tumor more than 0.75 mm but not more than 1.5 mm in thickness and/or invades to papillary-reticular dermal interface (Clark's level III)
pT3	Tumor more than 1.5 mm but not more than 4 mm in thickness and/or invades the reticular dermis (Clark's level IV)
pT3a	Tumor more than 1.5 mm but not more than 3 mm in thickness
pT3b	Tumor more than 3 mm but not more than 4 mm in thickness
pT4	Tumor more than 4 mm in thickness and/or invades the subcutaneous tissue (Clark's level V) and/or satellite(s) within 2 cm of the primary tumor
pT4a	Tumor more than 4 mm in thickness and/or invades the subcutaneous tissue
pT4b	Satellite(s) within 2 cm of primary tumor

Lymph node (N)

NX	Regional lymph nodes cannot be assessed
N0	No regional lymph node metastasis
N1	Metastasis 3 cm or less in greatest dimension in any regional lymph node(s)
N2	Metastasis more than 3 cm in greatest dimension in any regional lymph node(s) and/or in-transit metastasis
N2a	Metastasis more than 3 cm in greatest dimension in any regional lymph node(s)
N2b	In-transit metastasis

N2c   Both (N2a and N2b)

Distant metastasis (M)

MX   Presence of distant metastasis cannot be assessed
M0   No distant metastasis
M1   Distant metastasis
M1a   Metastasis in skin or subcutaneous tissue or lymph node(s) beyond the regional lymph nodes
M1b   Visceral metastasis

Stage grouping

0	pTis	N0	M0
I	pT1	N0	M0
	pT2	N0	M0
II	pT3	N0	M0
	pT4	N0	M0
III	Any pT	N1	M0
	Any pT	N2	M0
IV	Any pT	Any N	M1

Lip and oral cavity

Primary tumor (T)

TX   Primary tumor cannot be assessed
T0   No evidence of primary tumor
Tis   Carcinoma in situ
T1   Tumor 2 cm or less in greatest dimension
T2   Tumor more than 2 cm but not more than 4 cm in greatest dimension
T3   Tumor more than 4 cm in greatest dimension
T4   (lip) Tumor invades adjacent structures (e.g., through cortical bone, tongue, skin of neck)
T4   (oral cavity) Tumor invades adjacent structures (e.g., through cortical bone, into deep [extrinsic] muscle of tongue, maxillary sinus, skin)

Lymph node (N)

NX   Regional lymph nodes cannot be assessed
N0   No regional lymph node metastasis
N1   Metastasis in a single ipsilateral lymph node, 3 cm or less in greatest dimension
N2   Metastasis in a single ipsilateral lymph node, more than 3 cm but not more than 6 cm in greatest dimension, or multiple ipsilateral lymph nodes, none more than 6 cm in greatest dimension, or bilateral or contralateral lymph nodes, none more than 6 cm in greatest dimension
N2a   Metastasis in a single ipsilateral lymph node more than 3 cm but not more than 6 cm in greatest dimension
N2b   Metastasis in multiple ipsilateral lymph nodes, none more than 6 cm in greatest dimension
N2c   Metastasis in bilateral or contralateral lymph nodes, none more than 6 cm in greatest dimension
N3   Metastasis in a lymph node more than 6 cm in greatest dimension

Distant metastasis (M)

MX   Presence of distant metastasis cannot be assessed
M0   No distant metastasis
M1   Distant metastasis

Stage grouping

0	Tis	N0	M0
I	T1	N0	M0
II	T2	N0	M0
III	T3	N0	M0
	T1	N1	M0
	T2	N1	M0
	T3	N1	M0
IV	T4	N0	M0
	T4	N1	M0
	Any T	N2	M0
	Any T	N3	M0
	Any T	Any N	M1

Pharynx (including base of tongue, soft palate, and uvula)
Primary tumor (T)

TX   Primary tumor cannot be assessed
T0   No evidence of primary tumor
Tis   Carcinoma in situ

Oropharynx

T1   Tumor 2 cm or less in greatest dimension
T2   Tumor more than 2 cm but not more than 4 cm in greatest dimension
T3   Tumor more than 4 cm in greatest dimension
T4   Tumor invades adjacent structures (e.g., through cortical bone, soft tissues of neck, deep [extrinsic] muscle of tongue)

Nasopharynx

T1   Tumor limited to one subsite of nasopharynx
T2   Tumor invades more than one subsite of nasopharynx
T3   Tumor invades nasal cavity and/or oropharynx
T4   Tumor invades skull and/or cranial nerve(s)

Hypopharynx

T1   Tumor limited to one subsite of hypopharynx
T2   Tumor invades more than one subsite of hypopharynx or an adjacent site, without fixation of hemilarynx
T3   Tumor invades more than one subsite of hypopharynx or an adjacent site, with fixation of hemilarynx
T4   Tumor invades adjacent structures (e.g., cartilage or soft tissues of neck)

Lymph node (N)

NX   Regional lymph nodes cannot be assessed
N0   No regional lymph node metastasis
N1   Metastasis in a single ipsilateral lymph node, 3 cm or less in greatest dimension
N2   Metastasis in a single ipsilateral lymph node, more than 3 cm but not more than 6 cm in greatest dimension, or multiple ipsilateral lymph nodes, none more than 6 cm in greatest dimension, or bilateral or contralateral lymph nodes, none more than 6 cm in greatest dimension
N2a   Metastasis in a single ipsilateral lymph node more than 3 cm but not more than 6 cm in greatest dimension

N2b   Metastasis in multiple ipsilateral lymph nodes, none more than 6 cm in greatest dimension

N2c   Metastasis in bilateral or contralateral lymph nodes, none more than 6 cm in greatest dimension

N3   Metastasis in a lymph node more than 6 cm in greatest dimension

Distant metastasis (M)

MX   Presence of distant metastasis cannot be assessed

M0   No distant metastasis

M1   Distant metastasis

Stage grouping

0	Tis	N0	M0
I	T1	N0	M0
II	T2	N0	M0
III	T3	N0	M0
	T1	N1	M0
	T2	N1	M0
	T3	N1	M0
IV	T4	N0	M0
	T4	N1	M0
	Any T	N2	M0
	Any T	N3	M0
	Any T	Any N	M1

Maxillary sinus

Primary tumor (T)

TX   Primary tumor cannot be assessed

T0   No evidence of primary tumor

Tis   Carcinoma in situ

T1   Tumor limited to the antral mucosa with no erosion or destruction of bone

T2   Tumor with erosion or destruction of the infrastructure including the hard palate and/or the middle nasal meatus

T3   Tumor invades any of the following: skin of cheek, posterior wall of the maxillary sinus, floor or medial wall of orbit, anterior ethmoid sinus

T4   Tumor invades orbital contents and/or any of the following: cribriform plate, posterior ethmoid or sphenoid sinuses, nasopharynx, soft palate, pterygomaxillary or temporal fossae, or base of skull

Lymph node (N)

NX   Regional lymph nodes cannot be assessed

N0   No regional lymph node metastasis

N1   Metastasis in a single ipsilateral lymph node, 3 cm or less in greatest dimension

N2   Metastasis in a single ipsilateral lymph node, more than 3 cm but not more than 6 cm in greatest dimension, or multiple ipsilateral lymph nodes, none more than 6 cm in greatest dimension, or bilateral or contralateral lymph nodes, none more than 6 cm in greatest dimension

N2a   Metastasis in a single ipsilateral lymph node more than 3 cm but not more than 6 cm in greatest dimension

N2b   Metastasis in multiple ipsilateral lymph nodes, none more than 6 cm in greatest dimension

N2c   Metastasis in bilateral or contralateral lymph nodes, none more than 6 cm in greatest dimension

N3   Metastasis in a lymph node more than 6 cm in greatest dimension

Distant metastasis (M)

MX   Presence of distant metastasis cannot be assessed
M0   No distant metastasis
M1   Distant metastasis

Stage grouping

0	Tis	N0	M0
I	T1	N0	M0
II	T2	N0	M0
III	T3	N0	M0
	T1	N1	M0
	T2	N1	M0
	T3	N1	M0
IV	T4	N0	M0
	T4	N1	M0
	Any T	N2	M0
	Any T	N3	M0
	Any T	Any N	M1

Larynx

Primary tumor (T)

TX   Primary tumor cannot be assessed
T0   No evidence of primary tumor
Tis   Carcinoma in situ

Supraglottis

T1   Tumor limited to one subsite of supraglottis with normal vocal cord mobility
T2   Tumor invades more than one subsite of supraglottis or glottis, with normal vocal cord mobility
T3   Tumor limited to larynx with vocal cord fixation and/or invades postcricoid area, medial wall of piriform sinus, or pre-epiglottic tissues
T4   Tumor invades through thyroid cartilage, and/or extends to other tissues beyond the larynx (e.g., to oropharynx, soft tissues of neck)

Glottis

T1   Tumor limited to vocal cord(s) (may involve anterior or posterior commissures) with normal mobility
T1a   Tumor limited to one vocal cord
T1b   Tumor involves both vocal cords
T2   Tumor extends to supraglottis and/or subglottis, and/or with impaired vocal cord mobility
T3   Tumor limited to the larynx with vocal cord fixation
T4   Tumor invades through thyroid cartilage and/or extends to other tissues beyond the larynx (e.g., oropharynx, soft tissues of neck)

Subglottis

T1   Tumor limited to the subglottis
T2   Tumor extends to vocal cord(s) with normal or impaired mobility
T3   Tumor limited to the larynx with vocal cord fixation

T4   Tumor invades through thyroid cartilage and/or extends to other tissues beyond the larynx (e.g., oropharynx, soft tissues of the neck)

Lymph node (N)

NX   Regional lymph nodes cannot be assessed

N0   No regional lymph node metastasis

N1   Metastasis in a single ipsilateral lymph node, 3 cm or less in greatest dimension

N2   Metastasis in a single ipsilateral lymph node, more than 3 cm but not more than 6 cm in greatest dimension, or multiple ipsilateral lymph nodes, none more than 6 cm in greatest dimension, or bilateral or contralateral lymph nodes, none more than 6 cm in greatest dimension

   N2a   Metastasis in a single ipsilateral lymph node more than 3 cm but not more than 6 cm in greatest dimension

   N2b   Metastasis in multiple ipsilateral lymph nodes, none more than 6 cm in greatest dimension

   N2c   Metastasis in bilateral or contralateral lymph nodes, none more than 6 cm in greatest dimension

N3   Metastasis in a lymph node more than 6 cm in greatest dimension

Distant metastasis (M)

MX   Presence of distant metastasis cannot be assessed

M0   No distant metastasis

M1   Distant metastasis

Stage grouping

0	Tis	N0	M0
I	T1	N0	M0
II	T2	N0	M0
III	T3	N0	M0
	T1	N1	M0
	T2	N1	M0
	T3	N1	M0
IV	T4	N0	M0
	T4	N1	M0
	Any T	N2	M0
	Any T	N3	M0
	Any T	Any T	M1

Pleural Mesothelioma
Primary tumor (T)

TX   Primary tumor cannot be assessed

T0   No evidence of primary tumor

T1   Tumor limited to ipsilateral parietal and/or visceral pleura

T2   Tumor invades any of the following: Ipsilateral lung, endothoracic fascia, diaphragm, or pericardium

T3   Tumor invades any of the following: Ipsilateral chest wall muscle, ribs, or mediastinal organs or tissues

T4   Tumor directly extends to any of the following: contralateral pleura, lung, peritoneum, intraabdominal organs, or cervical tissues

Lymph node (N)

NX   Regional lymph nodes cannot be assessed

N0   No regional lymph node metastasis

N1   Metastasis in ipsilateral peribronchial and/or ipsilateral hilar lymph nodes, including direct extension

N2   Metastasis in ipsilateral mediastinal and/or subcarinal lymph node(s)

N3   Metastasis in contralateral mediastinal, contralateral hilar, ipsilateral or contralateral scalene, or supraclavicular lymph node(s)

Distant metastasis (M)

MX   Distant metastasis cannot be assessed

M0   No evidence of distant metastasis

M1   Distant metastasis

Stage grouping

Stage 1	T1	N0	M0
	T2	N0	M0
Stage II	T1	N1	M0
	T2	N1	M0
Stage III	T1	N2	M0
	T2	N2	M0
	T3	N0	M0
	T3	N1	M0
	T3	N2	M0
Stage IV	Any T	N3	M0
	T4	Any N	M0
	Any T	Any N	M1

Lung

Primary tumor (T)

TX   Primary tumor cannot be assessed, or tumor proven by presence of malignant cells in sputum or bronchial washings but not visualized by imaging or bronchoscopy

T0   No evidence of primary tumor

Tis   Carcinoma in situ

T1   Tumor 3 cm or less in greatest dimension, surrounded by lung or visceral pleura, without bronchoscopic evidence of invasion more proximal than the lobar bronchus (i.e., not in main bronchus)

T2   Tumor with any of the following features of size or extent: More than 3 cm in greatest dimension. Involves main bronchus, 2 cm or more distal to the carina. Invades the visceral pleura. Associated with atelectasis or obstructive pneumonitis which extends to the hilar region but does not involve the entire lung

T3   Tumor of any size that directly invades any of the following: chest wall (including superior sulcus tumors), diaphragm, mediastinal pleura, parietal pericardium; or tumor in the main bronchus less than 2 cm distal to the carina but without involvement of the carina; or associated atelectasis or obstructive pneumonitis of the entire lung

T4   Tumor of any size that invades any of the following: mediastinum, heart, great vessels, trachea, esophagus, vertebral body, carina; or tumor with a malignant pleural effusion

Lymph node (N)

NX   Regional lymph nodes cannot be assessed

N0   No regional lymph node metastasis

N1   Metastasis in ipsilateral peribronchial and/or ipsilateral hilar lymph nodes, including direct extension

N2   Metastasis in ipsilateral mediastinal and/or subcarinal lymph node(s)

N3   Metastasis in contralateral mediastinal, contralateral hilar, ipsilateral or contralateral scalene or supraclavicular lymph node(s)

Distant metastasis (M)

MX   Presence of distant metastasis cannot be assessed

M0   No distant metastasis

M1   Distant metastasis

Stage grouping

Occult	TX	N0	M0
0	Tis	N0	M0
I	T1	N0	M0
	T2	N0	M0
II	T1	N1	M0
	T2	N1	M0
IIIA	T1	N2	M0
	T2	N2	M0
	T3	N0	M0
	T3	N1	M0
	T3	N2	M0
IIIB	Any T	N3	M0
	T4	Any N	M0
IV	Any T	Any N	M1

Thyroid Gland
Primary tumor (T)

All categories may be subdivided: (a) solitary; (b) multifocal—measure the largest for classification

TX   Primary tumor cannot be assessed

T0   No evidence of primary tumor

T1   Tumor 1 cm or less in greatest dimension limited to the thyroid

T2   Tumor more than 1 cm but not more than 4 cm

T3   Tumor more than 4 cm in greatest dimension limited to the thyroid

T4   Tumor of any size extending beyond the thyroid capsule

Lymph node (N)

Regional nodes are the cervical and upper mediastinal lymph nodes

NX   Regional lymph nodes cannot be assessed

N0   No regional lymph node metastasis

N1   Regional lymph node metastasis

  N1a   Metastasis in ipsilateral cervical lymph nodes

  N1b   Metastasis in bilateral, midline, or contralateral cervical or mediastinal lymph nodes

Distant metastasis (M)

MX   Presence of distant metastasis cannot be assessed

M0   No distant metastasis

M1   Distant metastasis

Stage grouping

Separate stage groupings are recommended for papillary and follicular, medullary, and undifferentiated tumors.

Papillary or follicular

Under 45 Years

Stage I	Any T, Any N, M0
Stage II	Any T, Any N, M1

45 Years and Over

Stage I	T1, N0, M0
Stage II	T2, N0, M0
	T3, N0, M0
Stage III	T4, N0, M0
	Any T, N1, M0
Stage IV	Any T, Any N, M1

Medullary

Stage I	T1	N0	M0
Stage II	T2	N0	M0
	T3	N0	M0
	T4	N0	M0
Stage III	Any T	N1	M0
Stage IV	Any T	Any N	M1

Undifferentiated

All cases are Stage IV

Stage IV	Any T	Any N	Any M

Esophagus
Primary tumor (T)

TX	Primary tumor cannot be assessed
T0	No evidence of primary tumor
Tis	Carcinoma in situ
T1	Tumor invades lamina propria or submucosa
T2	Tumor invades muscularis propria
T3	Tumor invades adventitia
T4	Tumor invades adjacent structures

Lymph node (N)

NX	Regional lymph nodes cannot be assessed
N0	No regional lymph node metastasis
N1	Regional lymph node metastasis

Distant metastasis (M)

MX	Presence of distant metastasis cannot be assessed
M0	No distant metastasis
M1	Distant metastasis

Stage grouping

0	Tis	N0	M0
I	T1	N0	M0
IIA	T2	N0	M0
	T3	N0	M0
IIB	T1	N1	M0
	T2	N1	M0
III	T3	N1	M0
	T4	Any N	M0
IV	Any T	Any N	M1

Stomach

Primary tumor (T)

TX	Primary tumor cannot be assessed
T0	No evidence of primary tumor
Tis	Carcinoma in situ: intraepithelial tumor without invasion of lamina propria
T1	Tumor invades lamina propria or submucosa
T2	Tumor invades muscularis propria or subserosa
T3	Tumor penetrates serosa (visceral peritoneum) without invasion of adjacent structures
T4	Tumor invades adjacent structures

Lymph node (N)

NX	Regional lymph node(s) cannot be assessed
N0	No regional lymph node metastasis
N1	Metastasis in perigastric lymph node(s) within 3 cm of edge of primary tumor
N2	Metastasis in perigastric lymph node(s) more than 3 cm from edge of primary tumor, or in lymph nodes along left gastric, common hepatic, splenic, or celiac arteries

Distant metastasis (M)

MX	Presence of distant metastasis cannot be assessed
M0	No distant metastasis
M1	Distant metastasis

Stage grouping

0	Tis	N0	M0
1A	T1	N0	M0
IB	T1	N1	M0
	T2	N0	M0
II	T1	N2	M0
	T2	N1	M0
	T3	N0	M0
IIIA	T2	N2	M0
	T3	N1	M0
	T4	N0	M0
IIIB	T3	N2	M0
	T4	N1	M0
IV	T4	N2	M0
	Any T	Any N	M1

Small Intestine
Primary tumor (T)

TX	Primary tumor cannot be assessed
T0	No evidence of primary tumor
Tis	Carcinoma in situ
T1	Tumor invades lamina propria or submucosa
T2	Tumor invades muscularis propria
T3	Tumor invades through the muscularis propria into the subserosa or into the nonperitoneal- ized per muscular tissue (mesentery or retroperitoneum) with extension 2 cm or less
T4	Tumor perforates the visceral peritoneum, or directly invades other organs and structures (includes other loops of small intestine, mesentery, or retroperitoneum more than 2 cm, and the abdominal wall by way of the serosa; for the duodenum only includes invasion of the pancreas)

Regional lymph nodes (N)

NX	Regional lymph nodes cannot be assessed
N0	No regional lymph node metastasis
N1	Regional lymph node metastasis

Distant metastasis (M)

MX	Presence of distant metastasis cannot be assessed
M0	No distant metastasis
M1	Distant metastasis

Stage grouping

0	Tis	N0	M0
1	T1	N0	M0
	T2	N0	M0
II	T3	N0	M0
	T4	N0	M0
III	Any T	N1	M0
IV	Any T	Any N	M1

Colon and Rectum
Primary tumor (T)

TX	Primary tumor cannot be assessed
T0	No evidence of primary tumor
Tis	Carcinoma in situ intraepithelial or invasion of lamina propria
T1	Tumor invades submucosa
T2	Tumor invades muscularis propria
T3	Tumor invades through muscularis propria into subserosa, or into nonperitonealized pericolic or perirectal tissues
T4	Tumor directly invades other organs or structures, and/or perforates visceral peritoneum

Lymph node (N)

NX	Regional lymph nodes cannot be assessed
N0	No regional lymph node metastasis
N1	Metastasis in 1 to 3 pericolic or perirectal lymph nodes
N2	Metastasis in 4 or more pericolic or perirectal lymph nodes

N3   Metastasis in any lymph node along course of a named vascular trunk, and/or metastasis to apical node(s) (when marked by the surgeon)

Distant metastasis (M)

MX   Presence of distant metastasis cannot be assessed
M0   No distant metastasis
M1   Distant metastasis

Stage grouping

0	Tis	N0	M0
I	T1	N0	M0
	T2	N0	M0
II	T3	N1	M0
	T4	N0	M0
III	Any T	N2	M0
	Any T	N2	M0
	Any T	N3	M0
IV	Any T	Any N	M1

Anal Canal
Primary tumor (T)

TX   Primary tumor cannot be assessed
T0   No evidence of primary tumor
Tis   Carcinoma in situ
T1   Tumor 2 cm or less in greatest dimension
T2   Tumor more than 2 cm but not more than 5 cm in greatest dimension
T3   Tumor more than 5 cm in greatest dimension
T4   Tumor of any size invades adjacent organ(s): e.g., vagina, urethra, bladder (involvement of sphincter muscle[s] *alone* is not classified as T4)

Lymph node (N)

NX   Regional lymph nodes cannot be assessed
N0   No regional lymph node metastasis
N1   Metastasis in perirectal lymph node(s)
N2   Metastasis in unilateral internal iliac and/or inguinal lymph node(s)
N3   Metastasis in perirectal and inguinal lymph nodes and/or bilateral internal iliac and/or inguinal lymph nodes

Distant metastasis (M)

MX   Presence of distant metastasis cannot be assessed
M0   No distant metastasis
M1   Distant metastasis

Stage grouping

0	Tis	N0	M0
I	T1	N0	M0
II	T2	N0	M0
	T3	N0	M0
IIIA	T1	N1	M0
	T2	N1	M0

	T3	N1	M0
	T4	N0	M0
IIIB	T4	N1	M0
	Any T	N2	M0
	Any T	N3	M0
IV	Any T	Any N	M1

Salivary Glands

Primary tumor (T)

TX	Primary tumor cannot be assessed
T0	No evidence of primary tumor
T1	Tumor 2 cm or less in greatest dimension
T2	Tumor more than 2 cm but not more than 4 cm in greatest dimension
T3	Tumor more than 4 cm but not more than 6 cm in greatest dimension
T4	Tumor more than 6 cm in greatest dimension

Lymph node (N)

NX	Regional lymph nodes cannot be assessed
N0	No regional lymph node metastasis
N1	Metastasis in a single ipsilateral lymph node, 3 cm or less in greatest dimension
N2	Metastasis in a single ipsilateral lymph node, more than 3 cm but not more than 6 cm in greatest dimension, or in multiple ipsilateral lymph nodes, none more than 6 cm in greatest dimension or in bilateral or in contralateral lymph nodes, none more than 6 cm in greatest dimension
N2a	Metastasis in a single ipsilateral lymph node more than 3 cm but not more than 6 cm in greatest dimension
N2b	Metastasis in multiple ipsilateral lymph nodes, none more than 6 cm in greatest dimension
N2c	Metastasis in bilateral or contralateral lymph nodes, none more than 6 cm in greatest dimension
N3	Metastasis in a lymph node more than 6 cm in greatest dimension

Distant metastasis (M)

MX	Presence of distant metastasis cannot be assessed
M0	No distant metastasis
M1	Distant metastasis

Stage grouping

I	T1a	N0	M0
	T2a	N0	M0
II	T1b	N0	M0
	T2b	N0	M0
	T3a	N0	M0
III	T3b	N0	M0
	T4a	N0	M0
	Any T (except T4b)	N1	M0
IV	T4b	Any N	M0
	Any T	N2	M0
	Any T	N3	M0
	Any T	Any N	M1

Liver (Including Intrahepatic Bile Ducts)

Primary tumor (T)

TX	Primary tumor cannot be assessed
T0	No evidence of primary tumor
T1	Solitary tumor 2 cm or less in greatest dimension without vascular invasion
T2	Solitary tumor 2 cm or less in greatest dimension with vascular invasion, *or* Multiple tumors limited to one lobe, none more than 2 cm in greatest dimension without vascular invasion, *or* A solitary tumor more than 2 cm in greatest dimension without vascular invasion
T3	Solitary tumor more than 2 cm in greatest dimension with vascular invasion, *or* Multiple tumors limited to one lobe, none more than 2 cm in greatest dimension, with vascular invasion, *or* Multiple tumors limited to one lobe, any more than 2 cm in greatest dimension, with or without vascular invasion
T4	Multiple tumors in more than one lobe, *or* Tumor(s) involve(s) a major branch of portal or hepatic vein(s)

Lymph node (N)

NX	Regional lymph nodes cannot be assessed
N0	No regional lymph node metastasis
N1	Regional lymph node metastasis

Distant metastasis (M)

MX	Presence of distant metastasis cannot be assessed
M0	No distant metastasis
M1	Distant metastasis

Stage grouping

I	T1	N0	M0
II	T2	N0	M0
III	T1	N1	M0
	T2	N1	M0
	T3	N0	M0
	T3	N1	M0
IVA	T4	Any N	M0
IVB	Any T	Any N	M1

Gallbladder

Primary tumor (T)

TX	Primary tumor cannot be assessed
T0	No evidence of primary tumor
Tis	Carcinoma in situ
T1	Tumor invades mucosa or muscle layer
T1a	Tumor invades mucosa
T1b	Tumor invades muscle layer
T2	Tumor invades perimuscular connective tissue; no extension beyond serosa or into liver
T3	Tumor perforates the serosa (visceral peritoneum) or directly invades into one adjacent organ, or both (extension 2 cm or less into liver)

T4	Tumor extends more than 2 cm into liver, and/or into two or more adjacent organs (stomach, duodenum, colon, pancreas, omentum, extrahepatic bile ducts, any involvement of liver)

Lymph node (N)

NX	Regional lymph nodes cannot be assessed
N0	No regional lymph node metastasis
N1	Metastasis in cystic duct, pericholedochal, and/or hilar lymph nodes (i.e., in hepatoduodenal ligament)
N2	Metastasis in peripancreatic (head only), paraduodenal, periportal, celiac, and/or superior mesenteric lymph nodes

Distant metastasis (M)

MX	Presence of distant metastasis cannot be assessed
M0	No distant metastasis
M1	Distant metastasis

Stage grouping

0	Tis	N0	M0
I	T1	N0	M0
II	T2	N0	M0
III	T1	N1	M0
	T2	N1	M0
	T3	N0	M0
	T3	N1	M0
IVA	T4	N0	M0
	T4	N1	M0
IVB	Any T	N2	M0
	Any T	Any N	M1

Extrahepatic Bile Ducts
Primary tumor (T)

TX	Primary tumor cannot be assessed
T0	No evidence of primary tumor
Tis	Carcinoma in situ
T1	Tumor invades mucosa or muscle layer
T1a	Tumor invades mucosa
T1b	Tumor invades muscle layer
T2	Tumor invades perimuscular connective tissues
T3	Tumor invades adjacent structure(s), liver, pancreas, duodenum, gallbladder, colon, stomach

Lymph node (N)

NX	Regional lymph nodes cannot be assessed
N0	No regional lymph node metastasis
N1	Metastasis in cystic duct, pericholedochal and/or hilar lymph nodes
N2	Metastasis in peripancreatic (head only), periduodenal, periportal, celiac, and/or superior mesenteric and/or posterior pancreatic duodenal lymph nodes

Distant metastasis (M)

MX	Presence of distant metastasis cannot be assessed
M0	No distant metastasis
M1	Distant metastasis

Stage grouping

0	Tis	N0	M0
I	T1	N0	M0
II	T2	N0	M0
III	T1	N1	M0
	T1	N2	M0
	T2	N1	M0
	T2	N2	M0
IVA	T3	Any N	M0
IVB	Any T	Any N	M1

Exocrine Pancreas
Primary tumor (T)

TX	Primary tumor cannot be assessed
T0	No evidence of primary tumor
T1	Tumor limited to the pancreas
T1a	Tumor 2 cm or less in greatest dimension
T1b	Tumor more than 2 cm in greatest dimension
T2	Tumor extends directly to any of the following: duodenum, bile duct, or peripancreatic tissues
T3	Tumor extends directly to any of the following: stomach, spleen, colon, or adjacent large vessels

Lymph node (N)

NX	Regional lymph nodes cannot be assessed
N0	No regional lymph node metastasis
N1	Regional lymph node metastasis

Distant metastasis (M)

MX	Presence of distant metastasis cannot be assessed
M0	No distant metastasis
M1	Distant metastasis

Stage grouping

I	T1	N0	M0
	T2	N0	M0
II	T3	N0	M0
III	Any T	N1	M0
IV	Any T	Any N	M1

Ampulla of Vater
Primary tumor (T)

TX	Primary tumor cannot be assessed
T0	No evidence of primary tumor
Tis	Carcinoma in situ
T1	Tumor limited to ampulla of Vater
T2	Tumor invades duodenal wall
T3	Tumor invades 2 cm or less into pancreas
T4	Tumor invades more than 2 cm into pancreas and/or into other adjacent organs

Lymph node (N)

NX   Regional lymph nodes cannot be assessed
N0   No regional lymph node metastasis
N1   Regional lymph node metastasis

Distant metastasis (M)

MX   Presence of distant metastasis cannot be assessed
M0   No distant metastasis
M1   Distant metastasis

Stage grouping

0	Tis	N0	M0
I	T1	N0	M0
II	T2	N0	M0
	T3	N0	M0
III	T1	N1	M0
	T2	N1	M0
	T3	N1	M0
IV	T4	Any N	M0
	Any T	Any N	M1

Neuroblastoma

Primary tumor (T)

TX   Primary tumor cannot be assessed
T0   No evidence of primary tumor
T1   Single tumor 5 cm or less in greatest dimension
T2   Single tumor more than 5 cm but not more than 10 cm in greatest dimension
T3   Single tumor more than 10 cm in greatest dimension
T4   Multicentric tumors occurring simultaneously

Lymph node (N)

NX   Regional lymph nodes cannot be assessed
N0   No regional lymph node metastasis
N1   Regional lymph node metastasis

Distant metastasis (M)

MX   Presence of distant metastasis cannot be assessed
M0   No distant metastasis
M1   Distant metastasis

Primary tumor (pT)

pTX   Primary tumor cannot be assessed
pT0   No evidence of primary tumor
pT1   Excision of tumor complete and margins histologically free
pT2   The category does not apply to neuroblastoma
pT3   Residual tumor
    pT3a   Microscopic residual tumor

pT3b   Macroscopic residual tumor or grossly incomplete excision
pT3c   Surgical exploration tumor not resected
pT4   Multicentric tumors

Lymph node (pN)

pNX   Regional lymph nodes cannot be assessed
pN0   No regional lymph node metastasis
pN1   Regional lymph node metastasis
   pN1a   Regional lymph node metastases completely resected
   pN1b   Regional lymph node metastases incompletely resected

Distant metastasis (pM)

pMX   Presence of distant metastasis cannot be assessed
pM0   No distant metastasis
pM1   Distant metastasis

Carcinoma of the Kidney
Primary tumor (T)

TX   Primary tumor cannot be assessed
T0   No evidence of primary tumor
T1   Tumor 2.5 cm or less in greatest dimension limited to the kidney
T2   Tumor more than 2.5 cm in greatest dimension limited to the kidney
T3   Tumor extends into major veins or invades adrenal gland or perinephric tissues but not beyond Gerota's fascia
   T3a   Tumor invades adrenal gland or perinephric tissues but not beyond Gerota's fascia
   T3b   Tumor grossly extends into renal vein(s) or vena cava below diaphragm
   T3c   Tumor grossly extends into vena cava above diaphragm
T4   Tumor invades beyond Gerota's fascia

Lymph node (N)

NX   Regional lymph nodes cannot be assessed
N0   No regional lymph node metastasis
N1   Metastasis in a single lymph node, 2 cm or less in greatest dimension
N2   Metastasis in a single lymph node, more than 2 cm but not more than 5 cm in greatest dimension, or multiple lymph nodes, none more than 5 cm in greatest dimension
N3   Metastasis in a lymph node more than 5 cm in greatest dimension

Distant metastasis (M)

MX   Presence of distant metastasis cannot be assessed
M0   No distant metastasis
M1   Distant metastasis

Stage grouping

I	T1	N0	M0
II	T2	N0	M0
III	T1	N1	M0
	T2	N1	M0
	T3a	N0	M0
	T3a	N1	M0
	T3b	N0	M0

	T3b	N1	M0
	T3c	N0	M0
	T3c	N1	M0
IV	T4	Any N	M0
	Any T	N2	M0
	Any T	N3	M0
	Any T	Any N	M1

Nephroblastoma

Primary tumor (T)

TX	Primary tumor cannot be assessed
T0	No evidence of primary tumor
T1	Unilateral tumor 80 cm^2 or less in area (including kidney)*
T2	Unilateral tumor more than 80 cm^2 in area (including kidney)*
T3	Unilateral tumor rupture before treatment
T4	Bilateral tumors

*Note: The area is calculated by multiplying the vertical and horizontal dimensions of the radiologic shadow of the tumor and kidney.

Lymph node (N)

NX	Regional lymph nodes cannot be assessed
N0	No regional lymph node metastasis
N1	Regional lymph node metastasis

Distant metastasis (M)

MX	Presence of distant metastasis cannot be assessed
M0	No distant metastasis
M1	Distant metastasis

Primary tumor (pT)

pTX	Primary tumor cannot be assessed
pT0	No evidence of primary tumor
pT1	Intrarenal tumor completely encapsulated; excision complete and margins histologically free
pT2	Tumor invades beyond the capsule or renal parenchyma*; excision complete
pT3	Tumor invades beyond the capsule or renal parenchyma*; excision incomplete or preoperative or operative rupture
pT3a	Microscopic residual tumor limited to tumor bed
pT3b	Macroscopic residual tumor or spillage or malignant ascites
pT3c	Surgical exploration only, tumor not resected
pT4	Bilateral tumors

*Note: This includes breach of the renal capsule or tumor seen microscopically outside the capsule; tumor adhesions microscopically confirmed; infiltrations of or tumor thrombus within the renal vessels outside the kidney; and infiltration of the renal pelvis and/or ureter, peripelvic, and pericalyceal fat.

Lymph node (pN)

pNX	Regional lymph nodes cannot be assessed
pN0	No regional lymph node metastasis
pN1	Regional lymph node metastasis
pN1a	Regional lymph node metastasis completely resected
pN1b	Regional lymph node metastasis incompletely resected

Distant metastasis (pM)

pMX	Presence of distant metastasis cannot be assessed
pM0	No distant metastasis
pM1	Distant metastasis

Renal Pelvis and Ureter
Primary tumor (T)

TX	Primary tumor cannot be assessed
T0	No evidence of primary tumor
Ta	Papillary noninvasive carcinoma
Tis	Carcinoma in situ
T1	Tumor invades subepithelial connective tissue
T2	Tumor invades muscularis
T3	Tumor invades beyond muscularis into peripelvic fat or renal parenchyma (for renal pelvis only)
T3	Tumor invades beyond muscularis into periureteric fat (for ureter only)
T4	Tumor invades adjacent organs or through the kidney into perinephric fat

Lymph node (N)

NX	Regional lymph nodes cannot be assessed
N0	No regional lymph node metastasis
N1	Metastasis in a single lymph node, 2 cm or less in greatest dimension
N2	Metastasis in a single lymph node, more than 2 cm but not more than 5 cm in greatest dimension, or multiple lymph nodes, none more than 5 cm in greatest dimension
N3	Metastasis in a lymph node more than 5 cm in greatest dimension

Distant metastasis (M)

MX	Presence of distant metastasis cannot be assessed
M0	No distant metastasis
M1	Distant metastasis

Stage grouping

0a	Ta	N0	M0
0is	Tis	N0	M0
I	T1	N0	M0
II	T2	N0	M0
III	T3	N0	M0
IV	T4	N0	M0
	Any T	N1	M0
	Any T	N2	M0
	Any T	N3	M0
	Any T	Any N	M1

Urinary Bladder
Primary tumor (T)

TX	Primary tumor cannot be assessed
T0	No evidence of primary tumor
Ta	Noninvasive papillary carcinoma
Tis	Carcinoma in situ: "flat tumor"
T1	Tumor invades subepithelial connective tissue

T2	Tumor invades superficial muscle (inner half)
T3	Tumor invades deep muscle or perivesical fat
T3a	Tumor invades deep muscle (outer half)
T3b	Tumor invades perivesical fat
i.	Microscopically
ii.	Macroscopically (extravesical mass)
T4	Tumor invades prostate, uterus, vagina, pelvic wall, or abdominal wall
T4a	Tumor invades prostate, uterus, vagina
T4b	Tumor invades pelvic wall or abdominal wall

Lymph node (N)

NX	Regional lymph nodes cannot be assessed
N0	No regional lymph node metastasis
N1	Metastasis in a single lymph node, 2 cm or less in greatest dimension
N2	Metastasis in a single lymph node, more than 2 cm but not more then 5 cm in greatest dimension, or multiple lymph nodes, none more than 5 cm in greatest dimension
N3	Metastasis in a lymph node more than 5 cm in greatest dimension

Distant metastasis (M)

MX	Presence of distant metastasis cannot be assessed
M0	No distant metastasis
M1	Distant metastasis

Stage grouping

0a	Ta	N0	M0
0is	Tis	N0	M0
I	T1	N0	M0
II	T2	N0	M0
	T3a	N0	M0
III	T3b	N0	M0
	T4a	N0	M0
IV	T4b	N0	M0
	Any T	N1	M0
	Any T	N2	M0
	Any T	N3	M0
	Any T	Any N	M1

Urethra
Primary tumor (T)

TX	Primary tumor cannot be assessed
T0	No evidence of primary tumor
Ta	Noninvasive papillary, polypoid, or verrucous carcinoma
Tis	Carcinoma in situ
T1	Tumor invades subepithelial connective tissue
T2	Tumor invades corpus spongiosum or prostate or periurethral muscle
T3	Tumor invades corpus cavernosum or beyond prostatic capsule or the anterior vagina or bladder neck
T4	Tumor invades other adjacent organs

Lymph node (N)

NX	Regional lymph nodes cannot be assessed
N0	No regional lymph node metastasis
N1	Metastasis in a single lymph node, 2 cm or less in greatest dimension
N2	Metastasis in a single lymph node, more than 2 cm but not more than 5 cm in greatest dimension, or multiple lymph nodes, none more than 5 cm in greatest dimension
N3	Metastasis in a lymph node more than 5 cm in greatest dimension

Distant metastasis (M)

MX	Presence of distant metastasis cannot be assessed
M0	No distant metastasis
M1	Distant metastasis

Stage grouping

0a	Ta	N0	M0
0is	Tis	N0	M0
I	T1	N0	M0
II	T2	N0	M0
III	T1	N1	M0
	T2	N1	M0
	T3	N0	M0
	T3	N1	M0
IV	T4	N0	M0
	T4	N1	M0
	Any T	N2	M0
	Any T	N3	M0
	Any T	Any N	M1

Prostate

Primary tumor (T)

TX	Primary tumor cannot be assessed
T0	No evidence of primary tumor
T1	Clinically inapparent tumor not palpable or visible by imaging
T1a	Tumor incidental histologic finding in 5% or less of tissue resected
T1b	Tumor incidental histologic finding in more than 5% of tissue resected
T1c	Tumor identified by needle biopsy (e.g., because of elevated prostate-specific antigen [PSA])
T2	Palpable tumor confined within prostate*
T2a	Tumor involves half of a lobe or less
T2b	Tumor involves more than half of a lobe, but not both lobes
T2c	Tumor involves both lobes
T3	Tumor extends through the prostatic capsule†
T3a	Unilateral extracapsular extension
T3b	Bilateral extracapsular extension
T3c	Tumor invades seminal vesicle(s)
T4	Tumor is fixed or invades adjacent structures other than seminal vesicles
T4a	Tumor invades external sphincter and/or bladder neck and/or rectum
T4b	Tumor invades levator muscles and/or is fixed to pelvic wall

Lymph node (N)

NX   Regional lymph nodes cannot be assessed
N0   No regional lymph node metastasis
N1   Metastasis in a single lymph node, 2 cm or less in greatest dimension
N2   Metastasis in a single lymph node, more than 2 cm but not more than 5 cm in greatest dimension, or multiple lymph nodes, none more than 5 cm in greatest dimension
N3   Metastasis in a lymph node more than 5 cm in greatest dimension

Distant metastasis (M)‡

MX   Presence of distant metastasis cannot be assessed
M0   No distant metastasis
M1   Distant metastasis
  M1a   Nonregional lymph nodes
  M1b   Bone
  M1c   Other sites

---

*Tumor found in one or both lobes by needle biopsy, but not palpable or visible by imaging, is classified as T1c.
†Invasion into the prostatic apex or into (but not beyond) the prostatic capsule is not classified as T3, but as T2.
‡When more than one site of metastasis is present, the most advanced category (pM1c) is used.

Testis
Primary tumor (T)

pTX   Primary tumor cannot be assessed. (If no radical orchiectomy has been performed, TX is used)
pT0   No evidence of primary tumor (e.g., histologic scar in testis)
pTis   Intratubular tumor: preinvasive cancer
pT1   Tumor limited to testis, including rete testis
pT2   Tumor invades beyond tunica albuginea or into epididymis
pT3   Tumor invades spermatic cord
pT4   Tumor invades scrotum

Lymph node (N)

NX   Regional lymph nodes cannot be assessed
N0   No regional lymph node metastasis
N1   Metastasis in a single lymph node, 2 cm or less in greatest dimension
N2   Metastasis in a single lymph node, more than 2 cm but not more than 5 cm in greatest dimension, or multiple lymph nodes, none more than 5 cm in greatest dimension
N3   Metastasis in a lymph node more than 5 cm in greatest dimension

Distant metastasis (M)

MX   Presence of distant metastasis cannot be assessed
M0   No distant metastasis
M1   Distant metastasis

Stage grouping

0	pTis	N0	M0
I	Any pT	N0	M0
II	Any pT	N1	M0
	Any pT	N2	M0
	Any pT	N3	M0
III	Any pT	Any N	M1

Penis
Primary tumor (T)

TX	Primary tumor cannot be assessed
T0	No evidence of primary tumor
Tis	Carcinoma in situ
Ta	Noninvasive verrucous carcinoma
T1	Tumor invades subepithelial connective tissue
T2	Tumor invades corpus spongiosum or cavernosum
T3	Tumor invades urethra or prostate
T4	Tumor invades other adjacent structures

Lymph node (N)

NX	Regional lymph nodes cannot be assessed
N0	No regional lymph node metastasis
N1	Metastasis in a single, superficial inguinal lymph node
N2	Metastasis in multiple or bilateral superficial inguinal lymph nodes
N3	Metastasis in deep inguinal or pelvic lymph node(s), unilateral or bilateral

Distant metastasis

MX	Presence of distant metastasis cannot be assessed
M0	No distant metastasis
M1	Distant metastasis

Stage grouping

0	Tis	N0	M0
	Ta	N0	M0
I	T1	N0	M0
II	T1	N1	M0
	T2	N0	M0
	T2	N1	M0
III	T1	N2	M0
	T2	N2	M0
	T3	N0	M0
	T3	N1	M0
	T3	N2	M0
IV	T4	Any N	M0
	Any T	N3	M0
	Any T	Any N	M1

Vulva
Primary tumor (T)

TX	Primary tumor cannot be assessed
T0	No evidence of primary tumor
Tis	Preinvasive carcinoma (carcinoma in situ)
T1	Tumor confined to the vulva or to the vulva and perineum, 2 cm or less in greatest dimension
T2	Tumor confined to the vulva or to the vulva and perineum, more than 2 cm in greatest dimension
T3	Tumor involves any of the following: lower urethra, vagina, or anus

T4   Tumor invades any of the following: bladder mucosa, upper part of urethral mucosa, rectal mucosa, or tumor fixed to the bone

Lymph node (N)

Regional lymph nodes are the femoral and inguinal nodes

NX   Regional lymph nodes cannot be assessed
N0   No regional lymph node metastasis
N1   Unilateral regional lymph node metastasis
N2   Bilateral regional lymph node metastasis

Distant metastasis (M)

MX   Presence of distant metastasis cannot be assessed
M0   No distant metastasis
M1   Distant metastasis (pelvic lymph node metastasis is M1)

Stage grouping

AJCC/UICC				FIGO
0	Tis	N0	M0	
I	T1	N0	M0	I
II	T2	N0	M0	II
III	T1	N1	M0	III
	T2	N1	M0	
	T3	N0	M0	
	T3	N1	M0	
IVA	T1	N2	M0	IVA
	T2	N2	M0	
	T3	N2	M0	
	T4	Any N	M0	
IVB	Any T	Any N	M1	IVB

Vagina

Primary tumor (T)

TNM category	FIGO stage	
TX		Primary tumor cannot be assessed
T0		No evidence of primary tumor
Tis	0	Carcinoma in situ
T1	I	Tumor confined to vagina
T2	II	Tumor invades paravaginal tissues but not to pelvic wall
T3	III	Tumor extends to pelvic wall
T4*	IVA	Tumor invades mucosa of bladder or rectum and/or extends beyond the true pelvis
M2	IVB	Distant metastasis

Lymph node (N)

NX   Regional lymph nodes cannot be assessed
N0   No regional lymph node metastasis
            Upper two thirds of vagina
N1   Pelvic lymph node metastasis
            Lower one third of vagina
N1   Unilateral inguinal lymph node metastasis

| N2 | | | | Bilateral inguinal lymph node metastasis |

Distant metastasis (M)

MX		Presence of distant metastasis cannot be assessed
M0		No distant metastasis
M1	IVB	Distant metastasis

Stage grouping

AJCC/UICC				FIGO
0	Tis	N0	M0	Stage 0
I	T1	N0	M0	Stage I
II	T2	N0	M0	Stage II
III	T1	N1	M0	Stage III
	T2	N1	M0	
	T3	N0	M0	
	T3	N1	M0	
IVA	T1	N2	M0	Stage IVA
	T2	N2	M0	
	T3	N2	M0	
	T4	Any N	M0	
IVB	Any T	Any N	M1	Stage IVB

*The presence of bullous edema is not sufficient evidence to classify a tumor T4. If the mucosa is not involved, the tumor is stage III.

Cervix uteri
Primary tumor (T)

TNM category	FIGO stage	
TX		Primary tumor cannot be assessed
T0		No evidence of primary tumor
Tis		Carcinoma in situ
T1	I	Cervical carcinoma confined to uterus (extension to corpus should be disregarded)
T1a	IA	Preclinical invasive carcinoma, diagnosed by microscopy only
T1a1	IA1	Minimum microscopic stromal invasion
T1a2	IA2	Tumor with invasive component 5 mm or less in depth taken from the base of the epithelium and 7 mm or less in horizontal spread
T1b	IB	Tumor larger than T1a2
T2	II	Cervical carcinoma invades beyond uterus but not to pelvic wall or to the lower third of vagina
T2a	IIA	Tumor without parametrial invasion
T2b	IIB	Tumor with parametrial invasion
T3	III	Cervical carcinoma extends to pelvic wall and/or involves lower third of vagina and/or causes hydronephrosis or nonfunctioning kidney
T3a	IIIA	Tumor involves lower third of vagina, no extension to pelvic wall
T3b	IIIB	Tumor extends to pelvic wall and/or causes hydronephrosis or nonfunctioning kidney
T4*	IVA	Tumor invades mucosa of bladder or rectum and/or extends beyond the true pelvis

Lymph node (N)

| NX | | Regional lymph nodes cannot be assessed |
| N0 | | No regional lymph node metastasis |

N1   Regional lymph node metastasis

Distant metastasis (M)

MX   Presence of distant metastasis cannot be assessed
M0   No distant metastasis
M1   IVB   Distant metastasis

Stage grouping

AJCC/UICC				FIGO
0	Tis	N0	M0	
IA	T1a	N0	M0	IA
IB	T1b	N0	M0	IB
IIA	T2a	N0	M0	IIA
IIB	T2b	N0	M0	IIB
IIIA	T3a	N0	M0	IIIA
IIIB	T1	N1	M0	IIIB
	T2	N1	M0	
	T3a	N1	M0	
	T3b	Any N	M0	
IVA	T4	Any N	M0	IVA
IVB	Any T	Any N	M1	IVB

*Presence of bullous edema is not sufficient evidence to classify a tumor T4.

Corpus uteri
Primary tumor (T)

TNM category	FIGO stage	
TX		Primary tumor cannot be assessed
T0		No evidence of primary tumor
Tis		Carcinoma in situ
T1	I	Tumor confined to corpus uteri
T1a	IA	Tumor limited to endometrium
T1b	IB	Tumor invades up to or less than one half of the myometrium
T1c	IC	Tumor invades to more than one half of the myometrium
T2	II	Tumor invades cervix but does not extend beyond uterus
T2a	IIA	Endocervical glandular involvement only
T2b	IIB	Cervical stromal invasion
T3 &/or N1	III	Local and/or regional spread as specified in T3a, b, N1 and FIGO IIIA, B, and C below
T3a	IIIA	Tumor involves serosa and/or adnexae (direct extension or metastasis) and/or cancer cells in ascites or peritoneal washings
T3b	IIIB	Vaginal involvement (direct extension or metastasis)
N1	IIIC	Metastasis to the pelvic and/or para-aortic lymph nodes
T4*	IVA	Tumor invades bladder mucosa and/or bowel mucosa
M1	IVB	Distant metastasis (*excluding* metastasis to vagina, pelvic serosa, or adnexae; *including* metastasis to intra-abdominal lymph nodes other than para-aortic, and/or inguinal lymph nodes)

Lymph node (N)

NX	Regional lymph nodes cannot be assessed
N0	No regional lymph node metastasis
N1	Regional lymph node metastasis

Distant metastasis (M)

MX		Presence of distant metastasis cannot be assessed
M0		No distant metastasis
M1	IVB	Distant metastasis

Stage grouping

AJCC/UICC				FIGO
0	Tis	N0	M0	
IA	T1a	N0	M0	Stage IA
IB	T1b	N0	M0	Stage IB
IC	T1c	N0	M0	Stage IC
IIA	T2a	N0	M0	Stage IIA
IIB	T2b	N0	M0	Stage IIB
IIIA	T3a	N0	M0	Stage IIIA
IIIB	T3b	N0	M0	Stage IIIB
IIIC	T1	N1	M0	Stage IIIC
	T2	N1	M0	
	T3a	N1	M0	
	T3b	N1	M0	
IVA	T4	Any N	M0	Stage IVA
IVB	Any T	Any N	M1	Stage IVB

*The presence of bullous edema is not sufficient evidence to classify a tumor T4.

Ovary

Primary tumor (T)

TNM category	FIGO stage	
TX		Primary tumor cannot be assessed
T0		No evidence of primary tumor
T1	I	Tumor limited to ovaries (one or both)
T1a	IA	Tumor limited to one ovary; capsule intact, no tumor on ovarian surface. No malignant cells in ascites or peritoneal washings.
T1b	IB	Tumor limited to both ovaries; capsules intact, no tumor on ovarian surface. No malignant cells in ascites or peritoneal washings.
T1c	IC	Tumor limited to one or both ovaries with any of the following: capsule ruptured, tumor on ovarian surface, malignant cells in ascites, or peritoneal washings.
T2	II	Tumor involves one or both ovaries with pelvic extension
T2a	IIA	Extension and/or implants on uterus and/or tube(s). No malignant cells in ascites or peritoneal washings.
T2b	IIB	Extension to other pelvic tissues. No malignant cells in ascites or peritoneal washings.
T2c	IIC	Pelvic extension (2a or 2b) with malignant cells in ascites or peritoneal washings.
T3 &/or N1	III	Tumor involves one or both ovaries with microscopically confirmed peritoneal metastasis outside the pelvis and/or regional lymph node metastasis

T3a	IIIA	Microscopic peritoneal metastasis beyond pelvis		
T3b	IIIB	Macroscopic peritoneal metastasis beyond pelvis 2 cm or less in greatest dimension		
T3c &/or N1	IIIC	Peritoneal metastasis beyond pelvis more than 2 cm in greatest dimension and/or regional lymph node metastasis		
M1	IV	Distant metastasis (excludes peritoneal metastasis)		

Lymph node (N)

NX	Regional lymph nodes cannot be assessed
N0	No regional lymph node metastasis
N1	Regional lymph node metastasis

Distant metastasis (M)

MX		Presence of distant metastasis cannot be assessed
M0		No distant metastasis
M1	IV	Distant metastasis (excludes peritoneal metastasis)

Stage grouping

AJCC/UICC				FIGO
IVB	Any T	Any N	M1	IVB
IA	T1a	N0	M0	Stage IA
IB	T1b	N0	M0	Stage IB
IC	T1c	N0	M0	Stage IC
IIA	T2a	N0	M0	Stage IIA
IIB	T2b	N0	M0	Stage IIB
IIC	T2c	N0	M0	Stage IIC
IIIA	T3a	N0	M0	Stage IIIA
IIIB	T3b	N0	M0	Stage IIIB
IIIC	T3c	N0	M0	Stage IIIC
	Any T	N1	M0	
IV	Any T	Any N	M1	Stage IV

NOTE: Liver capsule metastasis is T3/stage III; liver parenchymal metastasis is M1/stage IV. Pleural effusion must have positive cytologic findings for M1/stage IV.

Breast
Primary tumor (T)

TX	Primary tumor cannot be assessed
T0	No evidence of primary tumor
Tis	Carcinoma in situ: intraductal carcinoma, lobular carcinoma in situ, or Paget's disease of the nipple with no tumor
T1	Tumor 2 cm or less in greatest dimension
T1a	0.5 cm or less in greatest dimension
T1b	More than 0.5 cm but not more than 1 cm in greatest dimension
T1c	More than 1 cm but not more than 2 cm in greatest dimension
T2	Tumor more than 2 cm but not more than 5 cm in greatest dimension
T3	Tumor more than 5 cm in greatest dimension
T4	Tumor of any size with direct extension to chest wall or skin

T4a	Extension to chest wall	
T4b	Edema (including peau d'orange) or ulceration of the skin of breast or satellite skin nodules confined to same breast	
T4c	Both T4a and T4b	
T4d	Inflammatory carcinoma	

Lymph node (N)

NX	Regional lymph nodes cannot be assessed (e.g., previously removed)
N0	No regional lymph node metastasis
N1	Metastasis to movable ipsilateral axillary lymph node(s)
N2	Metastasis to ipsilateral axillary lymph node(s) fixed to one another or to other structures
N3	Metastasis to ipsilateral internal mammary lymph node(s)

Pathologic classification (pN)

pNX Regional lymph nodes cannot be assessed (e.g., previously removed, or not removed for pathologic study)

pN0 No regional lymph node metastasis

pN1 Metastasis to movable ipsilateral axillary lymph node(s)

  pN1a Only micrometastasis (none larger than 0.2 cm)

  pN1b Metastasis to lymph nodes, any larger than 0.2 cm

    pN1bi Metastasis in 1 to 3 lymph nodes, any more than 0.2 cm and all less than 2 cm in greatest dimension

    pN1bii Metastasis to 4 or more lymph nodes, any more than 0.2 cm and all less than 2 cm in greatest dimension

    pN1biii Extension of tumor beyond the capsule of a lymph node metastasis less than 2 cm in greatest dimension

    pN1biv Metastasis to a lymph node 2 cm or more in greatest dimension

pN2 Metastasis to ipsilateral axillary lymph nodes that are fixed to one another or to other structures

pN3 Metastasis to ipsilateral internal mammary lymph nodes(s)

Distant metastasis (M)

MX	Presence of distant metastasis cannot be assessed
M0	No distant metastasis
M1	Distant metastasis (includes metastasis to ipsilateral supraclavicular lymph node[s])

Stage grouping

0	Tis	N0	M0
I	T1	N0	M0
IIA	T0	N1	M0
	T1	N1	M0
	T2	N0	M0
IIB	T2	N1	M0
	T3	N0	M0
IIIA	T0	N2	M0
	T1	N2	M0
	T2	N2	M0
	T3	N2	M0
IIIB	T4	Any N	M0
	Any T	N3	M0
IV	Any T	Any N	M1

Hodgkin's Disease
Stage grouping

Stage I — Involvement of single lymph node region (I) or localized involvement of a single extralymphatic organ or site (I_E).

Stage II — Involvement of two or more lymph node regions on the same side of the diaphragm (II) or localized involvement of a single associated extralymphatic organ or site and its regional lymph node(s) with or without involvement of other lymph node regions on the same side of the diaphragm (II_E).

NOTE: The number of lymph node regions involved may be indicated by a subscript (e.g., II_3).

Stage III — Involvement of lymph node regions on both sides of the diaphragm (III), which may also be accompanied by localized involvement of an associated extralymphatic organ or site (III_E), by involvement of the spleen (III_S), or both (III_{E+S}).

Stage IV — Disseminated (multifocal) involvement of one or more extralymphatic organs, with or without associated lymph node involvement, or isolated extralymphatic organ involvement with distant (nonregional) nodal involvement.

Non-Hodgkin's Lymphoma

Stage I — Involvement of single lymph node region (I) or localized involvement of a single extralymphatic organ or site (I_E).

Stage II — Involvement of two or more lymph node regions on the same side of the diaphragm (II), or localized involvement of a single associated extralymphatic organ or site and its regional nodes with or without other lymph node regions on the same side of the diaphragm (II_E).

NOTE: The number of lymph node regions involved may be indicated by a subscript (e.g., II_3).

Stage III — Involvement of lymph node regions on both sides of the diaphragm (III), which may also be accompanied by localized involvement of an extralymphatic organ or site (III_E), by involvement of the spleen (III_S), or both (III_{E+S}).

Stage IV — Disseminated (multifocal) involvement of one or more extralymphatic organs, with or without associated lymph node involvement, or isolated extralymphatic organ involvement with distant (nonregional) nodal involvement.

Bone
Primary tumor (T)

TX — Primary tumor cannot be assessed
T0 — No evidence of primary tumor
T1 — Tumor confined within the cortex
T2 — Tumor invades beyond the cortex

Lymph node (N)

NX — Regional lymph nodes cannot be assessed
N0 — No regional lymph node metastasis
N1 — Regional lymph node metastasis

Distant metastasis (M)

MX — Presence of distant metastasis cannot be assessed
M0 — No distant metastasis
M1 — Distant metastasis

Stage grouping

IVB	Any T	Any N	M1	IVB
IA	G1	T1	N0	M0

Lymph node (N)

This category does not apply to this site.

Distant metastasis (M)

MX	Presence of distant metastasis cannot be assessed
M0	No distant metastasis
M1	Distant metastasis

Stage grouping

IA	G1	T1	M0
IB	G1	T2	M0
	G1	T3	M0
IIA	G2	T1	M0
IIB	G2	T2	M0
	G2	T3	M0
IIIA	G3	T1	M0
IIIB	G3	T2	M0
	G3	T3	M0
IV	G1	T4	M0
	G2	T4	M0
	G3	T4	M0
	G4	Any T	M0
	Any G	Any T	M1

Carcinoma of the Eyelid
Primary tumor (T)

TX	Primary tumor cannot be assessed
T0	No evidence of primary tumor
Tis	Carcinoma in situ
T1	Tumor of any size, not invading the tarsal plate or the eyelid margin, 5 mm or less in greatest dimension
T2	Tumor invades tarsal plate or the eyelid margin, more than 5 mm but not more than 10 mm in greatest dimension
T3	Tumor involves full eyelid thickness or the eyelid margin, more than 10 mm in greatest dimension
T4	Tumor invades adjacent structures

Lymph node (N)

NX	Regional lymph nodes cannot be assessed
N0	No regional lymph node metastasis
N1	Regional lymph node metastasis

Distant metastasis (M)

MX	Presence of distant metastasis cannot be assessed
M0	No distant metastasis
M1	Distant metastasis

Malignant Melanoma of the Eyelid
Primary tumor (T)

No classification is recommended present.

Lymph node (N)

NX   Regional lymph nodes cannot be assessed

N0   No regional lymph node metastasis

N1   Metastasis 3 cm or less in greatest dimension in any regional lymph node(s)

N2   Metastasis more than 3 cm in greatest dimension in any regional lymph node(s) and/or in-transit metastasis

   N2a   Metastasis more than 3 cm in greatest dimension in any regional node(s)

   N2b   In-transit metastasis

   N2c   Both

Primary tumor (pT)

pTX   Primary tumor cannot be assessed

pT0   No evidence of primary tumor

pTis   Melanoma in situ (atypical melanocytic hyperplasia, severe melanocytic dysplasia), not an invasive malignant lesion (Clark's level I)

pT1   Tumor 0.75 mm or less in thickness and invades the papillary dermis (Clark's level II)

pT2   Tumor more than 0.75 mm but not more than 1.5 mm in thickness and/or invades the reticular dermis (Clark's level IV)

pT3   Tumor more than 1.5 mm but not more than 4 mm in thickness and/or invades the reticular dermis (Clark's level IV)

   pT3a   Tumor more than 1.5 mm but not more than 3 mm in thickness

   pT3b   Tumor more than 3 mm but not more than 4 mm in thickness

pT4   Tumor more than 4 mm in thickness and/or invades the subcutaneous tissue and/or satellite(s) within 2 cm of the primary tumor (Clark's level V)

   pT4a   Tumor more than 4 mm in thickness and/or invades the subcutaneous tissue

   pT4b   Satellite(s) within 2 cm of the primary tumor

Lymph node (pN)

pNX   Regional lymph nodes cannot be assessed

pN0   No regional lymph node metastasis

pN1   Metastasis 3 cm or less in greatest dimension in any regional lymph node(s)

pN2   Metastasis more than 3 cm in greatest dimension in any regional lymph node(s) and/or in-transit metastasis

   pN2a   Metastasis more than 3 cm in greatest dimension

   pN2b   In-transit metastasis

   pN2c   Both (pN2a and pN2b)

Distant metastasis (pM)

pMX   Presence of distant metastasis cannot be assessed

pM0   No distant metastasis

pM1   Distant metastasis

   pM1a   Metastasis in skin or subcutaneous tissue or lymph node(s) beyond the regional lymph nodes

   pM1b   Visceral metastasis

Stage grouping

I	pT1	N0	M0
	pT2	N0	M0
II	pT3	N0	M0
III	pT4	N0	M0
	Any pT	N1	M0

| I | Any pT | Any N | M1 |

Lacrimal Gland
Primary tumor (T)

TX	Primary tumor cannot be assessed
T0	No evidence of primary tumor
T1	Tumor 2.5 cm or less in greatest dimension limited to the lacrimal gland and mobile within the lacrimal fossa
T2	Tumor 2.5 cm or less in greatest dimension invading the periosteum of the fossa of the lacrimal gland
T3	Tumor more than 2.5 cm but not more than 5 cm in greatest dimension
T3a	Tumor limited to the lacrimal gland
T3b	Tumor invades the periosteum of the fossa of the lacrimal gland
T4	Tumor more than 5 cm in greatest dimension
T4a	With invasion of orbital soft tissues, optic nerve or globe, without bone invasion
T4b	With invasion of orbital soft tissues, optic nerve, or globe, with bone invasion

Lymph node (N)

NX	Regional lymph nodes cannot be assessed
N0	No regional lymph node metastasis
N1	Regional lymph node metastasis

Distant metastasis (M)

MX	Presence of distant metastasis cannot be assessed
M0	No distant metastasis
M1	Distant metastasis

Stage grouping

No stage grouping is presently recommended.

Sarcoma of the Orbit
Primary tumor (T)

TX	Primary tumor cannot be assessed
T0	No evidence of primary tumor
T1	Tumor 15 mm or less in greatest dimension
T2	Tumor more than 15 mm in greatest dimension
T3	Tumor of any size with diffuse invasion of orbital tissues and/or bony walls
T4	Tumor invades beyond the orbit to adjacent sinuses and/or to cranium

Lymph node (N)

NX	Regional lymph nodes cannot be assessed
N0	No regional lymph node metastasis
N1	Regional lymph node metastasis

Distant metastasis (M)

MX	Presence of distant metastasis cannot be assessed
M0	No distant metastasis
M1	Distant metastasis

Stage grouping

No stage grouping is presently recommended.

Carcinoma of the Conjunctiva
Primary tumor (T)

TX	Primary tumor cannot be assessed
T0	No evidence of primary tumor
Tis	Tumor in situ
T1	Tumor 5 mm or less in greatest dimension
T2	Tumor more than 5 mm in greatest dimension, without invasion of adjacent structures
T3	Tumor invades adjacent structures, excluding the orbit
T4	Tumor invades the orbit

Lymph node (N)

NX	Regional lymph nodes cannot be assessed
N0	No regional lymph node metastasis
N1	Regional lymph node metastasis

Distant metastasis (M)

MX	Presence of distant metastasis cannot be assessed
M0	No distant metastasis
M1	Distant metastasis

Stage grouping

No stage grouping is presently recommended.

Malignant Melanoma of the Conjunctiva
Primary tumor (T)

TX	Primary tumor cannot be assessed
T0	No evidence of primary tumor
T1	Tumor(s) of bulbar conjunctiva occupying one quadrant or less
T2	Tumor(s) of bulbar conjunctiva occupying more than one quadrant
T3	Tumor(s) of conjunctival fornix and/or palpebral conjunctiva and/or caruncle
T4	Tumor invades eyelid, cornea, and/or orbit

Lymph node (N)

NX	Regional lymph nodes cannot be assessed
N0	No regional lymph node metastasis
N1	Regional lymph node metastasis

Distant metastasis (M)

MX	Presence of distant metastasis cannot be assessed
M0	No distant metastasis
M1	Distant metastasis

Primary tumor (pT)

pTX	Primary tumor cannot be assessed
pT0	No evidence of primary tumor
pT1	Tumor(s) of bulbar conjunctiva occupying one quadrant or less and 2 mm or less in thickness
pT2	Tumor(s) of bulbar conjunctiva occupying more than one quadrant and 2 mm or less in thickness
pT3	Tumor(s) of conjunctival fornix and/or palpebral conjunctiva and/or caruncle and/or tumor of the bulbar conjunctiva, more than 2 mm in thickness
pT4	Tumor invades eyelid, cornea, and/or orbit

Lymph node (pN)

pNX   Regional lymph nodes cannot be assessed
pN0   No regional lymph node metastasis
pN1   Regional lymph node metastasis

Distant metastasis (pM)

pMX   Presence of distant metastasis cannot be assessed
pM0   No distant metastasis
pM1   Distant metastasis

Stage grouping

No stage grouping is presently recommended.

Malignant Melanoma of the Uvea
Iris
Primary tumor (T)

TX   Primary tumor cannot be assessed
T0   No evidence of primary tumor
T1   Tumor limited to the iris
T2   Tumor involves one quadrant or less, with invasion into the anterior chamber angle
T3   Tumor involves more than one quadrant, with invasion into the anterior chamber angle
T4   Tumor with extraocular extension

Lymph node (N)

NX   Regional lymph nodes cannot be assessed
N0   No regional lymph node metastasis
N1   Regional lymph node metastasis

Distant metastasis (M)

MX   Presence of distant metastasis cannot be assessed
M0   No distant metastasis
M1   Distant metastasis

Ciliary body
Primary tumor (T)

TX   Primary tumor cannot be assessed
T0   No evidence of primary tumor
T1   Tumor limited to ciliary body
T2   Tumor invades into anterior chamber and/or iris
T3   Tumor invades choroid
T4   Tumor with extraocular extension

Lymph node (N)

NX   Regional lymph nodes cannot be assessed
N0   No regional lymph node metastasis
N1   Regional lymph node metastasis

Distant metastasis (M)

MX   Presence of distant metastasis cannot be assessed
M0   No distant metastasis
M1   Distant metastasis

Choroid
Primary tumor (T)

TX	Primary tumor cannot be assessed
T0	No evidence of primary tumor
T1	Tumor 10 mm or less in greatest dimension with an elevation 3 mm or less
T1a	Tumor 7 mm or less in greatest dimension with an elevation 2 mm or less
T1b	Tumor more than 7 mm but not more than 10 mm in greatest dimension with an elevation more than 2 mm but not more than 3 mm
T2	Tumor more than 10 mm but not more than 15 mm in greatest dimension with an elevation of more than 3 mm but not more than 5 mm
T3	Tumor more than 15 mm in greatest dimension or with an elevation more than 5 mm
T4	Tumor with extraocular extension

Lymph node (N)

NX	Regional lymph nodes cannot be assessed
N0	No regional lymph node metastasis
N1	Regional lymph node metastasis

Distant metastasis (M)

MX	Presence of distant metastasis cannot be assessed
M0	No distant metastasis
M1	Distant metastasis

Stage grouping

Iris and ciliary body

I	T1	N0	M0
II	T2	N0	M0
III	T3	N0	M0
IVA	T4	N0	M0
IVB	Any T	N1	M0
	Any T	Any N	M1

Choroid

IA	T1a	N0	M0
IB	T1b	N0	M0
II	T2	N0	M0
III	T3	N0	M0
IVA	T4	N0	M0
IVB	Any T	N1	M0
	Any T	Any N	M1

Retinoblastoma
Primary tumor (T)

TX	Primary tumor cannot be assessed
T0	No evidence of primary tumor
T1	Tumor(s) limited to 25% or less of the retina
T2	Tumor(s) involve(s) more than 25% but not more than 50% of the retina
T3	Tumor(s) involve(s) more than 50% of the retina and/or invade(s) beyond the retina but remain(s) intraocular
T3a	Tumor(s) involve(s) more than 50% of the retina and/or tumor cells in the vitreous

T3b	Tumor(s) involve(s) optic disc
T3c	Tumor(s) involve(s) anterior chamber and/or uvea
T4	Tumor with extraocular invasion
T4a	Tumor invades retrobulbar optic nerve
T4b	Extraocular extension other than invasion of optic nerve

Lymph node (N)

NX	Regional lymph nodes cannot be assessed
N0	No regional lymph node metastasis
N1	Regional lymph node metastasis

Distant metastasis (M)

MX	Presence of distant metastasis cannot be assessed
M0	No distant metastasis
M1	Distant metastasis

Primary tumor (pT)

pTX	Primary tumor cannot be assessed
pT0	No evidence of primary tumor
pT1	Tumor(s) limited to 25% or less of the retina
pT2	Tumor(s) involve(s) more than 25% but not more than 50% of the retina
pT3	Tumor(s) involve(s) more than 50% of the retina and/or invade(s) beyond the retina but remain(s) intraocular
pT3a	Tumor(s) involve(s) more than 50% of the retina and/or tumor cells in the vitreous
pT3b	Tumor invades optic nerve as far as the lamina cribrosa
pT3c	Tumor in anterior chamber and/or invasion with thickening of the uvea and/or intrascleral invasion
pT4	Tumor with extraocular invasion
pT4a	Intraneural tumor beyond the lamina cribrosa but not the line of resection
pT4b	Tumor at the line of resection or other extraocular extension

Lymph node (pN)

pNX	Regional lymph nodes cannot be assessed
pN0	No regional lymph node metastasis
pN1	Regional lymph node metastasis

Distant metastasis (pM)

pMX	Presence of distant metastasis cannot be assessed
pM0	No distant metastasis
pM1	Distant metastasis

Stage grouping

IA	T1	N0	M0
IB	T2	N0	M0
IIA	T3a	N0	M0
IIB	T3b	N0	M0
IIC	T3c	N0	M0
IIIA	T4a	N0	M0
IIIB	T4b	N0	M0
IV	Any T	N1	M0
	Any T	Any N	M1

Appendix H
Guidelines for handling of most common and important surgical specimens

Some general guidelines for the procedure, description, and sampling of the most common and important surgical specimens received in the laboratory are set forth in the following pages. They are mainly derived from personal experience, although the *Gross Room Manual* used for years in the Surgical Pathology Laboratory at Barnes Hospital in St. Louis and considerably expanded by the surgical pathologists at Stanford University was freely used as a model for many of the procedures. These instructions can be used in the form of a manual, copied on microfiche cards to facilitate their reading by the prosector, or entered in the laboratory computer and made available through terminals in the gross room (see accompanying figures).

Naturally, not all types of specimens or eventualities can be covered. The guidelines presented herein will be useful only if they are taken as *general recommendations* for a typical specimen showing a typical lesion. All kinds of modifications need to be made according to the specific circumstances of the case. Each specimen is unique and thus requires variation in the dissection, description, and sampling procedures here recommended. To quote from a high source in connection with a somewhat related matter (i.e., the autopsy procedure)*:

> It is scarcely necessary to point out that there are many cases in which deviation from this method are not merely allowable, but also absolutely necessary. The individuality of the case must often determine the plan of the examination. But we must not begin with individualizing, nor make a rule of the exceptions. The expert may allow himself to make alterations, supposing that they are well founded, but he must be able to remember his motive for so doing, and also to state it.

Also, it should be pointed out that these guidelines deal with only one particular method for processing specimens. There are probably no two laboratories in the country that perform this task in exactly the same fashion. What we are describing here is a series of procedures that we have found useful and reliable over the years, fully realizing that they are not the only ones or necessarily the best.

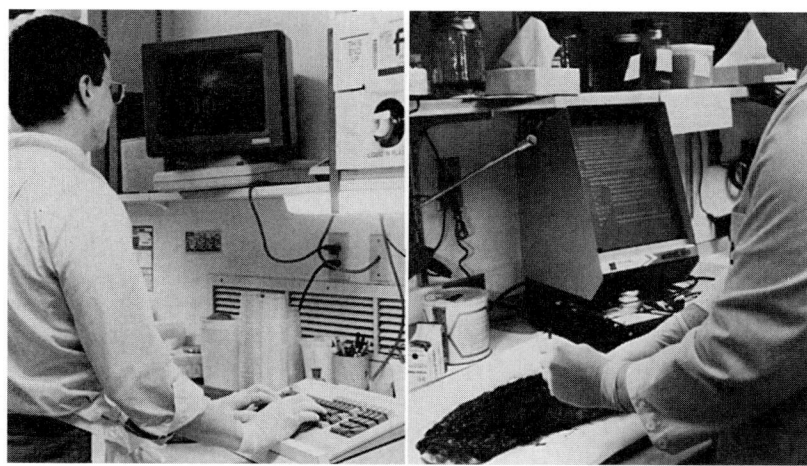

---

*Virchow R: Postmortem examinations and the position of pathology among biological sciences, with an introduction by Putschar WJ: The history of medicine, Series No 37, published under the auspices of the Library of the New York Academy of Medicine, Metuchen, NJ, 1973, Scarecrow.

Appendix—Appendectomy
Bladder—Cystectomy
Bladder—Stone removal
Bone—Biopsy
Bone—Femoral head excision
Bone marrow—Fragments from aspirate
Bone marrow—Needle biopsy
Bone marrow—Rib from thoracotomy
Breast—Biopsy and local excision for palpable mass
Breast—Mammographically directed excision
Breast—Mastectomy
Cell surface markers—Sampling
Chromosomal analysis—Sampling
Cultures—Bacterial, fungal, and viral
DNA ploidy and cell proliferation analysis by flow
    cytometry—Sampling
Ear—Temporal bone resection
Electron microscopy—Sampling
Esophagus—Esophagectomy
Extremities—Amputation for occlusive vascular disease
Extremities—Amputation for osseous tumor
Extremities—Amputation for soft tissue tumor
Eyes—Enucleation
Fallopian tubes—Ligation
Fallopian tubes—Salpingectomy
Fetus—Abortion
Gallbladder—Cholecystectomy
Heart—Valve replacement
Hormone receptor assays—Sampling
Imprints (touch preparations)
Injection of specimens—General guidelines
Jaw resection for tumor—Mandibulectomy
Jaw resection for tumor—Maxillectomy
Kidney—Needle biopsy
Kidney—Nephrectomy for nontumoral condition
Kidney—Nephrectomy for tumor
Large bowel—Colectomy for nontumoral condition
Large bowel—Colectomy for tumor
Large bowel—Polypectomy
Larynx—Laryngectomy
Lip—V excision
Liver—Excision
Lung—Biopsy
Lung—Resection for nontumoral condition
Lung—Resection for tumor
Lymph node—Biopsy

Lymph node dissection—General instructions
Lymph node dissection—Axillary
Lymph node dissection—Inguinal
Lymph node dissection—Radical neck
Lymph node dissection—Retroperitoneal
Molecular diagnosis—Sampling
Needle biopsies
Orbital exenteration
Orientation of specimens with agar
Ovary—Oophorectomy
Pancreas—Pancreatectomy
Parathyroid glands—Parathyroidectomy
Pelvic exenteration
Penis—Penectomy
Peripheral nerve—Biopsy
Placenta—Singleton
Placenta—Twin
Prostate gland—Radical prostatectomy for tumor
Prostate gland—Suprapubic prostatectomy for nodular
    hyperplasia
Prostate gland—Transurethral resection (TUR)
Salivary gland—Resection for tumor
Skeletal muscle—Biopsy
Skin—Excision for benign lesion
Skin—Excision for malignant tumor
Skin—Punch biopsy
Skin—Shave biopsy
Small bowel—Biopsy
Small bowel—Excision
Spleen—Splenectomy
Staging laparotomy for malignant lymphoma
Stomach—Gastrectomy for tumor
Stomach—Gastrectomy for ulcer
Testicle—Orchiectomy
Thymus gland—Thymectomy
Thyroid gland—Thyroidectomy
Uterus—Cervical biopsy
Uterus—Cervical conization
Uterus—Endometrial curettings or biopsy
Uterus—Hysterectomy (general instructions)
Uterus—Hysterectomy for cervical carcinoma
    (in situ or invasive)
Uterus—Hysterectomy for endometrial hyperplasia or
    carcinoma
Uterus—Tissue passed
Vulva—Vulvectomy

APPENDIX—APPENDECTOMY

Appendectomy consists of the removal of the entire appendix after dividing the mesoappendix and ligating the base of the appendix that connects to the cecum.

Procedure

1 Measure organ (length and greatest diameter).
2 Divide specimen in two by cutting a cross section 2 cm from tip.
3 Cut cross sections of proximal fragment at 5 mm intervals.
4 Divide distal fragment in two by a longitudinal cut.

Description

1 Length and greatest diameter
2 External surface: fibrin? pus? hemorrhage? hyperemia? perforation? condition of mesentery?
3 Wall: any localized lesions?
4 Mucosa: hyperemic? ulcerated?
5 Lumen: obliterated? dilated? Content: fecaliths? stones?

Sections for histology

1 Proximal one third, close to surgical margin: one cross section. If tumor is present in the specimen, paint the surgical margin with India ink and take an additional section from it.
2 Mid one third: one cross section
3 Distal one third: one longitudinal section

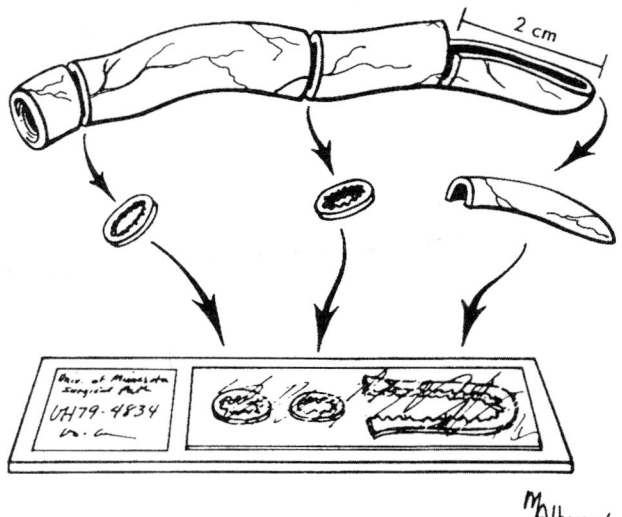

BLADDER—CYSTECTOMY

Cystectomy consists in removal of the bladder. In most instances the entire organ is removed (total cystectomy). In males this may be accompanied by removal of the prostate and seminal vesicles (cystoprostatectomy). The entire length of the urethra may also be excised (cystourethrectomy). The performance of partial cystectomies for carcinoma has fallen into disfavor.

Procedure

1 Paint the entire external surface (including the prostate, if present) with India ink.
2 Two options are available for the dissection depending on the type of lesion present and the status of the organ when received in the laboratory (see accompanying drawings):
 a Open with scissors in a Y shape through the anterior wall, pin on a corkboard, and fix overnight in formalin.
 b Fill with formalin; fix overnight and divide into anterior and posterior halves by first cutting the lateral bladder walls with scissors and then sectioning the prostate with a sharp knife, beginning at the bladder neck and being careful to make the cut through the urethra. See instructions for Injection of specimens—general guidelines. The injection can be performed through the urethra with a Foley catheter, with a 50-ml syringe with large-bore needle inserted through the bladder dome after the urethra has been clamped or tied, or by filling the bladder with formalin-soaked cotton.
3 Take two Polaroid photographs or photocopies and identify in one of them the site of the sections to be taken.

Description

1 Size of bladder; length of ureters; other organs present
2 Tumor characteristics: size (including thickness), location, extent of invasion, shape (papillary, ulcerated); multifocal lesions?
3 Appearance of non-neoplastic mucosa; thickness of bladder wall away from tumor

Sections for histology

1 Tumor: at least three sections, through bladder wall
2 Bladder neck: one section
3 Trigone: two sections
4 Anterior wall: two sections
5 Posterior wall: two sections
6 Dome: two sections
7 Any abnormal-looking area in bladder mucosa if not included in previous sections
8 Ureteral orifices, including intramural portion
9 Ureteral proximal margins
10 In males: prostate (two sections from each quadrant) and seminal vesicles (one section from each). If a prostatic carcinoma is identified, see instructions for Prostate gland—radical prostatectomy
11 Other organs present
12 Perivesical lymph nodes, if any

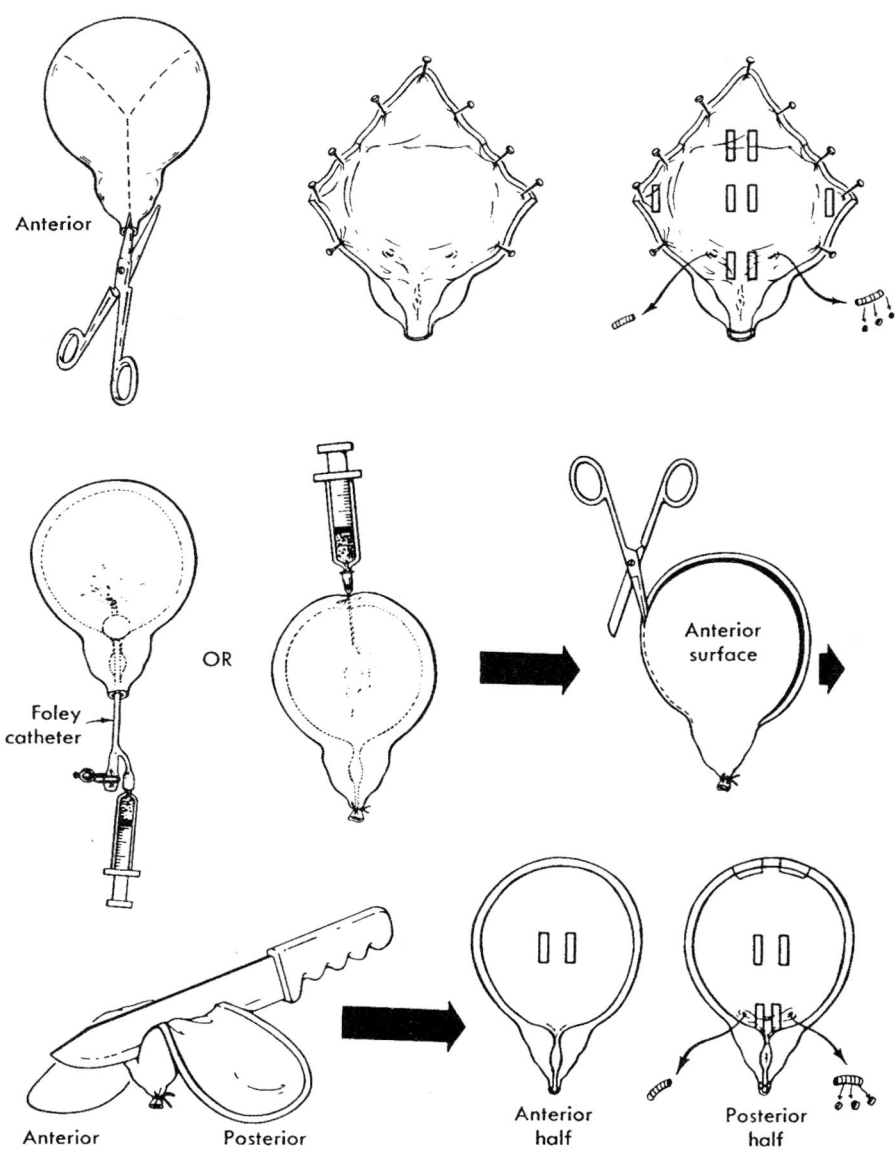

Anterior

Foley catheter

OR

Anterior surface

Anterior   Posterior

Anterior half   Posterior half

BLADDER—STONE REMOVAL

Procedure

1 Take Polaroid photographs or photocopies of all stones submitted.
2 Send a 1- to 2-g sample for crystallographic (often incorrectly referred to as chemical) analysis. *Specimens should be rinsed well in water and air dried. Formalin is to be avoided because uric acid is soluble therein. Heat should not be used to hasten drying because it will drive off the ammonium in magnesium ammonium phosphate, changing struvite into newberyite. Specimens should be shipped in protective containers rather than in plain envelopes. They should not be secured with a transparent tape.
3 The same procedure applies to stones removed from other portions of the urinary tract, such as the renal pelvis or ureter.

Description

1 Number of stones, shape, color, and consistency. *Phosphate* stones are gray or grayish white and may be hard or soft and friable. *Oxalate* stones are usually hard and smooth, rounded, or nodular (resembling mulberries) or irregularly spiculated. *Urate* stones are smooth, yellow or brown, and round or oval. *Cystine* stones are hard, smooth, and yellow, with a waxy appearance. Stones associated with local bleeding may be impregnated with blood and acquire a black or dark brown color.

Sections for histology

None

----

*The Laboratory for Stone Research, 81 Wyman Street, Newton, MA 02168 has had about 50 years' experience with this procedure.

BONE—BIOPSY

Procedure

1 Trocar or needle biopsy: divide longitudinally with a fine-toothed saw if specimen is over 5 mm in diameter. Look for any soft material, dissect from rest of specimen, and process separately without decalcification.
2 Open biopsy and curettage: divide calcified from noncalcified tissues and process separately.

Description

1 Number and size of fragments
2 Consistency, calcification, color, cystic changes, necrosis

Sections for histology

1 Submit all material received, except for unduly large specimens. Send, separately, material to be decalcified from the rest.

BONE—FEMORAL HEAD EXCISION

Procedure

1 Examine articular and cut surfaces.
2 Measure diameter and thickness.
3 Take photographs, if indicated.
4 Hold the specimen with a specially devised clamp (a meatball maker works quite well) or in a vise and cut through the center of the articular surface (fovea) with a band saw (see accompanying drawing).
5 Make a parallel cut about 3 mm from the first cut while holding the specimen in the same position.
6 Examine a cut section of the slice; take a photograph and roentgenogram. Make parallel cuts through remaining pieces, if indicated.

Description

1 Type of excision; side, if known
2 Diameter and thickness
3 Articular surface: smooth or irregular? osteophytic lipping at the periphery?
4 Synovial membrane at edges: hypertrophic? papillary?
5 Cut surface: thickness of articular cartilage; bone exposed? subchondral eburnation? cysts? (if so, size and content); areas of necrosis? (if so, size and appearance); appearance of bone away from the articular surface; evidence of previous fracture?

Sections for histology

1 Take two sections from the most abnormal areas, at least one including the articular surface and synovium (see accompanying drawing).
2 Two options are available for obtaining these sections. The first is more expeditious and quite adequate and is the one to be used in most instances. The second is more time consuming and requires extra care but provides slightly better results.
   a Cut the sections from the fresh slice with a fine band saw or strong knife, depending on the amount and hardness of the bone; fix thoroughly in formalin and decalcify.
   b Fix a whole slice in formalin for several hours or overnight; decalcify thoroughly; cut desired sections with a scalpel or submit material in its entirety, if facilities are available.

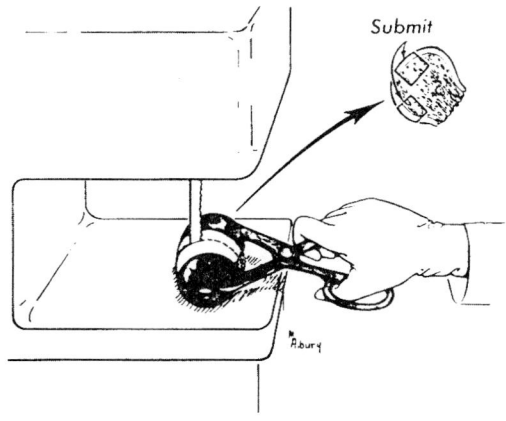

BONE MARROW—FRAGMENTS FROM ASPIRATE

Procedure

1 The material is obtained by aspiration and usually allowed to clot before fixation.
2 Alternatively, the marrow particles can be concentrated "by ejecting the aspirate, before it clots, onto a slanted slide and into a [fixative] solution. The latter is rapidly filtered, and the residue is processed by usual histologic technics."*

Description

1 Approximate amount of material
2 Appearance and relative amount of marrow particles in relation to blood clots

Sections for histology

1 Submit the material in its entirety unless blood clots are excessive.
2 If clots are excessive, select areas with largest concentration of marrow particles.
3 Decalcification is generally not needed for this material.

---

*From Rywlin AM, Marvan P, Robinson MJ: A simple technic for the preparation of bone marrow smears and sections. Am J Clin Pathol **53**:389-393, 1970.

BONE MARROW—NEEDLE BIOPSY

Procedure

The needle biopsy should be fixed immediately after it is obtained. Zenker's or B-5 fixative is preferable.

Description

1 Number, length, and diameter of fragments
2 Color and consistency; homogeneous?

Sections for histology

1 Submit the material in its entirety.
2 If bilateral biopsies were performed, submit them separately.
3 Decalcify only after the tissue is properly fixed and washed and for the shortest time that will allow proper sectioning.

BONE MARROW—RIB FROM THORACOTOMY

Procedure

Sometimes a rib is submitted together with a specimen of pneumonectomy or lobectomy. Gross examination alone is adequate if no gross abnormalities are detected. However, an opportunity to study the status of the patient's bone marrow should not be overlooked. Proceed as follows:

1 Measure the length and diameter of the rib.
2 With a saw cut a piece about 2 cm long, having bone marrow at both ends, from the fresh specimen.
3 Place between pliers longitudinally and squeeze until bone marrow is expressed from both ends (see accompanying drawing). Let the marrow fall in a container with fixative or scrape it out with a blade.
4 Fix and submit for microscopic examination; decalcification is not necessary.
5 Cut the remainder of the rib longitudinally along its entire length and examine cut sections.

Description

1 Identification of side and number of rib if information is provided
2 Length and greatest diameter
3 Appearance of bone marrow on cut section: color, amount; any focal changes?

Sections for histology

1 If no abnormalities are observed, submit only bone marrow preparation as described under Procedure (without decalcifying).
2 If gross abnormalities are present, cut blocks, fix, decalcify, and submit for histology.

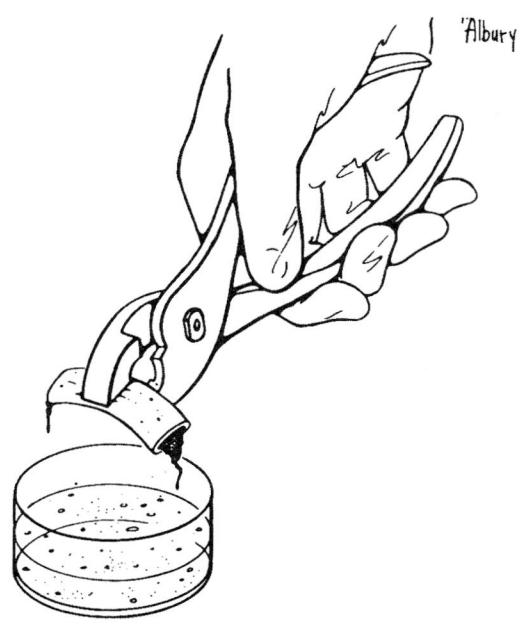

BREAST—BIOPSY AND LOCAL EXCISION FOR PALPABLE MASS

(Adapted from Schnitt SJ, Connolly JL: Processing and evaluation of breast excision specimens. A clinically oriented approach. Am J Clin Pathol **98**:125-137, 1992.)

Open breast biopsies are carried out after performing a circumareolar (preferable for cosmetic reasons) or a radial incision and removing the lesion either partially (incisional biopsy) or in its entirety with a rim of surrounding normal tissue (excisional biopsy). Excisional biopsy is essentially synonymous with lumpectomy and is sometimes combined with the sampling of axillary lymph nodes.

Procedure

1 Measure the specimen before cutting. Weigh if amount of material is substantial (over 50 g).
2 Blot dry, apply India ink to surface, and blot dry again.
3 If indicated, take a radiograph of the specimen.
4 Section specimen: if specimen is 3 cm or smaller, cut 3- to 4-mm slices; if it is larger, bisect specimen transversely, fix the residual hemispheres for 1 to 2 hours, place cut surface down, and take sagittal blocks through superior and inferior portions.
5 If indicated, take a sample for hormone receptor studies (see instructions for Hormone receptor assays—Sampling).

Description

1 Dimensions and consistency of specimen
2 Appearance of cut sections: fibrosis, cysts (size, number, content), calcification, tumor masses (size in three dimensions, color, borders, consistency, necrosis, distance from surgical margins)

Sections for histology

1 Small specimens: submit in their entirety (up to five cassettes).
2 Larger specimens: thorough sampling. At least two thirds of the breast tissue (exclusive of adipose tissue) should be processed. This should include any grossly visible lesions and the inked surgical margins.*

---

*For a description of two different procedures to submit tissue from surgical margins, the reader is referred to: Carter D: Margins of "lumpectomy" for breast cancer. Hum Pathol **17**:330-332, 1986. Connolly JL, Schnitt SJ: Evaluation of breast biopsy specimens in patients considered for treatment by conservative surgery and radiation therapy for early breast cancer. Pathol Annu **23**(Pt 1):1-23, 1988.

BREAST—MAMMOGRAPHICALLY DIRECTED EXCISION

(Adapted from Schnitt SJ, Connolly JL: processing and evaluation of breast excision specimens. A clinically oriented approach. Am J Clin Pathol **98:**125-137, 1992.)

Procedure

1 Obtain radiograph of intact specimen.

2 Measure specimen before cutting.

3 Blot dry, apply India ink to surface, and blot dry again.

4 Slice specimen through the equatorial plane at 3- to 4-mm intervals.

5 Obtain radiograph of sliced specimen. Some authors have found the use of a Perspex grid useful for the subsequent localization of the lesion.

6 Label slices on the radiograph.

7 Take a sample for hormone receptor analysis only if tumor is grossly visible and of sufficient size; do not submit tissue for this analysis if there is no grossly evident tumor.

Description

1 Dimension and consistency of specimen

2 Appearance of cut sections: fibrosis, cysts (size, number, content), calcification, tumor masses (size in three dimensions, color, borders, consistency, necrosis, distance from surgical margins)

Sections for histology

1 Submit in its entirety. Label cassettes as in the radiograph.

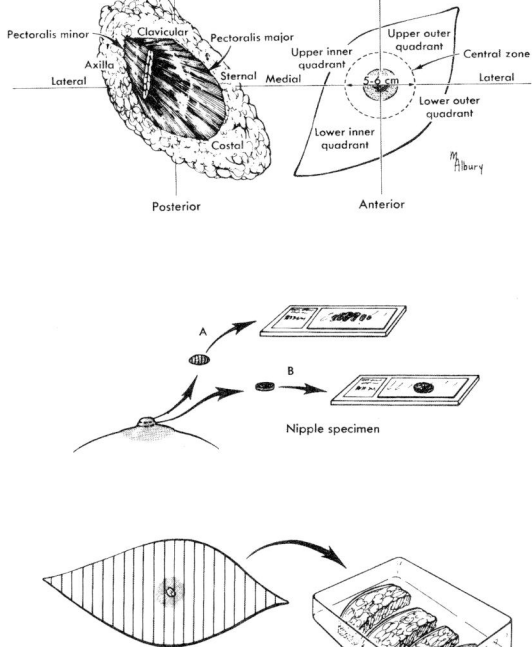

*Champ CS, Mason CH, Coghill SB, Robinson M: A Perspex grid for localization of non-palpable mammographic lesions in breast biopsies. Histopathology **124:**311-316, 1989.

Upper and middle drawings redrawn from National Cancer Institute: Standardized management of breast specimens recommended by Pathology Working Group, Breast Cancer Task Force. Am J Clin Pathol **60:**789-798, 1973.

BREAST—MASTECTOMY

(Adapted from National Cancer Institute: Standardized management of breast specimens recommended by Pathology Working Group, Breast Cancer Task Force. Am J Clin Pathol **60**:789-798, 1973.)

Several types of mastectomy procedures exist. The Halsted's type *radical mastectomy*, which has been all but abandoned, consists of removal of the entire breast parenchyma, the underlying and surrounding adipose tissue, the pectoralis major and minor muscles, and the axillary contents in continuity and en bloc. A *modified radical mastectomy* (also known as extended simple mastectomy and total mastectomy), consists in removal of all the mammary tissue, including the axillary tail, together with the nipple, the surrounding skin, and a variable amount of lymph node–bearing fat from the lower axilla; the pectoralis muscles are preserved. A *simple mastectomy* consists of all or almost all of the mammary tissue, the nipple, and a variable amount of surrounding skin. A *subcutaneous mastectomy* includes most of the mammary tissue, without overlying skin or nipple and often without the axillary tail. In a quadrantectomy a portion of the breast roughly corresponding to one of the four anatomic quadrants is excised, often in combination with removal of the axillary content. A *tylectomy* (lumpectomy; excisional biopsy) consists in removal of the entire mass and a variable amount of surrounding breast tissue. Finally, there is the *supraradical mastectomy*, mentioned here only for historical reasons. It contains all the components of a radical mastectomy specimen, plus a resected segment of chest wall, usually the sternal ends of the second, third, fourth, and fifth ribs, an adjacent segment of sternum, and the subpleural connective tissue that contains the internal mammary vessels and nodes; a segment of pleura also may be present.

Procedure
First day

1 Weigh the specimen.
2 Orient the specimen. In radical mastectomy cases, use the axillary fat as a marker for the lateral side and the surgical section of the muscle as a marker for the upper side. Place the specimen on the cutting board, posterior side up, with its most inferior point toward the dissector. The specimen is oriented as if the dissector were standing behind it. Note that at the junction of the upper and middle thirds of the pectoralis major, the muscle fibers run in a nearly horizontal direction.
3 Dissect lymph nodes groups as follows:
Radical mastectomy (rarely performed at present but included for historical reasons and completeness' sake):
  a Arrange the pectoral muscles and axillary contents in the anatomic positions, using the cut attachments of the pectoral muscle fibers as guides. The axillary contents, which are sometimes partially detached from the muscle during operation, when properly arranged will form a broadly linear fatty mass extending upward and laterally, crossing the posterior surface of the pectoralis minor muscle.
  b Using the pectoralis minor muscle as a guide, divide the axilla into three segments (see drawing, p. 2642):
   • Level I (low): inferior to lower border of muscle
   • Level II (middle): between upper and lower borders of muscle
   • Level III (high): superior to upper border of muscle
      Remove each separately and fix overnight; Carnoy's solution is preferred because, besides fixing, it clears the fat somewhat.
  c Remove the pectoralis minor muscle and search for the interpectoral (Rotter's) nodes; these are usually found near the lateral edge of the posterior surface of the pectoralis major. If no nodes are apparent, submit the adipose tissue from this site.
  d Remove the pectoralis major muscle and look for evidence of tumor invasion.

Modified radical mastectomy:

  a Separate the axillary tissue from the breast.
  b Since the landmarks used in radical mastectomy specimens are not present, divide the axillary tissue into a higher and lower half and fix overnight in separate containers.

BREAST—MASTECTOMY—cont'd

4 Turn the specimen around, with skin side up and the 6 o'clock position nearest the dissector (i.e., as if the dissector were facing the patient).

5 Evaluate features of the external appearance and measure. Palpate the specimen for masses or nodularity. With a water-resistant marker, draw a vertical line passing through the nipple and another perpendicular to it, also passing through the nipple. This will divide the breast specimen into four quadrants: upper outer, lower outer, lower inner, and upper inner.

6 Remove the nipple and areola, using scalpel, forceps, and scissors and fix the specimen thus obtained overnight.

7 With a long sharp knife, cut the entire breast longitudinally into slices about 2 cm thick. One of the cuts should be exactly through the level of the nipple, using as a guide the vertical line previously made in the skin; this will allow a precise separation of slices belonging to the inner and outer halves of the breast. Lay out the slices in order on a flat surface, maintaining orientation. Examine each slice carefully; take photographs and x-ray film, if indicated. Take a sample for hormone receptor studies, if indicated (see instructions for Hormone receptor assays-sampling). Fix all the slices overnight, keeping their orientation either by laying them flat sequentially in a long pan (preferable) or by stringing them together (see drawing, p. 2642).

Second day

1 Lymph node specimens (radical or modified radical mastectomies): shred the axillary tissue and dissect out all lymph nodes, which stand out as white nodules. A minimum of twenty lymph nodes should be found in the usual radical mastectomy.

2 Nipple specimen: if following fixation the nipple is erect, cut as indicated in the accompanying drawing. If it is retracted or inverted, cut several parallel sections, about 2 to 3 mm apart, perpendicular to the skin surface through the nipple and areola.

3 Breast specimen: reexamine the slices, make additional cuts, if necessary, and take sections for histology according to instructions that follow.

Description

It is preferable to make short notes at the time the specimen is examined the first day and to dictate the whole case the second day.

1 Side (right or left) and type of mastectomy

2 List of structures included in specimen: skin, nipple, breast, major and minor pectoralis muscles, fascia, axillary tissue, chest wall structures

3 Weight and dimensions (greatest length of skin and length perpendicular to it)

4 Features of external appearance:
   a Shape and color of skin
   b Location and extent of skin changes (scars, recent surgical incisions, erythema, edema, flattening, retraction, ulceration)
   c Appearance of nipple and areola (erosions, ulceration, retraction, inversion)
   d Location of lesions and other features, which can be designated by stating their distance from nipple and quadrant on their direction in clock face numerals
   e Description of abnormalities on palpation, if any

5 Features of cross sections:
   a Relative amounts of fat and parenchyma
   b Cysts and dilated ducts: size, number, location, content
   c Masses: quadrant and distance from nipple, depth beneath skin, size, shape, consistency, color; necrosis? hemorrhage? calcification? relation or attachment to skin, muscle, fascia, or nipple
   d Lymph nodes, if present: number of nodes in each group, size of largest node in each group, and sizes and locations of nodes containing grossly evident tumor

BREAST—MASTECTOMY—cont'd

Sections for histology

1 Breast: take three sections of tumor; sample all lesions noted grossly or radiographically; take at least one section from each quadrant (using as guidelines the previously made marks on the skin) in the following order:
   - Upper outer quadrant (UOQ)
   - Lower outer quadrant (LOQ)
   - Lower inner quadrant (LIQ)
   - Upper inner quadrant (UIQ)
2 Nipple: see under Procedure.
3 Pectoralis major muscle (in radical mastectomies): take one section from any grossly abnormal area or, if none is found, from the area closest to the tumor.
4 Lymph nodes: all identified nodes should be processed for histology. Small nodes are submitted entirely; nodes over 0.5 cm in diameter are sliced. If the axillary fat is grossly involved, a representative section should be taken. Label in the following order:

Radical mastectomy:

   - Low axillary (Level I)
   - Mid axillary (Level II)
   - High axillary (Level III)
   - Interpectoral (Rotter's) nodes or, if none found, adipose tissue from this site

Modified radical mastectomy:

   - Lower half
   - Upper half

(For this operation it is better not to use the terms low, mid, and high since these are used for radical mastectomies.)

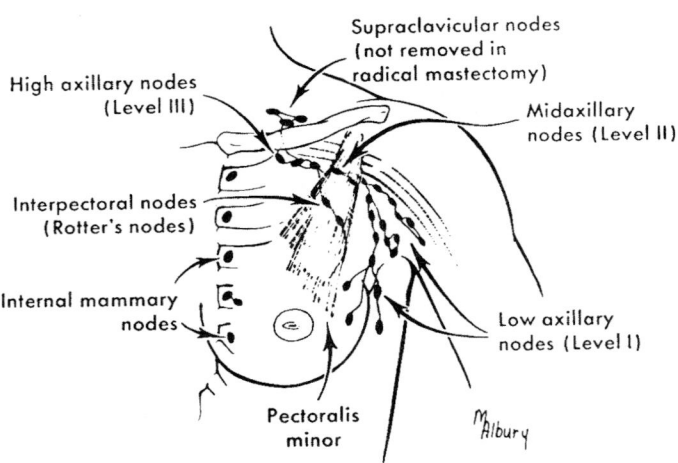

CELL SURFACE MARKERS—SAMPLING

This technique has become essential for the evaluation of lymphoid proliferations. It is useful in identifying a given proliferation as lymphoid, in distinguishing a reactive from a neoplastic process, and in identifying the specific cell type.

If facilities for the performance of this test are available, it should be used in:

- All specimens from lymph nodes, spleen, or thymus in which the possibility of a proliferative lymphoid process is considered
- All tumors with clinical or gross features suggestive of malignant lymphoma
- All tissues in patients with known malignant lymphoma or leukemia in which the possibility of involvement by the disease exists

Cell surface markers, detected with immunocytochemical reagents, can be evaluated quantitatively by flow cytometry or by microscopic examination of frozen sections. In either case the specimen should be received fresh. For flow cytometry a 0.5 cm^3 piece of tissue is sufficient. This should be dropped in a bottle containing culture medium (such as RPMI or DMEM) and submitted to the appropriate laboratory. If immediate transportation is not feasible, store temporarily in the refrigerator at 4° C.

For frozen section purposes, a 2 × 2 × 1 cm piece is desirable. This should be placed in a Petri dish having in its bottom a layer of filter paper wet (not overly soaked) with saline solution and submitted to the laboratory immediately. If the specimen is not large enough for a 2 × 2 × 1 cm piece to be taken, sample a fragment as large as feasible.

CHROMOSOMAL ANALYSIS—SAMPLING

Chromosomal analysis of surgically excised tissues (using direct and indirect techniques) can be useful in the differential diagnosis between reactive and neoplastic processes, and it can demonstrate specific chromosomal defects associated with particular tumor types.

Cut a piece of viable tissue in the fresh state as soon as possible after excision under sterile conditions, drop in a bottle containing culture medium (such as RPMI or DMEM), and submit to the genetics laboratory. The piece should be about 0.5 to 1 cm in diameter or as large a sample as allowable. If immediate transportation to the laboratory is not feasible, store temporarily in the refrigerator at 4° C.

CULTURES—BACTERIAL, FUNGAL, AND VIRAL

Whenever a fresh specimen is received in the laboratory and there is some indication (clinical, gross appearance, frozen section) that it may be involved by an infectious process, cultures should be taken, unless this has already been done in the operating room.*

Large specimens

Several techniques can be used for large operative specimens (lung, spleen) received intact in the fresh state. In general, technique 1 (following) is recommended over technique 2.

1 Technique 1
  a Burn the surface close to the area to be cultured with a red-hot spatula.
  b Make a deep cut through this sterilized surface with a sterile blade.
  c Cut a portion of tissue from the inside using sterile forceps and scalpel or scissors. A size of 1 × 1 × 1 cm is recommended.
  d Put the specimen in a sterile container.
2 Technique 2
  a Burn the surface close to the area to be cultured with a red-hot spatula.
  b Make a deep cut through this sterilized surface with a sterile blade.
  c Introduce a sterile swab stick (such as Culturette) through the opening, push beyond the cut into the tissue, remove, and place in appropriate transport medium.
3 For cystic processes that need to be cultured for anaerobic organisms: aspirate with a sterile syringe and needle (about 1 to 4 ml), expel air bubble from the syringe, and inject the sample into an anaerobic vial. If a vial is not available, put a rubber cork on the end of the needle.

Small specimens

1 If the specimen is submitted fresh in a sterile container with the request for bacteriologic studies to be carried out:
  a Open the container, cut a portion of tissue with sterile instruments, and transfer to a sterile container.
  b Use the rest of the specimen for histologic examination.
2 If the need for culture becomes evident after the fresh specimen has been handled in a nonsterile fashion, proceed as follows:
  a Cut a piece of the tissue (approximately 1 cm × 1 cm × 1 cm) with a sterile blade.
  b Sterilize a pair of clean forceps by dipping them in ethanol and flaming.
  c Holding the specimen with the sterilized forceps, wash thoroughly with sterile saline solution.
  d Lay specimen in a sterile container. Sterilize the forceps again and pick up the specimen in a different portion.
  e Repeat the washing with sterile solution.
  f Put the specimen in a sterile container.

All specimens

1 Send specimens to the microbiology laboratory as soon as possible after they have been obtained and properly identified with patient's name and surgical pathology number. If a specimen cannot be sent immediately, place it in the refrigerator at 4° C.
2 Specify the cultures desired and organisms suspected. The usual requests are the following:
  • Routine (includes aerobic and the less fastidious anaerobic)
  • Anaerobic
  • Acid-fast organisms
  • Fungi
  • Viruses
3 After a sample has been taken for cultures, it is advisable to make a smear from an adjacent area, fix in alcohol, and stain for the microorganisms suspected (Gram's, Ziehl-Neelsen).

*Braunstein H: The value of microbiologic culture of tissue samples in surgical pathology. Mod Pathol 2:217-221, 1989.

DNA PLOIDY AND CELL PROLIFERATION ANALYSIS BY FLOW CYTOMETRY—SAMPLING

Cut the viable tissue into 0.5 cm³ cubes in the fresh state as soon as possible after excision, drop in a bottle containing culture medium (such as RPMI or DMEM), and submit to the appropriate laboratory. If immediate transportation is not feasible, store temporarily in the refrigerator at 4° C.

EAR—TEMPORAL BONE RESECTION

Subtotal or total temporal bone resections can be carried out for carcinoma of the external auditory canal, middle ear, or mastoid.

Procedure

1 Review roentgenograms if available and obtain roentgenograms of the specimen if facilities are available.
2 Orient the specimen as to anteroposterior, superoinferior, and mediolateral planes.
3 Mark the margins with India ink.
4 Section longitudinally in two halves or in parallel cross sections, depending on location and size of tumor.

Description

1 Type of resection: subtotal or total
2 Tumor: size, gross features, and location: external ear, auditory canal, middle ear. If in the canal, does it involve the outer cartilaginous third or the inner osseous two thirds?
3 Location within the canal: floor, walls, roof, circumferential; invasion anteriorly toward the parotid gland? superiorly toward the cranial cavity?
4 Status of tympanic membrane
5 Parotid gland, if present: invaded by tumor?

Sections for histology

1 Tumor: in its entirety
2 Surgical margins
3 Parotid gland, if present

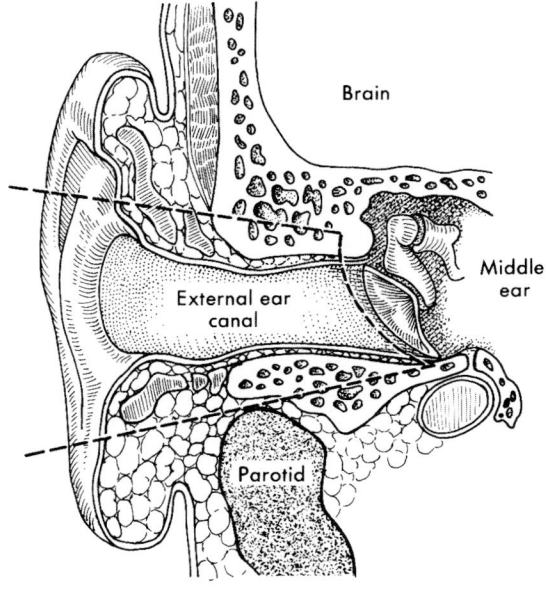

ELECTRON MICROSCOPY—SAMPLING

Fixative

Several fixatives are available for electron microscopy. The most commonly used is 2.5% glutaraldehyde in Millonig's phosphate buffer, in amounts of 3 to 4 ml per vial, which is kept refrigerated at 4° C. The working solution can be stored for up to 1 month.

Sampling from fresh tissue

Fresh tissue is highly preferable to routinely fixed material. It is imperative for tissue to be handled *immediately* after excision.

1 Put the specimen on a clear cutting board (such as a heavy plastic card) and cut 1-mm thick slices with a sharp razor blade.
2 Place several drops of electron microscopy fixative in another area of the cutting board, place the tissue slice on top, and cover with a few drops of fixative.
3 Chop the slide into 1-mm cubes with a sharp razor blade, and immerse them in cold (4° C) fixative. Five to fifteen fragments of tissue are adequate. If the specimen has grossly different areas, submit for electron microscopy in separate containers.
4 Submit to electron microscopy laboratory for processing; the tissue can remain in the electron microscopy fixative for several days at 4° C.

Sampling from routinely fixed tissue

In routinely fixed tissue, there is usually extensive fixation artifact, but at times recognizable diagnostic electron microscopy features are retained (such as desmosomes, neurosecretory granules, melanosomes).

1 Cut a 1-mm slice from an *edge* of the specimen that was in direct contact with the fixative.
2 Proceed as for fresh tissues.

ESOPHAGUS—ESOPHAGECTOMY

The extent of an *esophagectomy* depends on the type and location of the lesion. Most esophagectomies consist of removal of the distal portion of the organ, followed by an esophagogastric anastomosis.

Procedure

Two options are available. The first is used in most instances.

1 Dissect the specimen in the fresh state; open longitudinally from one end to the other after marking the deep margins with India ink, trying to cut on the side opposite the tumor (see accompanying drawing **A**). If a portion of stomach is included, open along the greater curvature in continuity with the esophageal cut (see accompanying drawing **B**).
  b Dissect the periesophageal fat and look for lymph nodes. Divide into three portions: adjacent, proximal, and distal to the tumor (the latter might include the cardioesophageal nodes).
  c Pin the specimen in a corkboard, mucosal side up, and float in a large formalin container with the specimen on the underside; fix overnight.
  d Take two Polaroid photographs or photocopies, and identify in one of them the sites of the sections to be taken.
  e Paint the surgical specimens with India ink after the specimens are fixed; this includes both mucosal ends and the soft tissue around the tumor.
2 Fill the lumen with gauze or cotton impregnated with formalin; fix overnight; cut with scissors longitudinally on the side opposite the tumor; complete the division by cutting with a long knife on the opposite side.

ESOPHAGUS—ESOPHAGECTOMY—cont'd

Description

1 Length and diameter or circumference of specimen; proximal stomach included? (if so, indicate length along lesser and greater curvature)
2 Tumor: size, appearance (fungating? rolled edges? ulcerated?); does it involve entire organ circumferentially? depth of invasion; extension into stomach and adjacent organs? distance from both lines of resection and from cardias, if present
3 Mucosa: appearance of non-neoplastic mucosa; recognizable esophageal mucosa *distal* to tumor? evidence of Barrett's esophagus? (if so, length of the segment and appearance of mucosa); lumen dilated proximal to tumor?
4 Wall: thickened? varices?
5 Stomach, if present: features of cardioesophageal junction and gastric mucosa
6 Lymph nodes: number found, size of largest; do they appear grossly involved by tumor?

Sections for histology

1 Tumor: four longitudinal sections, one including a portion of non-neoplastic mucosa proximal to tumor and another a portion distal to tumor
2 Non-neoplastic mucosa: two to three transverse sections, at different distances from tumor edge, proximally and/or distally, depending on location of tumor
3 Stomach, if present: two sections, one including gastroesophageal junction
4 Proximal line of resection
5 Distal line of resection
6 Lymph nodes:
    a Adjacent to tumor
    b Proximal to tumor
    c Distal to tumor

(Adapted from Rodriguez-Martinez HA, Cruz-Ortiz H, Alcantara-Vazquez A, Alcorta-Anguizola B, Burgos-Mendivil J: Dissecting technique for gangrenous lower limbs with vascular occlusions. Patología **10**:69-78, 1972.)

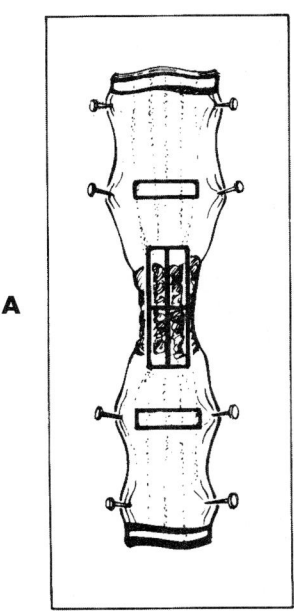

A

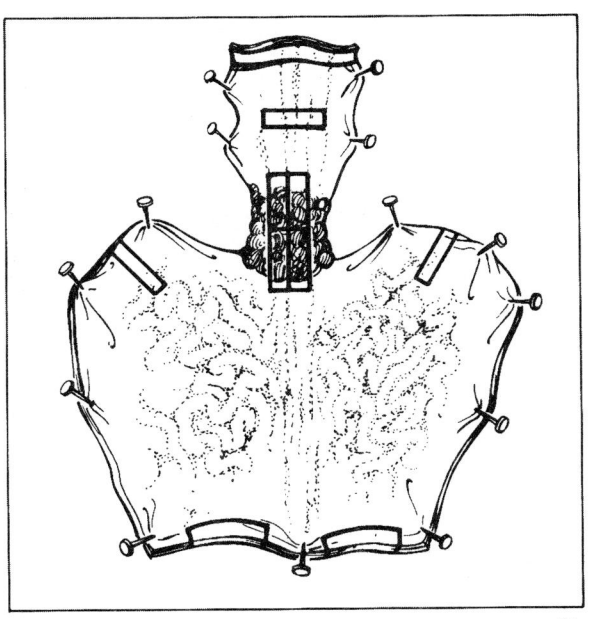

B

EXTREMITIES—AMPUTATION FOR OCCLUSIVE VASCULAR DISEASE

Procedure

1 Removal of femoral, popliteal, and posterior tibial neurovascular bundles and peroneal vessels:

   a Place the extremity on a dissecting board with the posterior surface upward. The dissection will be completed more rapidly if an assistant holds the specimen and helps retract flaps.

   b Incise longitudinally the skin over the midline of the popliteal region and the upper two thirds of the posterior tibial region (see accompanying diagram, p. 2649).

   c Incise obliquely the skin from the lower end of the first incision to 2 cm below the posterior border of the medial malleolus (see accompanying diagram, p. 2649).

   d With a scalpel or knife, cut through the subcutaneous tissue and superficial fascia of the entire incision.

   e In the posterior femoral and popliteal regions, separate, with blunt and sharp dissection, the semitendinous, semimembranous, and medial head of the gastrocnemius muscles from the biceps femoris and lateral head of the gastrocnemius. This maneuver will expose the sciatic and posterior tibial nerves and the femoral and popliteal vessels.

   f Deepen the incisions made in steps **b** and **c** in the posterior tibial regions, cutting through the gastrocnemius and soleus muscles and the tendo calcaneus. This will show, underneath the intermuscular fascial septum, the posterior tibial neurovascular bundle and the peroneal vessels.

   g Beginning at their upper end, dissect and excise the sciatic and posterior tibial nerves down to the place where the latter nerve joins the popliteal vessels.

   h Beginning at their upper end, dissect and excise the femoral and popliteal vessels down to the place where the latter vessels join the posterior tibial nerve.

   i Excise *en bloc* the popliteal vessels and the posterior tibial nerve.

   j Continue with the removal of the entire posterior tibial neurovascular bundle, down to the lowest portion of the skin incision, and transect it there. The bundle should be excised together with neighboring portions of muscle and fascia.

   k Last, remove the peroneal vessels together with contiguous muscle fibers. These vessels are chiefly located behind the fibula and the interosseous membrane and within the muscle fibers of the flexor hallucis longus.

2 Removal of the anterior tibial neurovascular bundle:

   a Place the extremity with its anterior surface upward.

   b Incise longitudinally the skin from a point located between the head of the fibula and the tibial tuberosity to a joint equidistant between both malleoli (see accompanying diagram).

   c With a scalpel or knife, cut through the subcutaneous tissue and superficial fascia of the whole incision.

   d In the middle portion of the incision, cut, with scissors or knife, through the fibers of the tibialis anterior muscle down to the interosseous membrane. This will uncover part of the anterior tibial neurovascular bundle.

   e With sharp or blunt dissection, separate partially the regional muscular masses in the upper portion and the tendons in the lower portion, so as to expose lengthwise the anterior tibial neurovascular bundle.

   f Cut across the lowest portion of the anterior tibial neurovascular bundle. Pull the bundle downward, and excise it together with portions of adjacent muscles and interosseous membrane. The upper end of the bundle becomes loose by just exerting traction downward.

3 Removal of the tissue block with dorsalis pedis vessels:

   a Trace a 3- to 4-cm wide rectangle over the dorsum of the foot, extending from the lowest part of the anterior tibial incision to the proximal portion of the first interosseous space.

   b Following the sides of the rectangle, cut through the skin, subcutaneous tissue, superficial fascia, regional muscles and tendons, and deep fascia. Actually, cut down to the very dorsal surface of the regional bones.

   c With a scalpel or knife, excise the whole tissue block, clearing away all the soft tissues from the underlying bones. The vessels lie very deep in this region.

4 Removal of the tissue blocks with the medial and lateral plantar vessels:

   a Place the extremity with the posterior surface upward.

   b Trace a rectangle on the sole with the following anatomic landmarks: posterior border of the medial malleolus, medial side of the foot, base of the metatarsal bones, and lateral side of the foot. The transverse limits can also be determined, approximately, dividing the sole in fifths.

   c Following the sides of the rectangle, cut through the skin, subcutaneous tissue, plantar aponeurosis and fascia, and regional muscles and tendons. In fact, cut down to the very plantar surfaces of the regional bones.

   d With sharp dissection, remove the entire tissue block so as to leave fully exposed the regional bones and ligaments.

   e Bisect longitudinally the tissue block. The medial half represents the tissue block of the medial plantar vessels, whereas the lateral half represents the tissue block of the lateral plantar vessels.

5 Take samples of skin and soft tissues from areas of ulceration, necrosis, or infection and from bone, if indicated. Now the extremity can be disposed of.

6 Fix all the excised tissues overnight in formalin. The neurovascular bundles should be pinned down on corkboard.

7 Once neurovascular bundles are well fixed, cut transversely every 4 to 5 mm and carefully examine the wall and lumen of vessels.

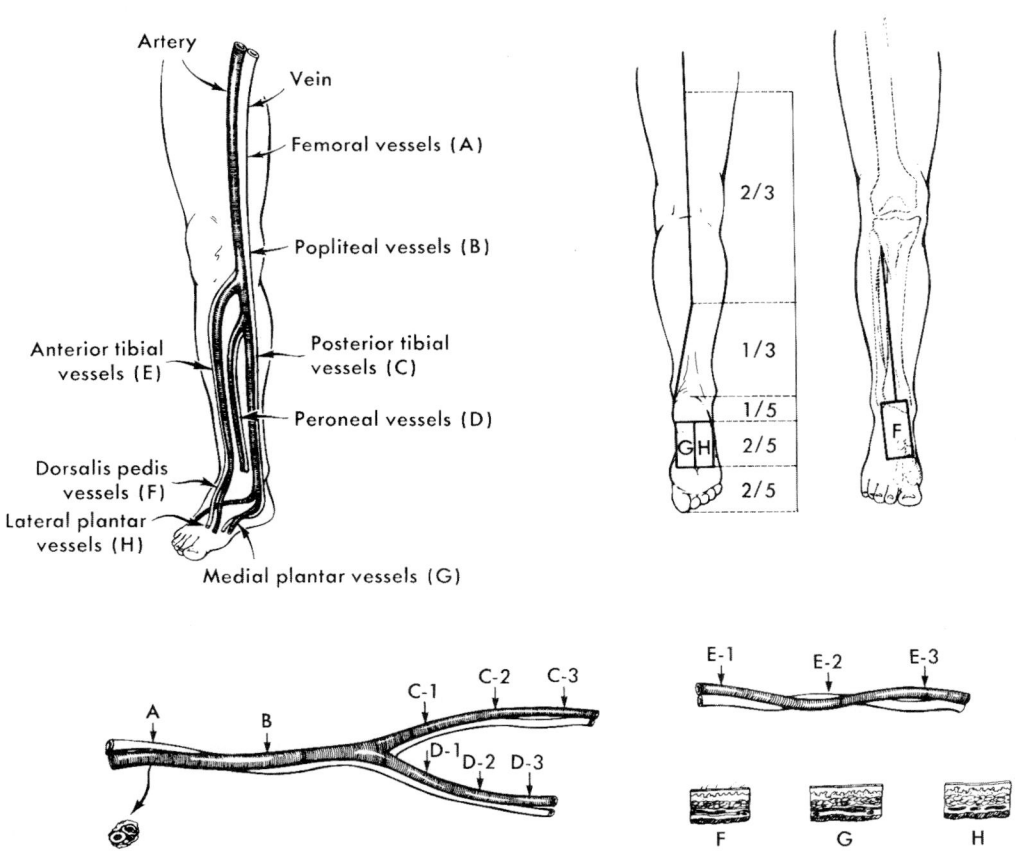

EXTREMITIES—AMPUTATION FOR OCCLUSIVE VASCULAR DISEASE—cont'd

Description

1 Type of amputation; side of extremity
2 Length and circumference
3 Appearance of skin: ulcers (size, extent), hemorrhage, stasis dermatitis
4 Subcutaneous tissue; muscle; bone and joints
5 Appearance of major arteries and veins: atherosclerosis (degree), thrombosis

Sections for histology

1 Skin
2 Major arteries, veins, and nerves according to accompanying diagram or an abbreviated version of it
3 Skeletal muscle
4 Bone and joint (when pertinent)

EXTREMITIES—AMPUTATION FOR OSSEOUS TUMOR

(Adapted from Weatherby RP, Unni KK: Practical aspects of handling orthopedic specimens in the surgical pathology laboratory. Pathol Annu 17[Pt 2]:1-31, 1982.)

Procedure

1 Review the x-ray studies taken before amputation.
2 Measure the length and circumference (including a measure of the circumference at the level of the tumor, if this is apparent or known).
3 Determine the presence, position, and dimensions of biopsy sites.
4 Search for the major lymph node groups; identify and place in separate containers.
5 Cut a cross section of the proximal bone margin with a band saw.
6 Dissect out all the soft tissues (down to the periosteum) around the involved bone with a scalpel, forceps, and scissors. Review the clinical and roentgenographic findings before proceeding. If there is any indication (from the roentgenograms or at the time of dissection) of soft tissue extension by the tumor, dissect *around* this area and keep it in continuity with the bone. If, from the x-ray studies, the tumor does not seem to involve the joint, cut through it; if it does, leave the joint intact and make a cross section with the band saw through the adjacent noninvolved bone, approximately 5 to 10 cm from the joint. If a previous incision site is present, take a sample for histology at this time, along the entire course of the incision.
7 Cut longitudinally the bone specimen thus obtained with a band saw. In most cases a section dividing the specimen into an anterior and a posterior half is preferable; in others, sagittal, lateralized, or even oblique cuts are to be recommended. The type of bone involved and the location of the tumor as seen radiographically will determine which plane of section will give the most information.
8 Examine the cut section, and take regular and two sets of Polaroid photographs or photocopies; identify in one set of the latter the site of the sections to be taken.
9 Examine under Wood's light if tetracycline had been administered before amputation (to detect satellite foci).
10 Cut a parallel section with the band saw, producing a slice about 5 mm thick. Use a saw guide for this purpose. Take a roentgenogram of the slice. Make additional cuts of the remaining bone pieces, if indicated. It might be desirable to take additional photographs (regular and Polaroid or photocopies) at this time.

EXTREMITIES—AMPUTATION FOR OSSEOUS TUMOR—cont'd

11 Quickly dissect the soft tissues that had been peeled off the involved bone; cut sagittally with the band saw all major bones that were left in this portion of the specimen and examine carefully for other foci of tumor or other lesions. Open the major joints and examine them.

Description

1 Type of amputation; side of extremity

2 Length and circumference of extremity, including circumference at level of tumor

3 Presence, position, and dimensions of biopsy sites

4 Tumor characteristics:

    a Location: bone involved; diaphysis, metaphysis, or epiphysis? medulla, cortex, or periosteum? epiphyseal line apparent? (if so, is the tumor crossing it)? does the tumor involve articular cartilage and joint cavity? does it extend into soft tissue? is the periosteum elevated by tumor? (if so, to what extent?) invaded by tumor? if previous incision present, is there evidence of tumor extension along it?

    b Features of tumor: size, shape, color, borders, consistency; does it appear to be bone forming, cartilaginous, fibrous, or myxoid? cystic changes, hemorrhage, or necrosis?

    c Distance of tumor to osseous margin of resection

5 Appearance of bone away from tumor; satellite lesions? any fluorescent foci seen if examined under Wood's light?

6 Appearance of remaining extremity if abnormal (if not, so state); skin, subcutaneous fat, muscles, major vessels and nerves, other bones, joints

7 Appearance and approximate number of lymph nodes found

Sections for histology

1 Tumor: four sections or more depending on size and extent

All grossly dissimilar areas should be sampled. Whenever possible, sections should be taken to include the periphery of the tumor *and* adjacent cortex, medulla, epiphyseal line, articular cartilage, periosteum, and soft tissues.

2 Previous incision site, if present, taken all along its course

3 Section from grossly noninvolved bone, midway between tumor and margin of resection

If the tumor involves upper end of a bone, take this section from midportion of proximally located bone.

4 Osseous margin of resection

5 Any abnormal-looking areas elsewhere in bone, soft tissues, or skin

6 Lymph nodes: if grossly normal, only representative ones; if grossly abnormal or if there is clinical suspicion of metastases, all of them

EXTREMITIES—AMPUTATION FOR SOFT TISSUE TUMOR

Procedure

1 Review any imaging studies (CT scans, MRIs) that may have been taken before amputation.

2 Measure the length and circumference of the extremity, including a measure of the circumference at the level of the tumor.

3 Determine the presence, position, and dimensions of biopsy sites.

4 Search for the major lymph node groups and identify and place in separate containers.

5 Cut through the skin and carefully dissect the subcutaneous fat, muscles, and major arteries, veins, and nerves *around* the tumor, avoiding cutting through the latter. Use an anatomy atlas as a guide, if necessary. Try to determine as accurately as possible the relationship of the tumor with the following structures: skin, subcutaneous fat, and specific muscles; arteries, veins, and nerves; and periosteum and bone. Mark some of the major anatomic landmarks with tags, if indicated.

6 As soon as all the margins of the tumor have been determined, remove the entire area with a good margin of normal tissues using a scalpel and scissors.

7 Two options, outlined later, are available for studying the specimen thus obtained. The first is used in most instances, but the second is preferable in selected cases. In either case, if a previous incision site is present, take a sample for histology at this time along the entire course of the incision.

  a Divide the tumor into slices with a large, sharp knife. Continue the dissection with the forceps, scissors, and scalpel to determine the tumor relationship with the structures previously mentioned. Place several pieces from different areas in formalin, fix for several hours or overnight, and trim to place in cassettes.

  b Place the entire specimen in a large pan containing formalin, cover with a towel, leave in the refrigerator at 4° C overnight, and cut parallel slices with a large, sharp knife. Take x-ray studies, if pertinent. Take two Polaroid photographs or photocopies, and identify in one of them the site of the sections to be taken.

8 Quickly dissect the soft tissues from the rest of the extremity, looking for other foci of tumor or other lesions.

9 Cut the major bones of the extremities longitudinally with a band saw. Make one of the sections through the area of bone closest to the soft tissue tumor. Examine for tumor extension or other lesions.

10 Open the major joints and examine them.

Description

1 Type of amputation; side of extremity

2 Length and circumference of extremity, including circumference at level of tumor

3 Presence, position, and dimensions of biopsy sites

4 Tumor characteristics:

  a Primary location: subcutaneous fat; muscle compartments(s) (specify which); fascial planes

  b Tumor extension into and relation with skin, subcutaneous fat, deep fascia, muscle, periosteum, bone, joint vessels, and nerves (specify which); presence of obvious vascular or neural involvement by tumor

  c If previous incision present, is there evidence of tumor extension along it?

  d Size (three dimensions), shape, color, borders (encapsulated? pushing? infiltrating?), consistency, secondary changes (cysts? necrosis? hemorrhage?)

  e Presence of myxoid changes, foci of calcification, cartilage, or bone

  f Shortest distance of tumor from margin of resection

5 Appearance of remaining extremity, if abnormal (if not, so state); skin, subcutaneous fat, muscles, major vessels and nerves, bone (tumor invasion? osteoporosis? bone marrow?), joints (osteoarthritis?)

6 Appearance and approximate number of lymph nodes found

EXTREMITIES—AMPUTATION FOR SOFT TISSUE TUMOR—cont'd

Sections for histology

1 Tumor: four sections or more, depending on size and extent

   All grossly dissimilar areas should be sampled. Whenever possible, sections should be taken to include the periphery of the tumor *and* adjacent fat, muscle, skin, periosteum, vessels, and/or nerves.

2 Previous incision site, if present, taken all along its course

3 Lymph nodes: if grossly normal, only representative ones; if grossly abnormal or if clinical suspicion of metastases, all of them

4 Proximal margins of resection: subcutaneous fat and muscle (plus skin and bone, if indicated)

EYES—ENUCLEATION*

Procedure

1 Fix the intact ocular globe in formalin for 24 hours before sectioning; it is not advisable to open the eye, to cut windows into the sclera, or to inject fixative into the vitreous.

2 Wash in running tap water for 1 or more hours and, optionally, place in 60% ethyl alcohol for a few more hours.

3 Review the summary of the clinical history and the results of the ophthalmologic examination prior to sectioning.

4 Measure anteroposterior, horizontal, and vertical dimensions of the globe, length of the optic nerve, and horizontal dimensions of the cornea.

5 Look for sites of accidental or surgical injuries.

6 Transilluminate the globe before opening it. A substage microscope lamp in a darkened room is satisfactory. Rotate the globe over the light source; if abnormal shadows are detected, mark them on the sclera with an indelible pencil.

7 Examination of the globe with a ×7 objective of a dissecting microscope can be carried out to detect minute lesions.

8 If intraocular foreign bodies or retinoblastoma is suspected, take a roentgenogram of the globe before it is opened.

9 If choroidal malignant melanoma is suspected, sample at least one of the vortex veins from each of the four quadrants (see accompanying drawing).

10 Open the eye with a sharp razor blade by holding the globe with the left hand, cornea down against the cutting block and the blade between the thumb and middle finger of the right hand. Open the eye with a sawing motion from back to front. The plane of section should begin adjacent to the optic nerve and end through the periphery of the cornea. The plane of section is dependent on whether a lesion has been detected in the previous steps. If it has not, cut the globe along a horizontal plane, using as surface landmarks the superior and inferior oblique insertions and the long postciliary vein (see accompanying drawing). If a lesion has been found, modify the plane of section so that the lesion will be included in the slab.

11 Examine the interior of the globe.

12 Place the eye flat on its cut surface, and make a second plane of section, parallel to the first, again passing from back to front.

13 Examine carefully the ~8-mm disc-shaped slab thus obtained, which should contain the cornea, pupils, lens, and optic nerve. Take regular and Polaroid photographs or photocopies, if indicated.

EYES—ENUCLEATION—cont'd

Description

Intact eye

1 Side of the globe (see accompanying drawing); anteroposterior, horizontal, and vertical dimensions
2 Length of optic nerve
3 Horizontal and vertical dimensions of cornea
4 Anterior segment: surgical incisions? corneal opacification? iris abnormalities? lens present?
5 Transillumination findings

Slab

1 Corneal thickness; anterior chamber depth; configuration of anterior chamber angle
2 Condition of iris, ciliary body, and lens
3 Condition of choroid, retina, vitreous body, and optic disc
4 If tumor present: location, size, color, edges, consistency, presence of hemorrhage or necrosis, ocular structures involved, extension into optic nerve

Sections for histology

1 Entire eye slab
2 Any (other) abnormal areas
3 In tumors, particularly retinoblastoma: cross section of surgical margin of optic nerve
4 In suspected malignant melanoma: sample from at least one of vortex veins from each of four quadrants

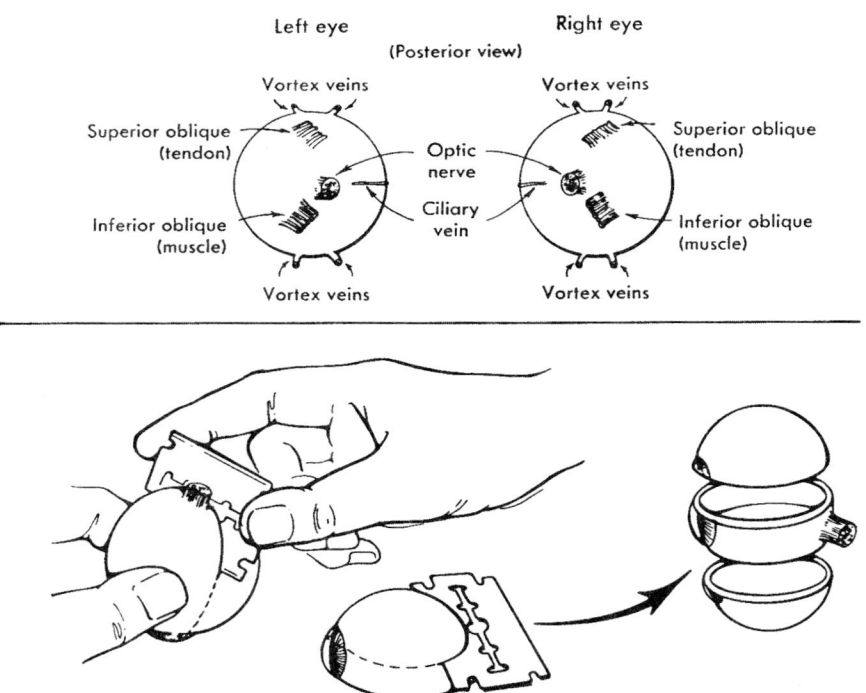

*Herreman R, De Buen S, Cortés T: Oftalmótomo: un nuevo apparato para secionar los ojos en el laboratorio de anatomía patológica. Rev Fac Med (Mexico) 7:157-167, 1965. Smith ME: A method for immediate gross sectioning of enucleated globes. Am J Ophthalmol 77:413-414, 1974. Yanoff M, Fine BS: Glutaraldehyde fixation of routine surgical eye tissue. Am J Ophthalmol 63:137-140, 1967.

FALLOPIAN TUBES—LIGATION

In tubal ligation, an avascular segment in the midisthmic portion of the tube is made into a loop, the base is ligated, and the top of the loop is excised.

Procedure

1 Separate specimens from right and left tubes.
2 Measure the length and diameter of each.

Description

1 Length and diameter of each specimen
2 Do they appear to be a complete segment of each tube? lumen present?

Sections for histology

1 All tissue received, identified as to right and left tube
2 Very important that tissue be sectioned on end; instructions to histotechnician or embedding in agar may be necessary.

Salpingectomy may be performed by itself in the case of fallopian tube pathology or—more often—as part of a total abdominal hysterectomy with unilateral or bilateral salpingo-oophorectomy.

FALLOPIAN TUBES—SALPINGECTOMY

Procedure

1 Fix the specimen before sectioning. If the tubes are attached to the uterus, they should be fixed in that position.
2 Measure the length and greatest diameter.
3 If the tube is relatively normal in size, serially section at 5-mm intervals and examine. Make the cuts incomplete so that the pieces remain attached by the serosa.
4 If the tube is obviously enlarged, make one complete longitudinal section, followed by parallel sections, if necessary.

Description

1 Length and greatest diameter
2 Serosa: fibrin? hemorrhage? fibrous adhesions to ovary or other organs?
3 Wall: abnormally thick? ruptured?
4 Mucosa: atrophic? hyperplastic? appearance of fimbriated end; inverted?
5 Lumen: patent? dilated? content; diameter, if abnormally large
6 Masses: size, appearance, invasion
7 Cysts in paraovarian region: diameter, thickness of wall, content; sessile or pedunculated?
8 In cases of suspected ectopic pregnancy: embryo or placenta identified? amount of hemorrhage; rupture?

Sections for histology

1 For incidental tubes without gross abnormalities: three cross sections of each tube, taken from the proximal, mid, and distal portions, submitted in the same cassette (see accompanying drawing).
2 For tubes with suspected ectopic pregnancy: submit any tissue with gross appearance of products of conception. If none is grossly identified, submit several sections from the wall in the area of hemorrhage as well as several from the *intraluminal clot*. If products of conception are not identified microscopically, submit additional sections.
3 For tubes with other lesions: as many as needed to adequately examine any abnormal areas. If tumor is present, at least three sections must be taken to include grossly uninvolved mucosa.

Procedure

Keep intact, cut sagittally, or dissect, depending on fetus size.

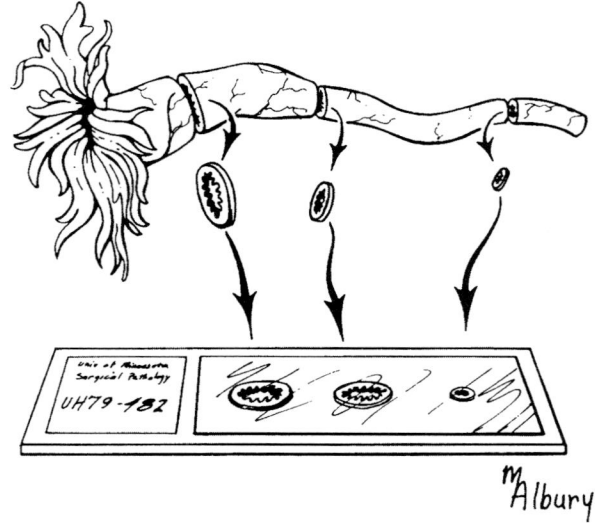

FETUS—ABORTION

Description

1 Sex; weight; crown-rump or crown-heel length or foot length (see accompany drawings)
2 Approximate length of gestation (see table, p. 2658, and figure below)
3 General condition: well preserved? macerated?
4 External and internal anomalies and other changes
5 Umbilical cord: appearance, number of vessels
6 Placental tissues accompanying fetuses:
   a Weight
   b Membranes: insertion, color, transparency, completeness; extramembranous pregnancy? marginal or membranous hemorrhage?
   c Umbilical cord: insertion, color, focal changes
   d Chorionic plate: vascular pattern, vessel caliber, color; subchorionic hemorrhage?
   e Villi: hydatidiform change? (note proportion of involved villi and size of cysts); focal lesions?

Sections for histology

1 Small embryos: submit whole embryo or one half, depending on size.
2 Large fetuses: submit one section from lungs, stomach (including gastric contents), kidneys, and other organs, as indicated.
3 Placental tissues:
   a Extraplacental membranes (one section)
   b Umbilical cord (one section)
   c Chorionic plate (one section)
   d Villi from chorion frondosum, including maternal surface (one section)

For a more thorough examination of specimens for fetal malformations and chromosomal abnormalities, see Klatt, EC: Pathologic examination of fetal specimens from dilation and evacuation procedures. Am J Clin Pathol **103:**415-418, 1995.

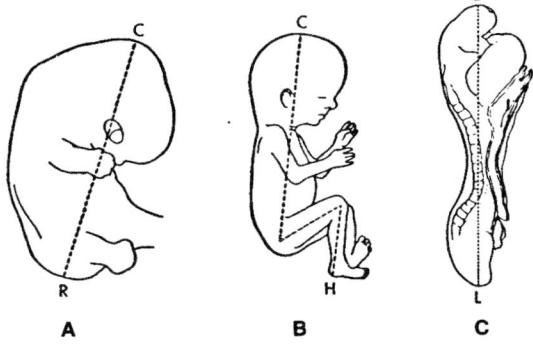

A   B   C

FETUS—ABORTION—cont'd

Cholecystectomy consists of removal of the entire gallbladder after dissecting it from the base of the liver and suturing the cystic duct and cystic artery. At present, a high number of cholecystectomies are performed through a laparoscopic route.

Table App H-1 Relations of age, size, and weight in the human embryo

Age of embryo	Crown-rump (CR) length (mm)	Crown-heel length (mm)	External diameter of chorionic sac (mm)	Weight in grams	Amount of increase each month when value at start of month equals unity	
					CR length	Weight
One week	0.1	—	0.2			
Two weeks	0.2	—	3			
Three weeks	2.0	—	10			
Four weeks	5.0	—	10	.02	49.0	40000.00
Five weeks	8.0	—	25			
Six weeks	12.0	—	30			
Seven weeks	17.0	19.0	40			
Two lunar months	25.0	30.0	50	1	3.6	49.00
Three lunar months	56.0	73.0	—	14	1.4	13.00
Four lunar months	112.0	157.0	—	105	1.0	6.50
Five lunar months	160.0	239.0	—	310	0.43	1.95
Six lunar months	203.0	296.0	—	640	0.26	1.07
Seven lunar months	242.0	355.0	—	1080	0.14	0.69
Eight lunar months	277.0	409.0	—	1670	0.14	0.55
Nine lunar months	313.0	458.0	—	2400	0.13	0.43
Full term (38 weeks)	350.0	500.0	—	3300	0.12	0.38

From Arey LB: Developmental anatomy, ed 7. Philadelphia, 1965, W.B. Saunders Co, p 104.
*Total length of embryonic disc.

GALLBLADDER—CHOLECYSTECTOMY

Procedure

1 Open the entire organ longitudinally as soon as feasible after excision; otherwise the mucosa will quickly undergo autolytic changes.

2 If stones are present, wash them, estimate the number and the size of the largest, and cut one or several of them with a scalpel.

3 Search for lymph nodes along the bladder neck.

4 In cases of carcinoma the organ also can be studied by extracting the bile with a syringe, filling the lumen with formalin, fixing overnight at 4° C, and cutting the specimen with scissors and a scalpel.

Description

1 Length and greatest diameter of gallbladder

2 Serosa: thickened? fibrous adhesions? fibrin?

3 Wall: thickened? (if so, focally or diffusely?) hemorrhage?

4 Mucosa: color, appearance, ulcerated? hyperplastic? cholesterosis

5 Cystic duct: dilated? impacted with stones? lymph nodes present? size and appearance

6 Approximate volume, color, and consistency of bile

7 Stones: approximate number, shape, and size range; color and appearance on cross section; type of stone (see accompanying table)

8 If tumor present: location, distance from fundus and neck, size; polypoid? ulcerated? infiltrative? serosal involvement?

Sections for histology

1 Three sections including entire wall, one from the fundus, one from the body, and one from the neck; additional sections from any area that appears grossly abnormal.

2 In cases of suspected carcinoma in situ, the organ can be studied by embedding the entire specimen by the Swiss roll method. In addition, the bile can be decanted into a breaker or centrifuge tube and studied cytologically.*

3 Cystic duct and lymph nodes, if they appear grossly abnormal or if the gallbladder contains a tumor.

*From Albores-Saavedra J, Henson DE: Tumors of the gallbladder and extrahepatic bile ducts. Atlas of tumor pathology, 2nd series, Fasc. 22. Washington, D.C., 1984, Armed Forces Institute of Pathology, p 151.

GALLBLADDER—CHOLECYSTECTOMY—cont'd

Table App H-2 Types of gallstones

Type of stone	Incidence	Composition	Appearance
Pure	10%	Cholesterol Calcium bilirubinate Calcium carbonate	Solitary; crystalline surface Multiple; jet black; crystalline or amorphous Grayish white; amorphous
Mixed	80%	Cholesterol and calcium bilirubinate Cholesterol and calcium carbonate Calcium bilirubinate and calcium carbonate Cholesterol, calcium bilirubinate, and calcium carbonate	Multiple, faceted or lobulated, laminated, and crystalline on cut surfaces Hue: Yellow—cholesterol Black—calcium bilirubinate White—calcium carbonate
Combined	10%	Pure gallstone nucleus with mixed gallstone shell Mixed gallstone nucleus with pure gallstone shell	Largest of gallstones when single Hue depends on composition of shell

Slightly modified from de Schryver-Kecskemet K: Gallbladder and biliary ducts. In Kissane JM, ed: Anderson's pathology, ed 9. St Louis, 1990, Mosby.

HEART—VALVE REPLACEMENT—cont'd

(Adapted from Roberts WC, Morrow AG: Cardiac valves and the surgical pathologist. Arch Pathol 82:309-313, 1996.)

Traditionally, valve replacement operations have entailed the removal of the entire diseased valve. However, in cases of mitral valve disease, there has been a tendency in recent years to remove only the anterior mitral leaflet during valve replacement and to remove only portions of the valve (usually from the posterior leaflet) during reparative procedures.

Procedure

1 Fix the specimen before sectioning.
2 Take Polaroid photographs or photocopies and a roentgenogram in every case. For atrioventricular valves, photograph from both atrial and ventricular aspects. For aortic valves, photograph from both aortic and ventricular aspects.

Description
Atrioventricular valves

1 Leaflets fibrotic, calcified, or normal?
2 Fibrosis or calcification focal or diffuse?
3 Fibrosis or calcification distributed on leaflets? (only at margins? on one surface? on both?)
4 Leaflets immobile, shortened, stretched, or normal?
5 Commissures fused? (if so, to what extent?)
6 Chordae tendineae intact, ruptured, shortened, elongated, fused, or normal?
7 Papillary muscles normal in number, scarred, hypertrophied, or elongated?
8 Valve incompetent, stenotic, or both?
9 If incompetent: because of scanty valvular tissue, dilated annulus, or ruptured chordae or because of ruptured, scarred, or shortened papillary muscle?

Semilunar valves

Same as for atrioventricular valves in most respects plus:
1 Number of cusps present?
2 Cusps of equal or unequal size?

Sections for histology

Several sections, including free edge; decalcify, if necessary

HORMONE RECEPTOR ASSAYS—SAMPLING

(Adapted from Keffer JH: Hormone-receptor assays and cancer of the breast. The pathologist's role [editorial]. Am J Clin Pathol **70:**719-720, 1978.)

Determination of receptors for different steroid hormones (estrogens, progesterone, androgens) has become an established technique for the evaluation of several surgically excised tissues, particularly breast carcinoma. It correlates with clinical response to hormone therapy and, according to some, also with clinical response to chemotherapeutic agents. In some cases of metastatic cancer, it may provide some indication of the site of origin of the primary lesion. Sampling should be taken of recurrent or metastatic carcinoma, even if the original tumor had been previously assayed, to establish the continued presence or absence of the receptor.

Two methods are available for the determination of hormone receptors in tissue: biochemical and immunohistochemical. The former, based on charcoal-dextran assay, has been the standard for many years, but it is being progressively replaced by the immunohistochemical method. The procedure for procuring tissue for the biochemical assay is the following:

1 Examine tissue in the fresh state, immediately after excision; select a sample carefully, avoiding areas of necrosis, adipose tissue, and other nonsuitable areas.
2 Cut a sample measuring approximately 1 cm in greatest diameter (or as large as allowable). The instruments should be clean but not necessarily sterile.
3 Freeze quickly in liquid nitrogen (-70° C) in isopentane or with freon spray.
4 Store in the deep freeze until the sample is ready to be delivered (in the frozen state) to the appropriate laboratory.
5 Submit for histology (for control purposes) a piece of tissue immediately adjacent to the one frozen and identify as such.
6 When the lesion is so small that a 1 cm sample for biochemical assay cannot be spared, cut frozen sections and store in the freezer (-70° C) for subsequent immunohistochemical staining for receptor.

IMPRINTS (TOUCH PREPARATIONS)

(Adapted from Berard CW, Bowling MC: Technical factors in evaluation of lymph node biopsies. Tutorial on Neoplastic Hematopathology, Henry Rappaport, M.D., Director, Pasadena, California, Feb. 5-9, 1979; presented in cooperation with The City of Hope National Medical Center and The University of Chicago Center for Continuing Education.)

1 Cut a block of tissue measuring approximately $10 \times 10 \times 3$ mm.

2 Hold the tissue gently with forceps with the freshly cut, flat surface upward.

3 With the other hand, lightly touch an alcohol-clean glass slide repeatedly in serial adjacent areas with the cut surface of the tissue. Just contact—do not compress the block. If the surface touched is excessively bloody or wet, discard the slide and repeat with another slide until the touch preparations are barely opaque. Prepare an average of four slides in this fashion.

4 As each slide is prepared, dry it rapidly by waving it in the air. Do not heat or blow on the slide. It should take no more than 30 to 60 seconds for the slide to dry; if it takes more, it means that the touches are too wet and that the resulting imprints will be unsatisfactory.

5 For standard purposes, fix (after drying) in methyl alcohol, and stain two with hematoxylin-eosin and two with Wright's or Giemsa stain.

6 After preparation of the imprints, fix and submit for histology the block used for this purpose to correlate its appearance with that of the imprint.

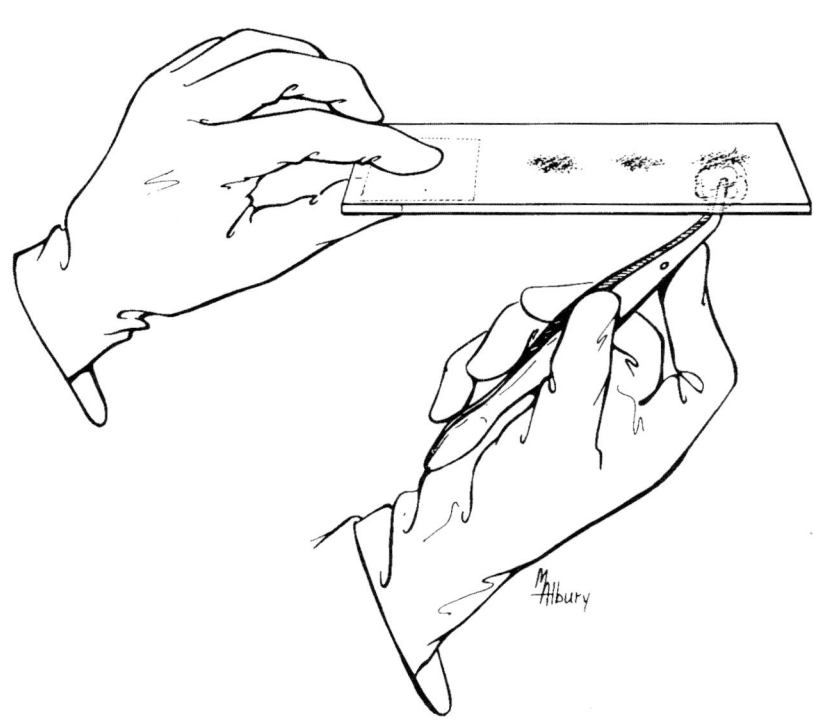

INJECTION OF SPECIMENS—GENERAL GUIDELINES

When feasible, the injection of surgical specimens may serve to illustrate more clearly the gross pathology present, as well as to ensure proper fixation. The procedure has been found most useful for lobectomies, pneumonectomies, cystectomies, colectomies, and pelvic exenterations.

1 Partially fill a large container with fixative.
2 Prepare the specimen properly (see specific instructions for the respective organs).
3 Place in container and inject with formalin.
4 Add additional fixative to the container to ensure that the entire specimen is covered by fixative.
5 Place a towel or several gauze pads of the free-floating specimen to prevent the surface from drying.
6 Cover the container with a lid.
7 Fix for 24 hours before dissecting.

JAW RESECTION FOR TUMOR—MANDIBULECTOMY

Procedure

1 Fix the whole specimen in formalin overnight in the refrigerator at 4° C.
2 Paint the surgical margins with India ink.
3 For bone tumors: make multiple parallel sections through bone and soft tissue with a band saw, fix further in formalin, and decalcify.
4 For mucosal or soft tissue tumors: separate soft tissue from the mandible with a scalpel. The direction of the dissection should be from the inferior to the superior and from the posterior to the anterior aspects.
5 Take two Polaroid photographs or photocopies and identify in one of them the site of the sections to be taken.
6 If the specimen includes a radical neck dissection, process according to instructions for Lymph node dissection—radical neck.

Description

1 Type of resection (partial or total) and side
2 Tumor: size, color, appearance, edges; bone invaded?
3 Non-neoplastic mucosa: leukoplakia?
4 Bone: appearance on cross sections
5 Teeth: number and appearance

Sections for histology

1 Tumor: three sections
2 Non-neoplastic mucosa
3 Mucosal surgical margins
4 Soft tissue surgical margins
5 Bone surgical margins
6 Mandibular nerve (surgical margins)
7 Bone, if grossly involved or suspicious

JAW RESECTION FOR TUMOR—MAXILLECTOMY

Procedure

1 Fix the specimen in formalin overnight in the refrigerator at 4° C.
2 Paint the surgical margins with India ink.
3 Take surgical margins (anterior, posterior, external, and superior); cut the specimen with the band saw in parallel slices 0.5 cm thick. Fix them overnight. Take photographs and x-ray studies, if indicated.
4 Take two Polaroid photographs or photocopies and identify in one of them the site of the sections to be taken.

Description

1 Extent of resection
2 Presence of following structures: hard and soft palates; superior, middle, and inferior turbinates; medial and lateral pterygoid plate of sphenoid bone; air cells of ethmoid; bony floor of orbit; orbital contents; zygoma, masseter, temporalis, external, and internal pterygoid muscles
3 Tumor characteristics: location, extent, size; limited to the maxillary sinus? arising from superior, medial, lateral, anterior, posterior, or inferior part of sinus? extending into intratemporal fossa, nasal cavity, ethmoid cells, or any other of aforementioned structures? presence of tumor at surgical margins?
4 Condition of ostium of maxillary sinus and any other sinuses present; fistulae present?

Sections for histology

1 Tumor: as many sections as necessary, with minimum of three
2 Surgical margins

KIDNEY—NEEDLE BIOPSY

Procedure

The examination and sampling of this material should be carried out at the bedside or *immediately* after the specimen is received in the pathology laboratory.

1 Measure the length and diameter.

2 Try to determine by gross inspection whether the cortex is present; this can be done by identifying glomeruli with a dissecting microscope or magnifying lenses. An experienced observer can do it most of the time with the naked eye on the basis of color.

3 If the cortex is grossly identified:

   a Take three pieces (1 mm thick each) from this area and fix in glutaraldehyde for electron microscopic examination.

   b Take one additional piece (2 mm thick) from this area and freeze in isopentane cooled with liquid nitrogen for immunofluorescence.

   c Place the remainder of the specimen in fixative for routine light microscopy. We use Zenker's fixative.

4 If the cortex cannot be identified with certainty on gross inspection, the operator may decide to perform another needle biopsy. Otherwise, the following should be done with the specimen:

   a Take two pieces (1 mm each) from *each* end and fix for electron microscopy.

   b Take two additional pieces (2 mm each) from *each* end and freeze for immunofluorescence.

   c Fix the remainder for routine histology.

5 If the amount of tissue is insufficient to divide for all these studies, electron microscopy and immunofluorescence have priority, one of the reasons being that a modified version of the light microscopic evaluation can be carried out on them.

6 If the specimen is an open wedge biopsy, the same guidelines apply, except for the fact that the cortex is always readily identifiable and therefore double sampling is not necessary.

Description

1 Number of fragments; length and diameter of each

2 Color: homogeneous or not?

3 Cortex recognizable? glomeruli; size, color; prominence

Sections for histology

1 See Procedure

2 Needle renal biopsies should be routinely stained with:

   a Hematoxylin-eosin

   b Alcian blue–PAS

   c Jones' silver methenamine

   d Masson's trichrome

KIDNEY—NEPHRECTOMY FOR NONTUMORAL CONDITION

Procedure

1 Measure and weigh the organ.
2 Two options are available depending on the type of abnormality present and the status of the organ when received in the laboratory:
   a Cut the kidney sagittally, strip the capsule, and carefully open the pelvis, calyces, and ureter.
   b Inject with formalin through the ureter and, if possible, through the renal artery, ligate the ureter (and artery), and submerge in formalin overnight. Cut sagittally the next day, strip the capsule, and open the pelvis, calyces, and ureter. This technique is especially useful in cases of hydronephrosis.
3 Take two Polaroid photographs or photocopies and identify in one of them the sites of the sections to be taken.
4 If stones are present, submit for chemical analysis, if indicated.

Description

1 Weight and size of kidney
2 Capsule: amount of pericapsular tissue, thickness of capsule, adherence to cortex
3 External surface: smooth? scars: number, size, shape (flat or V shaped?); cysts? (if so, number, size, location, content)
4 Cortex: color, width; glomeruli apparent? striations apparent and orderly?
5 Medulla: color, width; medullary rays apparent and orderly?
6 Pelvis: size; dilated? blunting of calyces? thickened? hemorrhage? crystalline deposits? stones: number, size, and shape (see Bladder—stone removal); amount of peripelvic fat
7 Ureter: diameter, length, evidence of dilatation or stricture
8 Renal artery and vein; appearance

KIDNEY—NEPHRECTOMY FOR NONTUMORAL CONDITION—cont'd

Sections for histology

1 Kidney: three sections, each including cortex and medulla
2 Pelvis: two sections
3 Ureter

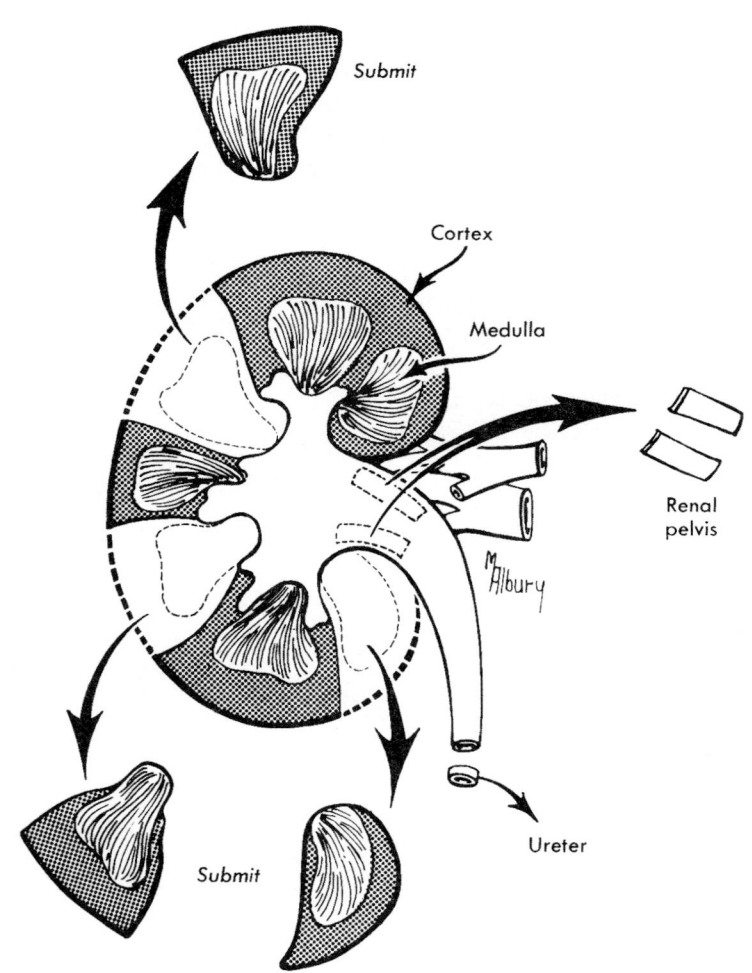

KIDNEY—NEPHRECTOMY FOR TUMOR

Procedure

1 Look for and dissect any perirenal lymph nodes.
2 Look for and open the renal vein longitudinally.
3 Cut the kidney sagittally and open the pelvis, calyces, and ureter.
4 Strip the capsule and look for capsular and perirenal tumor extension.
5 If stones are present, submit for chemical analysis.
6 Take two Polaroid photographs or photocopies and identify in one of them the sites of the sections to be taken.
7 Cut the kidney in thin slices searching for additional cortical or medullary lesions.

Description

1 Weight and dimensions of specimen; length and diameter of ureter
2 Tumor characteristics: size, shape, location, extent, homogenicity, necrosis, hemorrhage; invasion of capsule, perirenal tissues, calyces, pelvis, and renal vein
3 Uninvolved kidney: external surface, cortex, medulla; any additional focal lesions?
4 Pelvis: dilatated? blunting of calyces? stones?
5 Presence, number, size, and appearance of perirenal lymph nodes

Sections for histology

1 Tumor: for renal cell carcinoma: minimum of three sections (including one with adjacent kidney); for pediatric tumors: minimum of one section for each centimeter of tumor diameter; for carcinoma of renal pelvis: minimum of three sections with adjacent pelvis and/or renal parenchyma
2 Kidney not involved by tumor: two sections
3 Pelvis: one section in cases of renal cell carcinoma or pediatric tumors; two sections in cases of carcinoma of renal pelvis
4 Renal artery and vein
5 Ureter: one section in cases of renal cell carcinoma or pediatric tumors; one section of every centimeter of ureter resected (and any abnormal-looking area) in cases of carcinoma of renal pelvis
6 Lymph nodes, if present

LARGE BOWEL—COLECTOMY FOR NONTUMORAL CONDITION

Procedure

1 Sample a few lymph nodes, and remove the mesentery while the specimen is fresh.
2 Two options are available to study the bowel, depending on the type of abnormality present and the status of the specimen when received in the laboratory.
   a Open the bowel longitudinally, pin on a corkboard, and fix overnight in formalin.
   b Inject the specimen (see Injection of specimens—general guidelines). Evacuate gross fecal contents by gentle external massage of the specimen. Further cleansing my be accomplished by the use of a gentle stream of formalin or saline solution (*not* water) into the bowel lumen. One end of the specimen is tied off, the specimen is injected with formalin, and the other end is tied off. If a constricting lesion is present, be sure that adequate fixative can be easily passed through the point of constriction. If this cannot be achieved, the main mass will not be properly fixed; under these circumstances, it is better to open the specimen and fix as noted in **2a** rather than to inject on both sides of the lesion. Injection is especially demonstrative in cases of diverticulosis.
3 Take two Polaroid photographs or photocopies and identify in one of them the sites of the sections to be taken.
4 In general, take the sections *perpendicular* to the direction of the mucosal folds.

Description

1 Part of bowel removed, length of specimen, and amount of mesentery
2 Mucosa: type of lesions, extent, ulceration (linear or transverse), depth, pseudopolyps, hemorrhage, fissures
3 Wall: thickening (focal or diffuse), atrophy, fibrosis, necrosis
4 Serosa: fibrin, pus, fibrosis, adherence of mesentery
5 Diverticula: number, size, location in relation to teniae, content, evidence of inflammation, hemorrhage, or perforation

Sections for histology

1 As many as necessary to sample abnormal areas
2 Proximal and distal lines of resection in cases of colitis
3 Appendix, if included in specimen

LARGE BOWEL—COLECTOMY FOR TUMOR

The major types of large bowel resection are *total colectomy, right hemicolectomy* (which includes the colon up to the hepatic flexure, cecum, ileocecal valve, appendix, portion of terminal ileum, and the corresponding mesentery), *transverse colectomy* (from the hepatic to the splenic flexures), *left hemicolectomy* (from the splenic flexure to the sigmoid colon), *low anterior* (rectosigmoid) *resection,* and *abdominoperineal resection* (sigmoid colon, rectum, and anus).

Procedure

1 Dissect the lymph nodes and remove the mesentery while the specimen is fresh.
2 Two options are available to study the bowel, depending on the size and location of the tumor and the status of the specimen when received in the laboratory.
   a Open the bowel longitudinally through its entire length, trying not to cut through the tumor. Pin the intestine on a corkboard and fix overnight in formalin.
   b Inject the specimen (see Injection of specimens—general guidelines and **2b** under Procedure in the preceding section).
3 Take two Polaroid photographs or photocopies and identify in one of them the sites of the sections to be taken.
4 In cases with deep penetration by tumor, dissect the veins carefully for possible tumor invasion.
5 In general, take the sections *perpendicular* to the direction of the mucosal folds.

Description

1 Part of bowel removed, length of specimen, and amount of mesentery
2 a Tumor characteristics: size (including thickness); extent around bowel; shape (fungating, flat, ulcerating); presence of necrosis or hemorrhage; extent through bowel wall; serosal involvement, satellite nodules; evidence of blood vessel invasion; invasion of adjacent organs
   b Distance of tumor to pectinate line, peritoneal reflection, each line of resection
3 Other lesions in bowel and appearance of uninvolved mucosa; if polyps absent, so state
4 Estimate of number of lymph nodes found; whether or not nodes appear involved by tumor; size of largest node

LARGE BOWEL—COLECTOMY FOR TUMOR—cont'd

Sections for histology

1 Tumor: at least three sections (extending through the entire wall)
2 Representative section of subserosal connective tissue, fat, and blood vessel around tumor
3 Other lesions of bowel
4 Proximal line of resection
5 Distal line of resection
6 Bowel between tumor and distal line of resection (halfway or 5 cm, whichever suits case)
7 Appendix, if included in specimen
8 Lymph nodes:
    a Around tumor
    b Distal to tumor
    c Proximal to tumor
    d At high point of resection (areas surrounding ligated vessels)
9 In abdominoperineal resections: anorectal junction

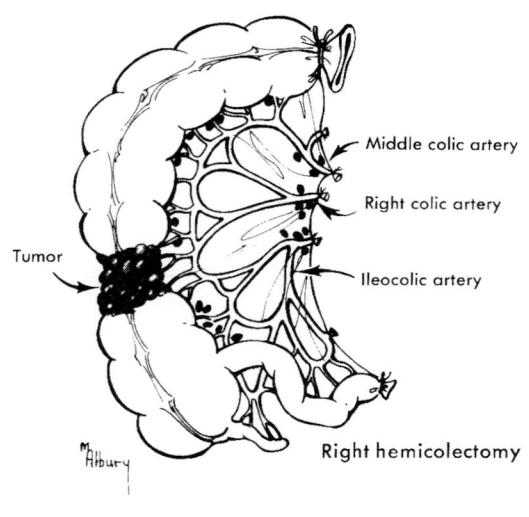

Right hemicolectomy

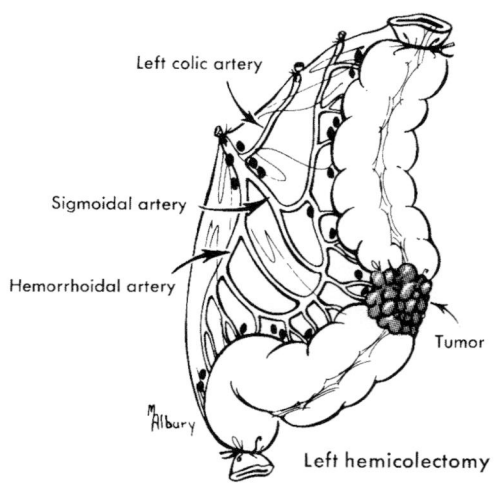

Left hemicolectomy

LARGE BOWEL—POLYPECTOMY

Procedure

1 Fix the specimen intact in formalin for several hours.
2 Measure the diameter of the head and length of the stalk.
3 For polyps with a short stalk or no stalk, identify the surgical section and cut in half longitudinally (see accompanying drawing **A**).
4 For polyps with a long stalk (1 cm or more), cut a cross section of the stalk near the surgical margin and then cut the polyp longitudinally, leaving as long a stalk as will fit in the cassette (see accompanying drawing **B**).
5 If half of the polyp head is over 3 mm, trim to this thickness on the convex side.

Description

1 Dimensions of polyp; diameter of head and length of stalk
2 Polyp sessile or pedunculated? ulcerated? surface smooth or papillary? any cysts on cross section? stalk appear normal?

Sections for histology

1 One longitudinal section (including surgical margin in polyps with short stalk or no stalk)
2 One cross section of base of stalk (in polyps with long stalk)
3 Appendix, if included in specimen

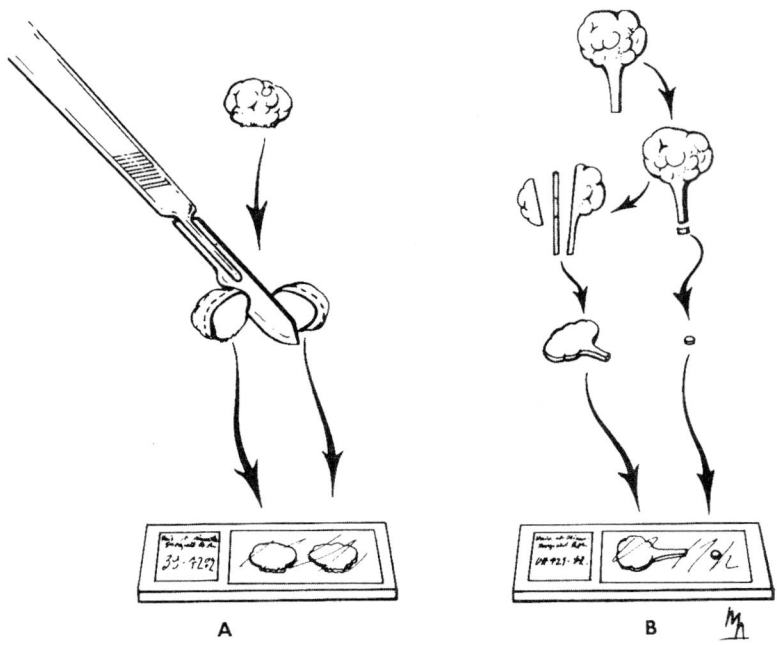

A   B

LARYNX—LARYNGECTOMY

(Adapted from Barnes L, Johnson JT: Pathologic and clinical consideration in the evaluation of major head and
neck specimens resected for cancer. Part I. Pathol Annu **21**[Pt 1]:173-250, 1986.

Three types of laryngectomy are performed: hemilaryngectomy, supraglottic laryngectomy, and total. *Hemilaryngectomy* consists of dividing the thyroid cartilage in the midline and resecting in continuity the thyroid cartilage along with the corresponding true and false vocal cords and ventricle. *Supraglottic laryngectomy* consists of excising the upper half of the larynx horizontally through the ventricle. *Total laryngectomy* consists of removal of the entire larynx, including upper laryngeal rings.

Procedure

1 Separate the larynx from the radical neck dissection if accompanied by the latter.
2 In total or supraglottic laryngectomy specimens, open the larynx along the posterior midline and keep it open with wires or by pinning to a corkboard.
3 Photograph, if indicated.
4 Fix overnight in formalin.
5 Remove the hyoid bone, thyroid cartilage, and cricoid cartilage, trying to keep the soft tissue as a single piece even if the bone and cartilage need to be fragmented in the process.
6 Take two Polaroid photographs or photocopies and identify in one of them the sites of the section to be taken.
7 Paint the surgical margins (lingual, pharyngeal, and tracheal) with India ink.
8 Orient as to superoinferior and anteroposterior axis.
10 Handle the radical neck dissection according to instructions for Lymph node dissection—radical neck.

Description

1 Type of laryngectomy: total laryngectomy, hemilaryngectomy, supraglottic laryngectomy; presence of pyriform sinus, hyoid bone, tracheal rings, thyroid and organs from neck dissection
2 Tumor characteristics: location (glottic, supraglottic, infraglottic, or transglottic?), side involved (wholly unilateral or encroaching on or crossing the midline?), size, pattern of growth (exophytic or endophytic?), ulceration, depth of invasion, presence of extralaryngeal spread, features of non-neoplastic mucosa (especially in true vocal cords)
  a For glottic tumors: length of cord involved; involvement of anterior or posterior commissures, extension to ventricle, and degree of subglottic extension as measured from the superior border of the true cord
  b For supraglottic tumors: if the hyoid bone is attached, is the tumor suprahyoid or infrahyoid? Does it involve the false cords, aryepiglottic folds, pyriform sinus (if present), or pre-epiglottic space?
  c If thyroid is included: weight, measurement, and appearance; invaded by tumor? parathyroid glands or perilaryngeal (delphian) node present? is there a tracheostomy? if so, is there any evidence of tumor involvement?
  d If thyroid is included: weight, measurement, and appearance; invaded by tumor? parathyroid glands or perilaryngeal (delphian) node present? is there a tracheostomy? if so, is there any evidence of tumor involvement?

Sections for histology

1 Entire tumor in properly identified longitudinal strips (unless massive, in which case representative sections should be taken)
2 Representative step section of larynx, including epiglottis
3 Thyroid cartilage at the site of maximum tumor invasion, if any
4 Thyroid, parathyroid, and tracheostomy site, if present
5 Lymph nodes (see under Lymph node dissection—radical neck)

LIP—V EXCISION

Procedure

1 Fix the specimen for several hours.
2 Paint all surgical margins with India ink.
3 Cut the specimen as shown in the accompanying drawing.

Description

1 Size of specimen
2 Tumor characteristics: size, shape (ulcerated, polypoid), location (vermilion border, skin), distance to margins

Sections for histology

1 Cross section through center (see accompanying drawing **A**)
2 Lateral margins, without trimming (see accompanying drawing **B** and **C**).

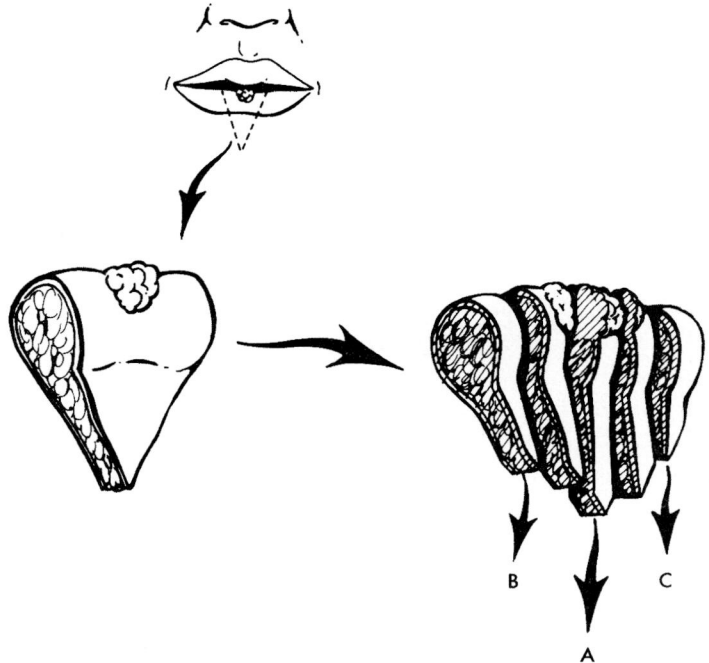

LIVER—EXCISION

Operations to remove liver masses include wedge resection, segmental resection, formal and extended right and left lobectomy, trisegmentectomy (which consists of resection of both right lobar segments and the medial segment of the left lobe), and total hepatectomy followed by liver transplant. The delineation of the various hepatic segments is difficult in the excised specimen and need not be attempted unless specifically requested by the surgeon, who may need to be consulted for assistance in the orientation of the specimen.

Procedure

1 Measure and weigh the specimen.

2 *For hepatic parenchymal tumors:* paint the hepatic surgical margin and cut parallel 1-cm slices in a plane roughly corresponding to the cut of the CT scan, if one was performed and is available.

3 *For tumors of major bile ducts:* identify all of the bile duct and vascular surgical margins (with the help of the surgeon, if necessary), and submit them *en face* (see later section); palpate the bile ducts for areas of induration; open the major bile ducts longitudinally with scissors; after taking photographs, serially section the bile ducts perpendicularly to their long axes; search for hilar lymph nodes.

Description

1 Size and weight of specimen

2 Appearance of the capsular surface

3 *For hepatic parenchymal tumors:* size; color; consistency; margins; relationship to capsular surface, major vessels (portal and hepatic veins) and biliary tree; distance to surgical margin; multiplicity; appearance of non-neoplastic liver (congested? signs of biliary obstruction? cirrhosis?)

4 *For tumors of major bile ducts:* same as for hepatic parenchymal tumors, plus: intraductal papillary component? areas of ductal stenosis or dilatation? presence of biliary stones?

5 Gallbladder: if present, describe as per instructions in Gallbladder—cholecystectomy; relationship with hepatic parenchymal or bile duct tumor

6 Hilar lymph nodes: number, size, and appearance

Sections for histology

1 Tumor: four sections or more depending on size and extent. All grossly dissimilar areas should be sampled. If several nodules are present, samples of up to five should be taken. Unless excessively large, tumors of major bile ducts should be submitted *in toto.*

2 Surgical margins: these should be taken from the areas that appear grossly closer to the tumor. In the case of the tumors of major bile ducts, one of these section should be an *en face* view of the bile duct and vascular surgical margin.

3 Non-neoplastic liver: include portions distal and proximal to the tumor, if feasible.

4 Gallbladder, if present: one section

5 Lymph nodes, if present: in their entirety

LUNG—BIOPSY

(Adapted from Brody Ar. Craighead JE: Preparation of human lung specimens by perfusion-fixation. Am Rev Respir Dis **112**:645-649, 1975; Carrington CB, Gaensler EA: Clinical-pathologic approach to diffuse interstitial lung disease. In Thurlbeck WM, ed: The lung. Baltimore, 1978, Waverly Press, pp 58-87; and Churg A: An inflation procedure for open lung biopsies. Am J Surg Pathol **7**:69-71. 1983.)

Procedure

1 Obtain cultures from lesions suspected of being infectious.
2 Take samples for electron microscopy and for deep freezing, if indicated.
3 Open biopsies obtained in patients with suspected interstitial lung disease are better evaluated micro-scopically if specimen has been fixed in the inflated state. This can be achieved by one of three methods:
   a The surgeon should take the biopsy from a lung that is held inflated and maintain inflation by clamp-ing the portion of the lung to be biopsied; the specimen should be placed in formalin immediately after excision.
   b The small airways and/or vessels are cannulated under a dissecting microscope. This is a tedious and somewhat complicated procedure.
   c The specimen is inflated slowly with formalin or other fixative (using a 25-gauge butterfly needle connected to a small syringe), sticking the needle through the pleura and gently infusing fixative until the specimen is well expanded. If specimen is large, several punctures with the needle may be nec-essary. After inflation, the specimen is dropped in formalin, allowed to fix for at least an hour, and then cut in parallel slices.

Description

1 Dimensions: weight, if specimen is large
2 Pleura: thickness; fibrosis? fibrin? other changes?
3 Lung parenchyma: consolidated? diffuse interstitial fibrosis or well-defined nodules?

Sections for histology

1 Submit entire biopsy

LUNG—RESECTION FOR NONTUMORAL CONDITION

Lung resections include *segmentectomy* (removal of one or more of the eighteen segments in which the various pulmonary lobes are divided), *lobectomy* (removal of one or more of the five pulmonary lobes), and *pneumonectomy* (removal of one entire lung).

Procedure

1 Obtain cultures from lesions suspected of being infectious.
2 Weigh the specimen.
3 Two options are available depending on the type of abnormality present and the status of the organ when received in the laboratory:
   a Open the bronchi longitudinally with scissors and cut the lung parenchyma (including the lesion) in slices with a sharp knife.
   b Inject with formalin through the main bronchus, tie off or clamp the bronchus, fix overnight, and section at 0.5- to 1-cm intervals with a sharp knife or meat cutter. The sections should be frontal, perpendicular to the hilum. The slices formed by this procedure can be kept in order by stringing them on a piece of twine.
4 For lungs with tuberculosis and other contagious diseases (proven or suspected): fix in formalin for 48 hours; keep the specimen in the same container while dissecting and cutting the sections; send the contaminated instruments for sterilization; carefully wrap the contaminated material in a plastic bag and place in a scrap bucket.
5 For lungs with suspected asbestosis: scrape vigorously the cut surface of the lung with a scalpel, layer twenty successive scrapings onto a glass slide, let the preparation dry, stain lightly with toluidine blue or leave unstained, apply a mounting medium and coverslip, and examine microscopically.*
6 If a rib was submitted as part of the thoracotomy, examine according to instructions under Bone marrow—rib from thoracotomy.

Description

1 Weight of specimen and type of resection (pneumonectomy, lobectomy, wedge resection)
2 Pleura: thickness; fibrosis? fibrin? other changes?
3 Bronchi: mucosa, lumen (diameter and content)
4 Parenchyma: appearance; if localized lesion is present: appearance; lobe and, if possible, bronchopulmonary segment in which located; relationships to bronchi, vessels, pleura, and lymph nodes
5 Lymph nodes: number, size, and appearance

Sections for histology

1 Main lesions: three sections
2 Uninvolved lung: one section per lobe
3 Bronchus
4 Lymph nodes, if present: at least one section

---

*Mark EJ: The second diagnosis. The role of the pathologist in identifying pneumoconioses in lungs excised for tumor. Hum Pathol **12**:585-587, 1981.

LUNG—RESECTION FOR TUMOR*

Procedure

1 Dissect hilar lymph nodes as a single group and take out a cross section from the bronchial line of resection while the specimen is fresh.

2 Two options are available depending on the location of the tumor and the status of the organ when received in the laboratory:

    a Open all major bronchi and their branches longitudinally with scissors and follow this by cutting parallel slices of the lung, including tumor.

    b Inject with formalin through the main bronchus, tie off or clamp the bronchus, fix overnight, and section at 0.5- to 1-cm intervals with a sharp knife or meat cutter. The sections should be frontal, perpendicular to the hilum. The slices formed by this procedure can be kept in order by stringing them on a piece of twine.

3 If tuberculosis, other infections, or asbestosis is suspected in the non-neoplastic lung, proceed according to instructions listed under Lung—resection for nontumoral condition.

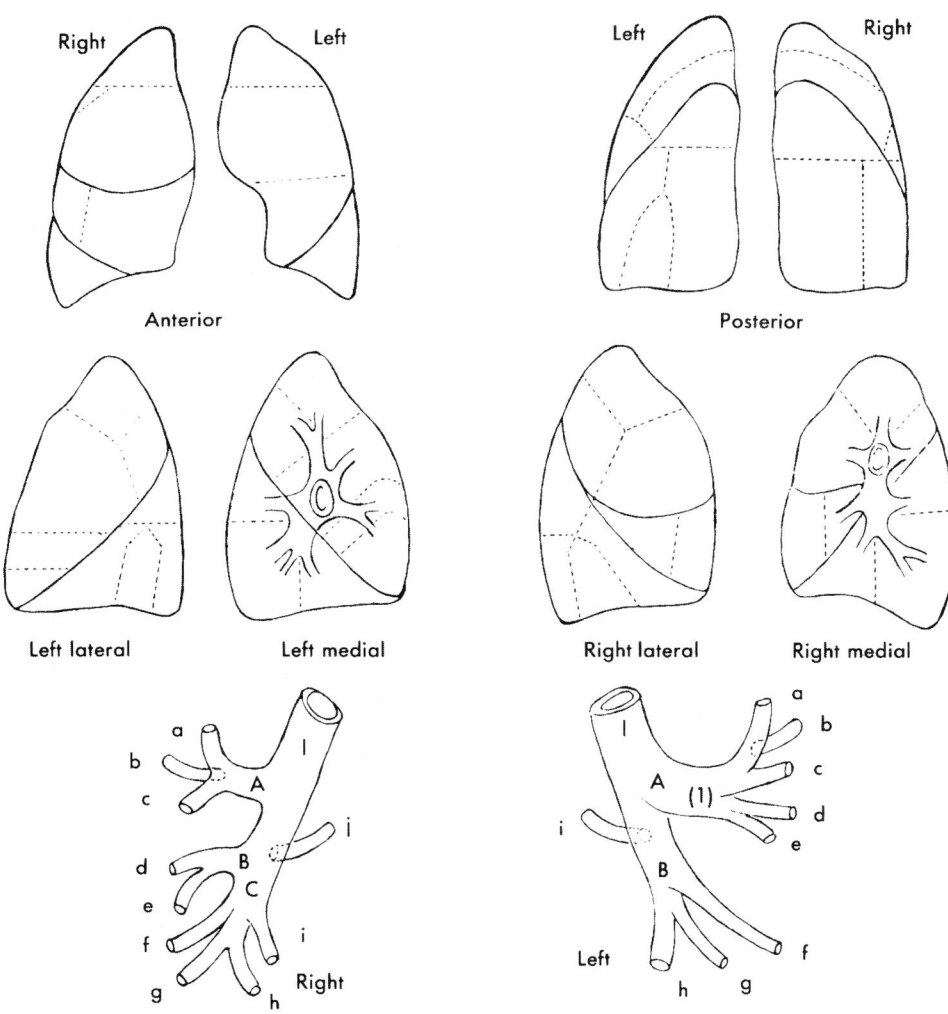

LUNG—RESECTION FOR TUMOR—cont'd

4 If a rib was submitted as part of the thoracotomy, examine according to instructions under Bone marrow—rib from the thoracotomy.

Description

1 Weight of fresh specimen and type of resection (pneumonectomy, lobectomy)
2 Pleura: fibrosis, fibrin, tumor invasion; parietal pleura present (identified by presence of fat)?
3 Tumor characteristics: size, location within lobe and segment, relation with bronchi, hemorrhage, necrosis, cavitation, blood vessel invasion, extension to pleura; distance to bronchial line of resection and pleura
4 Appearance of non-neoplastic lung
5 Number and appearance of regional lymph nodes

Sections for histology

1 Tumor: three sections, including one showing relationship to bronchus, if any
2 Non-neoplastic lung, including pleura: three sections, at least one from lung distal to tumor
3 Bronchial line of resection: one cross section comprising entire circumference
4 Lymph nodes: bronchopulmonary (hilar) and mediastinal
5 If rib submitted, process according to instructions under Bone marrow—rib from thoracotomy

*More detailed instructions are available from: Carler D: Pathologic examination of major pulmonary specimens resected for neoplastic disease. Pathol Annu **18**(Pt 2):315-332, 1983.

Brock's nomenclature	Jackson and Huber's nomenclature

Right bronchial tree (**I,** main bronchus; **A,** upper lobe bronchus; **B,** middle lobe bronchus; **C,** lower lobe bronchus)

a *Apical* bronchus, upper lobe	a *Apical* bronchus, upper lobe
b *Subapical* bronchus, upper lobe	b *Anterior* bronchus, upper lobe
c *Pectoral* bronchus, upper lobe	c *Posterior* bronchus, upper lobe
d *Medial* division, middle lobe	d *Medial* division, middle lobe
e *Lateral* division, middle lobe	e *Lateral* division, middle lobe
f *Anterior basal* bronchus, lower lobe	f *Anterior basal* bronchus, lower lobe
g *Middle basal* bronchus, lower lobe	g *Lateral basal* bronchus, lower lobe
h *Posterior basal* bronchus, lower lobe	h *Posterior basal* bronchus, lower lobe
I *Cardiac* bronchus, lower lobe	i *Medial basal* bronchus, lower lobe
j *Apical* bronchus, lower lobe	j *Superior* bronchus, lower lobe

Left bronchial tree (**I,** main bronchus; **A,** upper lobe bronchus; **B,** lower lobe bronchus; **(1),** lingular bronchus)

a *Apical* bronchus, upper lobe	a *Superior division,* upper lobe
b *Subapical* bronchus, upper lobe	b *Apical posterior,* upper lobe
c *Pectoral* bronchus, upper lobe	c *Anterior* bronchus, upper lobe
d *Upper division, lingular,* upper lobe	d *Superior lingular, inferior division,* upper lobe
e *Lower division, lingular,* upper lobe	e *Inferior lingular, inferior division,* upper lobe
f *Anterior basal* bronchus, lower lobe	f *Anterior-medial basal,* lower lobe
g *Middle basal* bronchus, lower lobe	g *Lateral basal,* lower lobe
h *Posterior basal* bronchus, lower lobe	h *Posterior basal,* lower lobe
i *Apical* bronchus, lower lobe	i *Superior bronchus,* lower lobe

LYMPH NODE—BIOPSY

Procedure

1 If the lymph node is received in the fresh state, cut 2- to 3-mm slices perpendicular to the long axis and:
   a Take a small portion for culture if an infectious disease is suspected or needs to be ruled out.
   b Make four imprints of the cut surface on alcohol-cleaned slides, fix in methanol, and stain two with hematoxylin-eosin and two with Wright's stain. See instructions for Imprints (touch preparations).
   c Place one of the slices in B5 fixative and submit for histology.
   d In cases of suspected hematolymphoid disorders, submit tissue for cell markers (by flow cytometry), cytogenetics, and molecular genetics (see respective sections for instructions).
   e If additional tissue is available, fix in formalin and submit for histology.
2 If the specimen is received already fixed in formalin, cut in 3-mm slices and submit representative sections.

Description

1 State whether node received fresh or fixed
2 Size of node and condition of capsule
3 Appearance of cut surface: color, nodularity, hemorrhage, necrosis

Sections for histology

Cross section of node, including at least portion of capsule: one to three sections depending on size of node

LYMPH NODE DISSECTION—GENERAL INSTRUCTIONS

Procedure

1 Dissect the node-containing fat from the organ in the fresh state, using forceps and sharp scissors. Make the fat dissection as close as possible to the wall of the organ; this is where most lymph nodes are located. Divide them in groups according to specific instructions.
2 Two options are available:
   a Search the fat for nodes while specimen is fresh, under a strong light and with the use of scissors, forceps, and scalpel. Avoid crushing the nodes by rough palpation. If not enough nodes are identified, contact the senior pathologist or surgeon.
   b Fix overnight in formalin or Carnoy's solution, and search for nodes the next day. The latter fixative is preferred because it clears the fat somewhat.

Description

1 Number of nodes in each group
2 Size of largest node in each group
3 Appearance; obvious involvement by tumor?

Sections for histology

1 *All* lymph nodes should be submitted for histology.
2 Small nodes (up to 3 mm in thickness after fat is removed) are submitted as a single piece.
3 Several small node groups may be submitted in the same cassette.
4 Larger nodes are bisected and, if necessary, further sectioned into 2- to 3-mm slices. A slice as large as will fit the cassette should be submitted for each one of these larger nodes.
5 Store the remainder in the formalin container, properly identified as belonging to lymph node group.

LYMPH NODE DISSECTION—AXILLARY

See under Breast—mastectomy.

LYMPH NODE DISSECTION—INGUINAL

1 All lymph nodes are submitted as a single group unless the surgeon has submitted the superficial and deep groups separately. A minimum of twelve lymph nodes should be found.
2 A cross section of the internal saphenous vein also should be submitted for histology.

LYMPH NODE DISSECTION—RADICAL NECK

The *standard* radical neck dissection includes removal of cervical lymph nodes, sternomastoid muscle, internal jugular vein, spinal accessory nerve, and submaxillary gland; the tail of the parotid is sometimes also included.

In the *modified* radical neck dissection (also known as functional or Bocca neck dissection), the sternomastoid muscle, spinal accessory nerve, and internal jugular vein are spared.

The *extended* radical neck dissection includes, in addition to the structures removed in the standard operation, the excision of retropharyngeal, paratracheal, parotid, suboccipital, and/or upper mediastinal lymph nodes.

In the *regional* (partial or selective) neck dissection, only the station of lymph nodes thought to represent the first metastatic station is removed.

The instructions following are devised for the standard radical neck dissection and need to be modified for the other three. Because of the lack of anatomic landmarks in the modified and regional procedures, the labeling of the lymph nodes according to groups needs to be done by the surgeon. The same applies to the extra lymph node groups removed in the extended operation.

Procedure

1 Orient the specimen and divide it into submaxillary gland, platysma, sternomastoid muscle, internal jugular veins, and node-containing fat.
2 Divide the lymph nodes into six groups depending on whether they are on the upper or lower portion of the specimen and on their relationship with the sternomastoid muscle (see accompanying drawing). A minimum of forty lymph nodes should be found.*

Description

1 Site and type of primary neoplasm (see specific instructions)
2 Length of sternomastoid muscle
3 Jugular vein included? length? invaded by tumor?
4 Presence of tumor in lymph nodes, submaxillary gland, soft tissue, or muscle
5 Size of the largest node

LYMPH NODE DISSECTION—RADICAL NECK—cont'd

Sections for histology

1 Superior anterior cervical lymph nodes
2 Superior jugular cervical lymph nodes
3 Superior posterior cervical lymph nodes
4 Inferior anterior cervical lymph nodes
5 Inferior jugular cervical lymph nodes
6 Inferior posterior cervical lymph nodes
7 Submaxillary gland
8 Jugular vein
9 Sternocleidomastoid muscle
10 Thyroid gland, if present

*Other pathologists use an alternative scheme in which lymph nodes are divided into five regions: anterior (submental and submandibular), superior jugular, middle jugular, inferior jugular, and posterior (posterior triangle).

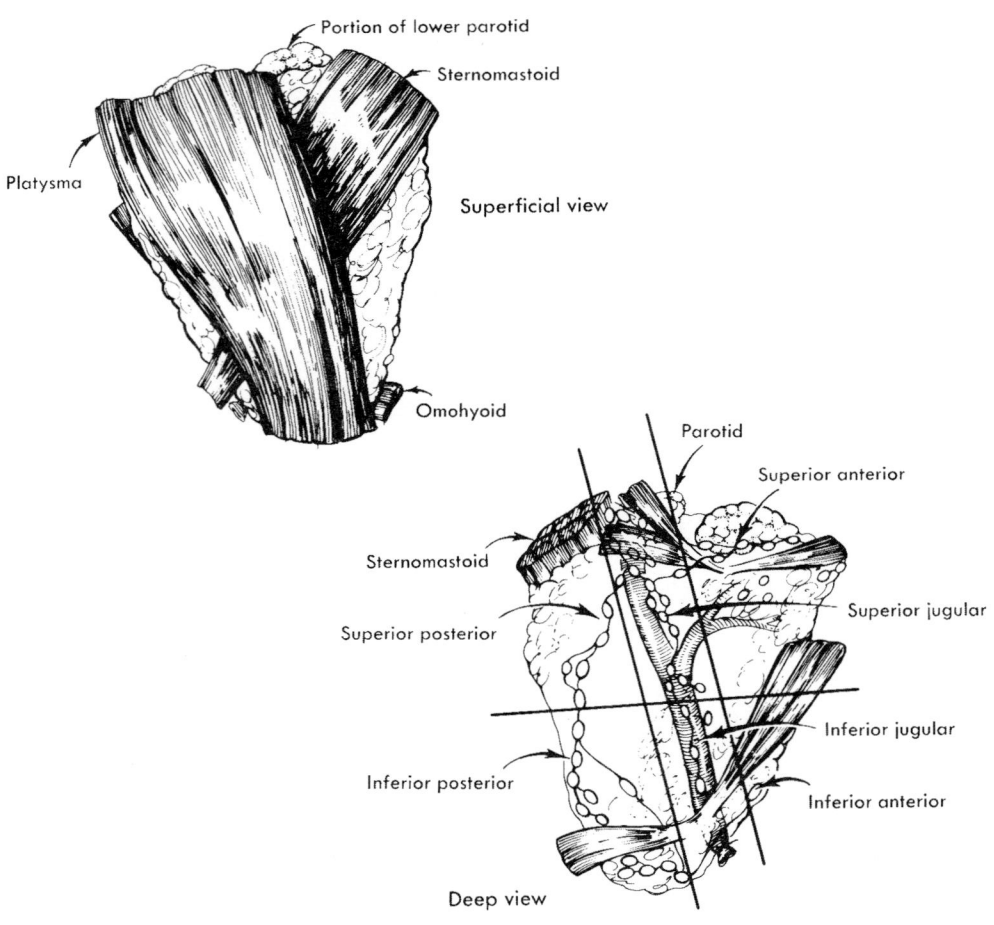

LYMPH NODE DISSECTION—RETROPERITONEAL

1 For the proper evaluation of this specimen, it is essential for the surgeon to divide the lymph nodes in groups at the time he is doing the dissection and submit them to the laboratory in separate containers. In most institutions, urologic surgeons divide the node groups as follows:
  - Suprahilar (above level of renal artery)
  - Superior interaortocaval
  - Pericaval
  - Periaortic
  - Common iliac (usually excised only on side of tumor)

2 If the specimen is submitted as a single piece, it is necessary to identify, with the help of the surgeon, the upper and lower borders and the periaortic and pericaval regions. When this is established, the lymph nodes can be divided in the following groups:
  - Superior periaortic
  - Middle periaortic
  - Inferior periaortic
  - Superior pericaval
  - Middle pericaval
  - Inferior pericaval
  - Common iliac (specify side)

3 If the surgeon is unavailable or unable to orient the specimen, all lymph nodes are submitted as one group. A minimum of twenty-five lymph nodes should be found.

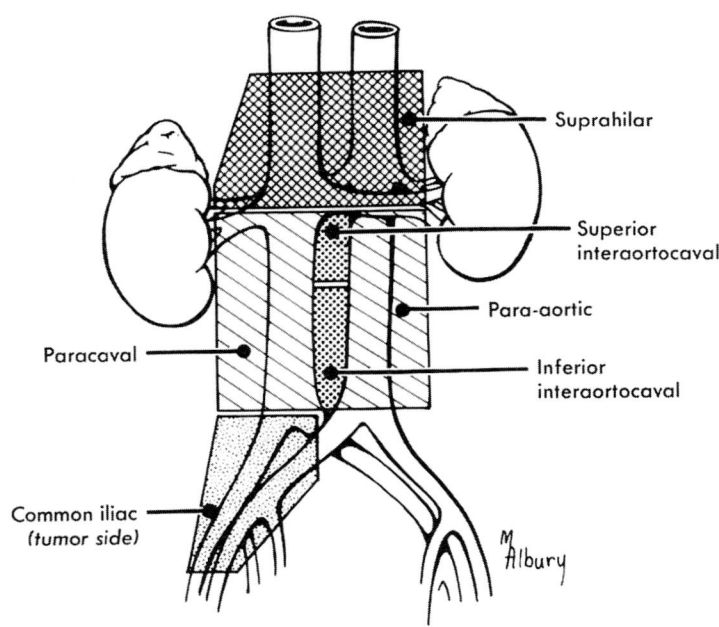

MOLECULAR DIAGNOSIS—SAMPLING

Evaluation of tissue using molecular techniques has rapidly become a very important diagnostic procedure, particularly for the evaluation of the hematolymphoid processes and pediatric malignancies, such as Ewing's sarcoma/PNET and neuroblastoma.

Sample 1 cm³ of fresh tumor tissue (or as much as available), drop in Petri dish having in its bottom a layer of filter paper wet (not overly soaked) with saline solution, and submit to appropriate laboratory immediately. If prompt transportation is not feasible, freeze at −70° C until time of use.

NEEDLE BIOPSIES

Procedure

1 Remove the tissue from the fixative without squeezing it with a forceps; do not use toothed forceps; handle the tissue in such a manner as to keep it intact; do not cut it transversely but rather coil it inside the cassette if overly long.
2 Always search the container, including the undersurface of the lid, for tiny fragments of tissue that may be overlooked.
3 Carefully wrap the tissue in a tea bag, without squeezing.
4 If the amount of the tissue core permits (a core over 1 cm long or two tissue cores) and if it would be anticipated that a fat stain may be useful, save a 3- to 5-mm portion in formalin.

Description

1 Length and diameter of core; number of fragments; color
2 Homogeneity or lack of it

Sections for histology

All material received (except if fat stains desired, see under Procedure)

ORBITAL EXENTERATION

Procedure

1 Pin down the elliptic piece of orbicular skin, and fix overnight at 4° C.
2 Paint the surgical margins with India Ink.
3 Take surgical margins: cutaneous, soft tissue, optic nerve.
4 Cut skin, soft tissue, and ocular globe.

Description

1 Skin: shape and length; appearance; if lesion present: size, shape, depth of invasion, color
2 Soft tissues
3 Ocular globe: dimensions, appearance, length of optic nerve (see under Eyes—enucleation)

Sections for histology
For skin tumors

1 Tumor: three sections
2 Cutaneous surgical margins (superior, inferior, internal, and external)
3 Soft tissue surgical margins
4 Ocular globe

For ocular tumors

1 Globe with tumor
2 Orbital soft tissue adjacent to tumor
3 Surgical margin of optic nerve

ORIENTATION OF SPECIMENS WITH AGAR

1 Prepare beforehand a 3% solution of "bacteriologic" agar, divide in 1- to 2-ml samples, and place in small test tubes. Keep these samples at 4° C in the refrigerator until the time of use.

2 Heat the test tube on a specially prepared hot plate until the agar acquires a semiviscid consistency. The temperature should be around 60° C, and it is important to keep it as close as possible to this figure (otherwise, the agar will not melt or will become too fluid). The melting of the agar should take no more than 1 to 2 minutes. It is convenient to heat as many test tubes in the morning as will be needed during the working day. However, it is advised not to keep the agar at 60° C longer than 24 to 48 hours.

3 Pick up the specimen gently with a small forceps and place it in the desired position ("on edge") on top of a glass slide (see accompanying drawing).

4 While holding the specimen in this position with one hand, use the other hand to drop a small amount of melted agar on top of the specimen with a Pasteur pipette. Do not use an excessive amount. The solidifying process can be speeded up by gently blowing in the agar. When the agar has solidified just enough for the tissue to remain in the desired position without support (it should take no more than 1 minute), remove the forceps and wait an additional 1 or 2 minutes.

5 Detach the tissue surrounded by the agar from the glass slide by sliding a blade beneath it (see accompanying drawing), and transfer the material to the cassette. If the size is very small, it may be necessary to wrap it in lens paper or a tea bag.

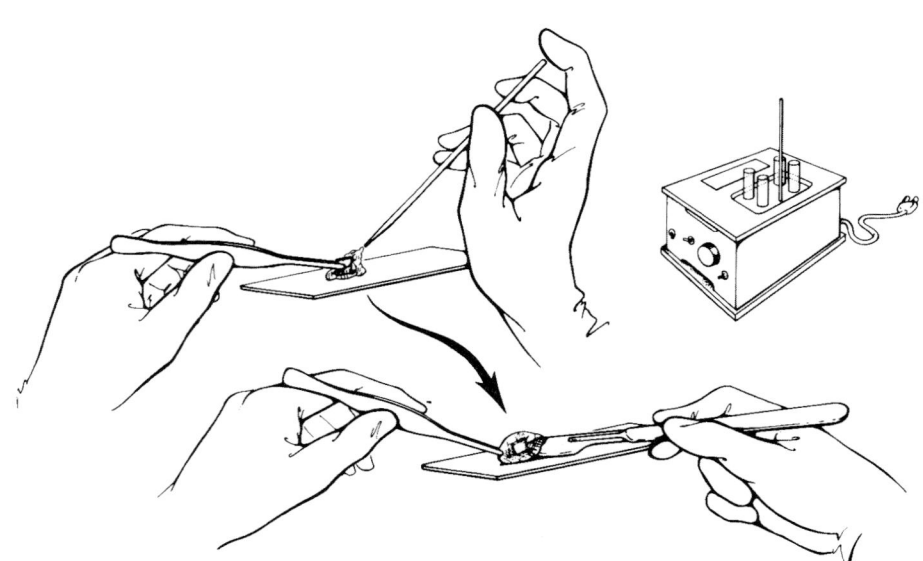

OVARY—OOPHORECTOMY

Oophorectomies may be total or partial. The most common type of conservative operation is the removal of an ovarian cyst with preservation of the uninvolved parenchyma (ovarian cystectomy).

Procedure

1 Measure the organ. Weigh it if it is obviously abnormal.
2 If the specimen is received fresh:
   a **Normal-sized** or nearly normal-sized organ: bivalve and fix for several hours.
   b **Enlarged** organ: Make several cuts and fix for several hours.

Description

1 Size and shape; weight, if enlarged
2 Capsule: thickened? adhesions? hemorrhage? rupture? external surface smooth or irregular?
3 Cut section: character of cortex, medulla, and hilum; cysts (size and content); corpus luteum? calcification? hemorrhage?
4 Tumors: size; external appearance: smooth or papillary? solid or cystic? content of cystic masses; hemorrhage, necrosis, or calcification?

Sections for histology

1 For incidental oophorectomies: one sagittal section of each entire ovary, labeled as to side
2 For cysts: up to three sections of cyst wall (particularly from areas with papillary appearance)
3 For tumors: three sections or one section for each centimeter of tumor, whichever is greater; also, one section of non-neoplastic ovary, if identifiable

PANCREAS—PANCREATECTOMY

The *Whipple's procedure* consists of partial pancreatectomy plus partial gastrectomy and duodenectomy. *Total pancreatectomy* consists of removal of the entire pancreas plus partial gastrectomy, duodenectomy, and splenectomy. *Regional pancreatectomy type I* consists of total pancreatectomy plus partial gastrectomy, cholecystectomy, duodenectomy, splenectomy, and resection of portal vein. It may also include transverse colectomy and removal of mesocolon, omentum, and regional lymph nodes. *Regional pancreatectomy type II* includes, in addition to the procedures listed under type I, the resection of mesenteric vessels, celiac axis vessels, and/or a segment of vena cava and aorta. *Distal pancreatectomy* consists in resection of the tail of the pancreas (often with a portion of the body) plus splenectomy.

Procedure

1 Dissect lymph nodes while the specimen is fresh and divide them according to groups (see accompanying drawing).
2 Fill the stomach and duodenum with gauze or cotton impregnated with formalin.
3 Pin the whole specimen on a corkboard, trying to preserve the anatomic relationships.
4 Place in a large container, cover with formalin, and fix overnight at 4° C.
5 Paint with India ink the common bile duct surgical margin, as well as the pancreatic surgical margin in a Whipple's procedure.
6 Divide the specimen into anterior and posterior halves as follows: with scissors, cut the lesser curvature of the stomach and the free border of the duodenum; with scissors, cut the gastric greater curvature up to the pancreas, as well as the fourth portion of the duodenum; with a large sharp knife, cut the peripancreatic border of the duodenum; and the pancreas. The orientation of the latter cut can be better controlled by introducing a catheter through the common bile duct and by cutting in front of it. It may be necessary to postfix the two halves overnight before proceeding to further dissection, as indicated.

Description

1 Type of operation: Whipple's procedure, total pancreatectomy, regional pancreatectomy type I or II, distal pancreatectomy
2 Organs present in specimen and their dimensions; weight of spleen
3 Tumor characteristics: involvement of ampulla, duodenal mucosa, stomach, common bile duct, pancreatic duct, and pancreas; size, shape (papillary? flat? ulcerated?), color, and consistency; if tumor is in the ampulla: intra-ampullary, periampullary, or mixed?
4 Common bile duct, main pancreatic duct, and accessory pancreatic duct: location and relationship with each other; dilated? stones? tumor?
5 Pancreas: tumor invasion? atrophy? fibrosis? ductal dilatation?
6 Spleen: tumor invasion? other features
7 Location, number, and appearance of regional lymph nodes

Sections for histology

1 Tumor: up to three sections
2 Pancreas: three sections, one from distal line of resection (or proximal, depending on the type of specimen)
3 Common bile duct: two cross sections, one from surgical margin
4 Uninvolved duodenum: two sections, one from distal line of resection
5 Stomach: two sections, including proximal line of resection
6 Lymph nodes*:

PANCREAS—PANCREATECTOMY—cont'd

- Peripancreatic (superior and inferior)
- Pancreaticoduodenal (anterior and posterior)
- Common bile duct and pericystic
- Lesser curvature
- Greater curvature
- Splenic
- Other groups, if present (jejunal, midcolic, omental)

7 Other organs, if present (gallbladder, spleen, portal vein, colon, omentum)

Other authors* divide these lymph nodes into the following five major groups:

1 Superior: superior margin of head and body of pancreas, common bile duct, and stomach (greater and lesser curvature and pylorus)

2 Inferior: inferior margin of head and body of pancreas, around mesenteric vessels, jejunal, gastrocolonic ligaments, pericolonic, and periaortic

3 Anterior (anterior pancreaticoduodenal): along the anterior surface of the head of the pancreas

4 Posterior (posterior pancreaticoduodenal): along the posterior surface of the head of the pancreas

5 Splenic: splenic hilum

---

*Cubilla AL, Fitzgerald PJ: Suggested technic for examining the resected pancreas. Tumors of the exocrine pancreas, appendix A. Atlas of tumor pathology, 2nd Series, Fasc 19. Washington, D.C., 1982, Armed Forces Institute of Pathology, pp 257-261.

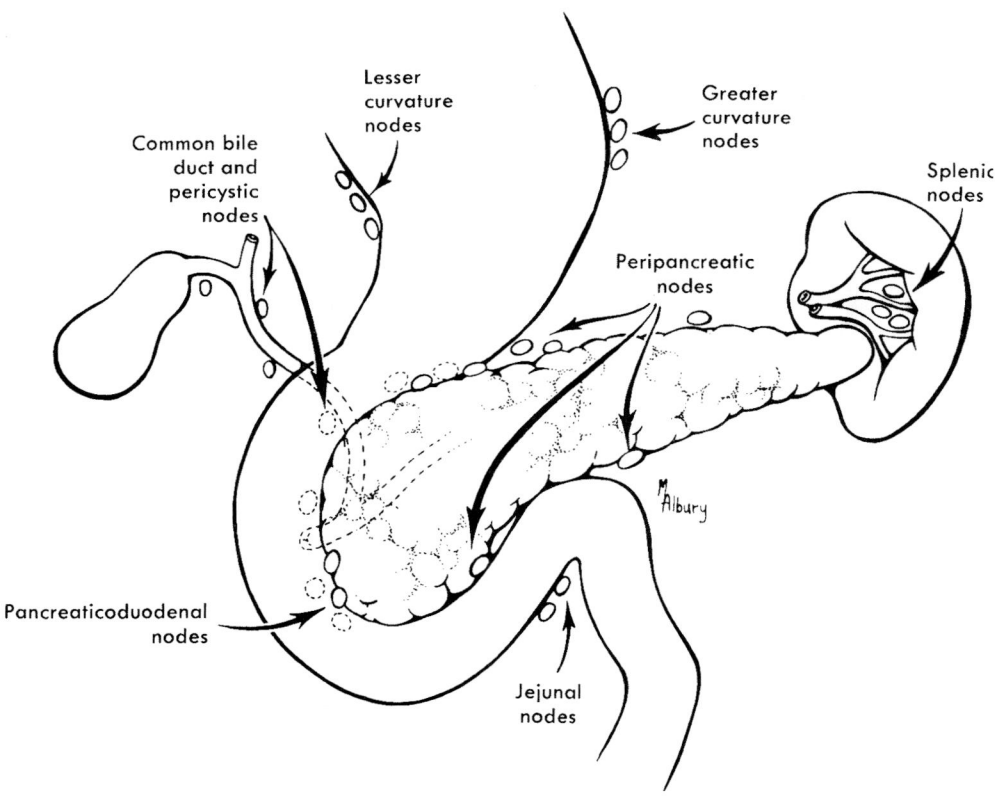

PARATHYROID GLANDS—PARATHYROIDECTOMY

Removal of diseased parathyroid glands is usually complete, but in cases of hyperplasia a portion (approximately one half) of one gland is retained, in situ or implanted in the forearm.

Procedure

1 Accurately weigh each gland on a delicate balance after removing the surrounding fat but *before* removing any parathyroid tissue for frozen or other sections.
2 Accurately label each parathyroid gland as to site.

Description

Weight, color, consistency, and external appearance of *each* gland

Sections for histology

All parathyroid tissue (except for markedly enlarged gland in which minimum of three sections should be taken) accurately labeled as to site

PELVIC EXENTERATION

Most pelvic exenterations are performed on females because of postradiation persistence of carcinoma of uterine cervix. Anterior pelvic exenteration consists of removal of the vagina, uterus and adnexa, bladder, distal ureters, and urethra. Posterior pelvic exenteration consists of removal of the vagina, uterus and adnexa, and rectum. Total pelvic exenteration is a combination of the two procedures. The operation also includes removal of the pelvic lymph nodes.

Procedure

1 Gently express content from the rectosigmoid, wash with formalin or saline solution, and fill with cotton or gauze impregnated in formalin.
2 Fill the vagina with the same material.
3 Inject the bladder with formalin with a Foley catheter or syringe after tying the urethra.
4 Suspend the specimen in anatomic position in a large container with abundant fixative.
5 Inject formalin in the uterine cavity with a syringe through the fundus.
6 Fix for 24 hours.
7 Removal all cotton and gauze and cut sagittally in equal halves. The sections of large bowel, bladder, and vagina are made with scissors; those of the uterus are made with a knife.
8 Take two Polaroid photographs or photocopies and identify in one of them the site of the sections to be taken.
9 Remove the lymph nodes in the following groups: right parametrial, left parametrial, retrorectal, and mesosigmoid.
10 Paint the surgical margins with India ink.

Description

1 Type of exenteration: total, anterior, posterior; organs included; length of ureters
2 Tumor characteristics: location, invasion of other structures, size, color, consistency; fistulae? signs of radiation change?
3 Number and appearance of lymph nodes

Sections for histology

1 Tumor: three sections or one section per centimeter of tumor, whichever is greater
2 Cervix and vagina
3 Cervix and bladder
4 Cervix and rectum
5 Surgical margins (parametrial, vaginal, vesical, and rectal)
6 *In females:* vulva, vagina, cervix endometrium, tubes, ovaries (in addition to sections from tumor)
7 *In males:* prostate
8 Lymph nodes:
   • Right parametrial
   • Left parametrial
   • Retrorectal
   • Mesosigmoid

PENIS—PENECTOMY

Procedure

1 If the specimen is accompanied by inguinal node dissections, separate them and handle according to specific instructions.
2 Introduce a catheter through the urethra.
3 Fix overnight at 4° C.
4 Paint the surgical margins (including the urethra) with India ink.
5 Cut longitudinally through the center; the section should cut the urethra in two.
6 Take two Polaroid photographs or photocopies and identify in one of them the site of the sections to be taken.

Description

1 Type of operation: partial, total, with or without scrotal skin, testicles, inguinal nodes
2 Length and diameter of specimen
3 Tumor: location in relations to glans, prepuce, skin, and urethra; size, color, borders, depth of invasion
4 Glans penis: balanitis? atrophy? leukoplakia?
5 Urethra: invaded by tumor?

Sections for histology

1 Tumor: three sections
2 Glans penis and urethra
3 Surgical margin (including urethra)

PERIPHERAL NERVE—BIOPSY

Procedure

1 The examination and sampling of this material should be carried out at the bedside or *immediately* after the specimen is received in the pathology laboratory. Be careful to avoid stretching or crushing.
2 Measure the length and diameter (biopsies of the sural nerve usually measure between 3 and 6 cm).
3 For paraffin embedding, cut a portion 2 to 4 mm long from either end, fix in B5, and postfix in formalin. Divide the specimen so that a cross section and a longitudinal section are obtained.
4 For "thick sections" and electron microscopy, fix a portion in 2.5% glutaraldehyde in 0.05M cacodylate buffer at pH 7.4 (osmolarity ≈340). After 2 hours of fixation, the nerve is placed under a dissecting microscope and divided into 3- to 4-mm segments. Four to five of these pieces are submitted in large blocks, whereas the others are sectioned along a longitudinal plane. Twenty to thirty pieces are thus obtained, each having two to three fascicles. For electron microscopy, 1- to 2-mm^3 fragments should be submitted.
5 If facilities are available for fiber teasing preparations, a 1- to 2-cm nerve segment should be dissected and, immediately after biopsy, fixed in formalin, postfixed in O_5O_4 in Millonig's buffer at pH 7.4 for 3 to 5 hours at room temperature, and passed through graded glycerine, where it can be kept until time of observation.
6 If indicated, a small piece of fresh nerve should be "snap frozen" for biochemical studies, lipid staining, and immunofluorescent techniques.

Description

1 Length and diameter
2 Color
3 Irregularities

Sections for histology

1 One cross section and one longitudinal section for paraffin embedding
2 For other portions of biopsy, see under Procedure

PLACENTA—SINGLETON

Procedure and description

1 Examine as soon as possible after delivery in the fresh state; handle the specimen with great care, avoiding lacerations.

2 Note the amount of blood and clots in the container and search for separate pieces of membranes, cord, or placenta.

3 Examine in this order: membranes, cord, fetal surface, and maternal surface.

4 Measure the distance from the placental margin to the nearest point of rupture (zero: marginal placenta previa).

5 Examine membranes for completeness (if a portion is missing, notify the obstetrician), insertion, decidual necrosis, edema, extra-amniotic pregnancy, retromembranous hemorrhage, meconium staining, color, and transparency.

6 Take a long, 2- to 3-cm wide section of membranes beginning with the point of rupture and extending to and including a small portion of placental margin. Roll the specimen with amniotic surface inward, fix for 24 hours, take a 3-mm section from the center (taking care not to strip the amnion off), and submit for histology. Take a second section including amnion, chorion, and decidua from the rim of the site rupture (in vaginal deliveries).

7 Trim the remaining membranes from the placental margin.

8 Measure the length of the cord and the shortest distance from the cord insertion to the placental margin.

9 Examine the cord: insertion (nonmembranous or membranous; if latter, are vessels intact?), number of umbilical vessels (by sectioning the cord transversely at two or more points), color, true knots, torsion, stricture, hematoma, thrombosis.

10 Remove the cord from the placenta 3 cm proximal to the insertion, and take a 2 - to 4-cm segment from its midpoint; fix this segment for 24 hours, take a 3-mm section, and submit for histology.

11 Examine the fetal surface: color, opacity, subchorionic fibrin, cysts (number and size), amnion nodosum, squamous metaplasia, thrombosis of fetal surface vessels, chorangioma.

12 Examine the maternal surface: completeness, normal fissures, laceration (extent), depressed areas, retroplacental hemorrhage (size and distance from margin).

13 Measure the maximum diameter, thickness in the center, weight (after trimming cord and membranes), shape.

14 Hold the placenta gently with one hand, maternal side up on a flat surface, and make parallel sections with a large sharp knife at 10-cm intervals. The fetal surface will not be cut through and will hold the specimen together.

15 Remove four 2-cm pieces that include the fetal surface and intact maternal surface, selecting tissues of the placenta (within 2 cm of placental margins). Take the piece so that the fetal surface vessels are cut at right angles to their long axis; fix for 24 hours, trim a 3-mm section (through and through), and submit for histology. One section should include the chorionic plate in an area with minimal subchorionic fibrin. The other sections should include the maternal surface. Submit similar sections of any lesions present.

16 Examine all cross sections for infarcts (location, size, number); intervillous thrombi (number); laminate, perivillous fibrin deposition, pallor, consistency, calcification (extent), cysts, tumors. Describe lesion location (central, lateral, or marginal), depth (parabasal, intermediate, or subchorionic), and age (recent or old).

Sections for histology

1 Placenta (as indicated previously plus abnormal areas, if present)
2 Membranes
3 Cord

PLACENTA—TWIN

Procedure and description

1 If placentas are separate (nonfused): examine each placenta as a singleton.

2 If placentas are fused:

   a Note whether the two cords are labeled twin A and twin B. If not, label them arbitrarily and make a statement to that effect.

   b Determine the presence and type of dividing membranes:

   (1) If absent (monochorionic-monoamniotic), so state.

   (2) If present:

   (a) Remove a square of the dividing membrane, roll it, fix it for 24 hours, take a 3-mm section, and submit for histology.

   (b) Attempt to determine grossly whether the dividing membrane has chorion or not, according to the accompanying tables.

   (c) Record the kind and number of vascular anastomoses in monochorionic-diamniotic placentas: artery-to-artery, vein-to-vein, artery-to-vein (arteriovenous shunts). The latter can be better demonstrated by injecting the artery of one twin along the plane of fusion of the placenta with 30 to 50 ml of saline solution containing a dye and noting whether the fluid emerges from the vein of the other twin through one or more common villous lobules. The placenta must be intact to perform this test. Arteries always run over veins.

   c Divide the fused twin placenta along the "vascular equator" (rather than through the base of the dividing membrane).

   d Examine each half as a singleton placenta.

Sections for histology

1 Placenta from twin A

2 Membranes from twin A

3 Cord from twin A

4 Placenta from twin B

5 Membranes from twin B

6 Cord from twin B

7 Dividing membrane, if present

PLACENTA—TWIN—cont'd

Table App H-3 Dividing membrane in twin placentas

Features	Dichorionic-diamniotic (fused)	Monochorionic-diamniotic
Appearance	Thick and opaque	Thin and transparent
Separation of membranes by stripping	Difficult	Easy
Point of attachment to fetal surface	Ridge or tearing of chorion	Smooth and continuous, without ridge
Vascular anastomoses	Very rare	Numerous

Table App H-4 Types of twin placentas

Type	Incidence	Gross	Twin type
Dichorionic-diamniotic (separate)	35%		Monozygotic or dizygotic
Dichorionic-diamniotic (fused)	34%		Monozygotic or dizygotic
Monochorionic-diamniotic	30%		Monozygotic
Monochorionic-monoamniotic	1%		Monozygotic

PROSTATE GLAND—RADICAL PROSTATECTOMY FOR TUMOR

This procedure can carried out through the retropubic or the perineal route.

Procedure

1 Fix the whole specimen in formalin at 4° C overnight.
2 Paint the surgical margins with India ink.
3 Amputate the distal 5 mm of the gland, divide cone thus obtained into right and left halves, and serially section (see under Sections for histology)
4 Shave off the bladder neck area (see under Sections for histology)
5 Make parallel transverse slices, about 3 mm thick, and examine the cut surfaces carefully.
6 Take two Polaroid photographs or photocopies of the slices to be submitted for histology and identify in one of them the site of the sections taken.

Description

1 Weight and dimensions of specimen
2 Organs present: whole prostate? urethra (length), seminal vesicles, vas, lymph nodes
3 **a** Prostate: tumor (location in lobes, size, color, borders, capsular and periprostatic extension)
  b Non-neoplastic prostate: nodular hyperplasia?
4 Urethra: patent? impinged by tumor?
5 Seminal vesicles: involved by tumor?

Sections for histology

1 Tumor: minimum of three sections, including capsule and urethra
2 Non-neoplastic prostate: at least two sections from each quadrant
3 Seminal vesicles: proximal, mid, and distal portions from each side
4 Urethral (apical) surgical margin: distal 5 mm of the gland divided into right and left, serially sectioned, and submitted in toto
5 Bladder neck: shave from the bladder neck area, submitted in toto

PROSTATE GLAND—SUPRAPUBIC PROSTATECTOMY FOR NODULAR HYPERPLASIA

Procedure

1 Step section the specimen 3-mm slices, either in the fresh state or after formalin fixation.
2 Examine *each slice* carefully for areas suspicious of carcinoma (yellow areas or foci that are harder or softer than the rest of the specimen).

Description

1 Weight of specimen
2 Shape, color, and consistency
3 Presence of hyperplastic nodules, cysts, calculi, areas suspicious of carcinoma

Sections for histology

1 Left lobe: three sections
2 Right lobe: three sections
3 Middle lobe

PROSTATE GLAND—TRANSURETHRAL RESECTION (TUR)

Procedure

1 Weigh with accurate balance.
2 Carefully examine all the fragments. Carcinoma of the prostate is often yellow and/or hard; submit for histology chips with these gross characteristics.

Description

1 Weight of specimen
2 Size, shape, and color of chips

Sections for histology

1 *If all fragments received in a single container*
   a All of specimen until four cassettes filled
   b If an excess, one additional cassette for each additional 10 g of tissue (each cassette holds approximately 2 g)
2 *If fragments received are identified as to lobe from which they were taken,* submit as follows for each specimen (lobe) received:
   a All of specimen until four cassettes filled
   b If an excess, one additional cassette for each additional 10 g of tissue
   c Identify in following order (not all lobes may have been biopsied in some cases):
   • Anterior lobe
   • Middle lobe
   • Posterior lobe
   • Left lateral lobe
   • Right lateral lobe
   d If carcinoma is identified microscopically in a specimen that was not entirely submitted, the remainder of the tissue should be processed in its entirety, regardless of amount.

SALIVARY GLAND—RESECTION FOR TUMOR

The three most common types of operation performed because of salivary gland tumors are superficial parotidectomy (also known as lateral lobectomy, consisting of removal of the superficial lobe of the gland with preservation of the facial nerve), total parotidectomy (removal of both superficial and deep lobes, usually with sacrifice of the facial nerve), and total submaxillectomy.

Procedure

1 Paint surgical margins with India ink.
2 Fix *in toto* or bisect in the fresh state, depending on size of specimen.
3 Cut parallel sections.
4 Look for intraparotid lymph nodes and for major nerves in total parotidectomy specimens.
5 If the specimen includes a radical neck dissection, process according to instructions for Lymph node dissection—radical neck.

Description

1 Type of specimen: parotid lobectomy, total parotidectomy without facial nerve, total parotidectomy with facial nerve, total submandibulectomy; side of operation
2 Tumor: size, location, shape, distance from closet margin; solitary or multiple? cystic or solid? encapsulated, circumscribed, or poorly defined? hemorrhage or necrosis? extraglandular extension?
3 Appearance of non-neoplastic gland
4 Appearance of intraparotid and other lymph nodes

Sections for histology

1 Tumor: four or more, depending on size; capsule or tumor margins should be included
2 Non-neoplastic gland
3 Surgical margins
4 Facial nerve margins, if included
5 Lymph nodes, if included

SKELETAL MUSCLE—BIOPSY

Procedure

The proper evaluation of a skeletal muscle biopsy includes routine processing and staining, enzyme histochemistry, and electron microscopic examination.

1 *Routine processing:* The specimen is usually received stretched on a special muscle biopsy clamp. It should remain on the clamp for overnight fixation. If the specimen is received fresh, pin it to a corkboard and fix overnight.

2 *Enzyme histochemistry:* Freeze a small fragment in liquid nitrogen. It is important for this to be a cross section. Freeze also a longitudinal section if enough tissue is available.

3 *Electron microscopy:* See instructions under Electron microscopy—sampling.

Description

1 Dimensions of specimen
2 Color and consistency; fibrosis? edema? necrosis?

Sections for histology

1 One longitudinal section
2 One cross section

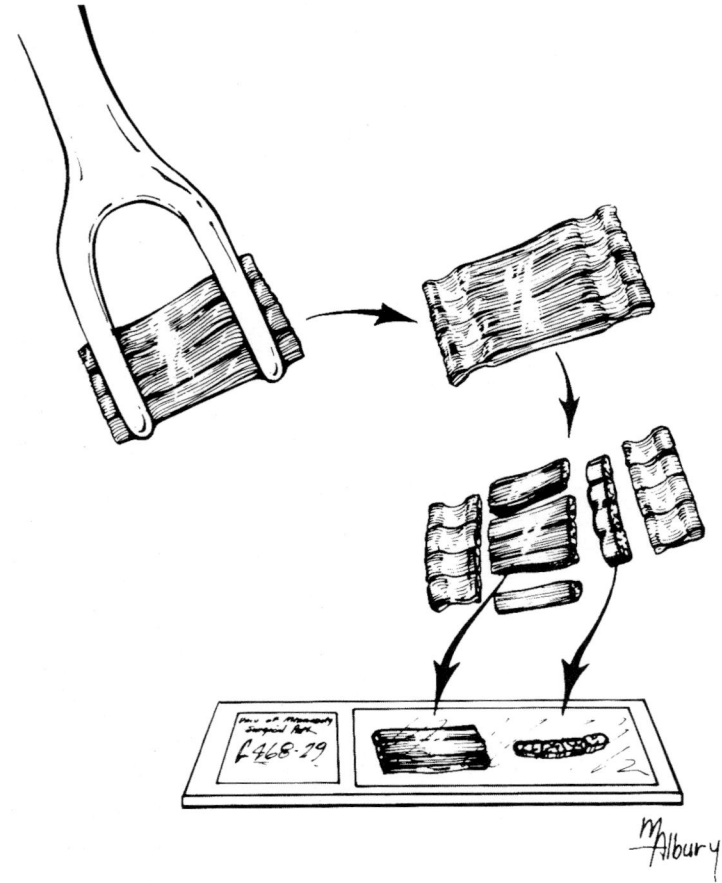

SKIN—EXCISION FOR BENIGN LESION

Procedure

1 Pigmented nevi, seborrheic keratoses, and other benign skin conditions (as well as small basal cell carcinomas) are usually removed with narrow margins, and the size of the specimen depends mainly on the size of the lesion.

2 Fix well before processing.

3 If there is any clinical or gross suggestion that the tumor may be malignant, paint margins with India ink.

Description

1 Size and shape of specimen; features of surface; lesion present? size, color, other features; margin grossly involved?

2 If specimen transected, description of appearance of cross section

Sections for histology

Note: In specimens from vesicular diseases, the vesicle should be submitted intact. Do not cut through the vesicle under any circumstances.

1 For specimens measuring 3 mm or less (see accompanying drawing **A**): submit *in toto* without cutting.

2 For specimens measuring between 4 and 6 mm in width (see accompanying drawing **B**): cut through the center and submit both halves.

3 For specimens with a width of 7 mm or more (see accompanying drawing **C**): cut a 2- to 3-mm slice from the center for histology and save the remainder in formalin.

4 Make sure that sections will be embedded on edge.

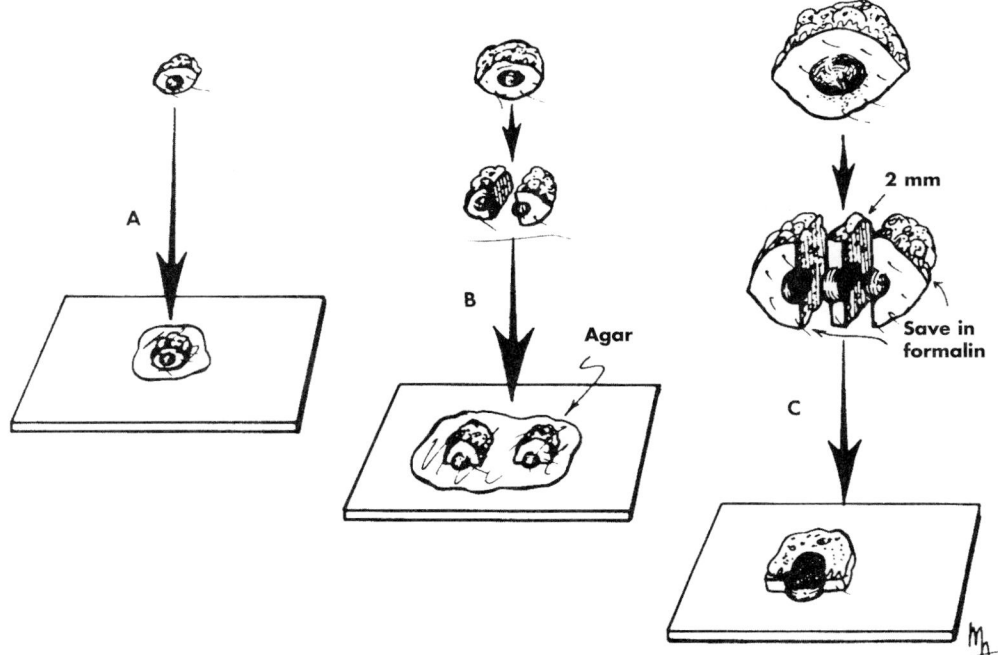

SKIN—EXCISION FOR MALIGNANT TUMOR

Procedure

1 Paint all excision margins with India ink.
2 Take two Polaroid photographs or photocopies in cases of large tumors and identify in one of them the site of the sections to be taken.

Description

1 Shape and dimensions of specimen
2 Characteristics of lesion: size, shape, color or colors, configuration; elevated or depressed? ulceration? types of margins (sharp or ill-defined? flat or elevated?); distance from margins of resection; satellite nodules?

Sections for histology

1 *Small specimens*—up to 5 cm in greatest length (see accompanying drawing **I**):
Cut parallel 3-mm slices of the entire specimen, making sure that the initial section goes from the center of the lesion to what grossly appears the narrowest surgical margin.
2 *Larger specimens* (see accompanying drawing **II**):
  a Tumor: parallel 3-mm slices of the entire lesion *(T)*
  b Surgical margins: tangential sections along the entire edge *(M)**

---

*For alternate methods to evaluate surgical margins, see:

Gormley DE: Evaluation of a method for controlled tissue embedding for histologic evaluation of tumor margins. Am J Dermatopathol **9**:308-315, 1987.
Hurt MA: The rule of halves. A method of controlling the uniform "cutting-in" of skin biopsies. Am J Dermatopathol **13**:7-10, 1991.
Rapini RP: Comparison of methods for checking surgical margins. J Am Acad Dermatol **23**:288-294, 1990.
Woods JE, Farrow GM: Peripheral tissue examination for malignant lesions of the skin. Mayo Clin Proc **66**:207-209, 1991.

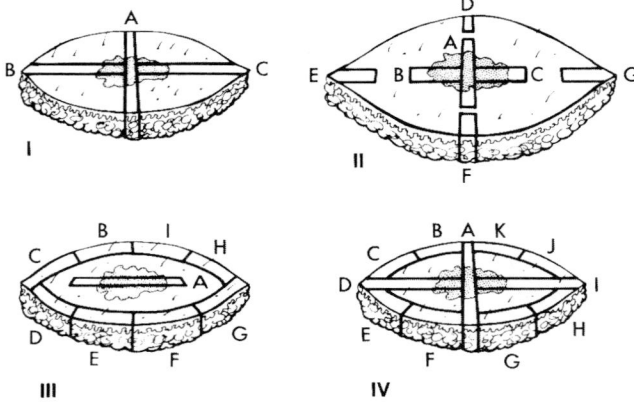

SKIN—PUNCH BIOPSY

Procedure

1 Submit *in toto,* if 4 mm in diameter or smaller (see accompanying drawing **A**). This prevents loss of tissue during the facing-up of the block and allows better microscopic sampling; cut in half longitudinally only if 5 mm or larger, and submit both halves for histology (see accompanying drawing **B**).

2 If the specimen is from a vesicular disease, the vesicle should be submitted *intact* for histology.

Description

1 Diameter and thickness of biopsy
2 Appearance of surface; subcutis included?

Sections for histology

1 Entire biopsy (see under Procedure)
2 Make sure section oriented on edge

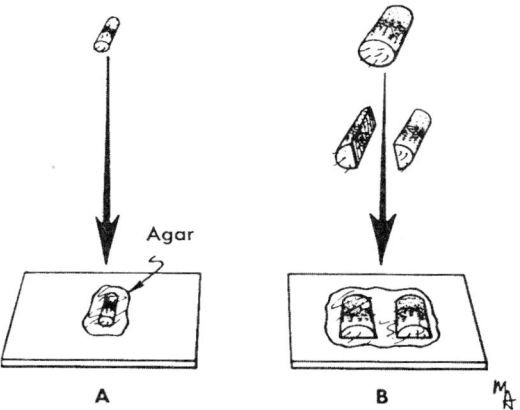

SKIN—SHAVE BIOPSY

Procedure

Shave biopsies of the skin, usually done for keratoses or basal cell carcinomas, can be quite thin, often of round or oval shape.

Description

1 Size of specimen
2 Number of fragments
3 Features of surface

Sections for histology

1 If width is 3 mm or less: submit *in toto* without cutting.
2 If width is 4 mm or more: cut in parallel slices, about 2 to 3 mm thick, and submit all for histology.
3 Make sure all sections are oriented on edge.

SMALL BOWEL—BIOPSY

Procedure

1 The specimen is usually received attached to a piece of filter paper or Gelfoam, mucosal side up; let it fix well before processing.
2 Examine with dissecting microscope and determine mucosal pattern; avoid drying of the specimen and traumatizing the mucosa during this procedure. Performance of this step has lost some of the popularity it had years ago, but it still retains some usefulness as a quick predictor of the histologic appearance and as an aid for proper orientation of the specimen.

Description

1 Size and color of specimen
2 Mucosal pattern with dissecting microscope (see accompanying drawings)

Sections for histology

1 The entire specimen is submitted. It is essential for it to be oriented on edge.
2 If the specimen comes attached to Gelfoam, the latter can be processed together with the specimen.

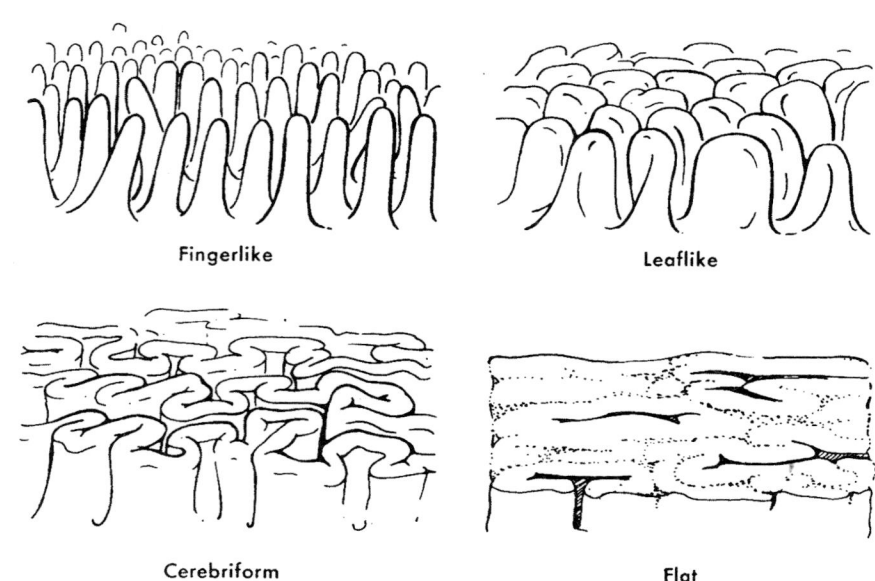

Fingerlike   Leaflike

Cerebriform   Flat

SMALL BOWEL—EXCISION

Small bowel resections vary a great deal in length and location depending on the characteristics of the lesion. They include the regional mesentery and are usually followed by an end-to-end anastomosis.

Procedure

1 Two options are available depending on the length of the bowel and the type of pathology present:
   a Cut longitudinally through the antimesenteric border, pin on corkboard, and fix overnight.
   b Wash out contents gently with formalin or saline solution (not with water), tie one end, fill the lumen with formalin, and tie the other end. Fix overnight and open longitudinally along the antimesenteric border.

Description

1 Length and diameter of specimen
2 Mucosa: appearance; edema? hemorrhage? ulcerations? tumor? (size, location, circumferential involvement? depth of invasion)
3 Wall: thickness, abnormalities
4 Serosa: fibrosis, peritonitis, adhesions
5 Lymph nodes: size and appearance
6 Mesentery; mesenteric blood vessels

Sections for histology

1 Depends on pathology present
2 In cases of infarct: several cross sections of mesenteric vessels

SPLEEN—SPLENECTOMY

Splenectomy consists of removal of the entire spleen after ligating the splenic artery and vein.

Procedure

1 Measure and weigh the specimen.
2 Cut parallel slices as thin as possible with a sharp knife or meat cutter while the specimen is fresh and examine each slice carefully for focal lesions; do not wash the cut surface in tap water. Fix each slice flat in a large container.
3 Take cultures if an inflammatory condition is suspected.
4 Prepare four imprints of the cut surface in all cases in which splenic pathology is suspected; stain two with hematoxylin-eosin and two with Wright's stain.
5 If sickle cell disease is suspected, fix a block of tissue in formalin *immediately* after it has been cut from the interior of the organ.
6 Look for lymph nodes and accessory spleens in the splenic hilum.
7 For the evaluation of the red pulp in diseases associated with hypersplenism, the specimen can be injected with formalin through the splenic artery. A sharp distinction between sinuses and chords will thus be obtained in the microscopic preparations.
8 For the spleen removed as part of a staging procedure, see under Staging laparotomy for malignant lymphoma.

Description

1 Weight and dimensions
2 Hilum: nature of vessels, presence of lymph nodes, presence of accessory spleens
3 Capsule: color, thickness, focal changes, adhesions, lacerations (location, length and depth)
4 Cut surface: color; consistency; bulging; malpighian corpuscles (size; color; conspicuous?); fibrous trabeculae; nodules or masses; diffuse infiltration?

Sections for histology

1 For incidental splenectomy: one section, including capsule
2 For traumatically ruptured spleen: one section through tear and one away from it
3 For diseased spleen: at least three sections, one to include hilum and two to include capsule

STAGING LAPAROTOMY FOR MALIGNANT LYMPHOMA

Procedure

1 Spleen: handle as described under Spleen—splenectomy except that *the entire spleen* should be sliced carefully, 3 to 4 mm apart, and each slice should be carefully examined. Any nodules, no matter how small, that differ from the adjacent normal malpighian corpuscles should be processed for histology. Square blocks containing these suspicious nodules, in addition to other obvious lesions, should be cut out and fixed separately for several hours or overnight in formalin.

2 Lymph nodes: these will usually include splenic hilar, para-aortic, and possible mesenteric nodes. Dissect carefully the splenic hilum for the former.

3 Liver wedge biopsy (right and left lobes): keep separate; trim into several slices, if necessary.

4 Open iliac crest biopsy: fix, decalcify, and trim, if necessary.

Description

1 Proceed as per instructions for the respective organs.

2 Presence or absence of grossly identifiable nodes in the splenic hilum must be noted.

Sections for histology

1 Spleen: all grossly abnormal or suspicious areas; if no gross abnormalities seen, four random pieces

2 Lymph nodes: all, properly identified as to site

3 Liver: all, properly identified as to lobe

4 Bone marrow: all

STOMACH—GASTRECTOMY FOR TUMOR

Gastrectomy for tumor can be *total* (including cardia and pylorus), *subtotal* (including the pylorus), and *proximal* or *inverted subtotal* (including the cardia).

Procedure

1 Open the specimen along the greater curvature (unless the lesion is in this location; if it is, open the specimen along the lesser curvature).
2 Dissect the lymph node groups according to the accompanying diagram and remove the omentum.
3 If a splenectomy is included, dissect the hilar lymph nodes, measure and weigh the spleen, and cut in 1-cm longitudinal slices.
4 Pin the stomach on a corkboard and fix overnight in formalin before sectioning.
5 Take two Polaroid photographs or photocopies and identify in one of them the sites of the sections to be taken.
6 Paint the surgical margins with India ink.
7 In general, take the sections *perpendicular* to the directions of the mucosal folds.
8 Another way to examine these specimens is as follows: inject the stomach with formalin (in cases of total gastrectomy) or fill it with gauze or cotton impregnated in formalin (in partial gastrectomies). Fix overnight. Cut the side opposite the tumor with scissors and the tumor side with a long knife.
9 If a thorough mapping of the mucosal abnormalities is desired, the entire specimen can be submitted, or the Swiss roll technique can be used (see Chapter 11, Stomach).

Description

1 Type of resection (total or subtotal); length of greater curvature, lesser curvature, and duodenal cuff
2 Tumor characteristics: location, size (including thickness), shape (fungating, spreading, ulcerated); depth of invasion; presence of serosal involvement; blood vessel invasion; extension into duodenum; distance from both lines of resection
3 Appearance of non-neoplastic mucosa

STOMACH—GASTRECTOMY FOR TUMOR—cont'd

Sections for histology (see accompanying drawings)

1 Tumor: four sections through wall and including tumor border and adjacent mucosa
2 Non-neoplastic mucosa; midstomach, two sections
3 Proximal line of resection along lesser curvature: two sections
4 Proximal line of resection along greater curvature: two sections
5 Distal line of resection (along pylorus and duodenum, if present): two sections
6 Spleen, if present
7 Pancreas, if present
8 Lymph nodes:
    a Pyloric
    b Lesser curvature
    c Greater curvature
    d Omentum
    e Perisplenic

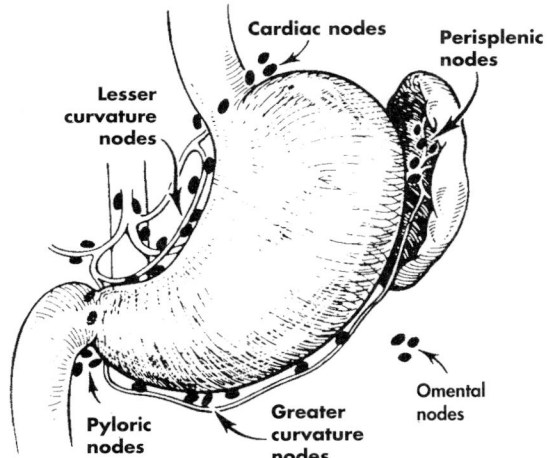

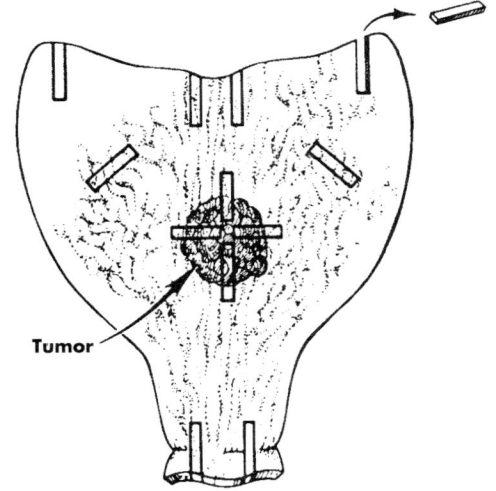

STOMACH—GASTRECTOMY FOR ULCER

Gastric resection for peptic ulcer includes removal of the antrum with the pylorus and a small portion of the first portion of the duodenum. For duodenal peptic ulcers, this is routinely combined with truncal vagotomy.

Procedure

1 Examine specimen in the fresh state.
2 Open the specimen along the greater curvature (unless the lesion is in this location; if it is, open the specimen along the lesser curvature).
3 Dissect the lymph node groups and remove the omentum.
4 Look carefully for small mucosal erosions and irregularities and for intramural or subserosal nodules.
5 Pin the stomach on a corkboard and fix overnight in formalin before sectioning.
6 Take two Polaroid photographs or photocopies and identify in one of them the sites of the sections to be taken.

Description

1 Type of resection; length of greater curvature, lesser curvature, and duodenal cuff
2 Ulcer characteristics: location, size, depth of penetration, shape, and color of edges (flat or elevated? converging folds?); presence of large vessels and/or perforation at ulcer base; appearance of serosa. (If the clinicoradiographic diagnosis is peptic ulcer but no ulcer is identified in the specimen, contact the surgeon or assistant to find out whether the ulcer was not resected. Record this information as part of the gross dictation.)
3 Appearance of uninvolved mucosa: atrophy, edema, hemorrhage

Sections for histology

1 Ulcer: at least four sections
2 Lesser curvature: two sections cut from proximal margin of excision (Paint line of resection with India ink.)
3 Greater curvature: two sections cut from proximal margin of excision (Paint line of resection with India ink.)
4 Pylorus and duodenum: two sections, including distal line of resection
5 Other lesions, if present
6 Lymph nodes: up to three sections

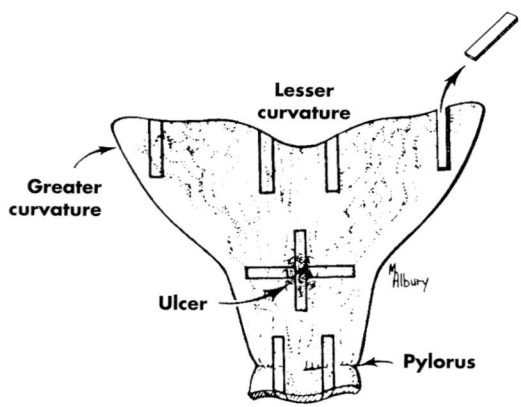

TESTICLE—ORCHIECTOMY

Procedure

1 Open the tunica vaginalis; weigh and measure the testicle.
2 Cut the testicle sagittally while it is in the fresh state and fix in formalin.
3 Take two Polaroid photographs or photocopies and identify in one of them the sites of the sections to be taken.
4 Cut serial slices, about 3 mm thick, of each testicular half, perpendicular to the original section, stopping just at the level of the tunica albuginea (to keep them together), and examine each surface carefully.
5 Cut the epididymis longitudinally throughout its entire length.
6 Make several cross sections of the spermatic cord at several levels.

Description

1 Weight and dimensions of testicle
2 Length of spermatic cord
3 Features of tumor, if present: size, color; consistency; homogeneity or lack of it; presence of cysts, necrosis, hemorrhage, bone, or cartilage; tumor extension to tunica albuginea, epididymis, cord, and other structures
4 Features of non-neoplastic testicle: atrophy? fibrosis? nodules?
5 Features of rete testis and epididymis

Sections for histology

1 Tumor: at least three sections or one section for each centimeter of tumor, whichever is greater, at least one of which should include some uninvolved testicle. Most of the sections should include tunica albuginea. (Always submit sections from hemorrhagic or necrotic areas of tumor, as well as from solid or fleshy areas.)
2 Uninvolved testicle: two sections
3 Epididymis
4 Spermatic cord and surrounding soft tissue at point about 1 cm from testicle: one cross section
5 Spermatic cord and surrounding soft tissue at line of resection: one cross section

THYMUS GLAND—THYMECTOMY

Procedure

1 Weigh the total organ. Cut parallel slices, either in the fresh specimen or after formalin fixation.
2 Look carefully for lymph nodes around the thymus.

Description

1 Weight and dimensions; both lobes identifiable?
2 Relative amount of fat and thymic parenchyma
3 Tumor characteristics: size, shape, external appearance (lobulated or smooth), cut section, color, necrosis, hemorrhage, fibrous bands, calcification, cysts (size, content)
4 Attached structures (pleura, pericardium, lung, lymph nodes)

Sections for histology

1 Tumor: three or more sections, at least two of which should include capsule
2 Uninvolved thymus: two sections
3 Other organs, if present (lung, lymph nodes)

THYROID GLAND—THYROIDECTOMY

Operations on the thyroid gland include *nodulectomy* (a procedure largely abandoned that consists of enucleation of a thyroid nodule), *lobectomy* (often combined for cosmetic reasons with removal of the isthmus), *subtotal thyroidectomy* (in which the posterior capsule and a small portion of thyroid tissue—1 to 2 g—are left on the side opposite to the lesion), and *total thyroidectomy* (in which the entire gland—including the posterior capsule—is removed)

Procedure

1 Weight and measure the specimen.
2 Orient the specimen and cut parallel longitudinal slices 5 mm each either in the fresh state or after formalin fixation.
3 Search for parathyroid glands in the surrounding fat.

Description

1 Type of specimen: lobectomy, isthmectomy, subtotal thyroidectomy, total thyroidectomy
2 Weight, shape, color, and consistency of specimen
3 Cut surface: smooth or nodular? if nodular: number, size, and appearance of nodules (cystic? calcified? hemorrhagic? necrotic?); encapsulated or invasive? distance to line of resection

Sections for histology

1 For diffuse and/or inflammatory lesions: three sections from each lobe and one from isthmus
2 For a solitary encapsulated nodule measuring up to 5 cm: entire circumference; take one additional section for each additional centimeter in diameter. Most of these sections should include the tumor capsule and adjacent thyroid tissue, if present.
3 For multinodular thyroid glands: one section of each nodule (up to five nodules), including rim and adjacent normal gland; more than one section for larger nodules
4 For papillary carcinoma: block entire thyroid gland and (separately) line of resection
5 For grossly invasive carcinoma other than papillary: three sections of tumor, three of non-neoplastic gland, and one from line of resection
6 For all cases: submit parathyroid glands if found on gross inspection

UTERUS—CERVICAL BIOPSY

Procedure

1 Do not cut the specimen unless the individual pieces are greater than 4 mm in diameter.
2 It is essential that *all of the tissue* received be processed, no matter how small.
3 Always carefully search the container and the underside of the lid for tiny fragments of tissue.

Description

1 Number of pieces received, shape and color
2 Measurement in aggregate
3 Presence or absence of epithelium; epithelial erosions or ulcers? irregularity in epithelial thickness?
4 Any evidence of tumors or cysts?

Sections for histology

1 Submit the material in its entirety.
2 If specimens are received with a specific identification (e.g., anterior lip, posterior lip), label and submit them separately.
3 If a specimen from endocervical scraping is received, submit as a separate specimen in its entirety (including the endocervical mucus).

UTERUS—CERVICAL CONIZATION

Specimens from cervical conizations have the shape of a cone with the base toward the portio. In the *leep procedure* (loop electroexcision procedure), the cone is much smaller than that obtained with the conventional method. Orientation of the specimen is more difficult but just as important.

Procedure

1 Ideally the specimen should be received intact, in the fresh state, and with a suture or other material identifying the 12 o'clock position.
2 Open the specimen by inserting a sharp pointed scissors into the cervical canal and cutting longitudinally along the 12 o'clock position. If the specimen has not been oriented as to position, open at any site.
3 Pin on a corkboard with the mucosal side up and fix in formalin for several hours.
4 Paint both surgical margins with India ink, taking special care that the epithelial side of the margins is well stained along its entire length.
5 Cut the entire cervix by making parallel sections, 2 to 3 mm apart, along the plane of the endocervical canal starting at the 12 o'clock position (or left-hand side of the specimen) and moving clockwise. Sections should be taken in such a way that the epithelium (including the squamocolumnar junction) is present in each section; some trimming of the stroma may be necessary (see accompanying drawing).

Description

1 Size (diameter and depth) and shape of cone; complete cast of cervix or fragmented?
2 Epithelium: color; presence of irregularities, erosions, healed or recent lacerations, masses (size, shape, location), cysts (size, content), previous biopsy sites

Sections for histology

1 All of the tissue must be submitted (except for trimming of the stroma).
2 If the cone has been oriented to the 12 o'clock position, identify separately:
   a Sections from 12 to 3 o'clock (**A-1** on accompanying drawings)
   b Sections from 3 to 6 o'clock (**A-2** on accompanying drawings)
   c Sections from 6 to 9 o'clock (**A-3** on accompanying drawings)
   d Sections from 9 to 12 o'clock (**A-4** on accompanying drawings)
3 If an accurate mapping of the lesions is desired, identify sequentially each section with a letter, beginning from the 12 o'clock position.

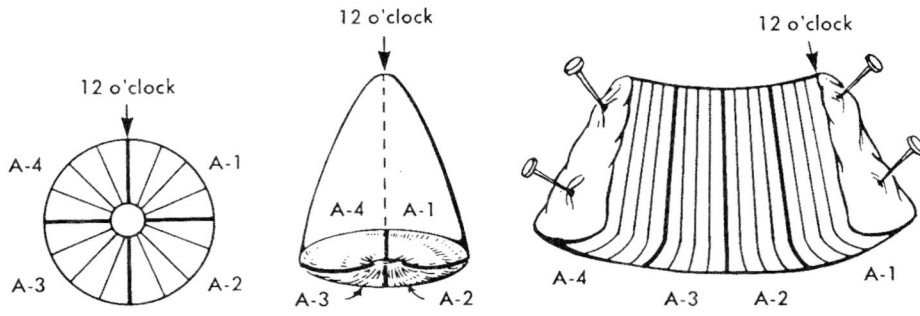

UTERUS—ENDOMETRIAL CURETTINGS OR BIOPSY

Procedure

1 Use a metal strainer or a filter paper in a funnel to collect the specimens.
2 In cases of suspected abortion, search for chorionic villi, if necessary, under a dissecting microscope.
3 In cases of recurrent abortion, save a sample of villi for possible cytogenetic evaluation. Clean the forceps, other instruments, and the table carefully before handling the next case.

Description

1 Measurement in the aggregate
2 Color and consistency; blood clots present? proportion of clots in relation to whole specimen; any unusually large for firm pieces? globular tissue? evidence of necrosis? tissue suggestive of products of conception? if so, describe the appearance of chorionic villi (a dissecting microscope may be necessary); presence or absence of villous vessels, shape of villi (tubular, clubbed, cystic, hydatidiform); if gestational sac is present, describe as indicated under Uterus—tissue passed.

Sections for histology

1 For endometrial biopsy or diagnostic curettage: submit *all* tissue. Do not fill the cassettes more than half full.
2 For endometrial curettage for incomplete abortion: submit representative sections of tissue with the appearance of placenta, fetal parts, and decidua unless the entire specimen is small enough to fit into three cassettes. If the microscopic sections do not show products of conception, submit the rest of the material.

UTERUS—HYSTERECTOMY (GENERAL INSTRUCTIONS)

Hysterectomies can be performed by either the abdominal or the vaginal route, the latter reserved for benign conditions. They consist of removal of the entire organ. Supracervical hysterectomies (in which the corpus is separated from the cervix and the latter is left in place) are no longer performed. Depending on the age of the patient and the nature of the disease, abdominal hysterectomies may be accompanied by unilateral or bilateral adnexectomy and by the removal of regional lymph nodes.

Abdominal hysterectomies are divided into simple and radical. The radical procedure includes removal of the upper third of the vagina and parametrium, in addition to regional node excision.

Procedure

1 If operation was done for endometrial hyperplasia, endometrial carcinoma, or cervical (in situ or invasive) carcinoma, read specific instructions before proceeding.
2 Measure and weigh the specimen.
3 If the uterus is received fresh and intact:
   a Open it by cutting with scissors through both lateral walls, from the cervix to the uterine cornua.
   b Make a mark as to which half is anterior (e.g., by cutting a small wedge on one side) and complete the division by cutting with a sharp knife horizontally through the fundus. The uterus can be oriented by examining the level of peritoneal reflection (lower in the posterior side) and, if the tubes are attached, by the fact that their insertion is anterior to that of the round ligament.
   c Make additional cuts through any large mass in the wall.
   d Fix for several hours or overnight.
   e Make parallel transverse sections through each half, about 1 cm apart, beginning at the upper level of the endocervical canal and stopping short of completing them on one side to keep them together, and examine carefully each surface.
   f Make several sections of the cervix along the endocervical canal.
   g Make at least one cross section of every myoma present and examine carefully; larger myomas need additional cuts.
   h If tubes and/or ovary accompanies the specimen, follow instructions for these organs.

Description

1 Type of hysterectomy: total? radical? with salpingo-oophorectomy?
2 Shape of uterus: deformed? subserosal bulges?
3 Serosa: fibrous adhesions?
4 Wall: thickness, abnormalities
5 Endometrium: appearance; thickness; polyps? (size, shape); cysts?
6 Cervix: appearance of exocervix, squamocolumnar junction, endocervical canal; erosions? polyps? cysts?
7 Myomas: number, location (subserosal, intramural, submucosal); size; sessile or pedunculated? hemorrhage, necrosis, or calcification? ulceration of overlying endometrium?

Sections for histology

1 Cervix: one section from anterior half and one from posterior half
2 Corpus: at least two sections taken close to fundus and including endometrium, good portion of myometrium, and, if thickness permits, serosa; additional sections from any grossly abnormal areas
3 Myomas: at least one section per myoma, up to three; sections from any grossly abnormal area (e.g., soft, fleshy, necrotic, cystic)
4 Cervical or endometrial polyps: to be submitted in entirety unless extremely large

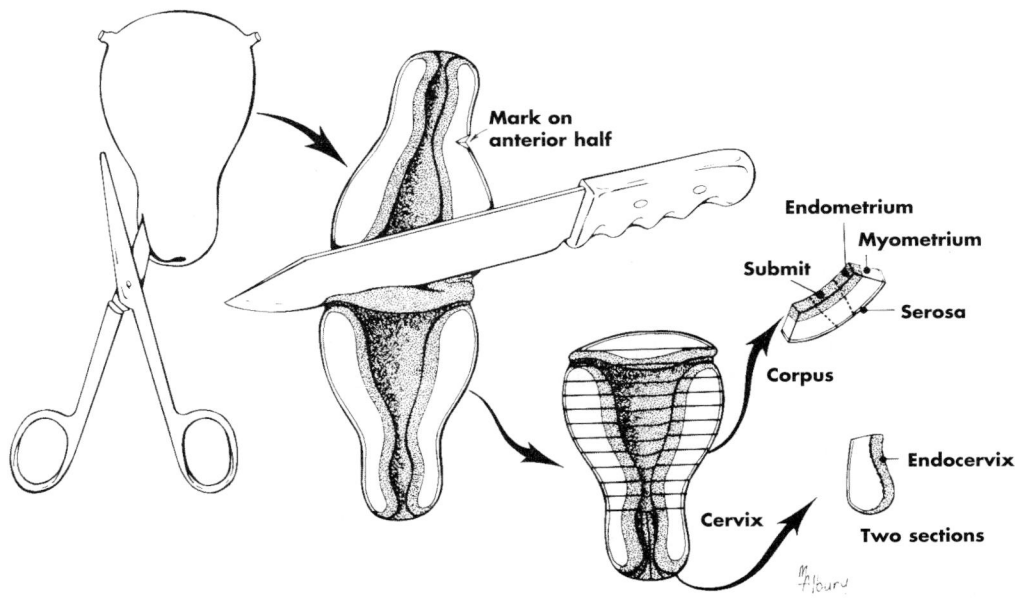

UTERUS—HYSTERECTOMY FOR CERVICAL CARCINOMA
(IN SITU OR INVASIVE)

Procedure

1 If lymph nodes are included (radical hysterectomy), dissect while fresh and separate into left and right obturator, interiliac, and left and right iliac (high nodes) groups (not all of these groups will be present in every specimen).

2 Measure and weigh the specimen; orient as to anterior and posterior sides; see under Uterus—hysterectomy (general instructions).

3 Amputate the cervix from the corpus about 2.5 cm above the external os with a sharp knife.

4 Handle the uterus as described under Uterus—hysterectomy (general instructions) and the tubes and ovaries, if present, according to instructions for these organs.

5 Open the cervix with scissors through the endocervical canal at the 12 o'clock position and carefully pin stretched specimen on a corkboard with the mucosal side up. Be careful to avoid tearing or rubbing the epithelial surface.

6 Fix by floating for several hours or overnight with the tissue on the underside of the corkboard in a formalin container.

7 Paint the vaginal surgical margin with India ink.

8 Cut the entire cervix by making parallel longitudinal sections, 2 to 3 mm apart, along the plane of the endocervical canal starting at the 12 o'clock position and moving clockwise. Sections should be taken in such a way that the epithelium (including the squamocolumnar junction) is present in each section; some trimming of the stroma may be necessary (see accompany drawing).

Description

1 Cervix: color of epithelium; presence of irregularities, erosions, healed or recent lacerations, masses (size, shape, location), cysts (size, content), previous biopsy, or conization sites

2 Rest of uterus: see under Uterus—hysterectomy (general instructions)

3 Ovaries and tubes, if present: see instructions for respective organs

4 Lymph nodes, if present: approximate number; gross appearance; seem involved by tumor?

Sections for histology

1 Cervix: all tissue is submitted (except for trimming of stroma) and identified separately as follows:
   a Sections from 12 to 3 o'clock (**A-1** on accompany drawings)
   b Sections from 3 to 6 o'clock (**A-2** on accompanying drawings)
   c Sections from 6 to 9 o'clock (**A-3** on accompanying drawings)
   d Sections from 9 to 12 o'clock (**A-4** on accompanying drawings)
      (If accurate mapping of lesions is desired, identify sequentially each section with a letter, beginning from 12 o'clock position)

2 Vaginal cuff (entire line of resection)

3 Left soft tissue (for invasive cases only)

4 Right soft tissue (for invasive cases only)

5 Rest of uterus: see under Uterus—hysterectomy (general instructions)

6 Ovaries and tubes: see Instructions for respective organs

7 Lymph nodes, if present
   • Left obturator
   • Right obturator
   • Interiliac
   • Left iliac (high nodes)
   • Right iliac (high nodes)

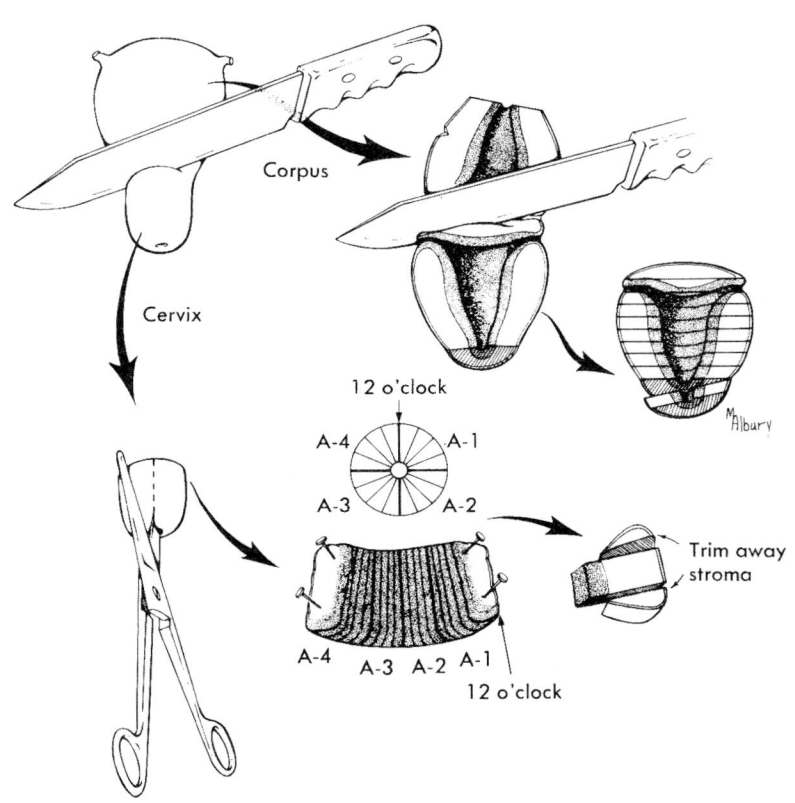

Corpus

Cervix

12 o'clock

A-4   A-1

A-3   A-2

12 o'clock

A-4   A-3 A-2 A-1

Trim away
stroma

M. Albury

UTERUS—HYSTERECTOMY FOR ENDOMETRIAL HYPERPLASIA OR CARCINOMA

Procedure

1 If lymph nodes are included (radical hysterectomy), dissect while fresh and separate into left and right obturator, interiliac, and left and right iliac (high nodes) groups (not all of these groups will be present in every specimen).
2 Open and fix the uterus as indicated under Uterus—hysterectomy (general instructions).
3 If ovaries and tubes are present, handle according to respective instructions.

Description

1 Type of operation: radical? total? with salpingectomy and oophorectomy?
2 Tumor: exact location; size; appearance (solid, papillary, ulcerated, necrotic, hemorrhagic); color; extent of endometrial extension; presence of myometrial, serosal, parametrial (soft tissue), venous, cervical, or tubal extension
3 Rest of uterus: see under Uterus—hysterectomy (general instructions)
4 Ovaries and tubes: see respective instructions
5 Lymph nodes, if present: approximate number; gross appearance; seem involved by tumor?

Sections for histology

1 If obvious tumor present:
   a Three sections, one of which should be through area of deepest invasion and be complete sections from surface of endometrium through serosa (If too thick for a cassette, divide in half and identify both halves appropriately.)
   b Two sections from non-neoplastic endometrium; do not need to be through entire wall.
2 Soft tissue from left and eighth parametria
3 If no obvious tumor present (previous irradiation, very superficial carcinoma, endometrial hyperplasia):
   a Sample entire endometrium by making complete transverse parallel sections, 2 to 3 mm part, of both uterine halves; one section should comprise entire thickness of organ, from mucosa to serosa; trim away from all others deepest two thirds of myometrium. Label separately as anterior and posterior halves.
   b Rest of uterus: see under Uterus—hysterectomy (general instructions)
   c Ovaries and tubes: see respective instructions
   d Lymph nodes, if present:
   • Left obturator
   • Right obturator
   • Interiliac
   • Left iliac (high nodes)
   • Right iliac (high nodes)

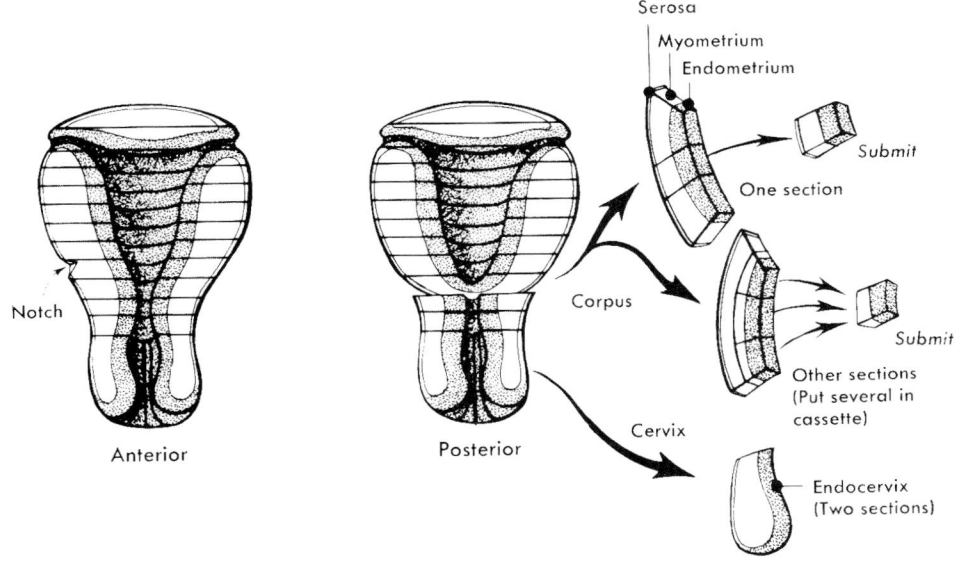

UTERUS*—TISSUE PASSED

Procedure

1 Examine for presence of gestational sac and other evidence of conception. Use dissecting microscope, if necessary.

Description

1 Measurement in the aggregate; color, consistency, appearance; decidual cast present? if so, note whether intact or ruptured, diameter, presence and size of amniotic sac, yolk sac, and embryo. If latter is present, measure and state whether it appears normal, malformed, or rudimentary, and whether there is evidence of maceration. If only fragments of the fetus are present, try to identify a foot and measure its length to estimate gestational age (see diagram).

Sections for histology

1 If identifiable products of conception are present: submit representative sections of the various components.
2 If identifiable products of conception are absent: submit entire material.

*Berry CL, ed: Correlation of foot length with crown-rump length of human fetuses. In Pediatric pathology. New York, 1981, Springer-Verlag, p 3.

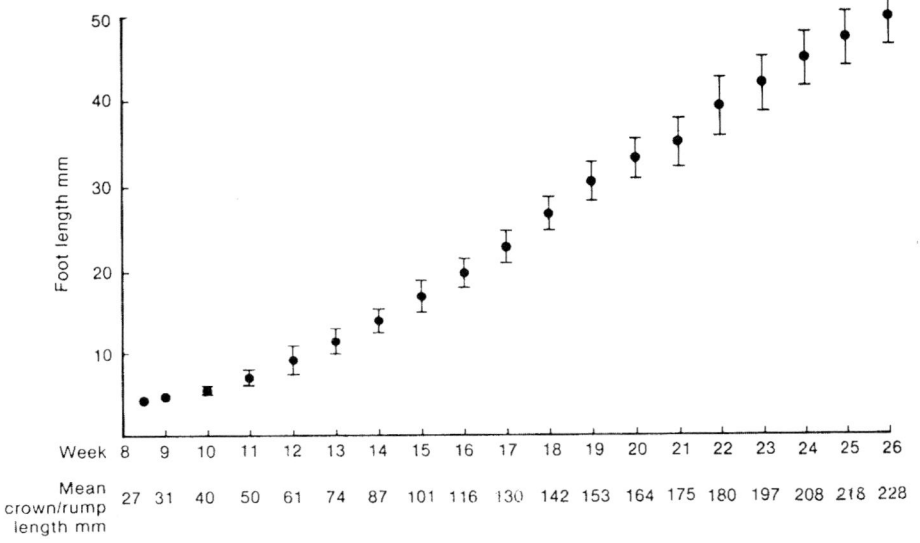

VULVA—VULVECTOMY

Procedure

1 Measure size of the specimen, including the inguinal region, if present; also measure the size of the lesion.
2 In radical vulvectomy specimens, separate lymph nodes into groups and fix overnight in separate jars; Carnoy's fluid is preferable.
3 Pin on a corkboard and fix overnight; be careful to pin down the entire external borders and the vaginal margins. the latter is better preserved when it is pinned down on a cork placed in the introitus.
4 Take two Polaroid photographs or photocopies, and identify in one of them the sites of the sections to be taken.

Description

1 Type of vulvectomy: simply, subcutaneous, radical; lymph node groups present
2 Size of specimen
3 Lesion: size, location, extent, invasion into adjacent structures or vessels, color, surface (verrucous? ulcerated?), borders (distinct? rolled?), depth of stromal invasion
4 Appearance of non-neoplastic surface: atrophy, keratosis, ulceration
5 Lymph nodes: size of largest appearing grossly involved?

Appendix I
Information systems in surgical pathology

Properly implemented, the ability of computers to store, organize, process, and retrieve prodigious amounts of information can measurably enhance the efficiency of the surgical pathology laboratory, improve the quality of the pathologist's service, monitor turnaround times and other quality assurance parameters, aid in research and teaching, and reduce the costs of operation.[5] However, the realization of these benefits is not automatic; it requires that the level of automation in a given installation be carefully matched to the needs of the pathologists, the institution, and the budget. Unfortunately, many surgical pathologists are poorly prepared to make the decisions required to design or choose a suitable automated system. The result, therefore, has too often been the implementation of systems that are little more than word processors with rudimentary patient registration features, or the initiation of extensive but poorly planned "in-house" software development efforts, usually by computer programmers with a limited understanding of what features are required. In the former situation, the laboratory is denied most of the benefits of automation; in the latter case, it is likely to experience endless development costs for capabilities that may never materialize and, at the same time, sacrifice most of the benefits of effective automation. Compounding the problem is the relative paucity of information in the literature specifically addressing the problem of automation in surgical pathology, a deficiency that began to be corrected only recently.[3,8]

Automation of surgical pathology laboratories has lagged far behind automation of the clinical laboratory for several reasons: (1) the relatively low volume of specimens, (2) the complexity of the tasks involved, (3) the nonquantitative (textual) nature of the data, and (4) the reluctance of many pathologists to alter their work habits to accommodate automation. Thus, although automated record-keeping systems that are able to file coded specimen information have been relatively easy to design and introduce, only the most comprehensive systems, beginning with the CAPER system developed at the Massachusetts General Hospital,[1] have been able to offer any degree of practical automation of the routine reporting and administrative tasks of the surgical pathology laboratory. Several technical advances during the past two decades have contributed to the increasing sophistication of such systems. The rapid development of microcomputer technology has made the necessary hardware affordable by any surgical pathology laboratory. Improvements in mass information storage technology (e.g., hard disks) now make the storage of enormous amounts of textual information practical for the periods of time routinely required (5 to 10 years). Finally, the development of high-level programming languages especially designed for database and string variable (text) manipulation have allowed the incremental development of sophisticated systems that retain the ability to be easily altered or enhanced to meet new user demands. Thus pathologists may now reasonably expect that an automated surgical pathology system will "talk" to them in their own language, will not require that they change the way diagnoses are worded or recorded, will not ask them to remember "codes," will accept the information they provide in almost any format, will store this information permanently and reliably, will automatically organize it for recall by any combination of criteria, and will unobtrusively attend to most of the routine administrative chores. More sophisticated systems are also now providing storage of both visual and textual information and "expert" consultative support such as on-line assistance with specimen preparation, grading, staging, diagnosis, and bibliographic retrieval.

Regardless of the level of automation chosen, certain features of the system design become very important if the system is to be both effective and acceptable to the user (see box). The introduction of an automated system into the diagnostic laboratories inevitably causes concern among the staff, whether they are professional, technical, or administrative. Many of the fears that accompany automation are widely recognized because the introduction of computer technology into any work environment significantly redefines "essential" tasks and shifts the balance of authority toward those with computer literacy. Some of these changes are unavoidable and perhaps not altogether undesirable. However, the best systems minimize the level of computer prowess needed to effectively use the system. This is essential at the professional level.

BASIC DESIGN CRITERIA FOR AN AUTOMATED SYSTEM IN SURGICAL PATHOLOGY

1 Pathologist participation unnecessary
2 Elimination of redundant data entry
3 Real-time integration of all data

4 On-line permanent and safe storage of all primary data
5 Rapid response time
6 Flexible and easily modified design

Few pathologists would welcome a system that asked them to alter the way they phrase their reports, and many would resist systems that force them to use the computer to complete their tasks.[4] Thus the first and paramount design requirement of any system must be to allow the pathologist to work independently of the computer if desired without sacrificing the advantages of the system. Although this requirement may become less important as familiarity with computers among anatomic pathologists grows, it remains the single most important feature of successful anatomic pathology systems.

A second feature desirable for effective automation is the rigorous avoidance of redundant data entry. Each data item relating to a case, be it patient name, number of blocks processed, special stains prepared, diagnosis or billing codes, should ideally involve only a single human intervention. All derivative information, including diagnosis codes, should be automatically assigned by the computer whenever possible. This principle should apply even to the inquiry of patient data, to make it possible to retrieve information on a patient by identifying only a portion of the name or to locate a case by providing only a portion of the diagnostic terms used or any one of an unlimited number of synonyms. A corollary to this requirement is that the system must independently track each data item to allow complete flexibility in the compilation of reports, searches, and inquiries using arbitrary formats. It follows that systems that capture data from paper records after case processing has begun (rather than in "real time") only give the illusion of automation and can offer little or no significant savings in the workload. Similarly, systems that capture most or all of the patient data as text documents in word processing files are highly limited in their reporting and searching capabilities and are also unlikely to eliminate much redundant data entry.

Real-time integration of information from all aspects of the diagnostic pathology operation is also required. For example, specimens for a patient may be simultaneously received in the cytology and surgical pathology laboratories, as well as in other laboratories for specialized diagnostic tests involving electron microscopy, cell markers, flow cytometry, and so on. Information on previous material may also exist. Good practice demands that the information from all current and previous examinations be considered by the pathologist when rendering an opinion. The system must therefore automatically bring to the attention of each user information on all previous specimens, as well as information on all current specimens that are being processed, regardless of their stage of completion. Thus an adequate pathology information system must be able to simultaneously correlate the input from multiple users, whether they are all working on different aspects of the same case or different specimens for the same patient, and will automatically inform each user of all pertinent patient information regardless of where or when the information was entered. The practical consequence of this requirement is that (except for the smallest institutions) all users are likely to share a common device (file server) on which the bulk of the relevant data is kept.

A related design requirement is that the system be able to retain *on-line* permanently all primary information about a case. This includes all demographic and clinical information, the full text of the gross and microscopic descriptions, the full text of the diagnosis and any diagnosis codes, all addenda and special procedures, and all billing and histology laboratory data. Permanent on-line storage of all data is practical and cost effective with current technology and eliminates the need for redundant hard copy storage of patient records if adequate precautions are taken to safeguard the data (see the following discussion). Conversely, any system that purges patient data (e.g., the gross description or other text fields) becomes an incomplete archive and sacrifices many of the advantages of automation since in such a system neither inquiry nor database searches can be relied on to return all available information on a case. Such crippled systems should be avoided.

If all primary information on every case is to be retained permanently on-line, adequate precautions must be built into the system to prevent permanent loss or corruption of the data. Security checks must prevent unauthorized access to the database, all transactions must be simultaneously recorded on two physically separate storage devices (journaling), copies of all data must be made (backed up) daily or as frequently as possible, complete machine-readable copies of the data must be stored off-site, and archival copies of the data on magnetic tape or a similar medium must be saved permanently off-site at regular intervals. Such precautions ensure that data will not be lost even with major system failures (e.g., disk crash) and that only a minimal amount of data will be corrupted or lost even if the whole computer facility were to be destroyed. The permanent storage or archival copies of the data are needed only to ensure against unauthorized database tampering. Although these precautions may seem excessive, they are easily implemented and provide a level of database security that in most institutions far exceeds that provided by hard copy (paper, microfiche) records.

An acceptable automated pathology computer system must also provide very rapid response times for all routine tasks. Any system that requires more than 1 second for routine inquiries of any patient-related information or more than a few seconds for simple diagnosis-based searches of all of the patient files is frustrating in daily use. Excellent response times require adequate equipment and well-designed software. Thus it is doubtful whether an adequate fully automated surgical pathology system can be developed on hardware that is already dedicated to operating a clinical pathology laboratory, unless the clinical laboratory has significant excess disk and computer capacity. The peaks of computer activity in a clinical laboratory occur around 10:30 AM to 12:00 PM and 2:00 to 3:30 PM, times that correlate closely with peak activity of the surgical pathology laboratory. Therefore the total capacity of a combined system must far exceed the initial expectation of the capacity thought to be appropriate to ensure adequate system performance at all times. Similarly, the software must be designed to minimize the number of disk operations required to find the data needed on a patient. The best systems make extensive use of "inverted files" or indices, which allow the system to immediately identify the information it is seeking without performing time-consuming searches of the database.

A final design criterion must be the ability of the system to be easily modified to accept changing user needs. Obsolescence will come early to any system without this feature, since the need to accommodate new or altered tasks will inevitably arise. This is particularly true when a system designed for one institution is adapted to another.

A MODEL FOR AN AUTOMATED ANATOMIC PATHOLOGY SYSTEM

An overview of the system currently used at Memorial Sloan-Kettering Cancer Center (MSKCC) is presented only as an example. Other institutions use other systems that offer similar features.

The system at MSKCC operates on a computer that is dedicated to anatomic pathology. There are numerous peripheral devices interfaced to the system, including dial-up modems and printers. Terminals linked to the system have been installed in the following places: staff offices; sign-out areas; secretarial areas; administration, cytology, histology, and special laboratories; and surgical pathology gross room, autopsy suite, and autopsy room. Similar terminals have also been strategically placed throughout the hospital to facilitate inquiry from authorized users. All functions are available from virtually any terminal; access to specific functions for each user is controlled by password at the time of log-on.

Organization

Overall, the system is organized into eight major sections: (1) surgical pathology, (2) cytology, (3) autopsy, (4) billing, (5) department-wide options (primarily data searches and administrative tasks), (6) system manager, (7) histology laboratory, and (8) miscellaneous (such as a grading and staging manual for major tumor types).

Surgical pathology

This system accomplishes all of the obvious tasks performed in a surgical pathology laboratory. During accessioning of a new specimen, information on the patient, specimen, submitting physician, billing agency, initial billing codes, and so forth is collected. Because all redundant entries are eliminated, it is usually unnecessary to enter the entire physician's name or address, billing agency, billing codes, towns, cities, ZIP codes in the area, any state, any hospital address or patient floor, most dates, or even the patient's name or demographic information (unless the patient is new). Information is also captured at accessioning on the "type of specimen" to allow the computer to obtain preliminary information about the specimen being processed. This data field is designed to allow a secretary to correctly identify broad categories of specimens. For example, if the specimen were a breast resection, the secretary might enter "BRE," to which the computer would respond by asking the user to select from:

1 BREAST: BIOPSY
2 BREAST: RESECTION FOR CANCER
3 BREAST: REDUCTION MAMMOPLASTY (NOT CANCER)

These three categories can be easily distinguished. Yet, this information allows the computer to seek additional information of the user via type-specific questions (e.g., "LUNG: CANCER" would elicit questions about the patient's smoking or asbestos history), to anticipate the proper procedure for cutting the specimen, to generate customized data labels for tissue embedding and later the microscope slides, and to provide specific instructions to pathologists and technicians at the time of the gross room examination. All of the information and protocols that are triggered by the selection of a specimen type are derived from user-defined "dictionaries" and may therefore be easily changed at any time. It is also possible to trigger billing code assignments from the specimen type.

All text entries, such as "gross description" or "final diagnosis," are made directly into the appropriate data field using either a simple text editor or a full screen-oriented word processor. The two editors may be used interchangeably at the discretion of the user. All aspects of each case can be edited simultaneously by different users, although the system does not allow editing of the same data item for a particular case by more than one user at a time. All text fields allow free text entry, as well as many choices of user-defined "canned" text. The latter includes the forms for the standardized reporting of surgical pathology diagnoses for the major tumor types that have been developed at MSKCC.[7,13] Free text and canned descriptions can be easily intermingled and edited. The diagnosis entered may be either "preliminary" or "final." Preliminary reports are generally used for cases requiring special studies and may read as follows: "Poorly differentiated carcinoma, specific type pending immunohistochemistry." Entering of the final diagnosis results in erasure of the preliminary report.

An *inquiry* is fundamentally different from a report. Thus the STANDARD INQUIRY option not only displays the full text of the gross description, diagnosis, information on special procedures, amendments to the diagnosis, and the date each task was completed but also gives detailed information about several other events such as the names of the staff pathologists, whether gross photographs were taken, frozen or gross tissue saved, special fixatives used, and whether the preparation of microscope slides has been completed. Separate inquiry options for use outside the department provide a simplified presentation of the diagnostic information, while other options provide detailed information on the status of the microscopic slides and special stains that are being prepared in a given case. This latter option (HISTOLOGY CASSETTE STATUS INQUIRY) allows immediate inquiry into the stage of preparation of all slides and all special stains on the case.

Many standard reports are generated by the system, the two most common being the WORKING DRAFT and the FINISHED FORMAT REPORT. The working draft is printed on completion of the gross dictation. This report contains a synopsis of all previous or current related case material, including cytology, clinical history, demographic and other data, and full text of the gross description (double-spaced for ease of editing). The reviewing pathologist may then record the diagnosis on this sheet for later transcription or enter it directly into the terminal. The finished format report is then signed electronically by the pathologist and made immediately available to the clinicians. This is done by mailing the hard copy of the report, by distributing it by a computer-driven fax device,[17] and by having it displayed on request in the various terminals located in the clinics and physicians' offices.

Most other standard reports, such as overdue case lists, conference lists, and consultation logs, are of an administrative nature.

Cytology

In many ways, the operation of the CYTOLOGY section is similar to that of the SURGICAL PATHOLOGY section. The major difference is that it makes extensive use of case/type-specific questionnaires, so that only relevant questions are asked at the time of accessioning. For example, routine Papanicolaou smears elicit questions on menstrual history, birth control medication, and previous cancer history; a sputum sample activates a different set of questions.

Reporting of routine gynecologic specimens such as Papanicolaou smears is also facilitated by using a "checklist," whereby the cytotechnologist may simply select any number of predefined features that are recognized in the smear. This may be done using the printed checklist for later entry, or the information may be entered directly into the computer as the smear is evaluated. From these checklists the computer will automatically SNOMED-code (see later section) the specimen, decide which specimens need to be reviewed by a pathologist (based on predefined user criteria), capture a percentage of the cases for quality control review, and generate a completed full text report ready for mailing.

At the time of cytology accessioning, slide labels are automatically generated. These contain the slide designation, cytology number, and patient name. Additional labels with any desired information can also be generated at will.

Autopsy

The AUTOPSY section of the system provides a complete morgue registration system and handles all aspects of autopsy report preparation. As with SURGICAL PATHOLOGY and CYTOLOGY, the AUTOPSY section supports unlimited text and "canned text" entries. The "specimen type" concept is also used in the AUTOPSY section to generate case-specific and informative autopsy worksheets, which enhance the training experience of the pathology residents and provide a measure of increased quality control in the autopsy suite.

Billing

The BILLING feature of the system allows automatic capture of charges for all specimens, including special procedures such as electron microscopy. These are compiled into charge batches sorted by user-defined tables into technical and professional components. These charge batches are delivered to the hospital via magnetic tape or to other group practice plans as printed hard copies. The system allows an unlimited number of separate billing groups, each with separate charge codes and fees.

Department-wide options

In the DEPARTMENT-WIDE OPTIONS, one finds the most general search capabilities of the system. Basically, two search options are provided. One type of search that is used frequently by the pathologists involves finding cases with certain diagnoses or combinations of diagnoses. This is most easily done using the SNOMED SEARCH option. Because SNOMED (*S*ystematized *N*omenclature *O*f *MED*icine) is a carefully constructed and rational coding system, indices based on SNOMED-coded cases provide a very accurate and rapid way to search by diagnosis categories.[2,14] Although not generally conceded, under most circumstances SNOMED has proved to be the superior system for this purpose.[10,11] The one drawback to using SNOMED has been the labor involved in properly coding the cases. Increasingly, however, SNOMED coding has been automated. The searches made using SNOMED coding are rapid and precise and are difficult to achieve with less precise coding schemes or by free-text searching. They also have the advantage that they can be conducted without clerical assistance at any time.

The other search option uses a "report generator." This software package allows arbitrary searches over virtually any of the data items captured by the system, as well as over many derived data items such as words or free-text phrases or intervals between accession and signout. The search may use any unlimited combination of Boolean logic. The output format is also user defined, so that almost any type of report can be compiled with this option. These searches are designed to be run in background. They are usually performed overnight when system load is reduced so that the many disk accesses required by such searches will not adversely affect overall system performance.

Systems manager

The SYSTEMS MANAGER section allows editing of all dictionaries used in the system and provides a number of other maintenance and administrative features. Almost all transactions in the system leave an audit trail, which may be examined by means of the options in this module. Access to the SYSTEMS MANAGER section is strictly limited to a few staff members at the managerial level.

Histology laboratory

The HISTOLOGY LABORATORY section handles all functions related to the preparation of slides from the specimen. The interaction begins in the gross room, where the pathologist enters directly into a terminal the information on the number of blocks and tissue pieces submitted to the histology laboratory, as well as any special requests for stains, recuts, altered processing, and so on. This task is simplified in the case of routine specimens because much of the information needed has already been anticipated by the computer on the basis of the "specimen type" and only needs to be verified by the pathologist. If at any point in the gross handling of a specimen the resident or histotechnologist needs help, the entry of "??" will gain access to the entire gross room manual (Appendix H of this book), which is maintained on-line.

All worksheets in the histology laboratory are generated automatically from the entries in the gross room. These worksheets are sorted in numeric order and contain all information necessary for slide preparation. All requests for special stains, recuts, and so on are entered directly into the system and appear immediately on the SPECIAL STAIN LOG, which is a perpetual log of unfinished stain requests. All slide labels are printed automatically in the histology laboratory; these include patient name, block designation, case and part number, and a computer-assigned block number (which eliminates redundant block labeling). For special stains, the label also contains the type of stain and the date the procedure was done, to facilitate comparison with control slides.

Future trends in automation

It is likely that the surgical pathology systems of the very near future will offer several additional features. High-quality digital images of gross and microscopic material can already be automatically linked to individual cases or teaching collections.[15] These images can also be transmitted to other computers anywhere in the world for diagnostic or teaching purposes (telepathology).[6,12]

Reporting by digital speech recognition is currently being tested in several institutions, at the same time that the speech recognition systems themselves are being developed and perfected. The successful implementation of a "continuous speech recognition" system (i.e., one that does not require a pause between words when dictating) would undoubtedly have a great impact on the practice of anatomic pathology.[9,16]

REFERENCES

1 Aller RD, Robboy SJ, Poitras JW, Altshuler BS, Cameron M, Prior MC, Miao S, Barnett GO: Computer-Assisted Pathology Encoding and Reporting System (CAPER). Am J Clin Pathol **68:**715-720, 1977.

2 Berman JJ, Moore GW, Donnelly WH, Massey JK, Craig B: A SNOMED analysis of three years' accessioned cases (40,124) of a surgical pathology department. Implications for pathology-based demographic studies. In Ozbolt JG, ed: Proceedings of the Eighteenth Annual Symposium on computer applications in medical care. Philadelphia, 1994, Hanley & Belfus, Inc., pp. 188-192.

3 Buffone GJ, Beck JR: Informatics. A subspecialty in pathology. Am J Clin Pathol **100:**75-81, 1993.

4 Cote RA, Rothwell DJ: The classification-nomenclature issues in medicine. A return to natural language. Med Inf (Lond) **14:**25, 1989.

5 Friedman BA: The impact of new features of laboratory information systems on quality assurance in anatomic pathology (editorial). Arch Pathol Lab Med **112:**1189-1191, 1988.

6 Ito H, Adachi H, Taniyama K, Fukuda Y, Dohi K: Telepathology is available for transplantation-pathology. Experience in Japan using an integrated, low-cost, and high-quality system. Mod Pathol **7:**801-805, 1994.

7 Leslie KO, Rosai J: Standardization of the surgical pathology report. Formats, templates, and synoptic reports. Semin Diagn Pathol **11:**253-257, 1994.

8 McNeely MDD: Advances in medical informatics during the 1980's. Am J Clin Pathol **96:**S33-S39, 1991.

9 Meijer GA, Baak JPA: Reporting by digital speech recognition (editorial). Hum Pathol **26:**813-815, 1995.

10 Moore GW, Berman JJ: Performance analysis of manual and automated systemized nomenclature of medicine (SNOMED) coding. Am J Clin Pathol **101:**253-256, 1994.

11 Moore GW, Berman JJ: Automatic SNOMED coding. JAMA **1:**S225, 1994.

12 Oberholzer M, Fischer HR, Christen H, Gerber S, Bruhlmann M, Mihatsch MJ, Gahm T, Famos M, Winkler C, Fehr P, Hosch HJ: Telepathology. Frozen section diagnosis at a distance. Virchows Arch **426:**3-9, 1995.

13 Rosai J and members of the Department of Pathology, Memorial Sloan-Kettering Cancer Center: Standardized reporting of surgical pathology diagnoses for the major tumor types. A proposal. Am J Clin Pathol **100:**240-255, 1993.

14 Rothwell DJ, Cote RA, Brochu L: The systematized nomenclature of human and veterinary medicine, SNOMED International Microglossary for pathology. Northfield, IL, 1993, College of American Pathologists.

15 Schubert E, Gross W, Siderits RH, Deckenbaugh L, He F, Beich MJ: A pathologist-designed imaging system for anatomic pathology signout, teaching, and research. Semin Diagn Pathol **11:**263-273, 1994.

16 Teplitz C, Cipriani M, Dicostanzo D, Sarlin J: Automated Speech-recognition Anatomic Pathology (ASAP) reporting. Semin Diagn Pathol **11:**245-252, 1994.

17 Wick MR, Archer JB, Isaacs HM, Gross W: Distribution of surgical pathology reports by a computer-driven telephone facsimile (FAX) device. Semin Diagn Pathol **11:**258-262, 1994.

Index

Page references in *italics* indicate figures. Page references followed by *t* or *b* indicate tables or boxes, respectively.

I-1

Index

I-23

Inflammatory pseudotumors
bladder, 1193, *1193*
cervix, 1381
dermal, 196
esophageal, 606-607
liver, 922
lung, 398-400, *399, 400*
lymph nodes, 1747, *1748*
mesentery, 2152
orbit, 2459, *2460*
prostate, 1227
salivary glands, 820
small bowel, 696
spleen, 1783, 1792, *1792*
subglottic, 319
Influenza pneumonia, 366
Information systems, 2727-2732
automated
basic design criteria for, 2728b
model, 2729-2732
Inguinal lymph node dissection, 2682
Injection of specimens, 2664
Injuries
acute pulmonary, 358
arteries, 2204-2207, *2206*
Inner ear, 2513-2516
adenocarcinoma of, 2515
non-neoplastic disorders of, 2513-2514
schwannoma (acoustic neuroma) of, 2514
tumors of, 2514-2516
Innominate bone
peripheral chondrosarcoma of, 1952-1953, *1954*
Insect bites, 75, *75*
Institutional consultations, 2567
Insulin, 43, *43*
Insulin-like growth factor II, 2087
Insulinoma
pancreatic, 994
Integrins, 40
Interdepartmental conferences
quality control and quality assurance program, 2579
recommendations, 2570
Interdigitating dendritic cell tumors, 1743
Interinstitutional review
quality control and quality assurance program, 2579
recommendations, 2570-2571
Interleukins, 40
Intermediate squamous metaplasia
cervix, 1355
International Lymphoma Study Group
lymphoid neoplasms recognized by, 1712b
Interosseous carcinoma
jaw, 274
Interstitial cystitis, 1187, *1187*
Interstitial pneumonia, *358*, 359
acute, 358-359
desquamative, 361, *362*
giant cell, 362
lymphoid or lymphocytic, 361
nonspecific, 362
usual, 359-361, *360, 361*
Intervertebral disk prolapse, 1997
Intervillositis
chronic, 1555
Intestinal epithelium
heterotopic, 224
Intestinal metaplasia
bladder, 1189
cervix, 1355
in chronic gastritis, 619, *619*
endometrium, 1401
Intestinal musculature
congenital defects in, 668
Intestinal neuronal dysplasia, 732
Intestinal-type adenocarcinoma
gastric, 633
Intestine; *see* Large bowel; Small bowel
Intimal fibroplasia
renal, 1129
Intimectomy, 2201
Intra-abdominal desmoplastic small cell tumors, 2145-2146, *2146, 2147*
Intracranial aneurysms, 2237-2238
Intracystic papillary carcinoma
breast, 1597
Intradepartmental conferences and consultations
quality control and quality assurance program, 2579
recommendations, 2570
Intraductal carcinoma
breast, 1596
pancreatic, 987-988
mucous hypersecreting, *986*, 987
papillary, *986*, 987
Intraductal epithelial hyperplasia
breast, 1583, *1585*
Intraductal papilloma
breast, 1576-1577
male breast, 1638
Intraepidermal epithelioma, 124-125

Intraepithelial glands
penile, 1305
Intraepithelial neoplasia
anal, 805
cervical, 1359-1363, *1360*
conjunctival or corneal, 2470
oral, 230
pancreatic, 977
penile, 1308
prostatic, 1235, *1238*
vaginal, 1344
vulvar, 1323-1324
Intrahepatic bile duct carcinoma
TNM staging, 2601
Intrahepatic cholestasis of pregnancy, 886
Intramedullary osteosarcoma
well-differentiated (low-grade), 1942
Intramucosal carcinoma
esophagus, 601
gastric, 641
Intramural esophageal diverticulosis
diffuse, 591
Intramural papilloma
vagina, 1341
Intramuscular hemangioma, 2063-2064
Intranodal leiomyoma, 1747
Intranuclear helioid inclusions
in breast, 1583
Intraocular tissues, 2450, 2475-2503
cytology, 2502-2503
degeneration of, 2484-2489
developmental anomalies of, 2476-2478
inflammation of, 2479-2484
acute, *2478*, 2479
chronic nongranulomatous, 2479, *2480*
granulomatous, 2479-2482
lymphoid tumors of, 2502
malignant melanoma of, 2489-2497
general and clinical features, 2489-2493, *2492, 2493, 2494, 2495*
microscopic features, 2494-2497, *2495, 2496*
prognostic factors, 2497
spread and metastases, 2497
therapy for, 2497
metastatic tumors to, 2502, *2502*
retinoblastoma of, 2497-2502
trauma to, *2478*, 2478-2479
tumors of, 2489-2502
Intraoperative consultations
recommendations, 2570
Intraoral tumors
metastatic, 248
Intraosseous osteosarcoma
well-differentiated (low-grade), 1942
Intrasellar gangliocytoma, 2309
Intrasellar mixed gangliocytoma-adenoma, 2435, *2436*
Intraspinal cysts, 2232
Intratubular germ cell neoplasia
classification of, 1279-1280
with extratubular extension, 1280
forms, 1280
testis, 1279-1280
unclassified, 1279-1280, *1280*
Intrauterine devices, 1397-1399
Intravagal paraganglioma, 1048
Intravascular coagulation
glomerular disease with, 1104-1108
Intravascular fasciitis, 2029
Intravascular lymphoma, 194
intranasal, 303
Intravascular lymphomatosis
lung, 406
malignant, 2337, *2338*
Intravascular papillary endothelial hyperplasia, *2063*, 2064
oral, 247
Intravenous leiomyomatosis
uterine, *1434*, 14321-1433
Intravenous pyogenic granuloma
conjunctiva, 2473
Intussusception
appendix, 724
small bowel, 681-682, *682*
Invasive carcinoma
breast, 1603-1620
hormone receptors in, *1620*, 1620-1621
standardized reports, 2532-2533, 2534-2535
cervical
hysterectomy for, 2720-2721
Invasive ductal carcinoma
breast, 1603-1618, *1604*
cytology, 1593, *1595*
Invasive hydatidiform mole, *1546*, 1549
Invasive lobular carcinoma
breast, 1618-1620
Inverted follicular keratosis, 131, *132*
oral, 246
Inverted papilloma
bladder, 1193-1194, *1194*

Inverted papilloma—cont'd
male urethra, 1312
Inverted transitional cell papilloma
cervix, 1359
Involucrin, 40
Iriditis
in diabetes, 2487, *2488*, 2489
Iridocyclitis, 2479, *2480*
Iris
malignant melanoma of, 2487, *2487*
staging, 2625
melanoma of, 2493, *2494*
tumor of, 2492, *2492*
Iritis
nongranulomatous, 2479, *2480*
Iron deposits
placental, 1555
Irradiation effects; *see* Radiation injury; Radiation therapy
Irritation fibromas, 225
ISH; *see* In situ hybridization
Islet cell tumors, 990, *990*, *992-993*, 994
Islets of Langerhans; *see* Langerhans' islets
Isolated event reports, 2571
Ito's nevus, 144

J

Jack straws, 2077
Jackson and Huber's nomenclature for lung, 2680
Jadassohn
nevus sebaceous of, 129, *130*
Jakob-Creutzfeldt disease, 2267-2268, *2268*
Jaws; *see* Mandible and maxilla
JC virus, 2259
J-chain, 40
Jejunal diverticula, 669
Jejunitis
acute (phlegmonous), 679
ulcerative, 680
Jejunum
smooth muscle tumors of, *692*, 692-694
Jelly roll syndrome, 2373, *2374*
Jelly-belly syndrome, 2149
Jessner's lymphocytic infiltration
dermal, 190
Joints, 1987-2002
anatomy, 1987
arthritis of, 1989-1997
articular and periarticular diseases of, 1997
Baker's cyst in, 1988, *1989*
bursae of, 1987-1988, *1988*
Charcot's, 1991, *1994*, *1995*
degenerative disease (osteoarthritis) of, 1989-1991, *1990, 1991-1993*
ganglia of, 1987, *1987, 1988*
gout in, 1996-1997, *1997*
infectious arthritis of, 1996, *1996, 1997*
intervertebral disk prolapse, 1997
non-neoplastic diseases of, 1987-1997
rheumatoid arthritis of, 1991-1996, *1994, 1995, 1996*
tumors of, 1997-2002
Junctional nevus, 140, *140*
Juvenile carcinoma
breast, *1612*, 1613
Juvenile fibromatosis, 2033
Juvenile granulosa cell tumors
ovary, 1508, *1508, 1509*
testis, 1286
Juvenile hemangioma, 2062
Juvenile laryngeal papillomas, 317, *317, 318*
Juvenile nephronophthisis-medullary cystic disease complex, 1134-1135
Juvenile ossifying fibroma, 261
Juvenile papillomatosis, 1636, *1636*
Juvenile polyposis
multiple, 760
Juvenile polyps
large bowel, 760, *763*
Juvenile xanthogranuloma, 174-177, *176, 177*
intraocular, 2502
soft tissue, 2037
testis, 1265
Juxtacortical chondroma, 1946-1947
Juxtacortical chondrosarcoma
bone, 1953-1956, *1955*
Juxtacortical osteosarcoma, 1942, *1942, 1943*
classification and distribution, 1933t
Juxtaglomerular cell tumors, 1157, *1158*

K

Kaposiform hemangioma, 2062
Kaposi-like hemangioma, 2062
Kaposi's sarcoma
appendix, 726
dermal, *184*, 184-188, *185, 186*
heart, 2186
jaw, 279
large bowel, 781
lung, 402

Skeletal muscle—cont'd
  drug-induced myopathies of, 2411-2412
  dystrophy of, 2404-2407
  fiber type grouping, 2400
  hemangioma of, 2063-2064
  histochemistry, 2398-2400, *2399*
  inflammatory myopathies of, 2400, 2402-2404
  metabolic myopathies of, 2408-2411
  neurogenic atrophy (denervation) of, 2400-2401,
    2401
  neuromuscular junction disorders of, 2412-2413
  perifascicular atrophy of, 2404, *2404*
  ragged red fibers, 2400, *2400*
  target fibers, 2400, *2401*
  working classification of, 2400-2412
Skenoid fibers, 645, 693
Skin, 63-221
  anatomy, 63-65
  bacterial diseases of, 67-69
  carcinoma metastatic to, 197, *197*
  carcinoma of
    TNM staging, 2587-2588
  degenerative diseases of, 93-98
  excision for benign lesion specimen, 2703
  excision for malignant tumor specimen, 2704
  foreign body reaction, 75, *75*
  fungal diseases of, 72-73
  granulomatous diseases of, 73-75
  histiocytic proliferations of, 177-178
  inflammatory diseases of known etiology of, 65-75
  malignant melanoma of
    TNM staging, 2588-2589
  mastocytosis of, 84, *84*, *85*
  meningioma-like tumors, 196
  Paget's disease of, 128-129, *129*
  punch biopsy, 2705
  resection for melanoma
    standardized reports, 2553
  sarcoidosis of, 73-75, *74*
  sebaceous carcinoma of, 131, *131*
  shave biopsy, 2705
  spirochetal diseases of, 69-72
  synovial metaplasia of, 196
  tumors of, 106-221
    orbital exenteration for, 2687
    sarcoma-like, 174
  verrucous carcinoma of, 109, *110*
  vesiculobullous diseases of, 89-93
  viral diseases of, 65-67
Skin adnexal tumors, 118-166
  oral, 246
  vulvar, 1329
Skin tags, 169
Skin tumors, 106-221
  orbital exenteration for, 2687
  sarcoma-like, 174
Skull
  osteolytic lesion of, 1985, *1986*
Slide review, 5-6
Slides delivery, 2583
Sloughing
  testicular, 1263
Small accessory urethral canals, 1305
Small bowel, 667-710
  adenocarcinoma of, *686*, 686-687
    in cervix, 1375
  AIDS-related inflammatory diseases of, 678-679
  anatomy, 667
  atresia of, 668
  benign epithelial tumors of, 683
  biopsy, *670*, 671, 2706
  carcinoid tumors of, 687-691
    general and clinical features of, 687
    immunohistochemical features, 689, *690*
    microscopic types, 689
    morphologic features, 687, *687*, *688*
    spread and metastases, 689
    treatment and prognosis, 689
  carcinoma of, 687
    TNM staging, 2598
  congenital defects, 667-671
  diverticula of, 669
  duplication of, 668, *668*
  endocrine tumors, 687-691
  excision of, 2707
  immunoproliferative disease of, 694
  inflammatory diseases of, 679-681
  intussusception of, 681-682, *682*
  irradiation effects, 681, *681*, *682*
  malabsorption in, 671-672
  malignant lymphoma of, 693-696, *694*, *696*
  Meckel's diverticulum of, 669, *669*
  non-neoplastic diseases of, 682-683
  resection for multiple diverticula, 17, *17*
  stromal tumors of, 691-693
  tumors metastatic to, 699, *699*
  tumors of, 683-699
    primary malignant, 699
  ulcers of, 673-675

Small bowel—cont'd
  vascular diseases of, 675
Small cell anaplastic carcinoma
  esophageal, 605
Small cell carcinoma, 397
  anus, 808
  bladder, 1207, *1207*
  cervix, 1365, *1365*
  classic form, 383, *383*
  combined, 384
  dermal, 169
  endometrial, 1415
  esophageal, 605
  extrapulmonary, 1375
  gallbladder, 957, *958*
  gastric, 637, 641
  kidney, 1155
  large bowel, 773, *774*
  lung, 383-384, *384*, *388*
    bone marrow biopsy, 1891, *1892*
  nasal cavity, *300*, 301
  oral, 239
  ovarian, 1513, *1514*
  prostate, 1234
  pulmonary, 1513
  rectum, 776, *776*
  renal, 25, *27*
  salivary glands, 842, *842*
  subclassification, 383
  thymic, 461, *462*
  thyroid, 543
  true cord, 321, *322*
  vagina, 1346-1347
Small cell lymphoma
  types of, 1724*t*
Small cell neuroendocrine carcinoma
  laryngeal, 325
  nasal, 301
  tracheal, 331
Small cell osteosarcoma, 1941
Small cell tumors
  intra-abdominal desmoplastic, 2145-2146, *2146*,
    2147
  malignant, *2104*, 2105-2106
Small centrocytic lymphoma
  diffuse, 1721, *1722*
Small cleaved cell lymphoma
  bone marrow, 1863, *1865*
  bone marrow biopsy, 1852, *1854*
  diffuse, 1721, *1722*
  follicular, 1852, *1855*
Small intestine; *see* Small bowel
Small lymphocytic infiltrations
  orbit, 2464-2467, *2465*, *2466*
Small lymphocytic lymphoma, 1711-1717, *1713*, *1714*,
    1715
  bone marrow, 1863
  with plasmacytoid differentiation, 1712
  spleen, *1783*, 1784, *1785*
  with Waldenstrom's macroglobulinemia, *1714*
Small lymphocytic proliferations
  lung, 403-405, *404*
  orbit, 2464, *2465*
Small noncleaved cell lymphoma, 1732-1734
  bone marrow biopsy, 1863, *1864*
Small vessel arteritis, 2211, *2211*
Smooth muscle proliferations
  in hilum, 1746
  lymph nodes, 1746-1747
Smooth muscle tumors
  cervix, *1380*, 1381
  clear cell (epithelioid), 2077, *2078*
  dermal, 177-178
  esophagus, 606
  jejunum, *692*, 692-693
  large bowel, 780
  oral, 247
  soft tissue, 2075-2077
  uterine, 1436*b*
Smooth muscle-stromal tumor or stromomyoma, 1421
SNCL; *see* Small noncleaved cell lymphoma
Sneddon's syndrome, 2211
Soft fibroma, 169
Soft palate, 223
Soft palate carcinoma
  TNM staging, 2590-2591
Soft part sarcoma
  alveolar
    orbital, 2461
    retroperitoneal, 2161
Soft parts
  malignant giant cell tumor of, *2102*, 2103
  malignant melanoma of, 2099-2101
  ossifying fibromyxoid tumor of, *2103*, 2103-2104
Soft tissue, 2021-2133
  alveolar soft part sarcoma of, *2098*, 2098-2099, *2099*,
    2100
  anatomy, 2021-0222
  chondroma of, 2087, *2087*, *2088*

Soft tissue—cont'd
  chondrosarcoma of, 2087-2088
  clear cell sarcoma of, *2100*, 2101
  clear cell (epithelioid) smooth muscle tumors of,
    2077
  elastofibroma of, 2030-2031, *2031*
  epithelioid sarcoma of, *2101*, 2101-2103, *2102*
  fibrous hamartoma of infancy in, 2094-2095
  hemangiopericytoma of, 2065-2068, *2066*, *2067*
  histiocytoma of, 2037
    benign fibrous, 2037, *2037*
    intermediate (borderline) fibrous, 2037
    malignant fibrous, 2038
  infections of, 2022-2023, *2023*
  leiomyoma of, 2075-2076
  leiomyosarcoma of, *2076*, 2076-2077, *2078*
  lymphangioma of, 2070-2072, *2073*
  lymphangiomyoma of, 2072-2073, *2073*
  lymphangiosarcoma of, *2074*, 2074-2075
  metastatic carcinoma to, 2107
  myxoma of, 2095-2096, *2096*
  nerve sheath myxoma of, 2049, *2050*
  neurofibroma of, 2041, 2045-2049, *2046*, *2047*
  neuroma of, 2042
  osteosarcoma of, 2088-2090, *2089*
  perineurioma of, 2049, *2049*, *2050*
  rhabdomyoma of, 2077-2080, *2078*
  rhabdomyosarcoma of, 2080-2087
    cytogenetics and molecular pathology, 2087
    DNA ploidy, 2087
    electron microscopy, 2083, *2084*
    immunohistochemical features, 2083-2087
  sarcoma of
    adult staging, 2619
    AJC staging, 2024*b*, 2025
    chromosomal alterations in, 2024, 2024*t*
    Enneking staging system, 2025, 2025*b*
    pediatric staging, 2619-2620
    pleural, 343
  schwannoma (neurilemoma) of, 2041, *2042*, 2042-
    2045, *2043*, *2044*, *2045*
  tumorlike conditions of, 2109
Soft tissue tumors, 2023-2109
  and age, 2023
  amputation for, 2652-2653
  classification of, 2023
  diagnosis of, 2023-2024
  extragonadal germ cell, 2093
  fibrohistiocytic, 2036-2041
  grading and staging, 2024-2025
  granular cell, 2096-2098, *2097*, *2098*
  hematopoietic tissue, 2094
  malignant peripheral nerve, 2041, 2049-2053, *2051*,
    2052
  metaplastic mesenchyme, 2087-2093
  nasal, 307
  neural, 2093-2094
  oral cavity, 248
  ossifying fibromyxoid, *2103*, 2103-2105
  pathogenesis of, 2026
  penis, 1312
  peripheral nerve, 2041-2053, *2042*
  phosphaturic mesenchymal, *2106*, 2107
  pigmented neuroectodermal, of infancy, *2093*, 2093-
    2094
  pluripotential mesenchyme, 2087
  prognostic factors, 2025
  retroperitoneal, 2157-2161
  rhabdoid, *2105*, *2106*, 2106-2107
  smooth muscle, 2075-2077
  striated muscle, 2077-2087
  therapy for, 2025-2026
  uncertain cell type, 2094-2107
Solar lentigo, 164, *165*
Solid cell nests
  thyroid, 494
Solid epithelial neoplasms
  pancreas, 988-989, *989*
Solid teratoma
  ovary, 1500
Solid tumors
  mesentery, 2153, *2153*
  omentum, 2152
Solitary bone cysts, *1976*, 1977
  classification and distribution, 1933*t*
Solitary circumscribed neuroma
  skin, 178-181
Solitary cysts
  peritoneal, 2137, *2137*
Solitary fibrous tumors
  bone, 1969
  kidney, 1158
  laryngeal, 331
  liver, 919
  lung, 409
  mediastinal, 480, *481*
  nasopharyngeal, *306*, 307
  orbit, 2461, *2461*
  peritoneum, 2146